西医经典名著集成

尼尔森儿科学

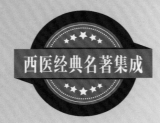

Nelson
TEXTBOOK OF
PEDIATRICS

KLIEGMAN | ST GEME
BLUM | SHAH | TASKER | WILSON

第21版（影印中文导读版）

编译委员会名誉主任委员　张金哲

编译委员会主任委员　王天有

上册

EDITION

21

VOLUME 1

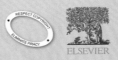

ELSEVIER

CNS | K 湖南科学技术出版社

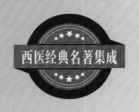

《西医经典名著集成》丛书编译委员会

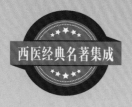

尼尔森儿科学
第21版（影印中文导读版）

编译委员会

名誉主任委员	张金哲	首都医科大学附属北京儿童医院
主 任 委 员	王天有	首都医科大学附属北京儿童医院
副主任委员	刘　钢	首都医科大学附属北京儿童医院
	姜玉武	北京大学医学部
	罗小平	华中科技大学同济医学院附属同济医院
	文飞球	汕头大学医学院附属深圳市儿童医院
委　　员	（按姓氏拼音排序）	
	崔永华	首都医科大学附属北京儿童医院
	杜军保	北京大学医学部
	方　方	首都医科大学附属北京儿童医院
	龚四堂	广州市妇女儿童医疗中心
	巩纯秀	首都医科大学附属北京儿童医院
	郭　东	首都医科大学附属北京儿童医院
	郝婵娟	首都医科大学附属北京儿童医院
	黑明燕	首都医科大学附属北京儿童医院
	胡　艳	首都医科大学附属北京儿童医院
	冀石梅	首都医科大学附属北京儿童医院
	姜玉武	北京大学医学部
	李彩凤	首都医科大学附属北京儿童医院
	李　莉	首都医科大学附属北京儿童医院
	李晓峰	首都医科大学附属北京儿童医院
	李在玲	北京大学第三医院
	刘　钢	首影医科大学附属北京儿童医院
	刘小荣	首都医科大学附属北京儿童医院
	罗小平	华中科技大学同济医学院附属同济医院
	马　琳	首都医科大学附属北京儿童医院
	马晓莉	首都医科大学附属北京儿童医院
	毛华伟	重庆医科大学附属儿童医院
	米　杰	首都医科大学附属北京儿童医院
	彭晓霞	首都医科大学附属北京儿童医院
	齐可民	首都医科大学附属北京儿童医院
	钱素云	首都医科大学附属北京儿童医院
	孙锦华	复旦大学附属儿科医院
	王天有	首都医科大学附属北京儿童医院

编 译 人 员	李乐乐	首都医科大学附属北京儿童医院
	李　莉	首都医科大学附属北京儿童医院
	李木生	广州市妇女儿童医疗中心
	李勤静	首都医科大学附属北京儿童医院
	李偲圆	首都医科大学附属北京儿童医院
	刘　畅	首都医科大学附属北京儿童医院
	刘定武	首都医科大学附属北京儿童医院
	刘昊楠	首都医科大学附属北京儿童医院
	刘　虎	首都医科大学附属北京儿童医院
	刘　明	首都医科大学附属北京儿童医院
	刘淑平	首都医科大学附属北京儿童医院
	刘　曦	首都医科大学附属北京儿童医院
	刘　雪	首都医科大学附属北京儿童医院
	马玉平	首都医科大学附属北京儿童医院
	施　维	首都医科大学附属北京儿童医院
	宋宝健	首都医科大学附属北京儿童医院
	田晓娟	首都医科大学附属北京儿童医院
	王佳平	首都医科大学附属北京儿童医院
	王晓东	汕头大学医学院附属深圳市儿童医院
	王　毅	首都医科大学附属北京儿童医院
	伍　妘	首都医科大学附属北京儿童医院
	谢　悦	首都医科大学附属北京儿童医院
	徐曼婷	首都医科大学附属北京儿童医院
	晏红改	首都医科大学附属北京儿童医院
	姚子明	首都医科大学附属北京儿童医院
	张军燕	首都医科大学附属北京儿童医院
	张　燕	首都医科大学附属北京儿童医院
	赵　丹	首都医科大学附属北京儿童医院
	赵俊红	广州市妇女儿童医疗中心
	周安娜	首都医科大学附属北京儿童医院
	周　季	首都医科大学附属北京儿童医院
	周　玲	首都医科大学附属北京儿童医院
	朱丹江	首都医科大学附属北京儿童医院
	卓秀伟	首都医科大学附属北京儿童医院
	左华欣	首都医科大学附属北京儿童医院

EDITION
21

Nelson
TEXTBOOK OF
PEDIATRICS

ROBERT M. KLIEGMAN, MD
Professor and Chair Emeritus
Department of Pediatrics
Medical College of Wisconsin
Milwaukee, Wisconsin

NATHAN J. BLUM, MD
William H. Bennett Professor of Pediatrics
University of Pennsylvania Perelman School of Medicine
Chief, Division of Developmental and Behavioral Pediatrics
Children's Hospital of Philadelphia
Philadelphia, Pennsylvania

SAMIR S. SHAH, MD, MSCE
Professor of Pediatrics
University of Cincinnati College of Medicine
Director, Division of Hospital Medicine
Chief Metrics Officer
James M. Ewell Endowed Chair
Cincinnati Children's Hospital Medical Center
Cincinnati, Ohio

JOSEPH W. ST GEME III, MD
Professor of Pediatrics and Microbiology and Chair of
    the Department of Pediatrics
University of Pennsylvania Perelman School of Medicine
Chair of the Department of Pediatrics and
    Physician-in-Chief
Leonard and Madlyn Abramson Endowed Chair in
    Pediatrics
Children's Hospital of Philadelphia
Philadelphia, Pennsylvania

ROBERT C. TASKER, MBBS, MD
Professor of Neurology
Professor of Anesthesia
Harvard Medical School
Senior Associate, Critical Care Medicine
Director, Pediatric NeuroCritical Care Program
Boston Children's Hospital
Boston, Massachusetts

KAREN M. WILSON, MD, MPH
Professor of Pediatrics
Debra and Leon Black Division Chief of General Pediatrics
Vice-Chair for Clinical and Translational Research
Kravis Children's Hospital at the Icahn School of Medicine at
    Mount Sinai
New York, New York

Editor Emeritus

RICHARD E. BEHRMAN, MD
Nonprofit Healthcare and Educational
Consultants to Medical Institutions
Santa Barbara, California

ELSEVIER

To the Child's Physician who through their expressed confidence in past editions of this book have provided the stimulus for this revision. May we continue to be a resource of helpful information for clinicians who care for all of our children.

R.M. Kliegman

Contributors

Nadia Y. Abidi, MD
Resident Physician
Department of Dermatology
University of Missouri School of Medicine
Columbia, Missouri
Cutaneous Defects
Ectodermal Dysplasias

Mark J. Abzug, MD
Professor of Pediatrics
Vice Chair for Academic Affairs
University of Colorado School of Medicine
Section of Pediatric Infectious Diseases
Children's Hospital Colorado
Aurora, Colorado
Nonpolio Enteroviruses

David R. Adams, MD, PhD
Associate Investigator, Undiagnosed Diseases
    Program
Senior Staff Clinician
National Human Genome Research Institute
National Institutes of Health
Bethesda, Maryland
Genetic Approaches to Rare and Undiagnosed
    Diseases

Nicholas S. Adams, MD
Plastic Surgery Resident
Spectrum Health Hospitals
Michigan State University
Grand Rapids, Michigan
Deformational Plagiocephaly

Stewart L. Adelson, MD
Assistant Clinical Professor
Department of Psychiatry
Columbia University College of Physicians and
    Surgeons
Adjunct Clinical Assistant Professor
Weill Cornell Medical College of Cornell
    University
New York, New York
Gay, Lesbian, and Bisexual Adolescents

Shawn K. Ahlfeld, MD
Assistant Professor of Pediatrics
University of Cincinnati College of Medicine
Attending Neonatologist, Perinatal Institute
Cincinnati Children's Hospital Medical Center
Cincinnati, Ohio
Respiratory Tract Disorders

Osman Z. Ahmad, MD
Fellow in Pediatric Gastroenterology
University of Alabama at Birmingham School of
    Medicine
Birmingham, Alabama
Clostridium difficile Infection

John J. Aiken, MD, FACS, FAAP
Professor of Surgery
Division of Pediatric General and Thoracic
    Surgery
Medical College of Wisconsin
The Children's Hospital of Wisconsin
Milwaukee, Wisconsin
Acute Appendicitis
Inguinal Hernias
Epigastric Hernia
Incisional Hernia

Cezmi A. Akdis, MD
Professor of Immunology
Swiss Institute of Allergy and Asthma Research
Christine Kühne Center for Allergy Research and
    Education
Davos, Switzerland;
Medical Faculty, University of Zurich
Zurich, Switzerland
Allergy and the Immunologic Basis of Atopic
    Disease

Evaline A. Alessandrini, MD, MSCE
Professor of Clinical Pediatrics
University of Cincinnati College of Medicine
Division of Emergency Medicine
Director, Quality Scholars Program in Health
    Care Transformation
Cincinnati Children's Hospital Medical Center
Cincinnati, Ohio
Outcomes and Risk Adjustment of Emergency
    Medical Services

Michael A. Alexander, MD
Professor of Pediatrics and Rehabilitation
    Medicine
Thomas Jefferson Medical College
Philadelphia, Pennsylvania;
Emeritus Medical Staff
Nemours Alfred I. duPont Hospital for Children
Wilmington, Delaware
Evaluation of the Child for Rehabilitative Services

Omar Ali, MD
Pediatric Endocrinology
Valley Children's Hospital
Madera, California
Hyperpituitarism, Tall Stature, and Overgrowth
    Syndromes
Hypofunction of the Testes
Pseudoprecocity Resulting from Tumors of
    the Testes
Gynecomastia

Karl E. Anderson, MD, FACP
Professor of Preventive Medicine and Community
    Health and Internal Medicine
Director, Porphyria Laboratory and Center
University of Texas Medical Branch
Galveston, Texas
The Porphyrias

Kelly K. Anthony, PhD, PLLC
Assistant Professor
Department of Psychiatry and Behavioral
    Sciences
Duke University Medical Center
Durham, North Carolina
Musculoskeletal Pain Syndromes

Alia Y. Antoon, MD, DCH
Senior Fellow
American Academy of Pediatrics
Honorary Pediatrician
MassGeneral Hospital for Children
Boston, Massachusetts
Burn Injuries
Cold Injuries

Susan D. Apkon, MD
Professor
Department of Physical Medicine and
    Rehabilitation
University of Colorado
Denver, Colorado;
Chief, Pediatric Rehabilitation
Children's Hospital Colorado
Aurora, Colorado
Ambulation Assistance

Stacy P. Ardoin, MD, MHS
Associate Professor of Clinical Medicine
Division of Adult and Pediatric Rheumatology
The Ohio State University Wexner Medical
    Center
Nationwide Children's Hospital
Columbus, Ohio
Systemic Lupus Erythematosus
Vasculitis Syndromes

Alexandre Arkader, MD
Attending Orthopaedic Surgeon
Children's Hospital of Philadelphia
Philadelphia, Pennsylvania
Common Fractures

Thaís Armangué, MD, PhD
Pediatric Neurologist
Neuroimmunology Program
IDIBAPS—Hospital Clinic–Hospital Sant Joan de
    Déu (Barcelona)
University of Barcelona
Barcelona, Spain
Autoimmune Encephalitis

Carola A.S. Arndt, MD
Professor of Pediatrics
Department of Pediatrics and Adolescent
    Medicine
Division of Pediatric Hematology-Oncology
Mayo Clinic
Rochester, Minnesota
Soft Tissue Sarcomas

Paul L. Aronson, MD
Associate Professor of Pediatrics and Emergency
    Medicine
Yale School of Medicine
New Haven, Connecticut
Fever in the Older Child

David M. Asher, MD
Supervisory Medical Officer and Chief
Laboratory of Bacterial and Transmissible
    Spongiform Encephalopathy Agents
Division of Emerging and Transfusion-
    Transmitted Diseases
US Food and Drug Administration
Silver Spring, Maryland
Transmissible Spongiform Encephalopathies

Ann Ashworth, PhD, Hon FRCPCH
Professor Emeritus
Department of Population Health
Nutrition Group
London School of Hygiene and Tropical Medicine
London, United Kingdom
Nutrition, Food Security, and Health

Amit Assa, MD
Associate Professor of Pediatrics
Sackler Faculty of Medicine
Tel Aviv University
Tel Aviv, Israel;
Head, IBD Unit
Institute of Gastroenterology, Nutrition, and Liver
    Diseases
Schneider Children's Medical Center
Petah Tikva, Israel
Immunodeficiency Disorders

Barbara L. Asselin, MD
Professor of Pediatrics and Oncology
Department of Pediatrics
University of Rochester School of Medicine and
    Dentistry
Golisano Children's Hospital and Wilmot Cancer
    Institute
Rochester, New York
Epidemiology of Childhood and Adolescent Cancer

Christina M. Astley, MD, ScD
Instructor in Pediatrics
Harvard Medical School
Attending Physician
Division of Endocrinology
Boston Children's Hospital
Boston, Massachusetts
Autoimmune Polyglandular Syndromes

Joann L. Ater, MD
Professor
Department of Pediatrics Patient Care
University of Texas MD Anderson Cancer Center
Houston, Texas
Brain Tumors in Childhood
Neuroblastoma

Norrell Atkinson, MD, FAAP
Assistant Professor of Pediatrics
Drexel University College of Medicine
Child Protection Program
St. Christopher's Hospital for Children
Philadelphia, Pennsylvania
Adolescent Sexual Assault

Erika U. Augustine, MD
Associate Professor of Neurology and Pediatrics
Associate Director, Center for Health +
    Technology
University of Rochester Medical Center
Rochester, New York
Dystonia

Marilyn C. Augustyn, MD
Professor of Pediatrics
Boston University School of Medicine
Boston Medical Center
Boston, Massachusetts
Impact of Violence on Children

Yaron Avitzur, MD
Associate Professor
Department of Pediatrics
University of Toronto Faculty of Medicine
Division of Gastroenterology, Hepatology,
    and Nutrition
The Hospital for Sick Children
Toronto, Canada
Short Bowel Syndrome

Carlos A. Bacino, MD
Professor and Vice Chair of Clinical Affairs
Department of Molecular and Human Genetics
Baylor College of Medicine
Director, Pediatrics Genetics Clinic
Texas Children's Hospital
Houston, Texas
Cytogenetics

Zinzi D. Bailey, ScD, MSPH
Assistant Scientist
University of Miami Miller School of Medicine
Miami, Florida
Racism and Child Health

Binod Balakrishnan, MBBS
Assistant Professor
Department of Pediatrics
Medical College of Wisconsin
Division of Pediatric Critical Care
Children's Hospital of Wisconsin
Milwaukee, Wisconsin
Brain Death

Frances B. Balamuth, MD, PhD, MSCE
Assistant Professor of Pediatrics
University of Pennsylvania Perelman School of
    Medicine
Associate Director of Research
Division of Emergency Medicine
Co-Director, Pediatric Sepsis Program
Children's Hospital of Philadelphia
Philadelphia, Pennsylvania
Triage of the Acutely Ill Child

Robert N. Baldassano, MD
Colman Family Chair in Pediatric Inflammatory
    Bowel Disease and Professor of Pediatrics
University of Pennsylvania Perelman School of
    Medicine
Director, Center for Pediatric Inflammatory
    Bowel Disease
Children's Hospital of Philadelphia
Philadelphia, Pennsylvania
Inflammatory Bowel Disease
Eosinophilic Gastroenteritis

Keith D. Baldwin, MD, MSPT, MPH
Assistant Professor
Department of Orthopaedic Surgery
University of Pennsylvania Perelman School of
    Medicine
Attending Physician
Neuromuscular Orthopaedics and Orthopaedic
    Trauma
Children's Hospital of Philadelphia
Philadelphia, Pennsylvania
Growth and Development
Evaluation of the Child
Torsional and Angular Deformities
Common Fractures

Christina Bales, MD
Associate Professor of Clinical Pediatrics
University of Pennsylvania Perelman School of
    Medicine
Medical Director, Intestinal Rehabilitation
    Program
Division of Gastroenterology, Hepatology,
    and Nutrition
Children's Hospital of Philadelphia
Philadelphia, Pennsylvania
Intestinal Atresia, Stenosis, and Malrotation

William F. Balistreri, MD
Medical Director Emeritus, Pediatric Liver Care
    Center
Division of Pediatric Gastroenterology,
    Hepatology, and Nutrition
Cincinnati Children's Hospital Medical Center
Cincinnati, Ohio
Morphogenesis of the Liver and Biliary System
Manifestations of Liver Disease
Cholestasis
Metabolic Diseases of the Liver
Viral Hepatitis
Liver Disease Associated with Systemic Disorders
Mitochondrial Hepatopathies

Allison Ballantine, MD, MEd
Associate Professor of Clinical Pediatrics
University of Pennsylvania Perelman School of
    Medicine
Co-Director Med Ed Program, Graduate School
    of Education
Section Chief, Inpatient Services
Division of General Pediatrics
Children's Hospital of Philadelphia
Philadelphia, Pennsylvania
Malnutrition

Robert S. Baltimore, MD
Professor of Pediatrics and Epidemiology
Clinical Professor of Nursing
Professor of Pediatrics and Epidemiology
Clinical Professor of Nursing
Yale School of Medicine
Associate Director of Hospital Epidemiology
    (for Pediatrics)
Yale–New Haven Hospital
New Haven, Connecticut
Listeria monocytogenes
Pseudomonas, Burkholderia, and
    Stenotrophomonas
Infective Endocarditis

Manisha Balwani, MBBS, MS
Associate Professor of Medicine and Genetics and
    Genomic Sciences
Kravis Children's Hospital at the Icahn School of
    Medicine at Mount Sinai
New York, New York
The Porphyrias

Vaneeta Bamba, MD
Associate Professor of Clinical Pediatrics
University of Pennsylvania Perelman School of
    Medicine
Medical Director, Diagnostic and Research
    Growth Center
Children's Hospital of Philadelphia
Philadelphia, Pennsylvania
Assessment of Growth

Brenda L. Banwell, MD
Professor of Neurology
Grace R. Loeb Endowed Chair in Neurosciences
University of Pennsylvania Perelman School of
    Medicine
Chief, Division of Neurology
Director, Pediatric Multiple Sclerosis Clinic
Children's Hospital of Philadelphia
Philadelphia, Pennsylvania
Central Nervous System Vasculitis

Sarah F. Barclay, PhD
Department of Medical Genetics
Cumming School of Medicine at University of
    Calgary
Alberta Children's Hospital Research Institute
Calgary, Alberta, Canada
*Rapid-Onset Obesity with Hypothalamic
    Dysfunction, Hypoventilation, and Autonomic
    Dysregulation (ROHHAD)*

Maria E. Barnes-Davis, MD, PhD
Assistant Professor of Pediatrics
University of Cincinnati College of Medicine
Attending Neonatologist
Division of Neonatology and Pulmonary Biology
Cincinnati Children's Hospital Medical Center
Cincinnati, Ohio
The High-Risk Infant

Karyl S. Barron, MD
Deputy Director
Division of Intramural Research
National Institute of Allergy and Infectious
    Diseases
National Institutes of Health
Bethesda, Maryland
Amyloidosis

Donald Basel, MBBCh
Associate Professor of Pediatrics and Genetics
Chief, Medical Genetics Division
Medical College of Wisconsin
Milwaukee, Wisconsin
Ehlers-Danlos Syndrome

Dorsey M. Bass, MD
Associate Professor of Pediatrics
Stanford University School of Medicine
Division of Pediatric Gastroenterology
Lucile Salter Packard Children's Hospital
Palo Alto, California
Rotaviruses, Caliciviruses, and Astroviruses

Mary T. Bassett, MD, MPH
FXB Professor of the Practice of Public Health
    and Human Rights
Harvard T.H. Chan School of Public Health
Boston, Massachusetts
Racism and Child Health

Christian P. Bauerfeld, MD
Assistant Professor of Pediatrics
Wayne State University School of Medicine
Division of Pediatric Critical Care Medicine
Children's Hospital of Michigan
Detroit, Michigan
Mechanical Ventilation

Rebecca A. Baum, MD
Clinical Associate Professor of Pediatrics
The Ohio State University College of Medicine
Chief, Developmental Behavioral Pediatrics
Nationwide Children's Hospital
Columbus, Ohio
Positive Parenting and Support

Michael J. Bell, MD
Professor, Pediatrics and Critical Care Medicine
Chief, Critical Care Medicine
Children's National Medical Center
The George Washington University School of
    Medicine
Washington, DC
Neurologic Emergencies and Stabilization

Nicole R. Bender, MD
Resident Physician
Department of Dermatology
Medical College of Wisconsin
Milwaukee, Wisconsin
Morphology of the Skin
Dermatologic Evaluation of the Patient
Eczematous Disorders
Photosensitivity
Diseases of the Epidermis

**Daniel K. Benjamin Jr, MD, PhD,
MPH**
Kiser-Arena Professor of Pediatrics
Duke Clinical Research Institute
Duke University Medical Center
Durham, North Carolina
Principles of Antifungal Therapy
Candida

**Michael J. Bennett, PhD, FRCPath,
FACB**
Professor of Pathology and Laboratory Medicine
University of Pennsylvania Perelman School of
    Medicine
Director, Michael J. Palmieri Metabolic Disease
    Laboratory
Children's Hospital of Philadelphia
Philadelphia, Pennsylvania
Disorders of Mitochondrial Fatty Acid β-Oxidation

Daniel Bernstein, MD
Alfred Woodley Salter and Mabel G. Salter
    Endowed Professor in Pediatrics
Associate Dean for Curriculum and Scholarship
Stanford University School of Medicine
Palo Alto, California
Cardiac Development
The Fetal to Neonatal Circulatory Transition
*History and Physical Examination in Cardiac
    Evaluation*
Laboratory Cardiac Evaluation
*Epidemiology and Genetic Basis of Congenital
    Heart Disease*
*Evaluation and Screening of the Infant or Child
    with Congenital Heart Disease*
*Acyanotic Congenital Heart Disease: Left-to-Right
    Shunt Lesions*
*Acyanotic Congenital Heart Disease: The
    Obstructive Lesions*
*Acyanotic Congenital Heart Disease: Regurgitant
    Lesions*
*Cyanotic Congenital Heart Disease: Evaluation of
    the Critically Ill Neonate with Cyanosis and
    Respiratory Distress*
*Cyanotic Congenital Heart Lesions: Lesions
    Associated with Decreased Pulmonary Blood
    Flow*
*Cyanotic Congenital Heart Disease: Lesions
    Associated with Increased Pulmonary Blood
    Flow*
*Other Congenital Heart and Vascular
    Malformations*
Pulmonary Hypertension
*General Principles of Treatment of Congenital
    Heart Disease*
*Diseases of the Blood Vessels (Aneurysms and
    Fistulas)*

**Henry H. Bernstein, DO, MHCM,
FAAP**
Professor of Pediatrics
Zucker School of Medicine at Hofstra/Northwell
Cohen Children's Medical Center of New York
New Hyde Park, New York
Immunization Practices

Diana X. Bharucha-Goebel, MD
Assistant Professor, Neurology and Pediatrics
Children's National Medical Center
Washington, DC;
Clinical Research Collaborator
National Institutes of Health/NINDS
Neurogenetics Branch/NNDCS
Bethesda, Maryland
Muscular Dystrophies
Myasthenia Gravis
Giant Axonal Neuropathy

Holly M. Biggs, MD, MPH
Medical Epidemiologist
Respiratory Viruses Branch, Division of Viral
    Diseases
National Center for Immunization and
    Respiratory Diseases
Centers for Disease Control and Prevention
Atlanta, Georgia
Parainfluenza Viruses

Samra S. Blanchard, MD
Associate Professor
Department of Pediatrics
University of Maryland School of Medicine
Baltimore, Maryland
Peptic Ulcer Disease in Children

Joshua A. Blatter, MD, MPH
Assistant Professor of Pediatrics, Allergy,
    Immunology, and Pulmonary Medicine
Researcher, Patient Oriented Research Unit
Washington University School of Medicine in
    St. Louis
St. Louis, Missouri
Congenital Disorders of the Lung

Archie Bleyer, MD, FRCP (Glasg)
Clinical Research Professor
Knight Cancer Center
Oregon Health & Science University
Chair, Institutional Review Board for St. Charles
    Health System
Portland, Oregon;
Professor of Pediatrics
University of Texas MD Anderson Cancer Center
Houston, Texas
Principles of Cancer Treatment
The Leukemias

Nathan J. Blum, MD
William H. Bennett Professor of Pediatrics
University of Pennsylvania Perelman School of
    Medicine
Chief, Division of Developmental and Behavioral
    Pediatrics
Children's Hospital of Philadelphia
Philadelphia, Pennsylvania

**Steven R. Boas, MD, FAAP,
FACSM**
Director, The Cystic Fibrosis Center of Chicago
President and CEO, The Cystic Fibrosis Institute
Glenview, Illinois;
Clinical Professor of Pediatrics
Northwestern University Feinberg School of
    Medicine
Chicago, Illinois
Emphysema and Overinflation
α1-Antitrypsin Deficiency and Emphysema
Other Distal Airway Diseases
Skeletal Diseases Influencing Pulmonary Function

Walter O. Bockting, PhD
Professor of Medical Psychology (in Psychiatry
    and Nursing)
Research Scientist, New York State Psychiatric
    Institute
Division of Gender, Sexuality, and Health
Department of Psychiatry
Columbia University Vagelos College of
    Physicians and Surgeons
New York, New York
Gender and Sexual Identity
Transgender Care

Mark Boguniewicz, MD
Professor of Pediatrics
Division of Allergy-Immunology
Department of Pediatrics
University of Colorado School of Medicine
National Jewish Health
Denver, Colorado
Ocular Allergies

Michael J. Boivin, PhD, MPH
Professor of Psychiatry and of Neurology and
    Ophthalmology
Michigan State University College of Osteopathic
    Medicine
East Lansing, Michigan
Nodding Syndrome

Daniel J. Bonthius, MD, PhD
Professor of Pediatrics and Neurology
University of Iowa Carver College of Medicine
Iowa City, Iowa
Lymphocytic Choriomeningitis Virus

Brett J. Bordini, MD, FAAP
Associate Professor of Pediatrics
Division of Hospital Medicine
Nelson Service for Undiagnosed and Rare
    Diseases
Director, Medical Spanish Curriculum
Medical College of Wisconsin
Milwaukee, Wisconsin
Plastic Bronchitis

Kristopher R. Bosse, MD
Instructor in Pediatrics
University of Pennsylvania Perelman School of
    Medicine
Attending Physician
Division of Oncology
Children's Hospital of Philadelphia
Philadelphia, Pennsylvania
Molecular and Cellular Biology of Cancer

Bret L. Bostwick, MD
Assistant Professor
Department of Molecular and Human Genetics
Baylor College of Medicine
Houston, Texas
Genetics of Common Disorders

Kenneth M. Boyer, MD
Professor and Woman's Board Chair, Emeritus
Department of Pediatrics
Rush University Medical Center
Chicago, Illinois
Toxoplasmosis (Toxoplasma gondii)

Jennifer M. Brady, MD
Assistant Professor of Pediatrics
University of Cincinnati College of Medicine
Perinatal Institute
Division of Neonatology
Cincinnati Children's Hospital Medical Center
Cincinnati, Ohio
The High-Risk Infant
Transport of the Critically Ill Newborn
*Neonatal Resuscitation and Delivery Room
    Emergencies*

Patrick W. Brady, MD, MSc
Associate Professor of Pediatrics
University of Cincinnati College of Medicine
Attending Physician, Division of Hospital
    Medicine
Cincinnati Children's Hospital Medical Center
Cincinnati, Ohio
Safety in Healthcare for Children

Rebecca C. Brady, MD
Professor of Pediatrics
University of Cincinnati College of Medicine
Cincinnati Children's Hospital Medical Center
Cincinnati, Ohio
Congenital and Perinatal Infections
Coccidioidomycosis (Coccidioides Species)

Samuel L. Brady, MS, PhD
Clinical Medical Physicist
Cincinnati Children's Hospital
Associate Professor of Radiology
University of Cincinnati
Cincinnati, Ohio
Biologic Effects of Ionizing Radiation on Children

Amanda M. Brandow, DO, MS
Associate Professor
Department of Pediatrics
Division of Pediatric Hematology/Oncology
Medical College of Wisconsin
Milwaukee, Wisconsin
Enzymatic Defects
*Hemolytic Anemias Resulting from Extracellular
    Factors—Immune Hemolytic Anemias*
*Hemolytic Anemias Secondary to Other
    Extracellular Factors*
Polycythemia
Nonclonal Polycythemia

David T. Breault, MD, PhD
Associate Professor of Pediatrics
Harvard Medical School
Division of Endocrinology
Boston Children's Hospital
Boston, Massachusetts
Diabetes Insipidus
*Other Abnormalities of Arginine Vasopressin
    Metabolism and Action*

Cora Collette Breuner, MD, MPH
Professor of Pediatrics
Adjunct Professor of Orthopedics and Sports
    Medicine
University of Washington School of Medicine
Division of Adolescent Medicine
Department of Orthopedics and Sports Medicine
Seattle Children's Hospital
Seattle, Washington
Substance Abuse
Adolescent Pregnancy

Carolyn Bridgemohan, MD
Associate Professor of Pediatrics
Harvard Medical School
Co-Director Autism Spectrum Center
Division of Developmental Medicine
Boston Children's Hospital
Boston, Massachusetts
Autism Spectrum Disorder

William J. Britt, MD
Charles A. Alford Professor of Pediatrics
Professor of Microbiology and Neurobiology
University of Alabama Birmingham School of
    Medicine
Division of Pediatric Infectious Diseases
Children's of Alabama
Birmingham, Alabama
Cytomegalovirus

Laura Brower, MD
Assistant Professor of Pediatrics
University of Cincinnati College of Medicine
Division of Hospital Medicine
Cincinnati Children's Hospital Medical Center
Cincinnati, Ohio
*Fever Without a Focus in the Neonate and Young
    Infant*

Rebeccah L. Brown, MD
Professor of Clinical Surgery and Pediatrics
University of Cincinnati College of Medicine
Co-Director of Pectus Program
Associate Director of Trauma Services
Cincinnati Children's Hospital Medical Center
Cincinnati, Ohio
*Meconium Ileus, Peritonitis, and Intestinal
    Obstruction*
Necrotizing Enterocolitis

J. Naylor Brownell, MD
Division of Gastroenterology, Hepatology, and
Nutrition
Children's Hospital of Philadelphia
Philadelphia, Pennsylvania
Feeding Healthy Infants, Children, and Adolescents

Meghen B. Browning, MD
Associate Professor of Pediatrics
The Medical College of Wisconsin
Division of Pediatric Hematology-Oncology
Children's Hospital of Wisconsin
Milwaukee, Wisconsin
Pancreatic Tumors

Nicola Brunetti-Pierri, MD
Associate Professor
Department of Translational Medicine
University of Naples Federico II
Associate Investigator, Telethon Institute of
Genetics and Medicine (TIGEM)
Naples, Italy
Management and Treatment of Genetic Disorders

Phillip R. Bryant, DO
Professor
Department of Pediatrics
University of Pennsylvania Perelman School of
Medicine
Division of Rehabilitation Medicine
Children's Hospital of Philadelphia
Philadelphia, Pennsylvania
Rehabilitation for Severe Traumatic Brain injury
Spinal Cord Injury and Autonomic Dysreflexia
Management

Rebecca H. Buckley, MD
J. Buren Sidbury Professor of Pediatrics
Professor of Immunology
Duke University School of Medicine
Durham, North Carolina
Evaluation of Suspected Immunodeficiency
The T-, B-, and NK-Cell Systems
T Lymphocytes, B Lymphocytes, and Natural Killer
Cells
Primary Defects of Antibody Production
Treatment of B-Cell Defects
Primary Defects of Cellular Immunity
Immunodeficiencies Affecting Multiple Cell Types

**Cynthia Etzler Budek, MS,
APN/NP, CPNP-AC/PC**
Pediatric Nurse Practitioner
Department of Pulmonary and Critical Care
Medicine
Transitional Care/Pulmonary Habilitation Unit
Ann & Robert H. Lurie Children's Hospital of
Chicago
Chicago, Illinois
Other Conditions Affecting Respiration

**Supinda Bunyavanich, MD, MPH,
MPhil**
Associate Professor
Associate Director, Jaffe Food Allergy Institute
Department of Pediatrics
Department of Genetics and Genomic Sciences
Kravis Children's Hospital at the Icahn School of
Medicine at Mount Sinai
New York, New York
Diagnosis of Allergic Disease

**Carey-Ann D. Burnham,
PhD D(ABMM), FIDSA, F(AAM)**
Professor of Pathology and Immunology,
Molecular Microbiology, Pediatrics, and
Medicine
Washington University School of Medicine in
St. Louis
Medical Director, Microbiology
Barnes Jewish Hospital
St. Louis, Missouri
Diagnostic Microbiology

Gale R. Burstein, MD, MPH
Clinical Professor
Department of Pediatrics
University at Buffalo Jacobs School of Medicine
and Biomedical Sciences
Commissioner, Erie County Department of
Health
Buffalo, New York
The Epidemiology of Adolescent Health Problems
Transitioning to Adult Care
The Breast
Menstrual Problems
Contraception
Sexually Transmitted Infections

**Amaya L. Bustinduy, MD, PhD,
MPH**
Associate Professor in Tropical Pediatrics
Department of Clinical Research
London School of Hygiene and Tropical Medicine
London, United Kingdom
Schistosomiasis (Schistosoma)
Flukes (Liver, Lung, and Intestinal)

Jill P. Buyon, MD
Professor of Medicine (Rheumatology)
Director, Division of Rheumatology
New York University School of Medicine
NYU Langone Medical Center
New York, New York
Neonatal Lupus

Miguel M. Cabada, MD, MSc
Assistant Professor
Division of Infectious Diseases
The University of Texas Medical Branch at
Galveston
Galveston, Texas
Echinococcosis (Echinococcus granulosus and
Echinococcus multilocularis)

**Michaela Cada, MD, FRCPC,
FAAP, MPH**
Assistant Professor
Department of Pediatrics
University of Toronto Faculty of Medicine
Director, Education Training Program
Division of Hematology/Oncology
The Hospital for Sick Children
Toronto, Ontario, Canada
Inherited Bone Marrow Failure Syndromes with
Pancytopenia

Derya Caglar, MD
Associate Professor
Fellowship Director, Pediatric Emergency
Medicine
Department of Pediatrics
University of Washington School of Medicine
Attending Physician
Division of Emergency Medicine
Seattle Children's Hospital
Seattle, Washington
Drowning and Submersion Injury

Mitchell S. Cairo, MD
Professor
Departments of Pediatrics, Medicine, Pathology,
Microbiology, and Immunology and Cell
Biology and Anatomy
New York Medical College
Chief, Division of Pediatric Hematology,
Oncology and Stem Cell Transplantation
Maria Fareri Children's Hospital at Westchester
Medical Center
New York Medical College
Valhalla, New York
Lymphoma

Diane P. Calello, MD
Associate Professor of Emergency Medicine
Rutgers University New Jersey Medical School
Executive and Medical Director
New Jersey Poison Information and Education
System
Newark, New Jersey
Nonbacterial Food Poisoning

Lauren E. Camarda, MD
Pediatric Pulmonology
Advocate Children's Hospital
Park Ridge, Illinois
Bronchitis

**Lindsay Hatzenbuehler Cameron,
MD, MPH**
Assistant Professor of Pediatrics
Baylor College of Medicine
Pediatric Infectious Diseases
Texas Children's Hospital
Houston, Texas
Tuberculosis (Mycobacterium tuberculosis)

Bruce M. Camitta, MD
Rebecca Jean Slye Professor of Pediatrics
Division of Pediatric Hematology/Oncology
Medical College of Wisconsin
Midwest Children's Cancer Center
Milwaukee, Wisconsin
Polycythemia
Nonclonal Polycythemia
Anatomy and Function of the Spleen
Splenomegaly
Hyposplenism, Splenic Trauma, and Splenectomy
Anatomy and Function of the Lymphatic System
Abnormalities of Lymphatic Vessels
Lymphadenopathy

Angela J.P. Campbell, MD, MPH
Medical Officer
Epidemiology and Prevention Branch, Influenza
Division
National Center for Immunization and
Respiratory Diseases
Centers for Disease Control and Prevention
Atlanta, Georgia
Influenza Viruses
Parainfluenza Viruses

Rebecca F. Carlin, MD
Attending Physician
Division of General and Community Pediatrics
Children's National Health System
Assistant Professor of Pediatrics
George Washington University School of
Medicine and Health Sciences
Washington, DC
Sudden Infant Death Syndrome

Michael R. Carr, MD
Assistant Professor of Pediatrics
Division of Cardiology
Northwestern University Feinberg School of
Medicine
Ann & Robert H. Lurie Children's Hospital of
Chicago
Chicago, Illinois
Rheumatic Heart Disease

Robert B. Carrigan, MD
Assistant Clinical Professor
Department of Orthopaedic Surgery
University of Pennsylvania Perelman School of
Medicine
Pediatric Hand Surgeon
Children's Hospital of Philadelphia
Philadelphia, Pennsylvania
The Upper Limb

Michael S. Carroll
Research Assistant Professor of Pediatrics
Northwestern University Feinberg School of
Medicine
Chicago, Illinois
Congenital Central Hypoventilation Syndrome

Rebecca G. Carter, MD
Assistant Professor
Department of Pediatrics
University of Maryland School of Medicine
Baltimore, Maryland
The Second Year
The Preschool Years

Mary T. Caserta, MD
Professor of Pediatrics
University of Rochester School of Medicine and
Dentistry
Division of Pediatric Infectious Diseases
Golisano Children's Hospital
Rochester, New York
Roseola (Human Herpesviruses 6 and 7)
Human Herpesvirus 8

Jennifer I. Chapman, MD
Assistant Professor of Pediatrics
George Washington University School of
Medicine and Health Sciences
Program Director, Pediatric Emergency Medicine
Fellowship
Children's National Medical Center
Washington, DC
Principles Applicable to the Developing World

**Ira M. Cheifetz, MD, FCCM,
FAARC**
Professor of Pediatrics and Anesthesiology
Duke University School of Medicine
Executive Director and Chief Medical Officer
Duke Children's Hospital
Associate Chief Medical Officer
Duke University Hospital
Durham, North Carolina
Pediatric Emergencies and Resuscitation
Shock

Gisela G. Chelimsky, MD
Professor of Pediatrics
Medical College of Wisconsin
Division of Pediatric Gastroenterology
Children's Hospital Milwaukee
Milwaukee, Wisconsin
Chronic Overlapping Pain Conditions
Postural Tachycardia Syndrome

Thomas C. Chelimsky, MD
Professor of Neurology
Medical College of Wisconsin
Milwaukee, Wisconsin
Chronic Overlapping Pain Conditions
Postural Tachycardia Syndrome

Wassim Chemaitilly, MD
Associate Member and Director
Division of Endocrinology
Department of Pediatric Medicine
St. Jude Children's Research Hospital
Memphis, Tennessee
Physiology of Puberty
Disorders of Pubertal Development

Yuan-Tsong Chen, MD, PhD
Professor of Pediatrics and Genetics
Duke University Medical Center
Durham, North Carolina
Defects in Metabolism of Carbohydrates

Jennifer A. Chiriboga, PhD
Pediatric and School Psychologist
Assistant Professor
Department of Counseling, Psychology, and
Special Education
Duquesne University School of Psychology
Pittsburgh, Pennsylvania
Anxiety Disorders

Yvonne E. Chiu, MD
Associate Professor of Dermatology and
Pediatrics
Medical College of Wisconsin
Department of Dermatology
Division of Pediatric Dermatology
Children's Hospital of Wisconsin
Milwaukee, Wisconsin
Morphology of the Skin
Dermatologic Evaluation of the Patient
Eczematous Disorders
Photosensitivity
Diseases of the Epidermis

Christine B. Cho, MD
Assistant Professor of Pediatrics
Division of Allergy-Immunology
Department of Pediatrics
University of Colorado School of Medicine
National Jewish Health
Denver, Colorado
Ocular Allergies
Adverse Reactions to Drugs

Hey Jin Chong, MD, PhD
Assistant Professor of Pediatrics
University of Pittsburgh School of Medicine
Chief, Division of Pediatric Allergy and
Immunology
UPMC Children's Hospital of Pittsburgh
Pittsburgh, Pennsylvania
Infections in Immunocompromised Persons

Stella T. Chou, MD
Associate Professor
Department of Pediatrics
University of Pennsylvania Perelman School of
Medicine
Children's Hospital of Philadelphia
Philadelphia, Pennsylvania
Development of the Hematopoietic System

John C. Christenson, MD
Professor of Clinical Pediatrics
Ryan White Center for Pediatric Infectious
Diseases and Global Health
Indiana University School of Medicine
Indianapolis, Indiana
*Health Advice for Children Traveling
Internationally*

Robert H. Chun, MD
Associate Professor of Pediatric Otolaryngology
Department of Otolaryngology and
Communication Sciences
Medical College of Wisconsin
Milwaukee, Wisconsin
Acute Mastoiditis

Michael J. Chusid, MD
Professor (Infectious Disease)
Department of Pediatrics
Medical College of Wisconsin
Medical Director, Infection Prevention and
Control
Children's Hospital of Wisconsin
Milwaukee, Wisconsin
Infection Prevention and Control
Other Anaerobic Infections

**Theodore J. Cieslak, MD, MPH,
FAAP, FIDSA**
Associate Professor of Epidemiology
Associate Director, Center for Biosecurity,
Biopreparedness, and Emerging Infectious
Diseases
University of Nebraska Medical Center
College of Public Health
Omaha, Nebraska
Biologic and Chemical Terrorism

**Donna J. Claes, MD, MS,
BS Pharm**
Assistant Professor of Pediatrics
University of Cincinnati College of Medicine
Division of Pediatric Nephrology
Cincinnati Children's Hospital Medical Center
Cincinnati, Ohio
Chronic Kidney Disease
End-Stage Renal Disease

Jeff A. Clark, MD
Associate Professor
Department of Pediatrics
Wayne State University School of Medicine
Children's Hospital of Michigan
Detroit, Michigan
Respiratory Distress and Failure

**John David Clemens, MD,
PhD (Hon)**
Professor and Vice Chair
Department of Epidemiology
Founding Director, Center for Global Infectious
Diseases
UCLA Fielding School of Public Health
Los Angeles, California;
International Centre for Diarrhoeal Disease
Research
Dhaka, Bangladesh
International Immunization Practices

Thomas D. Coates, MD
Professor of Pediatrics and Pathology
University of Southern California Keck School of
    Medicine
Head, Section of Hematology
Children's Center for Cancer and Blood Diseases
Children's Hospital of Los Angeles
Los Angeles, California
Neutrophils
Disorders of Phagocyte Function

Susan E. Coffin, MD, MPH
Professor of Pediatrics
Distinguished Chair in the Department of
    Pediatrics
University of Pennsylvania Perelman School of
    Medicine
Associate Chief, Division of Infectious Diseases
Children's Hospital of Philadelphia
Philadelphia, Pennsylvania
Childcare and Communicable Diseases

Joanna S. Cohen, MD
Associate Professor of Pediatrics and Emergency
    Medicine
George Washington University School of
    Medicine
Division of Pediatric Emergency Medicine
Children's National Medical Center
Washington, DC
Care of Abrasions and Minor Lacerations

Mitchell B. Cohen, MD
Katharine Reynolds Ireland Endowed Chair in
    Pediatrics
Professor and Chair, Department of Pediatrics
University of Alabama at Birmingham School of
    Medicine
Physician-in-Chief
Children's of Alabama
Birmingham, Alabama
Clostridium difficile Infection

Michael Cohen-Wolkowiez, MD
Professor of Pediatrics
Duke Clinical Research Institute
Duke University Medical Center
Durham, North Carolina
Principles of Antifungal Therapy

Robert A. Colbert, MD, PhD
Acting Clinical Director
National Institute of Arthritis and
    Musculoskeletal and Skin Diseases
Chief, Pediatric Translational Branch
National Institutes of Health
Bethesda, Maryland
Ankylosing Spondylitis and Other
    Spondylarthritides
Reactive and Postinfectious Arthritis

F. Sessions Cole III, MD
Assistant Vice-Chancellor for Children's Health
Park J. White Professor of Pediatrics
Professor of Cell Biology and Physiology
Washington University School of Medicine in
    St. Louis
Chief Medical Officer
Vice-Chairman, Department of Pediatrics
Director of Newborn Medicine
St. Louis Children's Hospital
St. Louis, Missouri
Inherited Disorders of Surfactant Metabolism
Pulmonary Alveolar Proteinosis

J. Michael Collaco, MD, MS, MBA,
MPH, PhD
Associate Professor of Pediatrics
Eudowood Division of Pediatric Respiratory
    Sciences
Johns Hopkins University School of Medicine
Baltimore, Maryland
Bronchopulmonary Dysplasia

John L. Colombo, MD
Professor of Pediatrics
University of Nebraska College of Medicine
Division of Pediatric Pulmonology
Nebraska Regional Cystic Fibrosis Center
University of Nebraska Medical Center
Omaha, Nebraska
Aspiration Syndromes
Chronic Recurrent Aspiration

Joseph A. Congeni, MD
Director, Sports Medicine Center
Akron Children's Hospital
Akron, Ohio;
Associate Professor of Pediatrics and Sports
    Medicine
Northeast Ohio Medical University
Rootstown, Ohio;
Clinical Associate Professor of Pediatrics and
    Sports Medicine
Ohio University College of Osteopathic Medicine
Athens, Ohio
Sports-Related Traumatic Brain Injury
    (Concussion)
Cervical Spinal Spine Injuries

Lindsay N. Conner, MD, MPH
Department of Obstetrics and Gynecology
Benefis Health System
Great Falls, Montana
Breast Concerns

Sarah M. Creighton, MBBS
Professor and Consultant Gynaecologist
Department of Women's Health
University College London Hospitals
London, United Kingdom
Female Genital Mutilation

James E. Crowe Jr, MD
Ann Scott Carell Chair and Professor of
    Pediatrics
Division of Pediatric Infectious Diseases
Professor of Pathology, Microbiology, and
    Immunology
Director, Vanderbilt Vaccine Center
Vanderbilt University School of Medicine
Nashville, Tennessee
Respiratory Syncytial Virus
Human Metapneumovirus

Steven J. Czinn, MD
Professor and Chair
Department of Pediatrics
University of Maryland School of Medicine
Baltimore, Maryland
Peptic Ulcer Disease in Children

Aarti S. Dalal, DO
Assistant Professor of Pediatrics
Washington University School of Medicine in
    St. Louis
Division of Pediatric Cardiology
St Louis Children's Hospital
St. Louis, Missouri
Syncope
Disturbances of Rate and Rhythm of the Heart
Sudden Death

Josep O. Dalmau, MD, PhD
Research Professor ICREA-IDIBAPS
Service of Neurology
Hospital Clinic
University of Barcelona
Barcelona, Spain;
Adjunct Professor of Neurology
University of Pennsylvania Perelman School of
    Medicine
Philadelphia, Pennsylvania
Autoimmune Encephalitis

Lara A. Danziger-Isakov, MD, MPH
Professor of Pediatrics
University of Cincinnati College of Medicine
Director, Immunocompromised Host Infectious
    Disease
Cincinnati Children's Hospital Medical Center
Cincinnati, Ohio
Histoplasmosis (Histoplasma capsulatum)

Toni Darville, MD
Professor of Pediatrics and Microbiology and
    Immunology
University of North Carolina at Chapel Hill
Chief, Division of Infectious Diseases
Vice-Chair of Pediatric Research
North Carolina Children's Hospital
Chapel Hill, North Carolina
Neisseria gonorrhoeae (Gonococcus)

Robert S. Daum, MD, CM, MSc
Professor of Medicine
Center for Vaccine Development and Global
    Health
University of Maryland School of Medicine
Baltimore, Maryland
Haemophilus influenzae

Loren T. Davidson, MD
Clinical Professor
Department of Physical Medicine and
    Rehabilitation
University of California, Davis School of
    Medicine
Davis, California;
Director, Spinal Cord Injury
Shriners Hospital for Children
Sacramento, California
Spasticity

Richard S. Davidson, MD
Emeritus Professor of Orthopaedic Surgery
University of Pennsylvania Perelman School of
    Medicine
Attending Orthopaedic Surgeon
Children's Hospital of Philadelphia
Philadelphia, Pennsylvania
The Foot and Toes
Leg-Length Discrepancy
Arthrogryposis

H. Dele Davies, MD, MS, MHCM
Vice-Chancellor for Academic Affairs
Dean for Graduate Studies
University of Nebraska Medical Center
Omaha, Nebraska
Chancroid (Haemophilus ducreyi)
Syphilis (Treponema pallidum)
Nonvenereal Treponemal Infections
Leptospira
Relapsing Fever (Borrelia)

Najat C. Daw, MD
Professor
Division of Pediatrics
University of Texas MD Anderson Cancer Center
Houston, Texas
Neoplasms of the Kidney

Shannon L. Dean, MD, PhD
Instructor in Neurology and Pediatrics
University of Rochester Medical Center
Rochester, New York
Dystonia

Helen M. Oquendo Del Toro, MD
Pediatric and Adolescent Gynecology
Clinical Assistant Professor
University of New Mexico
Department of Obstetrics and Gynecology
Albuquerque, New Mexico
Vulvovaginitis

David R. DeMaso, MD
Psychiatrist-in-Chief
The Leon Eisenberg Chair in Psychiatry
Boston Children's Hospital;
George P. Gardner and Olga E. Monks Professor
    of Child Psychiatry
Professor of Pediatrics
Harvard Medical School
Boston, Massachusetts
Psychosocial Assessment and Interviewing
Psychopharmacology
Psychotherapy and Psychiatric Hospitalization
Somatic Symptom and Related Disorders
Rumination and Pica
Motor Disorders and Habits
Anxiety Disorders
Mood Disorders
Suicide and Attempted Suicide
Disruptive, Impulse-Control, and Conduct
    Disorders
Tantrums and Breath-Holding Spells
Lying, Stealing, and Truancy
Aggression
Self-Injurious Behavior
Childhood Psychoses

Mark R. Denison, MD
Craig-Weaver Professor of Pediatrics
Professor of Pathology, Microbiology, and
    Immunology
Vanderbilt University Medical Center
Monroe Carell Jr Children's Hospital at Vanderbilt
Nashville, Tennessee
Coronaviruses

Arlene E. Dent, MD, PhD
Associate Professor of Pediatrics
Center for Global Health and Diseases
Case Western Reserve University School of
    Medicine
Cleveland, Ohio
Ascariasis (Ascaris lumbricoides)
Trichuriasis (Trichuris trichiura)
Enterobiasis (Enterobius vermicularis)
Strongyloidiasis (Strongyloides stercoralis)
Lymphatic Filariasis (Brugia malayi, Brugia
    timori, and Wuchereria bancrofti)
Other Tissue Nematodes
Toxocariasis (Visceral and Ocular Larva Migrans)
Trichinellosis (Trichinella spiralis)

Robert J. Desnick, MD, PhD
Dean for Genetics and Genomic Medicine
Professor and Chair Emeritus, Genetics and
    Genomic Sciences
Professor, Departments of Pediatrics, Oncological
    Sciences, and Obstetrics, Gynecology and
    Reproductive Science
Kravis Children's Hospital at the Icahn School of
    Medicine at Mount Sinai
New York, New York
Lipidoses (Lysosomal Storage Disorders)
Mucolipidoses
Disorders of Glycoprotein Degradation and
    Structure
The Porphyrias

Robin R. Deterding, MD
Professor of Pediatrics
University of Colorado School of Medicine
Chief, Pediatric Pulmonary Medicine
Director, Breathing Institute
Co-Chair, Children's Interstitial and Diffuse Lung
    Disease Research Network
Medical Director, Children's Colorado Innovation
    Center
Children's Hospital Colorado
Aurora, Colorado
Fibrotic Lung Disease

Prasad Devarajan, MD, FAAP
Louise M. Williams Endowed Chair
Professor of Pediatrics and Developmental
    Biology
University of Cincinnati College of Medicine
Director of Nephrology and Hypertension
CEO, Dialysis Unit
Cincinnati Children's Hospital Medical Center
Cincinnati, Ohio
Multisystem Disease Associated with Hematuria
Tubulointerstitial Disease Associated with
    Hematuria
Vascular Disease Associated with Hematuria
Anatomic Abnormalities Associated with
    Hematuria
Lower Urinary Tract Causes of Hematuria
Acute Kidney Injury

Gabrielle A. deVeber, MD, MHSc
Professor of Pediatrics
University of Toronto Faculty of Medicine
Children's Stroke Program
Division of Neurology
Senior Scientist Emeritus, Research Institute
Hospital for Sick Children
Toronto, Ontario, Canada
Pediatric Stroke

Vineet Dhar, BDS, MDS, PhD,
Clinical Professor and Chairman
Department of Orthodontics and Pediatric
    Dentistry
Director, Advanced Specialty Education Program,
    Pediatric Dentistry
Diplomate, American Board of Pediatric
    Dentistry
University of Maryland School of Dentistry
Baltimore, Maryland
Development and Developmental Anomalies of
    the Teeth
Disorders of the Oral Cavity Associated with Other
    Conditions
Malocclusion
Cleft Lip and Palate
Syndromes with Oral Manifestations
Dental Caries
Periodontal Diseases
Dental Trauma
Common Lesions of the Oral Soft Tissues
Diseases of the Salivary Glands and Jaws
Diagnostic Radiology in Dental Assessment

Anil Dhawan, MD, FRCPCH
Professor of Pediatric Hepatology
Pediatric Liver GI and Nutrition Centre
MowatLabs King's College London School of
    Medicine at King's College Hospital NSH
    Foundation Trust
London, United Kingdom
Liver and Biliary Disorders Causing Malabsorption

André A.S. Dick, MD, MPH, FACS
Associate Professor of Surgery
Division of Transplantation
University of Washington School of Medicine
Section of Pediatric Transplantation
Seattle Children's Hospital
Seattle, Washington
Intestinal Transplantation in Children with
    Intestinal Failure

Harry C. Dietz III, MD
Victor A. McKusick Professor of Medicine and
    Genetics
Departments of Pediatrics, Medicine, and
    Molecular Biology and Genetics
Investigator, Howard Hughes Medical Institute
Institute of Genetic Medicine
Johns Hopkins University School of Medicine
Baltimore, Maryland
Marfan Syndrome

Daren A. Diiorio, MD
Resident Physician
Department of Dermatology
Medical College of Wisconsin
Milwaukee, Wisconsin
Principles of Dermatologic Therapy
Cutaneous Bacterial Infections
Cutaneous Fungal Infections
Cutaneous Viral Infections
Arthropod Bites and Infestations

Linda A. DiMeglio, MD, MPH
Professor
Department of Pediatrics
Indiana University School of Medicine
Indiana University Clinical and Translational
    Science Institute
Riley Hospital for Children
Indianapolis, Indiana
Hypophosphatasia
Hyperphosphatasia

Bradley P. Dixon, MD, FASN
Associate Professor of Pediatrics and Medicine
Renal Section, Department of Pediatrics
University of Colorado School of Medicine
Kidney Center
Children's Hospital Colorado
Aurora, Colorado
Tubular Function
Renal Tubular Acidosis
Nephrogenic Diabetes Insipidus
Inherited Tubular Transport Abnormalities

Nomazulu Dlamini, MBBS, PhD
Assistant Professor of Pediatrics
University of Toronto Faculty of Medicine
Staff Physician in Neurology
Director, Children's Stroke Program
Hospital for Sick Children
Toronto, Ontario, Canada
Pediatric Stroke

Sonam N. Dodhia, MD
Resident Physician
New York-Presbyterian Hospital
New York, New York
Congenital Disorders of the Nose
Acquired Disorders of the Nose
Nasal Polyps
General Considerations and Evaluation of the Ear
Hearing Loss
Congenital Malformations of the Ear
External Otitis (Otitis Externa)
The Inner Ear and Diseases of the Bony Labyrinth
Traumatic Injuries of the Ear and Temporal Bone
Tumors of the Ear and Temporal Bone

Patricia A. Donohoue, MD
Professor of Pediatrics
Chief, Pediatric Endocrinology
Medical College of Wisconsin
Medical Director, Pediatric Endocrinology
Children's Hospital of Wisconsin
Milwaukee, Wisconsin
Development and Function of the Gonads
Hypofunction of the Testes
Pseudoprecocity Resulting from Tumors of
the Testes
Gynecomastia
Hypofunction of the Ovaries
Pseudoprecocity Resulting from Lesions of
the Ovary
Disorders of Sex Development

Kevin J. Downes, MD
Assistant Professor of Pediatrics
University of Pennsylvania Perelman School of
Medicine
Attending Physician, Division of Infectious
Diseases
Children's Hospital of Philadelphia
Philadelphia, Pennsylvania
Tularemia (Francisella tularensis)
Brucella

**Alexander J. Doyle, MBBS,
MDRes, FRCA**
William Harvey Research Institute
Barts and The London School of Medicine
Queen Mary University of London
London, United Kingdom
Marfan Syndrome

Daniel A. Doyle, MD
Associate Professor of Pediatrics
Thomas Jefferson University Sidney Kimmel
Medical College
Philadelphia, Pennsylvania;
Chief, Division of Pediatric Endocrinology
Nemours Alfred I. duPont Hospital for Children
Wilmington, Delaware
Hormones and Peptides of Calcium Homeostasis
and Bone Metabolism
Hypoparathyroidism
Pseudohypoparathyroidism (Albright Hereditary
Osteodystrophy)
Hyperparathyroidism

**Jefferson J. Doyle, MBBChir, PhD,
MHS**
Assistant Professor of Ophthalmology
Wilmer Eye Institute
Johns Hopkins Hospital
Affiliate Member, Institute of Genetic Medicine
Johns Hopkins University School of Medicine
Baltimore, Maryland
Marfan Syndrome

Stephen C. Dreskin, MD, PhD
Professor of Medicine and Immunology
Division of Allergy and Clinical Immunology
Department of Medicine
University of Colorado School of Medicine
Aurora, Colorado
Urticaria (Hives) and Angioedema

Sherilyn W. Driscoll, MD
Division Chair, Pediatric Rehabilitation
Departments of Physical Medicine and
Rehabilitation and Pediatric and Adolescent
Medicine
Mayo Clinic Children's Center
Rochester, Minnesota
Specific Sports and Associated Injuries

Yigal Dror, MD, FRCPC
Professor
Department of Pediatrics
University of Toronto Faculty of Medicine
Head, Hematology Section
Director, Marrow Failure and Myelodysplasia
Program
The Hospital for Sick Children
Toronto, Ontario, Canada
The Inherited Pancytopenias

Jill N. D'Souza, MD
Assistant Professor
Baylor College of Medicine
Division of Pediatric Otolaryngology – Head and
Neck Surgery
Texas Children's Hospital
Houston, Texas
Congenital Anomalies of the Larynx, Trachea, and
Bronchi

Howard Dubowitz, MD, MS, FAAP
Professor of Pediatrics
Head, Division of Child Protection
Director, Center for Families
University of Maryland School of Medicine
Baltimore, Maryland
Abused and Neglected Children

J. Stephen Dumler, MD
Professor and Chair
Joint Department of Pathology
Uniformed Services University of the Health
Sciences
Walter Reed National Military Medical Center
Bethesda, Maryland
Spotted Fever Group Rickettsioses
Scrub Typhus (Orientia tsutsugamushi)
Typhus Group Rickettsioses
Ehrlichioses and Anaplasmosis
Q Fever (Coxiella burnetii)

Janet Duncan, MSN, CPNP
Department of Psychosocial Oncology and
Palliative Care
Boston Children's Hospital
Dana-Farber Cancer Institute
Boston, Massachusetts
Pediatric Palliative Care

Jeffrey A. Dvergsten, MD
Assistant Professor of Pediatrics
Duke University School of Medicine
Division of Pediatric Rheumatology
Duke University Health System
Durham, North Carolina
Treatment of Rheumatic Diseases

Michael G. Earing, MD
Professor of Internal Medicine and Pediatrics
Division of Adult Cardiovascular Medicine and
Division of Pediatric Cardiology
Medical College of Wisconsin
Director, Wisconsin Adult Congenital Heart
Disease Program (WAtCH)
Children's Hospital of Wisconsin
Milwaukee, Wisconsin
Congenital Heart Disease in Adults

Matthew D. Eberly, MD
Associate Professor of Pediatrics
Program Director, Pediatric Infectious Diseases
Fellowship
Uniformed Services University of the Health
Sciences
Bethesda, Maryland
Primary Amebic Meningoencephalitis

S. Derrick Eddy, MD
Sports Medicine Education Director
Akron Children's Hospital
Clinical Assistant Professor of Pediatrics
Northeast Ohio Medical University
Akron, Ohio
Cervical Spinal Spine Injuries

Marie E. Egan, MD
Professor of Pediatrics (Respiratory) and Cellular
and Molecular Physiology
Director, Cystic Fibrosis Center
Vice Chair for Research
Department of Pediatrics
Yale School of Medicine
New Haven, Connecticut
Cystic Fibrosis

Jack S. Elder, MD, FACS
Chief of Pediatric Urology
Massachusetts General Hospital
Boston, Massachusetts
*Congenital Anomalies and Dysgenesis of
the Kidneys*
Urinary Tract Infections
Vesicoureteral Reflux
Obstruction of the Urinary Tract
Anomalies of the Bladder
Neuropathic Bladder
Enuresis and Voiding Dysfunction
Anomalies of the Penis and Urethra
Disorders and Anomalies of the Scrotal Contents
Trauma to the Genitourinary Tract
Urinary Lithiasis

Elizabeth Englander, PhD
Professor of Psychology
Founder and Director, Massachusetts Aggression
Reduction Center
Bridgewater State University
Bridgewater, Massachusetts
Bullying, Cyberbullying, and School Violence

Elizabeth Enlow, MD, MS
Assistant Professor of Pediatrics
University of Cincinnati College of Medicine
Division of Neonatology
Cincinnati Children's Hospital Medical Center
Cincinnati, Ohio
*Clinical Manifestations of Diseases in the Newborn
Period*

Stephen C. Eppes, MD
Professor of Pediatrics
Sidney Kimmel Medical College at Thomas
Jefferson University
Philadelphia, Pennsylvania;
Vice Chair, Department of Pediatrics
Division of Pediatric Infectious Diseases
Christiana Care Health System
Newark, Delaware
Lyme Disease (Borrelia burgdorferi)

Jessica Ericson, MD
Assistant Professor of Pediatrics
Pennsylvania State University College of Medicine
Division of Pediatric Infectious Disease
Milton S. Hershey Medical Center
Hershey, Pennsylvania
Candida

Elif Erkan, MD, MS
Associate Professor of Pediatrics
University of Cincinnati College of Medicine
Division of Pediatric Nephrology
Cincinnati Children's Hospital Medical Center
Cincinnati, Ohio
Nephrotic Syndrome

Yokabed Ermias, MPH
Fellow, Division of Reproductive Health
Centers for Disease Control and Prevention
Atlanta, Georgia
Contraception

Ashley M. Eskew, MD
Fellow, Reproductive Endocrinology and
Infertility
Department of Obstetrics and Gynecology
Washington University School of Medicine in
St. Louis
St. Louis, Missouri
Vulvovaginal and Müllerian Anomalies

Ruth A. Etzel, MD, PhD
Milken Institute School of Public Health
George Washington University
Washington, DC
Overview of Environmental Health and Children

Matthew P. Fahrenkopf, MD
Plastic Surgery Resident
Spectrum Health Hospitals
Michigan State University
Grand Rapids, Michigan
Deformational Plagiocephaly

Marni J. Falk, MD
Associate Professor of Pediatrics
University of Pennsylvania Perelman School of
Medicine
Executive Director, Mitochondrial Medicine
Frontier Program
Children's Hospital of Philadelphia
Philadelphia, Pennsylvania
Mitochondrial Disease Diagnosis

John J. Faria, MD
Assistant Professor of Otolaryngology and
Pediatrics
University of Rochester
Rochester, New York
Acute Mastoiditis

John H. Fargo, DO
Division of Pediatric Hematology/Oncology
Showers Family Center for Childhood Cancer
and Blood Disorders
Akron Children's Hospital
Akron, Ohio
The Acquired Pancytopenias

**Kristen A. Feemster, MD, MPH,
MSPHR**
Director of Research for the Vaccine Education
Center
Children's Hospital of Philadelphia
Medical Director of the Immunization Program
and Acute Communicable Diseases
Philadelphia Department of Public Health
Adjunct Associate Professor of Pediatrics
University of Pennsylvania Perelman School of
Medicine
Philadelphia, Pennsylvania
Human Papillomaviruses

Susan Feigelman, MD
Professor, Department of Pediatrics
University of Maryland School of Medicine
Baltimore, Maryland
Developmental and Behavioral Theories
Assessment of Fetal Growth and Development
The First Year
The Second Year
The Preschool Years
Middle Childhood

Jeffrey A. Feinstein, MD, MPH
Dunlevie Family Professor of Pulmonary Vascular
Disease
Division of Pediatric Cardiology
Stanford University School of Medicine
Professor, by courtesy, of Bioengineering
Medical Director, Pediatric Pulmonary
Hypertension Program
Lucile Packard Children's Hospital at Stanford
Palo Alto, California
Pulmonary Hypertension

Amy G. Feldman, MD, MSCS
Assistant Professor of Pediatrics
University of Colorado School of Medicine
Denver, Colorado;
Program Director, Liver Transplant Fellowship
Children's Hospital Colorado Research Institute
Aurora, Colorado
Drug- and Toxin-Induced Liver Injury
Acute Hepatic Failure

Eric I. Felner, MD, MS
Professor of Pediatrics
Division of Pediatric Endocrinology
Director, Pediatric Clerkships
Emory University School of Medicine
Atlanta, Georgia
Hormones of the Hypothalamus and Pituitary
Hypopituitarism

Edward C. Fels, MD
Clinical Assistant Professor of Medicine
Tufts University School of Medicine
Boston, Massachusetts;
Maine Medical Center
Portland, Maine
Vasculitis Syndromes

Sing-Yi Feng, MD, FAAP
Associate Professor
Division of Emergency Medicine
Department of Pediatrics
Children's Medical Center of Dallas
Medical Toxicologist
North Texas Poison Center
Parkland Memorial Hospital
The University of Texas Southwestern Medical
Center at Dallas
Dallas, Texas
Envenomations

Thomas W. Ferkol Jr, MD
Alexis Hartmann Professor of Pediatrics
Director, Division of Pediatric Allergy,
Immunology, and Pulmonary Medicine
Washington University School of Medicine in
St. Louis
St. Louis, Missouri
*Primary Ciliary Dyskinesia (Immotile Cilia
Syndrome, Kartagener Syndrome)*

Karin E. Finberg MD, PhD
Assistant Professor
Department of Pathology
Yale School of Medicine
New Haven, Connecticut
Iron-Refractory Iron-Deficiency Anemia

Jonathan D. Finder, MD
Professor of Pediatrics
The University of Tennessee Health Science
Center
Attending Pediatric Pulmonologist
Division of Pediatric Pulmonology
Le Bonheur Children's Hospital
Memphis, Tennessee
Bronchomalacia and Tracheomalacia
Congenital Disorders of the Lung

Laura H. Finkelstein, MD
Assistant Professor, Department of Pediatrics
University of Maryland School of Medicine
Baltimore, Maryland
Assessment of Fetal Growth and Development
Middle Childhood

Kristin N. Fiorino, MD
Associate Professor of Clinical Pediatrics
Suzie and Scott Lustgarten Motility Center
Gastroenterology, Hepatology, and Nutrition
Children's Hospital of Philadelphia
University of Pennsylvania Perelman School of
  Medicine
Motility Disorders and Hirschsprung Disease

Philip R. Fischer, MD
Professor of Pediatrics
Department of Pediatric and Adolescent Medicine
Mayo Clinic
Rochester, Minnesota
Adult Tapeworm Infections
Cysticercosis
Echinococcosis (Echinococcus granulosus *and*
  Echinococcus multilocularis)

Brian T. Fisher, DO, MSCE
Assistant Professor of Pediatrics and
  Epidemiology
University of Pennsylvania Perelman School of
  Medicine
Fellowship Program Director
Division of Infectious Diseases
Children's Hospital of Philadelphia
Philadelphia, Pennsylvania
Actinomyces
Nocardia

Veronica H. Flood, MD
Associate Professor
Department of Pediatrics
Division of Pediatric Hematology/Oncology
Medical College of Wisconsin
Milwaukee, Wisconsin
Hemostasis
Hereditary Clotting Factor Deficiencies (Bleeding
  Disorders)
von Willebrand Disease
Postneonatal Vitamin K Deficiency
Liver Disease
Acquired Inhibitors of Coagulation
Platelet and Blood Vessel Disorders

Francisco X. Flores, MD
Associate Professor of Pediatrics
University of Cincinnati College of Medicine
Medical Director, Clinical Services and MARS
  Program
Division of Nephrology and Hypertension
Cincinnati Children's Hospital Medical Center
Cincinnati, Ohio
Clinical Evaluation of the Child with Hematuria
Isolated Renal Disease Associated with Hematuria
Clinical Evaluation of the Child with Proteinuria
Conditions Associated with Proteinuria

Joseph T. Flynn, MD, MS
Dr. Robert O. Hickman Endowed Chair in
  Pediatric Nephrology
Professor of Pediatrics
University of Washington School of Medicine
Chief, Division of Nephrology
Seattle Children's Hospital
Seattle, Washington
Systemic Hypertension

Patricia M. Flynn, MD
Senior Vice President and Medical Director of
  Quality and Patient Care
Deputy Clinical Director
Member, Department of Infectious Diseases
Arthur Ashe Chair in Pediatric AIDS Research
St. Jude Children's Research Hospital
Memphis, Tennessee
Infection Associated with Medical Devices
Cryptosporidium, Isospora, Cyclospora, and
  Microsporidia

Joel A. Forman, MD
Associate Professor of Pediatrics and Preventive
  Medicine
Vice-Chair for Education
Department of Pediatrics
Kravis Children's Hospital at the Icahn School of
  Medicine at Mount Sinai
New York, New York
Chemical Pollutants

Michael M. Frank, MD
Professor Emeritus of Pediatrics, Medicine, and
  Immunology
Duke University School of Medicine
Durham, North Carolina
Urticaria (Hives) and Angioedema

Robert W. Frenck Jr, MD
Professor of Pediatrics
University of Cincinnati College of Medicine
Medical Director, Division of Infectious Diseases
Cincinnati Children's Hospital Medical Center
Cincinnati, Ohio
Liver Abscess

Deborah M. Friedman, MD
Pediatric Cardiology
New York Medical College
Maria Fareri Children's Hospital
Westchester Medical Center
Valhalla, New York
Neonatal Lupus

Erika Friehling, MD
Assistant Professor of Pediatrics
University of Pittsburgh School of Medicine
Division of Pediatric Hematology/Oncology
UPMC Children's Hospital of Pittsburgh
Pittsburgh, Pennsylvania
Principles of Cancer Diagnosis
Principles of Cancer Treatment
The Leukemias

Stephanie A. Fritz, MD, MSCI
Associate Professor of Pediatrics
University of Washington School of Medicine in
  St. Louis
Division of Infectious Diseases
St. Louis Children's Hospital
St. Louis, Missouri
Diphtheria (Corynebacterium diphtheriae)

Donald P. Frush, MD, FACR, FAAP
Professor of Radiology
Lucile Packard Children's Hospital at Stanford
Stanford University School of Medicine
Stanford, California
Biologic Effects of Ionizing Radiation on Children

Anne M. Gadomski, MD, MPH
Director, Bassett Research Institute
Bassett Medical Center
Cooperstown, New York;
Associate Professor of Pediatrics
Columbia University Medical Center
New York, New York
Strategies for Health Behavior Change

James T. Gaensbauer, MD, MScPH
Assistant Professor of Pediatrics
University of Colorado School of Medicine
Pediatric Infectious Diseases
Denver Health Medical Center and Children's
  Hospital Colorado
Denver, Colorado
Staphylococcus

Sheila Gahagan, MD, MPH
Professor of Clinical Pediatrics
Chief, Division of Academic General Pediatrics,
  Child Development, and Community Health
Martin Stein Endowed Chair, Developmental-
  Behavioral Pediatrics
University of California, San Diego School of
  Medicine
La Jolla, California
Overweight and Obesity

William A. Gahl, MD, PhD
Clinical Director, National Human Genome
  Research Institute
Director, NIH Undiagnosed Diseases Program
National Institutes of Health
Bethesda, Maryland
Genetic Approaches to Rare and Undiagnosed
  Diseases

Patrick G. Gallagher, MD
Professor of Pediatrics, Genetics, and Pathology
Yale University School of Medicine
Attending Physician
Yale New Haven Children's Hospital
New Haven, Connecticut
Definitions and Classification of Hemolytic Anemias
Hereditary Spherocytosis
Hereditary Elliptocytosis, Hereditary
  Pyropoikilocytosis, and Related Disorders
Hereditary Stomatocytosis
Paroxysmal Nocturnal Hemoglobinuria and
  Acanthocytosis

Hayley A. Gans, MD
Clinical Professor of Pediatrics
Stanford University School of Medicine
Division of Pediatric Infectious Diseases
Stanford, California
Measles
Rubella
Mumps

Cristina Garcia-Mauriño, MD
Physician Scientist
Center for Vaccines and Immunity
The Research Institute at Nationwide Children's
  Hospital
Columbus, Ohio
Hansen Disease (Mycobacterium leprae)

Paula M. Gardiner, MD, MPH
Associate Professor
Associate Research Director
Department of Family Medicine and Community
  Health
University of Massachusetts Medical School
Worcester, Massachusetts
Complementary Therapies and Integrative
  Medicine

Luigi R. Garibaldi, MD
Professor of Pediatrics
University of Pittsburgh School of Medicine
Clinical Director
Division of Pediatric Endocrinology
Children's Hospital of UPMC
Pittsburgh, Pennsylvania
Physiology of Puberty
Disorders of Pubertal Development

Gregory M. Gauthier, MD, MS
Associate Professor of Medicine
Division of Infectious Diseases
University of Wisconsin School of Medicine and
  Public Health
Madison, Wisconsin
Blastomycosis (Blastomyces dermatitidis)

Jeffrey S. Gerber, MD, PhD
Associate Professor of Pediatrics and
  Epidemiology
University of Pennsylvania Perelman School of
  Medicine
Division of Infectious Diseases
Children's Hospital of Philadelphia
Philadelphia, Pennsylvania
Legionella

Anne A. Gershon, MD
Professor of Pediatrics
Columbia University College of Physicians and
  Surgeons
Division of Pediatric Infectious Diseases
NewYork-Presbyterian Morgan Stanley Children's
  Hospital
New York, New York

Saied Ghadersohi, MD
Resident Physician
Department of Otolaryngology – Head and Neck
  Surgery
Northwestern University Feinberg School of
  Medicine
Chicago, Illinois
Neoplasms of the Larynx, Trachea, and Bronchi

Mark Gibson, MD
Professor (Clinical) Emeritus
Department of Obstetrics and Gynecology
Chief, Division of Reproductive Endocrinology
University of Utah School of Medicine
Salt Lake City, Utah
Polycystic Ovary Syndrome and Hirsutism

Francis Gigliotti, MD
Professor and Chief of Pediatric Infectious
  Diseases and Microbiology and Immunology
Vice Chair for Academic Affairs
University of Rochester Medical Center
School of Medicine and Dentistry
Rochester, New York
Pneumocystis jirovecii

Walter S. Gilliam, MSEd, PhD
Professor of Child Psychiatry and Psychology
Child Study Center
Director, The Edward Zigler Center in Child
  Development and Social Policy
Yale School of Medicine
New Haven, Connecticut
Childcare

Salil Ginde, MD, MPH
Assistant Professor of Pediatrics
Division of Pediatric Cardiology
Medical College of Wisconsin
Milwaukee, Wisconsin
Congenital Heart Disease in Adults

John A. Girotto, MD
Section Chief
Pediatric Plastic Surgery and Dermatology Center
Helen DeVos Children's Hospital
Grand Rapids, Michigan
Deformational Plagiocephaly

Samuel B. Goldfarb, MD
Medical Director
Pediatric Lung and Heart/Lung Transplant
  Programs
Division of Pulmonary Medicine
Medical Director, Solid Organ Transplant Center
Children's Hospital of Philadelphia
Professor of Clinical Pediatrics
University of Pennsylvania
Perelman School of Medicine
Philadelphia, Pennsylvania
Heart-Lung and Lung Transplantation

David L. Goldman, MD
Associate Professor of Pediatrics and
  Microbiology and Immunology
Albert Einstein College of Medicine
Division of Pediatric Infectious Disease
Montefiore Medical Center
Bronx, New York
*Cryptococcus neoformans and Cryptococcus
  gattii*

Stanton C. Goldman, MD
Division of Pediatric Hematology, Oncology, and
  Stem Cell Transplant
Medical City Children's Hospital
Texas Oncology, PA
Dallas, Texas

Neal D. Goldstein, PhD, MBI
Assistant Research Professor of Epidemiology and
  Biostatistics
Drexel University Dornsife School of Public
  Health
Philadelphia, Pennsylvania;
Infectious Disease Epidemiologist
Christiana Care Health System
Newark, Delaware
Lyme Disease (Borrelia burgdorferi)

**Stuart L. Goldstein, MD, FAAP,
FNKF**
Clark D. West Endowed Chair and Professor of
  Pediatrics
University of Cincinnati College of Medicine
Director, Center for Acute Care Nephrology
Cincinnati Children's Hospital Medical Center
Cincinnati, Ohio
End-Stage Renal Disease

Joseph Gonzalez-Heydrich, MD
Associate Professor of Psychiatry
Harvard Medical School
Senior Attending Psychiatrist
Boston Children's Hospital
Boston, Massachusetts
Childhood Psychoses

Denise M. Goodman, MD, MS
Professor of Pediatrics
Northwestern University Feinberg School of
  Medicine
Attending Physician, Division of Critical Care
  Medicine
Ann & Robert H. Lurie Children's Hospital of
  Chicago
Chicago, Illinois
Bronchitis
*Chronic Respiratory Failure and Long-Term
  Mechanical Ventilation*

Tracy S. Goodman, MA
Technical Officer, Expanded Programme on
  Immunization
Department of Immunization, Vaccines, and
  Biologicals
World Health Organization
Geneva, Switzerland
International Immunization Practices

Catherine M. Gordon, MD, MSc
Professor
Department of Pediatrics
Harvard Medical School
Chief, Division of Adolescent/Young Adult
  Medicine
Robert P. Masland Jr. Chair of Adolescent
  Medicine
Boston Children's Hospital
Boston, Massachusetts
Bone Structure, Growth, and Hormonal Regulation
Osteoporosis

Leslie B. Gordon, MD, PhD
Professor of Pediatrics Research
Hasbro Children's Hospital and Warren Alpert
  Medical School of Brown University
Providence, Rhode Island;
Department of Pediatrics
Boston Children's Hospital and Harvard Medical
  School
Boston, Massachusetts;
Medical Director, The Progeria Research
  Foundation
Peabody, Massachusetts
Hutchinson-Gilford Progeria Syndrome (Progeria)

Collin S. Goto, MD
Professor of Pediatrics
The University of Texas Southwestern Medical
  Center
Attending Physician
Division of Pediatric Emergency Medicine
Children's Medical Center
Dallas, Texas
Envenomations

W. Adam Gower, MD, MS
Associate Professor of Pediatrics
University of North Carolina School of Medicine
Chapel Hill, North Carolina
Neuroendocrine Cell Hyperplasia of Infancy

Neera K. Goyal, MD
Associate Professor of Pediatrics
Sidney Kimmel College of Medicine at Thomas
  Jefferson University
Philadelphia, Pennsylvania
The Newborn Infant
Jaundice and Hyperbilirubinemia in the Newborn
Kernicterus

Nicholas P. Goyeneche, MD
Department of Physical Medicine and
  Rehabilitation
Ochsner Health Center–Covington
Covington, Louisiana
Management of Musculoskeletal Injury

Kevin W. Graepel, PhD
Medical Scientist Training Program
Vanderbilt University School of Medicine
Vanderbilt University Medical Center
Nashville, Tennessee
Coronaviruses

Robert J. Graham, MD
Associate Professor
Department of Anesthesiology, Critical Care, and
Pain Medicine
Harvard Medical School
Division of Pediatric Critical Care Medicine
Boston Children's Hospital
Boston, Massachusetts
*Home Mechanical Ventilation and Technology
Dependence*

**John M. Greally, DMed, PhD,
FACMG**
Professor of Genetics, Medicine, and Pediatrics
Albert Einstein College of Medicine
Department of Genetics
Children's Hospital at Montefiore
Bronx, New York
Epigenome-Wide Association Studies and Disease

Cori M. Green, MD, MSc
Assistant Professor of Clinical Pediatrics
Weill Cornell Medicine
New York-Presbyterian Komansky Children's
Hospital
New York, New York
Strategies for Health Behavior Change

Michael Green, MD, MPH
Professor of Pediatrics, Surgery, and Clinical and
Translational Science
University of Pittsburgh School of Medicine
Division of Infectious Diseases
Director, Antimicrobial Stewardship and Infection
Prevention
UPMC Children's Hospital of Pittsburgh
Pittsburgh, Pennsylvania
Infections in Immunocompromised Persons

Larry A. Greenbaum, MD, PhD
Marcus Professor of Pediatrics
Director, Division of Pediatric Nephrology
Emory University School of Medicine
Children's Healthcare of Atlanta
Atlanta, Georgia
*Vitamin D Deficiency (Rickets) and Excess
Vitamin E Deficiency
Vitamin K Deficiency
Micronutrient Mineral Deficiencies
Electrolyte and Acid-Base Disorders
Maintenance and Replacement Therapy
Deficit Therapy*

V. Jordan Greenbaum, MD
International Centre for Missing and Exploited
Children
Alexandria, Virginia
Child Trafficking for Sex and Labor

James M. Greenberg, MD
Professor of Pediatrics
Director, Division of Neonatology
University of Cincinnati College of Medicine
Co-Director, Perinatal Institute
Cincinnati Children's Hospital Medical Center
Cincinnati, Ohio
*Overview of Morbidity and Mortality
Clinical Manifestations of Diseases in the Newborn
Period*

Anne G. Griffiths, MD
Pediatric Pulmonologist
Children's Respiratory and Critical Care
Specialists
Director, Primary Ciliary Dyskinesia Center
Children's Minnesota
Minneapolis, Minnesota
Chronic or Recurrent Respiratory Symptoms

Kenneth L. Grizzle, PhD
Associate Professor of Pediatrics
Medical College of Wisconsin
Child Development Center
Children's Hospital of Wisconsin
Milwaukee, Wisconsin
*Math and Writing Disabilities
Child-Onset Fluency Disorder*

Judith A. Groner, MD
Clinical Professor of Pediatrics
The Ohio State University College of Medicine
Section of Ambulatory Pediatrics
Nationwide Children's Hospital
Columbus, Ohio
Tobacco

Alfredo Guarino, MD
Professor of Pediatrics
Department of Translational Medical Sciences
University of Naples Federico II
Napoli, Italy
*Intestinal Infections and Infestations Associated
with Malabsorption*

Juan P. Gurria, MD
Fellow in Pediatric Trauma
Cincinnati Children's Hospital Medical Center
Cincinnati, Ohio
*Meconium Ileus, Peritonitis, and Intestinal
Obstruction*

Anat Guz-Mark, MD
Attending Physician
Institute of Gastroenterology, Nutrition and Liver
Disease
Schneider Children's Medical Center of Israel
Petah Tikva, Israel;
Sackler Faculty of Medicine
Tel Aviv University
Tel Aviv, Israel;
Chronic Diarrhea

Gabriel G. Haddad, MD
Distinguished Professor of Pediatrics and
Neuroscience
Chairman, Department of Pediatrics
University of California, San Diego School of
Medicine
Physician-in-Chief and Chief Scientific Officer
Rady Children's Hospital–San Diego
Diagnostic Approach to Respiratory Disease

Joseph Haddad Jr, MD
Lawrence Savetsky Professor Emeritus
Columbia University Irving Medical Center
New York, New York
*Congenital Disorders of the Nose
Acquired Disorders of the Nose
Nasal Polyps
General Considerations and Evaluation of the Ear
Hearing Loss
Congenital Malformations of the Ear
External Otitis (Otitis Externa)
The Inner Ear and Diseases of the Bony Labyrinth
Traumatic Injuries of the Ear and Temporal Bone
Tumors of the Ear and Temporal Bone*

Joseph F. Hagan Jr, MD, FAAP
Clinical Professor
Department of Pediatrics
The Robert Larner College of Medicine at the
University of Vermont College of Medicine
Hagan, Rinehart, and Connolly Pediatricians,
PLLC
Burlington, Vermont
*Maximizing Children's Health: Screening,
Anticipatory Guidance, and Counseling*

James S. Hagood, MD
Professor of Pediatrics (Pulmonology)
Director, Program in Rare and Interstitial Lung
Disease
University of North Carolina at Chapel Hill
Chapel Hill, North Carolina
Diagnostic Approach to Respiratory Disease

Suraiya K. Haider, MD
Sleep Physician
Fairfax Neonatal Associates
Fairfax, Virginia
Pleurisy, Pleural Effusions, and Empyema

Goknur Haliloglu, MD
Professor of Pediatrics
Department of Pediatric Neurology
Hacettepe University Children's Hospital
Ankara, Turkey
*Nemaline Rod Myopathy
Core Myopathies
Myofibrillar Myopathies
Brain Malformations and Muscle Development
Arthrogryposis
Spinal Muscular Atrophies
Other Motor Neuron Diseases*

Scott B. Halstead, MD
Adjunct Professor
Department of Preventive Medicine and
Biostatistics
Uniformed Services University of the Health
Sciences
Bethesda, Maryland
*Arboviral Infections
Dengue Fever, Dengue Hemorrhagic Fever, and
Severe Dengue
Yellow Fever
Ebola and Other Viral Hemorrhagic Fevers
Hantavirus Pulmonary Syndrome*

**Allison R. Hammer, MSN, APRN,
CPNP-PC**
Advanced Practice Nurse
Department of Otolaryngology – Head and Neck
Surgery
Ann & Robert H. Lurie Children's Hospital of
Chicago
Chicago, Illinois
Foreign Bodies in the Airway

Margaret R. Hammerschlag, MD
Professor of Pediatrics and Medicine
Director, Pediatric Infectious Disease Fellowship
Program
SUNY Down State Medical Center
Brooklyn, New York
*Chlamydia pneumoniae
Chlamydia trachomatis
Psittacosis (Chlamydia psittaci)*

Aaron Hamvas, MD
Raymond and Hazel Speck Barry Professor of
Neonatology
Northwestern University Feinberg School of
Medicine
Head, Division of Neonatology
Ann & Robert H. Lurie Children's Hospital of
Chicago
Chicago, Illinois
*Inherited Disorders of Surfactant Metabolism
Pulmonary Alveolar Proteinosis*

James C. Harris, MD
Professor of Pediatrics, Psychiatry and Behavioral
    Sciences, Mental Health, and History of
    Medicine
Division of Child and Adolescent Psychiatry
Director, Developmental Neuropsychiatry
Johns Hopkins University School of Medicine
Baltimore, Maryland
Disorders of Purine and Pyrimidine Metabolism

Douglas J. Harrison, MD, MS
Associate Professor of Pediatrics
Director of Patient Care and Programs
Co-Chair Pediatric Solid Tumor and Sarcoma
    Team
The Children's Cancer Hospital of MD Anderson
The University of Texas MD Anderson Cancer
    Center
Houston, Texas
Neuroblastoma

Corina Hartman, MD
Pediatric Gastroenterology and Nutrition Unit
Lady Davis Carmel Medical Center
Haifa, Israel
Other Malabsorptive Syndromes

Mary E. Hartman, MD, MPH
Assistant Professor of Pediatrics
Washington University School of Medicine in
    St. Louis
Division of Pediatric Critical Care Medicine
St. Louis Children's Hospital
St. Louis, Missouri
Pediatric Emergencies and Resuscitation

David B. Haslam, MD
Associate Professor of Pediatrics
University of Cincinnati College of Medicine
Director, Antimicrobial Stewardship Program
Cincinnati Children's Hospital Medical Center
Cincinnati, Ohio
Epidemiology of Infections
Healthcare-Acquired Infections
Non–Group A or B Streptococci
Enterococcus

**H. Hesham Abdel-Kader Hassan,
MD, MSc**
Professor of Pediatrics
Chief, Division of Pediatric Gastroenterology and
    Nutrition
The University of Arizona College of Medicine
Tucson, Arizona
Cholestasis

Fern R. Hauck, MD, MS
Spencer P. Bass MD Twenty-First Century
    Professor of Family Medicine
Departments of Family Medicine and Public
    Health Sciences
University of Virginia School of Medicine
Charlottesville, Virginia
Sudden Infant Death Syndrome

Fiona P. Havers, MD, MHS
Medical Epidemiologist
Epidemiology and Prevention Branch, Influenza
    Division
National Center for Immunization and
    Respiratory Diseases
Centers for Disease Control and Prevention
Atlanta, Georgia
Influenza Viruses

Ericka V. Hayes, MD
Associate Professor
Department of Pediatrics
Division of Infectious Diseases
Washington University School of Medicine in
    St. Louis
Medical Director, Pediatric and Adolescent HIV
    Program
Medical Director, Infection Prevention
St. Louis Children's Hospital
St. Louis, Missouri
Campylobacter
Yersinia
Nontuberculous Mycobacteria
Human Immunodeficiency Virus and Acquired
    Immunodeficiency Syndrome

Jacqueline T. Hecht, PhD
Professor and Division Head
Pediatric Research Center
Vice-Chair for Research
Leah L. Lewis Distinguished Chair
Department of Pediatrics
McGovern Medical School at UTHealth
Associate Dean for Research
UTHealth School of Dentistry
Houston, Texas
General Considerations in Skeletal Dysplasias
Disorders Involving Cartilage Matrix Proteins
Disorders Involving Transmembrane Receptors
Disorders Involving Ion Transporters
Disorders Involving Transcription Factors
Disorders Involving Defective Bone Resorption
Other Inherited Disorders of Skeletal Development

Sabrina M. Heidemann, MD
Professor
Department of Pediatrics
Wayne State University School of Medicine
Director, Intensive Care Unit
Co-Director of Transport
Children's Hospital of Michigan
Detroit, Michigan
Respiratory Distress and Failure

Jennifer R. Heimall, MD
Assistant Professor of Clinical Pediatrics
University of Pennsylvania Perelman School of
    Medicine
Attending Physician
Division of Allergy and Immunology
Children's Hospital of Philadelphia
Philadelphia, Pennsylvania
Immunodeficiencies Affecting Multiple Cell Types

Cheryl Hemingway, MBChB, PhD
Consultant Pediatric Neurologist
Great Ormond Street Hospital for Children
London, United Kingdom
Demyelinating Disorders of the Central Nervous
    System

†J. Owen Hendley, MD
Professor of Pediatric Infectious Diseases
University of Virginia School of Medicine
Charlottesville, Virginia
Sinusitis
Retropharyngeal Abscess, Lateral Pharyngeal
    (Parapharyngeal) Abscess, and Peritonsillar
    Cellulitis/Abscess

Michelle L. Hernandez, MD
Associate Professor of Pediatrics
University of North Carolina School of Medicine
Chief Medical Officer
UNC Center for Environmental Medicine,
    Asthma, and Lung Biology
Chapel Hill, North Carolina
Hypersensitivity Pneumonia
Occupational and Environmental Lung Disease

**Andrew D. Hershey, MD, PhD,
FAAN, FAHS**
Professor of Pediatrics
University of Cincinnati College of Medicine
Endowed Chair and Director, Division of
    Neurology
Headache Medicine Specialist
Cincinnati Children's Medical Center
Cincinnati, Ohio
Headaches

Cynthia E. Herzog, MD
Professor of Pediatrics
University of Texas MD Anderson Cancer Center
Houston, Texas
Retinoblastoma
Gonadal and Germ Cell Neoplasms
Neoplasms of the Liver
Benign Vascular Tumors
Melanoma
Nasopharyngeal Carcinoma
Adenocarcinoma of the Colon and Rectum
Desmoplastic Small Round Cell Tumor

Jesse P. Hirner, MD
Resident Physician
Department of Dermatology
University of Missouri School of Medicine
Columbia, Missouri
Tumors of the Skin

Jessica Hochberg, MD
Assistant Professor of Clinical Pediatrics
Division of Pediatric Hematology, Oncology, and
    Stem Cell Transplant
New York Medical College
Maria Fareri Children's Hospital at Westchester
    Medical Center
Valhalla, New York
Lymphoma

**Deborah Hodes, MBBS, BSc,
DRCOG, FRCPCH**
Consultant Community Paediatrician
Department of Paediatrics
University College London Hospitals
London, United Kingdom
Female Genital Mutilation

Holly R. Hoefgen, MD
Assistant Professor
Pediatric and Adolescent Gynecology
Washington University School of Medicine in
    St. Louis
Co-Director, Integrated Care and Fertility
    Preservation Program
St. Louis Children's Hospital
St. Louis, Missouri
Vulvovaginitis

---

†Deceased

Lauren D. Holinger, MD, FAAP, FACS
Paul H. Holinger MD Professor
Division of Pediatric Otolaryngology
Northwestern University Feinberg School of
    Medicine
Ann & Robert H. Lurie Children's Hospital of
    Chicago
Chicago, Illinois
Other Laryngeal Neoplasms
Tracheal Neoplasms

Cynthia M. Holland-Hall, MD, MPH
Associate Professor of Clinical Pediatrics
The Ohio State University College of Medicine
Section of Adolescent Medicine
Nationwide Children's Hospital
Columbus, Ohio
Adolescent Physical and Social Development
Transitioning to Adult Care
The Breast

David K. Hooper, MD, MS
Associate Professor of Pediatrics
University of Cincinnati College of Medicine
Medical Director of Kidney Transplantation
Cincinnati Children's Hospital Medical Center
Cincinnati, Ohio
Renal Transplantation

Julie E. Hoover-Fong, MD, PhD
Associate Professor
Department of Pediatrics
McKusick-Nathans Institute of Genetic Medicine
Director, Greenberg Center for Skeletal
    Dysplasias
Johns Hopkins University School of Medicine
Baltimore, Maryland
General Considerations in Skeletal Dysplasias
Disorders Involving Transmembrane Receptors

Jeffrey D. Hord, MD
The LOPen Charities and Mawaka Family Chair
    in Pediatric Hematology/Oncology
Director, Showers Family Center for Childhood
    Cancer and Blood Disorders
Akron Children's Hospital
Akron, Ohio
The Acquired Pancytopenias

B. David Horn, MD
Associate Professor
Department of Orthopaedic Surgery
University of Pennsylvania Perelman School of
    Medicine
Attending Orthopaedic Surgeon
Children's Hospital of Philadelphia
Philadelphia, Pennsylvania
The Hip

Helen M. Horstmann, MD
Associate Professor
Department of Orthopaedic Surgery
University of Pennsylvania Perelman School of
    Medicine
Attending Physician
Children's Hospital of Philadelphia
Philadelphia, Pennsylvania
Arthrogryposis

William A. Horton, MD
Professor
Department of Molecular Medical Genetics
Oregon Health & Science University
Director Emeritus of Research
Shriners Hospitals for Children
Portland, Oregon
General Considerations in Skeletal Dysplasias
Disorders Involving Cartilage Matrix Proteins
Disorders Involving Transmembrane Receptors
Disorders Involving Ion Transporters
Disorders Involving Transcription Factors
Disorders Involving Defective Bone Resorption
Other Inherited Disorders of Skeletal Development

Peter J. Hotez, MD, PhD
Dean, National School of Tropical Medicine
Professor, Pediatrics and Molecular Virology and
    Microbiology
Head, Section of Pediatric Tropical Medicine
Baylor College of Medicine;
Endowed Chair of Tropical Pediatrics
Center for Vaccine Development
Texas Children's Hospital;
Professor, Department of Biology
Baylor University
Waco, Texas;
Baker Institute Fellow in Disease and Poverty
Rice University
Houston, Texas
Hookworms (Necator americanus *and*
    Ancylostoma spp.)

Samantha A. House, DO
Assistant Professor of Pediatrics
Geisel School of Medicine at Dartmouth and The
    Dartmouth Institute
Hanover, New Hampshire
Wheezing in Infants: Bronchiolitis

Evelyn Hsu, MD
Associate Professor of Pediatrics
University of Washington School of Medicine
Medical Director, Liver Transplantation
Seattle Children's Hospital
Seattle, Washington
Liver Transplantation

Katherine Hsu, MD, MPH, FAAP
Associate Professor of Pediatrics
Section of Pediatric Infectious Diseases
Boston University Medical Center
Boston, Massachusetts;
Medical Director, Division of STD Prevention
    and HIV/AIDS Surveillance
Director, Ratelle STD/HIV Prevention Training
    Center
Bureau of Infectious Disease and Laboratory
    Sciences
Massachusetts Department of Public Health
Jamaica Plain, Massachusetts
Neisseria gonorrhoeae (Gonococcus)

Felicia A. Scaggs Huang, MD
Clinical Fellow
Division of Infectious Diseases
Cincinnati Children's Hospital Medical Center
Cincinnati, Ohio
Congenital and Perinatal Infections

Heather G. Huddleston, MD
Assistant Professor
Department of Obstetrics, Gynecology, and
    Reproductive Sciences
University of California, San Francisco School of
    Medicine
San Francisco, California
Polycystic Ovary Syndrome and Hirsutism

Sarah P. Huepenbecker, MD
Resident Physician
Department of Obstetrics and Gynecology
Washington University School of Medicine in
    St. Louis
St. Louis, Missouri
Gynecologic Neoplasms and Adolescent Prevention
    Methods for Human Papillomavirus

Vicki Huff, PhD
Professor
Department of Genetics
University of Texas MD Anderson Cancer Center
Houston, Texas
Neoplasms of the Kidney

Winston W. Huh, MD
Assistant Professor of Clinical Care
Children's Hospital of Los Angeles
Los Angeles, California
Gonadal and Germ Cell Neoplasms
Adenocarcinoma of the Colon and Rectum

Stephen R. Humphrey, MD
Assistant Professor
Department of Dermatology
Medical College of Wisconsin
Children's Hospital of Wisconsin
Milwaukee, Wisconsin
Principles of Dermatologic Therapy
Cutaneous Bacterial Infections
Cutaneous Fungal Infections
Cutaneous Viral Infections
Arthropod Bites and Infestations

Stephen P. Hunger, MD
Professor and Jeffrey E. Perelman Distinguished
    Chair
Department of Pediatrics
University of Pennsylvania Perelman School of
    Medicine
Chief, Division of Pediatric Oncology
Director, Center for Childhood Cancer Research
Children's Hospital of Philadelphia
Philadelphia, Pennsylvania
Molecular and Cellular Biology of Cancer

David A. Hunstad, MD
Professor of Pediatrics and Molecular
    Microbiology
Washington University School of Medicine in
    St. Louis
St. Louis, Missouri
Central Nervous System Infections
Animal and Human Bites
Rat Bite Fever
Monkeypox

Carl E. Hunt, MD
Research Professor of Pediatrics
Uniformed Services University of the Health
    Sciences
Division of Neonatology
Walter Reed National Military Medical Center
Bethesda, Maryland;
Adjunct Professor of Pediatrics
George Washington University School of
    Medicine and Health Sciences
Washington, DC
Sudden Infant Death Syndrome

Stacey S. Huppert, PhD
Associate Professor of Pediatrics
University of Cincinnati College of Medicine
Division of Gastroenterology, Hepatology, and
 Nutrition
Division of Developmental Biology
Cincinnati Children's Hospital Medical Center
Cincinnati, Ohio
Morphogenesis of the Liver and Biliary System

Anna R. Huppler, MD
Assistant Professor
Pediatric Infectious Diseases
Medical College of Wisconsin
Children's Hospital of Wisconsin
Milwaukee, Wisconsin
*Infectious Complications of Hematopoietic Stem
 Cell Transplantation*

Patricia I. Ibeziako, MBBS
Assistant Professor of Psychiatry
Harvard Medical School
Director, Psychiatry Consultation Service
Boston Children's Hospital
Boston, Massachusetts
Somatic Symptom and Related Disorders

Samar H. Ibrahim, MBChB
Assistant Professor of Pediatrics
Division of Pediatric Gastroenterology and
 Hepatology
Mayo Clinic
Rochester, Minnesota
Mitochondrial Hepatopathies

**Allison M. Jackson, MD, MPH,
FAAP**
Division Chief, Child and Adolescent Protection
 Center
Children's National Health System
Washington Children's Foundation
Professor of Child and Adolescent Protection
Associate Professor of Pediatrics
The George Washington University School of
 Medicine and Health Sciences
Washington, DC
Adolescent Sexual Assault

Elizabeth C. Jackson, MD
Professor Emerita of Pediatrics
University of Cincinnati College of Medicine
Division of Nephrology
Cincinnati Children's Hospital Medical Center
Cincinnati, Ohio
Urinary Tract Infections

Mary Anne Jackson, MD
Clinical Professor of Pediatrics
University of Missouri–Kansas City School of
 Medicine
Department of Pediatric Infectious Diseases
Children's Mercy Hospitals and Clinics
Kansas City, Missouri
Orbital Infections

Ashlee Jaffe, MD, MEd
Assistant Professor of Clinical Pediatrics
Department of Pediatrics
University of Pennsylvania Perelman School of
 Medicine
Attending Physician, Division of Rehabilitation
 Medicine
Children's Hospital of Philadelphia
Philadelphia, Pennsylvania
*Spinal Cord Injury and Autonomic Dysreflexia
 Management*

Andrew B. Janowski, MD
Instructor in Infectious Diseases
Department of Pediatrics
Washington University School of Medicine in
 St. Louis
St. Louis, Missouri
Central Nervous System Infections

Tara C. Jatlaoui, MD, MPH
Medical Epidemiologist
Division of Reproductive Health
Centers for Disease Control and Prevention
Atlanta, Georgia
Contraception

Elena J. Jelsing, MD
Assistant Professor
Departments of Physical Medicine and
 Rehabilitation and Division of Sports Medicine
Mayo Clinic Sports Medicine Center
Minneapolis, Minnesota
Specific Sports and Associated Injuries

M. Kyle Jensen, MD
Associate Professor
Department of Pediatrics
University of Utah School of Medicine
Division of Pediatric Gastroenterology
Primary Children's Hospital
Salt Lake City, Utah
Viral Hepatitis

Brian P. Jenssen, MD, MSHP
Assistant Professor
Department of Pediatrics
University of Pennsylvania Perelman School of
 Medicine
Division of General Pediatrics
Children's Hospital of Philadelphia
Philadelphia, Pennsylvania
Tobacco and Electronic Nicotine Delivery Systems

Karen E. Jerardi, MD, MEd
Associate Professor of Pediatrics
University of Cincinnati College of Medicine
Attending Physician, Division of Hospital
 Medicine
Cincinnati Children's Hospital Medical Center
Cincinnati, Ohio
Urinary Tract Infections

Chandy C. John, MD, MS
Ryan White Professor of Pediatrics
Director, Ryan White Center for Pediatric
 Infectious Diseases and Global Health
Indiana University School of Medicine
Indianapolis, Indiana
*Health Advice for Children Traveling
 Internationally*
Giardiasis and Balantidiasis
Malaria (Plasmodium)

Brian D. Johnston, MD, MPH
Professor of Pediatrics
Associate Chief of Clinical Services
Division of General Pediatrics
University of Washington School of Medicine
Chief of Service, Department of Pediatrics
Harborview Medical Center
Seattle, Washington
Injury Control

Michael V. Johnston, MD
Executive Vice President and Chief Medical
 Officer
Kennedy Krieger Institute
Professor of Pediatrics and Neurology
Johns Hopkins University School of Medicine
Baltimore, Maryland
*Congenital Anomalies of the Central Nervous
 System*
Encephalopathies

Richard B. Johnston Jr, MD
Professor Emeritus of Pediatrics
University of Colorado School of Medicine
Aurora, Colorado;
National Jewish Health
Denver, Colorado
Monocytes, Macrophages, and Dendritic Cells
The Complement System
Disorders of the Complement System

Bridgette L. Jones, MD
Associate Professor of Pediatrics
Division of Allergy, Asthma, and Immunology
University of Missouri – Kansas City School of
 Medicine
Division of Allergy, Asthma, and Immunology
Division of Clinical Pharmacology, Toxicology,
 and Therapeutic Innovation
Children's Mercy
Kansas City, Missouri
Principles of Drug Therapy

Marsha Joselow, MSW, LICSW
Department of Psychosocial Oncology and
 Palliative Care
Boston Children's Hospital
Dana-Farber Cancer Institute
Boston, Massachusetts
Pediatric Palliative Care

Cassandra D. Josephson, MD
Professor of Pathology and Pediatrics
Emory University School of Medicine
Director of Clinical Research, Center for
 Transfusion and Cellular Therapies
Program Director, Transfusion Medicine
Fellowship Medical Director
Children's Healthcare of Atlanta Blood, Tissue,
 and Apheresis Services
Atlanta, Georgia
*Red Blood Cell Transfusions and Erythropoietin
 Therapy*
Platelet Transfusions
Neutrophil (Granulocyte) Transfusions
Plasma Transfusions
Risks of Blood Transfusions

Nicholas Jospe, MD
Professor of Pediatrics
University of Rochester School of Medicine and
 Dentistry
Chief, Division of Pediatric Endocrinology
Golisano Children's Hospital
Rochester, New York
Diabetes Mellitus

Joel C. Joyce, MD
Pediatric Dermatologist
NorthShore University Health System
Skokie, Illinois;
Clinical Assistant Professor of Dermatology
University of Chicago Pritzker School of
 Medicine
Chicago, Illinois
Hyperpigmented Lesions
Hypopigmented Lesions
Vesiculobullous Disorders
Nutritional Dermatoses

Marielle A. Kabbouche, MD, FAHS
Professor of Pediatrics
University of Cincinnati College of Medicine
Director, Acute and Inpatient Headache Program
Division of Neurology
Cincinnati Children's Medical Center
Cincinnati, Ohio
Headaches

Joanne Kacperski, MD, FAHS
Assistant Professor of Pediatrics
University of Cincinnati College of Medicine
Headache Medicine Specialist, Division of
  Neurology
Director, Post-Concussion Headache Program
Director, Headache Medicine Fellowship
Cincinnati Children's Medical Center
Cincinnati, Ohio
Headaches

Deepak Kamat, MD, PhD
Professor of Pediatrics
Vice Chair for Education
Wayne State University School of Medicine
Designated Institutional Official
Detroit, Michigan
Fever

Beena D. Kamath-Rayne, MD, MPH
Associate Professor of Pediatrics
University of Cincinnati College of Medicine
Attending Neonatologist, Division of Neonatology
  and Pulmonary Biology
Cincinnati Children's Hospital Medical Center
Cincinnati, Ohio
*Neonatal Resuscitation and Delivery Room
  Emergencies*

Alvina R. Kansra, MD
Associate Professor of Pediatrics
Medical College of Wisconsin
Division of Pediatric Endocrinology
Children's Hospital of Wisconsin
Milwaukee, Wisconsin
Hypofunction of the Ovaries
*Pseudoprecocity Resulting From Lesions of
  the Ovary*

David M. Kanter, MD
Assistant Professor
Department of Physical Medicine and
  Rehabilitation
State University of New York
SUNY Upstate Medical University
Syracuse, New York
Health and Wellness for Children With Disabilities

Aaron M. Karlin, MD
Clinical Associate Professor
Department of Physical Medicine and
  Rehabilitation
Louisiana State University School of Medicine
Chair, Department of Physical Medicine and
  Rehabilitation
Section Head, Pediatric Rehabilitation
Ochsner Clinic Medical Center
Ochsner Children's Health Center
New Orleans, Louisiana
Management of Musculoskeletal Injury

Jacob Kattan, MD, MSCR
Assistant Professor
Department of Pediatrics
Jaffe Food Allergy Institute
Kravis Children's Hospital at the Icahn School of
  Medicine at Mount Sinai
New York, New York
Diagnosis of Allergic Disease

James W. Kazura, MD
Distinguished University Professor
Adel A. Mahmoud Professorship in Global Health
  and Vaccines
Director, Center for Global Health and Diseases
Case Western Reserve University School of
  Medicine
Cleveland, Ohio
Ascariasis (Ascaris lumbricoides)
Trichuriasis (Trichuris trichiura)
Enterobiasis (Enterobius vermicularis)
Strongyloidiasis (Strongyloides stercoralis)
Lymphatic Filariasis (Brugia malayi, Brugia
  timori, *and* Wuchereria bancrofti)
Other Tissue Nematodes
Toxocariasis (Visceral and Ocular Larva Migrans)
Trichinellosis (Trichinella spiralis)

Gregory L. Kearns, PharmD, PhD, FAAP
President, Arkansas Children's Research Institute
Senior Vice President and Chief Research Officer
Arkansas Children's
Ross and Mary Whipple Family Distinguished
  Research Scientist
Professor of Pediatrics
University of Arkansas for Medical Sciences
Little Rock, Arkansas
Principles of Drug Therapy

Andrea Kelly, MD, MSCE
Associate Professor of Pediatrics
University of Pennsylvania Perelman School of
  Medicine
Attending Physician
Children's Hospital of Philadelphia
Philadelphia, Pennsylvania
Assessment of Growth

Desmond P. Kelly, MD
Professor of Pediatrics
University of South Carolina School of Medicine
  Greenville
Chief Medical Research Officer
Health Sciences Center
Prisma Health-Upstate
Greenville, South Carolina
*Neurodevelopmental and Executive Function and
  Dysfunction*

Kevin J. Kelly, MD
Professor of Pediatrics (Emeritus)
Department of Pediatrics
University of North Carolina School of Medicine
Chapel Hill, North Carolina
Hypersensitivity Pneumonia
Occupational and Environmental Lung Disease
Granulomatous Lung Disease
Eosinophilic Lung Disease
Interstitial Lung Disease

Matthew S. Kelly, MD, MPH
Assistant Professor of Pediatrics
Division of Infectious Diseases
Duke University School of Medicine
Durham, North Carolina
Community-Acquired Pneumonia

Michael Kelly, MD, PhD
Chief Research Officer
Akron Children's Hospital
Akron, Ohio
Anatomy and Function of the Lymphatic System
Abnormalities of Lymphatic Vessels
Lymphadenopathy

Kimberly M. Ken, MD
Resident Physician
Department of Dermatology
University of Missouri School of Medicine
Columbia, Missouri
Disorders of the Sweat Glands
Disorders of Hair
Disorders of the Nails

Melissa A. Kennedy, MD
Assistant Professor of Clinical Pediatrics
Division of Gastroenterology, Hepatology, and
  Nutrition
University of Pennsylvania Perelman School of
  Medicine
Children's Hospital of Philadelphia
Philadelphia, Pennsylvania
*Intestinal Duplications, Meckel Diverticulum, and
  Other Remnants of the Omphalomesenteric
  Duct*

Eitan Kerem, MD
Professor and Chair
Department of Pediatrics
Hadassah University Medical Center
Jerusalem, Israel
Effects of War on Children

Joseph E. Kerschner, MD
Dean of the Medical School, Provost and
  Executive Vice President
Professor of Otolaryngology and Microbiology
  and Immunology
Medical College of Wisconsin
Milwaukee, Wisconsin
Otitis Media

Seema Khan, MD
Associate Professor of Pediatrics
Division of Gastroenterology and Nutrition
George Washington University School of
  Medicine and Health Sciences
Children's National Medical Center
Washington, DC
*Embryology, Anatomy, and Function of the
  Esophagus*
Congenital Anomalies
*Obstructing and Motility Disorders of the
  Esophagus*
Dysmotility
Hiatal Hernia
Gastroesophageal Reflux Disease
*Eosinophilic Esophagitis, Pill Esophagitis, and
  Infective Esophagitis*
Esophageal Perforation
Esophageal Varices
Ingestions

Ameneh Khatami, BHB, MBChB, MD
Clinical Senior Lecturer
Discipline of Child and Adolescent Health
University of Sydney
Department of Microbiology and Infectious
  Diseases
The Children's Hospital at Westmead
Sydney, Australia
Aeromonas and Plesiomonas

Soumen Khatua, MD
Associate Professor of Pediatrics
Section Chief, Neuro-Oncology
Department of Pediatrics Patient Care
The University of Texas MD Anderson Cancer
    Center
Houston, Texas
Brain Tumors in Childhood

Alexandra Kilinsky, DO
Fellow, Pediatric Hospital Medicine
Department of Pediatrics
Cohen Children's Medical Center of New York
New Hyde Park, New York
Immunization Practices

Chong-Tae Kim, MD, PhD
Associate Professor
Department of Pediatrics
University of Pennsylvania Perelman School of
    Medicine
Division of Rehabilitation Medicine
Children's Hospital of Philadelphia
Philadelphia, Pennsylvania
Rehabilitation for Severe Traumatic Brain Injury

Wendy E. Kim, DO
Assistant Professor of Internal Medicine and
    Pediatrics
Division of Pediatric Dermatology
Loyola University Chicago Stritch School of
    Medicine
Evanston, Illinois
Diseases of the Dermis
Diseases of Subcutaneous Tissue
Disorders of the Mucous Membranes
Acne

Charles H. King, MD
Professor Emeritus of International Health
Center for Global Health and Diseases
Case Western Reserve University School of
    Medicine
Cleveland, Ohio
Schistosomiasis (Schistosoma)
Flukes (Liver, Lung, and Intestinal)

Paul S. Kingma, MD, PhD
Associate Professor of Pediatrics
University of Cincinnati of College of Medicine
Neonatal Director, Cincinnati Fetal Center
Co-Director, Cincinnati Bronchopulmonary
    Dysplasia Center
The Perinatal Institute
Cincinnati Children's Hospital Medical Center
Cincinnati, Ohio
Fetal Intervention and Surgery

Stephen L. Kinsman, MD
Associate Professor of Pediatrics
Medical University of South Carolina
Charleston, South Carolina
*Congenital Anomalies of the Central Nervous
    System*

Priya S. Kishnani, MD, MBBS
C.L. and Su Chen Professor of Pediatrics
Chief, Division of Medical Genetics
Duke University Medical Center
Durham, North Carolina
Defects in Metabolism of Carbohydrates

Bruce L. Klein, MD
Associate Professor of Pediatrics
Johns Hopkins University School of Medicine
Interim Director, Pediatric Emergency Medicine
Director, Pediatric Transport
Johns Hopkins Children's Center
Baltimore, Maryland
*Interfacility Transport of the Seriously Ill or Injured
    Pediatric Patient*
Acute Care of Multiple Trauma
Care of Abrasions and Minor Lacerations

Bruce S. Klein, MD
Professor of Pediatrics, Internal Medicine, and
    Medical Microbiology and Immunology
Chief, Pediatric Infectious Disease Division
University of Wisconsin School of Medicine and
    Public Health
Madison, Wisconsin
Blastomycosis (Blastomyces dermatitidis)

Robert M. Kliegman, MD
Professor and Chairman Emeritus
Department of Pediatrics
Medical College of Wisconsin
Children's Hospital of Wisconsin
Milwaukee, Wisconsin
Culture-Specific Beliefs
Refeeding Syndrome
*Generalized Arterial Calcification of Infancy/
    Idiopathic Infantile Arterial Calcification*
Arterial Tortuosity

William C. Koch, MD
Associate Professor of Pediatrics
Virginia Commonwealth University School of
    Medicine
Division of Pediatric Infectious Diseases
Children's Hospital of Richmond at VCU
Richmond, Virginia
Parvoviruses

Patrick M. Kochanek, MD, MCCM
Ake N. Grenvik Professor of Critical Care
    Medicine
Vice Chair, Department of Critical Care Medicine
Professor of Anesthesiology, Pediatrics,
    Bioengineering, and Clinical and Translational
    Science
Director, Safar Center for Resuscitation Research
UPMC Children's Hospital of Pittsburgh
John G. Rangos Research Center
Pittsburgh, Pennsylvania
Neurologic Emergencies and Stabilization

Eric Kodish, MD
Professor of Pediatrics
Lerner College of Medicine
Cleveland Clinic
Cleveland, Ohio
Ethics in Pediatric Care

Stephan A. Kohlhoff, MD
Associate Professor of Pediatrics and Medicine
Chief, Pediatric Infectious Diseases
SUNY Downstate Medical Center
Brooklyn, New York
Chlamydia pneumoniae
Psittacosis (Chlamydia psittaci)

Mark A. Kostic, MD
Professor of Emergency Medicine and Pediatrics
Medical College of Wisconsin
Associate Medical Director
Wisconsin Poison Center
Milwaukee, Wisconsin
Poisoning

Karen L. Kotloff, MD
Professor of Pediatrics
Division Head, Infectious Disease and Tropical
    Pediatrics
Center for Vaccine Development and Global
    Health
University of Maryland School of Medicine
Baltimore, Maryland
Acute Gastroenteritis in Children

Elliot J. Krane, MD, FAAP
Professor of Pediatrics, and Anesthesiology,
    Perioperative, and Pain Medicine
Stanford University School of Medicine
Chief, Pediatric Pain Management
Stanford Children's Health
Lucile Packard Children's Hospital at Stanford
Stanford, California
Pediatric Pain Management

Peter J. Krause, MD
Senior Research Scientist in Epidemiology
    (Microbial Diseases), Medicine (Infectious
    Diseases), and Pediatrics (Infectious Diseases)
Lecturer in Epidemiology (Microbial Diseases)
Yale School of Public Health
New Haven, Connecticut
Babesiosis (Babesia)

**Richard E. Kreipe, MD, FAAAP,
FSAHM, FAED**
Dr. Elizabeth R. McArnarney Professor in
    Pediatrics funded by Roger and Carolyn
    Friedlander
Department of Pediatrics, Division of Adolescent
    Medicine
University of Rochester Medical Center
Golisano Children's Hospital
Director, New York State ACT for Youth Center
    of Excellence
Medical Director, Western New York
    Comprehensive Care Center for Eating
    Disorders
Rochester, New York
Eating Disorders

Steven E. Krug, MD
Professor of Pediatrics
Northwestern University Feinberg School of
    Medicine
Division of Pediatric Emergency Medicine
Ann & Robert H. Lurie Children's Hospital of
    Chicago
Chicago, Illinois
Emergency Medical Services for Children

Janet L. Kwiatkowski, MD, MSCE
Professor
Department of Pediatrics
University of Pennsylvania Perelman School of
    Medicine
Division of Hematology
Children's Hospital of Philadelphia
Philadelphia, Pennsylvania
Hemoglobinopathies

Jennifer M. Kwon, MD
Professor of Child Neurology
Department of Neurology
University of Wisconsin School of Medicine and
    Public Health
Madison, Wisconsin
Neurodegenerative Disorders of Childhood

Catherine S. Lachenauer, MD
Assistant Professor of Pediatrics
Harvard Medical School
Director, Infectious Diseases Outpatient Practice
Boston Children's Hospital
Boston, Massachusetts
Group B Streptococcus

Stephan Ladisch, MD
Professor of Pediatrics and Biochemistry/
　Molecular Biology
George Washington University School of
　Medicine
Center for Cancer and Immunology Research and
Center for Cancer and Blood Disorders
Children's Research Institute
Children's National Medical Center
Washington, DC
Histiocytosis Syndromes of Childhood

Oren J. Lakser, MD
Assistant Professor of Pediatrics
Northwestern University Feinberg School of
　Medicine
Associate Clinician Specialist
Division of Pulmonary Medicine
Ann & Robert H. Lurie Children's Hospital of
　Chicago
Chicago, Illinois
Bronchiectasis
Pulmonary Abscess

Philip J. Landrigan, MD, MSc, FAAP
Director, Global Public Health Program
Schiller Institute for Integrated Science and
　Society
Professor of Biology
Boston College
Chestnut Hill, Massachusetts
Chemical Pollutants

Gregory L. Landry, MD
Professor Emeritus
Department of Pediatrics
University of Wisconsin – Madison
School of Medicine and Public Health
Madison, Wisconsin
Epidemiology and Prevention of Injuries
Heat Injuries
Female Athletes: Menstrual Problems and the Risk
　of Osteopenia
Performance-Enhancing Aids

Wendy G. Lane, MD, MPH, FAAP
Associate Professor
Department Epidemiology and Public Health
Department of Pediatrics
University of Maryland School of Medicine
Baltimore, Maryland
Abused and Neglected Children

A. Noelle Larson, MD
Associate Professor, Orthopedic Surgery
Division of Pediatric Orthopedic Surgery
Mayo Clinic
Rochester, Minnesota
Benign Tumors and Tumor-Like Processes of Bone

Phillip S. LaRussa, MD
Professor of Pediatrics
Columbia University College of Physicians and
　Surgeons
Division of Pediatric Infectious Diseases
NewYork-Presbyterian Morgan Stanley Children's
　Hospital
New York, New York
Varicella-Zoster Virus

Oren J. Lakser, MD
Assistant Professor of Pediatrics
Northwestern University Feinberg School of
　Medicine
Division of Pulmonary Medicine
Ann & Robert H. Lurie Children's Hospital of
　Chicago
Chicago, Illinois
Bronchiectasis
Pulmonary Abscess

J. Todd R. Lawrence, MD, PhD
Assistant Professor
Department of Orthopaedic Surgery
University of Pennsylvania Perelman School of
　Medicine
Attending Orthopaedic Surgeon
Children's Hospital of Philadelphia
Philadelphia, Pennsylvania
The Knee

Brendan Lee, MD, PhD
Robert and Janice McNair Endowed Chair
in Molecular and Human Genetics
Professor and Chairman
Department of Molecular and Human Genetics
Baylor College of Medicine
Houston, Texas
Integration of Genetics into Pediatric Practice
The Genetic Approach in Pediatric Medicine
The Human Genome
Patterns of Genetic Transmission
Cytogenetics
Genetics of Common Disorders

K. Jane Lee, MD, MA
Associate Professor
Department of Pediatrics
Medical College of Wisconsin
Division of Pediatric Special Needs
Children's Hospital of Wisconsin
Milwaukee, Wisconsin
Brain Death

J. Steven Leeder, PharmD, PhD
Marion Merrell Dow / Missouri Endowed Chair
in Pediatric Pharmacology
Chief, Division of Pediatric Pharmacology and
　Medical Toxicology
Children's Mercy Hospitals and Clinics
Kansas City, Missouri;
Adjunct Professor
Department of Pharmacology, Toxicology, and
　Therapeutics
Kansas University School of Medicine
Kansas City, Kansas
Pediatric Pharmacogenetics, Pharmacogenomics,
　and Pharmacoproteomics

Jennifer W. Leiding, MD
Assistant Professor of Pediatrics
University of South Florida College of Medicine
St. Petersburg, Florida
Immunodeficiencies Affecting Multiple Cell Types

Michael J. Lentze, MD
Professor Emeritus of Pediatrics
Zentrum für Kinderheilkunde
Universitätsklinikum Bonn
Bonn, Germany
Enzyme Deficiencies

Steven O. Lestrud, MD
Assistant Professor of Pediatrics
Northwestern University Feinberg School of
　Medicine
Medical Director, Respiratory Care
Ann & Robert H. Lurie Children's Hospital of
　Chicago
Chicago, Illinois
Bronchopulmonary Dysplasia
Chronic Respiratory Failure and Long-Term
　Mechanical Ventilation

Donald Y. M. Leung, MD, PhD
Edelstein Family Chair of Pediatric
　Allergy-Immunology
National Jewish Health
Professor of Pediatrics
University of Colorado School of Medicine
Denver, Colorado
Atopic Dermatitis (Atopic Eczema)

Michael N. Levas, MD
Associate Professor of Pediatrics
Medical College of Wisconsin
Division of Pediatric Emergency Medicine
Children's Hospital of Wisconsin
Milwaukee, Wisconsin
Violent Behavior

Rona L. Levy, MSW, PhD, MPH
Professor and Director
Behavioral Medicine Research Group
Assistant Dean for Research
School of Social Work
University of Washington
Seattle, Washington
Pediatric Pain Management

B U.K. Li, MD
Clinical Professor of Pediatrics
Medical College of Wisconsin
Division of Pediatric Gastroenterology
Children's Hospital of Wisconsin
Milwaukee, Wisconsin
Cyclic Vomiting Syndrome

Chris A. Liacouras, MD
Professor of Pediatrics
University of Pennsylvania Perelman School of
　Medicine
Co-Director, Center for Pediatric Eosinophilic
　Disorders
Children's Hospital of Philadelphia
Philadelphia, Pennsylvania
Normal Digestive Tract Phenomena
Major Symptoms and Signs of Digestive Tract
　Disorders
Normal Development, Structure, and Function of
　the Stomach and Intestines
Pyloric Stenosis and Other Congenital Anomalies
　of the Stomach
Intestinal Atresia, Stenosis, and Malrotation
Intestinal Duplications, Meckel Diverticulum, and
　Other Remnants of the Omphalomesenteric
　Duct
Motility Disorders and Hirschsprung Disease
Ileus, Adhesions, Intussusception, and Closed-Loop
　Obstructions
Foreign Bodies and Bezoars
Functional Abdominal Pain
Cyclic Vomiting Syndrome
Malformations
Ascites
Peritonitis

Christopher W. Liebig, MD
Clinical Assistant Professor of Pediatrics
Northeast Ohio Medical University
Rootstown, Ohio;
Director, Sports Medicine in Mahoning Valley
Akron Children's Hospital
Boardman, Ohio
*Sports-Related Traumatic Brain Injury
    (Concussion)*

Paul H. Lipkin, MD
Associate Professor of Pediatrics
Director, Medical Informatics
Director, Interactive Autism Network
Kennedy Krieger Institute
Johns Hopkins University School of Medicine
Baltimore, Maryland
*Developmental and Behavioral Surveillance and
    Screening*

Deborah R. Liptzin, MD, MS
Assistant Professor of Pediatrics
University of Colorado School of Medicine
Associate Director, Colorado chILD
Children's Hospital Colorado
Aurora, Colorado
Fibrotic Lung Disease

Andrew H. Liu, MD
Professor
Department of Pediatrics
Children's Hospital Colorado
University of Colorado School of Medicine
Aurora, Colorado
Childhood Asthma

Lucinda Lo, MD
Clinical Assistant Professor of Pediatrics
Physician Advisor, CDI and CM
University of Pennsylvania Perelman School of
    Medicine
Children's Hospital of Philadelphia
Philadelphia, Pennsylvania
Malnutrition

Stanley F. Lo, PhD
Associate Professor of Pathology
Medical College of Wisconsin
Technical Director, Clinical Chemistry, POCT,
    and Biochemical Genetics
Director, Reference Standards Library
Children's Hospital of Wisconsin
Milwaukee, Wisconsin
*Laboratory Testing in Infants and Children
Reference Intervals for Laboratory Tests and
    Procedures*

Kathleen A. Long, MD
Department of Child Health
University of Missouri School of Medicine
Columbia, Missouri
Dermatologic Diseases of the Neonate

Sarah S. Long, MD
Professor of Pediatrics
Drexel University College of Medicine
Division of Infectious Diseases
St. Christopher's Hospital for Children
Philadelphia, Pennsylvania
*Pertussis (Bordetella pertussis and Bordetella
    parapertussis)*

Anna Lena Lopez, MD, MPH
Director, Institute of Child Health and Human
    Development
Research Associate Professor
University of the Philippines Manila–National
    Institutes of Health
Manila, Philippines
Cholera

Santiago M.C. Lopez, MD
Assistant Professor of Pediatrics
University of South Dakota School of Medicine
Pediatric Infectious Diseases
Sanford Children's Hospital/Specialty Clinic
Sioux Falls, South Dakota
The Common Cold

Steven V. Lossef, MD
Associate Professor of Radiology
George Washington University School of
    Medicine and Health Sciences
Head, Pediatric Interventional Radiology
Division of Diagnostic Imaging and Radiology
Children's National Medical Center
Washington, DC
*Pertussis (Bordetella pertussis and Bordetella
    parapertussis)*
Pleurisy, Pleural Effusions, and Empyema

Jennifer A. Lowry, MD
Professor of Pediatrics
University of Missouri – Kansas City School of
    Medicine
Director, Division of Clinical Pharmacology,
    Toxicology, and Therapeutic Innovation
Children's Mercy
Kansas City, Missouri
Principles of Drug Therapy

Ian R. Macumber, MD, MS
Assistant Professor of Pediatrics
University of Connecticut School of Medicine
Division of Nephrology
Connecticut Children's Medical Center
Hartford, Connecticut
Systemic Hypertension

Mark R. Magnusson, MD, PhD
Co-Director, Diagnostic and Complex Care
    Center
Medical Director, Spina Bifida Program
Children's Hospital of Philadelphia
Philadelphia, Pennsylvania
Chronic Fatigue Syndrome

Pilar L. Magoulas, MS
Assistant Professor, Clinical Program
Department of Molecular and Human Genetics
Baylor College of Medicine
Houston, Texas
Genetic Counseling

**Prashant V. Mahajan, MD, MPH,
MBA**
Professor of Emergency Medicine and Pediatrics
Vice-Chair, Department of Emergency Medicine
Division Chief, Pediatric Emergency Medicine
University of Michigan
Ann Arbor, Michigan
Heavy Metal Intoxication

Joseph A. Majzoub, MD
Thomas Morgan Rotch Professor of Pediatrics
Harvard Medical School
Division of Endocrinology
Boston Children's Hospital
Boston, Massachusetts
Diabetes Insipidus
*Other Abnormalities of Arginine Vasopressin
    Metabolism and Action*

Robert J. Mann, MD
The Karl and Patricia Betz Family
Endowed Director of Research
Helen DeVos Children's Hospital
Grand Rapids, Michigan
Deformational Plagiocephaly

Irini Manoli, MD, PhD
National Human Genome Research Institute
National Institutes of Health
Bethesda, Maryland
*Isoleucine, Leucine, Valine, and Related Organic
    Acidemias*

Asim Maqbool, MD
Associate Professor of Clinical Pediatrics
University of Pennsylvania Perelman School of
    Medicine
Division of Gastroenterology, Hepatology, and
    Nutrition
Children's Hospital of Philadelphia
Philadelphia, Pennsylvania
Nutritional Requirements
Normal Digestive Tract Phenomena
*Major Symptoms and Signs of Digestive Tract
    Disorders*
*Normal Development, Structure, and Function of
    the Stomach and Intestines*
*Pyloric Stenosis and Other Congenital Anomalies
    of the Stomach*
Intestinal Atresia, Stenosis, and Malrotation
*Intestinal Duplications, Meckel Diverticulum, and
    Other Remnants of the Omphalomesenteric
    Duct*
Motility Disorders and Hirschsprung Disease
*Ileus, Adhesions, Intussusception, and Closed-Loop
    Obstructions*
Foreign Bodies and Bezoars
Cyclic Vomiting Syndrome
Peritoneal Malformations
Ascites
Peritonitis

Ashley M. Maranich, MD
Program Director, Pediatrics Residency
Tripler Army Medical Center
Honolulu, Hawaii
Malassezia

Nicole Marcantuono, MD
Associate Professor
Department of Pediatrics
Thomas Jefferson Medical College
Philadelphia, Pennsylvania;
Attending Physician
Alfred I. du Pont Hospital for Children
Wilmington, Delaware
Evaluation of the Child for Rehabilitative Services

David Margolis, MD
Professor and Associate Chair
Department of Pediatrics
Medical College of Wisconsin
Program Director, Bone Marrow Transplantation
Children's Hospital of Wisconsin
Milwaukee, Wisconsin
*Principles and Clinical Indications of
    Hematopoietic Stem Cell Transplantation*
*Hematopoietic Stem Cell Transplantation from
    Alternative Sources and Donors*
*Graft-Versus-Host Disease, Rejection, and
    Venoocclusive Disease*
*Late Effects of Hematopoietic Stem Cell
    Transplantation*

Mona Marin, MD
Division of Viral Diseases
National Center for Immunization and
    Respiratory Diseases
Centers for Disease Control and Prevention
Atlanta, Georgia
Varicella-Zoster Virus

Joan C. Marini, MD, PhD
Chief, Bone and Extracellular Matrix Branch
National Institute for Child Health and
    Development
National Institutes of Health
Bethesda, Maryland
Osteogenesis Imperfecta

Thomas C. Markello, MD, PhD
Associate Staff Clinician,
Medical Genetics Branch
National Human Genome Research Institute
National Institutes of Health
Bethesda, Maryland
*Genetic Approaches to Rare and Undiagnosed
    Diseases*

Morri Markowitz, MD
Professor of Pediatrics and Medicine
Albert Einstein College of Medicine
Director, Lead Poisoning Prevention and
    Treatment Program
The Children's Hospital at Montefiore
Bronx, New York
Lead Poisoning

**Stacene R. Maroushek, MD, PhD,
MPH**
Assistant Professor of Pediatrics
Divisions of Pediatric Infectious Diseases and
    General Pediatrics
University of Minnesota Medical School
Hennepin County Medical Center
Minneapolis, Minnesota
Medical Evaluation of the Foreign-Born Child
Principles of Antimycobacterial Therapy

Justin D. Marsh, MD
Assistant Professor of Pediatric Ophthalmology
University of Missouri-Kansas City School of
    Medicine
Kansas City, Missouri
Growth and Development of the Eye
Examination of the Eye
Abnormalities of Refraction and Accommodation
Disorders of Vision
Abnormalities of Pupil and Iris
Disorders of Eye Movement and Alignment
Abnormalities of the Lids
Disorders of the Lacrimal System
Disorders of the Conjunctiva
Abnormalities of the Cornea
Abnormalities of the Lens
Disorders of the Uveal Tract
Disorders of the Retina and Vitreous
Abnormalities of the Optic Nerve
Childhood Glaucoma
Orbital Abnormalities
Orbital Infections
Injuries to the Eye

Kari L. Martin, MD
Assistant Professor of Dermatology and Child
    Health
University of Missouri School of Medicine
Columbia, Missouri
Dermatologic Diseases of the Neonate
Cutaneous Defects
Ectodermal Dysplasias
Vascular Disorders
Cutaneous Nevi
Disorders of Keratinization
Disorders of the Sweat Glands
Disorders of Hair
Disorders of the Nails
Tumors of the Skin

Maria G. Martinez, MD
Clinical Fellow, Pediatric Rehabilitation Medicine
Cincinnati Children's Hospital Medical Center
Cincinnati, Ohio
Health and Wellness for Children With Disabilities

Wilbert H. Mason, MD, MPH
Professor Emeritus of Clinical Pediatrics
University of Southern California Keck School of
    Medicine
Chief, Pediatric Infectious Diseases
Children's Hospital of Los Angeles
Los Angeles, California
Measles
Rubella
Mumps

Reuben K. Matalon, MD, PhD
Professor of Pediatrics and Genetics
University of Texas Medical Branch
University of Texas Children's Hospital
Galveston, Texas
*N-Acetylaspartic Acid Aspartic Acid (Canavan
    Disease)*

Sravan Kumar Reddy Matta, MD
Assistant Professor of Pediatrics
Division of Gastroenterology and Nutrition
Children's National Medical Center
Washington, DC
*Embryology, Anatomy, and Function of the
    Esophagus*
Congenital Anomalies
*Obstructing and Motility Disorders of the
    Esophagus*
Dysmotility
Hiatal Hernia
Gastroesophageal Reflux Disease

Aletha Maybank, MD, MPH
Deputy Commissioner
Founding Director, Center for Health Equity
New York City Department of Health and Mental
    Hygiene
Long Island City, New York
Racism and Child Health

Robert L. Mazor, MD
Clinical Associate Professor
Department of Pediatrics
University of Washington School of Medicine
Division of Critical Care and Cardiac Surgery
Clinical Director, CICU
Seattle Children's Hospital and Regional Medical
    Center
Seattle, Washington
Pulmonary Edema

Jennifer McAllister, MD, IBCLC
Assistant Professor of Pediatrics
University of Cincinnati College of Medicine
Medical Director, West Chester Hospital Special
    Care Nursery and University of Cincinnati
    Medical Center Newborn Nursery
Medical Director, NICU Follow Up Clinic–NAS
    Clinic
Cincinnati Children's Hospital Medical Center
Cincinnati, Ohio
*Maternal Selective Serotonin Reuptake Inhibitors
    and Neonatal Behavioral Syndromes*

Megan E. McCabe, MD, FAAP
Director, Pediatric Residency Program
Director, Pediatric Critical Care Fellowship
    Program
The Children's Hospital at Montefiore
The University Hospital for Albert Einstein
    College of Medicine
Bronx, New York
Loss, Separation, and Bereavement

Megan E. McClean, MD
Resident Physician
Department of Dermatology
University of Missouri School of Medicine
Columbia, Missouri
Cutaneous Nevi

Susanna A. McColley, MD
Professor of Pediatrics
Northwestern University Feinberg School of
    Medicine
Associate Chief Research Officer for Clinical
    Trials
Stanley Manne Children's Research Institute
Ann & Robert H. Lurie Children's Hospital of
    Chicago
Chicago, Illinois
*Extrapulmonary Diseases with Pulmonary
    Manifestations*
Pulmonary Tumors

Patrick T. McGann, MD, MS
Associate Professor of Pediatrics
University of Cincinnati College of Medicine
Division of Hematology
Cincinnati Children's Hospital Medical Center
Cincinnati, Ohio
Anemia in the Newborn Infant

Margaret M. McGovern, MD, PhD
Knapp Professor of Pediatrics
Physician-in-Chief
Stony Brook Children's Hospital
Dean for Clinical Affairs
Stony Brook University School of Medicine
Stony Brook, New York
Lipidoses (Lysosomal Storage Disorders)
Mucolipidoses
Disorders of Glycoprotein Degradation and
Structure

Sharon A. McGrath-Morrow, MD, MBA
Professor of Pediatrics
Eudowood Division of Pediatric Respiratory
Sciences
Johns Hopkins University School of Medicine
Baltimore, Maryland
Bronchopulmonary Dysplasia

Jeffrey S. McKinney, MD, PhD
Professor of Pediatrics
Vice Chair for Education
Harry W. Bass Jr. Professorship in Pediatric
Education
Distinguished Teaching Professor
Division of Pediatric Infectious Diseases
UT Southwestern Medical Center
Dallas, Texas
Salmonella

Matthew J. McLaughlin, MD
Assistant Professor of Pediatrics
University of Missouri–Kansas City School of
Medicine
Division of Pediatric Physical Medicine and
Rehabilitation
Children's Mercy Hospitals and Clinics
Kansas City, Missouri
Pediatric Pharmacogenetics, Pharmacogenomics,
and Pharmacoproteomics

Rima McLeod, MD
Professor of Ophthalmology and Visual Science
and Pediatrics
Medical Director, Toxoplasmosis Center
University of Chicago Medicine
Chicago, Illinois
Toxoplasmosis (Toxoplasma gondii)

Asuncion Mejias, MD, PhD, MSCS
Associate Professor of Pediatrics
Division of Infectious Diseases
The Ohio State University College of Medicine
Principal Investigator, Center for Vaccines and
Immunity
The Research Institute at Nationwide Children's
Hospital
Columbus, Ohio
Hansen Disease (Mycobacterium leprae)
Mycoplasma pneumoniae
Genital Mycoplasmas (Mycoplasma hominis,
Mycoplasma genitalium, and Ureaplasma
urealyticum)

Peter C. Melby, MD
Professor of Internal Medicine (Infectious
Diseases), Microbiology and Immunology, and
Pathology
Director, Division of Infectious Diseases
Director, Center for Tropical Diseases
University of Texas Medical Branch (UTMB)
Galveston, Texas
Leishmaniasis (Leishmania)

Marlene D. Melzer-Lange, MD
Professor of Pediatrics
Medical College of Wisconsin
Program Director, Project Ujima
Children's Hospital of Wisconsin
Milwaukee, Wisconsin
Violent Behavior

Matthew D. Merguerian, MD, PhD
Fellow, Division of Pediatric Oncology
Department of Oncology
Johns Hopkins Hospital
Pediatric Oncology Branch
National Cancer Institute
Baltimore, Maryland
Definitions and Classification of Hemolytic
Anemias
Hereditary Spherocytosis
Hereditary Elliptocytosis, Hereditary
Pyropoikilocytosis, and Related Disorders
Hereditary Stomatocytosis
Paroxysmal Nocturnal Hemoglobinuria and
Acanthocytosis

Stephanie L. Merhar, MD, MS
Assistant Professor of Pediatrics
University of Cincinnati College of Medicine
Attending Neonatologist, Division of Neonatology
and Pulmonary Biology
Research Director, NICU Follow-Up Clinic
Cincinnati Children's Hospital Medical Center
Cincinnati, Ohio
Nervous System Disorders

Diane F. Merritt, MD
Professor
Department of Obstetrics and Gynecology
Director, Pediatric and Adolescent Gynecology
Washington University School of Medicine in
St. Louis
St. Louis, Missouri
Gynecologic History and Physical Examination
Vaginal Bleeding in the Prepubertal Child
Breast Concerns
Neoplasms and Adolescent Prevention Methods for
Human Papillomavirus
Vulvovaginal and Müllerian Anomalies

Kevin Messacar, MD
Assistant Professor of Pediatrics
University of Colorado School of Medicine
Section of Pediatric Infectious Diseases
Section of Hospital Medicine
Children's Hospital Colorado
Aurora, Colorado
Nonpolio Enteroviruses

Marian G. Michaels, MD, MPH
Professor of Pediatrics and Surgery
University of Pittsburgh School of Medicine
UPMC Children's Hospital of Pittsburgh
Pittsburgh, Pennsylvania
Infections in Immunocompromised Persons

Thomas F. Michniacki
Pediatric Hematology/Oncology Fellow
Division of Pediatric Hematology/Oncology
University of Michigan Medical School
Ann Arbor, Michigan
Leukopenia
Leukocytosis

Mohamad A. Mikati, MD
Wilbur C. Davison Professor of Pediatrics
Professor of Neurobiology
Chief, Division of Pediatric Neurology
Duke University Medical Center
Durham, North Carolina
Seizures in Childhood
Conditions That Mimic Seizures

Henry Milgrom, MD
Professor of Pediatrics
National Jewish Health
University of Colorado School of Medicine
Denver, Colorado
Allergic Rhinitis

Jonathan W. Mink, MD, PhD
Frederick A. Horner MD Endowed Professor in
Pediatric Neurology
Professor of Neurology and Pediatrics
Chief, Division of Child Neurology
Vice-Chair, Department of Neurology
University of Rochester Medical Center
Rochester, New York
Mass Psychogenic Illness
Movement Disorders

R. Justin Mistovich, MD
Assistant Professor
Department of Orthopaedic Surgery
Case Western Reserve University School of
Medicine
MetroHealth Medical Center University Hospitals
Rainbow and Babies Children's Hospital
Cleveland, Ohio
The Spine
The Neck

Jonathan A. Mitchell, PhD, MsC
Research Assistant Professor of Pediatrics
University of Pennsylvania Perelman School of
Medicine
Division of Gastroenterology, Hepatology, and
Nutrition
Children's Hospital of Philadelphia
Nutritional Requirements
Feeding Healthy Infants, Children, and Adolescents

Mark M. Mitsnefes, MD, MS
Professor of Pediatrics
University of Cincinnati College of Medicine
Director, Clinical and Translational Research
Center
Division of Pediatric Nephrology
Cincinnati Children's Hospital Medical Center
Cincinnati, Ohio
Chronic Kidney Disease

Sindhu Mohandas, MD
Assistant Professor of Pediatrics
Division of Infectious Diseases
Keck School of Medicine
University of Southern California
Los Angeles, California
Other Anaerobic Infections

Rachel Y. Moon, MD
Professor of Pediatrics
Head, Division of General Pediatrics
University of Virginia School of Medicine
Charlottesville, Virginia
Sudden Infant Death Syndrome

Joan P. Moran, BSN, RN
Infection Preventionist
Infection Prevention and Control
Children's Hospital of Wisconsin
Milwaukee, Wisconsin
Infection Prevention and Control

Eva Morava, MD, PhD
Professor of Pediatrics
Tulane University Medical School
Clinical Biochemical Geneticist
Hayward Genetics Center
New Orleans, Louisiana
Congenital Disorders of Glycosylation

Megan A. Moreno, MD, MSEd, MPH
Professor of Pediatrics
Division Chief, General Pediatrics and Adolescent
 Medicine
Vice Chair of Digital Health
University of Wisconsin School of Medicine and
 Public Health
Madison, Wisconsin
Bullying, Cyberbullying, and School Violence
Media Violence

Esi Morgan, MD, MSCE
Associate Professor of Pediatrics
University of Cincinnati College of Medicine
Division of Rheumatology
James M. Anderson Center for Health Systems
 Excellence
Cincinnati Children's Hospital Medical Center
Cincinnati, Ohio
Treatment of Rheumatic Diseases

Peter E. Morrison, DO
Senior Instructor
Department of Neurology
University of Rochester Medical Center
Rochester, New York
Ataxias

Lovern R. Moseley, PhD
Clinical Assistant Professor of Psychiatry
Boston University School of Medicine
Boston, Massachusetts
Tantrums and Breath-Holding Spells
Lying, Stealing, and Truancy
Aggression
Self-Injurious Behavior

Yael Mozer-Glassberg, MD
Head, Pediatric Liver Transplant Program
Institute of Gastroenterology, Nutrition, and Liver
 Diseases
Schneider Children's Medical Center of Israel
Petah Tikva, Israel
Immunoproliferative Small Intestinal Disease

Louis J. Muglia, MD, PhD
Professor of Pediatrics
University of Cincinnati College of Medicine
Co-Director, Perinatal Institute
Director, Center for Prevention of Preterm Birth
Director, Division of Human Genetics
Cincinnati Children's Hospital Medical Center
Cincinnati, Ohio
The Endocrine System

Kevin P. Murphy, MD
Medical Director, Pediatric Rehabilitation
Sanford Health Systems
Bismarck, North Dakota;
Medical Director, Gillette Children's Specialty
 Healthcare
Duluth Clinic
Duluth, Minnesota
Management of Musculoskeletal Injury
Specific Sports and Associated Injuries

Timothy F. Murphy, MD
SUNY Distinguished Professor of Medicine
Senior Associate Dean for Clinical and
 Translational Research
Jacobs School of Medicine and Biomedical
 Sciences
University at Buffalo, State University of
 New York
Buffalo, New York
Moraxella catarrhalis

Karen F. Murray, MD
Professor and Interim-Chair
Chief, Division of Gastroenterology and
 Hepatology
Department of Pediatrics
University of Washington School of Medicine
Interim Pediatrician-In-Chief
Seattle Children's Hospital
Seattle, Washington
Tumors of the Digestive Tract

Thomas S. Murray, MD, PhD
Associate Professor of Medical Sciences
Quinnipiac University Frank H Netter MD
 School of Medicine
Hamden, Connecticut
Listeria monocytogenes
*Pseudomonas, Burkholderia, and
 Stenotrophomonas*
Infective Endocarditis

Sona Narula, MD
Assistant Professor of Clinical Neurology
Children's Hospital of Philadelphia
University of Pennsylvania Perelman School of
 Medicine
Philadelphia, Pennsylvania
Central Nervous System Vasculitis

Mindo J. Natale, PsyD
Assistant Professor of Psychology
University of South Carolina School of Medicine
Senior Staff Psychologist
GHS Children's Hospital
Greenville, South Carolina
*Neurodevelopmental and Executive Function and
 Dysfunction*

Amy T. Nathan, MD
Associate Professor of Pediatrics
University of Cincinnati College of Medicine
Medical Director, Perinatal Institute
Cincinnati Children's Hospital Medical Center
Cincinnati, Ohio
The Umbilicus

Dipesh Navsaria, MD, MPH, MSLIS, FAAP
Associate Professor of Pediatrics
University of Wisconsin School of Medicine and
 Public Health
Madison, Wisconsin
*Maximizing Children's Health: Screening,
 Anticipatory Guidance, and Counseling*

William A. Neal, MD
Professor Emeritus of Pediatrics
Division of Pediatric Cardiology
West Virginia University School of Medicine
Morgantown, West Virginia
Disorders of Lipoprotein Metabolism and Transport

Grace Nehme, MD
Fellow, Department of Pediatrics
University of Texas MD Anderson Cancer Center
Houston, Texas
Neoplasms of the Kidney

Edward J. Nehus, MD, MS
Assistant Professor of Clinical Pediatrics
University of Cincinnati College of Medicine
Division of Nephrology and Hypertension
Cincinnati Children's Hospital Medical Center
Cincinnati, Ohio
Introduction to Glomerular Diseases

Maureen R. Nelson, MD
Associate Professor of Physical Medicine &
 Rehabilitation and Pediatrics
Baylor College of Medicine
Medical Director, Physical Medicine &
 Rehabilitation
The Children's Hospital of San Antonio
San Antonio, Texas
Birth Brachial Plexus Palsy

Caitlin M. Neri, MD
Assistant Professor of Pediatrics
Boston University School of Medicine
Boston, Massachusetts
*Complementary Therapies and Integrative
 Medicine*

Mark I. Neuman, MD, MPH
Associate Professor of Pediatrics and Emergency
 Medicine
Harvard Medical School
Department of Emergency Medicine
Boston Children's Hospital
Boston, Massachusetts
Fever in the Older Child

Mary A. Nevin, MD, FAAP, FCCP
Associate Professor of Pediatrics
Northwestern University Feinberg School of
 Medicine
Department of Pediatrics, Division of Pulmonary
 Medicine
Ann & Robert H. Lurie Children's Hospital of
 Chicago
Chicago, Illinois
Pulmonary Hemosiderosis
Pulmonary Embolism, Infarction, and Hemorrhage

Jane W. Newburger, MD
Commonwealth Professor of Pediatrics
Harvard Medical School
Associate Cardiologist-in-Chief, Research and
 Education
Director, Cardiac Neurodevelopmental Program
Boston Children's Hospital
Boston, Massachusetts
Kawasaki Disease

Jonathan Newmark, MD, MM, FAAN
Adjunct Professor of Neurology
F. Edward Hebert School of Medicine
Uniformed Services University of the Health
  Sciences
Bethesda, Maryland;
Clinical Assistant Professor of Neurology
George Washington University School of
  Medicine and Health Sciences
Staff Neurologist
Washington DC VA Medical Center
Washington, DC
Biologic and Chemical Terrorism

Linda S. Nield, MD
Assistant Dean for Admissions
Professor of Medical Education and Pediatrics
West Virginia University School of Medicine
Morgantown, West Virginia
Fever

Omar Niss, MD
Assistant Professor of Pediatrics
University of Cincinnati College of Medicine
Division of Hematology
Cincinnati Children's Hospital Medical Center
Cincinnati, Ohio
Hemolytic Disease of the Newborn
Neonatal Polycythemia

Zehava L. Noah, MD
Associate Professor of Pediatrics
Northwestern University Feinberg School of
  Medicine
Division of Pediatric Critical Care Medicine
Ann & Robert H. Lurie Children's Hospital of
  Chicago
Chicago, Illinois
Other Conditions Affecting Respiration

James J. Nocton, MD
Professor of Pediatrics
Section of Pediatric Rheumatology
Medical College of Wisconsin
Milwaukee, Wisconsin
Mast Cell Activation Syndrome

Lawrence M. Nogee, MD
Professor of Pediatrics
Eudowood Neonatal Pulmonary Division
Johns Hopkins University School of Medicine
Baltimore, Maryland
Inherited Disorders of Surfactant Metabolism
Pulmonary Alveolar Proteinosis

Corina Noje, MD
Assistant Professor
Pediatric Critical Care Medicine
Department of Anesthesiology and Critical Care
  Medicine
Johns Hopkins University School of Medicine
Medical Director, Pediatric Transport
Johns Hopkins Bloomberg Children's Center
Baltimore, Maryland
Interfacility Transport of the Seriously Ill or Injured
  Pediatric Patient

Laura E. Norton, MD, MS
Assistant Professor of Pediatrics
Division of Pediatric Infectious Diseases and
  Immunology
University of Minnesota Medical School
Minneapolis, Minnesota
Botulism (Clostridium botulinum)

Anna Nowak-Węgrzyn, MD, PhD
Professor of Pediatrics
Jaffe Food Allergy Institute
Division of Allergy and Immunology
Department of Pediatrics
Kravis Children's Hospital at the Icahn School of
  Medicine at Mount Sinai
New York, New York
Serum Sickness
Food Allergy and Adverse Reactions to Foods

Stephen K. Obaro, MD, PhD
Professor of Pediatric Infectious Diseases
Director, Pediatric International Research
University of Nebraska Medical Center
Omaha, Nebraska
Nonvenereal Treponemal Infections
Relapsing Fever (Borrelia)

Makram M. Obeid, MD
Assistant Professor of Pediatrics and Adolescent
  Medicine
Pediatric Epileptologist, Division of Child
  Neurology
Department of Pediatrics and Adolescent
  Medicine
Department of Anatomy, Cell Biology and
  Physiology
American University of Beirut
Beirut, Lebanon
Conditions That Mimic Seizures

Hope L. O'Brien, MD, MBA, FAHS, FAAN
Associate Professor of Pediatrics
University of Cincinnati College of Medicine
Program Director, Headache Medicine Education
Co-Director Young Adult Headache Program
Cincinnati Children's Medical Center
Cincinnati, Ohio
Headaches

Jean-Marie Okwo-Bele, MD, MPH
Director, Department of Immunization, Vaccines,
  and Biologicals
World Health Organization
Geneva, Switzerland
International Immunization Practices

Joyce L. Oleszek, MD
Associate Professor
Department of Physical Medicine and
  Rehabilitation
University of Colorado School of Medicine
Children's Hospital Colorado
Denver, Colorado
Spasticity

Scott E. Olitsky, MD
Professor of Ophthalmology
University of Kansas School of Medicine
University of Missouri – Kansas City School of
  Medicine
Section Chief, Ophthalmology
Children's Mercy Hospitals and Clinics
Kansas City, Missouri
Growth and Development of the Eye
Examination of the Eye
Abnormalities of Refraction and Accommodation
Disorders of Vision
Abnormalities of Pupil and Iris
Disorders of Eye Movement and Alignment
Abnormalities of the Lids
Disorders of the Lacrimal System
Disorders of the Conjunctiva
Abnormalities of the Cornea
Abnormalities of the Lens
Disorders of the Uveal Tract
Disorders of the Retina and Vitreous
Abnormalities of the Optic Nerve
Childhood Glaucoma
Orbital Abnormalities
Orbital Infections
Injuries to the Eye

John M. Olsson, MD, CPE
Professor of Pediatrics
Medical Director, Well Newborn Services
Division of General Pediatrics
University of Virginia School of Medicine
Charlottesville, Virginia
The Newborn

Amanda K. Ombrello, MD
Associate Research Physician
National Human Genome Research Institute
National Institutes of Health
Bethesda, Maryland
Amyloidosis

Meghan E. O'Neill, MD
Fellow in Neurodevelopment Disabilities
Kennedy Krieger Institute
Baltimore, Maryland
Developmental Delay and Intellectual Disability

Mutiat T. Onigbanjo, MD
Assistant Professor
Department of Pediatrics
University of Maryland School of Medicine
Baltimore, Maryland
The First Year

Walter A. Orenstein, MD, DSc (Hon)
Professor of Medicine, Pediatrics, and Global
  Health
Emory University
Associate Director, Emory Vaccines Center
Atlanta, Georgia;
Former Deputy Director for Immunization
  Programs
Bill & Melinda Gates Foundation
Seattle, Washington;
Former Director, National Immunization
  Program
Centers for Disease Control and Prevention
Atlanta, Georgia
Immunization Practices

Rachel C. Orscheln, MD
Associate Professor of Pediatrics
Washington University School of Medicine in
 St. Louis
Director, Ambulatory Pediatric Infectious
 Diseases
Director, International Adoption Center
St. Louis Children's Hospital
St. Louis, Missouri
Bartonella

Marisa Osorio, DO
Assistant Professor
Department of Rehabilitation Medicine
University of Washington School of Medicine
Seattle Children's Hospital
Seattle, Washington
Ambulation Assistance

Christian A. Otto, MD, MMSc
Director of TeleOncology
Associate Attending Physician
Memorial Sloan Kettering Cancer Center
New York, New York
*Altitude-Associated Illness in Children (Acute
 Mountain Sickness)*

Judith A. Owens, MD, MPH
Professor of Neurology
Harvard Medical School
Director of Sleep Medicine
Boston Children's Hospital
Boston, Massachusetts
Sleep Medicine

Seza Özen, MD
Professor of Paediatrics
Divisions of Paediatric Rheumatology
Hacettepe University
Ankara, Turkey
Behçet Disease

Lee M. Pachter, DO
Professor of Pediatrics and Population Health
Sidney Kimmel Medical College and Jefferson
 College of Population Health
Thomas Jefferson University
Director, Community and Clinical Integration
Nemours Alfred I. duPont Hospital for Children
Wilmington, Delaware;
Director, Health Policy Program
Jefferson College of Population Health
Philadelphia, Pennsylvania
Overview of Pediatrics
Child Health Disparities
Cultural Issues in Pediatric Care

Amruta Padhye, MD
Assistant Professor of Clinical Child Health
Division of Pediatric Infectious Diseases
University of Missouri School of Medicine
Columbia, Missouri
Diphtheria (Corynebacterium diphtheriae)

**Suzinne Pak-Gorstein, MD, PhD,
MPH**
Associate Professor of Pediatrics
Adjunct Associate Professor of Global Health
University of Washington School of Medicine
Seattle, Washington
Global Child Health

Jennifer Panganiban, MD
Assistant Professor of Clinical Pediatrics
University of Pennsylvania Perelman School of
 Medicine
Director, Non Alcoholic Fatty Liver Disease
 Clinic
Division of Gastroenterology, Hepatology, and
 Nutrition
Children's Hospital of Philadelphia
Philadelphia, Pennsylvania
Nutritional Requirements

Diane E. Pappas, MD, JD
Professor of Pediatrics
Director of Child Advocacy
University of Virginia School of Medicine
Charlottesville, Virginia
Sinusitis
*Retropharyngeal Abscess, Lateral Pharyngeal
 (Parapharyngeal) Abscess, and Peritonsillar
 Cellulitis/Abscess*

John J. Parent, MD, MSCR
Assistant Professor of Pediatrics
Indiana University School of Medicine
Section of Cardiology
Riley Hospital for Children at Indiana University
 Health
Indianapolis, Indiana
Diseases of the Myocardium
Diseases of the Pericardium
Tumors of the Heart

**Alasdair P.J. Parker, MBBS (Lond),
MRCP, MD, MA (Camb)**
Consultant in Pediatric Neurology
Addenbrooke's Hospital
Associate Lecturer
University of Cambridge School of Clinical
 Medicine
Cambridge, United Kingdom
*Idiopathic Intracranial Hypertension (Pseudotumor
 Cerebri)*

Elizabeth Prout Parks, MD, MSCE
Assistant Professor of Pediatrics
University of Pennsylvania Perelman School of
 Medicine
Division of Gastroenterology, Hepatology, and
 Nutrition
Children's Hospital of Philadelphia
Philadelphia, Pennsylvania
Nutritional Requirements
Feeding Healthy Infants, Children, and Adolescents

Briana C. Patterson, MD, MS
Associate Professor of Pediatrics
Division of Pediatric Endocrinology
Director, Pediatric Endocrine Fellowship Program
Emory University School of Medicine
Atlanta, Georgia
Hormones of the Hypothalamus and Pituitary
Hypopituitarism

Maria Jevitz Patterson, MD, PhD
Professor Emeritus of Microbiology and
 Molecular Genetics
Michigan State University College of Human
 Medicine
East Lansing, Michigan
Syphilis (Treponema pallidum)

Anna L. Peters, MD, PhD
Clinical Fellow
Division of Gastroenterology, Hepatology, and
 Nutrition
Cincinnati Children's Hospital Medical Center
Cincinnati, Ohio
Metabolic Diseases of the Liver

Timothy R. Peters, MD
Professor of Pediatrics
Wake Forest School of Medicine
Division of Pediatric Infectious Diseases
Wake Forest Baptist Medical Center
Winston-Salem, North Carolina
Streptococcus pneumoniae (Pneumococcus)

Rachel A. Phelan, MD, MPH
Assistant Professor of Pediatrics
Medical College of Wisconsin
Division of Hematology/Oncology/BMT
Children's Hospital of Wisconsin
Milwaukee, Wisconsin
*Principles and Clinical Indications of
 Hematopoietic Stem Cell Transplantation*
*Hematopoietic Stem Cell Transplantation from
 Alternative Sources and Donors*
*Graft-Versus-Host Disease, Rejection, and
 Venoocclusive Disease*
*Late Effects of Hematopoietic Stem Cell
 Transplantation*

Anna Pinto, MD, PhD
Lecturer of Neurology
Harvard Medical School
Co-Director, Sturge Weber Clinic
Department of Neurology
Boston Children's Hospital
Boston, Massachusetts
Neurocutaneous Syndromes

Brenda B. Poindexter, MD, MS
Professor of Pediatrics
University of Cincinnati College of Medicine
Director of Clinical and Translational Research
Perinatal Institute
Cincinnati Children's Hospital Medical Center
Cincinnati, Ohio
The High-Risk Infant
Transport of the Critically Ill Newborn

**Andrew J. Pollard, FRCPCH, PhD,
FMedSci**
Professor of Paediatric Infection and Immunity
Department of Paediatrics
University of Oxford
Children's Hospital
Oxford, United Kingdom
Neisseria meningitidis (Meningococcus)

Diego Preciado, MD, PhD
Professor of Pediatrics, Surgery, and Integrative
 Systems Biology
George Washington University School of
 Medicine and Health Sciences
Vice-Chief, Division of Pediatric Otolaryngology
Children's National Health System
Washington, DC
Otitis Media

Mark R. Proctor, MD
Franc D. Ingraham Professor of Neurosurgery
Harvard Medical School
Neurosurgeon-in-Chief
Boston Children's Hospital
Boston, Massachusetts
Spinal Cord Injuries in Children
Spinal Cord Disorders

Howard I. Pryor II, MD
Instructor of Surgery
Division of Pediatric Surgery
Johns Hopkins University School of Medicine
Johns Hopkins Children's Center
Baltimore, Maryland
Acute Care of Multiple Trauma

Lee A. Pyles, MD, MS
Associate Professor of Pediatrics
Division of Pediatric Cardiology
West Virginia University School of Medicine
Morgantown, West Virginia
Disorders of Lipoprotein Metabolism and Transport

Molly Quinn, MD
Fellow, Reproductive Endocrinology and
   Infertility
Department of Obstetrics, Gynecology, and
   Reproductive Sciences
University of California, San Francisco
San Francisco, California
Polycystic Ovary Syndrome and Hirsutism

Elisabeth H. Quint, MD
Professor of Obstetrics and Gynecology
Director, Fellowship in Pediatric and Adolescent
   Gynecology
University of Michigan Medical School
Ann Arbor, Michigan
Gynecologic Care for Girls with Special Needs

Amy E. Rabatin, MD
Fellow, Pediatric Rehabilitation and Board
   Certified Sports Medicine
Department of Physical Medicine and
   Rehabilitation
Mayo Clinic Children's Center
Rochester, Minnesota
Specific Sports and Associated Injuries

C. Egla Rabinovich, MD, MPH
Professor of Pediatrics
Duke University School of Medicine
Co-Chief, Division of Pediatric Rheumatology
Duke University Health System
Durham, North Carolina
Evaluation of Suspected Rheumatic Disease
Treatment of Rheumatic Diseases
Juvenile Idiopathic Arthritis
Scleroderma and Raynaud Phenomenon
Sjögren Syndrome
Miscellaneous Conditions Associated With Arthritis

Leslie J. Raffini, MD
Associate Professor
Department of Pediatrics
University of Pennsylvania Perelman School of
   Medicine
Division of Hematology
Children's Hospital of Philadelphia
Philadelphia, Pennsylvania
Hemostasis
Hereditary Predisposition to Thrombosis
Thrombotic Disorders in Children
Disseminated Intravascular Coagulation

Shawn L. Ralston, MD, MS
Associate Professor and Vice Chair for Clinical
   Affairs
Department of Pediatrics
Geisel School of Medicine at Dartmouth
Chief, Section of Pediatric Hospital Medicine
Children's Hospital at Dartmouth-Hitchcock
Hanover, New Hampshire
Wheezing in Infants: Bronchiolitis

Sanjay Ram, MD
Professor of Medicine
University of Massachusetts Medical School
Division of Infectious Diseases and Immunology
UMass Memorial Medical Center
Worcester, Massachusetts
Neisseria gonorrhoeae (Gonococcus)

Octavio Ramilo, MD
Professor of Pediatrics
Henry G. Cramblett Chair in Medicine
The Ohio State University College of Medicine
Chief, Division of Infectious Diseases
Nationwide Children's Hospital
Columbus, Ohio
Mycoplasma pneumoniae

Kacy A. Ramirez, MD
Assistant Professor of Pediatrics
Wake Forest School of Medicine
Division of Pediatric Infectious Diseases
Wake Forest Baptist Medical Center
Winston-Salem, North Carolina
Streptococcus pneumoniae (Pneumococcus)

Casey M. Rand, BS
Project Manager, Center for Autonomic Medicine
   in Pediatrics
Ann & Robert H. Lurie Children's Hospital of
   Chicago
Chicago, Illinois
*Rapid-Onset Obesity with Hypothalamic
   Dysfunction, Hypoventilation, and Autonomic
   Dysregulation (ROHHAD)*
Congenital Central Hypoventilation Syndrome

Adam J. Ratner, MD, MPH
Associate Professor of Pediatrics and
   Microbiology
New York University School of Medicine
Chief, Division of Pediatric Infectious Diseases
New York University Langone Medical Center
New York, New York
Aeromonas and Plesiomonas

Lee Ratner, MD, PhD
Professor of Medicine
Professor of Molecular Microbiology and of
   Pathology and Immunology
Washington University School of Medicine in
   St. Louis
St. Louis, Missouri
Human T-Lymphotropic Viruses (1 and 2)

Gerald V. Raymond, MD
Professor of Neurology
University of Minnesota School of Medicine
Chief of Pediatric Neurology
University of Minnesota Medical Center, Fairview
Minneapolis, Minnesota
*Disorders of Very-Long-Chain Fatty Acids and
   Other Peroxisomal Functions*

Ann M. Reed, MD
Professor of Pediatrics
Chair, Department of Pediatrics
Physician-in-Chief
Duke Children's
Duke University
Durham, North Carolina
Juvenile Dermatomyositis

Shimon Reif, MD
Chairman, Department of Pediatrics
Hadassah Medical Center
Hebrew University
Jerusalem, Israel
Diarrhea From Neuroendocrine Tumors

Megan E. Reller, MD, PhD, MPH
Associate Professor of Medicine
Associate Research Professor of Global Health
Duke University Medical Center
Durham, North Carolina
Spotted Fever Group Rickettsioses
Scrub Typhus (Orientia tsutsugamushi)
Typhus Group Rickettsioses
Ehrlichioses and Anaplasmosis
Q Fever (Coxiella burnetii)

Caroline H. Reuter, MD, MSCI
Associate Medical Director, Pharmacovigilance
Bioverativ
Waltham, Massachusetts
Group A Streptococcus

Jorge D. Reyes, MD
Professor and Roger K. Giesecke Distinguished
   Chair
Department of Surgery
University of Washington School of Medicine
Chief, Division of Transplant Surgery
Seattle Children's Hospital
Seattle, Washington
*Intestinal Transplantation in Children with
   Intestinal Failure*
Liver Transplantation

Firas Rinawi, MD
Attending Physician
Institute of Gastroenterology, Nutrition, and Liver
   Diseases
Schneider Children's Medical Center of Israel
Petah Tikva, Israel
*Evaluation of Children with Suspected Intestinal
   Malabsorption*

A. Kim Ritchey, MD
Professor and Vice-Chair of International Affairs
Department of Pediatrics
University of Pittsburgh School of Medicine
Division of Hematology/Oncology
UPMC Children's Hospital of Pittsburgh
Pittsburgh, Pennsylvania
Principles of Cancer Diagnosis
Principles of Cancer Treatment
The Leukemias

Frederick P. Rivara, MD, MPH
Seattle Children's Guild Endowed Chair in
   Pediatrics
Professor and Vice-Chair, Department of
   Pediatrics
University of Washington School of Medicine
Seattle, Washington
Injury Control

Eric Robinette, MD
Attending Physician in Infectious Diseases
Akron Children's Hospital
Akron, Ohio
Osteomyelitis
Septic Arthritis

Angela Byun Robinson, MD, MPH
Associate Professor
Cleveland Clinic Lerner College of Medicine
Staff, Pediatrics Institute
Cleveland Clinic Children's
Cleveland, Ohio
Juvenile Dermatomyositis
Miscellaneous Conditions Associated with Arthritis

Kristine Knuti Rodrigues, MD, MPH
Assistant Professor of Pediatrics
University of Colorado School of Medicine
Department of Pediatrics
Denver Health Medical Center
Denver, Colorado
Acute Inflammatory Upper Airway Obstruction (Croup, Epiglottitis, Laryngitis, and Bacterial Tracheitis)

David F. Rodriguez-Buritica, MD
Assistant Professor
Department of Pediatrics
Division of Medical Genetics
McGovern Medical School at UTHealth
Houston, Texas
Disorders Involving Ion Transporters
Disorders Involving Transcription Factors
Disorders Involving Defective Bone Resorption

Rosa Rodríguez-Fernández, MD, PhD
Hospital General Universitario Gregorio Marañón
Instituto de Investigación Sanitaria Gregorio Marañón (IISGM)
Madrid, Spain;
Center for Vaccines and Immunity
The Research Institute at Nationwide Children's Hospital
The Ohio State University College of Medicine
Columbus, Ohio
Genital Mycoplasmas (Mycoplasma hominis, Mycoplasma genitalium, *and* Ureaplasma urealyticum)

Genie E. Roosevelt, MD, MPH
Professor of Emergency Medicine
University of Colorado School of Medicine
Department of Emergency Medicine
Denver Health Medical Center
Denver, Colorado
Acute Inflammatory Upper Airway Obstruction (Croup, Epiglottitis, Laryngitis, and Bacterial Tracheitis)

David R. Rosenberg, MD
Chair, Department of Psychiatry and Behavioral Neurosciences
Chief of Child Psychiatry and Psychology
Wayne State University School of Medicine
Detroit, Michigan
Anxiety Disorders

Cindy Ganis Roskind, MD
Program Director
Pediatric Emergency Medicine Fellowship
Children's Hospital of New York–Presbyterian
Associate Professor of Pediatrics
Columbia University Irving Medical Center
Columbia University College of Physicians and Surgeons
New York, New York
Acute Care of Multiple Trauma

A. Catharine Ross, PhD
Professor and Dorothy Foehr Huck Chair
Department of Nutritional Sciences
The Pennsylvania State University
College of Health and Human Development
University Park, Pennsylvania
Vitamin A Deficiencies and Excess

Joseph W. Rossano, MD, MS
Chief, Division of Cardiology
Co-Executive Director, The Cardiac Center
Jennifer Terker Endowed Chair in Pediatric Cardiology
Associate Professor of Pediatrics
Children's Hospital of Philadelphia
University of Pennsylvania Perelman School of Medicine
Philadelphia, Pennsylvania
Heart Failure
Pediatric Heart and Heart-Lung Transplantation

Jennifer A. Rothman, MD
Associate Professor
Department of Pediatrics
Division of Pediatric Hematology/Oncology
Duke University Medical Center
Durham, North Carolina
Iron-Deficiency Anemia
Other Microcytic Anemias

Ranna A. Rozenfeld, MD
Professor of Pediatrics
The Warren Alpert Medical School
Brown University
Division of Pediatric Critical Care Medicine
Hasbro Children's Hospital
Providence, Rhode Island
Atelectasis

Colleen A. Ryan, MD
Instructor in Psychiatry
Harvard Medical School
Boston Children's Hospital
Boston, Massachusetts
Motor Disorders and Habits

Monique M. Ryan, M Med BS, FRACP
Professor of Paediatric Neurology
Director, Department of Neurology
Honorary Fellow, Murdoch Children's Research Institute
University of Melbourne
Royal Children's Hospital
Parkville, Victoria, Australia
Autonomic Neuropathies
Guillain-Barré Syndrome
Bell Palsy

Julie Ryu, MD
Professor of Pediatrics
University of California, San Diego School of Medicine
Interim Chief, Division of Respiratory Medicine
Chief Research Informatics Officer
Department of Pediatrics
Rady Children's Hospital–San Diego
San Diego, California

H.P.S. Sachdev, MD, FIAP, FAMS, FRCPCH
Senior Consultant
Departments of Pediatrics and Clinical Epidemiology
Sitaram Bhartia Institute of Science and Research
New Delhi, India
Vitamin B Complex Deficiencies and Excess
Vitamin C (Ascorbic Acid)

Manish Sadarangani, MRCPCH, DPHIL, BM.BCh, MA
Assistant Professor of Pediatrics
Sauder Family Chair in Pediatric Infectious Diseases
University of British Columbia Faculty of Medicine
Director, Vaccine Evaluation Center
British Columbia Children's Hospital
Vancouver, British Columbia, Canada
Neisseria meningitidis (Meningococcus)

Rebecca E. Sadun, MD, PhD
Assistant Professor of Adult and Pediatric Rheumatology
Departments of Medicine and Pediatrics
Duke University School of Medicine
Durham, North Carolina
Systemic Lupus Erythematosus

Mustafa Sahin, MD, PhD
Professor of Neurology
Harvard Medical School
Director, Translational Neuroscience Center
Boston Children's Hospital
Boston, Massachusetts
Neurocutaneous Syndromes

Nina N. Sainath, MD
Division of Gastroenterology, Hepatology, and Nutrition
Children's Hospital of Philadelphia
Philadelphia, Pennsylvania
Feeding Healthy Infants, Children, and Adolescents

Robert A. Salata, MD
Professor and Chairman, Department of Medicine
Case Western Reserve University School of Medicine
Physician-in-Chief
University Hospitals Case Medical Center
Cleveland, Ohio
Amebiasis
Trichomoniasis (Trichomonas vaginalis)
African Trypanosomiasis (Sleeping Sickness; Trypanosoma brucei complex)
American Trypanosomiasis (Chagas Disease; Trypanosoma cruzi)

Edsel Maurice T. Salvana, MD
Clinical Associate Professor of Medicine
University of the Philippines College of Medicine
Director, Institute of Molecular Biology and Biotechnology
National Institutes of Health
Manila, The Philippines;
Adjunct Professor of Global Health
University of Pittsburgh School of Medicine
Pittsburgh, Pennsylvania
Amebiasis
Trichomoniasis (Trichomonas vaginalis)
African Trypanosomiasis (Sleeping Sickness; Trypanosoma brucei complex)
American Trypanosomiasis (Chagas Disease; Trypanosoma cruzi)

Hugh A. Sampson, MD
Kurt Hirschhorn Professor of Pediatrics
Jaffe Food Allergy Institute
Kravis Children's Hospital at the Icahn School of Medicine at Mount Sinai
New York, New York
Anaphylaxis
Food Allergy and Adverse Reactions to Foods

Chase B. Samsel, MD
Instructor in Psychiatry
Harvard Medical School
Boston Children's Hospital
Boston, Massachusetts
Rumination and Pica

Thomas J. Sandora, MD, MPH
Associate Professor of Pediatrics
Harvard Medical School
Hospital Epidemiologist
Division of Infectious Diseases
Boston Children's Hospital
Boston, Massachusetts
Community-Acquired Pneumonia

Tracy L. Sandritter, PharmD
Division of Clinical Pharmacology, Toxicology,
    and Therapeutic Innovation
Children's Mercy
Adjunct Clinical Professor
University of Missouri – Kansas City School of
    Pharmacy
Kansas City, Missouri
Principles of Drug Therapy

Wudbhav N. Sankar, MD
Associate Professor
Department of Orthopaedic Surgery
University of Pennsylvania Perelman School of
    Medicine
Attending Orthopaedic Surgeon
Children's Hospital of Philadelphia
Philadelphia, Pennsylvania
The Hip

Eric J. Sarkissian, MD
Resident Physician
Department of Orthopaedic Surgery
Stanford University School of Medicine
Stanford, California
*Osgood-Schlatter Disease and Sinding-Larsen-
    Johansson Syndrome*

Ajit A. Sarnaik, MD
Associate Professor of Pediatrics
Wayne State University School of Medicine
Director, Pediatric Critical Care Medicine
    Fellowship Program
Children's Hospital of Michigan
Detroit, Michigan
Mechanical Ventilation

Ashok P. Sarnaik, MD
Professor and Former Interim Chair
Department of Pediatrics
Wayne State University School of Medicine
Former Pediatrician-in-Chief
Children's Hospital of Michigan
Detroit, Michigan
Respiratory Distress and Failure

Harvey B. Sarnat, MD, MS, FRCPC
Professor of Pediatrics, Pathology
    (Neuropathology), and Clinical Neurosciences
University of Calgary Cumming School of
    Medicine
Division of Pediatric Neurology
Alberta Children's Hospital Research Institute
Calgary, Alberta, Canada
*Evaluation and Investigation of Neuromuscular
    Disorders*
Developmental Disorders of Muscle
Endocrine and Toxic Myopathies
Metabolic Myopathies
Hereditary Motor-Sensory Neuropathies
Toxic Neuropathies

Joshua K. Schaffzin, MD, PhD
Assistant Professor of Pediatrics
University of Cincinnati College of Medicine
Director, Infection Prevention and Control
Cincinnati Children's Hospital Medical Center
Cincinnati, Ohio
Liver Abscess

Laura E. Schanberg, MD
Professor of Pediatrics
Duke University School of Medicine
Division of Pediatric Rheumatology
Duke University Medical Center
Durham, North Carolina
Systemic Lupus Erythematosus
Musculoskeletal Pain Syndromes

Michael S. Schechter, MD, MPH
Professor of Pediatrics
Virginia Commonwealth University School of
    Medicine
Chief, Division of Pulmonary Medicine
Director, Cystic Fibrosis Center
Director, UCAN Community Asthma Program
Children's Hospital of Richmond at VCU
Richmond, Virginia
Cystic Fibrosis

Mark R. Schleiss, MD
Professor of Pediatrics
American Legion and Auxiliary Heart Research
    Foundation Endowed Chair
Division of Pediatric Infectious Diseases and
    Immunology
University of Minnesota Medical School
Minneapolis, Minnesota
Principles of Antibacterial Therapy
Botulism (Clostridium botulinum)
Tetanus (Clostridium tetani)
Principles of Antiviral Therapy
Principles of Antiparasitic Therapy

Nina F. Schor, MD, PhD
Deputy Director
National Institute of Neurological Disorders and
    Stroke
National Institute of Health
Bethesda, Maryland
Neurologic Evaluation

**James W. Schroeder Jr, MD,
FACS, FAAP**
Associate Professor
Department of Otolaryngology – Head and Neck
    Surgery
Northwestern University Feinberg School of
    Medicine
Ann & Robert H. Lurie Children's Hospital of
    Chicago
Chicago, Illinois
*Congenital Anomalies of the Larynx, Trachea, and
    Bronchi*
Foreign Bodies in the Airway
Laryngotracheal Stenosis and Subglottic Stenosis
Neoplasms of the Larynx, Trachea, and Bronchi

Elaine E. Schulte, MD, MPH
Professor of Pediatrics
Albert Einstein College of Medicine
Vice Chair, Academic Affairs and Faculty
    Development
Division of Academic General Pediatrics
The Children's Hospital at Montefiore
Bronx, New York
Domestic and International Adoption

Mark A. Schuster, MD, PhD
Founding Dean and CEO
Professor
Kaiser Permanente School of Medicine
Pasadena, California
Gay, Lesbian, and Bisexual Adolescents

Daryl A. Scott, MD, PhD
Assistant Professor
Department of Molecular and Human Genetics
Baylor College of Medicine
Houston, Texas
The Genetic Approach in Pediatric Medicine
The Human Genome
Patterns of Genetic Transmission

J. Paul Scott, MD
Professor
Department of Pediatrics
Division of Pediatric Hematology/Oncology
Medical College of Wisconsin
Blood Center of Southeastern Wisconsin
Milwaukee, Wisconsin
Hemostasis
*Hereditary Clotting Factor Deficiencies (Bleeding
    Disorders)*
von Willebrand Disease
Hereditary Predisposition to Thrombosis
Thrombotic Disorders in Children
Postneonatal Vitamin K Deficiency
Liver Disease
Acquired Inhibitors of Coagulation
Disseminated Intravascular Coagulation
Platelet and Blood Vessel Disorders

John P. Scott, MD
Associate Professor of Anesthesiology and
    Pediatrics
Divisions of Pediatric Anesthesiology and
    Pediatric Critical Care
Medical College of Wisconsin
Children's Hospital of Wisconsin
Milwaukee, Wisconsin
Anesthesia and Perioperative Care
Procedural Sedation

**Patrick C. Seed, MD, PhD, FAAP,
FIDSA**
Children's Research Fund Chair in Basic Science
Professor of Pediatrics, Microbiology and
    Immunology
Northwestern University Feinberg School of
    Medicine
Division Head, Pediatric Infectious Diseases
Associate Chief Research Officer of Basic Science
Stanley Manne Children's Research Institute
Director, Host-Microbial Interactions,
    Inflammation, and Immunity (HMI3) Program
Ann & Robert H. Lurie Children's Hospital
Chicago, Illinois
The Microbiome and Pediatric Health
Shigella
Escherichia coli

Janet R. Serwint, MD
Professor
Department of Pediatrics
Johns Hopkins University School of Medicine
Baltimore, Maryland
Loss, Separation, and Bereavement

Apurva S. Shah, MD, MBA
Assistant Professor
Department of Orthopedic Surgery
University of Pennsylvania Perelman School of
    Medicine
Attending Orthopaedic Surgeon
Children's Hospital of Philadelphia
Philadelphia, Pennsylvania
Common Fractures

Dheeraj Shah, MD, FIAP, MAMS
Professor
Department of Pediatrics
University College of Medical Sciences
Guru Teg Bahadur Hospital
New Delhi, India
Vitamin B Complex Deficiencies and Excess
Vitamin C (Ascorbic Acid)

Samir S. Shah, MD, MSCE
Professor of Pediatrics
University of Cincinnati College of Medicine
Director, Division of Hospital Medicine
Chief Metrics Officer
James M. Ewell Endowed Chair
Cincinnati Children's Hospital Medical Center
Cincinnati, Ohio
Quality and Value in Healthcare for Children
Fever Without a Focus in the Neonate and Young
    Infant
Osteomyelitis
Septic Arthritis

Ala Shaikhkhalil, MD
Pediatric Nutrition Fellow
Division of Gastroenterology, Hepatology, and
    Nutrition
Children's Hospital of Philadelphia
Philadelphia, Pennsylvania
Nutritional Requirements
Feeding Healthy Infants, Children, and Adolescents

Raanan Shamir, MD
Professor of Pediatrics
Sackler Faculty of Medicine
Tel-Aviv University
Tel Aviv, Israel;
Chairman, Institute of Gastroenterology,
    Nutrition, and Liver Diseases
Schneider Children's Medical Center of Petah
Tikva, Israel
Disorders of Malabsorption
Chronic Diarrhea

Christina M. Shanti, MD
Chief, Division of Pediatric Surgery
Children's Hospital of Michigan
Detroit, Michigan
Surgical Conditions of the Anus and Rectum

Bruce K. Shapiro, MD
Professor of Pediatrics
The Arnold J. Capute MD, MPH Chair in
    Neurodevelopmental Disabilities
The Johns Hopkins University School of Medicine
Vice-President, Training
Kennedy Krieger Institute
Baltimore, Maryland
Developmental Delay and Intellectual Disability

Erin E. Shaughnessy, MD, MSHCM
Division Chief, Hospital Medicine
Phoenix Children's Hospital
Phoenix, Arizona
Jaundice and Hyperbilirubinemia in the Newborn
Kernicterus

Bennett A. Shaywitz, MD
Charles and Helen Schwab Professor in Dyslexia
    and Learning Development
Co-Director, Center for Dyslexia and Creativity
Chief, Child Neurology
Yale University School of Medicine
New Haven, Connecticut
Dyslexia

Sally E. Shaywitz, MD
Audrey G. Ratner Professor in Learning
    Development
Co-Director, Center for Dyslexia and Creativity
Department of Pediatrics
Yale University School of Medicine
New Haven, Connecticut
Dyslexia

Oleg A. Shchelochkov, MD
Medical Genomics and Metabolic Genetics
    Branch
National Human Genome Research Institute
National Institutes of Health
Bethesda, Maryland
An Approach to Inborn Errors of Metabolism

Nicole M. Sheanon, MD, MS
Assistant Professor of Pediatrics
University of Cincinnati College of Medicine
Division of Endocrinology
Cincinnati Children's Hospital Medical Center
Cincinnati, Ohio
The Endocrine System

Benjamin L. Shneider, MD
Professor of Pediatrics
Texas Children's Hospital
Baylor College of Medicine
Houston, Texas
Autoimmune Hepatitis

Stanford T. Shulman, MD
Virginia H. Rogers Professor of Pediatric
    Infectious Diseases
Northwestern University Feinberg School of
    Medicine
Chief Emeritus, Division of Pediatric Infectious
    Diseases
Ann & Robert H. Lurie Children's Hospital of
    Chicago
Chicago, Illinois
Group A Streptococcus
Rheumatic Heart Disease

Scott H. Sicherer, MD
Elliot and Roslyn Jaffe Professor of Pediatrics,
    Allergy, and Immunology
Director, Jaffe Food Allergy Institute
Department of Pediatrics
Kravis Children's Hospital at the Icahn School of
    Medicine at Mount Sinai
New York, New York
Allergy and the Immunologic Basis of Atopic
    Disease
Diagnosis of Allergic Disease
Allergic Rhinitis
Childhood Asthma
Atopic Dermatitis (Atopic Eczema)
Insect Allergy
Ocular Allergies
Urticaria (Hives) and Angioedema
Anaphylaxis
Serum Sickness
Food Allergy and Adverse Reactions to Foods
Adverse Reactions to Drugs

Mark D. Simms, MD, MPH
Professor of Pediatrics
Medical College of Wisconsin
Medical Director
Child Development Center
Children's Hospital of Wisconsin
Milwaukee, Wisconsin
Language Development and Communication
    Disorders
Adoption

Jeffery M. Simmons, MD, MSc
Associate Professor of Pediatrics
University of Cincinnati College of Medicine
Associate Division Director for Quality
Division of Hospital Medicine
Safety Officer
Cincinnati Children's Hospital Medical Center
Cincinnati, Ohio
Quality and Value in Healthcare for Children
Safety in Healthcare for Children

Eric A.F. Simões, MBBS, DCH, MD
Professor of Pediatrics
University of Colorado School of Medicine
Division of Pediatric Infectious Diseases
Children's Hospital Colorado
Aurora, Colorado
Polioviruses

Kari A. Simonsen, MD
Professor of Pediatrics
Division of Pediatric Infectious Disease
University of Nebraska Medical Center
Omaha, Nebraska
Leptospira

Keneisha Sinclair-McBride, PhD
Assistant Professor of Psychology
Department of Psychiatry
Harvard Medical School
Staff Psychologist
Boston Children's Hospital
Boston, Massachusetts
Tantrums and Breath-Holding Spells
Lying, Stealing, and Truancy
Aggression
Self-Injurious Behavior

Vidya Sivaraman, MD
Clinical Assistant Professor of Pediatrics
Division of Adult and Pediatric Rheumatology
The Ohio State University Wexner Medical
  Center
Nationwide Children's Hospital
Columbus, Ohio
Vasculitis Syndromes

Anne M. Slavotinek, MB BS, PhD
Professor of Clinical Pediatrics
University of California San Francisco School of
  Medicine
Director, Medical Genetics and Genomics
UCSF Benioff Children's Hospital
San Francisco, California
Dysmorphology

Jessica R. Smith, MD
Assistant Professor of Pediatrics
Harvard Medical School
Clinical Director, Thyroid Program
Boston Children's Hospital
Boston, Massachusetts
Thyroid Development and Physiology
Disorders of Thyroxine-Binding Globulin
Hypothyroidism
Thyroiditis
Goiter
Thyrotoxicosis
Carcinoma of the Thyroid
Autoimmune Polyglandular Syndromes
Multiple Endocrine Neoplasia Syndrome

Stephanie H. Smith, MD
Resident Physician
Department of Obstetrics and Gynecology
Washington University School of Medicine in
  St. Louis
St. Louis, Missouri
*Gynecologic Neoplasms and Adolescent Prevention
  Methods for Human Papillomavirus*

Kim Smith-Whitley, MD
Professor, Department of Pediatrics
University of Pennsylvania Perelman School of
  Medicine
Clinical Director, Division of Hematology
Director, Comprehensive Sickle Cell Center
Children's Hospital of Philadelphia
Philadelphia, Pennsylvania
Hemoglobinopathies

Mary Beth F. Son, MD
Assistant Professor in Pediatrics
Harvard Medical School
Staff Physician, Division of Immunology
Boston Children's Hospital
Boston, Massachusetts
Kawasaki Disease

Laura Stout Sosinsky, PhD
Research Scientist
Research and Evaluation Group
Public Health Management Corporation
Philadelphia, Pennsylvania
Childcare

Emily Souder, MD
Drexel University College of Medicine
St. Christopher's Hospital for Children
Philadelphia, Pennsylvania
Pertussis (Bordetella pertussis *and* Bordetella
  parapertussis)

Joseph D. Spahn, MD
Professor
Department of Pediatrics
University of Colorado School of Medicine
Aurora, Colorado
Childhood Asthma

Paul Spearman, MD
Albert B. Sabin Professor of Pediatrics
University of Cincinnati College of Medicine
Director, Division of Infectious Diseases
Cincinnati Children's Hospital Medical Center
Cincinnati, Ohio
Human T-Lymphotropic Viruses (1 and 2)

Mark A. Sperling, MD
Professor Emeritus and Chair
Department of Pediatrics
University of Pittsburgh School of Medicine
Professorial Lecturer
Department of Pediatrics
Division of Endocrinology and Diabetes
Kravis Children's Hospital at the Icahn School of
  Medicine at Mount Sinai
New York, New York
Hypoglycemia

David A. Spiegel, MD
Professor
Department of Orthopaedic Surgery
University of Pennsylvania Perelman School of
  Medicine
Attending Orthopaedic Surgeon
Pediatric Orthopaedic Surgeon
Children's Hospital of Philadelphia
Philadelphia, Pennsylvania
The Spine
The Neck

Jaclyn B. Spitzer, PhD
Professor Emerita of Audiology and Speech
  Pathology in Otolaryngology
Columbia University Irving Medical Center
New York, New York

Jürgen W. Spranger, MD
Professor Emeritus of Pediatrics
University of Mainz School of Medicine
Children's Hospital
Mainz, Germany
Mucopolysaccharidoses

James E. Squires, MD, MS
Assistant Professor in Pediatrics
Children's Hospital of Pittsburgh
Pittsburgh, Pennsylvania
Manifestations of Liver Disease

Siddharth Srivastava, MD, PhD
Instructor in Neurology
Harvard Medical School
Department of Neurology
Boston Children's Hospital
Boston, Massachusetts
Neurocutaneous Syndromes

Joseph W. St Geme III, MD
Professor of Pediatrics and Microbiology and
  Chair of the Department of Pediatrics
University of Pennsylvania Perelman School of
  Medicine
Chair of the Department of Pediatrics and
  Physician-in-Chief
Leonard and Madlyn Abramson Endowed Chair
  in Pediatrics
Children's Hospital of Philadelphia
Philadelphia, Pennsylvania

Amy P. Stallings, MD
Assistant Professor of Pediatrics
Division of Pediatric Allergy and Immunology
Duke University School of Medicine
Durham, North Carolina
Urticaria (Hives) and Angioedema

Virginia A. Stallings, MD
Professor of Pediatrics
University of Pennsylvania Perelman School of
  Medicine
Director, Nutrition Center
Division of Gastroenterology, Hepatology, and
  Nutrition
Children's Hospital of Philadelphia
Philadelphia, Pennsylvania
Nutritional Requirements
Feeding Healthy Infants, Children, and Adolescents

Kathryn C. Stambough, MD
Resident Physician
Department of Obstetrics and Gynecology
Washington University School of Medicine in
  St. Louis
St. Louis, Missouri
Gynecologic History and Physical Examination

Lawrence R. Stanberry, MD, PhD
Associate Dean for International Programs
Department of Pediatrics
Columbia University Vagelos College of
  Physicians and Surgeons
New York, New York
Herpes Simplex Virus

Charles A. Stanley, MD
Professor of Pediatrics
University of Pennsylvania Perelman School of
  Medicine
Division of Endocrinology
Children's Hospital of Philadelphia
Philadelphia, Pennsylvania
Disorders of Mitochondrial Fatty Acid β-Oxidation

Jeffrey R. Starke, MD
Professor of Pediatrics
Baylor College of Medicine
Pediatric Infectious Diseases
Texas Children's Hospital
Houston, Texas
Tuberculosis (Mycobacterium tuberculosis)

Taylor B. Starr, DO, MPH
Associate Professor of Pediatrics
Division of Adolescent Medicine
University of Rochester Medical Center
Rochester, New York
Eating Disorders

**Andrew P. Steenhoff, MBBCh,
DCH, FAAP**
Assistant Professor of Pediatrics
University of Pennsylvania Perelman School of
  Medicine
Medical Director, Global Health Center
Children's Hospital of Philadelphia
Philadelphia, Pennsylvania
Fever of Unknown Origin
Paracoccidioides brasiliensis
Sporotrichosis (Sporothrix schenckii)

Ronen E. Stein, MD
Assistant Professor of Clinical Pediatrics
University of Pennsylvania Perelman School of
    Medicine
Attending Physician
Division of Gastroenterology, Hepatology, and
    Nutrition
Children's Hospital of Philadelphia
Philadelphia, Pennsylvania
Inflammatory Bowel Disease
Eosinophilic Gastroenteritis

William J. Steinbach, MD
Professor of Pediatrics, Molecular Genetics, and
    Microbiology
Chief, Pediatric Infectious Diseases
Duke University Medical Center
Durham, North Carolina
Principles of Antifungal Therapy
Aspergillus
Mucormycosis

Janet Stewart, MD
Associate Professor Emerita
Department of Pediatrics
University of Colorado School of Medicine
Spina Bifida Clinic
Children's Hospital Colorado
Denver, Colorado
Meningomyelocele (Spina Bifida)

Gregory A. Storch, MD
Ruth L. Siteman Professor of Pediatrics
Washington University School of Medicine in
    St. Louis
St. Louis Children's Hospital
St. Louis, Missouri
Diagnostic Microbiology
Polyomaviruses

Ronald G. Strauss, MD
Professor Emeritus
Departments of Pediatrics and Pathology
University of Iowa Carver College of Medicine
Iowa City, Iowa;
Medical Director, Vitalant (formerly LifeSource)
Rosemont, Illinois
Red Blood Cell Transfusions and Erythropoietin
    Therapy
Platelet Transfusions
Neutrophil (Granulocyte) Transfusions
Plasma Transfusions
Risks of Blood Transfusions

Gina S. Sucato, MD, MPH
Director, Adolescent Center
Washington Permanente Medical Group
Adjunct Investigator, Kaiser Permanente
    Washington Health Research Institute
Seattle, Washington
Menstrual Problems

Frederick J. Suchy, MD
Professor of Pediatrics
Associate Dean for Child Health Research
University of Colorado School of Medicine
Denver, Colorado;
Chief Research Officer and Director
Children's Hospital Colorado Research Institute
Aurora, Colorado
Autoimmune Hepatitis
Drug- and Toxin-Induced Liver Injury
Acute Hepatic Failure
Fulminant Hepatic Failure
Cystic Diseases of the Biliary Tract and Liver
Diseases of the Gallbladder
Portal Hypertension and Varices

Kristen R. Suhrie, MD
Assistant Professor
Department of Pediatrics
University of Cincinnati College of Medicine
Neonatologist, Perinatal Institute
Division of Neonatology
Cincinnati Children's Hospital Medical Center
Cincinnati, Ohio
High-Risk Pregnancies
The Fetus

Kathleen E. Sullivan, MD, PhD
Professor of Pediatrics
University of Pennsylvania Perelman School of
    Medicine
Chief, Division of Allergy and Immunology
Frank R. Wallace Endowed Chair in Infectious
    Diseases
Children's Hospital of Philadelphia
Philadelphia, Pennsylvania
Evaluation of Suspected Immunodeficiency
The T-, B-, and NK-Cell Systems
Primary Defects of Antibody Production
Treatment of B-Cell Defects
Primary Defects of Cellular Immunity
Immunodeficiencies Affecting Multiple Cell Types

Moira Szilagyi, MD, PhD
Professor of Pediatrics
David Geffen School of Medicine at UCLA
Section Chief, Developmental Studies
UCLA Mattel Children's Hospital
Los Angeles, California
Foster and Kinship Care

Sammy M. Tabbah, MD
Assistant Professor of Obstetrics and Gynecology
University of Cincinnati College of Medicine
Maternal-Fetal Medicine Specialist, Cincinnati
    Fetal Center
Cincinnati Children's Hospital Medical Center
Cincinnati, Ohio
High-Risk Pregnancies
The Fetus

Robert R. Tanz, MD
Professor of Pediatrics
Division of Academic General Pediatrics and
    Primary Care
Northwestern University Feinberg School of
    Medicine
Ann & Robert H. Lurie Children's Hospital of
    Chicago
Chicago, Illinois
Acute Pharyngitis

Cristina Tarango, MD
Associate Professor of Pediatrics
University of Cincinnati College of Medicine
Medical Director, Hemophilia Treatment Center
Clinical Director, Hematology Program
Cincinnati Children's Hospital Medical Center
Cincinnati, Ohio
Hemorrhage in the Newborn Infant
Nonimmune Hydrops

Nidale Tarek, MD
Assistant Professor of Pediatrics
Department of Pediatrics and Adolescent
    Medicine
American University of Beirut
Beirut, Lebanon
Retinoblastoma
Neoplasms of the Liver
Desmoplastic Small Round Cell Tumor

Robert C. Tasker, MBBS, MD
Professor of Neurology
Professor of Anesthesia
Harvard Medical School
Senior Associate, Critical Care Medicine
Director, Pediatric NeuroCritical Care Program
Boston Children's Hospital
Boston, Massachusetts
Outcomes and Risk Adjustment of Pediatric
    Emergency Medical Services

Dmitry Tchapyjnikov, MD
Assistant Professor of Pediatrics and Neurology
Duke University Medical Center
Durham, North Carolina
Seizures in Childhood

Brenda L. Tesini, MD
Assistant Professor of Medicine and Pediatrics
University of Rochester Medical Center
Division of Pediatric Infectious Diseases
Golisano Children's Hospital
Rochester, New York
Roseola (Human Herpesviruses 6 and 7)

Jillian L. Theobald, MD, PhD
Assistant Professor of Emergency Medicine
Medical College of Wisconsin
Toxicologist, Wisconsin Poison Center
Milwaukee, Wisconsin
Poisoning

Beth K. Thielen, MD, PhD
Fellow, Infectious Diseases and International
    Medicine
Department of Medicine
Fellow, Pediatric Infectious Diseases and
    Immunology
Department of Pediatrics
University of Minnesota Medical School
Minneapolis, Minnesota
Principles of Antiparasitic Therapy

Anita A. Thomas, MD, MPH
Assistant Professor
Department of Pediatrics
University of Washington School of Medicine
Attending Physician
Division of Emergency Medicine
Seattle Children's Hospital
Seattle, Washington
Drowning and Submersion Injury

Cameron W. Thomas, MD, MS
Assistant Professor of Pediatrics and Neurology
University of Cincinnati College of Medicine
Fetal and Neonatal Neurology Specialist, Division
    of Neurology
Cincinnati Children's Hospital Medical Center
Cincinnati, Ohio
Nervous System Disorders

Courtney D. Thornburg, MD, MS
Professor of Clinical Pediatrics
University of California San Diego School of
  Medicine
La Jolla, California;
Medical Director, Hemophilia and Thrombosis
  Treatment Center
Rady Children's Hospital, San Diego
San Diego, California
The Anemias
Congenital Hypoplastic Anemia (Diamond-
  Blackfan Anemia)
Pearson Syndrome
Acquired Pure Red Blood Cell Anemia
Anemia of Chronic Disease and Renal Disease
Congenital Dyserythropoietic Anemias
Physiologic Anemia of Infancy
Megaloblastic Anemias

Joel S. Tieder, MD, MPH
Associate Professor of Pediatrics
Seattle Children's Hospital
University of Washington School of Medicine
Division of Hospital Medicine
Seattle Children's Hospital
Seattle, Washington
Brief Resolved Unexplained Events and Other
  Acute Events in Infants

Cynthia J. Tifft, MD, PhD
Director, Pediatric Undiagnosed Diseases
  Program
Senior Staff Clinician
Medical Genetics Branch
National Human Genome Research Institute
National Institutes of Health
Bethesda, Maryland
Genetic Approaches to Rare and Undiagnosed
  Diseases

James K. Todd, MD
Professor Emeritus of Pediatrics
Jules Amer Chair in Community Pediatrics
University of Colorado School of Medicine
Section Head, Epidemiology (Pediatrics)
Director, Epidemiology, Clinical Outcomes, and
  Clinical Microbiology
Children's Hospital Colorado
Denver, Colorado
Staphylococcus

**Victor R. Tolentino Jr, JD, MPH,
NP**
Healthcare Consultant
Jackson Heights, New York
Principles Applicable to the Developing World

Camilo Toro, MD
Senior Staff Clinician
Director, Adult Undiagnosed Diseases Program
National Human Genome Research Institute
National Institutes of Health
Bethesda, Maryland
Genetic Approaches to Rare and Undiagnosed
  Diseases

Richard L. Tower II, MD, MS
Assistant Professor
Department of Pediatrics
Division of Pediatric Hematology/Oncology
Medical College of Wisconsin
Children's Hospital of Wisconsin
Milwaukee, Wisconsin
Anatomy and Function of the Lymphatic System
Abnormalities of Lymphatic Vessels
Lymphadenopathy

Joseph M. Trapasso, MD
Resident Physician
Department of Pediatrics
University of Texas Medical Branch
University of Texas Children's Hospital
Galveston, Texas
N-Acetylaspartic Acid (Canavan Disease)

Riccardo Troncone, MD
Professor and Director
Department of Pediatrics
University of Naples Federico II
Napoli, Italy
Celiac Disease

Elaine Tsao, MD
Assistant Professor
Department of Rehabilitation Medicine
University of Washington School of Medicine
Seattle Children's Hospital
Seattle, Washington
Ambulation Assistance

David G. Tubergen, MD
Medical Director, Host Program
MD Anderson Physicians Network
Houston, Texas
The Leukemias

Lisa K. Tuchman, MD, MPH
Associate Professor of Pediatrics
Chief, Division of Adolescent and Young Adult
  Medicine
Center for Translational Science, Children's
  Research Institute
Children's National Health System
Washington, DC
Transitioning to Adult Care

Margaret A. Turk, MD
Professor
Departments of Physical Medicine and
  Rehabilitation and Pediatrics
State University of New York
SUNY Upstate Medical University
Syracuse, New York
Health and Wellness for Children With Disabilities

David A. Turner, MD
Associate Professor
Department of Pediatrics
Duke University School of Medicine
Director, Pediatric Critical Care Fellowship
  Program
Medical Director, Pediatric Intensive Care Unit
Duke University Medical Center
Durham, North Carolina
Shock

Christina Ullrich, MD, PhD
Assistant Professor in Pediatrics
Department of Psychosocial Oncology and
  Palliative Care
Harvard Medical School
Boston Children's Hospital
Dana-Farber Cancer Institute
Boston, Massachusetts
Pediatric Palliative Care

Nicole Ullrich, MD, PhD
Associate Professor of Neurology
Harvard Medical School
Director, Neurologic Neuro-Oncology
Associate Director, Clinical Trials
Neurofibromatosis Program
Boston Children's Hospital
Boston, Massachusetts
Neurocutaneous Syndromes

Krishna K. Upadhya, MD, MPH
Assistant Professor
Division of Adolescent and Young Adult
  Medicine
Children's National Health System
Washington, DC
Menstrual Problems

David K. Urion, MD
Associate Professor and Charles F. Barlow Chair
  of Neurology
Harvard University Medical School
Director, Behavioral Neurology Clinics and
  Programs
Boston Children's Hospital
Boston, Massachusetts
Attention-Deficit/Hyperactivity Disorder

Taher Valika, MD
Clinical Instructor of Otolaryngology – Head and
  Neck Surgery
Northwestern University Feinberg School of
  Medicine
Attending Physician, Otorhinolaryngology
  – Head and Neck Surgery
Ann & Robert H. Lurie Children's Hospital of
  Chicago
Chicago, Illinois
Laryngotracheal Stenosis and Subglottic Stenosis

George F. Van Hare, MD
Professor of Pediatrics
Washington University School of Medicine in
  St Louis
Division of Pediatric Cardiology
St Louis Children's Hospital
St. Louis, Missouri
Syncope
Disturbances of Rate and Rhythm of the Heart
Sudden Death

Heather A. Van Mater, MD, MS
Associate Professor of Pediatrics
Duke University School of Medicine
Division of Pediatric Rheumatology
Duke University Health System
Durham, North Carolina
Scleroderma and Raynaud Phenomenon

Charles D. Varnell Jr, MD, MS
Instructor of Pediatrics
University of Cincinnati College of Medicine
Cincinnati Children's Hospital Medical Center
Cincinnati, Ohio
Renal Transplantation

Ana M. Vaughan, MD, MPH, FAAP
Assistant in Medicine
Division of Infectious Diseases
Associate Hospital Epidemiologist
Boston Children's Hospital
Instructor in Pediatrics
Harvard Medical School
Boston, Massachusetts
Childcare and Communicable Diseases

Timothy J. Vece, MD
Associate Professor of Pediatrics
University of North Carolina School of Medicine
Medical Director, Airway Center
North Carolina Children's Hospital
Chapel Hill, North Carolina
Granulomatous Lung Disease
Eosinophilic Lung Disease
Interstitial Lung Disease

Aarthi P. Vemana, MD
Pediatric Sleep Physician
Fairfax Neonatal Associates
Fairfax, Virginia
Pleurisy, Pleural Effusions, and Empyema

Charles P. Venditti, MD, PhD
Head, Organic Acid Research Section
Senior Investigator, National Human Genome
    Research Institute
National Institutes of Health
Bethesda, Maryland
An Approach to Inborn Errors of Metabolism

Sarah Vepraskas, MD
Assistant Professor of Pediatrics
Section of Hospital Medicine
Medical College of Wisconsin
Milwaukee, Wisconsin
Sudden Unexpected Postnatal Collapse

James W. Verbsky, MD, PhD
Associate Professor of Pediatrics (Rheumatology)
    and Microbiology and Immunology
Medical Director, Clinical Immunology Research
    Laboratory
Medical Director, Clinical and Translational
    Research
Medical College of Wisconsin
Milwaukee, Wisconsin
*Hereditary Periodic Fever Syndromes and Other
    Systemic Autoinflammatory Diseases*

Jennifer A. Vermilion, MD
Instructor in Neurology and Pediatrics
University of Rochester Medical Center
Rochester, New York
Chorea, Athetosis, Tremor

Brian P. Vickery, MD
Associate Professor of Pediatrics
Emory University School of Medicine
Director, Food Allergy Center at Emory and
    Children's Healthcare of Atlanta
Atlanta, Georgia
Eosinophils

Bernadette E. Vitola, MD, MPH
Associate Professor of Pediatrics
Medical College of Wisconsin
Children's Hospital of Wisconsin
Milwaukee, Wisconsin
Liver Disease Associated with Systemic Disorders

Judith A. Voynow, MD
Professor of Pediatrics
Virginia Commonwealth University School of
    Medicine
Edwin L. Kendig Jr. Professor of Pediatric
    Pulmonology
Children's Hospital of Richmond at VCU
Richmond, Virginia
Cystic Fibrosis

Jonathan B. Wagner, DO
Assistant Professor of Pediatrics
University of Missouri–Kansas City School of
    Medicine
Division of Pediatric Cardiology
Children's Mercy Hospitals and Clinics
Kansas City, Missouri
*Pediatric Pharmacogenetics, Pharmacogenomics,
    and Pharmacoproteomics*

Steven G. Waguespack, MD, FACE
Professor
Department of Endocrine Neoplasia and
    Hormonal Disorders
University of Texas MD Anderson Cancer Center
Houston, Texas
Thyroid Tumors
Adrenal Tumors

David M. Walker, MD
Chief, Pediatric Emergency Medicine
Department of Pediatrics
Joseph M. Sanarzi Children's Hospital
Hackensack University Medical Center
Hackensack, New Jersey
Principles Applicable to the Developing World

Kelly J. Walkovich, MD
Clinical Associate Professor of Pediatrics and
    Communicable Diseases
Division of Pediatric Hematology/Oncology
University of Michigan Medical School
Ann Arbor, Michigan
Leukopenia
Leukocytosis

Heather J. Walter, MD, MPH
Professor of Psychiatry and Pediatrics
Boston University School of Medicine
Senior Attending Psychiatrist
Boston Children's Hospital
Senior Lecturer on Psychiatry
Harvard Medical School
Boston, Massachusetts
Psychosocial Assessment and Interviewing
Psychopharmacology
Psychotherapy and Psychiatric Hospitalization
Somatic Symptom and Related Disorders
Rumination and Pica
Motor Disorders and Habits
Anxiety Disorders
Mood Disorders
Suicide and Attempted Suicide
*Disruptive, Impulse-Control, and Conduct
    Disorders*
Tantrums and Breath-Holding Spells
Lying, Stealing, and Truancy
Aggression
Self-Injurious Behavior
Childhood Psychoses

Jennifer A. Wambach, MD
Assistant Professor of Pediatrics
Washington University School of Medicine in
    St. Louis
Division of Newborn Medicine
St. Louis Children's Hospital
St. Louis, Missouri
Inherited Disorders of Surfactant Metabolism
Pulmonary Alveolar Proteinosis

Julie Wang, MD
Professor of Pediatrics
Jaffe Food Allergy Institute
Kravis Children's Hospital at the Icahn School of
    Medicine at Mount Sinai
New York, New York
Insect Allergy
Anaphylaxis

Michael F. Wangler, MD
Assistant Professor of Molecular and Human
    Genetics
Baylor College of Medicine
Jan and Dan Duncan Neurological Research
    Institute
Texas Children's Hospital
Houston, Texas
*Disorders of Very-Long-Chain Fatty Acids and
    Other Peroxisomal Functions*

Russell E. Ware, MD, PhD
Professor of Pediatrics
University of Cincinnati College of Medicine
Director, Division of Hematology
Co-Director, Cancer and Blood Diseases Institute
Director, Global Health Center
Marjory J. Johnson Chair of Hematology
    Translational Research
Cincinnati Children's Hospital Medical Center
Cincinnati, Ohio
Hemolytic Disease of the Newborn
Neonatal Polycythemia
Hemorrhage in the Newborn Infant
Nonimmune Hydrops

**Stephanie M. Ware, MD, PhD,
FACMG**
Professor of Pediatrics and Medical and
    Molecular Genetics
Vice Chair of Clinical Affairs in Medical and
    Molecular Genetics
Program Leader in Cardiovascular Genetics
Herman B Wells Center for Pediatric Research
Indiana University School of Medicine
Indianapolis, Indiana
Diseases of the Myocardium
Diseases of the Pericardium
Tumors of the Heart

Matthew C. Washam, MD, MPH
Assistant Professor of Pediatrics
The Ohio State University
Nationwide Children's Hospital
Columbus, Ohio
Histoplasmosis (Histoplasma capsulatum)

Ari J. Wassner, MD
Assistant Professor of Pediatrics
Harvard Medical School
Director, Thyroid Program
Boston Children's Hospital
Boston, Massachusetts
Thyroid Development and Physiology
Disorders of Thyroxine-Binding Globulin
Hypothyroidism
Thyroiditis
Goiter
Thyrotoxicosis
Carcinoma of the Thyroid
Autoimmune Polyglandular Syndromes
Multiple Endocrine Neoplasia Syndrome

Rachel Wattier, MD, MHS
Assistant Professor of Pediatrics
University of California San Francisco School of
    Medicine
San Francisco, California
Mucormycosis

David R. Weber, MD, MSCE
Assistant Professor of Pediatrics
University of Rochester School of Medicine and
  Dentistry
Division of Endocrinology and Diabetes
Pediatric Bone Health Program
Golisano Children's Hospital
Rochester, New York
Diabetes Mellitus

Debra E. Weese-Mayer, MD
Beatrice Cummings Mayer Professor of Pediatrics
  and Pediatric Autonomic Medicine
Northwestern University Feinberg School of
  Medicine
Chief, Division of Pediatric Autonomic Medicine
Ann & Robert H. Lurie Children's Hospital of
  Chicago
Chicago, Illinois
*Rapid-Onset Obesity with Hypothalamic
  Dysfunction, Hypoventilation, and Autonomic
  Dysregulation (ROHHAD)*
Congenital Central Hypoventilation Syndrome

Jason B. Weinberg, MD
Associate Professor of Pediatrics
Associate Professor of Microbiology and
  Immunology
University of Michigan Medical School
Division of Pediatric Infectious Diseases
C. S. Mott Children's Hospital
Ann Arbor, Michigan
Epstein-Barr Virus
Adenoviruses

Jason P. Weinman, MD
Associate Professor of Radiology
University of Colorado School of Medicine
Aurora, Colorado
Fibrotic Lung Disease

Kathryn L. Weise, MD, MA
Program Director, Cleveland Fellowship in
  Advanced Bioethics
Department of Bioethics
The Cleveland Clinic Foundation
Cleveland, Ohio
Ethics in Pediatric Care

Anna K. Weiss, MD, MSEd
Assistant Professor of Clinical Pediatrics
University of Pennsylvania Perelman School of
  Medicine
Director of Pediatric Resident Education
Division of Emergency Medicine
Children's Hospital of Philadelphia
Philadelphia, Pennsylvania
Triage of the Acutely Ill Child

Pamela F. Weiss, MD, MSCE
Associate Professor of Pediatrics and
  Epidemiology
University of Pennsylvania Perelman School of
  Medicine
Division of Rheumatology
Children's Hospital of Philadelphia
Philadelphia, Pennsylvania
*Ankylosing Spondylitis and Other
  Spondylarthritides*
Reactive and Postinfectious Arthritis

Carol Weitzman, MD
Professor of Pediatrics
Director, Developmental-Behavioral Pediatrics
  Program
Yale School of Medicine
New Haven, Connecticut
Fetal Alcohol Exposure

Morgan P. Welebir, MD
Department of Obstetrics and Gynecology
Providence Saint Joseph Medical Center
Burbank, California
Vaginal Bleeding in the Prepubertal Child

Lawrence Wells, MD
Associate Professor
Department of Orthopaedic Surgery
University of Pennsylvania Perelman School of
  Medicine
Attending Orthopaedic Surgeon
Children's Hospital of Philadelphia
Philadelphia, Pennsylvania
Growth and Development
Evaluation of the Child
Torsional and Angular Deformities
The Hip
Common Fractures

Jessica W. Wen, MD
Associate Professor of Clinical Pediatrics
University of Pennsylvania Perelman School of
  Medicine
Children's Hospital of Philadelphia
Philadelphia, Pennsylvania
Ascites
Peritonitis

Danielle Wendel, MD
Assistant Professor
Division of Gastroenterology and Hepatology
Department of Pediatrics
University of Washington School of Medicine
Seattle Children's Hospital
Seattle, Washington
Tumors of the Digestive Tract

Steven L. Werlin, MD
Professor Emeritus of Pediatrics
The Medical College of Wisconsin
Milwaukee, Wisconsin
*Embryology, Anatomy, and Physiology of the
  Pancreas*
Pancreatic Function Tests
Disorders of the Exocrine Pancreas
Treatment of Pancreatic Insufficiency
Pancreatitis
Pseudocyst of the Pancreas
Pancreatic Tumors

Michael R. Wessels, MD
John F. Enders Professor of Pediatrics
Professor of Medicine (Microbiology)
Harvard Medical School
Division of Infectious Diseases
Boston Children's Hospital
Boston, Massachusetts
Group B Streptococcus

Ralph F. Wetmore, MD
Professor
Department of Otorhinolaryngology–Head and
  Neck Surgery
University of Pennsylvania Perelman School of
  Medicine
E. Mortimer Newlin Professor and Chief
Division of Pediatric Otolaryngology
Children's Hospital of Pennsylvania
Philadelphia, Pennsylvania
Tonsils and Adenoids

Scott L. Wexelblatt, MD
Associate Professor
Department of Pediatrics
University of Cincinnati College of Medicine
Medical Director Regional Newborn Services
Cincinnati Children's Hospital Medical Center
Cincinnati, Ohio
Neonatal Abstinence (Withdrawal)

Isaiah D. Wexler, MD, PhD
Associate Professor
Department of Pediatrics
Hadassah University Medical Center
Jerusalem, Israel
Effects of War on Children

A. Clinton White Jr, MD
Professor of Medicine
Division of Infectious Diseases
The University of Texas Medical Branch at
  Galveston
Galveston, Texas
Adult Tapeworm Infections
Cysticercosis
Echinococcosis (Echinococcus granulosus *and*
  Echinococcus multilocularis)

Perrin C. White, MD
Professor of Pediatrics
Audre Newman Rapoport Distinguished Chair in
  Pediatric Endocrinology
Chief, Division of Pediatric Endocrinology
University of Texas Southwestern Medical Center
Dallas, Texas
Physiology of the Adrenal Gland
Adrenocortical Insufficiency
*Congenital Adrenal Hyperplasia and Related
  Disorders*
Cushing Syndrome
Primary Aldosteronism
Adrenocortical Tumors and Masses
Virilizing and Feminizing Adrenal Tumors
Cushing Syndrome
Primary Aldosteronism
Pheochromocytoma

John V. Williams, MD
Henry L. Hillman Professor of Pediatrics
Professor of Microbiology and Molecular
  Genetics
University of Pittsburgh School of Medicine
Chief, Division of Pediatric Infectious Diseases
UPMC Children's Hospital of Pittsburgh
Pittsburgh, Pennsylvania
Adenoviruses
Rhinoviruses
The Common Cold

Rodney E. Willoughby Jr, MD
Professor of Pediatrics
Medical College of Wisconsin
Division of Pediatric Infectious Diseases
Children's Hospital of Wisconsin
Milwaukee, Wisconsin
Rabies

Michael Wilschanski, MBBS
Professor of Pediatrics
The Hebrew University–Hadassah School of
  Medicine
Director, Pediatric Gastroenterology Unit
Hadassah University Hospitals
Jerusalem, Israel
*Embryology, Anatomy, and Physiology of
  the Pancreas*
Pancreatic Function Tests
Disorders of the Exocrine Pancreas
Treatment of Pancreatic Insufficiency
Pancreatitis
Pseudocyst of the Pancreas
Pancreatic Tumors

Karen M. Wilson, MD, MPH
Professor of Pediatrics
Debra and Leon Black Division Chief of General
  Pediatrics
Vice-Chair for Clinical and Translational
  Research
Kravis Children's Hospital at the Icahn School of
  Medicine at Mount Sinai
New York, New York

Pamela Wilson, MD
Associate Professor
Department of Physical Medicine and
  Rehabilitation
University of Colorado School of Medicine
Children's Hospital Colorado
Denver, Colorado
Meningomyelocele (Spina Bifida)

Jennifer J. Winell, MD
Clinical Assistant Professor of Orthopaedic
  Surgery
University of Pennsylvania Perelman School of
  Medicine
Attending Orthopaedic Surgeon
Children's Hospital of Philadelphia
Philadelphia, Pennsylvania
The Foot and Toes

Glenna B. Winnie, MD
Director, Pediatric and Adolescent Sleep Center
Fairfax Neonatal Associates, PC
Fairfax, Virginia
Emphysema and Overinflation
α1-Antitrypsin Deficiency and Emphysema
Pleurisy, Pleural Effusions, and Empyema
Pneumothorax
Pneumomediastinum
Hydrothorax
Hemothorax
Chylothorax

Lawrence Wissow, MD, MPH
James P. Connaughton Professor of Community
  Psychiatry
Division of Child and Adolescent Psychiatry
Johns Hopkins School of Medicine
Baltimore, Maryland
Strategies for Health Behavior Change

Peter Witters, MD
Professor of Pediatrics
Metabolic Center
University Hospitals Leuven
Leuven, Belgium
Congenital Disorders of Glycosylation

Joshua Wolf, MBBS
Assistant Member, St. Jude Faculty
St. Jude Children's Research Hospital
Memphis, Tennessee
Infection Associated with Medical Devices

Peter M. Wolfgram, MD
Assistant Professor
Medical College of Wisconsin
Division of Endocrinology
Children's Hospital of Wisconsin
Milwaukee, Wisconsin
Delayed or Absent Puberty

Joanne Wolfe, MD, MPH
Professor of Pediatrics
Harvard Medical School
Chief, Division of Pediatric Palliative Care
Dana-Farber Cancer Institute
Director, Pediatric Palliative Care
Boston Children's Hospital
Boston, Massachusetts
Pediatric Palliative Care

Brandon T. Woods, MD
Fellow, Critical Care Medicine
Department of Pediatrics
University of Washington School of Medicine
Seattle, Washington
Pulmonary Edema

Benjamin L. Wright, MD
Assistant Professor
Department of Allergy, Asthma, and Clinical
  Immunology
Mayo Clinic
Scottsdale, Arizona;
Phoenix Children's Hospital
Phoenix, Arizona
Eosinophils

Joseph L. Wright, MD, MPH
Adjunct Research Professor
Department of Family Science
University of Maryland School of Public Health
Adjunct Professor of Emergency Medicine and
  Health Policy
George Washington University
Washington, DC
Emergency Medical Services for Children

Terry W. Wright, PhD
Associate Professor of Pediatrics (Infectious
  Diseases)
University of Rochester Medical Center
School of Medicine and Dentistry
Rochester, New York
Pneumocystis jirovecii

Eveline Y. Wu, MD
Assistant Professor
Department of Pediatrics
Division of Allergy, Immunology, and
  Rheumatology
University of North Carolina at Chapel Hill
Chapel Hill, North Carolina
Juvenile Idiopathic Arthritis
Sarcoidosis

Pablo Yagupsky, MD
Professor of Pediatrics and Clinical Microbiology
  (Emeritus)
Ben-Gurion University of the Negev
Department of Pediatrics
Soroka Medical Center
Beer-Sheva, Israel
Kingella kingae

E. Ann Yeh, MD, MA
Associate Professor of Pediatrics (Neurology)
University of Toronto Faculty of Medicine
Director, MS and Demyelinating Disorders
  Program
Hospital for Sick Children
Toronto, Ontario, Canada
*Spinal Cord Lesions Associated with Vascular
  Processes*

Anusha K. Yeshokumar, MD
Assistant Professor
Departments of Neurology and Pediatrics
Kravis Children's Hospital at the Icahn School of
  Medicine at Mount Sinai
New York, New York
Central Nervous System Vasculitis

Wafik Zaky, MD
Professor
Department of Pediatrics Patient Care
The University of Texas MD Anderson Cancer
  Center
Houston, Texas
Brain Tumors in Childhood

Lauren B. Zapata, PhD
Epidemiologist, Division of Reproductive Health
Centers for Disease Control and Prevention
Atlanta, Georgia
Contraception

Lonnie K. Zeltzer, MD
Distinguished Research Professor
Departments of Anesthesiology, Psychiatry, and
  Biobehavioral Science
David Geffen School of Medicine at UCLA
Los Angeles, California
Pediatric Pain Management

Amy Zhou, BA
Clinical Research Coordinator
Center for Autonomic Medicine in Pediatrics
Ann & Robert H. Lurie Children's Hospital of
  Chicago
Chicago, Illinois
*Rapid-Onset Obesity with Hypothalamic
  Dysfunction, Hypoventilation, and Autonomic
  Dysregulation (ROHHAD)*
Congenital Central Hypoventilation Syndrome

Barry S. Zuckerman, MD
Professor of Pediatrics and Chair Emeritus
Boston University School of Medicine
Boston Medical Center
Boston, Massachusetts
Impact of Violence on Children

Preface

Whoever saves one life it is considered as if they saved an entire world.
— Babylonian Talmud

The 21st edition of *Nelson Textbook of Pediatrics* continues its tradition of being an essential resource for general pediatric providers and pediatric subspecialists as they diagnose and treat infants, children, and adolescents throughout the world. The 21st edition has been thoroughly revised, updated, and edited to keep up with the huge advances in clinical care derived from basic, clinical, and population-based research. The promise that translational medicine will improve the lives of children has become a daily reality for most but not all children. Knowledge of human development, behavior, and diseases from the molecular to sociologic levels has led to greater understanding of health and illness in children and substantial improvements in health quality for those who have access to health care. These exciting scientific advances also provide hope to effectively address prevention and treatment of new and emerging diseases threatening children and their families.

The field of pediatrics encompasses advocacy for all children throughout the world and must address societal inequalities of important resources required for normal development, as well as protection from natural and man-made disasters. Unfortunately, many children throughout the world have not benefited from the significant advances in the prevention and treatment of health-related problems. For our increasing knowledge to benefit all children and youth, medical advances and good clinical practice must always be coupled with effective advocacy to overcome unconscious bias, lack of political will, and misplaced priorities.

This new edition of *Nelson Textbook of Pediatrics* attempts to provide the essential information that practitioners, house staff, medical students, and all other care providers involved in pediatric health care throughout the world need to understand to effectively address the enormous range of biologic, psychologic, and social problems that our children and youth face. In addition, pediatric subspecialists will benefit from the details of coexisting disorders often seen in their patients. Our goal is to be comprehensive yet concise and reader friendly, embracing both new advances in clinical science and the time-honored art of pediatric practice.

The 21st edition is reorganized and revised from the previous edition. There are many additions of new diseases and new chapters, as well as substantial expansion or significant modification of others. In addition, many more tables, photographs, imaging studies, and illustrative figures, as well as up-to-date references, have been added. This new edition has greatly benefited by the addition of four new associate editors with an extremely broad base of clinic experiences: Dr. Nathan Blum, Chief, Division of Developmental and Behavioral Pediatrics at the Children's Hospital of Philadelphia; Dr. Samir S. Shah, Director, Division of Hospital Medicine and Chief Metrics Officer, Cincinnati Children's Hospital Medical Center; Dr. Robert Tasker, Director, Pediatric NeuroCritical Care Medicine, Boston Children's Hospital; and Dr. Karen Wilson, Division Chief of General Pediatrics, Vice-Chair for Clinical and Translational Research, Kravis Children's Hospital at the Icahn School of Medicine at Mount Sinai, have all contributed to the planning and editing of the 21st edition.

Although, to an ill child and their family and physician, even the rarest disorder is of central importance, all health problems cannot possibly be covered with the same degree of detail in one general textbook of pediatrics. Thus, leading articles and subspecialty texts are referenced and should be consulted when more information is desired. In addition, as new recommendations or policies are developed, they will be updated on our website.

The outstanding value of the 21st edition of the textbook is due to its many expert and authoritative contributors. We are all indebted to these dedicated authors for their hard work, knowledge, thoughtfulness, and good judgment. Our sincere appreciation also goes to Jennifer Shreiner and Sarah Barth at Elsevier and to Carolyn Redman in the Pediatric Department of the Medical College of Wisconsin. We have all worked hard to produce an edition that will be helpful to those who provide care for children and youth and to those desiring to know more about children's health worldwide.

In this edition we have had informal assistance from many faculty and house staff of the department of pediatrics at the Medical College of Wisconsin, University of Pennsylvania Perelman School of Medicine, University of Cincinnati College of Medicine, Harvard Medical School, and the Kravis Children's Hospital at the Icahn School of Medicine at Mount Sinai. The help of these individuals and of the many practicing pediatricians from around the world who have taken the time to offer thoughtful feedback and suggestions is always greatly appreciated and helpful.

Last and certainly not least, we especially wish to thank our families for their patience and understanding about the great time commitment we as editors have spent reading and editing this edition.

Robert M. Kliegman, MD
Joseph W. St. Geme III, MD
Nathan J. Blum, MD
Samir S. Shah, MD, MSCE
Robert C. Tasker, MBBS, MD
Karen M. Wilson, MD, MPH

Contents 目 录

Volume 1
上 册

PART III

Behavioral and Psychiatric Disorders
第三部分 行为和精神障碍

PART IV

Learning and Developmental Disorders
第四部分 学习及发育障碍

PART V

Nutrition
第五部分 营养

PART VI

Fluid and Electrolyte Disorders
第六部分 水和电解质紊乱

PART VII

Pediatric Drug Therapy
第七部分 儿科药物治疗

Volume 2
中 册

PART XIV

Allergic Disorders
第十四部分　过敏性疾病

PART XVIII

The Respiratory System
第十八部分　呼吸系统

Section 1 DEVELOPMENT AND FUNCTION
第一篇　发育与功能

Section 2 DISORDERS OF THE RESPIRATORY TRACT
第二篇　呼吸道疾病

---

†Deceased.

Volume 3
下　册

PART XIX
The Cardiovascular System
第十九部分　心血管系统

Section 1 DEVELOPMENTAL BIOLOGY OF THE CARDIOVASCULAR SYSTEM
第一篇　心血管系统发育生理学

PART XXV
The Endocrine System
第二十五部分 内分泌系统

PART **XXXI**

Bone and Joint Disorders
第三十一部分 骨骼和关节疾病

Section **1** ORTHOPEDIC PROBLEMS
第一篇 矫形骨科常见问题

PART **XXXII**

Rehabilitation Medicine
第三十二部分　康复医学

PART XXXIII

Environmental Health
第三十三部分 环境卫生

Chapter **1**
Overview of Pediatrics
Lee M. Pachter
第一章
儿科学绪论

中文导读

本章主要介绍了全球儿童健康生存状态统计、变化中的儿科世界、新病种和疾病谱、慢性病和有特殊保健需求的儿童，以及医疗保健体系。其中在新病种和疾病谱中涉及不良童年经历、毒性压力与非稳态负荷，以及生态环境–身心发展的框架模式；医疗保健体系中分别介绍了群体健康管理方式、医疗之家和医疗卫生及相关机构一站式服务等。

Pediatrics is the only discipline dedicated to all aspects of the care and well-being of infants, children, and adolescents, including their health—their physical, mental, social, and psychological growth and development—and their ability to achieve full potential as adults. Pediatricians must be concerned not only with specific organ systems, genetics, and biologic processes, but also with environmental, psychosocial, cultural, and political influences, all of which may have major impacts on the health and well-being of children and their families.

Children cannot advocate wholly for themselves. As the professionals whose purpose is to advance the well-being of children, pediatricians must be advocates for the individual child and for all children, irrespective of culture, religion, gender, sexual orientation, race, or ethnicity or of local, state, or national boundaries. The more politically, economically, or socially disenfranchised a population is, the greater the need for advocacy for its children and for those who support children. Youth are often among the most vulnerable persons in society, and thus their needs require special attention. As segmentation between nations blur through advances in media, transportation, technology, communication, and economics, a *global*, rather than a national or local, perspective for the field of pediatrics becomes both a reality and a necessity. The interconnectedness of health issues across the world has achieved widespread recognition in the wake of the Zika, Ebola, SARS, and AIDS epidemics; war and bioterrorism; the tsunami of 2004; the earthquake in Haiti in 2010; the displacement of families during the Syrian refugee crisis in 2016–2018; and the growing severity of drought, hurricanes, and cyclones brought about by climate change.

More than a century ago, pediatrics emerged as a medical specialty in response to increasing awareness that the health problems of children differ from those of adults, and that a child's response to disease and stress varies with age and development. In 1959 the United Nations issued the **Declaration of the Rights of the Child**, articulating the universal presumption that children everywhere have fundamental needs and rights. Today, an affirmation of those rights and an effort to satisfy those needs are more important than ever.

VITAL STATISTICS ABOUT CHILDREN'S HEALTH GLOBALLY

From 1990 to 2010, the world population grew at an annual rate of 1.3% per year, down from 1.8% during the prior 20 yr. This rate continues to decline; in 2016 the growth rate was 1.13%. Worldwide, there are 2.34 billion children 18 yr and younger, which accounts for approximately one third (32%) of the world's population of 7.4 billion persons. In 2016 the average birthrate in the world was 18.5 births per 1,000 population, with a high of 44.8/1,000 in Niger to the lowest in Monaco at 6.6/1,000. The most populous countries—China, India, and the United States—have rates of 12.4, 19.3, and 12.5 per 1,000 population, respectively.

Despite global interconnectedness, the health of children and youth varies widely between and within regions and nations of the world, depending on several interrelated factors. These include (1) economic conditions; (2) educational, social, and cultural considerations; (3) health and social welfare infrastructure; (4) climate and geography; (5) agricultural resources and practices, which account for nutritional resources;

(6) stage of industrialization and urbanization; (7) gene frequencies for certain disorders; (8) the ecology of infectious agents and their hosts; (9) social stability; and (10) political focus and stability. Although genetics, biology, and access to affordable and quality healthcare are important determinants, it has been shown that the *social* determinants of health—the physical environment, political and economic conditions, social and cultural considerations, and behavioral psychology—play as great a role, if not greater, in health outcomes.

To ensure that the needs of children and adults worldwide were not obscured by local needs, in 2000 the international community established 8 **Millennium Development Goals** (MDGs) to be achieved by 2015. Although all 8 MDGs impact child well-being, **MDG 4** was exclusively focused on children: to reduce the **under-five mortality rate (U5MR)** by two-thirds between 1990 and 2015. It was estimated that poor nutrition contributed to more than one third of the deaths worldwide in children <5 yr old, so many of the efforts to reach this goal centered on increasing household food security. Increasing measles vaccination, particularly in sub-Saharan Africa, was another strategy to reduce the U5MR.

There was some progress in achieving MDG 4; the worldwideU5MR decreased by 50% between 1990 and 2015. Although the goal of a two-thirds reduction was not achieved, deaths in children under5 dropped from 12.7 million in 1990 to about 6 million in 2015, despite growth in world population during the same period.

The U5MR can be further divided into neonatal (<1 mo of age), infant (<1 yr of age), and after infancy (1-5 yr of age) (Fig. 1.1). The leading causes of worldwide U5MR are preterm birth complications, pneumonia, perinatal asphyxia, diarrheal diseases, and malaria. Many of these causes are linked to **malnutrition**. Children in sub-Saharan Africa are 14 times more likely to die before age 5 yr than children in the developed areas of the world.

Causes of under-5 mortality differ greatly between developed and developing nations. In developing countries, 66% of deaths in children <5 yr old resulted from infectious and parasitic diseases. Among the 42 countries having 90% of childhood deaths, diarrheal disease accounted for 22% of deaths, pneumonia 21%, malaria 9%, AIDS 3%, and measles 1%. Neonatal causes contributed 33%. In the United States, pneumonia

(and influenza) accounted for only 2% of under-5 deaths, with only negligible contributions from diarrheal diseases and malaria. **Unintentional injury** is the most common cause of death among U.S. children age 1-4 yr, accounting for approximately 33% of deaths, followed by congenital anomalies (11%), homicides (9%), and malignant neoplasms (8%). Other causes accounted for <5% of total mortality within this age-group (Table 1.1). **Violence** is a significant contributor to injury-related mortality in all child age-groups (Tables 1.2 and 1.3). Although unintentional injuries in developing countries are proportionately less important causes of mortality than in developed countries, the absolute rates and contributions of these injuries to morbidity are substantially greater.

The **infant mortality rate** (deaths of children <1 yr old) accounts for 85% of the U5MR in industrialized countries, but only 70% in the least developed nations. Neonatal (<1 mo) death contributes substantially as well, growing in proportion as the U5MR decreases. Globally, the **neonatal mortality rate** of 19/1,000 live births represents 60% of the infant mortality rate and 45% of the U5MR. The neonatal mortality rate is responsible for 56% of the U5MR in industrialized nations, 45% in developing countries, but only 38% in the least-developed countries. More children <5 yr old in developing countries die from non–birth-related causes.

Across the globe, there are significant variations in child mortality rates by nation, by region, by economic status, and by level of industrial development, the categorizations employed by the World Bank (http://wdi.worldbank.org/table/2.18). As of 2015, 8 nations have a U5MR of ≥100 per 1,000 live births (all in the WHO African region) (Fig. 1.2). The average U5MR in low-income countries was 76/1,000 live births, and in high-income countries, 6/1,000. Income and wealth, however, are not the only determinants of mortality. For example, the United States has the 10th highest gross national income per capita, but ranked 57th in lowest infant mortality rate in 2016.

In addition to mortality rates, causes of death vary by developmental status of the nation. In the United States the 3 leading causes of death among children <5 yr old were congenital anomalies, disorders related to gestation and low birthweight, and unintentional injuries. By contrast, in developing countries, most infant deaths are caused by pneumonia, diarrheal disease, and malaria.

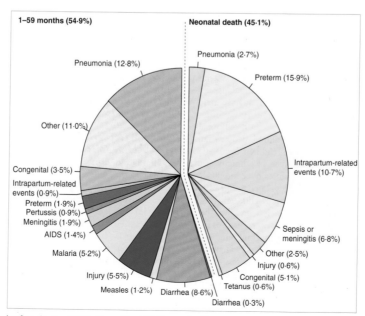

Fig. 1.1 Global causes of under-five deaths, 2015. (*From Oza LLS, Hogan D, Chu Y, et al: Global, regional, and national causes of under-5-mortality in 2000–15: an updated systematic analysis with implications for the sustainable development goals, Lancet 388:3027–3034, 2016, Fig 1, p 3029.*)

| **Table 1.1** | Ten Leading Causes of Death by Age Group, United States, 2015 |

10 Leading Causes of Death by Age Group, United States – 2015

Rank	<1	1-4	5-9	10-14	15-24	25-34	35-44	45-54	55-64	65+	Total
1	Congenital Anomalies 4,825	Unintentional Injury 1,235	Unintentional Injury 755	Unintentional Injury 763	Unintentional Injury 12,514	Unintentional Injury 19,795	Unintentional Injury 17,818	Malignant Neoplasms 43,054	Malignant Neoplasms 116,122	Heart Disease 507,138	Heart Disease 633,842
2	Short Gestation 4,084	Congenital Anomalies 435	Malignant Neoplasms 437	Malignant Neoplasms 428	Suicide 5,491	Suicide 6,947	Malignant Neoplasms 10,909	Heart Disease 34,248	Heart Disease 76,872	Malignant Neoplasms 419,389	Malignant Neoplasms 595,930
3	SIDS 1,568	Homicide 369	Congenital Anomalies 181	Suicide 409	Homicide 4,733	Homicide 4,863	Heart Disease 10,387	Unintentional Injury 21,499	Unintentional Injury 19,488	Chronic Low. Respiratory Disease 131,804	Chronic Low. Respiratory Disease 155,041
4	Maternal Pregnancy Comp.	Malignant Neoplasms 354	Homicide 140	Homicide 158	Malignant Neoplasms 1,469	Malignant Neoplasms 3,704	Suicide 6,936	Liver Disease 8,874	Chronic Low. Respiratory Disease 17,457	Cerebro-vascular 120,156	Unintentional Injury 146,571
5	Unintentional Injury 1,291	Heart Disease 147	Heart Disease 85	Congenital Anomalies 156	Heart Disease 997	Heart Disease 3,522	Homicide 2,895	Suicide 8,751	Diabetes Mellitus 14,166	Alzheimer's Disease 109,495	Cerebro-vascular 140,323
6	Placenta Cord. Membranes 910	Influenza & Pneumonia 88	Chronic Low. Respiratory Disease 80	Heart Disease 125	Congenital Anomalies 386	Liver Disease 844	Liver Disease 2,861	Diabetes Mellitus 6,212	Liver Disease 13,278	Diabetes Mellitus 56,142	Alzheimer's Disease 110,561
7	Bacterial Sepsis 599	Septicemia 54	Influenza & Pneumonia 44	Chronic Low Respiratory Disease 93	Chronic Low Respiratory Disease 202	Diabetes Mellitus 798	Diabetes Mellitus 1,986	Cerebro-vascular 5,307	Cerebro-vascular 12,116	Unintentional Injury 51,395	Diabetes Mellitus 79,535
8	Respiratory Distress 462	Perinatal Period 50	Cerebro-vascular 42	Cerebro-vascular 42	Diabetes Mellitus 196	Cerebro-vascular 567	Cerebro-vascular 1,788	Chronic Low. Respiratory Disease 4,345	Suicide 7,739	Influenza & Pneumonia 48,774	Influenza & Pneumonia 57,062
9	Circulatory System Disease 428	Cerebro-vascular 42	Benign Neoplasms 39	Influenza & Pneumonia 39	Influenza & Pneumonia 184	HIV 529	HIV 1,055	Septicemia 2,542	Septicemia 5,774	Nephritis 41,258	Nephritis 49,959
10	Neonatal Hemorrhage 406	Chronic Low Respiratory Disease 40	Septicemia 31	Two Tied: Benign Neo./Septicemia 33	Cerebro-vascular 166	Congenital Anomalies 443	Septicemia 829	Nephritis 2,124	Nephritis 5,452	Septicemia 30,817	Suicide 44,193

Data Source: National Vital Statistics System, National Center for Health Statistics, CDC.
Produced by: National Center for Injury Prevention and Control, CDC using WISQARS™.

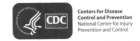

Centers for Disease Control and Prevention
National Center for Injury
Prevention and Control

Courtesy Centers for Disease Control and Prevention, Atlanta.

THE CHANGING PEDIATRIC WORLD

A profound improvement in child health within industrialized nations occurred in the 20th century with the introduction of vaccines, antibiotic agents, and improved hygienic practices. Efforts to control infectious diseases were complemented by better understanding of the role of nutrition in preventing illness and maintaining health. In the United States, Canada, and parts of Europe, new and continuing discoveries in these areas led to establishment of publicly funded **well-child clinics** for low-income families. Although the timing of infectious disease control was uneven around the globe, this focus on *control* was accompanied by significant decreases in morbidity and mortality in all countries.

In the later 20th century, with improved control of infectious diseases through more effective prevention and treatment (including the eradication of polio in the Western hemisphere), pediatric medicine in industrialized nations increasingly turned its attention to a broad spectrum of noninfectious acute and chronic conditions. These included potentially lethal conditions as well as temporarily or permanently handicapping conditions. Advances occurred in the diagnosis, care, and treatment of leukemia and other neoplasms, cystic fibrosis, sickle cell disease, diseases of the newborn infant, congenital heart disease, genetic defects, rheumatic diseases, renal diseases, and metabolic and endocrine disorders.

Until the 1970s and early 1980s, children affected with **sickle cell disease** often died within the 1st 3 yr of life often from overwhelming sepsis caused by encapsulated bacteria. In the 1980s a multicenter study showed that early initiation of *penicillin prophylaxis* led to an 84% risk reduction for pneumococcal sepsis. Life expectancy for those with sickle cell disease increased when penicillin prophylaxis was initiated early in life. The use of prophylactic penicillin became the standard of care, increasing the importance of early detection of sickle cell disease (which led to expanding universal *newborn screening*) and paving the way for advances in the chronic management of the disease, including transfusion therapy, radiographic screening for silent cerebral infarctions, and hydroxyurea as a disease-modifying therapy. The success of penicillin prophylaxis likely led to a more rapid rate of innovation in the diagnosis and management of the disease, since children with the condition now had increased life expectancy. Whereas in the preprophylaxis era children often died by age 3, now 95% of individuals born with sickle cell disease will live to their 18th birthday, and most will survive until their 5th decade.

The treatment of **acute lymphoblastic leukemia** (ALL), the most common pediatric malignancy, has also shown amazing advances. Five-year survival rates have increased from <10% in the 1960s to >90% in 2000–2005. **Cystic fibrosis** has shown improvements in survival as well. In the 1960s, most children with cystic fibrosis did not live until school age. With advances in pulmonary and nutritional therapies, as well as earlier initiation of these therapies secondary to earlier identification through newborn screening, a child born with cystic fibrosis in 2010 has a projected life expectancy of 39-56 yr.

Table 1.2 Ten Leading Causes of Injury Deaths by Age Group Highlighting Unintentional Injury Deaths, United States, 2015

10 Leading Causes of Injury Deaths by Age Group Highlighting Unintentional Injury Deaths, United States – 2015

Rank	<1	1-4	5-9	10-14	15-24	25-34	35-44	45-54	55-64	65+	Total
1	Unintentional Suffocation 1,125	Unintentional Drowning 390	Unintentional MV Traffic 351	Unintentional MV Traffic 412	Unintentional MV Traffic 6,787	Unintentional Poisoning 11,231	Unintentional Poisoning 10,580	Unintentional Poisoning 11,670	Unintentional Poisoning 7,782	Unintentional Fall 28,486	Unintentional Poisoning 47,478
2	Homicide Unspecified 135	Unintentional MV Traffic 332	Unintentional Drowning 129	Suicide Suffocation 234	Homicide Firearm 4,140	Unintentional MV Traffic 6,327	Unintentional MV Traffic 4,686	Unintentional MV Traffic 5,329	Unintentional MV Traffic 5,008	Unintentional MV Traffic 6,860	Unintentional MV Traffic 36,161
3	Homicide Other Spec., Classifiable 69	Homicide Unspecified 153	Unintentional Fire/Burn 72	Suicide Firearm 139	Unintentional Poisoning 3,920	Homicide Firearm 3,996	Suicide Firearm 2,952	Suicide Firearm 3,882	Suicide Firearm 3,951	Suicide Firearm 5,511	Unintentional Fall 33,381
4	Unintentional MV Traffic 64	Unintentional Suffocation 131	Homicide Firearm 69	Homicide Firearm 121	Suicide Firearm 2,461	Suicide Firearm 3,118	Suicide Suffocation 2,219	Suicide Suffocation 2,333	Unintentional Fall 2,504	Unintentional Unspecified 5,204	Suicide Firearm 22,018
5	Undetermined Suffocation 50	Unintentional Fire/Burn 100	Unintentional Other Land Transport 32	Unintentional Drowning 87	Suicide Suffocation 2,119	Suicide Suffocation 2,504	Homicide Firearm 2,197	Suicide Poisoning 1,835	Suicide Poisoning 1,593	Unintentional Suffocation 3,837	Homicide Firearm 12,979
6	Unintentional Drowning 30	Unintentional Pedestrian, Other 75	Unintentional Suffocation 31	Unintentional Other Land Transport 51	Unintentional Drowning 504	Suicide Poisoning 769	Suicide Poisoning 1,181	Homicide Firearm 1,299	Suicide Suffocation 1,535	Unintentional Poisoning 2,198	Suicide Suffocation 11,855
7	Homicide Suffocation 24	Homicide Other Spec., Classifiable 73	Unintentional Natural/ Environment 24	Unintentional Fire/Burn 41	Suicide Poisoning 409	Undetermined Poisoning 624	Undetermined Poisoning 699	Unintentional Fall 1,298	Unintentional Suffocation 777	Adverse Effects 1,721	Unintentional Unspecified 6,930
8	Unintentional Fire/Burn 22	Homicide Firearm 50	Unintentional Pedestrian, Other 20	Unintentional Poisoning 36	Homicide Cut/Pierce 312	Unintentional Drowning 445	Unintentional Fall 492	Undetermined Poisoning 828	Unintentional Unspecified 696	Unintentional Fire/Burn 1,171	Unintentional Suffocation 6,914
9	Undetermined Unspecified 21	Homicide Suffocation 31	Unintentional Poisoning 17	Unintentional Suffocation 26	Undetermined Poisoning 234	Homicide Cut/Pierce 399	Unintentional Drowning 374	Unintentional Suffocation 469	Homicide Firearm 681	Suicide Poisoning 1,005	Suicide Poisoning 6,816
10	Four Tied 12	Unintentional Fall 30	Unintentional Struck by or Against 17	Suicide Poisoning 23	Unintentional Fall 217	Unintentional Fall 324	Homicide Cut/Pierce 291	Unintentional Drowning 450	Two Tied: Undet. Poisoning, Unint. Fire/Burn 565	Suicide Suffocation 908	Unintentional Drowning 3,602

Data Source: National Center for Health Statistics (NCHS), National Vital Statistics System.
Produced by: National Center for Injury Prevention and Control, CDC using WISQARS ™.

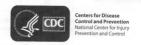

Centers for Disease Control and Prevention
National Center for Injury Prevention and Control

Courtesy Centers for Disease Control and Prevention, Atlanta.

These major advances in the management of chronic diseases of childhood were accomplished when significant improvement occurred in the prevention and treatment of acute infectious diseases, at least in industrial countries. This allowed human and economic resources to shift toward addressing chronic disease.

THE NEW MORBIDITIES

Given the advances in public health aimed at decreasing morbidity and mortality in infectious diseases (immunization, hygiene, antibiotics), along with the rise of technologic advances in clinical care, attention was given to the **new morbidities**—behavioral, developmental, and psychosocial conditions and problems shown to be increasingly associated with suboptimal health outcomes and quality of life. The American Academy of Pediatrics (AAP) **Committee on Psychosocial Aspects of Child and Family Health** asserted that the prevention, early detection, and management of these types of child health problems should be a central focus of the field of pediatrics, and that it would require an expansion in the knowledge base regarding (1) physical and environmental factors affecting behavior, (2) normal child behavior and development, (3) health behaviors as they pertain to child health, and (4) mild, moderate, and severe behavioral and developmental disorders. Accomplishing this would require reconceptualizing professional training, improving clinical communication and interviewing skills, expanding mental health resources for children, and shifting time allocation during child health supervision visits to address these concerns. In 2001 the Committee revisited this issue and reemphasized the need to address environmental and social aspects in addition to developmental and behavioral issues (Table 1.4). These included violence, firearms, substance use, and school problems, as well as poverty, homelessness, single-parent families, divorce, media, and childcare. Although this expanding list seems daunting and beyond the scope of what pediatricians typically addressed (i.e., physical health and development), many of these behavioral, environmental, and psychosocial issues (which fall under the category of social determinants of health) account for a large proportion of variance in health outcomes in children and youth. The role of pediatrics and the boundaries of clinical practice needed to change in order to address these salient contributors to child health and well-being. Newer models of clinical care that rely on close collaboration and coordination with other professionals committed to child welfare (e.g., social workers, psychologists, mental health providers, educators) were developed. As this model expanded, so did the role of the family, in particular the child's caregiver, from a passive recipient of professional services to a more equitable and inclusive partner in identifying the issues that needed to be addressed, as well as helping decide which therapeutic options had the "best fit" with the child, the family, and the condition.

The framing of salient child health issues under the "new morbidity" concept acknowledges that the determinants of health are heterogeneous but interconnected. Biology, genetics, healthcare, behaviors, social conditions, and environmental influences should not be viewed as

| Table 1.3 | Ten Leading Causes of Injury Deaths by Age Group Highlighting Violence-Related Injury Deaths, United States, 2015 |

10 Leading Causes of Injury Deaths by Age Group Highlighting Violence-Related Injury Deaths, United States – 2015

Rank	<1	1-4	5-9	10-14	15-24	25-34	35-44	45-54	55-64	65+	Total
1	Unintentional Suffocation 1,125	Unintentional Drowning 390	Unintentional MV Traffic 351	Unintentional MV Traffic 412	Unintentional MV Traffic 6,787	Unintentional Poisoning 11,231	Unintentional Poisoning 10,580	Unintentional Poisoning 11,670	Unintentional Poisoning 7,782	Unintentional Fall 28,486	Unintentional Poisoning 47,478
2	Homicide Unspecified 135	Unintentional MV Traffic 332	Unintentional Drowning 129	Suicide Suffocation 234	Homicide Firearm 4,140	Unintentional MV Traffic 6,327	Unintentional MV Traffic 4,686	Unintentional MV Traffic 5,329	Unintentional MV Traffic 5,008	Unintentional MV Traffic 6,860	Unintentional MV Traffic 36,161
3	Homicide Other Spec., Classifiable 69	Homicide Unspecified 153	Unintentional Fire/Burn 72	Suicide Firearm 139	Unintentional Poisoning 3,920	Homicide Firearm 3,996	Suicide Firearm 2,952	Suicide Firearm 3,882	Suicide Firearm 3,951	Suicide Firearm 5,511	Unintentional Fall 33,381
4	Unintentional MV Traffic 64	Unintentional Suffocation 131	Homicide Firearm 69	Homicide Firearm 121	Suicide Firearm 2,461	Suicide Firearm 3,118	Suicide Suffocation 2,219	Suicide Suffocation 2,333	Unintentional Fall 2,504	Unintentional Unspecified 5,204	Suicide Firearm 22,018
5	Unintentional Suffocation 50	Unintentional Fire/Burn 100	Unintentional Other Land Transport 32	Unintentional Drowning 87	Suicide Suffocation 2,119	Suicide Suffocation 2,504	Homicide Firearm 2,197	Suicide Poisoning 1,835	Suicide Poisoning 1,593	Unintentional Suffocation 3,837	Homicide Firearm 12,979
6	Unintentional Drowning 30	Unintentional Pedestrian, Other 75	Unintentional Suffocation 31	Unintentional Other Land Transport 51	Unintentional Drowning 504	Suicide Poisoning 769	Suicide Poisoning 1,181	Homicide Firearm 1,299	Suicide Suffocation 1,535	Unintentional Poisoning 2,198	Suicide Suffocation 11,855
7	Homicide Suffocation 24	Homicide Other Spec., Classifiable 73	Unintentional Natural/Environment 24	Unintentional Fire/Burn 41	Suicide Poisoning 409	Undetermined Poisoning 624	Undetermined Poisoning 699	Unintentional Fall 1,298	Unintentional Suffocation 777	Adverse Effects 1,721	Unintentional Unspecified 6,930
8	Unintentional Fire/Burn 22	Homicide Firearm 50	Unintentional Pedestrian, Other 20	Unintentional Poisoning 36	Homicide Cut/Pierce 312	Unintentional Drowning 445	Unintentional Fall 492	Undetermined Poisoning 828	Unintentional Unspecified 696	Unintentional Fire/Burn 1,171	Unintentional Suffocation 6,914
9	Undetermined Unspecified 21	Homicide Suffocation 31	Unintentional Poisoning 17	Unintentional Suffocation 26	Undetermined Poisoning 234	Homicide Cut/Pierce 399	Unintentional Drowning 374	Unintentional Suffocation 469	Homicide Firearm 681	Suicide Poisoning 1,005	Suicide Poisoning 6,816
10	Four Tied 12	Unintentional Fall 30	Unintentional Struck by or Against 17	Suicide Poisoning 23	Unintentional Fall 217	Unintentional Fall 324	Homicide Cut/Pierce 291	Unintentional Drowning 450	Two Tied: Undet. Poisoning, Unint. Fire/Burn 565	Suicide Suffocation 908	Unintentional Drowning 3,602

Data Source: National Center for Health Statistics (NCHS), National Vital Statistics System.
Produced by: National Center for Injury Prevention and Control, CDC using WISQARS ™.

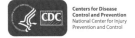 Centers for Disease Control and Prevention National Center for Injury Prevention and Control

Courtesy Centers for Disease Control and Prevention, Atlanta.

mutually exclusive determinants; they exert their influences through complex interactions on multiple levels. For example, epigenetic changes that result from specific social and environmental conditions illustrate the influence of context on gene expression.

Studies have demonstrated that while each of these interrelated determinants are important for optimal health, development, and well-being, the greatest contributions to health outcomes occur in the behavioral, social, and environmental domains—the **social determinants of health**. From 40% to 70% of the relative variation in certain health outcomes is caused by social and economic conditions, health behaviors, and environmental factors. Whereas traditional medical education and clinical practice emphasized the biologic, genetic, and healthcare-related determinants of health, the recognition of the new morbidities as a focus of child healthcare provision reinforced the need to address social determinants as a key component of pediatric care, training, and research.

The "New" New Morbidities

The new morbidities concept brought into perspective the importance of addressing the social determinants of health, as well as the increasing prevalence and salience of chronic physical and behavioral health conditions in pediatric healthcare. Since then, advances in epidemiology, physiology, and epigenetics have expanded the scope of inquiry into the effects of a broad range of health determinants and provided more sophisticated explanatory models for the mechanisms that explain their effects (Table 1.4).

Adverse Childhood Experiences

Adverse childhood experiences (**ACEs**) are stressful events experienced during childhood that can have profound health consequences in childhood and throughout the life course into adulthood. ACEs were initially defined as *abuse* (physical, emotional, sexual), *neglect* (physical and emotional), and *household challenges/family dysfunction* (parental spousal abuse, mental illness in household, household substance abuse, incarceration of household member, parental separation or divorce). Retrospective studies have shown a graded dose-response effect of ACEs experienced in childhood on the future adult health of the child who experience the ACEs. For example, more childhood adversity was associated with significantly increased risk in later life of ischemic heart disease, chronic obstructive pulmonary disease, liver disease, depression, obesity, and cancer. People who suffered ≥6 ACEs as a child died almost 20 yr earlier than those who experienced no ACEs.

While the original conceptualization of ACEs included family-level psychosocial trauma, recent attempts have been made to expand the concept to include "macro" level stressors, such as those encountered in the neighborhood and community (Table 1.5). These include witnessing violence in the community, poverty, bullying and peer victimization, peer isolation, living in unsafe neighborhoods, low neighborhood social capital, living in foster care, and experiencing discrimination or racism.

ACEs and other psychosocial traumas may influence health through a number of mechanisms. ACEs are associated with adoption of risky

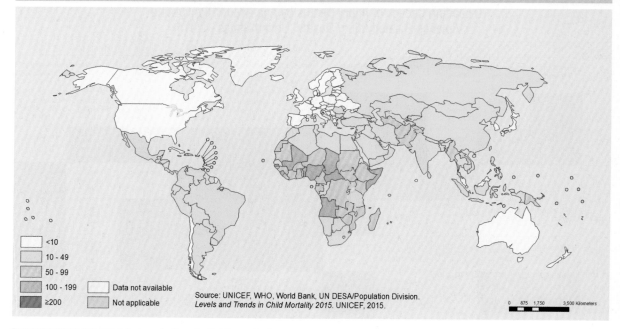

Fig. 1.2 Under-five mortality rate, 2015. Probability of dying by age 5 per 1000 live births. *(Courtesy World Health Organization, Geneva, 2015.)*

Table 1.4	A Developmental History of the New Morbidities in Child Health*	
THE NEW MORBIDITIES (1982–1993)	**THE NEW MORBIDITIES REVISITED (2001)**	**THE "NEW" NEW MORBIDITIES (2010 to Present)**
Behavioral disorders/mental health	School problems	Adverse childhood experiences (ACEs)
Family crisis	Mood and anxiety disorders	Toxic stress
Abuse & neglect	Adolescent suicide/homicide	Allostatic load
Long term disease	Firearms in home	Chronic illnesses of lifestyle (e.g., obesity, type-2 diabetes, hypertension)
Substance abuse	School violence	Behavioral conditions (autism, ADHD, depression, anxiety)
School difficulties	Drug and alcohol abuse HIV infection Effects of media Poverty Homelessness Single-parent families Effects of divorce Struggle of working parents Childcare quality & policy	Food insecurity Oral health Witnessing community/interpersonal violence Peer victimization/bullying Discrimination

*Each column adds further categories and refinements to prior columns.
  ADHD, Attention-deficit/hyperactivity disorder; HIV human immunodeficiency virus.

behaviors such as substance use and early initiation of sexual activity, which in turn may increase the risk of chronic diseases such as lung cancer, liver disease, obesity, human papillomavirus (HPV) infection and cervical cancer, chronic lung disease, and premature mortality. Childhood trauma can also disrupt neurodevelopment during critical stages and contribute to social, emotional, and cognitive impairment. Finally, ACEs can result in toxic stress and lead to the dysregulation of

normal physiologic processes.

Toxic Stress and Allostatic Load

The effects of stress are moderated by the intensity of the stress, the biologic response to the stress, and the social and physical environment in which the stress is experienced. **Toxic stress** occurs when a child experiences stressful events that are chronic, intense, or prolonged and are inadequately buffered by the child's social support system (most importantly, parents and adult caregivers). Toxic psychosocial stress influences physical health by producing **allostatic load**, or pathophysiologic dysregulation of normal regulatory systems. Allostatic load is the "wear and tear" that the body and its regulatory mechanisms experience in response to chronic, unbuffered stress. The systems that can be affected through allostatic load include the neuroendocrine, cardiovascular, immune, and metabolic systems. Dysregulation of stress hormones in the hypothalamic-pituitary-adrenal (HPA) and sympathetic-adrenal-medullary (SAM) systems, inflammatory cytokines, hormones (e.g., insulin), immune factors (e.g., fibrinogen, C-reactive protein), and cardiovascular biomarkers (e.g., blood pressure) can occur from chronic stress and result in pathophysiologic conditions associated with chronic diseases. Chronic stress can also have effects at the genetic level. Studies of cellular aging have shown that chronic stress decreases telomere length, a determinant of aging on the cellular level. Epigenetic changes, including differential immune system DNA methylation, have been shown to occur after child abuse and posttraumatic stress disorder (PTSD), contributing to inflammatory and immune dysregulation.

Pediatrics, developmental psychology, basic sciences, and public health have contributed significant advances to the study of the behavioral, developmental, and social determinants of child health. The influence of psychosocial stress brought about by environmental challenges, while always acknowledged as important, has taken on a new level of salience as epidemiologists have linked its occurrence to significant morbidities throughout the life course, and as basic and clinical neuroscience has provided a multilevel framework for understanding how behavioral and psychosocial issues "get under the skin" to cause physiologic dysfunction and dysregulation.

Ecobiodevelopmental Framework
An ecobiodevelopmental framework has been proposed to integrate the environmental, biologic, and developmental factors into a model of health and illness (Fig. 1.3). This model posits that the ecology (or the physical and social environment) effects biology through the epigenetic and allostatic load mechanisms discussed above. The environment also influences development through life course science, which includes the effects of toxic exposures and childhood adversity on cognitive, behavioral, and physical health throughout the life course. Biology influences development though brain maturation and neuroplasticity, which in turn are also affected by inputs from the social and physical environment. The ecobiodevelopmental framework is consistent with the biopsychosocial model while adding a life course developmental dimension.

CHRONIC ILLNESS AND CHILDREN WITH SPECIAL HEALTH CARE NEEDS
The care of children with chronic conditions has become an increasingly larger part of clinical pediatrics, for both the pediatric subspecialist and the general pediatrician. **Children and youth with special health care needs (CSHCN)** are defined by the U.S. Maternal and Child Health Bureau as "those who have or are at increased risk for a chronic physical, developmental, behavioral, or emotional condition and who also require health and related services of a type or amount beyond that required by children generally." According to the 2011/12 **National Survey of Children's Health** (NSCH), >14.5 million, or 20% of U.S. children, have a special health need. The 2009–2010 **National Survey of Children with Special Health Care Needs** (NS-CSHCN) reports that almost one quarter (23%) of U.S. households with children have a child with a special need. The conditions these children have are extremely heterogeneous and include cerebral palsy, asthma, obesity, sickle cell disease, diabetes, learning disability, communication disorders, Down syndrome, heart conditions, migraine headaches, depression, conduct disorder, autism, and attention-deficit/hyperactivity disorder (Table 1.6). Most of these children need specialty care in addition to primary care. In the United States, 0.4–0.7% of children fall into the category of "highest medical complexity"; these children account for 15–33% of all healthcare spending for children. Children with medical complexity account for >70% of hospital readmissions.

Table 1.5	Classification of Adverse Childhood Experiences (ACEs)
CATEGORY	**ITEMS**
Abuse & neglect	Physical abuse* Physical neglect* Emotional abuse* Emotional neglect* Sexual abuse*
Family dysfunction	Intimate partner violence* Substance use in household* Mental illness in household* Parental separation or divorce* Family member incarcerated* Parental discord
Community-level adversity	Witnessing community violence Neighborhood safety Lack of neighborhood connectedness/trust Experiencing discrimination
Others	Being bullied/peer victimization Living in foster care Social isolation Low socioeconomic status/poverty

*Items included in original Kaiser ACE study.

Nine of 10 CSHCN have functional difficulties in the sensory, cognitive, movement, emotional, or behavioral domains (Table 1.7). More than 65% (7.2 million) of CSHCN have conditions that affect their daily activities, and >2.3 million families experience financial difficulties because of their children's special health needs. The fact that 25% of family members of CSHCN cut back work hours or stop working because of their child's special needs highlights the social and economic impact of child chronic illness, at both the individual and the national economic level.

Pediatricians are typically the "point persons" in the professional care of these children and provide data and expert opinion to procure needed services and resources to the child in the clinic, home, schools, and community. Such demands require an efficient model of chronic care.

SYSTEMS OF CARE
Population Health Approach
Because pediatric practice is increasingly spent working with patients and families who have chronic issues and conditions, new approaches to healthcare services delivery have been proposed. Whereas traditional practice models concentrate efforts toward the preventive and therapeutic needs of those patients who present for care, a **population health** approach to care refocuses efforts to emphasize the need to address health from a community- or population-level perspective, with emphasis on identifying and addressing the needs of individuals and families who do not seek regular care, or whose care is episodic and suboptimal from a prevention or management standpoint. Effectiveness of such a system would increase with advances in collaboration between healthcare providers and payers (insurance companies) to identify gaps in care, data surveillance systems, and electronic health records (EHRs), and with an expanded cadre of health care personnel such as care coordinators, nurse practitioners and physician assistants, social workers, health navigators, and community health workers. Healthcare reimbursement modifications, such as incorporating value-based and quality-of-care–based models, if implemented correctly, may further advance a population health approach to care.

Medical Home
The concept of the **patient and family–centered medical home (PFCMH)** approach to providing care has its origins in pediatrics in the late 20th century. As defined by AAP, a medical home provides care that is accessible, continuous, comprehensive, family centered,

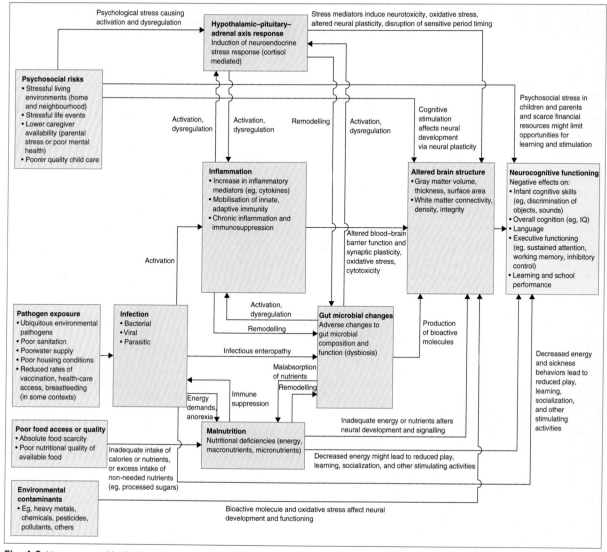

Fig. 1.3 New proposed biologic pathways that mediate effects of selected stressful or adversarial poverty-associated risks to neurocognitive outcomes in children. Complex interactions among key poverty-related risk factors, focusing on primary biologic pathways related to malnutrition, infection and inflammation, and neuroendocrine responses to stress. *(From Jensen SKG, Berens AE, Nelson CA: Effects of poverty on interacting biological systems underlying child development, Lancet 1:225–238, 2017, Fig 1, p 228.)*

coordinated, compassionate, and culturally effective. Patients and family members are key active participants, working with clinicians to identify priorities for and approaches to care. A key aspect of the PFCMH is care coordination. According to AAP, *care coordination* "addresses interrelated medical, social, developmental, behavioral, educational and financial needs to achieve optimal health and wellness outcomes." A *care coordinator* in the "point person" on the team who prospectively identifies the patient's and family's needs, concerns, and priorities for the healthcare visit, gathers pertinent information (lab results, consultations, educational plans, screening/testing results), communicates with subspecialists, and relays all important information to the clinical team before the patient/family visit. After a healthcare visit, the care coordinator works with the family to address any ongoing concerns, directs efforts to schedule follow up appointments and referrals, and communicates information to all necessary parties. The care coordinator typically is *not* a physician. The intended result of care coordination is an efficient and comprehensive interaction between the pediatric team and the

family, between primary care and specialty care, between ambulatory and inpatient care teams, and between the pediatric care team and the community-based supports on which the patient and family depend.

Provision of care consistent with the elements of a medical home has been associated with more accurate and early diagnosis, fewer emergency department visits and inpatient hospitalizations, lower costs, fewer unmet needs, lower out-of-pocket medical costs, less impact on parental employment, fewer school absences, and better patient satisfaction. According to the 2011/12 National Survey of Children's Health, 54.4% of U.S. children received coordinated, comprehensive care within a medical home.

Medical and Health Neighborhood

While the medical home concept relates to practice transformation specific to primary care, a broadening of this concept has been proposed along 2 separate dimensions. The **medical neighborhood** expands the medical home concept and refers to coordinated and efficient integration

Table 1.6	Heath Conditions in Children With Special Health Care Needs (CSHCN)*

Attention-deficit/hyperactivity disorder
Depression
Anxiety problems
Behavioral or conduct problems
Autism, pervasive developmental disorder, autism spectrum disorder
Developmental delay
Intellectual disability
Communication disorder
Asthma
Diabetes
Epilepsy or seizure disorder
Migraines or frequent headaches
Head injury, traumatic brain injury
Heart problems, including congenital heart disease
Blood problems, including anemia or sickle cell disease
Cystic fibrosis
Cerebral palsy
Muscular dystrophy
Down syndrome
Arthritis or joint problems
Allergies

*List is not comprehensive and does not include all conditions that CSHCN may have.
  Adapted from Child and Adolescent Health Measurement Initiative (2012). 2009/10 NS-CSHCN: Health Conditions and Functional Difficulties, Data Resource Center, supported by Cooperative Agreement 1-U59-MC06980-01 from the US Department of Health and Human Services, Health Resources and Services Administration (HRSA), Maternal and Child Health Bureau (MCHB). www.childhealthdata.org. Revised 01/27/2012.

Table 1.7	Functional Difficulties in Children With Special Health Care Needs (CSHCN)*

Experiencing Difficulty With ...
Breathing, or respiratory problem
Swallowing, digesting food, or metabolism
Blood circulation
Repeated or chronic physical pain, including headaches
Seeing, even when wearing glasses or contact lenses
Hearing, even when using a hearing aid or other devise
Taking care of self, such as eating, dressing, or bathing
Coordination or moving around
Using his/her hands
Learning, understanding, or paying attention
Speaking, communicating, or being understood
Feeling anxious or depressed
Behavior problems such as acting out, fighting, bullying, or arguing
Making and keeping friends

*List is not comprehensive and does not include all functional difficulties that CSHCN may have.
  Adapted from Child and Adolescent Health Measurement Initiative (2012). 2009/10 NS-CSHCN: Health Conditions and Functional Difficulties, Data Resource Center, supported by Cooperative Agreement 1-U59-MC06980-01 from the US Department of Health and Human Services, Health Resources and Services Administration (HRSA), Maternal and Child Health Bureau (MCHB). www.childhealthdata.org. Revised 01/27/2012.

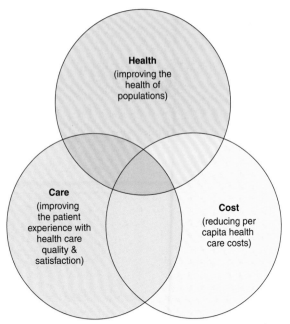

Fig. 1.4 The triple aim for healthcare. *(Adapted from Berwick DM, Nolan TW, Whittington J: The triple aim: care, health, and cost, Health Affairs 27:759–769, 2008.)*

between primary care pediatricians and the subspecialists, including integrated EHRs, efficient coordinated appointment scheduling, and enhanced communication. Such a system has the potential to provide a less stressful patient and family experience and could also lead to cost reduction and a decrease in medical errors.

Another expansion and modification of the medial home is the **health neighborhood** concept. The health neighborhood is based on the recognition of the importance of coordination with community-based and nonmedical providers to address comprehensively and efficiently the social determinants of health. Health neighborhoods include the healthcare providers (consistent with the medical home and neighborhood) but also involves services such as early intervention programs, the education system, childcare, community-based behavioral and mental health services, legal services, nutritional support services, and other clinical and community-based services that the patient and family need to access. The health neighborhood team helps families identify the needs of the patient, assists with referrals to appropriate agencies outside the healthcare system, and coordinates care.

Some nonmedical services may be co-located at the medical office. **Medical-legal partnerships** (MLPs) are collaborations between the healthcare and legal systems and embed legal aid personnel in the medical clinic. These lawyers and legal paraprofessionals can provide direct services to patients and families who have legal issues that may be affecting the child's health (e.g., housing code violations, utility shutoff, food insecurity, immigration issues, educational accommodations, guardianship). In addition to providing direct services, MLPs also train healthcare personnel in the legal and social determinants of health and work with physicians and others to advocate for policy change. Other nonmedical health neighborhood services that could be co-located in the medical center include supplemental nutrition assistance programs, parenting programs, behavioral health services, and family financial counseling.

Many, if not most, other services are located in the community. The health neighborhood model links families to these services and provides efficient on ongoing coordination and communication. Community health workers or health navigators are paraprofessional team members who are community and culturally informed and serve as a coordinating link between the family, the medical home, and needed community services. Community health workers and health navigators can also provide patient and family education.

Expanded care models such as these have the potential to achieve what the Institute for Healthcare Improvement calls the "triple aim" for healthcare, focusing on **care** (improving the patient experience with healthcare, quality care, and satisfaction), **health** (improving the health of populations), and **cost** (reducing per-capita healthcare costs) (Fig. 1.4).

Bibliography is available at Expert Consult.

Chapter **2**

Child Health Disparities

Lee M. Pachter

第二章

儿童卫生健康的不公平性

中文导读

本章主要介绍了决定健康和决定健康差异性的因素、儿童健康与医疗保健的差异，以及消除差异的干预方式三个主题。前两个主题详细论述了心理社会压力与非稳态负荷、拉美裔美国人的矛盾心态、儿童健康的差异、行为健康的差异和医疗保健状况的差异。第三个主题论述了种族主义与儿童健康，其中包括作为社会层面决定健康差异因素的种族主义（歧视）、对种族歧视类型的解读，以及回应和反对种族歧视的时机等。

Health and illness are not distributed equally among all members in most societies. Differences exist in risk factors, prevalence and incidence, manifestations, severity, and outcome of health conditions, as well as in the availability and quality of healthcare. When these differences are modifiable and avoidable, they are referred to as **disparities** or **inequities**. The U.S. Department of Health and Human Services (DHHS) *Healthy People 2020* report defines *health disparity* as "a particular type of health difference that is closely linked with social, economic, and/or environmental disadvantage. Health disparities adversely affect groups of people who have systematically experienced greater obstacles to health based on their racial or ethnic group; religion; socioeconomic status; gender; age; mental health; cognitive, sensory, or physical disability; sexual orientation or gender identity; geographic location; or other characteristics historically linked to discrimination or exclusion." The U.S. Centers for Disease Control and Prevention (CDC) define *health disparities* as "preventable differences in the burden of disease, injury, violence, or opportunities to achieve optimal health that are experienced by socially disadvantaged populations." Health and healthcare disparities occur by nature of unequal distribution of resources that are inherent in societies that exhibit *social stratification*, which occurs in social systems that rank and categorize people into a hierarchy of unequal status and power. There exists a hierarchy of "haves and have nots" based on group classifications.

Although there are many differences regarding health status, not all these differences are considered disparities. The increased prevalence of sickle cell disease in people of African descent, or the increased prevalence of cystic fibrosis in white individuals of Northern European descent, would not be considered a disparity because—at least at present—the genetic risk is not easily modifiable. However, in 2003, funding was 8-fold greater per patient for cystic fibrosis than for sickle cell disease, which could be considered a disparity because it is modifiable.

Health and healthcare disparities have existed for centuries. A critical mass of research building in the mid-2000s corresponded to the U.S. Institute of Medicine's 2003 book, *Unequal Treatment: Confronting Racial and Ethnic Disparities in Healthcare.* It reviewed the literature on racial and ethnic disparities in health and healthcare and found 600 citations.

DETERMINANTS OF HEALTH AND HEALTH DISPARITIES

Fig. 2.1 displays a categorization of the multiple determinants of health and well-being. Applying this categorization to health disparities, conceptualizations of the root causes of health disparities emphasize the most modifiable determinants of health: the physical and social environment, psychology and health behaviors, socioeconomic position and status, and access to and quality of healthcare. Differential access to these resources result in differences in *material* resources (e.g., money, education, healthcare) or *psychosocial* factors (e.g., locus of control, adaptive or risky behaviors, stress, social connectedness) that may contribute to differences in health status.

Fig. 2.2 illustrates the complex relationships among multileveled factors and health outcomes. **Social stratification** factors such as socioeconomic status (SES), race, and gender have profound influences on environmental resources available to individuals and groups, including neighborhood factors (e.g., safety, healthy spaces), social connectedness and support, work opportunities, and family environment. Much of the differential access to these resources results from discrimination, on a systematic or interpersonal level. **Discrimination** is defined as negative beliefs, attitudes, or behaviors resulting from categorizing individuals based on perceived group affiliation, such as gender (sexism) or race/ethnicity (racism).

SES, race/ethnicity, gender, and other social stratification factors also have effects on psychological functioning, including sense of control over one's life, expectations, resiliency, negative affect, and perceptions of and response to discrimination. Environmental and psychological context then have influence over more proximal determinants of health, including health-promoting or risk-promoting behaviors; access to and quality of healthcare and health education; exposure to pathogens, toxins, and carcinogens; pathophysiologic (biologic) and epigenetic response to stress; and the resources available to support optimal child development. Variability in these factors in turn results in differential health outcomes.

Psychosocial Stress and Allostatic Load

An understanding has emerged that helps explain how psychosocial stress influences disease and health outcomes (Fig. 2.3). This theory, **allostatic load**, provides insight into the processes and mechanisms that may contribute to health disparities. *Allostasis* refers to the normal physiologic changes that occur when individuals experience a stressful event. These internal reactions to an external stressor includes activation of the stress-response systems, such as increases in cortisol and epinephrine, changes in levels of inflammatory and immune mediators, cardiovascular reactivity, and metabolic and hormone activation. These are normal and adaptive responses to stress and result in physiologic

stability in the face of an external challenge. After an acute external stress or challenge, these systems revert to normal baseline states. However, when the stressor becomes chronic and unbuffered by social supports, dysregulation of these systems may occur, resulting in pathophysiologic alterations to these responses, such as hyperactivation of the allostatic systems, or *burnout*. Over time this dysregulation contributes to increased risk of disease and dysfunction. This pathophysiologic response is called *allostatic load*.

Given the systems affected (e.g., metabolic, immune, inflammatory, cardiovascular), allostatic load may contribute to increase incidence of chronic diseases such as cardiovascular disease, stroke, diabetes, asthma, and depression. It is notable that these specific chronic diseases have increased prevalence in racial and ethnic minority groups. Racial and ethnic minorities experience significantly higher degrees of chronic psychosocial stress (see Fig. 2.2), which over time contributes to allostatic load and the resultant disparities in these chronic diseases. Many of these conditions are noted to occur in adulthood, demonstrating the life course consequences of chronic psychosocial stress and adversity that begins in childhood.

The allostatic load model provides a pathophysiologic mechanism through which social determinants of health contribute to health disparities. It complements other mechanisms noted in Fig. 2.2, such as differential access to healthcare, increase in health risk behaviors, and increased exposure to pathogens, toxins, and other unhealthy agents.

The Hispanic Paradox

Whereas data suggest that minority racial and ethnic groups typically have worse health outcomes than the majority white group, this is not always the case. This finding demonstrates the complex interrelationship among race/ethnicity, minority status, and other factors that contribute to disparities, such as social class and SES.

Studies suggest that for many health outcomes, Hispanic/Latino populations do significantly better than other minority racial/ethnic groups and sometimes as well as the majority non-Hispanic white population. This finding has been called the *Hispanic Paradox* (also known as the Latino Paradox, Epidemiologic Paradox, Immigrant Paradox, and Health Immigrant Effect). Hispanic life expectancy is about 2 yr higher than for non-Hispanic whites, and mortality rates are lower for 7 of the 10 leading causes of death. Among child health issues, Hispanics in general have lower rates of prematurity and low birthweight than African Americans, and Mexican Americans have lower rates of asthma than African Americans and non-Hispanic whites.

Several hypotheses may explain these epidemiological findings. First, the relative advantages seen in Hispanic health are *greatest for non–U.S.-born Hispanics*, and many of the health advantages become nonsignificant in second- or third-generation U.S. Hispanics (as individuals spend

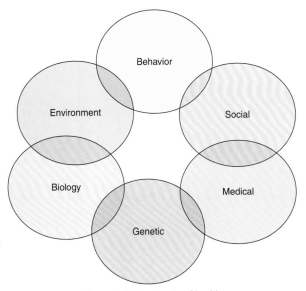

Fig. 2.1 Determinants of health.

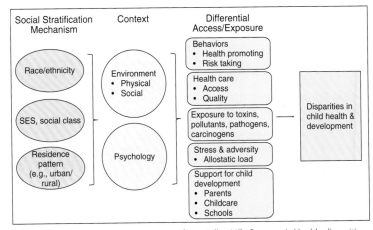

Fig. 2.2 Child health disparities. SES, Socioeconomic status. *(Data from Adler NE, Stewart J: Health disparities across the lifespan: meaning, methods, and mechanisms, Ann NY Acad Sci 1186(1):5–23, 2010.)*

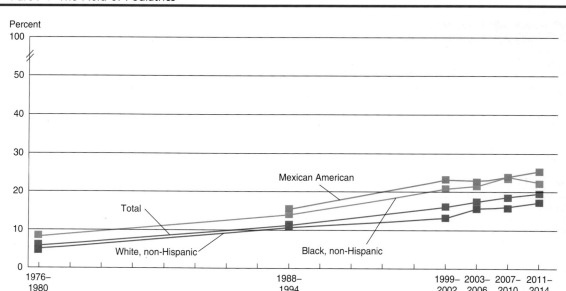

Fig. 2.3 Percentage of children age 6-17 yr who are obese by race and Hispanic origin, selected years 1976–2014 *(From National Center for Health Statistics, National Health and Nutrition Examination Survey. https://www.childstats.gov/americaschildren/health_fig.asp#health7. Accessed July 2018.)*

more time in the United States). Thus, indigenous cultural beliefs and lifestyles brought over by Hispanic immigrants may provide a selective health advantage, including low rates of tobacco and illicit drug use, strong family support and community ties, and healthy eating habits. Health advantages disappear as immigrants become more acculturated to U.S. standards—poorer nutritional habits and tobacco, alcohol, and illicit drug use—supporting this theory. It is also hypothesized that those who immigrate to the United States are younger and healthier than those Hispanics who do not immigrate and stay in their country of origin, so there may be a *selection* bias; Hispanic immigrants may start out healthier on arrival. Recent immigrants also tend to reside in ethnic enclaves, and socially supportive residential environments are associated with better health outcomes. When immigrants acculturate to U.S. lifestyles, not only do they acquire unhealthy behaviors, but they also tend to lose the protective aspects of their original culture and lifestyle.

There are also differences in outcomes among different Hispanic/Latino subgroups. Selective advantages in Hispanics are usually found among Hispanics from Mexico or South/Central America. Puerto Rican Hispanics typically have *worse* outcomes, compared to other Hispanic groups and non-Hispanic whites. Puerto Rico is a U.S. territory (Puerto Ricans are *not* immigrants) and has many of the negative health profiles seen in the mainland (e.g., high rates of tobacco rates and other health risk behaviors), which further supports the importance of indigenous, healthy, cultural behaviors and lifestyle as an explanation for the healthy immigrant profile seen in Central and South American Hispanics.

DISPARITIES IN CHILD HEALTH AND HEALTHCARE:
Tables 2.1 and 2.2 display some of the known disparities in child health and healthcare. As previously noted, health disparities may occur as a result of race/ethnicity, socioeconomic status (often operationalized through family income, sometimes using insurance status as a proxy), and residency patterns, such as urban and rural locale.

Child Health Disparities
Asthma
Disparities in asthma prevalence are seen by racial/ethnic group and SES. According to the 2015 U.S. National Health Interview Survey (NHIS), American Indian/Alaskan Native, Mainland Puerto Rican, and African American children have the highest prevalence of childhood

asthma (14.4%, 13.9%, and 13.4%, respectively), followed non-Hispanic white (7.4%) and Asian (5.4%). The prevalence of childhood asthma in Hispanics is 8%, but when the Hispanic category is disaggregated, Mexican Americans have a prevalence of 7.3%, which is lower than that for non-Hispanic whites; Puerto Rican children have among the highest rates of asthma. The cause of this difference among Hispanic/Latino subgroups is debatable, but some data suggest that bronchodilator response may be different in the 2 groups, possibly based on genetic variants. Data also suggest that within the Mexican American population, differences in prevalence exist based on birthplace or generation (see earlier, The Hispanic Paradox): immigrant and first-generation Mexican American children have lower prevalence of asthma than Mexican American children who have lived in the United States longer. This may reflect the changes that occur as Latinos become more acculturated to U.S. behavioral norms the longer they reside in the United States (e.g., tobacco use, dietary patterns, environmental exposures).

Regarding SES, children living at <100% the federal poverty level have a childhood asthma prevalence of 10.7%, whereas those living at ≥200% the poverty level have a prevalence of 7.2%.

Obesity
In 2014 the percentage of Hispanic/Latino children in the National Health and Nutrition Examination Survey (NHANES) age 6-17 yr who were obese was 24.3%. The percentage of African American children who were obese was 22.5%. This compares to non-Hispanic whites (17.1%) and Asian (9.8%) (see Fig. 2.3). Dietary patterns, access to nutritious foods, and differing cultural norms regarding body habitus may account for some of these differences. The relationship between SES and childhood obesity is less clear. Some studies suggest that the racial and ethnic differences in childhood obesity become nonsignificant when factoring in family income, whereas other national survey studies suggest a relationship between family income and obesity rates in non-Hispanic whites but not among black or Mexican American children.

Infant Mortality
Highest rates of infant mortality are seen in non-Hispanic black infants. According to data from the 2007–2008 National Center for Health Statistics (NCHS)–linked Live Birth–Infant Death Cohort Files, the odds ratio for non-Hispanic black infant mortality is 2.32, compared

Table 2.1	Child Health Disparities		
HEALTH INDICATOR	**RACE/ETHNICITY**	**FAMILY INCOME**	**RESIDENCE**
Child health status fair or poor	Black & Hispanic > White & Asian	Poor > Not Poor	
Children with special health care needs (CSHCN)	Black > White > Hispanic	Poor > Not Poor	
One or more chronic health conditions	Black > White > Hispanic > Asian	Poor > Not Poor	
Asthma	Mainland Puerto Rican > Black > White & Mexican American	Poor > Not Poor	Urban > Rural
Obesity	Hispanic & Black > White and Asian	Poor > Not Poor	Rural > Urban
Infant mortality	Black > Hispanic > White	Poor > Not Poor	
Low birthweight (<2,500 g.)	Black > White, Hispanic, American Indian/Native Alaskan, Asian/Pacific Islander Mainland Puerto Rican > Mexican American	Poor > Not Poor	
Preterm birth (<37 wk)	Black > American Indian/Native Alaskan, Hispanic, White, Asian/Pacific Islander Mainland Puerto Rican > Mexican American	Poor > Not Poor	
Seizure disorder, epilepsy	Black > White, Hispanic	Poor > Not Poor	
Bone, joint, or muscle problem	White > Black, Hispanic	Poor > Not Poor	
Ever breastfed	White, Hispanic, Asian > Black	Not Poor > Poor	Urban > Rural
No physical activity in the past week	Hispanic > Black, Asian > White Poor > Not Poor	Poor > Not Poor	
Hearing problem		Poor > Not Poor	
Vision problem		Poor > Not Poor	
Oral health problems (including caries and untreated caries)	Hispanic > Black > White, Asian	Poor > Not Poor	Rural > Urban
Attention-deficit/hyperactivity disorder (ADHD)	White, Black > Hispanic	Poor > Not Poor	Rural > Urban
Have ADHD but not taking medication	Hispanic, Black > White		
Anxiety problems	White > Black, Hispanic	Poor > Not Poor	
Depression		Poor > Not Poor	Rural > Urban
Behavior or conduct problem (ODD, conduct disorder)	Black > White, Hispanic	Poor > Not Poor	
Autism Spectrum Disorder	White > Black > Hispanic	Poor > Not Poor	
Learning disability	Black > White, Hispanic	Poor > Not Poor	Rural > Urban
Developmental delay	Black > White > Hispanic, Asian	Poor > Not Poor	
Risk of developmental delay, by parental concern	Hispanic > Black & White	Poor > Not Poor	
Speech or language problems		Poor > Not Poor	
Adolescent suicide attempts (consider, attempt, needed medical attention for an attempt)	Girls: Hispanic > Black & White Boys: Hispanic & Black > White		
Adolescent suicide rate	Girls: American Indian > White, Asian/Pacific Islander, Hispanic, Black Boys: American Indian & White > Hispanic, Black, Asian/Pacific Islander		
Child maltreatment (reported)	Black, American Indian/Alaskan Native, Multiracial > White, Hispanic, Asian, Pacific islander	Poor > Not Poor	
AIDS (adolescents)	Black > Hispanic > White		

AIDS, Acquired immunodeficiency syndrome; ODD, oppositional defiant disorder.

to non-Hispanic white rates, and remains significant after controlling for maternal age, education, marital status, parity, plurality, nativity, tobacco use, hypertension, and diabetes. Compared with non-Hispanic whites, higher infant mortality is also seen in Hispanic black and Hispanic white infants as well.

In 2012 the infant mortality rate for black, non-Hispanic (11.2/1,000 live births) and American Indian/Alaskan Native (8.4/1,000) infants was higher than for white, non-Hispanic (5.0/1,000), Hispanic (5.1/1,000), and Asian/Pacific Islander (4.1/1,000) (Fig. 2.4). There was variation in the U.S. Hispanic population: the Puerto Rican infant mortality rate was 6.9/1,000, compared to 5.0/1,000 for Mexican Americans and 4.1/1,000 for Central and South American origin.

Prematurity and Low Birthweight
There are significant black-white differences in preterm birth and low birthweight (LBW) (Fig. 2.5). According to the 2014 NCHS National

Table 2.2	Child Healthcare Disparities

HEALTHCARE INDICATOR	RACE/ETHNICITY	FAMILY INCOME	RESIDENCE
Did not receive any type of medical care in past 12 mo	Hispanic, Black, Asian > White	Poor > Not Poor	Rural > Urban
No well-child checkup or preventive visit in past 12 mo	Hispanic > White & Black	Poor > Not Poor	Rural > Urban
Delay in medical care	Hispanic > Black > White	Poor > Not Poor	
Unmet need in healthcare due to cost	Black > Hispanic > White > Asian	Poor > Not Poor	
No coordinated, comprehensive, or ongoing care in a medical home	Hispanic > Black & Asian > White	Poor > Not Poor	Rural > Urban
Problem accessing specialist care when needed	Hispanic & Black > White	Poor > Not Poor	
No preventative dental care visit in past 12 mo	Hispanic & Asian > Black > White	Poor > Not Poor	Rural > Urban
No vision screening in past 2 yr	Hispanic & Asian > Black & White	Poor > Not Poor	
Did not receive needed mental health treatment or counseling in past 12 mo	Black & Hispanic > White	Poor > Not Poor	
Not receiving a physician recommendation for HPV vaccination among 13-17-yr- old girls	Black & Hispanic > White		
Immunization rates: adolescent HPV vaccine	Girls: White > Black & Hispanic Boys: Black & Hispanic > White		

HPV, Human papillomavirus.

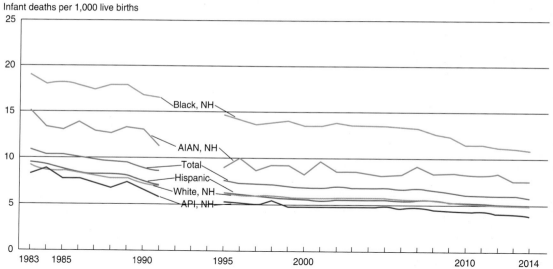

Fig. 2.4 Death rates among infants by race and Hispanic origin of mother, 1983–1991 and 1995–2014. AIAN, American Indian or Alaska Native; API, Asian or Pacific Islander; NH, non-Hispanic. *(From National Center for Health Statistics, National Vital Statistics System. https://www.childstats .gov/americaschildren/health_fig.asp#health2. Accessed July 2018.)*

Vital Statistics System, LBW births (<2500 g) were significantly higher among black non-Hispanic women (13.2%) than white non-Hispanic (7.0%), American Indian/Alaskan Native (7.6%), Asian/Pacific Islander (8.1%), or Hispanic (7.1%) women. Among Hispanics, Puerto Rican women had higher rates of LBW births than Mexican Americans (9.5% vs 6.6%).

Regarding preterm births (<37 wk), the black non-Hispanic rate was 13.2%, compared to 8.9% for white non-Hispanics, 8.5% for Asian/Pacific Islanders, 10.2% for American Indian/Alaskan Native, and 9% for Hispanics. Within the Hispanic group, the Puerto Rican preterm rate was higher than for Mexican Americans (11% vs 8.8%).

There are many hypotheses for the increased rates of preterm birth and LBW in black births. Risk factors such as inadequate prenatal care, genitourinary tract infections, increased exposure to environmental toxins, and increased tobacco use may account for some of the disparity, but not all, and neither do SES differences, since high-SES black women still have higher rates of premature and LBW births.

Increased **stress** has been presented as a potential mechanism. Studies have shown that minority women who experience perceptions of racism and discrimination have higher odds of delivering a preterm or LBW child than do minority women who have not perceived experiences with discrimination. **Residential segregation** is also a potential source of differences in preterm and LBW outcomes. Living in hypersegregated neighborhoods can decrease access to prenatal care, increased exposure to environmental pollutants, and increase psychosocial stress, all of which may contribute to increased risk.

Increased age at delivery in African American women does not lessen the risk of preterm or LBW delivery (as it does in white mothers). This

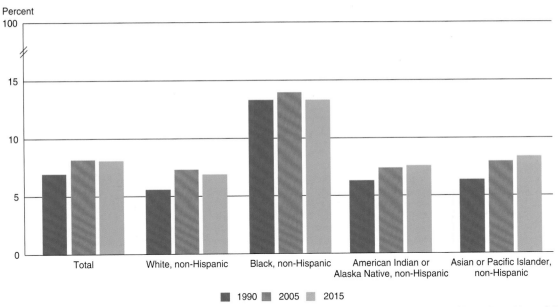

Fig. 2.5 Percentage of infants born with low birthweight by race and Hispanic origin of mother, 1990, 2005, and 2015 *(From National Center for Health Statistics, National Vital Statistics System. https://www.childstats.gov/americaschildren/health_fig.asp#health1b. Accessed July 2018.)*

has led to the theory that cumulative stress in black women, related to chronic exposure to factors such as socioeconomic deprivation and racial discrimination, leads to declining health at an earlier age compared with white women, and thus increases the risk for poor pregnancy outcomes. Called the **weathering hypothesis**, this has been proposed as an explanation for racial variations in pregnancy outcomes.

Oral Health

Significant differences exist in oral health status as well as preventive oral healthcare according to race/ethnicity, SES, and residency locale. Data from the 1994–2004 NHANES show that compared to non-Hispanic white children, black and Mexican American children had higher rates of caries and untreated caries and lower rates of receiving dental sealants. Children living at or below the federal poverty level also had higher rates of caries and untreated caries and lower rates of dental sealant applications, compared with nonpoor children.

Preventive oral healthcare may improve rates of caries and treat caries before further impairment ensues. Data from the 2004 Medical Expenditure Panel Survey revealed that only 34.1% of black and 32.9% of Hispanic children had a yearly visit to a dentist, compared to 52.5% of white children. Likewise, only 33.9% of low-income children had dentist visits, compared to 46.5% of middle-income children and 61.8% of high-income children.

According to the 2011/12 **National Survey of Children's Health (NSCH)**, parents reported fair to poor teeth condition at a higher rate in Asian non-Hispanic children (8.5%), black non-Hispanic children (7.6%), and Hispanic children (15.2%), compared to white children (4.2%). Hispanic and black non-Hispanic children had higher rates of oral health problems than white non-Hispanic and Asian non-Hispanic children as well.

Hearing Care

No data suggest that the prevalence of hearing loss (either congenital or acquired) is different among racial/ethnic or SES categories, but follow-up care after diagnosis of a hearing problem has been shown to be worse in certain groups. Higher "lost to follow-up" rates have been noted in children living in rural areas as well as with publically insured and nonwhite children. Much of this disparity is reduced when families have access to specialists.

Vision Problems

The parent-reported 2011/12 NSCH found no differences in the prevalence of correctable vision problem among white non-Hispanic, black non-Hispanic, Hispanic, and "other" racial/ethnic groups, or with regard to SES or urban/rural residence.

Immunization

Immunization against infectious agents was one of the major clinical and public health successes of the 20th century. Rates of life-threatening infectious diseases plummet after effective vaccines are introduced. The primary series of childhood immunizations against diphtheria, tetanus, pertussis, polio, rotavirus, measles, mumps, rubella, hepatitis A and B, *Haemophilus influenzae* type b, varicella, and *Streptococcus pneumoniae* have significantly decreased the incidence of illness caused by these agents.

Disparities in immunization rates had been noted regarding household income status, insurance status, and residential location. In response to these socioeconomic disparities, as well as higher rates of measles cases in the 1980s among racial and ethnic minority groups, a number of interventions were initiated, including the creation of the **Vaccines for Children program** (VFC), which eliminated the financial barrier to immunization by providing free immunizations to at-risk groups (Medicaid-eligible, uninsured, American Indian/Alaskan Native, or underinsured and vaccinated at a federally qualified health center or rural health clinic). Since VFC inception, disparities in immunization rates have either been eliminated or have significantly narrowed, showing that targeted public health programs can successfully eliminate health disparities.

Although rates of initial primary vaccine series demonstrate no or decreasing disparities, other vaccination rates do show differences. For example, black and Hispanic adolescent females have lower human papillomavirus (HPV) vaccination rates than whites. Reasons for this disparity include parental concerns about safety and no provider recommendation. Of interest, studies of HPV vaccination in adolescent males show that black and Hispanic male adolescents have higher rates of HPV vaccine coverage than whites.

Adolescent Suicide

In 2014 the highest rate of suicide for male adolescents was seen in American Indian (20 per 100,000 population) and white (17/100,000) teens, compared to Hispanic (9/100,000), black (7/100,000), and Asian/Pacific Islander (6/100,000) teens. For female adolescents, highest suicide rates were seen in American Indian (12/100,000), compared to white (5/100,000), Asian/Pacific Islander (5/100,000), Hispanic (3/100,000), and Black (2/100,000) teens.

Hispanic female students in grades 9-12 were more likely to consider suicide (26%), report attempting suicide (15%), and require medical attention for a suicide attempt (5%), compared to black (19%, 10%, 4%) or White (23%, 10%, 3%) female students. Among male students, Hispanic and black students, compared to white students, were more likely to attempt suicide (8% and 7% vs 4%, respectively) and require medical attention for a suicide attempt (4% and 3% vs 1%).

Child Maltreatment
In 2014, reports of child abuse and neglect were higher in black (15.3 per 1,000 children), American Indian/Alaskan Native (13.4/1,000), and multiracial (10.6/1,000) children, compared to Hispanic (8.8/1,000), Pacific Islander (8.6/1,000), white (8.4/1,000), and Asian (1.7/1,000) children. **Poverty**, measured at the family as well as community level, is also a significant risk factor for maltreatment. Counties with high poverty concentration had >3 times the rate of child abuse deaths than counties with the lowest concentration of poverty. Nonetheless, race itself *should not be a marker* for child abuse or neglect.

Behavioral Health Disparities
Attention-Deficit/Hyperactivity Disorder (ADHD)
White and black children are more often diagnosed with ADHD (10.7% and 8.4%, respectively) than are Hispanic children (6.3%), according to NHIS data. Other studies have shown that both black and Hispanic children have lower odds of having an ADHD diagnosis than white children. Children reared in homes that are below the federal poverty level are diagnosed more often (11.6%) that those at or above the FPL (8.1%).

Children diagnosed with ADHD have different medication practices. Hispanic (43.8%) and black (40.9%) children with ADHD are more likely than white children (25.5%) *not* to be taking medication. The causes of this disparity are unknown but may include different patient and parental beliefs and perceptions about medication side effects and different prescribing patterns by clinicians.

Depression and Anxiety Disorders
According to the 2011/12 NSCH, there were no parent-reported differences in rates of childhood depression (2-17 yr) among racial/ethnic groups. Children living in poverty, as well as children living in rural areas, had higher rates of parent-reported depression. According to the 2015 **Youth Risk Behavior Survey** of adolescent in grades 9-12, Hispanic students had higher rates of reporting that they felt sad or hopeless (35.3%) compared to white (28.6%) and black (25.2%) students. This relationship existed for both male and female students.

The NSCH data noted that white children ages 2-17 yr had higher rates of anxiety than black or Hispanic children. "Poor" children had higher rates of anxiety than "not poor" children.

Autism Spectrum Disorder (ASD)
Compared with white children, black and Hispanic children are less likely to be diagnosed with ASD, and when diagnosed, are typically diagnosed at a later age and with more severe symptoms. This disparity in diagnosis and timing of diagnosis is concerning given that early diagnosis provides access to therapeutic services that are best initiated as early as possible. Reasons for these disparities may include differences in cultural behavioral norms, stigma, differences in parental knowledge of typical and atypical child development, poorer access to quality healthcare and screening services, differences in the quality of provider–patient communication, trust in providers, as well as differential access to specialists.

Behavioral or Conduct Problems
According to the 2011/12 NSCH, black children age 2-17 yr have higher rates of **oppositional defiant disorder** (ODD) or **conduct disorder**

than white and Hispanic children. Children living in poverty have higher rates than those not living in poverty.

Developmental Delay
The 2011/12 NSCH found that black and white children age 2-17 yr had higher rates of developmental delay than Hispanic children (4.5% and 3.8% vs 2.7%, respectively). However, when parents of children age 4 mo to 5 yr were asked if they had concerns about their child's development (highly correlated with risk of developmental, behavioral, or social delays), Hispanic children had higher rates of moderate or high risk for developmental delay (32.5%) than did black (29.7%) or white (21.2%) children. This discrepancy may result from either overestimation of concerns in Hispanic mothers or underdiagnosis of Hispanic children by clinicians.

Children living below the poverty level have higher rates of developmental delay as well.

Disparities in Healthcare
In almost all areas, minority children have been identified as having worse access to needed healthcare, including receipt of any type of medical care within the past 12 mo, well-child or preventive visits, delay in care, having an unmet need due to healthcare cost, lack of care in a medical home, problems accessing specialist care when needed, lack of preventive dental care, vision screening, mental health counseling, and recommendations for adolescent immunizations (see Table 2.2). In addition, many of these healthcare indicators are found to be worse for children living in poverty, as well as those living in a rural area, compared to urban-dwelling children.

APPROACHES TO ERADICATING DISPARITIES: INTERVENTIONS
Much of the information regarding health disparities over the past 10-20 yr has focused on the identification of areas where health disparities exist. Additional work has expanded on simple description and acknowledged the multivariable nature of disparities. This has provided a more nuanced understanding of the complex interrelationships among factors such as race/ethnicity, socioeconomic status, social class, generation, acculturation, gender, and residency.

An example of a successful intervention that closed the disparity gap is the implementation of the VFC program, which, as noted earlier, significantly decreased the disparity in underimmunization rates noted among racial/ethnic groups and poor/underinsured children. This is an example of a **public health policy** approach to intervention.

Interventions need to occur at the **clinical** level as well. The almost universal use of electronic health records (EHR) provides a unique opportunity for collecting clinical and demographic data that can be helpful in identify disparities and monitor the success of interventions. All EHR platforms should use a standardized approach to gathering information on patient race/ethnicity, SES, primary language preferences, and health literacy. The Institute of Medicine's 2009 report *Race, Ethnicity, and Language Data: Standardization for Health Care Quality Improvement* provides best practices information about capturing these data in the health record.

The advancing science of clinical **quality improvement** can also provide a framework for identifying clinical strategies to reduce disparities in care. Use of **PDSA** (Plan-Do-Study-Act) cycles targeting specific clinical issues where health disparities exist can result in practice transformation and help reduce differential outcomes.

Another practice-level intervention that has the potential to reduce disparities in care and outcomes is the **medical home** model, providing care that is accessible, family centered, continuous, comprehensive, compassionate, coordinated, and culturally effective. The use of care coordinators and community-based health navigators is an effective tool in helping to break down the multiple social and health system barriers that contribute to disparities.

Population health strategies have the advantage of addressing the determinants of disparities at both the clinic and the community levels. Techniques such as "hotspotting," "cold-casing" (finding patients and families lost to follow up and not receiving care), and "geocoding," combined with periodic community health needs assessments, identify the structural, systemic, environmental, and social factors that contribute to disparities and help guide interventions that are tailored to the local setting.

When developing strategies to address disparities, it is imperative to include patients and community members from the beginning of any process aimed at identification and intervention. Many potential interventions seem appropriate and demonstrate efficacy under ideal circumstances. However, if the intervention does not address the concerns of the end users—patients and communities—or fit the social or cultural context, it will likely be ineffective in the "real world." Only by involving the community from the beginning, including defining the issues and problems, can the likelihood of success be optimized.

Health disparities are a consequence of the social stratification mechanisms inherent in many modern societies. Health disparities mirror other societal disparities in education, employment opportunities, and living conditions. While society grapples with the broader issues contributing to disparities, healthcare and public health can work to understand the multiple causes of these disparities and develop interventions that address the structural, clinical, and social root causes of these inequities.

Bibliography is available at Expert Consult.

2.1 Racism and Child Health
Mary T. Bassett, Zinzi D. Bailey, and Aletha Maybank

RACISM AS SOCIAL DETERMINANT
An emerging body of evidence supports the role of racism in a range of adverse physical, behavioral, developmental, and mental health outcomes. Racial/ethnic patterning of health in the United States is long-standing, apparent from the first collection of vital statistics in the colonial period. However, the extensive data that document racial disparities have not settled the question of why groups of people, particularly of African and Native American Indian ancestry, face increased odds of shorter lives and poorer health (Table 2.3). The role of societal factors,

Table 2.3	New Social and Health Inequities in the United States					
	TOTAL	**WHITE NON-HISPANIC**	**ASIAN***	**HISPANIC OR LATINO**	**BLACK NON-HISPANIC[†]**	**NATIVE AMERICAN OR ALASKA NATIVE**
Wealth: median household assets (2011)	$68,828	$110,500	$89,339	$7,683	$6,314	NR
Poverty: proportion living below poverty level, all ages (2014); children <18 yr (2014)	14.8%; 21.0%	10.1%; 12.0%	12.0%; 12.0%	23.6%; 32.0%	26.2%; 38.0%	28.3%; 35.0%
Unemployment rate (2014)	6.2%	5.3%	5.0%	7.4%	11.3%	11.3%
Incarceration: male inmates per 100,000 (2008)	982	610	185	836	3,611	1,573
Proportion with no health insurance, age <65 yr (2014)	13.3%	13.3%	10.8%	25.5%	13.7%	28.3%
Infant mortality per 1000 live births (2013)	6.0	5.1	4.1	5.0	10.8	7.6
Self-assessed health status (age-adjusted): proportion with fair or poor health (2014)	8.9%	8.3%	7.3%	12.2%	13.6%	14.1%
Potential life lost: person-years per 100,000 before age 75 yr (2014)	6621.1	6659.4	2954.4	4676.8	9490.6	6954.0
Proportion reporting serious psychological distress[‡] in past 30 days, age ≥18 yr, age-adjusted (2013–14)	3.4%	3.4%	3.5%	1.9%	4.5%	5.4%
Life expectancy at birth (2014), yr	78.8	79.0	NR	81.8	75.6	NR
Diabetes-related mortality: age-adjusted mortality per 100,000 (2014)	20.9	19.3	15.0	25.1	37.3	31.3
Mortality related to heart disease: age-adjusted mortality per 100,000 (2014)	167.0	165.9	86.1	116.0	206.3	119.1

*Economic data and data on self-reported health and psychological distress are for Asians only; all other health data reported combine Asians and Pacific Islanders.
[†]Wealth, poverty, and potential life lost before age 75 yr are reported for the black population only; all other data are for the black non-Hispanic population.
[‡]Serious psychological distress in the past 30 days among adults 18 yr and older is measured using the Kessler 6 scale (range: 0–24; serious psychological distress ≥13).
NR, Not reported.
Wealth data from the US Census; poverty data for adults from National Center for Health Statistics (NCHS), and poverty data for children from National Center for Education Statistics; unemployment data from US Bureau of Labor Statistics; incarceration data from Kaiser Family Foundation; data on uninsured individuals from NCHS; data on infant mortality, self-assessed health status, potential life lost, serious psychological distress, life expectancy, diabetes-related mortality, and mortality related to heart disease from NCHS.
From Bailey ZD, Krieger N, Agénor M, et al: Structural racism and health inequities in the USA: evidence and interventions, *Lancet* 389:1453–463, 2017 (Table, p 1455).

not only factors related to the individual, is increasingly recognized in determining population health, but often omits racism among social determinants of health. This oversight occurs in the face of a long history of racial and ethnic subjugation in the United States that has been justified both explicitly and implicitly by racism. From the early 18th century, colonial America established racial categories that enshrined the superiority of whites, conferring rights specifically on white men, while denying these rights to others. Similar, perhaps less explicit, discrimination has continued through the centuries and remains a primary contributor to racial inequities in children's health.

For generations, racial/ethnic disparities have been documented beginning at birth and extending across life. In 2014, life expectancy at birth for blacks was almost 4 yr shorter than life expectancy of non-Hispanic whites, influenced heavily by disparities starting at birth (Table 2.3). The **infant mortality rate** (IMR), arguably the most important measure of national health, has shown a persistent relative black-white gap. Despite the substantial decline in U.S. IMR for all racial/ethnic groups, there is still at least a 2-fold higher risk of death in the 1st yr of life for black infants than for white infants (Table 2.3). NCHS data in 2014 showed a double-digit IMR *only* among non-Hispanic blacks, with 11.8 deaths per 1,000 live births, compared to 4.89/1,000 for non-Hispanic whites. In 2016 the black IMR slightly increased after many years of progressive decline, which may portend a further rise in the relative black-white gap. A troubling stagnation in IMR, with no recent decline, is found among Alaska Natives and American Indians. The 2005 IMR in American Indian or Alaskan Native women, 8.06 deaths/1000 live births, has remained essentially unchanged for a decade, with the 2014 IMR at 7.59/1,000.

Exposures that affect infant survival occur before birth. Prenatal maternal exposures to pesticides, lead, and other environmental toxins vary by race. Additionally, a higher prevalence of maternal obesity, diabetes, and substance/alcohol use before conception also adversely affects birth outcomes. A California study of maternal obesity based on claims data and vital records found that 22.3% of pregnant black women and 20.3% of Latina women had a body mass index (BMI) of 30-40, compared to 14.9% of white and 5.6% of Asian women. BMI >40 was more than twice as prevalent in black (5.7%) than white (2.6%) women.

The effects of racism are also stressful and toxic to the body, and evidence supports biologic effects of discrimination across the life span, especially for pregnant women. Racism can increase cortisol levels and lead to a cascade of effects, including impaired cell function, altered fat metabolism, increased blood glucose and blood pressure, and decreased bone formation (see Chapter 1, Fig. 1.3). This can affect a growing fetus, leading to increased infant cortisol levels, lower birthweight (LBW), and prematurity. In New York City, white women had lower rates of adverse birth outcomes: 1.3% had preeclampsia, less than half the rate for black women (2.9%).

Although infant deaths occur more frequently among low-income groups of all race/ethnicities, these birth outcome disparities by race/ethnicity are found also in blacks with higher socioeconomic status (SES). College-educated black women are more likely than white high school–educated women to have a LBW infant, a principal risk factor for infant death. Another study examined California birth certificates of pregnant Arab American women after the September 11, 2001, terrorist attacks and found that those who experienced discrimination immediately after the 9/11 attacks had a higher relative risk of giving birth to an LBW infant in the following 6 mo than seen in births before this date.

The increased risk for populations of color continues from infancy into childhood; racial/ethnic disparities are seen across almost all health indicators, with most relative gaps remaining stagnant or worsening over the last 2 decades. Black children are about twice as likely to be diagnosed with **asthma**, more likely to be hospitalized for its treatment, and more likely to have fatal attacks. The black-white disparity in asthma has grown steadily over time. Native American children and youth (≤19 yr) also experience negative health outcomes, with the highest rates of **unintentional injury** and mortality rates at least twice as high as for other racial/ethnic groups. Additionally, according to a 2015 NCHS brief, Latino youth age 2-19 have the highest rates of **obesity**, defined as a BMI ≥95th percentile in the 2000 CDC sex/age-specific growth charts. The NCHS data show that 21.9% of Latino (followed by black) children qualified as obese from 2011 to 2014. Black children are more likely to be exposed to witnessed, personal, or family **violence** and have several-fold higher prevalence of **psychiatric distress** than their white counterparts, a racial difference that continues into adulthood.

EXPLAINING RACIAL DISPARITIES: A TAXONOMY OF RACISM

Explanations of these ubiquitous racial gaps have focused on individual factors, including variation in individual genetic constitution, behavioral risks, poverty, and access to (and use of) healthcare services. Scientists agree that "race" is a social construct that is not based on biology, despite the persistence of the idea that racial categories reflect a racially distinctive genetic makeup that has a bearing on health. In fact, the genetic variation between individuals within a particular racial/ethnic group is far greater than the variability between "races." Despite the genetic data, many groups have been "racialized" over time. Notably, the U.S. Census Bureau's demographic classifications reflect this process. In the mid-late 1800s the census counted "mulattos," those of white and black ancestry, as another race.

Starting in the late 19th century, Eastern European immigrants and Jews were considered different races. As early as 1961, the U.S. Census identified Mexicans and Puerto Ricans as "white," even as racial classification varied by geography. All states collected birth records by 1919, but there was little uniformity on how race was collected, if at all, across states. It was not until 1989, when the National Center for Health Statistics (NCHS) recommended assigning "infant race" as that of the mother, that standard guidance and categories were issued for states on collecting racial data at birth. Existing categories were changed and continue to change based on the economic, cultural, or political utility of the time, rather than actual genetic distinction.

Defining Racism

Racism has consistently structured U.S. society and is based on "white supremacy," a hierarchical idea that whites, the *dominant* group, are intrinsically superior to other groups who are not classified as "white." No single definition of racism exists, but one useful description is *racial prejudice backed by power and resources*. This conceptualization asserts that not only must there be prejudice, but also an interlocking system of institutions to produce and reproduce inequities in access to and utilization of resources and decision-making power. Even when considering variations in health behavior, lifestyles, economic status, and healthcare utilization, individual-level behavioral factors do not capture how broader shared social experiences shape outcomes. **Racial domination** or racism contributes to variation in the population's access to resources and exposure to disease, as well as the group experience of fair treatment and opportunity. Although many groups in the United States may encounter discrimination based on race/ethnicity, most of the modest literature on health effects of racism has focused on people of African descent, leaving a need to better understand the impact of racism on other nonwhite groups. Table 2.4 describes various pathways through which racism affects health.

While the empirical data on disparities for nonblack populations of color deserve greater research, useful frameworks exist to understand the disparities that public health has documented to date. A useful taxonomy of how racism operates in society has 4 categories: internalized racism, interpersonal racism, institutional racism, and structural racism. Each is relevant in considering the impact of racism on child health.

Internalized Racism

When the larger society characterizes marginalized racialized groups as "inferior," these negative assessments may be accepted by members of those groups themselves, either consciously or unconsciously. The result is *devaluation* of personal abilities and intrinsic worth, as well as the capacity, of others also classified as being a part of a marginalized racialized group. The best-known documentation of *internalized racism* comes from the study of Kenneth and Mamie Clark known as the **doll experiment**, conducted in the 1940s. Black children, both boys and girls, were asked to choose between a black doll and a white doll

Table 2.4	Pathways Between Racism and Health and Examples

Economic injustice and social deprivation
　Residential, educational, and occupational segregation to lower-quality neighborhoods, schools, and jobs (both historical de jure discrimination and contemporary de facto discrimination)
　Lower salary for same work
　Lower promotion rate despite comparable evaluations
Environmental and occupational health inequities
　Placement of bus garages and toxic waste sites
　Selective government failure to prevent lead in drinking water (per Flint, Michigan, 2015–2016)
　Disproportionate exposure of workers of color to occupational hazards
Psychosocial trauma
　Interpersonal racial discrimination, including microaggressions*
　Exposure to racist media, including social media
Targeted marketing of health-harming substances
　Legal: cigarettes; sugar sweetened beverages
　Illegal: heroin; illicit opioids
Inadequate healthcare
　Inadequate access to health insurance and healthcare facilities
　Inadequate treatment caused by implicit or explicit racial bias
State-sanctioned violence and alienation from property and traditional lands
　Police violence
　Forced urban "renewal" (use of eminent domain to force relocation of urban communities of color)
　Genocide and forced removal of Native Americans
Political exclusion
　Voter restrictions (e.g. for ex-felons, ID requirements)
Maladaptive coping behaviors
　Increased tobacco and alcohol consumption
Stereotype threat
　Stigma of inferiority leading to physiologic arousal
　Impaired patient-provider relationship

*Small, often unintentional racial slights/insults (e.g., a judge asking a black defense attorney, "Can you wait outside until your attorney gets here?")
From Bailey ZD, Krieger N, Agénor M, et al: Structural racism and health inequities in the USA: evidence and interventions, *Lancet* 389:1453–1463, 2017 (Panel 2, p 1546).

according to attributes described by the interviewer. In response to positive attributes (e.g., *pretty, good, smart*), most children chose the white doll. The Clarks interpreted this finding to mean that black children had internalized the societal views of black inferiority and white superiority, even at the expense of their personal self-image. Repeated by a New York City high school student several decades later, the findings were much the same, with 15 of 21 children endorsing positive attributes to light-skinned dolls. Multiple studies confirm that racial identity is established in young children, both black and white, along with negative views of blackness. Developmentally, however, nonwhite youth often explore racial identity earlier than their white counterparts. In terms of health outcomes, depending on perceived inferiority or superiority of the group, racial identification is associated with self-esteem, mastery, and depressive symptoms. Low self-esteem is independently implicated in mental health disorders and may contribute to the phenomenon of **stereotype threat**, in which personal expectation of underperformance correlates with prevailing social stereotypes and adversely affects actual performance.

Interpersonal Racism

How racial beliefs affect interactions between individuals has been the most studied aspect of racism. *Interpersonal racism* refers to situations where one person from society's privileged racial group acts in a discriminatory manner that adversely affects another person or group of people. Such actions may be based on explicit beliefs or on implicit beliefs of which the perpetrating individual is not consciously aware. A burgeoning field is examining how experience of unfair treatment

has *biologic* consequences, reflected in measurable increases in stress responses.

Such effects of interpersonal racism are best documented for **mental health**, where perceived unfair treatment serves as psychosocial stressors, and are weaker for physical health outcomes. A 2009 study of 5,147 5th-grade students found that compared to only 7% of whites who reported experiencing racial discrimination, 15% of Latinos and 20% of blacks self-reported enduring racial discrimination. Furthermore, discriminatory experiences have been strongly and consistently linked to greater risk for anxiety, depression, conduct disorder, psychological distress, ADHD, ODD, self-esteem, self-worth, and psychological adaptation and adjustment. Perceived racial discrimination can affect behavioral, mental, and physical health outcomes and is associated with: increased alcohol and drug use among Native Americans (age 9-16 yr), increased tobacco smoking for black youth (11-19 yr), higher depressive symptoms among Puerto Rican children, and insulin resistance among young females.

Understanding the enduring impact of childhood experience on adult health has increased with the study of **adverse childhood experiences** (ACEs) (see Chapter 1). ACEs have well-documented cumulative negative health effects that occur across the life span and are patterned by race/ethnicity. Early experience of racism is a proxy measure for **toxic stress**. The question, "Was [child's name] ever treated or judged unfairly because of [his/her] race or ethnic group?" is included in the U.S. Census Bureau's National Survey of Children's Health, a random sample of 91,000-102,000 households (depending on the year) to assess the health of children up to 17 yr old. Children of color from low-income households, especially Latino children, were reported to have the lowest level of health. However, exposure to racism among higher SES did not protect children from experiencing relatively poorer health. Children exposed to racism were also more likely (by 3.2%) to have a diagnosis of ADHD. Children exposed to racism were 2 times more likely to experience anxiety and depression.

Toxic stress increases cortisol levels in the body, increasing the risk of chronic disease. A 2010 study revealed that Mexican adolescents who perceived racism experienced greater cortisol output, after controlling for other stressors. Adolescents who experience racism with no support have been shown to have higher levels of blood pressure and obesity than those with emotional support, which can be protective.

Medical practice has not been exempt from these occurrences of interpersonal racism. Using variation in adherence to established clinical standards in diagnostic and treatment decisions across racialized groups, researchers have been assessing interpersonal racism in physician–patient interactions. The most comprehensive review of such bias in clinical care remains the 2003 study by the U.S. Institute of Medicine, in which the discriminatory treatment was inferred from examination of clinical decision-making rather than from directly observed interactions. For virtually every condition studied, black patients were less likely to receive recommended care. Such racial bias has been most extensively established in adults but also extends to children. A study conducted in an emergency department found pediatric patients (<21 yr) were less likely to receive medically indicated pain medication if they were black, mirroring the historical misconception of reduced pain sensitivity among blacks. Within this context, it is unsurprising that perceived interpersonal racism has been linked to healthcare utilization, including delays in seeking care or filling prescriptions and distrust of the health system.

Institutional Racism

Interpersonal racism clearly inflicts harms, but even if completely eliminated, racial inequities would persist because of institutional and structural racism. Broadly, *institutional racism* refers to patterns of discrimination based on policy, culture, or practice and carried out by state and nonstate institutions (e.g., corporations, universities, legal systems, cultural institutions) within various sectors (e.g., housing, education, criminal justice). Key to current residential segregation are banking practices dating to the post-Depression era. As an institution, the education system has been another tragic case of how racism impacts children's health. In addition, mass incarceration by the criminal justice system has dramatically increased in the United States while remaining

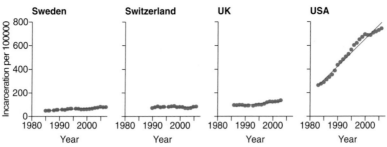

Fig. 2.6 Trends in incarceration prevalence in developed democracies, 1981–2007. *(Adapted from Wilderman C, Wang EA: Mass incarceration, public health, and widening inequality in the USA, Lancet 389:1464–1472, 2017, Fig 1.)*

relatively flat in other developed countries (Fig. 2.6). Over a lifetime, approximately 30% of African American men have been imprisoned.

In school, children of color can experience not only individual racism but also institutional racism, as documented by higher rates of disciplinary actions such as suspensions, and at younger ages than white children. According to a 2016 U.S. Department of Education civil rights survey, black children, who represent only 19% of national preschool students, account for a staggering 47% of at least 1 out-of-school suspension. Black preschoolers are 3.6 times more likely to be suspended than their white peers. Black females, representing 20% of female preschool population, account for 54% of out-of-school suspensions.

Unfortunately, this disparity persists as children continue through the school system: for kindergarten to grade 12 (K-12) students, black children are 3.8 times more likely to face out-of-school suspension than white peers. This inequity is particularly harmful because the educational system feeds into the criminal justice system. Black students are 2.2 times more likely to have either school-related arrests or law enforcement referrals than their white peers. The U.S. Department of Education survey also reveals racial inequities among children with disabilities. For K-12 children with disabilities covered under the Individuals with Disability in Education Act, 21% of multiracial females were issued with at least 1 out-of-school suspension, compared to 5% of white females.

In addition to the threat to educational and employment prospects, school suspensions also risk children's health. A 2016 brief from the Yale Child Study Center states that early suspensions and expulsions of children harm behavioral and social-emotional development, weakening a child's overall development. Furthermore, these forms of punishment may prevent the treatment of underlying health issues, such as mental health issues or disabilities, and cause increased stress for the entire family.

Institutional racism can function without apparent individual involvement and has powerful repercussions that persist centuries later. Both medical professional organizations and educational institutions have legacies of racial discrimination rooted in *scientific racism*. In 2008 the American Medical Association (AMA) issued a formal apology for its long history, dating to the 1870s, of endorsing explicitly racist practices, including exclusion of black physicians, silence on civil rights, and refusal to make any public statement on federally sponsored hospital segregation. Despite a focus on medical school desegregation in the 1960s and 1970s, the presence of black students in medical schools is actually declining. Low enrollment has become especially critical for black men, who in 2014 accounted for about 500 of the 20,000 medical students nationwide. If physicians hold stereotyped views about race that affect their clinical decision-making, the declining diversity of medical student bodies may well have consequences for the quality of medical care. This history of institutional racism on people of color contributes to the mistrust, apprehension, and fear projected toward the entire medical establishment.

Structural Racism

The institutional racism within medical institutions reinforces institutional racism in other sectors, creating a larger system of discrimination, *structural racism*. Structural racism can be described as "the totality of ways

in which societies foster racial discrimination via mutually reinforcing systems of housing, education, employment, earnings, benefits, credit, media, healthcare, and criminal justice. These patterns and practices in turn reinforce discriminatory beliefs, values, and distribution of resources, which together affect risk of adverse health outcomes." Institutional racism and structural racism are sometimes used interchangeably, but structural racism refers to overarching patterns beyond a single or even collection of institutions. Historically, government policies and practices have been largely responsible for the creation of these structures.

De facto and de jure urban residential segregation serves as a case study for how the mechanisms of structural racism operate across multiple sectors and can impact child health and development across the life course. In the 20th century, urban residential racial segregation was reinforced by the government-sanctioned policy and practice of *redlining*. This now-illegal practice was initiated by the U.S. Federal Housing Administration in 1934. Surveyors literally demarcated city maps with red ink to indicate those urban neighborhoods to be made ineligible for home loans. *Racial composition* was the most important driver of this categorization, and thus black neighborhoods were excluded from the federally financed, post-Depression home ownership boom and remained segregated. Through this segregation, existing resources were systematically removed (*disinvestment*) and led to further impoverished communities of color.

The effects of residential segregation were not restricted to the banking or housing sectors. **Residential segregation** ties together multiple systems, driving children's access to and quality of healthcare, education, and justice, as follows

◆ *Residential segregation and the healthcare system.* Healthcare institutions were explicitly racially segregated by law and inequitably resourced until passage of the 1964 Civil Rights Act. Vestiges of this segregation continue in recent hospital-level segregation and racial composition by hospital. In addition, institutions that provide mainly for uninsured or underserved residents are often financially unstable, leading to higher risk of closure in disinvested neighborhoods of color. On the provider level, fewer primary care and specialty physicians practice in disinvested, segregated neighborhoods, and those who are present are less likely to participate in Medicaid.

◆ *Residential segregation and the education system.* Schools have a similar history of racial segregation and, after a brief respite of integration peaking in 1980, the rates of segregation now resemble pre–Civil Rights levels of segregation. School segregation is related to high-risk health behaviors. Within these schools and in their neighborhoods, black children experience disproportionate penalization and criminalization in the educational and criminal justice systems, reinforcing institutional racism in other sectors and other forms of racism. A low-income black child is much more likely than a low-income white child to live in a segregated neighborhood. The result is that the black child will face not only the cumulative disadvantage in both family and neighborhood resources and experiences over time, but also the initiation of chains of disadvantage during sensitive periods of childhood key for development and adult transition (e.g., early childhood, adolescence).

◆ *Residential segregation and the criminal justice system.* Incarceration is concentrated in overpoliced and criminalized black communities. In the NCHS, almost 13% of black children had a parent imprisoned during their childhood (to age 17 yr), compared to about 6% of white children. Parental incarceration, which may start with a traumatic arrest in the home and later disrupt caregiving, create social stigma, deepen financial disadvantage, disconnect parents emotionally from children, and disrupt children's psychological development, has been independently associated with higher risk of children's antisocial behavior.

Most notably, experiences directly related to institutional and structural racism, operating through residential segregation (including financial hardship, parental imprisonment, and neighborhood violence), result in higher levels of ACEs for blacks and Latinos than whites. There has been growing, consistent evidence of the lifelong association between ACEs and a range of negative physical and mental health outcomes across the life course.

Structural racism, shown here with the example of residential segregation, affects child health through various direct and indirect, overlapping pathways, including the concentration of dilapidated housing, inferior quality of the social and built environment, exposure to pollutants and toxins, limited access to high-quality primary and secondary education, few well-paying jobs, overpolicing and criminalization, adverse experiences, and limited access to quality healthcare.

OPPORTUNITIES TO ADDRESS RACISM

Racism as a determinant of health has strong empirical support, and there is promising evidence for community-wide approaches to its mitigation. Less is known about effective interventions in clinical settings. Most medical schools and subsequent training will not have prepared practitioners to examine the role of racism in their patients' lives or clinical care settings. Nonetheless, it is reasonable to expect that pediatricians can help address racism and promote racial justice in at least 3 ways: during individual patient encounters and at their practice sites, as members of institutions that provide medical care and training, and as respected community members.

Clinical Settings

A first step is understanding that racism affects everyone and personally assessing **implicit bias**. Such biases reflect reflexive patterns of thinking often using racial stereotypes stemming from living in a racially stratified society. The **Project Implicit Race Implicit Association Test** (https://implicit.harvard.edu/implicit/takeatest.html) is available online, and its results are confidential. The purpose of such tests is to create awareness, not apportion blame. Nonetheless, results are usually jarring for all participants, no matter their racial identity, many of whom will uncover negative racial biases of which they were unaware. Such individual assessments may contribute to addressing interpersonal racism as it triggers self-reflection. Further, a growing number of organizations offer training in understanding common behaviors associated with implicit bias, including microaggressions (see later) and inequitable hiring practices. Recognizing and undoing personal biases as pediatricians requires training to challenge existing thought processes and actions that are often difficult to see.

Pediatricians and other health workers have an entrusted role in families that requires a partnership. Recognizing the strengths of families and valuing their lived experiences of internalized and interpersonal racism as expertise fosters a more collaborative clinical interaction and relationship. This expertise cannot be readily captured by pedagogy or acquired by a pediatrician in training or clinical practice. Such an approach emphasizes respect for the expertise that caregivers bring to raising their child and begins with the presumption that caregivers want to do what is best for the child. By doing this, physicians can form a collaborative relationship, rather than one based on racial stereotypes and blame. Cultural competence is a widespread concept recognizing that *other cultures* exist that the dominant culture must learn to decode. In contrast, the concept of **cultural humility**, for which training is increasingly available, considers equality among cultures and a partnership approach to differences.

During clinical encounters with children and families, healthcare workers can use their authority to acknowledge racism. Pediatricians should broach "The Talk" with their patients who are black, young adolescent, and male. "The Talk" is the conversation that black parents typically initiate with their sons regarding interactions with police. In doing so, the pediatrician affirms the need for such conversations to promote safety and may provide opportunities to connect families to community resources. For all young children and youth of color, pediatricians should ask patients if they have they been treated unfairly because of their race, recognizing this can by a form of **bullying**. The experience of racism at all levels can be traumatic. Trauma consists of experiences or situations that are emotionally painful and distressing, and that overwhelm people's ability to cope, leaving them powerless. Pediatricians must consider adopting trauma-informed care practices that shift the paradigm from, "What is wrong with you?" to, "What has happened to you?"

In addition, healthcare providers must strive for **structural competency**, which is the "trained ability to discern how a host of issues defined clinically as symptoms, attitudes, or diseases also represent the downstream implications of a number of upstream decisions," according to Johnathan M. Metzl and Helena Hansen. Consequently, it is helpful to ensure that clinical practices are aware of other social services that may enhance health and engagement with clinical care, such as need for legal counsel to address substandard housing, counter landlord harassment, or negotiate threatened evictions (http://medical-legalpartnership.org/), or the support of literacy by *prescribing* or distributing children's books in order to encourage parents to read to children (http://www.reachoutandread.org/).

Institutional Settings

The healthcare institution more broadly is also a setting where racial dynamics occur. Introducing conversations about race may uncover experiences that would not otherwise be apparent. A common outcome of implicit racial bias is **microaggressions**, actions and attitudes that may seem trivial or unimportant to the perpetrators but create a cumulative burden for those who perceive them. A physician of color might be asked for identification on entering a hospital, while white colleagues are not so queried. These microaggressions occur in interactions among staff as well with patients and may contribute to an unspoken and uncomfortable racial climate. While such interactions rarely would violate federal discrimination standards, interaction between co-workers shapes an entire practice and can be perceived by families.

Encouraging institutions to assess the impact of race among patients and staff is a first step. Healthcare delivery institutional settings can use both data and patient accounts to examine racial effects in the practice and experience by routinely disaggregating assessment measures by race/ethnicity. Patient-reported satisfaction or quality of care might be disaggregated by race. In addition, it is important to consider racial equity within the practice's employment structure: Are there discrepancies in hiring, retention, and salaries by race? Are there proper supervision and grievance procedures, particularly around issues related to racial microaggressions? Also, consider the images and language used to discuss and represent both patients and staff, particularly when alluding to race/ethnicity. Organizations such as **Race Forward** (https://www.raceforward.org) and organizational assessment tools developed by the **Race Matters Institute** can help to guide institutional assessments and internal change processes. Several local health departments have already incorporated antiracism training into staff professional development and introduced internal reforms to drive organizational change. Since institutional reform is closely associated with other models of productive practices, including quality improvement, collective impact, community engagement, and community mobilization, application of an antiracism lens should be judged by its contributions to organizational effectiveness as well as on its moral merits.

Education or training institutions have a special role in ensuring a workforce that is both diverse and informed. Patterns of student admissions should be scrutinized, as should the curriculum. Although many medical schools now include diversity training and provide instruction on cultural competency, such instruction is often brief (and sometimes delivered online). By contrast, approaches based on structural competency, cultural humility, and **cultural safety** have been implemented in health professionals' training in such countries as Canada and New Zealand. These approaches emphasize the value of gaining knowledge about structural racism, internalized scripts of racial superiority and inferiority, and the cultural and power contexts of health professionals and their patients or clients. Health professionals benefit from the scholarship of diverse disciplines about the origins and perpetuation of, as well as remedies to counter, racism. Finding class time for these topics encounters a *biomedical bias* that is widespread in medical education, although arguably successful medical practice also requires a host of skills in addition a firm grounding in pathophysiology and recommended treatments. Racism results in damaging disparities that cause ill health and shorten lives, which justifies the teaching hours committed to its understanding.

Pediatricians as Advocates for Antiracist Practices and Systems

Physicians are respected members of communities and wield the power,

privilege, and responsibility for dismantling structural racism. A conceptual review of structural racism highlights the promise of place-based interventions that target geographically defined communities, to engage residents and a range of institutions (across sectors) in order to ensure equitable access to resources and services, remediating the processes set in motion decades earlier. Clinicians play a role in linking patients to services, programming, and other resources and advocating for responsiveness in addressing gaps. Over time, concentrated efforts across sectors in targeted areas have shown improvement in a host of social outcomes, including health outcomes. Similarly, providing access to higher-quality housing, either with housing vouchers or housing lotteries, had unexpected positive health impacts. These findings are encouraging, as are the social policy interventions and systemic change, including legislation such as the Civil Rights Act, the advent of Medicare and Medicaid, and tenement regulations, associated with the narrowing of racial gaps.

Bibliography is available at Expert Consult.

Chapter 3
Global Child Health
Suzinne Pak-Gorstein

第三章
全球儿童健康

中文导读

　　本章主要介绍了全球儿童健康负担和趋势、社会层面儿童健康的决定因素、运用基于循证的干预和创新措施解决儿童健康的不公平性，以及全球卫生健康挑战。具体阐述了导致全球卫生健康不均衡的社会经济和政治根源、可持续发展目标、疫苗可防犯疾病、

有效的支持和保障（即：儿童疾病的综合治疗）、社会保障项目（即：有条约和无条件的现金调拨）、青少年健康和全球气候变化，还涉及冲突、紧急状况和移民，以及信息和通信技术等。

GLOBAL BURDEN AND TRENDS IN CHILD HEALTH

The **under-five mortality rate (U5MR)**, also known as the **child mortality rate**, serves as a reliable gauge of child well-being. It measures the outcome of a country's health system and reflects a nation's social and economic development. The global U5MR fell by 53% between 1990 and 2015. Despite these gains, in 2016 an estimated 5.6 million children <5 yr old died worldwide, equivalent to *41 deaths per 1,000 live births,* or almost *15,000 child deaths each day.* The burden of the world's child mortality disproportionately falls on low- and middle-income regions of Africa and Asia (Fig. 3.1), with 86% of child deaths occurring in these regions and <1% in high-income countries. Consequently, a child

born in sub-Saharan Africa is >15 times more likely to die by age 5 yr than a child born in a high-income country.

Improvements in child mortality have been uneven globally, regionally, and nationally. Rates of change in U5MR range from a decrease of 8.9% in the Maldives to an increase of 2.5% in Syria during 2000–2016. Significant disparities in child mortality persist and have become increasingly concentrated in specific regions of Africa and Asia, with one third of these deaths occurring in South Asia and half in sub-Saharan Africa.

While the number of child deaths has decreased dramatically over the past 2 decades, the early years of life remain one of a child's most vulnerable periods. Among the under-5 child deaths, almost half occurred

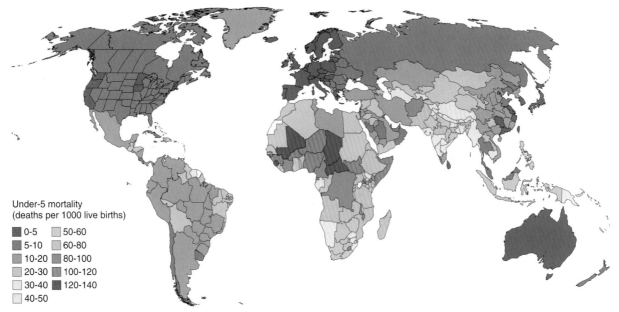

Fig. 3.1 Global under-five mortality rates, 2015. *(Data from Global Burden of Disease 2016 Causes of Death Collaborators: Global, regional, and national age-sex specific mortality for 264 causes of death, 1980–2016: a systematic analysis for the Global Burden of Disease Study 2016, Lancet 388:1151–1210, 2017.)*

Under-5 mortality
(deaths per 1000 live births)

0-5	50-60
5-10	60-80
10-20	80-100
20-30	100-120
30-40	120-140
40-50	

within the 1st mo of life (2.7 million deaths in 2016). This estimate of **neonatal deaths** (<1 mo) translates into 19 per 1,000 live births. Declines in neonatal mortality occurred at slower rates, so that in 2015 the neonatal deaths made up 46% of all under-5 deaths (Fig. 3.2).

Neonatal deaths account for a smaller percentage of child mortality in low- and middle-income countries compared to high-income countries (Fig. 3.3), but the absolute risk of death remains significantly higher. A child in sub-Saharan Africa or South Asia is 9 times more likely to die in the 1st mo of life than a child born in a high-income country.

An estimated 1.7 million **stillborn** deaths (≥28 completed wk of gestation) burden families worldwide every year, which correlates to 13.1 deaths per 1,000 births. Global and national estimates of stillbirths vary widely because of inadequate data collection, reflecting the low prioritization of this vulnerable age-group. Progress to reduce stillbirth rates during the MDG era (UN Millennium Development Goals) has been slow, with the annual rate of reduction estimated to be half that for neonatal deaths between 2000 and 2015. Almost all stillbirths occur in low- and middle-income countries (98%), with three-quarters in sub-Saharan Africa and South Asia.

Most childhood deaths are caused by conditions that could be prevented or managed through improved access to simple, low-cost interventions. The most common causes of child death are *pneumonia* (13%), *diarrhea* (9%), and *malaria* (5%), which account for almost one third of all under-5 deaths and about 40% of under-5 deaths in sub-Saharan Africa (see Chapter 1, Fig. 1.1). Neonatal deaths are caused by prematurity (16%), intrapartum-related complications such as birth asphyxia (11%), and neonatal sepsis (7%). In contrast, child deaths from infections in developed countries are less common, and injuries and congenital malformations account for higher proportions of under-5 deaths. **Undernutrition**, including fetal growth restriction, stunting and wasting, and micronutrient deficiencies, contributes up to 45% of under-5 deaths and leads to poor childhood development in low- and middle-income countries. Undernutrition has an enormous impact on child mortality because of the vicious cycle between nutrition and infection. Lowered immunity and mucosal damage from inadequate dietary intake leads to increased susceptibilty to pathogen invasion. Recurrent infections and immature microbiome impairs the child's ability to absorb nutrients.

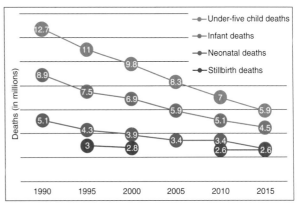

Fig. 3.2 Deaths for under-5 children, infants, neonates, and stillbirths, 1990–2015. *(Adapted with data from United Nations Interagency Group for Child Mortality Estimation 2017. Stillbirth estimates for 1995 and 2009 from Cousens, 2011 [2010 rate from 2009]; 2000 rates from Lawn, 2012; and 2015 rate of 2.6 million from Blencow, 2016.)*

Infants who start out life with a **low birthweight** (LBW) are at high risk of death, contributing 60–80% of all neonatal deaths. Most of these infants are premature (<37 wk of pregnancy) or had fetal growth restriction. About half of stillbirths take place during labor, ranging from 10.0% in developed regions to 59.3% in South Asia, which reflects the extent that timely, high-quality care at delivery can prevent many of these deaths.

Mortality among older children (5-14 yr) is low compared with the younger cohort, although 1 million children in this age-group died in 2016, equivalent to 3,000 children dying every day. Infectious diseases play a smaller role in deaths among these older children, with injuries from external causes such as drowning and motor vehicle crashes accounting for more than one quarter of the deaths and noncommunicable diseases for another quarter.

Child health should not be assessed based on mortality rates alone. Children surviving illness are often left with **lifelong disabilities**, burdening their families and impacting their economic productivity. Approximately 1 in 10 children are born with or acquire a disability, and 80% of these disabled children live in low- or middle-income countries. Neonatal disorders, infectious diseases, protein-energy and micronutrient deficiencies, hemoglobinopathies, and injuries are leading causes of disability in children. Child deaths can also lead to disability in the surviving mother. A woman who has a stillbirth is at risk of an obstetric fistula or death, with an estimated 78–98% of women with obstetric fistula having had a stillbirth. Also, perinatal loss with child death is a psychological trauma. Stillbirth, neonatal death, and child loss can lead to posttraumatic stress disorder, depression, anxiety, guilt, and in some settings, shame and social stigma, particularly in the mother, with significant impact on the health and well-being of the family.

Adolescents age 10-19 yr, who have benefited from the gains in child survival, grow up to find themselves in social settings where less attention and fewer resources are devoted to their well-being compared to their earlier years of growth. The paucity of support during this time of transition into adulthood diminishes the impact that child survival can have on their lives. Adolescents make up 18% of the world's population, approximately 1.8 billion in 2010, which is expected to increase to >2 billion by 2050. The vast majority of adolescents, 88%, live in low- and middle-income countries. In 2050, sub-Saharan Africa is projected to have more adolescents than any other region. While adolescent mortality rates are much lower than their younger-age cohorts, in low-income countries they face a lack of educational and employment opportunities, risk of injuries and violence, HIV/AIDS, mental health problems, marriage, and teenage pregnancy, preventing them from attaining their potential as they transition into adulthood. The decade of adolescence is a critical period when poverty and inequity frequently transfer to the next generation. The intergenerational transmission of poverty is most apparent among undereducated adolescent females. In many parts of the world, poor teenage females are likely to be married early, risking premature childbearing and higher rates of maternal mortality, and leading to infant and child undernutrition.

SOCIAL DETERMINANTS OF CHILD HEALTH

The gross national income level accounts for much of the difference in child mortality observed between countries, but other significant factors impact child health. Although the wealth of the United States places it in the 8th position with respect to gross domestic product (GDP) per capita (2016) in the world, the U.S. child mortality rate is ranked 56th in the world, at 5.8 deaths per 1,000 live births, which is higher than the United Kingdom (4.3), Cuba (4.4), Canada (4.5), Czech Republic (2.6), and Japan (2.0). *National estimates of mortality mask differences in health status among subpopulations within the same country.* In Burkina Faso the child mortality rate is 43.7/1,000 live births among children born to mothers with no education, whereas it is 16.7 per 1,000 among children born to mothers with at least secondary education. Similarly, in 2013, the infant mortality rate in the Dominican Republic was 14.0/1,000 live births for children in the highest wealth quintile, but 40.0/1,000 for children living in the lowest quintile.

Child health is influenced by socioeconomic factors that operate at multiple levels of the society. Disparities in these socioeconomic factors translate into child health inequities, as reflected by high rates of disease, poor nutrition, and disability. Fig. 3.4 outlines the immediate, underlying, and basic structural determinants of disease, malnutrition, and disability. Preventive and curative medical interventions focus on the immediate causes of poor health. However, inequities in child mortality and morbidity will persist unless the basic and underlying determinants of health are addressed.

Socioeconomic and Political Roots of Disparities in Global Health

The root causes of a child's health lie in the economic and political environments in which the child is born (Fig. 3.4). Growth of economies during the 1st half of the 20th century was associated with dramatic

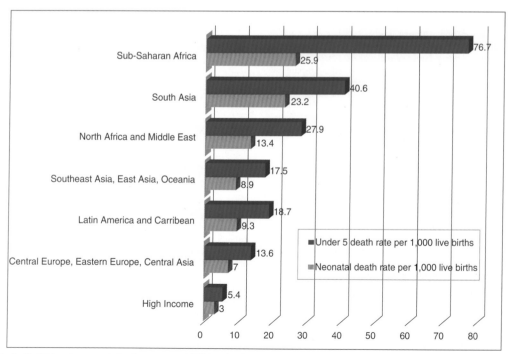

Fig. 3.3 Under-5 child and neonatal death rates per 1,000 live births, 2016. *(Data from Global Burden of Disease 2016: Global, regional, and national under-5 mortality, adult mortality, Lancet 390:1084–1150, 2017.)*

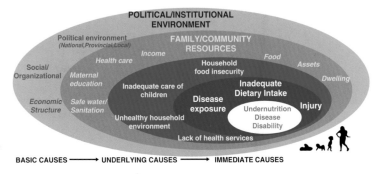

Fig. 3.4 Socioecologic model: basic, underlying, and immediate determinants of child health. *(Adapted with data from World Health Organization and Maternal and Child Epidemiology Estimation Group, 2017.)*

health improvements with falling mortality rates and rising life expectancy across all regions. However, the 2nd half observed significant disparities in global economies and health among and within many countries.

Between 1980 and 2016, the richest 1% of the world reaped twice as much of the world's income as the poorest 50% of the world (27% of income growth vs 12%) (World Inequality Report, 2018, http://wir2018.wid.world/). Almost all countries report income inequalities among its population, but a few countries, such as the United States, have seen income disparities at historical proportions (Fig. 3.5). Since 1980 the bottom half of Americans captured only 3% of the total growth. Growing income inequalities translates into greater differences in health outcomes, such as life expectancy, between the rich and the poor in the United States (Fig. 3.6). More aggressive redistribution of wealth through taxes and transfers has spared Europe from such glaring disparities.

Evidence supports that income inequality is not just a human rights issue, but also detrimental to economic growth. Wealthier households spend a smaller percentage of their own income, thereby dampening demand and slowing down economies. Poorer households face greater challenges to invest in health and educational opportunities, translating into less human capital, and obstacles to be productive and contribute to the economy. In extreme cases, inequalities can threaten social unrest, which further undermines economic activity.

Global disparities have grown between many wealthy and low-income countries, in large part from "austerity" measures, including structural adjustment programs, imposed on many postcolonial countries by the International Monetary Fund (IMF) and World Bank. In order to receive loans and pay off their debt, many of these countries were required to take on austerity measures that transformed their economies to produce cash crops and export natural resources to higher-income countries, rather than supporting local industries and investing in human capital and providing social services.

Foreign aid for healthcare programs has led to significant health improvements, with countries receiving more health aid demonstrating a more rapid rise in life expectancy and larger declines in child mortality than countries that received less health aid. National security concerns continue to drive U.S. assistance policy, which aims to reinforce ally countries, provide stability in conflict regions, promote democracy, and contribute to counterterrorism and law enforcement efforts abroad. Other goals, such as contributing humanitarian relief during natural disasters, poverty reduction, and health promotion, also drive assistance.

Sustainable Development Goals

The prioritization and planning of global development and international aid has been guided by international goals. In 2015, world leaders agreed to 17 goals, the **Sustainability Development Goals (SDGs)**, to improve global well-being by 2030 (Fig. 3.7). The SDGs were built on the eight **Millennium Development Goals (MDGs)**, which were concrete, specific, and measurable targets set by the United Nations in 2000 to eradicate poverty, hunger, illiteracy, and disease by 2015. Significant, although uneven, progress had been made toward meeting the MDGs, falling short in improving the lives of the poorest and most disadvantaged

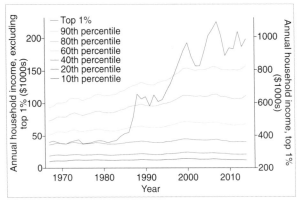

Fig. 3.5 Inflation-adjusted annual household income at selected percentiles, 1967–2014. All series show percentiles of the distribution except for top 1%, which shows the mean of the top 1%. All income series except for the top 1% are plotted against the left vertical axis, displaying incomes from $0 to $200,000. The top 1% is plotted against the right vertical axis, displaying incomes from $200,000 to $1,000,000. Income is expressed in 2014 US$. *(Data from US Census Bureau Current Population Survey, 1968–2015, Annual Social and Economic Supplements and World Wealth and Income Database. From Bor J, Cohen GH, Galea S: Population health in an era of rising income inequality: USA, 1980–2015, Lancet 389:1475–1490, 2017, Fig 1.)*

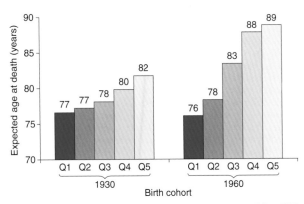

Fig. 3.6 Projected life expectancy for U.S. men at age 50 for 1930 and 1960 birth cohorts. By income quintile: Q1 (poorest) to Q5 (richest). *(From Bor J, Cohen GH, Galea S: Population health in an era of rising income inequality: USA, 1980–2015, Lancet 389:1475–1490, 2017, Fig 5b; with data from National Academies of Sciences, Engineering, and Medicine: The growing gap in life expectancy by income: implications for federal programs and policy responses, Washington, DC, 2015, National Academies Press.)*

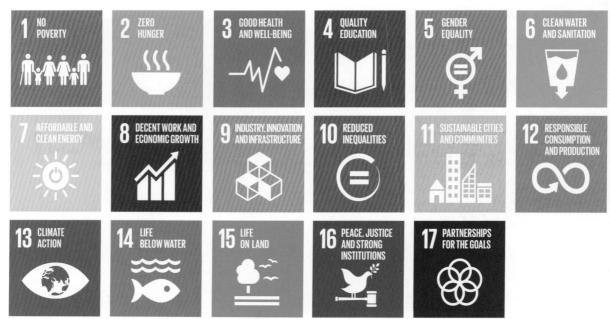

Fig. 3.7 Sustainable development goals (SDGs 1-17). *(Courtesy United Nations Department of Public Information, 2016.* http://www.un.org/sustainabledevelopment/sustainable-development-goals/*)*

countries, and bypassing social groups because of gender, age, disability, or ethnicity.

Unlike the MDGs, in which health was prominently featured in 3 of the goals, the SDG-3 is the primary SDG that focuses on health-related subtargets, including the reduction of U5MR to 25 deaths per 1,000 live births and neonatal mortality rate to 12 deaths per 1,000 live births by 2030. The other 16 SDGs focus mainly on social and economic determinants and the environment. This reflects an important shift to broaden the global targets to include upstream determinants of health, including health systems and socioeconomic, gender-based, political, and environmental factors. As a social movement to support sustainable development, the SDGs were founded on the recognition that the world's environment, socioeconomic development, and human health are interconnected and dependent. Therefore the SDGs were formulated with core principles and values for **economic development, environmental sustainability**, and **social inclusion** for all.

The **Global Strategy for Women's, Children's and Adolescent's Health** 2016–2030 maps out the strategies to achieve the SDGs by centering on the goal of health for all women, children, and adolescents using evidence-based approaches, backed by innovative and sustainable financing mechanisms. An important component of the Global Strategy is the inclusion of adolescents as central to the 2030 Agenda for Sustainable Development. In alignment with the SDGs, the Global Strategy focuses on 3 pillars of action: (1) *ending preventable deaths* among women, children, and adolescents; (2) *ensuring their health and well-being* by ending malnutrition and ensuring access to family planning, reducing exposure to pollution, and achieving universal health coverage; and (3) *expanding enabling environments* by efforts such as eradicating extreme poverty, ensuring good-quality education, eliminating violence against women and girls, enhancing research and technologic capabilities, and encouraging innovation.

In addition to being much broader in scope, the Global Strategy focuses on *equity* in that the strategy is meant to apply to all people, including the marginalized and difficult-to-reach populations, in all situations, including during crisis. Thus, for example, health insurance coverage would not be assessed based simply on the national average of coverage, but also by how well the increases in coverage benefit *all* population groups, regardless of income or educational level.

EVIDENCE-BASED INTERVENTIONS AND INNOVATIONS TO ADDRESS CHILD HEALTH INEQUITIES

Estimates indicate that most of the 5.6 million annual deaths in children <5 yr old could be averted by increasing coverage of proven low-cost interventions (Table 3.1). Childhood deaths from diarrheal illness and pneumonia can be prevented by simple measures such as vaccinations and exclusive breastfeeding until 6 mo of age. Deaths related to undernutrition, which predisposes children to infectious diseases, may be prevented by proper infant and young child feeding practices, micronutrient supplementation, and community-based screening and management of malnutrition.

Addressing the SDGs to improve health of mothers, children, and adolescents takes a life course approach. Fig. 3.8 displays estimates of coverage for essential interventions across the continuum of care, indicating the wide range of coverage rates within countries that will need to be addressed if SDGs are to be attained.

Vaccine-Preventable Diseases

In 2002 an estimated 1.5 million under-5 deaths were caused by vaccine-preventable diseases. Top contributors were pneumococcus and rotavirus, followed by *Haemophilus influenzae* B (Hib), measles, pertussis, and tetanus. The World Health Organization (WHO) **Expanded Program on Immunization** (EPI) has resulted in a dramatic reduction in deaths, illness, and disability from many of these diseases, as well as the near-elimination of poliomyelitis. Recommendations for routine immunizations have continued to grow with the development of new vaccines that have demonstrated significant lifesaving potential in industrialized countries (Table 3.2).

In 2015, 86% of the world's infants were vaccinated with 3 doses of diphtheria-tetanus-pertussis (DTP). Although vaccines are very effective in improving child survival, rates of coverage are low in many countries. In 2016 a total of 19.5 million children did not receive all routine lifesaving vaccinations, and 90,000 deaths were reported from measles. Although coverage rates are still improving, and lifesaving vaccines are still not available in many countries, progress has been made to expand availability to new countries every year. The lowest number of wild poliovirus cases (37) was reported in 2016.

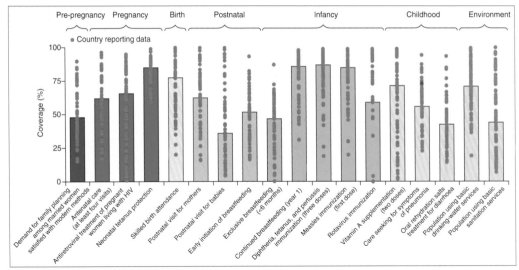

Fig. 3.8 Coverage of interventions across the continuum of care based on the most recent data since 2012 in Countdown countries. *Bars show median national coverage of interventions; dots show country-specific data. (From Countdown to 2030 Collaboration: Tracking progress towards universal coverage for reproductive, maternal, newborn, and child health, Lancet 391:1538-1548, 2018. Fig 1.)*

Reaching Every Child, Everywhere

Global vaccine organizations aim for universal coverage of immunizations but face challenges within countries to attain this goal. Other lifesaving interventions have met barriers to attain universal coverage. Oral rehydration therapy (ORT) has been the evidence-based intervention recommended to prevent dehydration from diarrheal disease since the 1970s, yet only 2 in 5 children <5 yr with diarrheal illness receive this treatment. Many factors determine whether a child receives a lifesaving intervention. Characteristics of the healthcare system, social attitudes and practices, and the political climate impact whether universal coverage can be reached for evidence-based essential interventions. Innovations to strengthen vaccine coverage to reach every child in every district of a country range from programs such as **Reaching Every Child through Quality Improvement** (REC-QI) using community mapping techniques, to integrating service delivery mechanisms and strengthening the health system with improved surveillance.

Effective Delivery Strategies: Integrated Management of Childhood Illness

Weak health systems impede the ability of countries to deliver cost-effective interventions and lifesaving health messages for children. Such systems are characterized by insufficient numbers of health workers, low-quality training and supervision, and poorly functioning supply chains. The provision of child health services may focus on a single level, such as the health facility, but effective and lasting improvements can only be achieved with the integration of delivery at all levels, such as adequate referrals and follow-up between community, clinic, and health facility. Other important lifesaving strategies include outreach services (e.g., mass immunization, vitamin A campaigns) and community-based health promotion activities (Fig. 3.9).

The **Integrated Management of Childhood Illnesses** (IMCI) was launched in the mid-1990s by the United Nations Children's Fund (UNICEF) and WHO as an approach to reduce child mortality, illness, and disability and to promote improved growth and development in countries struggling with high child mortality rates. The IMCI was designed to increase coverage of evidence-based, high-impact interventions that address the top causes of child mortality by integrating health promotion, illness prevention, and disease treatment. The IMCI contains both preventive and curative elements, set forth through a series of clinical algorithms and guidelines for case management (see Fig. 3.10

for an example) and implemented by health care workers in collaboration with families and communities. One key component of the IMCI strategy involves training frontline healthcare workers to use the algorithms to identify signs of common childhood illness and to decide when a child needs referral to a hospital. In early 2003, guidelines for newborn care were added to create the **Integrated Management of Neonatal and Childhood Illnesses** (IMNCI).

As facility-based services alone do not provide adequate access to timely treatment of childhood illnesses, in early 2000 the **Integrated Community Case Management** (i-CCM) was implemented to train community health workers to instruct parents on home management of ill children, including ORS and zinc for diarrhea, antimalarial medicine for febrile children who test positive for malaria, and antibiotics for children with signs of pneumonia. **Community health workers** (CHWs) are members of communities that have selected them to provide basic health care with support and training from the health system. CHWs carry out health promotional activities such as promotion of proper infant and young child feeding, hand-hygiene practices, and use of bed nets. The i-CCM strategy involved training CHWs to screen and manage diseases, including mild to moderate cases of undernutrition, diarrheal disease, and pneumonia. CHWs schedule follow-up visits for ill children managed in the community, and refer serious cases in a timely manner to healthcare facilities. Community-based interventions are effective in extending healthcare delivery, are low cost, improve healthcare-seeking behavior, and can reduce infant and child mortality and morbidity.

Over 100 countries have adopted IMNCI and implement some or all of its components, not only improving health workers' skills but also strengthening health systems and improving family and community practices. After 20 yr of implementation, a review noted that IMNCI was associated with a 15% reduction in child mortality when activities were properly implemented in health facilities and communities. However, the implementation of IMNCI was found to be uneven between and within countries. In many countries the resources for CHW training and supervision, supply of medications, and referrals were limited or absent. IMNCI was only successful in countries with strong government leadership and a commitment to implement IMNCI in partnership with support groups such as UNICEF and WHO. In addition, the success of IMNCI required an adequate health system and a systematic approach to planning and implementation.

Table 3.1	Essential Interventions Across the Continuum of Care to Improve Child Survival

HEALTH AND MULTISECTOR ACTIONS
- Ensuring food security for the family (or mother and child)
- Maternal education
- Safe drinking water and sanitation
- Handwashing with soap
- Reduced household air pollution
- Health education in schools

AGE-SPECIFIC ACTIONS	
Prevention	**Treatment**
ADOLESCENCE AND PRE-PREGNANCY • Family planning • Preconception care	
PREGNANCY • Appropriate care for normal and high-risk pregnancies (maternal tetanus vaccination)	• Antenatal steroids for premature births • Intermittent preventive treatment for malaria

CHILDBIRTH
• Maternal intrapartum care and monitoring
• Skilled delivery
  • Thermal care for all newborns
  • Clean cord and skin care
  • Early initiation and exclusive breastfeeding within 1st hr
	• Newborn resuscitation (e.g., Healthy Babies Breathe)
	• Premature: surfactant administration, continuous positive airway pressure (CPAP), treatment of jaundice
	• Feeding support for small/preterm infants

PRENATAL PERIOD • Appropriate postnatal visits	• Extra care for small and sick babies (kangaroo mother care, treatment of infection, support for feeding, management of respiratory complications) • Antibiotics for newborns at risk and for treatment of bacterial infections (PROM, sepsis, meningitis, pneumonia)

INFANCY AND CHILDHOOD
• Exclusive breastfeeding for 6 mo and continued breastfeeding up to at least 2 yr with appropriate complementary feeding from 6 mo
• Monitoring and care for child growth and development
• Routine immunization childhood diseases
• Micronutrient supplementation, including vitamin A from 6 mo
• Prevention of childhood diseases
  • Malaria (insecticide-treated bed nets)
  • Pneumonia
  • Diarrhea (rotavirus immunization)
  • Meningitis (meningococcal/Hib/pneumococcal vaccination)
  • Measles (vaccination)
• Prevention of mother-to-child HIV transmission
	• Case management of severe acute malnutrition
	
	• Management of childhood diseases
	  • Malaria (antimalarials)
	  • Pneumonia (case management, antibiotics)
	  • Diarrhea (ORS, zinc supplement, continued feeding)
	  • Meningitis (case management, antibiotics)
	  • Measles (vitamin A suppl)
	• Comprehensive care of children exposed to or infected with HIV (HAART)

HAART, Highly active antiretroviral therapy; ORS, oral rehydration solution (salts).
Adapted from Were W, Daelmans B, Bhutta ZA, et al. Children's health priorities and interventions, *BMJ* 351:h4300, 2015.

Social Protection Programs: Conditional and Unconditional Cash Transfers

Financial incentives are becoming widely used to improve healthcare coverage, alleviate poverty, and improve access to child health services. In industrialized countries, **cash transfers** is a common mechanism for ensuring that the poorest, most marginalized subgroups of the population, particularly with children, receive adequate support to meet their basic needs. Cash transfer programs are increasingly being used in low- and middle-income countries to support vulnerable populations.

Out-of-pocket expenses by households form the major share of total health expenditure in most low- and middle-income countries. Many social protection programs work to serve a dual purpose of reducing financial barriers and strengthening service delivery. Financial incentives may include cash transfers, microcredit, vouchers, and user fee removal and health insurance. Financial incentive programs may be unconditional, provided to eligible families without any requirements or expectations, based on the belief that families will use this type of financial support for their children's best interests. Other incentives are conditional on health promotion behavior targeting child health, such as providing cash or vouchers only to families who participate in preventive health

behaviors, such as attending mother groups to learn about breastfeeding practices, visiting clinics for child vaccinations and growth monitoring, engaging in deworming, and ensuring their children receive vitamin A and iron supplementation. Some social protection programs are also directed toward education improvement by making cash transfers conditional on child school enrollment, attendance, and occasionally some measure of academic performance.

CHALLENGES IN GLOBAL HEALTH
Adolescent Health

The Global Strategy, which directs countries to attain their SDGs, has called on nations to focus efforts to support adolescent health given their potential role in breaking the *intergenerational cycle* of poverty. The challenge to attain these health goals will be to effectively advocate governments to invest in this age-group as a means to improve the national productivity and economy. Considerable gaps in data on adolescents pose one of the greatest challenges to promoting their health and their rights.

Strategies to address the unmet needs of adolescent health efforts must highlight improving completion of secondary school education,

Table 3.2 Routine Immunizations Recommended by the World Health Organization (2017)

VACCINE (ANTIGEN)	AGE AT 1st DOSE	DOSES IN PRIMARY SERIES	INTERVAL BETWEEN DOSES			BOOSTER DOSE	ADOLESCENT	CONSIDERATIONS
			1st to 2nd	2nd to 3rd	3rd to 4th			
BCG (bacille Calmette-Guérin)	Birth	1						Prevents severe TB and TB meningitis. Recommended in TB-endemic countries. Contraindicated if HIV positive
Hepatitis B	Birth	3 (or 4)	4 wk w/ DTP2	4 wk w/ DTP3	(or 4 wk)		3 doses for high-risk groups if not previously immunized	Birth dose recommended for prevention of perinatal transmission. Premature infants <2 kg may not respond well. 3 doses needed for immunity, but can receive 4 if necessary when combined with other routine vaccinations
OPV (oral polio vaccine)	bOPV + IPV / IPV/bOPV / IPV	4 / 1-2 IPV/2 bOPV / 3	4 wk w/ DTP2 / 4-8 wk / 4-8 wk	4 wk w/ DTP3 / 4-8 wk / 4-8 wk	4-8 wk			OPV is used in many developing countries due to low cost, ease of administration, and resulting herd immunity. Different schedule exists for IPV, which creates less herd immunity; recommended only in low-risk countries. Additional birth dose (bOPV) is recommended in high-risk countries.
DTP (diphtheria, tetanus, and pertussis)	6 wk	3	4-8 wk	4-8 wk		3 boosters: 12-23 mo; 4-7 yr (Td); and 9-15 yr Td)	1 booster: 9-15 yr (Td)	Whole cell pertussis vaccine is still used in many countries. "DTP3" (receiving all 3 doses in the primary series) is common marker of vaccination coverage.
Hib (Haemophilus influenzae B)	6 wk-59 mo	3 / 2-3	4 wk w/ DTP2 / 8 wk if only 2 doses / 4 wk if 3 doses	4 wk w/ DTP3 / 4 wk if 3 doses		At least 6 mo after last dose		Important cause of pneumonia and meningitis, especially in children <2 yr old. Single dose if >12 mo old. Not recommended for children >5 yr
Pneumococcus (PCV10 or 13)	6 wk / 6 wk	3 / 2-3	4 wk / 8 wk	4 wk		Yes, if not given at 10 wk 9-15 mo		Important cause of pneumonia, sepsis, and meningitis. Not for children >5 yr old
Rotavirus	6 wk w/ DTP1 / 6 wk w/ DTP1	Rotarix: 6 wk w/ DTP1 / Rota Teq: 6 wk w/ DTP1	4 wk w/ DTP2 / 4-10 wk w/ DTP2	4 wk w/ DTP3				Not recommended if >24 mo old
Measles	9 or 12 mo	2	4 wk					All children should have 2 doses of measles vaccine. High-transmission, high-mortality countries should start at 9 mo to decrease mortality.
Rubella	9 or 12 mo (w/ measles-containing vaccines)	1					1 dose (adolescent girls and/or childbearing-age women, if not previously vaccinated)	Goal is to prevent CRS. >80% coverage is needed to avoid increasing risk for CRS by continued presence of unimmunized pregnant women who were not exposed as children.
HPV	9 yr (female)	2	6 mo				2 doses (female)	Target 9-14 yr old girls, pregnancy 15 yr: 3 doses. HIV infection and immunocompromised

CRS, Congenital rubella syndrome; IPV, inactivated polio vaccine; TB, tuberculosis.
Adapted from WHO Routine Guidelines for Immunization. http://www.who.int/immunization/policy/Immunization_routine_table2.pdf?ua=1.

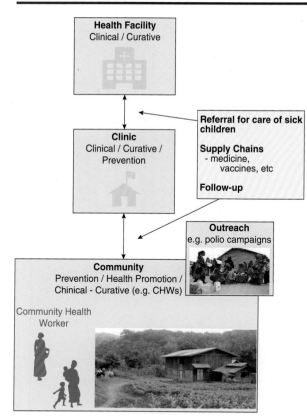

Fig. 3.9 Health services delivery systems.

is the single largest contributor to the global burden of disease for individuals age 15-19, and **suicide** is 1 of the 3 leading causes of mortality among people age 15-35. Efforts to tackle these problems will require an interdisciplinary approach, with more research needed to identify and evaluate interventions and effectively influence adolescent behavior in low- and middle-income countries.

Global Climate Change

Global climate change is currently the most urgent and alarming challenge to the environment. Contributing to environmental degradation, the loss of natural resources and change in climate undermine food and water sources. Climate change and increased frequency and severity of humanitarian crises adversely impact children health and nutrition, as well as threaten their education and development by disrupting school and home.

Conflict, Emergency Situations, and Migration

During times of crisis, children and adolescents are most vulnerable. Although the youngest are most likely to perish from disease or injuries, all children suffer as a result of food shortages, poor water and sanitation, interrupted education, and family separation or displacement. Approximately 214 million migrants live outside their countries of birth, which includes 33 million young children and adolescents under age 20 who have migrated either with their parents or unaccompanied. Many other children are directly or indirectly affected by migration, by parental separation, from deportation, or emigration.

Children and adolescents crossing borders may not be entitled to the same protection and rights as those who reside in a given country, leaving them at greater risk of discrimination and exploitation. A *rights-based* approach to migration is required to reinforce the steady buildup of national and international support. This approach must also address the root causes of migration (e.g., instability, inequality, discrimination, poverty) in the country of origin and should incorporate policies specifically targeted for young children and adolescents, girls and young women, and vulnerable populations, including those left behind when family members migrate.

Information and Communications Technology

Social network sites, mobile phones, programmers, and other stakeholders are implementing methods to appeal to youth in middle-income countries, harnessing this technology and their attention to increase awareness and build health skills. Parents and educators raise concern about the well-being and safety of children and adolescents who use these tools. The exposure to the immense amount of information on the internet places their privacy and psychological well-being at risk, since adults have not caught up to fully understand the implications.

Bibliography is available at Expert Consult.

particularly among females. The development of adolescents' capacities and values through education can empower an entire generation to become economically independent, positive contributors to society and break the cycle of poverty.

Other threats to adolescent health include mental health, substance abuse, sexual and reproductive health, and noncommunicable diseases (NCDs), such as obesity, which vary depending on country type (Fig. 3.11). A common theme for these threats is that interventions to combat these issues must attempt to influence individual behavior and attitudes while promoting healthy lifestyles. It is estimated that 20% of the world's adolescents have a mental health or behavioral problem. **Depression**

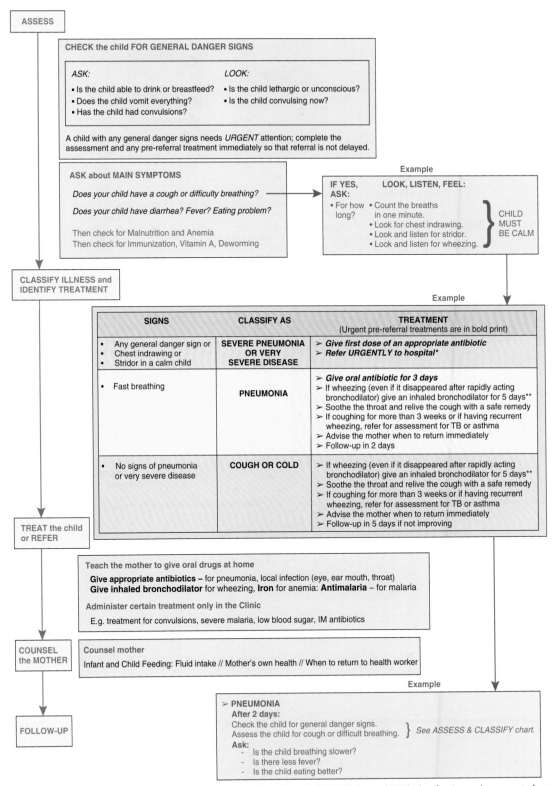

Fig. 3.10 Integrated Management of Childhood Illness (IMCI). (*Adapted from WHO 2014. Revised WHO classification and treatment of pneumonia in children at health facilities: evidence summaries; and WHO 2008. Integrated Management of Childhood Illness Booklet* http://apps.who.int/iris/bitstream/handle/10665/43993/9789241597289_eng.pdf;jsessionid=43EF43A92BDA8FBD35A835842F7280E4?sequence=1)

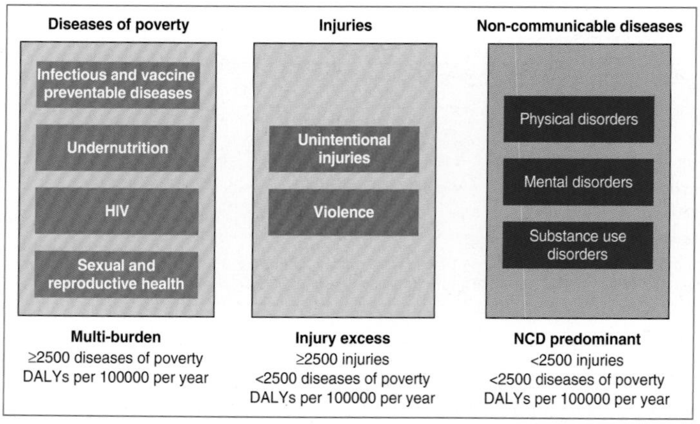

Fig. 3.11 Country categorization based on adolescent burden of disease. Categorization into 3 groups according to adolescent burden of disease and reflecting passage through epidemiologic transition. DALYs, Disability-adjusted life-years; HIV, human immunodeficiency virus; NCD, noncommunicable diseases. (*From Patton GC, Sawyer SM, Santelli JS, et al: Our future: a Lancet commission on adolescent health and wellbeing, Lancet 387:2423–2478, 2016, Fig 7.*)

Chapter 4
Quality and Value in Healthcare for Children
Jeffrey M. Simmons and Samir S. Shah

第四章
儿童医疗健康的性价比

中文导读

本章主要介绍了提高质量和效益（性价比）的必要性、质量的内涵、质量框架、建立与制定质量标准相关的指南、质量优化、质量测量、质量分析、质量对比和报告、美国医疗改革对医疗质量产生的影响、信息技术与质量改进，以及将个人质量改进计划向规模化扩展。在质量优化中具体阐述了质量优化模型、六个西格玛、精益方法、管理学，以及建设质量改进理论和措施所使用的工具。

THE NEED FOR IMPROVEMENT IN QUALITY AND VALUE

Adults and children only receive recommended evidence-based care about half the time. The gap between knowledge and practice widens to a *chasm* in part because of variations in practice and disparities in care from doctor to doctor, institution to institution, geographic region to geographic region, and socioeconomic group to socioeconomic group.

Furthermore, it is estimated that it takes about 17 yr for new knowledge to be adopted into clinical practice.

In addition to appropriate care that patients do not receive, U.S. healthcare systems also deliver much care that is unnecessary and waste many resources in doing so. This overuse and waste is one **key driver** of the disproportionate costs of care in the United States compared with other developed countries' delivery systems (in 2016, the United

States spent about twice as much per capita, adjusting for gross domestic product (GDP), on healthcare compared to the average of peer wealthy nations). It is estimated that more than one quarter of all U.S. healthcare spending is waste. Gaps in appropriate care, combined with overuse and high costs, have driven conversations about the need to improve the value of care, which would mean better quality at lower overall costs. **Choosing Wisely**, an initiative initially sponsored by the American Board of Internal Medicine and subsequently endorsed by the American Academy of Pediatrics (AAP), asked medical societies to identify practices typically overused that clinicians could then make collective efforts to address.

Quality improvement (QI) science has become a predominant method utilized to close gaps and improve value. Initially focused on improving performance and reliability in care processes, more recently, in part inspired by the Institute for Healthcare Improvement's **Triple Aim** approach, QI is being used to improve value for *populations* of patients by focusing more on *outcomes* defined by patients' needs. The **Quadruple Aim** approach adds the 4th dimension of healthcare worker experience or *joy in work* to focus delivery systems on the need to enhance the resiliency of the clinical workforce in order to sustain high-value care approaches.

WHAT IS QUALITY?

The Institute of Medicine (IOM) defines *quality* of healthcare as "the degree to which healthcare services for individuals and populations increases the likelihood of desired health outcomes and are consistent with current professional knowledge." This definition incorporates 2 key concepts related to healthcare quality: the direct relationship between the provision of healthcare services and health outcomes, and the need for healthcare services to be based on current evidence.

To measure healthcare quality, the IOM has identified *Six Dimensions of Quality*: **effectiveness, efficiency, equity, timeliness, patient safety**, and **patient-centered care**. Quality of care needs to be *effective*, which means that healthcare services should result in benefits and outcomes. Healthcare services also need to be *efficient*, which incorporates the idea of avoiding waste and improving system cost efficiencies. Healthcare quality should improve *patient safety*, which incorporates the concept of patient safety as 1 of the key elements in the Six Dimensions of Quality. Healthcare quality must be *timely*, thus incorporating the need for appropriate access to care (see Chapter 5). Healthcare quality should be *equitable*, which highlights the importance of minimizing variations as a result of ethnicity, gender, geographic location, and socioeconomic status (SES). Healthcare quality should be *patient centered*, which underscores the importance of identifying and incorporating individual patient needs, preferences, and values in clinical decision-making. In pediatrics, the patient-centered dimension extends to family-centeredness, so that the needs, preferences, and values of parents and other child caregivers are considered in care decisions and system design.

The IOM framework emphasizes the concept that all Six Dimensions of Quality need to be met for the provision of *high-quality* healthcare. Collectively, these concepts represent *quality* in the overall *value* proposition of quality per cost. From the standpoint of the practicing physician, these 6 dimensions can be categorized into *clinical quality* and *operational quality*. To provide high-quality care to children, both aspects of quality—clinical and operational—must be met. Historically, physicians have viewed quality to be limited in scope to clinical quality, with the goal of improving clinical outcomes, while considering improving efficiency and patient access to healthcare as the role of healthcare plans, hospitals, and insurers. Healthcare organizations, which are subject to regular accreditation requirements, viewed the practice of clinical care delivery as the responsibility of physicians and limited their efforts to improve quality largely to process improvement to enhance efficiencies.

The evolving healthcare system requires physicians, healthcare providers, hospitals, and healthcare organizations to partner together and with patients to define, measure, and improve the overall quality of care delivered. Concrete examples of the evolving U.S. perspective include the widespread adoption of **Maintenance of Certification** (MOC) requirements by medical-certifying bodies, which require providers to engage in activities that improve care in their practices, and the core quality measurement features and population health incentives of the **Patient Protection and Affordable Care Act (ACA)** of 2010. The ACA also established the **Patient-Centered Outcomes Research Institute (PCORI)** to develop a portfolio of effectiveness and implementation research that requires direct engagement of patients and families to partner in setting research priorities, formulating research questions, and designing studies that will directly impact the needs of patients to improve the value of the research.

FRAMEWORK FOR QUALITY

Quality is broader in scope than QI. The approach to quality includes 4 building blocks. *First*, the **standard for quality** must be defined (i.e., developing evidence-based guidelines, best practices, or policies that guide the clinician for the specific clinical situation). These guidelines should change based on new evidence. In 2000–2001 the AAP had published guidelines for care of children with attention-deficit/hyperactivity disorder (ADHD). Subsequently, in 2011, these were updated to highlight a greater emphasis on *behavioral interventions* rather than pharmacologic options based on new evidence. Similarly, the AAP has emphasized that guidelines evolve to include greater consideration of value in care, an example being the update to the clinical practice guideline for urinary tract infection in 2011, which called for a decrease in the use of screening radiologic tests and prophylactic antibiotics in certain populations of children due to a lack of cost-effectiveness. *Second*, **gaps in quality** need to be closed. One key gap is the difference between the recommended care and the actual care delivered to a patient. *Third*, quality needs to be **measured**. Quality measures can be developed as measures for accountability and measures for improvement. Accountability measures are developed with a high level of demonstrated rigor because these are used for measuring and comparing the quality of care at the state, regional, or health system (macro) level. Often, accountability measures are linked to **pay-for-performance (P4P)** incentive arrangements for enhanced reimbursement at the hospital and individual physician level. In contrast, improvement measures are metrics that can demonstrate the improvement accompanying a discrete QI project or program. These metrics need to be locally relevant, nimble, and typically have not had rigorous field testing. *Fourth*, the quality measurement approach should be used to **advocate** for providers and patients. For providers, meeting quality goals should be a key aspect of reimbursement if the system is designed to incentivize high-value care. At the population level, quality measurement strategies should advocate for preventive and early childhood healthcare, improving the value of care by decreasing costs across a patient's life span.

Lastly, many quality measurement systems have attempted to be more transparent with clinicians and patients about **costs** of care. Because more direct costs have been shifted to patients and families through widespread adoption of high-deductible insurance plans (i.e., families experience lower up-front insurance coverage costs but pay for certain acute healthcare expenses out-of-pocket until the preset deductible is met), better awareness of costs has become a more effective driver of improvement in value, in part by reducing overuse.

DEVELOPING GUIDELINES TO ESTABLISH THE STANDARD FOR QUALITY

Guidelines need to be developed based on accepted recommendations, such as the Grading of Recommendations Assessment, Development and Evaluation (**GRADE**) system for rating the quality and strength of the evidence, which is crucial for guideline development. Guidelines must adopt a high level of transparency in the development process. This is particularly relevant in the pediatric setting, where there may be limited research using methods such as randomized controlled trials (RCTs), which would have a high level of rating from an evidence standpoint. Because guidelines and policies related to quality need to be interpreted for specific settings, they should not be interpreted as "standards of care."

IMPROVING QUALITY

The applied science of QI currently in use in healthcare is also firmly grounded in the classic scientific method of observation, hypothesis, and planned experimentation. There are 4 key features of the applied science of quality improvement: appreciation of systems, understanding variation, knowledge theory, and psychology of change. In addition to this theoretical framework, statistical analytic techniques evolved to better evaluate variable systems over time. While each derives key features from this applied scientific foundation, multiple QI methodologies are currently in use in healthcare. At their most parsimonious level, each method can be described as a 3-step model: *Data → Information → Improvement*. Quality needs to be measured. Data obtained from measurement needs to be converted into meaningful information that can be analyzed, compared, and reported. Information must then be *actionable* to achieve improvements in clinical practice and health systems' processes.

Model for Improvement

The Model for Improvement is structured around 3 key questions: (1) What are we trying to accomplish? (2) How will we know that a change is an improvement? and (3) What change can we make that will result in improvement? Clarifying the first question, the *goal*, is critical and is often a step skipped by clinicians, who typically already have change ideas in mind. The second question is about defining measures, with an emphasis on practicality and efficiency. The third question is about defining testable ideas for improvement, which are subsequently tested using a framework of rapid cycle improvement, also known as the **plan-do-study-act (PDSA) cycle** (Fig. 4.1A). The PDSA cycle is typically aimed at testing small, care process changes in iterative, rapid cycles. After discrete testing periods, results are analyzed, and the next cycle of change testing is planned and implemented (i.e., multiple PDSA cycles, often called a PDSA *ramp*, build on previous learning from PDSAs; Fig. 4.1B). Valuable information can be obtained from PDSA cycles that are successful, and those that are not, to help plan the next iteration of the PDSA cycle. The PDSA cycle specifically requires that improvements be data driven. Many clinicians attempt to make changes for improvement in their practice based on clinical intuition rather than on interpretation of empirical data.

The Model for Improvement has been successfully used in the Vermont Oxford Network (VON) to achieve improvements in care in the neonatal intensive care unit (NICU) setting. The VON is a global network of collaborating NICUs involved in several studies that have favorably impacted the care of newborns. An example of a successful VON QI effort is a project aimed at reducing rates of chronic lung disease in extremely-low-birthweight infants. Clinical teams participating in this improvement effort used special reports from the VON database, reviewed the available evidence with content faculty experts, and then identified improvement goals. The teams received QI training through conference calls and emails for 1 yr. This effort resulted in a 37% increase in early surfactant administration for preterm infants.

One successful QI collaborative using the improvement model in the outpatient setting is related to improvement in remission rates and reduction in systemic corticosteroid use among children with inflammatory bowel disease (IBD, Crohn disease or ulcerative colitis). This work was supported by the **ImproveCareNow Network** (https://improvecarenow.org/), a learning health system. A *learning health system* is a collaborative endeavor organized around communities of patients, clinicians, and researchers working together to integrate research with QI (i.e., knowledge dissemination and implementation) to improve care delivery while advancing clinical research. The network model leverages the inherent motivation of participants to engage and contribute in a collaborative manner. Participants are supported by development of standard processes, such as common approaches to data transfer, measurement, and reporting, as well as emphasis on data transparency, and share knowledge, tools, and resources to accelerate learning and facilitate uptake of useful innovations. For the IBD network, outpatient gastroenterology practices standardized treatment approaches to align with existing evidence though QI interventions adapted to local circumstances, and therapeutic decisions for individual patients remained at the discretion of physicians and their patients. This network also developed methods to more fully engage patients, particularly adolescents,

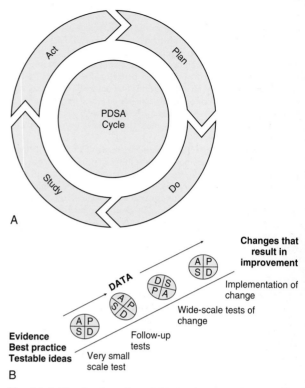

Fig. 4.1 **A,** The plan-do-study-act (PDSA) cycle. **B,** Use of PDSA cycles: a ramp. *(From Langley GJ: The improvement guide: a practical guide to enhancing organizational performance, San Francisco, 1996, Jossey-Bass. © 1996 by Gerald J. Langley, Kevin M. Nolan, Thomas W. Nolan, L. Norman, and Lloyd P. Provost.)*

and their caregivers through the use of social media, which helped drive improvement in some of the clinical behavior change aspects of the work.

Six Sigma

Six Sigma is related to the reduction in *undesirable variation in processes*. There are 2 types of variations in a process. **Random variation** refers to the variation that is inherent in a process simply because the process occurs within a system. Random variation in processes is expected in any system. In contrast, **special cause variation** refers to nonrandom variation that can impact a process and implies something in the system has been perturbed. For example, when tracking infection rates in a nursery, a sudden increase in the infection rates may be secondary to poor handwashing techniques by a new healthcare provider in the system. This would represent a special cause variation; once this provider's practice is improved, the system perturbation is resolved, and the infection rates will likely go back to the baseline level. Alternatively, improvement ideas are intended to perturb the system positively such that outcomes improve, ideally without exacerbating the variation in the system (Fig. 4.2). Six Sigma attempts to provide a structured approach to unwanted variations in healthcare processes. Six Sigma approaches have been successfully used in healthcare to improve processes in both clinical and nonclinical settings.

Lean Methodology

Lean methodology focuses on reducing waste within a process in a system. Fig. 4.3A illustrates the steps in the process of a patient coming to the emergency department (ED). After the initial registration, the patient is seen by a nurse and then the physician. In a busy ED, a patient may need to wait for hours before registration is complete and

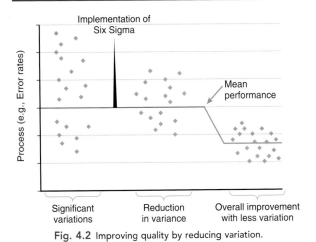

Fig. 4.2 Improving quality by reducing variation.

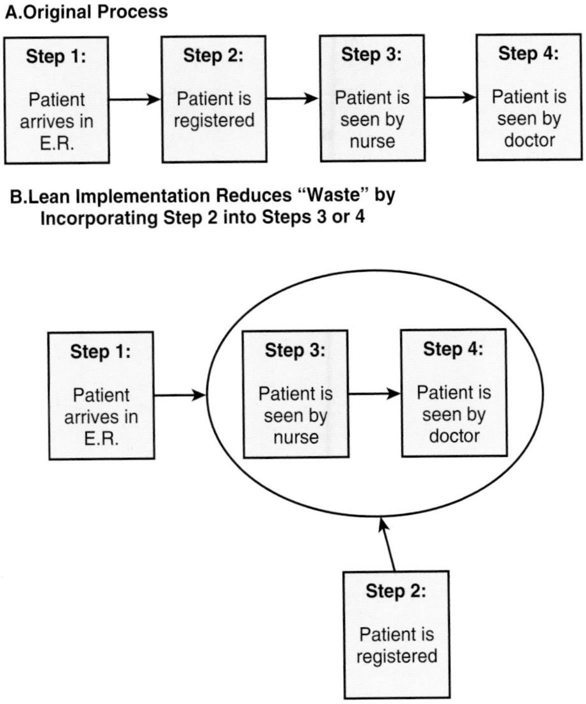

A. Original Process

Step 1: Patient arrives in E.R. → Step 2: Patient is registered → Step 3: Patient is seen by nurse → Step 4: Patient is seen by doctor

B. Lean Implementation Reduces "Waste" by Incorporating Step 2 into Steps 3 or 4

Step 1: Patient arrives in E.R. →

Step 3: Patient is seen by nurse → Step 4: Patient is seen by doctor

Step 2: Patient is registered

Fig. 4.3 A and B, Lean methodology—waste reduction.

the patient is placed in the examination room. This wait time is a waste from the perspective of the patient and the family. Incorporating the registration process after placing the patient in the physician examination room can save time and minimize waste (Fig. 4.3B). Lean methods have been successfully used in several outpatient and inpatient settings with resulting improvements in efficiency. Lean principles have also been adopted as a core strategy for many children's hospitals and health systems with the goal of improving efficiencies and reducing waste. These efforts can improve aspects of quality while also typically reducing costs.

Management Sciences

Management sciences, also known as *operations management*, stems from operations research and refers to the use of mathematical principles to maximize efficiencies within systems. Management sciences principles have been successful in many European healthcare settings to optimize efficiencies in outpatient primary care office settings, inpatient acute care hospital settings, and surgical settings including operating rooms, as well as for effective planning of transport and hospital expansion policies. Management sciences principles are being explored for use in the U.S. healthcare system; one technique, **discrete event simulation**, was used at the Children's Hospital of Wisconsin to plan the expansion of the pediatric critical care services with the goal of improving quality and safety. The discrete event simulation model illustrated in Fig. 4.4 depicts the various steps of the process in a pediatric intensive care unit (PICU). Patients stratified across 3 levels of severity (low, medium, high) are admitted to the PICU, are initially seen by a nurse and physician, then stay in the PICU with ongoing care provided by physicians and nurses, and finally are discharged from the PICU. The discrete event simulation model is a computer model developed using real estimates of numbers of patients, number of physicians and nurses in a PICU, and patient outcomes. Discrete event simulation models are created using real historical data, which allows testing the *what if* scenarios, such as the impact on patient flow and throughput by increasing the number of beds and/or changing nurse and physician staffing.

Another management sciences technique, **cognitive mapping**, measures the soft aspects of management sciences, as illustrated in Fig. 4.5. Cognitive mapping highlights the importance of perceptions and constructs of healthcare providers and the way these constructs are linked in a hierarchical manner. Goals and aspirations of individual healthcare providers are identified by structured interviews and are mapped to strategic issues and problems, and options. By using specialized computer software, complex relationships can be identified to better understand the relationships between different constructs in a system. A discrete event simulation model views patient throughput based on numbers of beds, physicians, and nurses, and accounts for differences

in patient mix. It does not account for many other factors, such as individual unit characteristics related to culture. By interviewing healthcare providers, cognitive maps can be developed that can help to better inform decision-making.

Tools for Organizing Quality Improvement Theory and Execution

QI efforts need to be organized around a theory of how the desired changes in outcome will be achieved. Multiple tools are available to help organize a QI team's thinking and execution. These tools typically help teams organize work into discrete projects or phases, and some of them also help teams develop change ideas.

Key driver diagrams (KDDs) are a tool to organize the theory of learning that underpins a QI project (Fig. 4.6), using the Model for Improvement. Important aspects of a KDD include a statement of the specific aim or improvement goal, a list of the key themes, or drivers, that are theorized to require improvement in order to achieve the aim, and lastly a list of the discrete change ideas or initiatives to be tested to determine whether or not they affect discrete drivers, and therefore the overall aim. Since most system outcomes are driven by multiple factors, a KDD allows a QI team to depict a theory that addresses multiple factors. Similarly, Lean and Six Sigma projects use a tool called an A3, that in addition to organizing the theory of a project, also prompts teams to assess the current state, and consider timelines and personnel for planned change (examples available at https://www.lean.org/common/display).

There are additional QI tools to help assess the current state of a system to better understand how to improve it. One, the **failure modes and effects analysis (FMEA)**, also helps teams develop change ideas (Fig. 4.7). Starting with a map of the processes in the current system, FMEA then asks teams to investigate and brainstorm the many ways discrete processes can go wrong—the *failure modes*. Once failure modes are identified, teams begin to develop discrete interventions or countermeasures to address the failures (see Chapter 5). A similar tool, the **fishbone** or **cause-and-effect** diagram, is organized around key

DES Model

- Mathematically depicts a 24-bed PICU
- Depicts the patient experience from admission to discharge
- Factors the staffing of physicians and nurses in the PICU using historical experience
- DES Model starts with baseline and runs computer iterations to identify predicted outcomes with changing patient flow and staffing
- Results of DES Model provide insight into predicted outcomes of changing bed/staffing assumptions

Illustration of DES Model

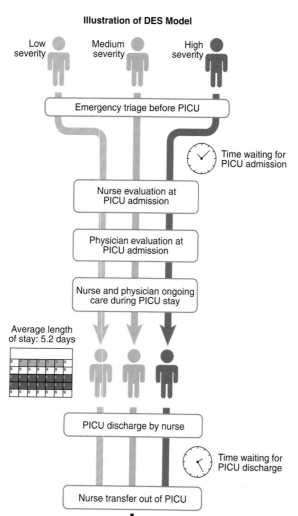

Conclusions

- Simply adding new PICU beds will not improve patient flow in itself
- Critical ratio between MDs, RNs, and beds in PICU adjusted for patient severity is needed to maximize patient flow, safety, and outcomes

Fig. 4.4 Management sciences—discrete event stimulation. PICU, Pediatric intensive care unit.

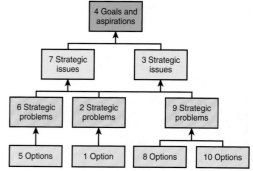

Fig. 4.5 Management sciences—cognitive mapping.

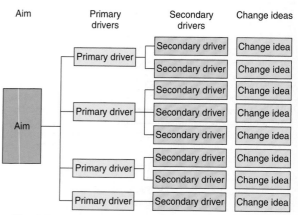

Fig. 4.6 Key driver diagram: theory of how to achieve an aim.

(Fig. 4.8). A Pareto chart typically displays the individual prevalence of discrete problems, determined by baseline analysis of data, as well as the cumulative prevalence, helping teams see which problems should be addressed first, to maximize impact on the overall outcome.

MEASURING QUALITY

Robust quality indictors should have clinical and statistical relevance. *Clinical relevance* ensures that the indicators are meaningful to patient care from the standpoint of patients and clinicians. *Statistical relevance* ensures that the indicators have measurement properties to allow an acceptable level of accuracy and precision. These concepts are captured in the national recommendations that quality measures must meet the criteria of being valid, reliable, feasible, and usable (Table 4.1). **Validity** of quality measures refers to the measure being an estimate of the true concept of interest. **Reliability** refers to the measure being reproducible and providing the same result if retested. It is important that quality measures are **feasible** in practice, with an emphasis on how the data to support the measures are collected. Quality measures must be **usable**, which means that they should be clinically meaningful. The **Agency for Healthcare Research and Quality** and the **National Quality Forum** have provided specific criteria to be considered when developing quality measures.

Quality indicators can be used to measure the performance within 3 components of healthcare delivery: structure, process, and outcome. **Structure** refers to the *organizational characteristics* in healthcare delivery. Examples of organizational characteristics are the number of physicians and nurses in an acute care setting and the availability and use of systems such as electronic health records. **Process** measures estimate how services

components in a system (e.g., people, material, machines) and helps teams catalog how deficiencies in each component can affect the overall outcome of a system.

A final key tool to help teams prioritize action is a **Pareto chart**, which organizes system deficiencies in terms of their prevalence

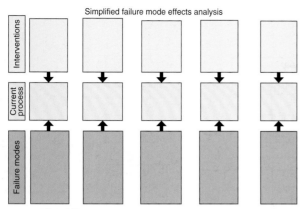

Fig. 4.7 Failure modes and effects analysis (FMEA).

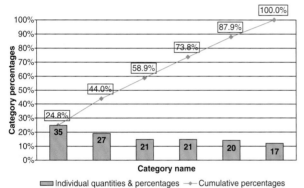

Fig. 4.8 Pareto chart.

Table 4.1	Properties of Robust Quality Measures
ATTRIBUTE	**RELEVANCE**
Validity	Indicator accurately captures the concept being measured.
Reliability	Measure is reproducible.
Feasibility	Data can be collected using paper or electronic records.
Usability	Measure is useful in clinical practice.

time. Sources of data vary in terms of reliability and accuracy, which will influence *rigor* and therefore appropriate-use cases for the data; many national databases invest significant resources in implementing processes to improve data reliability and accuracy.

It is important to distinguish between databases and data registries. *Databases* are data repositories that can be as simple as a Microsoft Excel spreadsheet or as complex as relational databases using sophisticated servers and information technology platforms. Databases can provide a rich source of aggregated data for both quality measurement and research. *Data registries* allow tracking individual patients over time; this dynamic and longitudinal characteristic is important for population health management and QI.

Data quality can become a significant impediment when using data from secondary sources, which can adversely impact the overall quality evaluation. Once data on the quality indicator have been collected, quality measurement can occur at 3 levels: (1) measuring quality status at one point in time (e.g., percent of children seen in a primary care office setting who received the recommended 2-year immunizations); (2) tracking performance over time (e.g., change in immunization rates in the primary care office setting for children 2 yr of age); and (3) comparing performance across clinical settings after accounting for epidemiologic confounders (e.g., immunization rates for children <2 yr of age in a primary care office setting stratified by race and SES as compared to the rates of other practices in community and national rates).

Pediatric quality measures are being developed nationally. Table 4.2 lists some currently endorsed pediatric national quality indicators.

ANALYZING QUALITY DATA

Three approaches have been used for analyzing and reporting data. The classic approach from a research paradigm has been applied to quality data for statistically comparing trends over time, and differences before and after an intervention. P-values are interpreted as being significant if ≤0.05, which suggests that the likelihood of seeing a difference as extreme as observed has a probability of ≤5% (type I error). Another approach from an improvement science paradigm uses techniques such as run charts and control charts to identify special cause variation. In the context of quality improvement, special cause variation in the desired direction is the intent, and these analytic techniques allow improvers to quickly recognize statistically significant changes in system performance over time. Lastly, quality data also have been reported on an individual patient level. This has gained popularity in the patient safety arena, where identifying individual patient events in the form of descriptive analysis (*stories*) may be more powerful in motivating a culture of change than statistical reporting of aggregate data in the form of rates of adverse patient safety events (see Chapter 5).

COMPARING AND REPORTING QUALITY

There is an increasing emphasis on quality reporting in the United States. Many states have mandatory policies for the reporting of quality data. This reporting may be tied to reimbursement using the policy of P4P, which implies that reimbursements by insurers to hospitals and physicians will be partially based on the quality metrics. P4P can include both incentives and disincentives. *Incentives* relate to additional payments for meeting certain quality thresholds. *Disincentives* relate to withholding

are provided; examples are the percentage of families of children with asthma who receive an asthma action plan as part of their office visit and percentage of hospitalized children who have documentation of pain assessments as part of their care. **Outcome** measures refer to the final health status of the child; examples are risk-adjusted survival in an intensive care unit setting, birthweight-adjusted survival in the NICU setting, and functional status of children with chronic conditions such as cystic fibrosis.

It is important to distinguish between measures for accountability and measures for improvement. Measures, particularly measures for accountability that may be linked to attribution and payment must be based on a rigorous process (Fig. 4.9). This can be resource intensive and time-consuming. In contrast, measures for improvement serve a different purpose—to track incremental improvements linked to specific QI efforts. These may not undergo rigorous testing, but they have limited applicability beyond the specific QI setting.

Quality data can be quantitative and qualitative. *Quantitative* data includes numerical data, which can be *continuous* (patient satisfaction scores represented as a percentage with higher numbers indicating better satisfaction) or *categorical* (patient satisfaction scores from a survey using a Likert scale indicating satisfactory, unsatisfactory, good, or superior care). Data can also be *qualitative* in nature, which includes nonnumerical data. Examples of qualitative data can include results from open-ended surveys related to the satisfaction of care in a clinic or hospital setting.

Data measuring quality of care can be obtained from a variety of sources, which include chart reviews, patient surveys, existing administrative data sources (billing data from hospitals), disease and specialty databases, and patient registries, which track individual patients over

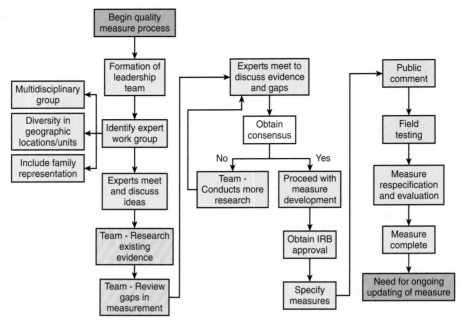

Fig. 4.9 Development of a rigorous quality measure.

Table 4.2	Examples of National Pediatric Quality Measures			
NQF PEDIATRIC QUALITY INDICATORS	**NQF-ENDORSED INPATIENT MEASURES AMONG PICUs**	**NQF-ENDORSED INPATIENT PEDIATRIC CARE MEASURES**	**NQF-ENDORSED OUTPATIENT PEDIATRIC CARE MEASURES**
Neonatal bloodstream infection rate Transfusion reaction Gastroenteritis admission rate	PICU standardized mortality ratio PICU severity-adjusted length of stay PICU unplanned readmission rate	CAC-1 relievers for inpatient asthma CAC-2 systemic corticosteroids for inpatient asthma Admit decision time to ED departure time for admitted patients Follow-up after hospitalization for mental illness (FUH) NHSN Catheter-Associated Urinary Tract Infection (CAUTI) outcome measure NHSN Central Line-Associated Bloodstream Infection (CLABSI) outcome measure Percent of residents or patients assessed and appropriately given the pneumococcal vaccine (short stay) Restraint prevalence (vest and limb) Validated family-centered survey questionnaire for parents' and patients' experiences during inpatient pediatric hospital stay Nursing hours per patient day Preventive care and screening: screening for clinical depression and follow-up plan Skill mix (RN, LVN/LPN, UAP, and contract)	Appropriate testing for children with pharyngitis CAHPS clinician/group surveys (adult primary care, pediatric care, and specialist care surveys) Child and adolescent major depressive disorder: diagnostic evaluation Child and adolescent major depressive disorder: suicide risk assessment Follow-up after hospitalization for mental illness (FUH) Median time from ED arrival to ED departure for discharged ED patients Pediatric symptom checklist (PSC)

CAC, Children's Asthma Care; CAHPS, Consumer Assessment of Healthcare Providers and Systems; ED, emergency department; HBIPS, hospital-based inpatient psychiatric services; LVN/LPN, licensed vocational/practical nurse; NHSN, National Healthcare Safety Network; NQF, National Quality Forum; PICU, pediatric intensive care unit; RACHS-1, risk adjustment for congenital heart surgery; RN, registered nurse; UAP, unlicensed assistive personnel.

certain payments for not meeting those quality thresholds. An extension of the P4P concept relates to the implementation of the policy of **nonreimbursable hospital-acquired conditions**, formerly called *never events* by the Centers for Medicare and Medicaid Services. CMS has identified a list of hospital-acquired conditions, which are specific quality events that will result in no payment for care provided to patients, such as wrong-site surgery, catheter-associated bloodstream infection (CA-BSI), and decubitus ulcers. This approach has not yet been widely implemented for pediatric patients.

Quality reporting is also being used in a voluntary manner as a business growth strategy. Leading U.S. children's hospitals actively compete to have high ratings in national quality evaluations that are reported in publications such as *Parents* (formerly *Child*) magazine and *US News & World Report*. Many children's hospitals have also developed their own websites for voluntarily reporting their quality information for greater transparency. Although greater transparency may provide a competitive advantage to institutions, the underlying goal of transparency is to improve the quality of care being delivered, and for families to be able to make informed choices in selecting hospitals and physicians for their children.

Quality measures may also be used for purposes of certifying individual physicians as part of the Maintenance of Certification process. In the past, specialty and subspecialty certification in medicine, including pediatrics, was largely based on demonstrating a core fund of knowledge by being successful in an examination. No specific evidence of competency in actual practice needed to be demonstrated beyond successful completion of a training program. There continues to be significant variations in practice patterns even among physicians who are board certified, which highlights the concept that medical knowledge is important, but not sufficient for the delivery of high-quality care. Subsequently, the American Board of Medical Specialties, including its member board, the American Board of Pediatrics, implemented the MOC process in 2010. Within the MOC process, there is a specific requirement (Part IV) for the physician to demonstrate the assessment of quality of care and implementation of improvement strategies as part of recertification in pediatrics and pediatric subspecialties. Lifelong learning and the translation of learning into practice are the basis for the MOC process and an essential competency for physicians' professionalism. There are also discussions to adopt a similar requirement for Maintenance of Licensure for physicians by state medical regulatory boards.

The Accreditation Council for Graduate Medical Education requires residency programs to incorporate QI curriculum to ensure that systems-based practice and QI are part of the overall competencies within accredited graduate medical training programs. One form of continuing medical education, **performance improvement**, is used for ongoing physician education. These initiatives require physicians to measure the quality of care they deliver to their patients, to compare their performance to peers or known benchmarks, and to work toward improving their care by leveraging QI methods. This forms a feedback loop for continued learning and improvement in practice.

Prior to comparing quality measures data both within and across clinical settings, it is important to perform risk adjustment to the extent that is feasible. **Risk adjustment** is the statistical concept that utilizes measures of underlying severity or risk so that the outcomes can be compared in a meaningful manner. The importance of risk adjustment was highlighted in the PICU setting many years ago. The unadjusted mortality rate for large tertiary care centers was significantly higher than that for smaller hospital settings. By performing **severity of illness** risk adjustment, it was subsequently shown that the risks in tertiary care, large PICUs were higher because patients had higher levels of severity of illness. Although this concept is now intuitive for most clinicians, the use of severity of illness models in this study allowed a mathematical estimate of patient severity using physiologic and laboratory data, which allowed for the statistical adjustment of outcomes. This permits meaningful comparisons of the outcomes of large and small critical care units. Severity of illness models and the concepts of statistical risk adjustment are most developed in pediatric critical care. However, these concepts are relevant for all comparisons of outcomes in the hospital settings where sicker patients may be transferred to the larger institutions for care, and therefore would be expected to have poorer outcomes than other settings with less sick patients.

Risk adjustment can be performed at 3 levels. First, patients who are sicker can be excluded from the analysis, thereby allowing the comparisons to be within homogeneous groups. Although this approach is relatively simple to use, it is limited in that it would result in patient groups being excluded from the analysis. Second, risk stratification can be performed using measures of patient acuity; for example, in the **All-Patient Refined Diagnosis-Related Group** system, patients can be grouped or stratified into different severity criteria based on acuity weights. This approach may provide more homogeneous strata within which comparisons can be performed. Third, severity of illness risk adjustment can use clinical data to predict the outcomes for patient groups, such as the **Pediatric Risk of Mortality (PRISM)** scoring system in the PICU setting. In the PRISM score and its subsequent iterations, physiologic and laboratory perimeters are weighted on a statistical logistic

scale to predict mortality risk within that PICU admission. By comparing the observed and expected outcomes (i.e., mortality or survival), a quantitative estimate of the performance of that PICU can be established, which can then be used to compare outcomes with other PICUs (standardized mortality ratio).

Risk adjustment systems have been effectively incorporated into specialty databases. For example, the **Virtual Pediatric Intensive Care Unit System (VPS)** represents the pediatric critical care database system in the United States. Comprising >100 PICUs and pediatric cardiac ICUs across the United States, as well as international PICUs, the VPS currently has >300,000 patients within its database. The VPS database emphasizes data validity and reliability to ensure that the resulting data are accurate. Data validity has been established using standard data definitions with significant clinical input. Data reliability is established using interrater reliability to ensure that the manual data collection that involves several data collectors within pediatric institutions is consistent. The PRISM scoring system is programmed into the VPS software to allow the rapid estimation of the severity of illness of individual patients. This in turn allows risk adjustment of the various outcomes, which are compared within institutions over time and across institutions for purposes of QI.

IMPLICATIONS OF THE U.S. HEALTHCARE REFORM FOR QUALITY

Regarding quality of healthcare for children, healthcare reform had 3 key implications. First, expanded insurance coverage optimized access and include expanded coverage for young adults to age 26 yr. Second, various initiatives related to quality, safety, patient-centered outcomes research, and innovation were implemented and funded. For example, the **Agency for Healthcare Research and Quality** (AHRQ) funded a national effort to establish 7 centers of excellence through the **Pediatric Quality Measurement Program** (PQMP) to improve existing pediatric quality measures and create new measures that can be used by states and in a variety of other settings to evaluate quality of care for children. Third, reform advocated a paradigm shift in the existing model of healthcare delivery from vertical integration toward a model of *horizontal* integration. This has led to the creation and rapid growth of integrated delivery systems and risk-sharing relationships of **accountable care organizations (ACOs)**. Population health outcomes from these changes remain uncertain, although it appears healthcare cost inflation may have slowed somewhat.

Another area of increasing emphasis is **population health**. This is important because it expands the traditional role of physicians to improve quality of care for individual patients also to improve the quality of care for larger populations. Populations can be defined by geographic constraints or disease/patient condition. Efforts to link payment and reimbursement for care delivery by physicians and health systems are being increasingly tied to measurable improvements in population health. To achieve a meaningful improvement in population outcome, physician practices will need to embrace the emerging paradigm of practice transformation, whose many facets include the adoption of a **medical home**, the seamless connectivity across the primary care and subspecialty continuum, and a strong connection between the medical and social determinants of healthcare delivery. To implement successful practice transformation, hospitals are increasingly adopting a broader view to evolve into healthcare systems that serve children across the entire range of the care continuum, including preventive and primary care, acute hospital care, and partnerships with community organizations for enhancing the social support structure. In addition, new risk-sharing payment models are evolving, resulting in the growth of entities such as ACOs, which represent a financial risk-sharing model across primary and subspecialty care and hospitals.

INFORMATION TECHNOLOGY AND QUALITY IMPROVEMENT

Health information technology (HIT) is a critical component in the effort to improve quality. HIT includes electronic health records, personal health records, and health information exchange. The purpose of a well-functioning **electronic health record** is to allow collection and

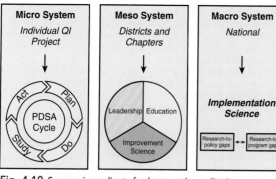

Fig. 4.10 Success ingredients for large-scale quality improvement.

storage of patient data in an electronic form, to allow this information to be efficiently provided to clinicians and healthcare providers, to have the ability to allow clinicians to enter patient care orders through the computerized physician order entry, and to have the infrastructure to provide clinical decision support that will improve physician decision-making at the individual patient level. The **personal health record** allows patients and families to be more actively engaged in managing their own health by monitoring their clinical progress and laboratory information, as well as to communicate with their physicians to make appointments, obtain medications, and have questions answered. Appropriate, timely, and seamless sharing of patient information across physician networks and healthcare organizations is critical to quality care and to achieve the full vision of a medical home for children. **Health information exchange** allows the sharing of healthcare information in an electronic format to facilitate the appropriate connections between providers and healthcare organizations within a community or region.

EXPANDING INDIVIDUAL QUALITY IMPROVEMENT INITIATIVES TO SCALE

Despite the success of individual QI projects, the overall progress to achieve large-scale improvements to reach all children across the spectrum of geographic location and SES remains limited. This contributes to the health disparities that persist for children, with significant differences in access and quality of care. A potential factor that limits the full impact of QI is the lack of strategic alignment of improvement efforts with hospitals, health systems, and across states.

This challenge can be viewed from a system standpoint in being able to conduct and expand QI from a micro level (individual projects), to the meso level (regional), to the macro level (national and international). The learning from individual QI projects for addressing specific challenges can be expanded to the regional level by ensuring that there is optimal leadership, opportunity for education, and adoption of improvement science (Fig. 4.10). To further expand the learning to a national and international level, it is important to leverage implementation science to allow a strategic approach to the identification of the key factors that influence success. To leverage fully the synergies in order to impact the quality of care delivered to children, it is important for national and international healthcare organizations to collaborate effectively from a knowledge management and improvement standpoint (Table 4.3).

Bibliography is available at Expert Consult.

Table 4.3	National Organizations Involved in Pediatric Quality Improvement (QI)	
ORGANIZATION	**ROLE**	**ACTIVITIES**
American Academy of Pediatrics (AAP)	Represents more than 60,000 pediatricians and pediatric subspecialists worldwide	Resources for QI to improve health for all children, best practices, advocacy, policy, research and practice, and medical home
American Board of Pediatrics (ABP)	Certifying board for pediatrics and pediatric subspecialties	Certification policies and resources for activities such as Maintenance of Certification (MOC)
American Medical Association (AMA)	Physician member association	Physician Consortium for Performance Improvement (PCPI)—physician-led initiative
Children's Hospital Association (CHA)	Formerly the National Association of Children's Hospitals and Related Institutions; and the Child Health Corporation of America	Databases, QI collaboratives, and policy
Institute for Healthcare Improvement (IHI)	QI organization for adult and pediatric care	QI collaboratives, QI educational workshops and materials
National Initiative for Child Health Quality (NICHQ)	QI organization for pediatric care	QI training, improvement networks
The Joint Commission	Hospital accreditation organization	Unannounced surveys to evaluate quality of care in hospitals
National Committee for Quality Assurance (NCQA)	QI organization	Healthcare Effectiveness Data and Information Set (HEDIS) and quality measures for improvement
National Quality Forum (NQF)	Multidisciplinary group including healthcare providers, purchases, consumers, and accrediting bodies	Endorsing national quality measures, convening expert groups, and setting national priorities

Chapter **5**
Safety in Healthcare for Children
Patrick W. Brady and Jeffrey M. Simmons
第五章
儿童医疗健康安全

中文导读

本章主要介绍了差错和伤害、安全框架，介绍了如何识别和分析伤害、差错和潜在危险，介绍了安全文化素养、可靠性科学性与高可靠性组织、严重事故与相关医疗状况、安全的把握和疏漏以及医疗安全研究与改进的新兴领域等。具体阐述了事故报告系统、模拟演练和事件回顾分析等识别和分析伤害、差错和潜在危险的手段；具体阐述了在下列情况下安全的把握和疏漏：病情进行性恶化时、在I-PASS病人交接程序中、在外科医疗环境中和针对流动病人时，以及整体职业安全等。

Children may be harmed by the healthcare that aims to make them better. Such harms include central line–associated bloodstream infections (CLA-BSIs) and medication overdoses. In 1991 the Harvard Medical Practice Study reviewed a large sample of adult medical records from New York State and found that adverse events occurred in an estimated 3.7% of hospitalizations. Most events gave rise to serious disability, and 13.6% led to death. The Institute of Medicine (IOM) estimated that as many as 98,000 Americans per year die in the hospital from medical errors.

Although fewer data are available for children, it is clear that children experience substantial healthcare-related harm. Nationally, hospitalized children experience approximately 1,700 CLA-BSIs and 84,000 adverse drug events each year. While the evidence is less robust, and not without controversy, substantial progress has been reported, particularly in **healthcare-associated conditions (HACs)**. Less strong epidemiologic estimates are available for adverse events in the ambulatory environment, but these events are likely more common than reported.

The **Solutions for Patient Safety (SPS)** collaborative started with the 8 children's hospitals in Ohio and has expanded to include >130 hospitals across the United States and Canada (http://www.solutionsforpatientsafety.org). The collaborative uses a learning network model to pursue the aim of eliminating serious harm across all children's hospitals. The American Academy of Pediatrics (AAP), Children's Hospital Association, and The Joint Commission (TJC) also have convened improvement collaboratives in pediatric safety. In addition, healthcare has recognized the high rates of healthcare worker injury and the critical role that the safety of healthcare providers plays in outcomes, burnout, and safe patient care.

ERROR VS HARM

Clinical leaders, improvers, and researchers often employ measures of error and harm to understand and improve safety, but the differences between these 2 measures can lead to confusion. **Errors** occur when a physician, nurse, or other member of the healthcare team does the wrong thing (*error of commission*) or fails to do the right thing (*error of omission*); errors of omission (e.g., not arriving at the right diagnosis) are considerably more difficult to measure. **Harm**, as defined by the Institute for Healthcare Improvement, is "unintended physical injury resulting from or contributed to by medical care (including the absence of indicated medical treatment), that requires additional monitoring, treatment, or hospitalization, or that results in death." Most errors in healthcare do not lead to harm; harm may be both preventable and nonpreventable (Fig. 5.1). A physician may erroneously fail to add a decimal point in a medication order for an aminoglycoside antibiotic, ordering a dose of 25 mg/kg rather than the intended dose of 2.5 mg/kg of gentamicin. If this error is caught by the computerized order entry system or the pharmacist, this would be an error with no resultant harm. If this error was not reviewed and caught by a pharmacist and reached the patient, who suffered acute kidney injury, this would be *preventable* harm since evidence shows that pharmacist review can reduce the risk of these errors 10-fold. Alternatively, if a patient received a first lifetime dose of amoxicillin and had anaphylaxis requiring treatment and hospital admission, this harm would be considered *nonpreventable* since no valid predictive tests are available for antibiotic allergy. Furthermore, the concept of **latent risk**, independent of any actual error, is inherent in any system where patients can be harmed. Among errors that do not lead to harm, **near misses** that do not reach

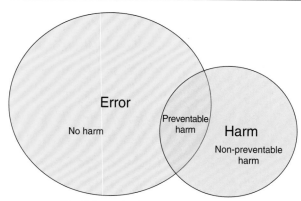

Fig. 5.1 Overlap between error and harm.

patients—or high-risk situations that do not lead to harm because of good fortune or mitigation—are important learning opportunities about safety threats.

Several classification systems exist to rate harm severity, including the NCC-MERP for medication-related harm and the severity scales for all-cause harm. **Serious safety events (SSEs)** are deviations from expected practice followed by death or severe harm. The SPS collaborative has SSE elimination as its primary goal. **Sentinel events** or **never events**, such as a wrong-site surgery, are also targets of external reporting as well as for elimination through quality improvement (QI) initiatives (see Chapter 4). Increasingly, health systems are using a *composite serious harm index*, which combines a variety of preventable HACs (e.g., CLA-BSIs) to examine system safety performance over time across various patient populations and sites of care.

SAFETY FRAMEWORKS

Safety frameworks are conceptual models and tools to help clinicians, improvers, and researchers understand the myriad contributors to safe healthcare and safety events. Healthcare is delivered in a complex system with many care providers and technologies, such as electronic health records and continuous physiologic monitors. The Donabedian framework, which links structure, process, and outcome, can be a very useful tool. The **Systems Engineering Initiative for Patient Safety (SEIPS)** model, developed by human factors engineers and cognitive psychologists at the University of Wisconsin–Madison, provides more detailed tools to understand the work system and the complex interactions between people and task work and technology and the environment. The SEIPS 2.0 model more prominently includes the patient and family in co-producing care outcomes. Other available safety frameworks include those from the Institute for Healthcare Improvement. The "Swiss cheese" model illustrates how an organization's defenses prevent failures from leading to harm, but only when the holes of the Swiss cheese slices, representing different components of the system, do not line up properly.

Traditionally, safety science and improvement have focused on identifying *what went wrong* (near misses, errors, and harm) and then tried to understand and improve the system of care that led these events. There is increasing focus on *what goes right*. This framework, called **Safety-II** to contrast with Safety-I and its focus on learning from what goes wrong, brings focus on the much greater number of things that go right and how people act every day to create safety in complex and unpredictable systems. Safety-II seeks to learn from people, the greatest source of system resilience, particularly in the midst of high levels of risk and stress, as often seen in healthcare.

IDENTIFYING AND ANALYZING HARM, ERRORS, AND LATENT THREATS

Health systems use a toolbox of processes to discover, understand, and mitigate unsafe conditions.

Incident Reporting Systems

Many health systems and hospitals offer employees access to a system to report errors, harms, or near misses. Most frequently, these are anonymous so that healthcare workers feel safe to submit an event in which they may have been involved, or when the harm involved someone in a position of authority. Ideally, these systems would facilitate smooth and efficient entry of enough information for further review but avoid excessive burden of time or cognitive load on the reporter. **Incident reporting** systems likely work best in the presence of a strong safety culture and when employees have some confidence that the event will be reviewed and actions taken. From studies that use more proactive assessment of harm and error, it is clear that incident reports dramatically *underreport* safety events. With this being the chief limitation, other mechanisms must also be in place to learn about safety. **Trigger tool** systems have been evaluated in pediatrics with encouraging results. These systems use *triggers*, such as the need for an antidote to an opioid overdose or the transfer of a patient to higher-level care, to facilitate targeted medical record review by trained nurses and physicians and elucidate any errors or system risks.

Simulation

Simulation is an excellent tool to better understand system and latent threats. *High-fidelity simulation* can allow clinicians to practice technical skills such as intubation in a safe environment; perhaps more importantly, simulation can help clinical teams improve non-technical skills such as using closed-loop communication and sharing a mental model (e.g., a team leader states, "I believe this patient has septic shock. We are rapidly infusing fluids and giving antibiotics. Blood pressure is normal for age. What other thoughts does the team have?"). It is often easier and more feasible to give feedback in a simulated scenario vs a real event.

Low-fidelity simulation on the hospital unit or in the clinic does not require costly simulated patients and may have advantages in identifying latent threats in the system. For example, a simulated scenario on a medical-surgical unit might identify that nurses do not know where to find a mask for continuous positive airway pressure (CPAP) to support an infant with respiratory failure. Identifying—and then mitigating—this latent threat in a simulated environment is preferable to doing so in an acutely deteriorating child.

Event Analysis

Several types of event analysis, including root cause analysis, apparent cause analysis, and common cause analysis, can help teams understand—and later mitigate—the causes of adverse events. Each model has its own strengths and weaknesses. **Root cause analysis (RCA)** is a useful, robust, and time-intensive process to ascertain the most fundamental, or *root*, causes of a safety event. TJC has required the use of RCA on sentinel events since 1997. Most health systems reserve this methodology primarily for sentinel events because RCAs can take months to complete and require convening a multidisciplinary team of experts. The safety event and its antecedents are reviewed in detail with a focus not on human behavior but instead on systems, hazards, and latent errors. The RCA team works to go beyond the event (e.g., enteral formula feeds connected to and administered through central line) to the proximal causes (e.g., "feeding tube and intravenous tubing are visually identical and are easily attached") and root cause (e.g., "organization lacks a system to assess human factors risks as new equipment is procured and put into practice"). When root causes are identified and tied to robust improvement action plans, safety can be substantially improved. In addition to the time-intensive nature of RCAs, *hindsight bias* is a risk and needs to be managed carefully by the team. Additional challenges with RCAs include the potential to *overfit solutions*—designing protocols or procedures that may have reduced the risk of the specific safety event reviewed but also introduce new problems and increase the probability of other safety threats—as well as difficulties in spreading solutions to different care areas that often have different needs, processes, and goals.

Apparent cause analysis, common cause analysis, and failure modes and effects analysis are complementary learning methods. **Apparent cause analysis** is performed by a smaller team and is feasible for events that occur often (e.g., the wrong medication is sent from pharmacy). Apparent cause analysis uses a multidisciplinary team to look for proximal causes. Importantly, in each analysis the team works to determine how likely it is that such an event will occur in the future and how widespread the proximate causes are in the microsystem. As with apparent cause analysis, **common cause analysis** seeks to aggregate learning across events. A similar common cause, such as poor handoff procedures, may lead to different safety events (e.g., a missed lab check and a delayed diagnosis); common cause analysis aids leaders in determining this. **Failure mode and effects analysis (FMEA)** is a powerful tool that clinicians use to describe a process and identify *failure modes*, or ways in which each step might fail. A more robust and quantitative form of FMEA rates potential failure modes in 3 categories: probability of event occurring, its severity, and its ability to be detected. The product of these, called the *risk priority number*, can help a team identify which failure modes may lead to the greatest harm and thus which to target first.

SAFETY CULTURE

A broad and supportive safety culture likely drives both patient and employee safety outcomes. An organization with a mature safety culture fosters a culture of learning and treats errors as opportunities to improve the system, rather than as the personal failures of individual clinicians. *Just culture* differentiates the mistakes and wrong decisions that a clinician makes commensurate with their training and experience from willful violations and gross or repeated patterns of negligence. A safety culture prioritizes clear and consistent communication and teamwork. Several tools are available to measure safety culture, including the Safety Attitudes Questionnaire and the Agency for Healthcare Research and Quality (AHRQ) surveys on Patient Safety Culture. A strong safety culture supports transfer of responsibility within disciplines at handoffs and across disciplines (e.g., when a nurse is calling a physician with a new concern). Structured communication tools such as the **Situation-Background-Assessment-Recommendation** (SBAR) approach are valued in a safety culture, as are safety behaviors such as "repeat back or write back," when a critical lab result is shared and repeated back by the receiving clinician. A safety culture also promotes teamwork and aims to ease authority gradients. Teamwork training can occur in simulation or in the clinical system. TeamSTEPPS (**Strategies and Tools to Enhance Performance and Patient Safety**) is a set of teamwork tools developed by AHRQ and the U.S. Department of Defense. It is an evidence-based training that facilitates learning in communication, leadership, situation monitoring, and mutual support.

Authority gradients are quite real in healthcare, and traditional medical culture may have done much to drive these. In a culture of safety, both junior and senior clinicians work together across disciplines to speak up when concerns are identified, to ask questions, and not to proceed if there is uncertainty about safe patient care. Unit/clinic and health system leaders have a critical role in supporting this culture, orienting new employees to its importance, and stepping in if authority gradients or disruptive behaviors contribute to safety events or unsafe conditions.

RELIABILITY SCIENCE AND HIGH-RELIABILITY ORGANIZATIONS

Reliability in healthcare is defined as the measurable capability of a process, procedure, or health service to perform its intended function in the required time under commonly occurring conditions. Most processes in healthcare organizations currently perform at **Level 1** reliability, meaning a success rate of only 80–90%. To achieve **Level 2** performance (≤5 failures/100 opportunities), processes must be *intentionally designed* with tools and concepts based on the principles of **human factors engineering** and **reliability science**. These processes include creating intentional redundancy, such as independent verification on high-risk medication dosing, and making the default action the desired action based on evidence, such as a default to an influenza vaccination for high-risk patients with asthma. Performance at **Level 3** (≤5 failures/1,000 opportunities), requires a well-designed system with low variation and cooperative relationships and a state of "mindfulness," with attention to processes, structure, and their relationship to outcomes.

Healthcare can learn important safety lessons from disciplines such as human factors engineering and cognitive psychology. Industries that better leverage learnings from these disciplines—and robustly identify and mitigate threats and use simulation—include commercial aviation and nuclear power, termed *high-reliability organizations*. These organizations achieve exemplary safety records under dynamic and high-risk conditions through consistent application of 5 tenets: (1) a preoccupation with failure—surprises and errors are thought of as learning opportunities, and learnings spread quickly through the organization; (2) reluctance to simplify interpretations—serious safety events receive an RCA; perspective of multiple stakeholders solicited on other safety events; (3) sensitivity to operations—proactive assessments and huddles target risks to patients and the organization; (4) a commitment to resilience—errors do not disable, and high-risk, uncommon scenarios are negotiated; and (5) deference to expertise—leaders defer to front-line experts when their knowledge is required.

SERIOUS HARM EVENTS AND HEALTHCARE-ASSOCIATED CONDITIONS

Substantial improvement in patient safety has occurred through improvement teams targeting *serious harm* events. The **serious harm event rate** is a composite metric that groups preventable HACs into 1 number (usually a rate per at-risk patient-days), so that an organization or collaborative can track progress on a variety of conditions with 1 metric and chart. Table 5.1 lists frequently targeted HACs. Commonalities among successful improvement teams targeting these HACs include multidisciplinary team membership, clear outcome definitions and measurement, learning systems around each HAC, and attention to both process and outcome measures. Much of the successes with CLA-BSIs was associated with targeted improvements to reliably adhere to a line insertion bundle and a line maintenance bundle. Fig. 5.2 illustrates coincident improvements in process measures and outcomes measure in a hypothetical CLA-BSI project. In this case, after improvement interventions targeted 2 process measures known to be important in CLA-BSI risk—the line insertion and the line maintenance bundles—the QI team saw improvement in both measures and coincident reduction in CLA-BSIs.

A safety culture and experienced improvement teams are consistent drivers of success. A **learning network model**, as used in SPS, is effective in bringing project teams (e.g., groups with shared charters to reduce catheter-associated urinary tract infections) together from different hospitals to discuss lessons learned and common barriers faced and negotiated.

SAFETY OPPORTUNITIES AND GAPS

In addition to HACs, several other safety events are the targets of active study and improvement. Both the unrecognized clinical deterioration of hospitalized children and the poor handoffs across multiple stakeholders lead to substantial and preventable harm. Human factors interventions, such as *timeouts*, are also improving surgical safety.

Clinical Deterioration

The deterioration of hospitalized patients is rarely a sudden and unpredictable event; rather, it is preceded by abnormal vital signs and concerns from patients, families, and providers. **Rapid response systems** are designed to detect deterioration and then deploy teams with critical care expertise to provide treatment or escalate care to an intensive care unit (ICU). While there remains variation in how these teams are activated and how the rapid response teams are staffed (e.g., nurse vs physician led), all U.S. children's hospitals have some version of a rapid response system. The initiation of rapid response teams is associated with a significant reduction in codes outside the ICU and in-hospital mortality.

Pediatric early warning scores (PEWS) are used in most large children's hospitals to identify deteriorating patients by assigning scores based on the degree of abnormality in different body systems. Different versions of PEWS are often employed, but all include scores driven by age-based vital signs as well as nursing assessments in areas such as mental status and perfusion. Importantly, PEWS take these diverse exam

Table 5.1	Common Healthcare-Associated Conditions (HACs) Targeted in Quality Improvement Efforts with Interventions			
HAC	**DEFINITION**	**COST PER EVENT**	**POTENTIALLY EFFECTIVE INTERVENTIONS**	
Central line–associated bloodstream infections	Laboratory-confirmed bloodstream infection with central line in place at time of or 48 hr before onset of event (details at https://www.cdc.gov/nhsn)	$55,646	Line insurance bundle (e.g., handwashing, chlorhexidine scrub), maintenance bundle (catheter care, change dressing, discuss daily if catheter is needed)	
Catheter-associated urinary tract infections	Urinary tract infection where an indwelling urinary catheter was in place >2 days on day of event (details at https://www.cdc.gov/nhsn)	$7,200	Protocols for reviewing and removing catheters daily, clear indications for inserting catheters, physician champions, audit and feedback of data	
Adverse drug events	Harm associated with any dose of a drug (details at http://www.nccmerp.org/types-medication-errors)	$3,659	Pharmacist review of medication order, computerized physician order entry, co-ordering of laxatives in patients on opiates	
Peripheral IV infiltrates	Moderate or serious harm (e.g., diminished pulses, >30% swelling) associated with a peripheral IV infiltrate (details at http://www.solutionsforpatientsafety.org)	—	Hourly reviews of IV status, limitations on use of desiccants through peripheral IVs, remove IVs when no longer needed	
Pressure injuries	Localized damage to skin and/or underlying soft tissue usually over a bony prominence or related to a device (details at http://www.solutionsforpatientsafety.org)	—	Screening of high-risk patients (e.g., Braden Q Scale), regular turning of low-mobility patients, regular inspection and skin care; specialized device padding	
Surgical site infections	Infection of incision or deep tissue space after operative procedure (details at https://www.cdc.gov/nhsn)	—	Surgical checklist, antimicrobial prophylaxis within 60 min before incision, preoperative baths, postoperative antibiotic redosing	
Venous thromboembolism	Blood clot in deep vein, stratified as central line–associated vs not (details at https://www.cdc.gov/nhsn)	$27,686	Screening for high-risk patients, removal of central line catheters when no longer needed, targeted prophylaxis	

IV, Intravenous line.

elements and combine them into a single score, which when coupled with clear, expected actions (e.g., evaluation by physician at score of 5, evaluation by rapid response team at score of 7) may better detect deterioration and improve safety outcomes.

PEWS are one method of improving a clinician's *situation awareness,* the sense of what is going on around the clinician, the notion of what is important, and the anticipation of future consequences. Maintaining situation awareness can be challenging in dynamic, high-risk environments such as healthcare. Work at several children's hospitals to improve situation awareness has been associated with sustained and significant reductions in unrecognized clinical deterioration. This improvement work first designed systematic and proactive identification of high-risk *watcher* patients, those a nurse or physician felt were close to the edge of deterioration. High-risk patients are discussed at multidisciplinary bedside "huddles" and specific treatment plans and predictions outlined. Concerns are more fully addressed through the rapid response team as well as hospital-wide safety huddles and safety rounds. To gain a better sense of organization safety and performance threats, many hospitals in the SPS collaborative employ a daily safety or operations brief, where leaders from a variety of service lines (e.g., inpatient, pharmacy, perioperative care) can discuss unexpected events and rapidly develop solutions and follow-up plans to mitigate emerging threats that cross disciplines.

Handoffs/I-PASS
There is a growing evidence base on the consequences of poor handoffs and on complex interventions to improve handoffs and resultant safety outcomes. The best-studied handoff is resident-to-resident shift handoff in teaching hospitals. Use of the **I-PASS** mnemonic—*i*llness severity, *p*atient summary, *a*ction list, *s*ituation awareness and contingency planning, and *s*ynthesis by receiver—and the surrounding educational quality improvement curriculum was associated with a significant 23% reduction in medical errors and 30% reduction in adverse events in a 9-hospital study. Related work has described improved communication

with work targeting ICU-to-floor, operating room–to-ICU, and inpatient medical team–to–primary care handoffs.

Surgical Safety
Initially, in response to the problem of wrong-patient or wrong-site surgeries, perioperative leaders have developed a set of safety strategies often termed the *tenets of surgical safety,* which are endorsed by the World Health Organization (http://www.who.int/patientsafety/safesurgery). The tenets are implemented as several discrete checklists at key points, or "timeouts," in the workflow around a procedure or surgery. Several studies have demonstrated reduced harm to patients, and surgical checklists are adopted widely throughout developed and developing world surgical and procedural environments. Typically, checklists are used at 3 key times during a procedure: before induction of anesthesia, before skin incision or insertion of a device into any body cavity or orifice, and before a patient leaves the procedural area or operating room. Key aspects of the impact of this approach include multidisciplinary active participation, visual display of the checklist or other key tools as references, and attention to hierarchies and team-based communication. An evolving area of surgical and procedural safety is the use of simulation and video-based procedure review to improve surgical technique and perioperative team function and identify latent threats.

Ambulatory Safety
Adverse drug events and medication dosing errors are the best-studied safety events in the outpatient environment. A study of children receiving chemotherapy used direct observation by a trained nurse at home and found approximately 70 errors per 100 patients, many of which were serious or significant. Families often make dosing errors in administering liquid medications, particularly when using kitchen spoons rather than dosing syringes. A health literacy–informed pictogram reduces the rates of these errors. Dosing errors and nonadherence also can occur in cancer care, epilepsy, and transplant settings. Additional ambulatory safety threats include delays in diagnosis or treatment caused by mis-

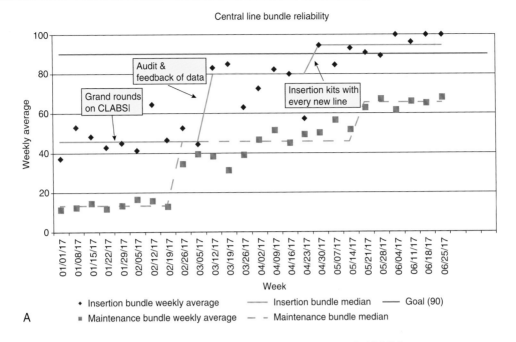

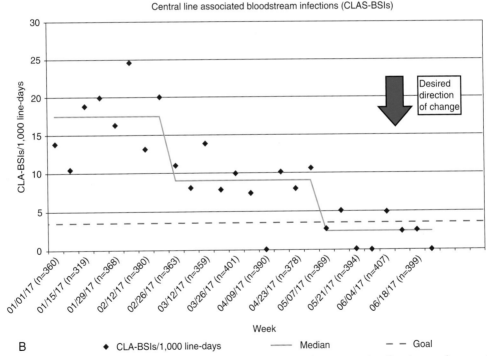

Fig. 5.2 Quality improvement interventions targeted process improvement in the **A,** line insertion bundle, where performance improved from 46% to 95%), and **B,** line maintenance bundle, where performance improved from 13% to 66%. Coincident with the improved bundle performance, the rate of CLA-BSIs fell from 17.6 to 2.5 per 1,000 line-days.

handling of lab or imaging results and failures in care coordination.

Occupational Safety

The provision of healthcare can be a dangerous profession, with injury rates that surpass those of coal miners. The magnitude of this challenge and efforts to improve workplace safety have gained considerable attention

the last several years. Nurses and physicians still typically view a needlestick injury or back strain from lifting a patient as simply "part of the job." A culture of safety should include employee safety, and health systems should have mechanisms for employees to report injuries, near misses, and threats. Focused improvement efforts might include the roll-out of safer needle systems, education on safe processes, and easy access to lifts for larger children with limited mobility. Violence and patient interaction injuries, often from children with psychiatric disease or developmental disabilities, are a growing source of harm to clinicians.

EMERGING AREAS OF SAFETY RESEARCH AND IMPROVEMENT

Diagnostic error is recognized as an increasingly common and impactful event. There are 2 systems of clinical decision-making. **System 1** is fast, instinctual, and largely unconscious. **System 2** is slow, effortful, and calculating. System 1 and its *heuristics* or *biases* allows for quick—almost automatic—decision-making, often by associating new information with existing patterns or beliefs (e.g., that red object on right side of road is a stop sign; I should stop). However, system 1 thinking can be dangerous in diagnostic thinking, particularly when new data are unconsciously made to fit the preconceived pattern, and are not seen as disconfirming. Many current efforts aim to better understand how well-described cognitive biases (e.g., premature closure, availability bias) play out in clinical care, and what system-based strategies can mitigate their effects (Tables 5.2 to 5.4). Diagnostic error is often an error of omission, making it difficult to measure or to produce valid epidemiologic estimates of its incidence. Despite this, many health systems are pursuing research

and improvement to move clinicians from system 1 to system 2 thinking, such as being explicit on uncertainty (e.g., patients admitted from ED as "diagnosis unknown") or using decision aids to prompt revisiting provisional diagnoses (Table 5.5).

Alarm fatigue, when a healthcare provider is subject to so many interruptions that a potentially relevant alarm is not heard, is also an area of active research and improvement. In the hospital, many physiologic monitor alarms occur each day (up to 400 per patient in some environments), and nurses exposed to a high volume of alarms respond more slowly to them. Interventions currently being studied include removing monitors from patients unlikely to benefit from them and designing smart alarms that alert only when certain scenarios occur (e.g., bradycardia in context of hypoxia). Particularly in the case of bronchiolitis, the overuse of pulse oximetry monitors likely contributes to **overdiagnosis**—the identification of an existing abnormality but whose detection will have no net benefit for the patient. Overdiagnosis of hypoxemia in children with bronchiolitis may contribute to hospital admissions, prolong length of stay, and subject children to hospital-related harm.

Alert fatigue is related to alarm fatigue but refers to clinicians not processing an alert, such as a medication interaction from the electronic health record, when receiving a large burden of alerts often regarded as nonactionable.

Table 5.2	Cognitive Biases Related to Heuristic Failure
BIASES	**DEFINITION**
Anchoring	Locking into a diagnosis based on initial presenting features, failing to adjust diagnostic impressions when new information becomes available.
Confirmation bias	Looking for and accepting only evidence that confirms a diagnostic impression, rejecting or not seeking contradictory evidence.
Diagnostic momentum	Perpetuating a diagnostic label over time, usually by multiple providers both within and across healthcare systems, despite the label being incomplete or inaccurate.
Expertise bias/yin-yang out	Believing that a patient who has already undergone an extensive evaluation will have nothing more to gain from further investigations, despite the possibility that the disease process or diagnostic techniques may have evolved so as to allow for appropriate diagnosis.
Overconfidence bias	Believing one knows more than one does, acting on incomplete information or hunches, and prioritizing opinion or authority, as opposed to evidence.
Premature closure	Accepting the first plausible diagnosis before obtaining confirmatory evidence or considering all available evidence. "When the diagnosis is made, thinking stops."
Unpacking principle	Failing to explore primary evidence or data in its entirety and subsequently failing to uncover important facts or findings, such as accepting a biopsy report or imaging study report without reviewing the actual specimen or image; especially important in undiagnosed and rare diseases.

From Bordini BJ, Stephany A, Kliegman R: Overcoming diagnostic errors in medical practice, *J Pediatr* 185:19–25, 2017 (Table I, p 20).

Table 5.3	Cognitive Biases Related to Errors of Attribution
BIASES	**DEFINITION**
Affective bias	Allowing emotions to interfere with a diagnosis, either positively or negatively; dislikes of patient types ("frequent flyers").
Appeal to authority	Deferring to authoritative recommendations from senior, supervising, or "expert" clinicians, independent of the evidentiary support for such recommendations.
Ascertainment bias	Maintaining preconceived expectations based on patient or disease stereotypes.
Attribution error	Placing undue importance on the perceived internal characteristics or motivations of others, whether they are the patient, the patient's family, or other members of the evaluation team.
Countertransference	Being influenced by positive or negative subjective feelings toward a specific patient.
Outcome bias	Minimizing or overemphasizing the significance of a finding or result, often based on subjective feelings about a patient, a desired outcome, or personal confidence in one's own clinical skills. The use of "slightly" to describe abnormal results.
Psych-out bias	Maintaining biases about people with presumed mental illness.

From Bordini BJ, Stephany A, Kliegman R: Overcoming diagnostic errors in medical practice, *J Pediatr* 185:19–25, 2017 (Table II, p 21).

Table 5.4	Cognitive Biases Related to Errors of Context
BIASES	**DEFINITION**
Availability bias	Basing decisions on the most recent patient with similar symptoms, preferentially recalling recent and more common diseases.
Base-rate neglect	Prioritizing specific information (e.g., a lab value) pertaining to a case while ignoring general base rate information about the prevalence of disease in populations (pre-test probability).
Framing effect	Being influenced by how or by whom a problem is described or by the context in which the evaluation takes place.
Frequency bias	Believing that common things happen commonly and usually are benign in general practice.
Hindsight bias	Reinforcing diagnostic errors once a diagnosis is discovered despite these errors. May lead to a clinician overestimating the efficacy of his or her clinical reasoning and may reinforce ineffective techniques.
Posterior probability error	Considering the likelihood of a particular diagnosis in light of a patient's chronic illness. New headaches in a patient with a history of migraines may in fact be a tumor.
Representative bias	Basing decisions on an expected typical presentation. Not effective for atypical presentations. Overemphasis on disease-diagnostic criteria or "classic" presentations. "Looks like a duck, quacks like a duck."
Sutton's slip	Ignoring alternate explanations for "obvious" diagnoses (Sutton's law is that one should first consider the obvious).
Thinking in silo	Restricting diagnostic considerations to a particular specialty or organ system. Each discipline has a set of diseases within its comfort zone, which reduces diagnostic flexibility or team-based communication.
Zebra retreat	Lacking conviction to pursue rare disorders even when suggested by evidence.

From Bordini BJ, Stephany A, Kliegman R: Overcoming diagnostic errors in medical practice, *J Pediatr* 185:19–25, 2017 (Table III, p 21).

Table 5.5	Solutions to Avoid Diagnostic Errors

1. Enhancing foundational knowledge in medical education
   - Teach symptoms and their differential pathophysiology, not just diseases.
   - Emphasize red flags and must-not-miss diagnoses.
2. Minimizing errors related to heuristic failure
   - Build understanding of system 1 and system 2 thought processes and the risks of heuristic failure.
   - Actively model and encourage counterfactual reasoning and hypothesis generation to enhance system 2 skills.
3. Mitigating errors of attribution
   - Increase awareness of biases toward specific patients by promoting self-reflection.
   - Use a team-based approach and diagnostic strategies that actively dispel biases.
4. Avoiding errors of context
   - Solicit input across a variety of specialties when appropriate.
   - Consciously acknowledge the risk of thinking in silo and actively seek explanations outside one's specialty.
5. Optimizing data gathering, analysis, and hypothesis generation
   - Develop differential diagnoses based on pathophysiology; consider alternatives and competing options.
   - Realize that diagnostic criteria for certain diseases do not account for atypical disease manifestations.
   - Rely on objective individual data, not just disease prevalence rates, when considering the pretest likelihood of a particular diagnosis.
   - Avoid diagnostic momentum and question-accumulated diagnostic labels, regardless of who applied the label.
6. Improving hypothesis testing
   - Know the limitations of laboratory tests (i.e., false positives and negatives).
   - Do not be so quick to "rule out" a diagnosis: consider the posttest likelihood of disease in terms of a probabilistic analysis that applies specifically to the patient.

- Acknowledge that the initial "working" diagnosis may not always be the final diagnosis.
- Rely on evidence-based data and avoid authority- or overconfidence-based errors.
- Recognize that diagnosis is an iterative and interactive process that should not be bounded by premature closure or anchoring. Be open to both confirmatory and nonconfirmatory data.
- Both know and accept what you do not know.
7. Critical solutions for complex and undiagnosed and rare disease patients
   - Maintain healthy skepticism, especially with patients who come prediagnosed.
   - Analyze historical diagnostic data methodically and thoroughly and unpack all data completely. Examine actual studies, such as tissue specimens and imaging investigations, and do not rely on written reports.
   - Question the working diagnosis when findings or the clinical course does not fit.
   - Realize that patients can have more than one disease process.
   - Incorporate all data and avoid minimizing the significance of abnormal results. Do not ignore contradictory clinical, laboratory, or imaging data.
   - Never say "never" or "it cannot be."
   - Use a systematic team-based approach to enhance debiasing, broaden the collective knowledge base, and minimize context-related errors.
   - Be aware that patients with undiagnosed and rare diseases may have an atypical or rare manifestation of a recognizable common disease, or may have a rare disease.
   - Use extensive literature review and search strategies based on the patient's phenotype and individual findings and hypotheses.

From Bordini BJ, Stephany A, Kliegman R: Overcoming diagnostic errors in medical practice. J Pediatr 185:19-25, 2017 (Table V, p. 24).

The most important area of current and growing research may be how health care providers can partner with patients and families to improve the safety of care. Families often identify a wide number of errors and safety events that clinicians fail to report. More important than families simply reporting mistakes are early efforts to engage families more broadly and deeply to co-produce healthcare that is efficient, effective, and safe.

Bibliography is available at Expert Consult.

Chapter 6
Ethics in Pediatric Care
Eric Kodish and Kathryn L. Weise

第六章
儿童医疗健康伦理

中文导读

本章主要介绍了何谓"患儿同意"和"父母允许"，介绍了危重症儿童的治疗、新生儿伦理、宣布死亡和器官捐献、宗教或文化的治疗抵触、儿科伦理委员会和伦理咨询、新生儿筛查、遗传学基因组学和精准医学、青春期健康保健、研究工作、平衡母亲和胎儿利益、公平性与儿科伦理、新事物新问题。在

危重症儿童的治疗中，具体阐述了如何调整医疗护理目标以及如何对待保留和撤除维持生命的治疗；另外还阐述了神经系统指标鉴定脑死亡、鉴定循环死亡。针对青春期健康保健，阐述了青少年的"本人同意"和"家长允许"、慢性疾病和涉及绝症青少年的决策等。

Pediatric ethics is the branch of bioethics that analyzes moral aspects of decisions made relating to the healthcare of children. In general terms, the **autonomy**-driven framework of adult medical ethics is replaced by a **beneficent** paternalism (or parentalism) in pediatrics. Pediatric ethics is distinctive because the pediatric clinician has an independent fiduciary obligation to act in a younger child's **best interest** that takes moral precedence over the wishes of the child's parent(s). For older children, the concept of **assent** suggests that the voice of the patient must be heard. These factors create the possibility of conflict among child, parent, and clinician. The approach to the ethical issues that arise in pediatric practice *must* include respect for parental responsibility and authority balanced with a child's developing capacity and autonomy. Heterogeneity of social, cultural, and religious views about the role of children adds complexity.

ASSENT AND PARENTAL PERMISSION

The doctrine of *informed consent* has limited direct application to children and adolescents who lack decisional capacity. The capacity for informed decision-making in healthcare involves the ability to understand and communicate, to reason and deliberate, and to analyze conflicting elements of a decision using a set of personal values. The age at which a competent patient may legally exercise voluntary and informed consent for medical care varies from state to state and may be limited to specific conditions (sexually transmitted infections, family planning, drug or alcohol abuse).

In contrast to decisions about one's own care, a parent's right to direct a child's medical care is more limited. For this reason, the term *parental consent* is misleading. The concept of parental permission (rather than consent) reflects a *surrogate* or *proxy* decision made by a parent on behalf of a child. It is constrained both by the child's best interest and the independent obligation of clinicians to act in the child's best interest, even if this places them in conflict with a parent. In any given instance,

the decision of what is or is not in a child's best interest may be difficult, especially given the diverse views of acceptable child rearing and child welfare. Parents are (and should be) granted wide discretion in raising their children. In cases involving a substantial risk of harm, the moral focus should be on avoiding or preventing harm to the child, not on a parental right to decide. While the term *best interests* may be too high of a threshold requirement, a minimum standard of *basic interests* is ethically obligatory.

Respect for children must account for both a child's vulnerability and developing capacity. This respect encompasses both the protective role of parental permission and the developmental role of **child assent** (the child's affirmative agreement). Understanding the concept of assent is one of the major conceptual challenges in pediatric ethics. The **dissent** (or disagreement) of a child is the opposite of assent and is also morally relevant. Pediatric ethics *requires* clinicians and parents to override a child's dissent when a proposed intervention is essential to the child's welfare. Otherwise, assent should be solicited and dissent honored. In seeking younger children's assent, a clinician should help them understand their condition, tell them what they can expect, assess their understanding and whether they feel pressured to assent, and solicit their willingness to participate. All efforts must be made to delineate situations in which the test or procedure will be done regardless of the child's assent/dissent, and in such cases the charade of soliciting assent should be avoided. There is an important distinction between soliciting assent and respectfully informing a child that a test or procedure will take place regardless of the child's decision. Optimally, an educational process can transpire (if time allows) to gain the trust and assent of the child-patient. When this cannot occur, pediatric ethics requires that clinicians apologize to a child for acting to override dissent.

Older children or adolescents may have the cognitive and emotional capacity to participate fully in healthcare decisions. If so, the adolescent should be provided with the same information given to an adult patient.

In such situations the patient may be able to provide informed consent ethically but not legally. The adolescent's parent(s) remain in a guiding and protective role. The process of communication and negotiation will be more complex should disagreement arise between the parent and adolescent. Pediatricians can be effective intercessors when these situations arise, making use of communication skills in a respectful way that uses an ethical framework as recently described by Sisk et al.

TREATMENT OF CRITICALLY ILL CHILDREN

Infants, children, and adolescents who become critically ill may recover fully, may die, or may survive with new or worsened limitations of function. Uncertainty about outcomes can make planning goals of care difficult, or if misunderstandings between patient, families, and medical staff occur, may drive conflict over treatment proposals. *Ethical issues* that arise during critical illness include balancing benefits, burdens, and harms of therapy in the face of uncertainty; maintaining a helpful degree of transparency and communication about medical standards of care at an institution; understanding and respecting religious and cultural differences that impact requests for or refusal of treatments; defining limits of therapy based on assessments of medical futility; recognizing the moral equivalence of not starting an ineffective treatment and stopping (although the 2 acts may seem very different to families and providers); and controversies such as withholding medically administered nutrition and hydration.

Transitioning the Goals of Care

Most acutely ill children who die in an intensive care unit do so after a decision has been made to forgo or withdraw **life-sustaining medical treatment (LSMT)**, and the same may apply in the chronically ill population. LSMT is justified when the anticipated benefit outweighs the burdens to the patient; the availability of technology does not in and of itself obligate its use. Decisions to use, limit, or withdraw LSMT should be made after careful consideration of all pertinent factors recognizable by both family and medical staff, including medical likelihood of particular outcomes, burdens on the patient and family, religious and cultural decision-making frameworks, and input by the patient when possible. Although fear of legal repercussions may sometimes drive treatment and medical advice, ultimately decisions should be based on what is thought to be best for the patient rather than based on fears of litigation.

The concept of **futility** has been used to support unilateral forgoing of LSMT against the wishes of patients and families by holding that clinicians should not provide futile (or useless) interventions. If *medical futility* is defined narrowly as the impossibility of achieving a desired physiologic outcome, forgoing a particular intervention is ethically justified. However, this approach may not adequately engage professionals and families in understanding facts and values that might allow the same therapy to reach other goals, and may leave medical and family stakeholders in permanent conflict. Guidance from critical care groups recommend restricting use of the word *futility* to situations of strict physiologic futility, and instead use process guidelines to evaluate and manage situations of *potentially inappropriate treatment*. If agreement cannot be reached through clear and compassionate communication efforts, further input should be sought from an ethics consultant or committee.

Communication about life-threatening or life-altering illness is challenging and requires skills learned through both modeling and practice. These *skills* include choosing a setting conducive to what may become one or more long conversations; listening carefully to children's and families' hopes, fears, understanding, and expectations; explaining medical information and uncertainties simply and clearly without complicated terms and concepts; conveying concern and openness to discussion; and being willing to share the burdens of decision-making with families by giving clear recommendations. Discussing difficult topics with children requires an understanding of child development and can be aided by professionals such as child psychologists or child life specialists. Such conversations and their outcomes have a major impact on the future care of the patient, on families, and on medical staff. For this reason, ongoing evaluation of goals and communication

about them is needed with families and within complex medical teams as the course of the illness unfolds.

Experts recognize that good medical care involves providing for communication, symptom management, and a range of supportive services from the onset of acute illness. In this way, if an illness proves to be life-limiting despite aggressive therapies, the elements of palliative care are already in place. This concept has had difficulty gaining traction, especially in critical care settings, because of the mistaken conflation of broadly defined palliative measures with hospice care. **Palliative care** interventions focus on the relief of symptoms and conditions that may detract from quality of life regardless of the impact on a child's underlying disease process, and as such are important whether care is focused on cure or on transitioning to end-of-life care (see Chapter 7). Some interventions regarded as life-sustaining, such as chemotherapy, may be ethically acceptable in the end-of-life setting if their use decreases pain and suffering rather than only prolonging dying.

Withholding and Withdrawing Life-Sustaining Treatment

Limitation of interventions or withdrawal of existing therapies are ethically acceptable if they are congruent with a plan of care focused on **comfort** and **improved quality** at the end of life rather than cure. The prevailing view in Western, traditional medical ethics is that there is no moral distinction between withholding or withdrawing interventions that are not medically indicated. Uncertainty in predicting a child's response to treatment may drive the initiation and continuation of interventions that are subsequently determined to be no longer supportive of shared goals of care. It is necessary to evaluate continually the results of these treatments and the evolution of the illness to recognize whether such interventions continue to be the best medical and moral choices. Maintaining the focus on the child rather than on the interests of parents or medical staff will help guide decision-making.

The decision about whether to attempt **cardiopulmonary resuscitation** (CPR) may become an issue to discuss with parents of children living with life-threatening or terminal conditions. All elements of end-of-life care approaches, including resuscitation status, should be supportive of agreed-on goals of care. It is imperative that decisions and plans are effectively communicated to all caregivers in order to avoid denying medically effective interventions and measures to ensure comfort. Orders about resuscitation status should clarify the plan regarding intubation and mechanical ventilation, the use of cardiac medications, chest compressions, and cardioversion. Because goals of care may change over time, a medical order regarding resuscitation is not irrevocable. Clinicians may assume that the absence of a **do-not-attempt-resuscitation (DNAR)** order obligates them to perform a prolonged resuscitation. This action may not be ethically supportable if resuscitative efforts will not achieve the desired physiologic end-point. In all cases, treatments should be tailored to the child's clinical condition, balancing benefits and burdens to the patient. Resuscitation should not be performed solely to mollify parental distress at the tragic time of the loss of their child.

Advance Directives

An *advance directive* is a mechanism that allows patients and/or appropriate surrogates to designate the desired medical interventions under applicable circumstances. Discussion and clarification of resuscitation status should be included in advance care planning, and for children attending school despite advanced illness, may need to be addressed in that setting. Decisions regarding resuscitation status in the out-of-hospital setting can be an important component of providing comprehensive care.

The 1991 federal Patient Self-Determination Act requires that healthcare institutions ask adult (>18 yr) patients whether they have completed an **advance directive** and, if not, inform them of their right to do so. Few states support creation of broad advance directives for minors because advance directives are traditionally created for persons with legal decision-making capacity. Some have moved in this direction, however, because it is recognized that minors may be capable of participating in decision-making, especially if they have experienced chronic disease. Most states have approved the implementation of **prehospital** or **portable DNAR orders**, through which adults may indicate their desire not to be resuscitated by emergency personnel. On a state-by-state basis, portable orders regarding resuscitation status may also apply to children. If DNAR orders exist for an infant or a child, it is important to communicate effectively about their intent among all potential caregivers, because nonmedical stakeholders such as teachers or sitters may not want to be in the position of interpreting or honoring them. Some institutions have established local policies and procedures by which an appropriately executed, outpatient DNAR order can be honored on a child's arrival in the emergency department. Key features may include a standardized document format, review by an attending physician, ongoing education, and involvement of a pediatric palliative medicine service.

In cases involving prenatal diagnosis of a lethal or significantly burdensome anomaly, parents may choose to carry their fetus/unborn child to term in order to cherish a short time with the infant after birth, but they do not feel that resuscitation or certain other aggressive measures would support their well-considered goals of care. In this setting, a birth plan explaining the reasons for each choice can be developed by the parents and medical staff before delivery and shared with involved medical staff. This approach gives staff a chance to find other caregivers if they are uncomfortable with the approach, without abandoning the care of the child. If, after evaluation at birth, the infant's condition is as had been expected, honoring the requested plan is ethically supportable and should be done in a way that optimizes comfort of the infant and family.

Many states use **Physician Orders for Life-Sustaining Treatment** or **Medical Orders for Life-Sustaining Treatment** approaches to communicating a patient or surrogates wishes regarding advance care planning. Other tools, such as **Five Wishes**, have been adapted for use by adolescent patients to elicit values and desires. It is important for pediatricians to learn which pathways for communicating goals of care are available in their own states.

Artificial Hydration and Nutrition

Issues surrounding withholding or withdrawing artificial hydration and nutrition are controversial, and interpretations are affected by parental, religious, and medical beliefs. Any adult or child who is fully dependent on the care of others will die as a result of not receiving hydration and nutrition. Case law has supported the withholding of artificially administered nutrition and hydration in the setting of adult vegetative or permanently unconscious patients who can be shown to have previously expressed a wish not to be maintained in such a state. This requires a valid advance directive, or for a surrogate decision maker to speak on behalf of the patient's known wishes. Because infants and many children have not reached a developmental stage in which such discussions would have been possible, decisions about stopping artificially administered nutrition and hydration as a limitation of treatment are more problematic. These decisions should be based on what families and caregivers decide best support comfort. In the child who is imminently dying, unaware of hunger, does not tolerate enteral feedings, and in whom family and staff agree that IV nutrition and hydration only prolong the dying process, it may be ethically supportable to withhold or withdraw these treatments based on a benefit-burden analysis.

The Doctrine of Double Effect

Treatment decisions at the end of life may include limitations of certain LSMT or may involve the use of analgesic or sedative medications that some fear may shorten life, thereby causing death. The doctrine of double effect (**DDE**) holds that an action with both good and bad effects is morally justifiable if the good effect is the only one intended, and the bad effect is foreseen and accepted, but not desired. In pediatrics, DDE is most commonly applied in end-of-life cases, when upward titration of medication (opiates) necessary to relieve pain, anxiety, or air hunger can be expected to result in a degree of respiratory depression. In such cases, meeting a provider's obligation to relieve suffering is the intended effect, and this obligation to the patient outweighs the acknowledged but unavoidable side effect. Choosing medications that

adequately relieve symptoms with minimal adverse effects would be ethically preferable, but the obligation to provide comfort at the end of life outweighs the foreseeable occurrence of unavoidable side effects. Hastening death as a primary intention is not considered to be morally acceptable.

Providing pain medication guided by the DDE should not be confused with active euthanasia. The distinction is clear:

◆ In **active euthanasia**, causing death is chosen as a means of relieving the symptoms that cause suffering.
◆ Under DDE, adequate management of pain, anxiety, or air hunger is recognized as an obligation to dying patients, and is provided by careful titration of medications in response to symptoms. If death occurs sooner as a result, this is accepted.

In both cases the patient dies, and in both cases suffering ends, but immediate death is the intended consequence only in the case of euthanasia. Codes of ethics and legislation in many states support the obligation to provide pain and symptom relief at the end of life, even if this requires increasing doses of medication.

NEONATAL ETHICS

As neonatal care has evolved, the limits of viability of extremely premature infants are continuing to change. This introduces new elements of uncertainty to decision-making, often in emotionally fraught circumstances such as a precipitous premature delivery. In cases of uncertain prognosis, the American Academy of Pediatrics (AAP) supports parental desires as driving decision-making, while encouraging providers to recognize when treatments are inappropriate, and using a careful shared decision-making approach to developing plans of care.

The federal **Child Abuse Prevention and Treatment Act** of 1984 (CAPTA), which became known as "Baby Doe Regulations," required state child protective services agencies to develop and implement mechanisms to report to a specific government agency treatment that providers believed was withheld from infants on the basis of disability. Exceptions were (1) an infant is chronically and irreversibly comatose, (2) if providing a treatment would merely prolong dying, would not be effective in ameliorating or correcting all the infant's life-threatening conditions, or would be futile in terms of the infant's survival, and (3) if the treatment would be virtually futile and inhumane. This legislation pertains *only* to infants and is intended to prevent discrimination on the basis of disability alone. One consequence of the legislation was a shift from potential undertreatment to widespread overtreatment (LSMT that does not serve the interests of the child) of severely disabled newborns. As parental involvement in decisions-making is again taking a more central role, and as palliative care approaches in infants have become more available and skilled, balanced approaches to valuing lives of disabled infants should be considered. Understanding institutional, regional, state, and national regulations related to care of infants is important in order to practice within regulatory frameworks while respecting family values and pursuing the interests of the patient.

Active euthanasia of severely suffering disabled newborns has been legalized in The Netherlands and Belgium, using protocols designed to minimize risk of abuse and maximize transparency. It is currently illegal in the United States, and although controversy surrounds the subject, the predominant view is that active euthanasia is not ethically acceptable in the care of infants and children, instead favoring palliative treatment and potential limitation of escalation.

DECLARING DEATH AND ORGAN DONATION

Donation of solid organs necessary to support life can occur after a patient is declared dead based on either irreversible cessation of neurologic function of the brain and brainstem (death by neurologic criteria, or *brain death*) or a predetermined period of cardiac asystole called *circulatory death*. To avoid a potential conflict of interest by surgeons or others caring for a potential organ recipient, the request for organ donation should be separated from the clinical discussion of either brain death or withdrawal of LSMT. Although clinicians may be the first providers to enter discussion about death and organ donation with family members during conversations about outcomes and options, detailed discussion of organ donation should be done by other individuals who are specifically trained for this purpose. This decoupling of clinical decision-making from a request for organ donation by trained individuals, perhaps by providing families with expert information without a perceived conflict of interest, has been associated with improved donation rates.

Death by Neurologic Criteria

Death by neurologic criteria (**DBNC**), commonly referred to as "brain death," may be difficult for families to understand when the child appears to be breathing (although on a ventilator), pink, and warm to the touch, and when language such as "life support" is used at the bedside by staff. Studies also document clinician misunderstanding of the diagnosis of DBNC. For these reasons, strict criteria adhering to nationally accepted guidelines must be used to determine when irreversible cessation of brain and brainstem function has occurred and adequately document these findings (see Chapter 85).

The states of New York and New Jersey allow families to object on "religious grounds" to the declaration of DBNC. In this situation the clinical determination of DBNC sets the stage for a discussion of forgoing LSMT, rather than the death of the patient. A unilateral decision not to initiate new or *escalate* existing interventions is ethically supportable under these circumstances, given the documented death of the patient. Even though it would seem to follow that a similar unilateral decision to withdraw existing interventions would also be supportable, this act is not in accordance with the intent of the state laws. Institutional procedures for conflict resolution, including involvement of the courts if necessary, should be followed.

Circulatory Death

Protocols allowing for **organ donation after determination of circulatory death (DDCD)** rather than after DBNC have been developed. DDCD can occur under either controlled (after planned withdrawal of LSMT) or uncontrolled (after failed CPR) circumstances, but in both cases require rapid removal of organs in order for subsequent transplantation to be successful. An increasing number of programs are pursuing DDCD protocols after federal legislation began requiring accredited hospitals to address the issue in hopes of decreasing organ shortages. Hospitals can make policy that either allows or disallows the process. In adults, consent for donation by either means can be obtained from patients or surrogates; for children, parents or guardians would make the decision to donate.

Ethical concerns about DDCD protocols focus on 2 principles that have served as the basis for organ donation: (1) the *dead donor* rule limiting the donation of vital organs to those who are irreversibly dead (either by circulatory or neurologic criteria, not both), and (2) the absence of conflict of interest between clinical care and organ procurement. With DDCD protocols, *irreversibility* has been declared at varying times after asystole occurs (usually 2-5 min), to avoid spontaneous return of circulation after forgoing CPR. To avoid a potential conflict of interest during the DDCD process, there is a requirement for strict decoupling of end-of-life care after discontinuation of LSMT and presence of the transplant team. Unlike in the setting of DBNC, a patient who is being considered for DDCD remains alive until after asystole has occurred. Careful evaluation by the transplantation team and organ procurement agency is performed before discontinuation of LSMT. Then, in most DDCD protocols, the medical caregivers from the ICU continue to care for the patient until after death by cardiac criteria has been declared, and only then is the surgical transplant team allowed into the room to procure organs.

It is *ethically imperative* to correctly diagnose the state of death, whether by neurologic criteria or prior to organ donation after cardiac death. Doing so avoids the danger of removing life-sustaining organs from a living person. Strict adherence to an ethically sound protocol is the best way to prevent both the perception and the potential reality of mistakes related to the pronunciation of death and organ procurement.

RELIGIOUS OR CULTURAL OBJECTIONS TO TREATMENT

Differences in religious beliefs or ethic-based cultural norms may lead to conflict between patients, families, and medical caregivers over the approach to medical care. Pediatricians need to remain sensitive to and maintain an attitude of respect for these differences, yet recognize that an independent obligation exists to provide effective medical treatment to the child. An adult with decision-making capacity is recognized as having the right to refuse treatment on religious or cultural grounds, but children who have not yet developed this capacity are considered a vulnerable population who has a right to treatment. In situations that threaten the life of the child or that may result in substantial harm, legal intervention should be sought if reasonable efforts toward collaborative decision-making are ineffective. If a child's life is imminently threatened, medical intervention is ethically justified despite parental objections.

PEDIATRIC ETHICS COMMITTEES AND ETHICS CONSULTATION

Most hospitals have *institutional ethics committees* to assist with policy development, education, and case consultation. When these committees serve institutions caring for children, they may be referred to as *pediatric ethics committees*. Because of the important differences in approach between adult and pediatric ethics, member expertise on this committee should include those with special insight into the unique ethical issues arising in the care of children. Such committees generally provide ethics consultation advice without mandating action or being determinative. For the vast majority of decisions involving the medical treatment of children (including forgoing LSMT), pediatric clinicians and parents are in agreement about the desirability of the proposed intervention. Because of the ethical importance of assent, the views of older children should also be given considerable weight.

Pediatric ethics committees typically perform at least 3 different functions: (1) the drafting and review of institutional policy on such issues as DNAR orders and forgoing LSMT; (2) the education of healthcare professionals, patients, and families about ethical issues in healthcare; and (3) case consultation and conflict resolution. Although the process of *case consultation* may vary, ideally the committee (or consultant) should adopt a collaborative approach that uncovers all the readily available and relevant facts, considers the values of those involved, and balances the relevant interests, while arriving at a recommendation based on a consistent ethical analysis. One helpful approach involves consideration of the 4 following elements: (1) medical indications, (2) patient preferences, (3) quality of life, and (4) contextual features. Another framework based on principles would suggest attention to respect for persons, beneficence/nonmaleficence, and justice.

Pediatric ethics committees often play a constructive role when parents and medical staff cannot agree on the proper course of action. Over the past several decades, these committees have acquired considerable influence and are increasingly recognized by state courts as an important aid in decision-making. The membership, policies, and procedures of a pediatric ethics committee should conform to accepted professional standards.

NEWBORN SCREENING

The *Oxford Dictionary of Public Health* defines screening as "the identification of a previously unrecognized disease or disease precursor, using procedures or tests that can be conducted rapidly and economically on large numbers of people with the aim of sorting them into those who may have the condition(s)… and those who are free from evidence of the condition(s)." Several programs, such as newborn screening for inborn errors of metabolism (see Chapter 102; e.g., phenylketonuria and hypothyroidism), are rightly counted among the triumphs of contemporary pediatrics. The success of such programs sometimes obscures serious ethical issues that continue to arise in proposals to screen for other conditions for which the benefits, risks, and costs have not been clearly established. Advances in genetics and technology have led to exponential growth in the number of conditions for which screening programs might be considered, with insufficient opportunity to study each proposed testing program (see Chapter 95).

The introduction of screening efforts should be done in a carefully controlled manner that allows for the evaluation of the costs (financial, medical, and psychological) and benefits of screening, including the effectiveness of follow-up and treatment protocols. New programs should be considered *experimental* until the risks and benefits can be carefully evaluated. Screening tests that identify candidates for treatment must have demonstrated sensitivity, specificity, and high predictive value, lest individuals be falsely labeled and subject to possibly toxic treatments or to psychosocial risks. As newborn screening tests are being developed, parents should be given the opportunity to exercise informed parental permission or refusal. However, once a particular screening test has been clearly demonstrated to benefit the individual or public health, a formal, active parental permission process may not be ethically obligatory.

A persistent ethical issue is whether screening should be (1) voluntary ("opt in"), (2) routine, with the ability to "opt out" or refuse, or (3) mandatory. A **voluntary** approach entails an informed decision by parents before screening. Concern is often expressed that seeking parental permission is ethically misguided for tests of clear benefit, such as phenylketonuria screening, because refusal would constitute neglect. **Routine** testing with an opt-out approach requires an explicit refusal of screening by parents who object to this intervention. The principal ethical justification for **mandatory** screening is the claim that society's obligation to promote child welfare through early detection and treatment of selected conditions supersedes any parental right to refuse this simple and low-risk medical intervention. Parental permission is clearly required when there is a research agenda (i.e., for incorporating experimental tests into established screening programs).

GENETICS, GENOMICS, AND PRECISION MEDICINE

Genetics refers to the study of particular genes, and **genomics** describes the entirety of an individual's genetic material. Genomics has been made possible by technologic advances that allowed the rapid and inexpensive sequencing now used in clinical care. The development of **precision medicine** is in large part predicated on genomic science and may have a major impact on the practice of pediatrics in the future. Efforts to undertake whole genome sequencing of newborns may yield actionable information to benefit the child, but also carry the risk of stigmatization, false positives, and unwanted information that could lead to anxiety and psychological distress.

Genetic testing of young children for late-onset disorders such as the *BRCA1* and *BRCA2* breast cancer risk genes has also been the subject of some ethical controversy. Knowledge of increased risk status may lead to lifestyle changes that can reduce morbidity and the risk of mortality, or may precipitate adverse emotional and psychological responses and discrimination. Because many adults choose not to be tested for late-onset disorders, one cannot assume that a child would want or will benefit from similar testing. Genetic testing of young children for late-onset disorders is generally inappropriate unless such testing will result in interventions that have been shown to reduce morbidity and mortality when initiated in childhood. Otherwise, such testing should be deferred until the child has the capacity to make an informed and voluntary choice.

ADOLESCENT HEALTHCARE
Adolescent Assent and Consent
Many adolescents are more like adults than children in their capacity to understand healthcare issues and to relate them to their life goals (see Chapter 132). Teenagers may lack legally defined competency, yet they may have developed the capacity meet the elements of informed consent for many aspects of medical care (see Chapter 137). There are also public health reasons for allowing adolescents to consent to their own healthcare with regard to reproductive decisions, such as contraception, abortion, and treatment of sexually transmitted infections. Strict requirements for parental permission may deter adolescents from seeking healthcare, with serious implications for their health and other community interests.

Counterbalancing these arguments are legitimate parental interests to maintain responsibility and authority for child rearing, including the opportunity to influence the sexual attitudes and practices of their children. Others claim that access to treatment such as contraception, abortion, or needle exchange programs implicitly endorses sexual activity

or drug use during adolescence. Pediatricians should not impose their own moral beliefs in these disputes. Rather, they should provide unbiased evidence-based information and nonjudgmental support. One guiding principle should be encouragement of children and adolescents to begin taking responsibility, with guidance, for their own health. This requires some input from parents or guardians but also some privacy during decision-making as adolescents achieve developmentally anticipated separation from parental control.

Chronic Illness
The normal process of adolescent development involves gradually separating from parents, establishing self-confidence, asserting individuality, developing strong peer relationships, solidifying an ability to function independently outside the family, and taking on increasing autonomy in healthcare decisions. Most developmentally normal children older than age 14 yr understand the implications of well-explained medical options as well as the average adult, and their input into their own care should be respected. For children living with chronic illness, the ability to make medical decisions for themselves may either occur earlier than for those who have been previously healthy, or may occur later if, because of illness, they have not been able to achieve normal developmental milestones or psychological maturity. The clinician's role involves assessment of the individual adolescent patient's ability to understand the medical situation, to support the patient's efforts to express wishes regarding medical treatment, to value and encourage parental support and involvement, and to foster cooperation and mutual understanding. This may be difficult in situations in which parents and adolescents disagree about life-sustaining treatments such as organ transplantation or chemotherapy, but many such conflicts may be resolved by exploring the reasons for the disagreement. Overriding an adolescent's wishes should be done very infrequently, and only after careful consideration of the potential consequences of unwanted interventions.

Decisions in Terminally Ill Adolescents
Most adolescents share end-of-life decision making with family members, although communication may be challenging because of a growing sense of independence. Open communication and flexibility about treatment preferences may help teens cope with fears and uncertainties. Development of an age-appropriate advance directive may support the patient's emerging autonomy by clarifying the adolescent's wishes, while fostering a collaborative process among the patient, family, and medical caregivers. From the time of diagnosis of a life-threatening condition through the end-of-life phase, children should be included in a developmentally tailored process of communication and shared decision-making that builds a foundation of mutual respect and trust. Some experts believe that most adolescents are not yet fully capable of making a decision to forgo life-sustaining treatment. Careful case-by-case evaluation is required to make this determination, and assistance from developmental psychologists and ethics consultants may be helpful.

RESEARCH
The central ethical challenge of pediatric research is the need to balance protection of children from research risk against the ethical imperative of conducting studies to better the lives of future children. *Research* is defined in the federal regulations as "a systematic investigation designed to develop or contribute to generalizable knowledge." For any research to be performed, the risks should be minimized and reasonable with respect to any anticipated benefits to the participants and the importance of the resulting knowledge. That some children derive a direct benefit from participation in research must also be considered, making it important to distinguish research with the prospect of direct benefit from nontherapeutic pediatric research. *Because children are a vulnerable population, there are restrictions on the research risks to which a child may be exposed,* in contrast to the risk level acceptable for research with consenting adults. These restrictions function by limiting the type of research that institutional review boards (IRBs) are permitted to approve and by specifying the conditions under which parents have the moral

and legal authority to permit a child to participate in research.

Nontherapeutic research in children is the most ethically controversial because it holds no expected direct benefit for the individual. The prohibition against using a person (especially a child) solely as a means to an end has led some to argue that children should *never* be used in nontherapeutic research. The more widely held opinion is that children may be exposed to a limited degree of risk with IRB approval, parental permission, and assent if the child is capable. The federal regulations allow healthy children to participate in minimal-risk research regardless of the potential benefit to the child. More controversially, the regulations also state that children with a disorder or condition may be exposed to slightly more than minimal risk in nontherapeutic research if the child's experience is similar to everyday life with the condition and the anticipated knowledge is of vital importance for understanding the condition.

In pediatric research with the prospect of direct benefit, the risks must be justified by the anticipated benefit to the child, and the balance of anticipated benefit to the risk should be at least as favorable as that presented by available alternatives. *The welfare of an individual child must always come before the scientific goals of the research study.*

U.S. regulations for the protection of human research participants rest on 2 foundations: (1) independent review of the ethics and science of the research by an IRB **prior to** (2) voluntary and informed consent of the participant. Although it is not amenable to regulation, the *integrity* of the investigator is probably the most important element contributing to the protection of human research participants. The standard for informed consent in a research setting is higher than for clinical care because the risks and benefits are typically less clear, the investigator has a conflict of interest, and humans have historically been subjected to unauthorized risks when strict requirements for consent were not respected.

Adolescents who are competent may sometimes consent to be research participants. Younger children may participate in a process of assent, but this does not imply that a child's signature on an assent document is necessarily a legal or ethical requirement. Children should be given the opportunity to dissent, particularly for nontherapeutic research, when there cannot be a claim that participation is in the child's interest. In the United States, national regulations require that reasonable efforts be made at least to inform children who are capable of understanding that participation is *not* part of their care, and therefore they are free to refuse to participate. In the rare case that the research offers a direct benefit to the child that would not otherwise be available, the regulations do not require child assent but only parental permission.

In addition to the protection that informed consent or parental permission is intended to provide, virtually all research involving humans in the United States is reviewed by an IRB, as required by federal regulations for institutions receiving federal research funds and for drug research regulated by the U.S. Food and Drug Administration. For research that carries more than a minor increase over minimal risk without prospect of benefit to the child such that a local IRB cannot provide approval, there is a process for federal review of research that "presents a reasonable opportunity to further the understanding, prevention, or alleviation of a serious problem affecting the health or welfare of children." Ultimately, the U.S. Secretary of Health and Human Services has the authority to approve such research.

BALANCING MATERNAL AND FETAL INTERESTS

Some situations require balancing of maternal health and well-being with those of the fetus/unborn child to reach an ethically sound decision. For instance, innovative surgical treatment of a prenatally diagnosed anomaly may help the fetus/unborn child survive, but in the process place the mother at risk of injury or of loss of the pregnancy. Alternatively, a pregnant woman may object to cesarean delivery for various reasons despite advice that it may protect the fetus/unborn child during birth. Another important situation involves risk-taking behaviors during pregnancy that are known to injure the developing fetus/unborn child, such as drug or alcohol use. These issues raise conflicts over clinicians' responsibility to the living, competent decision-maker—the pregnant mother—as opposed to the interests of the fetus/unborn child.

In certain cases, U.S. courts have decided that a woman can be required to undergo cesarean birth against her will when the risk to her health is minimal and the benefit to the otherwise normal, near-term fetus/unborn child is clear, as in a case of placenta previa. Other factors, such as prematurity, have led to the opposite legal conclusion in otherwise similar situations, because the benefit of intervention was less clear. In general, a clinician should not oppose a pregnant woman's refusal of a recommended intervention unless (1) the risk to the pregnant woman is minimal, (2) the intervention is clearly effective, and (3) the harm to the fetus/unborn child without the intervention would be certain, substantial, and irrevocable. Attempts should be made to persuade the pregnant woman to comply with recommendations in the interest of the fetus/unborn child when these 3 conditions exist, using support strategies such as the influence of other trusted caregivers, clergy, and ethics consultation or committee involvement. If these approaches fail and there is time, a clinician may seek judicial intervention as a last resort in the attempt to prevent harm to the fetus/unborn child.

Obstetricians and pediatricians may consider reporting women under child abuse or neglect statutes if ingesting alcohol or illicit drugs during pregnancy is believed to place the fetus/unborn child at risk of injury. However, clinicians must consider the likelihood of benefit from reporting, the harm to the child as well as to the mother if criminal charges or custody changes are sought, and the possible effects of reporting on driving pregnant women away from prenatal or postnatal care. The U.S. Supreme Court has held that drug testing of pregnant women without consent was a violation of the Fourth Amendment, which provides protection from unreasonable searches.

JUSTICE AND PEDIATRIC ETHICS

The most serious ethical problem in U.S. healthcare may be *inequality* in access to healthcare. Children are particularly vulnerable to this disparity, and pediatricians have a moral obligation to advocate for children as a class. Because children do not vote and do not have financial resources at their disposal, they are subject to a greater risk of being uninsured or underinsured. This lack of adequate and affordable healthcare has serious consequences in terms of death, disability, and suffering. The per capita proportion of healthcare funding spent on adults greatly exceeds that spent on children, and Medicare is available to all adults who turn 65 yr old, whereas Medicaid is limited to those beneath a specific income level. Pediatricians should be familiar with policy issues around the economics of childcare so that they will be better able to advocate for their own patients.

EMERGING ISSUES

The ready availability of information on the internet and disease-specific social media support groups have encouraged parents to become more involved in advocating for specific approaches to the healthcare of their children, requiring physicians to remain aware of the quality of these information sources in order to counsel parents on treatment choices. Because the range of aggressive, innovative, or exceedingly expensive therapies has increased, without necessarily providing clear benefit to the patient, pediatricians must exercise care and judgment before agreeing to pursue these interventions. In addition, the growth of social media has presented expectations for clinicians to be quickly responsive, as well as challenges in maintaining privacy of medical information and professional boundaries. This will be an evolving issue, since the use of telemedicine is also gaining traction in certain sectors of healthcare, including the care of children and adolescents.

A growing number of parents are refusing to immunize their children because of fear of adverse reaction to vaccine. This raises the ethical problem of the *free rider*, in which a child may benefit from herd immunity because others have been immunized without contributing to this public good. Outbreaks of preventable infectious disease have been detected in communities where vaccine refusal is prevalent. Pediatricians should manage this issue with ethical sensitivity, educating parents about the safety profile of vaccines and encouraging appropriate immunization. More confrontational approaches are not generally effective or ethically warranted. Another emerging issue is children as stem cell or solid-organ donors. Here the risk/benefit balance should be carefully weighed, but in general, a permissive policy with regard to stem cell donation and a more restrictive approach to solid-organ donation are ethically justified.

Lastly, controversial medical and surgical interventions have raised awareness of situations in which families and children may not be in agreement with approaches that were recommended as "standard of care" in the past. Examples include delaying surgical treatment of sexual development disorders to determine the child's gender identity and arresting puberty through hormonal treatment to allow transgender or questioning children or adolescents to make decisions about gender identity before developing enduring secondary sexual characteristics. Attitudes about emerging technologies and treatments may be influenced by media coverage, special interest groups, and efforts by understandably desperate families to help their children. The clinician attempting to practice ethically must carefully consider all relevant facts in each case and try to focus families and caregivers on a reasonable *best interest* assessment for the child. The tension between finding optimal policy for groups of children and doing the right thing for an individual child raises formidable ethical challenges in this context. Ethics consultation may be helpful to frame the issues and design ethically supportable approaches to care.

Bibliography is available at Expert Consult.

Chapter 7
Pediatric Palliative Care
Christina Ullrich, Janet Duncan, Marsha Joselow, and Joanne Wolfe

第七章
儿科姑息治疗

中文导读

本章主要介绍了儿科适于进行姑息治疗的状况；介绍了临终前医疗护理地点的选择，可以在医院、家庭、门诊或儿科护理机构；介绍了沟通、预订临终照顾计划和先期辅导，分别针对的是患儿父母、患儿本人、兄弟姐妹、医务人员、临终护理目标的制定和相关决策、临终的抢救复苏、对症处理、高强度对症处理、临终关怀以及儿科医师。还运用图表分别介绍了处于不同疾病状态下，危重病儿童典型的疾病轨迹；不同年龄段在临终前的自发的提问或表述、对死亡的认识，以及适宜采取的对策和回应等。

According to the World Health Organization (WHO), "Palliative care for children is the active total care of the child's body, mind and spirit and also involves giving support to the family. Optimally, this care begins when a life-threatening illness or condition is diagnosed and continues regardless of whether or not a child receives treatment directed at the underlying illness." Provision of palliative care applies to children with a wide variety of diagnoses, including cancer, cystic fibrosis, complex or severe cardiac disease, neurodegenerative disorders, severe malformations, and trauma with life-threatening sequelae (Table 7.1). Medical and technologic advances have resulted in children living longer, often with significant dependence on expensive technologies. These children have *complex chronic conditions* across the spectrum of congenital and acquired life-threatening disorders. Children with complex chronic conditions benefit from integration of palliative care strategies. These children, who often survive near-death crises followed by the renewed need for rehabilitative and life-prolonging treatments, are best served by a system that is flexible and responsive to changing needs and blended goals of care.

Although often mistakenly understood as equivalent to *end-of-life care*, the scope and potential benefits of palliative care are applicable *throughout the illness trajectory*. Palliative care emphasizes optimization of quality of life, communication, and symptom control, goals that may be congruent with maximal treatment aimed at sustaining or prolonging life.

The mandate of the pediatrician and other pediatric clinicians to attend to children's physical, mental, and emotional health and development includes the provision of palliative care for those who live with a significant possibility of death before adulthood (Fig. 7.1). Such comprehensive physical, psychological, social, and spiritual care requires an interdisciplinary approach.

Table 7.1	Conditions Appropriate for Pediatric Palliative Care

Conditions for Which Curative Treatment Is Possible but May Not Succeed

Advanced or progressive cancer or cancer with a poor prognosis
Complex and severe congenital or acquired heart disease

Conditions for Which There Is Intensive Long-Term Treatment Aimed at Prolonging Life and Maintaining Quality of Life, but Premature Death Is Still Possible

Cystic fibrosis
Severe immunodeficiency
High-risk solid-organ transplant candidates and/or recipients (e.g., lung, multivisceral)
Chronic or severe respiratory failure
Muscular dystrophy
Complex multiple congenital malformation syndromes
Primary pulmonary hypertension
Severe chromosomal disorders (aneuploidy, deletions, duplications)

Progressive Conditions for Which There Is No Curative Option and in Which Treatment Is Almost Exclusively Palliative After Diagnosis

Progressive metabolic disorders (Tay-Sachs disease)
Batten disease
Severe forms of osteogenesis imperfecta

Conditions Involving Severe, Nonprogressive Disability, Causing Extreme Vulnerability to Health Complications

Severe cerebral palsy with recurrent infection or difficult-to-control symptoms
Severe neurologic sequelae of infectious disease
Hypoxic or anoxic brain injury
Brain malformations (e.g., holoprosencephaly, lissencephaly)

Adapted from The Together for Short Lives [formerly the Association for Children's Palliative Care (ACT)] Life-limiting/Life-threatening Condition Categories. http://www.togetherforshortlives.org.uk/professionals/childrens_palliative_care_essentials/approach.

In the United States the healthcare and reimbursement structure, combined with frequent use of medical technology (e.g., home ventilatory support) or continuous home nursing, historically precluded formal enrollment of children on the hospice benefit when they were otherwise eligible (i.e., had estimated prognosis of ≤6 mo). Section 2302 of the Patient Protection and Affordable Care Act (ACA), the **Concurrent Care for Children Requirement (CCCR)**, eliminated the requirement that Medicaid patients <21 yr old forgo curative or life-prolonging therapies to be eligible for hospice. Although Medicaid programs in every state are now required to provide concurrent curative/life-prolonging treatment and hospice services for hospice-eligible children, development of systems to make such concurrent care a reality has been slow. A limitation of the CCCR is that it does not expand access to hospice for children with life-threatening illness who do not meet hospice eligibility criteria (i.e., have a prognosis that cannot be estimated to be <6 mo) or those not receiving Medicaid.

A number of state-based pediatric palliative care coalitions have formed in recent years to improve access to home-based pediatric hospice/palliative care services, using strategies such as Medicaid waivers or state plan amendments to increase coverage for hospice services. A growing number of home care agencies have also developed palliative care programs that serve as a bridge to hospice services for children not yet meeting hospice eligibility criteria. Some hospices have adopted an **open hospice** model with more flexible eligibility criteria. However, provision of hospice or palliative care for children is often also limited by the availability of clinicians who have training or experience in caring for seriously ill children.

CARE SETTINGS

Pediatric palliative care should be provided across settings, including hospital, outpatient, and home, as well as pediatric nursing facilities and sometimes inpatient hospice houses. **Home care** for the child with a life-threatening illness requires 24 hr/day access to experts in pediatric palliative care, a team approach, and an identified coordinator who serves as a link among hospitals, the community, and specialists and who may assist in preventing or arranging for hospital admissions,

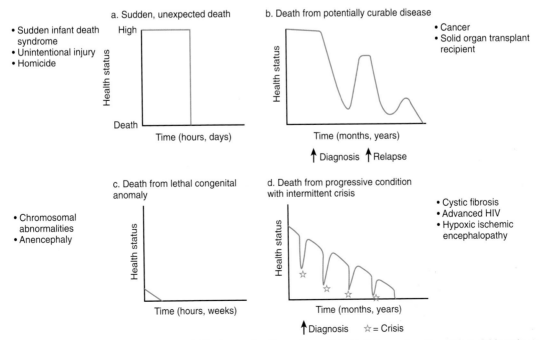

Fig. 7.1 Typical illness trajectories for children with life-threatening illness. *(From Field M, Behrman R, editors: When children die: improving palliative and end-of-life care for children and their families, Washington, DC, 2003, National Academies Press, p 74.)*

respite care, and increased home care support as needed. Adequate home care support and respite care, although sorely needed, is often not readily available because staffing or the high-tech skill required to care for these children is lacking. Furthermore, families may view using respite care as a personal failure, or they may worry that others cannot adequately care for their child's special needs or potential rapid escalation of symptoms.

At the end of life, children and families may need intensive support. About half of pediatric deaths occur in acute care hospitals, and end-of-life care may thus be provided in the home, hospital, pediatric nursing facility, or hospice house. Families need to feel safe and well cared for and given permission, if possible, to choose location of care. In tertiary care hospitals, most children die in the neonatal and pediatric intensive care units (ICUs). In some instances, when death at home for a child in the ICU is preferred, transport and even extubation at home may be possible, if clinical and logistical circumstances permit it.

The philosophy of palliative care can be successfully integrated into any hospital setting, including the ICU, when the focus of care also includes the prevention or amelioration of suffering and improving comfort and quality of life. All interventions that affect the child and family need to be assessed in relationship to these goals. This proactive approach asks the question, "What can we offer that will improve the quality of this child's life and provide the most meaning and sense of control and choice for their family?" instead of, "What therapies are we no longer going to offer this patient?" Staff may benefit from education, support, and guidance because pediatric palliative care, as with other types of intensive care, is an area of specialty. Regardless of the care setting, comprehensive palliative care requires an interdisciplinary approach that may include nurses, physicians, psychologists, psychiatrists, social workers, chaplains/clergy, child life specialists, and trained volunteers.

COMMUNICATION, ADVANCE CARE PLANNING, AND ANTICIPATORY GUIDANCE

Although accurate prognostication is a particular challenge in pediatrics, the medical team often recognizes a terminal prognosis before the prognosis is understood by parents or the child. This delay may impede informed decision-making about how the child lives at the end of life. Given the inherent prognostic uncertainty of a life-threatening diagnosis, discussions concerning resuscitation, symptom control, and end-of-life care planning should be initiated when the physician recognizes that a significant possibility of patient mortality exists. Having these conversations in the midst of a crisis is not ideal. Whenever possible, they should occur well in advance of the crisis or when the patient has recovered from a crisis but is at high risk for others.

Patients and families are most comfortable being cared for by physicians and other care providers with whom they have an established relationship. Even in the face of long-standing and highly connected relationships, *clinicians often hold assumptions about parent prognostic awareness, as well as parent readiness and willingness to have such discussions.* In an attempt to protect families, clinicians may avoid conversations that they perceive as promoting distress or hopelessness. However, parents greatly value honesty, and in fact such conversations can promote parent hopefulness, as well as trust and connection with the care team. At times, therefore, a *consultative* palliative care team provides the family with an opportunity to engage in sensitive conversations that do not as readily occur with the primary team, at least initially.

The population of individuals who die before reaching adulthood includes a disproportionate number of nonverbal and preverbal children and adolescents who are developmentally unable to make autonomous care decisions. Although parents are usually the primary decision-makers, these youth should be as fully involved in discussions and decisions about their care as appropriate for their developmental status. Using communication experts, child life therapists, chaplains, social workers, psychologists, or psychiatrists to allow children to express themselves through art, play, music, talk, and writing will enhance the provider's knowledge of the child's understanding and hopes. Tools such as **Five Wishes** (for adults), **Voicing My Choices** (for adolescents), and **My Wishes** (for school-age children), have in practice been useful in helping

to introduce advance care planning to children, adolescents, and their families (www.agingwithdignity.org/index.php).

The Parents

For parents, **compassionate communication** with medical providers who understand their child's illness, treatment options, and family beliefs and goals are the cornerstone of caring for children with life-threatening illness. During this time, one of the most significant relationships is that with the child's pediatrician, who often has an enduring relationship with the child and family, including healthy siblings. Parents need to know that their child's pediatrician will not abandon them as the goals of care evolve. A family's goals may change with the child's evolving clinical condition and other variable factors. A flexible approach rooted in ongoing communication and guidance that incorporates understanding of the family's values, goals, and religious, cultural, spiritual, and personal beliefs is of paramount importance.

Pediatricians should recognize the important role they have in continuing to care for the child and family, since the primary goal of treatment may simultaneously be prolongation of life and comfort, relief of suffering, and promoting quality of life. Regular meetings between caregivers and the family are essential to reassess and manage symptoms, explore the impact of illness on immediate family members, and provide anticipatory guidance. At these meetings, important issues with lifelong implications for parents and their child may be discussed. Such discussions should be planned with care, ensuring that adequate time for in-depth conversation is allotted; a private, physical setting is arranged; devices are silenced; and that both parents and others who might be identified by the family as primary supports are present. Strategies for facilitating conversations related to goals of care and decision-making are detailed later.

Families may look to their pediatrician for assurance that all treatment options have been explored. Assisting a patient's family to arrange a second opinion may be helpful. Listening to families and children speak about the future even in the face of poor prognosis may help keep the focus on living even while the child may be dying. Hoping for a miracle can coexist for parents even as they are facing and accepting the more likely reality of death.

Parents also need to know about the availability of home care, respite services, web-based support (e.g., www.courageousparentsnetwork.org), educational materials, and support groups. Responding to parental requests or need for counseling referrals for themselves, other children, or family is essential. Also, attending to the concrete needs of families (e.g., financial, insurance, housing) can be paramount in freeing them of worries that might interfere or compete with their ability to be fully present in their child's care.

When closer to the patient's end of life, although broaching the topic may seem daunting, exploration of how parents envision their child's death, addressing their previous loss experiences (most often with death of an adult relative) and any misconceptions, is often a great relief to parents. Learning about cultural, spiritual, and family values regarding pain management, suffering, and the preferred place of end-of-life care is essential. Even mentioning funeral arrangements, possible autopsy, and organ/tissue donation can be helpful to give parents choices and know that these considerations can be discussed without fear. A major worry of many parents is how to involve and communicate with siblings, as well as the child, about the likelihood of impending death.

Ratings of "high satisfaction" with physician care have been directly correlated with receiving **clear communication** around end-of-life issues, delivered with sensitivity and caring; such communication included speaking directly to the child when appropriate. Communication is complicated by an assumed need for mutual protection in which the child wants to protect his or her parents, and likewise the parents want to protect their child, from painful information or sadness. Honoring the uniqueness of the child, as well as understanding and respecting the family's communication style, values, spirituality, and culture, is critical in these highly sensitive conversations. Evidence shows that parents who have open conversations with their child about death and dying do not regret having done so.

In communications with the child and family, the physician should avoid giving specific estimates of survival length, even when the child or family explicitly asks for them. These predictions are invariably inaccurate because population-based statistics do not predict the course for individual patients. A more honest approach may be to explore *ranges of time in general terms* (weeks to months, months to years) while recognizing that children with serious illness are also susceptible to acute events that cause rapid deterioration. The physician can also ask parents what they might do differently if they knew how long their child would live, then assist them in thinking through the options relating to their specific concerns (e.g., suggest celebrating upcoming holidays or important events earlier to take advantage of times when the child may be feeling better). It is generally wise to suggest that relatives who wish to visit might do so earlier rather than later, given the unpredictable trajectory of many conditions.

For the child and family, the integration of "bad news" is a *process*, not an event, and when done sensitively, does not take away hope or alter the relationship between the family and physician. The physician should expect that some issues previously discussed may not be fully resolved for the child and parents (e.g., do-not-resuscitate [DNR] orders, artificial nutrition or hydration) and may need to be revisited over time. Parents of a child with chronic illness may reject the reality of an impending death because past predictions may not have been accurate. Whether they are parents of a child with a chronic illness or a child whose death is the result of accident or sudden catastrophic illness, they may experience great anxiety, guilt, or despair.

The Child

Truthful communication that takes into account the child's developmental stage and unique lived experience can help to address the fear and anxiety commonly experienced among children with life-threatening illness. Responding in a developmentally appropriate fashion (Table 7.2) to a child's questions about death (e.g., "What's happening to me?" or "Am I dying?") requires a careful exploration of what is already known by the child, what is really being asked (*the question behind the question*), and why the question is being asked at this particular time and in this setting. It may signal a need to be with someone who is comfortable listening to such unanswerable questions. Many children find nonverbal expression much easier than talking; art, play therapy, and storytelling may be more helpful than direct conversation.

A child's perception of death depends on his or her conceptual understanding of *universality* (that all things inevitably die), *irreversibility* (that dead people cannot come back to life), *nonfunctionality* (that being dead means that all biologic functions cease), and *causality* (that there are objective causes of death).

Very young children may struggle with the concepts of irreversibility and nonfunctionality. For young school-age children, who are beginning to understand the finality of death, worries may include *magical thinking* in which their thoughts, wishes, or bad behavior might be the underlying cause for their illness. Older children seek more factual information to gain some control over the situation.

Children's fears of death are often centered on the concrete fear of being separated from parents and other loved ones and what will happen to their parents rather than themselves. This can be true for teens and young adults as well. This fear may be responded to in different ways: some families may give reassurance that loving relatives will be waiting, while others use religious concepts to refer to an eternal spiritual connection.

Adolescents may have a conceptual understanding of death similar to that of adults, but working with the adolescent with life-threatening illness presents unique concerns and issues. The developmental work of adolescence includes separating from their parents, developing strong peer relationships, and moving towards independent adulthood. For this population, the teenager's developmental need to separate is complicated by the increasing dependence both physically and emotionally on their parents.

In addition to developmental considerations, understanding related to the child's life experiences, the length of the child's illness, the understanding of the nature and prognosis of the illness, the child's role in the family (peacemaker, clown, troublemaker, the good child)

should be considered in communication with children.

The question of whether and when to involve adolescents in decision-making arises particularly often. There is no one answer to this question. Instead, numerous considerations should be taken into account, including the adolescent's chronological age, developmental stage, adolescent preference with regard to such participation, and the family's preferred approach to communication and decision-making.

Parents have an instinctive and strong desire to protect their children from harm. When facing the death of their child, many parents attempt to keep the reality of impending death hidden from their child, hoping the child can be *protected* from the harsh reality. Although it is important to respect parental wishes, it is also true that most children already have a sense of what is happening to their bodies, even when it has been purposely left unspoken. Children may blame themselves for their illness and the resulting hardships for their loved ones. Perpetuating the myth that "everything is going to be all right" takes away the chance to explore fears and provide reassurance. Assisting parents to understand that the key to honest communication is not telling a child he or she is dying but opening the door to conversation and validating what the child *already knows*. Honest communication also allows opportunities for memory and legacy making and saying goodbye.

School is the work of childhood and adolescence and is important in optimizing quality of life for a child seeking normalcy in the face of illness. Finding ways to help children and their families to maintain these connections through modification of the school day, and exploring options to promote educational and social connections into the home or into the hospital room, can be meaningful in the event that a child is not well enough to attend school. Video conferencing now can be readily arranged from almost any setting.

The Siblings

Brothers and sisters are at special risk both during their sibling's illness and after the death. Because of the extraordinary demands placed on parents to meet the needs of their ill child, healthy siblings may feel that their own needs are not being acknowledged or fulfilled. These feelings of neglect may then trigger guilt about their own good health and resentment toward their parents and ill sibling. Younger siblings may react to the stress by becoming seemingly oblivious to the turmoil around them. Some younger siblings may feel guilty for wishing the affected child would die so they could get their parents back (magical thinking). Parents need to know that these are normal responses, and siblings should be encouraged to maintain the typical routines of daily living. Siblings who are most involved with their sick brothers or sisters before death usually adjust better both at the time of and after the death. Acknowledging and validating sibling feelings, being honest and open, and appropriately involving them in the life of their sick sibling provide a good foundation for the grief process. It is often helpful to identify a person in the family (e.g., caring aunt) or school (e.g., counselor) to offer confidential and supportive opportunities for the sibling to reflect on their family experience, particularly as parents may be too overwhelmed to provide this at crucial times.

The Staff

Inadequate support for the staff providing palliative care can result in depression, emotional withdrawal, and other symptoms. Offering educational opportunities and emotional support for staff at various stages of caring for a child with life-threatening illness can be helpful in bettering patient/family care and preventing staff from experiencing compassion fatigue, burnout, and long-term repercussions, including leaving the field.

Goals of Care and Decision-Making

In the course of a child's life-limiting illness, a series of important decisions may arise in relation to location of care, medications with risks and benefits, not starting or discontinuing life-prolonging treatments, experimental treatments in research protocols, and use of integrative therapies (see Chapter 78). Such family decisions are greatly facilitated by opportunities for in-depth and guided discussions around **goals of care** for the child. This is often accomplished by eliciting parent (and child)

Table 7.2 | Developmental Questions, Thoughts, and Concepts of Dying, With Responsive Strategies

TYPICAL QUESTIONS AND STATEMENTS ABOUT DYING	THOUGHTS THAT GUIDE BEHAVIOR	DEVELOPMENTAL UNDERSTANDING OF DEATH	STRATEGIES AND RESPONSES
MONTHS TO 3 YR OF AGE "Mommy, don't cry." "Daddy, will you still tickle me when I'm dead?"	Child has limited understanding of events, future and past, and of the difference between living and nonliving.	Child may have "sense" that something is wrong. Death is often viewed as continuous with life (analogous to being awake and being asleep).	Optimize comfort, and consistency; familiar persons, objects, routines. Use soothing songs, words, and touch. "I will always love you." "I will always take care of you." "I will tickle you forever."
AGE 3-5 YR "I did something bad and so I will die." "Can I eat anything I want in heaven?"	Concepts are simple and reversible. Variations between reality and fantasy.	Child may see death as temporary and reversible and not universal. Child may feel responsible for illness. Death may be perceived as an external force that can get you.	Assure child that illness not her fault. Provide consistent caregivers. Promote honest simple language. Use books to explain the life cycle and promote questions and answers. "You did not do anything to cause this." "You are so special to us, and we will always love you." "We know (God, Jesus, Grandma, Grandpa) are waiting to see you."
AGE 5-10 YR "How will I die?" "Will it hurt?" "Is dying scary?"	Child begins to demonstrate organized, logical thought. Thinking becomes less esoteric. Child begins to problem-solve concretely, reason logically, and organize thoughts coherently. However, child has limited abstract reasoning.	Child begins to understand death as real and permanent. Death means that your heart stops, your blood does not circulate, and you do not breathe. It may be viewed as a violent event. Child may not accept death could happen to himself or to anyone he knows but starts to realize that people that he knows will die.	Be honest and provide specific details if they are requested. Help and support the child's need for control. Permit and encourage the child's participation in decision making. "We will work together to help you feel comfortable. It is very important that you let us know how you are feeling and what you need. We will always be with you, so you do not need to be afraid."
AGE 10-18 YR "I'm afraid if I die my mom will just break down." "I'm too young to die. I want to get married and have children." "Why is God letting this happen?"	Abstract thoughts and logic possible. Body image is important. Child needs peer relationships for support and for validation. Child expresses altruistic values, such as staying alive for family (parents, siblings) and donating organs/tissue. Disbelief that she is dying.	Understand death as irreversible, inevitable and universal. Child needs reassurance of continued care and love. Search for meaning and purpose of life.	Reinforce child/adolescent's self-esteem, sense of worth, and self-respect. Allow need for privacy, independence, access to friends and peers. Tolerate expression of strong emotions and permit participation in decision-making. "I can't imagine how you must be feeling. Despite it all, you are doing an incredible job. I wonder how I can help?" "What's most important to you now?" "What are your hopes … your worries?" "You have taught me so much; I will always remember you."

Adapted from Hurwitz C, Duncan J, Wolfe J: Caring for the child with cancer at the close of life, JAMA 292:2141–2149, 2003.

understanding of the child's condition and asking open-ended questions that explore the parent's and child's hopes, worries, and family values. Goals-of-care conversations include what is most important for them as a family, considerations of their child's clinical condition, and their values and beliefs, including cultural, religious, and spiritual considerations. Table 7.3 presents specific questions that can effectively guide these discussions. The conversation should also include a review of previous discussions, active listening to concerns and issues as they are raised, opportunities to repeat back elements of the discussion to ensure clarity, and provision of honest, factual answers even in areas of uncertainty.

Decision-making should be focused on the goals of care, as opposed to limitations of care; "This is what we can offer," instead of, "There is nothing more we can do." Rather than meeting specifically to discuss withdrawing support or a do-not-resuscitate (DNR) order, a more general discussion centered on the goals of care will naturally lead to considering which interventions are in the child's best interests and can present an opportunity for the clinicians to make recommendations based on these

goals. By offering medical recommendations based on family goals and the clinical reality, the team can decrease the burden of responsibility for decision-making that parents carry.

Resuscitation Status

Many parents do not understand the legal mandate requiring attempted resuscitation for cardiorespiratory arrest unless a written DNR order is in place. In broaching this topic, rather than asking parents if they want to forgo cardiopulmonary resuscitation (CPR) for their child (and placing the full burden of decision-making on them), it is preferable to discuss whether or not resuscitative interventions are likely to benefit the child. *It is important to make recommendations based on overall goals of care and medical knowledge of potential benefit and/or harm of these interventions.* Once the goals of therapy are agreed on, the physician is required to write a formal order. Out-of-hospital DNR verification forms are available in many states, which if completed on behalf of the child, affirm that rather than initiating resuscitative efforts, emergency

Table 7.3	Five Basic Questions to Guide "Goals of Care" Conversation

PHRASING FOR ADULT OR OLDER ADOLESCENT	PHRASING FOR CHILD
Tell us about your child as a person. What does your child enjoy?	Tell me about yourself before you got sick.
What is your understanding of your child's illness/condition?	Why are you in the hospital? What do you understand about your illness?
In light of your understanding, what is most important to you regarding your child's care?	What do you want others to know or do for you when taking care of you?
What are you hoping for? What are your worries?	I wonder if there is anything that is worrying you or that is keeping you up at night. Is there anything you wish you could talk about?
What gives you strength in the face of your child's illness/condition?	What helps you get through the day? What helps you feel good?

Table 7.4	Key Elements of Effective Symptom Management

SETTING THE STAGE
- Establish and periodically revisit goals of care and ensure that goals are communicated to entire care team.
- Plan for symptoms (including unanticipated ones) before they occur.

ASSESSMENT
- Assess the child for symptoms regularly, using consistent and developmentally appropriate assessment tools.
  - Utilize self-report, if the child is able to reliably report symptoms.
- Evaluate all aspects of the symptom, including quality, frequency, duration, and intensity.
- Consider the holistic nature of symptoms.
- Explore the meaning that symptoms may have for families in their social, cultural, and religious context.
- Assess distress caused by the symptom.
- Evaluate the degree of functional impairment from the symptom.

TREATMENT
- Understand the pathophysiology of the symptom, and establish a complete differential diagnosis.
- Treat the underlying cause if possible, weighing benefits and risks, in the context of goals of care.
- Choose the least invasive route for medications—by mouth whenever possible.
- Prescribe regular medications for constant symptoms, and consider prn doses for breakthrough or uncontrolled symptoms.
- Consider all approaches (i.e., pharmacologic/nonpharmacologic and local/systemic).
- Partner with families to identify and address any barriers to optimal control of symptoms.
- Address spiritual, emotional, and existential suffering in addition to physical suffering since these are often interrelated.

ONGOING CARE
- Reassess the symptom and response to interventions regularly.
- For refractory symptoms, revisit the differential diagnosis and review potentially contributing factors.
- Effective interventions relieve the symptom and reduce distress and functional impairment.

response teams are obligated to provide appropriate symptom management with comfort and relief of suffering with appropriate interventions when called to the scene.

Almost half of all states have implemented the **physician orders for life treatment (POLST) system**. A POLST order is completed for children with life-threatening illness, translating the expressed parent's and/or child's wishes for interventions to do or not do into actionable orders (www.polst.org). It is usually helpful to frame discussions about POLST as ways for parents to maintain some control, by communicating their goals and care preferences, so that they may be honored, irrespective of the setting. It may also be beneficial to write a letter that delineates decisions regarding resuscitation interventions and supportive care measures to be undertaken for the child, particularly if POLST are not available. The letter should be as detailed as possible, including recommendations for comfort medications and contact information for caregivers best known to the patient. Such a letter, given to the parents, with copies to involved caregivers and institutions, can be a useful communication aid, especially in times of crisis. In any case, if a child may die in the home setting, and the parents opt to use on out-of-hospital DNR verification form or POLST, plans to pronounce the child and provide support for the family must be in place. If the child has been referred to hospice, the hospice usually fulfills those responsibilities.

Conflicts in decision-making can occur within families, within healthcare teams, between the child and family, and between the family and professional caregivers (see Chapter 6). For children who are developmentally unable to provide guidance in decision-making (neonates, very young children, or children with cognitive impairment), parents and healthcare professionals may come to different conclusions as to what is in the child's best interests. Decision-making around the care of adolescents presents specific challenges, given the shifting boundary that separates childhood from adulthood. In some families and cultures, truth-telling and autonomy are secondary to maintaining the integrity of the family (see Chapter 11). Although frequently encountered, differences in opinion are often manageable for all involved when lines of communication are kept open, team and family meetings are held, and the goals of care are clear.

Symptom Management

Intensive symptom management is another cornerstone of pediatric palliative care. Alleviation of symptoms reduces suffering of the child and family and allows them to focus on other concerns and participate in meaningful experiences. Despite increasing attention to symptoms, and pharmacologic and technical advances in medicine, children often suffer from multiple symptoms. Table 7.4 provides key elements and general approaches to managing symptoms.

Pain is a complex sensation triggered by actual or potential tissue damage and influenced by cognitive, behavioral, emotional, social, and cultural factors. Effective pain relief is essential to prevent *central sensitization*, a central hyperexcitation response that may lead to hypersensitivity and escalating pain, and to diminish a stress response that may have a variety of physiologic effects. Assessment tools include self-report tools for children who are able to communicate their pain verbally, as well as tools based on behavioral cues for children who are unable to do so because of their medical condition or a neurodevelopmental disorder. Tables 7.5 to 7.7 address management of pain (see also Chapter 76).

Many children with life-threatening illness experience pain that requires **opioids** for adequate relief at some point in their illness trajectory. The WHO pain guidelines recommend the first step for mild pain and the second step for moderate to severe pain. Although it was previously recommended, prescribing *codeine* should generally be avoided because of its side effect profile and lack of superiority over nonopioid analgesics. Furthermore, relatively common genetic polymorphisms in the *CYP2D6* gene lead to wide variation in codeine metabolism. Specifically, 10–40% of individuals carry polymorphisms causing them to be *poor metabolizers* who cannot convert codeine to its active form, *morphine*, and therefore are at risk for inadequate pain control. Others

Table 7.5	Guidelines for Pain Management

- Use nonopioid analgesics as monotherapy for mild pain, and together with opioids for more severe pain.
  Nonopioid analgesics include acetaminophen, nonsteroidal antiinflammatory drugs (NSAIDs), salicylates, and selective cyclooxygenase (COX-2) inhibitors.
- For moderate or severe pain, start with a short-acting opioid at regular intervals.
  When dose requirements have stabilized, consider converting opioid to a long-acting formulation with doses available for breakthrough or uncontrolled pain, as needed.
  - For uncontrolled pain, increase opioid dose by 30–50%; for severe pain, increase by 50–100%.
  - Avoid codeine and opioids with mixed-agonist activity (e.g., butorphanol, pentazocine).
- Administer medications by the simplest, most effective, and least distressing route.
- Dispel the myth that strong medications should be saved for extreme situations or the very end of life.
  Opioids do not have a "ceiling effect," and escalating symptoms can usually be treated with an increase in dose. If further titration does not provide adequate analgesia, the opioid may be rotated to another (see below).
- Clarify for families the differences among tolerance, physical dependence, and addiction.

- Anticipate and treat/prevent common analgesic side effects (gastritis with NSAIDs; constipation, pruritus, nausea, and sedation with opioids).
  Always initiate a bowel regimen to prevent constipation when starting opioids.
  Consider a stimulant for opioid-induced somnolence.
  Pruritus rarely indicates a true allergy. If not responsive to an antihistamine, consider low-dose naloxone or switching opioids.
  Consider switching to a different opioid for intolerable side effects or neurotoxicity (e.g., myoclonus).
  Use an equianalgesic conversion table when switching opioids, and account for incomplete cross-tolerance with dose reduction.
- Consider the use of adjuvant drugs for specific pain syndromes, and for their opioid-sparing effect:
  Antidepressants (e.g., amitriptyline, nortriptyline) and anticonvulsants (e.g., gabapentin, carbamazepine, topiramate) for neuropathic pain
  Steroids or NSAIDs for bone pain
  Sedatives and hypnotics for anxiety and muscle spasm
  To enhance analgesia from opioids, consider clonidine or ketamine.
- Use topical local anesthetics (lidocaine, prilocaine, bupivacaine) when possible
- Consider anesthetic blocks for regional pain.
- Consider palliative radiation therapy.
- Consider psychological approaches (e.g., cognitive or behavioral therapy) and integrative therapies (e.g., acupuncture, massage).

are *ultrametabolizers* who may even experience respiratory depression from rapid generation of morphine from codeine. It is therefore preferable to use a known amount of the active agent, morphine.

It is important to explore with families, as well as members of the care team, misconceptions that they may have regarding respiratory suppression, addiction, dependence, the symbolic meaning of starting an opioid such as methadone or morphine and/or a morphine drip, and the potential for opioids to hasten death. *There is no association between administration or escalation of opioids and length of survival.* Evidence supports longer survival in individuals with symptoms that are well controlled.

Children also often experience a multitude of **nonpain symptoms**. A combination of both pharmacologic (Table 7.6) and nonpharmacologic (Table 7.7) interventions is often optimal. **Fatigue** is one of the most common symptoms in children with advanced illness. Children may experience fatigue as a physical symptom (e.g., weakness or somnolence), a decline in cognition (e.g., diminished attention or concentration), and impaired emotional function (e.g., depressed mood or decreased motivation). Because of its multidimensional and incapacitating nature, fatigue can prevent children from participating in meaningful or pleasurable activities, thereby impairing quality of life. Fatigue is usually multifactorial in etiology. A careful history may reveal contributing physical factors (uncontrolled symptoms, medication side effects), psychological factors (anxiety, depression), spiritual distress, or sleep disturbance. Interventions to reduce fatigue include treatment of contributing factors, exercise, pharmacologic agents, and behavior modification strategies. Challenges to effectively addressing fatigue include the common belief that fatigue is inevitable, lack of communication between families and care teams about it, and limited awareness of potential interventions for fatigue.

Dyspnea (the subjective sensation of shortness of breath) results from a mismatch between afferent sensory input to the brain and the outgoing motor signal from the brain. It may stem from respiratory causes (e.g., airway secretions, obstruction, infection) or other factors (e.g., cardiac) and may also be influenced by psychological factors (e.g., anxiety). Respiratory parameters such as respiratory rate and oxygen saturation correlate unreliably with the degree of dyspnea. Therefore,

giving oxygen to a cyanotic or hypoxic child who is otherwise quiet and relaxed may relieve staff discomfort while having no impact on patient distress and may also add burden if the child cannot tolerate the mask or cannula. Dyspnea can be relieved with the use of regularly scheduled plus as-needed doses of opioids. Opioids work *directly* on the brainstem to reduce the sensation of respiratory distress, as opposed to relieving dyspnea by sedation. The dose of opioid needed to reduce dyspnea is as little as 25% of the amount that would be given for analgesia. Nonpharmacologic interventions, including guided imagery or hypnosis to reduce anxiety, or cool, flowing air, aimed toward the face, are also frequently helpful in alleviating dyspnea. While oxygen may relieve hypoxemia-related headaches, it is no more effective than blowing room air in reducing the distressing sensation of shortness of breath.

As death approaches, a buildup of secretions may result in noisy respiration sometimes referred to as a "death rattle." Patients at this stage are usually unconscious, and noisy respirations are often more distressing for others than for the child. It is often helpful to discuss this anticipated phenomenon with families in advance, and if it occurs, to point out the child's lack of distress from it. If treatment is needed, an anticholinergic medication, such as glycopyrrolate, may reduce secretions.

Neurologic symptoms include **seizures** that are often part of the antecedent illness but may increase in frequency and severity toward the end of life. A plan for managing seizures should be made in advance, and anticonvulsants should be readily available in the event of seizure. Parents can be taught to use rectal diazepam at home. Increased **neuroirritability** accompanies some neurodegenerative disorders; it may be particularly disruptive because of the resultant break in normal sleep–wake patterns and the difficulty in finding respite facilities for children who have prolonged crying. Such neuroirritability may respond to gabapentin. Judicious use of sedatives, benzodiazepines, clonidine, nortriptyline, or methadone may also reduce irritability without inducing excessive sedation; such treatment can dramatically improve the quality of life for both child and caregivers. Increased **intracranial pressure** and **spinal cord compression** are most often encountered in children with brain tumors or metastatic and solid tumors. Depending on the

| Table 7.6 | Pharmacologic Approach to Symptoms Commonly Experienced by Children With Life-Threatening Illness |

SYMPTOM	MEDICATION	STARTING DOSE	COMMENTS
Pain—mild	Acetaminophen	15 mg/kg PO q4h, max 4 g/day	Available PO (including liquid), PR, or IV
	Ibuprofen	10 mg/kg PO q6h	PO (including liquid) only; avoid if risk of bleeding; use only in infants ≥6 mo. Use with caution in congestive heart failure. Chewable tablets contain phenylalanine.
	Choline magnesium trisalicylate	10-20 mg/kg PO tid (max 500-1000 mg/dose)	Trilisate may have less antiplatelet activity and therefore pose less risk for bleeding than other salicylates. Salicylates, however, have been associated with Reye syndrome in children <2 yr.
	Celecoxib	1-2 mg/kg (max 100 mg) PO q12-24h	Selective cyclooxygenase (COX-2) inhibitor has low risk of gastritis and low antiplatelet activity.
Pain—moderate/severe	Morphine immediate release (i.e., MSIR)	0.3 mg/kg PO q4h if <50 kg 5-10 mg PO q4h if >50 kg[*†]	Also available in IV/SQ formulation.[‡§]
	Oxycodone	0.1 mg/kg PO q4h if <50 kg 5-10 mg PO q4h if >50 kg[*†]	No injectable formulation.[‡§]
	Hydromorphone	0.05 mg/kg PO q4h if <50 kg 1-2 mg PO q4h if >50 kg[*†]	Also available in IV/SQ formulation. Injectable form very concentrated, facilitating subcutaneous delivery.[‡§]
	Fentanyl	0.5-1.5 µg/kg IV/SQ q30min[*†]	Rapid infusion may cause chest wall rigidity.[‡§]
	Methadone	Starting dose 0.1-0.2 mg/kg PO bid. May give tid if needed. Recommend consultation with experienced clinician for equivalence dosing from other opioids.[*†]	Only opioid with immediate and prolonged effect available as a liquid; do not adjust dose more often than every 72 hr because prolonged biologic half-life > therapeutic half-life. Knowledge of methadone pharmacokinetics is needed for converting to and from doses of other opioids. Also available IV/SQ. May cause QT interval prolongation (consider ECG), especially in adults on >200 mg/day or in those at risk for QT prolongation. Interacts with several antiretroviral agents.[§]
Pain—sustained release	MS Contin Kadian (contains sustained release pellets) Avinza (contains immediate and extended release beads) Oramorph	Total daily dose of MSIR divided bid-tid	Do not crush MS Contin. For those unable to swallow pills, Kadian and Avinza capsules may be opened and contents mixed with food but *cannot be chewed*. Kadian contents may be mixed in 10 mL water and given via 16-French G-tube. Avoid alcohol with Avinza. Larger-dose formulation may not be suitable for small children.[§]
	Oxycontin	Total daily dose of oxycodone divided bid-tid	Do not crush.[§]
	Transdermal fentanyl patch	Divide 24 hr PO morphine dose by 2 to determine starting dose of transdermal fentanyl. No data exist on the equianalgesic conversion from transdermal fentanyl to any oral opioid.	Smallest patch size may be too high for small children. For children >2 yr. Apply to upper back in young children. Patch may **not** be cut. Typically for patients taking at least 60 mg morphine/day or its equivalent. Not appropriate when dosage changes are frequent or for opioid-naïve patients. Fever >40°C results in higher serum concentrations.[§]
Pain—neuropathic	Nortriptyline	0.5 mg/kg PO at bedtime (max 150 mg/day)	Fewer anticholinergic side effects than amitriptyline. May cause constipation, sedation, postural hypotension, and dry mouth. May cause QT interval prolongation (consider ECG). At higher doses, monitor ECG and plasma levels.
	Gabapentin	Start at 5 mg/kg/day at bedtime and gradually increase to 10-15 mg/kg/day divided tid; titrate up by 5 mg/kg/day q 3-4 days as needed but not to exceed 50-75 mg/kg/day (3600 mg/day)	May cause neuropsychiatric events in children (aggression, emotional lability, hyperkinesia), usually mild but may require discontinuation of gabapentin. May cause dizziness, drowsiness, tremor, nystagmus, ataxia, and swelling.
	Pregabalin	Start at 1 mg/kg/dose PO at bedtime for 3 days, then increase to 1 mg/kg/dose bid. Increase every 3 days to 3 mg/kg/dose PO bid (max 6 mg/kg/dose).	
	Methadone	See previous listing	See previous listing.
Dyspnea	Morphine, immediate release (i.e., MSIR)	0.1 mg/kg PO q4h prn[*†]	All opioids may relieve dyspnea. For dyspnea, the starting dose is 30% of the dose that would be administered for pain.[§]
	Lorazepam	0.025-0.05 mg/kg IV/PO q6h, up to 2 mg/dose	See previous listing

Continued

Table 7.6	Pharmacologic Approach to Symptoms Commonly Experienced by Children With Life-Threatening Illness—cont'd		
SYMPTOM	**MEDICATION**	**STARTING DOSE**	**COMMENTS**
Respiratory secretions	Scopolamine patch	1.5 mg patch, change q72h (for children >8-12 yr old)	Excessive drying of secretions can cause mucus plugging of airways. Good for motion-induced nausea and vomiting. Handling patch and contacting eye may cause anisocoria and blurry vision. May fold patches, but do not cut them. Anticholinergic side effects possible.
	Glycopyrrolate	0.04-0.1 mg/kg PO q4-8h	Powerful antisialagogue. Excessive drying of secretions can cause mucus plugging of airways. Anticholinergic side effects possible. Quaternary ammonium structure limits its ability to cross lipid membranes, such as the blood-brain barrier (in contrast to atropine, scopolamine, and hyoscyamine sulfate), so may exert fewer central anticholinergic effects.
	Hyoscyamine sulfate	4 gtt PO q4h prn if <2 yr 8 gtt PO q4h prn if 2-12 yr Do not exceed 24 gtt/24 hr.	Anticholinergic side effects possible, including sedation. May be given sublingually.
	Atropine	1-2 gtt SL q4-6h prn	Give 0.5% ophthalmic drops sublingually.
Nausea	Metoclopramide	0.1-0.2 mg/kg/dose q6h, up to 10 mg/dose (prokinetic and mild nausea dosing). For chemotherapy-associated nausea, 0.5-1 mg/kg q6h prn PO/IV/SC; give with diphenhydramine and continue diphenhydramine for 24 hr after last dose of high-dose metoclopramide to prevent extrapyramidal reaction.	Helpful when dysmotility is an issue; may cause extrapyramidal reactions, particularly in children following IV administration of high doses. Contraindicated in complete bowel obstruction or pheochromocytoma. Avoid concomitant use with olanzapine.
	Ondansetron	0.15 mg/kg dose IV/PO q8h prn. No single IV dose should exceed 16 mg due to risk of QT prolongation.	Significant experience in pediatrics. Good empirical therapy for nausea in palliative care population. Oral dissolving tablet contains phenylalanine. Higher doses used with chemotherapy although single 32 mg IV dose is no longer available (risk for QT prolongation). Consider ECG monitoring in patients with electrolyte abnormalities, congestive heart failure, bradyarrhythmias, or in patients taking other medications with potential to cause QT prolongation.
	Dexamethasone	0.1 mg/kg/dose tid PO/IV; max dose 10 mg/day	Also helpful with hepatic capsular distension, bowel wall edema, anorexia, increased ICP. May cause mood swings or psychosis.
	Lorazepam	See previous listing.	See previous listing
	Dronabinol	2.5-5 mg/m²/dose q3-4h	Available in 2.5 and 5 mg capsules. May remove liquid contents from capsules for children who cannot swallow capsules. Avoid in patients with sesame oil hypersensitivity or history of schizophrenia. May cause euphoria, dysphoria, or other mood changes. Tolerance to CNS side effects usually develops in 1-3 days of continuous use. Avoid in patients with depression or mania.
	Scopolamine patch	See previous listing.	See previous listing
	Olanzapine	4-6 yr: 1.25 mg PO daily 6-12 yr: 2.5 mg PO daily ≥12 yr: 5 mg daily	Little evidence to guide antiemetic dosing. Ranges largely derived from olanzapine dosing for other purposes. Avoid concomitant use with metoclopramide.
Anxiety	Lorazepam	See previous listing.	See previous listing.
Agitation	Haloperidol	0.01 mg/kg PO tid prn for acute onset: 0.025-0.050 mg/kg PO, may repeat 0.025 mg/kg in 1 hr prn	May cause extrapyramidal reactions, which can be reversed with diphenhydramine or Cogentin. Safety not established in children <3 yr.
Sleep disturbance/insomnia	Lorazepam	See previous listing.	See previous listing.
	Trazodone	Children 6-18 yr: 0.75-1 mg/kg/dose, given bid-tid if needed If >18 yr, start at 25-50 mg/dose, given bid-tid if needed	Potentially arrhythmogenic
Fatigue	Methylphenidate	0.3 mg/kg/dose titrated as needed, up to 60 mg/day	Rapid antidepressant effect; also improves cognition. Administer before meals to avoid appetite suppression. Use with caution in children at risk for cardiac arrhythmia. Available as liquid and chewable tablet.

Continued

| **Table 7.6** | Pharmacologic Approach to Symptoms Commonly Experienced by Children With Life-Threatening Illness—cont'd |

SYMPTOM	MEDICATION	STARTING DOSE	COMMENTS
Pruritus	Diphenhydramine	0.5-1 mg/kg q6h IV/PO (100 mg max per day)	May reverse phenothiazine-induced dystonic reactions. Topical formulation on large areas of the skin or open area may cause toxic reactions. May cause paradoxical reaction in young children.
	Hydroxyzine	0.5-1 mg/kg q6h IV/PO (600 mg max per day)	
Constipation	Docusate	40-150 mg/day PO in 1-4 divided doses	Stool softener available as liquid or capsule
	Miralax	<5 yr: ½ scoop (8.5 g) in 4 oz water daily >5 yr: 1 scoop (17 g) in 8 oz water daily	Tasteless powder may be mixed in beverage of choice. Now available over the counter.
	Lactulose	5-10 mL PO up to q2h until bowel movement	Bowel stimulant; dosing q2h may cause cramping.
	Senna	2.5 mL PO daily (for children >27 kg)	Bowel stimulant; available as granules
	Dulcolax	3-12 yr: 5-10 mg PO daily >12 yr 5-15 mg PO daily	Available in oral or rectal formulation
	Pediatric Fleets Enema	2.5 oz pediatric enema for children 2-11 yr; adult enema for children ≥12 yr	May repeat ×1 if needed. Do not use in neutropenic patients.
	Methylnaltrexone	10-20 kg: 2 mg SC 21-33 kg: 4 mg SC 34-46 kg: 6 mg SC 47.62 kg: 8 mg SC 63-114 kg: 12 mg SC ≥155 kg: 0.15 mg/kg SC Administer 1 dose every other day as needed; max 1 dose/24 hr	Peripherally acting opioid antagonist for opioid-induced constipation. Usually works within 30-60 min of administration.
Muscle spasm	Diazepam	0.5 mg/kg/dose IV/PO q6h prn Initial dose for children <5 yr: 5 mg dose; for children ≥5 yr: 10 mg/dose	May be irritating if given by peripheral IV line.
	Baclofen	5 mg PO tid, increase by 5 mg/dose as needed.	Helpful with neuropathic pain and spasticity; abrupt withdrawal may result in hallucinations and seizures; not for children <10 yr
Seizures	Lorazepam	0.1 mg/kg IV/PO/SL/PR; repeat q10min ×2	
	Diazepam	0.1 mg/kg q6h (max 5 mg/dose if <5 yr; max 10 mg/dose if >5 yr)	May be given PR as Diastat (0.2 mg/kg/dose q15min ×3 doses)
Neuroirritability	Gabapentin	See previous listing.	
	Clonidine	Starting dose: 0.05 mg/day. May increase every 3-5 days by 0.05 mg/day to 3-5 µg/kg/day given in divided doses 3-4 times/day; max dose 0.3 mg/day. May switch from oral to transdermal route once optimal oral dose is established. Transdermal dose is equivalent to the total oral daily dose (e.g., if total oral dose is 0.1 mg/day, apply 1 patch (delivers 0.1 mg/day). Change patch every 7 days.	Transdermal patch may contain metal (e.g., aluminum) that may cause burns if worn during MRI scan. Remove patch prior to MRI. Patch may be cut into ¼ or ½ fractions based on dose needed.
	Clonazepam	<10 yr or <30 kg: initial dose 0.01-0.03 mg/kg/day divided tid ≥10 yr (≥30 kg): initial dose up to 0.25 mg PO tid; may increase by 0.5-1 mg/day every 3 days Maintenance dose: 0.05-0.2 mg/kg/day up to 20 mg/day	
Anorexia	Megestrol acetate	10 mg/kg/day in 1-4 divided doses, may titrate up to 15 mg/kg/day or 800 mg/day	For children >10 yr. Acute adrenal insufficiency may occur with abrupt withdrawal after long-term use. Use with caution in patients with diabetes mellitus or history of thromboembolism. May cause photosensitivity.
	Dronabinol	See previous listing.	See previous listing.
	Cyproheptadine	Children ≥2 yr and adolescents: 0.08 mg/kg PO q8h; if no benefit in 5 days, increase dose by 0.04-0.08 mg/kg/dose Max daily dose: ≤6 yr: 12 mg/day; 7-14 yr: 16 mg/day; ≥15 yr: 32 mg/day	Potent antihistamine and serotonin antagonist

Note: **Some medications or dosing may not apply to infants (≤12 mo). Verify suitability and dosing of all medications before administering to neonates.**
*Infants <6 mo should receive 25–30% of the usual opioid starting dose.
†Although the usual opioid starting dose is presented, dose may be titrated as needed. There is no ceiling/maximum dose for opioids.
‡Breakthrough dose is 10% of 24 hr dose. See Chapter 76 for information regarding titration of opioids.
§Side effects from opioids include constipation, respiratory depression, pruritus, nausea, urinary retention, physical dependence.
IV, Intravenous(ly); PO, by mouth; PR, rectally; prn, as needed; gtt, drops; SC, subcutaneously; bid, twice daily; tid, 3 times daily; q4h, every 4 hours; q30min, every 30 minutes; CNS, central nervous system; ECG, electrocardiogram; ICP, intracranial pressure.
Adapted from Ullrich C, Wolfe J: Pediatric pain and symptom control. In Walsh TD, Caraceni AT, Fainsinger R, et al: *Palliative medicine*, Philadelphia, 2008, Saunders.

Table 7.7	Nonpharmacologic Approach to Symptoms Commonly Experienced by Children With Life-Threatening Illness
SYMPTOM	**APPROACH TO MANAGEMENT**
Pain	Prevent pain when possible by limiting unnecessary painful procedures, providing sedation, and giving preemptive analgesia before a procedure (e.g., including sucrose for procedures in neonates). Address coincident depression, anxiety, sense of fear or lack of control. Consider guided imagery, relaxation, hypnosis, art/pet/play therapy, acupuncture/acupressure, biofeedback, massage, heat/cold, yoga, transcutaneous electric nerve stimulation, distraction.
Dyspnea or air hunger	Suction oral secretions if present; positioning, comfortable loose clothing, fan to provide cool, blowing air. Limit volume of intravenous fluids; consider diuretics if fluid overload/pulmonary edema present. Behavioral strategies, including breathing exercises, guided imagery, relaxation, music, distraction.
Fatigue	Sleep hygiene (establish a routine, promote habits for restorative sleep). Regular, gentle exercise; prioritize or modify activities. Address potentially contributing factors (e.g., anemia, depression, side effects of medications). Aromatherapy*: peppermint, rosemary, basil.
Nausea/vomiting	Consider dietary modifications (bland, soft, adjust timing/volume of foods or feeds). Aromatherapy*: ginger, peppermint, lavender, acupuncture/acupressure.
Constipation	Increase fiber in diet, encourage fluids, ambulation (if possible).
Oral lesions/dysphagia	Oral hygiene and appropriate liquid, solid and oral medication formulation (texture, taste, fluidity). Treat infections, complications (mucositis, pharyngitis, dental abscess, esophagitis). Oropharyngeal motility study and speech (feeding team) consultation.
Anorexia/cachexia	Manage treatable lesions causing oral pain, dysphagia, or anorexia. Support caloric intake during phase of illness when anorexia is reversible. Acknowledge that anorexia/cachexia is intrinsic to the dying process and may not be reversible. Prevent/treat coexisting constipation.
Pruritus	Moisturize skin. Trim child's nails to prevent excoriation. Try specialized anti-itch lotions. Apply cold packs. Counterstimulation, distraction, relaxation.
Diarrhea	Evaluate/treat if obstipation. Assess and treat infection. Dietary modification.
Depression	Psychotherapy, behavioral techniques, setting attainable daily goals. Aromatherapy*: bergamot, lavender.
Anxiety	Psychotherapy (individual and family), behavioral techniques. Aromatherapy*: clary sage, angelica, mandarin, lavender.
Agitation/terminal restlessness	Evaluate for organic or drug causes. Educate family. Orient and reassure child; provide calm, nonstimulating environment, use familiar music, verse, voice, touch. Aromatherapy*: frankincense, ylang ylang.

*Best if aromatherapy is administered by a practitioner trained in aromatherapy use and safety and if child has choice of essential oil aroma that stimulates positive response.

From Sourkes B, Frankel L, Brown M, et al: Food, toys, and love: pediatric palliative care, *Curr Probl Pediatr Adolesc Health Care* 35:345–392, 2005.

clinical situation and the goals of care, radiation therapy, surgical interventions, and steroids are potential therapeutic options.

Delirium is an underrecognized brain disorder characterized by waxing-and-waning attention, confusion, and disorientation. Agitation may occur, as well as features of hypomania. Although delirium as a whole is often not diagnosed, the hypomanic form is particularly underrecognized. Delirium has a range of causes, including medications such as anticholinergics and benzodiazepines. Environmental strategies to calm and orient the child while addressing potentially contributing factors are helpful. In some patients, antipsychotic/neuroleptic medications are indicated (see Chapter 33 and 47).

Feeding and hydration issues can raise ethical questions that evoke intense emotions in families and medical caregivers alike. Options that may be considered to artificially support nutrition and hydration in a child who can no longer feed by mouth include nasogastric and gastrostomy feedings or intravenous nutrition or hydration (see Chapter 55). These complex decisions require evaluating the risks and benefits of artificial feedings and taking into consideration the child's functional level and prognosis. At times, it may be appropriate to initiate a trial of tube feedings, with the understanding that they may be discontinued at a later stage of the illness. A commonly held but unsubstantiated belief is that artificial nutrition and hydration are comfort measures, without which a child may suffer from starvation or thirst. This may result in well-meaning but disruptive and invasive attempts to administer nutrition or fluids to a dying child. In dying adults, the sensation of thirst may be alleviated by careful efforts to keep the mouth moist and clean. There may also be deleterious side effects to artificial hydration in the form of increased secretions, need for frequent urination, edema, and exacerbation of dyspnea. For these reasons, it is important to educate families about anticipated decreases in appetite/thirst and therefore little need for nutrition and hydration as the child approaches death. In addition, exploring the meaning that provision of nutrition and hydration may hold for families, as well as helping families anticipate the changes in their child's appearance and exploring alternative ways that they may love and nurture their child, may ease distress around this issue.

Nausea and vomiting may be caused by medications or toxins, irritation to or obstruction of the gastrointestinal tract, motion, and emotions. Drugs such as metoclopramide, 5-hydroxytryptamine antagonists, corticosteroids, olanzapine, and aprepitant may be used and should be chosen depending on the underlying pathophysiology and neurotransmitters involved. Vomiting may accompany nausea but may also occur without nausea, as with increased intracranial pressure. **Constipation** is commonly encountered in children with neurologic impairment or children receiving medications that impair gastrointestinal motility (most notably opioids). Stool frequency and quantity should be evaluated in the context of the child's diet and usual bowel pattern. Children taking regular opioids should routinely be placed on stool softeners (docusate) in addition to a laxative agent (e.g., senna). For some patients, parenteral methylnaltrexone is also helpful in relieving opioid-induced constipation. **Diarrhea** may be particularly difficult for the child and family and may be treated with loperamide (an opioid that does not cross the blood-brain barrier), and in some cases, colestyramine or octreotide may be indicated. Paradoxical diarrhea, a result of overflow resulting from constipation, should also be included in the differential diagnosis.

Hematologic issues include consideration of anemia and thrombocytopenia or bleeding. If the child has symptomatic anemia (weakness, dizziness, shortness of breath, tachycardia), red blood cell transfusions may be considered. Platelet transfusions may be an option if the child has symptoms of bleeding. Life-ending hemorrhage is disturbing for all concerned, and a plan involving the use of fast-acting sedatives should be prepared in advance if such an event is a possibility.

Skin care issues include primary prevention of problems by ongoing and timely assessment (including observation of indwelling lines and tubes) and frequent turning and repositioning and alleviating pressure wherever possible (e.g., elevating heels off the bed with pillows). Pruritus may be secondary to systemic disorders or drug therapy. Treatment includes avoiding excessive use of drying soaps, using moisturizers, trimming fingernails, and wearing loose-fitting clothing, in addition to administering topical or systemic corticosteroids. Oral antihistamines and other specific therapies may also be indicated (e.g., cholestyramine in biliary disease). Opioids can cause histamine release from mast cells, but this does not account for most of the pruritus caused by opioids. A trial of diphenhydramine may provide relief; alternatively, rotating opioids or instituting a low dose of opioid antagonist may be needed for refractory pruritus.

Children with life-threatening illness may experience psychological symptoms such as **anxiety** and **depression.** Such symptoms are frequently multifactorial and sometimes interrelated with uncontrolled symptoms such as pain and fatigue. Diagnosing depression in the context of serious illness may pose challenges because neurovegetative symptoms may not be reliable indicators. Instead, expressions of hopelessness, helplessness, worthlessness, and guilt may be more useful. Pharmacologic agents such as antidepressants may be helpful, although their effect is often preceded by a significant lag phase. Because of its immediate and positive effect on mood, *methylphenidate* may be an effective antidepressant for children at end of life, when there may not be time for a traditional antidepressant to take effect. Interventions and opportunities for children to explore worries, hopes, and concerns in an open, supportive, and nonjudgmental setting are equally if not more important approaches to psychological distress. Skilled members from a variety of disciplines, including psychology, social work, chaplaincy, child life, and expressive therapy, may help children and their families in this regard. Such opportunities may create positive moments in which meaning, connection, and new definitions of hope are found.

Discussions with adolescent patients, or with the parents of any ill child, about possible therapies or interventions should include **integrative therapies** such as massage therapy, Reiki, acupuncture, clinical aromatherapy, prayer, and nutritional supplements. Many families use integrative therapy but do not bring it up with their physician unless explicitly asked (see Chapter 78). Although largely unproven, some of these therapies are inexpensive and provide relief to individual patients. Other therapies may be expensive, painful, intrusive, and even toxic. By initiating conversation and inviting discussion in a nonjudgmental way, the clinician can offer advice on the safety of different therapies and may help avoid expensive, dangerous, or burdensome interventions. Medical marijuana (**cannabis**) for pediatric use has been legalized by some states, and

pediatricians are increasingly asked about it. In such cases, it is most helpful to use this opportunity to engage in a broader conversation about symptoms and symptom management, even in states where use of cannabis for pediatric medicinal purposes is legal.

Intensive Symptom Management

At the end of life, when intensive efforts to relieve the symptom have been exhausted, or when efforts to address suffering are incapable of providing relief with acceptable toxicity/morbidity or in an acceptable time frame, **palliative sedation** may be considered. Palliative sedation may relieve suffering from refractory symptoms by reducing a child's level of consciousness. It is most often used for intractable pain, dyspnea, or agitation, but is not limited to these distressing indications. Palliative sedation provides opportunities for parents, staff, and primary clinicians to discuss the indications and goals for sedation, as well as questions or concerns about this therapy, both before and after initiation of sedation.

The doctrine of double effect (DDE) is often invoked to justify escalation of symptom-relieving medications or palliative sedation for uncontrolled symptoms at the end of life. Use of DDE emphasizes the risk of hastening death posed by escalating opioids or sedation, which is theoretical and unproven (see Chapter 6). There is mounting evidence that patients with well-controlled symptoms live longer.

Approaching End of Life

As death seems imminent, the major task of the physician and team are to help the child have as many good days as possible and not suffer. If not already in place, a referral **for hospice care** (usually provided in the *home*, not a hospice house for children) may provide the most comprehensive care for the child and family. Gently preparing the family for what to expect and offering choices, when possible, will allow them a sense of control in the midst of tragic circumstances. Before death, it can be very helpful to discuss the following:

◆ Support of siblings or other family members
◆ Resuscitation status
◆ Limiting technology when no longer beneficial to the child
◆ Cultural, spiritual, or religious needs
◆ Location of death
  Who will pronounce if death occurs at home
◆ Funeral arrangements
  Offering siblings choice and appropriate support to attend
◆ Autopsy and/or tissue/organ donation
  Legacy building, benefits others, informs science and family

Offered the opportunity, families will often tolerate thinking and speaking about their hopes and fears regarding their child's end of life, and some even express relief when the door to such conversation in opened by the care team. It may help to let the family know these conversations are not about *whether* the child will die but *how* the child may die.

Families gain tremendous support from having a physician and team who will continue to stay involved in the child's care. If the child is at home or hospitalized, regular phone calls or visits, assisting with symptom management, and offering emotional support is invaluable for families.

In an intensive care setting, where technology can be overwhelming and put distance between the child and parent, the physician can offer discontinuation of that which is not benefiting the child or adding to quality of life. Less invasive ways to control symptoms, such as subcutaneous infusions or topical applications, may be helpful. Parents may be afraid to ask about holding or sleeping next to their child. They may need reassurance and assistance in holding, touching, and speaking with their child, despite tubes and technology, even if the child appears unresponsive.

It is believed that hearing and the ability to sense touch are often present until death; all family members should be encouraged to continue interacting with their loved one through the dying process. Parents may be afraid to leave the bedside so that their child will not die alone. Offering parents other supports such as chaplaincy/clergy, social work, and extended family members may be helpful. In most instances the moment of death cannot be predicted. Some propose that children wait to die until their parents are ready, an important event has passed, or they are given permission. Caregivers need not dispute this, nor the hope for a miracle often held by families until the child takes the last breath.

For the family, the moment of death is an event that is recalled in detail for years to come, and thus enhancing opportunity for dignity and limited suffering is essential. Research suggests that improved symptom control and easing of difficult moments at the time of death may lessen the long-term distress of bereaved parents. Clinical experience has shown that families often find solace in clinician presence, whether at home or in the hospital. After death, families should be given the option of remaining with their child for as long as they would like and should be prepared for changes in the child's body. During this time, physicians and other professionals may ask permission to say goodbye. The family may be invited to bathe and dress the body as a final act of caring for the child.

The physician's decision to attend the funeral is a personal one. Participation may serve the dual purpose of showing respect and helping the clinician cope with a personal sense of loss. If unable to attend

services, families report highly valuing the importance of receiving a call, card, or note from the physician. To know that their child made a difference and will not be forgotten is often very important to families in their bereavement.

The Pediatrician

Although optimal palliative care for children entails caregivers from a variety of disciplines, pediatricians are well positioned to support children and their families, particularly if they have a long-standing relationship with multiple family members. A pediatrician who has cared for a family over time may already know and care for other family members, understand preexisting stressors for the family, and may be familiar with coping strategies used by family members. Pediatricians are familiar with the process of eliciting concerns and providing anticipatory guidance for parents, as well as developmentally appropriate explanations for children.

Bibliography is available at Expert Consult.

Chapter **8**
Domestic and International Adoption
Elaine E. Schulte
第八章
本土收养和跨国收养

中文导读

本章主要介绍了国内收养、跨国收养、儿科医师在其中的角色。具体阐述了《收养和安全家庭法》、同性夫妇收养和公开领养等相关问题，阐述了儿科医师在涉及领养前的病史回顾和领养后的医疗保健事务中所起的作用，如针对：跨国收养抵达目的地的访视、生长落后、发育落后、语言发育问题、饮食问题、睡眠问题、社交和情感发育、种族认同感的形成、毒性压力、家庭支持以及指导收养者如何进行对收养史的讲述。

Adoption is a social, emotional, and legal process that provides a new family for a child when the birth family is unable or unwilling to parent. In the United States, about 1 million children <18 yr of age are adopted; 2-4% of all American families have adopted. Annually across the globe, approximately 250,000 children are adopted, with 30,000 of these between nations. In the United States, approximately 120,000 children are adopted every year. Of these, 49% are from private agencies, American Indian Tribes, stepparent, or other forms of kinship care. The remaining 51% of adoptions include public and international adoptions. Public adoptions account for the majority of these. Because of changing policies toward

adoption and social change in several of the sending countries, the number of international adoptions has decreased dramatically over the last 10 yr. Public agencies support approximately 50% of total annual adoptions in the United States, private agencies facilitate 25% of adoptions, and independent practitioners (e.g., lawyers) handle 15% of adoptions. Compared to 19% of the general population, approximately 39% of adopted children have special healthcare needs.

DOMESTIC ADOPTION
The **Adoption and Safe Families Act** (P.L. 105-89) requires children

in foster care to be placed with adoptive families if they cannot be safely returned to their families within a reasonable time. In fiscal year (FY) 2014, there were an estimated 415,129 children in foster care, and 107,918 were waiting for adoption. Of the 238,230 children who exited foster care, 51% were reunited with parent(s) or primary caretakers(s), and 21% were adopted (see Chapter 9).

Many children awaiting adoption are less likely to be adopted because they are of school age, part of a sibling group, members of historically oppressed racial/ethnic groups, or because they have considerable physical, emotional, or developmental needs. A number of policy efforts are aimed at increasing adoption opportunities for these children, including federal adoption subsidies, tax credits, recruitment efforts to identify ethnically diverse adults willing to adopt, increased preplacement services, and expanding adoption opportunities to single adults, older couples, and gay/lesbian partners.

Although **same-sex couple adoption** is legal in more than a dozen countries worldwide, it is actively debated in the United States. Although legislation regarding same-sex couple adoption varies by state, increasing numbers of gay and lesbian partners have been able to adopt. Current estimates suggest that almost 2 million children, including 5% of all adopted children, are raised by gay and lesbian parents. Adopted children include those adopted domestically, those from foster care, and internationally adopted children. There is increasing evidence that children raised by same-sex couples are as physically or psychologically healthy, capable, and successful as those raised by opposite-sex couples. Pediatricians can advocate for adopted children by supporting gay and lesbian parents.

Open adoption, usually through an agency or privately, occurs when the birth mother arranges to continue to be involved, although in a limited manner, with the legally adopted family. This may occur through surrogacy or more often in an unplanned pregnancy.

INTERCOUNTRY ADOPTION

Along with foster care adoptions, **international adoptions** are a way of providing stable, long-term care to vulnerable children throughout the world. There is concern that in some countries of origin, the rapid growth of international adoption has outpaced regulation and oversight to protect vulnerable children and families. Opportunities for financial gain have led to abuses, including the sale and abduction of children, bribery, and financial coercion of families, but the extent and scope of the potential concern is difficult to ascertain. Increasing global efforts, such as the **Hague Convention on Protection of Children and Co-operation in Respect of Intercountry Adoption**, have promoted political cooperation between nations and established international law to reduce potential for child abduction and child trafficking and to ensure that the best interests of the child are paramount in decision making. Participating nations, including the United States, are working to address the myriad of sociopolitical conditions that create the need for out-of-family care, and are working to support children within their nation's borders. International adoption is increasingly considered a measure of last resort if the child cannot be cared for within his or her birth family (including extended relatives), the immediate community, or the larger national culture. As a result, children adopted internationally into the United States are more likely to enter their families at older ages or with complex medical, developmental, or social-emotional needs.

Although the vast majority of children adopted internationally *enter* the United States for purposes of adoption, a small but growing number of children *exit* the United States for adoption into other countries. For example, in FY 2014, 96 children exited the United States for adoption by families in other countries (e.g., Canada, Netherlands, Ireland, United Kingdom). Little is known about the circumstances surrounding these adoptions and the eventual outcomes of the children who are adopted internationally *from* the United States.

In 2015, U.S. families adopted 5,647 children from other countries (compared with a peak of 22,884 in 2004). Children from China, Ethiopia, South Korea, Ukraine, Bulgaria, and the Congo represented 65% of children adopted internationally into the United States in 2015; 42% were from China alone. Although individual experiences vary, most children placed for international adoption have some history of poverty

and social hardship in their home countries, and most are adopted from orphanages or institutional settings. Many young infants are placed into **orphanage care** shortly after birth. Some older children have experienced family disruption resulting from parental illness, war, or natural disasters. Still others enter orphanage care after determination of significant abuse or neglect within their biological families. The effects of **institutionalization** and other life stresses may impact all areas of growth and development. As a result, many children require specialized support and understanding to overcome the impact of stress and early adversity and to reach their full potential.

ROLE OF PEDIATRICIANS
Preadoption Medical Record Reviews

Preadoption medical record reviews are important for both domestic and international adoptions. Adoption agencies are making increased efforts to obtain biological family health information and genetic histories to share with adoptive families prior to adoption. Such information is often becomes increasingly relevant as the child ages. Pediatricians can help prospective adoptive parents understand the health and developmental history of a child and available background information from birth families in order to assess actual and potential medical risk factors to support adult decision-making about the family's ability to parent the waiting child.

Under the Hague Convention, U.S. agencies that arrange international adoptions must make efforts to obtain accurate and complete health histories on children awaiting adoption. The nature and quality of medical and genetic information, when available, vary greatly. Poor translation and use of medical terminology and medications that are unfamiliar to U.S.-trained physicians are common. Results of specific diagnostic studies and laboratory tests performed outside the United States should not be relied on and *should be repeated* once the child arrives in the United States. Paradoxically, review of the child's medical records may raise more questions than provide answers. Each medical diagnosis should be considered carefully before being rejected or accepted. Country-specific growth curves should be avoided because they may be inaccurate or may reflect a general level of poor health and nutrition in the country of origin. Instead, *serial growth* data should be plotted on U.S. standard growth curves; this may reveal a pattern of poor growth because of malnutrition or other chronic illness. Photographs or video files may provide the only objective information from which medical status can be determined. Full-face photographs may reveal dysmorphic features consistent with **fetal alcohol syndrome** (see Chapter 126.3) or findings suggestive of other congenital disorders.

Frank interpretations of available information should be shared with the prospective adoptive parents. The role of the healthcare provider is not to comment on the advisability of an adoption, but to inform the prospective parents of any significant health needs identified now or anticipated in the future.

Postadoption Medical Care
Arrival Visit–International Adoption

All internationally adopted children should have a thorough medical evaluation shortly after arriving in the United States. Many children may have acute or chronic medical problems that are not always immediately evident, including malnutrition, growth deficiencies; stool pathogens, anemia, elevated blood lead, dental decay, strabismus, birth defects, developmental delay, feeding and sensory difficulty, and social-emotional concerns. *All children who are adopted from other countries undergo comprehensive screening for infectious diseases and disorders of growth, development, vision, and hearing* (Tables 8.1 and 8.2). Regardless of test results before arrival, all children should be screened for **tuberculosis** with either a tuberculin skin test (TST) or interferon-γ release assays (IGRA). If the child's purified protein derivative (PPD) skin test is negative, it should be repeated in 4-6 mo; children may have false-negative tests because of poor nutrition. Additional tests (e.g., malaria) should be ordered depending on the prevalence of disease in the child's country of origin (see Chapter 10). **Immunization records** should be carefully reviewed. Internationally adopted children frequently have incomplete records or have been vaccinated using alternative schedules. Pediatricians may choose to check titers to determine which vaccines need to be given, or they can *choose to reimmunize* the child. The unique medical and developmental needs of internationally adopted children have led to the creation of specialty clinics throughout the United States, which may be a valuable resource for adoptive families at all stages in the adoption process and throughout the adopted child's life.

Growth Delays

Physical growth delays are common in internationally adopted children and may represent the combined result of many factors, such as unknown/untreated medical conditions, malnutrition, and psychological deprivation. It is more important to monitor growth over time, including preplacement measurements, since trend data may provide a more objective assessment of the child's nutritional and medical status. Children

Table 8.1	Recommended Screening Tests for International Adoptees on U.S. Arrival

SCREENING TESTS
Complete blood cell count
Blood lead level
Newborn screening (young infants)
Vision and hearing screening
Dental screening
Developmental testing

OTHER SCREENING TESTS TO CONSIDER BASED ON CLINICAL FINDINGS AND AGE OF CHILD
Stool cultures for bacterial pathogens
Glucose-6-phosphate dehydrogenase deficiency screening
Sickle cell test
Urine pregnancy test

INFECTIOUS DISEASE SCREENING (see Table 8.2)

Table 8.2	Screening Tests for Infectious Diseases in International Adoptees

RECOMMENDED TESTS
Hepatitis A total Ig (with reflex testing for IgM if total Ig is positive)
Hepatitis B virus serologic testing*
- Hepatitis B surface antigen (HBsAg)
- Antibody to hepatitis B surface antigen (anti-HBs)
- Antibody to hepatitis B core antigen (anti-HBc)
Hepatitis C virus serologic testing*†
Syphilis serologic testing
- Nontreponemal test (RPR, VDRL, or ART)
- Treponemal test (MHA-TP or FTA-ABS)
HIV-1 and HIV-2 testing (ELISA if >18 mo, PCR if <18 mo)*
Complete blood cell count with red blood cell indices and differential (if eosinophilia, see Chapter 10)
Stool examination for ova and parasites (optimal: 3 specimens) with specific requests for *Giardia lamblia* and *Cryptosporidium* spp. testing
Tuberculin skin test (with CXR if >5 mm induration) or interferon-γ release assay*†

OPTIONAL TESTS (FOR SPECIAL POPULATIONS OR CIRCUMSTANCES)
GC/Chlamydia
Strongyloides spp.
Schistosoma spp.
Trypanosoma cruzi

*Repeat 3-6 mo after arrival.
†See Chapter 10.
ART, Automated reagin test; CXR, chest radiograph; ELISA, enzyme-linked immunosorbent assay; FTA-ABS, fluorescent treponemal antibody absorption; GC, gonococcus; HIV, human immunodeficiency virus; MHA-TP, microhemagglutination test for *Treponema pallidum*; PCR, polymerase chain reaction; RPR, rapid plasma reagin; VDRL, Venereal Disease Research Laboratories.

who present with low height-for-age (**growth stunting**) may have a history of inadequate nutrition as well as chronic adversity. Although most children experience a significant catch-up in physical growth following adoption, many remain shorter than their U.S. peers.

Developmental Delays

Many children adopted internationally exhibit delays in at least 1 area of development, but most exhibit significant gains within the 1st 12 mo after adoption. Children adopted at older ages are likely to have more variable outcomes. In the immediate post-adoption period, it may be impossible to determine with any certainty whether developmental delays will be transient or long-lasting. Careful monitoring of development within the first years of adoption can identify a **developmental trend** over time that may be more predictive of long-term functioning than assessment at any specific point in time. When in doubt, it is better to *refer early* for developmental intervention, rather than wait to see if the children will catch up.

Language Development

For both domestic and international adoptees, genetic or biologic risk factors for poor language development may be identified preadoptively, but it is unlikely that international adoptees will have had these delays identified before adoption. These children typically have not had an assessment in their native language and have had little exposure to English. It may not be possible to fully assess their language abilities until they have had a chance to learn English. Regardless of the age at adoption, most internationally adopted children will reach age-expected language skills over time.

If a child has language delays, referral to early intervention or the school district should be made. Clinicians may need to work with these groups to help them understand the unique circumstances surrounding an adopted child's language development. For example, English language acquisition in internationally adopted children depends on the age of adoption and native language skills. Placing the recently adopted, school-age child in an English as a Second Language class may not be sufficient if the child's language development in the primary language has been atypical.

Eating Concerns

Initial concerns about eating, sleep regulation, and repetitive (e.g., self-stimulating or self-soothing) behaviors are common, especially among children adopted following a high degree of neglect or developmental trauma. Feeding behaviors of international adoptees may be linked to orphanage feeding practices, or limited exposure to textured or solid foods during later infancy/toddlerhood. Children who have experienced chronic lack of food may not have developed an awareness of *satiation cues*, leading to hoarding or frequent vomiting. **Feeding concerns** often subside gradually with introduction of age-appropriate foods and parental support for positive feeding practices. Many children who were adopted after significant malnutrition may eat an excessive amount of food. Unless the child is eating to the point of vomiting (which would indicate little awareness of satiation cues), it is generally best to allow the child to eat until satiation. Typically, within several months, the child will regulate food intake appropriately. Occasionally, additional support from a speech pathologist or feeding specialist is warranted to address possible sensory, physical, or psychological issues around proper feeding.

Sleep Concerns

Sleep is often disrupted as the child reacts to changes in routines and environments. Efforts to create continuity between the preadoption and postadoption environment can be helpful. Within the 1st 3-6 mo, as the child's emotional self-regulation improves, many sleep concerns subside. Similarly, stereotypical behaviors, such as rocking or head banging, often diminish within the 1st few mo after adoption.

Social and Emotional Development

Dyadic interactions between child and caretaker are a critical component to later regulatory functioning and social-emotional development. The amount and quality of individualized caretaking that children have received before their adoption, whether international, domestic, or through the foster care system, is usually unknown. In many cases, entry into a secure, stable home setting with consistent childcare routines is sufficient to support the child's emerging social-emotional development. Pediatricians can help parents remember that adoption is part of a child's history. Throughout one's childhood, prior experiences or biologic disposition may result in behavior that is confusing to the adoptive parents. The child's reactions may be subtle or difficult to interpret, interfering with the parents' ability to respond in a sensitive manner. In these circumstances, additional support may be helpful to foster the emerging relationships and behavioral regulation in the newly formed family.

Racial Identity Development

Transracial adoption (where the racial background of the child differs from that of the parent/parents) accounts for a significant percentage of adoptions each year in the United States. In most of these adoptive placements, children of color have been adopted by white parents. Racial identity development, including ways to understand and respond to discrimination, is increasingly recognized as important in the overall development of children. Surveys of adults adopted transracially indicate that racial identity is of central importance at many ages and tends to increase in significance during young adulthood. Integrating race/ethnicity into identity can be a complex process for all children, but it may be especially complicated when they are raised in a family where racial differences are noted. Adults raised within interracial families have noted the value of attending racially diverse schools and of having adult role models (e.g., teachers, doctors, coaches) who share their racial background. Parents who adopt transracially are often encouraged to support interactions within diverse communities (and associated discrimination) often within the family. Black children raised by white families in white communities may have been sheltered from overt racism but need to be taught that many others (including law enforcement officers) will regard them as black with all the intense biases associated with race (see Chapter 2.1).

Toxic Stress

The cumulative amount of early adversity (e.g., numerous years within international orphanage care, extensive abuse/neglect prior to removal from biological family, or multiple foster care placements) experienced by a child before adoption, referred to as *toxic stress*, can impact both immediate placement stability and long-term functioning (see Chapter 2). The degree of presumed toxic stress may be helpful in interpreting a child's behavior and supporting family functioning.*

Family Support

The unique aspects to adoptive family formation can create familial stress and impact child and family functioning. Some adoptive families may have to address infertility, creation of a multiracial family, disclosure of adoptive status, concerns and questions the child may have about their biologic origins, and ongoing scrutiny by adoption agencies. With gay/lesbian parents, there are often additional psychosocial stressors, including continued barriers to legal recognition of both parents in a gay/lesbian partnership that can negatively impact family functioning. Although most families acclimate well to adoption-related stressors, some parents experience postadoption depression and may benefit from additional support to ease the family's transition.

Adoption Narrative

Families are encouraged to speak openly and repeatedly about adoption with their child, beginning in the toddler years and continuing through adolescence. Creating a *Lifebook* for the adopted child provides a way to support family communication about the child's history and significant relationships (including birth family members) and to document the child's important life transitions (e.g., through foster care or immigration to the United States). It is common, and normal, for children to have questions about adoption and their biological family throughout their development. An increase in cognitive understanding between ages 7 and 10 yr can sometimes increase adoption-related questions and distress. Youth who have questions about biological family members are increasingly able to access information via social media and web-based searching, raising the importance of ongoing open communication about adoption. Pediatricians may need to respond to increased concerns/questions when the adoptee's health and genetic history is incomplete or unknown. At any time, concerns about development, behavior, and social-emotional functioning may or may not be related to the child's adoption history.

The vast majority of adopted children and families adjust well and lead healthy, productive lives. Adoptions infrequently disrupt; disruption rates are higher among children adopted from foster care, which research associates with their age at adoption and a history of multiple placements before adoption. With increased understanding of the needs of families who adopt children from foster care, agencies are placing greater emphasis on the preparation of adoptive parents and ensuring the availability of a full range of postadoption services, including physical health, mental health, and developmental services for their adopted children.

Bibliography is available at Expert Consult.

---

*See video at http://developingchild.harvard.edu/resources/multimedia/videos/three_core_concepts/toxic_stress/.

Chapter **9**

Foster and Kinship Care

Moira Szilagyi

第九章
寄养和亲属照顾

中文导读

　　本章主要介绍了由美国收养和寄养的分析报告系统（AFCARS）提供的寄养情况统计；涉及美国相关的法律法规，如美国《收养和安全家庭法案》《促进沟通和促成收养法案》以及《家庭一级预防服务法》等；介绍了儿童早期创伤所导致的不良健康结果，以及相关健康问题，如在寄养儿童中，诸如注意广度缩短、注意缺陷多动障碍、认知功能差、攻击性和记忆问题等是经常遇到的异常情况，且普遍存在慢性健康问题、心理健康问题、发育问题、牙科和教育问题；最后介绍了寄养儿童和青少年的保健。

The placement of children in out-of-home care has served the needs of children in many societies worldwide throughout history. The institution of **foster care** was developed in the United States as a temporary resource for children during times of family crisis and is rooted in the principle that children fare best when raised in family settings. The mission of foster care is to provide for the safety, permanency, and well-being of children while assisting their families with services to promote reunification.

EPIDEMIOLOGY

The number of children in foster care worldwide is unknown, although it has been estimated that 8 million may be in foster and residential care. On September 11, 2015, approximately 427,910 children in the United States resided in foster care, representing a slight increase since the nadir of 397,301 reached in 2012. Early in the millennium, foster care numbers decreased despite an increase in maltreatment reports, as child welfare offered families more preventive services and alternative placement with relatives or nonrelative caregivers (**kinship care**) as an alternative to court-ordered removal. The more recent increase in numbers appears to be related to the opioid epidemic. Over the last 15 years, reunification rates have stabilized while adoption of children from foster care has increased. Nationally, approximately 45% of children live with a nonrelative foster parent, 30% of children are in placement with a relative who is a certified foster parent, and just under 15% are in **congregate** (group) **care**.

Approximately 33% of children in foster care in the United States are younger than 5 yr, and 34% are older than 12 yr. Most children are white (41%); 24% are black, 21% are Hispanic of any race, and 7% are identified as ≥2 races. As foster care numbers declined by 25% beginning in 1999, the reduction in African American children was even greater as child welfare made efforts to reduce the disparities in investigation and removal. The average length of stay in foster care continues to

decline (median in 2015, 20.4 mo), with a significant drop in the number who spend ≥2 yr from 31% in 2011 to 26% in 2015. Only approximately half of children achieve reunification, while 22% (53,000) are adopted and 6% reside with relatives. Among remaining children, 9% (20, 800) emancipate between ages 18 and 21 yr, 9% enter into long-term state guardianship, <1% run away, and 2% transfer to other institutions. There were 336 deaths reported in foster care in fiscal year 2015.

Only 4% of children reside in a preadoptive home, although they represent 12% of children awaiting adoption; 52% of children awaiting adoption reside with a foster parent who is a relative. The average number of placements a child experiences in foster care is not included in **Adoption and Foster Care Analysis and Reporting System (AFCARS)**, but important predictors of an increased number of different placements include severe behavioral and developmental problems, larger sibling group size, and longer time spent in foster care. Within 12 mo, almost all emancipated youth have at least 1 homeless night. Within a decade, less than half have achieved a high school degree, most are living in poverty, and many have psychiatric disorders, including posttraumatic stress disorder and depression.

LEGISLATION IN THE UNITED STATES

In the **United States the Adoption and Safe Families Act** (P.L. 105-89) requires that a permanency plan be made for each child no later than 12 mo after entry into foster care, and that a petition to terminate parental rights typically be filed when a child has been in foster care for at least 15 of the previous 22 mo. The **Fostering Connections and Promoting Adoptions Act** of 2009 (P.L. 110-351) focused on incentives for guardianship and adoption, supports for the young adults at the age of emancipation, and rights of Native American children to care within their tribe. This act also contained a clause requiring states to develop and coordinate healthcare systems for children in foster care in collaboration with Medicaid and pediatricians. In 2018 the **Family**

First Prevention Services Act was signed into law. This legislation emphasizes providing evidence-based mental health and substance abuse services for families whose children are at imminent risk of entering foster care.

EARLY CHILDHOOD TRAUMA LEADS TO POOR HEALTH OUTCOMES

Children in foster care have high rates of early childhood trauma and adversity. More than 60% are placed for neglect, 13% for physical abuse, and 5% are abandoned. Parental **substance abuse** is a factor in 32% of removals, and parent alcohol abuse in 6%. **Violence** in the home is common, with >80% having experienced domestic and/or community violence, but domestic violence is not included in the AFCARS reporting system as a reason for removal. Parental **mental illness** is also not reported as a reason for removal in AFCARS, but the literature indicates that birth parents have high rates of mental illness, criminal justice system involvement, substance abuse, unemployment, and cognitive impairment. Many children, particularly infants entering care, have had prenatal substance exposure, multiple caregivers of varying quality, and are from families with long involvement with child protective services.

Removal from the family of origin may compound prior trauma experiences, although some children experience relief at removal from a chaotic, abusive, or dangerous home. Most children miss their family, worry about their parents and siblings, and long for reunification. Separation, loss and grief, unpredictable contact with birth parents, placement changes, the process of terminating parental rights, and the sheer uncertainty of foster care may further erode a child's well-being.

Childhood trauma is correlated with poor developmental, behavioral, and health outcomes. Early trauma and chronic stress adversely affect the neurobiology of the developing brain, especially those areas involved in attention, emotional regulation, memory, executive function, and cognition. As a result, shortened attention span, hyperactivity, poorer cognitive function, aggression, and memory issues are problems encountered frequently among children in foster care. However, evidence shows that specific interventions, such as specially trained foster parents for children or youth and mentoring for adolescents in foster care, can improve outcomes, although replication and dissemination of these evidence-based interventions are limited.

HEALTH ISSUES

Experiencing multiple childhood adversities and receiving fragmented and inadequate health services before placement into foster care mean that children enter foster care with a high prevalence of chronic medical, mental health, developmental, dental, and educational problems (Table 9.1). Thus they are defined as *children with special health care needs* (CSHCN). The greatest single healthcare need of this population is for high-quality, evidence-based trauma-informed mental health services to address the impacts of prior and ongoing trauma, loss, and unpredictability. In addition, children in foster care have higher rates of asthma, growth failure, obesity, vertically transmitted infections, and neurologic conditions than the general pediatric population. Adolescents need access to reproductive health and substance abuse services. Up to 60% of children <5 yr old have a developmental delay in at least 1 domain and >40% of school-age children qualify for special education services. Unfortunately, educational difficulties persist despite improvements in school attendance and performance after placement in foster care. Each placement change that is accompanied by a change in school sets children back academically by about 4 mo. Federal legislation requires child welfare to maintain children in their school of origin when possible, even if child welfare has to provide transportation to ensure this.

Although children in foster care are CSHCN, they often lack access to the services they need. Most public and private child welfare agencies do not have formal arrangements for accessing the needed array of health services and rely on local physicians and health clinics funded by Medicaid. Health histories are often sparse at admission because many have lacked regular care, or their biological parents may not be available or forthcoming. Once children enter foster care, there is often a diffusion of responsibility across caregivers and child welfare. Foster parents usually receive little information about a child's healthcare needs, but they are typically expected to decide when and where children receive healthcare services. Child welfare caseworkers are responsible for ensuring that a child's health needs are addressed but coordination across multiple healthcare providers may be daunting. Uncertainty about who is legally responsible for making healthcare treatment decisions and who may have access to health information may delay or result in the denial of healthcare services.

HEALTHCARE FOR CHILDREN AND ADOLESCENTS IN FOSTER CARE

The American Academy of Pediatrics (AAP) has published detailed healthcare standards for children in foster care, available on the *Healthy Foster Care America* website. The AAP recommends that children receive healthcare services in a medical home setting, where comprehensive healthcare is continuous over time (Table 9.2). Compassionate, culturally competent healthcare that is **trauma informed** means that health staff should understand, recognize, and respond to symptoms and risk factors of traumatic stress and provide an environment that offers physical, emotional, and psychological safety for children and caregivers. In foster care, attention must be paid to the effects of past trauma and the impact of ongoing uncertainty and loss on a child's health and well-being, as well as that of their birth and foster/kinship families.

Table 9.1	Health Issues of Children in Foster Care

CHRONIC MEDICAL PROBLEMS
Affect 40–60% of children.
Asthma, dermatologic, neurologic, obesity, growth failure, hearing, and vision problems are most common.

ABUSE AND NEGLECT
>70% of children have a history of abuse and neglect at entry into foster care.
Monitor at all health visits for abuse or neglect or poor care in the home.

COMPLEX CHRONIC MEDICAL PROBLEMS
Involves up to 10% of children in foster care.
Children may be dependent on medical technologies or may have multiple disabilities.

MENTAL HEALTH CONCERNS
Affects 80% of children >4 yr of age.
Result of childhood trauma and adversity.
Most common diagnoses are adjustment disorder, posttraumatic stress disorder, attention-deficit/hyperactivity disorder, oppositional defiant disorder, and conduct disorder.
Externalizing problems are more likely to result in therapy.
Minority children and those in kinship care have less access to mental health services.

DEVELOPMENTAL PROBLEMS
60% of children <5 yr of age have at least 1 documented delay.
Typically affect communication, cognition, problem-solving, and personal-social domains, including emotional self-regulation.

DENTAL PROBLEMS
20–35% of children have significant dental disease.

ADOLESCENT HEALTH ISSUES
High rates of sexually transmitted infections, high-risk behaviors, and substance abuse.

EDUCATIONAL PROBLEMS
Half of special education placements relate to behavioral or emotional issues, not cognitive.
Only 32% of adolescents eventually graduate from high school; 32% obtain a general equivalency diploma; 1–2% complete any amount of college.

FAMILY RELATIONSHIP PROBLEMS
100% of children have family relationship problems.

Table 9.2	Trauma-Informed Pediatric Medical Home for Children in Foster Care
CHARACTERISTIC	**APPLICATION IN FOSTER CARE**
Comprehensive healthcare	Perform comprehensive admission assessment within 30 days of entry. Ensure access to mental health, developmental, and dental evaluation and services. Screen and refer as needed for abuse and neglect.
Coordination of care	Make timely referrals and follow up subspecialist visits. Communicate with caseworkers, foster parents, and legal professionals. Maintain a comprehensive medical record despite changes in placement.
Compassionate care	Understand and educate children, families, and other healthcare professionals on the impact of early childhood adversities, trauma, and ongoing uncertainties of foster care on the developing child. Promote positive purposeful parenting strategies and minimizing conflict among caregivers.
Child-centered and family-focused care	Prioritize the needs of children first and foremost. Partner with families to increase understanding of a child's needs. Focus on the strengths of children and caregivers. Understand the conflicts for the child of belonging in multiple families.
Continuity of care	Invite children to remain patients throughout their stay in foster care, and beyond when feasible.
Cultural competence	Extend this concept to include the microculture of foster care and the multiple transitions that can further erode a child's well-being. Understand the roles of caseworkers, foster parents, law guardians, etc. Understand the importance of quality visitation for family reunification.
Accessibility	Create a welcoming environment for children and all their families (birth, foster, kin, preadoptive).

Table 9.3	Trauma-Informed Anticipatory Guidance for Children in Foster Care
SITUATION	**ANTICIPATORY GUIDANCE FOR FOSTER PARENTS**
Preparing for visits	Educate foster/kinship parents about impact of visitation on children and ways to improve the experience for children. Send familiar object with child to visit. Have child draw picture to give birth parent. Reassure child that foster parent will be there when child returns from visits. Advise all caregivers to minimize conflict with and negativity toward each other. Ideally, visits are coached by trained professionals.
Returning from visits and other transitions	Greet child warmly and help with unpacking. Establish reentry rituals, such as quiet play, reading together, active play, having a healthy snack.
Relationship with birth parent(s)	Encourage caseworker to have birth parents keep child's rituals and routines consistent with those in foster/kinship home (vice versa when appropriate). Focus on birth parent's positive qualities; maintain a neutral or positive affect;.
Building on child's strengths	Encourage participation in child-directed play. Time-in with child. Encourage participation in normalizing activities (e.g., hobbies, sports) "Catch the child being good." Give specific praise. Practice attentive listening. Provide child with words for emotions. Ignore negative behavior or redirect unless there is a safety issue.
Preparing for court dates	Foster/kinship parent, caseworker or law guardian should explain purpose of court hearings to child in simple terms.
School	If changing schools, visit school together a few times, and meet teacher. Check in regularly (weekly or monthly depending on need) with child's teacher.
Adolescent	Decide what issues demand firm limits and guidelines (e.g., curfews, no smoking, party at a friend's house), what issues are not important and can be left up to teen (e.g., hair length and color), and what issues are ideal for negotiation (e.g., transportation to school function, style of dress). Encourage responsible decision-making by recognizing and complimenting it. Encourage after-school activities. Teach driving when age and developmentally appropriate. Encourage teen to seek employment and teach job skills. Help teen to identify mentors and focus on the future.

The trauma-informed office is one in which symptoms such as dysregulation of sleep, behavioral problems, developmental delays, poor school function, and somatic complaints are recognized as potential effects of childhood trauma. Understanding the child's psychosocial context and history, as well as that of the caregiver, and exploring their strengths, assets, and challenges are the foundation of a trauma-informed approach. The office should have print resources for education of families and child welfare professionals and a list of helpful local community resources. Referral to trauma-informed pediatric mental health services, when available, should be considered in collaboration with caregivers, child welfare, and educators. **Continuity of care** is very important for the child in foster care and includes ongoing monitoring and management of progress and care. The AAP has several resources for caring for traumatized children.*

Several recommendations are specific to the care of children and youth in foster care. Children should be seen early and often when they first enter a new placement to identify all their health issues, and to support the child and caregivers through a major transition that involves considerable loss and adjustment, including the development of an attachment relationship with a new caregiver, for the child and many challenges for the foster/kinship parent.

The AAP recommends that every child in foster care have comprehensive medical, dental, developmental, and mental health assessments within 30 days of entering foster care. Almost every child in foster care deserves a full mental health evaluation to assess for the impact of trauma and loss on emotional well-being. *Psychotropic medication* should only be considered, if at all, after a thorough high-quality trauma-informed mental health evaluation by a pediatric-trained mental health professional. The pediatrician should remember that inattention, impulsivity, and hyperactivity may reflect the impact of past trauma on the developing brain rather than attention-deficit/hyperactivity disorder (see Chapter 49). Childhood trauma may impair cognition and memory (see Chapter 16), so that children <6 yr of age benefit from a comprehensive developmental assessment, whereas older children often benefit from a comprehensive educational assessment. The caseworker should provide consents for healthcare and any available

health history and encourage the appropriate involvement of the birth parent. The primary care provider can help caseworkers and caregivers by obtaining and interpreting the results of these assessments. Pediatricians, caregivers, and caseworkers should share health information.

Foster/kinship parents are the major therapeutic intervention of the foster care system, and pediatricians are in a unique position to provide them with appropriate education and support. Important topics include positive parenting strategies, supporting children through transitions, providing a consistent and nurturing environment, and helping children heal from past trauma and adversity (Table 9.3). All caregivers may need extensive education about behavioral and emotional problems within the context of the child's trauma history to remove blame and promote healing. Minimizing conflict among caregivers is extremely important because children ideally have affection and loyalty for all their caregivers. Pediatricians can promote resilience by focusing on both caregiver and child strengths. For teens and young adults in foster care, the pediatrician can provide anticipatory guidance around education, identifying formation in the face of past trauma, independent decision-making, health promotion including reproductive health, healthy relationships, and developing the skills and competencies needed for a successful future life. The pediatrician can advocate for placement stability in a nurturing and responsive foster family where caregivers possess the appropriate skills to help children and youth heal.

Bibliography is available at Expert Consult.

Chapter **10**
Medical Evaluation of the Foreign-Born Child
Stacene R. Maroushek

第十章
境外出生儿童的医疗评估

中文导读

本章主要介绍了常见感染和免疫接种。常见感染包括B 型肝炎（见第三百八十五章）、A 型肝炎（见第三百八十五章）、C 型肝炎（见第三百八十五章）、肠道病原体、结核（见第二百四十二章）、先天性梅毒（见第二百四十五章）和HIV感染（见第三百零二章）等；免疫接种见第一百九十七章。

---

*https://www.aap.org/en-us/advocacy-and-policy/aap-health-initiatives/resilience/Pages/Becoming-a-Trauma-Informed-Practice.aspx.

More than 210,000 foreign-born children (≤16 yr old) enter the United States each year as asylees (asylum seekers), refugees, and immigrants, including international adoptees (see Chapter 8). This number does not include undocumented children living and working in the United States, the U.S.-born children of foreign-born parents, or the approximately 2.7 million nonimmigrant visitors ≤16 yr old who legally enter the United States annually with temporary visas. With the exception of internationally adopted children, pediatric guidelines for screening these newly arrived children are sparse. The diverse countries of origin and patterns of infectious disease, the possibility of previous high-risk living circumstances (e.g., refugee camps, orphanages, foster care, rural/urban poor), the limited availability of reliable healthcare in many economically developing countries, the generally unknown past medical histories, and interactions with parents who may have limited English proficiency and/or varied educational and economic experiences, make the medical evaluation of immigrant children a challenging but important task.

Before admission into the United States, all immigrant children are required to have a medical examination performed by a physician designated by the U.S. Department of State in their **country of origin**. This examination is limited to completing legal requirements for screening for certain communicable diseases and examination for serious physical or mental problems that would prevent issuing a permanent residency visa. This evaluation is *not* a comprehensive assessment of the child's health, and except in limited circumstances, laboratory or radiographic screening for infectious diseases *is not required* for children <15 yr old. After entry into the United States, health screenings of refugees, but not other immigrants, are recommended to be done by the resettlement state. There is limited tracking of refugees as they move to different cities or states. Thus, many foreign-born children have had minimal pre- or postarrival screening for infectious diseases or other health issues.

Immunization requirements and records also vary depending on entry status. Internationally adopted children who are younger than 10 yr are exempt from Immigration and Nationality Act regulations pertaining to immunization of immigrants before arrival in the United States. Adoptive parents are required to sign a waiver indicating their intention to comply with U.S.-recommended immunizations, whereas older immigrants need only show evidence of up-to-date, not necessarily complete, immunizations before application for permanent resident (green card) status after arrival in the United States.

Infectious diseases are among the most common medical diagnoses identified in immigrant children after arrival in the United States. Children may be asymptomatic; therefore, diagnoses must be made by screening tests in addition to history and physical examination. Because of inconsistent perinatal screening for hepatitis B and hepatitis C viruses, syphilis, and HIV, and the high prevalence of certain intestinal parasites and tuberculosis, all foreign-born children should be screened for these infections on arrival in the United States. Table 10.1 lists suggested screening tests for infectious diseases. Table 10.2 lists incubation periods of common internationally acquired diseases. In addition to these infections, other medical and developmental issues, including hearing, vision, dental, and mental health assessments; evaluation of growth and development; nutritional assessment; lead exposure risk; complete blood cell count with red blood cell indices; microscopic urinalysis; newborn screening (this could also be done in non-neonates) and/or measurement of thyroid-stimulating hormone concentration; and examination for congenital anomalies (including fetal alcohol syndrome) should be considered as part of the initial evaluation of any immigrant child.*

Children should be examined within 1 mo of arrival in the United States, or earlier if there are immediate health concerns, but foreign-born parents may not access the healthcare system with their children unless prompted by illness, school vaccination, or other legal requirements. *It is important to assess the completeness of previous medical screenings at any first visit with a foreign-born child.*

Clinicians should be aware of potential diseases in high-risk immigrant children and their clinical manifestations. Some diseases, such as central

---

*For the most up-to-date guidelines, see: https://www.cdc.gov/immigrantrefugeehealth/guidelines/domestic/domestic-guidelines.html.

Table 10.1	Screening Tests for Infectious Diseases in International Adoptees and Foreign-Born (Immigrant) Children

RECOMMENDED TESTS

Hepatitis B virus serologic testing*
- Hepatitis B surface antigen (HBsAg)
- Antibody to hepatitis B surface antigen (anti-HBs)

Hepatitis C virus serologic testing*†
Hepatitis A virus serologic testing†
Varicella virus serologic testing†
Syphilis serologic testing
- Nontreponemal test (RPR, VDRL, or ART)
- Treponemal test (MHA-TP or FTA-ABS)

Human immunodeficiency viruses 1 *and* 2 testing (ELISA if >18 mo, PCR if <18 mo)*
Complete blood cell count with red blood cell indices and differential (if eosinophilia, see text)
Strongyloides serology
Stool examination for O&P (2-3 specimens)†
Stool examination for *Giardia lamblia* and *Cryptosporidium* antigen (1 specimen)†
Tuberculin skin test (with CXR if >5 mm induration) or interferon-γ release assay*†

OPTIONAL TESTS (FOR SPECIAL POPULATIONS OR CIRCUMSTANCES)

GC/Chlamydia
Chagas disease serology (endemic areas)
Malaria, thick and thin smears (endemic areas)
Filaria testing (endemic areas)
Urine for O&P for schistosomiasis, if hematuria present
Stool testing for enteric bacteria and viruses in children with diarrhea

*Repeat 3-6 mo after arrival.
†See text.
ART, Automated reagin test; CXR, chest radiograph; ELISA, enzyme-linked immunosorbent assay; FTA-ABS, fluorescent treponemal antibody absorption; GC, gonococcus; MHA-TP, microhemagglutination test for *Treponema pallidum*; O&P, ova and parasites; PCR, polymerase chain reaction; RPR, rapid plasma reagin; VDRL, Venereal Disease Research Laboratories.

---

nervous system cysticercosis, may have incubation periods as long as several years, and thus may not be detected during initial screening. On the basis of findings at the initial evaluation, consideration should be given to a repeat evaluation 6 mo after arrival. In most cases, the longer the interval from arrival to development of a clinical syndrome, the less likely the syndrome can be attributed to a pathogen acquired in the country of origin.

COMMONLY ENCOUNTERED INFECTIONS
Hepatitis B
See also Chapter 385.

The prevalence of hepatitis B surface antigen (HBsAg) in refugee children ranges from 4–14%, depending on the country of origin, age, and year studied. Prevalence of markers of past hepatitis B virus (HBV) infection is higher. HBV infection is most prevalent in immigrants from Asia, Africa, and some countries in Central and Eastern Europe, as well as the former Soviet Union (e.g., Bulgaria, Romania, Russia, Ukraine), but also occurs in immigrants born in other countries. All immigrant children, even if previously vaccinated, coming from high-risk countries (HBsAg seropositivity >2%) should undergo serologic testing for HBV infection, including both HBsAg and antibody to HBsAg (anti-HBs), to identify current or chronic infection, past resolved infection, or evidence of previous immunization. Because HBV has a long incubation period (6 wk–6 mo), the child may have become infected at or near the time of migration, and initial testing might be falsely negative. Therefore, strong consideration should be given to a repeated evaluation 6 mo after arrival for all children, especially those from highly endemic countries. Chronic HBV infection is indicated by persistence of HBsAg

Table 10.2	Incubation Periods of Common Travel-Related Infections*		
SHORT INCUBATION (<10 DAYS)		**MEDIUM INCUBATION (10-21 DAYS)**	**LONG INCUBATION (>21 DAYS)**
Malaria		Malaria	Malaria
Arboviruses including dengue, yellow fever, Japanese encephalitis, Zika, chikungunya		Flaviviruses: tick-borne encephalitis and Japanese encephalitis	Schistosomiasis
Hemorrhagic fevers: Lassa, Ebola, South American arenaviruses		Hemorrhagic fevers: Lassa, Ebola, Crimean-Congo	Tuberculosis
Respiratory viruses including severe acute respiratory syndrome		Acute HIV infection	Acute HIV infection
Typhoid and paratyphoid		Typhoid and paratyphoid	Viral hepatitis
Bacterial enteritis		*Giardia*	Filariasis
Rickettsia: spotted fever group—Rocky Mountain spotted fever, African tick typhus, Mediterranean spotted fever, scrub typhus, Q fever		*Rickettsia*: flea-borne, louse-borne, and scrub typhus, Q fever, spotted fevers (rare)	*Rickettsia*: Q fever
		Cytomegalovirus	Secondary syphilis
		Toxoplasma	Epstein-Barr virus including mononucleosis
Bacterial pneumonia including *Legionella*		Amoebic dysentery	Amoebic liver disease
Relapsing fever		Histoplasmosis	Leishmaniasis
Amoebic dysentery		*Brucella*	*Brucella*
Meningococcemia		Leptospirosis	Bartonellosis (chronic)
Brucella (rarely)		Babesiosis	Babesiosis
Leptospirosis		Rabies	Rabies
Fascioliasis		East African trypanosomiasis (acute)	West African trypanosomiasis (chronic)
Rabies (rarely)		Hepatitis A (rarely)	Cytomegalovirus
African trypanosomiasis (acute), East African (rarely)		Measles	

HIV, Human immunodeficiency virus.

*Diseases that commonly have variable incubation periods are shown more than once. However, most diseases may rarely have an atypical incubation period, and this is not shown here.

From Freedman DO: Infections in returning travelers. In Bennett JE, Dolin R, Blaser MJ, editors: *Mandell, Douglas, and Bennett's principles and practice of infectious diseases*, ed 8, Philadelphia, 2015, Elsevier (Table 324-2).

for >6 mo. Children with HBsAg-positive test results should be evaluated to identify the presence of chronic HBV infection, which occurs in >90% of infants infected at birth or in the 1st yr of life and in 30% of children exposed at ages 1-5 yr. Once identified as being infected, additional testing should be done to assess for biochemical evidence of severe or chronic liver disease or liver cancer.

Hepatitis A
See Chapter 385.

Hepatitis C
See also Chapter 385.

The decision to screen children should depend on history (e.g., receipt of blood products; traditional percutaneous procedures such as tattooing, body piercing, circumcisions, or other exposures to reused, unsterile medical devices) and the prevalence of hepatitis C virus (HCV) infection in the child's country of origin. Children from Eastern Mediterranean and Western Pacific countries, Africa, China, and Southeast Asia should be considered for HCV infection screening. All children coming from Egypt, which has the highest known HCV seroprevalence (12% nationally and 40% in some villages), should be tested for hepatitis C.

Intestinal Pathogens
Fecal examinations for ova and parasites (O&P) by an experienced laboratory will identify a pathogen in 8–86% of immigrants and refugees The prevalence of intestinal parasites varies by country of origin, time period when studied, previous living conditions (including water quality, sanitation, and access to footwear) and age, with toddler/young school-age children being most affected. If documented predeparture treatment was given, an eosinophil count should be performed. An absolute eosinophil count of >400 cells/μL, if persistently elevated for 3-6 mo after arrival, should prompt further investigation for tissue-invasive parasites such as *Strongyloides* (see Chapter 321) and *Schistosoma* (Chapter 326) species (if no predeparture praziquantel given). If no documented predeparture treatment was given, 2 stool O&P specimens obtained from separate morning stools should be examined by the concentration method, and an eosinophil count performed. If the child is symptomatic, including evidence of poor physical growth, but no

eosinophilia is present, a single stool specimen should also be sent for *Giardia lamblia* (see Chapter 308.1) and *Cryptosporidium parvum* (Chapter 309) antigen detection. All potentially pathogenic parasites found should be treated appropriately. All nonpregnant refugees >2 yr of age coming from sub-Saharan Africa and Southeast Asia should be presumptively treated with predeparture albendazole.

Tuberculosis
See also Chapter 242.

Tuberculosis (TB) commonly is encountered in immigrants from all countries because *Mycobacterium tuberculosis* infects approximately 30% of the world's population. Latent TB infection rates can be up to 60% in some refugee children from North Africa and the Middle East. Prior to 2007, chest radiographs or tuberculin skin tests were generally not administered in children <15 yr of age, and reports indicate that 1–2% of these unscreened children may enter the United States with undiagnosed active TB disease.

Since 2007, TB *Technical Instructions for Medical Evaluation of Aliens* have required that children ages 2-14 yr undergo a TB skin test or interferon-γ release assay if they are medically screened in countries where the TB rate is ≥20 cases per 100,000 population. If the testing is positive, a chest radiograph is required. If the chest film suggests TB, cultures and 3 sputum smears are required, all before arrival in the United States. Check with the Centers for Disease Control and Prevention, Division of Global Migration and Quarantine, for the latest information (www.cdc.gov/ncidod/dq/technica.htm).

Congenital Syphilis
See Chapter 245.

HIV Infection
See Chapter 302.

IMMUNIZATIONS
See Chapter 197.

Immigrant children and adolescents should receive immunizations according to the recommended schedules in the United States for healthy children and adolescents. Some immigrants will have written documenta-

tion of immunizations received in their birth or home country. Although immunizations such as bacille Calmette-Guérin, diphtheria and tetanus toxoids and pertussis (DTP), poliovirus, measles, and HBV vaccines often are documented, other immunizations, such as *Haemophilus influenzae* type b, mumps, and rubella vaccines, are given less frequently, and *Streptococcus pneumoniae*, human papillomavirus, meningococcal, and varicella vaccines are given rarely. When doubt exists, an equally acceptable alternative is to reimmunize the child. Because the rate of more serious local reactions after diphtheria, tetanus toxoid, and acellular pertussis vaccine increases with the number of doses administered, serologic testing for antibody to tetanus and diphtheria toxins before reimmunizing, or if a serious reaction occurs, can decrease risk.

In children older than 6 mo with or without written documentation of immunization, testing for antibodies to diphtheria and tetanus toxoid and poliovirus may be considered to determine whether the child has protective antibody concentrations. If the child has protective concentrations, the immunization series should be completed as appropriate for that child's age. In children older than 12 mo, measles, mumps, rubella, and varicella antibody concentrations may be measured to determine whether the child is immune; these antibody tests should not be performed in children younger than 12 mo because of the potential presence of maternal antibody.

Bibliography is available at Expert Consult.

Chapter 11
Cultural Issues in Pediatric Care
Lee M. Pachter

第十一章
儿科卫生保健服务中的文化

中文导读

本章主要介绍了何谓文化，其中阐述了关于文化认同的问题和相同文化群体内部存在着差异；还介绍了关于文化习俗相关的护理告知，其中具体阐述了在医疗保健工作中理解文化习俗以及在实际操作中运用的知晓–判断–协商模式；最后介绍了具有文化特异性的信仰，即：文化相关、具有群体特异性的风俗习惯（如斋戒、净身、死亡、父权、上帝意志等）影响着该群体维护健康的理念。

Pediatricians live and work in a multicultural world. Among the world's 7 billion people residing in over 200 countries, more than 6,000 languages are spoken. As the global population becomes more mobile, population diversity increases in all countries. In the United States, sources of ethnic and cultural diversity come from indigenous cultural groups such as Native Americans and Alaskan and Hawaiian natives, groups from U.S. territories such as Puerto Rico, recent immigrant groups, those whose heritage originates from the African diaspora, as well as others whose families and communities migrated to the United States from Europe and Asia generations ago but who have retained cultural identification. U.S. census estimates suggest that in 2016, almost 40% of the U.S. population self-identified as belonging to a racial/ethnic group other than non-Hispanic white. Recent immigrants comprise 13.5% of the U.S. population, but if U.S.-born children of these immigrants are included,

27% of the population are either new immigrants or first-generation Americans. Immigrants from China and India account for the largest groups coming to the United States, followed by those from Mexico. This national and international diversity allows for a heterogeneity of experience that enriches the lives of everyone. Much of this diversity is based on varied cultural orientation.

WHAT IS CULTURE?
The concept of *culture* does not refer exclusively to racial and ethnic categorizations. A common definition of **cultural group** is a *collective that shares common heritage, worldviews, beliefs, values, attitudes, behaviors, practices, and identity.* Cultural groups can be based on identities such as gender orientation (gay/lesbian, bisexual, transgender), age (teen culture), being deaf or hearing impaired (deaf culture), and

having neurodevelopmental differences (neurodiversity; neurotypical and neuroatypical). All these groups to a certain extent share common worldviews, attitudes, beliefs, values, practices, and identities.

Medical professionals can also be considered as belonging to a specific cultural group. Those who identify with the **culture of medicine** share common theories of well-being and disease, acceptance of the biomedical and biopsychosocial models of health, and common practices and rituals. As with other cultural groups, physicians and other healthcare professionals have a distinct language and share a common history, the same preparatory courses that must be mastered for entrance into training for the profession (a rite of passage). Medical professionals subscribe to common norms in medical practice. Young physicians learn a new way to describe health and illness that requires a new common vocabulary and an accepted structure for communicating a patient's history. These common beliefs, orientations, and practices are often not shared by those outside medicine. Therefore, *any* clinical interaction between a healthcare provider and a patient can be a potential *cross-cultural interaction*—between the culture of medicine and the culture of the patient—regardless of the race or ethnicity of the participants. A culturally informed and sensitized approach to clinical communication is a fundamental skill required of all medical professionals, regardless of the demographic makeup of one's patient population.

Culture and Identity

We are all members of multiple cultural groups. Our identification or affiliation with different groups is not fixed or unchangeable. With whom we self-identify may depend on specific situations and contexts and may change over time. A gay Latino physician may feel, at different times and in different situations, greatest affinity as a member of Latino culture, a member of the culture of medicine, a minority in the United States, or a gay man. An immigrant from India may initially feel great connection with her Indian culture and heritage, which may wane during periods of assimilation into American cultural life, then increase again in later life. Culturally informed clinicians should never assume that they know or understand the cultural identity of a person based solely on perception of ethnic, racial, or other group affiliation.

Intracultural Variability

There can be significantly different beliefs, values, and behaviors among members of the same cultural group. Often, there is as much variability *within* cultures as there is *between* cultures. The sources of this variability include differences in personal psychology and philosophy, family beliefs and practices, social context, and other demographic differences, as well as **acculturation**, defined as the changes in beliefs and practices resulting from continuous interactions with another culture. The literature on acculturation and health outcomes shows varied effects of cultural change on health and well-being. These differences are in part caused by overly simplistic ways of measuring acculturation in public health and health services research. The use of *proxies,* such as generational status (recent immigration, first generation) and socioeconomic status, as measures of acculturation does not allow for an understanding of the complex behavioral changes that occur during shifts in cultural orientation. Often, acculturation is seen as a *linear process* where individuals move from unacculturated to acculturated or assimilated into the host culture. This simplistic view does not take into account the reality that acculturation is **bidimensional**: the degree to which an individual continues to identify with her original cultural identity, and the degree to which the host cultural orientation is adopted. These are separate and independent processes. One can become *bicultural* (adopting the host culture while retaining aspects of the original culture), *assimilated* (host culture is adopted, but original culture is not retained), *separated* (original cultural orientation is retained, but host culture is not greatly adopted), or *marginalized* (does not adopt host culture and does not retain original culture). These variations in the acculturation process are determined not only by the individual going through the cultural change process but also by the degree of acceptance of diversity in the host culture. In theory, individuals who best adapt to the multicultural society are those who are **bicultural**, since they retain the strengths and assets of their heritage culture while being able to positively adjust

to host cultural norms. Likewise, members of the majority culture who are able to take a bicultural perspective will have relative advantage in the multicultural society. This type of perspective is a foundation of cultural awareness and culturally informed practice.

CULTURALLY INFORMED CARE

Physicians and patients bring to their interactions diverse orientations from multiple cultural systems. These different belief systems and practices could have significant implications for the delivery of healthcare (Table 11.1). Consequently, physician cultural awareness, sensitivity, and humility is critical to successful patient–provider interaction.

The culturally informed physician (1) attempts to understand and respect the beliefs, values, attitudes, and lifestyles of patients; (2) understands that health and illness are influenced by ethnic and cultural orientation, religious and spiritual beliefs, and linguistic considerations; (3) has insight into own cultural biases and does not see cultural issues as something that only affects the patient; (4) is sensitive to how differences in power and privilege may affect the quality of the clinical encounter; (5) recognizes that in addition to the physiologic aspects of disease, the culturally and psychologically constructed meaning of illness and health is a central clinical issue; and (6) is sensitive to intragroup variations in beliefs and practices and avoids stereotyping based on any group affiliation. These core components of culturally-informed care are important for interactions with *all* patients, regardless of race or ethnicity. Culturally sensitive clinical care is essentially *generally sensitive* clinical care.

Becoming culturally informed is a developmental process. Fig. 11.1 displays a framework that includes a continuum of perceptions and orientations to cultural awareness. Individuals in the *denial* stage perceive their own cultural orientation as the true one, with other cultures either undifferentiated or unnoticed. In the *defensive* stage, other cultures are acknowledged but regarded as inferior to one's own culture. The *minimization* stage is characterized by beliefs that fundamental similarities among people outweigh any differences, and downplays the role of culture as a source of human variation. The idea that one should be "color blind" is an example of a common belief of individuals in the minimization stage.

As one moves to the *acceptance* stage, cultural differences are acknowledged. Further expansion and understanding lead to *adaptation*, where one not only acknowledges differences but can shift frames of reference and have a level of comfort outside one's own cultural frame. This eventually leads to further comfort with different worldviews seen at the *integration* stage, where individuals respect cultural differences and can comfortably interact across cultures, even incorporating aspects of different cultural orientations into their own.

Understanding Culture in the Context of Healthcare

Cultural orientation is just one of many different perspectives that individuals draw on as they make health and healthcare decisions. Individual psychology, past experiences, religious and spiritual views, social position, socioeconomic status, and family norms all can contribute

Table 11.1	Culturally Informed Care

1. Respects the beliefs, values, and lifestyles of patients
2. Understands that health and illness are influenced by ethnic and cultural orientation, religious and spiritual beliefs, and linguistic considerations
3. Has insight into one's own cultural biases; doesn't see "cultural issues" as something that only affects the patient
4. Is sensitive to how differences in power and privilege affect the clinical encounter
5. Recognizes that the culturally constructed meaning of illness and health is as important a clinical issue as the biomedical aspects of disease
6. Sensitive to within group variations in beliefs and practices; avoids stereotyping

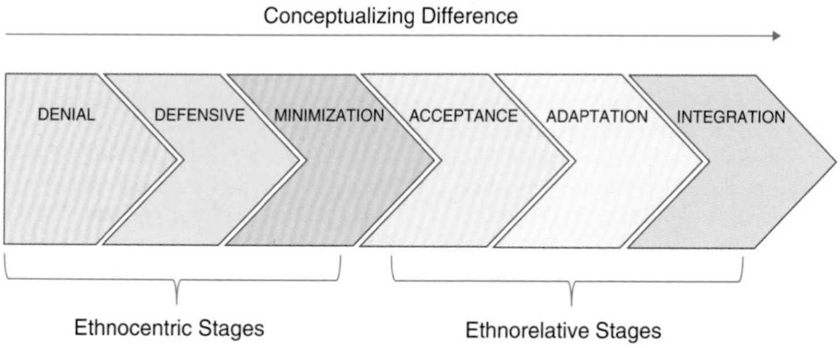

Fig. 11.1 Development of intercultural sensitivity. *(Adapted from Bennett MJ: A developmental approach to training for intercultural sensitivity, Int J Intercultural Relations 10(2):179–196, 1986.)*

to a person's health beliefs and practices. These beliefs and practices can also change over time and may be expressed differently in different situations and circumstances. Because of the significant variability in health beliefs and behaviors seen among members of the same cultural group, an approach to cultural competency that emphasizes a knowledge set of specific cultural health practices in different cultural groups could lead to false assumptions and stereotyping. Knowledge is important, but it only goes so far. Instead, an approach that focuses on the healthcare provider acquiring skills and attitudes relating to open and effective communication styles is a preferable approach to culturally effective and informed care. Such an approach does not rely on rote knowledge of facts that may change depending on time, place, and individuals. Instead, it provides a skills toolbox that can be used in all circumstances. The following skills can lead to a culturally informed approach to care:

1. *Don't assume.* Presupposing that a particular patient may have certain beliefs, or may act in a particular way based on their cultural group affiliation, could lead to incorrect assumptions. Sources of intracultural diversity are varied.
2. *Practice humility.* Cultural humility has been described by Hook et al. (2013) as "the ability to maintain an interpersonal stance that is other-oriented (or open to the other) in relation to aspects of cultural identity." Cultural humility goes beyond cultural competency in that it requires the clinician to self-reflect and acknowledge that one's *own* cultural orientation enters into any transaction with a patient (see Chapter 2.1).

   Cultural humility aims to fix power imbalances between the dominant (hospital-medical) culture and the patient. It recognizes the value of the patient's culture and incorporates the patient's life experiences and understanding outside the scope of the provider; it creates a collaboration and a partnership.

   Cultural competency is an approach that typically focuses on the patient's culture, whereas cultural humility acknowledges that both physicians and patients have cultural orientations, and that a successful relationship requires give and take among those differing perspectives. It also includes an understanding that differences in social power, which are inherent in the physician–patient relationship, need to be understood and addressed so that open communication can occur.
3. *Understand privilege.* Members of the majority culture have certain privileges and benefits that are often unrecognized and unacknowledged. For example, they can have high expectations that they will be positively represented in media such as movies and television. Compared with minority groups, those in the majority culture have less chance of being followed by security guards at stores, or having their bags checked. They have a greater chance of having a positive reception in a new neighborhood, or of finding food in the supermarket that is consistent with one's heritage. These privileges typically go unnoticed by members of the majority culture, but their absence is painfully recognized by members of nonmajority cultural groups. The culturally informed physician should try to be mindful of these

Table 11.2	The Health Beliefs History

- What do you think is wrong with your child?
- Why do you think your child has gotten it [the illness]?
- What do you think caused it?
- Why do you think it started when it did?
- What do you think is happening inside the body?
- What are the symptoms that make you know your child has this illness?
- What problems does this illness cause your child?
- What are you most worried about with this illness?
- How long do you think it will last?
- How do you treat it?
- What will happen if it is not treated?
- What do you expect from the treatments?

Adapted from Kleinman A, Eisenberg L, Good B: Culture, illness, and care: clinical lessons from anthropologic and cross-cultural research, *Ann Intern Med* 88(2):251–258, 1978.

privileges, and how they may influence the interaction between physicians and patients.

4. *Be inquisitive.* Because of the significant amount of intracultural diversity of beliefs and practices, the only way to know a particular patient's approach to issues concerning health and illness is through direct and effective communication. Asking about the patient's/family's perspective in an inquisitive and respectful manner will usually be met with open and honest responses, as long as the patient does not feel looked down on and the questions are asked in genuine interest. Obtaining a **health beliefs history** is an effective way of understanding clinical issues from the patient's and family's perspective (Table 11.2). The health beliefs history gathers information on the patient's views on the identification of health problems, causes, susceptibility, signs and symptoms, concerns, treatment, and expectations. Responses gathered from the health beliefs history can be helpful in guiding care plans and health education interventions.
5. *Be flexible.* As members of the culture of medicine, clinicians have been educated and acculturated to the biomedical model as the optimal approach to health and illness. Patients and families may have health beliefs and practices that do not fully fit the biomedical model. Traditional beliefs and practices may be used in tandem with biomedical approaches. An individual's approach to health rarely is exclusively biomedical or traditional, and often a combination of multiple approaches. The health beliefs history provides clinicians with information regarding the nonbiomedical beliefs and practices that may be held by the patient. Culturally informed physicians should be flexible and find ways of integrating nonharmful traditional beliefs and practices into the medical care plan to make that plan fit the patient's needs and worldview. This will likely result in better adherence to treatment and prevention.

Obtaining a health beliefs history for a child with asthma, for example, may reveal that the family uses an alternative remedy when the symptoms first occur. If the symptoms do not resolve after giving the remedy, the family administers standard medical care. In this case, if the alternative remedy is safe and has no significant likelihood of causing adverse effects, the culturally informed physician might say, "I'm not sure if the remedy you're using is helpful or not, but I can say that if used as directed, it's not likely to be harmful. So if you think it may work, feel free to try it. But instead of waiting to give the prescription medicine until after you see if the remedy works, why don't you give it at the same time you give the remedy? Maybe they'll work well together." This approach shows respect for the family-held beliefs and practices while increasing timely adherence to the biomedical therapy.

At times, an alternative therapy the patient is using may be contraindicated or may have adverse effects. In this case it is advisable to recommend against the therapy, but whenever possible, one should attempt to replace the therapy with another, safer, culturally acceptable treatment. If a parent is giving a child tea containing harmful ingredients to treat a cold, the culturally informed physician could recommend stopping the practice and explain the concerns, but then recommend replacing the harmful tea with something safer that fits the family's cultural belief system, such as a weak herbal tea with no harmful ingredients. This requires an awareness and background knowledge of the cultural belief system, but this approach increases the chances that the family will follow through on the recommendation and feel that their beliefs are respected.

Awareness-Assessment-Negotiation Model

Providing care in the multicultural context can be challenging, but it offers opportunities for creativity and can result in improved long-term physician–patient relationships, which will ultimately improve the quality and outcomes of healthcare. Culturally informed care combines knowledge with effective communication skills, an open attitude, and the qualities of flexibility and humility.

The culturally informed physician should first become aware of common health beliefs and practices of patients in the practice. Reading literature on the particular groups could increase awareness, but with the caution that such information may be outdated (cultural beliefs and practices change over time) and not specific to the local context. The best approach to becoming aware of specific health beliefs and practices is to ask—enter into conversations with patients, families, and community members. One might say, "I've heard that there are ways of treating this illness [or staying healthy] that people believe work, but doctors don't know about. Sometimes they're recommended by grandparents or others in your community. They may be effective. Have you heard of any of these?" This approach shows genuine interest and openness, is not based on presumptions, and does not ask about behaviors or practices, only if the patient has *heard* of these practices. If the question elicits a positive response, the conversation can then continue, including asking whether the patient has personally tried any of the therapies, under what circumstances, and if they thought it was helpful. This approach shows respect for the patient as an individual and avoids stereotyping all members of a particular group as having a uniform set of cultural beliefs and practices.

The information obtained should be seen only as common ways that members of a community *may* interpret health-related issues. Assuming that all members subscribe to similar beliefs and practices would be incorrect and potentially damaging by promoting stereotypes. Since the unit of measurement in clinical care is the individual patient and family, clinicians must assess to what extent a specific patient may act on these general beliefs and under what circumstances. The health beliefs history can help the physician become aware of the specific beliefs and practices that a patient holds, and allow one to tailor the care to the individual patient.

Once the patient's explanatory model is elicited and understood, the clinician should be able to assess the congruity of this model and the biomedical model, finding similarities. Then the process of negotiating can occur. Integrating patient-held approaches to health with evidence-based biomedical standards of care will help place care within the lifestyle and worldview of patients, leading to increased adherence to medical care plans, better physician–patient communication, enhanced long-term therapeutic relationship, and improved patient (and physician) satisfaction.

Bibliography is available at Expert Consult.

11.1 Culture-Specific Beliefs

Robert M. Kliegman

Cultural group-specific practices that affect health-seeking behaviors are noted in Tables 11.3 and 11.4.

Table 11.3	Cultural Values* Relevant to Health and Health-Seeking Behavior	
CULTURAL GROUP	**RELEVANT CULTURAL NORMS**	
	Description of Norm	**Consequences of Failure to Appreciate**
Latino	*Fatalismo:* Fate is predetermined, reducing belief in the importance of screening and prevention.	Less preventive screening
	Simpática: Politeness/kindness in the face of adversity—expectation that the physician should be polite and pleasant, not detached.	Nonadherence to therapy, failure to make follow-up visits
	Personalismo: Expectation of developing a warm, personal relationship with the clinician, including introductory touching.	Refusal to divulge important parts of medical history, dissatisfaction with treatment
	Respeto: Deferential behavior on the basis of age, social stature, and economic position, including reluctance to ask questions.	Mistaking a deferential nod of the head/not asking questions for understanding; anger at not receiving due signs of respect
	Familismo: Needs of the extended family outrank those of the individual, and thus family may need to be consulted in medical decision-making.	Unnecessary conflict, inability to reach a decision
Muslim	*Fasting* during the holy month of Ramadan: fasting from sunrise to sundown, beginning during the teen years. Women are exempted during pregnancy, lactation, and menstruation, and there are exemptions for illness, but an exemption may be associated with a sense of personal failure.	Inappropriate therapy; will not take medicines during daytime misinterpreted as noncompliance; misdiagnosed

Continued

Table 11.3	Cultural Values* Relevant to Health and Health-Seeking Behavior—cont'd	
CULTURAL GROUP	**RELEVANT CULTURAL NORMS**	
	Description of Norm	**Consequences of Failure to Appreciate**
	Modesty: Women's body, including hair, body, arms, and legs, not to be seen by men other than in immediate family. Female chaperone and/or husband must be present during exam, and only that part of the body being examined should be uncovered.	Deep personal outrage, seeking alternative care
	Touch: Forbidden to touch members of the opposite sex other than close family. Even a handshake may be inappropriate.	Patient discomfort, seeking care elsewhere
	After death, body belongs to God. Postmortem examination will not be permitted unless required by law; family may wish to perform after-death care.	Unnecessary intensification of grief and loss
	Cleanliness essential before prayer. Individual must perform ritual ablutions before prayer, especially elimination of urine and stool. Nurse may need to assist in cleaning if patient is incapable.	Affront to religious beliefs
	God's will: God causes all to happen for a reason, and only God can bring about healing.	Allopathic medicine will be rejected if it conflicts with religious beliefs, family may not seek healthcare.
	Patriarchal, extended family. Older male typically is head of household, and family may defer to him for decision-making.	Child's mother or even both parents may not be able to make decisions about child's care; emergency decisions may require additional time.
	Halal (permitted) vs *haram* (forbidden) foods and medications. Foods and medicine containing alcohol (some cough and cold syrups) or pork (some gelatin-coated pills) are not permitted.	Refusal of medication, religious effrontery
Native American	*Nature* provides the spiritual, emotional, physical, social, and biologic means for human life; by caring for the earth, Native Americans will be provided for. Harmonious living is important.	Spiritual living is required of Native Americans; if treatments do not reflect this view, they are likely not to be followed.
	Passive forbearance: Right of the individual to choose his or her path. Another family member cannot intervene.	Mother's failure to intervene in a child's behavior and/or use of noncoercive disciplinary techniques may be mistaken for neglect.
	Natural unfolding of the individual. Parents further the development of their children by limiting direct interventions and viewing their natural unfolding.	Many pediatric preventive practices will run counter to this philosophy.
	Talking circle format to decision-making. Interactive learning format including diverse tribal members.	Lecturing, excluding the views of elders, is likely to result in advice that will be disregarded.
African-American	Great heterogeneity in beliefs and culture among African-Americans.	Risk of stereotyping and/or making assumptions that do not apply to a specific patient or family.
	Extended family and variations in family size and childcare arrangements are common; matriarchal decision-making regarding healthcare.	Advice/instructions given only to the parent and not to others involved in health decision-making may not be effective.
	Parenting style often involves stricter adherence to rules than seen in some other cultures.	Advice regarding discipline may be disregarded if it is inconsistent with perceived norms; other parenting styles may not be effective.
	History-based widespread mistrust of medical profession and strong orientation toward culturally specific alternative/complementary medicine.	In patient noncompliance, physicians will be consulted as a last resort.
	Greater orientation toward others; the role of an individual is emphasized as it relates to others within a social network.	Compliance may be difficult if the needs of 1 individual are stressed above the needs of the group.
	Spirituality/religiosity important; church attendance central in most African American families.	Loss of opportunity to work with the church as an ally in healthcare
East and Southeast Asian	Long history of Eastern medicines (e.g., Chinese medicine) as well as more localized medical traditions.	May engage with multiple health systems (Western biomedical and traditional) for treatment of symptoms and diseases
	Extended families and care networks. Grandparents may provide day-to-day care for children while parents work outside of the home.	Parents may not be the only individuals a physician needs to communicate with in regard to symptoms, follow-through on treatments, and preventive behaviors.
	Sexually conservative. Strong taboos for premarital sexual relationships, especially for women.	Adolescents may be reluctant to talk about issues of sexuality, pregnancy, and birth control with physicians. Recent immigrants or native populations may have less knowledge regarding pregnancy prevention, sexually transmitted infections, and HIV.
	Infant/child feeding practices may overemphasize infant's or child's need to eat a certain amount of food to stay "healthy."	Guidelines for child nutrition and feeding practices may not be followed out of concern for child's well-being.
	Saving face. This is a complex value whereby an individual may lose prestige or respect of a 3rd party when a 2nd individual makes negative or contradictory statements.	Avoid statements that are potentially value laden or imply a criticism of an individual. Use statements such as, "We have now found that it is better to …," rather than criticizing a practice.

*Adherence to these or other beliefs will vary among members of a cultural group based on nation of origin, specific religious sect, degree of acculturation, age of patient, etc.

Table 11.4	Examples of Disease Beliefs and Health Practices in Select Cultures
CULTURAL GROUP	**BELIEF OR PRACTICE**
Latino	Use of traditional medicines (*nopales*, or cooked prickly pear cactus, as a hypoglycemic agent) along with allopathic medicine. Recognition of disorders not recognized in Western allopathic medicine (*empacho*, in which food adheres to the intestines or stomach), which are treated with folk remedies but also brought to the pediatrician. Cultural interpretation of disease (*caida de mollera* or "fallen fontanel") as a cultural interpretation of severe dehydration in infants.
Muslim	Female genital mutilation: practiced in some Muslim countries; the majority do not practice it, and it is not a direct teaching of the Koran. Koranic faith healers: use verses from the Koran, holy water, and specific foods to bring about recovery.
Native American	Traditional "interpreters" or "healers" interpret signs and answers to prayers. Their advice may be sought in addition or instead of allopathic medicine. Dreams are believed to provide guidance; messages in the dream will be followed.
East and Southeast Asian	Concepts of "hot" and "cold," whereby a combination of hot and cold foods and other substances (e.g., coffee, alcohol) combine to cause illness. One important aspect is that Western medicines are considered "hot" by Vietnamese, and therefore nonadherence may occur if it is perceived that too much of a medicine will make their child's body "hot." *Note:* Hot and cold do not refer to temperatures but are a typology of different foods; for example, fish is hot and ginger is cold. Foods, teas, and herbs are also important forms of medicine because they provide balance between hot and cold.

Chapter 12

Maximizing Children's Health: Screening, Anticipatory Guidance, and Counseling

Joseph F. Hagan Jr and Dipesh Navsaria

第十二章

儿童健康最大化：筛查、预期指导和咨询

中文导读

　　本章主要介绍了儿童健康管理周期表和指南、正常儿童的保健服务、婴幼儿时期和学龄期及青春期管理、保健门诊对行为和心理健康问题的干预、尊重客观证据的意义以及在家庭和社区范围内进行儿童和青少年的保健服务。具体阐述了基于儿童身体健康的前提下采取的措施和方案，以及与质量改进相关的办公系统的改进完善。用表格呈现了在预防性儿科保健中推荐的内容。

Routine, scheduled care of well infants, children, and adolescents is an essential prevention effort for children and youth worldwide. Children's constantly changing development lends added value to regular and periodic encounters between children and their families and practitioners of pediatric healthcare. Health supervision visits from birth to age 21 yr are the platform for a young person's healthcare. The provision of **well care** in the medical home fosters strong relationships between the clinic or practice and the child and family, enabling the provision of appropriate surveillance, screening, and sick care.

To ensure the optimal health of the developing child, pediatric care in the United States and other countries evolved into regularly-scheduled visits to ensure adequate nutrition, to detect and immunize against infectious diseases, and to observe the child's development. Assessment of these key arenas remains essential to the well-child **health supervision** visit. However, contemporary analysis of changes in the population's health, coupled with the recognition that early life experiences and social factors impact health along the entire life course, have led to the addition of other components to the content of today's well-child encounter.

Stressful circumstances impair development, and **adverse childhood experiences** (ACEs) early in life increase the risk of disease (see Chapter 2). Adults who experienced abuse, violence, or other stressors as children have an increased risk for depression, heart disease, and other morbidities. Biology informs us that **stress** leads to increased heart rate and blood pressure and increased levels of inflammatory cytokines, cortisol, and other stress hormones, all of which impair brain activity, immune status, and cardiovascular function. There are both a causal model and evidence that ACEs, including those that could have been prevented, negatively impact the life course.

Preventive care for children and youth is a component of contemporary U.S. health reform activities and offers great opportunity for health cost savings. A healthy economy requires educated and healthy workers. For children to have a successful, meaningful, and useful educational experience, they must have physical, cognitive, and emotional health. Educational success, in particular, is tied to early childhood developmental competence. Thus, well-child care plays a vital role in promoting adult health, a concept endorsed by business leaders as essential to building the human infrastructure of the U.S. economy and society.

Although well-child care focuses on the health and well-being of the child, the reality is that children live in families. The context of the child within the family unit is also key to this primary goal and therefore also may necessitate the *addressing of needs* in the family, including the parents or other adults. Addressing of needs may be as straightforward as supportive listening, validation, and referral to an appropriate resource, whether in the community or the adult's own medical home. The importance of dual-generation approaches that benefit both the parent and the child is immense.

PERIODICITY SCHEDULE AND GUIDELINES

The frequency and content for well-child care activities are derived from evidence-based practice and research. In addition, federal agencies and professional organizations, such as the American Academy of Pediatrics (AAP), have developed evidence-informed, expert consensus guidelines for care. The *Recommendations for Preventive Pediatric Health Care* or **Periodicity Schedule** is a compilation of recommendations listed by age-based visits (Fig. 12.1). It is intended to guide practitioners of pediatric primary care to perform certain services and intentionally make observations at age-specific visits; it designates the standard for *preventive services* for U.S. children and youth and is referred to as such in some legislation. It is updated regularly and is available online.

Comprehensive guides for care of well infants, children, and adolescents have been developed based on the Periodicity Schedule to expand and further recommend how practitioners might accomplish the tasks outlined. The current guideline standard is *The Bright Futures Guidelines for Health Supervision of Infants, Children, and Adolescents*, 4th edition (https://brightfutures.aap.org/Pages/default.aspx). These guidelines were developed by AAP under the leadership of the Maternal Child Health Bureau of the U.S. Department of Health and Human Services, in collaboration with the National Association of Pediatric Nurse Practitioners, American Academy of Family Physicians, American

Medical Association, American Academy of Pediatric Dentistry, Family Voices, and others.

TASKS OF WELL-CHILD CARE

The well-child encounter aims to promote the physical and emotional well-being of children and youth. Child health professionals, including pediatricians, family medicine physicians, nurse practitioners, and physician assistants, take advantage of the opportunity well-child visits provide to elicit parental questions and concerns, gather relevant family and individual health information, perform a physical examination, and initiate screening tests. The tasks of each well-child visit include the following:

1. Disease detection
2. Disease prevention
3. Health promotion
4. Anticipatory guidance

To achieve these outcomes, healthcare professionals employ techniques to screen for disease—or for the risk of disease—and provide advice about healthy behaviors. These activities lead to the formulation of appropriate anticipatory guidance and health advice.

Clinical detection of disease in the well-child encounter is accomplished by a careful physical examination and both surveillance and screening. In well-child care, **surveillance** occurs in every health encounter and is enhanced by repeated visits and observations with advancing developmental stages. It relies on the experience of a skilled clinician performing intentional observation over time. **Screening** is a more formal process using some form of validated assessment tool and has known sensitivity and specificity. For example, anemia *surveillance* is accomplished through taking a dietary history and seeking signs of anemia in the physical examination. Anemia *screening* is done by hematocrit or hemoglobin tests. Developmental *surveillance* relies on the observations of parents and the assessment of clinicians in pediatric healthcare who are experienced in child development. Developmental *screening* uses a structured developmental screening tool by personnel trained in its use or in the scoring and interpretation of parent report questionnaires.

The 2nd essential action of the well-child encounter, **disease prevention**, may include both *primary prevention* activities applied to a whole population and *secondary prevention* activities aimed at patients with specific factors of risk. For example, counseling about reducing fat intake is appropriate for all children and families. However, counseling is intensified for overweight and obese youth or in the presence of a family history of hyperlipidemia and its sequelae. The child and adolescent healthcare professional needs to individualize disease prevention strategies to the specific patient, family, and community.

Health promotion and **anticipatory guidance** activities distinguish the well-child health supervision visit from all other encounters with the healthcare system. Disease detection and disease prevention activities are germane to all interactions of children with physicians and other healthcare clinicians, but health promotion and anticipatory guidance shift the focus to wellness and to the strengths of the family (e.g., what is being done well and how this might be improved). This approach is an opportunity to help the family address relationship issues, broach important safety topics, access needed services, and engage with extended family, school, neighborhood, and community and spiritual organizations.

It is not possible to cover all the topics suggested by comprehensive guidelines such as *Bright Futures* in the average 18 min well-child visit. Child health professionals must prioritize the most important topics to cover. Consideration should be given to a discussion of the following:

◆ First and foremost, the agenda the parent or child brings to the health supervision visit.
◆ The topics where evidence suggests counseling is effective in behavioral change.
◆ The topics where there is a clear rationale for the issue's critical importance to health, such as sleep environment to prevent sudden unexpected infant death (SUID) or attention to diet and physical activity.

Recommendations for Preventive Pediatric Health Care

Bright Futures/American Academy of Pediatrics

American Academy of Pediatrics
DEDICATED TO THE HEALTH OF ALL CHILDREN®

Bright Futures
prevention/health promotion for infants, children, adolescents, and their families®

Each child and family is unique; therefore, these Recommendations for Preventive Pediatric Health Care are designed for the care of children who are receiving competent parenting, have no manifestations of any important health problems, and are growing and developing in a satisfactory fashion. Developmental, psychosocial, and chronic disease issues for children and adolescents may require frequent counseling and treatment visits separate from preventive care visits. Additional visits also may become necessary if circumstances suggest variations from normal.

These recommendations represent a consensus by the American Academy of Pediatrics (AAP) and Bright Futures. The AAP continues to emphasize the great importance of continuity of care in comprehensive health supervision and the need to avoid fragmentation of care.

Refer to the specific guidance by age as listed in the *Bright Futures Guidelines* (Hagan JF, Shaw JS, Duncan PM, eds. *Bright Futures: Guidelines for Health Supervision of Infants, Children, and Adolescents.* 4th ed. Elk Grove Village, IL: American Academy of Pediatrics; 2017).

The recommendations in this statement do not indicate an exclusive course of treatment or standard of medical care. Variations, taking into account individual circumstances, may be appropriate.

Copyright © 2017 by the American Academy of Pediatrics, updated February 2017.

No part of this statement may be reproduced in any form or by any means without prior written permission from the American Academy of Pediatrics except for one copy for personal use.

Fig. 12.1 Recommendations for preventive pediatric healthcare. *(From Bright Futures/American Academy of Pediatrics. Copyright 2017, American Academy of Pediatrics, Elk Grove Village, IL. https://www.aap.org/en-us/documents/periodicity_schedule.pdf.)*

- A summary of the child's progress in emotional, cognitive, and social development, physical growth, and strengths.
- Issues that address the questions, concerns, or specific health problems relevant to the individual family.
- Community-specific problems that could significantly impact the child's health (e.g., neighborhood violence from which children need protection, absence of bike paths that would promote activity).

This approach must be directed at *all children*, including children and youth with special health care needs. CSHCN are no different from other children in their need for guidance about healthy nutrition, physical activity, progress in school, connection with friends, a healthy sense of self-efficacy, and avoidance of risk-taking behaviors. The existence of frequent visits to the medical home or specialists to address the special health needs sometimes masks the lack of general health supervision care. The coordination of specialty consultation, medication monitoring, and functional assessment, which should occur in their periodic visits, needs to be balanced with a discussion of the child's unique ways of accomplishing the emotional, social, and developmental tasks of childhood and adolescence. Comprehensive, integrated care planning for CSHCN should support partnerships between medical homes and families and youth through goal setting and negotiating next steps. In this process, chronic condition management and health surveillance (including adolescent engagement and planning for transition to adult care) occur within an effective patient care relationship, partnering to improve health outcomes and efficiencies of care provision.

INFANCY AND EARLY CHILDHOOD

Nutrition, physical activity, sleep, safety, and emotional, social, and physical growth, along with parental well-being, are critical for all children. For each well-child visit, there are topics specific to individual children based on their age, family situation, chronic health condition, or a parental concern, such as sleep environment to prevent SUID, activities to lose weight, and fences around swimming pools. Attention should also be focused on the family milieu and other social determinants of health, including screening for parental depression (especially maternal postpartum depression) and other mental illness, family violence, substance abuse, nutritional inadequacy, and lack of housing. It is equally important to identify, acknowledge, and empower family strengths. These issues are essential to the care of young children.

Answering parents' questions while creating an environment where parents feel comfortable asking is the most important priority of the well-child visit. Promoting family-centered care and partnership with parents increases the ability to elicit parental concerns, especially about their child's development, learning, and behavior. Evidence-based approaches such as early literacy assessment and promotion (e.g., Reach Out and Read) provide a structure for enquiry, surveillance, and parent coaching efficiently within the health supervision visit.

It is important to identify children with developmental disorders as early as possible. Developmental surveillance at every visit combined with a structured developmental screening, neuromuscular screening, and autism screening at certain visits is a way to improve diagnosis, especially for some of the subtler delays or autism spectrum disorders for which early intervention is believed to be associated with reduced morbidity.

MIDDLE CHILDHOOD AND ADOLESCENCE

As the child enters school-age years, additional considerations emerge. Attention to their developing autonomy requires fostering a clinician–patient relationship separate from the clinician–child-family relationship, with increasing needs for privacy and confidentiality as the child ages. The 6 health behaviors that most significantly impact adolescent and adult morbidity and mortality are inadequate physical activity, poor nutrition, sexuality-related behaviors, substance use and abuse (including tobacco and vaporized nicotine), unintentional injury–related behaviors, and intentional injury–related behaviors. Emotional well-being and early diagnosis and treatment of mental health problems are equally important, with attention to the developmental tasks of adolescence: competence at school and other activities, connection to friends and family, autonomy, empathy, and a sense of self-worth.

OFFICE INTERVENTION FOR BEHAVIORAL AND MENTAL HEALTH ISSUES

One fifth of primary care encounters with children are for a behavioral or mental health problem or sickness visits complicated by a mental health issue. Pediatricians and other primary care clinicians seeing children must have reasonable comfort and knowledge for diagnosis, treatment, and referral criteria for attention-deficit/hyperactivity disorder (see Chapter 49), depression and other mood disorders (Chapter 39), anxiety (Chapter 38), and conduct disorder (Chapter 42), as well as an understanding of the pharmacology of the frequently prescribed psychotropic medications. Familiarity with available local mental health services and clinicians and knowledge of the types of services indicated are important for effective consultation or referral. With new understanding of the impact of lifestyle on mood disorders and anxiety, encouragement of behavioral change to implement regular exercise, a healthy diet, avoidance of substances, and judicious use of media has become an important responsibility of the primary care clinician. **Motivational interviewing** provides a structured approach that has been designed to help patients and parents identify the discrepancy between their desire for health and the outcomes of their current behavioral choices. It also allows the clinician to use proven strategies that lead to a patient-initiated plan for change.

Strength-Based Approaches and Framework

Questions about school or extracurricular accomplishments or competent personal characteristics should be integrated into the content of the well-child visit. Such inquiries set a positive context for the visit, deepen the partnership with the family, acknowledge the child's healthy development, and facilitate discussing social-emotional development with children and their parents. There is a strong relationship between appropriate social-emotional development (e.g., children's strong connection to their family, social friends, and mentors; competence; empathy; appropriate autonomy) and decreased participation in all the risk behaviors of adolescence (related to drugs, sex, and violence). An organized approach to the identification and encouragement of a child's strengths during health supervision visits provides both the child and the parent with an understanding of how to promote healthy achievement of the developmental tasks of childhood and adolescence. It also provides an opportunity to assess and comment on the relational health in the family. CSHCN often have a different timetable, but they have an equal need to be encouraged to develop strong family and peer connections, competence in a variety of arenas, ways to do things for others, and appropriate independent decision-making.

Office System Change for Quality Improvement

To facilitate the effective delivery of preventive services for children and youth, screening schedules and parent handouts, flow sheets, registries, and parent and youth previsit questionnaires are available in *The Bright Futures Guidelines Toolkit*; online previsit tools are under construction. These efforts are part of a larger national effort that is built on a coordinated team approach in the office setting and the use of continuous measurement for improvement.

EVIDENCE

Available evidence should be utilized in developing health-promotion and disease-detection recommendations. Revisions to the AAP Periodicity Schedule undergo rigorous evidence assessment; however, many highly valued well-child care activities have not been evaluated for efficacy. Lack of evidence is most often related to absence of systematic study and does not necessarily mean lack of benefit. Thus the clinical encounter with the well child is also guideline and recommendation driven and requires the integration of clinician goals, family needs, and community realities in seeking better health for the child. The evidence and rationale for recommendations in the Periodicity Schedule (see Fig. 12.1) and *Bright Futures Guidelines* regarding well-child care activities are a balance of evidence from research, clinical practice guidelines, professional recommendations, expert opinion, experience, and knowledge of the needs of the patient population in the context of community assets and challenges. Clinical or counseling decisions and recommendations may also be based on local legislation (e.g., seat belts), on commonsense measures not likely to be studied experimentally (e.g., lowering water heater temperatures, use of car seats), or on the basis of relational evidence (e.g., television watching associated with violent behavior in young children). Most important, sound clinical and counseling decisions are responsive to family needs and desires and support patient-centered decision-making.

CARING FOR THE CHILD AND YOUTH IN THE CONTEXT OF THE FAMILY AND COMMUNITY

A successful primary care practice for children incorporates families, is family centered, and embraces the concept of the medical home. A **medical home** is defined as primary care that is accessible, continuous, comprehensive, family centered, coordinated, compassionate, and culturally effective. In a medical home, a clinician works in partnership with the family and patient to ensure that all medical and nonmedical needs of the child are met. Through this partnership, the child healthcare professional helps the family/patient access and coordinate specialty care, educational services, out-of-home care, family support, and other public and private community services that are important to the overall health of the child and family.

Ideally, health promotion activities occur not only in the medical home, but also through community members and other health and education professionals. To be most effective, communication and coordination around providing accurate, consistent information is key, with a clear understanding of the important role that the community plays in supporting healthy behaviors among families. Communities where children and families feel safe and valued and have access to positive activities and relationships provide the important base that the healthcare professional can build on and refer to for needed services that support health but are outside the realm of the healthcare system or primary care medical home. It is important for the medical home and community agencies to identify mutual resources, communicate well with families and each other, and partner in designing service delivery systems. This interaction is the practice of **community pediatrics**, whose unique feature is its concern for all the population: those who remain well but need preventive services, those who have symptoms but do not receive effective care, and those who do seek medical care in a physician's office or hospital.

Bibliography is available at Expert Consult.

Chapter **13**

Injury Control

Brian D. Johnston and Frederick P. Rivara

第十三章

创伤管理

中文导读

本章首先概述了儿童创伤的死亡率、非致命性伤害和全球性的儿童创伤；而后主要介绍了创伤处理原则、儿童创伤的危险因素、创伤的发生机制以及创伤在社会心理层面造成的后果；具体阐述了年龄、性别、种族和伦理、社会经济地位、城乡结合部和环境等创伤的危险因素；阐述了骑摩托车和自行车受伤、行人受伤、滑雪和滑雪板相关的头部损伤、枪伤、坠落伤，以及暴力行为和攻击性等方式致伤的发生机制。用表格分别呈现了美国2015年0~29岁创伤死亡的原因分类、用于儿科医师宣教的创伤防范要素，以及推荐的儿童约束方法。

In all high-income countries of the world, and increasingly in many low- and middle-income countries, injuries are the most common cause of death during childhood and adolescence beyond the 1st few mo of life (Table 13.1 and Fig. 13.1). Injuries represent one of the most important causes of preventable pediatric morbidity and mortality in the United States. Identification of risk factors for injuries has led to the development of successful programs for prevention and control. Strategies for injury prevention and control should be pursued by the pediatrician in the office, emergency department (ED), hospital, and community setting and should be done in a multidisciplinary, multifaceted way.

Injuries have identifiable risk and protective factors that can be used to define prevention strategies. The term *accidents* implies a chance event occurring without pattern or predictability. In fact, most injuries occur under fairly predictable circumstances to high-risk children and families. *Most injuries are preventable.*

Reduction of morbidity and mortality from injuries can be accomplished not only through *primary* prevention (averting the event or injury), but also through *secondary* and *tertiary* prevention. The latter

Table 13.1	Injury Deaths in the United States, 2015* [N (Rate per 100,000)]					
CAUSE OF DEATH	<1 yr	1-4 yr	5-9 yr	10-14 yr	15-19 yr	0-19 yr
ALL CAUSES	23,161 (583.4)	4045 (25.3)	2490 (12.2)	3013 (14.6)	10,812 (51.2)	43,521 (53.0)
ALL INJURIES	1616 (40.70)	1660 (10.40)	960 (4.70)	1468 (7.12)	8148 (39.03)	13,952 (16.99)
All unintentional	1219 (30.70)	1261 (7.90)	787 (3.85)	847 (4.11)	4152 (19.65)	8266 (10.07)
Motor vehicle occupant	26 (0.65)	80 (0.50)	111 (0.54)	144 (0.70)	748 (3.54)	1109 (1.35)
Pedestrian	12 (0.30)	175 (1.10)	98 (0.48)	117 (0.57)	329 (1.56)	731 (0.89)
Drowning	38 (0.96)	425 (2.66)	147 (0.72)	103 (0.50)	253 (1.20)	966 (1.18)
Fire and burn	13 (0.33)	107 (0.67)	78 (0.38)	52 (0.25)	35 (0.17)	285 (0.35)
Poisoning	9 (0.23)	34 (0.21)	13 (0.06)	28 (0.14)	771 (3.65)	855 (1.04)
Bicycle	0 (0.00)	6 (0.04)	15 (0.07)	38 (0.18)	45 (0.21)	104 (0.13)
Firearm	1 (0.03)	34 (0.21)	16 (0.08)	23 (0.11)	53 (0.25)	127 (0.15)
Fall	7 (0.16)	19 (0.12)	5 (0.02)	14 (0.07)	66 (0.31)	111 (0.14)
Suffocation	1023 (25.77)	118 (0.74)	35 (0.17)	39 (0.19)	43 (0.20)	1258 (1.53)
All intentional	276 (6.95)	339 (2.12)	146 (0.71)	585 (2.84)	3959 (18.74)	5305 (6.46)
Suicide	0 (0.00)	0 (0.00)	7 (0.03)	436 (2.11)	2117 (10.02)	2560 (3.12)
Firearm suicide	0 (0.00)	0 (0.00)	0 (0.00)	160 (0.78)	942 (4.46)	1102 (1.34)
Homicide	276 (6.95)	339 (2.12)	139 (0.68)	147 (0.71)	1816 (8.59)	2717 (3.13)
Firearm homicide	11 (0.28)	64 (0.40)	68 (0.33)	95 (0.46)	1611 (7.62)	1849 (2.25)
Undetermined intent	121 (3.05)	60 (0.38)	27 (0.13)	36 (0.17)	137 (0.65)	381 (0.46)

*Injury data from US Centers for Disease Control and Prevention (CDC): Web-based Injury Statistics Query and Reporting System (WISQARS) (website). National Center for Injury Prevention and Control, CDC (producer). https://www.cdc.gov/injury/wisqars/.
   All-cause data from CDC, National Center for Health Statistics: Compressed Mortality File 1999–2015, Series 20, No 2U, 2016, as compiled from data provided by the 57 vital statistics jurisdictions through the Vital Statistics Cooperative Program, CDC WONDER online database, October 2018.

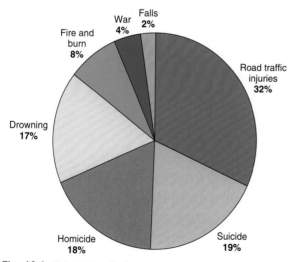

Fig. 13.1 Global injury deaths to children, adolescents, and young adults, 0-29 yr of age, 2012. *(From WHO: Injuries and Violence: The Facts 2012. Geneva: World Health Organization, 2014.)*

2 approaches include appropriate **emergency medical services** (EMS) for injured children; **regionalized trauma care** for the child with multiple injuries, severe burns, or traumatic brain injury; and **specialized pediatric rehabilitation** services that attempt to return children to their previous level of functioning.

Injury control also encompasses *intentional injuries* (assaults and self-inflicted injuries). These injuries are important in adolescents and young adults, and in some populations, these rank 1st or 2nd as causes of death in these age-groups. Many of the same principles of injury control can be applied to these problems; for example, limiting access to firearms may reduce both unintentional shootings, homicides, and suicides.

SCOPE OF THE PROBLEM
Mortality

In the United States, injuries cause 42% of deaths among 1-4 yr old children and 3.5 times more deaths than the next leading cause, congenital anomalies. For the rest of childhood and adolescence up to age 19 yr, 64% of deaths are a result of injuries, more than all other causes combined. In 2016, injuries caused 13,952 deaths (16.78 deaths per 100,000 population) among individuals ≤19 yr old in the United States, resulting in more years of potential life lost than any other cause. **Unintentional injuries** remained the leading cause of death among those <24 yr old in 2016 (see Table 13.1 and Fig. 13.1).

Motor vehicle injuries lead the list of injury deaths among school-age children and adolescents and are the 2nd leading cause of injury death for those age 1-4 yr. In children and adults, motor vehicle *occupant* injuries account for the majority of these deaths. During adolescence, occupant injuries are the leading cause of injury death, accounting for >50% of unintentional trauma mortality in this age-group.

Drowning ranks 2nd overall as a cause of unintentional injury deaths among those age 1-19 yr, with peaks in the preschool and later teenage years (see Chapter 91). In some areas of the United States, drowning is the leading cause of death from trauma for preschool-age children. The causes of drowning deaths vary with age and geographic area. In young children, bathtub and swimming pool drowning predominates, whereas in older children and adolescents, drowning occurs predominantly in natural bodies of water while the victim is swimming or boating.

Fire- and burn-related deaths account for 3% of all unintentional trauma deaths, with the highest rates among those <5 yr of age (see Chapter 92). Most deaths are a result of house fires and are caused by smoke inhalation or asphyxiation rather than severe burns. Children and elderly persons are at greatest risk for these deaths because of difficulty in escaping from burning buildings.

Suffocation accounts for approximately 87% of all unintentional deaths in children <1 yr old. Some cases result from choking on food items, such as hot dogs, candy, grapes, and nuts. Nonfood items that can cause choking include undersize infant pacifiers, small balls, and latex balloons. An increasing number of infant suffocation deaths represent sleep-related mortality in the presence of unsafe bedding, crib bumpers, or cosleeping with an impaired adult. In previous years these might have been classified as sudden infant death syndrome (see Chapter 402).

Homicide is the 3rd leading cause of injury death in children 1-4 yr old and the 3rd leading cause of injury death in adolescents (15-19 yr old) (Fig. 13.2). Homicide in the pediatric age-group falls into 2 patterns: infant (child) and adolescent. Child homicide involves children <5 yr old and represents child abuse (see Chapter 16). The perpetrator is usually a caretaker; death is generally the result of blunt trauma to the head and/or abdomen. The adolescent pattern of homicide involves peers and acquaintances and is caused by firearms in 88% of cases. The majority of these deaths involve handguns. Children between these 2 age-groups experience homicides of both types.

Suicide is rare in children <10 yr old; only 1% of all suicides occur in children <15 yr. The suicide rate increases greatly after age 10 yr, with the result that suicide is now the 2nd leading cause of death for 15-19 yr olds. Native American teenagers are at the highest risk, followed by white males; black females have the lowest rate of suicide in this age-group. Approximately 40% of teenage suicides involve firearms (see Chapter 40).

There has been a sharp and substantial increase in unintentional **poisoning** deaths among teens and young adults. In 2016, unintentional poisonings were the 2nd leading cause of injury deaths among 15-24 yr olds. Many of these were from prescription analgesic and opioid medications such as fentanyl.

Nonfatal Injuries

Most childhood injuries do not result in death. Approximately 12% of children and adolescents receive medical care for an injury each year in hospital EDs, and at least as many are treated in physicians' offices. Of these, 2% require inpatient care, and 55% have at least short-term temporary disability as a result of their injuries.

The distribution of nonfatal injuries is very different from that of fatal trauma (Fig. 13.3). **Falls** are the leading cause of both ED visits and hospitalizations. **Bicycle-related trauma** is the most common type of sports and recreational injury, accounting for approximately 300,000 ED visits annually. **Nonfatal injuries**, such as anoxic encephalopathy from near-drowning, scarring and disfigurement from burns, and persistent neurologic deficits from head injury, may be associated with severe morbidity, leading to substantial changes in the quality of life for victims and their families. In 2010, nonfatal injuries to U.S. children <19 yr old resulted in >$32 billion in direct medical and lifetime work loss costs.

Global Child Injuries

Child injuries are a global public health issue, and prevention efforts are necessary in low-, middle-, and high-income countries. Between 1990 and 2010 there was a 53% decrease in mortality of people of all ages from communicable, maternal, neonatal, and nutritional disorders, while injury mortality decreased by only 16% (Fig. 13.4).

Worldwide, almost 1 million children and adolescents die from injuries and violence each year, and >90% of these deaths are in low- and middle-income countries. As child mortality undergoes an epidemiologic transition because of better control of infectious diseases and malnutrition, injuries have and will increasingly become the leading cause of death for children in the developing world, as it now is in all industrialized countries. Drowning is the 5th most common cause of death for 5-9 yr

old children globally, and in some countries, such as Bangladesh, it is the leading cause of death among children beyond the 1st yr of life, with a rate 22 times greater than that in the Americas. An estimated 1 billion people do not currently have immediate access to roads; as industrialization and motorization spreads, the incidence of motor vehicle crashes, injuries, and fatalities will climb. The rate of child injury death in low- and middle-income countries is 3-fold higher than that in high-income countries and reflects both a higher incidence of many types of injuries and a much higher case fatality rate in those injured because of a lack of access to emergency and surgical care. As in high-income countries, prevention of child injuries and consequent morbidity and mortality is feasible with multifaceted approaches, many of which are low cost and of proven effectiveness.

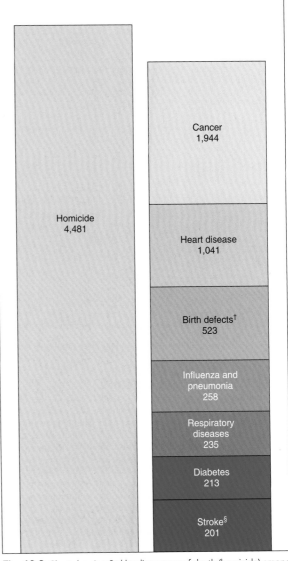

Fig. 13.2 Chart showing 3rd leading cause of death (homicide) among persons age 10-24 yr compared with 4th through 10th leading causes of death in the same age-group in the United States in 2013. *Does not include the 2 leading causes of death among persons age 10-24 yr in 2013: unintentional injuries (12,394 deaths) and suicide (5,264); [†]congenital anomalies; [§]cerebrovascular diseases. *(From David-Ferdon C, Simon TR, Spivak H, et al: CDC grand rounds: preventing youth violence, MMWR 64(7):172, 2015.)*

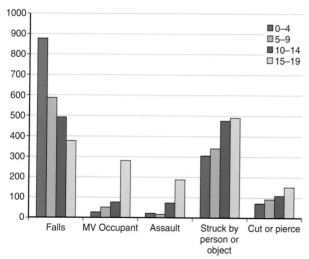

Fig. 13.3 Emergency department visits for injuries, United States 2016. *(Data from NEISS All Injury Program operated by the Consumer Product Safety Commission for numbers of injuries. U.S. Bureau of Census for population estimates.)*

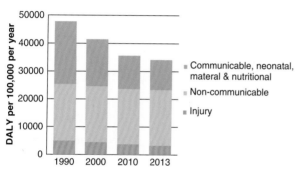

Fig. 13.4 Rates of disability-adjusted life-years (DALYs) loss per 100,000 per year by major grouping of cause. *(Data from Institute for Health Metrics and Evaluation; GBD data visualization site. From Johnston BD: A safer world, Injury Prev 22(1):1–2, 2016.)*

PRINCIPLES OF INJURY CONTROL

Injury prevention once centered on attempts to pinpoint the innate characteristics of a child that result in greater frequency of injury. Most discount the theory of the "accident-prone child." Although longitudinal studies have demonstrated an association between attention-deficit/hyperactivity disorder (ADHD) and increased rates of injury, the sensitivity and specificity of these traits as a test to identify individuals at high risk for injury are extremely low. The concept of *accident proneness* is counterproductive in that it shifts attention away from potentially more modifiable factors, such as product design or the environment. It is more appropriate to examine the physical and social environment of children with frequent rates of injury than to try to identify particular personality traits or temperaments, which are difficult to modify. Children at high risk for injury are likely to be relatively poorly supervised, to have disorganized or stressed families, and to live in hazardous environments.

Efforts to control injuries include education or persuasion, changes in product design, and modification of the social and physical environment. Efforts to persuade individuals, particularly parents, to change their behaviors have constituted the greater part of injury control efforts. Speaking with parents specifically about using child car-seat restraints and bicycle helmets, installing smoke detectors, and checking the tap water temperature is likely to be more successful than offering

well-meaning but too-general advice about supervising the child closely, being careful, and childproofing the home. This information should be geared to the developmental stage of the child and presented in moderate doses in the form of anticipatory guidance at well-child visits. Table 13.2 lists important topics to discuss at each developmental stage. It is important to acknowledge that there are many barriers to prevention adherence beyond simple knowledge acquisition; pediatricians should be familiar with low-cost sources for safety equipment such as bicycle helmets, smoke detectors, trigger locks, and car seats in their community.

The most successful injury prevention strategies generally are those involving **changes in product design**. These passive interventions protect all individuals in the population, regardless of cooperation or level of skill, and are likely to be more successful than active measures that require repeated behavior change by the parent or child. The most important and effective product changes have been in motor vehicles, in which protection of the passenger compartment and use of airbags have had large effects on injury risk. Turning down the water heater temperature, installing smoke detectors, and using child-resistant caps on medicines and household products are other examples of effective product modifications. Many interventions require both active and passive measures. Smoke detectors provide passive protection when fully functional, but behavior change is required to ensure periodic battery changes and proper testing.

Modification of the environment often requires greater changes than individual product modification but may be very effective in reducing injuries. Safe roadway design, decreased traffic volume and speed limits in neighborhoods, and elimination or safe storage of guns in households are examples of such interventions. Included in this concept are changes in the social environment through legislation, such as laws mandating child seat restraint and seatbelt use, bicycle helmet use, and graduated driver's licensing laws.

Prevention campaigns combining 2 or more of these approaches have been particularly effective in reducing injuries. The classic example is the combination of legislation/regulation and education to increase child seat restraint and seatbelt use; other examples are programs to promote bike helmet use among school-aged children and improvements in occupant protection in motor vehicles.

RISK FACTORS FOR CHILDHOOD INJURIES

Major factors associated with an increased risk of injuries to children include age, sex, race and ethnicity, socioeconomic status, rural-urban location, and the environment.

Age

Toddlers are at the greatest risk for burns, drowning, and falling. Poisonings become another risk as these children acquire mobility and exploratory behavior. Young school-age children are at greatest risk for pedestrian injuries, bicycle-related injuries (the most serious of which usually involve motor vehicles), motor vehicle occupant injuries, burns, and drowning. During the teenage years, there is a greatly increased risk from motor vehicle occupant trauma, a continued risk from drowning and burns, and the new risk of intentional trauma. Sports- and recreation-related injuries, including concussion, become more common, and more serious, as children age. Work-related injuries associated with child labor, especially for 14-16 yr olds, are an additional risk.

Injuries occurring at a particular age represent a period of vulnerability during which a child or an adolescent encounters a new task or hazard that they may not have the developmental skills to handle successfully. Toddlers do not have the judgment to know that medications can be poisonous or that some houseplants are not to be eaten; they do not understand the hazard presented by a swimming pool or an open second-story window. For young children, parents may inadvertently set up this mismatch between the skills of the child and the demands of the task. Many parents expect young school-age children to walk home from school, the playground, or the local convenience store, tasks for which most children are not developmentally ready. Likewise, the lack of skills and experience to handle many tasks during the teenage years contributes to an increased risk of injuries, particularly motor

| Table 13.2 | Injury Prevention Topics for Anticipatory Guidance by the Pediatrician |

NEWBORN
Car seats
Tap water temperature
Smoke detectors
Sleep safe environments

INFANT
Car seats
Tap water temperature
Bath safety
Choking prevention

TODDLER AND PRESCHOOLER
Car seats and booster seats
Water safety
Poison prevention
Fall prevention

PRIMARY SCHOOL CHILD
Pedestrian skills training
Water skills training
Booster seats and seat belts
Bicycle helmets
Safe storage of firearms in the home

MIDDLE SCHOOL CHILD
Seatbelts
Safe storage of firearms in the home
Water skills training
Sports safety and concussion prevention

HIGH SCHOOL AND OLDER ADOLESCENT
Seatbelts
Alcohol and drug use, especially while driving and swimming
Mobile phone use while driving
Safe storage of firearms
Sports safety and concussion prevention
Occupational injuries

vehicle injuries. The high rate of motor vehicle crashes among 15-17 yr olds is caused in part by inexperience but also appears to reflect their level of cognitive development and emotional maturity. Alcohol, other drugs, and mobile phone use substantially add to these limitations.

Age also influences the severity of injury and the risk of long-term disability. Young school-age children have an incompletely developed pelvis. In a motor vehicle crash the seatbelt does not anchor onto the pelvis, but rides up onto the abdomen, resulting in the risk of serious abdominal injury. Proper restraint for 4-8 yr old children requires the use of booster seats. Children <2 yr old have much poorer outcomes from traumatic brain injuries than older children and adolescents, partly related to the severity of abusive head trauma.

Gender
Beginning at 1-2 yr of age and continuing throughout the life span, males have higher rates of fatal injury than females. During childhood, this does *not* appear to be primarily a result of developmental differences between the sexes, differences in coordination, or differences in muscle strength. Variation in *exposure* to risk may account for the male predominance in some types of injuries. Although males in all age-groups have higher rates of bicycle-related injuries, adjusting for exposure reduces this excess rate. Sex differences in rates of pedestrian injuries do *not* appear to be caused by differences in the amount of walking, but rather reflect differences in *behavior* between young females and males; whether these are genetic or the result of gender socialization is uncertain. Greater risk-taking behavior, combined with greater frequency of alcohol use, may lead to the disproportionately high rate of

motor vehicle crashes among teenage males. The rate of violence-related injuries is higher among males because of their risk-taking behavior.

Race and Ethnicity
In the United States, Native Americans have the highest death rate from unintentional injuries, reflecting both the increased incidence and the poorer access to trauma care because of their rural location. African American children and adolescents have higher rates of fatal injuries than whites, whereas Asians have lower rates; rates for Hispanic children and adolescents are intermediate between those for blacks and those for whites. These discrepancies are even more pronounced for some injuries. The homicide rate for African Americans age 15-19 yr was 32.74 per 100,000 population in 2016, compared with 5.59/100,000 for American Indians and Alaskan Natives and 3.91/100,000 for whites and 2.18/100,000 for Asians. The suicide rate for Native American youth was 1.5 times the rate for whites and 2.7 times rates for blacks. The rate of firearm homicide deaths for African American youth ages 15-19 is 10-fold higher than that for whites and 17 times that of Asian American youth.

These disparities appear to be primarily related to poverty, the educational status of parents, and the presence of hazardous environments. Homicide rates among blacks are nearly equivalent to those among whites, when adjusted for socioeconomic status. *It is important to acknowledge racial disparities in injury rates and the importance of racism at all levels in society, but inappropriate to ascribe the etiology of these differences solely to the effect of race or ethnicity.*

Socioeconomic Status
Poverty is one of the most important risk factors for childhood injury. Mortality from fires, motor vehicle crashes, and drowning is 2-4 times higher in poor children. Death rates among both blacks and whites have an inverse relationship to income level: the higher the income level, the lower the death rate. Native Americans have especially high mortality rates. Other factors are single-parent families, teenage mothers, multiple care providers, family stress, and multiple siblings; these are primarily a function of poverty rather than independent risk factors.

Rural-Urban Location
Injury rates are generally higher in rural than in urban areas. Homicide rates are higher in urban areas, as is violent crime in general. However, suicide among adolescents is higher in rural than urban areas. Case fatality from injury is generally twice as high in rural areas than in urban areas, reflecting both the increased severity of some injuries (e.g., motor vehicle crashes occurring at higher speeds) and poorer access to EMS and definitive trauma care in rural areas. Some injuries are unique to rural areas, such as agricultural injuries to children and adolescents.

Environment
Poverty increases the risk of injury to children, at least in part through its effect on the environment. Children who are poor are at increased risk for injury because they are exposed to more hazards in their living environments. They may live in poor housing, which is more likely to be dilapidated and less likely to be protected by smoke detectors. The roads in their neighborhoods are more likely to be major thoroughfares. Their neighborhoods are more likely to experience higher levels of violence, and they are more likely to be victims of assault than children and adolescents living in the suburbs. The focus on the environment is also important because it directs attention away from relatively immutable factors, such as family dynamics, poverty, and race, and directs efforts toward factors that can be changed through interventions.

MECHANISMS OF INJURY
Motor Vehicle Injuries
Motor vehicle injuries are the leading cause of serious and fatal injuries for children and adolescents. Large and sustained reductions in motor vehicle crash injuries can be accomplished by identifiable interventions.

Occupants
Injuries to passenger vehicle occupants are the predominant cause of motor vehicle deaths among children and adolescents. The peak injury

Table 13.3	Recommended Child-Restraint Methods		
	INFANTS	**TODDLERS (1-3)**	**YOUNG CHILDREN**
Recommended age/weight requirements	Birth to 1 yr or below weight limit of seat.	Older than 1 yr and weight 20-40 lb.	Weight 40-80 lb and height under 4 ft 9 in; generally between 4 and 8 yr of age.
Type of seat	Infant-only or rear-facing convertible.	Convertible or forward-facing harness seat.	Belt-positioning booster seat.
Seat position	Rear-facing only. Place in back seat of vehicle.	Can be rear-facing until 30 lb if seat allows; generally forward-facing. Place in back seat of vehicle.	Forward-facing. Place in back seat of vehicle.
Notes	Children should use rear-facing seat until at least 1 yr and at least 20 lb.	Harness straps should be at or above shoulder level.	Belt-positioning booster seats must be used with both lap and shoulder belts.
	Harness straps should be at or below shoulder level.	Most seats require top strap for forward-facing use.	Make sure that lap belt fits low and tightly across lap/upper thigh area, and that shoulder belt fits snugly, crossing chest and shoulder to avoid abdominal injuries.

Data from http://www.safercar.gov/parents/CarSeats.htm.

and death rate for both males and females in the pediatric age-group occurs between 15 and 19 yr (see Table 13.1). Proper restraint use in vehicles is the single most effective method for preventing serious or fatal injury. Table 13.3 shows the recommended restraints at different ages. Fig. 13.5 provides examples of car safety seats.

Much attention has been given to child occupants <8 yr old. Use of child-restraint devices, infant car seats, and booster seats can be expected to reduce fatalities by 71% and the risk of serious injuries by 67% in this age-group. All 50 states and the District of Columbia have laws mandating their use, although the upper age limit for booster seat requirements varies by state. Physician reinforcement of the positive benefits of child seat restraints has been successful in improving parent acceptance. Pediatricians should point out to parents that toddlers who normally ride restrained behave better during car trips than children who ride unrestrained.

A detailed guide and list of acceptable devices is available from the American Academy of Pediatrics (AAP)* and the National Highway Traffic Safety Administration (NHTSA).† Children weighing <20 lb may use an infant seat or may be placed in a convertible infant-toddler child-restraint device. Infants and toddlers <4 yr should be placed in the rear seat facing backward; older toddlers and young children can be placed in the rear seat in a forward-facing child harness seat until it is outgrown. Emphasis must be placed on the correct use of these seats, including placing the seat in the right direction, routing the belt properly, and ensuring that the child is buckled into the seat correctly. Government regulations specific to automobile and product design have made the fit between car seats and the car easier, quicker, and less prone to error. *Children <13 yr old should never sit in the front seat. Inflating airbags can be lethal to infants in rear-facing seats and to small children in the front passenger seat.*

Older children are often not adequately restrained. Many children ride in the rear seat restrained with lap belts only. **Booster seats** have been shown to decrease the risk of injury by 59% and should be used by children who weigh between 40 lb (about 4 yr of age) and 80 lb, are <8 yr of age, and are <4 ft 9 in (145 cm) tall. Many states have extended their car seat laws to include children of booster seat age as well. Shoulder straps placed behind the child or under the arm do not provide adequate crash protection and may increase the risk of serious injury. The use of lap belts alone has been associated with an increased risk of seatbelt-related injuries, especially fractures of the lumbar spine and hollow-viscus injuries of the abdomen. These flexion-distraction injuries of the spine are often accompanied by injuries to the abdominal organs.

The rear seat is clearly much safer than the front seat for both children and adults. One study of children <15 yr old found that the risk of injury in a crash was 70% lower for children in the rear seat compared with those sitting in the front seat. Frontal **airbags** present a risk of serious or fatal injury from the airbag itself for children <13 yr. Side airbags also pose a risk for children who are in the front seat and are leaning against the door at the time of a crash. The safest place for children is in the rear middle seat, properly restrained for their age and size. Educational and legislative interventions to increase the number of children traveling in the rear seat have been successful.

Transportation of **premature infants** presents special problems. The possibility of oxygen desaturation, sometimes associated with bradycardia, among premature infants while in child seat restraints has led the AAP to recommend an observed trial of infants born at <37 wk of gestational age in the seat before discharge and the use of oxygen or alternative restraints for infants who experience desaturation or bradycardia, such as seats that can be reclined and used as a car bed.

Children riding in the rear bed of pickup trucks are at special risk for injury because of the possibility of ejection from the truck and resultant serious injury.

Teenage Drivers

Drivers 15-17 yr old have more than twice the rate of collisions compared with motorists 18 yr and older. Formal driver education courses for young drivers appear to be ineffective as a primary means of decreasing the number of collisions, and in fact may increase risk by allowing younger teens to drive. The risk of serious injury and mortality is directly related to the speed at the time of the crash and inversely related to the size of the vehicle. Small, fast cars greatly increase the risk of a fatal outcome in the event of a crash.

The number of passengers traveling with teen drivers influences the risk of a crash. The risk of death for 17 yr old drivers is 50% greater when driving with 1 passenger compared with driving alone; this risk is 2.6-fold higher with 2 passengers and 3-fold higher with 3 or more passengers.

Teens driving at night are overrepresented in crashes and fatal crashes, with nighttime crashes accounting for >33% of teen motor vehicle fatalities. Almost 50% of fatal crashes involving drivers <18 yr old occur in the 4 hours before or after midnight. Teens are 5-10 times more likely to be in a fatal crash while driving at night compared with driving during the day. The difficulty of driving at night combined with the inexperience of teen drivers appears to be a deadly combination.

Another risk factor for motor vehicle crashes for people of all ages, including teens, is **distracted driving**. Distracting events can include *visual* distraction (taking eyes from the forward roadway), *manual* distraction (removing hands from vehicle controls), or *cognitive* distraction (taking attention from navigating the vehicle or responding to critical events). **Electronic devices** present all 3 modes of distraction

---

*http://www.healthychildren.org/english/safety-prevention/on-the-go/pages/car-safety-seats-information-for-families.aspx.
†https://www.nhtsa.gov/equipment/car-seats-and-booster-seats.

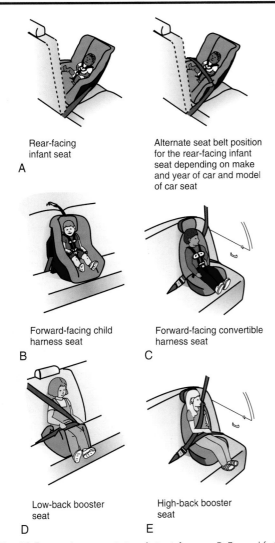

Rear-facing infant seat

A

Alternate seat belt position for the rear-facing infant seat depending on make and year of car and model of car seat

Forward-facing child harness seat

B

Forward-facing convertible harness seat

C

Low-back booster seat

D

High-back booster seat

E

Fig. 13.5 Car safety seats. **A,** Rear-facing infant seat. **B,** Forward-facing child harness seat. **C,** Forward-facing convertible harness seat. **D,** Low-back booster seat. **E,** High-back booster seat. *(From Ebel BE, Grossman DC: Crash proof kids? An overview of current motor vehicle child occupant safety strategies,* Curr Probl Pediatr Adolesc Health Care *33:33–64, 2003. Source: NHTSA.)*

in combination and are increasingly recognized as a major threat to driver safety, especially among teens. The uptick in motor vehicle fatality rates per vehicle mile driven is generally believed to be caused by distracted driving.

In 2017, 39.2% of teen drivers reported they had texted or emailed while driving in the last 30 days. Dialing on a cell phone increases the risk of a crash almost 3-fold, and texting may increase the risk as much as 6-fold. Although most states have banned text messaging for all drivers, the effect of state laws on prohibiting such behavior while driving is unknown. Parents should set limits on the use of these devices by their teens; technologic interventions that can block cell phone signals in a moving vehicle are also be available and should be considered by parents for their teens.

Graduated driver's licensing (GDL) programs consist of a series of steps over a designated period before a teen can receive full, unrestricted driving privileges. In a 3-stage graduated license, the student driver must first pass vision and knowledge-based tests, followed by obtaining a learner's permit, and once a specific age has been achieved and driving

skills advanced, the student driver is eligible to take the driving test. Once given a provisional license, the new driver will have a specified time to do low-risk driving. GDL usually places initial restrictions on the number of passengers (especially teenage) allowed in the vehicle and limits driving at night. The number of crashes decreased 10–30% among the youngest drivers in states with a GDL system. The characteristics of GDL programs vary substantially across states. Optimal safety benefits depend on parent monitoring and engagement with teens around driving restrictions and responsibilities. Parent-teen driving contracts are available and help to facilitate these discussions.

Alcohol use is a major cause of motor vehicle trauma among adolescents. The combination of inexperience in driving and inexperience with alcohol is particularly dangerous. Approximately 20% of all deaths from motor vehicle crashes in this age-group are the result of alcohol intoxication, with impairment of driving seen at blood alcohol concentrations (BACs) as low as 0.05 g/dL. In 2017, approximately 16.5% of adolescents reported riding with a driver who had been drinking, and 5.5% reported driving after drinking. All states have adopted a *zero tolerance policy* to adolescent drinking while driving, which defines any measurable alcohol content as legal intoxication. All adolescent motor vehicle injury victims should have their BAC measured in the ED and should be screened for high-risk alcohol use with a validated screening test (e.g., CRAFFT, Alcohol Use Disorders Identification Test [AUDIT]) to identify those with alcohol abuse problems (see Chapter 140.1). Individuals who have evidence of alcohol abuse should not leave the ED or hospital without plans for appropriate alcohol abuse treatment. Interventions for problem drinking can be effective in decreasing the risk of subsequent motor vehicle crashes. Even brief interventions in the ED using motivational interviewing can be successful in decreasing adolescent problem drinking.

Another cause of impaired driving is **marijuana use**. In 2017, nearly 20% of high school students reported using marijuana in the prior 30 days. Marijuana is currently legal (2018) for adult use in 9 U.S. states and for medical use in 30 states, while being considered in many others; the effects of this on adolescent injury remains to be determined. Marijuana is often co-ingested with alcohol or other drugs, and blood thresholds for biologic impairment have not been standardized. It is therefore difficult to estimate the independent effect of marijuana on crash risk.

All-Terrain Vehicles

All-terrain vehicles (ATVs) in many parts of the United States are an important cause of injuries to children and adolescents. These vehicles can attain high speeds, especially with low-weight children, and are prone to rollover because of their high center of gravity. Orthopedic and head injuries are the most common serious injuries seen among children involved in ATV crashes. Helmets can significantly decrease the risk and severity of head injuries among ATV riders, but current use is very low. Voluntary industry efforts to decrease the risk of injuries appear to have had little effect in making ATVs safer. The AAP recommends that children <16 yr old should not ride on ATVs.

Bicycle Injuries

Each year in the United States, approximately 161,000 children and adolescents are treated in EDs for bicycle-related injuries, making this one of the most common reasons that children with trauma visit EDs. The majority of severe and fatal bicycle injuries involve **head trauma**. A logical step in the prevention of these head injuries is the use of helmets. **Helmets** are very effective, reducing the risk of all head injury by 85% and the risk of traumatic brain injury by 88%. Helmets also reduce injuries to the mid and upper face by as much as 65%. Pediatricians can be effective advocates for the use of bicycle helmets and should incorporate this advice into their anticipatory guidance schedules for parents and children. Appropriate helmets are those with a firm polystyrene liner that fit properly on the child's head. Parents should avoid buying a larger helmet to give the child "growing room."

Promotion of helmet use can and should be extended beyond the pediatrician's office. Community education programs spearheaded by coalitions of physicians, educators, bicycle clubs, and community service organizations have been successful in promoting the use of bicycle helmets to children across the socioeconomic spectrum, resulting in helmet use rates of ≥70% with a concomitant reduction in the number of head injuries. Passage of bicycle helmet laws also leads to increased helmet use.

Consideration should also be given to other types of preventive activities, although the evidence supporting their effectiveness is limited. Bicycle paths are a logical method for separating bicycles and motor vehicles.

Pedestrian Injuries

Pedestrian injuries are a major cause of traumatic death for children and adolescents in the United States and in most high-income countries. In low-income countries, a much higher proportion of road traffic fatalities are pedestrians, especially among 5-14 yr olds. Although case fatality rates are <5%, serious nonfatal injuries constitute a much larger problem, resulting in 34,498 ED visits annually for children and adolescents. Pedestrian injuries are the most important cause of traumatic coma in children and a frequent cause of serious lower-extremity fractures, particularly in school-age children.

Most injuries occur during the day, with a peak in the after-school period. Improved lighting or reflective clothing would be expected to prevent few injuries. Surprisingly, approximately 30% of pedestrian injuries occur while the individual is in a marked crosswalk, perhaps reflecting a false sense of security and decreased vigilance in these areas. The risk of pedestrian injury is greater in neighborhoods with high traffic volumes, speeds >25 miles/hr, absence of play space adjacent to the home, household crowding, and low socioeconomic status.

One important risk factor for childhood pedestrian injuries is the developmental level of the child. Children <5 yr old are at risk for being run over in the driveway. Few children <9 or 10 yr of age have the developmental skills to successfully negotiate traffic 100% of the time. Young children have poor ability to judge the distance and speed of traffic and are easily distracted by playmates or other factors in the environment. Many parents are not aware of this potential mismatch between the abilities of the young school-age child and the skills needed to cross streets safely. The use of mobile phones and devices has become increasingly common while walking and can increase the risk of being struck by a motor vehicle.

Prevention of pedestrian injuries is difficult but should consist of a multifaceted approach. Education of the child in pedestrian safety should be initiated at an early age by the parents and continue into the school-age years. Younger children should be taught never to cross streets when alone; older children should be taught (and practice how) to negotiate quiet streets with little traffic. Major streets should not be crossed alone until the child is at least 10 yr of age and has been observed to follow safe practices.

Legislation and police enforcement are important components of any campaign to reduce pedestrian injuries. Right-turn-on-red laws increase the hazard to pedestrians. In many cities, few drivers stop for pedestrians in crosswalks, a special hazard for young children. Engineering changes in roadway design are extremely important as passive prevention measures. Most important are measures to slow the speed of traffic and to route traffic away from schools and residential areas; these efforts are endorsed by parents and can decrease the risk of injuries and death by 10–35%. Other modifications include networks of 1-way streets, proper placement of transit or school bus stops, sidewalks in urban and suburban areas, stripping in rural areas to delineate the edge of the road, and curb parking regulations. Comprehensive traffic "calming" schemes using these strategies have been very successful in reducing child pedestrian injuries in Sweden, The Netherlands, Germany, and increasingly, the United States.

Ski- and Snowboard-Related Head Injuries

The increasing use of helmets in snow sports, such as skiing and snowboarding, is encouraging since head injuries are the most common cause of death in these sports, and helmets reduce the risk of head injury by ≥50%. Use of helmets does not result in skiers or snow boarders taking more risks and should be encouraged in all snow sports at all ages, not just for young children.

Fire- and Burn-Related Injuries

See Chapter 92.

Poisoning
See Chapter 77.

Drowning
See Chapter 91.

Traumatic Brain Injury
See Chapter 85.

Firearm Injuries

Injuries to children and adolescents involving firearms occur in 3 different situations: unintentional injury, suicide attempt, and assault. The injury may be fatal or may result in permanent sequelae. **Unintentional firearm injuries** and deaths have continued to decrease and accounted for 127 deaths in 2016, representing only a very small fraction of all firearm injuries among children and adolescents. The majority of these deaths occur to teens during hunting or recreational activities. **Suicide** is the 2nd most common cause of death from all causes in both males and females age 10-19 yr. During the 1950s to 1970, suicide rates for children and adolescents more than doubled; firearm suicide rates peaked in 1994 and decreased by 59% from this peak by 2010 before gradually increasing, paralleling increases in the overall suicide rate. The difference in the rate of suicide death between males and females is related to the differences in method used during attempts. Girls die less often in suicide attempts because they use less lethal means (mainly drugs) and perhaps have a lower degree of intent. The use of firearms in a suicidal act confers an approximately 90% case fatality rate.

Homicides are 3rd only to motor vehicle crashes and suicide among causes of death in teenagers >15 yr old. In 2016, 1816 adolescents age 15-19 yr were homicide victims; African American teenagers accounted for 63% of the total, making homicides the most common cause of death among black teenagers. Over 85% of homicides among teenage males involved firearms, mostly handguns.

In the United States, approximately 36% of households owned guns in 2016. Handguns account for approximately 30% of the firearms in use today, yet they are involved in 80% of criminal and other firearm misuse. Home ownership of guns increases the risk of adolescent suicide 3- to 10-fold and the risk of adolescent homicide up to 4-fold. In homes with guns, the risk to the occupants is far greater than the chance that the gun will be used against an intruder; for every death occurring in self-defense, there may be 1.3 unintentional deaths, 4.6 homicides, and 37 suicides.

Of all firearms, **handguns** pose the greatest risk to children and adolescents. Access to handguns by adolescents is surprisingly common and is not restricted to those involved in gang or criminal activity. Stricter approaches to reduce youth access to handguns, rather than all firearms, would appear to be the most appropriate focus of efforts to reduce shooting injuries in children and adolescents.

Locking and unloading guns as well as storing ammunition locked in a different location substantially reduces the risk of a suicide or unintentional firearm injury among youth by up to 73%. Because up to 30% of handgun-owning households have at least 1 firearm stored unsafely, one potential approach to reducing these injuries could focus on improving household firearm storage practices where children and youth reside or visit. The evidence regarding the effectiveness of office-based counseling to influence firearm storage practice is mixed; the most effective programs are those in which devices are dispensed along with advice.

Adolescents with mental health conditions and alcoholism are at particularly high risk for firearm injury. In the absence of conclusive evidence, physicians should continue to work with families to eliminate access to guns in these households.

Falls

Falls are the leading cause of **nonfatal injury** in children and adolescents. Altogether, there were 2.3 million falls that led to ED visits in 2016 for children and adolescents; approximately 2.9% of these visits led to a hospitalization or transfer. There have been relatively few in-depth analytic studies of falls, except in particular circumstances, such as playground injuries. Strategies to prevent falls depend on the environmental circumstances and social context in which they occur. *Window falls* have been successfully prevented with the use of devices that prevent egress, and injuries from *playground falls* can be mitigated through the use of proper surfacing, such as woodchips or other soft, energy-absorbing materials. Alcohol may also contribute to falls among teenagers, and these injuries can be reduced by general strategies to reduce teen alcohol use.

Violent Behavior and Aggression

Although the current rates of homicide are much lower than at their peak in the late 1980s and early 1990s, the problem of violence and assault remains large. The origins of adult and teen violence occur during childhood. Almost all adults who commit violent acts have a history of violent behavior during childhood or adolescence. Longitudinal studies following groups of individuals from birth have found that aggression occurs early and that most children learn to control this aggression in childhood. Children who later become violent adolescents and adults do not learn to control this aggressive behavior.

The most successful interventions for violence target young children and their families. These include home visits by nurses and paraprofessionals beginning in the prenatal period and continuing for the 1st few yr of life to provide support and guidance to parents, especially parents without other resources. Enrollment in early childhood education programs (e.g., Head Start) beginning at age 3 yr has been shown to be effective in improving school success, keeping children in school, and decreasing the chance that the child will be a delinquent adolescent. School-based interventions, including curricula to increase the social skills of children and improve the parenting skills of caregivers, have long-term effects on violence and risk-taking behavior. Early identification of behavior problems by primary care pediatricians can best be accomplished through the routine use of formal screening tools. Interventions in adolescence, such as family therapy, multisystemic therapy, and therapeutic foster care, can decrease problem behavior and a subsequent decline into delinquency and violence.

PSYCHOSOCIAL CONSEQUENCES OF INJURIES

Many children and their parents have substantial psychosocial sequelae from trauma. Studies in adults indicate that 10–40% of hospitalized injured patients will have **posttraumatic stress disorder** (PTSD; see Chapter 38). Among injured children involved in motor vehicle crashes, 90% of families will have symptoms of acute stress disorder after the crash, although the diagnosis of acute stress disorder is poorly predictive of later PTSD. Standardized questionnaires that collect data from the child, the parents, and the medical record at the time of initial injury can serve as useful screening tests for later development of PTSD. Early mental health intervention, with close follow-up, is important for the treatment of PTSD and for minimizing its effect on the child and family.

Bibliography is available at Expert Consult.

Chapter **14**

Impact of Violence on Children

Marilyn C. Augustyn and Barry S. Zuckerman

第十四章

暴力对儿童的影响

中文导读

　　本章主要介绍了针对暴力结果的诊断和随访。具体阐述了恐吓、网络欺凌和校园暴力，其中涉及这三类暴力的不良后果和术语、分布流行情况、危险因素，以及在治疗和预防方面如何辨别症状体征，如何进行对恐吓的筛查等；还阐述了媒介暴力，其中涉及对媒介的甄别筛选和推荐介绍等；最后阐述了战争对儿童的影响，涉及战时儿童的脆弱、战争的心理冲击、努力保护儿童免受战争影响的国际公约和人道主义举措，以及儿科医师和相关卫生专业人员的作用。

The reach of violence, whether as the victim, perpetrator, or witness, whether in person or through the media, is far, deep, and long-standing across the globe. In the home, it is estimated that 80–95% of such aggression is witnessed by a child. *Exposure to violence* disrupts the healthy development of children in a myriad of ways. Pediatric clinicians must be competent to address these issues in impacted children and families under their care (**trauma-informed care**). Clinicians also have a wider responsibility to advocate on local, state, national, and international levels for safer environments in which all children can grow and thrive.

Witnessing violence is detrimental to children. Because their scars as bystanders are emotional and not physical, the pediatric clinician may not fully appreciate their distress and thereby miss an opportunity to provide needed interventions. For children not living in war zones, the source of first exposure to violence is often **intimate partner violence (IPV)**. In the United States alone, >1 in 15 children witness IPV each year, and worldwide approximately 275 million children are exposed to IPV yearly. Exposure to IPV in infancy and toddlerhood impacts attachment relationships, and school-age children who witness IPV have difficulties in developing and maintaining friendships, as well as an increased likelihood of developing maladaptive peer relations.

Another source of witnessed violence is **community violence**, a serious problem in the United States that disproportionately affects children from low-income areas. Approximately 22% of children witness violence in their family or in their community each year; *witnessed violence* includes assaults and bullying, sexual victimization, maltreatment by a caregiver, and theft or vandalism. Almost 60% of children will experience or witness violence during childhood. Witnessing acts of violence may be a significant stressor in children's lives. Witnessed community violence is related to internalizing problems such as depression and posttraumatic stress disorder (PTSD) as well as externalizing problems, including delinquent behavior, aggression, and substance abuse.

The most ubiquitous source of witnessing violence for U.S. children is **media violence**, sometimes referred to as **virtual violence**. This form of violence is not experienced physically; rather it is experienced in realistic ways through technology and ever more intense and realistic games. There is an ever-widening array of screens that are part of children's everyday lives, including computers, tablets, and cell phones, in addition to long-standing platforms, such as televisions and movies. Recent tragic events, including mass shootings and acts of terrorism, have increased the specter of fear among children as these events are reenacted for them on the multiple screens they encounter. Although exposure to media/virtual violence cannot be equated to exposure to real-life violence, many studies confirm that media/virtual violence *desensitizes* children to the meaning and impact of violent behavior. Violent video game exposure is associated with: an increased composite aggression score; increased aggressive behavior; increased aggressive cognitions; increased aggressive affect, increased desensitization, and decreased empathy; and increased physiological arousal. Violent video game use is a risk factor for adverse outcomes; however, insufficient data exist to examine any potential link between violent video game use and delinquency or criminal behavior. Table 14.1 lists interventions to reduce exposure to media violence.

IMPACTS OF VIOLENCE

All types of violence have a profound impact on health and development both psychologically and behaviorally; it may influence how children view the world and their place in it. Children can come to see the world as a dangerous and unpredictable place. This fear may thwart their exploration of the environment, which is essential to learning in childhood. Children may experience overwhelming terror, helplessness, and fear, even if they are not immediately in danger. Preschoolers are most vulnerable to threats that involve the safety (or perceived safety) of their caretakers. High exposure to violence in older children correlates with poorer performances in school, symptoms of anxiety and depression, and lower self-esteem. Violence, particularly IPV, can also teach children especially powerful early lessons about the role of violence in

Table 14.1	Public Health Recommendations to Reduce Effects of Media Violence on Children and Adolescents

Parents should:
- Be made aware of the risks associated with children viewing violent imagery, as it promotes aggressive attitudes, antisocial behavior, fear, and desensitization.
- Review the nature, extent, and context of violence in media available to their children before children view.
- Assist children's understanding of violent imagery appropriate to their developmental level.

Professionals should:
- Offer support and advice to parents who allow their children unsupervised access to extreme violent imagery, as this could be seen as a form of emotional abuse and neglect.
- Educate all young people in critical film appraisal, in terms of realism, justification, and consequences.
- Exercise greater control over access to inappropriate violent media entertainment by young people in secure institutions.
- Use violent film material in anger management programs under guidance.

Media producers should:
- Reduce violent content, and promote antiviolence themes and publicity campaigns.
- Ensure that when violence is presented, it is in context and associated with remorse, criticism, and penalty.
- Ensure that violent action is not justified, or its consequences understated.

Policymakers should:
- Monitor the nature, extent, and context of violence in all forms of media, and implement appropriate guidelines, standards, and penalties.
- Ensure that education in media awareness is a priority and a part of school curricula.

From Browne KD, Hamilton-Giachritsis C: The influence of violent media on children and adolescents: a public-health approach, *Lancet* 365:702–710, 2005.

relationships. Violence may change the way that children view their future; they may believe that they could die at an early age and thus take more risks, such as drinking alcohol, abusing drugs, not wearing a seatbelt, and not taking prescribed medication.

Some children exposed to severe and/or chronic violence may suffer from PTSD, exhibiting constricted emotions, difficulty concentrating, autonomic disturbances, and reenactment of the trauma through play or action (see Chapter 38). Based on *Diagnostic and Statistical Manual of Mental Disorders, Fifth Edition* (DSM-5) criteria for PTSD in children ≤6 yr old, >50% of preschoolers may experience clinically significant symptoms of PTSD after exposure to IPV. Although young children may not fully meet these criteria, certain behavioral changes are associated with exposure to trauma, such as sleep disturbances, aggressive behavior, new fears, and increased anxiety about separations (clinginess). A challenge in treating and diagnosing pediatric PTSD is that a child's caregiver exposed to the same trauma may be suffering from it as well.

Diagnosis and Follow-Up

The simplest way to recognize whether violence has become a problem in a family is to screen both the parents and the children (after approximately 8 yr of age) on a regular basis. This practice is particularly important during pregnancy and the immediate postpartum period, when women may be at highest risk for being abused. It is important to assure families that they are not being singled out, but that all families are asked about their exposure to violence. A direct approach may be useful: "Violence is a major problem in our world today and one that impacts everyone in our society. So I ask all my patients and families about violence that they are experiencing in their lives. …" In other cases, beginning with general questions and then moving to the specific may be helpful: "Do you feel safe in your home and neighborhood? Has anyone ever hurt you or your child?" When violence has impacted the child, it is important to gather details about symptoms and behaviors.

The pediatric clinician can effectively counsel many parents and children who have been exposed to violence. Regardless of the type of violence to which the child has been exposed, the following components are part of the guidance: (1) careful review of the facts and details of the event, (2) gaining access to support services, (3) providing information about the symptoms and behaviors common in children exposed to violence, (4) assistance in restoring a sense of stability to the family in order to enhance the child's feelings of safety, and (5) helping parents talk to their children about the event. When the symptoms are chronic (>6 mo) or not improving, if the violent event involved the death or departure of a parent, if the caregivers are unable to empathize with the child, or if the ongoing safety of the child is a concern, it is important that the family be referred to mental health professionals for additional treatment.

Bibliography is available at Expert Consult.

14.1 Bullying, Cyberbullying, and School Violence
Megan A. Moreno and Elizabeth Englander

BULLYING AND CYBERBULLYING
Bullying behavior affects people throughout the life span, but much of the focus has been on children and adolescents. In the past, bullying was sometimes considered a rite of passage, or was written off as "kids being kids." It is now recognized that bullying can have profound short- and long-term negative consequences on all those involved, including perpetrators, targets, and bystanders. The consequences of bullying can affect a child's social experiences, academic progress, and health.

Bullying is defined as any unwanted aggressive behavior by another youth or group of youths that involves an observed or perceived power imbalance and is repeated multiple times or is highly likely to be repeated. Generally, sibling aggression and dating violence are excluded, but research has associated these problems with *peer bullying*. Digital technology was initially viewed as a context in which bullying can occur. Further research studies have suggested that **cyberbullying** is not merely bullying that occurs through electronic communications, but rather a type of bullying with distinct elements, such as the potential for a single event to "go viral" and the use of technology as a tool to achieve power imbalance.

It is thought that bullying and cyberbullying are more alike than dissimilar, and that surveillance efforts, as well as prevention and intervention approaches, should address both types of bullying.

Bullying Roles and Nomenclature
Bullying represents a dynamic social interaction in which an individual may play different roles at different stages. A child can be a perpetrator of bullying, a target of bullying, a witness or bystander, or simply a child whose environment is affected by pervasive bullying. In any bullying experience, the roles that each child plays may be fluid; such that a target of bullying may then become a perpetrator, or vice versa. Thus, common nomenclature has evolved to refer to children as *perpetrators* of bullying or *targets* of bullying to represent a present state, rather than labeling a child as a bully or a victim, which suggests a static role and may impact that child's self-image.

Epidemiology
Bullying is a widespread problem during childhood and adolescence. Current estimates suggest that school-based bullying likely affects 18–31% of children and youth and that cyberbullying affects 7–15% of youth. Apparent rates of bullying are influenced by the questions that are asked; the word "bully" is stigmatized, and absent that label, youth are more willing to acknowledge having engaged in activities that can be categorized as bullying. Estimates of bullying prevalence are typically based on self-reported victimization (not perpetration), but here too, language can influence results. Targets of other types of social conflict may overestimate or underestimate their bullying victimization unless precise language is used during assessment.

Risk Factors
Certain groups are more vulnerable to bullying, including youth who are lesbian, gay, bisexual, transgender, and questioning (LGBTQ); immigrant and racial minority youth; obese youth; and youth with disabilities. However, it is important to recognize that while these individual risk factors exist, the context and situation can also present unique risk factors. Some studies have found that African Americans are bullied more often than Latinos, whereas other studies have found no group differences. Contextual factors, such as the school climate or prevalence of a particular ethnic group in a school setting, may be important factors in a given bullying situation. The 2015 **Youth Risk Behavior Survey** found that white students were much more likely than black teens to report being bullied at school or online. Thus, it is important to recognize that in any bullying situation, an individual is embedded within a situation that is within a larger social context. This *person by situation by context* approach is useful to consider in identifying why bullying takes place in some situations but not others.

Bullying may occur with other high-risk behaviors. Students who carry weapons, smoke, and drink alcohol >5-6 days/wk are at greatest risk for moderate bullying. Those who carry weapons, smoke, have >1 alcoholic drink/day, have above-average academic performance, moderate/high family affluence, and feel irritable or bad-tempered daily are at greatest risk for engaging in frequent bullying. Negative parenting behavior is related to a moderately increased risk of becoming a *bully/victim* (youth who are both perpetrators and targets) and small to moderate effects on being targeted for bullying at school.

Some risk factors may be specific to cyberbullying. Among preadolescent children, more access to technology (e.g., cell phone ownership) predicts cyberbullying behaviors and some types of digital victimization. Also, communications through digital technology can be misperceived as hostility, and those misperceptions can in turn increase electronic forms of bullying.

Consequences of Bullying
Involvement in any type of bullying is associated with poorer psychosocial adjustment; perpetrators, targets, and those both perpetrator and target report greater health problems and poorer emotional and social adjustment. Bullying consequences of both traditional and cyber forms of bullying are particularly significant in the areas of physical health, mental health, and academic achievement. Being the target of bullying is typically viewed as particularly stressful. The impact of this stress has been shown to affect the developing brain and to be associated with changes to the stress response system, which confers an increased risk for future health and academic difficulties. The long-term consequences of being bullied as a child include increased risk for depression, poor self-esteem, and abusive relationships. Negative outcomes for perpetrating bullying include higher risks of depression as well as substance abuse. Mental health consequences for both perpetrator and target include, across types of bullying, increased risks of depression, poor-self-esteem, increased suicidality, and anxiety. Academic difficulties include increased risk of poor school performance, school failure, and dropping out.

SCHOOL VIOLENCE
Epidemiology
School violence is a significant problem in the United States. Almost 40% of U.S. schools report a least 1 violent incident to police, with >600,000 victims of violent crime per year. Among 9th to 12th graders, 8% were threatened or injured on school property in the last 12 mo, and 14% were involved in a physical fight over the last year. Still,

school-associated violent deaths are rare. Seventeen homicides of children age 5-18 yr occurred at school during the 2009–2010 school year. Of all youth homicides, <2% occur at school. While urban schools experience more episodes of violence, the rare rampage gun violence that happens in rural and suburban schools demonstrates that no region is immune to lethal violence.

Risk Factors

Bullying and weapon carrying may be important precursors to more serious school violence. Among perpetrators of violent deaths at school, 20% had been bullying victims, and 6% carried a weapon to school in the last 30 days. Nonlethal violence, mental health problems, racial tensions, student attacks on teachers, and the effects of rapid economic change in communities can all lead to school violence. Individual risk factors for violence include prior history of violence, drug, alcohol, or tobacco use, association with delinquent peers, poor family functioning, poor grades in school, and poverty in the community.

Family risk factors include early childbearing, low parental attachment and involvement, authoritarian or permissive parenting styles (see Chapter 19), and poverty. There is more school violence in areas with higher crime rates and more street gangs, which take away students' ability to learn in a safe environment and leave many children with traumatic stress and grief reactions.

TREATMENT AND PREVENTION OF BULLYING AND SCHOOL VIOLENCE

Pediatric providers are in a unique position to screen, treat, and advocate for reducing the impact of bullying and school violence by assisting those affected and seeking to prevent further occurrences.

Signs and Symptoms

Signs of a child being involved in bullying or exposed to school violence include physical complaints such as insomnia, stomachaches, headaches, and new-onset enuresis. **Psychological symptoms,** such as depression (see Chapter 39), loneliness, anxiety (see Chapter 38), and suicidal ideation, may occur. **Behavioral changes,** such as irritability, poor concentration, school avoidance, and substance abuse, are common. **School problems,** such as academic failure, social problems, and lack of friends, can also occur. Additional vigilance is warranted for those children who represent vulnerable groups for bullying and aggression, including youth with disabilities, obesity, or minority, immigrant, or LGBTQ status.

Screening for Bullying

Assessing bullying and cyberbullying involvement is an important part of pediatric visits. Several tools can be helpful for clinicians, including the *Bright Futures Guidelines,* which recommend screening at each well-child visit. In these discussions, begin by normalizing the discussion; for example, practitioners can let the patient know that bullying is a topic they discuss with all their patients. It is advisable to define bullying based on the Uniform Definition, but using readily understandable and developmentally appropriate language. Physicians can ask patients if they have had experiences where there was repeated cruelty between peers, either as a target of that cruelty or seeing the cruelty, or even being angry or mean toward others. Asking a patient if he or she is a bully is not likely to generate either trust or an honest answer. Asking about exposures to peer victimization or school violence is also important. Throughout these discussions, it is critical to provide support and empathy while engaging the patient.

One tool to help providers begin and navigate these discussions is a *Practice Enhancement Tool* developed by the **Massachusetts Aggression Reduction Center** (MARC) and Children's Hospital Boston (Fig. 14.1). It begins by defining bullying in readily understandable language and then asks, "Is there any one kid, or a bunch of kids, that pick on you or make feel bad over and over again?" The Tool also guides the practitioner in asking about problematic digital experiences and asks whom the child has spoken to about the problem, and whether that has helped. Finally, it guides the practitioner through emphasizing the usefulness of talking about social problems and discusses how the physician can assist the patient.

Children who are aggressive, overly confident, lacking in empathy, or having persistent conduct problems may need careful screening. It is important to bear in mind that bullying is a dynamic process, and a child may be involved as both a perpetrator and a target at different time points. The physical, behavioral, psychological, and academic symptoms of bullying may overlap with other conditions, such as medical illness, learning problems, and psychological disorders. Thus, labeling the behavior as *bullying* rather than the child as a "bully" is recommended.

Management of bullying and school violence involves several steps. First, ensure that all parties understand the relevant information (the patient, parents, and school). Second, assess a child's need for specialized counseling or social skills interventions. Extracurricular activities, (e.g., drama clubs, mentoring programs, sports) can be discussed as avenues to help to increase the child's social skills and self-esteem. Third, ensure that the patient has adequate support, including at home and at school. Peers are a particularly effective source of support, and patients can be encouraged to spend time with friends, but parents and educators are also important sources of emotional support. Many children benefit from planning their actions in unstructured settings (e.g., discussing where they could sit during lunch), while some benefit from role-playing. Finally, the clinician should identify safety issues, such as suicidal ideation and plans, substance abuse, and other high-risk behaviors.

When bullying or cyberbullying is suspected or confirmed, the parents and child should be offered education and resources. Some resources include the government-supported website www.stopbullying.gov, as well as MARC. Both provide free downloadable literature that can be offered to parents and families.

Addressing cases of bullying or exposure to violence in clinic often requires a cross-disciplinary approach. Involving teachers or school counselors, as well as outside referrals to psychologists, social workers, or counselors, may be warranted. Parental mental health and resource risk factors should also be addressed.

Prevention

Pediatric clinicians can reasonably expect their patients' schools to provide violence and bullying prevention programs. Rather than focusing on only changing a target of bullying, successful interventions use whole school approaches that involve multiple stakeholders. **School climate** has been shown to have significant effects on bullying prevalence, so these approaches are essential to primary prevention. These broad-based programs simultaneously include school-wide rules and sanctions, teacher training, classroom curriculum, and high levels of student engagement. Addressing access to firearms, involving community organizations and parents, and supporting youth mental health are important in creating a safe school climate.

Prevention programs for cyberbullying are at a nascent stage, reflecting uncertainty about the prevalence of the practice, who is perpetrating it and from where, and how students respond when they are victimized. Many schools have established cyberbullying policies and are increasingly involved with teaching youth about guidelines for appropriate online interactions and monitoring for cyberbullying problems. As of 2016, 23 states included cyberbullying in their state antibullying laws, while 48 states included "electronic harassment." Although legal remedies are frequently not the most productive answer to bullying and cyberbullying incidents, pediatric physicians should be aware of local laws and be prepared to refer parents to more information about these laws when necessary. Studies suggest that preventive interventions designed to address bullying have effects on cyberbullying, and vice versa.

The American Academy of Pediatrics (AAP) provides a free online **Family Media Use Plan** that allows families to develop rules for digital media use and prompts for discussions about safety and online relationships with the goal of preventing negative consequences of online behavior and interactions. The tool is designed for ongoing discussions with family members about online experiences and family rules and values.

Bibliography is available at Expert Consult.

MARC/BACPAC Pediatric Questionnaire: **Bullying & Cyberbullying**

Massachusetts MARC Aggression Reduction Center at Bridgewater State University

Boston Children's Hospital Until every child is well

Date of office visit:__________

Child's name: ______________	Gender: ☐Male ☐Female	Parent present during interview? ☐Yes ☐No
Child's grade: ______________	Child's age: ________ years ________ months	Subjective complaints (eg, H/A, tics, sleep): ______________ ______________
IEP? ☐Yes ☐No	Neurodev / Psych Dx (if established): ______________	

BEGIN BY STATING:

"You probably know that grownups today are very worried about bullying. I'd like to ask you a little bit about that, but I want to make sure you understand what I mean. When I ask about bullying, I mean another kid (or group of kids) who picks on someone or is mean to them on purpose, over and over again – not just one time."

1. Do you see bullying happen at your school?

☐ **Yes** ☐ **No**

2. Is there any one kid or a bunch of kids that pick on you or make you feel bad over and over again?

☐ **Yes** (inquire as to the frequency):

(_____ times daily; _____ times a week; _____ times a month; _____ times a year).

IF NO, SKIP TO **#3**

If YES:
Where does this happen? (check all that apply):

☐ classroom ☐ lunchroom ☐ hallways

☐ stairwell ☐ bathroom ☐ locker-room

☐ playground ☐ bus ☐ other: ______________

What did he or she do to you? (check all that apply):

☐ made fun of me ☐ kids laughed ☐ name-calling

☐ rumors ☐ made up lies ☐ got me in trouble

☐ pushed, shoved, hit, threw stuff ☐ other:______________

3. How about on the computer at home? Has anyone been mean to you or made fun of you on the internet?

☐ **Yes** (Details):

____

____

If **NO** to both **#2** and **#3, END HERE.** Otherwise, continue.

Fig. 14.1 MARC/BACPAC* pediatric questionnaire on bullying and cyberbullying. *Massachusetts Aggression Reduction Center and Bullying And Cyberbullying Prevention and Advocacy Collaborative. *(Copyright ©2013 Peter C. Raffalli, MD, and Elizabeth Englander, PhD.)*

Continued

MARC/BACPAC Pediatric Questionnaire:
Bullying & Cyberbullying

---

4. It's very important that you understand that if you are being bullied that it is _never_ your fault. Bullying is wrong and people should _never_ bully others. Have you told any adults about the kids that are bothering you?

☐ **Yes** (Who have you told?)

    ☐ Parent

    ☐ Teacher

    ☐ Other: _____

If Yes.....Were the adults able to stop the bullying?

    ☐ **Yes** ☐ **No**

If Yes.....Did talking about it make you feel better?

    ☐ **Yes** ☐ **No** ("That's ok. Sometimes talking does help though.")

---

5. "Sometimes it feels good just to talk about things. I wish you and I had more time to talk about it today. Would you like to have a chance to talk about it sometime soon?"

☐ **Yes** (if YES, refer to):

_____

_____

☐ **No**

IF NO...

    ..."Would you like me to try to help? As your doctor, I can talk with the school officials and try to make sure that the bullying stops. While I cannot promise that everything will be better, I know that if we do nothing the bullying will likely continue and probably get worse. I want you to be happy and safe at school — is it okay with you if I talk to your school about this?"

☐ **Yes**
    (Who would you like me to talk to? Principal / Nurse / Counselor / Teacher / Other: _____)

☐ **No**

Fig. 14.1, cont'd

MARC/BACPAC Pediatric Questionnaire:
Bullying & Cyberbullying

Guide to the bullying/cyberbullying checklist/interview

"Warm up" questions: briefly acknowledge these but do not discuss at length. No need to note the child's answers.

> Are the kids in your school friendly?

> Tell me about one child at your school who you like.

> Tell me about one child at your school who is not friendly.

(Brief acknowledgement, e.g.: "Ok" or "that's good.")

Note: It's fine to skip the warm-up questions if you have already chatted with the child.

Websites for parents/ teachers/students:

The Massachusetts Aggression Reduction Center (MARC): MARCcenter.org

Bullying And Cyberbullying Prevention and Advocacy Collaborative (BACPAC) at Boston Children's Hospital: bostonchildrens.org/BACPAC

Stop Bullying Now from the U.S. government: stopbullying.gov

When a child is being bullied

There are three venues through which you can help this child:

1. **BY GIVING THEM A "SAFE ADULT" AT SCHOOL THEY CAN ALWAYS SPEAK WITH (EG, THE SCHOOL NURSE, THE SCHOOL ADJUSTMENT COUNSELOR);**

2. **BY GIVING THEIR PARENTS GUIDANCE ABOUT HOW TO COPE (THROUGH HANDOUTS, WEBSITES); AND**

3. **BY OFFERING THEM SUPPORT FROM YOURSELF.**

If child consents to your involvement, seek written parental consent to share information with the school in writing. The more details the child can provide as to who, what, where, how, the more power the school will have to act. Explain this to the child/parent and do your best to gently get details for your letter to the school. If child or parent will not consent to communication with school, provide advice / handouts (MARCcenter.org) to help the parent advocate themselves for their child with the school. Always document in your note the conversation in the office.

Fig. 14.1, cont'd

14.2 Media Violence

Megan A. Moreno

Today's youth are growing up in a media-rich environment of both traditional and digital media. *Traditional* media includes television (TV), radio, and periodicals; *digital* media includes online content that promote interactive and social engagement. The online world allows youth instant access to entertainment, information, and knowledge; social contact; and marketing. Social and interactive media allow media users to act as both creators and consumers of content. Examples include applications (apps), multiplayer video games, YouTube videos, and video blogs (vlogs).

One of the earliest studies that has been linked to media effects on aggression and violence was the "bobo doll" experiment in which children who observed an aggressive adult model were more likely to be aggressive toward a doll afterward. It has been widely accepted that media exposure can affect behavior; the advertising industry is grounded in the concept that media exposure can change purchasing behavior. Exposure to sexual content in media has been linked to earlier sexual initiation. However, applying these same constructs to media violence has been controversial. Some suggest that other concepts may be important to consider, such as "dose-response" effects of media, or gene-environment interactions.

There are 3 main types of media in which children may be exposed to violence: video games, traditional media, and social media. **Violent video game** exposure is associated with several outcomes, including increases in composite aggression score, aggressive behavior, aggressive cognitions, aggressive affect, and desensitization; decreased empathy; and increased physiological arousal.

Movies and TV often model violent behavior for the purposes of entertainment. Media violence does not always portray the real human cost or suffering caused by violence. Special effects can make virtual violence more believable and appealing than in the real world. For some children, exposure to media violence can lead to anxiety, depression, posttraumatic stress disorder, or sleep disorders and nightmares. Repeated exposure to the behavioral scripts provided by entertainment media can lead to increased feelings of hostility, expectations for aggression, desensitization to violence, and increased likelihood of interacting and responding to others with violence.

Social media presents similar risks of exposure to virtual violence, but because of the interactive nature of the medium, this content can feel more personal or targeted. Social media combines peer and media effects and thereby represents a powerful motivator of behavior, whether content created by adolescents themselves or content they find and share with peers. The Facebook Influence Model describes 13 distinct constructs in which social media may influence users, such as establishing *social norms* and connection to identity. Thus, exposure to violent content on social media may have influence in promoting a social norm, or connecting this type of content to one's own identity.

SCREENING

It is important for pediatricians to screen and counsel patients and families about media use and exposure to violent content. Both the quantity and the quality of media are critical factors in media effects on children. When heavy media use by a child is identified, pediatricians should evaluate the child for aggressive behaviors, fears, or sleep disturbances and intervene appropriately.

RECOMMENDATIONS (see Table 14.1)

Pediatricians can counsel parents to help their children *avoid exposure to any form of media violence under age 8 yr*. These younger children do not have the capacity to distinguish fantasy from reality.

Parents should *select and co-view media with their children*, including playing video games with them, watching movies together, and co-viewing social media content. Parents can then assess these games and shows in regard to what they are teaching about communication and interactions with others.

Parents should *feel empowered to place restrictions* on games or shows that reward shooting, killing, or harming other people. Media are

powerful teachers, and parents can make choices about how much violence they want their children to learn. Parents can use industry ratings, such as from the Motion Picture Association of America and the Entertainment Software Ratings Board, as well as resources such as Commonsense Media, to guide media selections.

Bibliography is available at Expert Consult.

14.3 Effects of War on Children

Isaiah D. Wexler and Eitan Kerem

The adverse consequences of war on children are devastating and long-lasting—death, injury, disfigurement, pain and other physical and cognitive disabilities, acute and chronic psychological suffering, temporary and permanent loss of family members, abduction, rape, conscription into armed service, forced relocation, epidemics, famine, drought, and residual trauma lasting decades after hostilities have ceased. The impact of war on children is detailed annually by the Secretary General of the United Nations, and in the 2016 report he described the increasing intensity of human rights violations in a large number of armed conflict situations throughout the world that included mass abduction of children, coercive conscription, death of children or their parents, attacks on schools, and sexual violence. Exploitation in the form of human trafficking has significantly increased in areas of conflict. Slavery, forced marriages, prostitution, and child labor are often a consequence of displacement, which has seen an increase in the past decade due to the increasing number of intrastate conflicts, especially in the Middle East and Northern Africa. In 2017, UNHCR (**Office of the United Nations High Commissioner for Refugees**), the UN Refugee Agency, reported the astounding statistic of 65.6 million people forcibly displaced worldwide.

Mortality and morbidity related to the long-term effects of war and civil strife are often higher than that occurring during actual fighting. War and violence are not listed as leading causes of childhood mortality, but the regions with the highest levels of child mortality, especially among children <5 yr of age, are the same locations involved in military conflicts. Nations experiencing conflict devote substantial portions of their budgets to military expenditures at the expense of the healthcare infrastructure; a substantial proportion of deaths attributed to malnutrition, environmentally related infectious disease, or inadequate immunization are related to the effects of war. Children experiencing the trauma of wartime violence are at risk for long-term health sequelae, with greater risk for obesity, hypertension, stroke, and cardiovascular disease.

During wartime, customary patterns of behavior are forced to change, overcrowding is frequent, and essential resources, such as water and food staples, may be polluted or contaminated. War is associated with plagues and epidemics, and novel disease entities can develop. Reemergence of polio or cholera and the increased virulence of tuberculosis have been associated with conflict-affected regions and large population displacements.

The morbidity of children exposed to conflicts is significant (Table 14.2). Many more children are physically harmed than killed. Children bear the psychological scars of war resulting from exposure to violent events, loss of primary caregivers, and forced removal from their homes. Impressment of children into service as **soldiers** or agents is a form of *exploitation* associated with long-term problems of adjustment, because child soldiers often lack the appropriate education and socialization and thus their moral compass is often misaligned. They are often incapable of understanding the sources of conflict or why they have been targeted. Their thought processes are more concrete; it is easier for them to dehumanize their adversaries. Children, who themselves are exposed to violence and cruelty, frequently become the worst perpetrators of atrocities.

After cessation of hostilities, children are still at risk for life-endangering injuries from **landmines**, unexploded ordnance, and other explosive remnants of war. Prior to the signing of the international treaty to ban landmines in 1997, an estimated 20,000-25,000 casualties occurred

Table 14.2	Impact of War on Children

PHYSICAL
Death
Rape
Abduction
Injuries
Amputations and fractures
Head trauma
Ballistic wounds
Blast injuries
Burns
Chemical and biologic induced
Malnutrition and starvation
Infectious disease
Displacement

PSYCHOSOCIAL
Loss of caregivers and family members
Separation from community
Lack of education
Inappropriate socialization
Acute stress reaction
Posttraumatic stress disorder
Depression
Maladaptive behavior

EXPLOITATION
Conscription as soldiers
Coerced involvement in terrorist activities
Prostitution
Slavery
Forced adoption

The changing nature of war has adversely affected children. Conventional warfare in which armies of professional soldiers representing different countries battle each other has become less common. **Intrastate conflicts** in the form of civil war are more frequent. In 2013, there were 33 active intrastate armed conflicts in the world as documented by the Uppsala Conflict Data Program (UCDP). These conflicts are often rooted in factious ethnic, political, or religious ideologies, and the participants are frequently nonprofessional irregulars who lack discipline and accountability to higher echelons, and are directed by those who do not acknowledge or respect international accords governing warfare. Often the military resources of the antagonists are disproportionate, leading the weaker protagonist to develop compensatory tactics that can include guerrilla, paramilitary, and terrorist activities, while the stronger side often resorts to the disproportionate use of force. Low-intensity conflicts have become more common. These types of conflicts are often characterized by military activities targeting civilian populations with the goal of disrupting normal routines and generating publicity for the perpetrators. Sites of violence can be remote from the battleground when one or both parties to a conflict resort to terrorist activities.

Terrorism and organized urban-based **gang warfare** have become prevalent. Violence perpetrated by terrorists groups or gangs is designed to coerce and intimidate both individuals and entire societies. Children are often intended victims of political- or religious-motivated violence because this serves to maximize the impact of terrorism. The destruction of the New York City World Trade Center Towers in 2001 and the nearly 3,000 fatalities showed that highly organized and motivated terrorists have few inhibitions and can strike anywhere. **Biologic** and **chemical** weapons of mass destruction have been employed, with the most recent example being the use of poisonous gases in the Syrian civil war. Children are more susceptible to chemical and biologic toxins because of their higher respiratory rates, more permeable skin, and other developmental vulnerabilities (see Chapter 741).

The media and internet have had a significant role in exacerbating the effects of war on children. Media coverage of war and terrorist events is extensive and visual, and social media promulgated via the internet is a convenient tool for disseminating **propaganda** and graphic video material designed to recruit volunteers and shock opponents. Children, more impressionable than adults, often view this material uncontrolled. Uncensored pictures of victims, unbridled violence, people in shock, or family members searching through ruins for relatives may traumatize children and even encourage inappropriate behavior. Overt broadcast propaganda glorifying war and violence may sway children to participate in militaristic or antisocial activities.

annually from landmines. Since the ban, the number of casualties from landmines and explosive devices had been declining until 2015, when there was a significant increase in causalities attributed to the increasing number of conflicts. Approximately 40% of these casualties occur in children. Injuries and death tended to occur while children were either playing or involved in household chores, and in contrast to adults, a large proportion of the injuries involved upper-extremity amputation. After the end of armed conflict, the continued proliferation of small arms and light weapons, which are easily handled by children, continues to take its toll on human life and hinders stabilization in postconflict societies.

SUSCEPTIBILITY OF CHILDREN IN TIMES OF WAR

Children do not have the physical or intellectual capabilities to defend themselves. It is easier for adults to victimize children than other adults. Older children's curiosity, desire for adventure, and imperfect assessment of risk often lead them to participate in dangerous behavior. Younger children, because of their small size and immature physiology, are more susceptible to disease and starvation and are more likely to sustain fatal injuries from ballistic projectiles and explosive devices such as mines. **Blast injuries**, a common cause of violence-related injuries, have a more devastating impact on children than adults. Specific types of military engagement can have a disproportionate effect on children. In a survey of war-related mortality in Iraq from 2003–2008, it was found that approximately 10% of the violence-related fatalities were children. Most children succumbed to either small arms gunfire or suicide bombs (35%). Compared with adults, a proportionately higher rate of children died as a result of the indiscriminant use of weaponry such as mortars, missiles, and aircraft-delivered bombs; 40% of the total casualties in these types of attacks were children.

During times of war, there is a breakdown of social inhibitions and cultural norms. Exploitation of children, such as forced marriages or involuntary conscription, are rationalized as being beneficial for the greater cause. Aberrant behavior such as rape, torture, and pillaging, which would be inconceivable in times of peace, is common during war. Children may be attacked, kidnapped, or used as human shields.

PSYCHOLOGICAL IMPACT OF WAR

Exposure to war and violence can have a significant impact on a child's psychosocial development. Displacement, loss of caregivers, physical suffering, and the lack of appropriate socialization all contribute to abnormal child development (see Table 14.2). Often the reactions are age specific (Table 14.3). Preschoolers may have an increase in somatic complaints and sleep disturbances and display acting-out behaviors such as tantrums or excessively clinging behavior. School-age children may show regressive behavior such as enuresis and thumb sucking. They, too, have an increase in somatic complaints; there is often a negative impact on school performance. For teenagers, psychological withdrawal and depression are common. Adolescents often exhibit trauma-stimulated acting-out behavior. Motivated by the desire for revenge, they may be quick to join in the violence and contribute to the continuation of conflict.

There is an increased incidence of both **acute stress reactions** and **posttraumatic stress disorder** (PTSD; see Chapter 38). The true incidence is difficult to assess because of the heterogeneous nature of war, degree of exposure to violence, and methodologic challenges related to the precise characterization of PTSD. Risk factors for having a more serious psychological response to a violent event include severity of the incident, personal involvement (physical injury, proximity, loss of a relative), prior history of exposure to traumatic events, female gender, and a dysfunctional parental response to the same event. Children may develop PTSD many years after the traumatic event. Children do not have to

Table 14.3	Manifestations of Stress Reactions in Children and Adolescents Exposed to War, Terrorism, and Urban Violence

CHILDREN ≤6 YR
Excessive fear of separation
Clinging behavior
Uncontrollable crying or screaming
Freezing (persistent immobility)
Sleep disorders
Terrified affect
Regressive behavior
Expressions of helplessness and passivity

CHILDREN 7-11 YR
Decline in school performance
Truancy
Sleep disorders
Somatization
Depressive affect
Abnormally aggressive or violent behavior
Irrational fears
Regressive and childish behavior
Expressions of fearfulness, withdrawal, and worry

ADOLESCENTS 12-17 YR
Decline in school performance
Sleep disturbances
Flashbacks
Emotional numbness
Antisocial behavior
Substance abuse
Revenge fantasies
Suicidal ideation
Withdrawal

be directly exposed to violent activity, and media coverage of terrorist events may be sufficient to trigger PTSD.

The trauma experienced by children during war can have lifelong effects. Studies on children imprisoned in concentration camps or evacuated from their homes in London during the Battle of Britain show that these individuals were at greater risk for PTSD, anxiety disorders, and a higher level of dissatisfaction with life when surveyed decades after the traumatic events. Trauma may have a **transgenerational effect** with epigenetic alterations and environmental influences causing children of PTSD victims to display a wide variety of psychological disorders. On the positive side, children are more resilient than adults. With appropriate support from family and community, together with timely and intensive psychological intervention, children can recover and lead normal, productive lives despite the searing trauma that they may have experienced.

EFFORTS TO PROTECT CHILDREN FROM THE EFFECTS OF WAR
International Conventions
War and terror violate the human rights of children, including the right to life, the right to be nurtured and protected, the right to develop appropriately, the right to be with family and community, and the right to a healthy existence. Several international treaties and conventions have been ratified, beginning with the **Fourth Geneva Convention** (1949) that set forth guidelines regarding appropriate treatment of children in times of war. The **United Nations Convention on the Rights of the Child** (1990) delineated specific human rights inherent to every child (defined as any individual younger than 18 yr), and the subsequent **First Optional Protocol** (2000), which prohibits conscripting or recruiting children for military activities. The **Third Optional Protocol** in 2014 established methods for communicating complaints of human rights violations involving children to the United Nations Committee on the Rights of the Child and sets up procedures by which the Committee can conduct inquiries into alleged human rights violations among

signatory nations. The **Rome Statute of the International Criminal Court** enacted in 2002 declared that the conscription or enlistment of children younger than 15 yr is a prosecutable war crime. A decade since the ratification of the Rome Statute, the number of armed conflicts in which children were serving as soldiers had decreased from 36 to 16 worldwide.

Although these treaties and conventions define the extent of protection afforded to children, the means of enforcement available to the international community is limited. Individuals, motivated by religious fervor, nationalistic zeal, or ethnic xenophobia, are unlikely to curb their activities because of fear of prosecution. These treaties better serve in heightening awareness regarding the protected status of children in wartime, and perhaps deter high-ranking leaders who fear being held accountable for war crimes.

Humanitarian Efforts
Several organizations, either nongovernmental or under UN auspices, are involved in mitigating the effects of war on children. The International Red Cross, UNICEF, UNHCR, International Rescue Committee, World Health Organization, and Médicins Sans Frontières (Doctors Without Borders), have had a significant impact on reducing violence-related casualties in war-torn regions. The infusion of humanitarian aid into developing countries often improves overall mortality and morbidity by increasing the level of medical and social services available to the general population. Other organizations, such as Amnesty International, Stockholm International Peace Research Institute, and Physicians for Human Rights, actively monitor human rights abuses involving children and other civilian groups. In 2005 the UN Security Council approved the establishment of a monitoring and reporting system designed to protect children exposed to war. UN-led task forces conduct active surveillance in war-stricken regions reporting on the *6 grave violations against children during armed conflict*: the killing or injuring of children, recruitment of child soldiers, attacks directed against schools or hospitals, sexual violence against children, abduction of children, and denial of humanitarian access for children.

ROLE OF PEDIATRICIANS AND ALLIED HEALTH PROFESSIONALS
War is a chronic condition, and health providers need to be prepared to treat childhood casualties resulting from military or terrorist activity, as well as caring for children suffering from the aftermath of war or related violence. Community and hospital pediatricians need to be involved in community disaster planning. General disaster planning should not ignore the unique needs and requirements of children; in planning for a possible chemical attack, appropriate resuscitation equipment suitable for children needs to be stockpiled. The signs of biologic infection, chemical intoxication, or radiation injury are different for children, and pediatricians and emergency personnel need to be aware of these differences (see Chapters 736 and 741). Surveys of pediatricians and other healthcare providers indicate that many feel unprepared for bioterrorism attacks. Professional organizations (e.g., AAP, CDC) have published position papers; there is a special section in the AAP *Red Book* that presents guidelines for treating specific pathogens likely to be used in **biologic warfare**. In regions where violent terrorist activity is likely, pediatricians, nurses, and rescue personnel should consider becoming certified in the Red Cross Basic and Advanced Trauma Life Support programs.

Pediatricians need to be aware of the potential effects of war and terror on parents and children. Loss or separation from parents or caregivers has a devastating impact on children (see Chapter 30). Parents, who themselves are under tremendous strain, may not be sensitive to the effects that the same stressors have on their children. Parents and caregivers must be made cognizant of the effect that media coverage can have on their children and their role in the intermediation of the repetitive broadcast of real-time acts of violence and incendiary communications designed to enlist support for specific causes. Pediatricians should draw out both parents and children and encourage them to talk freely about their feelings. Child healthcare providers can be instrumental in educating parents to be more aware of inappropriate responses by children to war and violence. When necessary, pediatricians can serve their families by referring them to appropriate support services.

Just as it is important to administer first aid for physical trauma, it is also critical to provide psychologic first aid to victims of trauma. An excellent source of online information for both providers and caregivers is the **National Child Traumatic Stress Network** (www.nctsn.org). In day-to-day patient interactions, a pediatrician is most likely to confront situations related to stress reactions such as PTSD or depressive disorders. Recognition of PTSD is essential so that early treatment can be initiated. The *Diagnostic and Statistical Manual of Mental Disorders, Fifth Edition* (DSM-5) stipulates that for a diagnosis of PTSD, there has to be manifestations from each of 4 symptom clusters: *intrusion, avoidance, negative alterations in cognitions and mood*, and *alterations in arousal and reactivity*. DSM-5 also established a special preschool subtype of PTSD that has the same 4 symptom clusters but with specific manifestations typical of preschoolers exposed to trauma. Clues to the presence of PTSD and acute anxiety reactions include changes in behavior, school performance, affect, and sleep patterns and an increase in somatic complaints. Even when the triggering event is neither temporally nor physically proximate, it should not dissuade the pediatrician from making an appropriate referral to mental health professionals who are expert in childhood stress disorders.

Medical professional standards demand that the physician treat all patients equitably without regard to their background. Both international law and professional medical societies ban physicians from actively participating in **torture** or other activities that infringe on human rights, including those of children. It is difficult to countenance any situation in which a health professional, even acting as a representative of his country, might directly or indirectly injure a minor. On the positive side, many pediatricians and other physicians have treated children during war either as members of the armed services or volunteers, often under adverse conditions, refusing to abandon their patients even when it has put their own life at risk. Pediatricians and pediatric organizations have been at the forefront in advocating for peaceful coexistence, assisting in relief efforts, and attempting to alleviate the disparities in healthcare resulting from war.

Health professionals have an important role in preventing the atrocities that occur to children. In their role as advocates for the rights of children, pediatricians can be instrumental in focusing public attention on the precarious situation of children exposed to the brutality and mayhem of organized violence. They can promulgate the message that war and terror should not be allowed to rob children of their childhood.

Bibliography is available at Expert Consult.

Chapter **15**
Child Trafficking for Sex and Labor

V. Jordan Greenbaum

第十五章
贩卖儿童为奴为娼

中文导读

本章主要介绍了此类儿童的临床表现；介绍了医务人员如何以了解伤情、维护人权、符合文化风俗和规避性别敏感的方式接近被贩卖的儿童；介绍了以上有关的体格检查和诊断性检验；特别阐述了如何在受害者知情同意的情况下进行移交和寻求援助。用表格分别呈现了所贩卖儿童被剥削的类型、有利于贩卖儿童的潜在条件、被贩卖儿童的潜在特征，以及以人权和深谙创伤为前提的诊疗要素。

Human trafficking violates the fundamental human rights of child and adult victims and impacts families, communities, and societies. Trafficked persons originate from countries worldwide and may belong to any racial, ethnic, religious, socioeconomic, or cultural group. They may be of any gender. According to the United Nations *Protocol to Prevent,* *Suppress and Punish Trafficking in Persons*, **child trafficking** refers to the "recruitment, transportation, transfer, harboring or receipt of a person" under 18 yr old for purposes of exploitation. Two major types of trafficking involve **forced labor** and **sexual exploitation** (Table 15.1). While adult sex trafficking requires demonstration of force, fraud,

Table 15.1	Types of Exploitation Included in Child Trafficking

Sexual Exploitation
Prostitution of a child
Production of child sexual exploitation materials (child pornography)
Exploitation in context of travel and tourism
Engaging child in sex-oriented business
Child marriage or forced marriage
Live online sexual abuse

Labor Exploitation
Occurs in a variety of sectors, such as agriculture, manufacturing, textiles, food/hospitality services; domestic work; construction, magazine sales, health and beauty, and cleaning services

Forced Begging

Forced Criminality

Forced Engagement in Armed Conflict

Illegal Adoption

Table 15.2	Vulnerability Factors for Child Trafficking

INDIVIDUAL
Member of marginalized group (racial, ethnic, sexual minority, caste, etc.)
History of sexual/physical abuse or neglect
Limited education
Substance misuse
Homeless status; runaway; told to leave home
History of child welfare and/or juvenile justice involvement (U.S., sex trafficking)
Untreated mental health or behavioral condition
Significantly older intimate partner

FAMILY
Poverty
Violence, substance misuse, other dysfunction
Migration

COMMUNITY
Limited resources (economic, educational, social support)
Tolerance of trafficking/exploitation
Social or political upheaval
Natural disaster
Violence
Limited knowledge of trafficking/exploitation
Increased tourism, travel to area

SOCIETAL
Cultural beliefs about roles and rights of children
Gender bias/discrimination
Tolerance of marginalization, exploitation
Sexual objectification of girls
Tolerance of violence
Economic disparities

coercion, deception, or the abuse of power as a means of exploitation, these are *not* required for persons younger than 18 yr. Interpretation of the international protocol varies across the globe; U.S. law does not require movement of a victim to qualify as human trafficking. In addition, minors who "consent" to commercial sex in the absence of a third party (trafficker) are victims of commercial sexual exploitation, because their age precludes true informed consent.

The word *victim* is used in this chapter in the legal sense and refers to a person who has been harmed as a result of a crime or other event. It is not intended to imply any subjective interpretation of the person's feelings about his/her situation or imply any judgment about that person's resilience.

Child trafficking may occur within the confines of the child's home country (*domestic* trafficking) or may cross national borders (*international*, or *transnational*, trafficking). Globally, victims tend to be trafficked within their own country or to a country in the same region. In the United States, most identified *child sex trafficking* victims are U.S. citizens or legal residents; few statistical data exist on victims of child labor trafficking. Variations in definitions of terms, problems with data collection, and underrecognition of victims complicate estimates of the prevalence of human trafficking, but the International Labour Organization estimates that 5.5 million of the world's children are victims of forced labor (this includes human trafficking). In a study of 55,000 officially identified trafficking victims, the United Nations Office on Drugs and Crime estimated that approximately 17% were girls and 10% boys. However, laws that define sexual exploitation in terms of girls and women, as well as cultural views regarding gender roles, lead to underreporting of boys, especially as victims of sex trafficking, so their numbers may be higher than estimated.

Factors creating vulnerability to human trafficking exist at the individual, family, community, and societal levels (Table 15.2). **Age** is an important risk factor for adolescents since they are at a stage in their development at which they have limited life experience, a desire to demonstrate their independence from parental control, and a level of brain maturation that favors risk-taking and impulsive behaviors over careful situational analysis and other executive functions. They are also very interested in social media and are savvy at internet use, which render them susceptible to online recruitment and solicitation.

Recruitment of child victims for labor or sex trafficking often involves false promises of romance, job opportunities, or a better life. Children may remain in their exploitative situation for a number of reasons, including **fear of violence** to themselves or their loved ones should they attempt escape; **guilt and shame** for believing the fraudulent recruitment scheme or engaging in illegal and/or socially condemned activities; **humiliation** and fear of criticism by authorities; **debt bondage** (believing they owe the trafficker exorbitant amounts of money and cannot leave until the debt is paid), and fear of **arrest** and/or deportation. Many children do not recognize their victimization. Girls who believe their trafficker is a boyfriend may view their commercial sexual activities as demonstrations of their love; boys engaging in commercial sex to obtain shelter or food while living on the street may feel they are exploiting buyers rather than being victimized. Traffickers may use violence, economic manipulation, and psychological manipulation to control their victims.

CLINICAL PRESENTATION

Trafficked persons may seek medical care for any of the myriad physical and emotional consequences of exploitation. They may present with traumatic injuries inflicted by traffickers, buyers, or others or injuries related to unsafe working conditions. They may present with a history of sexual assault, or symptoms/signs of sexually transmitted infections (STIs) and infections related to overcrowded, unsanitary conditions. They may request testing for HIV or complain of signs/symptoms of HIV or infections endemic to the victim's home country (e.g., malaria, schistosomiasis, tuberculosis). Other clinical presentations may involve pregnancy and complications of pregnancy or abortion; malnutrition and/or dehydration; exhaustion; conditions related to exposure to toxins, chemicals, and dust; and signs and symptoms of posttraumatic stress disorder (PTSD), major depression, suicidality, behavioral problems with aggression, and somatization. Some children may have preexisting chronic medical conditions that have been inadequately treated before or during the exploitation (e.g., diabetes, seizure disorder, asthma). Trafficked persons may also seek care for medical issues related to their children.

Many of the same factors that keep victims trapped in their exploitative conditions also preclude them from disclosing their situation to others.

Table 15.3	Possible Indicators of Child Trafficking

INDICATORS AT PRESENTATION

Chief complaint of acute physical or sexual assault
Chief complaint of suicide attempt
Child accompanied by unrelated adult or juvenile
Child or parent accompanied by domineering person who appears in hurry to leave; child/parent appears intimidated, fearful
Child or accompanying person provides inconsistent or unlikely history of events
Child does not know city he or she is in, or address where staying

PHYSICAL FINDINGS

Child withdrawn and with flat affect; fearful; very anxious; intoxicated; or with inappropriate affect
Motel key(s), multiple cell phones, large amounts of cash, or a few expensive items (clothing, nails, etc.)
Tattoos (especially with street names or sexual innuendo)
Evidence of remote or acute inflicted injury (suspicious burns, bruising, signs of strangulation, fractures, closed head injury, thoracoabdominal trauma)
Malnutrition and/or poor hygiene
Poor dentition and/or dental trauma
Late presentation of illness/injury

Table 15.4	Elements of Human Rights–Based, Trauma-Informed Approach to Patient Care

BASIC RIGHTS

Best interest of the child to be primary concern in all actions involving the child
Protection from discrimination because of gender, race, ethnicity, culture, socioeconomic status, disability, religion, language, country of origin, or other status
Right to express views and be heard, appropriate to child's age and development
Right to obtain information relevant to child, to be given in a way that children understand
Right to privacy and confidentiality
Right to highest attainable standard of health and to access healthcare services
Right to dignity, self-respect
Right to consideration of special needs (age, disability, etc.)
Right to respect of cultural and religious beliefs and practices

TRAUMA-INFORMED CARE

Strength-based approach; facilitate patient resilience and empowerment.
Obtain medical history in private, safe place, outside presence of persons accompanying child to visit.
Explain all processes in way child understands, and obtain assent for each step; discuss limits of confidentiality and mandated reporting.
Encourage patient to express views and to participate in decision-making regarding referrals and care.
Foster patient's sense of control during evaluation.
Ask only the questions needed to assess safety, health, and well-being. Avoid asking irrelevant questions about trauma, to avoid unnecessarily triggering anxiety and distress.
Minimize retraumatization during history, examination, and diagnostic testing (avoid triggers of stress when possible).
Monitor for signs of distress, both verbal and nonverbal.
Allow patient option to choose gender of provider, if feasible.
Have trained personnel present during examination to assist with providing support and reassurance.
Avoid making promises provider cannot fulfill.
Put information gathered to good use.
Conduct safety assessment and create plan.
Be prepared to make referrals and offer resources.

Most victims presenting for medical care at clinics, hospitals, and emergency departments do not self-identify as trafficked persons. Consequently, it is incumbent on the medical professional to be aware of risk factors so that potential victims may be recognized and offered services. A trafficked child may present to a medical facility alone, in the company of a parent/guardian (who may or may not be aware of the trafficking situation), a friend or other person not involved in the trafficking, a person working for the trafficker (who may pose as a friend or relative), or the trafficker. Traffickers may be male or female, adult or juvenile, and they may be family members, acquaintances, friends, or strangers. On occasion, children are brought in by law enforcement or child protective services, as known or suspected victims. Table 15.3 lists possible indicators of labor or sex trafficking. In some cases, the best indicator is the **chief complaint**, which may be a condition frequently associated with trafficking (e.g., teen pregnancy, STI symptoms/signs (especially with history of prior STI), preventable work-related injury). The practitioner may become concerned about possible trafficking on recognizing the presence of 1 or more **risk factors** (runaway status; recent migration and current work in sector known for labor trafficking).

APPROACH TO THE POTENTIALLY TRAFFICKED CHILD

When interacting with a possible victim of trafficking, the medical provider should use a **trauma-informed, human rights–based, culturally appropriate, and gender-sensitive approach** (Table 15.4). This involves being aware that trauma experienced by children may influence their thoughts about themselves and others, their beliefs and perceptions of the world, and their behavior. Hostility, withdrawal, or distrust may be reactions to trauma and should be met with a sensitive, nonjudgmental, empathic response by the provider. Physical safety of the patient and staff are critical, and protocols should be in place to address security issues that may arise if the trafficker is on the premises. Psychological safety of the patient may be facilitated by separating them from any accompanying person when obtaining the medical history, conducting the visit in a warm, child-friendly environment, taking adequate time to build rapport and begin to establish trust, and ensuring that any interpreter used is not from the same community as the patient and is trained in human trafficking.

Respect for the **patient's rights** is essential, including the right to an explanation of the purpose of the questions being asked, and the reasons for, and elements of, the examination and diagnostic evaluation. Informed assent by the patient for all steps of the process should be obtained when possible. The limits of confidentiality should be explained in a way the child understands so that they are able to choose what information to disclose. A **risk assessment** should include a discussion with the patient of safety concerns (involving current risks and perceived risks after discharge). While many trafficked persons have committed crimes during their period of exploitation, it is critical to treat the child with respect and compassion, viewing the patient as a victim of exploitation rather than a criminal offender. Every attempt should be made to understand and respect cultural and religious influences that may affect the child's views of their bodies, their condition, and their desired treatment.

In some cases the provider may become concerned about the possibility of human trafficking only after speaking with the child and obtaining the medical history. Social or other vulnerability factors may come to light, prompting concern about exploitation. In such cases the provider may consider asking additional questions, if this can be done in a nontraumatizing manner. Such questions might include the following:

◆ "Many children who have to live on the street have a hard time getting money for food and shelter. Sometimes they have to exchange sex to get what they need. Has this ever happened to you or anyone you know?"
◆ When asking about sexual history: "Has anyone ever asked you or forced you to have sex when you really didn't want to? Do you feel comfortable telling me about it?"

◆ "If you feel comfortable, can you tell me a little bit about your job? Who offered you the job? Is the work you do what you expected when you agreed to the job? Are you allowed to keep all of the money you earn, or send it home? Where, and with whom, do you live? When you are not working, are you allowed to come and go from the place you stay?"

Such questions may open the door to a discussion of exploitation and facilitate the provider identifying appropriate resources and referrals.

All elements of the medical history and review of systems are important, but special attention should be paid to reproductive history (including sexual orientation and identity, prior history of sex partners, STIs, pregnancy/abortions, condom use); injury history; substance use/misuse; and mental health history and current symptoms. Rates of substance misuse, depression, PTSD, depression, and suicidality are very high, and questioning may highlight the need for emergency care or nonurgent referrals. It also provides an opportunity for anticipatory guidance aimed at harm reduction: a discussion of condom use, STIs, HIV/AIDS, and substance use may prove invaluable, since many victims lack accurate information on these topics. It is important to identify any chronic conditions, especially if untreated, and to assess vaccination status. Many trafficked persons have had very poor healthcare in the past and lack basic primary care. It is important to ask questions about signs/symptoms of infections endemic to the child's home country or to countries in which the child has been trafficked (e.g., tuberculosis, dengue, malaria; see Chapter 10).

EXAMINATION AND DIAGNOSTIC TESTING

A thorough physical examination allows the provider to assess and treat acute and chronic medical conditions, collect forensic evidence (as appropriate), assess nutritional and developmental status, and document recent and remote injuries. Diagnostic testing may identify pregnancy, STIs, HIV, non–sexually transmitted infections, vitamin and mineral deficiencies, anemia, toxic exposures, drugs, or alcohol. A sexual assault evidence kit may reveal trace evidence or DNA from offenders. Informed assent for the exam, assault kit, and diagnostic tests is important, as is careful explanation of each step during the process, and monitoring of the patient for signs of distress and anxiety. Those who have been sex-trafficked may experience particular distress during the anogenital examination, the oral exam, and when injuries are photographed. A trauma-trained chaperone is very helpful in providing comfort and support to the patient. The examination should be conducted outside the presence of anyone suspected of being involved in the trafficking situation. After the exam the provider should explain the results, ask the child if they have any questions about the exam, and give them the opportunity to discuss concerns about their bodies. Trafficked persons may harbor anxiety about a variety of issues, including possible infertility, future health, or possible permanent damage from work-related injuries and toxic conditions.

Providers may follow U.S. Centers for Disease Control and Prevention (CDC) guidelines on STI testing and prophylaxis. Additional resources on laboratory testing for sexually and non–sexually transmitted diseases may be obtained from the CDC (https://www.cdc.gov/) or World Health Organization (WHO) websites (http://www.who.int/en/). In general, STIs of greatest relevance include *Neisseria gonorrhoeae*, *Chlamydia trachomatis*, *Trichomonas vaginalis*, HIV, syphilis, and hepatitis B and C viruses. Methods of testing and decisions to treat (e.g., positive test results vs prophylaxis vs syndromic treatment) will depend on national guidelines as well as on medical resources, which may be limited in some countries or regions. However, consideration should be given to the high likelihood that the patient may be lost to follow-up after the visit, so the decision to delay treatment until test results are available may lead to lack of needed medication. Testing and treatment decisions need to be outlined in a protocol. Emergency contraception and other methods of birth control (especially long-acting reversible contraception) should be discussed with the patient as feasible.

Many child victims of trafficking (and children of trafficked adults) have experienced nutritional deprivation, lack of immunizations, and general poor health, especially if they are from low-resource countries or are born into the trafficking situation. Guidance on **medical screening** and care for immigrant children (see Chapter 10) may also be obtained from the CDC or American Academy of Pediatrics (AAP) *Red Book* or *Immigrant Child Health Toolkit*.* Consideration should be given to vaccine-preventable diseases (including tetanus if there are open wounds) and common diseases in the child's home country. Domestic or international victims may have iron deficiency, hemoglobinopathies, vitamin D deficiency, and undiagnosed vision or hearing problems. Crowded, unhygienic living conditions during the trafficking period raise the risks of tuberculosis, scabies, and diarrheal illnesses. Toxic levels of lead or chemicals may be present, and vitamin/mineral deficiencies should be considered. A **developmental assessment** is important, given the high likelihood of poor primary care in the past and possible harsh living conditions.

Documentation of health and injuries is extremely important and should be detailed and accurate. Body diagrams and photographs (if not traumatizing to the child) are helpful, as are written descriptions of injury location, type (e.g., contusion, laceration), size, shape, and color. All photographs should include patient identifiers and a measuring instrument when possible. Distance photographs to establish injury location may be supplemented with close-up photographs from various angles. Physical signs of untreated illness, malnutrition, and other conditions need to be documented carefully. When documenting the medical history, direct quotes should be used when possible (quotes of provider and of victim statements). Records, including written, video, audio, and photographic records, should be stored in a secure health information system, with limited access and password protection. Strict protocols for patient confidentiality and privacy should be established and followed.

REFERRALS AND RESOURCES

Healthcare providers must comply with mandatory reporting laws in their state or country, but in doing so, should make every effort to avoid causing harm to the child or their family. In the event the parent is the trafficking victim rather than the child, care should be taken to make reports and referrals only with the victim's consent (unless child's safety/health are at risk). For those practicing within the United States, assistance on interpreting laws, working with suspected victims, making reports to authorities, and identifying local referral sources may be obtained by contacting the **National Human Trafficking Resource Center** (1-888-3737-888). The NHTRC has trained staff to assist victims and professionals alike, including interpreters for over 100 languages. Additional assistance may be obtained by contacting state or local law enforcement and antitrafficking task forces or local child advocacy centers. In some countries, "helplines" and "hotlines" may be used to seek assistance for suspected trafficking victims. It is important for the healthcare provider to be aware of local, state, and national resources for trafficking victims. Exploited persons have numerous needs that extend beyond the range of the healthcare provider's ability to respond. A multidisciplinary team approach is needed to ensure the child is provided with necessary food, shelter, crisis management, language interpretation, immigration assistance, mental health and medical care, educational needs, and other services. Such a team may include local victim service providers, shelter staff, behavioral health professionals, child protective services (CPS) workers, law enforcement, child advocacy center staff, sexual assault providers, and victim advocates. Table 15.5 lists potential health-related referrals.

Trafficked victims may face considerable **social stigma** and **discrimination**. They may be viewed as consenting participants, illegal immigrants who deserve maltreatment, or "bad kids" who are responsible for their own actions. In some countries, laws on sexual exploitation do not include boys, and cultural beliefs foster the attitude that males cannot be victimized. Variations in the age of consent may result in a child being considered an adult in one country and a child in another. For these reasons and others, it is important for the healthcare provider to advocate for the child's victim status when interacting with other

---

*https://www.aap.org/en-us/about-the-aap/Committees-Councils-Sections/Council-on-Community-Pediatrics/Pages/Section-1-Clinical-Care.aspx#q1.

Table 15.5	Potential Health Referrals for Trafficked Persons

Behavioral health assessment and treatment (emergent or nonurgent): trauma-focused, preferably conducted by professional trained in trauma therapies*
Substance abuse assessment/treatment
Obstetrician/gynecologist
Specialized medical service
Primary medical home (for immunizations including HPV, periodic STI testing, monitoring of growth and development, family planning, anticipatory guidance, nutrition/hygiene counseling, etc.)
Physical therapy, occupational therapy
Developmental assessment
Dentist
Optometrist or audiologist
Resources for LGBTQ
HIV clinic
Child advocacy center (for 2nd opinion on exam; forensic interview, behavioral health services)

*Appropriate therapy may differ with victims from varied cultures; there is a very limited evidence-base for effectiveness of behavioral health therapy for trafficked children. However, therapies with an evidence base for child sexual assault/abuse are often used in the U.S.
HPV, Human papillomavirus; HIV, human immunodeficiency virus; LGBTQ, lesbian, gay, bisexual, transgender, and questioning; STI, sexually transmitted infection.

professionals and emphasize the need for comprehensive, sustained, trauma-informed services.

Prior to discharge, the provider should ensure the patient understands the results of the evaluation and the treatment plan, has a safety plan, and is aware of options for future care. When referrals are being made, it is helpful for the provider to take steps to ensure services are actually obtained by following up with the referral staff, sending medical records (as appropriate and with victim consent), and assisting the victim with arrangements as feasible. It is also helpful to counsel the victim on their basic human rights, including their right to medical care. If responsible for long-term care of the child, the provider should consider that treatment needs change over time, so treatment plans must be reevaluated periodically. Continuity of care is important but can be challenging when the child is moved to another city, is transported back to the home country, or is re-trafficked. Communication and collaboration with external agencies and healthcare providers can be extremely helpful, along with assignment of a case manager to help ensure referrals are in place in destination towns or villages.

Bibliography is available at Expert Consult.

Chapter 16
Abused and Neglected Children
Howard Dubowitz and Wendy G. Lane

第十六章
虐待和疏于照顾

中文导读

　　本章主要介绍了虐待和疏于照顾的定义、在全球范围和美国本土发生和分布的情况、判断可疑虐待和疏忽的一般原则、处理虐待儿童问题的一般原则、遭受虐待和被疏于照顾的儿童的结局，以及如何预防、如何进行宣传支持。具体阐述了性虐待，内容包括定义、性虐待的表现、全科儿科医师在判断和处理可疑性虐待案例中的作用、可疑性虐待案例中的体格检查、其他如HIV抗体检测等的处理，以及如何防范性虐待；另外，还介绍了针对儿童的医疗虐待（代理型虚构疾病，代理型孟乔森综合征），内容包括临床表现、诊断和治疗。

The abuse and neglect (**maltreatment**) of children are pervasive problems worldwide, with short- and long-term physical and mental health and social consequences. Child healthcare professionals have an important role in helping address this problem. In addition to their responsibility to identify maltreated children and help ensure their protection and health, child healthcare professionals can also play vital roles related to prevention, treatment, and advocacy. Rates and policies vary greatly among nations and, often, within nations. Rates of maltreatment and provision of services are affected by the overall policies of the country, province, or state governing recognition and responses to child abuse and neglect. Two broad approaches have been identified: a *child and family welfare* approach and a *child safety* approach. Although overlapping, the focus in the former is the family as a whole, and in the latter, on the child perceived to be at risk. The United States has primarily had a child safety approach.

DEFINITIONS

Abuse is defined as acts of commission and **neglect** as acts of omission. The U.S. government defines *child abuse* as "any recent act or failure to act on the part of a parent or caretaker, which results in death, serious physical or emotional harm, sexual abuse or exploitation, or an act or failure to act which presents an imminent risk of serious harm." Some states also include other household members. Children may be found in situations in which no actual harm has occurred, and no imminent risk of serious harm is evident, but potential harm may be a concern. Many states include *potential harm* in their child abuse laws. Consideration of potential harm enables preventive intervention, although predicting potential harm is inherently difficult. Two aspects should be considered: the likelihood of harm and the severity of that harm.

Physical abuse includes beating, shaking, burning, and biting. **Corporal punishment**, however, is increasingly being prohibited. The Global Initiative to End All Corporal Punishment of Children reported that 52 countries have prohibited corporal punishment in all settings, including the home. Governments in 55 other countries have expressed a commitment to full prohibition. In the United States, corporal punishment in the home is lawful in all states, but 31 states have banned corporal punishment in public.

The threshold for defining corporal punishment as abuse is unclear. One can consider any injury beyond transient redness as abuse. If parents spank a child, it should be limited to the buttocks, should occur over clothing, and should never involve the head and neck. When parents use objects other than a hand, the potential for serious harm increases. Acts of serious violence (e.g., throwing a hard object, slapping an infant's face) should be seen as abusive even if no injury ensues; significant risk of harm exists. While some child healthcare professionals think that **hitting** is acceptable under limited conditions, almost all know that more constructive approaches to discipline are preferable. The American Academy of Pediatrics clearly opposed the use of corporal punishment in a recent policy statement. Although many think that hitting a child should never be accepted, and many studies have documented the potential harm, there remains a reluctance in the United States to label hitting as abuse, unless there is an injury. It is clear that the emotional impact of being hit may leave the most worrisome scar, long after the bruises fade and the fracture heals.

Sexual abuse has been defined as "the involvement of dependent, developmentally immature children and adolescents in sexual activities which they do not fully comprehend, to which they are unable to give consent, or that violate the social taboos of family roles." Sexual abuse includes exposure to sexually explicit materials, oral-genital contact, genital-to-genital contact, genital-to-anal contact, and genital fondling. Any touching of *private parts* by parents or caregivers in a context other than necessary care is inappropriate.

Neglect refers to omissions in care, resulting in actual or potential harm. *Omissions* include inadequate healthcare, education, supervision, protection from hazards in the environment, and unmet physical needs (e.g., clothing, food) and emotional support. A preferable alternative to focusing on caregiver omissions is to instead consider the *basic needs* (or rights) of children (e.g., adequate food, clothing, shelter, healthcare, education, nurturance). Neglect occurs when a need is not adequately met and results in actual or potential harm, whatever the reasons. A child whose health is jeopardized or harmed by not receiving necessary care experiences **medical neglect**. Not all such situations necessarily require a report to child protective services (CPS); less intrusive initial efforts may be appropriate.

Psychological abuse includes verbal abuse and humiliation and acts that scare or terrorize a child. Although this form of abuse may be extremely harmful to children, resulting in depression, anxiety, poor self-esteem, or lack of empathy, CPS seldom becomes involved because of the difficulty in proving such allegations. Child healthcare professionals should still carefully consider this form of maltreatment, even if the concern fails to reach a legal or agency threshold for reporting. These children and families can benefit from counseling and social support. Many children experience more than one form of maltreatment; CPS are more likely to address psychological abuse in the context of other forms of maltreatment.

Within in the United States and internationally, problems of **trafficking** in children, for purposes of cheap labor and sexual exploitation, expose children to all the forms of abuse just noted (see Chapter 15).

INCIDENCE AND PREVALENCE
Global
Child abuse and neglect are not rare and occur worldwide. Based on international studies, the World Health Organization (WHO) has estimated that 18% of girls and 8% of boys experience sexual abuse as children, while 23% of children report being physically abused (Figs. 16.1 and 16.2). In addition, many children experience emotional abuse and neglect. Surveys reported by United Nations Children's Fund (UNICEF) confirm these reports; one survey conducted in the Middle East reported that 30% of children had been beaten or tied up by parents, and in a survey in a Southeast Asian country, 30% of mothers reported having hit their child with an object in the past 6 mo.

United States
Abuse and neglect mostly occur behind closed doors and often are a well-kept secret. Nevertheless, there were 4 million reports to CPS involving 7.2 million children in the United States in 2015. Of the 683,000 children with substantiated reports (9.2 per 1,000 children), 78.3% experienced neglect (including 1.9% medical neglect), 17.2% physical abuse, 8.4% sexual abuse, and 6.2% psychological maltreatment. While there had been a decline in rates beginning in the early 1990s, rates increased in 2014 and 2015 from prior years. Likewise, the rate of hospitalized children with serious physical abuse has not declined in recent years. Medical personnel made 9.1% of all reports.

Other sources independent from the official CPS statistics cited above confirm the prevalence of child maltreatment. In a community survey, 3% of parents reported using very severe violence (e.g., hitting with fist, burning, using gun or knife) against their child in the prior year. Considering a natural disinclination to disclose socially undesirable information, such rates are both conservative and alarming.

ETIOLOGY
Child maltreatment seldom has a single cause; rather, multiple and interacting biopsychosocial **risk factors** at 4 levels usually exist. To illustrate, at the *individual level*, a child's disability or a parent's depression or substance abuse predispose a child to maltreatment. At the *familial level*, intimate partner (or domestic) violence presents risks for children. Influential *community factors* include stressors such as dangerous neighborhoods or a lack of recreational facilities. Professional inaction may contribute to neglect, such as when the treatment plan is not clearly communicated. Broad *societal factors*, such as poverty and its associated burdens, also contribute to maltreatment. WHO estimates the rate of homicide of children is approximately 2-fold higher in low-income compared to high-income countries (2.58 vs 1.21 per 100,000 population), but clearly homicide occurs in high-income countries too. Children in all social classes can be maltreated, and child healthcare professionals need to guard against biases concerning low-income families.

In contrast, **protective factors**, such as family supports, or a mother's concern for her child, may buffer risk factors and protect children from

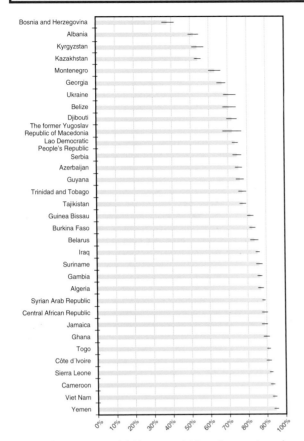

Fig. 16.1 Percentage of children ages 2-14 yr who experienced any violent discipline (physical punishment and/or psychological aggression) in the past month, by country. *(United Nations Children's Fund, Hidden in Plain Sight: A statistical analysis of violence against children. UNICEF, New York, 2014, Fig 2.* http://www.data.unicef.org/resources/hidden-in-plain-sight.)

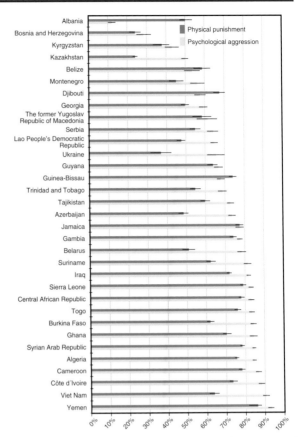

Fig. 16.2 Percentage of children ages 2-14 yr who experienced psychological aggression and percentage of children ages 2-14 yr who experienced physical punishment in the past month, by country, 2005–2006. *(United Nations Children's Fund, Hidden in Plain Sight: A statistical analysis of violence against children. UNICEF, New York, Fig 2.* http://www.data.unicef.org/resources/hidden-in-plain-sight.)

maltreatment. Identifying and building on protective factors can be vital to intervening effectively. One can say to a parent, "I can see how much you love [child's name]. What can we do to keep her out of the hospital?" Child maltreatment results from a complex interplay among risk and protective factors. A single mother who has a colicky baby and who recently lost her job is at risk for maltreatment, but a loving grandmother may be protective. A good understanding of factors that contribute to maltreatment, as well as those that are protective, should guide an appropriate response.

CLINICAL MANIFESTATIONS

Child abuse and neglect can manifest in many ways. A critical element of physical abuse is the lack of a plausible history other than inflicted trauma. The onus is on the clinician to carefully consider the differential diagnosis and not jump to conclusions.

Bruises are the most common manifestation of physical abuse. Features suggestive of inflicted bruises include (1) bruising in a preambulatory infant (occurring in just 2% of infants), (2) bruising of padded and less exposed areas (buttocks, cheeks, ears, genitalia), (3) patterned bruising or burns conforming to shape of an object or ligatures around the wrists, and (4) multiple bruises, especially if clearly of different ages (Fig. 16.3 and Table 16.1). Earlier suggestions for estimating the age of bruises have been discredited. It is very difficult to precisely determine the ages of bruises.

Other conditions such as birthmarks and congenital dermal melanocytosis (e.g., mongolian spots) can be confused with bruises and

abuse. These skin markings are not tender and do not rapidly change color or size. An underlying medical explanation for bruises may exist, such as blood dyscrasias (hemophilia) or connective tissue disorders (Ehlers-Danlos syndrome). The history or examination usually provides clues to these conditions. Henoch-Schönlein purpura, the most common vasculitis in young children, may be confused with abuse. The pattern and location of bruises caused by abuse are usually different from those due to a coagulopathy. Noninflicted bruises are characteristically anterior and over bony prominences, such as shins and forehead. The presence of a medical disorder does not preclude abuse.

Cultural practices can cause bruising. Cao gio, or *coining*, is a Southeast Asian folkloric therapy. A hard object is vigorously rubbed on the skin, causing petechiae or purpura. *Cupping* is another approach, popular in the Middle East. A heated glass is applied to the skin, often on the back. As it cools, a vacuum is formed, leading to perfectly circular bruises. The context here is important, and such circumstances should not be considered abusive (see Chapter 11).

A careful history of bleeding problems in the patient and first-degree relatives is needed. If a bleeding disorder is suspected, a complete blood count including platelet count, prothrombin time, and partial thromboplastin time should be obtained. More extensive testing, such as factors VIII, IX and XIII activity and von Willebrand evaluation, should be considered in consultation with a hematologist.

Bites have a characteristic pattern of 1 or 2 opposing arches with multiple bruises. They can be inflicted by an adult, another child, an animal, or the patient. Forensic odontologists have previously developed

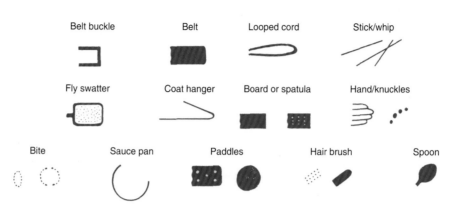

Fig. 16.3 A variety of instruments may be used to inflict injury on a child. Often the choice of an instrument is a matter of convenience. Marks tend to silhouette or outline the shape of the instrument. The possibility of intentional trauma should prompt a high degree of suspicion when injuries to a child are geometric, paired, mirrored, of various ages or types, or on relatively protected parts of the body. Early recognition of intentional trauma is important to provide therapy and prevent escalation to more serious injury.

Table 16.1	Injury Patterns
METHOD OF INJURY/ IMPLEMENT	**PATTERN OBSERVED**
Grip/grab	Relatively round marks that correspond to fingertips and/or thumb
Closed-fist punch	Series of round bruises that correspond to knuckles of the hand
Slap	Parallel, linear bruises (usually petechial) separated by areas of central sparing
Belt/electrical cord	Loop marks or parallel lines of petechiae (the width of the belt/cord) with central sparing; may see triangular marks from the end of the belt, small circular lesions caused by the holes in the tongue of the belt, and/or a buckle pattern
Rope	Areas of bruising interspersed with areas of abrasion
Other objects/household implements	Injury in shape of object/implement (e.g., rods, switches, and wires cause linear bruising)
Human bite	Two arches forming a circular or oval shape, may cause bruising and/or abrasion
Strangulation	Petechiae of the head and/or neck, including mucous membranes; may see subconjunctival hemorrhages
Binding/ligature	Marks around the wrists, ankles, or neck; sometimes accompanied by petechiae or edema distal to the ligature mark Marks adjacent to the mouth if the child has been gagged
Excessive *hincar**	Abrasions/burns, especially to knees
Hair pulling	Traumatic alopecia; may see petechiae on underlying scalp, or swelling or tenderness of the scalp (from subgaleal hematoma)
Tattooing or intentional scarring	Abusive cases have been described, but can also be a cultural phenomenon (e.g., Maori body ornamentation)

*Punishment by kneeling on salt or other rough substance.

guidelines for distinguishing adult from child and human from animal bites. However, several studies have identified problems with the accuracy and consistency of bite mark analysis.

Burns may be inflicted or caused by inadequate supervision. Scalding burns may result from immersion or splash. *Immersion burns*, when a child is forcibly held in hot water, show clear delineation between the burned and healthy skin and uniform depth. They may have a sock or glove distribution. Splash marks are usually absent, unlike when a child inadvertently encounters hot water. Symmetric burns are especially suggestive of abuse, as are burns of the buttocks and perineum (Fig. 16.4). Although most often accidental, splash burns may also result from abuse. Burns from hot objects such as curling irons, radiators, steam irons, metal grids, hot knives, and cigarettes leave patterns representing the object (Fig. 16.5). A child is likely to draw back rapidly

from a hot object; thus burns that are extensive and deep reflect more than fleeting contact and are suggestive of abuse.

Several conditions mimic abusive burns, such as brushing against a hot radiator, car seat burns, hemangiomas, and folk remedies such as moxibustion. Impetigo may resemble cigarette burns. *Cigarette burns* are usually 7-10 mm across, whereas impetigo has lesions of varying size. Noninflicted cigarette burns are usually oval and superficial.

Neglect frequently contributes to childhood burns. Children, home alone, may be burned in house fires. A parent taking drugs may cause a fire and may be unable to protect a child. Exploring children may pull hot liquids left unattended onto themselves. Liquids cool as they flow downward so that the burn is most severe and broad proximally. If the child is wearing a diaper or clothing, the fabric may absorb the hot water and cause burns worse than otherwise expected. Some circumstances are

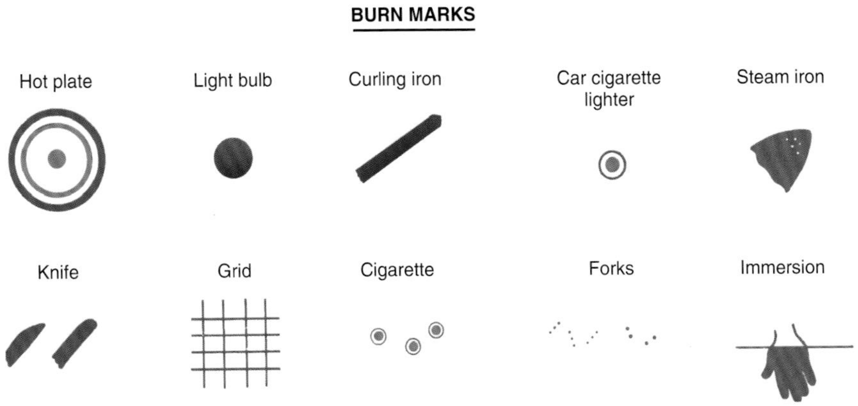

BURN MARKS

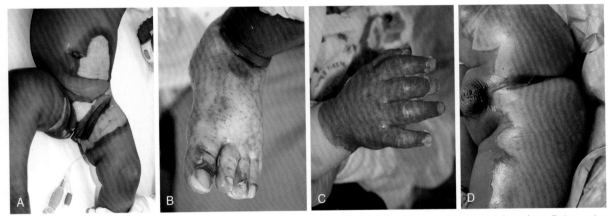

Hot plate   Light bulb   Curling iron   Car cigarette lighter   Steam iron

Knife   Grid   Cigarette   Forks   Immersion

Fig. 16.4 Marks from heated objects cause burns in a pattern that duplicates that of the object. Familiarity with the common heated objects that are used to traumatize children facilitates recognition of possible intentional injuries. The location of the burn is important in determining its cause. Children tend to explore surfaces with the palmar surface of the hand and rarely touch a heated object repeatedly for long.

Fig. 16.5 Immersion injury patterns. **A,** Sparing of the flexoral creases. **B,** Immersion "stocking" burn. **C,** Immersion "glove" burn. **D,** Immersion buttocks burn. *(From Jenny C: Child abuse and neglect: diagnosis, treatment, and evidence, Philadelphia, 2011, Saunders, p. 225, Fig 28-3)*

difficult to foresee, and a single burn resulting from a momentary lapse in supervision should not automatically be seen as neglectful parenting.

Concluding whether a burn was inflicted depends on the history, burn pattern, and the child's capabilities. A delay in seeking healthcare may result from the burn initially appearing minor, before blistering or becoming infected. This circumstance may represent reasonable behavior and should not be automatically deemed neglectful. A home investigation is often valuable (e.g., testing the water temperature).

Fractures that strongly suggest abuse include classic metaphyseal lesions, posterior rib fractures, and fractures of the scapula, sternum, and spinous processes, especially in young children (Table 16.2). These fractures all require more force than would be expected from a minor fall or routine handling and activities of a child. Rib and sternal fractures rarely result from cardiopulmonary resuscitation (CPR), even when performed by untrained adults. The recommended 2-finger or 2-thumb technique recommended for infants since 2005 may produce anterolateral rib fractures. In abused infants, rib (Fig. 16.6), metaphyseal (Fig. 16.7), and skull fractures are most common. Femoral and humeral fractures in nonambulatory infants are also very worrisome for abuse. With increasing mobility and running, toddlers can fall with enough rotational force to cause a spiral, femoral fracture. Multiple fractures in various stages of healing are suggestive of abuse; nevertheless, underlying conditions need to be considered. Clavicular, femoral, supracondylar humeral, and distal extremity fractures in children older than 2 yr are most likely noninflicted unless they are multiple or accompanied by

Table 16.2	Specificity of Radiologic Findings for Fractures

HIGH SPECIFICITY*
Classic metaphyseal lesions
Rib fractures, especially posteromedial
Scapular fractures
Spinous process fractures
Sternal fractures

MODERATE SPECIFICITY
Multiple fractures, especially bilateral
Fractures of different ages
Epiphyseal separations
Vertebral body fractures and subluxations
Digital fractures
Complex skull fractures
Pelvic fractures

COMMON BUT LOW SPECIFICITY
Subperiosteal new bone formation
Clavicular fractures
Long-bone shaft fractures
Linear skull fractures

*Highest specificity applies in infants.
From Kleinman PK: *Diagnostic imaging of child abuse,* ed 3, Cambridge, UK, 2015, Cambridge University Press, p 24.

other signs of abuse. Few fractures are pathognomonic of abuse; all must be considered in light of the history and the child's developmental level. Fractures may present as an irritable fussy child.

The differential diagnosis includes conditions that increase susceptibility to fractures, such as osteopenia and osteogenesis imperfecta, metabolic and nutritional disorders (e.g., scurvy, rickets), renal osteodystrophy, osteomyelitis, congenital syphilis, and neoplasia. Some have pointed to possible rickets and low but subclinical levels of vitamin D as being responsible for fractures thought to be abusive. The evidence to date does not support this supposition. Features of congenital or metabolic conditions associated with nonabusive fractures include family history

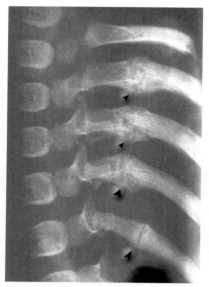

Fig. 16.6 High-detail oblique view of the ribs of a 6 mo old infant shows multiple healing posteromedial rib fractures (*arrowheads*). The level of detail in this image is far greater than what would be present on a standard chest radiograph. (*From Dwek JR: The radiographic approach to child abuse, Clin Orthop Relat Res 469:776–789, 2011, p 780, Fig 4.*)

of recurrent fractures after minor trauma, abnormally shaped cranium, dentinogenesis imperfecta, blue sclera, craniotabes, ligamentous laxity, bowed legs, hernia, and translucent skin. *Subperiosteal new bone formation* is a nonspecific finding seen in infectious, traumatic, and metabolic disorders. In young infants, new bone formation may be a normal physiologic finding, usually bilateral, symmetric, and <2 mm in depth.

The evaluation of a fracture should include a skeletal radiologic survey in children <2 yr old when abuse seems possible (Table 16.3). Multiple radiographs with different views are needed; "babygrams" (1 or 2 films of the entire body) should be avoided. If the survey is normal, but concern for an occult injury remains, a radionucleotide bone scan should be performed to detect a possible acute injury. Follow-up films after 2 wk may also reveal fractures not apparent initially.

In corroborating the history and the injury, the age of a fracture can be crudely estimated (Table 16.4). Soft tissue swelling subsides in 2-21 days. Subperiosteal new bone is visible within 6-21 days. Loss of definition of the fracture line occurs in 10-21 days. Soft callus can be visible after 9 days and hard callus at 14-90 days. These ranges are shorter in infancy and longer in children with poor nutritional status or a chronic underlying disease. Fractures of flat bones such as the skull do not form callus and cannot be aged, although soft tissue swelling indicates approximate recency (within the prior week).

Abusive head trauma (AHT) results in the most significant morbidity and mortality. Abusive injury may be caused by direct impact, asphyxia, or shaking. Subdural hematomas (Fig. 16.8), retinal hemorrhages, especially when extensive and involving multiple layers, and diffuse axonal injury strongly suggest AHT, especially when they occur together. The poor neck muscle tone and relatively large heads of infants make them vulnerable to acceleration-deceleration forces associated with shaking, leading to AHT. Children may lack external signs of injury, even with serious intracranial trauma. Signs and symptoms may be nonspecific, ranging from lethargy, vomiting (without diarrhea), changing neurologic status or seizures, and coma. In all preverbal children, an index of suspicion for AHT should exist when children present with these signs and symptoms.

Acute intracranial trauma is best evaluated by initial and follow-up CT. MRI is helpful in differentiating extra axial fluid, determining timing of injuries, assessing parenchymal injury, and identifying vascular anomalies. MRI is best obtained 5-7 days after an acute injury. Glutaric aciduria type 1 can present with intracranial bleeding and should be considered. Other causes of subdural hemorrhage in infants include

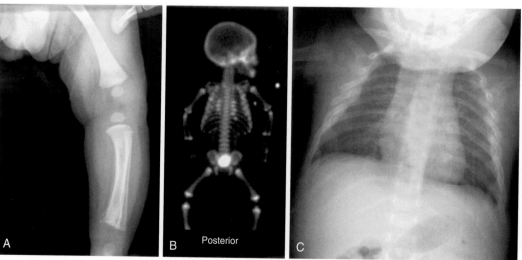

Fig. 16.7 A, Metaphyseal fracture of the distal tibia in a 3 mo old infant admitted to the hospital with severe head injury. There is also periosteal new bone formation of the tibia, perhaps from previous injury. **B,** Bone scan of same infant. Initial chest radiograph showed a single fracture of the right posterior 4th rib. A radionuclide bone scan performed 2 days later revealed multiple previously unrecognized fractures of the posterior and lateral ribs. **C,** Follow-up radiographs 2 wk later showed multiple healing rib fractures. This pattern of fracture is highly specific for child abuse. The mechanism of these injuries is usually violent squeezing of the chest.

Table 16.3	Radiologic Skeletal Survey for Infants and Children Under 2 Yr of Age*

- Anteroposterior (AP) and lateral views of skull (Townes view optional; add if any fracture seen)
- Lateral spine (cervical spine [C-spine] may be included on skull radiographs; AP spine is included on AP chest and AP pelvis views to include entire spine)
- AP view, right posterior oblique, left posterior oblique view of chest—rib technique
- AP pelvis
- AP view of each femur
- AP view of each leg
- AP view of each humerus
- AP view of each forearm
- Posteroanterior (PA) view of each hand
- AP (dorsoventral) view of each foot

*Images are checked by a radiologist before the patient leaves. Poorly positioned or otherwise suboptimal images should be repeated. Lateral views are added for positive or equivocal findings in the extremities. Coned views of positive or equivocal findings (i.e., at ends of long bones, ribs) may be obtained.

Adapted from Coley BD: *Caffey's pediatric diagnostic imaging*, ed 12, vol 2, Philadelphia, 2013, Mosby/Elsevier, p 1588 (Box 144-1).

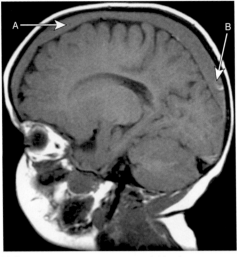

Fig. 16.8 CT scan indicating intracranial bleeding. *A arrow*, Older blood. *B arrow*, New blood.

Table 16.4	Timetable of Radiologic Changes in Children's Fractures* (in Days)		
CATEGORY	**EARLY**	**PEAK**	**LATE**
1. Subperiosteal new bone formation	4-10	10-14	14-21
2. Loss of fracture line definition		10-14	14-21
3. Soft callus		10-14	14-21
4. Hard callus	14-21	21-42	42-90

*Repetitive injuries may prolong all categories. The time points tend to increase from early infancy into childhood.

Adapted from Kleinman PK: *Diagnostic imaging of child abuse*, ed 3, Cambridge, UK, 2015, Cambridge University Press, p 215.

arteriovenous malformations, coagulopathies, birth trauma, tumor, and infections. When AHT is suspected, injuries elsewhere—skeletal and abdominal—should be ruled out.

Retinal hemorrhages are an important marker of AHT (Fig. 16.9). Whenever AHT is being considered, a dilated indirect eye examination by a pediatric ophthalmologist should be performed. Although retinal hemorrhages can be found in other conditions, hemorrhages that are multiple, involve >1 layer of the retina, and extend to the periphery are very suspicious for abuse. The mechanism is likely repeated acceleration-deceleration from shaking. Traumatic retinoschisis points strongly to abuse.

With other causes of retinal hemorrhages, the pattern is usually different than seen in child abuse. After birth, many newborns have them, but they disappear in 2-6 wk. Coagulopathies (particularly leukemia), retinal diseases, carbon monoxide poisoning, or glutaric aciduria may be responsible. Severe, noninflicted, direct crush injury to the head can rarely cause an extensive hemorrhagic retinopathy. CPR rarely, if ever, causes retinal hemorrhage in infants and children; if present, there a few hemorrhages in the posterior pole. Hemoglobin-opathies, diabetes mellitus, routine play, minor noninflicted head trauma, and vaccinations do not appear to cause retinal hemorrhage in children. Severe coughing or seizures rarely cause retinal hemorrhages that could be confused with AHT.

The dilemma frequently posed is whether minor, everyday forces can explain the findings seen in AHT. Simple linear skull fractures in the absence of other suggestive evidence can be explained by a short fall, although even that is rare (1-2%), and underlying brain injury from short falls is exceedingly rare. Timing of brain injuries in cases of abuse is not precise. In fatal cases, however, the trauma most likely occurred very soon before the child became symptomatic.

Other manifestations of AHT may be seen. *Raccoon eyes* occur in association with subgaleal hematomas after traction on the anterior hair and scalp, or after a blow to the forehead. Neuroblastoma can present similarly and should be considered. Bruises from attempted strangulation may be visible on the neck. Choking or suffocation can cause hypoxic brain injury, often with no external signs.

Abdominal trauma accounts for significant morbidity and mortality in abused children. Young children are especially vulnerable because of their relatively large abdomens and lax abdominal musculature. A forceful blow or kick can cause hematomas of solid organs (liver, spleen, kidney) from compression against the spine, as well as hematoma (duodenal) or rupture (stomach) of hollow organs. Intraabdominal bleeding may result from trauma to an organ or from shearing of a vessel. More than 1 organ may be affected. Children may present with cardiovascular failure or an acute condition of the abdomen, often after a delay in care. Bilious vomiting without fever or peritoneal irritation suggests a duodenal hematoma, often caused by abuse.

The manifestations of abdominal trauma are often subtle, even with severe injuries. Bruising of the abdominal wall is unusual, and symptoms may evolve slowly. Delayed perforation may occur days after the injury; bowel strictures or a pancreatic pseudocyst may occur weeks or months later. Child healthcare professionals should consider screening for occult abdominal trauma when other evidence of physical abuse exists. Screening should include liver and pancreatic enzyme levels, and testing urine for blood. Children with lab results indicating possible injury should have abdominal CT performed. CT or ultrasound should also be performed if there is concern about possible splenic, adrenal, hepatic, or reproductive organ injury.

Oral lesions may present as bruised lips, bleeding, torn frenulum, and dental trauma or caries (neglect).

Neglect

Neglect is the most prevalent form of child maltreatment, with potentially severe and lasting sequelae. It may manifest in many ways, depending on which needs are not adequately met. Nonadherence to medical treatment, for example, may aggravate the condition, as may a delay in seeking care. Inadequate food may manifest as impaired growth; inattention to obesity may compound that problem. Poor hygiene may contribute to infected cuts or lesions. Inadequate supervision contributes to injuries and ingestions. Children's needs for mental healthcare, dental

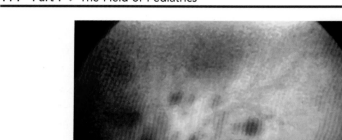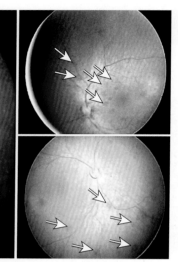

Fig. 16.9 Retinal hemorrhages. *Arrows* point to hemorrhages of various sizes.

care, and other health-related needs may be unmet, manifesting as neglect in those areas. Educational needs, particularly for children with learning disabilities, are often not met.

The evaluation of possible neglect requires addressing critical questions: "Is this neglect?" and "Have the circumstances harmed the child, or jeopardized the child's health and safety?" For example, suboptimal treatment adherence may lead to few or no clear consequences. Inadequacies in the care that children receive naturally fall along a continuum, requiring a range of responses tailored to the individual situation. Legal considerations or CPS policies may discourage physicians from labeling many circumstances as neglect. Even if neglect does not meet a threshold for reporting to CPS, child healthcare professionals can still help ensure children's needs are adequately met.

GENERAL PRINCIPLES FOR ASSESSING POSSIBLE ABUSE AND NEGLECT

The heterogeneity of circumstances in situations of child maltreatment precludes specific detailing of varied assessments. The following are useful general principles.

◆ Given the complexity and possible ramifications of determining child maltreatment, an **interdisciplinary assessment** is optimal, with input from all involved professionals. Consultation with a physician expert in child maltreatment is recommended.

◆ A thorough **history** should be obtained from the parent(s) optimally via separate interviews.

◆ Verbal children should be interviewed separately, in a developmentally appropriate manner. **Open-ended questions** (e.g., "Tell me what happened") are best. Some children need more directed questioning (e.g., "How did you get that bruise?"); others need multiple-choice questions. Leading questions must be avoided (e.g., "Did your daddy hit you?").

◆ A thorough **physical examination** is necessary.

◆ Careful **documentation** of the history and physical is essential. Verbatim quotes are valuable, including the question that prompted the response. Photographs are helpful.

◆ For **abuse**: What is the evidence for concluding abuse? Have other diagnoses been ruled out? What is the likely mechanism of the injury? When did the injury likely occur?

◆ For **neglect**: Do the circumstances indicate that the child's needs have not been adequately met? Is there evidence of actual harm? Is there evidence of potential harm and on what basis? What is the nature of the neglect? Is there a pattern of neglect?

◆ Are there indications of other forms of maltreatment? Has there been prior CPS involvement?

◆ A child's **safety** is a paramount concern. What is the risk of imminent harm, and of what severity?

◆ What is contributing to the maltreatment? Consider the categories described in the section on etiology.

◆ What **strengths/resources** are there? This is as important as identifying problems.

◆ What **interventions** have been tried, with what results? Knowing the nature of these interventions can be useful, including from the parent's perspective.

◆ What is the **prognosis**? Is the family motivated to improve the circumstances and accept help, or resistant? Are suitable resources, formal and informal, available?

◆ Are there other children in the home who should be assessed for maltreatment?

GENERAL PRINCIPLES FOR ADDRESSING CHILD MALTREATMENT

The heterogeneity of circumstances also precludes specific details regarding how to address different types of maltreatment. The following are general principles.

◆ Treat any medical problems.

◆ Help ensure the child's **safety**, often in conjunction with CPS; this is a priority.

◆ Convey concerns of maltreatment to parents, kindly but forthrightly. Avoid blaming. It is natural to feel anger toward parents of maltreated children, but they need support and deserve respect.

◆ Have a means of addressing the difficult emotions child maltreatment can evoke.

◆ Be empathic, and state interest in helping or suggest another pediatrician.

◆ Know your national and state laws and/or local CPS policies on reporting child maltreatment. In the United States, the legal threshold for reporting is typically "reason to believe" (or similar language such as "reason to suspect"); one does not need to be certain. Physical abuse and moderate to severe neglect warrant a report. In less severe, less intrusive interventions may be an appropriate initial response. For example, if an infant's mild failure to thrive is caused by an error in mixing the formula, parent education and perhaps a visiting nurse should be tried. In contrast, severe failure to thrive may require hospitalization, and if the contributing factors are particularly serious (e.g., psychotic mother), out-of-home placement may be needed. CPS can assess the home environment, providing valuable insights.

◆ Reporting child maltreatment is never easy. Parental inadequacy or culpability is at least implicit, and parents may express considerable anger. Child healthcare professionals should supportively inform families directly of the report; it can be explained as an effort to clarify the situation and provide help, as well as a professional (and legal) responsibility. Explaining what the ensuing process is likely to entail (e.g., a visit from a CPS worker and sometimes a police officer) may ease a parent's anxiety. Parents are frequently concerned that they might lose their child. Child healthcare professionals can cautiously reassure parents that CPS is responsible for helping children and families and that, in most instances, children remain with their parents. When CPS does not accept a report or when a report is not substantiated, they may still offer voluntary supportive services such as food, shelter, parenting resources, and childcare. Child healthcare professionals can be a useful liaison between the family and the public agencies and should try to remain involved after reporting to CPS.

◆ Help address contributory factors, prioritizing those most important and amenable to being remedied. Concrete needs should not be overlooked; accessing nutrition programs, obtaining health insurance, enrolling children in preschool programs, and help finding safe housing can make a valuable difference. Parents may need their own problems addressed to enable them to provide adequate care for their children.

◆ Establish specific **objectives** (e.g., no hitting, diabetes will be adequately controlled), with measurable **outcomes** (e.g., urine dipsticks, hemoglobin A1c). Similarly, advice should be specific and limited to a few reasonable steps. A written contract can be very helpful.

◆ Engage the family in developing the plan, solicit their input and agreement.

◆ Build on **strengths**; there are always some. These provide a valuable way to engage parents.

◆ Encourage informal supports (e.g., family, friends; invite fathers to office visits). This is where most people get their support, not from professionals. Consider support available through a family's religious affiliation.

◆ Consider children's **specific needs**. Too often, maltreated children do not receive direct services.

◆ Be knowledgeable about community resources, and facilitate appropriate referrals.

◆ Provide support, follow-up, review of progress, and adjust the plan if needed.

◆ Recognize that maltreatment often requires long-term intervention with ongoing support and monitoring.

OUTCOMES OF CHILD MALTREATMENT

Child maltreatment often has significant short- and long-term medical, mental health, and social sequelae. Physically abused children are at risk for many problems, including conduct disorders, aggressive behavior, posttraumatic stress disorder (PTSD), anxiety and mood disorders, decreased cognitive functioning, and poor academic performance. Neglect is similarly associated with many potential problems. Even if a maltreated child appears to be functioning well, healthcare professionals and parents need to be sensitive to the possibility of later problems. Maltreatment is associated with increased risk in adolescence and adulthood for health risk behaviors (e.g., smoking, alcohol/drug abuse), mental health problems (e.g., anxiety, depression, suicide attempt), physical health problems (e.g., heart disease, arthritis), and mental health problems. Maltreated children are at risk for becoming abusive parents. The neurobiologic effects of child abuse and neglect on the developing brain may partly explain some of these sequelae.

Some children appear to be resilient and may not exhibit sequelae of maltreatment, perhaps because of protective factors or interventions. The benefits of intervention have been found in even the most severely neglected children, such as those from Romanian orphanages, who were adopted—the earlier the better.

PREVENTION OF CHILD ABUSE AND NEGLECT

An important aspect of prevention is that many of the efforts to strengthen families and support parents should promote children's health, development, and safety, as well as prevent child abuse and neglect. Medical responses to child maltreatment have typically occurred after the fact;

preventing the problem is preferable. Child healthcare professionals can help in several ways. An ongoing relationship offers opportunities to develop trust and knowledge of a family's circumstances. Astute observation of parent–child interactions can reveal useful information.

Parent and child education regarding medical conditions helps to ensure implementation of the treatment plan and to prevent neglect. Possible barriers to treatment should be addressed. Practical strategies such as writing down the plan can help. In addition, anticipatory guidance may help with child rearing, diminishing the risk of maltreatment. Hospital-based programs that educate parents about infant crying and the risks of shaking the infant may help prevent abusive head trauma.

Screening for major psychosocial risk factors for maltreatment (depression, substance abuse, intimate partner violence, major stress), and helping address identified problems, often through referrals, may help prevent maltreatment. The primary care focus on prevention offers excellent opportunities to screen briefly for psychosocial problems. The traditional organ system–focused review of systems can be expanded to probe areas such as feelings about the child, the parent's own functioning, possible depression, substance abuse, intimate partner violence, disciplinary approaches, stressors, and supports. The **Safe Environment for Every Kid** (SEEK) model offers a promising approach for pediatric primary care to identify and help address prevalent psychosocial problems. This can strengthen families; support parents; promote children's health, development, and safety; and help prevent child maltreatment.

Obtaining information directly from children or youth is also important, especially given that separate interviews with teens have become the norm. Any concerns identified on such screens require at least brief assessment and initial management, which may lead to a referral for further evaluation and treatment. More frequent office visits can be scheduled for support and counseling while monitoring the situation. Other key family members (e.g., fathers) might be invited to participate, thereby encouraging informal support. Practices might arrange parent groups through which problems and solutions are shared.

Child healthcare professionals also need to recognize their limitations and facilitate referrals to other community resources. Finally, the problems underpinning child maltreatment, such as poverty, parental stress, substance abuse, and limited child-rearing resources, require policies and programs that enhance families' abilities to care for their children adequately. Child healthcare professionals can help advocate for such policies and programs.

ADVOCACY

Child healthcare professionals can assist in understanding what contributed to the child's maltreatment. When advocating for the best interest of the child and family, addressing risk factors at the individual, family, and community levels is optimal. At the individual level, an example of advocating on behalf of a child is explaining to a parent that an active toddler is behaving normally and not intentionally challenging the parent. Encouraging a mother to seek help dealing with a violent spouse (e.g., saying, "You and your life are very important"), asking about substance abuse, and helping parents obtain health insurance for their children are all forms of advocacy.

Efforts to improve family functioning, such as encouraging fathers' involvement in child care, are also examples of advocacy. Remaining involved after a report to CPS and helping ensure appropriate services are provided is advocacy as well. In the community, child health professionals can be influential advocates for maximizing resources devoted to children and families. These include parenting programs, services for abused women and children, and recreational facilities. Lastly, child healthcare professionals can play an important role in advocating for policies and programs at the local, state, and national levels to benefit children and families. Child maltreatment is a complex problem that has no easy solutions. Through partnerships with colleagues in child protection, mental health, education, and law enforcement, child health professionals can make a valuable difference in the lives of many children and families.

Bibliography is available at Expert Consult.

16.1 Sexual Abuse

Wendy G. Lane and Howard Dubowitz

See also Chapter 145.

Approximately 18% of females and 7% of males in the United States will be sexually abused at some point during their childhood. Whether children and families share this information with their pediatrician will depend largely on the pediatrician's comfort with and openness to discussing possible sexual abuse with families. Pediatricians may play a number of different roles in addressing sexual abuse, including identification, reporting to child protective services (CPS), testing for and treating sexually transmitted infections (STIs), and providing support and reassurance to children and families. Pediatricians may also play a role in the prevention of sexual abuse by advising parents and children about ways to help keep safe from sexual abuse. In many U.S. jurisdictions, general pediatricians will play a *triage* role, with the definitive medical evaluation conducted by a child abuse specialist.

DEFINITION

Sexual abuse may be defined as any sexual behavior or action toward a child that is unwanted or exploitative. Some legal definitions distinguish sexual abuse from **sexual assault**: abuse being committed by a caregiver or household member, and assault being committed by someone with a noncustodial relationship or no relationship with the child. For this chapter, the term *sexual abuse* will encompass both abuse and assault. It is important to note that sexual abuse does not have to involve direct touching or contact by the perpetrator. Showing pornography to a child, filming or photographing a child in sexually explicit poses, and encouraging or forcing one child to perform sex acts on another all constitute sexual abuse.

PRESENTATION OF SEXUAL ABUSE

Children who have been sexually abused sometimes provide a clear, spontaneous disclosure to a trusted adult. Often the signs of sexual abuse are subtle. For some children, behavioral changes are the first indication that something is amiss. **Nonspecific behavior changes** such as social withdrawal, acting out, increased clinginess or fearfulness, distractibility, and learning difficulties may be attributed to a variety of life changes or stressors. Regression in developmental milestones, including new-onset bed-wetting or encopresis, is another behavior that caregivers may overlook as an indicator of sexual abuse. Teenagers may respond by becoming depressed, experimenting with drugs or alcohol, or running away from home. Because nonspecific symptoms are very common among children who have been sexually abused, it should almost always be included in one's differential diagnosis of child behavior changes.

Some children may not exhibit behavioral changes or provide any other indication that something is wrong. For these children, sexual abuse may be discovered when another person witnesses the abuse or discovers evidence such as sexually explicit photographs or videos. Pregnancy may be another way that sexual abuse is identified. Other children, some with and some without symptoms, will not be identified at any point during their childhood.

Caregivers may become concerned about the possibility of sexual abuse when children exhibit **sexually explicit behavior**. This behavior includes that which is outside the norm for a child's age and developmental level. For preschool and school-age children, sexually explicit behavior may include compulsive masturbation, attempting to perform sex acts on adults or other children, or asking adults or children to perform sex acts on them. Teenagers may become sexually promiscuous and even engage in prostitution. Older children and teenagers may respond by sexually abusing younger children. It is important to recognize that this behavior could also result from accidental exposure (e.g., child enters parents' bedroom at night and sees them having sex), or from neglect (e.g., adults watching pornographic movies where a child can see them).

ROLE OF GENERAL PEDIATRICIAN IN ASSESSMENT AND MANAGEMENT OF POSSIBLE SEXUAL ABUSE

Before determining where and how a child with suspected sexual abuse is evaluated, it is important to assess for and rule out any medical problems that can be confused with abuse. A number of **genital findings** may raise concern about abuse but often have alternative explanations. Genital redness in a prepubertal child is more often caused by nonspecific vulvovaginitis, eczema, or infection with staphylococcus, group A streptococcus, *Haemophilus*, or yeast. Lichen sclerosis is a less common cause of redness. Vaginal discharge can be caused by STIs, but also by poor hygiene, vaginal foreign body, early in the onset of puberty, or infection with *Salmonella*, *Shigella*, or *Yersinia*. Genital ulcers can be caused by herpes simplex virus (HSV) and syphilis, but also by Epstein-Barr virus, varicella-zoster virus, Crohn disease, and Behçet disease. Genital bleeding can be caused by urethral prolapse, vaginal foreign body, accidental trauma, and vaginal tumor.

Although other medical conditions may need to be evaluated, any possible sexual abuse should be investigated (Fig. 16.10). Where and how a child with suspected sexual abuse is evaluated should be determined by duration since the last incident of abuse likely occurred, and whether the child is prepubertal or postpubertal. For the *prepubertal child*, if abuse has occurred in the previous 72 hr, and history suggests direct contact, forensic evidence collection (e.g., external genital, vaginal, anal, and oral swabs, sometimes referred to as a "rape kit") is indicated, and the child should be referred to a site equipped to collect forensic evidence. Depending on the jurisdiction, this site may be an emergency department (ED), a child advocacy center, or an outpatient clinic. If the last incident of abuse occurred >72 hr prior, the likelihood of recovering forensic evidence is extremely low, making forensic evidence collection unnecessary. For *postpubertal females*, many experts recommend forensic evidence collection up to 120 hr following the abuse—the same time limit as for adult women. The extended time frame is justified because some studies have demonstrated that semen can remain in the postpubertal vaginal vault for >72 hr.

The site to which a child is referred may be different when the child does not present until after the cutoff for an acute examination. Because

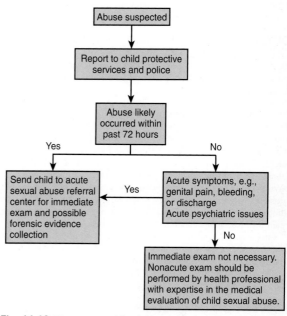

Fig. 16.10 Triage protocol for children with suspected sexual abuse.

EDs may not have a child abuse expert and can be busy, noisy, and lacking in privacy, examination at an alternate location such as a child advocacy center or outpatient clinic is recommended. If the exam is not urgent, waiting until the next morning is recommended because it is easier to interview and examine a child who is not tired and cranky. Referring physicians should be familiar with the triage procedures in their communities, including the referral sites for both acute and chronic exams, and whether there are separate referral sites for prepubertal and postpubertal children.

Children with suspected sexual abuse may present to the pediatrician's office with a clear disclosure of abuse or subtler indicators. A private, brief conversation between pediatrician and child can provide an opportunity for the child to speak in his or her own words without the parent speaking for the child. Doing this may be especially important when the caregiver does not believe the child, or is unwilling or unable to offer emotional support and protection. Telling caregivers that a private conversation is part of the routine assessment for the child's concerns can help comfort a hesitant parent.

When speaking with the child, experts recommend establishing rapport by starting with general and open-ended questions, such as, "Tell me about school," and "What are your favorite things to do?" Questions about sexual abuse should be nonleading (e.g., "Who touched you there?"). A pediatrician should explain that sometimes children are hurt or bothered by others, and that he or she wonders whether that might have happened to the child. Open-ended questions, such as, "Can you tell me more about that?" allow the child to provide additional information and clarification in his or her own words. It is not necessary to obtain extensive information about what happened because the child will usually have a forensic interview once a report is made to CPS and an investigation begins. Very young children and those with developmental delay may lack the verbal skills to describe what happened. In this situation the caregiver's history may provide enough information to warrant a report to CPS without interviewing the child.

All 50 U.S. states mandate that professionals report suspected maltreatment to CPS. The specific criteria for "reason to suspect" are generally not defined by state law. It is clear that *reporting does not require certainty that abuse has occurred.* Therefore, it may be appropriate to report a child with sexual behavior concerns when no accidental sexual exposure can be identified, and when the child does not clearly confirm or deny abuse.

PHYSICAL EXAMINATION OF THE CHILD WITH SUSPECTED SEXUAL ABUSE

Unfortunately, many physicians are unfamiliar with genital anatomy and examination, particularly in the prepubertal child (Figs. 16.11 and 16.12). Because about 95% of children who undergo a medical evaluation following sexual abuse have normal examinations, the role of the primary care provider is often simply to be able to distinguish a normal exam from findings indicative of common medical concerns or trauma. The absence of physical findings can often be explained by the type and timing of sexual contact that has occurred. Abusive acts such as fondling, or even digital penetration, can occur without causing injury. In addition, many children do not disclose abuse until days, weeks, months, or even years after the abuse has occurred. Because genital injuries usually heal rapidly, injuries are often completely healed by the time a child presents for medical evaluation. A normal genital examination does not rule out the possibility of abuse and should not influence the decision to report to CPS.

Even with the high proportion of normal genital exams, there is value in conducting a thorough physical examination. Unsuspected injuries or medical problems, such as labial adhesions, imperforate hymen, or urethral prolapse, may be identified. In addition, reassurance about the child's physical health may allay anxiety for the child and family.

Few findings on the genital examination are diagnostic for sexual abuse. In the acute time frame, lacerations or bruising of the labia, penis, scrotum, perianal tissues, or perineum are indicative of trauma. Likewise, hymenal bruising and lacerations and perianal lacerations extending deep to the external anal sphincter indicate penetrating trauma. In the nonacute time frame, perianal scars and scars of the posterior fourchette or fossa indicate trauma and/or sexual activity. A complete transection of the hymen to the base between the 4 and 8 o'clock in the supine position (i.e., absence of hymenal tissue in the posterior rim) is considered diagnostic for trauma (Fig. 16.12). For these findings, the cause of injury must be elucidated through the child and caregiver history. If there is any concern that the finding may be the result of sexual abuse, CPS should be notified and a medical evaluation performed by an experienced child abuse pediatrician.

Testing for STIs is not indicated for all children but is warranted in certain situations (Table 16.5). *Culture* was once considered the gold standard for the diagnosis of vaginal gonorrhea (see Chapter 219) and

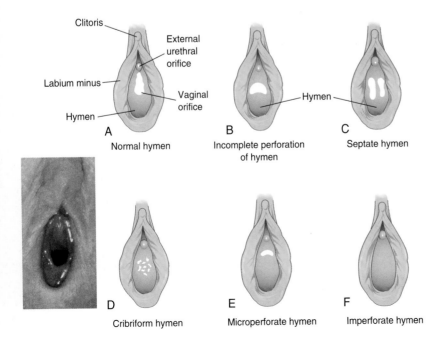

Fig. 16.11 Congenital anomalies of the hymen. **A-F,** Different types of hymen abnormalities. Photograph shows a normal hymen, as in **A.** (*From Moore KL, Persaud TVN. The developing human, ed 7, Philadelphia, 2003, Elsevier.*)

Clitoris

External urethral orifice

Labium minus

Hymen

Vaginal orifice

Hymen

A Normal hymen

B Incomplete perforation of hymen

C Septate hymen

D Cribriform hymen

E Microperforate hymen

F Imperforate hymen

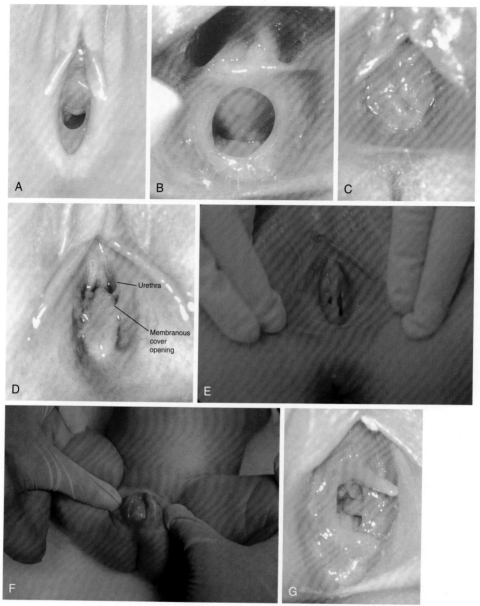

Fig. 16.12 Types of hymens. **A,** Crescentic. **B,** Annular. **C,** Redundant. **D,** Microperforate. **E,** Septated. **F,** Imperforate. **G,** Hymeneal tags. (*A-F, From Perlman SE, Nakajima ST, Hertweck SP. Clinical protocols in pediatric and adolescent gynecology, London, 2004, Parthenon Publishing Group; **G,** From McCann JJ, Kerns DL. The anatomy of child and adolescent sexual abuse, St. Louis, 1999, InterCorp.*)

chlamydia (Chapter 252) infections in children. However, several studies demonstrated that *nucleic acid amplification testing* (NAAT) for gonorrhea and chlamydia by either vaginal swab or urine in prepubertal females is as sensitive, and possibly more sensitive, than culture. Current guidelines from the Centers for Disease Control and Prevention (CDC) allow for NAAT testing by vaginal swab or urine as an alternative to culture in females. Because obtaining vaginal swabs can be uncomfortable for prepubertal children, urine testing is preferable. Culture remains the preferred method for testing of rectal and pharyngeal specimens in males and females. Few data are available on the use of urine NAAT testing in prepubertal boys. Therefore the CDC continues to recommend urine or urethral culture for boys. Many child abuse experts perform urine NAAT testing on prepubertal boys because urethral swabs are

uncomfortable, and good data support urine NAAT testing in females. For all NAAT testing in both genders, the child should *not* receive presumptive treatment at testing. Instead, a positive NAAT should be confirmed by culture or an alternate NAAT test before treatment. Because gonorrhea and chlamydia in prepubertal children do not typically cause ascending infection, waiting for a definitive diagnosis before treatment will not increase the risk for pelvic inflammatory disease. Testing for *Trichomonas vaginalis* is by culture (Diamond media or InPouch; Biomed Diagnostics, White City, OR) or wet mount. *Wet mount* requires the presence of vaginal secretions, viewing must be immediate for optimal results, and sensitivity is only 44–68%; therefore false-negative tests are common. Experts have determined that insufficient data exist to recommend commercially available *Trichomonas* NAATs

Table 16.5	Indications for STI Screening in Children With Suspected Sexual Abuse

1. Child has experienced penetration or has evidence of recent or healed penetrative injury to the genitals, anus, or oropharynx.
2. Child has been abused by a stranger.
3. Child has been abused by a perpetrator known to be infected with a sexually transmitted infection (STI) or at high risk for STIs (e.g., intravenous drug abusers, men who have sex with men, persons with multiple sexual partners, those with a history of STIs).
4. Child has a sibling, other relative, or another person in the household with an STI.
5. Child lives in an area with a high rate of STI in the community.
6. Child has signs or symptoms of STIs (e.g., vaginal discharge or pain, genital itching or odor, urinary symptoms, genital lesions or ulcers).
7. Child or parent requests STI testing.

From Centers for Disease Control and Prevention: Sexually transmitted diseases treatment guidelines, 2015, *MMWR* 64(RR3):1–137, 2015.

Table 16.6	Implications of Commonly Encountered Sexually Transmitted or Sexually Associated Infections for Diagnosis and Reporting of Sexual Abuse Among Infants and Prepubertal Children

ST/SA CONFIRMED	EVIDENCE FOR SEXUAL ABUSE	SUGGESTED ACTION
Gonorrhea*	Diagnostic	Report[†]
Syphilis*	Diagnostic	Report[†]
HIV[‡]	Diagnostic	Report[†]
Chlamydia trachomatis*	Diagnostic	Report[†]
Trichomonas vaginalis*	Highly suspicious	Report[†]
Genital herpes	Highly suspicious (HSV-2 especially)	Report[†,§]
Condylomata acuminata (anogenital warts)*	Suspicious	Consider report[†,§,**]
Bacterial vaginosis	Inconclusive	Medical follow-up

*If not likely to be perinatally acquired, and rare vertical transmission is excluded.
[†]Reports should be made to the agency in the community mandated to receive reports of suspected child abuse or neglect.
[‡]If not likely to be acquired perinatally or through transfusion.
[§]Unless a clear history of autoinoculation exists.
[**]Report if evidence exists to suspect abuse, including history, physical examination, or other identified infections.
HIV, Human immunodeficiency virus; HSV, herpes simplex virus; SA, sexually associated; ST, sexually transmitted.
From Centers for Disease Control and Prevention: Sexually transmitted diseases treatment guidelines, 2015, *MMWR* 64(RR3):1-137, 2015 (Table 6).

for prepubertal children. However, there is also no reason to suspect that test performance in children would be different from adults.

A number of STIs should raise concern for abuse (Table 16.6). In a prepubertal child, **gonorrhea** or **syphilis** beyond the neonatal period indicates that the child has had some contact with infected genital secretions, almost always as a result of sexual abuse. There is some evidence to indicate that **chlamydia** in children up to 3 yr of age may be perinatally acquired. Chlamydia in children >3 yr old is diagnostic of contact with infected genital secretions, almost always a result of sexual abuse. In children <3 yr old, sexual abuse should still be strongly considered beyond the neonatal period. **HIV** is diagnostic for sexual abuse if other means of transmission have been excluded. Because of the potential for transmission either perinatally or through nonsexual contact, the presence of **genital warts** has a low specificity for sexual abuse. The possibility of sexual abuse should be considered and addressed with the family, especially in children whose warts first appear beyond 5 yr of age. Type 1 or 2 genital herpes is concerning for sexual abuse, but not diagnostic given other possible routes of transmission. For human papillomavirus (HPV) and HSV, the American Academy of Pediatrics (AAP) recommends reporting to CPS unless perinatal or horizontal transmission is considered likely.

ADDITIONAL MANAGEMENT

Because HIV testing identifies antibodies to the virus and not the human immunodeficiency virus itself, and because it may take several months for seroconversion, repeat testing at 6 wk and 3 mo after the last suspected exposure is indicated. Repeat testing for syphilis is also recommended. Hepatitis B and HPV vaccination (for children ≥9 yr) should be given if the child has not been previously vaccinated or vaccination is incomplete.

SEXUAL ABUSE PREVENTION

Pediatricians can play a role in the prevention of sexual abuse by educating parents and children about sexual safety at well-child visits. During the genital exam the pediatrician can inform the child that only the doctor and select adult caregivers should be permitted to see their private parts, and that a trusted adult should be told if anyone else attempts to do so. Pediatricians can raise parental awareness that older kids or adults may try to engage in sexual behavior with children. The pediatrician can teach parents how to minimize the opportunity for perpetrators to access children, for example, by limiting one-adult/one-child situations and being sensitive to any adult's unusual interest in young children. In addition, pediatricians can help parents talk to children about what to do if confronted with a potentially abusive situation. Some examples include telling children to say "no," to leave, and to tell a parent and/or another adult. If abuse does occur, the pediatrician can tell parents how to recognize possible signs and symptoms, and how to reassure the child that she or he was not at fault. Lastly, pediatricians can provide

parents with suggestions about how to maintain open communication with their children so that these conversations can occur with minimal parent and child discomfort.

Bibliography is available at Expert Consult.

16.2 Medical Child Abuse (Factitious Disorder by Proxy, Munchausen Syndrome by Proxy)
Howard Dubowitz and Wendy G. Lane

The term *Munchausen syndrome* is used to describe situations in which adults falsify their own symptoms. In *Munchausen syndrome by proxy*, a parent, typically a mother, simulates or causes disease in her child. Several terms have been suggested to describe this phenomenon: factitious disorder by proxy, pediatric condition falsification, and currently, **medical child abuse (MCA)**. In some instances, such as partial suffocation, child abuse may be most appropriate.

The core dynamic of MCA is that a parent falsely presents a child for medical attention. This may occur by fabricating a history, such as reporting seizures that never occurred. A parent may directly cause a child's illness, by exposing a child to a toxin, medication, or infectious agent (e.g., injecting stool into an intravenous line). Signs or symptoms may also be manufactured, such as when a parent smothers a child, or alters laboratory samples or temperature measurements. Each of these actions may lead to unnecessary medical care, sometimes including intrusive tests and surgeries. The "problems" often recur repeatedly over several years. In addition to the physical concomitants of testing and treatment, there are potentially serious and lasting social and psychological sequelae.

Child healthcare professionals are typically misled into thinking that the child really has a medical problem. Parents, sometimes working in a medical field, may be adept at constructing somewhat plausible presentations. A convincing seizure history may be offered, and a normal electroencephalogram (EEG) cannot fully rule out the possibility of a seizure disorder. Even after extensive testing fails to lead to a diagnosis or treatment proves ineffective, health professionals may think they are confronting a new or rare disease. Unwittingly, this can lead to continued testing (leaving no stone unturned) and interventions, thus perpetuating the MCA. Pediatricians generally rely on and trust parents to provide an accurate history. As with other forms of child maltreatment, an accurate diagnosis of MCA requires that the pediatrician maintain a healthy skepticism under certain circumstances.

CLINICAL MANIFESTATIONS

The presentation of MCA may vary in nature and severity. Consideration of MCA should be triggered when the reported symptoms are repeatedly noted by only 1 parent, appropriate testing fails to confirm a diagnosis, and seemingly appropriate treatment is ineffective. At times, the child's symptoms, their course, or the response to treatment may be incompatible with any recognized disease. Preverbal children are usually involved, although older children may be convinced by parents that they have a particular problem and become dependent on the increased attention; this may lead to feigning symptoms.

Symptoms in young children are mostly associated with proximity of the offending caregiver to the child. The mother may present as a devoted or even model parent who forms close relationships with members of the healthcare team. While appearing very interested in her child's condition, she may be relatively distant emotionally. She may have a history of Munchausen syndrome, although not necessarily diagnosed as such.

Bleeding is a particularly common presentation. This may be caused by adding dyes to samples, adding blood (e.g., from the mother) to the child's sample, or giving the child an anticoagulant (e.g., warfarin).

Seizures are another common manifestation, with a history easy to fabricate, and the difficulty of excluding the problem based on testing. A parent may report that another physician diagnosed seizures, and the myth may be continued if there is no effort to confirm the basis for the "diagnosis." Alternatively, seizures may be induced by toxins, medications (e.g., insulin), water, or salts. Physicians need to be familiar with the substances available to families and the possible consequences of exposure.

Apnea is also a common presentation. The observation may be falsified or created by partial suffocation. A history of a sibling with the same problem, perhaps dying from it, should be cause for concern. Parents of children hospitalized for brief resolved unexplained events (or apparent life-threatening events) have been videotaped attempting to suffocate their child while in the hospital.

Gastrointestinal signs or symptoms are another common manifestation. Forced ingestion of medications such as ipecac may cause chronic vomiting, or laxatives may cause diarrhea.

The **skin**, easily accessible, may be burned, dyed, tattooed, lacerated, or punctured to simulate acute or chronic skin conditions. **Recurrent sepsis** may be caused by infectious agents being administered; intravenous lines during hospitalization may provide a convenient portal. Urine and blood samples may be contaminated with foreign blood or stool.

DIAGNOSIS

In assessing possible MCA, several explanations should be considered in addition to a true medical problem. Some parents may be extremely anxious and genuinely concerned about possible problems. This anxiety may result from a personality trait, the death of neighbor's child, or something read on the internet. Alternatively, parents may believe something told to them by a trusted physician despite subsequent evidence to the contrary and efforts to correct the earlier misdiagnosis. Physicians may unwittingly contribute to a parent's belief that a real problem exists by, perhaps reasonably, persistently pursuing a medical diagnosis. There is a need to discern commonly used hyperbole (e.g., exaggerating height of fever) in order to evoke concern and perhaps justify an ED visit. In the end, a diagnosis of MCA rests on clear evidence of a child repeatedly being subjected to unnecessary medical tests and treatment, primarily stemming from a parent's actions. Determining the parent's underlying psychopathology is the responsibility of mental health professionals.

Once MCA is suspected, gathering and reviewing **all** the child's medical records from all sources is an onerous but critical first step. It is often important to confer with other treating physicians about what specifically was conveyed to the family. A mother may report that the child's physician insisted that a certain test be done, when instead it was the mother who demanded the test. It is also necessary to confirm the basis for a given diagnosis, rather than simply accepting a parent's account.

Pediatricians may face the dilemma of when to accept that all plausible diagnoses have been reasonably ruled out, the circumstances fit MCA, and further testing and treatment should cease. The likelihood of MCA must be balanced with concerns about possibly missing an important diagnosis. Consultation with a pediatrician expert in child abuse is recommended. In evaluating possible MCA, specimens should be carefully collected, with no opportunity for tampering with them. Similarly, temperature measurements should be closely observed.

Depending on the severity and complexity, hospitalization may be needed for careful observation to help make the diagnosis. In some instances, such as repeated apparent life-threatening events, covert video surveillance accompanied by close monitoring (to rapidly intervene in case a parent attempts to suffocate a child) can be valuable. Close coordination among hospital staff is essential, especially since some may side with the mother and resent even the possibility of MCA being raised. Parents should not be informed of the evaluation for MCA until the diagnosis is made. Doing so could naturally influence their behavior and jeopardize establishing the diagnosis. All steps in making the diagnosis and all pertinent information should be very carefully documented, perhaps using a "shadow chart" to which the parent does not have access.

TREATMENT

Once the diagnosis is established, the medical team and CPS should determine the treatment plan, which may require out-of-home placement and should include mental healthcare for the offending parent as well as for other affected children. Further medical care should be carefully organized and coordinated by one primary care provider. CPS should be encouraged to meet with the family only after the medical team has informed the offending parent of the diagnosis; their earlier involvement may hamper the evaluation. Parents often respond with resistance, denial, and threats. It may be prudent to have hospital security in the vicinity.

Bibliography is available at Expert Consult.

Chapter 17
Strategies for Health Behavior Change

Cori M. Green, Anne M. Gadomski,
and Lawrence Wissow

第十七章
统筹设计实现健康行为的改观

中文导读

本章主要介绍了行为变化的统一理论、健康行为变化的跨理论模型、共同因素的运用、富有启发诱导的会谈以及决策共享。在共同因素的运用中阐述了人际交往技巧（寄予希望、善解人意、语言亲和、态度诚恳、避免唐突、伙伴关系和精心安排），运用有计划有条理并就问题达成一致的会谈明确患者的忧虑所在、周密安排、如何应对愤怒和士气低落、如何强调成功。

To improve the health of children, pediatricians often ask patients and caregivers to make behavioral changes. These may be lifestyle changes to manage a chronic condition (e.g., obesity, asthma), adherence with the recommended timing and frequency of medications, or recommendations to seek assistance from other health providers (e.g., dieticians, mental health providers, physical, occupational, or speech therapists). However, change is difficult and can cause distress, and families often express reluctance or ambivalence to change due to perceived barriers. When families do not believe change is needed or possible, pediatricians may become discouraged or uncomfortable in providing care. This can make it difficult for clinicians to form an alliance with families, which is central to finding a solution to most problems identified in the medical setting.

Many healthcare problems may require complex, multifaceted interventions, but the first step is always to engage the family in identifying the healthcare problem driving the need for behavior change. Once a problem is identified and agreed on, clinicians and families need to set an achievable goal and identify specific behaviors that can help families reach their goal. It is important to be specific and precise about the actual behavior and not simply identify the *category* of the behavior. When counseling a patient on weight loss for obesity, for example, one might discuss 3 possible approaches: making dietary changes, increasing exercise, and decreasing screen time. The choice of which behavior to focus on should come from the patient but needs to be specific. It is not enough for the patient to state he will exercise more. Instead, the clinician should help the patient identify a more specific goal, such as playing basketball with his friends 3 times a week at the park near home. This takes in to account the action, context, setting, and time of the new behavioral goal. Specific examples of problems that would necessitate a behavior change to improve outcomes are used throughout the chapter.

UNIFIED THEORY OF BEHAVIOR CHANGE

There are several theories of health-related behavior change. Each highlights a different concept, but frameworks that unite these theories suggest that the factor most predictive of whether one will perform a behavior is the *intention* to do so. The **unified theory of behavior change** examines behavior along 2 dimensions: influences on intent and moderators of the intention-behavior relationship (Fig. 17.1). Five main factors that influence one's decision to perform a behavior are expectancies, social norms/normative influences, self-concept/self-image, emotions, and self-efficacy. Table 17.1 provides specific examples on how to explore influences of intent when guiding families in decision-making, such as deciding to start a stimulant medication for a child diagnosed with attention-deficit/hyperactivity disorder (ADHD). It is not necessary to ask about each influence, but these principles are particularly useful when guiding patients who may be resistant to change.

Once a decision to make a change is made, 4 factors determine whether an intention leads to carrying out the behavior: knowledge and skills, environmental facilitators and constraints, salience of the behavior, and habits. The pediatrician can help ensure intent leads to behavior change by addressing these factors during the visit. In the ADHD example, the clinician can help the family build their knowledge by providing handouts on stimulants, nutritional pamphlets on how to minimize the appetite-suppressant effects of the medication on weight, and information on how the family can explain to others the need for medication. Asking about morning routines will help identify potential barriers in remembering to take the medication. Lastly, clinicians can

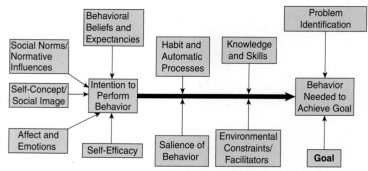

Fig. 17.1 The 5 constructs that influence one's intent to perform a behavior and the 4 influences that determine whether an intent will lead to performing the behavior. Problem identification (*box at upper right*) is where the process of thinking about health behavior changes begins. A clinician can then help the patient decide on which behavior can help the patient to meet the health goal. Once this is decided, to help with behavior change, clinicians should think about intent, influences of intent, and the factors that may facilitate or impede intent from leading to action.

Table 17.1	Influences of Intent and Possible Use During a Patient Encounter (Specifically, Starting Stimulant for ADHD)	
INFLUENCE OF INTENT	**STRATEGIES TO ENGAGE FAMILIES USING INFLUENCES OF INTENT**	**POSSIBLE FACTORS INFLUENCING THE DECISION**
Beliefs and expectancies Perceived advantages and disadvantages of performing a behavior.	Ask questions about their beliefs and experiences. "What do you know already know about stimulants?" "Have you heard about other children's experiences taking stimulants?" "What do you expect will happen if your child takes a stimulant?" Ask permission to give information addressing their prior beliefs or experiences. "Is it all right if I give you some information addressing your concerns?"	"I know that stimulants helped my nephew do better in school." "I heard stimulants stunt children's growth."
Social norms Pressures to (or not) perform a behavior because of what is standard among social groups.	Share information about the normative nature of the behavior and ways to cope if performing a behavior that is not the social norm. "I have a lot of patients who have improved in school after starting a stimulant."	"Do other parents give their children stimulants if they are diagnosed with ADHD?" "What would my mother think if she found out my child was taking a stimulant?"
Self-concept/self-image Overall sense of self and whether behavior is congruent with that and with the image they want to project to others.	Interact with family in a partnering, supportive, respectful manner. Identify strengths. Reframe any negative images they foresee may happen with the behavior. "I am sure your in-laws will be so happy when your child is doing better in school."	"Am I a good parent if I give my child medications that affect his brain?" "What will other parents at school think if I allow my child to start a stimulant? What will my in-laws think?"
Emotions Emotional reactions to performing behaviors, in intensity and direction (positive or negative).	Allow patients to express their feelings. Suggest ways to manage negative or avoidant feelings. "Many parents are scared to start stimulants at first. However, once their child is succeeding in school, they realize the benefits outweighed the risks. Let's talk more about your fears."	"I am so nervous about my child starting to take a stimulant." "I am so upset with how my child is doing in school and really do not know what to do next." "I am so relieved that there is a medication that may help improve my child's grades and chance of going to college."
Self-efficacy Perceived confidence they can perform the behavior.	Provide information, model the behavior, encourage success, and teach skills. Explore what obstacles they foresee and how confident they are they can overcome obstacles. Help strategize ways to overcome obstacles. "Do you feel confident you will be able to get your child to take the medication?" "Let's brainstorm how we can prevent any of the side effects." "Many of my patients have a large breakfast before taking the medication. Can I help you figure out how to fit that into your schedule?"	"Will I be able to remember to give my child his medication every day?" "Will I be able to make sure my child has a large breakfast in the morning before taking her medication?"

ADHD, Attention-deficit/hyperactivity disorder.

Table 17.2	Stages of Change and Strategies for Counseling*

STAGE/DEFINITION	GOAL AND STRATEGY	SPECIFIC EXAMPLES
Precontemplation Not considering change. May be unaware that a problem exists.	Establish a therapeutic relationship. Increase awareness of need to change.	"I understand you are only here because your parents are worried and that you don't feel that smoking marijuana is a big deal." "Can I ask if smoking marijuana has created any problems for you now? I know your parents were worried about your grades." "It's up to you to decide if and when you are ready to cut back on smoking marijuana." "Is it okay if I give you some information about marijuana use?" "I know it can be hard to change a habit when you feel under pressure. It is totally up to you to decide if cutting back is right for you. Is it okay if I ask you about this during our next visit?"
Contemplation Beginning to consider making a change, but still feeling ambivalent about making a change.	Identify ambivalence. Help develop discrepancy between goals and current behaviors. Ask about pros and cons of changing problem behavior. Support patient toward making a change.	"I'm hearing that you do agree that sometimes your marijuana use does get in the way, especially with school. However, it helps relax you and it would be hard to make a change right now." "What would be one benefit of cutting back? What would be a drawback to cutting back? Do you think your smoking will cause problems in the future?" "After talking about this, if you feel you want to cut back, the next step would be to think about how to best do that. We wouldn't need to jump right into a plan. Why don't you think about what we discussed, and we can meet next week if you are ready to make a plan?"
Preparation Preparing for action. Reduced ambivalence and exploration of options for change.	Help patient set a goal and prepare a concrete plan. Offer a menu of choices. Identify supports and barriers.	"It's great that you are thinking about ways to cut back on your smoking. I understand your initial goal is to stop smoking during the week." "I can give you some other options of how to relax and reduce stress during the week." "We need to figure out how to react to your friends after school who you normally smoke with." "Do you have other friends who you can see after school instead, who would support this decision?"
Action Taking action; actively implementing plan.	Provide positive feedback. Identify unexpected barriers and create coping strategies.	"Congratulations on cutting back. Have you noticed any differences in your schoolwork? I'm so happy to hear your grades improved." "Has it been difficult to not see your friends after school? How have you reacted when they get annoyed you don't want to smoke with them?" "Let's continue to track your progress."
Maintenance Continues to change behavior and maintains healthier lifestyle.	Reinforce commitment and affirm ability to change. Create coping plans when relapse does occur. Manage triggers.	"You really are committed to going to a good college and improving your grades. I'm so happy the hard work has paid off." "I understand that it was hard to say no to smoking with your friends last week when it was someone's birthday. How did you feel after? Are there triggers that we can think about preventing in the future?"

*This table uses an example of an adolescent who is initially resistant to cutting back on smoking marijuana. His parents caught him smoking in his room and arranged for him to see the pediatrician.

Adapted from *Implementing mental health priorities in practice: substance use*, American Academy of Pediatrics. https://www.aap.org/en-us/advocacy-and-policy/aap-health-initiatives/Mental-Health/Pages/substance-use.aspx.

help families think about cues for remembering to give the medication in the morning, since their morning routines, or habits, will have to be adjusted to adhere to this medication.

By using these principles of behavior change, pediatricians can guide their patients toward change during an encounter by ensuring they leave with (1) a strong positive intention to perform the behavior; (2) the perception that they have the skills to accomplish it; (3) a belief that the behavior is socially acceptable and consistent with their self-image; (4) a positive feeling about the behavior; (5) specific strategies in overcoming potential barriers in performing the behavior; and (6) a set of identified cues and enablers to help build new habits.

TRANSTHEORETICAL MODEL OF HEALTH BEHAVIOR CHANGE

It is difficult to counsel families to change a behavior when they may not agree there is a problem or when they are not ready to build an intention to change. The **transtheoretical model of health behavior change** places an individual's motivation and readiness to change on a continuum. The premise of this model is that behavior change is a process, and as someone attempts to change, they move through 5 stages (although not always in a linear fashion): *precontemplation* (no current intention of making a change), *contemplation* (considering change), *preparation* (creating an intention, planning, and committing

to change), *action* (has changed behavior for a short time), and *maintenance* (sustaining long-term change). Assessing a patient's stage of change and then targeting counseling toward that stage can help build a *therapeutic alliance*, in contrast to counseling a patient to do something she is not ready for, which can disrupt therapeutic alliance and lead to resistance. Table 17.2 further describes stages of change and gives examples for counseling that targets the adolescent's stage of change in reducing marijuana smoking.

COMMON FACTORS APPROACH

Conversations around behavior change are most effective when they take place in a context of a trusting, mutually respectful relationship. The traditional medical model assumes that patients and their families come with questions and needs, and that the pediatrician's job is to offer specific advice and advocate for its acceptance. This approach fails when families are reluctant, ambivalent, demoralized, or unfamiliar with the healthcare system or the treatment choices offered. A context more supportive of behavior change can be developed when pediatricians use communication strategies that facilitate collaboration and building therapeutic alliance.

The **common factors approach** is an evidence-based communication strategy that is effective in facilitating behavior change. The skills central to a common factors approach are consistent across multiple forms of psychotherapy and can be viewed as generic aspects of treatment that can be used across a wide range of symptoms to build a therapeutic alliance between the physician and patient. This alliance predicts outcomes of counseling more than the specific modality of treatment. The common factors approach has been implemented and studied in pediatric primary care for children with mental health problems. Children who were treated by pediatricians trained in the common factors approach had improved functioning compared to those who saw pediatricians without this training.

A common factors approach distinguishes between the impact of the patient–provider alliance and the pediatrician's use of skills that influence patient behavior change across a broad range of conditions. Interpersonal skills that help build alliances with patients include showing empathy, warmth, and positive regard. Skills that influence behavior change include a clinician's ability to provide optimism, facilitate treatment engagement, and maintain the focus on achievable goals. This can be done by clearly explaining the condition and treatment approaches while keeping the discussion focused on immediate and practical concerns.

Interpersonal Skills: HEL²P³

The interpersonal skills that facilitate an affective bond between the patient and clinician can be remembered by the HEL²P³ mnemonic (Table 17.3). These skills include providing **hope, empathy**, and **loyalty**; using the patient's **language**; **partnering** with the family; asking **permission** to raise more sensitive questions or to give advice; and creating a **plan** that is initiated by the family. These interpersonal skills should help operationalize the common factors approach by increasing a patient's optimism, feelings of well-being, and willingness to work toward improved health, while also targeting feelings of anger, ambivalence, and hopelessness.

Structuring a patient encounter using common factors to facilitate behavior change uses these steps: eliciting concerns while setting an agenda and agreeing on the nature of the problem; establishing a plan; and responding to anger and demoralization and emphasizing hope.

Table 17.3	Hope, Empathy, Language, Loyalty, Permission, Partnership, Plan (HEL²P³)*
SKILL	**EXAMPLES**
Hope for improvement: Develop strengths.	"I have seen other children like you with similar feelings of sadness, and they have gotten better."
Empathy: Listen attentively.	"It must be hard for you that you no longer get pleasure in playing soccer."
Language: Use family's language. Check understanding.	"Let me make sure I understand what you are saying. You no longer feel like doing things that make you happy in the past?"
Loyalty: Express support and commitment.	"You are free to talk to me about anything while we work through this."
Permission: Ask permission to explore sensitive subjects. Offer advice.	"I would like to ask more questions that you may find more sensitive, is that okay?"
Partnership: Identify and overcome barriers.	"Is it okay with you if I give you my opinion on what may be the problem here?"
Plan: Establish a plan, or at least a first step family can take.	"If we work together, maybe we can think through solutions for the problems you identified."

*This table illustrates the **interpersonal skills** highlighted in the common factors approach. In this example the clinician is responding to an adolescent struggling with depression and resistant to seeking help.

Adapted with data from Foy JM, Kelleher KJ, Laraque D; American Academy of Pediatrics: Enhancing pediatric mental health care: strategies for preparing a primary care practice, *Pediatrics* 125(Suppl 3):S87–S108, 2010.

Elicit Concerns: Set the Agenda and Agree on the Problem

The first step of the visit is to elicit both the child's and the parent's concerns and agree on the focus for the visit. This can be accomplished by using open-ended questions and asking "anything else?" until nothing else is disclosed. It is important to show you have time and are interested in their concerns by making eye contact, listening attentively, minimizing distractions, and responding with empathy and interest. Engage both the child and the parent by taking turns eliciting their concerns. It is helpful to summarize their story to reassure them you have heard and understand what they are saying. Keep the session organized, and manage rambling by gently interrupting, paraphrasing, asking for additional concerns, and refocusing the conversation.

By the end of this step in the visit, all parties should feel reassured that their problems were heard and accurately described. The next step is to agree on the problem to be addressed during that visit. If the parent and child do not agree on the issue, try to find a common thread that will address the concerns of both.

Establish a Plan

Once a problem is agreed on, the pediatrician can partner with families to develop acceptable and achievable plans for treatment or further evaluation. Families should take the lead in developing goals and the strategies to attain them, and information should be given in response to patients' expressed needs. Pediatricians can involve families by offering choices and asking for feedback. Advice should be given only after asking a family's permission to do so. If the family asks for advice, the clinician should respond by considering principles of behavior change, as described earlier. Advice should be tailored toward the family's willingness to act, concerns for barriers, and attitudes and should be as specific and practical as possible. Once an initial plan is established, it is important to partner in monitoring responses and to provide continued support.

Respond to Anger and Demoralization and Emphasize Hope

The common factors approach is particularly helpful in engaging families in situations where anger and demoralization could prevent patients from being able to use the clinician's advice. Focusing the conversation on goals for the future and how to achieve them is more productive than discussing how problems began. This "solution-focused therapy" approach grew out of the need for clinicians to help people in a brief encounter. Hopelessness can be relieved by pediatricians helping patients to identify and build on strengths and past success, reframing events and feelings, and breaking down overwhelming goals into small, concrete steps that are more readily accomplished. In general, pediatricians can use the **elicit-provide-elicit model**. First, ask if they want to hear your thoughts about the situation. Provide guidance in a neutral way, and then ask the family what they think about what you just stated.

Table 17.4 provides an example of how to use common factors in practice using a scenario of an adolescent female who has been teased for using albuterol before physical education class for her exercise-induced asthma. The clinician in the scenario attempts to address both the patient's and her mother's concerns.

MOTIVATIONAL INTERVIEWING

Motivational interviewing (MI) is a goal-oriented, supportive counseling style that complements the HEL²P³ framework and is useful when patients or families remain ambivalent about making health-related behavior changes. MI is designed to enhance intrinsic motivation in patients by exploring their perspectives and ambivalence. It is also aligned with the transtheoretical model's continuum of change, where the pediatrician not only tailors counseling to a patient's stage of change, but does so with the goal of moving the patient toward the next stage. It is particularly effective for those not interested in change or not ready to make a commitment. MI has been shown to be an effective intervention strategy for decreasing high-risk behaviors, improving chronic disease control, and increasing adherence to preventive health measures.

Table 17.4	Common Factors Approach in Practice*	
GOAL	**SPECIFIC SKILLS**	**EXAMPLES**
Elicit child and parents' concerns.	Use open-ended questions and ask, "What else?" until nothing else is listed, while engaging both parties and demonstrating empathy.	"Hi, Jacqueline and Mrs. Smith. How have things been since last time? What are your biggest concerns for today?" "What else do you think we should put on the agenda for today?" "I am sorry to hear that you have had more asthma symptoms around gym time, Jacqueline. I'd like to ask you a few more questions to get a better understanding of what has changed, if that's okay with you." "I understand this is upsetting you, Mrs. Smith, and that you worry that Jacqueline is not going to the nurse before gym to use her inhaler pump anymore. Let's hear from Jacqueline."
	Agree on the problem.	"Can we all agree that managing the asthma symptoms around gym time is the most pressing issue for today? Should we focus on that today?"
	Manage rambling.	"What you're saying is really important, but I want to be sure we have time to talk about controlling your daughter's asthma symptoms during gym. Is it okay if we go back to that topic?"
Partner with families to find acceptable forms of treatment.	Develop acceptable plans for treatment of further diagnoses.	"I believe we can develop a plan to help deal with this. Is it okay to start talking about next steps?" "I know these asthma symptoms are concerning to your mom. But, Jacqueline, is this something you can act on now?" "I am happy to give suggestions on how to more easily use your inhaler before gym, without the other kids noticing. But what were you thinking, Jacqueline?" "Let's make a specific plan on where you can keep your inhaler so the other kids don't see it."
	Address barriers to treatment.	"Is there anything that makes you worry that this may not work?"
Increase expectations that treatment will be helpful.	Respond to hopelessness, anger, and frustration.	"I realize it wasn't your choice to come here, Jacqueline, but I'm interested in hearing how you feel about this issue." "It must be really hard for you, Jacqueline, when the kids tease you about your inhaler." "It must be frustrating for the school nurse to call you in the middle of the day at work, Mrs. Smith." "I would be angry, too, if I felt my mom didn't understand how it felt when I got teased for going to the nurse's office."
	Emphasize hope.	"We've managed difficult things before. Remember when Jacqueline kept getting admitted for her asthma when she was younger? We have come a long way since then, and I'm sure we can manage this as well."

*Jacqueline is an adolescent female who has had asthma since she was an infant. Despite multiple hospitalizations as an infant, her asthma had been under control except for during exercise, including physical education (PE) class. She had been going to the nurse's office to take albuterol before PE class, but recently she had been teased for having to take medication before PE. She has begun to skip treatments to avoid the teasing. However, her mother has now been called a few times to pick her up from school due to her asthma symptoms. Mrs. Smith is a single mother who cannot miss work and is very frustrated. She was not aware of the bullying Jacqueline has undergone.

This scenario is adapted from the American Academy of Pediatrics curricula on common factors. https://www.aap.org/en-us/advocacy-and-policy/aap-health -initiatives/Mental-Health/Pages/Module-1-Brief-Intervention.aspx.

MI is a collaborative approach in which the pediatrician respects patients' perspective and treats them as the "expert" on their values, beliefs, and goals. *Collaboration, acceptance, compassion,* and *evocation* are the foundation of MI and are referred to as the "spirit" of the approach. The clinician is a "guide," respecting patients' autonomy and their ability to make their own decision to change. The pediatrician expresses genuine concern and demonstrates that he or she understands and validates the patient's or family's struggle. Using open-ended questions, the pediatrician evokes the patient's own motivation for change.

Expressing empathy facilitates behavior change by accepting the patient's beliefs and behaviors. This contrasts to *direct persuasion*, which often leads to resistance. The pediatrician must reinforce that ambivalence is normal and use skillful reflective listening, showing the patient an understanding of the situation.

Developing a discrepancy between current behaviors (or treatment choices) and treatment goals motivates change and helps move the patient from the precontemplative stage to the contemplative stage or from the contemplative stage to preparation, as described in the transtheoretical model. Through MI the clinician can guide patients in understanding that their current behaviors may not be consistent with their stated goals and values.

Rolling with resistance, or not pushing back when suggestions are declined, is a strategy again to align with the patient. Resistance is usually a sign that a different approach is needed. As necessary, the clinician can ask permission to give new perspectives.

Self-efficacy, or a patient's belief in her ability to perform the behavior, is a key element for change and a powerful motivator. Clinicians can express confidence in the patient's ability to achieve change and support the patient's self-efficacy.

The process by which MI is used in a patient encounter involves the following 4 parts:
1. *Engagement* is the rapport-building part of the encounter. In addition to using the skills presented in the HEL²P³ framework, the MI approach highlights the use of open-ended questions, affirmations, reflective listening, and summaries (**OARS**). **Open-ended questions** should be inviting and probing enabling the patient to think through and come to a better understanding of the problem and elicit their internal motivation. **Affirmations** provide positive feedback, express appreciation about a patient's strengths and can reinforce autonomy and self-efficacy. **Reflective listening** demonstrates that the clinician understands the patient's thoughts and feelings without judgement or interruption. It should be done frequently and can encourage the patient to be more open. **Summarizing** the conversation in a succinct way reinforces that you are listening, pulls together all information, and allows the patient to hear his own motivations and ambivalence.

Table 17.5	Counseling for Obesity Using a Motivational Interviewing (MI) Approach	
ACTION	**SPECIFIC SKILLS**	**EXAMPLES**
Engagement*	Open-ended questions	"Now that we have finished the majority of the visit, I'd like to talk about your weight. Is that okay? How do you feel about your size?" "Mrs. Smith, how do you feel about Jimmy's weight?"
	Affirmations	"You definitely have shown how strong you are having dealt with kids teasing you about your size." "Remember when you were having difficulty with school? You were able to make a few changes, and now you are doing well. I am confident we can do the same with your weight."
	Reflective listening	"You are feeling like your son is the same size as everyone in your family, and you aren't concerned right now." "Having your family watch TV before bed really works for your family, Mrs. Smith." "You're not terribly excited about having to think of ways to cook differently."
	Summary statements	"So far, we have discussed how challenging it would be to lose weight and make changes for the whole family, but you are willing to consider some simple changes."
Focusing	Set the agenda.	"We could talk about increasing the amount of exercise Jimmy has every week, reducing screen time, or making a dietary change. What do you think would work best?" "Great, so we will talk about soda. What do you like about it? How many times a week do you drink it?"
Evocation	Reinforce any change talk. Change ruler.	"Those are great reasons for thinking about cutting back on soda." "On a scale of 1 to 10, how confident are you (or important is it) that you can cut back on soda?" "A 5. Why didn't you answer a 3?" "What would it take to bring it to a 7?"
Planning	Focus on how to make the change, not "why" anymore. Be concrete.	"Maybe completely eliminating soda is too difficult right now. Do you want to think of a couple of times during the week where you can reward yourself with a soda?" "What will you drink after school instead of soda?"

*OARS is used to engage the patient and build rapport.
Adapted from *Changing the conversation about childhood obesity*, American Academy of Pediatrics, Institute for Healthy Childhood Weight. https://www.aap.org/en-us/about-the-aap/aap-press-room/pages/Changing-the-conversation-about-Childhood-Obesity.aspx.

2. *Focusing* the visit is done to clarify the patient's priorities, stage of readiness, and to identify the problem where there is ambivalence. If a patient remains resistant to change, ask permission to give information or share ideas and then ask for feedback on what they think about what you said. In the **elicit-ask-elicit model**, a clinician can deliver information about an unhealthy behavior or lifestyle decision in a nonpaternalistic manner.

3. *Evocation* is when the clinician assesses their patients' reasons for change and helps them to explore advantages, disadvantages, and barriers to change. It is important to reinforce the patient's **change talk.** Examples of change talk include an expression of desire ("I want to…"), ability ("I can…"), reasons ("There are good reasons to…"), or a need for change ("I need to…"). Clinician can use "readiness rulers" by asking their patients to rate on a scale from 1 to 10 how important and confident they are in making change. The clinician should then respond by asking why the patient did not choose a lower number and should follow up asking what it would take to bring it to a higher number.

4. The *planning* stage is similar to that described in the discussion of a common factors approach and occurs once a patient is in the preparation stage on the continuum of change. A clinician can guide their patient through this stage by having them write down responses to statements such as, "The changes I want to make are…," "The most important reasons to make this change are…," "Some people who can support me are…," and "They can help me by …." A concrete plan should include specific actions and a way to factor in accountability and rewards. Table 17.5 uses a visit for counseling about obesity to demonstrate the process of motivational interviewing.

SHARED DECISION-MAKING

Shared decision-making has many similarities to the processes previously described in that it emphasizes moving physicians away from a paternalistic approach in dictating treatment to one where patients and clinicians collaborate in making a medical decision, particularly when multiple evidence-based treatments options exist. The pediatrician or clinician offers different treatment options and describes the risks and benefits for each one. The patient or caregiver expresses their values, preferences, and treatment goals, and a decision is made together.

Shared decision-making is often facilitated by using evidence-based decision aids such as pamphlets, videos, web-based tools, or educational workshops. Condition-specific or more generic decision aids have been created and facilitate the process of shared decision-making. Studies in adults show that such aids improve knowledge and satisfaction, reduce decisional conflict, and increase the alignment between patient preferences and treatment options. More study is needed to assess behavioral and physiologic outcomes specifically when involving children in the decision-making process.

Bibliography is available at Expert Consult.

Growth, Development, and Behavior
生长、发育及行为

Chapter **18**

Developmental and Behavioral Theories

Susan Feigelman

第十八章
发育与行为理论

中文导读

　　本章主要介绍了生物–心理–社会模型和生态生物发展框架，以及生物学因素、心理学因素和社会学因素对儿童健康的影响。具体描述了遗传、致畸物质暴露、低出生体重、疾病等生物学因素对儿童健康的影响，儿童气质与养育方式的相互作用；描述了依恋关系、相倚等心理学因素和生态模式系统中家庭系统对儿童发展的重要的作用；描述了交互模型、复原力的概念及儿童发展的风险因素评估；描述了儿童发展领域和精神分析理论、认知理论、道德发展理论、行为理论等经典的发展阶段理论；描述了相关统计学指标。

The field of pediatrics is dedicated to optimizing the growth and development of each child. Pediatricians require knowledge of normal growth, development, and behavior in order to effectively monitor children's progress, identify delays or abnormalities in development, help obtain needed services, and counsel parents and caretakers. To alter factors that increase or decrease risk, pediatricians need to understand how biologic and social forces interact within the parent–child relationship, within the family, and between the family and the larger society. Growth is an indicator of overall well-being, status of chronic disease, and interpersonal and psychologic stress. By monitoring children and families over time, pediatricians are uniquely situated to observe the interrelationships between physical growth and cognitive, motor, and emotional development. Observation is enhanced by familiarity with developmental and behavioral theories that inform one about typical patterns of development and provide guidance for prevention or intervention for behavior problems. Familiarity with theories of health behavior may assist in guiding patients and families in disease management and wellness care.

BIOPSYCHOSOCIAL MODEL AND ECOBIODEVELOPMENTAL FRAMEWORK: MODELS OF DEVELOPMENT

The **medical model** presumes that a patient presents with signs and symptoms and a physician focuses on diagnosing and treating diseases of the body. This model neglects the psychologic aspect of a person who exists in the larger realm of the family and society. In the **biopsychosocial model**, societal and community systems are simultaneously considered along with more proximal systems that make up the person and the person's environment (Fig. 18.1). A patient's symptoms are examined and explained in the context of the patient's existence. This basic model can be used to understand health and both acute and chronic disease.

With the advances in neurology, genomics (including epigenetics), molecular biology, and the social sciences, a more accurate model, the **ecobiodevelopmental framework**, has emerged. This framework emphasizes how the ecology of childhood (social and physical environments) interacts with biologic processes to determine outcomes and life trajectories. Early influences, particularly those producing **toxic levels of stress**, affect the individual through modification of gene expression, without change in DNA sequencing. These **epigenetic changes**, such as DNA methylation and histone acetylation (see Chapter 100), are influenced by the early life experiences (the environment).

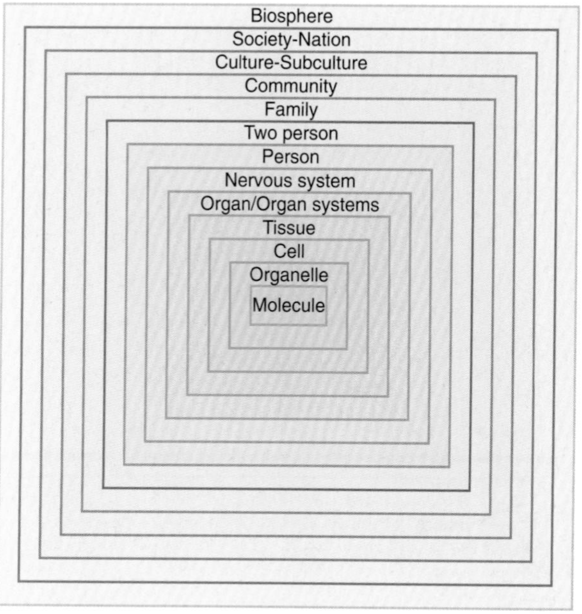

Stress responses may produce alterations in brain structure and function, leading to disruption of later coping mechanisms. These changes will produce long-lasting effects on the health and well-being of the individual and may be passed on to future generations (Fig. 18.2).

Critical to learning and remembering (and therefore development) is **neuronal plasticity**, which permits the central nervous system to reorganize neuronal networks in response to environmental stimulation, both positive and negative. An overproduction of neuronal precursors eventually leads to about 100 billion neurons in the adult brain. Each neuron develops on average 15,000 synapses by 3 yr of age. During early childhood, synapses in frequently used pathways are preserved, whereas less-used ones atrophy, a process termed "pruning." Changes in the strength and number of synapses and reorganization of neuronal circuits also play important roles in brain plasticity. Increases or decreases in synaptic activity result in persistent increases or decreases in synaptic strength. Thus experience (**environment**) has a direct effect on the physical and therefore functional properties of the brain. Children with different talents and temperaments (already a combination of genetics and environment) further elicit different stimuli from their (differing) environments.

Periods of rapid development generally correlate with periods of great changes in synaptic numbers in relevant areas of the brain. Accordingly, sensory deprivation during the time when synaptic changes should be occurring has profound effects. For example, the effects of strabismus leading to amblyopia in one eye may occur quickly during early childhood; likewise, patching the eye with good vision to reverse amblyopia in the other eye is less effective in late childhood (see Chapter 641). Early experience is particularly important because learning proceeds more efficiently along established synaptic pathways.

Early traumatic experiences modify the expression of stress mediators (in particular the hypothalamic-pituitary-adrenal axis) and neurotransmitters, leading to changes in brain structure and function. These effects may be persistent, leading to alterations and dysfunction in the stress response throughout life. Chronic stress has negative effects on cognitive functions, including memory and emotional regulation. Positive and negative experiences do not determine the ultimate outcome, but shift

Fig. 18.1 Continuum and hierarchy of natural systems in the biopsychosocial model. *(From Engel GL: The clinical application of the biopsychosocial model, Am J Psychiatry 137:535–544, 1980.)*

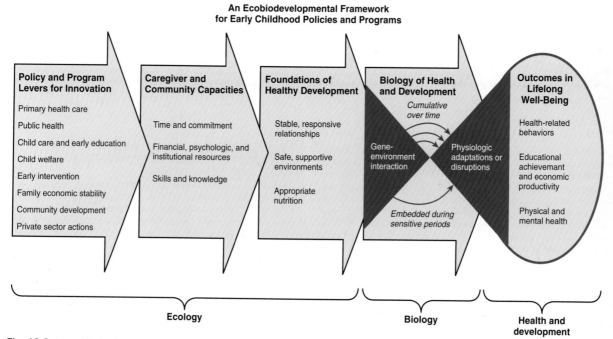

An Ecobiodevelopmental Framework for Early Childhood Policies and Programs

Fig. 18.2 An ecobiodevelopmental framework for early childhood policies and programs. *(Adapted from Center on the Developing Child (2010). The foundations of lifelong health are built in early childhood. Available at: http://developingchild.harvard.edu/.)*

the probabilities by influencing the child's ability to respond adaptively to future stimuli. The plasticity of the brain continues into adolescence, with further development of the prefrontal cortex, which is important in decision-making, future planning, and emotional control; neurogenesis persists in adulthood in certain areas of the brain.

Biologic Influences

Biologic influences on development include genetics, in utero exposure to teratogens, the long-term negative effects of low birthweight (neonatal morbidities plus increased rates of subsequent adult-onset obesity, coronary heart disease, stroke, hypertension, and type 2 diabetes), postnatal illnesses, exposure to hazardous substances, and maturation. Adoption and twin studies consistently show that heredity accounts for approximately 40% of the variance in IQ and in other personality traits, such as sociability and desire for novelty, whereas shared environment accounts for another 50%. The negative effects on development of prenatal exposure to teratogens, such as mercury and alcohol, and of postnatal insults, such as meningitis and traumatic brain injury, have been extensively studied (see Chapters 115 and 120). Any chronic illness can affect growth and development, either directly or through changes in nutrition, parenting, school attendance, or peer interactions.

Most children follow similar motor developmental sequences; the age at which children walk independently is similar around the world, despite great variability in child-rearing practices. The attainment of other skills, such as the use of complex sentences, is less tightly bound to a maturational schedule. Maturational changes also generate behavioral challenges at predictable times. Decrements in growth rate and sleep requirements around 2 yr of age often generate concern about poor appetite and refusal to nap. Although it is possible to accelerate many developmental milestones (toilet-training a 12 mo old or teaching a 3 yr old to read), *the long-term benefits of such precocious accomplishments are questionable.*

In addition to physical changes in size, body proportions, and strength, maturation brings about hormonal changes. Sexual differentiation, both somatic and neurologic, begins in utero. Both stress and reproductive hormones affect brain development as well as behavior throughout development. Steroid production by the fetal gonads leads to differences in brain structures between males and females.

Temperament describes the stable, early-appearing individual variations in behavioral dimensions, including emotionality (crying, laughing, sulking), activity level, attention, sociability, and persistence. The classic theory proposes 9 dimensions of temperament (Table 18.1). These characteristics lead to 3 common constellations: (1) the easy, highly adaptable child, who has regular biologic cycles; (2) the difficult child, who is inflexible, moody, and easily frustrated; and (3) the slow-to-warm-up child, who needs extra time to adapt to new circumstances. Various combinations of these clusters also occur. Temperament has long been described as biologic or "inherited." Monozygotic twins are rated by their parents as temperamentally similar more often than are dizygotic twins. Estimates of heritability suggest that genetic differences account for approximately 20–60% of the variability of temperament within a population. The remainder of the variance is attributed to the child's environment. Maternal prenatal stress and anxiety is associated with child temperament, possibly through stress hormones. However, certain polymorphisms of specific genes moderate the influence of maternal stress on infant temperament. Children who are easily frustrated, fearful, or irritable may elicit negative parental reactions, making these children even more susceptible to negative parenting behaviors and to poor adjustment to adversity. Longitudinal twin studies of adult personality indicate that changes in personality over time largely result from nonshared environmental influences, whereas stability of temperament appears to result from genetic factors.

The concept of temperament can help parents understand and accept the characteristics of their children without feeling responsible for having caused them. Children who have difficulty adjusting to change may have behavior problems when a new baby arrives or at the time of school entry. In addition, pointing out the child's temperament may allow for adjustment in parenting styles. Behavioral and emotional problems may develop when the temperamental characteristics of children and parents are in conflict. For example, if parents who keep an irregular schedule have a child who is not readily adaptable, behavioral difficulties are more likely than if the child has parents who have predictable routines.

Psychologic Influences: Attachment and Contingency

The influence of the child-rearing environment dominates most current models of development. Infants in hospitals and orphanages, devoid of opportunities for attachment, have severe developmental deficits. **Attachment** refers to a biologically determined tendency of a young child to seek proximity to the parent during times of stress and also to the relationship that allows securely attached children to use their parents to reestablish a sense of well-being after a stressful experience. Insecure attachment may be predictive of later behavioral and learning problems.

Table 18.1	Temperamental Characteristics: Descriptions and Examples	
CHARACTERISTIC	**DESCRIPTION**	**EXAMPLES***
Activity level	Amount of gross motor movement	"She's constantly on the move." "He would rather sit still than run around."
Rhythmicity	Regularity of biologic cycles	"He's never hungry at the same time each day." "You could set a watch by her nap."
Approach and withdrawal	Initial response to new stimuli	"She rejects every new food at first." "He sleeps well in any place."
Adaptability	Ease of adaptation to novel stimulus	"Changes upset him." "She adjusts to new people quickly."
Threshold of responsiveness	Intensity of stimuli needed to evoke a response (e.g., touch, sound, light)	"He notices all the lumps in his food and objects to them." "She will eat anything, wear anything, do anything."
Intensity of reaction	Energy level of response	"She shouts when she is happy and wails when she is sad." "He never cries much."
Quality of mood	Usual disposition (e.g., pleasant, glum)	"He does not laugh much." "It seems like she is always happy."
Distractibility	How easily diverted from ongoing activity	"She is distracted at mealtime when other children are nearby." "He doesn't even hear me when he is playing."
Attention span and persistence	How long a child pays attention and sticks with difficult tasks	"He goes from toy to toy every minute." "She will keep at a puzzle until she has mastered it."

*Typical statements of parents, reflecting the range for each characteristic from very little to very much.
Based on data from Chess S, Thomas A: *Temperament in clinical practice*, New York, 1986, Guilford.

At all stages of development, children progress optimally when they have adult caregivers who pay attention to their verbal and nonverbal cues and respond accordingly. In early infancy, such contingent responsiveness to signs of overarousal or underarousal helps maintain infants in a state of quiet alertness and fosters autonomic self-regulation. **Contingent responses** (reinforcement depending on the behavior of the other) to nonverbal gestures create the groundwork for the shared attention and reciprocity that are critical for later language and social development. Children learn best when new challenges are just slightly more difficult than what they have already mastered, a degree of difficulty dubbed the "zone of proximal development." Psychologic forces, such as attention problems (see Chapter 49) or mood disorders (see Chapter 39), will have profound effects on many aspects of an older child's life.

Social Factors: Family Systems and the Ecologic Model

Contemporary models of child development recognize the critical importance of influences outside the mother–child dyad. Fathers play critical roles, both in their direct relationships with their children and in supporting mothers. As traditional nuclear families become less dominant, the influence of other family members (grandparents, foster and adoptive parents, same-sex partners) becomes increasingly important. Children are increasingly raised by unrelated caregivers while parents work or while they are in foster care.

Families function as systems, with internal and external boundaries, subsystems, roles, and rules for interaction. In families with rigidly defined parental subsystems, children may be denied any decision-making, exacerbating rebelliousness. In families with poorly defined parent–child boundaries, children may be required to take on responsibilities beyond their years or may be recruited to play a spousal role.

Family systems theory recognizes that individuals within systems adopt implicit roles. Although birth order does not have long-term effects on personality development, within families the members take on different roles. One child may be the troublemaker, whereas another is the negotiator and another is quiet. Changes in one person's behavior affects every other member of the system; roles shift until a new equilibrium is found. The birth of a new child, attainment of developmental milestones such as independent walking, the onset of nighttime fears, and the death of a grandparent are all changes that require renegotiation of roles within the family and have the potential for healthy adaptation or dysfunction.

The family system, in turn, functions within the larger systems of extended family, subculture, culture, and society. Bronfenbrenner's ecologic model depicts these relationships as concentric circles, with the parent–child dyad at the center (with associated risks and protective factors) and the larger society at the periphery. Changes at any level are reflected in the levels above and below. The shift from an industrial economy to one based on service and information is an obvious example of societal change with profound effects on families and children.

Unifying Concepts: The Transactional Model, Risk, and Resilience

The **transactional model** proposes that a child's status at any point in time is a function of the interaction between biologic and social influences. The influences are bidirectional: biologic factors, such as temperament and health status, both affect the child-rearing environment and are affected by it. A premature infant may cry little and sleep for long periods; the infant's depressed parent may welcome this behavior, setting up a cycle that leads to poor nutrition and inadequate growth. The child's failure to thrive may reinforce the parent's sense of failure as a parent. At a later stage, impulsivity and inattention associated with early, prolonged undernutrition may lead to aggressive behavior. The cause of the aggression in this case is not the prematurity, the undernutrition, or the maternal depression, but the interaction of all these factors (Fig. 18.3). Conversely, children with biologic risk factors may nevertheless do well developmentally if the child-rearing environment is supportive. Premature infants with electroencephalographic evidence of neurologic immaturity may be at increased risk for cognitive delay. This risk may only be realized when the quality of parent–child interaction is poor. When parent–child interactions are optimal, prematurity carries a reduced risk of developmental disability.

An estimate of developmental risk can begin with risk factors, such as low income, limited parental education, and lack of neighborhood resources. Stress and anxiety in pregnancy are associated with cognitive, behavioral, and emotional problems in the child. Early stress may have effects on aging mediated by shortening of telomere length, a link to health disparities. Risk for negative outcomes over time increases exponentially as a result of declining plasticity and accumulation of risk factors (both behavioral and environmental). Interventions are most effective in young children; over time, risk increases as the ability to change decreases.

Children growing up in poverty experience multiple levels of developmental risk: increased exposure to biologic risk factors, such as environmental lead and undernutrition; lack of stimulation in the home; and decreased access to interventional education and therapeutic experiences. As they respond by withdrawal or acting out, they further discourage positive stimulation from those around them. Children of adolescent mothers are also at risk. When early intervention programs provide timely, intensive, comprehensive, and prolonged services, at-risk children show marked and sustained upswings in their developmental trajectory. Early identification of children at developmental risk, along with early intervention to support parenting, is critically important.

Children can have appropriate developmental trajectories despite childhood trauma. **Resilience** is the ability to withstand, adapt to, and recover from adversities. There are several resilience factors that can be modified: a positive appraisal or outlook and good executive functioning (see Chapter 48); nurturing parenting (see Chapter 19); good maternal mental health, good self-care skills, and consistent household routines; and an understanding of trauma. The personal histories of children who overcome poverty often include at least one trusted adult (parent,

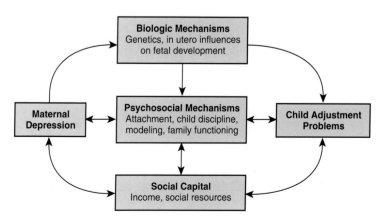

Fig. 18.3 Theoretical model of mutual influences on maternal depression and child adjustment. *(From Elgar FJ, McGrath PJ, Waschbusch DA, et al: Mutual influences on maternal depression and child adjustment problems, Clin Psychol Rev 24:441–459, 2004.)*

Table 18.2	Classic Developmental Stage Theories				
	INFANCY (0-1 YR)	**TODDLERHOOD (2-3 YR)**	**PRESCHOOL (3-6 YR)**	**SCHOOL AGE (6-12 YR)**	**ADOLESCENCE (12-20 YR)**
Freud: psychosexual	Oral	Anal	Phallic/oedipal	Latency	Genital
Erikson: psychosocial	Basic trust vs mistrust	Autonomy vs shame and doubt	Initiative vs guilt	Industry vs inferiority	Identity vs role diffusion
Piaget: cognitive	Sensorimotor	Sensorimotor	Preoperational	Concrete operations	Formal operations
Kohlberg: moral	—	Preconventional: avoid punishment/obtain rewards (stages 1 and 2)	Conventional: conformity (stage 3)	Conventional: law and order (stage 4)	Postconventional: moral principles

grandparent, teacher) with whom the child has a special, supportive, close relationship. Pediatric providers are positioned to target and bolster resilience in their patients and families.

Developmental Domains and Theories of Emotion and Cognition

Child development can also be tracked by the child's developmental progress in particular domains, such as gross motor, fine motor, social, emotional, language, and cognition. Within each of these categories are *developmental lines* or sequences of changes leading up to particular attainments. Developmental lines in the gross motor domain, from rolling to creeping to independent walking, are clear. Others, such as the line leading to the development of conscience, are subtler.

The concept of a developmental line implies that a child passes through successive stages. Several psychoanalytic theories are based on stages as qualitatively different epochs in the development of emotion and cognition (Table 18.2). In contrast, behavioral theories rely less on qualitative change and more on the gradual modification of behavior and accumulation of competence.

Psychoanalytic Theories

At the core of **Freudian theory** is the idea of body-centered (or broadly, "sexual") drives; the emotional health of both the child and the adult depends on adequate resolution of these conflicts. Although Freudian ideas have been challenged, they opened the door to subsequent theories of development.

Erikson recast Freud's stages in terms of the emerging personality (see Table 18.2). The child's sense of basic trust develops through the successful negotiation of infantile needs. As children progress through these psychosocial stages, different issues become salient. It is predictable that a toddler will be preoccupied with establishing a sense of autonomy, whereas a late adolescent may be more focused on establishing meaningful relationships and an occupational identity. Erikson recognized that these stages arise in the context of Western European societal expectations; in other cultures, the salient issues may be quite different.

Erikson's work calls attention to the intrapersonal challenges facing children at different ages in a way that facilitates professional intervention. Knowing that the salient issue for school-age children is industry vs inferiority, pediatricians inquire about a child's experiences of mastery and failure and (if necessary) suggest ways to ensure adequate successes.

Cognitive Theories

Cognitive development is best understood through the work of **Piaget**. A central tenet of Piaget's work is that cognition changes in *quality*, not just quantity (see Table 18.2). During the sensorimotor stage, an infant's thinking is tied to immediate sensations and a child's ability to manipulate objects. The concept of "in" is embodied in a child's act of putting a block into a cup. With the arrival of language, the nature of thinking changes dramatically; symbols increasingly take the place of objects and actions. Piaget described how children actively construct knowledge for themselves through the linked processes of **assimilation** (taking in new experiences according to existing schemata) and **accommodation** (creating new patterns of understanding to adapt to new information).

In this way, children are continually and actively reorganizing cognitive processes.

Piaget's basic concepts have held up well. Challenges have included questions about the timing of various stages and the extent to which context may affect conclusions about cognitive stage. Children's understanding of cause and effect may be considerably more advanced in the context of sibling relationships than in the manipulation and perception of inanimate objects. In many children, logical thinking appears well before puberty (even in toddlers), the age postulated by Piaget. Of undeniable importance is Piaget's focus on cognition as a subject of empirical study, the universality of the progression of cognitive stages, and the image of a child as actively and creatively interpreting the world.

Piaget's work is of special importance to pediatricians for 3 reasons: (1) Piaget's observations provide insight into many puzzling behaviors of infancy, such as the common exacerbation of sleep problems at 9 and 18 mo of age; (2) Piaget's observations often lend themselves to quick replication in the office, with little special equipment; and (3) open-ended questioning, based on Piaget's work, can provide insights into children's understanding of illness and hospitalization.

Based on cognitive development, **Kohlberg** developed a theory of moral development in 6 stages, from early childhood through adulthood. Preschoolers' earliest sense of right and wrong is egocentric, motivated by externally applied controls. In later stages, children perceive equality, fairness, and reciprocity in their understanding of interpersonal interactions through perspective taking. Most youth will reach stage 4, conventional morality, by mid- to late adolescence. The basic theory has been modified to distinguish morality from social conventions. Whereas moral thinking considers interpersonal interactions, justice, and human welfare, social conventions are the agreed-on standards of behavior particular to a social or cultural group. Within each stage of development, children are guided by the basic precepts of moral behavior, but they also may take into account local standards, such as dress code, classroom behavior, and dating expectations. Additional studies have even demonstrated some protomorality in infants.

Behavioral Theory

This theoretical perspective distinguishes itself by its lack of concern with a child's inner experience. Its sole focus is on observable behaviors and measurable factors that either increase or decrease the frequency with which these behaviors occur. No stages are implied; children, adults, and indeed animals all respond in the same way. In its simplest form, the behaviorist orientation asserts that behaviors that are reinforced occur more frequently; behaviors that are punished or ignored occur less frequently. Reinforcement may be further divided into *positive* reinforcement, when a reward or attention increases the chance of a behavior occurring, and *negative* reinforcement, when removal of an aversive stimulus increases the frequency of the behavior. For example, a teacher who allows students who do the homework Monday through Thursday not to do the assignment on Friday, is using negative reinforcement to motivate homework completion during the week.

The strengths of behavioral theory are its simplicity, wide applicability, and conduciveness to scientific verification. A behavioral approach lends

Table 18.3 Similar or Identical Elements Within 5 Theories of Health Behavior

CONCEPT	GENERAL TENET OF THE CONCEPT "ENGAGING IN THE BEHAVIOR IS LIKELY IF ..."	HEALTH BELIEF MODEL	THEORY OF REASONED ACTION	THEORY OF PLANNED BEHAVIOR	SOCIAL COGNITIVE THEORY	TRANSTHEORETICAL MODEL
ATTITUDINAL BELIEFS						
Appraisal of positive and negative aspects of the behavior and its expected outcome	The positive aspects outweigh the negative aspects.	Benefits, barriers/health motive	Behavioral beliefs and evaluation of those beliefs (attitudes)	Behavioral beliefs and evaluation of those beliefs (attitudes)	Outcome expectations/expectancies	Pros, cons (decisional balance)
SELF-EFFICACY BELIEFS/BELIEFS ABOUT CONTROL OVER THE BEHAVIOR						
Belief in one's ability to perform the behavior; confidence	One believes in one's ability to perform the behavior.	Self-efficacy	—	Perceived behavioral control	Self-efficacy	Self-efficacy/temptation
NORMATIVE AND NORM-RELATED BELIEFS AND ACTIVITIES						
Belief that others want one to engage in the behavior (and one's motivation to comply); may include actual support of others	One believes that people important to one want one to engage in the behavior; person has others' support.	Cues from media, friends (cues to action)	Normative beliefs and motivation to comply (subjective norms)	Normative beliefs and motivation to comply (subjective norms)	Social support	Helping relationships (process of change)
Belief that others (e.g., peers) are engaging in the behavior	One believes that other people are engaging in the behavior.	—	—	—	Social environment/norms; modeling	Social liberation (process of change)
Responses to one's behavior that increase or decrease the likelihood one will engage in the behavior; may include reminders	One receives positive reinforcement from others or creates positive reinforcements for oneself.	Cues from media, friends (cues to action)	—	—	Reinforcement	Reinforcement management/stimulus control (processes of change)
RISK-RELATED BELIEFS AND EMOTIONAL RESPONSES						
Belief that one is at risk if one does not engage in the behavior, and that the consequences may be severe; may include actually experiencing negative emotions or symptoms and coping with them	One feels at risk with regard to a negative outcome or disease.	Perceived susceptibility/severity (perceived threat)	—	—	Emotional coping responses/expectancies about environmental cues	Dramatic relief (process of change)
INTENTION/COMMITMENT/PLANNING						
Intending or planning to perform the behavior; setting goals or making a commitment to perform the behavior	One has formed strong behavioral intentions to engage in the behavior; one has set realistic goals or made a firm commitment to engage in the behavior.	—	Behavioral intentions	Behavioral intentions	Self-control/self-regulation	Contemplation/preparation (stages of change); self-liberation (process of change)

From Noar SM, Zimmerman RS: Health behavior theory and cumulative knowledge regarding health behaviors: are we moving in the right direction? *Health Educ Res* 20:275–290, 2005, Table 1.

itself to interventions for various common problems, such as temper tantrums, aggressive preschool behavior, and eating disorders in which behaviors are broken down into discrete units. In cognitively limited children and children with autism spectrum disorder, behavioral interventions using **applied behavior analysis** approaches have demonstrated the ability to teach new, complex behaviors. Applied behavior analysis has been particularly useful in the treatment of early-diagnosed autism (see Chapter 54). However, when misbehavior is symptomatic of an underlying emotional, perceptual, or family problem, an exclusive reliance on behavior therapy risks leaving the cause untreated. Behavioral approaches can be taught to parents for application at home.

Theories Used in Behavioral Interventions

An increasing number of programs or interventions (within and outside the physician's office) are designed to influence health behaviors; some of these models are based on behavioral or cognitive theory or may have attributes of both. The most commonly employed models are the Health Belief Model, Theory of Reasoned Action, Theory of Planned Behavior, Social Cognitive Theory, and Transtheoretical Model, also known as Stages of Change Theory (see Chapter 17). Pediatricians should be aware of these models and their similarities and differences (Table 18.3). Interventions based on these theories have been designed for children and adolescents in community, clinic, and hospital-based settings.

Motivational interviewing is a technique often used in clinical settings to bring about behavior change, as discussed in detail in Chapter 17. Briefly, the goal is to enhance an individual's motivation to change behavior by exploring and overcoming ambivalence. The therapist is a partner rather than an authority figure and recognizes that, ultimately, the patient has control over his or her choices.

Statistics Used in Describing Growth and Development

(See Chapter 27.)

In everyday use, the term *normal* is synonymous with *healthy*. In a statistical sense, *normal* means that a set of values generates a normal (bell-shaped or gaussian) distribution. This is the case with anthropometric quantities, such as height and weight, and with many developmental measures, such as intelligence quotient (IQ). For a **normally distributed measurement**, a histogram with the quantity (height, age) on the *x* axis and the frequency (the number of children of that height, or the number who stand on their own at that age) on the *y* axis generates a bell-shaped curve. In an ideal bell-shaped curve, the peak corresponds to the arithmetic **mean** (average) of the sample, as well as to the median and the mode. The **median** is the value above and below which 50% of the observations lie; the **mode** is the value having the highest number of observations. Distributions are termed *skewed* if the mean, median, and mode are not the same number.

The extent to which observed values cluster near the mean determines the width of the bell and can be described mathematically by the **standard deviation (SD)**. In the ideal normal curve, a range of values extending from 1 SD below the mean to 1 SD above the mean includes approximately 68% of the values, and each "tail" above and below that range contains 16% of the values. A range encompassing ±2 SD includes 95% of the values (with the upper and lower tails each comprising approximately 2.5% of the values), and ±3 SD encompasses 99.7% of the values (Table 18.4 and Fig. 18.4).

For any single measurement, its distance away from the mean can be expressed in terms of the number of SDs (also called a **z score**); one can then consult a table of the normal distribution to find out what

Table 18.4	Relationship Between Standard Deviation (SD) and Normal Range for Normally Distributed Quantities	

OBSERVATIONS INCLUDED IN THE NORMAL RANGE		PROBABILITY OF A "NORMAL" MEASUREMENT DEVIATING FROM THE MEAN BY THIS AMOUNT	
SD	%	SD	%
±1	68.3	≥1	16.0
±2	95.4	≥2	2.3
±3	99.7	≥3	0.13

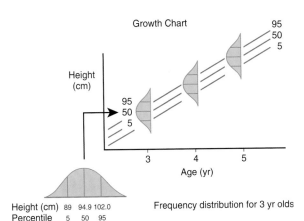

Fig. 18.4 Relationship between percentile lines on the growth curve and frequency distributions of height at different ages.

percentage of measurements fall within that distance from the mean. Software to convert anthropometric data into z scores for epidemiologic purposes is available. A measurement that falls "outside the normal range"—arbitrarily defined as 2, or sometimes 3, SDs on either side of the mean—is atypical, but not necessarily indicative of illness. The further a measurement (height, weight, IQ) falls from the mean, the greater is the probability that it represents not simply normal variation, but rather a different, potentially pathologic condition.

Another way of relating an individual to a group uses percentiles. The **percentile** is the percentage of individuals in the group who have achieved a certain measured quantity (e.g., height of 95 cm) or a developmental milestone (e.g., walking independently). For anthropometric data, the percentile cutoffs can be calculated from the mean and SD. The 5th, 10th, and 25th percentiles correspond to −1.65 SD, −1.3 SD, and −0.7 SD, respectively. Fig. 18.4 demonstrates how frequency distributions of a particular parameter (height) at different ages relate to the percentile lines on the growth curve.

Bibliography is available at Expert Consult.

Chapter **19**

Positive Parenting and Support

Rebecca A. Baum

第十九章
积极养育与支持

中文导读

本章主要介绍了积极养育的重要性，家庭环境、父母教养方式、子女的气质类型、儿童行为问题等因素对儿童健康发展的影响，介绍了积极养育的概念以及儿科医师在养育支持中所起的作用。具体描述了亲子关系和父母的教养对儿童认知技能、社会情感等方面的影响；描述了家庭环境对养育方式的影响，权威型、独裁型和宽容型的父母在教养方式上的差异；描述了儿童气质与父母的养育实践的相互作用，儿童行为问题产生的危险因素；描述了积极养育的属性和特征，以及积极养育作为一种干预措施的效果；描述了儿科医师对积极养育的支持及支持的途径。

No force may be more important to a child's development than the family. Many factors contribute to the family's influence, including family structure, functioning, economics, and stress. Parenting provides the foundation to promote healthy child development and to protect against adverse outcomes. The term **positive parenting** describes an approach to parenting that achieves these goals.

THE IMPORTANCE OF PARENTING

Interactions between parents and their children provide stimulation that promotes the development of language, early cognitive skills, and school readiness. Less frequent participation in interactive parenting practices, such as reading aloud to children, eating family meals, and participating in family outings, predicts an increased risk of developmental delay in low-income families. Interventions that increase parents' reading to children promote positive developmental outcomes such as early language and literacy development.

The affective nature of the parent–child interaction is important for both cognitive and social emotional development. Persistent maternal depression has been linked to decreases in child IQ scores at school entry. Early exposure to positive parenting has been associated with lower rates of childhood depression, risky behavior, delinquency, injuries, behavior problems, and bullying, with increased likelihood of empathy and prosocial behavior. The beneficial effects of early maternal sensitivity on social competence have been found to persist into adulthood, suggesting that early life experiences have a long-term impact.

Positive parenting practices, such as using a warm, supporting approach during conflict, and negative practices, such as maternal aggression, have been associated with MRI changes in adolescent brain development in boys. Animal models have been used to demonstrate the detrimental effects of stressful early life experiences, characterized by maternal separation or decreased maternal responsiveness. Offspring raised in these environments were more likely to exhibit fearful behavior. Differences were noted in brain architecture and epigenetic changes that alter gene expression (see Chapter 100). Importantly in these animal models, increased maternal nurturing could protect against these changes.

THE ROLE OF THE FAMILY

Parenting occurs in the context of a family unit, and there is significant diversity among families. Family makeup has changed greatly over the last several decades in the United States, with increases in cultural, ethnic, and spiritual diversity and in single-parent families. In 2014, based on U.S. Census Bureau data, 26% of children lived in single-parent families, and 62% lived in households with 2 married parents. These patterns differ when race and ethnicity are considered; the majority of children in white and Asian American families live in households with married parents, whereas only 31% of black children do, with about half (57%) living in single-parent households. Although children can thrive in all types of family environments, data suggest that, on average, children living in single-parent families fare less well than their counterparts. Children in single-parent households are 3 times more likely to be living below the poverty line than those in families with 2 married parents. Mothers are the primary breadwinner in 40% of families, an increase from 10% in 1960, yet families led by unmarried mothers tend to fare worse than those led by unmarried fathers.

Families are also changing how they spend time together. Media use for both parents and children has increased dramatically with the advent of tablets and smartphones. Over the last several decades, as women have entered the workforce, increasing numbers of children participate in childcare, and in after-school activities. Racial, ethnic, and economic disparities are found in those participating in these activities as well. More children from economically advantaged families participate in extracurricular activities; low-income and black families worry more about the availability of high-quality programming for their children.

The U.S. Census Bureau projects that by 2040 the majority of the U.S. population will consist of minorities, with steady increases in foreign-born populations and individuals reporting 2 or more ethnicities. This diversity will impact family composition, as well as family values and approaches to parenting. *Culture* refers to a pattern of social norms, values, language, and behavior shared by a group of individuals, and parents are thus affected by their culture. Parenting approaches to self-regulation vary across cultures with respect to promoting attention, compliance, delayed gratification, executive function, and effortful control.

PARENTING STYLES

Three styles of parenting are authoritative, authoritarian, and permissive, each with varying approaches to parental control and responsiveness. A fourth style, neglectful parenting, has also been suggested. **Authoritative parenting** describes a parenting style that is warm, responsive, and accepting but that also sets expectations for behavior and achievement. Differences are approached with reasoning and discussion rather than by exerting control. **Authoritarian parenting** is characterized by a high degree of parental control in which obedience is expected. Punishment is often employed to foster compliance rather than verbal discussion. **Permissive parenting** refers to an approach characterized by warmth and acceptability but with few rules or expectations, and the child's autonomy is highly valued. This contrasts with **neglectful parenting**, similarly characterized by few rules or expectations, but also by limited parental warmth or responsiveness.

Studies have found that an authoritative parenting style is most likely to be associated with positive child outcomes across multiple domains, including educational achievement and social-emotional competence. Parental supervision, consistency, and open communication reduce risky behaviors in adolescents. Harsh, inconsistent, and coercive discipline and physical punishment have been associated with increases in emotional and behavioral problems and may be a risk factor for child maltreatment. Much of the initial research on parenting styles was based on select U.S. populations (white middle-class families). Some suggest that an authoritarian parenting style may be beneficial in certain environments, and further work is needed to account for the economic and demographic changes in U.S. families.

CHILD TEMPERAMENT

As evidenced by the effects of family structure, culture/ethnicity, and economics, parenting does not occur in isolation. The child also brings to the parent–child relationship their own personality, or **temperament,** a collection of traits that stay relatively constant over time (see Chapter 18). Nine traits have been identified in child temperament: activity level, predictability of behavior, reaction to new environments, adaptability, intensity, mood, distractibility, persistence, and sensitivity. Most infants (65%) fit into 1 of 3 groups: easy (40%), difficult (10%), and slow to warm up (15%), and these patterns are relatively stable over time. Although variations in temperament traits are part of normal human variations, certain behavioral difficulties have been associated with certain temperament types. For example, a difficult temperament has been associated with the development of externalizing behavior (e.g., acting-out, disruptive, and aggressive behavior) and not surprisingly, a slow-to-warm-up temperament with internalizing behavior (e.g., anxious and moody behavior).

Temperament traits are relatively stable, but how the child functions is affected by the environment, especially by parenting and the "goodness of fit" between the parent and child. Children with difficult temperament

characteristics respond more negatively to neglectful parenting, and children of all temperament groups respond positively to responsive and sensitive parenting. Moreover, childhood traits such as low adaptability, impulsivity, and low frustration tolerance may lead some parents to engage in more negative parenting practices. These findings illustrate the interactive nature between parent and child, with parental behavior shaping child behavior, and vice versa.

CHILD BEHAVIORAL PROBLEMS

Emotional and behavioral problems are common in childhood. Indeed, many patterns of challenging behavior are normative in childhood, such as the tantrums and negativism seen in toddlers. Approximately 7.4% of children 4-17 yr of age have emotional and behavioral problems, defined as either elevated symptoms or serious overall difficulties. Emotional and behavioral problems have been associated with mother-only households, poverty, and developmental disorders. In preschool children, rates of clinically significant challenging behavior have been estimated at 8–17%, again with an increased prevalence among children living in poverty. The association between challenging behavior and poverty is likely multifactorial, mediated by increases in family stress, more negative parenting behaviors, lower-quality childcare, parental mental health issues, and community violence. Evidence also suggests that some types of challenging behavior apparent at a young age may persist. In one study, a high percentage of preschoolers identified as having both internalizing and externalizing behavior at age 3 yr continued to have similar difficulties at 6 yr.

Other risk factors for the development of challenging behavior include trauma and developmental problems. **Adverse childhood experiences**

Table 19.1	Components of Purposeful Parenting
ATTRIBUTE	**DEFINING ACTIONS**
Protective	Ensure the child's emotional, developmental, and physiologic needs are met. Provide a safe environment. Balance the need for safety with the child's need for exploration and independence.
Personal	Show unconditional love and acceptance. Be kind and gentle. Avoid name-calling and harsh language. Label emotions and behaviors to help children understand their feelings. Teach and model helpful behavior rather than just saying "no."
Progressive	Adapt parenting skills and discipline to meet the child's developmental needs. Learn about child development to know what to expect. Notice and praise new skills and desirable behaviors.
Positive	Be warm, supportive, and optimistic, even during times of misbehavior. Avoid harsh or physical punishments. Provide encouragement and reward effort, not just a positive result.
Playful	Enjoy child-led time together to encourage exploration, foster creativity, and learn new skills. Read together.
Purposeful	Take care of your needs as a parent. Keep the long-terms goals of parenting in mind. Preferentially use teaching instead of punishment to encourage desirable behavior. Be consistent with routines and expectations. Try to understand the reason behind the child's behavior.

Adapted from the work of Andrew Garner and the Ohio Chapter, American Academy of Pediatrics. http://ohioaap.org/wp-content/uploads/2013/07/BPoM_PurposefulParenting.pdf.

(ACEs), defined as abuse and neglect, caregiver substance use, caregiver depression, and domestic violence or criminality, are often present during childhood. In the National Survey of Child and Adolescent Well-Being, 42% of children under 6 yr of age in the child welfare system had experienced 4 or more ACEs. Further, there was a cumulative relationship between emotional and behavioral problems and ACE exposure, with children exposed to 4 or more ACEs almost 5 times more likely to have internalizing problems than children not exposed to ACEs. A similar relationship was found for externalizing problems. Studies involving children with developmental disabilities suggest emotional and behavioral problems occur more frequently in this group than in typically developing children. These children may have delays in self-regulation and communication skills as well as increased family stress, which contribute to the increased likelihood of behavioral challenges.

DEFINING POSITIVE PARENTING

The precise definition of the components of positive parenting are lacking. Positive parenting must ensure the child's safety, health, and nutrition as well as developmental promotion. Common attributes of positive parenting include: caring, leading, providing, teaching, and communicating with the child in a consistent and unconditional manner. To account for the long-term goals of successful parenting in promoting optimal emotional, behavioral, and developmental outcomes, some suggest the term **purposeful parenting** and related characteristics (Table 19.1). The characterization of an ideal approach to parenting will evolve with ever-changing societal norms, but key components such as those in Table 19.1 will likely remain fundamental.

PARENTING AS AN INTERVENTION

The influence of parenting practices on child behavior, development, and overall adjustment has led to efforts to teach parenting as a method of primary prevention. The Video Interaction Project (VIP) uses a coaching and education model with recorded parent–child interactions to foster positive parenting behavior. These parenting behaviors range from reading aloud to encouraging interactive play. In an urban, low-income, primary care setting, parent and child outcomes for the VIP group were compared to those from a lower-intensity intervention (parent mailings encouraging positive parenting behaviors) and a control group. VIP produced the most robust impacts on socioemotional outcomes, including increased attention and decreased distress with separation, hyperactivity, and externalizing behavior in toddlers.

Positive parenting as a public health intervention has resulted in decreased rates of substantiated child maltreatment cases, out-of-home placements, and child maltreatment injuries. Other effective public health approaches include home-visiting programs, which have been deployed to at-risk families in an effort to improve maternal and child outcomes. The Maternal, Infant and Early Childhood Home Visiting Program, authorized as part of the Affordable Care Act of 2010 and again in 2015, is part of the Medicare Access and Children's Health Insurance Program (CHIP) Reauthorization Act. A key component of home-visiting programs is the promotion of positive parenting behavior to foster child developmental and school readiness. Group parenting programs have been deployed as primary prevention to promote emotional and behavioral adjustment in young children. There is moderate-quality evidence that group-based parenting programs may improve parent–child interactions. These programs typically employ praise, encouragement, and affection and have been associated with improved self-esteem and social and academic competence.

Parenting behaviors have also been employed as an *intervention* to treat emotional and behavioral problems in young children. Parenting interventions such as Incredible Years, Triple P Positive Parenting Program, and New Forrest Parenting Program are effective for at least short-term improvements in child conduct problems, parental mental health, and parenting practices. Also called *parent training programs*, most teach the importance of play, rewards, praise, and consistent discipline and allow parents to practice new skills. This active-learning component distinguishes parent training programs from educational programs, which have been shown to be less effective.

Teaching emotional communication skills and positive parent–child

Table 19.2	Parent Training Program Components	
COMPONENT	**ACTIVITIES**
Knowledge about child development and behavior	Providing developmentally-appropriate environment Learning about child development Promoting positive emotional development
Positive parent–child interactions	Learning the importance of positive, non–discipline-focused interactions Using skills that promote positive interactions Providing positive attention
Responsiveness and warmth	Responding sensitively to the child's emotional needs Providing appropriate physical contact and affection
Emotional communication	Using active listening to foster communication Helping children identify and express emotion
Disciplinary communication	Setting clear, appropriate, and consistent expectations Establishing limits and rules Choosing and following through with appropriate consequences
Discipline and behavior management	Understanding child misbehavior Understanding appropriate discipline strategies Using safe and appropriate monitoring and supervision practices Using reinforcement techniques Using problem solving for challenging behavior Being consistent
Promoting children's social skills and prosocial behavior	Teaching children to share, cooperate, and get along with others Using good manners
Promoting children's cognitive or academic skills	Fostering language and literacy development Promoting school readiness

Adapted from US Centers for Disease Control and Prevention: Parent training programs: insight for practitioners, Atlanta, 2009, CDC.

interaction skills are associated with parent training programs that demonstrate a greater increase in parenting skills (Table 19.2). Several components are associated with programs that show greater improvements in child externalizing behavior: teaching parents to use time-out correctly, respond consistently, and interact positively with their children. All successful programs require parents to practice parenting skills during the program.

Parents have been found to benefit from participation in parenting programs. Before their participation, parents experienced a loss of control, self-blame, social isolation, and difficulty dealing with their child's emotional and behavioral problems, all of which improved after participation. The few studies that have assessed the long-term efficacy of parent-training programs suggest overall positive child outcomes, but also periods of relapse during which the use of positive parenting skills decreased. Use of social supports is associated with positive child outcomes and may be an important program component when considering long-term success.

THE ROLE OF THE PEDIATRICIAN

Pediatricians and other pediatric practitioners have a primary responsibility to support the needs of parents and their children. Numerous programs and interventions have been developed to be delivered effectively and efficiently in the primary care setting.

The American Academy of Pediatrics published Bright Futures and the associated Guidelines for Preventive Care to standardize child health promotion and prevention in primary care. A substantial amount of the content in Bright Futures maps to the positive-parenting domains of safety, feeding, developmental promotion, and protection. Implementing Bright Futures guidelines in health supervision visits is an important way for pediatric practitioners to support the promotion of positive parenting in practice.

Reading aloud to children is a powerful strategy to promote language development, early literacy, and positive parent–child interaction. The Reach Out and Read program is a primary care–based intervention that trains practitioners to encourage parents to read with their child and provides books to at-risk families. In the absence of a formal partnership with Reach Out and Read, practitioners should promote the benefits of reading aloud to children and support parents in their efforts to develop habits that incorporate reading into daily routines.

In addition to VIP described earlier, other primary care models to promote parenting have been studied. The Healthy Steps for Young Children program is a strengths-based approach delivered in the primary care setting from infancy to age 3 yr. Healthy Steps promotes changes in parents' knowledge, beliefs, and psychologic health and changes in parenting behaviors using a variety of methods delivered in the office setting by the practitioner and Healthy Steps specialists and through home visits. Extensive evaluations have shown improvements in parental well-being, parenting practices, and parent–child attachment and decreased child behavior problems. Another promising approach uses community health workers and nurses to provide parenting education and allow mothers to practice parenting skills outside the office setting.

If participation in a formal parenting program is not possible, pediatric practitioners can still implement a systematic approach to support the needs of parents and their children. Practitioners can take advantage of materials in the public domain from national organizations devoted to child and family health, such as ZERO TO THREE (https://www.zerotothree.org/ and the American Academy of Pediatrics https://www.aap.org/). The U.S. Centers for Disease Control and Prevention (CDC) also provides evidenced-based parenting resources (https://www.cdc.gov/parents/essentials/index.html). Additional components include early identification of parents' concerns, addressing concerns in a supportive and nonjudgmental way, and providing linkage to treatment services when appropriate.

Parents want more information about child development, but parents of children with behavior problems often feel stigmatized and isolated. Practitioners are encouraged to be supportive and optimistic in their interactions with families, to develop a partnership aimed at promoting parent and child health (see Chapter 17). Practitioners may also encourage parents to practice new skills briefly in the office setting before trying a new skill at home. Active modeling by the practitioner using "teachable moments" may also be effective.

Bibliography is available at Expert Consult.

Chapter 20

Assessment of Fetal Growth and Development

Susan Feigelman and Laura H. Finkelstein

第二十章

胎儿生长发育评估

中文导读

本章主要介绍了胎儿的生长发育，包括体细胞的发育、神经系统的发育及行为的发展，介绍了妊娠期父母的心理变化以及影响胎儿发育的危险因素。具体描述了胚胎期和胎儿期的生长，组织、器官的形成以及发育里程碑；描述了神经系统发育的生理学基础，神经功能行为的出现和胎儿的运动模式等内容；描述了影响胎儿发育的危险因素，包括染色体异常、传染病、化学制剂、高温和辐射、尼古丁、乙醇、可卡因、胎儿宫内营养状况及心理创伤等。

The developing fetus is affected by social and environmental influences, including maternal nutritional status; substance use (both legal and illicit); and psychologic trauma. Correspondingly, the psychologic alterations experienced by the parents during the gestation profoundly impact the lives of all members of the family. Growing evidence implicates the importance of these and other maternal and paternal experiences that occur during and prior to the pregnancy (and even among members of earlier generations) on the subsequent development of the individual (epigenetic effects; see Chapter 100). The complex interplay among these forces and the somatic and neurologic transformations occurring in the fetus influence growth and behavior at birth, through infancy, and potentially throughout the individual's life.

SOMATIC DEVELOPMENT
Embryonic Period
Table 20.1 lists milestones of prenatal development. By 6 days postconception age, as implantation begins, the embryo consists of a spherical mass of cells with a central cavity (the *blastocyst*). By 2 wk, implantation is complete and the uteroplacental circulation has begun; the embryo has 2 distinct layers, *endoderm* and *ectoderm*, and the amnion has started to form. By 3 wk, the 3rd primary germ layer (*mesoderm*) has appeared, along with a primitive neural tube and blood vessels. Paired heart tubes have begun to pump.

During wk 4-8, lateral folding of the embryologic plate, followed by growth at the cranial and caudal ends and the budding of arms and legs, produces a human-like shape. Precursors of skeletal muscle and vertebrae (somites) appear, along with the branchial arches that will form the mandible, maxilla, palate, external ear, and other head and neck structures. Lens placodes appear, marking the site of future eyes; the brain grows rapidly. By the end of wk 8, as the embryonic period closes, the rudiments of all major organ systems have developed; the crown-rump length is 3 cm.

Fetal Period
From the 9th wk on (fetal period), somatic changes consist of rapid body growth as well as differentiation of tissues, organs, and organ systems. Fig. 20.1 depicts changes in body proportion. By wk 10, the face is recognizably human. The midgut returns to the abdomen from the umbilical cord, rotating counterclockwise to bring the stomach, small intestine, and large intestine into their normal positions. By wk 12, the gender of the external genitals becomes clearly distinguishable. Lung development proceeds, with the budding of bronchi, bronchioles, and successively smaller divisions. By wk 20-24, primitive alveoli have formed and surfactant production has begun; before that time, the absence of alveoli renders the lungs useless as organs of gas exchange.

During the 3rd trimester, weight triples and length doubles as body stores of protein, fat, iron, and calcium increase.

NEUROLOGIC DEVELOPMENT
During the 3rd wk, a neural plate appears on the ectodermal surface of the trilaminar embryo. Infolding produces a neural tube that will become the central nervous system and a neural crest that will become the peripheral nervous system. Neuroectodermal cells differentiate into neurons, astrocytes, oligodendrocytes, and ependymal cells, whereas microglial cells are derived from mesoderm. By the 5th wk, the 3 main subdivisions of forebrain, midbrain, and hindbrain are evident. The dorsal and ventral horns of the spinal cord have begun to form, along with the peripheral motor and sensory nerves. Myelinization begins at midgestation and continues for years.

By the end of the embryonic period (wk 8), the gross structure of the nervous system has been established. On a cellular level, neurons migrate outward to form the 6 cortical layers. Migration is complete by the 6th mo, but differentiation continues. Axons and dendrites form synaptic connections at a rapid pace, making the central nervous system vulnerable to teratogenic or hypoxic influences throughout gestation. Fig. 20.2 shows rates of increase in DNA (a marker of cell number), overall brain weight, and cholesterol (a marker of myelinization). The prenatal and postnatal peaks of DNA probably represent rapid growth of neurons and glia, respectively. The glial cells are important in shaping

Table 20.1	Milestones of Prenatal Development
WK	**DEVELOPMENTAL EVENTS**
1	Fertilization and implantation; beginning of *embryonic* period
2	Endoderm and ectoderm appear (bilaminar embryo)
3	First missed menstrual period; mesoderm appears (trilaminar embryo); somites begin to form
4	Neural folds fuse; folding of embryo into human-like shape; arm and leg buds appear; crown-rump length 4-5 mm
5	Lens placodes, primitive mouth, digital rays on hands
6	Primitive nose, philtrum, primary palate
7	Eyelids begin; crown-rump length 2 cm
8	Ovaries and testes distinguishable
9	*Fetal* period begins; crown-rump length 5 cm; weight 8 g
12	External genitals distinguishable
20	Usual lower limit of viability; weight 460 g; length 19 cm
25	Third trimester begins; weight 900 g; length 24 cm
28	Eyes open; fetus turns head down; weight 1,000-1,300 g
38	Term

the brain and neuronal circuits. The various types of glial cells are needed for the formation of axonal myelin sheaths, a range of functions in the formation and maintenance of neural pathways, and removal of waste (the brain has no lymphoid system for this task).

By the time of birth, the structure of the brain is complete. However, many cells will undergo *apoptosis* (cell death). Synapses will be pruned back substantially, and new connections will be made, largely as a result of experience. Many psychiatric and developmental disorders are thought to result at least in part from disruptions in the **functional connectivity** of brain networks. Disorders of connectivity may begin during fetal life; MRI studies provide a developmental timetable for such connections that lend support to the possible role of disruptions in the establishment of such connections.

BEHAVIORAL DEVELOPMENT
No behavioral evidence of neural function is detectable until the 3rd mo. Reflexive responses to tactile stimulation develop in a craniocaudal sequence. By wk 13-14, breathing and swallowing motions appear. The grasp reflex appears at 17 wk and is well developed by 27 wk. Eye opening occurs around 26-28 wk. By midgestation, the full range of neonatal movements can be observed.

During the 3rd trimester, fetuses respond to external stimuli with heart rate elevation and body movements, which can be observed with ultrasound (see Chapter 115). Reactivity to auditory (vibroacoustic) and visual (bright light) stimuli vary, depending on their behavioral state, which can be characterized as quiet sleep, active sleep, or awake. Individual differences in the level of fetal activity are usually noted by mothers. Fetuses will preferentially turn to light patterns in the configuration of the human face. Fetal movement is affected by maternal medications and diet, increasing after ingestion of caffeine. Behavior may be entrained to the mother's diurnal rhythms: asleep during the day, active at night. Abnormal fetal movement patterns are found in neonates with subsequent muscular or neurologic abnormalities.

Fetal movement increases in response to a sudden auditory tone but decreases after several repetitions. This demonstrates **habituation**, a basic form of learning in which repeated stimulation results in a response decrement. If the tone changes in pitch, the movement increases again, which is evidence that the fetus distinguishes between a familiar, repeated tone and a novel tone. Habituation improves in older fetuses and decreases in neurologically impaired or physically stressed fetuses. Similar responses to visual and tactile stimuli have been observed.

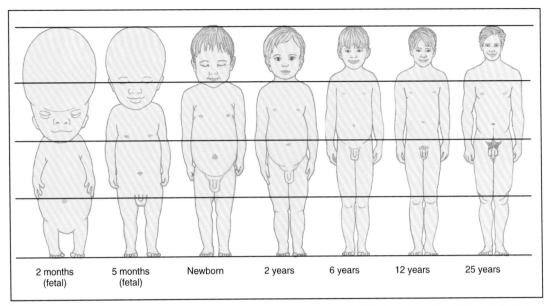

Fig. 20.1 **Changes in body proportions.** Approximate changes in body proportions from fetal life through adulthood. *(From Leifer G: Introduction to maternity & pediatric nursing, Philadelphia, 2011, WB Saunders, pp 347–385, Fig. 15-2.)*

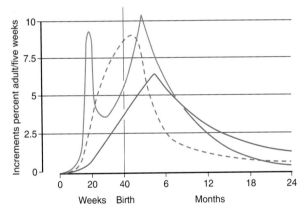

Fig. 20.2 **Velocity curves of the various components of human brain growth.** *Blue line,* DNA; *red line,* brain weight; *green line,* cholesterol. *(From Brasel JA, Gruen RK. In Falkner F, Tanner JM, editors: Human growth: a comprehensive treatise, New York, 1986, Plenum Press, pp 78–95.)*

PSYCHOLOGIC CHANGES IN PARENTS

Many psychologic changes occur during pregnancy. An unplanned pregnancy may be met with anger, denial, or depression. Ambivalent feelings are the norm, whether or not the pregnancy was planned. Elation at the thought of producing a baby and the wish to be the perfect parent compete with fears of inadequacy and of the lifestyle changes that parenting will impose. Parents of an existing child may feel protective of the child, worried that the child may feel less valued. Old conflicts may resurface as a woman psychologically identifies with her own mother and with herself as a child. The father-to-be faces similar mixed feelings, and problems in the parental relationship may intensify.

Tangible evidence that a fetus exists as a separate being, whether as a result of ultrasonic visualization or awareness of fetal movements known as *quickening* (at 16-20 wk), often heightens a woman's feelings.

Parents worry about the fetus's healthy development and mentally rehearse what they will do if the child is malformed, including their response to evidence of abnormality through ultrasound, amniocentesis, or other fetal laboratory tests. Toward the end of pregnancy, a woman becomes aware of patterns of fetal activity and reactivity and begins to ascribe to her fetus an individual personality and an ability to survive independently. Appreciation of the psychologic vulnerability of the expectant parents and of the powerful contribution of fetal behavior facilitates supportive clinical intervention.

THREATS TO FETAL DEVELOPMENT

Mortality and morbidity are highest during the prenatal period (see Chapter 112). An estimated 50% of all pregnancies end in spontaneous abortion, including 10–15% of all clinically recognized pregnancies. The majority occur in the 1st trimester. Some occur as a result of chromosomal or other abnormalities.

Teratogens associated with gross physical and mental abnormalities include various infectious agents (e.g., toxoplasmosis, rubella, syphilis, Zika virus); chemical agents (e.g., mercury, thalidomide, antiepileptic medications, ethanol), high temperature, and radiation (see Chapters 115.6 and 736).

Teratogenic effects may also result in decreased growth and cognitive or behavioral deficits that only become apparent later in life. Nicotine has vasoconstrictor properties and may disrupt dopaminergic and serotonergic pathways. Prenatal exposure to cigarette smoke is associated with lower birthweight, stunting, and smaller head circumference, as well as changes in neonatal neurodevelopmental assessments. Later, these children are at increased risk for learning problems, attention and behavior disorders, and long-term health effects. Alcohol is a significant teratogen affecting physical development, cognition, and behavior (see Chapter 126.3). The effects of prenatal exposure to cocaine, also occurring through alternations in placental blood flow and in direct toxic effects to the developing brain, have been followed in several cohorts and are less dramatic than previously believed. Exposed adolescents show small but significant effects in behavior and functioning but may not show cognitive impairment. The associated risk factors, including other prenatal exposures (alcohol and cigarette co-use) as well as "toxic" postnatal environments frequently characterized by instability, multiple caregivers, and violence exposure remain significant (see Chapters 14 and 16).

The association between an inadequate nutrient supply to the fetus and low birthweight has been recognized for decades; this adaptation on the part of the fetus presumably increases the likelihood that the fetus will survive until birth. For any potential fetal insult, the extent and nature of its effects are determined by characteristics of the host as well as the dose and timing of the exposure. Inherited differences in the metabolism of ethanol, timing of exposure, and the mother's diet may explain the variability in fetal alcohol effects. Organ systems are most vulnerable during periods of maximum growth and differentiation, generally during the 1st trimester (**organogenesis**) (http://www2.epa.gov/children/children-are-not-little-adults details critical periods and specific developmental abnormalities).

Fetal adaptations or responses to an adverse situation in utero, termed **fetal programming** or **developmental plasticity**, have lifelong implications for the individual. Fetal programming may prepare the fetus for an environment that matches that experienced in utero. Fetal programming in response to some environmental and nutritional signals in utero increases the risk of cardiovascular disease, diabetes, and obesity in later life. These adverse long-term effects appear to represent a mismatch between fetal and neonatal environmental conditions and the conditions that the individual will confront later in life; a fetus deprived of adequate calories may or may not as a child or teenager face famine. One proposed mechanism for fetal programming is **epigenetic imprinting**, in which 1 of 2 alleles is turned off through environmentally induced epigenetic modification (see Chapters 97 and 100). Exposure to psychoactive drugs in utero produces drug–protein receptor interactions, affecting both nervous system development and neurotransmitter function. This dysregulation causes long-lasting effects on fetal growth and adult function and may have effects on future generations through these epigenetic changes.

Just as the fetal adaptations to the in utero environment may increase the likelihood of later metabolic conditions, the fetus adapts to the mother's psychologic distress. In response to the stressful environment, physiologic changes involving the hypothalamic-pituitary-adrenal axis and the autonomic nervous system occur. Dysregulation of these systems may explain the associations observed in some but not all studies between maternal distress and negative infant outcomes, including low birthweight, spontaneous abortion, prematurity, and decreased head circumference. In addition, children born to mothers experiencing high stress levels have been found to have higher rates of inattention, impulsivity, conduct disorders, and cognitive changes. Although these changes may have been adaptive in primitive cultures, they are maladaptive in modern societies, leading to psychopathology. Genetic variability, timing of stress during sensitive periods, and the quality of postnatal parenting can attenuate or exacerbate these associations.

Bibliography is available at Expert Consult.

Chapter **21**
The Newborn
John M. Olsson

第二十一章
新生儿

中文导读

本章主要介绍了父母、婴儿在母婴依恋中的角色和儿科医师在新生儿健康发展中所起到的作用。具体描述了促进母婴依恋的产前、产后的影响因素；描述了新生儿体格检查、新生儿互动能力的发展、新生儿唤醒状态调节、新生儿行为状态、新生儿与父母的互动调节；描述了儿科医师在产前评估、促进母乳喂养、新生儿访视、父母–婴儿互动评估及新生儿行为评估中所起的作用。

(See also Chapter 113.)

Regardless of gestational age, the newborn (neonatal) period begins at birth and includes the 1st mo of life. During this time, marked physiologic transitions occur in all organ systems, and the infant learns to respond to many forms of external stimuli. Because infants thrive physically and psychologically only in the context of their social relationships, any description of the newborn's developmental status has to include consideration of the parents' role as well.

PARENTAL ROLE IN MOTHER–INFANT ATTACHMENT

Parenting a newborn infant requires dedication because a newborn's needs are urgent, continuous, and often unclear. Parents must attend to an infant's signals and respond empathically. Many factors influence parents' ability to assume this role.

Prenatal Factors

Pregnancy is a period of psychologic preparation for the profound demands of parenting. Women may experience ambivalence, particularly (but not exclusively) if the pregnancy was unplanned. If financial concerns, physical illness, prior miscarriages or stillbirths, or other crises interfere with psychologic preparation, the neonate may not be welcomed. For adolescent mothers, the demand that they relinquish their own developmental agenda, such as an active social life, may be especially burdensome.

The early experience of being mothered may establish unconsciously held expectations about nurturing relationships that permit mothers to "tune in" to their infants. These expectations are linked with the quality of later infant–parent interactions. Mothers whose early childhoods were marked by traumatic separations, abuse, or neglect may find it especially difficult to provide consistent, responsive care. Instead, they may reenact their childhood experiences with their own infants, as if unable to conceive of the mother–child relationship in any other way. **Bonding** may be adversely affected by several risk factors during pregnancy and in the postpartum period that undermine the mother–child relationship and may threaten the infant's cognitive and emotional development (Table 21.1).

Social support during pregnancy, particularly support from the father and close family members, is also important. Conversely, conflict with or abandonment by the father during pregnancy may diminish the mother's ability to become absorbed with her infant. Anticipation of an early return to work may make some women reluctant to fall in love with their babies because of anticipated separation. Returning to work should be delayed for at least 6 wk, by which time feeding and basic behavioral adjustments have been established.

Many decisions have to be made by parents in anticipation of the birth of their child. One important choice is that of how the infant will be nourished. Among the important benefits of **breastfeeding** is its promotion of bonding. Providing breastfeeding education for the parents at the prenatal visit by the pediatrician and by the obstetrician during prenatal care can increase maternal confidence in breastfeeding after delivery and reduce stress during the newborn period (see Chapter 56).

Peripartum and Postpartum Influences

The continuous presence during labor of a woman trained to offer friendly support and encouragement (a **doula**) results in shorter labor, fewer obstetric complications (including cesarean section), and reduced postpartum hospital stays. Early skin-to-skin contact between mothers and infants immediately after birth may correlate with an increased rate and longer duration of breastfeeding. Most new parents value even a brief period of uninterrupted time in which to get to know their new infant, and increased mother–infant contact over the 1st days of life may improve long-term mother–child interactions. Nonetheless, early separation, although predictably very stressful, does not inevitably impair a mother's ability to bond with her infant. Early discharge home from the maternity ward may undermine bonding, particularly when a new mother is required to resume full responsibility for a busy household.

Postpartum depression may occur in the 1st wk or up to 6 mo after delivery and can adversely affect neonatal growth and development.

Table 21.1	Prenatal Risk Factors for Attachment

Recent death of a loved one
Previous loss of or serious illness in another child
Prior removal of a child
History of depression or serious mental illness
History of infertility or pregnancy loss
Troubled relationship with parents
Financial stress or job loss
Marital discord or poor relationship with the other parent
Recent move or no community ties
No friends or social network
Unwanted pregnancy
No good parenting model
Experience of poor parenting
Drug and/or alcohol abuse
Extreme immaturity

From Dixon SD, Stein MT: *Encounters with children: pediatric behavior and development*, ed 4, Philadelphia, 2006, Mosby, p 131.

Screening tools, such as the **Edinburgh Postnatal Depression Scale (EPDS)**, are available for use during neonatal and infant visits to the pediatric provider. On the EPDS, scores of 0-8 indicate a low likelihood of depression (Table 21.2). Cutoff-score recommendations for further evaluation of depression have ranged from 9 to 13; thus any woman scoring 9 or above should be evaluated further. If postpartum depression is present, referral for mental healthcare will greatly accelerate recovery.

THE INFANT'S ROLE IN MOTHER–INFANT ATTACHMENT

The in utero environment contributes greatly but not completely to the future growth and development of the fetus. Abnormalities in maternal-fetal placental circulation and maternal glucose metabolism or the presence of maternal infection can result in abnormal fetal growth. Infants may be small or large for gestational age as a result. These abnormal growth patterns not only predispose infants to an increased requirement for medical intervention, but also may affect their ability to respond behaviorally to their parents.

Physical Examination

Examination of the newborn should include an **evaluation of growth** (see Chapter 20) and an **observation of behavior**. The average term newborn weighs approximately 3.4 kg (7.5 lb); boys are slightly heavier than girls. Average weight does vary by ethnicity and socioeconomic status. The average length and head circumference are about 50 cm (20 in) and 35 cm (14 in), respectively, in term infants. Each newborn's growth parameters should be plotted on growth curves specific for that infant's gestational age to determine the appropriateness of size. Likewise, specific growth charts for conditions associated with variations in growth patterns have also been developed. The infant's response to being examined may be useful in assessing its vigor, alertness, and tone. Observing how the parents handle their infant, their comfort and affection, is also important. The order of the physical examination should be from the least to the most intrusive maneuver. Assessing visual tracking and response to sound and noting changes of tone with level of activity and alertness are very helpful. Performing this examination and sharing impressions with parents is an important opportunity to facilitate bonding (see Chapter 113).

Interactional Abilities

Soon after birth, neonates are alert and ready to interact and nurse. This first alert-awake period may be affected by maternal analgesics and anesthetics or fetal hypoxia. Neonates are nearsighted, having a fixed focal length of 8-12 inches, approximately the distance from the breast to the mother's face, as well as an inborn visual preference for faces. Hearing is well developed, and infants preferentially turn toward a female voice. These innate abilities and predilections increase the likelihood that when a mother gazes at her newborn, the baby will gaze back. The initial period of social interaction, usually lasting about 40 minutes, is followed by a period of somnolence. After that, briefer periods of alertness or excitation alternate with sleep. If a mother misses her baby's first alert-awake period, she may not experience as long a period of social interaction for several days. The hypothalamic-midbrain-limbic-paralimbic-cortical circuit of the parents interacts to support responses to the infants that are critical for effective parenting (e.g., emotion, attention, motivation, empathy, decision-making).

Modulation of Arousal

Adaptation to extrauterine life requires rapid and profound physiologic changes, including aeration of the lungs, rerouting of the circulation, and activation of the intestinal tract. The necessary behavioral changes are no less profound. To obtain nourishment, to avoid hypo- and hyperthermia, and to ensure safety, neonates must react appropriately to an expanded range of sensory stimuli. Infants must become aroused in response to stimulation, but not so overaroused that their behavior

becomes disorganized. Underaroused infants are not able to feed and interact; overaroused infants show signs of **autonomic instability**, including flushing or mottling, perioral pallor, hiccupping, vomiting, uncontrolled limb movements, and inconsolable crying.

Behavioral States

The organization of infant behavior into discrete behavioral states may reflect an infant's inborn ability to regulate arousal. *Six states* have been described: quiet sleep, active sleep, drowsy, alert, fussy, and crying. In the **alert state**, infants visually fixate on objects or faces and follow them horizontally and (within a month) vertically; they also reliably turn toward a novel sound, as if searching for its source. When overstimulated, they may calm themselves by looking away, yawning, or sucking on their lips or hands, thereby increasing parasympathetic activity and reducing sympathetic nervous activity. The behavioral state determines an infant's muscle tone, spontaneous movement, electroencephalogram pattern, and response to stimuli. In **active sleep**, an

---

Table 21.2	Edinburgh Postnatal Depression Scale

INSTRUCTIONS FOR USERS
1. The mother is asked to underline the response that comes closest to how she has been feeling in the previous 7 days.
2. All 10 items must be completed.
3. Care should be taken to avoid the possibility of the mother discussing her answers with others.
4. The mother should complete the scale herself, unless she has limited English or has difficulty with reading.
5. The Edinburgh Postnatal Depression Scale may be used at 6-8 wk to screen postnatal women. The child health clinic, a postnatal checkup, or a home visit may provide a suitable opportunity for its completion.

EDINBURGH POSTNATAL DEPRESSION SCALE
Name:
Address:
Baby's age:
Because you have recently had a baby, we would like to know how you are feeling. Please underline the answer that comes closest to how you have felt in the past 7 days, not just how you feel today.
Here is an example, already completed.
I have felt happy:
    Yes, all the time
    Yes, most of the time
    No, not very often
    No, not at all
This would mean: "I have felt happy most of the time" during the past week. Please complete the other questions in the same way.
In the past 7 days:

1. I have been able to laugh and see the funny side of things
    As much as I always could
    Not quite so much now
    Definitely not so much now
    Not at all
2. I have looked forward with enjoyment to things
    As much as I ever did
    Rather less than I used to
    Definitely less than I used to
    Hardly at all
*3. I have blamed myself unnecessarily when things went wrong
    Yes, most of the time
    Yes, some of the time
    Not very often
    No, never
4. I have been anxious or worried for no good reason
    No, not at all
    Hardly ever
    Yes, sometimes
    Yes, very often
*5. I have felt scared or panicky for no very good reason
    Yes, quite a lot
    Yes, sometimes
    No, not much
    No, not at all

*6. Things have been getting on top of me
    Yes, most of the time I haven't been able to cope at all
    Yes, sometimes I haven't been coping as well as usual
    No, most of the time I have coped quite well
    No, I have been coping as well as ever
*7. I have been so unhappy that I have had difficulty sleeping
    Yes, most of the time
    Yes, sometimes
    Not very often
    No, not at all
*8. I have felt sad or miserable
    Yes, most of the time
    Yes, quite often
    Not very often
    No, not at all
*9. I have been so unhappy that I have been crying
    Yes, most of the time
    Yes, quite often
    Only occasionally
    No, never
*10. The thought of harming myself has occurred to me
    Yes, quite often
    Sometimes
    Hardly ever
    Never

Response categories are scored 0, 1, 2, and 3 according to increased severity of the symptom. Items marked with an asterisk (*) are reverse-scored (i.e., 3, 2, 1, and 0). The total score is calculated by adding the scores for each of the 10 items. Users may reproduce the scale without further permission provided they respect copyright (which remains with the *British Journal of Psychiatry*) by quoting the names of the authors, the title, and the source of the paper in all reproduced copies.
From Currie ML, Rademacher R: The pediatrician's role in recognizing and intervening in postpartum depression, *Pediatr Clin North Am* 51:785–801, 2004.

infant may show progressively less reaction to a repeated heelstick (habituation), whereas in the **drowsy state**, the same stimulus may push a child into fussing or crying.

Mutual Regulation

Parents actively participate in an infant's state regulation, alternately stimulating and soothing. In turn, they are regulated by the infant's signals, responding to cries of hunger with a letdown of milk (or with a bottle). Such interactions constitute a system directed toward furthering the infant's physiologic homeostasis and physical growth. At the same time, they form the basis for the emerging psychologic relationship between parent and child. Infants come to associate the presence of the parent with the pleasurable reduction of tension (as in feeding) and show this preference by calming more quickly for their mother than for a stranger. This response in turn strengthens a mother's sense of efficacy and her connection with her baby.

IMPLICATIONS FOR THE PEDIATRICIAN

The pediatrician can support healthy newborn development in several ways.

Optimal Practices

A **prenatal pediatric visit** allows pediatricians to assess potential threats to bonding (e.g., tense spousal relationship) and sources of social support. **Supportive hospital policies** include the use of birthing rooms rather than operating suites and delivery rooms; encouraging the father or a trusted relative or friend to remain with the mother during labor or the provision of a professional doula; the practice of giving the newborn infant to the mother immediately after drying and a brief assessment; placement of the newborn in the mother's room rather than in a central nursery; and avoiding in-hospital distribution of infant formula. Such policies ("Baby Friendly Hospital") have been shown to significantly increase breastfeeding rates (see Chapter 113.3). After discharge, **home visits** by nurses and lactation counselors can reduce early feeding problems and identify emerging medical conditions in either mother or baby. Infants requiring transport to another hospital should be brought to see the mother first, if at all possible. On discharge home, fathers can shield mothers from unnecessary visits and calls and take over household duties, allowing mothers and infants time to get to know each other without distractions. The **first office visit** should occur during the 1st 2 wk after discharge to determine how smoothly the mother and infant are making the transition to life at home. Babies who are discharged early, those who are breastfeeding, and those who are at risk for jaundice should be seen 1-3 days after discharge.

Assessing Parent–Infant Interactions

During a feeding or when infants are alert and face-to-face with their parents, it is normal for the dyad to appear absorbed in one another. Infants who become overstimulated by the parent's voice or activity may turn away or close their eyes, leading to a premature termination of the encounter. Alternatively, the infant may be ready to interact, but the parent may appear preoccupied. Asking a new mother about her own emotional state, and inquiring specifically about a history of depression, facilitates referral for therapy, which may provide long-term benefits to the child. Pediatricians may detect postpartum depression using the EPDS at well-child visits during the 1st yr (see Table 21.2).

Teaching About Individual Competencies

The **Newborn Behavior Assessment Scale (NBAS)** provides a formal measure of an infant's neurodevelopmental competencies, including state control, autonomic reactivity, reflexes, habituation, and orientation toward auditory and visual stimuli. This examination can also be used to demonstrate to parents an infant's capabilities and vulnerabilities. Parents might learn that they need to undress their infant to increase the level of arousal or to swaddle the infant to reduce overstimulation by containing random arm movements. The NBAS can be used to support the development of positive early parent–infant relationships. Demonstration of the NBAS to parents in the 1st wk of life has been shown to correlate with improvements in the caretaking environment months later.

Bibliography is available at Expert Consult.

Chapter 22
The First Year
Mutiat T. Onigbanjo and Susan Feigelman

第二十二章
婴儿期

中文导读

本章主要介绍了0~2月龄、2~6月龄、6~12月龄3个年龄阶段婴儿的体格发育,认知、情绪及交流能力的发展,父母和儿科医师的角色。具体描述了婴儿身高、体重、头围、脑容量的变化;描述了婴儿期出现的行为模式和发展领域里关键的里程碑,睡眠–觉醒的周期模式,社会性依恋、分离和陌生人焦虑等内容;阐述了婴儿哭闹可能的医学问题以及对哭闹的管理;阐述了肠绞痛的特点、诊断、治疗及父母采取的应对策略。

The prenatal period and the 1st yr of life provide the platform for remarkable growth and development, setting the trajectory for a child's life. **Neural plasticity**, the ability of the brain to be shaped by experience, both positive and negative, is at its peak. Total brain volume doubles in the 1st yr of life and increases by an additional 15% over the 2nd yr. Total brain volume at age 1 mo is approximately 36% of adult volume but by age 1 yr is approximately 72% (83% by 2 yr) (Fig. 22.1).

The acquisition of seemingly "simple" skills, such as swallowing, reflect a series of intricate and highly coordinated processes involving multiple levels of neural control distributed among several physiologic systems whose nature and relationships mature throughout the 1st yr of life. Substantial learning of the basic tools of language (phonology, word segmentation) occurs during infancy. Speech processing in older individuals requires defined and precise neuronal networks; the infant brain possesses a structural and functional organization similar to that of adults, suggesting that structural neurologic processing of speech may guide infants to discover the properties of their native language. Myelination of the cortex begins at 7-8 mo gestation and continues into adolescence and young adulthood. It proceeds posterior to anterior, allowing progressive maturation of sensory, motor, and finally associative pathways. Given the importance of iron, cholesterol, and other nutrients in myelination, adequate stores throughout infancy are critical (see Chapter 56). Insufficient interactions with caregivers or the wider environment may alter experience-dependent processes that are critical to brain structure development and function during infancy. Although for some processes, subsequent stimulation may allow catch-up, as the periods of plasticity close during the rapid developmental changes occurring in infancy, more permanent deficits may result.

The infant acquires new competences in all developmental domains. The concept of **developmental trajectories** recognizes that complex skills build on simpler ones; it is also important to realize how development in each domain affects functioning in all the others. All growth parameters should be plotted using the World Health Organization charts, which show how children from birth through 72 mo "should" grow under optimal circumstances (see Chapter 23, Figs. 23.1 and 23.2). Table 22.1 presents an overview of key milestones by domain; Table 22.2 presents similar information arranged by age. Table 22.3 presents age at time of x-ray appearance of centers of ossification. Parents often seek information about "normal development" during this period and should be directed to reliable sources, including the American Academy of Pediatrics website (healthychildren.org).

AGE 0-2 MONTHS

In the full-term infant, **myelination** is present by the time of birth in the dorsal brainstem, cerebellar peduncles, and posterior limb of the internal capsule. The cerebellar white matter acquires myelin by 1 mo of age and is well myelinated by 3 mo. The subcortical white matter of the parietal, posterior frontal, temporal, and calcarine cortex is partially myelinated by 3 mo of age. In this period the infant experiences tremendous growth. Physiologic changes allow the establishment of effective feeding routines and a predictable sleep–wake cycle. The social interactions that occur as parents and infants accomplish these tasks lay the foundation for cognitive and emotional development.

Physical Development

A newborn's weight may initially decrease 10% (vaginal delivery) to

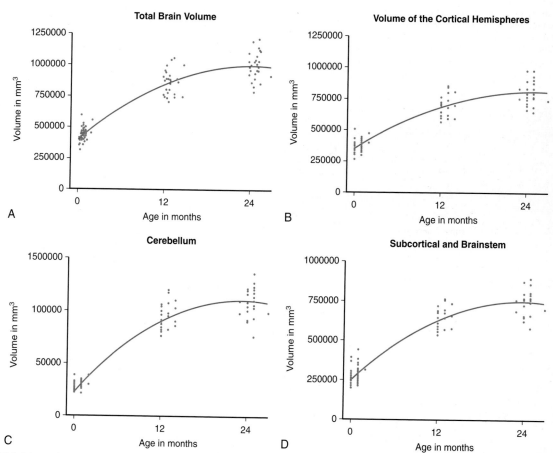

Fig. 22.1 Scatterplots showing brain growth in the 1st 2 yr of life. **A,** Total brain volume by age at scan. **B,** Cortical hemispheres. **C,** Cerebellum. **D,** Subcortical region and brainstem. *(From Knickmeyer RC, Gouttard S, Kang C, et al: A structural MRI study of human brain development from birth to 2 years, J Neurosci 28(47):12176–12182, 2008.)*

Table 22.1	Developmental Milestones in 1st 2 Yr of Life	
MILESTONE	**AVERAGE AGE OF ATTAINMENT (MO)**	**DEVELOPMENTAL IMPLICATIONS**
GROSS MOTOR		
Holds head steady while sitting	2	Allows more visual interaction
Pulls to sit, with no head lag	3	Muscle tone
Brings hands together in midline	3	Self-discovery of hands
Asymmetric tonic neck reflex gone	4	Can inspect hands in midline
Sits without support	6	Increasing exploration
Rolls back to stomach	6.5	Truncal flexion, risk of falls
Walks alone	12	Exploration, control of proximity to parents
Runs	16	Supervision more difficult
FINE MOTOR		
Grasps rattle	3.5	Object use
Reaches for objects	4	Visuomotor coordination
Palmar grasp gone	4	Voluntary release
Transfers object hand to hand	5.5	Comparison of objects
Thumb-finger grasp	8	Able to explore small objects
Turns pages of book	12	Increasing autonomy during book time
Scribbles	13	Visuomotor coordination
Builds tower of 2 cubes	15	Uses objects in combination
Builds tower of 6 cubes	22	Requires visual, gross, and fine motor coordination
COMMUNICATION AND LANGUAGE		
Smiles in response to face, voice	1.5	More active social participant
Monosyllabic babble	6	Experimentation with sound, tactile sense
Inhibits to "no"	7	Response to tone (nonverbal)
Follows 1-step command with gesture	7	Nonverbal communication
Follows 1-step command without gesture	10	Verbal receptive language (e.g., "Give it to me")
Says "mama" or "dada"	10	Expressive language
Points to objects	10	Interactive communication
Speaks first real word	12	Beginning of labeling
Speaks 4-6 words	15	Acquisition of object and personal names
Speaks 10-15 words	18	Acquisition of object and personal names
Speaks 2-word sentences (e.g., "Mommy shoe")	19	Beginning grammatization, corresponds with 50-word vocabulary
COGNITIVE		
Stares momentarily at spot where object disappeared	2	Lack of object permanence (out of sight, out of mind; e.g., yarn ball dropped)
Stares at own hand	4	Self-discovery, cause and effect
Bangs 2 cubes	8	Active comparison of objects
Uncovers toy (after seeing it hidden)	8	Object permanence
Egocentric symbolic play (e.g., pretends to drink from cup)	12	Beginning symbolic thought
Uses stick to reach toy	17	Able to link actions to solve problems
Pretend play with doll (e.g., gives doll bottle)	17	Symbolic thought

12% (cesarean section) below birthweight in the 1st wk as a result of excretion of excess extravascular fluid and limited nutritional intake. Nutrition improves as colostrum is replaced by higher-fat content breast milk, and when infants learn to latch on and suck more efficiently, and as mothers become more comfortable with feeding techniques. Infants regain or exceed birthweight by 2 wk of age and should grow at approximately 30 g (1 oz) per day during the 1st mo (see Table 27.1). This is the period of fastest postnatal growth. Arms are held to the sides. Limb movements consist largely of uncontrolled writhing, with apparently purposeless opening and closing of the hands. Smiling occurs involuntarily. Eye gaze, head turning, and sucking are under better control and thus can be used to demonstrate infant perception and cognition. An infant's preferential turning toward the mother's voice is evidence of recognition memory.

Six **behavioral states** have been described (see Chapter 21). Initially, sleep and wakefulness are evenly distributed throughout the 24 hr day (Fig. 22.2). Neurologic maturation accounts for the consolidation of sleep into blocks of 5 or 6 hr at night, with brief awake, feeding periods. Learning also occurs; infants whose parents are consistently more interactive and stimulating during the day learn to concentrate their sleeping during the night.

Cognitive Development
Infants can differentiate among patterns, colors, and consonants. They can recognize facial expressions (smiles) as similar, even when they appear on different faces. They also can match abstract properties of stimuli, such as contour, intensity, or temporal pattern, across sensory modalities. Infants at 2 mo of age can discriminate rhythmic patterns in native vs non-native language. Infants appear to seek stimuli actively, as though satisfying an innate need to make sense of the world. These phenomena point to the integration of sensory inputs in the central nervous system. Caretaking activities provide visual, tactile, olfactory, and auditory stimuli, all of which support the development of cognition. Infants **habituate** to the familiar, attending less to repeated stimuli and increasing their attention to novel stimuli.

Emotional Development
The infant is dependent on the environment to meet his or her needs. The consistent availability of a trusted adult to meet the infant's urgent needs creates the conditions for **secure attachment**. Basic **trust vs mistrust,** the first of Erikson's psychosocial stages (see Chapter 18), depends on attachment and reciprocal maternal bonding. Crying occurs in response to stimuli that may be obvious (a soiled diaper) but are

Table 22.2	Emerging Patterns of Behavior During the 1st Yr of Life*

NEONATAL PERIOD (1ST 4 WK)

Prone:	Lies in flexed attitude; turns head from side to side; head sags on ventral suspension
Supine:	Generally flexed and a little stiff
Visual:	May fixate face on light in line of vision; doll's eye movement (oculocephalic reflex) of eyes on turning of the body
Reflex:	Moro response active; stepping and placing reflexes; grasp reflex active
Social:	Visual preference for human face

AT 1 MO

Prone:	Legs more extended; holds chin up; turns head; head lifted momentarily to plane of body on ventral suspension
Supine:	Tonic neck posture predominates; supple and relaxed; head lags when pulled to sitting position
Visual:	Watches person; follows moving object
Social:	Body movements in cadence with voice of other in social contact; beginning to smile

AT 2 MO

Prone:	Raises head slightly farther; head sustained in plane of body on ventral suspension
Supine:	Tonic neck posture predominates; head lags when pulled to sitting position
Visual:	Follows moving object 180 degrees
Social:	Smiles on social contact; listens to voice and coos

AT 3 MO

Prone:	Lifts head and chest with arms extended; head above plane of body on ventral suspension
Supine:	Tonic neck posture predominates; reaches toward and misses objects; waves at toy
Sitting:	Head lag partially compensated when pulled to sitting position; early head control with bobbing motion; back rounded
Reflex:	Typical Moro response has not persisted; makes defensive movements or selective withdrawal reactions
Social:	Sustained social contact; listens to music; says "aah, ngah"

AT 4 MO

Prone:	Lifts head and chest, with head in approximately vertical axis; legs extended
Supine:	Symmetric posture predominates, hands in midline; reaches and grasps objects and brings them to mouth
Sitting:	No head lag when pulled to sitting position; head steady, tipped forward; enjoys sitting with full truncal support
Standing:	When held erect, pushes with feet
Adaptive:	Sees raisin, but makes no move to reach for it
Social:	Laughs out loud; may show displeasure if social contact is broken; excited at sight of food

AT 7 MO

Prone:	Rolls over; pivots; crawls or creep-crawls (Knobloch)
Supine:	Lifts head; rolls over; squirms
Sitting:	Sits briefly, with support of pelvis; leans forward on hands; back rounded
Standing:	May support most of weight; bounces actively
Adaptive:	Reaches out for and grasps large object; transfers objects from hand to hand; grasp uses radial palm; rakes at raisin
Language:	Forms polysyllabic vowel sounds
Social:	Prefers mother; babbles; enjoys mirror; responds to changes in emotional content of social contact

AT 10 MO

Sitting:	Sits up alone and indefinitely without support, with back straight
Standing:	Pulls to standing position; "cruises" or walks holding on to furniture
Motor:	Creeps or crawls
Adaptive:	Grasps objects with thumb and forefinger; pokes at things with forefinger; picks up pellet with assisted pincer movement; uncovers hidden toy; attempts to retrieve dropped object; releases object grasped by other person
Language:	Repetitive consonant sounds ("mama," "dada")
Social:	Responds to sound of name; plays peek-a-boo or pat-a-cake; waves bye-bye

AT 1 YR

Motor:	Walks with one hand held; rises independently, takes several steps (Knobloch)
Adaptive:	Picks up raisin with unassisted pincer movement of forefinger and thumb; releases object to other person on request or gesture
Language:	Says a few words besides "mama," "dada"
Social:	Plays simple ball game; makes postural adjustment to dressing

*Data are derived from those of Gesell (as revised by Knobloch), Shirley, Provence, Wolf, Bailey, and others.
Data from Knobloch H, Stevens F, Malone AF: *Manual of developmental diagnosis,* Hagerstown, MD, 1980, Harper & Row.

often obscure (see Chapter 22.1). Infants who are consistently picked up and held in response to distress cry less at 1 yr and show less aggressive behavior at 2 yr. Infants cry in response to the cry of another infant, which has been interpreted as an early sign of empathy.

Implications for Parents and Pediatricians

Success or failure in establishing feeding and sleep cycles influences parents' feelings of competence. When things go well, the parents' anxiety and ambivalence, as well as the exhaustion of the early weeks, decrease. Infant issues (e.g., colic) or familial conflict may prevent this from occurring. With physical recovery from delivery and hormonal normalization, the mild postpartum "blues" that affects many mothers passes. If the mother continues to feel sad, overwhelmed, and anxious, the possibility of moderate to severe **postpartum depression,** found in 10–15% of postpartum women, needs to be considered. Major depression that arises during pregnancy or in the postpartum period threatens the mother–child relationship and is a risk factor for later cognitive and behavioral problems. The pediatrician may be the first professional to encounter the depressed mother and should be instrumental in assisting her in seeking treatment (see Chapter 21).

AGE 2-6 MONTHS

At about age 2 mo, the emergence of voluntary (social) smiles and increasing eye contact mark a change in the parent–child relationship,

Table 22.3	Time of Radiographic Appearance of Centers of Ossification in Infancy and Childhood	
BOYS—AGE AT APPEARANCE*	**BONES AND EPIPHYSEAL CENTERS**	**GIRLS—AGE AT APPEARANCE***
HUMERUS, HEAD		
3 wk		3 wk
CARPAL BONES		
2 mo ± 2 mo	Capitate	2 mo ± 2 mo
3 mo ± 2 mo	Hamate	2 mo ± 2 mo
30 mo ± 16 mo	Triangular[†]	21 mo ± 14 mo
42 mo ± 19 mo	Lunate[†]	34 mo ± 13 mo
67 mo ± 19 mo	Trapezium[†]	47 mo ± 14 mo
69 mo ± 15 mo	Trapezoid[†]	49 mo ± 12 mo
66 mo ± 15 mo	Scaphoid[†]	51 mo ± 12 mo
No standards available	Pisiform[†]	No standards available
METACARPAL BONES		
18 mo ± 5 mo	II	12 mo ± 3 mo
20 mo ± 5 mo	III	13 mo ± 3 mo
23 mo ± 6 mo	IV	15 mo ± 4 mo
26 mo ± 7 mo	V	16 mo ± 5 mo
32 mo ± 9 mo	I	18 mo ± 5 mo
FINGERS (EPIPHYSES)		
16 mo ± 4 mo	Proximal phalanx, 3rd finger	10 mo ± 3 mo
16 mo ± 4 mo	Proximal phalanx, 2nd finger	11 mo ± 3 mo
17 mo ± 5 mo	Proximal phalanx, 4th finger	11 mo ± 3 mo
19 mo ± 7 mo	Distal phalanx, 1st finger	12 mo ± 4 mo
21 mo ± 5 mo	Proximal phalanx, 5th finger	14 mo ± 4 mo
24 mo ± 6 mo	Middle phalanx, 3rd finger	15 mo ± 5 mo
24 mo ± 6 mo	Middle phalanx, 4th finger	15 mo ± 5 mo
26 mo ± 6 mo	Middle phalanx, 2nd finger	16 mo ± 5 mo
28 mo ± 6 mo	Distal phalanx, 3rd finger	18 mo ± 4 mo
28 mo ± 6 mo	Distal phalanx, 4th finger	18 mo ± 5 mo
32 mo ± 7 mo	Proximal phalanx, 1st finger	20 mo ± 5 mo
37 mo ± 9 mo	Distal phalanx, 5th finger	23 mo ± 6 mo
37 mo ± 8 mo	Distal phalanx, 2nd finger	23 mo ± 6 mo
39 mo ± 10 mo	Middle phalanx, 5th finger	22 mo ± 7 mo
152 mo ± 18 mo	Sesamoid (adductor pollicis)	121 mo ± 13 mo
HIP AND KNEE		
Usually present at birth	Femur, distal	Usually present at birth
Usually present at birth	Tibia, proximal	Usually present at birth
4 mo ± 2 mo	Femur, head	4 mo ± 2 mo
46 mo ± 11 mo	Patella	29 mo ± 7 mo
FOOT AND ANKLE[‡]		

Values represent mean ± standard deviation, when applicable.

*To nearest month.

[†]Except for the capitate and hamate bones, the variability of carpal centers is too great to make them very useful clinically.

[‡]Standards for the foot are available, but normal variation is wide, including some familial variants, so this area is of little clinical use.

The norms present a composite of published data from the Fels Research Institute, Yellow Springs, OH (Pyle SI, Sontag L: *AJR Am J Roentgenol* 49:102, 1943), and unpublished data from the Brush Foundation, Case Western Reserve University, Cleveland, OH, and the Harvard School of Public Health, Boston, MA. Compiled by Lieb, Buehl, and Pyle.

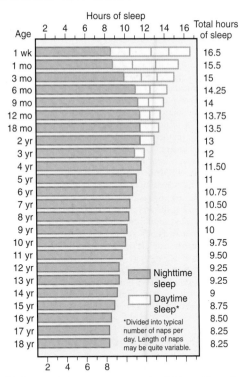

Fig. 22.2 Typical sleep requirements in children. *(From Ferber R: Solve your child's sleep problems, New York, 1985, Simon & Schuster.)*

primitive reflexes; see Chapter 608). Disappearance of the asymmetric tonic neck reflex means that infants can begin to examine objects in the midline and manipulate them with both hands. Waning of the early grasp reflex allows infants both to hold objects and to let them go voluntarily. A novel object may elicit purposeful, although inefficient, reaching. The quality of spontaneous movements also changes, from larger writhing to smaller, circular movements that have been described as "fidgety." Abnormal or absent fidgety movements may constitute a risk factor for later neurologic abnormalities.

Increasing control of truncal flexion makes intentional rolling possible. Once infants can hold their heads steady while sitting, they can gaze across at things rather than merely looking up at them, opening up a new visual range. They can begin taking food from a spoon. At the same time, maturation of the visual system allows greater depth perception.

In this period, infants achieve stable state regulation and regular sleep–wake cycles. Total sleep requirements are approximately 14-16 hr/24 hr, with about 9-10 hr concentrated at night and 2 naps/day. Approximately 70% of infants sleep for a 6-8 hr stretch by age 6 mo (see Fig. 22.2). By 4-6 mo, the sleep electroencephalogram shows a mature pattern, with demarcation of rapid eye movement and 3 stages of non–rapid eye movement sleep. The sleep cycle remains shorter than in adults (50-60 min vs approximately 90 min). As a result, infants arouse to light sleep or wake frequently during the night, setting the stage for behavioral sleep problems (see Chapter 31).

Cognitive Development

The overall effect of these developments is a qualitative change. At 4 mo of age, infants are described as "hatching" socially, becoming interested in a wider world. During feeding, infants no longer focus exclusively on the mother, but become distracted. In the mother's arms, the infant may literally turn around, preferring to face outward.

Infants at this age also explore their own bodies, staring intently at their hands, vocalizing, blowing bubbles, and touching their ears, cheeks, and genitals. These explorations represent an early stage in the understanding of cause and effect as infants learn that voluntary

heightening the parents' sense of being loved reciprocally. During the next months, an infant's range of motor and social control and cognitive engagement increases dramatically. Mutual regulation takes the form of complex social interchanges, resulting in strong mutual attachment and enjoyment. Routines are established. Parents are less fatigued.

Physical Development

Between 3 and 4 mo of age, the rate of growth slows to approximately 20 g/day (see Table 27.1 and Figs. 23.1 and 23.2). By age 4 mo, birthweight is doubled. Early reflexes that limited voluntary movement recede (e.g., muscle movements generate predictable tactile and visual sensations. They also have a role in the emergence of a sense of self, separate from the mother. This is the 1st stage of personality development. Infants come to associate certain sensations through frequent repetition. The proprioceptive feeling of holding up the hand and wiggling the fingers always accompanies the sight of the fingers moving. Such "self" sensations are consistently linked and reproducible at will. In contrast, sensations that are associated with "other" occur with less regularity and in varying combinations. The sound, smell, and feel of the mother sometimes appear promptly in response to crying, but sometimes do not. The satisfaction that the mother or another loving adult provides continues the process of attachment.

Emotional Development and Communication

Babies interact with increasing sophistication and range. The primary **emotions** of anger, joy, interest, fear, disgust, and surprise appear in appropriate contexts as distinct facial expressions. When face-to-face, the infant and a trusted adult can match affective expressions (smiling or surprise) approximately 30% of the time. Initiating games (singing, hand games) increases social development. Such face-to-face behavior reveals the infant's ability to share emotional states, the 1st step in the development of communication. Infants of depressed parents show a different pattern, spending less time in coordinated movement with their parents and making fewer efforts to reengage. Rather than anger, they show sadness and a loss of energy when the parents continue to be unavailable.

Implications for Parents and Pediatricians

Motor and sensory maturation makes infants at 3-6 mo exciting and interactive. Some parents experience their 4 mo old child's outward turning as a rejection, secretly fearing that their infants no longer love them. For most parents, this is a happy period. Most parents excitedly report that they can hold conversations with their infants, taking turns vocalizing and listening. Pediatricians share in the enjoyment, as the baby coos, makes eye contact, and moves rhythmically. Infants who do not show this reciprocal language and movements are at risk for autism spectrum disorders or other developmental disabilities (see Chapters 52 and 54). If this visit does not feel joyful and relaxed, causes such as social stress, family dysfunction, parental mental illness, or problems in the infant–parent relationship should be considered. Parents can be reassured that responding to an infant's emotional needs cannot spoil the infant. Giving vaccines and drawing blood while the child is seated on the parent's lap or nursing at the breast increases pain tolerance.

AGE 6-12 MONTHS

With achievement of the sitting position, increased mobility, and new skills to explore the world around them, 6-12 mo old infants show advances in cognitive understanding and communication, and new tensions arise in regard to attachment and separation. Infants develop will and intentions, characteristics that most parents welcome but still find challenging to manage.

Physical Development

Growth slows more (see Table 27.1 and Figs. 23.1 and 23.2). By the 1st birthday, birthweight has tripled, length has increased by 50%, and head circumference has increased by 10 cm (4 in). The ability to sit unsupported (6-7 mo) and to pivot while sitting (around 9-10 mo) provides increasing opportunities to manipulate several objects at a time and to experiment with novel combinations of objects. These explorations are aided by the emergence of a thumb–finger grasp (8-9 mo) and a neat pincer grasp by 12 mo. Voluntary release emerges at 9 mo. Many infants begin crawling and pulling to stand around 8 mo, followed by cruising. Some walk by 1 yr. Motor achievements correlate with increasing myelinization and cerebellar growth. These gross motor skills expand infants' exploratory range and create new physical dangers, as well as opportunities for learning. Tooth eruption occurs, usually starting with the mandibular central incisors. Tooth development reflects skeletal maturation and bone age, although there is wide individual variation (see Table 22.3 and Chapter 333).

Cognitive Development

The 6 mo old infant has discovered his hands and will soon learn to manipulate objects. At first, everything is mouthed. In time, novel objects are picked up, inspected, passed from hand to hand, banged, dropped, and then mouthed. Each action represents a nonverbal idea about what things are for (in Piagetian terms, a *schema*; see Chapter 18). The complexity of an infant's play, how many different schemata are brought to bear, is a useful index of cognitive development at this age. The pleasure, persistence, and energy with which infants tackle these challenges suggest the existence of an intrinsic drive or mastery motivation. Mastery behavior occurs when infants feel secure; those with less secure attachments show limited experimentation and less competence.

A major milestone is the achievement by 9 mo of **object permanence** (**constancy**), the understanding that objects continue to exist, even when not seen. At 4-7 mo of age, infants look down for a yarn ball that has been dropped but quickly give up if it is not seen. With object constancy, older infants persist in searching. They will find objects hidden under a cloth or behind the examiner's back. Peek-a-boo brings unlimited pleasure as the child magically brings back the other player. Events seem to occur as a result of the child's own activities.

Emotional Development

The advent of object permanence corresponds with qualitative changes in social and communicative development. Infants look back and forth between an approaching stranger and a parent and may cling or cry anxiously, demonstrating **stranger anxiety**. Separations often become more difficult. Infants who have been sleeping through the night for months begin to awaken regularly and cry, as though remembering that the parents are nearby or in the next room.

A new demand for **autonomy** also emerges. Poor weight gain at this age often reflects a struggle between an infant's emerging independence and parent's control of the feeding situation. Use of the 2-spoon method of feeding (1 for the child and 1 for the parent), finger foods, and a high chair with tray table can avert potential problems. Tantrums make their first appearance as the drives for autonomy and mastery come in conflict with parental controls and the infant's still-limited abilities.

Communication

Infants at 7 mo of age are adept at nonverbal communication, expressing a range of emotions and responding to vocal tone and facial expressions. About 9 mo of age, infants become aware that emotions can be shared between people; they show parents toys as a way of sharing their happy feelings. Between 8 and 10 mo of age, babbling takes on a new complexity, with multisyllabic sounds ("ba-da-ma") called **canonical babbling**. Babies can discriminate between languages. Infants in bilingual homes learn the characteristics and rules that govern 2 different languages. Social interaction (attentive adults taking turns vocalizing with the infant) profoundly influences the acquisition and production of new sounds. The first true word (i.e., a sound used consistently to refer to a specific object or person) appears in concert with an infant's discovery of object permanence. Picture books now provide an ideal context for verbal language acquisition. With a familiar book as a shared focus of attention, a parent and child engage in repeated cycles of pointing and labeling, with elaboration and feedback by the parent. The addition of sign language may support infant development while enhancing parent–infant communication.

Implications for Parents and Pediatricians

With the developmental reorganization that occurs around 9 mo of age, previously resolved issues of feeding and sleeping reemerge. Pediatricians can prepare parents at the 6 mo visit so that these problems can be understood as the result of developmental progress and not regression. Parents should be encouraged to plan ahead for necessary, and inevitable, separations (e.g., babysitter, daycare). Routine preparations may make these separations easier. Dual parent employment has not been consistently found to be harmful or beneficial for long-term cognitive or social-emotional outcomes. Introduction of a **transitional object** may allow the infant to self-comfort in the parents' absence. The object cannot have any potential for asphyxiation or strangulation.

Infants' wariness of strangers often makes the 9 mo examination difficult, particularly if the infant is temperamentally prone to react negatively to unfamiliar situations. Initially, the pediatrician should avoid direct eye contact with the child. Time spent talking with the parent and introducing the child to a small, washable toy will be rewarded with more cooperation. The examination can be continued on the parent's lap when feasible.

Bibliography is available at Expert Consult.

22.1 Infant Crying and Colic
Susan Feigelman

Crying or fussiness is present in all babies but reaches medical attention in about 20% of infants younger than 2 mo. Although usually a transient and normal infant behavior, crying is often associated with parental concern and distress. On average, babies cry 2 hr/day, peaking at 6 wk of age. Premature infants will have peak crying at 6 wk corrected age (Fig. 22.3). Small-for-gestational-age and premature babies may be at higher risk. The peak period of infant crying usually occurs in the evenings and early part of the night. Excessive crying or fussiness persisting longer than 3-5 mo may be associated with behavioral problems in an older child (anxiety, aggression, hyperactivity), decreased duration of breastfeeding, or postnatal depression, but it is uncertain which is the cause or effect. Most infants with crying/fussiness do not have gastroesophageal reflux, lactose intolerance, constipation, or cow's milk protein allergy.

Acute-onset uncontrollable crying could be caused by a medical condition. Potentially overlooked conditions to consider include corneal abrasion, tourniquet effect of a hair wrapped around a digit or penis, occult fracture, urinary tract infection, acute abdomen including inguinal hernia, or anomalous coronary artery. Breastfeeding mothers should be questioned about medications, drugs, and diet. Gastrointestinal distress can result from a maternal diet high in cruciferous vegetables. Most of the time, the etiology of a serious problem can be discovered with a careful history and physical examination.

Crying is a normal part of neurobehavioral development. Infants have various signals for their needs and for getting attention from a caregiver. These behaviors progressively increase in intensity in many infants, from changes in breathing and color, to postural and movement changes, and then to calm vocalizations. These precry cues, if not attended to, will eventually lead to active crying. Some infants may go directly

to crying, perhaps based on temperament; these infants may be less easily consolable, more intense, or more responsive to sensory stimuli. Management of crying/fussiness should include teaching caregivers about precry cues and responding to the signal for feeding in a calm, relaxed manner. If sensory overstimulation is a factor, creating a nondistracting, calm environment may help, as well as swaddling. When lack of sensory stimulation is present, mother–infant skin-to-skin contact and carrying the infant may be beneficial. In all situations, reassurance that this is both normal and transient, with only 5% of infants persisting beyond 3 mo of age, helps the family cope. Teaching families about expectations for normal crying behavior can reduce emergency department visits.

The emotional significance of any experience depends on both the individual child's temperament and the parent's responses (see Table 18.1); differing feeding schedules produce differing reactions. Hunger generates increasing tension; as the urgency peaks, the infant cries, the parent offers the breast or bottle, and the tension dissipates. Infants fed "on demand" consistently experience this link among their distress, the arrival of the parent, and relief from hunger. Most infants fed on a fixed schedule quickly adapt their hunger cycle to the schedule. Those who cannot adapt, because they are temperamentally prone to irregular biologic rhythms, experience periods of unrelieved hunger as well as unwanted feedings when they already feel full. Similarly, infants who are fed at the parents' convenience, with neither attention to the infant's hunger cues nor a fixed schedule, may not consistently experience feeding as the pleasurable reduction of tension. Infants with early dysregulation often show increased irritability and physiologic instability (spitting, diarrhea, poor weight gain) as well as later behavioral problems. Infants with excess crying after 4-6 mo may have neurobehavioral dysregulation and may be at higher risk of other behavior problems (sleep, behavior, feeding).

Colic is characterized by the "rule of 3." It occurs in a healthy, thriving infant beginning in the 2nd or 3rd week of life, lasts about 3 hr/day, occurs 3 days/wk, lasts for more than 3 wk, and resolves by 3 or 4 mo of age. It is equally common in breast- and bottle-fed infants, although prevalence is variable (up to 20%). There is no racial, socioeconomic status, or gender risk for colic. Colic is a diagnosis of exclusion following a careful history and physical examination. Few cases will be found to have an organic etiology. Although all babies have crying episodes, colicky babies cry excessively and are difficult to settle. The fussiness is not associated with hunger or any other form of discomfort. Colicky babies may be more reactive to the same stimulus and may cry louder than other babies. Although crying periods are a normal developmental phenomenon, babies with colic can cause parents to become anxious, distraught, frustrated, and sleep deprived. Mothers are at higher risk for postpartum depression if they report inconsolable crying episodes lasting more than 20 min. Depression may lead to cessation of breastfeeding. The risk of abuse increases as parents may use aggressive means to quiet the child, resulting in the **shaken baby syndrome**.

There is no specific treatment for colic, but practitioners should provide advice and reassurance to parents. Parents must be counseled about the problem, the importance of implementing a series of calm, systematic steps to sooth the infant, and having a plan for stress relief, such as time-out for parents and substitute caregivers. Parents can be advised that that colic is self-limited with no adverse effects on the child. Public health programs, such as the **Period of PURPLE Crying** (http://purplecrying.info/) and **Take 5 Safety Plan for Crying**, are invaluable tools for parents. These programs inform parents that all babies go through periods of crying, deflecting parental guilt and self-recrimination. Most importantly, parents are reminded that it is better to allow the baby to cry than engage in shaking that leads to head trauma. Although babies with colic will have inconsolable periods when there is no relief, parents can try some simple steps. Predictable daily schedules may help, ensuring the baby has adequate sleep. Parents should provide appropriate stimulation throughout the day when baby is in an alert/awake period. The sleep environment should be free of stimulation. Swaddling, rocking, white noise, and movement (e.g., stroller, car ride) help some babies settle. Infants who are carried by a parent show different physiologic changes than when held in a sitting position, although there is no evidence

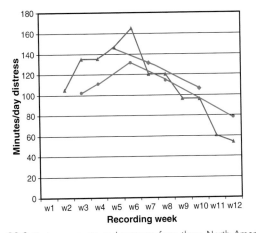

Fig. 22.3 Crying amounts and patterns from three North American studies illustrating similarities in crying pattern. (*From Barr RG, Trent RB, Cross J: Age-related incidence curve of hospitalized shaken baby syndrome cases: convergent evidence for crying as a trigger to shaking,* Child Abuse Neglect 30(1):7–16, 2006.)

that continuous carrying is effective in colic management. A study in a hunter–gatherer society showed that children who are continuously carried by their mothers display similar crying periods as those in Western societies.

Some studies have found differences in **fecal microflora** between babies with excess crying and controls. Results include fewer bifidobacteria and lactobacilli and more coliform bacteria such as *Escherichia coli*. None has been conclusive, however, and each study was found to have limitations such as lack of precise inclusion criteria, lack of blinded observers, and variability in outcome measurements.

If the child appears to have gastrointestinal symptoms, breastfeeding mothers may try elimination of milk, beans, and cruciferous vegetables. In allergic families, mothers may try a stricter elimination of food allergens (milk, egg, wheat, nuts, soy, and fish), although nutritional status should be monitored. For formula-fed infants, changing from milk-based to soy-based or other lactose-free formulas had no effect in most studies. A protein hydrolysate formula may moderately improve symptoms.

The cause of colic in not known, and no medical intervention has been consistently effective. Colic has been described as a "functional gastrointestinal disorder" and has been associated with later development of **migraine**. Simethicone has not been shown to be better than placebo. Anticholinergic medications should not be used in infants younger than 6 mo. Early studies of probiotics look promising, but evidence is insufficient to recommend their routine use. Among various complementary therapies, certain **herbal teas**, sugar solutions, Gripe water (containing herbal supplements), and fennel extract may have benefit, but the evidence is weak. Baby massage may be helpful, but chiropractic manipulation should not be performed in young children. Acupuncture was effective in 1 trial, and singing while in utero may produce babies who cry less.

Bibliography is available at Expert Consult.

Chapter 23
The Second Year
Rebecca G. Carter and Susan Feigelman
第二十三章
生后第二年

中文导读

本章主要介绍了12~18月龄、18~24月龄两个年龄阶段幼儿的体格发育，以及认知、情绪、交流及语言的发展。具体描述了身高、体重、头围、骨骼的生长，行走姿势的变化；描述了幼儿的认知、情绪、语言方面的发展水平，父母和儿科医师在幼儿发展中所起到的作用；描述了幼儿对环境的探索，感觉运动阶段的结束，逐渐形成物体永久性的意识，解决问题的能力不断提高，象征性游戏、自觉意识和内化行为的出现。此阶段是语言发展最迅速的时期。

The 2nd year of life is a time of rapid growth of development, particularly in the realms of social-emotional and cognitive skills as well as motor development. The toddler's newly found ability to walk allows separation and independence; however, the toddler continues to need secure attachment to the parents. At approximately 18 mo of age, the emergence of symbolic thought and language causes a reorganization of behavior, with implications across many developmental domains.

AGE 12-18 MONTHS
Physical Development
While overall rate of growth continues to decline, the toddler continues to experience considerable brain growth and myelination in the 2nd yr of life, resulting in an increase in head circumference of 2 cm over the year (Figs. 23.1 and 23.2). Toddlers have relatively short legs and long torsos, with exaggerated lumbar lordosis and protruding abdomens.

Text continued on p. 155

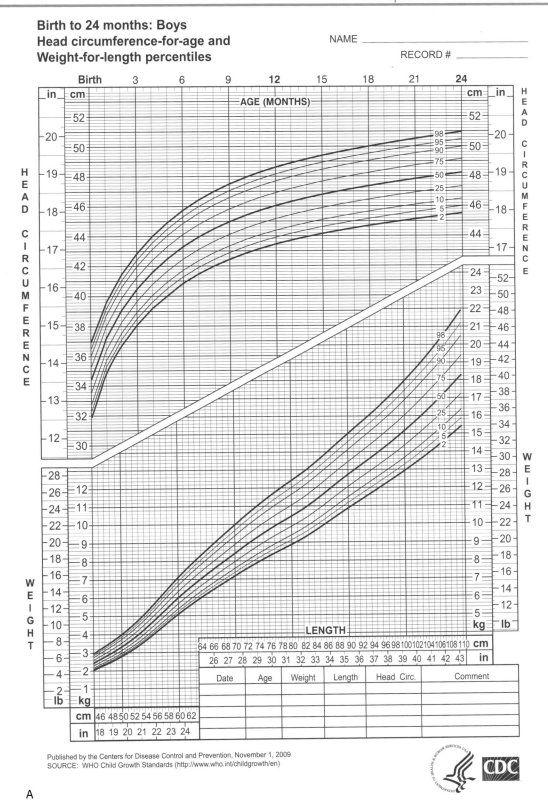

A

Fig. 23.1 The World Health Organization Growth Charts. **A,** Weight for length and head circumference for age for boys, birth to 24 mo. *(Courtesy World Health Organization: WHO Child Growth Standards, 2014.)*

Birth to 24 months: Girls
Head circumference-for-age and
Weight-for-length percentiles

NAME _____

RECORD # _____

Published by the Centers for Disease Control and Prevention, November 1, 2009
SOURCE: WHO Child Growth Standards (http://www.who.int/childgrowth/en)

B

Fig. 23.1, cont'd B, Weight for length and head circumference for age for girls, birth to 24 mo. *(Courtesy World Health Organization: WHO Child Growth Standards, 2014.)*

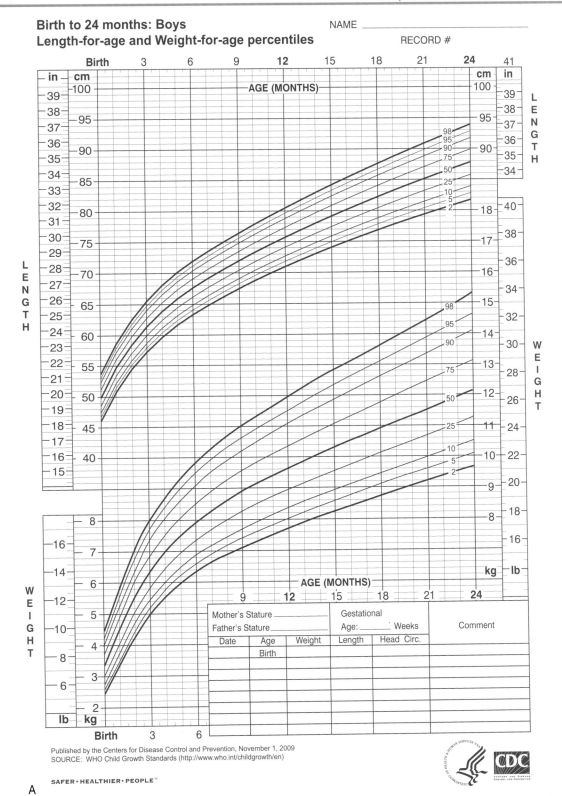

Fig. 23.2 The World Health Organization Growth Charts. **A,** Length for age and weight for age for boys, birth to 24 mo. *(Courtesy World Health Organization: WHO Child Growth Standards, 2014.)*

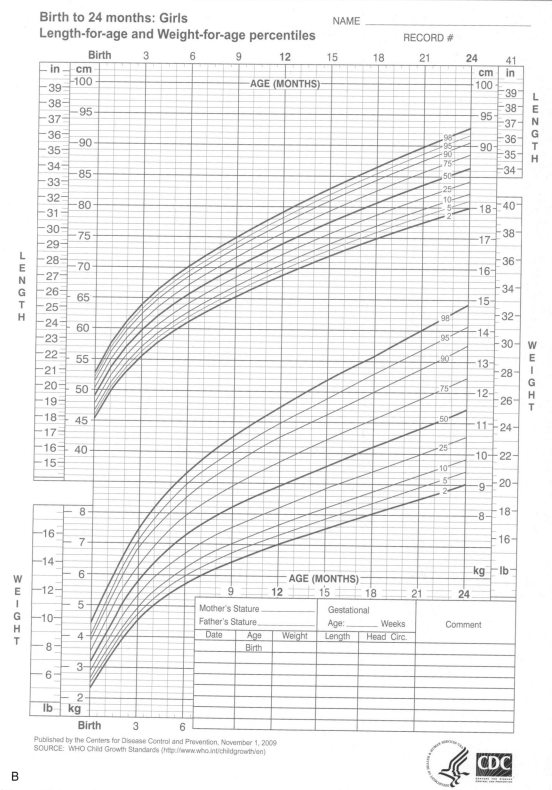

Birth to 24 months: Girls
Length-for-age and Weight-for-age percentiles

NAME _____

RECORD # _____

Published by the Centers for Disease Control and Prevention, November 1, 2009
SOURCE: WHO Child Growth Standards (http://www.who.int/childgrowth/en)

B

Fig. 23.2, cont'd B, Length for age and weight for age for girls, birth to 24 mo. *(Courtesy World Health Organization: WHO Child Growth Standards, 2014.)*

Most children begin to walk independently at about 12-15 mo of age. Early walking is not associated with advanced development in other domains. Infants initially toddle with a wide-based gait, with the knees bent and the arms flexed at the elbow; the entire torso rotates with each stride; the toes may point in or out, and the feet strike the floor flat. The appearance is that of genu varum (**bowleg**). Subsequent refinement leads to greater steadiness and energy efficiency. After several months of practice, the center of gravity shifts back and the torso stabilizes, while the knees extend and the arms swing at the sides for balance. The feet are held in better alignment, and the child is able to stop, pivot, and stoop without toppling over (see Chapters 692 and 693).

Cognitive Development

Exploration of the environment increases in parallel with improved dexterity (reaching, grasping, releasing) and mobility. Learning follows the precepts of Piaget's **sensorimotor stage** (see Chapter 18). Toddlers manipulate objects in novel ways to create interesting effects, such as stacking blocks or filling and dumping buckets. Playthings are also more likely to be used for their intended purposes (combs for hair, cups for drinking). Imitation of parents and older siblings or other children is an important mode of learning. Make-believe play (**symbolic play**) centers on the child's own body, such as pretending to drink from an empty cup (Table 23.1; see also Table 22.1).

Emotional Development

Infants who are approaching the developmental milestone of taking their 1st steps may be irritable. Once they start walking, their predominant mood changes markedly. Toddlers are often elated with their new ability and with the power to control the distance between themselves and their parents. Exploring toddlers orbit around their parents, moving away and then returning for a reassuring touch before moving away again. A child with **secure attachment** will use the parent as a secure base from which to explore independently. Proud of her or his accomplishments, the child illustrates Erikson's **stage of autonomy and separation** (see Chapter 18). The toddler who is overly controlled and discouraged from active exploration will feel doubt, shame, anger, and insecurity. All children will experience tantrums, reflecting their inability to delay gratification, suppress or displace anger, or verbally communicate their emotional states. The quality of the parent–child relationship may moderate negative behavioral effects of childcare arrangements when parents work.

Linguistic Development

Receptive language precedes *expressive* language. By the time infants speak their first words around 12 mo of age, they already respond appropriately to several simple statements, such as "no," "bye-bye," and "give me." By 15 mo, the average child points to major body parts and uses 4-6 words spontaneously and correctly. Toddlers also enjoy **polysyllabic jargoning** (see Tables 22.1 and 23.1) and do not seem upset that no one understands. Most communication of wants and ideas continues to be nonverbal.

Implications for Parents and Pediatricians

Parents who cannot recall any other milestone tend to remember when their child began to walk, perhaps because of the symbolic significance of walking as an act of independence and because of the new demands that the ambulating toddler places on the parent. All toddlers should be encouraged to explore their environment; however, a child's ability to wander out of sight also increases the risks of injury and the need for supervision, making **childproofing** an integral focus of physician visits.

In the office setting, many toddlers are comfortable exploring the examination room, but cling to the parents under the stress of the examination. Performing most of the physical examination in the parent's lap may help allay fears of separation. Infants who become more, not less, distressed in their parents' arms or who avoid their parents at times of stress may be insecurely attached. Young children who, when distressed, turn to strangers rather than parents for comfort are particularly worrisome. Children raised in **toxic stressful environments** have increased

Table 23.1	Emerging Patterns of Behavior From 1-5 Yr of Age*
15 MO	
Motor:	Walks alone; crawls up stairs
Adaptive:	Makes tower of 3 cubes; makes a line with crayon; inserts raisin in bottle
Language:	Jargon; follows simple commands; may name a familiar object (e.g., ball); responds to his/her name
Social:	Indicates some desires or needs by pointing; hugs parents
18 MO	
Motor:	Runs stiffly; sits on small chair; walks up stairs with 1 hand held; explores drawers and wastebaskets
Adaptive:	Makes tower of 4 cubes; imitates scribbling; imitates vertical stroke; dumps raisin from bottle
Language:	10 words (average); names pictures; identifies 1 or more parts of body
Social:	Feeds self; seeks help when in trouble; may complain when wet or soiled; kisses parent with pucker
24 MO	
Motor:	Runs well, walks up and down stairs, 1 step at a time; opens doors; climbs on furniture; jumps
Adaptive:	Makes tower of 7 cubes (6 at 21 mo); scribbles in circular pattern; imitates horizontal stroke; folds paper once imitatively
Language:	Puts 3 words together (subject, verb, object)
Social:	Handles spoon well; often tells about immediate experiences; helps to undress; listens to stories when shown pictures
30 MO	
Motor:	Goes up stairs alternating feet
Adaptive:	Makes tower of 9 cubes; makes vertical and horizontal strokes, but generally will not join them to make cross; imitates circular stroke, forming closed figure
Language:	Refers to self by pronoun "I"; knows full name
Social:	Helps put things away; pretends in play
36 MO	
Motor:	Rides tricycle; stands momentarily on 1 foot
Adaptive:	Makes tower of 10 cubes; imitates construction of "bridge" of 3 cubes; copies circle; imitates cross
Language:	Knows age and sex; counts 3 objects correctly; repeats 3 numbers or a sentence of 6 syllables; most of speech intelligible to strangers
Social:	Plays simple games (in "parallel" with other children); helps in dressing (unbuttons clothing and puts on shoes); washes hands
48 MO	
Motor:	Hops on 1 foot; throws ball overhand; uses scissors to cut out pictures; climbs well
Adaptive:	Copies bridge from model; imitates construction of "gate" of 5 cubes; copies cross and square; draws man with 2-4 parts besides head; identifies longer of 2 lines
Language:	Counts 4 pennies accurately; tells story
Social:	Plays with several children, with beginning of social interaction and role-playing; goes to toilet alone
60 MO	
Motor:	Skips
Adaptive:	Draws triangle from copy; names heavier of 2 weights
Language:	Names 4 colors; repeats sentence of 10 syllables; counts 10 pennies correctly
Social:	Dresses and undresses; asks questions about meaning of words; engages in domestic role-playing

*Data derived from those of Gesell (as revised by Knobloch), Shirley, Provence, Wolf, Bailey, and others. After 6 yr, the Wechsler Intelligence Scales for Children (WISC-IV) and other scales offer the most precise estimates of cognitive development. To have their greatest value, they should be administered only by an experienced and qualified person.

vulnerability to disease. The conflicts between independence and security manifest in issues of discipline, temper tantrums, toilet training, and changing feeding behaviors. Parents should be counseled on these matters within the framework of normal development.

Parents may express concern about poor food intake as growth slows. The growth chart should provide reassurance. Many children still take 2 daytime naps, although the duration steadily decreases and may start to condense to 1 longer nap (see Fig. 22.2).

AGE 18-24 MONTHS
Physical Development
Motor development during this period is reflected in improvements in balance and agility and the emergence of running and stair climbing. Height and weight increase at a steady rate during this year, with a gain of 5 in and 5 lb. By 24 mo, children are about half their ultimate adult height. Head growth slows slightly, with 85% of adult head circumference achieved by age 2 yr, leaving only an additional 5 cm (2 in) gain over the next few years (see Fig. 23.1 and Table 27.1).

Cognitive Development
At approximately 18 mo of age, several cognitive changes coalesce, marking the conclusion of the sensorimotor period. These can be observed during *self-initiated play*. **Object permanence** is firmly established; toddlers anticipate where an object will end up, even though the object was not visible while it was being moved. Cause and effect are better understood, and toddlers demonstrate flexibility in problem solving (e.g., using a stick to obtain a toy that is out of reach, figuring out how to wind a mechanical toy). Symbolic transformations in play are no longer tied to the toddler's own body; thus a doll can be "fed" from an empty plate. As with the reorganization that occurs at 9 mo (see Chapter 22), the cognitive changes at 18 mo correlate with important changes in the emotional and linguistic domains (see Table 23.1).

Emotional Development
The relative independence of the preceding half-year often gives way to increased clinginess about 18 mo. This stage, described as "rapprochement," may be a reaction to growing awareness of the possibility of separation. Many parents report that they cannot go anywhere without having a small child attached to them. **Separation anxiety** will manifest at bedtime. Many children use a special blanket or stuffed toy as a **transitional object**, which functions as a symbol of the absent parent. The transitional object remains important until the transition to symbolic thought has been completed and the symbolic presence of the parent fully internalized. Despite the attachment to the parent, the child's use of "no" is a way of declaring independence. Individual differences in **temperament**, in both the child and the parents, play a critical role in determining the balance of conflict vs cooperation in the parent–child relationship. As effective language emerges, conflicts often become less frequent.

Self-conscious awareness and internalized standards of behavior first appear at this age. Toddlers looking in a mirror will, for the first time, reach for their own face rather than the mirror image if they notice something unusual on their nose. They begin to recognize when

toys are broken and may hand them to their parents to fix. Language becomes a means of impulse control, early reasoning, and connection between ideas. When tempted to touch a forbidden object, they may tell themselves "no, no." This is the very beginning of the formation of a conscience. The fact that they often go on to touch the object anyway demonstrates the relative weakness of **internalized inhibitions** at this stage.

Linguistic Development
Perhaps the most dramatic developments in this period are linguistic. Labeling of objects coincides with the advent of symbolic thought. After the realization occurs that words can stand for objects or ideas, a child's vocabulary grows from 10-15 words at 18 mo to between 50 and 100 at 2 yr. After acquiring a vocabulary of about 50 words, toddlers begin to combine them to make simple sentences, marking the beginning of grammar. At this stage, toddlers understand **2-step commands**, such as "Give me the ball and then get your shoes." Language also gives the toddler a sense of control over the surroundings, as in "night-night" or "bye-bye." The emergence of verbal language marks the end of the sensorimotor period. As toddlers learn to use symbols to express ideas and solve problems, the need for cognition based on direct sensation and motor manipulation wanes.

Implications for Parents and Pediatricians
With children's increasing mobility, physical limits on their explorations become less effective; words become increasingly important for behavior control as well as cognition. Children with delayed language acquisition often have greater behavior problems and frustrations due to problems with communication. Language development is facilitated when parents and caregivers use clear, simple sentences; ask questions; and respond to children's incomplete sentences and gestural communication with the appropriate words. Television viewing, as well as television as background noise, decreases parent–child verbal interactions, whereas looking at picture books and engaging the child in 2-way conversations stimulates language development. In the world of constant access to tablets, phones, and screens, parents and children have more distractions from direct language engagement.

In the office setting, certain procedures may lessen the child's **stranger anxiety**. Avoid direct eye contact initially. Perform as much of the examination as feasible with the child on the parent's lap. Pediatricians can help parents understand the resurgence of problems with separation and the appearance of a transitional object as a developmental phenomenon. Parents must understand the importance of exploration. Rather than limiting movement, parents should place toddlers in safe environments or substitute one activity for another. Methods of discipline, including **corporal punishment** (which is not recommended), should be discussed; effective alternatives will usually be appreciated. Helping parents to understand and adapt to their children's different temperamental styles can constitute an important intervention (see Table 18.1). Developing daily routines is helpful to all children at this age. Rigidity in those routines reflects a need for mastery over a changing environment.

Bibliography is available at Expert Consult.

Chapter **24**
The Preschool Years

Rebecca G. Carter and Susan Feigelman

第二十四章
学龄前期

中文导读

本章主要介绍了2~5岁学龄前儿童脑结构的发育、体格发育以及语言、认知和游戏的发展。具体描述了学龄前儿童大脑的解剖和生理特征；具体描述了体格发育，包括体格生长、睡眠需求、运动发育、优势手的发展、膀胱肠道控制能力等；描述了语言的发展水平、语言习得的影响因素、语言与认知情感发展的关联、双语儿童语言的发展及口吃等；描述了认知发展的前运算阶段、模仿行为等；描述了游戏能力的发展；描述了情绪和道德的发展；具体描述了父母和儿科医师在儿童体格发育以及语言、认知、游戏、情绪和道德的发展中所起到的作用。

The emergence of language and exposure of children to an expanding social sphere represent the critical milestones for children ages 2-5 yr. As toddlers, children learn to walk away and come back to the secure adult or parent. As preschoolers, they explore emotional separation, alternating between stubborn opposition and cheerful compliance, between bold exploration and clinging dependence. Increasing time spent in classrooms and playgrounds challenges a child's ability to adapt to new rules and relationships. Emboldened by their growing array of new skills and accomplishments, preschool children also are increasingly cognizant of the constraints imposed on them by the adult world and their own limited abilities.

STRUCTURAL DEVELOPMENT OF THE BRAIN
The preschool brain experiences dramatic changes in its anatomic and physiologic characteristics, with increases in cortical area, decreases in cortical thickness, and changing cortical volume. These changes are not uniform across the brain and vary by region. Gray and white matter tissue properties change dramatically, including diffusion properties in the major cerebral fiber tracts. Dramatic increases occur in brain metabolic demands. In general, more brain regions are required in younger than in older children to complete the same cognitive task. This duplication has been interpreted as a form of "scaffolding," which is discarded with increasing age. The preschool brain is characterized by growth and expansion that will be followed in later years by "pruning."

PHYSICAL DEVELOPMENT
Somatic and brain growth slows by the end of the 2nd yr of life, with corresponding decreases in nutritional requirements and appetite, and the emergence of "picky" eating habits (see Table 27.1). Increases of approximately 2 kg (4-5 lb) in weight and 7-8 cm (2-3 in) in height per year are expected. Birthweight quadruples by 2.5 yr of age. An average 4 yr old weighs 40 lb and is 40 in tall. The head will grow only an additional 5-6 cm between ages 3 and 18 yr. Current growth charts, with growth parameters, can be found on the U.S. Centers for Disease Control and Prevention website (http://www.cdc.gov/growthcharts/) and in Chapter 27. Children with early **adiposity rebound** (increase in body mass index) are at increased risk for adult obesity.

The preschooler has genu valgum (**knock-knees**) and mild pes planus (**flatfoot**). The torso slims as the legs lengthen. Growth of sexual organs is commensurate with somatic growth. Physical energy peaks, and the need for sleep declines to 11-13 hr/24 hr, with the child eventually dropping the nap (see Fig. 22.2). Visual acuity reaches 20/30 by age 3 yr and 20/20 by age 4 yr. All 20 primary teeth should have erupted by 3 yr of age (see Chapter 333).

Most children walk with a mature gait and run steadily before the end of their 3rd yr (see Table 23.1). Beyond this basic level, there is wide variation in ability as the range of motor activities expands to include throwing, catching, and kicking balls; riding on bicycles; climbing on playground structures; dancing; and other complex pattern behaviors. Stylistic features of gross motor activity, such as tempo, intensity, and cautiousness, also vary significantly. Although toddlers may walk with different styles, **toe walking** should not persist.

The effects of such individual differences on cognitive and emotional development depend in part on the demands of the social environment. Energetic, coordinated children may thrive emotionally with parents or teachers who encourage physical activity; lower-energy, more cerebral children may thrive with adults who value quiet play.

Handedness is usually established by the 3rd yr. Frustration may result from attempts to change children's hand preference. Variations in fine motor development reflect both individual proclivities and different opportunities for learning. Children who are restricted from drawing with crayons, for example, develop a mature pencil grasp later.

Bowel and bladder control emerge during this period, with "readiness" for toileting having large individual and cultural variation. Girls tend to potty "train" faster and earlier than boys. Bed-wetting is common up to age 5 yr (see Chapter 558). Many children master toileting with ease, particularly once they are able to verbalize their bodily needs. For others, **toilet training** can involve a protracted power struggle. Refusal to defecate in the toilet or potty is relatively common, associated with constipation, and can lead to parental frustration. Defusing the issue with a temporary cessation of training (and a return to diapers) often allows toilet mastery to proceed.

Implications for Parents and Pediatricians

The normal decrease in appetite at this age may cause parental concern about nutrition; growth charts should reassure parents that the child's intake is adequate. Children normally modulate their food intake to match their somatic needs according to feelings of hunger and satiety. Daily intake fluctuates, at times widely, but intake over a week is relatively stable. Parents should provide a predictable eating schedule, with 3 meals and 2 snacks per day, allowing the child to choose how much to eat in order to avoid power struggles and to allow the child to learn to respond to satiety cues. However, it is important to obtain thorough diet histories for children at this age to advise parents about healthy choices and encourage physical activity to decrease long-term obesity risks and improve learning and cognitive development.

Highly active children face increased risks of injury, and parents should be counseled about safety precautions. Parental concerns about possible hyperactivity may reflect inappropriate expectations, heightened fears, or true overactivity. Children who engage in ongoing impulsive activity with no apparent regard for personal safety or those harming others on a regular basis should be evaluated further.

LANGUAGE, COGNITION, AND PLAY

These 3 domains all involve **symbolic function**, a mode of dealing with the world that emerges during the preschool period.

Language

Our understanding of the acquisition of language is evolving. Preschool children command significant computational skills and understanding of statistical patterns that allow them to learn about both language and causation. The 2 and 3 yr old child employs frequency distributions to identify phonetic units distinguishing words in his or her native language from other languages.

Language development occurs most rapidly between 2 and 5 yr of age. Vocabulary increases from 50-100 words to more than 2,000. Sentence structure advances from telegraphic phrases ("Baby cry") to sentences incorporating all the major grammatical components. As a rule of thumb, between ages 2 and 5 yr, the number of words the child puts in a typical sentence should, at a minimum, equal the child's age (2 by age 2 yr, 3 by age 3 yr, and so on). By 21-24 mo, most children are using possessives ("My ball"), progressives (the "-ing" construction, as in "I playing"), questions, and negatives. By age 4 yr, most children can count to 4 and use the past tense; by age 5 yr, they can use the future tense. Young children do not use figurative speech; they will only comprehend the literal meaning of words. Referring to an object as "light as a feather" may produce a quizzical look on a child.

It is important to distinguish between **speech** (the production of intelligible sounds) and **language**, which refers to the underlying mental act. Language includes both expressive and receptive functions. *Receptive* language (understanding) varies less in its rate of acquisition than does *expressive* language; therefore, it has greater prognostic importance (see Chapters 28 and 52).

Language acquisition depends critically on environmental input. Key determinants include the amount and variety of speech directed toward children and the frequency with which adults ask questions and encourage verbalization. Children raised in poverty typically perform lower on measures of language development than children from economically advantaged families, who tend to be exposed to many more words in the preschool period.

Although experience influences the rate of language development, many linguists believe that the basic mechanism for language learning is "hard-wired" in the brain. Children do not simply imitate adult speech; they abstract the complex rules of grammar from the ambient language, generating implicit hypotheses. Evidence for the existence of such implicit rules comes from analysis of grammatical errors, such as the overgeneralized use of "-s" to signify the plural and "-ed" to signify the past ("We seed lots of mouses.").

Language is linked to both cognitive and emotional development. Language delays may be the 1st indication of an intellectual disability, autism spectrum disorder, or child neglect or maltreatment. Language plays a critical part in the regulation of behavior through internalized "private speech" in which a child repeats adult prohibitions, first audibly and then mentally. Language also allows children to express feelings, such as anger or frustration, without acting them out; consequently, language-delayed children show higher rates of tantrums and other externalizing behaviors.

Preschool language development lays the foundation for later success in school. Approximately 35% of U.S. children may enter school lacking the language skills that are the prerequisites for acquiring literacy. Children from socially and economically disadvantaged backgrounds have an increased risk of school problems, making early detection, along with referral and enrichment, highly crucial for later development. Although children typically learn to read and write in elementary school, critical foundations for literacy are established during the preschool years. Through repeated early exposure to written words, children learn about the uses of writing (telling stories or sending messages) and about its form (left to right, top to bottom). Early errors in writing, like errors in speaking, reveal that literacy acquisition is an active process involving the generation and revision of hypotheses. Programs such as Head Start are especially important for improving language skills for children from bilingual homes. Such parents should be reassured that although **bilingual children** may initially appear to lag behind their monolingual peers in acquiring language, they learn the differing rules governing both languages, and generally have the same number of total words between the languages. Bilingual children do not follow the same course of language development as monolingual children, but rather create a different system of language cues. Several cognitive advantages have been repeatedly demonstrated among bilingual compared to monolingual children.

Picture books have a special role in familiarizing young children with the printed word and in the development of verbal language. Children's vocabulary and receptive language improve when their parents or caregivers consistently read to them. Reading aloud with a young child is an interactive process in which a parent repeatedly focuses the child's attention on a particular picture, asks questions, and then gives the child feedback (**dialogic reading**). The elements of shared attention, active participation, immediate feedback, repetition, and graduated difficulty make such routines ideal for language learning. Programs in which physicians provide books to preschool children have shown improvement in language skills among the children (e.g., Reach Out and Read).

The period of rapid language acquisition is also when **developmental dysfluency** and **stuttering** are most likely to emerge (see Chapter 52.1); these can be traced to activation of the cortical motor, sensory, and cerebellar areas. Common difficulties include pauses and repetitions of initial sounds. Stress or excitement exacerbates these difficulties, which generally resolve on their own. Although 5% of preschool children will stutter, it will resolve in 80% of those children by age 8 yr. Children with stuttering should be referred for evaluation if it is severe, persistent, or associated with anxiety, or if parental concern is elicited. Treatment includes guidance to parents to reduce pressures associated with speaking.

Cognition

The preschool period corresponds to Piaget's **preoperational** (prelogical) **stage,** characterized by magical thinking, egocentrism, and thinking that is dominated by perception, not abstraction (see Table

18.2). **Magical thinking** includes confusing coincidence with causality, *animism* (attributing motivations to inanimate objects and events), and unrealistic beliefs about the power of wishes. A child might believe that people cause it to rain by carrying umbrellas, that the sun goes down because it is tired, or that feeling resentment toward a sibling can actually make that sibling sick. **Egocentrism** refers to a child's inability to take another's point of view and does not connote selfishness. A child might try to comfort an adult who is upset by bringing the adult a favorite stuffed animal. After 2 yr of age, the child develops a concept of herself or himself as an individual and senses the need to feel "whole."

Piaget demonstrated the dominance of **perception** over logic. In one experiment, water is poured back and forth between a tall, thin vase and a low, wide dish, and children are asked which container has more water. Invariably, they choose the one that looks larger (usually the tall vase), even when the examiner points out that no water has been added or taken away. Such misunderstandings reflect young children's developing hypotheses about the nature of the world, as well as their difficulty in attending simultaneously to multiple aspects of a situation.

Recent work indicating that preschool children do have the ability to understand **causal relationships** has modified our understanding of the ability of preschool children to engage in abstract thinking (see Chapter 18).

Imitation, central to the learning experience of preschool children, is a complex act because of differences in the size of the operators (the adult and the child), different levels of dexterity, and even different outcomes. A child who watches an adult unsuccessfully attempt a simple act (unscrew a lid) will imitate the action—but often with the intended outcome, not the demonstrated but failed outcome. Thus "imitation" goes beyond the mere repetition of observed movements.

By age 3, children have self-identified their sex and are actively seeking understanding of the meaning of **gender identification**. There is a developmental progression from rigidity (boys and girls have strict gender roles) in the early preschool years to a more flexible realistic understanding (boys and girls can have a variety of interests).

Play

Play involves learning, physical activity, socialization with peers, and practicing adult roles. Play increases in complexity and imagination, from simple imitation of common experiences, such as shopping and putting baby to bed (2 or 3 yr of age), to more extended scenarios involving singular events, such as going to the zoo or going on a trip (3 or 4 yr of age), to the creation of scenarios that have only been imagined, such as flying to the moon (4 or 5 yr of age). By age 3 yr, **cooperative play** is seen in activities such as building a tower of blocks together; later, more structured **role-play activity**, as in playing house, is seen. Play also becomes increasingly governed by rules, from early rules about asking (rather than taking) and sharing (2 or 3 yr of age), to rules that change from moment to moment, according to the desires of the players (4 and 5 yr of age), to the beginning of the recognition of rules as relatively immutable (5 yr of age). Electronic forms of play (games) are best if interactive and educational and should remain limited in duration.

Play also allows for resolution of conflicts and anxiety and for creative outlets. Children can vent anger safely (spanking a doll), take on superpowers (dinosaur and superhero play), and obtain things that are denied in real life (an imaginary friend or stuffed animal). Creativity is particularly apparent in drawing, painting, and other artistic activities. Themes and emotions that emerge in a child's drawings often reflect the emotional issues of greatest importance for the child.

Difficulty distinguishing fantasy from reality colors a child's perception of what the child views in the media, through programming and advertising. One fourth of young children have a television set in their bedroom; a TV in the bedroom is associated with more hours of watching. The number of hours that most preschoolers watch TV exceeds guidelines (1 hr/day for 2-5 year olds). Interactive quality educational programming in which children develop social relationships with the characters can increase learning if paired with adult interaction around the storyline. However, exposure to commercial TV with violent content is associated with later behavior problems, and because children younger than 8 yr are not able to comprehend the concept of persuasive intent, they are more vulnerable to TV advertising.

Implications for Parents and Pediatricians

The significance of language as a target for assessment and intervention cannot be overestimated, because of its central role as an indicator of cognitive and emotional development and a key factor in behavioral regulation and later school success. As language emerges, parents can support emotional development by using words that describe the child's feeling states ("You sound angry right now") and urging the child to use words to express rather than act out feelings. Active imaginations will come into play when children offer explanations for misbehavior. A parent's best way of dealing with untruths is to address the event, not the child, and have the child participate in "making things right."

Parents should have a regular time each day for reading or looking at books with their children. Programs such as **Reach Out and Read,** in which pediatricians give out picture books along with appropriate guidance during primary care visits, have been effective in increasing reading aloud and thereby promoting language development, particularly in lower-income families. TV and similar media should be limited to 1 hr/day of quality programming for children aged 2-5 yr, and parents should be watching the programs with their children and debriefing their young children afterward. At-risk children, particularly those living in poverty, can better meet future school challenges if they have early high-quality child care and learning experiences (e.g., Head Start).

Preoperational thinking constrains how children understand experiences of illness and treatment. Children begin to understand that bodies have "insides" and "outsides." Children should be given simple, concrete explanations for medical procedures and given some control over procedures if possible. Children should be reassured that they are not to blame when receiving a vaccine or venipuncture. An adhesive bandage will help to make the body "whole" again in a child's mind.

The active imagination that fuels play and the magical, animist thinking characteristic of preoperational cognition can also generate intense fears. More than 80% of parents report at least 1 fear in their preschool children. Refusal to take baths or to sit on the toilet may arise from the fear of being washed away or flushed away, reflecting a child's immature appreciation of relative size. Attempts to demonstrate rationally that there are no monsters in the closet often fail, inasmuch as the fear arises from preoperational thinking. However, this same thinking allows parents to be endowed with magical powers that can banish the monsters with "monster spray" or a night-light. Parents should acknowledge the fears, offer reassurance and a sense of security, and give the child some sense of control over the situation. Use of the **Draw-a-Person**, in which a child is asked to draw the best person he or she child can, may help elucidate a child's viewpoint.

Emotional and Moral Development

Emotional challenges facing preschool children include accepting limits while maintaining a sense of self-direction, reigning in aggressive and sexual impulses, and interacting with a widening circle of adults and peers. At 2 yr of age, behavioral limits are predominantly external; by 5 yr of age, these controls need to be internalized if a child is to function in a typical classroom. Success in achieving this goal relies on prior emotional development, particularly the ability to use internalized images of trusted adults to provide a secure environment in times of stress. The love a child feels for important adults is the main incentive for the development of self-control.

Children learn what behaviors are acceptable and how much power they wield vis-à-vis important adults by testing limits. **Limit testing** increases when it elicits attention, even though that attention is often negative, and when limits are inconsistent. Testing often arouses parental anger or inappropriate solicitude as a child struggles to separate, and it gives rise to a corresponding parental challenge: letting go. Excessively tight limits can undermine a child's sense of initiative, whereas overly loose limits can provoke anxiety in a child who feels that no one is in control.

Control is a central issue. Young children cannot control many aspects of their lives, including where they go, how long they stay, and what they take home from the store. They are also prone to lose internal control, that is, to have **temper tantrums**. Fear, overtiredness, hunger, inconsistent expectations, or physical discomfort can also evoke tantrums. Tantrums normally appear toward the end of the 1st yr of life and peak in prevalence between 2 and 4 yr of age. Tantrums lasting more than 15 min or regularly occurring more than 3 times/day may reflect underlying medical, emotional, developmental, or social problems.

Preschool children normally experience complicated feelings toward their parents that can include strong attachment and possessiveness toward the parent of the opposite sex, jealousy and resentment of the other parent, and fear that these negative feelings might lead to abandonment. These emotions, most of which are beyond a child's ability to comprehend or verbalize, often find expression in highly labile moods. The resolution of this crisis (a process extending over years) involves a child's unspoken decision to identify with the parents rather than compete with them. Play and language foster the development of emotional controls by allowing children to express emotions and role-play.

Curiosity about genitals and adult sexual organs is normal, as is **masturbation**. Excessive masturbation interfering with normal activity, acting out sexual intercourse, extreme modesty, or mimicry of adult seductive behavior all suggest the possibility of sexual abuse or inappropriate exposure (see Chapter 16.1). Modesty appears gradually between 4 and 6 yr of age, with wide variations among cultures and families. Parents should begin to teach children about "private" body areas before school entry.

Moral thinking is constrained by a child's cognitive level and language abilities but develops as the child continues her or his identity with the parents. Beginning before the 2nd birthday, the child's sense of right and wrong stems from the desire to earn approval from the parents and avoid negative consequences. The child's impulses are tempered by external forces; the child has not yet internalized societal rules or a sense of justice and fairness. Over time, as the child internalizes parental admonitions, words are substituted for aggressive behaviors. Finally, the child accepts personal responsibility. Actions will be viewed by damage caused, not by intent. Empathic responses to others' distress arise during the 2nd yr of life, but the ability to consider another child's point of view remains limited throughout this period. In keeping with a child's inability to focus on more than one aspect of a situation at a time, fairness is taken to mean equal treatment, regardless of circumstance. A 4 yr old will acknowledge the importance of taking turns, but will complain if he or she "didn't get enough time." Rules tend to be absolute, with guilt assigned for bad outcomes, regardless of intentions.

Implications for Parents and Pediatricians

The importance of the preschooler's sense of control over his or her body and surroundings has implications for practice. Preparing the patient by letting the child know how the visit will proceed is reassuring. Tell the child what will happen, but do not ask permission unless you are willing to deal with a "no" answer. A brief introduction to "private parts" is warranted before the genital examination.

The visit of the 4 or 5 yr old should be entertaining, because of the child's ability to communicate, as well as the child's natural curiosity. Physicians should realize that all children are occasionally difficult. Guidance emphasizing appropriate expectations for behavioral and emotional development and acknowledging normal parental feelings of anger, guilt, and confusion should be part of all visits at this time. Parents should be queried about daily routines and their expectations of child behavior. Providing children with **acceptable choices** (all options being acceptable to the parent) and encouraging independence in self-care activities (feeding, dressing, and bathing) will reduce conflicts.

Although some cultures condone the use of **corporal punishment** for disciplining of young children, it is not a consistently effective means of behavioral control. As children habituate to repeated spanking, parents have to spank ever harder to achieve the desired response, increasing the risk of serious injury. Sufficiently harsh punishment may inhibit undesired behaviors, but at great psychologic cost. Children mimic the corporal punishment that they receive; children who are spanked will have more aggressive behaviors later. Whereas spanking is the use of force, externally applied, to produce behavior change, **discipline** is the process that allows the child to internalize controls on behavior. Alternative discipline strategies should be offered, such as the "countdown" for transitions along with consistent limit setting, "time-outs" or "time-ins" (breaks from play with caregiver present and interacting), clear communication of rules, and frequent approval with positive reinforcement of productive play and behavior (see Chapter 19). Punishment should be immediate, specific to the behavior, and time-limited. *Time-out for approximately 1 min/yr of age is very effective.* A kitchen timer allows the parent to step back from the situation; the child is free when the timer rings. Although one strategy might not work for all children uniformly, consistency is integral to healthy learning and growth.

Bibliography is available at Expert Consult.

Chapter **25**
Middle Childhood
Laura H. Finkelstein and Susan Feigelman
第二十五章
学龄期

中文导读

本章主要介绍了6~11岁学龄儿童的体格发育及认知、社交、情感和道德的发展。具体描述了儿童体格生长，儿童对体形和性别差异的认知；具体描述了认知发展的具体运算阶段以及学校对儿童认知发展水平的要求；描述了社会交往、性别认同、解决冲突、遵守规范、内化的社会规则等社交、情感、道德方面的发展；具体描述了父母和儿科医师在儿童体格发育，以及认知、社交、情感和道德的发展中所起到的作用。

Middle childhood (6-11 yr of age) is the period in which children increasingly separate from parents and seek acceptance from teachers, other adults, and peers. Children begin to feel under pressure to conform to the style and ideals of the peer group. Self-esteem becomes a central issue, as children develop the cognitive ability to consider their own self-evaluations and their perception of how others see them. For the first time, they are judged according to their ability to produce socially valued outputs, such as getting good grades, playing a musical instrument, or hitting home runs.

PHYSICAL DEVELOPMENT
Growth occurs *discontinuously,* in 3-6 irregularly timed spurts each year, but varies both within and among individuals. Growth during the period averages 3-3.5 kg (6.6-7.7 lb) and 6-7 cm (2.4-2.8 in) per year (Fig. 25.1). The head grows only 2 cm in circumference throughout the entire period, reflecting a slowing of brain growth. Myelination continues into adolescence, with peak gray matter at 12-14 yr. Body habitus is more erect than previously, with long legs compared with the torso.

Growth of the midface and lower face occurs gradually. Loss of deciduous (baby) teeth is a more dramatic sign of maturation, beginning around 6 yr of age. Replacement with adult teeth occurs at a rate of about 4 per year, so that by age 9 yr, children will have 8 permanent incisors and 4 permanent molars. Premolars erupt by 11-12 yr of age (see Chapter 333). Lymphoid tissues hypertrophy and reach maximal size, often giving rise to impressive tonsils and adenoids.

Muscular strength, coordination, and stamina increase progressively, as does the ability to perform complex movements, such as dancing or shooting baskets. Such higher-order motor skills are the result of both maturation and training; the degree of accomplishment reflects wide variability in innate skill, interest, and opportunity.

Physical fitness has declined among school-age children. Sedentary habits at this age are associated with increased lifetime risk of obesity, cardiovascular disease, lower academic achievement, and lower self-esteem . The number of overweight children and the degree of overweight have been increasing, although recently at a slower rate (see Chapter 60). Only 15% of middle and junior high schools require physical education class at least 3 days/wk. One quarter of youth do not engage in any free-time physical activity, despite the recommendation for at least 1 hr of physical activity per day.

Perceptions of **body image** develop early during this period; children as young as 5 and 6 yr express dissatisfaction with their body image; by ages 8 and 9 yr many of these youth report trying to diet, often using ill-advised regimens. Loss-of-control (binge) eating occurs among approximately 6% of children at this age.

Prior to puberty, the sensitivity of the hypothalamus and pituitary changes, leading to increased gonadotropin synthesis. Interest in gender differences and sexual behavior increases progressively until puberty. Although this is a period when sexual drives are limited, masturbation is common, and children may be interested in differences between genders. Rates of maturation differ by geography, ethnicity, and country. Sexual maturity occurs earlier for both genders in the United States. Differences in maturation rates have implications for differing expectations of others based on sexual maturation.

Implications for Parents and Pediatricians
Middle childhood is generally a time of excellent health. However, children have variable sizes, shapes, and abilities. Children of this age compare themselves with others, eliciting feelings about their physical attributes and abilities. Fears of being "abnormal" can lead to avoidance of situations in which physical differences might be revealed, such as gym class or medical examinations. Children with actual physical disabilities may face special stresses. Medical, social, and psychologic risks tend to occur together.

Children should be asked about risk factors for **obesity**. Participation in physical activity, including organized sports or other organized activities, can foster skill, teamwork, and fitness as well as a sense of accomplishment, but pressure to compete when the activity is no longer enjoyable has negative effects. Counseling on establishing healthy eating

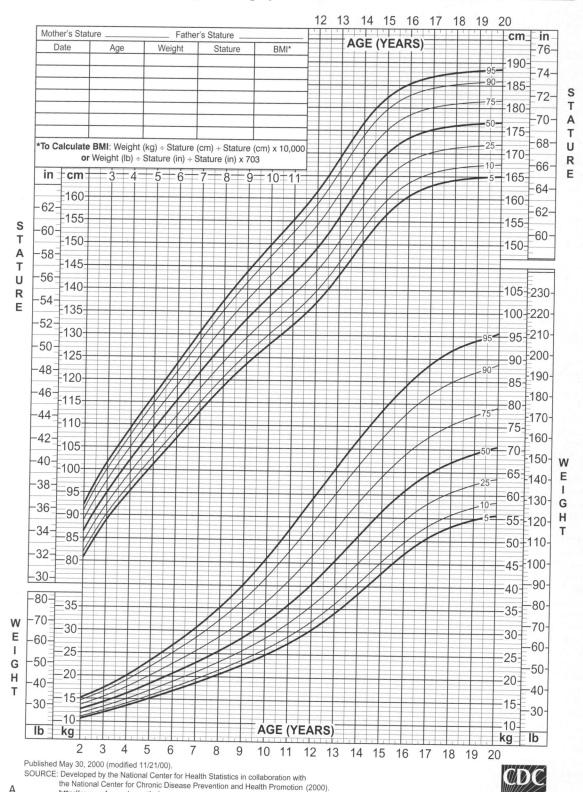

2 to 20 years: Boys
Stature-for-age and Weight-for-age percentiles

NAME _____

RECORD # _____

Fig. 25.1 A, Stature (height) for age and weight for boys age 2-20 yr. *(Courtesy National Center for Health Statistics, in collaboration with the National Center for Chronic Disease Prevention and Health Promotion, 2000. http://www.cdc.gov/growthcharts.)*

Continued

2 to 20 years: Girls
Stature-for-age and Weight-for-age percentiles

To Calculate BMI: Weight (kg) ÷ Stature (cm) ÷ Stature (cm) x 10,000
or Weight (lb) ÷ Stature (in) ÷ Stature (in) x 703

Published May 30, 2000 (modified 11/21/00).
SOURCE: Developed by the National Center for Health Statistics in collaboration with
the National Center for Chronic Disease Prevention and Health Promotion (2000).
http://www.cdc.gov/growthcharts

CDC

SAFER · HEALTHIER · PEOPLE™

B

Fig. 25.1, cont'd B, Stature (height) for age and weight for girls, age 2-20 yr. (*Courtesy National Center for Health Statistics, 2000.*)

Table 25.1	Selected Perceptual, Cognitive, and Language Processes Required for Elementary School Success	
PROCESS	**DESCRIPTION**	**ASSOCIATED PROBLEMS**
PERCEPTUAL		
Visual analysis	Ability to break a complex figure into components and understand their spatial relationships	Persistent letter confusion (e.g., between b, d, and g); difficulty with basic reading and writing and limited "sight" vocabulary
Proprioception and motor control	Ability to obtain information about body position by feel and unconsciously program complex movements	Poor handwriting, requiring inordinate effort, often with overly tight pencil grasp; special difficulty with timed tasks
Phonologic processing	Ability to perceive differences between similar-sounding words and to break down words into constituent sounds	Delayed receptive language skill; attention and behavior problems secondary to not understanding directions; delayed acquisition of letter-sound correlations (phonetics)
COGNITIVE		
Long-term memory, both storage and recall	Ability to acquire skills that are "automatic" (i.e., accessible without conscious thought)	Delayed mastery of the alphabet (reading and writing letters); slow handwriting; inability to progress beyond basic mathematics
Selective attention	Ability to attend to important stimuli and ignore distractions	Difficulty following multistep instructions, completing assignments, and behaving well; problems with peer interaction
Sequencing	Ability to remember things in order; facility with time concepts	Difficulty organizing assignments, planning, spelling, and telling time
LANGUAGE		
Receptive language	Ability to comprehend complex constructions, function words (e.g., if, when, only, except), nuances of speech, and extended blocks of language (e.g., paragraphs)	Difficulty following directions; wandering attention during lessons and stories; problems with reading comprehension; problems with peer relationships
Expressive language	Ability to recall required words effortlessly (word finding), control meanings by varying position and word endings, and construct meaningful paragraphs and stories	Difficulty expressing feelings and using words for self-defense, with resulting frustration and physical acting out; struggling during "circle time" and in language-based subjects (e.g., English)

habits and limited screen time should be given to all families. Prepubertal children should not engage in high-stress, high-impact sports, such as power lifting or tackle football, because skeletal immaturity increases the risk of injury (see Chapter 713).

COGNITIVE DEVELOPMENT

The thinking of early elementary school-age children differs qualitatively from that of preschool children. In place of magical, egocentric, and perception-bound cognition, school-age children increasingly apply rules based on observable phenomena, factor in multiple dimensions and points of view, and interpret their perceptions using physical laws. Piaget documented this shift from preoperational to **concrete** (logical) **operations**. When 5 yr olds watch a ball of clay being rolled into a snake, they might insist that the snake has "more" because it is longer. In contrast, 7 yr olds typically reply that the ball and the snake must weigh the same because nothing has been added or taken away or because the snake is both longer and thinner. This cognitive reorganization occurs at different rates in different contexts. In the context of social interactions with siblings, young children often demonstrate an ability to understand alternate points of view long before they demonstrate that ability in their thinking about the physical world. Understanding time and space constructs occurs in the later part of this period.

The concept of **school readiness** has evolved. The American Academy of Pediatrics recommends following an "interactional relational" model in which the focus is on the child, the environment, and the resulting interactions. This model explicitly asserts that all children can learn and that the educational process is reciprocal between the child and the school. It is developmentally based, recognizing the importance of early experiences for later development. Rather than delaying school entry, high-quality early-education programs may be the key to ultimate school success.

School makes increasing cognitive demands on the child. Mastery of the elementary curriculum requires that many perceptual, cognitive, and language processes work efficiently (Table 25.1), and children are expected to attend to many inputs at once. The 1st 2-3 yr of elementary school are devoted to acquiring the fundamentals: reading, writing, and basic mathematics skills. By 3rd grade, children need to be able to sustain attention through a 45 min period, and the curriculum requires more complex tasks. The goal of reading a paragraph is no longer to decode the words, but to understand the content; the goal of writing is no longer spelling or penmanship, but composition. The volume of work increases along with the complexity.

Cognitive abilities interact with a wide array of attitudinal and emotional factors in determining classroom performance. These factors include *external rewards* (eagerness to please adults and approval from peers) and *internal rewards* (competitiveness, willingness to work for a delayed reward, belief in one's abilities, and ability to risk trying when success is not ensured). Success predisposes to success, whereas failure impacts self-esteem and reduces self-efficacy, diminishing a child's ability to take future risks.

Children's intellectual activity extends beyond the classroom. Beginning in the 3rd or 4th grade, children increasingly enjoy strategy games and wordplay (puns and insults) that exercise their growing cognitive and linguistic mastery. Many become experts on subjects of their own choosing, such as sports trivia, or develop hobbies, such as special card collections. Others become avid readers or take on artistic pursuits. Whereas board and card games were once the usual leisure-time activity of youth, video, computer, and other electronic games currently fill this need.

Implications for Parents and Pediatricians

Pediatricians have an important role in preparing their patients for school entrance by promoting health through immunizations, adequate nutrition, appropriate recreation, and screening for physical, developmental, and cognitive disorders. The American Academy of Pediatrics recommends that pediatric providers promote the "5 Rs" of early education: (1) reading as a daily family activity; (2) rhyming, playing, and cuddling together; (3) routines and regular times for meals, play, and sleep; (4) reward through praise for successes; and (5) reciprocal nurturing relationships.

Concrete operations allow children to understand simple explanations for illnesses and necessary treatments, although they may revert to prelogical thinking when under stress. A child with pneumonia may be able to explain about white cells fighting the "germs" in the lungs, but may still secretly harbor the belief that the sickness is a punishment for disobedience.

As children are faced with more abstract concepts, academic and classroom behavior problems emerge and come to the pediatrician's attention. Referrals may be made to the school for remediation or to community resources (medical or psychologic) when appropriate. The causes may be one or more of the following: deficits in perception (vision and hearing); specific learning disabilities (see Chapters 50 and 51); global cognitive delay (intellectual disability; Chapter 53); deficits in attention and executive function (Chapters 48 and 49); and attention deficits secondary to family dysfunction, depression, anxiety, or chronic illness. Children whose learning style does not fit the classroom culture may have academic difficulties and need assessment before failure sets in. Simply having a child repeat a failed grade rarely has any beneficial effect and often seriously undercuts the child's self-esteem. In addition to finding the problem areas, identifying each child's strengths is important. Educational approaches that value a wide range of talents ("multiple intelligences") beyond the traditional reading, writing, and mathematics may allow more children to succeed.

The change in cognition allows the child to understand "if/when" clauses. Increased responsibilities and expectations accompany increased rights and privileges. Discipline strategies should move toward negotiation and a clear understanding of consequences, including removal of privileges for infringements.

SOCIAL, EMOTIONAL, AND MORAL DEVELOPMENT
Social and Emotional Development
In middle childhood, energy is directed toward creativity and productivity. Changes occur in 3 spheres: the home, the school, and the neighborhood. Of these, the home and family remains the most influential. Increasing independence is marked by the first sleepover at a friend's house and the first time at overnight camp. Parents should make demands for effort in school and extracurricular activities, celebrate successes, and offer unconditional acceptance when failures occur. Regular chores, associated with an allowance, provide an opportunity for children to contribute to family functioning and learn the value of money. These responsibilities may be a testing ground for psychologic separation, leading to conflict. Siblings have critical roles as competitors, loyal supporters, and role models.

The beginning of school coincides with a child's further separation from the family and the increasing importance of teacher and peer relationships. Social groups tend to be same-sex, with frequent changing of membership, contributing to a child's growing social development and competence. Popularity, a central ingredient of self-esteem, may be won through possessions (having the latest electronic gadgets or the right clothes), as well as through personal attractiveness, accomplishments, and actual social skills. Children are aware of racial differences and are beginning to form opinions about racial groups that impact their relationships. **Gender identification**, which began in early childhood, continues to evolve and can have significant implications for peer relationships and self-awareness.

Some children conform readily to the peer norms and enjoy easy social success. Those who adopt individualistic styles or have visible differences may be teased or bullied. Such children may be painfully aware that they are different, or they may be puzzled by their lack of popularity. Children with deficits in social skills may go to extreme lengths to win acceptance, only to meet with repeated failure. Attributions conferred by peers, such as funny, stupid, bad, or fat, may become incorporated into a child's self-image and affect the child's personality, as well as school performance. Parents may have their greatest effect indirectly, through actions that change the peer group (moving to a new community or insisting on involvement in structured after-school activities). Children who identify with a gender different from their sex of birth, or whose manner and dress reflect those more typically seen as "opposite" their birth sex, may be subject to teasing or, **bullying**. This can magnify the confusion for these children, who are formulating their own concept of "self."

In the neighborhood, real dangers, such as busy streets, bullies, violence, and strangers, tax school-age children's common sense and resourcefulness (see Chapter 14). Interactions with peers without close adult supervision call on increasing conflict resolution skills. Media exposure to adult materialism, sexuality, substance use, and violence may be frightening, reinforcing children's feeling of powerlessness in the larger world. Compensatory fantasies of being powerful may fuel the fascination with heroes and superheroes. A balance between fantasy and an appropriate ability to negotiate real-world challenges indicates healthy emotional development.

Moral Development
Although by age 6 yr most children will have a **conscience** (internalized rules of society), they vary greatly in their level of moral development. For the younger youth, many still subscribe to the notion that rules are established and enforced by an authority figure (parent or teacher), and decision-making is guided by self-interest (avoidance of negative and receipt of positive consequences). The needs of others are not strongly considered in decision-making. As they grow older, most will recognize not only their own needs and desires but also those of others, although personal consequences are still the primary driver of behavior. Social behaviors that are socially undesirable are considered wrong. By age 10-11 yr, the combination of peer pressure, a desire to please authority figures, and an understanding of **reciprocity** (treat others as you wish to be treated) shapes the child's behavior.

Implications for Parents and Pediatricians
Children need unconditional support as well as realistic demands as they venture into a world that is often frightening. A daily query from parents over the dinner table or at bedtime about the good and bad things that happened during the child's day may uncover problems early. Parents may have difficulty allowing the child independence or may exert excessive pressure on their children to achieve academic or competitive success. Children who struggle to meet such expectations may have behavior problems or psychosomatic complaints.

Many children face stressors that exceed the normal challenges of separation and success in school and the neighborhood. Divorce affects almost 50% of children. Domestic violence, parental substance abuse, and other mental health problems may also impair a child's ability to use home as a secure base for refueling emotional energies. In many neighborhoods, random violence makes the normal development of independence extremely dangerous. Older children may join gangs as a means of self-protection and a way to attain recognition and to belong to a cohesive group. Children who bully others and those who are victims of bullying should be evaluated, since bullying is associated with mood disorders, family problems, and school adjustment problems. Parents should reduce exposure to hazards where possible. Because of the risk of unintentional firearm injuries to children, parents should be encouraged to ask parents of playmates whether a gun is kept in their home and, if so, how it is secured. The high prevalence of adjustment disorders among school-age children attests to the effects of such overwhelming stressors on development.

Pediatrician visits are infrequent in this period; therefore each visit is an opportunity to assess children's functioning in all contexts (home, school, neighborhood). Maladaptive behaviors, both internalizing and externalizing, occur when stress in any of these environments overwhelms the child's coping responses. Because of continuous exposure and the strong influence of media (programming and advertisements) on children's beliefs and attitudes, parents must be alert to exposures from television and Internet. An average American youth spends over 6 hr/day with a variety of media, and 65% of these children have a TV in their bedrooms. Parents should be advised to remove the TV from their children's rooms, limit viewing to 2 hr/day, and monitor what programs children watch. The **Draw-a-Person** (for ages 3-10 yr, with instructions to "draw a complete person") and **Kinetic Family Drawing** (beginning at age 5 yr, with instructions to "draw a picture of everyone in your family doing something") are useful office tools to assess a child's functioning.

Bibliography is available at Expert Consult.

Chapter **26**

Adolescence

第二十六章
青春期

中文导读

见第十二部分，第一百三十二章。

See Part XII, Chapter 132, Adolescent Physical and Social Development.

Chapter **27**

Assessment of Growth

Vaneeta Bamba and Andrea Kelly

第二十七章
生长评估

中文导读

本章主要介绍了生长测量、生长曲线以及与生长相关的其他发育情况。具体描述了生长指标的测量方法、生长指标的监测、不同年龄的生长速度和生长特征；具体描述了生长曲线的评价指标和评价方法，世界卫生组织和美国CDC的生长曲线图的差异；具体描述了正常生长、生长异常以及对生长异常的评估；描述了儿童肥胖和牙齿的发育。

Growth can be considered a vital sign in children, and aberrant growth may be the first sign of an underlying pathologic condition. The most powerful tool in growth assessment is the **growth chart** (Figs. 23.1, 23.2, 25.1, and 27.1), used in combination with accurate measurements of height, weight, head circumference, and calculation of the body mass index.

TECHNIQUES TO MEASURE GROWTH

Growth assessment requires accurate and precise measurements. For infants and toddlers age <2 yr, weight, length, and head circumference are obtained. **Head circumference** is measured with a flexible tape measure starting at the supraorbital ridge around to the occipital prominence in the back of the head, locating the maximal circumference. **Height** and **weight** measures should be performed with the infant naked, and ideally, repeated measures will be performed on the same equipment. **Recumbent length** is most accurately measured by two examiners (one to position the child). Hair ornaments and hairstyles that interfere with measurements and positioning should be removed. The child's head is positioned against an inflexible measuring board in the **Frankfurt plane**, in which the outer canthi of the eyes are in line with the external auditory meatus and are perpendicular to the long axis of the trunk. Legs should be fully extended, and feet are maintained perpendicular to the plane of the supine infant. For older children (>2 yr) who can stand unassisted, standing heights should be obtained without shoes, using a stadiometer with the head in the Frankfurt plane, and the back of the head, thoracic spine, buttocks, and heels approximating the vertical axis of one another and the stadiometer.

Measurements obtained using alternative means, such as marking examination paper at the foot and head of a supine infant or using a tape measure or wall growth chart with a book or ruler on the head can lead to inaccuracy and render the measurement useless.

Measurements for height and weight should be plotted on the age-appropriate growth curve. Comparing measurements with previous growth trends, repeating measures that are inconsistent, and plotting results longitudinally are essential for monitoring growth. Calculation of interim linear height velocity, such as centimeters per year (cm/yr), allows more precise comparison of growth rate to the norm (Table 27.1).

If a child is growing faster or more slowly than expected, measurement of body proportions, which follow a predictable sequence of changes with development, are useful. The head and trunk are relatively large at birth, with progressive lengthening of the limbs throughout development, particularly during puberty. The **upper-to-lower body segment ratio** (**U/L ratio**) provides an assessment of truncal growth relative to limb growth. The **lower-body segment** is defined as the length from the top of the symphysis pubis to the floor, and the **upper-body segment** is the total height minus the lower-body segment. The U/L ratio equals approximately 1.7 at birth, 1.3 at 3 yr, and 1.0 after 7 yr. Higher U/L ratios are characteristic of short-limb dwarfism, as occurs with Turner syndrome or bone disorders, whereas lower ratios suggest hypogonadism or Marfan syndrome.

Arm span also provides assessment of proportionality and is measured as the distance between the tips of the middle fingers while the patient stands with the back against the wall with arms outstretched horizontally at a 90-degree angle to the trunk. This span should be close to height, although the proportion changes with age.

GROWTH CURVES

The American Academy of Pediatrics (AAP) and the U.S. Centers for Disease Control and Prevention (CDC) recommend use of the 2006 World Health Organization (WHO) growth curves for children age 0-24 mo and the 2000 CDC growth curves for children age 2-19 yr (https://www.cdc.gov/growthcharts). There are 5 standard gender-specific charts: (1) weight for age, (2) height (length and stature) for age, (3) head circumference for age, (4) weight for height (length and stature) for infants, and (5) body mass index for age (Fig. 27.1; see also Figs. 23.1, 23.2, and 25.1). Clinicians should confirm that the correct CDC and WHO growth charts are used in electronic medical records to ensure accurate characterization of growth.

Table 27.1	Growth Velocity and Other Growth Characteristics by Age		
INFANCY		**CHILDHOOD**	**ADOLESCENCE**
Birth-12 mo: 24 cm/yr 12-24 mo: 10 cm/yr 24-36 mo: 8 cm/yr		6 cm/yr Slowly decelerates before pubertal onset Height typically does not cross percentile lines	Sigmoid-shaped growth Adolescent growth spurt accounts for about 15% of adult height Peak height velocity Girls: 8 cm/yr Boys: 10 cm/yr

The WHO curves describe growth differently than the CDC curves (Fig. 27.2). The WHO curves are **growth standards** that describe how children grow under optimal conditions, whereas the CDC curves are **growth references** that describe how children grew in a specific time and place. The WHO growth curves are based on longitudinal growth studies in which cohorts of newborns were chosen from six countries (Brazil, Ghana, India, Norway, Oman, United States) using specific inclusion and exclusion criteria; all infants were breastfed for at least 12 months and were predominantly breastfed for the first 4 mo of life. They were measured regularly from birth to 23 mo during 1997–2003. In contrast, the CDC curves are based on cross-sectional data from different studies during different time points. Growth curves for children age 2-59 mo were based on the National Health and Nutrition Examination Survey (NHANES), which included a cross section of the U.S. population. These data were supplemented with additional participants in a separate nutrition surveillance study.

Several deficiencies of the older charts have been corrected, such as the overrepresentation of bottle-fed infants and the reliance on a local dataset for the infant charts. The disjunction between length and height when transitioning from the infant curves to those for older children is improved.

Each chart is composed of percentile curves, which indicate the percentage of children at a given age on the x axis whose measured value falls below the corresponding value on the y axis. The 2006 WHO growth curves include values that are 2 standard deviations (SD) above and below median (2nd and 98th percentiles), whereas the 2000 CDC growth curves include 3rd and 97th percentiles. On the WHO weight chart for boys age 0-24 mo (see Fig. 23.2A), the 9 mo age line intersects the 25th percentile curve at 8.3 kg, indicating that 25% of 9 mo old boys in the WHO cohorts weigh less than 8.3 kg (75% weigh more). Similarly, a 9 mo old boy weighing more than 11 kg is heavier than 98% of his peers. The median or 50th percentile is also termed the **standard value**, in the sense that the standard length for a 7 mo old girl is 67.3 cm (see Fig. 23.2B). The weight-for-length charts (see Fig. 23.1) are constructed in an analogous fashion, with length or stature in place of age on the x axis; the median or standard weight for a girl measuring 100 cm is 15 kg.

Extremes of height or weight can also be expressed in terms of the age for which they would represent the standard or median. For instance, an 18 mo old girl who is 74.9 cm (2nd percentile) is at the 50th percentile for a 13 mo old. Thus the height age is 13 mo. Weight age can also be expressed this way.

In assessing adolescents, caution must be used in applying cross-sectional charts. Growth during adolescence is linked temporally to the onset of puberty, which varies widely. Normal variations in the timing of the growth spurt can lead to misdiagnosis of growth abnormalities. By using cross-sectional data based on chronological age, the charts combine youth who are at different stages of maturation. Data for 12 yr old boys include both earlier-maturing boys who are at the peak of their growth spurts and later-maturing ones who are still growing at their prepubertal rate. The net results are an artificially blunted growth peak, and the appearance that adolescents grow more gradually and for a longer duration than in actuality.

When additional insight is necessary, growth charts derived from longitudinal data, such as the **height velocity charts** of Tanner and colleagues, are recommended. The longitudinal component of these

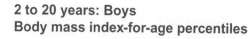

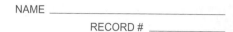

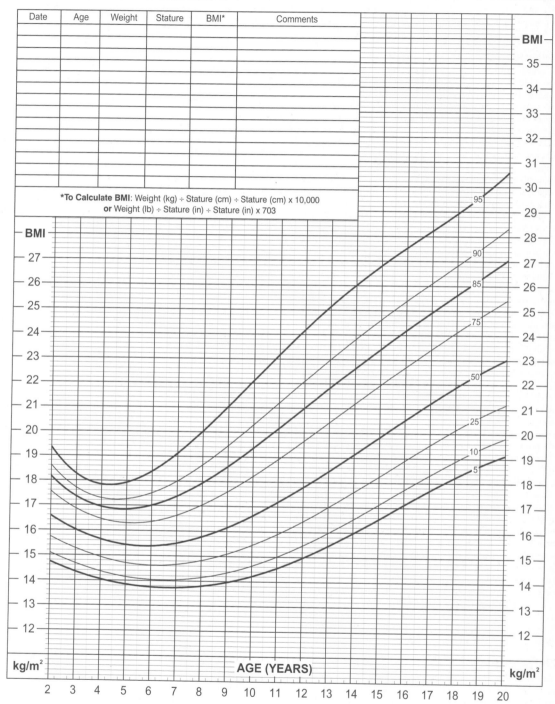

Published May 30, 2000 (modified 10/16/00).

SOURCE: Developed by the National Center for Health Statistics in collaboration with
the National Center for Chronic Disease Prevention and Health Promotion (2000).
http://www.cdc.gov/growthcharts

A

SAFER·HEALTHIER·PEOPLE™

Fig. 27.1 **A,** Body mass index (BMI) percentiles for boys, age 2-20 yr. *(Official Centers for Disease Control [CDC] growth charts, as described in this chapter. The 85th to 95th percentile is at risk for overweight; >95th percentile is overweight; <5th percentile is underweight. Technical information and interpretation and management guides are available at www.cdc.gov/nchs. Developed by the National Center for Health Statistics in collaboration with the National Center for Chronic Disease Prevention and Health Promotion, 2000. http://www.cdc.gov/growthcharts)*

2 to 20 years: Girls
Body mass index-for-age percentiles

NAME _____

RECORD # _____

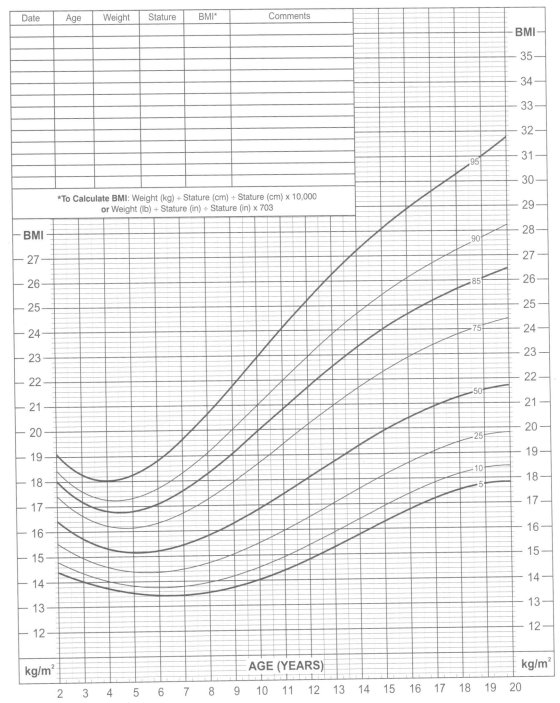

Date	Age	Weight	Stature	BMI*	Comments

*To Calculate BMI: Weight (kg) ÷ Stature (cm) ÷ Stature (cm) x 10,000
or Weight (lb) ÷ Stature (in) ÷ Stature (in) x 703

AGE (YEARS)

Published May 30, 2000 (modified 10/16/00).
SOURCE: Developed by the National Center for Health Statistics in collaboration with
the National Center for Chronic Disease Prevention and Health Promotion (2000).
http://www.cdc.gov/growthcharts

SAFER · HEALTHIER · PEOPLE™

B

Fig. 27.1, cont'd B, Body mass index (BMI) percentiles for girls, age 2-20 yr.

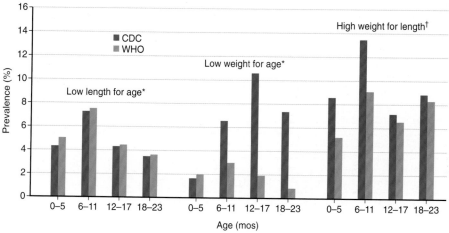

Fig. 27.2 Comparison of WHO and CDC growth chart prevalence of low length for age, low weight for age, and high weight for length among children age <24 mo, United States, 1999–2004. *, ≤5th percentile on the CDC charts; ≤2.3rd percentile on the WHO charts. †, ≥95th percentile on the CDC charts; ≥97.7th percentile on the WHO charts. *(Data from the National Health and Nutrition Examination Survey, 1999–2004; from Grummer-Strawn LM, Reinold C, Krebs NF; Centers for Disease Control and Prevention: Use of World Health Organization and CDC growth charts for children aged 0-59 months in the United States, MMWR Recomm Rep 59(RR-9):1–15, 2010.)*

velocity curves are based on British children from the 1950s–1960s, and cross-sectional data from U.S. children were superimposed. More recently, height velocity curves based on longitudinal data from a multiethnic study conducted at five U.S. sites included standard deviation scores for height velocity for earlier- and later-maturing adolescents to facilitate the identification of poor or accelerated linear growth.

Specialized growth charts have been developed for U.S. children with various conditions, including very low birthweight, small for gestational age, trisomy 21, Turner syndrome, and achondroplasia, and should be used when appropriate.

Facilitating identification of obesity, the charts include curves for plotting **body mass index (BMI)** for ages 2-20 yr rather than weight for height (see Fig. 27.1). Methodological steps have ensured that the increase in the prevalence of obesity has not unduly raised the upper limits of normal. BMI can be calculated as weight in kilograms/(height in meters)^2 or weight in pounds/(height in inches)$^2 \times 703$, with fractions of pounds and inches expressed as decimals. Because of variable weight and height gains during childhood, BMI must be interpreted relative to age and sex; BMI percentile provides a more standardized comparison. For example, a 6 yr old girl with BMI of 19.7 kg/m^2 (97th percentile) is obese, whereas a 15 yr old girl with BMI of 19.7 kg/m^2 (50th percentile) is normal weight.

Normal Growth

Height is highly correlated with genetics, specifically parental height. Calculation of sex-adjusted **midparental height** is important when assessing growth in a child to avoid misclassification of abnormal growth. The average difference in stature between men and women is 5 inches (13 cm); therefore 5 inches (13 cm) is subtracted from father's height before averaging with mother's height in a female, whereas 5 inches (13 cm) is added to mother's height before averaging with father's height in a male:

◆ Boys: [(Maternal height + 5 inches) + Paternal height]/2
◆ Girls: [Maternal height + (Paternal height − 5 inches)]/2

Furthermore, generally 4 inches (2 SD) is applied above and below this value to provide a *genetic target height range*. For example, if the mother is 63 inches tall and the father 70 inches tall, the daughter's sex-adjusted midparental height is 64 inches ± 4 inches, for a target height range of 60-68 inches. The son of these same parents would have a sex-adjusted midparental height of 69 inches, with a range of 65-73 inches. Note that these general guidelines do not address extreme

differences between parental heights that may affect individual target height range.

Growth can be divided into four major phases: fetal, infantile, childhood, and adolescence. Growth rate varies by age (see Table 27.1). Different factors are of different importance in each phase, and the various contributors to poor growth may feature more in one phase than another. Long-term height may be permanently compromised if one entire phase is characterized by poor growth. Therefore, early detection and prevention are critical. **Fetal growth** is the fastest growth phase, with maternal, placental, fetal, and environmental factors playing key roles. Birthweight does not necessarily correlate with adult height, although factors that inhibit fetal growth may have long-lasting effects, as seen in children with intrauterine growth retardation. **Infantile growth** is particularly sensitive to nutrition as well as congenital conditions. Genetic height gradually becomes influential; indeed, crossing of percentiles in the 1st 2 yr of life is common as children begin to approach their genetic potential. **Childhood growth** is often the most steady and predictable. During this phase the height percentile channel is fairly consistent in otherwise healthy children.

Adolescent growth is associated with a decrease in growth velocity prior to the onset of puberty; this deceleration tends to be more pronounced in males. During pubertal development, sex hormones (testosterone and estrogen) are the primary drivers of growth and enhance growth hormone secretion, thereby facilitating pubertal growth acceleration. Girls typically experience growth acceleration during Tanner Stage 3 for breast development, whereas this acceleration occurs during Tanner Stage 4 for pubic hair development in boys. Boys not only achieve greater height velocities than girls during puberty, but also grow approximately 2 yr longer than girls, both of which contribute to the taller average height of adult men compared with adult women.

Abnormal Growth

Growth is a dynamic process. A child measured at the 5th percentile for stature may be growing normally, may be failing to grow, or may be recovering from growth failure, depending on the trajectory of the growth curve (Fig. 27.3). Growth failure must be distinguished from short stature. **Growth failure** is defined as achievement of height velocity that is less than expected for a child's age and sex (and pubertal development if relevant) or a downward crossing of more than 2 percentile lines for height on the growth chart. **Short stature** is defined as growing either below expected genetic potential or growing below −2 SD for

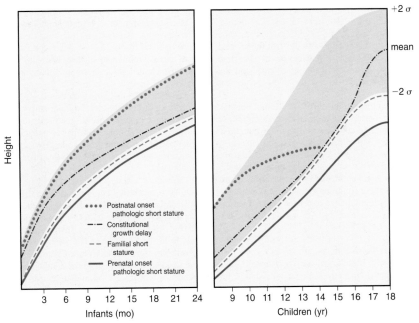

Fig. 27.3 Height-for-age curves of the 4 general causes of proportional short stature: postnatal onset pathologic short stature, constitutional growth delay, familial short stature, and prenatal onset short stature. *(From Mahoney CP: Evaluating the child with short stature, Pediatr Clin North Am 34:825, 1987.)*

age and sex. For some children, however, growth parameters <−2 SD may be normal, and differentiating appropriately small vs pathologically small is crucial. Midparental height, ethnicity, and other factors that may be inherent in the child's genetic potential for growth are important considerations in the assessment of growth. For children with particularly tall or short parents, overdiagnosing and underdiagnosing growth disorders are risks if parental heights are not taken into account. In the setting of familial short stature or tall status, more specialized charts can help determine if a child is even shorter or taller than expected for parental heights, to prevent misdiagnosis of growth disorders.

For **premature infants**, overdiagnosis of growth failure can be avoided by using growth charts developed specifically for this population. A cruder method, subtracting the weeks of prematurity from the postnatal age when plotting growth parameters, does not capture the variability in growth velocity that very-low-birthweight (VLBW) infants demonstrate. Although VLBW infants may continue to show **catch-up growth** through early school age, most achieve weight catch-up during the 2nd year and height catch-up by 3-4 yr, barring medical complications (see Chapter 117).

Abnormal growth may be caused by a variety of factors, including congenital conditions, systemic disease, endocrine disorders, nutritional deficiency (see Chapter 57), psychosocial conditions, constitutional delay, or familial disorders (Tables 27.2 and 27.3). In congenital pathologic short stature, an infant may or may not be born small, but growth gradually tapers throughout infancy (Fig. 27.3). Causes include chromosome or genetic abnormalities (Turner syndrome, skeletal dysplasia, trisomy 21; see Chapter 98), perinatal infection, extreme prematurity, and teratogens (phenytoin, alcohol) (see Chapter 115.5). Linear growth deceleration with or without changes in weight can occur at the onset or as a result of a systemic illness or chronic inflammation. Medications such as high-dose glucocorticoids may also impact growth. Analysis of growth patterns requires consideration of weight status. Poor linear growth in the setting of decreasing BMI suggests a nutritional or gastrointestinal issue, whereas poor linear growth in the context of good or robust BMI suggests a hormonal condition (hypothyroidism, growth hormone deficiency, cortisol excess).

Table 27.2	Common Causes of Decreased Growth and Short Stature

Variation of normal
   Familial short stature
   Constitutional delay
   Delayed puberty
Nutrition and gastrointestinal conditions
   Malnutrition
   Celiac disease
   Inflammatory bowel disease
Genetic conditions
   Turner syndrome
   Prader-Willi syndrome
   22q deletion syndrome
   Trisomy 21
   Skeletal dysplasias: achondroplasia, SHOX haploinsufficiency, osteogenesis imperfecta
Endocrine conditions
   Hypothyroidism
   Growth hormone deficiency
   Poorly controlled diabetes mellitus
   Poorly controlled diabetes insipidus
   Metabolic bone disease: rickets, hypophosphatasia
   Glucocorticoid excess
Psychosocial causes
Renal conditions
   Renal tubular acidosis
   Nephrotic syndrome
Medications
   Glucocorticoids
   Inappropriate sex steroid exposure
   Antiepileptic medications

Not all decreased growth is abnormal; variations of growth include constitutional growth (and pubertal) delay and familial short stature. In **constitutional growth delay**, weight and height decrease near the end of infancy, parallel the norm through middle childhood, and accelerate toward the end of adolescence with achievement of normal adult height. In **familial short stature**, both the infant/child and the parent(s) are small; growth runs parallel to and just below the normal curves.

Although **tall or accelerated growth** may be a variation of normal, unexpected increase in growth may also signal an underlying condition (Table 27.3). Typically, obese individuals grow more quickly than their peers because of peripheral aromatization of estrogen and effects on bone maturation. Despite early taller stature, obese children are not ultimately taller than anticipated for genetic height. Early onset of puberty, growth hormone excess, and sex steroid exposure can also lead to accelerated growth. Several of these conditions may ultimately lead to short stature in adulthood. Genetic conditions associated with tall stature and overgrowth include Sotos, Klinefelter, and Marfan syndromes (see Chapter 576).

Evaluation of Abnormal Growth

Evaluation of abnormal growth should include confirmation that the data are accurate and plotted correctly. Comparisons should be made with previous measurements. If poor or rapid growth or short or tall stature is a concern, a radiograph of the left hand and wrist,

Table 27.3	Common Causes of Increased Growth and Tall Stature

Variation of normal
    Constitutional tall stature
    Familial tall stature
Endocrine conditions
    Growth hormone excess
    Precocious puberty
    Congenital adrenal hyperplasia
Obesity
Genetic conditions
    Marfan syndrome
    Klinefelter syndrome
    Sotos syndrome

the **bone age**, can provide information about skeletal maturation. Skeletal development represents physiologic rather than chronological age. Reference standards for bone maturation facilitate estimation of bone age (see Table 22.3). A delayed bone age (skeletal age younger than chronological age) suggests catch-up potential for linear growth. Advanced bone age suggests a rapid maturation of the skeleton that may lead to earlier cessation of growth. Bone age should be interpreted with the guidance of a pediatric endocrinologist. Skeletal age correlates well with stage of pubertal development and may be helpful in predicting adult height in early- or late-maturing adolescents. In familial short stature the bone age is normal (comparable to chronological age), whereas constitutional delay, endocrinologic short stature, and under-nutrition may be associated with delay in bone age comparable to the height age.

Laboratory testing is also useful in assessment of growth and may be tailored to suspected etiology based on the patient history and physical examination. Initial assessment includes comprehensive metabolic panel, complete blood count, sedimentation rate, C-reactive protein, thyroid-stimulating hormone, thyroxine, celiac panel, and insulin-like growth factor (IGF)-I and IGF-BP3, which are surrogate markers for growth hormone secretion (see Chapter 573). A karyotype to exclude Turner syndrome is an essential component of the evaluation of short stature in females and should be performed even in the absence of characteristic physical features (see Chapter 604). If there is concern for abnormal timing of puberty contributing to growth pattern, gonadotropins (luteinizing hormone, follicle-stimulating hormone), and estradiol or testosterone may also be assessed. A urinalysis can provide additional information about renal function. Evaluation by a (pediatric) nutritionist for caloric needs assessment may be useful in patients with malnutrition, underweight status, or slow weight gain. Additional testing and referral to specialists should be performed as indicated.

OTHER GROWTH CONSIDERATIONS
Obesity

Obesity affects large numbers of children (see Chapter 60). The CDC defines *obesity* as BMI ≥95th percentile for age and sex, and *overweight* as BMI 85th to <95th percentile for age and sex. Although widely accepted as the best clinical measure of underweight and overweight, BMI may not provide an accurate index of adiposity because it does not differentiate lean tissue and bone from fat. In otherwise healthy individuals, lean body mass is largely represented by BMI at lower percentiles. BMI >80–85% largely reflects increased body fat with a nonlinear relationship

Table 27.4	Chronology of Human Dentition of Primary (Deciduous) and Secondary (Permanent) Teeth					
	CALCIFICATION		**AGE AT ERUPTION**		**AGE AT SHEDDING**	
	Begins at	**Complete at**	**Maxillary**	**Mandibular**	**Maxillary**	**Mandibular**
PRIMARY TEETH						
Central incisors	5th fetal mo	18-24 mo	6-8 mo	5-7 mo	7-8 yr	6-7 yr
Lateral incisors	5th fetal mo	18-24 mo	8-11 mo	7-10 mo	8-9 yr	7-8 yr
Cuspids (canines)	6th fetal mo	30-36 mo	16-20 mo	16-20 mo	11-12 yr	9-11 yr
First molars	5th fetal mo	24-30 mo	10-16 mo	10-16 mo	10-12 yr	10-12 yr
Second molars	6th fetal mo	36 mo	20-30 mo	20-30 mo	10-12 yr	11-13 yr
SECONDARY TEETH						
Central incisors	3-4 mo	9-10 yr	7-8 yr	6-7 yr		
Lateral incisors	Max, 10-12 mo	10-11 yr	8-9 yr	7-8 yr		
	Mand, 3-4 mo					
Cuspids (canines)	4-5 mo	12-15 yr	11-12 yr	9-11 yr		
First premolars (bicuspids)	18-21 mo	12-13 yr	10-11 yr	10-12 yr		
Second premolars (bicuspids)	24-30 mo	12-14 yr	10-12 yr	11-13 yr		
First molars	Birth	9-10 yr	6-7 yr	6-7 yr		
Second molars	30-36 mo	14-16 yr	12-13 yr	12-13 yr		
Third molars	Max, 7-9 yr	18-25 yr	17-22 yr	17-22 yr		
	Mand, 8-10 yr					

Mand, Mandibular; Max, maxillary.
Adapted from a chart prepared by P.K. Losch, Harvard School of Dental Medicine, who provided the data for this table.

between BMI and adiposity. In the setting of chronic illness, increased body fat may be present at low BMI, whereas in athletes, high BMI may reflect increased muscle mass. Measurement of the triceps, subscapular, and suprailiac skinfold thickness have been used to estimate adiposity. Other methods of measuring fat, such as hydrodensitometry, bioelectrical impedance, and total body water measurement, are used in research, but not in clinical evaluation, but whole body dual-energy x-ray absorptiometry (DXA) is beginning to emerge as a tool for measuring body fat and lean body mass.

Dental Development

Dental development includes mineralization, eruption, and exfoliation (Table 27.4). Initial mineralization begins as early as the 2nd trimester (mean age for central incisors, 14 wk) and continues through 3 yr of age for the primary (deciduous) teeth and 25 yr of age for the secondary (permanent) teeth. Mineralization begins at the crown and progresses toward the root. Eruption begins with the central incisors and progresses laterally. Exfoliation begins at about 6 yr of age and continues through 12 yr. Eruption of the permanent teeth may follow exfoliation immediately or may lag by 4-5 mo. The timing of dental development is poorly correlated with other processes of growth and maturation. **Delayed eruption** is usually considered when no teeth have erupted by approximately 13 mo of age (mean + 3 SD). Common causes include congenital or genetic disorders, endocrine disorders (e.g., hypothyroidism, hypoparathyroidism), familial conditions, and (the most common) idiopathic conditions. Individual teeth may fail to erupt because of mechanical blockage (crowding, gum fibrosis). Causes of **early exfoliation** include hypophosphatasia, histiocytosis X, cyclic neutropenia, leukemia, trauma, and idiopathic factors. Nutritional and metabolic disturbances, prolonged illness, and certain medications (tetracycline) frequently result in discoloration or malformations of the dental enamel. A discrete line of pitting on the enamel suggests a time-limited insult.

Bibliography is available at Expert Consult.

Chapter **28**
Developmental and Behavioral Surveillance and Screening
Paul H. Lipkin

第二十八章
发育行为监测和筛查

中文导读

本章主要介绍了儿童发育与行为的监测和筛查，以及监测和筛查后的综合评估、转诊和干预，并进行管理和实施的具体内容。具体描述了发育与行为的病史采集，观察儿童的发育技能、行为互动等内容；具体描述了儿童发育与行为筛查使用的标准化筛查工具，筛查测试的特征；具体描述了通过监测和筛查，识别发育与行为问题的儿童，进行多专业综合评估，以及转诊、干预、管理和具体实施中出现的问题。

In healthy development, a child will acquire new skills beginning prenatally and extending into at least young adulthood. The roots of this acquisition of skills lie in the development of the nervous system, with additional influences from the health status of other organ systems and the physical and social environment in which the development occurs. *Development* and its milestones are divided into the "streams" of gross motor, fine motor, verbal language (expressive and receptive), social language, and self-help. *Behavior* can be categorized into observable, spontaneous, and responsive behaviors in the settings of home, school, and community.

Although typical development is associated with a wide variability of skill acquisition in each of these streams, specific developmental and behavioral disorders are seen in approximately 1 of every 6 children and may affect the health, function, and well-being of the child and family for a lifetime. These disorders include rare conditions that often cause severe impairments, such as cerebral palsy and autism, and relatively

Table 28.1	Key Components of Developmental and Behavioral Surveillance

HISTORY

1. Parental developmental concerns
2. Developmental history
   a. Streams of developmental milestone achievement
      i. Gross motor
      ii. Fine motor
      iii. Verbal speech and language
         (1) Expressive
         (2) Receptive
      iv. Social language and self-help
   b. Patterns of abnormality
      i. Delay
      ii. Dissociation
      iii. Deviancy or deviation
      iv. Regression
3. Behavior history
   a. Interactions
      i. Familiar settings (e.g. home, school): parents, siblings, other familiar people, peers, other children
      ii. Interaction in unfamiliar settings (e.g., community): unfamiliar adults and children
   b. Patterns of abnormality
      i. Noncompliance, disruption (including tantrums), aggression, impulsivity, increased activity, decreased attention span, decreased social engagement, decreased auditory or visual attention
      ii. Deviation or atypical behaviors
         (1) Repetitive play, rituals, perseverative thought or action, self-injury
4. Risk factor identification: medical, family, and social history (including social determinants of health)
5. Protective factor identification (also including social determinants)

DEVELOPMENTAL OBSERVATION

1. Movement: gross and fine motor skills
2. Verbal communication: expressive speech and language, language understanding
3. Social engagement and response
4. Behavior: spontaneous and responsive with caregiver and with staff
5. Related neurologic function on physical examination

Table 28.2	"Red Flags" in Developmental Screening and Surveillance*

These indicators suggest that development is seriously disordered and that the child should be promptly referred to a developmental or community pediatrician.

POSITIVE INDICATORS
Presence of Any of the Following:

Loss of developmental skills at any age
Parental or professional concerns about vision, fixing, or following an object or a confirmed visual impairment at any age (simultaneous referral to pediatric ophthalmology)
Hearing loss at any age (simultaneous referral for expert audiologic or ear, nose, and throat assessment)
Persistently low muscle tone or floppiness
No speech by 18 mo, especially if the child does not try to communicate by other means, such as gestures (simultaneous referral for urgent hearing test)
Asymmetry of movements or other features suggestive of cerebral palsy, such as increased muscle tone
Persistent toe walking
Complex disabilities
Head circumference above the 99.6th centile or below 0.4th centile; also, if circumference has crossed 2 centiles (up or down) on the appropriate chart or is disproportionate to parental head circumference
An assessing clinician who is uncertain about any aspect of assessment but thinks that development may be disordered

NEGATIVE INDICATORS
Activities That the Child Cannot Do:

Sit unsupported by 12 mo
Walk by 18 mo (boys) or 2 yr (girls) (check creatine kinase urgently)
Walk other than on tiptoes
Run by 2.5 yr
Hold object placed in hand by 5 mo (corrected for gestation)
Reach for objects by 6 mo (corrected for gestation)
Point at objects to share interest with others by 2 yr

*Most children do not have "red flags" and thus require quality screening to detect any problems.
Adapted from Horridge KA. Assessment and investigation of the child with disordered development. *Arch Dis Child Educ Pract Ed* 96:9–20, 2011.

common conditions such as attention-deficit/hyperactivity disorder, speech language disorders, and behavioral and emotional disorders that affect as many as 1 in 4 children. The more common conditions are generally perceived as "less severe," but these too can have major short-term and long-term impact on the child's health and daily functioning in the home, school, and community and can affect lifelong well-being. Because of their high prevalence in children; their impact on health, social, and economic status; and their effect on the child, the home, and the community, these disorders require the attention of the pediatrician throughout childhood. In addition, both the child and the family benefit from the early identification and treatment of many of these conditions, including the most severe. It is therefore incumbent on the pediatric clinician to conduct regular **developmental surveillance** and periodic **developmental screening** at primary care health supervision visits aimed at early identification and treatment.

Among the many types of developmental or behavioral conditions, the most common include *language problems,* affecting at least 1 in 10 children (see Chapter 52); *behavior or emotional disorders,* affecting up to 25% of children, with 6% considered serious; *attention-deficit/hyperactivity disorder,* affecting 1 in 10 children (Chapter 49); and *learning disabilities,* affecting up to 10% (Chapters 50 and 51). Less common and more disabling are the *intellectual disabilities* (1–2%; Chapter 53); *autism spectrum disorders* (1 in 59 children; Chapter 54); *cerebral palsy* and related *motor impairments* (0.3%, or 1 in 345 children; Chapter 616); *hearing impairment,* also referred to as deafness, hard-of-hearing,

or hearing loss (0.12%; Chapter 655); and nonrefractive *vision impairment* (0.8%; Chapter 639).

DEVELOPMENTAL AND BEHAVIORAL SURVEILLANCE

General health surveillance is a critical responsibility of the primary care clinician and is a key component of health supervision visits. Regular developmental and behavioral surveillance should be performed at every health supervision visit from infancy through young adulthood. Surveillance of a child's development and behavior includes both obtaining historical information on the child and family and making observations at the office visit (Tables 28.1 and 28.2).

Key historical elements include (1) eliciting and attending to the parents' or caregivers' concerns around the child's development or behavior; (2) obtaining a history of the child's developmental skills and behavior at home, with peers, in school, and in the community; and (3) identifying the risks, strengths, and protective factors for development and behavior in the child and family, including the social determinants of health. During the office visit, the clinician should make and document direct observations of the child's developmental skills and behavioral interactions. Skills in all streams of development should be considered along with observations of related neurologic functioning made on physical examination.

With this history and observation, the clinician should create and maintain a longitudinal record of the child's development and behavior for tracking the child across visits. It is often helpful to obtain information from and share information with other professionals involved with the child, including childcare professionals, home visitors, teachers, after-school providers, and developmental therapists. This provides a complete picture of the child's development and behavior and allows collaborative tracking of the child's progress.

The Developmental and Behavioral Histories

Developmental surveillance includes tracking a child's achievement of milestones, which represent key readily recognizable skills that usually occur in a predictable sequence and at predictable age ranges during childhood. The developmental skill areas can be divided into **gross motor**, **fine motor**, **verbal speech and language** (expressive and receptive), **social language**, and **self-help**. Tracking milestones will reveal that most children achieve the milestones in a typical pattern and within typical age ranges. However, the pediatrician or the parent may recognize concerning patterns of development, such as delay, dissociation, deviancy or deviation, or regression.

Developmental delay occurs when development is occurring in its usual sequence but at a slower rate, with milestones achieved later than the normal range (see Chapter 53). Delay can occur in a single area of development or across several streams and can be expressed as a *developmental quotient* (DQ). The DQ is calculated by dividing the age at which the child is functioning developmentally (*developmental age*; DA) by *chronologic age* (CA) and multiplying by 100 (DQ = DA/CA × 100). A DQ of 100 indicates that the child is developing at the mean or average rate, whereas a DQ below 70 is approximately 2 standard deviations (SD) below the mean and suggests a significant delay that requires evaluation.

Developmental dissociation indicates delay in a single stream with typical development in other streams. A child with autism may have delays in verbal or social language but normal motor skills. *Deviancy* or *deviation* is defined by development occurring out of sequence, as when a child stands before sitting (as in diplegic cerebral palsy) or has better expressive vocabulary than receptive understanding of words (language and autism spectrum disorders). *Regression* refers to a loss of skills. It may also be identified earlier or more subtly by a slowing or lack of advancement in skills. Although uncommon, regression is described in as many as 1 in 4 children with autism and is also seen in rarer neurologic disorders, such as Rett syndrome and Duchenne muscular dystrophy (see Chapter 53.1).

Behavioral surveillance is conducted by obtaining a history of a child's behavior and interactions across settings, including home, daycare, school, and community, and in situations such as eating, sleeping, and play. In addition, interactions may differ based on who the child is with (parent or guardian, sibling, peers, strangers). Concerns may include limited engagement or socializing, compliance, tantrums, aggression, impulsivity, activity level, auditory or visual attention, and attention span. Deviations from usual behavior may also occur, including repetitive play, ritualistic behaviors, perseverative thoughts or actions, and self-injury.

Observation

Observations of the child's developmental skills and behavioral interactions should be made in the examining room, with documentation in the medical record, and combined with the examination of other neurologic functioning, such as muscle tone, reflexes, and posture.

Developmental observations may include a child's gross and fine motor movements, both on the floor and on the examination table. Spoken language and response to others' communications, as well as interactions and engagement with the parent or guardian, should be noted. If siblings are in the room, the interaction between the child and a sibling may also be informative. Impulsivity, attention problems, tantrums, noncompliance, oppositionality, and aggression may be observed along with interactions with the clinician, but one should inquire about whether these behaviors are seen in *other settings*, given the possible unfamiliarity or discomfort of the child with the healthcare professional or in healthcare settings.

If inquiring about and observing the child's development and behavior

suggests normal or typical patterns of development and behavior, discussions can be held about future milestones and usual behavior management strategies employable at home. If problems or concerns are identified by the parent or clinician, however, formal developmental screening, evaluation, or management should be considered, along with early follow-up and review.

DEVELOPMENTAL AND BEHAVIORAL SCREENING

Periodic episodic screening for developmental and behavioral conditions should be conducted on every child, as done for other health conditions such as anemia, lead poisoning, hearing, and congenital metabolic disorders. Developmental and behavioral screenings are centered on administration of low-cost, brief, and standardized tests designed for such purposes in the primary care office setting. These tests can be implemented by health assistants at age-determined visits, with interpretation of the results and referral or treatment initiation by the pediatric healthcare clinician as indicated.

The American Academy of Pediatrics provides recommendations and guidelines on age-specific developmental screening for implementation in the primary care medical home. Developmental screening using a formal, validated, and standardized test is recommended during the 1st 3 yr of life at the preventive care visit at 9 m, 18 mo, and 30 mo. Tests recommended at these ages screen development across all the streams. In addition, an autism screening test is recommended at the 18 and 24 mo visits. Table 28.3 provides recommended screening tests for general development and for autism. It is also recommended that a child have a screening test administered any time that a parent, guardian, or child health or early childhood professional has concerns identified during developmental surveillance, or through screening performed at early childhood programs. Although routine formal screening before the child's entry into elementary school is not included in current guidelines, the primary care clinician should be vigilant about surveillance regarding development at the 4 or 5 yr old visit and perform formal screening if concerns are identified, because of the potential impact on learning and school services.

Each of the screening visits offers special opportunities to identify specific developmental conditions. At the 9 mo screening, critical areas of development are vision, hearing, gross motor, fine motor, and receptive language. It is at this age that disabilities may be identified in vision or hearing, as well as cerebral palsy and other neuromotor disorders. At 18 mo, expressive language and social language development are particularly important areas. Conditions identified at this age may include those considered at 9 mo, although in milder forms, as well as autism spectrum, language, and intellectual disorders. By the 30 mo visit, the child's behavioral interactions become an additional area of focus, with problems emerging tied to attention and disruptive behavior disorders. While universal screening is not recommended at later ages, developmental surveillance may identify children in need of screening or evaluation for problems in learning, attention, and behavior.

Additional screening for *behavioral conditions* should be considered, although there is currently no recommended consensus on the ages at which behavioral screening should occur. One possibility would be to provide behavioral screening at the 30 mo, 4 or 5 yr, and 8 yr visits to identify problems emerging in the toddler, preschool, and early elementary years. For older children, visits during preadolescent or adolescent ages also offer an opportunity for surveillance and possible screening for behavioral and emotional problems meriting professional assistance or intervention. Table 28.4 provides recommended behavior screening tools.

Evidence-Based Tools

Tables 28.3, 28.4, and 28.5 show a range of measures useful for early identification of developmental and behavioral problems, including autism spectrum disorders. Because well-child visits are brief and with broad agendas (health surveillance and screening, physical examination, immunization, anticipatory guidance, safety and injury prevention, and developmental promotion), tools relying on parent completion with office staff administration and scoring are well suited for primary care settings. Such tests may be completed in advance of appointments,

Table 28.3 Standardized Tools for General Developmental Screening

SCREENING TEST	AGE RANGE	NUMBER OF ITEMS	ADMINISTRATION TIME	PUBLICATION INFORMATION	REF*
Ages & Stages Questionnaires-3 (ASQ3)	2-60 mo	30	10-15 min	Paul H. Brookes Publishing 800-638-3775 www.brookespublishing.com	1
Parents' Evaluation of Developmental Status (PEDS)	0-8 y	10	2-10 min	Ellsworth & Vandermeer Press 888-729-1697 www.pedstest.com	2
Parents' Evaluation of Developmental Status: Developmental Milestones (PEDS:DM) Screening Version	0-8 y	6-8 items at each age level	4-6 min	Ellsworth & Vandermeer Press 888/729-1697 or www.pedstest.com	2
Survey of Well-being of Young Children (SWYC)†	Dev: 1-65 mo Autism: 16-35 mo	Dev: 10 Autism: 7	Dev: <5 min Autism: <5 min	www.theswyc.org	3-6

*Key reference sources:
1. Squires J, Potter L, Bricker D: The ASQ user's guide, ed 3, Baltimore, MD, 2009, Paul H Brookes Publishing.
2. Glascoe FP, Marks KP, Poon JK, et al, editors: Identifying and addressing developmental-behavioral problems: a practical guide for medical and non-medical professionals, trainees, researchers and advocates, Nolensville, TN, 2013, PEDStest.com.
3. Sheldrick RC, Perrin EC: Evidence-based milestones for surveillance of cognitive, language, and motor development, Acad Pediatr 13(6):577–586, 2013.
4. Smith N, Sheldrick R, Perrin E: An abbreviated screening instrument for autism spectrum disorders, Infant Ment Health J 34(2):149–155, 2012.
5. Salisbury LA, Nyce JD, Hannum CD, et al: Sensitivity and specificity of 2 autism screeners among referred children between 16 and 48 months of age, J Dev Behav Pediatr 39(3):254–258, 2018.
6. Publications and user's manual available at www.theswyc.org.
†Initial validation studies have been completed. Further validation on large populations is currently in progress. Dev, Development.

Table 28.4 Standardized Tools for General Behavioral Screening

SCREENING TEST	AGE RANGE	NUMBER OF ITEMS	ADMINISTRATION TIME	PUBLICATION INFORMATION	REF*
Ages & Stages Questionnaire: Social-Emotional-2 (ASQ:SE-2) (2015)	2-60 mo	9 age-specific forms with 19-33 items	10 min	Paul H. Brookes Publishing, 800-638-3775 www.agesandstages.com	1, 2
Brief Infant Toddler Social Emotional Assessment (BITSEA)	12-36 mo	42	7-10 min	Pearson Assessments†	3
Pediatric Symptom Checklist–17 items (PSC-17b)	4-16 yr PSC-35 Youth self-report: ≥11 yr	17	<5 min	Website‡	4
Strengths and Difficulties Questionnaire (SDQ)	4-17 yr 3-4 yr old version available Youth self-report 11-16 yr	25; 22 for 3-4 yr olds	5-10 min	www.sdqinfo.org	5

*Key reference sources:
1. Squires J, Bricker DD, Twombly E: Ages & Stages Questionnaires: Social-Emotional-2 (ASQ:SE-2): a parent-completed, child-monitoring system for social-emotional behaviors, Baltimore, MD, 2016, Paul H Brookes Publishing.
2. Briggs RD, Stettler EM, Johnson Silver, et al: Social-emotional screening for infants and toddlers in primary care, Pediatrics 129(2):1–8, 2012.
3. Briggs-Gowan MJ, Carter AS, Irwin JR, et al: The Brief-Infant Toddler Social and Emotional Assessment: screening for social-emotional problems and delays in competence, J Pediatr Psychol 29:143–155, 2004.
4. Gardner W, Lucas A, Kolko DJ, Campo JV: Comparison of the PSC-17 and alternative mental health screens in an at-risk primary care sample, J Am Acad Child Adolesc Psychiatry 46:611–618, 2007.
5. Stone LL, Otten R, Engels RC, et al: Psychometric properties of the parent and teacher versions of the Strengths and Difficulties Questionnaire for 4- to 12-year-olds: a review. Clin Child Fam Psychol Rev 13(3):254–274, 2010.
†http://www.pearsonassessments.com/HAIWEB/Cultures/en-us/Productdetail.htm?Pid=015-8007-352.
‡http://www.massgeneral.org/psychiatry/services/psc_about.aspx.

either online or in writing, whether at home or while waiting for the pediatric visit to begin. If a test is scored in advance of the visit, the pediatric clinician can enter the room with results in hand for review and discussion, including a description of the child's development and behavior compared with peers, general information on child development and behavior, any areas of concern, referrals needed, and information to share with the child's daycare, preschool, or other community providers, when applicable.

Screening Test Properties

Each of the tests provided in Tables 28.3 to 28.5 meets accepted psychometric test criteria. The test has norms, with standardized questions

or milestones based on administration to parents of a large sample of children with typical development. These norms are used for comparing an individual child's performance on the test with that of the large sample of typically developing children. In addition, the tests demonstrate accepted standards of *reliability*, or the ability to produce consistent results; *predictive validity*, or the ability to predict later test performance or development; *sensitivity*, or accuracy in the identification of delayed development or disability; and *specificity*, or accuracy in the identification of children who are not delayed. Some of the screening tests are general, evaluating multiple areas of development or behavior (sometimes referred to as "broad band"). Others are domain specific, evaluating one area of development (e.g., language), or disorder specific, aimed at

Table 28.5	Standardized Tools for Language and Autism Screening				
SCREENING TEST	**AGE RANGE**	**NUMBER OF ITEMS**	**ADMINISTRATION TIME**	**PURCHASE/ OBTAINMENT INFORMATION**	**REF***
LANGUAGE					
Communication and Symbolic Behavior Scales: Developmental Profile (CSBS-DP): Infant Toddler Checklist	6-24 mo	24	5-10 min	Paul H. Brookes Publishing Co 800/638-3775 www.brookespublishing.com	1
AUTISM					
Modified Checklist for Autism in Toddlers, Revised with Follow-up (M-CHAT-R/F)	16-48 mo	20 (avg)	5-10 min	www.m-chat.org/ Follow up interview†	2
Social Communication Questionnaire (SCQ)	4+ yr	40 (avg)	5-10 min	Western Psychological Services www.wpspublish.com	3, 4

*Key reference sources:
1. Wetherby AM, Prizant BM: Communication and Symbolic Behavior Scales: Developmental Profile, Baltimore, MD, 2002, Paul H Brookes Publishing.
2. Robins DL, Casagrande K, Barton M, et al: Validation of the Modified Checklist for Autism in Toddlers, Revised with Follow-up (M-CHAT-R/F), Pediatrics 133(1):37–45, 2014.
3. Rutter M, Bailey A, Lord C: The Social Communication Questionnaire (SCQ) manual, Los Angeles, 2003, Western Psychological Services.
4. Corsello C, Hus V, Pickles A, et al: Between a ROC and a hard place: decision making and making decisions about using the SCQ, J Child Psychol Psychiatry 48(9):932–940, 2007.
†http://www2.gsu.edu/~psydlr/Diana_L._Robins,_Ph.D._files/M-CHATInterview.pdf.

identifying a specific developmental disorder (sometimes referred to as "narrow band").

BEYOND SURVEILLANCE AND SCREENING
Comprehensive Evaluation
When a developmental or behavioral concern is identified through surveillance or screening, the primary care physician's role is to ensure that the child receives an appropriate diagnostic evaluation, related medical testing, and indicated developmental interventions and medical treatment. When a concern is identified, a full diagnostic evaluation should be performed by a professional with appropriate training and experience. In the case of developmental concerns, this may be a pediatric specialist, such as a neurodevelopmental pediatrician/neurologist or a developmental-behavioral pediatrician, or a related developmental professional, depending on resources in the local community. Related professionals may include early childhood educators, psychologists, speech/language pathologists, audiologists, physical therapists, and occupational therapists, many of whom are available through the local early intervention system. Such an evaluation would typically include more detailed standardized developmental testing. The primary care physician should ensure that hearing and vision assessments are completed. For the child with motor concerns, the physician should pay particular attention to the motor and neurologic evaluation. Children with language delays should have hearing, speech, language, and learning skills (e.g., reading, phonics) evaluated.

The primary care pediatrician should also perform a comprehensive medical evaluation of the child to identify any related health conditions. Physical examination including head circumference should be reviewed to identify growth abnormalities and dysmorphic features. For the child with motor delay and decreased or normal muscle tone, serum creatine kinase and thyroid function testing are recommended to rule out muscular dystrophy and thyroid disease, respectively. When there is increased tone, MRI or referral to a neurologist should be considered. For the child with suspected autism or intellectual disability (or global developmental delay), chromosomal microarray and fragile X testing are recommended (see Chapter 53).

Referral and Intervention
Children with significant developmental delays or an identified developmental disability are entitled to and usually benefit from early intervention with therapy services directed at delayed or atypical development. The U.S. Individuals with Disabilities Education Act (IDEA) entitles any child with a disability or developmental delay to receive local education and related services, including therapy, from as early as birth, for known or high-risk conditions that lead to such delay or disability, through age 21 yr. These interventions enhance the child's development through early intervention and family support as well as individualized public education with the goal of reducing public costs. The pediatric clinician should therefore refer every child with developmental concerns to the local early intervention program or agency (ages 0-3 yr), public school program (≥3 yr), or local therapy providers. Typical service needs include special education for the child with intellectual or learning concerns, physical or occupational therapy for children with motor delays, speech language therapy for the child with language or social communication difficulties, and behavioral therapy services for the child with social engagement or other behavior problems.

Likewise, the child with specific behavior concerns should be referred to an appropriate pediatric or mental health professional who can perform a thorough evaluation and assist the family to alleviate the problems or concerns. Such professionals may include those trained in developmental-behavioral pediatrics, neurodevelopmental disabilities, adolescent medicine, child and adolescent psychiatry, pediatric psychology, psychiatric advanced practice nursing, and social work. Such an evaluation is similar to developmental evaluation in its aim of determining a diagnosis, as well as developing a treatment program that may include psychotherapeutic and medication management. Associated medical or developmental disorders should be considered and further evaluated as needed.

Ongoing Management
Children with developmental or behavioral disorders should be identified as *children with special healthcare needs* in the medical home, with a program of chronic condition management initiated by the clinical program staff, including its medical and nonmedical staff. In doing so, the clinician and family should work together to outline the child's short- and long-term goals and management plan. This includes a program of regular monitoring and follow-up of the child's development and behavior, referrals, treatment, and surveillance for identification and treatment of related medical, developmental, or behavioral comorbidities that may arise. Some children and families may warrant assignment of a case manager either within the medical home or in a related local agency. The pediatric clinician or other medical home staff should participate in care coordination activities as needed and assist the family and other professionals in decision-making on medical care, therapies, and educational services.

The family can be further assisted during the screening and referral phases or later with ongoing care by referral to support service programs, such as respite care, parent-to-parent programs, and advocacy organizations. Some children may qualify for additional state or federal benefit programs, including insurance, supplemental security income, and state programs for children with special healthcare needs. Families often seek out information, support, or connection to other families with similarly affected children and find benefit in local or national networks (e.g., Family Voices, Family to Family Health Information centers) and condition-specific associations.

Implementation

The principles and professional guidelines for developmental-behavioral surveillance and screening have been solidified to identify children with developmental disabilities, including the specific conditions of intellectual disability, autism, motor disorders, and behavioral-emotional problems. Specific algorithms are included in these guidelines to assist the clinician with implementation. However, pediatricians have reported difficulties in putting these into practice, with obstacles and barriers identified and policy changes made to ensure that screening and referral can be implemented. (See Bibliography online for specific guidelines.)

Implementation projects have identified key factors for successful incorporation of developmental surveillance and screening into practice.

Successful office-based screening requires development of a comprehensive office-based system that extends from the child's home to the front office and into the clinic visit, rather than solely centered on the time in the clinic room. This requires utilizing office and medical support staff for scheduling, advance test distribution, and initiation of the surveillance and screening procedures before the preventive care visit. The pediatric staff must choose screening tests that are not only valid for screening of the specific condition at the recommended ages, but also appropriate to the population being served (including reading level and language). The tests chosen should be able to be completed by the caregiver in a short time and at low cost. Staff training on billing and coding for these procedures ensures appropriate payment.

Practice systems should also be developed for referral and tracking of children who have problems identified through screening. This should include systems for referral to early intervention, community therapy, developmental professionals, and medical consultants. Office representatives or the clinician should establish working relationships with local community programs and resources to assist the child and family.

Bibliography is available at Expert Consult.

Chapter **29**
Childcare
Laura Stout Sosinsky and Walter S. Gilliam
第二十九章
儿童保健

中文导读

本章主要介绍了美国儿童保育服务的提供、使用和监管，儿童保育在儿童健康和发展中的作用以及儿科医师在儿童保育中的作用。具体描述了儿童保育场所，儿童保育许可、监管和认证；具体描述了儿童保育的特点、儿童保育与儿童发展的联系、患病儿童的保育、儿童保育与儿童健康、以及特殊需求儿童保育的相关内容；具体描述了儿科医师就儿童保育选择及儿童健康问题向父母提供咨询，帮助有特殊需求的儿童，为儿童保育人员提供咨询与合作。

In the United States, approximately half of all children under the age of 3 yr and 60–75% of children age 3-5 yr had at least 1 regular nonparental childcare arrangement in 2012. Young children of employed mothers spend on average 36 hr per week in a childcare arrangement.

Childcare provision is affected by many factors, derived from family demand, childcare supply, and child/family policy. With increasing movement of mothers into the workplace across the globe, the prime reason most families use childcare is to support employment of both parents. At childbirth, unpaid maternity leave is the typical solution among U.S. mothers. The U.S. Federal leave program allows for 12 wk of unpaid job-protected leave during pregnancy or after childbirth, but only covers approximately 50% of the workforce because companies with <50 employees, with part-time employees, and those working in informal labor markets are exempt. Four states and several cities have passed paid family leave laws.

In part because of the financial burden of an unpaid maternity leave, many mothers return to work, and their children may begin childcare in the 1st few weeks after birth. In a 2000 Family and Medical Leave Act survey, only 10% of respondents reported taking more than 60 days for maternity leave. Approximately 44% of mothers in 2005–2007 were working by the time their 1st child was 3-4 mo of age, and approximately 63% of mothers were working by the time their 1st child was 12 mo. Some mothers face work requirements if they are receiving public benefits because of the reforms to welfare passed by the U.S. Congress in 1996. Many mothers feel strong financial motivation or even pressure to work, especially in single-parent households, or have strong incentive to work for short- and long-term financial security, or because interest and preference, or all these. Employment is not the only factor driving childcare use; young children of unemployed mothers spend on average 21 hr/wk in childcare. Many parents want their children to have childcare experiences for the potential benefits that early learning environments can give to their children, particularly preschoolers. Given these realities, childcare quality is of great concern, yet the quality of childcare and early education environments varies widely, and the supply of high-quality childcare is largely deemed inadequate.

PROVISION, REGULATION, AND USE OF CHILDCARE IN AMERICA
Childcare Settings

Childcare settings vary widely and fall into 4 broad categories, listed here from the least to the most formal: (1) relative care; (2) in-home nonrelative care, such as nannies, babysitters, or au pairs; (3) family childcare, in which the caregiver provides care in her own home for up to 6 young children, often including children of mixed ages, siblings, or the provider's own children; and (4) center-based care, provided in nonresidential facilities for children grouped by age.

Parents more often use home-based care for infants and toddlers, partly because of greater preference, flexibility, and availability, and sometimes because of lower cost. Use of center-based childcare is greater among preschoolers (children 3-5 yr old). Childcare centers and early education programs are administered by a wide array of businesses and organizations, including for-profit independent companies and chains, religious organizations, public and private schools, nonprofit community organizations, cooperatives, and public agencies. **Preschool** programs (e.g., Head Start, **prekindergarten**) also may play an important role in childcare. Although early education programs may have a greater focus on educational activities and often provide only limited hours of care daily, the health and safety issues involved with preschool programs are similar to those presented by other group childcare settings.

Childcare Licensing, Regulation, and Accreditation

Poor-quality childcare settings and unsafe environments that do not meet children's basic physical and emotional needs can result in neglect, toxic stress, injury, or even death. Licensing and regulatory requirements establish the minimum requirements necessary to protect the health and safety of children in childcare. For the most part, licensing standards mandate basic health and safety standards, such as sanitary practices, child and provider vaccinations, access to a healthcare professional, and facilities and equipment safety, as well as basic structural and caregiver characteristics, such as the ratio of children to staff, group sizes, and minimum caregiver education and training requirements. Most childcare centers and preschools and many family daycare providers are subject to state **licensing and regulation**. All states regulate centers, as does the District of Columbia, and most states regulate family childcare providers.* Childcare programs that are subject to licensing must comply with their state's requirements to legally operate. Many early care and

education providers are subject to monitoring by multiple agencies and organizations.

Many providers are legally exempt from licensing standards. However, the 2014 Child Care Development Block Grant (CCDBG) reauthorization required states and territories to expand their monitoring of legally exempt providers to protect the health and safety of children receiving subsidized childcare. Exemptions for various types of programs vary by state. The smallest homes (3-4 children in care) are typically license exempt, encompassing relative, friend, and neighbor caregivers as well as babysitters, nannies, and au pairs. These providers may fall outside of any regulatory scrutiny, and some may not even think of themselves as offering "childcare." Fewer children (≥4) are cared for in large home-based settings, typically by nonrelatives. Depending on the state, small family childcare homes may be exempt if there are few children in care, and large/group family childcare homes may be exempt if they are open part-day. Unlike exemption rules for homecare providers, which typically are based on size, centers are often exempted if overseen by other organizations such as schools, churches, or local governments, and thus have some external oversight. Many of these entities provide part-day or part-week Head Start or preschool programs, and about half the states also explicitly exempt such part-time programs.

Homes and centers that fall under state-licensing guidelines face different requirements, which can have a direct impact on the quality of children's experiences. Size differs greatly between the 2 types of contexts, and such size differences are built into regulations in terms of the maximum number of children who can be cared for in a group and the number of adults that must be present. The most common state-required maximum group size in **centers** is 8 for infants, 12 for toddlers, and 20 for preschoolers; centers may have numerous classrooms of these sizes. For centers, regulations explicitly state an allowable ratio of children to adults. The most common ratios are 4:1 for infants, 6:1 for toddlers, and 10:1 for preschoolers, meaning that typically there would be 2 adults in a group. However, other states permit ratios that are 5:1 or 6:1 for infants ≤9 mo of age. Furthermore, most states' child/staff ratio requirements increase as children age; for children 27 mo old, only a handful of states have ratios of 4:1.

States license **homes** in 2 categories, small and large, with typical maximums of 6 and 12, respectively (including the provider's own children). More than 75% of licensed homes fall within the small category. Thus the total size of a typical home is smaller than just 1 classroom in a center. States less often explicitly lay out child/adult ratios for homes, given that many homes involve one provider caring for all the children. Some states restrict the number of younger children who may be in care or explicitly provide ratios (especially for large homes), although these restrictions vary greatly across states.

Health and safety conditions may be unsatisfactory in unlicensed settings. In most states, licensing and regulatory standards have been found to be inadequate to promote optimal child development, and in many states, standards are so low as to endanger child health and safety. Therefore, even licensed providers may be providing care at quality levels far below professional recommendations. A small portion of providers become accredited by National Association for the Education of Young Children (NAEYC), National Association for Family Child Care (NAFCC), or other organizations by voluntarily meeting high-quality, developmentally appropriate, professionally recommended standards. The accreditation process goes well beyond health and safety practices and structural and caregiver characteristics, to examine the quality of child–caregiver interactions, which are crucial for child development, as described in the next section. Evidence indicates that childcare programs that complete voluntary accreditation through NAEYC improve in quality and provide an environment that better facilitates children's overall development. Only 10% of childcare centers and 1% of family childcare homes are accredited. This is partly the result of a lack of knowledge, resources, and incentives for providers to improve quality, but also because of expenses providers incur in the process of becoming accredited.

State childcare licensing agencies are playing a larger role in various initiatives designed to improve the quality of childcare, working through the infrastructure of the early care and education system. Several states

---

*For the most recent state and territory licensing regulations, see https://childcareta.acf.hhs.gov/resource/state-and-territory-licensing-agencies-and-regulations.

have quality initiatives called *quality ratings and improvement systems (QRIS)*, such as tiered quality strategies (e.g., tiered reimbursement systems for participating providers who achieve levels of quality beyond basic licensing requirements), public funding to facilitate accreditation, professional development systems, and program assessments and technical assistance.

CHILDCARE'S ROLE IN CHILD HEALTH AND DEVELOPMENT
Characteristics of Childcare and Associations With Child Developmental Outcomes

High-quality childcare is characterized by warm, responsive, and stimulating interactions between children and caregivers. In high-quality interactions, caregivers express positive feelings toward their children; are emotionally involved, engaged, and aware of the child's needs and sensitive and responsive to their initiations; speak directly with children in a manner that is elaborative and stimulating while being age appropriate; and ask questions and encourage children's ideas and verbalizations. Structural quality features of the setting, including ratio of children to adults, group size, and caregiver education and training, act indirectly on child outcomes by facilitating high-quality child–caregiver interactions. It would be difficult for even the most sensitive and stimulating provider to engage in high-quality interactions with each child, if the provider was the sole caregiver of 10 toddlers.

Practices in childcare centers can support or undermine the potential for caregivers to provide high-quality individualized interactions with young children in their care and support development. **Primary caregiving** is the practice of assigning 1 teacher the primary responsibility for the care of a small group of children within a larger group setting; this teacher takes the lead role in providing intentional and individual care for the child's routine needs and establishes relationships with the children and families in their care. This practice is consistent with research showing that infants who experience stable, consistent, sensitive, and responsive care from their primary caregivers develop more **secure attachment** relationships (see Chapters 18, 19, and 22) and more positive developmental outcomes. To enact primary caregiving, centers need to have child-to-staff ratios and staffing arrangements consistent with this practice. Several states' child/staff ratio licensing requirements (e.g., 4:1 for 6 or 9 mo old infants) are consistent with staffing arrangements conducive to creating and maintaining primary caregiving relationships, but other states' ratios are much larger and rise even higher during the infant/toddler years.

The quality, quantity, type of setting, and stability of childcare experienced by young children contribute to child development. Childcare use by itself does not affect mother–child attachment. Only when combined with low maternal sensitivity and responsiveness does poor-quality childcare, larger quantities of childcare, or multiple childcare arrangements predict greater likelihood of insecure attachment.

Adjusting for family factors (parental income, education, race/ethnicity, family structure, parental sensitivity), the quality of childcare has a unique and consistent but small association with child outcomes across most domains of development. The type of childcare setting has unique effects, controlling for quality, with results from numerous studies demonstrating that center-based care is associated with better language and preacademic performance than home-based care. Quantity of care (hours per week) may also have unique effects, but findings are mixed, with some studies demonstrating small associations between greater quantity and elevated behavior problems, and other studies finding no associations with most children. **Instability** in childcare—over the course of a day, such as with rotating staff or multiple arrangements, or over time, with frequent staff turnover or changes in arrangements—does have negative effects on children's language and internalizing problems. Also, since childcare settings naturally have packages of quality characteristics, which are a mix of lower- and higher-quality indicators, the bundle of features in a childcare arrangement may be another meaningful way for a parent to consider the potential effects of an arrangement on their child.

When a healthcare provider talks with a parent about the childcare arrangement, it is also important to consider the individual child's characteristics, health concerns, dispositions, and even physiologic responses to the environment. As with all environments, childcare is experienced differently by different children. An average environment can often sufficiently compensate for the typical regulatory capacities of most children, but when an environment lacks adequate support for a child's unique needs, healthy development can be further compromised. Some children may be more vulnerable to poor childcare (or particularly responsive to good childcare), such as children with difficult or fearful temperaments, especially if their home environments are characterized by more risk factors, such as poverty or high conflict with a parent.

Several large studies have found that most U.S. childcare is of "poor to mediocre" quality. In one study, only 14% of centers (8% of center-based infant care) were found to provide developmentally appropriate care, while 12% scored at minimal levels that compromised health and safety (40% for infant care). In another study, 58% of family daycare homes provided adequate or custodial care, and only 8% provided good care. Children with the greatest amount of family risk may be the most likely to receive childcare that is substandard in quality. Many children from lower-risk families also receive lower-quality care, and despite their advantages at home, these children may not be protected from the negative effects of poor-quality care.

Affordable, accessible, high-quality childcare is difficult to find. Middle-class families spend approximately 6% of their annual income on childcare expenses, whereas poor families spend approximately 33% (on par with housing expenses). Infant and toddler care is particularly expensive, with fewer available slots. For a married couple with children, the average cost of full-time center care for 1 infant ranges from 7% to approximately 19% of the state median income, depending on the state. In 38 states the cost of infant care exceeds 10% of the state's median income for a 2-parent family. The average cost of center care for one 4 yr old exceeds 10% of the median household income in 21 states and the District of Columbia. For single parents, the average cost of center-based infant care exceeds 25% of median income in every state. The average cost of family childcare is only slightly lower.

In addition to the stress of meeting such a high expense, many parents worry that their child will feel unhappy in group settings, will suffer from separation from the parents, or will be subjected to neglect or abuse. This worry is especially likely among low-income parents with more risk factors, fewer resources, and fewer high-quality options available. Parents are the purchasers but not the recipients of care and are not in the best position to judge its quality. Many parents are 1st-time purchasers of childcare with little experience and very immediate needs, selecting care in a market that does little to provide them with useful information about childcare arrangements. In many states, efforts are underway to improve quality and provide parents with this information, but several states do not have a quality rating and information system, and programs in states that do are still emerging, and testing of effectiveness is still underway. To inform their care decisions, parents may turn to their child's pediatrician as the only professional with expertise in child development with whom they have regular and convenient contact.

Pediatricians may frequently be asked to provide input regarding child health in out-of-home childcare settings. **Standards and guidelines** are provided by the American Academy of Pediatrics, the American Public Health Association, and the National Resource Center for Health and Safety in Child Care and Early Education, in *Stepping Stones to Caring for Our Children: National Health and Safety Performance Standards—Guidelines for Early Care and Education Programs* (3rd edition, 2013). *Caring for our Children Basics* (2014), which is based on the larger resource document, represents the **minimum** health and safety standards experts believe should be in place where children are cared for outside their homes. The intent is for the guidelines to serve as a resource for states and other entities as they work to improve health and safety standards in licensing and quality rating improvement systems. The guidelines include sections on program activities for healthy development (e.g., monitoring children's development, obtaining consent for age-appropriate developmental and behavioral screenings), health promotion and protection (e.g., active opportunities for physical activity; safe sleep practices and SIDS risk reduction; diaper-changing and hand hygiene procedures; emergency procedures; recognizing and reporting suspected child abuse, neglect, and exploitation), and nutrition and food service (e.g., care for children with food allergies; preparing, feeding, and storing human milk).

Pediatricians most often may encounter questions from parents and caregivers regarding sick children, exposure to and prevention of risks in childcare, and support for children with special needs in childcare. Guidelines in these areas are summarized in the next sections.

Sick Children

When children are ill, they may be excluded from out-of-home arrangements, and settings under state licensure are required to exclude children with certain conditions. *Stepping Stones* offers guidelines and recommendations regarding the conditions under which sick children should and should not be excluded from group programs. State laws typically mirror these guidelines but may be stricter in some states. *Caring for Our Children Basics* (2014) summarizes guidelines for inclusion, exclusion, or dismissal of children based on signs or symptoms or illness (Table 29.1).

The caregiver/teacher should determine if the illness (1) prevents the child from participating comfortably in activities; (2) results in a need for care that is greater than the staff can provide without compromising the health and safety of other children; (3) poses a risk of spread of harmful diseases to others; or (4) causes a fever and behavior change or other signs and symptoms (e.g., sore throat, rash, vomiting, diarrhea). An unexplained temperature above 100°F (37.8°C) (armpit) in a child <6 mo old should be medically evaluated. Any infant <2 mo old with fever should receive immediate medical attention.

Most families need to arrange to keep sick children at home, such as staying home from work or having backup plans with an alternative caregiver. Alternative care arrangements outside the home for sick children are relatively rare but may include either (1) care in the child's own center, if it offers special provisions designed for the care of ill children (sometimes called the **infirmary model** or **sick daycare**), or (2) care in a center that serves only children with illness or temporary conditions. Although it is important that such arrangements emphasize preventing further spread of disease, one study found no occurrence of additional transmission of communicable disease in children attending a sick center. The impact of group care of ill children on their subsequent health and on the health of their families and community is unknown.

Caring for Our Children Basics also provides guidelines for control of infectious disease outbreaks and for exclusion of any child or staff member who is suspected of contributing to transmission of the illness, who is not adequately immunized when there is an outbreak of a vaccine-preventable disease, or when the circulating pathogen poses an increased risk to the individual.

Childcare and Child Health

A disproportionate number of **sudden infant death syndrome (SIDS)** deaths occur in childcare centers or family-based childcare homes (approximately 20%). Infants who are back-sleepers at home but are put to sleep on their front in childcare settings have a higher risk of SIDS. Providers and parents should be made aware of the importance of placing infants on their backs to sleep (see Chapter 402).

Children enrolled in childcare are also of an age that places them at increased risk for acquiring **infectious diseases**. Participation in group settings elevates exposure. Children enrolled in such settings have a higher incidence of illness (upper respiratory tract infections, otitis media, diarrhea, hepatitis A infections, skin conditions, and asthma) than those cared for at home, especially in the preschool years; these illnesses have no long-term adverse consequences. Childcare providers who follow childcare licensure guidelines for handwashing, diapering, and food handling, and who manage child illness appropriately, can reduce communicable illnesses.

Debate surrounds whether childcare exposure serves as a risk or protective factor for asthma. One cross-sectional study found that preschoolers in childcare had increased risk of the common cold and otitis media, and children who began childcare before age 2 yr had increased risk of developing recurrent otitis media and asthma. However, a longitudinal study found that children exposed to older children at home or to other children at childcare during the 1st 6 mo of life were less likely to have frequent wheezing from ages 6-13 yr, suggesting that childcare exposure may protect against the development of asthma and frequent wheezing later in childhood. A 10 yr follow-up of a birth cohort found no association between childcare attendance and respiratory infections, asthma, allergic rhinitis, or skin-prick test reactivity. Another study found that in the 1st yr of elementary school, children who had attended childcare had fewer absences from school, half as many episodes of asthma, and less acute respiratory illness than their peers who had never attended childcare. These results may be related to protection against respiratory illness as a result of early exposure or a shift in the age-related peak of illness, although selection of illness-prone children into homecare may play a role. Other factors may also be relevant to this issue, such as children in childcare potentially being less exposed to passive smoking than children at home.

Childcare and Children With Special Needs

The needs of children with mental, physical, or emotional disabilities who, because of their chronic illness, require special care and instruction may require particular attention when it comes to their participation in most childcare settings. Guiding principles of services for children with disabilities advocate supporting children in natural environments, including childcare. Furthermore, the Americans with Disabilities Act and Section 504 of the Rehabilitation Act of 1973 prohibit discrimination against children and adults with disabilities by requiring equal access to offered programs and services.

Although many childcare providers and settings are unprepared to identify or administer services for children with special needs, childcare could be utilized for delivery of support services to these children and for linking families to services, such as early intervention and physician referrals. Furthermore, pediatricians can draw on childcare providers for important evaluative data regarding a child's well-being, since these providers have extensive daily contact with the child and may have broad, professional understanding of normative child development. A childcare provider may be the first to identify a child's potential language delay. Childcare providers are also necessary and valuable partners in the development and administration of early intervention service plans.

Children with special needs may be eligible for services under the **Individuals with Disabilities Education Act (IDEA; see Chapters 48 and 51)**. The purpose of this law is to provide "free appropriate public education," regardless of disability or chronic illness, to all eligible children, birth to 21 yr, in a natural and/or least restrictive environment. Eligible children include those with mental, physical, or emotional disabilities who, because of their disability or chronic illness, require special instruction to learn. As a part of these services, a formal plan of intervention is to be developed by the service providers, families, and the children's healthcare providers. Federal funds are available to implement a collaborative early intervention system of services for eligible infants and toddlers from birth to 3 yr and their families. These services include screening, assessment, service coordination, and collaborative development of an **individualized family service plan (IFSP)**. The IFSP describes early intervention services for the infant or toddler and family, including family support and the child's health, therapeutic, and educational needs. An understanding of the child's routines and real-life opportunities and activities, such as eating, playing, interacting with others, and working on developmental skills, is crucial to enhancing a child's ability to achieve the functional goals of the IFSP. Therefore it is critical that childcare providers be involved in IFSP development or revision, with parental consent. Childcare providers should also become familiar with the child's IFSP and understand the providers' role and the resources available to support the family and childcare provider.

Additionally, IDEA provides support for eligible preschool-age children to receive services through the local school district. This includes development of a written **individualized education program (IEP)**, with implementation being the responsibility of the local education agency in either a public or a private preschool setting. As with IFSPs, childcare providers should become familiar with the preschooler's special

Table 29.1	Conditions That Do and Do Not Require Exclusion From Group Childcare Settings

CONDITIONS THAT REQUIRE EXCLUSION	COMMENTS
If any of these 3 key criteria for exclusion of children who are ill are met, the child should be temporarily excluded, regardless of the type of illness:	
Illness preventing the child from participating comfortably in activities, as determined by the childcare provider	Providers should specify in their policies, approved by the facility's healthcare consultant, what severity level of illness the facility can manage, and how much and what types of illness will be addressed: • Severity level 1 consists of children whose health condition is accompanied by high interest and complete involvement in activity, associated with an absence of symptoms of illness (e.g., children recovering from pinkeye, rash, or chickenpox) but who need further recuperation time. • Severity level 2 encompasses children whose health condition is accompanied by a medium activity level because of symptoms (e.g., children with low-grade fever, children at beginning of illness, children in early recovery period of illness) • Severity level 3 consists of children whose health condition is accompanied by a low activity level because of symptoms that preclude much involvement.
Illness resulting in a greater need for care than the childcare staff can provide without compromising the health and safety of the other children, as determined by the childcare provider	
Illness that poses a risk of spread of harmful diseases to others	
In addition to the above key criteria, temporary exclusion is recommended when the child has any of the following conditions:	
Fever (temperature above 38°C [101°F] orally, above 38.9°C [102°F] rectally, or above 37.8°C [100°F] or higher taken axillary [armpit] or measured by an equivalent method) and behavior change or other signs and symptoms (e.g., sore throat, rash, vomiting, diarrhea)	Accompanied by behavior changes or other signs or symptoms of illness until medical professional evaluation finds the child able to be included at the facility
Acute change in behavior including lethargy/lack of responsiveness, inexplicable irritability or persistent crying, difficult breathing, or having a quickly spreading rash	Until evaluation by a medical professional finds the child able to be included at the facility
Diarrhea (defined by watery stools or decreased form of stool that is not associated with changes of diet). Exclusion is required for all diapered children whose stool is not contained in the diaper and toilet-trained children if the diarrhea is causing soiled pants or clothing.	Readmission after diarrhea can occur when diapered children have their stool contained by the diaper (even if the stools remain loose) and when toilet-trained children are continent. Special circumstances that require specific exclusion criteria include the following: • Toxin-producing *Escherichia coli* or *Shigella* infection, until stools are formed and test results of 2 stool cultures obtained from stools produced 24 hr apart do not detect these organisms • *Salmonella* serotype Typhi infection, until diarrhea resolves and, in children <5 yr old, 3 negative stool cultures obtained at 24 hr intervals
Blood or mucus in stool	Not explained by dietary change, medication, or hard stools
Vomiting illness	More than 2 times in previous 24 hr, unless vomiting is determined to be caused by a noninfectious condition and child remains adequately hydrated
Abdominal pain	Persistent (continues >2 hr) or intermittent associated with fever or other signs or symptoms
Mouth sores with drooling	Unless the child's primary care provider or local health department authority states that the child is noninfectious
Rash with fever or behavior changes	Until the primary care provider has determined that the illness is not an infectious disease
Active tuberculosis	Until the child's primary care provider or local health department states child is on appropriate treatment and can return
Impetigo	Until treatment has been started
Streptococcal pharyngitis (i.e., strep throat or other streptococcal infection)	Until 24 hr after treatment has been started
Purulent conjunctivitis	Defined as pink or red conjunctiva with white or yellow eye discharge, until after treatment has been initiated
Pediculosis (head lice)	Until after 1st treatment *Note:* Exclusion is not necessary before end of the program day.
Scabies	Until after treatment has been given
Varicella-zoster virus (chickenpox)	Until all lesions have dried or crusted (usually 6 days after onset of rash)
Rubella	Until 6 days after onset of rash

Continued

Table 29.1	Conditions That Do and Do Not Require Exclusion From Group Childcare Settings—cont'd
CONDITIONS THAT REQUIRE EXCLUSION	**COMMENTS**
Pertussis	Until 5 days of appropriate antibiotic treatment
Mumps	Until 5 days after onset of parotid gland swelling
Measles	Until 4 days after onset of rash
Hepatitis A virus	Until 1 wk after onset of illness or jaundice if child's symptoms are mild or as directed by health department
Any child determined by the local health department to be contributing to the transmission of illness during an outbreak	
CONDITIONS THAT DO NOT REQUIRE EXCLUSION	**COMMENTS**
Common colds, runny noses	Regardless of color or consistency of nasal discharge
A cough not associated with an infectious disease or a fever	
Watery, yellow or white discharge or crusting eye discharge without fever, eye pain, or eyelid redness	
Presence of bacteria or viruses in urine or feces in the absence of illness symptoms (e.g., diarrhea)	Exceptions include children infected with highly contagious organisms capable of causing serious illness.
Pinkeye (bacterial conjunctivitis), indicated by pink or red eyelids after sleep	If 2 unrelated children in the same program have conjunctivitis, the organism causing the conjunctivitis may have a higher risk for transmission, and a child healthcare professional should be consulted.
Fever without any signs or symptoms of illness in children >6 mo old regardless of whether acetaminophen or ibuprofen was given	If the child is behaving normally but has fever <38.9°C (102°F) rectally or the equivalent, child should be monitored but does not need to be excluded for fever alone.
Rash without fever and without behavioral changes	
Lice or nits	Exclusion for treatment of an active lice infestation may be delayed until end of the day.
Ringworm	Exclusion for treatment may be delayed until end of the day.
Molluscum contagiosum	Do not require exclusion or covering of lesions
Thrush (i.e., white spots or patches in mouth or on cheeks or gums)	
Fifth disease	Once the rash has appeared
Methicillin-resistant *Staphylococcus aureus* (MRSA) without an infection or illness that would otherwise require exclusion	Known MRSA carriers or colonized individuals should not be excluded.
Cytomegalovirus infection	
Chronic hepatitis B infection	
HIV infection	
Asymptomatic children who have been previously evaluated and found to be shedding potentially infectious organisms in the stool	Children who are continent of stool or who are diapered with formed stools that can be contained in the diaper may return to care
Children with chronic infections conditions who can be accommodated in the program according to federal legal requirement in Americans with Disabilities Act (ADA)	ADA requires that childcare programs make reasonable accommodations for children with disabilities and/or chronic illnesses, considering each child individually.

Adapted from American Academy of Pediatrics (AAP), American Public Health Association, National Resource Center for Health and Safety in Child Care and Early Education: *Stepping stones to caring for our children: national health and safety performance standards—guidelines for early care and education programs*, ed 3, Elk Grove Village, IL, 2013, AAP, pp 46–52. http://nrckids.org/index.cfm/products/stepping-stones-to-caring-for-our-children-3rd-edition-ss3/stepping-stones-to-caring-for-our-children-3rd-edition-ss3/.

needs as identified in the IEP and may become involved, with parental consent, in IEP development and review meetings. For children who have or may be at risk for developmental delay, a diagnosis is important for obtaining and coordinating services and further evaluation. To this end, pediatricians can partner with childcare providers to screen and monitor children's behavior and development.

ROLE OF PEDIATRIC PROVIDERS IN CHILDCARE
Advising Parents on Childcare Selection
Organized professional guidance in choosing childcare is insufficient. Pediatricians can help parents understand the importance of high-quality care for their child's development by describing this care and providing referrals and advice on finding and selecting high-quality childcare (Table 29.2). In addition, pediatricians can help parents determine how

to adjust childcare arrangements to best meet their child's specific needs (e.g., allergies, eating and sleeping habits, temperament and stress-regulation capacities). For most parents, finding childcare that they can afford, access, manage, and accept as a good environment for their child is a difficult and often distressing process. Many parents also worry about how their child will fare in childcare (e.g., Will their child feel distressed by group settings, suffer from separation from the parents, or even be subjected to neglect or abuse?). These worries are especially likely among low-income parents with fewer family and community resources. A few parents may think of childcare only as "babysitting" and may not consider the consequences for their child's cognitive, linguistic, and social development, focusing solely on whether the child is safe and warm. These parents may be less likely to select a high-quality childcare arrangement, which is especially problematic if the family is

Table 29.2	Childcare Information Resources	
ORGANIZATION	**SPONSOR**	**WEBSITE AND CONTACT INFORMATION**
Child Care Aware	Child Care Aware of America (formerly National Association of Child Care Resource and Referral Agencies)	http://www.childcareaware.org
Healthy Child Care America	American Academy of Pediatrics (AAP)	http://www.healthychildcare.org
National Association for the Education of Young Children (NAEYC)		http://www.naeyc.org
National Association for Sick Child Daycare (NASCD)		http://www.nascd.com
National Resource Center for Health and Safety in Child Care and Early Education (NRC)		http://www.nrckids.org For 2013 report from AAP, APHA, NRC, *Stepping Stones to Caring for Our Children: National Health and Safety Performance Standards—Guidelines for Early Care and Education Programs*, ed 3, go to: http://nrckids.org/index.cfm/products/stepping-stones-to-caring-for-our-children-3rd-edition-ss3/stepping-stones-to-caring-for-our-children-3rd-edition-ss3/
Office of Child Care (OCC)	U.S. Department of Health and Human Services, Administration for Children and Families	http://www.acf.hhs.gov/programs/occ
Office of Child Care Technical Assistance Network (CCTAN)	U.S. Department of Health and Human Services, Administration for Children and Families, Office of Child Care	https://childcareta.acf.hhs.gov/

facing socioeconomic challenges that already place them at risk of receiving lower-quality care for their children. For these parents, it is vital to stress the importance of quality and its implications for their child's cognitive, language, and behavioral development and school readiness.

Advising Parents on Childcare Health Issues
Parents of infants should be advised to ensure that childcare providers put infants on their back to sleep to prevent SIDS. Also, pediatricians should emphasize the importance of following vaccination schedules; most states require compliance for children to participate in licensed group childcare settings.

When children are ill, parents should be advised to follow guidelines for inclusion and exclusion (see Table 29.1). Parents may disagree with childcare staff about whether a child meets or does not meet the exclusion criteria. However, professional guidelines state that "if ... the reason for exclusion relates to the child's ability to participate or the caregiver's/teacher's ability to provide care for the other children, the caregiver/teacher should not be required to accept responsibility for the care of the child."*

Helping Children With Special Needs
Pediatricians should work with parents and communicate with other service providers and early intervention staff to identify problems, remove access barriers, and coordinate service delivery for children with special needs. They should also encourage involvement of parents and childcare providers in IFSP or IEP plan development.

Consulting and Partnering With Childcare Providers
Most state regulations mandate that licensed programs have a formal relationship with a healthcare provider. Additional state efforts include mental health consultation models to support providers, who are often not well trained in managing child behavior, and build capacity to raise quality for all children. Early childhood mental health consultation links a mental health professional with an early education and care provider in an ongoing problem-solving and capacity-building relationship.

Pediatricians can provide consultation to childcare providers about measures to protect and maintain the health and safety of children and staff. This may include consultation regarding promoting practices to prevent SIDS; preventing and reducing the spread of communicable disease; reducing allergen, toxin, and parasite exposure; ensuring vaccinations for children and staff; removing environmental hazards; and preventing injuries.

Bibliography is available at Expert Consult.

---

*http://nrckids.org/index.cfm/products/stepping-stones-to-caring-for-our-children-3rd-edition-ss3/.

Chapter **30**
Loss, Separation, and Bereavement
Megan E. McCabe and Janet R. Serwint
第三十章
丧失、分离和丧亲

中文导读

本章主要介绍了分离和丧失、父母离异、搬迁、移民、住院、父母服役、父母或同胞的死亡对儿童的影响，介绍了儿童悲伤反应、对死亡的认知发展、儿科医师在悲伤中的角色、干预治疗，以及对患者及其家庭成员信仰的回应等内容。具体描述了分离、丧亲等对儿童的心理、行为、情绪产生的不利影响；描述了随年龄增长儿童在理解死亡和悲伤反应方面的发展变化；介绍了家庭、学校、社区、儿科医师、专业人员所提供的支持、评估、干预、心理和药物治疗等。

All children will experience involuntary separations, whether from illness, death, or other causes, from loved ones at some time in their lives. Relatively brief separations of children from their parents, usually produce minor transient effects, but more enduring and frequent separation may cause sequelae. The potential impact of each event must be considered in light of the age, stage of development, and experiences of the child, the particular relationship with the absent person, and the nature of the situation.

SEPARATION AND LOSS

Separations may be from temporary causes, such as vacations, parental job requirements, natural disasters or civil unrest, or parental or sibling illness requiring hospitalization. More long-term separations occur as a result of divorce, placement in foster care, or immigration, whereas permanent separation may occur because of death. The initial reaction of young children to separation of any duration may involve crying, either of a tantrum-like, protesting type, or of a quieter, sadder type. Children's behavior may appear subdued, withdrawn, fussy, or moody, or they may demonstrate resistance to authority. Specific problems may include poor appetite, behavior issues such as acting against caregiver requests, reluctance to go to bed, sleep problems, or regressive behavior, such as requesting a bottle or bed-wetting. School-age children may experience impaired cognitive functioning and poor performance in school. Some children may repeatedly ask for the absent parent and question when the absent parent will return. The child may go to the window or door or out into the neighborhood to look for the absent parent; a few may even leave home or their place of temporary placement to search for their parents. Other children may not refer to the parental absence at all.

A child's response to reunion may surprise or alarm an unprepared parent. A parent who joyfully returns to the family may be met by wary or cautious children. After a brief interchange of affection, children may seem indifferent to the parent's return. This response may indicate anger at being left or wariness that the event will happen again, or the young child may feel, as a result of **magical thinking** (see Chapter 24), as if the child caused the parent's departure. For example, if the parent who frequently says "Stop it, or you'll give me a headache" is hospitalized, the child may feel at fault and guilty. Because of these feelings, children may seem more closely attached to the present parent than to the absent one, or even to the grandparent or babysitter who cared for them during their parent's absence. Some children, particularly younger ones, may become more clinging and dependent than they were before the separation, while continuing any regressive behavior that occurred during the separation. Such behavior may engage the returned parent more closely and help to reestablish the bond that the child felt was broken. Such reactions are usually transient, and within 1-2 wk, children will have recovered their usual behavior and equilibrium. Recurrent separations may tend to make children wary and guarded about reestablishing the relationship with the repeatedly absent parent, and these traits may affect other personal relationships. Parents should be advised not to try to modify a child's behavior by threatening to leave.

DIVORCE

More sustained experiences of loss, such as divorce or placement in foster care, can give rise to the same kinds of reactions noted earlier, but they are more intense and possibly more lasting. Currently in the United States, approximately 40% of marriages end in divorce. Divorce has been found to be associated with negative parent functioning, such as parental depression and feelings of incompetence; negative child behavior, such as noncompliance and whining; and negative parent–child interaction, such as inconsistent discipline, decreased communication, and decreased affection. Greater childhood distress is associated with greater parental distress. Continued parental conflict and loss of contact with the noncustodial parent, usually the father, is common.

Two of the most important factors that contribute to morbidity of the children in a divorce include *parental psychopathology* and *disrupted parenting* before the separation. The year following the divorce is the period when problems are most apparent; these problems tend to dissipate over the next 2 yr. Depression may be present up to 5 yr later, and educational or occupational decline may occur even 10 yr later. It is difficult to sort out all confounding factors. Children may suffer when exposed to parental conflict that continues after divorce and that in some cases may escalate. The degree of *interparental conflict* may be the most important factor associated with child morbidity. A continued relationship with the noncustodial parent when there is minimal interparental conflict is associated with more positive outcomes.

School-age children may become depressed, may seem indifferent, or may be extremely angry. Other children appear to deny or avoid the issue, behaviorally or verbally. Most children cling to the hope that the actual placement or separation is not real and only temporary. The child may experience guilt by feeling that the loss, separation, or placement represents rejection and perhaps punishment for misbehavior. Children may protect a parent and assume guilt, believing that their own "badness" caused the parent to depart. Children who feel that their misbehavior caused their parents to separate may have the fantasy that their own trivial or recurrent behavioral patterns caused their parents to become angry at each other. A child might perceive that outwardly blaming parents is emotionally risky; parents who discover that a child harbors resentment might punish the child further for these thoughts or feelings. Some children have behavioral or psychosomatic symptoms and unwittingly adopt a "sick" role as a strategy for reuniting their parents.

In response to divorce of parents and the subsequent separation and loss, older children and adolescents usually show intense anger. Five years after the breakup, approximately 30% of children report intense unhappiness and dissatisfaction with their life and their reconfigured family; another 30% show clear evidence of a satisfactory adjustment; and the remaining children demonstrate a mixed picture, with good achievement in some areas and faltering achievement in others. After 10 yr, approximately 45% do well, but 40% may have academic, social, or emotional problems. As adults, some are reluctant to form intimate relationships, fearful of repeating their parents' experience.

Parental divorce has a moderate long-term negative impact on the adult mental health status of children, even after controlling for changes in economic status and problems before divorce. Good adjustment of children after a divorce is related to ongoing involvement with two psychologically healthy parents who minimize conflict and to the siblings and other relatives who provide a positive support system. Divorcing parents should be encouraged to avoid adversarial processes and to use a trained mediator to resolve disputes if needed. Joint-custody arrangements may reduce ongoing parental conflict, but children in joint custody may feel overburdened by the demands of maintaining a strong presence in two homes.

When the primary care provider is asked about the effects of divorce, parents should be informed that different children may have different reactions, but that the parents' behavior and the way they interact will have a major and long-term effect on the child's adjustment. The continued presence of both parents in the child's life, with minimal interparental conflict, is most beneficial to the child.

MOVE/FAMILY RELOCATION

A significant proportion of the U.S. population changes residence each year. The effects of this movement on children and families are frequently overlooked. For children, the move is essentially involuntary and out of their control. When changes in family structure such as divorce or death precipitate moves, children face the stresses created by both the precipitating events and the move itself. Parental sadness surrounding the move may transmit unhappiness to the children. Children who move lose their old friends, the comfort of a familiar bedroom and house, and their ties to school and community. They not only must sever old relationships, but also are faced with developing new ones in new neighborhoods and new schools. Children may enter neighborhoods with different customs and values, and because academic standards and curricula vary among communities, children who have performed well in one school may find themselves struggling in a new one. Frequent moves during the school years are likely to have adverse consequences on social and academic performance.

Migrant children and children who emigrate from other countries present with special circumstances. These children not only need to adjust to a new house, school, and community, but also need to adjust to a new culture and in many cases a new language. Because children have faster language acquisition than adults, they may function as translators for the adults in their families. This powerful position may lead to role reversal and potential conflict within the family. In the evaluation of migrant children and families, it is important to ask about the circumstances of the migration, including legal status, violence or threat of violence, conflict of loyalties, and moral, ethical, and religious differences.

Parents should prepare children well in advance of any move and allow them to express any unhappy feelings or misgivings. Parents should acknowledge their own mixed feelings and agree that they will miss their old home while looking forward to a new one. Visits to the new home in advance are often useful preludes to the actual move. Transient periods of regressive behavior may be noted in preschool children after moving, and these should be understood and accepted. Parents should assist the entry of their children into the new community, and whenever possible, exchanges of letters and visits with old friends should be encouraged.

SEPARATION BECAUSE OF HOSPITALIZATION

Potential challenges for hospitalized children include coping with separation, adapting to the new hospital environment, adjusting to multiple caregivers, seeing very sick children, and sometimes experiencing the disorientation of intensive care, anesthesia, and surgery. To help mitigate potential problems, a preadmission visit to the hospital can help by allowing the child to meet the people who will be offering care and ask questions about what will happen. Parents of children <5-6 yr old should room with the child if feasible. Older children may also benefit from parents staying with them while in the hospital, depending on the severity of their illness. Creative and active recreational or socialization programs with child life specialists, chances to act out feared procedures in play with dolls or mannequins, and liberal visiting hours, including visits from siblings, are all helpful. Sensitive, sympathetic, and accepting attitudes toward children and parents by the hospital staff are very important. Healthcare providers need to remember that parents have the best interest of their children at heart and know their children the best. Whenever possible, school assignments and tutoring for hospitalized children should be available to engage them intellectually and prevent them from falling behind in their scholastic achievements.

The psychologic aspects of illness should be evaluated from the outset, and physicians should act as a model for parents and children by showing interest in a child's feelings, allowing them a venue for expression, and demonstrating that it is possible and appropriate to communicate about discomfort. Continuity of medical personnel may be reassuring to the child and family.

MILITARY FAMILIES

More than 2 million children live in military families in the United States, and approximately 50% of them obtain medical care in the community rather than at a military medical facility. Children whose parents are serving in the military may experience loss and separation in multiple ways. These include frequent relocations, relocation to foreign countries, and duty-related separation from parents. In recent years the most impactful experiences have been repeated wartime deployments of parents and the death of parents during military service. All branches of the military have increased their focus on preparing and supporting military families for a service member's deployment in order to improve family coping. Military families composed of young parents and young children are at risk for child maltreatment in the context of repeated or prolonged deployments.

PARENTAL/SIBLING DEATH

Approximately 5–8% of U.S. children will experience parental death; rates are much higher in other parts of the world more directly affected by war, AIDS, and natural disasters. Anticipated deaths from chronic illness may place a significant strain on a family, with frequent bouts of illness, hospitalization, disruption of normal home life, absence of the ill parent, and perhaps more responsibilities placed on the child. Additional strains include changes in daily routines, financial pressures, and the need to cope with aggressive treatment options.

Children can and should continue to be involved with the sick parent or sibling, but they need to be prepared for what they will see in the home or hospital setting. The stresses that a child will face include visualizing the physical deterioration of the family member, helplessness, and emotional lability. Forewarning the child that the family member may demonstrate physical changes, such as appearing thinner or losing hair, will help the child to adjust. These warnings combined with simple yet specific explanations of the need for equipment, such as a nasogastric tube for nutrition, an oxygen mask, or a ventilator, will help lessen the child's fear. Children should be honestly informed of what is happening, in language they can understand, allowing them choices, but with parental involvement in decision-making. They should be encouraged, but not forced, to see their ill family member. Parents who are caring for a dying spouse or child may be too emotionally depleted to be able to tend to their healthy child's needs or to continue regular routines. Children of a dying parent may suffer the loss of security and belief in the world as a safe place, and the surviving parent may be inclined to impose his or her own need for support and comfort onto the child. However, the well parent and caring relatives must keep in mind that children need to be allowed to remain children, with appropriate support and attention. Sudden, unexpected deaths lead to more anxiety and fear because there is no time for preparation, and explanations for the death can cause uncertainty.

GRIEF AND BEREAVEMENT

Grief is a personal, emotional state of bereavement or an anticipated response to loss, such as a death. Common reactions include sadness, anger, guilt, fear, and at times, relief. The normality of these reactions needs to be emphasized. Most bereaved families remain socially connected and expect that life will return to some new, albeit different, sense of normalcy. The pain and suffering imposed by grief should never be automatically deemed "normal" and thus neglected or ignored. In **uncomplicated grief** reactions, the steadfast concern of the pediatrician can help promote the family's sense of well-being. In more distressing reactions, as seen in traumatic grief of sudden death, the pediatrician may be a major, first-line force in helping children and families address their loss.

Participation in the care of a child with a life-threatening or terminal illness is a profound experience. Parents experience much anxiety and worry during the final stages of their child's life. In one study, 45% of children dying from cancer died in the pediatric intensive care unit, and parents report that 89% of their children suffered "a lot" or "a great deal" during the last month of life. Physicians consistently underreport children's symptoms in comparison to parents' reports. Better ways are needed to provide care for dying children. Providers need to maintain honest and open communication, provide appropriate pain management, and meet the families' wishes as to the preferred location of the child's death, in some cases in their own home. Inclusion of multiple disciplines, such as hospice, clergy, nursing, pain service, child life specialists, and social work, often helps to support families fully during this difficult experience.

The practice of withholding information from children and parents regarding a child's diagnosis and prognosis has generally been abandoned, because physicians have learned that protecting parents and patients from the seriousness of their child's condition does not alleviate concerns

and anxieties. Even very young children may have a real understanding of their illness. Children who have serious diseases and are undergoing aggressive treatment and medication regimens, but who are told by their parents that they are okay, are not reassured. These children understand that something serious is happening to them, and they are often forced to suffer in silence and isolation because the message they have been given by their parents is to not discuss it and to maintain a cheerful demeanor. Children have the right to know their diagnosis and should be informed early in their treatment. The content and depth of the discussion needs to be tailored to the child's personality and developmental level of understanding. Parents have choices as to how to orchestrate the disclosure. Parents may want to be the ones to inform the child themselves, may choose for the pediatric healthcare provider to do so, or may do it in partnership with the pediatrician.

A **death**, especially the death of a family member, is the most difficult loss for a child. Many changes in normal patterns of functioning may occur, including loss of love and support from the deceased family member, a change in income, the possible need to relocate, less emotional support from surviving family members, altering of routines, and a possible change in status from sibling to only child. Relationships between family members may become strained, and children may blame themselves or other family members for the death of a parent or sibling. Bereaved children may exhibit many of the emotions discussed earlier as a result of the loss, in addition to behaviors of withdrawal into their own world, sleep disturbances, nightmares, and symptoms such as headache, abdominal pains, or possibly similar to those of the family member who has died. Children 3-5 yr of age who have experienced a family bereavement may show regressive behaviors such as bed-wetting and thumb sucking. School-age children may exhibit nonspecific symptoms, such as headache, abdominal pain, chest pain, fatigue, and lack of energy. Children and adolescents may also demonstrate enhanced anxiety if these symptoms resemble those of the family member who died. The presence of secure and stable adults who can meet the child's needs and who permit discussion about the loss is most important in helping a child to grieve. The pediatrician should help the family understand this necessary presence and encourage the protective functioning of the family unit. More frequent visits to the healthcare professional may be necessary to address these symptoms and provide reassurance when appropriate. Suggested availability of clergy or mental health providers can provide additional support and strategies to facilitate the transitions after the death.

Death, separation, and loss as a result of **natural catastrophes** and **human-made disasters** have become increasingly common events in children's lives. Exposure to such disasters occurs either directly or indirectly, where the event is experienced through the media. Examples of **indirect exposure** include televised scenes of earthquakes, hurricanes, tsunamis, tornadoes, and domestic and international terrorist attacks. Children who experience personal loss in disasters tend to watch more television coverage than children who do not. Children without a personal loss watch as a way of participating in the event and may thus experience repetitive exposure to traumatic scenes and stories. The loss and devastation for a child who personally lives through a disaster are significant; the effect of the simultaneous occurrence of disaster and personal loss complicates the bereavement process as grief reactions become interwoven with posttraumatic stress symptoms (see Chapter 38). After a death resulting from aggressive or traumatic circumstances, access to expert help may be required. Under conditions of threat and fear, children seek proximity to safe, stable, protective figures.

It is important for parents to grieve with their children. Some parents want to protect their children from their grief, so they put on an outwardly brave front or do not talk about the deceased family member or traumatic event. Instead of the desired protective effect, the child receives the message that demonstrating grief or talking about death is wrong, leading the child to feel isolated, grieve privately, or delay grieving. The child may also conclude that the parents did not really care about the deceased because they seem to have forgotten the person so easily or demonstrate no emotion. The parents' efforts to avoid talking about the death may cause the parents to isolate themselves from their children at a time when the children most need them. Children need to know that their parents love them and will continue to protect them. Children need opportunities to talk about their relative's death and associated memories. A surviving sibling may feel guilty simply because he or she survived, especially if the death was the result of an accident that involved both children. Siblings' grief, especially when compounded by feelings of guilt, may manifest as regressive behavior or anger. Parents should be informed of this possibility and encouraged to discuss it with their children.

DEVELOPMENTAL PERSPECTIVE

Children's responses to death reflect the family's current culture, their past heritage, their experiences, and the sociopolitical environment. Personal experience with terminal illness and dying may also facilitate children's comprehension of death and familiarity with mourning. Developmental differences exist in children's efforts to make sense of and master the concept and reality of death and profoundly influence their grief reactions.

Children younger than 3 yr have little or no understanding of the concept of death. Despair, separation anxiety, and detachment may occur at the withdrawal of nurturing caretakers. Young children may respond in reaction to observing distress in others, such as a parent or sibling who is crying, withdrawn, or angry. Young children also express signs and symptoms of grief in their emotional states, such as irritability or lethargy, and in severe cases, mutism. If the reaction is severe, failure to thrive may occur.

Preschool children are in the preoperational cognitive stage, in which communication takes place through play and fantasy (see Chapter 24). They do not show well-established cause-and-effect reasoning. They feel that death is reversible, analogous to someone going away. In attempts to master the finality and permanence of death, preschoolers frequently ask unrelenting, repeated questions about when the person who died will be returning. This makes it difficult for parents, who may become frustrated because they do not understand why the child keeps asking and do not like the constant reminders of the person's death. The primary care provider has a very important role in helping families understand the child's struggle to comprehend death. Preschool children typically express magical explanations of death events, sometimes resulting in guilt and self-blame ("He died because I wouldn't play with him"; "She died because I was mad at her"). Some children have these thoughts but do not express them verbally because of embarrassment or guilt. Parents and primary care providers need to be aware of magical thinking and must reassure preschool children that their thoughts had nothing to do with the outcome. Children of this age are often frightened by prolonged, powerful expressions of grief by others. Children conceptualize events in the context of their own experiential reality, and therefore consider death in terms of sleep, separation, and injury. Young children express grief intermittently and show marked affective shifts over brief periods.

Younger school-age children think concretely, recognize that death is irreversible, but believe it will not happen to them or affect them, and begin to understand biologic processes of the human body ("You'll die if your body stops working"). Information gathered from the media, peers, and parents forms lasting impressions. Consequently, they may ask candid questions about death that adults will have difficulty addressing ("He must have been blown to pieces, huh?").

Children approximately 9 yr and older do understand that death is irreversible and that it may involve them or their families. These children tend to experience more anxiety, overt symptoms of depression, and somatic complaints than do younger children. School-aged children are often left with anger focused on the loved one, those who could not save the deceased, or those presumed responsible for the death. Contact with the pediatrician may provide great reassurance, especially for the child with somatic symptoms, and particularly when the death followed a medical illness. School and learning problems may also occur, often linked to difficulty concentrating or preoccupation with the death. Close collaboration with the child's school may provide important diagnostic information and offer opportunities to mobilize intervention or support.

At **12-14 yr of age**, children begin to use symbolic thinking, reason abstractly, and analyze hypothetical, or "what if," scenarios systematically.

Death and the end of life become concepts rather than events. Teenagers are often ambivalent about dependence and independence and may withdraw emotionally from surviving family members, only to mourn in isolation. Adolescents begin to understand complex physiologic systems in relationship to death. Since they are often egocentric, they may be more concerned about the impact of the death on themselves than about the deceased or other family members. Fascination with dramatic, sensational, or romantic death sometimes occurs and may find expression in *copycat behavior,* such as cluster suicides, as well as *competitive behavior,* to forge emotional links to the deceased person ("He was my best friend"). Somatic expression of grief may revolve around highly complex syndromes such as eating disorders (see Chapter 41) or conversion reactions (Chapter 35), as well as symptoms limited to the more immediate perceptions (stomachaches). *Quality of life* takes on meaning, and the teenager develops a focus on the future. Depression, resentment, mood swings, rage, and risk-taking behaviors can emerge as the adolescent seeks answers to questions of values, safety, evil, and fairness. Alternately, adolescents may seek philosophic or spiritual explanations ("being at peace") to ease their sense of loss. The death of a peer may be especially traumatic.

Families often struggle with how to inform their children of the death of a family member. The answer depends on the child's developmental level. It is best to avoid misleading euphemisms and metaphor. A child who is told that the relative who died "went to sleep" may become frightened of falling asleep, resulting in sleep problems or nightmares. Children can be told that the person is "no longer living" or "no longer moving or feeling." Using examples of pets that have died sometimes can help children gain a more realistic idea of the meaning of death. Parents who have religious beliefs may comfort their children with explanations, such as, "Your sister's soul is in heaven," or "Grandfather is now with God," provided those beliefs are honestly held. If these are not religious beliefs that the parents share, children will sense the insincerity and experience anxiety rather than the hoped-for reassurance. Children's books about death can provide an important source of information, and when read together, these books may help the parent to find the right words while addressing the child's needs.

ROLE OF THE PEDIATRICIAN IN GRIEF

The pediatric healthcare provider who has had a longitudinal relationship with the family will be an important source of support in the disclosure of bad news and in critical decision-making, during both the dying process and the bereavement period. The involvement of the healthcare provider may include being present at the time the diagnosis is disclosed, at the hospital or home at the time of death, being available to the family by phone during the bereavement period, sending a sympathy card, attending the funeral, and scheduling a follow-up visit. Attendance at the funeral sends a strong message that the family and their child are important, respected by the healthcare provider, and can also help the pediatric healthcare provider to grieve and reach personal closure about the death. A family meeting 1-3 mo later may be helpful because parents may not be able to formulate their questions at the time of death. This meeting allows the family time to ask questions, share concerns, and review autopsy findings (if one was performed), and allows the healthcare provider to determine how the parents and family are adjusting to the death.

Instead of leaving the family feeling abandoned by a healthcare system that they have counted on, this visit allows them to have continued support. This is even more important when the healthcare provider will be continuing to provide care for surviving siblings. The visit can be used to determine how the mourning process is progressing, detect evidence of marital discord, and evaluate how well surviving siblings are coping. This is also an opportunity to evaluate whether referrals to support groups or mental health providers may be of benefit. Continuing to recognize the child who has died is important. Families appreciate the receipt of a card on their child's birthday, around holidays, or the anniversary of their child's death.

The healthcare provider needs to be an *educator* about disease, death, and grief. The pediatrician can offer a safe environment for the family to talk about painful emotions, express fears, and share memories. By giving families permission to talk and modeling how to address children's concerns, the pediatrician demystifies death. Parents often request practical help. The healthcare provider can offer families resources, such as literature (both fiction and nonfiction), referrals to therapeutic services, and tools to help them learn about illness, loss, and grief. In this way the physician reinforces the sense that other people understand what they are going through and helps to normalize their distressing emotions. The pediatrician can also facilitate and demystify the grief process by sharing basic tenets of **grief therapy**. There is no single right or wrong way to grieve. Everyone grieves differently; mothers may grieve differently than fathers, and children mourn differently than adults. Helping family members to respect these differences and reach out to support each other is critical. Grief is not something to "get over," but a lifelong process of adapting, readjusting, and reconnecting.

Parents may need help in knowing what constitutes **normal grieving**. Hearing, seeing, or feeling their child's presence may be a normal response. Vivid memories or dreams may occur. The pediatrician can help parents to learn that, although their pain and sadness may seem intolerable, other parents have survived similar experiences, and their pain will lessen over time.

Pediatricians are often asked whether children should attend the **funeral** of a parent or sibling. These rituals allow the family to begin their mourning process. Children >4 yr old should be given a choice. If the child chooses to attend, the child should have a designated, trusted adult who is not part of the immediate family and who will stay with the child, offer comfort, and be willing to leave with the child if the experience proves to be overwhelming. If the child chooses not to attend, the child should be offered additional opportunities to share in a ritual, go to the cemetery to view the grave, tell stories about the deceased, or obtain a keepsake object from the deceased family member as a remembrance.

In the era of regionalized tertiary care medicine, the primary care provider and medical home staff may not be informed when one of their patients dies in the hospital. Yet, this communication is critically important. Families assume their pediatrician has been notified and often feel hurt when they do not receive some symbol of condolence. Because of their longitudinal relationship with the family, primary care providers may offer much needed support. There are practical issues, such as the need to cancel previously made appointments and to alert office and nursing staff so that they are prepared should the family return for a follow-up visit or for ongoing health maintenance care with the surviving siblings. Even minor illnesses in the surviving siblings may frighten children. Parents may contribute to this anxiety because their inability to protect the child who has died may leave them with a sense of guilt or helplessness. They may seek medical attention sooner or may be hypervigilant in the care of the siblings because of guilt over the other child's death, concern about their judgment, or the need for continued reassurance. A visit to the pediatrician can do much to allay their fears.

Clinicians must remain vigilant for risk factors in each family member and in the family unit as a whole. Primary care providers, who care for families over time, know bereft patients' premorbid functioning and can identify those at current or future risk for physical and psychiatric morbidity. Providers must focus on symptoms that interfere with a patient's normal activities and compromise a child's attainment of developmental tasks. Symptom duration, intensity, and severity, in context with the family's culture, can help identify **complicated grief** reactions in need of therapeutic attention. Descriptive words such as "unrelenting," "intense," "intrusive," or "prolonged" should raise concern. Total absence of signs of mourning, specifically an inability to discuss the loss or express sadness, also suggests potential problems.

No specific sign, symptom, or cluster of behaviors identifies the child or family in need of help. Further assessment is indicated if the following occur: (1) persistent somatic or psychosomatic complaints of undetermined origin (headache, stomachache, eating and sleeping disorders, conversion symptoms, symptoms related to the deceased's condition, hypochondriasis); (2) unusual circumstances of death or loss (sudden, violent, or traumatic death; inexplicable, unbelievable, or particularly senseless death; prolonged, complicated illness; unexpected separation);

(3) school or work difficulties (declining grades or school performance, social withdrawal, aggression); (4) changes in home or family functioning (multiple family stresses, lack of social support, unavailable or ineffective functioning of caretakers, multiple disruptions in routines, lack of safety); and (5) concerning psychologic factors (persistent guilt or blame, desire to die or talk of suicide, severe separation distress, disturbing hallucinations, self-abuse, risk-taking behaviors, symptoms of trauma such as hyperarousal or severe flashbacks, grief from previous or multiple deaths). Children who are intellectually impaired may require additional support.

Finally, pediatric healthcare providers need to recognize that the loss of a patient will have an impact on them, both as a health professional and as a caring individual. Identifying one's responses to the loss (grief, guilt, anger, sadness) and finding time to process these feelings is important. Providers cope with these experiences in many ways. Strong coping mechanisms foster resilience and allow providers to continue to engage with patients and families in meaningful ways even in the face of grief and loss.

TREATMENT

Suggesting interventions outside the natural support network of family and friends can often prove useful to grieving families. Bereavement counseling should be readily offered if needed or requested by the family. Interventions that enhance or promote attachments and security, as well as give the family a means of expressing and understanding death, help to reduce the likelihood of future or prolonged disturbance, especially in children. Collaboration between pediatric and mental health professionals can help determine the timing and appropriateness of services.

Interventions for children and families who are struggling to cope with a loss in the community include gestures such as sending a card or offering food to the relatives of the deceased and teaching children the etiquette of behaviors and rituals around bereavement and mutual support. Performing community service or joining charitable organizations, such as fund-raising in memory of the deceased, may be useful. In the wake of a disaster, parents and older siblings may give blood or volunteer in search and recovery efforts. When a loss does not involve an actual death (e.g., parental divorce, geographic relocation), empowering the child to join or start a "divorced kids' club" in school or planning a "new kids in town" party may help. Participating in a constructive activity moves the family away from a sense of helplessness and hopelessness and helps them find meaning in their loss.

Psychotherapeutic services may benefit the entire family or individual members. Many support or self-help groups focus on specific types of losses (sudden infant death syndrome, suicide, widow/widowers, AIDS) and provide an opportunity to talk with other people who have experienced similar losses. Family, couple, sibling, or individual counseling may be useful, depending on the nature of the residual coping issues. Combinations of approaches may work well for children or parents with evolving needs. A child may participate in family therapy to deal with the loss of a sibling and use individual treatment to address issues of personal ambivalence and guilt related to the death.

The question of **pharmacologic intervention** for grief reactions often arises. Explaining that medication does not cure grief and often does not reduce the intensity of some symptoms (separation distress) can help. Although medication can blunt reactions, the psychologic work of grieving still must occur. The pediatrician must consider the patient's premorbid psychiatric vulnerability, current level of functioning, other available supports, and the use of additional therapeutic interventions. Medication as a first line of defense rarely proves useful in normal or uncomplicated grief reactions. In certain situations (severe sleep disruption, incapacitating anxiety, intense hyperarousal), an anxiolytic or antidepressant may help to achieve symptom relief and provide the patient with the emotional energy to mourn. Medication used in conjunction with some form of psychotherapy, and in consultation with a psychopharmacologist, has optimal results.

Children who are **refugees** and may have experienced war, violence, or personal torture, while often resilient, may experience posttraumatic stress disorder if exposures were severe or repeated (see Chapter 14.3). Sequelae such as depression, anxiety, and grief need to be addressed, and mental health therapy is indicated. Cognitive-behavioral therapy, use of journaling and narratives to bear witness to the experiences, and use of translators may be essential.

SPIRITUAL ISSUES

Responding to patients' and families' spiritual beliefs can help in comforting them during family tragedies. Offering to call members of pastoral care teams or their own spiritual leader can provide needed support and can aid in decision-making. Families have found it important to have their beliefs and their need for hope acknowledged in end-of-life care. The majority of patients report welcoming discussions on spirituality, which may help individual patients cope with illness, disease, dying, and death. In addressing spirituality, physicians need to follow certain

guidelines, including maintaining respect for the patient's beliefs, following the patient's lead in exploring how spirituality affects the patient's decision-making, acknowledging the limits of their own expertise and role in spirituality, and maintaining their own integrity by not saying or doing anything that violates their own spiritual or religious views. Healthcare providers should not impose their own religious or nonreligious beliefs on patients, but rather should listen respectfully to their patients. By responding to spiritual needs, physicians may better aid their patients and families in end-of-life care and bereavement and take on the role of healers.

Bibliography is available at Expert Consult.

Chapter **31**
Sleep Medicine
Judith A. Owens
第三十一章
睡眠医学

中文导读

本章主要介绍了睡眠和时间生物学基础知识、睡眠发展变化、常见的睡眠障碍、保健管理以及儿童睡眠问题评估。具体描述了常见的睡眠障碍，包括儿童失眠、阻塞性睡眠呼吸暂停综合征、睡眠相关性运动障碍（不宁腿综合征、周期性肢体运动障碍和与睡眠相关的节律性运动障碍）、发作性睡病以及睡眠觉醒时相延迟障碍的病因学、流行病学、临床表现、诊断和治疗。

BASICS OF SLEEP AND CHRONOBIOLOGY

Sleep, with its counterpart of wakefulness, is a highly complex and intricately regulated neurobiologic system that both influences and is influenced by all physiologic systems in the body, as well as by the environment and sociocultural practices. The concept of **sleep regulation** is based on what is usually referred to as the "2-process model" because it requires the simultaneous operation of 2 basic, highly coupled processes that govern sleep and wakefulness. The **homeostatic process** ("Process S"), regulates the length and depth of sleep and is thought to be related to the accumulation of adenosine and other sleep-promoting chemicals ("somnogens"), such as cytokines, during prolonged periods of wakefulness. This sleep pressure appears to build more quickly in infants and young children, thus limiting the duration that wakefulness can be sustained during the day and necessitating periods of daytime sleep (i.e., naps). The endogenous **circadian rhythms** ("Process C") influence the internal organization of sleep and the timing and duration of daily

sleep–wake cycles and govern predictable patterns of alertness throughout the 24 hr day.

The "master circadian clock" that controls sleep–wake patterns, of which melatonin secretion is the principal biomarker, is located in the suprachiasmatic nucleus in the ventral hypothalamus. In addition, "circadian clocks" are present in virtually every cell in the body, which in turn govern the timing of multiple other physiologic systems (e.g., cardiovascular reactivity, hormone levels, renal and pulmonary functions). Because the human circadian clock is slightly longer than 24 hr, intrinsic circadian rhythms must be synchronized or "entrained" to the 24 hr day cycle by environmental cues called *zeitgebers*. The **dark–light cycle** is the most powerful of the zeitgebers; light signals are transmitted to the suprachiasmatic nucleus via the circadian photoreceptor system within the retina (functionally and anatomically separate from the visual system), which switch the pineal gland's production of the hormone melatonin off (light) or on (dark). Circadian rhythms are also synchronized by other external time cues, such as timing of meals and alarm clocks.

Sleep propensity, the relative level of sleepiness or alertness experienced at any given time during a 24 hr period, is partially determined by the homeostatic *sleep drive,* which in turn depends on the duration and quality of previous sleep and the amount of time awake since the last sleep period. Interacting with this *sleep homeostat* is the 24 hr cyclic pattern or rhythm characterized by clock-dependent periods of maximum sleepiness (*circadian troughs*) and maximum alertness (*circadian nadirs*). There are two periods of maximum sleepiness, one in the late afternoon (approximately 3:00-5:00 PM) and one toward the end of the night (around 3:00-5:00 AM), and two periods of maximum alertness, one in mid-morning and one in the evening just before the onset of natural sleep, the so-called forbidden zone or second-wind phenomenon, which allows for the maintenance of wakefulness in the face of accumulated sleep drive.

There are significant health, safety, and performance consequences of failure to meet basic sleep needs, termed *insufficient/inadequate sleep* or **sleep loss.** Sufficient sleep is a biologic imperative, necessary for optimal brain and body functioning. **Slow-wave sleep (SWS)** (i.e., N3, delta, or deep sleep) appears to be the most restorative form of sleep; it is entered relatively quickly after sleep onset, is preserved in the face of reduced total sleep time, and increases (rebounds) after a night of restricted total sleep time. These restorative properties of sleep may be linked to the "glymphatic system," which increases clearance of metabolic waste products, including β-amyloid, produced by neural activity in the awake brain. **Rapid eye movement (REM)** sleep (stage R or "dream" sleep) appears to be involved in numerous important brain processes, including completion of vital cognitive functions (e.g., consolidation of memory), promoting the plasticity of the central nervous system (CNS), and protecting the brain from injury. Sufficient amounts of these sleep stages are necessary for optimal cognitive functioning and emotional and behavioral self-regulation.

Partial sleep loss (i.e., sleep restriction) on a chronic basis accumulates in a **sleep debt** and over several days produces deficits equivalent to those seen under conditions of 1 night of total sleep deprivation. If the sleep debt becomes large enough and is not voluntarily repaid by obtaining sufficient recovery sleep, the body may respond by overriding voluntary control of wakefulness. This results in periods of decreased alertness, dozing off, and unplanned napping, recognized as *excessive daytime sleepiness.* The sleep-restricted individual may also experience very brief (several seconds) repeated daytime microsleeps, of which the individual may be completely unaware, but which nonetheless may result in significant lapses in attention and vigilance. There is also a relationship between the amount of sleep restriction and performance on cognitive tasks, particularly those requiring sustained attention and higher-level cognitive skills (*executive functions;* see Chapter 48), with a decay in performance correlating with declines in sleep amounts.

It has also been increasingly recognized that what may be globally described as "deficient" sleep involves alterations in both amount and *timing* of sleep. Misalignment of intrinsic circadian rhythms with extrinsic societal demands, such a shift work and early school start times, is associated with deficits in cognitive function and self-regulation, increased emotional and behavioral problems and risk-taking behaviors, and negative impacts on health, such as increased risk of cardiovascular disease, obesity, and metabolic dysfunction.

Insufficient quantity of sleep, mistimed sleep, and poor-quality sleep in children and adolescents frequently result in excessive daytime sleepiness and decreased daytime alertness levels. **Sleepiness** in children may be recognizable as drowsiness, yawning, and other classic "sleepy behaviors," but can also manifest as mood disturbance, including complaints of moodiness, irritability, emotional lability, depression, and anger; fatigue and daytime lethargy, including increased somatic complaints (headaches, muscle aches); cognitive impairment, including problems with memory, attention, concentration, decision-making, and problem solving; daytime behavior problems, including hyperactivity, impulsivity, and noncompliance; and academic problems, including chronic tardiness related to insufficient sleep and school failure resulting from chronic daytime sleepiness.

DEVELOPMENTAL CHANGES IN SLEEP

Sleep disturbances, as well as many characteristics of sleep itself, have some distinctly different features in children from sleep and sleep disorders in adults. Changes in sleep architecture and the evolution of sleep patterns and behaviors reflect the physiologic/chronobiologic, developmental, and social/environmental changes that are occurring across childhood. These trends may be summarized as the gradual assumption of more adult sleep patterns as children mature:

1. Sleep is *the* primary activity of the brain during early development; for example, by age 2 yr, the average child has spent 9500 hr (approximately 13 mo) asleep vs 8000 hr awake, and between 2 and 5 yr, the time asleep is equal to the time awake.

2. There is a gradual decline in the average 24 hr sleep duration from infancy through adolescence, which involves a decrease in both diurnal and nocturnal sleep amounts. The decline in daytime sleep (scheduled napping) results in termination of naps typically by age 5 yr. There is also a gradual continued decrease in nocturnal sleep amounts into late adolescence; however, the typical adolescent still requires 8-10 hr of sleep per night.

3. There is also a decline in the relative percentage of REM sleep from birth (50% of sleep) through early childhood into adulthood (25–30%), and a similar initial predominance of SWS that peaks in early childhood, drops off abruptly after puberty (40–60% decline), and then further decreases over the life span. This SWS preponderance in early life has clinical significance; for example, the high prevalence of partial arousal parasomnias (sleepwalking and sleep terrors) in preschool and early school-age children is related to the relative increased percentage of SWS in this age-group.

4. The within-sleep **ultradian cycle** lengthens from about 50 min in the term infant to 90-110 min in the school-age child. This has clinical significance in that typically a brief arousal or awakening occurs during the night at the termination of each ultradian cycle. As the length of the cycles increase, there is a concomitant decrease in the number of these end-of-cycle arousals (night wakings).

5. A gradual shift in the circadian sleep–wake rhythm to a delayed (later) sleep onset and offset time, linked to pubertal stage rather than chronological age, begins with pubertal onset in middle childhood and accelerates in early to mid-adolescence. This biologic phenomenon often coincides with environmental factors, which further delay bedtime and advance wake time and result in insufficient sleep duration, including exposure to electronic "screens" (television, computer) in the evening, social networking, academic and extracurricular demands, and early (before 8:30 AM) high school start times.

6. Increasing irregularity of sleep–wake patterns is typically observed across childhood into adolescence; this is characterized by increasingly larger discrepancies between school night and non–school night bedtimes and wake times, and increased "weekend oversleep" in an attempt to compensate for chronic weekday sleep insufficiency. This phenomenon, often referred to as "social jet lag," not only fails to adequately address performance deficits associated with insufficient sleep on school nights, but further exacerbates the normal adolescent phase delay and results in additional circadian disruption (analogous to that experienced by shift workers).

Table 31.1 lists normal developmental changes in children's sleep.

COMMON SLEEP DISORDERS

Childhood sleep problems may be conceptualized as resulting from (1) inadequate duration of sleep for age and sleep needs (insufficient sleep quantity); (2) disruption and fragmentation of sleep (poor sleep quality) as a result of frequent, repetitive, and brief arousals during sleep; and (3) misalignment of sleep–wake timing with circadian rhythms or CNS-mediated **hypersomnia** (excessive daytime sleepiness and increased sleep needs). Insufficient sleep is usually the result of difficulty initiating (*delayed sleep onset*) or maintaining sleep (*prolonged night wakings*), but, especially in older children and adolescents, may also represent a conscious lifestyle decision to sacrifice sleep in favor of competing priorities, such as homework and social activities. The underlying causes of delayed sleep onset/prolonged night wakings or sleep fragmentation may in turn be related to primarily behavioral factors (e.g., bedtime

Table 31.1	Normal Developmental Changes in Children's Sleep		
AGE CATEGORY	**SLEEP DURATION* AND SLEEP PATTERNS**	**ADDITIONAL SLEEP ISSUES**	**SLEEP DISORDERS**
Newborn (0-2 mo)	Total sleep: 10-19 hr per 24 hr (average, 13-14.5 hr), may be higher in premature babies Bottle-fed babies generally sleep for longer periods (2-5 hr bouts) than breastfed babies (1-3 hr). Sleep periods are separated by 1-2 hr awake. No established nocturnal-diurnal pattern in 1st few wk; sleep is evenly distributed throughout the day and night, averaging 8.5 hr at night and 5.75 hr during day.	American Academy of Pediatrics issued a revised recommendation in 2016 advocating against bed-sharing in the 1st yr of life, instead encouraging proximate but separate sleeping surfaces for mother and infant for at least the 1st 6 mo and preferably 1st yr of life. Safe sleep practices for infants: • Place baby on his or her back to sleep at night and during nap times. • Place baby on a firm mattress with well-fitting sheet in safety-approved crib. • Do not use pillows or comforters. • Standards require crib bars to be no farther apart than 2⅜ in. • Make sure baby's face and head stay uncovered and clear of blankets and other coverings during sleep.	Most sleep issues perceived as problematic at this stage represent a discrepancy between parental expectations and developmentally appropriate sleep behaviors. Newborns who are extremely fussy and persistently difficult to console, as noted by parents, are more likely to have underlying medical issues such as colic, gastroesophageal reflux, and formula intolerance.
Infant (2-12 mo)	Recommended sleep duration (4-12 mo) is 12-16 hr (note that there is great individual variability in sleep times during infancy).	Sleep regulation or self-soothing involves the infant's ability to negotiate the sleep–wake transition, both at sleep onset and following normal awakenings throughout the night. The capacity to self-soothe begins to develop in the 1st 12 wk of life and is a reflection of both neurodevelopmental maturation and learning. Sleep consolidation, or "sleeping through the night," is usually defined by parents as a continuous sleep episode without the need for parental intervention (e.g., feeding, soothing) from the child's bedtime through the early morning. Infants develop the ability to consolidate sleep between 6 wk and 3 mo.	Behavioral insomnia of childhood; sleep-onset association type Sleep-related rhythmic movements (head banging, body rocking)
Toddler (1-2 yr)	Recommended sleep amount is 11-14 hr (including naps). Naps decrease from 2 to 1 nap at average age of 18 mo.	Cognitive, motor, social, and language developmental issues impact sleep. Nighttime fears develop; transitional objects and bedtime routines are important.	Behavioral insomnia of childhood, sleep-onset association type Behavioral insomnia of childhood, limit-setting type
Preschool (3-5 yr)	Recommended sleep amount is 10-13 hr (including naps). Overall, 26% of 4 yr olds and just 15% of 5 yr olds nap.	Persistent cosleeping tends to be highly associated with sleep problems in this age-group. Sleep problems may become chronic.	Behavioral insomnia of childhood, limit-setting type Sleepwalking, sleep terrors, nighttime fears/nightmares, obstructive sleep apnea syndrome
Middle childhood (6-12 yr)	Recommended sleep amount is 9-12 hr.	School and behavior problems may be related to sleep problems. Media and electronics, such as television, computer, video games, and the Internet, increasingly compete for sleep time. Irregularity of sleep–wake schedules reflects increasing discrepancy between school and non–school night bedtimes and wake times.	Nightmares Obstructive sleep apnea syndrome Insufficient sleep
Adolescence (13-18 yr)	Recommended sleep amount is 8-10 hr. Later bedtimes; increased discrepancy between sleep patterns on weekdays and weekends	Puberty-mediated phase delay (later sleep onset and wake times), relative to sleep-wake cycles in middle childhood Earlier required wake times Environmental competing priorities for sleep	Insufficient sleep Delayed sleep–wake phase disorder Narcolepsy Restless legs syndrome/periodic limb movement disorder

*All recommended sleep amounts from Paruthi S, Brooks LJ, D'Ambrosio C, et al: Recommended amount of sleep for pediatric populations: a consensus statement of the American Academy of Sleep Medicine. *J Clin Sleep Med* 12:785–786, 2016.

resistance resulting in shortened sleep duration) or medical causes (e.g., obstructive sleep apnea causing frequent, brief arousals).

Certain pediatric populations are relatively more vulnerable to acute or chronic sleep problems. These include children with medical problems, such as chronic illnesses or pain conditions (e.g., cystic fibrosis, asthma, idiopathic juvenile arthritis) and acute illnesses (e.g., otitis media); children taking stimulants s (e.g., psychostimulants, caffeine), sleep-disrupting medications (e.g., corticosteroids), or daytime-sedating

medications (some anticonvulsants, α-agonists); hospitalized children; and children with a variety of psychiatric disorders, including attention-deficit/hyperactivity disorder (ADHD), depression, bipolar disorder, and anxiety disorders. Children with neurodevelopmental disorders such as autism, intellectual disability, blindness, and some chromosomal syndromes (e.g., Smith-Magenis, fragile X) have especially high rates of sleep disturbances for a wide variety of reasons. They may have comorbid medical issues or may be taking sleep-disrupting medications, may be more prone to nocturnal seizures, may be less easily entrained by environmental cues and thus more vulnerable to circadian disruption, and are more likely to have psychiatric and behavioral comorbidities that further predispose them to disrupted sleep.

Insomnia of Childhood

Insomnia is defined as difficulty initiating and/or maintaining sleep that occurs despite age-appropriate time and opportunity for sleep and results in some degree of impairment in daytime functioning for the child and/or family (ranging from fatigue, irritability, lack of energy, and mild cognitive impairment to effects on mood, school performance, and quality of life). Insomnia may be of a short-term and transient nature (usually related to an acute event) or may be characterized as long-term and chronic. Insomnia is a set of *symptoms* with many possible etiologies (e.g., pain, medication, medical/psychiatric conditions, learned behaviors). As with many behavioral issues in children, insomnia is often primarily defined by parental concerns rather than by objective criteria, and therefore should be viewed in the context of family (maternal depression, stress), child (temperament, developmental level), and environmental (cultural practices, sleeping space) considerations.

While current terminology (*Diagnostic and Statistical Manual of Mental Disorders*, 5th edition, 2015; *International Classification of Sleep Disorders*, 3rd edition, 2014) groups most types of insomnia in children and adults under a single category of Chronic Insomnia Disorder, the descriptor of Behavioral Insomnia of Childhood and its subtypes (Sleep Onset Association and Limit Setting) remains a useful construct, particularly for young children (0-5 yr) in clinical practice. One of the most common presentations of insomnia found in infants and toddlers is the **sleep-onset association type.** In this situation the child learns to fall asleep only under certain conditions or associations, which typically require parental presence, such as being rocked or fed, and does not develop the ability to self-soothe. During the night, when the child experiences the type of brief arousal that normally occurs at the end of an ultradian sleep cycle or awakens for other reasons, the child is not able to get back to sleep without those same associations being present. The infant then "signals" the parent by crying (or coming into the parents' bedroom, if the child is ambulatory) until the necessary associations are provided. The presenting complaint is typically one of prolonged night waking requiring caregiver intervention and resulting in insufficient sleep (for both child and parent).

Management of **night wakings** should include establishment of a set sleep schedule and bedtime routine and implementation of a behavioral program. The treatment approach typically involves a program of rapid withdrawal (extinction) or more gradual withdrawal (graduated extinction) of parental assistance at sleep onset and during the night. **Extinction** ("cry it out") involves putting the child to bed at a designated bedtime, "drowsy but awake," to maximize sleep propensity and then systematically ignoring any protests by the child until a set time the next morning. Although it has considerable empirical support, extinction is often not an acceptable choice for families. **Graduated extinction** involves gradually weaning the child from dependence on parental presence; typically, the parent leaves the room at "lights out" and then returns or "checks" periodically at fixed or successively longer intervals during the sleep–wake transition to provide brief reassurance until the child falls asleep. The exact interval between checks is generally determined by the parents' tolerance for crying and the child's temperament. The goal is to allow the infant or child to develop skills in self-soothing during the night, as well as at bedtime. In older infants and young children, the introduction of more appropriate sleep associations that will be readily available to the child during the night (transitional objects, such as a blanket or toy), in addition to positive reinforcement (stickers for remaining in bed), is often beneficial. If the child has become habituated to awaken for nighttime feedings (learned hunger), these feedings should be slowly eliminated. Parents must be consistent in applying behavioral programs to avoid inadvertent, intermittent reinforcement of night wakings. They should also be forewarned that crying behavior often temporarily escalates at the beginning of treatment (*postextinction burst*).

Bedtime problems, including stalling and refusing to go to bed, are more common in preschool-age and older children. This type of insomnia is frequently related to inadequate **limit setting** and is often the result of parental difficulties in setting limits and managing behavior in general and the inability or unwillingness to set consistent bedtime rules and enforce a regular bedtime. The situation may be exacerbated by the child's oppositional behavior. In some cases the child's resistance at bedtime is the result of an underlying problem in falling asleep that is caused by other factors (medical conditions such as asthma or medication use; a sleep disorder such as restless legs syndrome; anxiety) or a mismatch between the child's intrinsic circadian rhythm ("night owl") and parental expectations regarding an "appropriate" bedtime.

Successful treatment of limit-setting sleep problems generally involves a combination of parent education regarding appropriate limit setting, decreased parental attention for bedtime-delaying behavior, establishment of bedtime routines, and positive reinforcement (sticker charts) for appropriate behavior at bedtime. Other behavioral management strategies that have empirical support include **bedtime fading**, or temporarily setting the bedtime closer to the actual sleep-onset time and then gradually advancing the bedtime to an earlier target bedtime. Older children may benefit from being taught relaxation techniques to help themselves fall asleep more readily. Following the principles of healthy sleep practices for children is essential (Table 31.2).

A 3rd type of childhood insomnia is related to a mismatch between parental expectations regarding time in bed and the child's intrinsic sleep needs. If, as illustrated in Fig. 31.1, a child's typical sleep time is 10 hr but the "sleep window" is set for 12 hr (7 PM to 7 AM), the result is likely to be a prolonged sleep onset of 2 hr, an extended period of wakefulness during the night, or early morning waking (or a combination); these periods are usually characterized by "normal" wakefulness in the child that is not accompanied by excessive distress. This situation is important to recognize because the solution—reducing the time in bed to actual sleep time—is typically simple and effective.

Another form of insomnia that is more common in older children and adolescents is often referred to as *psychophysiologic, primary,* or *learned* insomnia. **Primary insomnia** occurs mainly in adolescents and is characterized by a combination of learned sleep-preventing associations and heightened physiologic arousal resulting in a complaint of sleeplessness and decreased daytime functioning. A hallmark of primary insomnia is excessive worry about sleep and an exaggerated concern of the potential daytime consequences. The physiologic arousal can be in the form of cognitive **hypervigilance**, such as "racing" thoughts; in many individuals

Table 31.2	Basic Principles of Healthy Sleep for Children

1. Have a set bedtime and bedtime routine for your child.
2. Bedtime and wake-up time should be about the same time on school nights and non–school nights. There should not be more than about 1 hr difference from one day to another.
3. Make the hour before bed shared quiet time. Avoid high-energy activities, such as rough play, and stimulating activities, such as watching television or playing computer games, just before bed.
4. Don't send your child to bed hungry. A *light* snack (e.g., milk and cookies) before bed is a good idea. Heavy meals within 1 hr or 2 of bedtime, however, may interfere with sleep.
5. Avoid products containing caffeine for at least several hours before bedtime. These include caffeinated sodas, coffee, tea, and chocolate.
6. Make sure your child spends time outside every day, whenever possible, and is involved in regular exercise.
7. Keep your child's bedroom quiet and dark. A low-level night light is acceptable for children who find completely dark rooms frightening.
8. Keep your child's bedroom at a comfortable temperature during the night (<24°C [75°F]).
9. Don't use your child's bedroom for time-out or punishment.
10. Keep the television set out of your child's bedroom. Children can easily develop the bad habit of "needing" the television to fall asleep. It is also much more difficult to control your child's viewing if the set is in the bedroom.

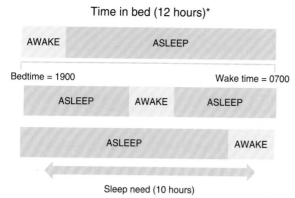

Time in bed (12 hours)*

Bedtime = 1900   Wake time = 0700

Sleep need (10 hours)

Fig. 31.1 Mismatch between sleep needs/duration and time in bed, resulting in insomnia.

Table 31.3	Basic Principles of Healthy Sleep for Adolescents

1. **Wake up and go to bed at about the same time** every night. Bedtime and wake-up time should not differ from school to non–school nights by more than approximately 1 hr.
2. **Avoid sleeping in on weekends** to "catch up" on sleep. This makes it more likely that you will have problems falling asleep.
3. If you take **naps**, they should be **short** (no more than 1 hr) and **scheduled in the early to mid-afternoon**. However, if you have a problem with falling asleep at night, napping during the day may make it worse and should be avoided.
4. **Spend time outside** every day. Exposure to sunlight helps to keep your body's internal clock on track.
5. **Exercise regularly.** Exercise may help you fall asleep and sleep more deeply.
6. **Use your bed for sleeping only.** Don't study, read, listen to music, or watch television on your bed.
7. **Make the 30-60 minutes before bedtime a quiet or wind-down time.** Relaxing, calm, enjoyable activities, such as reading a book or listening to calm music, help your body and mind slow down enough to let you get to sleep. Don't study, watch exciting/scary movies, exercise, or get involved in "energizing" activities just before bed.
8. Eat regular meals, and **don't go to bed hungry.** A light snack before bed is a good idea; eating a full meal within 1 hr before bed is not.
9. **Avoid** eating or drinking products containing **caffeine** from dinnertime to bedtime. These include caffeinated sodas, coffee, tea, and chocolate.
10. **Do not use alcohol.** Alcohol disrupts sleep and may cause you to awaken throughout the night.
11. Smoking (e.g., cigarettes) disturbs sleep. Although you should not smoke at all, if you do, **do not smoke at least 2 hr before bed.**
12. **Do not use sleeping pills, melatonin, or other nonprescription sleep aids** to help you sleep unless specifically recommended by your doctor. These can be dangerous, and the sleep problems often return when you stop taking the medicine.

with insomnia, an increased baseline level of arousal is further intensified by this secondary anxiety about sleeplessness. Treatment usually involves educating the adolescent about the principles of healthy sleep practices (Table 31.3), institution of a consistent sleep–wake schedule, avoidance of daytime napping, instructions to use the bed for sleep only and to get out of bed if unable to fall asleep (*stimulus control*), restricting time in bed to the actual time asleep (*sleep restriction*), addressing maladaptive cognitions about sleep, and teaching relaxation techniques to reduce anxiety.

Behavioral treatments for insomnia, even in young children, appear to be highly effective and well tolerated. Several studies have failed to demonstrate long-term negative effects of behavioral strategies such as "sleep training" on parent–child relationships and attachment, psychosocial-emotional functioning, and chronic stress. In general, hypnotic medications or supplements such as melatonin are infrequently needed as an adjunct to behavioral therapy to treat insomnia in typically developing and healthy children.

Obstructive Sleep Apnea Syndrome

Sleep-related breathing disorder (SRBD) in children encompasses a broad spectrum of respiratory disorders that occur exclusively in sleep or that are exacerbated by sleep, including primary snoring and upper airway resistance syndrome, as well as apnea of prematurity (see Chapter 122.2) and central apnea (see Chapter 446.2). **Obstructive sleep apnea syndrome (OSAS)**, the most important clinical entity within the SRBD spectrum, is characterized by repeated episodes of prolonged upper airway obstruction during sleep despite continued or increased respiratory effort, resulting in complete (*apnea*) or partial (*hypopnea*; ≥30% reduction in airflow accompanied by ≥3% O_2 desaturation and/or arousal) cessation of airflow at the nose and/or mouth, as well as in disrupted sleep. Both intermittent hypoxia and the multiple arousals resulting from these obstructive events likely contribute to significant metabolic, cardiovascular, and neurocognitive-neurobehavioral morbidity.

Primary snoring is defined as snoring without associated ventilatory abnormalities on overnight polysomnogram (e.g., apneas or hypopneas, hypoxemia, hypercapnia) or respiratory-related arousals and is a manifestation of the vibrations of the oropharyngeal soft tissue walls that occur when an individual attempts to breathe against increased upper airway resistance during sleep. Although generally considered nonpathologic, primary snoring in children may still be associated with subtle breathing abnormalities during sleep, including evidence of increased respiratory effort, which in turn may be associated with adverse neurodevelopmental outcomes.

Etiology

OSAS results from an anatomically or functionally narrowed upper airway; this typically involves some combination of decreased upper airway patency (upper airway obstruction and/or decreased upper airway diameter), increased upper airway collapsibility (reduced pharyngeal muscle tone), and decreased drive to breathe in the face of reduced upper airway patency (reduced central ventilatory drive) (Table 31.4). Upper airway obstruction varies in degree and level (i.e., nose, nasopharynx/oropharynx, hypopharynx) and is most frequently caused by adenotonsillar hypertrophy, although tonsillar size does not necessarily correlate with degree of obstruction, especially in older children. Other causes of airway obstruction include allergies associated with chronic rhinitis or nasal obstruction; craniofacial abnormalities, including hypoplasia or displacement of the maxilla and mandible; gastroesophageal reflux with resulting pharyngeal reactive edema (see Chapter 349); nasal septal deviation (Chapter 404); and velopharyngeal flap cleft palate repair. Reduced upper airway tone may result from neuromuscular diseases, including hypotonic cerebral palsy and muscular dystrophies (see Chapter 627), or hypothyroidism (Chapter 581). Reduced central ventilatory drive may be present in some children with Arnold-Chiari malformation (see Chapter 446); rapid-onset obesity with hypothalamic dysfunction, hypoventilation, and autonomic dysregulation (Chapter 60.1); and meningomyelocele (Chapter 609.4). In other situations the etiology is mixed; individuals with Down syndrome (see Chapter 98.2), because of their facial anatomy, hypotonia, macroglossia, and central adiposity, as well as the increased incidence of hypothyroidism, are at particularly high risk for OSAS, with some estimates of prevalence as high as 70%.

Although many children with OSAS are of normal weight, an increasingly large percentage are overweight or obese, and many of these children are school-age or younger (see Chapter 60). There is a significant correlation between weight and SRBD (e.g., habitual snoring, OSAS, sleep-related hypoventilation). Although adenotonsillar hypertrophy also plays an important etiologic role in overweight/obese children with

Table 31.4	Anatomic Factors That Predispose to Obstructive Sleep Apnea Syndrome and Hypoventilation in Children

NOSE
Anterior nasal stenosis
Choanal stenosis/atresia
Deviated nasal septum
Seasonal or perennial rhinitis
Nasal polyps, foreign body, hematoma, mass lesion

NASOPHARYNGEAL AND OROPHARYNGEAL
Adenotonsillar hypertrophy
Macroglossia
Cystic hygroma
Velopharyngeal flap repair
Cleft palate repair
Pharyngeal mass lesion

CRANIOFACIAL
Micrognathia/retrognathia
Midface hypoplasia (e.g., trisomy 21, Crouzon disease, Apert syndrome)
Mandibular hypoplasia (Pierre Robin, Treacher Collins, Cornelia de Lange syndromes)
Craniofacial trauma
Skeletal and storage diseases
Achondroplasia
Storage diseases (e.g., glycogen; Hunter, Hurler syndromes)

OSAS, mechanical factors related to an increase in the amount of adipose tissue in the throat (pharyngeal fat pads), neck (increased neck circumference), and chest wall and abdomen can increase upper airway resistance, worsen gas exchange, and increase the work of breathing, particularly in the supine position and during REM sleep. A component of blunted central ventilatory drive in response to hypoxia/hypercapnia and hypoventilation may occur as well (see Chapter 446.3), particularly in children with morbid or syndrome-based (e.g., Prader-Willi) obesity. Overweight and obese children and adolescents are at particularly high risk for metabolic and cardiovascular complications of SRBD, such as insulin resistance and systemic hypertension. Morbidly obese children are also at increased risk for postoperative complications as well as residual OSAS after adenotonsillectomy.

Epidemiology
Overall prevalence of parent-reported snoring in the pediatric population is approximately 8%; "always" snoring is reported in 1.5–6%, and "often" snoring in 3–15%. When defined by parent-reported symptoms, the prevalence of OSAS is 4–11%. The prevalence of pediatric OSAS as documented by overnight sleep studies using ventilatory monitoring procedures (e.g., in-lab polysomnography, home studies) is 1–4% overall, with a reported range of 0.1–13%. Prevalence is also affected by the demographic characteristics such as age (increased prevalence between 2 and 8 yr), gender (more common in boys, especially after puberty), race/ethnicity (increased prevalence in African American and Asian children), history of prematurity, and family history of OSAS.

Pathogenesis
The upregulation of inflammatory pathways, as indicated by an increase in peripheral markers of inflammation (e.g., C-reactive protein, interleukins), appears to be linked to metabolic dysfunction (e.g., insulin resistance, dyslipidemia, alterations in neurohormone levels such as leptin) in both obese and nonobese children with OSAS. Systemic inflammation and arousal-mediated increases in sympathetic autonomic nervous system activity with altered vasomotor tone may be key contributors to increased cardiovascular risk due to alterations in vascular endothelium in both adults and children with OSA. Other potential mechanisms that may mediate cardiovascular sequelae in adults and children with OSA include elevated systemic blood pressure and

ventricular dysfunction. Mechanical stress on the upper airway induced by chronic snoring may also result in both local mucosal inflammation of adenotonsillar tissues and subsequent upregulation of inflammatory molecules, most notably leukotrienes. .

One of the primary mechanisms by which OSAS is believed to exert negative influences on cognitive function appears to involve repeated episodic arousals from sleep leading to sleep fragmentation and sleepiness. Equally important, intermittent hypoxia may lead directly to systemic inflammatory vascular changes in the brain. Levels of inflammatory markers such as C-reactive protein and interleukin-6 are elevated in children with OSAS and are also associated with cognitive dysfunction.

Clinical Manifestations
The clinical manifestations of OSAS may be divided into sleep-related and daytime symptoms. The most common nocturnal manifestations of OSAS in children and adolescents are loud, frequent, and disruptive snoring; breathing pauses; choking or gasping arousals; restless sleep; and nocturnal diaphoresis. Many children who snore do not have OSAS, but few children with OSAS do not snore (caregivers may not be aware of snoring in older children and adolescents). Children, like adults, tend to have more frequent and more severe obstructive events in REM sleep and when sleeping in the supine position. Children with OSAS may adopt unusual sleeping positions, keeping their necks hyperextended to maintain airway patency. Frequent arousals associated with obstruction may result in nocturnal awakenings but are more likely to cause fragmented sleep.

Daytime symptoms of OSAS include mouth breathing and dry mouth, chronic nasal congestion or rhinorrhea, hyponasal speech, morning headaches, difficulty swallowing, and poor appetite. Children with OSAS may have *secondary enuresis,* postulated to result from the disruption of the normal nocturnal pattern of atrial natriuretic peptide secretion by changes in intrathoracic pressure associated with OSAS. Partial arousal parasomnias (sleepwalking and sleep terrors) may occur more frequently in children with OSAS, related to the frequent associated arousals and an increased percentage of SWS.

One of the most important but frequently overlooked sequelae of OSAS in children is the effect on mood, behavior, learning, and academic functioning. The neurobehavioral consequences of OSAS in children include daytime sleepiness with drowsiness, difficulty in morning waking, and unplanned napping or dozing off during activities, although evidence of frank hypersomnolence tends to be less common in children compared to adults with OSA (except in very obese children or those with severe disease). Mood changes include increased irritability, mood instability and emotional dysregulation, low frustration tolerance, and depression or anxiety. Behavioral issues include both "internalizing" (i.e., increased somatic complaints and social withdrawal) and "externalizing" behaviors, including aggression, impulsivity, hyperactivity, oppositional behavior, and conduct problems. There is substantial overlap between the clinical impairments associated with OSAS and the diagnostic criteria for ADHD, including inattention, poor concentration, and distractibility (see Chapter 49).

Many of the studies that have looked at changes in behavior and neuropsychologic functioning in children after treatment (usually adenotonsillectomy) for OSAS have largely documented significant improvement in outcomes, both short term and long term, including daytime sleepiness, mood, behavior, academics, and quality of life. However, most studies failed to find a dose-dependent relationship between OSAS in children and specific neurobehavioral-neurocognitive deficits, suggesting that other factors may influence neurocognitive outcomes, including individual genetic susceptibility, racial/ethnic background, environmental influences (e.g., passive smoking exposure), and comorbid conditions, such as obesity, shortened sleep duration, and other sleep disorders.

Diagnosis
The 2012 revised American Academy of Pediatrics clinical practice guidelines provide excellent information for the evaluation and management of uncomplicated childhood OSAS (Table 31.5). No physical examination findings are truly pathognomonic for OSAS, and most

Table 31.5	American Academy of Pediatrics Clinical Practice Guideline: Diagnosis and Management of Childhood Obstructive Sleep Apnea Syndrome (OSAS)

Key Action Statement 1: Screening for OSAS

As part of routine health maintenance visits, clinicians should inquire whether the child or adolescent snores. If the answer is affirmative or if a child or adolescent presents with signs or symptoms of OSAS, clinicians should perform a more focused evaluation. (Evidence Quality: Grade B; Recommendation Strength: Recommendation.)

Key Action Statement 2A: Polysomnography

If a child or adolescent snores on a regular basis and has any of the complaints or findings of OSAS, clinicians should either (1) obtain a polysomnogram (Evidence Quality: Grade A; Recommendation Strength: Recommendation) or (2) refer the patient to a sleep specialist or otolaryngologist for a more extensive evaluation (Evidence Quality: Grade D; Recommendation Strength: Option.)

Key Action Statement 2B: Alternative Testing

If polysomnography is not available, clinicians may order alternative diagnostic tests, such as nocturnal video recording, nocturnal oximetry, daytime nap polysomnography, or ambulatory polysomnography. (Evidence Quality: Grade C; Recommendation Strength: Option.)

Key Action Statement 3: Adenotonsillectomy

If a child is determined to have OSAS, has a clinical examination consistent with adenotonsillar hypertrophy, and does not have a contraindication to surgery, the clinician should recommend adenotonsillectomy as the first line of treatment. If the child has OSAS but does not have adenotonsillar hypertrophy, other treatment should be considered (see Key Action Statement 6). Clinical judgment is required to determine the benefits of adenotonsillectomy compared with other treatments in obese children with varying degrees of adenotonsillar hypertrophy. (Evidence Quality: Grade B; Recommendation Strength: Recommendation.)

Key Action Statement 4: High-Risk Patients Undergoing Adenotonsillectomy

Clinicians should monitor high-risk patients undergoing adenotonsillectomy as inpatients postoperatively. (Evidence Quality: Grade B; Recommendation Strength: Recommendation.)

Key Action Statement 5: Reevaluation

Clinicians should clinically reassess all patients with OSAS for persisting signs and symptoms after therapy to determine whether further treatment is required. (Evidence Quality: Grade B; Recommendation Strength: Recommendation.)

Key Action Statement 5B: Reevaluation of High-Risk Patients

Clinicians should reevaluate high-risk patients for persistent OSAS after adenotonsillectomy, including those who had a significantly abnormal baseline polysomnogram, have sequelae of OSAS, are obese, or remain symptomatic after treatment, with an objective test (see Key Action Statement 2), or refer such patients to a sleep specialist. (Evidence Quality: Grade B; Recommendation Strength: Recommendation.)

Key Action Statement 6: Continuous Positive Airway Pressure (CPAP)

Clinicians should refer patients for CPAP management if symptoms/signs or objective evidence of OSAS persists after adenotonsillectomy or if adenotonsillectomy is not performed. (Evidence Quality: Grade B; Recommendation Strength: Recommendation.)

Key Action Statement 7: Weight Loss

Clinicians should recommend weight loss in addition to other therapy if a child/adolescent with OSAS is overweight or obese. (Evidence Quality: Grade C; Recommendation Strength: Recommendation.)

Key Action Statement 8: Intranasal Corticosteroids

Clinicians may prescribe topical intranasal corticosteroids for children with mild OSAS in whom adenotonsillectomy is contraindicated or for children with mild postoperative OSAS. (Evidence Quality: Grade B; Recommendation Strength: Option.)

Adapted from Marcus CL, Brooks LJ, Draper KA, et al: Diagnosis and management of childhood obstructive sleep apnea syndrome. *Pediatrics* 130:576–584, 2012.

healthy children with OSAS appear normal; however, certain physical examination findings may suggest OSAS. Growth parameters may be abnormal (obesity, or less frequently, failure to thrive), and there may be evidence of chronic nasal obstruction (hyponasal speech, mouth breathing, septal deviation, "adenoidal facies") as well as signs of atopic disease (i.e., "allergic shiners"). Oropharyngeal examination may reveal enlarged tonsils, excess soft tissue in the posterior pharynx, and a narrowed posterior pharyngeal space, as well as dental features consistent with obstruction (e.g., teeth crowding, narrow palate, short frenulum). Any abnormalities of head position, such as forward head posture, and facial structure, such as retrognathia, micrognathia, and midfacial hypoplasia, best appreciated by inspection of the lateral facial profile, increase the likelihood of OSAS and should be noted. In severe cases the child may have evidence of pulmonary hypertension, right-sided heart failure, and cor pulmonale; systemic hypertension may occur, especially in obese children.

Because no combination of clinical history and physical findings can accurately predict which children with snoring have OSAS, the gold standard for diagnosing OSAS remains an in-lab overnight **polysomnogram (PSG)**. Overnight PSG is a technician-supervised, monitored study that documents physiologic variables during sleep; sleep staging, arousal measurement, cardiovascular parameters, and body movements (electroencephalography, electrooculography, chin and leg electromyography, electrocardiogram, body position sensors, and video recording), and a combination of breathing monitors (oronasal thermal sensor and nasal air pressure transducer for airflow), chest/abdominal monitors (e.g., inductance plethysmography for respiratory effort, pulse oximeter for O_2 saturation, end-tidal or transcutaneous CO_2 for CO_2 retention, snore microphone). The PSG parameter most often used in evaluating for sleep-disordered breathing is the **apnea-hypopnea index (AHI)**, which indicates the number of apneic and hypopneic (both obstructive and central) events per hour of sleep. Currently, there are no universally accepted PSG normal reference values or parameters for diagnosing OSAS in children, and it is still unclear which parameters best predict morbidity. Normal preschool and school-age children generally have a total AHI <1.5 (obstructive AHI <1), and this is the most widely used cutoff value for OSA in children ≤12 yr old; in older adolescents the adult cutoff of an AHI ≥5 is generally used. When AHI is between 1 and 5 obstructive events per hour, assessment of additional PSG parameters (e.g., elevated CO_2 indicating obstructive hypoventilation, O_2 desaturation, respiratory-related arousals), clinical judgment regarding risk factors for SRBD, presence and severity of clinical symptoms, and evidence of daytime sequelae should determine further management.

Treatment

At present, no universally accepted guidelines exist regarding the indications for treatment of pediatric SRBD, including primary snoring and OSAS. Current recommendations largely emphasize weighing what is known about the potential cardiovascular, metabolic, and neurocognitive sequelae of SRBD in children in combination with the individual healthcare professional's clinical judgment. The decision of whether and how to treat OSAS specifically in children depends on several parameters, including severity (nocturnal symptoms, daytime sequelae, sleep study results), duration of disease, and individual patient variables such as age, comorbid conditions, and underlying etiologic factors. In the case of moderate (AHI 5-10) to severe (AHI >10) disease, the decision to treat is usually straightforward, and most pediatric sleep experts recommend that any child with AHI >5 should be treated. However, a large randomized trial of early adenotonsillectomy vs watchful waiting with supportive care demonstrated that 46% of the control group children normalized on PSG (vs 79% of early adenotonsillectomy group) during the 7 mo observation period.

In the majority of cases of pediatric OSAS, adenotonsillectomy is the first-line treatment in any child with significant adenotonsillar hypertrophy, even in the presence of additional risk factors such as obesity. Adenotonsillectomy in uncomplicated cases generally (70–90% of children) results in complete resolution of symptoms; regrowth of adenoidal tissue after surgical removal occurs in some cases. Groups considered at high risk include young children (<3 yr) as well as those with severe OSAS documented by PSG, significant clinical sequelae of OSAS (e.g., failure to thrive), or associated medical conditions, such as craniofacial syndromes, morbid obesity, and hypotonia. All patients should be reevaluated postoperatively to determine whether additional evaluation, a repeat PSG, and treatment are required. The American Academy of Sleep Medicine recommends that in high-risk groups (children with obesity, craniofacial anomalies, Down syndrome, or moderate-severe OSAS) or in children with continued symptoms of OSAS, a follow-up sleep study about 6 wk after adenotonsillectomy is indicated. Also, a number of studies have suggested that children who are underweight, normal weight, or overweight/obese at baseline all tend to *gain weight* after AT, and thus clinical vigilance is required during follow-up.

Additional treatment measures that may be appropriate include weight loss, **positional therapy** (attaching a firm object, such as a tennis ball, to the back of a sleep garment to prevent the child from sleeping in the supine position) and aggressive treatment of additional risk factors when present, such as asthma, seasonal allergies, and gastroesophageal reflux. Evidence suggests that intranasal corticosteroids and leukotriene inhibitors may be helpful in reducing upper airway inflammation in mild OSAS. Other surgical procedures (e.g., uvulopharyngopalatoplasty) and maxillofacial surgery (e.g., mandibular distraction osteogenesis) are seldom performed in children. Oral appliances, such as mandibular advancing devices and palatal expanders, may be considered in select cases; consultation with a pediatric dentist or orthodontist is recommended. Neuromuscular reeducation or repatterning of the oral and facial muscles with exercises to address abnormal tongue position and low upper airway tone (i.e., **myofunctional therapy**) have been shown to be beneficial in addressing pediatric OSAS as well as alleviating chewing and swallowing problems in children able to cooperate with the behavioral program.

Continuous or **bilevel positive airway pressure (CPAP** or **BiPAP)** is the most common treatment for OSAS in adults and can be used successfully in children and adolescents. Positive airway pressure (PAP) may be recommended if removing the adenoids and tonsils is not indicated, if there is residual disease following adenotonsillectomy, or if there are major risk factors not amenable to surgery (obesity, hypotonia). PAP delivers humidified, warmed air through an interface (mask, nasal pillows) that, under pressure, effectively "splints" the upper airway open. Optimal pressure settings (that abolish or significantly reduce respiratory events without increasing arousals or central apneas) are determined in the sleep lab during a full-night PAP titration. Careful attention should be paid to education of the child and family, and desensitization protocols should usually be implemented to increase the likelihood of adherence. Efficacy studies at the current pressure and retitrations should be conducted periodically with long-term use (at least annually) or in association with significant weight changes or resurgence of SRBD symptoms.

Parasomnias

Parasomnias are episodic nocturnal behaviors that often involve cognitive disorientation and autonomic and skeletal muscle disturbance. Parasomnias may be further characterized as occurring primarily during non-REM sleep (partial arousal parasomnias) or in association with REM sleep, including nightmares, hypnogogic hallucinations, and sleep paralysis; other common parasomnias include sleep-talking and hypnic jerks or "sleep starts."

Etiology

Partial arousal parasomnias represent a dissociated sleep–wake state, the neurobiology of which remains unclear, although genetic factors and an intrinsic oscillation of subcortical-cortical arousal with sleep have been proposed. These episodic events, which include sleepwalking, sleep terrors, and confusional arousals, are more common in preschool and school-age children because of the relatively higher percentage of SWS in younger children. Partial arousal parasomnias typically occur when SWS predominates, in the 1st third of the night. In contrast, **nightmares**, which are much more common than partial arousal parasomnias but are often confused with them, tend to be concentrated in the last third of the night, when REM sleep is most prominent. Any factor associated with an increase in the relative percentage of SWS (certain medications, previous sleep restriction) may increase the frequency of events in a predisposed child. There appears to be a genetic predisposition for both sleepwalking and night terrors. Partial arousal parasomnias may also be difficult to distinguish from nocturnal seizures. Table 31.6 summarizes similarities and differences among these nocturnal arousal events.

Epidemiology

Many children sleepwalk on at least one occasion; the lifetime prevalence by age 10 yr is 13%. **Sleepwalking** (somnambulism) may persist into adulthood, with the prevalence in adults of approximately 4%. The prevalence is approximately 10 times greater in children with a family history of sleepwalking. The peak prevalence of **sleep terrors** is 34% at age 1-5 yr, decreasing to 10% by age 7; the age at onset is usually between 4 and 12 yr. Because of the common genetic predisposition, the likelihood of developing sleepwalking after age 5 is almost 2-fold higher in children with a history of sleep terrors. Although sleep terrors can occur at any age from infancy through adulthood, most individuals outgrow sleep terrors by adolescence. **Confusional arousals** (sleep drunkenness, sleep inertia) usually occur with sleepwalking and sleep terrors; prevalence rates have been estimated at >15% in children age 3-13 yr.

Clinical Manifestations

The partial arousal parasomnias have several features in common. Because they typically occur at the transition out of "deep" sleep or SWS, partial arousal parasomnias have clinical features of both the *awake* (ambulation, vocalizations) and the *sleeping* (high arousal threshold, unresponsiveness to environment) states, usually with amnesia for the events. External (noise) or internal (obstruction) factors may trigger events in some individuals. The duration is typically a few minutes (sleep terrors) up to 30-40 min (confusional arousals). Sleep terrors are sudden in onset and characteristically involve a high degree of autonomic arousal (tachycardia, dilated pupils). Confusional arousals typically arise more gradually from sleep, may involve thrashing around but usually not displacement from bed, and are often accompanied by slow mentation, disorientation, and confusion on forced arousal from SWS or on waking in the morning. Sleepwalking may be associated with safety concerns (e.g., falling out of windows, wandering outside). The child's avoidance of, or increased agitation with, comforting by parents or attempts at awakening is also common to all partial arousal parasomnias.

Table 31.6	Key Similarities and Differentiating Features Between Non-REM and REM Parasomnias as Well as Nocturnal Seizures				
	CONFUSIONAL AROUSALS	**SLEEP TERRORS**	**SLEEPWALKING**	**NIGHTMARES**	**NOCTURNAL SEIZURES**
Time	Early	Early	Early-mid	Late	Any
Sleep stage	SWA	SWA	SWA	REM	Any
EEG discharges	–	–	–	–	+
Scream	–	++++	–	++	+
Autonomic activation	+	++++	+	+	+
Motor activity	–	+	+++	+	++++
Awakens	–	–	–	+	+
Duration (min)	0.5-10; more gradual offset	1-10; more gradual offset	2-30; more gradual offset	3-20	5-15; abrupt onset and offset
Postevent confusion	+	+	+	–	+
Age	Child	Child	Child	Child, young adult	Adolescent, young adult
Genetics	+	+	+	–	±
Organic CNS lesion	–	–	–	–	++++

CNS, Central nervous system; EEG, electroencephalogram; REM, rapid eye movement; SWA, slow-wave arousal.
From Avidan A, Kaplish N: The parasomnias: epidemiology, clinical features and diagnostic approach. *Clin Chest Med* 31:353–370, 2010.

Treatment

Management of partial arousal parasomnias involves some combination of parental education and reassurance, healthy sleep practices, and avoidance of exacerbating factors such as sleep restriction and caffeine. Particularly in the case of sleepwalking, it is important to institute safety precautions such as use of gates in doorways and at the top of staircases, locking of outside doors and windows, and installation of parent notification systems such as bedroom door alarms. **Scheduled awakenings** is a behavioral intervention that involves having the parent wake the child 15-30 min before the time of night that the 1st parasomnia episode occurs and is most likely to be successful in situations where partial arousal episodes occur on a nightly basis. Pharmacotherapy is rarely necessary but may be indicated in cases of frequent or severe episodes, high risk of injury, violent behavior, or serious disruption to the family. The primary pharmacologic agents used are potent SWS suppressants, primarily benzodiazepines and tricyclic antidepressants.

Sleep-Related Movement Disorders: Restless Legs Syndrome/Periodic Limb Movement Disorder and Rhythmic Movements

Restless legs syndrome (**RLS**), also termed *Willis-Ekbom disease*, is a chronic neurologic disorder characterized by an almost irresistible urge to move the legs, often accompanied by uncomfortable sensations in the lower extremities. Both the urge to move and the sensations are usually worse at rest and in the evening and are at least partially relieved by movement, including walking, stretching, and rubbing, but only if the motion continues. RLS is a clinical diagnosis that is based on the presence of these key symptoms (Table 31.7).

Periodic limb movement disorder (**PLMD**) is characterized by periodic, repetitive, brief (0.5-10 sec), and highly stereotyped limb jerks typically occurring at 20-40 sec intervals. These movements occur primarily during sleep, usually occur in the legs, and frequently consist of rhythmic extension of the big toe and dorsiflexion at the ankle. The diagnosis of **periodic limb movements (PLMs)** requires overnight PSG to document the characteristic limb movements with anterior tibialis electromyography leads.

Etiology

"Early-onset" RLS (onset of symptoms before 35-40 yr of age), often termed *primary* RLS, appears to have a particularly strong genetic component, with a 6-7–fold increase in prevalence in first-degree relatives

Table 31.7	Diagnostic Criteria for Restless Legs Syndrome

A. An urge to move legs, usually accompanied by or in response to uncomfortable and unpleasant sensations in the legs, characterized by the following:
  1. The urge to move the legs begins or worsens during periods of rest or inactivity.
  2. The urge to move the legs is partially or totally relieved by movement.
  3. The urge to move the legs is worse in the evening or at night than during the day, or occurs only in the evening or at night.
B. The symptoms in Criterion A occur at least three times per week and have persisted for at least 3 months.
C. The symptoms in Criterion A are accompanied by significant distress or impairment in social, occupational, educational, academic, behavioral, or other important areas of functioning.
D. The symptoms in Criterion A are not attributable to another mental disorder or medical condition (e.g., arthritis, leg edema, peripheral ischemia, leg cramps) and are not better explained by a behavioral condition (e.g., positional discomfort, habitual foot tapping).
E. The symptoms are not attributable to the physiological effects of a drug or abuse or medication (e.g., akathisia).

From American Psychiatric Association: *Diagnostic and Statistical Manual of Mental Disorders*, 5th ed, 2013, p 410.

of RLS patients. The mode of inheritance is complex, and several genetic loci have been identified (*MEIS1, BTBD9, MAP2K5*). Low serum iron levels (even without anemia) in both adults and children may be an important etiologic factor for the presence and severity of both RLS symptoms and PLMs. As a marker of decreased iron stores, serum ferritin levels in both children and adults with RLS are frequently low; (<50 μg/mL). The postulated underlying mechanism is related to the role of iron as a cofactor in tyrosine hydroxylation, a rate-limiting step in dopamine synthesis; in turn, dopaminergic dysfunction has been implicated, particularly in the genesis of the sensory component of RLS, as well as in PLMD. Certain medical conditions, including diabetes mellitus, end-stage renal disease, cancer, idiopathic juvenile arthritis, hypothyroidism, and pregnancy, may also be associated with RLS/PLMD, as are specific medications (e.g., antihistamines such as diphenhydramine, antidepressants, H_2 blockers such as cimetidine) and substances (notably, caffeine).

Epidemiology
Previous studies found prevalence rates of RLS in the pediatric population ranging from 1–6%; approximately 2% of 8-17 yr olds meet the criteria for "definite" RLS. Prevalence rates of PLMs >5 per hour in clinical populations of children referred for sleep studies range from 5–27%; in survey studies of PLM symptoms, rates are 8–12%. About 40% of adults with RLS have symptoms before age 20 yr; 20% report symptoms before age 10. Familial cases usually have a younger age of onset. Several studies in referral populations have found that PLMs occur in as many as 25% of children diagnosed with ADHD.

Clinical Manifestations
In addition to the urge to move the legs and the sensory component (paresthesia-like, tingling, burning, itching, crawling), most RLS episodes are initiated or exacerbated by rest or inactivity, such as lying in bed to fall asleep or riding in a car for prolonged periods. A unique feature of RLS is that the timing of symptoms also appears to have a circadian component, in that they often peak in the evening hours. Some children may complain of "growing pains," although this is considered a nonspecific feature. Because RLS symptoms are usually worse in the evening, bedtime struggles and difficulty falling asleep are two of the most common presenting complaints. In contrast to patients with RLS, individuals with PLMs are usually unaware of these movements, but children may complain of morning muscle pain or fatigue; these movements may result in arousals during sleep and consequent significant sleep disruption. Parents of children with RLS/PLMD may report that their child is a restless sleeper, moves around, or even falls out of bed during the night.

The differential diagnosis includes growing pains, leg cramps, neuropathy, arthritis, myalgias, nerve compression ("leg fell asleep"), and dopamine antagonist–associated akathisia.

Treatment
The decision of whether and how to treat RLS depends on the level of severity (intensity, frequency, and periodicity) of sensory symptoms, the degree of interference with sleep, and the impact of daytime sequelae in a particular child or adolescent. With PLMs, for an index (PLMs/hr) <5, usually no treatment is recommended; for an index >5, the decision to specifically treat PLMs should be based on the presence or absence of nocturnal symptoms (restless or nonrestorative sleep) and daytime clinical sequelae.

The acronym **AIMS** represents a comprehensive approach to the treatment of RLS: **avoidance** of exacerbating factors, such as caffeine and drugs, that increase symptoms; **iron** supplementation when appropriate; **muscle** activity, with increased physical activity, muscle relaxation, and application of heat/cold compresses; and **sleep**, with a regular sleep schedule and sufficient sleep for age. Iron supplements should be instituted if serum ferritin levels are <50 μg/L; it should be kept in mind that ferritin is an acute-phase reactant and thus may be falsely elevated (i.e., normal) in the setting of a concomitant illness. The recommended dose of oral ferrous sulfate is typically 3-6 mg/kg/day for 3 mo. If there is no response to oral iron, intravenous iron compounds may be needed. Medications that increase dopamine levels in the CNS, such as ropinirole and pramipexole, are effective in relieving RLS/PLMD symptoms in adults; data in children are extremely limited. Dopaminergic therapy may lead to a loss of therapeutic response. Some recommend gabapentin enacarbil or other related alpha-2 delta ligands that bind to the alpha-2 delta subunit of the voltage-activated calcium channel.

Sleep-related rhythmic movements, including head banging, body rocking, and head rolling, are characterized by repetitive, stereotyped, and rhythmic movements or behaviors that involve large muscle groups. These behaviors typically occur with the transition to sleep at bedtime, but also at nap times and after nighttime arousals. Children typically engage in these behaviors as a means of soothing themselves to (or back to) sleep; these are much more common in the 1st yr of life and usually disappear by preschool age. In most cases, rhythmic movement behaviors are benign, because sleep is not significantly disrupted, and associated significant injury is rare. These behaviors typically occur in normally developing children and in the majority of cases do not indicate some underlying neurologic or psychologic problem. Usually, the most important aspect in management of sleep-related rhythmic movements is reassurance to the family that this behavior is normal, common, benign, and self-limited.

Narcolepsy
Hypersomnia is a clinical term that is used to describe a group of disorders characterized by recurrent episodes of **excessive daytime sleepiness (EDS)**, reduced baseline alertness, and/or prolonged nighttime sleep periods that interfere with normal daily functioning (Table 31.8). The many potential causes of EDS can be broadly grouped as "extrinsic" (e.g., secondary to insufficient and/or fragmented sleep) or "intrinsic" (e.g., resulting from an increased need for sleep). **Narcolepsy** is a chronic, lifelong CNS disorder, typically presenting in adolescence and early adulthood, characterized by profound daytime sleepiness resulting in significant functional impairment. More than half of patients with narcolepsy also present with **cataplexy** (type 1), defined as the sudden, brief, partial or complete loss of skeletal muscle tone, typically triggered by strong emotion (e.g., laughter, surprise, anger), with retained consciousness. Other symptoms frequently associated with narcolepsy, including hypnogogic/hypnopompic (immediately before falling asleep/awakening) typically visual hallucinations and sleep paralysis, may be conceptualized as representing the "intrusion" of REM sleep features into the waking state. Other REM-related features include observance of eye movements and twitches at sleep onset and vivid dreams. Rapid weight gain, especially near symptom onset, is frequently observed, and young children with narcolepsy have been reported to develop precocious puberty.

Etiology
The genesis of narcolepsy with cataplexy (type 1) is thought to be related to a specific deficit in the hypothalamic orexin/hypocretin neurotransmitter system involving the selective loss of cells that secrete hypocretin/orexin in the lateral hypothalamus. *Hypocretin* neurons stimulate a range of wake-promoting neurons in the brainstem, hypothalamus, and cortex and basal forebrain that produce neurochemicals to sustain the wake state and prevent lapses into sleep.

The development of narcolepsy most likely involves autoimmune mechanisms, possibly triggered by streptococcal, influenza virus, H1N1, and other viral infections, likely in combination with a genetic predisposition and environmental factors. A 12-13–fold increase in narcolepsy type 1 cases, especially in children, was reported in parts of Europe in 2009–2010 following immunization with the AS03 adjuvanted H1N1 influenza vaccine. Human leukocyte antigen testing also shows a strong association with narcolepsy; the majority of individuals with this antigen do not have narcolepsy, but most (>90%) patients with narcolepsy with cataplexy are HLA-DQB1*0602–positive. Patients with narcolepsy without cataplexy (type 2) are increasingly thought to have a significantly different pathophysiology; they are much less likely to be HLA-DQB1*0602–positive (4–50%), and cerebrospinal fluid (CSF) hypocretin levels are normal in most patients.

Although the majority of cases of narcolepsy are considered idiopathic (autoimmune), secondary narcolepsy can be caused by lesions to the posterior hypothalamus induced by traumatic brain injury, tumor, stroke, and neuroinflammatory processes such as post-streptococcal PANDAS (see Chapter 210), as well as by neurogenetic diseases such as Prader-Willi syndrome (Chapter 98.8), Niemann-Pick type C (Chapter 104.4), myotonic dystrophy (Chapter 627.6), and Norrie disease.

Epidemiology
Narcolepsy is a rare disorder with a prevalence of approximately 0.025–0.05%. The risk of developing narcolepsy with cataplexy in a first-degree relative of a narcoleptic patient is estimated at 1–2%. This represents an increase of 10-40–fold compared to the general population, but the risk remains very low, reinforcing the likely role for other etiologic factors.

Table 31.8	Diagnostic Criteria for Narcolepsy

A. Recurrent periods of an irrepressible need to sleep, lapsing into sleep, or napping occurring within the same day. These must have been occurring at least three times per week over the past 3 months.
B. The presence of at least one of the following:
1. Episodes of cataplexy, defined as either (a) or (b), occurring at least a few time per month:
    a. In individuals with long-standing disease, brief (seconds to minutes) episodes of sudden bilateral loss of muscle tone with maintained consciousness that are precipitated by laughter or joking.
    b. In children or individuals within 6 months of onset, spontaneous grimaces or jaw-opening episodes with tongue thrusting or a global hypotonia, without any obvious emotional triggers.
2. Hypocretin deficiency, as measured using cerebrospinal fluid (CSF) hypocretin-1 immunoreactivity values (less than or equal to one-third of values obtained in healthy subjects tested using the same assay, or less than or equal to 110 pg/mL). Low CSF levels of hypocretin-1 must not be observed in the context of acute brain injury, inflammation, or infection.
3. Nocturnal sleep polysomnography showing rapid eye movement (REM) sleep latency less than or equal to 15 minutes, or a multiple sleep latency test showing a mean sleep latency less than or equal to 8 minutes and two or more sleep-onset REM periods.
Specify whether:
Narcolepsy without cataplexy but with hypocretin deficiency: Criterion B requirements of low CSF hypocretin-1 levels and positive polysomnography/multiple sleep latency test are met, but no cataplexy is present (Criterion B1 not met).
Narcolepsy with cataplexy but without hypocretin deficiency: In this rare sub-type (less than 5% of narcolepsy cases), Criterion B requirements of cataplexy and positive polysomnography/ multiple sleep latency test are met, but CSF hypocretin-1 levels are normal (Criterion B2 not met).
Autosomal dominant cerebellar ataxia, deafness, and narcolepsy: This sub-type is caused by exon 21 DNA (cytosine-5)-methyltransferase-1 mutations and is characterized by late-onset (age 30-40 years) narcolepsy (with low or intermediate CSF hypocretin-1 levels), deafness, cerebellar ataxia, and eventually dementia.
Autosomal dominant narcolepsy, obesity, and type 2 diabetes: Narcolepsy, obesity, and type 2 diabetes are low CSF hypocretin-1 levels have been described in rare cases and are associated with a mutation in the myelin oligodendrocyte glycoprotein gene.
Narcolepsy without cataplexy but with hypocretin deficiency: This sub-type is for narcolepsy that develops secondary to medical conditions that cause infectious (e.g., Whipple's disease, sarcoidosis), traumatic, or tumoral destruction of hypocretin neurons.
Severity:
Mild: Infrequent cataplexy (less than once per week), need for naps only once or twice per day, and less disturbed nocturnal sleep.
Moderate: Cataplexy once daily or every few days, disturbed nocturnal sleep and need for multiple naps daily.
Severe: Drug-resistant cataplexy with multiple attacks daily, nearly constant sleepiness, and disturbed nocturnal sleep (i.e., movements, insomnia, and vivid dreaming).

From American Psychiatric Association: *Diagnostic and Statistical Manual of Mental Disorders*, 5th ed, 2013, pp 372–373.

Clinical Manifestations and Diagnosis

The typical onset of symptoms of narcolepsy is in adolescence and early adulthood, although symptoms may initially present in school-age and even younger children. The early manifestations of narcolepsy are often ignored, misinterpreted, or misdiagnosed as other medical, neurologic, or psychiatric conditions, and the appropriate diagnosis is frequently delayed for years. The onset may be abrupt or slowly progressive.

The most prominent clinical manifestation of narcolepsy is profound daytime sleepiness, characterized by both an increased baseline level of daytime drowsiness and the repeated occurrence of sudden and unpredictable sleep episodes. These "sleep attacks" are often described as "irresistible," in that the child or adolescent is unable to stay awake despite considerable effort, and occur even in the context of normally stimulating activities (e.g., during meals, in conversation). Very brief (several seconds) sleep attacks may also occur in which the individual may "stare off," appear unresponsive, or continue to engage in an ongoing activity (*automatic behavior*). EDS may also be manifested by increased nighttime sleep needs and extreme difficulty waking in the morning or after a nap.

Cataplexy is considered virtually pathognomonic for narcolepsy but can develop several years after the onset of EDS. Manifestations are triggered by strong positive (laughing, joy) or negative (fright, anger, frustration) emotions and predominantly include facial slackening, head nodding, jaw dropping, and less often, knees buckling or complete collapse with falling to the ground. The cataplectic attacks are typically brief (seconds to minutes), the patient is awake and aware, and episodes are fully reversible, with complete recovery of normal tone when the episode ends. A form of cataplexy unique to children known as **cataplectic facies** is characterized by prolonged tongue protrusion, ptosis, slack jaw, slurred speech, grimacing, and gait instability. Additionally, children may have positive motor phenomenon similar to dyskinesias or motor tics, with repetitive grimacing and tongue thrusting. The cataplectic attacks are typically brief (seconds to minutes) but in children may last for hours or days (**status cataplecticus**).

Hypnogogic/hypnopompic hallucinations usually involve vivid visual but also auditory and sometimes tactile sensory experiences during transitions between sleep and wakefulness, either at sleep offset (hypnopompic) or sleep onset (hypnogogic). **Sleep paralysis** is the inability to move or speak for a few seconds or minutes at sleep onset or offset and often accompanies the hallucinations. Other symptoms associated with narcolepsy include disrupted nocturnal sleep, impaired cognition, inattention and ADHD-like symptoms, and behavioral and mood dysregulation.

Several pediatric screening questionnaires for EDS, including the modified Epworth Sleepiness Scale, help to guide the need for further evaluation in clinical practice when faced with the presenting complaint of daytime sleepiness. Physical examination should include a detailed neurologic assessment. Overnight PSG and a multiple sleep latency test (MSLT) are strongly recommended components in the evaluation of a patient with profound unexplained daytime sleepiness or suspected narcolepsy. The purpose of the overnight PSG is to evaluate for primary sleep disorders (e.g., OSAS) that may cause EDS. The MSLT involves a series of 5 opportunities to nap (20 min long), during which patients with narcolepsy demonstrate a pathologically shortened mean sleep-onset latency (≤8 min, typically <5 min) as well as at least 2 periods of REM sleep occurring immediately after sleep onset. Alternatively, a diagnosis can be made by findings of low CSF hypocretin-1 concentration (typically ≤110 pg/mL) with a standardized assay.

Treatment

An individualized narcolepsy treatment plan usually involves education, good sleep hygiene, behavioral changes, and medication. Scheduled naps during the day are often helpful. Wake-promoting medications such as modafinil or armodafinil may be prescribed to control the EDS, although they are not approved for use in children by the U.S. Food and Drug Administration (FDA), and potential side effects include rare reports of Stevens-Johnson syndrome and reduced efficacy of hormone-based contraceptives. Psychostimulants are approved for ADHD in children and can be used for EDS; side effects include appetite suppression, mood lability, and cardiovascular effects. Antidepressants (serotonin reuptake inhibitors, venlafaxine) may be used to reduce cataplexy. Sodium oxybate, also not currently FDA-approved for use in children, is a unique drug that appears to have a positive impact on daytime sleepiness, cataplexy, and nocturnal sleep disruption; reported side effects include dizziness, weight loss, enuresis, exacerbation of OSAS, depression, and risk of respiratory depression, especially when combined with CNS depressants, including alcohol. Pitolisant, a histamine (H_3) receptor agonist, has been shown to improve cataplexy and EDS in adult patients with narcolepsy. The goal for the child should be to allow the fullest possible return of normal functioning in school, at home, and in social situations.

Delayed Sleep–Wake Phase Disorder

Delayed sleep–wake phase disorder (**DSWPD**), a circadian rhythm disorder, involves a significant, persistent, and intractable phase shift in sleep–wake schedule (later sleep onset and wake time) that conflicts with the individual's normal school, work, and lifestyle demands. DSWPD may occur at any age but is most common in adolescents and young adults.

Etiology

Individuals with DSPD may start out as "night owls"; that is, they have an underlying predisposition or circadian "eveningness" preference for staying up late at night and sleeping late in the morning, especially on weekends, holidays, and summer vacations. The underlying pathophysiology of DSWPD is still unknown, although some theorize that it involves an intrinsic abnormality in the circadian oscillators that govern the timing of the sleep period.

Epidemiology

Studies indicate that the prevalence of DSWPD may be as high as 7–16% in adolescents and young adults.

Clinical Manifestations

The most common clinical presentation is sleep-initiation insomnia when the individual attempts to fall asleep at a "socially acceptable" desired bedtime and experiences very delayed sleep onset (often after 1-2 AM), accompanied by daytime sleepiness. Patients may have extreme difficulty arising in the morning even for desired activities, with pronounced confusion on waking (*sleep inertia*). Sleep maintenance is generally not problematic, and no sleep-onset insomnia is experienced if bedtime coincides with the preferred sleep-onset time (e.g., on weekends, school vacations). School tardiness and frequent absenteeism with a decline in academic performance often occur. Patients may also develop "secondary" psychophysiologic insomnia as a result of spending prolonged time in bed attempting to fall asleep at bedtime.

Treatment

The treatment of DSWPD usually has three components, all directed toward the goals of shifting the sleep–wake schedule to an earlier, more desirable time and maintaining the new schedule. The initial step involves shifting the sleep–wake schedule to the desired earlier times, usually with gradual (i.e., 15-30 min increments every few days) advancement of bedtime in the evening and rise time in the morning. More significant phase delays (i.e., larger difference between current sleep onset and desired bedtime) may require *chronotherapy*, which involves delaying bedtime and wake time by 2-3 hr every 24 hr "forward around the clock" until the target bedtime is reached. Because melatonin secretion is highly sensitive to light, exposure to light in the morning (either natural light or a "light box," which typically produces light at around 10,000 lux) and avoidance of evening light exposure (especially from screens emitting predominantly blue light, such as computers and laptops) are often beneficial. Exogenous oral melatonin supplementation may also be used; larger, mildly sedating doses (5 mg) are typically given at bedtime, but some studies have suggested that physiologic doses of oral melatonin (0.3-0.5 mg) administered in the afternoon or early evening (5-7 hr before the habitual sleep-onset time) may be more effective in advancing the sleep phase.

HEALTH SUPERVISION

It is especially important for pediatricians to screen for and recognize sleep disorders in children and adolescents during healthcare encounters. The well-child visit is an opportunity to educate parents about normal sleep in children and to teach strategies to prevent sleep problems from developing (primary prevention) or becoming chronic, if problems already exist (secondary prevention). Developmentally appropriate screening for sleep disturbances should take place in the context of every well-child visit and should include a range of potential sleep problems; Table 31.9 outlines a simple sleep screening algorithm, the

Table 31.9	BEARS Sleep Screening Algorithm

The BEARS instrument is divided into 5 major sleep domains, providing a comprehensive screen for the major sleep disorders affecting children 2-18 yr old. Each sleep domain has a set of age-appropriate "trigger questions" for use in the clinical interview.
B = Bedtime problems
E = Excessive daytime sleepiness
A = Awakenings during the night
R = Regularity and duration of sleep
S = Snoring

	EXAMPLES OF DEVELOPMENTALLY APPROPRIATE TRIGGER QUESTIONS		
	Toddler/Preschool Child (2-5 yr)	**School-Age Child (6-12 yr)**	**Adolescent (13-18 yr)**
1. Bedtime problems	Does your child have any problems going to bed? Falling asleep?	Does your child have any problems at bedtime? (P) Do you any problems going to bed? (C)	Do you have any problems falling asleep at bedtime? (C)
2. Excessive daytime sleepiness	Does your child seem overtired or sleepy a lot during the day? Does your child still take naps?	Does your child have difficulty waking in the morning, seem sleepy during the day, or take naps? (P) Do you feel tired a lot? (C)	Do you feel sleepy a lot during the day? In school? While driving? (C)
3. Awakenings during the night	Does your child wake up a lot at night?	Does your child seem to wake up a lot at night? Any sleepwalking or nightmares? (P) Do you wake up a lot at night? Do you have trouble getting back to sleep? (C)	Do you wake up a lot at night? Do you have trouble getting back to sleep? (C)
4. Regularity and duration of sleep	Does your child have a regular bedtime and wake time? What are they?	What time does your child go to bed and get up on school days? Weekends? Do you think your child is getting enough sleep? (P)	What time do you usually go to bed on school nights? Weekends? How much sleep do you usually get? (C)
5. Snoring	Does your child snore a lot or have difficulty breathing at night?	Does your child have loud or nightly snoring or any breathing difficulties at night? (P)	Does your teenager snore loudly or nightly? (P)

C, Child; P, parent.

"BEARS." Because parents may not always be aware of sleep problems, especially in older children and adolescents, it is also important to question the child directly about sleep concerns. The recognition and evaluation of sleep problems in children require both an understanding of the association between sleep disturbances and daytime consequences (e.g., irritability, inattention, poor impulse control) and familiarity with the developmentally appropriate differential diagnoses of common presenting sleep complaints (difficulty initiating and maintaining sleep, episodic nocturnal events). An assessment of sleep patterns and possible sleep problems should be part of the initial evaluation of every child presenting with behavioral or academic problems, especially ADHD.

Effective preventive measures include educating parents of newborns about normal sleep amounts and patterns. The ability to regulate sleep, or control internal states of arousal to fall asleep at bedtime and to fall back asleep during the night, begins to develop in the 1st 8-12 wk of life. Thus it is important to recommend that parents put their 2-4 mo old infants to bed "drowsy but awake" if they want to avoid dependence on parental presence at sleep onset and foster the infant's ability to self-soothe. Other important sleep issues include discussing the importance of regular bedtimes, bedtime routines, and transitional objects for toddlers, and providing parents and children with basic information about healthy sleep practices, recommended sleep amounts at different ages, and signs that a child is not getting sufficient sleep (wakes with difficulty at required time in morning, sleeps longer given opportunity on weekends and vacation days).

The cultural and family context within which sleep problems in children occur should be considered. For example, bed-sharing of infants and parents is a common and accepted practice in many racial/ethnic groups, and these families may not share the goal of independent self-soothing in young infants. *Anticipatory guidance* needs to balance cultural awareness with the critical importance of "safe sleep" conditions in sudden infant death syndrome prevention (i.e., sleeping in the supine position, avoidance of bed-sharing but encouragement of room-sharing in the 1st yr of life) (see Chapter 402). On the other hand, the institution of cosleeping by parents as an attempt to address a child's underlying sleep problem (so-called reactive cosleeping), rather than as a conscious family decision, is likely to yield only a temporary respite from the problem and may set the stage for more significant sleep issues.

EVALUATION OF PEDIATRIC SLEEP PROBLEMS

The clinical evaluation of a child presenting with a sleep problem involves obtaining a careful medical history to assess for potential medical causes of sleep disturbances, such as allergies, concomitant medications, and acute or chronic pain conditions. A developmental history is important because of the increased risk of sleep problems in children with neurodevelopmental disorders. Assessment of the child's current level of functioning (school, home) is a key part of evaluating possible mood, behavioral, and neurocognitive sequelae of sleep problems. Current sleep patterns, including the usual sleep duration and sleep–wake schedule, are often best assessed with a **sleep diary,** in which a parent (or adolescent) records daily sleep behaviors for an extended period (1-2 wk). A review of sleep habits, such as bedtime routines, daily caffeine intake, and the sleeping environment (e.g., temperature, noise level), may reveal environmental factors that contribute to the sleep problems. Nocturnal symptoms that may be indicative of a medically based sleep disorder, such as OSAS (loud snoring, choking or gasping, sweating) or PLMs (restless sleep, repetitive kicking movements), should be elicited. Home video recording may be helpful in the evaluation of potential parasomnia episodes and the assessment of snoring and increased work of breathing in children with OSAS. An overnight sleep study (PSG) is not routinely warranted in the evaluation of a child with sleep problems unless there are symptoms suggestive of OSAS or PLMs, unusual features of episodic nocturnal events, or unexplained daytime sleepiness.

Bibliography is available at Expert Consult.

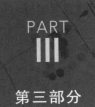

Behavioral and Psychiatric Disorders
行为和精神障碍

Chapter 32
Psychosocial Assessment and Interviewing
Heather J. Walter and David R. DeMaso

第三十二章
心理社会评估和访谈

中文导读

　　本章主要介绍了心理社会评估的目的、儿童青少年各时期出现的心理问题、心理社会访谈的一般原则、转诊指征、精神障碍诊断性评估、婴幼儿诊断评估中的特殊考虑。其中，在"心理社会访谈的一般原则"这一节中，介绍了11项心理健康行为观察指征（见原文表32.1）和用于青少年心理问题筛查的HEADSS量表（见原文表32.2），它们可用于家庭、学校、同龄人和社区人群筛查。并选择性地列举了公共卫生领域使用的心理健康评定量表（见原文表32.3）。这些可作为临床一线医师识别精神障碍早期症状的工具。

It is estimated that 20% of children living in the United States experience a mental illness in a given year, at a cost of almost $14 billion. In children, mental illness is more prevalent than leukemia, diabetes, and AIDS combined; more money is spent on mental disorders than on any other childhood illness, including asthma, trauma, and infectious diseases. Although nearly 1 in 5 youths suffers from a psychiatric disorder, 75–85% do not receive specialty mental health services. Those who do, primarily receive services in nonspecialty sectors (primary care, schools, child welfare, juvenile justice), where mental health expertise may be limited. Untreated or inadequately treated psychiatric disorders persist over decades, become increasingly intractable to treatment, impair adherence to medical treatment regimens, and incur progressively greater social, educational, and economic consequences over time.

AIMS OF ASSESSMENT
A psychosocial assessment in the pediatric setting should determine whether there are signs and symptoms of cognitive, developmental, emotional, behavioral, or social difficulties and characterize these signs and symptoms sufficiently to determine their appropriate management. The focus of the assessment varies with the nature of the presenting problem and the clinical setting. Under emergency circumstances, the focus may be limited to an assessment of "dangerousness to self or others" for the purpose of determining the safest level of care. In routine circumstances (well-child visits), the focus may be broader, involving a screen for symptoms and functional impairment in the major psychosocial domains. The challenge for the pediatric practitioner will be to determine as accurately as possible whether the presenting signs and symptoms are likely to meet criteria for a psychiatric disorder and whether the severity and complexity of the disorder suggest referral to a mental health specialist or management in the pediatric setting.

PRESENTING PROBLEMS
Infants may come to clinical attention because of problems with eating and/or sleep regulation, concerns about failure to gain weight and length, poor social responsiveness, limited vocalization, apathy or disinterest, and response to strangers that is excessively fearful or overly familiar. Psychiatric disorders most commonly diagnosed during this period are rumination and reactive attachment disorders.

　　Toddlers are assessed for concerns about sleep problems, language delay, motor hyperactivity, extreme misbehavior, extreme shyness, inflexible adherence to routines, difficulty separating from parents, struggles over toilet training, dietary issues, and testing limits. Developmental delays and more subtle physiologic, sensory, and motor processing problems can be presented as concerns. Problems with "goodness of fit" between the child's temperament and the parents' expectations can create relationship difficulties that also require assessment (see Chapter 19). Psychiatric disorders most commonly diagnosed during this period are autism spectrum disorder (ASD) and reactive attachment disorders.

Presenting problems in **preschoolers** include elimination difficulties, sibling jealousy, lack of friends, self-destructive impulsiveness, multiple fears, nightmares, refusal to follow directions, somatization, speech that is difficult to understand, and temper tantrums. Psychiatric disorders most commonly diagnosed in this period are ASD communication, oppositional, attention-deficit/hyperactivity disorder (ADHD), anxiety (separation, selective mutism), reactive attachment, gender dysphoria, and sleep disorders.

Older children are brought to clinical attention because of concerns about angry or sad mood, bedwetting, overactivity, impulsiveness, distractibility, learning problems, arguing, defiance, nightmares, school refusal, bullying or being bullied, worries and fears, somatization, communication problems, tics, and withdrawal or isolation. Psychiatric disorders most commonly diagnosed during this period are ADHD, oppositional, anxiety (generalized, phobias), elimination, somatic symptom, specific learning, and tic disorders.

Adolescents are assessed for concerns about the family situation, experimentation with sexuality and drugs, delinquency and gang involvement, friendship patterns, issues of independence, identity formation, self-esteem, and morality. Psychiatric disorders most often diagnosed during this period are anxiety (panic, social anxiety), depressive, bipolar, psychotic, obsessive-compulsive, impulse control, conduct, substance-related, and eating disorders.

GENERAL PRINCIPLES OF THE PSYCHOSOCIAL INTERVIEW

Psychosocial interviewing in the context of a routine pediatric visit requires adequate time and privacy. The purpose of this line of inquiry should be explained to the child and parents ("to make sure things are going OK at home, at school, and with friends"), along with the limits of **confidentiality**. Thereafter, the first goal of the interview is to build **rapport** with both the child and the parents (see Chapters 17 and 34 for further discussion of strategies for engaging families).

With the parents, this rapport is grounded in respect for the parents' knowledge of their child, their role as the central influence in their child's life, and their desire to make a better life for their child. Parents often feel anxious or guilty because they believe that problems in a child imply that their parenting skills are inadequate. Parents' experiences of their own childhood influence the meaning a parent places on a child's feelings and behavior. A good working alliance allows mutual discovery of the past as it is active in the present and permits potential distortions to be modified more readily. Developmentally appropriate overtures can facilitate rapport with the child. Examples include playing peek-a-boo with an infant, racing toy cars with a preschooler, commenting on sports with a child who is wearing a baseball cap, and discussing music with a teenager who is wearing a rock band T-shirt.

After an overture with the child, it is helpful to begin with **family-centered interviewing**, in which the parent is invited to present any psychosocial concerns (learning, feelings, behavior, peer relationships) about the child. With adolescent patients, it is important to conduct a separate interview to give the adolescent an opportunity to confirm or refute the parent's presentation and to present the problem from his or her perspective. Following the family's undirected presentation of the primary problem, it is important to shift to direct questioning to clarify the duration, frequency, and severity of symptoms, associated distress or functional impairment, and the developmental and environmental context in which the symptoms occur.

Because of the high degree of comorbidity of psychosocial problems in children, after eliciting the presenting problem, the pediatric practitioner should then briefly screen for problems in all the major developmentally appropriate categories of cognitive, developmental,

Table 32.1	Mental Health Action Signs

- Feeling very sad or withdrawn for more than 2 weeks
- Seriously trying to harm or kill yourself, or making plans to do so
- Sudden overwhelming fear for no reason, sometimes with a racing heart or fast breathing
- Involvement in many fights, using a weapon, or wanting to badly hurt others
- Severe out-of-control behavior that can hurt yourself or others
- Not eating, throwing up, or using laxatives to make yourself lose weight
- Intense worries or fears that get in the way of your daily activities
- Extreme difficulty in concentrating or staying still that puts you in physical danger or causes school failure
- Repeated use of drugs or alcohol
- Severe mood swings that cause problems in relationships
- Drastic changes in your behavior or personality

From The Action Signs Project, Center for the Advancement of Children's Mental Health at Columbia University.

emotional, behavioral, and social disturbance, including problems with mood, anxiety, attention, behavior, thinking and perception, substance use, social relatedness, eating, elimination, development, language, and learning. This can be preceded by a transition statement such as, "Now I'd like to ask about some other issues that I ask all parents and kids about."

A useful guide for this area of inquiry is provided by the **11 Action Signs** (Table 32.1), designed to give frontline clinicians the tools needed to recognize early symptoms of mental disorders. *Functional impairment* can be assessed by inquiring about symptoms and function in the major life domains, including home and family, school, peers, and community. These domains are included in the **HEADSS** (Home, Education, Activities, Drugs, Sexuality, Suicide/Depression) Interview Guide, often used in the screening of adolescents (Table 32.2).

The nature and severity of the presenting problem(s) can be further characterized through a standardized self-, parent-, or teacher-informant symptom rating scale; Table 32.3 lists selected scales in the public domain. A *rating scale* is a type of measure that provides a relatively rapid assessment of a specific construct with an easily derived numerical score that is readily interpreted. The use of symptom rating scales can ensure efficient, systematic coverage of relevant symptoms, quantify symptom severity, and document a baseline against which treatment effects can be measured. Functional impairment also can be assessed with self- and other-reported rating scales.

Clinical experience and methodological studies suggest that parents and teachers are more likely than the child to report externalizing problems (disruptive, impulsive, overactive, or antisocial behavior). Children may be more likely to report anxious or depressive feelings, including suicidal thoughts and acts, of which the parents may be unaware. Discrepancies across informants are common and can shed light on whether the symptoms are pervasive or contextual. Although concerns have been raised about children's competence as self-reporters (because of limitations in linguistic skills; self-reflection; emotional awareness; ability to monitor behavior, thoughts, and feelings; tendency toward social desirability), children and adolescents can be reliable and valid self-reporters.

Clinicians are encouraged to become familiar with the psychometric characteristics and appropriate use of at least 1 broad-band symptom rating scale, such as the *Strengths and Difficulties Questionnaire* (SDQ),* the *Pediatric Symptom Checklist* (PSC),† or the *Swanson, Nolan, and Pelham–IV* (SNAP-IV).‡ These measures are available in multiple languages. If the clinical interview or broad-band rating scale suggests difficulties in one or more specific symptom areas, the clinician can follow with a psychometrically sound, relevant narrow-band instrument, such as the *Vanderbilt ADHD Diagnostic Rating Scale* for attention,

---

*http://www.sdqinfo.org/py/sdqinfo/b0.py.
†http://www.brightfutures.org/mentalhealth/pdf/professionals/ped_sympton_chklst.pdf.
‡http://psychiatryassociatespc.com/doc/SNAP-IV_Parent&Teacher.pdf.

Table 32.2	HEADSS* Screening Interview for Taking a Rapid Psychosocial History

PARENT INTERVIEW

Home
- How well does the family get along with each other?

Education
- How well does your child do in school?

Activities
- What does your child like to do?
- Does your child do anything that has you really concerned?
- How does your child get along with peers?

Drugs
- Has your child used drugs or alcohol?

Sexuality
- Are there any issues regarding sexuality or sexual activity that are of concern to you?

Suicide/Depression
- Has your child ever been treated for an emotional problem?
- Has your child ever intentionally tried to hurt him/herself or made threats to others?

ADOLESCENT INTERVIEW

Home
- How do you get along with your parents?

Education
- How do you like school and your teachers?
- How well do you do in school?

Activities
- Do you have a best friend or group of good friends?
- What do you like to do?

Drugs
- Have you used drugs or alcohol?

Sexuality
- Are there any issues regarding sexuality or sexual activity that are of concern to you?

Suicide/Depression
- Everyone feels sad or angry some of the time. How about you?
- Did you ever feel so upset that you wished you were not alive or so angry you wanted to hurt someone else badly?

*HEADSS, Home, Education, Activities, Drugs, Sexuality, Suicide/Depression. From Cohen E, MacKenzie RG, Yates GL: HEADSS, a psychosocial risk assessment instrument: implications for designing effective intervention programs for runaway youth, *J Adolesc Health* 12:539–544, 1991.

behavior, and learning problems; the *Center for Epidemiological Studies Depression Scale for Children* (CES-DC), *Mood and Feelings Questionnaire* (MFQ), or *Patient Health Questionnaire-9* (PHQ-9) for depression; or the *Screen for Child Anxiety Related Emotional Disorders* (SCARED) for anxiety.

Children and adolescents scoring above standardized rating scale cutpoints in most cases should be referred to a qualified mental health professional for assessment and treatment, because scores above cutpoint are highly correlated with clinically significant psychiatric disorders. Youths scoring just below or only slightly above cutpoints (e.g., subsyndromal or mild mood, anxiety, or disruptive behavior disorders) may be appropriate for management in the pediatric primary care or subspecialty settings, as may youths scoring well above cutpoints for certain neurodevelopmental disorders (ADHD, autism spectrum, tic).

The safety of the child in the context of the home and community is of paramount importance. The interview should sensitively assess whether the child has been exposed to any frightening events, including abuse, neglect, bullying, marital discord, or domestic or community violence; whether the child shows any indication of dangerousness to self or others or a severely altered mental status (psychosis, intoxication, delirium, rage, hopelessness); or whether the child (if age appropriate) has been involved in any risky behavior, including running away, staying out without permission, truancy, gang involvement, experimentation with substances, and unprotected sexual encounters. The interview also should assess the capacity of the parents to adequately provide for the child's physical, emotional, and social needs or whether parental capacity has been diminished by psychiatric disorder, family dysfunction, or the sequelae of disadvantaged socioeconomic status. Any indications of threats to the child's safety should be immediately followed by thorough assessment and protective action.

INDICATIONS FOR REFERRAL

There is variability in the level of **confidence** pediatric practitioners perceive in diagnosing psychosocial problems in children and adolescents. Pediatric practitioners who have familiarity with psychiatric diagnostic criteria may feel confident diagnosing certain disorders, particularly the neurodevelopmental and other biologically based disorders (ADHD, ASD, tic disorders, enuresis, encopresis, insomnia, anorexia). The disorders about which some pediatric practitioners might have less diagnostic confidence include the disruptive/impulse control/conduct, depressive, bipolar, anxiety, psychotic, obsessive-compulsive, trauma-related, somatic symptom, and substance-related disorders. Pediatric practitioners should refer to a mental health practitioner whenever they experience diagnostic uncertainty with a child who has distressing or functionally impairing psychosocial symptoms. Children found to have indicators of dangerousness on initial assessment always should be immediately referred to a mental health professional.

PSYCHIATRIC DIAGNOSTIC EVALUATION

The objectives of the psychiatric diagnostic evaluation of the child and adolescent are to determine whether *psychopathology* or *developmental risk* is present and if so, to establish an explanatory formulation and a differential diagnosis, and to determine whether treatment is indicated and if so, to develop a treatment plan and facilitate the parents' and child's involvement in the plan. The aims of the diagnostic evaluation are to clarify the reasons for the referral; to obtain an accurate accounting of the child's developmental functioning and the nature and extent of the child's psychosocial difficulties, functional impairment, and subjective distress; and to identify potential individual, family, or environmental factors that might account for, influence, or ameliorate these difficulties. The issues relevant to diagnosis and treatment planning can span genetic, constitutional, and temperamental factors; individual psychodynamics; cognitive, language, and social skills; family patterns of interaction and child-rearing practices; and community, school, and socioeconomic influences.

The focus of the evaluation is *developmental*; it seeks to describe the child's functioning in various realms and to assess the child's adaptation in these areas relative to that expected for the child's age and phase of development. The developmental perspective extends beyond current difficulties to vulnerabilities that can affect future development and as such are important targets for preventive intervention. Vulnerabilities may include subthreshold or subsyndromal difficulties that, especially when manifold, often are accompanied by significant distress or impairment and as such are important as potential harbingers of future problems.

Throughout the assessment, the clinician focuses on identifying a realistic balance of vulnerabilities and strengths in the child, in the parents, and in the parent–child interactions. From this strength-based approach, over time a hopeful family narrative is co-constructed to frame the child's current developmental progress and predict the child's ongoing progress within the scope of current risk and protective factors.

Although the scope of the evaluation will vary with the clinical circumstance, the comprehensive psychiatric diagnostic evaluation has 12 major components: the presenting problem(s) and the context in which they occur; a review of psychiatric symptoms; a history of psychiatric treatment; a medical history, a developmental history; an educational history; a family history; a mental status examination; a biopsychosocial clinical formulation; a *Diagnostic and Statistical Manual*

Table 32.3	**Select List of Mental Health Rating Scales in the Public Domain**			
INSTRUMENTS	**FOR AGES (yr)**	**INFORMANT: NUMBER OF ITEMS**	**TIME TO COMPLETE (min)**	**AVAILABLE AT**
BROAD BAND				
Pediatric Symptom Checklist (PSC)	4-18	Parent: 35, 17 Youth: 35, 17	5-10	www.massgeneral.org/psychiatry/services/ psc_home.aspx
SNAP-IV Rating Scale	6-18	Parent, Teacher: 90	10	http://www.crfht.ca/files/8913/7597/8069/ SNAPIV_000.pdf
Strengths and Difficulties Questionnaire (SDQ)	4-18	Parent, Teacher, Child: 25	5	www.sdqinfo.com
NARROW BAND				
Anxiety				
Self-Report for Childhood Anxiety Related Emotional Disorders (SCARED)	8-18	Parent, Child: 41	5	http://www.pediatricbipolar.pitt.edu/ content.asp?id=2333#3304
Attention and Behavior				
Vanderbilt ADHD Diagnostic Rating Scale	6-12	Parent: 55 Teacher: 43	10	http://www.nichq.org/childrens-health/ adhd/resources/vanderbilt-assessment -scales
Autism				
Modified Checklist for Autism in Toddlers (M-CHAT)	16-30 mo	Parent: 23	5-10	https://www.m-chat.org/index.php
Depression				
Center for Epidemiological Studies Depression Scale for Children (CES-DC)	6-18	Child: 20	5	https://www.brightfutures.org/mentalhealth/ pdf/professionals/bridges/ces_dc.pdf
Mood and Feelings Questionnaire (MFQ)–Short Version	7-18	Parent: 34 Child: 33	<5	www.devepi.duhs.duke.edu/mfq.html
Patient Health Questionnaire–9 (PHQ-9)	12/13+	9	<5	http://www.phqscreeners.com/sites/g/files/ g10016261/f/201412/PHQ-9_English.pdf

ADHD, Attention-deficit/hyperactivity disorder.

of Mental Disorders, Fifth Edition (DSM-5) diagnosis; a risk assessment; and a treatment plan. For infants and young children, the presenting problem and historical information is derived from parents and other informants. As children mature, they become increasingly important contributors to the information base, and they become the primary source of information in later adolescence. Information relevant to formulation and differential diagnosis is derived in multiple ways, including directive and nondirective questioning, interactive play, and observation of the child alone and together with the caregiver(s).

The explication of the **presenting problem(s)** includes information about onset, duration, frequency, setting, and severity of symptoms; associated distress and/or functional impairment; and predisposing, precipitating, perpetuating, and ameliorating contextual factors. The **symptom review** assesses potential comorbidity in the major domains of child and adolescent psychopathology, including problems with intellectual, communication, motor, learning, and developmental capabilities; attention deficits; angry, sad, or elated mood; anxiety; obsessions or compulsions; trauma or stress reactions; somatic symptoms; eating, elimination, sleep, or gender disturbances; disruptive, impulse-control, or conduct problems; psychosis; or substance abuse or addiction. The **history of psychiatric treatment** includes gathering information about prior emergency mental health assessments, psychiatric hospitalizations, day treatment, psychotherapy, pharmacotherapy, and nontraditional treatments.

The **medical history** includes information about the source of primary care, the frequency of health supervision, past and current medical illnesses and treatments, and the youth and family's history of adherence to medical treatment. A systematic review of organ or functional systems facilitates the identification of abnormalities that require investigation or monitoring by the pediatric practitioner, as well as the identification of cautionary factors related to the prescription of psychotropic medication. The **developmental history** includes information about the circumstances of conception, pregnancy, or adoption; pre-, peri-, or postnatal insults; attachment and temperament; cognitive, motor,

linguistic, emotional, social, and moral development; health habits, sexuality, and substance use (as age appropriate), coping and defensive structure, future orientation, and perceived strengths. The **educational history** includes schools attended; typical grades, attendance, and behavior; classroom accommodations; special education services; disciplinary actions; social relationships; extracurricular activities; and barriers to learning. The **family history** assesses family composition; sociodemographic and neighborhood characteristics; domiciliary arrangements; parenting capacities; family function; medical/psychiatric histories of family members; and cultural/religious affiliations.

Orientation is tested by the ability to correctly identify time (date, month, year, season), place (hospital, clinic, city, state, country), and name, as well as remember (recall) 3 objects. **Attention/calculation** testing is age dependent and includes counting forward by 3s, or more classically, counting backward from 100 by 7 ("serial 7s") or 5. **Language** is tested by pointing to familiar objects (clock, pen) and asking the patient to name them, as well as having the patient follow a 3-step command. Language is also tested by having the patient write a sentence, as well as having the patient read another sentence and perform the command in that sentence.

The **mental status examination** assesses appearance, relatedness, cognition, communication, mood, affective expression, behavior, memory, orientation, and perception.

The evaluation culminates in a biopsychosocial formulation, diagnosis, and risk assessment. The **biopsychosocial formulation** is derived from an assessment of *vulnerabilities* and *strengths* in the biologic, psychological, and social domains and serves to identify targets for intervention and treatment. In the *biologic* domain, major vulnerabilities include a family history of psychiatric disorder and personality or behavior problems, as well as a personal history of pre-, peri-, or postnatal insults; cognitive or linguistic impairments; chronic physical illness; and a difficult temperament. In the *psychological* domain, major vulnerabilities include failure to achieve developmental tasks, unresolved unconscious conflicts, and maladaptive coping and defensive styles. In the *social* domain, major vulnerabilities include parental incapacity; unskilled parenting; family dysfunction; social isolation; unfavorable school setting; unsupportive community structures; and sociodemographic disadvantage. Major strengths include cognitive and linguistic capability; physical health and attractiveness; stable, moderate temperamental characteristics; and stable supportive parenting, family, peer, and community structures. The biopsychosocial formulation can be organized to reflect predisposing, precipitating, perpetuating, and protective (ameliorating) factors (the "4 Ps") influencing the development of the observed psychopathology.

The **diagnosis** must be made in accordance with the nomenclature in DSM-5. This nomenclature categorizes cross-sectional phenomenology into discrete clinical syndromes and seeks to improve diagnostic accuracy at the expense of theories of causation and dimensional presentations. By DSM-5 convention, if diagnostic criteria are met, the diagnosis is given (except where hierarchical rules apply); consequently, psychiatric comorbidity is a common occurrence. The **risk assessment** includes a careful assessment of risk status, including suicidality, homicidality, assaultiveness, self-injuriousness, and involvement in risky behavior or situations.

The psychiatric diagnostic evaluation culminates in a **treatment plan** that brings the broad array of targeted psychosocial interventions to the service of the child. Diagnoses drive the choice of evidence-based psychotherapeutic and psychopharmacologic treatments. The formulation drives the selection of interventions targeted at biologic, psychological, and social vulnerabilities and strengths. Many of these treatments and interventions are described in the succeeding chapters.

SPECIAL CONSIDERATIONS IN THE DIAGNOSTIC EVALUATION OF INFANTS AND YOUNG CHILDREN

Psychiatric evaluation of infants and young children includes the domains of physiology, temperament, language and motor development, affective behavior, social behavior, and communication. Although much of the information in these domains will be derived from parent report, much also can be gleaned from nonverbal behavior and observation of the parent–child interaction. Observations should include predominant affective tone of parent and child (positive, negative, apathetic); involvement in the situation (curiosity, disinterest); social responsiveness (mutuality of gaze, auditory responsiveness); and reactions to transitions (including separation).

A screen for maternal depression* is critical at this stage, as is an assessment of the mother's (or other caregiver's) ability to respond rapidly on a contingent basis to the child's expressed needs, regulate the child's rapid shifts of emotion and behavior, and provide a stimulus shelter to prevent the child from being overwhelmed.

Standardized screening instruments—*Ages and Stages Questionnaires, Brief Infant-Toddler Social & Emotional Assessment, Early Childhood Screening Assessment, Modified Checklist for Autism in Toddlers, Parents' Evaluation of Developmental Status,* and *Survey of Well-being of Young Children*—designed for this age-group can be helpful in systematizing the evaluation. In addition, the *Infant, Toddler and Preschool Mental Status Exam* (ITP-MSE) is a reference tool that describes how traditional categories of the mental status examination can be adapted to observations of young children. Additional categories, including sensory and state regulation, have been added that reflect important areas of development in young children.

Diagnostic systems that are more age appropriate than DSM-5 have been developed for infants and young children. These systems include the *Research Diagnostic Criteria–Preschool Age* (RDC-PA) and *Zero to Three Diagnostic Classification of Mental Health and Developmental Disorders of Infancy and Early Childhood-Revised* (DC: 0-3R). The DC: 0-3R includes a relationship classification that assesses the range of interactional adaptation in each parent–child relationship and regulation disorders of sensory processing that identify a range of constitutionally and maturationally based sensory reactivity patterns, motor patterns, and behavior patterns that together can dysregulate a child internally and impact the child's interactions with caregivers.

Bibliography is available at Expert Consult.

---

*See http://www.medicalhomeportal.org/clinical-practice/screening-and-prevention/maternal-depression for several examples.

Chapter **33**
Psychopharmacology
David R. DeMaso and Heather J. Walter

第三十三章
精神药理学

中文导读

　　本章主要介绍了兴奋剂和其他治疗注意缺陷多动障碍（ADHD）的药物、抗抑郁药、抗精神病药物、心境稳定剂等几种药物和同时患有躯体疾病的精神科药物使用要点。列举了治疗ADHD症状、儿童青少年抑郁和焦虑（见原文表33.4）、精神病性症状、躁狂、易激惹、激越、攻击症状和Tourette障碍等可供选择的各种治疗药物（见原文表33.3）；对同时伴有躯体疾病的儿童精神科药物使用这一节，介绍了当患有肝脏疾病、胃肠道疾病、肾脏疾病、呼吸道疾病、神经系统疾病时精神科药物的使用原则。并特别介绍了初级保健中精神药物处方的原则　（见原文表33.8）。

Psychopharmacology is the first-line treatment for several child and adolescent psychiatric disorders (e.g., ADHD, schizophrenia, bipolar) and is used adjunctively with psychosocial treatments for other disorders (or coexisting conditions), including anxiety, depression, autism spectrum, tic, trauma-related, and obsessive-compulsive disorders. Although pediatric primary care practitioners (PCPs) may routinely manage medications for attention-deficit/hyperactivity disorder (ADHD), anxiety, and depression, they may be called on to manage psychotropic medications with which they have had less experience. As such, it is useful for PCPs to be familiar with basic information about child and adolescent psychopharmacology. Before prescribing a psychotropic medication, PCPs should review full prescribing information for each medication (in package inserts or at reliable websites such as the National Institutes of Health *DailyMed**) to obtain complete and up-to-date information about indications, contraindications, warnings, interactions, and precautions.

Pediatric prescribers should be aware of "best practice" principles that underlie medication assessment and management by child and adolescent psychiatrists (Table 33.1), so as to consider extrapolation of these principles to prescribing in the primary care setting. The use of medication involves a series of interconnected steps, including performing an assessment, constructing working diagnoses and an explanatory formulation, deciding on treatment and a monitoring plan, obtaining treatment assent/consent, and implementing treatment.

Questions remain about the quality of the evidence supporting the use of many psychotropic medications in children and adolescents. Therefore, cognitive, emotional, and behavioral symptoms are targets for medication treatment when (1) there is no or insufficient response to available evidence-based psychosocial interventions, (2) the patient's symptoms convey significant risk of harm, or (3) the patient is experiencing significant distress or functional impairment. Common target symptoms include agitation, aggression, anxiety, depression, hyperactivity, inattention, impulsivity, mania, obsessions, compulsions, and psychosis (Table 33.2). All these can be quantitatively measured with standardized symptom rating scales to establish baseline symptom severity and facilitate "treating to target."

STIMULANTS AND OTHER ADHD MEDICATIONS

Stimulants are sympathomimetic drugs that act both in the central nervous system (CNS) and peripherally by enhancing dopaminergic and noradrenergic transmission (Table 33.3). Strong evidence exists for the effectiveness of these medications for the treatment of ADHD and aggression, as well as moderate evidence for the treatment of hyperactivity in autism spectrum disorder (ASD). In some cases, stimulants are used adjunctively with antidepressants in the treatment of depression and as monotherapy for fatigue or malaise associated with chronic physical illnesses.

No major differences in efficacy or tolerability have been found between different classes of stimulants, and no consistent patient profile identifies those who will respond preferentially to one class over another. The most common (generally dose-dependent) side effects of stimulants include headache, stomachache, appetite suppression, weight loss, blood pressure (BP) and heart rate increases, and delayed sleep onset. Less common side effects include irritability (particularly prominent in younger children), aggression, social withdrawal, and hallucinations (visual or tactile). Amphetamine preparations prescribed concurrently with serotonergic antidepressants can be associated with the development of serotonin syndrome.

Stimulants have been associated with elevations in mean BP (<5 mm Hg) and pulse (<10 beats/min); a subset of individuals (5–10%) may have greater increases. The rate of sudden death in pediatric patients taking stimulants is comparable to children in the general population;

Table 33.1	Best Principles for Use of Psychotropic Medications With Children and Adolescents

1. Before initiating pharmacotherapy, a psychiatric evaluation is completed.
2. Before initiating pharmacotherapy, a medical history is obtained, and a medical evaluation is considered when appropriate.
3. The prescriber communicates with other professionals to obtain collateral history and collaborate in the monitoring of outcome and side effects during the medication trial.
4. The prescriber develops a psychosocial and psychopharmacologic treatment plan based on the best available evidence.
5. The prescriber develops a plan to monitor the patient during the medication trial.
6. The prescriber is cautious when the medication trial cannot be appropriately monitored.
7. The prescriber educates the patient and family about the patient's diagnosis and treatment plan.
8. The prescriber obtains and documents informed consent before initiating the medication trial and at appropriate intervals during the trial.
9. The informed-consent process focuses on the risks and benefits of the proposed and alternative treatments.
10. The medication trial should involve an adequate dose of medication for an adequate duration.
11. The prescriber reassesses the patient if the patient fails to respond to the medication trial as expected.
12. The prescriber has a clear rationale for using medication combinations.
13. The prescriber has a specific plan for medication discontinuation.

Adapted from American Academy of Child and Adolescent Psychiatry: Practice parameter on the use of psychotropic medication in children and adolescents. *J Am Acad Child Adolesc Psychiatry* 48(9):961–973, 2009.

Table 33.2	Target Symptom Approach to Psychopharmacologic Management
TARGET SYMPTOM	**MEDICATION CONSIDERATIONS**
Agitation	Atypical antipsychotic Typical antipsychotic Anxiolytic
Aggression	Stimulant Atypical antipsychotic
Anxiety	Antidepressant Anxiolytic (only situational anxiety)
Depression	Antidepressant
Hyperactivity, inattention, impulsivity	Stimulant α-Agonist Atomoxetine
Mania	Atypical antipsychotic Lithium
Obsessions, compulsions	Antidepressant
Psychosis	Atypical antipsychotic Typical antipsychotic
Tics	α-Agonist Atypical antipsychotic Typical antipsychotic

Adapted from Shaw RJ, DeMaso DR: *Clinical manual of pediatric psychosomatic medicine: mental health consultation with physically ill children and adolescents,* Washington, DC, 2006, American Psychiatric Press, p 306.

Table 33.3 | Select Medications for Attention-Deficit/Hyperactivity Disorder (ADHD) Symptoms

GENERIC (BRAND) APPROXIMATE DURATION OF ACTION	FDA APPROVED (Pediatric age range in years)	TARGET SYMPTOMS	DAILY STARTING DOSE	DAILY THERAPEUTIC DOSAGE RANGE*	SELECT MEDICAL MONITORING AND PRECAUTIONS
STIMULANTS					
Long Acting					
OROS methylphenidate (Concerta) 12 hr	ADHD (6+)	Inattention Hyperactivity Impulsivity	18 mg	Age 6-12: 18-54 mg Age >12: 18-72 mg	Personal and family CV history; personal seizure history; Ht, Wt, BP, P; bipolar or psychotic symptoms; substance abuse; potential for GI obstruction
Dexmethylphenidate (Focalin XR)† 10-12 hr	ADHD (6+)	Inattention Hyperactivity Impulsivity	5 mg	5-30 mg	Personal and family CV history; personal seizure history; Ht, Wt, BP, P; bipolar or psychotic symptoms; substance abuse
Amphetamine combination (Adderall XR)† 12 hr	ADHD (6+)	Inattention Hyperactivity Impulsivity	5 mg	5-30 mg	Personal and family CV history; personal seizure history; Ht, Wt, BP, P; bipolar or psychotic symptoms; substance abuse
Lisdexamfetamine (capsule† and chewable) (Vyvanse) 12 hr	ADHD (6+)	Inattention Hyperactivity Impulsivity	20 mg	20-70 mg	Personal and family CV history; personal seizure history; Ht, Wt, BP, P; bipolar or psychotic symptoms; substance abuse
Methylphenidate transdermal (Daytrana) 12 hr	ADHD (6+)	Inattention Hyperactivity Impulsivity	10 mg	10-30 mg	Personal and family CV history; personal seizure history; Ht, Wt, BP, P; bipolar or psychotic symptoms; substance abuse; skin reactions
Methylphenidate suspension (Quillivant XR) 12 hr	ADHD (6+)	Inattention Hyperactivity Impulsivity	20 mg	20-60 mg	Personal and family CV history; personal seizure history; Ht, Wt, BP, P; bipolar or psychotic symptoms; substance abuse
Intermediate Acting					
Methylphenidate (Metadate CD, Ritalin LA) 8 hr	ADHD (6+)	Inattention Hyperactivity Impulsivity	10 mg	10-60 mg	Personal and family CV history; personal seizure history; Ht, Wt, BP, P; bipolar or psychotic symptoms; substance abuse
Dextroamphetamine (Dexedrine Spansule) 8 hr	ADHD (6+)	Inattention Hyperactivity Impulsivity	5 mg	5-40 mg	Personal and family CV history; personal seizure history; Ht, Wt, BP, P; bipolar or psychotic symptoms; substance abuse
Methylphenidate chewable (Quillichew ER) 8 hr	ADHD (6+)	Inattention Hyperactivity Impulsivity	20 mg	20-60 mg	Personal and family CV history; personal seizure history; Ht, Wt, BP, P; bipolar or psychotic symptoms; substance abuse
Short Acting					
Dexmethylphenidate (Focalin) 4-5 hr	ADHD (6+)	Inattention Hyperactivity Impulsivity	5 mg	5-20 mg	Personal and family CV history; personal seizure history; Ht, Wt, BP, P; bipolar or psychotic symptoms; substance abuse
Methylphenidate (Ritalin, Methylin) 4 hr	ADHD (6+)	Inattention Hyperactivity Impulsivity	5 mg	5-60 mg	Personal and family CV history; personal seizure history; Ht, Wt, BP, P; bipolar or psychotic symptoms; substance abuse
Amphetamine combination (Adderall) 4-5 hr	ADHD (3+)	Inattention Hyperactivity Impulsivity	Age 3-5: 2.5 mg Age ≥6: 5 mg	5-40 mg	Personal and family CV history; personal seizure history; Ht, Wt, BP, P; bipolar or psychotic symptoms; substance abuse
Dextroamphetamine (Dexedrine) 4 hr	ADHD (3+)	Inattention Hyperactivity Impulsivity	Age 3-5: 2.5 mg Age ≥6: 5 mg	5-40 mg	Personal and family CV history; personal seizure history; Ht, Wt, BP, P; bipolar or psychotic symptoms; substance abuse
SELECTIVE NOREPINEPHRINE REUPTAKE INHIBITOR					
Atomoxetine (Strattera) 24 hours	ADHD (6+)	Inattention Hyperactivity Impulsivity	<70 kg: 0.5 mg/ kg/day >70 kg: 40 mg	<70 kg: 0.5-1.2 mg/kg/day >70 kg: 40-100 mg	Personal and family CV history; BP, P; liver injury; suicidal ideation; bipolar or psychotic symptoms

Continued

Table 33.3 | Select Medications for Attention-Deficit/Hyperactivity Disorder (ADHD) Symptoms—cont'd

GENERIC (BRAND) APPROXIMATE DURATION OF ACTION	FDA APPROVED (Pediatric age range in years)	TARGET SYMPTOMS	DAILY STARTING DOSE	DAILY THERAPEUTIC DOSAGE RANGE*	SELECT MEDICAL MONITORING AND PRECAUTIONS
ALPHA (α)-AGONISTS					
Short Acting					
Clonidine (Catapres) 4 hr	None	Inattention Hyperactivity Impulsivity	0.05 mg	27-40.5 kg: 0.05-0.2 mg 40.5-45 kg: 0.05-0.3 mg >45 kg: 0.05-0.4 mg	CV history; BP, P; rebound hypertension; cardiac conduction abnormalities
Guanfacine (Tenex) 6 hr	None	Inattention Hyperactivity Impulsivity	0.5 mg	27-40.5 kg: 0.5-2 mg 40.5-45 kg: 0.5-3 mg >45 kg: 0.5-4 mg	CV history; BP, P; rebound hypertension; cardiac conduction abnormalities
Long Acting					
Clonidine (Kapvay) 12 hr	ADHD (6+)	Inattention Hyperactivity Impulsivity	0.1 mg	0.1-0.4 mg	CV history; BP, P; rebound hypertension; cardiac conduction abnormalities
Guanfacine (Intuniv) 24 hr	ADHD (6+)	Inattention Hyperactivity Impulsivity	1 mg	*Monotherapy:* 25-33.9 kg: 2-3 mg 34-41.4 kg: 2-4 mg 41.5-49.4 kg: 3-5 mg 49.5-58.4 kg: 3-6 mg 58.5-91 kg: 4-7 mg >91 kg: 5-7 mg *Adjunctive* (with stimulant): 0.05-0.12 mg/kg/day	CV history; BP, P; rebound hypertension, cardiac conduction abnormalities

*Doses shown in table may exceed maximum recommended dose for some children.
†Capsule contents may be sprinkled on soft food.
FDA, U.S. Food and Drug Administration; CV, cardiovascular; Ht, height; Wt, weight; BP, blood pressure; P, pulse; GI, gastrointestinal.

the hazard ratio for serious cardiovascular (CV) events is 0.75 (although up to a 2-fold increase in risk could not be ruled out). Moreover, a case series analysis of children with a CV incident and treatment with methylphenidate demonstrated an increased risk of arrhythmia (incidence rate ratio, 1.61) that was highest in the presence of congenital heart disease. The U.S. Food and Drug Administration (FDA) recommends that stimulants should be avoided in the presence of structural cardiac abnormalities (e.g., postoperative tetralogy of Fallot, coronary artery abnormalities, subaortic stenosis, hypertrophic cardiomyopathy) and patient symptoms (syncope, palpitations, arrhythmias) or family history (e.g., unexplained sudden death) suggestive of CV disease. In these circumstances, cardiology consultation is recommended before prescribing. Routine electrocardiograms (ECGs) are not recommended in the absence of cardiac risk factors.

Atomoxetine is a selective inhibitor of presynaptic norepinephrine reuptake; it increases dopamine and norepinephrine in the prefrontal cortex (Table 33.3). It is less effective for the treatment of ADHD and aggression than stimulants, but atomoxetine has a longer duration of action (approximately 24 hr). Atomoxetine can have an onset of action within 1-2 wk of starting treatment, but there is an incrementally increasing response for up to 24 wk or longer. Common side effects of atomoxetine include nausea, headache, abdominal pain, insomnia, somnolence, erectile dysfunction, irritability, fatigue, decreased appetite, weight loss, and dizziness, along with nonclinical increases in heart rate and BP. Potential serious neuropsychiatric reactions include psychosis, mania, panic attacks, aggressive behavior, depression, seizures, and suicidal thinking. Atomoxetine carries an FDA warning regarding the risk of suicidal thinking and the need to monitor this closely. Atomoxetine also has been associated with hepatotoxicity and should be discontinued in patients with jaundice or laboratory evidence of liver injury, and should not be restarted. Because of the risk of sudden death, atomoxetine generally should be avoided in youth with known serious structural cardiac abnormalities, cardiomyopathy, heart rhythm abnormalities, or other serious cardiac problems.

The α-adrenergic agents **clonidine** and **guanfacine**, along with the longer-acting preparation of each, are presynaptic adrenergic agonists

that appear to stimulate inhibitory presynaptic autoreceptors in the CNS (Table 33.3). The extended-release formulation of guanfacine has moderate to strong evidence for the monotherapy of ADHD and weaker evidence as adjunctive therapy to stimulant medication. Combination stimulant/α-agonist therapy is superior to monotherapy with either and to placebo for improving inattention and working memory. Extended-release guanfacine also has moderate evidence for effective treatment of ADHD with comorbid oppositional defiant disorder (ODD), favorably affecting both symptom clusters, as well as for the treatment of agitation in autism.

Sedation, somnolence, headache, abdominal pain, hypotension, bradycardia, cardiac conduction abnormalities, dry mouth, depression, and confusion are potential side effects of clonidine and guanfacine. Abrupt withdrawal can result in rebound hypertension; overdose can result in death.

ANTIDEPRESSANTS

Antidepressant drugs act on pre- and postsynaptic receptors affecting the release and reuptake of brain neurotransmitters, including norepinephrine, serotonin, and dopamine (Table 33.4). There is strong evidence for the effectiveness of antidepressant medications in the treatment of anxiety and obsessive-compulsive disorders and weaker evidence for the treatment of depressive disorders. Suicidal thoughts have been reported during treatment with all antidepressants. The overall risk difference of suicidal ideation/attempts across all randomized controlled trials (RCTs) of antidepressants and indications has been reported as 0.7%, corresponding to a *number needed to harm* of 143. All antidepressants carry an FDA warning for suicidality; careful monitoring is recommended during the initial stages of treatment and following dose adjustments.

The **selective serotonin reuptake inhibitor (SSRI)** fluoxetine outperforms all other antidepressants (both SSRI and non-SSRI) studied and is the only SSRI separating from placebo in studies of depressed *preadolescents*. SSRIs have a large margin of safety. Side effects of SSRIs generally manifest in the first few weeks of treatment, and many will resolve with time. More common side effects include nausea, irritability,

| Table 33.4 | Select Medications for Depression and Anxiety in Children and Adolescents |

GENERIC (BRAND)	FDA APPROVED (Pediatric age range in years)	TARGET SYMPTOMS	DAILY STARTING DOSE	DAILY THERAPEUTIC DOSAGE RANGE*	SELECT MEDICAL MONITORING AND PRECAUTIONS
SELECTIVE SEROTONIN REUPTAKE INHIBITORS					
Citalopram (Celexa)	None	Depression Anxiety Obsessions/ compulsions	10 mg	10-40 mg	Suicidal ideation; QT prolongation at doses >40 mg; abnormal bleeding; mania; SS, DS
Escitalopram (Lexapro)	Depression (12-17)	Depression Anxiety Obsessions/ compulsions	5 mg	5-20 mg	Suicidal ideation; abnormal bleeding; mania; SS, DS
Fluoxetine (Prozac)	Depression (8-17) OCD (7-17)	Depression Anxiety Obsessions/ compulsions	Age 6-12: 10 mg Age 13-17: 20 mg	Depression: 10-20 mg Anxiety, OCD: 10-60 mg	Suicidal ideation; abnormal bleeding; mania; SS
Sertraline (Zoloft)	OCD (6-17)	Depression Anxiety Obsessions/ compulsions	Age 6-12: 12.5-25 mg Age 13-17: 25-50 mg	12.5-200 mg	Suicidal ideation; abnormal bleeding; mania; SS, DS
ATYPICAL ANTIDEPRESSANTS					
Bupropion (Wellbutrin XL)	None	Depression	150 mg	150-300 mg	Suicidal ideation; neuropsychiatric reaction, seizures (>300 mg/day), BP; mania; contraindicated in patients with seizure and eating disorders
Duloxetine (Cymbalta)	Anxiety (7-17)	Depression Anxiety	30 mg	30-60 mg	Suicidal ideation; BP, P; liver damage; severe skin reactions; abnormal bleeding; mania; SS, DS
Mirtazapine (Remeron)	None	Depression	7.5 mg	7.5-45 mg	Suicidal ideation; weight; somnolence; agranulocytosis; QT prolongation; mania; SS, DS
Venlafaxine (Effexor XR)	None	Depression Anxiety	37.5 mg	37.5-225 mg	Suicidal ideation; BP; abnormal bleeding; mania; SS, DS
TRICYCLIC ANTIDEPRESSANTS					
Clomipramine (Anafranil)	OCD (10-17)	Obsessions Compulsions	25 mg	25-200 mg	Suicidal ideation; BP; P; ECG; blood level; mania; SS; seizures; DS
ANXIOLYTIC AGENTS (SITUATIONAL USE)					
Lorazepam (Ativan)	None	Anxiety	0.5 mg	0.5-2 mg	Respiratory depression; sedation; physical and psychological dependence; paradoxical reactions
Clonazepam (Klonopin)	None	Panic	0.5 mg	0.5-1 mg	Respiratory depression; sedation; physical and psychological dependence; paradoxical reactions; suicidal ideation
Hydroxyzine (Atarax, Vistaril)	Anxiety	Anxiety	50 mg	Age <6: 50 mg Age >6: 50-100 mg	QT prolongation

*Doses shown in table may exceed maximum recommended dose for some children.
OCD, Obsessive-compulsive disorder; BP, blood pressure; P, pulse; ECG, electrocardiogram; SS, serotonin syndrome; DS, discontinuation syndrome.

insomnia, appetite changes, weight loss/gain, headaches, dry mouth, dizziness, bruxism, diaphoresis, tremors, akathisia, restlessness, and behavioral activation. Approximately 5% of youth taking SSRIs, particularly children, develop **behavioral activation** (increased impulsivity, agitation, and irritability) that can be confused with mania, but the activation symptoms typically resolve when the dose is decreased or the medication discontinued. Sexual side effects are common, including decreased libido, anorgasmia, and erectile dysfunction. There is an increased risk of bleeding, especially when used with aspirin or nonsteroidal antiinflammatory drugs (NSAIDs).

SSRIs can be associated with abnormal heart rhythms, and citalopram causes dose-dependent QT-interval prolongation, contraindicating doses >40 mg/day. Patients with diabetes may experience hypoglycemia during SSRI treatment and hyperglycemia on discontinuation. **Discontinuation symptoms** (e.g., dysphoric mood, irritability, agitation, dizziness, sensory disturbances, anxiety, confusion, headache, lethargy, emotional lability,

insomnia, hypomania) are common with short-acting SSRIs (sertraline, citalopram, escitalopram), leading to a recommendation for divided doses if these medications are used at higher doses and graduated reduction if discontinued.

The **serotonin syndrome** is characterized by the triad of mental status changes (e.g., agitation, hallucinations, delirium, coma), autonomic instability (e.g., tachycardia, labile BP, dizziness, diaphoresis, flushing, hyperthermia), and neuromuscular symptoms (e.g., tremor, rigidity, myoclonus, hyperreflexia, incoordination). Serotonin syndrome results from excessive agonism of the CNS and peripheral nervous system serotonergic receptors and can be caused by a range of drugs, including SSRIs, valproate, and lithium. Interactions that can cause serotonin syndrome include SSRIs with linezolid (antibiotic with monoamine oxidase inhibitor properties) and with antimigraine preparations, as well as with amphetamine preparations, trazodone, buspirone, and venlafaxine. Serotonin syndrome is generally self-limited and can resolve spontaneously after the serotonergic agents are discontinued. Patients with severe disease require the control of agitation, autonomic instability, and hyperthermia as well as administration of 5-hydroxytryptamine (5-HT$_{2A}$, serotonin) antagonists (e.g., cyproheptadine).

The **non-SSRI antidepressants** include bupropion, duloxetine, venlafaxine, and mirtazapine (Table 33.4). These medications all lack rigorous evidence to support their effectiveness in children and adolescents, and as such should not be considered first-line options. *Bupropion*, a **norepinephrine-dopamine reuptake inhibitor (NDRI)**, appears to have an indirect mixed-agonist effect on dopamine and norepinephrine transmission. No rigorous studies of bupropion for anxiety or depression have been conducted with children or adolescents, although some evidence suggests that bupropion may be effective for smoking cessation and ADHD in youth. Common side effects include irritability, nausea, anorexia, headache, and insomnia. Dose-related seizures (0.1% risk at 300 mg/day and 0.4% risk at 400 mg/day) have occurred with bupropion, so it is contraindicated in those with epilepsy, eating disorders, or at risk for seizures.

Duloxetine and *venlafaxine* are **serotonin-norepinephrine reuptake inhibitors (SNRIs)**. *Duloxetine* has FDA approval for treatment of generalized anxiety disorder in children and adolescents, but studies of duloxetine for depression in youth have been negative. There is some evidence in adults that duloxetine can be useful for fibromyalgia and chronic musculoskeletal pain, an effect that has also been observed in children and adolescents. Common side effects of duloxetine include nausea, diarrhea, decreased weight, and dizziness. Increases in heart rate and BP have been noted, and BP should be monitored at each visit and with each dosage change. In addition, there have been reports of hepatic failure, sometimes fatal; duloxetine should be discontinued and not resumed in patients who develop jaundice or other evidence of liver dysfunction. Duloxetine also has been associated with severe skin reactions (erythema multiforme and Stevens-Johnson syndrome).

Venlafaxine has only negative trials for the treatment of depression in children and adolescents, but does have favorable evidence for the treatment of anxiety. Side effects are similar to SSRIs, including hypertension, irritability, insomnia, headaches, anorexia, nervousness, and dizziness, and dropout rates are high in clinical trials of venlafaxine. BP should be monitored at each visit and with each dosage change. Discontinuation symptoms (e.g., dysphoric mood, irritability, agitation, dizziness, sensory disturbances, anxiety, confusion, headache, lethargy, emotional lability, insomnia, hypomania, tinnitus, seizures) are more pronounced with venlafaxine than the other non-SSRI antidepressants. In addition, suicidal thinking and agitation may be more common with venlafaxine than with other antidepressants, requiring close monitoring. In light of the substantial adverse effects, venlafaxine likely should be considered to be a third-line medication.

Mirtazapine is both a noradrenergic and a specific serotonergic antidepressant. Mirtazapine has only negative trials for the treatment of depression in youth and has no rigorous evidence of effectiveness for any other child or adolescent psychiatric disorder. Mirtazapine is associated with a risk for substantial weight gain and more rarely, hypotension, elevated liver enzymes, agranulocytosis, and QT prolongation. While its sedating properties have led to its adjunctive use for insomnia in adults with depressive/anxiety disorders, there is no evidence for use of mirtazapine in childhood sleep disorders.

The **tricyclic antidepressants (TCAs)** have mixed mechanisms of action; for example, clomipramine is primarily serotonergic, and imipramine is both noradrenergic and serotonergic. With the advent of the SSRIs, the lack of efficacy studies, particularly in depression, and more serious side effects, the use of TCAs in children has declined. *Clomipramine* is used in the treatment of obsessive-compulsive disorder (Table 33.4). Unlike the SSRIs, the TCAs may be helpful in pain disorders. They have a narrow therapeutic index, with overdoses being potentially fatal. Anticholinergic symptoms (e.g., dry mouth, blurred vision, constipation) are the most common side effects. TCAs can have cardiac conduction effects in doses >3.5 mg/kg. BP and ECG monitoring is indicated at doses above this level.

Anxiolytic agents, including lorazepam, clonazepam, and hydroxyzine, have been effectively used for the short-term relief of the symptoms of acute anxiety (Table 33.4). They are less effective as chronic (>4 mo) anxiolytic medications, particularly when one is used as monotherapy. Chronic use carries a significant risk of physical and psychological dependence.

ANTIPSYCHOTICS

Based on their mechanism of action, antipsychotic medications can be divided into first-generation (blocking dopamine D$_2$ receptors) and second-generation (mixed dopaminergic and serotonergic antagonists) agents (Table 33.5).

The **second-generation** (or **atypical**) **antipsychotics (SGAs)** have relatively strong antagonistic interactions with 5-HT$_2$ receptors and perhaps more variable activity at central adrenergic, cholinergic, and histaminic sites, which might account for the varying side effects, particularly metabolic, noted among these agents. The SGAs have moderate evidence for the treatment of agitation in autism and for the treatment of schizophrenia, bipolar disorder, and aggression. Haloperidol is a high-potency antipsychotic that is the **first-generation** (or **typical**) **antipsychotic** most commonly used in treatment of agitation and schizophrenia.

The SGAs have significant side effects, including sedation, extrapyramidal symptoms, weight gain, metabolic syndrome, diabetes, hyperlipidemia, hyperprolactinemia, hematologic effects (e.g., leukopenia, neutropenia), elevated liver transaminases, seizures, and CV effects (Table 33.6). They have an FDA warning for increased risk of diabetes. Youth appear to be more sensitive to sedation, extrapyramidal side effects (except akathisia), withdrawal dyskinesia, prolactin abnormalities, weight gain, hepatotoxicity, and metabolic abnormalities. The development of diabetes or tardive dyskinesia appears less prevalent than in adults, although this may be a function of short follow-up periods because these side effects may not emerge until adulthood.

The management of adverse effects should be proactive with baseline assessment and ongoing monitoring (Table 33.7). Abnormal movements (dystonia, akathisia, tardive dyskinesia) need periodic assessment using a standardized instrument such as the *Abnormal Involuntary Movement Scale* (AIMS). Valbenazine is FDA approved for the treatment of tardive dyskinesia in adults. The need for antiparkinsonian agents may be a consideration, particularly for patients at risk for acute dystonia or who have a previous history of dystonic reactions. CV effects of SGAs include prolongation of the QTc interval, tachycardia, orthostatic hypertension, and pericarditis. In patients with a personal or family history of cardiac abnormalities, including syncope, palpitations, arrhythmias, or sudden unexplained death, a baseline ECG with subsequent monitoring should be considered, along with cardiology consultation before prescribing. Alternative pharmacology should be considered if the resting heart rate exceeds 130 beats/min, or the PR, QRS, and QTc exceed 200, 120, and 460 milliseconds (msec), respectively.

The cytochrome P450 (CYP) enzymes metabolize the antipsychotics and as such necessitate that the PCP and psychiatrist are alert for potential drug-drug interactions that may impact the serum levels of all patient medications. CYP3A4 is mainly relevant to lurasidone, quetiapine, olanzapine, and haloperidol, whereas CYP2D6 predominately clears aripiprazole and risperidone. Asenapine is metabolized by CYP1A2 as well as direct glucuronidation by UGT1A4. Because <10% of paliperidone undergoes CYP first-pass metabolism, there is a lower likelihood of drug-drug interactions.

Primary prevention strategies to manage weight and metabolic dysfunction include educating the youth and family about healthy lifestyle behaviors and selecting an agent that has the lowest likelihood of impacting metabolic status. Secondary strategies would include intensifying healthy lifestyle instructions, consideration of switching agents, and a weight loss treatment program. Consideration of weight management interventions and increased monitoring of blood glucose and lipid levels should be implemented if weight gain exceeds the 90th percentile of body mass index (BMI) for age, or a change of 5 BMI units in youth who were obese at the initiation of treatment. Tertiary strategies, where diabetes, hypertension, obesity, or another metabolic abnormality has occurred, require more intensive weight reduction interventions, changing medication, and consultation with a medical subspecialist. Metformin

Table 33.5	Select Medications for Psychosis, Mania, Irritability, Agitation, Aggression, and Tourette Disorder in Children and Adolescents

GENERIC (BRAND)	FDA APPROVED (Pediatric age range in years)	TARGET SYMPTOMS	DAILY STARTING DOSE	DAILY THERAPEUTIC DOSAGE RANGE*	SELECT MEDICAL MONITORING AND PRECAUTIONS
SECOND-GENERATION ANTIPSYCHOTICS					
Aripiprazole (Abilify) Available in liquid preparation	Bipolar (10-17) Schizophrenia (13-17) Irritability in autism (6-17) Tourette (6-17)	Mania Psychosis Irritability Aggression Agitation Vocal/motor tics	Bipolar, schizophrenia: 2 mg Autism: 2 mg Tourette: 2 mg	Bipolar, schizophrenia: 10-30 mg Autism: 5-15 mg Tourette: 5-20 mg	BMI, BP, P, fasting glucose and lipids, abnormal movements; compulsive behaviors; neuroleptic malignant syndrome; leukopenia, neutropenia, agranulocytosis; seizures
Olanzapine (Zyprexa) Available in liquid, dissolvable, and IM preparations	Bipolar (13-17) Schizophrenia (13-17)	Mania Psychosis Agitation	2.5 mg	2.5-20 mg	BMI, BP, P, fasting glucose and lipids, abnormal movements; skin rash (DRESS); neuroleptic malignant syndrome; leukopenia, neutropenia, agranulocytosis; seizures
Quetiapine (Seroquel)	Bipolar (10-17) Schizophrenia (13-17)	Mania Psychosis Agitation	25 mg bid	Bipolar: 400-600 mg Schizophrenia: 400-800 mg	BMI, BP, P, fasting glucose and lipids, abnormal movements; ophthalmologic exam; neuroleptic malignant syndrome; leukopenia, neutropenia, agranulocytosis; seizures; QT prolongation
Risperidone (Risperdal) Available in liquid and dissolvable preparations	Bipolar (10-17) Schizophrenia (13-17) Irritability in autism (5-17)	Mania Psychosis Irritability Aggression Agitation	Bipolar, schizophrenia: 0.5 mg Autism: <20 kg: 0.25 mg ≥20 kg: 0.5 mg	Bipolar, schizophrenia: 1-6 mg Autism: 0.5-3 mg	BMI, BP, P, fasting glucose and lipids, prolactin, abnormal movements; neuroleptic malignant syndrome; leukopenia, neutropenia, agranulocytosis; seizures
Paliperidone (Invega) Available in liquid and IM preparations	Schizophrenia (12-17)	Psychosis	3 mg	<51 kg: 3-6 mg ≥51 kg: 3-12 mg	BMI, BP, P, fasting glucose and lipids, prolactin, abnormal movements, QT prolongation; neuroleptic malignant syndrome; potential for GI obstruction; leukopenia, neutropenia, agranulocytosis; seizures
Lurasidone (Latuda)	Schizophrenia (13-17)	Psychosis	40 mg	40-80 mg	BMI, BP, P, fasting glucose and lipids, prolactin, abnormal movements; neuroleptic malignant syndrome; leukopenia, neutropenia, agranulocytosis; seizures
Asenapine (Saphris)	Bipolar (10-17)	Mania Psychosis	2.5 mg twice daily	5-20 mg	BMI, BP, P, fasting glucose and lipids, prolactin, abnormal movements; QT prolongation; neuroleptic malignant syndrome; leukopenia, neutropenia, agranulocytosis; seizures
FIRST-GENERATION ANTIPSYCHOTIC					
Haloperidol (Haldol) Available in liquid and IM preparations	Psychosis Tourette disorder Severe behavioral disorders Agitation (3-17)	Mania Psychosis Irritability Aggression Agitation Vocal/motor tics	0.05 mg/kg/day	0.05-0.15 mg/kg/day	BP, P; abnormal movements; QT prolongation; neuroleptic malignant syndrome; encephalopathy when combined with lithium; leukopenia, neutropenia, agranulocytosis
MOOD STABILIZER					
Lithium carbonate Available in liquid preparation	Bipolar (12-17)	Mania	Acute mania: 1800 mg/day Target level: 1.0-1.5 mEq/L	Long-term control: 900-1200 mg/day Target level: 0.6-1.2 mEq/L	Serum level, CBC/diff, thyroid function, BUN/creatine, UA, electrolytes, FBS; ECG; encephalopathy when combined with haloperidol

*Doses shown in table may exceed maximum recommended dose for some children.
BMI, Body mass index; BP, blood pressure; P, pulse; IM, intramuscular; GI, gastrointestinal; CBC/diff, complete blood count with differential; BUN, blood urea nitrogen; UA, urinalysis; FBS, fasting blood sugar; ECG, electrocardiogram.

has been used to treat severe weight gain associated with antipsychotic medication. Extrapyramidal adverse effects are generally dose and titration rate dependent and may respond to dose or titration rate reductions. More disabling effects may benefit from adjunctive treatment (e.g., anticholinergics, antihistamines).

Neuroleptic malignant syndrome is a rare, potentially fatal reaction that can occur during antipsychotic therapy. The syndrome generally manifests with fever, muscle rigidity, autonomic instability, and delirium. It is associated with elevated serum creatine phosphokinase levels, a metabolic acidosis, and high end-tidal CO_2 excretion. It has been estimated to occur in 0.2–1% of patients treated with dopamine-blocking agents. Malnutrition and dehydration in the context of an organic brain syndrome and simultaneous treatment with lithium and antipsychotic agents (particularly haloperidol) can increase the risk. Mortality rates may be as high as 20–30% as a result of dehydration, aspiration, kidney failure, and respiratory collapse. Differential diagnosis of neuroleptic malignant syndrome includes infections, heat stroke, malignant hyperthermia, lethal catatonia, agitated delirium, thyrotoxicosis, serotonin

Table 33.6	Adverse Effects for Select Antipsychotic Medications						
ADVERSE EFFECT	**ARIPIPRAZOLE (ABILIFY)**	**OLANZAPINE (ZYPREXA)**	**QUETIAPINE (SEROQUEL)**	**RISPERIDONE (RISPERDAL)**	**PALIPERIDONE (INVEGA)**	**LURASIDONE (LATUDA)**	**HALOPERIDOL (HALDOL)**
Weight gain	0/+	+++	++	++	++	0/+	+
QTc interval	0/+	0/+	+	+	+	0/+	0/+
Sedation	0/+	+/++	++	+	0/+	+/++	+
Prolactin increase	0	+	0	+++	+++	+	++/+++
Lipid increase	0/+	+++	++	+	+	0/+	0/+
Diabetes	0/+	+++	++	+	+	0/+	0/+
Anticholinergic	0	++	+/++	0	0	0	0
Acute parkinsonism	+	0/+	0	++	++	+/++	+++
Akathisia	++	+	+	+	+	+/++	+++
Tardive dyskinesia	0/+	0/+	0/+	0/+	0/+	0/+	++
Withdrawal dyskinesia	+/++	0/+	0/+	+	+	+	++
Orthostasis	0/+	++	++	+	+	0/+	0
Seizures	0/+	0/+	0/+	0/+	0/+	0/+	0/+

0 = none; 0/+ = minimal; + = mild; ++ = moderate; +++ = severe.
Adapted from Correll CU: Antipsychotic medications. In Dulcan MK, editor: *Dulcan's textbook of child and adolescent psychiatry*, ed 2, Washington, DC, 2016, American Psychiatric Press, pp 795–846.

Table 33.7	Metabolic Monitoring Parameters Based on ADA/APA Consensus Guidelines					
	BASELINE	**WEEK 4**	**WEEK 8**	**WEEK 12**	**EVERY 3 MO THEREAFTER**	**ANNUALLY**
Medical history*	X			X		X
Weight (BMI)	X	X	X	X	X	X
Waist circumference	X			X		X
Blood pressure	X			X		X
Fasting glucose/HbA₁c	X			X		X
Fasting lipids	X			X		X

*Personal and family history of obesity, hypertension, and cardiovascular disease.
BMI, Body mass index; Hb, hemoglobin.
From American Diabetes Association (ADA), American Psychiatric Association (APA), American Association of Clinical Endocrinologists, North American Association for the Study of Obesity. Consensus development conference on antipsychotic drugs and obesity and diabetes, *Diabetes Care* 27:596–601, 2004.

syndrome, drug withdrawal, and anticholinergic or amphetamine, ecstasy, and salicylate toxicity.

MOOD STABILIZERS
Because of their limited evidence of effectiveness and concerns about safety, mood-stabilizing medications (see Table 33.5) have limited use in the treatment of child and adolescent psychiatric disorders. For the treatment of bipolar mania in adolescents, atypical antipsychotics are considered first-line therapy.

Of the mood stabilizers, **lithium** alone has rigorous support for the treatment of bipolar mania. Lithium's mechanism of action is not well understood; proposed theories relate to neurotransmission, endocrine effects, circadian rhythm, and cellular processes. Common side effects include polyuria and polydipsia, hypothyroidism, hyperparathyroidism, weight gain, nausea, abdominal pain, diarrhea, acne, and CNS symptoms (sedation, tremor, somnolence, memory impairment). Periodic monitoring of lithium levels along with thyroid and renal function is needed. Lithium serum levels of 0.8-1.2 mEq/L are targeted for acute episodes and 0.6-0.9 mEq/L are targeted for maintenance therapy. Acute overdose (level > 1.5 mEq/L) manifests with neurologic symptoms (e.g., tremor, ataxia, nystagmus, hyperreflexia, myoclonus, slurred speech, delirium, coma, seizures), and altered renal function. Toxicity is enhanced when dehydrated or with drugs that affect renal function, such as NSAIDs or angiotensin-converting enzyme (ACE) inhibitors. Neuroleptic

malignant syndrome has been reported in patients concurrently taking antipsychotic drugs and lithium.

MEDICATION USE IN PHYSICAL ILLNESS
There are special considerations in the use of psychotropic medications with physically ill children. Between 80% and 95% of most psychotropic medications are protein bound, the exceptions being lithium (0%), methylphenidate (10–30%), and venlafaxine (25–30%). As a result, psychotropic levels may be directly affected because albumin binding is reduced in many physical illnesses. Metabolism is primarily through the liver and gastrointestinal (GI) tract, with excretion via the kidney. Therefore, dosages may need to be adjusted in children with hepatic or renal impairment.

Hepatic Disease
Lower doses of medications may be required in patients with hepatic disease. Initial dosing of medications should be reduced, and titration should proceed slowly. In steady-state situations, changes in protein binding can result in elevated unbound medication, resulting in increased drug action even in the presence of normal serum drug concentrations. Because it is often difficult to predict changes in protein binding, it is important to maintain attention to the clinical effects of psychotropic medications and not rely exclusively on serum drug concentrations.

In acute hepatitis, there is generally no need to modify dosing because metabolism is only minimally altered. In chronic hepatitis and cirrhosis, hepatocytes are destroyed, and doses may need to be modified.

Medications with high baseline rates of liver clearance (e.g., haloperidol, sertraline, venlafaxine, TCAs) are significantly affected by hepatic disease. For drugs that have significant hepatic metabolism, intravenous administration may be preferred because parenteral administration avoids first-pass liver metabolic effects, and the dosing and action of parenteral medications are similar to those in patients with normal hepatic function. Valproic acid can impair the metabolism of the hepatocyte disproportionate to the degree of hepatocellular damage. In patients with valproate-induced liver injury, low albumin, high prothrombin, and high ammonia levels may be seen without significant elevation in liver transaminases.

Gastrointestinal Disease
Medications with anticholinergic side effects can slow GI motility, affecting absorption and causing constipation. SSRIs increase gastric motility and can cause diarrhea. SSRIs can increase the risk of GI bleeding, especially when administered with NSAIDs. Extended-release or controlled-release preparations of medications can reduce GI side effects, particularly where gastric distress is related to rapid increases in plasma drug concentrations.

Renal Disease
With the exceptions of lithium and gabapentin, psychotropic medications do not generally require significant dosing adjustments in kidney failure. It is important to monitor serum concentrations in renal insufficiency, particularly for medications with a narrow therapeutic index; cyclosporine can elevate serum lithium levels by decreasing lithium excretion. Patients with kidney failure and those on dialysis appear to be more sensitive to TCA side effects, possibly because of the accumulation of hydroxylated tricyclic metabolites.

Because most psychotropic medications are highly protein bound, they are not significantly cleared by dialysis. Lithium is essentially completely removed by dialysis, and the common practice is to administer lithium after dialysis. Patients on dialysis often have significant fluid shifts and are at risk for dehydration, with neuroleptic malignant syndrome more likely in these situations.

Cardiac Disease
Antipsychotics, TCAs, and citalopram (>40 mg/day) can lead to prolongation of the QTc interval, with increased risk of ventricular tachycardia and ventricular fibrillation, particularly in patients with structural heart disease. Patients with a baseline QTc interval of >440 msec should be particularly considered at risk. The normal QTc value in children is 400 msec (±25-30 msec). A QTc value that exceeds 2 SD (>450-460 msec) is considered too long and may be associated with increased mortality. An increase in the QTc from baseline of >60 msec is also associated with increased mortality.

There is increased risk of morbidity and mortality in patients with preexisting cardiac conduction problems. Some of the calcium channel–blocking agents (e.g., verapamil) can slow atrioventricular conduction and can theoretically interact with TCAs. Patients with Wolff-Parkinson-White syndrome who have a short PR interval (<0.12 sec) and widened QRS interval associated with paroxysmal tachycardia are at high risk for life-threatening ventricular tachycardia that may be exacerbated by the use of antipsychotics, TCAs, and citalopram.

Respiratory Disease
Anxiolytic agents can increase the risk of respiratory suppression in patients with pulmonary disease. In these situations, SSRIs and buspirone are good alternative medications to consider in treating disabling anxiety. Possible airway compromise caused by acute laryngospasm should be considered when dopamine-blocking antipsychotic agents are used.

Neurologic Disease
Psychotropic medications can be used safely with epilepsy following consideration of potential interactions among the medication, the seizure

Table 33.8	Principles for Psychotropic Prescribing in Primary Care

1. Identify potential target symptoms through the systematic use (e.g., at all well-child visits) of broad-band mental health screening instruments, such as the Pediatric Symptom Checklist or the Strengths and Difficulties Questionnaire.
2. Establish the baseline severity of identified target symptom(s) through the use of narrow-band symptom rating scales, such as the following (selected from instruments in the public domain):
   a. Depression
      - Mood and Feelings Questionnaire
      - Centers for Epidemiologic Studies Depression Scale
      - Patient Health Questionnaire-9
   b. Anxiety
      - Screen for Child Anxiety Related Disorders
   c. ADHD, Behavior Problems
      - Vanderbilt ADHD Diagnostic Rating Scale
      - SNAP-IV 19
   d. Aggression
      - Outburst Monitoring Scale
3. Select a medication that is FDA approved for the target symptom and age range; titrate as tolerated from starting dose to therapeutic dosage range.
4. *Treat to target:* Readminister baseline symptom rating scale at regular intervals (at least monthly) to assess treatment response (reduction in rating scale score), with the goal of remission (rating scale score below clinical cutpoint).
5. If medication trial is unsuccessful after adherence to therapeutic dose for adequate duration (typically 1-2 mo), consider 2nd trial of alternative medication with FDA approval for target symptom and age range, following same principles as for 1st trial.
6. If 2nd medication trial is unsuccessful, consultation with a child and adolescent psychiatrist is recommended before resorting to medication doses outside therapeutic range, polypharmacy, or non–FDA-approved medications.

ADHD, Attention-deficit/hyperactivity disorder; FDA, U.S. Food and Drug Administration.

disorder, and the anticonvulsant. Any behavioral toxicity of anticonvulsants used either alone or in combination should be considered before proceeding with psychotropic treatment. Simplification of combination anticonvulsant therapy or a change to another agent can result in a reduction of behavioral or emotional symptoms and obviate the need for psychotropic intervention. Clomipramine and bupropion possess significant seizure-inducing properties and should be avoided when the risk of seizures is present.

Principles for Psychotropic Prescribing in Primary Care
Because nonpsychiatrist physicians (predominantly pediatricians) provide three quarters and two thirds, respectively, of all child and adolescent mental health visits in which new psychotropic medications are initiated, it can be helpful for PCPs to develop consultative relationships with child and adolescent psychiatrists who can advise about safe and effective psychotropic prescribing. If such consultation is not readily available, PCPs may benefit from following a standardized approach to prescribing that is feasible in the primary care setting (Table 33.8). This approach emphasizes baseline assessment with standardized rating scales to identify target symptoms and their level of severity; selection of FDA-approved medications for the target symptom and patient age range; adherence to recommendations regarding therapeutic dosage ranges; follow-up rating scale assessment to monitor medication response; sufficient duration of the medication trial; and switching to an alternative FDA-approved medication if the first medication trial is ineffective. Generally, consultation with a physician experienced in managing the child's disorder should occur if one is considering using multiple psychotropic medications, doses outside of therapeutic range, or non-FDA-approved medications.

Bibliography is available at Expert Consult.

Chapter **34**

Psychotherapy and Psychiatric Hospitalization

Heather J. Walter and David R. DeMaso

第三十四章

心理治疗和精神科住院

中文导读

本章介绍了心理治疗的概念，提出心理治疗是大多数儿童青少年精神障碍治疗的一线治疗选择。对行为治疗、认知行为治疗、人际关系治疗、精神动力性心理治疗、支持性心理治疗、家庭治疗的治疗原理和适应人群做了介绍；也介绍了针对父母的心理干预（在第十九章作了具体介绍）。详细阐述了有循证证据的心理治疗所需要具备的常见要素、模块化治疗包、治疗保持连续性干预常涉及的一些要素、在医疗场所里的心理治疗；本章还介绍了精神科住院的评估要求和指征。

PSYCHOTHERAPY

Psychotherapy is the first-line treatment for most child and adolescent psychiatric disorders, because this type of treatment generally produces outcomes similar to pharmacotherapy, with less risk of harm. Even with disorders such as schizophrenia, bipolar disorder, and attention-deficit/hyperactivity disorder (ADHD) for which *medication is the first-line treatment*, adjunctive psychotherapy can convey considerable additional benefit. Because pediatric primary care practitioners (PCPs) likely will be referring youth with psychiatric disorders for psychotherapy, they should be familiar with basic information about child and adolescent psychotherapy.

Overall, psychotherapy is moderately effective in reducing psychiatric symptomatology and achieving remission of illness. In a 2017 multilevel meta-analysis of almost 500 randomized trials over 5 decades, there was a 63% probability that a youth receiving psychotherapy fared better than a youth in a control condition. Effects varied across multiple moderators, including the problem targeted in treatment. Thus, the mean posttreatment and follow-up effect sizes were highest for anxiety, followed by behavior/conduct, ADHD, and depression, and lowest for multiple concurrent comorbidities. Effect sizes varied according to outcome measure informant, with youth and parents generally reporting larger effects than teachers. Ethnicity moderator tests showed no significant differences in treatment benefit between majority Caucasian samples and majority non-Caucasian samples.

A variety of psychotherapeutic programs have been developed, with varying levels of effectiveness (Table 34.1). Differences between therapeutic approaches may be less pronounced in practice than in theory. The quality of the therapist–patient alliance is consistently an important predictor of treatment outcome. A positive working relationship, expecting change to occur, facing problems assertively, increasing mastery, and attributing change to the participation in the therapy have all been connected to effective therapy.

All psychotherapy interventions involve a series of interconnected steps, including performing an assessment, constructing working diagnoses and an explanatory formulation, deciding on treatment and a monitoring plan, obtaining treatment assent/consent, and implementing treatment. Psychotherapists ideally develop a treatment plan by combining known evidence-based therapies with clinical judgment and patient/family preference to arrive at a specific intervention plan for the individual patient.

Behavior Therapy

Behavior therapy is based on both classic (Pavlovian) and operant (Skinnerian) conditioning. Both approaches do not concern themselves with the inner motives of the individual, but instead address the antecedent stimuli and consequent responses. The treatment begins with a behavioral assessment with interview, observation, diary, and rating scale components, along with a functional analysis of the setting context, immediately preceding external events, and real-world consequences of the behavior. A treatment plan is developed to modify the maladaptive functions of the behavior, using tools such as positive and negative reinforcement, social and tangible rewards, shaping, modeling, and prompting to increase positive behavior, and extinction, stimulus control, punishment, response cost, overcorrection, differential reinforcement of incompatible behavior, graded exposure/systematic desensitization, flooding, modeling, and role-playing to decrease negative behavior.

Behavior therapy has shown applicability to anxiety disorders, obsessive-compulsive and related disorders, behavior disorders, **ADHD**, and autism spectrum disorder.

Table 34.1	Effective Psychotherapies for Specific Behavioral Health Disorders	
DISORDER	**WELL ESTABLISHED***	**PROBABLY EFFICACIOUS†**
Anorexia	Family therapy: behavioral	Family therapy: systemic Individual insight-oriented psychotherapy
Anxiety	Individual CBT	CBT + parent component CBT + medication
ADHD	Behavioral parent training Behavioral classroom management Behavioral peer interventions Organization (executive function) training	Combined training interventions
Autism	Individual, comprehensive ABA Teacher-implemented ABA + DSP	Individual, focused ABA + DSP Focused DSP parent training
Bipolar	None	Family psychoeducation + skill building
Depression, child	Group CBT Group CBT + parent component	Behavior therapy
Depression adolescent	Group CBT Individual interpersonal psychotherapy	Group CBT + parent component Individual CBT Individual CBT + parent/family component
Insomnia	Individual CBT	
ODD and CD, child	Individual/parent management training Individual CBT Problem-solving skill training Group assertiveness training Multidimensional treatment foster care Multisystemic therapy	Group CBT Group/parent management training
ODD and CD, adolescent	Combined behavioral therapy, CBT, and family therapy Treatment foster care	CBT
OCD	None	Individual CBT Family-focused individual CBT
Personality Disorders	None	Dialectical behavioral therapy
PTSD	Trauma-focused CBT	Group CBT
Social phobia	None	Group CBT
Specific phobia	None	None
Substance use	Group CBT Individual CBT Family-based treatment, ecologic	Family-based treatment, behavioral Motivational interviewing
Self-injury	Individual + family CBT + parent training Psychodynamic individual + family	Family-based therapy

ADHD, Attention-deficit/hyperactivity disorder CBT, cognitive-behavioral therapy; ABA, applied behavioral analysis; DSP, developmental social-pragmatic; ODD, oppositional defiant disorder; CD, conduct disorder; OCD, obsessive-compulsive disorder; PTSD, posttraumatic stress disorder.

*Two or more consistent randomized controlled trials demonstrating superiority of treatment over control groups; conducted by independent investigators working at different research settings.

†Same as above, but lacking independent investigator criterion.

Adapted from Society of Clinical Child and Adolescent Psychology: Effective child psychotherapy. http://effectivechildtherapy.org/content/ebp-options-specific-disorders. Accessed March 5, 2017.

Cognitive-Behavioral Therapy

Cognitive-behavioral therapy (CBT) is based on social and cognitive learning theories and extends behavior therapy to address the influence of cognitive processes on behavior. CBT is a problem-oriented treatment centered on correcting problematic patterns in *thinking* and *behavior* that lead to emotional difficulties and functional impairments. The CBT therapist seeks to identify and change cognitive distortions (e.g., learned helplessness, irrational fears), identify and avoid distressing situations, and identify and practice distress-reducing behavior. Self-monitoring (daily thought records), self-instruction (brief sentences asserting thoughts that are comforting and adaptive), and self-reinforcement (rewarding oneself) are key tools used to facilitate achievement of the CBT goals. Table 34.2 outlines the key descriptive features of CBT that can be used by PCPs when describing CBT to patients and their family members.

Table 34.2	Core Components and Characteristics of Cognitive-Behavioral Therapy

- One 60- to 90-minute session each week, typically for 6-12 weeks
- Symptom measures typically are collected frequently.
- Treatment is goal-oriented and collaborative with patient as an active participant.
- Treatment is focused on changing current problematic thoughts or behaviors.
- Weekly homework typically is assigned.

From Coffey SF, Banducci AN, Vinci C: Common questions about cognitive behavior therapy for psychiatric disorders. *Am Fam Physician* 92:807–812, 2015.

CBT has good-quality evidence for the treatment of depression, anxiety, obsessive-compulsive disorders (OCDs), behavior disorders, substance abuse, and insomnia (see Table 34.1). For many childhood psychiatric disorders, CBT alone provides outcomes comparable to psychotropic medication alone, and the combination of both may convey additional benefit in symptom and harm reduction.

Modified versions of CBT have shown applicability to the treatment of other disorders. **Trauma-focused cognitive-behavioral therapy (TF-CBT)** involves a combination of psychoeducation; teaching effective relaxation, affective modulation, and cognitive coping and processing skills; engaging in a trauma narrative; mastering trauma reminders; and enhancing future safety and development. TF-CBT is considered the first-line treatment for posttraumatic stress disorder (PTSD).

Dialectical behavioral therapy (DBT) is a CBT approach targeted at emotional and behavioral dysregulation by synthesizing or integrating the seemingly opposite strategies of acceptance and change. Dialectic conflicts (wanting to die vs wanting to live) often exist in the same patient and are important to address. The 4 skills modules—*mindfulness* (the practice of being fully aware and present in the moment), *distress tolerance* (how to tolerate emotional pain), *interpersonal effectiveness* (how to maintain self-respect and effective communication in relationships with others), and *emotion regulation* (how to manage complex emotions)—are balanced in terms of acceptance and change. Patients who receive DBT typically have multiple problems; the treatment targets, in order of priority within a given session, are *life-threatening* behaviors, such as suicidal and self-injurious behaviors or communications; *therapy-interfering* behaviors, such as coming late to sessions, cancelling appointments, and being noncollaborative in working toward treatment goals; *quality-of-life* behaviors, including relationship and occupational problems and financial crises; and skills acquisition to help patients achieve their goals. DBT has shown promise for the treatment of personality disorders, suicidal behavior, bipolar disorder, and other manifestations of emotional-behavioral dysregulation.

Interpersonal Psychotherapy

Interpersonal psychotherapy (IPT) focuses on interpersonal issues that lead to psychological distress. Patients are viewed to having biopsychosocial strengths and vulnerabilities that determine the manner in which they cope or respond to an interpersonal crisis (**stressor**). Symptom resolution, improved interpersonal functioning, and increased social support are the IPT targets. IPT has proved to be a well-established treatment for adolescent depression.

Psychodynamic Psychotherapy

At the core of psychodynamic psychotherapy lies a *dynamic* interaction between different dimensions of the mind. This approach is based on the belief that much of one's mental activity occurs outside one's awareness. The patient is often unaware of internal conflicts because threatening or painful emotions, impulses, and memories are repressed. Behavior is then controlled by what the patient does not know about himself or herself. Therapy objectives are to increase self-understanding, increase acceptance of feelings, and develop realistic relationships between self and others. This therapy is nondirective to allow a patient's characteristic patterns to emerge, so that self-understanding and a corrective emotional experience can then be fostered.

Psychodynamic psychotherapy has shown applicability for the treatment of anxiety and depression as well as maladaptive aspects of personality. Brief, time-limited psychodynamic psychotherapy can be appropriate for youth who are in acute situational distress. Long-term therapy can be appropriate when the biologic or social factors destabilizing the child's adaptation and development are chronic, or the psychological difficulties caused by comorbidities are complex, or if entrenched conflicts and developmental interferences are present.

Supportive Psychotherapy

Supportive psychotherapy aims to minimize levels of emotional distress through the provision of individual and contextual support. The goal is to reduce symptoms, and treatment is focused on the "here and now." The therapist is active and helpful in providing the patient with symptomatic relief by helping the patient to contain and manage anxiety, sadness, and anger. The therapist provides support and encouragement to bolster a patient's existing coping mechanisms, facilitates problem-solving, and provides social and instrumental support for ameliorating or lessening contextual precipitants. CBT-informed techniques are often combined with supportive psychotherapy. Probably the most common psychotherapy employed by therapists, supportive psychotherapy has shown comparable results to CBT in a number of research studies.

Family Therapy

The core premise in family therapy is that dysfunctional family interaction patterns precipitate and/or perpetuate an individual's emotional or behavioral difficulties. Family dysfunction can take a variety of forms, including enmeshment, disengagement, role-reversal or confusion, and maladaptive communication patterns. Family therapy begins with an assessment of the family system, including observing patterns of interaction, assessing family beliefs and the meanings attached to behaviors, defining social and cultural contexts, exploring the presenting problem in the context of individual and family development, assessing the family's style of dealing with problems, and identifying family strengths and weaknesses.

Family therapy techniques are drawn from 2 major theoretical models: structural and behavioral. *Structural* family therapy develops structures believed to foster well-functioning families, including clear and flexible boundaries between individuals, well-defined roles, and an appropriate balance between closeness and independence. *Behavioral* family therapy focuses on behavioral sequences that occur in daily life and attempts to interrupt unhelpful patterns and strengthen positive patterns through effective communication and problem solving.

Family therapy has shown established applicability in anorexia nervosa and substance use and may be a promising treatment for depression.

Parenting Interventions
(See Chapter 19 for more details)

Parenting interventions seek to improve both the parent–child relationship and parenting skills using the principles of behavior therapy previously described. They can be provided in individual or group therapy formats. Core relationship recommendations include spending quality time with the child, increasing verbal interaction, showing physical affection, providing contingent praise, and engaging in child-directed play. Core parenting skills include increasing reinforcement of positive behaviors, decreasing reinforcement of negative behaviors, ignoring merely annoying behaviors, applying consequences for dangerous/destructive behaviors, and making parental responses predictable, contingent, and immediate. Parenting interventions have shown applicability for behavior disorders and ADHD.

Common Elements of Evidence-Based Psychotherapies

A major challenge for the practitioner is selecting the "right intervention" for the "right person" in the "right setting," and delivering the intervention in the "right way" (to meet the needs of patients and families). This challenge has led to interest in identifying common **practice elements** across efficacious evidence-based therapies that could be "matched" in a flexible way to patients of a certain age, gender, and race/ethnicity who have certain psychiatric disorders. Table 34.3 provides the major practice elements for 3 of the most common child and adolescent psychiatric disorders: anxiety, depression, and disruptive behaviors. These practice elements, when made available to patients with psychiatric disorders in a system of care, are estimated to be relevant to approximately two thirds of the patients. Six of the practice elements—problem-solving skills, psychoeducation of the parent, relaxation skills, self-monitoring, cognitive/coping skills, and psychoeducation of the child—are applicable to all 3 disorders and as such could be considered "core skills" for the child and adolescent psychotherapist.

Psychoeducation is the education of the parent and child about the cause, course, prognosis, and treatment of the disorder. **Problem solving** is techniques, discussions, or activities designed to bring about solutions to targeted problems, with the intention of imparting a skill for how

Table 34.3	Practice Elements in Interventions for 3 Common Child and Adolescent Psychiatric Disorders		
	ANXIETY DISORDERS	**DEPRESSION**	**DISRUPTIVE BEHAVIOR**
Directed play			X
Limit setting			X
Time-out			X
Cost response			X
Activity scheduling		X	
Maintenance		X	X
Skill building		X	
Social skills training		X	X
Therapist praise/ rewards			X
Natural and logical consequences	X		X
Communication skills	X		X
Assertiveness training	X		
Parent monitoring	X		X
Modeling	X		
Ignoring	X		X
Parent praise	X		X
Problem solving	X	X	X
Parent coping	X		X
Psychoeducation, parent	X	X	X
Relaxation	X	X	X
Tangible rewards	X		X
Self-monitoring	X	X	X
Cognitive/coping	X	X	X
Psychoeducation, child	X	X	X
Exposure	X		

Adapted from Chorpita BF, Daleiden EL, Weisz JR: Identifying and selecting the common elements of evidence based interventions: a distillation and matching model, *Ment Health Serv Res* 7(1):5–20, 2005.

to approach and solve future problems in a similar manner. **Relaxation** is techniques designed to create and maintain the physiologic relaxation response. **Self-monitoring** is the repeated measurement of a target metric by the child. **Cognitive/coping** skills consist of techniques designed to alter interpretations of events through examination of the child's reported thoughts, accompanied by exercises designed to test the validity of the reported thoughts. PCPs can incorporate some of these elements into their anticipatory guidance work with pediatric patients.

Modular Therapy Packages

Of considerable importance to day-to-day clinical work is the manner in which common therapy practice elements are selected, sequenced, repeated, or selectively applied. This **coordination** of psychotherapeutic elements is particularly relevant for patients presenting with multiple concurrent psychiatric disorders. The *Modular Approach to Therapy for Children* (MATCH) is a multidisorder intervention system that incorporates treatment procedures (practice elements) and treatment logic (coordination) corresponding to efficacious interventions for childhood anxiety, depression, and behavior problems, with modifications to allow the system to operate as a single protocol. Compared with standard manualized treatments for individual disorders and with usual care, the modular package outperformed both comparators on multiple clinical and service outcome measures when assessed over a 2-yr period, although additional, independently derived evidence is needed to categorize this treatment approach as well established.

Common Elements of Treatment Engagement Interventions

Treatment engagement is conceptualized as a multidimensional construct targeting *cognitive, attendance,* and *adherence* domains. Research has identified several key factors addressing these domains that are associated with treatment engagement: accessibility promotion, psychoeducation about services, appointment reminders, assessment of treatment barriers, patient assessment, expectation setting, modeling, and homework assignments (Table 34.4). To promote treatment engagement, the first 7 of these factors can be addressed by the PCP and the medical home team as soon as a mental health problem is identified that would benefit from treatment (see Chapter 17 for further discussion).

Psychotherapy in the Medical Home

Recognizing that up to one half of visits to PCPs involve a mental health problem, and that an estimated one fifth of pediatric patients have a functionally impairing psychiatric disorder, in the context of limited access to specialty mental health services in community or hospital settings, a number of models have been developed to deliver psychotherapy in primary care. Two prominent models, both originally developed for adult populations, are collaborative care and primary care behavioral health.

Collaborative care integrates physical and mental healthcare for patients who have a psychiatric disorder in a treatment model that provides both psychotropic medication and psychotherapy delivered by an interdisciplinary care team of PCPs, social workers, and care managers supported by a consulting psychiatrist. The role of the consulting psychiatrist is to advise the PCPs about psychotropic medication management and the therapists about brief psychotherapeutic interventions. The 4 critical elements of collaborative care are team-driven, population-focused, measurement-guided, and evidence-based. These elements guide a treatment approach in which evidence-based, measurement-guided (e.g., symptom rating scale scores as treatment targets) mental healthcare is delivered by the multidisciplinary team to the entire patient population as indicated, such that the patient perceives a seamless integration of medical and mental healthcare.

In children and adolescents, randomized controlled trials (RCT) have shown that collaborative care for behavior problems, adolescent depression, and adolescent substance use is associated with more favorable treatment adherence, symptom reduction, disorder remission, and consumer satisfaction outcomes than usual care, with or without specialty referral. In a meta-analysis and systematic review, overall integrated medical-mental healthcare for children and adolescents led to improved mental health outcomes compared with usual care. Larger effects were observed for treatment trials targeting diagnoses and elevated symptoms relative to prevention trials, as well as for collaborative care models relative to other integrated mental healthcare.

Primary care behavioral health employs an on-site mental health professional (psychologist, social worker, mental health counselor) to provide focused assessment of patients with mental health, health behavior, and substance use problems and short-term therapy as well as health/mental health promotion and prevention interventions. Mental health clinicians typically collaborate with primary care physicians to develop treatment plans, monitor patient progress, and flexibly provide care to meet patients' changing needs. The model uses a "wide net" approach aimed at serving the entire primary care population, with emphasis on brief, focused interventions. Key features of the model include "warm handoffs," in which the physician introduces the mental health clinician directly to the patient, and "curbside consultations," in

Table 34.4	Select Psychotherapy Engagement Elements
ELEMENT	**DEFINITION**
Accessibility promotion	Any strategy used to make services convenient and accessible in order to proactively encourage and increase participation in treatment; e.g., hiring a co-located therapist or referring to a local community-based therapist with whom the practice has an ongoing collaborative relationship
Psychoeducation about services	Provision of information about services or the service delivery system; e.g., type of therapy being recommended, information about the therapist, session frequency and duration
Appointment reminders	Providing information about the day, time, and location of the therapy office for the initial appointment via mail, text, phone, email, etc., to increase session attendance
Assessment of treatment barriers	Discussion to elicit and identify barriers that hinder participation in treatment; e.g. transportation, scheduling, childcare, previous experiences with therapy, stigma
Assessment	Measurement of the patient's strengths/needs through a variety of methods; e.g., mental health screening instruments, interviews, recorded reviews during which the referring practitioner can motivate treatment engagement
Modeling	Vehicle to convey information about specific roles of the therapist; e.g., introductory video or brochure
Expectation setting	Instillation of hope regarding the efficacy of therapy and the patient's ability to participate successfully in treatment
Homework assignment	Therapeutic tasks given to the patient to complete outside the therapy session to reinforce or facilitate knowledge or skills that are consistent with the treatment plan

Adapted from Lindsey MA, Brandt NE, Becker KD, et al: Identifying the common elements of treatment engagement interventions in children's mental health services, *Clin Child Fam Psychol Rev* 17:283–298, 2014; and Becker KD, Lee BR, Daleiden EL, et al: The common elements of engagement in children's mental health services: which elements for which outcomes? *J Clin Child Adolesc Psychol* 44(1):30–43, 2015.

which the physician and mental health clinician have frequent informal interactions to discuss patients.

A limited evidence base supports the primary care behavioral health model, but the research literature on brief intervention is increasing and encouraging. Brief interventions lasting only 1 session are effective for multiple child psychiatric disorders, particularly anxiety and behavior problems and among children (vs adolescents), and are most effective for CBT approaches. Psychosocial interventions delivered by PCPs (rather than behavioral health clinicians) have not been found to be effective in a Cochrane review.

PSYCHIATRIC HOSPITALIZATION

Youth with severe psychiatric disorders require initial evaluation, treatment planning, and stabilization by child-trained behavioral health clinicians. Psychiatric hospital programs address the serious risks and severe impairments caused by the most acute and complex forms of psychiatric disorder that cannot be managed effectively at any other level of care. The goal is to produce rapid clinical stabilization that allows an expeditious, safe, and appropriate treatment transition to a less intensive level of mental healthcare outside the hospital.

High levels of illness severity combined with significant functional impairment signal a need for hospitalization. Admission criteria must include significant signs and symptoms of active psychiatric disorder. Functional admission indicators generally include a significant risk of self-harm or harm to others, although in some cases the patient is unable to meet basic self-care or healthcare needs, jeopardizing well-being. Serious emotional disturbances that prevent participation in family, school, or community life can also rise to a level of global impairment that can only be addressed on an inpatient basis.

Discharge planning begins at admission, when efforts are made to coordinate care with services and resources that are already in place for the child or adolescent in the community. Step-down care might be needed in partial hospital or residential settings if integrated services in a single location are still indicated after sufficient clinical stabilization has occurred in the hospital setting. Transition from the hospital entails active collaboration and communication with PCPs in the child's medical home. In some cases the PCP resumes the pharmacologic treatment of these youth once stabilized.

Bibliography is available at Expert Consult.

Chapter **35**

Somatic Symptom and Related Disorders

Patricia I. Ibeziako, Heather J. Walter, and David R. DeMaso

第三十五章
躯体症状和相关障碍

中文导读

本章主要介绍了躯体症状和相关障碍的流行病学、风险因素、评估和处理。风险因素包括个体因素（气质类型、应对方式、习得的行为、精神病共病、儿童期躯体疾病）和家庭与环境因素（症状模型、父母亲的反应、学校和家庭中的应激源、创伤、遗传和生物易感性）。评估需要对躯体状况、心理社会因素进行评估，包括需要加以鉴别诊断。至于临床上如何处理躯体症状及相关障碍，本章重点介绍了常规治疗方案和治疗的设置，提出一个综合的多学科康复模型可为治疗提供一个有用的框架；药物治疗、物理治疗和心理干预的综合治疗则被证明是有效的。

Pediatric psychosomatic medicine deals with the relation between physical and psychological factors in the causation or maintenance of disease states. The process whereby distress is experienced and expressed in physical symptoms is referred to as **somatization** or **psychosomatic illness**. Even though present in virtually every psychiatric disorder, physical symptoms are most prominent in the various somatic symptom and related disorders.

In the *Diagnostic and Statistical Manual of Mental Disorders, Fifth Edition* (DSM-5), illnesses previously referred to as "somatoform disorders" are classified as **somatic symptom and related disorders (SSRDs).** In children and adolescents, the SSRDs include **somatic symptom disorder** (Table 35.1), **conversion disorder** (Table 35.2), **factitious disorders** (Table 35.3), **illness anxiety disorder** (Table 35.4), and other **specified/unspecified somatic symptom disorders** (Table 35.5), as well as psychological factors affecting other medical conditions (Table 35.6).

With the exception of illness anxiety disorder, in which there is a high level of anxiety about health in the absence of significant somatic symptoms, and psychological factors affecting other medical conditions, in which psychological and/or behavioral factors adversely affect a medical condition, SSRDs are classified on the basis of physical symptoms associated with significant distress and impairment, with or without the presence of a diagnosed medical condition. The symptoms form a continuum that can range from pain to disabling neurologic symptoms and generally interfere with school/home life and peer relationships.

Most patients with SSRDs are seen by primary care practitioners or by pediatric subspecialists, who may make specialty-specific diagnoses

Table 35.1	DSM-5 Diagnostic Criteria for Somatic Symptom Disorder

A. One or more somatic symptoms that are distressing or result in significant disruption of daily life.
B. Excessive thoughts, feelings, or behaviors related to the somatic symptoms or associated health concerns, as manifested by at least one of the following:
  1. Disproportionate and persistent thoughts about the seriousness of one's symptoms.
  2. Persistent high level of anxiety about health and symptoms.
  3. Excessive time and energy devoted to these symptoms or health concerns.
C. Although any one somatic symptom may not be continuously present, the state of being symptomatic is persistent (typically >6 mo).
Specify if:
With predominant pain (previously known as "pain disorder" in DSM IV-TR): for individuals whose somatic symptoms predominantly involve pain.
Persistent: A persistent course is characterized by severe symptoms, marked impairment, and long duration (>6 mo).

Adapted from the *Diagnostic and Statistical Manual of Mental Disorders, Fifth Edition,* (Copyright 2013). American Psychiatric Association, p 311.

Table 35.2	DSM-5 Diagnostic Criteria for Conversion Disorder or Functional Neurologic Symptom Disorder

A. One or more symptoms of altered voluntary motor or sensory function.
B. Clinical findings provide evidence of incompatibility between the symptom and recognized neurologic or medical conditions.
C. The symptom is not better explained by another medical or mental disorder.
D. The symptom causes clinically significant distress or impairment in social, occupational, or other important areas of functioning or warrants medical evaluation.
Specify symptom type: weakness or paralysis, abnormal movements, swallowing symptoms, speech symptom, attacks/seizures, anesthesia/sensory loss, special sensory symptom (e.g., visual, olfactory, hearing), or mixed symptoms.

Adapted from the *Diagnostic and Statistical Manual of Mental Disorders, Fifth Edition,* (Copyright 2013). American Psychiatric Association, p 318.

Table 35.3	DSM-5 Diagnostic Criteria for Factitious Disorders

Factitious Disorder Imposed on Self
A. Falsification of physical or psychological signs or symptoms, or induction of injury or disease, associated with identified deception.
B. The individual presents himself or herself to others as ill, impaired, or injured.
C. The deceptive behavior is evident even in the absence of obvious external rewards.
D. The behavior is not better explained by another mental disorder, such as delusional disorder or another psychotic disorder.
Specify if: single episode or recurrent episodes.

Factitious Disorder Imposed on Another (Previously "Factitious Disorder by Proxy")
A. Falsification of physical or psychological signs or symptoms, or induction of injury or disease, in another, associated with identified deception.
B. The individual presents another individual (victim) to others as ill, impaired, or injured.
C. The deceptive behavior is evident even in the absence of obvious external rewards.
D. The behavior is not better explained by another mental disorder, such as delusional disorder or another psychotic disorder.
Note: The perpetrator, not the victim, receives this diagnosis.
Specify if: single episode or recurrent episodes.

Adapted from the *Diagnostic and Statistical Manual of Mental Disorders, Fifth Edition,* (Copyright 2013). American Psychiatric Association, p 324.

Table 35.4	DSM-5 Diagnostic Criteria for Illness Anxiety Disorder

A. Preoccupation with having or acquiring a serious illness.
B. Somatic symptoms are not present, or, if present, are only mild in intensity. If another medical condition is present or there is a high risk for developing a medical condition (e.g., strong family history is present), the preoccupation is clearly excessive or disproportionate.
C. There is a high level of anxiety about health, and the individual is easily alarmed about personal health status.
D. The individual performs excessive health-related behaviors (e.g., repeatedly checks his or her body for signs of illness) or exhibits maladaptive avoidance (e.g., avoids doctor appointments and hospitals).
E. Illness preoccupation has been present for at least 6 mo, but the specific illness that is feared may change over that time.
F. The illness-related preoccupation is not better explained by another mental disorder.
Specify whether: care-seeking type or care-avoidant type.

Adapted from the *Diagnostic and Statistical Manual of Mental Disorders, Fifth Edition,* (Copyright 2013). American Psychiatric Association, p 315.

Table 35.5	DSM-5 Diagnostic Criteria for Other Specified/Unspecified Somatic Symptom and Related Disorders

Other Specified
This category applies to presentations in which symptoms characteristic of a somatic symptom and related disorder that cause clinically significant distress or impairment in social, occupational, or other important areas of functioning predominate but do not meet full criteria for any of the disorders in the *somatic symptom and related disorders* diagnostic class.
Examples of presentations that can be specified using the "other specified" designation include the following:
1. Brief somatic symptom disorder: duration of symptoms is <6 mo.
2. Brief illness anxiety disorder: duration of symptoms is <6 mo.
3. Illness anxiety disorder without excessive health-related behaviors: Criterion D for illness anxiety disorder is not met (see Table 35.4).
4. *Pseudocyesis:* a false belief of being pregnant that is associated with objective signs and reported symptoms of pregnancy.

Unspecified
This category applies to presentations in which symptoms characteristic of a somatic symptom and related disorder that cause clinically significant distress or impairment in functioning predominate but do not meet criteria for any of the other disorders in the *somatic symptom and related disorders* diagnostic class.

Adapted from the *Diagnostic and Statistical Manual of Mental Disorders, Fifth Edition,* (Copyright 2013). American Psychiatric Association, p 327.

such as visceral hyperalgesia, chronic fatigue syndrome, psychogenic syncope, or noncardiac chest pain. Even within psychiatry, SSRDs are variously referred to as **functional** or **psychosomatic disorders** or as **medically unexplained symptoms**. The nosologic heterogeneity across the pediatric subspecialties contributes to the varying diagnostic labels. There is a significant overlap in the symptoms and presentation of patients with somatic symptoms who have received different diagnoses from different specialties. Moreover, SSRDs share similarities in etiology, pathophysiology, neurobiology, psychological mechanisms, patient characteristics, and management and treatment response, which is indicative of a single spectrum of somatic disorders.

It is helpful for healthcare providers to avoid the dichotomy of approaching illness using a medical model in which diseases are considered physically or psychologically based. In contrast, a *biobehavioral continuum* of disease better characterizes illness as occurring across a spectrum ranging from a predominantly biologic to a predominantly psychosocial etiology.

EPIDEMIOLOGY

Between 10% and 30% of children worldwide experience physical symptoms that are seemingly unexplained by a physical illness. Estimated prevalence varies greatly between studies based on the type of symptoms and the study methodology. The frequency and heterogeneity of complaints increase with age, with symptoms occurring more frequently in girls than boys.

Many children with persistent complaints of abdominal pain meet criteria for somatic symptom disorder with predominant pain in DSM-5. Headaches and back, limb, and chest pain are also frequently occurring pain symptoms in adolescents. Prevalence rates of conversion disorder in adolescents are 0.3–10%. Nonepileptic seizures, loss of consciousness, and motor symptoms are common conversion symptoms across cultures.

Table 35.6	DSM-5 Diagnostic Criteria for Psychological Factors Affecting Other Medical Conditions

A. A medical symptom or condition (other than a mental disorder) is present.
B. Psychological or behavioral factors adversely affect the medical condition in one of the following ways:
   1. The factors have influenced the course of the medical condition, as shown by a close temporal association between the psychological factors and the development or exacerbation of, or delayed recovery from, the medical condition.
   2. The factors interfere with the treatment of the medical condition (e.g., poor adherence).
   3. The factors constitute additional well-established health risks for the individual.
   4. The factors influence the underlying pathophysiology, precipitating or exacerbating symptoms or necessitating medical attention.
C. The psychological and behavioral factors in Criterion B are not better explained by another mental disorder (e.g., panic disorder, major depressive disorder, posttraumatic stress disorder).
Specify if: mild, moderate, severe, or extreme.

Adapted from the *Diagnostic and Statistical Manual of Mental Disorders, Fifth Edition,* (Copyright 2013). American Psychiatric Association, p 322.

RISK FACTORS
Individual
Temperament/Coping Styles

Somatic symptoms have been found to be more common in children who are conscientious, sensitive, insecure, internalizers, and anxious, and in those who strive for high academic achievement. Somatization may also occur in children who are unable to verbalize emotional distress. Somatic symptoms are often seen as a form of psychological defense against intrapsychic distress that allows the child to avoid confronting anxieties or conflicts, a process referred to as "primary gain." The symptoms may also lead to what is described as "secondary gain" if the symptom results in the child being allowed to avoid unwanted responsibilities or consequences.

Learned Behavior

Somatic complaints may be reinforced through a decrease in responsibilities or expectations by others and through receiving attention and sympathy. Many children may have an antecedent underlying general medical condition that may then be reinforced by parental and peer attention as well as additional medical attention in the form of unnecessary tests and investigations.

Psychiatric Comorbidity

There is an association between somatization and other psychiatric illness, in particular depressive and anxiety disorders. A familial link exists between SSRDs and other psychiatric disorders (e.g., higher rates of anxiety and depression in family members).

Childhood Physical Illness

There appears to be a connection between childhood physical illness and the later development of somatization. Many children with an SSRD have other medical conditions. An antecedent history (e.g., accident, viral illness) may trigger onset of symptoms and lead to prolonged recovery or recurrence of symptoms after illness should have subsided. Children who tend to somatize may have a tendency to experience normal somatic sensations as "intense, noxious, and disturbing," referred to as *somatosensory amplification.*

Family and Environmental
Symptom Modeling

Multiple studies have found evidence that a significant proportion of patients with SSRD had recently encountered similar symptoms in their local environment or live with family members who complain of similar physical symptoms (e.g., child with nonepileptic seizures who has parent or sibling with seizure disorder).

Parental Responses

Parent beliefs about the significance of symptoms influence the extent of symptoms the child reports. Having a somatic complaint may be more acceptable or noticed in some households than the expression of strong emotions (e.g., anxiety, fear, anger). In such an environment, a child may garner minimal attention for emotional distress, but obtain more attention and sympathy for physical symptoms. Multiple studies have shown that parental protectiveness predicts child functional disability and parental responses (e.g., discouraging activity, expressing concern, providing comfort) may serve inadvertently to reinforce and maintain illness behaviors.

School and Family Stressors

External environmental factors (e.g., school stress, change in family situation) are common in children presenting with an SSRD. Common school stressors include bullying, beginning the school year, fear of academic failure, or participation in extracurricular school activities. Dysfunction and less support within the family system are common. Transitions within the family system, including death of a family member, birth of a sibling, parental divorce, physical punishment by parents, and increased arguments between parents, have all been linked to somatic symptoms. Nevertheless, a significant minority of patients with SSRD do not appear to have obvious psychosocial precipitants for their symptoms. It is unclear whether recorded stressful events are absent in these patients because they were unwilling or unable to report relevant stressors or because the stressors were simply absent.

Trauma

Elevated rates of childhood trauma (e.g., sexual, physical, or emotional abuse) have been found in patients with SSRD, although the trauma prevalence rates in studies vary widely.

Genetic and Biologic Vulnerabilities

Genetic and biologic vulnerabilities (e.g., increased pain sensitivity) are thought to contribute to SSRDs. Research has suggested some unifying mechanisms, including aberrant functions of efferent neural pathways, such as the autonomic nervous system and hypothalamic-pituitary axis, and alterations in central processing of sensory input. Hyperactivity of the anterior cingulate cortex has been found in patients with conversion disorder, along with impaired activity of the dorsolateral prefrontal cortex. In chronic pain studies, including migraine and tension-type headaches, there appears to be progressive loss of gray matter density in brain structures involved in registering pain, such as the somatosensory cortex, anterior cingulate cortex, and insula. Additionally, when there is a strong expectation of pain, the anterior insular cortex is activated in proportion to this expectation.

ASSESSMENT

The majority of patients with SSRD present in the pediatric setting rather than the mental health setting. It is important for pediatric practitioners to make their diagnosis based on positive symptoms and signs (distressing somatic symptoms plus abnormal thoughts, feelings, and behaviors in response to these symptoms) rather than the absence of a medical explanation. As such, the evaluation of suspected disorders should include an assessment of biologic, psychological, social, and developmental realms, both separately and in relation to each other. An integrated approach in which both pediatric and mental health clinicians are involved in the assessment, management, and treatment is indicated.

Medical

The presence of a physical illness does not exclude the possibility of somatization playing an important role in the child's presentation. Somatic symptoms early in a disease course that can be directly attributed to a specific physical illness (e.g., acute respiratory illness) may evolve into psychologically based symptoms, particularly in situations where the child may experience benefit from adopting the sick role. Somatic symptoms may also occur in excess of what would be expected of the symptoms experienced in an existing physical illness. Physical findings may occur secondary to the effects of the somatic symptom disorder, especially when chronic or severe (e.g., deconditioning, disuse atrophy and contractures from prolonged immobilization, nutritional deficiency, gastroparesis and constipation from chronic poor oral intake).

A comprehensive medical workup to rule out serious physical illness must be carefully balanced with efforts to avoid unnecessary and potentially harmful tests and procedures. The physical examination will find that the child's symptoms may fluctuate in different contexts, may be anatomically inconsistent, or may be in excess of what would be expected from the physical findings.

Psychosocial

If somatization is suspected, mental health consultation should be included early in the diagnostic workup. The reason for consultation should be carefully explained to the family to help avoid the perception that their child's symptoms are not being taken seriously by the pediatric team (i.e., "it's in her head"). It should be explained that a complete workup involves a thorough assessment of the physical and psychological domains of the child, and that the psychiatric consultation can provide further understanding of the origins of the child's distress, what perpetuates it, and which treatments are likely to be most effective.

The mental health evaluation should include a careful assessment of the psychological and social stressors and risk factors, including a thorough family psychiatric and medical history. The nature of current physical symptoms and any history of prior episodes of somatic symptoms should be included in the assessment, in addition to the child's emotional, social, and academic functioning; coping strategies; and family functioning. The evaluation should provide the clinical team with a biopsychosocial explanation of the child's symptoms, which will inform the treatment plan.

Differential Diagnoses

The primary differential diagnosis is between an SSRD and a physical illness. Importantly, however, these disorders are not mutually exclusive and often coexist. Mood and anxiety disorders frequently include the presence of physical symptoms, which tend to remit with treatment of the primary mood or anxiety symptoms, and which appear distinct from physical complaints seen in SSRDs. Chronic pain syndromes may be caused by fibromyalgia and small fiber autonomic neuropathy.

MANAGEMENT

With the completion of medical and psychological assessments, a multidisciplinary team meeting of pediatric and mental health clinicians should be arranged to review all the specialty evaluations and tests and discuss diagnostic impressions and treatment recommendations. This should occur to ensure consensus on the diagnosis and treatment plan and facilitate adequate and consistent communication among all providers.

An informing meeting or conference with the family should be facilitated after the team meeting to convey the multidisciplinary team's diagnostic impressions and treatment recommendations to the patient and family. Pediatric and mental health clinicians together should communicate the diagnosis (or diagnoses) in a way that families can understand using a comprehensive biopsychosocial formulation. Medical and psychosocial findings should be acknowledged and discussed.

Patients and families with SSRD often present with the belief that there is primarily a medical cause for their problem, and psychosocial contributors are often resisted. After exhaustive medical investigations yield no unifying results, labeling the symptoms as "psychiatric" can effectively shift the search for the cause onto family functioning, resulting in children and parents feeling blamed for the symptoms. The team should help the family move toward an understanding of the mind–body connection and shift their approach from searching for the cause of the symptoms to increasing family functioning. Providing education about the benefits of treatment and risks of no treatment is helpful to move the family through the treatment steps.

Treatment

An integrated multidisciplinary rehabilitation model provides a useful framework for treatment that shifts the focus away from finding a cure for symptoms, and instead emphasizes a return to normal adaptive functioning. This includes increased activities of daily living, improved nutrition, enhanced mobility, return to school and socialization with peers.

Cognitive behavioral therapy (CBT) is the evidence-based intervention of choice. CBT interventions modify symptom experience (including pain perception) and restore central nervous system abnormalities associated with functional impairment. CBT techniques (e.g., relaxation training, biofeedback, hypnosis) can be used to teach patients the control they can have over certain physiologic processes, such as autonomic system activity. Cognitive restructuring is effective in addressing and altering dysfunctional thoughts regarding symptoms and their implications for functioning. Treatments that encourage active coping strategies and emotional expression and modulation, and that limit patient reliance on emotional support provided by parents, are helpful in reducing symptoms and improving functioning. Modifying parental response patterns that are overprotective and potentially reinforcing (e.g., allowing the child to sleep late or to stay home from school in response to symptoms) help to decrease disability.

Psychopharmacologic treatment may be considered when psychiatric comorbidities are present, specifically, depressive and anxiety disorders. A combination of pharmacotherapy, physical therapy, and psychological interventions in multicomponent management programs has been shown to be effective.

Treatment Setting

The majority of patients can be managed in the outpatient setting with appropriate mental health follow-up. Scheduled follow-up visits with the primary care provider are important to maintain alliance and investment in treatment, prevent "doctor shopping," and avoid unnecessary invasive tests and procedures.

Because of the nature of their symptoms, most patients with SSRD do not present in mental health settings for their physical complaints, and only patients who display prominent emotional symptoms or who have a concurrent mental disorder are referred to mental health services. Pediatric specialists treat "their own" specialty somatic syndromes within their service, as a natural consequence of the large number of patients with these disorders presenting at their clinics. The management in these clinics is often monodisciplinary and comprises primarily medically based treatments and interventions. The existence of various syndrome-specific clinics perpetuates the separate, specialty-dominated approach to SSRDs and can perpetuate fragmented care rather than moving toward a more integrated model. Although specialized clinics play an important role in providing the expertise needed in the evaluation of these patients, these clinics are often not prepared to manage patients who have symptoms involving multiorgan systems. These patients may attend several clinics simultaneously and receive several parallel, uncoordinated treatments.

A **medical home model** with mental health clinicians working in collaboration with pediatric practitioners and/or different pediatric specialists may prove to be the most suitable approach for patients with SSRD. Integrated pediatric and mental health services improve communication, decrease fragmentation of services, and decrease the stigma and resistance some families may have with attending mental health clinics. A treatment program with comprehensive multidisciplinary services and CBT showed immediate, clinically relevant benefits that were sustained at the 1 yr follow-up in a randomized controlled trial.

Patients with profound and pervasive functional impairment likely will need more intensive psychiatric treatment (e.g., medical-psychiatric partial hospital program or inpatient unit). Multidisciplinary inpatient rehabilitation programs have much to offer these patients because they are designed to support both physical and psychological recovery. Families feel reassured that multidisciplinary staff can continue to monitor symptoms, thus ensuring that any missed diagnoses will be recognized quickly.

Children with a high level of impairment often miss a significant amount of school; communication with the school is often crucial in helping a successful transition back and improving overall functioning.

In addition to discussions with the school guidance counselor and nurse, a letter for the school providing education and recommended approaches for the patient's symptoms is often beneficial. These interventions can be formalized by having the school work with the family and medical team to develop either a 504 plan for accommodations needed in regular education settings, or an individualized educational plan (IEP) if the child needs special education services. Ongoing communication between the school and the primary care provider for monitoring of further symptoms is recommended.

Bibliography is available at Expert Consult.

Chapter **36**
Rumination and Pica
第三十六章
反刍和异食癖

<hr>

中文导读

本章分两节详细介绍了反刍障碍和异食癖。详细阐述了反刍障碍的流行病学、病因和鉴别诊断、治疗。具体描述了婴幼儿反刍障碍的危险因素，包括与主要照料者的关系紊乱、缺乏适当的环境刺激、被忽视、紧张的生活环境、愉悦感强化的学习行为、消极情绪的干扰，以及来自主要护理者的无意强化。对于治疗，则需要对反刍行为进行分析和开展行为治疗。

行为治疗的中心是加强正确的饮食行为，同时尽量减少对反刍症状的注意。成功的行为治疗则需要孩子的主要照顾者参与到治疗中来。

本章还重点介绍了异食癖的流行病学、病因和鉴别诊断、治疗。详细描述了该症的一些病因，包括心理社会因素对生理因素的影响、营养缺乏、文化和家庭环境因素等。

36.1 Rumination Disorder
Chase B. Samsel, Heather J. Walter, and David R. DeMaso

Rumination disorder is the repeated regurgitation of food, where the regurgitated food may be rechewed, reswallowed, or spit out, for a period of at least 1 mo following a period of normal functioning. Regurgitation is typically frequent and daily; it does not occur during sleep. It is not caused by an associated gastrointestinal illness or other medical conditions (e.g., gastroesophageal reflux, pyloric stenosis). It does not occur exclusively during the course of anorexia nervosa, bulimia nervosa, binge-eating disorder, or avoidant/restrictive food intake disorder. If the symptoms occur in the context of an intellectual developmental disorder or another neurodevelopmental disorder, the symptoms must be sufficiently severe to warrant additional clinical attention.

Weight loss and failure to make expected weight are common features in infants with rumination disorder. Infants may display a characteristic position of straining and arching the back with the head held back, making sucking movements with their tongue. In infants and older individuals with intellectual disability, the rumination behavior may appear to have a self-soothing or self-stimulating function. Malnutrition may occur in older children and adults, particularly when the regurgitation is associated with restricted food intake (which may be designed to avoid regurgitation in front of others). They may attempt to hide the regurgitation behavior or avoid eating among others.

EPIDEMIOLOGY
Originally thought of as a disorder predominantly seen in infants and those with intellectual disability, rumination disorder has also been recognized in healthy individuals across the life span and can be overlooked in adolescents. In otherwise healthy children, rumination disorder typically appears in the 1st year of life, generally between ages 3 and 12 mo. The disorder can have an episodic course or can occur continuously until treatment is initiated. In infants the disorder frequently remits spontaneously but can be protracted with problematic and even life-threatening malnutrition. Additional complications related to the

secondary effects of malnutrition include growth delay and negative effects on development and learning potential.

ETIOLOGY AND DIFFERENTIAL DIAGNOSIS

Risk factors for rumination disorder in infants and young children include a disturbed relationship with primary caregivers, lack of an appropriately stimulating environment, neglect, stressful life situations, learned behavior reinforced by pleasurable sensations, distraction from negative emotions, and inadvertent reinforcement (attention) from primary caregivers. Risk factors for rumination disorder in adolescents include similar early childhood factors along with female gender and comorbid anxiety and depression. The differential diagnosis includes congenital gastrointestinal system anomalies, pyloric stenosis, Sandifer syndrome, gastroparesis, hiatal hernia, increased intracranial pressure, diencephalic tumors, adrenal insufficiency, and inborn errors of metabolism. Older children and adults with anorexia nervosa or bulimia nervosa may also engage in regurgitation because of concerns about weight gain. The diagnosis of rumination disorder is appropriate only when the severity of the disturbance exceeds that routinely associated with a concurrent physical illness or mental disorder.

TREATMENT

The 1st step in treatment begins with a behavioral analysis to determine if the disorder serves as a self-stimulation purpose and/or is socially motivated. The behavior may begin as self-stimulation, but it subsequently becomes reinforced and maintained by the social attention given to the behavior. The central focus of behavioral treatment is to reinforce correct eating behavior while minimizing attention to rumination. Diaphragmatic breathing and postprandial gum chewing, when used as a competing response, have been shown to be helpful. **Aversive conditioning** techniques (e.g., withdrawal of positive attention, introducing bitter/sour flavors when regurgitating) are considered when a child's health is jeopardized but can be more reasonable and useful in adolescents. Additional techniques shown to be useful in adolescents include reswallowing all regurgitation, use of paradoxical intention, and guided progressive food trials.

Successful behavioral treatment requires the child's primary caregivers to be involved in the intervention. The caretakers need education and counseling on responding adaptively to the child's behavior as well as altering any maladaptive responses. No current evidence supports a psychopharmacologic intervention for rumination disorder. In more severe or intractable cases (e.g., severe dehydration, malnutrition), an intensive integrated medical-behavioral treatment program on a medical or medical-psychiatric unit may be necessary.

Bibliography available at Expert Consult.

36.2 Pica

Chase B. Samsel, Heather J. Walter, and David R. DeMaso

Pica involves the persistent eating of nonnutritive, nonfood substances (e.g., paper, soap, plaster, charcoal, clay, wool, ashes, paint, earth) over a period of at least 1 mo. The eating behavior is inappropriate to the developmental level (e.g., the normal mouthing and tasting of objects in infants and toddlers), and therefore a minimum age of 2 yr is suggested. The eating behavior is not part of a culturally supported or socially normative practice. A diagnosis of pica may be assigned in the presence of any other feeding and eating disorder.

EPIDEMIOLOGY

Pica can occur throughout life but occurs most frequently in childhood. It appears to be more common in those with intellectual disability and autism spectrum disorders, and to a lesser degree in obsessive-compulsive and schizophrenic disorders. The prevalence of pica is unclear, although it appears to increase with the severity of an intellectual disability. It usually remits in childhood but can continue into adolescence and adulthood. **Geophagia** (eating earth) is associated with pregnancy and is not seen as abnormal in some cultures (e.g., rural or preindustrial societies in parts of Africa and India). Children with pica are at increased risk for lead poisoning, iron-deficiency anemia, mechanical bowel problems, intestinal obstruction, intestinal perforations, dental injury, and parasitic infections. Pica can be fatal based on substances ingested.

ETIOLOGY AND DIFFERENTIAL DIAGNOSIS

Numerous etiologies have been proposed but not proved, ranging from psychosocial causes to physical ones. They include nutritional deficiencies (e.g., iron, zinc, calcium), low socioeconomic factors (e.g., lead paint exposure), child abuse and neglect, family disorganization (e.g., poor supervision), mental disorder, learned behavior, underlying (but undetermined) biochemical disorder, and cultural and familial factors. The differential diagnosis includes anorexia nervosa, factitious disorder, and nonsuicidal self-injury in personality disorders. A separate diagnosis of pica should be made only if the eating behavior is sufficiently severe enough to warrant additional clinical attention.

TREATMENT

Combined behavioral, social, and medical approaches are generally indicated for pica. Assessment for neglect and family supervision combined with psychiatric assessment for concurrent mental disorders and developmental delay are important in developing an effective intervention strategy for pica. Behavioral interventions, particularly applied behavioral analysis in patients with intellectual disability or autism spectrum disorders, are increasingly found to be helpful. The sequelae related to an ingested item can require specific treatment (e.g., lead toxicity, iron-deficiency anemia, parasitic infestation). Ingestion of hair can require medical or surgical intervention for a gastric bezoar.

Bibliography available at Expert Consult.

Chapter **37**
Motor Disorders and Habits

Colleen A. Ryan, Heather J. Walter, and David R. DeMaso

第三十七章
运动障碍和习惯

中文导读

本章介绍了抽动障碍和习惯等临床特征和诊疗策略。抽动障碍章节描述了抽动障碍、抽动的概念，对抽动障碍的临床病程、流行病学、鉴别诊断、共病、病因、结局与转归、筛查、评估和治疗进行了详细介绍。

本章还简要介绍了刻板性运动障碍的特征，对刻板性运动障碍的临床病程、流行病学、共病、鉴别诊断、治疗进行了详细介绍。列举了几种常见的行为习惯，并对吮吸拇指、磨牙等习惯的临床表现和处理进行了专门介绍。

Motor disorders are interrelated sets of psychiatric symptoms characterized by abnormal motor movements and associated phenomena. In the *Diagnostic and Statistical Manual of Mental Disorders, Fifth Edition* (DSM-5), **motor disorders** include tic, stereotypic movement, and developmental coordination disorders. **Tic disorders** (Tourette, persistent motor or vocal tic, provisional tic, other specified/unspecified tic) and **stereotypic movement disorder** are addressed in this chapter, along with habits. Although not DSM-5 motor disorders, **habits** present as repetitive and often problematic motor behaviors (e.g., thumb sucking, teeth grinding).

37.1 Tic Disorders

Colleen A. Ryan, Heather J. Walter, and David R. DeMaso

Tourette disorder (TD), **persistent (chronic) motor or vocal tic disorder (PTD)**, and **provisional tic disorders** are characterized by involuntary, rapid, repetitive, single or multiple motor and/or vocal/phonic tics that wax and wane in frequency but have persisted for >1 yr since first tic onset (<1 yr for provisional tic disorder) (Table 37.1). PTD is differentiated from TD in that PTD is limited to either motor or vocal tics (not both), whereas TD has both motor and vocal tics at some point in the illness (although not necessarily concurrently). The tic disorders are hierarchical in order (i.e., TD followed by PTD followed by provisional tic disorder), such that once a tic disorder at one level of the hierarchy is diagnosed, a lower-hierarchy diagnosis cannot be made. **Other specified/unspecified tic disorders** are presentations in which symptoms characteristic of a tic disorder that cause significant distress or impairment

predominate but do not meet the full criteria for a tic or other neurodevelopmental disorder.

DESCRIPTION

Tics are sudden, rapid, recurrent, nonrhythmic motor movements or vocalizations. *Simple motor tics* (e.g., eye blinking, neck jerking, shoulder shrugging, extension of the extremities) are fast, brief movements involving one or a few muscle groups. *Complex motor tics* involve sequentially and/or simultaneously produced, relatively coordinated movements that can seem purposeful (e.g., brushing back one's hair bangs, tapping the foot, imitating someone else's movement [**echopraxia**], or making a sexual or obscene gesture [**copropraxia**]). *Simple vocal tics* (e.g., throat clearing, sniffing, coughing) are solitary, meaningless sounds and noises. *Complex vocal tics* involve recognizable word or utterances (e.g., partial words [syllables], words out of context, coprolalia [obscenities or slurs], **palilalia** [repeating one's own sounds or words], or **echolalia** [repeating the last heard word or phrase]).

Sensory phenomena (premonitory urges) that precede and trigger the urge to tic have been described. Individuals with tics can suppress them for varying periods of time, particularly when external demands exert their influence, when deeply engaged in a focused task or activity, or during sleep. Tics are often suggestible and are worsened by anxiety, excitement, or exhaustion. Parents have described increasing frequency of tics at the end of the day. Research has not supported volitional suppressing of tics leading to tic rebound.

CLINICAL COURSE

Onset of tics is typically between ages 4 and 6 yr. The frequency of tics tends to wax and wane with peak tic severity between ages 10 and 12 yr and marked attenuation of tic severity in most individuals (65%) by

Table 37.1	DSM-5 Diagnostic Criteria for Tic Disorders

Note: A tic is a sudden, rapid, recurrent, nonrhythmic motor movement or vocalization.

TOURETTE DISORDER
A. Both multiple motor and one or more vocal tics have been present at some time during the illness, although not necessarily concurrently.
B. The tics may wax and wane in frequency but have persisted for >1 yr since first tic onset.
C. Onset is before age 18 yr.
D. The disturbance is not attributable to the physiologic effects of a substance (e.g., cocaine) or another medical condition (e.g., Huntington disease, postviral encephalitis).

PERSISTENT (CHRONIC) MOTOR OR VOCAL TIC DISORDER
A. Single or multiple motor or vocal tics have been present during the illness, but not both motor and vocal.
B. The tics may wax and wane in frequency but have persisted for >1 yr since first tic onset.
C. Onset is before age 18 yr.
D. The disturbance is not attributable to the physiologic effects of a substance (e.g., cocaine) or another medical condition (e.g., Huntington disease, postviral encephalitis).
E. Criteria have never been met for Tourette disorder.
Specify if:
With motor tics only
With vocal tics only

PROVISIONAL TIC DISORDER
A. Single or multiple motor and/or vocal tics.
B. The tics have been present for <1 yr since first tic onset.
C. Onset is before age 18 yr.
D. The disturbance is not attributable to the physiologic effects of a substance (e.g., cocaine) or another medical condition (e.g., Huntington disease, postviral encephalitis).
E. Criteria have never been met for Tourette disorder or persistent (chronic) motor or vocal tic disorder.

Adapted from the *Diagnostic and Statistical Manual of Mental Disorders, Fifth Edition,* (Copyright 2013). American Psychiatric Association, p. 81.

age 18-20 yr. A small percentage will have worsening tics into adulthood. New onset of tics in adulthood is very rare and most often is associated with exposure to drugs or insults to the central nervous system. Tics manifest similarly in all age-groups and changes in affected muscle groups and vocalizations occur over time. Some individuals may have tic-free periods of weeks to months.

EPIDEMIOLOGY
Prevalence rates for all tics range from 6–18% for boys and 3–11% for girls, with the rate of TD alone estimated as 0.8%. In general, PTD/TD has a male preponderance with a gender ratio varying from 2:1 to 4:1. Evidence supports higher rates in white youth than black or Hispanic youth.

DIFFERENTIAL DIAGNOSIS
The differential diagnosis includes the repetitive movements of childhood (Table 37.2). Tics may be difficult to differentiate from stereotypies. Although stereotypies may resemble tics, **stereotypies** are typically rhythmic movements and do not demonstrate the change in body location or movement type over time that is typical of tics. **Compulsions** may be difficult to differentiate from tics when tics have premonitory urges. Tics should be differentiated from a variety of developmental and benign movement disorders (e.g., benign paroxysmal torticollis, Sandifer syndrome, benign jitteriness of newborns, shuddering attacks). Tics may present in various neurologic illnesses (e.g., Wilson disease, neuroacanthocytosis, Huntington syndrome, various frontal-subcortical brain lesions), but it is rare for tics to be the only manifestation of these disorders.

Individuals presenting with tics in the context of declining motor or cognitive function should be referred for neurologic assessment. Substances/medications that are reported to worsen tics include selective serotonin reuptake inhibitors (SSRIs), lamotrigine, and cocaine. If tics develop in close temporal relationship to the use of a substance or medication and then remit when use of the substance is discontinued, a causal relationship is possible. Although a long-standing clinical concern, controlled studies show no evidence that stimulants commonly increase tics.

COMORBIDITIES
Comorbid psychiatric disorders are common, often with both patient and family viewing the accompanying condition as more problematic than the tics. There is a bidirectional association between PTD/TD (especially TD) and obsessive-compulsive disorder (OCD), with 20–60% of TD patients meeting OCD criteria and 20–40% of OCD patients reporting tics (Fig. 37.1). Attention-deficit/hyperactivity disorder (ADHD) occurs in approximately 50% of all childhood PTD/TD, but estimates in clinically referred patients suggest much higher rates (60–80%). PTD/TD is often accompanied by behavior problems, including poor frustration tolerance, temper outbursts, and oppositionality. Learning disabilities have been found in >20% of these patients. Concurrent anxiety and depression have also been observed. Some patients with PTD/TD will display symptoms of autism spectrum disorder (ASD); careful assessment is required to determine which disorder is primary.

ETIOLOGY
Tics are proposed to be the result of dysfunctional corticostriatal-thalamocortical motor pathways in the basal ganglia, striatum, and frontal lobes associated with abnormalities in the dopamine, serotonin, and norepinephrine neurotransmitter systems. Male predominance in PTD/TD may be attributable to influences of sex hormones on the neurodevelopment of these motor pathways, as reflected by the effects of antiandrogens in the treatment of TD.

Family studies suggest a 10-100–fold increased risk of PTD/TD among first-degree relatives compared to rates in the general population. Twin studies also support a genetic link, with approximately 80% of monozygotic twins and 30% of dizygotic twins showing concordance for PTD/TD. Candidate-gene association and nonparametric linkage studies have not identified specific susceptibility genes for PTD/TD.

Autoimmune-mediated mechanisms have been hypothesized as having a potential etiologic role in some tic disorders. The **pediatric autoimmune neuropsychiatric disorder associated with streptococcal infection (PANDAS)** designation has been used to describe cases of acute childhood onset of OCD and/or tics following a streptococcal infection. **Pediatric acute-onset neuropsychiatric syndrome (PANS)** has been used to describe a subtype of acute childhood-onset OCD (tics are not a required feature) in which a link to a prior streptococcal infection is not evident, suggesting that other infectious agents may also be responsible. In addition to a diagnosis of OCD and tics, children with PANS/PANDAS have been reported with symptoms of separation anxiety, nightmares, personality change, oppositional behaviors, and deterioration in math skills and handwriting. Although some studies suggest a prior history of infections may increase the risk for developing tic disorder, this remains controversial.

Premorbid stress has been hypothesized to act as a sensitizing agent in the pathogenesis of TD among susceptible individuals by affecting stress-responsive biologic systems such as the hypothalamic-pituitary-adrenal axis.

SEQUELAE
Many individuals with mild to moderate tics express minimal to no distress or functional impairment and may even be unaware of their tics. Even individuals with moderate to severe tics can experience minimal functional impairment, but psychological distress may occur. Infrequently, the presence of tics can lead to social isolation, social victimization, inability to work or attend school, or impaired quality of life.

Table 37.2	Repetitive Movements of Childhood	
MOVEMENT	**DESCRIPTION**	**TYPICAL DISORDERS WHERE PRESENT**
Tics	Sudden rapid, recurrent, nonrhythmic, stereotyped, vocalization or motor movement	Transient tics, Tourette disorder, persistent tic disorder
Dystonia	Involuntary, sustained, or intermittent muscle contractions that cause twisting and repetitive movements, abnormal postures, or both	DYT1 gene, Wilson disease, myoclonic dystonia, extrapyramidal symptoms caused by dopamine-blocking agents
Chorea	Involuntary, random, quick, jerking movements, most often of the proximal extremities, that flow from joint to joint. Movements are abrupt, nonrepetitive, and arrhythmic and have variable frequency and intensity	Sydenham chorea, Huntington chorea
Stereotypies	Stereotyped, rhythmic, repetitive movements or patterns of speech, with lack of variation over time	Autism, stereotypic movement disorder, intellectual disability
Compulsions	A repetitive, excessive, meaningless activity or mental exercise that a person performs in an attempt to avoid distress or worry	Obsessive-compulsive disorder, anorexia, body dysmorphic disorder, trichotillomania, excoriation disorder
Myoclonus	Shock-like involuntary muscle jerk that may affect a single body region, one side of the body, or the entire body; may occur as a single jerk or repetitive jerks	Hiccups, hypnic jerks, Lennox-Gastaut syndrome, juvenile myoclonic epilepsy, mitochondrial encephalopathies, metabolic disorders
Akathisia	Unpleasant sensations of "inner" restlessness, often prompting movements in an effort to reduce the sensations	Extrapyramidal adverse effects from dopamine-blocking agents; anxiety
Volitional behaviors	Behavior that may be impulsive or caused by boredom, such as tapping peers or making sounds (animal noises)	Attention-deficit/hyperactivity disorder, oppositional defiant disorder, sensory integration disorders

Adapted from Murphy TK, Lewin AB, Storch EA, et al: Practice parameter for the assessment and treatment of children and adolescents with chronic tic disorders, *J Am Acad Child Adolesc Psychiatry* 52(12):1341–1359, 2013.

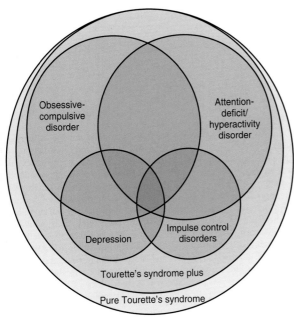

Fig. 37.1 Schematic representation of the behavioral spectrum in Tourette's syndrome. The size of each area is proportional to the estimated prevalence of the symptoms; the background color intensity is proportional to the complexity of the clinical presentation. *(From Cavanna AE, Seri S: Tourette's syndrome. BMJ 347:f4964, 2013.)*

SCREENING

Pediatricians should routinely screen for unusual movements and vocalizations. As an adjunct to a verbal screen, commonly used broadband symptom rating scales such as the *Child Behavior Checklist* (CBCL) and the *Swanson, Nolan, and Pelham* (SNAP) include specific tic questions. Often families are unaware that frequent sniffing, coughing, or blinking may be indicative of tics, attributing these behaviors to medical problems (e.g., allergies, visual problems). A careful assessment of the timing, triggers, and specific characteristics may differentiate tics from other medical problems. If differentiation is difficult, a referral to a pediatric specialist in the affected system is warranted.

ASSESSMENT

If the screening suggests the presence of a tic disorder, a more comprehensive evaluation should ensue, including the age of onset, types of tics, tic frequency, alleviating and aggravating factors, and a family history of tics. Symptom rating scales specific for tics (e.g., the *Motor Tic, Obsessions and Compulsions, Vocal Tic Evaluation Survey* [MOVES], *Tic Self Report Scale, Tourette's Disorder Scale, Parent Tic Questionnaire* [PTQ], and *Child Tourette's Disorder Impairment Scale–Parent Version* can supplement the assessment. For clinician-rated tic severity, the most commonly used instruments are the *Yale Global Tic Severity Scale* (YGTSS), *Tourette Syndrome Severity Scale* (TSSS), and *Tourette Syndrome Global Scale* (TSGS).

A medical workup should be considered for new-onset tics, particularly for presentations characterized by sudden onset, atypicality, or mental status abnormalities. Basic laboratory measures (hemogram, renal/hepatic function panel, thyroid panel, and ferritin, along with urine drug screen for adolescents) should be considered. For new, sudden onset or severe symptom exacerbation, pediatric practitioners may assess for concurrent acute infection (e.g., culture, rapid viral tests). Electroencephalography and brain imaging are not routinely recommended and should be reserved for patients with other neurologic findings that might suggest an autoimmune encephalitis syndrome (limbic encephalitis). Comorbid psychiatric disorders (e.g., OCD, ADHD, ASD) should be investigated.

TREATMENT

The decision to treat tics is made with the child and family based on the level of impairment and distress caused by the tics. If tics are mild in severity, there may be no need for intervention after psychoeducation is provided.

Psychoeducation should include common symptom presentations, implications of concurrent conditions, course and prognosis, and treatment options (including no treatment). The youth's typical exacerbating and alleviating factors should be reviewed. The clinician can direct the family and youth to informational websites, including the Tourette Association of America (www.tourette.org).

Almost 75% of children with TD/PTD receive some form of classroom accommodation (most often ignoring the tics and permission to leave the room as needed). The accommodations may need to be formalized in an individualized education plan (IEP) if a child needs special education services or a 504 plan if the child just needs accommodations in the regular classroom.

Referral to a behavioral treatment specialist should be considered when tics are distressing or functionally impairing. The behavioral interventions with the strongest empirical support are **habit reversal therapy (HRT)** and **comprehensive behavioral intervention for tics (CBIT)**. The basic components of HRT include premonitory urge awareness training and building a competing response to the urge to tic (Table 37.3). Based on HRT, CBIT also includes relaxation training and a functional intervention designed to mitigate against tic-generating situations. A course of HRT/CBIT treatment typically takes several months or 8-10 sessions. In children and adolescents with TD, CBIT has been found to reduce significantly the severity of tics compared to education and supportive therapy. This finding has been supported by a meta-analysis of behavior therapy (HRT/CBIT) for TD, in which a medium to large effect size has been shown for behavioral therapy relative to comparison conditions.

Medications should be considered when the tics are causing severe impairment in the quality of life, or when psychiatric comorbidities are present. The only U.S. Food and Drug Administration (FDA)–approved medications to treat TD in children and adolescents are 2 first-generation (typical) antipsychotics (haloperidol, pimozide) and 1 second-generation (atypical) antipsychotic (aripiprazole). Alpha-agonists (clonidine, guanfacine) are also a consideration as first-line agents because of their more favorable side effect profile than the first- or second-generation antipsychotics (see Chapter 33).

Both antipsychotic and α-adrenergic medications have significant benefit compared with placebo for the pharmacologic treatment of youth with tic disorders. There have been no significant differences between the first- and second-generation antipsychotic agents tested.

Children with tic disorders may benefit from SSRIs for the treatment of comorbid OCD, anxiety, or depressive disorders. Augmentation of SSRIs with an atypical antipsychotic has been a consideration in patients with concurrent tic disorders and OCD responding poorly to an SSRI alone. The presence of tics does not preclude the use of stimulants to address comorbid ADHD. However, close clinical monitoring is required for possible exacerbation of tics during stimulant treatment. Anger and rage outbursts are not uncommon among youth with tics (up to 80% in clinically referred samples). Behavioral therapies (CBT, parent management training) that address anger management may be useful. There are no controlled pharmacologic studies in youth with tic disorders with anger outbursts. There also is no rigorous scientific evidence to support the use of deep brain stimulation, repetitive magnetic stimulation, or dietary supplements in the treatment of TD or PTD.

37.2 Stereotypic Movement Disorder

Colleen A. Ryan, Heather J. Walter, and David R. DeMaso

In DSM-5, **stereotypic movement disorder (SMD)** is defined as a neurodevelopmental disorder characterized by repetitive, seemingly driven, and apparently purposeless motor behavior *(stereotypy)* that interferes with social, academic, or other activities and may result in self-injury. The onset of SMD is the early developmental period (often before age 3 yr), and the symptoms are not attributable to the physiologic effects of a substance or neurologic condition and are not better explained by another neurodevelopmental or mental disorder. The disorder is considered *mild* if symptoms are easily suppressed by sensory stimulus or distraction, and *severe* if continuous monitoring and protective

Table 37.3	Components of Habit Reversal Procedure

Increase Individual's Awareness of Habit

Response description—have individual describe behavior to therapist in detail while reenacting the behavior and looking in a mirror.

Response detection—inform individual of each occurrence of the behavior until each occurrence is detected without assistance.

Early warning—have individual practice identifying earliest signs of the target behavior.

Situation awareness—have individual describe all situations in which the target behavior is likely to occur.

Teach Competing Response to Habit

The competing response must result in isometric contraction of muscles involved in the habit, be capable of being maintained for 3 min, and be socially inconspicuous and compatible with normal ongoing activities but incompatible with the habit (e.g., clenching one's fist, grasping and clenching an object). For vocal tics and stuttering, deep relaxed breathing with a slight exhale before speech has been used as the competing response.

Sustain Compliance

Habit inconvenience review—have individual review in detail all problems associated with target behavior.

Social support procedure—family members and friends provide high levels of praise when a habit-free period is noted.

Public display—individual demonstrates to others that he or she can control the target behavior in situations in which the behavior occurred in the past.

Facilitate Generalization—Symbolic Rehearsal Procedure

For each situation identified in situation awareness procedure, individual imagines himself or herself beginning the target behavior but stopping and engaging in the competing response.

From Carey WB, Crocker AC, Coleman WL, et al, editors: *Developmental-behavioral pediatrics,* ed 4, Philadelphia, 2009, Elsevier/Saunders, p 639.

measures are required to prevent serious injury, with *moderate* falling between mild and severe.

DESCRIPTION

Examples of stereotypic movements include hand shaking or waving, body rocking, head banging, self-biting, and hitting one's own body. The presentation depends on the nature of the stereotypic movement and level of the child's awareness of the behavior. Among typically developing children, the repetitive movements may be stopped when attention is directed to the movements or when the child is distracted from performing them. Among children with intellectual disability, the behaviors may be less responsive to such efforts. Each individual presents with his or her own uniquely patterned behavior. Stereotypic movements may occur many times during a day, lasting a few seconds to several minutes or longer. The behaviors may occur in multiple contexts, including when the individual is excited, stressed, fatigued, or bored.

CLINICAL COURSE

Stereotypic movements typically begin within the 1st 3 yr of life. In children who develop complex motor stereotypies, the great majority exhibit symptoms before 24 mo of age. In most typically developing children, these movements resolve over time. Among individuals with intellectual disability, the stereotyped behaviors may persist for years, although the pattern may change over time.

EPIDEMIOLOGY

Simple stereotypic movements are common in typically developing young children. Some children may bang their head on their mattress as they are falling asleep or may sit and rock when bored or overstimulated. Self-injurious habits, such as self-biting or head banging, can occur in up to 25% of typically developing toddlers (often during tantrums), but they are *almost invariably* associated with developmental delay in children older than age 5 yr. *Complex* stereotypic movements are much less common (occurring in approximately 3–4% of children). Between 4% and 16% of individuals with intellectual disability engage in stereotypic movements.

COMORBIDITY

Stereotypic movements are a common manifestation of a variety of neurogenetic disorders, such as Lesch-Nyhan, Rett, fragile X, Cornelia de Lange, and Smith-Magenis syndromes.

DIFFERENTIAL DIAGNOSIS

According to DSM-5, stereotypic movements must be differentiated from normal development, ASDs, tic disorders, OCDs, and other neurologic and medical conditions. Simple stereotypic movements occurring in the context of typical development usually resolve with age. Stereotypic movements may be a presenting symptom of ASD, but SMD does not include the deficits in social communication characteristic of ASD. When ASD is present, SMD is diagnosed only when there is self-injury or when the stereotypic behaviors are sufficiently severe to become a focus of treatment. Typically, SMD has an earlier age of onset than the tic disorders, and the movements are fixed in their pattern. SMD is distinguished from OCD by the absence of obsessions as well as the nature of the repetitive behaviors, which in OCD are purposeful (e.g., in response to obsessions). The diagnosis of stereotypic movements requires the exclusion of habits, mannerisms, paroxysmal dyskinesias, and benign hereditary chorea. A neurologic history and examination are required to assess features suggestive of other disorders, such as myoclonus, dystonia, and chorea.

ETIOLOGY

There is a possible evolutionary link between repetitive abnormal grooming-like behaviors and early human experience with adversity. Brain regions implicated in this model (e.g., amygdala, hippocampus) are those involved in navigating human experience through unpredictable, anxiety-provoked emotional states, as well as regions (e.g., nucleus accumbens) related to pleasure and reward seeking. The latter involves the hypothesis that individuals experience some level of gratification from performing the habit behavior.

Social isolation with insufficient stimulation (e.g., severe neglect) is a risk factor for self-stimulation that may progress into stereotypies, particularly repetitive rocking or spinning. Environmental stress may trigger stereotypic behaviors. Repetitive self-injurious behavior may be a behavioral phenotype in neurogenetic syndromes (e.g., Lesch-Nyhan, Rett, and Cornelia de Lange syndromes). Lower cognitive functioning is also linked to greater risk of stereotypic behaviors.

TREATMENT

The initial approach to helping children with mild stereotypy is for parents to ignore the undesired behavior, encourage substitute behavior, and not convey worry to their child. These behaviors may disappear with time and elimination of attention in young children. However, in children with intellectual disability or ASDs, stereotypies may be more refractory to treatment than in typically developing children and may necessitate referral to a behavioral psychologist, developmental-behavioral pediatrician, or child and adolescent psychiatrist for behavioral and psychopharmacologic management. The pediatrician should consider and rule out neglect of the child, which can be associated with repetitive rocking, spinning, or other stereotypic movements.

Behavior therapy is the mainstay of treatment, using a variety of strategies, including habit reversal, relaxation training, self-monitoring, contingency management, competing responses, and negative practice. The environment should also be modified to reduce risk of injury to those engaging in self-injurious behavior.

Atypical antipsychotic medications appear to be helpful in reducing stereotypic movements in youth with ASD. Patients with anxiety and obsessive-compulsive behaviors treated with SSRIs may show improvement in their stereotypic movements.

HABITS

Habits involve an action or pattern of behavior that is repeated often. Habits are common in childhood and range from usually benign and transient behaviors (e.g., thumb sucking, nail biting) to more problematic (e.g., trichotillomania, bruxism). In DSM-5, habits are not included as a diagnostic category because they are not viewed as disorders causing clinically significant distress or impairment in functioning. Treatment with HRT has been effective as a first-line approach (see Table 37.3).

Thumb Sucking

Thumb sucking is common in infancy and in as many as 25% of children age 2 yr and 15% of children age 5 yr. Thumb sucking beyond 5 yr may be associated with sequelae (e.g., paronychia, anterior open bite). As with other rhythmic patterns of behavior, thumb sucking is self-soothing. Basic behavioral management, including encouraging parents to ignore thumb sucking and instead focus on praising the child for substitute behaviors, is often effective treatment. Simple reminders and reinforcers can also be considered, such as giving the child a sticker (or other reward) for each block of time that he or she does not suck the thumb. In rare cases, mechanical devices placed on the thumb or in the mouth to prevent thumb sucking or noxious agents (bitter salves) placed on the thumb may be part of the treatment plan.

Bruxism

Bruxism or teeth grinding is common (5–30% of children), can begin in the first 5 yr of life, and may be associated with daytime anxiety. Persistent bruxism can manifest as muscular or temporomandibular joint pain. Untreated bruxism can cause problems with dental occlusion. Helping the child find ways to reduce anxiety might relieve the problem; bedtime can be made more relaxing by reading or talking with the child and allowing the child to discuss fears. Praise and other emotional support are useful. Persistent bruxism requires referral to a dentist given the risk for dental occlusion.

Bibliography available at Expert Consult.

Chapter **38**

Anxiety Disorders

David R. Rosenberg and
Jennifer A. Chiriboga

第三十八章
焦虑障碍

中文导读

本章介绍了焦虑障碍的概念、流行病学、发生原因、临床表现和治疗，对病理性的焦虑和生理性的焦虑反应进行了鉴别。原文以表格的形式列举了美国DSM-5焦虑障碍的诊断标准与鉴别诊断，以及特定性恐惧障碍、社交焦虑障碍、惊恐障碍、广场恐怖症、广泛性焦虑障碍、强迫谱系障碍、创伤后应激障碍的诊断标准（见原文表38.1~表38.8），对各种焦虑障碍亚型临床特征和治疗方案分别进行了阐述。最后对与焦虑相关的躯体状况、SSRIs抗抑郁药的有效性和安全性进行了介绍。

Anxiety, defined as dread or apprehension, is not considered pathologic, is seen across the life span, and can be adaptive (e.g., the anxiety one might feel during an automobile crash). Anxiety has both a cognitive-behavioral component, expressed in worrying and wariness, and a physiologic component, mediated by the autonomic nervous system. Anxiety disorders are characterized by **pathologic anxiety,** in which anxiety becomes disabling, interfering with social interactions, development, and achievement of goals or quality of life, and can lead to low self-esteem, social withdrawal, and academic underachievement. The average age of onset of anxiety disorder is 11 yr. Diagnosis of a particular anxiety disorder in a child requires significant interference in the child's psychosocial and academic or occupational functioning, which can occur even with subthreshold symptoms that do not meet criteria in the *Diagnostic and Statistical Manual of Mental Disorders, Fifth Edition* (DSM-5). Anxiety may have physical manifestations such as weight loss, pallor, tachycardia, tremors, muscle cramps, paresthesias, hyperhidrosis, flushing, hyperreflexia, and abdominal tenderness.

Separation anxiety disorder (SAD), childhood-onset social phobia or social anxiety disorder, generalized anxiety disorder (GAD), obsessive-compulsive disorder (OCD), phobias, posttraumatic stress disorder (PTSD), and panic disorder (PD) are all defined by the occurrence of either diffuse or specific anxiety, often related to predictable situations or cues. Anxiety disorders are the most common psychiatric disorders of childhood, occurring in 5–18% of all children and adolescents, prevalence rates comparable to physical disorders such as asthma and diabetes. Anxiety disorders are often comorbid with other psychiatric and medical disorders (including a second anxiety disorder); significant impairment in day-to-day functioning is common. High levels of fear in adolescence are also a significant risk factor for experiencing later episodes of major depression in adulthood. Anxiety and depressive disorder in adolescence predict increased risk of anxiety and depressive symptoms (including suicide attempts) in adulthood, underscoring the need to diagnose and treat these underreported, yet prevalent, conditions early.

Because anxiety is both a normal phenomenon and, when highly activated, strongly associated with impairment, the pediatrician must be able to differentiate normal anxiety from abnormal anxiety across development (Fig. 38.1 and Table 38.1). Anxiety has an identifiable developmental progression for most children; most infants exhibit stranger wariness or anxiety beginning at 7-9 mo of age. **Behavioral inhibition** to the unfamiliar (withdrawal or fearfulness to novel stimuli associated with physiologic arousal) is evident in approximately 10–15% of the population at 12 mo of age and is moderately stable. Most children who show behavioral inhibition do not develop impairing levels of anxiety. A family history of anxiety disorders and maternal overinvolvement or enmeshment predicts later clinically significant anxiety in behaviorally inhibited infants. The infant who is excessively clingy and difficult to calm during pediatric visits should be followed for signs of increasing levels of anxiety.

Preschoolers typically have specific fears related to the dark, animals, and imaginary situations, in addition to normative separation anxiety. Preoccupation with orderliness and routines (*just right* phenomena) often takes on a quality of anxiety for preschool children. Parents' reassurance is usually sufficient to help the child through this period. Although most school-age children abandon the imaginary fears of early childhood, some replace them with fears of bodily harm or other worries (Table 38.2). In adolescence, general worrying about school performance and worrying about social competence are common and remit as the teen matures.

Genetic or temperamental factors contribute more to the development of some anxiety disorders, whereas environmental factors are closely linked to the cause of others. Specifically, behavioral inhibition appears to be a heritable tendency and is linked with social phobia, generalized anxiety, and selective mutism. OCD and other disorders associated with OCD-like behaviors, such as Tourette syndrome and other tic disorders, tend to have high genetic risk as well (see Chapter 37.1). Environmental factors, such as parent–infant attachment and exposure to trauma, contribute more to SAD and PTSD. Parental anxiety disorder is associated with an increased risk of anxiety disorder in offspring. Differences in the size of the amygdala and hippocampus are noted in patients with anxiety symptoms.

Separation anxiety disorder is one of the most common childhood anxiety disorders, with a prevalence of 3.5–5.4%. Approximately 30% of children presenting to an outpatient anxiety disorder clinic have SAD as a primary diagnosis. Separation anxiety is developmentally normal when it begins about 10 mo of age and tapers off by 18 mo. By 3 yr of age, most children can accept the temporary absence of their mother or primary caregiver.

SAD is more common in prepubertal children, with an average age of onset of 7.5 yr. Girls are more frequently affected than boys. SAD is characterized by unrealistic and persistent worries about separation from the home or a major attachment figure. Concerns include possible harm befalling the affected child or the child's primary caregivers, reluctance to go to school or to sleep without being near the parents, persistent avoidance of being alone, nightmares involving themes of separation, numerous somatic symptoms, and complaints of subjective distress. The first clinical sign might not appear until 3rd or 4th grade, typically after a holiday or a period where the child has been home

Table 38.1	Differential Diagnosis of Anxiety Disorders

Shyness
Substance use
Substance use withdrawal
Hyperthyroidism
Arrhythmias
Pheochromocytoma
Mast cell disorders
Carcinoid syndrome
Anaphylaxis
Hereditary angioedema
Lupus
Autoimmune encephalitis
Body dysmorphic disorder
Autism spectrum disorder
Major depressive disorder
Delusional disorder
Oppositional defiant disorder
Embarrassing medical condition

because of illness, or when the stability of the family structure has been threatened by illness, divorce, or other psychosocial stressors.

Symptoms vary depending on the child's age: Children <8 yr often have associated school refusal and excessive fear that harm will come to a parent; children 9-12 yr have excessive distress when separated from a parent; and those 13-16 yr often have school refusal and physical complaints. SAD may be more likely to develop in children with lower levels of psychosocial maturity. Parents are often unable to be assertive in returning the child to school. Mothers of children with SAD often have a history of an anxiety disorder. In these cases the pediatrician should screen for parental depression or anxiety. Often, referral for parental treatment or family therapy is necessary before SAD and concomitant school refusal can be successfully treated.

Comorbidity is common in SAD. In children with comorbid tic disorders and anxiety, SAD is especially associated with tic severity. SAD is a predictor for early onset of PD. Children with SAD compared to those without SAD are 3 times more likely to develop PD in adolescence.

When a child reports recurring acute severe anxiety, antidepressant or anxiolytic medication is often necessary. Controlled studies of tricyclic antidepressants (TCAs, imipramine) and benzodiazepines (clonazepam) show that these agents are not generally effective. Data support the use of cognitive-behavioral therapy (CBT) *and* selective serotonin reuptake inhibitors (SSRIs) (see Chapter 33, Table 33.4). Adverse events with SSRI treatment, including suicidal and homicidal ideation, are uncommon. CBT alone is associated with less insomnia, fatigue, sedation, and restlessness than SSRIs. Combining SSRIs with CBT may be the best approach to achieving a positive response; long-term SSRI treatment can provide additional benefit.

Childhood-onset social phobia (social anxiety disorder) is characterized by excessive anxiety in social settings (including the presence of unfamiliar peers, or unfamiliar adults) or performance situations, leading to social isolation, and is associated with social scrutiny and fear of doing something embarrassing (Table 38.3). Fear of social settings can also occur in other disorders, such as GAD. Avoidance or escape from the situation usually dissipates anxiety in **social phobia (SP)**, unlike GAD, where worry persists.

Children and adolescents with SP often maintain the desire for involvement with family and familiar peers. When severe, the anxiety can manifest as a panic attack. SP is associated with a decreased quality of life, with increased likelihood of having failed at least 1 grade, and a 38% likelihood of not graduating from high school. Its onset is typically during or before adolescence and is more common in girls. A family history of SP or extreme shyness is common. Approximately 70–80% of patients with SP have at least 1 comorbid psychiatric disorder. Most shy patients do not have SP.

Social effectiveness therapy for children (SET-C), alone or with SSRIs, is considered the treatment of choice for SP (see Table 33.4). SSRI and SET-C are superior to placebo in reducing social distress and

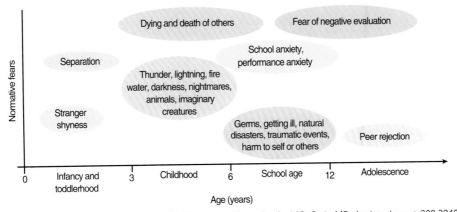

Fig. 38.1 Normative fears throughout childhood and adolescence. *(From Craske MG, Stein MB: Anxiety. Lancet 388:3048–3058, 2016.)*

Table 38.2	DSM-5 Diagnostic Criteria for Specific Phobia

A. Marked fear or anxiety about a specific object or situation (e.g., flying, heights, animals, receiving an injection, seeing blood).
  Note: In children, the fear or anxiety may be expressed by crying, tantrums, freezing, or clinging.
B. The phobic object or situation almost always provokes immediate fear or anxiety.
C. The phobic object or situation is actively avoided or endured with intense fear or anxiety.
D. The fear or anxiety is out of proportion to the actual danger posed by the specific object or situation and to the sociocultural context.
E. The fear, anxiety, or avoidance is persistent, typically lasting for 6 mo or more.
F. The fear, anxiety, or avoidance causes clinically significant distress or impairment in social, occupational, or other important areas of functioning.
G. The disturbance is not better explained by the symptoms of another mental disorder, including fear, anxiety and avoidance or situations associated with panic-like symptoms or other incapacitating symptoms (as in agoraphobia); objects or situations related to obsessions (as in obsessive-compulsive disorder); remainders of traumatic events (as in posttraumatic stress disorder); separation from home or attachment figures (as in separation anxiety disorder); or social situations (as in social anxiety disorder).
Specify if:
Code based on the phobic stimulus:
  Animal (e.g., spiders, insects, dogs).
  Natural environment (e.g., heights, storms, water).
  Blood-injection-injury (e.g., needles, invasive medical procedures).
  Situational (e.g., airplanes, elevators, enclosed places).
  Other (e.g., situations that may lead to choking or vomiting; in children, e.g., loud sounds or costumed characters).

From the *Diagnostic and Statistical Manual of Mental Disorders, Fifth Edition,* (Copyright 2013). American Psychiatric Association, pp 197–198.

Table 38.3	DSM-5 Diagnostic Criteria for Social Anxiety Disorder (Social Phobia)

A. Marked fear or anxiety about 1 or more social situations in which the individual is exposed to possible scrutiny by others. Examples include social interactions (e.g., having a conversation, meeting unfamiliar people), being observed (e.g., eating or drinking), and performing in front of others (e.g., giving a speech).
B. The individual fears that he or she will act in a way or show anxiety symptoms that will be negatively evaluated (i.e., will be humiliating or embarrassing; will lead to rejection or offend others).
C. The social situations almost always provoke fear or anxiety.
  Note: In children, the fear or anxiety may be expressed by crying, tantrums, freezing, clinging, shrinking, or failing to speak in social situations.
D. The social situations are avoided or endured with intense fear or anxiety.
E. The fear or anxiety is out of proportion to the actual threat posed by the social situation and to the sociocultural context.
F. The fear, anxiety, or avoidance is persistent, typically lasting for 6 mo or more.
G. The fear, anxiety, or avoidance causes clinically significant distress or impairment in social, occupational, or other important areas of functioning.
H. The fear, anxiety, or avoidance is not attributable to the physiologic effects of a substance (e.g., a drug of abuse, a medication) or another medical condition.
I. The fear, anxiety, or avoidance is not better explained by the symptoms of another mental disorder, such as panic disorder, body dysmorphic disorder, or autism spectrum disorder.
J. If another medical condition (e.g., Parkinson disease, obesity, disfigurement from burns or injury) is present, the anxiety or avoidance is clearly unrelated or is excessive.
Specify if:
Performance only: If the fear is restricted to speaking or performing in public.

From the *Diagnostic and Statistical Manual of Mental Disorders, Fifth Edition,* (Copyright 2013). American Psychiatric Association, pp 202–203.

behavioral avoidance and increasing general functioning. SET-C may be better than SSRI in reducing these symptoms. SET-C, but not SSRI, may be superior to placebo in improving social skills, decreasing anxiety in specific social interactions, and enhancing social competence. SSRIs have a maximum effect by 8 wk; SET-C provides continued improvement through 12 wk. A combination of SSRI and CBT is superior to either treatment alone in reducing severity of anxiety in children with SP and other anxiety disorders. β-Adrenergic blocking agents are used to treat SP, particularly the subtype with performance anxiety and stage fright. β-Blockers are not approved by the U.S. Food and Drug Administration (FDA) for SP.

School refusal, which occurs in approximately 1–2% of children, is associated with anxiety in 40–50% of cases, depression in 50–60% of cases, and oppositional behavior in 50% of cases. Younger anxious children who refuse to attend school are more likely to have SAD, whereas older anxious children usually refuse to attend school because of SP. Somatic symptoms, especially abdominal pain and headaches, are common. There may be increasing tension in the parent–child relationship or other indicators of family disruption (domestic violence, divorce, or other major stressors) contributing to school refusal.

Management of school refusal typically requires parent management training and family therapy. Working with school personnel is always indicated; anxious children often require special attention from teachers, counselors, or school nurses. Parents who are coached to calmly send the child to school and to reward the child for each completed day of school are usually successful. In cases of ongoing school refusal, referral to a child and adolescent psychiatrist and psychologist is indicated. SSRI treatment may be helpful. Young children with affective symptoms have a good prognosis, whereas adolescents with more insidious onset or with significant somatic complaints have a more guarded prognosis.

Selective mutism is conceptualized as a disorder that overlaps with SP. Children with selective mutism talk almost exclusively at home, although they are reticent in other settings, such as school, daycare, or even relatives' homes. The mutism must be present for ≥1 mo. Often, one or more stressors, such as a new classroom or conflicts with parents or siblings, drive an already shy child to become reluctant to speak. It may be helpful to obtain history of normal language use in at least one situation to rule out any communication disorder (fluency disorder), neurologic disorder, or pervasive developmental disorder (autism, schizophrenia) as a cause of mutism. Fluoxetine in combination with behavioral therapy is effective for children whose school performance is severely limited by their symptoms (see Chapter 52). Other SSRIs may also be effective.

Panic disorder is a syndrome of recurrent, discrete episodes of marked fear or discomfort in which patients experience abrupt onset of physical and psychological symptoms called *panic attacks* (Table 38.4). Physical symptoms can include palpitations, sweating, shaking, shortness of breath, dizziness, chest pain, and nausea. Children can present with acute respiratory distress but without fever, wheezing, or stridor, ruling out organic causes of the distress. The associated psychological symptoms include fear of death, impending doom, loss of control, persistent concerns about having future attacks, and avoidance of settings where attacks have occurred (agoraphobia, Table 38.5).

PD is uncommon before adolescence, with the peak age of onset at 15-19 yr, occurring more often in girls. The postadolescence prevalence of PD is 1–2%. Early-onset PD and adult-onset PD do not differ in symptom severity or social functioning. *Early-onset PD* is associated with greater comorbidity, which can result from greater familial loading for anxiety disorders in the early-onset subtype. Children of parents with PD are much more likely to develop PD. A predisposition to react to autonomic arousal with anxiety may be a specific risk factor leading to PD. Twin studies suggest that 30–40% of the variance is

Table 38.4	DSM-5 Diagnostic Criteria for Panic Disorder

A. Recurrent unexpected panic attacks. A panic attack is an abrupt surge of intense fear or intense discomfort that reaches a peak within minutes, and during which time 4 (or more) of the following symptoms occur:

Note: The abrupt surge can occur from a calm state or an anxious state.

1. Palpitations, pounding heart, or accelerated heart rate.
2. Sweating.
3. Trembling or shaking.
4. Sensations of shortness of breath or smothering.
5. Feelings of choking.
6. Chest pain or discomfort.
7. Nausea or abdominal distress.
8. Feeling dizzy, unsteady, light-headed, or faint.
9. Chills or heart sensations.
10. Paresthesias (numbness or tingling sensations).
11. Derealizations (feeling or unreality) or depersonalization (being detached from one-self).
12. Fear of losing control or "going crazy."
13. Fear of dying.

Note: Culture-specific symptoms (e.g., tinnitus, neck soreness, headache, uncontrollable screaming or crying) may be seen. Such symptoms should not count as 1 of the 4 required symptoms.

B. At least 1 of the attacks has been followed by 1 mo (or more) of 1 or both of the following:
1. Persistent concern or worry about additional panic attacks or their consequences (e.g., losing control, having a heart attack, "going crazy").
2. A significant maladaptive change in behavior related to the attacks (e.g., behaviors designed to avoid having panic attacks, such as avoidance of exercise or unfamiliar situations).

C. The disturbance is not attributable to the physiologic effects of a substance (e.g., a drug of abuse, a medication) or another medical condition (e.g., hyperthyroidism, cardiopulmonary disorders).

D. The disturbance is not better explained by another mental disorder (e.g., the panic attacks do not occur only in response to feared social situations, as in social anxiety disorder; in response to circumscribed phobic objects or situations, as in specific phobia; in response to obsessions, as in obsessive-compulsive disorder; or in response to reminders of traumatic events, as in posttraumatic stress disorder; or in response to separation from attachment figures, as in separation anxiety disorder).

From the *Diagnostic and Statistical Manual of Mental Disorders, Fifth Edition,* (Copyright 2013). American Psychiatric Association, pp 208–209.

Table 38.5	DSM-5 Diagnostic Criteria for Agoraphobia

A. Marked fear or anxiety about 2 (or more) if the following 5 situations:
1. Using public transportation (e.g., automobiles, buses, trains, ships, planes).
2. Being in open spaces (e.g., parking lots, marketplaces, bridges).
3. Being in enclosed places (e.g., shops, theaters, cinemas).
4. Standing in line or being in a crowd.
5. Being outside of the home alone.

B. The individual fears or avoids these situations because of thoughts that escape might be difficult or help might not be available in the event of a developing panic-like symptoms or other incapacitating or embarrassing symptoms (e.g., fear or falling in the elderly, fear of incontinence).

C. The agoraphobic situations almost always provoke fear or anxiety.

D. The agoraphobic situations are actively avoided, require the presence of a companion, or are endured with intense fear or anxiety.

E. The fear or anxiety is out of proportion to the actual danger posed by the agoraphobic situations and to the sociocultural context.

F. The fear, anxiety, or avoidance is persistent, typically lasting for 6 mo or more.

G. The fear, anxiety, or avoidance causes clinically significant distress or impairment in social, occupational, or other important area of functioning.

H. If another medical condition (e.g., inflammatory bowel disease, Parkinson disease) is present, the fear, anxiety, or avoidance is clearly excessive.

I. The fear, anxiety, or avoidance is not better explained by the symptoms or another mental disorder—for example, the symptoms are not confined to specific phobia, situational type; do not involve only social situations (as in social anxiety disorder); and are not related exclusively to obsessions (as in obsessive-compulsive disorder), reminders or traumatic events (as in posttraumatic stress disorder), or fear of separation (as in separation anxiety disorder).

Note: Agoraphobia is diagnosed irrespective of the presence of panic disorder. If an individual's presentation meets criteria for panic disorder and agoraphobia, both diagnoses should be assigned.

From the *Diagnostic and Statistical Manual of Mental Disorders, Fifth Edition,* (Copyright 2013). American Psychiatric Association, pp 217–218.

attributed to genetics. The increasing rates of panic attack are also directly related to earlier sexual maturity. Cued panic attacks can be present in other anxiety disorders and differ from the uncued "out-of-the-blue" attacks in PD.

No randomized controlled trials (RCTs) have evaluated the effectiveness of antidepressant medication in youth with PD. Open-label studies with SSRIs appear to show effectiveness in the treatment of adolescents (see Table 33.4). CBT may also be helpful. The recovery rate is approximately 70%.

Generalized anxiety disorder occurs in children who often experience unrealistic worries about different events or activities for at least 6 mo with at least 1 somatic complaint (Table 38.6). The diffuse nature of the anxiety symptoms differentiates it from other anxiety disorders. Worries in children with GAD usually center around concerns about competence and performance in school and athletics. GAD often manifests with somatic symptoms, including restlessness, fatigue, problems concentrating, irritability, muscle tension, and sleep disturbance. Given the somatic symptoms characteristic of GAD, the differential diagnosis must consider other medical causes. Excessive use of caffeine or other stimulants in adolescence is common and should be determined with a careful history. When the history or physical examination is suggestive, the pediatrician should rule out hyperthyroidism, hypoglycemia, lupus, pheochromocytoma, and other disorders (see Table 38.1; Fig. 38.2).

Children with GAD are extremely self-conscious and perfectionistic and struggle with more intense distress than is evident to parents or others around them. They often have other anxiety disorders, such as simple phobia and PD. Onset may be gradual or sudden, although GAD seldom manifests until puberty. Boys and girls are equally affected before puberty, when GAD becomes more prevalent in girls. The prevalence of GAD ranges from 2.5–6% of children. Hypermetabolism in frontal precortical area and increased blood flow in the right dorsolateral prefrontal cortex may be present.

Children with GAD are good candidates for CBT, an SSRI, or their combination (see Table 33.4). Buspirone may be used as an adjunct to SSRI therapy. The combination of CBT and SSRI often results in a superior response in pediatric patients with anxiety disorders, including GAD. The recovery rate is approximately 80%.

It is important to distinguish children with GAD from those who present with specific repetitive thoughts that invade consciousness (**obsessions**) or repetitive rituals or movements that are driven by anxiety (**compulsions**). The most common obsessions are concerned with bodily wastes and secretions, the fear that something calamitous will happen, or the need for sameness. The most common compulsions are handwashing, continual checking of locks, and touching. At times of stress (bedtime, preparing for school), some children touch certain objects, say certain words, or wash their hands repeatedly.

Obsessive-compulsive disorder is diagnosed when the thoughts or rituals cause distress, consume time, or interfere with occupational or social functioning (Table 38.7). In the DSM-5, OCD and related disorders, such as trichotillomania, excoriation, body dysmorphic disorder, and hoarding, are listed separately and are no longer included under anxiety disorders.

OCD is a chronically disabling illness characterized by repetitive, ritualistic behaviors over which the patient has little or no control. OCD has a lifetime prevalence of 1–3% worldwide, and as many as 80% of all cases have their onset in childhood and adolescence. Common

obsessions include contamination (35%) and thoughts of harming loved ones or oneself (30%). Washing and cleaning compulsions are common in children (75%), as are checking (40%) and straightening (35%). Many children are observed to have visuospatial irregularities, memory problems, and attention deficits, causing academic problems not explained by OCD symptoms alone.

The *Children's Yale-Brown Obsessive-Compulsive Scale* (C-YBOCS) and the *Anxiety Disorders Interview Schedule for Children* (ADIS-C) are reliable and valid methods for identifying children with OCD. The C-YBOCS is helpful in following the progression of symptoms with treatment. The *Leyton Obsessional Inventory* (LOI) is a self-report measure of OCD symptoms that is quite sensitive. Patients with OCD have consistently identified abnormalities in the frontostriatal-thalamic circuitry associated with severity of illness and treatment response. Comorbidity is common in OCD, with 30% of patients having comorbid tic disorders, 26% comorbid major depression, and 24% comorbid developmental disorders.

Consensus guidelines recommend that children and adolescents with OCD begin treatment with either CBT alone or CBT in combination with SSRI, when symptoms are moderate to severe (YBOCS >21). In OCD patients with comorbid tics, SSRIs are no more effective than placebo, and the combination of CBT and SSRI is superior to CBT; CBT alone is superior to placebo. Pediatric OCD patients with comorbid tics should begin treatment with CBT alone or combined CBT and SSRI. Pediatric patients with OCD who have a family history of OCD may be significantly less responsive to CBT alone than patients without a family history.

There are 4 FDA-approved medications for pediatric OCD: fluoxetine, sertraline, fluvoxamine, and clomipramine. *Clomipramine*, a heterocyclic antidepressant and nonselective serotonin and norepinephrine reuptake inhibitor, is only indicated when a patient has failed 2 or more SSRI trials. There may be a role for glutamate-modulating medications in the treatment of OCD. The glutamate inhibitor *riluzole* (Rilutek) is FDA approved for amyotrophic lateral sclerosis (see Chapter 630.3) and has a good safety record. The most common adverse event with riluzole is transient increase in liver transaminases. Riluzole in children with treatment-resistant OCD may be beneficial and is well tolerated. Other glutamate-modulating agents, such as memantine, N-acetylcysteine, and D-cycloserine, have been used with some success in patients with OCD. Referral of patients with OCD to a mental health professional is always indicated.

In 10% of children with OCD, symptoms are triggered or exacerbated by group A β-hemolytic streptococcal infection (see Chapter 210). Group A β-hemolytic streptococci trigger antineuronal antibodies that cross-react with basal ganglia neural tissue in genetically susceptible hosts, leading to swelling of this region and resultant obsessions and compul-

Table 38.6	DSM-5 Diagnostic Criteria for Generalized Anxiety Disorder

A. Excessive anxiety and worry (apprehensive expectation), occurring more days than not for at least 6 mo, about a number of events or activities (such as work or school performance).
B. The individual finds it difficult to control the worry.
C. The anxiety and worry are associated with 3 (or more) of the following 6 symptoms (with at least some symptoms having been present for more days than not for the past 6 mo):
Note: Only 1 item is required in children.
  1. Restlessness or feeling keyed up or on edge.
  2. Being easily fatigued.
  3. Difficulty concentrating or mind going blank.
  4. Irritability.
  5. Muscle tension.
  6. Sleep disturbance (difficulty falling or staying asleep, or restless, unsatisfying sleep).
D. The anxiety, worry, or physical symptoms cause clinically significant distress or impairment in social, occupational, or other important areas of functioning.
E. The disturbance is not attributable to the physiologic effects of a substance (e.g., a drug of abuse, a medication) or other medical condition (e.g., hyperthyroidism).
F. The disturbance is not better explained by another mental disorder (e.g., anxiety or worry about having panic attacks in panic disorder, negative evaluation in social anxiety disorder [social phobia], contamination or other obsessions in obsessive-compulsive disorder, separation from attachment figures in separation anxiety disorder, remainders of traumatic events in posttraumatic stress disorder, gaining weight in anorexia nervosa, physical complaints in somatic symptom disorder, perceived appearance flaws in body dysmorphic disorder, having a serious illness in illness anxiety disorder, or the content of delusional beliefs in schizophrenia or delusional disorder).

From the *Diagnostic and Statistical Manual of Mental Disorders, Fifth Edition,* (Copyright 2013). American Psychiatric Association, p 222.

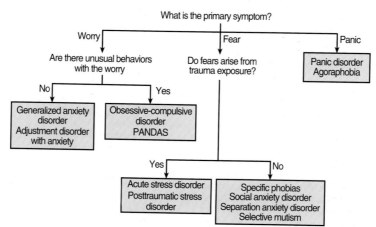

Fig. 38.2 Evaluation of worry, fear, and panic. *PANDAS,* Pediatric autoimmune neuropsychiatric disorders associated with *Streptococcus pyogenes.* *(From Kliegman RM, Lye PS, Bordini B, et al, editors:* Nelson pediatric symptom-based diagnosis, *Philadelphia, 2018, Elsevier, p 429).*

Table 38.7	DSM-5 Diagnostic Criteria for Obsessive-Compulsive Disorder

A. Presence of obsessions, compulsions, or both:

Obsessions are defined by (1) and (2):

1. Recurrent and persistent thoughts, urges, or images that are experienced, at some time during the disturbance, as intrusive and unwanted, and that in most individuals cause marked anxiety or distress.
2. The individual attempts to ignore or suppress such thoughts, urges, or images, or to neutralize them with some other thought or action (i.e., by performing a compulsion).

Compulsions are defined by (1) and (2):

1. Repetitive behaviors (e.g., hand washing, ordering, checking) or mental acts (e.g., praying, counting, repeating words silently) that the individual feels driven to perform in response to an obsession or according to rules that must be applied rigidly.
2. The behaviors or mental acts are aimed at preventing or reducing anxiety or distress, or preventing some dreaded event or situation; however, these behaviors or mental acts are not connected in a realistic way with what they are designed to neutralize or prevent, or are clearly excessive.

B. The obsessions or compulsions are time-consuming (e.g., take more than 1 hr per day) or cause clinically significant distress or impairment in social, occupational, or other important areas of functioning.

C. The obsessive-compulsive symptoms are not attributable to the physiologic effects of a substance (e.g., a drug of abuse, a medication) or another medical condition.

D. The disturbance is not better explained by the symptoms of another mental disorder (e.g., excessive worries, as in generalized anxiety disorder; preoccupation with appearance, as in body dysmorphic disorder; difficulty discarding or parting with possessions, as in hoarding disorder; hair pulling, as in trichotillomania [hair-pulling disorder]; skin picking, as in excoriation [skin-picking] disorder; stereotypies, as in stereotypic movement disorder; ritualized eating behavior, as in eating disorders; preoccupation with substances or gambling, as in substance-related and addictive disorders; preoccupation with having an illness, as in illness anxiety disorder; sexual urges or fantasies, as in paraphilic disorders; impulses, as in disruptive, impulse-control, and conduct disorders; guilty ruminations, as in schizophrenia spectrum and other psychotic disorders; or repetitive patterns of behavior, as in autism spectrum disorder).

Specify if:

With good or fair insight: The individual recognizes that obsessive-compulsive disorder beliefs are definitely or probably not true or that they may or may not be true.

With poor insight: The individual thinks obsessive-compulsive disorder beliefs are probably true.

With absent insight/delusional beliefs: The individual is completely convinced that obsessive-compulsive disorder beliefs are true.

Specify if:

Tic-related: The individual has a current or past history of a tic disorder.

From the *Diagnostic and Statistical Manual of Mental Disorders, Fifth Edition,* (Copyright 2013). American Psychiatric Association, p 237.

sions. This subtype of OCD, called **pediatric autoimmune neuropsychiatric disorder associated with streptococcal infection (PANDAS),** is characterized by sudden and dramatic onset or exacerbation of OCD or tic symptoms, associated neurologic findings, and a recent streptococcal infection. Increased antibody titers of antistreptolysin O and antideoxyribonuclease B correlates with increased basal ganglia volumes. Plasmapheresis is effective in reducing OCD symptoms in some patients with PANDAS and also decreasing enlarged basal ganglia volume. OCD has also followed episodes of acute disseminated encephalomyelitis (see Chapter 618.4) The pediatrician should be aware of the infectious cause of some cases of tic disorders, and OCD and follow management guidelines (see Chapter 37).

Children with **phobias** avoid specific objects or situations that reliably trigger physiologic arousal (e.g., dogs, spiders) (see Table 38.2). The fear is excessive and unreasonable and can be cued by the presence or anticipation of the feared trigger, with anxiety symptoms occurring immediately. Neither obsessions nor compulsions are associated with the fear response; phobias only rarely interfere with social, educational, or interpersonal functioning. Assault by a relative and verbal aggression between parents can influence the onset of specific phobias. The parents of phobic children should remain calm in the face of the child's anxiety or panic. Parents who become anxious themselves may reinforce their children's anxiety, and the pediatrician can usefully interrupt this cycle by calmly noting that phobias are not unusual and rarely cause impairment. The prevalence of specific phobias in childhood is 0.5–2%.

Systematic desensitization is a form of behavior therapy that gradually exposes the patient to the fear-inducing situation or object, while simultaneously teaching relaxation techniques for anxiety management. Successful repeated exposure leads to extinguishing anxiety for that stimulus. When phobias are particularly severe, SSRIs can be used with behavioral intervention. Low-dose SSRI treatment may be especially effective for some children with severe, refractory choking phobia.

Posttraumatic stress disorder is typically precipitated by an extreme stressor (see Chapter 14). PTSD is an anxiety disorder resulting from the long- and short-term effects of trauma that cause behavioral and physiologic sequelae in toddlers, children, and adolescents (Table 38.8). Another diagnostic category, **acute stress disorder,** reflects that traumatic events often cause acute symptoms that may or may not resolve. Previous trauma exposure, a history of other psychopathology, and symptoms

of PTSD in parents predict childhood-onset PTSD. Many adolescent and adult psychopathologic conditions, such as conduct disorder, depression, and some personality disorders, might relate to previous trauma. PTSD is also linked to mood disorders and disruptive behavior. Separation anxiety is common in children with PTSD. The lifetime prevalence of PTSD by age 18 yr is approximately 6%. Up to 40% show symptoms, but do not fulfill the diagnostic criteria.

Events that pose actual or threatened physical injury, harm, or death to the child, child's caregiver, or others close to the child, and that produce considerable stress, fear, or helplessness, are required to make the diagnosis of PTSD. Three clusters of symptoms are also essential for diagnosis: reexperiencing, avoidance, and hyperarousal. Persistent **reexperiencing** of the stressor through intrusive recollections, nightmares, and reenactment in play are typical responses in children. Persistent **avoidance** of reminders and numbing of emotional responsiveness, such as isolation, amnesia, and avoidance, constitute the 2nd cluster of behaviors. Symptoms of **hyperarousal,** such as hypervigilance, poor concentration, extreme startle responses, agitation, and sleep problems, complete the symptom profile of PTSD. Occasionally, children regress in some of their developmental milestones after a traumatic event. Avoidance symptoms are usually observable in younger children, whereas older children may better describe reexperiencing and hyperarousal symptoms. Repetitive play involving the event, psychosomatic symptoms, and nightmares may also be observed.

Initial interventions after a trauma should focus on reunification with a parent and attending to the child's physical needs in a safe place. Aggressive treatment of pain, and facilitating a return to comforting routines, including regular sleep, is indicated. Long-term treatment may include individual, group, school-based, or family therapy, as well as pharmacotherapy, in selected cases. *Individual* treatment involves transforming the child's concept of himself or herself as victim to that of survivor and can occur through play therapy, psychodynamic therapy, or CBT. *Group* work is also helpful for identifying which children might need more intensive assistance. Goals of *family* work include helping the child establish a sense of security, validating the child's emotions, and anticipating situations when the child will need more support from the family.

Clonidine or *guanfacine* may be helpful for sleep disturbance, persistent arousal, and exaggerated startle response. Recent RCTs in children and adolescents with PTSD found no significant difference between SSRI and placebo. SSRIs may be considered in pediatric patients with PTSD who have comorbid conditions responsive to SSRIs, including depression, affective numbing, and anxiety (see Table 33.4). As for many other anxiety disorders, CBT is the psychotherapeutic intervention with the most empirical support.

ANXIETY ASSOCIATED WITH MEDICAL CONDITIONS

It is prudent to rule out organic conditions such as hyperthyroidism, caffeinism (carbonated beverages), hypoglycemia, central nervous system disorders (delirium, encephalopathy, brain tumors), migraine, asthma, lead poisoning, cardiac arrhythmias, and rarely, pulmonary embolism, hyperparathyroidism, systemic lupus erythematosus, anaphylaxis, porphyria, or pheochromocytoma, before making a diagnosis of an anxiety disorder (see Table 38.1). Some *prescription* drugs with side effects that can mimic anxiety include antiasthmatic agents, corticosteroids, sympathomimetics, SSRIs (initiation), anticholinergic agents, and antipsychotics. *Nonprescription* drugs causing anxiety include diet pills, antihistamines, stimulant drugs of abuse, drug withdrawal, and cold medicines.

Chronic illness is also an underlying cause of anxiety. Children are not often emotionally and cognitively competent to understand the implications of a serious and prolonged illness. In addition to the physiologic implications of illness, they must also attend to the hospitalizations, procedures, and medications that permeate their everyday schedule. This experience affects their schooling, friendships, activities, and dynamics of the nuclear family, including the experiences of their well siblings.

School issues surrounding both prolonged absences and school reentry following a medical condition can cause or reinforce and escalate existing anxiety. School is a foundation not only for learning, but it is central to children's social experiences and feelings of normalcy. It is often impeded and stunted by illness. Academic struggles can result from missing classes, medication use, and emotional status. Children with chronic conditions are also socially disadvantaged, with friendship networks hampered by unstable attendance or social rejection for being different. Consulting with the school psychologist can be beneficial in preparing teachers and classmates before the child returns to school. An agreement between the student and school staff should be implemented, outlining a plan for taking medication, needing rest, or consulting on other needs. If the child and family agree, an informational meeting with students and teachers can normalize the situation. Explaining the condition makes it less scary for children who *catastrophize* or worry about contagion. Classmates and teachers are a natural accessible resource and can be a valuable support community. Medication may also be warranted to supplement social supports.

The experiences of the **siblings** of children with chronic illness are often forgotten, with familial resources focused on medical-financial consequences and the emotional and physical functioning of the ill child. It is not uncommon for the siblings of ill children to experience depression and anxiety as well. Assessing their social support systems, communication opportunities with parents and emotional outlets are critical to maintaining healthy functioning. Maintaining a redefined schedule of after-school activities and social engagements are helpful in allowing siblings to continue in school.

SAFETY AND EFFICACY CONCERNS ABOUT SSRIS

No empirical evidence suggests the superiority of one SSRI over another. Data are limited on combining medications. SSRIs are usually well tolerated by most children and adolescents. The FDA issued a "black box" warning of increased agitation and suicidality among adolescents and children taking SSRIs. This warning was based on review of studies in children and adolescents with major depression and not anxiety disorders. Close monitoring is always warranted.

Bibliography is available at Expert Consult.

Table 38.8	DSM-5 Diagnostic Criteria for Posttraumatic Stress Disorder

POSTTRAUMATIC STRESS DISORDER

Note: The following criteria apply to adults, adolescents, and children older than 6 yr. For children 6 yr and younger, see corresponding criteria below.

A. Exposure to actual or threatened death, serious injury, or sexual violence in 1 (or more) of the following ways:
1. Directly experiencing the traumatic event(s).
2. Witnessing, in person, the event(s) as it occurred to others.
3. Learning that the traumatic event(s) occurred to a close family member or close friend. In cases of actual or threatened death of a family member or friend, the event(s) must have been violent or accidental.
4. Experiencing repeated or extreme exposure to aversive details of the traumatic event(s) (e.g., 1st responders collecting human remains; police officers repeatedly exposed to details of child abuse).

Note: Criterion A4 does not apply to exposure through electronic media, television, movies, or pictures, unless this exposure is work related.

B. Presence of 1 (or more) of the following intrusion symptoms associated with the traumatic event(s), beginning after the traumatic event(s) occurred:
1. Recurrent, involuntary, and intrusive distressing memories of the traumatic event(s).

Note: In children older than 6 yr, repetitive play may occur in which themes or aspects of the traumatic event(s) are expressed.
2. Recurrent distressing dreams in which the content and/or effect of the dream are related to the traumatic event(s).

Note: In children, there may be frightening dreams without recognizable content.
3. Dissociative reactions (e.g., flashbacks) in which the individual feels or acts as if the traumatic event(s) were recurring. (Such reactions may occur on a continuum, with the more extreme expression being a complete loss or awareness of present surroundings.)

Note: In children, trauma-specific reenactment may occur in play.
4. Intense or prolonged psychological distress at exposure to internal or external cues that symbolize or resemble an aspect of the traumatic event(s).
5. Marked physiologic reactions to internal or external cues that symbolize or resemble an aspect of the traumatic event(s).

C. Persistent avoidance of stimuli associated with the traumatic event(s), beginning after the traumatic event(s) occurred, as evidenced by 1 or both of the following:
1. Avoidance of or efforts to avoid distressing memories, thoughts, or feelings about or closely associated with the traumatic event(s).
2. Avoidance of or efforts to avoid external reminders (people, places, conversations, activities, objects, situations) that arouse distressing memories, thoughts, or feelings about or closely associated with the traumatic event(s).

D. Negative alterations in cognitions and mood associated with the traumatic event(s), beginning or worsening after the traumatic event(s) occurred, as evidenced by 2 (or more) of the following:
1. Inability to remember an important aspect of the traumatic event(s) (typically due to dissociative amnesia and not to other factors such as head injury, alcohol, or drugs).
2. Persistent and exaggerated negative beliefs or expectations about oneself, others, or the world (e.g., "I am bad," "No one can be trusted," "The world is completely dangerous," "My whole nervous system is permanently ruined").
3. Persistent, distorted cognitions about the cause or consequences of the traumatic event(s) that lead the individual to blame himself/herself or others.

Continued

Table 38.8 | DSM-5 Diagnostic Criteria for Posttraumatic Stress Disorder—cont'd

4. Persistent negative emotional state (e.g., fear, horror, anger, guilt, or shame).
5. Markedly diminished interest or participation in significant activities.
6. Feelings of detachment or estrangement from others.
7. Persistent inability to experience positive emotions (e.g., inability to experience happiness, satisfaction, or loving feelings).
E. Marked alterations in arousal and reactivity associated with the traumatic event(s), beginning or worsening after the traumatic event(s) occurred, as evidenced by 2 (or more) of the following:
   1. Irritable behavior and angry outbursts (with little or no provocation) typically expressed by verbal or physical aggression toward people or objects.
   2. Reckless or self-destructive behavior.
   3. Hypervigilance.
   4. Exaggerated startle response.
   5. Problems with concentration.
   6. Sleep disturbance (e.g., difficulty falling or staying asleep or restless sleep).
F. Duration of the disturbance (Criteria B, C, D, and E) is more than 1 mo.
G. The disturbance causes clinically significant distress or impairment in social, occupational, or other important areas of functioning.
H. The disturbance is not attributable to the physiologic effects of a substance (e.g., medication, alcohol) or another medical condition.
Specify whether:
With dissociative symptoms: The individual's symptoms meet the criteria for posttraumatic stress disorder, and in addition, in response to the stressor, the individual experiences persistent or recurrent symptoms of either of the following:
   1. **Depersonalization:** Persistent or recurrent experiences of feeling detached from, and as if one were an outside observer of, one's mental processes or body (e.g., feeling as though one were in a dream; feeling a sense of unreality of self or body or of time moving slowly).
   2. **Derealization:** Persistent or recurrent experiences of unreality of surroundings (e.g., the world around the individual is experienced as unreal, dreamlike, distant, or distorted).
Note: To use this subtype, the dissociative symptoms must not be attributable to the physiologic effects of a substance (e.g., blackouts, behavior during alcohol intoxication) or another medical condition (e.g., complex partial seizures).
Specify if:
With delayed expression: If the full diagnostic criteria are not met until at least 6 mo after the event (although the onset and expression of some symptoms may be immediate).

POSTTRAUMATIC STRESS DISORDER FOR CHILDREN 6 YR AND YOUNGER
A. In children 6 yr and younger, exposure to actual or threatened death, serious injury, or sexual violence in 1 (or more) of the following ways:
   1. Directly experiencing the traumatic event(s).
   2. Witnessing, in person, the event(s) as it occurred to others, especially primary caregivers.
Note: Witnessing does not include events that are only in electronic media, television, movies, or pictures.
   3. Learning that the traumatic event(s) occurred to a parent or caregiving figure.
B. Presence of 1 (or more) of the following intrusion symptoms associated with the traumatic event(s), beginning after the traumatic event(s) occurred:
   1. Recurrent, involuntary, and intrusive distressing memories of the traumatic event(s).
Note: Spontaneous and intrusive memories may not necessarily appear distressing and may be expressed as play reenactment.
   2. Recurrent distressing dreams in which the content and/or effect of the dream is related to the traumatic event(s).

Note: It may not be possible to ascertain that the frightening content is related to the traumatic event.
   3. Dissociative reactions (e.g., flashbacks) in which the child feels or acts as if the traumatic event(s) were recurring. (Such reactions may occur on a continuum, with the most extreme expression being a complete loss of awareness of present surroundings.) Such trauma-specific reenactment may occur in play.
   4. Intense or prolonged psychological distress at exposure to internal or external cues that symbolize or resemble an aspect of the traumatic event(s).
C. One (or more) of the following symptoms, representing either persistent avoidance of stimuli associated with the traumatic event(s) or negative alterations in cognitions and mood associated with the traumatic event(s), must be present, beginning after the event(s) or worsening after the event(s):
Persistent Avoidance of Stimuli
   1. Avoidance of or efforts to avoid activities, places, or physical reminders that arouse recollections or the traumatic event(s).
   2. Avoidance of or efforts to avoid people, conversations, or interpersonal situations that around recollections of the traumatic event(s).
Negative Alterations in Cognitions
   3. Substantially increased frequency of negative emotional states (e.g., fear, guilt, sadness, shame, confusion).
   4. Markedly diminished interest or participation in significant activities, including constriction of play.
   5. Socially withdrawn behavior.
   6. Persistent reduction in expression of positive emotions.
D. Alterations in arousal and reactivity associated with the traumatic event(s), beginning or worsening after the traumatic event(s) occurred, as evidenced by 2 (or more) of the following:
   1. Irritable behavior and angry outbursts (with little or no provocation), typically expressed as verbal and physical aggression toward people or objects (including extreme temper tantrums).
   2. Hypervigilance.
   3. Exaggerated startle response.
   4. Problems with concentration.
   5. Sleep disturbance (e.g., difficulty falling asleep or staying asleep or restless sleep).
E. The duration of the disturbance is more than 1 mo.
F. The disturbance causes clinically significant distress or impairment in relationships with parents, siblings, peers, or other caregivers or with school behavior.
G. The disturbance is not attributable to the physiologic effects of a substance (e.g., medication or alcohol) or another medical condition.
Specify whether:
With dissociative symptoms: The individual's symptoms meet the criteria for posttraumatic stress disorder, and the individual experiences persistent or recurrent symptoms of either of the following:
   1. **Depersonalization:** Persistent or recurrent experiences of feeling detached from, and as if one were an outside observer of, one's mental processes or body (e.g., feeling as though one were in a dream; feeling a sense of unreality of self or body or of time moving slowly).
   2. **Derealization:** Persistent or recurrent experiences of unreality of surroundings (e.g., the world around the individual is experienced as unreal, dreamlike, distant, or distorted).
Note: To use this subtype, the dissociative symptoms must not be attributable to the physiologic effects of a substance (e.g., blackouts, behavior during alcohol intoxication) or another medical condition (e.g., complex partial seizures).
Specify if:
With delayed expression: If the full diagnostic criteria are not met until at least 6 mo after the event (although the onset and expression of some symptoms may be immediate).

From the *Diagnostic and Statistical Manual of Mental Disorders, Fifth Edition,* (Copyright 2013). American Psychiatric Association, pp 271–274.

Chapter **39**
Mood Disorders
Heather J. Walter and David R. DeMaso

第三十九章
心境障碍

中文导读

本章分重性抑郁和其他抑郁障碍、双相及相关障碍两个章节进行了具体介绍。其中，重性抑郁和其他抑郁障碍这一节，介绍了重性抑郁障碍和持续性抑郁障碍的概念和诊断标准，详细描述了重性抑郁障碍的流行病学、临床病程、鉴别诊断、共病、结局与转归、病因和风险因素、预防、筛查/个案发现、早期干预、治疗和照料的分级处置原则。

在双相及相关障碍这一节中，对双相障碍各临床特征进行了描述，列举了躁狂发作和轻躁狂发作的诊断标准。详细阐述了双相障碍的流行病学、临床病程、鉴别诊断、共病、结局与转归、病因和风险因素、预防、筛查/个案发现、早期干预、治疗和照料的分级处置原则。

Mood disorders are interrelated sets of psychiatric symptoms characterized by a core deficit in emotional self-regulation. Classically, the mood disorders have been divided into depressive and bipolar disorders, representing the two emotional polarities, *dysphoric* ("low") and *euphoric* ("high") mood.

39.1 Major and Other Depressive Disorders
Heather J. Walter and David R. DeMaso

The depressive disorders include major depressive, persistent depressive, disruptive mood dysregulation, other specified/unspecified depressive, premenstrual dysphoric, and substance/medication-induced disorders, as well as depressive disorder caused by another medical condition (Fig. 39.1).

DESCRIPTION
Major depressive disorder (MDD) is characterized by a distinct period of at least 2 wk (an *episode*) in which there is a depressed or irritable mood and/or loss of interest or pleasure in almost all activities that is present for most of the day, nearly every day (Table 39.1). Major depression is associated with characteristic vegetative and cognitive symptoms, including disturbances in appetite, sleep, energy, and activity level; impaired concentration; thoughts of worthlessness or guilt; and suicidal thoughts or actions. Major depression is considered *mild* if few or no symptoms in excess of those required to make the diagnosis are present, and the symptoms are mildly distressing and manageable and result in minor functional impairment. Major depression is considered *severe* if

symptoms substantially in excess of those required to make the diagnosis are present, and the symptoms are highly distressing and unmanageable and markedly impair function. *Moderate* major depression is intermediate in severity between mild and severe.

Persistent depressive disorder is characterized by depressed or irritable mood for more days than not, for at least 1 yr (in children and adolescents). As with major depression, this chronic form of depression is associated with characteristic vegetative and cognitive symptoms; however, the cognitive symptoms of persistent depression are less severe (e.g., low self-esteem rather than worthlessness, hopelessness rather than suicidality). As with major depression, persistent depressive disorder is characterized as mild, moderate, or severe (Table 39.2).

Overall, the clinical presentation of major and persistent depressive disorders in children and adolescents is similar to that in adults. The prominence of the symptoms can change with age: irritability and somatic complaints may be more common in children, and energy, activity level, appetite, and sleep disturbances may be more common in adolescents. Because of the cognitive and linguistic immaturity of young children, symptoms of depression in that age-group may be more likely to be observed than self-reported.

The core feature of **disruptive mood dysregulation disorder (DMDD)** is severe, persistent irritability evident most of the day, nearly every day, for at least 12 mo in multiple settings (at home, at school, with peers). The irritable mood is interspersed with frequent (≥3 times/wk) and severe (verbal rages, physical aggression) temper outbursts (Table 39.3). This diagnosis is intended to characterize more accurately the extreme irritability that some investigators had considered a developmental presentation of bipolar disorder, and to distinguish extreme irritability from the milder presentations characteristic of oppositional

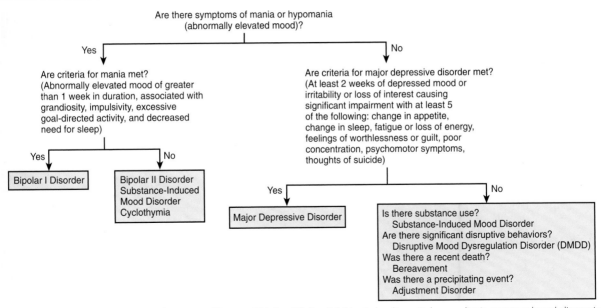

Fig. 39.1 Evaluation of mood disorders. *(From Kliegman RM, Lye PS, Bordini BJ, et al, editors: Nelson pediatric symptom-based diagnosis, Philadelphia, 2018, Elsevier, p 426.)*

Table 39.1	DSM-5 Diagnostic Criteria for Major Depressive Episode

A. Five (or more) of the following symptoms have been present during the same 2 wk period and represent a change from previous functioning; at least 1 of the symptoms is either (1) depressed mood or (2) loss of interest or pleasure.
1. Depressed most of the day, nearly every day, as indicated by either subjective report (e.g., feels sad, empty, hopeless) or observation made by others (e.g., appears tearful).
Note: In children and adolescents, can be irritable mood.
2. Markedly diminished interest or pleasure in all, or almost all, activities most of the day, nearly every day (as indicated by either subjective account or observation).
3. Significant weight loss when not dieting or weight gain (e.g., a change of more than 5% of body weight in a month), or decrease or increase in appetite nearly every day.
Note: In children, consider failure to make expected weight gain.
4. Insomnia or hypersomnia nearly every day.
5. Psychomotor agitation or retardation nearly every day (observable by others, not merely subjective feelings of restlessness or being slowed down).
6. Fatigue or loss of energy nearly every day.

7. Feelings of worthlessness or excessive or inappropriate guilt (which may be delusional) nearly every day (not merely self-reproach or guilt about being sick).
8. Diminished ability to think or concentrate, or indecisiveness, nearly every day (either by subjective account or as observed by others).
9. Recurrent thoughts of death (not just fear of dying), recurrent suicidal ideation without a specific plan, or a suicide attempt or a specific plan for committing suicide.
B. The symptoms cause clinically significant distress or impairment in social, occupational, or other important areas of functioning.
C. The episode is not attributable to the physiologic effects of a substance or to another medical condition.
Note: Criteria A-C represent a major depressive episode.
D. The occurrence of the major depressive episode is not better explained by schizoaffective disorder, schizophrenia, schizophreniform disorder, delusional disorder, or other specified and unspecified schizophrenia spectrum and other psychotic disorders.
E. There has never been a manic episode or a hypomanic episode.

From the *Diagnostic and Statistical Manual of Mental Disorders, Fifth Edition,* (Copyright 2013). American Psychiatric Association, pp 125–126.

defiant disorder (ODD) and intermittent explosive disorder.

Other specified/unspecified depressive disorder (subsyndromal depressive disorder) applies to presentations in which symptoms characteristic of a depressive disorder are present and cause clinically significant distress or functional impairment, but do not meet the full criteria for any of the disorders in this diagnostic class.

EPIDEMIOLOGY
The overall prevalence of parent-reported diagnosis of depressive disorder in the United States (excluding DMDD) among 3-17 yr old children is approximately 2.1% (current) and 3.9% (ever); the prevalence rate increases to 12.8% (lifetime) for 12-17 yr olds. The male:female ratio (excluding DMDD) is approximately 1:1 during childhood and beginning in early adolescence rises to 1:1.5-3.0 in adulthood.

Based on rates of chronic and severe persistent irritability, which is the core feature of DMDD, the overall 6 mo to 1 yr prevalence has been estimated in the 2–5% range. In 3 community samples, the 3 mo prevalence rate of DMDD ranged from 0.8–3.3%, with the highest rates occurring in preschoolers (although DSM-5 does not permit this diagnosis until age 6 yr). Approximately 5–10% of children and adolescents are estimated to have **subsyndromal (unspecified) depression**.

CLINICAL COURSE
Major depression may first appear at any age, but the likelihood of onset greatly increases with puberty. Incidence appears to peak in the 20s. The median duration of a major depressive episode is about 5-8 mo for clinically referred youth and 3-6 mo for community samples. The course is quite variable in that some individuals rarely or never experience remission, whereas others experience many years with few or no symptoms between episodes. Persistent depressive disorder often has an early and insidious onset and by definition, a chronic course (average untreated duration in both clinical and community samples: 3.5 yr).

Table 39.2	DSM-5 Diagnostic Criteria for Persistent Depressive Disorder

A. Depressed mood for most of the day, for more days than not, as indicated either by subjective account or observation by others, for at least 2 yr.
Note: In children and adolescents, mood can be irritable and duration must be at least 1 yr.
B. Presence, while depressed, of 2 (or more) of the following:
  1. Poor appetite or overeating.
  2. Insomnia or hypersomnia.
  3. Low energy or fatigue.
  4. Low self-esteem.
  5. Poor concentration or difficulty making decisions.
  6. Feelings of hopelessness.
C. During the 2 yr period (1 yr for children or adolescents) of the disturbance, the individual has never been without the symptoms in Criteria A and B for more than 2 mo at a time.
D. Criteria for a major depressive disorder may be continuously present for 2 yr.
E. There has never been a manic episode or a hypomanic episode, and criteria have never been met for cyclothymic disorder.
F. The disturbance is not better explained by a persistent schizoaffective disorder, schizophrenia, delusional disorder, or other specified or unspecified schizophrenia spectrum and other psychotic disorder.
G. The symptoms are not attributable to the physiologic effects of a substance (e.g., a drug of abuse, a medication) or another medical condition (e.g., hypothyroidism).
H. The symptoms cause clinically significant distress or impairment in social, occupational, or other important areas of functioning.
Note: Because the criteria for a major depressive episode include 4 symptoms that are absent from the symptom list for persistent depressive disorder (dysthymia), a very limited number of individuals will have depressive symptoms that have persisted longer than 2 yr but will not meet criteria for persistent depressive disorder. If full criteria for a major depressive episode have been met at some point during the current episode of illness, they should be given a diagnosis of major depressive disorder. Otherwise, a diagnosis of other specified depressive disorder or unspecified depressive disorder is warranted.

From the *Diagnostic and Statistical Manual of Mental Disorders, Fifth Edition,* (Copyright 2013). American Psychiatric Association, pp 168–169.

Table 39.3	DSM-5 Diagnostic Criteria for Disruptive Mood Dysregulation Disorder

A. Severe recurrent temper outbursts manifested verbally (e.g., verbal rages) and/or behaviorally (e.g., physical aggression toward people or property) that are grossly out of proportion in intensity or duration to the situation or provocation.
B. The temper outbursts are inconsistent with developmental level.
C. The temper outbursts occur, on average, 3 or more times per week.
D. The mood between temper outbursts is persistently irritable or angry most of the day, nearly every day, and is observable by others (e.g., parents, teachers, peers).
E. Criteria A-D have been present for 12 or more months. Throughout that time, the individual has not had a period lasting 3 or more consecutive months without all of the symptoms in Criteria A-D.
F. Criteria A and D are present in at least 2 of 3 settings (i.e., at home, at school, with peers) and are severe in at least 1 of these.
G. The diagnosis should not be made for the first time before age 6 yr or after age 18 yr.
H. By history or observation, the age at onset of Criteria A-E is before 10 yr.
I. There has never been a distinct period lasting more than 1 day during which the full symptom criteria, except duration, for a manic or hypomanic episode have been met.
Note: Developmentally appropriate mood elevation, such as occurs in the context of a highly positive event or its anticipation, should not be considered as a symptom of mania or hypomania.
J. The behaviors do not occur exclusively during an episode of major depressive disorder and are not better explained by another mental disorder (e.g., autism spectrum disorder, posttraumatic stress disorder, separation anxiety disorder, persistent depressive disorder [dysthymia]).
Note: The diagnosis cannot coexist with oppositional defiant disorder, intermittent explosive disorder, or bipolar disorder, though it can coexist with others, including major depressive disorder, attention-deficit/hyperactivity disorder, conduct disorder, and substance use disorders. Individuals whose symptoms meet criteria for both disruptive mood dysregulation disorder and oppositional defiant disorder should only be given the diagnosis of disruptive mood dysregulation disorder. If an individual has ever experienced a manic or hypomanic episode, the diagnosis of disruptive mood dysregulation disorder should not be assigned.
K. The symptoms are not attributable to the physiologic effects of a substance or to another medical or neurologic condition.

From the *Diagnostic and Statistical Manual of Mental Disorders, Fifth Edition,* (Copyright 2013). American Psychiatric Association, p. 156.

Prepubertal depressive disorders exhibit more heterotypic than homotypic continuity; depressed children appear to be more likely to develop nondepressive psychiatric disorders in adulthood than depressive disorders. Adolescents exhibit greater homotypic continuity, with the probability of recurrence of depression reaching 50–70% after 5 yr. The persistence of even mild depressive symptoms during remission is a powerful predictor of recurrence; other negative prognostic factors include more severe symptoms, longer time to remission, history of maltreatment, and comorbid psychiatric disorders. Up to 20% of depressed adolescents develop a bipolar disorder; the risk is higher among adolescents who have a high family loading for bipolar disorder, who have psychotic depression, or who have had pharmacologically induced mania.

DIFFERENTIAL DIAGNOSIS

A number of psychiatric disorders, general medical conditions, and medications can generate symptoms of depression or irritability and must be distinguished from the depressive disorders. The psychiatric disorders include autism spectrum disorder (ASD), attention-deficit/hyperactivity disorder (ADHD), and bipolar, anxiety, trauma- and stressor-related, disruptive/impulse control/conduct, and substance-related disorders. Medical conditions include neurologic disorders (including autoimmune encephalitis), endocrine disorders (including hypothyroidism and Addison disease), infectious diseases, tumors, anemia, uremia, failure to thrive, chronic fatigue disorder, and pain disorder. Medications include narcotics, chemotherapy agents, β-blockers, corticosteroids, and contraceptives. The diagnosis of a depressive disorder

should be made after these and other potential explanations for the observed symptoms have been ruled out.

COMORBIDITY

Major and persistent depressive disorders often co-occur with other psychiatric disorders. Depending on the setting and source of referral, 40–90% of youths with a depressive disorder have other psychiatric disorders, and up to 50% have ≥2 comorbid diagnoses. The most common comorbid diagnosis is an **anxiety disorder** and as such may reflect a common diathesis; other common comorbidities include ADHD and disruptive behavior, eating, and substance use disorders. The development of depressive disorders can both lead to and follow the development of the comorbid disorders.

Preliminary data suggest that DMDD occurs with other psychiatric disorders, including other depressive disorders, ADHD, conduct disorder, and substance use disorders, from 60–90% of the time. Because the symptoms of DMDD overlap in part with symptoms of bipolar disorder, ODD, and intermittent explosive disorder, by *Diagnostic Statistical Manual of Mental Disorders, Fifth Edition* (DSM-5) convention, hierarchical diagnostic rules apply. Thus, bipolar disorder takes precedence over DMDD if a manic/hypomanic episode has ever occurred, and DMDD takes precedence over ODD and intermittent explosive disorder if full criteria for DMDD are met.

SEQUELAE

Approximately 60% of youths with MDD report thinking about **suicide,** and 30% attempt suicide. Youths with depressive disorders are also at high risk of substance abuse, impaired family and peer relationships, early pregnancy, legal problems, educational and occupational underachievement, and poor adjustment to life stressors, including physical illness.

Children with DMDD have displayed elevated rates of social impairments, school suspension, and service use. Irritability in adolescence has predicted the development of major depressive and dysthymic disorders and generalized anxiety disorder (but not bipolar disorder) 20 yr later, as well as lower educational attainment and income.

ETIOLOGY AND RISK FACTORS

Current models of vulnerability to depressive disorders are grounded in gene and environment pathways. Genetic studies have demonstrated the heritability of depressive disorders, with monozygotic twin studies finding concordance rates of 40–65%. In families, both bottom-up (children to parents) and top-down (parents to children) studies have shown a 2-4–fold bidirectional increase in depression among first-degree relatives. The exact nature of genetic expression remains unclear. Cerebral variations in structure and function (particularly serotonergic), the function of the hypothalamic-pituitary-adrenal axis, difficult temperament/personality (i.e., negative affectivity), and ruminative, self-devaluating cognitive style have been implicated as components of biologic vulnerability. The great majority of depressive disorders arise in youths with long-standing psychosocial difficulties, among the most predictive of which are physical/sexual abuse, neglect, chronic illness, school difficulties (bullying, academic failure), social isolation, family or marital disharmony, divorce/separation, parental psychopathology, and domestic violence. Longitudinal studies demonstrate the greater importance of environmental influences in children who become depressed than in adults who become depressed. Factors shown to be protective against the development of depression include a positive relationship with a parent; better family function; closer parental supervision, monitoring, and involvement; a prosocial peer group; higher IQ; and greater educational aspirations.

PREVENTION

Numerous experimental trials have sought to demonstrate the effectiveness of psychological or educational strategies in preventing the onset of depressive disorders in children and adolescents. These programs generally have provided information about the link between depressed mood and depressogenic thoughts and behaviors, as well as training in skills intended to modify these thoughts and behaviors. A Cochrane review found small effects of these programs on depression symptoms when implemented universally vs no intervention, with selective programs (targeted at high-risk groups) performing better than universal programs; however, the effect of prevention programs was null compared with attention controls.

SCREENING/CASE FINDING

Adolescents presenting in the primary care setting should be queried, along with their parent(s), about depressed mood as part of the routine clinical interview. A typical screening question would be, "Everyone feels sad or angry some of the time, how about you (or your teen)?" The parents of younger children can be queried about overt signs of depression, such as tearfulness, irritability, boredom, or social isolation. A number of standardized screening instruments widely used in the primary care setting (e.g., *Pediatric Symptom Checklist, Strengths and Difficulties Questionnaire, Vanderbilt ADHD Diagnostic Rating Scales*) have items specific to sad mood, and as such can be used to focus the interview.

The role of universal depression screening using standardized depression-specific instruments is unclear. A Cochrane review found that the use of depression screening in primary care has little or no impact on the recognition, management, or outcome of depression. Nonetheless, the U.S. Preventive Services Task Force (PSTF) recommends the universal use of depression screening instruments, but only among adolescents and only when systems are in place to ensure adequate follow-up. Targeted screening of known high-risk groups (e.g., youth who are homeless, refugees, attracted to the same sex, involved with child welfare or juvenile justice), or youth experiencing known psychosocial adversities (see Etiology and Risk Factors earlier) or self-reporting a dysphoric mood, may be a higher-yield case-finding strategy than universal screening.

EARLY INTERVENTION

Youth (and/or their parents) presenting in the primary care setting who self-report, or respond affirmatively to queries about, a distressing life experience or a depressed or irritable mood should be offered the opportunity to talk about the situation with the pediatric practitioner (separately with the older youth as indicated). By engaging in active listening (e.g., "I hear how upset you have been feeling, tell me more about what happened to make you feel that way"), the pediatric practitioner can begin to assess the onset, duration, context, and severity of the symptoms and associated dangerousness, distress, and functional impairment. In the absence of acute dangerousness (e.g., suicidality, psychosis, substance abuse) and significant distress or functional impairment, the pediatric practitioner (or co-located behavioral health therapist) can schedule a follow-up appointment within 1-2 wk to conduct a depression assessment. At this follow-up visit, to assist with decision-making about appropriate level of care, a depression-specific screening standardized rating scale can be administered to assess symptom severity (Table 39.4), and additional risk factors can be explored (see Etiology and Risk Factors earlier).

Treatment decisions should be guided by the understanding that depression in youth is highly responsive to placebo (50–60%) or brief nonspecific intervention (15–30%). The goal of treatment is **remission,** defined as a period of at least 2 wk with no or very few depressive symptoms, and ultimately **recovery,** defined as a period of at least 2 mo with no or very few depressive symptoms. Assessment of remission and recovery can be aided using the depression-specific standardized rating scales, in which remission is defined as scores below the scale-specific clinical cutpoint.

For mild symptoms (manageable and not functionally impairing) and in the absence of major risk factors (e.g., suicidality; psychosis; substance use; history of depression, mania, or traumatic exposures; parental psychopathology, particularly depression; severe family dysfunction), **guided self-help** (anticipatory guidance) with watchful waiting and scheduled follow-up may suffice. Guided self-help can include provision of educational materials (e.g., pamphlets, books, workbooks, apps, internet sites) that provide information to the youth about coping adaptively with depressogenic situations, as well as advice to parents about strengthening the parent–child relationship and modifying depressogenic exposures (e.g., taking action against bullying, increasing opportunities for social interaction and support, protecting child from exposure to marital discord). Additional self-help activities that have shown promise in improving mild depressive symptoms include physical exercise, relaxation therapy (e.g., yoga, mindfulness), and a regular sleep schedule.

For youths who continue to have mild depression after a few weeks of guided self-help, supportive therapy by a mental health professional (ideally co-located in the primary care, school, or community setting) may be an appropriate subsequent step. **Supportive psychotherapy,** which can be delivered in individual or group formats, focuses on teaching thoughts (e.g., positive self-talk) and behaviors (e.g., pleasurable activities, relaxation, problem solving, effective communication) known to ameliorate depressive symptoms, as well as providing concrete social or material problem-solving assistance to the youth or family as needed.

TREATMENT

For youths who have not responded to approximately 4-8 wk of supportive psychotherapy, or who from the outset exhibit moderate to severe, comorbid, or recurrent depression or suicidality, or who have

Table 39.4	Depression-Specific Rating Scales		
NAME OF INSTRUMENT	**INFORMANT(S)**	**AGE RANGE**	**NUMBER OF ITEMS**
Beck Depression Inventory	Youth	13+ yr	21
Beck Depression Inventory for Youth	Youth	7-14 yr	20
Center for Epidemiologic Studies-Depression-Children	Youth	6-18 yr	20
Children's Depression Rating Scale-Revised	Youth, Parent, Clinician	6-18 yr	47
Children's Depression Inventory, Second Edition	Youth, Parent, Teacher	7-17 yr	28/17/12
Depression Self-Rating Scale	Youth	7-13 yr	18
Mood and Feelings Questionnaire	Youth, Parent	7-18 yr	33-34
Patient Health Questionnaire-9	Youth	12/13+ yr	9
Preschool Feelings Checklist	Parent	3-5.6 yr	20
PROMIS Emotional Distress-Depressive Symptoms	Youth, Parent	Youth: 8-17 yr Parent: 5-17 yr	8/6
Reynolds Child Depression Scale	Youth	8-13 yr	30
Reynolds Adolescent Depression Scale, Second Edition	Youth	11-20 yr	30

a history of mania, traumatic exposures, or severe family dysfunction or psychopathology, assessment and treatment in the specialty mental health setting by a child-trained mental health clinician should be considered.

For moderate to severe depression, specific manualized psychotherapies, antidepressant medication, or a combination of both should be considered. At present, there is insufficient evidence on which to base definitive conclusions about the relative effectiveness of these treatments.

Clinical trials of acute treatments have generated support for the efficacy of cognitive-behavioral therapy (CBT)/behavioral activation therapy and interpersonal therapy as monotherapies in depressed youth, but overall effect sizes are modest (0.35 and 0.26, respectively). For children age 12 and younger, meta-analyses suggest no benefit of CBT over no treatment. CBT focuses on identifying and correcting cognitive distortions that may lead to depressed mood and teaches problem-solving, behavior activation, social communication, and emotional regulation skills to combat depression. Interpersonal therapy focuses on enhancing interpersonal problem solving and social communication to decrease interpersonal conflicts. Each of these therapies typically involves 8-12 weekly visits. Limited evidence suggests that family therapy may be more effective than no treatment in decreasing depression and improving family functioning.

Two selective serotonin reuptake inhibitors (SSRIs), **fluoxetine** and **escitalopram,** are the only antidepressants approved by the U.S. Food and Drug Administration (FDA) for the treatment of depression in youth, and fluoxetine alone is approved for preadolescents. Randomized controlled trials (RCTs) of the effectiveness of antidepressants are mixed, but meta-analyses of RCTs have been fairly consistent in their disappointing findings.

Based on a 2007 meta-analysis, approximately 60% of youths with MDD responded to antidepressants from multiple medication classes (vs 50% for placebo), but only about 30% of medicated depressed youths experienced symptom remission. Fluoxetine consistently demonstrated greater efficacy and was the only SSRI separating from placebo in studies of depressed preadolescents. The absolute risk for suicidal thoughts in youths treated with antidepressant medication was approximately 3%, vs 2% of those given placebo.

In another Cochrane review, antidepressants from multiple classes decreased symptom severity in children and adolescents with depressive disorders and increased remission/response in adolescents, but the effects were small and may not have been clinically significant. Fluoxetine and escitalopram possibly outperformed other antidepressants for safety and effectiveness.

In a 2016 meta-analysis of all classes of antidepressants prescribed for MDD in children and adolescents, only fluoxetine was statistically significantly more effective than placebo. Duloxetine and venlafaxine had adverse tolerability profiles, and youths taking venlafaxine were suggested to have a significantly increased risk for suicidality.

These findings converge in the suggestion that fluoxetine should be considered first-line therapy among antidepressants unless other factors (e.g., comorbidities, side effect profiles, personal/family history of response to a specific medication) favor an alternative antidepressant. Considering both efficacy and tolerability findings, next-best choices may be escitalopram (for adolescents) and sertraline (for children and adolescents). In light of the accumulated findings, antidepressants should be used cautiously in youth and likely should limited to patients (especially adolescents) with moderate to severe depression for whom psychosocial interventions are either ineffective or not feasible.

Clinical severity, comorbidity, family conflict, low drug concentration, nonadherence, anhedonia, sleep difficulties, subsyndromal manic symptoms, and child maltreatment have all been related to treatment resistance. Approximately 50% of depressed youth failing to respond to the 1st SSRI respond after switching to a 2nd antidepressant plus CBT, vs approximately 40% who respond to a 2nd medication alone. For youth with psychotic depression, augmenting the antidepressant with an atypical antipsychotic medication should be considered, while monitoring closely for side effects.

Before initiating antidepressant medication, baseline symptom severity should be assessed using a standardized rating scale (see Table 39.4). The initial dose of fluoxetine for moderate to severe major depressive disorder generally would be 10 mg for children age 6-12 yr and 20 mg for adolescents age ≥13. Clinical response, tolerability, and emergence of behavioral activation, mania, or suicidal thoughts should be assessed weekly (per FDA recommendation) for the 1st 4 wk. If the youth has safely tolerated the antidepressant, the baseline standardized symptom rating scale should be readministered to assess response to treatment. Because the findings from a recent meta-analysis suggest that treatment gains in response to SSRI medications are greatest early in treatment and minimal after 4 wk, if substantial improvement in the rating scale score has not occurred at 4 wk despite confirmation of adherence to the medication regimen, consultation from a child and adolescent psychiatrist should be considered.

Because of the high rate of recurrence, successful treatment should continue for 6-12 mo. The findings from one RCT suggested that the addition of relapse-prevention CBT to ongoing medication management reduces the risk of relapse more than medication management alone, even after the end of treatment. When treatment concludes, all antidepressants (except possibly fluoxetine because of long half-life) should be discontinued gradually to avoid withdrawal symptoms (gastrointestinal upset, disequilibrium, sleep disruption, flulike symptoms, sensory disturbances). Patients with recurrent (≥2 episodes), chronic, or severe major depression may require treatment beyond 12 mo.

To date, there are no rigorous studies evaluating the effectiveness of pharmacologic or psychosocial treatment approaches to persistent depressive disorder or DMDD. The aforementioned treatments for MDD may prove helpful in persistent depressive disorder. In suspected cases of DMDD, child and adolescent psychiatry consultation may be helpful to clarify diagnosis and suggest treatment approaches.

LEVEL OF CARE

Most children and adolescents with mild to moderate depressive disorders can be safely and effectively treated as outpatients, provided that a clinically appropriate schedule of visits can be maintained through the phases of treatment. Inpatient treatment should be considered for youth who present with a high risk of suicide, serious self-harm, or self-neglect, or when the family is not able to provide an appropriate level of supervision or follow-up with outpatient treatment recommendations, or when comprehensive assessment for diagnostic clarity is needed. When considering inpatient admission for a young person with depression, the benefits of inpatient treatment needs to be balanced against potential detrimental effects, such as the loss of family and community support.

Bibliography is available at Expert Consult.

39.2 Bipolar and Related Disorders
Heather J. Walter and David R. DeMaso

DESCRIPTION

The bipolar and related disorders include bipolar I, bipolar II, cyclothymic, and other specified/unspecified bipolar and related disorders, as well as bipolar and related disorder caused by another medical condition.

A **manic episode** is characterized by a distinct period of at least 1 wk in which there is an abnormally and persistently elevated, expansive, or irritable mood and abnormally and persistently increased goal-directed activity or energy that is present for most of the day, nearly every day (or any duration if hospitalization is necessary). The episode is associated with characteristic cognitive and behavioral symptoms, including disturbances in self-regard, speech, attention, thought, activity, impulsivity, and sleep (Table 39.5). To diagnose **bipolar I disorder**, criteria must be met for at least 1 manic episode, and the episode must not be better explained by a psychotic disorder. The manic episode may have been preceded and may be followed by hypomanic or major depressive episodes. Bipolar I disorder is rated as mild, moderate, or severe in the same way as the depressive disorders (see Description section of Chapter 39.1).

To diagnose **bipolar II disorder**, criteria must be met for at least 1 hypomanic episode and at least 1 major depressive episode. A **hypomanic episode** is similar to a manic episode but is briefer (at least 4 days) and less severe (causes less impairment in functioning, is not associated with psychosis, and would not require hospitalization) (Table 39.6). In bipolar II disorder, there must never have been a manic disorder, the episodes must not be better explained by a psychotic disorder, and the symptoms of depression or the unpredictability caused by frequent alternation between periods of depression and hypomania must cause clinically significant distress or functional impairment. Bipolar II disorder is also rated as mild, moderate, or severe.

Cyclothymic disorder is characterized by a period of at least 1 yr (in children and adolescents) in which there are numerous periods with hypomanic and depressive symptoms that do not meet criteria for a hypomanic episode or a major depressive episode, respectively.

Other specified/unspecified bipolar and related disorders (**subsyndromal bipolar disorder**) applies to presentations in which symptoms characteristic of a bipolar and related disorder are present and cause distress or functional impairment, but do not meet the full criteria for

Table 39.5	DSM-5 Diagnostic Criteria for a Manic Episode

A. A distinct period of abnormally and persistently elevated, expansive, or irritable mood and abnormally and persistently increased goal-directed activity or energy, lasting at least 1 wk and present most of the day, nearly every day (or any duration if hospitalization is necessary).

B. During the period of mood disturbance and increased energy or activity, 3 (or more) of the following symptoms (4 if the mood is only irritable) are present to a significant degree and represent a noticeable change from usual behavior:
1. Inflated self-esteem or grandiosity.
2. Decreased need for sleep (e.g., feels rested after only 3 hr of sleep).
3. More talkative than usual or pressure to keep talking.
4. Flight of ideas or subjective experience that thoughts are racing.
5. Distractibility (i.e., attention too easily drawn to unimportant or irrelevant external stimuli), as reported or observed.
6. Increase in goal-directed activity (either socially, at work or school, or sexually) or psychomotor agitation (i.e., purposeless non-goal-directed activity).
7. Excessive involvement in activities that have a high potential for painful consequences (e.g., engaging in unrestrained buying sprees, sexual indiscretions, or foolish business investments).

C. The mood disturbance is sufficiently severe to cause marked impairment in social or occupational functioning or to necessitate hospitalization to prevent harm to self or others, or there are psychotic features.

D. The episode is not attributable to the physiologic effects of a substance (e.g., a drug of abuse, a medication, other treatment) or to another medical condition.

Note: A full manic episode that emerges during antidepressant treatment (e.g., medication, electroconvulsive therapy) but persists at a fully syndromal level beyond the physiologic effect of that treatment is sufficient evidence for a manic episode and, therefore, a bipolar I diagnosis.

Note: Criteria A-D constitute a manic episode. At least 1 lifetime manic episode is required for the diagnosis of bipolar I disorder.

From the *Diagnostic and Statistical Manual of Mental Disorders, Fifth Edition,* (Copyright 2013). American Psychiatric Association, p 124.

any of the disorders in this diagnostic class. Although this diagnosis (formerly known as "bipolar disorder, not otherwise specified") had frequently been applied to children with severe and chronic mood and behavioral dysregulation who did not precisely fit other diagnostic categories, the empirical support for the validity of this practice has been sparse. Children who formerly received this diagnosis may meet criteria for DMDD (see Chapter 39.1).

In adolescents, the clinical manifestations of mania are similar to those in adults, and **psychosis** (delusions, hallucinations) often is an associated symptom. Mood in a manic episode is often described as euphoric, excessively cheerful, high, or "feeling on top of the world." During the episode, the adolescent may engage in multiple new projects that are initiated with little knowledge of the topic and often at unusual hours (middle of the night). Inflated self-esteem is usually present, ranging from uncritical self-confidence to marked grandiosity, and may reach delusional proportions. The adolescent may sleep little if at all for days and still feel rested and full of energy. Speech can be rapid, pressured, and loud and characterized by jokes, puns, amusing irrelevancies, and theatricality. Frequently there is a "flight of ideas," evidenced by an almost continuous flow of accelerated speech, with abrupt shifts from one topic to another. Distractibility is evidenced by an inability to censor irrelevant extraneous stimuli, which often prevents an individual with mania from engaging in a rational conversation. The expansive mood, grandiosity, and poor judgment often lead to reckless involvement in activities with high potential for personal harm.

Controversy surrounds the applicability of the diagnostic criteria for mania to *prepubertal* children. It may be developmentally normal for

Table 39.6	DSM-5 Diagnostic Criteria for a Hypomanic Episode

A. A distinct period of abnormally and persistently elevated, expansive, or irritable mood and abnormally and persistently increased goal-directed activity or energy, lasting at least 4 consecutive days and present most of the day, nearly every day.

B. During the period of mood disturbance and increased energy or activity, 3 (or more) of the following symptoms (4 if the mood is only irritable) have persisted, represent a noticeable change from usual behavior, and have been present to a significant degree:
  1. Inflated self-esteem or grandiosity.
  2. Decreased need for sleep (e.g., feels rested after only 3 hr of sleep).
  3. More talkative than usual or pressure to keep talking.
  4. Flight of ideas or subjective experience that thoughts are racing.
  5. Distractibility (i.e., attention too easily drawn to unimportant or irrelevant external stimuli), as reported or observed.
  6. Increase in goal-directed activity (either socially, at work or school, or sexually) or psychomotor agitation (i.e., purposeless non-goal-directed activity).
  7. Excessive involvement in activities that have a high potential for painful consequences (e.g., engaging in unrestrained buying sprees, sexual indiscretions, or foolish business investments).

C. The episode is associated with an unequivocal change in functioning that is uncharacteristic of the individual when not symptomatic.

D. The disturbance in mood and the change in functioning are observable by others.

E. The disturbance is not severe enough to cause marked impairment in social or occupational functioning or to necessitate hospitalization. If there are psychotic features, the episode is, by definition, manic.

F. The episode is not attributable to the physiologic effects of a substance (e.g., a drug of abuse, a medication, other treatment) or to another medical condition.

Note: A full hypomanic episode that emerges during antidepressant treatment (e.g., medication, electroconvulsive therapy) but persists at a fully syndromal level beyond the physiologic effect of that treatment is sufficient evidence for a hypomanic episode diagnosis. However, caution is indicated so that 1 or 2 symptoms (particularly increased irritability, edginess, or agitation following antidepressant use) are not taken as sufficient for diagnosis of a hypomanic episode, nor necessarily indicative of a bipolar diathesis.

Note: Criteria A-F constitute a hypomanic episode. Hypomanic episodes are common in bipolar I disorder but are not required for the diagnosis of bipolar I disorder.

From the *Diagnostic and Statistical Manual of Mental Disorders, Fifth Edition*, (Copyright 2013). American Psychiatric Association, p 124.

visits of youth with a diagnosis of bipolar disorder increased from 25 per 100,000 population in 1994–1995 to 1,003/100,000 in 2002–2003. U.S. hospital discharge diagnoses increased from 1.4 to 7.3/10,000 in 9-13 yr old children and from 5.1 to 20.4/10,000 in 14-19 yr olds. These increases were not found in U.K. hospital discharges, questioning whether bipolar disorder was being overdiagnosed in the United States, with resultant increases in prescribing of antipsychotic and mood-stabilizing medications.

CLINICAL COURSE

The mean age of onset of the 1st manic episode is approximately 18 yr for bipolar I disorder. Premorbid problems are common in bipolar disorder, especially temperamental difficulties with mood and behavioral regulation. Premorbid anxiety also is common. The early course of adolescent-onset bipolar I disorder appears to be more chronic and refractory to treatment than adult-onset bipolar disorder. Comorbidity predicts functional impairment, and age at onset predicts duration of episodes. Sleep impairment and family conflict are inversely related to favorable treatment response, suggesting important targets for treatment. The bipolar disorders are highly recurrent, and 70–80% of bipolar I patients will have additional mood episodes. Recurrent episodes can approximate 4 in 10 years, with the interepisode interval shortening as the patient ages. Although the majority of patients with bipolar I return to a fully functional level between episodes, approximately one-third continue to be symptomatic and functionally impaired between episodes.

The initial presentation of bipolar I disorder is often an MDD. Switching from a depressive episode to a manic episode by adulthood may occur in 10–20% of youth, both spontaneously and during depression treatment. Factors that predict the eventual development of mania in depressed youth include a depressive episode characterized by rapid onset, psychomotor retardation, and psychotic features; a family history of affective disorders, especially bipolar disorder; and a history of mania or hypomania after antidepressant therapy.

The mean age of onset of bipolar II disorder is 20 yr. The illness most often begins with a depressive episode and is not recognized as bipolar II disorder until a hypomanic episode occurs, in about 12% of individuals with the initial diagnosis of major depression. Many individuals experience several episodes of major depression before experiencing the first recognized hypomanic episode. Anxiety, substance misuse, or eating disorders may also precede the onset of bipolar II, complicating its detection. About 5–15% of individuals with bipolar II disorder will ultimately develop a manic episode, which changes the diagnosis to bipolar I disorder.

Depression in bipolar I or II usually has an earlier age of onset, more frequent episodes of shorter duration, an abrupt onset and offset, is linked to comorbid substance misuse, and is triggered by stressors. Atypical symptoms such as hypersomnia, lability, and weight instability are also common in bipolar depression, reported in up to 90% of cases vs 50% in unipolar depression. Psychosis, psychomotor retardation, and catatonia are also more characteristic of bipolar depression, whereas somatic complaints are more frequent in unipolar depression. A family history of mania is also a relevant discriminating factor.

Provision of clinical services is poor for youth with bipolar disorder. In one healthcare system study spanning 2 yr follow-up after diagnosis, despite complex drug regimens, medication appointments were infrequent, averaging 1 visit every 2 mo. More than half of patients needed 1 or more hospitalizations, and almost half had psychiatric emergency department visits. In a national study, 38% of youths diagnosed with bipolar disorder had received no treatment at all.

DIFFERENTIAL DIAGNOSIS

Numerous psychiatric disorders, general medical conditions, and medications can generate manic-like symptoms and must be distinguished from the bipolar and related disorders. The psychiatric disorders include ADHD, ODD, and intermittent explosive, posttraumatic stress, depressive, anxiety, substance abuse, and borderline personality disorders. Medical conditions include neurologic disorders, endocrine disorders, infectious diseases, tumors, anemia, uremia, and vitamin deficiencies. Medications include androgens, bronchodilators, cardiovascular medications,

children to be elated, expansive, grandiose, or talkative, reducing the specificity of these symptoms to this disorder. In addition, the distractibility, overactivity, impulsivity, and irritability formerly ascribed to bipolar disorder by some investigators may be better explained by a diagnosis of ADHD, with or without comorbid ODD. The presentation of severe and pervasive irritability formerly diagnosed as "bipolar disorder" may be better captured by the diagnosis of DMDD.

EPIDEMIOLOGY

The lifetime prevalence of bipolar disorder I among adults worldwide is approximately 0.6% for bipolar I disorder, 0.4% for bipolar II disorder, and 1.4% for subsyndromal bipolar disorder. Bipolar I disorder affects men and women equally, whereas bipolar II disorder is more common in women. Lifetime rates of mania among youth have ranged from 0.1% to 1.7%. Since the 1990s, there has been a significant increase in the diagnosis of bipolar disorder in the United States that was not mirrored in the United Kingdom. The estimated annual number of U.S. office-based corticosteroids, chemotherapy agents, thyroid preparations, and certain psychiatric medications (benzodiazepines, antidepressants, stimulants). The diagnosis of a bipolar disorder should be made after these other explanations for the observed symptoms have been ruled out.

For bipolar II disorder, the main differential is unipolar depression (MDD) or cyclothymic disorder.

COMORBIDITY

The most common simultaneous comorbidities (ADHD, ODD, conduct disorder, anxiety) may be difficult to distinguish from mania because of considerable symptom overlap. Substance use also is a common comorbidity in adolescents, and presentations that appear to be manic may remit when the substances of abuse are discontinued.

SEQUELAE

The lifetime risk of **suicide** in individuals with bipolar disorder is estimated to be at least 15 times that of the general population. Factors associated with suicide attempts include female gender, young age at illness onset, depressive polarity of first illness episode or of current or most recent episode, comorbid anxiety disorder, any comorbid substance use disorder, borderline personality disorder, and first-degree family history of suicide. By contrast, completed suicides are associated with male sex and a first-degree family history of suicide. Despite patients with bipolar disorder having normal or even superior cognition before diagnosis, bipolar disorder has been associated with decrements in executive function and verbal memory. Youths with bipolar disorder are also at high risk for substance abuse, antisocial behavior, impaired academic performance, impaired family and peer relationships, and poor adjustment to life stressors.

ETIOLOGY AND RISK FACTORS

Twin studies of adults suggest the heritability of bipolar disorder may be 60–90%, while shared and unique environmental factors may account for 30–40% and 10–20%, respectively. Offspring of parents with bipolar disorders are at high risk for early-onset bipolar disorders as well as anxiety and behavioral disorders and mood dysregulation. There is an average 10-fold increased risk among adult relatives of individuals with bipolar disorder, with the magnitude of risk increasing with the degree of kinship. Bipolar disorder and schizophrenia likely share a genetic origin, reflected in familial co-aggregation of the two disorders.

Studies to date suggest key roles for the amygdala, anterior paralimbic cortices, and their connections in the emotional dysregulation of bipolar disorder. Some of these abnormalities are apparent by adolescence, whereas others appear to progress over adolescence into young adulthood.

Dysthymic (sad), *cyclothymic* (labile), or *hyperthymic* (irritable) temperaments may presage eventual bipolar disorder. Premorbid anxiety and dysphoria also are common. Environmental factors such as irritable and negative parenting styles, physical and sexual abuse, poor social support, and prenatal alcohol exposure may interact with genetic vulnerability to produce early onset of bipolar illness as well as negative prognostic indicators. *Affective lability* in particular has been associated with high levels of childhood trauma, and gradual sensitization to stressors has been linked to episode recurrence.

PREVENTION

Although empirical support is sparse, one study demonstrated the effectiveness of family-focused treatment vs an educational control in hastening and sustaining recovery from mood symptoms in a high-familial-risk cohort of youths with subsyndromal symptoms of mania. Family-focused treatment is a manualized psychoeducational intervention designed to reduce family stress, conflict, and affective arousal by enhancing communication and problem solving between youths and their caregivers. Pharmacologic interventions for subsyndromal mania have produced equivocal results.

CASE FINDING

Cardinal manic symptoms of elation, increased energy, and grandiosity occurring in adolescents as a discrete episode representing an unequivocal and uncharacteristic change in functioning should alert pediatric practitioners to the possibility of bipolar disorder. High scores on parent-completed versions of mania-specific rating scales (e.g., *General Behavior Inventory, Child Mania Rating Scale, Young Mania Rating Scale*) have been associated with increased likelihood of a bipolar diagnosis. However, in general, screening tools for bipolar disorder have suboptimal psychometric properties when applied to young people. Because of the complexity of diagnosing and treating bipolar disorders, any suspected cases should be referred to the specialty mental health setting for comprehensive assessment and treatment.

TREATMENT

For mania in bipolar I disorder, medication is the primary treatment. Studies have demonstrated the superiority of **antipsychotics** over mood stabilizers in the treatment of mania, with haloperidol, risperidone, and olanzapine ranked as the most efficacious agents and quetiapine, risperidone, and olanzapine ranked as the most tolerable agents. Taken together, risperidone and olanzapine may have the best overall efficacy and tolerability. Asenapine has also been found to be effective and well tolerated. The FDA has approved aripiprazole, risperidone, quetiapine, and asenapine for the treatment of bipolar disorder from age 10 yr, and olanzapine from age 13 years. The choice of antipsychotic medication is based on factors such as side effect profiles, comorbidities, adherence, and positive response of a family member.

Among traditional **mood stabilizers**, only lithium is FDA approved for the treatment of bipolar disorder from age 12 yr, and its efficacy and tolerability compared to placebo has been demonstrated in RCTs. There also is meta-analytic evidence that lithium reduces the risk of suicide and total deaths in patients with both unipolar and bipolar depressive disorder.

No published RCT evidence supports the efficacy of other mood stabilizers (e.g., divalproex sodium, topiramate, carbamazepine, oxcarbazepine, lamotrigine) in the treatment of youth with bipolar disorder, and retrospective cohort studies suggest that those who receive antipsychotics are less likely to discontinue treatment and less likely to receive treatment augmentation than youth who receive mood stabilizers. None of the mood-stabilizing medications (other than lithium) have FDA approval for the treatment of bipolar disorder in youth, and as such, likely should not be first-line treatments.

Medication trials should be systematic and their duration sufficient (generally 6-8 wk) to determine the agent's effectiveness. Care should be taken to avoid unnecessary polypharmacy, in part by discontinuing agents that have not demonstrated significant benefit. Because these medications are associated with significant side effects, careful monitoring of baseline and follow-up indices is imperative.

The regimen needed to stabilize acute mania should be maintained for 12-24 mo. Maintenance therapy is often needed for adolescents with bipolar I disorder, and some patients need lifelong medication. Any attempts to discontinue prophylactic medication should be done gradually while closely monitoring the patient for relapse.

Antidepressants *alone* should not be prescribed for depressive symptoms in bipolar I disorder because of the risk of manic switch. However, in an RCT, olanzapine/fluoxetine combination was superior to placebo in youth with depression in bipolar I and has been FDA approved for this indication in patients age 10-17 yr. For treatment of depression in bipolar II, antidepressant medication (preferably SSRIs or bupropion) may be used cautiously. Comorbid ADHD can be treated with a stimulant once a mood-stabilizer has been initiated.

Psychotherapy is a potentially important adjunctive treatment for the bipolar disorders. Therapies with some evidence of efficacy, primarily as adjunctive to pharmacotherapy, include multifamily psychoeducational psychotherapy and family-focused treatment (probably efficacious), child and family-focused CBT (possibly efficacious), dialectical behavioral therapy, and interpersonal and social rhythm therapy (experimental). Active components of these therapies include family involvement and psychoeducation, along with self-regulation, cognitive restructuring, communication, problem-solving, and emotion regulation skills. Factors that adversely influence response to therapy include high-conflict families and sleep impairment, suggesting the importance of targeting these factors in treatment.

LEVEL OF CARE

Most youths with bipolar disorders can be safely and effectively treated as outpatients, provided that an appropriate schedule of visits and laboratory monitoring can be maintained through the course of treatment. Youths who are suicidal or psychotic typically require inpatient care.

Bibliography is available at Expert Consult.

Chapter 40
Suicide and Attempted Suicide
David R. DeMaso and Heather J. Walter

第四十章
自杀和自杀未遂

中文导读

　　本章主要介绍了青少年自杀的流行病学情况，分别从自杀意念、自杀企图、自杀成功各自发生率来分别描述。还介绍了引起自杀的风险因素，如包括自杀发生前有无精神障碍、认知歪曲、生物学因素，社会、文化和环境因素及保护性因素，介绍了自杀风险模型。对自杀如何评估、如何干预和预防进行了详细阐述，原文列举了自杀发生前的一些警示信号（见原文表40.2），供读者参考。

Youth suicide is a major public health problem. In 2014 for all youth between ages 10 and 19 yr in the United States, suicide was the 2nd leading cause of death, with approximately 5,500 lives lost each year. The suicide rate for youth age 15-19 yr was 9.8 per 100,000 persons (14.2 for males, 5.1 for females), while the rate for youth age 10-14 yr was 2.0/100,000 (2.4 for males, 1.6 for females). There are numerous psychiatric, social, cultural, and environmental risk factors for suicidal behavior, and knowledge of these risk factors can facilitate identification of youths at highest risk (Fig. 40.1).

EPIDEMIOLOGY
Suicidal Ideation and Attempts
Based on the 2015 Youth Risk Behavior Survey, almost one third of 9th through 12th grade students in the United States felt so sad or hopeless almost every day for ≥2 wk in a row during the previous year that they stopped doing usual activities. During that same period, 18% of the students reported that they had seriously considered attempting suicide, and 9% reported that they had actually attempted suicide one or more times. A suicide attempt in the previous year that resulted in an injury, poisoning, or overdose that had to be treated by a physician or nurse was reported by 3% of students.

It is estimated that for every completed youth suicide, as many as 200 suicide attempts are made. Poisoning, suffocation, and firearms are the most common causes of suicide, whereas ingestion of medication is the most common method of *attempted* suicide (Fig. 40.2). The 15-19 yr old age-group is the most likely to intentionally harm themselves by ingestion, receive treatment in the emergency department (ED), and survive. Attempts are more common in adolescent females than males (approximately 3:1-4:1) and in Hispanic females than their non-Hispanic counterparts. Gay, lesbian, bisexual, transgender, and bullied youths also have disproportionately high rates of suicide attempts. Attempters who have made prior suicide attempts, who used a method other than ingestion, who have a plan (nonimpulsive), who have no regret, and who still want to die are at increased risk for completed suicide.

Suicide Completions
In the United States, *completed* suicide is very rare before age 10. Rates of completed suicide increase steadily across adolescence into young adulthood, peaking in the early 20s. The male:female ratio for completed suicide rises with age from 3:1 in children to approximately 4:1 in 15-24 yr olds, and to >6:1 among 20-24 yr olds.

In 2015 among 10-19 yr olds, the highest suicide rates, 21.8 and 16.6 per 100,000, were among Native American males and females, respectively, followed by white males (10.6/100,000). The groups with the lowest rates were Asian/Pacific Islander females, Hispanic females, and black females (2.4, 2.3, and 1.9/100,000, respectively). **Firearms** are the most common method used to complete suicide in the United States, accounting for 50% of all suicide deaths in 2015 (Fig. 40.2). The next

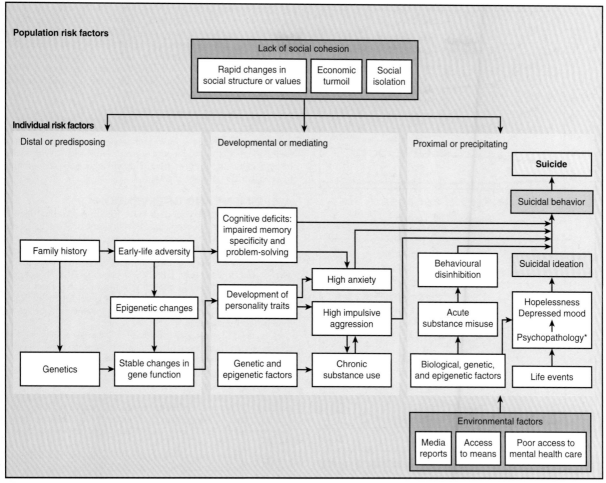

Fig. 40.1 Model for suicide risk. Suicide risk is modulated by a range of factors at both the population and the individual levels. Individual risk factors can be grouped into *distal* (or predisposing), *developmental* (or mediating), and *proximal* (or precipitating) factors, and many of these factors interact to contribute to the risk of developing suicidal behaviors. *Any single mental illness associated with suicide risk, or a combination of mental illnesses, including major depressive disorder, bipolar disorder, schizophrenia, and personality disorders; the presence of a depressive episode is often a sign of increased risk of suicide. (From Turecki D, Brent DA: Suicide and suicidal behaviours. Lancet 387:1227–1238, 2016.)

most prevalent methods are **suffocation** (27%) and **poisoning** (15%). Firearms are the most lethal method of suicide completion; the death rate with respect to firearms is approximately 80–90%, whereas the death rate is only 1.5–4% for overdoses. Among males, firearms are the most frequently used method of suicide (55%); among females, poisoning is the most common method (34%).

From 1999 through 2014, the age-adjusted suicide rate in the United States increased 24%, from 10.5 to 13.0/100,000, with the pace of increase greater after 2006. Rates increased for both males and females and for all ages 10-74; the percent increase among females was greatest for those age 10-14, and for males, those age 45-64.

RISK FACTORS
In addition to age, race/ethnicity, and a history of a previous suicide attempt, multiple risk factors predispose youths to suicide (see Fig. 40.1).

Preexisting Mental Disorder
Approximately 90% of youths who complete suicide have a preexisting psychiatric illness, most often major depression. Among females, chronic anxiety, especially panic disorder, also is associated with suicide attempts and completion. Among males, conduct disorder and substance use convey increased risk. Comorbidity of a substance use disorder, a

depressive disorder, and conduct disorder are linked to suicide by firearm. Schizophrenia spectrum disorders are linked to suicide attempts and completions.

Cognitive Distortions
Negative self-attributions can contribute to the hopelessness typically associated with suicidality; hopelessness may contribute to approximately 55% of the explained variance in continued suicidal ideation. Many youth who are suicidal hold negative views of their own competence, have poor self-esteem, engage in catastrophic thinking, and have difficulty identifying sources of support or reasons to live. Many young people lack the coping strategies necessary to manage strong emotions and instead tend to *catastrophize* and engage in *all-or-nothing* thinking.

Biologic Factors
Postmortem studies show observable differences between the brains of individuals who have completed suicide and those who died from other causes. The brain systems that may be related to suicide completion are the serotonergic system, adrenergic system, and the hypothalamic-pituitary axis. Family history of mental disorders also is linked to completed suicide.

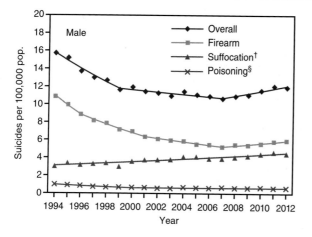

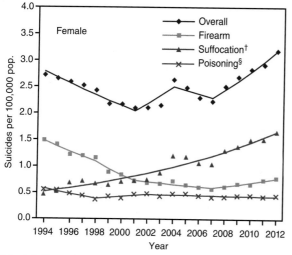

* Symbols (diamond, square, triangle, x) representing joinpoints are displayed on the line graphs because, for both males and females, some of the suicide rates were best fitted by multiple segments of lines (number of joinpoints >0).
† Including hanging.
§ Including drug overdose.

Fig. 40.2 Age-adjusted suicide rates among persons aged 10-24 yr, by sex and mechanism—United States, 1994–2012; **top**, males; **bottom**, females. *Symbols,* * See footnotes on figure. *(From Sullivan EM, Annest JL, Simon TR, et al: Suicide trends among persons aged 10-24 years – United States, 1994-2012. MMWR 64(8):201-205, 2015. Fig, p. 203.)*

Social, Environmental, and Cultural Factors

Of youths who attempt suicide, 65% can name a precipitating event for their action. Most adolescent suicide attempts are precipitated by **stressful life events** (e.g., academic or social problems; being bullied; trouble with the law; questioning one's sexual orientation or gender identify; newly diagnosed medical condition; recent or anticipated loss).

Suicide attempts may also be precipitated by exposure to news of another person's suicide or by reading about or viewing a suicide portrayed in a romantic light in the media. Media coverage of suicide is linked to fluctuating incidence rates of suicides, particularly among adolescents. Glorification or sensationalization of suicide in the media has found to be associated with an increase in suicides. When media coverage includes a detailed description of specific means used, the use of that particular method may increase in the overall population.

For some immigrants, suicidal ideation can be associated with high levels of acculturative stress, especially in the context of family separation

and limited access to supportive resources. Physical and sexual abuse can also increase one's risk of suicide, with 15–20% of female suicide attempters having had a history of abuse. The general association between family conflict and suicide attempts is strongest in children and early adolescents. Family psychopathology and a family history of suicidal behavior also convey excess risk. The lack of supportive social relations with peers, parents, and school personnel interacts in increasing the risk of suicide among youth.

Protective Factors

Protective factors can provide a counterbalance for those contemplating suicide. These may include a sense of family responsibility, life satisfaction, future orientation, social support, coping and problem-solving skills, religious faith, intact reality testing, and solid therapeutic relationships (e.g., pediatrician, teacher, therapist).

ASSESSMENT AND INTERVENTION

The U.S. Preventive Services Task Force has concluded that there is insufficient evidence to recommend universal suicide screening in the primary care setting for children and adolescents. Pediatric practitioners should consider suicide potential and the need for mental health assessment in the context of concerning information elicited in child/parent psychosocial histories (e.g., HEADSS Psychosocial Risk Assessment; see Chapter 32, Table 32.2), general screening measure scores out of the normal range (e.g., Pediatric Symptom Checklist Internalizing Sub-Scale; see Chapter 28), or self-reported statements or behaviors from patients and parents.

All suicidal ideation and attempts should be taken seriously and require a thorough assessment by a child-trained mental health clinician to evaluate the youth's current state of mind, underlying psychiatric conditions, and ongoing risk of harm. **Emergency** mental health assessment is needed for immediate threat to self (i.e., suicidal intent and plan); **urgent** mental health assessment (48-72 hr) is needed for severe psychiatric symptoms, significant change in overall functioning, and suicidal ideation without intent or plan. **Routine** mental health assessment is appropriate for mild to moderate psychiatric symptoms without suicidal ideation.

Pediatric practitioners should expect the mental health clinician to evaluate the presence and degree of suicidality and underlying risk factors. The reliability and validity of child interviewing are affected by children's level of cognitive development as well as their understanding of the relationship between their emotions and behavior. Confirmation of the youth's suicidal behavior can be obtained from information gathered by interviewing others who know the child or adolescent. A discrepancy between patient and parent reports is not unusual, with both children and adolescents being more likely to disclose suicidal ideation and suicidal actions than their parents.

In the mental health assessment, **suicidal ideation** can be assessed by explicit questions posed in a nonjudgmental, noncondescending, matter-of-fact approach. The *Ask Suicide-Screening Questionnaire* (ASQ) is a validated 4-item measure shown in the ED setting to have high sensitivity and negative predictive value in identifying youth at risk for suicide ideation and behavior: (1) "In the past few weeks, have you felt that you or your family would be better off if you were dead?" (2) "In the past few weeks, have you wished you were dead?" (3) "In the past few weeks, have you been having thoughts about killing yourself?" and (4) "Have you ever tried to kill yourself?" If a "yes" response is given to any of these 4 questions, the patient is asked, (5) "Are you having thoughts of killing yourself right now?" Another common screening test is the *Columbia Suicide Severity Rating Scale (C-SSRS) Screener* (Table 40.1).

The assessment of a suicidal attempt should include a detailed exploration of the hours immediately preceding the attempt to identify precipitants as well as the circumstances of the attempt itself, to understand fully the patient's intent and potential lethality. The calculation of the level of suicide concern is complex, requiring a determination across a spectrum of risk. At the low end of the risk spectrum are youth with thoughts of death or wanting to die, but without suicidal thoughts, intent, or plan. Those with highly specific suicide plans, preparatory

Table 40.1	Columbia Suicide Severity Rating Scale Screener

1. Have you wished you were dead or wished you could go to sleep and not wake up?
2. Have you actually had any thoughts about killing yourself?
   If "Yes" to 2, answer questions 3, 4, 5, and 6.
   If "No" to 2, go directly to question 6.
3. Have you thought about how you might do this?
4. Have you had any intention of acting on these thoughts of killing yourself, as opposed to you having the thoughts but you definitely would not act on them?
5. Have you started to work out or worked out the details of how to kill yourself? Do you intend to carry out this plan?
6. Have you done anything, started to do anything, or prepared to do anything to end your life?

Response Protocol to Screening (based on last item answered "Yes")

Item 1—Mental Health Referral at discharge
Item 2—Mental Health Referral at discharge
Item 3—Care Team Consultation (Psychiatric Nurse) and Patient Safety Monitor/Procedures
Item 4—Psychiatric Consultation and Patient Safety Monitor/Procedures
Item 5—Psychiatric Consultation and Patient Safety Monitor/Procedures
Item 6—If over 3 months ago, Mental Health Referral at discharge
   If 3 months ago or less, Psychiatric Consultation and Patient Safety Monitor

From Posner K. Columbia Lighthouse Project. The Columbia-Suicide Severity Rating Scale (C-SSRS) Screener–Recent. http://www.cssrs.columbia.edu/scales_practice_cssrs.html.

Table 40.2	Warning Signs of Suicide

Seek help as soon as possible by contacting a mental health professional or by calling the National Suicide Prevention Lifeline at **1-800-273-TALK** if you or someone you know exhibits any of the following signs:
- Threatening to hurt or kill oneself or talking about wanting to hurt or kill oneself.
- Looking for ways to kill oneself by seeking access to firearms, available pills, or other means.
- Talking or writing about death, dying, or suicide when these actions are out of the ordinary for the person.
- Feeling hopeless.
- Feeling rage or uncontrolled anger or seeking revenge.
- Acting reckless or engaging in risky activities, seemingly without thinking.
- Feeling trapped, "like there's no way out."
- Increasing alcohol or drug use.
- Withdrawing from friends, family, and society.
- Feeling anxious, agitated, or unable to sleep, or sleeping all the time.
- Experiencing dramatic mood changes.
- Seeing no reason for living, or having no sense of purpose in life.

Developed by the US Department of Health and Human Services, Substance Abuse and Mental Health Services Administration (SAMHSA). https://www.nimh.nih.gov/health/topics/suicide-prevention/suicide-prevention-studies/warning-signs-of-suicide.shtml.

acts or suicide rehearsals, and clearly articulated intent are at the high end. A suicidal history, presently impaired judgment (as seen in altered mental states including depression, mania, anxiety, intoxication, substance abuse, psychosis, trauma-reactive, hopelessness, rage, humiliation, impulsivity), as well as poor social support, further exacerbates the heightened risk. Among adolescents who consider self-harm, those who carry out (**enactors**) self-injury are more likely to have family or friends (or think that their peers) engaged in self-harm, and are more impulsive than those who only have thoughts of self-harm (**ideators**).

For youth who are an imminent danger to themselves (i.e, have *active* ["I want to die"] or *implied* ["I can't see any reason to go on living"] suicidal intent), inpatient level of psychiatric care is necessary to ensure safety, clarify diagnoses, and comprehensively plan treatment. These patients can be hospitalized voluntarily or involuntarily. It is helpful for the pediatric practitioner to have an office protocol to follow in these situations. This protocol should take into consideration state laws regarding involuntary hospitalization, transportation options, nearest emergency assessment site, necessary forms for hospitalization, and available emergency mental health consultants.

For those youth suitable for treatment in the outpatient setting (e.g., suicidal ideation without intent, intact mental status, few or no other risk factors for suicidality, willing and able to participate in outpatient treatment; has caregivers able to provide emotional support, supervision, safeguarding, and adherence to follow-up), an appointment should be scheduled within a few days with a mental health clinician. Ideally, this appointment should be scheduled before leaving the assessment venue, because almost 50% of those who attempt suicide fail to follow through with the mental health referral. A procedure should be in place to contact the family if the family fails to complete the referral.

Through follow-up office visits, pediatric practitioners can help support and facilitate the implementation of psychotherapies (e.g., cognitive-behavioral therapy, dialectical behavioral therapy, mentalization-based treatment, family therapy) that target the specific psychiatric disorders and the emotional dysphoria or behavioral dysregulation that accompany suicidal ideation or behavior. In conjunction with a child and adolescent child psychiatrist, psychotropic medications may be used as indicated

to treat underlying psychiatric disorders. Pediatric practitioners also can encourage social connectedness to peers and to community organizations (e.g., school or church), as well as promote help-seeking (e.g., talking to a trusted adult when distressed) and wellness (e.g., sleep, exercise, relaxation, nutrition) behaviors. In the event of a completed suicide, pediatricians can offer support to the family, particularly by monitoring for adverse bereavement responses in siblings and parents.

PREVENTION

The aforementioned risk factors associated with suicide are relatively common and individually not strong predictors of suicide. The assessment is complicated by patients who may attempt to conceal their suicide thoughts and by those who express suicidal thoughts without serious intent. Suicide screening has been challenging because most screening instruments have variable sensitivity and specificity. In addition, the burden of follow-up mental health evaluations for those who screen positive has been daunting. Although primary care–feasible screening tools may be help to identify some adults at increased risk for suicide, they have, to date, demonstrated limited ability to detect suicide risk in adolescents.

Prevention strategies in the **pediatric medical home** include training staff to recognize and respond to the *warning signs* of suicide (Table 40.2), screening for and treating depression, educating patients/parents about warning signs for suicide, and restricting access to modes of lethal self-harm. Young people have increased rates of suicide attempts and completions if they live in homes where firearms are present and available. When recommended by their primary care providers, most parents restrict access of their children to guns and medications. Pediatric practitioners should consider counseling parents to remove firearms from the home entirely or securely lock guns and ammunition in separate locations. Anecdotal evidence suggests youths frequently know where guns and keys to gun cabinets are kept, even though parents may think they do not. The same recommendation applies to restricting access to potentially lethal prescription and nonprescription medications (e.g., containers of >25 acetaminophen tablets) and alcohol. These approaches emphasize the importance of restriction of access to means for suicide to prevent self-harm.

Screening for suicide in **schools** is also fraught with problems related to low specificity of the screening instrument and paucity of referral sites, as well as poor acceptability among school administrators. **Gatekeeper** (e.g., student support personnel) **training** appears effective in improving skills among school personnel and is highly acceptable to administrators but has not been shown to prevent suicide. School curricula (e.g., *Signs of Suicide*) have shown some preventive potential by teaching students to recognize the signs of depression and suicide in themselves and others and providing them with specific action steps necessary for responding to these signs. Peer helpers have not generally been shown to be efficacious.

Bibliography is available at Expert Consult.

Chapter 41
Eating Disorders
Richard E. Kreipe and Taylor B. Starr

第四十一章
进食障碍

中文导读

　　本章首先对进食障碍的概念进行了描述，对神经性厌食、神经性贪食、非典型神经性厌食和回避限制性摄食障碍、暴食障碍和未特定的进食障碍的概念进行了界定，并列举了各自的诊断标准。后对进食障碍的流行病学、病理和发病机制、临床表现、鉴别诊断、实验室检查、并发症和治疗策略进行了详细阐述。在治疗这一节中，介绍了初级保健治疗的基本原则指南、营养与体力活动、初级保健治疗等方法，包括如果需要，可转介开展精神卫生服务（如是否要采取SSRIs药物治疗、认知行为治疗、辩证行为治疗、团体治疗、家庭治疗），转介到一个内在整合的进食障碍团队和开展支持性照料的策略，最后，对该疾病的预后与预防进行了简要介绍。

Eating disorders (EDs) are characterized by body dissatisfaction related to overvaluation of a thin body ideal, associated with dysfunctional patterns of cognition and weight control behaviors that result in significant biologic, psychological, and social complications. Although usually affecting white, adolescent females, EDs also affect males and cross all racial, ethnic, and cultural boundaries. Early intervention in EDs improves outcome.

DEFINITIONS

Anorexia nervosa (AN) involves significant overestimation of body size and shape, with a relentless pursuit of thinness that, in the **restrictive** subtype, typically combines excessive dieting and compulsive exercising. In the **binge-purge** subtype, patients might intermittently overeat and then attempt to rid themselves of calories by vomiting or taking laxatives, still with a strong drive for thinness (Table 41.1).

Bulimia nervosa (BN) is characterized by episodes of eating large amounts of food in a brief period, followed by compensatory vomiting, laxative use, exercise, or fasting to rid the body of the effects of overeating in an effort to avoid obesity (Table 41.2).

Children and adolescents with EDs may not fulfill criteria for AN or BN in the *Diagnostic and Statistical Manual of Mental Disorders, Fifth Edition* (DSM-5) and may fall into a subcategory of **atypical anorexia nervosa,** or a more appropriately defined category of **avoidant/restrictive food intake disorder (ARFID).** In these conditions, food intake is restricted or avoided because of adverse feeding or eating experiences or the sensory qualities of food, resulting in significant unintended weight loss or nutritional deficiencies and problems with social interactions (Table 41.3).

Binge eating disorder (BED), in which binge eating is not followed regularly by any compensatory behaviors (vomiting, laxatives), is a stand-alone category in DSM-5 but shares many features with obesity (see Chapter 60). **Eating disorder–not otherwise specified (ED-NOS),** often called "disordered eating," can worsen into full syndrome EDs.

EPIDEMIOLOGY

The classic presentation of AN is an early to middle adolescent female of above-average intelligence and socioeconomic status who is a conflict-avoidant, risk-aversive perfectionist and is struggling with disturbances of anxiety and/or mood. BN tends to emerge in later adolescence, sometimes evolving from AN, and is typified by impulsivity and features of borderline personality disorder associated with depression and mood swings. The 0.5–1% and 3–5% incidence rates among younger and older adolescent females for AN and BN, respectively, probably reflect ascertainment bias in sampling and underdiagnosis in cases not fitting the common profile. The same may be true of the significant gender disparity, in which female patients account for approximately 85% of

Table 41.1	DSM-5 Diagnostic Criteria for Anorexia Nervosa

A. Restriction of energy intake relative to requirements, leading to a significantly low body weight in the context of age, sex, developmental trajectory, and physical health. Significantly low weight is defined as a weight that is less than minimally normal or, for children and adolescents, less than that minimally expected.

B. Intense fear of gaining weight or of becoming fat, or persistent behavior that interferes with weight gain, even though at a significantly low weight.

C. Disturbance in the way in which one's body weight or shape is experienced, undue influence of body weight or shape on self-evaluation, or persistent lack of recognition of the seriousness of the current low body weight.

Specify whether:

Restricting type (ICD-10-CM code F50.01): During the last 3 mo, the individual has not engaged in recurrent episodes of binge eating or purging behavior (i.e., self-induced vomiting or the misuse of laxatives, diuretics, or enemas). This subtype describes presentations in which weight loss is accomplished primarily through dieting, fasting, and/or excessive exercise.

Binge-eating/purging type (ICD-10-CM code F50.02): During the last 3 mo, the individual has engaged in recurrent episodes of binge eating or purging behavior (i.e., self-induced vomiting or the misuse of laxatives, diuretics, or enemas).

Specify if:

In partial remission: After full criteria for anorexia nervosa were previously met, Criterion A (low body weight) has not been met for a sustained period, but either Criterion B (intense fear of gaining weight or becoming fat or behavior that interferes with weight gain) or Criterion C (disturbances in self-perception of weight and shape) is still met.

In full remission: After full criteria for anorexia nervosa were previously met, none of the criteria has been met for a sustained period of time.

Specify current severity:

The minimum level of severity is based, for adults, on current body mass index (BMI) (see below) or, for children and adolescents, on BMI percentile. **The ranges below are derived from World Health Organization categories for thinness in adults; for children and adolescents, corresponding BMI percentiles should be used.** The level of severity may be increased to reflect clinical symptoms, the degree of functional disability, and the need for supervision.

Mild: BMI $\geq$ 17 kg/m^2

Moderate: BMI 16-16.99 kg/m^2

Severe: BMI 15-15.99 kg/m^2

Extreme: BMI < 15 kg/m^2

From the *Diagnostic and Statistical Manual of Mental Disorders, Fifth Edition,* (Copyright 2013). American Psychiatric Association, pp 338–339.

Table 41.2	DSM-5 Diagnostic Criteria for Bulimia Nervosa

A. Recurrent episodes of binge eating. An episode of binge eating is characterized by both of the following:
   1. Eating, in a discrete period of time (e.g., within any 2 hr period), an amount of food that is definitely larger than what most individuals would eat in a similar period of time under similar circumstances.
   2. A sense of lack of control over eating during the episode (e.g., a feeling that one cannot stop eating or control what or how much one is eating).

B. Recurrent inappropriate compensatory behaviors in order to prevent weight gain, such as self-induced vomiting; misuse of laxatives, diuretics, or other medications; fasting; or excessive exercise.

C. The binge eating and inappropriate compensatory behaviors both occur, on average, at least once a week for 3 mo.

D. Self-evaluation is unduly influenced by body shape and weight.

E. The disturbance does not occur exclusively during episodes of anorexia nervosa.

Specify if:

In partial remission: After full criteria for bulimia nervosa were previously met, some, but not all, of the criteria have been met for a sustained period of time.

In full remission: After full criteria for bulimia nervosa were previously met, none of the criteria has been met for a sustained period of time.

Specify current severity:

The minimum level of severity is based on the frequency of inappropriate compensatory behaviors (see below). The level of severity may be increased to reflect other symptoms and the degree of functional disability.

Mild: An average of 1-3 episodes of inappropriate compensatory behaviors per week.

Moderate: An average of 4-7 episodes of inappropriate compensatory behaviors per week.

Severe: An average of 8-13 episodes of inappropriate compensatory behaviors per week.

Extreme: An average of 14 or more episodes of inappropriate compensatory behaviors per week.

From the *Diagnostic and Statistical Manual of Mental Disorders, Fifth Edition,* (Copyright 2013). American Psychiatric Association, p 345.

patients with diagnosed EDs. In some adolescent female populations, $\geq$10% have ED-NOS.

No single factor causes the development of an ED; sociocultural studies indicate a complex interplay of culture, ethnicity, gender, peers, and family. The **gender** dimorphism is presumably related to females having a stronger relationship between body image and self-evaluation, as well as the influence of the Western culture's thin body ideal. Race and ethnicity appear to moderate the association between risk factors and disordered eating, with African American and Caribbean females reporting lower body dissatisfaction and less dieting than Hispanic and non-Hispanic white females. Because peer acceptance is central to healthy adolescent growth and development, especially in early adolescence, when AN tends to have its initial prevalence peak, the potential influence of peers on EDs is significant, as are the relationships among peers, body image, and eating. Teasing by peers or by family members (especially males) may be a contributing factor for overweight females.

Family influence in the development of EDs is even more complex because of the interplay of environmental and genetic factors; shared elements of the family environment and immutable genetic factors account for approximately equal amounts of the variance in disordered eating. There are associations between parents' and children's eating behaviors; dieting and physical activity levels suggest parental reinforcement of body-related societal messages. The influence of inherited genetic factors on the emergence of EDs during adolescence is also significant, but not directly. Rather, the risk for developing an ED appears to be mediated through a genetic predisposition to *anxiety* (see Chapter 38), *depression* (see Chapter 39), or *obsessive-compulsive traits* that may be modulated through the internal milieu of puberty. There is no evidence to support the outdated notion that parents or family dynamics cause an ED. Rather, the family dynamics may represent responses to having a family member with a potentially life-threatening condition. The supportive influence on recovery of parents as nurturing caregivers cannot be overestimated.

PATHOLOGY AND PATHOGENESIS

The emergence of EDs coinciding with the processes of adolescence (e.g., puberty, identity, autonomy, cognition) indicates the central role of development. A history of sexual trauma is not significantly more common in EDs than in the population at large, but when present makes recovery more difficult and is more common in BN. EDs may be viewed as a final common pathway, with a number of *predisposing* factors that increase the risk of developing an ED, *precipitating* factors often related to developmental processes of adolescence triggering the emergence of the ED, and *perpetuating* factors that cause an ED to persist. EDs often begin with dieting but gradually progress to unhealthy habits that lessen the negative impact of associated psychosocial problems to which the affected person is vulnerable because of premorbid biologic and psychological

Table 41.3	DSM-5 Diagnostic Criteria for Avoidant/Restrictive Food Intake Disorder

A. An eating or feeding disturbance (e.g., apparent lack of interest in eating or food; avoidance based on the sensory characteristics of food; concern about aversive consequences of eating) as manifested by persistent failure to meet appropriate nutritional and/or energy needs associated with one (or more) of the following:
1. Significant weight loss (or failure to achieve expected weight gain or faltering growth in children).
2. Significant nutritional deficiency.
3. Dependence on enteral feeding or oral nutritional supplements.
4. Marked interference with psychosocial functioning.
B. The disturbance is not better explained by lack of available food or by an associated culturally sanctioned practice.
C. The eating disturbance does not occur exclusively during the course of anorexia nervosa or bulimia nervosa, and there is no evidence of a disturbance in the way in which one's body weight or shape is experienced.
D. The eating disturbance is not attributable to a concurrent medical condition or not better explained by another mental disorder. When the eating disturbance occurs in the context of another condition or disorder, the severity of the eating disturbance exceeds that routinely associated with the condition or disorder and warrants additional clinical attention.

Specify if:

In remission: After full criteria for avoidant/restrictive food intake disorder were previously met, the criteria have not been met for a sustained period of time.

From the *Diagnostic and Statistical Manual of Mental Disorders, Fifth Edition,* (Copyright 2013). American Psychiatric Association, p 334.

characteristics, family interactions, and social climate. When persistent, the biologic effects of starvation and malnutrition (e.g., true loss of appetite, hypothermia, gastric atony, amenorrhea, sleep disturbance, fatigue, weakness, depression), combined with the psychological rewards of increased sense of mastery and reduced emotional reactivity, actually maintain and reward pathologic ED behaviors.

This positive reinforcement of behaviors and consequences, generally viewed by parents and others as negative, helps to explain why persons with an ED characteristically deny that a problem exists and resist treatment. Although noxious, purging can be reinforcing because of a reduction in anxiety triggered by overeating; purging also can result in short-term, but reinforcing, improvement in mood related to changes in neurotransmitters. In addition to an imbalance in neurotransmitters, most notably serotonin and dopamine, alterations in functional anatomy also support the concept of EDs as brain disorders. The cause-and-effect relationship in central nervous system (CNS) alterations in EDs is not clear, nor is their reversibility.

CLINICAL MANIFESTATIONS

Except for ARFID, in which weight loss is *unintentional*, a central feature of EDs is the overestimation of body size, shape, or parts (e.g., abdomen, thighs) leading to intentional weight control practices to reduce weight (AN) or prevent weight gain (BN). Associated practices include severe restriction of caloric intake and behaviors intended to reduce the effect of calories ingested, such as compulsive exercising or purging by inducing vomiting or taking laxatives. Eating and weight loss habits commonly found in EDs can result in a wide range of energy intake and output, the balance of which leads to a wide range in weight, from extreme loss of weight in AN to fluctuation around a normal to moderately high weight in BN. Reported eating and weight control habits thus inform the initial primary care approach (Table 41.4).

Although weight control patterns guide the initial pediatric approach, an assessment of common symptoms and findings on physical examination is essential to identify targets for intervention. When reported symptoms of excessive weight loss (feeling tired and cold; lacking energy;

orthostasis; difficulty concentrating) are explicitly linked by the clinician to their associated physical signs (hypothermia with acrocyanosis and slow capillary refill; loss of muscle mass; bradycardia with orthostasis), it becomes more difficult for the patient to deny that a problem exists. Furthermore, awareness that bothersome symptoms can be eliminated by healthier eating and activity patterns can increase a patient's motivation to engage in treatment. Tables 41.5 and 41.6 detail common symptoms and signs that should be addressed in a pediatric assessment of a suspected ED.

DIFFERENTIAL DIAGNOSIS

In addition to identifying symptoms and signs that deserve targeted intervention for patients who have an ED, a comprehensive history and physical examination are required to rule out other conditions in the differential diagnosis. Weight loss can occur in any condition with increased *catabolism* (e.g., hyperthyroidism, malignancy, occult chronic infection) or *malabsorption* (e.g., inflammatory bowel disease, celiac disease) or in other disorders (Addison disease, type 1 diabetes mellitus, stimulant abuse), but these illnesses are generally associated with other findings and are not usually associated with decreased caloric intake. Patients with **inflammatory bowel disease** can reduce intake to minimize abdominal cramping; eating can cause abdominal discomfort and early satiety in AN because of gastric atony associated with significant weight loss, not malabsorption. Likewise, signs of weight loss in AN might include hypothermia, acrocyanosis with slow capillary refill, and neutropenia similar to some features of sepsis, but the overall picture in EDs is one of relative cardiovascular stability compared with sepsis. **Endocrinopathies** are also in the differential of EDs. With BN, voracious appetite in the face of weight loss might suggest diabetes mellitus, but blood glucose levels are normal or low in EDs. Adrenal insufficiency mimics many physical symptoms and signs found in restrictive AN but is associated with elevated potassium levels and hyperpigmentation. Thyroid disorders may be considered, because of changes in weight, but the overall presentation of AN includes symptoms of both underactive and overactive thyroid, such as hypothermia, bradycardia, and constipation, as well as weight loss and excessive physical activity, respectively.

In the CNS, craniopharyngiomas and Rathke pouch tumors can mimic some of the findings of AN, such as weight loss and growth failure, and even some body image disturbances, but the latter are less fixed than in typical EDs and are associated with other findings, including evidence of increased intracranial pressure. **Mitochondrial neurogastrointestinal encephalomyopathy,** caused by a mutation in the *TYMP* gene, presents with gastrointestinal dysmotility, cachexia, ptosis, peripheral neuropathy, ophthalmoplegia, and leukoencephalopathy. Symptoms begin during the 2nd decade of life and are often initially diagnosed as AN. Early satiety, vomiting, cramps, constipation, and pseudoobstruction result in weight loss often before the neurologic features are noticed (see Chapter 616.2). Acute or chronic oromotor dysfunction and obsessive-compulsive disorder may mimic an eating disorder. Fear of choking may lead to **avoidance-restrictive food intake disorder.**

Any patient with an atypical presentation of an ED, based on age, sex, or other factors not typical for AN or BN, deserves a scrupulous search for an alternative explanation. In ARFID, disturbance in the neurosensory processes associated with eating, not weight loss, is the central concern and must be recognized for appropriate treatment. Patients can have both an underlying illness and an ED. The core features of dysfunctional eating habits—body image disturbance and change in weight—can coexist with conditions such as diabetes mellitus, where patients might manipulate their insulin dosing to lose weight.

LABORATORY FINDINGS

Because the diagnosis of an ED is made clinically, there is no confirmatory laboratory test. Laboratory abnormalities, when found, are the result of malnutrition, weight control habits, or medical complications; studies should be chosen based on history and physical examination. A routine screening battery typically includes complete blood count, erythrocyte sedimentation rate (should be normal), and biochemical profile. Common abnormalities in ED include low white blood cell count with normal hemoglobin and differential; hypokalemic, hypochloremic metabolic alkalosis from severe vomiting; mildly elevated liver enzymes, cholesterol,

Table 41.4	Eating and Weight Control Habits Commonly Found in Children and Adolescents With an Eating Disorder (ED)			
	PROMINENT FEATURE		**CLINICAL COMMENTS REGARDING ED HABITS**	
HABIT	**Anorexia Nervosa**	**Bulimia Nervosa**	**Anorexia Nervosa**	**Bulimia Nervosa**
Overall intake	Inadequate energy (calories), although volume of food and beverages may be high because of very low caloric density of intake as a result of "diet" and nonfat choices	Variable, but calories normal to high; intake in binges is often "forbidden" food or drink that differs from intake at meals	Consistent inadequate caloric intake leading to wasting of the body is an essential feature of diagnosis	Inconsistent balance of intake, exercise and vomiting, but severe caloric restriction is short-lived
Food	Counts and limits calories, especially from fat; emphasis on "healthy food choices" with reduced caloric density. Monotonous, limited "good" food choices, often leading to vegetarian or vegan diet. Strong feelings of guilt after eating more than planned leads to exercise and renewed dieting	Aware of calories and fat, but less regimented in avoidance than AN. Frequent dieting interspersed with overeating, often triggered by depression, isolation, or anger	Obsessive-compulsive attention to nutritional data on food labels and may have "logical" reasons for food choices in highly regimented pattern, such as sports participation or family history of lipid disorder	Choices less structured, with more frequent diets
Beverages	Water or other low- or no-calorie drinks; nonfat milk	Variable, diet soda common; may drink alcohol to excess	Fluids often restricted to avoid weight gain	Fluids ingested to aid vomiting or replace losses
Meals	Consistent schedule and structure to meal plan. Reduced or eliminated caloric content, often starting with breakfast, then lunch, then dinner. Volume can increase with fresh fruits, vegetables, and salads as primary food sources	Meals less regimented and planned than in AN; more likely impulsive and unregulated, often eliminated following a binge-purge episode	Rigid adherence to "rules" governing eating leads to sense of control, confidence, and mastery	Elimination of a meal following a binge-purge only reinforces the drive for binge later in the day
Snacks	Reduced or eliminated from meal plan	Often avoided in meal plans, but then impulsively eaten	Snack foods removed early because "unhealthy"	Snack "comfort foods" can trigger a binge
Dieting	Initial habit that becomes progressively restrictive, although often appearing superficially "healthy". Beliefs and "rules" about the patient's idiosyncratic nutritional requirements and response to foods are strongly held	Initial dieting gives way to chaotic eating, often interpreted by the patient as evidence of being "weak" or "lazy"	Distinguishing between healthy meal planning with reduced calories and dieting in ED may be difficult	Dieting tends to be impulsive and short-lived, with "diets" often resulting in unintended weight gain
Binge eating	None in restrictive subtype, but an essential feature in binge-purge subtype	Essential feature, often secretive. Shame and guilt prominent afterward	Often "subjective" (more than planned but not large)	Relieves emotional distress, may be planned
Exercise	Characteristically obsessive-compulsive, ritualistic, and progressive. May excel in dance, long-distance running	Less predictable. May be athletic, or may avoid exercise entirely	May be difficult to distinguish active thin vs ED	Males often use exercise as means of "purging"
Vomiting	Characteristic of binge-purge subtype. May chew, then spit out, rather than swallow, food as a variant	Most common habit intended to reduce effects of overeating. Can occur after meal as well as a binge	Physiologic and emotional instability prominent	Strongly "addictive" and self-punishing, but does not eliminate calories ingested—many still absorbed
Laxatives	If used, generally to relieve constipation in restrictive subtype, but as a cathartic in binge-purge subtype	Second most common habit used to reduce or avoid weight gain, often used in increasing doses for cathartic effect	Physiologic and emotional instability prominent	Strongly "addictive," self-punishing, but ineffective means to reduce weight (calories are absorbed in small intestine, but laxatives work in colon)
Diet pills	Very rare, if used; more common in binge-purge subtype	Used to either reduce appetite or increase metabolism	Use of diet pills implies inability to control eating	Control over eating may be sought by any means

AN, Anorexia nervosa; BN, bulimia nervosa.

Table 41.5	Symptoms Commonly Reported by Patients With an Eating Disorder (ED)		
	DIAGNOSIS		**CLINICAL COMMENTS REGARDING ED SYMPTOMS**
SYMPTOMS	**Anorexia Nervosa**	**Bulimia Nervosa**	
Body image	Feels fat, even with extreme emaciation, often with specific body distortions (e.g., stomach, thighs); strong drive for thinness, with self-efficacy closely tied to appraisal of body shape, size, and/or weight	Variable body image distortion and dissatisfaction, but drive for thinness is less than desire to avoid gaining weight	Challenging patient's body image is both ineffective and countertherapeutic clinically Accepting patient's expressed body image but noting its discrepancy with symptoms and signs reinforces concept that patient can "feel" fat but also "be" too thin and unhealthy
Metabolism	Hypometabolic symptoms include feeling cold, tired, and weak and lacking energy May be both bothersome and reinforcing	Variable, depending on balance of intake and output and hydration	Symptoms are evidence of body's "shutting down" in an attempt to conserve calories with an inadequate diet Emphasizing reversibility of symptoms with healthy eating and weight gain can motivate patients to cooperate with treatment
Skin	Dry skin, delayed healing, easy bruising, gooseflesh Orange-yellow skin on hands	No characteristic symptom; self-injurious behavior may be seen	Skin lacks good blood flow and ability to heal in low weight Carotenemia with large intake of β-carotene foods; reversible
Hair	Lanugo-type hair growth on face and upper body Slow growth and increased loss of scalp hair	No characteristic symptom	Body hair growth conserves energy Scalp hair loss can worsen during refeeding "telogen effluvium" (resting hair is replaced by growing hair) Reversible with continued healthy eating
Eyes	No characteristic symptom	Subconjunctival hemorrhage	Caused by increased intrathoracic pressure during vomiting
Teeth	No characteristic symptom	Erosion of dental enamel erosion Decay, fracture, and loss of teeth	Intraoral stomach acid resulting from vomiting etches dental enamel, exposing softer dental elements
Salivary glands	No characteristic symptom	Enlargement (no to mild tenderness)	Caused by chronic binge eating and induced vomiting, with parotid enlargement more prominent than submandibular; reversible
Heart	Dizziness, fainting in restrictive subtype Palpitations more common in binge-purge subtype	Dizziness, fainting, palpitations	Dizziness and fainting due to postural orthostatic tachycardia and dysregulation at hypothalamic and cardiac level with weight loss, as a result of hypovolemia with binge-purge Palpitations and arrhythmias often caused by electrolyte disturbance Symptoms reverse with weight gain and/or cessation of binge-purge
Abdomen	Early fullness and discomfort with eating Constipation Perceives contour as "fat," often preferring well-defined abdominal musculature	Discomfort after a binge Cramps and diarrhea with laxative abuse	Weight loss is associated with reduced volume and tone of GI tract musculature, especially the stomach Laxatives may be used to relieve constipation or as a cathartic Symptom reduction with healthy eating can take weeks to occur
Extremities and musculoskeletal	Cold, blue hands and feet	No characteristic symptoms Self-cutting or burning on wrists or arms	Energy-conserving low body temperature with slow blood flow most notable peripherally Quickly reversed with healthy eating
Nervous system	No characteristic symptom	No characteristic symptom	Neurologic symptoms suggest diagnosis other than ED
Mental status	Depression, anxiety, obsessive-compulsive symptoms, alone or in combination	Depression; PTSD; borderline personality disorder traits	Underlying mood disturbances can worsen with dysfunctional weight control practices and can improve with healthy eating AN patients might report emotional "numbness" with starvation preferable to emotionality associated with healthy eating

AN, Anorexia nervosa; BN, bulimia nervosa; ED, eating disorder; GI, gastrointestinal; PTSD, posttraumatic stress disorder.

and cortisol levels; low gonadotropins and blood glucose with marked weight loss; and generally normal total protein, albumin, and renal function. An electrocardiogram may be useful when profound bradycardia or arrhythmia is detected; the ECG usually has low voltage, with nonspecific ST or T-wave changes. Although prolonged QTc has been reported, prospective studies have not found an increased risk for this. Nonetheless, when a prolonged QTc is present in a patient with ED, it may increase the risk for ventricular dysrhythmias.

Table 41.6	Signs Commonly Found in Patients With Eating Disorder (ED) Relative to Prominent Feature of Weight Control		
	PROMINENT FEATURE		
PHYSICAL SIGN	**Restrictive Intake**	**Binge Eating/Purging**	**CLINICAL COMMENTS RELATED TO ED SIGNS**
General appearance	Thin to cachectic, depending on balance of intake and output Might wear bulky clothing to hide thinness and might resist being examined	Thin to overweight, depending on the balance of intake and output through various means	Examine in hospital gown Weight loss more rapid with reduced intake and excessive exercise Binge eating can result in large weight gain, regardless of purging behavior Appearance depends on balance of intake and output and overall weight control habits
Weight	Low and falling (if previously overweight, may be normal or high); may be falsely elevated if patient drinks fluids or adds weights to body before being weighed	Highly variable, depending on balance of intake and output and state of hydration Falsification of weight is unusual	Weigh in hospital gown with no underwear, after voiding (measure urine SG) Remain in gown until physical exam completed to identify possible fluid loading (low urine SG, palpable bladder) or adding weights to body
Metabolism	Hypothermia: temp <35.5°C (95.9°F), pulse <60 beats/min Slowed psychomotor response with very low core temperature	Variable, but hypometabolic state is less common than in AN	Hypometabolism related to disruption of hypothalamic control mechanisms as a result of weight loss Signs of hypometabolism (cold skin, slow capillary refill, acrocyanosis) most evident in hands and feet, where energy conservation is most active
Skin	Dry Increased prominence of hair follicles Orange or yellow hands	Calluses over proximal knuckle joints of hand (Russell's sign)	Carotenemia with large intake of β-carotene foods Russell's sign: maxillary incisors abrasion develops into callus with chronic digital pharyngeal stimulation, usually on dominant hand
Hair	Lanugo-type hair growth on face and upper body Scalp hair loss, especially prominent in parietal region	No characteristic sign	Body hair growth conserves energy Scalp hair loss "telogen effluvium" can worsen weeks after refeeding begins, as hair in resting phase is replaced by growing hair
Eyes	No characteristic sign	Subconjunctival hemorrhage	Increased intrathoracic pressure during vomiting
Teeth	No characteristic sign	Eroded dental enamel and decayed, fractured, missing teeth	Perimolysis, worse on lingual surfaces of maxillary teeth, is intensified by brushing teeth without preceding water rinse
Salivary glands	No characteristic sign	Enlargement, relatively nontender	Parotid > submandibular involvement with frequent and chronic binge eating and induced vomiting
Throat	No characteristic sign	Absent gag reflex	Extinction of gag response with repeated pharyngeal stimulation
Heart	Bradycardia, hypotension, and orthostatic pulse differential >25 beats/min	Hypovolemia if dehydrated	Changes in AN resulting from central hypothalamic and intrinsic cardiac function Orthostatic changes less prominent if athletic, more prominent if associated with purging
Abdomen	Scaphoid, organs may be palpable but not enlarged, stool-filled left lower quadrant	Increased bowel sounds if recent laxative use	Presence of organomegaly requires investigation to determine cause Constipation prominent with weight loss
Extremities and musculoskeletal system	Cold, acrocyanosis, slow capillary refill Edema of feet Loss of muscle, subcutaneous, and fat tissue	No characteristic sign, but may have rebound edema after stopping chronic laxative use	Signs of hypometabolism (cold) and cardiovascular dysfunction (slow capillary refill and acrocyanosis) in hands and feet Edema, caused by capillary fragility more than hypoproteinemia in AN, can worsen in early phase of refeeding
Nervous system	No characteristic sign	No characteristic sign	Water loading before weigh-ins can cause acute hyponatremia
Mental status	Anxiety about body image, irritability, depressed mood, oppositional to change	Depression, evidence of PTSD, more likely suicidal than AN	Mental status often improves with healthier eating and weight; SSRIs only shown to be effective for BN

AN, Anorexia nervosa; BN, bulimia nervosa; PTSD, posttraumatic stress disorder; SG, specific gravity; SSRIs, selective serotonin reuptake inhibitors.

COMPLICATIONS

No organ is spared the harmful effects of dysfunctional weight control habits, but the most concerning targets of medical complications are the heart, brain, gonads, and bones. Some **cardiac** findings in EDs (e.g., sinus bradycardia, hypotension) are *physiologic* adaptations to starvation that conserve calories and reduce afterload. Cold, blue hands and feet with slow capillary refill that can result in tissue perfusion insufficient to meet demands also represent energy-conserving responses associated with inadequate intake. All these acute changes are reversible with restoration of nutrition and weight. Significant orthostatic pulse changes, ventricular dysrhythmias, or reduced myocardial contractility reflect myocardial impairment that can be lethal. In addition, with extremely low weight, **refeeding syndrome** (a result of the rapid drop in serum phosphorus, magnesium, and potassium with excessive reintroduction of calories, especially carbohydrates), is associated with acute tachycardia and heart failure and neurologic symptoms. With long-term malnutrition, the myocardium appears to be more prone to tachyarrhythmias, the second most common cause of death in these patients after suicide. In BN, dysrhythmias can also be related to electrolyte imbalance.

Clinically, the primary CNS area affected acutely in EDs, especially with weight loss, is the **hypothalamus.** Hypothalamic dysfunction is reflected in problems with thermoregulation (warming and cooling), satiety, sleep, autonomic cardioregulatory imbalance (orthostasis), and endocrine function (reduced gonadal and excessive adrenal cortex stimulation), all of which are reversible. Anatomic studies of the brain in ED have focused on AN, with the most common finding being increased ventricular and sulcal volumes that normalize with weight restoration. Persistent gray matter deficits following recovery, related to the degree of weight loss, have been reported. Elevated medial temporal lobe cerebral blood flow on positron emission tomography, similar to that found in psychotic patients, suggests that these changes may be related to body image distortion. Also, visualizing high-calorie foods is associated with exaggerated responses in the visual association cortex that are similar to those seen in patients with specific phobias. Patients with AN might have an imbalance between serotonin and dopamine pathways related to neurocircuits in which dietary restraint reduces anxiety.

Reduced **gonadal** function occurs in male and female patients; it is clinically manifested in AN as amenorrhea in female patients and erectile dysfunction in males. It is related to understimulation from the hypothalamus as well as cortical suppression related to physical and emotional stress. Amenorrhea precedes significant dieting and weight loss in up to 30% of females with AN, and most adolescents with EDs perceive the absence of menses positively. The primary health concern is the negative effect of decreased ovarian function and estrogen on **bones.** Decreased bone mineral density (BMD) with osteopenia or the more severe osteoporosis is a significant complication of EDs (more pronounced in AN than BN). Data do not support the use of sex hormone replacement therapy because this alone does not improve other causes of low BMD (low body weight, lean body mass, low insulin-like growth factor-1, high cortisol).

TREATMENT
Principles Guiding Primary Care Treatment
The approach in primary care should facilitate the acceptance by the ED patient (and parents) of the diagnosis and initial treatment recommendations. A **nurturant-authoritative** approach using the biopsychosocial model is useful. A pediatrician who explicitly acknowledges that the patient may disagree with the diagnosis and treatment recommendations and may be ambivalent about changing eating habits, while also acknowledging that recovery requires strength, courage, willpower, and determination, demonstrates *nurturance*. Parents also find it easier to be nurturing once they learn that the development of an ED is neither a willful decision by the patient nor a reflection of poor parenting. Framing the ED as a "coping mechanism" for a complex variety of issues with both positive and negative aspects avoids blame or guilt and can prepare the family for professional help that will focus on strengths and restoring health, rather than on the deficits in the adolescent or the family.

The *authoritative* aspect of a physician's role comes from expertise in health, growth, and physical development. A goal of primary care treatment should be attaining and maintaining health—not merely weight gain—although weight gain is a means to the goal of wellness. Providers who frame themselves as consultants to the patient with authoritative knowledge about health can avoid a countertherapeutic authoritarian stance. Primary care health-focused activities include monitoring the patient's physical status, setting limits on behaviors that threaten the patient's health, involving specialists with expertise in EDs on the treatment team, and continuing to provide primary care for health maintenance, acute illness, or injury.

The **biopsychosocial model** uses a broad ecologic framework, starting with the biologic impairments of physical health related to dysfunctional weight control practices, evidenced by symptoms and signs. Explicitly

linking ED behaviors to symptoms and signs can increase motivation to change. In addition, there are usually unresolved psychosocial conflicts in both the intrapersonal (self-esteem, self-efficacy) and the interpersonal (family, peers, school) domains. Weight control practices initiated as coping mechanisms become reinforced because of positive feedback. That is, external rewards (e.g., compliments about improved physical appearance) and internal rewards (e.g., perceived mastery over what is eaten or what is done to minimize the effects of overeating through exercise or purging) are more powerful to maintain behavior than negative feedback (e.g., conflict with parents, peers, and others about eating) is to change it. Thus, when definitive treatment is initiated, more productive alternative means of coping must be developed.

Nutrition and Physical Activity
The primary care provider generally begins the process of prescribing nutrition, although a dietitian should be involved eventually in the meal planning and nutritional education of patients with AN or BN. Framing food as fuel for the body and the source of energy for daily activities emphasizes the health goal of increasing the patient's energy level, endurance, and strength. For patients with AN and low weight, the nutrition prescription should work toward gradually increasing weight at the rate of about 0.5-1 lb/wk, by increasing energy intake by 100-200 kcal increments every few days, toward a target of approximately 90% of average body weight for sex, height, and age. Weight gain will not occur until intake exceeds output, and eventual intake for continued weight gain can exceed 4,000 kcal/day, especially for patients who are anxious and have high levels of thermogenesis from nonexercise activity. Stabilizing intake is the goal for patients with BN, with a gradual introduction of "forbidden" foods while also limiting foods that might trigger a binge.

When initiating treatment of an ED in a primary care setting, the clinician should be aware of common cognitive patterns. Patients with AN typically have all-or-none thinking (related to perfectionism) with a tendency to overgeneralize and jump to catastrophic conclusions, while assuming that their body is governed by rules that do not apply to others. These tendencies lead to the dichotomization of foods into good or bad categories, having a day ruined because of one unexpected event, or choosing foods based on rigid self-imposed restrictions. These thoughts may be related to neurocircuitry and neurotransmitter abnormalities associated with executive function and rewards. Weight loss in the absence of body shape, size, or weight concerns should raise suspicion about ARFID, because the emotional distress associated with "forced" eating is not associated with gaining weight, but with the neurosensory experience of eating.

A standard nutritional balance of 15-20% calories from protein, 50-55% from carbohydrate, and 25-30% from fat is appropriate. The fat content may need to be lowered to 15-20% early in the treatment of AN because of continued fat phobia. With the risk of low BMD in patients with AN, calcium and vitamin D supplements are often needed to attain the recommended 1,300 mg/day intake of calcium. Refeeding can be accomplished with frequent small meals and snacks consisting of a variety of foods and beverages (with minimal diet or fat-free products), rather than fewer high-volume high-calorie meals. Some patients find it easier to take in part of the additional nutrition as canned supplements (medicine) rather than food. Regardless of the source of energy intake, the risk for refeeding syndrome (see Complications earlier) increases with the degree of weight loss and the rapidity of caloric increases. Therefore, if the weight has fallen below 80% of expected weight for height, refeeding should proceed carefully (not necessarily slowly) and possibly in the hospital (Table 41.7).

Patients with AN tend to have a highly structured day with restrictive intake, in contrast to BN, which is characterized by a lack of structure, resulting in chaotic eating patterns and binge-purge episodes. All patients with AN, BN, or ED-NOS benefit from a daily structure for healthy eating that includes 3 meals and at least 1 snack a day, distributed evenly over the day, based on balanced meal planning. Breakfast deserves special emphasis because it is often the first meal eliminated in AN and is often avoided the morning after a binge-purge episode in BN. In addition to structuring meals and snacks, patients should plan structure

Table 41.7	Potential Indications for Inpatient Medical Hospitalization of Patients With Anorexia Nervosa

PHYSICAL AND LABORATORY

Heart rate <50 beats/min
Other cardiac rhythm disturbances
Blood pressure <80/50 mm Hg
Postural hypotension resulting in >10 mm Hg decrease or >25 beats/min increase
Hypokalemia
Hypophosphatemia
Hypoglycemia
Dehydration
Body temperature <36.1°C (97°F)
<80% healthy body weight
Hepatic, cardiac, or renal compromise

PSYCHIATRIC

Suicidal intent and plan
Very poor motivation to recover (in family and patient)
Preoccupation with ego-syntonic thoughts
Coexisting psychiatric disorders

MISCELLANEOUS

Requires supervision after meals and while using the restroom
Failed day treatment

---

in their activities. Although overexercising is common in AN, completely prohibiting exercise can lead to further restriction of intake or to surreptitious exercise; inactivity should be limited to situations in which weight loss is dramatic or there is physiologic instability. Also, healthy exercise (once a day, for no more than 30 min, at no more than moderate intensity) can improve mood and make increasing calories more acceptable. Because patients with AN often are unaware of their level of activity and tend toward progressively increasing their output, exercising without either a partner or supervision is not recommended.

Primary Care Treatment

Follow-up primary care visits are essential in the management of EDs. Close monitoring of the response of the patient and the family to suggested interventions is required to determine which patients can remain in primary care treatment (patients with early, mildly disordered eating), which patients need to be referred to individual specialists for co-management (mildly progressive disordered eating), and which patients need to be referred for interdisciplinary team management (EDs). Between the initial and subsequent visits, the patient can record daily caloric intake (food, drink, amount, time, location), physical activity (type, duration, intensity), and emotional state (e.g., angry, sad, worried) in a journal that is reviewed jointly with the patient in follow-up. Focusing on the recorded data helps the clinician to identify dietary and activity deficiencies and excesses, as well as behavioral and mental health patterns, and helps the patient to become objectively aware of the relevant issues to address in recovery.

Given the tendency of patients with AN to overestimate their caloric intake and underestimate their activity level, before reviewing the journal record it is important at each visit to measure weight, without underwear, in a hospital gown after voiding; urine specific gravity; temperature; and blood pressure and pulse in supine, sitting, and standing positions as objective data. In addition, a targeted physical examination focused on hypometabolism, cardiovascular stability, and mental status, as well as any related symptoms, should occur at each visit to monitor progress (or regression).

Referral to Mental Health Services

In addition to referral to a registered dietitian, mental health and other services are important elements of treatment of ED patients. Depending on availability and experience, these services can be provided by a psychiatric social worker, psychologist, or psychiatrist, who should team

with the primary care provider. ARFID presents the challenge of working with patients' negative experience of eating, or fear of trauma such as vomiting or choking, while also addressing inadequate nutritional needs. Although patients with AN often are prescribed a selective serotonin reuptake inhibitor (SSRI) because of depressive symptoms, there is no evidence of efficacy for patients at low weight; **food** remains the initial treatment of choice to treat depression in AN. **SSRIs**, very effective in reducing binge-purge behaviors regardless of depression, are considered a standard element of therapy in BN. SSRI dosage in BN, however, may need to increase to an equivalent of >60 mg of fluoxetine to maintain effectiveness.

Cognitive-behavioral therapy, which focuses on restructuring "thinking errors" and establishing adaptive patterns of behavior, is more effective than interpersonal or psychoanalytic approaches in ED patients. **Dialectical behavioral therapy**, in which distorted thoughts and emotional responses are challenged, analyzed, and replaced with healthier ones, with an emphasis on "mindfulness," requires adult thinking skills and is useful for older patients with BN. **Group therapy** can provide much needed support, but it requires a skilled clinician. Combining patients at various levels of recovery who experience variable reinforcement from dysfunctional coping behaviors can be challenging if group therapy patients compete with each other to be "thinner" or take up new behaviors such as vomiting.

The younger the patient, the more intimately the parents need to be involved in therapy. The only treatment approach with evidence-based effectiveness in the treatment of AN in children and adolescents is **family-based treatment**, exemplified by the Maudsley approach. This 3-phase intensive outpatient model helps parents play a positive role in restoring their child's eating and weight to normal, then returns control of eating to the child, who has demonstrated the ability to maintain healthy weight, and then encourages healthy progression in the other domains of adolescent development. Features of effective family treatment include (1) an agnostic approach in which the cause of the disease is unknown and irrelevant to weight gain, emphasizing that parents are *not* to blame for EDs; (2) parents being actively nurturing and supportive of their child's healthy eating while reinforcing limits on dysfunctional habits, rather than an authoritarian "food police" or complete hands-off approach; and (3) reinforcement of parents as the best resource for recovery for almost all patients, with professionals serving as consultants and advisors to help parents address challenges.

Referral to an Interdisciplinary Eating Disorder Team

The treatment of a child or adolescent diagnosed with an ED is ideally provided by an interdisciplinary team (physician, nurse, dietitian, mental health provider) with expertise treating pediatric patients. Because such teams, often led by specialists in adolescent medicine at medical centers, are not widely available, the primary care provider might need to convene such a team. Adolescent medicine–based programs report encouraging treatment outcomes, possibly related to patients entering earlier into care and the stigma that some patients and parents may associate with psychiatry-based programs. Specialty centers focused on treating EDs are generally based in psychiatry and often have separate tracks for younger and adult patients. The elements of treatment noted earlier (cognitive-behavioral, dialectical behavioral, family-based), as well as individual and group treatment, should all be available as part of interdisciplinary team treatment. Comprehensive services ideally include intensive outpatient and partial hospitalization as well as inpatient treatment. Regardless of the intensity, type, or location of the treatment services, the patient, parents, and primary care provider are essential members of the treatment team. A recurring theme in effective treatment is helping patients and families reestablish connections that are disrupted by the ED.

Inpatient medical treatment of EDs is generally limited to patients with AN, to stabilize and treat life-threatening starvation and to provide supportive mental health services. Inpatient medical care may be required to avoid refeeding syndrome in severely malnourished patients, provide nasogastric tube feeding for patients unable or unwilling to eat, or initiate mental health services, especially family-based treatment, if this has not occurred on an outpatient basis (see Table 41.7). Admission to a general pediatric unit is advised only for short-term stabilization in preparation for transfer to a medical unit with expertise in treating pediatric EDs. Inpatient psychiatric care of EDs should be provided on a unit with expertise in managing the often challenging behaviors (e.g., hiding or discarding food, vomiting, surreptitious exercise) and emotional problems (e.g., depression, anxiety). Suicidal risk is small, but patients with AN might threaten suicide if made to eat or gain weight in an effort to "get their parents to back off."

An ED **partial hospital program** offers outpatient services that are less intensive than round-the-clock inpatient care. Generally held 4-5 days/wk for 6 to 9 hr each session, partial hospital program services typically are group-based and include eating at least 2 meals as well as opportunities to address issues in a setting that more closely approximates "real life" than inpatient treatment. That is, patients sleep at home and are free-living on weekends, exposing them to challenges that can be processed during the 25-40 hr each week in program, as well as sharing group and family experiences.

Supportive Care
In relation to pediatric EDs, support groups are primarily designed for parents. Because their daughter or son with an ED often resists the diagnosis and treatment, parents often feel helpless and hopeless. Because of the historical precedent of blaming parents for causing EDs, parents often express feelings of shame and isolation (www.maudsleyparents.org). Support groups and multifamily therapy sessions bring parents together with other parents whose families are at various stages of recovery from an ED in ways that are educational and encouraging. Patients often benefit from support groups after intensive treatment or at the end of treatment because of residual body image or other issues after eating and weight have normalized.

PROGNOSIS
With early diagnosis and effective treatment, ≥80% of youth with AN recover: They develop normal eating and weight control habits, resume menses, maintain average weight for height, and function in school, work, and relationships, although some still have poor body image. With weight restoration, fertility returns as well, although the weight for resumption of menses (approximately 92% of average body weight for height) may be lower than the weight for ovulation. The prognosis for BN is less well established, but outcome improves with multidimensional treatment that includes SSRIs and attention to mood, past trauma, impulsivity, and any existing psychopathology. Since the diagnosis of ARFID was only established in 2013, little is known about its long-term prognosis, although anecdotal evidence suggests that weight restoration is not actively resisted as it is in AN. Atypical AN and ED-NOS may still have significant morbidity.

PREVENTION
Given the complexity of the pathogenesis of EDs, prevention is difficult. Targeted preventive interventions can reduce risk factors in older adolescents and college-age women. Universal prevention efforts to promote healthy weight regulation and discourage unhealthy dieting have not shown effectiveness in middle school students. Programs that include recovered patients or focus on the problems associated with EDs can inadvertently normalize or even glamorize EDs and should be discouraged.

Bibliography is available at Expert Consult.

Chapter **42**

Disruptive, Impulse-Control, and Conduct Disorders

Heather J. Walter and David R. DeMaso

第四十二章

破坏性、冲动控制和品行障碍

中文导读

　　本章对破坏性行为障碍的概念进行了描述，对对立违抗障碍、间歇性暴怒障碍和品行障碍各自的临床特征和诊断标准进行了描述。详细阐述了该疾病各临床亚型的流行病学、临床病程、共病、结局与转归、病因与风险因素、预防、筛查/案例发现、早期干预、治疗（多学科联合培育性保健干预）和分级照料策略。列举了可供父母或教师使用的愤怒/攻击特定筛查工具（见原文表42.4）。

The disruptive, impulse-control, and conduct disorders are interrelated sets of psychiatric symptoms characterized by a core deficit in self-regulation of anger, aggression, defiance, and antisocial behaviors. The disruptive, impulse-control, and conduct disorders include oppositional defiant, intermittent explosive, conduct, other specified/unspecified disruptive/impulse control/conduct, and antisocial personality disorders, as well as pyromania and kleptomania.

DESCRIPTION

Oppositional defiant disorder (ODD) is characterized by a pattern lasting at least 6 mo of angry, irritable mood, argumentative/defiant behavior, or vindictiveness exhibited during interaction with at least 1 individual who is not a sibling (Table 42.1). For preschool children, the behavior must occur on most days, whereas in school-age children, the behavior must occur at least once a week. The severity of the disorder is considered *mild* if symptoms are confined to only 1 setting (e.g., at home, at school, at work, with peers), *moderate* if symptoms are present in at least 2 settings, and *severe* if symptoms are present in ≥4 settings.

Intermittent explosive disorder (IED) is characterized by recurrent verbal or physical aggression that is grossly disproportionate to the provocation or to any precipitating psychosocial stressors (Table 42.2). The outbursts, which are impulsive and/or anger-based rather than premeditated and/or instrumental, typically last <30 min and frequently occur in response to a minor provocation by a close intimate.

Conduct disorder (CD) is characterized by a repetitive and persistent pattern over at least 12 mo of serious rule-violating behavior in which the basic rights of others or major societal norms or rules are violated (Table 42.3). The symptoms of CD are divided into 4 major categories: aggression to people and animals, destruction of property, deceitfulness or theft, and serious rule violations (e.g., truancy, running away). Three subtypes of CD (which have different prognostic significance) are based on the age of onset: childhood-onset type, adolescent-onset type, and unspecified. A small proportion of individuals with CD exhibit characteristics (lack of remorse/guilt, callous/lack of empathy, unconcerned about performance, shallow/deficient affect) that qualify for the "with limited prosocial emotions" specifier. CD is classified as *mild* when few if any symptoms over those required for the diagnosis are present, and the symptoms cause relatively minor harm to others. CD is classified as *severe* if many symptoms over those required for the diagnosis are present, and the symptoms cause considerable harm to others. *Moderate* severity is intermediate between mild and severe.

Other specified/unspecified disruptive/impulse-control/CD (sub-syndromal disorder) applies to presentations in which symptoms characteristic of the disorders in this class are present and cause clinically significant distress or functional impairment, but do not meet full diagnostic criteria for any of the disorders in this class.

EPIDEMIOLOGY

The prevalence of ODD is approximately 3%, and in preadolescents is more common in males than females (1.4:1). One-year prevalence

Table 42.1	DSM-5 Diagnostic Criteria for Oppositional Defiant Disorder

A. A pattern of angry/irritable mood, argumentative/defiant behavior, or vindictiveness lasting at least 6 mo as evidenced by at least 4 symptoms from any of the following categories, and exhibited during interaction with at least 1 individual who is not a sibling:

Angry/Irritable Mood
1. Often loses temper.
2. Is often touchy or easily annoyed.
3. Is often angry and resentful.

Argumentative/Defiant Behavior
4. Often argues with authority figures or, for children and adolescents, with adults.
5. Often actively defies or refuses to comply with requests from authority figures or with rules.
6. Often deliberately annoys others.
7. Often blames others for his or her mistakes or misbehavior.

Vindictiveness
8. Has been spiteful or vindictive at least twice within the past 6 mo.

Note: The persistence and frequency of these behaviors should be used to distinguish a behavior that is within normal limits from a behavior that is symptomatic. For children younger than 5 yr, the behavior should occur on most days for a period of at least 6 mo unless otherwise noted (Criterion A8). For individuals 5 yr or older, the behavior should occur at least once per week for at least 6 mo, unless otherwise noted (Criterion A8). While these frequency criteria provide guidance on a minimal level of frequency to define symptoms, other factors should be considered, such as whether the frequency and intensity of the behaviors are outside a range that is normative for the individual's developmental level, gender, and culture.

B. The disturbance in behavior is associated with distress in the individual or others in his or her immediate social context (e.g., family, peer group, work colleagues), or it impacts negatively on social, educational, occupational, or other important areas of functioning.

C. The behaviors do not occur exclusively during the course of a psychotic, substance use, depressive, or bipolar disorder. Also, the criteria are not met for disruptive mood dysregulation disorder.

From the *Diagnostic and Statistical Manual of Mental Disorders, Fifth Edition,* (Copyright 2013). American Psychiatric Association, pp 462–463.

Table 42.2	DSM-5 Diagnostic Criteria for Intermittent Explosive Disorder

A. Recurrent behavioral outbursts representing a failure to control aggressive impulses as manifested by either of the following:
1. Verbal aggression (e.g., temper tantrums, tirades, verbal arguments or fights) or physical aggression toward property, animals, or other individuals, occurring twice weekly, on average, for a period of 3 mo. The physical aggression does not result in damage or destruction of property and does not result in physical injury to animals or other individuals.
2. Three behavioral outbursts involving damage or destruction of property and/or physical assault involving physical injury against animals or other individuals occurring with a 12 mo period.

B. The magnitude of aggressiveness expressed during the recurrent outbursts is grossly out of proportion to the provocation or to any precipitating psychosocial stressors.

C. The recurrent aggressive outbursts are not premeditated (i.e., they are impulsive and/or anger-based) and are not committed to achieve some tangible objective (e.g., money, power, intimidation).

D. The recurrent aggressive outbursts cause either marked distress in the individual or impairment in occupational or interpersonal functioning, or as associated with financial or legal consequences.

E. Chronological age is at least 6 yr (or equivalent developmental level).

F. The recurrent aggressive outbursts are not better explained by another mental disorder (e.g., major depressive disorder, bipolar disorder, disruptive mood dysregulation disorder, a psychotic disorder, antisocial personality disorder, borderline personality disorder) and are not attributable to another medical condition (e.g., head trauma, Alzheimer disease) or to the physiologic effects of a substance (e.g., a drug of abuse, a medication). For children ages 6-18 yr, aggressive behavior that occurs as part of an adjustment disorder should not be considered for this diagnosis.

Note: This diagnosis can be made in addition to the diagnosis of attention-deficit/hyperactivity disorder, conduct disorder, oppositional defiant disorder, or autism spectrum disorder when recurrent impulsive aggressive outbursts are in excess of those usually seen in these disorders and warrant clinical attention.

From the *Diagnostic and Statistical Manual of Mental Disorders, Fifth Edition,* (Copyright 2013). American Psychiatric Association, p 466.

Table 42.3	DSM-5 Diagnostic Criteria for Conduct Disorder

A. A repetitive and persistent pattern of behavior in which the basic rights of others or major age-appropriate societal norms or rules are violated, as manifested by the presence of at least 3 of the following 15 criteria in the past 12 mo from any of the categories below, with at least 1 criterion present in the past 6 mo:

Aggression to People and Animals
1. Often bullies, threatens, or intimidates others.
2. Often initiates physical fights.
3. Has used a weapon that can cause serious physical harm to others (e.g., a bat, brick, broken bottle, knife, gun).
4. Has been physically cruel to people.
5. Has been physically cruel to animals.
6. Has stolen while confronting a victim (e.g., mugging, purse snatching, extortion, armed robbery).
7. Has forced someone into sexual activity.

Destruction of Property
8. Has deliberately engaged in fire setting with the intention of causing serious damage.
9. Has deliberately destroyed others' property (other than by fire setting).

Deceitfulness or Theft
10. Has broken into someone else's house, building, or car.
11. Often lies to obtain good or favors or to avoid obligations (i.e., "cons" others).
12. Has stolen items of nontrivial value without confronting a victim (e.g., shoplifting, but without breaking and entering; forgery).

Serious Violations of Rules
13. Often stays out at night despite parental prohibitions, beginning before age 13 yr.
14. Has run away from home overnight at least twice while living in the parental or parental surrogate home, or once without returning for a lengthy period.
15. Is often truant from school, beginning before age 13 yr.

B. The disturbance in behavior causes clinically significant impairment in social, academic, or occupational functioning.
C. If the individual is age 18 yr or older, criteria are not met for antisocial personality disorder.

From the *Diagnostic and Statistical Manual of Mental Disorders, Fifth Edition*, (Copyright 2013). American Psychiatric Association, pp 469–471.

rates for IED and CD approximate 3% and 5%, respectively. For CD, prevalence rates rise from childhood to adolescence and are higher among males than females. The prevalence of these disorders has been shown to be higher in lower socioeconomic classes. This class of disorders constitutes the most frequent referral problem for youth, accounting for one third to one half of all cases seen in mental health clinics. Racial/ethnic minority youth with these disorders utilize specialty mental health services at lower rates than their white peers.

CLINICAL COURSE

Oppositional *behavior* can occur in all children and adolescents at times, particularly during the toddler and early teenage periods when establishing autonomy and independence are normative developmental tasks. Oppositional behavior becomes a concern when it is intense, persistent, and pervasive and when it affects the child's social, family, and academic life.

Some of the earliest manifestations of oppositionality are stubbornness (3 yr), defiance and temper tantrums (4-5 yr), and argumentativeness (6 yr). Approximately 65% of children with ODD exit from the diagnosis after a 3 yr follow-up; earlier age at onset of oppositional symptoms conveys a poorer prognosis. ODD often precedes the development of CD (approximately 30% higher likelihood with comorbid attention-deficit/hyperactivity disorder [ADHD]), but also increases the risk for the development of depressive and anxiety disorders. The defiant and vindictive symptoms carry most of the risk for CD, whereas the angry, irritable mood symptoms carry most of the risk for anxiety and depression.

IED usually begins in late childhood or adolescence and appears to follow a chronic and persistent course over many years.

The onset of CD may occur as early as the preschool years, but the first significant symptoms usually emerge during the period from middle childhood through middle adolescence; onset is rare after age 16 yr. Symptoms of CD vary with age as the individual develops increased physical strength, cognitive abilities, and sexual maturity. Symptoms that emerge first tend to be less serious (e.g., lying), while those emerging later tend to be more severe (e.g., sexual or physical assault). Severe behaviors emerging at an early age convey a poor prognosis. In the majority of individuals, the disorder remits by adulthood; in a substantial fraction, antisocial personality disorder develops. Individuals with CD also are at risk for the later development of mood, anxiety, posttraumatic stress, impulse control, psychotic, somatic symptom, and substance-related disorders.

DIFFERENTIAL DIAGNOSIS

The disorders in this diagnostic class share a number of characteristics with each other as well as with disorders from other classes, and as such must be carefully differentiated. ODD can be distinguished from CD by the absence of physical aggression and destructiveness and by the presence of angry, irritable mood. ODD can be distinguished from IED by the lack of serious aggression (physical assault). IED can be distinguished from CD by the lack of predatory aggression and other, nonaggressive symptoms of CD.

The **oppositionality** seen in ODD must be distinguished from that seen in ADHD, depressive and bipolar disorders (including disruptive mood dysregulation disorder), language disorders, intellectual disability, and social anxiety disorder. ODD should not be diagnosed if the behaviors occur exclusively during the course of a psychotic, substance use, depressive, or bipolar disorder, or if criteria are met for disruptive mood dysregulation disorder. IED should not be diagnosed if the behavior can be better explained by a depressive, bipolar, disruptive mood dysregulation, psychotic, antisocial personality, or borderline personality disorder. The **aggression** seen in CD must be distinguished from that seen in ADHD and intermittent explosive, depressive, bipolar, and adjustment disorders.

COMORBIDITY

Rates of ODD are much higher in children with ADHD, which suggests shared temperamental risk factors. Depressive, anxiety, and substance use disorders are most often comorbid with IED. ADHD and ODD are both common in individuals with CD, and this comorbid presentation predicts worse outcomes. CD also may occur with anxiety, depressive, bipolar, learning, language, and substance-related disorders.

SEQUELAE

The disruptive, impulse-control, and conduct disorders are associated with a wide range of psychiatric disorders in adulthood and with many other adverse outcomes, such as suicidal behavior, physical injury, delinquency and criminality, legal problems, substance use, unplanned pregnancy, social instability, marital failure, and academic and occupational underachievement.

ETIOLOGY AND RISK FACTORS

At the individual level, a number of neurobiologic markers (lower heart rate and skin conductance reactivity, reduced basal cortisol reactivity, abnormalities in the prefrontal cortex and amygdala, serotonergic abnormalities) have been variously associated with aggressive behavior disorders. Other biologic risk factors include pre-, peri-, and postnatal insults; cognitive and linguistic impairment, particularly language-based learning deficits; difficult temperamental characteristics, particularly negative affectivity, poor frustration tolerance, and impulsivity; certain personality characteristics (novelty seeking, reduced harm avoidance, and reward dependence); and certain cognitive characteristics (cognitive rigidity, hostile attributions for ambiguous social cues).

At the family level, a consistently demonstrated risk factor is **ineffective parenting**. Parents of behaviorally disordered children are more inconsistent in their use of rules; issue more and unclear commands; are more likely to respond to their child based on their own mood rather than the child's behavior; are less likely to monitor their children's whereabouts; and are relatively unresponsive to their children's prosocial behavior. Complicating this association is the consistent finding that *temperamentally difficult children are more likely to elicit negative parenting responses*, including physical punishment, which can exacerbate anger and oppositionality in the child. Other important family-level influences include impaired parent–child attachment, child maltreatment (physical and sexual abuse), exposure to marital conflict and domestic violence, family poverty and crime, and **family genetic liability** (family history of the disorders in this class along with substance use, depressive, bipolar, schizophrenic, somatization, and personality disorders, as well as ADHD, have all been shown to be associated with the development of behavior disorders).

Peer-level influence on the development of behavior problems include peer rejection in childhood and antisocial peer groups. Neighborhood influences include social processes such as collective efficacy and social control.

PREVENTION

A useful conduct problem prevention program is the *Fast Track* (http://fasttrackproject.org), a multicomponent school-based intervention comprising a classroom curriculum targeted at conflict resolution and interpersonal skills, parent training, and interventions targeted at the school environment. Implemented in 1st through 10th grade, former program participants at age 25 had a lower prevalence of any externalizing, internalizing, or substance abuse problem than program nonparticipants. Program participants also had lower violent and drug crime conviction scores, lower risky sexual behavior scores, and higher well-being scores. Another useful prevention program, the *Seattle Social Development Project* (http://ssdp-tip.org/SSDP/index.html), is also a multicomponent school-based intervention of teacher, parent, and student components targeting classroom management, interpersonal problem-solving, child behavior management, and academic support skills. Implemented in 1st through 6th grades, outcomes at age 19 yr demonstrated that the intervention decreased lifetime drug use and delinquency for participant males compared with males in comparator communities, but had no significant effects on females.

SCREENING/CASE FINDING

The parents of children presenting in the primary care setting should be queried about angry mood or aggressive, defiant, or antisocial behavior as part of the routine clinical interview. A typical screening question would be, "Does [name] have a lot of trouble controlling [his/her] anger or behavior?" A number of standardized broad-band screening instruments widely used in the primary care setting *(Pediatric Symptom Checklist, Strengths and Difficulties Questionnaire, Vanderbilt ADHD Diagnostic Rating Scales)* have items specific to angry mood and aggressive behavior, and as such can be used to focus the interview.

EARLY INTERVENTION

Youth (and/or their parents) presenting in the primary care setting who self-report or respond affirmatively to queries about difficulties managing angry mood or aggressive or antisocial behavior should be afforded the opportunity to talk about the situation with the pediatric practitioner (separately with the older youth as indicated). By engaging in active listening (e.g., "I hear how you have been feeling. Tell me more about what happened to make you feel that way"), the pediatric practitioner can establish a therapeutic rapport and begin to assess the onset, duration, context, and severity of the symptoms, and associated dangerousness, distress, and functional impairment. In the absence of acute dangerousness (e.g., homicidality, assaultiveness, psychosis, substance abuse) and significant distress or functional impairment, the pediatric practitioner can schedule a follow-up appointment within 1-2 wk to conduct a behavior assessment. At this follow-up visit, to assist with decision-making about appropriate level of care, a behavior screening instrument can be administered (Table 42.4) and additional risk factors explored (see Etiology and Risk Factors earlier).

For mild symptoms (manageable by the parent and not functionally impairing) and in the absence of major risk factors (homicidality, assaultiveness, psychosis, substance use, child maltreatment, parental psychopathology, or severe family dysfunction), **guided self-help** (anticipatory guidance) with watchful waiting and scheduled follow-up may suffice. Guided self-help can include provision of educational materials (pamphlets, books, videos, workbooks, internet sites) that provide information to the youth about dealing with anger-provoking situations, and advice to parents about strengthening the parent–child relationship, effective parenting strategies, and the effects of adverse environmental exposures on the development of behavior problems. In a Cochrane review, media-based parenting interventions had a moderate positive effect on child behavior problems, either alone or as an adjunct to medication. An example of a self-help program for parents is the *Positive Parenting Program* (Triple P; www.triplep.net), online version, in which parents can purchase 4 modules of instruction addressing techniques for positive parenting and strategies for encouraging good behavior, teaching new emotional and behavioral skills, and managing misbehavior (see Chapter 19).

If the problematic behavior is occurring predominantly at school, the parent can be advised about the role of a special education evaluation in the assessment and management of the child's misbehavior, including the development of a behavioral intervention plan to prevent disciplinary actions that is formalized in an individualized educational plan (IEP) or 504 plan.

If a mental health clinician has been co-located or integrated into the primary care setting, all parents of young children (universal prevention), as well as the parents of youth with mild behavior problems (indicated prevention), can be provided with a brief version of **parent training**. Programs targeted at toddlers through 12 yr olds have been found to be effective in improving parenting skills, parental mental health, and child emotional and behavior problems. For example, *Incredible Years* (http://www.incredibleyears.com) has a 6-8 session

Table 42.4	Anger/Aggression-Specific Screening Instruments			
NAME OF INSTRUMENT		**INFORMANT(S)**	**AGE RANGE**	**NUMBER OF ITEMS**
Children's Aggression Scale		Parent, Teacher	5-18 yr	33 (P), 23 (T)
Eyberg Child Behavior Inventory		Parent	2-16 yr	36
Outburst Monitoring Scale		Parent	12-17 yr	20
Sutter-Eyberg Student Behavior Inventory–Revised		Teacher	2-16 yr	38
Vanderbilt ADHD Diagnostic Rating Scales		Parent, Teacher	6-12 yr	55 (P), 43 (T)

universal prevention version to help parents promote their 2-6 yr old children's emotional regulation, social competence, problem solving, and reading readiness. A 12-20 session version is designed to strengthen parent–child interactions, reduce harsh discipline, and foster parents' ability to promote children's social, emotional, and language development in their toddler to school-age children. A randomized trial in pediatric practices found that Incredible Years significantly improved parenting practices and 2-4 yr olds' disruptive behaviors compared to a wait-list control. Similarly, for children with behavior problems, the Triple P program has seminar (three 90 min sessions), brief (15-30 min consultations), and primary care (four 20-30 min consultations) versions for the parents of youth from birth to the teenage years, specifically designed for implementation in the primary care setting. The Triple P interventions, supported by an extensive evidence base, focus on strengthening the parent–child relationship, identifying and monitoring the frequency of a problem behavior, and implementing and reviewing the effects of a targeted behavior plan.

TREATMENT

For youth who continue to have mild to moderate behavior problems after several weeks of guided self-help or a brief course of parent training, or who from the outset exhibit moderate to severe or comorbid aggression, homicidality, assaultiveness, psychosis, or substance use, or who have a history of child maltreatment or severe family dysfunction or psychopathology, assessment and treatment in the specialty mental health setting by a child-trained mental health clinician should be provided.

The youth's problem behavior may predominantly occur at home, at school, with peers, or in the community, or it may be pervasive. If possible, interventions need to address each context specifically, rather than assuming generalizability of treatment. Thus, for behaviors mostly manifested in the home setting, parent training would be the treatment of choice, whereas for behaviors manifested mostly at school, consultation with the teacher and recommendation of a special education evaluation for service eligibility can be useful. When there are pervasive problems, including aggression toward peers, cognitive-behavioral therapy with the child/teen can be employed in addition to the other interventions.

Parent training has been extensively studied for the treatment of youth problem behavior. These programs, typically 10-15 wk in duration, focus on some combination of the following components: understanding social learning principles, developing a warm supportive relationship with the child, encouraging child-directed interaction and play, providing a predictable structured household environment, setting clear simple household rules, consistently praising and materially rewarding positive behavior, consistently ignoring annoying behavior (followed by praise when the annoying behavior ceases), and consistently giving consequences (e.g., time-out, loss of privileges) for dangerous or destructive behavior. Other important targets for parenting training include understanding developmentally appropriate moods and behavior, managing difficult temperamental characteristics, fostering the child's social and emotional development, and protecting the child from traumatic exposures. Specific parent training programs include *Parent–Child Interaction Therapy, Triple P, Helping the Noncompliant Child, Incredible Years,* and *Parent Management Training Oregon.* Predictors of nonresponse to these interventions have included greater initial symptom severity as well as involvement of the parent with child protection services.

Adherence to the complete treatment regimen has limited the effectiveness of parent training programs. Estimates of premature termination are as high as 50–60%, and termination within 5 treatment sessions is not uncommon. Predictors of premature termination of parent training programs have included single-parent status, low family income, low parental education levels, young maternal age, minority group status, and life stresses.

Cognitive behavioral therapy (CBT) for youth with disruptive behavior also has been extensively studied. Common CBT techniques for disruptive behavior include identifying the antecedents and consequences of disruptive or aggressive behavior, learning strategies for recognizing and regulating anger expression, problem-solving and cognitive restructuring (perspective-taking) techniques, and modeling and rehearsing social appropriate behaviors that could replace angry or aggressive reactions. Programs typically are delivered in 16-20 weekly sessions.

Multicomponent treatments for serious behavior disorders such as CD target the broader social context. **Multidimensional Treatment Foster Care**, delivered in a foster care setting for 6-9 mo, typically includes foster parent training and support; family therapy for biologic parents; youth anger management, social skills, and problem-solving training; school-based behavioral interventions and academic support; and psychiatric consultation and medication management, when needed. **Multisystemic Therapy**, typically lasting 3-5 mo, generally includes social competence training, parent and family skills training, medications, academic engagement and skills building, school interventions and peer mediation, mentoring and after-school programs, and involvement of child-serving agencies. These multicomponent programs have been designated "probably efficacious" because of the limited rigorous supporting evidence. Predictors of nonresponse to multicomponent treatments have included higher frequency of rule-breaking behavior and predatory aggression, higher psychopathy scores, and comorbid mood disorders.

Two classes of medication, **stimulants** and **atypical antipsychotics**, have strong evidence for the management of impulsive, anger-driven aggressive behavior, although neither is approved by the U.S. Food and Drug Administration (FDA) for this indication. Resource limitations may necessitate provision of pharmacotherapy in the primary care setting; the safety and efficacy of this practice can be enhanced by regular consultation with a child and adolescent psychiatrist. Several studies have shown favorable effects of stimulants on oppositional behavior and aggression in youths with ADHD. The doses of stimulants used for aggression are similar to those used for ADHD (average dose for methylphenidate, approximately 1 mg/kg/day). There is evidence for efficacy of risperidone in reducing aggression and conduct problems in children age 5-18 yr. The suggested usual daily dose of risperidone for severe aggression is 1.5-2 mg for children and 2-4 mg for adolescents. The initial starting doses are 0.25 mg for children and 0.5 mg for adolescents, titrating upward to the usual daily dose, as indicated and tolerated.

Medication trials should be systematic, and the duration of trials should be sufficient (generally 6-8 wk for atypical antipsychotics) to determine the agent's effectiveness. The short-term goal of treatment is to achieve at least a 50% reduction in aggressive symptoms, as assessed by a standardized rating scale (see Table 42.4); the ultimate goal is to achieve symptom remission (below clinical cutpoint on rating scale). A 2nd medication of the same class can be considered if there is insufficient evidence of response to the maximal tolerated dose by 8 weeks. Care should be taken to avoid unnecessary polypharmacy, in part by discontinuing agents that have not demonstrated significant benefit. Discontinuation of the medication should be considered after a symptom-free interval.

LEVEL OF CARE

Most children and adolescents with a behavior disorder can be safely and effectively treated in the outpatient setting. Youths with intractable CD may benefit from residential or specialized foster care treatment, where more intensive treatments can be provided.

Bibliography is available at Expert Consult.

Chapter 43
Tantrums and Breath-Holding Spells

Lovern R. Moseley,
Keneisha Sinclair-McBride,
David R. DeMaso, and Heather J. Walter

第四十三章
发脾气和屏气发作

中文导读

本章主要介绍了发脾气和屏气发作各自发生的病因学、临床表现、诊断和治疗要点。介绍了不同年龄儿童发脾气的心理成因和父母提供心理支持的要点。在屏气发作这部分内容，介绍了屏气发作的临床亚型、各自临床表现和父母该如何采取措施提供心理支持。详细描述了父母如何与孩子建立关系、如何保持平静的心情，与孩子保持有效沟通，作为榜样，提供心理支持，改善亲子关系。

Temper tantrums are common during the first few years of life. They are typically developmentally normative expressions of children's frustration with their own limitations or anger about not being able to get their way. It is important for parents to recognize the differences between tantrum types and precipitants in order to determine the best course of action to manage the ensuing behavior. Dealing with tantrum behavior can become very frustrating for parents, but many tantrums can be averted by a parent's awareness or attunement to certain cues given by their child, particularly in the early years. In particular, parents should be aware that when a child is tired, hungry, or feeling ill or has to make a transition, it can be expected that the child will be more likely to have a tantrum because children are more easily overwhelmed. In this case, it is advised that parents plan ahead and take a preventive stance by being aware of *triggers* and minimizing the potential for a tantrum. For example, parents should not make a tired or hungry child accompany them on an extended outing unless absolutely necessary. Additionally, depending on the child's developmental level, it is helpful to have a clear discussion ahead of time about the expectations in certain scenarios. When children are able to demonstrate good control, their behavior should be acknowledged and praised. This will increase the likelihood that they will engage in the desired response more often, even in frustrating situations.

In the case of children who engage in tantrum behavior to get their way, parents may feel more inclined to respond to such defiance with yelling or threats, which can reinforce and even escalate the oppositional behavior. Parents should attempt to avert defiance by giving the child choices; once the child has begun a tantrum, he or she can be placed in time-out. If the tantrum was to avoid a task, the child should be required to complete the task once time-out is over. Parents should state the reason the child is being placed in time-out, but they should not discuss the reasons before or during time-out. Once the time-out is over and the child is calm, it may be helpful for parents to discuss with the child the reasons for the child's frustration and their expectations for how the child will respond in the future.

Breath-holding spells occasionally occur during a tantrum and can be frightening to parents. These are reflexive events in which the crying child becomes apneic, pale, or cyanotic, may lose consciousness, and occasionally will have a brief seizure. Parents are best advised to ignore breath holding once it has started. Without reinforcement, breath holding generally disappears.

Subtypes of breath-holding spells include cyanotic, pallid, or mixed episodes. *Cyanotic spells* are the dominant type. *Pallid spells* may be similar to vasovagal-related syncopal events in older children and may be initiated by similar stimuli. *Iron deficiency* with or without anemia may be present, and some children with breath-holding spells respond to iron therapy. There is no increased risk of seizure disorders in children who have had a short seizure during a breath-holding spell. Medical conditions to rule-out in breath-holding spells (usually pallid) include seizures, Chiari crisis, dysautonomia, cardiac arrhythmias, and central nervous system lesions.

The first key to the office **management** of temper tantrums and breath-holding spells is to help parents intervene before the child is highly distressed. The parent can be instructed to calmly remind the child of the expected behavior and the potential consequence if the expected behavior does not occur. If the child does not comply, he or she should be placed in time-out for a period approximating 1 min for each year of age. Time-out can be effectively used in children up to age 10 yr. Parents should also be advised to be mindful of their own reactions to their child's tantrum behavior, to avoid an escalation of the child's behavior caused by an angry parental response.

If behavioral measures such as time-out fail, pediatricians must assess other aspects of parent–child interactions, such as the frequency of positive interactions, the consistency of parental responses to child behavior, and the way that parents handle anger, before making further recommendations. In the absence of frequent positive parent–child interactions, time-out may not be effective, and inconsistent responding to problem behavior increases the likelihood of the behavior continuing. Children can be frightened by the intensity of their own angry feelings and by angry feelings they arouse in their parents. Parents should model the anger control that they want their children to exhibit. Some parents are unable to see that if they lose control themselves, their own angry behavior does not help their children to internalize appropriate behavior.

Advising parents to calmly provide simple choices will help the child to feel more in control and to develop a sense of *autonomy*. Providing the child with options also typically helps reduce the child's feelings of anger and shame, which can later have adverse effects on social and emotional development. Providing choice also reduces power struggles between the parent and child and can aid in enhancing the parent–child relationship and building problem-solving skills.

When tantrum behavior, including breath holding, does not respond to parent coaching or is accompanied by head banging or high levels of aggression, referral for a mental health evaluation is indicated. Further evaluation is also recommended if tantrum behavior persists into the latency period and preteen years.

Bibliography is available at Expert Consult.

Chapter **44**

Lying, Stealing, and Truancy

Lovern R. Moseley,
Keneisha Sinclair-McBride,
David R. DeMaso, and Heather J. Walter

第四十四章
说谎、偷窃和逃学

中文导读

本章主要介绍了说谎、偷窃和逃学各自发生的病因学、临床表现、诊断和治疗要点。在说谎这一节中，介绍了不同年龄儿童说谎的心理成因，并对父母如何处置孩子的说谎行为给出了建议，提出评估的重要性。

在偷窃行为这一节中，介绍了不同年龄儿童出现偷窃行为的心理成因，介绍了不同年龄儿童出现偷窃行为后家长如何处置，如果存在其他精神卫生问题，建议进行心理评估。

在逃学行为这一节中，介绍了逃学发生的心理社会因素，学生在该年龄段可能存在的压力。介绍了处理逃学问题的干预策略和加强心理卫生评估的必要性。

LYING

There are various reasons why a child might lie. For children between ages 2 and 4 yr, lying can be used as a method of playing with language. By observing the reactions of parents, preschoolers learn about expectations for honesty in communication. Lying can also be a form of fantasy for children, who describe things as they wish them to be rather than as they are. To avoid an unpleasant confrontation, a child who has not done something that a parent wanted may say that it has been done.

The child's sense of time and reason does not permit the realization that this only postpones a confrontation. It is important for the parent to keep in mind that lying behavior in this age-group is rarely malicious or premeditated.

In **older children**, lying is generally an effort to cover up something that they do not want to accept in their own behavior. The lie is invented to achieve a temporary good feeling and to protect the child against a loss of self-esteem. Lying in this age-group is also an attempt to avoid a negative consequence for misbehavior. Older children are also more likely to intentionally leave out critical parts of a story in an attempt to deceive or avoid a negative consequence. **Habitual lying** can also be promoted by poor adult modeling. Many adolescents lie to avoid adults' disapproval. Alternatively, lying may be used as a method of rebellion. **Chronic lying** can occur in combination with several other antisocial behaviors and is a sign of underlying psychopathology or family dysfunction.

Parents should address lying by giving the child a clear message of what is acceptable. Sensitivity and support combined with limit setting are necessary for a successful intervention. While habitual lying can become frustrating for parents, they should be discouraged from making accusations or focusing on catching their child in a lie and instead should work toward creating an atmosphere that makes it easier for their child to tell the truth. Parents should let the child know that telling the truth about a difficult situation will allow the parents to help them better problem-solve the issue at hand. Should a situation arise where the parents are aware of the details, the lie should be confronted while providing the facts of what is known and also stating the desired or expected behavior. If a parent is aware that a child took a cookie without permission and the child denies it, the parent can state, "I am disappointed that you took the cookie without permission. I need you to ask me first." The child is then reminded of how he can get things that he desires in an acceptable way; an appropriate consequence can then be given. Parents should be encouraged to address the expectations for their home and children in a family meeting or in regular discussions with their child outside the context of the child's lying.

Regardless of age or developmental level, when lying becomes a common way of managing conflict, intervention is warranted. If this behavior cannot be resolved through the parents' understanding of the situation and the child's understanding that lying is not a reasonable alternative, a mental health evaluation is indicated.

STEALING

Many children steal something at some point in their lives. Often, when very young children steal, the behavior is an impulsive action to acquire something they want. A common example is the child who takes candy or a toy from the store shelf. If a parent notices this behavior, the situation is a teaching opportunity and should be used to talk with the child about having to pay for things at the store and not taking things without permission. It should not be expected that a very young child will be aware of all the rules around shopping or stealing. It may also be difficult for a child who has been used to being able to freely take whatever she wants to be aware of all the expected behaviors across different settings. When preschoolers and school-age children begin to steal frequently even after they have been told not to, the behavior may be a response to stressful environmental circumstances and requires further exploration and evaluation.

For some **older children**, stealing can be an expression of anger or revenge for perceived frustrations with parents or other authority figures. In such instances, stealing becomes one way the child and adolescent can manipulate and attempt to control their world. Stealing can also be learned from adults. Some children will report that the behavior is "exciting" for them, and they may also engage in the behavior for peer approval. In some cases, youth living in poverty may engage in the behavior as a survival mechanism.

It is important for parents to help the child undo the theft through some form of restitution. The child should be made to return the stolen articles or render their equivalent either in money that the child can earn or in services. When stealing is part of a pattern of broader conduct problems, referral for a mental health evaluation is warranted.

TRUANCY

Truancy and running away are never developmentally appropriate. **Truancy** may represent disorganization within the home, caretaking needs of younger siblings, developing conduct problems, or emotional problems including depression or anxiety. When truancy occurs in **younger children**, there are usually psychosocial concerns with the parents or adult caretakers in the home that prevent them from following through with the regular demands for their children. It is important to consider whether parents are struggling with housing and food insecurity, making school attendance less of a priority. Parents with intellectual disability or their own mental health or substance abuse problems may become overwhelmed with managing the home and caring for their children, and thus might not consistently ensure their child gets to school. Also, children might decide to remain at home to take care of parents who are impaired.

Truancy is more common in **older children** and can be a function of multiple factors, including but not limited to learning difficulties, social anxiety, depression, traumatic exposure, bullying, peer pressure, and substance use. In any of these cases, the child should be referred for further evaluation to assess the barriers to returning to school. Best practices for dealing with truancy resulting from *school avoidance* and *anxiety* include addressing the underlying psychological symptoms causing the school avoidance and empowering parents, children, and school staff to work on a consistent plan for a return to school.

Younger children may threaten **running away** out of frustration or a desire to "get back at" parents. Older children who run away are almost always expressing a serious underlying problem within themselves or their family, including violence, abuse, and neglect. Adolescent runaways are at high risk for substance abuse, unsafe sexual activity (e.g., sexual exploitation), and other risk-taking behaviors.

Youth exhibiting truancy or running away should be referred for a mental health evaluation.

Bibliography is available at Expert Consult.

Chapter **45**
Aggression
Lovern R. Moseley,
Keneisha Sinclair-McBride,
David R. DeMaso, and Heather J. Walter

第四十五章
攻击

中文导读

　　本章描述了攻击行为的定义，介绍了儿童青少年攻击行为的表现形式、流行病学特征（如性别差异、年龄差异）、攻击行为发生的相关因素（如校园霸凌、网络欺凌、家庭环境因素）、攻击行为常伴发的心理障碍，并针对攻击行为如何评估和干预，给出了针对个体、家庭、学校的综合评估和干预的建议。

Aggressive behavior is a serious symptom associated with significant morbidity and mortality. Early intervention is indicated for persistent aggressive behavior, because children may not simply "grow out of it." Aggressive tendencies are heritable, although environmental factors can promote aggression in susceptible children. Both enduring and temporary stressors affecting a family can increase aggressive behavior in children. Aggression in childhood is correlated with both poverty and chaotic family situations, including chronic unemployment, family discord, and exposure to community and domestic violence, criminality, and psychiatric disorders. Children born to teenage mothers and parents with limited resources and support are also at risk. Boys are almost universally reported to be more aggressive than girls. A *difficult temperament* and later aggressiveness are related. When children with temperament difficulties elicit punitive caregiving within the family environment, it can set up a cycle of increasing aggression. Aggressive children often misinterpret social cues in such a way that they perceive hostile intent in ambiguous or benign interactions, and then may react with verbal or physical aggression toward peers and parents.

It is important to differentiate the causes and motives for childhood aggression. Intentional aggression may be primarily instrumental, i.e. to achieve an end, primarily hostile, i.e. to inflict physical or psychological pain, or primarily angry and impulsive. Children who are callous, not empathetic, and often aggressive require mental health intervention. These children are at high risk for suspension from school and eventual school failure. Because learning disorders are common in this population, aggressive children should be referred for screening. Aggressive behavior is often present in a variety of other psychological conditions, including attention-deficit/hyperactivity, oppositional defiant, intermittent explosive, conduct, and disruptive mood dysregulation disorders (see Chapters 39 and 42).

Aggressive behavior in **boys** is relatively consistent from the preschool period through adolescence. Without effective intervention, a boy with a high level of aggressive behavior between 3 and 6 yr of age has a high probability of carrying this behavior into adolescence. The developmental progression of aggression among **girls** is less well studied. Fewer girls show physically aggressive behavior in early childhood. However, **interpersonal coercive behavior**, especially in peer relationships, is seen in girls. This behavior may be related to the development of physical aggression for girls in adolescence (e.g., fighting) or other conduct problems (e.g., stealing).

Children exposed to aggressive models on television, in video games, or in play have more aggressive behavior compared with children not exposed to these models. Parents' anger and aggressive or harsh punishment can model behavior that children may imitate when they are physically or psychologically hurt. Parents' abuse may be transmitted to the next generation by several modes: children imitate aggression that they have witnessed; abuse can cause brain injury, which itself predisposes the child to violence; and internalized rage often results from abuse.

Aggressive behavior in youth is often oriented toward peers through **bullying** (see Chapter 14.1). While it is developmentally normative for children to engage in some teasing behavior, bullying has a more serious tone. Bullying is defined as *unwanted aggressive behavior* in which there is a real or perceived *imbalance of power or strength* between the bully and the victim. Typically, it involves a pattern of behavior repeated over time. Although most often perceived as physical aggression, bullying can take on a variety of forms, including **relational bullying**, the most common form engaged in by girls. **Cyberbullying** is a particular risk during the middle and high school years because of increased exposure and access to multiple social media platforms at this developmental stage. Parents should be advised to closely monitor their child's social media exposure through both smartphone- and internet-based platforms and maintain open communication with their children. Children may bully others because of impulse control and social skills deficits, strong need for power and negative dominance, satisfaction in causing harm to others, or psychological or material rewards. Children who bully are at risk for a variety of negative school and psychological outcomes.

Victims of bullying are particularly at risk for negative outcomes, especially if the behavior is not addressed by adults. Victimization experiences are associated with school avoidance and school dropout, social isolation, somatic symptoms, and increased psychological problems such as depression and anxiety. There have been numerous cases of suicide in children who reported a prior history of being bullied. Should a concern arise around bullying in the school setting, parents should be advised to reach out to their child's teacher, school counselor, and school administrative staff to have the bullying behavior addressed. Many schools also have a *bullying intervention protocol* that can be implemented, and state departments of education have antibullying policies with formal protocols to address concerns. Given the significant psychological risks for victims of bullying, it is essential that victims be referred for mental health evaluation.

Bibliography is available at Expert Consult.

Chapter **46**
Self-Injurious Behavior

Lovern R. Moseley,
Keneisha Sinclair-McBride,
David R. DeMaso, and Heather J. Walter

第四十六章
自伤行为

中文导读

　　本章主要对自伤行为的定义进行描述，介绍了青少年常见的自伤类型、最常见的受伤部位、自伤的流行病学资料、自伤的成因、风险因素和发生的相关因素，并对自杀和非自杀故意自我伤害的临床特征进行鉴别，推荐了非自杀性故意自我伤害的诊断条目。最后，该章对自伤的干预列出了一些建议，包括家庭和媒体该如何提供支持，如保持开放性沟通等。

Self-injurious behavior can be defined as intentional self-inflicted damage to the surface of an individual's body of a type likely to induce bleeding, bruising, or pain, with the expectation that the injury will lead to only minor or moderate physical harm.

Self-injurious behaviors and **cutting** in particular have been documented in children as young as 7 yr, with increasing rates among preteens, adolescents, and young adults. Rates of self-injury are generally higher in females than in males, but cutting and other self-injurious behaviors occur in both sexes. It is estimated that in the United States, approximately 20% or more of adolescents have engaged in some form of self-injury at some point in their lives. There are no significant race, ethnicity, or class differences among youth who engage in self-injurious behavior. Youth identified as those with the highest risk include females age 15-19 and males 20-24, with cutting being the most common form of self-injury. For those youth who engage in self-injurious behavior for the first time, approximately 20% will repeat the behavior within the same year, with cutting being the most likely repeated self-injurious behavior.

Common types of self-injury include cutting, scratching, burning, carving, piercing, hitting or punching, biting, picking at wounds, and digging nails into the skin. The most common areas of injury are the arms, legs, and torso. Females with significant psychiatric symptomatology have been found to cut on parts of their body other than their arms (breasts, genitals, groin, neck). Objects used in cutting include razors, scissors, broken glass, hard plastic, knives, staples, paperclips, or any other object sharp enough to cause injury.

Usually, self-injurious behavior does not occur with the intention of **suicide** but can unintentionally result in significant harm or even death. Although self-injury and suicide are often seen as distinct behaviors, research exploring the attitudes of youth who have engaged in self-injury indicates that there is a strong identification with suicide and death for this population, making self-injurious behavior a significant clinical issue that cannot be ignored or minimized. Some youth engage in repeated self-injury without ever attempting suicide, but studies suggest that 50–75% of adolescents who have a history of self-injurious behavior will make a suicide attempt at some point.

Youth have reported many avenues of exposure before engaging in self-injurious behavior. They often report that they have **friends** who cut to attempt to alleviate negative emotions, so they try it as well. Youth may also share their stories of self-injury on websites and **social media**, possibly contributing to experimentation in those who view the postings. Impressionable youth have also reported learning about cutting for the first time from hearing reports of celebrities who have engaged in the behavior.

Self-injurious behavior is associated with depression, anxiety, peer victimization, social isolation, low self-esteem, substance abuse, eating disorders, impulsivity, poor school performance, delinquency, and neglectful or highly punitive parenting practices, as well as a history of physical or sexual abuse. The behavior may begin as an impulsive response to internal distress for younger adolescents, but for those who are older, the behavior can take on a self-reinforcing function. Youth may feel a sense of *relief* or *mastery* over negative emotions once the behavior has been completed. Some youth report that they engage in self-injurious behavior when feeling overwhelmed or in a state of panic, in order to feel that they can "breathe again," or when they are feeling numb, the self-injury pain allows them to "feel something" again. Cutting may also serve as a *distraction* from emotional pain, provide a sense of *control* over the body, or be used as a form of *self-punishment* for a perceived wrongdoing. Youth often report that they are unable to resist the urge to engage in the behavior and will continue to feel increasing levels of distress until they have completed the self-injury; they view it as a way to regulate affect. Others also look forward to and enjoy the behavior and tend to plan and think about when they will be able to do it again. Youth who view the cutting behavior as an enjoyable, private, and positive coping strategy tend to have more dependence on the behavior and more resistance to stopping it.

Some adolescents and young adults have engaged in repeated acts of self-injury for years without sharing this behavior with others or without the behavior being known. They will often go to great lengths to keep the behavior a secret. Some individuals wear bracelets to cover scars on their arms or wear long sleeves in summer to hide the scarring. They report feeling ashamed of the behavior and fear rejection or disappointment from family and friends should they find out. At times, fear of being rejected or a disappointment to others can increase feelings of depression and anxiety and can serve to perpetuate the behavior. There is also a cohort of adolescents who are more open about showing their scars and sharing their behavior with others;

their discussion about the behavior can tend to seem provocative. In either case, the behavior is a way to communicate or manage some level of *distress*. Many youth who engage in self-injurious behavior may never be seen in a hospital emergency department or by a mental health professional.

Parents should be advised to monitor their child's and adolescent's media access and be aware of their peer group. Maintaining open communication can assist parents in recognizing an increase in concerning behaviors and patterns of behaviors. Parents should also be encouraged to talk with their child about their use of and exposure to drugs and alcohol, because substance use can accompany involvement in self-injurious behavior. Learning that their child has been engaging in self-injury can be frightening for parents because they are unsure of what to do or why their child is engaging in this behavior. It is important that they seek mental health services for their child. It is also recommended that the adolescent receive a full assessment for risk of suicide when self-injury is a concern.

The *Diagnostic and Statistical Manual of Mental Disorders, Fifth Edition* (DSM-5) has classified **nonsuicidal self-injury (NSSI)** as a condition requiring further study before consideration for possible placement in forthcoming editions of DSM. Proposed diagnostic criteria include self-inflicted injury without suicidal intent occurring on 5 or more days in the past year, with lack of suicidal intent either stated by the individual or inferred by the individual's repeated engagement in a behavior that he knows is not likely to result in death. The individual expects that the self-injurious behavior will relieve a negative feeling or thought, resolve an interpersonal difficulty, or induce a positive feeling state. The self-injurious behavior is associated with interpersonal difficulties or negative feelings or thoughts, preoccupation with the intended behavior that is difficult to control, or frequent thoughts about the intended behavior. The proposed criteria also specify that the behavior is not socially sanctioned (e.g., body piercing, tattooing) and is not restricted to skin picking or nail biting. Finally, the behavior must be associated with significant *distress* or functional impairment.

Self-injurious behavior in individuals with developmental disabilities often occurs in association with stereotypic movement disorder (see Chapter 37.2).

Bibliography is available at Expert Consult.

Chapter **47**
Childhood Psychoses

Joseph Gonzalez-Heydrich,
Heather J. Walter, and David R. DeMaso

第四十七章
儿童期精神病

中文导读

　　本章主要介绍了儿童期精神病的概念，对精神性性症状如幻觉、妄想等概念进行了描述。选择了精神分裂症谱系障碍和其他精神病性障碍重点阐述，在这一节重点介绍了短暂精神病性障碍、精神分裂症样障碍、精神分裂症等疾病的流行病学状况、临床病程、鉴别诊断、共病、结局与转归、病因与风险因素（如包括遗传因素、环境因素）、神经解剖异常、预防、筛查/案例发现、评估和治疗（包括心理健康教育、药物治疗和电抽搐治疗等）。

在与癫痫相关的精神病性障碍、儿童青少年紧张症、儿童期急性恐怖性幻觉症各节中，对这几种精神病性障碍的诊断和治疗策略分别进行了介绍。列举了由于其他状况继发的精神病性障碍诊断标准（见原文表47.7）、与紧张症相关的情况诊断标准（见原文表47.8）。

Psychosis is a severe disruption of thought, perception, and behavior resulting in **loss of reality testing.** Psychosis can occur as part of a mood disorder, such as major depressive disorder or bipolar I disorder; between mood disorder episodes, as in schizoaffective disorder; or without mood disorder episodes, as in schizophrenia. Transient psychotic episodes can arise during times of psychological or physiologic stress in patients who are vulnerable because of personality, developmental, or genetic disorders. Delusions, hallucinations, disorganized thinking, and grossly disorganized behavior (positive symptoms) are key features that define psychoses across disorders, likely because of shared pathophysiologic mechanisms. Negative symptoms, on the other hand, are most typical of schizophrenia.

Delusions are fixed, unchangeable, false beliefs held despite conflicting evidence. They may include a variety of themes (persecutory, referential, somatic, religious, grandiose). Delusions are considered bizarre if they are clearly implausible. **Hallucinations** are vivid, clear, perceptual-like experiences that occur without external stimulus and have the full force and impact of normal perceptions. They may occur in any sensory modality; auditory hallucinations are the most common. **Disorganized thinking** is typically inferred from an individual's speech (loose associations, tangentiality, or incoherence). **Grossly disorganized behavior** may range from childlike silliness to catatonic behavior. **Negative symptoms** include diminished emotional expression, avolition, alogia (lack of speech), anhedonia (inability to experience pleasure), and asociality. Negative symptoms generally account for a substantial portion of the long-term morbidity associated with schizophrenia.

Given the centrality of hallucinations and delusions in making a diagnosis of a psychotic illness, their differentiation from developmentally normal *fantasy* is essential. When children are *imagining,* they control the fantasy and do not have the perceptual experience of seeing and hearing. When children are *hallucinating,* they do not control the hallucination. Almost two thirds of children will endorse at least 1 psychotic-like experience, most often a hallucination, and when not persistent or accompanied by distress, these experiences are not usually a cause for concern. The largest population-based study to date evaluating psychotic symptoms and neurocognition in youth 11-21 yr old found that those who endorsed more psychotic-like experiences than is typical for their age had reduced accuracy across neurocognitive domains, reduced global functioning, and increased risk of depression, anxiety, behavioral disorders, substance use, and suicidal ideation. Thus, psychotic-like symptoms that are frequent, distressing, and cause impairment signal a need for further evaluation and monitoring; however, only a small minority of these children will develop full-blown psychotic illnesses.

47.1 Schizophrenia Spectrum and Other Psychotic Disorders

Joseph Gonzalez-Heydrich, Heather J. Walter, and David R. DeMaso

Schizophrenia spectrum and other psychotic disorders as described in the *Diagnostic and Statistical Manual of Mental Disorders, Fifth Edition* (DSM-5) include brief psychotic disorder, schizophreniform disorder, schizophrenia, schizoaffective disorder, substance/medication-induced psychotic disorder, psychotic disorder caused by another medical condition, catatonia associated with another mental disorder, catatonic disorder due to another medical condition, unspecified catatonia, delusional disorder, schizotypal personality disorder, and other specified/unspecified schizophrenia spectrum and other psychotic disorders.

DESCRIPTION

The **schizophrenia spectrum** and other psychotic disorders are primarily characterized by the active (or positive) symptoms of psychosis, specifically delusions, hallucinations, disorganized speech, or grossly disorganized or catatonic behavior. **Brief psychotic disorder** is characterized by the duration of 1 or more of these symptoms for at least 1 day but <1 mo followed by complete resolution. Emergence of symptoms may or may not be preceded by an identifiable stressor (Table 47.1). Although brief, the level of impairment in this disorder may be severe enough that supervision is required to ensure that basic needs are met and the individual is protected from the consequences of poor judgment and cognitive impairment.

If 2 or more psychotic symptoms persist from 1 mo up to 6 mo, the condition is called **schizophreniform disorder** (Table 47.2). To meet DSM-5 criteria for **schizophrenia,** 2 or more psychotic symptoms must

Table 47.1	DSM-5 Diagnostic Criteria for Brief Psychotic Disorder

A. Presence of 1 (or more) of the following symptoms. At least 1 of these must be (1), (2), or (3):
  1. Delusions.
  2. Hallucinations.
  3. Disorganized speech (e.g., frequent derailment or incoherence).
  4. Grossly disorganized or catatonic behavior.
Note: Do not include a symptom if it is a culturally sanctioned response.
B. Duration of an episode of the disturbance is at least 1 day but less than 1 mo, with eventual full return to premorbid level of functioning.
C. The disturbance is not better explained by major depressive or bipolar disorder with psychotic features or another psychotic disorder such as schizophrenia or catatonia, and is not attributable to the physiologic effects of a substance (e.g., a drug of abuse, a medication) or another medical condition.
Specify if:
With marked stressor(s) (brief reactive psychosis): If symptoms occur in response to events that, singly or together, would be markedly stressful to almost anyone in similar circumstances in the individual's culture.
Without marked stressor(s): If the symptoms do not occur in response to events that, singly or together, would be would be markedly stressful to almost anyone in similar circumstances in the individual's culture.
With postpartum onset: If onset is during pregnancy or within 4 wk postpartum.

From the *Diagnostic and Statistical Manual of Mental Disorders, Fifth Edition,* (Copyright 2013). American Psychiatric Association, p 94.

have been present for a significant time during 1 mo (unless suppressed by treatment), and the level of psychosocial functioning must be markedly below the level achieved before the onset (or there is failure in children to achieve the expected level of functioning). In addition, there must be continuous signs of the disturbance (prodromal, active, or residual symptoms) for at least 6 mo (Table 47.3).

Individuals with schizophrenia can display inappropriate affect, dysphoric mood, disturbed sleep patterns, and lack of interest in eating, or food refusal. Depersonalization, derealization, somatic concerns, and anxiety and phobias are common. Cognitive deficits are observed, including decrements in declarative memory, working memory, language function, and other executive functions, as well as slower processing speed. These individuals may have no insight or awareness of their disorder, which is a predictor of nonadherence to treatment, higher relapse rates, and poorer illness course. Hostility and aggression can be associated with schizophrenia, although spontaneous or random assault is uncommon. Aggression is more frequent for younger males and for individuals with a past history of violence, non-adherence with treatment, substance abuse, and impulsivity.

The essential features of schizophrenia are the same in childhood as in adulthood, but it is more difficult to make the diagnosis. In children, delusions and hallucinations may be less elaborate, visual hallucinations may be more common, and disorganized speech may be better attributed to an autism spectrum or communication disorder. In a review of 35 studies of youth with schizophrenia, the most frequent psychotic symptoms were auditory hallucinations (82%), delusions (78%), thought disorder (66%), disorganized or bizarre behavior (53%), and negative symptoms (50%).

EPIDEMIOLOGY

Brief psychotic disorders have been reported to account for 9% of first-onset psychosis in the United States, with a 2:1 ratio in favor of

females. The incidence of schizophreniform disorders in the United States appears as much as 5-fold less than that of schizophrenia. The lifetime prevalence of schizophrenia is approximately 0.3–0.7%, although variations are reported by race/ethnicity, across countries, and by geographic origin for immigrants. The male:female ratio is approximately 1.4:1. Males generally have worse premorbid adjustment, lower educational achievement, more prominent negative symptoms, and more cognitive impairment than females.

CLINICAL COURSE

Brief psychotic disorder most often appears in adolescence or early adulthood, with the average age of onset in the mid-30s, but can occur throughout the life span. A diagnosis of brief psychotic disorder requires full remission within 1 mo of onset and gradual return to premorbid level of function. The age of onset of schizophreniform disorder is similar to that of schizophrenia. Recovery from an episode of the disorder is within 6 mo; however, about two thirds of patients relapse and eventually receive a diagnosis of schizophrenia or schizoaffective disorder. Abrupt onset, confusion, absence of blunted affect, and good premorbid functioning predict a better outcome in schizophreniform disorder.

Schizophrenia typically develops between the late teens and the mid-30s; onset before adolescence is rare. The peak age at onset for the first psychotic episode is in the early to mid-20s for males and in the late 20s for females. The onset may be abrupt or insidious, but the majority of individuals manifest a slow and gradual development of

Table 47.2	DSM-5 Diagnostic Criteria for Schizophreniform Disorder

A. Two (or more) of the following, each present for a significant portion of time during a 1 mo period (or less if successfully treated). At least 1 of these must be (1), (2), or (3):
1. Delusions.
2. Hallucinations.
3. Disorganized speech (e.g., frequent derailment or incoherence).
4. Grossly disorganized or catatonic behavior.
5. Negative symptoms (i.e., diminished emotional expression or avolition).
B. An episode of the disorder lasts at least 1 mo but less than 6 mo. When the diagnosis must be made without waiting for recovery, it should qualified as "provisional."
C. Schizoaffective disorder and depressive or bipolar disorder with psychotic features have been ruled out because either (1) no major depressive or manic episodes have occurred concurrently with the active-phase symptoms; or (2) if mood episodes have occurred during active-phase symptoms, they have been present for a minority of the total duration of the active and residual periods of the illness.
D. The disturbance is not attributable to the physiologic effects of a substance (e.g., a drug of abuse, a medication) or another medical condition.
Specify if:
With good prognostic features: This specifier requires the presence of at least 2 of the following features: onset of prominent psychotic symptoms within 4 wk of the first noticeable change in usual behavior or functioning; confusion or perplexity; good premorbid social and occupational functioning; and absence of blunted or flat affect.
Without good prognostic features: This specifier is applied if 2 or more of the above features have not been present.

From the *Diagnostic and Statistical Manual of Mental Disorders, Fifth Edition,* (Copyright 2013). American Psychiatric Association, pp 96–97.

Table 47.3	DSM-5 Diagnostic Criteria for Schizophrenia

A. Two (or more) of the following, each present for a significant portion of time during a 1 mo period (or less if successfully treated). At least 1 of these must be (1), (2), or (3):
1. Delusions.
2. Hallucinations.
3. Disorganized speech (e.g., frequent derailment or incoherence).
4. Grossly disorganized or catatonic behavior.
5. Negative symptoms (i.e., diminished emotional expression or avolition).
B. For a significant portion of the time since the onset of the disturbance, level of functioning in 1 or more major areas, such as work, interpersonal relations, or self-care, is markedly below the level achieved prior to the onset (or when the onset is in childhood or adolescence, there is failure to achieve expected level of interpersonal, academic, or occupational functioning).
C. Continuous signs of the disturbance persist for at least 6 mo. This 6 mo period must include at least 1 mo of symptoms (or less if successfully treated) that meet Criterion A (i.e., active-phase symptoms) and may include periods of prodromal or residual symptoms. During these prodromal or residual periods, the signs of the disturbance may be manifested by only negative symptoms or by 2 or more symptoms listed in Criterion A present in an attenuated form (e.g., odd beliefs, unusual perceptual experiences).
D. Schizoaffective disorder and depressive or bipolar disorder with psychotic features have been ruled out because either (1) no major depressive or manic episodes have occurred concurrently with the active-phase symptoms; or (2) if mood episodes have occurred during active-phase symptoms, they have been present for a minority of the total duration of the active and residual periods of the illness.
E. The disturbance is not attributable to the physiologic effects of a substance (e.g., a drug of abuse, a medication) or another medical condition.
F. If there is a history of autism spectrum disorder or a communication disorder of childhood onset, the additional diagnosis of schizophrenia is made only if prominent delusions or hallucinations, in addition to the other required symptoms of schizophrenia, are also present for at least a month (or less if successfully treated).

From the *Diagnostic and Statistical Manual of Mental Disorders, Fifth Edition,* (Copyright 2013). American Psychiatric Association, pp 99–100.

symptoms, with about half of individuals complaining of depressive symptoms. The predictors of course and outcome are largely unexplained. The course appears to be favorable in approximately 20% of cases, and a small number of individuals are reported to recover completely. However, many remain chronically ill, with exacerbations and remissions of active symptoms, whereas others experience progressive deterioration. Most individuals diagnosed with schizophrenia require daily living supports. Positive symptoms tend to diminish over time, and negative symptoms are the most persistent, along with cognitive deficits.

DIFFERENTIAL DIAGNOSIS

The differential diagnosis for the psychotic disorders is broad and includes reactions to substances/medications (dextromethorphan, LSD, hallucinogenic mushrooms, psilocybin, peyote, cannabis, stimulants, inhalants; corticosteroids, anesthetics, anticholinergics, antihistamines, amphetamines); medical conditions causing psychotic-like symptoms (Table 47.4); and other psychiatric disorders (depressive, bipolar, obsessive-compulsive, factitious, body dysmorphic, posttraumatic stress, autism spectrum, communication, personality). The differential diagnosis can be difficult because many conditions that can be mistaken for psychosis also increase the risk for it.

Autoimmune encephalitis caused by anti–N-methyl-D-aspartate (NMDA) receptor or other autoantibodies may manifest with psychosis, anxiety, depression, agitation, aggression, delusions, catatonia, visual or auditory hallucinations, disorientation, and paranoia in combination with sleep disturbances, autonomic dysfunction (hypoventilation), dyskinesias, movement disorders, seizures, memory loss, and a depressed level of consciousness (Fig. 47.1). The electroencephalogram (EEG), cerebrospinal fluid (CSF), and MRI are usually, but not always, abnormal. The constellation of psychosis and encephalitic features should suggest the diagnosis, although at presentation, behavioral problems may be the dominant feature (see Chapter 616.4).

Determining when identifiable medical conditions are causing delirium with prominent psychotic symptoms may be difficult (Table 47.5 and Table 47.6). In general, delirium due to medical causes is often associated with abnormalities in vital signs and the neurologic examination (including level of consciousness). A positive family or prior personal history of serious psychiatric illness is less likely. When psychotic symptoms are caused by identifiable medical conditions, there are often impairments in attention, orientation, recent memory, and intellectual function. Hallucinations may be caused by medical illness, but are often tactile, visual, or olfactory, whereas auditory hallucinations are more common in primary psychotic disorders. Patients whose hallucinations are caused by medical illness are more likely than patients with primary psychotic disorders to be aware that the hallucinations do not represent reality.

The diagnosis of a psychotic disorder should be made only after other explanations for the observed symptoms have been thoroughly considered. Mistakenly diagnosing psychosis when it is not present can lead to inappropriate use of antipsychotics with all their attendant risks, and mistakenly dismissing psychotic symptoms as nonpsychotic manifestations of, for example, autism or trauma can lead to long delays in treatment of the psychosis. The persistence, frequency, and form of possible psychotic symptoms, as well the degree of accompanying distress and functional regression, need to be considered in determining the likelihood of an underlying psychotic pathophysiology.

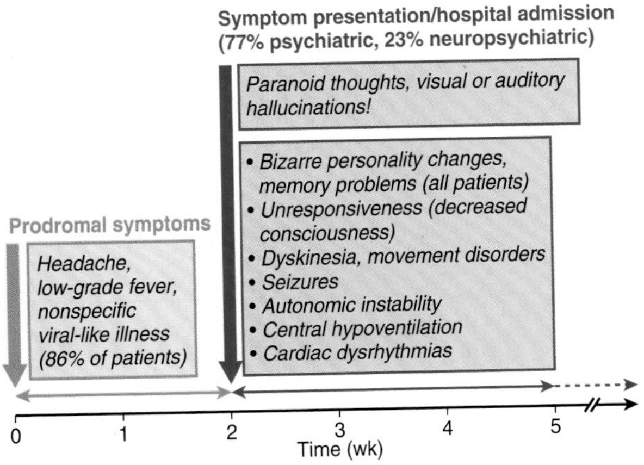

COMORBIDITY

In a review of 35 studies of youth with schizophrenia, rates of comorbidity approximated 34% for posttraumatic stress disorder, 34% for attention-deficit/hyperactivity and/or disruptive behavior disorders, and 32% for substance abuse/dependence.

SEQUELAE

Follow-up studies of early-onset schizophrenia suggest moderate to severe impairment across the life span. Poor outcome is predicted by low premorbid functioning, insidious onset, higher rates of negative symptoms, childhood onset, and low intellectual functioning. When followed into adulthood, youth with schizophrenia demonstrated greater social deficits, lower levels of employment, and were less likely to live independently, relative to those with other childhood psychotic disorders.

Approximately 5–6% of individuals with schizophrenia die by suicide, approximately 20% attempt suicide on one or more occasions, and many more have suicidal ideation. Life expectancy is reduced in individuals with schizophrenia because of associated medical conditions; a shared vulnerability for psychosis and medical disorders may explain some of the medical comorbidity of schizophrenia.

ETIOLOGY AND RISK FACTORS

Etiologic evidence for schizophrenia supports a neurodevelopmental and neurodegenerative model, with multiple genetic and environmental exposures playing important roles. It has been hypothesized that although psychotic disorders likely have their origins in early development, it is not until youth are in their mid-teens that the underlying neural structures manifest the disabling functional deficits and resultant psychotic symptoms.

Genetic Factors

The lifetime risk of developing schizophrenia is 5-20 times higher in first-degree relatives of affected probands than the general population. Concordance rates of 40–60% and 5–15% have been reported, respectively, in monozygotic and dizygotic twins. Genome-wide association studies have implicated variants in >100 different genes as leading to statistically significant but small increases in the risk for schizophrenia (odds ratios of about 1.4). The risk for schizophrenia increases with increasing burden of these common risk alleles, and approximately 30% of the risk of schizophrenia is attributable to common genetic variants. Rare variants of larger effect have also been implicated as increasing risk. Some rare copy number variants where stretches of the genome encompassing many genes are either duplicated or deleted have been shown to increase the risk of schizophrenia more markedly, with odds ratios of 2-25. Although these copy number variants, including such "hot spots" as 1q21.1, 15q13.3, and 22q11.2, may be responsible for 0.5–1.0% of typical adolescent/adult-onset schizophrenia, data indicate that they are responsible for about 12% of schizophrenia cases with onset before age 13 yr. There is increasing evidence that the same genetic risk alleles impart risk for multiple disorders (e.g., depression).

Environmental Factors

In utero exposure to maternal famine, advanced paternal age, prenatal infections, obstetric complications, marijuana use, and immigration have been hypothesized to contribute to the development of schizophrenia.

Symptom presentation/hospital admission (77% psychiatric, 23% neuropsychiatric)

Paranoid thoughts, visual or auditory hallucinations!

- *Bizarre personality changes, memory problems (all patients)*
- *Unresponsiveness (decreased consciousness)*
- *Dyskinesia, movement disorders*
- *Seizures*
- *Autonomic instability*
- *Central hypoventilation*
- *Cardiac dysrhythmias*

Prodromal symptoms

Headache, low-grade fever, nonspecific viral-like illness (86% of patients)

Time (wk) — 0 1 2 3 4 5

Fig. 47.1 Clinical characteristics of patients with anti–NMDA receptor encephalitis. (*Modified from Wandinger KP, Saschenbrecker S, Stoecker W, Dalmau J: Anti-NMDA-receptor encephalitis: a severe multistage, treatable disorder presenting with psychosis, J Neuroimmunol 231:86-91, 2011, Fig 2.*)

Table 47.4	Select Neurologic and Systemic Causes of Depression and/or Psychosis			

CATEGORY	DISORDERS	CATEGORY	DISORDERS
Head trauma	Traumatic brain injury Subdural hematoma	Inherited metabolic	Wilson disease Posterior horn syndrome Tay-Sachs disease Neuronal ceroid lipofuscinosis Niemann-Pick disease type C Acute intermittent porphyria Mitochondrial encephalopathy, lactic acidosis, and stroke-like episodes (MELAS) Cerebrotendinous xanthomatosis Homocystinuria Ornithine transcarbamylase deficiency
Infectious	Lyme disease Prion diseases Neurosyphilis Viral infections/encephalitides (HIV infection/encephalopathy, herpes encephalitis, cytomegalovirus. Epstein-Barr virus) Whipple disease Cerebral malaria Systemic infection		
Inflammatory	Autoimmune encephalitis Celiac disease Systemic lupus erythematosus Sjögren syndrome Temporal arteritis Hashimoto encephalopathy Sydenham chorea Sarcoidosis	Syndromes	Williams Prader-Willi Fragile X Deletion 22q11.2 ROHHAD
		Epilepsy	Ictal Interictal Postictal Forced normalization Postepilepsy surgery Lafora progressive myoclonic epilepsy
Neoplastic	Primary or secondary cerebral neoplasm Systemic neoplasm Paraneoplastic encephalitis		
Endocrine or acquired metabolic	Hepatic encephalopathy Uremic encephalopathy Dialysis dementia Hypo/hyperparathyroidism Hypo/hyperthyroidism Addison disease, Cushing disease Postpartum Vitamin deficiency: vitamin B_{12}, folate, niacin, vitamin C. thiamine Gastric bypass–associated nutritional deficiencies Hypoglycemia Hyponatremia	Medications	Analgesics Androgens (anabolic steroids) Antiarrhythmics Anticonvulsants Anticholinergics Antibiotics Antihypertensives Antineoplastic agents β-Blocking agents Corticosteroids Cyclosporin Dopamine agonists Oral contraceptives Sedatives/hypnotics Selective serotonin reuptake inhibitors (SSRIs) (serotonin syndrome)
Vascular	Stroke Cerebral autosomal dominant aneriopathy with subcortical infarcts and leukoencephalopathy (CADASIL)		
		Drugs of abuse	Alcohol Amphetamines Cocaine Hallucinogens Marijuana and synthetic cannabinoids Methylenedioxymethamphetamine (MDMA, Ecstasy) Phencyclidine
Degenerative	Progressive supranuclear palsy Huntington disease Corticobasal ganglionic degeneration Multisystem atrophy, striatonigral degeneration, olivopontocerebellar atrophy Idiopathic basal ganglia calcifications, Fahr disease Neuroacanthosis Neurodegeneration with brain iron accumulation (NBIA) Adrenoleukodystrophy Metachromatic leukodystrophy		
		Drug withdrawal syndromes	Alcohol Barbiturates Benzodiazepines Amphetamines SSRIs
		Toxins	Heavy metals Inhalants
Demyelinating, dysmyelinating	Multiple sclerosis Acute disseminated encephalomyelitis Adrenoleukodystrophy Metachromatic leukodystrophy	Other	Normal-pressure hydrocephalus Ionizing radiation Decompression sickness

ROHHAD, Rapid-onset obesity with hypothalamic dysfunction, hypoventilation, autonomic dysregulation.
Modified from Perez DL, Murray ED, Price BH: Depression and psychosis in neurological practice. In Daroff RB, Jankovic J, Mazziotta JC, et al, editors: *Bradley's neurology in clinical practice*, 7th ed, Philadelphia, 2015, Elsevier.

Environmental exposures may mediate disease risk through direct neurologic damage, gene-environment interactions, epigenetic effects, or de novo mutations. There is no evidence that psychological or social factors alone cause schizophrenia. Rather, environmental factors potentially interact with biologic risk factors to mediate the timing of onset, course, and severity of the disorder. Expressed emotion within the family setting can influence the onset and exacerbation of acute episodes and relapse rates.

NEUROANATOMIC ABNORMALITIES

Increased lateral ventricle volumes, along with reductions in hippocampus, thalamus, and frontal lobe volumes, have been reported in

| Table 47.5 | Special Problems in the Differential Diagnosis of Delirium* | | | |

CLINICAL FEATURE	DELIRIUM	DEMENTIAS	SCHIZOPHRENIA	DEPRESSION
Course	Acute onset; hours, days, or more	Insidious onset, months or years, progressive	Insidious onset, ≥6 mo, acute psychotic phases	Insidious onset, at least 2 wk, often months
Attention	Markedly impaired attention and arousal	Normal early; impairment later	Normal to mild impairment	Mild impairment
Fluctuation	Prominent in attention arousal; disturbed day/night cycle	Prominent fluctuations absent; lesser disturbances in day/night cycle	Absent	Absent
Perception	Misperceptions; hallucinations, usually visual, fleeting; paramnesia	Perceptual abnormalities much less prominent; paramnesia	Hallucinations, auditory with personal reference	May have mood-congruent hallucinations
Speech and language	Abnormal clarity, speed, and coherence; disjointed and dysarthric; misnaming; characteristic dysgraphia	Early anomia; empty speech; abnormal comprehension	Disorganized, with a bizarre theme	Decreased amount of speech
Other cognition	Disorientation to time, place; recent memory and visuospatial abnormalities	Disorientation to time, place; multiple other higher cognitive deficits	Disorientation to person; concrete interpretations	Mental slowing; indecisiveness; memory retrieval difficulty
Behavior	Lethargy or delirium; nonsystematized delusions; emotional lability	Disinterested; disengaged; disinhibited; delusions and other psychiatric symptoms	Systematized delusions; paranoia; bizarre behavior	Depressed mood; anhedonia; lack of energy; sleep and appetite disturbances
Electroencephalogram	Diffuse slowing; low-voltage fast activity; specific patterns	Normal early; mild slowing later	Normal	Normal

*The characteristics listed are the usual ones and not exclusive.
From Mendez MF, Padilla CR: Delirium. In Daroff RB, Jankovic J, Mazziotta JC, et al, editors: *Bradley's neurology in clinical practice*, 7th ed, Philadelphia, 2015, Elsevier.

| Table 47.6 | Features Suggesting Neurologic Disease in Patients With Psychiatric Symptoms |

ATYPICAL PSYCHIATRIC FEATURES
Late or very early age of onset
Acute or subacute onset
Lack of significant psychosocial stressors
Catatonia
Diminished comportment
Cognitive decline
Intractability despite adequate therapy
Progressive symptoms

HISTORY OF PRESENT ILLNESS
New or worsening headache
Inattention
Somnolence
Incontinence
Focal neurologic complaints such as weakness, sensory changes, incoordination, or gait difficulty
Neuroendocrine changes
Anorexia/weight loss

PATIENT MEDICAL HISTORY
Risk factors for cerebrovascular disease or central nervous system infections
Malignancy
Immunocompromised status
Significant head trauma
Seizures
Movement disorder
Hepatobiliary disorders
Abdominal crises of unknown cause
Biologic relatives with similar diseases or complaints

UNEXPLAINED DIAGNOSTIC ABNORMALITIES
Screening laboratory tests
Neuroimaging studies or possibly imaging of other systems
Electroencephalogram
Cerebrospinal fluid

From Perez DL Murray ED, Price BH: Depression and psychosis in neurological practice. In Daroff RB, Jankovic J, Mazziotta JC, editors: *Bradley's neurology in clinical practice*, 7th ed, Philadelphia, 2015, Elsevier.

schizophrenia. Youth in particular have reductions in gray matter volumes and reduced cortical folding. Neurotransmitter systems, particularly central nervous system dopamine circuits, are hypothesized to have a key role in the pathophysiology of schizophrenia. The dopamine hypothesis is derived in part from the identification of D_2 receptor blockade as the mechanism for the action of antipsychotic medications.

PREVENTION

There has been significant interest in prospectively identifying youth at risk for schizophrenia spectrum and other psychotic disorders in an effort to provide early intervention before the development of a full-blown psychotic disorder. Various names, including *attenuated psychosis syndrome* (APS), *clinical high risk* (CHR), psychosis risk syndrome,

ultrahigh risk, at-risk mental state, and prodromal stage, have been used to describe patients who present with troubling symptoms suggestive of early psychosis.

APS or CHR is characterized by the presence of delusions, hallucinations, or disorganized speech in attenuated forms. Affected individuals may express a variety of unusual or odd beliefs or may have unusual perceptual experiences, including frank hallucinations, but retain insight into their unreality; their speech may be generally understandable but vague; and their behavior may be unusual but not grossly disorganized. Individuals who had been socially active may become withdrawn. The symptoms are described as present at least once per week for the past month and have begun or worsened over the past year. Although the symptoms are less severe and more transient than in a psychotic disorder,

20–40% with these attenuated symptoms appear to go on to a psychotic disorder within several years of symptom presentation. There is evidence that premorbid lower cognitive and social skills as well as a history of substance abuse contribute to the risk of developing a full-blown psychotic disorder in individuals with APS/CHR.

Some evidence indicates that antipsychotic medication may delay conversion of attenuated to full-blown psychosis and ameliorate attenuated symptoms in active treatment, yet there appear to be no lasting effects after the medication is withdrawn. Additionally, the known adverse effects of antipsychotics argue against their being used broadly to prevent psychosis in patients with APS/CHR, given that about two thirds of them do not go on to develop a psychotic disorder.

Antidepressants have been associated with symptomatic improvement in adolescents with APS/CHR. Psychological interventions, including social skills, cognitive, and interaction training programs, as well as educational family interventions and cognitive-behavioral therapy (CBT), are reported to improve symptoms and psychosocial functioning in youth with early symptoms and decrease the rate of conversion to psychosis.

Despite improvements in diagnostic predictive validity, significant concern remains regarding a high *false-positive* rate (identifying an individual as prodromal who does not go on to develop psychosis) that may cause individuals to be stigmatized or exposed to unnecessary treatment. In this context, youth with early symptoms suggestive of psychosis should be referred to a child and adolescent psychiatrist or other qualified mental health specialist, and/or a specialized research program.

SCREENING/CASE FINDING

Pediatric practitioners can make general inquiries of youth and their parents regarding problems with thinking or perceptions. For the older youth, such questions as "Does your mind ever play tricks on you?," "Do you hear voices talking to you when no one is there?," and "Does your mind ever feel confused?" can help elicit symptoms. For younger children, the clinician must ensure that the child understands the questions. True psychotic symptoms are generally confusing to the individual. Highly descriptive, detailed, organized, and situation-specific reports are less likely to represent true psychosis. Overt evidence of psychosis is not always present on mental status examination, but in the absence of this, the validity of symptom reports should be scrutinized. Youth presenting with possible psychosis warrant assessment and treatment by a child and adolescent psychiatrist or other qualified mental health specialist.

ASSESSMENT

The diagnostic assessment of schizophrenia in youth is uniquely complicated, and misdiagnosis is common. Most children who report hallucinations do not meet criteria for schizophrenia, and many do not have a psychotic illness. The persistence, frequency, and form of possible psychotic symptoms; the presence of distress; functional impairment; and insight need to be considered in arriving at a diagnosis. Expertise in childhood psychopathology and experience in assessing reports of psychotic symptoms in youth are important prerequisite skills for clinicians evaluating youth for possible psychosis. Comprehensive diagnostic assessments, which reconcile mental status findings with the rigorous application of diagnostic criteria, help improve accuracy.

There are no neuroimaging, psychological, or laboratory tests that establish a diagnosis of schizophrenic spectrum disorders. The medical evaluation focuses on ruling out nonpsychiatric causes of psychosis, while also establishing baseline laboratory parameters for monitoring medication therapy. Routine laboratory testing typically includes blood counts, basic metabolic panel, and liver, renal, and thyroid function. More extensive evaluation is indicated for atypical presentations, such as a gross deterioration in cognitive and motor abilities, focal neurologic symptoms, or delirium. Neuroimaging may be indicated when neurologic symptoms are present, or an EEG may be indicated for a clinical history suggestive of seizures. Toxicology screens are indicated for acute onset or exacerbations of psychosis, when exposure to drugs of abuse cannot be ruled out. Genetic testing is indicated if there are associated dysmorphic or syndromic features. Tests to rule out specific syndromes or diseases are indicated for clinical presentations suggestive of a specific syndrome (e.g., amino acid screens for inborn errors of metabolism, ceruloplasmin for Wilson disease, porphobilinogen for acute intermittent porphyria, NMDA receptor antibodies for autoimmune encephalitis). Neuropsychological testing cannot establish the diagnosis but may be important for documenting cognitive deficits for academic planning.

TREATMENT

It is important to recognize hallmark phases in the assessment and management of schizophrenia. In the **prodrome phase**, most patients experience functional deterioration (i.e., social withdrawal, idiosyncratic preoccupations, unusual behaviors, academic failure, deteriorating self-care skills, and/or dysphoria) before the onset of psychotic symptoms. The **acute phase** is characterized by prominent positive symptoms and deterioration in functioning. The **recuperative/recovery phase** is marked by a several-month period of impairment and predominantly negative symptoms. The **residual phase** (if reached) has no positive symptoms, although negative symptoms may cause continued impairment.

Treatment goals include decreasing psychotic symptomatology, directing the child toward a developmentally typical trajectory, and reintegrating the child into the home and community. Children and families facing schizophrenia spectrum disorders require an array of mental health services to address their psychological, social, educational, and cultural needs. Given the insidious onset and chronic course of these disorders, the patient must be followed longitudinally, with periodic reassessment to hone diagnostic accuracy and tailor services to meet the patient's and family's needs. Integrated psychopharmacologic, psychotherapeutic, psychoeducational, and case management services are often necessary.

Psychoeducation about the illness with an assessment of the potential role of stigma in treatment participation is critical for improving adherence with treatment recommendations. Assessing a child's strengths and vulnerabilities as well as available environmental resources is critical in devising an effective treatment plan. School and community liaison work to develop and maintain a day-to-day schedule for the patient is important. Specialized educational programs should be considered within the school system. Cognitive remediation has led to some promising gains in planning ability and cognitive flexibility. Effective and collaborative communication among the family, the pediatrician, a child and adolescent psychiatrist, and other mental health providers increases the potential for the patient's optimal functioning.

Pharmacotherapy

First-generation (typical) and second-generation (atypical) antipsychotic medications have been shown to be effective in reducing psychotic symptoms. These antipsychotics appear to outperform placebo and to have approximately equal effectiveness, except for *ziprasidone* and *clozapine*, which may be less and more effective than the others, respectively. Risperidone, aripiprazole, quetiapine, olanzapine, and lurasidone are FDA-approved second-generation antipsychotics for treating schizophrenia in patients 13 yr and older, and *paliperidone* for those 12 yr and older. Several of the first-generation antipsychotics are also FDA approved for children and adolescents. The choice of which agent to use first is typically based on U.S. Food and Drug Administration approval status, side effect profile, patient and family preference, clinician familiarity, and cost. *Depot* antipsychotics have not been studied in pediatric age groups and have inherent risks with long-term exposure to side effects. Although clozapine is effective in treating both positive and negative symptoms, its risk for agranulocytosis and seizures limits its use to those patients with treatment-resistant disorders. Ziprasidone and paliperidone are associated with QT prolongation; this finding along with the inferior effectiveness of ziprasidone limits its use with children and adolescents.

Most patients require long-term treatment and are at significant risk for relapse if their medication is discontinued, and more than three quarters of youth with schizophrenia discontinue their medication within 180 days. As such, the goal is to maintain the medication at the lowest effective dose to minimize potential adverse events. Many patients will continue to experience some degree of positive or negative symptoms, requiring ongoing treatment. Patients should maintain regular physician contact to monitor symptom course, side effects, and adherence.

Electroconvulsive therapy (ECT) may be used with severely impaired adolescents if medications are either not helpful or cannot be tolerated. It has not been systematically studied in children.

Bibliography is available at Expert Consult.

47.2 Psychosis Associated With Epilepsy
Joseph Gonzalez-Heydrich, Heather J. Walter, and David R. DeMaso

Schizophrenia spectrum and other psychotic disorders include psychotic disorder due to another medical condition (Table 47.7). **Psychosis associated with epilepsy** has been reported in children and adults. Also called *schizophrenic-like psychosis of epilepsy,* the disorder manifests with delusions or hallucinations associated with poor insight. The characterization is complicated by the fact that anticonvulsant drugs can cause psychosis and antipsychotic drugs can lower the seizure threshold, producing seizures.

Psychosis associated with epilepsy can be further differentiated into ictal, interictal, and postictal psychosis. Ictal-induced psychosis is a form of **nonconvulsive status epilepticus**, usually complex partial status that can last for hours to days and is associated with periods of impaired consciousness. Brief interictal psychosis can last days to weeks and is associated with paranoia, delusions, and auditory hallucinations. Chronic interictal psychosis resembles schizophrenia and manifests with paranoia, visual hallucinations, and catatonia. Postictal psychosis is the most common type (observed in 2–7% of patients with epilepsy) and lasts up to 1 wk and then spontaneously remits.

The diagnosis requires a strong index of suspicion and EEG monitoring. Treatment requires appropriate anticonvulsant drugs and, if the psychosis persists, initiating low-dose antipsychotic medication.

Bibliography is available at Expert Consult.

47.3 Catatonia in Children and Adolescents
Joseph Gonzalez-Heydrich, Heather J. Walter, and David R. DeMaso

Catatonia is a poorly defined state presenting as an unusual manifestation of decreased or increased muscle tone and decreased responsiveness (although agitation may be present) occurring in association with a broad array of conditions affecting children, adolescents, and adults.

These conditions include psychosis, autism spectrum disorder, developmental disorders, drug-induced conditions, mood disorders, and a wide range of medical disorders (Table 47.8). Not surprising given its ill-defined nature, the prevalence of catatonia in children and adolescents is unknown, although it is generally believed to be significantly underdiagnosed. Recognition of catatonia by a clinician is important because the disorder is generally very responsive to treatment with benzodiazepines and/or ECT.

DIAGNOSIS AND TREATMENT
Catatonia is defined as 3 or more of the 12 symptoms listed in Table 47.9. An important next step is the evaluation (and possible elimination) of medications being administered to the child for their potential to induce catatonic symptoms, a not-infrequent side effect of many medical and psychiatric medications. Of particular importance, antipsychotics should be discontinued because they have been associated with an increased incidence of malignant catatonia or neuroleptic malignant syndrome.

Benzodiazepines (typically lorazepam) and ECT are effective in adults and appear to be effective in children. Fig. 47.2 shows a treatment algorithm using a lorazepam challenge test (oral, intravenous, or intramuscular lorazepam, 1-2 mg). If the challenge test does reverse symptoms, increasing doses of lorazepam are indicated, with careful monitoring to avoid side effects. ECT may be indicated alone (if no improvement with lorazepam) or in combination with lorazepam if some but incomplete improvement is noted.

The outlook for catatonia is greatly impacted by that of the associated condition(s). The long-term outcome for patients treated with ECT is unknown, but mortality rates in catatonic patients declined after the introduction of ECT in treatment.

Bibliography is available at Expert Consult.

47.4 Acute Phobic Hallucinations of Childhood
Joseph Gonzalez-Heydrich, Heather J. Walter and David R. DeMaso

Among adults, hallucinations are viewed as synonymous with "psychosis" and as harbingers of serious psychopathology. In children, hallucinations can be part of normal development and more often than in adults can be associated with nonpsychotic psychopathology, psychosocial stressors, drug intoxication, or physical illness. The first clinical task in evaluating youth who report hallucinations is to sort out those associated with severe mental illness from those derived from other causes (Fig. 47.3).

Table 47.7	DSM-5 Diagnostic Criteria for Psychotic Disorder Due to Another Medical Condition

A. Prominent hallucinations or delusions.
B. There is evidence from the history, physical examination, or laboratory findings that the disturbance is the direct pathophysiologic consequence of another medical condition.
C. The disturbance is not better explained by another mental disorder.
D. The disturbance does not occur exclusively during the course of a delirium.
E. The disturbance causes clinically significant distress or impairment in social, occupational, or other important areas of functioning.
Specify whether:
With delusions: If delusions are the predominant symptom.
With hallucinations: If hallucinations are the predominant symptom.

From the *Diagnostic and Statistical Manual of Mental Disorders, Fifth Edition,* (Copyright 2013). American Psychiatric Association, pp 115–116.

Table 47.8	Conditions Associated With Catatonia

Psychotic disorders
   Paranoid schizophrenia, catatonic schizophrenia, psychosis, autism, Prader-Willi syndrome, intellectual impairment
Mood disorders
   Bipolar disorder: manic or mixed episodes
Major depressive disorder
Medical conditions
   Endocrine abnormalities, infections, electrolyte imbalances, mutations in *SCN2A* gene
Neurologic conditions
   Epilepsy, strokes, traumatic brain injury, multiple sclerosis, infectious and autoimmune encephalitis
Drugs
   Withdrawal: benzodiazepines, L-dopa, gabapentin
   Overdose: LSD, phencyclidine (PCP), cocaine, MDMA (Ecstasy), disulfiram, levetiracetam

Adapted from Weder ND, Muralee S, Penland H, Tampi RR: Catatonia: a review, *Ann Clin Psychiatry* 20(2):97–107, 2008, Table 2.

Table 47.9	DSM-5 Diagnostic Criteria for Catatonic Disorder Due to Another Medical Condition

A. The clinical picture is dominated by 3 (or more) of the following symptoms:
  1. Stupor (i.e., no psychomotor activity; not actively relating to environment).
  2. Catalepsy (i.e., passive induction of a posture held against gravity).
  3. Waxy flexibility (i.e., slight, even resistance to positioning by examiner).
  4. Mutism (i.e., no, or very little, verbal response [*Note*: not applicable if there is an established aphasia]).
  5. Negativism (i.e., opposing or not responding to instructions or external stimuli).
  6. Posturing (i.e., spontaneous and active maintenance of a posture against gravity).
  7. Mannerism (i.e., odd, circumstantial caricature of normal actions).
  8. Stereotypy (i.e., repetitive, abnormally frequent, non–goal-directed movements).
  9. Agitation, not influenced by external stimuli.

  10. Grimacing.
  11. Echolalia (i.e., mimicking another's speech).
  12. Echopraxia (i.e., mimicking another's movements).
B. There is evidence from the history, physical examination, or laboratory findings that the disturbance is the direct pathophysiologic consequence of another medical condition.
C. The disturbance is not better explained by another mental disorder (e.g., a manic episode).
D. The disturbance does not occur exclusively during the course of a delirium.
E. The disturbance causes clinically significant distress or impairment in social, occupational, or other areas of functioning.
Coding note: Include the name of the medical condition in the name of the mental disorder (e.g., F06.1 catatonic disorder due to hepatic encephalopathy). The other medical condition should be coded and listed separately immediately before the catatonic disorder due to the medical condition (e.g., K71.90 hepatic encephalopathy; F06.1 catatonic disorder due to hepatic encephalopathy).

From the *Diagnostic and Statistical Manual of Mental Disorders, Fifth Edition,* (Copyright 2013). American Psychiatric Association, pp 120–121.

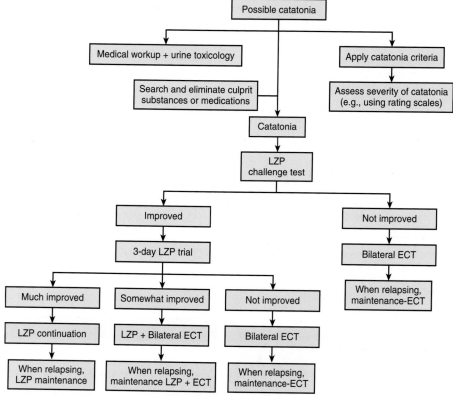

Fig. 47.2 Evaluation, diagnosis, and treatment of catatonia in children and adolescents. ECT, Electroconvulsive therapy; LZP, lorazepam. *(From Dhossche DM, Wilson C, Wachtel LE: Catatonia in childhood and adolescents: implications for the DSM-5, Prim Psychiatry 17(4):23–26, 2010.)*

CLINICAL MANIFESTATIONS

Hallucinations are perceptions (typically auditory, visual, tactile, or olfactory) that occur in the absence of identifiable external stimuli. Hallucinations can be further categorized as *nondiagnostic* (hearing footsteps, knocking, or one's name) and *diagnostic* (hearing one or more voices saying words other than one's own name).

In children with nonpsychotic hallucinations, the other symptoms of psychosis are absent. *Nonpsychotic* hallucinations typically occur in the context of severe traumatic stress, developmental difficulties, social and emotional deprivation, parents whose own psychopathology promotes a breakdown in the child's sense of reality, cultural beliefs in mysticism, and unresolved mourning. *Auditory* hallucinations of voices telling the child to do "bad things" may be more often associated with disruptive behavior disorders than psychotic diagnoses. Hearing a voice invoking suicide is often associated with depression. Trauma-related auditory hallucinations are commonly associated with posttraumatic stress disorder

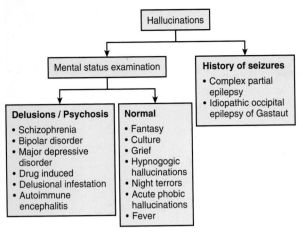

Fig. 47.3 Evaluation of hallucinations.

is unknown. The differential diagnosis includes drug overdose or poisoning, high fever, encephalitis, and psychosis. The child's fear is not alleviated by reassurance by the parents or physician, and the child is not amenable to reason. Findings on physical and mental status examinations are otherwise normal. Symptoms can persist for 1-3 days, slowly abating over 1-2 wk.

The differential diagnosis of hallucinations comprises a broad range of mental disorders, including diagnoses in which hallucinations are not the hallmark feature, but may be viewed as associated symptoms (posttraumatic stress disorder, nonpsychotic mood disorders, and disruptive, impulse-control, and conduct disorders); diagnoses that are defined by psychotic features (brief psychotic disorder, schizophrenia, major depressive or bipolar disorder with psychotic features); and at-risk clinical states (poor reality testing). In addition, other medical conditions can manifest with hallucinations, including drug intoxications (cannabis, LSD, cocaine, amphetamines, barbiturates), medication side effects (e.g., corticosteroids, anticholinergics, stimulants), and physical illnesses (e.g., thyroid, parathyroid, and adrenal disorders; Wilson disease; electrolyte imbalances; infections; migraines; seizures; neoplasms).

TREATMENT

The evaluation of the underlying condition directs the type of treatment needed. Nonpsychotic hallucinations suggest the need for disorder-specific psychotherapy (e.g., trauma-focused CBT for posttraumatic stress disorder) and perhaps adjunctive medication (e.g., antidepressant for depression or anxiety, brief trial of antipsychotic for agitation). CBT focused on helping the youth understand the origin of the hallucinations and on developing coping strategies for stressful situations may be helpful for older children and adolescents. True psychotic hallucinations suggest the need for antipsychotic medication.

Bibliography is available at Expert Consult.

or a brief psychotic disorder with marked stressors. The content of the hallucinations may be relevant in understanding the underlying psychopathology and developmental issues.

DIAGNOSIS AND DIFFERENTIAL DIAGNOSIS

Acute phobic hallucinations are benign and common and occur in previously healthy preschool children. The hallucinations are often visual or tactile, last 10-60 min, and occur at any time but most often at night. The child is quite frightened and might complain that bugs or snakes are crawling over him or her and attempt to remove them. The cause

Learning and Developmental Disorders
学习及发育障碍

Chapter **48**
Neurodevelopmental and Executive Function and Dysfunction

Desmond P. Kelly and Mindo J. Natale

第四十八章
神经发育、执行功能和功能障碍

中文导读

　　本章主要介绍了神经发育功能和执行功能，以及相关功能障碍的临床表现、评估和治疗。神经发育功能具体描述了感觉和运动功能、语言、视觉空间/视觉感知功能、智力功能、记忆、社会认知和执行功能；执行功能具体描述了注意力、抑制控制、工作记忆、任务启动、计划、组织、情绪控制和动机。同时主要介绍了神经发育功能和执行功能的

功能障碍的临床表现、评估与诊断和治疗。临床表现中描述了学习相关问题和学习非相关问题；治疗中分别描述了神经发育功能障碍的治疗和执行功能障碍的治疗，并详细阐述了治疗方法，包括发展疗法、个体化课程、提高能力、个体及家庭咨询、非标准疗法和药物治疗等内容。

TERMINOLOGY AND EPIDEMIOLOGY

A **neurodevelopmental function** is a basic brain process needed for learning and productivity. **Executive function (EF)** is an umbrella term used to describe specific neurocognitive processes involved in the regulating, guiding, organizing, and monitoring of thoughts and actions to achieve a specific goal. Processes considered to be "executive" in nature include inhibition/impulse control, cognitive/mental flexibility, emotional control, initiation skills, planning, organization, working memory, and self-monitoring. **Neurodevelopmental and/or executive dysfunctions** reflect any disruptions or weaknesses in these processes, which may result from neuroanatomic or psychophysiologic malfunctioning. **Neurodevelopmental variation** refers to differences in neurodevelopmental functioning. Wide variations in these functions exist within

and between individuals. These differences can change over time and need not represent pathology or abnormality.

Neurodevelopmental and/or executive dysfunction places a child at risk for developmental, cognitive, emotional, behavioral, psychosocial, and adaptive challenges. Preschool-age children with neurodevelopmental or executive dysfunction may manifest delays in developmental domains such as language, motor, self-help, or social-emotional development and self-regulation. For the school-age child, an area of particular focus is academic skill development. The *Diagnostic and Statistical Manual of Mental Disorder, Fifth Edition* (DSM-5) classifies **academic disorder** within the group of neurodevelopmental disorders as **specific learning disorder (SLD)**, with broadened diagnostic criteria recognizing impairments in reading, written expression, and mathematics. In the

International Classification of Diseases, Tenth Edition (ICD-10), neurodevelopmental disorders include **specific developmental disorders of scholastic skills** with specific reading disorder, mathematics disorder, and disorder of written expression. **Dyslexia** is categorized separately in ICD-10 under "Symptoms and Signs Not Elsewhere Classified." **Frontal lobe and executive function deficit** is also included in this category. **Disorders of executive function** have traditionally been viewed as a component of **attention-deficit/hyperactivity disorder (ADHD)**, which is also classified in DSM-5 as a neurodevelopmental disorder.

There are no prevalence estimates specifically for neurodevelopmental dysfunction, but overall estimates for learning disorders range from 3–10% with a similar range reported for ADHD. These disorders frequently co-occur. The range in prevalence is likely related to differences in definitions and criteria used for classification and diagnosis, as well as differences in methods of assessment.

ETIOLOGY AND PATHOGENESIS

Neurodevelopmental and executive dysfunction may result from a broad range of etiologic factors, including genetic, medical, psychological, environmental, and sociocultural influences.

There is a high degree of **heritability** reported in learning and attention disorders, with estimates ranging from 45–80%. Specific genes have been identified that are associated with reading disorders, including the *DYX2* locus on chromosome 6p22 and the *DYX3* locus on 2p12. Neuroimaging studies have confirmed links between gene variations and variations in cortical thickness in areas of the brain known to be associated with learning and academic performance, such as the temporal regions. Chromosomal abnormalities can lead to unique patterns of dysfunction, such as visual-spatial deficits in girls diagnosed with Turner syndrome (see Chapter 98.4) or executive and language deficits in children with fragile X syndrome (Chapter 98.5). Chromosome 22q11.2 deletion syndrome (velocardiofacial-DiGeorge syndrome; Chapter 98.3) has been associated with predictable patterns of neurodevelopmental and executive dysfunction that can be progressive, including a higher prevalence of intellectual disability, as well as deficits in visual-spatial processing, attention, working memory, verbal learning, arithmetic, and language.

Genetic vulnerabilities may be further influenced by **perinatal** factors, including very low birthweight, severe intrauterine growth restriction, perinatal hypoxic-ischemic encephalopathy, and prenatal exposure to substances such as alcohol and drugs. Increased risk of neurodevelopmental and executive dysfunction has also been associated with environmental toxins, including lead (see Chapter 739); drugs such as cocaine; infections such as meningitis, HIV, and Zika; and brain injury secondary to intraventricular hemorrhage, periventricular leukomalacia, or head trauma. The academic effects of concussion in children and adolescents, although usually temporary, have been well characterized, including impaired concentration and slowed processing speed. Repeated injuries have a much higher likelihood of long-term negative neurocognitive effects.

Early **psychological trauma** may result in both structural and neurochemical changes in the developing brain, which may contribute to neurodevelopmental and executive dysfunction. Findings suggest that the effects of exposure to trauma or abuse early in the developmental course can induce disruption of the brain's regulatory system and may influence right hemisphere function with associated risk for problems with information processing, memory, focus, and self-regulation. Environmental and sociocultural deprivation can lead to, or potentiate, neurodevelopmental and executive dysfunction, and numerous studies have indicated that parent/caregiver executive functioning impacts the development of EFs in offspring.

With regard to **pathogenesis**, investigations of neuroanatomic substrates have yielded important information about the underlying mechanisms in neurodevelopmental and executive dysfunction. Multiple neurobiologic investigations have identified differences in the left parietotemporal and left occipitotemporal brain regions of individuals with dyslexia compared to those without reading difficulties (see Chapter 50). Studies have also described the neural circuitry, primarily in the parietal cortex, underlying mathematical competencies such as the

processing of numerical magnitude and mental arithmetic. The associations between executive dysfunction and the *prefrontal/frontal cortex* have been well established, and insults to the frontal lobe regions often result in dysfunction of executive abilities (e.g., poor inhibitory control). Although the prefrontal/frontal cortex may be the primary control region for EFs, there is considerable interconnectivity between the brain's frontal regions and other areas, such as *arousal* systems (reticular activating system), *motivational and emotional* systems (limbic system), *cortical association* systems (posterior/anterior; left/right hemispheres), and *input/output* systems (frontal motor/posterior sensory areas).

CORE NEURODEVELOPMENTAL FUNCTIONS

The neurodevelopmental processes that are critical to a child's successful functioning may best be understood as falling within **core neurodevelopmental domains**. Notwithstanding such classification of domains, the clinical distinctions often made regarding "cognitive" processes (e.g., intelligence, EF, attention, language, memory) are relatively artificial because these brain functions are highly integrated.

Sensory and Motor Function

Sensory development (e.g., auditory, visual, tactile, proprioceptive) begins well before birth. This neurodevelopmental process is crucial in helping children experience, understand, and manipulate their environments. Sensory development progresses in association with environmental exposure and with the development of other cognitive processes, such as motor development. Through sensory experiences, children's brains mature as new neuronal pathways are created and existing pathways are strengthened.

There are three distinct, yet related, forms of neuromotor ability: fine motor, graphomotor, and gross motor coordination. **Fine motor function** reflects the ability to control the muscles and bones to produce small, exact movements. Deficits in fine motor function can disrupt the ability to communicate in written form, to excel in artistic and crafts activities, and can interfere with learning a musical instrument or mastering a computer keyboard. The term **dyspraxia** relates to difficulty in developing an ideomotor plan and activating coordinated and integrated visual-motor actions to complete a task or solve a motor problem, such as assembling a model. **Graphomotor function** refers to the specific motor aspects of written output. Several subtypes of graphomotor dysfunction can significantly impede writing. Children who harbor weaknesses of visualization during writing have trouble picturing the configurations of letters and words as they write (orthographics), with poorly legible written output with inconsistent spacing between words. Others have weaknesses in orthographic memory and may labor over individual letters and prefer printing (manuscript) to cursive writing. Some exhibit signs of finger agnosia and have trouble localizing their fingers while they write, needing to keep their eyes very close to the page and applying excessive pressure to the pencil. Others struggle producing the highly coordinated motor sequences needed for writing, a phenomenon also described as **dyspraxic dysgraphia**. It is important to emphasize that a child may show excellent fine motor dexterity (as revealed in mechanical or artistic domains) but very poor graphomotor fluency (with labored or poorly legible writing).

Gross motor function refers to control of large muscles. Children with gross motor incoordination often have problems in processing "outer spatial" information to guide gross motor actions. Affected children may be inept at catching or throwing a ball because they cannot form accurate judgments about trajectories in space. Others demonstrate diminished body position sense. They do not efficiently receive or interpret proprioceptive and kinesthetic feedback from peripheral joints and muscles. They are likely to evidence difficulties when activities demand balance and ongoing tracking of body movement. Others are unable to satisfy the motor praxis demands of certain gross motor activities. It may be difficult for them to recall or plan complex motor procedures such as those needed for dancing, gymnastics, or swimming.

Language

Language is one of the most critical and complex cognitive functions and can be broadly divided into **receptive** (auditory comprehension/ understanding) and **expressive** (speech and language production and/ or communication) functions. Children who primarily experience receptive language problems may have difficulty understanding verbal information, following instructions and explanations, and interpreting what they hear. Expressive language weaknesses can result from problems with speech production and/or problems with higher-level language development. **Speech production difficulties** include oromotor problems affecting articulation, verbal fluency, and naming. Some children have trouble with sound sequencing within words. Others find it difficult to regulate the rhythm or prosody of their verbal output. Their speech may be dysfluent, hesitant, and inappropriate in tone. Problems with word retrieval can result in difficulty finding exact words when needed (as in a class discussion) or substituting definitions for words (circumlocution).

The basic components of language include **phonology** (ability to process and integrate the individual sounds in words), **semantics** (understanding the meaning of words), **syntax** (mastery of word order and grammatical rules), **discourse** (processing and producing paragraphs and passages), **metalinguistics** (ability to think about and analyze how language works and draw inferences), and **pragmatics** (social understanding and application of language). Children who evidence higher-level expressive language impediments have trouble formulating sentences, using grammar acceptably, and organizing spoken (and possibly written) narratives.

To one degree or another, all academic skills are taught largely through language, and thus it is not surprising that children who experience language dysfunction often experience problems with academic performance. In fact, some studies suggest that up to 80% of children who present with a specific learning disorder also experience language-based weaknesses. Additionally, the role of language in executive functioning cannot be understated, since language serves to guide cognition and behavior.

Visual-Spatial/Visual-Perceptual Function

Important structures involved in the development and function of the visual system include the retina, optic cells (e.g., rods and cones), the optic chiasm, the optic nerves, the brainstem (control of automatic responses, e.g., pupil dilation), the thalamus (e.g., lateral geniculate nucleus for form, motion, color), and the primary (visual space and orientation) and secondary (color perception) visual processing regions located in and around the occipital lobe. Other brain areas, considered to be outside of the primary visual system, are also important to visual function, helping to process *what* (temporal lobe) is seen and *where* it is located in space (parietal lobe). It is now well documented that the left and right cerebral hemispheres interact considerably in visual processes, with each hemisphere possessing more specialized functions, including left hemisphere processing of details, patterns, and linear information and right hemisphere processing of the gestalt and overall form.

Critical aspects of visual processing development in the child include appreciation of **spatial relations** (ability to perceive objects accurately in space in relation to other objects), **visual discrimination** (ability to differentiate and identify objects based on their individual attributes, e.g., size, shape, color, form, position), and **visual closure** (ability to recognize or identify an object even when the entire object cannot be seen). Visual-spatial processing dysfunctions are rarely the cause of reading disorders, but some investigations have established that deficits in orthographic coding (visual-spatial analysis of character-based systems) can contribute to reading disorders. Spelling and writing can emerge as a weakness because children with visual processing problems usually have trouble with the precise visual configurations of words. In mathematics, these children often have difficulty with visual-spatial orientation, with resultant difficulty aligning digits in columns when performing calculations and difficulty managing geometric material. In the social realm, intact visual processing allows a child to make use of visual or physical cues when communicating and interpreting the paralinguistic aspects of language. Secure visual functions are also necessary to process proprioceptive and kinesthetic feedback and to coordinate movements during physical activities.

Intellectual Function

A useful definition of **intellectual function** is the capacity to think in the abstract, reason, problem-solve, and comprehend. The concept of intelligence has had many definitions and theoretical models, including Spearman's unitary concept of "the g-factor," the "verbal and nonverbal" theories (e.g., Binet, Thorndike), the 2-factor theory from Catell (crystallized vs fluid intelligence), Luria's simultaneous and successive processing model, and more recent models that view intelligence as a global construct composed of more-specific cognitive functions (e.g., auditory and visual-perceptual processing, spatial abilities, processing speed, working memory).

The expression of intellect is mediated by many factors, including language development, sensorimotor abilities, genetics, heredity, environment, and neurodevelopmental function. When an individual's measured intelligence is >2 standard deviations below the mean (a standard score of <70 on most IQ tests) and accompanied by significant weaknesses in adaptive skills, the diagnosis of **intellectual disability** may be warranted (see Chapter 53).

Functionally, some common characteristics distinguish children with deficient intellectual functioning from those with average or above-average abilities. Typically, those at the lowest end of the spectrum (e.g., profound or severe intellectual deficiencies) are incapable of independent function and require a highly structured environment with constant aid and supervision. At the other end of the spectrum are those with unusually well-developed intellect ("gifted"). Although this level of intellectual functioning offers many opportunities, it can also be associated with functional challenges related to socialization and learning and communication style. Individuals whose intellect falls in the below-average range (sometimes referred to as the "borderline" or "slow learner" range) tend to experience greater difficulty processing and managing information that is abstract, making connections between concepts and ideas, and generalizing information (e.g., may be able to comprehend a concept in one setting but are unable to carry it over and apply it in different situation). In general, these individuals tend to do better when information is presented in more concrete and explicit terms, and when working with rote information (e.g., memorizing specific material). Stronger intellect has been associated with better-developed concept formation, critical thinking, problem solving, understanding and formulation of rules, brainstorming and creativity, and *metacognition* (ability to "think about thinking").

Memory

Memory is a term used to describe the cognitive mechanism by which information is acquired, retained, and recalled. Structurally, some major brain areas involved in memory processing include the hippocampus, fornix, temporal lobes, and cerebellum, with connections in and between most brain regions. The memory system can be partitioned into subsystems based on processing sequences; the form, time span, and method of recall; whether memories are conscious or unconsciously recalled; and the types of memory impairments that can occur.

Once information has been identified (through auditory, visual, tactile, and/or other sensory processes), it needs to be **encoded and registered**, a mental process that constructs a representation of the information into the memory system. The period (typically seconds) during which this information is being held and/or manipulated for registration, and ultimately encoded, consolidated, and retained, is referred to as **working memory**. Other descriptors include **short-term memory** and **immediate memory**. **Consolidation** and **storage** represent the process by which information in short-term memory is transferred into **long-term memory**. Information in long-term memory can be available for hours or as long as a life span. Long-term memories are generally thought to be housed, in whole or in part, in specific brain regions (e.g., cortex, cerebellum). Ordinarily, consolidation in long-term memory is accomplished in 1 or more of 4 ways: pairing 2 bits of information (e.g., a group of letters and the English sound it represents); storing procedures (consolidating new skills, e.g., the steps in solving mathematics problems); classifying data in categories (filing all insects together in memory); and linking new information to established rules, patterns, or systems of organization (rule-based learning).

Once information finds its way into long-term memory, it must be accessed. In general, information can be retrieved spontaneously (a process known as **free recall**) or with the aid of cues (**cued or recognition recall**). Some other common descriptors of memory include **anterograde memory** (capacity to learn from a single point in time forward), **retrograde memory** (capacity to recall information that was already learned), and **explicit memory** (conscious awareness of recall), **implicit memory** (subconscious recall: no awareness that the memory system is being activated), **procedural memory** (memory for how to do things), and **prospective memory** or *remembering to remember*. **Automatization** reflects the ability to instantaneously access what has been learned in the past with no expenditure of effort. Successful students are able to automatically form letters, master mathematical facts, and decode words.

Social Cognition

The development of effective social skills is heavily dependent on secure **social cognition,** which consists of mental processes that allow an individual to understand and interact with the social environment. Although some evidence shows that social cognition exists as a discrete area of neurodevelopmental function, multiple cognitive processes are involved with social cognition. These include the ability to recognize, interpret, and make sense of the thoughts, communications (verbal and nonverbal), and actions of others; the ability to understand that others' perceptions, perspectives, and intentions might differ from one's own (commonly referred to as "theory of mind"); the ability to use language to communicate with others socially (pragmatic language); and the ability to make inferences about others and the environment based on contextual information. It can also be argued that social cognition involves processes associated with memory and EFs such as flexibility.

Executive Function

The development of EFs begins very early on in the developmental course (early indications of inhibitory control and even working memory have been found in infancy), matures significantly during the preschool years, and continues to develop through adolescence and well into adulthood. Some studies suggest that secure EF may be more important than intellectual ability for academic success and have revealed that a child's ability to delay gratification early in life predicts competency, attention, self-regulation, frustration tolerance, aptitude, physical and mental health, and even substance dependency in adolescence and adulthood. Conversely, deficits in other areas of neurodevelopment, such as language development, impact EF.

Attention is far from a unitary, independent, or specific brain function. This may be best illustrated through the phenotype associated with ADHD) (see Chapter 49). Disordered attention can result from faulty mechanisms in and across subdomains of attention. These subdomains include *selective* attention (ability to focus attention on a particular stimulus and to discriminate relevant from irrelevant information), *divided* attention (ability to orient to more than one stimulus at a given time), *sustained* attention (ability to maintain one's focus), and *alternating* attention (capacity to shift focus between stimuli).

Attention problems in children can manifest at any point, from arousal through output. Children with diminished alertness and arousal can exhibit signs of mental fatigue in a classroom or when engaged in any activity requiring sustained focus. They are apt to have difficulty allocating and sustaining their concentration, and their efforts may be erratic and unpredictable, with extreme performance inconsistency. Weaknesses of determining saliency often result in focusing on the wrong stimuli, at home, in school, and socially, and missing important information. **Distractibility** can take the form of listening to extraneous noises instead of a teacher, staring out the window, or constantly thinking about the future. Attention dysfunction can affect the output of work, behavior, and social activity. It is important to appreciate that most children with attentional dysfunction also harbor other forms of neurodevelopmental dysfunction that can be associated with academic disorders (with some estimates suggesting up to 60% comorbidity).

Inhibitory control (IC) can be described as one's ability to restrain, resist, and not act (cognitively or behaviorally/emotionally) on a thought. IC may also be seen as one's ability to stop thoughts or ongoing actions. Deficits in this behavioral/impulse regulation mechanism are a core feature of the **combined** or **hyperactive impulsive** presentation of ADHD and have a significant adverse impact on a child's overall functioning. In everyday settings, children with weak IC may exhibit difficulties with self-control and self-monitoring of their behavior and output (e.g., impulsivity), may not recognize their own errors or mistakes, and often act prematurely and without consideration of the potential consequences of their actions. In the social context, disinhibited children may interrupt others and demonstrate other impulsive behaviors that often interfere with interpersonal relationships. The indirect consequences of poor IC often lead to challenges with behavior, emotional, and academic functioning and social interaction (Table 48.1).

Working memory (WM) can be defined as the ability to hold, manipulate, and store information for short periods. This function is critical to be able to complete multistep problems and more complex instructions and tasks. In its simplest form, WM involves the interaction of short-term verbal and visual processes (e.g., memory, phonologic, awareness, and spatial skills) with a centralized control mechanism that is responsible for coordinating all the cognitive processes involved (e.g., temporarily suspending information in memory while working with it). Developmentally, WM capacity can double or triple between the preschool years and adolescence. When doing math, a child with WM dysfunction might carry a number and then forget what he intended to do after carrying that number. WM is an equally important underlying function for reading, where it enables the child to remember the beginning of a paragraph when she arrives at the end of it. In writing, WM helps children remember what they intend to express in written form while they are performing another task, such as placing a comma or working on spelling a word correctly. WM also enables the linkage between new incoming information in short-term memory with prior

Table 48.1	Symptom Expression of Executive Dysfunction
EXECUTIVE FUNCTION DEFICIT	**SYMPTOM EXPRESSION**
Disinhibition	Impulsivity/poor behavioral regulation Interrupts "Blurts things out"
Shifting	Problems with transitioning from one task/activity to another Unable to adjust to unexpected change Repeats unsuccessful problem-solving approaches
Initiation	Difficulty independently beginning tasks/activities Lacks initiative Difficulty developing ideas or making decisions
Working memory	Challenges following multistep instruction (e.g., only completes 1 of 3 steps) Forgetfulness
Organization and planning	Fails to plan ahead Work is often disorganized Procrastinates and does not complete tasks "Messy" child
Self-monitoring	Fails to recognize errors and check work Does not appreciate impact of actions on others Poor self-awareness
Affect control	Experiences behavioral and emotional outbursts (e.g., tantrums) Easily upset/frustrated Frequent mood changes

knowledge or skills held in longer-term memory.

Initiation refers to the ability to independently begin an activity, a task, or thought process (e.g., problem-solve). Children who present with initiation difficulties often have trouble "getting going" or "getting started." This can be exhibited behaviorally, such that the child struggles to start on physical activities such as getting out of bed or beginning chores. Cognitively, weaknesses in initiation may manifest as difficulty coming up with ideas or generating plans. In school, children who have poor initiation abilities may be delayed in or unable to start homework assignments or tests. In social situations, initiation challenges may cause a child to have difficulty beginning conversations, calling on friends, or going out to be with friends.

Deficits in "primary" initiation are relatively rare and are often associated with significant neurologic conditions and treatments (e.g., traumatic brain injury, anoxia, effects of radiation treatment in childhood cancer). More often, initiation deficits are secondary to other executive problems (e.g., disorganization) or behavioral (e.g., oppositional/defiant behaviors), developmental (e.g., autism spectrum disorder), or emotional (e.g., depression, anxiety) disorders.

Planning refers to the ability to effectively generate, sequence, and put into motion the steps and procedures necessary to realize a specific goal. In real-world settings, children who struggle with planning are typically described by caregivers and teachers as being inept at independently gathering what is required to solve a problem, or as unable to complete more weighty assignments. Another common complaint is that these children exhibit poor time management skills. **Organization** is an ability that represents a child's proficiency in arranging, ordering, classifying, and categorizing information. Common daily life challenges associated with organizational difficulties in childhood include problems with gathering and managing materials or items. When children struggle with organization, indirect consequences may include becoming overwhelmed with information and being unable to complete a task or activity. Effective organization is a vital component in learning (more specifically, in memory/retention); many studies along with clinical experience have shown that poor organization significantly impacts how well a child recalls information. Planning and organizing depend on **discrimination** ability, which refers to the child's ability to determine what is and is not valuable when trying to problem-solve or organize.

Emotional control is the ability to regulate emotions in order to realize goals and direct one's behavior, thoughts, and actions. It has been well established that affective/emotional states have an impact on many aspects of functioning. Conversely, executive function or dysfunction often contributes to modulation or affect. While emotional control is highly interrelated with different EFs (e.g., disinhibition, self-monitoring), separating it conceptually facilitates an appreciation for and recognition of the often-overlooked role that a child's emotional state plays in cognitive and behavioral functioning. Children with weak emotional control may exhibit explosive outbursts, poor temper/anger control, and oversensitivity. Clearly, understanding a child's emotional state is vital to understanding its impact not only on executive functioning, but also on functioning as a whole (e.g., socially, mentally, behaviorally, academically).

Any discussion involving emotional control should also recognize **motivation**. *Motivation/effort* may be defined as the reason or reasons one acts or behaves in a certain way. Less motivated children are less likely to engage and utilize all their abilities. Such a disposition not only interferes with application of executive skills, but also results in less than optimal performance and functioning. The less success a child feels, the less likely the child is to put forth effort and to persevere when things become more challenging. If a child's initial efforts are met with a negative reaction, the likelihood that the child will continue putting forth adequate effort diminishes. If left unchecked, a child's overall level of functioning will likely be compromised. More importantly, the child's sense of personal efficacy (e.g., self-esteem) and competence may suffer.

CLINICAL MANIFESTATIONS

The symptoms and clinical manifestations of neurodevelopmental and executive dysfunction differ with age. **Preschool-age children** might

present with delayed language development, including problems with articulation, vocabulary development, word finding, and rhyming. They often experience early challenges with learning colors, shapes, letters, and numbers; the alphabet; and days of the week. Children with visual processing deficits may have difficulty learning to draw and write and have problems with art activities. These children might also have trouble discriminating between left and right. They might encounter problems recognizing letters and words. Difficulty following instructions, overactivity, and distractibility may be early symptoms of emerging executive dysfunction. Difficulties with fine motor development (e.g., grasping crayons/pencils, coloring, drawing) and social interaction may develop.

School-age children with neurodevelopmental and executive dysfunctions can vary widely in clinical presentations. Their specific patterns of academic performance and behavior represent final common pathways of neurodevelopmental strengths and deficits interacting with environmental, social, or cultural factors; temperament; educational experience; and intrinsic resilience (Table 48.2). Children with language weaknesses might have problems integrating and associating letters and sounds, decoding words, deriving meaning, and being able to comprehend passages. Children with early signs of a mathematics weakness might have difficulty with concepts of quantity or with adding or subtracting without using concrete representation (e.g., their fingers when calculating). Difficulty learning time concepts and confusion with directions (right/left) might also be observed. Poor fine motor control and coordination and poor planning can lead to writing problems. Attention and behavioral regulation weaknesses observed earlier can continue, and together with other executive functioning weaknesses (e.g., organization, initiation skills), further complicate the child's ability to acquire and generalize new knowledge. Children with weaknesses in WM may struggle to remember the steps necessary to complete an activity or problem-solve. In social settings, these children often have difficulty keeping up with more complex conversations.

Table 48.2	Neurodevelopmental Dysfunction Underlying Academic Disorders*
ACADEMIC DISORDER	**POTENTIAL UNDERLYING NEURODEVELOPMENTAL DYSFUNCTION**

Reading	Language
	    Phonologic processing
	    Verbal fluency
	    Syntactic and semantic skills
	Memory
	    Working memory
	Sequencing
	Visual-spatial
	Attention

Written expression, spelling	Language
	    Phonologic processing
	    Syntactic and semantic skills
	Graphomotor
	Visual-spatial
	Memory
	    Working memory
	Sequencing
	Attention

Mathematics	Visual-spatial Memory Working memory Language Sequencing Graphomotor Attention

*Isolated neurodevelopmental dysfunction can lead to a specific academic disorder, but more often there is a combination of factors underlying weak academic performance. In addition to the dysfunction in neurodevelopmental domains as listed in the table, the clinician must also consider the possibility of limitations of intellectual and cognitive abilities or associated social and emotional problems.

In **middle school children** the shift in cognitive, academic, and regulatory demands can cause further difficulties for those with existing neurodevelopmental and executive challenges. In reading and writing, middle school children might present with transposition and sequencing errors; might struggle with root words, prefixes, and suffixes; might have difficulty with written expression; and might avoid reading and writing altogether. Challenges completing word problems in math are common. Difficulty with recall of information might also be experienced. Although observable in both lower and more advanced grades, behavioral, emotional, and social difficulties tend to become more salient in middle school children who experience cognitive or academic problems.

High school students can present with deficient reading comprehension, written expression, and slower processing efficiency. Difficulty in answering open-ended questions, dealing with abstract information, and producing executive control (e.g., self-monitoring, organization, planning, self-starting) is often reported.

Academic Problems

Reading disorders (see Chapter 50) can stem from any number of neurodevelopmental dysfunctions, as described earlier (see Table 48.2). Most often, language and auditory processing weaknesses are present, as evidenced by poor phonologic processing that results in deficiencies at the level of decoding individual words and, consequently, a delay in *automaticity* (e.g., acquiring a repertoire of words readers can identify instantly) that causes reading to be slow, laborious, and frustrating. Deficits in other core neurodevelopmental domains might also be present. Weak WM might make it difficult for a child to hold sounds and symbols in mind while breaking down words into their component sounds, or might cause reading comprehension problems. Some children experience temporal-ordering weaknesses and struggle with reblending phonemes into correct sequences. Memory dysfunction can cause problems with recall and summarization of what was read. Some children with higher-order cognitive deficiencies have trouble understanding what they read because they lack a strong grasp of the concepts in a text. Although relatively rare as a cause of reading difficulty, problems with visual-spatial functions (e.g., visual perception) can cause children difficulty in recognizing letters. It is not unusual for children with reading problems to avoid reading practice, and a delay in reading proficiency becomes increasingly pronounced and difficult to remediate.

Spelling and writing impairments share many related underlying processing deficits with reading, so it is not surprising that the 2 disorders often occur simultaneously in school-age children (see Table 48.2). Core neurodevelopmental weaknesses that underlie *spelling difficulties* include phonologic and decoding difficulties, orthographic problems (coding letters and words into memory), and morphologic deficits (use of suffixes, prefixes, and root words). Problems in these areas can manifest as phonetically poor, yet visually comparable approximations to the actual word (*faght* for *fight*), spelling that is phonetically correct but visually incorrect (*fite* for *fight*), and inadequate spelling patterns (*played* as *plade*). Children with memory disorders might misspell words because of coding weaknesses. Others misspell because of poor auditory WM that interferes with their ability to process letters. Sequencing weaknesses often result in transposition errors when spelling.

Writing difficulties have been classified as **disorder of written expression**, or **dysgraphia** (see Table 48.2). Although many of the same dysfunctions described for reading and spelling can contribute to problems with writing, written expression is the most complex of the language arts, requiring synthesis of many neurodevelopmental functions (e.g., auditory, visual-spatial, memory, executive; see Chapter 51.2). Weaknesses in these functions can result in written output that is difficult to comprehend, disjointed, and poorly organized. The child with WM challenges can lose track of what the child intended to write. Attention deficits can make it difficult for a child to mobilize and sustain the mental effort, pacing, and self-monitoring demands necessary for writing. In many cases, writing is laborious because of an underlying *graphomotor dysfunction* (e.g., fluency does not keep pace with ideation and language production). Thoughts may also be forgotten or underdeveloped during writing because the mechanical effort is so taxing.

Weaknesses in mathematical ability, known as **mathematics disorder** or **dyscalculia**, require early intervention because math involves the assimilation of both procedural knowledge (e.g., calculations) and higher-order cognitive processes (e.g., WM) (see Table 48.2). There are many reasons why children experience failure in mathematics (see Chapter 51.1). It may be difficult for some to grasp and apply math concepts effectively and systematically; good mathematicians are able to use both verbal and perceptual conceptualization to understand such concepts as fractions, percentages, equations, and proportion. Children with language dysfunctions have difficulty in mathematics because they have trouble understanding their teachers' verbal explanations of quantitative concepts and operations and are likely to experience frustration in solving word problems and in processing the vast network of technical vocabulary in math. Mathematics also relies on visualization. Children who have difficulty forming and recalling visual imagery may be at a disadvantage in acquiring mathematical skills. They might experience problems writing numbers correctly, placing value locations, and processing geometric shapes or fractions. Children with executive dysfunction may be unable to focus on fine detail (e.g., operational signs), might take an impulsive approach to problem solving, engage in little or no self-monitoring, forget components of the problem, or commit careless errors. When a child's memory system is weak, the child might have difficulty recalling appropriate procedures and automatizing mathematical facts (e.g., multiplication tables). Moreover, children with mathematical disabilities can have superimposed mathematics **phobias**; anxiety over mathematics can be especially debilitating.

Nonacademic Problems

The impulsivity and lack of effective self-monitoring of children with executive dysfunction can lead to unacceptable actions that were unintentional. Children struggling with neurodevelopmental dysfunction can experience excessive performance anxiety, sadness, or clinical depression; declining self-esteem; and chronic fatigue. Some children lose motivation. They tend to give up and exhibit **learned helplessness**, a sense that they have no control over their destiny. Therefore they feel no need to exert effort and develop future goals. These children may be easily led toward dysfunctional interpersonal relationships, detrimental behaviors (e.g., delinquency), and the development of mental health disorders, such as mood disorders (see Chapter 39) or conduct disorder (Chapter 42).

ASSESSMENT AND DIAGNOSIS

Pediatricians have a critical role in identifying and treating the child with neurodevelopmental or executive dysfunction (Fig. 48.1). They have knowledge of the child's medical and family history and social-environmental circumstances and have the benefit of longitudinal contact over the course of routine health visits. Focused **surveillance and screening** will lead to early identification of developmental-behavioral and preacademic difficulties and interventions to facilitate optimal outcomes.

A **family history** of a parent who still struggles with reading or time management, or an older sibling who has failed at school, should spur an increased level of monitoring. **Risk factors** in the medical history, such as extreme prematurity or chronic medical conditions, should likewise be flagged. Children with low birthweight and those born prematurely who appear to have been spared more serious neurologic problems might only manifest academic problems later in their school career. **Nonspecific physical complaints** or unexpected **changes in behavior** might be presenting symptoms. Warning signs might be subtle or absent, and parents might have concerns about their child's learning progress but may be reluctant to share these with the pediatrician unless prompted, such as through completion of **standardized developmental screening questionnaires** or direct questioning regarding possible concerns. There should be a low threshold for initiating further school performance screening and assessment if there are any "red flags."

Review of **school report cards** can provide very useful information. In addition to patterns of grades in the various academic skill areas, it is also important to review ratings of classroom behavior and work habits. Group-administered **standardized tests** provide further

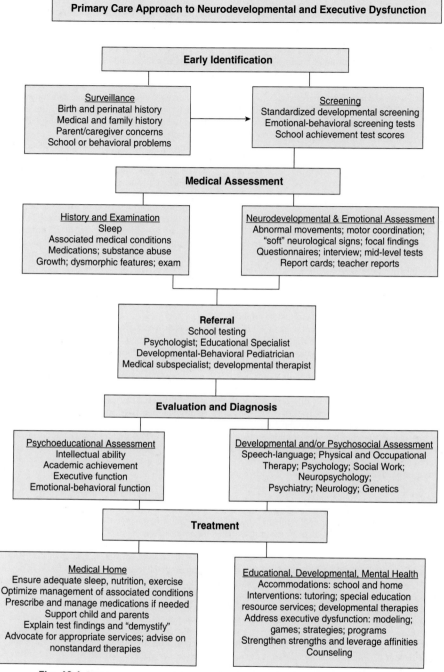

Fig. 48.1 Primary care approach to neurodevelopmental and executive dysfunction.

information, although interpretation is required because poor scores could result from a learning disorder, ADHD, anxiety, lack of motivation, or some combination. Conversely, a discrepancy between above-average scores on standardized tests and unsatisfactory classroom performance could signal motivation or adjustment issues. Challenges related to **homework** can provide further insight regarding executive, academic skill, and behavioral factors.

Underlying or associated medical problems should be ruled out. Any suspicion of sensory difficulty should warrant referral for **vision or hearing testing**. The influence of chronic medical problems or potential side effects of medications should be considered. **Sleep deprivation** is increasingly being recognized as a contributor to academic problems, especially in middle and high school. **Substance abuse** must always be a consideration as well, especially in the adolescent previously achieving well who has shown a rapid decline in academic performance.

The physician should be alert for dysmorphic physical features, minor congenital anomalies, or constellations of physical findings (e.g., cardiac and palatal anomalies in velocardiofacial syndrome) and should perform a detailed neurologic examination, including an assessment of fine and gross motor coordination and any involuntary movements or soft neurologic signs. Special investigations (e.g., genetic deletion-duplication microarray, electroencephalogram, MRI) are not always indicated in the absence of specific medical findings or a family history. Measures of brain function, such as functional MRI, offer insight into possible areas of neurodevelopmental dysfunction but remain primarily research tools.

Early signs of executive dysfunction can also be subtle and easily overlooked or misinterpreted. Informal inquiry might include questions about how children complete schoolwork or tasks, how organized or disorganized they are, how much guidance they need, whether they think through problems or respond and react too quickly, what circumstances or individuals affect their ability to employ EFs, how easily they begin tasks and activities, and how well they plan, manage belongings, and control their emotions.

Pediatricians who are interested in performing further assessment before referral, or who are practicing in areas where psychological testing resources are limited, can utilize standardized rating scales and inventories or brief, individually administered tests to narrow potential diagnoses and guide next steps in diagnosis and treatment. Such instruments, completed by the parents, teachers, and the child (if old enough), can provide information about emotions and behavior, patterns of academic performance, and traits associated with specific neurodevelopmental dysfunctions (see Chapter 32). Screening instruments such as the *Pediatric Symptom Checklist* and behavioral questionnaires such as the *Child Behavior Checklist* (CBCL) and *Behavior Assessment System for Children, Second Edition* (BASC-2) can aid in evaluation. Instruments more specifically focused on academic disorders, such as the *Learning Disabilities Diagnostic Inventory,* can be completed by the child's teacher to reveal the extent to which skill patterns in a particular area (e.g., reading, writing) are consistent with those of individuals known to have a learning disability.

Executive functions can be further assessed by instruments such as the *Behavior Rating Inventory of Executive Function, Second Edition* (BRIEF2), which provides a comprehensive measure of real-world behaviors that are closely tied to executive functioning in children age 5-18 yr. An alternative rating inventory of EF in children is the *Comprehensive Executive Function Inventory* (CEFI). Tests that can be directly administered to gauge intellectual functioning include the *Kaufman Brief Intelligence Test, Second Edition* (KBIT-2) and *Peabody Picture Vocabulary Test, Fourth Edition* (PPVT 4; assessing receptive vocabulary). A relatively brief test of academic skills is the *Wide Range Achievement Test 4* (WRAT4). It should be recognized that these are midlevel tests that can provide descriptive estimates of function but are not diagnostic.

Children who are struggling academically are entitled to evaluations in school. Such assessments are guaranteed in the United States under Public Law 101-476, the **Individuals with Disabilities Education Act (IDEA)**. One increasingly common type of evaluation supported by IDEA is referred to as a **response to intervention (RtI)** model (see Chapter 51.1). In this model, students who are struggling with academic skills are initially provided research-based instruction. If a child does not respond to this instruction, an individualized evaluation by a multidisciplinary team is conducted. Children found to have attentional dysfunction and other disorders might qualify for educational accommodations in the regular classroom under Section 504 of the Rehabilitation Act of 1973 (**504 plan**).

The pediatrician should advise and support parents regarding steps to request evaluations by the school. Multidisciplinary evaluations are focused primarily on determining whether a student meets the eligibility criteria for special education services and to assist in developing an **individualized educational plan (IEP)** for those eligible for these services. Independent evaluations can provide second opinions outside the school setting. The multidisciplinary team should include a psychologist and preferably an educational diagnostician who can undertake a detailed analysis of academic skills and subskills to pinpoint where breakdowns are occurring in the processes of reading, spelling, writing, and mathematics. Other professionals should become involved, as needed,

such as a speech-language pathologist, occupational therapist, and social worker. A mental health specialist can be valuable in identifying family-based issues or psychiatric disorders that may be complicating or aggravating neurodevelopmental dysfunctions.

In some cases, more in-depth examination of a child's **neurocognitive status** is warranted. This is particularly true for children who present with developmental or cognitive difficulties in the presence of a medical condition (e.g., epilepsy, traumatic brain injury, childhood cancers/brain tumors, genetic conditions). A **neuropsychological evaluation** involves comprehensive assessment to understand brain functions across domains. Neuropsychological data are often analyzed together with other tests, such as MRI, to look for supporting evidence of any areas of difficulty (e.g., memory weaknesses associated with temporal lobe anomalies). Neuropsychologists can also provide more in-depth evaluation of EFs. Assessment of EFs is typically completed in an examination setting using tools specifically designed to identify any weaknesses in these functions. Although few tools are currently available to assess EF in preschool-age children, the assessment of school-age children is better established. Problems with EFs should be evaluated across measures and in different settings, particularly within the context of the child's daily demands.

TREATMENT

In addition to addressing any underlying or associated medical problems, the pediatrician can play an important role as a **consultant and advocate** in overseeing and monitoring the implementation of a comprehensive multidisciplinary management plan for children with neurodevelopmental dysfunctions. Most children require several of the following forms of intervention.

Demystification

Many children with neurodevelopmental dysfunctions have little or no understanding of the nature or sources of their academic difficulties. Once an appropriate descriptive assessment has been performed, it is important to explain to the child the nature of the dysfunction while delineating the child's strengths. This explanation should be provided in nontechnical language, communicating a sense of optimism and a desire to be helpful and supportive.

Bypass Strategies (Accommodations)

Numerous techniques can enable a child to circumvent neurodevelopmental dysfunctions. Such bypass strategies are ordinarily used in the regular classroom. Examples of bypass strategies include using a calculator while solving mathematical problems, writing essays with a word processor, presenting oral instead of written reports, solving fewer mathematical problems, being seated near the teacher to minimize distraction, presenting correctly solved mathematical problems visually, and taking standardized tests untimed. These bypass strategies do not cure neurodevelopmental dysfunctions, but they minimize their academic and nonacademic effects and can provide a scaffold for more successful academic achievement.

Treatment of Neurodevelopmental Dysfunctions

Interventions can be implemented at home and in school to strengthen the weak links in academic skills. Reading specialists, mathematics tutors, and other professionals can use diagnostic data to select techniques that use a student's neurodevelopmental strengths to improve decoding skills, writing ability, or mathematical computation skills. **Remediation** need not focus exclusively on specific academic areas. Many students need assistance in acquiring study skills, cognitive strategies, and productive organizational habits.

Early identification is critical so that appropriate instructional interventions can be introduced to minimize the long-term effects of academic disorders. Any interventions should be empirically supported (e.g., phonologically based reading intervention has been shown to significantly improve reading skills in school-age children). Remediation may take place in a resource room or learning center at school and is usually limited to children who have met the educational criteria for special education resource services described earlier.

Interventions that can be implemented at home could include drills to aid the automatization of subskills, such as arithmetic facts or letter formations, or the use of phonologically based reading programs.

Treatment of Executive Dysfunction

Interventions to strengthen EFs can be implemented throughout childhood but are most effective if started at a young age. Preschool-age children first experience EFs by way of the **modeling, boundaries, and rules** observed and put in place by their parents/caregivers, and this modeled behavior must gradually become "internalized" by the child. Early **play** has been shown to be effective in promoting executive skills in younger children with games such as peek-a-boo (WM); pat-a-cake (WM and IC); follow the leader, Simon says, and "ring around the rosie" (self-control); imitation activities (attention and impulse control); matching and sorting games (organization and attention); and imaginary play (attention, WM, IC, self-monitoring, cognitive flexibility).

In school-age children it is crucial to establish consistent **cognitive and behavioral routines** that foster and maximize independent, goal-oriented problem solving and performance through mechanisms that include modification of the child's environment, modeling and guidance with the child, and positive reinforcement strategies. Interventions should promote **generalization** (teaching executive routines in the context of a problem, not as a separate skill) and should move from the external to the internal (from "external support" with active and directive modeling to an "internal process"). An intervention could proceed from external modeling of multistep problem-solving routines and external guidance in developing and implementing everyday routines, to practicing application and use of routines in everyday situations, to a gradual fading of external support and cueing of internal generation and use of executive skills. Such approaches should make the child a part of

intervention planning, should avoid labeling, reward effort not outcomes, make interventions positive, and hold the child responsible for his or her efforts. Studies have consistently shown that a combination of medication and behavioral treatments are most effective, although evidence for long term efficacy is lacking. It is important that any treatment plans aimed at bolstering attention and executive functioning also include interventions that address the specific deficits associated with any comorbid diagnoses.

In addition to behavioral approaches, computerized **training programs** have been shown to strengthen WM skills in children using a computer game model. Generalized and lasting improvements in WM have been reported. Also evidencing positive outcomes are curriculum-based **classroom programs**, such as the *Tools of the Mind* (Tools) and *Promoting Alternative Thinking Strategies* (PATHS). Other promising approaches to EF intervention include **aerobic exercise,** shown to improve EFs through prefrontal cortex stimulation. **Martial arts** such as tae kwon do, which stresses discipline and self-regulation, has demonstrated improvements that generalize in many aspects of EFs and attention (e.g., sustained focus). Approaches that use **mindfulness techniques** are also gaining prominence. Formal **parenting interventions** have also demonstrated strong evidence for effectiveness. Four programs that have the most empirical support are the *Triple P, Parent-Child Interaction Therapy* (PCIT), *Incredible Years,* and *New Forest Parenting Programme.*

Table 48.3 outlines interventions to target the specific components of EF. Although interventions may target each component separately, success will be determined by how well treatments can be integrated across settings and generalized to other areas of function. Whenever possible, working with more than one EF simultaneously is encouraged as a means of scaffolding intervention and building on previously mastered skills.

Table 48.3	Executive Function Categories: Presenting Symptoms, Suggested Dysfunction, and Potential Interventions	
SYMPTOM/PRESENTING COMPLAINT	**SUSPECTED AREA OF DYSFUNCTION**	**POSSIBLE "REAL WORLD" INTERVENTIONS**
Acts before thinking Interrupts Poor behavioral and/or emotional control	Disinhibition/impulsivity	Increase structure in environment to set limits for inhibition problems. Make behavior and work expectations clear and explicit; review with child. Post rules in view; point to them when child breaks rule. Teach response-delay techniques (e.g., counting to 10 before acting).
Cannot follow multistep instructions Forgetful	Working memory	Repeat instructions as needed. Keep instructions clear and concise. Provide concrete references.
Struggles starting assignments/tasks Lacks initiative/motivation Has trouble developing ideas/ strategies	Initiation	Increase structure of tasks. Establish and rely on routine. Break tasks into smaller, manageable steps. Place child with partner or group for modeling and cuing from peers.
Does not plan ahead Uses trial-and-error approach	Planning	Practice with tasks with only a few steps first. Teach simple flow charting as a planning tool. Practice with planning tasks (e.g., mazes). Ask child to verbalize plan before beginning work. Ask child to verbalize second plan if first does not work. Ask child to verbalize possible consequences of actions before beginning. Review incidents of poor planning/anticipation with child.
Work/belongings is/are "messy" Random/haphazard problem solving Procrastinates/does not complete tasks	Organization	Increase organization of classroom and activities to serve as model, and help child grasp structure of new information. Present framework of new information to be learned at the outset, and review again at the end of a lesson. Begin with tasks with only few steps and increase gradually.
Gets "stuck" Trouble transitioning Does not adapt to change	Flexibility/shifting	Increase routine to the day. Make schedule clear and public. Forewarn of any changes in schedule. Give "2-minute warning" of time to change. Make changes from one task to the next or one topic to the next, clear and explicit. Shifting may be a problem of inhibiting, so apply strategies for inhibition problems.

Developmental Therapy

Speech-language pathologists offer intervention for children with various forms of language disability. Occupational therapists focus on sensorimotor skills, including the motor skills of students with writing problems, and physical therapists address gross motor incoordination.

Curriculum Modifications

Many children with neurodevelopmental dysfunctions require alterations in the school curriculum to succeed, especially as they progress through secondary school. Students with memory weaknesses might need to have their courses selected for them so that they do not have an inordinate cumulative memory load in any single semester. The timing of foreign language learning, the selection of a mathematics curriculum, and the choice of science courses are critical issues for many of these struggling adolescents.

Strengthening of Strengths

Affected children need to have their affinities, potentials, and talents identified clearly and exploited widely. It is as important to augment strengths as it is to attempt to remedy deficiencies. Athletic skills, artistic inclinations, creative talents, and mechanical abilities are among the potential assets of certain students who are underachieving academically. Parents and school personnel need to create opportunities for such students to build on these assets and to achieve respect and praise for their efforts. These well-developed personal assets can ultimately have implications for the transition into young adulthood, including career or college selection.

Individual and Family Counseling

When academic difficulties are complicated by family problems or identifiable psychiatric disorders, **psychotherapy** may be indicated. Mental health professionals may offer long-term or short-term therapy. Such intervention may involve the child alone or the entire family. Cognitive-behavioral therapy is especially effective for mood and anxiety disorders. It is essential that the therapist have a firm understanding of the nature of a child's neurodevelopmental dysfunctions.

Nonstandard Therapies

A variety of treatment methods for neurodevelopmental dysfunctions have been proposed that currently have little to no known scientific evidence of efficacy. This list includes dietary interventions (vitamins, elimination of food additives or potential allergens), neuromotor programs or medications to address vestibular dysfunction, eye exercises, filters, tinted lenses, and various technologic devices. Parents should be cautioned against expending the excessive amounts of time and financial resources usually demanded by these remedies. In many cases, it is difficult to distinguish the nonspecific beneficial effects of increased support and attention paid to the child from the supposed target effects of the intervention.

Medication

Psychopharmacologic agents may be helpful in lessening the toll of some neurodevelopmental dysfunctions. Most often, **stimulants** are used in the treatment of children with attention deficits. Although most children with attention deficits have other associated dysfunctions, such as language disorders, memory problems, motor weaknesses, or social skill deficits, medications such as methylphenidate, dextroamphetamine, lisdexamfetamine, and mixed amphetamine salts, as well as nonstimulants such as α_2-**adrenergic agonists** and **atomoxetine**, can be important adjuncts to treatment by helping some children focus more selectively and control their impulsivity. When depression or excessive anxiety is a significant component of the clinical picture, **antidepressants** or **anxiolytics** may be helpful. Other drugs may improve behavioral control (see Chapter 33). Children receiving medication need regular follow-up visits that include a history to check for side effects, a review of current behavioral checklists, a complete physical examination, and appropriate modifications of the medication dose. Periodic trials off medication are recommended to establish whether the medication is still necessary.

Bibliography is available at Expert Consult.

Chapter **49**
Attention-Deficit/ Hyperactivity Disorder
David K. Urion

第四十九章
注意缺陷多动障碍

中文导读

本章主要介绍了注意缺陷多动障碍（ADHD）的病因学、流行病学、发病机制、临床表现、诊断及鉴别诊断、治疗、预后和预防。其中诊断及鉴别诊断主要包括临床问诊及病史分析、行为评定量表（行为评定量表在确定症状的严重程度和广泛性方面是有用的，但仅凭行为评定量表还不足以进行ADHD的诊断）、身体检查和实验室检查及鉴别诊断；治疗包括　心理治疗、行为治疗和药物治疗。

Attention-deficit/hyperactivity disorder (ADHD) is the most common neurobehavioral disorder of childhood, among the most prevalent chronic health conditions affecting school-aged children, and one of the most extensively studied neurodevelopmental disorders of childhood. ADHD is characterized by inattention, including increased distractibility and difficulty sustaining attention; poor impulse control and decreased self-inhibitory capacity; and motor overactivity and motor restlessness (Table 49.1 and Fig. 49.1). Definitions vary in different countries (Table 49.2). Affected children usually experience academic underachievement, problems with interpersonal relationships with family members and peers, and low self-esteem. ADHD often co-occurs with other emotional, behavioral, language, and learning disorders (Table 49.3). Evidence also suggests that for many people, the disorder continues with varying manifestations across the life cycle, leading to significant under- and unemployment, social dysfunction and increased risk of antisocial behaviors (e.g., substance abuse), difficulty maintaining relationships, encounters with the law, death from suicide, and, if untreated, accidents (Figs. 49.2 and 49.3).

ETIOLOGY
No single factor determines the expression of ADHD; ADHD may be a final common pathway for a variety of complex brain developmental processes. Mothers of children with ADHD are more likely to experience birth complications, such as toxemia, lengthy labor, and complicated delivery. Maternal drug use has also been identified as a risk factor in the development of ADHD. Maternal smoking, alcohol use during pregnancy, and prenatal or postnatal exposure to lead are frequently linked to the attentional difficulties associated with development of ADHD, but less clearly to hyperactivity. Food coloring and preservatives have inconsistently been associated with increased hyperactivity in children with ADHD.

There is a strong genetic component to ADHD. Genetic studies have primarily implicated 2 candidate genes, the dopamine transporter gene (*DAT1*) and a particular form of the dopamine 4 receptor gene (*DRD4*), in the development of ADHD. Additional genes that might contribute to ADHD include *DOCK2*, associated with a pericentric inversion 46N inv(3)(p14:q21) involved in cytokine regulation; a sodium-hydrogen exchange gene; and *DRD5, SLC6A3, DBH, SNAP25, SLC6A4*, and *HTR1B*.

Structural and functional abnormalities of the brain have been identified in children with ADHD. These include dysregulation of the frontal subcortical circuits, small cortical volumes in this region, widespread small-volume reduction throughout the brain, and abnormalities of the

Table 49.1	DSM-5 Diagnostic Criteria for Attention-Deficit/Hyperactivity Disorder (ADHD)

A. A persistent pattern of inattention and/or hyperactivity/impulsivity that interferes with functioning or development, as characterized by (1) and/or (2):
  1. **Inattention:** Six (or more) of the following symptoms of inattention have persisted for ≥6 mo to a degree that is inconsistent with development level and that negatively impacts directly on social and academic/occupational activities:
    a. Often fails to give close attention to details or makes careless mistakes in schoolwork, at work, or during other activities (e.g., overlooks or misses details, work is inaccurate).
    b. Often has difficulty sustaining attention in tasks or play activities.
    c. Often does not seem to listen when spoken to directly.
    d. Often does not follow through on instructions and fails to finish schoolwork, chores, or duties in the workplace (not due to oppositional behavior or failure to understand instructions).
    e. Often has difficulty organizing tasks and activities.
    f. Often avoids, dislikes, or is reluctant to engage in tasks that require sustained mental effort (e.g., schoolwork, homework).
    g. Often loses things necessary for tasks or activities (e.g., toys, school assignments, pencils, books, tools).
    h. Is often easily distracted by extraneous stimuli.
    i. Is often forgetful in daily activities.
  2. **Hyperactivity/impulsivity:** Six (or more) of the following symptoms of inattention have persisted for ≥6 mo to a degree that is inconsistent with development level and that negatively impacts directly on social and academic/occupational activities.
    a. Often fidgets with hands or feet or squirms in seat.
    b. Often leaves seat in classroom or in other situations in which remaining seated is expected.
    c. Often runs about or climbs excessively in situations in which it is inappropriate (in adolescents or adults, may be limited to subjective feelings of restlessness).
    d. Often has difficulty playing or engaging in leisure activities quietly.
    e. Is often "on the go" or often acts as if "driven by a motor."

f. Often talks excessively.
  Impulsivity.
    g. Often blurts out answers before questions have been completed.
    h. Often has difficulty awaiting turn.
    i. Often interrupts or intrudes on others (e.g., butts into conversations or games).
B. Several inattentive or hyperactive/impulsive symptoms were present before 12 yr of age.
C. Several inattentive or hyperactive/impulsive symptoms are present in 2 or more settings (e.g., at school [or work] or at home) and is documented independently.
D. There is clear evidence of clinically significant impairment in social, academic, or occupational functioning.
E. Symptoms do not occur exclusively during the course of schizophrenia, or another psychotic disorder, and are not better accounted for by another mental disorder (e.g., mood disorder, anxiety disorder, dissociative disorder, personality disorder, substance intoxication or withdrawal).

CODE BASED ON TYPE
314.01 Attention-deficit/hyperactivity disorder, combined presentation: if both Criteria A1 and A2 are met for the past 6 mo.
314.00 Attention-deficit/hyperactivity disorder, predominantly inattentive presentation: if Criterion A1 is met but Criterion A2 is not met for the past 6 mo.
314.01 Attention-deficit/hyperactivity disorder, predominantly hyperactive-impulsive presentation: if Criterion A2 is met but Criterion A1 is not met for the past 6 mo.
Specify if:
Mild: Few, if any, symptoms in excess of those required to make the diagnosis are present, and if the symptoms result in no more than minor impairments in social and occupational functioning.
Moderate: Symptoms or functional impairment between "mild" and "severe" are present.
Severe: Many symptoms in excess of those required to make the diagnosis, or several symptoms that are particularly severe, are present, or the symptoms result in marked impairment in social or occupational functioning.

From the *Diagnostic and Statistical Manual of Mental Disorders, Fourth Edition, Text Revision,* Washington, DC, 2000, and *Fifth Edition,* (Copyright 2013). American Psychiatric Association.

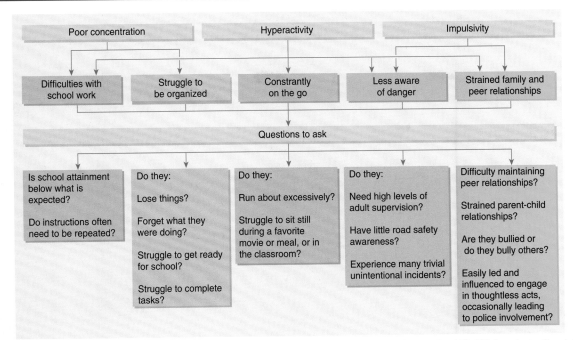

Fig. 49.1 How to assess children for attention-deficit/hyperactivity disorder. (*From Verkuijl N, Perkins M, Fazel M: Childhood attention-deficit/ hyperactivity disorder, BMJ 350:h2168, 2015, Fig 2, p 146.*)

Table 49.2	Differences Between U.S. and European Criteria for ADHD or HKD

DSM-5 ADHD	ICD-10 HKD
SYMPTOMS	
Either or both of the following: At least 6 of 9 inattentive symptoms At least 6 of 9 hyperactive or impulsive symptoms	*All of the following:* At least 6 of 8 inattentive symptoms At least 3 of 5 hyperactive symptoms At least 1 of 4 impulsive symptoms
PERVASIVENESS	
Some impairment from symptoms is present in >1 setting	Criteria are met for >1 setting

ADHD, Attention-deficit/hyperactivity disorder; HKD, hyperkinetic disorder; DSM-5, *Diagnostic and Statistical Manual of Mental Disorders, Fifth Edition*; ICD-10, *International Classification of Diseases, Tenth Edition.*
From Biederman J, Faraone S: Attention-deficit hyperactivity disorder, *Lancet* 366:237–248, 2005.

Table 49.3	Differential Diagnosis of Attention-Deficit/ Hyperactivity Disorder (ADHD)

PSYCHOSOCIAL FACTORS
Response to physical or sexual abuse
Response to inappropriate parenting practices
Response to parental psychopathology
Response to acculturation
Response to inappropriate classroom setting

DIAGNOSES ASSOCIATED WITH ADHD BEHAVIORS
Fragile X syndrome
Fetal alcohol syndrome
Pervasive developmental disorders
Obsessive-compulsive disorder
Gilles de la Tourette syndrome
Attachment disorder with mixed emotions and conduct

MEDICAL AND NEUROLOGIC CONDITIONS
Thyroid disorders (including general resistance to thyroid hormone)
Heavy metal poisoning (including lead)
Adverse effects of medications
Effects of abused substances
Sensory deficits (hearing and vision)
Auditory and visual processing disorders
Neurodegenerative disorder, especially leukodystrophies
Posttraumatic head injury
Postencephalitic disorder

Note: Coexisting conditions with possible ADHD presentation include oppositional defiant disorder, anxiety disorders, conduct disorder, depressive disorders, learning disorders, and language disorders. Presence of one or more of the symptoms of these disorders can fall within the spectrum of normal behavior, whereas a range of these symptoms may be problematic but fall short of meeting the full criteria for the disorder.
From Reiff MI, Stein MT: Attention-deficit/hyperactivity disorder evaluation and diagnosis: a practical approach in office practice, *Pediatr Clin North Am* 50:1019–1048, 2003. Adapted from Reiff MI: Attention-deficit/hyperactivity disorders. In Bergman AB, editor: *20 Common problems in pediatrics*, New York, 2001, McGraw-Hill, p 273.

cerebellum, particularly midline/vermian elements (see Pathogenesis). Brain injury also increases the risk of ADHD. For example, 20% of children with severe traumatic brain injury are reported to have subsequent onset of substantial symptoms of impulsivity and inattention. However, ADHD may also increase the risk of traumatic brain injury.

Psychosocial family stressors can also contribute to or exacerbate the symptoms of ADHD, including poverty, exposure to violence, and undernutrition or malnutrition.

EPIDEMIOLOGY
Studies of the prevalence of ADHD worldwide have generally reported that 5–10% of school-age children are affected, although rates vary considerably by country, perhaps in part because of differing sampling

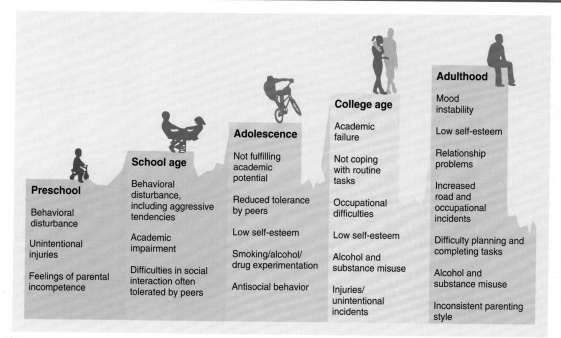

Fig. 49.2 Possible developmental impacts of attention-deficit/hyperactivity disorder. *(From Verkuijl N, Perkins M, Fazel M: Childhood attention-deficit/hyperactivity disorder, BMJ 350:h2168, 2015, Fig 1, p 145.)*

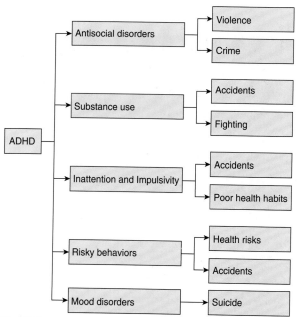

Fig. 49.3 Pathways to premature death in persons with attention-deficit/hyperactivity disorder (ADHD). *(From Faraone SV: Attention deficit hyperactivity disorder and premature death, Lancet 385:2132–2133, 2015.)*

and testing techniques. Rates may be higher if symptoms (inattention, impulsivity, hyperactivity) are considered in the absence of functional impairment. The prevalence rate in adolescent samples is 2–6%. Approximately 2% of adults meet criteria for ADHD. ADHD is often underdiagnosed in children and adolescents. Youth with ADHD are often undertreated with respect to what is known about the needed and appropriate doses of medications. Many children with ADHD also

present with comorbid neuropsychiatric diagnoses, including oppositional defiant disorder, conduct disorder, learning disabilities, and anxiety disorders. The incidence of ADHD appears increased in children with neurologic disorders such as the epilepsies, neurofibromatosis, and tuberous sclerosis (see Table 49.3).

PATHOGENESIS

Brain MRI studies in children with ADHD indicate a reduction or even loss of the normal hemispheric asymmetry in the brain, as well as smaller brain volumes of specific structures, such as the prefrontal cortex and basal ganglia. Children with ADHD have approximately a 5–10% reduction in the volume of these brain structures. MRI findings suggest low blood flow to the striatum. Functional MRI data suggest deficits in dispersed functional networks for selective and sustained attention in ADHD that include the striatum, prefrontal regions, parietal lobe, and temporal lobe. The prefrontal cortex and basal ganglia are rich in dopamine receptors. This knowledge, plus data about the dopaminergic mechanisms of action of medication treatment for ADHD, has led to the **dopamine hypothesis,** which postulates that disturbances in the dopamine system may be related to the onset of ADHD. Fluorodopa positron emission tomography (PET) scans also support the dopamine hypothesis through the identification of low levels of dopamine activity in adults with ADHD.

CLINICAL MANIFESTATIONS

Development of the *Diagnostic and Statistical Manual of Mental Disorders, Fifth Edition* (DSM-5) criteria leading to the diagnosis of ADHD has occurred mainly in field trials with children 5-12 yr of age (see Table 49.1 and Fig. 49.1). The DSM-5 notably expanded the accepted age of onset for symptoms of ADHD, and studies utilizing these broader criteria demonstrate a good correlation with data from DSM-IV criteria–based studies. The current DSM-5 criteria state that the behavior must be developmentally inappropriate (substantially different from that of other children of the same age and developmental level), must begin before age 12 yr, must be present for at least 6 mo, must be present in 2 or more settings and reported as such by independent observers, and must not be secondary to another disorder. DSM-5 identifies three presentations of ADHD. The **inattentive** presentation is more common in females and is associated with relatively high rates of internalizing symptoms (anxiety and low mood). The other two presentations, **hyperactive-impulsive** and **combined**, are more often diagnosed in males (see Fig. 49.1).

Clinical manifestations of ADHD may change with age (see Fig. 49.2). The symptoms may vary from motor restlessness and aggressive and disruptive behavior, which are common in preschool children, to disorganized, distractible, and inattentive symptoms, which are more typical in older adolescents and adults. ADHD is often difficult to diagnose in preschoolers because distractibility and inattention are often considered developmental norms during this period.

DIAGNOSIS AND DIFFERENTIAL DIAGNOSIS

A diagnosis of ADHD is made primarily in clinical settings after a thorough evaluation, including a careful history and clinical interview to rule in or to identify other causes or contributing factors; completion of behavior rating scales by different observers from at least 2 settings (e.g., teacher and parent); a physical examination; and any necessary or indicated laboratory tests that arise from conditions suspected based on history and/or physical examination. It is important to systematically gather and evaluate information from a variety of sources, including the child, parents, teachers, physicians, and when appropriate, other caretakers, over the course of both diagnosis and subsequent management.

Clinical Interview and History

The clinical interview allows a comprehensive understanding of whether the symptoms meet the diagnostic criteria for ADHD. During the interview, the clinician should gather information pertaining to the history of the presenting problems, the child's overall health and development, and the social and family history. The interview should emphasize factors that might affect the development or integrity of the central nervous system or reveal chronic illness, sensory impairments, sleep disorders, or medication use that might affect the child's functioning. Disruptive social factors, such as family discord, situational stress, and abuse or neglect, can result in hyperactive or anxious behaviors. A family history of first-degree relatives with ADHD, mood or anxiety disorders, learning disability, antisocial disorder, or alcohol or substance abuse might indicate an increased risk of ADHD and comorbid conditions.

Behavior Rating Scales

Behavior rating scales are useful in establishing the magnitude and pervasiveness of the symptoms, but are not sufficient alone to make a diagnosis of ADHD. A variety of well-established behavior rating scales have obtained good results in discriminating between children with ADHD and controls. These measures include, but are not limited to, the *Vanderbilt ADHD Diagnostic Rating Scale*, the *Conner Rating Scales* (parent and teacher), *ADHD Rating Scale 5*, the *Swanson, Nolan, and Pelham Checklist* (SNAP), and the *ADD-H: Comprehensive Teacher Rating Scale* (ACTeRS). Other broad-band checklists, such as the *Achenbach Child Behavior Checklist* (CBCL) or *Behavioral Assessment Scale for Children* (BASC), are useful, particularly when the child may be experiencing coexisting problems in other areas (anxiety, depression, conduct problems). Some, such as the BASC, include a validation scale to help determine the reliability of a given observer's assessment of the child.

Physical Examination and Laboratory Findings

No laboratory tests are available to identify ADHD in children. The presence of hypertension, ataxia, or symptoms of a sleep or thyroid disorder should prompt further neurologic or endocrine diagnostic evaluation. Impaired fine motor movement and poor coordination and other subtle neurologic motor signs (difficulties with finger tapping, alternating movements, finger-to-nose, skipping, tracing a maze, cutting paper) are common but not sufficiently specific to contribute to a diagnosis of ADHD. The clinician should also identify any possible vision or hearing problems. The clinician should consider testing for elevated lead levels in children who present with some or all of the diagnostic criteria, if these children are exposed to environmental factors that might put them at risk (substandard housing, old paint, proximity

to highway with deposition of lead in topsoil from automobile exhaust years ago). Behavior in the structured laboratory setting might not reflect the child's typical behavior in the home or school environment. Thus, computerized attentional tasks and electroencephalographic assessments are not needed to make the diagnosis, and compared to the clinical gold standard, these are subject to false-positive and false-negative errors. Similarly, observed behavior in a physician's office is not sufficient to confirm or rule-out the diagnosis of ADHD.

Differential Diagnosis

Chronic illnesses, such as migraine headaches, absence seizures, asthma/allergies, hematologic disorders, diabetes, and childhood cancer, affect up to 20% of U.S. children and can impair children's attention and school performance, because of either the disease itself or the medications used to treat or control the underlying illness (medications for asthma, corticosteroids, anticonvulsants, antihistamines) (see Table 49.3). In older children and adolescents, **substance abuse** can result in declining school performance and inattentive behavior (see Chapter 140).

Sleep disorders, including those secondary to chronic upper airway obstruction from enlarged tonsils and adenoids, often result in behavioral and emotional symptoms that can resemble or exacerbate ADHD (see Chapter 31). Periodic leg movements of sleep/restless leg syndrome has been associated with attentional symptoms, and inquiry regarding this should be made during the history. Behavioral and emotional disorders can cause disrupted sleep patterns as well.

Depression and anxiety disorders can cause many of the same symptoms as ADHD (inattention, restlessness, inability to focus and concentrate on work, poor organization, forgetfulness) but can also be comorbid conditions (see Chapters 38 and 39). Obsessive-compulsive disorder can mimic ADHD, particularly when recurrent and persistent thoughts, impulses, or images are intrusive and interfere with normal daily activities. Adjustment disorders secondary to major life stresses (death of a close family member, parents' divorce, family violence, parents' substance abuse, a move, shared social trauma such as bombings or other attacks) or parent–child relationship disorders involving conflicts over discipline, overt child abuse and/or neglect, or overprotection can result in symptoms similar to those of ADHD.

Although ADHD is believed to result from primary impairment of attention, impulse control, and motor activity, there is a high prevalence of comorbidity with other neuropsychiatric disorders (see Table 49.3). Of children with ADHD, 15–25% have learning disabilities, 30–35% have developmental language disorders, 15–20% have diagnosed mood disorders, and 20–25% have coexisting anxiety disorders. Children with ADHD can also have concurrent diagnoses of sleep disorders, memory impairment, and decreased motor skills.

TREATMENT
Psychosocial Treatments

Once the diagnosis of ADHD has been established, the parents and child should be educated with regard to the ways ADHD can affect learning, behavior, self-esteem, social skills, and family function. The clinician should set goals for the family to improve the child's interpersonal relationships, develop study skills, and decrease disruptive behaviors. Parent support groups with appropriate professional consultation to such groups can be very helpful.

Behaviorally Oriented Treatments

Treatments geared toward behavioral management often occur in the time frame of 8-12 sessions. The goal of such treatment is for the clinician to identify targeted behaviors that cause impairment in the child's life (disruptive behavior, difficulty in completing homework, failure to obey home or school rules) and for the child to work on progressively improving his or her skill in these areas. The clinician should guide the parents and teachers in setting appropriate expectations, consistently implementing rewards to encourage desired behaviors and consequences to discourage undesired behaviors. In short-term comparison trials, stimulants have been more effective than behavioral treatments used alone in improving core ADHD symptoms for most children. Behavioral interventions are modestly successful at improving core ADHD symptoms and are considered the first-line treatment in preschool-age children with ADHD. In addition, behavioral treatment may be particularly useful for children with comorbid anxiety, complex comorbidities, family stressors, and when combined with medication.

Medications

The most widely used medications for the treatment of ADHD are the presynaptic dopaminergic agonists, commonly called **psychostimulant** medications, including methylphenidate, dexmethylphenidate, amphetamine, and various amphetamine and dextroamphetamine preparations. Longer-acting, once-daily forms of each of the major types of stimulant medications are available and facilitate compliance with treatment and coverage over a longer period (see Table 49.3). When starting a stimulant, the clinician can select either a methylphenidate-based or an amphetamine-based compound. If a full range of methylphenidate dosages is used, approximately 25% of patients have an optimal response on a low dose (<0.5 mg/kg/day for methylphenidate, <0.25 mg/kg/day for amphetamines), 25% on a medium dose (0.5-1.0 mg/kg/day for methylphenidate, 0.25-0.5 mg/kg/day for amphetamines), and 25% on a high dose (1.0-1.5 mg/day for methylphenidate, 0.5-0.75 mg/kg/day for amphetamine); another 25% will be unresponsive or will have side effects, making that drug particularly unpalatable for the family (See Table 33.2 for more information on dosing).

Over the first 4 wk of treatment, the physician should increase the medication dose as tolerated (keeping side effects minimal to absent) to achieve maximum benefit. If this strategy does not yield satisfactory results, or if side effects prevent further dose adjustment in the presence of persisting symptoms, the clinician should use an alternative class of stimulants that was not used previously. If a methylphenidate compound is unsuccessful, the clinician should switch to an amphetamine product. If satisfactory treatment results are not obtained with the 2nd stimulant, clinicians may choose to prescribe *atomoxetine*, a noradrenergic reuptake inhibitor that has been approved by the U.S. Food and Drug Administration (FDA) for the treatment of ADHD in children, adolescents, and adults. Atomoxetine should be initiated at a dose of 0.3 mg/kg/day and titrated over 1-3 wk to a maximum total daily dosage of 1.2-1.4 mg/kg/day. The dose should be divided into twice-daily portions. Once-daily dosing appears to be associated with a high incidence of treatment failure. Long-acting *guanfacine* and *clonidine* are also FDA approved for the treatment of ADHD (see Chapter 33). These medications can also treat motor and vocal tics and so may be a reasonable choice in a child with a comorbid tic disorder. Drugs to treat ADHD do not increase the incidence of tics in children predisposed to a tic disorder. In the past, tricyclic antidepressants have been used to treat ADHD, but TCAs are rarely used now because of the risk of sudden death, particularly if an overdose is taken.

The clinician should consider careful monitoring of medication a necessary component of treatment in children with ADHD. When physicians prescribe medications for the treatment of ADHD, they tend to use lower-than-optimal doses. Optimal treatment usually requires somewhat higher doses than tend to be found in routine practice settings. All-day preparations are also useful to maximize positive effects and minimize side effects, and regular medication follow-up visits should be offered (≥4 times/yr) as opposed to the twice-yearly medication visits often used in standard community care settings.

Medication alone may not be sufficient to treat ADHD in children, particularly when children have multiple psychiatric disorders or a stressed home environment. When children do not respond to medication, it may be appropriate to refer them to a mental health specialist. Consultation with a child psychiatrist, developmental-behavioral pediatrician, or psychologist can also be beneficial to determine the next steps for treatment, including adding other components and supports to the overall treatment program. Evidence suggests that children who receive careful medication management, accompanied by frequent treatment follow-up, all within the context of an educative, supportive relationship with the primary care provider, are likely to experience behavioral gains.

Stimulant drugs used to treat ADHD may be associated with an increased risk of adverse cardiovascular events, including sudden cardiac death, myocardial infarction, and stroke, in young adults and rarely in

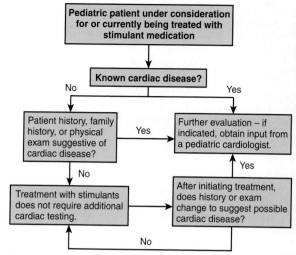

Fig. 49.4 Cardiac evaluation of children and adolescents with ADHD receiving or being considered for stimulant medications. *(From Perrin JM, Friedman RA, Knilans TK: Cardiovascular monitoring and stimulant drugs for attention-deficit/hyperactivity disorder, Pediatrics 122:451–453, 2008.)*

children. In some of the reported cases, the patient had an underlying disorder, such as hypertrophic obstructive cardiomyopathy, which is made worse by sympathomimetic agents. These events are rare but nonetheless warrant consideration before initiating treatment and during monitoring of therapy with stimulants. Children with a positive personal or family history of cardiomyopathy, arrhythmias, or syncope require an electrocardiogram and possible cardiology consultation before a stimulant is prescribed (Fig. 49.4).

PROGNOSIS

A childhood diagnosis of ADHD often leads to persistent ADHD throughout the life span. From 60–80% of children with ADHD continue to experience symptoms in adolescence, and up to 40–60% of adolescents exhibit ADHD symptoms into adulthood. In children with ADHD, a reduction in hyperactive behavior often occurs with age. Other symptoms associated with ADHD can become more prominent with age, such as inattention, impulsivity, and disorganization, and these exact a heavy toll on young adult functioning. Risk factors in children with untreated ADHD as they become adults include engaging in risk-taking behaviors (sexual activity, delinquent behaviors, substance use), educational underachievement or employment difficulties, and relationship difficulties. With proper treatment, the risks associated with ADHD, including injuries, can be significantly reduced. Consistent treatment with medication and adjuvant therapies appears to lower the risk of adverse outcomes, such as substance abuse.

PREVENTION

Parent training can lead to significant improvements in preschool children with ADHD symptoms, and parent training for preschool youth with ADHD can reduce oppositional behavior. To the extent that parents, teachers, physicians, and policymakers support efforts for earlier detection, diagnosis, and treatment, prevention of long-term adverse effects of ADHD on affected children's lives should be reconsidered within the lens of prevention. Given the effective treatments for ADHD now available, and the well-documented evidence about the long-term effects of untreated or ineffectively treated ADHD on children and youth, prevention of these consequences should be within the grasp of physicians and the children and families with ADHD for whom we are responsible.

Bibliography is available at Expert Consult.

Chapter 50
Dyslexia
Sally E. Shaywitz and Bennett A. Shaywitz

第五十章
阅读障碍

中文导读

本章主要介绍了阅读障碍的病因学、流行病学、发病机制、临床表现、诊断、治疗（管理）和预后。其中特别指出，阅读障碍是一种临床诊断，病史尤其重要，阅读障碍的诊断应反映所有综合的临床数据；

阅读障碍的治疗是全生命周期的治疗，有效的干预计划可在五个关键领域提供系统的指导：音素意识、语音、流利度、词汇量和理解策略。

The most current definition of *dyslexia* is now codified in U.S. Federal law (First Step Act of 2018, PL: 115–391): "The term *dyslexia* means an unexpected difficulty in reading for an individual who has the intelligence to be a much better reader, most commonly caused by a difficulty in the phonological processing (the appreciation of the individual sounds of spoken language), which affects the ability of an individual to speak, read, and spell." In typical readers, development of reading and intelligence quotient (IQ) are dynamically linked over time. In dyslexic readers, however, a developmental uncoupling occurs between reading and IQ (Fig. 50.1), such that reading achievement is significantly below what would be expected given the individual's IQ. The discrepancy between reading achievement and IQ provides the long-sought empirical evidence for the seeming paradox between cognition and reading in individuals with developmental dyslexia, and this discrepancy is now recognized in the Federal definition as unexpected difficulty in reading.

ETIOLOGY

Dyslexia is familial, occurring in 50% of children who have a parent with dyslexia, in 50% of the siblings of dyslexic persons, and in 50% of the parents of dyslexic persons. Such observations have naturally led to a search for genes responsible for dyslexia, and at one point there was hope that heritability would be related to a small number of genes. Genome-wide association studies (GWAS), however, have demonstrated that a large number of genes are involved, each producing a small effect. Advances in genetics have confirmed what the GWAS suggested, that complex traits such as reading are the work of thousands of genetic variants, working in concert (see Chapter 99). Thus, pediatricians should be wary of recommending any genetic test to their patients that purports to diagnose dyslexia in infancy or before language and reading have even emerged. It is unlikely that a single gene or even a few genes will reliably identify people with dyslexia. Rather, dyslexia is best explained by **multiple genes**, each contributing a small amount toward the expression of dyslexia.

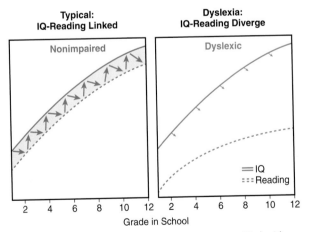

Fig. 50.1 Uncoupling of reading and IQ over time: empirical evidence for a definition of dyslexia. **Left,** In typical readers, reading and IQ development are dynamically linked over time. **Right,** In contrast, reading and IQ development are dissociated in dyslexic readers, and one does not influence the other. *(Data adapted from Ferrer E, Shaywitz BA, Holahan JM, et al: Uncoupling of reading and IQ over time: empirical evidence for a definition of dyslexia, Psychol Sci 21(1):93–101, 2010.)*

EPIDEMIOLOGY

Dyslexia is the most common and most comprehensively studied of the learning disabilities, affecting 80% of children identified as having a learning disability. Dyslexia may be the most common neurobehavioral disorder affecting children, with prevalence rates ranging from 20% in unselected population-based samples to much lower rates in school-identified samples. The low prevalence rate in school-identified samples may reflect the reluctance of schools to identify dyslexia. Dyslexia occurs with equal frequency in boys and girls in survey samples in which *all* children are assessed. Despite such well-documented findings, schools continue to identify more boys than girls, probably reflecting the more rambunctious behavior of boys who come to the teacher's attention because of misbehavior, while girls with reading difficulty, who are less likely to be misbehaving, are also less likely to be identified by the schools. Dyslexia fits a dimensional model in which reading ability and disability occur along a *continuum,* with dyslexia representing the lower tail of a normal distribution of reading ability.

PATHOGENESIS

Evidence from a number of lines of investigation indicates that dyslexia reflects deficits within the language system, and more specifically, within the **phonologic component** of the language system engaged in processing the sounds of speech. Individuals with dyslexia have difficulty developing an awareness that spoken words can be segmented into smaller elemental units of sound (phonemes), an essential ability given that reading requires that the reader map or link printed symbols to sound. Increasing evidence indicates that disruption of attentional mechanisms may also play an important role in reading difficulties.

Functional brain imaging in both children and adults with dyslexia demonstrates an inefficient functioning of left hemisphere posterior brain systems, a pattern referred to as the *neural signature of dyslexia* (Fig. 50.2). Although functional magnetic resonance imaging (fMRI) consistently demonstrates differences between *groups* of dyslexic compared to typical readers, brain imaging is not able to differentiate an *individual* case of a dyslexic reader from a typical reader and thus is not useful in diagnosing dyslexia.

CLINICAL MANIFESTATIONS

Reflecting the underlying phonologic weakness, children and adults with dyslexia manifest problems in both spoken and written language. Spoken language difficulties are typically manifest by mispronunciations, lack of glibness, speech that lacks fluency with many pauses or hesitations and "ums," word-finding difficulties with the need for time to summon an oral response, and the inability to come up with a verbal response quickly when questioned; these reflect *sound-based,* not semantic or knowledge-based, difficulties.

Struggles in decoding and word recognition can vary according to age and developmental level. The cardinal signs of dyslexia observed in school-age children and adults are a labored, effortful approach to reading involving decoding, word recognition, and text reading. Listening comprehension is typically robust. Older children improve reading accuracy over time, but without commensurate gains in reading fluency; they remain slow readers. Difficulties in spelling typically reflect the phonologically based difficulties observed in oral reading. Handwriting is often affected as well.

History often reveals early subtle language difficulties in dyslexic children. During the preschool and kindergarten years, at-risk children display difficulties playing rhyming games and learning the names for letters and numbers. Kindergarten assessments of these language skills can help identify children at risk for dyslexia. Although a dyslexic child enjoys and benefits from being read to or reading independently, the child might avoid reading aloud to the parent or reading independently.

Dyslexia may coexist with attention-deficit/hyperactivity disorder (see Chapter 49); this comorbidity has been documented in both referred samples (40% comorbidity) and nonreferred samples (15% comorbidity).

DIAGNOSIS

A large achievement gap between typical and dyslexic readers is evident as early as 1st grade and persists (Fig. 50.3). These findings provide strong evidence and impetus for early screening and identification of and early intervention for young children at risk for dyslexia. One source of potentially powerful and highly accessible screening information is the teacher's judgment about the child's reading and reading-related skills. Evidence-based screening can be carried out as early as kindergarten, and also in grades 1-3, by the child's teacher. The teachers' responses to a small set of questions (10-12 questions) predict a pool of children who are at risk for dyslexia with a high degree of accuracy. Screening takes less than 10 minutes, is completed on a tablet, and is extremely efficient and economical. Children found to be at-risk will then have further assessment and, if diagnosed as dyslexic, should receive evidence-based intervention.

Dyslexia is a clinical diagnosis, and history is especially critical. The clinician seeks to determine through history, observation, and psychometric assessment, if there are unexpected difficulties in reading (based on the person's intelligence, chronological/grade, level of education or professional status) and associated linguistic problems at the level of phonologic processing. No single test score is pathognomonic of dyslexia. The diagnosis of dyslexia should reflect a thoughtful synthesis of all clinical data available.

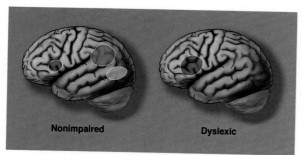

Fig. 50.2 A neural signature for dyslexia. The *left* side of the figure shows a schematic of left hemisphere brain systems in in typical (nonimpaired) readers. The 3 systems for reading are an anterior system in the region of the inferior frontal gyrus (Broca's area), serving articulation and word analysis, and 2 posterior systems, 1 in the occipitotemporal region serving word analysis, and a 2nd in the occipitotemporal region (the word-form area) serving the rapid, automatic, fluent identification of words. In dyslexic readers (*right* side of figure), the 2 posterior systems are functioning inefficiently and appear underactivated. This pattern of underactivation in left posterior reading systems is referred to as the neural signature for dyslexia. (*Adapted from Shaywitz S: Overcoming dyslexia: a new and complete science-based program for reading problems at any level. New York, 2003, Alfred A. Knopf. Copyright 2003 by S. Shaywitz. Adapted with permission.*)

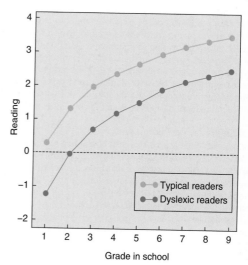

Fig. 50.3 Reading from grades 1 through 9 in typical and dyslexic readers. The achievement gap between typical and dyslexic readers is evident as early as 1st grade and persists through adolescence. (*Adapted from Ferrer E, Shaywitz BA, Holahan JM, et al: Achievement gap in reading is present as early as first grade and persists through adolescence, J Pediatr 167:1121–1125, 2015.*)

Dyslexia is distinguished from other disorders that can prominently feature reading difficulties by the unique, circumscribed nature of the *phonologic deficit*, one that does not intrude into other linguistic or cognitive domains. A core assessment for the diagnosis of dyslexia in children includes tests of language, particularly phonology; reading, including real and pseudowords; reading fluency; spelling; and tests of intellectual ability. Additional tests of memory, general language skills, and mathematics may be administered as part of a more comprehensive evaluation of cognitive, linguistic, and academic function. Some schools use a **response to intervention (RtI)** approach to identifying reading disabilities (see Chapter 51.1). Once a diagnosis has been made, dyslexia is a permanent diagnosis and need not be reconfirmed by new assessments.

For informal screening, in addition to a careful history, the primary care physician in an office setting can listen to the child read aloud from the child's own grade-level reader. Keeping a set of graded readers available in the office serves the same purpose and eliminates the need for the child to bring in schoolbooks. **Oral reading** is a sensitive measure of reading accuracy and fluency. The most consistent and telling sign of a reading disability in an accomplished young adult is slow and laborious reading and writing. In attempting to read aloud, most children and adults with dyslexia display an effortful approach to decoding and recognizing single words, an approach in children characterized by hesitations, mispronunciations, and repeated attempts to sound out unfamiliar words. In contrast to the difficulties they experience in decoding single words, persons with dyslexia typically possess the vocabulary, syntax, and other higher-level abilities involved in comprehension.

The failure either to recognize or to measure the lack of fluency in reading is perhaps the most common error in the diagnosis of dyslexia in older children and accomplished young adults. Simple word identification tasks will not detect dyslexia in a person who is accomplished enough to be in honors high school classes or to graduate from college or obtain a graduate degree. Tests relying on the accuracy of word identification alone are inappropriate to use to diagnose dyslexia because they show little to nothing of the *struggle* to read. Because they assess reading accuracy but not automaticity (speed), the types of reading tests used for school-age children might provide misleading data on bright adolescents and young adults. The most critical tests are those that are *timed*; they are the most sensitive in detecting dyslexia in a bright adult. Few standardized tests for young adult readers are administered under timed and untimed conditions; the *Nelson-Denny Reading Test* is an exception. The helpful *Test of Word Reading Efficiency* (TOWRE) examines simple word reading under timed conditions. Any scores obtained on testing must be considered relative to peers with the same degree of education or professional training.

MANAGEMENT

The management of dyslexia demands a life-span perspective. Early in life the focus is on **remediation** of the reading problem. Applying knowledge of the importance of early language, including vocabulary and phonologic skills, leads to significant improvements in children's reading accuracy, even in predisposed children. As a child matures and enters the more time-demanding setting of middle and then high school, the emphasis shifts to the important role of providing accommodations. Based on the work of the National Reading Panel, evidence-based reading intervention methods and programs are identified. Effective intervention programs provide systematic instruction in 5 key areas: phonemic awareness, phonics, fluency, vocabulary, and comprehension strategies. These programs also provide ample opportunities for writing, reading, and discussing literature.

Taking each component of the reading process in turn, effective interventions improve phonemic awareness: the ability to focus on and manipulate phonemes (speech sounds) in spoken syllables and words. The elements found to be most effective in enhancing **phonemic awareness**, reading, and spelling skills include teaching children to manipulate phonemes with letters; focusing the instruction on 1 or 2 types of phoneme

manipulations rather than multiple types; and teaching children in small groups. Providing instruction in phonemic awareness is necessary but not sufficient to teach children to read. Effective intervention programs include teaching **phonics**, or making sure that the beginning reader understands how letters are linked to sounds (phonemes) to form letter-sound correspondences and spelling patterns. The instruction should be explicit and systematic; phonics instruction enhances children's success in learning to read, and systematic phonics instruction is more effective than instruction that teaches little or no phonics or teaches phonics casually or haphazardly. Important but often overlooked is starting children on reading connected text early on, optimally at or near the beginning of reading instruction.

Fluency is of critical importance because it allows the automatic, rapid recognition of words, and while it is generally recognized that fluency is an important component of skilled reading, it has proved difficult to teach. Interventions for vocabulary development and reading comprehension are not as well established. The most effective methods to teach reading comprehension involve teaching vocabulary and strategies that encourage active interaction between the reader and the text. Emerging science indicates that it is not only teacher content knowledge but the teacher's skill in engaging the student and focusing the student's attention on the reading task at hand that is required for effective instruction.

For those in high school, college, and graduate school, provision of **accommodations** most often represents a highly effective approach to dyslexia. Imaging studies now provide neurobiologic evidence of the need for extra time for dyslexic students; accordingly, college students with a childhood history of dyslexia require extra time in reading and writing assignments as well as examinations. Many adolescent and adult students have been able to improve their reading accuracy, but without commensurate gains in reading speed. The accommodation of extra time reconciles the individual's often high cognitive ability and slow reading, so that the exam is a measure of that person's ability rather than his disability. Another important accommodation is teaching the dyslexic student to listen to texts. Excellent text-to-speech programs and apps available for Apple and Android systems include Voice Dream Reader, Immersive Reader (in OneNote as part of Microsoft Office), Kurzweil Firefly, Read & Write Gold, Read: OutLoud, and Natural Reader. Voice-to-text programs are also helpful, often part of the suite of programs as well as the popular Dragon Dictate. Voice to text is found on many smartphones. Other helpful accommodations include the use of laptop computers with spelling checkers, access to lecture notes, tutorial services, and a separate quiet room for taking tests.

In addition, the impact of the primary phonologic weakness in dyslexia mandates special consideration during oral examinations so that students are not graded on their lack of glibness or speech hesitancies but on their content knowledge. Unfortunately, speech hesitancies or difficulties in word retrieval often are wrongly confused with insecure content knowledge. The major difficulty in dyslexia, reflecting problems accessing the sound system of spoken language, causes great difficulty learning a 2nd language. As a result, an often-necessary accommodation is a waiver or partial waiver of the foreign language requirement; the dyslexic student may enroll in a course on the history or culture of a non–English-speaking country.

PROGNOSIS

Application of evidence-based methods to young children (kindergarten to grade 3), when provided with sufficient intensity and duration, can result in improvements in reading accuracy and, to a much lesser extent, fluency. In older children and adults, interventions result in improved accuracy, but not an appreciable improvement in fluency. Accommodations are critical in allowing the dyslexic child to demonstrate his or her knowledge. Parents should be informed that with proper support, dyslexic children can succeed in a range of future occupations that might seem out of their reach, including medicine, law, journalism, and writing.

Bibliography is available at Expert Consult.

Chapter 51

Math and Writing Disabilities

第五十一章
数学和书写障碍

中文导读

本章主要介绍了数学障碍和书写障碍。数学障碍部分具体描述了数学障碍的定义、流行病学、病因、治疗及干预。其中流行病学中详细阐述了发病率、危险因素及合并症；病因中详细阐述了综合认知过程和特定数学过程。书写障碍部分具体描述了流行病学、与书写障碍相关的技能缺陷及治疗。其中与书写障碍相关的技能缺陷详细阐述了抄写、口语、执行功能、工作记忆。

51.1 Math Disabilities

Kenneth L. Grizzle

Data from the U.S. National Center for Educational Statistics for 2009 showed that 69% of U.S. high school graduates had taken algebra 1, 88% geometry, 76% algebra 2/trigonometry, and 35% precalculus. These percentages are considerably higher than those for 20 years earlier. However, concerns remain about the limited literacy level in mathematics for children, adolescents, and those entering the workforce; poor math skills predict numerous social, employment, and emotional challenges. The need for number and math literacy extends beyond the workplace and into daily lives, and weaknesses in this area can negatively impact daily functioning. Research into the etiology and treatment of **math disabilities** falls far behind the study of reading disabilities (see Chapter 50). Therefore the knowledge needed to identify, treat, and minimize the impact of math challenges on daily functioning and education is limited.

MATH LEARNING DISABILITY DEFINED

Understanding learning challenges associated with mathematics requires a basic appreciation of domain-specific terminology and operations. The *Diagnostic and Statistical Manual for Mental Disorders, Fifth Edition* (DSM-5) has published diagnostic criteria for learning disorders. Specific types of learning challenges are subsumed under the broad term of **specific learning disorder (SLD).** The DSM identifies the following features of a SLD with an **impairment in math:** difficulties mastering number sense, number facts, or fluent calculation and difficulties with math reasoning. Symptoms must be present for a minimum of 6 mo and persist despite interventions to address the learning challenges. **Number sense** refers to a basic understanding of quantity, number, and operations and is represented as nonverbal and symbolic. Examples of

number sense include an understanding that each number is 1 more or 1 less than the previous or following number; knowledge of number words and symbols; and the ability to compare the relative magnitude of numbers and perform simple arithmetic calculations.

The DSM-5 definition can be contrasted with an **education-defined learning disability in mathematics.** Two math-related areas are identified as part of the **Individuals with Disabilities Education Act (IDEA):** mathematics calculation and mathematics problem solving. Operationally, this is reflected in age-level competency in arithmetic and math calculation, word problems, interpreting graphs, understanding money and time concepts, and applying math concepts to solve quantitative problems. The federal government allows states to choose the way a *learning disability* (LD) is identified if the procedure is "research based." Referred to specifically in IDEA as methods for identifying an LD are a **discrepancy model** and "use of a process based on the child's response to scientific, research-based intervention." The former refers to identifying a LD based on a pronounced discrepancy between intellectual functioning and academic achievement. The latter, referred to as a **response to intervention (RtI)** model, requires school systems to screen for a disability, intervene using empirically supported treatments for the identified disability, closely monitor progress, and make necessary adjustments to the intervention as needed. If a child is not responding adequately, a multidisciplinary team evaluation is used to develop an **individualized educational plan (IEP).**

It is important that primary care providers understand the RtI process because many states require or encourage this approach to identifying LDs. Confusion can be avoided by helping concerned parents understand that a school may review their child's records, screen the skills of concern, and provide intervention with close progress monitoring, before initiating the process for an IEP. Traditional psychoeducation testing (IQ and achievement) may only be completed if a child has not responded well to specific interventions. The RtI approach is a valuable, empirically supported way to approach and identify a potential learning disability, but very different from a medical approach to diagnosis and treatment.

Terminology

The term **dyscalculia**, often used in medicine and research but seldom used by educators, is reserved for children with a SLD in math when there is a pattern of deficits in learning arithmetic facts and accurate, fluent calculations. The term **math learning disability (MLD)** is used generically here, with dyscalculia used when limiting the discussion to children with deficient math calculation skills. A distinction is also made between children with a MLD and those who are **low achieving (LA) in math;** both groups have received considerable research focus. Although not included in either definition above, research into math deficits typically requires that individuals identified with MLD have math achievement scores below the 10th percentile across multiple grade levels. These children start out poorly in math and continue poor performance across grades, despite interventions. LA math students consistently score below the 25th percentile on math achievement tests across grades, but show more typical entry-level math skills.

EPIDEMIOLOGY
Prevalence

Depending on how MLD is defined and assessed, the prevalence varies. Based on findings from multiple studies, approximately 7% of children will show a MLD profile before high school graduation. An additional 10% of students will be identified as LA. Because research in the area typically requires that individuals show deficits for consecutive years, the respective prevalence estimates are lower than the 10th percentile cutoff for being identified as MLD or the 25th percentile cutoff for being identified as LA. It is not unusual for children to score below the criterion one year and above the criterion in subsequent years. These children do not show the same cognitive deficits associated with a MLD. Unlike dyslexia, boys are at greater risk to experience MLD. This is found in epidemiologic research in the United States (risk ratio, 1.6-2.2:1) and various European countries.

Risk Factors
Genetics

The heritability of math skills is estimated to be approximately 0.50. The heritability or genetic influence on math skills is consistent across the continuum from high to low math skills. This research emphasizes that although math skills are learned across time, the stability of math performance is the result of genetic influences. Math heritability appears to be the product of multiple genetic markers, each having a small effect.

Medical/Genetic Conditions

Numerous genetic syndromes are associated with math problems. Although most children with **fragile X syndrome** have an *intellectual disability* (ID), approximately 50% of girls with the condition do not. Of those without an ID, ≥75% have a math disability by the end of 3rd grade and are already scoring below average in mathematics in kindergarten and 1st grade. For girls with fragile X MLD, weak working memory seems to play an important role. The frequency of MLD in girls with **Turner syndrome (TS)** is the same as found in girls with fragile X syndrome. A consistent finding is girls with TS complete math calculations at significantly slower speed than typically developing students. Although girls with TS have weak calculation skills, their ability to complete math problems not requiring explicit calculation is similar to that of their peers. The percentage of children with the **22q11.2 deletion syndrome** (22q11.2ds) with MLD is not clear. Younger children with this genetic condition (6-10 yr old) showed similar number sense and calculation skills as typically developing children but weaker math problem solving. Older children with 22q11.2ds showed slower speed in their general number sense and calculations, but accuracy was maintained. Weak counting skills and magnitude comparison have been found in this group of children, suggesting weak visual-spatial

processing. Children with **myelomeningocele** are at greater risk for math difficulties than their unaffected peers. Almost 30% of these children have MLD without an additional diagnosed learning disorder, and >50% have both math and reading learning disorders. While broad, deficits are most pronounced in speed of math calculation and written computation.

Comorbidities

It is estimated that 30–70% of those with MLD will also have reading disability. This is especially important because children with MLD are less likely to be referred for additional educational assistance and intervention than students with reading problems. Unfortunately, children identified with both learning challenges perform poorer across psychosocial and academic measures than children with MLD alone. Having a MLD places a child at greater risk for not only other learning challenges but also psychiatric disorders, including attention-deficit/hyperactivity disorder, oppositional defiant disorder, conduct disorder, generalized anxiety disorder, and major depressive disorder. Individuals with MLD have been found to have increased social isolation and difficulties developing social relationships in general.

CAUSES OF MATH LEARNING DISABILITY

There is a consensus that individuals with MLD are a heterogeneous group, with multiple potential broad and specific deficits driving their learning difficulties. Research into the causes of MLD has focused on math-specific processes and broad cognitive deficits, with an appreciation that these two factors are not always independent.

Broad Cognitive Processes
Intelligence

Intelligence affects learning, but if intellectual functioning were the primary driver of poor math performance, the math skills of low-IQ children would be similar or worse than individuals with MLD. On the contrary, children with MLD have significantly poorer math achievement than children with low IQ. Children with MLD have severe deficits in math not accounted for by their cognitive functioning. Individuals with lower cognition may have difficulty learning mathematics, but their math skills are likely to be commensurate with their intelligence.

Working Memory

Working memory refers to the ability to keep information in mind while using the information in other mental processes. Working memory is composed of 3 core systems: the central executive, the language-related phonologic loop, and the visual-based sketch pad. The central executive coordinates the functioning of the other two systems. All three play a role in various aspects of learning and in the development and application of math skills in particular; children with MLD have shown deficits in each area.

Processing Speed

Individuals with MLD are often slower to complete math problems than their typically developing peers, a result of their poor fact retrieval rather than broader speed of processing deficits. However, young children later identified with a MLD when beginning school have number-processing speed that is considerably slower than same-age same-grade peers.

Math-Specific Processes
Procedural Errors

The type of errors made by children with a MLD are typical for any child, the difference being that children with a learning disability show a 2-3 yr lag in understanding the concept. An example of a common error a 1st grade child with a MLD might make when "counting on" is to undercount: "6 + 2= ?;" "6, 7" rather than starting at 6 and counting an additional 2 numbers. As children with math deficits get older, it is common to subtract a larger number from a smaller number. For example, in the problem "63 − 29 = 46," the child makes the mistake of subtracting 3 from 9. Another common error is not decreasing the number in the

Table 51.1	Parent Resources for the Child With Math Learning Disability

Let's Talk About Math. Available from: http://www.zerotothree.org/parenting-resources/early-math-video-series. Accessed January 2, 2017.

Mixing in Math. Available from: https://mixinginmath.terc.edu/aboutMiM/what_isMiM.php. Accessed January 2, 2017.

PBS Parents. Math resources available to parents through the Public Broadcasting Service website. Accessed January 28, 2017: http://www.pbs.org/parents/earlymath/index.html http://www.pbs.org/parents/education/math/

US Department of Education: *Helping your child learn mathematics.* Available from: https://www2.ed.gov/parents/academic/help/math/index.html. Accessed January 28, 2017.

Table 51.2	Risk Factors for a Specific Learning Disability Involving Mathematics

The child is at or below the 20th percentile in any math area, as reflected by standardized testing or ongoing measures of progress monitoring.

The teacher expresses concerns about the child's ability to "take the next step" in math.

There is a positive family history for math learning disability (this alone will not initiate an intervention).

Parents think they have to "reteach" math concepts to their child.

10s column when borrowing: "64 − 39 = 35." For both adding and subtracting, there is a lack of understanding of the commutative property of numbers and a tendency to use repeated addition rather than fact retrieval. It is not that children with a MLD do not develop these skills, it is that they develop them much later than their peers, thereby making the transition to complicated math concepts much more challenging.

Memory for Math Facts

Committing math facts to or retrieving facts from memory have consistently been found to be problematic for children with MLD. Weak fact encoding or retrieval alone do not determine a MLD diagnosis. Many math curricula in the United States do not include development of math facts as a part of the instructional process, resulting in children not knowing basic facts.

Unlike dyslexia, in which deficits have been isolated and identified as causal (see Chapter 50), factors involved in the development of a MLD are much more heterogeneous. Alone, none of the processes previously outlined fully accounts for MLD, although all have been implicated as problematic for those struggling with math.

TREATMENT AND INTERVENTIONS

The most effective interventions for MLD are those that include explicit instruction on solving specific types of problems and that take place over several weeks to several months. Skill-based instruction is a critical component; general math problem solving will not carry over across various math skills, unless the skill is part of a more complex math concept. Clear, comprehensive guidelines for effective interventions for students struggling with math have been provided by the U.S. Department of Education in the form of a *Practice Guide* released through the What Works Clearinghouse. This document gives excellent direction in the identification and treatment of children with math difficulties in the educational system. Although not intended for medical personnel or parents, the guide is available free of charge and can be helpful for parents when talking to teachers about their child's learning. Table 51.1 lists additional resources for parents concerned about their young child's development of math facts.

Awareness that most public school systems have implemented some form of a RtI to identify learning disabilities allows the primary care physician to encourage parents to return to the school seeking an intervention to address their child's concern. Receiving special education services in the form of an IEP may be necessary for some children. However, the current approach to identifying children with a learning disability allows school systems to intervene earlier, when problems arise, and potentially avoid the need for an IEP. Pediatricians with patients whose parents have received feedback from school with any of the risk factors outlined in Table 51.2 should encourage the parents to discuss an intervention plan with the child's teacher.

Bibliography is available at Expert Consult.

51.2 Writing Disabilities
Kenneth L. Grizzle

Oral language is a complex process that typically develops in the absence of formal instruction. In contrast, *written language* requires instruction in acquisition (word reading), understanding (reading comprehension), and expression (spelling and composition). Unfortunately, despite reasonable pedagogy, a subset of children struggle with development in one or several of these areas. The disordered output of written language is currently referred to within the *Diagnostic and Statistical Manual for Mental Disorders, Fifth Edition* (DSM-5) as a **specific learning disorder with impairment in written expression** (Table 51.3).

Various terminology has been used when referring to individuals with writing deficits; this subchapter uses the term **impairment in written expression (IWE)** rather than "writing disorder" or "disorder of written expression." **Dysgraphia** is often used when referring to children with writing problems, sometimes synonymously with IWE, although the two are related but distinct conditions. Dysgraphia is primarily a deficit in motor output (paper/pencil skills), and IWE is a conceptual weakness in developing, organizing, and elaborating on ideas in writing.

The diagnoses of a IWE and dysgraphia are made largely based on phenotypical presentation; spelling, punctuation, grammar, clarity, and organization are factors to consider with IWE concerns. Aside from these potentially weak writing characteristics, however, no other guidelines are offered. Based on clinical experience and research into the features of writing samples of children with disordered writing skills, one would expect to see limited output, poor organization, repetition of content, and weak sentence structure and spelling, despite the child taking considerable time to produce a small amount of content. For those with comorbid dysgraphia, the legibility of their writing product will also be poor, sometimes illegible.

EPIDEMIOLOGY

The incidence of IWE is estimated at 6.9–14.7%, with the relative risk for IWE 2-2.9 times higher for boys than girls. One study covering three U.S. geographic regions found considerably higher rates of IWE in the Midwest and Southeast than in the West.

The risk for writing problems is much greater among select populations; >50% of children with oral language disorders reportedly have IWE. The relationship between attention-deficit/hyperactivity disorder (ADHD) and learning disorders in general is well established, including IWE estimates in the 60% range for the combined and inattentive presentations of ADHD. Because of the importance of working memory and other executive functions in the writing process, any child with weakness in these areas will likely find the writing process difficult (see Chapter 48).

SKILL DEFICITS ASSOCIATED WITH IMPAIRED WRITING

Written language, much like reading, occurs along a developmental trajectory that can be seamless as children master skills critical to the next step in the process. Mastery of motor control that allows a child

Table 51.3	DSM-5 Diagnostic Criteria for Specific Learning Disability With Impairment in Written Expression

A. Difficulties learning and using academic skills that have persisted for at least 6 mo, despite the provision of interventions that target those difficulties.

Difficulties with written expression (e.g., makes multiple grammatical or punctuation errors within sentences; employs poor paragraph organization; written expression of ideas lacks clarity).

B. The affected academic skills are substantially and quantifiably below those expected for the individual's chronological age, and cause significant interference with academic or occupational performance, or with activities of daily living, as confirmed by individually administered standardized achievement measures and comprehensive clinical assessment. For individuals age 17 yr and older, a documented history of impairing learning difficulties may be substituted for the standardized assessment.

C. The learning difficulties begin during school-age years but may not become fully manifest until the demands for those affected academic skills exceed the individual's limited capacities (e.g., as in timed tests, reading or writing lengthy complex reports for a tight deadline, excessively heavy academic loads).

D. The learning difficulties are not better accounted for by intellectual disabilities, uncorrected visual or auditory acuity, other mental or neurologic disorders, psychosocial adversity, lack of proficiency in the language of academic instruction, or inadequate educational instruction.

315.2 (F81.81) With impairment in written expression:
Spelling accuracy
Grammar and punctuation accuracy
Clarity or organization of written expression

Specify current severity:

Mild: Some difficulties learning skills in 1 or 2 academic domains, but of mild enough severity that the individual may be able to compensate or function well when provided with appropriate accommodations or support services, especially during the school years.

Moderate: Marked difficulties learning skills in ≥1 academic domain(s), so that the individual is unlikely to become proficient without some intervals of intensive and specialized teaching during the school years. Some accommodations or supportive services at least part of the day at school, in the workplace, or at home may be needed to complete activities accurately and efficiently.

Severe: Severe difficulties learning skills, affecting several academic domains, so that the individual is unlikely to learn those skills without ongoing intensive individualized and specialized teaching for most of the school years. Even with an array of appropriate accommodations or services at home, at school, or in the workplace, the individual may not be able to complete all activities efficiently.

Adapted from the *Diagnostic and Statistical Manual of Mental Disorders, Fifth Edition,* (Copyright 2013). American Psychiatric Association, pp 66–67.

to produce letters and letter sequences frees up cognitive energy to devote to spelling words and eventually stringing words into sentences, paragraphs, and complex composition. Early in the development of each individual skill, considerable cognitive effort is required, although ideally the lower-level skills of motor production, spelling, punctuation, and capitalization (referred to as **writing mechanics** or **writing conventions**) will gradually become automatic and require progressively less mental effort. This effort can then be devoted to higher-level skills, such as planning, organization, application of knowledge, and use of varied vocabulary. For children with writing deficits, breakdowns can occur at one, some, or every stage.

Transcription

Among preschool and primary grade children, there is a wide range of what is considered "developmentally typical" as it relates to letter production and spelling. However, evidence indicates that poor writers in later grades are slow to produce letters and write their name in preschool and kindergarten. Weak early spelling and reading skills (letter identification and phonologic awareness; see Chapter 50) and weak oral language have also been found to predict weak writing skills in later elementary grades. Children struggling to master early **transcription** skills tend to write slowly, or when writing at reasonable speed, the legibility of their writing degrades. Output in quantity and variety is limited, and vocabulary use in poor spellers is often restricted to words they can spell.

As children progress into upper elementary school and beyond, a new set of challenges arise. They are now expected to have mastered lower-level transcription skills, and the focus turns to the application of these skills to more complex text generation. In addition to transcription, this next step requires the integration of additional cognitive skills that have yet to be tapped by young learners.

Oral Language

Language, although not speech, has been found to be related to writing skills. Writing difficulties are associated with deficits in both expression and comprehension of oral language. Writing characteristics of children with **specific language impairment (SLI)** can differ from their unimpaired peers early in the school experience, and persist through high school (see Chapter 52). In preschool and kindergarten, as a group, children with language disorders show poorer letter production and ability to print their name. Poor spelling and weak vocabulary also contribute to the poor writing skills. Beyond primary grades, the written narratives of SLI children tend to be evaluated as "lower quality with poor organization" and weaker use of varied vocabulary.

Pragmatic language and higher-level language deficits also negatively impact writing skills. **Pragmatic language** refers to the social use of language, including, though not limited to greeting and making requests; adjustments to language used to meet the need of the situation or listener; and following conversation rules verbally and nonverbally. **Higher-level language** goes beyond basic vocabulary, word form, and grammatical skills and includes making inferences, understanding and appropriately using figurative language, and making cause-and-effect judgments. Weaknesses in these areas, with or without intact foundational language, can present challenges for students in all academic areas that require writing. For example, whether producing an analytic or narrative piece, the writer must understand the extent of the reader's background knowledge and in turn what information to include and omit, make an argument for a cause-and-effect relationship, and use content-specific vocabulary or vocabulary rich in imagery and nonliteral interpretation.

Executive Functions

Writing is a complicated process and, when done well, requires the effective integration of multiple processes. Executive functions (EFs) are a set of skills that include planning, problem solving, monitoring and making adjustments as needed (see Chapter 48). Three recursive processes have consistently been reported as involved in the writing process: *translation* of thought into written output, *planning,* and *reviewing.* Coming up with ideas, while challenging for many, is simply the first step when writing a narrative (story). Once an idea has emerged, the concept must be developed to include a plot, characters, and story line and then coordinated into a coherent whole that is well organized and flows from beginning to end. Even if one develops ideas and begins to write them down, *persistence* is required to complete the task, which requires *self-regulation.* Effective writers rely heavily on EFs, and children with IWE struggle with this set of skills. Poor writers seldom engage in the necessary planning and struggle to self-monitor and revise effectively.

Working Memory

Working memory (WM) refers to the ability to hold, manipulate, and store information for short periods. The more space available, the more memory can be devoted to problem solving and thinking tasks. Nevertheless, there is limited space in which information can be held, and the more effort devoted to one task, the less space is available to devote to other tasks. WM has consistently been shown to play an important role in the writing process, because weak WM limits the

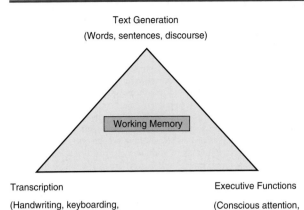

Fig. 51.1 Simple view of writing. *(From Berninger VW: Preventing written expression disabilities through early and continuing assessment and intervention for handwriting and/or spelling problems: research into practice. In Swanson HL, Harris KR, Graham S, editors: Handbook of learning disabilities, New York, 2003, The Guilford Press.)*

space available. Further, when writing skills that are expected to be *automatic* continue to require effort, precious memory is required, taking away what would otherwise be available for higher-level language.

The *Simple View of Writing* is an approach that integrates each of the 4 ideas just outlined to describe the writing process (Fig. 51.1). At the base of the triangle are transcription and executive functions, which support, within WM, the ability to produce text. Breakdowns in any of these areas can lead to poor writing, and identifying where the deficit(s) are occurring is essential when deciding to treat the writing problem. For example, children with weak **graphomotor** skills (e.g., dysgraphia) must devote considerable effort to the accurate production of written language, thereby increasing WM use devoted to lower-level transcription and limiting memory that can be used for developing discourse. The result might be painfully slow production of a legible story, or a passage that is largely illegible. If, on the other hand, a child's penmanship and spelling have developed well, but their ability to persist with challenging tasks or to organize their thoughts and develop a coordinated plan for their paper is limited, one might see very little information written on the paper despite considerable time devoted to the task. Lastly, even when skills residing at the base of this triangle are in place, students with a language disorder will likely produce text that is more consistent with their language functioning than their chronological grade or age (Fig. 51.1).

TREATMENT

Poor writing skills can improve with effective treatment. Weak graphomotor skills may not necessarily require intervention from an **occupational therapist (OT),** although *Handwriting Without Tears* is a curriculum frequently used by OTs when working with children with poor penmanship. An empirically supported writing program has been developed by Berninger, but it is not widely used inside or outside school systems (*PAL Research-Based Reading and Writing Lessons*). For children with dysgraphia, lower-level transcription skills should be emphasized to the point of becoming automatic. The connection between transcription skills and composition should be included in the instructional process; that is, children need to see how their work at letter production is related to broader components of writing. Further, because of WM constraints that frequently impact the instructional process for students with learning disorders, all components of writing should be taught within the same lesson.

Explicit instruction of writing strategies combined with implementation and coaching in self-regulation will likely produce the greatest gains for students with writing deficits. Emphasis will vary depending on the deficit specific to the child. A well-researched and well-supported intervention for poor writers is **self-regulated strategy development (SRSD)**. The 6 stages in this model include developing and activating a child's background knowledge; introducing and discussing the strategy that is being taught; modeling the strategy for the student; assisting the child in memorization of the strategy; supporting the child's use of the strategy during implementation; and independent use of the strategy. SRSD can be applied across various writing situations and is supported until the student has developed mastery. The model can emphasize or deemphasize the areas most needed by the child.

Educational Resources

Children with identified learning disorders can potentially qualify for formal education programming through special education or a section 504 plan. **Special education** is guided on a federal level by the **Individual with Disabilities Education Act (IDEA)** and includes development of an **individual education plan** (see Chapter 48). A **504 plan** provides accommodations to help children succeed in the regular classroom. Accommodations that might be provided to a child with IWE, through an IEP or a 504 plan, include dictation to a scribe when confronted with lengthy writing tasks, additional time to complete exams that require writing, and use of technology such as keyboarding, speech-to-text software, and writing devices that record teacher instruction. When recommending that parents pursue assistive technology for their child as a potential accommodation, the physician should emphasize the importance of instruction to mastery of the device being used. Learning to use technology effectively requires considerable time and is initially likely to require additional effort, which can result in frustration and avoidance.

Bibliography is available at Expert Consult.

Chapter 52
Language Development and Communication Disorders

Mark D. Simms

第五十二章
语言发育和交流障碍

中文导读

　　本章主要介绍了正常的语言发展、语言和沟通障碍、运动性言语障碍、听力受损、脑积水、语言障碍的罕见原因、不明原因的语言延迟、治疗、预后、共患病。正常的语言发展具体描述了语言接收能力的发展、语言表达能力的发展及正常模式的变化；语言和沟通障碍具体描述了流行病学、病因、发病机制、临床表现等；运动性言语障碍具体描述了构音障碍、儿童言语失用症、语音障碍；共患病具体描述了情绪和行为困难、运动和协调延迟。

Most children learn to communicate in their native language without specific instruction or intervention other than exposure to a language-rich environment. Normal development of speech and language is predicated on the infant's ability to hear, see, comprehend, remember, and socially interact with others. The infant must also possess sufficient motor skills to imitate oral motor movements.

NORMAL LANGUAGE DEVELOPMENT

Language can be subdivided into several essential components. **Communication** consists of a wide range of behaviors and skills. At the level of basic verbal ability, **phonology** refers to the correct use of speech sounds to form words, **semantics** refers to the correct use of words, and **syntax** refers to the appropriate use of grammar to make sentences. At a more abstract level, verbal skills include the ability to link thoughts together coherently and to maintain a topic of conversation. **Pragmatic** abilities include verbal and nonverbal skills that facilitate the exchange of ideas, including the appropriate choice of language for the situation and circumstance and the appropriate use of body language (i.e., posture, eye contact, gestures). Social pragmatic and behavioral skills also play an important role in effective interactions with communication partners (i.e., engaging, responding, and maintaining reciprocal exchanges).

It is customary to divide language skills into **receptive** (hearing and understanding) and **expressive** (talking) abilities. Language development usually follows a fairly predictable pattern and parallels general intellectual development (Table 52.1).

Receptive Language Development

The peripheral auditory system is mature by 26 wk gestation, and the fetus responds to and discriminates speech sounds. Anatomic asymmetry in the *planum temporale*, the structural brain region specialized for language processing, is present by 31 wk gestation. At birth, the full-term newborn appears to have functionally organized neural networks that are sensitive to different properties of language input. The normal newborn demonstrates preferential response to human voices over inanimate sound and recognizes the mother's voice, reacting stronger to it than to a stranger's voice. Even more remarkable is the ability of the newborn to discriminate sentences in their "native" (mother's) language from sentences in a "foreign" language. In research settings, infants of monolingual mothers showed a preference for only that language, whereas infants of bilingual mothers showed a preference for both exposed languages over any other language.

Between 4 and 6 mo, infants visually search for the source of sounds, again showing a preference for the human voice over other environmental sounds. By 6 mo, infants can passively follow the adult's line of visual regard, resulting in a "joint reference" to the same objects and events in the environment. The ability to share the same experience is critical to the development of further language, social, and cognitive skills as the infant "maps" specific meanings onto his or her experiences. By 8-9 mo, the infant can actively show, give, and point to objects. Comprehension of words often becomes apparent by 9 mo, when the infant selectively responds to his or her name and appears to comprehend the

Table 52.1	Normal Language Milestones: Birth to 5 Years

HEARING AND UNDERSTANDING	**TALKING**
BIRTH TO 3 MONTHS	
Startles to loud sounds Quiets or smiles when spoken to Seems to recognize your voice and quiets if crying Increases or decreases sucking behavior in response to sound	Makes pleasure sounds (cooing, gooing) Cries differently for different needs Smiles when sees you
4-6 MONTHS	
Moves eyes in direction of sounds Responds to changes in tone of your voice Notices toys that make sounds Pays attention to music	Babbling sounds more speech-like, with many different sounds, including *p, b,* and *m* Vocalizes excitement and displeasure Makes gurgling sounds when left alone and when playing with you
7 MONTHS TO 1 YEAR	
Enjoys games such as peek-a-boo and pat-a-cake Turns and looks in direction of sounds Listens when spoken to Recognizes words for common items, such as *cup, shoe,* and *juice* Begins to respond to requests (*Come here; Want more?*)	Babbling has both long and short groups of sounds, such as *tata upup bibibibi.* Uses speech or noncrying sounds to get and keep attention Imitates different speech sounds Has 1 or 2 words (*bye-bye, dada, mama*), although they might not be clear
1-2 YEARS	
Points to a few body parts when asked Follows simple commands and understands simple questions (*Roll the ball; Kiss the baby; Where's your shoe?*) Listens to simple stories, songs, and rhymes Points to pictures in a book when named	Says more words every month Uses some 1-2 word questions (*Where kitty? Go bye-bye? What's that?*) Puts 2 words together (*more cookie, no juice, mommy book*) Uses many different consonant sounds at the beginning of words
2-3 YEARS	
Understands differences in meaning (e.g., go–stop, in–on, big–little, up–down) Follows 2-step requests (*Get the book and put it on the table.*)	Has a word for almost everything Uses 2-3 word "sentences" to talk about and ask for things Speech is understood by familiar listeners most of the time Often asks for or directs attention to objects by naming them
3-4 YEARS	
Hears you when you call from another room Hears television or radio at the same loudness level as other family members Understands simple *who, what, where, why* questions	Talks about activities at school or at friends' homes Usually understood by people outside the family Uses a lot of sentences that have ≥4 words Usually talks easily without repeating syllables or words
4-5 YEARS	
Pays attention to a short story and answers simple questions about it Hears and understands most of what is said at home and in school	Voice sounds as clear as other children's Uses sentences that include details (*I like to read my books*) Tells stories that stick to a topic Communicates easily with other children and adults Says most sounds correctly except a few, such as *l, s, r, v, z, ch, sh,* and *th* Uses the same grammar as the rest of the family

Adapted from American Speech-Language-Hearing Association, 2005. http://www.asha.org/public/speech/development/chart.htm.

word "no." Social games, such as "peek-a-boo," "so big," and waving "bye-bye" can be elicited by simply mentioning the words. At 12 mo, many children can follow a simple, 1-step request without a gesture (e.g., "Give it to me").

Between 1 and 2 yr, comprehension of language accelerates rapidly. Toddlers can point to body parts on command, identify pictures in books when named, and respond to simple questions (e.g., "Where's your shoe?"). The 2 yr old is able to follow a 2-step command, employing unrelated tasks (e.g., "Take off your shoes, then go sit at the table"), and can point to objects described by their use (e.g., "Give me the one we drink from"). By 3 yr, children typically understand simple "wh-" question forms (e.g., who, what, where, why). By 4 yr, most children can follow adult conversation. They can listen to a short story and answer simple questions about it. A 5 yr old typically has a receptive vocabulary of more than 2000 words and can follow 3- and 4-step commands.

Expressive Language Development

Cooing noises are established by 4-6 wk of age. Over the 1st 3 mo of life, parents may distinguish their infant's different vocal sounds for pleasure, pain, fussing, tiredness, and so on. Many 3 mo old infants vocalize in a reciprocal fashion with an adult to maintain a social interaction ("vocal tennis"). By 4 mo, infants begin to make bilabial ("raspberry") sounds, and by 5 mo, monosyllables and laughing are noticeable. Between 6 and 8 mo, polysyllabic *babbling* ("lalala" or "mamama") is heard, and the infant might begin to communicate with gestures. Between 8 and 10 mo, babbling makes a phonologic shift toward the particular sound patterns of the child's native language (i.e., they produce more native sounds than nonnative sounds). At 9-10 mo, babbling becomes truncated into specific words (e.g., "mama," "dada") for their parents.

Over the next several months, infants learn 1 or 2 words for common objects and begin to imitate words presented by an adult. These words might appear to come and go from the child's repertoire until a stable group of 10 or more words is established. The rate of acquisition of new words is approximately 1 new word per week at 12 mo, but it accelerates to approximately 1 new word per day by 2 yr. The first words to appear are used primarily to label objects (nouns) or to ask for objects and people (requests). By 18-20 mo, toddlers should use a minimum of 20 words and produce *jargon* (strings of word-like sounds) with language-like inflection patterns (rising and falling speech patterns). This jargon usually contains some embedded true words. Spontaneous

2-word phrases (pivotal speech), consisting of the flexible juxtaposition of words with clear intention (e.g., "Want juice!" or "Me down!"), is characteristic of 2 yr olds and reflects the emergence of grammatical ability (syntax).

Two-word, combinational phrases do not usually emerge until children have acquired 50-100 words in their lexicon. Thereafter, the acquisition of new words accelerates rapidly. As knowledge of grammar increases, there is a proportional increase in verbs, adjectives, and other words that serve to define the relation between objects and people (predicates). By 3 yr, sentence length increases, and the child uses pronouns and simple present-tense verb forms. These 3-5 word sentences typically have a subject and verb but lack conjunctions, articles, and complex verb forms. The *Sesame Street* character Cookie Monster ("Me want cookie!") typifies the "telegraphic" nature of the 3 yr old's sentences. By 4-5 yr, children should be able to carry on conversations using adult-like grammatical forms and use sentences that provide details (e.g., "I like to read my books").

Variations of Normal

Language milestones have been found to be largely universal across languages and cultures, with some variations depending on the complexity of the grammatical structure of individual languages. In Italian (where verbs often occupy a prominent position at the beginning or end of sentences), 14 mo olds produce a greater proportion of verbs compared with English speaking infants. Within a given language, development usually follows a predictable pattern, paralleling general cognitive development. Although the sequences are predictable, the exact timing of achievement is not. There are marked variations among normal children in the rate of development of babbling, comprehension of words, production of single words, and use of combinational forms within the first 2-3 yr of life.

Two basic patterns of language learning have been identified, analytic and holistic. The *analytic* pattern is the most common and reflects the mastery of increasingly larger units of language form. The child's analytic skills proceed from simple to more complex and lengthy forms. Children who follow a *holistic* or gestalt learning pattern might start by using relatively large chunks of speech in familiar contexts. They might memorize familiar phrases or dialog from movies or stories and repeat them in an overgeneralized fashion. Their sentences often have a formulaic pattern, reflecting inadequate mastery of the use of grammar to flexibly and spontaneously combine words appropriately in the child's own unique utterance. Over time, these children gradually break down the meanings of phrases and sentences into their component parts, and they learn to analyze the linguistic units of these memorized forms. As this occurs, more original speech productions emerge, and the child is able to assemble thoughts in a more flexible manner. Both analytic and holistic learning processes are necessary for normal language development to occur.

LANGUAGE AND COMMUNICATION DISORDERS
Epidemiology
Disorders of speech and language are very common in preschool-age children. Almost 20% of 2 yr olds are thought to have delayed onset of language. By age 5 yr, approximately 6% of children are identified as having a speech impairment, 5% as having both speech and language impairment, and 8% as having language impairment. Boys are nearly twice as likely to have an identified speech or language impairment as girls.

Etiology
Normal language ability is a complex function that is widely distributed across the brain through interconnected neural networks that are synchronized for specific activities. Although clinical similarities exist between acquired aphasia in adults and childhood language disorders, unilateral focal lesions acquired in early life do not seem to have the same effects in children as in adults. Risk factors for **neurologic injury** are absent in the vast majority of children with language impairment.

Genetic factors appear to play a major role in influencing how children learn to talk. Language disorders cluster in families. A careful family history may identify current or past speech or language problems in up to 30% of first-degree relatives of proband children. Although children exposed to parents with language difficulty might be expected to experience poor language stimulation and inappropriate language modeling, studies of twins have shown the concordance rate for low language test score and/or a history of speech therapy to be approximately 50% in dizygotic pairs, rising to over 90% in monozygotic pairs. Despite strong evidence that language disorders have a genetic basis, consistent genetic mutations have not been identified. Instead, multiple genetic regions and epigenetic changes may result in heterogeneous genetic pathways causing language disorders. Some of these genetic pathways disrupt the timing of early prenatal neurodevelopmental events affecting migration of nerve cells from the germinal matrix to the cerebral cortex. Several single nucleotide polymorphisms (SNPs) involving noncoding regulatory genes, including *CNTNAP2* (contactin-associated-protein-like-2) and *KIAA0319*, are strongly associated with early language acquisition and are also believed to affect early neuronal structural development.

In addition, other environmental, hormonal, and nutritional factors may exert **epigenetic** influences by dysregulating gene expression and resulting in aberrant sequencing of the onset, growth, and timing of language development.

Pathogenesis
Language disorders are associated with a fundamental deficit in the brain's capacity to process complex information rapidly. Simultaneous evaluation of words (semantics), sentences (syntax), *prosody* (tone of voice), and social cues can overtax the child's ability to comprehend and respond appropriately in a verbal setting. Limitations in the amount of information that can be stored in verbal working memory can further limit the rate at which language information is processed. Electrophysiologic studies show abnormal latency in the early phase of auditory processing in children with language disorders. Neuroimaging studies identify an array of anatomic abnormalities in regions of the brain that are central to language processing. MRI scans in children with **specific language impairment (SLI)** may reveal white matter lesions and volume loss, ventricular enlargement, focal gray matter heterotopia within the right and left parietotemporal white matter, abnormal morphology of the inferior frontal gyrus, atypical patterns of asymmetry of language cortex, or increased thickness of the corpus callosum in a minority of affected children. Postmortem studies of children with language disorders found evidence of atypical symmetry in the plana temporale and cortical dysplasia in the region of the sylvian fissure. In support of a genetic mechanism affecting cerebral development, a high rate of atypical perisylvian asymmetries has also been documented in the parents of children with SLI.

Clinical Manifestations
Primary disorders of speech and language development are often found in the absence of more generalized cognitive or motor dysfunction. However, disorders of communication are also the most common comorbidities in persons with generalized cognitive disorders (intellectual disability or autism), structural anomalies of the organs of speech (e.g., velopharyngeal insufficiency from cleft palate), and neuromotor conditions affecting oral motor coordination (e.g., dysarthria from cerebral palsy or other neuromuscular disorders).

Classification
Each professional discipline has adopted a somewhat different classification system, based on cluster patterns of symptoms. The American Psychiatric Association (APA) *Diagnostic and Statistical Manual of Mental Disorders, Fifth Edition* (DSM-5) organized communication disorders into: (1) language disorder (which combines expressive and mixed receptive-expressive language disorders), speech sound disorder (phonologic disorder), and childhood-onset fluency disorder (stuttering); and (2) social (pragmatic) communication disorder, which is characterized by persistent difficulties in the social uses of verbal and nonverbal communication (Table 52.2). In clinical practice, childhood speech and language disorders occur as a number of distinct entities.

Table 52.2	DSM-5 Diagnostic Criteria for Communication Disorders

Language Disorder

A Persistent difficulties in the acquisition and use of language across modalities (i.e., spoken, written, sign language, or other) due to deficits in comprehension or production that include the following:
 1. Reduced vocabulary (word knowledge and use).
 2. Limited sentence structure (ability to put words and word endings together to form sentences based on the rules of grammar and morphology).
 3. Impairments in discourse (ability to use vocabulary and connect sentences to explain or describe a topic or series of events or have a conversation).
B. Language abilities are substantially and quantifiably below those expected for age, resulting in functional limitations in effective communication, social participation, academic achievement, or occupational performance, individually or in any combination.
C. Onset of symptoms is in the early developmental period.
D. The difficulties are not attributable to hearing or other sensory impairment, motor dysfunction, or another medical or neurologic condition and are not better explained by intellectual disability (intellectual developmental disorder) or global developmental delay.

Speech Sound Disorder

A. Persistent difficulty with speech sound production that interferes with speech intelligibility or prevents verbal communication of messages.
B. The disturbance causes limitations in effective communication that interfere with social participation, academic achievement, or occupational performance, individually or in any combination.
C. Onset of symptoms is in the early developmental period.
D. The difficulties are not attributable to congenital or acquired conditions, such as cerebral palsy, cleft palate, deafness or hearing loss, traumatic brain injury, or other medical or neurologic conditions.

Social (Pragmatic) Communication Disorder

A. Persistent difficulties in the social use of verbal and nonverbal communication as manifested by all of the following:
 1. Deficits in using communication for social purposes, such as greeting and sharing information, in a manner that is appropriate for the social context.
 2. Impairment of the ability to change communication to match context or the needs of the listener, such as speaking differently in a classroom than on a playground, talking differently to a child than to an adult, and avoiding use of overly formal language.
 3. Difficulties following rules for conversation and storytelling, such as taking turns in conversation, rephrasing when misunderstood, and knowing how to use verbal and nonverbal signals to regulate interaction.
 4. Difficulties understanding what is not explicitly stated (e.g., making inferences) and nonliteral or ambiguous meanings of language (e.g., idioms, humor, metaphors, multiple meanings that depend on the context for interpretation).
B. The deficits result in functional limitations in effective communication, social participation, social relationships, academic achievement, or occupational performance, individually or in combination.
C. The onset of the symptoms is in the early developmental period (but deficits may not become fully manifest until social communication demands exceed limited capacities).
D. The symptoms are not attributable to another medical or neurologic condition or to low abilities in the domains of word structure and grammar, and are not better explained by autism spectrum disorder, intellectual disability (intellectual developmental disorder), global developmental delay, or another mental disorder.

From the *Diagnostic and Statistical Manual of Mental Disorders, Fifth Edition*, (Copyright 2013). American Psychiatric Association, pp 42, 44, 47–48.

Language Disorder or Specific Language Impairment

The condition DSM-5 refers to as **language disorder** is also referred to as **specific language impairment (SLI)**, **developmental dysphasia**, or **developmental language disorder**. SLI is characterized by a significant discrepancy between the child's overall cognitive level (typically nonverbal measures of intelligence) and functional language level. These children also follow an atypical pattern of language acquisition and use. Closer examination of the child's skills might reveal deficits in understanding and use of word meaning (semantics) and grammar (syntax). Often, children are delayed in starting to talk. Most significantly, they usually have difficulty understanding spoken language. The problem may stem from insufficient understanding of single words or from the inability to deconstruct and analyze the meaning of sentences. Many affected children show a *holistic* pattern of language development, repeating memorized phrases or dialog from movies or stories (echolalia). In contrast to their difficulty with spoken language, children with SLI appear to learn visually and demonstrate their ability on nonverbal tests of intelligence.

After children with SLI become fluent talkers, they are generally less proficient at producing oral narratives than their peers. Their stories tend to be shorter and include fewer propositions, main story ideas, or story grammar elements. Older children include fewer mental state descriptions (e.g., references to what their characters think and how they feel). Their narratives contain fewer cohesive devices, and the story line may be difficult to follow.

Many children with SLI show difficulties with **social interaction**, particularly with same-age peers. Social interaction is mediated by oral communication, and a child deficient in communication is at a distinct disadvantage in the social arena. Children with SLI tend to be more dependent on older children or adults, who can adapt their communication to match the child's level of function. Generally, social interaction

skills are more closely correlated with language level than with nonverbal cognitive level. Using this as a guide, one usually sees a developmental progression of increasingly more sophisticated social interaction as the child's language abilities improve. In this context, social ineptitude is not necessarily a sign of asocial distancing (e.g., autism) but rather a delay in the ability to negotiate social interactions.

Higher-Level Language Disorder

As children mature, the ability to communicate effectively with others depends on mastery of a range of skills that go beyond basic understanding of words and rules of grammar. Higher-level language skills include the development of advanced vocabulary, the understanding of word relationships, reasoning skills (including drawing correct inferences and conclusions), the ability to understand things from another person's perspective, and the ability to paraphrase and rephrase with ease. In addition, higher-order language abilities include pragmatic skills that serve as the foundation for social interactions. These skills include knowledge and understanding of one's conversational partner, knowledge of the social context in which the conversation is taking place, and general knowledge of the world. Social and linguistic aspects of communication are often difficult to separate, and persons who have trouble interpreting these relatively abstract aspects of communication typically experience difficulty forming and maintaining relationships.

DSM-5 identified **social (pragmatic) communication disorder (SPCD)** as a category of communication disorder (Table 52.2). Symptoms of pragmatic difficulty include extreme literalness and inappropriate verbal and social interactions. Proper use and understanding of humor, slang, and sarcasm depend on correct interpretation of the meaning and the context of language and the ability to draw proper inferences. Failure to provide a sufficient referential base to one's conversational partner—to take the perspective of another person—results in the appearance of talking or behaving randomly or incoherently. SPCD often occurs in the context of another language disorder and has been recognized as a symptom of a wide range of disorders, including right-hemisphere damage to the brain, Williams syndrome, and nonverbal learning disabilities. SPCD can also occur independently of other disorders. Children with **autism spectrum disorder (ASD)** often have symptoms of SPCD, but SPCD is not diagnosed in these children because the symptoms are a component of ASD. In school settings, children with SPCD may be socially ostracized and bullied.

Intellectual Disability
Most children with a mild degree of intellectual disability learn to talk at a slower-than-normal rate; they follow a normal sequence of language acquisition and eventually master basic communication skills. Difficulties may be encountered with higher-level language concepts and use. Persons with moderate to severe degrees of intellectual disability can have great difficulty in acquiring basic communication skills. About half of persons with an intelligence quotient (IQ) of <50 can communicate using single words or simple phrases; the rest are typically nonverbal.

Autism Spectrum Disorder
A disordered pattern of language development is one of the core features of ASD (see Chapter 54). The language profile of children with ASD is often indistinguishable from that in children with SLI or SPCD. The key characteristics of ASD that distinguish it from SLI or SPCD are lack of reciprocal social relationships; limitation in the ability to develop functional, symbolic, or pretend play; hyper- or hyporeactivity to sensory input; and an obsessive need for sameness and resistance to change. Approximately 40% of children with ASD also have intellectual disability, which can limit their ability to develop functional communication skills. Language abilities can range from absent to grammatically intact, but with limited pragmatic features and odd prosody patterns. Some individuals with ASD have highly specialized, but isolated, "savant" skills, such as calendar calculations and **hyperlexia** (the precocious ability to recognize written words beyond expectation based on general intellectual ability). Parents report regression in language and social skills (**autistic regression**) in approximately 20–25% of children with ASD, usually between 12 and 36 mo of age. The cause of the regression is not known, but it tends to be associated with an increased risk for comorbid intellectual disability and more severe ASD (Fig. 52.1).

Asperger Syndrome
Asperger syndrome is characterized by difficulties in social interaction, eccentric behaviors, and abnormally intense and circumscribed interests despite normal cognitive and verbal ability. Affected individuals may engage in long-winded, verbose monologs about their topics of special interest, with little regard to the reaction of others. Adults with Asperger syndrome generally have a more favorable prognosis of than those with "classic" autism. Prior to 2013, Asperger syndrome was classified as distinct from autism; however, DSM-5 no longer recognizes Asperger as a separate neurodevelopmental disorder. More severely affected individuals are now considered to be at the "high functioning" end of the autism spectrum (see Chapter 54), whereas mildly impaired individuals may be diagnosed with SPCD.

Selective Mutism
Selective mutism is defined as a failure to speak in specific social situations despite speaking in other situations, and it is typically a symptom of an underlying **anxiety disorder**. Children with selective mutism can speak normally in certain settings, such as within their home or when they are alone with their parents. They fail to speak in other social settings, such as at school or at other places outside their home. Other symptoms associated with selective mutism can include excessive shyness, withdrawal, dependency on parents, and oppositional behavior. Most cases of selective mutism are not the result of a single traumatic event, but rather the manifestation of a chronic pattern of anxiety. Mutism is not passive-aggressive behavior. Selectively mute children often report that they want to speak in social settings but are afraid to do so. Often, one or both parents of a child with selective mutism has a history of

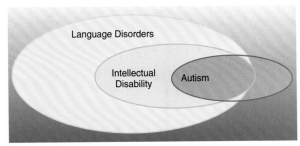

Fig. 52.1 Relationship of autism, language disorders, and intellectual disability. (*From Simms MD, Schum RL: Preschool children who have atypical patterns of development, Pediatr Rev 21:147–158, 2000.*)

anxiety symptoms, including childhood shyness, social anxiety, or panic attacks. Mutism is highly functional for the child in that it reduces anxiety and protects the child from the perceived challenge of social interaction. Treatment of selective mutism should utilize cognitive behavioral strategies focused on reducing the general anxiety and increasing speaking in social situation (see Chapter 38). Occasionally, selective serotonin reuptake inhibitors are helpful in conjunction with cognitive-behavioral therapy. Selective mutism reflects a difficulty of *social interaction*, not a disorder of language processing.

Isolated Expressive Language Disorder
More often seen in boys than girls, **isolated expressive language disorder** ("late talker syndrome") is a diagnosis best made in retrospect. These children have age-appropriate receptive language and social ability. Once they start talking, their speech is clear. There is no increased risk for language or learning disability as they progress through school. A family history of other males with a similar developmental pattern is often reported. This pattern of language development likely reflects a variation of normal.

MOTOR SPEECH DISORDERS
Dysarthria
Motor speech disorders can originate from neuromotor disorders such as cerebral palsy, muscular dystrophy, myopathy, and facial palsy. The resulting **dysarthria** affects both speech and nonspeech functions (smiling and chewing). Lack of strength and muscular control manifests as slurring of words and distorting of vowels. Speech patterns are often slow and labored. Poor velopharyngeal function can result in mixed nasal resonance (hyper- or hyponasal speech). In many cases, feeding difficulty, drooling, open-mouth posture, and protruding tongue accompany the dysarthric speech.

Childhood Apraxia of Speech
Difficulty in planning and coordinating movements for speech production can result in inconsistent distortion of speech sounds. The same word may be pronounced differently each time. Intelligibility tends to decline as the length and complexity of the child's speech increases. Consonants may be deleted and sounds transposed. As they try to talk spontaneously, or imitate other's speech, children with **childhood apraxia of speech** may display oral groping or struggling behaviors. Children with childhood apraxia of speech frequently have a history of early feeding difficulty, limited sound production as infants, and delayed onset of spoken words. They may point, grunt, or develop an elaborate gestural communication system in an attempt to overcome their verbal difficulty. Apraxia may be limited to oral-motor function, or it may be a more generalized problem affecting fine and/or gross motor coordination.

Speech Sound Disorder
Children with **speech sound disorder (SSD)**, previously called *phonologic disorder,* are often unintelligible, even to their parents. Articulation errors are not the result of neuromotor impairment, but rather seem

to reflect an inability to correctly process the words they hear (Table 52.2). As a result, they lack understanding of how to fit sounds together properly to create words. In contrast to children with childhood apraxia of speech, those SSD are fluent, although unintelligible, and produce a consistent, highly predictable pattern of articulation errors. Children with SSD are at high risk for later reading and learning disability.

HEARING IMPAIRMENT

Hearing loss can be a major cause of delayed or disordered language development (see Chapter 655). Approximately 16-30 per 1,000 children have mild to severe hearing loss, significant enough to affect educational progress. In addition to these "hard of hearing" children, approximately another 1 : 1,000 are **deaf** (profound bilateral hearing loss). Hearing loss can be present at birth or acquired postnatally. Newborn screening programs can identify many forms of congenital hearing loss, but children can develop progressive hearing loss or acquire deafness after birth.

The most common types of hearing loss are attributable to conductive (middle ear) or sensorineural deficit. Although it is not possible to accurately predict the impact of hearing loss on a child's language development, the type and degree of hearing loss, the age of onset, and the duration of the auditory impairment clearly play important roles. Children with significant hearing impairment often have problems developing facility with language and often have related academic difficulties. Presumably, the language impairment is caused by lack of exposure to fluent language models, starting in infancy.

Approximately 30% of hearing-impaired children have at least 1 other disability that affects development of speech and language (e.g., intellectual disability, cerebral palsy, craniofacial anomalies). Any child who shows developmental warning signs of a speech or language problem should have a hearing assessment by an audiologist.

HYDROCEPHALUS

Some children with **hydrocephalus** may be described as having "cocktail-party syndrome." Although they may use sophisticated words, their comprehension of abstract concepts is limited, and their pragmatic conversational skills are weak. As a result, they speak superficially about topics and appear to be carrying on a monolog (see Chapter 609.11).

RARE CAUSES OF LANGUAGE IMPAIRMENT
Hyperlexia

Hyperlexia is the precocious development of reading single words that spontaneously occurs in some young children (2-5 yr) without specific instruction. It is often associated with ASD or SLI. It stands in contrast to precocious reading development in young children who do not have any other developmental disorders. A typical manifestation is a child with SLI orally reading single words or matching pictures with single words. Although hyperlexic children show early and well-developed word-decoding skills, they usually do not have precocious ability for comprehension of text. Rather, text comprehension is closely intertwined with oral comprehension, and children who have difficulty decoding the syntax of language are also at risk for having reading comprehension problems.

Landau-Kleffner Syndrome (Verbal Auditory Agnosia)

Children with Landau-Kleffner syndrome have a history of normal language development until they experience a regression in their ability to comprehend spoken language, **verbal auditory agnosia.** The regression may be sudden or gradual, and it usually occurs between 3 and 7 yr of age. Expressive language skills typically deteriorate, and some children may become mute. Despite their language regression, these children typically retain appropriate play patterns and the ability to interact in a socially appropriate manner. An electroencephalogram (EEG) might show a distinct pattern of status epilepticus in sleep (continuous spike wave in slow-wave sleep), and up to 80% of children with Landau-Kleffner syndrome eventually exhibit clinical seizures. A number of treatment approaches have been reported, including antiepileptic medication, corticosteroids, and intravenous gamma globulin, with varying results. The prognosis for return of normal language ability is uncertain, even

with resolution of the EEG abnormality. Epileptic interictal discharges are more frequently found on EEGs of children with language impairments than in otherwise normally developing children, even in those without any history of language regression. However, this phenomenon is believed to represent a manifestation of an underlying disorder of brain structure or function that is distinct from the language impairment, because there has been little evidence of improvement in language function when the EEG was normalized after antiepileptic administration. Unless there is a clear pattern of either seizure symptoms or regression in language ability, a routine EEG is not recommended as part of the evaluation for a child with speech and/or language impairment.

Metabolic and Neurodegenerative Disorders
(See also Part X.)

Regression of language development may accompany loss of neuromotor function at the outset of a number of metabolic diseases, including lysosomal storage disorders (metachromatic leukodystrophy), peroxisomal disorders (adrenal leukodystrophy), ceroid lipofuscinosis (Batten disease), and mucopolysaccharidosis (Hunter disease, Hurler disease). Recently, creatine transporter deficiency was identified as an X-linked disorder that manifests with language delay in boys and with mild learning disability in female carriers.

Screening

Developmental surveillance at each well child visit should include specific questions about normal language developmental milestones and observations of the child's behavior. **Clinical judgment,** defined as eliciting and responding to parents' concerns, can detect the majority of children with speech and language problems. The AAP recommends clinicians employ standardized developmental screening questionnaires and observation checklists at select well child visits. (see Chapter 28).

In 2015 the U.S. Preventive Services Task Force reviewed screening for SLI in young children in primary care settings and found inadequate evidence to support screening in the absence of parental or clinician concern about children's speech, language, hearing, or development. When either parents or physicians are concerned about speech or language development for reasons such as highlighted in Table 52.3, the child should be referred for further evaluation and intervention (see Diagnostic Evaluation).

NONCAUSES OF LANGUAGE DELAY

Twinning, birth order, "laziness," exposure to multiple languages (bilingualism), tongue-tie (ankyloglossia), or otitis media are not adequate explanations for significant language delay. Normal twins learn to talk at the same age as normal single-born children, and birth-order effects on language development have not been consistently found. The drive to communicate and the rewards for successful verbal interaction are so strong that children who let others talk for them usually cannot talk for themselves and are not "lazy." Toddlers exposed to more than one language can show a mild delay in starting to talk, and they can initially mix elements (vocabulary and syntax) of the different languages they are learning (code switching). However, they learn to segregate each language by 24-30 mo and are equal to their monolingual peers by 3 yr of age. An extremely tight lingual frenulum (tongue-tie) can affect feeding and speech articulation but does not prevent the acquisition of language abilities. Prospective studies also show that frequent ear infections and serous otitis media in early childhood do not result in persisting language disorder.

Diagnostic Evaluation

It is important to distinguish developmental delay (abnormal timing) from abnormal patterns or sequences of development. A child's language and communication skills must also be interpreted within the context of the child's overall cognitive and physical abilities. It is also important to evaluate the child's use of language to communicate with others in the broadest sense (communicative intent). Thus a multidisciplinary evaluation is often warranted. At a minimum, this should include psychologic evaluation, neurodevelopmental pediatric assessment, and speech-language examination.

Table 52.3	Speech and Language Screening	

REFER FOR SPEECH–LANGUAGE EVALUATION IF:

AT AGE	RECEPTIVE	EXPRESSIVE
15 mo	Does not look/point at 5-10 objects	Is not using 3 words
18 mo	Does not follow simple directions ("get your shoes")	Is not using Mama, Dada, or other names
24 mo	Does not point to pictures or body parts when they are named	Is not using 25 words
30 mo	Does not verbally respond or nod/shake head to questions	Is not using unique 2-word phrases, including noun–verb combinations
36 mo	Does not understand prepositions or action words; does not follow 2-step directions	Has a vocabulary of <200 words; does not ask for things; echolalia to questions; language regression after attaining 2-word phrases

Psychologic Evaluation

There are two main goals for the psychologic evaluation of a young child with a communication disorder. Nonverbal cognitive ability must be assessed to determine if the child has an intellectually disability, and the child's social behaviors must be assessed to determine whether ASD is present. Additional diagnostic considerations may include emotional disorders such as anxiety, depression, mood disorder, obsessive-compulsive disorder, academic learning disorders, and attention-deficit/hyperactivity disorder (ADHD).

Cognitive Assessment

Intellectual disability is defined as deficits in cognitive abilities and adaptive behaviors. In this context, children with intellectual disability show delayed development of communication skills; however, delayed communication does not necessarily signal intellectual disability. Therefore, a broad-based cognitive assessment is an important component to the evaluation of children with language delays, including evaluation of both verbal and nonverbal skills. If a child has intellectual disability, both verbal and nonverbal scores will be low compared to norms (≤2nd percentile). In contrast, a typical cognitive profile for a child with SLI includes a significant difference between nonverbal and verbal abilities, with nonverbal IQ being greater than verbal IQ and the nonverbal score being within an average range.

Evaluation of Social Behaviors

Social interest is the key difference between children with a primary language disorder (SLI) and those with a communication disorder secondary to ASD. Children with SLI have an interest in social interaction, but they may have difficulty enacting their interest because of their limitations in communication. In contrast, autistic children show little social interest.

Relationship of Language and Social Behaviors to Mental Age

Cognitive assessment provides a mental age for the child, and the child's behavior must be evaluated in that context. Most 4 yr old children typically engage peers in interactive play, but most 2 yr olds are playful but primarily focused on interactions with adult caretakers. A 4 yr old with mild to moderate intellectual disability and a mental age of 2 yr might not yet play with peers because of cognitive limitation, not a lack of desire for social interaction.

Speech and Language Evaluation

A certified **speech-language pathologist** should perform a speech and language evaluation. A typical evaluation includes assessment of language, speech, and the physical mechanisms associated with speech production. Both expressive and receptive language is assessed by a combination of standardized measures and informal interactions and observations. All components of language are assessed, including syntax, semantics, pragmatics, and fluency. Speech assessment similarly uses a combination of standardized measures and informal observations. Assessment of physical structures includes oral structures and function, respiratory

function, and vocal quality. In many settings, a speech-language pathologist works in conjunction with an **audiologist**, who can do appropriate hearing evaluation of the child. If an audiologist is not available in that setting, a separate referral should be made. No child is too young for a speech-language or hearing evaluation. A referral for evaluation is appropriate whenever there is suspicion of language impairment.

Medical Evaluation

Careful history and physical examination should focus on the identification of potential contributors to the child's language and communication difficulties. A **family history** of delay in talking, need for speech and language therapy, or academic difficulty can suggest a genetic predisposition to language disorders. **Pregnancy history** might reveal risk factors for prenatal developmental anomalies, such as polyhydramnios or decreased fetal movement patterns. Small size for gestational age at birth, symptoms of neonatal encephalopathy, or early and persistent oral-motor feeding difficulty may presage speech and language difficulty. **Developmental history** should focus on the age when various language skills were mastered and the sequences and patterns of milestone acquisition. Regression or loss of acquired skills should raise immediate concern.

Physical examination should include measurement of height (length), weight, and head circumference. The skin should be examined for lesions consistent with phakomatosis (e.g., tuberous sclerosis, neurofibromatosis, Sturge-Weber syndrome) and other disruptions of pigment (e.g., hypomelanosis of Ito). Anomalies of the head and neck, such as white forelock and hypertelorism (Waardenburg syndrome), ear malformations (Goldenhar syndrome), facial and cardiac anomalies (Williams syndrome, velocardiofacial syndrome), retrognathism of the chin (Pierre Robin anomaly), or cleft lip/palate, are associated with hearing and speech abnormalities. **Neurologic examination** might reveal muscular hypertonia or hypotonia, both of which can affect neuromuscular control of speech. Generalized muscular hypotonia, with increased range of motion of the joints, is frequently seen in children with SLI. The reason for this association is not clear, but it might account for the fine and gross motor clumsiness often seen in these children. However, mild hypotonia is not a sufficient explanation for the impairment of expressive and receptive language.

No routine diagnostic studies are indicated for SLI or isolated language disorders. When language delay is a part of a generalized cognitive or physical disorder, referral for further genetic evaluation, chromosome testing (e.g., fragile X testing, microarray comparative genomic hybridization), neuroimaging studies, and EEG may be considered, if clinically indicated.

TREATMENT

The federal Individuals with Disabilities Education Act (IDEA) requires that schools provide early intervention and **special education** services to children who have learning difficulties. This includes children with speech and language disorders. Services are provided to children from birth through 21 yr of age. States have various methods for providing services, including speech and language therapy for young children, such as *Birth-to-Three*, *Early Childhood*, and *Early Learning* programs. Children can also receive therapy from nonprofit service agencies, hospital and rehabilitation centers, and speech pathologists in private practice.

Of concern is that many children with identified speech and language deficits do not receive appropriate intervention services. Population-based surveys in both the United States and Canada have found that less than half of children identified by kindergarten entry receive **speech and language interventions**, even when their parents have been educated about the nature of their child's condition. In one study, children with deficits in speech sound production were much more likely to receive services (41%) than those who had problems with language alone (9%). These findings are troubling because poor educational outcome, especially in reading, and impaired social-behavioral adjustment are more highly associated with language than with speech sound disorders. Therefore the children at greatest risk are least likely to receive intervention services. Boys were twice as likely to receive speech intervention as girls, regardless of their speech-language diagnosis. Social and demographic factors did not appear to influence whether identified children received interventions services.

Speech-language therapy includes a variety of goals. Sometimes both speech and language activities are incorporated in therapy. The speech goals focus on development of more intelligible speech. Language goals can focus on expanding vocabulary (lexicon) and understanding of the meaning of words (semantics), improving syntax by using proper forms or learning to expand single words into sentences, and social use of language (pragmatics). Therapy can include individual sessions, group sessions, and mainstream classroom integration. **Individual** sessions may use drill activities for older children or play activities for younger children to target specific goals. **Group** sessions can include several children with similar language goals to help them practice peer communication activities and to help them bridge the gap into more naturalistic communication situations. **Classroom** integration might include the therapist team-teaching or consulting with the teacher to facilitate the child's use of language in common academic situations.

For children with severe language impairment, alternative methods of communication are often included in therapy, such as manual sign language, use of pictures (e.g., Picture Exchange Communication System), and computerized devices for speech output. Often the ultimate goal is to achieve better spoken language. Early use of **signs** or **pictures** can help the child establish better functional communication and understand the symbolic nature of words to facilitate the language process. There is no evidence that use of signs or pictures interferes with development of oral language if the child has the capacity to speak. Many clinicians believe that these alternative methods accelerate the learning of language. These methods also reduce the frustration of parents and children who cannot communicate for basic needs.

Parents can consult with their child's speech-language therapist about home activities to enhance language development and extend therapy activities through appropriate language-stimulating activities and recreational reading. Parents' language activities should focus on emerging communication skills that are within the child's repertoire, rather than teaching the child new skills. The speech pathologist can guide parents on effective modeling and eliciting communication from their child.

Recreational **reading** focuses on expanding the child's comprehension of language. Sometimes the child's avoidance of reading is a sign that the parent is presenting material that is too complex for the child. The speech-language therapist can guide the parent in selecting an appropriate level of reading material.

PROGNOSIS

Children with mild isolated expressive language disorder ("late talkers") have an excellent prognosis for both language, learning, and social-emotional adjustment.

Over time, children with SLI respond to therapeutic/educational interventions and show a trend toward improvement of communication skills. Adults with a history of childhood language disorder continue to show evidence of impaired language ability, even when surface features

of the communication difficulty have improved considerably. This suggests that many persons find successful ways of adapting to their impairment. Although the majority of children improve their communication ability with time, 50–80% of preschoolers with language delay and normal nonverbal intelligence continue to experience difficulty with language and social development up to 20 yr beyond the initial diagnosis. Language disorders often interfere with the child's ability to conceptualize the increasingly complex and ambiguous worlds of social relationship and emotions. Consequently, in later childhood and adolescence, children with persisting symptoms of SLI are about twice as likely as their typical-language peers to show clinical levels of emotional problems and twice as likely to show behavioral difficulties.

A Danish study found that adults with SLI were less likely to have completed formal education beyond high school, and that they had lower occupational and socioeconomic success than the general population; 56% had a paid job (vs 84% of same-age general population), of whom 35% were unskilled and 40% skilled workers. About 80% of the adults reported difficulty reading while in school, most had received remedial teaching, and 50% continued to report reading difficulty as adults (vs 5% of Danish adults). Lower nonverbal intelligence and comorbid psychiatric or neurologic disorders independently contributed to a worse prognosis. These results were consistent with previous reports of adult outcomes of children with SLI from Canada and the United Kingdom.

Academic Disorders

Early language difficulty is strongly related to later **reading disorder**. Approximately 50% of children with early language difficulty develop reading disorder, and 55% of children with reading disorder have a history of impaired early oral language development. By the time they enter kindergarten, many children with early language deficits may have improved significantly, and they may begin to show early literacy skills, identifying and sounding out letters. However, as they progress through school, they are often unable to keep up with the increasing demands for both oral and written language. Despite their ability to read words, these children lack oral and reading comprehension, may read slowly, and struggle with a wide range of academic subjects. This "illusory recovery" of early language skill may result in children losing speech-language services or other special education support in early grades, only to be identified later with academic problems. In addition, children with subtle but persisting language impairments may appear inattentive or anxious in language-rich classroom environments and may be misdiagnosed as having an attention disorder.

A study from Australia found that at 7-9 yr of age, children with communication impairments were reported by their parents and teachers to be making slower progress in reading, writing, and overall school achievement than other children their age. The children reported a higher incidence of bullying, poorer peer relationships, and less overall enjoyment of school than their typically developing peers.

COMORBID DISORDERS
Emotional and Behavioral Difficulty

Early language disorder, particularly difficulty with auditory comprehension, appears to be a specific risk factor for later emotional dysfunction. Boys and girls with language disorder have a higher-than-expected rate of **anxiety disorder** (principally social phobia). Boys with language disorder are more likely to develop symptoms of ADHD, conduct disorder, and antisocial personality disorder compared with normally developing peers. Language disorders are common in children referred for psychiatric services, but they are often underdiagnosed, and their impact on children's behavior and emotional development is often overlooked.

Preschoolers with language difficulty frequently express their frustration through anxious, socially withdrawn, or aggressive behavior. As their ability to communicate improves, parallel improvements are usually noted in their behavior, suggesting a cause-and-effect relationship between language and behavior. However, the persistence of emotional and behavioral problems over the life span of persons with early language disability suggests a strong biologic or genetic connection between language development and subsequent emotional disorders.

The full impact of environmental and education support on these emotional and behavioral difficulties is not known at this time, but many children with SLI need psychologic support. Efforts should be made to support the child's resilience, emotional competency, and coping abilities. Parents and teachers should be encouraged to strengthen the child's prosocial behavior and reduce noncompliant and aggressive behaviors.

Motor and Coordination Delays

Approximately one third to one half of children with speech and/or language disorders have some degree of motor coordination impairment that may have an important impact on their ability to carry out activities of daily living (dressing, eating, bathing), school tasks (writing, drawing, coloring), and social/recreational activities (participation in sports and other playground activities). Motor difficulties are not related to the type of language impairment (i.e., they are found both in children with only receptive delays and in those with both expressive and receptive delays). The patterns of motor difficulty seen in children with language impairment are not distinctly "abnormal," and the motor profiles of children with language impairment resemble those of younger children, suggesting that they result from delayed maturation of motor development rather than from a neurologic impairment. Several researchers have postulated that language impairments and motor difficulties may have a common neurodevelopmental basis. Because attention may be focused on the child's language delays, the need for intervention and support for the child's comorbid motor impairment may be overlooked.

Bibliography is available at Expert Consult.

52.1 Childhood-Onset Fluency Disorder

Kenneth L. Grizzle

Developmental stuttering is a childhood speech disorder that is not associated with stroke, traumatic brain injury, or other possible medical conditions and that interrupts the normal flow of speech through repeated or prolonged sounds, syllables, or single-syllable words. (Table 52.4 lists definitions of terminology.) All speakers experience **speech dysfluencies**. During the toddler and preschool years, children often make repetitions of sounds, syllables, or words, particularly at the beginning of sentences (normal dysfluencies). However, dysfluencies found in individuals who stutter are distinct from those experienced by typically developing speakers. Specifically, children who stutter show greater part-word repetition ("b-b-b-b-but"), single-syllable word repetition ("My, my, my"), and sound prolongation ("MMMMMM-an"), and the frequency of their stuttering is much greater than found in normal dysfluencies. Other types of dysfluency that are not exclusive to children who stutter include *interjections* ("well, uhh, umm"), *revisions* ("I thought…I mean"), and *phrase repetitions* ("Did you say–Did you say"). The perspective of the speaker also characterizes differences between those children who stutter and a typical dysfluency. Children who stutter have decided on a word to use but are unable to "get the word out," while a typically developing child may struggle to express herself because she is unable to retrieve the word, changes thought, or is distracted.

Multiple nonspeech features can accompany stuttering. **Physical concomitants** that occur at the onset and as the condition persists include movements of the head (head turning or jerking), face (eye blinking/squinting, grimacing, opening or tightly closing the jaw), and neck (tightening) and irregular inhalations and exhalations. *Fear and anxiety* about speaking in a large-group setting, such as in front of a class or in interpersonal social interactions, are **emotional symptoms** associated with stuttering. As with all social beings, children closely monitor the reactions of those with whom they associate, especially as they get older. It is not difficult to imagine the impact a single or series of negative interactions or comments could have on a child's future attempts to interact verbally with another or in a large social setting. Consider also the potential **social challenges** associated with entering a classroom for the first time, transitioning to middle/high school/

Table 52.4	Terminology Related to Childhood-Onset Fluency Disorder
TERM	**DEFINITION**
Stuttering	A speech disorder manifested through abnormal speech patterns referred to as *dysfluencies*
Childhood-onset fluency disorder	Term used in DSM-5 that is synonymous with *stuttering*
Stammering	The clinical term used in the United Kingdom rather than stuttering; stammering also used informally to describe halting speech
Cluttering	A speech disorder characterized by excessively rapid and irregular rate of speech
Dysfluency	Speech disruptions that can occur in normal or disordered speech

college, beginning a job, dating, and so on. Not surprisingly, *avoidance* is a common way of coping with the anxiety created by the fear of stuttering.

In the *Diagnostic and Statistical Manual for Mental Disorders, Fifth Edition* (DSM-5), the term *stuttering* has been removed from the diagnostic classification, and the disorder is referred to as **childhood-onset fluency disorder** (Table 52.5). Note that impact on functional behavior is a component of the psychiatric diagnosis of this condition. In contrast, communication disorder specialists would consider possible anxiety and avoidance of various activities and situations a common concomitant of childhood-onset fluency disorder (stuttering) and not necessarily a requirement for the diagnosis to be made.

Stuttering is distinct from other disordered speech output conditions such as cluttering in several ways. Unlike stuttering, for which distinct episodes can be identified and even counted, **cluttering** affects the entire speech output. In addition to elevated repetitions of partial words (as in stuttering), whole words, and phrases, those who clutter show speech bursts that are often choppy, and articulation can be slurred and imprecise. The level of awareness of how their speech affects those listening, unlike children who stutter, is minimal for those who clutter. **Stammering** and stuttering are terms used interchangeably, although the former is used in the United Kingdom and the latter in the United States. "Stammer" is also used informally to describe when an individual is struggling to express himself and may speak in a halting or "bumbling" manner.

EPIDEMIOLOGY

Although prevalence studies have produced a range of estimates for developmental stuttering, it appears that 0.75–1% of the population is experiencing this condition at any one time. Incidence rates are considerably higher: Estimates to date suggest an incidence rate of approximately 5%, with rates considerably higher among young children than older children or adolescents. Seldom does a child begin stuttering before 2 yr of age or after 12 yr; in fact, the mean age of onset is 2-4 yr, and most children stop stuttering within 4 yr of onset. Symptoms will disappear within 4 wk for a minority of children. Although studies have consistently shown that the male:female ratio favors males, the magnitude of the pattern increases as children get older. The ratio among children <5 yr is approximately 2:1 and jumps to 4:1 among adolescents and young adults.

GENETICS

There is convergent evidence of a genetic link for childhood-onset fluency disorder. Concordance rates among MZ twins range from 20–83%, and for DZ twins, 4–19%. Family aggregation studies suggest increased incidence rate of approximately 15% among first-degree relatives of those affected, 3 times higher than the 5% rate for the general population. The variance in risk for stuttering attributed to genetic effects is high,

Table 52.5	DSM-5 Diagnostic Criteria for Childhood-Onset Fluency Disorder (Stuttering)

A. Disturbances in the normal fluency and time patterning of speech that are inappropriate for the individual's age and language skills, persist over time, and are characterized by frequent and marked occurrences of one (or more) of the following:
  1. Sound and syllable repetitions.
  2. Sound prolongations of consonants as well as vowels.
  3. Broken words (e.g., pauses within a word).
  4. Audible or silent blocking (filled or unfilled pauses in speech).
  5. Circumlocutions (word substitutions to avoid problematic words).
  6. Words produced with an excess of physical tension.
  7. Monosyllabic whole-word repetitions (e.g., "I-I-I-I see him").
B. The disturbance causes anxiety about speaking or limitations in effective communication, social participation, or academic or occupational performance, individually or in any combination.
C. The onset of symptoms is in the early developmental period.
  Note: Later-onset cases are diagnosed as 307.0 [F98.5] adult-onset fluency disorder.
D. The disturbance is not attributable to a speech-motor or sensory deficit, dysfluency associated with neurologic insult (e.g., stroke, tumor, trauma), or another medical condition and is not better explained by another mental disorder.

From the *Diagnostic and Statistical Manual of Mental Disorders, Fifth Edition,* (Copyright 2013). American Psychiatric Association, pp 45–46.)

ranging from 70–85%. Although evidence is limited, stuttering appears to be a polygenic condition, and several genes increase susceptibility.

ETIOLOGY

Brain structure and function abnormalities found in stutterers include deficits in white matter in the left hemisphere, overactivity in the right cortical region, and underactivity in the auditory cortex. Abnormal basal ganglia activation has also been identified among stutterers.

COMORBIDITIES

Despite the widely held belief in a high degree of comorbidity between childhood-onset fluency disorder and other communication disorders, research to date does not necessarily support this assertion. Speech-language pathologists (SLPs) consistently report higher rates of comorbidity on their caseload, although this would be expected in clinical samples. Speech sound (phonologic) disorders are the most commonly reported comorbidities, and 30–40% of children on SLP caseloads are also experiencing problems with phonology. However, studies have not found greater incidence of phonologic disorders among those who stutter compared to a control group. Similarly, SLPs report a much higher percentage of children with language disorders among their patients who stutter than the approximately 7% expected in the population at large, yet the language functioning among stutters apparently is no different than in the general population. The same pattern holds for learning disorder (LD). The incidence of various types of LDs associated with a language disorder is well documented, so one would expect to see increased frequency within a clinical population.

The perception of communication disorder professionals and people in general is that children who stutter experience more **anxiety** than their nonstuttering peers. This in fact is supported by clinical research that has found considerably higher rates of psychopathology, specifically social anxiety and generalized anxiety disorder, among adolescents who stutter. The frequency of reported anxiety increases with age. To date, however, the lack of controlled studies should not lead to the assumption

that stuttering itself places a child or adolescent at greater risk for a psychiatric disorder of any type. This is not meant to suggest that anxiety has no impact on a stuttering child's behavior in specific situations; as indicated earlier in this chapter, children who stutter frequently avoid situations that demand speaking.

Children who stutter have consistently been found to be bullied more than peers. In one study, stutterers were almost 4 times more likely to be bullied than their nonstuttering counterparts. About 45% of those who stuttered reported being the victim of bullying.

DEVELOPMENTAL PROGRESSION

Onset of stuttering typically occurs between 2 and 4 yr of age. Severity of symptoms vary, from pronounced stuttering within a few days of onset to gradual worsening of symptoms across months. Symptoms may ebb and flow, including disappearing for weeks before returning, especially among young children. From 40–75% of young children who stutter will stop spontaneously, typically within months of starting. Although predicting which child will stop stuttering is difficult, risk factors for persisting include stuttering for >1 yr, continued stuttering after age 6 yr, and experiencing other speech or language problems.

TREATMENT

Several factors should be considered when deciding to refer a younger child with childhood-onset fluency disorder for therapy. If there is a positive family history for stuttering, if symptoms have been present for >4 wk, and if the dysfluencies are impacting the child's social, behavioral, and emotional functioning, referral is warranted. Although there is no cure for stuttering, behavioral therapies are available that are developed and implemented by SLPs. Treatment emphasizes managing stuttering while speaking by regulating rate of speech and breathing and helping the child gradually progress from the fluent production of syllables to more complex sentences. Approaches to treatment may include parents directly in the process, although even if not active participants, parents play an important role in the child coping with stuttering. Treatment in preschool-age children has been shown to improve stuttering. Management of stuttering is also emphasized in older children. For school-age children, treatment includes improving not only fluency but also concomitants of the condition. This includes recognizing and accepting stuttering and appreciating others' reaction to the child when stuttering, managing secondary behaviors, and addressing avoidance behaviors. The broad focus allows for minimizing the adverse effects of the condition. To date, no evidence supports the use of a pharmacologic agent to treat stuttering in children and adolescents.

Preschool children with normal developmental dysfluency can be observed with parental education and reassurance. Parents should not reprimand the child or create undue anxiety.

Preschool or older children with stuttering should be referred to a speech pathologist. Therapy is most effective if started during the preschool period. In addition to the risks noted in Table 52.5, indications for referral include 3 or more dysfluencies per 100 syllables (b-b-but; th-th-the; you, you, you), avoidances or escapes (pauses, head nod, blinking), discomfort or anxiety while speaking, and suspicion of an associated neurologic or psychotic disorder.

Most preschool children respond to interventions taught by speech pathologists and to behavioral feedback by parents. Parents should not yell at the child, but should calmly praise periods of fluency ("That was smooth") or nonjudgmentally note episodes of stuttering ("That was a bit bumpy"). The child can be involved with self-correction and respond to requests ("Can you say that again?") made by a calm parent. Such treatment greatly improves dysfluency, but it may never be eliminated.

Bibliography is available at Expert Consult.

Chapter **53**

Developmental Delay and Intellectual Disability

Bruce K. Shapiro and Meghan E. O'Neill

第五十三章

发育迟缓和智力障碍

中文导读

本章主要介绍了发育迟缓和智力障碍的定义、病因学、流行病学、病理学及发病机制、临床表现、诊断评估、鉴别诊断、诊断心理学测试、共患病、预防、治疗、支持性保健和管理以及预后。其中支持性保健和管理部分具体描述了发育迟缓和智力障碍的初级保健、跨学科管理、定期重新评估、联邦和教育服务、康乐活动、家庭咨询、过渡到成年等内容。

Intellectual disability (ID) refers to a group of disorders that have in common deficits of adaptive and intellectual function and an age of onset before maturity is reached.

DEFINITION

Contemporary conceptualizations of ID emphasize functioning and social interaction rather than test scores. The definitions of ID by the World Health Organization (WHO) *International Classification of Diseases, Tenth Edition* (ICD-10), the U.S. Individuals with Disabilities Education Act (IDEA), the American Psychiatric Association (APA) *Diagnostic and Statistical Manual of Mental Disorders, Fifth Edition* (DSM-5), and the American Association on Intellectual and Developmental Disabilities (AAIDD) all include significant impairment in general intellectual function (reasoning, learning, problem solving), social skills, and adaptive behavior. This focus on conceptual, social, and practical skills enables the development of individual treatment plans designed to enhance functioning. Consistent across these definitions is onset of symptoms before age 18 yr or adulthood.

Significant impairment in general intellectual function refers to performance on an individually administered test of intelligence that is approximately 2 standard deviations (SD) below the mean. Generally these tests provide a standard score that has a mean of 100 and SD of 15, so that intelligence quotient (IQ) scores <70 would meet these criteria. If the standard error of measurement is considered, the upper limits of significantly impaired intellectual function may extend to an IQ of 75. Using a score of 75 to delineate ID might double the number of children with this diagnosis, but the requirement for impairment of adaptive skills limits the false positives. Children with ID often show a variable pattern of strengths and weaknesses. Not all their subtest scores on IQ tests fall into the significantly impaired range.

Significant impairment in adaptive behavior reflects the degree that the cognitive dysfunction impairs daily function. **Adaptive behavior** refers to the skills required for people to function in their everyday lives. The AAIDD and DSM-5 classifications of adaptive behavior addresses three broad sets of skills: conceptual, social, and practical. **Conceptual skills** include language, reading, writing, time, number concepts, and self-direction. **Social skills** include interpersonal skills, personal and social responsibility, self-esteem, gullibility, naiveté, and ability to follow rules, obey laws, and avoid victimization. Representative **practical skills** are performance of activities of daily living (dressing, feeding, toileting/bathing, mobility), instrumental activities of daily living (e.g., housework, managing money, taking medication, shopping, preparing meals, using phone), occupational skills, and maintenance of a safe environment. For a deficit in adaptive behavior to be present, a significant delay in at least 1 of the 3 skill areas must be present. The rationale for requiring only 1 area is the empirically derived finding that people with ID can have varying patterns of ability and may not have deficits in all 3 areas.

The requirement for adaptive behavior deficits is the most controversial aspect of the diagnostic formulation. The controversy centers on two broad areas: whether impairments in adaptive behavior are necessary for the construct of ID, and what to measure. The adaptive behavior criterion may be irrelevant for many children; adaptive behavior is impaired in virtually all children who have IQ scores <50. The major utility of the adaptive behavior criterion is to confirm ID in children with IQ scores in the 65-75 range. It should be noted that deficits in adaptive behavior are often found in disorders such as autism spectrum disorder (ASD; see Chapter 54) and attention-deficit/hyperactivity disorder (ADHD; see Chapter 49) in the presence of typical intellectual function.

The issues of measurement are important as well. The independence of the 3 domains of adaptive behavior has not been validated. The relationship between adaptive behavior and IQ performance is insufficiently explored. Most adults with mild ID do not have significant impairments in practical skills. Adaptive behavior deficits also must be distinguished from *maladaptive behavior* (e.g., aggression, inappropriate sexual contact).

Onset before age 18 yr or adulthood distinguishes dysfunctions that originate during the developmental period. The diagnosis of ID may be made after 18 yr of age, but the cognitive and adaptive dysfunction must have been manifested before age 18.

The term "mental retardation" should not be used because it is stigmatizing, has been used to limit the achievements of the individual, and has not met its initial objective of assisting people with the disorder. The term *intellectual disability* is increasingly used in its place, but has not been adopted universally. In the United States, Rosa's law (Public Law 111-256) was passed in 2010 and now mandates that the term mental retardation be stripped from federal health, education, and labor policy. As of 2013, at least 9 states persist in using the outdated terminology. In Europe the term *learning disability* is often used to describe ID.

Global developmental delay (GDD) is a term often used to describe young children whose limitations have not yet resulted in a formal diagnosis of ID. In DSM-5, GDD is a diagnosis given to children <5 yr of age who display significant delay (>2 SD) in acquiring early childhood developmental milestones in 2 or more domains of development. These domains include receptive and expressive language, gross and fine motor function, cognition, social and personal development, and activities of daily living. Typically, it is assumed that delay in 2 domains will be associated with delay across all domains evaluated, but this is not always the case. Furthermore, not all children who meet criteria for a GDD diagnosis at a young age go on to meet criteria for ID after age 5 yr. Reasons for this might include maturational effects, a change in developmental trajectory (possibly from an intervention), reclassification to a different disability category, or imprecise use of the GDD diagnosis initially. Conversely, in patients with more severe delay, the GDD term is often inappropriately used beyond the point when the child clearly has ID, often by 3 yr of age.

It is important to distinguish the medical diagnosis of GDD from the federal disability classification of "developmental delay" that may be used by education agencies under IDEA. This classification requires that a child have delays in only 1 domain of development with subsequent need for special education. Each state determines its own precise definition and terms of eligibility under the broader definition outline by IDEA, and many states use the label for children up to age 9 yr.

ETIOLOGY

Numerous identified causes of ID may occur prenatally, during delivery, postnatally, or later in childhood. These include infection, trauma, prematurity, hypoxia-ischemia, toxic exposures, metabolic dysfunction, endocrine abnormalities, malnutrition, and genetic abnormalities. However, more than two thirds of persons with ID will not have a readily identifiable underlying diagnosis that can be linked to their clinical presentation, meriting further medical evaluation. For those who then undergo further genetic and metabolic workup, about two thirds will have an etiology that is subsequently discovered. There does appear to be 2 overlapping populations of children with ID with differing corresponding etiologies. *Mild ID* (IQ 50-70) is associated more with environmental influences, with the highest risk among children of low socioeconomic status. *Severe ID* (IQ <50) is more frequently linked to biologic and genetic causes. Accordingly, diagnostic yield is generally higher among persons with more severe disability (>75%) than among those with mild disability (<50%). With continued advancement of technologic standards and expansion of our knowledge base, the number of identified biologic and genetic causes is expected to increase.

Nongenetic risk factors that are often associated with mild ID include low socioeconomic status, residence in a developing country, low maternal education, malnutrition, and poor access to healthcare. The most common biologic causes of mild ID include genetic or chromosomal syndromes with multiple, major, or minor congenital anomalies (e.g., velocardiofacial, Williams, and Noonan syndromes), intrauterine growth restriction, prematurity, perinatal insults, intrauterine exposure to drugs of abuse (including alcohol), and sex chromosomal abnormalities. Familial clustering is common.

Table 53.1	Identification of Cause in Children With Significant Intellectual Disability	
CAUSE	**EXAMPLES**	**% OF TOTAL**
Chromosomal disorder	Trisomies 21, 18, 13; Deletions 1p36, 4p, 5p, 11p, 12q, 17p; Microdeletions; 47,XXX; Klinefelter and Turner syndromes	~20
Genetic syndrome	Fragile X, Prader-Willi, Angelman, and Rett syndromes	~20
Nonsyndromic autosomal mutations	Variations in copy number; de novo mutations in *SYNGAP1*, *GRIK2*, *TUSC3*, oligosaccharyl transferase, and others	~10
Developmental brain abnormality	Hydrocephalus ± meningomyelocele; schizencephaly, lissencephaly	~8
Inborn errors of metabolism or neurodegenerative disorder	Phenylketonuria, Tay-Sachs disease, various storage diseases	~7
Congenital infections	HIV, toxoplasmosis, rubella, cytomegalovirus, syphilis, herpes simplex	~3
Familial intellectual disability	Environment, syndromic, or genetic	~5
Perinatal causes	Hypoxic-ischemic encephalopathy, meningitis, intraventricular hemorrhage, periventricular leukomalacia, fetal alcohol syndrome	4
Postnatal causes	Trauma (abuse), meningitis, hypothyroidism	~4
Unknown		20

Adapted from Stromme P, Hayberg G: Aetiology in severe and mild mental retardation: a population based study of Norwegian children, *Dev Med Child Neurol* 42:76–86, 2000.

In children with severe ID, a biologic cause (usually prenatal) can be identified in about three fourths of all cases. Causes include chromosomal (e.g., Down, Wolf-Hirschhorn, and deletion 1p36 syndromes) and other genetic and epigenetic disorders (e.g., fragile X, Rett, Angelman, and Prader-Willi syndromes), abnormalities of brain development (e.g., lissencephaly), and inborn errors of metabolism or neurodegenerative disorders (e.g., mucopolysaccharidoses) (Table 53.1). *Nonsyndromic* severe ID may be a result of inherited or de novo gene mutations, as well as microdeletions or microduplications not detected on standard chromosome analysis. Currently, >700 genes are associated with nonsyndromic ID. Inherited genetic abnormalities may be mendelian (autosomal dominant de novo, autosomal recessive, X-linked) or nonmendelian (imprinting, methylation, mitochondrial defects; see Chapter 97). De novo mutations may also cause other phenotypic features such as seizures or autism; the presence of these features suggests more pleiotropic manifestations of genetic mutations. Consistent with the finding that disorders altering early embryogenesis are the most common and severe, the earlier the problem occurs in development, the more severe its consequences tend to be.

Etiologic workup is recommended in all cases of GDD or ID. Although there are only about 80 disorders (all of which are metabolic in nature) for which treatment may ameliorate the core symptoms of ID, several reasons beyond disease modification should prompt providers to seek etiologic answers in patients with ID. These include insight into possible associated medical or behavioral comorbidities; information on prognosis and life expectancy; estimation of recurrence risk for family planning counseling, potential validation, and closure for the family; increased access to services or specific supports; and better understanding of underlying pathology with the hope of new eventual treatment options. When surveyed, families of children with ID with no identified underlying etiology almost universally report that they would want to know of an etiologic diagnosis if given the choice.

EPIDEMIOLOGY

The prevalence of ID depends on the definition, method of ascertainment, and population studied, both in terms of geography and age. According to the statistics of a normal distribution, 2.5% of the population should have ID (based on IQ alone), and 75% of these individuals should fall into the mild to moderate range. Variability in rates across populations likely results from the heavy influence of external environmental factors on the prevalence of mild ID. The prevalence of severe ID is relatively stable. Globally, the prevalence of ID has been estimated to be approximately 16.4 per 1,000 persons in low-income countries, approximately 15.9/1,000 for middle-income countries, and approximately 9.2/1,000 in high-income countries. A meta-analysis of worldwide studies from 1980–2009 yielded an overall prevalence of 10.4/1000. ID occurs more in boys than in girls, at 2:1 in mild ID and 1.5:1 in severe ID. In part this may be a consequence of the many X-linked disorders associated with ID, the most prominent being fragile X syndrome (see Chapter 98.5).

In 2014–2015 in the United States, approximately 12/1000 students 3-5 yr old and 6.2/1000 students 6-21 yr old received services for ID in federally supported school programs. In 2012 the National Survey of Children's Health reported an estimated prevalence of ID among American children (age 2-17 yr) of 1.1%. For several reasons, fewer children than predicted are identified as having mild ID. Because it is more difficult to diagnose mild ID than the more severe forms, professionals might defer the diagnosis and give the benefit of the doubt to the child. Other reasons that contribute to the discrepancy are use of instruments that underidentify young children with mild ID, children diagnosed as having ASD without their ID being addressed, misdiagnosis as a language disorder or specific learning disability, and a disinclination to make the diagnosis in poor or minority students because of previous overdiagnosis. In some cases, behavioral disorders may divert the focus from the cognitive dysfunction.

Beyond potential underdiagnosis of mild ID, the number of children with mild ID may be decreasing as a result of public health and education measures to prevent prematurity and provide early intervention and Head Start programs. However, although the number of schoolchildren who receive services under a federal disability classification of ID has decreased since 1999, when *developmental delay* is included in analysis of the data, the numbers have not changed appreciably.

The prevalence of severe ID has not changed significantly since the 1940s, accounting for 0.3–0.5% of the population. Many of the causes of severe ID involve genetic or congenital brain malformations that can neither be anticipated nor treated at present. In addition, new populations with severe ID have offset the decreases in the prevalence of severe ID that have resulted from improved healthcare. Although prenatal diagnosis and subsequent pregnancy terminations could lead to a decreasing incidence of Down syndrome (see Chapter 98.2), and newborn screening with early treatment has virtually eliminated ID caused by phenylketonuria and congenital hypothyroidism, continued high prevalence of fetal exposure to illicit drugs and improved survival of very-low-birthweight premature infants has counterbalanced this effect.

PATHOLOGY AND PATHOGENESIS

The limitations in our knowledge of the neuropathology of ID are exemplified by 10–20% of brains of persons with severe ID appearing entirely normal on standard neuropathologic study. Most of these brains show only mild, nonspecific changes that correlate poorly with the degree of ID, including microcephaly, gray matter heterotopias in the subcortical white matter, unusually regular columnar arrangement of the cortex, and neurons that are more tightly packed than usual. Only a minority of the brain shows more specific changes in dendritic and synaptic organization, with dysgenesis of dendritic spines or cortical pyramidal neurons or impaired growth of dendritic trees. The

programming of the central nervous system (CNS) involves a process of *induction*; CNS maturation is defined in terms of genetic, molecular, autocrine, paracrine, and endocrine influences. Receptors, signaling molecules, and genes are critical to brain development. The maintenance of different neuronal phenotypes in the adult brain involves the same genetic transcripts that play a crucial role in fetal development, with activation of similar intracellular signal transduction mechanisms.

As the ability to identify genetic aberrations that correspond to particular phenotypes expands through the use of next-generation sequencing, more will be elucidated about the pathogenesis of ID at a genetic and molecular level. This expanding pathophysiologic knowledge base may serve as a framework with which to develop targeted therapies to bypass or correct newly identified defects. For example, use of histone deacetylase (HDAC) inhibitors has been shown to rescue structural and functional neural deficits in mouse models of Kabuki syndrome, a disorder of histone methylation that leads to variable levels of ID and characteristic facial features (see Chapter 100).

CLINICAL MANIFESTATIONS

Early diagnosis of ID facilitates earlier intervention, identification of abilities, realistic goal setting, easing of parental anxiety, and greater acceptance of the child in the community. Most children with ID first come to the pediatrician's attention in infancy because of dysmorphisms, associated developmental disabilities, or failure to meet age-appropriate developmental milestones (Tables 53.2 and 53.3). There are no specific physical characteristics of ID, but dysmorphisms may be the earliest signs that bring children to the attention of the pediatrician. They might fall within a genetic syndrome such as Down syndrome or might be isolated, as in microcephaly or failure to thrive. Associated developmental disabilities include seizure disorders, cerebral palsy, and ASD.

Most children with ID do not keep up with their peers' developmental skills. In early infancy, failure to meet age-appropriate expectations can include a lack of visual or auditory responsiveness, unusual muscle tone (hypo- or hypertonia) or posture, and feeding difficulties. Between 6 and 18 mo of age, gross motor delay (lack of sitting, crawling, walking) is the most common complaint. Language delay and behavior problems are common concerns after 18 mo (Table 53.4). For some children with mild ID, the diagnosis remains uncertain during the early school years. It is only after the demands of the school setting increase over the years, changing from "learning to read" to "reading to learn," that the child's limitations are clarified. Adolescents with mild ID are typically up to date on current trends and are conversant as to "who," "what," and "where." It is not until the "why" and "how" questions are asked that their limitations become apparent. If allowed to interact at a superficial level, their mild ID might not be appreciated, even by professionals, who may be their special education teachers or healthcare providers. Because of the stigma associated with ID, adolescents may use euphemisms to avoid being thought of as "stupid" or "retarded" and may refer to themselves as learning disabled, dyslexic, language disordered, or slow learners. Some people with ID emulate their social milieu to be accepted. They may be social chameleons and assume the morals of the group to whom they are attached. Some would rather be thought "bad" than "incompetent."

Children with ID have a nonprogressive disorder; loss of developmental milestones or progressive symptoms suggest another disorder (see Chapter 53.1).

DIAGNOSTIC EVALUATION

Intellectual disability is one of the most frequent reasons for referral to pediatric genetic providers, with separate but similar diagnostic evaluation guidelines put forth by the American College of Medical Genetics, the American Academy of Neurology, the American Academy of Pediatrics (AAP), and the American Academy of Child and Adolescent Psychiatry. ID is a diagnosis of great clinical heterogeneity, with only a subset of syndromic etiologies identifiable through classic dysmorphology. If diagnosis is not made after conducting an appropriate history and physical examination, chromosomal microarray is the recommended first step in the diagnostic evaluation of ID. Next-generation sequencing

Table 53.2	Physical Examination of a Child With Suspected Developmental Disabilities
ITEM	**POSSIBLE SIGNIFICANCE**
General appearance	May indicate significant delay in development or obvious syndrome
Stature	
Short stature	Malnutrition, many genetic syndromes are associated with short stature (e.g., Turner, Noonan)
Obesity	Prader-Willi syndrome
Large stature	Sotos syndrome
Head	
Macrocephaly	Alexander syndrome, Canavan disease, Sotos syndrome, gangliosidosis, hydrocephalus, mucopolysaccharidosis, subdural effusion
Microcephaly	Virtually any condition that can restrict brain growth (e.g., malnutrition, Angelman syndrome, Cornelia de Lange syndrome, fetal alcohol effects)
Face	
Coarse, triangular, round, or flat face; hypotelorism or hypertelorism; slanted or short palpebral fissure; unusual nose, maxilla, and mandible	Specific measurements may provide clues to inherited, metabolic, or other diseases such as fetal alcohol syndrome, cri du chat (5p–) syndrome, or Williams syndrome.
Eyes	
Prominent	Crouzon, Seckel, and fragile X syndromes
Cataract	Galactosemia, Lowe syndrome, prenatal rubella, hypothyroidism
Cherry-red spot in macula	Gangliosidosis (GM₁), metachromatic leukodystrophy, mucolipidosis, Tay-Sachs disease, Niemann-Pick disease, Farber lipogranulomatosis, sialidosis type III
Chorioretinitis	Congenital infection with cytomegalovirus, toxoplasmosis, Zika virus, or rubella
Corneal cloudiness	Mucopolysaccharidosis types I and II, Lowe syndrome, congenital syphilis
Ears	
Low-set or malformed pinnae	Trisomies such as Down syndrome, Rubinstein-Taybi syndrome, CHARGE syndrome, cerebrooculofacioskeletal syndrome, fetal phenytoin effects
Hearing	Loss of acuity in mucopolysaccharidosis; hyperacusis in many encephalopathies
Heart	
Structural anomaly or hypertrophy	CHARGE syndrome, velocardiofacial syndrome, glycogenosis type II, fetal alcohol effects, mucopolysaccharidosis type I; chromosomal anomalies such as Down syndrome; maternal PKU; chronic cyanosis may impair cognitive development.
Liver	
Hepatomegaly	Fructose intolerance, galactosemia, glycogenosis types I-IV, mucopolysaccharidosis types I and II, Niemann-Pick disease, Tay-Sachs disease, Zellweger syndrome, Gaucher disease, ceroid lipofuscinosis, gangliosidosis
Genitalia	
Macroorchidism	Fragile X syndrome
Hypogenitalism	Prader-Willi, Klinefelter, and CHARGE syndromes
Extremities	
Hands, feet; dermatoglyphics, creases	May indicate a specific entity such as Rubinstein-Taybi syndrome or may be associated with chromosomal anomaly
Joint contractures	Signs of muscle imbalance around the joints; e.g., with meningomyelocele, cerebral palsy, arthrogryposis, muscular dystrophy; also occurs with cartilaginous problems such as mucopolysaccharidosis
Skin	
Café au lait spots	Neurofibromatosis, tuberous sclerosis, chromosomal aneuploidy, ataxia-telangiectasia, multiple endocrine neoplasia type 2b
	Fanconi anemia, Gaucher disease
	Syndromes: basal cell nevus, McCune-Albright, Silver-Russell, Bloom, Chediak-Higashi, Hunter, Bannayan-Riley-Ruvalcaba, Maffucci
Seborrheic or eczematoid rash	PKU, histiocytosis
Hemangiomas and telangiectasia	Sturge-Weber syndrome, Bloom syndrome, ataxia-telangiectasia
Hypopigmented macules, streaks, adenoma sebaceum	Tuberous sclerosis, hypomelanosis of Ito
Hair	
Hirsutism	De Lange syndrome, mucopolysaccharidosis, fetal phenytoin effects, cerebrooculofacioskeletal syndrome, trisomy 18, Wiedemann-Steiner syndrome (hypertrichosis cubiti)
Neurologic	
Asymmetry of strength and tone	Focal lesion, hemiplegic cerebral palsy
Hypotonia	Prader-Willi, Down, and Angelman syndromes; gangliosidosis; early cerebral palsy; muscle disorders (dystrophy or myopathy)
Hypertonia	Neurodegenerative conditions involving white matter, cerebral palsy, trisomy 18
Ataxia	Ataxia-telangiectasia, metachromatic leukodystrophy, Angelman syndrome

CHARGE, Coloboma, heart defects, atresia choanae, retarded growth, genital anomalies, ear anomalies (deafness); CATCH-22, cardiac defects, abnormal face, thymic hypoplasia, cleft palate, hypocalcemia—defects on chromosome 22; PKU, phenylketonuria.

From Simms M: Intellectual and developmental disability. In Kliegman RM, Lye PS, Bordini BJ, et al, editors: *Nelson pediatric symptom-based diagnosis,* Philadelphia, 2018, Elsevier, Table 24.11, p 376.

| Table 53.3 | Examples of Minor Anomalies and Associated Syndromes*† |

AREA	ANOMALY/SYNDROME	AREA	ANOMALY/SYNDROME
Head	Flat occiput: Down syndrome, Zellweger syndrome; prominent occiput: trisomy 18 Delayed closure of sutures: hypothyroidism, hydrocephalus Craniosynostosis: Crouzon syndrome, Pfeiffer syndrome Delayed fontanel closure: hypothyroidism, Down syndrome, hydrocephalus, skeletal dysplasias	Teeth	Anodontia: ectodermal dysplasia Notched incisors: congenital syphilis Late dental eruption: Hunter syndrome, hypothyroidism Talon cusps: Rubinstein-Taybi syndrome Wide-spaced teeth: Cornelia de Lange syndrome, Angelman syndrome
Face	Midface hypoplasia: fetal alcohol syndrome, Down syndrome Triangular facies: Russell-Silver syndrome, Turner syndrome Coarse facies: mucopolysaccharidoses, Sotos syndrome Prominent nose and chin: fragile X syndrome Flat facies: Apert syndrome, Stickler syndrome Round facies: Prader-Willi syndrome	Hair	Hirsutism: Hurler syndrome Low hairline: Klippel-Feil sequence, Turner syndrome Sparse hair: Menkes disease, argininosuccinic acidemia Abnormal hair whorls/posterior whorl: chromosomal aneuploidy (e.g., Down syndrome) Abnormal eyebrow patterning: Cornelia de Lange syndrome
Eyes	Hypertelorism: fetal hydantoin syndrome, Waardenburg syndrome Hypotelorism: holoprosencephaly sequence, maternal phenylketonuria effect Inner canthal folds/Brushfield spots: Down syndrome; slanted palpebral fissures: trisomies Prominent eyes: Apert syndrome, Beckwith-Wiedemann syndrome Lisch nodules: neurofibromatosis Blue sclera: osteogenesis imperfecta, Turner syndrome, hereditary connective tissue disorders	Neck	Webbed neck/low posterior hairline: Turner syndrome, Noonan syndrome
		Chest	Shield-shaped chest: Turner syndrome
		Genitalia	Macroorchidism: fragile X syndrome Hypogonadism: Prader-Willi syndrome
Ears	Large pinnae/simple helices: fragile X syndrome Malformed pinnae/atretic canal: Treacher Collins syndrome, CHARGE syndrome Low-set ears: Treacher Collins syndrome, trisomies, multiple disorders	Extremities	Short limbs: achondroplasia, rhizomelic chondrodysplasia Small hands: Prader-Willi syndrome Clinodactyly: trisomies, including Down syndrome Polydactyly: trisomy 13, ciliopathies Broad thumb: Rubinstein-Taybi syndrome Syndactyly: de Lange syndrome Transverse palmar crease: Down syndrome Joint laxity: Down syndrome, fragile X syndrome, Ehlers-Danlos syndrome Phocomelia: Cornelia de Lange syndrome
Nose	Anteverted nares/synophrys: Cornelia de Lange syndrome; broad nasal bridge: fetal drug effects, fragile X syndrome Low nasal bridge: achondroplasia, Down syndrome Prominent nose: Coffin-Lowry syndrome, Smith-Lemli-Opitz syndrome	Spine	Sacral dimple/hairy patch: spina bifida
		Skin	Hypopigmented macules/adenoma sebaceum: tuberous sclerosis Café au lait spots and neurofibromas: neurofibromatosis Linear depigmented nevi: hypomelanosis of Ito Facial port-wine hemangioma: Sturge-Weber syndrome Nail hypoplasia or dysplasia: fetal alcohol syndrome, trisomies
Mouth	Long philtrum/thin vermilion border: fetal alcohol effects Cleft lip and palate: isolated or part of a syndrome Micrognathia: Pierre Robin sequence, trisomies, Stickler syndrome Macroglossia: hypothyroidism, Beckwith-Wiedemann syndrome		

CHARGE, Coloboma, heart defects, atresia choanae, retarded growth, genital anomalies, ear anomalies (deafness).
*Increased incidence of minor anomalies have been reported in cerebral palsy, intellectual disability, learning disabilities, and autism.
†The presence of 3 or more minor anomalies implies a greater chance that the child has a major anomaly and a diagnosis of a specific syndrome.
Modified from Levy SE, Hyman SL. Pediatric assessment of the child with developmental delay, *Pediatr Clin North Am* 40:465-477, 1993.

represents the new diagnostic frontier, with extensive gene panels (exome or whole genome) that increase the diagnostic yield and usefulness of genetic testing in ID. Other commonly used medical diagnostic testing for children with ID includes neuroimaging, metabolic testing, and electroencephalography (Fig. 53.1).

Decisions to pursue an etiologic diagnosis should be based on the medical and family history, physical examination, and the family's wishes. Table 53.5 summarizes clinical practice guidelines and the yields of testing to assist in decisions about evaluating the child with GDD or ID. Yield of testing tends increase with worsening severity of delays.

Microarray analysis has replaced a karyotype as first-tier testing given that it discerns abnormalities that are far below the resolution of a karyotype. Microarray analysis may identify variants of unknown significance or benign variants and therefore should be used in conjunction with a genetic consultation. Karyotyping has a role when concerns for inversions, balanced insertions, and reciprocal translocations are present. Fluorescence in situ hybridization (FISH) and subtelomeric

analysis have been largely replaced by microarray analysis but are occasionally used for specific indications. If microarray analysis is not diagnostic, whole exome sequencing increases the diagnostic yield in many children with nonsyndromic severe ID. Starting with whole exome sequencing may be more cost-effective and may substantially reduce time to diagnosis with higher ultimate yields compared with the traditional diagnostic pathway.

Molecular genetic testing for fragile X syndrome is recommended for all children presenting with GDD. Yields are highest in males with moderate ID, unusual physical features, and/or a family history of ID, or for females with more subtle cognitive deficits associated with severe shyness and a relevant family history, including premature ovarian failure or later-onset ataxia-tremor symptoms. For children with a strong history of X-linked ID, specific testing of genes or the entire chromosome may be revealing. Testing for Rett syndrome (MECP2, methyl CpG–binding protein 2) should be considered in girls with moderate to severe disability.

A child with a progressive neurologic disorder, developmental regression, or acute behavioral changes needs metabolic investigation as shown in Figure 53.1. Some are advocating that metabolic testing should be done more frequently in children with ID because of the possibility of detecting a condition that could be treatable (Fig. 53.2 and Table 53.6). A child with seizure-like episodes should have an electroencephalogram (EEG), although this testing is generally not helpful outside the scope

of ruling out seizures. **MRI of the brain** may provide useful information in directing the care of a child with micro- or macrocephaly, change in head growth trajectory, asymmetric head shape, new or focal neurologic findings, or seizure. MRI can detect a significant number of subtle markers of cerebral dysgenesis in children with ID, but these markers do not usually suggest a specific etiologic diagnosis.

Some children with subtle physical or neurologic findings can also have determinable biologic causes of their ID (see Tables 53.2 and 53.3). How intensively one investigates the cause of a child's ID is based on the following factors:

- What is the degree of delay, and what is the age of the child? If milder or less pervasive delays are present, especially in a younger child, etiologic yield is likely to be lower.
- Is the medical history, family history, or physical exam suggestive of a specific disorder, increasing the likelihood that a diagnosis will be made? Are the parents planning on having additional children, and does the patient have siblings? If so, one may be more likely to intensively seek disorders for which prenatal diagnosis or a specific early treatment option is available.
- What are the parents' wishes? Some parents have little interest in searching for the cause of the ID, whereas others become so focused on obtaining a diagnosis that they have difficulty following through on interventions until a cause has been found. The entire spectrum of responses must be respected, and supportive guidance should be provided in the context of the parents' education.

DIFFERENTIAL DIAGNOSIS

One of the important roles of pediatricians is the early recognition and diagnosis of cognitive deficits. The developmental surveillance approach to early diagnosis of ID should be multifaceted. Parents' concerns and observations about their child's development should be listened to

Table 53.4	Common Presentations of Intellectual Disability by Age
AGE	**AREA OF CONCERN**
Newborn	Dysmorphic syndromes, (multiple congenital anomalies), microcephaly Major organ system dysfunction (e.g., feeding, breathing)
Early infancy (2-4 mo)	Failure to interact with the environment Concerns about vision and hearing impairments
Later infancy (6-18 mo)	Gross motor delay
Toddlers (2-3 yr)	Language delays or difficulties
Preschool (3-5 yr)	Language difficulties or delays Behavior difficulties, including play Delays in fine motor skills: cutting, coloring, drawing
School age (>5 yr)	Academic underachievement Behavior difficulties (e.g., attention, anxiety, mood, conduct)

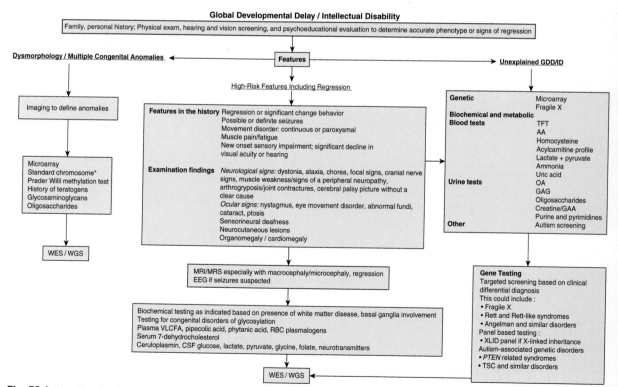

Fig. 53.1 Algorithm for the evaluation of the child with unexplained global developmental delay (GDD) or intellectual disability (ID). AA, amino acids; ASD, autistic spectrum disorder; CK, creatine kinase; CSF, cerebrospinal fluid; FBC, full blood count; GAA, guanidinoacetic acid; GAG, glycosaminoglycans; LFT, liver function test; OA, organic acids; TFT, thyroid function tests; TSC, tuberous sclerosis complex; U&E, urea and electrolytes; VLCFA, very long chain fatty acids; WES, whole exome sequencing; WGS, whole genome sequencing; X-linked intellectual disability genes.

TEST	COMMENT
Table 53.5	**Suggested Evaluation of the Child With Intellectual Disability (ID) or Global Developmental Delay (GDD)**
In-depth history	Includes pre-, peri-, and postnatal events (including seizures); developmental attainments; and 3-generation pedigree in family history (focusing on neurologic or developmental abnormalities, miscarriages, consanguinity, etc.)
Physical examination	Particular attention to minor or subtle dysmorphisms; growth issues; neurocutaneous findings; eye and skull abnormalities; hepatosplenomegaly; and neurologic examination for focality Behavioral phenotype
Vision and hearing evaluation	Essential to detect and treat; can mask as developmental delay
Gene microarray analysis	A 15% yield overall Better resolution than with karyotype; may identify up to twice as many abnormalities as karyotyping
Karyotype	Yield of 4% in ID/GDD (18.6% if syndromic features, 3% excluding trisomy 21) Best for inversions and balanced insertions, reciprocal translocations, and polyploidy
Fragile X screen	Combined yield of 2% Preselection on clinical grounds can increase yield to 7.6%
Next-generation gene sequencing	Detects inherited and de novo point mutations, especially in nonsyndromic severe intellectual disability Whole exome sequencing (WES, introduced in 2010) gives an additional yield of about 30–40%. Although not yet used clinically, pilot studies of whole genome sequencing (WGS) reveal additional yield of about 15%.
Neuroimaging	MRI preferred; positive findings increased by abnormalities of skull contour or microcephaly and macrocephaly, or focal neurologic examination (30–40% if indicated, 10–14% if screening). Identification of specific etiologies is rare; most conditions that are found do not alter the treatment plan; need to weigh risk of sedation against possible yield.
Thyroid (T_4, TSH)	Near 0% in settings with universal newborn screening program
Serum lead	If there are identifiable risk factors for excessive environmental lead exposure (e.g., low socioeconomic status, home built before 1950)
Metabolic testing	Yield of 0.2–4.6% based on clinical indicators and tests performed Urine organic acids, plasma amino acids, ammonia, lactate, and capillary blood gas Focused testing based on clinical findings is warranted if lack of newborn screen results or suggestive history/exam (e.g., regression, consanguinity, hepatosplenomegaly, course facies). Tandem mass spectrometry newborn screening has allowed for identification of many disorders in perinatal period and have decreased yield in older children; other disorders have emerged, such as congenital disorders of glycosylation (yield 1.4%) and disorders of creatine synthesis and transport (yield 2.8%).
MECP2 for Rett syndrome	1.5% of females with criteria suggestive of Rett (e.g., acquired microcephaly, loss of skills) 0.5% of males
EEG	May be deferred in absence of history of seizures
Repeated history and physical examination	Can give time for maturation of physical and behavioral phenotype; new technology may be available for evaluation.

EEG, Electroencephalogram; CGH, comparative genomic hybridization; MECP2, methyl CpG–binding protein 2; T_4, thyroxine; TSH, thyroid-stimulating hormone.
Data from Michelson DJ et al: Evidence report. Genetic and metabolic testing on children with global developmental delay: report of the Quality Standards Subcommittee of the American Academy of Neurology and the Practice Committee of Child Neurology, Neurology 77:1629-35, 2011; Curry CJ et al: Evaluation of mental retardation: recommendations of a Consensus Conference: American College of Medical Genetics, Am J Med Genet 12:72:468-477, 1997; Shapiro BK, Batshaw ML: Mental retardation. In Burg FD et al: *Gellis and Kagan's current pediatric therapy*, ed 18, Philadelphia, 2005, Saunders; and Shevell M et al: Practice parameter: evaluation of the child with global developmental delay, *Neurology* 60:367–380, 2003.

carefully. Medical, genetic, and environmental risk factors should be recognized. Infants at high risk (prematurity, maternal substance abuse, perinatal insult) should be registered in newborn follow-up programs in which they are evaluated periodically for developmental lags in the 1st 2 yr of life; they should be referred to early intervention programs as appropriate. Developmental milestones should be recorded routinely during healthcare maintenance visits. The AAP has formulated a schema for developmental surveillance and screening (see Chapter 28).

Before making the diagnosis of ID, other disorders that affect cognitive abilities and adaptive behavior should be considered. These include conditions that mimic ID and others that involve ID as an associated impairment. Sensory deficits (severe hearing and vision loss), communication disorders, refractory seizure disorders, poorly controlled mood disorders, or unmanaged severe attention deficits can mimic ID; certain progressive neurologic disorders can appear as ID before regression is appreciated. Many children with cerebral palsy (see Chapter 616.1) or ASD (Chapter 54) also have ID. Differentiation of isolated **cerebral palsy** from ID relies on motor skills being more affected than cognitive skills and on the presence of pathologic reflexes and tone changes. In **autism spectrum disorders,** language and social adaptive skills are more affected than nonverbal reasoning skills, whereas in ID, there are usually more equivalent deficits in social, fine motor, adaptive, and cognitive skills.

DIAGNOSTIC PSYCHOLOGIC TESTING

The formal diagnosis of ID requires the administration of individual tests of intelligence and adaptive functioning.

The *Bayley Scales of Infant and Toddler Development* (BSID-III), the most commonly used infant intelligence test, provides an assessment of cognitive, language, motor, behavior, social-emotional, and general adaptive abilities between 1 mo and 42 mo of age. Mental Developmental Index (MDI) and Psychomotor Development Index (PDI, a measure of motor competence) scores are derived from the results. The BSID-III permits the differentiation of infants with severe ID from typically developing infants, but it is less helpful in distinguishing between a typical child and one with mild ID.

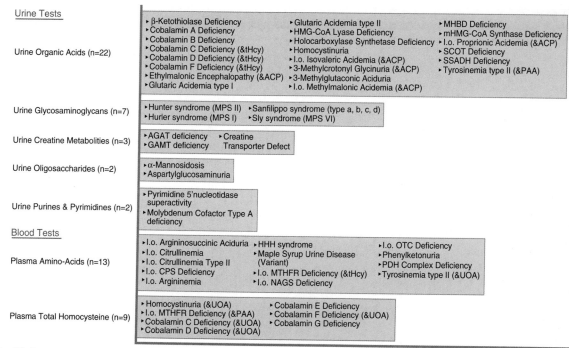

Fig. 53.2 Summary of treatable inherent errors of metabolism (IEM) that can be detected by metabolic tests in affected children, each of which is affordable and accessible and has the potential to identify at least 2 IEM (and up to 22). Each bar represents the yield of the specific screening test and lists the number and types of treatable IEM it can identify. PAA, Plasma amino acids; tHcy, total homocysteine; ACP, plasma acylcarnitine profile; UOA, urine organic acids. *(From van Karnebeek CD, Stockler S: Treatable inborn errors of metabolism causing intellectual disability: a systematic literature review,* Mol Genet Metab *105:368–381, 2012, Fig 1, p 374.)*

Table 53.6	Treatable Intellectual Disability Endeavor (TIDE) Diagnostic Protocol

Tier 1: Nontargeted Metabolic Screening to Identify 54 (60%) Treatable IEM

Blood
  Plasma amino acids
  Plasma total homocysteine
  Acylcarnitine profile
  Copper, ceruloplasmin
Urine
  Organic acids
  Purines and pyrimidines
  Creatine metabolites
  Oligosaccharides
  Glycosaminoglycans
  Amino acids (when indicated)

Tier 2: Current Practice Adhering to International Guidelines* (1 or more of:)

Audiology
Ophthalmology
Cytogenetic testing (array CGH)
Thyroid studies
Complete blood count (CBC)
Lead
Metabolic testing
Brain MRI and 1H spectroscopy (where available)
Fragile X

Targeted gene sequencing/molecular panel
Other

Tier 3: Targeted Workup to Identify 35 (40%) Treatable IEM Requiring Specific Testing

According to patient's symptomatology and clinician's expertise
Utilization of digital tools (www.treatable-id.org)
Specific biochemical/gene test
Whole blood manganese
Plasma cholestanol
Plasma 7-dehydroxycholesterol:cholesterol ratio
Plasma pipecolic acid and urine α-amino adipic semialdehyde (AASA)
Plasma very-long-chain fatty acids
Plasma vitamin B_{12} and folate
Serum and CSF lactate to pyruvate ratio
Enzyme activities (leukocytes): arylsulfatase A, biotinidase, glucocerebrosidase, fatty aldehyde dehydrogenase
Urine deoxypyridinoline
CSF amino acids
CSF neurotransmitters
CSF-to-plasma glucose ratio
CoQ measurement: fibroblasts
Molecular analysis: CA5A, NPC1, NPC2, SC4MOL, SLC18A2, SLC19A3, SLC30A10, SLC52A2, SLC52A3, PDHA1, DLAT, PDHX, SPR, TH genes

*Low threshold for ordering tests.

IEM, Inborn errors of metabolism; CSF, cerebrospinal fluid; CGH, comparative genomic hybridization; CoQ, coenzyme Q (ubiquinone).
Adapted from Van Karnebeek CD, Stockler-Ipsiroglu S. Early identification of treatable inborn errors of metabolism in children with intellectual disability: The Treatable Intellectual Disability Endeavor protocol in British Columbia, *Paediatr Child Health* 19(9):469–471, 2014.

The most commonly used psychologic tests for children older than 3 yr are the Wechsler Scales. The *Wechsler Preschool and Primary Scale of Intelligence, Fourth Edition* (WPPSI-IV) is used for children with mental ages of 2.5-7.6 yr. The *Wechsler Intelligence Scale for Children, Fifth Edition* (WISC-V) is used for children who function above a 6 yr mental age. Both scales contain numerous subtests in the areas of verbal and performance skills. Although children with ID usually score below average on all subscale scores, they occasionally score in the average range in one or more performance areas.

Several normed scales are used in practice to evaluate adaptive functioning. For example, the *Vineland Adaptive Behavior Scale* (VABS-3) uses semistructured interviews with parents and caregivers/teachers to assess adaptive behavior in 4 domains: communication, daily living skills, socialization, and motor skills. Other tests of adaptive behavior include the *Woodcock-Johnson Scales of Independent Behavior–Revised*, the AAIDD Diagnostic *Adaptive Behavior Scale* (DABS), and the *Adaptive Behavior Assessment System* (ABAS-3). There is usually (but not always) a good correlation between scores on the intelligence and adaptive scales. However, it is important to recognize that adaptive behavior can by influenced by environmentally based opportunities as well as family or cultural expectations. Basic practical adaptive skills (feeding, dressing, hygiene) are more responsive to remedial efforts than is the IQ score. Adaptive abilities are also more variable over time, which may be related to the underlying condition and environmental expectations.

COMPLICATIONS

Children with ID have higher rates of vision, hearing, neurologic, orthopedic, and behavioral or emotional disorders than typically developing children. These other problems are often detected later in children with ID. If untreated, the associated impairments can adversely affect the individual's outcome more than the ID itself.

The more severe the ID, the greater are the number and severity of associated impairments. Knowing the cause of the ID can help predict which associated impairments are most likely to occur. Fragile X syndrome and fetal alcohol syndrome (see Chapter 126.3) are associated with a high rate of behavioral disorders; Down syndrome has many medical complications (hypothyroidism, obstructive sleep apnea, congenital heart disease, atlantoaxial subluxation). Associated impairments can require ongoing physical therapy, occupational therapy, speech-language therapy, behavioral therapy, adaptive and mobility equipment, glasses, hearing aids, and medication. Failure to identify and treat these impairments adequately can hinder successful habilitation and result in difficulties in the school, home, and neighborhood environment.

PREVENTION

Examples of primary programs to prevent ID include the following:
- Increasing the public's awareness of the adverse effects of alcohol and other drugs of abuse on the fetus (the most common preventable cause of ID in the Western world is fetal alcohol exposure).
- Encouraging safe sexual practices, preventing teen pregnancy, and promoting early prenatal care with a focus on preventive programs to limit transmission of diseases that may cause congenital infection (syphilis, toxoplasmosis, cytomegalovirus, HIV).
- Preventing traumatic injury by encouraging the use of guards, railings, and window locks to prevent falls and other avoidable injuries in the home; using appropriate seat restraints when driving; wearing a safety helmet when biking or skateboarding; limiting exposure to firearms.
- Preventing poisonings by teaching parents about locking up medications and potential poisons.
- Implementing immunization programs to reduce the risk of ID caused by encephalitis, meningitis, and congenital infection.

Presymptomatic detection of certain disorders can result in treatment that prevents adverse consequences. State newborn screening by tandem mass spectrometry (now including >50 rare genetic disorders in most states), newborn hearing screening, and preschool lead poisoning prevention programs are examples. Additionally, screening for comorbid conditions can help to limit the extent of disability and maximize level of functioning in certain populations. Annual thyroid, vision, and hearing screening in a child with Down syndrome is an example of presymptomatic testing in a disorder associated with ID.

TREATMENT

Although the core symptoms of ID itself are generally not treatable, many associated impairments are amenable to intervention and therefore benefit from early identification. Most children with an ID do not have a behavioral or emotional disorder as an associated impairment, but challenging behaviors (aggression, self-injury, oppositional defiant behavior) and mental illness (mood and anxiety disorders) occur with greater frequency in this population than among children with typical intelligence. These behavioral and emotional disorders are the primary cause for out-of-home placements, increased family stress, reduced employment prospects, and decreased opportunities for social integration. Some behavioral and emotional disorders are difficult to diagnose in children with more severe ID because of the child's limited abilities to understand, communicate, interpret, or generalize. Other disorders are masked by the ID. The detection of ADHD (see Chapter 49) in the presence of moderate to severe ID may be difficult, as may be discerning a thought disorder (psychosis) in someone with autism and ID.

Although mental illness is generally of biologic origin and responds to medication, **behavioral disorders** can result from a mismatch between the child's abilities and the demands of the situation, organic problems, and family difficulties. These behaviors may represent attempts by the child to communicate, gain attention, or avoid frustration. In assessing the challenging behavior, one must also consider whether it is inappropriate for the child's *mental age*, rather than the *chronological age*. When intervention is needed, an environmental change, such as a more appropriate classroom setting, may improve certain behavior problems. Behavior management techniques are useful; psychopharmacologic agents may be appropriate in certain situations.

No medication has been found that improves the core symptoms of ID. However, several agents are being tested in specific disorders with known biologic mechanisms (e.g., mGluR5 inhibitors in fragile X syndrome, mTOR inhibitors in tuberous sclerosis), with the hope for future pharmacologic options that could alter the natural course of cognitive impairment seen in patients with these disorders. Currently, medication is most useful in the treatment of associated behavioral and psychiatric disorders. Psychopharmacology is generally directed at specific symptom complexes, including ADHD (stimulant medication), self-injurious behavior and aggression (antipsychotics), and anxiety, obsessive-compulsive disorder, and depression (selective serotonin reuptake inhibitors). Even if a medication proves successful, its use should be reevaluated at least yearly to assess the need for continued treatment.

SUPPORTIVE CARE AND MANAGEMENT

Each child with ID needs a medical home with a pediatrician who is readily accessible to the family to answer questions, help coordinate care, and discuss concerns. Pediatricians can have effects on patients and their families that are still felt decades later. The role of the pediatrician includes involvement in prevention efforts, early diagnosis, identification of associated deficits, referral for appropriate diagnostic and therapeutic services, interdisciplinary management, provision of primary care, and advocacy for the child and family. The management strategies for children with an ID should be multimodal, with efforts directed at all aspects of the child's life: health, education, social and recreational activities, behavior problems, and associated impairments. Support for parents and siblings should also be provided.

Primary Care

For children with an ID, primary care has the following important components:
- Provision of the same primary care received by all other children of similar chronological age.
- Anticipatory guidance relevant to the child's level of function: feeding, toileting, school, accident prevention, sexuality education.
- Assessment of issues that are relevant to that child's disorder, such as dental examination in children who exhibit bruxism, thyroid

function in children with Down syndrome, and cardiac function in Williams syndrome (see Chapter 454.5).

The AAP has published a series of guidelines for children with specific genetic disorders associated with ID (Down syndrome, fragile X syndrome, and Williams syndrome). Goals should be considered and programs adjusted as needed during the primary care visit. Decisions should also be made about what additional information is required for future planning or to explain why the child is not meeting expectations. Other evaluations, such as formal psychologic or educational testing, may need to be scheduled.

Interdisciplinary Management

The pediatrician has the responsibility for consulting with other disciplines to make the diagnosis of ID and coordinate treatment services. Consultant services may include psychology, speech-language pathology, physical therapy, occupational therapy, audiology, nutrition, nursing, and social work, as well as medical specialties such as neurodevelopmental disabilities, neurology, genetics, physical medicine and rehabilitation, psychiatry, developmental-behavioral pediatricians, and surgical specialties. Contact with early intervention and school personnel is equally important to help prepare and assess the adequacy of the child's individual family service plan or individual educational plan. The family should be an integral part of the planning and direction of this process. Care should be family centered and culturally sensitive; for older children, their participation in planning and decision-making should be promoted to whatever extent possible.

Periodic Reevaluation

The child's abilities and the family's needs change over time. As the child grows, more information must be provided to the child and family, goals must be reassessed, and programming needs should be adjusted. A periodic review should include information about the child's health status as well as the child's functioning at home, at school, and in other community settings. Other information, such as formal psychologic or educational testing, may be helpful. Reevaluation should be undertaken at routine intervals (every 6-12 mo during early childhood), at any time the child is not meeting expectations, or when the child is moving from one service delivery system to another. This is especially true during the transition to adulthood, beginning at age 16, as mandated by the IDEA Amendments of 2004, and lasting through age 21, when care should be transitioned to adult-based systems and providers.

Federal and Education Services

Education is the single most important discipline involved in the treatment of children with an ID. The educational program must be relevant to the child's needs and address the child's individual strengths and weaknesses. The child's developmental level, requirements for support, and goals for independence provide a basis for establishing an **individualized education program (IEP)** for school-age children, as mandated by federal legislation.

Beyond education services, families of children with ID are often in great need of federal or state-provided social services. All states offer developmental disabilities programs that provide home and community-based services to eligible children and adults, potentially including in-home supports, care coordination services, residential living arrangements, and additional therapeutic options. A variety of Medicaid waiver programs are also offered for children with disabilities within each state. Children with ID who live in low socioeconomic status households should qualify to receive supplemental security income (SSI). Of note, in 2012, an estimated >40% of children with ID did not receive SSI benefits for which they would have been eligible, indicating an untapped potential resource for many families.

Leisure and Recreational Activities

The child's social and recreational needs should be addressed. Although young children with ID are generally included in play activities with children who have typical development, adolescents with ID often do not have opportunities for appropriate social interactions. Community participation among adults with ID is much lower than that of the typical population, stressing the importance of promoting involvement in social activities such as dances, trips, dating, extracurricular sports, and other social-recreational events at an early age. Participation in sports should be encouraged (even if the child is not competitive) because it offers many benefits, including weight management, development of physical coordination, maintenance of cardiovascular fitness, and improvement of self-image.

Family Counseling

Many families adapt well to having a child with ID, but some have emotional or social difficulties. The risks of parental depression and child abuse and neglect are higher in this group of children than in the general population. The factors associated with good family coping and parenting skills include stability of the marriage, good parental self-esteem, limited number of siblings, higher socioeconomic status, lower degree of disability or associated impairments (especially behavioral), parents' appropriate expectations and acceptance of the diagnosis, supportive extended family members, and availability of community programs and respite care services. In families in whom the emotional burden of having a child with ID is great, family counseling, parent support groups, respite care, and home health services should be an integral part of the treatment plan.

Transition to Adulthood

Transition to adulthood in adolescents with intellectual disabilities can present a stressful and chaotic time for both the individual and the family, just as it does among young adults of typical intelligence. A successful transition strongly correlates to later improved quality of life but requires significant advanced planning. In moving from child to adult care, families tend to find that policies, systems, and services are more fragmented, less readily available, and more difficult to navigate. Several domains of transition must be addressed, such as education and employment, health and living, finances and independence, and social and community life. Specific issues to manage include transitioning to an adult healthcare provider, determining the need for decision-making assistance (e.g., guardianship, medical power of attorney), securing government benefits after aging out of youth-based programs (e.g., SSI, medical assistance), agreeing on the optimal housing situation, applying for state disability assistance programs, and addressing caretaker estate planning as it applies to the individual with ID (e.g., special needs trusts).

Following graduation from high school, options for continued education or entry into the workforce should be thoroughly considered, with the greater goal of ultimate community-based employment. Although employment is a critical element of life adaptation for persons with ID, only 15% are estimated to have jobs, with significant gaps in pay and compensation compared to workers without disability. Early planning and expansion of opportunities can help to reduce barriers to employment. Post–secondary education possibilities might involve community college or vocational training. Employment selection should be "customized" to the individual's interests and abilities. Options may include participation in competitive employment, supported employment, high school–to–work transition programs, job-coaching programs, and consumer-directed voucher programs.

PROGNOSIS

In children with severe ID, the prognosis is often evident by early childhood. Mild ID might not always be a lifelong disorder. Children might meet criteria for GDD at an early age, but later the disability can evolve into a more specific developmental disorder (communication disorder, autism, specific learning disability, or borderline normal intelligence). Others with a diagnosis of mild ID during their school years may develop sufficient adaptive behavior skills that they no longer fit the diagnosis as adolescents or young adults, or the effects of maturation and plasticity may result in children moving from one diagnostic category to another (from moderate to mild ID). Conversely, some children who have a diagnosis of a specific learning disability or communication disorder might not maintain their rate of cognitive growth and may fall into the range of ID over time.

The apparent higher prevalence of ID in low- and middle-income countries is of concern given the limitations in available resources. **Community-based rehabilitation (CBR)** is an effort promoted by WHO over the past 4 decades as a means of making use of existing community resources for persons with disabilities in low-income countries with the goal of increasing inclusion and participation within the community. CBR is now being implemented in >90 countries, although the efficacy of such programs has not been established.

The long-term outcome of persons with ID depends on the underlying cause, degree of cognitive and adaptive deficits, presence of associated medical and developmental impairments, capabilities of the families, and school and community supports, services, and training provided to the child and family (Table 53.7). As adults, many persons with mild ID are capable of gaining economic and social independence with functional literacy, but they may need periodic supervision (especially when under social or economic stress). Most live successfully in the community, either independently or in supervised settings.

For persons with moderate ID, the goals of education are to enhance adaptive abilities and "survival" academic and vocational skills so they are better able to live and function in the adult world (Table 53.7). The concept of supported employment has been very beneficial to these individuals; the person is trained by a coach to do a specific job in the setting where the person is to work, bypassing the need for a "sheltered workshop" experience and resulting in successful work adaptation in the community. These persons generally live at home or in a supervised setting in the community.

As adults, people with severe to profound ID usually require extensive to pervasive supports (Table 53.7). These individuals may have associated impairments, such as cerebral palsy, behavioral disorders, epilepsy, or sensory impairments, that further limit their adaptive functioning. They can perform simple tasks in supervised settings. Most people with this level of ID can live in the community with appropriate supports.

The life expectancy of people with mild ID is similar to the general population, with a mean age at death in the early 70s. However, persons with severe and profound ID have a decreased life expectancy at all ages, presumably from associated serious neurologic or medical disorders, with a mean age at death in the mid-50s. Given that persons with ID are living longer and have high rates of comorbid health conditions in adulthood (e.g., obesity, hypertension, diabetes), ID is now one of the costliest ICD-10 diagnoses, with an average lifetime cost of 1-2 million dollars per person. Thus the priorities for pediatricians are to improve healthcare delivery systems during childhood, facilitate the transition of care to adult providers, and ensure high-quality, integrated community-based services for all persons with ID.

Bibliography is available at Expert Consult.

53.1 Intellectual Disability With Regression
Bruce K. Shapiro and Meghan E. O'Neill

The patients discussed in Chapter 53 with intellectual disability (ID) usually have a static and nonprogressive disease course. They may acquire new developmental milestones, although at a slower rate than unaffected children, or they may remain fixed at a particular developmental stage. Regression of milestones in these children may be caused by increasing spasticity or contractures, new-onset seizures or a movement disorder, or the progression of hydrocephalus.

Nonetheless, **regression** or loss of milestones should suggest a **progressive encephalopathy** caused by an *inborn error of metabolism,* including disorders of energy metabolism and storage disorders, or a *neurodegenerative disorder,* including disorders of the whole brain (diffuse encephalopathies), white matter (leukodystrophies), cerebral cortex, and basal ganglia as well as spinocerebellar disorders (Table 53.8) (see Chapters 616 and 617).

Bibliography is available at Expert Consult.

Table 53.7	Severity of Intellectual Disability and Adult-Age Functioning	
LEVEL	**MENTAL AGE AS ADULT**	**ADULT ADAPTATION**
Mild	9-11 yr	Reads at 4th-5th grade level; simple multiplication and division; writes simple letter, lists; completes job application; basic independent job skills (arrive on time, stay at task, interact with coworkers); uses public transportation, might qualify for driver's license; keeps house, cooks using recipes
Moderate	6-8 yr	Sight-word reading; copies information (e.g., address from card to job application); matches written number to number of items; recognizes time on clock; communicates; some independence in self-care; housekeeping with supervision or cue cards; meal preparation, can follow picture recipe cards; job skills learned with much repetition; uses public transportation with some supervision
Severe	3-5 yr	Needs continuous support and supervision; might communicate wants and needs, sometimes with augmentative communication techniques
Profound	<3 yr	Limitations of self-care, continence, communication, and mobility; might need complete custodial or nursing care

Data from World Health Organization: *International Statistical Classification of Diseases and Related Health Problems,* 10th revision, Geneva, 2011, WHO.

Table 53.8	Causes of Progressive Encephalopathy

ONSET BEFORE AGE 2 YEARS
Acquired Immunodeficiency Syndrome Encephalopathy*

Disorders of Amino Acid Metabolism
Guanidinoacetate methyltransferase deficiency*
Homocystinuria (21q22)*
Maple syrup urine disease (intermediate and thiamine response forms)*
Phenylketonuria

Guanidinoacetate methyltransferase deficiency*
Hyperammonemic disorders

Disorders of Lysosomal Enzymes
Ganglioside storage disorders
    GM₁ gangliosidosis
    GM₂ gangliosidosis (Tay-Sachs disease, Sandhoff disease)
Gaucher disease type II (glucosylceramide lipidosis)*
Globoid cell leukodystrophy (Krabbe disease)

Continued

Table 53.8	Causes of Progressive Encephalopathy—cont'd

Glycoprotein degradation disorders
I-cell disease
   Mucopolysaccharidoses*
   Type I (Hurler Syndrome)*
   Type III (Sanfilippo disease)
Niemann-Pick disease type A (sphingomyelin lipidosis)
Sulfatase deficiency disorders
Metachromatic leukodystrophy (sulfatide lipidoses)
Multiple sulfatase deficiency

Carbohydrate-Deficient Glycoprotein Syndromes

Hypothyroidism*

Mitochondrial Disorders
Alexander disease
Mitochondrial myopathy, encephalopathy, lactic acidosis, stroke
Progressive infantile poliodystrophy (Alpers disease)
Subacute necrotizing encephalomyelopathy (Leigh disease)
Trichopoliodystrophy (Menkes disease)

Neurocutaneous Syndromes
Chediak-Higashi syndrome
Neurofibromatosis*
Tuberous sclerosis*

Other Disorders of Gray Matter
Infantile ceroid lipofuscinosis (Santavuori-Haltia disease)
Infantile neuroaxonal dystrophy
Lesch-Nyhan disease*
Progressive neuronal degeneration with liver disease
Rett syndrome

Progressive Hydrocephalus*

Other Disorders of White Matter
Aspartoacylase deficiency (Canavan disease)
Galactosemia: Transferase deficiency*
Neonatal adrenoleukodystrophy
Pelizaeus-Merzbacher disease
Progressive cavitating leukoencephalopathy

ONSET AFTER AGE 2 YEARS
Disorders of Lysosomal Enzymes
Gaucher disease type III (glucosylceramide lipidosis)
Globoid cell leukodystrophy (late-onset Krabbe disease)
Glycoprotein degradation disorders
Aspartylglycosaminuria
Mannosidosis type II
GM_2 gangliosidosis (juvenile Tay-Sachs disease)
Metachromatic leukodystrophy (late-onset sulfatide lipidoses)
Mucopolysaccharidoses types II and VII
Niemann-Pick type C (sphingomyelin lipidosis)

Infectious Disease
Acquired immunodeficiency syndrome encephalopathy*
Congenital syphilis*
Subacute sclerosing panencephalitis

Other Disorders of Gray Matter
Ceroid lipofuscinosis
   Juvenile
   Late infantile (Bielschowsky-Jansky disease)
Huntington disease
Mitochondrial disorders
   Late-onset poliodystrophy
   Myoclonic epilepsy and ragged-red fibers
Progressive neuronal degeneration with liver disease
Xeroderma pigmentosum

Other Disorders of White Matter
Adrenoleukodystrophy
Alexander disease
Cerebrotendinous xanthomatosis
Progressive cavitating leukoencephalopathy

Other Diseases
Wilson disease
Friedreich ataxia
Pantothenate kinase neurodegeneration
Neurodegeneration with brain iron accumulation

*Denotes the most common conditions and those with disease-modifying treatment.
From Pina-Garza JE: *Fenichel's clinical pediatric neurology*, ed 7, Philadelphia, 2013, Elsevier, Boxes 5-2 and 5-5, pp 114, 121.

Chapter **54**
Autism Spectrum Disorder
Carolyn F. Bridgemohan
第五十四章
孤独症谱系障碍

中文导读

本章主要介绍了孤独症谱系障碍的定义、诊断标准和症状、流行病学、病因学、鉴别诊断、共患病、筛查、评估、治疗和管理以及预后。诊断标准和症状部分具体描述了社会交往和社会互动，发展、维持和理解关系，限制性和重复性行为，DSM-5中定义的严重性级别，DSM-5中定义的特殊说明；治疗和管理部分具体描述了教育、共患病的处理、药物治疗、补充和替代医学、过渡等内容。

DEFINITION

Autism spectrum disorder (ASD) is a neurobiologic disorder with onset in early childhood. The key features are impairment in social communication and social interaction accompanied by restricted and repetitive behaviors. The presentation of ASD can vary significantly from one individual to another, as well as over the course of development for a particular child. There is currently no diagnostic biomarker for ASD. Accurate diagnosis therefore requires careful review of the history and direct observation of the child's behavior.

DIAGNOSTIC CRITERIA AND SYMPTOMS

The diagnostic criteria in the *Diagnostic and Statistical Manual, Fifth Edition* (DSM-5) focus on symptoms in two primary domains (Table 54.1). To meet criteria for ASD, the symptoms need to have been present since the early developmental period, significantly impact functioning, and not be better explained by the diagnoses of intellectual disability (ID) or global developmental delay (GDD; Chapter 53). Table 54.2 provides associated features not included in DSM-5 criteria.

Previously, ASD was grouped under the heading of *pervasive developmental disorders* (PDDs) and included a variety of subdiagnoses, including autistic disorder, PDD not otherwise specified (PDD-NOS), and **Asperger disorder**. Research did not support these as distinct conditions; in the current diagnostic framework, any individual previously diagnosed with 1 of these conditions should be diagnosed with ASD.

Symptoms can present early in infancy, with reduced response to name and unusual use of objects being strong predictors for risk of ASD. However, symptoms before age 12 mo are not as reliably predictive of later diagnosis. Individuals with milder severity may not present until preschool or school age, when the social demands for peer interaction and group participation are higher.

Social Communication and Social Interaction

Individuals with ASD have difficulty understanding and engaging in social relationships. The problems are pervasive and impact 3 major areas: reciprocal social interactions (social-emotional reciprocity), nonverbal communication, and understanding of social relationships. The presentation can vary with severity and developmental functioning. Diagnosis of ASD requires the presence of symptoms from all 3 categories (Table 54.3).

Social-Emotional Reciprocity

Reduced social interactions in ASD may range from active avoidance or reduced social response to having an interest in, but lacking ability to initiate or sustain, an interaction with peers or adults. A young child with ASD may not respond when his name is called, may exhibit limited showing and sharing behaviors, and may prefer solitary play. In addition, the child may avoid attempts by others to play and may not participate in activities that require taking turns, such as peek-a-boo and ball play. An older child with ASD may have an interest in peers but may not know how to initiate or join in play. The child may have trouble with the rules of conversation and may either talk at length about an area of interest or abruptly exit the interaction. Younger children often have limited capacity for imaginative or pretend play skills. Older children may engage in play but lack flexibility and may be highly directive to peers. Some children with ASD interact well with adults but struggle to interact with same-age peers.

Table 54.1	DSM-5 Diagnostic Criteria for Autism Spectrum Disorder

A. Persistent deficits in social communication and social interaction across multiple contexts, as manifested by the following, currently or by history:
  1. Deficits in social-emotional reciprocity.
  2. Deficits in nonverbal communicative behaviors used for social interaction.
  3. Deficits in developing, maintaining, and understanding relationships.
B. Restricted, repetitive patterns of behavior, interests, or activities, as manifested by at least 2 of the following, currently or by history:
  1. Stereotyped or repetitive motor movements, use of objects, or speech.
  2. Insistence on sameness, inflexible adherence to routines, or ritualized patterns of verbal or nonverbal behavior.
  3. Highly restricted, fixated interests that are abnormal in intensity or focus.
  4. Hyper- or hyporeactivity to sensory input or unusual interest in sensory aspects of the environment.
C. Symptoms must be present in the early developmental period (may not become fully manifest until social demands exceed limited capacities, or may be masked by learned strategies in later life).
D. Symptoms cause clinically significant impairment in social, occupational, or other important areas of current functioning.
E. These disturbances are not better explained by intellectual disability (intellectual developmental disorder) or global developmental delay.

From the *Diagnostic and Statistical Manual of Mental Disorders, Fifth Edition,* (Copyright 2013). American Psychiatric Association, pp 50–51.

Table 54.2	Associated Features of Autism Not in DSM-5 Criteria

Atypical language development and abilities
  Age <6 yr: frequently disordered and delayed in comprehension; two-thirds have difficulty with expressive phonology and grammar
  Age ≥6 yr: disordered pragmatics, semantics, and morphology, with relatively intact articulation and syntax (i.e., early difficulties are resolved)
Motor abnormalities: motor delay; hypotonia; catatonia; deficits in coordination, movement preparation and planning, praxis, gait, and balance

For version with full references, see *Diagnostic and Statistical Manual of Mental Disorders, Fifth Edition,* Washington DC, 2013, American Psychiatric Association. Adapted from Lai MC, Lombardo MV, Baron-Cohen S: Autism, *Lancet* 383: 896–910, 2014.

Nonverbal Communicative Behavior

Difficulties with nonverbal communication may manifest as reduced use of eye contact and gestures such as pointing. Children may also show reduced awareness or response to the eye gaze or pointing of others. They may use eye contact only when communicating a highly preferred request or may have difficulty coordinating the use of nonverbal

Table 54.3	Signs and Symptoms of Possible Autism in Preschool Children (or Equivalent Mental Age)

SOCIAL INTERACTION AND RECIPROCAL COMMUNICATION BEHAVIORS

Spoken Language

Language delay (in babbling or using words; e.g., using <10 words by age 2 yr).

Regression in, or loss of, use of speech.

Spoken language (if present) may include unusual features, such as vocalizations that are not speech-like; odd or flat intonation; frequent repetition of set words and phrases (echolalia); reference to self by name or "you" or "she" or "he" beyond age 3 yr.

Reduced and/or infrequent use of language for communication; e.g., use of single words, although able to speak in sentences.

Responding to Others

Absent or delayed response to name being called, despite normal hearing.

Reduced or absent responsive social smiling.

Reduced or absent responsiveness to other people's facial expressions or feelings.

Unusually negative response to the requests of others ("demand avoidance" behavior).

Rejection of cuddles initiated by parent or caregiver, although the child may initiate cuddles.

Interacting With Others

Reduced or absent awareness of personal space, or unusually intolerant of people entering their personal space.

Reduced or absent social interest in others, including children of own age—may reject others; if interested in others, child may approach others inappropriately, seeming to be aggressive or disruptive.

Reduced or absent imitation of others' actions.

Reduced or absent initiation of social play with others; plays alone.

Reduced or absent enjoyment of situations that most children like; e.g., birthday parties.

Reduced or absent sharing of enjoyment.

Eye Contact, Pointing, and Other Gestures

Reduced or absent use of gestures and facial expressions to communicate (although may place an adult's hand on objects).

Reduced and poorly integrated gestures, facial expressions, body orientation, eye contact (looking at people's eyes when speaking), and speech used in social communication.

Reduced or absent social use of eye contact (assuming adequate vision).

Reduced or absent "joint attention" (when 1 person alerts another to something by means of gazing, finger pointing, or other verbal or nonverbal indication for the purpose of sharing interest). This would be evident in the child from lack of:

Gaze switching

Following a point (looking where the other person points to—may look at hand)

Using pointing at or showing objects to share interest

Ideas and Imagination

Reduced or absent imagination and variety of pretend play.

Unusual or Restricted Interests and/or Rigid and Repetitive Behaviors

Repetitive "stereotypic" movements such as hand flapping, body rocking while standing, spinning, and finger flicking.

Repetitive or stereotyped play; e.g., opening and closing doors.

Over focused or unusual interests.

Excessive insistence on following own agenda.

Extremes of emotional reactivity to change or new situations; insistence on things being "the same."

Overreaction or underreaction to sensory stimuli, such as textures, sounds, or smells.

Excessive reaction to the taste, smell, texture, or appearance of food, or having extreme food fads.

Adapted from Baird G, Douglas HR, Murphy MS: Recognizing and diagnosing autism in children and young people: summary of NICE guidance. *BMJ* 343:d6360, 2011, Box 1, p 901.

with verbal communication. Children with ASD may have limited range of facial expression or expressed emotion.

Developing, Maintaining, and Understanding Relationships

Children with ASD have limited insight regarding social relationships. They have difficulty understanding the difference between a true friend and a casual acquaintance. They have trouble picking up on the nuances of social interactions and understanding social expectations for polite behavior. They may have reduced understanding of personal boundaries and may stand too close to others. In addition, they can have trouble understanding and inferring others' emotions and are less likely to share emotion or enjoyment with others. Adolescents and young adults have difficulty engaging in group interactions and navigating romantic relationships.

Restrictive and Repetitive Behavior

Diagnosis of ASD requires the presence of 2 of the 4 symptoms of restrictive and repetitive patterns of behavior discussed next.

Stereotyped Motor Movements or Speech

Stereotyped (or stereotypic) movements and repetitive behaviors may include hand flapping, finger movements, body rocking and lunging, jumping, running and spinning, and repetitive speech such as echoing words immediately after they are said. Repetitive patterns of play may be present, such as lining up objects, repetitively turning light switches on and off or opening and closing doors, spinning objects, or arranging toys in a specific manner. These repetitive patterns may not be seen in very young toddlers but may develop as they get older. Stereotyped

movements can change over time and in older children are seen more often in individuals with lower cognitive functioning.

Insistence on Sameness

Children with ASD have difficulty tolerating transitions or change. They may insist on certain routines or schedules and can become very distressed with unexpected events or new situations. They may repeat scripts from shows or movies or watch the same portion of a video repeatedly. Intolerance for change causes significant impairment and impact on child and family function.

Restricted Interests

This symptom may manifest as intense interests that seem out of the norm in comparison to same-age peers. Younger children may play with a limited range of toys or may insist on retaining a small object in each hand. Older children may have a strong preference for a particular story or movie. The area of interest may be shared by peers (e.g., Disney movies, Legos, Thomas the Train) but *unusual* in its intensity. Other affected children may have interests that are both intense and odd, such as an interest in brands of vehicles, license plate numbers, or fans and heating systems. These interests interfere with social interactions; a child may only want to talk about her area of interest or may insist that peers act out a particular story in a rigid and inflexible manner.

Hypo- or Hyperreactivity to Sensory Input

Children with ASD may be overly sensitive to sensory input, such as noise, smells, or texture. Children may scream when they hear a siren or vacuum and may gag and choke with certain foods or odors. They may refuse to wear certain clothing or may become very distressed with bathing or with cutting nails and hair. Conversely, some affected children seem to crave sensory input. They may engage in repetitive jumping or hugging and may smell or lick objects or people. Young children may inappropriately touch the face or hair of others.

Diagnosing ASD with DSM-5 criteria can be challenging in very young children because of reduced expression of repetitive behaviors, particularly stereotyped behavior and intense interests. Studies monitoring development in high-risk young children who have an older sibling with ASD indicate these additional symptoms may emerge over time. This creates a dilemma for specialty clinicians evaluating very young children for ASD, because they may not be able to endorse sufficient symptoms to make an early diagnosis and access specialized intervention services.

Severity Levels Defined in DSM-5

Severity level in ASD is based on the level of support the individual requires in each of the major domains impacted—social communication and restricted and repetitive behavior. Levels range from –"needing support" (level 1), to –"needing substantial support" (level 2), to –"needing very substantial support" (level 3) (Table 54.4).

Specifiers Defined in DSM-5

Formal diagnosis of ASD also includes documenting associated conditions including whether the individual has cognitive and/or language impairment, any related medical, genetic or environmental factors and any other neurodevelopmental or behavioral health conditions, including catatonia (Table 54.5). This process helps to better characterize the presentation in an individual child and ensures that the diagnosis has been made by considering the symptoms in the context of the child's current cognitive and language abilities.

EPIDEMIOLOGY

The prevalence of ASD is estimated at 1 in 59 persons by the U.S. Centers for Disease Control and Prevention (CDC). The prevalence increased significantly over the past 25 years, primarily because of improved diagnosis and case finding as well as inclusion of less severe presentations within the **autism** spectrum. There is a 4:1 male predominance. The prevalence is increased in siblings (up to 10% recurrence rate) and particularly in identical twins. There are no racial or ethnic differences in prevalence. Individuals from racial minorities and lower socioeconomic status are at risk for later diagnosis.

ETIOLOGY

The etiology of ASD is thought to result from disrupted neural connectivity and is primarily impacted by genetic variations affecting early brain development. Animal models and studies of individuals with ASD indicate changes in brain volume and neural cell density in the limbic system, cerebellum, and frontotemporal regions. One study documented changes in early brain development, characterized as "hyperexpansion of cortical surface area," at age 6-12 mo on brain MRI, which correlated with later development of impaired social skills. Functional studies show abnormalities of processing information, particularly related to foundational social skills such as facial recognition. The disruptions in early brain development likely are responsive the treatment. Early developmental therapies in young children with ASD have demonstrated the capacity for normalization of electrophysiologic response to visual stimuli, including faces.

Numerous **genes** involved in brain development and synaptic function have been associated with ASD. Mutations that include large genetic deletions or duplications and small sequencing changes have been implicated; these can be inherited or occur de novo. Heterozygous mutations in genes, such as present in deletion or duplication of 15q11.2 or 16p11.2, may have variable expression within a family. Rare recessive mutations have been implicated in some populations with high levels of consanguinity. Patients with a number of genetic syndromes (e.g., fragile X, Down, Smith-Lemli-Opitz, Rett, Angelman, Timothy, Joubert) as well as disorders of metabolism and mitochondrial function have higher rates of ASD than the general population (Table 54.5).

There is also evidence for **environmental** contributions to ASD. Older maternal or paternal age may increase the risk of ASD. In addition, factors influencing the intrauterine environment, such as maternal obesity or overweight, short interval from prior pregnancy, premature birth, and certain prenatal infections (e.g., rubella, cytomegalovirus) are associated with ASD. An epigenetic model is considered one explanation for the etiology; individuals with genetic vulnerability may be more sensitive to environmental factors influencing early brain development.

Despite frequent concerns from families that **vaccines** or the preservatives in vaccines lead to ASD, *there is no evidence to support this claim.* Multiple research studies and meta-analyses have failed to show an association of vaccines with ASD.

DIFFERENTIAL DIAGNOSIS

The differential diagnosis of ASD is complex because many conditions in the differential can also occur with ASD. The most important conditions to consider in young children are language disorder (see Chapter 52), intellectual disability or global developmental delay (Chapter 53), and hearing loss (Chapter 655). Children with **language disorder** may have impairments in social communication and play; their social and play skills, however, are typically on par with their language level. In addition, they do not have associated restricted and repetitive behavior or atypical use of language, such as scripting. The diagnosis of **social communication disorder** is also distinguished from ASD by the lack of restrictive and repetitive behaviors. Children with **intellectual disability (ID)** or **global developmental delay (GDD)** may have delays in social and communication skills as well as stereotyped behavior. However, social and communication skills are typically commensurate with their cognitive and adaptive functioning. Children with **hearing loss** may present with some "red flags" for ASD, such as poor response to name. However, they typically develop nonverbal communication and play skills as expected and do not have stereotyped or restricted behavior patterns.

In older children, disorders of attention, learning, and mood regulation must be considered in the differential diagnosis of ASD. Children with **attention-deficit/hyperactivity disorder (ADHD)** may present with reduced eye contact and response to name caused by poor attention rather than lack of social awareness. Children with ADHD, however, do not have associated impairments in shared enjoyment and social reciprocity or repetitive behaviors. Children with **social anxiety** or other anxiety disorders may present with some symptoms suggestive of ASD. Shy children may have reduced eye contact and social initiation. Anxious children can be resistant to change and prefer familiar routines. Children with anxiety, however, typically will have preserved social interest and insight and will not exhibit high levels of stereotyped behaviors. **Reactive attachment disorder** can be difficult to distinguish from ASD, particularly in younger children with history of trauma. However, social behaviors in these children generally improve with positive caretaking.

The differentiation of ASD from **obsessive-compulsive disorder (OCD)**, tics, and stereotyped behaviors can sometimes be challenging. In general, stereotyped behaviors may be calming or preferred, whereas tics and compulsive routines are distressing to the individual. Children with OCD have intense interests as well as repetitive behaviors and rituals but do not have impairment in social communication or interaction. Children with **stereotypic movement disorder** will not have impaired social skills or other types of restricted and repetitive behaviors. Children with **Landau Kleffner syndrome (LKS)** present with loss of skills in language comprehension (auditory verbal agnosia) and verbal expression (aphasia) associated with onset of epileptic seizures during sleep (see Chapter 52). In contrast to ASD, children with LKS present with typical early development followed by loss of language function at age 3-6 yr.

COMORBID CONDITIONS

Up to 50% of individuals with ASD have intellectual disability, ranging in severity from mild to severe (Table 54.5). Intellectual disability is associated with higher rates of both identified genetic conditions and epilepsy. Children with ASD often have associated language impairments, including delays in expressive, receptive, and pragmatic (social) language skills. Language function can range widely from nonverbal status to age appropriate. Gastrointestinal (GI) problems such as constipation, esophagitis, and gastroesophageal reflux disease (GERD) are reported

Table 54.4	DSM-5 Severity Levels for Autism Spectrum Disorder

SEVERITY LEVEL	SOCIAL COMMUNICATION	RESTRICTED, REPETITIVE BEHAVIORS
Level 3 "Requiring very substantial support"	Severe deficits in verbal and nonverbal social communication skills cause severe impairments in functioning, very limited initiation of social interactions, and minimal response to social overtures from others. *For example,* a person with few words of intelligible speech who rarely initiates interaction and, when he or she does, makes unusual approaches to meet needs only and responds to only very direct social approaches	Inflexibility of behavior, extreme difficulty coping with change, or other restricted/repetitive behaviors markedly interfere with functioning in all spheres. Great distress/difficulty changing focus or action.
Level 2 "Requiring substantial support"	Marked deficits in verbal and nonverbal social communication skills; social impairments apparent even with supports in place; limited initiation of social interactions; and reduced or abnormal responses to social overtures from others. *For example,* a person who speaks simple sentences, whose interaction is limited to narrow special interests, and who has markedly odd nonverbal communication	Inflexibility of behavior, difficulty coping with change, or other restricted/repetitive behaviors appear frequently enough to be obvious to the casual observer and interfere with functioning in a variety of contexts. Distress and/or difficulty changing focus or action.
Level 1 "Requiring support"	Without supports in place, deficits in social communication cause noticeable impairments. Difficulty initiating social interactions, and clear examples of atypical or unsuccessful responses to social overtures of others. May appear to have decreased interest in social interactions. *For example,* a person who is able to speak in full sentences and engages in communication but whose to-and-fro conversation with others fails, and whose attempts to make friends are odd and typically unsuccessful	Inflexibility of behavior causes significant interference with functioning in one or more contexts. Difficulty switching between activities. Problems of organization and planning hamper independence.

From the *Diagnostic and Statistical Manual of Mental Disorders, Fifth Edition,* (Copyright 2013). American Psychiatric Association, p 52.

Table 54.5	Common Co-occurring Conditions in Autism Spectrum Disorder (ASD)

COMORBIDITY	INDIVIDUALS WITH AUTISM AFFECTED	COMMENTS
DEVELOPMENTAL DISORDERS		
Intellectual disability	~45%	Prevalence estimate is affected by the diagnostic boundary and definition of intelligence (e.g., whether verbal ability is used as a criterion). In individuals, discrepant performance between subtests is common.
Language disorders	Variable	In DSM-IV, language delay was a defining feature of autism (autistic disorder), but is no longer included in DSM-5. An autism-specific language profile (separate from language disorders) exists, but with substantial interindividual variability.
Attention-deficit/ hyperactivity disorder	28–44%	In DSM-IV, not diagnosed when occurring in individuals with autism, but no longer so in DSM-5.
Tic disorders	14–38%	~6.5% have Tourette syndrome.
Motor abnormality	≤79%	See Table 54.2.
GENERAL MEDICAL DISORDERS		
Epilepsy	8–35%	Increased frequency in individuals with intellectual disability or genetic syndromes. Two peaks of onset: early childhood and adolescence. Increases risk of poor outcome.
Gastrointestinal problems	9–70%	Common symptoms include chronic constipation, abdominal pain, chronic diarrhea, and gastroesophageal reflux. Associated disorders include gastritis, esophagitis, gastroesophageal reflux disease, inflammatory bowel disease, celiac disease, Crohn disease, and colitis.
Immune dysregulation	≤38%	Associated with allergic and autoimmune disorders.
Genetic disorders	10–20%	Collectively called *syndromic autism.* Examples include fragile X syndrome (21–50% of individuals affected have autism), Rett syndrome (most have autistic features but with profiles different from idiopathic autism), tuberous sclerosis complex (24–60%), Down syndrome (5–39%), phenylketonuria (5–20%), CHARGE syndrome* (15–50%), Angelman syndrome (50–81%), Timothy syndrome (60–70%), and Joubert syndrome (~40%).
Sleep disorders	50–80%	Insomnia is the most common.
PSYCHIATRIC DISORDERS		
Anxiety	~40%	Common across all age-groups. Most common are social anxiety disorder (13–29% of individuals with autism) and generalized anxiety disorder (13–22%). High-functioning individuals are more susceptible (or symptoms are more detectable).
Depression	12–70%	Common in adults, less common in children. High-functioning adults who are less socially impaired are more susceptible (or symptoms are more detectable).

Continued

Table 54.5	Common Co-occurring Conditions in Autism Spectrum Disorder (ASD)—cont'd	
COMORBIDITY	**INDIVIDUALS WITH AUTISM AFFECTED**	**COMMENTS**
Obsessive-compulsive disorder (OCD)	7–24%	Shares the repetitive behavior domain with autism that could cut across nosologic categories. Important to distinguish between repetitive behaviors that do not involve intrusive, anxiety-causing thoughts or obsessions (part of autism) and those that do (and are part of OCD).
Psychotic disorders	12–17%	Mainly in adults. Most commonly recurrent hallucinosis. High frequency of autism-like features (even a diagnosis of ASD) preceding adult-onset (52%) and childhood-onset schizophrenia (30–50%).
Substance use disorders	≤16%	Potentially because individual is using substances as self-medication to relieve anxiety.
Oppositional defiant disorder	16–28%	Oppositional behaviors could be a manifestation of anxiety, resistance to change, stubborn belief in the correctness of own point of view, difficulty seeing another's point of view, poor awareness of the effect of own behavior on others, or no interest in social compliance.
Eating disorders	4–5%	Could be a misdiagnosis of autism, particularly in females, because both involve rigid behavior, inflexible cognition, self-focus, and focus on details.
PERSONALITY DISORDERS[†]		
Paranoid personality disorder	0–19%	Could be secondary to difficulty understanding others' intentions and negative interpersonal experiences.
Schizoid personality disorder	21–26%	Partly overlapping diagnostic criteria.
Schizotypal personality disorder	2–13%	Some overlapping criteria, especially those shared with schizoid personality disorder.
Borderline personality disorder	0–9%	Could have similarity in behaviors (e.g., difficulties in interpersonal relationships, misattributing hostile intentions, problems with affect regulation), which requires careful differential diagnosis. Could be a misdiagnosis of autism, particularly in females.
Obsessive-compulsive personality disorder	19–32%	Partly overlapping diagnostic criteria.
Avoidant personality disorder	13–25%	Could be secondary to repeated failure in social experiences.
BEHAVIORAL DISORDERS		
Aggressive behaviors	≤68%	Often directed toward caregivers rather than noncaregivers. Could be a result of empathy difficulties, anxiety, sensory overload, disruption of routines, and difficulties with communication.
Self-injurious behaviors	≤50%	Associated with impulsivity and hyperactivity, negative affect, and lower levels of ability and speech. Could signal frustration in individuals with reduced communication, as well as anxiety, sensory overload, or disruption of routines. Could also become a repetitive habit. Could cause tissue damage and need for restraint.
Pica	~36%	More likely in individuals with intellectual disability. Could be a result of a lack of social conformity to cultural categories of what is deemed edible, or sensory exploration, or both.
Suicidal ideation or attempt	11–14%	Risks increase with concurrent depression and behavioral problems, and after being teased or bullied.

*Coloboma of the eye; heart defects; atresia of the choanae; retardation of growth and development, or both; genital and urinary abnormalities, or both; and ear abnormalities and deafness.
[†]Particularly in high-functioning adults.
DSM-IV, *Diagnostic and Statistical Manual of Mental Disorders, 4th edition*; DSM-5, *Diagnostic and Statistical Manual of Mental Disorders, Fifth edition*.
Adapted from Lai MC, Lombardo MV, Baron-Cohen S: Autism, *Lancet* 383:896–910, 2014.

in up to 70% of children with ASD. Epilepsy occurs in up to 35% of children with ASD and presents in 2 peaks, in early childhood and in adolescence. Epilepsy or electrical seizures without motor manifestations may be a cause of **regression** in young children with ASD.

Children with ASD are at higher risk for disorders of attention, including reduced attention for nonpreferred activities and excessive attention for preferred activities. A subset of children will also meet full criteria for a diagnosis of ADHD. There are higher rates of anxiety (~40%) and mood disorders in ASD, particularly during adolescence. Children with ASD are also at increased risk for being bullied and may present with secondary irritability, anxiety, or depression.

Sleep problems, including delayed sleep onset, frequent night waking, and abnormal sleep architecture, are reported in 50–80% of children with ASD. There is some evidence for baseline abnormalities in melatonin secretion. The use of screen-based activities such as television, computers, or tablets before bedtime can inhibit melatonin secretion. Children

with ASD also have higher rates of feeding and toileting problems resulting from resistance to change, sensory sensitivity, and repetitive behavior patterns. Many children with ASD have restrictive feeding patterns and food selectivity. They also have higher rates of overweight, possibly because of diets higher in carbohydrates, reduced physical activity, use of food rewards to regulate behavior, and side effects from medications used for managing mood and behavior.

Disruptive behaviors such as self-injury and aggression are common in ASD patients, but most common in individuals with lower cognitive function and limited language. Sleep deprivation, nutritional deficits, pain, epilepsy, and medication side effects may contribute to disruptive behaviors.

SCREENING

The American Academy of Pediatrics recommends screening for ASD for *all* children at age 18 mo and 24 mo (see Chapter 28). Screening should also occur when there is increased risk for ASD, such as a child with an older sibling who has ASD, or concern for possible ASD. Screening can be done by parent checklist or direct assessment. The most frequently used screening tool is the *Modified Checklist for Autism, Revised/Follow-Up Interview* (MCHAT-R/FU), a 20-item parent report measure, with additional parent interview completed for intermediate scores. The MCHAT-R/FU can be used from age 16-30 mo.

ASSESSMENT

Diagnostic assessment should include medical evaluation and assessment of the child's cognitive, language, and adaptive function. Assessment may occur in a single multidisciplinary visit or through a series of visits with different developmental specialists. Multidisciplinary evaluation with clinicians who have expertise with ASD is optimal for diagnostic accuracy and treatment planning. Developmental-behavioral pediatricians, neurodevelopmental disability specialists, neurologists, psychiatrists, and psychologists are qualified to make a formal diagnosis of ASD. Other specialists, including speech-language pathologists and occupational therapists, should also be included depending on the child's age and the presenting concerns.

Assessment of ASD includes direct observation of the child to evaluate social skills and behavior. Informal observation can be supplemented with structured diagnostic tools such as the *Autism Diagnostic Observation Schedule, Second Edition* (ADOS-2) and *Autism Diagnostic Observation Schedule, Toddler module* (ADOS-T). These structured play-based assessments provide social prompts and opportunities to evaluate the frequency and quality of a child's social responsiveness to, initiation, and maintenance of social interactions; the capacity for joint attention and shared enjoyment; the child's behavioral flexibility; and presence of repetitive patterns of behavior. The ADOS-2 and ADOS-T are not required for accurate diagnosis and do not stand alone, but rather can be used to augment a careful history and observation. The *Childhood Autism Rating Scale, Second Edition* (CARS-2) is a 15-item direct clinical observation instrument that can assist clinicians in the diagnosis of ASD. The *Autism Diagnostic Interview-Revised* (ADI-R) is a lengthy clinical interview tool that is used primarily in research settings since it takes several hours to administer. Other tools include standardized rating scales that parents and teachers can complete to report on the child's social skills and behaviors.

Medical evaluation should include a thorough history and detailed physical examination of the child, including direct behavioral observations of communication and play. In addition, the examination should include measurement of head circumference, careful evaluation for dysmorphic features, and screening for tuberous sclerosis with Wood lamp exam. Children with ASD should have genetic testing (described later), an audiology examination to rule out hearing loss, and in children with pica, a lead test (Table 54.6).

There are currently several specialty-specific clinical guidelines for genetic evaluation of children diagnosed with ASD. Genetic testing is shown to impact clinical decision-making, but no studies have evaluated the impact of genetic testing on the outcome for the child. The American College of Medical Genetics recommends a tiered approach to genetic testing.

First Tier

All children with ASD should have a **chromosomal microarray (CMA)**. CMA will be positive in 10–15% of individuals with ASD. The rate is increased to almost 30% in individuals who have complex presentations, such as associated microcephaly, dysmorphic features, congenital anomalies, or seizures. CMA technology will identify copy number variants but not DNA sequencing errors, balanced translocations, or abnormalities in trinucleotide repeat length. *Fragile X DNA testing is therefore recommended for all boys with ASD.* Fragile X testing should also be considered in girls with physical features suggestive of fragile X syndrome or with a family history of fragile X, X-linked pattern of intellectual disability, tremor/ataxia, or premature ovarian failure.

Second Tier

Girls with ASD should have testing for mutation in the *MeCP2* gene if

CMA is normal. Boys who have hypotonia, drooling, and frequent respiratory infections should have *MeCP2* deletion/duplication testing. All individuals with ASD and a head circumference greater than 2.5 standard deviations (SD) above the mean should have testing for mutation in the *PTEN* gene because there is a risk for hamartoma tumor disorders (Cowden, Proteus-like, Bannayan-Riley-Ruvakaba syndromes) in these individuals. Cytogenetic testing (karyotype) has a lower yield than CMA. Karyotype is recommended if microarray is not available and in children with suspected balanced translocation, such as history of multiple prior miscarriages.

Further medical diagnostic testing is indicated by the child's history and presentation. Brain imaging is indicated in cases of microcephaly, significant developmental regression, or focal findings on neurologic examination. Because of the high rate (up to 25%) of macrocephaly in ASD, imaging is not indicated for macrocephaly alone. MRI is not recommended for minor language regression (loss of a few words) during the 2nd year of life that is often described in toddlers with ASD. Children with concern for seizures, spells, or developmental regression should have an electroencephalogram (EEG). Metabolic screening is indicated for children with signs of a metabolic or mitochondrial disorder, such as developmental regression, weakness, fatigue, lethargy, cyclic vomiting, or seizures (see Chapters 53 and 102).

TREATMENT AND MANAGEMENT
Educational

The primary treatment for ASD is done outside the medical setting and includes developmental and educational programming. Numerous resources have been developed that can help families in the complex process of treatment planning (Table 54.7). Intensive behavioral therapies have the strongest evidence to date. Earlier age at initiation of treatment

Table 54.6	Medical and Genetic Evaluation of Children With Autism Spectrum Disorder

Physical Examination
Dysmorphic physical features
Muscle tone and reflexes
Head circumference
Wood lamp examination for tuberous sclerosis

Diagnostic Testing
Chromosomal microarray (CMA) in all individuals
Fragile X DNA test in males
Audiology evaluation
Lead test in children with pica

Additional Targeted Genetic Testing
Fragile X DNA test in females with symptoms suggestive of fragile X, family history of X-linked intellectual disability, tremor, ataxia, or premature ovarian failure
MeCP2 sequencing in females
PTEN mutation testing if head circumference >2.5 SD above the mean
MeCP2 deletion/duplication testing in males with significant developmental regression, drooling, respiratory infections, and hypotonia
Karyotype if unable to obtain CMA or if balanced translocation suspected

Additional Targeted Diagnostic Testing
EEG in children with seizures, staring spells, or developmental regression
Brain MRI in children with microcephaly, focal neurologic findings, or developmental regression
Metabolic testing in children with developmental regression, hypotonia, seizures, food intolerance, hearing loss, ataxia, or course facial features

Data from Schaefer GB, Mendelsohn NJ: Clinical genetics evaluation in identifying the etiology of autism spectrum disorders: 2013 guideline revisions, *Genet Med* 15(5):399–407, 2013.

and higher intensity of treatment are associated with better outcomes. Programming must be individualized, and no approach is successful for all children. In addition, research treatments are often conducted with a high level of intensity and fidelity that are difficult to scale up or reproduce in community settings. Higher cognitive, play, and joint attention skills and lower symptom severity at baseline are predictors for better outcomes in core symptoms, intellectual function, and language function.

Behavioral approaches based on the principles of **applied behavioral analysis (ABA)** involve direct incremental teaching of skills within a traditional behavioral framework using reinforcement of desired behavior, careful data collection, and analysis and adjustment of the treatment program based on review of data. Comprehensive models integrating behavioral and developmental approaches that build on key foundational skills, such as joint attention, shared enjoyment, and reciprocal communication, show strong evidence of efficacy for young children, particularly toddlers, with ASD. Examples include the *Early Start Denver Model* (ESDM), *Joint Attention Symbolic Play Engagement and Regulation* (JASPER), and *Social Communication/Emotional Regulation/Transactional Support* (SCERTS). Parent training models also show promise for younger children.

Educational approaches such as the *Treatment and Education of Autistic and Communication Handicapped Children* (TEACCH) incorporate structured teaching, visual supports, and adjustment of the environment to the individual needs of students with ASD, such as difficulty with communication, understanding time, and need for routine. These approaches have demonstrated efficacy for improved cognitive and adaptive skills. For older children with more severe symptoms, approaches that use behavioral principles in addition to adjusting the environment may be most effective.

Speech and language therapy can help build vocabulary, comprehension, and pragmatic skills. Children with ASD benefit from visual supports for comprehension, understanding expectations, and communicating their needs. **Augmentative communication** approaches using photographs or picture icons can improve comprehension and ability to communicate. There are a range of options with varying levels of complexity, flexibility, and technology. Using augmentative communication does not inhibit acquisition of verbal language. On the contrary, supporting a child's language development with augmentative supports can facilitate the development of spoken language, even in older children.

Additional strategies to build social skills are used for school age children and adolescents and may be administered in the school or community setting by a variety of specialists, including speech therapists, psychologists, and counselors. **Social skills programs** that include training peer mentors have higher rates of efficacy. Occupational and physical therapy may be indicated for individuals with motor delay and difficulty acquiring adaptive skills such as dressing and toileting.

For some high school students with ASD, training in life skills and vocational skills is critical for maximizing independence in adulthood. Training may focus on basic self-care (e.g., dressing, hygiene), functional academics (e.g., money management, banking skills), learning to fill out a job application, and understanding how to behave with strangers and in work settings. Social skills and job coaching may be needed even for adolescents with strong cognitive and academic function,

because they may struggle with social perception and may be vulnerable to exploitation by others.

Co-occurring Conditions

Additional medical or behavioral health treatment is often required for management of co-occurring conditions in ASD. Seizures occur in up to 35% of children with ASD and should be managed with appropriate antiepileptic therapy (see Chapter 611). GI problems (e.g., constipation, esophagitis, GERD) may present with nonspecific irritability, sleep disturbance, self-injury, aggression, and signs of pain or discomfort, such as crying, and can be managed with the same approaches used in typically developing children.

Management of co-occurring attention and mood disorders is similar to that for typically developing children. Strategies to increase structure and organization in the environment and use of visual supports (e.g., schedules) can improve attention and reduce anxiety. Some children with ASD benefit from modified cognitive-behavioral therapy to address anxiety and OCD.

Strategies to promote **sleep hygiene** and use of behavioral approaches, such as structured bedtime routines, can address delayed sleep onset. Other medical problems, such as epilepsy or GERD, can also contribute to poor sleep and should be treated directly. In cases refractory to behavioral approaches, medications may be used. (For further discussion of management of sleep problems, see Chapter 31.)

Structured behavioral approaches for delayed toilet training in concert with treatment to prevent constipation are often needed for children with ASD. For children with highly restrictive diets, nutrition counseling and behaviorally based feeding therapy may be needed to address poor caloric intake or lack of nutritional quality. Because of limited diets, children with ASD may be at risk for low levels of calcium, vitamin D, and iron. Children who are overweight may have poor nutrition as a result of restrictive diets.

Irritability is a nonspecific symptom and can be a reflection of pain, anxiety, distress, or lack of sleep. Children with ASD are prone to irritability because of their difficulty tolerating change and their limited communication skills. Management of irritability includes evaluating carefully for medical problems that may be causing pain, as well as for any factors in the child's home or school environment that may be causing distress. Possible causes of distress range from common experiences such as changes in the routine to undisclosed abuse or bullying. Treatment should be targeted first at any underlying cause. Medications are often used to treat irritability in ASD but should only be used after appropriate behavioral and communication supports have been implemented.

Pharmacology

There are currently no medications that treat the core symptoms of ASD. Medications can be used to target specific co-occurring conditions or symptoms (Table 54.8; see also Table 54.5). Families should be cautioned, however, that the effect size may be lower and the rate of medication side effects higher in children with ASD.

Preliminary data suggest that intranasal therapy with neuropeptide oxytocin may improve social functioning in children with ASD, particularly those with low pretreatment oxytocin levels.

There is evidence to support use of stimulant medication, **atomoxetine** and α-agonists for ADHD in ASD. Selective serotonin reuptake inhibitors (SSRI) can be used for anxiety and OCD and in adolescents may also be useful for depression. Benzodiazepines may be useful for situational anxiety, for example, triggered by dental and medical procedures or air travel. Medications used to treat ADHD and anxiety may result in activation or irritability in ASD and require careful monitoring.

Melatonin can be used to improve sleep onset but will not address night waking. **Clonidine** or **trazodone** may be used for sleep onset and maintenance. No medications are specifically labeled for treatment of insomnia in ASD.

The α-adrenergic agonists may be helpful in children who present with significant behavioral dysregulation. There are two atypical antipsychotic medications that have U.S. Food and Drug Administration (FDA) recommendation for irritability and aggression in children with

Table 54.8	Common Pharmacologic Treatments in Autism Spectrum Disorder (ASD)			
TARGET SYMPTOM	**MEDICATION CLASS***	**EFFECTS**	**SIDE EFFECTS**	**MONITORING**
Hyperactivity and/or Inattention	Stimulants	Decreased hyperactivity, impulsivity, improved attention	Activation, irritability, emotional lability, lethargy/social withdrawal, stomach ache, reduced appetite, insomnia, increased stereotypy	Height, weight, BP, HR
	α₂-Agonists	Decreased hyperactivity, impulsivity, improved attention	Drowsiness, irritability, enuresis, decreased appetite, dry mouth, hypotension	Height, weight, BP, HR
	Selective norepinephrine reuptake inhibitor	Decreased hyperactivity, impulsivity, improved attention	Irritability, decreased appetite, fatigue, stomach ache, nausea, vomiting, racing heart rate	Height, weight, BP, HR
Anxiety	Selective serotonin reuptake inhibitors	Decreased anxiety	Activation, hyperactivity, inattention, sedation, change in appetite, insomnia, stomach ache, diarrhea Citalopram: prolonged QTc interval	Weight, BP, HR
Irritability	Atypical antipsychotics (risperidone, aripiprazole)	Decreased irritability, aggression, self-injurious behavior, repetitive behavior, hyperactivity	Somnolence, weight gain, extrapyramidal movements, drooling, tremor, dizziness, vomiting, gynecomastia	Weight, BP, HR Monitor CBC, cholesterol, ALT, AST, prolactin, glucose or hemoglobin A₁c
Insomnia	Melatonin	Shortened sleep onset	Nightmares, enuresis	—

*Specific medications names are provided in parentheses when there is a FDA-approved indication for the use of the medication to treat the symptom in children with ASD. Further information about these medications is available in Chapter 33.

BP, Blood pressure; HR, heart rate; CBC, complete blood count; ALT, alanine transaminase; AST, aspartate transaminase.

ASD. Both **risperidone** and **aripiprazole** have several studies documenting efficacy for reducing irritability, aggression, and self-injury. Secondary improvements in attention and repetitive behavior were also noted. Side effects include weight gain and metabolic syndrome as well as tardive dyskinesia and extrapyramidal movements. Careful laboratory monitoring is recommended. Mood-stabilizing antiepileptic medications have also been used to treat irritability.

Complementary and Alternative Medicine

Families of children with ASD often use complementary and alternative medicine (CAM) approaches. These treatments can include supplements, dietary changes, and body or physical treatments. There is a limited evidence to inform families, who often learn about these treatments from friends and family members, alternative medicine providers, or the internet. For most therapies, evidence is insufficient to show benefit. There is strong evidence that secretin and facilitated communication are not effective. Some therapies, such as hyperbaric oxygen, chelation, and high-dose vitamins, are potentially harmful. For children with restrictive diets, taking a daily multivitamin and 400 IU vitamin D may be indicated, although there is no evidence to support megadoses of vitamins. Similarly, for children with evidence of gluten sensitivity, a trial of gluten-free diet may be indicated. However, current evidence does not support this as a treatment for all children with ASD.

When discussing CAM with a family, it is best to use open and collaborative communication, encouraging them to share their current practices and any questions. Specifically ask if they use any herbal treatments, supplements, or other therapies, such as acupuncture, massage, or chiropractic treatment, and what they have observed since trying the treatment. Provide accurate information regarding potential benefit and risk for any treatment. Educate about "red flags" such as treatments that are marketed as a cure for multiple conditions, that report no risk of side effects, or that are marketed by the clinician recommending the treatment. Encourage families to identify a target symptom, "try one thing at a time," and monitor response carefully.

Transition

Navigating a successful transition to adult care is a key role for the pediatric provider. This process should ideally start as early as age 12-13 yr. Parents are faced with a complex and disconnected system of diverse agencies that they need to navigate. Use of structured-visit templates and care coordinators can help ensure that families and their youth with ASD are able to make appropriate decisions about secondary and postsecondary educational programming, vocational training, guardianship, finances, housing, and medical care. High school educational programming should include individualized and meaningful vocational training, as well as instruction regarding sexuality, relationships, safety and abuse prevention, finances, travel training, and general self-advocacy. Individuals with ASD who are higher functioning will need help accessing supports for college or postsecondary skills training and may benefit from referral to their state vocational rehabilitative services as well as personal life coaches or counselors. Families who have adult children with more significant cognitive disability need information about the range of adult disability services, how to apply for supplemental security income (SSI), and the process for considering guardianship or medical and financial conservatorship for their adult child. These decisions are complex and must be individualized for the adult with ASD and the family.

OUTCOME

Autism spectrum disorder is a lifelong condition. Although a minority of individuals respond so well to therapy that they no longer meet criteria for the diagnosis, most will make progress but continue to have some impairment in social and behavioral function as adults. Adult outcome studies are sobering, indicating that many adults with ASD are socially isolated, lack gainful employment or independent living, and have higher rates of depression and anxiety. It is not clear if these data can be extrapolated to younger children currently receiving intensive educational therapies. There is a growing network of adult self-advocates who promote the unique strengths in individuals with ASD. Outcome as measured by developmental progress and functional independence is better for individuals who have higher cognitive and language skills and lower ASD severity at initial diagnosis.

Bibliography is available at Expert Consult.

Nutrition
营养

Chapter 55
Nutritional Requirements

Asim Maqbool, Elizabeth Prout Parks,
Ala Shaikhkhalil, Jennifer Panganiban,
Jonathan A. Mitchell, and
Virginia A. Stallings

第五十五章
营养需求

中文导读

　　本章主要介绍了膳食参考摄入量、能量、脂肪、蛋白质、碳水化合物、纤维素、微量营养素、水以及其营养状况评估，并深入描述了各大类营养素的推荐摄入量、食物来源以及过量危害。进而具体描述了微量元素中的铁、维生素D、钙、维生素K和电解质的推荐摄入量、食物来源以及过量危害。

Nutrition for infants, children, and adolescents should maintain current weight and support normal growth and development. Growth during infancy is rapid, critical for neurocognitive development, and has the highest energy and nutrient requirements relative to body size than any other period of growth. It is followed by growth during childhood, when 60% of total growth occurs, and finally by puberty. Nutrition and growth during the 1st 3 yr of life predict adult stature and some health outcomes. The major risk period for **growth stunting** (impaired linear growth) is between 4 and 24 mo of age. Therefore, it is critical to identify nutrient deficiencies promptly and to address them aggressively early in life, because missing them can impart lasting adverse effects on later growth and development.

Dietary intake should provide energy requirements as well as the essential macronutrient and micronutrient needs for sustaining the function of multiple vital processes. Nutrient deficiencies can limit growth, impair immune function, affect neurodevelopment, and increase morbidity and mortality. Worldwide, malnutrition and undernutrition are the leading causes of acquired immunodeficiency, and a major factor underlying morbidity and mortality in children <5 yr of age.

The transition in food supply and type of nutrition chosen in many developing countries, coincident with population change, from traditional to Western diet has resulted in increased life expectancy and adult stature. Unfortunately, the Western diet in these populations is also frequently accompanied by decreased physical activity and, in parallel, decreases in the incidence and prevalence of communicable (infectious) diseases along with increases in the incidence and prevalence of noncommunicable diseases such as type 2 diabetes, cardiovascular (CV) disease, obesity, inflammatory bowel disease (IBD), and certain cancers. Consequently, it is important to view the impact of nutrition on health from various perspectives: to prevent deficiency, to promote adequacy, and to prevent or reduce the risk for acquiring diseases associated with excess intakes, such as obesity, diabetes, and CV disease.

Advances in our understanding of the roles of some nutrients such as vitamin D, polyunsaturated fatty acids (PUFAs), and fiber have changed our focus from recommendations about preventing deficiency to recommendations about nutritional intake associated with optimal health. The 2006 World Health Organization (WHO) growth charts, which now are recommended *for all children until age 2 yr,* are not only descriptive but also proscriptive on how children with adequate nutrition and health care should grow. Therefore, identifying and providing appropriate and adequate nutrition in infancy and childhood are critical to supporting normal growth and development as well as providing the foundation for lifelong health and well-being.

DIETARY REFERENCE INTAKES
The **dietary reference intake (DRI)** established by the Food and Nutrition Board of the U.S. Institutes of Medicine (IOM) provides guidance on

the nutrient needs for individuals and groups across different life stages and by gender (see Tables 55.1 to 55.4).

Key concepts on DRI concepts include the **estimated average requirement (EAR)**, the **recommended dietary allowance (RDA)**, and the tolerable **upper limit** of intake **(UL)** (Fig. 55.1). The EAR is the average level of daily nutrient intake that is estimated to meet the requirements for 50% of the population, assuming normal distribution. The RDA is an estimate of the daily average nutrient intake that meets the nutritional needs of >97% of the individuals in a population, and it can be used as a guideline for individuals to avoid deficiency. When an EAR cannot be derived, an RDA cannot be calculated; therefore, an **adequate intake (AI)** is developed as a guideline for individuals based on the best available data and scientific consensus. The UL denotes the highest average daily intake with no associated adverse health effects for almost all individuals in a particular group. Fig. 55.2 shows the relationships among EAR, RDA, and UL.

ENERGY

Energy includes both food intake *and* metabolic expenditure. Deficits and excesses of energy intake yield undesirable health consequences. *Inadequate* energy intake can lead to growth faltering, catabolism of body tissues, and inability to provide adequate energy substrate. *Excess* energy intakes can increase the risk for obesity. Adequacy of energy

intake in adults is associated with maintenance of a healthy weight. The three components of energy expenditure in adults are the *basal metabolic rate* (BMR), *thermal effect* of food (e.g., energy required for digestion and absorption), and *energy* for physical activity. In children, additional energy intake is required to support growth and development.

Estimated energy requirement (EER) is the average dietary energy intake predicted to maintain energy balance in a healthy individual and takes into account age, gender, weight, stature, and level of physical activity (Table 55.1). The 2015–2020 **Dietary Guidelines for Americans** refer to the 2008 Physical Activity Guidelines for Americans. These guidelines recommend ≥60 min of moderate- or vigorous-intensity aerobic physical daily for children and adolescents. This activity should include vigorous intensity physical activity at least 3 days per week. In addition, as part of their ≥60 min of daily physical activity, children and adolescents are advised to incorporate muscle- and bone-strengthening activity for ≥3 days a week, to maintain a healthy weight

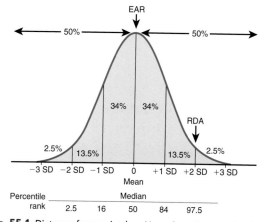

Fig. 55.1 Dietary reference intakes. Normal requirement distribution of hypothetical nutrient showing percentile rank and placement of the estimated average requirement (EAR) and the recommended dietary allowance (RDA) on the distribution; SD, standard deviation.

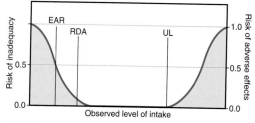

Fig. 55.2 Dietary reference intakes: the relationship among the estimated average requirement (EAR), the recommended dietary allowance (RDA), and the tolerable upper limit of intake (UL). This figure shows that the EAR is the intake at which the risk of inadequacy is estimated to be 0.5 (50%). The RDA is the intake at which the risk of inadequacy would be very small, only 0.02-0.03 (2–3%). At intakes between the RDA and the UL, the risk of inadequacy and of excess are estimated to be close to 0.0. At intakes above the UL, the potential risk of adverse effects can increase.

Table 55.1	Equations to Estimate Energy Requirement

INFANTS AND YOUNG CHILDREN: EER (kcal/day) = TEE + ED

0-3 mo	EER = (89 × weight [kg] − 100) + 175
4-6 mo	EER = (89 × weight [kg] − 100) + 56
7-12 mo	EER = (89 × weight [kg] − 100) + 22
13-36 mo	EER = (89 × weight [kg] − 100) + 20

CHILDREN AND ADOLESCENTS 3-18 YR: EER (kcal/day) = TEE + ED

Boys

3-8 yr	EER = 88.5 − (61.9 × age [yr] + PA × [(26.7 × weight [kg] + (903 × height [m])] + 20
9-18 yr	EER = 88.5 − (61.9 × age [yr] + PA × [(26.7 × weight [kg] + (903 × height [m])] + 25

Girls

3-8 yr	EER = 135.3 − (30.8 × age [yr] + PA [(10 × weight [kg] + (934 × height [m])] + 20
9-18 yr	EER = 135.3 − (30.8 × age [yr] + PA [(10 × weight [kg] + (934 × height [m])] + 25

EER, Estimated energy requirement; TEE, total energy expenditure; ED, energy deposition (energy required for growth /new tissue accretion).
PA indicates the physical activity coefficient:
For boys:
  PA = 1.00 (sedentary, estimated physical activity level 1.0-1.4)
  PA = 1.13 (low active, estimated physical activity level 1.4-1.6)
  PA = 1.26 (active, estimated physical activity level 1.6-1.9)
  PA = 1.42 (very active, estimated physical activity level 1.9-2.5)
For girls:
  PA = 1.00 (sedentary, estimated physical activity level 1.0-1.4)
  PA = 1.16 (low active, estimated physical activity level 1.4-1.6)
  PA = 1.31 (active, estimated physical activity level 1.6-1.9)
  PA = 1.56 (very active, estimated physical activity level 1.9-2.5)
Adapted from Kleinman RE, editor: *Pediatric nutrition handbook*, ed 7, Elk Grove Village, IL, 2013, American Academy of Pediatrics.

Table 55.2	Acceptable Macronutrient Distribution Ranges

AMDA (% OF ENERGY)		
Macronutrient	**Age 1-3 yr**	**Age 4-18 yr**
Fat	30-40	25-35
ω6 PUFAs (linoleic acid)	5-10	5-10
ω3 PUFAs (α-linolenic acid)	0.6-1.2	0.6-1.2
Carbohydrate	45-65	45-65
Protein	5-20	10-30

PUFAs, Polyunsaturated fatty acids.
Adapted from Otten JJ, Hellwig JP, Meyers LD, editors; Institute of Medicine: *Dietary reference intakes: the essential guide to nutrient requirements*, Washington, DC, 2006, National Academies Press.

| Table 55.3 | Dietary Reference Intakes: Macronutrients |

FUNCTION	LIFE STAGE GROUP	RDA OR AI* (g/day)	SELECTED FOOD SOURCES	ADVERSE EFFECTS OF EXCESSIVE CONSUMPTION
TOTAL DIGESTIBLE CARBOHYDRATE RDA based on its role as the primary energy source for the brain AMDR based on its role as a source of kcal to maintain body weight	*Infants* 0-6 mo 7-12 mo *Children* >1 yr *Pregnancy* ≤18 yr 19-30 yr	60* 95* 130 175 175	Major types: starches and sugars, grains, and vegetables (corn, pasta, rice, potatoes, and breads) are sources of starch. Natural sugars are found in fruits and juices. Sources of added sugars: soft drinks, candy, fruit drinks, desserts, syrups, and sweeteners[†]	No defined intake level for potential adverse effects of total digestible carbohydrate is identified, but the upper end of the AMDR was based on decreasing risk of chronic disease and providing adequate intake of other nutrients. It is suggested that the maximal intake of added sugars be limited to providing no more than 10% of energy.
TOTAL FIBER Improves laxation, reduces risk of coronary artery (heart) disease, assists in maintaining normal blood glucose levels	*Infants* 0-6 mo 7-12 mo *Children* 1-3 yr 4-8 yr *Males* 9-13 yr 14-18 yr 19-21 yr *Females* 9-13 yr 14-18 yr 19-21 yr *Pregnancy* ≤18 yr 19-21 yr	ND ND 190* 25* 31* 38* 38* 26* 26* 25* 28* 28*	Includes dietary fiber naturally present in grains (e.g., oats, wheat, unmilled rice) and functional fiber synthesized or isolated from plants or animals and shown to be of benefit to health	Dietary fiber can have variable compositions; therefore it is difficult to link a specific source of fiber with a particular adverse effect, especially when phytate is also present in the natural fiber source. As part of an overall healthy diet, a high intake of dietary fiber will not produce deleterious effects in healthy persons. Occasional adverse GI symptoms are observed when consuming some isolated or synthetic fibers, but serious chronic adverse effects have not been observed because of the bulky nature of fibers. Excess consumption is likely to be self-limiting; therefore, UL was not set for individual functional fibers.
TOTAL FAT Energy source When found in foods, is a source of ω3 and ω6 PUFAs Facilitates absorption of fat-soluble vitamins	*Infants* 0-6 mo 7-12 mo 1-18 yr	31* 30* Insufficient evidence to determine AI or EAR; see AMDR, Table 55.2.	*Infants:* Human milk or infant formula *Older children:* Butter, margarine, vegetable oils, whole milk, visible fat on meat and poultry products, invisible fat in fish, shellfish, some plant products such as seeds and nuts, bakery products	UL is not set because there is no defined intake of fat at which adverse effects occur. High fat intake will lead to obesity. Upper end of AMDR is also based on reducing risk of chronic disease and providing adequate intake of other nutrients.[†] Low fat intake (with high carbohydrate) has been shown to increase plasma triacylglycerol concentrations and decrease HDL cholesterol.
ω6 POLYUNSATURATED FATTY ACIDS Essential component of structural membrane lipids, involved with cell signaling Precursor of eicosanoids Required for normal skin function	*Infants* 0-6 mo 7-12 mo *Children* 1-3 yr 4-8 yr *Males* 9-13 yr 14-18 yr 19-21 yr *Females* 9-13 yr 14-18 yr 19-21 yr *Pregnancy* ≤18 yr 19-21 yr *Lactation* ≤18 yr 19-21 yr	4.4* 4.6* 7* 10* 12* 16* 17* 10* 11* 12* 13* 13* 13* 13*	Nuts, seeds; vegetable oils such as soybean, safflower, corn oil	There is no defined intake of ω6 level at which adverse effects occur. Upper end of AMDR is based on the lack of evidence that demonstrates long-term safety and human in vitro studies that show increased free radical formation and lipid peroxidation with higher amounts of ω6 fatty acids. Lipid peroxidation is thought to be a component of atherosclerotic plaques.

Continued

Table 55.3	Dietary Reference Intakes: Macronutrients—cont'd

FUNCTION	LIFE STAGE GROUP	RDA OR AI* (g/day)	SELECTED FOOD SOURCES	ADVERSE EFFECTS OF EXCESSIVE CONSUMPTION
ω3 POLYUNSATURATED FATTY ACIDS				
Involved with neurologic development and growth Precursor of eicosanoids	*Infants* 0-6 mo 7-12 mo *Children* 1-3 yr 4-8 yr *Males* 9-13 yr 14-18 yr 19-21 yr *Females* 9-13 yr 14-18 yr 19-21 yr *Pregnancy* ≤18 yr 19-21 yr *Lactation* ≤18 yr 19-21 yr	 0.5* 0.5* 0.7* 0.9* 1.2* 1.6* 1.6* 1.0* 1.1* 1.1* 1.4* 1.4* 1.3* 1.3*	Vegetable oils, e.g., soybean, canola, flax seed oil; fish oils, fatty fish, walnuts;[†] smaller amounts in meats and eggs	No defined intake levels for potential adverse effects of ω3 PUFAs are identified. Upper end of AMDR is based on maintaining appropriate balance with ω6 fatty acids and the lack of evidence that demonstrates long-term safety, along with human in vitro studies that show increased free radical formation and lipid peroxidation with higher amounts of PUFAs. Because the longer-chain *n-3* fatty acids, eicosapentaenoic acid (EPA) and docosahexaenoic acid (DHA), are biologically more potent than their precursor, linolenic acid, much of the work on adverse effects of this group of fatty acids has been on DHA and EPA. Lipid peroxidation is thought to be a component in the development of atherosclerotic plaques.
SATURATED AND *TRANS* FATTY ACIDS				
The body can synthesize its needs for saturated fatty acids from other sources.		No dietary requirement	Saturated fatty acids are present in animal fats (meat fats and butter fat), and coconut and palm kernel oils. *Trans* fat: stick margarines, foods containing hydrogenated or partially hydrogenated vegetable shortenings	There is an incremental increase in plasma total and LDL cholesterol concentrations with increased intake of saturated or *trans* fatty acids; therefore, saturated fat intake should be limited to <10% with no *trans* fat.[†‡]
CHOLESTEROL				
		No dietary requirement	Sources: liver, eggs, foods that contain eggs, e.g., cheesecake, custard pie	
PROTEIN AND AMINO ACIDS[‡]				
Major structural component of all cells in the body Functions as enzymes, in membranes, as transport carriers, and as some hormones During digestion and absorption, dietary protein is broken down to amino acids, which become the building blocks of these structural and functional compounds. Nine indispensable amino acids must be provided in the diet; the body can make the other amino acids needed to synthesize specific structures from other amino acids.	*Infants* 0-6 mo 7-12 mo *Children* 1-3 yr 4-8 yr *Males* 9-13 yr 14-18 yr ≥19 yr *Females* 9-13 yr ≥14 yr ≤18 yr 19-21 yr	 9.1* **11.0** **13** **19** **34** **52** **56** **34** **46** **71**	Proteins from animal sources, e.g., meat, poultry, fish, eggs, milk, cheese, yogurt, provide all 9 indispensable amino acids in adequate amounts and are considered "complete protein." Protein from plants, legumes, grains, nuts, seeds, and vegetables tend to be deficient in ≥1 of the indispensable amino acids and are called "incomplete protein." Vegan diets adequate in total protein content can be "complete" by combining sources of incomplete protein, which lack different indispensable amino acids.	No defined intake levels for potential adverse effects of protein are identified. Upper end of AMDR was based on complementing AMDR for carbohydrate and fat for the various age-groups. Lower end of AMDR is set at approximately the RDA.

Note: Starred (*) numbers are AI; **bold** numbers are RDA. RDAs and AIs may both be used as goals for individual intake. RDAs are set to meet the needs of 97-98% of members in a group. For healthy breastfed infants, the AI is the mean intake. The AI for other life stage and gender groups is believed to cover the needs of all members of the group, but lack of data prevents specifying with confidence the percentage covered by this intake.

AMDR is the range of intake for a particular energy source that is associated with reduced risk of chronic disease while providing intakes of essential nutrients. With consumption in excess of the AMDR, there is a potential for increasing the risk of chronic diseases and/or insufficient intakes of essential nutrients.

ND amounts are not determinable because of a lack of data regarding adverse effects in this age-group and concern with regard to a lack of ability to handle excess amounts. Source of intake should be from food only to prevent high levels of intake.

*Adequate intake.

[†]2015–2020 Dietary Guidelines for Americans. US Department of Health and Human Services. https://health.gov/dietaryguidelines/2015/.

[‡]Based on 1.5 g/kg/day for infants, 1.1 g/kg/day for 1-3 yr, 0.95 g/kg/day for 4-13 yr, 0.85 g/kg/day for 14-18 yr, 0.8 g/kg/day for adults, and 1.1 g/kg/day for pregnant (using pre-pregnancy weight) and lactating women.

AI, Adequate intake; AMDR, acceptable macronutrient distribution range; EAR, estimated average requirement; GI, gastrointestinal; HDL, high-density lipoprotein; LDL, low-density lipoprotein; ND, not determinable; PUFAs, polyunsaturated fatty acids; RDA, recommended dietary allowance; UL, upper limit of normal.

Adapted from Food and Nutrition Board, Institute of Medicine: *Dietary reference intakes for, energy, carbohydrate fiber, fat, fatty acids, cholesterol, protein, and amino acids.* https://www.nap.edu/read/10490/chapter/32.

and to prevent or delay progression of chronic noncommunicable diseases such as obesity and CV disease.

The EER was determined based on empirical research in healthy persons at different levels of physical activity, including levels different from recommended levels. They do not necessarily apply to children with acute or chronic diseases. EER is estimated by equations that account for *total energy expenditure* (TEE) and *energy deposition* (ED) for healthy growth. EERs for infants, relative to body weight, are approximately twice those for adults because of the increased metabolic rate and requirements for weight maintenance and tissue accretion (growth).

Dietary nutrients that provide energy include *fats* (approximately 9 kcal/g), *carbohydrates* (4 kcal/g), and *protein* (4 kcal/g). These nutrients are called **macronutrients**. If alcohol is consumed, it also contributes to energy intake (7 kcal/g). The EER does not specify the relative energy contributions of macronutrients. Once the minimal intake of each macronutrient is attained (e.g., sufficient protein intake to meet specific amino acid requirements, sufficient fat intake to meet linoleic acid and α-linolenic acid needs for brain development), the remainder of the intake is used to meet energy requirements, with some degree of freedom and interchangeability among fat, carbohydrate, and protein. This argument forms the basis for the **acceptable macronutrient distribution ranges (AMDRs)**, expressed as a function of total energy intake (Table 55.2).

FAT

Fat is the most calorically dense macronutrient, providing approximately 9 kcal/g. For infants, human milk and formula are the main dietary sources of fat, whereas older children obtain fat from animal products, vegetable oils, and margarine. The AMDR for fats is 30–40% of total energy intake for children 1-3 yr and 25–35% for children 4-18 yr of age. In addition to being energy dense, fats provide essential fatty acids that have body structural and functional roles (e.g., cholesterol moieties are precursors for cell membranes, hormones, and bile acids). Fat intake facilitates absorption of fat-soluble vitamins (vitamins A, D, E, and K). Both roles are relevant to neurologic and ocular development (Table 55.3).

Triglycerides are the most common form of dietary fat and are composed of 1 glycerol molecule with 3 fatty acids. Triglycerides are found in animal and vegetable fats. Simple sugars (i.e., refined grains and high sugar drinks) are converted to triglycerides in the liver. Elevated serum triglycerides are a risk factor for CV disease and metabolic syndrome. Decreasing simple sugars and increasing complex carbohydrate intake reduces serum triglyceride levels.

Dietary saturated fatty acids (found primarily in animal fat and dairy products), *trans* fats (found in hydrogenated margarines and oils), and **cholesterol** increase the low-density lipoprotein (LDL) fraction of serum cholesterol, which is a risk factor for the development of atherosclerosis (Fig. 55.3). Autopsy studies demonstrate that atherosclerosis begins early in childhood, even in infancy. Therefore, dietary advice to optimize CV health should be given starting from age 2 yr, when sufficient fat intake to sustain growth and brain development is less of a concern.

Because saturated and monounsaturated fats can be synthesized endogenously to support adequate structural and physiologic requirements, there is no AI or RDA set for these dietary components. *Trans* fats, a by-product of the hydrogenation of vegetables oils to form margarine, *have no known health benefits in humans. Trans* fats do not have an AI or RDA defined. In fact, *trans* fats behave like saturated fats. An UL has not been set for cholesterol, saturated, or *trans* fats because there is a continuous positive linear association between intake of these fats and increased risk for CV disease, without a threshold level. Diets low in saturated fats and cholesterol without *trans* fats are therefore preferred.

Efforts continue to reduce or eliminate *trans* fats from the diet. For optimal CV health in the general population, rather than limiting fat intake, advice should focus in most cases on changing the type of fat consumed. With respect to preventing obesity, all types of fatty acids have the same energy content and can contribute to increasing the risk for obesity. The current 2015–2020 Dietary Guidelines for Americans no longer restrict how much energy should come from fat intake, but

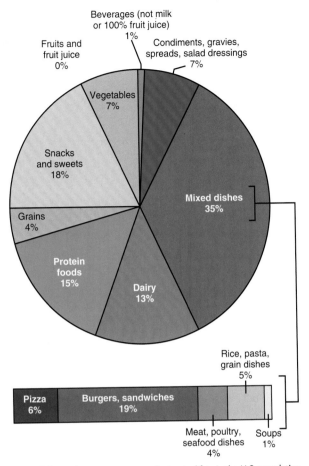

Saturated Fats

- Beverages (not milk or 100% fruit juice) 1%
- Fruits and fruit juice 0%
- Condiments, gravies, spreads, salad dressings 7%
- Vegetables 7%
- Snacks and sweets 18%
- Grains 4%
- Protein foods 15%
- Dairy 13%
- Mixed dishes 35%
- Rice, pasta, grain dishes 5%
- Pizza 6%
- Burgers, sandwiches 19%
- Meat, poultry, seafood dishes 4%
- Soups 1%

Fig. 55.3 Food category sources of saturated fats in the U.S. population age 2 yr and older. Estimates based on day 1 dietary recalls from WWEIA, National Health and Nutrition Examination Survey (NHANES), 2009–2010. *(From What We Eat in America (WWEIA) category analysis for the 2015 Dietary Guidelines Advisory Committee.* https://health .gov/dietaryguidelines/2015/guidelines/chapter-2/a-closer-look-at -current-intakes-and-recommended-shifts/#figure-2-12.)

continue to recommend that <10% of total daily calories come from saturated fat, with no *trans* fat intake. Furthermore, these guidelines do not specify limits on dietary cholesterol intake, because there is no clear strong evidence of the relationship between dietary and blood cholesterol.

Humans are incapable of synthesizing the precursor omega (ω) 3 (α-linolenic acid; ALA) and ω6 (linoleic acid; LA) PUFAs and depend on diet for these 2 essential fatty acids (EFAs). Safflower and sunflower oil are good sources of linoleic acid. Walnut and flaxseed oil are good sources of ALA. **Essential fatty acid deficiency** with LA is associated with desquamating skin rashes, alopecia, thrombocytopenia, impaired immunity, and growth deficits but is rare in the general population. EFAs are enzymatically elongated and desaturated into longer-chain fatty acids; ALA can be converted to eicosapentaenoic acid (EPA) and docosahexaenoic acid (DHA) ω3 PUFAs. LA is converted to arachidonic acid (ARA). Long-chain PUFAs such as DHA and ARA have a variety of cellular structural and functional roles; they influence membrane fluidity and function in gene expression and modulate the inflammatory response. ARA and DHA are present in breast milk, often supplemented in infant formulas, and are required for normal growth and development.

Table 55.4	Indispensable, Dispensable, and Conditionally Indispensable Amino Acids in the Human Diet			
INDISPENSABLE	**DISPENSABLE**	**CONDITIONALLY INDISPENSABLE***	**PRECURSORS OF CONDITIONALLY INDISPENSABLE**
Histidine†	Alanine	Arginine	Glutamine/glutamate, aspartate
Isoleucine	Aspartic acid	Cysteine	Methionine, serine
Leucine	Asparagine	Glutamine	Glutamic acid/ammonia
Lysine	Glutamic acid	Glycine	Serine, choline
Methionine	Serine	Proline	Glutamate
Phenylalanine		Tyrosine	Phenylalanine
Threonine			
Tryptophan			
Valine			

*Conditionally indispensable is defined as requiring a dietary source when endogenous synthesis cannot meet metabolic need.
†Although histidine is considered indispensable, unlike the other 8 indispensable amino acids, it does not fulfill the criteria of reducing protein deposition and inducing negative nitrogen balance promptly on removal from the diet.
Adapted from Otten JJ, Hellwig JP, Meyers LD, editors; Institute of Medicine: *Dietary reference intakes: the essential guide to nutrient requirements*, Washington, DC, 2006, National Academies Press.

DHA is present in the retina and is involved in the visual evoked response in infants.

The conversion of ALA to EPA and DHA and of LA to ARA is influenced by many factors, including type and amounts of dietary fats, and by enzymatic substrate affinity among competing ω3, ω6, ω9, saturated, and *trans* fatty acids. Approximately 0.5% of dietary ALA is converted to DHA, and 5% of ALA intake is converted to EPA; therefore, dietary intake of longer-chain PUFAs is an important determinant of serum and tissue long-chain PUFA status. The biologic activity and health benefits of ALA are thought to be derived from the longer-chain PUFA products EPA and DHA. Consistent with these findings of limited conversion of ALA to EPA and DHA, and that EPA and DHA appear to confer the biologic role and health benefits, the dietary reference intake (DRI) stipulates that up to 10% of the AI for ω3 PUFA (ALA being the major dietary constituent) can be replaced by DHA and EPA to support normal neural development and growth.

The ratio of dietary intake of each type of PUFA influences their relative amounts in different tissue compartments. A dietary ω6:ω3 PUFA ratio of 4-5:1 may be beneficial in reducing risk of disease and may be associated with improved health outcomes, compared with the current 15-30:1 ratio observed in U.S. diets.

PROTEIN
Protein and amino acids have structural and functional roles in every cell in the body. Dietary protein intake is required to replenish the turnover of protein and to meet amino acid needs for growth. Dietary protein also provides approximately 4 kcal/g as an energy substrate when intake is in excess of needs, or during periods of catabolism. Inadequate energy intake or inadequate protein intake increases catabolism of body protein reservoirs (i.e., lean body mass) for energy and free amino acids required to support normal physiologic function. Nitrogen from protein turnover is excreted in urine, stool, and other bodily excretions. Increased protein intake may be required for rare hypermetabolic states, such as extensive burn injury. Protein-energy malnutrition, although relatively rare in the noninstitutionalized U.S. population, is more common in the developing world. Protein-energy malnutrition impairs brain, immune system, and intestinal mucosal functions (see Chapter 59).

The DRI for protein is provided in Table 55.3. According to the 2015–2020 Dietary Guidelines for Americans, the average intake of protein from poultry, meat, eggs, nuts, seeds, and soy products are close to the recommended amounts for all ages. Protein intake is higher than recommended amounts in adolescent males (mostly from meats, poultry, and eggs). Intake of seafood protein is low across all age and sex groups. An UL for protein has not been set. Some athletes may have increased protein needs, of approximately 2 g/kg/day, to prevent loss of fat-free mass or lean body mass. Certain conditions may require a modest increase in protein intake, including conditions with high protein turnover, inflammatory conditions, or postsurgical states, as well as

with cystic fibrosis, critical illnesses, burn injuries, compensated liver disease, and bariatric surgery (e.g., laparoscopic sleeve gastrectomy and Roux-en-Y gastric bypass). Intake of protein or specific amino acids needs to be limited in some health conditions, such as renal disease and decompensated liver disease, and metabolic diseases such as phenylketonuria and maple syrup urine disease, in which specific amino acids can be toxic.

The amino acid content of dietary protein is also important. Certain amino acids are **indispensable**, and humans depend on dietary sources to meet adequacy and prevent deficiency. Certain amino acids are termed **conditional essential/indispensable**, meaning they become essential in patients affected by some diseases or during a certain life stage, such as with cysteine, tyrosine, and arginine in newborns because of enzyme immaturity (Table 55.4). Human milk contains both the indispensable and conditionally indispensable amino acids and therefore meets the protein requirements for infants. Breast milk is considered the optimal protein source for infants and is the reference amino acid composition by which biologic quality is determined for infants. If a single amino acid in a food protein source is low or absent but is required to support normal metabolism, that specific amino acid becomes the limiting nutrient in that food. For soy-based infant formula, supplementing the formula with the limiting amino acid (methionine) is necessary. Certain amino acid–like substances, such as creatinine, are used by some athletes and may enhance performance. Such supplementation should be monitored for potential side effects.

To ensure appropriate growth and to promote satiety, children should consume the recommended amount of protein. Specific recommendations for appropriate dietary protein sources to meet indispensable amino acid requirements are available for groups adopting specific diets, such as vegetarians and vegans. Inclusion of legumes and corn, as well as the use of a variety of food sources to provide all of the required amino acids is a strategy advocated for vegetarians and vegans (see Chapter 56).

CARBOHYDRATES
Carbohydrates are abundant in many foods, including cereals, grains, fruits, and vegetables, and provide approximately 4 kcal/g. Dietary carbohydrates include *monosaccharides*, which contain 1 sugar molecule (glucose, fructose); *disaccharides*, which contain 2 sugar molecules (sucrose, lactose); *oligosaccharides* or *polysaccharides*, which contain multiple sugar molecules in a chain or complex configuration (e.g., starch); and *sugar alcohols*. **Glucose** serves as the essential energy source for erythrocytes and the central nervous system and a major energy source for all other cells. The requirements for carbohydrates are based on the average minimum amount of glucose utilized by the brain. Chronic low carbohydrate intake results in ketosis. Although an UL for carbohydrates has not been set, a maximal intake of <10% of total energy intake from added sugars has been proposed in the 2015–2020 Dietary Guidelines for Americans. Added sugars include syrups and other caloric sweeteners (Fig. 55.4). These added sugars do not contribute essential

nutrients and function to sweeten foods and beverages to which they are added. Naturally occurring sugars, such as in milk (lactose) or fruits, are not included. Higher intakes of added sugar can displace other macro- and micronutrients and increase risk for nutrient deficiency and excessive energy intake. There is no advantage or benefit from discretionary calorie intake such as consuming added sugars. In fact, the excess calories from added sugars may make it difficult to meet nutrient needs while remaining within recommended total calorie intake.

The recommended AMDR for carbohydrates is based on data suggesting a risk for coronary artery disease (CAD) with diets high in carbohydrates and low in fat (see Table 55.2). These diets, compared to diets with higher fat intake, result in high triglyceride levels, low high-density lipoprotein (HDL) cholesterol, and small LDL cholesterol particles, and are associated with a high risk of CAD, especially in sedentary overweight individuals. Diets within the AMDR for carbohydrates and fats minimize the risks of diabetes, obesity, and CAD. Diets with less than the minimum AMDR for carbohydrate most likely do not meet the AI for fiber (see Table 55.3).

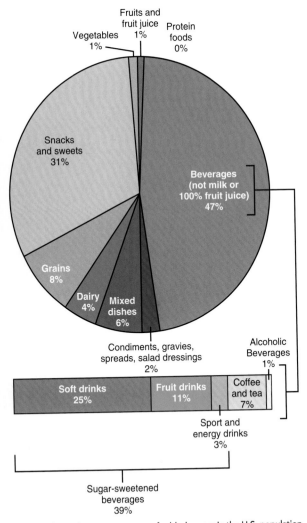

Added Sugars

Fig. 55.4 Food category sources of added sugars in the U.S. population age 2 yr and older. Estimates based on day 1 dietary recalls from WWEIA, NHANES, 2009–2010. (From *What We Eat in America (WWEIA) category analysis for the 2015 Dietary Guidelines Advisory Committee.* https://health.gov/dietaryguidelines/2015/guidelines/chapter-2/a-closer-look-at-current-intakes-and-recommended-shifts/#figure-2-10.)

Most carbohydrates are present as starches or sugars in food. Simple sugars (monosaccharides and disaccharides) are often added to foods and beverages during food preparation, processing, and packaging to enhance their palatability, as well as acting as preservatives. Nondiet soft drinks, juice drinks, iced tea, and sport drinks are among the major contributors to added sugars in the diet of U.S. children and adolescents. Added sugars increase the risk for obesity, diabetes, and dental caries. Fructose is one such added sugar in the form of high-fructose corn syrup, which is ubiquitous in the U.S. diet. Fructose increases HDL and triglyceride production in the liver and serum uric acid, which increases systolic blood pressure and is associated with nonalcoholic fatty liver disease and metabolic syndrome. Excessive fructose intake, such as in the form of fruit juices, is associated with diarrhea, abdominal pain, and failure to thrive in children.

The **glycemic index** is a measure of peak blood glucose concentration 2 hr after ingestion of a given food compared with a reference standard (slice of white bread). The glycemic index has predictable effects on blood glucose, hemoglobin A_{1c}, insulin, triglycerides, and HDL cholesterol. Lower–glycemic index foods are recommended and may reduce the risk of insulin resistance and CV disease (e.g., oat bran, muesli, barley carrots, nonstarchy vegetables, most fruits).

FIBER

Fiber consists of *nondigestible* carbohydrates mostly derived from plant sources, such as whole grains, fruits, and vegetables, that escape digestion and reach the colon almost 100% intact. These compounds were previously classified as being *water soluble* vs *insoluble*, which may be a less meaningful health distinction but still commonly used. The DRI classification lists **dietary fiber** (nondigestible carbohydrates and lignin that are intrinsic and intact in plants), **functional fiber** (fiber with known physiologic benefits in humans), and **total fiber** (dietary plus functional).

Although fiber intake does not contribute significantly to energy intake, it does have several important roles. The metabolic fate of fiber is influenced primarily by colonic bacteria, which render it susceptible to fermentation, depending on the structure of the fiber (e.g., pectin, oat bran). Common by-products of colonic fermentation include carbon dioxide, methane (in addition to other gases), **oligofructose** (also known as a *prebiotic*, a substrate that nourishes beneficial commensurate gastrointestinal microbiota), and **short-chain fatty acids (SCFAs)**. The common SCFAs produced by fermentation include acetate, butyrate, and propionate. There is dynamic interplay between the colonic bacterial milieu and the diet. SCFAs influence colonic physiology by stimulating colonic blood flow and fluid and electrolyte uptake. Butyrate is the preferred fuel for the colonocyte and may have a role in maintaining the normal phenotype in these cells.

Dietary fiber may have an important role in reducing dysplasia risk by diluting toxins, carcinogens, and tumor promoters; decreasing transit time, thereby decreasing colonic mucosal exposure; and promoting toxin expulsion in the fecal stream. Dietary fiber that is resistant to colonic degradation may also play a role in maintaining and promoting stool bulk and in regulating intraluminal pressure and colonic wall resistance, disordered colonic motility, or both. Lack of certain types of dietary fiber is associated with constipation and diverticulosis.

All types of dietary fiber slow gastric emptying and promote satiety, and thus may help to regulate appetite. Dietary fiber may decrease the rate of release and absorption of simple sugars and may help regulate blood sugar concentration, with lower postprandial level. Dietary fiber has a low glycemic index and may have a beneficial effect on insulin sensitivity. Fiber also binds luminal cholesterol and reduces absorption and enterohepatic circulation of the cholesterol in bile salts (with the intake of more viscous forms of dietary fiber, such as pectin). Guar gum, oat products, and pectin (previously categorized as soluble fiber) lower serum cholesterol, whereas insoluble fiber (e.g., flax, wheat bran) may reduce serum triglycerides. However, fiber such as psyllium, resistant dextrins, and resistant starch may lower both serum LDL cholesterol and triglycerides. The older classifications of the benefits of soluble vs insoluble fiber types are thus not always consistent. Decreased fiber intake

Text continued on p. 347

Table 55.5 Dietary Reference Intakes for Vitamins

NUTRIENT	FUNCTION	LIFE-STAGE GROUP	RDA OR AI	UL	SELECTED FOOD SOURCES	ADVERSE EFFECTS OF EXCESSIVE CONSUMPTION	SPECIAL CONSIDERATIONS
Biotin (vitamin B₇)	Coenzyme in synthesis of fat, glycogen, and amino acids	*Infants (µg/day)*			Liver	No adverse effects of biotin in humans or animals have been found; this does not mean there is no potential for adverse effects resulting from high intakes.	None
		0-6 mo	5*	ND	Smaller amounts in fruits and meats		
		7-12 mo	6*	ND			
		Children (µg/day)				Because data on the adverse effects of biotin are limited, caution may be warranted.	
		1-3 yr	8*	ND			
		4-8 yr	12*	ND			
		Males (µg/day)					
		9-13 yr	20*	ND			
		14-18 yr	25*	ND			
		19-21 yr	30*	ND			
		Females (µg/day)					
		9-13 yr	20*	ND			
		14-18 yr	25*	ND			
		19-21 yr	30*	ND			
		Pregnancy (µg/day)					
		≤18 yr	30*	ND			
		19-21 yr	30*	ND			
		Lactation (µg/day)					
		≤18 yr	35*	ND			
		19-21 yr	35*	ND			
Choline	Precursor for acetylcholine, phospholipids, and betaine	*Infants (mg/day)*			Milk, liver, eggs, peanuts	Fishy body odor, sweating, salivation, hypotension, hepatotoxicity	Patients with trimethylaminuria, renal disease, liver disease, depression, and Parkinson disease may be at risk for adverse effects with choline intakes at the UL.
		0-6 mo	125*	ND			
		7-12 mo	150*	ND			AIs have been set for choline, but there are little data to assess whether a dietary supply of choline is needed at all stages of the life cycle, and the choline requirement might be met by endogenous synthesis at some of these stages.
		Children (mg/day)					
		1-3 yr	200*	1,000			
		4-8 yr	250*	1,000			
		Males (mg/day)					
		9-13 yr	375*	2,000			
		14-18 yr	550*	3,000			
		19-21 yr	550*	3,500			
		Females (mg/day)					
		9-13 yr	375*	2,000			
		14-18 yr	400*	3,000			
		19-21 yr	425*	3,500			
		Pregnancy (mg/day)					
		≤18 yr	450*	3,000			
		19-21 yr	450*	3,500			
		Lactation (mg/day)					
		≤18 yr	550*	3,000			
		19-21 yr	550*	3,500			

Continued

Nutrient and Function	Life Stage Group	RDA/AI	UL	Selected Food Sources	Comments
Folate (folic acid, vitamin B_9, folacin); pteroyl-polyglutamates given as dietary folate equivalents (DFEs) Coenzyme in metabolism of nucleic and amino acids Prevents megaloblastic anemia 1 DFE = 1 μg food folate = 0.6 μg folate from fortified food, or as supplement consumed with food = 0.5 μg of supplement taken on empty stomach	*Infants (μg/day)* 0-6 mo 7-12 mo *Children (μg/day)* 1-3 yr 4-8 yr *Males (μg/day)* 9-13 yr 14-18 yr 19-21 yr *Females (μg/day)* 9-13 yr 14-18 yr 19-21 yr *Pregnancy (μg/day)* ≤18 yr 19-21 yr *Lactation (μg/day)* ≤18 yr 19-21 yr	65* 80* 150 200 300 400 400 300 400 400 600 600 500 500	ND ND 300 400 600 800 1,000 600 800 1,000 800 1,000 800 1,000	Enriched cereal, grains, dark leafy vegetables, enriched and whole-grain breads and bread products, fortified ready-to-eat cereals	Masks neurologic complications in people with vitamin B_{12} deficiency No adverse effects associated with folate from food or supplements have been reported; this does not mean that there is no potential for adverse effects resulting from high intakes. Because data on adverse effects of folate are limited, caution may be warranted. UL for folate applies to synthetic forms obtained from supplements and/or fortified foods. In view of evidence linking poor folate intake with neural tube defects, all women who can become pregnant should consume 400 μg/day from supplements or fortified foods in addition to intake of food folate from a varied diet.
Niacin (vitamin B_3) Includes nicotinic acid amide, nicotinic acid (pyridine-3 carboxylic acid), and derivatives that exhibit biologic activity of nicotinamide Coenzyme or cosubstrate in many biologic reduction and oxidation reactions, thus required for energy metabolism Given as niacin equivalents (NE) 1 mg niacin = 60 mg tryptophan Age 0-6 mo: preformed niacin (not NE).	*Infants (mg/day)* 0-6 mo 7-12 mo *Children (mg/day)* 1-3 yr 4-8 yr *Males (mg/day)* 9-13 yr 14-18 yr 19-21 yr *Females (mg/day)* 9-13 yr 14-18 yr 19-21 yr *Pregnancy (mg/day)* ≤18 yr 19-21 yr *Lactation (mg/day)* ≤18 yr 19-21 yr	2* 4* 6 8 12 16 16 12 14 14 18 18 17 17	ND ND 10 15 20 30 35 20 30 35 30 35 30 35	Meat, fish, poultry, enriched and whole-grain breads and bread products, fortified ready-to-eat cereals	No evidence of adverse effects from consuming naturally occurring niacin in food Adverse effects from niacin-containing supplements can include flushing and GI distress. UL for niacin applies to synthetic forms obtained from supplements, fortified food, or a combination of these. Extra niacin may be required by persons treated with hemodialysis or peritoneal dialysis or those with malabsorption syndrome.

Continued

Table 55.5 | Dietary Reference Intakes for Vitamins—cont'd

NUTRIENT	FUNCTION	LIFE-STAGE GROUP	RDA OR AI	UL	SELECTED FOOD SOURCES	ADVERSE EFFECTS OF EXCESSIVE CONSUMPTION	SPECIAL CONSIDERATIONS
Pantothenic acid (vitamin B$_5$)	Coenzyme in fatty acid metabolism	*Infants (mg/day)*			Chicken, beef, potatoes, oats, cereals, tomato products, liver, kidney, yeast, egg yolk, broccoli, whole grains	No adverse effects associated with pantothenic acid from food or supplements have been reported; this does not mean there is no potential for adverse effects resulting from high intakes. Because data on adverse effects of pantothenic acid are limited, caution may be warranted.	None
		0-6 mo	1.7*	ND			
		7-12 mo	1.8*	ND			
		Children (mg/day)					
		1-3 yr	2*	ND			
		4-8 yr	3*	ND			
		Males (mg/day)					
		9-13 yr	4*	ND			
		14-18 yr	5*	ND			
		19-21 yr	5*	ND			
		Females (mg/day)					
		9-13 yr	4*	ND			
		14-18 yr	5*	ND			
		19-21 yr	5*	ND			
		Pregnancy (mg/day)					
		≤18 yr	6*	ND			
		19-21 yr	6*	ND			
		Lactation (mg/day)					
		≤18 yr	7*	ND			
		19-21 yr	7*	ND			
Riboflavin (vitamin B$_2$)	Coenzyme in numerous redox reactions	*Infants (mg/day)*			Organ meats, milk, bread products, fortified cereals	No adverse effects associated with vitamin B$_2$ consumption from food or supplements have been reported; this does not mean there is no potential for adverse effects resulting from high intake. Because data on adverse effects of vitamin B$_2$ are limited, caution may be warranted.	None
		0-6 mo	0.3*	ND			
		7-12 mo	0.4*	ND			
		Children (mg/day)					
		1-3 yr	0.5	ND			
		4-8 yr	0.6	ND			
		Males (mg/day)					
		9-13 yr	0.9	ND			
		14-18 yr	1.3	ND			
		19-21 yr	1.3	ND			
		Females (mg/day)					
		9-13 yr	0.9	ND			
		14-18 yr	1.0	ND			
		19-21 yr	1.1	ND			
		Pregnancy (mg/day)					
		≤18 yr	1.4	ND			
		19-21 yr	1.4	ND			
		Lactation (mg/day)					
		≤18 yr	1.6	ND			
		19-21 yr	1.6	ND			

Continued

Nutrient and function	Life stage group	RDA/AI	UL	Food sources	Adverse effects of excessive consumption	Special considerations
Thiamin (vitamin B₁, aneurin) Coenzyme in metabolism of carbohydrates and branched-chain amino acids	*Infants (mg/day)* 0-6 mo / 7-12 mo	0.2* / 0.3*	ND / ND	Enriched, fortified, or whole-grain products, bread and bread products, mixed foods whose main ingredient is grain, ready-to-eat cereals	No adverse effects associated with vitamin B₁ consumption from food or supplements have been reported; this does not mean there is no potential for adverse effects resulting from high intake. Because data on adverse effects of vitamin B₁ are limited, caution may be warranted.	Persons who might have increased need for vitamin B₁ include those being treated with hemodialysis or persons with a malabsorption syndrome.
	Children (mg/day) 1-3 yr / 4-8 yr	0.5 / 0.6	ND / ND			
	Males (mg/day) 9-13 yr / 14-18 yr / 19-21 yr	0.9 / 1.2 / 1.2	ND / ND / ND			
	Females (mg/day) 9-13 yr / 14-18 yr / 19-21 yr	0.9 / 1.0 / 1.1	ND / ND / ND			
	Pregnancy (mg/day) ≤18 yr / 19-21 yr	1.4 / 1.4	ND / ND			
	Lactation (mg/day) ≤18 yr / 19-21 yr	1.4 / 1.4	ND / ND			
Vitamin A Includes provitamin A carotenoids that are dietary precursors of retinol. Given as retinol activity equivalents (RAEs) 1 RAE = 1 µg retinol, 12 µg β-carotene, 24 µg α-carotene, or 24 µg β-cryptoxanthin. To calculate RAEs from REs of provitamin A carotenoids in food, divide REs by 2. For preformed vitamin A in food or supplements and for provitamin A carotenoids in supplements, 1 RE = 1 RAE. Required for normal vision, gene expression, reproduction, embryonic development, and immune function	*Infants (µg/day)* 0-6 mo / 7-12 mo	400* / 500*	600 / 600	Liver, dairy products, fish, dark-colored fruit, leafy vegetable	Teratologic effects, liver toxicity (from preformed vitamin A only)	Persons with high alcohol intake, preexisting liver disease, hyperlipidemia, or severe protein malnutrition may be distinctly susceptible to the adverse effects of excess preformed vitamin A intake. β-Carotene supplements are advised only to serve as a provitamin A source for persons at risk for vitamin A deficiency.
	Children (µg/day) 1-3 yr / 4-8 yr	300 / 400	600 / 900			
	Males (µg/day) 9-13 yr / 14-18 yr / 19-21 yr	600 / 900 / 900	1,700 / 2,800 / 3,000			
	Females (µg/day) 9-13 yr / 14-18 yr / 19-21 yr	600 / 700 / 700	1,700 / 2,800 / 3,000			
	Pregnancy (µg/day) ≤18 yr / 19-21 yr	750 / 770	2,800 / 3,000			
	Lactation (µg/day) ≤18 yr / 19-21 yr	1,200 / 1,300	2,800 / 3,000			

Continued

Table 55.5 Dietary Reference Intakes for Vitamins—cont'd

NUTRIENT	FUNCTION	LIFE-STAGE GROUP	RDA OR AI	UL	SELECTED FOOD SOURCES	ADVERSE EFFECTS OF EXCESSIVE CONSUMPTION	SPECIAL CONSIDERATIONS
Pyridoxine (vitamin B_6) Comprises a group of 6 related compounds: pyridoxal, pyridoxine, pyridoxamine, and 5'-phosphates (PLP, PNP, PMP)	Coenzyme in metabolism of amino acids, glycogen, and sphingoid bases	*Infants (mg/day)*			Fortified cereals, organ meats, fortified soy-based meat substitutes	No adverse effects associated with vitamin B_6 from food have been reported; this does not mean there is no potential for adverse effects resulting from high intake. Because data on adverse effects of vitamin B_6 are limited, caution may be warranted. Sensory neuropathy has occurred from high intakes of supplemental forms.	None
		0-6 mo	0.1*	ND			
		7-12 mo	0.3*	ND			
		Children (mg/day)					
		1-3 yr	0.5	30			
		4-8 yr	0.6	40			
		Males (mg/day)					
		9-13 yr	1.0	60			
		14-18 yr	1.3	80			
		19-21 yr	1.3	100			
		Females (mg/day)					
		9-13 yr	1.0	60			
		14-18 yr	1.2	80			
		19-21 yr	1.3	100			
		Pregnancy (mg/day)					
		≤18 yr	1.9	80			
		19-21 yr	1.9	100			
		Lactation (mg/day)					
		≤18 yr	2.0	80			
		19-21 yr	2.0	100			
Cobalamin (vitamin B_{12})	Coenzyme in nucleic acid metabolism Prevents megaloblastic anemia	*Infants (µg/day)*			Fortified cereals, meat, fish, poultry	No adverse effects have been associated with consumption of the amounts of vitamin B_{12} normally found in food or supplements; this does not mean there is no potential for adverse effects resulting from high intake. Because data on adverse effects of vitamin B_{12} are limited, caution may be warranted.	Because 10–30% of older people malabsorb food-bound vitamin B_{12}, those >50 yr are advised to meet their RDA mainly by consuming foods fortified with vitamin B_{12} or a supplement containing vitamin B_{12}.
		0-6 mo	0.4*	ND			
		7-12 mo	0.5*	ND			
		Children (µg/day)					
		1-3 yr	0.9	ND			
		4-8 yr	1.2	ND			
		Males (µg/day)					
		9-13 yr	1.8	ND			
		14-18 yr	2.4	ND			
		19-21 yr	2.4	ND			
		Females (µg/day)					
		9-13 yr	1.8	ND			
		14-18 yr	2.4	ND			
		19-21 yr	2.4	ND			
		Pregnancy (µg/day)					
		≤18 yr	2.6	ND			
		19-21 yr	2.6	ND			
		Lactation (µg/day)					
		≤18 yr	2.8	ND			
		19-21 yr	2.8	ND			

Continued

Vitamin C (ascorbic acid, dehydroascorbic acid)

Cofactor for reactions requiring reduced copper or iron metalloenzyme and as a protective antioxidant

Life stage	RDA/AI (mg/day)	UL (mg/day)
Infants (mg/day)		
0-6 mo	40*	ND
7-12 mo	50*	ND
Children (mg/day)		
1-3 yr	15	400
4-8 yr	25	650
Males (mg/day)		
9-13 yr	45	1,200
14-18 yr	75	1,800
19-21 yr	90	2,000
Females (mg/day)		
9-13 yr	45	1,200
14-18 yr	65	1,800
19-21 yr	75	2,000
Pregnancy (mg/day)		
≤18 yr	80	1,800
19-21 yr	85	2,000
Lactation (mg/day)		
≤18 yr	115	1,800
19-21 yr	120	2,000

Sources: Citrus fruit, tomatoes, tomato juice, potatoes, Brussels sprouts, cauliflower, broccoli, strawberries, cabbage, spinach

Adverse effects: GI disturbances, kidney stones, excess iron absorption

Comments: Smokers require additional 35 mg/day of vitamin C over that needed by nonsmokers. Nonsmokers regularly exposed to tobacco smoke should ensure they meet the RDA for vitamin C.

Vitamin E (α-tocopherol)

α-Tocopherol includes RRR-α-tocopherol, the only form of α-tocopherol that occurs naturally in foods, and the 2R-stereoisomeric forms of α-tocopherol (RRR-, RSR-, RRS-, and RSS-α-tocopherol) that occur in fortified foods and supplements

It does not include the 2S-stereoisomeric forms of α-tocopherol (SRR-, SSR-, SRS-, and SSS-α-tocopherol), also found in fortified foods and supplements

A metabolic function has not yet been identified. Vitamin E's major function appears to be as a nonspecific chain-breaking antioxidant.

Life stage	RDA/AI (mg/day)	UL (mg/day)
Infants (mg/day)		
0-6 mo	4*	ND
7-12 mo	5*	ND
Children (mg/day)		
1-3 yr	6	200
4-8 yr	7	300
Males (mg/day)		
9-13 yr	11	600
14-18 yr	15	800
19-21 yr	15	1,000
Females (mg/day)		
9-13 yr	11	600
14-18 yr	15	800
19-21 yr	15	1,000
Pregnancy (mg/day)		
≤18 yr	15	800
19-21 yr	15	1,000
Lactation (mg/day)		
≤18 yr	19	800
19-21 yr	19	1,000

Sources: Vegetable oil, unprocessed cereal grains, nuts, fruit, vegetables, meat

Adverse effects: No evidence of adverse effects from consuming vitamin E naturally occurring in food. Adverse effects from vitamin E-containing supplements may include hemorrhagic toxicity. UL for vitamin E applies to any form of α-tocopherol obtained from supplements, fortified foods, or a combination of these.

Comments: Patients receiving anticoagulant therapy should be monitored when taking vitamin E supplements.

Continued

Table 55.5 Dietary Reference Intakes for Vitamins—cont'd

NUTRIENT	FUNCTION	LIFE-STAGE GROUP	RDA OR AI	UL	SELECTED FOOD SOURCES	ADVERSE EFFECTS OF EXCESSIVE CONSUMPTION	SPECIAL CONSIDERATIONS
Vitamin K	Coenzyme during synthesis of many proteins involved in blood clotting and bone metabolism	*Infants (µg/day)*			Green vegetables (collards, spinach, salad greens, broccoli), Brussels sprouts, cabbage, plant oil, margarine	No adverse effects associated with vitamin K consumption from food or supplements have been reported in humans or animals; this does not mean there is no potential for adverse effects resulting from high intake. Because data on adverse effects of vitamin K are limited, caution may be warranted.	Patients receiving anticoagulant therapy should monitor vitamin K intake.
		0-6 mo	2.0*	ND			
		7-12 mo	2.5*	ND			
		Children (µg/day)					
		1-3 yr	30*	ND			
		4-8 yr	55*	ND			
		Males (µg/day)					
		9-13 yr	60*	ND			
		14-18 yr	75*	ND			
		19-21 yr	120*	ND			
		Females (µg/day)					
		9-13 yr	60*	ND			
		14-18 yr	75*	ND			
		19-21 yr	90*	ND			
		Pregnancy (µg/day)					
		≤18 yr	75*	ND			
		19-21 yr	90*	ND			
		Lactation (µg/day)					
		≤18 yr	75*	ND			
		19-21 yr	90*	ND			

Note: Starred (*) numbers are AI, and **bold** numbers are RDA. RDAs and AIs may both be used as goals for individual intake. RDAs are set to meet the needs of 97–98% of members in a group. For healthy breastfed infants, the AI is the mean intake. The AI for other life stage and gender groups is believed to cover the needs of all members of the group, but lack of data prevents specifying with confidence the percentage covered by this intake.

UL is the maximum level of daily nutrient intake that is likely to pose no risk of adverse effects. Unless otherwise specified, the UL represents total intake from food, water, and supplements. Because of a lack of suitable data, ULs could not be established for potassium, water, or inorganic sulfate. In the absence of ULs, extra caution may be warranted in consuming levels above recommended intakes.

ND amounts are not determinable because of a lack of data of adverse effects in this age-group and concern with regard to lack of ability to handle excess amounts. Source of intake should be from food only to prevent high levels of intake.

*Adequate intake. *RDA for vitamin D in IU/day: 400 if <1 yr age, 600 if >1 yr, lactating, or pregnant.

AI, Adequate intake; GI, gastrointestinal; ND, not determinable; PLP, pyridoxal phosphate; PMP, pyridoxamine phosphate; PNP, pyridoxine phosphate; RDA, recommended dietary allowance; UL, upper limit of normal.

Data from Dietary reference intakes for calcium, phosphorus, magnesium, vitamin D, and fluoride, 1997; Dietary reference intakes for thiamin, riboflavin, niacin, vitamin B₆, folate, vitamin B₁₂, pantothenic acid, biotin, and choline, 1998; Dietary reference intakes for vitamin C, vitamin E, selenium, and carotenoids, 2000; Dietary reference intakes for vitamin A, vitamin K, arsenic, boron, chromium, copper, iodine, iron, manganese, molybdenum, nickel, silicon, vanadium, and zinc, 2001; Dietary reference intakes for energy, carbohydrate, fiber, fat, fatty acids, cholesterol, protein, and amino acids, 2002/2005; Dietary reference intakes for calcium and vitamin D, 2011. These reports may be accessed via www.nap.edu. Accessed on January 18, 2017.

in Western society has been associated with the increasing incidence and prevalence of diabetes, obesity, CV disease, colon cancer, and IBD.

Data are insufficient to establish an EAR for dietary fiber. AI for dietary fiber has been established based on the intake levels associated with reducing risk for CV disease and in lowering or normalizing serum cholesterol (see Table 55.3). A UL has not been established for fiber, which is not thought to be harmful to human health. Several recommendations address dietary fiber intake in children based on body weight or as a proportion of daily calories consumed. The prevailing approach, however, is based on expert consensus and uses a rule of thumb guided by safety considerations, with improved laxation and reduced risk of future chronic diseases as goals. The equation for fiber intake in children follows:

Range of grams of fiber per day = Age [yr] + 5 to Age [yr] + 10.

It is noteworthy that the recommendation does not specify type of fiber, and it predates the newer definition of fiber. Difficulties in making better recommendations for fiber intake goals in children include the lack of consensus on defining fiber and inadequate randomized double-blinded placebo-controlled trials with well-defined, clinically meaningful end-points.

Certain types of fiber intake are associated with increased risk for gastrointestinal (GI) symptoms along the functional abdominal pain, functional GI disorders, and IBD spectrum. Some fiber types may exert symptoms on the basis of their digestibility, by-product formation, and interactions with GI microbiota. Restriction of **fermentable** (i.e., to produce methane, CO_2, and hydrogen) **oligosaccharides** (e.g., fructooligosaccharides such as onions), **disaccharides** (e.g., lactose), **monosaccharides** (e.g., fructose), **and polyols** (e.g., sorbitol) (**FODMAP**) or substitution with lower-FODMAP foods may be beneficial. Substitutions within the same food groups can shift from a high-FODMAP diet to a low-FODMAP diet, which may provide GI symptom relief. For example, substituting cucumber for celery would be exchanging a high-FODMAP food for a low-FODMAP food.

Lastly, dietary management in certain diseases may put such children at risk of low fiber intake. For example, children with celiac disease are advised gluten-free diets. As such, these children are at risk of inadequate fiber intake, for which alternative, gluten-free sources of fiber should be recommended, such as tapioca, flax, corn, rice, sorghum, and quinoa.

MICRONUTRIENTS

(See Chapters 61-67.)

Vitamins and trace minerals, the dietary **micronutrients**, are essential for growth and development and contribute to a host of physiologic functions. Many U.S. children have suboptimal intake of iron, zinc, potassium, calcium, vitamin D, and vitamin K, and excess intake of sodium. Dietary recommendations for micronutrients were originally established to prevent deficiency and currently also include the impact of micronutrients on long-term health outcomes (Table 55.5). Food fortification is an effective strategy to prevent some nutrient deficiencies and has been successfully implemented to prevent iodine and folate deficiency.

Breast milk provides optimal intake of most nutrients, including iron and zinc. Although present in lower amounts compared with infant formula, iron and zinc are more bioavailable and are sufficient to meet infant needs until approximately 4-6 mo of age. After 4-6 mo, iron and zinc are required from complementary foods, such as iron-fortified cereal and pureed meats.

Iron

Iron requirements are relatively higher during infancy and childhood than later in life and are higher for menstruating females than for males of similar age-groups (see Chapter 67). Iron present in animal protein is more bioavailable than that found in vegetables and other foods because it is already incorporated into heme moieties in blood and muscle. **Iron deficiency** is the most common micronutrient deficiency in the world and is associated with iron-deficiency anemia and neurocognitive deficits in some children. **Zinc deficiency** affects millions of children and is associated with increased risk for impaired linear growth

(stunting), impaired immune function, and increased risk for respiratory and diarrheal diseases.

Vitamin D

Breast milk is a poor source of vitamin D. Vitamin D insufficiency is more common than previously thought in infants and children. Vitamin D is central to calcium and bone metabolism but is also an important determinant of various nonosseous health outcomes (see Chapter 64). Children of all ages with darker skin and those who do not consume fortified dairy products should be screened for vitamin D deficiency. The DRI for vitamin D is based on its effects on calcium status and bone health. The goal is to achieve serum 25-hydroxyvitamin D levels >50 nmol/L (30 ng/dL). The American Academy of Pediatrics (AAP) recommends total vitamin D intake of 400 IU/day for infants and children. A supplement is recommended for all breastfed infants to ensure sufficient intake. In 2010, IOM increased the RDA of vitamin D to 600 units daily for healthy children 1-18 yr of age.

Calcium

Calcium is key to bone health. Adequacy is determined in part by bone mineral content and bone mineral density (BMD). The main storage organs for calcium are the bones and teeth. Bone mineral accretion occurs primarily during childhood, with peak bone mass being achieved by the 2nd to 3rd decade of life. Calcium recommendations vary by age and were updated in 2011. These changes include a change from an AI to RDA, in terms of strength of evidence for recommendations, and increased UL in 9-18 yr olds (Table 55.6). There are no adequate biomarkers to assess calcium status in healthy children, because serum calcium is tightly regulated (regardless of intake and total body calcium) by changes in parathyroid hormone and calcitriol levels. Maintaining adequate serum calcium level despite inadequate intake could come at the expense of BMD. Therefore, in the long term, reduced BMD could serve as a surrogate marker of calcium intake and status. It is important to note that other variables influence BMD. Assessments of calcium status should include calcium intake in the diet. It is also important to educate families on additional and alternative sources of calcium (including calcium supplementation) if calcium intake is determined to be low.

Vitamin K

Vitamin K is an important determinant of bone health and an important cofactor for coagulation factors (factors II, VII, IX, and X; protein C and S) (see Chapter 66).

Electrolytes

Potassium (K^+) and sodium (Na^+) are the main intra- and extracellular cations, respectively, and are involved in transport of fluids and nutrients across the cellular membrane. The AI for **potassium** is related to its effects in maintaining a healthy blood pressure, reducing risk for nephrolithiasis, and supporting bone health. Moderate potassium deficiency occurs even in the absence of hypokalemia and can result in increased blood pressure, stroke, and other CV disease.

Most American children have potassium intake below the current recommendations, and blacks have lower potassium intake than whites. For people at increased risk of hypertension and who are salt sensitive, reducing sodium intake and increasing potassium intake is advised. Leafy green vegetables, vine fruit (e.g., tomatoes, eggplant, zucchini, pumpkin) and root vegetables (e.g., yams, beets) are good sources of potassium (see Table 55.6).

People with impaired renal function may need to reduce potassium intake, because hyperkalemia can increase risk for fatal cardiac arrhythmias among these patients.

Most dietary **sodium** (as sodium chloride, or table salt) in the United States is found in processed foods, breads, and condiments (Fig. 55.5). Sodium salt is added to foods to serve as a food preservative and enhance palatability. Sodium has an AI, but given the risk of table salt–related hypertension, an UL has also been set. The UL threshold may be even lower in blacks, who on average are more sodium salt sensitive, and for those with hypertension or preexisting renal disease. Dietary sodium

Table 55.6 Dietary Reference Intakes for Select Micronutrients and Water

NUTRIENT	FUNCTION	LIFE-STAGE GROUP	AI (mg/day)	UL (mg/day)	SELECTED FOOD SOURCES	ADVERSE EFFECTS OF EXCESSIVE CONSUMPTION	SPECIAL CONSIDERATIONS
Sodium	Maintains fluid volume outside of cells and thus normal cell function	*Infants*			Processed foods with added sodium chloride (salt), benzoate, phosphate; salted meats, bread, nuts, cold cuts; margarine; butter; salt added to foods in cooking or at the table. Salt is about 40% sodium by weight.	Hypertension Increased risk of cardiovascular disease and stroke	AI is set based on ability to obtain a nutritionally adequate diet for other nutrients and to meet the needs for sweat losses for persons engaged in recommended levels of physical activity. Persons engaged in activity at higher levels or in humid climates resulting in excessive sweat might need more than the AI. UL applies to apparently healthy persons without hypertension; it thus may be too high for persons who already have hypertension or who are under the care of a health professional.
		0–6 mo	120	ND			
		7–12 mo	370	ND			
		Children					
		1–3 yr	1,000	1,500			
		4–8 yr	1,200	1,900			
		Males					
		9–13 yr	1,500	2,200			
		14–21 yr	1,500	2,300			
		Females					
		9–13 yr	1,500	2,200			
		13–21 yr	1,500	2,300			
		Pregnancy and Lactation					
		≥14 yr	1,500	2,300			
Chloride	With sodium, maintains fluid volume outside of cells and thus normal cell function	*Infants*			Processed foods with added sodium chloride (salt), benzoate, phosphate; salted meats, nuts, cold cuts; margarine; butter; salt added to foods in cooking or at the table. Salt is about 60% chloride by weight.	In concert with sodium, results in hypertension	Chloride is lost, usually with sodium, in sweat, as well as in vomiting and diarrhea. AI and UL are equimolar in amount to sodium because most of sodium in diet comes as sodium chloride (salt).
		0–6 mo	180	ND			
		7–12 mo	570	ND			
		Children					
		1–3 yr	1,500	2,300			
		4–8 yr	1,900	2,900			
		Males					
		9–13 yr	2,300	3,400			
		14–21 yr	2,300	3,600			
		Females					
		9–13 yr	2,300	3,400			
		13–21 yr	2,300	3,600			
		Pregnancy and Lactation					
		≥14 yr	2,300	3,600			
Potassium	Maintains fluid volume inside/outside of cells and thus normal cell function; acts to blunt the rise of blood pressure in response to excess sodium intake, and decrease markers of bone turnover and recurrence of kidney stones	*Infants*			Fruits and vegetables, dried peas, dairy products, meats, nuts	None documented from food alone, but potassium from supplements or salt substitutes can result in hyperkalemia and possibly sudden death if excess is consumed by persons with chronic renal insufficiency (kidney disease) or diabetes.	Persons taking drugs for cardiovascular disease such as ACE inhibitors, ARBs, or potassium-sparing diuretics should be careful not to consume supplements containing potassium and might need to consume less than the AI.
		0–6 mo	400	None set			
		7–12 mo	700	No UL			
		Children					
		1–3 yr	3,000				
		4–8 yr	3,800				
		Males					
		9–13 yr	4,500				
		14–21 yr	4,700				
		Females					
		9–13 yr	4,500				
		13–21 yr	4,700				
		Pregnancy					
		≥14 yr	4,700				
		Lactation					
		≥14 yr	5,100				

Continued

Nutrient	Function	Life Stage		RDA/AI	UL	Food Sources	Adverse Effects of Excessive Consumption	Comments
Vitamin D (calciferol) 1 μg calciferol = 40 IU vitamin D. DRI values are based on absence of adequate exposure to sunlight.	Maintains serum calcium and phosphorus concentrations	Infants (μg/day)*	0-6 mo	10	25	Fish liver oils, flesh of fatty fish, liver and fat from seals and polar bears, eggs from hens that have been fed vitamin D, fortified milk products, fortified cereals	Elevated plasma 25(OH)D concentration causing hypercalcemia	Patients receiving glucocorticoid therapy might require additional vitamin D.
			7-12 mo	10	38			
		Children (μg/day)*	1-3 yr	15	63			
			4-8 yr	15	75			
		Males (μg/day)*	9-21 yr	15	100			
		Females (μg/day)*	9-21 yr	15	100			
		Pregnancy (μg/day)*	≤18 yr	15	100			
			19-21 yr	15	100			
		Lactation (μg/day)	≤18 yr	15	100			
			19-21 yr	15	100			
Calcium	Essential role in blood clotting, muscle contraction, nerve transmission, and bone and tooth formation	Infants	0-6 mo	200	1,000	Milk, cheese, yogurt, corn tortillas, calcium-set tofu, Chinese cabbage, kale, broccoli	Kidney stones, hypercalcemia, milk alkali syndrome, renal insufficiency	Amenorrheic women (exercise or anorexia nervosa induced) have reduced net calcium absorption.
			7-12 mo	260	1,500			
		Children	1-3 yr	700	2,500			
			4-8 yr	1,000	2,500			
		Males	9-18 yr	1,300	3,000			
			19-21 yr	1,000	2,500			
		Females	9-18 yr	1,300	3,000			
		Pregnancy	≤18 yr	1,300	3,000			
			19-21 yr	1,000	2,500			
		Lactation	≤18 yr	1,300	3,000			
			19-21 yr	1,000	2,500			
Iron	Critical component of enzymes, cytochromes, myoglobin, and hemoglobin	Infants	0-6 mo	0.27	40	Heme sources: meat, poultry, fish. Nonheme sources: dairy, eggs, plant-based foods, breads, cereals, breakfast foods	GI distress	Persons with decreased gastric acidity may be at increased risk for deficiency. Cow's milk is a poor source of bioavailable iron and is not recommended for children <1 yr old. Neurocognitive deficits have been reported in infants with iron deficiency. RDA for females increases with menarche related to increased losses during menstruation. Vegans and vegetarians might require iron supplementation or intake of iron-fortified foods. GI parasites can increase iron losses via GI bleeds. Iron supplements can interfere with zinc absorption, and vice versa; if supplements are being used, the doses should be staggered.
			7-12 mo	11	40			
		Children	1-3 yr	7	40			
			4-8 yr	10	40			
		Males	9-13 yr	8	40			
			14-18 yr	11	45			
			19-21 yr	8	45			
		Females	9-13 yr	8	40			
			14-18 yr	15	45			
			19-21 yr	18	45			
		Pregnancy	≤18 yr	27	45			
			19-21 yr	27	45			
		Lactation	≤18 yr	10	45			
			19-21 yr	9	45			

Continued

Table 55.6 | Dietary Reference Intakes for Select Micronutrients and Water—cont'd

NUTRIENT	FUNCTION	LIFE-STAGE GROUP	AI (mg/day)	UL (mg/day)	SELECTED FOOD SOURCES	ADVERSE EFFECTS OF EXCESSIVE CONSUMPTION	SPECIAL CONSIDERATIONS
Zinc	Essential for proper growth and development; important catalyst for 100 specific enzymes	Infants			Meats, shellfish, legumes, fortified cereals, whole grains	Acutely, zinc supplements cause GI irritation and headache; chronic effects of zinc supplementation include impaired immune function, changes in lipoprotein and cholesterol levels, and reduced copper status.	Zinc supplements interfere with iron absorption, and vice versa; therefore, if supplements are being used, the doses should be staggered. Zinc deficiency can be associated with stunting or impaired linear growth.
		0-6 mo	2	4			
		7-12 mo	3	5			
		Children					
		1-3 yr	3	7			
		4-8 yr	5	12			
		Males					
		9-13 yr	8	23			
		14-18 yr	11	34			
		19-21 yr	11	40			
		Females					
		9-13 yr	8	23			
		14-18 yr	9	34			
		19-21 yr	8	40			
		Pregnancy					
		≤18 yr	12	34			
		19-21 yr	11	40			
		Lactation					
		≤18 yr	13	34			
		19-21 yr	12	40			
Water	Maintains homeostasis in the body Allows transport of nutrients to cells and removal and excretion of waste products of metabolism	Infants (L/day)		None set	All beverages, including water Moisture in foods High-moisture foods include watermelon, meats, and soups	No UL because normally functioning kidneys can handle >0.7 L (24 oz) of fluid per hour Symptoms of water intoxication include hyponatremia, which can result in heart failure, and rhabdomyolysis (skeletal muscle tissue injury), which can lead to kidney failure.	Recommended intakes for water are based on median intakes of generally healthy persons who are adequately hydrated. Persons can be adequately hydrated at levels above or below the AIs provided; AIs provided are for total water in temperate climates. All sources can contribute to total water needs: beverages (tea, coffee, juice, soda, drinking water) and moisture found in foods. Moisture in food accounts for about 20% of total water intake. Thirst and consumption of beverages at meals are adequate to maintain hydration.
		0-6 mo	0.7				
		7-12 mo	0.8				
		Children					
		1-3 yr	1.3				
		4-8 yr	1.7				
		Males (L/day)					
		9-13 yr	2.4				
		14-18 yr	3.3				
		≥19 yr	3.7				
		Females (L/day)					
		9-13 yr	2.1				
		14-18 yr	2.3				
		≥19 yr	2.7				
		Pregnancy (L/day)					
		≥14 yr	3.0				
		Lactation (L/day)					
		≥14 yr	3.8				

Note: **Bold** numbers are RDA. RDAs and AIs may both be used as goals for individual intake. RDAs are set to meet the needs of 97–98% of members in a group. For healthy breastfed infants, the AI is the mean intake. The AI for other life stage and gender groups is believed to cover the needs of all members of the group, but lack of data prevents specifying with confidence the percentage covered by this intake. UL is the maximum level of daily nutrient intake that is likely to pose no risk of adverse effects. Unless otherwise specified, the UL represents total intake from food, water, and supplements. Because of a lack of suitable data, ULs could not be established for potassium, water, or inorganic sulfate. In the absence of ULs, extra caution may be warranted in consuming levels above recommended intakes. ND amounts are not determinable because of a lack of data on adverse effects in this age-group and concern with regard to lack of ability to handle excess amounts. Source of intake should be from food only to prevent high levels of intake.

*Vitamin D RDA in IU/day: 40 if <1 yr, 600 if >1 yr of age or pregnant or lactating.

ACE, Angiotensin-converting enzyme; AI, adequate intake; ARB, angiotensin receptor blocker; GI, gastrointestinal; ND, not determinable; RDA, recommended dietary allowance; UL, upper limit of normal.

Adapted from Food and Nutrition Board, US Institute of Medicine: Dietary reference intakes for water, potassium, sodium, chloride, and sulfate (website). http://www.nap.edu/openbook.php?record_id=10925; and Ross AC, US Institute of Medicine, Committee to Review Dietary Reference Intakes for Vitamin D and Calcium: Dietary reference intakes: calcium, vitamin D, Washington, DC, 2011, National Academies Press, pp xv, 536.

intake also displaces potassium intake. Elevated sodium:potassium ratios can increase the risk for nephrolithiasis. Intakes of <2,300 mg (approximately 1 tsp) per day are recommended. The average daily salt intake for most people in the United States and Canada exceeds both the AI and UL. For populations with or at risk for hypertension and renal disease, *sodium intake should be decreased to <1,500 mg/day and potassium*

intake increased to >4,700 mg/day. For persons with hypertension, additional dietary guidelines are available from the Dietary Approaches to Stop Hypertension (DASH) eating plan.

WATER

The daily water requirement and water content as a proportion of body weight are highest in infants and decrease with age. Water intake is achieved with liquid and food intake, and losses include excretion in the urine and stool as well as insensible and evaporative losses through the skin and respiratory tract. An AI has been established for water (see Table 55.6). Special considerations are required by life stages and by BMR, physical activity, body proportions (surface area to volume), environment, and underlying medical conditions. Breast milk and infant formula provide adequate water, and additional water or other fluid intake is not required until complementary foods are introduced. Water contains no calories; the concern is that water intake will decrease breast milk intake and displace the intake of essential nutrients during this phase of rapid rate of growth and metabolically very active life stage. The relatively higher fluid needs of infants and young children can be explained in part by the high ratio of body surface area to volume in infancy, high respiratory rate, and period of rapid growth.

The consequences of inadequate fluid intake include impaired thermoregulation and heat dissipation, reduced activity tolerance and performance, and reduced intravascular fluid and dehydration. This inadequate fluid intake may be reflected by decreased urine input. These deficits can result in an increased compensatory heart rate, hypotension, and syncope, and if uncorrected, renal injury or nephrolithiasis. "Free water" is defined as water in the body that can be removed by ultrafiltration and in which substances can be dissolved. Excess free water intake is usually better tolerated by healthy adults than by younger children, who are at increased risk for **water intoxication**. Hyponatremia can result from excess free water intake coupled with inadequate sodium intake. Fluid intake requirements and restrictions are also influenced by any underlying renal and hormonal disorders, including diabetes, the syndrome of inappropriate antidiuretic hormone secretion, and diabetes insipidus.

MEASURING NUTRITIONAL ADEQUACY

The U.S. Centers for Disease Control and Prevention (CDC) and AAP recommend the use of the WHO charts to monitor growth of all infants and children (breastfed and bottle-fed or infant formula–fed) from birth to 2 yr, and the use of the CDC 2000 growth charts for children 2-20 yr (see Chapters 18 and 27). The WHO growth charts are derived from longitudinal and cross-sectional data obtained from a sample of healthy breastfed infants and children (0-5 yr) who were receiving adequate nutritional intake and medical care in Brazil, Ghana, India, Norway, Oman, and the United States. Consequently, the WHO growth charts are not only descriptive of population average and distribution, but also describe growth of adequately nourished healthy children under best-care practices.

In the clinical setting, the 2.3rd and 97.7th percentiles on the WHO growth charts are used to identify *insufficient* and *excessive* growth from birth to 2 yr, respectively. In contrast, the 5th and 95th percentiles are

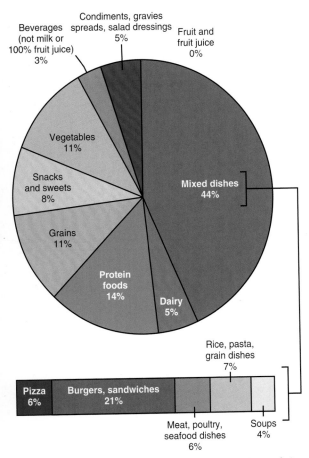

Sodium

Fig. 55.5 Food category sources of sodium in the U.S. population age 2 yr and older. Estimates based on day 1 dietary recalls from WWEIA, NHANES, 2009–2010. *(From What We Eat in America (WWEIA) category analysis for the 2015 Dietary Guidelines Advisory Committee. https://health.gov/dietaryguidelines/2015/guidelines/chapter-2/a-closer -look-at-current-intakes-and-recommended-shifts/#figure-2-14.)*

Table 55.7	Growth Chart Comparisons for Measuring Growth from Birth to 20 Years				
GROWTH CHART	**AGE RANGE**	**GROWTH METRICS**	**INSUFFICIENT GROWTH PERCENTILE**	**EXCESSIVE GROWTH PERCENTILE**	**BMI STATUS PERCENTILE**
World Health Organization, 2006	Birth to 2 yr	Weight, length, weight-for-length, and head circumference	<2.3rd	>97.7th	—
US Centers for Disease Control and Prevention, 2000	2-20 yr	Weight, height, body mass index (BMI)	<5th	>95th	Under (<5th) Normal (5–85th) Over (85–95th) Obese (>95th) Severe Obesity (≥120% of 95th, or ≥35 kg/m²)

recommended for the equivalent identification in the CDC growth charts from 2-20 yr (Table 55.7). Note that length, weight, and weight-for-length are used in the WHO growth charts from birth to 2 yr. *Body mass index* (BMI) can be calculated but is not recommended for use in children <2 yr. Stature, weight, and BMI are used in the CDC 2000 growth charts from 2-20 yr of age. These charts can be used to categorize children 2-20 yr as *underweight* (<5th BMI percentile), normal weight (5–85th), overweight (85–95th), and obese (≥95th BMI percentile). Severe obesity is defined as BMI ≥120% of the 95th percentile, or BMI ≥35 kg/m² (whichever is lower). This assessment corresponds to approximately the 99th percentile or a BMI *z* score ≥2.33. Severe obesity that exceeds the 99th percentile is tracked on a specialized percentile curve for obesity. Furthermore, adult classification is used for BMI ≥27 kg/m² in adolescents over age 18 for consideration of medication and bariatric surgery.

Bibliography is available at Expert Consult.

Chapter 56
Feeding Healthy Infants, Children, and Adolescents

Elizabeth Prout Parks, Ala Shaikhkhalil, Nina N. Sainath, Jonathan A. Mitchell, J. Naylor Brownell, and Virginia A. Stallings

第五十六章
健康婴幼儿、儿童、青少年的喂养和膳食

中文导读

本章主要介绍了婴儿期喂养、牛奶源配方奶粉、大豆配方奶粉、蛋白水解配方、氨基酸配方、婴幼儿期奶和其他液体食物、辅食添加、幼儿和学龄前儿童喂养、学龄期儿童和青少年的饮食以及不同年龄阶段营养的重要性。具体描述了婴儿期喂养相关的母乳喂养、乳头疼痛、乳房肿胀、乳腺炎、母乳摄入不足、黄疸、母乳收集与保存、母乳喂养婴儿的生长以及奶粉喂养；具体描述了幼儿和学龄前儿童的喂养方法和措施以及托幼机构的饮食；具体描述了学龄期儿童和青少年的饮食指导，包括我的盘子膳食指南、家庭和学校就餐、家庭和学校外就餐；具体描述了不同年龄阶段的重要营养问题中的食物环境、食物作为奖赏、营养与喂养的文化因素、素食饮食、有机食物、补充和替代医学中的营养（功能食品、膳食和维生素补充剂、植物和草药制剂）、食物安全、初级儿童保健中的预防营养咨询以及美国食物帮助计划。

Early feeding and nutrition are of importance in the origin of adult diseases such as type 2 diabetes, hypertension, obesity, and the metabolic syndrome. Therefore, appropriate feeding practices should be established in the neonatal period and continued throughout childhood and adolescence to adulthood. Healthful feeding in children requires partnerships between family members, the healthcare system, schools, the community, and the government.

FEEDING DURING THE FIRST YEAR OF LIFE
Breastfeeding
The American Academy of Pediatrics (AAP) and World Health Organization (WHO) have declared breastfeeding and the administration of human milk to be the normative practice for infant feeding and nutrition. **Breastfeeding** has documented short- and long-term medical and neurodevelopmental advantages and rare contraindications (Tables 56.1 and 56.2 and Table 56.3). Thus the decision to breastfeed should be considered a public health issue and not only a lifestyle choice. The AAP and the WHO recommend that infants should be exclusively breastfed or given breast milk for 6 mo. Breastfeeding should be continued with the introduction of complementary foods for 1 yr or longer, as mutually desired by mother and infant. The success of breastfeeding initiation and continuation depends on multiple factors, such as education about breastfeeding, hospital breastfeeding practices and policies, routine and timely follow-up care, and family and societal support (Table 56.4

Table 56.1	Selected Beneficial Properties of Human Milk Compared With Infant Formula
FACTOR	**ACTION**
ANTIBACTERIAL FACTORS	
Secretory IgA	Specific antigen-targeted antiinfective action
Lactoferrin	Immunomodulation, iron chelation, antimicrobial action, antiadhesive, trophic for intestinal growth
κ-Casein	Antiadhesive, bacterial flora
Oligosaccharides	Prevention of bacterial attachment
Cytokines	Antiinflammatory, epithelial barrier function
GROWTH FACTORS	
Epidermal growth factor	Luminal surveillance, repair of intestine
Transforming growth factor (TGF)	Promotes epithelial cell growth (TGF-β) Suppresses lymphocyte function (TGF-β)
Nerve growth factor	Promotes neural growth
ENZYMES	
Platelet-activating factor (PAF)–acetylhydrolase	Blocks action of PAF
Glutathione peroxidase	Prevents lipid oxidation
Nucleotides	Enhance antibody responses, bacterial flora

Adapted from Hamosh M: Bioactive factors in human milk, *Pediatr Clin North Am* 48:69–86, 2001.

and Table 56.5).

Feedings should be initiated soon after birth unless medical conditions preclude them. Mothers should be encouraged to nurse at each breast at each feeding starting with the breast offered second at the last feeding. It is not unusual for an infant to fall asleep after the 1st breast and refuse the 2nd. It is preferable to empty the 1st breast before offering the 2nd to allow complete emptying of both breasts and therefore better milk production. Table 56.6 summarizes patterns of milk supply in the 1st week.

New mothers should be instructed about infant hunger cues, correct nipple latch, positioning of the infant on the breast, and feeding frequency. It is also suggested that someone trained in lactation observe a feeding to evaluate positioning, latch, milk transfer, maternal responses, and infant satiety. Attention to these issues during the birth hospitalization allows dialog with the mother and family and can prevent problems that could occur with improper technique or knowledge of breastfeeding. As part of the discharge teaching process, issues on infant feeding, elimination patterns, breast engorgement, breast care, and maternal nutrition should be discussed. A follow-up appointment is recommended within 24-48 hr after hospital discharge.

Nipple Pain

Nipple pain is one of the most common complaints of breastfeeding mothers in the immediate postpartum period. Poor infant positioning and improper latch are the most common reasons for nipple pain beyond the mild discomfort felt early in breastfeeding. If the problem persists and the infant refuses to feed, evaluation for nipple candidiasis is indicated. If candidiasis is present, the mother should be treated with an antifungal cream that is wiped off of the breast before feeding, and the infant treated with an oral antifungal medication.

Tongue-tie (ankyloglossia) has been associated with nipple pain, poor latching, and poor weight gain in breastfed and bottle-fed infants. *Frenotomy* is a minor surgical procedure with few complications and has been suggested as a treatment option for ankyloglossia. Nonetheless, there is considerable disagreement about the significance of ankyloglossia and the value of frenotomy. It is often difficult to assess the severity of ankyloglossia on physical examination; a combination of physical assessment and functional feeding difficulty is more useful. Nonetheless, about 50% of infants with ankyloglossia have no feeding problems, and most infants with nursing problems do not have ankyloglossia. Lactation

Table 56.2	Absolute and Relative Contraindications to Breastfeeding Because of Maternal Health Conditions
MATERNAL HEALTH CONDITION	**DEGREE OF RISK**
HIV and HTLV infection	In the United States, breastfeeding is contraindicated. In other settings, health risks of not breastfeeding must be weighed against the risk of transmitting virus to the infant.
Tuberculosis infection	Breastfeeding is contraindicated until completion of approximately 2 wk of appropriate maternal therapy.
Varicella-zoster infection	Infant should not have direct contact to active lesions. Infant should receive immune globulin.
Herpes simplex infection	Breastfeeding is contraindicated with active herpetic lesions of the breast.
CMV infection	May be found in milk of mothers who are CMV seropositive. Transmission through human milk causing symptomatic illness in term infants is uncommon.
Hepatitis B infection	Infants routinely receive hepatitis B immune globulin and hepatitis B vaccine if mother is HBsAg positive. No delay in initiation of breastfeeding is required.
Hepatitis C infection	Breastfeeding is not contraindicated.
Alcohol intake	Limit maternal alcohol intake to <0.5 g/kg/day (for a woman of average weight, this is the equivalent of 2 cans of beer, 2 glasses of wine, or 2 oz of liquor).
Cigarette smoking	Discourage cigarette smoking, but smoking is not a contraindication to breastfeeding.
Chemotherapy, radiopharmaceuticals	Breastfeeding is generally contraindicated.

CMV, Cytomegalovirus; HBsAg, hepatitis B surface antigen; HIV, human immunodeficiency virus; HTLV, human T-lymphotropic virus.
Data from Schanler RJ, Krebs NF, Mass SB, editors: *Breastfeeding handbook for physicians*, ed 2, Elk Grove Village, IL, 2014, American Academy of Pediatrics, pp 223–226.

Table 56.3	Conditions for Which Human Milk May Have a Protective Effect	
Diarrhea	Crohn disease	
Otitis media	Childhood cancer	
Urinary tract infection	Lymphoma	
Necrotizing enterocolitis	Leukemia	
Septicemia	Recurrent otitis media	
Infant botulism	Allergy	
Insulin-dependent diabetes mellitus	Hospitalizations	
Celiac disease	Infant mortality	

consultants often recommend frenotomy, whereas pediatricians provide lactation management approaches and wait at least 2-3 wk before considering frenotomy. During that time many feeding issues resolve, thus avoiding frenotomy.

Engorgement

In the 2nd stage of lactogenesis, physiologic fullness of the breast occurs. Breasts may become engorged: firm, overfilled, and painful as the pattern

Table 56.4	Ten Hospital Practices to Encourage and Support Breastfeeding*‡

1. Have a written breastfeeding policy that is routinely communicated to all health care staff.
2. Train all health care staff in the skills necessary to implement this policy.
3. Inform all pregnant women about the benefits and management of breastfeeding.
4. Help women initiate breastfeeding within 1 hour of birth.
5. Show women how to breastfeed and how to maintain lactation, even if they are separated from their newborns.
6. Give newborns no food or drink other than breast milk unless medically indicated.
7. Practice rooming-in; allow mothers and newborns to remain together 24 hours a day.
8. Encourage breastfeeding on demand.
9. Give no pacifiers or artificial nipples to breastfeeding infants.†
10. Foster the establishment of breastfeeding support groups and refer to them on discharge from the hospital or birth center.

COMPONENTS OF SAFE POSITIONING FOR THE NEWBORN WHILE SKIN-TO-SKIN

1. Infant's face can be seen.
2. Infant's head is in "sniffing" position.
3. Infant's nose and mouth are not covered.
4. Infant's head is turned to one side.
5. Infant's neck is straight, not bent.
6. Infant's shoulders and chest face mother.
7. Infant's legs are flexed.
8. Infant's back is covered with blankets.
9. Mother-infant dyad is monitored continuously by staff in the delivery environment and regularly on the postpartum unit.
10. When mother wants to sleep, infant is placed in bassinet or with another support person who is awake and alert.

*The 1994 report of the Healthy Mothers, Health Babies National Coalition Expert Work Group recommend that the UNICEF-WHO Baby Friendly Hospital Initiative be adapted for use in the United States as the United States Breastfeeding Health Initiative, using the adapted ten hospital practices above.
†The American Academy of Pediatrics endorsed the UNICEF-WHO Ten Steps to Successful Breastfeeding, but does not support a categorical ban on pacifiers because of their role in reducing the risk of sudden infant death syndrome and their analgesic benefit during painful procedures when breastfeeding cannot provide the analgesia.
‡Data from Baby-Friendly USA. Guidelines and evaluation criteria for facilities seeking baby-friendly designation. Sandwich (MA): Baby Friendly USA, 2010. Available at https://www.babyfriendlyusa.org/for-facilities/practice-guidelines/. Accessed 10 December 2018. From ACOG Committee Opinion: Optimizing support for breastfeeding as part of obstetric practice. Obstet Gynecol 132(4):e187-e195, 2018 (Box 1, p. e191 and Box 2, p. e192).
**Data from Ludington-Hoe SM, Morgan K. Infant assessment and reduction of sudden unexpected postnatal collapse risk during skin-to-skin contact. Newborn Infant Nurs Rev 2014;14:28-33.

Table 56.5	Recommendations on Breastfeeding Management for Healthy Term Infants

1. Exclusive breastfeeding for about 6 months
   • Breastfeeding preferred; alternatively expressed mother's milk, or donor breast milk
   • To continue for at least the first year and beyond as long as mutually desired by mother and child
   • Complementary foods rich in iron and other micronutrients should be introduced at about 6 mo of age
2. Peripartum policies and practices that optimize breastfeeding initiation and maintenance should be compatible with the AAP and Academy of Breastfeeding Medicine Model Hospital Policy and include the following:
   • Direct skin-to-skin contact with mothers immediately after delivery until the first feeding is accomplished and encouraged throughout the postpartum period
   • Delay in routine procedures (weighing, measuring, bathing, blood tests, vaccines, and eye prophylaxis) until after the first feeding is completed
   • Delay in administration of intramuscular vitamin K until after the first feeding is completed but within 6 hr of birth
   • Ensure 8-12 feedings at the breast every 24 hr
   • Ensure formal evaluation and documentation of breastfeeding by trained caregivers (including position, latch, milk transfer, examination) at least once for each nursing shift
   • Give no supplements (water, glucose water, commercial infant formula, or other fluids) to breastfeeding newborn infants unless medically indicated using standard evidence-based guidelines for the management of hyperbilirubinemia and hypoglycemia
   • Avoid routine pacifier use in the postpartum period
   • Begin daily oral vitamin D drops (400 IU) at hospital discharge
3. All breastfeeding infants should be seen by a pediatrician within 48 to 72 hr after discharge from the hospital
   • Evaluate hydration and elimination patterns
   • Evaluate body weight gain (body weight loss no more than 7% from birth and no further weight loss by day 5: assess feeding and consider more frequent follow-up)
   • Discuss maternal/infant issues
   • Observe feeding
4. Mother and infant should sleep in proximity to each other to facilitate breastfeeding
5. Pacifier should be offered, while placing infant in back-to-sleep-position, no earlier than 3 to 4 weeks of age and after breastfeeding has been established

From American Academy of Pediatrics (AAP): Breast-feeding and the use of human milk, Pediatrics 129:e827–e841, 2012.

Table 56.6	Patterns of Milk Supply	
DAY OF LIFE		**MILK SUPPLY**
Day 1		Some milk (~5 mL) may be expressed.
Days 2-4		Lactogenesis; milk production increases.
Day 5		Milk present; fullness and leaking are felt.
Day 6 onward		Breasts should feel "empty" after feeding.

Adapted from Neifert MR: Clinical aspects of lactation: promoting breastfeeding success, Clin Perinatol 26:281–306, 1999.

and volume of milk production adjusts to the infant's feeding schedule. Incomplete removal of milk as a result of poor breastfeeding technique or infant illness can cause engorgement. Breastfeeding immediately at signs of infant hunger will eventually prevent this from occurring. To reduce engorgement, breasts should be softened before infant feeding with a combination of hot compresses and expression of milk. To reduce inflammation and pain, between feedings a supportive bra should be worn, cold compresses applied, and oral nonsteroidal antiinflammatory drugs (NSAIDs) administered.

Mastitis

Mastitis occurs in 2–3% of lactating women and is usually unilateral, manifesting with localized warmth, tenderness, edema, and erythema after the 2nd postdelivery week. Sudden onset of breast pain, myalgia, and fever with fatigue, nausea, vomiting, and headache can also occur. Organisms implicated in mastitis include *Staphylococcus aureus, Escherichia coli,* group A streptococcus, *Haemophilus influenzae, Klebsiella pneumoniae,* and *Bacteroides* species. Diagnosis is confirmed by physical examination. Oral antibiotics and analgesics, while promoting breastfeeding or emptying of the affected breast, usually resolve the infection.

A **breast abscess** is a less common complication of mastitis, but it is a more serious infection that requires intravenous antibiotics and incision and drainage, along with temporary cessation of feeding from that breast.

Inadequate Milk Intake

Insufficient milk intake, dehydration, and jaundice in the infant can occur within the 1st week of life. Signs include lethargy, delayed stooling, decreased urine output, weight loss >7–10% of birth weight, hypernatremic dehydration, inconsolable crying, and increased hunger. Insufficient milk intake may be caused by insufficient milk production, failure of established breastfeeding, and health conditions in the infant that prevent proper breast stimulation. Parents should be counseled that breastfed neonates feed 8-12 times/day with a minimum of 8 times/day. Careful attention to prenatal history can identify maternal factors associated with this problem (failure of breasts to enlarge during pregnancy or within the 1st few days after delivery). Direct observation of breastfeeding can help identify improper technique. If a large volume of milk is expressed manually after breastfeeding, the infant might not be extracting enough milk, eventually leading to decreased milk output. Late preterm infants (34-36 wk) are at risk for insufficient milk syndrome because of poor suck and swallow patterns or medical issues.

Jaundice

Breastfeeding jaundice is related to insufficient fluid intake during the 1st week of life and is a common reason for hospital readmission of healthy breastfed infants (see Chapter 123.3). Breastfeeding jaundice is associated with dehydration and hypernatremia. **Breast milk jaundice** is a different disorder that causes persistently high serum indirect bilirubin in thriving healthy well-fed infants. Breast milk contains inhibitors of glucuronyl transferase and causes enhanced absorption of bilirubin from the gut. Breast milk jaundice becomes evident later than breastfeeding jaundice and generally declines in the 2nd to 3rd wk of life. Infants with severe or persistent jaundice should be evaluated for other medical causes. Persistently high bilirubin levels may require changing from breast milk to infant formula for 24-48 hr and/or treatment with phototherapy without cessation of breastfeeding. Breastfeeding should resume after the decline in serum bilirubin. Parents should be reassured and encouraged to continue collecting breast milk during the period the infant is taking formula.

Breast Milk Collection

The pumping of breast milk is a common practice when the mother and baby are separated. Good handwashing and hygiene should be emphasized. Electric breast pumps are generally more efficient and better tolerated by mothers than mechanical pumps or manual expression. Collection kits should be cleaned with hot soapy water, rinsed, and air-dried after each use. Glass or plastic containers should be used to collect the milk, and milk should be refrigerated and then used within 48 hr. Expressed breast milk can be frozen and used for up to 6 mo. Milk should be thawed rapidly by holding under running tepid water and used completely within 24 hr after thawing. *Milk should never be microwaved.*

Growth of the Breastfed Infant

The rate of weight gain of the breastfed infant differs from that of the formula-fed infant; the infant's risk for excess weight gain during late infancy may be associated with bottle feeding. The WHO growth charts are based on growth patterns of healthy breastfed infants through the 1st year of life. These standards (http://www.who.int/childgrowth) are the result of a study in which >8,000 children were selected from 6 countries. The infants were selected based on being breastfed, having good health care, high socioeconomic status, and nonsmoking mothers, so that they reflect the growth pattern of breastfed infants in optimal conditions and can be used as prescriptive rather than normative curves. Charts are available for growth monitoring. The U.S. Centers for Disease Control and Prevention (CDC) recommend use of the WHO growth charts for infants 0-23 mo of age and CDC growth charts for ages 24 mo to 20 yr (see Chapter 27).

Formula Feeding (Fig. 56.1)

Despite efforts to promote exclusive breastfeeding through 6 mo, <50% of women continue to breastfeed at 6 mo. Most women make their

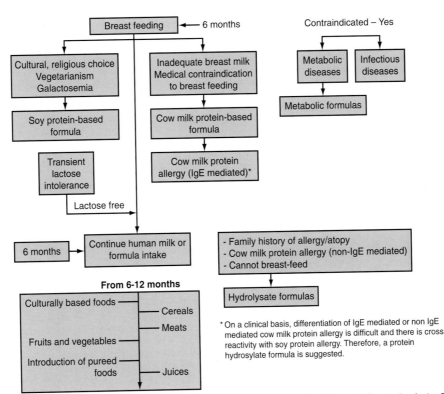

Fig. 56.1 Feeding algorithm for term infants. (*From Gamble Y, Bunyapen C, Bhatia J: Feeding the term infant. In Berdanier CD, Dwyer J, Feldman EB, editors:* Handbook of nutrition and food, *Boca Raton, FL, 2008, CRC Press, pp 271–284, Fig 15-3.*)

infant feeding choices early in pregnancy. Parental preference is the most common reason for using infant formula. However, infant formula is also indicated for infants whose intake of breast milk is contraindicated for infant factors (e.g., inborn errors of metabolism) and maternal factors (see Table 56.2). In addition, infant formula is used as a supplement to support inadequate weight gain in breastfed infants.

Infant formulas marketed in the United States are safe and nutritionally adequate as the sole source of nutrition for healthy infants for the 1st 6 mo of life. Infant formulas are available in ready-to-feed, concentrated liquid or powder forms. Ready-to-feed products generally provide 19-20 kcal/30 mL (1 oz) and approximately 64-67 kcal/dL. Concentrated liquid products, when diluted according to instructions, provide a preparation with the same concentration. Powder formulas come in single or multiple servings and when mixed according to instructions will result in similar caloric density.

Although infant formulas are manufactured in adherence to good manufacturing practices and are regulated by the U.S. Food and Drug Administration (FDA), there are potential safety issues. Ready-to-feed and concentrated liquid formulas are commercially sterile, but powder preparations are not. Although the number of bacterial colony-forming units per gram (CFU/g) of powder formula is generally lower than allowable limits, outbreaks of infections with *Cronobacter sakazakii* (previously *Enterobacter sakazakii*) have been documented, especially in premature infants. The powder preparations can contain other coliform bacteria but have not been linked to disease in healthy term infants. Care must be taken in following the mixing instructions to avoid over- or underdilution, to use boiled or sterilized water, and to use the specific scoops provided by the manufacturer because scoop sizes vary. Water that has been boiled should be allowed to cool fully to prevent degradation of heat-labile nutrients, specifically vitamin C. Well water should be tested regularly for bacteria and toxin contamination. Municipal water can contain variable concentrations of fluoride, and if the concentrations are high, bottled water that is defluoridated should be used to avoid toxicity.

Parents should be instructed to use proper handwashing techniques when preparing formula and feedings for the infant. Guidance on formula storage should also be given. Once opened, ready-to-feed and concentrated liquid containers can be covered with aluminum foil or plastic wrap and stored in the refrigerator for no longer than 48 hr. Powder formula should be stored in a cool, dry place; once opened, cans should be covered with the original plastic cap or aluminum foil, and the powdered product can be used within 4 wk. Once prepared, all bottles, regardless of type of formula, should be used within 24 hr. Formula should be used within 2 hr of removal from the refrigerator, and once a feeding has started, that formula should be used within 1 hr or be discarded. Prepared formula stored in the refrigerator should be warmed by placing the container in warm water for about 5 min. Formula should *not* be heated in a microwave because it can heat unevenly and result in burns, despite appearing to be at the right temperature when tested.

Formula feedings should be ad libitum, with the goal of achieving growth and development to the child's genetic potential. The usual intake to allow a weight gain of 25-30 g/day will be 140-200 mL/kg/day in the 1st 3 mo of life. The rate of weight gain declines from 3-12 mo of age.

COW'S MILK PROTEIN–BASED FORMULAS

Intact cow's milk protein–based formulas in the United States contain a protein concentration varying from 1.8-3 g/100 kcal (or 1.4-1.8 g/dL), considerably higher than in mature breast milk (1.2-1.3 g/100 kcal; 0.9-1.0 g/dL). This increased concentration is designed to meet the needs of the youngest infants, but leads to excess protein intake for older infants. In contrast, breast milk content varies over time to match protein needs at various ages. The whey:casein ratio varies in infant formula from 18:82 to 60:40; one manufacturer markets a formula that is 100% whey. The predominant whey protein is β-globulin in cow's milk and α-lactalbumin in human milk. This and other differences between human milk and cow's milk–based formulas result in different plasma amino acid profiles in infants on different feeding patterns, but clinical significance has not been demonstrated.

The primary source of fat in cow's milk protein–based infant formulas is plant or a mixture of plant and animal oils. Fat provides 40–50% of the energy in cow's milk–based formulas. Fat blends are better absorbed than dairy fat and provide saturated, monounsaturated, and polyunsaturated fatty acids (PUFAs). All infant formulas are supplemented with long-chain PUFAs, docosahexaenoic acid (DHA), and arachidonic acid (ARA) at varying concentrations. ARA and DHA are found at varying concentrations in human milk and vary by geographic region and maternal diet. DHA and ARA are derived from single-cell microfungi and microalgae and are classified as "generally recognized as safe" (GRAS) for use in infant formulas at approved concentrations and ratios. The routine supplementation of milk formula with long-chain PUFAs to improve the physical, neurodevelopmental, or visual outcomes of term infants cannot be recommended based on the current evidence.

Lactose is the major carbohydrate in breast milk and in standard cow's milk–based formulas for term infants. Formulas for term infants may also contain modified starch or other complex carbohydrates. Carbohydrates constitute 67-75 g/L of cow's milk–based formula.

SOY FORMULAS

Soy protein–based formulas on the market are all free of cow's milk–based protein and lactose. Carbohydrates are provided by sucrose, corn syrup solids, and maltodextrins to provide 67 kcal/dL. They meet the vitamin, mineral, and electrolyte guidelines from the AAP and the FDA for feeding term infants. The protein is a soy isolate supplemented with L-methionine, L-carnitine, and taurine to provide a protein content of 2.45-2.8 g/100 kcal, or 1.7-1.9 g/dL.

The quantity of specific fats varies by manufacturer and is usually similar to the manufacturer's corresponding cow's milk–based formula. The fat content is 5.0-5.5 g/100 kcal, or 3.4-3.6 g/dL. The oils used in both cow's milk and soy formula include soy, palm, sunflower, olein, safflower, and coconut. DHA and ARA are also added.

In term infants, although soy protein–based formulas have been used to provide nutrition resulting in normal growth patterns, there are few indications for use in place of cow's milk–based formula. Indications for soy formula include galactosemia, preference for a vegetarian diet, and hereditary lactase deficiency, because soy-based formulas are lactose free. Most healthy infants with acute gastroenteritis can be managed after rehydration with continued use of breast milk or cow's milk–based formulas and do not require a lactose-free formula, such as soy-based formula. However, soy protein–based formulas may be indicated when documented secondary lactose intolerance occurs. Soy protein–based formulas have no advantage over cow's milk protein–based formulas as a supplement for the breastfed infant, unless the infant has one of the indications noted previously, and are not recommended for preterm infants. The routine use of soy protein–based formula has no proven value in the prevention or management of infantile colic, fussiness, or atopic disease. Infants with documented cow's milk protein–induced enteropathy or enterocolitis often are also sensitive to soy protein. They should be provided formula derived from extensively hydrolyzed protein or synthetic amino acids. Soy formulas contain *phytoestrogens,* which have been shown to have physiologic activity in rodent models, but there is no conclusive evidence of adverse developmental effects in infants fed soy formula.

PROTEIN HYDROLYSATE FORMULAS

Protein hydrolysate formulas may be *partially hydrolyzed,* containing oligopeptides with a molecular weight of <5000 daltons (range 3,000-10,000 Da), or *extensively hydrolyzed,* containing peptides with a molecular weight <3000 Da. Partially hydrolyzed proteins formulas have fat blends similar to cow's milk–based formulas, and carbohydrates are supplied by corn maltodextrin or corn syrup solids. Because the protein is not extensively hydrolyzed, these formulas should not be fed to infants who are allergic to cow's milk protein. In studies of formula-fed infants who are at high risk of developing atopic disease, there is modest evidence that childhood atopic dermatitis may be delayed or prevented by the use of extensively or partially hydrolyzed formulas, compared with cow's milk–based formula. Comparative studies of the various hydrolyzed formulas have also indicated that not all formulas have the same protective benefit. Extensively hydrolyzed formulas may be more effective than partially hydrolyzed in preventing atopic disease. Extensively hydrolyzed formulas are recommended for infants intolerant to cow's milk or soy proteins. These formulas are lactose free and can include medium-chain triglycerides, making them useful in infants with gastrointestinal malabsorption as a consequence of cystic fibrosis, short gut syndrome, prolonged diarrhea, and hepatobiliary disease.

AMINO ACID FORMULAS

Amino acid formulas are peptide-free formulas that contain mixtures of essential and nonessential amino acids. They are designed for infants with cow's milk–based protein allergy who failed to thrive on extensively hydrolyzed protein formulas. The effectiveness of amino acid formulas to prevent atopic disease has not been studied.

MILK AND OTHER FLUIDS IN INFANTS AND TODDLERS

Neither breastfed nor formula-fed infants require additional water unless dictated by a specific condition involving excess water loss, such as diabetes insipidus. Vomiting and spitting up are common in infants. When weight gain and general well-being are noted, no change in formula is necessary.

Whole cow's milk should not be introduced until 12 mo of age. In children 12-24 mo of age for whom overweight or obesity is a concern or who have a family history of obesity, dyslipidemia, or cardiovascular disease, the use of reduced-fat milk is appropriate. Otherwise, whole milk is recommended until age 24 mo, changing to 1% milk at 24 mo for healthy children. Regardless of the type, all animal milk consumed should be pasteurized. Infants and young children are particularly susceptible to infections such as *E. coli*, *Campylobacter*, and *Salmonella* found in **raw or unpasteurized milk**. For cultural and other reasons, such as parental preference, **goat's milk** is sometimes given in place of formula, although this is not recommended. Goat's milk has been shown to cause significant electrolyte disturbances and anemia because it has low folic acid concentrations.

Nondairy alternatives to milk from plant-based (e.g., soy, hemp, pea, rice) and nut-based (e.g., almond, cashew, peanut) sources have become popular. When counseling parents, it is important to emphasize that the overall nutritional content of plant-based milk alternatives *is not* equivalent to cow's milk. Although most are fortified with vitamin D and calcium, with the exception of some soy-, hemp-, and pea-based milk alternatives, most products have a lower protein content. Concurrently, plant-based products such as soy and rice milk tend to have added oils and sugars, giving them a higher energy content than cow's milk. Secondary to a lower protein content, these alternative milks *should not be given to infants*. Nut-based milks may be suitable to toddlers ≥24 mo of age without allergies who have an otherwise adequate diet.

COMPLEMENTARY FEEDING

The timely introduction of **complementary foods** (solid and liquid foods other than breast milk or formula, also called **weaning foods**) during infancy is important for nutritional and developmental reasons (Table 56.7). The ability of exclusive breastfeeding to meet macronutrient and micronutrient requirements becomes limited with increasing age of the infant. The recommendation for timing of complementary food initiation is based on the benefits on neurodevelopment and prevention of future comorbidities from exclusive breastfeeding after 6 mo. The AAP, WHO, and European Society for Pediatric Gastroenterology, Hepatology, and Nutrition Committee on Nutrition all recommend exclusive breastfeeding for the 1st 6 mo. Similar data on the benefits of the exclusive use of formula for 6 mo have not been published.

Some foods are more nutritionally appropriate than others to complement breast milk or infant formula. The food consumption patterns of U.S. infants and toddlers demonstrate that almost all infants ≤12 mo consumed some form of milk every day; infants >4 mo consumed more formula than human milk, and by 9-11 mo, 20% consumed whole cow's milk and 25% consumed nonfat or reduced-fat milk.

Table 56.7	Important Principles for Weaning

Begin at 6 mo of age.
At the proper age, encourage a cup rather than a bottle.
Introduce 1 new food at a time.
Energy density should exceed that of breast milk.
Iron-containing foods (meat, iron-supplemented cereals) are required.
Zinc intake should be encouraged with foods such as meat, dairy products, wheat, and rice.
Phytate intake should be low to enhance mineral absorption.
Breast milk should continue to 12 mo of age; formula or cow's milk is then substituted.
Give no more than 24 oz/day of cow's milk.
Fluids other than breast milk, formula, and water should be discouraged.
Give no more than 4-6 oz/day of 100% fruit juice; no sugar-sweetened beverages.

Adapted from American Academy of Pediatrics: *Pediatric nutrition handbook*, ed 6, Elk Grove Village, IL, 2008, American Academy of Pediatrics.

The most common complementary foods between 4 and 11 mo of age are infant cereals. Almost 45% of infants between 9 and 11 mo of age consumed noninfant cereals. Infant eating patterns also vary, with up to 61% of infants 4-11 mo of age consuming no vegetables. French fries were the most frequently consumed vegetables in toddlers. Positive changes in the last decade include increased duration of breastfeeding, delayed introduction of complementary foods, and decreased juice consumption. Continuing concerns include lack of fruits and vegetables; diets low in iron, essential fatty acids, fiber, and whole grains; and diets high in saturated fat and sodium. Table 56.7 summarizes the AAP recommendations for initiating complementary foods.

The complementary foods should be varied to ensure adequate macro- and micronutrient intake. In addition to complementary foods introduced at 6 mo of age, continued breastfeeding or the use of infant formula for the entire 1st year of life should be encouraged. Overconsumption of energy-dense complementary foods can lead to excessive weight gain in infancy, resulting in an increased risk of obesity in childhood.

FEEDING TODDLERS AND PRESCHOOL-AGE CHILDREN

Toddlerhood is a period when eating behavior and healthful habits can be established and is often a confusing and anxiety-generating period for parents. Growth after the 1st year slows, motor activity increases, and appetite decreases. Birth weight triples during the 1st year of life and quadruples by the 2nd year, reflecting this slowing in growth velocity. Eating behavior is erratic, and the child appears distracted from eating as he explores the environment. Children consume a limited variety of foods and often only "like" a particular food for a period and then reject the favored food. The use of growth charts to demonstrate adequate growth and provide guidance about typical behavior and eating habits will help allay parents' concerns. Important goals of early childhood nutrition are to foster healthful eating habits and offer foods that are developmentally appropriate.

Feeding Practices

The period starting after 6 mo until 15 mo is characterized by the acquisition of self-feeding skills because the infant can grasp finger foods, learn to use a spoon, and eat soft foods (Table 56.8). Around 12 mo of age, the child learns to drink from a cup and may still breastfeed or desire formula bottle feeding. Bottle weaning should begin around 12-15 mo, and bedtime bottles should be discouraged because of the association with **dental carries**. Unless being used at mealtime, the sippy cup should only contain water to prevent caries. Sugar-sweetened beverages and 100% fruit juice should also be discouraged from being used in bottles in all infants at all times. Cups without a lid can be used for no more than 4-6 oz/day of 100% fruit juice for toddlers.

Table 56.8	Feeding Skills Birth to 36 Months
AGE (mo)	**FEEDING/ORAL SENSORIMOTOR SKILLS**
Birth to 4-6	Nipple feeding, breast or bottle Hand on bottle during feeding (2-4 mo) Maintains semiflexed posture during feeding Promotion of infant–parent interaction
6-9 (transition feeding)	Feeding more in upright position Spoon feeding thin, pureed foods Both hands to hold bottle Finger feeding introduced Vertical munching of easily dissolvable solids Preference for parents to feed
9-12	Cup drinking Eats lumpy, mashed food Finger feeding for easily dissolvable solids Chewing includes rotary jaw action
12-18	Self-feeding; grasps spoon with whole hand Holds cup with 2 hands Drinking with 4-5 consecutive swallows Holding and tipping bottle
>18-24	Swallowing with lip closure Self-feeding predominates Chewing broad range of food Up-down tongue movements
24-36	Circulatory jaw rotations Chewing with lips closed One-handed cup holding and open cup drinking with no spilling Using fingers to fill spoon Eating wide range of solid food Total self-feeding, using fork

Adapted from Arvedson JC: Swallowing and feeding in infants and young children. *GI Motility online*, 2006. doi:10.1038/gimo17.

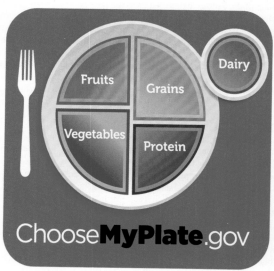

Fig. 56.2 MyPlate food guide. *(From US Department of Agriculture:* http://www.choosemyplate.gov/.)

Juices should not be given before 12 mo of age. The volume of juices should be limited to 4 oz/day in children 1-3 yr old, to 4-6 oz/day for 4-6 yr olds, and to 8 oz/day for 7-18 yr olds. Children taking medications metabolized by CYP3A4 must avoid grapefruit juices.

In the 2nd year of life, self-feeding becomes a norm and provides the opportunity for the family to eat together with less stress. Self-feeding allows the child to limit her intake. Child feeding is an interactive process. Children receive cues regarding appropriate feeding behaviors from parents. Parents should praise positive and ignore negative eating behaviors unless the behavior jeopardizes the health and safety of the child. In addition, parents should eat with their toddlers and not simply feed them, in order to model positive eating behaviors.

The 2 yr old child should progress from small pieces of soft food to prepared table foods with precautions. At this stage, the child is not capable of completely chewing and swallowing foods, and particular attention should be paid to foods with a choking risk. Hard candies, nuts, and raw carrots should be avoided. Hot dogs, sausages, and grapes should be sliced lengthwise. Caregivers should always be vigilant and present during feeding, and the child should be placed in a high chair or booster seat. The AAP discourages eating in the presence of distractions such as television, tablets, mobile devices, and other screens, or eating in a car where an adult cannot adequately observe the child.

Young children have a natural preference for sweetened foods and beverages that begins in infancy. Reluctance to accept new foods is a common developmental phase. A new food should be offered multiple times (8-15) over a period of months for acceptance by the child.

Toddlers need to eat 3 healthy meals and 2 snacks daily. Milk continues to be an important source of nutrition. Guidelines for vitamin D supplementation recommend a daily vitamin D intake of 600 IU/day for children and adolescents who are ingesting <1000 mL/day of vitamin

D–fortified milk or formula. Toddlers and preschool children often fail to meet the recommended servings of fruits, vegetables, and fiber, whereas intakes of food with fat and added sugar are high. Giving vegetables at the beginning of the meal and increasing the portion size of vegetables served during meals can be an effective strategy for increasing vegetable consumption in preschool children.

Eating in the Daycare Setting
Many U.S. toddlers and preschool children attend daycare and receive meals and snacks in this setting. There is a wide variation in the quality of the food offered and the level of supervision during meals. Parents are encouraged to assess the quality of the food served at daycare by asking questions, visiting the center, and taking part in parent committees. Free or reduced-price snacks and meals are provided in daycare centers for low- and medium-income communities through the U.S. Department of Agriculture (USDA) **Child and Adult Care Food Program**. Participating programs are required to provide meals and snacks that meet the meal regulations set by the USDA, guaranteeing a certain level of food quality. However, often for monetary reasons, many daycare centers still struggle to provide high-quality meals and snacks.

FEEDING SCHOOL-AGE CHILDREN AND ADOLESCENTS
MyPlate
The USDA MyPlate (www.choosemyplate.gov) is a basis for building an optimal diet for children and adults (Fig. 56.2). MyPlate is based on the 2010 **Dietary Guidelines for Americans** and replaced MyPyramid. MyPlate provides a visual representation of the different food groups and portion sizes designed for the general public. In addition to food group information, the website provides discretionary calorie information, weight management strategies, and tools to track calories and physical activity goals. A personalized eating plan based on these guidelines provides, on average over a few days, all the essential nutrients necessary for health and growth, while limiting nutrients associated with chronic disease development. MyPlate can also be used as an interactive tool that allows customization of recommendations, based on age, sex, physical activity, and for some populations, weight and height. Print materials from the USDA are also available for families without internet access.

Recommendations based on MyPlate emphasize making half the plate vegetables and fruits and half the plate protein and grains, with protein having the smallest section. Protein replaces the meat category since many protein sources are not from animals. A separate dairy section is included. Physical activity recommendations to achieve a healthful energy balance are not visually displayed but are provided on the website. MyPlate has removed foods that have low nutritional value, such as sweetened sugar beverages and sweetened bakery products.

In the United States and an increasing number of other countries, the vast majority of children and adolescents do not consume a diet that follows the recommendations of MyPlate. The intake of discretionary calories is much higher than recommended, with frequent consumption of sweetened sugar beverages (soda, juice drinks, iced tea, sport drinks), snack foods, high-fat meat (bacon, sausage), and high-fat dairy products (cheese, ice cream). Intake of dark-green and orange vegetables (vs fried white potatoes), whole fruits, reduced-fat dairy products, and whole grains is typically lower than recommended. Furthermore, unhealthful eating habits, such as larger-than-recommended portion sizes; food preparation that adds fat, sugar, or salt; skipping breakfast and/or lunch; grazing; or following fad diets are prevalent and associated with a poorer diet quality. MyPlate offers a helpful and customer-friendly tool to assist pediatricians counseling families on optimal eating plans for short- and long-term health.

Eating at Home
At home, much of what children and adolescents eat is under the control of their parents. Typically, parents shop for groceries and control, to some extent, what food is available in the house. Modeling of healthful eating behavior by parents is a critical determinant of the food choices of children and adolescents. Counseling to improve diet should include guiding parents in using their influence to make healthier food choices available and attractive at home.

Regular family meals sitting at a table, as opposed to eating alone or watching a TV or other screen, are associated with improved diet quality, perhaps because of increased opportunities for **positive parenting** during meals. Many families with busy schedules and other stressors are unable to provide the ideal meal setting. Another parenting challenge is to control the excess appetite of some children and adolescents. Children should be supported to eat at a slower pace and to chew their food properly. Conversation at the dinner table should be encouraged to prolong eating to at least 15 min. Offering vegetables while children are hungry at the beginning of the meal has been shown to increase vegetable consumption. Useful strategies, when the child is still hungry after a meal, include a 15-20 min pause (allow child to engage in another activity) before a 2nd serving or offering foods that are insufficiently consumed, such as vegetables, whole grains, or fruits.

Eating at School
The **National School Lunch Program** and the **School Breakfast Program** provide low-cost meals to more than 5 billion children nationwide. Guidelines for meals are taken from the Dietary Guidelines for Americans and the 2005 Dietary Reference. Recommendations include the use of age-grade portion sizes and the amounts of vegetables and fruits, grains, and fats (Table 56.9). The training and equipment for school food service staff, school community engagement, parent education, and food industry involvement are among the necessary components. The target year is 2020 for achieving recommendations for sodium. In the meantime, while schools are working on implementing changes, parents should be encouraged to examine the weekly menu with their child and assist with their choices. If children bring their lunch from home, recommendations for what constitutes a healthful lunch should be provided by the pediatrician. Parents can be directed to www.choosemyplate.org for healthful lunch ideas. In addition, parties within classrooms should be limited to once a month.

Eating Out
The number of meals eaten outside the home or brought home from takeout restaurants has increased in all age-groups of the U.S. population. The increased convenience of this meal pattern is undermined by the generally lower nutritional value of the meals, compared to home-cooked

Table 56.9	Revised National School Lunch Program and School Breakfast Program Recommendations

- Portion sizes of food are to be based on age-grade groups.
- School lunches and breakfasts will have a minimum and maximum calorie level, maximum saturated fat content, and a maximum sodium content.
- Foods must contain zero grams of *trans* fat per serving.
- The inclusion of unsaturated vegetable oils is encouraged within calorie limits.
- Vegetables and fruits are not interchangeable.
- Vegetable offerings at lunch must include ½ cup equivalent of the following: dark-green vegetables, bright-orange vegetables, and legumes.
- No more than half of fruit servings may be in the form of juice.
- At least one half of bread/grain offered must be whole grain.
- Milk must be fat free if flavored and either fat free or 1% fat if plain.
- Students must select a fruit option at breakfast with their meal, and either a fruit or a vegetable at lunch, for the meal to be reimbursable.

Adapted from the National Academies of Engineering, Science and Medicine: *School meals: building blocks for healthy children,* Washington, DC, 2010, National Academies Press.

meals. Typically, meals consumed or purchased in fast-food or casual restaurants are of large portion size, are dense in calories, and contain large amounts of saturated fat, salt, and sugar and low amounts of whole grains, fruits, and vegetables. Although still a problem currently, *trans* fat is being phased out of most commercial restaurants and prepared foods. Although an increasing number of restaurants offer healthier alternatives, the vast majority of what is consumed at restaurants does not fit MyPlate recommendations.

With increasing age, an increasing number of meals and snacks are also consumed during peer social gatherings at friends' houses and parties. When a large part of a child's or adolescent's diet is consumed on these occasions, the diet quality can suffer, because food offerings are typically of low nutritional value. Parents and pediatricians need to guide teens in navigating these occasions while maintaining a healthful diet and enjoying meaningful social interactions. These occasions often are also opportunities for teens to consume alcohol; consequently, adult supervision is important.

NUTRITION ISSUES OF IMPORTANCE ACROSS PEDIATRIC AGES
Food Environment
Most families have some knowledge of nutrition and intend to provide their children with a healthful diet. The discrepancy between this fact and the actual quality of the diet consumed by U.S. children is often explained by challenges in the environment for families to make healthful food choices. Because the final food choice is made by individual children or their parents, interventions to improve diet have focused on individual knowledge and behavior changes, but these have had limited success (Fig. 56.3). Understanding the context of food and lifestyle choices helps in understanding lack of changes or "poor compliance" and can decrease the frustration often experienced by the pediatricians who might "blame the victim" for behavior that is not entirely under their control. In recent time, national initiatives have been launched to increase access to vegetables and fruits and increase public awareness of healthful eating (e.g., Let's Move!).

While **taste** is the main determinant of food choice, many other complex determinants influence that choice including **cost** and marketing strategies. **Marketing** includes strategies as diverse as shelf placements, association of cartoon characters with food products, coupons, and special offers or pricing, all of which influence food purchase choices. Television advertising is an important part of how children and adolescents hear about food, with an estimated 40,000 TV commercials per year, as seen by the average U.S. child, many of which are for food,

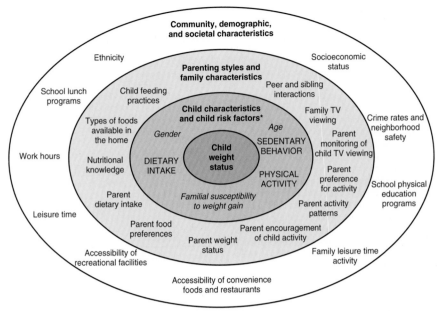

Fig. 56.3 A conceptual framework of the context of food and lifestyle choices. Child risk factors (shown in uppercase lettering) refer to child behaviors associated with the development of overweight. Characteristics of the child (shown in italic lettering) interact with child risk factors and contextual factors to influence the development of overweight (i.e., moderator variables). *(From Davison KK, Birch LL: Childhood overweight: a contextual model and recommendations for future research, Obes Rev 2:159–171, 2001. © 2001 The International Association for the Study of Obesity.)*

compared to the few hours of nutrition education they receive in school. Additional food advertisement increasingly occurs as brand placement in movies and TV shows, on websites, and even video games.

Using Food as Reward
It is a prevalent habit to use food as a reward or sometimes withdraw food as punishment. Most parents use this practice occasionally, and some use it almost systematically, starting at a young age. The practice is also commonly used in other settings where children spend time, such as daycare, school, or even athletic settings. Although it might be a good idea to limit some unhealthful but desirable food categories to special occasions, using food as a reward is problematic. Limiting access to some foods and making its access contingent on a particular accomplishment increases the desirability of that type of food. Conversely, encouraging the consumption of some foods renders them less desirable. Therefore, phrases such as, "Finish your vegetables, and you will get ice cream for dessert," can result in establishing unhealthful eating habits once the child has more autonomy in food choices. Parents should be counseled on such issues and encouraged to choose items other than food as reward, such as inexpensive toys or sporting equipment, family time, special family events, or collectible items. Similar types of behavior are also seen in schools and extracurricular events. Instead of rewards of food (e.g., pizza, candy), daycare providers, teachers, and counselors should be encouraged to use alternative rewards, such as minutes of free time, sitting in the teacher's chair, being the teacher's helper, and homework-free nights.

Cultural Considerations in Nutrition and Feeding
Food choices, food preparation, eating patterns, and infant feeding practices all have very deep cultural roots. In fact, beliefs, attitudes, and practices surrounding food and eating are some of the most important components of cultural identity. Therefore, it is not surprising that in multicultural societies, great variability exists in the cultural characteristics of the diet. Even in a world where global marketing forces tend to reduce geographic differences in the types of food, or even brands,

that are available, most families, especially during family meals at home, are still much influenced by their cultural background. Therefore, pediatricians should become familiar with the dietary characteristics of various cultures in their community, so that they can identify and address, in a nonjudgmental way and avoiding stereotypes, the potential nutritional issues related to the diet of their patients.

Vegetarianism
Vegetarianism is the practice of following a diet that excludes animal flesh foods, including beef, pork, poultry, fish, and shellfish. There are several variants of the diet, some of which also exclude eggs and/or some products produced from animal labor, such as dairy products and honey. It is important to understand different variations in vegetarianism, as follows:
◆ Veganism: excludes all animal products. It may be part of a larger practice of abstaining from the use of animal products for any purpose.
◆ Ovovegetarianism: includes eggs but not dairy products.
◆ Lactovegetarianism: includes dairy products but excludes eggs.
◆ Lactoovovegetarianism: includes eggs and dairy products.
◆ Flexitarian: a vegetarian who will occasionally eat meat.
◆ Pescatarian: consumes fish, but often self-labeled a vegetarian.
Another expression used for vegetarianism and veganism is "plant-based diets."

Other dietary practices commonly associated with vegetarianism include *fruitarian* diet (fruits, nuts, seeds, and other plant matter gathered without harm to the plant), *Su vegetarian* diet (excludes all animal products as well as onion, garlic, scallions, leeks, or shallots), *macrobiotic* diet (includes whole grains and beans and, in some cases, fish), and *raw vegan* diet (includes fresh and uncooked fruits, nuts, seeds, and vegetables). The safety of these restrictive diets has not been studied in children. These diets can be very limited in macro- and micronutrients and are not recommended for children. While being on a vegetarian or vegan diet does not appear to increase the risk of an eating disorder, some teenagers with disordered eating may choose such diets to aid in limiting their caloric intake.

Vegetarianism is considered a healthful and viable diet; both the U.S. Academy of Nutrition and Dietetics and the Dietitians of Canada have found that a properly planned and well-balanced vegetarian diet can satisfy the nutritional goals for all stages of life. Compared with non-vegetarian diets, vegetarian diets have lower intakes of saturated fat, cholesterol, and animal protein and relatively higher levels of complex carbohydrates, fiber, magnesium, potassium, folate, vitamins C and E, and phytochemicals. Vegetarians have a lower body mass index, cholesterol level, and blood pressure and are at decreased risk for cancer and ischemic heart disease. Specific nutrients of concern in vegetarian diets include the following:

◆ **Iron** (see Chapter 55): Vegetarian diets may have similar levels of iron as nonvegetarian diets, but iron from vegetable sources has lower bioavailability than iron from meat sources, and iron absorption may be inhibited by other dietary constituents, such as phytate (found in leafy green vegetables and whole grains). Iron stores are lower in vegetarians and vegans than in nonvegetarians; and iron deficiency is more common in vegetarian and vegan women and children. Foods rich in iron include iron-fortified cereals, black beans, cashews, kidney beans, lentils, oatmeal, raisins, black-eyed peas, soybeans, sunflower seeds, chickpeas, molasses, chocolate, and tempeh. Iron absorption can be increased by eating food containing ascorbic acid (vitamin C) along with foods containing iron.

◆ **Vitamin B$_{12}$:** Plants are not a good source of B$_{12}$ (see Chapter 62.7). Vitamin B$_{12}$ can be obtained through dairy products and eggs; vegans need fortified foods or supplements. Breastfeeding by vegan mothers can place an infant at risk for vitamin B$_{12}$ deficiency.

◆ **Fatty acids:** Vegetarians and vegans may be at risk for insufficient eicosapentaenoic acid (EPA) and DHA. The inclusion of sources of linolenic acid (precursor of EPA and DHA), such as walnuts, soy products, flaxseed oil, and canola oil, is recommended.

◆ **Calcium and vitamin D:** Without supplementation, vegan diets are low in calcium and vitamin D, putting vegans at risk for impaired bone mineralization (see Chapter 64). Serum hydroxyvitamin D levels should be monitored in vegans and supplemented for levels <30 dL. Calcium sources include leafy greens with low oxalate, such as broccoli, kale, and Chinese cabbage. Calcium and vitamin D are found in fortified almond, soy milk, and orange juice.

◆ **Zinc:** The bioavailability of zinc in plant sources tends to be low because of the presence of phytates and fiber that inhibit zinc absorption (see Chapter 67). Zinc is found in soy products, legumes, grains, cheese, and nuts.

◆ **Iodine:** Plant-based diets can be low in iodine, and therefore vegetarians and vegans who do not consume iodized salt or sea vegetables (which have variable iodine content) may be at risk of iodine deficiency. The exclusive use of sea salt or kosher salt could further increase that risk, because these are typically not iodized, and iodized salt is not used in processed foods.

Organic Foods

Parents may prefer organic foods to feed children secondary to concerns regarding chemical and hormonal content of animals and produce. **Organic food** is defined as produce and ingredients that are grown without the use of pesticides, synthetic fertilizers, sewage sludge, genetically modified organisms, or ionizing radiation. Animals that produce meat, poultry, eggs, and dairy products are not given antibiotics or growth hormones. In the United States, certification must be obtained, and USDA regulations must be followed to market food as "organic." The nutritional differences between organic and conventional foods may not be clinically relevant. Children consuming organic foods have lower or no detectable levels of pesticides in their urine compared to those consuming nonorganic foods. It remains unclear whether such a reduction in exposure to chemicals is clinically significant. Organic foods have higher levels of PUFAs (α-linolenic acid, very-long-chain n-3 fatty acids), α-tocopherol, and iron and lower levels of cadmium, selenium, and iodine. Similarly, despite concerns of parents, the amount of bovine growth hormone in conventional milk is thought to be neither significant nor biologically active in humans. Additionally, milk consumption from estrogen-treated cows does not result

in endocrine disruptions in infants. However, other chemicals in the environment, such as bisphenol-A (found in plastics), nitrates, endocrine disruptors, and phthalates, should be avoided. Organic certification of a food also suggests the food source is not from a genetically modified nutrient.

Genetically modified organisms (GMOs) in themselves may not be harmful. However, GMOs are modified to be resistant to the effects of herbicides, including glyphosate and 2,4-dichlorophenoxyacetic acid (2,4-D), which give GMOs a selective growth advantage. Nonetheless, glyphosate and 2,4-D have been designated by the International Agency for Research on Cancer as probable and possible human carcinogens, respectively.

Because the cost of organic foods is generally higher than that of other foods, a prudent approach is to explain to families that the scientific basis for choosing organic foods is uncertain, and that large-scale human studies to evaluate these issues will be difficult to carry out. If it is their preference, however, and they can afford the added cost, there is no reason not to eat organic foods.

Nutrition as Part of Complementary and Alternative Medicine, Functional Foods, Dietary Supplements, Vitamin Supplements, and Botanical and Herbal Products

The use of nutrition or nutritional supplements as complementary or alternative medicine is increasing, despite limited data on safety and efficacy, especially in children. Many parents assume that if a food or supplement is "natural" or "organic," there is no potential for risk and some potential for benefit. However, adverse effects of some dietary supplements have been documented, and some supplements have been discovered to contain common allergens. Dietary supplements, including botanical and herbal products, are regulated differently than medication in the United States. Manufacturers do not have to prove safety or efficacy before marketing the supplement; the potential for adverse effects or simply for inefficacy is therefore high. It is difficult for pediatricians to compete against the aggressive marketing through multimedia sources of food supplements to families of healthy and chronically ill children. Pediatricians must also compete against word of mouth, the internet, and advice from people without a scientific background and those with significant conflicts of interest.

Pediatricians are often asked by parents if their children need to receive a **daily multivitamin**. Unless the child follows a particular diet that may be poor in one or more nutrients for health, cultural, or religious reasons, or if the child has a chronic health condition that puts the child at risk for deficiency in one or more nutrients, multivitamins are not indicated. Many children do not follow all the guidelines of MyPlate, and parents and pediatricians may be tempted to use multivitamin supplements to ensure nutrient deficiencies are avoided. Use of a daily multivitamin supplement can result in a false impression that the child's diet is complete and in decreased efforts to meet dietary recommendations with food rather than the intake of supplements (see Chapter 55). The average U.S. diet provides more than a sufficient amount of most nutrients, including most vitamins. Therefore, multivitamins should not be routinely recommended.

Food Safety

Constantly keeping food safety issues in mind is an important aspect of feeding infants, children, and adolescents. In addition to choking hazards and food allergies, pediatricians and parents should be aware of food safety issues related to infectious agents and environmental contaminants. **Food poisoning** with bacteria, viruses, or their toxins is most common with raw or undercooked food, such as oysters, beef, and eggs, or cooked foods that have not been handled or stored properly. The specific bacteria and viruses involved in food poisoning are described in Chapter 740. Many chemical contaminants, such as heavy metals, pesticides, and organic compounds, are present in various foods, usually in small amounts. Because of concerns regarding their child's neurologic development and cancer risk, many questions arise from parents, especially after media coverage of isolated incidents. A recurring debate is the balance between the benefits of seafood for the growing brain and cardiovascular health and the risk of mercury contamination from consuming large, predatory fish species. Pediatricians need to become familiar with reliable sources of information, such as the websites of the U.S. Environmental Protection Agency (EPA), FDA, and CDC. The **Food Safety Modernization Act** provides the FDA with authority to have stricter control over food production and distribution. The FDA can require that manufacturers develop food safety plans. A good source of information for patients and parents can be found at www.foodsafety.gov.

Preventive Nutrition Counseling in Pediatric Primary Care

An important part of the primary care well child visit focuses on nutrition and growth because most families turn to pediatricians for guidance on child nutrition. Preventive nutrition is one of the cornerstones of preventive pediatrics and a critical aspect of anticipatory guidance. The first steps of nutrition counseling are nutritional status assessments, primarily done through growth monitoring and dietary intake assessment. Although **dietary assessment** is somewhat simple in infants who have a relatively monotonous diet, it is more challenging at older ages. The goals of dietary assessment in the primary care setting need to include an idea of the eating patterns (time, location, and environment) and usual diet by asking the parent to describe the child's dietary intake on a typical day or in the last 24 hr. Alternatively, a basic assessment of the child's consumption of vegetables, fruits, whole grains, low-fat or nonfat dairy products, 100% fruit juice, and sugar-sweetened beverages should be assessed. Pediatricians should encourage regularly scheduled meals and 1 or 2 healthy snacks (depending on the child's age). For more ambitious goals of dietary assessment, referral to a registered dietician with pediatric experience is recommended.

After understanding the child's usual diet, existing or anticipated nutritional problems should be addressed, such as diet quality, dietary habits, and portion size. For a few nutritional problems, a lack of knowledge can be addressed with nutrition education, but key nutritional issues, such as overeating or poor food choices, are not solely the result of lack of parents' knowledge. Therefore, nutrition education alone is insufficient in these situations, and pediatricians need to acquire training in behavior-modification techniques or refer to specialists to assist their patients in engaging in healthful feeding and eating behaviors. The physical, cultural, and family environment in which the child lives should always be considered so that nutrition counseling is relevant and changes are feasible.

One important aspect of nutrition counseling is providing families with sources of additional information and behavioral change tools. Although some handouts are available from government agencies, the AAP, and other professional organizations for families without internet access, an increasing number of families rely on the internet to find nutrition information. Therefore, pediatricians need to become familiar with common websites so that they can point families to reliable and unbiased sources of information. Perhaps the most useful websites for children are the AAP and USDA MyPlate sites and those of the CDC, FDA, National Institutes of Health, The National Academies, and Food and Nutrition Board for government sources. Other professional resources include the American Heart Association and Academy of Nutrition and Dietetics. Pediatricians should also be aware of sites that provide biased or even dangerous information so that they can warn families accordingly. Examples include dieting sites, sites that openly promote dietary supplements or other food products, and the sites of "nonprofit" organizations that are mainly sponsored by food companies or that have other social or political agendas.

U.S. Food Assistance Programs

Several programs exist in the United States to ensure sufficient and high-quality nutrition for children of families who cannot always afford optimal nutrition. One of the most utilized federal programs is the **Special Supplemental Nutrition Program for Women, Infants, and Children (WIC)**. This program provides nutrition supplements to a large proportion of pregnant women, postpartum women, and children up to their 5th birthday. One of its strengths is that in order to qualify, families need to regularly visit a WIC nutritionist, who can be a useful resource for nutritional counseling. For older children, federal programs provide school lunches, breakfasts, and after-school meals, as well as daycare and summer nutrition. Lower-income families are also eligible for the **Supplemental Nutrition Assistance Program (SNAP)**, formerly known as the Food Stamp Program. This program provides funds directly to families to purchase various food items in regular food stores.

Bibliography is available at Expert Consult.

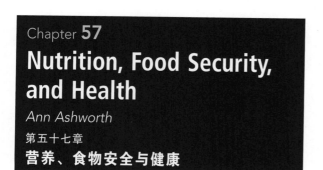

Chapter **57**

Nutrition, Food Security, and Health

Ann Ashworth

第五十七章
营养、食物安全与健康

中文导读

本章主要介绍了食物安全和健康威胁下的营养不　　良、食物安全、营养低下以及严重的急性营养不良。

具体描述了食物安全的监测、食物安全与贫穷、食物安全与营养目标以及食物安全未来规划；具体描述了营养低下的评估、流行病学、健康结局、临床表现与治疗；还具体描述了严重急性营养不良的临床表现、病理生理改变以及主要治疗措施。

MALNUTRITION AS THE INTERSECTION OF FOOD INSECURITY AND HEALTH INSECURITY

Undernutrition is usually an outcome of three factors, often in combination: household food supply, childcare practices, and access to health and water/sanitation services. In famine and emergency settings, food shortage is the foremost factor, but in many countries with widespread undernutrition, food production or access to food might not be the most limiting factor. More important causes might be repeated childhood infections, especially diarrheal diseases associated with an unsafe environment and lack of exclusive breastfeeding, or inadequate complementary feeding practices, or the lack of time families have available for appropriate infant or maternal care. Fig. 57.1 shows some of the many causal factors on the pathway to undernutrition and how they extend from household and community levels to national/international levels. Inequitable distribution of resources because of political, economic, and agricultural policies often denies families their right to adequate land, water, food, healthcare, education, and a safe environment, all of which can influence nutritional status.

Families with few economic resources who know how to care for their children and are enabled to do so can often use available food and health services to produce well-nourished children. If food resources and health services are not available in a community, not utilized, or not accessible to some families, children might become undernourished. Undernutrition is not confined to low-income countries. It has been noted in chronically ill patients in neonatal and pediatric intensive care units in high-income countries and among patients with burns, human immunodeficiency virus (HIV) infection, tuberculosis, cystic fibrosis, chronic diarrhea syndromes, malignancies, bone marrow transplantation, and inborn errors of metabolism. Severe malnutrition has been reported in affluent communities in infants whose families believe in fad diets, as well as in infants with food allergies fed nutritionally inadequate foods such as rice "milk," which has a very low protein and micronutrient content (Figs. 57.2 and 57.3).

FOOD SECURITY

Food security exists when all people, at all times, have access to sufficient, safe, nutritious food to maintain a healthy and active life. Four main dimensions of food security can be identified: availability, access, utilization, and stability. **Availability** refers to the *supply* of food, reflecting the level of food production, food stocks, and net trade. **Access** is at the household level, reflecting purchasing power, household food production, and food/cash transfers received through social "safety net" programs. The **utilization** dimension recognizes that even when a household has access to food, it is not necessarily shared equitably within a household. **Stability** refers to being "food secure" at all times: Examples of situations that affect stability are the "lean seasons" before a harvest, natural disasters, political unrest, and rising food prices. To be food secure, all four dimensions must be met simultaneously.

Measuring Food Insecurity

The most commonly used measurement of food insecurity is *undernourishment* (chronic hunger), which is the proportion of the population who are unable to meet daily energy requirements for light activities. It is an estimate calculated by the **Food and Agriculture Organization (FAO)** based on country-level food balance sheets. It does not take nutrient adequacy into account, but has the advantage of being available for almost all countries annually (although with a time lag) and assists

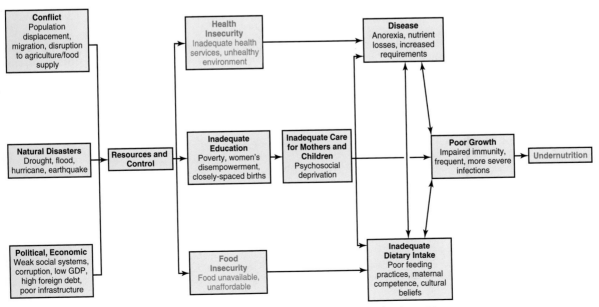

Fig. 57.1 Basic, underlying, and immediate causes of undernutrition.

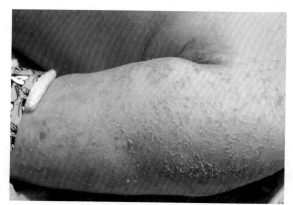

Fig. 57.2 A 14 mo old girl with "flaky paint" dermatitis. *(From Katz KA, Mahlberg MH, Honig PJ, et al: Rice nightmare: kwashiorkor in 2 Philadelphia-area infants fed Rice Dream beverage, J Am Acad Dermatol 52(5 Suppl 1):S69–S72, 2005.)*

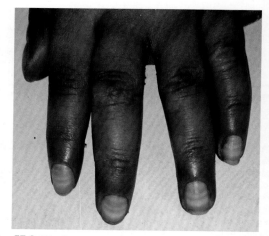

Fig. 57.3 Paired, transverse, homogeneous, and smooth bordered lines noted in all finger nails suggestive of Muehrcke lines in an infant fed diluted cow's milk since birth. *(From Williams V, Jayashree M: Muehrcke lines in an infant, J Pediatr 189:234, 2017.)*

in monitoring global trends. In addition, FAO measures food access by asking individuals about their experiences over the last 12 mo, such as whether they ran out of food or skipped meals. The responses are graded from mild to severe food insecurity. This relatively simple monitoring tool, the **Food Insecurity Experience Scale**, provides timely information to guide decision-making at national and local levels.

In 2017, FAO estimated that about 821 million people, or 10.9% of the world's population, were undernourished, 98% of whom were in developing countries. The majority are rural poor people subsisting on small plots of land or hired as laborers, and urban poor people who lack the means to grow or buy food. Alongside the 0.82 billion people who are underfed are 1.9 billion who are overfed, reflecting global inequalities and the "double burden of malnutrition" in low- and middle-income countries.

Nutrition, Food Security, and Poverty

Household food security tracks income closely. With rising incomes, very poor households first increase their dietary energy intake to avert hunger. If incomes rise further, there is a shift to more expensive staple foods and then to a more varied diet with a greater proportion of energy from animal sources, fruits/vegetables, and fats/sugars, and less from cereals, roots, and tubers. National economic growth tends to be accompanied by reductions in stunting, but economic growth can pass by poor persons if they work in unaffected sectors, or are unable to take advantage of new opportunities because of lack of education, access to credit, or transportation, or if governments do not channel resources accruing from economic growth to healthcare, education, social protection, and other public services and infrastructure. There is good evidence that economic growth reduces poverty but does not necessarily reduce undernutrition.

Food Security and Nutrition Targets

The period of Millennium Development Goals (MDGs) ended in 2015. All developing regions except sub-Saharan Africa achieved the target to halve the proportion of people living in extreme poverty, with the proportion falling from 47% in 1990 to 14% in 2015. Reductions in hunger were broadly consistent with those of poverty reduction, and rates of undernourishment in developing regions fell from 23% in 1990 to 13% in 2015. The prevalence of underweight children (another MDG indicator of "hunger") fell from 29% in 1990 to 15% in 2015 for the developing regions combined. Rural children are almost twice as likely to be underweight as urban children, and the poorest quintile is almost 3 times as likely to be underweight as the richest quintile.

Eradicating poverty and hunger continue to be core targets of the **Sustainable Development Goals**, as agreed by 193 countries of the

Table 57.1	Global Food Security and Nutrition Targets
ZERO HUNGER CHALLENGE OBJECTIVES	**WORLD HEALTH ASSEMBLY GLOBAL NUTRITION TARGETS FOR 2025**
1. Access to an adequate and stable food supply for all 2. Elimination of stunting in children <2 yr, and no malnutrition in pregnancy and early childhood 3. Sustainable food systems 4. Doubling of smallholder productivity and income, particularly for women 5. No loss or waste of food, and responsible consumption	1. A 40% reduction in the number of stunted children <5 yr 2. A 50% reduction in anemia in women of reproductive age 3. A 30% reduction in low birthweight 4. No increase in childhood overweight 5. Increase exclusive breastfeeding rates to at least 50% in the 1st 6 mo 6. Reduce and maintain childhood wasting to <5%

United Nations General Assembly in September 2015, and are to be achieved by 2030. In addition, in 2012 the World Health Assembly agreed to 6 global nutrition targets to be reached by 2025, measured against a 2010 baseline, and the United Nations Secretary-General launched the **Zero Hunger Challenge** with 5 objectives that "would boost economic growth, reduce poverty and safeguard the environment" and "would foster peace and stability" (Table 57.1).

Future Food Security

Between now and 2050 the world's population is expected to exceed 9 billion, and an increase in food supply of 70–100% will be needed to feed this larger, more urban, and more affluent populace. Over this same period, the world's food supply is expected to diminish unless action is taken. Accelerating the decline in fertility rates and reducing overconsumption are basic but difficult actions to bridge the gap between increasing demand and diminishing supply. Equally challenging actions include limiting climate disruption, increasing the efficiency of food production, reducing waste, and reducing the demand for meat and dairy foods.

◆ *Limit climate disruption.* Drought, floods, and other extreme weather events are becoming more prevalent and destroy crops and livestock, often on a huge scale. Rising sea levels will lead to loss of productive land through inundation and salinization. Acidification of oceans will reduce marine harvests. Because curbing greenhouse gas emissions is essential to minimize climate disruption, the goals are (1) to cut fossil fuel use by at least half of present levels by 2050 so as to reduce carbon dioxide (CO_2) emissions and (2) change livestock husbandry and agronomic practices to reduce methane and nitrous oxide (N_2O) emissions.

◆ *Increase efficiency of food production.* Expanding the area of agricultural land to any large extent (e.g., by deforestation) is not a sustainable option because of adverse consequences on ecosystems and biodiversity, although some expansion of food production could be achieved by switching good-quality land away from first-generation biofuels. For example, almost 40% of the U.S. corn harvest in 2016–2017 went to biofuels. Efforts to increase the intensity of production need to be environmentally sustainable. These include optimizing yields by soil and water conservation, removal of technical and financial constraints faced by farmers, and breeding resource-efficient crops and livestock that are also climate resilient and pest/disease resistant.

◆ *Reduce waste.* From 30–40% of food is wasted, between harvesting and the market, during retail, at home, and in the food service industry. Better transport and storage facilities in developing countries, less stringent sell-by dates, lower cosmetic standards for fruits and vegetables, and ending supersized portions would help reduce waste.

◆ *Change diets.* As wealth increases, so does the demand for processed foods, meat, dairy products, and fish. About one third of global cereal production is fed to animals, so reducing consumption of meat from grain-fed livestock and increasing the proportion derived from the most efficient sources (pigs and poultry) would allow more people to be fed from the same amount of land.

UNDERNUTRITION

The greatest risk of undernutrition (underweight, stunting, wasting, and micronutrient deficiencies) occurs in the first 1000 days, from conception to 24 mo of age, and this early damage to growth and development can have adverse consequences in later life on health, intellectual ability, school achievement, work productivity, and earnings. Governments and agencies are therefore advised to focus interventions on this critical window of opportunity. For folate deficiency, which increases the risk of birth defects, this particular window is before conception.

Measurement of Undernutrition

The term **malnutrition** encompasses both ends of the nutrition spectrum, from undernutrition to overweight. Many poor nutritional outcomes begin in utero and are manifest as low birthweight (LBW, <2,500 g). Preterm delivery and fetal growth restriction are the 2 main causes of LBW, with prematurity relatively more common in richer countries and fetal growth restriction relatively more common in poorer countries.

Nutritional status is often assessed in terms of anthropometry (Table 57.2). International standards of normal child growth under optimum conditions from birth to 5 yr have been established by the World Health Organization (WHO). To compile the standards, longitudinal data from birth to 24 mo of healthy, breastfed, term infants were combined with cross-sectional measurements of children ages 18-71 mo. The standards allow normalization of anthropometric measures in terms of z scores (standard deviation [SD] scores). A z-score is the child's height (weight) minus the median height (weight) for the child's age and sex divided by the relevant SD. The standards are applicable to all children everywhere, having been derived from a large, multicountry study reflecting diverse ethnic backgrounds and cultural settings.

Height-for-age (or length-for-age for children <2 yr) is a measure of linear growth, and a deficit represents the cumulative impact of adverse events, usually in the first 1000 days from conception, that result in *stunting*, or chronic malnutrition. A low height-for-age typically reflects socioeconomic disadvantage. A low **weight-for-height**, or *wasting*, usually indicates acute malnutrition. Conversely, a high weight-for-height indicates *overweight*. **Weight-for-age** is the most commonly used index of nutritional status, although a low value has limited clinical significance because it does not differentiate between wasting and stunting. Weight-for-age has the advantage of being somewhat easier to measure than indices that require height measurements. In humanitarian emergencies and some community or outpatient settings, **mid-upper arm circumference** is used for screening wasted children (Fig. 57.4).

Body mass index (BMI) is calculated by dividing weight in kilograms by the square of height in meters. For children, BMI is age and gender specific. **BMI-for-age** can be used from birth to 20 yr and is a screening tool for *thinness* (less than −2 SD), *overweight* (between +1 SD and +2 SD), and *obesity* (greater than +2 SD). To diagnose obesity, additional measures of adiposity are desirable because a high BMI can result from high muscularity, and not only from excess subcutaneous fat.

Micronutrient deficiencies are another dimension of undernutrition. Those of particular public health significance are vitamin A, iodine, iron, and zinc deficiencies.

Vitamin A deficiency is caused by a low intake of retinol (in animal foods) or its carotenoid precursors, mainly beta carotene (in orange-colored fruits and vegetables and dark-green leaves) (see Chapter 61).

Table 57.2	Classification of Undernutrition	
CLASSIFICATION	**INDEX**	**GRADING**
Gomez (underweight)	90–75% of median weight-for-age	Grade 1 (mild)
	75-60%	Grade 2 (moderate)
	<60%	Grade 3 (severe)
Waterlow (wasting)	90–80% of median weight-for-height	Mild
	80–70%	Moderate
	<70%	Severe
Waterlow (stunting)	95–90% of median height-for-age	Mild
	90–85%	Moderate
	<85%	Severe
WHO (wasting)	< −2 to > −3 SD weight-for-height	Moderate
	< −3	Severe
WHO (stunting)	< −2 to > −3 SD height-for-age	Moderate
	<−3	Severe
WHO (wasting) (for age-group 6-59 mo)	115-125 mm mid-upper arm circumference	Moderate
	<115 mm	Severe

SD, Standard deviation; WHO, World Health Organization.

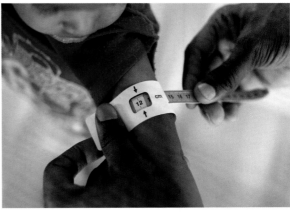

Fig. 57.4 Measuring mid-upper arm circumference. (*Courtesy of Nyani Quarmyne/Panos Pictures.*)

The prevalence of *clinical deficiency* is assessed from symptoms and signs of xerophthalmia (principally night blindness and Bitot spots). *Subclinical deficiency* is defined as serum retinol concentration ≤0.70 μmol/L. Vitamin A deficiency is the leading cause of preventable blindness in children. It is also associated with a higher morbidity and mortality among young children.

Iodine deficiency is the main cause of preventable intellectual impairment (see Chapter 67). An enlarged thyroid (goiter) is a sign of deficiency. Severe deficiency in pregnancy causes fetal loss and permanent damage to the brain and central nervous system in surviving offspring (cretinism). It can be prevented by iodine supplementation before conception or during the 1st trimester of pregnancy. Postnatal iodine deficiency is associated with impaired mental function and growth retardation. The median urinary iodine concentration in children age 6-12 yr is used to assess the prevalence of deficiency in the general population, and a median of <100 μg/L indicates insufficient iodine intake.

Iron-deficiency anemia is common in childhood either from low iron intakes or poor absorption, or as a result of illness or parasite infestation (see Chapter 67). Women also have relatively high rates of anemia as a result of menstrual blood loss, pregnancy, low iron intake, poor absorption, and illness. Hemoglobin cutoffs to define anemia are 110 g/L for children 6-59 mo, 115 g/L for children 5-11 yr, and 120 g/L for children 12-14 yr. Cutoffs to define anemia for nonpregnant women are 120 g/L, 110 g/L for pregnant women, and 130 g/L for men.

Zinc deficiency increases the risk of morbidity and mortality from diarrhea, pneumonia, and possibly other infectious diseases (see Chapter 67). Zinc deficiency also has an adverse effect on linear growth. Deficiency at the population level is assessed from dietary zinc intakes or serum zinc concentrations.

Prevalence of Undernutrition

It is estimated that approximately 16% of births worldwide in 2013 were LBW. Rates of LBW are highest (28%) in southern Asia, which are twice those of sub-Saharan Africa. Globally, in 2015, 14% of children <5 yr of age were *underweight* (weight-for-age < −2 SD). The global prevalence of *stunting* (height-for-age < −2 SD) has declined from 33% in 2000 to 22% in 2017, with the greatest reductions occurring in Asia. Stunting prevalence is highest in the African region (30%). *Wasting* (weight-for-height < −2 SD) affects 7% of children <5 yr, with minimal change in prevalence over the past 2 decades. These figures represent 151 million stunted children, and 51 million wasted children.

Asia carries most of the global burden of underweight children because of the combination of large population size and high prevalence. In 2017, 55% of all stunted children and 69% of all wasted children lived in Asia. Africa carries most of the remaining global burden. For children <5 yr, the global prevalence is estimated to be 33% for *vitamin A deficiency*, 29% for *iodine deficiency*, 17% for *zinc deficiency*, and 18% for *iron-deficiency anemia*. Prevalence of micronutrient deficiencies tends to be highest in Africa. For pregnant women, the estimated prevalence of vitamin A deficiency is 15% and for iron-deficiency anemia, 19%.

Rates of clinical deficiency of vitamin A in children <5 yr have been declining, probably as a result of high-dose vitamin A supplementation programs and measles vaccination (because measles leads to sizable urinary loss of vitamin A), but subclinical deficiency remains widespread (>90 million children). Large-scale availability of iodized salt has reduced rates of iodine deficiency substantially, and iodized salt reaches an estimated 75% of households. In contrast, progress in reducing rates of iron-deficiency anemia is slow, and rates remain largely static.

Consequences of Undernutrition

The most profound consequence of undernutrition is premature death (Table 57.3). Fetal growth restriction together with suboptimal breastfeeding in the 1st month of life contribute to 19% of all deaths in children <5 yr (1.3 million deaths/yr). When the effects of stunting, wasting, and deficiencies of vitamin A and zinc are also considered, these 6 items jointly contribute to 45% of global child deaths (3.1 million deaths/ yr), and many more are disabled or stunted for life. Anemia contributes to over one quarter of maternal deaths.

The risk of child death from infectious diseases increases even with mild undernutrition, and as the severity of undernutrition increases, the risk increases exponentially (Table 57.4). Undernutrition impairs immune function and other host defenses; consequently, childhood infections are more severe and longer-lasting in undernourished children and more likely to be fatal than the same illnesses in well-nourished children. Infections can adversely affect nutritional status, and young children can quickly enter a cycle of repeated infections and ever-worsening malnutrition. Even for the survivors, physical and cognitive damage as a result of undernutrition can impact their future health and economic well-being. For girls, the cycle of undernutrition is passed on to the next generation when undernourished women give birth to LBW babies.

Fetal growth restriction and early childhood undernutrition have consequences for adult chronic illness. LBW is associated with an increased risk of hypertension, stroke, and type 2 diabetes in adults. The increased risk is thought to reflect "fetal programming," a process by which fetal undernutrition leads to permanent changes in the structure and metabolism of organs and systems that manifest as disease in later life. The risk is exacerbated by low weight gain during the first 2 yr of life. The increased risk of adult chronic disease from undernutrition early in life is a particular challenge to low-income countries with rapid economic growth.

Stunting before age 3 yr is associated with poorer motor and cognitive development and altered behavior in later years. The effect is 6-13 DQ (developmental quotient) points. Iodine and iron deficiencies also lead to loss of cognitive potential. Indications are that children living in areas of chronic iodine deficiency have an average reduction in IQ (intelligence quotient) of 12-13.5 points compared with children in iodine-sufficient areas. Iron deficiency has a detrimental effect on the motor development of children <4 yr and on cognition of school-age children. The estimated deficit is 1.73 IQ points for each 10 g/L decrease in hemoglobin concentration.

Undernutrition can have substantial economic consequences for survivors and their families. The consequences can be quantified in 5 categories: (1) increased costs of healthcare, either neonatal care for LBW babies or treatment of illness for infants and young children; (2) productivity losses (and thus reduced earnings) associated with smaller stature and muscle mass; (3) productivity losses from reduced cognitive ability and poorer school performance; (4) increased costs of chronic diseases associated with fetal and early child malnutrition; and (5) consequences of maternal undernutrition on future generations. The

Table 57.3	Global Deaths in Children <5 yr Attributed to Nutritional Conditions	
CONDITION	**ATTRIBUTABLE DEATHS**	**% OF TOTAL DEATHS <5 YR**
(a) Fetal growth restriction (<1 mo)	817,000	11.8
(b) Stunting (1-59 mo)	1,017,000	14.7
(c) Wasting (1-59 mo)	875,000	12.6
(d) Zinc deficiency (12-59 mo)	116,000	1.7
(e) Vitamin A deficiency (6-59 mo)	157,000	2.3
(f) Suboptimal breastfeeding (0-23 mo)	804,000	11.6
Joint effects of (a) + (f)	1,348,000	19.4
Joint effects of all 6 factors	3,097,000	44.7

From Black RE, Victora CG, Walker SP, et al: Maternal and child undernutrition and overweight in low- and middle-income countries, *Lancet* 382:427–451, 2013.

| Table 57.4 | Hazard Ratios for All-Cause and Cause-Specific Deaths Associated With Stunting, Wasting, and Underweight in Children <5 yr | | | | |

STANDARD DEVIATION (SD) SCORE	DEATHS				
	All	Pneumonia	Diarrhea	Measles	Other Infections
Height/length-for-age					
< −3	5.5	6.4	6.3	6.0	3.0
−3 to < −2	2.3	2.2	2.4	2.8	1.9
−2 to < −1	1.5	1.6	1.7	1.3	0.9
≥ −1	1.0	1.0	1.0	1.0	1.0
Weight-for-length					
< −3	11.6	9.7	12.3	9.6	11.2
−3 to < −2	3.4	4.7	3.4	2.6	2.7
−2 to < −1	1.6	1.9	1.6	1.0	1.7
≥ −1	1.0	1.0	1.0	1.0	1.0
Weight-for-age					
< −3	9.4	10.1	11.6	7.7	8.3
−3 to < −2	2.6	3.1	2.9	3.1	1.6
−2 to < −1	1.5	1.9	1.7	1.0	1.5
≥ −1	1.0	1.0	1.0	1.0	1.0

From Black RE, Victora CG, Walker SP, et al: Maternal and child undernutrition and overweight in low- and middle-income countries, *Lancet* 382:427–451, 2013.

impact of nutrition on earnings appears to be independent of the effects of childhood deprivation.

Key Interventions

Interventions to address child undernutrition can be divided into those that address immediate causes (*nutrition-specific interventions*) and those that address underlying causes (*nutrition-sensitive interventions*) (Table 57.5). In the short-term, nutrition-specific interventions (e.g., salt iodization) can have substantial impact even in the absence of economic growth, and micronutrient interventions (supplementation and fortification) are consistently ranked as the most cost-effective investment. There is increased attention to nutrition-sensitive interventions as the best means of sustainably eliminating malnutrition, and to multisectoral policies that harness the synergism between the two types of intervention (e.g., cross-sectoral linkages among agriculture, nutrition, and health).

To reduce the adverse consequences of undernutrition on mortality, morbidity, and cognitive development, interventions must encompass both fetal and postnatal periods. Preventing LBW is essential, with emphasis on prevention of low maternal BMI and anemia, and in the longer term, prevention of low maternal stature. Other measures include smoking cessation, birth spacing, delaying pregnancy until after 18 yr of age, and intermittent preventive treatment of malaria. In the postnatal period, promotion and support of exclusive breastfeeding is a high priority. Although the Baby Friendly Hospital Initiative has a marked benefit on rates of exclusive breastfeeding in hospital, postnatal counseling from community workers or volunteers is needed to facilitate continuation of exclusive breastfeeding at home for 6 mo (see Chapter 56). Most studies show a lower risk of HIV transmission with exclusive breastfeeding than with mixed breastfeeding. The risk of HIV transmission by breastfeeding is approximately 5–20%, depending on duration, but can be reduced to <2% with antiretroviral drugs. Even without antiretroviral drugs, exclusively breastfed children of HIV-infected mothers in low-income countries have lower mortality than non-breastfed children, because the latter are at increased risk of death from diarrhea and pneumonia.

Interventions to improve infant feeding must be designed for the local setting and thus require careful formative research during their development. Messages should be few, feasible, and culturally appropriate.

Table 57.5	Examples of Nutrition-Specific and Nutrition-Sensitive Interventions
NUTRITION-SPECIFIC INTERVENTIONS	**NUTRITION-SENSITIVE INTERVENTIONS**
• Promotion and support for exclusive breastfeeding for 6 mo, and continued breastfeeding for at least 2 yr • Promotion of adequate, timely, and safe complementary feeding from 6 mo • Increased micronutrient intake through dietary diversity • Micronutrient supplements for pregnant women (iron/folate) and young children (vitamin A, iron, zinc) in deficient areas • Zinc supplements to children during and after diarrhea (10-20 mg/day for 2 wk) • Prevention and treatment of severe acute malnutrition • Crop biofortification, food fortification, salt iodization • Reduced heavy physical activity in pregnancy	• Increased access to affordable, nutritious food; smallholder agriculture; credit and microfinance • Postharvest food processing and preservation • Vaccination against neonatal and childhood illness; access to healthcare • Improved water/sanitation and hygiene (e.g., handwashing with soap) • Education; women's empowerment; gender equality • Social protection (e.g., cash transfers) • Malaria prevention (vector control/bednets); intermittent preventive treatment during pregnancy and in children 3-59 mo • Birth spacing; delaying pregnancy until after 18 yr of age

For complementary feeding, nutrient-rich energy-dense mixtures of foods and responsive feeding are often emphasized. Where adequate complementary feeding is difficult to achieve and subclinical deficiencies are common, high-dose vitamin A supplementation every 6 mo in children 6-59 mo of age reduces all-cause mortality and death due to diarrhea by 12%, and zinc supplementation can reduce 1-4 yr mortality by 18%, diarrhea incidence by 13%, and pneumonia by 19%. Monitoring of child growth provides an early alert to a nutrition or health problem but is only worthwhile if accompanied by good counseling and growth promotion activities. The impact of growth monitoring and promotion will depend on coverage, intensity of contact, health worker performance and communication skills, adequacy of resources, and the motivation and ability of families to follow agreed actions.

Clinical Manifestations and Treatment of Undernutrition

Treatment of vitamin and mineral deficiencies is discussed in Chapters 61-67. Treatment of LBW and intrauterine growth restriction is discussed in Chapter 117.

SEVERE ACUTE MALNUTRITION

Severe acute malnutrition is defined as severe wasting and/or bilateral edema.

Severe wasting is extreme thinness diagnosed by a weight-for-length (or height) < −3 SD of the WHO Child Growth Standards. In children ages 6-59 mo, a mid-upper arm circumference <115 mm also denotes extreme thinness: a color-banded tape (see Fig. 57.4) is a convenient way of screening children in need of treatment.

Bilateral edema is diagnosed by grasping both feet, placing a thumb on top of each, and pressing gently but firmly for 10 sec. A pit (dent) remaining under each thumb indicates bilateral edema.

This definition of severe acute malnutrition distinguishes wasted/edematous children from those who are stunted, since stunted children (although underweight) are not a priority for acute clinical care because their deficits in height and weight cannot be corrected in the short term. The previous name *protein-energy malnutrition* is avoided because it oversimplifies the complex, multideficiency etiology. Other terms are *marasmus* (severe wasting), *kwashiorkor* (characterized by edema), and *marasmic-kwashiorkor* (severe wasting and edema).

Children with severe acute malnutrition have had a diet insufficient in energy and nutrients relative to their needs. The magnitude of the deficits will differ depending on the duration of inadequacy, quantity and diversity of food consumed, presence of antinutrients (e.g., phytate), individual variation in requirements, and number and severity of coexisting infections and their duration. Infections can lead to profound nutrient deficits and imbalances: For example, amino acids are diverted to form acute-phase proteins, and potassium, magnesium, vitamin A, and zinc are lost through diarrhea, and losses of glycine and taurine are linked to small bowel bacterial overgrowth. Ingested microbes can cause villous atrophy and loss of nutrients from maldigestion and malabsorption, as well as disruption of gut barrier function leading to microbial translocation, chronic immune activation, and altered gut microbiome (environmental enteric dysfunction). Deficits can also arise from increased nutrient utilization in response to noxae (e.g., cysteine and methionine to detoxify dietary cyanogens).

Heterogeneity in the extent and nature of the deficits and imbalances, reflecting the diverse pathways to severe acute malnutrition, helps explain why affected children differ in their clinical presentation and degree of metabolic disturbance. Children who develop edematous malnutrition are more likely than nonedematous children to have been exposed to noxae that generate oxidative stress and/or to have greater deficits in free radical–scavenging antioxidants (glutathione, vitamins A, C, and E, and essential fatty acids) or cofactors (zinc, copper, selenium).

Clinical Manifestations of Severe Acute Malnutrition (Table 57.6)

Severe wasting is most visible on the thighs, buttocks, and upper arms, as well as over the ribs and scapulae, where loss of fat and skeletal muscle is greatest (Fig. 57.5). Wasting is preceded by failure to gain weight and then by weight loss. The skin loses turgor and becomes loose as subcutaneous tissues are broken down to provide energy. The face may retain a relatively normal appearance, but eventually becomes wasted and wizened. The eyes may be sunken from loss of retroorbital fat, and lacrimal and salivary glands may atrophy, leading to lack of tears and a dry mouth. Weakened abdominal muscles and gas from bacterial overgrowth of the upper gut may lead to a distended abdomen. Severely wasted children are often fretful and irritable.

In **edematous malnutrition** the edema is most likely to appear first in the feet and then in the lower legs. It can quickly develop into generalized edema affecting also the hands, arms, and face (Fig. 57.6). Skin changes typically occur over the swollen limbs and include dark, crackled peeling patches ("flaky paint" dermatosis) with pale skin underneath that is easily infected (see Figs. 57.2 and 57.6). The hair is sparse and easily pulled out and may lose its curl. In dark-haired children the hair may turn pale or reddish. The liver is often enlarged with fat. Children with edema are miserable and apathetic, and often refuse to eat.

Pathophysiology

When a child's intake is insufficient to meet daily needs, physiologic and metabolic changes take place in an orderly progression to conserve energy and prolong life. This process is called *reductive adaptation*. Fat stores are mobilized to provide energy. Later, protein in muscle, skin, and the gastrointestinal tract is mobilized. Energy is conserved by reducing physical activity and growth, reducing basal metabolism and the functional reserve of organs, and reducing inflammatory and immune responses. These changes have important consequences:

◆ The liver makes glucose less readily, making the child more prone to hypoglycemia. It produces less albumin, transferrin, and other transport proteins. It is less able to cope with excess dietary protein and to excrete toxins.
◆ Heat production is less, making the child more vulnerable to hypothermia.
◆ The kidneys are less able to excrete excess fluid and sodium, and fluid easily accumulates in the circulation, increasing the risk of fluid overload.

Table 57.6	Clinical Signs of Malnutrition
SITE	**SIGNS**
Face	Moon face (kwashiorkor), simian facies (marasmus)
Eye	Dry eyes, pale conjunctiva, Bitot spots (vitamin A), periorbital edema
Mouth	Angular stomatitis, cheilitis, glossitis, spongy bleeding gums (vitamin C), parotid enlargement
Teeth	Enamel mottling, delayed eruption
Hair	Dull, sparse, brittle hair; hypopigmentation; flag sign (alternating bands of light and normal color); broomstick eyelashes; alopecia
Skin	Loose and wrinkled (marasmus); shiny and edematous (kwashiorkor); dry, follicular hyperkeratosis; patchy hyper- and hypopigmentation ("crazy paving" or "flaky paint" dermatoses); erosions; poor wound healing
Nails	Koilonychia; thin and soft nail plates, fissures, or ridges
Musculature	Muscle wasting, particularly buttocks and thighs; Chvostek or Trousseau sign (hypocalcemia)
Skeletal	Deformities, usually as a result of calcium, vitamin D, or vitamin C deficiencies
Abdomen	Distended: hepatomegaly with fatty liver; ascites may be present
Cardiovascular	Bradycardia, hypotension, reduced cardiac output, small vessel vasculopathy
Neurologic	Global developmental delay, loss of knee and ankle reflexes, impaired memory
Hematologic	Pallor, petechiae, bleeding diathesis
Behavior	Lethargic, apathetic, irritable on handling

From Grover Z, Ee LC: Protein energy malnutrition, *Pediatr Clin North Am* 56:1055–1068, 2009.

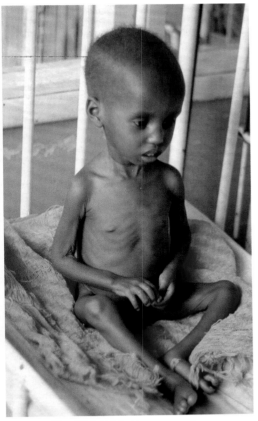

Fig. 57.5 Child with severe wasting.

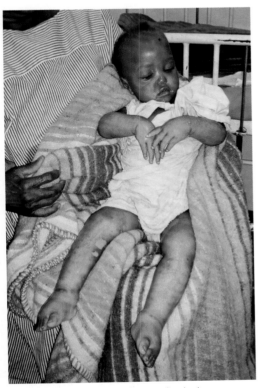

Fig. 57.6 Child with generalized edema.

- The heart is smaller and weaker and has a reduced output, and fluid overload readily leads to death from cardiac failure.
- Sodium builds up inside cells due to leaky cell membranes and reduced activity of the sodium-potassium pump, leading to excess body sodium, fluid retention, and edema.
- Potassium leaks out of cells and is excreted in urine, contributing to electrolyte imbalance, fluid retention, edema, and anorexia.
- Loss of muscle protein is accompanied by loss of potassium, magnesium, zinc, and copper.
- The gut produces less gastric acid and enzymes. Motility is reduced, and bacteria may colonize the stomach and small intestine, damaging the mucosa and deconjugating bile salts. Digestion and absorption are impaired.
- Cell replication and repair are reduced, increasing the risk of bacterial translocation through the gut mucosa.
- Immune function is impaired, especially cell-mediated immunity. The usual responses to infection may be absent, even in severe illness, increasing the risk of undiagnosed infection.
- Red blood cell mass is reduced, releasing iron, which requires glucose and amino acids to be converted to ferritin, increasing the risk of hypoglycemia and amino acid imbalances. If conversion to ferritin is incomplete, unbound iron promotes pathogen growth and formation of free radicals.
- Micronutrient deficiencies limit the body's ability to deactivate free radicals, which cause cell damage. Edema and hair/skin changes are outward signs of cell damage.

When prescribing treatment, it is essential to take these changes in function into account. Otherwise, organs and systems will be overwhelmed, and death will rapidly ensue.

Principles of Treatment
Fig. 57.7 shows the 10 steps of treatment, which are separated into 2 phases, stabilization and rehabilitation. These steps apply to all clinical forms and all geographic locations, including North America and Europe. The aim of the **stabilization** phase is to repair cellular function, correct fluid and electrolyte imbalance, restore homeostasis, and prevent death from the interlinked triad of hypoglycemia, hypothermia, and infection. The aim of the **rehabilitation** phase is to restore wasted tissues (i.e., catch-up growth). It is essential that treatment proceeds in an ordered progression and that the metabolic machinery is repaired before any attempt is made to promote weight gain. Pushing ahead too quickly risks inducing the potentially fatal "refeeding syndrome" (see Chapter 58).

Caregivers bring children to health facilities because of illness, rarely because of their malnutrition. A common mistake among healthcare providers is to focus on the illness and treat as for a well-nourished child. This approach ignores the deranged metabolism in malnourished children and can be fatal. Such children should be considered as severely malnourished with a complication, and treatment should follow the 10 steps. Two other potentially fatal mistakes are to treat edema with a diuretic and to give a high-protein diet in the early phase of treatment.

Emergency Treatment
Table 57.7 summarizes the therapeutic directives for malnourished children with shock and other emergency conditions. Note that treatment of shock in these children is different (less rapid, smaller volume, different fluid) from treatment of shock in well-nourished children, because shock from dehydration and shock from sepsis often coexist and are difficult to differentiate on clinical grounds. Thus the physician must be guided by the response to treatment: children with dehydration respond to intravenous (IV) fluid, whereas those with septic shock will not respond. Since severely malnourished children can quickly succumb to fluid overload, they must be monitored closely.

Stabilization
Table 57.8 summarizes the therapeutic directives for stabilization steps 1-7 (Fig. 57.7). Giving broad-spectrum antibiotics (Table 57.9) and feeding frequent small amounts of F75 (a specially formulated low-lactose

milk with 75 kcal and 0.9 g protein per 100 mL to which potassium, magnesium, and micronutrients are added), will reestablish metabolic control, treat edema, and restore appetite. The parenteral route should be avoided; children who lack appetite should be fed by nasogastric tube, because nutrients delivered within the gut lumen help in its repair. Table 57.10 provides recipes for preparing the special feeds and their nutrient composition. Of the 2 recipes for F75, one requires no cooking, and the other is cereal based and has a lower osmolality, which may benefit children with persistent diarrhea. F75 is also available commercially; maltodextrins replace some of the sugar, and potassium, magnesium, minerals, and vitamins are already added.

Dehydration status is easily misdiagnosed in severely wasted children, because the usual signs (e.g., slow skin pinch, sunken eyes) may be present even without dehydration. Rehydration must therefore be closely monitored for signs of fluid overload. Serum electrolyte levels can be misleading because of sodium leaking from the blood into cells and potassium leaking out of cells. Keeping the intake of electrolytes and nutrients constant (see Table 57.8) allows systems to stabilize more quickly than adjusting intake in response to laboratory results.

Table 57.11 provides a recipe for the special rehydration solution used in severe malnutrition (ReSoMal). Therapeutic **Combined Mineral Vitamin mix (CMV)** contains electrolytes, minerals, and vitamins and is added to ReSoMal and feeds. If unavailable, potassium, magnesium, zinc, and copper can be added as an electrolyte/mineral stock solution (Table 57.12 provides a recipe), and a multivitamin supplement can be given separately.

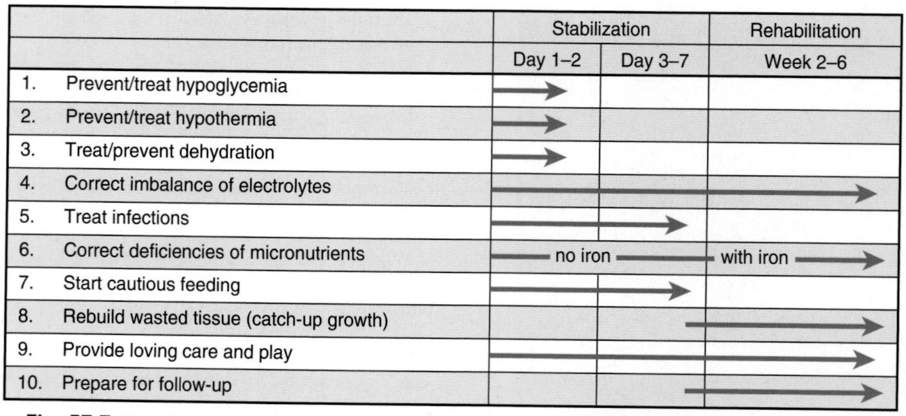

		Stabilization		Rehabilitation
		Day 1–2	Day 3–7	Week 2–6
1.	Prevent/treat hypoglycemia	→		
2.	Prevent/treat hypothermia	→		
3.	Treat/prevent dehydration	→		
4.	Correct imbalance of electrolytes	→—————————————————→		
5.	Treat infections	—————————→		
6.	Correct deficiencies of micronutrients	— no iron —	— with iron —————→	
7.	Start cautious feeding	———————————→		
8.	Rebuild wasted tissue (catch-up growth)		————————————→	
9.	Provide loving care and play	——————————————————→		
10.	Prepare for follow-up		—————→	

Fig. 57.7 The 10 steps of treatment for severe acute malnutrition and their approximate time frames.

Table 57.7	Emergency Treatment in Severe Malnutrition

CONDITION	IMMEDIATE ACTION

Shock
• Lethargic or unconscious *and*
• Cold hands
Plus either:
• Slow capillary refill (>3 sec) *or*
• Weak fast pulse
	1. Give oxygen.
	2. Give sterile 10% glucose (5 mL/kg) rapidly by IV injection.
	3. Give IV fluid at 15 mL/kg over 1 hr, using:
	  • Ringer lactate with 5% dextrose *or*
	  • Half-normal saline* with 5% dextrose *or*
	  • Half-strength Darrow solution with 5% dextrose
	  • If all the above are unavailable, Ringer lactate
	4. Measure and record pulse and respirations at the start and every 10 min.
	If there are signs of improvement (pulse and respiration rates fall) repeat IV drip, 15 mL/kg for 1 more hr. Then switch to oral or nasogastric rehydration with ReSoMal, 5-10 mL/kg in alternate hr (see Table 57.8 step 3).
	If there are no signs of improvement, assume septic shock and:
	1. Give maintenance fluid IV (4 mL/kg/hr) while waiting for blood.
	2. Order 10 mL/kg fresh whole blood and transfuse slowly over 3 hr. If signs of heart failure, give 5-7 mL/kg packed cells rather than whole blood.
	3. Give furosemide, 1 mL/kg IV at start of transfusion.

Hypoglycemia Blood glucose <3 mmol/L	See Table 57.8 step 1 for treatment.
Severe dehydration	Do *not* give IV fluids except in shock. See Table 57.8 step 3 for treatment.
Very severe anemia Hgb <4 g/dL	If very severe anemia (or Hgb 4-6 g/dL *and* respiratory distress): 1. Give whole blood 10 mL/kg slowly over 3 hr. If signs of heart failure, give 5-7 mL/kg packed cells rather than whole blood. 2. Give furosemide 1 mL/kg IV at the start of the transfusion.
Emergency eye care Corneal ulceration	If corneal ulceration: 1. Give vitamin A immediately (age <6 mo: 50,000 IU; 6-12 mo: 100,000 IU; >12 mo: 200,000 IU) 2. Instill 1 drop atropine (1%) into affected eye to relax the eye and prevent the lens from pushing out.

Hgb, Hemoglobin; IV, intravenous(ly).
*Some would recommend 5% dextrose in normal saline.

Table 57.8	Therapeutic Directives for Stabilization of Malnourished Children	
STEP	**PREVENTION**	**TREATMENT**
1. Prevent/treat hypoglycemia blood glucose <3 mmol/L.	Avoid long gaps without food and minimize need for glucose: 1. Feed immediately. 2. Feed every 3 hr day and night (2 hr if ill). 3. Feed on time. 4. Keep warm. 5. Treat infections (they compete for glucose). *Note:* Hypoglycemia and hypothermia often coexist and are signs of severe infection.	If conscious: 1. Give 10% glucose (50 mL), or a feed (see step 7), or 1 tsp sugar under tongue, whichever is quickest. 2. Feed every 2 hr for at least 1st day. Initially give ¼ of feed every 30 min. 3. Keep warm. 4. Start broad-spectrum antibiotics. If unconscious: 1. Immediately give sterile 10% glucose (5 mL/kg) rapidly by IV. 2. Feed every 2 hr for at least 1st day. Initially give ¼ of feed every 30 min. Use nasogastric (NG) tube if unable to drink. 3. Keep warm. 4. Start broad-spectrum antibiotics.
2. Prevent/treat hypothermia axillary <35°C (95°F); rectal <35.5°C (95.9°F).	Keep warm and dry and feed frequently. 1. Avoid exposure. 2. Dress warmly, including head and cover with blanket. 3. Keep room hot; avoid drafts. 4. Change wet clothes and bedding. 5. Do not bathe if very ill. 6. Feed frequently day and night. 7. Treat infections.	Actively rewarm. 1. Feed. 2. Skin-to-skin contact with caregiver ("kangaroo technique") or dress in warmed clothes, cover head, wrap in warmed blanket and provide indirect heat (e.g., heater; transwarmer mattress; incandescent lamp). 3. Monitor temperature hourly (or every 30 min if using heater). 4. Stop rewarming when rectal temperature is 36.5°C (97.7°F).
3. Prevent/treat dehydration.	Replace stool losses. 1. Give ReSoMal after each watery stool. ReSoMal (37.5 mmol Na/L) is a low-sodium rehydration solution for malnutrition.	Do *not* give IV fluids unless the child is in shock. 1. Give ReSoMal 5 mL/kg every 30 min for 1st 2 hr orally or NG tube. 2. Then give 5-10 mL/kg in alternate hours for up to 10 hr. Amount depends on stool loss and eagerness to drink. Feed in the other alternate hour. 3. Monitor hourly and stop if signs of overload develop (pulse rate increases by 25 beats/min and respiratory rate by 5 breaths/min; increasing edema; engorged jugular veins). 4. Stop when rehydrated (≥3 signs of hydration: less thirsty, passing urine, skin pinch less slow, eyes less sunken, moist mouth, tears, less lethargic, improved pulse and respiratory rate).
4. Correct electrolyte imbalance—deficit of potassium and magnesium, excess sodium.		1. Give extra potassium (4 mmol/kg/day) and magnesium (0.6 mmol/kg/day) for at least 2 wk (see Table 57.12). *Note:* Potassium and magnesium are already added in Nutriset F75 and F100 packets.
5. Prevent/treat infections.	Minimize risk of cross-infection. 1. Avoid overcrowding. 2. Wash hands. 3. Give measles vaccine to unimmunized children age >6 mo.	Infections are often silent. Starting on 1st day, give broad-spectrum antibiotics to all children. 1. For antibiotic choices/schedule, see Table 57.9. 2. Ensure all doses are given, and given on time. 3. Cover skin lesions so that they do not become infected. *Note:* Avoid steroids because they depress immune function.
6. Correct micronutrient deficiencies.	*Note:* Folic acid, multivitamins, zinc, copper, and other trace minerals are already added in Nutriset F75 and F100 packets.	Do *not* give iron in the stabilization phase. 1. Give vitamin A on day 1 (<6 mo 50,000 units; 6-12 mo 100,000 units; >12 mo 200,000 units) if child has any eye signs of vitamin A deficiency or has had recent measles. Repeat this dose on days 2 and 14. 2. Give folic acid, 1 mg (5 mg on day 1). 3. Give zinc (2 mg/kg/day) and copper (0.3 mg/kg/day). These are in the electrolyte/mineral solution and Combined Mineral Vitamin mix (CMV) and can be added to feeds and ReSoMal. 4. Give multivitamin syrup or CMV.
7. Start cautious feeding.		1. Give 8-12 small feeds of F75 to provide 130 mL/kg/day, 100 kcal/kg/day, and 1-1.5 g protein/kg/day. 2. If gross edema, reduce volume to 100 mL/kg/day. 3. Keep a 24-hr intake chart. Measure feeds carefully. Record leftovers. 4. If child has poor appetite, coax and encourage to finish the feed. If unfinished, reoffer later. Use NG tube if eating ≤80% of the amount offered. 5. If breastfed, encourage continued breastfeeding but also give F75. 6. Transfer to F100 when appetite returns (usually within 1 wk) and edema has been lost or is reduced. 7. Weigh daily and plot weight.

Table 57.9	Recommended Antibiotics for Malnourished Children*	
		GIVE
If no complications		Amoxicillin, 25 mg/kg PO twice daily for 5 days
If complications (shock, hypoglycemia, hypothermia, skin lesions, respiratory or urinary tract infections, or lethargy/sickly)		Gentamicin, 7.5 mg/kg IV or IM once daily for 7 days *and* Ampicillin, 50 mg/kg IV or IM every 6 hr for 2 days, then amoxicillin, 25-40 mg/kg PO every 8 hr for 5 days

*Local resistance patterns may require these to be adjusted: Ensure that there is Gram-negative cover.
If specific infections are identified, add appropriate antibiotics.
For persistent diarrhea or small bowel overgrowth, add metronidazole, 7.5 mg/kg PO every 8 hr for 7 days.
PO, Orally; IM, intramuscularly; IV, intravenously.

Table 57.10	Recipes for Milk Formulas F75 and F100		
	F75[b] **(STARTER)**	**F75**[c] **(STARTER) (CEREAL-BASED)**	**F100**[d] **(CATCH-UP)**
Dried skimmed milk (g)	25	25	80
Sugar (g)	100	70	50
Cereal flour (g)	—	35	—
Vegetable oil (g)	30	30	60
Electrolyte/mineral solution (mL)[a]	20	20	20
Water: make up to (mL)	1000	1000	1000
Content/100 mL			
Energy (kcal)	75	75	100
Protein (g)	0.9	1.1	2.9
Lactose (g)	1.3	1.3	4.2
Potassium (mmol)	4.0	4.2	6.3
Sodium (mmol)	0.6	0.6	1.9
Magnesium (mmol)	0.43	0.46	0.73
Zinc (mg)	2.0	2.0	2.3
Copper (mg)	0.25	0.25	0.25
% Energy from protein	5	6	12
% Energy from fat	32	32	53
Osmolality (mOsm/L)	413	334	419

Whisk at high speed to prevent oil from separating out.
[a]See Table 57.12 for recipe, or use commercially available therapeutic Combined Mineral Vitamin mix (CMV).
[b]A comparable F75 can be made from 35 g dried whole milk, 100 g sugar, 20 g oil, 20 mL electrolyte/mineral solution, and water to 1000 mL; or from 300 mL full-cream cow's milk, 100 g sugar, 20 g oil, 20 mL electrolyte/mineral solution, and water to 1000 mL.
[c]This lower-osmolality formula may be helpful for children with dysentery or persistent diarrhea. Cook for 4 min.
[d]A comparable F100 can be made from 110 g dried whole milk, 50 g sugar, 30 g oil, 20 mL electrolyte/mineral solution, and water to 1000 mL; or from 880 mL full-cream cow's milk, 75 g sugar, 20 g oil, 20 mL electrolyte/mineral solution, and water to 1000 mL.

Table 57.11	Recipe for Rehydration Solution for Malnutrition (ReSoMal)	
INGREDIENT		**AMOUNT**
Water		2 L
WHO ORS		One 1-L sachet*
Sucrose		50 g
Electrolyte/mineral solution[†]		40 mL

ReSoMal contains 37.5 mmol sodium and 40 mmol potassium/L.
*Sachet contains 2.6 g sodium chloride, 2.9 g trisodium citrate dihydrate, 1.5 g potassium chloride, and 13.5 g glucose.
[†]See Table 57.12 for recipe, or use commercially available therapeutic Combined Mineral Vitamin mix (CMV).
WHO ORS, World Health Organization Oral Rehydration Solution.

Rehabilitation

The signals for entry to the rehabilitation phase are reduced or minimal edema and return of appetite.

A controlled transition over 3 days is recommended to prevent refeeding syndrome (see Chapter 58). After the transition, unlimited amounts should be given of a high-energy, high-protein milk formula such as F100 (100 kcal and 3 g protein per 100 mL), or a **ready-to-use therapeutic food (RUTF)**, or family foods modified to have comparable energy and protein contents.

To make the transition, for 2 days replace F75 with an equal volume of F100, then increase each successive feed by 10 mL until some feed remains uneaten (usually at about 200 mL/kg/day). After this transition, give 150-220 kcal/kg/day and 4-6 g protein/kg/day, and continue to give potassium, magnesium, and micronutrients. Add iron (3 mg/kg/day). If breastfed, encourage continued breastfeeding. Children with

Table 57.12	Recipe for Concentrated Electrolyte/ Mineral Solution*	
INGREDIENT	**g**	**mol/20 mL**
Potassium chloride: KCl	224.0	24 mmol
Tripotassium citrate	81.0	2 mmol
Magnesium chloride: $MgCl_2 \cdot 6H_2O$	76.0	3 mmol
Zinc acetate: Zn acetate $\cdot 2H_2O$	8.2	300 μmol
Copper (cupric) sulfate: $CuSO_4 \cdot 5H_2O$	1.4	45 μmol
Water: make up to	2500 mL	

Add 20 mL when preparing 1 L of feed or ReSoMal.
*Make fresh each month. Use cooled boiled water.

severe malnutrition have developmental delays, so loving care, structured play, and sensory stimulation during and after treatment are essential to aid recovery of brain function.

Community-Based Treatment

Many children with severe acute malnutrition can be identified in their communities before medical complications arise. If these children have a good appetite and are clinically well, they can be rehabilitated at home through community-based therapeutic care, which has the added benefit of reducing their exposure to nosocomial infections and providing continuity of care after recovery. It also reduces the time caregivers spend away from home and their opportunity costs and can be cost-effective for health services.

Fig. 57.8 shows the criteria for inpatient and outpatient care. To maximize coverage and compliance, community-based therapeutic care has 4 main elements: community mobilization and sensitization, active case finding, therapeutic care, and follow-up after discharge.

Community-based therapeutic care comprises steps 8-10 (Fig. 57.7), plus a broad-spectrum antibiotic (step 5). RUTF is usually provided, especially in times of food shortage. RUTF is specially designed for rehabilitating children with severe acute malnutrition at home. It is high in energy and protein and has electrolytes and micronutrients

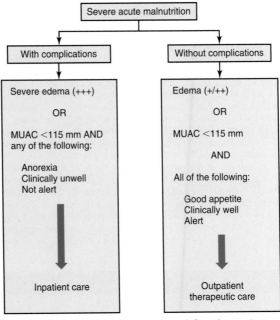

Fig. 57.8 Flow diagram for inpatient care (*left*) and outpatient care (*right*) in the child with severe acute malnutrition. MUAC, Mid-upper arm circumference.

added. The most widely used RUTF is a thick paste that contains milk powder, peanuts, vegetable oil, and sugar. Pathogens cannot grow in it because of its low moisture content. Hospitalized children who have completed steps 1-7 and the transition can be transferred to community-based care for completion of their rehabilitation, thereby reducing their hospital stay to about 7-10 days.

Bibliography is available at Expert Consult.

Chapter **58**
Refeeding Syndrome
Robert M. Kliegman

第五十八章
再喂养综合征

中 文 导 读

本章主要介绍了再喂养综合征的临床表现，包括低磷血症、低钾血症、低镁血症、维生素/维生素B1缺乏、钠潴留和高血糖以及其导致的心血管系统、呼吸系统、神经系统、血液系统、胃肠道等方面的临床症状和体征。

The **refeeding syndrome** may occur if high-energy feeding is started too soon or too vigorously, and it may lead to sudden death with signs of heart failure. Early accounts of the syndrome were among starved survivors of wartime sieges and concentration camps and among prisoners of war when given sudden access to unlimited food. The refeeding syndrome occurs in malnourished individuals as a result of untimely, overzealous oral, enteral, or parenteral (highest risk) feeding, and the risk is not widely recognized. Refeeding syndrome has also been seen among malnourished patients with anorexia nervosa with a body mass index (BMI) <70% median values. Onset is usually 24-48 hr after the start of high-energy feeding and is characterized by breathlessness, rapid pulse, increased venous pressure, rapid enlargement of the liver, and watery diarrhea. Other features are noted in Table 58.1.

An increase in the supply of energy (usually carbohydrates) is accompanied by an increase in sodium pump activity, and too sudden a supply risks causing a rapid release of accumulated sodium from cells, causing expansion of extracellular and plasma volumes. At the same time there is increased uptake by cells of glucose, potassium, magnesium, and phosphate. A sudden lowering of serum potassium, magnesium, and phosphate concentrations is an important feature of the refeeding syndrome.

The key to preventing the syndrome is to minimize the risk of its occurrence. It can be avoided by following the World Health Organization (WHO) guidelines for the treatment of malnutrition (see Chapter 57). Of particular relevance to minimizing the risk is the initial **stabilization phase**, which includes providing maintenance amounts of energy and protein and correcting electrolyte imbalances and micronutrient deficiencies, followed by a controlled transition to high-energy feeding. Milk-based diets are desirable because milk is a good source of phosphate. No or minimal edema and return of appetite are signs of readiness for the transition. Monitoring for sudden increases in pulse and respiration rates during the transition to high-energy feeding is advisable to detect these early warning signs. Should refeeding syndrome occur, prompt treatment with a single parenteral dose of digoxin and furosemide has been useful.

Bibliography is available at Expert Consult.

Table 58.1	Clinical Signs and Symptoms of Refeeding Syndrome					
HYPOPHOSPHATEMIA	**HYPOKALEMIA**	**HYPOMAGNESEMIA**	**VITAMIN/THIAMINE DEFICIENCY**	**SODIUM RETENTION**	**HYPERGLYCEMIA**
Cardiac Hypotension Decreased stroke volume	*Cardiac* Arrhythmias	*Cardiac* Arrhythmias	Encephalopathy Lactic acidosis Death	Fluid overload Pulmonary edema Cardiac compromise	*Cardiac* Hypotension
Respiratory Impaired diaphragm contractility Dyspnea Respiratory failure	*Respiratory* Failure	*Neurologic* Weakness Tremor Tetany Seizures Altered mental status Coma			*Respiratory* Hypercapnia Failure
Neurologic Paresthesia Weakness Confusion Disorientation Lethargy Areflexic paralysis Seizures Coma	*Neurologic* Weakness Paralysis	*Gastrointestinal* Nausea Vomiting Diarrhea			*Other* Ketoacidosis Coma Dehydration Impaired immune function
Hematologic Leukocyte dysfunction Hemolysis Thrombocytopenia	*Gastrointestinal* Nausea Vomiting Constipation	*Other* Refractory hypokalemia and hypocalcemia Death			
Other Death	*Muscular* Rhabdomyolysis Muscle necrosis				
	Other Death				

Data from Kraft MD, Btaiche IF, Sacks GS: Review of RFS, *Nutr Clin Pract* 20:625–633, 2005. From Fuentebella J, Kerner JA: Refeeding syndrome, *Pediatr Clin North Am* 56:1201–1210, 2009.

Chapter **59**
Malnutrition
Lucinda Lo and Allison Ballantine
第五十九章
营养不良

中文导读

　　本章主要介绍了营养不良的临床表现、病因与诊断、治疗以及预后。其中病因包括婴儿生长迟缓的心理、中枢神经系统、心血管、肺、胃肠道、肾脏、内分泌等系统或器官以及遗传方面的原因；诊断包括临床症状、体征和体格发育指标以及住院患儿营养不良的识别；治疗包括营养支持和心理社会支持。

Failure to thrive (FTT) has classically been the term used to describe children who are not growing as expected. Studies have advocated using the term **malnutrition** to describe this cohort of children with specifically defined classification based on anthropometric measurements. In this chapter, malnutrition refers to **undernutrition** and is defined as an imbalance between nutrient requirements and intake or delivery that then results in deficits—of energy, protein, or micronutrients—that may negatively affect growth and development. Malnutrition may be illness related or non–illness related, or both. Illness-related malnutrition may be caused by one or more diseases, infections, or congenital anomalies, as well as by injury or surgery. Non–illness-related causes include environmental, psychosocial, or behavioral factors. Often, one cause may be primary and exacerbated by another. Patients with malnutrition may present with growth deceleration, faltering growth, or even weight loss, as measured by anthropometric parameters, including weight, height/length, skinfolds, and mid-upper arm circumference (see Chapter 57).

CLINICAL MANIFESTATIONS

Inadequate weight-for–corrected age, failure to gain adequate weight over a period of time (weight gain velocity), height velocity, weight-for-height, body mass index (BMI), and developmental outcomes help define malnutrition (see Chapter 57). These growth and anthropometric parameters should be measured serially and plotted on growth charts appropriate for the child's sex, age (corrected if premature), and, if known, genetic disorders, such as trisomy 21. The American Academy of Pediatrics (AAP) and U.S. Centers for Disease Control and Prevention (CDC) recommend the 2006 World Health Organization (WHO) charts for children up to 2 yr of age who are measured supine for length. The CDC 2000 growth charts are recommended for children and adolescents (age 2-20 yr) when measured with a standing height. The severity of malnutrition (mild, moderate, or severe) may be determined by plotting the z score (standard deviation [SD] from the mean) for each of these anthropometric values (Table 59.1).

ETIOLOGY AND DIAGNOSIS

The most common mechanisms for illness-related causes of insufficient growth include (1) failure to ingest sufficient calories, or starvation (e.g., cardiac failure, fluid restriction), (2) increased nutrient losses (e.g., protein-losing enteropathy, chronic diarrhea), (3) increased metabolic demands, as seen in extensive burn injuries, and (4) altered nutrient absorption or utilization (e.g., cystic fibrosis, short bowel syndrome). More than one mechanism can exist simultaneously (Fig. 59.1). *Acute malnutrition* is defined as having a duration of <3 mo (see Chapter 57).

A complete history should include a detailed nutritional, family, and prenatal history; the quantity, quality, and frequency of meals; and further information regarding the onset of the growth failure (Table 59.2). A comprehensive physical examination is necessary to elicit underlying etiologies (Table 59.3). Puberty is often delayed or stalled in malnutrition, so Tanner stage should be carefully noted during the initial evaluation of preteens and adolescents. Tanner staging cannot be used as a marker for nutritional status, but it is influenced by malnourishment. Puberty will usually resume progression when the malnourished state improves. Laboratory evaluation of children with malnutrition should be judicious and based on findings from the history and physical examination. Obtaining the state's newborn screening results, a complete blood count, and urinalysis represent a reasonable initial screen.

Additional measurements that are useful for following the progress of the acutely malnourished child are mid-upper arm circumference (MUAC) and hand-grip strength. MUAC is a particularly useful anthropometric measure when weight may be distorted by use of corticosteroids or fluid status (e.g., ascites, edema).

For children 6 yr and older, **hand-grip strength** may be a more acute measurement of response to nutritional intervention than MUAC, because muscle function reacts earlier to changes in nutritional status than does muscle mass. The *dynamometer* is a simple, noninvasive, and low-cost instrument for measuring baseline functional status and tracking progress

Table 59.1	Comprehensive Malnutrition Indicators		
INDICATORS*	**SEVERE MALNUTRITION**	**MODERATE MALNUTRITION**	**MILD MALNUTRITION**
Weight-for-length z score	≥ −3 z score or worse	−2.0 to 2.99 z score	−1.0 to −1.99 z score†
BMI-for-age z score	≥ −3 z score or worse	−2.0 to 2.99 z score	−1.0 to −1.99 z score†
Weight-for-length/height z score	≥ −3 z score or worse	No data available	No data available
Mid-upper arm circumference (<5 yr of age)	≥ −3 z score or worse	−2.0 to 2.99 z score	−1.0 to −1.99 z score
Weight gain velocity (≤2 yr of age)	≤25% of norm	26–50% of norm	51–75% of the norm
Weight loss (2-20 yr of age)	>10% of UBW	>7.5% UBW	>5% UBW
Deceleration in weight-for-length/height or BMI-for-age	Deceleration across 3 z score lines	Deceleration across 2 z score lines	Deceleration across 1 z score line
Inadequate nutrient intake	≤25% of estimated energy – protein need	26–50% of estimated energy – protein need	51–75% of estimated energy – protein need

*It is recommended that when a child meets more than one malnutrition acuity level, the provider should document the severity of the malnutrition at the highest acuity level to ensure that an appropriate treatment plan and appropriate intervention, monitoring, and evaluation are provided.
†Needs additional positive diagnostic criteria to make a malnutrition diagnosis.
BMI, Body mass index; UBW, usual body weight.
Use clinical judgment when applying these diagnostic criteria.
Adapted from Becker PJ, Carney LN, Corkins MR, et al: Consensus Statement of the Academy of Nutrition and Dietetics/American Society for Parenteral and Enteral Nutrition: Indicators recommended for the identification and documentation of pediatric malnutrition (undernutrition). *J Acad Nutr Diet* 114(12): 1988-2000, 2014.

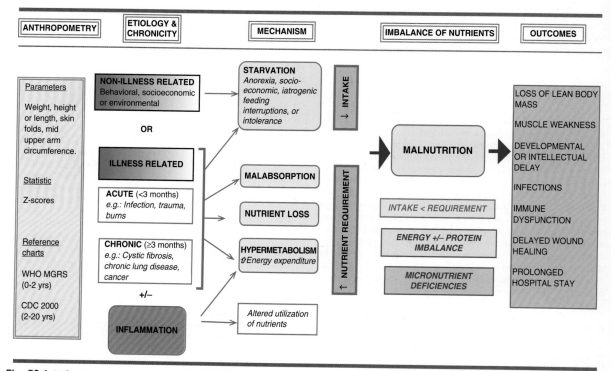

Fig. 59.1 Defining malnutrition in hospitalized children (ASPEN). CDC, Centers for Disease Control and Prevention; MGRS, Multicenter Growth Reference Study; WHO, World Health Organization. *From Mehta NM, Corkins MR, Lyman B, et al: Defining pediatric malnutrition: A paradigm shift toward etiology-related definitions. JPEN J Parenter Enteral Nutr 37(4):460-481, 2013.*

throughout the therapeutic course. Hand-grip strength can help to identify the presence of malnutrition, but the current lack of reference ranges for mild, moderate, and severe malnutrition in large populations limit the ability to use hand-grip strength to quantify the degree of malnutrition.

TREATMENT

While an illness-related etiology of mild malnutrition is being investigated, caloric supplementation should occur simultaneously. Both the medical workup and the initiation of supplemental oral feeds should occur in the outpatient setting with close follow-up. Consider including

Table 59.2	Approach to Malnutrition Based on Signs and Symptoms
HISTORY/PHYSICAL EXAMINATION	**DIAGNOSTIC CONSIDERATION**
Spitting, vomiting, food refusal	Gastroesophageal reflux, chronic tonsillitis, food allergies, eosinophilic esophagitis
Diarrhea, fatty stools	Malabsorption, intestinal parasites, milk protein intolerance, pancreatic insufficiency, celiac disease, immunodeficiency, inflammatory bowel disease
Snoring, mouth breathing, enlarged tonsils	Adenoid hypertrophy, obstructive sleep apnea
Recurrent wheezing, pulmonary infections	Asthma, aspiration, food allergy, cystic fibrosis, immunodeficiency
Recurrent infections	HIV or congenital primary immunodeficiency diseases, anatomic defects
Travel to/from developing countries	Parasitic or bacterial infections of gastrointestinal tract

Table 59.3	Findings in Failure to Thrive in Infancy			
CAUSE	**APPROXIMATE PERCENTAGE OF ALL CASES**	**HISTORY**	**SYSTEM-SPECIFIC PHYSICAL FINDINGS**	**SYSTEM-SPECIFIC LABORATORY STUDIES**
Psychosocial	Up to 50% or more	Vague, inconsistent feeding history, history of bottle propping	None, may have soft neurologic signs	None
CNS	13%	Poor feeding, gross developmental delay, vomiting	Grossly abnormal neurologic findings	Frequent gross abnormalities on EEG and MRI scan or grossly abnormal tests of neuromuscular function
Gastrointestinal	10%	Chronic vomiting and/or diarrhea, abnormal stools, crying with feedings, nocturnal cough/snoring	Often negative, may have abdominal distention	Abnormal barium, pH probe, or endoscopic study; abnormal stool findings (pH, reducing substances, fat stain, Wright stain)
Cardiac	9%	Slow feeding, dyspnea and diaphoresis with feeding, restlessness and diaphoresis during sleep	Often cyanotic or have signs of congestive heart failure	Abnormal echocardiogram, ECG, catheterization findings
Genetic	8%	May have positive family history or a history of developmental delay	Often have facies typical of a syndrome, skeletal abnormalities, neurologic abnormalities, or visceromegaly	May have typical radiographic findings, chromosomal abnormalities, abnormal metabolic screens
Pulmonary	3.5%	Chronic or recurrent dyspnea with feedings, tachypnea	Grossly abnormal chest examination findings	Abnormal chest radiographs
Renal	3.5%	May be negative or may have history of polyuria	Often negative, may have flank masses	Abnormal urinalysis, frequently elevated BUN and creatinine, signs of renal osteodystrophy on radiographs
Endocrine	3.5%	With hypothyroidism, constipation and decreased activity level; with diabetes, polyuria, polydipsia	With hypothyroidism, no wasting but mottling, umbilical hernia, often open posterior fontanelle. With diabetes, often without specific abnormality, but may have signs of dehydration, ketotic breath, and hyperpnea. With hypopituitarism and isolated growth hormone deficiency, growth normal until 9 mo or later, then plateaus, but normal weight for height; delayed tooth eruption	Decreased T_4, increased TSH; glucosuria and hyperglycemia; abnormal pituitary function study results

BUN, Blood urea nitrogen; *CNS*, central nervous system; *CT*, computed tomography; *ECG*, electrocardiogram; *EEG*, electroencephalogram; T_4, thyroxine; *TSH*, thyroid-stimulating hormone.
From Carrasco MM, Wolford JE: Child abuse and neglect. In Zitelli BJ, McIntire SC, Nowalk AJ, editors: Atlas of pediatric physical diagnosis, ed 7, Philadelphia, 2018, Elsevier, Table 6.6.

a speech therapist for a suck-and-swallow evaluation if the history suggests difficulty with oral feeds. If a child has not responded after 2-3 mo of outpatient management. consider hospitalization for potential initiation of nasogastric tube feeds, further diagnostic and laboratory evaluation, assessment and observed implementation of adequate nutrition, and evaluation of the parent–child feeding interaction. Additional indications for hospitalization include moderate or severe malnutrition, since the potential for refeeding syndrome requires close monitoring (see Chapter 58). The type of caloric supplementation is based on the severity of malnutrition and the underlying medical condition. The response to feeding depends on the specific diagnosis, medical treatment, and severity of malnutrition.

The same anthropometric measures used to diagnosis malnutrition should be used to measure progress and recovery from the malnourished state. Multivitamin supplementation should be given to all children with malnutrition to meet the recommended dietary allowance, because these children usually have iron, zinc, and vitamin D deficiencies, as well as increased micronutrient demands with catch-up growth.

Therapy for the psychosocial factors should be specific for the underlying issue, such as maternal depression or insufficient funds for food. In addition, parent education should focus on what is normal infant development and on correcting any parental misconceptions about feeding and temperament, as well as learning the infant cues for hunger, satiety, and sleep. Some children who develop feeding aversion behaviors will require treatment by a specialized feeding team. If abuse or purposeful neglect is a concern, the family should be referred to the child protective services team.

PROGNOSIS

Malnutrition, regardless of cause, is concerning because of the detrimental effect on physical and intellectual growth and development. Early diagnosis and treatment of acute malnutrition allow children to catch up to and sometimes even surpass their peers who were not malnourished. The long-term sequelae of malnutrition in young infants and children have been conflicting, and there is no clear consensus regarding the long-term emotional, cognitive, and metabolic effects. Despite inconclusive long-term outcomes in children who have malnutrition, investigators support early nutritional interventions for children who have poor growth.

Bibliography is available at Expert Consult.

Chapter 60

Overweight and Obesity

Sheila Gahagan

第六十章
超重和肥胖

中文导读

　　本章主要介绍了超重和肥胖的流行病学、体质指数、病因、并发症、识别、评估、干预和预防。具体描述了病因的环境因素、遗传因素、肠道微生态变化以及内分泌和神经变化方面的因素；详细阐述了ROHHAD综合征的临床表现、诊断、治疗、病因研究和假说以及鉴别诊断。

EPIDEMIOLOGY

Obesity is an important pediatric public health problem associated with risk of complications in childhood and increased morbidity and mortality throughout adult life. Obesity is now linked to more deaths than underweight. In 2014, according to the World Health Organization (WHO), more than 1.9 billion persons ≥20 yr old were overweight or obese.

In the United States, 37% of adults are obese, and 35% are overweight. In children the prevalence of obesity increased 300% over approximately 40 yr. According to the National Health and Nutrition Examination Survey (NHANES), 2013–2014, 34% of children 2-19 yr old were overweight or obese, with 17% in the obese range. Risk for obesity in children 2-19 yr old varies significantly by race/ethnicity, with >20% for minority children compared with 15% for white children. Across all racial groups, higher maternal education confers protection against childhood obesity.

The first 1000 days, the period from conception to age 2 yr, are increasingly recognized as a modifiable period related to risk for childhood obesity. Parental obesity correlates with a higher risk for obesity in the children. Prenatal factors, including high preconceptual weight, gestational weight gain, high birthweight, and maternal smoking, are associated with increased risk for later obesity. Paradoxically, intrauterine growth restriction with early infant catch-up growth is associated with the development of central adiposity and adult-onset cardiovascular (CV) risk. Breastfeeding is modestly protective for obesity based on dose and duration. Infants with high levels of negative reactivity (temperament) are more at risk for obesity than those with better self-regulation.

BODY MASS INDEX

Obesity or increased adiposity is defined using the **body mass index (BMI)**, an excellent proxy for more direct measurement of body fat. BMI = weight in kg/(height in meters)². Adults with a BMI ≥30 meet the criterion for obesity, and those with a BMI 25-30 fall in the overweight range. During childhood, levels of body fat change beginning with high adiposity during infancy. Body fat levels decrease for approximately 5.5 yr until the period called *adiposity rebound*, when body fat is typically at the lowest level. Adiposity then increases until early adulthood (Fig. 60.1). Consequently, obesity and overweight are defined using BMI percentiles for children ≥2 yr old and weight/length percentiles for infants <2 yr old. The criterion for **obesity** is BMI ≥95th percentile and for **overweight** is BMI between 85th and 95th percentiles.

ETIOLOGY

Humans have the capacity to store energy in adipose tissue, allowing improved survival in times of famine. Simplistically, obesity results from an imbalance of caloric intake and energy expenditure. Even incremental but sustained caloric excess results in excess adiposity. Individual adiposity is the result of a complex interplay among genetically determined body habitus, appetite, nutritional intake, **physical activity (PA)**, and energy expenditure. Environmental factors determine levels of available food, preferences for types of foods, levels of PA, and preferences for types of activities. Food preferences play a role in consumption of energy-dense foods. Humans innately prefer sweet and salty foods and tend initially to reject bitter flavors, common to many vegetables. Repeated exposure to healthy foods promotes their acceptance and liking, especially in early life. This human characteristic to adapt to novel foods can be used to promote healthy food selection.

Environmental Changes

Over the last 4 decades, the food environment has changed dramatically related to urbanization and the food industry. As fewer families routinely prepare meals, foods prepared by a food industry have higher levels of calories, simple carbohydrates, and fat. The price of many foods has declined relative to the family budget. These changes, in combination with marketing pressure, have resulted in larger portion sizes and increased snacking between meals. The increased consumption of high-carbohydrate beverages, including sodas, sport drinks, fruit punch, and juice, adds to these factors.

Fast food is consumed by one third of U.S. children each day and by two thirds of children every week. A typical fast food meal can contain 2000 kcal and 84 g of fat. Many children consume 4 servings of high-carbohydrate beverages per day, resulting in an additional 560 kcal of low nutritional value. Sweetened beverages have been linked to increased risk for obesity. The dramatic increase in the use of high-fructose corn syrup to sweeten beverages and prepared foods is another important environmental change, leading to availability of inexpensive calories.

Since World War II, levels of PA in children and adults have declined. According to the 2012 NHANES survey, 25% of 12-15 yr olds met PA guidelines of 60 min of PA per day. Decline in PA is related to many factors, including changes in the built environment, more reliance on cars, lower levels of active transportation, safety issues, and increasingly sedentary lifestyles. Many sectors of society do not engage in PA during leisure time. For children, budgetary constraints and pressure for academic performance have led to less time devoted to physical education in schools. Perception of poor neighborhood safety also leads to lower levels of PA. Furthermore, screens (televisions, tablets, smartphones, computers) offer compelling sedentary activities that do not burn calories.

Sleep plays a role in risk for obesity. Over the last 4 decades, children and adults have decreased the amount of time spent sleeping. Reasons for these changes may relate to increased time at work, increased time watching television, and a generally faster pace of life. Chronic partial sleep loss can increase risk for weight gain and obesity, with the impact possibly greater in children than in adults. In studies of young, healthy, lean men, short sleep duration was associated with decreased leptin levels and increased ghrelin levels, along with increased hunger and appetite. *Sleep debt* also results in decreased glucose tolerance and insulin sensitivity related to alterations in glucocorticoids and sympathetic activity. Some effects of sleep debt might relate to *orexins*, peptides synthesized in the lateral hypothalamus that can increase feeding, arousal, sympathetic activity, and neuropeptide Y activity.

Genetics

Genetic determinants also have a role in individual susceptibility to obesity (Table 60.1). Findings from genome-wide association studies explain a very small portion of interindividual variability in obesity. One important example, the *FTO* gene at 16q12, is associated with adiposity in childhood, probably explained by increased energy intake. Monogenic forms of obesity have also been identified, including **melanocortin-4 receptor (MC4R)** deficiency, associated with early-onset obesity and food-seeking behavior. Mutations in *MC4R* are a common cause of monogenetic obesity but a rare cause of obesity in general. Deficient activation of *MC4R* is seen in patients with **proopiomelanocortin (POMC)** deficiency, a prohormone precursor of adrenocorticotropic hormone (ACTH) and melanocyte-stimulating hormone (MSH), resulting in adrenal insufficiency, light skin, hyperphagia, and obesity.

In addition, evidence suggests that appetitive traits are moderately heritable. For example, some genes associated with appetite also relate to weight, and vice-versa. In addition, there are genetic conditions associated with obesity, such as **Prader-Willi syndrome,** which results from absence of paternally expressed imprinted genes in the 15q11.2–q13 region. Prader-Willi syndrome is characterized by insatiable appetite and food seeking. In the era of genomic medicine, it will be increasingly possible to identify risks according to specific genes and consider gene-environment interactions. Epigenetic environmental modification of genes may have a role in the development of obesity, especially during fetal and early life.

Microbiome

It is increasingly recognized the human gut microbiota play a role in regulating metabolism. This novel area of research raises questions about the role of antibiotics in the pathway to obesity and the possibility that probiotics could be therapeutic for certain individuals.

Endocrine and Neural Physiology

Monitoring of "stored fuels" and short-term control of food intake (appetite and satiety) occurs through neuroendocrine feedback loops linking adipose tissue, the gastrointestinal (GI) tract, and the central nervous system (CNS) (Figs. 60.2 and 60.3). GI hormones, including cholecystokinin, glucagon-like peptide 1, peptide YY, and vagal neuronal feedback promote satiety. *Ghrelin* stimulates appetite. Adipose tissue provides feedback regarding energy storage levels to the brain through hormonal release of adiponectin and leptin. These hormones act on the arcuate nucleus in the hypothalamus and on the solitary tract nucleus in the brainstem and in turn activate distinct neuronal networks. Adipocytes secrete *adiponectin* into the blood, with reduced levels in response to obesity and increased levels in response to fasting. Reduced adiponectin levels are associated with lower insulin sensitivity and adverse CV outcomes. *Leptin* is directly involved in satiety; low leptin levels stimulate food intake, and high leptin levels inhibit hunger in animal models and in healthy human volunteers. However, the negative feedback loop from leptin to appetite may be more adapted to preventing starvation than excess intake.

Numerous neuropeptides in the brain, including peptide YY (PYY), agouti-related peptide, and orexin, appear to affect appetite stimulation, whereas melanocortins and α-melanocortin–stimulating hormone are

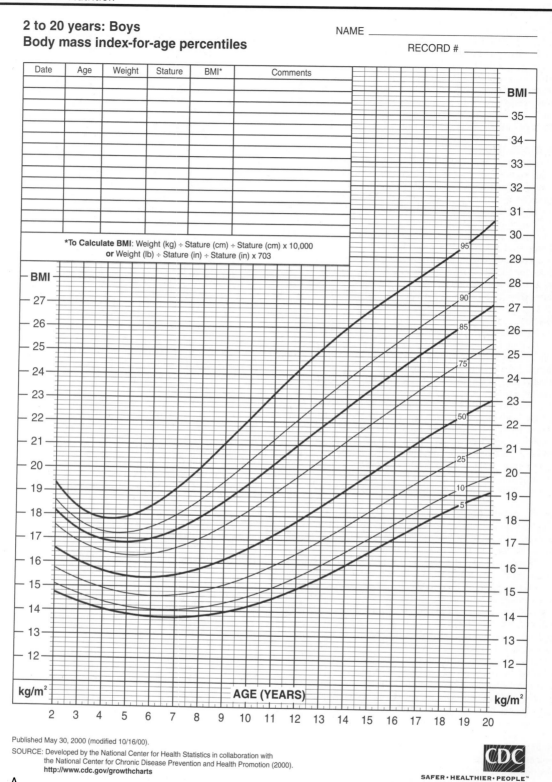

2 to 20 years: Boys
Body mass index-for-age percentiles

NAME _____

RECORD # _____

Fig. 60.1 A, Body mass index (BMI)-for-age profiles for boys and men. *(Developed by the National Center for Health Statistics in collaboration with the National Center for Chronic Disease Prevention and Health Promotion, 2000. See www.cdc.gov/growthcharts.)*

Continued

2 to 20 years: Girls
Body mass index-for-age percentiles

NAME _____

RECORD # _____

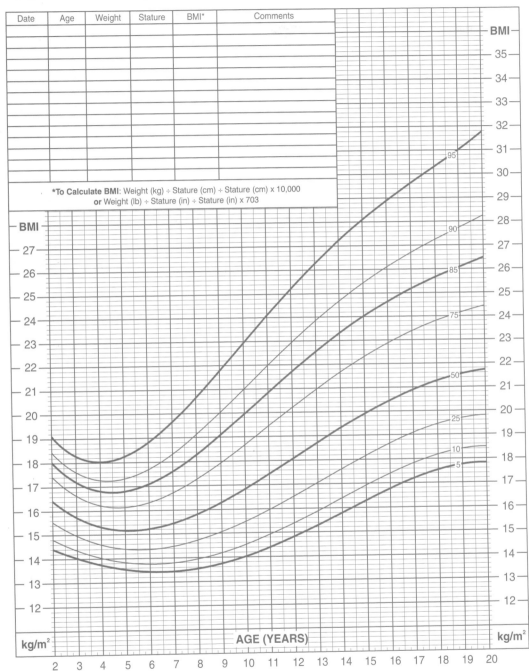

*To Calculate BMI: Weight (kg) ÷ Stature (cm) ÷ Stature (cm) x 10,000
or Weight (lb) ÷ Stature (in) ÷ Stature (in) x 703

Published May 30, 2000 (modified 10/16/00).
SOURCE: Developed by the National Center for Health Statistics in collaboration with
the National Center for Chronic Disease Prevention and Health Promotion (2000).
http://www.cdc.gov/growthcharts

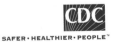

B

Fig. 60.1, cont'd B, BMI-for-age profiles for girls and women.

Table 60.1	Endocrine and Genetic Causes of Obesity	
DISEASE	**SYMPTOMS**	**LABORATORY**
ENDOCRINE		
Cushing syndrome	Central obesity, hirsutism, moon face, hypertension	Dexamethasone suppression test
GH deficiency	Short stature, slow linear growth	Evoked GH response, IGF-1
Hyperinsulinism	Nesidioblastosis, pancreatic adenoma, hypoglycemia, Mauriac syndrome	Insulin level
Hypothyroidism	Short stature, weight gain, fatigue, constipation, cold intolerance, myxedema	TSH, FT$_4$
Pseudohypoparathyroidism	Short metacarpals, subcutaneous calcifications, dysmorphic facies, mental retardation, short stature, hypocalcemia, hyperphosphatemia	Urine cAMP after synthetic PTH infusion
GENETIC		
Albright hereditary osteodystrophy	Short stature, skeletal defects, PTH resistance	GNAS gene
Alström syndrome	Cognitive impairment, retinitis pigmentosa, diabetes mellitus, hearing loss, hypogonadism, cardiomyopathy	ALMS1 gene
Bardet-Biedl syndrome	Retinitis pigmentosa, renal abnormalities, polydactyly, syndactyly, hypogonadism	BBS1 gene
BDNF/TrkB deficiency	Hyperactivity, impaired concentration, limited attention span, impaired short-term memory and pain sensation	BDNF/TrkB gene
Biemond syndrome	Cognitive impairment, iris coloboma, hypogonadism, polydactyly	
Carpenter syndrome	Polydactyly, syndactyly, cranial synostosis, mental retardation	Mutations in RAB23 gene, located on chromosome 6 in humans
Cohen syndrome	Mid-childhood-onset obesity, short stature, prominent maxillary incisors, hypotonia, mental retardation, microcephaly, decreased visual activity	Mutations in VPS13B gene (often called COH1) at locus 8q22
Deletion 9q34	Early-onset obesity, mental retardation, brachycephaly, synophrys, prognathism, behavior and sleep disturbances	Deletion 9q34
Down syndrome	Short stature, dysmorphic facies, mental retardation	Trisomy 21
ENPP1 gene mutations	Insulin resistance, childhood obesity	Gene mutation on chromosome 6q
Fröhlich syndrome	Hypothalamic tumor	
FTO gene polymorphism, plus upstream regulatory and downstream activation genes	Dysregulation of orexigenic hormone acyl-ghrelin, poor postprandial appetite suppression	Homozygous for FTO AA allele
KSR2 deficiency	Mild hyperphagia and reduced basal metabolic rate, insulin resistance often with acanthosis nigricans, irregular menses, early development of type 2 diabetes mellitus	KSR2 gene
Leptin or leptin receptor gene deficiency	Early-onset severe obesity, infertility (hypogonadotropic hypogonadism), hyperphagia, infections	Leptin
Melanocortin 4 receptor gene mutation	Early-onset severe obesity, increased linear growth, hyperphagia, hyperinsulinemia Most common known genetic cause of obesity Homozygous worse than heterozygous	MC4R mutation
PCSK1 deficiency	Small bowel enteropathy, hypoglycemia, hypothyroidism, ACTH deficiency, diabetes insipidus	PCSK1 gene
Prader-Willi syndrome	Neonatal hypotonia, slow infant growth, small hands and feet, mental retardation, hypogonadism, hyperphagia leading to severe obesity, paradoxically elevated ghrelin	Partial deletion of chromosome 15 or loss of paternally expressed genes
Proopiomelanocortin (POMC) deficiency	Obesity, red hair, adrenal insufficiency due to ACTH deficiency, hyperproinsulinemia, hyperphagia, pale skin, cholestatic jaundice	Loss-of-function mutations of POMC gene
Rapid-onset obesity with hypothalamic dysfunction, hypoventilation, and autonomic dysregulation (ROHHAD)	Often confused with congenital central hypoventilation syndrome (CCHS); presentation ≥1.5 yr with weight gain, hyperphagia, hypoventilation, cardiac arrest, central diabetes insipidus, hypothyroidism, GH deficiency, pain insensitivity, hypothermia, precocious puberty, neural crest tumors	Unknown genes May be a paraneoplastic disorder
SH2B1 deficiency	Hyperphagia, disproportionate hyperinsulinemia, early speech and language delay that often resolves, behavioral problems including aggression	SH2B1 gene
SIM1 deficiency	Hyperphagia with autonomic dysfunction (characterized by low systolic blood pressure), speech and language delay, neurobehavioral abnormalities including autistic-type behaviors	SIM1 gene
TUB deficiency	Retinal dystrophy, deafness	TUB gene
Turner syndrome	Ovarian dysgenesis, lymphedema, web neck, short stature, cognitive impairment	XO chromosome

ACTH, Adrenocorticotropic hormone; cAMP, cyclic adenosine monophosphate; FT$_4$, free thyroxine; GH, growth hormone; IGF, insulin-like growth factor; PTH, parathyroid hormone; TSH, thyroid-stimulating hormone.

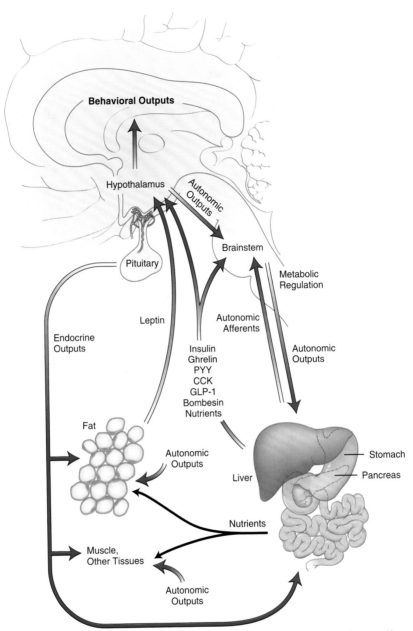

Fig. 60.2 Regulation of energy homeostasis by the brain-gut-adipose axis. CCK, Cholecystokinin; GLP-1, glucagon-like peptide 1; PYY, peptide YY. *(From Melmed S, Polonsky KS, Larsen PR, Kronenberg HM, editors: Williams textbook of endocrinology, ed 13, Philadelphia, 2016, Elsevier, p 1610.)*

involved in satiety (Fig. 60.3). The neuroendocrine control of appetite and weight involves a negative-feedback system, balanced between short-term control of appetite and long-term control of adiposity (including leptin). PYY reduces food intake via the vagal-brainstem-hypothalamic pathway. Developmental changes in PYY are evident as infants have higher PYY levels than school-age children and adults. Obese children have lower fasting levels of PYY than adults. Weight loss may restore PYY levels in children, even though this does not happen in adults. In addition, patients homozygous for the *FTO* obesity-risk allele demonstrate poor regulation of the orexigenic hormone acyl-ghrelin and have poor postprandial appetite suppression.

COMORBIDITIES

Complications of pediatric obesity occur during childhood and adolescence and persist into adulthood. An important reason to prevent and treat pediatric obesity is the increased risk for morbidity and mortality later in life. The Harvard Growth Study found that boys who were overweight during adolescence were twice as likely to die from CV disease as those who had normal weight. More immediate comorbidities include type 2 diabetes, hypertension, hyperlipidemia, and **nonalcoholic fatty liver disease** (NAFLD) (Table 60.2). Insulin resistance increases with increasing adiposity and independently affects lipid metabolism and CV health. The **metabolic syndrome** (central obesity,

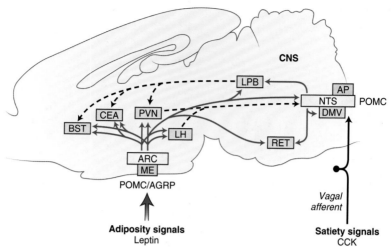

Fig. 60.3 Brain structures involved in energy homeostasis. Receipt of long-term adipostatic signals and acute satiety signals by neurons in arcuate nucleus and brainstem, respectively. *Pale-blue boxes* indicate nuclei containing proopiomelanocortin (POMC) neurons; *tan boxes* indicate nuclei containing melanocortin-4 receptor (MC4R) neurons that may serve to integrate adipostatic and satiety signals; and *darker-blue boxes* show some circumventricular organs involved in energy homeostasis. *Magenta arrows* designate a subset of projections of POMC neurons; *blue arrows* show a subset of projections of agouti-related peptide (AGRP) neurons. AP, Area postrema; ARC, arcuate nucleus; BST, bed nucleus of stria terminalis; CCK, cholecystokinin; CEA, central nucleus of amygdala; CNS, central nervous system; DMV, dorsal motor nucleus of vagus; LH, lateral hypothalamic area; LPB, lateral parabrachial nucleus; ME, median eminence; NTS, nucleus tractus solitarius; PVN, paraventricular nucleus of hypothalamus; RET, reticular formation. *(Modified from Fan W, Ellacott KL, Halatchev IG, et al: Cholecystokinin-mediated suppression of feeding involves the brainstem melanocortin system,* Nat Neurosci 7:335–336, 2004.)

hypertension, glucose intolerance, and hyperlipidemia) increases risk for CV morbidity and mortality. NAFLD has been reported in 34% of patients treated in pediatric obesity clinic. NAFLD is now the most common chronic liver disease in U.S. children and adolescents. It can present with advanced fibrosis or nonalcoholic steatohepatitis and may result in cirrhosis and hepatocellular carcinoma. Insulin resistance is often associated. Furthermore, NAFLD is independently associated with increased risk of CV disease.

Obesity may also be associated with chronic inflammation. Adiponectin, a peptide with antiinflammatory properties, occurs in reduced levels in obese patients compared to insulin-sensitive, lean persons. Low adiponectin levels correlate with elevated levels of free fatty acids and plasma triglycerides as well as a high BMI, and high adiponectin levels correlate with peripheral insulin sensitivity. Adipocytes secrete peptides and cytokines into the circulation, and proinflammatory peptides such interleukin (IL)-6 and tumor necrosis factor (TNF)-α occur in higher levels in obese patients. Specifically, IL-6 stimulates production of C-reactive protein (CRP) in the liver. CRP is a marker of inflammation and might link obesity, coronary disease, and subclinical inflammation.

Some complications of obesity are mechanical, including obstructive sleep apnea and orthopedic complications. Orthopedic complications include Blount disease and slipped femoral capital epiphysis (see Chapters 697 and 698.4).

Mental health problems can coexist with obesity, with the possibility of bidirectional effects. These associations are modified by gender, ethnicity, and socioeconomic status. Self-esteem may be lower in obese adolescent girls than in nonobese peers. Some studies have found an association between obesity and adolescent depression. There is considerable interest in the co-occurrence of eating disorders and obesity. Obese youth are also at risk for bullying based on their appearance.

IDENTIFICATION

Overweight and obese children are often identified as part of routine medical care. The child and family may be unaware that the child has increased adiposity. They may be unhappy with the medical provider for raising this issue and may respond with denial or apparent lack of concern. It is often necessary to begin by helping the family understand

the importance of healthy weight for current and future health. Forging a good therapeutic relationship is important because obesity intervention requires a chronic disease management approach. Intervention and successful resolution of this problem require considerable effort by the family and the child over an extended period in order to change eating and activity behaviors.

EVALUATION

The evaluation of the overweight or obese child begins with examination of the growth chart for weight, height, and BMI trajectories; consideration of possible medical causes of obesity; and detailed exploration of family eating, nutritional, and activity patterns. A complete pediatric history is used to uncover comorbid disorders. The family history focuses on the adiposity of other family members and the family history of obesity-associated disorders. The physical examination adds data that can lead to important diagnoses. Laboratory testing is guided by the need to identify comorbidities.

Examination of the **growth chart** reveals the severity, duration, and timing of obesity onset. Children who are overweight (BMI in 85–95th percentile) are less likely to have developed comorbid conditions than those who are obese (BMI ≥95th percentile). Those with a BMI ≥99th percentile are more likely to have coexisting medical problems. Once obesity severity is determined, the BMI trajectory is examined to elucidate when the child became obese. Several periods during childhood are considered *sensitive* periods, or times of increased risk for developing obesity, including infancy, adiposity rebound (when body fat is lowest at approximately age 5.5 yr), and adolescence. An abrupt change in BMI might signal the onset of a medical problem or a period of family or personal stress for the child. Examination of the weight trajectory can further reveal how the problem developed. A young child might exhibit high weight and high height because linear growth can increase early in childhood if a child consumes excess energy. At some point the weight percentile exceeds the height percentile, and the child's BMI climbs into the obese range. Another example is a child whose weight rapidly increases when she reduces her activity level and consumes more meals away from home. Examination of the height trajectory can reveal endocrine problems, which often occur with slowing of linear growth.

Table 60.2	Obesity-Associated Comorbidities	
DISEASE	**POSSIBLE SYMPTOMS**	**LABORATORY CRITERIA**
CARDIOVASCULAR		
Dyslipidemia	HDL <40, LDL >130, total cholesterol >200 mg/dL	Fasting total cholesterol, HDL, LDL, triglycerides
Hypertension	SBP >95% for sex, age, height	Serial testing, urinalysis, electrolytes, blood urea nitrogen, creatinine
ENDOCRINE		
Type 2 diabetes mellitus	Acanthosis nigrans, polyuria, polydipsia	Fasting blood glucose >110, hemoglobin A_{1c}, insulin level, C-peptide, oral glucose tolerance test
Metabolic syndrome	Central adiposity, insulin resistance, dyslipidemia, hypertension, glucose intolerance	Fasting glucose, LDL and HDL cholesterol
Polycystic ovary syndrome	Irregular menses, hirsutism, acne, insulin resistance, hyperandrogenemia	Pelvic ultrasound, free testosterone, LH, FSH
GASTROINTESTINAL		
Gallbladder disease	Abdominal pain, vomiting, jaundice	Ultrasound
Nonalcoholic fatty liver disease (NAFLD)	Hepatomegaly, abdominal pain, dependent edema, ↑ transaminases. Can progress to fibrosis, cirrhosis	AST, ALT, ultrasound, CT, or MRI
NEUROLOGIC		
Pseudotumor cerebri	Headaches, vision changes, papilledema	Cerebrospinal fluid opening pressure, CT, MRI
Migraines	Hemicrania, headaches	None
ORTHOPEDIC		
Blount disease (tibia vara)	Severe bowing of tibia, knee pain, limp	Knee radiographs
Musculoskeletal problems	Back pain, joint pain, frequent strains or sprains, limp, hip pain, groin pain, leg bowing	Radiographs
Slipped capital femoral epiphysis	Hip pain, knee pain, limp, decreased mobility of hip	Hip radiographs
PSYCHOLOGIC		
Behavioral complications	Anxiety, depression, low self-esteem, disordered eating, signs of depression, worsening school performance, social isolation, problems with bullying or being bullied	Child Behavior Checklist, Children's Depression Inventory, Peds QL, Eating Disorder Inventory 2, subjective ratings of stress and depression, Behavior Assessment System for Children, Pediatric Symptom Checklist
PULMONARY		
Asthma	Shortness of breath, wheezing, coughing, exercise intolerance	Pulmonary function tests, peak flow
Obstructive sleep apnea	Snoring, apnea, restless sleep, behavioral problems	Polysomnography, hypoxia, electrolytes (respiratory acidosis with metabolic alkalosis)

ALT, Alanine transaminase; AST, aspartate transaminase; CT, computed tomography; FSH, follicle-stimulating hormone; HDL, high-density lipoprotein; LDL, low-density lipoprotein; LH, luteinizing hormone; MRI, magnetic resonance imaging; Peds QL, Pediatric Quality of Life Inventory; SBP, systolic blood pressure.

Consideration of possible medical causes of obesity is essential, even though endocrine and genetic causes are rare (see Table 60.1). Growth hormone deficiency, hypothyroidism, and Cushing syndrome are examples of endocrine disorders that can lead to obesity. In general, these disorders manifest with slow linear growth. Because children who consume excessive amounts of calories tend to experience accelerated linear growth, short stature warrants further evaluation. Genetic disorders associated with obesity may manifest extreme hyperphagia, or they can have coexisting dysmorphic features, cognitive impairment, vision and hearing abnormalities, or short stature. In some children with congenital disorders such as myelodysplasia or muscular dystrophy, lower levels of PA can lead to secondary obesity. Some medications, such as atypical antipsychotics, can cause excessive appetite and hyperphagia, resulting in obesity (Table 60.3). Rapid weight gain in a child or adolescent taking one of these medications might require its discontinuation. Poor linear growth and rapid changes in weight gain are indications for evaluation of possible medical causes.

Exploration of family eating, nutritional, and activity patterns begins with a description of regular meal and snack times and family habits for walking, bicycle riding, active recreation, and **screen time** (TV, computer, video games). It is useful to request a 24-hr dietary recall with special attention to intake of fruits, vegetables, and water, as well as high-calorie foods and high-carbohydrate beverages. When possible, evaluation by a nutritionist is extremely helpful. This information will

Table 60.3	Medications Associated With Obesity

Prednisone and other glucocorticoids
Thioridazine
Olanzapine
Clozapine
Quetiapine
Risperidone
Lithium
Amitriptyline and other tricyclic antidepressants
Paroxetine
Valproate
Carbamazepine
Gabapentin
Cyproheptadine
Propranolol and other β-blockers

form the basis for incremental changes in eating behavior, caloric intake, and PA during the intervention.

Initial assessment of the overweight or obese child includes a complete review of bodily systems focusing on the possibility of comorbid conditions (see Table 60.2). Developmental delay and visual and hearing impairment can be associated with genetic disorders. Difficulty sleeping, snoring, or daytime sleepiness suggests sleep apnea. Abdominal pain might suggest NAFLD. Symptoms of polyuria, nocturia, or polydipsia may be the result of type 2 diabetes. Hip or knee pain can be caused by secondary orthopedic problems, including Blount disease and slipped capital femoral epiphysis. Irregular menses may be associated with polycystic ovary syndrome. Acanthosis nigricans can suggest insulin resistance and type 2 diabetes (Fig. 60.4).

The family history begins with identifying other obese family members. Parental obesity is an important risk for child obesity. If all family members are obese, focusing the intervention on the entire family is reasonable. The child may be at increased risk for developing type 2 diabetes if a family history exists. Patients of African American, Hispanic, or Native American heritage are also at increased risk for developing type 2 diabetes. Identification of a family history of hypertension, CV disease, or metabolic syndrome indicates increased risk for developing these obesity-associated conditions. If the clinician helps the family to understand that childhood obesity increases risk for developing these chronic diseases, this educational intervention might serve as motivation to improve their nutrition and PA.

Physical examination should be thorough, focusing on possible comorbidities (see Table 60.2). Careful screening for hypertension using an appropriately sized blood pressure cuff is important. Systematic examination of the skin can reveal acanthosis nigricans, suggesting insulin resistance, or hirsutism, suggesting polycystic ovary syndrome. Tanner staging can reveal premature adrenarche secondary to advanced sexual maturation in overweight and obese girls.

Laboratory testing for fasting plasma glucose, triglycerides, low-density lipoprotein and high-density lipoprotein cholesterol, and liver function tests are recommended as part of the initial evaluation for newly identified pediatric obesity (Table 60.4). Overweight children (BMI 85–95th percentile) who have a family history of diabetes mellitus or signs of insulin resistance should also be evaluated with a fasting plasma glucose test. Other laboratory testing should be guided by history or physical examination findings. Fig. 60.5 provides a recommended approach to categorization, evaluation, and treatment.

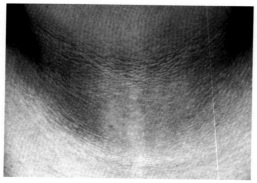

Fig. 60.4 Acanthosis nigricans. *(From Gahagan S: Child and adolescent obesity, Curr Probl Pediatr Adolesc Health Care 34:6–43, 2004.)*

INTERVENTION

Evidence shows that some interventions result in modest but significant and sustained improvement in body mass. Based on behavior change theories, treatment includes specifying **target behaviors**, **self-monitoring**, **goal setting**, **stimulus control**, and promotion of **self-efficacy** and **self-management** skills. **Behavior changes** associated with improving BMI include drinking lower quantities of sugar-sweetened beverages, consuming higher-quality diets, increasing exercise, decreasing screen time, and self-weighing. Most successful interventions have been *family based* and consider the child's developmental age. "Parent-only" treatment can be as effective as "parent–child" treatment. Because obesity is multifactorial, not all children and adolescents will respond to the same approach. For example, *loss-of-control eating*, associated with weight gain and obesity, predicts poor outcome in response to family-based treatment. Furthermore, clinical treatment programs are expensive and not widely available. Therefore, interest has grown in novel approaches such as internet-based treatments and guided self-help.

It is important to begin with clear recommendations about **appropriate caloric intake** for the obese child (Table 60.5). Working with a dietitian is essential. Meals should be based on fruits, vegetables, whole grains, lean meat, fish, and poultry. Prepared foods should be chosen for their nutritional value, with attention to calories and fat. Foods that provide excessive calories and low nutritional value should be reserved for infrequent treats.

Table 60.4	Normal Laboratory Values for Recommended Tests
LABORATORY TEST	**NORMAL VALUE**
Glucose	<110 mg/dL
Insulin	<15 mU/L
Hemoglobin A_{1c}	<5.7%
AST (age 2-8 yr)	<58 U/L
AST (age 9-15 yr)	<46 U/L
AST (age 15-18 yr)	<35 U/L
ALT	<35 U/L
Total cholesterol	<170 mg/dL
LDL	<110 mg/dL
HDL	>45 mg/dL
Triglycerides (age 0-9 yr)	<75 mg/dL
Triglycerides (age 10-19 yr)	<90 mg/dL

AST, Aspartate transaminase; ALT, alanine transaminase; LDL, low-density lipoprotein; HDL, high-density lipoprotein.

From Children's Hospital of Wisconsin: *The NEW (nutrition, exercise and weight management) kids program* (PDF file). http://www.chw.org/display/displayFile.asp?docid=33672&filename=/Groups/NEWKids/NewKidsReferral .PDF.

Table 60.5	Recommended Caloric Intake Designated by Age and Gender			
LIFE-STAGE GROUP	**AGE (yr)**	**RELATIVELY SEDENTARY LEVEL OF ACTIVITY (kcal)**	**MODERATE LEVEL OF ACTIVITY (kcal)**	**ACTIVE (kcal)**
Child	2-3	1,000	1,000-1,400	1,000-1,400
Female	4-8	1,200	1,400-1,600	1,400-1,800
	9-13	1,600	1,600-2,000	1,800-2,200
	14-18	1,800	2,000	2,400
Male	4-8	1,400	1,400-1,600	1,600-2,000
	9-13	1,800	1,800-2,200	2,000-2,600
	14-18	2,200	2,400-2,800	2,800-3,200

Adapted from U.S. Department of Agriculture: *Dietary guidelines for Americans*, 2005. http://www.health.gov/DIETARYGUIDELINES/dga2005/document/html/chapter2.htm.

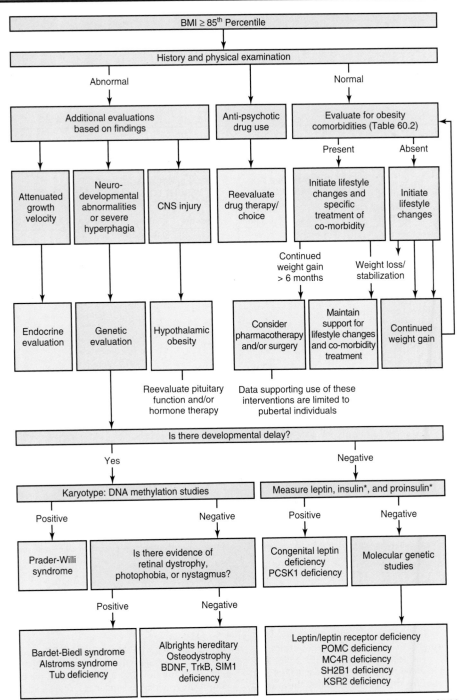

Fig. 60.5 Diagnosis and management flow chart. *Measure insulin and proinsulin in patients with clinical features of PCSK1 deficiency. BMI, Body mass index; CNS, central nervous system. (From Farooqi SOR, O'Rahilly S: Genetic obesity syndromes. In Grant S, editor: The genetics of obesity, New York, 2014, Springer, pp 23–32; originally adapted from August GP, Caprio S, Fennoy I, et al: Prevention and treatment of pediatric obesity: an Endocrine Society clinical practice guideline based on expert opinion, J Clin Endocrinol Metab 93:4576–4599, 2008.)*

Weight reduction diets in adults generally do not lead to sustained weight loss. Therefore the focus should be on changes that can be maintained for life. Attention to eating patterns is helpful. Families should be encouraged to plan *family meals,* including breakfast. It is almost impossible for a child to make changes in nutritional intake and eating patterns if other family members do not make the same changes. Dietary needs also change developmentally; adolescents require greatly increased calories during their growth spurts, and adults who lead inactive lives need fewer calories than active, growing children.

Psychologic strategies are helpful. The **"traffic light" diet** groups foods into those that can be consumed without any limitations (green), in moderation (yellow), or reserved for infrequent treats (red) (Table 60.6). The concrete categories are very helpful to children and families. This approach can be adapted to any ethnic group or regional cuisine.

Table 60.6	"Traffic Light" Diet Plan		
FEATURE	**GREEN LIGHT FOODS**	**YELLOW LIGHT FOODS**	**RED LIGHT FOODS**
Quality	Low-calorie, high-fiber, low-fat, nutrient-dense	Nutrient-dense, but higher in calories and fat	High in calories, sugar, and fat
Types of food	Fruits, vegetables	Lean meats, dairy, starches, grains	Fatty meats, sugar, sugar-sweetened beverages, fried foods
Quantity	Unlimited	Limited	Infrequent or avoided

Table 60.7	Medications for Weight Management With Mechanism of Action, Availability, and Dosing						
		AVAILABLE FOR CHRONIC USE		**MEAN PERCENTAGE WEIGHT LOSS**			
MEDICATION	**MECHANISM OF ACTION**	**USA**	**European Union**	**Placebo**	**Drug**	**ADVANTAGES**	**DISADVANTAGES**
Phentermine, 15-30 mg PO	Sympathomimetic	For short-term use	No	Not stated in label	Not stated in label	Inexpensive	Side effect profile; no long-term data*
Orlistat, 120 mg PO tid before meals	Pancreatic lipase inhibitor	Yes	Yes	−2.6%†	−6.1%†	Not absorbed; long-term data*	Modest weight loss; side effect profile
Lorcaserin, 10 mg PO bid	5-HT$_{2c}$ serotonin agonist with little affinity for other serotonergic receptors	Yes	No	−2.5%	−5.8%	Mild side effects; long-term data*	Expensive; modest weight loss
Phentermine/topiramate ER, 7.5 mg/46 mg or 15 mg/92 mg PO indicated as rescue (requires titration)	Sympathomimetic anticonvulsant (GABA receptor modulation, carbonic anhydrase inhibition, glutamate antagonism)	Yes	No	−1.2%	−7.8% (mid-dose) −9.8% (full dose)	Robust weight loss; long-term data*	Expensive; teratogen
Naltrexone SR/bupropion SR, 32 mg/360 mg PO (requires titration)	Opioid receptor antagonist; dopamine and noradrenaline reuptake inhibitor	Yes	Yes	−1.3%	−5.4%	Reduces food craving; long-term data*	Moderately expensive; side effect profile
Liraglutide, 3.0 mg injection (requires titration)	GLP-1 receptor agonist	Yes	Yes	−3%	−7.4% (full dose)	Side effect profile; long-term data*	Expensive; injectable

Information is from U.S. product labels, except where noted. The data supporting these tables are derived from the prescribing information labeling approved by the US Food and Drug Administration.
*Data from randomized controlled trials lasting >52 wk.
†Assuming the average patient in the orlistat and placebo groups weighed 100 kg at baseline.
ER, Extended release; SR, sustained release; PO, orally; bid, twice daily; tid, 3 times daily.
Adapted from Bray GA, Frühbeck G, Ryan DH, Wilding JPH: Management of obesity, *Lancet* 387:1947–1965, 2016, p 1950.

Motivational interviewing begins with assessing how ready the patient is to make important behavioral changes. The professional then engages the patient in developing a strategy to take the next step toward the ultimate goal of healthy nutritional intake. This method allows the professional to take the role of a coach, helping the child and family reach their goals. Other behavioral approaches include family rules about where food may be consumed (e.g., "not in the bedroom").

Increasing PA without decreasing caloric intake is unlikely to result in weight loss. However, **aerobic exercise** training has been shown to improve metabolic profiles in obese children and adolescents. Furthermore, it can increase aerobic fitness and decrease percent body fat even without weight loss. Therefore, increasing PA can decrease risk for CV disease, improve well-being, and contribute to weight loss. Increased PA can be accomplished by walking to school, engaging in PA during leisure time with family and friends, or enrolling in organized sports. Children are more likely to be active if their parents are active. As with

family meals, family PA is recommended. When adults lose significant weight, they may regain that weight despite eating fewer calories. The body may adapt to weight loss by reducing the basal metabolic rate (BMR), thus requiring fewer calories. One approach to this phenomenon is to increase PA.

Active pursuits can replace more sedentary activities. The American Academy of Pediatrics recommends that screen time be restricted to no more than 2 hr/day for children >2 yr old and that children <2 yr old not watch television. TV watching is often associated with eating, and many highly caloric food products are marketed directly to children during child-oriented television programs.

Pediatric healthcare providers should assist families to develop goals to change nutritional intake and PA. They can also provide the child and family with needed information. The family should not expect immediate lowering of BMI percentile related to behavioral changes, but can instead count on a gradual decrease in the rate of BMI percentile increase until it stabilizes, followed by a gradual decrease. Referral to multidisciplinary, comprehensive pediatric weight management programs is ideal for obese children whenever possible.

Pharmacotherapy for weight loss in the pediatric population is understudied. Randomized controlled trials (RCTs) have evaluated many medications, including metformin, orlistat, sibutramine, and exanatide (Table 60.7). Available medications result in modest weight loss or BMI improvement, even when combined with behavioral interventions. Various classes of drugs are of interest, including those that decrease energy intake or act centrally as **anorexiants**, those that affect the availability of nutrients through intestinal or renal tubular reabsorption, and those that affect metabolism. The only U.S. Food and Drug Administration (FDA)–approved medication for obesity in children <16 yr old is *orlistat,* which decreases absorption of fat, resulting in modest weight loss. This agent offers little benefit to severely obese adolescents. Because multiple redundant neural mechanisms act to protect body weight, promoting weight loss is extremely difficult. Thus there is considerable interest in combining therapies that simultaneously target multiple weight-regulating pathways. One example, approved for adults, combines *phentermine,* a noradrenergic agent, with *topiramate,* a γ-aminobutyric acid (GABA)–ergic medication. This combination resulted in a mean 10.2-kg weight loss vs 1.4 kg in the placebo group. Side effects are common and include dry mouth, constipation, paresthesias, insomnia, and cognitive dysfunction. Another promising example is the combination of amylin (decreases food intake and slows gastric emptying) with leptin, which has no anorexigenic effects when given alone. This combination

requires injection and is in clinical trials in adults. Another FDA-approved drug for adults is *lorcaserin,* a selective serotonin 2C receptor agonist. Establishing long-term safety and tolerability in children is a challenge because medications of interest have CNS effects or interfere with absorption of nutrients. Teratologic effects must be considered for use in adolescent girls.

Hormone replacement therapy is available for patients with leptin deficiency and may become available for patients with POMC deficiency. Setmelanotide binds to and activates MC4R and may be useful for patients with POMC deficiency–associated obesity.

In some cases it is reasonable to refer adolescents for **bariatric surgery** evaluation. The American Pediatric Surgical Association guidelines recommends that surgery be considered only in children with complete or near-complete skeletal maturity, a BMI ≥40, and a medical complication resulting from obesity, *after* they have failed 6 mo of a multidisciplinary weight management program. Surgical approaches include the Roux-en-Y and the adjustable gastric band (Fig. 60.6). In obese adults, bariatric surgery reduces the risk of developing type 2 diabetes mellitus. In obese adult patients with existing type 2 diabetes, bariatric surgery improves diabetic control. Nutritional complications of bariatric surgery include malabsorption and vitamin (A, B_1, B_2, B_6, B_{12}, D, E, K) and mineral (copper, iron) deficiencies that require supplementation.

PREVENTION

Prevention of child and adolescent obesity is essential for public health in the United States and most other countries (Tables 60.8 and 60.9).

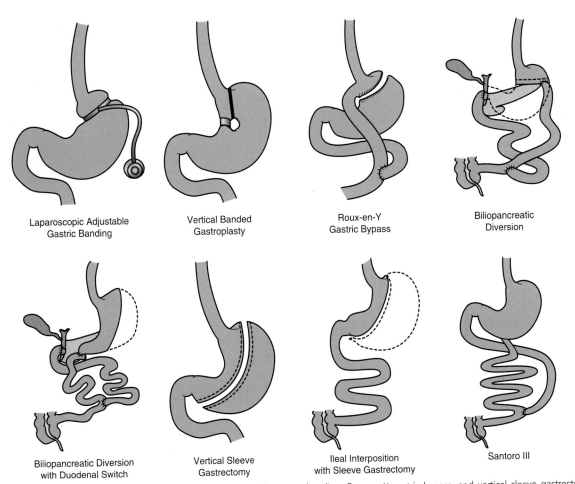

Laparoscopic Adjustable
Gastric Banding

Vertical Banded
Gastroplasty

Roux-en-Y
Gastric Bypass

Biliopancreatic
Diversion

Biliopancreatic Diversion
with Duodenal Switch

Vertical Sleeve
Gastrectomy

Ileal Interposition
with Sleeve Gastrectomy

Santoro III

Fig. 60.6 Bariatric surgical procedures. Laparoscopic adjustable gastric banding, Roux-en-Y gastric bypass, and vertical sleeve gastrectomy techniques.

Table 60.8	Proposed Suggestions for Preventing Obesity

PREGNANCY

Normalize body mass index (BMI) before pregnancy.

Do not smoke.

Maintain moderate exercise as tolerated.

In women with gestational diabetes, provide meticulous glucose control.

Monitor gestational weight gain within Institute of Medicine (IOM) recommendations.

POSTPARTUM AND INFANCY

Breastfeeding: exclusive for 4-6 mo; continue with other foods for 12 mo.

Postpone introduction of baby foods to 4-6 mo and juices to 12 mo.

FAMILIES

Eat meals as a family in a fixed place and time.

Do not skip meals, especially breakfast.

Do not allow television during meals.

Use small plates, and keep serving dishes away from the table.

Avoid unnecessary sweet or fatty foods and sugar-sweetened drinks.

Remove televisions from children's bedrooms; restrict times for TV viewing and video games.

Do not use food as a reward.

SCHOOLS

Eliminate candy and cookie sales as fundraisers.

Review the contents of vending machines, and replace with healthier choices; eliminate sodas.

Avoid financial support for sports teams from beverage and food industries.

Install water fountains and hydration stations.

Educate teachers, especially physical education and science faculty, about basic nutrition and the benefits of physical activity (PA).

Educate children from preschool through high school on appropriate diet and lifestyle.

Mandate minimum standards for physical education, including 60 min of strenuous exercise 5 times weekly.

Encourage "the walking school bus": groups of children walking to school with adult supervision.

COMMUNITIES

Increase family-friendly exercise and safe play facilities for children of all ages.

Develop more mixed residential-commercial developments for walkable and bicyclable communities.

Discourage the use of elevators and moving walkways.

Provide information on how to shop and prepare healthier versions of culture-specific foods.

HEALTHCARE PROVIDERS

Explain the biologic and genetic contributions to obesity.

Give age-appropriate expectations for body weight in children.

Work toward classifying obesity as a disease to promote recognition, reimbursement for care, and willingness and ability to provide treatment.

INDUSTRY

Mandate age-appropriate nutrition labeling for products aimed at children (e.g., "red light/green light" foods, with portion sizes).

Encourage marketing of interactive video games in which children must exercise to play.

Use celebrity advertising directed at children for healthful foods to promote breakfast and regular meals.

Reduce portion size (drinks and meals).

GOVERNMENT AND REGULATORY AGENCIES

Classify childhood obesity as a legitimate disease.

Find novel ways to fund healthy lifestyle programs (e.g., with revenues from food and drink taxes).

Subsidize government-sponsored programs to promote the consumption of fresh fruits and vegetables.

Provide financial incentives to industry to develop more healthful products and to educate the consumer on product content.

Provide financial incentives to schools that initiate innovative PA and nutrition programs.

Allow tax deductions for the cost of weight loss and exercise programs.

Provide urban planners with funding to establish bicycle, jogging, and walking paths.

Ban advertising of fast foods, non-nutritious foods, and sugar-sweetened beverages directed at preschool children, and restrict advertising to school-age children.

Ban toys as gifts to children for purchasing fast foods.

Adapted from Speiser PW, Rudolf MCJ, Anhalt H, et al: Consensus statement: childhood obesity, *J Clin Endocrinol Metab* 90:1871–1887, 2005.

Table 60.9	Anticipatory Guidance: Establishing Healthy Eating Habits in Children

Do not punish a child during mealtimes with regard to eating. The emotional atmosphere of a meal is very important. Interactions during meals should be pleasant and happy.

Do not use foods as rewards.

Parents, siblings, and peers should model healthy eating, tasting new foods, and eating a well-balanced meal.

Children should be exposed to a wide range of foods, tastes, and textures.

New foods should be offered multiple times. Repeated exposure leads to acceptance and liking.

Forcing a child to eat a certain food will decrease the child's preference for that food. Children's wariness of new foods is normal and should be expected. Offering a variety of foods with low-energy density helps children balance energy intake.

Parents should control what foods are in the home. Restricting access to foods in the home will increase rather than decrease a child's desire for that food.

Children tend to be more aware of satiety than adults, so allow children to respond to satiety, and stop eating. Do not force children to "clean their plate."

Adapted from Benton D: Role of parents in the determination of food preferences of children and the development of obesity, *Int J Obes Relat Metab Disord* 28:858–869, 2004. Copyright 2004. Reprinted by permission from Macmillan Publishers Ltd.

Efforts by pediatric providers can supplement national and community public health programs. The National Institutes of Health (NIH) and U.S. Centers for Disease Control and Prevention (CDC) recommend a variety of initiatives to combat the current obesogenic environment, including promotion of breastfeeding, access to fruits and vegetables, walkable communities, and 60 min/day of activity for children. The U.S. Department of Agriculture (USDA) sponsors programs promoting 5.5 cups of fruits and vegetables per day. Incentives for the food industry to promote consumption of healthier foods should be considered. Marketing of unhealthy foods to children is now being regulated. Changes in federal food programs are expected, including commodity foods, the Women, Infant, and Children Supplemental Food Program (WIC), and school lunch programs, to meet the needs of today's children.

Pediatric prevention efforts begin with careful monitoring of weight and BMI percentiles at healthcare maintenance visits. Attention to changes in BMI percentiles can alert the pediatric provider to increasing adiposity before the child becomes overweight or obese. All families should be counseled about healthy nutrition for their children, because the current prevalence of overweight and obesity in adults is 65%. Therefore, approximately two thirds of all children can be considered at risk for becoming overweight or obese at some time in their lives. Those who have an obese parent are at increased risk. Prevention efforts begin with promotion of *exclusive breastfeeding for 6 mo* and total breastfeeding for 12 mo. Introduction of infant foods at 6 mo should focus on cereals, fruits, and vegetables. Lean meats, poultry, and fish may be introduced later in the 1st year of life. Parents should be specifically counseled to *avoid introducing highly sugared beverages and foods in the 1st year* of life. Instead, they should expose their infants and young children to a rich variety of fruits, vegetables, grains, lean meats, poultry, and fish to facilitate acceptance of a diverse and healthy diet. Parenting matters, and **authoritative** parents are more likely to have children with a healthy weight than those who are authoritarian or permissive. Families who eat regularly scheduled meals together are less likely to have overweight or obese children. Child health professionals can address a child's nutritional status and provide expertise in child growth and development.

Child health professionals can also *promote PA* during regular healthcare maintenance visits. Parents who spend some of their leisure time in PA promote healthy weight in their children. Beginning in infancy, parents should be cognizant of their child's developmental capability and need for PA. Because TV, computer, and video game time can replace health-promoting PA, physicians should counsel parents to limit screen time for their children. Snacking during TV watching should be discouraged. Parents can help their children to understand that television commercials intend to sell a product. Children can learn that their parents will help them by responsibly choosing healthy foods.

Because obesity is determined by complex multifactorial conditions, prevention will take efforts at multiple levels of social organization. Successful programs include **EPODE** (Ensemble Prévenons l'Obésité Des Enfants), a multilevel prevention strategy that began in France and has been adopted by more than 500 communities in 6 countries. **Shape Up Somerville** is a citywide campaign to increase daily PA and healthy eating in Somerville, MA, since 2002. The **"Let's Move"** campaign was championed by former First Lady Michelle Obama. Since community and environmental factors are related to pediatric obesity risk, changes in local environments, daycare centers, schools, and recreational settings can have a public health impact. Programs can empower families to adopt practices that promote healthy lifestyles for children and adolescents. The most successful programs are comprehensive and rely on 4 strategies: political commitment to change, resources to support social marketing and changes, support services, and evidence-based practices. Community-wide programs are important because neighborhood environmental factors (e.g., poverty) have been associated with obesity in its residents. There is considerable interest in focusing these efforts early in the life cycle. Beginning obesity prevention during pregnancy and engaging health systems, early childhood programs, and community systems to support healthier life cycles is an approach with great promise.

Bibliography is available at Expert Consult.

60.1 Rapid-Onset Obesity With Hypothalamic Dysfunction, Hypoventilation, and Autonomic Dysregulation (ROHHAD)

Sarah F. Barclay, Amy Zhou, Casey M. Rand, and Debra E. Weese-Mayer

ROHHAD—rapid-onset obesity with hypothalamic dysfunction, hypoventilation, and autonomic dysregulation—is a rare, poorly understood disease of childhood onset, the first sign of which is sudden, rapid, and extreme weight gain in a previously healthy child. The acronym describes the presenting symptoms and the typical order in which they will manifest or unfold, as the condition evolves over months to years. Despite its rarity, ROHHAD must be considered whenever rapid-onset obesity is observed in a child, because in the absence of appropriate treatment, a high mortality rate is associated with the severe central hypoventilation that will invariably develop.

The diagnosis is initially considered after the observation of rapid-onset obesity (15-20 lb gain) after age 1.5 yr, accompanied by at least 1 additional sign of hypothalamic dysfunction. Central hypoventilation may not be present at diagnosis but will develop over time, and artificial ventilatory support will be required at least during sleep, if not 24 hr/day. Signs of autonomic nervous system dysregulation typically occur after the weight gain, hypothalamic dysfunction, and hypoventilation have been identified. Additionally, approximately 40% of ROHHAD patients will have a tumor of neural crest origin, typically ganglioneuroma or ganglioneuroblastoma.

ROHHAD is distinct from **late-onset congenital central hypoventilation syndrome (LO-CCHS;** see later and Chapter 446.2). ROHHAD is primarily distinguished from LO-CCHS by the presence of obesity and other signs of hypothalamic dysfunction and by the absence of CCHS-related *PHOX2B* mutation. Approximately 100 cases of ROHHAD have been described in the literature to date.

CLINICAL MANIFESTATIONS

Children with ROHHAD initially appear healthy, with an unremarkable history. The initial symptoms present between ages 18 mo and 7 yr. Typically, the 1st symptom observed is **rapid-onset obesity**, with weight gain of 15-20 lb in 6-12 mo. This is a sign of **hypothalamic dysfunction (HD)** in these patients. The 2nd common sign of HD, seen in most ROHHAD patients, is **disordered water balance**, including hyper- and hyponatremia and both adipsia and polydipsia. Growth hormone (GH) deficiency is also observed in most patients. In some this manifests clinically as slowed growth rate and short stature, whereas in others a failed GH stimulation test is the only evidence. Other symptoms of HD, occurring in >25–50% of ROHHAD patients, include hyperprolactinemia, poor thermoregulation, central hypothyroidism, adrenal insufficiency, and delayed or precocious puberty. The number of hypothalamic abnormalities that will be observed and the sequential order in which they will appear are variable, and some symptoms may not manifest for months to 1-2 yr after the initial diagnosis. However, all ROHHAD patients will present with at least 1 of these signs of HD.

Sleep-disordered breathing (SDB) is one of the key symptoms of ROHHAD, often manifesting as one of the most severe features of the phenotype, with the greatest potential for fatal complications. More than half of ROHHAD patients have initial **obstructive sleep apnea (OSA)**; although SDB is known to be associated with obesity, and OSA is often seen in obese individuals, the extent that SDB is tied to obesity in ROHHAD patients is not yet well defined. However, over time, as the ROHHAD phenotype unfolds, SDB will evolve beyond what could potentially be explained as obesity related. All ROHHAD patients will eventually develop **central alveolar hypoventilation**, requiring artificial ventilatory support, even when the upper airway obstruction is relieved as an intervention for OSA. About half of ROHHAD patients will require artificial ventilation only during sleep, while half will require continuous artificial ventilation (during sleep and wakefulness). More than 40% of children with ROHHAD will have a cardiorespiratory arrest before their hypoventilation is identified and treated. Unfortunately, many ROHHAD patients die from cardiorespiratory arrest because of unrecognized or inadequately managed hypoventilation. Thus, if a ROHHAD diagnosis is suspected, it is crucial that a comprehensive respiratory physiology evaluation is performed, including overnight polysomnography and awake physiologic recording in activities of daily living (ADLs).

All ROHHAD patients have symptoms of **autonomic nervous system (ANS) dysregulation**, but as described for signs of HD, the exact symptoms and the order and timing of their appearance will vary between patients. The most common manifestations of ANS dysregulation in ROHHAD are ophthalmologic, including pupillary dysfunction, strabismus, and alacrima. Many ROHHAD patients will have gastrointestinal dysmotility, presenting as either chronic constipation or chronic diarrhea. Other signs of ANS dysregulation include altered sweating, decreased body temperature, decreased sensitivity to pain, and cold hands and feet indicating altered vasomotor tone. Bradycardia is seen in some ROHHAD patients, typically related to extreme hypothermia.

Neural crest tumors are observed in at least 40% of ROHHAD patients, most frequently ganglioneuromas and ganglioneuroblastomas of the chest or abdomen; rarely a neuroblastoma has been reported. These tumors can occur at any age, so proactive imaging evaluation to identify the tumors is essential.

Most patients do not have **behavioral or psychologic disorders**. For those who do, however, the disorders can be quite severe, including anxiety, depression, rage, lethargy, irritability, aggressiveness, psychosis, and obsessive-compulsive disorder. Developmental disorders described include neurocognitive delay, developmental regression, attention-deficit/hyperactivity disorder, and pervasive developmental disorder. These disorders are most likely caused by poorly managed hypoventilation because the majority of ROHHAD patients have no behavioral issues and a normal IQ.

Seizures have been reported in some ROHHAD patients, likely caused by episodes of hypoxemia, when hypoventilation either has not yet been diagnosed or has been inadequately managed.

DIAGNOSIS

The diagnostic criteria for ROHHAD include **r**apid-onset obesity after 1.5 years of age, central hypoventilation beginning after age 1.5 yr, and ≥1 of the following signs of HD: disordered water balance, hyperprolactinemia, failed GH stimulation test, central hypothyroidism, corticotropin deficiency, and altered onset of puberty. Additionally, it should be confirmed that no CCHS-related *PHOX2B* gene mutation is present, to rule out a diagnosis of CCHS or LO-CCHS.

Since no single diagnostic test is currently available for ROHHAD, diagnosis must be based on observation of the clinical presentation and therefore requires expert consultation in several specialties, including respiratory physiology, endocrinology, autonomic medicine, cardiology, oncology, nutrition, critical care, and psychiatry. When a child with rapid-onset obesity is seen by a general pediatrician or family physician, the trajectory of weight gain should signal prompt consideration of a ROHHAD diagnosis, with immediate referral to a center with expertise in this unique constellation of symptoms. Early recognition is critical for a positive outcome in children with ROHHAD. If alveolar hypoventilation is not identified and aggressively managed, cardiorespiratory arrest can occur and has proved fatal in many cases.

Initial evaluations should include overnight polysomnography to identify OSA or central hypoventilation, awake comprehensive physiologic recording in activities of daily living, cardiac evaluation to evaluate for cor pulmonale, endocrine function evaluation, screening for neural crest tumors (chest radiograph, abdominopelvic ultrasound), and a psychiatric evaluation, especially if any behavioral, psychologic, or developmental disorders are seen or suspected. Brain imaging should be performed to rule out intracranial lesions that may account for the observed hypothalamic-pituitary abnormalities. If the criteria are met, and a ROHHAD diagnosis is made, successful management requires ongoing cooperation among the various specialists, with a team leader to orchestrate all testing, to provide integrated care for the child.

MANAGEMENT

There is currently no cure for ROHHAD. Rather, treatment consists of early identification, meticulous monitoring, and symptomatic management of the various symptoms as they develop. Comprehensive initial evaluations should determine the nature and severity of hypoventilation, HD, and ANS dysregulation, and appropriate interventions should be implemented. Obesity is very difficult to control, but in consultation with a nutritionist and endocrinologist, the trajectory of advancing weight gain can be diminished with moderate exercise and calorie restriction, leading to improved body mass index (BMI) with advancing age. Specific signs of HD and ANS dysregulation should be evaluated by a pediatric endocrinologist and expert in pediatric autonomic medicine, respectively, and treated as necessary. Such treatments or management strategies may

include hormone replacement; regimented fluid intake; ophthalmologic assessment and treatment; longitudinal monitoring of peripheral, core, and ambient temperature; and management of constipation with stool softeners. Disordered water balance to prevent dehydration should be addressed, as well as regulation of heart rate, since bradycardia is seen in some patients (usually with decreased core temperature).

Neural crest tumors should be assessed and resected by a pediatric surgeon together with a pediatric oncologist, because the sheer size of these benign tumors creates serious compromise to surrounding tissues. If no tumor is identified initially, screening should continue every 6 mo until age 7 yr and thereafter annually.

Most critical is the management of hypoventilation. Initial intervention for OSA will likely involve surgical relief of the upper airway obstruction. This will usually unveil central hypoventilation, and initiation of supported ventilation will be required. If no central hypoventilation is identified, the patient should continue to be vigilantly monitored by a respiratory physiologist because all ROHHAD patients will eventually develop central hypoventilation requiring artificial ventilation. Optimal oxygenation and ventilation can then be maintained using a mechanical ventilator with mask or tracheostomy. This should be accompanied by highly trained home nursing and continuous monitoring with oximetry and capnography during sleep, with spot checks during wakefulness. The goal should be to maintain hemoglobin saturation values of ≥95% and end-tidal CO_2 values of 35-45 mm Hg, with vigilant evaluation for awake hypoventilation necessitating artificial ventilation up to 24 hr/day as necessary.

Given that the ROHHAD phenotype evolves with advancing age, ongoing care requires regularly scheduled evaluation of all the systems involved to identify and treat further symptoms as they appear. Comprehensive evaluation should ideally occur at a **Center of Excellence** for ROHHAD and should include respiratory physiology assessment both asleep and awake (in ADLs including varied levels of exertion, concentrational tasks, quiet play, and eating), screening of chest and abdomen for neural crest tumors in the adrenals or along the sympathetic chain, evaluation of the hypothalamic-pituitary axis with hormonal replacement as necessary, age-appropriate noninvasive evaluation of ANS dysregulation, comprehensive cardiac evaluation for evidence of recurrent hypoxemia, and neurocognitive testing. These evaluations should initially occur at 3-6 mo intervals, but this schedule may be altered with advancing age, depending on each patient's clinical condition.

Without proper management, oxygen deprivation can lead to irreversible deterioration in patients. However, with prompt diagnosis and aggressive management, including careful attention to the child's airway, breathing, and circulation, complications can be minimized and the prognosis can be quite favorable, although long-term outcome remains unknown but the focus of an international registry (https://clinicaltrials.gov/show/NCT03135730).

ETIOLOGY: STUDIES AND HYPOTHESES

Despite advances made in the characterization of the ROHHAD phenotype and early identification, the cause of the disease is unknown. The interrelationships among the observed symptoms, as well as the mechanisms that underlie them, remain to be elucidated.

Genetic Studies

Because the related but seemingly distinct disorder CCHS has a genetic basis (*PHOX2B* mutation), ROHHAD may be genetic as well. ROHHAD patients do not have CCHS-related *PHOX2B* mutations, however, and no numerical or structural chromosomal rearrangements have been described. The sporadic occurrence of ROHHAD, without familial recurrence, is consistent with de novo mutations. Exome-sequencing analysis of 7 ROHHAD family trios did not identify any causative de novo protein-altering mutations, or any candidates under autosomal recessive or autosomal dominant inheritance models, even when a replication cohort of 28 additional ROHHAD probands was included.

Another genetic mutation model that can account for sporadic occurrence of a phenotype is a *somatic mutation* model, in which mutations occur postzygotically and are thus only present in a subset of an individual's cells. Consistent with a somatic mutation hypothesis, 2 pairs of monozygotic twins discordant for the ROHHAD phenotype have been reported. The exomes (from blood samples) of 1 twin pair were compared, but no discordant coding mutations were identified. The challenge is that the "correct" tissue needs to be sampled for the somatic mutation to be identified. In other phenotypes caused by somatic mutations, such as Proteus syndrome, the mutation causes overgrowth, so the affected (mutated) tissue is visible and can be sampled and sequenced. In ROHHAD, presumably the affected (mutated) cells are in the hypothalamus and/or ANS, which cannot be sampled and sequenced from living individuals. The neural crest tumors in many ROHHAD patients might represent an additional affected tissue. The exomes of neural crest tumors from 4 ROHHAD patients were compared to the exomes of blood samples from the same patients, but no tumor-specific mutations were identified.

The observation of monozygotic twins discordant for the ROHHAD phenotype could be consistent with a somatic genetic mutation, but could also suggest an alternative, nongenetic etiology. For example, epigenetic variation can account for some discordance between monozygotic twins and also can play a role in diseases involving respiratory and autonomic function, such as Prader-Willi syndrome (see later) and Rett syndrome.

Paraneoplastic/Autoimmune Hypothesis

Paraneoplastic syndromes are rare disorders caused by a neoplasm triggering an altered immune response that aberrantly attacks and destroys neurons, leading to the nervous system symptoms. An autoimmune or paraneoplastic basis for ROHHAD has been suggested based on neural crest tumors occurring in 40% of ROHHAD patients and 2 early cases with autopsies revealing low-density lesions in the basal ganglia and neuronal loss from lymphocytic infiltration of the hypothalamus, thalamus, midbrain, and pons. Autopsy of another ROHHAD patient revealed similar findings of hypothalamic inflammation with lymphocytic infiltrates and gliosis, although other autopsies have found no such pathology. Some cerebrospinal fluid (CSF) analyses have revealed pleocytosis, elevated neopterins, and oligoclonal bands consistent with intrathecal synthesis of oligoclonal immunoglobulin G. However, other studies report a lack of oligoclonal IgG and antineuronal antibodies, as well as clear CSF microscopies and cultures. Thus the evidence so far is conflicting, with some reports supporting the autoimmune hypothesis, while others do not. Further, the onset of ROHHAD symptoms often precedes the diagnosis of a neural crest tumor in ROHHAD patients, and in many cases, neural crest tumors have not been discovered with MRI or even an autopsy, although these tumors are often difficult to detect. However, this is also seen in other paraneoplastic syndromes, such as opsoclonus-myoclonus, where only some cases are associated with a neoplasm, the remainder being idiopathic.

After a patient with idiopathic HD was treated with immune globulin therapy, several other studies pursued similar treatments with immunoglobulins and corticosteroids in ROHHAD patients. After high-dose cyclophosphamide treatment, some ROHHAD patients reported symptomatic and neurophysiologic improvements while others had poor clinical results. Notably, reports indicate that immunotherapy has not consistently halted unfolding and advancing of the unique constellation of symptoms described in ROHHAD. Even with complete tumor resection and immunoablation, only partial recovery has been reported. The lack of return to baseline has been attributed to late treatment, where early rapid progressive disease left residual damage. This would be consistent with an immune-mediated hypothesis, in which an autoimmune process is initiated by a neural crest tumor but maintained in its absence, resulting in irreversible injury that prevents complete symptom resolution.

Neurocristopathy

Neurocristopathies are disorders caused by abnormal development of any of the tissues or systems that develop from the embryonic neural crest cell lineage. Given that the systems involved in the ROHHAD phenotype (hypothalamus, ANS, endocrine system) share a neural crest origin, ROHHAD fits into this class. One could then hypothesize that the observed symptoms are caused by abnormal development of neural crest cells at an early embryonic stage. This is indeed the case for the related disorder, CCHS, caused by mutations in the gene *PHOX2B*, which is important for the development of the ANS from neural crest cells. Under this hypothesis, the neural crest tumors seen in ROHHAD patients, rather than being the trigger for the rest of the phenotype (as proposed by the paraneoplastic theory), would be a result of the same abnormal development that caused the rest of the phenotype.

DIFFERENTIAL DIAGNOSIS

As noted earlier, **congenital central hypoventilation syndrome** is a rare pediatric disorder of the ANS and respiratory control. CCHS is caused by mutations in the *PHOX2B* gene, which plays an important role in the differentiation and development of the ANS from neural crest progenitor cells. The hallmark feature of CCHS is life-threatening hypoventilation while sleeping (and in some cases, also while awake). As with ROHHAD patients, CCHS patients require artificial ventilatory support, typically by tracheostomy and mechanical ventilator. Unlike ROHHAD, however, CCHS usually presents in the newborn period, although late-onset CCHS has been diagnosed in later childhood, adolescence, and even adulthood. CCHS also presents with other symptoms of ANS dysregulation, including altered heart rate regulation and altered vasomotor tone, altered temperature regulation, ophthalmologic manifestations, and reduced gastrointestinal motility. However, CCHS patients are not obese and do not typically have HD. When hypoventilation is observed, a simple blood test can confirm a CCHS diagnosis by looking for *PHOX2B* mutations. If *PHOX2B* mutations are not identified and the other features of the ROHHAD phenotype are identified, a ROHHAD diagnosis must be considered.

Prader-Willi syndrome (PWS) is similar to ROHHAD in that childhood obesity is one of the most prominent features; however, many important differences set these two conditions apart. PWS is caused by chromosomal abnormalities at chromosome 15q11-q13, specifically by a lack of the paternal contribution at this region (from genomic deletion, uniparental disomy, or imprinting error). Infants with PWS present with neonatal hypotonia and failure to thrive (malnutrition). Later, children with PWS develop extreme hyperphagia and obesity. Other major symptoms include mild intellectual impairment, maladaptive behaviors, short stature caused by GH insufficiency, hypogonadism, and SDB. In addition, many PWS patients show signs of ANS dysregulation, including altered temperature perception and regulation, strabismus, and high pain threshold. Although there are several apparently overlapping symptoms (pediatric obesity, SDB, ANS dysregulation), ROHHAD patients do not have the characteristic PWS genomic abnormality, hypogonadism, or consistent neurocognitive impairment. ROHHAD patients also are healthy in the neonatal period, showing none of the early PWS symptoms.

Bibliography is available at Expert Consult.

Chapter **61**

Vitamin A Deficiencies and Excess

A. Catharine Ross

第六十一章

维生素A缺乏和过量

中文导读

本章主要介绍了维生素A概述、维生素A代谢、维生素A的功能与机制、维生素A缺乏以及维生素A过量。针对维生素A代谢具体描述了新生儿维生素A营养状态和炎症引发维生素A缺乏；具体描述了维生素A缺乏的临床表现、诊断、治疗、维生素A缺乏流行病与公共卫生问题，以及正常人群维生素A参考摄入量。

OVERVIEW OF VITAMIN A

Vitamin A is a fat-soluble micronutrient that cannot be synthesized de novo by mammals; thus it is an obligatory dietary factor. The term **vitamin A** is generally used to refer to a group of compounds that possess the biologic activity of all-*trans* retinol (Fig. 61.1). As a fat-soluble micronutrient, vitamin A is recognized as being essential for all vertebrates for normal vision, reproduction, cell and tissue differentiation, and functions of the immune system. Vitamin A plays critical roles in neonatal development. It is required for normal embryonic development, hematopoiesis, immune response, metabolism, and growth and differentiation of many types of cells.

Vitamin A can be obtained from the diet from preformed vitamin A (retinyl esters, such as retinyl palmitate) primarily in foods of animal origin. Organ meats (especially liver, kidney) are very rich in vitamin A, whereas other meats, milk, and cheese contain moderate levels. Other sources of vitamin A include several provitamin A carotenoids, which are found naturally in many fruits and vegetables, especially yellow-orange vegetables (pumpkin, squash, sweet potato), and leafy green vegetables (chard, spinach, broccoli). One of the most abundant carotenoids is β-carotene. Several *cultivars* or biofortified forms of sweet potatoes have been introduced to elevate carotene intake in areas of the world where vitamin A deficiency still is prevalent. α-Carotene and oxygenated carotenoids, such as β-cryptoxanthin, found in oranges, also possess vitamin A activity, at a lower bioactivity. In the body, these precursors are used for the synthesis of 2 essential metabolites of vitamin A. **All-*trans* retinoic acid** is the form required for cell differentiation and regulation of gene transcription and is the most bioactive form of vitamin A; **11-*cis* retinal** is the form required for vision as the light-absorbing chromophore of the visual pigments rhodopsin and iodopsin.

METABOLISM OF VITAMIN A

Vitamin A compounds in foods must first be released through normal digestive processes. Retinyl esters must first be hydrolyzed in the intestinal lumen to liberate unesterified retinol for absorption across the mucosal barrier. Once in the enterocyte, most of the retinol is reesterified, forming new retinyl esters for inclusion in chylomicrons. Approximately 70–90% of dietary preformed vitamin A is absorbed provided there is ≥10 g fat in the meal; otherwise the absorption efficiency is lower. Chronic intestinal disorders or lipid malabsorption can result in vitamin A deficiency. Provitamin-A carotenoids are transported from the intestinal lumen into the enterocytes by specific transporters, then either incorporated intact into chylomicrons or cleaved to form *retinal*, a precursor for retinol; β-carotene becomes retinol through this process. The estimated efficiency of absorption of carotenoids is 20–50%, lower than for preformed vitamin A. Moreover, the efficiency is reduced when the body's vitamin A status is high, and because vitamin A status may vary, there is significant interindividual variability in absorption efficiency. The carotene cleavage enzyme β-carotene monooxygenase, present in the enterocyte and in other tissues at lower levels, exhibits certain single nucleotide polymorphisms (SNPs) that, at least in vitro, reduce the efficiency of conversion of β-carotene to retinol. Clinical studies suggest a similar effect in vivo.

Once retinol is esterified in the enterocyte, retinyl ester is then packaged into nascent chylomicrons, which are secreted into the lymphatic vessels, enter the systemic circulation, and are then transported to and taken up by various tissues. When vitamin A status is adequate, in most mammals, including humans, the liver is the major site of chylomicron vitamin A uptake and storage, with potentially high levels of retinyl

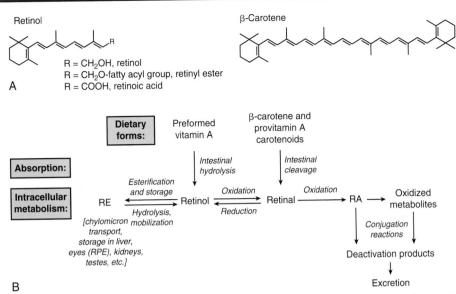

Fig. 61.1 A, Vitamin A structures. **B,** Overview of vitamin A metabolism. RA, All-*trans* retinoic acid; RE, retinyl ester; RPE, retinal pigment epithelium.

esters within hepatic stellate cells (HSCs). As vitamin A status deteriorates into the deficient range, vitamin A stores are mobilized from the HSCs, such that the released retinol can be taken up and utilized by extrahepatic tissues. Circulating retinol is bound to a specific transport protein, **retinol-binding protein (RBP)**, which in turn binds to the thyroid hormone transport protein, **transthyretin (TTR)**; this complex delivers plasma retinol (as well as the thyroid hormone) to a large number of vitamin A target tissues. The major physiologic mediator of retinol uptake by cells in many tissues is Stra6, a widely expressed multitransmembrane domain protein that functions as a cell surface receptor for retinol bound to RBP. Stra6 is not significantly expressed in the liver, but a homologous receptor may perform the similar function. Within target tissues, retinol is either esterified into retinyl esters for storage or oxidized into retinoic acid for function. In the eye, 11-*cis*-retinal is formed, bound to the protein rhodopsin (rods) or iodopsin (cones), where it functions as a light-sensing receptor.

Vitamin A Status in Neonates
Neonates begin life with low levels of vitamin A, in plasma, liver, and extrahepatic tissues, compared with those in adults. Normal plasma levels of retinol are 20-50 μg/dL in infants and increase gradually as children become older. Median serum retinol values are 1.19 μmol/L in both boys and girls ages 4-8 yr; 1.4 and 1.33 μmol/L in boys and girls, respectively, ages 9-13; and 1.71 and 1.57 μmol/L in boys and girls, ages 14-18 (for conversion, 1 μmol/L = 28.6 μg/dL). Values of 1.96 and 1.85 μmol/L are found in 19-30 yr old adult men and women, respectively. Fig. 61.2 shows the distribution of serum retinol concentrations in U.S. children.

Retinol levels are even lower in neonates in developing countries, where vitamin A intakes may be low and vitamin A deficiency is a common and significant nutritional problem. Lower vitamin A stores and plasma retinol concentrations are seen in low-birthweight infants and in preterm newborns. Malnutrition, particularly protein deficiency, can cause vitamin A deficiency because of the impaired synthesis of RBP.

Inflammation Causing Low Plasma Retinol
Inflammation is a cause of reduced levels of plasma retinol as a result of reduced synthesis of RBP and TTR. This condition may mimic a lack of vitamin A, but will not be corrected by supplementation. In U.S. adults, those with moderately elevated levels of C-reactive protein (CRP),

indicative of mild inflammation, had lower average plasma retinol levels. The extent to which inflammation is a factor in low plasma retinol in children is uncertain but likely significant in acute infectious diseases such as measles, and possibly in chronic inflammatory conditions such as cystic fibrosis.

FUNCTIONS OF VITAMIN A AND MECHANISMS OF ACTION
Except for its role in vision, the pleiotropic actions of this micronutrient are mediated by all-*trans*-retinoic acid (RA), which is a ligand for specific nuclear transcription factors, the **retinoid receptors**; RARs and RXRs regulate the expression of several hundred genes. When an RAR is activated by RA, an RAR-RXR complex is formed, which binds to and activates specific DNA sequences present in retinoid-responsive genes, RAREs and RXREs. Genes can be either induced or repressed, depending on additional co-activators or co-repressors recruited to the RAR-RXR complex. Retinoid-regulated genes are involved in several fundamental biologic activities, including regulation of cell division, death, and differentiation. The term *retinoids* applies to both natural and synthetic compounds with vitamin A activity and is most often used in the context of vitamin A acting at the gene level. Numerous synthetic retinoids have gained clinical acceptance in the treatment of skin disorders and certain cancers.

During embryonic development, retinoic acid is among the most important signaling molecules that determine body patterning (morphogenesis). Many physiologic processes are sensitive to a deficiency or excess of vitamin A or RA, including reproduction, growth, bone development, and the functions of the respiratory, gastrointestinal, hematopoietic, and immune systems. Vitamin A, presumably by enhancing immune function and host defense, is particularly important in developing countries; studies show that vitamin A supplementation or therapy reduces morbidity and mortality from various infectious diseases, including measles (see Chapter 273).

Vitamin A plays a critical role in vision, mediated by 11-*cis* retinal. The human retina contains 2 distinct photoreceptor systems: the *rods,* in which rhodopsin senses light of low-intensity, and the *cones,* in which iodopsins detect different colors; 11-*cis*-retinal is the prosthetic group on both these visual proteins. The mechanism of vitamin A action is similar for rods and cones, based on *photoisomerization* of 11-*cis* to all-*trans* retinal (change shape when exposed to light), which initiates signal transduction via the optic nerve to the brain, resulting in visual sensation. After isomerization (also known as photobleaching), a series of reactions serves to regenerate the 11-*cis* retinal for resynthesis of rhodopsin and iodopsin; accessory cells, including retinal pigment epithelium and Müller cells, are involved in this recycling process.

VITAMIN A DEFICIENCY

If the growing child has a well-balanced diet and obtains vitamin A from foods rich in vitamin A or provitamin A (Table 61.1), the risk of vitamin A deficiency is small. However, even subclinical vitamin A deficiency can have serious consequences.

Deficiency states in developed countries are rare, except in some impoverished populations (see Chapter 57), or after mistakes in food preparation or with fad diets, but are common in many developing countries and often associated with global malnutrition. In the clinical setting, vitamin deficiencies can also occur as complications in children with various chronic disorders or diseases. Information obtained in the medical history related to dietary habits can be important in identifying the risk of such nutritional problems. Except for vitamin A, toxicity

from excess intake of vitamins is rare. Table 61.1 summarizes the food sources, functions, and deficiency and excess symptoms of the vitamins.

Clinical Manifestations of Vitamin A Deficiency

The most obvious symptoms of vitamin A deficiency are associated with changes in epithelial cell morphology and functions. In the intestines, mucus-secreting goblet cells are affected, and loss of an effective barrier against pathogens can cause diarrhea or impairment of epithelial barrier function. Similarly, mucus secretion by the epithelium is essential in the respiratory tract for the disposal of inhaled pathogens and toxicants. Characteristic epithelial changes result from vitamin A deficiency, including proliferation of basal cells, hyperkeratosis, and formation of stratified cornified squamous epithelium. Squamous metaplasia of the renal pelves, ureters, vaginal epithelium, and the pancreatic and salivary ducts can lead to increased infections in these areas. In the urinary bladder, loss of epithelial integrity can result in pyuria and hematuria. In the skin, vitamin A deficiency manifests as dry, scaly, hyperkeratotic patches, typically on the arms, legs, shoulders, and buttocks. The combination of defective epithelial barriers to infection, low immune response, and lowered response to inflammatory stress, all from insufficient vitamin A, can cause poor growth and serious health problems in children.

The most characteristic and specific signs of vitamin A deficiency are *eye lesions*, but these may manifest rather late in the progression of vitamin A deficiency, develop insidiously, and rarely occur before age 2 yr. An earlier symptom of vitamin A deficiency is delayed dark adaptation, as a result of reduced resynthesis of rhodopsin; this may progress to **night blindness**. Photophobia is a common symptom. The retinal pigment epithelium (RPE), the structural element of the retina, undergoes keratinization. When the RPE degenerates, the rods and cones have no support and eventually break down, resulting in blindness.

As vitamin A deficiency progresses, the corneal and conjunctival epithelial tissues of the eye become severely altered because of a lack of sufficient RA for normal epithelial cell differentiation. The cornea protects the eye from the environment and is also important in light refraction. Stages in vitamin A deficiency include corneal keratinization and opacity, susceptibility to infection, and formation of dry, scaly layers of cells (**xerophthalmia**) (Figs. 61.3 and 61.4). The conjunctival membrane undergoes keratinization and may develop foamy-appearing plaques (**Bitôt spots**; Fig. 61.5). When lymphocytes infiltrate the cornea in later stages of infection, it degenerates irreversibly (**keratomalacia and corneal ulceration**), resulting in irreversible blindness. These eye lesions are primarily diseases of the young and are a major cause of blindness in developing countries. Although rates of xerophthalmia have fallen, the number of affected children is still too high. Treatment

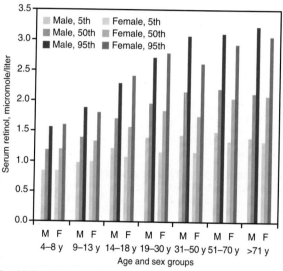

Fig. 61.2 Distribution of serum retinol concentrations in U.S. children and adults by age and sex in the National Health and Nutrition Examination Survey (NHANES).

Table 61.1	Vitamin A Characteristics				
NAMES AND SYNONYMS	**CHARACTERISTICS**	**BIOCHEMICAL ACTION**	**EFFECTS OF DEFICIENCY**	**EFFECTS OF EXCESS**	**SOURCES**
Retinol (vitamin A₁); 1 μg retinol = 3.3 IU vitamin A = 1 RAE Provitamins A: the plant pigments α-, β-, and γ-carotenes and cryptoxanthin have partial retinol activity: 12 μg β-carotene, or 24 μg other provitamin A carotenoids = 1 μg retinol	Fat-soluble; heat-stable; destroyed by oxidation, drying Bile necessary for absorption Stored in liver Protected by vitamin E	In vision, as retinal, for synthesis of the visual pigments rhodopsin and iodopsin In growth, reproduction, embryonic and fetal development, bone growth, immune and epithelial functions, via retinoic acid as a ligand for specific nuclear transcription factors, regulating genes involved in many fundamental cellular processes	Nyctalopia Photophobia, xerophthalmia, Bitôt spots, conjunctivitis, keratomalacia leading to blindness Faulty epiphyseal bone formation Defective tooth enamel Keratinization of mucous membranes and skin Retarded growth Impaired resistance to infection, anemia, reproductive failure, fetal abnormalities	Anorexia, slow growth, drying and cracking of skin, enlargement of liver and spleen, swelling and pain of long bones, bone fragility, increased intracranial pressure, alopecia, carotenemia Fetal abnormalities	Liver, fish liver oils Dairy products, except skim milk Egg yolk, fortified margarine, fortified skim milk Carotenoids from plants: green vegetables, yellow fruits, and vegetables

RAE, Retinol activity equivalent.

with vitamin A, up to the stage of keratomalacia, is effective in rapidly repleting the individual and saving vision.

Other clinical signs of vitamin A deficiency include poor overall growth, diarrhea, susceptibility to infections, anemia, apathy, intellectual impairment, and increased intracranial pressure, with wide separation of the cranial bones at the sutures. There may be vision problems as a consequence of bone overgrowth causing pressure on the optic nerve.

Malnutrition, particularly protein deficiency, can cause vitamin A deficiency through impaired synthesis of retinol transport protein. In developing countries, subclinical or clinical zinc deficiency can increase the risk of vitamin A deficiency. There is also some evidence of marginal zinc intakes in U.S. children.

Diagnosis

Dark adaptation tests can be used to assess early-stage vitamin A deficiency. Although Bitôt spots develop relatively early, those related to active vitamin A deficiency are usually confined to preschool-age children. Xerophthalmia is a very characteristic lesion of vitamin A deficiency. For detection of less severe deficiency (marginal vitamin A status), methods include conjunctival impression cytology, relative dose response, and modified relative dose response tests. A diet history is useful in suggesting or ruling out low intake as a cause of symptoms. Marginal vitamin A status is relatively prevalent among pregnant and lactating women in low-resource (and therefore poor dietary intake) areas of the world. Although plasma retinol level is not a completely accurate indicator of vitamin A status, various guidelines have been proposed for categorizing vitamin A status based on serum retinol. In children, plasma retinol <0.35 μmol/L is considered *very deficient*, 0.35-0.7 μmol/L *deficient*, 0.7-1.05 μmol/L *marginal*, and >1.05 μmol/L *adequate*. It has long been thought that a liver vitamin A concentration >20 μg/g is needed to support a normal rate of secretion of retinol-RBP into plasma, and therefore normal delivery of retinol to peripheral tissues.

Epidemiology and Public Health Issues

Vitamin A deficiency and xerophthalmia still occur throughout much of the developing, income-poor world and are linked to undernourishment and complicated by illness. Various public health programs to provide large doses of vitamin A periodically have been instituted. Vitamin A supplementation is considered part of the strategy of the World Health Organization (WHO) Millennium Development Goals to reduce <5 yr mortality. Neonatal supplementation may be most effective in populations with a high incidence of maternal vitamin A deficiency. Other strategies being tested include improving the content of β-carotene in staple foods through plant breeding (biofortification).

Dietary Reference Intakes for the Healthy Population

Table 61.2 summarizes the dietary reference intakes for infants and children. Dietary reference intake values include the estimated average requirement (EAR), which is the mean biologic requirement for the nutrient for the age-sex group of interest; the recommended dietary allowance (RDA), which is set to cover the physiological needs of >97% of the population (thus the needs of many people are more than met by consuming the RDA); and the upper level of normal (UL), an intake level above which risk of adverse effects may increase; the UL pertains only to chronic consumption of preformed vitamin A. The RDA is expressed as retinol activity equivalents (RAEs; 1 RAE = 1 μg all-*trans* retinol; equivalents for provitamin-A in foods = 12 μg β-carotene, 24 μg α-carotene, or 24 μg β-cryptoxanthin). From infancy to age 18 yr, the RDA increases as a result of increased body size, becoming higher for boys than girls during adolescence. During pregnancy the RDA is 750-770 μg, and during lactation it increases to 1,200-1,300 μg to ensure sufficient vitamin A content during breastfeeding.

It is noteworthy that, especially for young children, the UL is only about 2 times higher than the RDA. This suggests that for children whose diet is good, care should be taken not to overuse dietary supplements (vitamin-mineral supplements) containing preformed vitamin A, and/or to avoid excessive consumption of foods that are very rich in vitamin A, such as liver.

Vitamin A for Treatment of Deficiency

A daily supplement of 1,500 μg of vitamin A is sufficient for treating latent vitamin A deficiency, after which intake at the RDA level should be the goal. In children without overt signs of vitamin A deficiency but suspected low reserves of vitamin A, rates of morbidity and mortality, as from viral infections such as measles, have been reduced by a weekly doses of vitamin A at the RDA level. More often, higher doses of 30-60 mg of retinol (100,000-200,000 IU/child) are given once or twice, under careful monitoring to avoid toxicity associated with excess vitamin A. Xerophthalmia is treated by giving 1,500 μg/kg body weight orally for

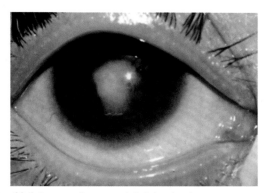

Fig. 61.4 Recovery from xerophthalmia, showing a permanent eye lesion. *(From Bloch CE: Blindness and other disease arising from deficient nutrition [lack of fat soluble A factor], Am J Dis Child 27:139, 1924.)*

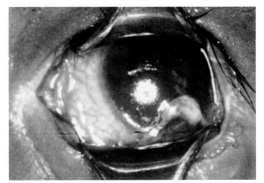

Fig. 61.3 Advanced xerophthalmia with an opaque, dull cornea and some damage to the iris in a 1 yr old boy. *(From Oomen HAPC: Vitamin A deficiency, xerophthalmia and blindness, Nutr Rev 6:161–166, 1974.)*

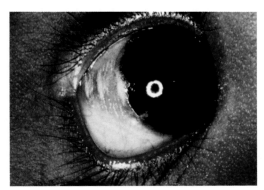

Fig. 61.5 Bitôt spots with hyperpigmentation seen in a 10 mo old Indonesian boy. *(From Oomen HAPC: Vitamin A deficiency, xerophthalmia and blindness, Nutr Rev 6:161–166, 1974.)*

Table 61.2	Dietary Reference Intakes for Vitamin A in Children		
AGE RANGE	**RECOMMENDED DIETARY ALLOWANCE (RDA) (μg retinol equivalents per day)**	**UPPER LEVEL (UL) (μg retinol equivalents per day)**	**COMMENTS**
0-6 mo	400	600	The recommended intake for infants is an adequate intake, based
7-12 mo	500	600	on the amount of vitamin A normally present in breast milk.
1-3 yr	300	600	The UL applies only to preformed vitamin A (retinol).
4-8 yr	400	900	
9-13 yr	600	1,700	
14-18 yr	900, male; 700, female	2,800	

5 days, followed by intramuscular injection of 7,500 μg of vitamin A in oil, until recovery. In neonatal rats, vitamin A given as a supplemental dose only transiently increased retinol levels in most tissues, although liver vitamin A remained higher more persistently.

Vitamin A is also used in preterm infants to improve respiratory function and prevent development of chronic lung disease. An analysis of 9 randomized controlled trials found that vitamin A appears to be beneficial in reducing death or oxygen requirement with no difference in neurodevelopmental outcomes.

HYPERVITAMINOSIS A

Chronic hypervitaminosis A results from excessive ingestion of preformed vitamin A (retinol or retinyl ester), generally for several weeks or months. Hypervitaminosis A is most often caused by vitamin A–containing supplements or food faddism, including high intakes of organ meats. Chronic daily intakes of 15,000 μg and 6,000 μg can be toxic in adults and children, respectively. Because there is no antidote for hypervitaminosis A, and vitamin A is readily stored in liver and other tissues, it is most important to prevent toxicity. Symptoms may subside rapidly on withdrawal of the vitamin, but the rate of improvement depends on the amount of vitamin A stored in tissues. Extreme hypervitaminosis A is fatal. Signs of subacute or chronic toxicity can include headache, vomiting (early signs), anorexia, dry itchy desquamating skin, and seborrheic cutaneous lesions. With chronic hypervitaminosis A, one may observe fissuring at the corners of the mouth, alopecia and coarsening of the hair, bone abnormalities and swelling, enlargement of the liver and spleen, diplopia, increased intracranial pressure, irritability, stupor, limited motion, dryness of the mucous membranes, and desquamation of the palms and the soles of the feet. Radiographs may show *hyperostosis* affecting several long bones, especially in the middle of the shafts (Fig. 61.6). Serum levels of vitamin A are elevated, mostly as retinyl esters carried in lipoproteins, which may result in tissue damage and release of liver enzymes into plasma. Hypercalcemia and/or liver cirrhosis may be present. Hypervitaminosis A is distinct from cortical hyperostosis (see Chapter 720).

In young children, signs of vitamin A toxicity include vomiting and bulging fontanels, neither of which is specific. Combined with anorexia, pruritus, and a lack of weight gain, vitamin A toxicity should be considered. Less common symptoms include diplopia, papilledema, cranial nerve palsies, and other symptoms suggesting **pseudotumor cerebri.**

If high levels of vitamin A or synthetic retinoids are taken early in pregnancy, **severe congenital malformations** may occur in the fetus. **Teratogenicity** has been associated with therapeutic doses (0.5-1.5 mg/kg) of oral 13-*cis*-retinoic acid (e.g., Accutane), generally taken for the treatment of acne or cancer, during the 1st trimester of pregnancy. A high incidence (>20%) of spontaneous abortions and birth defects, including characteristic craniofacial abnormalities, has prompted the U.S. Food and Drug Administration (FDA) to enact more stringent prescription regulations for such drugs in women of childbearing age, to attempt to reduce these birth defects.

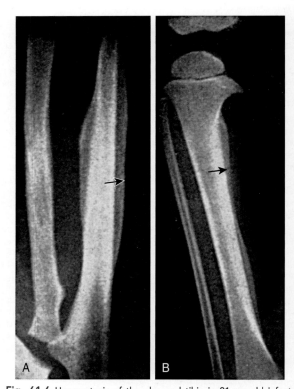

Fig. 61.6 Hyperostosis of the ulna and tibia in 21 mo old infant, resulting from vitamin A positioning. **A,** Long, wavy cortical hyperostosis of the ulna (*arrow*). **B,** Long, wavy cortical hyperostosis of the right tibia (*arrow*), with a striking absence of metaphyseal changes. *(From Caffey J: Pediatric x-ray diagnosis, ed 5, Chicago, 1967, Year Book, p 994.)*

Carotenoids, even in high doses, are not associated with toxicity but can cause yellowing of the skin (**carotenodermia**), including palms of the hands, and high levels in serum (carotenemia); this relatively benign state disappears slowly when carotene intake is reduced. Children with liver disease, diabetes mellitus, or hypothyroidism are more susceptible. Food faddism, such as excessive consumption of carotene-rich foods and juices, may be a cause of carotenodermia.

Bibliography is available at Expert Consult.

Chapter **62**
Vitamin B Complex Deficiencies and Excess
H.P.S. Sachdev and Dheeraj Shah

第六十二章
B族维生素缺乏和过量

中文导读

本章主要介绍了B族维生素的缺乏和过量。详细阐述了维生素B$_1$（硫胺素）、维生素B$_2$（核黄素）、维生素B$_3$（烟酸）、维生素B$_6$（吡多醇）、生物素、叶酸的缺乏与过量中毒以及维生素B$_{12}$（钴胺素）的缺乏。

Vitamin B complex includes a number of water-soluble nutrients, including thiamine (vitamin B$_1$), riboflavin (B$_2$), niacin (B$_3$), pyridoxine (B$_6$), folate, cobalamin (B$_{12}$), biotin, and pantothenic acid. *Choline* and *inositol* are also considered part of the B complex and are important for normal body functions, but specific deficiency syndromes have not been attributed to a lack of these factors in the diet.

B-complex vitamins serve as coenzymes in many metabolic pathways that are functionally closely related. Consequently, a lack of one of the vitamins has the potential to interrupt a chain of chemical processes, including reactions that are dependent on other vitamins, and ultimately can produce diverse clinical manifestations. Because diets deficient in any one of the B-complex vitamins are often poor sources of other B vitamins, manifestations of several vitamin B deficiencies usually can be observed in the same person. It is therefore a general practice in a patient who has evidence of deficiency of a specific B vitamin to treat with the entire B-complex group of vitamins.

62.1 Thiamine (Vitamin B$_1$)
H.P.S. Sachdev and Dheeraj Shah

Thiamine diphosphate, the active form of thiamine, serves as a cofactor for several enzymes involved in carbohydrate catabolism such as pyruvate dehydrogenase, transketolase, and α-ketoglutarate. These enzymes also play a role in the hexose monophosphate shunt that generates nicotinamide adenine dinucleotide phosphate (NADP) and pentose for nucleic acid synthesis. Thiamine is also required for the synthesis of acetylcholine (ACh) and γ-aminobutyric acid (GABA), which have important roles in nerve conduction. Thiamine is absorbed efficiently in the gastrointestinal (GI) tract and may be deficient in persons with GI or liver disease. The requirement of thiamine is increased when carbohydrates are taken in large amounts and during periods of increased metabolism, such as fever, muscular activity, hyperthyroidism, pregnancy, and lactation. Alcohol affects various aspects of thiamine transport and uptake, contributing to the deficiency in alcoholics.

Pork (especially lean), fish, and poultry are good nonvegetarian **dietary sources** of thiamine. Main sources of thiamine for vegetarians are rice, oat, wheat, and legumes. Most ready-to-eat breakfast cereals are enriched with thiamine. Thiamine is water soluble and heat labile; most of the vitamin is lost when the rice is repeatedly washed and the cooking water is discarded. The breast milk of a well-nourished mother provides adequate thiamine; breastfed infants of thiamine-deficient mothers are at risk for deficiency. Thiamine antagonists (coffee, tea) and thiaminases (fermented fish) may contribute to thiamine deficiency. Most infants and older children consuming a balanced diet obtain an adequate intake of thiamine from food and do not require supplements.

THIAMINE DEFICIENCY

Deficiency of thiamine is associated with severely malnourished states, including malignancy and following surgery. The disorder (or spectrum of disorders) is classically associated with a diet consisting largely of polished rice (oriental beriberi); it can also arise if highly refined wheat flour forms a major part of the diet, in alcoholic persons, and in food faddists (occidental beriberi). Thiamine deficiency has often been reported from inhabitants of refugee camps consuming the polished rice–based monotonous diets. Low thiamine concentrations are also noted during critical illnesses.

Thiamine-responsive megaloblastic anemia (TRMA) syndrome is a rare autosomal recessive disorder characterized by megaloblastic anemia, diabetes mellitus, and sensorineural hearing loss, responding in varying degrees to thiamine treatment. The syndrome occurs because of mutations in the *SLC19A2* gene, encoding a thiamine transporter protein, leading to abnormal thiamine transportation and cellular vitamin deficiency. Another dependency state, **biotin and thiamine–responsive basal ganglia disease**, results from mutations in the *SLC19A3* gene; presents with lethargy, poor contact, and poor feeding in early infancy; and responds to combined treatment with biotin and thiamine. Thiamine and related vitamins may improve the outcome in children with Leigh encephalomyelopathy and type 1 diabetes mellitus.

Clinical Manifestations

Thiamine deficiency can develop within 2-3 mo of a deficient intake. Early symptoms of thiamine deficiency are nonspecific, such as fatigue, apathy, irritability, depression, drowsiness, poor mental concentration, anorexia, nausea, and abdominal discomfort. As the condition progresses, more-specific manifestations of **beriberi** develop, such as peripheral neuritis (manifesting as tingling, burning, paresthesias of the toes and feet), decreased deep tendon reflexes, loss of vibration sense, tenderness and cramping of the leg muscles, heart failure, and psychologic disturbances. Patients can have ptosis of the eyelids and atrophy of the optic nerve. Hoarseness or aphonia caused by paralysis of the laryngeal nerve is a characteristic sign. Muscle atrophy and tenderness of the nerve trunks are followed by ataxia, loss of coordination, and loss of deep sensation. Later signs include increased intracranial pressure, meningismus, and coma. The clinical picture of thiamine deficiency is usually divided into a dry (**neuritic**) type and a wet (**cardiac**) type. The disease is wet or dry depending on the amount of fluid that accumulates in the body because of cardiac and renal dysfunction, even though the exact cause for this edema is unknown. Many cases of thiamine deficiency show a mixture of both features and are more properly termed **thiamine deficiency with cardiopathy and peripheral neuropathy**.

The classic clinical triad of **Wernicke encephalopathy**—mental status changes, ocular signs, and ataxia—is rarely reported in infants and young children with severe deficiency secondary to malignancies or feeding of defective formula. An epidemic of life-threatening thiamine deficiency was seen in infants fed a defective soy-based formula that had undetectable thiamine levels. Manifestations included emesis, lethargy, restlessness, ophthalmoplegia, abdominal distention, developmental delay, failure to thrive (malnutrition), lactic acidosis, nystagmus, diarrhea, apnea, seizures, and auditory neuropathy. An acute presentation with tachycardia, moaning, and severe metabolic acidosis responding to parenteral thiamine has been occasionally reported in infants of mothers consuming polished and frequently washed rice.

Death from thiamine deficiency usually is secondary to cardiac involvement. The initial signs are cyanosis and dyspnea, but tachycardia, enlargement of the liver, loss of consciousness, and convulsions can develop rapidly. The heart, especially the right side, is enlarged. The electrocardiogram (ECG) shows an increased QT interval, inverted T waves, and low voltage. These changes, as well as the cardiomegaly, rapidly revert to normal with treatment, but without prompt treatment, cardiac failure can develop rapidly and result in death. In fatal cases of beriberi, lesions are principally located in the heart, peripheral nerves, subcutaneous tissue, and serous cavities. The heart is dilated, and fatty degeneration of the myocardium is common. Generalized edema or edema of the legs, serous effusions, and venous engorgement are often present. Degeneration of myelin and axon cylinders of the peripheral nerves, with wallerian degeneration beginning in the distal locations, is also common, particularly in the lower extremities. Lesions in the brain include vascular dilation and hemorrhage.

Diagnosis

The diagnosis is often suspected based on clinical setting and compatible symptoms. A high index of suspicion in children presenting with unexplained cardiac failure may sometimes be lifesaving. Objective biochemical tests of thiamine status include measurement of erythrocyte transketolase activity and the thiamine pyrophosphate effect. The biochemical diagnostic criteria of thiamine deficiency consist of low erythrocyte transketolase activity and high thiamine pyrophosphate effect (normal range: 0–14%). Urinary excretion of thiamine or its metabolites (thiazole or pyrimidine) after an oral loading dose of thiamine may also be measured to help identify the deficiency state. MRI changes of thiamine deficiency in infants are characterized by bilateral symmetric

hyperintensities of the basal ganglia and frontal lobe, in addition to the lesions in the mammillary bodies, periaqueductal region, and thalami described in adults.

Prevention

A maternal diet containing sufficient amounts of thiamine prevents thiamine deficiency in breastfed infants, and infant formulas marketed in all developed countries provide recommended levels of intake. During complementary feeding, adequate thiamine intake can be achieved with a varied diet that includes meat and enriched or whole-grain cereals. When the staple cereal is polished rice, special efforts need to be made to include legumes and/or nuts in the ration. Thiamine and other vitamins can be retained in rice by *parboiling*, a process of steaming the rice in the husk before milling. Improvement in cooking techniques, such as not discarding the water used for cooking, minimal washing of grains, and reduction of cooking time helps to minimize the thiamine losses during the preparation of food. Thiamine supplementation should be ensured during total parenteral nutrition (TPN).

Treatment

In the absence of GI disturbances, oral administration of thiamine is effective. Children with cardiac failure, convulsions, or coma should be given 10 mg of thiamine intramuscularly (IM) or intravenously (IV) daily for the 1st wk. This treatment should then be followed by 3-5 mg/day of thiamine orally (PO) for at least 6 wk. The response is dramatic in infants and in those having predominantly cardiovascular manifestations, whereas the neurologic response is slow and often incomplete. Epilepsy, mental disability, and language and auditory problems of varying degree have been reported in survivors of severe infantile thiamine deficiency.

Patients with beriberi often have other B-complex vitamin deficiencies; therefore, all other B-complex vitamins should also be administered. Treatment of TRMA and other dependency states require higher dosages (100-200 mg/day). The anemia responds well to thiamine administration, and insulin for associated diabetes mellitus can also be discontinued in many patients with TRMA syndrome.

THIAMINE TOXICITY

There are no reports of adverse effects from consumption of excess thiamine by ingestion of food or supplements. A few isolated cases of pruritus and anaphylaxis have been reported in patients after parenteral administration of vitamin B_1.

Bibliography is available at Expert Consult.

62.2 Riboflavin (Vitamin B_2)
H.P.S. Sachdev and Dheeraj Shah

Riboflavin is part of the structure of the coenzymes flavin adenine dinucleotide (FAD) and flavin mononucleotide, which participate in oxidation-reduction (redox) reactions in numerous metabolic pathways and in energy production via the mitochondrial respiratory chain. Riboflavin is stable to heat but is destroyed by light. Milk, eggs, organ meats, legumes, and mushrooms are rich dietary sources of riboflavin. Most commercial cereals, flours, and breads are enriched with riboflavin.

RIBOFLAVIN DEFICIENCY

The causes of riboflavin deficiency (**ariboflavinosis**) are mainly related to malnourished and malabsorptive states, including GI infections. Treatment with some drugs, such as probenecid, phenothiazine, or oral contraceptives (OCs), can also cause the deficiency. The side chain of the vitamin is photochemically destroyed during phototherapy for hyperbilirubinemia, since it is involved in the photosensitized oxidation of bilirubin to more polar excretable compounds.

Isolated complex II deficiency, a rare mitochondrial disease manifesting in infancy and childhood, responds favorably to riboflavin supplementation and thus can be termed a dependency state. **Brown-Vialetto-Van Laere syndrome (BVVLS)**, a rare, potentially lethal neurologic disorder characterized by rapidly progressive neurologic deterioration, peripheral neuropathy, hypotonia, ataxia, sensorineural hearing loss, optic atrophy, pontobulbar palsy, and respiratory insufficiency, responds to treatment with high doses of riboflavin if treated early in the disease course. Mutations in *SLC52A2* gene (autosomal recessive), encoding riboflavin transporter proteins, have been identified in children with BVVLS.

Clinical Manifestations
Clinical features of nutritional riboflavin deficiency include cheilosis, glossitis, keratitis, conjunctivitis, photophobia, lacrimation, corneal vascularization, and seborrheic dermatitis. Cheilosis begins with pallor at the angles of the mouth and progresses to thinning and maceration of the epithelium, leading to fissures extending radially into the skin (Fig. 62.1). In glossitis the tongue becomes smooth, with loss of papillary structure (Fig. 62.2). Normochromic, normocytic anemia may also be seen because of the impaired erythropoiesis. A low riboflavin content of the maternal diet has been linked to congenital heart defects, but the evidence is weak.

Diagnosis
Most often, the diagnosis is based on the clinical features of angular cheilosis in a malnourished child, who responds promptly to riboflavin supplementation. A functional test of riboflavin status is done by measuring the activity of erythrocyte glutathione reductase (EGR), with and without the addition of FAD. An EGR activity coefficient (ratio of EGR activity with added FAD to EGR activity without FAD) of >1.4 is used as an indicator of deficiency. Urinary excretion of riboflavin <30 µg/24 hr also suggests low intakes.

Prevention
Table 62.1 lists the recommended daily allowance of riboflavin for infants, children, and adolescents. Adequate consumption of milk, milk products, and eggs prevents riboflavin deficiency. Fortification of cereal products is helpful for those who follow vegan diets or who are consuming inadequate amounts of milk products for other reasons.

Treatment
Treatment includes oral administration of 3-10 mg/day of riboflavin, often as an ingredient of a vitamin B–complex mix. The child should also be given a well-balanced diet, including milk and milk products.

RIBOFLAVIN TOXICITY
No adverse effects associated with riboflavin intakes from food or supplements have been reported, and the upper safe limit for consumption has not been established. Although the photosensitizing property of vitamin B_2 suggests some potential risks, limited absorption in high-intake situations precludes such concerns.

Bibliography is available at Expert Consult.

62.3 Niacin (Vitamin B_3)
H.P.S. Sachdev and Dheeraj Shah

Niacin (nicotinamide or nicotinic acid) forms part of two cofactors, nicotinamide adenine dinucleotide (NAD) and NADP, which are important in several biologic reactions, including the respiratory chain, fatty acid and steroid synthesis, cell differentiation, and DNA processing. Niacin is rapidly absorbed from the stomach and the intestines and can also be synthesized from tryptophan in the diet.

Major dietary sources of niacin are meat, fish, and poultry for nonvegetarians and cereals, legumes, and green leafy vegetables for vegetarians. Enriched and fortified cereal products and legumes also are major contributors to niacin intake. Milk and eggs contain little niacin but are good sources of tryptophan, which can be converted to NAD (60 mg tryptophan = 1 mg niacin).

NIACIN DEFICIENCY
Pellagra, the classic niacin deficiency disease, occurs chiefly in populations where corn (maize), a poor source of tryptophan, is the major foodstuff. A severe dietary imbalance, such as in anorexia nervosa and in war or famine conditions, also can cause pellagra. Pellagra can also develop in conditions associated with disturbed tryptophan metabolism, such as carcinoid syndrome and Hartnup disease.

Clinical Manifestations
The early symptoms of pellagra are vague: anorexia, lassitude, weakness, burning sensation, numbness, and dizziness. After a long period of deficiency, the classic triad of dermatitis, diarrhea, and dementia appears. **Dermatitis**, the most characteristic manifestation of pellagra, can develop suddenly or insidiously and may be initiated by irritants, including intense sunlight. The lesions first appear as symmetric areas of erythema on exposed surfaces, resembling sunburn, and might go unrecognized. The lesions are usually sharply demarcated from the surrounding healthy skin, and their distribution can change frequently. The lesions on the hands and feet often have the appearance of a glove or stocking (Fig. 62.3). Similar demarcations can also occur around the neck (**Casal necklace**) (Fig. 62.3). In some cases, vesicles and bullae develop (wet type). In others there may be suppuration beneath the scaly, crusted epidermis; in still others the swelling can disappear after a short time, followed by desquamation (Fig. 62.4). The healed parts of the skin might remain pigmented. The cutaneous lesions may be preceded by or accompanied by stomatitis, glossitis, vomiting, and diarrhea. Swelling and redness of the tip of the tongue and its lateral margins is often followed by intense redness, even ulceration, of the entire tongue and the papillae. Nervous symptoms include depression, disorientation, insomnia, and delirium.

The classic symptoms of pellagra usually are not well developed in infants and young children, but anorexia, irritability, anxiety, and apathy

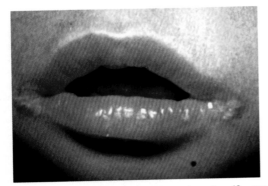

Fig. 62.1 Angular cheilosis with ulceration and crusting. *(Courtesy of National Institute of Nutrition, Indian Council of Medical Research, Hyderabad, India.)*

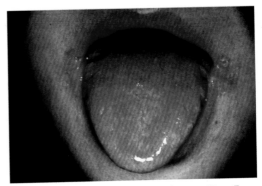

Fig. 62.2 Glossitis as seen in riboflavin deficiency. *(From Zappe HA, Nuss S, Becker K, et al: Riboflavin deficiency in Baltistan. http://www.rzuser.uni-heidelberg.de/%7Ecn6/baltista/riboﬂ_e.htm.)*

| Table 62.1 | Water-Soluble Vitamins | | | | | |

NAMES AND SYNONYMS	BIOCHEMICAL ACTION	EFFECTS OF DEFICIENCY	TREATMENT OF DEFICIENCY	CAUSES OF DEFICIENCY	DIETARY SOURCES	RDA* BY AGE
Thiamine (vitamin B₁)	Coenzyme in carbohydrate metabolism Nucleic acid synthesis Neurotransmitter synthesis	Neurologic (dry beriberi): irritability, peripheral neuritis, muscle tenderness, ataxia Cardiac (wet beriberi): tachycardia, edema, cardiomegaly, cardiac failure	3-5 mg/day PO thiamine for 6 wk	Polished rice–based diets Malabsorptive states Severe malnutrition Malignancies Alcoholism	Meat, especially pork; fish; liver Rice (unmilled), wheat germ; enriched cereals; legumes	0-6 mo: 0.2 mg/day 7-12 mo: 0.3 mg/day 1-3 yr: 0.5 mg/day 4-8 yr: 0.6 mg/day 9-13 yr: 0.9 mg/day 14-18 yr: Girls: 1.0 mg/day Boys: 1.2 mg/day
Riboflavin (vitamin B₂)	Constituent of flavoprotein enzymes important in redox reactions: amino acid, fatty acid, and carbohydrate metabolism and cellular respiration	Glossitis, photophobia, lacrimation, corneal vascularization, poor growth, cheilosis	3-10 mg/day PO riboflavin	Severe malnutrition Malabsorptive states Prolonged treatment with phenothiazines, probenecid, or OCPs	Milk, milk products, eggs, fortified cereals, green vegetables	0-6 mo: 0.3 mg/day 7-12 mo: 0.4 mg/day 1-3 yr: 0.5 mg/day 4-8 yr: 0.6 mg/day 9-13 yr: 0.9 mg/day 14-18 yr: Girls: 1.0 mg/day Boys: 1.3 mg/day
Niacin (vitamin B₃)	Constituent of NAD and NADP, important in respiratory chain, fatty acid synthesis, cell differentiation, and DNA processing	Pellagra manifesting as diarrhea, symmetric scaly dermatitis in sun-exposed areas, and neurologic symptoms of disorientation and delirium	50-300 mg/day PO niacin	Predominantly maize-based diets Anorexia nervosa Carcinoid syndrome	Meat, fish, poultry Cereals, legumes, green vegetables	0-6 mo: 2 mg/day 7-12 mo: 4 mg/day 1-3 yr: 6 mg/day 4-8 yr: 8 mg/day 9-13 yr: 12 mg/day 14-18 yr: Girls: 14 mg/day Boys: 16 mg/day
Pyridoxine (vitamin B₆)	Constituent of coenzymes for amino acid and glycogen metabolism, heme synthesis, steroid action, neurotransmitter synthesis	Irritability, convulsions, hypochromic anemia Failure to thrive Oxaluria	5-25 mg/day PO for deficiency states 100 mg IM or IV for pyridoxine-dependent seizures	Prolonged treatment with INH, penicillamine, OCPs	Fortified ready-to-eat cereals, meat, fish, poultry, liver, bananas, rice, potatoes	0-6 mo: 0.1 mg/day 7-12 mo: 0.3 mg/day 1-3 yr: 0.5 mg/day 4-8 yr: 0.6 mg/day 9-13 yr: 1.0 mg/day 14-18 yr: Girls: 1.2 mg/day Boys: 1.3 mg/day
Biotin	Cofactor for carboxylases, important in gluconeogenesis, fatty acid and amino acid metabolism	Scaly periorificial dermatitis, conjunctivitis, alopecia, lethargy, hypotonia, and withdrawn behavior	1-10 mg/day PO biotin	Consumption of raw eggs for prolonged periods Parenteral nutrition with infusates lacking biotin Valproate therapy	Liver, organ meats, fruits	0-6 mo: 5 µg/day 7-12 mo: 6 µg/day 1-3 yr: 8 µg/day 4-8 yr: 12 µg/day 9-13 yr: 20 µg/day 14-18 yr: 25 µg/day
Pantothenic acid (vitamin B₅)	Component of coenzyme A and acyl carrier protein involved in fatty acid metabolism	Experimentally produced deficiency in humans: irritability, fatigue, numbness, paresthesias (burning feet syndrome), muscle cramps		Isolated deficiency extremely rare in humans	Beef, organ meats, poultry, seafood, egg yolk Yeast, soybeans, mushrooms	0-6 mo: 1.7 mg/day 7-12 mo: 1.8 mg/day 1-3 yr: 2 mg/day 4-8 yr: 3 mg/day 9-13 yr: 4 mg/day 14-18 yr: 5 mg/day
Folic acid	Coenzymes in amino acid and nucleotide metabolism as an acceptor and donor of 1-carbon units	Megaloblastic anemia Growth retardation, glossitis Neural tube defects in progeny	0.5-1 mg/day PO folic acid	Malnutrition Malabsorptive states Malignancies Hemolytic anemias Anticonvulsant therapy	Enriched cereals, beans, leafy vegetables, citrus fruits, papaya	0-6 mo: 65 µg/day 7-12 mo: 80 µg/day 1-3 yr: 150 µg/day 4-8 yr: 200 µg/day 9-13 yr: 300 µg/day 14-18 yr: 400 µg/day

Continued

Table 62.1	Water-Soluble Vitamins—cont'd					
NAMES AND SYNONYMS	**BIOCHEMICAL ACTION**	**EFFECTS OF DEFICIENCY**	**TREATMENT OF DEFICIENCY**	**CAUSES OF DEFICIENCY**	**DIETARY SOURCES**	**RDA* BY AGE**
Cobalamin (vitamin B_{12})	As deoxyadenosylcobalamin, acts as cofactor for lipid and carbohydrate metabolism As methylcobalamin, important for conversion of homocysteine to methionine and folic acid metabolism	Megaloblastic anemia, irritability, developmental delay, developmental regression, involuntary movements, hyperpigmentation	1,000 µg IM vitamin B_{12}	Vegan diets Malabsorptive states Crohn disease Intrinsic factor deficiency (pernicious anemia)	Organ meats, sea foods poultry, egg yolk, milk, fortified ready-to-eat cereals	0-6 mo: 0.4 µg/day 7-12 mo: 0.5 µg/day 1-3 yr: 0.9 µg/day 4-8 yr: 1.2 µg/day 9-13 yr: 1.8 µg/day 14-18 yr: 2.4 µg/day
Ascorbic acid (vitamin C)	Important for collagen synthesis, metabolism of cholesterol and neurotransmitters Antioxidant functions and nonheme iron absorption	Scurvy manifesting as irritability, tenderness and swelling of legs, bleeding gums, petechiae, ecchymoses, follicular hyperkeratosis, and poor wound healing	100-200 mg/day PO ascorbic acid for up to 3 mo	Predominantly milk-based (non–human milk) diets Severe malnutrition	Citrus fruits and fruit juices, peppers, berries, melons, tomatoes, cauliflower, leafy green vegetables	0-6 mo: 40 mg/day 7-12 mo: 50 mg/day 1-3 yr: 15 mg/day 4-8 yr: 25 mg/day 9-13 yr: 45 mg/day 14-18 yr: Girls: 65 mg/day Boys: 75 mg/day

*For healthy breastfed infants, the values represent adequate intakes, that is, the mean intake of apparently "normal" infants.
  PO, Orally; IM, intramuscularly; IV, intravenously; INH, isoniazid; NAD, nicotinamide adenine dinucleotide; NADP, nicotinamide adenine dinucleotide phosphate; OCP, oral contraceptive pill; RDA, recommended dietary allowance.
  From Dietary reference intakes (DRIs): *Recommended dietary allowances and adequate intakes, vitamins,* Food and Nutrition Board, Institute of Medicine, National Academies. http://www.nationalacademies.org/hmd/~/media/Files/Activity%20Files/Nutrition/DRI-Tables/2_%20RDA%20and%20AI%20Values_Vitamin%20and%20Elements.pdf?la=en.

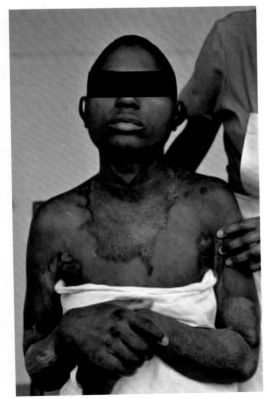

Fig. 62.3 Characteristic skin lesions of pellagra on hands and lesions on the neck (Casal necklace). *(Courtesy of Dr. J.D. MacLean, McGill Centre for Tropical Diseases, Montreal.)*

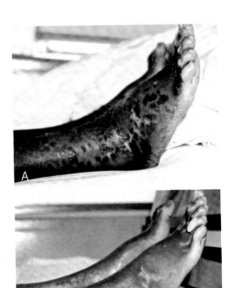

Fig. 62.4 Clinical manifestations of niacin deficiency before (**A**) and after (**B**) therapy. *(From Weinsier RL, Morgan SL: Fundamentals of clinical nutrition, St Louis, 1993, Mosby, p 99.)*

are common. Young patients might also have sore tongues and lips and usually have dry scaly skin. Diarrhea and constipation can alternate, and anemia can occur. Children who have pellagra often have evidence of other nutritional deficiency diseases.

Diagnosis

Because of lack of a good functional test to evaluate niacin status, the diagnosis of deficiency is usually made from the physical signs of glossitis, GI symptoms, and a symmetric dermatitis. Rapid clinical response to niacin is an important confirmatory test. A decrease in the concentration and/or a change in the proportion of the niacin metabolites N^1-methyl-nicotinamide and 2-pyridone in the urine provide biochemical evidence of deficiency and can be seen before the appearance of overt signs of deficiency. Histopathologic changes from the affected skin include dilated blood vessels without significant inflammatory infiltrates, ballooning of the keratinocytes, hyperkeratosis, and epidermal necrosis.

Prevention

Adequate intakes of niacin are easily met by consumption of a diet that consists of a variety of foods and includes meat, eggs, milk, and enriched or fortified cereal products. The **dietary reference intake (DRI)** is expressed in milligram niacin equivalents (NE) in which 1 mg NE = 1 mg niacin or 60 mg tryptophan. An intake of 2 mg of niacin is considered adequate for infants 0-6 mo of age, and 4 mg is adequate for infants 7-12 mo. For older children, the recommended intakes are 6 mg for 1-3 yr of age, 8 mg for 4-8 yr, 12 mg for 9-13 yr, and 14-16 mg for 14-18 yr of age.

Treatment

Children usually respond rapidly to treatment. A liberal and varied diet should be supplemented with 50-300 mg/day of niacin; in severe cases or in patients with poor intestinal absorption, 100 mg may be given IV. The diet should also be supplemented with other vitamins, especially other B-complex vitamins. Sun exposure should be avoided during the active phase of pellagra, and the skin lesions may be covered with soothing applications. Other coexisting nutrient deficiencies such as iron-deficiency anemia should be treated. Even after successful treatment, the diet should continue to be monitored to prevent recurrence.

NIACIN TOXICITY

No toxic effects are associated with the intake of naturally occurring niacin in foods. Shortly after the ingestion of large doses of nicotinic acid taken as a supplement or a pharmacologic agent, a person often experiences a burning, tingling, and itching sensation as well as flushing on the face, arms, and chest. Large doses of niacin also can have nonspecific GI effects and can cause cholestatic jaundice or hepatotoxicity. Tolerable upper intake levels for children are approximately double the recommended dietary allowance.

Bibliography is available at Expert Consult.

62.4 Vitamin B₆ (Pyridoxine)

H.P.S. Sachdev and Dheeraj Shah

Vitamin B_6 includes a group of closely related compounds: pyridoxine, pyridoxal, pyridoxamine, and their phosphorylated derivatives. **Pyridoxal 5'-phosphate (PLP)** and, to a lesser extent, pyridoxamine phosphate function as coenzymes for many enzymes involved in amino acid metabolism, neurotransmitter synthesis, glycogen metabolism, and steroid action. If vitamin B_6 is lacking, glycine metabolism can lead to oxaluria. The major excretory product in the urine is 4-pyridoxic acid.

The vitamin B_6 content of human milk and infant formulas is adequate. Good food sources of the vitamin include fortified ready-to-eat cereals, meat, fish, poultry, liver, bananas, rice, and certain vegetables. Large losses of the vitamin can occur during high-temperature processing of foods or milling of cereals, whereas parboiling of rice prevents its loss.

VITAMIN B₆ DEFICIENCY

Because of the importance of vitamin B_6 in amino acid metabolism, high protein intakes can increase the requirement for the vitamin; the recommended daily allowances are sufficient to cover the expected range of protein intake in the population. The risk of deficiency is increased in persons taking medications that inhibit the activity of vitamin B_6 (e.g., isoniazid, penicillamine, corticosteroids, phenytoin, carbamazepine), in young women taking oral progesterone-estrogen OCs, and in patients receiving maintenance dialysis.

Clinical Manifestations

The vitamin B_6 deficiency symptoms seen in infants are listlessness, irritability, seizures, vomiting, and failure to thrive. Peripheral neuritis is a feature of deficiency in adults but is not usually seen in children. Electroencephalogram (EEG) abnormalities have been reported in infants as well as in young adults in controlled depletion studies. Skin lesions include cheilosis, glossitis, and seborrheic dermatitis around the eyes, nose, and mouth. Microcytic anemia can occur in infants but is not common. Oxaluria, oxalic acid bladder stones, hyperglycinemia, lymphopenia, decreased antibody formation, and infections also are associated with vitamin B_6 deficiency.

Several types of vitamin B_6 **dependence syndromes**, presumably resulting from errors in enzyme structure or function, respond to very large amounts of pyridoxine. These syndromes include pyridoxine-dependent epilepsy, a vitamin B_6–responsive anemia, xanthurenic aciduria, cystathioninuria, and homocystinuria (see Chapter 103). Pyridoxine-dependent epilepsy involves mutations in the *ALDH7A1* gene causing deficiency of antiquitin, an enzyme involved in dehydrogenation of L-α-aminoadipic semialdehyde.

Diagnosis

The activity of aspartate (glutamic-oxaloacetic) transaminase (AST) and alanine (glutamic-pyruvic) transaminase (ALT) is low in vitamin B_6 deficiency; tests measuring the activity of these enzymes before and after the addition of PLP may be useful as indicators of vitamin B_6 status. Abnormally high xanthurenic acid excretion after tryptophan ingestion also provides evidence of deficiency. Plasma PLP assays are being used more often, but factors such as inflammation, renal function, and hypoalbuminemia can influence the results. Ratios between substrate-products pairs (e.g., PAr index, 3-hydroxykynurenine/xanthurenic acid ratio, oxoglutarate/glutamate ratio) may attenuate such influence. Quantification of a large number of metabolites, using mass spectrometry–based metabolomics, are being evaluated as functional biomarkers of pyridoxine status.

Vitamin B_6 deficiency or dependence should be suspected in all infants with **seizures**. If more common causes of infantile seizures have been eliminated, 100 mg of pyridoxine can be injected, with EEG monitoring if possible. If the seizure stops, vitamin B_6 deficiency should be suspected. In older children, 100 mg of pyridoxine may be injected IM while the EEG is being recorded; a favorable response of the EEG suggests pyridoxine deficiency.

Prevention

Deficiency is unlikely in children consuming diets that meet their energy needs and contain a variety of foods. Parboiling of rice prevents the loss of vitamin B_6 from the grains. The DRIs for vitamin B_6 are 0.1 mg/day for infants up to 6 mo of age; 0.3 mg/day for 6 mo to 1 yr; 0.5 mg/day for 1-3 yr; 0.6 mg/day for 4-8 yr; 1.0 mg/day for 9-13 yr; and 1.2-1.3 mg/day for 14-18 yr. Infants whose mothers have received large doses of pyridoxine during pregnancy are at increased risk for seizures from pyridoxine dependence, and supplements during the 1st few weeks of life should be considered. Any child receiving a pyridoxine antagonist, such as isoniazid, should be carefully observed for neurologic manifestations; if these develop, vitamin B_6 should be administered or the dose of the antagonist should be decreased.

Treatment

Intramuscular or intravenous administration of 100 mg of pyridoxine is used to treat convulsions caused by vitamin B_6 deficiency. One dose should be sufficient if adequate dietary intake follows. For pyridoxine-dependent children, daily doses of 2-10 mg IM or 10-100 mg PO may be necessary.

VITAMIN B₆ TOXICITY

Adverse effects have not been associated with high intakes of vitamin B_6 from food sources. However, ataxia and sensory neuropathy have been reported with dosages as low as 100 mg/day in adults taking vitamin B_6 supplements for several months.

Bibliography is available at Expert Consult.

62.5 Biotin
H.P.S. Sachdev and Dheeraj Shah

Biotin (vitamin B_7 or vitamin H) functions as a cofactor for enzymes involved in carboxylation reactions within and outside mitochondria. These biotin-dependent carboxylases catalyze key reactions in gluconeogenesis, fatty acid metabolism, and amino acid catabolism.

There is limited information on the biotin content of foods; biotin is believed to be widely distributed, making a deficiency unlikely. *Avidin* found in raw egg whites acts as a biotin antagonist. Signs of biotin deficiency have been demonstrated in persons who consume large amounts of raw egg whites over long periods. Deficiency also has been described in infants and children receiving enteral and parenteral nutrition formula that lack biotin. Treatment with valproic acid may result in a low biotinidase activity and/or biotin deficiency.

The clinical findings of biotin deficiency include scaly periorificial dermatitis, conjunctivitis, thinning of hair, and alopecia (Fig. 62.5). Central nervous system (CNS) abnormalities seen with biotin deficiency are lethargy, hypotonia, seizures, ataxia, and withdrawn behavior. Biotin deficiency can be successfully treated using 1-10 mg of biotin orally daily. The adequate dietary intake values for biotin are 5 μg/day for ages 0-6 mo, 6 μg/day for 7-12 mo, 8 μg/day for 1-3 yr, 12 μg/day for 4-8 yr, 20 μg/day for 9-13 yr, and 25 μg/day for 14-18 yr. No toxic effects have been reported with very high doses.

Biotin-responsive basal ganglia disease or **biotin and thiamine–responsive basal ganglia disease** is a rare childhood neurologic disorder characterized by encephalopathy, seizures, extrapyramidal manifestations, altered signals in basal ganglia (bilateral involvement of caudate nuclei and putamen with sparing of globus pallidus) on MRI, and homozygous missense mutation in the *SLC19A3* gene. Chapter 103 describes conditions involving deficiencies in the enzymes holocarboxylase synthetase and biotinidase that respond to treatment with biotin.

Bibliography is available at Expert Consult.

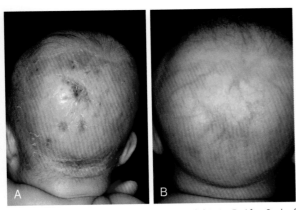

Fig. 62.5 **A,** Scalp rash before treatment with biotin. **B,** After 3 wk of biotin treatment. *(From Ito T, Nishie W, Fujita Y, et al: Infantile eczema caused by formula milk. Lancet 381:1958, 2013.)*

62.6 Folate
H.P.S. Sachdev and Dheeraj Shah

Folate exists in a number of different chemical forms. **Folic acid** (pteroylglutamic acid) is the synthetic form used in fortified foods and supplements. Naturally occurring folates in foods retain the core chemical structure of pteroylglutamic acid but vary in their state of reduction, the single-carbon moiety they bear, or the length of the glutamate chain. These polyglutamates are broken down and reduced in the small intestine to dihydro- and tetrahydrofolates, which are involved as coenzymes in amino acid and nucleotide metabolism as acceptors and donors of 1-carbon units. Folate is important for CNS development during embryogenesis.

Rice and cereals are rich dietary sources of folate, especially if enriched. Beans, leafy vegetables, and fruits such as oranges and papaya are good sources as well. The vitamin is readily absorbed from the small intestine and is broken down to monoglutamate derivatives by mucosal polyglutamate hydrolases. A high-affinity proton-coupled folate transporter (PCFT) seems to be essential for absorption of folate in intestine and in various cell types at low pH. The vitamin is also synthesized by colonic bacteria, and its half-life is prolonged by enterohepatic recirculation.

FOLATE DEFICIENCY

Because of folate's role in protein, DNA, and RNA synthesis, the risk of deficiency is increased during periods of rapid growth or increased cellular metabolism. Folate deficiency can result from poor nutrient content in diet, inadequate absorption (celiac disease, inflammatory bowel disease), increased requirement (sickle cell anemia, psoriasis, malignancies, periods of rapid growth as in infancy and adolescence), or inadequate utilization (long-term treatment with high-dose nonsteroidal antiinflammatory drugs; anticonvulsants such as phenytoin and phenobarbital; methotrexate). Rare causes of deficiency are hereditary folate malabsorption, inborn errors of folate metabolism (methylene tetrahydrofolate reductase, methionine synthase reductase, and glutamate formiminotransferase deficiencies), and cerebral folate deficiency. A loss-of-function mutation in the gene coding for PCFT is the molecular basis for hereditary folate malabsorption. A high-affinity blocking autoantibody against the membrane-bound folate receptor in the choroid plexus preventing its transport across the blood-brain barrier is the likely cause of the infantile cerebral folate deficiency.

Clinical Manifestations

Folic acid deficiency results in megaloblastic anemia and hypersegmentation of neutrophils. Nonhematologic manifestations include glossitis, listlessness, and growth retardation not related to anemia. An association exists between low maternal folic acid status and **neural tube defects**, primarily spina bifida and anencephaly, and the role of periconceptional folic acid in their prevention is well established (see Chapter 481.1).

Hereditary folate malabsorption manifests at 1-3 mo of age with recurrent or chronic diarrhea, failure to thrive (malnutrition), oral ulcerations, neurologic deterioration, megaloblastic anemia, and opportunistic infections. **Cerebral folate deficiency** manifests at 4-6 mo of age with irritability, microcephaly, developmental delay, cerebellar ataxia, pyramidal tract signs, choreoathetosis, ballismus, seizures, and blindness as a result of optic atrophy. 5-Methyltetrahydrofolate levels are normal in serum and red blood cells (RBCs) but greatly depressed in the cerebrospinal fluid (CSF).

Diagnosis

The diagnosis of folic acid deficiency anemia is made in the presence of macrocytosis along with low folate levels in serum or RBCs. Normal serum folic acid levels are 5-20 ng/mL; with deficiency, levels are <3 ng/mL. Levels of RBC folate are a better indicator of chronic deficiency. The normal RBC folate level is 150-600 ng/mL of packed cells. The bone marrow is hypercellular because of erythroid hyperplasia, and megaloblastic changes are prominent. Large, abnormal neutrophilic forms (giant metamyelocytes) with cytoplasmic vacuolation also are seen.

Cerebral folate deficiency is associated with low levels of 5-methyltetrahydrofolate in CSF and normal folate levels in the plasma and RBCs. Mutations in the *PCFT* gene are demonstrated in the hereditary folate malabsorption.

Prevention

Breastfed infants have better folate nutrition than nonbreastfed infants throughout infancy. Consumption of folate-rich foods and food fortification programs are important to ensure adequate intake in children and in women of childbearing age. The DRIs for folate are 65 μg of dietary folate equivalents (DFE) for infants 0-6 mo of age and 80 μg of DFE for infants 6-12 mo. (1 DFE = 1 μg food folate = 0.6 μg of folate from fortified food or as a supplement consumed with food = 0.5 μg of a supplement taken on an empty stomach.) For older children, the DRIs are 150 μg of DFE for ages 1-3 yr; 200 μg DFE for 4-8 yr; 300 μg DFE for 9-13 yr; and 400 μg DFE for 14-18 yr. All women desirous of becoming pregnant should consume 400-800 μg folic acid daily; the dose is 4 mg/day in those having delivered a child with neural tube defect. To be effective, supplementation should be started at least 1 mo before conception and continued through the 1st 2-3 mo of pregnancy. The benefit of periconceptional folate supplementation in prevention of congenital heart defects, orofacial clefts, and autistic spectrum disorders is unclear. Preconceptional folate supplementation continued throughout pregnancy may marginally reduce the risk of delivering a small-for-gestational-age infant. Providing iron and folic

acid tablets for prevention of anemia in children and pregnant women is a routine strategy in at-risk populations. Mandatory fortification of cereal flours with folic acid coupled with health-education programs has been associated with a substantial reduction in incidence of neural tube defects in many countries.

Treatment

When the diagnosis of folate deficiency is established, folic acid may be administered orally or parenterally at 0.5-1.0 mg/day. Folic acid therapy should be continued for 3-4 wk or until a definite hematologic response has occurred. Maintenance therapy with 0.2 mg of folate is adequate. Prolonged treatment with oral folinic acid is required in cerebral folate deficiency, and the response may be incomplete. High-dose intravenous folinic acid may help in refractory cases. Treatment of hereditary folate malabsorption may be possible with intramuscular folinic acid; some patients may respond to high-dose oral folinic acid therapy.

FOLATE TOXICITY

No adverse effects have been associated with consumption of the amounts of folate normally found in fortified foods. Excessive intake of folate supplements might obscure and potentially delay the diagnosis of vitamin B_{12} deficiency. Massive doses given by injection have the potential to cause neurotoxicity.

Bibliography is available at Expert Consult.

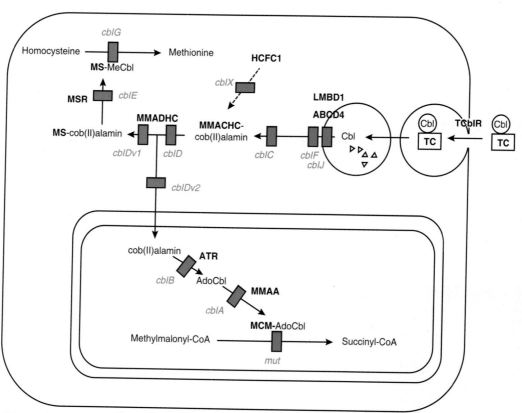

Fig. 62.6 Scheme of cobalamin (Cbl) metabolism. The sites affected by methylmalonyl-CoA mutase deficiency (*mut*) and the inborn errors of cobalamin metabolism (*cblA-cblG, cblJ,* and *cblX*) are shown in *red.* The cblA disorder is caused by defects in the MMAA protein; the cblB disorder by defects in the cob(I)alamin adenosyltransferase (MMAB) protein; the cblC disorder by defects in the MMACHC protein; the cblD, cblD variant 1 (*cblDv1*), and cblD variant 2 (*cblDv2*) disorders are caused by defects in the MMADHC protein; cblE disorder is caused by defects in the methionine synthase reductase (MSR) protein; cblG disorder by defects in the methionine synthase (MS) protein; cblJ disorder by mutations in the ABCD4 protein; cblX disorder by mutations in the HCFC1 protein, and the mut disorder by defects in methylmalonyl-CoA mutase (MCM) . The protein affected in the cblF disorder is unknown. MCM-AdoCbl, Holomethylmalonyl-CoA mutase (mutase with bound adenosylcobalamin); MS-cob(II) alamin, methionine synthase with bound cob(II)alamin; MS-MeCbl, holomethionine synthase (synthase with bound methylcobalamin; TC, transcobalamin. (*From* Nathan and Oski's hematology and oncology of infancy and childhood, ed 8, Vol 1, Philadelphia, 2015, Elsevier, p 318.)

62.7 Vitamin B₁₂ (Cobalamin)

H.P.S. Sachdev and Dheeraj Shah

Vitamin B_{12}, in the form of deoxyadenosylcobalamin, functions as a cofactor for isomerization of methylmalonyl-CoA to succinyl-CoA, an essential reaction in lipid and carbohydrate metabolism. Methylcobalamin is another circulating form of vitamin B_{12} and is essential for methyl group transfer during the conversion of homocysteine to methionine. This reaction also requires a folic acid cofactor and is important for protein and nucleic acid biosynthesis. Vitamin B_{12} is important for hematopoiesis, CNS myelination, and mental and psychomotor development (Fig. 62.6).

Dietary sources of vitamin B_{12} are almost exclusively from animal foods. Organ meats, muscle meats, seafood (mollusks, oysters, fish), poultry, and egg yolk are rich sources. Fortified ready-to-eat cereals and milk and their products are the important sources of the vitamin for vegetarians. Human milk is an adequate source for breastfeeding infants if the maternal serum B_{12} levels are adequate. Vitamin B_{12} is absorbed from ileum at alkaline pH after binding with intrinsic factor. Enterohepatic circulation, direct absorption, and synthesis by intestinal bacteria are additional mechanisms helping to maintain the vitamin B_{12} nutriture.

VITAMIN B₁₂ DEFICIENCY

Deficiency of vitamin B_{12} caused by inadequate dietary intake occurs primarily in persons consuming strict vegetarian or vegan diets. Prevalence of vitamin B_{12} deficiency is high in predominantly vegetarian or lactovegetarian populations. Breastfeeding infants of B_{12}-deficient mothers are also at risk for significant deficiency. Malabsorption of B_{12} occurs in celiac disease, ileal resections, Crohn disease, *Helicobacter pylori* infection, and autoimmune atrophic gastritis (pernicious anemia). Use of metformin, proton pump inhibitors, and histamine (H_2) receptor antagonists may increase the risk of deficiency. **Hereditary intrinsic factor deficiency** and **Imerslund-Gräsbeck disease** are inborn errors of metabolism leading to vitamin B_{12} malabsorption. Mutations in the hereditary intrinsic factor gene cause hereditary intrinsic factor deficiency, whereas mutations in any of the 2 subunits (cubilin and amnionless) of the intrinsic factor receptor cause Imerslund-Gräsbeck disease.

Clinical Manifestations

The hematologic manifestations of vitamin B_{12} deficiency are similar to manifestations of folate deficiency and are discussed in Chapter 481.2. Irritability, hypotonia, developmental delay, developmental regression, and involuntary movements (predominantly coarse tremors) are the common neurologic symptoms in infants. Older children with vitamin B_{12} deficiency may show poor growth and poor school performance, whereas sensory deficits, paresthesias, peripheral neuritis, and psychosis are seen in adults. Hyperpigmentation of the knuckles and palms is another common observation with B_{12} deficiency in children (Fig. 62.7). Maternal B_{12} deficiency may also be an independent risk factor for fetal neural tube defects.

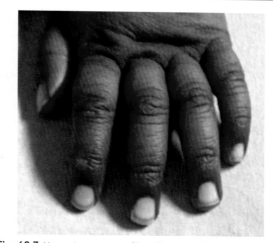

Fig. 62.7 Hyperpigmentation of knuckles in an infant with vitamin B_{12} deficiency and megaloblastic anemia.

Diagnosis

See Chapter 481.2.

Treatment

The hematologic symptoms respond promptly to parenteral administration of 250-1,000 µg vitamin B_{12}. Children with severe deficiency and those with neurologic symptoms need repeated doses, daily or on alternate days in first week, followed by weekly for the 1st 1-2 mo and then monthly. Children having only hematologic presentation recover fully within 2-3 mo, whereas those with neurologic disease need at least 6 mo of therapy. Children with a continuing malabsorptive state and those with inborn errors of vitamin B_{12} malabsorption need lifelong treatment. Prolonged daily treatment with high-dose (1,000-2,000 µg) oral vitamin B_{12} preparations is also equally effective in achieving hematologic and neurologic responses in elderly patients, but the data are inadequate in children and young adults.

Prevention

Vitamin B_{12} DRIs are 0.4 µg/day at age 0-6 mo, 0.5 µg/day at 6-12 mo, 0.9 µg/day at 1-3 yr, 1.2 µg/day at 4-8 yr, 1.8 µg/day at 9-13 yr, 2.4 µg/day at 14-18 yr and in adults, 2.6 µg/day in pregnancy, and 2.8 µg/day in lactation. Pregnant and breastfeeding women should ensure an adequate consumption of animal products to prevent cobalamin deficiency in infants. Strict vegetarians, especially vegans, should ensure regular consumption of vitamin B_{12}. Food fortification with the vitamin helps to prevent deficiency in predominantly vegetarian populations.

Bibliography is available at Expert Consult.

Chapter 63
Vitamin C (Ascorbic Acid) Deficiency and Excess
Dheeraj Shah and H.P.S. Sachdev

第六十三章
维生素C缺乏和过量

中文导读

　　本章主要介绍了维生素C的膳食需求与食物来源、维生素C缺乏和中毒。具体描述了维生素C缺乏的临床表现、实验室检查和诊断、鉴别诊断、治疗和预防。其中临床表现包括肌肉骨骼疼痛、肢体假性瘫痪、贫血与出血；实验室检查和诊断包括长骨X线检查和血液生化检查。

Vitamin C is important for synthesis of collagen at the level of hydroxylation of lysine and proline in precollagen. It is also involved in neurotransmitter metabolism (conversion of dopamine to norepinephrine and tryptophan to serotonin), cholesterol metabolism (conversion of cholesterol to steroid hormones and bile acids), and the biosynthesis of carnitine. Vitamin C functions to maintain the iron and copper atoms, cofactors of the metalloenzymes, in a reduced (active) state. Vitamin C is an important antioxidant (electron donor) in the aqueous milieu of the body. Vitamin C enhances nonheme iron absorption, the transfer of iron from transferrin to ferritin, and the formation of tetrahydrofolic acid and thus can affect the cellular and immunologic functions of the hematopoietic system.

DIETARY NEEDS AND SOURCES OF VITAMIN C
Humans depend on dietary sources for vitamin C. An adequate intake is 40 mg for ages 0-6 mo and 50 mg for 6-12 mo. For older children the recommended dietary allowance is 15 mg for ages 1-3 yr, 25 mg for 4-8 yr, 45 mg for 9-13 yr, and 65-75 mg for 14-18 yr. The recommended dietary allowances during pregnancy and lactation are 85 mg/day and 120 mg/day, respectively. The requirement for vitamin C is increased during infectious and diarrheal diseases. Children exposed to smoking or environmental tobacco smoke also require increased amounts of foods rich in vitamin C. The best food sources of vitamin C are citrus fruits and fruit juices, peppers, berries, melons, guava, kiwifruit, tomatoes, cauliflower, and green leafy vegetables. Vitamin C is easily destroyed by prolonged storage, overcooking, and processing of foods.

Absorption of vitamin C occurs in the upper small intestine by an active process or by simple diffusion when large amounts are ingested. Vitamin C is not stored in the body but is taken up by all tissues; the highest levels are found in the pituitary and adrenal glands. The brain ascorbate content in the fetus and neonate is markedly higher than the content in the adult brain, a finding probably related to its function in neurotransmitter synthesis.

When a mother's intake of vitamin C during pregnancy and lactation is adequate, the newborn will have adequate tissue levels of vitamin C related to active placental transfer, subsequently maintained by the vitamin C in breast milk or commercial infant formulas. Breast milk contains sufficient vitamin C to prevent deficiency throughout infancy. Infants consuming pasteurized or boiled animal milk are at significant risk of developing deficiency if the other sources of vitamin C are also lacking in the diet. Neonates whose feeding has been delayed because of a clinical condition can also have ascorbic acid deficiency. For patients receiving total parenteral nutrition (TPN), 80 mg/day is recommended for full-term infants and 25 mg/kg/day for preterm infants. Parents and children who choose a limited (selective) diet or those on fad diets are at risk for vitamin C deficiency.

VITAMIN C DEFICIENCY
A deficiency of vitamin C results in the clinical presentation of **scurvy**. Children fed predominantly heat-treated (ultrahigh-temperature or pasteurized) milk or unfortified formulas and not receiving fruits and fruit juices are at significant risk for symptomatic disease. Infants and children on highly restrictive diets, devoid of most fruits and vegetables, are at risk of acquiring severe vitamin C deficiency. Such diets are occasionally promoted with unsubstantiated claims of benefit in autism and other developmental disorders, In scurvy, there is defective formation of connective tissues and collagen in skin, cartilage, dentine, bone, and blood vessels, leading to their fragility. In the long bones, osteoid is not deposited by osteoblasts, cortex is thin, and the trabeculae become brittle and fracture easily.

Clinical Features
The early manifestations of vitamin C deficiency are irritability, loss of appetite, low-grade fever, musculoskeletal pain, and tenderness in the legs. These signs and symptoms are followed by leg swelling—most marked at the knees and the ankles—and **pseudoparalysis**. The infant might lie with

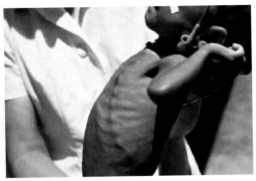

Fig. 63.1 Scorbutic "rosary." *(Courtesy of Dr. J.D. MacLean, McGill Centre for Tropical Diseases, Montreal.)*

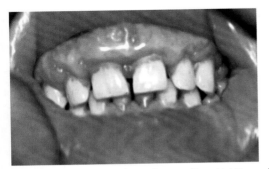

Fig. 63.2 Gingival lesions in advanced scurvy. *(From Nutrition, ed 4, Kalamazoo, MI, 1980, The Upjohn Company, p 80. Used with permission of Pfizer, Inc.)*

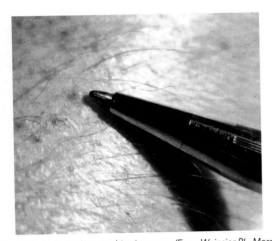

Fig. 63.3 Perifollicular petechiae in scurvy. *(From Weinsier RL, Morgan SL: Fundamentals of clinical nutrition, St Louis, 1993, Mosby, p 85.)*

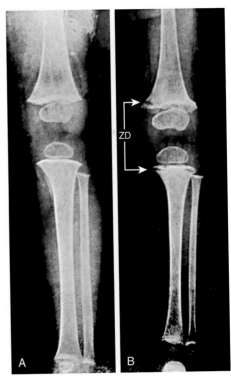

Fig. 63.4 Radiographs of a leg. **A,** An early scurvy "white line" is visible on the ends of the shafts of the tibia and fibula; sclerotic rings (Wimberger sign) are shown around the epiphyses of the femur and tibia. **B,** More advanced scorbutic changes; zones of destruction (ZD) are evident in the femur and tibia. Pelkan spur is also seen at the cortical end.

B_{12}, and folate. Hemorrhagic manifestations of scurvy include petechiae, purpura, and ecchymoses at pressure points; epistaxis; gum bleeding; and the characteristic perifollicular hemorrhages (Fig. 63.3). Other manifestations are poor wound and fracture healing, hyperkeratosis of hair follicles, arthralgia, and muscle weakness.

Laboratory Findings and Diagnosis

The diagnosis of vitamin C deficiency is usually based on the characteristic clinical picture, the radiographic appearance of the long bones, and a history of poor vitamin C intake. A high index of suspicion is required in children on restrictive diets, particularly those with autism and other developmental disorders, and they should be evaluated for scurvy whenever they present with difficulty in walking or bone pains. The typical radiographic changes occur at the distal ends of the long bones and are particularly common at the knees. The shafts of the long bones have a ground-glass appearance because of trabecular atrophy. The cortex is thin and dense, giving the appearance of *pencil outlining* of the diaphysis and epiphysis. The *white line of Fränkel*, an irregular but thickened white line at the metaphysis, represents the zone of well-calcified cartilage. The epiphyseal centers of ossification also have a ground-glass appearance and are surrounded by a sclerotic ring (Fig. 63.4). The more specific but late radiologic feature of scurvy is a zone of rarefaction under the white line at the metaphysis. This zone of rarefaction (*Trümmerfeld zone*), a linear break in the bone that is proximal and parallel to the white line, represents area of debris of broken-down bone trabeculae and connective tissue. A *Pelkan spur* is a lateral prolongation of the white line and may be present at cortical ends. Epiphyseal separation can occur along the line of destruction, with either linear displacement or compression of the epiphysis against the shaft (Fig. 63.5). Subperiosteal hemorrhages are not visible using plain radiographs during the active phase of scurvy. However, during healing the elevated periosteum

the hips and knees semiflexed and the feet rotated outward. Subperiosteal hemorrhages in the lower-limb bones sometimes acutely increase the swelling and pain, and the condition might mimic acute osteomyelitis or arthritis. A "rosary" at the costochondral junctions and depression of the sternum are other typical features (Fig. 63.1). The angulation of scorbutic beads is usually sharper than that of a rachitic rosary. Gum changes are seen in older children after teeth have erupted, manifested as bluish purple, spongy swellings of the mucous membrane, especially over the upper incisors (Fig. 63.2). **Anemia,** a common finding in infants and young children with scurvy, is related to impaired iron absorption and coexistent hematopoietic nutrient deficiencies, including iron, vitamin

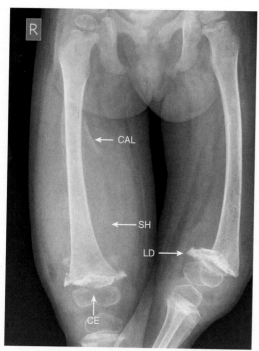

Fig. 63.5 Large subperiosteal hematoma (SH) with areas of calcification (CAL) is seen along the shaft of right femur of a child with advanced scurvy. Epiphyseal separation is seen in both knees, with linear displacement (LD) in left knee and compression (CE) against the shaft in right knee.

becomes calcified and radiopaque (Fig. 63.5), sometimes giving a dumbbell or club shape to the affected bone. MRI can demonstrate acute as well as healing subperiosteal hematomas along with periostitis, metaphyseal changes, and heterogeneous bone marrow signal intensity, even in absence of changes in plain radiographs. Gelatinous transformation of bone marrow, on aspiration, has been reported in children with suspected malignancy.

Biochemical tests are not very useful in the diagnosis of scurvy, because they do not reflect the tissue status. A plasma ascorbate concentration of <0.2 mg/dL usually is considered deficient. Leukocyte concentration of vitamin C is a better indicator of body stores, but this measurement is technically more difficult to perform. Leukocyte concentrations of

≤ 10 μg/10^8 white blood cells are considered deficient and indicate latent scurvy, even in the absence of clinical signs of deficiency. Saturation of the tissues with vitamin C can be estimated from the urinary excretion of the vitamin after a test dose of ascorbic acid. In healthy children, 80% of the test dose appears in the urine within 3-5 hr after parenteral administration. Generalized nonspecific aminoaciduria is common in scurvy, whereas plasma amino acid levels remain normal.

Differential Diagnosis

Scurvy is often misdiagnosed as arthritis, osteomyelitis, nonaccidental trauma (child abuse), malignancy, or acrodynia. The early irritability and bone pain are sometimes attributed to nonspecific pains or other nutritional deficiencies. Copper deficiency results in a radiographic picture similar to that of scurvy. Henoch-Schönlein purpura, thrombocytopenic purpura, or leukemia is sometimes suspected in children presenting with hemorrhagic manifestations.

Treatment

Vitamin C supplements of 100-200 mg/day orally or parenterally ensure rapid and complete cure. The clinical improvement is seen within 1 week in most cases, but the treatment should be continued for up to 3 mo for complete recovery.

Prevention

Breastfeeding protects against vitamin C deficiency throughout infancy. In children consuming milk formula, fortification with vitamin C must be ensured. Children consuming heat-treated milk or plant-based beverages (e.g., almond milk, soy milk) should consume adequate vitamin C–rich foods in infancy. Dietary or medicinal supplements are required in children on restrictive diets deficient in vitamin C, severely malnourished children, and those with chronic debilitating conditions (e.g., malignancies, neurologic disorders). Providing antenatal supplements of vitamin C to smoking mothers may mitigate some of the harmful effects of smoking on fetal and infant lung development and function.

VITAMIN C TOXICITY

Daily intake of <2 g of vitamin C is generally without adverse effects in adults. Larger doses can cause gastrointestinal problems, such as abdominal pain and osmotic diarrhea. Hemolysis has rarely been reported after high doses of ascorbic acid. Megadoses of vitamin C should be avoided in patients with a history of urolithiasis or conditions related to excessive iron accumulation, such as thalassemia and hemochromatosis. Data are sparse regarding vitamin C toxicity in children. The following values for tolerable upper intake levels are extrapolated from data for adults based on body weight differences: ages 1-3 yr, 400 mg; 4-8 yr, 650 mg; 9-13 yr, 1,200 mg; and 14-18 yr, 1,800 mg.

Bibliography is available at Expert Consult.

Chapter **64**
Vitamin D Deficiency (Rickets) and Excess
Larry A. Greenbaum

第六十四章
维生素D缺乏（佝偻病）和过量

中文导读

本章主要介绍了佝偻病、维生素D缺乏性疾病、钙缺乏、磷缺乏、早产儿佝偻病、远端肾小管酸中毒以及维生素D过量。具体描述了佝偻病的病因、临床表现、影像学、诊断和临床评估；维生素D缺乏性疾病中具体描述了维生素D的生理功能、营养性维生素D缺乏、先天性维生素D缺乏、继发性维生素D缺乏、维生素D依赖性佝偻病Ⅰ型和Ⅱ型以及慢性肾脏疾病；具体描述了钙缺乏的病理生理、临床表现、诊断和治疗；针对磷缺乏具体描述了磷摄入不足、纤维

生长因子23、X连锁低磷性佝偻病、常染色体显性低磷性佝偻病、常染色体隐性低磷性佝偻病、遗传性低磷性佝偻病伴高钙尿症、纤维生长因子23过量、范可尼综合征以及X连锁Dent病；具体描述了早产儿佝偻病的发病机制、临床表现、实验室检查、诊断、预防和治疗；具体描述了维生素D过量的病因、发病机制、临床表现、实验室检查、诊断与鉴别诊断、治疗和预后。

RICKETS

Bone consists of a protein matrix called *osteoid* and a mineral phase, principally composed of calcium and phosphate, mostly in the form of *hydroxyapatite*. **Osteomalacia** occurs with inadequate mineralization of bone osteoid in children and adults. **Rickets** is a disease of growing bone caused by unmineralized matrix at the growth plates in children only before fusion of the epiphyses. Because growth plate cartilage and osteoid continue to expand but mineralization is inadequate, the growth plate thickens. Circumference of the growth plate and metaphysis is also greater, increasing bone width at the growth plates and causing classic clinical manifestations, such as widening of the wrists and ankles. The general softening of the bones causes them to bend easily when subject to forces such as weight bearing or muscle pull. This softening leads to a variety of bone deformities.

Rickets is principally caused by vitamin D deficiency and was rampant in northern Europe and the United States during the early years of the 20th century. Although largely corrected through public health measures that provided children with adequate vitamin D, rickets remains a persistent problem in developed countries, with many cases still secondary to preventable nutritional vitamin D deficiency. It remains a significant problem in developing countries and may be secondary to nutritional vitamin D deficiency and inadequate intake of calcium (Table 64.1).

Etiology

There are many causes of rickets, including vitamin D disorders, calcium deficiency, phosphorus deficiency, and distal renal tubular acidosis (Table 64.2).

Clinical Manifestations

Most manifestations of rickets are a result of skeletal changes (Table 64.3). **Craniotabes** is a softening of the cranial bones and can be detected by applying pressure at the occiput or over the parietal bones. The sensation is similar to the feel of pressing into a Ping-Pong ball and then releasing. Craniotabes may also be secondary to osteogenesis imperfecta, hydrocephalus, and syphilis. It is a normal finding in many newborns, especially near the suture lines, but typically disappears within a few months of birth. Widening of the costochondral junctions results in a **rachitic "rosary,"** which feels like the beads of a rosary as the examiner's fingers move along the costochondral junctions from rib to rib (Fig. 64.1). Growth plate widening is also responsible for the enlargement at the wrists and ankles (Fig. 64.2). The horizontal depression along the lower anterior chest known as *Harrison groove* occurs from pulling of the softened ribs by the diaphragm during inspiration. Softening of the ribs also impairs air movement and predisposes patients to atelectasis and pneumonia. Valgus or varus deformities of the legs are

Table 64.1	Physical and Metabolic Properties and Food Sources of Vitamins D, E, and K				
NAMES AND SYNONYMS	**CHARACTERISTICS**	**BIOCHEMICAL ACTION**	**EFFECTS OF DEFICIENCY**	**EFFECTS OF EXCESS**	**SOURCES**
VITAMIN D Vitamin D_3 (3-cholecalciferol), which is synthesized in the skin, and vitamin D_2 (from plants or yeast) are biologically equivalent; 1 μg = 40 IU vitamin D.	Fat-soluble, stable to heat, acid, alkali, and oxidation; bile necessary for absorption; hydroxylation in the liver and kidney necessary for biologic activity	Necessary for GI absorption of calcium; also increases absorption of phosphate; direct actions on bone, including mediating resorption	Rickets in growing children; osteomalacia; hypocalcemia can cause tetany and seizures	Hypercalcemia, which can cause emesis, anorexia, pancreatitis, hypertension, arrhythmias, CNS effects, polyuria, nephrolithiasis, renal failure	Exposure to sunlight (UV light); fish oils, fatty fish, egg yolks, and vitamin D–fortified formula, milk, cereals, bread
VITAMIN E Group of related compounds with similar biologic activities; α-tocopherol is the most potent and most common form	Fat-soluble; readily oxidized by oxygen, iron, rancid fats; bile acids necessary for absorption	Antioxidant; protection of cell membranes from lipid peroxidation and formation of free radicals	Red cell hemolysis in premature infants; posterior column and cerebellar dysfunction; pigmentary retinopathy	Unknown	Vegetable oils, seeds, nuts, green leafy vegetables, margarine
VITAMIN K Group of naphthoquinones with similar biologic activities; K_1 (phylloquinone) from diet; K_2 (menaquinones) from intestinal bacteria	Natural compounds are fat-soluble; stable to heat and reducing agents; labile to oxidizing agent, strong acids, alkali, light; bile salts necessary for intestinal absorption	Vitamin K–dependent proteins include coagulation factors II, VII, IX, and X; proteins C, S, Z; matrix Gla protein, osteocalcin	Hemorrhagic manifestations; long-term bone and vascular health	Not established; analogs (no longer used) caused hemolytic anemia, jaundice, kernicterus, death	Green leafy vegetables, liver, certain legumes and plant oils; widely distributed

CNS, Central nervous system; GI, gastrointestinal; UV, ultraviolet.

Table 64.2	Causes of Rickets

VITAMIN D DISORDERS
Nutritional vitamin D deficiency
Congenital vitamin D deficiency
Secondary vitamin D deficiency
Malabsorption
Increased degradation
Decreased liver 25-hydroxylase
Vitamin D–dependent rickets types 1A and 1B
Vitamin D–dependent rickets types 2A and 2B
Chronic kidney disease

CALCIUM DEFICIENCY
Low intake
Diet
Premature infants (rickets of prematurity)
Malabsorption
Primary disease
Dietary inhibitors of calcium absorption

PHOSPHORUS DEFICIENCY
Inadequate intake
Premature infants (rickets of prematurity)
Aluminum-containing antacids

RENAL LOSSES
X-linked hypophosphatemic rickets*
Autosomal dominant hypophosphatemic rickets*
Autosomal recessive hypophosphatemic rickets types 1 and 2*
Hereditary hypophosphatemic rickets with hypercalciuria
Overproduction of fibroblast growth factor-23
Tumor-induced rickets*
McCune-Albright syndrome*
Epidermal nevus syndrome*
Neurofibromatosis*
Fanconi syndrome
Dent disease
Distal renal tubular acidosis

*Disorders secondary to excess fibroblast growth factor-23.

common; **windswept deformity** occurs when one leg is in extreme valgus and the other is in extreme varus (Fig. 64.3).

The clinical presentation of rickets may vary based on the etiology. Changes in the lower extremities tend to be the dominant feature in X-linked hypophosphatemic rickets. Symptoms secondary to hypocalcemia occur only in those forms of rickets associated with decreased serum calcium.

The chief complaint in a child with rickets is quite variable. Many children present because of skeletal deformities, whereas others have difficulty walking owing to a combination of deformity and weakness.

Other common presenting complaints include failure to thrive (malnutrition) and symptomatic hypocalcemia (see Chapters 588 to 590).

Radiology

Rachitic changes are most easily visualized on posteroanterior radiographs of the wrist, although characteristic rachitic changes can be seen at other growth plates (Figs. 64.4 and 64.5). Decreased calcification leads to thickening of the growth plate. The edge of the metaphysis loses its sharp border, which is described as *fraying*. The edge of the metaphysis changes from a convex or flat surface to a more concave surface. This

Table 64.3	Clinical Features of Rickets

GENERAL
Failure to thrive (malnutrition)
Listlessness
Protruding abdomen
Muscle weakness (especially proximal)
Hypocalcemic dilated cardiomyopathy
Fractures (pathologic, minimal trauma)
Increased intracranial pressure

HEAD
Craniotabes
Frontal bossing
Delayed fontanel closure (usually closed by 2 yr)
Delayed dentition
    No incisors by age 10 mo
    No molars by age 18 mo
Caries
Craniosynostosis

CHEST
Rachitic rosary
Harrison groove
Respiratory infections and atelectasis*

BACK
Scoliosis
Kyphosis
Lordosis

EXTREMITIES
Enlargement of wrists and ankles
Valgus or varus deformities
Windswept deformity (valgus deformity of one leg with varus
    deformity of other leg)
Anterior bowing of tibia and femur
Coxa vara
Leg pain

HYPOCALCEMIC SYMPTOMS†
Tetany
Seizures
Stridor caused by laryngeal spasm

*These features are most frequently associated with the vitamin D deficiency disorders.
    †These symptoms develop only in children with disorders that produce hypocalcemia (see Table 64.4).

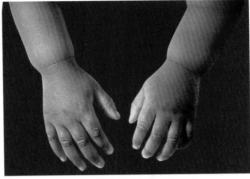

Fig. 64.2 Hands and forearms of a young child with rickets show prominence above the wrist, resulting from flaring and poor mineralization of lower end of the radius and ulna. *(From Bullough PG: Orthopaedic pathology, ed 5, St Louis, 2010, Mosby, Fig 8-31.)*

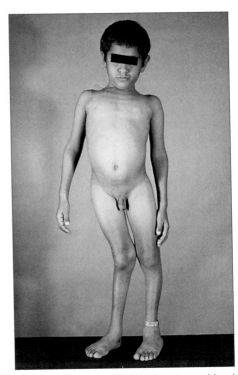

Fig. 64.3 Windswept deformity of the legs in an older child with rickets. *(From Rickets and osteomalacia. In Hochberg MC, Silman AJ, Smolen JS, et al, editors: Rheumatology, 4e. London, 2008, Mosby, Fig 192-6.)*

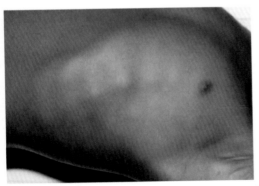

Fig. 64.1 Rachitic "rosary" in a child with rickets. *(Courtesy of Dr. Thomas D. Thacher, Rochester, MN.)*

change to a concave surface is termed *cupping* and is most easily seen at the distal ends of the radius, ulna, and fibula. There is widening of the distal end of the metaphysis, corresponding to the clinical observation of thickened wrists and ankles, as well as the rachitic rosary. Other

radiologic features include coarse trabeculation of the diaphysis and generalized rarefaction.

Diagnosis
The diagnosis of rickets is based on the presence of classic radiographic abnormalities. It is supported by physical examination findings, history, and laboratory results consistent with a specific etiology (Table 64.4).

Clinical Evaluation
Because the majority of children with rickets have a nutritional deficiency, the initial evaluation should focus on a **dietary history,** emphasizing

intake of both vitamin D and calcium. Most children in industrialized nations receive vitamin D from formula, fortified milk, or vitamin supplements. Along with the amount, the exact composition of the formula or milk is pertinent, because rickets has occurred in children given products that are called "milk" (e.g., soy milk) but are deficient in vitamin D and minerals.

Cutaneous synthesis mediated by sunlight exposure is an important source of vitamin D. It is important to ask about time spent outside, sunscreen use, and clothing, especially if there may be a cultural reason for increased covering of the skin. Because winter sunlight is ineffective at stimulating cutaneous synthesis of vitamin D, the season is an additional

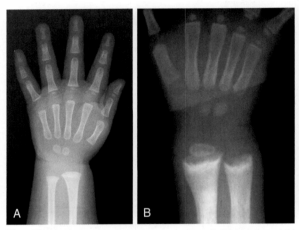

Fig. 64.4 Radiographs of the wrist in **A,** normal child; and **B,** child with rickets, who has metaphyseal fraying and cupping of the distal radius and ulna.

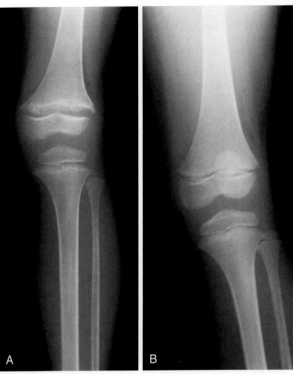

Fig. 64.5 Radiographs of the knees in 7 yr old girl with distal renal tubular acidosis and rickets. **A,** At initial presentation, there is widening of the growth plate and metaphyseal fraying. **B,** Dramatic improvement after 4 mo of therapy with alkali.

Table 64.4	Laboratory Findings in Various Disorders Causing Rickets

Disorder	Ca	Pi	PTH	25-(OH)D	1,25-(OH)₂D	ALP	URINE Ca	URINE Pi
Vitamin D deficiency	N, ↓	↓	↑	↓	↓, N, ↑	↑	↓	↑
VDDR, type 1A	N, ↓	↓	↑	N	↓	↑	↓	↑
VDDR, type 1B	N, ↓	↓	↑	↓	N	↑	↓	↑
VDDR, type 2A	N, ↓	↓	↑	N	↑↑	↑	↓	↑
VDDR, type 2B	N, ↓	↓	↑	N	↑↑	↑	↓	↑
Chronic kidney disease	N, ↓	↑	↑	N	↓	↑	N, ↓	↓
Dietary Pi deficiency	N	↓	N, ↓	N	↑	↑	↑	↓
XLH*	N	↓	N, ↑	N	RD	↑	↓	↑
ADHR*	N	↓	N	N	RD	↑	↓	↑
HHRH	N	↓	N, ↓	N	↑	↑	↑	↑
ARHR, type 1 or type 2*	N	↓	N	N	RD	↑	↓	↑
Tumor-induced rickets†	N	↓	N	N	RD	↑	↓	↑
Fanconi syndrome	N	↓	N	N	RD or ↑	↑	↓ or ↑	↑
Dent's disease	N	↓	N	N	N	↑	↑	↑
Dietary Ca deficiency	N, ↓	↓	↑	N	↑	↑	↓	↑

ADHR, Autosomal dominant hypophosphatemic rickets; ALP, alkaline phosphatase; ARHR, autosomal recessive hypophosphatemic rickets; Ca, calcium; HHRH, hereditary hypophosphatemic rickets with hypercalciuria; N, normal; Pi, inorganic phosphorus; PTH, parathyroid hormone; RD, relatively decreased (because it should be increased given the concurrent hypophosphatemia); VDDR, vitamin D–dependent rickets; XLH, X-linked hypophosphatemic rickets; 1,25-(OH)₂D, 1,25-dihydroxyvitamin D; 25-OHD, 25-hydroxyvitamin D; ↓, decreased; ↑, increased; ↑↑, extremely increased.
*Elevated fibroblast growth factor-23 (FGF-23).
†FGF-23 elevated in some patients.

consideration. Children with increased skin pigmentation are at increased risk for vitamin D deficiency because of decreased cutaneous synthesis.

The presence of **maternal** risk factors for nutritional vitamin D deficiency, including diet and sun exposure, is an important consideration when a neonate or young infant has rachitic findings, especially if the infant is breastfed (Table 64.5). Determining a child's intake of dairy products, the main dietary source of calcium, provides a general sense of calcium intake. High dietary fiber can interfere with calcium absorption.

The child's **medication** use is relevant, because certain medications, such as the anticonvulsants phenobarbital and phenytoin, increase degradation of vitamin D, and phosphate binders or aluminum-containing antacids interfere with the absorption of phosphate.

Malabsorption of vitamin D is suggested by a history of liver or intestinal disease. Undiagnosed liver or intestinal disease should be suspected if the child has gastrointestinal (GI) symptoms, although occasionally rickets is the presenting complaint. Fat malabsorption is often associated with diarrhea or oily stools, and there may be signs or symptoms suggesting deficiencies of other fat-soluble vitamins (A, E, and K; see Chapters 61, 65, and 66).

A history of **renal disease** (proteinuria, hematuria, urinary tract infections) is an additional significant consideration, given the importance of chronic kidney disease as a cause of rickets. Polyuria can occur in children with chronic kidney disease or Fanconi syndrome.

Children with rickets might have a history of dental caries, poor growth, delayed walking, waddling gait, pneumonia, and hypocalcemic symptoms.

The family history is critical, given the large number of **genetic causes** of rickets, although most of these causes are rare. Along with bone disease, it is important to inquire about leg deformities, difficulties with walking, or unexplained short stature, because some parents may be unaware of their diagnosis. Undiagnosed disease in the mother is not

unusual in X-linked hypophosphatemia. A history of an unexplained sibling death during infancy may be present in the child with cystinosis, the most common cause of Fanconi syndrome in children.

The physical examination focuses on detecting manifestations of rickets (see Table 64.3). It is important to observe the child's gait, auscultate the lungs to detect atelectasis or pneumonia, and plot the patient's growth. Alopecia suggests vitamin D–dependent rickets type 2.

The initial **laboratory tests** in a child with rickets should include serum calcium, phosphorus, alkaline phosphatase (ALP), parathyroid hormone (PTH), 25-hydroxyvitamin D, 1,25-dihydroxyvitamin D (1,25-D), creatinine, and electrolytes (see Table 64.4 for interpretation). Urinalysis is useful for detecting the glycosuria seen with Fanconi syndrome and low-molecular-weight proteinuria (positive dipstick for protein) in Fanconi syndrome or Dent disease. Evaluation of urinary excretion of calcium (24 hr collection for calcium or calcium:creatinine ratio) is helpful if hereditary hypophosphatemic rickets with hypercalciuria or Dent disease is suspected. Direct measurement of other fat-soluble vitamins (A, E, and K) or indirect assessment of deficiency (prothrombin time for vitamin K deficiency) is appropriate if malabsorption is a consideration.

VITAMIN D DISORDERS
Vitamin D Physiology

Vitamin D can be synthesized in skin epithelial cells and therefore technically is not a vitamin. Cutaneous synthesis is normally the most important source of vitamin D and depends on the conversion of 7-dehydrochlesterol to vitamin D_3 (3-cholecalciferol) by ultraviolet B (UVB) radiation from the sun. The efficiency of this process is decreased by melanin; therefore, more sun exposure is necessary for vitamin D synthesis in people with increased skin pigmentation. Measures to decrease sun exposure, such as covering the skin with clothing or applying sunscreen, also decrease vitamin D synthesis. Children who spend less time outside have reduced vitamin D synthesis. The winter sun away from the equator is ineffective at mediating vitamin D synthesis.

There are few natural dietary sources of vitamin D. Fish liver oils have a high vitamin D content. Other good dietary sources include fatty fish and egg yolks. Most children in industrialized countries receive vitamin D via fortified foods, especially formula and milk (both of which contain 400 IU/L) and some breakfast cereals and breads. Supplemental vitamin D may be vitamin D_2 (which comes from plants or yeast) or vitamin D_3. Breast milk has a low vitamin D content, approximately 12-60 IU/L.

Vitamin D is transported bound to vitamin D–binding protein to the liver, where 25-hydroxylase converts vitamin D into 25-hydroxyvitamin D (25-D), the most abundant circulating form of vitamin D. Because there is little regulation of this liver hydroxylation step, measurement of 25-D is the standard method for determining a patient's vitamin D status. The final step in activation occurs in the kidney, where the enzyme 1α-hydroxylase adds a second hydroxyl group, resulting in 1,25-D. The 1α-hydroxylase is upregulated by PTH and hypophosphatemia and inhibited by hyperphosphatemia and 1,25-D. Most 1,25-D circulates bound to vitamin D–binding protein.

1,25-Dihydroxyvitamin D acts by binding to an intracellular receptor, and the complex affects gene expression by interacting with vitamin D response elements. In the intestine, this binding results in a marked increase in calcium absorption, which is highly dependent on 1,25-D. There is also an increase in phosphorus absorption, but this effect is less significant because most dietary phosphorus absorption is vitamin D independent. 1,25-D also has direct effects on bone, including mediating resorption. 1,25-D directly suppresses PTH secretion by the parathyroid gland, thus completing a negative feedback loop. PTH secretion is also suppressed by the increase in serum calcium mediated by 1,25-D. 1,25-D inhibits its own synthesis in the kidney and increases the synthesis of inactive metabolites.

Nutritional Vitamin D Deficiency

Vitamin D deficiency remains the most common cause of rickets globally and is prevalent, even in industrialized countries. Because vitamin D can be obtained from dietary sources or from cutaneous synthesis, most

Table 64.5	Risk Factors for Nutritional Rickets and Osteomalacia and Their Prevention

MATERNAL FACTORS

Vitamin D deficiency
    Dark skin pigmentation
    Full body clothing cover
    High latitude during winter/spring season
    Other causes of restricted sun (UVB) exposure, e.g., predominant indoor living, disability, pollution, cloud cover
    Low–vitamin D diet
Low-calcium diet
    Poverty, malnutrition, special diets

INFANT/CHILDHOOD FACTORS

Neonatal vitamin D deficiency secondary to maternal deficiency/vitamin D deficiency
    Lack of infant supplementation with vitamin D
    Prolonged breastfeeding without appropriate complementary feeding from 6 mo
    High latitude during winter/spring season
    Dark skin pigmentation and/or restricted sun (UVB) exposure, e.g., predominant indoor living, disability, pollution, cloud cover
    Low–vitamin D diet
Low-calcium diet
    Poverty, malnutrition, special diets

PREVENTIVE MEASURES

Sun exposure (UVB content of sunlight depends on latitude and season)
Vitamin D supplementation
Strategic fortification of the habitual food supply
Normal calcium intake

Adapted from Munns CF, Shaw N, Kiely M, et al: Global consensus recommendations on prevention and management of nutritional rickets, *J Clin Endocrinol Metab* 101:394-415, 2016, p 401.

patients in industrialized countries have a combination of risk factors that lead to vitamin D deficiency.

Etiology

Vitamin D deficiency most frequently occurs in infancy because of a combination of poor intake and inadequate cutaneous synthesis. Transplacental transport of vitamin D, mostly 25-D, typically provides enough vitamin D for the 1st 2 mo of life unless there is severe maternal vitamin D deficiency. Infants who receive formula receive adequate vitamin D, even without cutaneous synthesis. Because of the low vitamin D content of breast milk, breastfed infants rely on cutaneous synthesis or vitamin supplements. Cutaneous synthesis can be limited because of the ineffectiveness of the winter sun in stimulating vitamin D synthesis; avoidance of sunlight because of concerns about cancer, neighborhood safety, or cultural practices; and decreased cutaneous synthesis because of increased skin pigmentation.

The effect of skin pigmentation explains why most cases of nutritional rickets in the United States and northern Europe occur in breastfed children of African descent or other dark-pigmented populations. The additional impact of the winter sun is supported by such infants more often presenting in the late winter or spring. In some groups, complete covering of infants or the practice of not taking infants outside has a significant role, explaining the occurrence of rickets in infants living in areas of abundant sunshine, such as the Middle East. Because the mothers of some infants can have the same risk factors, decreased maternal vitamin D can also contribute, both by leading to reduced vitamin D content in breast milk and by lessening transplacental delivery of vitamin D. Rickets caused by vitamin D deficiency can also be secondary to unconventional dietary practices, such as vegan diets that use unfortified soy milk or rice milk.

Clinical Manifestations

The clinical features are typical of rickets (see Table 64.3), with a significant minority presenting with symptoms of hypocalcemia. Prolonged laryngospasm is occasionally fatal. These children have an increased risk of pneumonia and muscle weakness leading to a delay in motor development.

Laboratory Findings

Table 64.4 summarize the principal laboratory findings. Hypocalcemia is a variable finding because the elevated PTH acts to increase the serum calcium concentration. The hypophosphatemia is caused by PTH-induced renal losses of phosphate, combined with a decrease in intestinal absorption.

The wide variation in 1,25-D levels (low, normal, or high) is secondary to the upregulation of renal 1α-hydroxylase caused by concomitant hypophosphatemia and hyperparathyroidism. Because serum levels of 1,25-D are much lower than the levels of 25-D, even with low levels of 25-D there is often enough 25-D still present to act as a precursor for 1,25-D synthesis in the presence of upregulated 1α-hydroxylase. The level of 1,25-D is only low when there is severe vitamin D deficiency.

Some patients have a metabolic acidosis secondary to PTH-induced renal bicarbonate wasting. There may also be generalized aminoaciduria.

Diagnosis and Differential Diagnosis

The diagnosis of nutritional vitamin D deficiency is based on the combination of a history of poor vitamin D intake and risk factors for decreased cutaneous synthesis, radiographic changes consistent with rickets, and typical laboratory findings (see Table 64.4). A normal PTH level almost never occurs with vitamin D deficiency and suggests a primary phosphate disorder.

Treatment

Children with nutritional vitamin D deficiency should receive vitamin D and adequate nutritional intake of calcium and phosphorus. There are 2 strategies for administration of vitamin D. With **stoss therapy**, vitamin D (300,000-600,000 IU) is administered orally (preferred) or intramuscularly as 2-4 doses over 1 day (vitamin D_3 is preferred to D_2 because of longer half-life of D_3). Since the doses are observed, stoss

therapy is ideal in patients in whom adherence to therapy is questionable. The alternative strategy is daily vitamin D with a minimum dose of 2,000 IU/day for a minimum of 3 mo. Either strategy should be followed by daily vitamin D intake of 400 IU/day if <1 yr old or 600 IU/day if >1 yr old. It is important to ensure that children receive adequate dietary calcium (minimum of 500 mg/day) and phosphorus; this dietary intake is usually provided by milk, formula, and other dairy products, although calcium supplements may be needed in some patients.

Children who have symptomatic hypocalcemia might need intravenous (IV) calcium acutely, followed by oral calcium supplements, which typically can be tapered over 2-6 wk in children who receive adequate dietary calcium. Transient use of IV or oral 1,25-D (**calcitriol**) is often helpful in reversing hypocalcemia in the acute phase by providing active vitamin D during the delay as supplemental vitamin D is converted to active vitamin D. Calcitriol doses are typically 0.05 µg/kg/day. IV calcium is initially given as an acute bolus for symptomatic hypocalcemia (20 mg/kg calcium chloride or 100 mg/kg calcium gluconate). Some patients require a continuous IV calcium drip, titrated to maintain the desired serum calcium level. These patients should transition to enteral calcium, and most infants require approximately 1,000 mg of elemental calcium.

Prognosis

Most children with nutritional vitamin D deficiency have an excellent response to treatment, with radiologic healing occurring within a few months. Laboratory test results should also normalize rapidly. Many of the bone malformations improve dramatically, but children with severe disease can have permanent deformities and short stature. Rarely, patients benefit from orthopedic intervention for leg deformities, although this is generally not done until the metabolic bone disease has healed, there is clear evidence that the deformity will not self-resolve, and the deformity is causing functional problems.

Prevention

Most cases of nutritional rickets can be prevented by universal administration of 400 IU of vitamin D to infants <1 yr old. Older children with risk factors for inadequate intake should receive 600 IU/day. Vitamin D may be administered as a component of a multivitamin or as a vitamin D supplement.

Congenital Vitamin D Deficiency

Congenital rickets is quite rare in industrialized countries and occurs when there is severe maternal vitamin D deficiency during pregnancy. Maternal risk factors include poor dietary intake of vitamin D, lack of adequate sun exposure, and closely spaced pregnancies. These newborns can have symptomatic hypocalcemia, intrauterine growth retardation, and decreased bone ossification, along with classic rachitic changes. Subtler maternal vitamin D deficiency can have an adverse effect on neonatal bone density and birthweight, cause a defect in dental enamel, and predispose infants to neonatal hypocalcemic tetany. Treatment of congenital rickets includes vitamin D supplementation and adequate intake of calcium and phosphorus. Use of prenatal vitamins containing vitamin D (600 IU) prevents this entity.

Secondary Vitamin D Deficiency
Etiology

Along with inadequate intake, vitamin D deficiency can result from inadequate absorption, decreased hydroxylation in the liver, and increased degradation. Because vitamin D is fat soluble, its absorption may be decreased in patients with a variety of liver and GI diseases, including cholestatic liver disease, defects in bile acid metabolism, cystic fibrosis and other causes of pancreatic dysfunction, celiac disease, and Crohn disease. Malabsorption of vitamin D can also occur with intestinal lymphangiectasia and after intestinal resection.

Severe liver disease, which usually is also associated with malabsorption, can cause a decrease in 25-D formation as a result of insufficient enzyme activity. Because of the large reserve of 25-hydroxlase activity in the liver, vitamin D deficiency caused by liver disease usually requires a loss of >90% of liver function. A variety of medications increase the degradation of vitamin D by inducing the cytochrome P450 (CYP) system. Rickets from vitamin D deficiency can develop in children receiving anticonvulsants (e.g., phenobarbital, phenytoin) or antituberculosis medications (e.g., isoniazid, rifampin).

Treatment

Treatment of vitamin D deficiency attributable to malabsorption requires high doses of vitamin D. Because of its better absorption, 25-D (25-50 μg/day or 5-7 μg/kg/day) is superior to vitamin D_3. The dose is adjusted based on monitoring of serum levels of 25-D. Alternatively, patients may be treated with 1,25-D, which also is better absorbed in the presence of fat malabsorption, or with parenteral vitamin D. Children with rickets as a result of increased degradation of vitamin D by the CYP system require the same acute therapy as indicated for nutritional deficiency (discussed earlier), followed by long-term administration of high doses of vitamin D (e.g., 1,000 IU/day), with dosing titrated based on serum levels of 25-D. Some patients require as much as 4,000 IU/day.

Vitamin D–Dependent Rickets, Type 1

Children with vitamin D–dependent rickets **type 1A**, an autosomal recessive disorder, have mutations in the gene encoding renal 1α-hydroxylase, preventing conversion of 25-D into 1,25-D. These patients normally present during the 1st 2 yr of life and can have any of the classic features of rickets (see Table 64.3), including symptomatic hypocalcemia. They have normal levels of 25-D but low levels of 1,25-D (see Table 64.4). Occasionally, 1,25-D levels are at the lower limit of normal, inappropriately low given the high PTH and low serum phosphorus levels, both of which should increase the activity of renal 1α-hydroxylase and cause elevated levels of 1,25-D. As in nutritional vitamin D deficiency, renal tubular dysfunction can cause a metabolic acidosis and generalized aminoaciduria.

Vitamin D–dependent rickets **type 1B** is secondary to a mutation in the gene for a 25-hydroxylase. Patients have low levels of 25-D but normal levels of 1,25-D (see Table 64.4).

Treatment

Vitamin D–dependent rickets type 1A responds to long-term treatment with 1,25-D (calcitriol). Initial doses are 0.25-2 μg/day, and lower doses are used once the rickets has healed. Especially during initial therapy, it is important to ensure adequate intake of calcium. The dose of calcitriol is adjusted to maintain a low-normal serum calcium level, a normal serum phosphorus level, and a high-normal serum PTH level. Targeting a low-normal calcium concentration and a high-normal PTH level avoids excessive dosing of calcitriol, which can cause hypercalciuria and nephrocalcinosis. Therefore, patient monitoring includes periodic assessment of urinary calcium excretion, with a target of <4 mg/kg/day.

Vitamin D–dependent rickets type 1B may respond to pharmacologic doses of vitamin D_2 (3,000 U/day) as a result of alternative enzymes with 25-hydroxylase activity or residual activity of the mutant protein.

Vitamin D–Dependent Rickets, Type 2

Patients with vitamin D–dependent rickets **type 2A** have mutations in the gene encoding the vitamin D receptor, preventing a normal physiologic response to 1,25-D. Levels of 1,25-D are extremely elevated in this autosomal recessive disorder (see Table 64.4). Most patients present during infancy, although rickets in less severely affected patients might not be diagnosed until adulthood. Less severe disease is associated with a partially functional vitamin D receptor. Approximately 50–70% of children have **alopecia**, which tends to be associated with a more severe form of the disease and can range from alopecia areata to alopecia totalis. Epidermal cysts are a less common manifestation.

Vitamin D–dependent rickets **type 2B** appears to result from overexpression of a hormone response element–binding protein that interferes with the actions of 1,25-D. Alopecia may be present.

Treatment

Some patients respond to extremely high doses of vitamin D_2 (25-D or 1,25-D), especially patients without alopecia. This response is caused by a partially functional vitamin D receptor in patients with vitamin D–dependent rickets type 2A, but may also occur in vitamin D–dependent

rickets type 2B. All patients should be given a 3-6 mo trial of high-dose vitamin D and oral calcium. The initial dose of 1,25-D should be 2 μg/day, but some patients require doses as high as 50-60 μg/day. Calcium doses are 1,000-3,000 mg/day. Patients who do not respond to high-dose vitamin D may be treated with long-term IV calcium, with possible transition to very high dose oral calcium supplements. Treatment of patients who do not respond to vitamin D is difficult.

Chronic Kidney Disease

With chronic kidney disease, there is decreased activity of 1α-hydroxylase in the kidney, leading to diminished production of 1,25-D. In chronic kidney disease, unlike the other causes of vitamin D deficiency, patients have hyperphosphatemia as a result of decreased renal excretion (see Table 64.4 and Chapter 550.2).

Treatment

Therapy requires the use of a form of vitamin D that can act without 1-hydroxylation by the kidney (calcitriol), which both permits adequate absorption of calcium and directly suppresses the parathyroid gland. Because hyperphosphatemia is a stimulus for PTH secretion, normalization of the serum phosphorus level through a combination of dietary phosphorus restriction and use of oral phosphate binders is as important as the use of activated vitamin D.

CALCIUM DEFICIENCY
Pathophysiology

Rickets secondary to inadequate dietary calcium is a significant problem in some countries in Africa, although there are cases in other regions of the world, including industrialized countries. Because breast milk and formula are excellent sources of calcium, this form of rickets develops after children have been weaned from breast milk or formula and is more likely to occur in children who are weaned early. Rickets develops because the diet has low calcium content, typically <200 mg/day if <12 mo old or <300 mg/day if >12 mo old. The child has minimal intake of dairy products or other sources of calcium. In addition, because of reliance on grains and green leafy vegetables, the diet may be high in phytate, oxalate, and phosphate, which decrease absorption of dietary calcium. In industrialized countries, rickets caused by calcium deficiency can occur in children who consume an unconventional diet. Examples include children with milk allergy who have low dietary calcium and children who transition from formula or breast milk to juice, soda, or a calcium-poor soy drink, without an alternative source of dietary calcium.

This type of rickets can develop in children who receive intravenous nutrition without adequate calcium. Malabsorption of calcium can occur in celiac disease, intestinal abetalipoproteinemia, and after small bowel resection. There may be concurrent malabsorption of vitamin D.

Clinical Manifestations

Children with calcium deficiency have the classic signs and symptoms of rickets (see Table 64.3). Presentation can occur during infancy or early childhood, although some cases are diagnosed in teenagers. Because calcium deficiency occurs after the cessation of breastfeeding, it tends to occur later than the nutritional vitamin D deficiency that is associated with breastfeeding. In Nigeria, nutritional vitamin D deficiency is most common at 4-15 mo of age, whereas calcium deficiency rickets typically occurs at 15-25 mo.

Diagnosis

Laboratory findings include increased levels of ALP, PTH, and 1,25-D (see Table 64.4). Calcium levels may be normal or low, although symptomatic hypocalcemia is uncommon. There is decreased urinary excretion of calcium, and serum phosphorus levels may be low as a result of renal wasting of phosphate from secondary hyperparathyroidism. In some children, there is coexisting nutritional vitamin D deficiency, with low 25-D levels.

Treatment

Treatment focuses on providing adequate calcium, typically as a dietary supplement (doses of 700 [age 1-3 yr], 1,000 [4-8 yr], and 1,300 [9-18 yr] mg/day of elemental calcium are effective). Vitamin D supplementation is necessary if there is concurrent vitamin D deficiency (discussed earlier). Prevention strategies include discouraging early cessation of breastfeeding and increasing dietary sources of calcium. In countries such as Kenya, where many children have diets high in cereal with negligible intake of cow's milk, school-based milk programs have been effective in reducing the prevalence of rickets.

PHOSPHORUS DEFICIENCY

Inadequate Intake

With the exception of starvation or severe anorexia, it is almost impossible to have a diet that is deficient in phosphorus, because phosphorus is present in most foods. Decreased phosphorus absorption can occur in diseases associated with malabsorption (celiac disease, cystic fibrosis, cholestatic liver disease), but if rickets develops, the primary problem is usually malabsorption of vitamin D and/or calcium.

Isolated malabsorption of phosphorus occurs in patients with long-term use of **aluminum-containing antacids**. These compounds are very effective at chelating phosphate in the GI tract, leading to decreased absorption. This decreased absorption results in hypophosphatemia with secondary osteomalacia in adults and rickets in children. This entity responds to discontinuation of the antacid and short-term phosphorus supplementation.

Fibroblast Growth Factor-23

Fibroblast growth factor-23 (**FGF-23**) is a humoral mediator that decreases renal tubular reabsorption of phosphate and therefore decreases serum phosphorus. FGF-23, synthesized by osteocytes, also decreases the activity of renal 1α-hydroxylase, resulting in a decrease in the production of 1,25-D. Increased levels of FGF-23 cause many of the renal phosphate-wasting diseases (see Table 64.2).

X-Linked Hypophosphatemic Rickets

Among the genetic disorders causing rickets because of hypophosphatemia, X-linked hypophosphatemic rickets (**XLH**) is the most common, with a prevalence of 1/20,000. The defective gene is on the X chromosome, but female carriers are affected, so it is an X-linked dominant disorder.

Pathophysiology

The defective gene is called *PHEX* because it is a *p*hosphate-regulating gene with homology to *e*ndopeptidases on the *X* chromosome. The product of this gene appears to have an indirect role in inactivating FGF-23. Mutations in *PHEX* lead to increased levels of FGF-23. Because the actions of FGF-23 include inhibition of phosphate reabsorption in the proximal tubule, phosphate excretion is increased. FGF-23 also inhibits renal 1α-hydroxylase, leading to decreased production of 1,25-D.

Clinical Manifestations

These patients have rickets, but abnormalities of the lower extremities and poor growth are the dominant features. Delayed dentition and tooth abscesses are also common. Some patients have hypophosphatemia and short stature without clinically evident bone disease.

Laboratory Findings

Patients have high renal excretion of phosphate, hypophosphatemia, and increased ALP; PTH and serum calcium levels are normal (see Table 64.4). Hypophosphatemia normally upregulates renal 1α-hydroxylase and should lead to an increase in 1,25-D, but these patients have low or inappropriately normal levels of 1,25-D.

Treatment

Patients respond well to a combination of oral phosphorus and 1,25-D (calcitriol). The daily need for phosphorus supplementation is 1-3 g of elemental phosphorus divided into 4 or 5 doses. Frequent dosing helps to prevent prolonged decrements in serum phosphorus because there is a rapid decline after each dose. In addition, frequent dosing decreases diarrhea, a complication of high-dose oral phosphorus. Calcitriol is administered at 30-70 ng/kg/day in 2 doses. Burosumab-twza is a

monoclonal antibody to FGF-23 that is an approved alternative approach for treating XLH in children >1 yr.

Complications of treatment occur when there is not an adequate balance between phosphorus supplementation and calcitriol. Excess phosphorus, by decreasing enteral calcium absorption, leads to secondary hyperparathyroidism, with worsening of the bone lesions. In contrast, excess calcitriol causes hypercalciuria and nephrocalcinosis and can even cause hypercalcemia. Therefore, laboratory monitoring of treatment includes serum calcium, phosphorus, ALP, PTH, and urinary calcium, as well as periodic renal ultrasound to evaluate patients for nephrocalcinosis. Because of variation in the serum phosphorus level and the importance of avoiding excessive phosphorus dosing, normalization of ALP levels is a more useful method of assessing the therapeutic response than measuring serum phosphorus. For children with significant short stature, growth hormone is an effective option. Children with severe deformities might need osteotomies, but these procedures should be done only when treatment has led to resolution of the bone disease.

Prognosis

The response to therapy is usually good, although frequent dosing can lead to problems with compliance. Girls generally have less severe disease than boys, probably because of the X-linked inheritance. Short stature can persist despite healing of the rickets. Adults generally do well with less aggressive treatment, and some receive calcitriol alone. Adults with bone pain or other symptoms improve with oral phosphorus supplementation and calcitriol.

Autosomal Dominant Hypophosphatemic Rickets

Autosomal dominant hypophosphatemic rickets (**ADHR**) is much less common than XLH. There is incomplete penetrance and variable age of onset. Patients with ADHR have a mutation in the gene encoding FGF-23 (*FGF23*). The mutation prevents degradation of FGF-23 by proteases, leading its level to increase. The actions of FGF-23 include decreased reabsorption of phosphate in the renal proximal tubule, which results in hypophosphatemia, and inhibition of the 1α-hydroxylase in the kidney, causing a decrease in 1,25-D synthesis.

In ADHR, as in XLH, abnormal laboratory findings are hypophosphatemia, elevated ALP level, and a low or inappropriately normal 1,25-D level (see Table 64.4). Treatment is similar to the approach used in XLH.

Autosomal Recessive Hypophosphatemic Rickets

Autosomal recessive hypophosphatemic rickets (**ARHR**) **type 1** is an extremely rare disorder caused by mutations in the gene encoding dentin matrix protein 1 (*DMP1*). ARHR **type 2** occurs in patients with mutations in the *ENPP1* gene. Mutations in *ENPP1* also cause generalized arterial calcification of infancy. Both types of ARHR are associated with elevated levels of FGF-23, leading to renal phosphate wasting, hypophosphatemia, and low or inappropriately normal levels of 1,25-D. Treatment is similar to the approach used in XLH, although monitoring for arterial calcification is prudent in patients with *ENPP1* mutations.

Hereditary Hypophosphatemic Rickets With Hypercalciuria

Hereditary hypophosphatemic rickets with hypercalciuria (**HHRH**) is a rare disorder that is mainly found in the Middle East.

Pathophysiology

This autosomal recessive disorder is caused by mutations in the gene for a sodium-phosphate co-transporter in the proximal tubule (*SLC34A3*). The renal phosphate leak causes hypophosphatemia, which then stimulates production of 1,25-D. The high level of 1,25-D increases intestinal absorption of calcium, suppressing PTH. Hypercalciuria ensues as a result of the high absorption of calcium and the low level of PTH, which normally decreases renal excretion of calcium.

Clinical Manifestations

The dominant symptoms of HHRH are rachitic leg abnormalities (see Table 64.3), muscle weakness, and bone pain. Patients can have short stature, with a disproportionate decrease in the length of the lower extremities. The severity of the disease varies, and some family members have no evidence of rickets but have kidney stones secondary to hypercalciuria.

Laboratory Findings

Laboratory findings include hypophosphatemia, renal phosphate wasting, elevated serum ALP levels, and elevated 1,25-D levels. PTH levels are low (see Table 64.4).

Treatment

Therapy for HHRH patients relies on oral phosphorus replacement (1-2.5 g/day of elemental phosphorus in 5 divided doses). Treatment of the hypophosphatemia decreases serum levels of 1,25-D and corrects the hypercalciuria. The response to therapy is usually excellent, with resolution of pain, weakness, and radiographic evidence of rickets.

Overproduction of FGF-23

Tumor-induced osteomalacia is more common in adults; in children it can produce classic rachitic findings. Most tumors are mesenchymal in origin and are usually benign, small, and located in bone. These tumors secrete FGF-23 and produce a biochemical phenotype similar to XLH, including urinary phosphate wasting, hypophosphatemia, elevated ALP levels, and low or inappropriately normal 1,25-D levels (see Table 64.4). Curative treatment is excision of the tumor. If the tumor cannot be removed, treatment is identical to that for XLH.

Renal phosphate wasting leading to hypophosphatemia and rickets (or osteomalacia in adults) is a potential complication in **McCune-Albright syndrome**, an entity that includes the triad of polyostotic fibrous dysplasia, hyperpigmented macules, and polyendocrinopathy (see Chapter 578.6). Affected patients have inappropriately low levels of 1,25-D and elevated ALP levels. The renal phosphate wasting and inhibition of 1,25-D synthesis are related to the polyostotic fibrous dysplasia. Patients have elevated FGF-23, presumably caused by the dysplastic bone. Hypophosphatemic rickets can also occur in children with isolated polyostotic fibrous dysplasia. Although it is rarely possible, removal of the abnormal bone can cure this disorder in children with McCune-Albright syndrome. Most patients receive the same treatment as children with XLH. Bisphosphonate treatment decreases the pain and fracture risk associated with the bone lesions.

Rickets is an unusual complication of **epidermal nevus syndrome** (see Chapter 670). Patients have hypophosphatemic rickets caused by renal phosphate wasting and an inappropriately normal or low level of 1,25-D from excessive production of FGF-23. The timing of presentation with rickets varies from infancy to early adolescence. Hypophosphatemia and rickets have resolved after excision of the epidermal nevi in some patients, but not in others. In most the skin lesions are too extensive to be removed, necessitating treatment with phosphorus supplementation and 1,25-D. Rickets caused by phosphate wasting is an extremely rare complication in children with **neurofibromatosis** (see Chapter 614.1).

Raine syndrome, an autosomal recessive disorder caused by mutations in the *FAM20C* gene, is an osteosclerotic bone dysplasia that is often fatal in the neonatal period. However, patients who survive into childhood may develop rickets from increased levels of FGF-23.

Fanconi Syndrome

Fanconi syndrome is secondary to generalized dysfunction of the renal proximal tubule (see Chapter 547.1). There are renal losses of phosphate, amino acids, bicarbonate, glucose, urate, and other molecules that are normally reabsorbed in the proximal tubule. Some patients have partial dysfunction, with less generalized losses. The most clinically relevant consequences are hypophosphatemia caused by phosphate losses and proximal renal tubular acidosis caused by bicarbonate losses. Patients have rickets as a result of hypophosphatemia, with exacerbation from the chronic metabolic acidosis, which causes bone dissolution. Failure to thrive (malnutrition) is a consequence of both rickets and renal tubular acidosis. Treatment is dictated by the etiology (see Chapter 547).

Dent Disease

Dent disease is an X-linked disorder usually caused by mutations in the gene encoding a chloride channel expressed in the kidney (*CLCN5*). Some patients have mutations in the *OCRL1* gene, which can also cause Lowe syndrome (see Chapter 549.3). Affected males have variable manifestations, including hematuria, nephrolithiasis, nephrocalcinosis, rickets, and chronic kidney disease. Almost all patients have low-molecular-weight proteinuria and hypercalciuria. Other, less universal abnormalities are aminoaciduria, glycosuria, hypophosphatemia, and hypokalemia. Rickets occurs in approximately 25% of patients, and it responds to oral phosphorus supplements. Some patients also need 1,25-D, but this treatment should be used cautiously because it can worsen the hypercalciuria.

RICKETS OF PREMATURITY

Rickets in very-low-birthweight infants has become a significant problem, as the survival rate for this group of infants has increased (see Chapter 117.2).

Pathogenesis

The transfer of calcium and phosphorus from mother to fetus occurs throughout pregnancy, but 80% occurs during the 3rd trimester. Premature birth interrupts this process, with rickets developing when the premature infant does not have an adequate supply of calcium and phosphorus to support mineralization of the growing skeleton.

Most cases of rickets of prematurity occur in infants with a birthweight <1,000 g. It is more likely to develop in infants with lower birthweight and younger gestational age. Rickets occurs because unsupplemented breast milk and standard infant formula do not contain enough calcium and phosphorus to supply the needs of the premature infant. Other risk factors include cholestatic jaundice, a complicated neonatal course, prolonged use of parenteral nutrition, the use of soy formula, and medications such as diuretics and corticosteroids.

Clinical Manifestations

Rickets of prematurity occurs 1-4 mo after birth. Infants can have nontraumatic fractures, especially of the legs, arms, and ribs. Most fractures are not suspected clinically. Because fractures and softening of the ribs lead to decreased chest compliance, some infants have respiratory distress from atelectasis and poor ventilation. This rachitic respiratory distress usually develops >5 wk after birth, distinguishing it from the early-onset respiratory disease of premature infants. These infants have poor linear growth, with negative effects on growth persisting beyond 1 yr of age. An additional long-term effect is enamel hypoplasia. Poor bone mineralization can contribute to dolichocephaly. There may be classic rachitic findings, such as frontal bossing, rachitic rosary (see Fig. 64.1), craniotabes, and widened wrists and ankles (see Table 64.3). Most infants with rickets of prematurity have no clinical manifestations, and the diagnosis is based on radiographic and laboratory findings.

Laboratory Findings

Because of inadequate intake, the serum phosphorus level is low or low-normal in patients with rickets of prematurity. The renal response is appropriate, with conservation of phosphate leading to a low urine phosphate level; tubular reabsorption of phosphate is >95%. Most patients have normal levels of 25-D, unless there has been inadequate intake or poor absorption (discussed earlier). The hypophosphatemia stimulates renal 1α-hydroxylase, so levels of 1,25-D are high or high-normal. These high levels can contribute to bone demineralization because 1,25-D stimulates bone resorption. Serum levels of calcium are low, normal, or high, and patients often have hypercalciuria. Elevated serum calcium levels and hypercalciuria are secondary to increased intestinal absorption and bone dissolution caused by elevated 1,25-D levels and inability to deposit calcium in bone because of an inadequate phosphorus supply. The hypercalciuria indicates that phosphorus is the limiting nutrient for bone mineralization, although increased provision of phosphorus alone often cannot correct the mineralization defect; increased calcium is also necessary. Thus there is an inadequate supply of calcium and phosphorus, but the deficiency in phosphorus is greater.

Alkaline phosphatase levels are often elevated, but some affected infants have normal levels. In some cases, normal ALP levels may be secondary to resolution of the bone demineralization because of an adequate mineral supply despite the continued presence of radiologic changes, which take longer to resolve. However, ALP levels may be normal despite active disease. No single blood test is 100% sensitive for the diagnosis of rickets. The diagnosis should be suspected in infants with ALP >5-6 times the upper limit of normal (UL) for adults (unless there is concomitant liver disease) or phosphorus <5.6 mg/dL. The diagnosis is confirmed by radiologic evidence of rickets, which is best seen on x-ray films of the wrists and ankles. Films of the arms and legs might reveal fractures. The rachitic rosary may be visible on chest radiograph. Unfortunately, x-ray films cannot show early demineralization of bone because changes are not evident until there is >20–30% reduction in the bone mineral content.

Diagnosis

Because many premature infants have no overt clinical manifestations of rickets, screening tests are recommended. These tests should include weekly measurements of calcium, phosphorus, and ALP. Periodic measurement of the serum bicarbonate concentration is also important, because metabolic acidosis causes dissolution of bone. At least 1 screening radiograph for rickets at 6-8 wk of age is appropriate in infants who are at high risk for rickets; additional films may be indicated in high-risk infants.

Prevention

Provision of adequate amounts of calcium, phosphorus, and vitamin D significantly decreases the risk of rickets of prematurity. Parenteral nutrition is often necessary initially in very premature infants. In the past, adequate parenteral calcium and phosphorus delivery was difficult because of limits secondary to insolubility of these ions when their concentrations were increased. Current amino acid preparations allow higher concentrations of calcium and phosphate, decreasing the risk of rickets. Early transition to enteral feedings is also helpful. These infants should receive either human milk fortified with calcium and phosphorus or preterm infant formula, which has higher concentrations of calcium and phosphorus than standard formula. Soy formula should be avoided because there is decreased bioavailability of calcium and phosphorus. Increased mineral feedings should continue until the infant weighs 3-3.5 kg. These infants should also receive approximately 400 IU/day of vitamin D through formula and vitamin supplements.

Treatment

Therapy for rickets of prematurity focuses on ensuring adequate delivery of calcium, phosphorus, and vitamin D. If mineral delivery has been good and there is no evidence of healing, it is important to screen for vitamin D deficiency by measuring serum 25-D. Measurement of PTH, 1,25-D, and urinary calcium and phosphorus may be helpful in some cases.

DISTAL RENAL TUBULAR ACIDOSIS

Distal renal tubular acidosis usually manifests with failure to thrive. Patients have a metabolic acidosis with an inability to acidify the urine appropriately. Hypercalciuria and nephrocalcinosis are typically present. The many etiologies include autosomal recessive and autosomal dominant forms. Rickets is variable and responds to alkali therapy (see Fig. 64.5 and Chapter 547.2).

HYPERVITAMINOSIS D
Etiology

Hypervitaminosis D is caused by excessive intake of vitamin D. It can occur with long-term high intake or with a substantial, acute ingestion (see Table 64.1). Most cases are secondary to misuse of prescribed or nonprescription vitamin D supplements, but other cases have been secondary to accidental overfortification of milk, contamination of table sugar, and inadvertent use of vitamin D supplements as cooking oil. The recommended upper limits for long-term vitamin D intake are 1,000 IU for children <1 yr old and 2,000 IU for older children and adults. Hypervitaminosis D can also result from excessive intake of synthetic vitamin D analogs (25-D, 1,25-D). Vitamin D intoxication is never secondary to excessive exposure to sunlight, probably because ultraviolet irradiation can transform vitamin D_3 and its precursor into inactive metabolites.

Pathogenesis

Although vitamin D increases intestinal absorption of calcium, the dominant mechanism of the hypercalcemia is excessive bone resorption.

Clinical Manifestations

The signs and symptoms of vitamin D intoxication are secondary to hypercalcemia. GI manifestations include nausea, vomiting, poor feeding, constipation, abdominal pain, and pancreatitis. Possible cardiac findings are hypertension, decreased QT interval, and arrhythmias. The central nervous system effects of hypercalcemia include lethargy, hypotonia, confusion, disorientation, depression, psychosis, hallucinations, and coma. Hypercalcemia impairs renal concentrating mechanisms, which can lead to polyuria, dehydration, and hypernatremia. Hypercalcemia can also lead to acute renal failure, nephrolithiasis, and nephrocalcinosis, which can result in chronic renal insufficiency. Deaths are usually associated with arrhythmias or dehydration.

Laboratory Findings

The classic findings in vitamin D intoxication are hypercalcemia, elevated levels of 25-D (>100 ng/mL), hypercalciuria, and suppressed PTH. Hyperphosphatemia is also common. Hypercalciuria can lead to nephrocalcinosis, which is visible on renal ultrasound. Hypercalcemia and nephrocalcinosis can lead to renal insufficiency.

Surprisingly, levels of 1,25-D are usually normal. This may result from downregulation of renal 1α-hydroxylase by the combination of low PTH, hyperphosphatemia, and a direct effect of 1,25-D. The level of free 1,25-D may be high because of displacement from vitamin D–binding proteins by 25-D. Anemia is sometimes present; the mechanism is unknown.

Diagnosis and Differential Diagnosis

The diagnosis is based on the presence of hypercalcemia and an elevated serum 25-D level, although children with excess intake of 1,25-D or another synthetic vitamin D preparation have normal levels of 25-D. With careful sleuthing, there is usually a history of excess intake of vitamin D, although in some situations (overfortification of milk by a dairy) the patient and family may be unaware.

The differential diagnosis of vitamin D intoxication focuses on other causes of **hypercalcemia**. Hyperparathyroidism produces hypophosphatemia, whereas vitamin D intoxication usually causes hyperphosphatemia. Williams syndrome is often suggested by phenotypic features and accompanying cardiac disease. Idiopathic infantile hypercalcemia occurs in children taking appropriate doses of vitamin D. Subcutaneous fat necrosis is a common cause of hypercalcemia in young infants; skin findings are usually present. The hypercalcemia of familial benign hypocalciuric hypercalcemia is mild, asymptomatic, and associated with hypocalciuria. Hypercalcemia of malignancy is an important consideration. High intake of calcium can also cause hypercalcemia, especially in the presence of renal insufficiency. Questioning about calcium intake should be part of the history in a patient with hypercalcemia. Occasionally, patients are intentionally taking high doses of calcium and vitamin D.

Treatment

The treatment of vitamin D intoxication focuses on control of hypercalcemia. Many patients with hypercalcemia are dehydrated as a result of polyuria from nephrogenic diabetes insipidus, poor oral intake, and vomiting. Rehydration lowers the serum calcium level by dilution and corrects prerenal azotemia. The resultant increased urine output increases urinary calcium excretion. Urinary calcium excretion is also increased by high urinary sodium excretion. The mainstay of the initial treatment is aggressive therapy with normal saline, often in conjunction with a loop diuretic to further increase calcium excretion; this is often adequate for treating mild or moderate hypercalcemia. More significant hypercalcemia usually requires other therapies. Glucocorticoids decrease intestinal absorption of calcium by blocking the action of 1,25-D. There is also a decrease in the levels of 25-D and 1,25-D. The usual dosage of prednisone is 1-2 mg/kg/24 hr.

Calcitonin, which lowers calcium by inhibiting bone resorption, is a useful adjunct, but its effect is usually not dramatic. There is an excellent response to IV or oral bisphosphonates in vitamin D intoxication. Bisphosphonates inhibit bone resorption through their effects on osteoclasts. Hemodialysis using a low or 0 dialsate calcium can rapidly lower serum calcium in patients with severe hypercalcemia that is refractory to other measures.

Along with controlling hypercalcemia, it is imperative to eliminate the source of excess vitamin D. Additional sources of vitamin D such as multivitamins and fortified foods should be eliminated or reduced. Avoidance of sun exposure, including the use of sunscreen, is prudent. The patient should also restrict calcium intake.

Prognosis
Most children make a full recovery, but hypervitaminosis D may be fatal or can lead to chronic kidney disease. Because vitamin D is stored in fat, levels can remain elevated for months, necessitating regular monitoring of 25-D, serum calcium, and urine calcium.

Bibliography is available at Expert Consult.

Chapter 65
Vitamin E Deficiency
Larry A. Greenbaum

第六十五章
维生素E缺乏

中文导读

　　本章主要介绍了维生素E缺乏的病因和发病机制、临床表现、实验室检查、诊断和鉴别诊断、治疗、预后和预防。其中病因和发病机制包括饮食摄入减少、疾病导致吸收障碍和遗传病（无β脂蛋白血症、维生素E缺乏性共济失调）；临床表现包括小脑病变、脊髓后角功能失调和视网膜病变。

Vitamin E is a fat-soluble vitamin and functions as an antioxidant, but its precise biochemical functions are not known. Vitamin E deficiency can cause hemolysis or neurologic manifestations and occurs in premature infants, in patients with malabsorption, and in an autosomal recessive disorder affecting vitamin E transport. Because of its role as an antioxidant, there is considerable research on vitamin E supplementation in chronic illnesses.

PATHOGENESIS
The term *vitamin E* denotes a group of 8 compounds with similar structures and antioxidant activity. The most potent member of these compounds is **α-tocopherol**, which is also the main form in humans. The best dietary sources of vitamin E are vegetable oils, seeds, nuts, green leafy vegetables, and margarine (see Table 64.1).

The majority of vitamin E is located within cell membranes, where it prevents lipid peroxidation and the formation of free radicals. Other antioxidants, such as ascorbic acid, enhance the antioxidant activity of vitamin E. The importance of other functions of vitamin E is still being delineated.

Premature infants are particularly susceptible to vitamin E deficiency, because there is significant transfer of vitamin E during the last trimester of pregnancy. Vitamin E deficiency in premature infants causes thrombocytosis, edema, and hemolysis, potentially causing anemia. The risk of symptomatic vitamin E deficiency was increased by the use of formulas for premature infants that had a high content of polyunsaturated fatty acids (PUFAs). These formulas led to a high content of PUFAs in red blood cell membranes, making them more susceptible to oxidative stress, which could be ameliorated by vitamin E. Oxidative stress was augmented by aggressive use of iron supplementation; iron increases the production of oxygen radicals. The incidence of hemolysis as a result of vitamin E deficiency in premature infants decreased secondary to the use of formulas with a lower content of PUFAs, less-aggressive use of iron, and provision of adequate vitamin E.

Because vitamin E is plentiful in common foods, primary dietary deficiency is rare except in premature infants and in severe, generalized malnutrition. Vitamin E deficiency does occur in children with fat malabsorption secondary to the bile acid needed for vitamin E absorption. Although symptomatic disease is most common in children with cholestatic liver disease, it can occur in patients with cystic fibrosis, celiac disease, short bowel syndrome, and Crohn disease. The autosomal recessive disorder **abetalipoproteinemia** causes fat malabsorption, and vitamin E deficiency is a common complication (see Chapter 104).

In **ataxia with isolated vitamin E deficiency (AVED)**, a rare autosomal recessive disorder, there are mutations in the gene for α-tocopherol transfer protein (*TTPA*). Patients with this disorder are unable to incorporate vitamin E into lipoproteins before their release from the liver, leading to reduced serum levels of vitamin E. There is no associated fat malabsorption, and absorption of vitamin E from the intestine occurs normally.

CLINICAL MANIFESTATIONS

A severe, progressive neurologic disorder occurs in patients with prolonged vitamin E deficiency. Clinical manifestations do not appear until after 1 yr of age, even in children with cholestasis since birth. Patients may have cerebellar disease, posterior column dysfunction, and retinal disease. Loss of deep tendon reflexes is usually the initial finding. Subsequent manifestations include limb ataxia (intention tremor, dysdiadochokinesia), truncal ataxia (wide-based, unsteady gait), dysarthria, ophthalmoplegia (limited upward gaze), nystagmus, decreased proprioception (positive Romberg test), decreased vibratory sensation, and dysarthria. Some patients have pigmentary retinopathy. Visual field constriction can progress to blindness. Cognition and behavior can also be affected. Myopathy and cardiac arrhythmias are less common findings.

In premature infants, hemolysis as a result of vitamin E deficiency typically develops during the 2nd mo of life. Edema may also be present.

LABORATORY FINDINGS

Serum vitamin E levels increase in the presence of high serum lipid levels, even when vitamin E deficiency is present. Therefore, vitamin E status is best determined by measuring the ratio of vitamin E to serum lipids; a ratio <0.8 mg/g is abnormal in older children and adults; <0.6 mg/g is abnormal in infants <1 yr. Premature infants with hemolysis caused by vitamin E deficiency also often have elevated platelet counts.

Neurologic involvement can cause abnormal somatosensory evoked potentials and nerve conduction studies. Abnormalities on electroretinography can precede physical examination findings in patients with retinal involvement.

DIAGNOSIS AND DIFFERENTIAL DIAGNOSIS

Premature infants with unexplained hemolytic anemia after the 1st mo of life, especially if thrombocytosis is present, either should be empirically treated with vitamin E or should have serum vitamin E and lipid levels measured. Children with neurologic findings and a disease that causes fat malabsorption should have their vitamin E status evaluated.

Because children with AVED do not have symptoms of malabsorption, a correct diagnosis requires a high index of suspicion. **Friedreich ataxia** has been misdiagnosed in some patients (see Chapter 615.1). Children with unexplained ataxia should be screened for vitamin E deficiency.

TREATMENT

For correction of deficiency in neonates, the dose of vitamin E is 25-50 units/day for 1 wk, followed by adequate dietary intake. Children with deficiency as a result of malabsorption should receive 1 unit/kg/day, with the dose adjusted based on levels; ongoing treatment is necessary. Children with AVED normalize their serum vitamin E levels with high doses of vitamin E and require ongoing treatment.

PROGNOSIS

The hemolytic anemia in infants resolves with correction of the vitamin E deficiency. Some neurologic manifestations of vitamin E deficiency may be reversible with early treatment, but many patients have little or no improvement. Importantly, treatment prevents progression.

PREVENTION

Premature infants should receive sufficient vitamin E through formula or breast milk fortifier and formula without a high content of PUFAs. Children at risk for vitamin E deficiency as a result of malabsorption should be screened for deficiency and given adequate vitamin E supplementation. Vitamin preparations with high content of all the fat-soluble vitamins are available.

Bibliography is available at Expert Consult.

Chapter **66**

Vitamin K Deficiency

Larry A. Greenbaum

第六十六章

维生素K缺乏

中文导读

本章主要介绍了维生素K缺乏的病因和发病机制、临床表现、诊断与鉴别诊断、治疗及预防。其中发病包括早发新生儿维生素K缺乏性出血、晚发新生儿维生素K缺乏性出血和出生时维生素K缺乏性出血；临床表现包括胃肠道和黏膜出血以及颅内出血；鉴别诊断包括肝脏疾病和抗凝血药应用。

Vitamin K is necessary for the synthesis of clotting factors II, VII, IX, and X; deficiency of vitamin K can result in clinically significant bleeding. Vitamin K deficiency typically affects infants, who experience a transient deficiency related to inadequate intake, or patients of any age who have decreased vitamin K absorption. Mild vitamin K deficiency can affect long-term bone and vascular health (see Chapters 124.4 and 507).

PATHOGENESIS

Vitamin K is a group of compounds that have a common naphthoquinone ring structure (see Table 64.1). **Phylloquinone**, called *vitamin K_1*, is present in a variety of dietary sources, with green leafy vegetables, liver, and certain legumes and plant oils having the highest content. Vitamin K_1 is the form used to fortify foods and as a medication in the United States. *Vitamin K_2* is a group of compounds called **menaquinones**, which are produced by intestinal bacteria. There is uncertainty regarding the relative importance of intestinally produced vitamin K_2. Menaquinones are also present in meat, especially liver, and cheese. A menaquinone is used pharmacologically in some countries.

Vitamin K is a cofactor for γ-glutamyl carboxylase, an enzyme that performs posttranslational carboxylation, converting glutamate residues in proteins to **γ-carboxyglutamate (Gla)**. The Gla residues, by facilitating calcium binding, are necessary for protein function.

The classic Gla-containing proteins involved in blood coagulation that are decreased in vitamin K deficiency are factors II (prothrombin), VII, IX, and X. Vitamin K deficiency causes a decrease in proteins C and S, which inhibit blood coagulation, and protein Z, which also has a role in coagulation. All these proteins are made only in the liver, except for protein S, a product of various tissues.

Gla-containing proteins are also involved in bone biology (osteocalcin and protein S) and vascular biology (matrix Gla protein and protein S). Based on the presence of reduced levels of Gla, these proteins appear more sensitive than the coagulation proteins to subtle vitamin K deficiency. Evidence suggests that mild vitamin K deficiency might have a deleterious effect on long-term bone strength and vascular health.

Because it is fat soluble, vitamin K requires the presence of bile salts for its absorption. Unlike other fat-soluble vitamins, there are limited body stores of vitamin K. In addition, there is high turnover of vitamin K, and the vitamin K–dependent clotting factors have a short half-life. Thus, symptomatic vitamin K deficiency can develop within weeks when there is inadequate supply because of low intake or malabsorption.

There are 3 forms of **vitamin K deficiency bleeding (VKDB)** of the newborn (see Chapter 124.4). *Early* VKDB was formerly called *classic hemorrhagic disease of the newborn* and occurs at 1-14 days of age. Early VKDB is secondary to low stores of vitamin K at birth as a result of the poor transfer of vitamin K across the placenta and inadequate intake during the 1st few days of life. In addition, there is no intestinal synthesis of vitamin K_2 because the newborn gut is sterile. Early VKDB occurs mostly in breastfed infants as a consequence of the low vitamin K content of breast milk (formula is fortified). Delayed feeding is an additional risk factor.

Late VKDB most often occurs at 2-12 wk of age, although cases can occur up to 6 mo after birth. Almost all cases are in breastfed infants because of the low vitamin K content of breast milk. An additional risk factor is occult malabsorption of vitamin K, as occurs in children with undiagnosed cystic fibrosis or cholestatic liver disease (e.g., biliary atresia, α_1-antitrypsin deficiency). Without vitamin K prophylaxis, the incidence is 4-10 per 100,000 newborns.

The third form of VKDB of the newborn occurs *at birth* or shortly thereafter. It is secondary to maternal intake of medications (warfarin, phenobarbital, phenytoin) that cross the placenta and interfere with vitamin K function.

VKDB as a result of fat malabsorption can occur in children of any age. Potential etiologies include cholestatic liver disease, pancreatic disease, and intestinal disorders (celiac sprue, inflammatory bowel disease, short bowel syndrome). Prolonged diarrhea can cause vitamin K deficiency, especially in breastfed infants. Children with cystic fibrosis are most likely to have vitamin K deficiency if they have pancreatic insufficiency and liver disease.

Beyond infancy, low dietary intake by itself never causes vitamin K deficiency. However, the combination of poor intake and the use of broad-spectrum antibiotics that eliminate the intestine's vitamin K_2–producing bacteria can cause vitamin K deficiency. This scenario is especially common in the intensive care unit. Vitamin K deficiency can also occur in patients who receive total parenteral nutrition (TPN) without vitamin K supplementation.

CLINICAL MANIFESTATIONS

In early VKDB, the most common sites of bleeding are the gastrointestinal (GI) tract, mucosal and cutaneous tissue, umbilical stump, and post-circumcision site; intracranial bleeding is less common. GI blood loss can be severe enough to require a transfusion. In contrast, the most common site of bleeding in late VKDB is intracranial, although cutaneous and GI bleeding may be the initial manifestation. Intracranial bleeding can cause convulsions, permanent neurologic sequelae, or death. In some patients with late VKDB, the presence of an underlying disorder may be suggested by jaundice or failure to thrive (malnutrition). Older children with vitamin K deficiency can present with bruising, mucocutaneous bleeding, or more serious bleeding.

Laboratory Findings

In patients with bleeding as a result of vitamin K deficiency, the prothrombin time (PT) is prolonged. The PT must be interpreted based on the patient's age, because it is normally prolonged in newborns (see Chapters 124.4 and 502). The partial thromboplastin time (PTT) is usually prolonged but may be normal in early deficiency. Factor VII has the shortest half-life of the coagulation factors and is the first to be affected by vitamin K deficiency, but isolated factor VII deficiency does not affect PTT. The platelet count and fibrinogen level are normal.

When there is mild vitamin K deficiency, the PT is normal, but there are elevated levels of the undercarboxylated forms of the proteins that are normally carboxylated in the presence of vitamin K. These undercarboxylated proteins are called *proteins induced by vitamin K absence* (PIVKA). Measurement of undercarboxylated factor II (PIVKA-II) can be used to detect mild vitamin K deficiency. Determination of blood vitamin K levels is less useful because of significant variation based on recent dietary intake; levels do not always reflect tissue stores.

DIAGNOSIS AND DIFFERENTIAL DIAGNOSIS

The diagnosis is established by the presence of a prolonged PT that corrects rapidly after administration of vitamin K, which stops the active bleeding. Other possible causes of bleeding and a prolonged PT include **disseminated intravascular coagulation (DIC)**, liver failure, and rare hereditary deficiencies of clotting factors. DIC, which is usually secondary to sepsis, is associated with thrombocytopenia, low fibrinogen, and elevated D-dimers. Severe liver disease results in decreased production of clotting factors; the PT does not fully correct with administration of vitamin K. Children with a hereditary disorder have a deficiency in a specific clotting factor (I, II, V, VII, X).

Coumarin derivatives inhibit the action of vitamin K by preventing its recycling to an active form after it functions as a cofactor for γ-glutamyl carboxylase. Bleeding can occur with overdosage of the common anticoagulant **warfarin** or with ingestion of rodent poison, which contains a coumarin derivative. High doses of salicylates also inhibit vitamin K regeneration, potentially leading to a prolonged PT and clinical bleeding.

TREATMENT

Infants with VKDB should receive 1 mg of parenteral vitamin K. The PT should decrease within 6 hr and normalize within 24 hr. For rapid correction in adolescents, the parenteral dose is 2.5-10 mg. In addition to vitamin K, a patient with severe, life-threatening bleeding should receive an infusion of fresh-frozen plasma (FFP), which corrects the coagulopathy rapidly. Children with vitamin K deficiency caused by malabsorption require chronic administration of high doses of oral vitamin K (2.5 mg twice/wk to 5 mg/day). Parenteral vitamin K may be necessary if oral vitamin K is ineffective.

PREVENTION

Administration of either oral or parenteral vitamin K soon after birth prevents early VKDB of the newborn. In contrast, a single dose of oral vitamin K does not prevent a substantial number of cases of late VKDB. However, a single intramuscular (IM) injection of vitamin K (1 mg), the current practice in the United States, is almost universally effective, except in children with severe malabsorption. This increased efficacy of the IM form is thought to be the result of a depot effect. Concerns about an association between parenteral vitamin K at birth and the later development of malignancy are unsubstantiated.

Discontinuing the offending medications before delivery can prevent VKDB attributable to maternal medications. If this is not possible, administration of vitamin K to the mother may be helpful. In addition, the neonate should receive parenteral vitamin K immediately after birth. If parenteral vitamin K does not correct the coagulopathy rapidly, the child should receive FFP.

Children who are at high risk for malabsorption of vitamin K should receive supplemental vitamin K and periodic measurement of the PT.

Bibliography is available at Expert Consult.

Chapter **67**
Micronutrient Mineral Deficiencies
Larry A. Greenbaum

第六十七章
微量元素缺乏

中文导读

本章主要介绍了铬、铜、氟、碘、铁、镁、钼、硒、锌的生理功能、食物来源以及缺乏和过量的主要临床表现。其中重点介绍了碘缺乏、硒缺乏和锌缺乏。微量元素缺乏导致的严重临床表现主要见于遗传性疾病如Menkes病、肠病性肢端皮炎等。

Micronutrients include vitamins (see Chapters 61-66) and trace elements. By definition, a **trace element** is <0.01% of the body weight. Trace elements have a variety of essential functions (Table 67.1). With the exception of iron deficiency, trace element deficiency is uncommon in developed countries, but some deficiencies (iodine, zinc, selenium) are important public health problems in a number of developing countries. Because of low nutritional requirements and plentiful supply, deficiencies of some of the trace elements are extremely rare in humans and typically occur in patients receiving unusual diets or prolonged total parenteral nutrition (TPN) without adequate delivery of a specific trace element. Trace element deficiencies can also occur in children with short bowel syndrome or malabsorption. Excess intake of trace elements is uncommon but can result from environmental exposure or overuse of supplements (Table 67.1).

For a number of reasons, children are especially susceptible to trace element deficiency. First, growth creates an increased demand for most trace elements. Second, some organs are more likely to sustain permanent damage because of trace element deficiency during childhood. The developing brain is particularly vulnerable to the consequences of certain deficiency states (iron, iodide). Similarly, adequate fluoride is most critical for dental health during childhood. Third, children, especially in the developing world, are more prone to gastrointestinal disorders that can cause trace element deficiencies because of malabsorption.

A normal diet provides adequate intake of most trace elements. However, the intake of certain trace elements varies significantly in different geographic locations. Iodide-containing food is plentiful near the ocean, but inland areas often have inadequate sources, leading to goiter and **hypothyroidism**. **Iodine deficiency** is not a problem in the United States because of the widespread use of iodized salt; however, symptomatic iodine deficiency (goiter, hypothyroidism) is common in many developing countries. Selenium content of the soil and consequently of food is also quite variable. Dietary **selenium deficiency** (associated with cardiomyopathy) occurs in certain locations, such as some parts of China.

The consequences of severe isolated trace mineral deficiency are illustrated in certain genetic disorders. The manifestations of **Menkes disease** are caused by a mutation in the gene coding for a protein that facilitates intestinal copper absorption (see Chapters 617.5 and 682).

Table 67.1	Trace Elements			
ELEMENT	**PHYSIOLOGY**	**EFFECTS OF DEFICIENCY**	**EFFECTS OF EXCESS**	**DIETARY SOURCES**
Chromium	Potentiates the action of insulin	Impaired glucose tolerance, peripheral neuropathy, and encephalopathy	Unknown	Meat, grains, fruits, and vegetables
Copper	Absorbed via specific intestinal transporter Circulates bound to ceruloplasmin Enzyme cofactor (superoxide dismutase, cytochrome oxidase, and enzymes involved in iron metabolism and connective tissue formation)	Microcytic anemia, osteoporosis, neutropenia, neurologic symptoms, depigmentation of hair and skin	Acute: nausea, emesis, abdominal pain, coma, and hepatic necrosis Chronic toxicity (liver and brain injury) occurs in **Wilson disease** (see Chapter 384.2) and secondary to excess intake (see Chapter 384.3).	Vegetables, grains, nuts, liver, margarine, legumes, corn oil
Fluoride	Incorporated into bone	Dental caries (see Chapter 338)	Chronic: dental fluorosis (see Chapter 333)	Toothpaste, fluoridated water
Iodine	Component of thyroid hormone (see Chapter 580)	Hypothyroidism (see Chapters 579 and 580)	Hypothyroidism and goiter (see Chapters 581 and 583); maternal excess can cause congenital hypothyroidism and goiter (see Chapter 584.1).	Saltwater fish, iodized salt
Iron	Component of hemoglobin, myoglobin, cytochromes, and other enzymes	Anemia (see Chapter 482), decreased alertness, impaired learning	Acute (see Chapter 77): nausea, vomiting, diarrhea, abdominal pain, and hypotension Chronic excess usually secondary to hereditary disorders (see Chapter 489); causes organ dysfunction.	Meat, fortified foods Deficiency can also result from blood loss (hookworm infestation, menorrhagia)
Manganese	Enzyme cofactor	Hypercholesterolemia, weight loss, decreased clotting proteins*	Neurologic manifestations, cholestatic jaundice	Nuts, meat, grains, tea
Molybdenum	Enzyme cofactor (xanthine oxidase and others)	Tachycardia, tachypnea, night blindness, irritability, coma*	Hyperuricemia and increased risk of gout	Legumes, grains, liver
Selenium	Enzyme cofactor (prevents oxidative damage)	Cardiomyopathy (**Keshan disease**), myopathy	Nausea, diarrhea, neurologic manifestations, nail and hair changes, garlic odor	Meat, seafood, whole grains, garlic
Zinc	Enzyme cofactor Constituent of zinc-finger proteins, which regulate gene transcription	Decreased growth, dermatitis of extremities and around orifices, impaired immunity, poor wound healing, hypogonadism, diarrhea Supplements are beneficial in diarrhea and improve neurodevelopmental outcomes.	Abdominal pain, diarrhea, vomiting Can worsen copper deficiency	Meat, shellfish, whole grains, legumes, cheese

*These deficiency states have been reported only in case reports associated with parenteral nutrition or highly unusual diets.

This mutation results in severe copper deficiency; subcutaneous copper is an effective treatment. The recessive disorder **acrodermatitis enteropathica** is secondary to malabsorption of zinc (see Chapter 691). These patients respond dramatically to zinc supplementation.

Children can have apparently asymptomatic deficiencies of certain trace elements but still benefit from supplementation. As an example, zinc is highly effective in treating children before or during diarrheal illnesses in the developing world.

Zinc deficiency is quite common in the developing world and is often associated with malnutrition or other micronutrient deficiencies (iron). Chronic zinc deficiency is associated with dwarfism, hypogonadism, dermatitis, and T-cell immunodeficiency. Diets rich in phytates bind zinc, impairing its absorption. Zinc supplementation in at-risk children reduces the incidence and severity of diarrhea, pneumonia, and possibly malaria. In developing countries, children who have diarrhea may benefit from zinc supplementation, especially if there is underlying malnutrition.

Bibliography is available at Expert Consult.

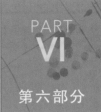

Fluid and Electrolyte Disorders

水和电解质紊乱

Chapter 68

Electrolyte and Acid-Base Disorders

第六十八章
电解质和酸碱失衡

中文导读

本章主要介绍了电解质和酸碱失衡。首先详细阐述了体液组成，包括机体水的总量、体液分布、电解质组成、渗透浓度和即时检测；还阐述了渗透压和容量的调节，包括渗透压调节和容量调节；并介绍了钠、钾、镁、磷的代谢及失衡；最后介绍了酸碱失衡，包括酸碱生理学、正常酸碱平衡、酸碱失衡的临床评估、代谢性酸中毒、代谢性碱中毒、呼吸性酸中毒和呼吸性碱中毒。

68.1 Composition of Body Fluids

Larry A. Greenbaum

TOTAL BODY WATER

Total body water (TBW) as a percentage of body weight varies with age (Fig. 68.1). The fetus has very high TBW, which gradually decreases to approximately 75% of birthweight for a term infant. Premature infants have higher TBW than term infants. During the 1st yr of life, TBW decreases to approximately 60% of body weight and remains at this level until puberty. At puberty, the fat content of females increases more than that in males, who acquire more muscle mass than females. Because fat has very low water content and muscle has high water content, by the end of puberty, TBW in males remains at 60%, but TBW in females decreases to approximately 50% of body weight. The high fat content in overweight children causes a decrease in TBW as a percentage of body weight. During dehydration, TBW decreases and thus is a smaller percentage of body weight.

FLUID COMPARTMENTS

TBW is divided between 2 main compartments: **intracellular fluid (ICF)** and **extracellular fluid (ECF)**. In the fetus and newborn, the ECF volume is larger than the ICF volume (Fig. 68.1). The normal postnatal diuresis causes an immediate decrease in the ECF volume. This is followed by continued expansion of the ICF volume, which results from cellular growth. By 1 yr of age, the ratio of ICF volume to ECF volume approaches adult levels. The ECF volume is approximately 20–25% of body weight, and the ICF volume is approximately 30–40% of body weight, close to twice the ECF volume (Fig. 68.2). With puberty, the increased muscle mass of males causes them to have a higher ICF volume than females. There is no significant difference in the ECF volume between postpubertal females and males.

The ECF is further divided into the plasma water and the interstitial fluid (see Fig. 68.2). The *plasma water* is 5% of body weight. The blood volume, given a hematocrit of 40%, is usually 8% of body weight, although it is higher in newborns and young infants; in premature newborns it is approximately 10% of body weight. The volume of plasma water can be altered by pathologic conditions, including dehydration, anemia, polycythemia, heart failure, abnormal plasma osmolality, and hypoalbuminemia. The *interstitial fluid*, normally 15% of body weight, can increase dramatically in diseases associated with edema, such as heart failure, protein-losing enteropathy, liver failure, nephrotic syndrome, and sepsis. An increase in interstitial fluid also occurs in patients with ascites or pleural effusions.

There is a delicate equilibrium between the intravascular fluid and the interstitial fluid. The balance between hydrostatic and oncotic forces

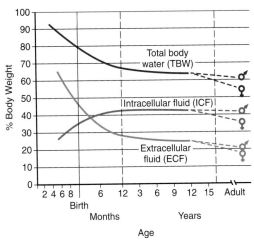

Fig. 68.1 Total body water, intracellular fluid, and extracellular fluid as a percentage of body weight as a function of age. *(From Winters RW: Water and electrolyte regulation. In Winters RW, editor: The body fluids in pediatrics, Boston, 1973, Little, Brown.)*

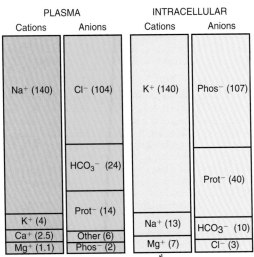

Fig. 68.3 Concentrations of the major cations and anions in the intracellular space and the plasma, expressed in mEq/L.

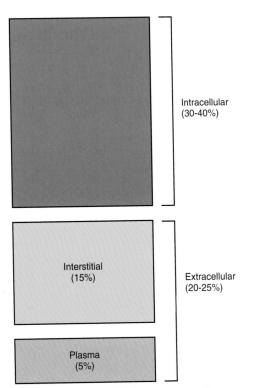

Fig. 68.2 Compartments of total body water, expressed as percentages of body weight, in an older child or adult.

regulates the intravascular volume, which is critical for proper tissue perfusion. The *intravascular fluid* has a higher concentration of albumin than the interstitial fluid, and the consequent oncotic force draws water into the intravascular space. The maintenance of this gradient depends on the limited permeability of albumin across the capillaries. The hydrostatic pressure of the intravascular space, which is caused by the pumping action of the heart, drives fluid out of the intravascular space. These forces favor movement into the interstitial space at the arterial ends of the capillaries. The decreased hydrostatic forces and increased

oncotic forces, which result from the dilutional increase in albumin concentration, cause movement of fluid into the venous ends of the capillaries. Overall, there is usually a net movement of fluid out of the intravascular space to the interstitial space, but this fluid is returned to the circulation via the *lymphatics*.

An imbalance in these forces may cause expansion of the interstitial volume at the expense of the intravascular volume. In children with hypoalbuminemia, the decreased oncotic pressure of the intravascular fluid contributes to the development of **edema**. Loss of fluid from the intravascular space may compromise the intravascular volume, placing the child at risk for inadequate blood flow to vital organs. This is especially likely in diseases in which capillary leak occurs because the loss of albumin from the intravascular space is associated with an increase in the albumin concentration in the interstitial space, further compromising the oncotic forces that normally maintain intravascular volume. In contrast, with **heart failure**, there is an increase in venous hydrostatic pressure from expansion of the intravascular volume, which is caused by impaired pumping by the heart, and the increase in venous pressure causes fluid to move from the intravascular space to the interstitial space. Expansion of the intravascular volume and increased intravascular pressure also cause the edema that occurs with acute glomerulonephritis.

ELECTROLYTE COMPOSITION

The composition of the solutes in the ICF and ECF are very different (Fig. 68.3). **Sodium** (Na^+) and **chloride** (Cl^-) are the dominant cation and anion, respectively, in the ECF. The sodium and chloride concentrations ($[Na^+]$, $[Cl^-]$) in the ICF are much lower. **Potassium** (K^+) is the most abundant cation in the ICF, and its concentration ($[K^+]$) within the cells is approximately 30 times higher than in the ECF. Proteins, organic anions, and phosphate are the most plentiful anions in the ICF. The dissimilarity between the anions in the ICF and the ECF is largely determined by the presence of intracellular molecules that do not cross the cell membrane, the barrier separating the ECF and the ICF. In contrast, the difference in the distribution of cations—Na^+ and K^+—relies on activity of the Na^+,K^+-adenosine triphosphatase (ATPase) pump and membrane ion channels.

The difference in the electrolyte compositions of the ECF and the ICF has important ramifications in the evaluation and treatment of electrolyte disorders. Serum concentrations of electrolytes—$[Na^+]$, $[K^+]$, and $[Cl^-]$—do not always reflect total body content. Intracellular $[K^+]$ is much higher than the serum concentration. A shift of K^+ from the **intracellular space (ICS)** can maintain a normal or even an elevated serum $[K^+]$ despite massive losses of K^+ from the ICS. This effect is seen in diabetic ketoacidosis, in which significant K^+ depletion is masked by transmembrane shift of K$^+$ from the ICF to the ECF. Therefore, for K$^+$ and phosphorus, electrolytes with a high intracellular concentration, serum level may not reflect total body content. Similarly, the serum **calcium** concentration ([Ca^{2+}]) does not reflect total body content of Ca^{2+}, which is largely contained in bone and teeth (see Chapter 64).

OSMOLALITY

The ICF and the ECF are in **osmotic equilibrium** because the cell membrane is permeable to water. If the osmolality in 1 compartment changes, then water movement leads to a rapid equalization of osmolality, with a shift of water between the ICS and **extracellular space (ECS)**. Clinically, the primary process is usually a change in the osmolality of the ECF, with resultant shift of water into the ICF if ECF osmolality decreases, or vice versa if ECF osmolality increases. The *ECF osmolality can be determined and usually equals ICF osmolality*. **Plasma osmolality**, normally 285-295 mOsm/kg, is measured by the degree of freezing-point depression. The plasma osmolality can also be *estimated* by a calculation based on the following formula:

$$\text{Osmolality} = 2 \times [\text{Na}] + [\text{glucose}]/18 + [\text{BUN}]/2.8$$

Glucose and blood urea nitrogen (BUN) are reported in mg/dL. Division of these values by 18 and 2.8, respectively, converts the units into mmol/L. Multiplication of the [Na$^+$] value by 2 accounts for its accompanying anions, principally Cl$^-$ and bicarbonate. The calculated osmolality is usually slightly lower than measured osmolality.

Urea is not only confined to the ECS because it readily crosses the cell membrane, and its intracellular concentration approximately equals its extracellular concentration. Whereas an elevated [Na$^+$] causes a shift of water from the ICS, with **uremia** there is no osmolar gradient between the two compartments and consequently no movement of water. The only exception is during **hemodialysis**, when the decrease in extracellular urea is so rapid that intracellular urea does not have time to equilibrate. This **disequilibrium syndrome** may result in shift of water into brain cells and leads to severe symptoms. Ethanol, because it freely crosses cell membranes, is another ineffective osmole. In the case of glucose, the effective osmolality can be calculated as follows:

$$\text{Effective osmolality} = 2 \times [\text{Na}] + [\text{glucose}]/18$$

The *effective osmolality* (also called the *tonicity*) determines the osmotic force that is mediating the shift of water between the ECF and the ICF.

Hyperglycemia causes an increase in the plasma osmolality because it is not in equilibrium with the ICS. During hyperglycemia, there is shift of water from the ICS to the ECS. This shift causes dilution of the Na$^+$ in the ECS, causing hyponatremia despite elevated plasma osmolality. The magnitude of this effect can be calculated as follows:

$$[\text{Na}]_{\text{corrected}} = [\text{Na}]_{\text{measured}} + 1.6 \times ([\text{glucose}] - 100\,\text{mg/dL})/100$$

where [Na]$_{\text{measured}}$ = Na$^+$ concentration measured by the clinical laboratory and [Na]$_{\text{corrected}}$ = corrected Na$^+$ concentration (the Na$^+$ concentration if the glucose concentration were normal and its accompanying water moved back into the cells). The [Na]$_{\text{corrected}}$ is the more reliable indicator of the ratio of total body Na$^+$ to TBW, the usual determinant of the [Na$^+$].

Normally, measured osmolality and calculated osmolality are within 10 mOsm/kg. However, there are some clinical situations in which this difference does not occur. The presence of **unmeasured osmoles** causes measured osmolality to be significantly elevated in comparison with the calculated osmolality. An **osmolal gap** is present when the difference between measured osmolality exceeds calculated osmolality by >10 mOsm/kg. Examples of unmeasured osmoles include ethanol, ethylene glycol, methanol, sucrose, sorbitol, and mannitol. These substances increase measured osmolality but are not part of the equation for calculating osmolality. The presence of an osmolal gap is a clinical clue to the presence of unmeasured osmoles and may be diagnostically useful when there is clinical suspicion of poisoning with methanol or ethylene glycol.

Pseudohyponatremia is a second situation in which there is discordance between measured osmolality and calculated osmolality. Lipids and proteins are the solids of the serum. In patients with elevated serum lipids or proteins, the water content of the serum decreases because water is displaced by the larger amounts of solids. Some instruments measure [Na$^+$] by determining the amount of Na$^+$ per liter of serum, including the solid component. When the solid component increases, there is a decrease in [Na$^+$] per liter of serum, despite a normal concentration when based on the amount of Na$^+$ per liter of serum water. *It is the concentration of Na$^+$ in serum water that is physiologically relevant.* A similar problem occurs when using instruments that require dilution of the sample prior to measurement of Na$^+$ (indirect potentiometry). In both situations, the plasma osmolality is normal despite the presence of pseudohyponatremia, because the method for measuring osmolality is not appreciably influenced by the percentage of serum that is composed of lipids and proteins. Pseudohyponatremia is diagnosed by the finding of a normal measured plasma osmolality despite hyponatremia. This laboratory artifact does not occur if the [Na$^+$] in water is measured directly with an ion-specific electrode, as with arterial blood gas (ABG) analyzers. **Pseudohypernatremia** may occur in patients with very low levels of serum proteins by a similar mechanism.

When there are no unmeasured osmoles and pseudohyponatremia is not a concern, the calculated osmolality provides an accurate estimate of the plasma osmolality. Measurement of plasma osmolality is useful for detecting or monitoring unmeasured osmoles and confirming the presence of true hyponatremia. Whereas many children with high plasma osmolality are dehydrated—as seen with hypernatremic dehydration or diabetic ketoacidosis—high osmolality does not always equate with dehydration. A child with salt poisoning or uremia has an elevated plasma osmolality but may be volume-overloaded.

POINT-OF-CARE TESTING

Point-of-care (POC) testing offers a number of advantages, including rapid turnaround and usually smaller blood sample volume required. POC devices may provide more accurate results in certain situations, such as pseudohyponatremia (see earlier) and pseudohyperkalemia (see Chapter 68.4). However, the agreement between POC and the laboratory is variable, and thus caution is needed when interpreting results. Because of bias, POC and laboratory results should not be used on an alternating basis when following critical trends (e.g., during correction of hypernatremia or hyponatremia; see Chapter 68.3).

Bibliography is available at Expert Consult.

68.2 Regulation of Osmolality and Volume
Larry A. Greenbaum

The regulation of plasma **osmolality** and the intravascular **volume** is controlled by independent systems for water balance, which determines osmolality, and sodium balance, which determines volume status. Maintenance of normal osmolality depends on control of water balance. Control of volume status depends on regulation of sodium balance. When present, volume depletion takes precedence over regulation of osmolality, and retention of water contributes to the maintenance of intravascular volume.

REGULATION OF OSMOLALITY

The plasma osmolality is tightly regulated and maintained at 285-295 mOsm/kg. Modification of water intake and excretion maintains normal plasma osmolality. In the steady state the combination of water intake and water produced by the body from oxidation balances water losses from the skin, lungs, urine, and gastrointestinal (GI) tract. Only water intake and urinary losses can be regulated.

Osmoreceptors in the hypothalamus sense plasma osmolality (see Chapter 572). An elevated effective osmolality leads to secretion of **antidiuretic hormone (ADH)** by neurons in the supraoptic and paraventricular nuclei in the hypothalamus. The axons of these neurons terminate in the posterior pituitary. Circulating ADH binds to its V$_2$ receptors in the collecting duct cells of the kidney, and causes insertion of water channels (aquaporin-2) into the renal collecting duct cells. This produces increased permeability to water, permitting resorption of water into the hypertonic renal medulla. Urine concentration increases and water excretion decreases. Urinary water losses cannot be eliminated because there is obligatory excretion of urinary solutes, such as urea and sodium. The regulation of ADH secretion is tightly linked to plasma osmolality, responses being detectable with a 1% change in osmolality. ADH secretion virtually disappears when plasma osmolality is low, allowing excretion of maximally dilute urine. The resulting loss of free water (i.e., water without Na^+) corrects plasma osmolality. ADH secretion is not an all-or-nothing response; there is a graded adjustment as the osmolality changes.

Water intake is regulated by hypothalamic osmoreceptors, which stimulate thirst when the serum osmolality increases. Thirst occurs with a small increase in the serum osmolality. *Control of osmolality is subordinate to maintenance of an adequate intravascular volume.* When volume depletion is present, both ADH secretion and thirst are stimulated, regardless of the plasma osmolality. The sensation of thirst requires moderate volume depletion but only a 1–2% change in the plasma osmolality.

A number of conditions can limit the kidney's ability to excrete adequate water to correct low plasma osmolality. In the **syndrome of inappropriate antidiuretic hormone (SIADH)**, ADH continues to be produced despite a low plasma osmolality (see Chapters 68.3 and 575).

The glomerular filtration rate (GFR) affects the kidney's ability to eliminate water. With a decrease in the GFR, less water is delivered to the collecting duct, limiting the amount of water that can be excreted. The impairment in the GFR must be quite significant to limit the kidney's ability to respond to an excess of water.

The **minimum urine osmolality** is approximately 30-50 mOsm/kg. This places an upper limit on the kidney's ability to excrete water; sufficient solute must be present to permit water loss. Massive water intoxication may exceed this limit, whereas a lesser amount of water is necessary in the child with a diet that has very little solute. This can produce severe hyponatremia in children who receive little salt and have minimal urea production as a result of inadequate protein intake. Volume depletion is an extremely important cause of decreased water loss by the kidney despite a low plasma osmolality. This "appropriate" secretion of ADH occurs because volume depletion takes precedence over the osmolality in the regulation of ADH.

The **maximum urine osmolality** is approximately 1,200 mOsm/kg. The obligatory solute losses dictate the minimum volume of urine that must be produced, even when maximally concentrated. Obligatory water losses increase in patients with high salt intake or high urea losses, as may occur after relief of a urinary obstruction or during recovery from acute kidney injury. An increase in urinary solute and thus water losses occurs with an **osmotic diuresis**, which occurs classically from glycosuria in diabetes mellitus as well as iatrogenically after mannitol administration. There are developmental changes in the kidney's ability to concentrate the urine. The maximum urine osmolality in a newborn, especially a premature newborn, is less than that in an older infant or child. This limits the ability to conserve water and makes such a patient more vulnerable to hypernatremic dehydration. Very high fluid intake, as seen with **psychogenic polydipsia**, can dilute the high osmolality in the renal medulla, which is necessary for maximal urinary concentration. If fluid intake is restricted in patients with this condition, the kidney's ability to concentrate the urine may be somewhat impaired, although this defect corrects after a few days without polydipsia. This may also occur during the initial treatment of central diabetes insipidus with desmopressin acetate; the renal medulla takes time to achieve its normal maximum osmolality.

REGULATION OF VOLUME

An appropriate intravascular volume is critical for survival; both volume depletion and volume overload may cause significant morbidity and mortality. Because sodium is the principal extracellular cation and is restricted to the ECF, adequate body sodium is necessary for maintenance of intravascular volume. The principal extracellular anion, Cl^-, is also necessary, but for simplicity, Na^+ balance is considered the main regulator of volume status because body content of sodium and that of chloride usually change proportionally, given the need for equal numbers of

cations and anions. In some situations, Cl^- depletion is considered the dominant derangement causing volume depletion (metabolic alkalosis with volume depletion).

The kidney determines sodium balance because there is little homeostatic control of sodium intake, even though **salt craving** does occasionally occur, typically in children with chronic renal salt loss. The kidney regulates Na^+ balance by altering the percentage of filtered Na^+ that is resorbed along the nephron. Normally, the kidney excretes <1% of the Na^+ filtered at the glomerulus. In the absence of disease, extrarenal losses and urinary output match intake, with the kidney having the capacity to adapt to large variations in sodium intake. When necessary, urinary sodium excretion can be reduced to virtually undetectable levels or increased dramatically.

The most important determinant of renal Na^+ excretion is the volume status of the child; it is the effective intravascular volume that influences urinary Na^+ excretion. The *effective intravascular volume* is the volume status that is sensed by the body's regulatory mechanisms. Heart failure is a state of volume overload, but the effective intravascular volume is low because poor cardiac function prevents adequate perfusion of the kidneys and other organs. This explains the avid renal Na^+ retention often present in patients with heart failure.

The **renin-angiotensin system** is an important regulator of renal Na^+ excretion. The juxtaglomerular apparatus produces renin in response to decreased effective intravascular volume. Specific stimuli for renin release are decreased perfusion pressure in the afferent arteriole of the glomerulus, decreased delivery of sodium to the distal nephron, and $β_1$-adrenergic agonists, which increase in response to intravascular volume depletion. Renin, a proteolytic enzyme, cleaves angiotensinogen, producing angiotensin I. Angiotensin-converting enzyme (ACE) converts angiotensin I into angiotensin II. The actions of angiotensin II include direct stimulation of the proximal tubule to increase sodium resorption and stimulation of the adrenal gland to increase aldosterone secretion. Through its actions in the distal nephron—specifically, the late distal convoluted tubule and the collecting duct—aldosterone increases sodium resorption. Aldosterone also stimulates potassium excretion, increasing urinary losses. Along with decreasing urinary loss of sodium, angiotensin II acts as a vasoconstrictor, which helps maintain adequate blood pressure in the presence of volume depletion.

Volume expansion stimulates the synthesis of **atrial natriuretic peptide (ANP)**, which is produced by the atria in response to atrial wall distention. Along with increasing the GFR, ANP inhibits Na^+ resorption in the medullary portion of the collecting duct, facilitating an increase in urinary Na^+ excretion.

Volume overload occurs when Na^+ intake exceeds output. Children with kidney failure have impaired ability to excrete Na^+. The GFR is low at birth, limiting a newborn's ability to excrete an Na^+ load. In other situations, there is a loss of the appropriate regulation of renal Na^+ excretion. This loss occurs in patients with excessive aldosterone, as seen in primary hyperaldosteronism or renal artery stenosis, where excess renin production leads to high aldosterone levels. In acute glomerulonephritis, even without significantly reduced GFR, the normal intrarenal mechanisms that regulate Na^+ excretion malfunction, causing excessive renal retention of Na^+ and volume overload.

Renal retention of Na^+ occurs during volume depletion, but this appropriate response causes the severe excess in total body Na^+ that is present in heart failure, liver failure, nephrotic syndrome, and other causes of hypoalbuminemia. In these diseases the effective intravascular volume is decreased, causing the kidney and the various regulatory systems to respond, leading to renal Na^+ retention and edema formation.

Volume depletion usually occurs when Na^+ losses exceed intake. The most common etiology in children is gastroenteritis. Excessive losses of sodium may also occur from the skin in children with burns, in sweat from patients with cystic fibrosis, or after vigorous exercise. Inadequate intake of Na^+ is uncommon except in neglect, in famine, or with an inappropriate choice of liquid diet in a child who cannot take solids. Urinary Na^+ wasting may occur in a range of renal diseases, from renal dysplasia to tubular disorders, such as Bartter syndrome. The neonate, especially if premature, has a mild impairment in the ability to conserve Na^+. Iatrogenic renal Na^+ wasting takes place during diuretic therapy. Renal Na^+ loss occurs as a result of derangement in the normal regulatory systems. An absence of aldosterone, seen most frequently in children with **congenital adrenal hyperplasia** caused by 21-hydroxylase deficiency, causes sodium wasting (see Chapter 594).

Isolated disorders of water balance can affect volume status and Na^+ balance. Because the cell membrane is permeable to water, changes in TBW influence both the extracellular volume and the intracellular volume. In isolated water loss, as occurs in diabetes insipidus, the impact is greater on the ICS because it has a greater volume than the ECS. Thus, compared with other types of dehydration, hypernatremic dehydration has less impact on plasma volume; most of the fluid loss comes from the ICS. Yet, significant water loss eventually affects intravascular volume and will stimulate renal Na^+ retention, even if total body Na^+ content is normal. Similarly, with acute water intoxication or SIADH, there is an excess of TBW, but most is in the ICS. However, there is some effect on the intravascular volume, which causes renal excretion of Na^+. Children with SIADH or water intoxication have high urine Na^+ concentration, despite hyponatremia. This finding reinforces the concept of independent control systems for water and Na^+, but the 2 systems interact when pathophysiologic processes dictate, and control of effective intravascular volume always takes precedence over control of osmolality.

Bibliography is available at Expert Consult.

68.3 Sodium

Larry A. Greenbaum

SODIUM METABOLISM
Body Content and Physiologic Function
Sodium is the dominant cation of the ECF (see Fig. 68.3), and it is the principal determinant of extracellular osmolality. Na^+ is therefore necessary for the maintenance of intravascular volume. Less than 3% of Na^+ is intracellular. More than 40% of total body Na^+ is in bone; the remainder is in the interstitial and intravascular spaces. The low intracellular $[Na^+]$, approximately 10 mEq/L, is maintained by Na^+,K^+-ATPase, which exchanges intracellular Na^+ for extracellular K^+.

Sodium Intake
A child's diet determines the amount of Na^+ ingested—a predominantly cultural determination in older children. An occasional child has salt craving because of an underlying salt-wasting renal disease or adrenal insufficiency. Children in the United States tend to have very high salt intakes because their diets include a large amount of "junk" food or fast food. Infants receive sodium from breast milk (approximately 7 mEq/L) and formula (7-13 mEq/L, for 20 calorie/oz formula).

Sodium is readily absorbed throughout the GI tract. Mineralocorticoids increase sodium transport into the body, although this effect has limited clinical significance. The presence of glucose enhances sodium absorption owing to the presence of a co-transport system. This is the rationale for including sodium and glucose in oral rehydration solutions (see Chapter 366).

Sodium Excretion
Sodium excretion occurs in stool and sweat, but the kidney regulates Na^+ balance and is the principal site of Na^+ excretion. There is some Na^+ loss in stool, but it is minimal unless diarrhea is present. Normally, sweat has 5-40 mEq/L of sodium. Sweat Na^+ concentration is increased in children with cystic fibrosis, aldosterone deficiency, or pseudohypoaldosteronism. The higher sweat losses in these conditions may cause or contribute to Na^+ depletion.

Sodium is unique among electrolytes because water balance, not Na^+ balance, usually determines its concentration. When the $[Na^+]$ increases, the resultant higher plasma osmolality causes increased thirst and increased secretion of ADH, which leads to renal conservation of water. Both these mechanisms increase the water content of the body, and the $[Na^+]$ returns to normal. During hyponatremia, the decrease in plasma

osmolality stops ADH secretion, and consequent renal water excretion leads to an increase in the $[Na^+]$. Even though water balance is usually regulated by osmolality, volume depletion does stimulate thirst, ADH secretion, and renal conservation of water. Volume depletion takes precedence over osmolality; volume depletion stimulates ADH secretion, even if a patient has hyponatremia.

The excretion of Na^+ by the kidney is not regulated by the plasma osmolality. The patient's effective plasma volume determines the amount of sodium in the urine. This is mediated by a variety of regulatory systems, including the renin-angiotensin-aldosterone system and intrarenal mechanisms. In hyponatremia or hypernatremia, the underlying pathophysiology determines the amount of urinary Na^+, not the serum $[Na^+]$.

HYPERNATREMIA
Hypernatremia is a $[Na^+]$ >145 mEq/L, although it is sometimes defined as >150 mEq/L. Mild hypernatremia is fairly common in children, especially among infants with gastroenteritis. Hypernatremia in hospitalized patients may be iatrogenic—caused by inadequate water administration or, less often, by excessive Na^+ administration. Moderate or severe hypernatremia has significant morbidity because of the underlying disease, the effects of hypernatremia on the brain, and the risks of overly rapid correction.

Etiology and Pathophysiology
There are 3 basic mechanisms of hypernatremia (Table 68.1). *Sodium intoxication* is frequently iatrogenic in a hospital setting as a result of correction of metabolic acidosis with sodium bicarbonate. Baking soda, a putative home remedy for upset stomach, is another source of sodium bicarbonate; the hypernatremia is accompanied by a profound metabolic alkalosis. In hyperaldosteronism, there is renal retention of sodium and resultant hypertension; hypernatremia may not be present or is usually mild.

The classic causes of hypernatremia from a *water deficit* are **nephrogenic** and **central diabetes insipidus** (see Chapters 548 and 574). Hypernatremia develops in diabetes insipidus only if the patient does not have access to water or cannot drink adequately because of immaturity, neurologic impairment, emesis, or anorexia. Infants are at high risk because of their inability to control their own water intake. Central diabetes insipidus and the genetic forms of nephrogenic diabetes insipidus typically cause massive urinary water losses and very dilute urine. The water losses are less dramatic, and the urine often has the same osmolality as plasma when nephrogenic diabetes insipidus is secondary to intrinsic renal disease (obstructive uropathy, renal dysplasia, sickle cell disease).

The other causes of a water deficit are also secondary to an imbalance between losses and intake. Newborns, especially if premature, have high insensible water losses. Losses are further increased if the infant is placed under a radiant warmer or with the use of phototherapy for hyperbilirubinemia. The renal concentrating mechanisms are not optimal at birth, providing an additional source of water loss. Ineffective breastfeeding, often in a primiparous mother, can cause severe hypernatremic dehydration. **Adipsia**, the absence of thirst, is usually secondary to damage to the hypothalamus, such as from trauma, tumor, hydrocephalus, or histiocytosis. Primary adipsia is rare.

When hypernatremia occurs in conditions with *deficits of sodium and water*, the water deficit exceeds the sodium deficit. This occurs only if the patient is unable to ingest adequate water. Diarrhea results in depletion of both Na^+ and water. Because diarrhea is hypotonic—typical Na^+ concentration of 35-65 mEq/L—water losses exceed Na^+ losses, potentially leading to hypernatremia. Most children with gastroenteritis do not have hypernatremia because they drink enough hypotonic fluid to compensate for stool water losses (see Chapter 366). Fluids such as water, juice, and formula are more hypotonic than the stool losses, allowing correction of the water deficit and potentially even causing hyponatremia. Hypernatremia is most likely to occur in the child with diarrhea who has inadequate intake because of emesis, lack of access to water, or anorexia.

Osmotic agents, including mannitol, and glucose in **diabetes mellitus**, cause excessive renal losses of water and Na^+. Because the urine is

Table 68.1	Causes of Hypernatremia

EXCESSIVE SODIUM
Improperly mixed formula
Excess sodium bicarbonate
Ingestion of seawater or sodium chloride
Intentional salt poisoning (child abuse or Munchausen syndrome by proxy)
Intravenous hypertonic saline
Hyperaldosteronism

WATER DEFICIT
Nephrogenic Diabetes Insipidus
Acquired
X-linked (OMIM 304800)
Autosomal recessive (OMIM 222000)
Autosomal dominant (OMIM 125800)

Central Diabetes Insipidus
Acquired
Autosomal recessive (OMIM 125700)
Autosomal dominant (OMIM 125700)
Wolfram syndrome (OMIM 222300/598500)

Increased Insensible Losses
Premature infants
Radiant warmers
Phototherapy
Inadequate intake:
    Ineffective breastfeeding
    Child neglect or abuse
    Adipsia (lack of thirst)

WATER AND SODIUM DEFICITS
Gastrointestinal Losses
Diarrhea
Emesis/nasogastric suction
Osmotic cathartics (lactulose)

Cutaneous Losses
Burns
Excessive sweating

Renal Losses
Osmotic diuretics (mannitol)
Diabetes mellitus
Chronic kidney disease (dysplasia and obstructive uropathy)
Polyuric phase of acute tubular necrosis
Postobstructive diuresis

OMIM, database number from the Online Mendelian Inheritance in Man (http://www.ncbi.nlm.nih.gov/omim).

hypotonic (Na^+ concentration of approximately 50 mEq/L) during an osmotic diuresis, water loss exceeds Na^+ loss, and hypernatremia may occur if water intake is inadequate. Certain chronic kidney diseases, such as renal dysplasia and obstructive uropathy, are associated with tubular dysfunction, leading to excessive losses of water and Na^+. Many children with such diseases have disproportionate water loss and are at risk for hypernatremic dehydration, especially if gastroenteritis supervenes. Similar mechanisms occur during the polyuric phase of acute kidney injury and after relief of urinary obstruction (postobstructive diuresis). Patients with either condition may have an osmotic diuresis from urinary losses of urea and an inability to conserve water because of tubular dysfunction.

Essential hypernatremia is rare in children and is thought to occur with injury to the hypothalamic-posterior pituitary axis. It is euvolemic, nonhypertensive, and associated with hypodipsia, possibly related to a reset osmol sensor.

Clinical Manifestations

Most children with hypernatremia are dehydrated and show the typical clinical signs and symptoms (see Chapter 70). Children with hypernatremic dehydration tend to have better preservation of intravascular volume because of the shift of water from the ICS to the ECS. This shift maintains blood pressure and urine output and allows hypernatremic infants to be less symptomatic initially and potentially to become more dehydrated before medical attention is sought. Breastfed infants with hypernatremia are often profoundly dehydrated, with failure to thrive (malnutrition). Probably because of intracellular water loss, the pinched abdominal skin of a dehydrated, hypernatremic infant has a "doughy" feel.

Hypernatremia, even without dehydration, causes central nervous system (CNS) symptoms that tend to parallel the degree of Na^+ elevation and the acuity of the increase. Patients are irritable, restless, weak, and lethargic. Some infants have a high-pitched cry and hyperpnea. Alert patients are very thirsty, even though nausea may be present. Hypernatremia may cause fever, although many patients have an underlying process that contributes to the fever. Hypernatremia is associated with hyperglycemia and mild hypocalcemia; the mechanisms are unknown. Beyond the sequelae of dehydration, there is no clear direct effect of hypernatremia on other organs or tissues, except the brain.

Brain hemorrhage is the most devastating consequence of untreated hypernatremia. As the extracellular osmolality increases, water moves out of brain cells, leading to a decrease in brain volume. This decrease can result in tearing of intracerebral veins and bridging blood vessels as the brain moves away from the skull and the meninges. Patients may have subarachnoid, subdural, and parenchymal hemorrhages. Seizures and coma are possible sequelae of the hemorrhage, although seizures are more common during correction of hypernatremia. The cerebrospinal fluid protein is often elevated in infants with significant hypernatremia, probably because of leakage from damaged blood vessels. Neonates, especially if premature, seem especially vulnerable to hypernatremia and excessive sodium intake. There is an association between rapid or hyperosmolar sodium bicarbonate administration and the development of intraventricular hemorrhages in neonates. Even though central pontine myelinolysis is classically associated with overly rapid correction of hyponatremia, both central pontine and extrapontine myelinolysis can occur in children with hypernatremia (see Treatment). Thrombotic complications occur in severe hypernatremic dehydration, including stroke, dural sinus thrombosis, peripheral thrombosis, and renal vein thrombosis. This is secondary to dehydration and possibly hypercoagulability associated with hypernatremia.

Diagnosis

The etiology of hypernatremia is usually apparent from the history. Hypernatremia resulting from water loss occurs only if the patient does not have access to water or is unable to drink. In the absence of dehydration, it is important to ask about sodium intake. Children with excess salt intake do not have signs of dehydration, unless another process is present. Severe Na^+ intoxication causes signs of volume overload, such as pulmonary edema and weight gain. **Salt poisoning** is associated with an elevated fractional excretion of Na^+, whereas hypernatremic dehydration causes a low fractional excretion of Na^+. Gastric sodium concentrations are often elevated in salt poisoning. In hyperaldosteronism, hypernatremia is usually mild or absent and is associated with edema, hypertension, hypokalemia, and metabolic alkalosis.

When there is isolated water loss, the signs of volume depletion are usually less severe initially because much of the loss is from the ICS. When pure water loss causes signs of dehydration, the hypernatremia and water deficit are usually severe. In the child with renal water loss, either central or nephrogenic diabetes insipidus, the urine is inappropriately dilute and urine volume is not low. The urine is maximally concentrated and urine volume is low if the losses are extrarenal or caused by inadequate intake. With extrarenal causes of loss of water, the urine osmolality should be >1,000 mOsm/kg. When diabetes insipidus is suspected, the evaluation may include measurement of ADH and a water deprivation test, including a trial of desmopressin acetate (synthetic ADH analog) to differentiate between nephrogenic diabetes insipidus and central diabetes insipidus (see Chapters 548 and 574). A water-deprivation test is unnecessary if the patient has simultaneous documentation of hypernatremia and poorly concentrated urine (osmolality lower than that of plasma). In children with central diabetes insipidus, administration of desmopressin acetate increases the urine osmolality above the plasma osmolality, although maximum osmolality does not occur immediately because of the decreased osmolality of the renal medulla as a result of the chronic lack of ADH. In children with nephrogenic diabetes insipidus, there is no response to desmopressin acetate. Hypercalcemia or hypokalemia may produce a nephrogenic diabetes insipidus–like syndrome.

With combined Na^+ and water deficits, analysis of the urine differentiates between renal and nonrenal etiologies. When the losses are extrarenal, the kidney responds to volume depletion with low urine volume, concentrated urine, and Na^+ retention (urine $[Na^+]$ <20 mEq/L, fractional excretion of Na^+ <1%). With renal causes, the urine volume is not appropriately low, the urine is not maximally concentrated, and the urine $[Na^+]$ may be inappropriately elevated.

Treatment

As hypernatremia develops, the brain generates **idiogenic osmoles** to increase the intracellular osmolality and prevent the loss of brain water. This mechanism is not instantaneous and is most prominent when hypernatremia has developed gradually. If the serum $[Na^+]$ is lowered rapidly, there is movement of water from the serum into the brain cells to equalize the osmolality in the 2 compartments. The resultant brain swelling manifests as seizures or coma.

Because of the associated dangers, *chronic hypernatremia should not be corrected rapidly.* The goal is to decrease the serum $[Na^+]$ by <10 mEq/L every 24 hr. The most important component of correcting moderate or severe hypernatremia is frequent monitoring of the serum $[Na^+]$ value so that fluid therapy can be adjusted to provide adequate correction, neither too slow nor too fast. If a child has seizures as a result of brain edema secondary to rapid correction, administration of hypotonic fluid should be stopped. An infusion of 3% saline can acutely increase the serum $[Na^+]$, reversing the cerebral edema.

Chapter 70 outlines a detailed approach to the child with hypernatremic dehydration. Acute, severe hypernatremia, usually secondary to sodium administration, can be corrected more rapidly with 5% dextrose in water (D5W) because idiogenic osmoles have not had time to accumulate. This fact balances the high morbidity and mortality rates associated with hypernatremia with the dangers of overly rapid correction. When hypernatremia is severe and is caused by sodium intoxication, it may be impossible to administer enough water to correct the hypernatremia rapidly without worsening the volume overload. In this situation, dialysis allows for removal of the excess Na^+, with the precise strategy dependent on the mode of dialysis. In less severe cases, the addition of a loop diuretic increases the removal of excess Na^+ and water, decreasing the risk of volume overload. With Na^+ overload, hypernatremia is corrected with Na^+-free intravenous (IV) fluid (D5W).

Hyperglycemia from hypernatremia is not usually a problem and is not treated with insulin because the acute decrease in glucose may precipitate cerebral edema by lowering plasma osmolality. Rarely, the glucose concentration of IV fluids must be reduced (from 5% to 2.5% dextrose in water). The secondary hypocalcemia is treated as needed.

It is important to address the underlying cause of the hypernatremia, if possible. The child with central diabetes insipidus should receive desmopressin acetate. Because this treatment reduces renal excretion of water, excessive intake of water must be avoided to prevent both overly rapid correction of the hypernatremia and the development of hyponatremia. Over the long term, reduced sodium intake and the use of medications can somewhat ameliorate the water losses in nephrogenic diabetes insipidus (see Chapter 548). The daily water intake of a child receiving tube feeding may need to be increased to compensate for high losses. The patient with significant ongoing losses, such as through diarrhea, may need supplemental water and electrolytes (see Chapter 69). Sodium intake is reduced if it contributed to the hypernatremia.

HYPONATREMIA

Hyponatremia, a very common electrolyte abnormality in hospitalized patients, is a serum sodium level <135 mEq/L. Both total body sodium and TBW determine the serum sodium concentration. Hyponatremia

exists when the ratio of water to Na^+ is increased. This condition can occur with low, normal, or high levels of body Na^+. Similarly, body water can be low, normal, or high.

Etiology and Pathophysiology

Table 68.2 lists the causes of hyponatremia. **Pseudohyponatremia** is a laboratory artifact present when the plasma contains very high concentrations of protein (multiple myeloma, IVIG infusion) or lipid (hypertriglyceridemia, hypercholesterolemia). It does not occur when a direct ion-selective electrode determines the $[Na^+]$ in undiluted plasma, a technique that is used by ABG analyzers or POC instruments (see Chapter 68.1). In true hyponatremia, the measured osmolality is low, whereas it is normal in pseudohyponatremia. **Hyperosmolality,** as may occur with hyperglycemia, causes a low $[Na^+]$ because water moves down its osmotic gradient from the ICS into the ECS, diluting the $[Na^+]$. However, because the manifestations of hyponatremia are a result of the low plasma osmolality, patients with hyponatremia resulting from hyperosmolality do not have symptoms of hyponatremia. When the etiology of the hyperosmolality resolves, such as hyperglycemia in diabetes mellitus, water moves back into the cells, and the $[Na^+]$ rises to its "true" value. Mannitol or sucrose, a component of intravenous immune globulin (IVIG) preparations, may cause hyponatremia because of hyperosmolality.

Classification of hyponatremia is based on the patient's volume status. In **hypovolemic hyponatremia** the child has lost Na^+ from the body. The water balance may be positive or negative, but Na^+ loss has been higher than water loss. The pathogenesis of the hyponatremia is usually a combination of Na^+ loss and water retention to compensate for the volume depletion. The patient has a pathologic increase in fluid loss, and this fluid contains Na^+. Most fluid that is lost has a lower $[Na^+]$ than that of plasma. Viral diarrhea fluid has an average $[Na^+]$ of 50 mEq/L. Replacing diarrhea fluid, which has $[Na^+]$ of 50 mEq/L, with formula, which has only approximately 10 mEq/L of Na^+, reduces $[Na^+]$. Intravascular volume depletion interferes with renal water excretion, the body's usual mechanism for preventing hyponatremia. The volume depletion stimulates ADH synthesis, resulting in renal water retention. Volume depletion also decreases the GFR and enhances water resorption in the proximal tubule, thereby reducing water delivery to the collecting duct.

Diarrhea as a result of gastroenteritis is the most common cause of hypovolemic hyponatremia in children. Emesis causes hyponatremia if the patient takes in hypotonic fluid, either intravenously or enterally, despite the emesis. Most patients with emesis have either a normal $[Na^+]$ or hypernatremia. Burns may cause massive losses of isotonic fluid and resultant volume depletion. Hyponatremia develops if the patient receives hypotonic fluid. Losses of sodium from sweat are especially high in children with cystic fibrosis, aldosterone deficiency, or pseudohypoaldosteronism, although high losses can also occur in a hot climate. Third space losses are isotonic and can cause significant volume depletion, leading to ADH production and water retention, which can cause hyponatremia if the patient receives hypotonic fluid. In diseases that cause volume depletion through extrarenal Na^+ loss, the urine Na^+ level should be low (<10 mEq/L) as part of the renal response to maintain the intravascular volume. The only exceptions are diseases that cause both extrarenal and renal Na^+ losses: adrenal insufficiency and pseudohypoaldosteronism.

Renal Na^+ loss may occur in a variety of situations. In some situations the urine $[Na^+]$ is >140 mEq/L; thus hyponatremia may occur without any fluid intake. In many cases the urine Na^+ level is less than the serum $[Na^+]$; thus the intake of hypotonic fluid is necessary for hyponatremia to develop. In diseases associated with urinary Na^+ loss, the urine Na^+ level is >20 mEq/L despite volume depletion. This may not be true if the urinary Na^+ loss is no longer occurring, as is frequently the case if diuretics are discontinued. Because loop diuretics prevent generation of a maximally hypertonic renal medulla, the patient can neither maximally dilute nor concentrate the urine. The inability to maximally retain water provides some protection against severe hyponatremia. The patient receiving thiazide diuretics can concentrate the urine and is at higher risk for severe hyponatremia. Osmotic agents, such as glucose during diabetic ketoacidosis, cause loss of both water and Na^+. Urea

Table 68.2	Causes of Hyponatremia

PSEUDOHYPONATREMIA
Hyperlipidemia
Hyperproteinemia

HYPEROSMOLALITY
Hyperglycemia
Iatrogenic (mannitol, sucrose, glycine)

HYPOVOLEMIC HYPONATREMIA

EXTRARENAL LOSSES
Gastrointestinal (emesis, diarrhea)
Skin (sweating or burns)
Third space losses (bowel obstruction, peritonitis, sepsis)

RENAL LOSSES
Thiazide or loop diuretics
Osmotic diuresis
Postobstructive diuresis
Polyuric phase of acute tubular necrosis
Juvenile nephronophthisis (OMIM 256100/606966/602088/604387/611498)
Autosomal recessive polycystic kidney disease (OMIM 263200)
Tubulointerstitial nephritis
Obstructive uropathy
Cerebral salt wasting
Proximal (type II) renal tubular acidosis (OMIM 604278)*
Lack of aldosterone effect (high serum potassium):
Absence of aldosterone (e.g., 21-hydroxylase deficiency [OMIM 201910])
Pseudohypoaldosteronism type I (OMIM 264350/177735)
Urinary tract obstruction and/or infection
Addison disease

EUVOLEMIC HYPONATREMIA
Syndrome of inappropriate antidiuretic hormone secretion
Nephrogenic syndrome of inappropriate antidiuresis (OMIM 304800)
Desmopressin acetate
Glucocorticoid deficiency
Hypothyroidism
Antidepressant medications
Water intoxication
Iatrogenic (excess hypotonic intravenous fluids)
Feeding infants excessive water products
Swimming lessons
Tap water enema
Child abuse
Psychogenic polydipsia
Diluted formula
Beer potomania
Exercise-induced hyponatremia

HYPERVOLEMIC HYPONATREMIA
Heart failure
Cirrhosis
Nephrotic syndrome
Acute, chronic kidney injury
Capillary leak caused by sepsis
Hypoalbuminemia caused by gastrointestinal disease (protein-losing enteropathy)

*Most cases of proximal renal tubular acidosis are not caused by this primary genetic disorder. Proximal renal tubular acidosis is usually part of Fanconi syndrome, which has multiple etiologies.
OMIM, database number from the Online Mendelian Inheritance in Man (http://www.ncbi.nlm.nih.gov/omim).

accumulates during renal failure and then acts as an osmotic diuretic after relief of urinary tract obstruction and during the polyuric phase of acute tubular necrosis. Transient tubular damage in these conditions further impairs Na^+ conservation. The serum $[Na^+]$ in these conditions depends on $[Na^+]$ of the fluid used to replace the losses. Hyponatremia develops when the fluid is hypotonic relative to the urinary losses.

Renal salt wasting occurs in hereditary kidney diseases, such as juvenile nephronophthisis and autosomal recessive polycystic kidney disease. Obstructive uropathy, most often a result of posterior urethral valves, produces salt wasting, but patients with the disease may also have hypernatremia as a result of impaired ability to concentrate urine and high-water loss. Acquired tubulointerstitial nephritis, usually secondary to either medications or infections, may cause salt wasting, along with other evidence of tubular dysfunction. CNS injury may produce cerebral salt wasting, which is theoretically caused by the production of a natriuretic peptide that causes renal salt wasting. In type II **renal tubular acidosis (RTA)**, usually associated with Fanconi syndrome (see Chapter 547.1), there is increased excretion of Na^+ and bicarbonate in the urine. Patients with Fanconi syndrome also have glycosuria, aminoaciduria, and hypophosphatemia because of renal phosphate wasting.

Aldosterone is necessary for renal Na^+ retention and for the excretion of K^+ and acid. In congenital adrenal hyperplasia caused by 21-hydroxylase deficiency, the block of aldosterone production results in hyponatremia, hyperkalemia, and metabolic acidosis. Decreased aldosterone secretion may be seen in Addison disease (adrenal insufficiency). In pseudohypoaldosteronism, aldosterone levels are elevated, but there is no response because of either a defective Na^+ channel or a deficiency of aldosterone receptors. A lack of tubular response to aldosterone may occur in children with urinary tract obstruction, especially during an acute urinary tract infection.

In **hypervolemic hyponatremia** there is an excess of TBW and Na^+, although the increase in water is greater than the increase in Na^+. In most conditions that cause hypervolemic hyponatremia, there is a decrease in the *effective blood volume*, resulting from third space fluid loss, vasodilation, or poor cardiac output. The regulatory systems sense a decrease in effective blood volume and attempt to retain water and Na^+ to correct the problem. ADH causes renal water retention, and the kidney, under the influence of aldosterone and other intrarenal mechanisms, retains sodium. The patient's sodium concentration decreases because water intake exceeds sodium intake and ADH prevents the normal loss of excess water.

In these disorders, there is low urine $[Na^+]$ (<10 mEq/L) and an excess of both TBW and Na^+. The only exception is in patients with renal failure and hyponatremia. These patients have an expanded intravascular volume, and hyponatremia can therefore appropriately suppress ADH production. Water cannot be excreted because very little urine is being made. Serum Na^+ is diluted through ingestion of water. Because of renal dysfunction, the urine $[Na^+]$ may be elevated, but urine volume is so low that urine Na^+ excretion has not kept up with Na^+ intake, leading to sodium overload. The urine $[Na^+]$ in renal failure varies. In patients with acute glomerulonephritis, because it does not affect the tubules, the urine Na^+ level is usually low, whereas in patients with acute tubular necrosis, it is elevated because of tubular dysfunction.

Patients with hyponatremia and no evidence of volume overload or volume depletion have **euvolemic hyponatremia.** These patients typically have an excess of TBW and a slight decrease in total body Na^+. Some of these patients have an increase in weight, implying that they are volume-overloaded. Nevertheless, from a clinical standpoint, they usually appear normal or have subtle signs of fluid overload. In SIADH the secretion of ADH is not inhibited by either low serum osmolality or expanded intravascular volume (see Chapter 575). The result is that the child with SIADH is unable to excrete water. This results in dilution of the serum Na^+ and hyponatremia. The expansion of the extracellular volume because of the retained water causes a mild increase in intravascular volume. The kidney increases Na^+ excretion to decrease intravascular volume to normal; thus the patient has a mild decrease in body Na^+. SIADH typically occurs with disorders of the CNS (infection, hemorrhage, trauma, tumor, thrombosis, Guillain-Barré syndrome), but lung disease (infection, asthma, positive pressure ventilation) and malignant tumors (producing ADH) are other potential causes. A variety of medications may cause SIADH, including recreational use of 3,4-methylenedioxymethylamphetamine (MDMA, or "Ecstasy"), opiates, antiepileptic drugs (carbamazepine, oxcarbazepine, valproate), tricyclic antidepressants, vincristine, cyclophosphamide, and selective serotonin reuptake inhibitors (SSRIs). The diagnosis of SIADH is one of exclusion,

Table 68.3	Diagnostic Criteria for Syndrome of Inappropriate Antidiuretic Hormone Secretion

- Absence of:
  Renal, adrenal, or thyroid insufficiency
  Heart failure, nephrotic syndrome, or cirrhosis
  Diuretic ingestion
  Dehydration
- Urine osmolality >100 mOsm/kg (usually > plasma)
- Serum osmolality <280 mOsm/kg and serum sodium <135 mEq/L
- Urine sodium >30 mEq/L
- Reversal of "sodium wasting" and correction of hyponatremia with water restriction

because other causes of hyponatremia must be eliminated (Table 68.3). Because SIADH is a state of intravascular volume expansion, low serum uric acid and BUN levels are supportive of the diagnosis. A rare gain-of-function mutation in the renal ADH receptor causes **nephrogenic syndrome of inappropriate antidiuresis.** Patients with this X-linked disorder appear to have SIADH but have undetectable levels of ADH.

Hyponatremia in hospitalized patients is frequently caused by inappropriate production of ADH and administration of hypotonic IV fluids (see Chapter 69). Causes of inappropriate ADH production include stress, medications such as narcotics or anesthetics, nausea, and respiratory illness. The synthetic analog of ADH, desmopressin acetate, causes water retention and may cause hyponatremia if fluid intake is not appropriately limited. The main uses of desmopressin acetate in children are for the management of central diabetes insipidus and nocturnal enuresis.

Excess water ingestion can produce hyponatremia. In these cases, [Na⁺] decreases as a result of dilution. This decrease suppresses ADH secretion, and there is a marked water diuresis by the kidney. Hyponatremia develops only because the intake of water exceeds the kidney's ability to eliminate water. This condition is more likely to occur in infants because their lower GFR limits their ability to excrete water.

Hyponatremia may develop in infants <6 mo of age when caregivers offer water to their infant as a supplement, during hot weather, or when they run out of formula. Hyponatremia may result in transient seizures, hypothermia, and poor tone. With cessation of water intake, the hyponatremia rapidly corrects. Infants <6 mo of age should not be given water to drink; infants 6-12 mo of age should not receive >1-2 ounces. If the infant appears thirsty, the parent should offer formula or breastfeed the child.

In some situations the water intoxication causes acute hyponatremia and is caused by a massive **acute water load.** Causes include infant swimming lessons, inappropriate use of hypotonic IV fluids, water enemas, and forced water intake as a form of child abuse. Chronic hyponatremia occurs in children who receive water but limited sodium and protein. The minimum urine osmolality is approximately 50 mOsm/kg, the kidney can excrete 1 L of water only if there is enough solute ingested to produce 50 mOsm for urinary excretion. Because Na⁺ and urea (a breakdown product of protein) are the principal urinary solutes, a lack of intake of Na⁺ and protein prevents adequate water excretion. This occurs with the use of diluted formula or other inappropriate diets. Subsistence on beer, a poor source of Na⁺ and protein, causes hyponatremia because of the inability to excrete the high water load ("beer potomania"). **Exercise-induced hyponatremia,** reported frequently during marathons, is caused by excessive water intake, salt losses from sweat, and secretion of ADH.

The pathogenesis of the hyponatremia in glucocorticoid deficiency (adrenal insufficiency) is multifactorial and includes increased ADH secretion. In hypothyroidism there is an inappropriate retention of water by the kidney, but the precise mechanisms are not clearly elucidated.

Cerebral salt wasting, an uncommon disorder in children, may be confused with SIADH and is often associated with CNS injury or lesions. Cerebral salt wasting produces renal salt losses and hypovolemia (orthostatic hypotension and elevated hematocrit, BUN, or creatinine).

Clinical Manifestations

Hyponatremia causes a decrease in the osmolality of the ECS. Because the ICS then has a higher osmolality, water moves from the ECS to the ICS to maintain osmotic equilibrium. The increase in intracellular water causes cells to swell. Although cell swelling is not problematic in most tissues, it is dangerous for the brain, which is confined by the skull. As brain cells swell, there is an increase in intracranial pressure, which impairs cerebral blood flow. Acute, severe hyponatremia can cause brainstem herniation and apnea; respiratory support is often necessary. Brain cell swelling is responsible for most of the symptoms of hyponatremia. Neurologic symptoms of hyponatremia include anorexia, nausea, emesis, malaise, lethargy, confusion, agitation, headache, seizures, coma, and decreased reflexes. Patients may have hypothermia and Cheyne-Stokes respirations. Hyponatremia can cause muscle cramps and weakness; rhabdomyolysis can occur with water intoxication.

The symptoms of hyponatremia are mostly a result of the decrease in extracellular osmolality and the resulting movement of water down its osmotic gradient into the ICS. Brain swelling can be significantly obviated if the hyponatremia develops gradually, because brain cells adapt to the decreased extracellular osmolality by reducing intracellular osmolality. This reduction is achieved by extrusion of the main intracellular ions (K⁺, Cl⁻) and a variety of small organic molecules. This process explains why the range of symptoms in hyponatremia is related to both the serum [Na⁺] and its rate of decrease. A patient with chronic hyponatremia may have only subtle neurologic abnormalities with a serum [Na⁺] of 110 mEq/L, but another patient may have seizures because of an acute decline in serum [Na⁺] from 140 to 125 mEq/L.

Diagnosis

The history usually points to a likely etiology of the hyponatremia. Most patients with hyponatremia have a history of volume depletion. Diarrhea and diuretic use are common causes of hyponatremia in children. A history of polyuria, perhaps with enuresis, and/or salt craving is present in children with primary kidney diseases or absence of aldosterone effect. Children may have signs or symptoms suggesting a diagnosis of hypothyroidism or adrenal insufficiency (see Chapters 581 and 593). Brain injury raises the possibility of SIADH or cerebral salt wasting, with the caveat that SIADH is much more likely. Liver disease, nephrotic syndrome, renal failure, or congestive heart failure may be acute or chronic. The history should include a review of the patient's intake, both intravenous and enteral, with careful attention to the amounts of water, Na⁺, and protein.

The traditional first step in the diagnostic process is determination of the plasma osmolality. This is done because some patients with a low serum [Na⁺] do not have low osmolality. The clinical effects of hyponatremia are secondary to the associated low osmolality. Without a low osmolality, there is no movement of water into the intracellular space.

A patient with hyponatremia can have a low, normal, or high osmolality. A normal osmolality in combination with hyponatremia occurs in pseudohyponatremia. Children with elevation of serum glucose concentration or of another effective osmole (mannitol) have a high plasma osmolality and hyponatremia. The presence of a low osmolality indicates "true" hyponatremia. Patients with low osmolality are at risk for neurologic symptoms and require further evaluation to determine the etiology of the hyponatremia.

In some situations, true hyponatremia is present despite a normal or elevated plasma osmolality. The presence of an ineffective osmole, usually urea, increases the plasma osmolality, but because the osmole has the same concentration in the ICS, it does not cause fluid to move into the ECS. There is no dilution of the serum Na⁺ by water, and the [Na⁺] remains unchanged if the ineffective osmole is eliminated. Most importantly, the ineffective osmole does not protect the brain from edema caused by hyponatremia. Therefore, a patient may have symptoms of hyponatremia despite having a normal or increased osmolality because of uremia.

In patients with true hyponatremia, the next step in the diagnostic process is to clinically evaluate the volume status. Patients with hyponatremia can be hypovolemic, hypervolemic, or euvolemic. The diagnosis of volume depletion relies on the usual findings with dehydration (see Chapter 70), although subtle volume depletion may not be clinically apparent. Children with hypervolemia are **edematous** on physical examination. They may have ascites, pulmonary edema, pleural effusion, or hypertension.

Hypovolemic hyponatremia can have renal or nonrenal causes. The urine [Na⁺] is very useful in differentiating between renal and nonrenal causes. When the losses are nonrenal and the kidney is working properly, there is renal retention of Na⁺, a normal homeostatic response to volume depletion. Thus the urinary [Na⁺] is low, typically <10 mEq/L, although Na⁺ conservation in neonates is less avid. When the kidney is the cause of the Na⁺ loss, the urine [Na⁺] is >20 mEq/L, reflecting the defect in renal Na⁺ retention. The interpretation of the urine Na⁺ level is challenging with diuretic therapy because it is high when diuretics are being used but low after the diuretic effect is gone. This becomes an issue only when diuretic use is surreptitious. The urine [Na⁺] is not useful if a metabolic alkalosis is present; the urine [Cl⁻] must be used instead (see Chapter 68.7).

Differentiating among the nonrenal causes of hypovolemic hyponatremia is usually facilitated by the history. Although the renal causes are more challenging to distinguish, a high serum [K⁺] is associated with disorders in which the Na⁺ wasting is caused by absence of or ineffectiveness of aldosterone.

In the patient with hypervolemic hyponatremia, the urine [Na⁺] is a helpful parameter. It is usually <10 mEq/L, except in the patient with renal failure.

Treatment

The management of hyponatremia is based on the pathophysiology of the specific etiology. The management of all causes requires judicious monitoring and avoidance of an overly quick normalization of the serum [Na⁺]. A patient with severe symptoms (seizures), no matter the etiology, should be given a bolus of hypertonic saline to produce a small, rapid increase in serum sodium. *Hypoxia worsens cerebral edema, and hyponatremia may exacerbate hypoxic cell swelling.* Therefore, pulse oximetry should be monitored and hypoxia aggressively corrected.

With all causes of hyponatremia, it is important to avoid overly rapid correction, which may cause **central pontine myelinolysis (CPM)**. This syndrome, which occurs within several days of rapid correction of hyponatremia, produces neurologic symptoms, including confusion, agitation, flaccid or spastic quadriparesis, and death. There are usually characteristic pathologic and radiologic changes in the brain, especially in the pons, but extrapontine lesions are quite common and may cause additional symptoms. Despite severe symptoms, full recovery does occur in some patients.

CPM is more common in patients who are treated for *chronic* hyponatremia than for acute hyponatremia. Presumably, this difference is based on the adaptation of brain cells to the hyponatremia. The reduced intracellular osmolality, an adaptive mechanism for chronic hyponatremia, makes brain cells susceptible to dehydration during rapid correction of the hyponatremia, which may be the mechanism of CPM. Even though CPM is rare in pediatric patients, it is advisable to avoid correcting the serum [Na⁺] by >10 mEq/L/24 hr or >18 mEq/L/48 hr. Desmopressin is a potential option if the serum [Na⁺] is increasing too rapidly. This guideline *does not* apply to acute hyponatremia, as may occur with water intoxication, because the hyponatremia is more often symptomatic, and the adaptive decrease in brain osmolality has not had time to occur. The consequences of brain edema in acute hyponatremia exceed the small risk of CPM.

Patients with hyponatremia can have severe neurologic symptoms, such as seizures and coma. The seizures associated with hyponatremia generally are poorly responsive to anticonvulsants. The child with hyponatremia and severe symptoms needs treatment that will quickly reduce cerebral edema. This goal is best accomplished by increasing the extracellular osmolality so that water moves down its osmolar gradient from the ICS to the ECS.

Intravenous hypertonic saline rapidly increases serum [Na⁺], and the effect on serum osmolality leads to a decrease in brain edema. Each mL/kg of 3% NaCl increases the serum [Na⁺] by approximately 1 mEq/L. A child with active symptoms often improves after receiving 4-6 mL/kg of 3% NaCl.

The child with **hypovolemic hyponatremia** has a deficiency in Na⁺ and may have a deficiency in water. The cornerstone of therapy is to replace the Na⁺ deficit and any water deficit present. The first step in treating any dehydrated patient is to restore the intravascular volume with isotonic saline. Ultimately, complete restoration of intravascular volume suppresses ADH production, thereby permitting excretion of the excess water. Chapter 70 discusses the management of hyponatremic dehydration.

The management of **hypervolemic hyponatremia** is difficult; patients have an excess of both water and Na⁺. Administration of Na⁺ leads to worsening volume overload and edema. In addition, patients are retaining water and Na⁺ because of their ineffective intravascular volume or renal insufficiency. The cornerstone of therapy is water and Na⁺ restriction, because patients have volume overload. Diuretics may help by causing excretion of both Na⁺ and water. Vasopressin antagonists (**vaptans**), by blocking the action of ADH and causing a water diuresis, are effective in correcting the hypervolemic hyponatremia caused by heart failure. Vaptans are contraindicated if there are moderate to severe CNS symptoms.

Hyponatremic patients with low albumin from nephrotic syndrome have a better response to diuretics after an infusion of 25% albumin; the [Na⁺] often normalizes as a result of expansion of the intravascular volume. A child with heart failure may have an increase in renal water and Na⁺ excretion if there is an improvement in cardiac output. This improvement will "turn off" the regulatory hormones causing renal water (ADH) and Na⁺ (aldosterone) retention. The patient with renal failure cannot respond to any of these therapies except fluid restriction. Insensible fluid losses eventually result in an increase in the [Na⁺] as long as insensible and urinary losses are greater than intake. A more definitive approach in children with renal failure is to perform dialysis, which removes water and Na⁺.

In **isovolumic hyponatremia** there is usually an excess of water and a mild Na⁺ deficit. Therapy is directed at eliminating the excess water. The child with acute excessive water intake loses water in the urine because ADH production is turned off as a result of the low plasma osmolality. Children may correct their hyponatremia spontaneously over 3-6 hr. For acute, symptomatic hyponatremia as a result of water intoxication, hypertonic saline may be needed to reverse cerebral edema. For chronic hyponatremia from poor solute intake, the child needs an appropriate formula, and excess water intake should be eliminated.

Children with **iatrogenic hyponatremia** caused by the administration of hypotonic IV fluids should receive 3% saline if symptomatic. Subsequent management is dictated by the patient's volume status. The hypovolemic child should receive isotonic IV fluids. The child with nonphysiologic stimuli for ADH production should undergo fluid restriction. Prevention of this iatrogenic complication requires judicious use of IV fluids (see Chapter 69).

Specific hormone replacement is the cornerstone of therapy for the hyponatremia of hypothyroidism or cortisol deficiency. Correction of the underlying defect permits appropriate elimination of the excess water.

SIADH is a condition of excess water, with limited ability of the kidney to excrete water. The mainstay of its therapy is fluid restriction with normal sodium intake. Furosemide and NaCl supplementation are effective in the patient with SIADH and *severe* hyponatremia. Even in a patient with SIADH, furosemide causes an increase in water and Na⁺ excretion. The loss of Na⁺ is somewhat counterproductive, but this Na⁺ can be replaced with hypertonic saline. Because the patient has a net loss of water and the urinary losses of Na⁺ have been replaced, there is an increase in the [Na⁺], but no significant increase in blood pressure. Vaptans, which block the action of ADH and cause a water diuresis, are effective at correcting **euvolemic hyponatremia**, but overly rapid correction is a potential complication. Vaptans are not appropriate for treating symptomatic hyponatremia because it can take a few hours before the water diuresis occurs.

Treatment of chronic SIADH is challenging. Fluid restriction in children is difficult for nutritional and behavioral reasons. Other options are long-term furosemide therapy with Na⁺ supplementation, an oral vaptan (tolvaptan), or oral urea.

Bibliography is available at Expert Consult.

68.4 Potassium

Larry A. Greenbaum

POTASSIUM METABOLISM
Body Content and Physiologic Function

The intracellular [K^+], approximately 150 mEq/L, is much higher than the plasma [K^+] (see Fig. 68.3). The majority of body K^+ is contained in muscle. As muscle mass increases, there is an increase in body K^+. Thus an increase in body K^+ occurs during puberty, and it is more significant in males. The majority of extracellular K^+ is in bone; <1% of total body K^+ is in plasma.

Because most K^+ is intracellular, the plasma concentration does not always reflect the total body K^+ content. A variety of conditions alter the distribution of K^+ between the intracellular and extracellular compartments. Na^+,K^+-ATPase maintains the high intracellular [K^+] by pumping Na^+ out of the cell and K^+ into the cell. This activity balances the normal leak of K^+ out of cells via potassium channels that is driven by the favorable chemical gradient. Insulin increases K^+ movement into cells by activating Na^+,K^+-ATPase. Hyperkalemia stimulates insulin secretion, which helps mitigate the hyperkalemia. Acid-base status affects K^+ distribution, probably via K^+ channels and the Na^+,K^+-ATPase. A decrease in pH drives potassium extracellularly; an increase in pH has the opposite effect. β-Adrenergic agonists stimulate the Na^+,K^+-ATPase, increasing cellular uptake of K^+. This increase is protective, in that hyperkalemia stimulates adrenal release of catecholamines. α-Adrenergic agonists and exercise cause a net movement of K^+ out of the ICS. An increase in plasma osmolality, as with mannitol infusion, leads to water movement out of the cells, and K^+ follows as a result of solvent drag. The serum [K^+] increases by approximately 0.6 mEq/L with each 10 mOsm rise in plasma osmolality.

The high intracellular concentration of K^+, the principal intracellular cation, is maintained through Na^+,K^+-ATPase. The resulting chemical gradient is used to produce the resting membrane potential of cells. K^+ is necessary for the electrical responsiveness of nerve and muscle cells and for the contractility of cardiac, skeletal, and smooth muscle. The changes in membrane polarization that occur during muscle contraction or nerve conduction make these cells susceptible to changes in serum [K^+]. The ratio of intracellular to extracellular K^+ determines the threshold for a cell to generate an action potential and the rate of cellular repolarization. The intracellular [K^+] affects cellular enzymes. K^+ is necessary for maintaining cell volume because of its important contribution to intracellular osmolality.

Potassium Intake

Potassium is plentiful in food. Dietary consumption varies considerably, even though 1-2 mEq/kg is the recommended intake. The intestines normally absorb approximately 90% of ingested K^+. Most absorption occurs in the small intestine, whereas the colon exchanges body K^+ for luminal Na^+. Regulation of intestinal losses normally has a minimal role in maintaining potassium homeostasis, although renal failure, aldosterone, and glucocorticoids increase colonic secretion of K^+. The increase in intestinal losses in the setting of renal failure and hyperkalemia, which stimulates aldosterone production, is clinically significant, helping to protect against hyperkalemia.

Potassium Excretion

Some loss of K^+ occurs in sweat but is normally minimal. The colon has the ability to eliminate some K^+. In addition, after an acute K^+ load, much of the K^+, >40%, moves intracellularly, through the actions of epinephrine and insulin, which are produced in response to hyperkalemia. This process provides transient protection from hyperkalemia, but most ingested K^+ is eventually excreted in the urine. The kidneys principally regulate long-term K^+ balance, and they alter excretion in response to a variety of signals. K^+ is freely filtered at the glomerulus, but 90% is resorbed before reaching the distal tubule and collecting duct, the principal sites of K^+ regulation that have the ability to absorb and secrete K^+. The amount of tubular secretion regulates the amount of K^+ that appears in the urine. The plasma [K^+] directly influences secretion in the distal nephron. As the [K^+] increases, secretion increases.

The principal hormone regulating potassium secretion is **aldosterone**, which is released by the adrenal cortex in response to increased plasma K^+. Its main site of action is the cortical collecting duct, where aldosterone stimulates Na^+ movement from the tubule into the cells. This movement creates a negative charge in the tubular lumen, facilitating K^+ excretion. In addition, the increased intracellular Na^+ stimulates the basolateral Na^+,K^+-ATPase, causing more K^+ to move into the cells lining the cortical collecting duct. Glucocorticoids, ADH, a high urinary flow rate, and high Na^+ delivery to the distal nephron also increase urinary K^+ excretion. Insulin, catecholamines, and urinary ammonia decrease K^+ excretion. Whereas ADH increases K^+ secretion, it also causes water resorption, decreasing urinary flow. The net effect is that ADH has little overall impact on K^+ balance. Alkalosis causes potassium to move into cells, including the cells lining the collecting duct. This movement increases K^+ secretion, and because acidosis has the opposite effect, it decreases K^+ secretion.

The kidney can dramatically vary K^+ excretion in response to changes in intake. Normally, approximately 10–15% of the filtered load is excreted. In an adult, excretion of K^+ can vary from 5-1,000 mEq/day.

HYPERKALEMIA

Hyperkalemia—because of the potential for lethal arrhythmias—is one of the most alarming electrolyte abnormalities.

Etiology and Pathophysiology

Three basic mechanisms cause hyperkalemia (Table 68.4). In the individual patient, the etiology is sometimes multifactorial.

Spurious hyperkalemia or **pseudohyperkalemia** is very common in children because of the difficulties in obtaining blood specimens. This laboratory result is usually caused by hemolysis during a heelstick or phlebotomy, but it can be the result of prolonged tourniquet application or fist clenching, either of which causes local potassium release from muscle.

The serum [K^+] is normally 0.4 mEq/L higher than the plasma value, secondary to K^+ release from cells during clot formation. This phenomenon is exaggerated with thrombocytosis because of K^+ release from platelets. For every 100,000/m^3 increase in the platelet count, the serum [K^+] rises by approximately 0.15 mEq/L. This phenomenon also occurs with the marked white blood cell (WBC) count elevations sometimes seen with leukemia. Elevated WBC counts, typically >200,000/m^3, can cause a dramatic elevation in the serum [K^+]. Analysis of a plasma sample usually provides an accurate result. It is important to analyze the sample promptly to avoid K^+ release from cells, which occurs if the sample is stored in the cold, or cellular uptake of K^+ and spurious hypokalemia, which occurs with storage at high temperatures. Pneumatic tube transport can cause pseudohyperkalemia if cell membranes are fragile (leukemia). Occasionally, heparin causes lysis of leukemic cells and a false elevation of the plasma sample; a blood gas syringe has less heparin and may provide a more accurate reading than a standard tube. There are rare genetic disorders causing in vitro leakage of K^+ from red blood cells (RBCs) that may causes familial pseudohyperkalemia.

Because of the kidney's ability to excrete K^+, it is unusual for excessive intake, by itself, to cause hyperkalemia. This condition can occur in a patient who is receiving large quantities of IV or oral K^+ for excessive losses that are no longer present. Frequent or rapid blood transfusions can acutely increase the [K^+] because of the K^+ content of blood, which is variably elevated. Increased intake may precipitate hyperkalemia if there is an underlying defect in K^+ excretion.

The ICS has a very high [K^+], so a shift of K^+ from the ICS to the ECS can have a significant effect on the plasma [K^+]. This shift occurs with metabolic acidosis, but the effect is minimal with an organic acid (lactic acidosis, ketoacidosis). A respiratory acidosis has less impact than a metabolic acidosis. Cell destruction, as seen with rhabdomyolysis, tumor lysis syndrome, tissue necrosis, or hemolysis, releases K^+ into the extracellular milieu. The K^+ released from RBCs in internal bleeding, such as hematomas, is resorbed and enters the ECS.

Normal doses of succinylcholine or β-blockers and fluoride or digitalis intoxication all cause a shift of K^+ out of the intracellular compartment. *Succinylcholine should not be used during anesthesia in patients at risk for hyperkalemia.* β-Blockers prevent the normal cellular uptake of K^+ mediated by binding of β-agonists to the $β_2$-adrenergic receptors. K^+

Table 68.4	Causes of Hyperkalemia

SPURIOUS LABORATORY VALUE
Hemolysis
Tissue ischemia during blood drawing
Thrombocytosis
Leukocytosis
Familial pseudohyperkalemia (OMIM 609153/611184/612126)

INCREASED INTAKE
Intravenous or oral
Blood transfusions

TRANSCELLULAR SHIFTS
Acidosis
Rhabdomyolysis
Tumor lysis syndrome
Tissue necrosis
Hemolysis/hematomas/gastrointestinal bleeding
Succinylcholine
Digitalis intoxication
Fluoride intoxication
β-Adrenergic blockers
Exercise
Hyperosmolality
Insulin deficiency
Malignant hyperthermia (OMIM 145600/601887)
Hyperkalemic periodic paralysis (OMIM 170500)

DECREASED EXCRETION
Renal failure
Primary adrenal disease
    Acquired Addison disease
    21-Hydroxylase deficiency (OMIM 201910)
    3β-Hydroxysteroid dehydrogenase deficiency (OMIM 201810)
    Lipoid congenital adrenal hyperplasia (OMIM 201710)
    Adrenal hypoplasia congenita (OMIM 300200)
    Aldosterone synthase deficiency (OMIM 203400/610600)
    Adrenoleukodystrophy (OMIM 300100)
Hyporeninemic hypoaldosteronism
    Urinary tract obstruction
    Sickle cell disease (OMIM 603903)
    Kidney transplant
    Lupus nephritis
Renal tubular disease
    Pseudohypoaldosteronism type I (OMIM 264350/177735)
    Pseudohypoaldosteronism type II (OMIM 145260)
    Bartter syndrome, type 2 (OMIM 241200)
    Urinary tract obstruction
    Kidney transplant
Medications
    Renin inhibitors
    Angiotensin-converting enzyme inhibitors
    Angiotensin II blockers
    Potassium-sparing diuretics
    Calcineurin inhibitors
    Nonsteroidal antiinflammatory drugs
    Trimethoprim
    Heparin
    Drospirenone (in some oral contraceptives)

OMIM, database number from the Online Mendelian Inheritance in Man (http://www.ncbi.nlm.nih.gov/omim).

release from muscle cells occurs during exercise, and levels can increase by 1-2 mEq/L with high activity. With an increased plasma osmolality, water moves from the ICS, and K^+ follows. This process occurs with hyperglycemia, although in nondiabetic patients the resultant increase in insulin causes K^+ to move intracellularly. In **diabetic ketoacidosis (DKA)**, the absence of insulin causes potassium to leave the ICS, and the problem is compounded by the hyperosmolality. The effect of hyperosmolality causes a transcellular shift of K^+ into the ECS after mannitol or hypertonic saline infusions. **Malignant hyperthermia**, which is triggered by some inhaled anesthetics, causes muscle release of potassium (see Chapter 629.2). **Hyperkalemic periodic paralysis** is an autosomal dominant disorder caused by a mutated Na^+ channel. It results in episodic cellular release of K^+ and attacks of paralysis (see Chapter 629.1).

The kidneys excrete most of the daily K^+ intake, so a decrease in kidney function can cause hyperkalemia. Newborn infants in general, and especially premature infants, have decreased kidney function at birth and thus are at increased risk for hyperkalemia despite an absence of intrinsic renal disease. Neonates also have decreased expression of K^+ channels, further limiting K^+ excretion.

A wide range of primary **adrenal disorders**, both hereditary and acquired, can cause decreased production of aldosterone, with secondary hyperkalemia (see Chapters 593 and 594). Patients with these disorders typically have metabolic acidosis and salt wasting with hyponatremia. Children with subtle adrenal insufficiency may have electrolyte problems only during acute illnesses. The most common form of **congenital adrenal hyperplasia**, 21-hydroxylase deficiency, typically manifests in male infants as hyperkalemia, metabolic acidosis, hyponatremia, and volume depletion. Females with this disorder usually are diagnosed as newborns because of their ambiguous genitalia; treatment prevents the development of electrolyte problems.

Renin, via angiotensin II, stimulates aldosterone production. A deficiency in renin, a result of kidney damage, can lead to decreased aldosterone production. **Hyporeninemia** occurs in many kidney diseases, with some of the more common pediatric causes listed in Table 68.4. These patients typically have hyperkalemia and a metabolic acidosis, without hyponatremia. Some of these patients have impaired renal function, partially accounting for the hyperkalemia, but the impairment in K^+ excretion is more extreme than expected for the degree of renal insufficiency.

A variety of **renal tubular disorders** impair renal excretion of K^+. Children with **pseudohypoaldosteronism type 1** have hyperkalemia, metabolic acidosis, and salt wasting (kidney, colon, sweat) leading to hyponatremia and volume depletion; aldosterone values are elevated. In the autosomal recessive variant, there is a defect in the renal Na^+ channel that is normally activated by aldosterone. Patients with this variant have severe symptoms (failure to thrive, diarrhea, recurrent respiratory infections, miliaria-rubra like rash), beginning in infancy. Patients with the autosomal dominant form have a defect in the aldosterone receptor, and the disease is milder, often remitting in adulthood. **Pseudohypoaldosteronism type 2 (familial hyperkalemic hypertension)**, also called **Gordon syndrome**, is an autosomal dominant disorder characterized by hypertension caused by salt retention and impaired excretion of K^+ and acid, leading to hyperkalemia and hyperchloremic metabolic acidosis. Activating mutations in either *WNK1* or *WNK4*, both serine-threonine kinases located in the distal nephron, cause Gordon syndrome. Patients may respond well to thiazide diuretics. In **Bartter syndrome**, caused by mutations in the potassium channel *ROMK* (type 2 Bartter syndrome), there can be transient hyperkalemia in neonates, but hypokalemia subsequently develops (see Chapter 549.1).

Acquired renal tubular dysfunction, with an impaired ability to excrete K^+, occurs in a number of conditions. These disorders, all characterized by **tubulointerstitial disease**, are often associated with impaired acid secretion and a secondary metabolic acidosis. In some affected children, the metabolic acidosis is the dominant feature, although a high K^+ intake may unmask the defect in K^+ handling. The tubular dysfunction can cause renal salt wasting, potentially leading to hyponatremia. Because of the tubulointerstitial damage, these conditions may also cause hyperkalemia as a result of hyporeninemic hypoaldosteronism.

The risk of hyperkalemia resulting from **medications** is greatest in patients with underlying renal insufficiency. The predominant mechanism of medication-induced hyperkalemia is impaired renal excretion, although ACE inhibitors may worsen hyperkalemia in anuric patients, probably by inhibiting GI potassium loss, which is normally upregulated in renal insufficiency. The hyperkalemia caused by trimethoprim generally occurs only at the very high doses used to treat *Pneumocystis jiroveci* pneumonia. Potassium-sparing diuretics may easily cause hyperkalemia, especially because they are often used in patients receiving oral K^+ supplements. Oral contraceptives containing drospirenone, which blocks the action of aldosterone, may cause hyperkalemia and should not be used in patients with decreased renal function.

Clinical Manifestations

The most important effects of hyperkalemia result from the role of K^+ in membrane polarization. The cardiac conduction system is usually the dominant concern. Changes in the electrocardiogram (ECG) begin with peaking of the T waves. This is followed, as K^+ level increases, by ST-segment depression, an increased PR interval, flattening of the P wave, and widening of the QRS complex. However, the correlation between K^+ level and ECG changes is poor. This process can eventually progress to ventricular fibrillation. Asystole may also occur. Some patients have paresthesias, fasciculations, weakness, and even an ascending paralysis, but cardiac toxicity usually precedes these clinical symptoms, emphasizing the danger of assuming that an absence of symptoms implies an absence of danger. Chronic hyperkalemia is generally better tolerated than acute hyperkalemia.

Diagnosis

The etiology of hyperkalemia is often readily apparent. Spurious hyperkalemia is very common in children, so obtaining a 2nd potassium measurement is often appropriate. If there is a significant elevation of WBC or platelet count, the 2nd measurement should be performed on a plasma sample that is evaluated promptly. The history should initially focus on potassium intake, risk factors for transcellular shifts of K^+, medications that cause hyperkalemia, and signs of renal insufficiency, such as oliguria and edema. Initial **laboratory evaluation** should include creatinine, BUN, and assessment of the acid-base status. Many etiologies of hyperkalemia cause **metabolic acidosis**, which worsens hyperkalemia through the transcellular shift of K^+ out of cells. Renal insufficiency is a common cause of the combination of metabolic acidosis and hyperkalemia, also seen in diseases associated with aldosterone insufficiency or aldosterone resistance. Children with absent or ineffective aldosterone often have hyponatremia and volume depletion because of salt wasting. Genetic diseases, such as congenital adrenal hyperplasia and pseudohypoaldosteronism, usually manifest in infancy and should be strongly considered in the infant with hyperkalemia and metabolic acidosis, especially if hyponatremia is present.

It is important to consider the various etiologies of a transcellular K^+ shift. In some of these disorders, the K^+ level continues to increase, despite the elimination of all K^+ intake, especially with concurrent renal insufficiency. This increase is potentially seen in tumor lysis syndrome, hemolysis, rhabdomyolysis, and other causes of cell death. All these entities can cause concomitant hyperphosphatemia and hyperuricemia. **Rhabdomyolysis** produces an elevated creatinine phosphokinase (CPK) value and hypocalcemia, whereas children with hemolysis have hemoglobinuria and a decreasing hematocrit. For the child with diabetes, elevated blood glucose suggests a transcellular shift of K^+.

Treatment

The plasma K^+ level, the ECG, and the risk of the problem worsening determine the aggressiveness of the therapeutic approach. High serum $[K^+]$ and the presence of ECG changes require vigorous treatment. An additional source of concern is the patient in whom plasma K^+ levels are rising despite minimal intake. This situation can happen if there is cellular release of K^+ (tumor lysis syndrome), especially in the setting of diminished excretion (renal failure).

The first action in a child with a concerning elevation of plasma $[K^+]$ is to stop all sources of additional K^+ (oral, intravenous). Washed RBCs can be used for patients who require blood transfusions. If the $[K^+]$ is >6.5 mEq/L, an ECG should be obtained to help assess the urgency of the situation. Peak T waves are the first sign of hyperkalemia, followed by a prolonged PR interval, and when most severe, prolonged QRS complex. Life-threatening ventricular arrhythmias may also develop. The treatment of hyperkalemia has 2 basic goals: (1) to stabilize the heart to prevent life-threatening arrhythmias and (2) to remove K^+ from the body. The treatments that acutely prevent arrhythmias all

have the advantage of working quickly (within minutes) but do not remove K^+ from the body. **Calcium** stabilizes the cell membrane of heart cells, preventing arrhythmias; it is given intravenously over a few minutes, and its action is almost immediate. Calcium should be given over 30 min in a patient receiving digitalis; otherwise the calcium may cause arrhythmias. **Bicarbonate** causes potassium to move intracellularly, lowering the plasma $[K^+]$; it is most efficacious in a patient with a metabolic acidosis. **Insulin** causes K^+ to move intracellularly but must be given with **glucose** to avoid hypoglycemia. The combination of insulin and glucose works within 30 min. Nebulized **albuterol**, by stimulation of β_1-adrenergic receptors, leads to rapid intracellular movement of K^+. This has the advantage of not requiring an IV route of administration, allowing it to be given concurrently with the other measures.

It is critical to begin measures that remove K^+ from the body. In patients who are not anuric, a **loop diuretic** increases renal excretion of K^+. A high dose may be required in a patient with significant renal insufficiency. **Sodium polystyrene sulfonate** (**SPS**; Kayexalate) is an exchange resin that is given either rectally or orally. **Patiromer** is an oral exchange resin for treating hyperkalemia. Some patients require **dialysis** for acute K^+ removal. Dialysis is often necessary if the patient has either severe renal failure or an especially high rate of endogenous K^+ release, as is sometimes present with tumor lysis syndrome or rhabdomyolysis. Hemodialysis rapidly lowers plasma $[K^+]$. Peritoneal dialysis is not nearly as quick or reliable, but it is usually adequate as long as the acute problem can be managed with medications and the endogenous release of K^+ is not high.

Long-term management of hyperkalemia includes reducing intake through dietary changes and eliminating or reducing medications that cause hyperkalemia (see Chapter 550). Some patients require medications to increase potassium excretion, such as SPS, patiromer and loop or thiazide diuretics. Some infants with chronic renal failure may need to start dialysis to allow adequate caloric intake without hyperkalemia. It is unusual for an older child to require dialysis principally to control chronic hyperkalemia. The disorders caused by aldosterone deficiency respond to replacement therapy with fludrocortisone.

HYPOKALEMIA

Hypokalemia is common in children, with most cases related to gastroenteritis.

Etiology and Pathophysiology

There are 4 basic mechanisms of hypokalemia (Table 68.5). **Spurious hypokalemia** occurs in patients with leukemia and very elevated WBC counts if plasma for analysis is left at room temperature, permitting the WBCs to take up K^+ from the plasma. With a transcellular shift, there is no change in total body K^+, although there may be concomitant potassium depletion resulting from other factors. Decreased intake, extrarenal losses, and renal losses are all associated with total body K^+ depletion.

Because the intracellular $[K^+]$ is much higher than the plasma level, a significant amount of K^+ can move into cells without greatly changing the intracellular $[K^+]$. **Alkalemia** is one of the more common causes of a transcellular shift. The effect is much greater with a *metabolic alkalosis* than with a *respiratory alkalosis*. The impact of exogenous insulin on K^+ movement into the cells is substantial in patients with DKA. Endogenous insulin may be the cause when a patient is given a bolus of glucose. Both endogenous (epinephrine in stress) and exogenous (albuterol) β-adrenergic agonists stimulate cellular uptake of K^+. Theophylline overdose, barium intoxication, administration of cesium chloride (a homeopathic cancer remedy), and toluene intoxication from paint or glue sniffing can cause a transcellular shift hypokalemia, often with severe clinical manifestations. Children with **hypokalemic periodic paralysis**, a rare autosomal dominant disorder, have acute cellular uptake of K^+ (see Chapter 629). **Thyrotoxic periodic paralysis**, which is more common in Asians, is an unusual initial manifestation of hyperthyroidism. Affected patients have dramatic hypokalemia as a result of a transcellular shift of potassium. Hypokalemia can occur during refeeding syndrome (see Chapters 58 and 364.8).

Inadequate K$^+$ intake occurs in **anorexia nervosa**; accompanying bulimia and laxative or diuretic abuse exacerbates the K$^+$ deficiency. Sweat losses of K$^+$ can be significant during vigorous exercise in a hot climate. Associated volume depletion and hyperaldosteronism increase renal losses of K$^+$ (discussed later). Diarrheal fluid has a high concentration of K$^+$, and hypokalemia as a result of diarrhea is usually associated with metabolic acidosis resulting from stool losses of bicarbonate. In contrast, normal acid-base balance or mild metabolic alkalosis is seen with laxative abuse. Intake of SPS or ingestion of clay because of pica increases stool losses of potassium.

Urinary potassium wasting may be accompanied by a metabolic acidosis (proximal or distal RTA). In DKA, although it is often associated with normal plasma [K$^+$] from transcellular shifts, there is significant total body K$^+$ depletion from urinary losses because of the osmotic diuresis, and the K$^+$ level may decrease dramatically with insulin therapy (see Chapter 607). Both the polyuric phase of acute tubular necrosis and postobstructive diuresis cause transient, highly variable K$^+$ wasting and may be associated with metabolic acidosis. Tubular damage, which occurs either directly from medications or secondary to interstitial nephritis, is often accompanied by other tubular losses, including magnesium, Na$^+$, and water. Such tubular damage may cause a secondary RTA with metabolic acidosis. Isolated magnesium deficiency causes renal K$^+$ wasting. **Penicillin** is an anion excreted in the urine, resulting in increased K$^+$ excretion because the penicillin anion must be accompanied by a cation. Hypokalemia from penicillin therapy occurs only with the *sodium* salt of penicillin, not with the potassium salt.

Urinary K$^+$ wasting is often accompanied by a metabolic alkalosis. This condition is usually associated with increased aldosterone, which increases urinary K$^+$ and acid losses, contributing to the hypokalemia and the metabolic alkalosis. Other mechanisms often contribute to both the K$^+$ losses and the metabolic alkalosis. With emesis or nasogastric suction, there is gastric loss of K$^+$, but this is fairly minimal, given the low K$^+$ content of gastric fluid, approximately 10 mEq/L. More important is the gastric loss of hydrochloric acid (HCl), leading to metabolic alkalosis and a state of volume depletion. The kidney compensates for metabolic alkalosis by excreting bicarbonate in the urine, but there is obligate loss of K$^+$ and Na$^+$ with the bicarbonate. The volume depletion raises aldosterone levels, further increasing urinary K$^+$ losses and preventing correction of metabolic alkalosis and hypokalemia until the volume depletion is corrected.

Urinary chloride (Cl$^-$) is low as a response to the volume depletion. Because the volume depletion is secondary to Cl$^-$ loss, this is a **state of Cl$^-$ deficiency**. There were cases of Cl$^-$ deficiency resulting from infant formula deficient in Cl$^-$, which caused a metabolic alkalosis with hypokalemia and low urine [Cl$^-$]. Current infant formula is not deficient in Cl$^-$. A similar mechanism occurs in cystic fibrosis because of Cl$^-$ loss in sweat. In **congenital chloride-losing diarrhea**, an autosomal recessive disorder, there is high stool loss of Cl$^-$, leading to metabolic alkalosis, an unusual sequela of diarrhea. Because of stool K$^+$ losses, Cl$^-$ deficiency, and metabolic alkalosis, patients with this disorder have hypokalemia. During respiratory acidosis, there is renal compensation, with retention of bicarbonate and excretion of Cl$^-$. After the respiratory acidosis is corrected, the patients have Cl$^-$ deficiency and post–hypercapnic alkalosis with secondary hypokalemia. Patients with Cl$^-$ deficiency, metabolic alkalosis, and hypokalemia have a urinary [Cl$^-$] of <10 mEq/L. Loop and thiazide diuretics lead to hypokalemia, metabolic alkalosis, and Cl$^-$ deficiency. During treatment, these patients have high urine chloride levels resulting from the effect of the diuretic. However, after the diuretics are discontinued, there is residual Cl$^-$ deficiency, the urinary [Cl$^-$] is appropriately low, and neither the hypokalemia nor the alkalosis resolves until the Cl$^-$ deficiency is corrected.

Table 68.5	Causes of Hypokalemia

SPURIOUS LABORATORY VALUE
High white blood cell count
 	
TRANSCELLULAR SHIFTS
Alkalemia
Insulin
α-Adrenergic agonists
Drugs/toxins (theophylline, barium, toluene, cesium chloride, hydroxychloroquine)
Hypokalemic periodic paralysis (OMIM 170400)
Thyrotoxic period paralysis
Refeeding syndrome
 	
DECREASED INTAKE
Anorexia nervosa
 	
EXTRARENAL LOSSES
Diarrhea
Laxative abuse
Sweating
Sodium polystyrene sulfonate (Kayexalate) or clay ingestion
 	
RENAL LOSSES
With Metabolic Acidosis
Distal renal tubular acidosis (OMIM 179800/602722/267300)
Proximal renal tubular acidosis (OMIM 604278)*
Ureterosigmoidostomy
Diabetic ketoacidosis
 	
Without Specific Acid–Base Disturbance
Tubular toxins: amphotericin, cisplatin, aminoglycosides
Interstitial nephritis
	Diuretic phase of acute tubular necrosis
	Postobstructive diuresis
	Hypomagnesemia
	High urine anions (e.g., penicillin or penicillin derivatives)
	
	With Metabolic Alkalosis
	Low urine chloride
	  Emesis or nasogastric suction
	  Chloride-losing diarrhea (OMIM 214700)
	  Cystic fibrosis (OMIM 219700)
	  Low-chloride formula
	  Posthypercapnia
	  Previous loop or thiazide diuretic use
	High urine chloride and normal blood pressure
	  Gitelman syndrome (OMIM 263800)
	  Bartter syndrome (OMIM 241200/607364/602522/601678/300971/
	    601198/613090)
	  Autosomal dominant hypoparathyroidism (OMIM 146200)
	  EAST syndrome (OMIM 612780)
	  Loop and thiazide diuretics (current)
	High urine chloride and high blood pressure
	  Adrenal adenoma or hyperplasia
	  Glucocorticoid-remediable aldosteronism (OMIM 103900)
	  Renovascular disease
	  Renin-secreting tumor
	  17β-Hydroxylase deficiency (OMIM 202110)
	  11β-Hydroxylase deficiency (OMIM 202010)
	  Cushing syndrome
	  11β-Hydroxysteroid dehydrogenase deficiency (OMIM 218030)
	  Licorice ingestion
	  Liddle syndrome (OMIM 177200)

*Most cases of proximal renal tubular acidosis are not caused by this primary genetic disorder. Proximal renal tubular acidosis is usually part of Fanconi syndrome, which has multiple etiologies.

EAST, Epilepsy, ataxia, sensorineural hearing loss, and tubulopathy; OMIM, database number from the Online Mendelian Inheritance in Man (http://www.ncbi.nlm.nih.gov/omim).

The combination of metabolic alkalosis, hypokalemia, high urine [Cl⁻], and normal blood pressure is characteristic of Bartter syndrome, Gitelman syndrome, and current diuretic use. Patients with any of these conditions have high urinary losses of Cl⁻ despite a state of relative volume depletion with secondary hyperaldosteronism (high plasma renin). Bartter and Gitelman syndromes are autosomal recessive disorders caused by defects in tubular transporters (see Chapter 549). **Bartter syndrome** is usually associated with hypercalciuria, and often with nephrocalcinosis, whereas children with **Gitelman syndrome** have low urinary calcium losses but hypomagnesemia because of urinary magnesium losses. Some patients with Bartter syndrome have hypomagnesemia. A transient antenatal form of Bartter syndrome is associated with severe polyhydramnios and mutations in *MAGED2*.

Some patients with hypoparathyroidism and hypocalcemia caused by an activating mutation of the calcium-sensing receptor (**autosomal dominant hypoparathyroidism**) have hypokalemia, hypomagnesemia, and metabolic alkalosis. The reason is that activation of the calcium-sensing receptor in the loop of Henle impairs tubular resorption of sodium and chloride, causing volume depletion and secondary hyperaldosteronism. **EAST syndrome**, an autosomal recessive disorder caused by mutations in the gene for a potassium channel in the kidney, inner ear, and brain, consists of *e*pilepsy, *a*taxia, *s*ensorineural hearing loss, and *t*ubulopathy (hypokalemia, metabolic alkalosis, hypomagnesemia, and hypocalciuria).

In the presence of high aldosterone levels, there is urinary loss of K⁺, hypokalemia, metabolic alkalosis, and elevated urinary [Cl⁻]. Also, renal retention of Na⁺ leads to hypertension. Primary hyperaldosteronism caused by adenoma or hyperplasia is much less common in children than in adults (see Chapters 597 and 598). **Glucocorticoid-remediable aldosteronism**, an autosomal dominant disorder that leads to high levels of aldosterone (but low renin levels), is often diagnosed in childhood, although hypokalemia is not always present.

Increased aldosterone levels may be secondary to increased renin production. Renal artery stenosis leads to hypertension from increased renin and secondary hyperaldosteronism. The increased aldosterone can cause hypokalemia and metabolic alkalosis, although most patients have normal electrolyte levels. Renin-producing tumors, which are extremely rare, can cause hypokalemia.

A variety of disorders cause hypertension and hypokalemia without increased aldosterone levels. Some are a result of increased levels of mineralocorticoids other than aldosterone. Such increases occur in two forms of **congenital adrenal hyperplasia** (see Chapter 594). In **11β-hydroxylase deficiency**, which is associated with virilization, the value of 11-deoxycorticosterone is elevated, causing variable hypertension and hypokalemia. A similar mechanism, increased 11-deoxycorticosterone, occurs in **17α-hydroxylase deficiency**, but patients with this disorder are more uniformly hypertensive and hypokalemic, and they have a defect in sex hormone production. **Cushing syndrome**, frequently associated with hypertension, less frequently causes metabolic alkalosis and hypokalemia, secondary to the mineralocorticoid activity of cortisol. In **11β-hydroxysteroid dehydrogenase deficiency**, an autosomal recessive disorder, the enzymatic defect prevents the conversion of cortisol to cortisone in the kidney. Because cortisol binds to and activates the aldosterone receptor, children with this deficiency have all the features of excessive mineralocorticoids, including hypertension, hypokalemia, and metabolic alkalosis. Patients with this disorder, which is also called **apparent mineralocorticoid excess**, respond to spironolactone therapy, which blocks the mineralocorticoid receptor. An acquired form of 11β-hydroxysteroid dehydrogenase deficiency occurs from the ingestion of substances that inhibit this enzyme. A classic example is glycyrrhizic acid, which is found in natural licorice. **Liddle syndrome** is an autosomal dominant disorder that results from an activating mutation of the distal nephron sodium channel that is normally upregulated by aldosterone. Patients have the characteristics of hyperaldosteronism—hypertension, hypokalemia, and alkalosis—but low serum renin and aldosterone levels. These patients respond to the potassium-sparing diuretics (triamterene and amiloride) that inhibit this sodium channel (see Chapter 549.3). Hypertension exacerbated by pregnancy and syndrome of apparent mineralocortical excess are associated with hypokalemia and low renin levels.

Clinical Manifestations

The heart and skeletal muscle are especially vulnerable to hypokalemia. ECG changes include a flattened T wave, a depressed ST segment, and the appearance of a U wave, which is located between the T wave (if still visible) and the P wave. Ventricular fibrillation and torsades de pointes may occur, although usually only in the context of underlying heart disease. Hypokalemia makes the heart especially susceptible to digitalis-induced arrhythmias, such as supraventricular tachycardia, ventricular tachycardia, and heart block (see Chapter 462).

The clinical consequences of hypokalemia in skeletal muscle include muscle weakness and cramps. Paralysis is a possible complication, generally only at [K⁺] <2.5 mEq/L. It usually starts in the legs and moves to the arms. Respiratory paralysis may require mechanical ventilation. Some patients have rhabdomyolysis; the risk increases with exercise. Hypokalemia slows GI motility. This effect manifests as constipation; with K⁺ levels <2.5 mEq/L, an ileus may occur. Hypokalemia impairs bladder function, potentially leading to urinary retention.

Hypokalemia causes **polyuria** and **polydipsia** by impairing urinary concentrating ability, which produces nephrogenic diabetes insipidus. Hypokalemia stimulates renal ammonia production, an effect that is clinically significant if hepatic failure is present, because the liver cannot metabolize the ammonia. Consequently, hypokalemia may worsen hepatic encephalopathy. Chronic hypokalemia may cause kidney damage, including interstitial nephritis and renal cysts.

Diagnosis

Most causes of hypokalemia are readily apparent from the history. It is important to review the child's diet, GI losses, and medications. Both emesis and diuretic use can be surreptitious. The presence of **hypertension** suggests excess mineralocorticoid effects or levels. Concomitant electrolyte abnormalities are useful clues. The combination of hypokalemia and metabolic acidosis is characteristic of diarrhea and distal and proximal RTA. A concurrent metabolic alkalosis is characteristic of emesis or nasogastric losses, aldosterone excess, use of diuretics, and Bartter and Gitelman syndromes. Fig. 68.4 shows an approach to persistent hypokalemia.

If a clear etiology is not apparent, the measurement of urinary K⁺ distinguishes between renal and extrarenal losses. The kidneys should conserve K⁺ in the presence of extrarenal losses. Urinary K⁺ losses can be assessed with a 24 hr urine collection, spot K⁺:creatinine ratio, fractional excretion of K⁺, or calculation of the *transtubular K⁺ gradient* (TTKG), which is the most widely used approach in children:

$$TTKG = [K]_{urine}/[K]_{plasma} \times (\text{plasma osmolality}/\text{urine osmolality})$$

where [K]ₐᵤᵣᵢₙₑ = urine potassium concentration and [K]ₚₗₐₛₘₐ = plasma potassium concentration.

The urine osmolality must be greater than the serum osmolality for the result of this calculation to be valid. A TTKG >4 in the presence of hypokalemia suggests excessive urinary losses of K⁺. The urinary K⁺ excretion value can be misleading if the stimulus for renal loss, such as a diuretic, is no longer present.

Treatment

Factors that influence the treatment of hypokalemia include the K⁺ level, clinical symptoms, renal function, the presence of transcellular shifts of K⁺, ongoing losses, and the patient's ability to tolerate oral K⁺. Severe, symptomatic hypokalemia requires aggressive treatment. Supplementation is more cautious if renal function is decreased because of the kidney's limited ability to excrete excessive K⁺. The plasma potassium level does not always provide an accurate estimation of the total body K⁺ deficit because there may be shifts of K⁺ from the ICS to the plasma. Clinically, such shifts occur most often with metabolic acidosis and the insulin deficiency of DKA; the plasma [K⁺] measurement underestimates the degree of total body K⁺ depletion. When these problems are corrected, K⁺ moves into the ICS, so more K⁺ supplementation is required to correct the hypokalemia. Likewise, the presence of a transcellular shift of K⁺ into the cells indicates that the total body K⁺ depletion is less severe. In an isolated transcellular shift, as in hypokalemic periodic paralysis, K⁺ supplementation should be used cautiously, given the risk

Chapter 70
Deficit Therapy
Larry A. Greenbaum

第七十章
液体疗法

中文导读

本章主要介绍了液体疗法。其中临床表现部分包括轻、中、重度脱水的症状和体征；实验室检查部分介绍了常用评估儿童水和电解质紊乱的实验室指标，如血清钠、碳酸氢盐、阴离子间隙、血清钾、血尿素氮和肌酐、尿相对密度、血细胞容积等；列举了计算水和电解质缺乏的方法；此外还介绍了严重脱水的治疗；监测和调整治疗包括脱水程度的评估、出入量的监测、体格检查的评估及监测电解质的必要性，最后阐述了低钠、高钠性脱水的处理原则。

Dehydration, most often caused by gastroenteritis, is a common problem in children. Most cases can be managed with oral rehydration (see Chapter 366). *Even children with mild to moderate hyponatremic or hypernatremic dehydration can be managed with oral rehydration.*

CLINICAL MANIFESTATIONS

The 1st step in caring for the child with dehydration is to assess the degree of dehydration (Table 70.1), which dictates both the urgency of the situation and the volume of fluid needed for rehydration. The infant with mild dehydration (3–5% of body weight dehydrated) has few clinical signs or symptoms. The infant may be thirsty; the alert parent may notice a decline in urine output. The history is most helpful. The infant with moderate dehydration has clear physical signs and symptoms. Intravascular space depletion is evident from an increased heart rate

Table 70.1	Clinical Evaluation of Dehydration

Mild dehydration (<5% in an infant; <3% in an older child or adult): Normal or increased pulse; decreased urine output; thirsty; normal physical findings
Moderate dehydration (5–10% in an infant; 3–6% in an older child or adult): Tachycardia; little or no urine output; irritable/lethargic; sunken eyes and fontanel; decreased tears; dry mucous membranes; mild delay in elasticity (skin turgor); delayed capillary refill (>1.5 sec); cool and pale
Severe dehydration (>10% in an infant; >6% in an older child or adult): Peripheral pulses either rapid and weak or absent; decreased blood pressure; no urine output; very sunken eyes and fontanel; no tears; parched mucous membranes; delayed elasticity (poor skin turgor); very delayed capillary refill (>3 sec); cold and mottled; limp, depressed consciousness

and reduced urine output. This patient needs fairly prompt intervention. The infant with severe dehydration is gravely ill. The decrease in blood pressure indicates that vital organs may be receiving inadequate perfusion. Immediate and aggressive intervention is necessary. If possible, the child with severe dehydration should initially receive intravenous (IV) therapy. For older children and adults, mild, moderate, or severe dehydration represents a lower percentage of body weight lost. This difference occurs because water accounts for a higher percentage of body weight in infants (see Chapter 68).

Clinical assessment of dehydration is only an estimate; thus the patient must be continually reevaluated during therapy. The degree of dehydration is underestimated in hypernatremic dehydration because the movement of water from the intracellular space (ICS) to the extracellular space (ECS) helps preserve the intravascular volume.

The history usually suggests the etiology of the dehydration and may predict whether the patient will have a normal sodium concentration (isotonic dehydration), hyponatremic dehydration, or hypernatremic dehydration. The neonate with dehydration caused by poor intake of breast milk often has hypernatremic dehydration. **Hypernatremic dehydration** is likely in any child with losses of hypotonic fluid and poor water intake, as may occur with diarrhea, and poor oral intake because of anorexia or emesis. **Hyponatremic dehydration** occurs in the child with diarrhea who is taking in large quantities of low-salt fluid, such as water or formula.

Some children with dehydration are appropriately thirsty, but in others the lack of intake is part of the pathophysiology of the dehydration. Even though decreased urine output is present in most children with dehydration, good urine output may be deceptively present if a child has an underlying renal defect, such as diabetes insipidus or a salt-wasting nephropathy, or in infants with hypernatremic dehydration.

Physical examination findings are usually proportional to the degree of dehydration. Parents may be helpful in assessment of the child for the presence of sunken eyes, because this finding may be subtle. Pinching and gently twisting the skin of the abdominal or thoracic wall detects tenting of the skin (turgor, elasticity). Tented skin remains in a pinched position rather than springing quickly back to normal. It is difficult to properly assess tenting of the skin in premature infants or severely malnourished children. Activation of the sympathetic nervous system causes **tachycardia** in children with intravascular volume depletion; diaphoresis may also be present. Postural changes in blood pressure are often helpful for evaluating and assessing the response to therapy in children with dehydration. **Tachypnea** in children with dehydration may be present secondary to a metabolic acidosis from stool losses of bicarbonate or lactic acidosis from shock (see Chapter 88).

LABORATORY FINDINGS

Several laboratory findings are useful for evaluating the child with dehydration. The serum sodium concentration determines the type of dehydration. **Metabolic acidosis** may be a result of stool bicarbonate losses in children with diarrhea, secondary renal insufficiency, or lactic acidosis from shock. The anion gap is useful for differentiating among the various causes of a metabolic acidosis (see Chapter 68). Emesis or nasogastric losses usually cause a **metabolic alkalosis**. The serum potassium (K^+) concentration may be low as a result of diarrheal losses. In children with dehydration as a result of emesis, gastric K^+ losses, metabolic alkalosis, and urinary K^+ losses all contribute to hypokalemia. Metabolic acidosis, which causes a shift of K^+ out of cells, and renal insufficiency may lead to hyperkalemia. A combination of mechanisms may be present; thus, it may be difficult to predict the child's acid-base status or serum K^+ level from the history alone.

The blood urea nitrogen (BUN) value and serum creatinine concentration are useful in assessing the child with dehydration. Volume depletion without parenchymal renal injury may cause a disproportionate increase in the BUN with little or no change in the creatinine concentration. This condition is secondary to increased passive resorption of urea in the proximal tubule as a result of appropriate renal conservation of sodium and water. The increase in the BUN with moderate or severe dehydration may be absent or blunted in the child with poor protein intake, because urea production depends on protein degradation. The BUN may be disproportionately increased in the child with increased urea production, as occurs with a gastrointestinal bleed or with the use of glucocorticoids, which increase catabolism. A significant elevation of the creatinine concentration suggests renal insufficiency, although a small, transient increase can occur with dehydration. **Acute kidney injury** (see Chapter 550.1) because of volume depletion is the most common etiology of renal insufficiency in a child with volume depletion, but occasionally the child may have previously undetected chronic renal insufficiency or an alternative explanation for the acute renal failure. **Renal vein thrombosis** is a well-described sequela of severe dehydration in infants; findings may include thrombocytopenia and hematuria (see Chapter 540.2).

Hemoconcentration from dehydration causes increases in hematocrit, hemoglobin, and serum proteins. These values normalize with rehydration. A normal hemoglobin concentration during acute dehydration may mask an underlying anemia. A decreased albumin level in a dehydrated patient suggests a chronic disease, such as malnutrition, nephrotic syndrome, or liver disease, or an acute process, such as capillary leak. An acute or chronic protein-losing enteropathy may also cause a low serum albumin concentration.

CALCULATION OF THE FLUID DEFICIT

Determining the fluid deficit necessitates clinical determination of the percentage of dehydration and multiplication of this percentage by the patient's weight; a child who weighs 10 kg and is 10% dehydrated has a fluid deficit of 1 L.

APPROACH TO SEVERE DEHYDRATION

The child with dehydration needs acute intervention to ensure that there is adequate tissue perfusion. This resuscitation phase requires rapid restoration of the circulating intravascular volume and treatment

of **shock** with an isotonic solution, such as normal saline (NS), Ringer lactate (lactated Ringer solution, LR), or PlasmaLyte (see Chapter 88). The child is given a fluid bolus, usually 20 mL/kg of the isotonic fluid, over approximately 20 min. The child with severe dehydration may require multiple fluid boluses and may need to receive the boluses as fast as possible. In a child with a known or probable metabolic alkalosis (e.g., child with isolated vomiting), LR or PlasmaLyte should not be used because the lactate or acetate would worsen the alkalosis. However, LR or PlasmaLyte may be preferable to NS in shock since it is a balanced solution (see Chapter 69); NS may cause a hyperchloremic metabolic acidosis.

Colloids, such as blood, 5% albumin, and plasma, are rarely needed for fluid boluses. A crystalloid solution (NS or LR) is satisfactory, with both lower risk of infection and lower cost. Blood is obviously indicated in the child with significant anemia or acute blood loss. Plasma is useful for children with a coagulopathy. The child with hypoalbuminemia may benefit from 5% albumin, although there is evidence that albumin infusions increase mortality in adults. The volume and the infusion rate for colloids are generally modified compared with crystalloids (see Chapter 500).

The initial resuscitation and rehydration phase is complete when the child has an adequate intravascular volume. Typically, the child shows clinical improvement, including a lower heart rate, normalization of blood pressure, improved perfusion, better urine output, and a more alert affect.

With adequate intravascular volume, it is appropriate to plan the fluid therapy for the next 24 hr. A general approach is outlined in Table 70.2, with the caveat that there are many different approaches to correcting dehydration. A balanced solution can be substituted for NS. In isonatremic or hyponatremic dehydration, the entire fluid deficit is corrected over 24 hr; a slower approach is used for hypernatremic dehydration (discussed later). The volume of isotonic fluids that the patient has received is subtracted from this total. The remaining fluid volume is then administered over 24 hr. The potassium concentration may need to be decreased or, less frequently, increased, depending on the clinical situation. Potassium is not usually included in the IV fluids until the patient voids and normal renal function is documented by measurement of BUN and creatinine. Children with significant ongoing losses need to receive an appropriate replacement solution (see Chapter 69).

MONITORING AND ADJUSTING THERAPY

The formulation of a plan for correcting a child's dehydration is only the beginning of management. *All calculations in fluid therapy are only approximations.* This statement is especially true for the assessment of percentage dehydration. It is equally important to monitor the patient during treatment and to modify therapy on the basis of the clinical situation. Table 70.3 lists the cornerstones of patient monitoring. The patient's vital signs are useful indicators of intravascular volume status. The child with decreased blood pressure and an increased heart rate will probably benefit from a fluid bolus.

The patient's intake and output are critically important in the dehydrated child. The child who, after 8 hr of therapy, has more output than input because of continuing diarrhea needs to be started on a replacement solution. See the guidelines in Chapter 69 for selecting an appropriate replacement solution. Urine output is useful for evaluating the success

Table 70.2	Fluid Management of Dehydration

Restore intravascular volume:
    Isotonic fluid (NS or LR): 20 mL/kg over 20 min
    Repeat as needed
Calculate 24 hr fluid needs: maintenance + deficit volume
Subtract isotonic fluid already administered from 24 hr fluid needs
Administer remaining volume over 24 hr using 5% dextrose NS + 20 mEq/L KCl
Replace ongoing losses as they occur

LR, Ringer lactate; NS, normal saline.

Table 70.3	Monitoring Therapy

Vital signs:
    Pulse
    Blood pressure
Intake and output:
    Fluid balance
    Urine output
Physical examination:
    Weight
    Clinical signs of depletion or overload
Electrolytes

of therapy. Good urine output indicates that rehydration has been successful.

Signs of dehydration on physical examination suggest the need for continued rehydration. Signs of fluid overload, such as edema and pulmonary congestion, are present in the child who is overhydrated. An accurate daily weight measurement is critical for the management of the dehydrated child. There should be a gain in weight during successful therapy.

Measurement of serum electrolyte levels at least daily is appropriate for any child who is receiving IV rehydration. Such a child is at risk for sodium, potassium, and acid-base disorders. It is always important to look at trends. For example, a sodium concentration ($[Na^+]$) of 144 mEq/L is normal; but if the $[Na^+]$ was 136 mEq/L 12 hr earlier, there is a distinct risk that the child will be hypernatremic in 12 or 24 hr. It is advisable to be proactive in adjusting fluid therapy.

Both hypokalemia and hyperkalemia are potentially serious (see Chapter 68). Because dehydration can be associated with acute renal failure and hyperkalemia, potassium is withheld from IV fluids until the patient has voided. The potassium concentration in the patient's IV fluids is not rigidly prescribed. Rather, the patient's serum K^+ level and underlying renal function are used to modify potassium delivery. The patient with an elevated creatinine value and K^+ level of 5 mEq/L does not receive any potassium until the serum K^+ level decreases. Conversely, the patient with a K^+ level of 2.5 mEq/L may require additional potassium.

Metabolic acidosis can be quite severe in dehydrated children. Although normal kidneys eventually correct this problem, a child with renal dysfunction may be unable to correct a metabolic acidosis, and a portion of the patient's IV sodium chloride may have to be replaced with sodium bicarbonate or sodium acetate.

The serum K^+ level is modified by the patient's acid-base status. Acidosis increases serum K^+ by causing intracellular K^+ to move into the ECS. Thus, as acidosis is corrected, the serum potassium concentration ($[K^+]$) decreases. Again, it is best to anticipate this problem and to monitor the serum $[K^+]$ and adjust potassium administration appropriately.

HYPONATREMIC DEHYDRATION

The pathogenesis of hyponatremic dehydration usually involves a combination of sodium and water loss and water retention to compensate for the volume depletion. The patient has a pathologic increase in fluid loss, and the lost fluid contains sodium. Most fluid that is lost has a lower sodium concentration, so patients with only fluid loss would have hypernatremia. Diarrhea has, on average, a sodium concentration of 50 mEq/L. Replacing diarrheal fluid with water, which has almost no sodium, causes a reduction in the serum $[Na^+]$. The volume depletion stimulates synthesis of antidiuretic hormone (ADH), resulting in reduced renal water excretion. Therefore, the body's usual mechanism for preventing hyponatremia, renal water excretion, is blocked. The risk of hyponatremia is further increased if the volume depletion is a result of loss of fluid with a higher sodium concentration, as may occur with renal salt wasting, third space losses, or diarrhea with high sodium content (cholera).

The initial goal in treating hyponatremia is correction of intravascular volume depletion with isotonic fluid. An overly rapid (>12 mEq/L over 1st 24 hr) or overcorrection in the serum $[Na^+]$ (>135 mEq/L) is associated with an increased risk of **central pontine myelinolysis** (see Chapter 68). Most patients with hyponatremic dehydration do well with the same basic strategy outlined in Table 70.2. Again, K^+ delivery is adjusted according to the initial serum K^+ level and the patient's renal function. Potassium is not given until the patient voids.

The patient's $[Na^+]$ is monitored closely to ensure appropriate correction, and the sodium concentration of the fluid is adjusted accordingly. Patients with ongoing losses require an appropriate replacement solution (see Chapter 69). Patients with neurologic symptoms (seizures) as a result of hyponatremia need to receive an acute infusion of hypertonic (3%) saline to increase the serum $[Na^+]$ rapidly (see Chapter 68).

HYPERNATREMIC DEHYDRATION

Hypernatremic dehydration is the most dangerous form of dehydration because of complications of hypernatremia itself and of its therapy. Hypernatremia can cause serious neurologic damage, including central nervous system hemorrhages and thrombosis. This damage appears to be secondary to the movement of water from the brain cells into the hypertonic extracellular fluid (ECF), causing brain cell shrinkage and tearing blood vessels within the brain (see Chapter 68).

The movement of water from the ICS to the ECS during hypernatremic dehydration partially protects the intravascular volume. Unfortunately, because the initial manifestations are milder, children with hypernatremic dehydration are often brought for medical attention with more profound dehydration.

Children with hypernatremic dehydration are often lethargic, and they may be irritable when touched. Hypernatremia may cause fever, hypertonicity, and hyperreflexia. More severe neurologic symptoms may develop if cerebral bleeding or thrombosis occurs.

Overly rapid treatment of hypernatremic dehydration may cause significant morbidity and mortality. **Idiogenic osmoles** are generated within the brain during the development of hypernatremia; they increase the osmolality within the cells of the brain, providing protection against brain cell shrinkage caused by movement of water out of the cells and into the hypertonic ECF. Idiogenic osmoles dissipate slowly during the correction of hypernatremia. With overly rapid lowering of the extracellular osmolality during the correction of hypernatremia, an osmotic gradient may be created that causes water movement from the ECS into the cells of the brain, producing cerebral edema. Symptoms of the resultant cerebral edema can range from seizures to brain herniation and death.

To minimize the risk of **cerebral edema** during the correction of hypernatremic dehydration, *the serum sodium concentration should not decrease by >10 mEq/L every 24 hr.* The deficits in severe hypernatremic dehydration may need to be corrected over 2-4 days (Table 70.4).

The initial resuscitation of hypernatremic dehydration requires restoration of the intravascular volume with NS. LR should not be used because it is more hypotonic than NS and may cause too rapid a decrease in the serum $[Na^+]$, especially if multiple fluid boluses are necessary.

To avoid cerebral edema during correction of hypernatremic dehydration, the fluid deficit is corrected slowly. The rate of correction depends on the initial sodium concentration (Table 70.4). There is no general agreement on the choice or the rate of fluid administration for correcting hypernatremic dehydration; these factors are not nearly as important as vigilant monitoring of the serum $[Na^+]$ and adjustment of the therapy according to the result. The rate of decrease of the serum $[Na^+]$ is roughly related to the "free water" delivery, although there is considerable variation between patients. Free water is water without sodium. NS contains no free water, half-normal saline ($\frac{1}{2}$ NS) is 50% free water, and water is 100% free water. Smaller patients, to achieve the same decrease in the sodium concentration, tend to need higher amounts of free water delivery per kilogram because of **higher insensible fluid losses**. Five percent dextrose (D5) with $\frac{1}{2}$ NS is usually an appropriate starting solution for

Table 70.4	Treatment of Hypernatremic Dehydration

Restore intravascular volume:
  Normal saline: 20 mL/kg over 20 min (repeat until intravascular
    volume restored)
  Determine time for correction on basis of initial sodium
    concentration:
  • [Na] 145-157 mEq/L: 24 hr
  • [Na] 158-170 mEq/L: 48 hr
  • [Na] 171-183 mEq/L: 72 hr
  • [Na] 184-196 mEq/L: 84 hr
Administer fluid at constant rate over time for correction:
  Typical fluid: 5% dextrose + half-normal saline (with 20 mEq/L
    KCl unless contraindicated)
  Typical rate: 1.25-1.5 times maintenance
Follow serum sodium concentration
Adjust fluid on basis of clinical status and serum sodium
  concentration:
  Signs of volume depletion: administer normal saline
    (20 mL/kg)
  Sodium decreases too rapidly; either:
  • Increase sodium concentration of IV fluid
  • Decrease rate of IV fluid
  Sodium decreases too slowly; either:
  • Decrease sodium concentration of IV fluid
  • Increase rate of IV fluid
Replace ongoing losses as they occur

correction of a patient with hypernatremic dehydration. Some patients, especially infants with ongoing high insensible water losses, may rarely need to receive D5 0.2NS, which should be used with great caution and constant monitoring. Others require D5 NS. A child with dehydration as a result of pure free water loss, as usually occurs with diabetes insipidus, usually needs a more hypotonic fluid than a child with depletion of both sodium and water from diarrhea.

Adjustment in the sodium concentration of the IV fluid is the most common approach to modify the rate of decrease in the serum concentration (see Table 70.4). For difficult-to-manage patients with severe hypernatremia, having two IV solutions (e.g., D5 ½NS and D5 NS, both with the same concentration of potassium) at the bedside can facilitate this approach by allowing for rapid adjustments of the rates of the 2 fluids. If the serum [Na⁺] decreases too rapidly, the rate

of D5 NS can be increased and the rate of D5 ½NS can be decreased by the same amount. Adjustment in the total rate of fluid delivery is another approach to modifying free water delivery. For example, if the serum [Na⁺] is decreasing too slowly, the rate of the IV fluid can be increased, thereby increasing the delivery of free water. There is limited flexibility in modifying the rate of the IV fluid because patients generally should receive 1.25-1.5 times the normal maintenance fluid rate. Nevertheless, in some situations, it can be a helpful adjustment.

Because increasing the rate of the IV fluid increases the rate of decline of the sodium concentration, signs of volume depletion are treated with additional isotonic fluid boluses. The serum [K⁺] and the level of renal function dictate the potassium concentration of the IV fluid; potassium is withheld until the patient voids. Patients with hypernatremic dehydration need an appropriate replacement solution if they have ongoing, excessive losses (see Chapter 69).

Seizures and a depressed level of consciousness are the most common manifestations of **cerebral edema** from an overly rapid decrease of the serum [Na⁺] during correction of hypernatremic dehydration. Signs of increased intracranial pressure or impending herniation may develop quite rapidly (see Chapter 85). Acutely, increasing the serum [Na⁺] through an infusion of 3% sodium chloride can reverse the cerebral edema. Each 1 mL/kg of 3% NaCl increases the serum [Na⁺] by approximately 1 mEq/L. An infusion of 4 mL/kg often results in resolution of the symptoms. This strategy is similar to that used for treating symptomatic hyponatremia (see Chapter 68).

Many patients with mild to moderate hypernatremic dehydration as a result of gastroenteritis can be managed with oral rehydration (see Chapter 366). In patients with severe hypernatremia, oral fluids must be used cautiously. Infant formula, because of its low sodium concentration, has a high free water content, and especially if added to IV therapy, it may contribute to a rapid decrease in the serum [Na⁺]. Less hypotonic fluid, such as an oral rehydration solution, may be more appropriate initially. If oral intake is allowed, its contribution to free water delivery must be taken into account, and adjustment in the IV fluid is usually appropriate. Judicious monitoring of the serum [Na⁺] is critical.

Bibliography is available at Expert Consult.

Chapter 71
Fluid and Electrolyte Treatment of Specific Disorders

第七十一章
特殊疾病的液体和电解质治疗

中文导读

急性腹泻（见第三百六十六章），幽门狭窄（见 原文355.1），围手术期液体（见第七十四章）。

ACUTE DIARRHEA
See Chapter 366.

PYLORIC STENOSIS
See Chapter 355.1.

PERIOPERATIVE FLUIDS
See Chapter 74.

Chapter 72

Pediatric Pharmacogenetics, Pharmacogenomics, and Pharmacoproteomics

Jonathan B. Wagner, Matthew J. McLaughlin, and J. Steven Leeder

第七十二章

儿科遗传药理学、药物基因组学和药物蛋白质组学

中文导读

本章主要介绍了儿科遗传药理学、药物基因组学和药物蛋白质组学。包括相关专业术语定义、儿科发育遗传药理学和药物基因组学、药物蛋白质组学和代谢组学、药物生物转化在儿科治疗中的应用、药物转运体的遗传药理学和药物受体的多态性。详细阐述了 CYP2D6、CYP2C9、CYP2C19、CYP3A4、CYP3A5 和 CYP3A7、葡萄糖醛酸转移酶和硫嘌呤甲基转移酶在药物生物转化中的作用，以及三磷酸腺苷结合盒超家族、有机阴离子转运多肽和有机阴离子转运体的遗传药理学特性。

Interindividual variability in the response to similar doses of a given medication is an inherent characteristic of both adult and pediatric populations. **Pharmacogenetics**, the role of genetic factors in drug disposition and response, has resulted in many examples of how variations in human genes can lead to interindividual differences in pharmacokinetics and drug response at the level of individual patients. Pharmacogenetic variability contributes to the broad range of drug responses observed in children at any given age or developmental stage. Therefore, it is expected that children will benefit from the promise of **personalized medicine**—identifying the right drug for the right patient at the right time (Fig. 72.1). However, pediatricians are keenly aware that children are not merely small adults. Numerous maturational processes occur from birth through adolescence such that utilization of information resulting from the Human Genome Project and related initiatives must take into account the changing patterns of gene expression that occur over development to improve pharmacotherapeutics in children.

DEFINITION OF TERMS

The terms pharmacogenomics and pharmacogenetics tend to be used interchangeably, and precise, consensus definitions are often difficult to determine. **Pharmacogenetics** classically is defined as the study or clinical testing of genetic variations that give rise to interindividual response to drugs. Examples of pharmacogenetic traits include specific adverse drug reactions, such as unusually prolonged respiratory muscle paralysis due to succinylcholine, hemolysis associated with antimalarial therapy, and isoniazid-induced neurotoxicity, all of which were found

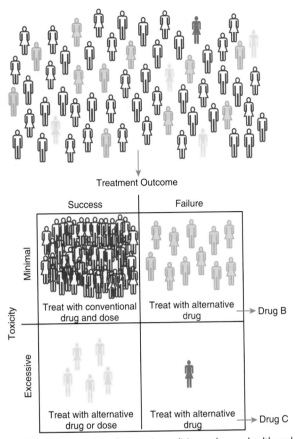

Fig. 72.1 The promise of genomic medicine to human health and disease. The goal of personalized medicine is to identify subgroups of patients who will respond favorably to a given drug with a minimum of side effects, as well as those who will not respond or who will show excessive toxicity with standard doses. A further benefit of pharmacogenomics is the ability to select the most appropriate alternative drug for patients who cannot be treated successfully with conventional drugs and doses. (*Adapted from Yaffe SJ, Aranda JV: Neonatal and pediatric pharmacology, ed 3, Philadelphia, 2004, Lippincott Williams & Wilkins.*)

to be a consequence of inherited variations in enzyme activity. The importance of pharmacogenetic differences has become better understood and is exemplified by the half-life of several drugs being more similar in monozygotic twins than in dizygotic twins. However, it is important to note that in addition to pharmacogenetic differences, environmental factors (diet, smoking status, concomitant drug or toxicant exposure), physiologic variables (age, sex, disease, pregnancy), and patient adherence all contribute to variations in drug metabolism and response. Likewise, ethnicity is another potential genetic determinant of drug variability. Chinese patients who are HLA-B*1502 positive have an increased risk of carbamazepine-induced Stevens-Johnson syndrome; white patients who are HLA-B*5701 positive have an increased risk of hypersensitivity to abacavir (Table 72.1).

Pharmacogenomics represents the marriage of pharmacology and genomics and can be defined as the broader application of genome-wide technologies and strategies to identify both disease processes that represent new targets for drug development and factors predictive of efficacy and risk of adverse drug reactions.

Pharmacokinetics describes what the body does to a drug. It is often studied in conjunction with **pharmacodynamics**, which explores what a drug does to the body. The **pharmacokinetic properties** of a drug are determined by the genes that control the drug's disposition in the body (absorption, distribution, metabolism, excretion).

Drug-metabolizing enzymes and drug transporters play a particularly important role in this process (Table 72.2), and the functional consequences of genetic variations in many drug-metabolizing enzymes have been described between individuals of both similar and different ethnic groups. The most common clinical manifestation of pharmacogenetic variability in drug biotransformation is an increased risk of concentration-dependent toxicity caused by reduced clearance and consequent drug accumulation. However, an equally important manifestation of this variability is lack of efficacy caused by variations in metabolism of prodrugs that require biotransformation to be converted into a pharmacologically active form of a medication. The pharmacogenetics of drug receptors and other target proteins involved in signal transduction or disease pathogenesis can also be expected to contribute significantly to interindividual variability in drug disposition and response.

Therapeutic drug monitoring (TDM) programs recognize that all patients are unique and that the serum concentration-time data for an individual patient theoretically can be used to optimize pharmacotherapy. TDM programs have been the earliest application of personalized medicine; however, routine TDM does not necessarily translate to improved patient outcome in all situations.

The concept of **personalized medicine** is based on the premise that the information explosion accompanying the application of genomic technologies to patient-related problems will allow (1) stratification of patient populations according to their response to a particular medication (e.g., lack of drug efficacy or excessive toxicity) and (2) stratification of diseases into specific subtypes that are categorized according to genomic criteria and by response to particular treatments. Personalized medicine has become supplanted by **individualized medicine**, which takes into consideration the vast amount of information that can be collected from an individual patient and applied to inform decisions for that patient. **Precision medicine** is an emerging approach for disease treatment and prevention that considers individual variability in genes, environment, and lifestyle for each person; it reflects the progression in delivery of care for more accurately diagnosing or treating a patient at an individual level. As the amount of data specific to an individual patient increases (e.g., genomic data, electronic health records), precision medicine can be further divided into **precision diagnosis** and **precision therapeutics**; pharmacokinetics, pharmacodynamics, and pharmacogenomics all represent tools that can be applied to implement precision therapeutics for children.

Genetic polymorphisms (variations) result when copies of a specific gene present within a population do not have identical nucleotide sequences. The term **allele** refers to one of a series of alternative DNA sequences for a particular gene. In humans, there are 2 copies of every gene. An individual's genotype for a given gene is determined by the set of alleles that the individual possesses. The most common form of genetic variation involves a single base change at a given location, referred to as a **single nucleotide polymorphism (SNP)** (see Chapter 95). At the other end of the spectrum are **copy number variations (CNVs)**, which refer to the deletion or duplication of identical or near-identical DNA sequences that may be thousands to millions of bases in size. CNVs occur less frequently than SNPs, but may constitute 0.5–1% of an individual's genome and thereby contribute significantly to phenotypic variation. **Haplotypes** are collections of SNPs and other allelic variations that are located close to each other; when inherited together, these create a catalog of haplotypes, or **HapMap**. When the alleles at a particular gene locus on both chromosomes are identical, a **homozygous** state exists, whereas the term **heterozygous** refers to the situation in which different alleles are present at the same gene locus. The term **genotype** refers to an individual's genetic constitution, whereas the observable characteristics or physical manifestations constitute the **phenotype**, which is the net consequence of genetic and environmental effects (see Chapters 94–101).

Pharmacogenetics focuses on the phenotypical consequences of allelic variation in single genes. **Pharmacogenetic polymorphisms** are monogenic traits that are functionally relevant to drug disposition and action and are caused by the presence (within one population) of >1 allele (at the same gene locus) and >1 phenotype with regard to drug interaction with the organism. The key elements of pharmacogenetic

Table 72.1	Examples of Effects of Gene Polymorphisms on Drug Response		
GENE	**ENZYME/TARGET**	**DRUG**	**CLINICAL RESPONSE**
BCHE	Butyrylcholinesterase	Succinylcholine	Prolonged paralysis
CYP2C9	Cytochrome P450 2C9	Warfarin	Individuals having ≥1 reduced function alleles require lower doses of warfarin for optimal anticoagulation, especially initial anticoagulant control.
CYP2C19	Cytochrome P450 2C19	Clopidogrel	Individuals having ≥1 loss-of-function alleles have reduced capacity to form pharmacologically active metabolite of clopidogrel and reduced antiplatelet effect.
CYP2D6	Cytochrome P450 2D6	Codeine	Poor metabolizers—individuals with 2 loss-of-function alleles—do not metabolize codeine to morphine and thus experience no analgesic effect. Ultrarapid metabolizers—individuals with ≥3 functional alleles—may experience morphine toxicity.
G6PD	Glucose-6-phosphate dehydrogenase	Primaquine (others)	Hemolysis
HLA-A*3101	Human leukocyte antigen A31	Carbamazepine	Carriers of HLA-A*3101 allele have increased risk of SJS and TEN from carbamazepine.
HLA-B*1502	Human leukocyte antigen B15	Allopurinol	Han Chinese carriers of HLA-B*1502 allele have increased risk of SJS and TEN from carbamazepine.
HLA-B*5701	Human leukocyte antigen B57	Abacavir Flucloxacillin	Carriers of HLA-B*5701 allele have increased risk of hypersensitivity reactions to abacavir- and flucloxacillin-induced liver injury.
HLA-B*5801	Human leukocyte antigen B58	Allopurinol	Carriers of HLA-B*5801 allele have increased risk of severe cutaneous adverse reactions to allopurinol, including hypersensitivity reactions, SJS, and TEN.
NAT2	N-Acetyltransferase 2	Isoniazid, hydralazine	Individuals homozygous for "slow acetylation" polymorphisms are more susceptible to isoniazid toxicity, or hydralazine-induced systemic lupus erythematosus.
SLCO1B1	Organic anion–transporting protein (OATP) 1B1	Simvastatin	Carriers of the SLCO1B1*5 allele are at increased risk for musculoskeletal side effects from simvastatin.
TPMT	Thiopurine S-methyltransferase	Azathioprine 6-Mercaptopurine	Individuals homozygous for an inactivating mutation have severe toxicity if treated with standard doses of azathioprine or 6-mercaptopurine; rapid metabolism causes undertreatment.
UGT1A1	Uridine diphospho-glucuronosyltransferase 1A1	Irinotecan	UGT1A1*28 allele is associated with decreased glucuronidation of SN-38, the active metabolite of irinotecan, and increased risk of neutropenia.
VKORC1	Vitamin K oxidoreductase complex 1	Warfarin	Individuals with a haplotype associated with reduced expression of VKORC1 protein (therapeutic target of warfarin) require lower doses of the drug for stable anticoagulation.

SJS, Stevens-Johnson syndrome; TEN, toxic epidermal necrolysis.

polymorphisms are heritability, the involvement of a single gene locus, functional relevance, and the fact that distinct phenotypes are observed within the population only after drug challenge.

DEVELOPMENTAL OR PEDIATRIC PHARMACOGENETICS AND PHARMACOGENOMICS

Our current understanding of pharmacogenetic principles involves enzymes responsible for **drug biotransformation**. Individuals are classified as being "fast," "rapid," or "extensive" metabolizers at one end and "slow" or "poor" metabolizers at the other end of the continuum. This may or may not also include an "intermediate" metabolizer group, depending on the particular enzyme. With regard to biotransformation, children are more complex than adults; fetuses and newborns may be phenotypically "slow" or "poor" metabolizers for certain drug-metabolizing pathways because of their stage of development and may acquire a phenotype consistent with their genotype at some point later in the developmental process as they mature. Examples of drug-metabolizing pathways that are significantly affected by **ontogeny** include glucuronidation and some of the **cytochrome P450 (CYP)** activities. It is also apparent that not all infants acquire drug metabolism activity at the same rate, a result of interactions between genetics and

environmental factors. Interindividual variability in the trajectory (i.e., rate and extent) of acquired drug biotransformation capacity may be considered a **developmental phenotype** (Fig. 72.2). This helps to explain the considerable variability in some CYP activities observed immediately after birth.

In contrast to pharmacogenetic studies that typically target single genes, **pharmacogenomic** analyses are considerably broader in scope and focus on complex and highly variable drug-related phenotypes with targeting of many genes. Genome-wide genotyping technologies and massively parallel "next-generation" sequencing platforms for genomic analyses continue to evolve and allow evaluation of genetic variation at more than 1 million sites throughout an individual genome for SNP and CNV analyses. Genome-wide association studies (GWAS) have been conducted in several pediatric settings, in part to identify novel genes involved in disease pathogenesis that can lead to new therapeutic targets. GWAS are also being applied to identify genetic associations with response to drugs, such as warfarin and clopidogrel, and risk for drug-induced toxicity, including statin-induced myopathy and flucloxacillin hepatotoxicity. The "Manhattan plot," a form of data presentation for GWAS, is becoming more common in many medical journals (Fig. 72.3A). Whole genome and exome sequencing have been applied in a diagnostic setting to identify disease-causing genetic

Table 72.2	Some Important Relationships Between Drugs and Cytochrome P450 (CYP) Enzymes* and P-Glycoprotein Transporter		
ENZYME	**DRUG SUBSTRATES**	**INHIBITORS**	**INDUCERS**
CYP1A2	Caffeine, clomipramine (*Anafranil*[†]), clozapine (*Clozaril*[†]), theophylline	Cimetidine (*Tagamet*[†]) Fluvoxamine (*Luvox*[†]) Ciprofloxacin (*Cipro*)	Omeprazole (*Prilosec*[†]) Tobacco
CYP2C9	Diclofenac (*Voltaren*[†]), ibuprofen (*Motrin*[†]), piroxicam (*Feldene*[†]), Losartan (*Cozaar*), irbesartan (*Avapro*), celecoxib (*Celebrex*), tolbutamide (*Orinase*[†]), warfarin (*Coumadin*[†]), phenytoin (*Dilantin*)	Fluconazole (*Diflucan*) Fluvastatin (*Lescol*) Amiodarone (*Cordarone*) Zafirlukast (*Accolate*)	Rifampin (*Rifadin*[†])
CYP2C19	Omeprazole, lansoprazole (*Prevacid*), pantoprazole (*Protonix*), (S)-mephenytoin, (S)-citalopram (*Lexapro*); nelfinavir (*Viracept*), diazepam (*Valium*[†]), voriconazole (*Vfend*)	Cimetidine Fluvoxamine	Rifampin
CYP2D6	**CNS-active agents:** Atomoxetine (*Strattera*), amitriptyline (*Elavil*[†]), desipramine (*Norpramin*[†]), imipramine (*Tofranil*[†]), paroxetine (*Paxil*), haloperidol (*Haldol*[†]), risperidone (*Risperdal*), thioridazine (*Mellaril*[†]) **Antiarrhythmic agents:** Mexiletine (*Mexitil*), propafenone (*Rythmol*) **β-Blockers:** Propranolol (*Inderal*[†]), metoprolol (*Lopressor*[†]), timolol (*Blocadren*[†]) **Narcotics:** Codeine, dextromethorphan, hydrocodone (*Vicodin*[†]) **Others:** Tamoxifen (*Nolvadex*)	Fluoxetine (*Prozac*[†]) Paroxetine (*Paxil*) Amiodarone (*Cordarone*[†]) Quinidine (*Quinidex*[†]) Terbinafine Cimetidine Ritonavir	
CYP3A4	**Calcium channel blockers:** Diltiazem (*Cardizem*[†]), felodipine (*Plendil*), nimodipine (*Nimotop*), nifedipine (*Adalat*[†]), nisoldipine (*Sular*), nitrendipine, verapamil (*Calan*[†]) **Immunosuppressive agents:** Cyclosporine A (*Sandimmune, Neoral*[†]), tacrolimus (*Prograf*) **Corticosteroids:** Budesonide (*Pulmicort*), cortisol, 17β-estradiol, progesterone, testosterone **Macrolide antibiotics:** Clarithromycin (*Biaxin*), erythromycin (*Erythrocin*[†]), troleandomycin (*TAO*) **Anticancer agents:** Cyclophosphamide (*Cytoxan*[†]), gefitinib (*Iressa*), ifosfamide (*Ifex*), tamoxifen, vincristine (*Oncovin*[†]), vinblastine (*Velban*[†]), **Benzodiazepines:** Alprazolam (*Xanax*[†]), midazolam (*Versed*[†]), triazolam (*Halcion*[†]) **Opioids:** Alfentanil (*Alfenta*[†]), fentanyl (*Sublimaze*[†]), sufentanil (*Sufenta*[†]) **HMG-CoA reductase inhibitors:** Lovastatin (*Mevacor*)[†], simvastatin (*Zocor*), atorvastatin (*Lipitor*) **HIV protease inhibitors:** Indinavir (*Crixivan*), nelfinavir, ritonavir (*Norvir*), saquinavir (*Invirase, Fortovase*), amprenavir (*Agenerase*) **Others:** Quinidine (*Quinidex*[†]), sildenafil (*Viagra*), eletriptan (*Relpax*), ziprasidone (*Geodon*)	Amiodarone Fluconazole Ketoconazole (*Nizoral*[†]) Itraconazole (*Sporanox*) Clarithromycin Erythromycin Troleandomycin Imatinib Ritonavir[‡] Indinavir Grapefruit juice Nefazodone (*Serzone*)	Barbiturates Carbamazepine (*Tegretol*[†]) Phenytoin (*Dilantin*[†]) Efavirenz (*Sustiva*) Nevirapine (*Viramune*) Rifampin Ritonavir[‡] St. John's wort
P-glycoprotein	Aldosterone, amprenavir, atorvastatin, cyclosporine, dexamethasone (*Decadron*[†]), digoxin (*Lanoxin*[†]), diltiazem, domperidone (*Motilium*), doxorubicin (*Adriamycin*[†]), erythromycin, etoposide (*VePesid*), fexofenadine (*Allegra*), hydrocortisone, indinavir, ivermectin (*Stromectol*), lovastatin, loperamide (*Imodium*[†]), nelfinavir, ondansetron (*Zofran*), paclitaxel (*Taxol*), quinidine, saquinavir, simvastatin, verapamil, vinblastine, vincristine	Amiodarone Carvedilol (*Coreg*) Clarithromycin Cyclosporine Erythromycin Itraconazole Ketoconazole Quinidine Ritonavir[‡] Tamoxifen Verapamil	Amprenavir Clotrimazole (*Mycelex*[†]) Phenothiazine Rifampin Ritonavir[‡] St. John's wort

*www.drug-interactions.com.
[†]Also available generically.
[‡]Can be both an inhibitor and an inducer.
CNS, Central nervous system.
From *Med Lett* 2003;45:47.

variation, usually in the context of rare, undiagnosed diseases that would otherwise require a "diagnostic odyssey" lasting several years before a definitive diagnosis is made (and thereby delaying therapeutic intervention). Contained within this genome sequence is the **pharmacogenome**, and an area of intense interest is the development of bioinformatics tools to determine a patient's drug metabolism and response genotype from whole genome sequence data.

Investigating differential gene expression before and after drug exposure has the potential to correlate gene expression with variable drug responses and uncover the mechanisms of tissue-specific drug

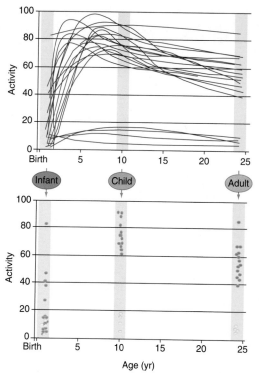

Fig. 72.2 "Developmental" phenotypes. Variability in developmental changes in gene expression and functional enzyme activity are superimposed on pharmacogenetic determinants. **Top,** Developmental profile of a theoretical drug-metabolizing enzyme over a 25 yr span in 20 individuals. **Bottom,** At maturity (adults), allelic variation within the coding region of the gene gives rise to 2 distinct phenotypes: high activity in 92% of the population ("extensive metabolizers"; *red circles*) and low activity in 8% of the population ("poor metabolizers"; *yellow circles*). However, there is also interindividual variability in the rate at which functional activity is acquired after birth. For example, the 2 phenotypes may not be readily distinguishable in newborn infants immediately after birth. Furthermore, there may be discrete periods during childhood in which the genotype-phenotype relationship may differ from that observed in adults (e.g., developmental stages at which enzyme activity appears to be greater in children than in adults). (*Adapted from Leeder JS: Translating pharmacogenetics and pharmacogenomics into drug development for clinical pediatric and beyond, Drug Discov Today 9:567–573, 2004.*)

toxicities. These types of studies use **microarray technology** to monitor global changes in expression of thousands of genes (the **transcriptome**) simultaneously. Genomic sequencing technologies can also be applied to RNA (RNA-Seq) and result in a more complete and quantitative assessment of the transcriptome. Gene expression profiling data from microarrays or RNA-Seq analyses are used to improve disease classification and risk stratification and are common in oncology. This approach has been widely used to address treatment resistance in acute lymphoblastic leukemia and has provided clinically relevant insights into the mechanistic basis of drug resistance and the genomic basis of interindividual variability in drug response. Subsets of transcripts, or gene expression "signatures," are being investigated as potential prognostic indicators for identifying patients at risk for treatment failure (Fig. 72.3B).

Pharmacoproteomic and Metabolomic Tools
Proteomic studies use many different techniques to detect, quantify, and identify proteins in a sample (**expression proteomics**) and to characterize protein function in terms of activity and protein-protein or protein–nucleic acid interactions (**functional proteomics**). Mass spectrometry–based analyses are able to provide quantitative data

regarding protein abundance, and several studies have been applied to pediatric liver samples, for example, to generate more accurate developmental trajectories for several drug-metabolizing enzymes and transporters.

Metabolomics and metabonomics utilize sophisticated analytical platforms, such as nuclear magnetic resonance (NMR) spectroscopy and liquid or gas chromatography coupled with mass spectral detection, to measure the concentrations of all small molecules present in a sample. **Metabolomics** refers to the complete set of low-molecular-weight molecules (metabolites) present in a living system (cell, tissue, organ or organism) at a particular developmental or pathologic state. **Metabonomics** is defined as the study of how the metabolic profile of biologic systems change in response to alterations caused by pathophysiologic stimuli, toxic exposures, or dietary changes. **Pharmacometabonomics** involves prediction of the outcome, efficacy, or toxicity of a drug or xenobiotic intervention in an individual patient based on a mathematical model of preintervention metabolite signatures.

DRUG BIOTRANSFORMATION: APPLICATIONS TO PEDIATRIC THERAPY
The major consequence of pharmacogenetic polymorphisms in drug-metabolizing enzymes is concentration-dependent toxicity caused by impaired drug clearance. In certain cases, reduced conversion of prodrug to therapeutically active compounds is also of clinical importance (see Table 72.2). Chemical modification of drugs by biotransformation reactions generally results in termination of biologic activity through decreased affinity for receptors or other cellular targets as well as more rapid elimination from the body. The process of drug biotransformation can be very complex but is characterized by 3 important features: (1) the concept of broad **substrate specificity**, in which a single isozyme may metabolize a large variety of chemically diverse compounds; (2) many different enzymes may be involved in the biotransformation of a single drug (**enzyme multiplicity**); and (3) a given drug may undergo several different types of reactions. One example of this **product multiplicity** occurs with racemic warfarin, in which at least 7 different hydroxylated metabolites are produced by different CYP isoforms.

Drug biotransformation reactions are conveniently classified into 2 main types, which occur sequentially and serve to terminate biologic activity and enhance elimination (see Chapter 73). **Phase I** reactions introduce or reveal (through oxidation, reduction, or hydrolysis) a functional group within the substrate drug molecule that serves as a site for a phase II conjugation reaction. **Phase II** reactions involve conjugation with endogenous substrates, such as acetate, glucuronic acid, glutathione, glycine, and sulfate. These reactions further increase the polarity of an intermediate metabolite, make the compound more water soluble, and thereby enhance its renal excretion. Interindividual variability in drug biotransformation activity (for both phase I and phase II reactions) is a consequence of the complex interplay among genetic (genotype, sex, race or ethnic background) and environmental (diet, disease, concurrent medication, other xenobiotic exposure) factors. The pathway and rate of a given compound's biotransformation are a function of each individual's unique phenotype with respect to the forms and amounts of drug-metabolizing enzymes expressed.

The CYP enzymes (CYPs) are quantitatively the most important of the **phase I enzymes**. These heme-containing proteins catalyze the metabolism of many lipophilic endogenous substances (steroids, fatty acids, fat-soluble vitamins, prostaglandins, leukotrienes, thromboxanes) as well as exogenous compounds, including a multitude of drugs and environment toxins. CYP nomenclature is based on evolutionary considerations and uses the root symbol *CYP* for *cytochrome P450*. CYPs that share at least 40% homology are grouped into families denoted by an Arabic number after the CYP root. Subfamilies, designated by a letter, appear to represent clusters of highly related genes. Members of the human CYP2 family, for example, have >67% amino acid sequence homology. Individual P450s in a subfamily are numbered sequentially (e.g., CYP3A4, CYP3A5). CYPs that have been identified as being important in human drug metabolism are predominantly found in the CYP1, CYP2, and CYP3 gene families. Importantly, enzyme activity may be induced or inhibited by various agents (see Table 72.2).

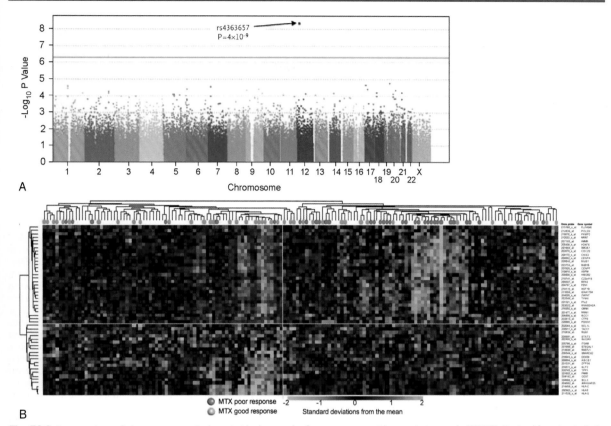

Fig. 72.3 Presentations of pharmacogenomic data. **A,** Manhattan plot from a genome-wide association study (GWAS). Derived from its similarity to the Manhattan skyline, the Manhattan plot presents the genome-wide significance of several hundred thousand single nucleotide polymorphisms (SNPs) distributed throughout the genome with the trait or phenotype of interest. In this example, each SNP included on the "chip" is plotted along the x axis according to its chromosomal coordinate, with each color representing an individual chromosome from chromosome 1 to the X chromosome. The y axis represents the inverse $\log_{10}$ of the p value for the association: the higher the value on the y-axis, the smaller the p value. A value of "15" corresponds to a p value of 10^{-15}. SNPs exceeding a particular threshold are subject to further verification and validation. **B,** "Heat map" constructed from gene expression data. In a heat map the level of expression of many genes, as obtained from microarray analysis, is presented as a 2-dimensional matrix of values. Each column represents an individual patient, and each row is an individual RNA transcript designated by the gene name. The level of gene expression is indicated by the color of each rectangle on a continuum from high expression *(red)* to low expression *(green)*. In this example, acute lymphoblastic leukemia (ALL) patients are clustered by their response to methotrexate (MTX); patients responding to MTX have markedly different patterns of gene expression compared to nonresponders. One of the goals of personalized medicine is to use genomic information (e.g., microarray data) to identify signatures of drug response (or risk of drug toxicity), to select the most appropriate drug among available options for each patient. (*A, Reprinted with permission from Search Collaborative Group. SLCO1B1 variants and statin-induced myopathy: a genome-wide study, N Engl J Med 359:789–799, 2008; B, from Sorich MJ et al. In vivo response to methotrexate forecasts outcome of acute lymphoblastic leukemia and has a distinct gene expression profile, PLoS Med 5(4):e83, 2008.*)

Phase II enzymes include arylamine *N*-acetyltransferases (NAT1, NAT2), uridine diphospho-glucuronosyltransferases (UGTs), epoxide hydrolase, glutathione *S*-transferases (GSTs), sulfotransferases (SULTs), and methyltransferases (catechol *O*-methyltransferase, thiopurine *S*-methyltransferase, several *N*-methyltransferases). As with the CYPs, UGTs, SULTs, and GSTs are gene families with multiple individual isoforms, each having its own preferred substrates, mode of regulation, and tissue-specific pattern of expression.

For most CYPs, genotype-phenotype relationships are influenced by development in that fetal expression is limited (with the exception of CYP3A7) and functional activity is acquired postnatally in isoform-specific patterns. Clearance of some compounds appears to be greater in children relative to adults, and the correlation between genotype and phenotype in neonatal life through adolescence may be obscured.

CYP2D6

The *CYP2D6* gene locus is highly polymorphic, with >110 allelic variants identified to date (http://www.imm.ki.se/CYPalleles/cyp2d6.htm; see Table 72.2). Individual alleles are designated by the gene name *(CYP2D6)*

followed by an asterisk, and an Arabic number. By convention, *CYP2D6*1* designates the fully functional wild-type allele. Allelic variants are the consequence of point mutations, single–base pair deletions or additions, gene rearrangements, or deletion of the entire gene, resulting in a reduction or complete loss of activity. Inheritance of 2 recessive, nonfunctional or "null" alleles results in the **poor-metabolizer (PM) phenotype**, which is found in approximately 5–10% of whites and approximately 1–2% of Asians. In whites the **3, *4, *5,* and **6* alleles are the most common loss-of-function alleles and account for approximately 98% of PM phenotypes. In contrast, CYP2D6 activity on a population basis tends to be lower in Asian and African American populations because of a lower frequency of nonfunctional alleles (**3, *4, *5,* and **6*) *and* a relatively high frequency of population-selective alleles associated with decreased activity ("reduced function" alleles) relative to the wild-type *CYP2D6*1* allele. The *CYP2D6*10* allele occurs at a frequency of approximately 50% in Asians, whereas *CYP2D6*17* and *CYP2D6*29* occur at relatively high frequencies in persons of black African origin.

In addition to nonfunctional and partial-function alleles, the presence of gene duplication and multiplication events (≥3 copies of *CYP2D6* gene in tandem on a single chromosome) further complicates the prediction of phenotype from genotype information. The concept of "activity score" has been developed to simplify translation of *CYP2D6* genotype information into a predicted phenotype of CYP2D6 activity for a particular patient. Fully functional alleles (*1, *2, *35, etc.) are assigned a value of "1", reduced-function alleles (*9, *10, *17, *29) are assigned a value of "0.5", and nonfunctional alleles (*3-*6, etc.) are assigned a value of "0"; for duplications/multiplication events, the allele score is multiplied by the number of copies detected (*10 × 2 = 0.5 × 2 = "1"). The activity score for an individual is the sum of the scores for each chromosome, with poor metabolizers (PMs) defined by a score of "0", whereas a score of "0.5" indicating an **intermediate-metabolizer (IM) phenotype**, and a score >2 indicating an **ultrarapid-metabolizer (UM) phenotype**; scores of 1 to 2 are referred to as **extensive metabolizers (EMs)**. The activity score classification system has been adopted by the Clinical Pharmacogenetics Implementation Consortium (CPIC; see below). In the past, individuals with an activity score of "1" have been referred to as "IMs," and any reference to IM status in literature before 2012 likely refers to a genotype with the equivalent of 1 functional allele, in contrast to the current definition (0.5).

CYP2D6 is involved in the biotransformation of >40 therapeutic entities, including several β-receptor antagonists, antiarrhythmics, antidepressants, antipsychotics, and morphine derivatives[†] (see Table 72.2). CYP2D6 substrates commonly encountered in pediatrics include selective serotonin reuptake inhibitors (SSRIs; fluoxetine, paroxetine), risperidone, atomoxetine, promethazine, tramadol, and codeine. Furthermore, over-the-counter cold remedies (e.g., dextromethorphan, diphenhydramine, chlorpheniramine) are also CYP2D6 substrates. An analysis of CYP2D6 ontogeny in vitro that utilized a relatively large number of samples revealed that CYP2D6 protein and activity remain relatively constant after 1 wk of age up to 18 yr. Similarly, results from an in vivo longitudinal phenotyping study involving >100 infants over the 1st year of life demonstrated considerable interindividual variability in CYP2D6 activity, but no relationship between CYP2D6 activity and postnatal age between 2 wk and 12 mo. Furthermore, a cross-sectional study involving 586 children reported that the distribution of CYP2D6 phenotypes in children was comparable to that observed in adults by at least 10 yr of age. Thus, both available in vitro and in vivo data, although based on phenotype data rather than information on drug clearance from pharmacokinetic studies, imply that genetic variation is more important than developmental factors as a determinant of CYP2D6 variability in children.

One consequence of CYP2D6 developmental pharmacogenetics may be the syndrome of irritability, tachypnea, tremors, jitteriness, increased muscle tone, and temperature instability in neonates born to mothers receiving SSRIs during pregnancy. Controversy exists as to whether these symptoms reflect a neonatal withdrawal (hyposerotonergic) state or represent manifestations of serotonin toxicity analogous to the hyperserotonergic state associated with the SSRI-induced serotonin syndrome in adults. Delayed expression of CYP2D6 (and CYP3A4) in the 1st few weeks of life is consistent with a hyperserotonergic state caused by delayed clearance of paroxetine and fluoxetine (CYP2D6) or sertraline (CYP3A4) in neonates exposed to these compounds during pregnancy. Furthermore, decreases in plasma SSRI concentrations and resolution of symptoms would be expected with increasing postnatal age and maturation of these pathways. Given that treatment of a "withdrawal" reaction may include administration of an SSRI, there is considerable potential for increased toxicity in affected neonates. Resolution of the question whether symptoms are caused by withdrawal vs a hyperserotonergic state is essential for appropriate management of SSRI-induced neonatal adaptation syndromes. Until further data are available, it would be prudent to consider newborns and infants <28 days of age as CYP2D6 PMs.

In older children, drug accumulation and resultant concentration-dependent toxicities in CYP2D6 genotypic poor metabolizers should be anticipated in the same way that they are in adults due to the risk of significant morbidity and mortality. Although a fluoxetine-related death has been reported in a 9 yr old child with a CYP2D6 PM genotype, experience with paroxetine indicates that the risk of drug accumulation may also occur, under certain conditions, in individuals at the opposite end of the activity spectrum. For example, chronic dosing of paroxetine may lead to greater-than-anticipated drug accumulation in children classified as CYP2D6 EMs. In fact, the largest decreases in paroxetine clearance observed with ascending doses are seen in patients who have the greatest clearance at the initial dose level (10 mg/day) and are predicted to have the greatest CYP2D6 activity based on CYP2D6 genotype. This seemingly paradoxical effect appears to involve oxidation of paroxetine within the CYP2D6 active site to form a reactive intermediate that is associated with irreversible modification of the CYP2D6 protein in or near the active site and loss of enzyme activity. As a consequence, CYP2D6 activity progressively declines such that drug accumulation may occur over time, placing CYP2D6 EM patients also at increased risk of concentration-dependent toxicity.

Theoretically, younger children may experience decreased efficacy or therapeutic failure with drugs such as codeine and tramadol that are dependent on functional CYP2D6 activity for conversion to the pharmacologically active species. CYP2D6 catalyzes the O-demethylation of codeine to morphine. Infants and children appear capable of converting codeine to morphine and achieving morphine:codeine ratios comparable to those of adults. However, in one study, morphine and its metabolites were not detected in 36% of children receiving codeine making the level of analgesia from codeine unreliable in the studied pediatric population. Interestingly, levels of morphine and its metabolites are not related to CYP2D6 phenotype. Finally, *ultrarapid* CYP2D6 metabolism of codeine may result in opiate intoxication, including maternal ultrarapid metabolism of codeine, which can result in high serum and breast milk concentrations of morphine and may have adverse effects in the breastfed neonate.

Rapid metabolism and clearance of CYP2D6 substrates may also contribute to poor therapeutic response because of an inability to achieve adequate plasma concentrations, even when medications are dosed at the maximum approved dose level. The product label for atomoxetine (Strattera) indicates that CYP2D6 PMs have a systemic exposure to the drug (e.g., amount of drug in body over time as determined by area under plasma concentration-time curve) that is 10 times greater than in typical individuals (EMs), and yet the same starting dose of 0.5 mg/kg is recommended for all patients. A genotype-stratified pharmacokinetic study of atomoxetine in children and adolescents with attention-deficit/hyperactivity disorder (ADHD) confirmed an 11-14-fold difference in average systemic exposure between PM and EM groups. However, the most informative finding was the 50-fold range in exposure (30-fold, if exposure corrected for actual mg dose administered) between the PM participant with the highest exposure and the UM participant (3 functional alleles) with the lowest exposure. Using the results of this single-dose study to simulate atomoxetine exposure at steady state for each study participant revealed that even at the maximum recommended dose of atomoxetine, exposure was likely to be subtherapeutic for the majority of patients with ≥1 functional *CYP2D6* alleles.

Avoiding ineffective treatment at one end of the spectrum and excessive toxicity at the other are potential benefits of individualizing doses based on genomic information for medications dependent on a polymorphic clearance pathway, such as CYP2D6. The CPIC has published several guidelines that include CYP2D6 substrates, such as the CPIC guideline for codeine,* SSRIs,[†] and tricyclic antidepressants.[‡] Although pediatric data are sparse, these links serve as valuable sources of information regarding the effect of genotype on the dose-exposure relationship for several CYP2D6 substrates.

[†]For an updated list, see http://www.mayomedicallaboratories.com/it-mmfiles/Pharmacogenomic_Associations_Tables.pdf.

*https://cpicpgx.org/guidelines/guideline-for-codeine-and-cyp2d6/.

[†]https://cpicpgx.org/guidelines/guideline-for-selective-serotonin-reuptake-inhibitors-and-cyp2d6-and-cyp2c19/.

[‡]https://cpicpgx.org/guidelines/guideline-for-tricyclic-antidepressants-and-cyp2d6-and-cyp2c19/.

CYP2C9

Although several clinically useful compounds are substrates for CYP2C9[§] (see Table 72.2), the effects of allelic variation are most profound for drugs with a narrow therapeutic index, such as phenytoin, warfarin, and tolbutamide. In vitro studies show a progressive increase in CYP2C9 expression from 1–2% of mature levels in the 1st trimester to approximately 30% at term. Considerable variability (approximately 35-fold) in expression is apparent over the 1st 5 mo of life, with about half the samples studied exhibiting values equivalent to those observed in adults. One interpretation of these data is that broad interindividual variability exists in the rate at which CYP2C9 expression is acquired after birth, and in general, the ontogeny of CYP2C9 activity in vivo, as inferred from pharmacokinetic studies of phenytoin in newborns, is consistent with the in vitro results. The apparent half-life of phenytoin is prolonged (approximately 75 hours) in preterm infants, but decreases to approximately 20 hr in term newborns. By 2 wk of age, the half-life has further declined to 8 hr. The appearance of concentration-dependent (saturable) metabolism of phenytoin, reflecting the functional acquisition of CYP2C9 activity, does not appear until approximately 10 days of age. The maximal velocity of phenytoin metabolism has been reported to decrease from an average of 14 mg/kg/day in infants to 8 mg/kg/day in adolescents, which may reflect changes in the ratio of liver mass to total body mass observed over this period of development, as has been observed for warfarin.

Several allelic variants of *CYP2C9* have been reported, but not all have been evaluated for their functional consequences. The *CYP2C9*2* allele is associated with approximately 5.5-fold decreased intrinsic clearance for *S*-warfarin relative to the wild-type enzyme. Allelic variations resulting in amino acid changes within the enzyme active site, such as the *CYP2C9*3*, *CYP2C9*4*, and *CYP2C9*5* alleles, are associated with activities that are approximately 5% of the wild-type protein. Approximately one third of the white population carries a variant *CYP2C9* allele (typically *2 and *3 alleles), whereas the *2 and *3 alleles are virtually nonexistent in African American, Chinese, Japanese, or Korean populations. In contrast, the *5 allele has been detected in blacks but not in whites. The risk of bleeding complications in patients treated with warfarin and with concentration-dependent toxicity in patients treated with phenytoin is most pronounced for individuals with a *CYP2C9*3/*3* genotype. Although the relationship between the *CYP2C9* genotype and warfarin dosing and pharmacokinetics has not been as extensively studied in children, consequences of allelic variation can be expected to be similar to those observed in adults. In adults, *CYP2C9* and *VKORC1* genotype and patient age, sex, and weight can account for 50–60% of the variation in warfarin dose requirements. A large part of the variation is still unknown, but may be at least partially attributed to interactions with other drugs and foods.

CYP2C19

In vitro, CYP2C19 protein and catalytic activity can be detected at levels representing 12–15% of mature values by 8 wk of gestation and remain essentially unchanged throughout gestation and at birth. Over the 1st 5 mo of postnatal age, CYP2C19 activity increases linearly. Adult levels are achieved by 10 yr of age, although variability in expression is estimated to be approximately 21-fold between 5 mo and 10 yr of age. The major source of this variability is likely pharmacogenetic in nature. The CYP2C19 PM phenotype (also known as *mephenytoin hydroxylase deficiency*) is present in 3–5% of the white population and 20–25% of Asians. Although 25 variant alleles have been reported to date, the 2 most common variant alleles, *CYP2C19*2* and *CYP2C19*3*, result from single-base substitutions that introduce premature stop codons and, consequently, truncated polypeptide chains that possess no functional activity. Despite consistent increases in CYP2C19 activity observed in vitro over the 1st 5 months of life, the results of an in vivo phenotyping study with omeprazole in Mexican children revealed a broad range of activity and implied that 17% of infants <4 mo of age could be classified as PMs (no PMs were detected beyond that point). In contrast, 20% of

children 3–9 mo old were classified as ultrarapid metabolizers (UMs) compared with 6% of infants 1-3 mo of age. For omeprazole, pharmacokinetic parameters comparable to those observed in adults are achieved by age 2 yr.

CYP2C19 also plays an important role in the metabolism of lansoprazole. In Japanese adults treated with lansoprazole, amoxicillin, and clarithromycin for *Helicobacter pylori* infection, the eradication rate for CYP2C19 PMs (97.8%) and heterozygous EMs (1 functional *CYP2C19* allele; 92.1%) was significantly greater than that observed in homozygous EMs (72.7%). Initial treatment did not eradicate *H. pylori* in 35 patients, 34 of whom had at least 1 functional *CYP2C19* allele, and eradication could be achieved with higher lansoprazole doses in almost all cases. Given that the frequency of the functional *CYP2C19*1* allele is considerably greater in whites (0.84 [84%]) than Japanese (0.55 [55%]), eradication failure can be expected to occur more frequently in whites. Because proton pump inhibitors are widely used in children, pharmacogenetic as well as developmental considerations should guide pediatric dosing strategies.

CYP3A4, CYP3A5, and CYP3A7

The CYP3A subfamily consists of four members in humans (CYPs 3A4, 3A5, 3A7, and 3A43) and is quantitatively the most important group of CYPs in terms of human hepatic drug biotransformation. These isoforms catalyze the oxidation of many different therapeutic entities, several of which are of potential importance to pediatric practice[†] (see Table 72.2). CYP3A7 is the predominant CYP isoform in fetal liver and can be detected in embryonic liver as early as 50–60 days' gestation. CYP3A4, the major CYP3A isoform in adults, is essentially absent in fetal liver, but increases gradually throughout childhood. Over the 1st 6 mo of life, CYP3A7 expression exceeds that of CYP3A4, although its catalytic activity toward most CYP3A substrates is rather limited compared with CYP3A4. CYP3A4 is also abundantly expressed in intestine, where it contributes significantly to the first-pass metabolism of oral drugs, which are substrates (e.g., midazolam). CYP3A5 is polymorphically expressed and is present in approximately 25% of adult liver samples studied in vitro.

Several methods have been proposed to measure CYP3A activity. Using these various phenotyping probes, CYP3A4 activity has been reported to vary widely (up to 50-fold) among individuals, but the population distributions of activity are essentially unimodal and evidence for polymorphic activity has been elusive. Although 20 allelic variants have been identified (http://www.imm.ki.se/CYPalleles/cyp3a4.htm), most occur relatively infrequently and do not appear to be of clinical importance. Of interest to pediatrics is the *CYP3A4*1B* allele present in the *CYP3A4* promoter region. The clinical significance of this allelic variant appears limited with respect to drug biotransformation activity, despite in vitro assays showing 2-fold increased activity over the wild-type *CYP3A4*1* allele. Although no association appears to exist between the *CYP3A4*1B* allele and age of menarche, a significant relationship does exist between the number of *CYP3A4*1B* alleles and the age at onset of puberty, as defined by Tanner breast score. In one study, 90% of 9 yr old girls with a *CYP3A4*1B/*1B* genotype had a Tanner breast score of ≥2 vs 56% of *CYP3A4*1A/*1B* heterozygotes and 40% of girls homozygous for the *CYP3A4*1A* allele. Because CYP3A4 plays an important role in testosterone catabolism, it was proposed that the estradiol:testosterone ratio may be shifted toward higher values in the presence of the *CYP3A4*1B* allele and might trigger the hormonal cascade that accompanies puberty. Intestinal CYP3A4 activity is inhibited by grapefruit juice and may result in higher levels of the many drugs metabolized by this enzyme; very large quantities of grapefruit juice may also inhibit the hepatic CYP3A4.

Polymorphic *CYP3A5* expression is largely caused by an SNP in intron 3 that creates a cryptic splice site and gives rise to messenger RNA splice variants that retain part of intron 3 with a premature stop codon. The truncated mRNA transcripts associated with this allele, *CYP3A5*3*, cannot be translated into a functional protein. Individuals with at least

---

[§]http://www.mayomedicallaboratories.com/it-mmfiles/Pharmacogenomic_Associations_Tables.pdf.

[†]For an updated list, see http://www.mayomedicallaboratories.com/it-mmfiles/Pharmacogenomic_Associations_Tables.pdf.

one wild-type *CYP3A5*1* allele express functional CYP3A5 protein, whereas those homozygous for *CYP3A5*3 (CYP3A5*3/*3)* do not express appreciable amounts of functional protein. Approximately 60% of African Americans show functional hepatic CYP3A5 activity, compared with only 33% of European Americans.

Clinically important consequences of *CYP3A5* allelic variation have been reported in children. In pediatric heart transplant patients with a *CYP3A5*1/*3* genotype, tacrolimus concentrations were approximately 25% of those observed in patients with *CYP3A5*3/*3* genotypes, when corrected for dose, in the highly vulnerable period immediately after transplant (≤2 wk), and 50% less at 3, 6, and 12 mo after transplant. Thus, larger doses of tacrolimus are required in patients with functional CYP3A5 protein to achieve comparable blood levels and to minimize the risk of rejection. Of concern, <15% of tacrolimus concentrations in the immediate posttransplant period were within the therapeutic target range, highlighting the need for prospective, precision-guided tacrolimus trials in the pediatric population. In addition to *CYP3A5* expressor genotype, younger age was associated with lower tacrolimus concentrations. The same age and genotype relationship is observed for renal transplantation. Conversely, the same age- and genotype-tailored treatment is more challenging in liver transplantation unless the donor *CYP3A5* is known. In pediatric liver transplant recipients, *CYP3A5* expressor genotype was not associated with tacrolimus concentrations and dosing. This implies that hepatic metabolism, from the donor liver and genotype status, plays a larger role in tacrolimus concentrations than intestinal metabolism or the recipient's *CYP3A5* genotype status. Collectively, these pediatric tacrolimus datasets have informed the CPIC to recommend a 1.5-2-fold increase in tacrolimus dosing, followed by close plasma drug monitoring, in children and adolescents with at least one *CYP3A5*1* allele (https://cpicpgx.org/guidelines/guideline-for-tacrolimus-and-cyp3a5/).

Glucuronosyl Transferases (UGTs)

The UGT gene superfamily catalyzes the conjugation (with glucuronic acid) of several drugs used clinically in pediatrics, including morphine, acetaminophen, nonsteroidal antiinflammatory drugs, and benzodiazepines. The effect of development on glucuronidation capacity has been well described and is illustrated by hyperbilirubinemia, **gray baby syndrome** (cardiovascular collapse associated with high doses of chloramphenicol in newborns), and the 3.5-fold increase in morphine clearance observed in premature neonates at 24-39 wk postconception age. As with the CYPs, there are multiple UGT isoforms, and the acquisition of functional UGT activity appears to be isoform and substrate specific.

UGT1A1 is the major UGT gene product responsible for bilirubin glucuronidation, and >100 genetic alterations have been reported (Table 72.3), most of which are rare and are more properly considered *mutations* rather than gene polymorphisms. Inheritance of 2 defective alleles is associated with reduced bilirubin-conjugating activity and gives rise to clinical conditions such as Crigler-Najjar and Gilbert syndromes. More frequently occurring polymorphisms involve a dinucleotide (TA) repeat in the atypical TATA box of the *UGT1A1* promoter. The wild-type *UGT1A1*1* allele has 6 repeats (TA$_6$), and the TA$_5$ (*UGT1A1*33*), TA$_7$ (*UGT1A1*28*), and TA$_8$ (*UGT1A1*34*) variants are all associated with reduced activity. *UGT1A1*28*, the most frequent variant, is a contributory factor to prolonged neonatal jaundice. This variant is also associated with impaired glucuronidation and thus toxicity of the active metabolite

Table 72.3	Internet Resources for Pharmacogenetics and Pharmacogenomics*

INTRODUCTION TO PHARMACOGENOMICS
http://www.pharmgkb.org/
http://www.mayoclinic.org/healthy-lifestyle/consumer-health/in-depth/personalized-medicine/art-20044300

PHARMACOGENETICS: ALLELIC VARIANTS OF DRUG-METABOLIZING ENZYMES

CYP2C9	http://www.cypalleles.ki.se/cyp2c9.htm
CYP2C19	http://www.cypalleles.ki.se/cyp2c19.htm
CYP2D6	http://www.cypalleles.ki.se/cyp2d6.htm
CYP3A4	http://www.cypalleles.ki.se/cyp3a4.htm
CYP3A5	http://www.cypalleles.ki.se/cyp3a5.htm
UGTs	https://www.pharmacogenomics.pha.ulaval.ca/ugt-alleles-nomenclature/
NAT1 and NAT2	http://nat.mbg.duth.gr/

PHARMACOGENETICS: SUBSTRATES OF DRUG-METABOLIZING ENZYMES
http://medicine.iupui.edu/clinpharm/ddis/clinical-table
http://www.mayomedicallaboratories.com/it-mmfiles/Pharmacogenomic_Associations_Tables.pdf

PHARMACOGENETICS-BASED DOSING GUIDELINES
Dosing guidelines incorporating pharmacogenetic data developed by the Clinical Pharmacogenetics Implementation Consortium are available on the CPIC web page https://cpicpgx.org/, which is mirrored at PharmGKB: https://www.pharmgkb.org/page/cpic, or through the National Guidelines Clearinghouse website, a publically accessible resource for evidence-based clinical guidelines sponsored by the Agency for Healthcare Research and Quality (AHRQ), U.S. Department of Health Services, at https://www.guideline.gov/search?q=CPIC.
CYP2D6, CYP2C19, and antidepressants:
https://cpicpgx.org/guidelines/guideline-for-tricyclic-antidepressants-and-cyp2d6-and-cyp2c19/
CYP2D6 and codeine:
https://cpicpgx.org/guidelines/guideline-for-codeine-and-cyp2d6/
CYP2D6, CYP2C19, and SSRIs:
https://cpicpgx.org/guidelines/guideline-for-selective-serotonin-reuptake-inhibitors-and-cyp2d6-and-cyp2c19/
CYP3A5 and tacrolimus:
https://cpicpgx.org/guidelines/guideline-for-tacrolimus-and-cyp3a5/
HLA-B and abacavir and allopurinol:
https://cpicpgx.org/guidelines/guideline-for-abacavir-and-hla-b/
https://cpicpgx.org/guidelines/guideline-for-allopurinol-and-hla-b/
https://cpicpgx.org/guidelines/guideline-for-carbamazepine-and-hla-b/
SLCO1B1 and simvastatin:
https://cpicpgx.org/guidelines/guideline-for-simvastatin-and-slco1b1/
TPMT and thiopurines:
https://cpicpgx.org/guidelines/guideline-for-thiopurines-and-tpmt/

*All sites were accessible on July 14, 2017.

SN-38 of the chemotherapeutic agent irinotecan. Allelic variations in *UGT1A7* and *UGT1A9* have also been associated with irinotecan toxicity in adults with colorectal cancer.

The consequences of allelic variation in the UGT2B family are less certain. The predominant routes of morphine elimination include biotransformation to the pharmacologically active 6-glucuronide (M6G) and the inactive 3-glucuronide (M3G). M6G formation is almost exclusively catalyzed by UGT2B7, whereas several UGTs in the UGT1A subfamily and UGT2B7, both contribute to M3G formation. Increased M6G:morphine ratios have been reported in individuals homozygous for the SNPs constituting the *UGT2B7*2* allele. Although individuals genotyped as *UGT2B7*2/*2* may produce higher-than-anticipated concentrations of pharmacologically active morphine and its metabolites, prospective studies addressing phenotype-genotype correlations and the consequences of morphine analgesia have had conflicting results.

Thiopurine S-Methyltransferase

Thiopurine S-methyltransferase (**TPMT**) is a cytosolic enzyme that catalyses the S-methylation of aromatic and heterocyclic sulfur-containing compounds, such as 6-mercaptopurine (6MP), azathioprine, and 6-thioguanine, used in the treatment of acute lymphoblastic leukemia (ALL), inflammatory bowel disease (IBD), and juvenile idiopathic arthritis and the prevention of renal allograft rejection. To exert its cytotoxic effects, 6MP requires metabolism to thioguanine nucleotides by a multistep process initiated by hypoxanthine guanine phosphoribosyl-transferase. TPMT prevents thioguanine nucleotide production by methylating 6MP (Fig. 72.4*A*). TPMT activity is usually measured in erythrocytes, with erythrocyte activity reflecting that found in other tissues, including liver and leukemic blasts. Although approximately 89% of whites and blacks have high TPMT activity and 11% have intermediate activity, 1 in 300 individuals inherits TPMT deficiency as an autosomal recessive trait (Fig. 72.4*B*). In newborn infants, peripheral blood TPMT activity is 50% greater than in race-matched adults and shows a distribution of activity consistent with the polymorphism characterized in adults. No data currently indicate how long this higher activity is maintained, although TPMT activities were comparable to previously reported adult values in a population of Korean schoolchildren age 7–9 yr. In patients with intermediate or low activity, more drug is shunted toward production of cytotoxic thioguanine nucleotides. TPMT can also methylate 6-thioinosine 5′-monophosphate to generate a methylated metabolite capable of inhibiting de novo purine synthesis (Fig. 72.4*C*).

Multiple SNP variants have been identified in the *TPMT* gene, and a GWAS from 2 independent pediatric ALL cohorts confirmed that TPMT activity is a monogenic pharmacogenetics trait; 3 variants (*TPMT*2, *3A, *3C*) account for 98% of whites with low activity and have high predictive capacity for TPMT phenotype. *TPMT*3A* is the most common and is characterized by 2 nucleotide transition mutations, G460A and A719G, that lead to 2 amino acid substitutions, Ala154Thr and Tyr240Cys (Fig. 72.4*D*). The *TPMT*3A* allele occurs more frequently in white (9.5%) and Hispanic (7.0%) patients and is absent in black patients. In contrast, *TPMT*3C* is reported to be the predominant variant allele in black patients (12.2%), and only rarely observed in white or Hispanic patients; overall, black patients have lower TPMT activities than nonblack patients. The **3A* and **3C* variants each result in loss of functional activity through the production of unstable proteins that are subject to accelerated proteolytic degradation.

The relatively few patients with low to absent TPMT activity (0.3%) are at increased risk for **severe myelosuppression** if treated with normal doses of thiopurines; thus they require a 10-15-fold reduction in dose to minimize this risk. Furthermore, if not dosed properly, patients may be at increased risk for relapse as a result of inadequate or a lack of treatment with thiopurines. Given the expanding use of 6MP and azathioprine in pediatrics to treat IBD and juvenile arthritis and to prevent renal allograft rejection, TPMT pharmacogenetics is not trivial, and a CPIC guideline assists with genotype-guided dosing.[†] However, *TPMT* genotype is not the only determinant of intolerance to thiopurines. Multiple

studies have also implicated genetic variation in *NUDT15*, a nucleotide diphosphatase that converts thioguanine triphosphate to thioguanine monophosphate, thereby reducing incorporation of thioguanine into DNA; reduction or loss of this activity results in greater-than-expected thioguanine incorporation into DNA and thus increased cytotoxicity. Reduced-function *NUDT15* alleles are more common in Hispanic patients and those with Asian ancestry, and patients who have inherited 2 reduced-function alleles tolerate thiopurine doses that are much lower (10%) than normal. Thus it is reasonable to expect that both *TPMT* and *NUDT15* genotype will need to be considered for individualized thiopurine treatment.

PHARMACOGENETICS OF DRUG TRANSPORTERS

There are several major types of membrane transporters, including organic anion transporters (OATs), organic anion–transporting polypeptides (OATPs), organic cation transporters (OCTs), and the adenosine triphosphate–binding cassette (ABC) transporters, such as P-glycoprotein and the multidrug-resistant proteins. Membrane transporters are heavily involved in drug disposition and actively transport substrate drugs between organs and tissues. Drug transporters are expressed at numerous epithelial cells, such as intestinal epithelial cells, hepatocytes, renal tubular cells, and the blood-brain barrier (BBB) (Fig. 72.5). Transporters often are also determinants of drug resistance, and many drugs work by affecting the function of transporters. As such, polymorphisms in the genes encoding these proteins may have a significant effect on the absorption, distribution, metabolism, and excretion as well as the pharmacodynamic effect of a wide variety of compounds.

Adenosine Triphosphate–Binding Cassette Superfamily

The ATP-binding cassette (ABC) transporters belong to the largest known transporter gene family and translocate a variety of substrates, including chemotherapy agents. ABC multidrug transporter expression has been implicated in tumor cell resistance to anticancer therapy, altered disposition of chemotherapy drugs, and toxic side effects associated with chemotherapy. More recently, the genetic heterogeneity of several ABC transporter genes has been described. Apart from having at least one ATP-binding domain, these transporters are characterized by a signature sequence of amino acid residues within the domain. In humans the ABC transporters function as efflux pumps, which together with detoxification enzymes, constitute a complex, integrated, "chemoimmunologic defense" system against drugs and other foreign chemicals. A variety of epithelial barriers, including the kidney, liver, and BBB have abundant expression of ABC transporters, such as P-glycoprotein (P-gp; also known as *MDR1*), and multidrug-resistant proteins (MRPs) 1, 2, and 3. Powered by ATP, these transporters actively extrude substrates from the respective cell and organ.

Considerable genetic variation has been reported in the superfamily of ABC transporter genes. Many studies have investigated the relationship between *ABCB1* genotype or haplotype and P-gp expression, activity, or drug response, yielding inconsistent results, largely due to methodological limitations. No association between genotype and drug disposition or response would be expected if the drug of interest were not substrate for P-gp. However, even when drugs are tested for transport by P-gp using in vitro systems, the results are not necessarily conclusive, as is the case for carbamazepine. On the other hand, an association between *ABCB1* genotype and drug response was observed in patients receiving antidepressants that were ABC substrates (e.g., citalopram, paroxetine, amitriptyline, venlafaxine)., but not in drugs that were not substrates (e.g., mirtazapine).

Studies conducted in children need to also consider the ontogeny of P-gp expression. Based on studies using human lymphocytes, it appears that P-gp activity is high at birth, decreases between 0 and 6 mo, and stabilizes between 6 mo and 2 yr of age. In contrast, P-gp can be detected in human neural stem/progenitor cells and decreases with differentiation. Furthermore, P-gp has been proposed as an endothelial marker for development of the BBB, and expression increases with postnatal age as the BBB matures. Proteomic analysis of the ontogeny of hepatic P-gp has demonstrated that P-gp expression increases through infancy,

[†]https://cpicpgx.org/guidelines/guideline-for-thiopurines-and-tpmt/.

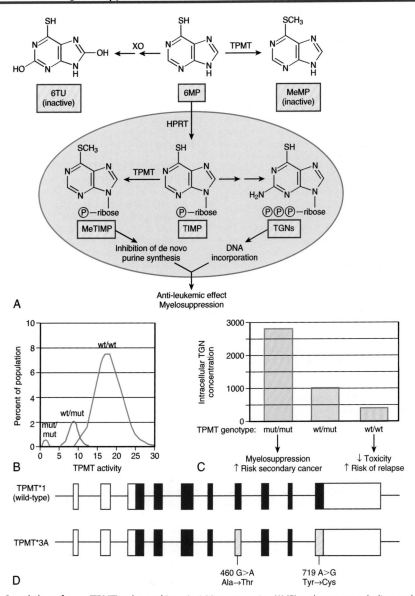

Fig. 72.4 Thiopurine *S*-methyltransferase (TPMT) polymorphism. **A,** 6-Mercaptopurine (6MP) undergoes metabolism to thioguanine nucleotides (TGNs) to exert its cytotoxic effects. TPMT and xanthine oxidase reduce the amount of 6MP available for the bioactivation pathway to TGNs. TPMT can also methylate 6-thioinosine 5′-monophosphate (TIMP) to generate a methylated compound capable of inhibiting de novo purine synthesis. **B,** Distribution of TPMT activity in humans. Of the population, 89% has high activity, whereas 11% has intermediate activity. Approximately 1 in 300 individuals homozygous for 2 loss-of-function alleles has very low activity. **C,** Correlation between the TPMT genotype and intracellular TGN concentrations. In TPMT poor metabolizers, more 6MP is available to go down the bioactivation pathway to form TGNs; this situation is associated with an increased risk of myelosuppression. **D,** The most common variant TPMT allele is the result of 2 mutations that give rise to an unstable protein product that undergoes proteolytic degradation. 6TU, 6-Thiouric acid; MeMP, 6-methylmercaptopurine; HPRT, 6-thiomethylinosine 5-monophosphate; MeTIMP, hypoxanthine-guanine phosphoribosyl transferase; wt, wild type; mut, mutant. *(Modified with permission from Relling MV, Dervieux T: Pharmacogenetics and cancer therapy, Nat Rev Cancer 11:99–108, 2001; copyright 2001, Macmillan Magazines Ltd.)*

achieving 50% of adult expression at approximately 3 yr and reaching a plateau during adolescence. Thus the developmental patterns of P-gp expression likely are tissue specific, but data still are sparse in this regard. Nevertheless, expression of P-gp at a young age in gut and liver likely represents a protective mechanism in which both endogenous and exogenous toxins are efficiently excreted from the body. However, developmental patterns of expression in tissues of drug response, such as lymphocytes and tumors, may also affect the efficacy of intracellular drugs. For example, polymorphisms in the gene have been shown to

be predictive of the ability to wean corticosteroids after heart transplantation, as well as the susceptibility to and clinical outcome of treatment for pediatric ALL. On the other hand, immaturity of P-gp expression in the developing BBB may contribute to discrete periods of increased susceptibility to drug toxicity in the central nervous system. However, for most other drugs, including immunosuppressants and protease inhibitors, studies investigating the effect of *ABCB1* polymorphisms in drug disposition and response have yielded conflicting results. In one study investigating the relationship between *ABCB1* genotype and

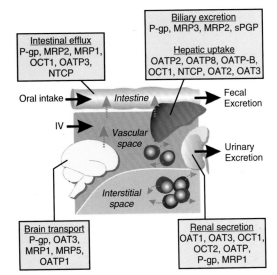

Fig. 72.5 Schematic diagram of important transport proteins and their known locations in humans. *Spheres correspond to drug molecules. (Reprinted with permission from American Pharmacists Association. Ritschel WA, Kearns GL, editors. Handbook of basic pharmacokinetics including clinical applications, ed 7, Washington, DC, 2009, American Pharmacists Association, p 45.)*

cyclosporin pharmacokinetics, an effect of genotype on oral availability was only apparent in children >8 yr of age. Although these results require further replication, the implication is that a better understanding of transporter ontogeny is required to properly design and interpret pharmacogenetic studies of *ABCB1* in pediatric populations.

Organic Anion–Transporting Polypeptides

Organic anion–transporting polypeptides (OATPs) in the solute carrier organic anion transporter (SLCO) are a family of glycoprotein transporters with 12 transmembrane-spanning domains expressed in various epithelial cells. There are 11 OATPs in humans, some of which are ubiquitously expressed and others whose expression is restricted to specific tissues. Typical substrates include bile salts, hormones and their conjugates, toxins, and various drugs. The solute carrier, human OATP 1A2 (OATP1A2, OATP-A, OATP1, and OATP) is highly expressed in the intestine, kidney, cholangiocytes, and BBB and may be important in the absorption, distribution, and excretion of a broad array of clinically important drugs. Several nonsynonymous polymorphisms have been identified in the gene encoding OATP1A2, SLCO1A2 (SLC21A3), with some of these variants demonstrating functional changes in the transport of OATP1A2 substrates.

OATP1B1 (SLCO1B1) and OATP1B3 (SLCO1B3) are liver-specific transporters and promote the cellular uptake of endogenous substrates, such as bilirubin, bile acids, DHEA-sulfate, and leukotriene C4, as well as various drugs, including several statins, methotrexate, and enalapril. Allelic variation in OATP1B1 (specifically the *SLCO1B1*5* allele) results in reduced clearance and increased systemic exposure of several statin drugs (atorvastatin, pravastatin, simvastatin) and has been associated with an increased risk of musculoskeletal side effects from simvastatin. The expression of OATP1B1 in human pediatric liver tissue was independent of age in all samples, but age dependency was demonstrated in samples homozygous for the *SLCO1B1* reference sequence (i.e., *SLCO1B1*1A/*1A* genotype). Therefore, not only genotype, but also growth and development, may influence OATP1B1 protein expression in the developing child. To date, only one study has investigated the effect of *SLCO1B1* genotype on statin disposition in children, reporting a genotype-phenotype relationship for pravastatin that was discordant with the relationship observed in adults. However, data with simvastatin in dyslipidemic children and adolescents (LDL >130 mg/dL) suggest

that the genotype-phenotype relationships observed in adults are also present in this population, but the magnitude of the genetic effect may be greater in pediatric patients.

Several studies have confirmed that the 2 SNPs determining the most common *SLCO1B1* haplotypes (**1a, *1b, *5,* and **15*), rs4149056 and rs2306283, are associated with decreased clearance of high-dose methotrexate in children with ALL. Genotyping for *SLCO1B1* may be helpful in identifying patients at increased risk of toxicity from reduced clearance or increased accumulation of methotrexate. In the pediatric liver proteomic analysis, OATP1B3 expression was age dependent, with a 3-fold difference observed between neonates and adults. Similar to P-gp, expression steadily increased during childhood; however, 50% of adult level expression was much earlier (6 mo) compared with P-gp.

Organic Cation Transporters

Organic cation transporters (OCTs) in the SCL22A subfamily are primarily expressed on the basolateral membrane of polarized epithelia and mediate the renal secretion of small organic cations. Originally, OCT1 (also known as SLC22A1) was thought to be primarily expressed in liver, but recent studies have also localized its expression to the apical side of proximal and distal renal tubules. Hepatic OCT1 expression was found to be age dependent with almost a 5-fold difference between neonates and adults. OCT2 (SLC22A2) is predominantly expressed on the basolateral surface of proximal renal tubules. In adults, allelic variation in OCT1 and OCT2 is associated with increased renal clearance of metformin. The role of genetic variation of OCT1 and OCT2 has not been studied in children, but developmental factors appear to be operative. Neonates possess very limited ability to eliminate organic cations, but this function increases rapidly during the 1st few months of life, and when standardized for body weight or surface area, it tends to exceed adult levels during the toddler stage.

POLYMORPHISMS IN DRUG RECEPTORS

Receptors are the targets for drugs and endogenous transmitters because of their inherent molecular recognition sites. Drugs and transmitters bind to the receptor to produce a pharmacologic effect. Variability in the receptor protein or the ion channel may determine the magnitude of the pharmacologic response. Polymorphisms of the β_2-adrenergic receptor gene (*ADRB2*) are associated with variable responses to bronchodilator drugs.

Drug responses are seldom monogenic events because multiple genes are involved in both drug binding to the pharmacologic target and the subsequent downstream signal transduction events that ultimately manifest collectively as a therapeutic effect. Although genotypes at a particular locus may show a statistically significant effect on the outcome of interest, they may account for only a relatively small amount of the overall population variability for that outcome. A particular group of SNPs in the corticotropin-releasing hormone receptor 1 gene (*CRHR1*) is associated with a statistically significant improvement in forced expiratory volume in 1 second (FEV_1), but accounts for only 6% of the overall variability in response to inhaled corticosteroids. A series of subsequent studies has determined that allelic variation in several genes in the steroid pathway contributes to overall response to this form of therapy.

The listing and classification of receptors is a major initiative of the International Union of Pharmacology (IUPHAR). The list of receptors and voltage-gated ion channels is available on the IUPHAR website (http://www.iuphar-db.org). The effect of growth and development on the activities and binding affinities of these receptors, effectors, and ion channels has been studied in animals to some extent but remains to be elucidated in humans.

CURRENT AND FUTURE APPLICATIONS IN PEDIATRICS

Progress in the treatment of acute lymphoblastic leukemia shows how the application of pharmacogenomic principles can improve pediatric drug therapy (see Chapter 522.1). Despite improved understanding of the genetic determinants of drug response, however, many complexities remain to be resolved. Patients with ALL who have 1 wild-type

Drug metabolism (degradation) genotype

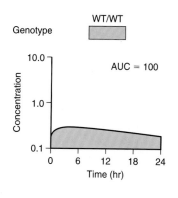 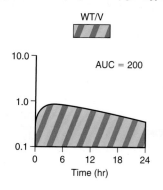 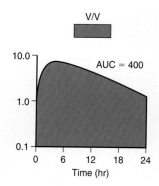

Drug receptor (efficacy) genotype

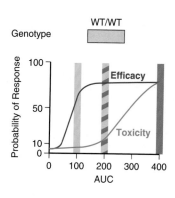 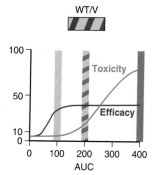 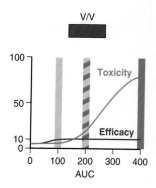

Polygenic drug response

Metabolism genotype		Receptor genotype	Probability of Response		Therapeutic Index	Individual risk : benefit assessment		
			Efficacy	Toxicity		Benefit	vs	risk
	+		65%	5%	13.0	Benefit	>>>>	Risk
	+		32%	5%	6.0	Benefit	>>>	Risk
	+		10%	5%	2.0	Benefit	>	Risk
	+		75%	15%	5.0	Benefit	>>	Risk
	+		40%	15%	2.7	Benefit	>	Risk
	+		10%	15%	0.7	Risk	>	Benefit
	+		80%	80%	1.0	Benefit	≈	Risk
	+		40%	80%	0.5	Risk	>>	Benefit
	+		10%	80%	0.1	Risk	>>>>	Benefit

Fig. 72.6 Polygenic determinants of drug response. The potential effects of 2 genetic polymorphisms are illustrated. In each panel, there is a profile for individuals who have 2 wild-type alleles (WT/WT), those who are heterozygous for 1 wild-type and 1 variant (V) allele (WT/V), and those who have 2 variant alleles (V/V) for the depicted gene. The **top panels** illustrate a potential polymorphism involving a drug-metabolizing enzyme where variant alleles result in decreased drug metabolism and greater exposure (as shown by the increasing area under the concentration-time curve [AUC]). The **middle panels** illustrate a potential polymorphism involving a drug receptor and depicts variant alleles which result in decreased receptor sensitivity. Note that for each receptor type, there are 3 possibilities for drug exposure. The **bottom table** shows the 9 resulting combinations of drug-metabolism and drug-receptor genotypes and the corresponding drug-response phenotypes calculated from data shown in the middle panels. These phenotypes allow for calculation of a therapeutic index (i.e., efficacy:toxicity; here this ranges from 13 [65%:5%] to 0.1 [10%:80%]), which results in the ability to perform an individualized risk/benefit assessment. (*Adapted from Evans WE, McLeod HL: Pharmacogenomics—drug disposition, drug targets, and side effects, N Engl J Med 348:538–549, 2003.*)

allele and intermediate TPMT activity tend to have a better response to 6MP therapy than patients with 2 wild-type alleles and full activity. Reduced TPMT activity also places patients at risk for irradiation-induced secondary brain tumors and etoposide-induced acute myeloid leukemia. Pharmacogenetic polymorphisms of several additional genes, such as *NUDT15*, also have the potential to influence successful treatment of ALL. Multiple genetic and treatment-related factors interact to create patient subgroups with varying degrees of risk. These represent an opportunity for pharmacogenomic approaches to identify subgroups of patients who will benefit from specific treatment regimens and those who will be at risk for short-term and long-term toxicities (Fig. 72.6).

Bibliography is available at Expert Consult.

Chapter 73
Principles of Drug Therapy
Tracy L. Sandritter, Bridgette L. Jones, Gregory L. Kearns, and Jennifer A. Lowry

第七十三章
药物治疗原则

中文导读

本章主要介绍了儿科药物治疗原则。具体描述了药代动力学和药效学的一般原则、个体发育对药物处置的影响、个体发育对药效学的影响、儿科治疗中的其他注意事项、药物剂型和给药、用药依从性、药物相互作用、药物不良反应和个体化给药。详细阐述了个体发育在药物处置中对药物吸收、药物分布、药物代谢和肾脏药物清除的影响，以及儿童剂量和方案选择和治疗药物监测等注意事项。

The clinical pharmacology of a given drug reflects a multifaceted set of properties that pertain to not only the disposition and action of drugs, but also the response (e.g., adverse effects, therapeutic effects, therapeutic outcomes) to their administration or use. The 3 most important facets of clinical pharmacology are pharmacokinetics, pharmacodynamics, and pharmacogenomics. **Pharmacokinetics** describes the movement of a drug throughout the body and the concentrations (or amounts) of a drug that reach a given body space or tissue and its residence time there. Pharmacokinetics of a drug are conceptualized by considering the characteristics that collectively are the determinants of the dose-concentration-effect relationship: absorption, distribution, metabolism, and excretion. **Pharmacodynamics** describes the relationship between drug dose or drug concentration and response. The response may be desirable (*effectiveness*) or untoward (*toxicity*). Although in clinical practice the response to drugs in different patient populations is often described by a standard dosing or concentration range, response is best conceptualized along a continuum where the relationship between dose and response(s) is not linear. **Pharmacogenomics** is the study of how variant forms of human genes contribute to interindividual variability in drug response. The finding that drug responses can be influenced by the patient's genetic profile has offered great hope for realizing individualized pharmacotherapy, in which the relationship between genotype and phenotype (either disease and/or drug response) is predictive of drug response (see Chapter 72). In the developing child, ontogeny has the potential to modulate drug response through altering both pharmacokinetics and pharmacodynamics.

GENERAL PHARMACOKINETIC AND PHARMACODYNAMIC PRINCIPLES

A drug effect is produced only when an exposure (both amount and duration) occurs that is sufficient to produce a drug-receptor interaction capable of modulating the cellular milieu and inducing a physiologic response. Thus, exposure-response relationships for a given drug represent an interface between pharmacokinetics and pharmacodynamics, which can be simply conceptualized by consideration of 2 profiles: plasma concentration vs effect (Fig. 73.1) and plasma concentration vs time (Fig. 73.2).

The relationship between drug concentration and effect for most drugs is not linear (Fig. 73.1). At a drug concentration of zero, the effect from the drug is generally zero or not perceptible (E_0). After drug administration and with dose escalation, the concentration increases, as does the effect, first in an apparent linear fashion (at low drug concentrations), followed by a nonlinear increase in effect to an asymptotic point in the relationship where a maximal effect (E_{max}) is attained that does not perceptibly change with further increases in drug

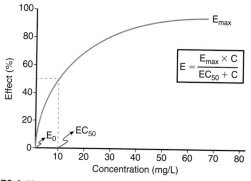

Fig. 73.1 Plasma concentration vs effect curve. The percent effect is measured as a function of increasing drug concentration in the plasma. E_0, Dose at which no effect is seen in the population; EC_{50}, dose of a drug required to produce a specified effect in 50% of the population; E_{max}, concentration associated with the maximal effect that can be produced by a drug. (From Abdel-Rahman SM, Kearns GL: The pharmacokinetic-pharmacodynamic interface: determinants of anti-infective drug action and efficacy in pediatrics. In Feigin RD, Cherry JD, Demmler-Harrison GJ, Kaplan SL, editors: Textbook of pediatric infectious disease, ed 6, Philadelphia, 2009, Saunders-Elsevier, pp 3156–3178; reproduced with permission.)

The equation shown in Fig. 73.1:

$$E = \frac{E_{max} \times C}{EC_{50} + C}$$

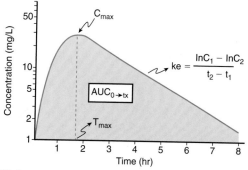

Fig. 73.2 Semilogarithmic plot of the plasma concentration vs time curve for a hypothetical drug following extravascular administration. The area under the plasma level-time curve (AUC) is a concentration- and time-dependent measure of systemic drug exposure. After administration, the drug is absorbed and reaches the maximal concentration (C_{max}) at its peak time (T_{max}). Following completion of drug absorption and distribution, plasma drug concentrations decline in an apparent monoexponential manner in which the slope of the apparent elimination phase represents the apparent elimination rate constant (ke). (From Abdel-Rahman SM, Kearns GL: The pharmacokinetic-pharmacodynamic interface: determinants of anti-infective drug action and efficacy in pediatrics. In Feigin RD, Cherry JD, Demmler-Harrison GJ, Kaplan SL, editors: Textbook of pediatric infectious disease, ed 6, Philadelphia, 2009, Saunders-Elsevier, pp 3156–3178; reproduced with permission.)

The elimination rate constant equation shown in Fig. 73.2:

$$ke = \frac{\ln C_1 - \ln C_2}{t_2 - t_1}$$

concentration. The point in the concentration-effect relationship where the observed effect represents 50% of the E_{max} is defined as **EC_{50}**, a common pharmacodynamic term used to compare concentration-effect relationships between patients (or research participants) and between drugs that may be in a given drug class.

Because it is rarely possible to measure drug concentrations at or near the receptor, it is necessary to utilize a surrogate measurement to assess **exposure-response relationships**. In most cases this surrogate is represented by the plasma drug concentration vs time curve. For drugs whose pharmacokinetic properties are best described by first-order (vs zero- or mixed-order) processes, a semilogarithmic plot of plasma drug concentration vs time data for an agent given by an extravascular route of administration (e.g., intramuscular, subcutaneous, intracisternal, peroral, transmucosal, transdermal, rectal) produces a pattern depicted

by Fig. 73.2. The ascending portion of this curve represents a time during which the liberation of a drug from its formulation, dissolution of the drug in a biologic fluid (e.g., gastric or intestinal fluid, interstitial fluid; a prerequisite for absorption), and absorption of the drug are rate limiting relative to its elimination. After the time (T_{max}) where maximal plasma concentrations (C_{max}) are observed, the plasma concentration decreases as metabolism and elimination become rate limiting; the terminal portion of this segment of the plasma concentration vs time curve is representative of drug elimination from the body. Finally, the area under the plasma concentration vs time curve (**AUC**), a concentration- and time dependent parameter reflective of the degree of systemic exposure from a given drug dose, can be determined by integrating the plasma concentration data over time.

Being able to characterize the pharmacokinetics of a specific drug allows the clinician to use the data to adjust "normal" dosing regimens and individualize them to produce the degree of systemic exposure associated with desired pharmacologic effects. For drugs where a therapeutic plasma concentration range or "target" systemic exposure (i.e., AUC) is known, a priori knowledge of pharmacokinetic parameters for a given population or patient within a population can facilitate the selection of a drug dosing regimen. Along with information on the pharmacodynamic behavior of a drug and the status of the patient (e.g., age, organ function, disease state, concomitant medications), the application of pharmacokinetics allows the practitioner to exercise a real degree of adaptive control over therapeutic decision-making through the selection of a drug and dosing regimen with the greatest likelihood of producing both efficacy and safety.

IMPACT OF ONTOGENY ON DRUG DISPOSITION

Development represents a continuum of biologic events that enable adaptation, somatic growth, neurobehavioral maturation, and eventually reproduction. The impact of development on the pharmacokinetics of a given drug is determined to a great degree by age-related changes in body composition and the acquisition of function in organs and organ systems important in determining drug metabolism and excretion. Although it is often convenient to classify pediatric patients on the basis of postnatal age in providing drug therapy, with neonates ≤1 mo of age, infants 1-24 mo, children 2-12 yr, and adolescents 12-18 yr, it is important to recognize that the changes in physiology are not linearly related to age and may not correspond to these age-defined breakpoints. In fact, the most dramatic changes in drug disposition occur during the 1st 18 mo of life, when the acquisition of organ function is most dynamic. It is important to note that the pharmacokinetics of a given drug may be altered in pediatric patients because of *intrinsic* (e.g., gender, genotype, ethnicity, inherited diseases) or *extrinsic* (e.g., acquired diseases, xenobiotic exposure, diet) factors that may occur during the 1st 2 decades of life.

Selection of an appropriate drug dose for a neonate, infant, child, or adolescent requires an understanding of the basic pharmacokinetic properties of a given compound and how the process of development impacts each facet of drug disposition. Accordingly, it is most useful to conceptualize pediatric pharmacokinetics by examining the impact of development on the physiologic variables that govern drug **absorption, distribution, metabolism, and elimination** (ADME).

Pediatrics encompasses a broad range of ages at which certain stages of life profoundly influence drug response and disposition. Dramatic pharmacokinetic, pharmacodynamic, and psychosocial changes occur as preterm infants mature toward term, as infants mature through the 1st few years of life, and as children reach puberty and adolescence (Fig. 73.3). To meet the needs of these different pediatric groups, different formulations are needed for drug delivery that can influence drug absorption and disposition, and different psychosocial issues influence compliance, timing of drug administration, and reactions to drug use. These additional factors must be considered in conjunction with known pharmacokinetic and pharmacodynamic influences of age when developing an optimal, patient-specific drug therapy strategy.

Drug Absorption

Drug absorption mainly occurs through passive diffusion, but active transport or facilitated diffusion may also be necessary for drug entry

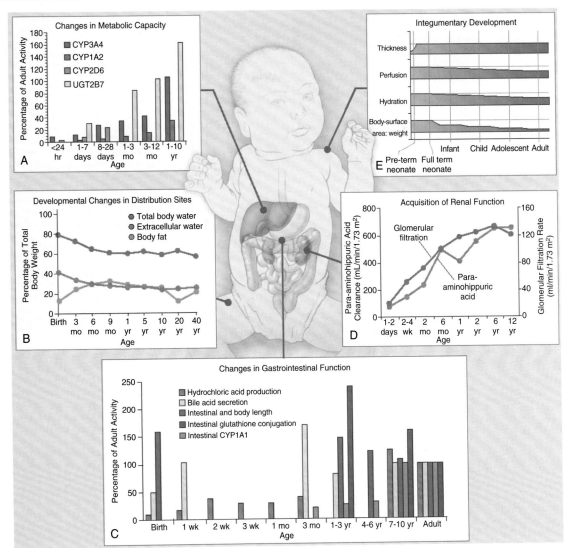

Fig. 73.3 Developmental changes in physiologic factors that influence drug disposition in infants, children, and adolescents. Physiologic changes in multiple organ systems during development are responsible for age-related differences in drug disposition. As reflected by panel **A**, the activity of many cytochrome P450 (CYP) isoforms and a single glucuronosyltransferase (UGT) isoform is markedly diminished during the 1st 2 mo of life. In addition, the acquisition of adult activity over time is enzyme and isoform specific. Panel **B** shows age-dependent changes in body composition, which influence the apparent volume of distribution of drugs. Infants in the 1st 6 mo of life have markedly expanded total-body water and extracellular water, expressed as a percentage of total body weight, compared with older infants and adults. Panel **C** summarizes the age-dependent changes in both structure and function of the gastrointestinal tract. As with hepatic drug-metabolizing enzymes (**A**), the activity of CYP1A1 in the intestine is low during early life. Panel **D** shows the effect of postnatal development on the processes of active tubular secretion, represented by the clearance of paraaminohippuric acid and the glomerular filtration rate, both of which approximate adult activity by 6-12 mo of age. Panel **E** shows age dependence in the thickness, extent of perfusion, and extent of hydration of the skin and the relative size of the skin-surface area (reflected by the ratio of body surface area to body weight). Although skin thickness is similar in infants and adults, the extent of perfusion and hydration diminishes from infancy to adulthood. (*From Kearns GL et al: Developmental pharmacology—drug disposition, action, therapy in infants and children, N Engl J Med 349:1160–1167, 2003. Copyright © 2003, reproduced with permission.*)

into cells. Several physiologic factors affect this process, one or more of which may be altered in certain disease states (e.g., inflammatory bowel disease, diarrhea), and thus produce changes in drug bioavailability. The rate and extent of absorption can be significantly affected by a child's normal growth and development.

Peroral Absorption

The most important factors that influence drug absorption from the gastrointestinal (GI) tract are related to the physiology of the stomach, intestine, and biliary tract (Fig. 73.3C and Table 73.1). The rate and

extent of peroral absorption of drugs depend primarily on the pH-dependent *passive diffusion* and *motility* of the stomach and intestinal tract, because both these factors will influence transit time of the drug. Gastric pH changes significantly throughout development, with the highest (alkaline) values occurring during the neonatal period. In the fully mature neonate the gastric pH ranges from 6-8 at birth and drops to 2-3 within a few hours of birth. However, after the 1st 24 hr of life, the gastric pH increases because of the immaturity of the parietal cells. As the parietal cells mature, the gastric acid secretory capacity increases (pH decreases) over the 1st few months of life, reaching adult levels by

Table 73.1 Developmental Alterations in Intestinal Drug Absorption

PHYSIOLOGIC ALTERATION	NEONATES	INFANTS	CHILDREN
Gastric pH	>5	4 to 2	Normal (2-3)
Gastric emptying time	Irregular	Increased	Slightly increased
Intestinal motility	Reduced	Increased	Slightly increased
Intestinal surface area	Reduced	Near adult	Adult pattern
Microbial colonization	Reduced	Near adult	Adult pattern
Biliary function	Immature	Near adult	Adult pattern

Direction of alteration given relative to expected normal adult pattern.
Data from Morselli PL: Development of physiological variables important for drug kinetics. In Morselli PL, Pippenger CE, Penry JK, editors: *Antiepileptic drug therapy in pediatrics*, New York, 1983, Raven Press.

Table 73.2 Influence of Ontogeny on Drug Absorption

PHYSIOLOGIC ALTERATION	NEONATES	INFANTS	CHILDREN
Oral absorption	Erratic	Increased	Near adult
Intramuscular absorption	Variable	Increased	Near adult
Percutaneous absorption	Increased	Increased	Near adult
Rectal absorption	Very efficient	Efficient	Near adult

Direction of alteration given relative to expected normal adult pattern.
Data from Morselli PL: Development of physiological variables important for drug kinetics. In Morselli PL, Pippenger CE, Penry JK, editors: *Antiepileptic drug therapy in pediatrics*, New York, 1983, Raven Press.

age 3-7 yr. As a result, the peroral bioavailability of acid-labile drugs (e.g., penicillin, ampicillin) is increased. In contrast, the absorption of weak organic acids (e.g., phenobarbital, phenytoin) is relatively decreased, a condition that may necessitate administration of larger doses in very young patients to achieve therapeutic plasma levels.

Gastric emptying time is prolonged throughout infancy and childhood as a result of reduced motility, which may impair drug passage into the intestine, where most absorption takes place. Gastric emptying rates reach or exceed adult values by 6-8 mo of life. As such, intestinal motility is important for the rate of drug absorption and, as with other factors, is dependent on the age of the child. Consequently, the rate of absorption of drugs with limited water solubility (e.g., phenytoin, carbamazepine) can be dramatically altered consequent to changes in GI motility. In older infants and young children, more rapid rates of intestinal drug transit can reduce the bioavailability for some drugs (e.g., phenytoin) and drug formulations (e.g., sustained-release) by reducing their residency time at the absorption surfaces in the small intestine.

Neonates, particularly premature neonates, have a reduced bile acid pool and biliary function, resulting in a decreased ability to solubilize and absorb lipophilic drugs. Biliary function develops in the 1st few months of life, but it may be difficult for the neonate and young infant to absorb fat-soluble vitamins because low concentrations of bile acids are necessary for their absorption.

Extravascular Drug Absorption

Intravenous (IV) drug administration is assumed to be the most dependable and accurate route for drug delivery, with a bioavailability of 100%. Absorption of drugs from tissues and organs (e.g., intramuscular, transdermal, rectal) can also be affected by development (Table 73.2). Intramuscular (IM) blood flow changes with age, which can result in variable and unpredictable absorption. Reduced muscular blood flow in the 1st few days of life, the relative inefficiency of muscular contractions

(useful in dispersing an IM drug dose), and an increased percentage of water per unit of muscle mass may delay the rate and extent of drugs given intramuscularly to the neonate. Muscular blood flow increases into infancy, and thus the bioavailability of drugs given by the IM route is comparable to that seen in children and adolescents.

In contrast, *mucosal* permeability (rectal and buccal) in the neonate is increased and thus may result in enhanced absorption by this route. *Transdermal* drug absorption in the neonate and very young infant is increased because of the thinner and more hydrated stratum corneum (Fig. 73.3E). In addition, the ratio of body surface area to body weight is greater in infants and children than in adults. Collectively, these developmental differences may predispose the child to increased exposure and risk for toxicity for drugs or chemicals placed on the skin (e.g., silver sulfadiazine, topical corticosteroids, benzocaine, diphenhydramine), with higher likelihood of occurrence during the 1st 8-12 mo of life.

Normal developmental differences in drug absorption from most all extravascular routes of administration can influence the dose–plasma concentration relationship in a manner sufficient to alter pharmacodynamics. The presence of disease states that influence a physiologic barrier for drug absorption or the time that a drug spends at a given site of absorption can further influence drug bioavailability and effect.

Drug Distribution

Drug distribution is influenced by a variety of drug-specific physiochemical factors, including the role of drug transporters, blood-tissue protein binding, blood-tissue pH, and perfusion. However, age-related changes in drug distribution are primarily related to developmental changes in body composition and the quantity of plasma proteins capable of drug binding. Age-dependent changes in the relative sizes of **body water**—*total body water* (TBW) and *extracellular water* (ECW) compartments may alter the apparent *volume of distribution* (VD) for a given drug. The absolute amounts and distribution of body water and fat depend on a child's age and nutritional status. Also, certain disease states (e.g., ascites, dehydration, burn injuries, skin disruption involving large surface area) can influence body water compartment sizes and thereby, further impact the VD for certain drugs.

Newborns have a much higher proportion of body mass in the form of water (approximately 75% TBW) than older infants and children (Fig. 73.3B). In addition, the percentage of ECW changes (decreases) from the newborn stage (approximately 45%) into adulthood (20–30%). In fact, the increase of TBW in the neonate is attributable to ECW. The reduction in TBW is rapid in the 1st year of life, with adult values (approximately 55%) achieved by approximately 12 yr of age. In contrast, the percentage of *intracellular water* (ICW) as a function of body mass remains stable from the 1st months of life through adulthood. The impact of developmental changes in body water spaces are exemplified by drugs such as the aminoglycoside antibiotics; compounds that distribute predominantly throughout the extracellular fluid space and have a higher VD (0.4-0.7 L/kg) in neonates and infants than in adults (0.2-0.3 L/kg).

Body fat percentage and composition increase during normal development. The body fat percentage in a neonate is approximately 16% (60% water and 35% lipid). Despite the relatively low body fat content in the neonate, it is important to note that the lipid content in the developing central nervous system (CNS) is high, which has implications for the distribution of lipophilic drugs (e.g., propranolol) and their CNS effects during this period. The body fat percentage tends to increase up to about age 10 yr, then changes composition with respect to puberty and sex to approach adult body fat composition (26% water and 71% lipid). In addition, a sex difference exists as the child transitions into adolescence. Whereas total body fat in males is reduced to 50% between 10 and 20 yr of life, the reduction in females is not as dramatic and decreases 28–25% during this same developmental stage.

Albumin, total proteins, and total globulins (e.g., α_1-acid glycoprotein) are the most important circulating proteins responsible for **drug binding** in plasma. The absolute concentration of these proteins is influenced by age, nutrition, and disease (Table 73.3). The concentrations of almost all circulating plasma proteins are reduced in the neonate and young infant (approximately 80% of adult) and reach adult values by 1 yr of age. A similar pattern of maturation is observed with α_1-acid glycoprotein

Table 73.3	Factors Influencing Drug Binding in Pediatric Patients		
PHYSIOLOGIC ALTERATION	**NEONATES**	**INFANTS**	**CHILDREN**
Plasma albumin	Reduced	Near adult	Near adult
Fetal albumin	Present	Absent	Absent
Total proteins	Reduced	Decreased	Near adult
Total globulins	Reduced	Decreased	Near adult
Serum bilirubin	Increased	Normal	Adult pattern
Serum free fatty acids	Increased	Normal	Adult pattern

Direction of alteration given relative to expected normal adult pattern.
Data from Morselli PL: Development of physiological variables important for drug kinetics. In Morselli PL, Pippenger CE, Penry JK, editors: *Antiepileptic drug therapy in pediatrics*, New York, 1983, Raven Press.

Table 73.4	Impact of Development on Drug Metabolism		
PHYSIOLOGIC ALTERATION	**NEONATE**	**INFANTS**	**CHILDREN**
Cytochrome P450 activity	Reduced	Increased	Slightly increased
Phase II enzyme activity	Reduced	Increased	Near adult
Blood esterase activity	Reduced	Normal (by 1 yr)	Adult pattern
Presystemic enzyme activity	Reduced	Increased	Near adult

Direction of alteration given relative to expected normal adult pattern.
Data from Morselli PL: Development of physiological variables important for drug kinetics. In Morselli PL, Pippenger CE, Penry JK, editors: *Antiepileptic drug therapy in pediatrics*, New York, 1983, Raven Press.

(an acute-phase reactant capable of binding basic drugs), for which neonatal plasma concentrations are approximately 3 times lower than in maternal plasma and attain adult values by approximately 1 yr of age.

The extent of drug binding to proteins in the plasma may influence distribution characteristics. Only free, unbound drug can be distributed from the vascular space into other body fluids and, ultimately, to tissues where drug-receptor interaction occurs. Drug protein binding depends on a number of age-related variables, including the absolute amount of proteins and their available binding sites, the conformational structure of the binding protein (e.g., reduced binding of acidic drugs to glycated albumin in patients with poorly controlled diabetes mellitus), the affinity constant of the drug for the protein, the influence of pathophysiologic conditions that either reduce circulating protein concentrations (e.g., ascites, major burn injury, chronic malnutrition, hepatic failure) or alter their structure (e.g., diabetes, uremia), and the presence of endogenous or exogenous substances that may compete for protein binding (i.e., protein displacement interactions).

Developmentally associated changes in drug binding can occur because of altered protein concentrations and binding affinity. Circulating fetal albumin in the neonate has significantly reduced binding affinity for acid drugs such as phenytoin, which is extensively (94–98%) bound to albumin in adults, compared to 80–85% in the neonate. The resultant 6-8-fold difference in the free fraction can result in CNS adverse effects in the neonate when total plasma phenytoin concentrations are within the generally accepted "therapeutic range" (10-20 mg/L). The importance of reduced drug-binding capacity of albumin in the neonate is exemplified by interactions between endogenous ligands (e.g., bilirubin, free fatty acids) and drugs with greater binding affinity (e.g., ability of sulfonamides to produce kernicterus).

Drug transporters such as P-glycoprotein and multidrug-resistant proteins 1 and 2 can influence drug distribution. These drug transporters can greatly influence the extent that drugs cross membranes in the body and whether drugs can penetrate or are secreted from the target sites (inside cancer cells or microorganisms or crossing the blood-brain barrier). Thus, drug resistance to cancer chemotherapy, antibiotics, or epilepsy may be conferred by these drug transport proteins and their effect on drug distribution. Growing evidence on the ontogeny of drug transport proteins demonstrates their presence as early as 12 wk gestation and low levels in the neonatal period, which rapidly increase to adult values by 1 to 2 yr of age, depending on the transporter. In addition, genetic variation can affect drug transporter expression and function but may not be readily apparent until adult levels are obtained (see Chapter 72).

Drug Metabolism

Metabolism reflects the biotransformation of an endogenous or exogenous molecule by one or more enzymes to moieties that are more hydrophilic and thus can be more easily eliminated by excretion, secretion, or exhalation. Although metabolism of a drug generally reduces its ability to produce a pharmacologic action, metabolism also can result in metabolites that have significant potency and thereby contribute to

the drug's overall pharmacodynamic profile (e.g., biotransformation of the tricyclic antidepressant amitriptyline to nortriptyline; codeine to morphine; cefotaxime to desacetyl cefotaxime; theophylline to caffeine). In the case of prodrugs (e.g., zidovudine, enalapril, fosphenytoin) or some drug salts or esters (e.g., cefuroxime axetil, clindamycin phosphate), biotransformation is required to produce a pharmacologically active moiety. Finally, for some drugs, cellular injury and associated adverse reactions are the result of drug metabolism (e.g., acetaminophen hepatotoxicity, Stevens-Johnson syndrome associated with sulfamethoxazole).

The primary organ responsible for drug metabolism is the liver, although the kidney, intestine, lung, adrenals, blood (phosphatases, esterases), and skin can also biotransform certain compounds. Drug metabolism occurs primarily in the endoplasmic reticula of cells through 2 general classes of enzymatic processes: phase I (nonsynthetic) and phase II (synthetic) reactions. **Phase I** reactions include oxidation, reduction, hydrolysis, and hydroxylation reactions. **Phase II** reactions primarily involve conjugation with an endogenous ligand (e.g., glycine, glucuronide, glutathione or sulfate). Many drug-metabolizing enzymes demonstrate an ontogenic profile with generally low activity at birth and maturation over months to years (Table 73.4 and Fig. 73.3A).

Many enzymes are capable of catalyzing the biotransformation of drugs and xenobiotics, but quantitatively the most important are represented by cytochrome P450 (**CYP**), a supergene family with at least 16 primary enzymes. The specific CYP isoforms responsible for the majority of human drug metabolism are represented by CYP1A2, CYP2C9, CYP2C19, CYP2D6, CYP2E1, and CYP3A4. These enzymes represent the products of genes that in some cases are polymorphically expressed, with allelic variants producing enzymes generally resulting in either no or reduced catalytic activity (a notable exception being the *17 allele of CYP2C19, which may have increased activity) (see Chapter 72). At birth the concentration of drug-oxidizing enzymes in fetal liver (corrected for liver weight) appears similar to that in adult liver. However, the activity of these oxidizing enzyme systems is reduced, which results in slow clearance (and prolonged elimination) of many drugs that are substrates for them (e.g., phenytoin, caffeine, diazepam). Postnatally, the hepatic CYPs appear to mature at different rates. Within hours after birth, CYP2E1 activity increases rapidly, with CYP2D6 being detectable soon thereafter. CYP2C (CYP2C9 and CYP2C19) and CYP3A4 are present within the 1st mo of life, a few months before CYP1A2. CYP3A4 activity in young infants may exceed that observed in adults, as reflected by the clearance of drugs that are substrates for this enzyme (e.g., cyclosporine, tacrolimus).

Compared to phase I drug-metabolizing enzymes, the impact of development on the activity of phase II enzymes (acetylation, glucuronidation, sulfation) is not characterized as well. Phase II enzyme activity is decreased in the newborn and increases into childhood. Conjugation of compounds metabolized by isoforms of glucuronosyltransferase (**UGT**) (e.g., morphine, bilirubin, chloramphenicol) is reduced at birth but can exceed adult values by 3-4 yr of age. Also, the ontogeny of UGT expression is isoform specific. Newborns and infants primarily metabolize the common analgesic acetaminophen by sulfate conjugation, since the UGT isoforms responsible for its glucuronidation (UGT1A1 and UGT1A9) have greatly reduced activity. As children age, the glucuronide conjugate becomes predominant in the metabolism of therapeutic doses of acetaminophen. In contrast, the glucuronidation of morphine (a UGT2B7 substrate) can be detected as early as 24 wk gestation.

The activity of certain hydrolytic enzymes, including blood esterases, is also reduced during the neonatal period. Blood esterases are important for the metabolic clearance of cocaine, and the reduced activity of these plasma esterases in the newborn may account for the delayed metabolism (prolonged effect) of local anesthetics in the neonate. In addition, this may account for the prolonged effect that cocaine has on the fetus with prenatal exposures. Adult esterase activity is achieved by 10-12 mo of age.

The development of **presystemic clearance** or "first-pass" metabolism is unclear given the involvement of multiple enzymes and transporters in the small intestine, many of which have patterns of developmental expression that may be more or less concordant. However, given that the activity of almost all drug-metabolizing enzymes is markedly reduced in the neonate, the extent of bioavailability of drugs given by the peroral route that may be subjected to significant presystemic clearance in older children and adults would appear to be greatly increased during the 1st days to weeks of life. It is important for the clinician to recognize that estimates of bioavailability for a host of drugs available in reference texts and therapeutic compendia are most often derived from studies conducted in young adults. Thus, estimates of the rate and extent of absorption (including a propensity to be affected by presystemic clearance) from adults cannot be accurately used to extrapolate how a peroral drug dose may need to be age-adjusted for a neonate or infant.

With regard to the impact of development on drug metabolism, it must be recognized that most therapeutic drugs are polyfunctional substrates for a host of enzymes and transporters. It is the isoform-specific ontogenic profile (Fig. 73.3) that must be considered in the context of deducing how development can affect the metabolic portion of drug clearance. True developmental dependence of drug clearance must also consider the role of pharmacogenetic constitution on the activity of enzymes and transporters (see Chapter 72) and the impact of ontogeny on the nonmetabolic routes (e.g., renal drug excretion, salivary/biliary drug excretion, pulmonary drug excretion), which contribute to the overall drug clearance (Total $CL = CL_{hepatic} + CL_{renal} + CL_{nonrenal}$).

Renal Drug Elimination

The kidney is the primary organ responsible for the elimination of drugs and their metabolites. The development of renal function begins during early fetal development and is complete by early childhood (Fig. 73.3D and Table 73.5). Total renal drug clearance (CL_{renal}) can be conceptualized by considering the following equation:

$$CL_{renal} = (GFR + ATS) - ATR$$

where glomerular filtration rate (GFR), active tubular secretion (ATS), and active tubular reabsorption (ATR) of drugs can contribute to overall clearance. As for hepatic drug metabolism, only free (unbound) drug and metabolite can be filtered by a normal glomerulus and secreted or reabsorbed by a renal tubular transport protein.

Renal clearance is limited in the newborn because of anatomic and functional immaturity of the nephron unit. In both the term and the preterm neonate, GFR averages 2-4 mL/min/1.73 m² at birth. During the 1st few days of life, a decrease in renal vascular resistance results in a net increase in renal blood flow and a redistribution of intrarenal blood flow from a predominantly medullary to a cortical distribution. All these changes are associated with a commensurate increase in GFR. In term neonates, GFR increases rapidly over the 1st few months of life and approaches adult values by 10-12 mo (Fig. 73.3D). The rate of GFR acquisition is blunted in preterm neonates because of continued nephrogenesis in the early postnatal period. In young children 2-5 yr of age, GFR may exceed adult values, especially during periods of increased metabolic demand (e.g., fever).

In addition, a relative glomerular/tubular imbalance results from a more advanced maturation of glomerular function. Such an imbalance may persist up to 6 mo of age and may account for the observed decrease in the ATS of drugs commonly used in neonates and young infants (e.g., β-lactam antibiotics). Finally, some evidence suggests that ATR is reduced in neonates and that it appears to mature at a slower rate than the GFR.

Altered renal drug clearance in the newborn and infants result in the different dosing recommendations seen in pediatrics. The aminoglycoside antibiotic gentamicin provides an illustrative example. In adolescents and young adults with normal values for GFR (85-130 mL/min/1.73 m²), the recommended dosing interval for gentamicin is 8 hours. In young children who may have a GFR >130 mL/min/1.73 m², a gentamicin dosing interval of every 6 hr may be necessary in selected patients who have serious infections that require maintaining steady-state peak and trough plasma concentrations near the upper boundary of the recommended therapeutic range. In contrast, to maintain "therapeutic" gentamicin plasma concentrations in neonates during the 1st few weeks of life, a dosing interval of 18-24 hr is required.

The impact of developmental differences in GFR on the elimination characteristics of a given drug can be assessed by estimating the apparent elimination rate constant (Kel) for a drug by using the following equation:

$$Kel\ (in\ reduced\ renal\ function)$$
$$= Kel_{normal}\ \{[(GFR_{observed}/GFR_{normal})-1]\ Fel\}+1$$

where the *Fel* represents the fraction of the drug excreted unchanged in an adult with normal renal function; $GFR_{observed}$ is the value calculated (from creatinine clearance or age-appropriate estimation equation) for the patient (in mL/min/1.73 m²); and GFR_{normal} is the average value considered for a healthy adult (120 mL/min/1.73 m²). Kel_{normal} is estimated from the average elimination $T_{1/2}$ for a drug taken from the medical literature using the following equation:

$$Kel_{normal}\ [hr^{-1}] = 0.693/T_{1/2\ normal}\ [hr]$$

Likewise, the elimination half-life ($T_{1/2}$) for a drug in patients with reduced renal function can be estimated as follows:

$$T_{1/2}\ (in\ reduced\ renal\ function) = 0.693/Kel\ (in\ reduced\ function)$$

An estimate of the drug elimination $T_{1/2}$ in patients with reduced renal function with knowledge of the desired interdose excursion in steady-state plasma concentrations can allow determination of the desired drug dosing interval.

IMPACT OF ONTOGENY ON PHARMACODYNAMICS

Although it is generally accepted that developmental differences exist in drug action, there is little evidence of true age related pharmacodynamic variation among children of differing age-groups and adults. **Drug action** is typically mediated by interaction of a small molecule with 1 or more receptors that may be located either on or in a cell. **Drug effect** is mediated at the receptor by 4 main biochemical

Table 73.5	Impact of Development on Renal Drug Elimination		
PHYSIOLOGIC ALTERATION	**NEONATE**	**INFANTS**	**CHILDREN**
Glomerular filtration	Reduced	Normal (by 1 yr)	Adult pattern
Active tubular secretion	Reduced	Near normal	Adult pattern
Active tubular reabsorption	Reduced	Near normal	Adult pattern
Active drug excretion	Reduced	Near normal	Adult pattern
Passive drug excretion	Reduced	Increased	Adult pattern
Excretion of basic drugs	Increased	Increased	Near normal

Direction of alteration given relative to expected normal adult pattern.
Data from Morselli PL: Development of physiological variables important for drug kinetics. In Morselli PL, Pippenger CE, Penry JK, editors: *Antiepileptic drug therapy in pediatrics*, New York, 1983, Raven Press.

mechanisms involved in cell signaling. *Binding* of the receptors on the cell surface or within the cell activates downstream pathways that mediate a specific cellular action. Some receptors act as *enzymes,* whereby on ligand binding the enzyme phosphorylates downstream effector proteins, thereby activating or inhibiting a cellular signal (e.g., guanosine triphosphate–binding regulatory protein, also known as G-protein–coupled receptors). Other receptors mediate their actions through *ion channels,* whereby on ligand binding the cell's membrane potential or ionic composition is altered, allowing cellular activation or inhibition. Lastly, some receptors act as *transcription factors,* which when bound by a ligand activate transcription of specific genes within the cell.

Drug action is concentration dependent, with onset and offset generally associated with appearance and disappearance, respectively, of the drug at the receptor(s) in an amount that is sufficient to initiate the cascade of biologic effects that terminate in drug action (see Fig. 73.1). The *minimum effective concentration* of a drug is that observed with the immediate onset of effect, whereas the duration of action is predicated on the maintenance of drug concentrations at the receptor within a range associated with the desirable pharmacologic action(s). Receptor binding by a drug may have varying consequences. Drugs that are **agonists** bind to and activate the receptor, directly or indirectly achieving the desired effect. An agonist binding to a receptor results in the same biologic effect as binding of the endogenous ligand. **Partial agonist** binding results in activation of the receptor, but maximal effect is not achieved, even in the presence of receptor saturation. **Antagonists** bind to a receptor, preventing binding of other molecules, thereby preventing activation of the receptor.

Evidence supports developmental differences in receptor number, density, distribution, function, and ligand affinity for some drugs. Human data are limited, so much of what is known has been derived from animal studies. In the CNS, unique developmental aspects of drug-receptor interaction affect therapeutic efficacy of both analgesics and sedatives in neonates. The number of γ-aminobutyric acid (GABA) receptors, which mediate inhibitory signal transduction in the CNS, is reduced in newborns compared to adults. Functional differences have also been observed between neonatal and adult brain on GABA receptor activation. These changes may explain observed differences in dosing of drugs such as midazolam in infants and in part may explain seizures experienced by infants on benzodiazepine exposure. Another CNS example is the μ-opioid receptor, whereby receptor number is reduced in newborns and receptor distribution also differs between newborns and adults.

For the clinician, consideration of age-dependent differences in pharmacodynamics is particularly relevant when associated with **adverse drug reactions** (e.g., higher incidence of valproic acid-associated hepatotoxicity in young infants; greater frequency of paradoxical CNS reactions to diphenhydramine in infants; weight gain associated with

atypical antipsychotic drugs in adolescents) or when drugs have a narrow therapeutic index (Fig. 73.4). The age-associated pharmacodynamics of warfarin observed in children with congenital heart disease is related to developmental differences in serum concentrations of vitamin K–dependent coagulation factors (II, VII, IX, X) between children and adults. Developmental differences in drug action have been observed between prepubertal children and adults in regard to warfarin action. Prepubertal children exhibit a more profound response, demonstrated by lower protein C concentration, prothrombin fragments 1 and 2, and greater rise in INR, to comparable doses of warfarin. Thus, when age-dependent pharmacodynamics of a given drug is evident, the use of simple allometric approaches for "scaling" the pediatric dose from the usual adult dose may not produce the desired pharmacologic effects. Pharmacokinetic and pharmacodynamic (PK/PD) modeling techniques that use known developmental changes in body composition, enzyme function, renal function, effector proteins, and receptors are being used to predict optimal dosing in children. However, data regarding differences in pharmacodynamic response across the age continuum remain lacking and limit the application of these techniques to accurately predict dose-response relationships in the pediatric population.

Surrogate Endpoints
Biomarkers and surrogate endpoints (markers) are ideally simple, reliable, inexpensive, and easily obtainable measures of a biologic response or disease phenotype that can be used to facilitate either clinical research or patient care. **Biomarkers** have been defined by the U.S. National Institutes of Health as "a characteristic that is objectively measured and evaluated as an indicator of normal biological processes, pathogenic processes, or pharmacologic responses to a therapeutic intervention." A **surrogate endpoint** is defined "as a biomarker that is intended to substitute for a specific clinical endpoint. A surrogate endpoint is expected to predict clinical benefit (or harm or lack of benefit or harm) based on epidemiologic, therapeutic, pathophysiologic, or other scientific evidence." Reliable surrogate endpoints predict a specific physiologic event (e.g., intraesophageal pH to assess gastroesophageal reflux) that may be used diagnostically, prognostically, or in predicting a specific drug response (therapeutic, subtherapeutic, or adverse) or potentially the impact of ontogeny on pharmacodynamics. Specific examples of surrogate endpoints used in pediatric pharmacology include measurement of esophageal pH to assess the action of prokinetic or acid-modifying drugs and pulmonary function tests (e.g., FEV_1) to evaluate the effect of drugs on pulmonary function in patients with conditions such as asthma and cystic fibrosis. Biomarkers used in pediatric studies to assess drug disposition or effect include hemoglobin A_{1c} plasma concentration (to assess efficacy of peroral hypoglycemic agents), urinary leukotriene concentrations (to assess effects of nonsteroidal antiinflammatory drugs), and minimal inhibitory concentration (MIC) and minimal bacteriocidal concentration (MBC) of drugs to select antiinfective agents.

ADDITIONAL CONSIDERATIONS IN PEDIATRIC THERAPEUTICS
Pediatric Dose and Regimen Selection
Incomplete developmental profiles for hepatic and extrahepatic drug-metabolizing enzymes and drug transporters that may influence drug clearance and bioavailability prevent the use of simple formulas or allometric scaling for effective pediatric dose prediction. Although these approaches may have some clinical utility in older children (>8 yr) and adolescents whose organ function and body composition approximate that of young adults, their utility is severely limited in neonates, infants, and young children, in whom ontogeny produces dramatic differences in drug disposition. This is especially problematic for therapeutic drugs whose doses cannot be easily individualized using patient-specific pharmacokinetic data obtained from therapeutic drug monitoring. In the absence of such pharmacokinetic data or established pediatric dosing guidelines, alternate methods must often be employed.

To date, >20 different approaches for initial selection of a drug dose for pediatric patients have been described. The majority use either total body weight (BW) or body surface area (BSA) as surrogates that reflect the developmental changes of body composition or organ function,

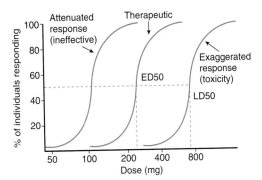

Fig. 73.4 Quantal dose–effect curve. Age-related pharmacokinetic variation may result in alterations in drug concentration at the receptor resulting in ineffective, therapeutic or toxic results. LD50, Dose at which 50% of the population is lethal. The ratio of the LD50 to the ED50 is an indication of the therapeutic index, which is a reflection of drug potency relative to its concentration.

which collectively are the major determinants of drug disposition. Selection based on BW or BSA will generally produce similar relationships between drug dose and resultant plasma concentration, except for those drugs whose apparent volume of distribution (VD) corresponds to the extracellular fluid pool (i.e., VD <0.3 L/kg), in which a BSA-based approach is preferable. In contrast, for drugs whose apparent VD exceeds the extracellular fluid space (i.e., VD >0.3 L/kg), a BW-based approach for dose selection is preferable, which is the most frequently used method in pediatrics. When the pediatric dose for a given drug is not known, these principles can be used to best approximate a proper dose for the initiation of treatment, as illustrated by the following equations:

$$\text{Child dose (if VD} < 0.3 \text{ L/kg)}$$
$$= (\text{Child BSA in m}^2/1.73 \text{ m}^2) * \text{Adult dose}$$

$$\text{Infant dose (if VD} \geq 0.3 \text{ L/kg)} = (\text{Infant BW in kg}/70 \text{ kg}) * \text{Adult dose}$$

It should be noted that this approach assumes that the child's weight, height, and body composition are age appropriate and normal, and that the "reference" normal adult has a BW and BSA of 70 kg and 1.73 m², respectively. It is useful only for selection of dose size and does not offer information regarding dosing interval, because the equations contain no specific variable that describes potential age-associated differences in drug clearance.

Similar to obese adults, **obesity in children** would be expected to result in to alterations in drug pharmacokinetics. Unfortunately, few data exist on drug dosing in obese pediatric patients. Alterations in VD, which is important for loading-dose calculations, is related to the lipophilicity or water solubility of the medication to be administered. Some limited data are available on the impact of obesity on VD in children with the antibiotics cefazolin and tobramycin. The impact of obesity in pediatric patients on absorption and drug metabolism (phase I and II pathways) is not known. No validated estimate of GFR in obese children exists, but current information suggests that serum creatinine concentration may be higher or no different in obese children than in those of normal weight. Drug dosing in normal-weight children typically uses age-based dosing, allometric scaling, BSA, or BW. These same estimates can be used in obese children, although use of an adjusted BW should be considered. Variations on weight used in adults include ideal body weight (IBW), lean body weight, adjusted body weight, and total body weight. However, in children, standards for calculating adjusted weights may not be standardized (e.g., IBW). When dosing medications in obese children, it is important to consider information regarding drug dosing in obese adults, recommended adult maximum doses, and the physiochemical properties of the drug to be given.

In neonates and young infants with developmental immaturity in GFR or ATS, it is often necessary to adjust the "normal" dosing interval (i.e., that used for older infants and children who have attained developmental competence of renal function) for drugs with significant (>50%) renal elimination, to prevent excessive drug accumulation (and possible associated toxicity) with administration of multiple doses. To accomplish this therapeutic goal, it is necessary to estimate the apparent elimination half-life ($T_{1/2}$) of the drug (see equations earlier).

Therapeutic Drug Monitoring

Clinically, systemic drug exposure is usually evaluated through assessing the plasma drug concentration, a surrogate measurement for a drug reaching its pharmacologic receptor(s). In the patient, drug level monitoring can be used to facilitate 2 approaches for evaluating the dose-concentration-effect relationship: single-concentration (e.g., trough or random level) therapeutic drug monitoring (TDM) and multilevel pharmacokinetic-based TDM. Both lead to dose individualization for a given patient.

Drug-level monitoring largely entails measurement of drug concentrations in plasma (primarily) or other biologic fluids at some point during a drug's dosing interval. These levels are then compared with those that are "desired" for a given drug based on published information and used to adjust the dose/dosing regimen. For *single* trough-level measurement (at the end of a dosing interval) or random-level measurement (nonspecific time point during a dosing interval), adjustment of the medications dose

is done empirically without pharmacokinetic parameters. In using a TDM approach, it should be recognized that for many drugs which are therapeutically monitored in the clinical setting (e.g., aminoglycoside antibiotics, vancomycin, phenytoin, phenobarbital, cyclosporine, tacrolimus, mycophenolate mofetil, selected antiretroviral drugs, acyclovir), "desired" plasma concentrations are generally determined from studies in adult patients where drug disposition and disease states may be quite different from those in infants and children.

Clinical pharmacokinetics represents a proactive approach where *multiple* plasma drug concentrations are used to estimate pharmacokinetic parameters for a specific patient to a specific drug at that point in time (e.g., apparent elimination rate constant, elimination $T_{1/2}$, apparent VD, total plasma clearance, AUC), which are then used to calculate a dosing regimen required to attain a desired level of systemic exposure (e.g., AUC, steady-state peak/trough plasma drug concentrations) that would portend a desired pharmacologic response. Of these 2 approaches, the use of drug-level data for performing clinical pharmacokinetics provides the better approach for individualizing dose/dosing regimen and maintaining some adaptive control over the dose-concentration-effect relationship. This approach is particularly useful for patients who may have "abnormal" pharmacokinetics because of their age and/or disease states. Approaches used to enable the performance of clinical pharmacokinetics include the manual use of established formulas for calculating pharmacokinetic parameters (generally using a simple 1-compartment open model consequent to the few plasma drug-level observations obtained in clinical patient care) or computer-based algorithms (e.g., bayesian estimation, population-based pharmacokinetic approaches).

Common to both of the aforementioned approaches is the need to accurately assess plasma drug concentrations in a given patient. Fig. 73.5 represents a hypothetical general steady-state plasma concentration vs time profile for a drug given by an extravascular route, illustrating the following general principles to recognize and follow when plasma drug-level monitoring is used in patients as a "tool" to individualize drug treatment:

◆ When a drug reaches a pharmacokinetic steady state (a period corresponding to 5 times the apparent elimination $T_{1/2}$ for a given drug), both the excursion between the peak (C_{max}) and trough (C_{min}) plasma concentration and the AUC are identical between dose intervals provided that (1) the dose is not changed; (2) an exact dose-to-dose interval is maintained for drug administration; and (3) the route or rate of drug administration between dosing intervals has not changed.

◆ Steady-state plasma drug concentrations provide the best surrogate for assessing exposure-response relationships for a given drug. These

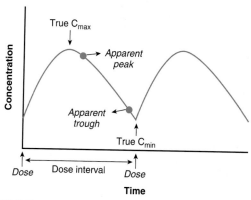

Fig. 73.5 Plasma concentration vs time profile for a hypothetical drug at steady state. When dose size, route of administration, time of administration, and dosing interval remain constant, the resultant true peak (C_{max}) and trough (C_{min}) plasma concentrations and AUC from dose to dose are identical. Apparent values for C_{max} and C_{min} are denoted to illustrate the potential difference from true values that can result when the actual times for obtaining samples for either therapeutic drug monitoring or clinical pharmacokinetic applications are not realized.

drug concentrations provide the most accurate estimation of patient-specific pharmacokinetic parameters. Plasma concentrations assessed before the attainment of steady state can be useful for evaluating exaggerated drug response or predicting eventual steady-state drug levels and exposure.

◆ To reliably interpret any drug plasma concentration, it is imperative that the clinician know and consider the following:

1. The expected pharmacokinetic profile for a given drug (e.g., time after dosing required for completion of drug absorption [for extravascularly administered drugs] and distribution)
2. The exact time that the drug was administered
3. For drugs given by IV infusion, the total duration of infusion (including time required to flush the dose from the IV tubing)
4. Pertinent limitations of the analytic method used to measure the plasma drug level (e.g., range of linearity, potential for analytic interference from concomitant drugs)
5. The method used to obtain the blood specimen(s) used for plasma level determination (e.g., venous puncture vs cutaneous puncture; use of vascular catheter different from one used for drug administration)
6. Whether the blood specimen was adequate for accurate drug-level measurement (e.g., sufficient volume, presence or absence of hemolysis or lipemia)
7. The *exact* time that the blood specimens were obtained in relationship to the time of drug administration and the drug dosing interval

This last point is illustrated by Fig. 73.5, which denotes the "true" peak (C_{max}) and trough (C_{min}) plasma concentrations in relationship to apparent values. This situation frequently occurs when "peak" and "trough" blood levels are ordered, and nursing/phlebotomy procedures allow some period of leeway as to when they can be obtained. When such a discrepancy is realized, and the exact timing of the samples relative to dose administration is known, corrections can be made to insure pharmacokinetic parameters estimated from the data are accurate. If such a discrepancy is not realized, errant parameter estimation and dose regimen calculation/determination may result, thereby compromising safety or efficacy of drug treatment.

DRUG FORMULATION AND ADMINISTRATION

One of the more unique challenges in pediatric therapeutics is the drug formulation itself. Despite the increasing sensitivity for the need to study pediatric drugs before their use in children and to have available "pediatric-friendly" formulations, many drug products formulated only for adult use are routinely given to pediatric patients. Their use can result in inaccurate dosing (e.g., administration of a fixed dose to children with widely varying body weights), loss of desired performance characteristics of the formulation (e.g., crushing sustained-release tablet, cutting transdermal patch), and exposure of infants and children to excipients (e.g., binding agents, preservatives) in amounts capable of producing adverse effects.

Peroral Drug Administration

One of the principal determinants of peroral drug administration in children is the ability to get the drug into the body. Peroral formulations are often expelled by children because of poor taste and texture. This is a significant issue, especially when considering that taste sensation differs because of development and on an interindividual basis. Solid peroral formulations such as tablets and capsules are not easily administered to the majority of infants and children because of their inability to swallow them easily and safely. Incomplete development of swallowing coordination may result in choking or aspiration when solid peroral formulations are given to infants and small children. Further, solid peroral formulations limit the ability for dose titration and dosing flexibility. Drug developers are working to address this limitation with new techniques suitable for both oral and peroral drug administration that encompass both products (e.g., dispersible peroral tablets, oral films, titratable granules, oral melts) and drug administration devices (e.g., dosing straws, graduated cylinders for peroral granules). With regard to dosing accuracy with peroral formulations, **liquids** (e.g., drops, solutions, syrups, suspensions, elixirs) are preferred for infants and young children. The utility of these formulations is often limited by palatability when taste-masking of the active ingredient(s) cannot be effectively achieved. In the case of suspension formulations, improper reconstitution and/or resuspension before dose administration can introduce problems related to accuracy of dosing. Other potential limitations of peroral liquid formulations (e.g., those that may be extemporaneously compounded by the pharmacist from drug powder or from solid peroral dosage forms of a given drug) include potential problems related to drug stability, contamination (chemical or bacterial), portability, and for some products the need for refrigeration.

Administration of liquid medications can be associated with risk if the device for administering the medication is not appropriate (e.g., use of a kitchen teaspoon vs 5.0 mL dosing spoon) or is used improperly to insure the drug dose is measured appropriately for the patient's age or weight. The low cost and convenience of hypodermic syringes has prompted many physicians and pharmacists to dispense them with liquid medications in order to improve accuracy. While this approach would seemingly be associated with greater accuracy in dosing, parents/caregivers can have difficulty in reading the graduations on a syringe, and the plastic caps on the plungers of syringes can produce a choking hazard for infants and young children. These problems can be obviated by education of parents/caregivers on how to reliably use peroral dosing syringes, which pharmacists should dispense with every liquid drug formulation.

Parenteral Drug Administration

In contrast to adults, in whom vascular access is relatively easy to obtain, difficulties are often present in the infant and young child, resulting from the smaller diameter of peripheral vessels (relative to size of IV cannula), developmentally associated differences in body composition (e.g., body fat distribution), and use of topical anesthetic agents, which can produce venous constriction. The small peripheral blood vessels in infants and young children can also limit the volume and rate of parenteral drug administration due to issues of capacity and with drugs capable of producing venous irritation, which induces infusion-related pain.

An underappreciated complicating issue for parenteral drug administration to infants is the relative lack of formulations in concentrations suitable for IV administration. Errors consequent to improper dilution of adult formulations necessary to ensure appropriate osmolarity and volume for IV administration (the most common resulting in a 10-fold overdose) are not uncommon. Morphine, a drug commonly used in neonates, infants, and children, is commonly available in an 8 mg/mL concentration. A usual 0.1 mg/kg morphine dose for a 1 kg infant using this formulation would require a nurse or pharmacist to accurately withdraw 0.013 mL and administer it into a length of IV tubing with a dead space volume that may exceed that of the dose by 100-fold. In this situation, accuracy of dose and infusion time can be significantly compromised. Although underdosing is often a serious problem when attempting to administer very small volumes, overdoses also occur from inaccurate extemporaneous dilutions. Moreover, attempts to compensate for the volumes present within the IV tubing further predispose the patient to receive an incorrect, possibly unsafe, dose. Whenever such concentrated drug formulations are the only source for use, appropriate alteration of the stock parenteral solution should be performed and manufactured by the pharmacy department. Also, many errors can be avoided by the use of standard dilutions that all practitioners are aware of and using standardized approaches for IV drug administration that minimize complications associated with unrealized drug dilution and errant infusion times (e.g., pediatric syringe pumps attached to low-volume tubing).

Although used rather infrequently, intramuscular (IM) drug administration offers a route of administration for many drugs when venous access is not immediately available or when a therapeutic drug regimen involves use of a single or limited number of doses. While appealing with respect to immediacy, this route of administration can be associated with problems (e.g., muscle/nerve damage, sterile abscess formation, variable rate of drug absorption because of developmental differences in vascular perfusion of muscle beds), especially in the neonate and small infant. Lastly, the decision to use the IM route must take into consideration the physicochemical properties (e.g., pH, osmolarity, solubility) of the drug formulation and any diluent used to prepare it.

Other Routes for Drug Administration

Neonates, infants, children, and adolescents with certain pulmonary conditions (e.g., reactive airway disease, viral-induced bronchiolitis, asthma, cystic fibrosis) frequently receive drugs (e.g., corticosteroids, β-adrenergic agonists, antimicrobial agents, mucolytic drugs) by **inhalation**. The pulmonary surface area in pediatric patients of all ages is a very effective, easily traversable barrier for drug absorption. Rate-limiting factors for pulmonary drug absorption include physicochemical factors associated with the drug and delivery system (e.g., particle size, diffusion coefficient, chemical stability of drug molecule in the lung) and physical factors that influence intrapulmonary drug disposition (e.g., active vs passive drug delivery to tracheobronchial tree, respiratory minute volume, internal airway diameter), many of which are developmentally determined. For drugs formulated for delivery using a metered-dose inhaler (either drug powder or suspended particles using a carrier gas), developmental factors (e.g., incoordination of device actuation with inhalation, inability to follow instructions for clearing of airway, passive inhalation with actuation of delivery device) either prevent their use (as in infants and small children) or limit the bioavailability of the drug to be administered. In these instances, specific devices (e.g., masks, spacer chambers) and methods of delivery (e.g., continuous aerosolization by mask) can be used to improve the efficiency of drug delivery and thus drug efficacy.

In pediatric patients, **percutaneous** drug administration is generally reserved for agents intended to produce a local effect within the dermis. Development has an impact on the barrier of the skin that, if not recognized and controlled for with proper drug administration techniques, can produce situations in which systemic toxicity can result. Similar therapeutic challenges occur when **transmucosal** routes (e.g., buccal, sublingual, rectal) are used for drug administration. Specifically, unpredictable systemic bioavailability may complicate treatment consequent to variability in the rate and/or extent of drug absorption. As a consequence, transmucosal drug administration to pediatric patients is no longer widely used as a matter of convenience but, rather, when the condition of the patient does not enable drug administration by the peroral or the parenteral routes. Direct **intraosseous** drug administration through puncture of the tibia is occasionally used in infants and small children for administration of drugs and crystalloid fluids given acutely during resuscitation efforts. It is particularly useful when vascular access sufficient for drug administration cannot be immediately accomplished, since the onset of action by the intraosseous route is comparable to that after IV administration.

ADHERENCE AND COMPLIANCE

The success of drug treatment in a pediatric patient depends on the successful administration of the drug. Physical and cognitive immaturity makes the infant and the child a dependent creature in almost all respects, including those related to therapeutic drug administration. Until a child reaches an age at which the child can physically self-administer a drug in an accurate, proficient manner and can mentally assume this responsibility (generally 7-14 yr of age, depending on the individual child), **compliance** with a drug regimen becomes the responsibility of an adult. In a hospital environment, compliance is ensured through the actions of physicians, nurses, and pharmacists who, collectively through an integrated system of medical care, assume this responsibility. On discharge, the responsibility is transferred to parents/guardians or other adult caregivers in an environment that is generally nonmedical. At this juncture, therapeutic compliance morphs into **adherence**, as defined by the potential for conflicting demands, such as multiple adult caregivers, different external environments (e.g., home, daycare, school), and parents tending to the needs of multiple children, to introduce variability (anticipated and unpredictable) in drug administration. Whether treatment is for a self-limiting (e.g., antibiotic administration) or chronic (e.g., asthma, diabetes) condition, challenges to therapeutic adherence can serve as rate-limiting events in the determination of drug safety and efficacy in infants and young children.

In contrast to the period encompassing infancy and childhood, adolescence poses its own unique challenges to therapeutic adherence. During this period, psychosocial maturation almost always lags behind physical maturation. Development of cognitive and physical skills in most adolescents enables them to self-administer a prescribed medication in a proper manner with little to no supervision. However, psychodynamic issues experienced by a substantial number of adolescents (e.g., complete understanding of the ramifications of undertreatment, disease progression, and roles of disease prevention and health maintenance; perceptions of immortality and associated lack of need for treatment; disorganized patterns of thinking capable of confounding treatment schedules; defiant/oppositional behavior toward authority figures) can often precipitate therapeutic failure, through either undertreatment or overtreatment, the latter occasionally leading to drug toxicity.

Unfortunately, the only approach that can be used to facilitate therapeutic compliance and adherence in the pediatric patient is the combination of *vigilance* (on behalf of all caregivers) and repetitive *education* coupled with positive reinforcement. When children reach the age of assent (generally by 7 yr in children who have normal neurobehavioral development), they have the beginning level of cognitive ability sufficient to engender understanding about their medical condition(s) and how effective treatment can be used to improve their life. Through diligent patient education and reeducation, older children and adolescents can assume a level of responsibility for active partnership in their overall medical management, one that will mature as educational efforts, driven by a shared desire for an optimal outcome, are regularly made.

DRUG-DRUG INTERACTIONS

Pharmacokinetic and pharmacodynamic properties of drugs may be altered when ≥2 drugs are administered to a patient (Table 73.6). Interactions largely occur at the level of drug *metabolism* but may occur at the level of drug *absorption* (e.g., inhibition of intestinal CYP3A4 activity by grapefruit juice or St. John's wort and consequent reduction in presystemic clearance of CYP3A4 substrates), distribution (e.g., displacement of warfarin plasma protein binding by ibuprofen with consequent increased hemorrhagic risk), or elimination (e.g., inhibition of ATS of β-lactam antibiotics by probenecid). Also, drug-drug interactions may occur at the level of the *receptor* (through competitive antagonism); many of which are intentional and produce therapeutic benefit in pediatric patients (e.g., antihistamine reversal of histamine effects, naloxone reversal of opiate adverse effects).

Drug interactions may also occur at a pharmaceutical level as a result of a physicochemical incompatibility of 2 medications when combined. Such interactions generally alter the chemical structure of one or both constituents and thereby renders them inactive and potentially dangerous (e.g., IV infusion of crystalline precipitate or unstable suspension). Ceftriaxone should be avoided in infants <28 days of age if they are receiving or expected to receive IV calcium-containing products, due to reports of neonatal deaths resulting from crystalline deposits in the lungs and kidneys. Alternatively, 2 drugs simultaneously administered perorally may form a complex that can inhibit drug absorption (eg., co-administration of doxycycline with a food or drug containing divalent cations).

Drug-drug interactions at the level of drug metabolism can be somewhat predictable based on a priori knowledge of a given drug's biotransformation profile. Although such information can be derived from the primary literature, it may not be immediately translated into a useful clinical context because of limitations associated with in vitro to in vivo extrapolation, including (1) use of animal models for characterizing metabolism; (2) extrapolating enzyme kinetics derived from pooled human liver microsomes or recombinant human drug-metabolizing enzymes to estimates of in vivo drug clearance; (3) extrapolating in vitro data obtained from fully competent (i.e., adult activity) hepatic microsomes to estimates of clearance in patients who may have developmental or disease-associated compromise in enzyme activity; (4) inaccurate accounting for pharmacogenetic variation in drug-metabolizing activity (i.e., constitutive activity) and the contribution of multiple different drug-metabolizing enzymes in overall drug biotransformation; and (5) the potential role of enzyme induction or inhibition in vivo that is not reflected by conditions used for in vitro metabolism studies.

Despite these limitations, information pertaining to a drug's impact on drug-metabolizing enzymes (e.g., substrate, inducer, inhibitor) can

Table 73.6	Mechanism of Drug Interactions[1]

EXAMPLE DRUG COMBINATION	RESULT
PHARMACODYNAMIC	
Additive	Use of multiple drugs with similar adverse effect profiles can lead to additive effects:
Fentanyl + midazolam	Increased sedation
Class 1A antiarrhythmic[2] + erythromycin[3]	Increased QT prolongation
Vancomycin + an aminoglycoside[4]	Increased potential for nephrotoxicity
Synergy Penicillin + an aminoglycoside[4]	Improved bactericidal efficacy against some gram-positive organisms; penicillin inhibits bacterial cell wall synthesis, which for some gram-positive organisms can improve the intracellular penetration of the aminoglycoside
Antagonism Opioid + naloxone	Competitive receptor antagonism; decreased efficacy of the opioid, reversal of sedation, respiratory depression, and hypotension
Donepezil + an anticholinergic	Oppositional effects; acetylcholinesterase inhibitors such as donepezil increase acetylcholine concentrations by slowing the degradation of acetylcholine, and anticholinergic drugs antagonize the effect of acetylcholine
PHARMACOKINETIC	
Absorption Inhibition of P-gp[5]:	
Amiodarone + digoxin	Increased digoxin concentration; gut P-gp is an efflux transporter that takes drugs from cell cytoplasm and transports them back into the intestinal lumen for excretion, limiting bioavailability
Complex formation: Oral quinolone and tetracycline antibiotics + divalent/trivalent cations (eg, Ca^{2+}, Mg^{2+}, Fe^{3+}, Al^{3+})	Decreased antibiotic concentrations due to binding in the gut
Distribution Ceftriaxone + endogenous bilirubin	Displacement of bilirubin from albumin binding site, increased risk of kernicterus in neonates
Metabolism Induction of CYP isozymes[5,6]: Rifampin + protease inhibitors[7]	Decreased serum concentrations of protease inhibitors metabolized by CYP3A4 due to induction of CYP3A4-mediated metabolism; may result in subtherapeutic levels and resistance
Inhibition of CYP isozymes[5,6]: Azole antifungals[8] + CYP3A4 substrates	Increased serum concentrations of CYP3A4 substrates due to inhibition of CYP3A4-mediated metabolism; may result in drug toxicity
Elimination Penicillin + probenecid	Decreased tubular secretion of penicillin resulting in increased serum concentrations
Methotrexate + aspirin	Inhibition of tubular secretion of methotrexate resulting in increased methotrexate concentrations

This table is not an all-inclusive list of drug interactions. The prescriber is encouraged to assess the possibility of drug interactions when prescribing medications. This table does not address the chemical compatibility of drugs (eg, IV-line compatibility).

[1] Drug interactions from The Medical Letter. Available at: www.medicalletter.org/subDIO.
[2] Disopyramide, procainamide, quinidine
[3] Woosley RL, Romero KA: QT drugs list. Available at: www.crediblemeds.org
[4] Gentamicin, tobramycin, amikacin, streptomycin, neomycin
[5] Inhibitors and inducers of CYP enzymes and P-glycoprotein. Med Lett Drugs Ther 2017; September 18 (epub). Available at: www.medicalletter.org/downloads/CYP_PGP_Tables.pdf
[6] Cytochrome P450 (CYP) isozymes that can affect drug metabolism include CYP1A2, 2C8, 2C9, 2C19, 2D6, and 3A4.
[7] Some protease inhibitors metabolized by CYP3A4 include atazanavir, darunavir, fosamprenavir, indinavir, lopinavir/ritonavir, nelfinavir, and saquinavir.
[8] Itraconazole, ketoconazole, posaconazole, and voriconazole are strong inhibitors of CYP3A4. Fluconazole is a moderate CYP3A4 inhibitor.
CYP = cytochrome P-450; P-gp = P-glycoprotein.
Modified from Rizack M, Hillman C: *The Medical Letter Handbook of Adverse Drug Interactions.* New Rochelle, NY, The Medical Letter, 1989. IBM Micromedex DRUGDEX, Copyright IBM Corporation 2018; Med Lett Drugs Ther 2018;60:e160.

be useful in understanding if the drug has the potential to compete for, induce, or inhibit the metabolism of another drug (e.g., enzyme inhibition enhanced effect or enzyme induction → diminished effect) of a drug-drug interaction. While multiple sources for this information exist (e.g., primary and secondary literature, drug product labeling), it may not be complete or updated. In examining multiple information sources pertaining to this topic, the authors have found the website https://www.pharmgkb.org/ (accessed 21 February 2017) to be the most complete and useful for understanding drug metabolism pathways.

Extensive databases of reported and/or potential (e.g., theoretical mechanism- or metabolism-based) drug interactions exist and are widely available via the internet,* some of which provide some assessment as to their potential significance. Also, many computer-based information systems used by hospital and community pharmacies will routinely screen a patient's medication profile (generally restricted to prescription drugs) against new prescriptions to evaluate the potential for drug-drug

interactions. When using drug-drug interaction databases or online resources, it is advisable to use multiple sources to check for complete information because information regarding interactions is evolving, and all databases may not be fully complete or may provide different information. The clinician is subsequently challenged with determining whether drug-drug or drug-food interactions found by searching these databases is of sufficient magnitude as to be clinically significant. Utilizing primary literature should be assessed when information is not available in online sources.

Over-the-counter (OTC) preparations, herbal supplements, and certain foods also have the potential to produce interactions with drugs. These are often quite challenging for the clinician, especially for alternative therapies, in that their composition (or potency) may not be completely discernible from the product labels, and the disposition of many natural products has not been studied in either children or adults. Further, many patients and their parents do not consider alternative therapies (including nutriceuticals) to be "medicines" (and consequently will not disclose their use during a routine medication history) but rather safe "nutritional supplements" despite absent regulation for their testing. An assessment

*For example, http://www.medscape.com/druginfo/druginterchecker; http://www.drugs.com/; http://www.umm.edu/adam/drug_checker.htm; all accessed 21 February 2017.

should therefore begin with a thorough medication history that includes discussions of which OTC medications and herbal products are used as well as the regularity of their use. This will allow the clinician to identify the primary ingredients contained in these products and query their potential for producing clinically significant drug-drug interactions.

The provision of individualized, optimal drug therapy requires that the clinician make an assessment of potential drug-drug interactions and their significance. This requires knowledge of the interaction, the patient's condition, concomitant treatments (prescriptions, OTC drugs, alternative medicines), the impact of development on the dose-concentration-response relationship and a consideration of the risk vs benefit profile of the drug being prescribed. The clinician must be cognizant that if he or she treats a potential drug-drug interaction as a contraindication to drug use, it is possible that an alternative drug choice could produce a treatment associated with either less benefit or greater risk. Although many drugs have the potential to cause drug interactions, not all cases are deemed clinically relevant. For patients with complex histories requiring multiple medications, consultation with a clinical pharmacologist or pharmacist can help provide guidance on drug-drug interactions and their potential to impact therapy.

ADVERSE DRUG REACTIONS

The World Health Organization has defined adverse drug reactions (ADRs) as "a response to a drug that is noxious and unintended and occurs at doses normally used in man for the prophylaxis, diagnosis or therapy of disease or for the modification of physiological function." There are 2 traditional pharmacologic classifications. **Type A**, generally referred to as "side effects," are dose-dependent and predictable reactions that account for 85–90% of all ADRs. **Type B** reactions, generally referred to as "idiosyncratic" or "allergies," are not dose dependent and are unpredictable and account for approximately 10–15% of all ADRs. Patients sometimes misinterpret some side effects as allergies (e.g., diarrhea with amoxicillin/clavulanate), which may be perpetuated through the patient's medical record.

In the pediatric population, ADRs are common occurrences that produce a major burden to patients and the healthcare system. While ADRs have not been as thoroughly studied in children as in adults, their significance has been widely recognized in pediatrics for >25 yr. Studies concerning ADRs in pediatric patients suggest the following:

1. Approximately 9% of all pediatric patients admitted to the hospital experience an ADR during their treatment.
2. The apparent incidence of ADRs in children in outpatient clinics is approximately 1.5%.
3. ADRs have been reported as being responsible for up to 10% of pediatric admissions to children's hospitals, with a pooled estimate data of about 3%.
4. Approximately 40% of ADRs occurring in hospitalized children are potentially life threatening.

In considering these "statistics," it should be recognized that the true incidence of ADRs in children is not known because of generalized underreporting by healthcare providers (physicians > nurses > pharmacists), parents/caregivers, and patients (who may not recognize signs/symptoms and/or may be unable to report them) and in many countries (including the United States) the lack of a standardized surveillance and real-time reporting system.

Despite the limitations associated with determining the incidence of ADRs in children, it is estimated that their occurrence in patients 0-4 yr of age (3.8%) is more than double that seen at any other time during childhood or adolescence. In the outpatient setting, children age 0-4 yr accounted for 43% of clinic and emergency department visits for ADRs. One study reported that 60% of the ADRs occurred in those <1 yr. The reasons for this are not currently known but may involve developmental differences in pharmacokinetics and pharmacodynamics (i.e., altered dose-concentration-effect relationship), age-associated differences in physiologic "systems" that modulate drug- and metabolite-mediated cellular injury (e.g., immune system), and therapeutic use of drugs known to have a relatively high incidence of producing ADRs (e.g., delayed hypersensitivity reactions associated with β-lactam antibiotics). Also, it is important to recognize that infants can experience ADRs from drugs that are not directly administered to them therapeutically, but rather from maternal drug exposure (transplacental, breastfeeding). Examples include neonatal abstinence syndrome associated with maternal opiate use, production of a hyperserotonergic state in neonates born to mothers who received selective serotonin reuptake inhibitors during pregnancy, and opiate toxicity in breastfed infants whose mothers were taking codeine for pain management. In these cases, drug accumulation caused by reduced activity of drug-metabolizing enzymes associated with development and, potentially, pharmacogenetically determined phenotypical changes, which in concert can produce a level of systemic drug exposure capable of producing an exaggerated response or frank toxicity.

Specific ADRs occur at a much greater frequency in infants and children than in adults. Examples include aspirin-associated Reye syndrome, cefaclor-associated serum sickness–like reactions, lamotrigine-induced cutaneous toxicity, and valproic acid (VPA)–induced hepatotoxicity in infants <2 yr of age. It is not clear whether the age predilection for these specific ADRs is associated with developmental differences in drug biotransformation, related to both metabolite formation and detoxification, or alternatively, has a pharmacogenetic basis. Also, children experience **hypersensitivity reactions** to drugs such as anticonvulsants (e.g., phenytoin, carbamazepine, phenobarbital), sulfonamides (e.g., sulfamethoxazole, sulfasalazine), minocycline, cefaclor, and abacavir. These specific ADRs are not characteristic of type I (i.e., immediate) hypersensitivity reactions (e.g., true penicillin allergy) or anaphylactoid reactions, but rather have been previously classified as *idiosyncratic* with respect to their origin. A relatively common constellation of symptoms (fever, rash, and lymphadenopathy) suggests that abnormal activation/regulation of the immune system is a predominant component of the pathogenesis. Data from in vitro studies of sulfamethoxazole hypersensitivity also support this assertion. In addition, a requisite role for metabolic bioactivation (for anticonvulsants, sulfamethoxazole, and cefaclor) and possibly genetic factors such as allelic variants in HLA-B (e.g., HLA-B*6001 and HLA-B*1502 associated with hypersensitivity reactions to abacavir and carbamazepine) appears also to be involved in their etiology.

PERSONALIZED MEDICINE

The general concept of personalized medicine involves the application of genomic information to predicting a disease, disease severity, and therapeutic response (see Chapter 72). This "new vision of medicine" has been described as the "3 Ps": predictive, personalized, and preventive. In children, however, ontogeny should also be considered when discussing personalizing therapy. Thus the aim of pediatric personalized medicine is uniquely to combine genetic variation with developmental stage to provide a tailored preventive, diagnostic, and therapeutic regimen.

Bibliography is available at Expert Consult.

Chapter **74**
Anesthesia and Perioperative Care

John P. Scott

第七十四章
麻醉和围手术期照护

中文导读

　　本章主要介绍了麻醉前评估、手术前准备、全身麻醉、全麻诱导、麻醉维持、麻醉恢复室、术后疼痛管理以及麻醉药品的神经毒性。其中麻醉前评估包括呼吸系统、气道评估、心血管系统、血液系统、神经系统、心理评估以及遗传评估；手术前准备主要包括术前禁食以及麻醉诱导时父母在场；全身麻醉主要包括镇痛、催眠与遗忘、失去活动能力、监测、具体药物以及静脉麻醉药；全麻诱导包括诱导时并发症；麻醉维持包括体温管理以及液体管理；麻醉恢复室包括麻醉后并发症；术后疼痛管理包括局部麻醉。

The continuum of anesthesia includes varying degrees of sedation (i.e., mild, moderate, or deep) and general anesthesia. All forms of **sedation** are characterized by some preservation of purposeful movement (see Chapter 75), whereas **general anesthesia** is defined by the complete loss of consciousness. Potent pharmacologic agents are required to suppress the perception and physiologic response to noxious stimuli. Perioperatively, the anesthesiologist is responsible for providing analgesia while preserving physiologic and metabolic stability (Table 74.1). This responsibility begins with the performance of a comprehensive preanesthesia history (Table 74.2). Although anesthetic risk has greatly decreased with advancements in pharmacology and monitoring technology, the persistent risk of perioperative morbidity and mortality demands vigilance. The risk is elevated in certain disease states (Table 74.3).

PREANESTHETIC EVALUATION
All children presenting for surgery should undergo a preanesthetic history and multiorgan system assessment with assignment of **American Society of Anesthesiologists Physical Status (ASA-PS)** (Table 74.4). Children of ASA-PS I-II generally require a brief history, notation of

medical allergies, and physical examination focusing on the neurologic and cardiorespiratory systems, with no additional testing. Patients with complex medical history of ASA-PS ≥III require a more comprehensive preanesthetic assessment often with ancillary preoperative testing. Children should be screened for anesthetic risks, including drug allergies, previous reactions to anesthetics, and family history of problems with anesthesia (e.g., sudden perioperative death, hyperthermia after surgery), which may indicate risk of malignant hyperthermia.

Respiratory System
Recent respiratory tract infections should be noted. *Clear rhinorrhea without fever is not associated with increased anesthetic risk.* Respiratory illnesses associated with fever, mucopurulent nasal discharge, productive cough, or lower respiratory symptoms (wheezing, rales) are associated with increased airway reactivity and anesthetic complications for up to 6 wk thereafter. There may also be increased risk of perioperative laryngospasm and bronchospasm, reduced mucociliary clearance, atelectasis, and hypoxemia. It is recommended that elective procedures requiring general anesthesia be postponed 4-6 wk in this setting.

Children with reactive airway disease require a thorough preanesthetic assessment. Acute, potentially fatal bronchospasm can occur during induction of anesthesia and endotracheal intubation for routine, minor surgery in children with asthma. Children at increased risk for anesthetic complications have experienced asthma exacerbations requiring (1) hospital admission within the previous year; (2) emergency department (ED) care within the last 6 mo; (3) previous intensive care unit (ICU) admission; or (4) previous parenteral systemic corticosteroids. Ideally, children should be free of wheezing for least several days before surgery, even if this necessitates increased controller medication administration

Table 74.1	Goals of Anesthesia

Analgesia
Amnesia
Hypnosis
Akinesia
Maintenance of physiologic homeostasis
Vigilance

Table 74.2	The Preanesthetic History

<table>
<tr><td>

Child's previous anesthetic and surgical procedures:
- Review previous anesthetic records:
  Ease of mask ventilation
  Grade of laryngoscopy; type and size of laryngoscope; endotracheal tube size
  Issues during emergence (awakening) from anesthesia (postoperative vomiting, emergence delirium)
  History of hyperthermia or acidosis in the child or family members.

Perinatal problems (especially for infants):
- Prematurity
- Need for supplemental oxygen or intubation and ventilation
- History of apnea and bradycardia
- History of cardiovascular compromise

Other major illnesses and hospitalizations

Family history of anesthetic complications, malignant hyperthermia, or pseudocholinesterase deficiency

Respiratory problems:
- Long-term exposure to environmental tobacco smoke
- Obstructive breathing score
- STBUR (snoring, trouble breathing, un-refreshed)
- Cyanosis (especially in infants <6 mo of age)
- Recurrent respiratory infections
- Recent lower respiratory tract infection
- Previous laryngotracheitis (croup) or laryngomalacia
- Reactive airway disease
- Airway abnormalities, facial anomalies, mucopolysaccharidosis

Cardiac problems:
- Murmur or history of congenital heart disease
- Dysrhythmia
- Exercise intolerance
- Syncope
- Cyanosis

Gastrointestinal problems:
- Reflux and vomiting
- Feeding difficulties

</td><td>

- Failure to thrive
- Liver disease

Exposure to infectious pathogens

Neuromuscular problems:
- Neuromuscular diseases
- Developmental delay
- Myopathy
- Seizure disorder

Hematologic problems:
- Anemia
- Bleeding diathesis
- Tumor
- Immunocompromise
- Prior blood transfusions and reactions

Renal problems:
- Renal insufficiency, oliguria, anuria
- Fluid and electrolyte abnormalities

Psychosocial considerations:
- Drug abuse, use of cigarettes or alcohol
- Physical or sexual abuse
- Family dysfunction
- Previous traumatic medical or surgical experience
- Psychosis, anxiety, depression

Gynecologic considerations:
- Sexual history (sexually transmitted infections)
- Possibility of pregnancy

Current medications:
- Prior administration of corticosteroids

Allergies:
- Drugs
- Iodine
- Latex products
- Surgical tape
- Food (especially soya and egg albumin)

Dental condition (loose or cracked teeth)

When and what the child last ate (especially in emergency procedures)

</td></tr>
</table>

(β-adrenergic agonist and corticosteroids). Active wheezing is an indication for delaying elective surgery. Chronic respiratory conditions such as bronchopulmonary dysplasia and cystic fibrosis are also associated with significant intraoperative risks. Every effort should be made to ensure that children with such disorders achieve optimal respiratory status before surgery.

Airway Evaluation
Induction of general anesthesia is associated with reduced spontaneous ventilation and airway reflexes. Prediction of difficult bag-mask ventilation and/or intubation before anesthesia is critical. Congenital anomalies associated with airway compromise include micrognathia, macroglossia, and thoracic anomalies (Table 74.5). Conditions that impair mouth opening (e.g., temporomandibular joint disease) should also be noted. A history of wheezing or stridor may indicate postoperative airway complications and difficult intraoperative airway management. It is also essential to ask about a history of sleep-disordered breathing using the **STBUR** (snoring, trouble breathing, un-refreshed) index, which may be predictive of perioperative respiratory complications.

Cardiovascular System
Most anesthetic agents possess myocardial depressant properties. All patients should be screened for the presence of heart disease. Important cardiovascular considerations include history of congenital heart disease (CHD), cyanosis, arrhythmias, or cardiomyopathy. Room-air pulse oximetry should be performed as part of the preanesthetic evaluation. Accurate diagnosis of cardiac murmurs in neonates is essential. A history of cardiac dysrhythmias should be investigated because inhalational anesthetics may be arrhythmogenic. A pediatric cardiologist should evaluate children with known CHD undergoing surgery. Preoperative ancillary studies may include electrocardiogram (ECG), echocardiogram,

or cardiac catheterization. Lesions associated with increased anesthetic risk include single-ventricle heart disease, fixed obstructive outflow tract lesions (aortic valve and pulmonary valve stenosis), and cardiomyopathy. Children with these conditions should be cared for by a **cardiac anesthesia service**. Antibiotic prophylaxis for the prevention of bacterial endocarditis may also be indicated, and the American Heart Association (AHA) guidelines should be followed.

Hematologic System
Evidence of coagulopathy should be sought. Easy bruising, familial bleeding disorders, and anticoagulant (e.g., aspirin, heparin, warfarin) use should be discussed. Preoperative adequacy of hemostatic function (e.g., platelet count, fibrinogen, prothrombin time, partial thromboplastin time) and correction of coagulopathic disorders may be indicated for complex procedures associated with significant risk of perioperative hemorrhage. In neonates, assurance of vitamin K prophylaxis and adequate coagulation status is critical before any major surgery. Although anemia may be well tolerated in healthy children, anesthesia and surgery increase oxygen consumption. Preoperative anemia should be corrected in the setting of reduced oxygen delivery or expected blood loss. In the patient with life threatening hemorrhage (trauma), massive transfusion protocols of 1 : 1 : 1 replacement of packed red blood cells:fresh-frozen plasma:platelets should be used.

Neurologic System
A history of neurologic and neuromuscular disorders should be sought. Preoperative developmental assessments may be helpful in interpreting age-dependent variation in the response to pain. Maintenance of appropriate perioperative anticonvulsant therapy is essential in children with seizure disorders because the seizure threshold may be lowered perioperatively. Children with obstructive hydrocephalus typically require

Table 74.3 Specific Pediatric Diseases and Their Anesthetic Implications

DISEASE	IMPLICATIONS	DISEASE	IMPLICATIONS
RESPIRATORY SYSTEM		**GASTROINTESTINAL**	
Asthma	Intraoperative bronchospasm that may be life threatening Pneumothorax or atelectasis Optimal preoperative medical management is essential.	Esophageal, gastric Liver	Potential for reflux and aspiration Altered metabolism of many anesthetic drugs Potential for coagulopathy and uncontrollable intraoperative bleeding
Difficult airway	Special equipment and personnel may be required. Should be anticipated with dysmorphic features or storage diseases Patients with trisomy 21 may require atlantooccipital joint evaluation. Increased risk with acute airway obstruction, epiglottitis, laryngotracheobronchitis, or airway foreign body	**RENAL**	Altered electrolyte and acid-base status Altered clearance of many anesthetic drugs Need for preoperative dialysis in selected cases Succinylcholine to be used with extreme caution and only when the serum potassium level has recently been shown to be normal
Bronchopulmonary dysplasia	Barotrauma with positive pressure ventilation Oxygen toxicity, pneumothorax a risk	**NEUROLOGIC**	
Cystic fibrosis	Airway reactivity, bronchorrhea, increased intraoperative pulmonary shunt and hypoxia Risk of pneumothorax, pulmonary hemorrhage Atelectasis, risk of prolonged postoperative ventilation Patient should be assessed for cor pulmonale.	Seizure disorder	Avoidance of anesthetics that may lower the seizure threshold Optimal control ascertained preoperatively Preoperative serum anticonvulsant measurements
Sleep apnea	Pulmonary hypertension and cor pulmonale must be excluded. Careful postoperative observation for obstruction required	Increased intracranial pressure	Avoidance of agents that increase cerebral blood flow Maintain cerebral perfusion pressure.
		Neuromuscular disease	Avoidance of depolarizing relaxants; at risk for hyperkalemia Patient may be at risk for malignant hyperthermia; avoid volatile anesthetics in myopathies.
CARDIAC	Bacterial endocarditis prophylaxis as indicated Use of air filters; careful purging of air from the intravenous equipment Physician must understand the effects of various anesthetics on the hemodynamics of specific lesions. Possible need for preoperative evaluation of myocardial function and pulmonary vascular resistance Provide information about pacemaker function and ventricular device function.	Developmental delay	Patient may be uncooperative during induction and emergence.
		Psychiatric	Monoamine oxidase inhibitor (or cocaine) may interact with meperidine, resulting in hyperthermia and seizures. Selective serotonin reuptake inhibitors may induce or inhibit various hepatic enzymes that may alter anesthetic drug clearance. Illicit drugs may have adverse effects on cardiorespiratory homeostasis and may potentiate the action of anesthetics.
HEMATOLOGIC		**ENDOCRINE**	
Sickle cell disease	Possible need for simple or exchange transfusion based on preoperative hemoglobin concentration and percentage of hemoglobin S Avoid hypoxemia, hypothermia, dehydration, and hyperviscosity states.	Diabetes	Greatest risk is unrecognized intraoperative hypoglycemia; intraoperative blood glucose level monitoring needed especially when insulin is administered.
Oncology	Pulmonary evaluation of patients who have received bleomycin, *bis*-chloroethyl-nitrosourea, chloroethyl-cyclohexyl-nitrosourea, methotrexate, or radiation to the chest Avoidance of high oxygen concentration Cardiac evaluation of patients who have received anthracyclines; risk of severe myocardial depression with volatile agents Potential for coagulopathy	**SKIN** Burns	Difficult airway Fluid shifts Bleeding Risk of rhabdomyolysis and hyperkalemia from succinylcholine following burns for many months
RHEUMATOLOGIC	Limited mobility of the temporomandibular joint, cervical spine, arytenoid cartilages Careful preoperative evaluation required Possible difficult airway	**IMMUNOLOGIC**	Retroviral drugs may inhibit benzodiazepine clearance. Immunodeficiency requires careful infection control practices. Cytomegalovirus-negative blood products, irradiation, or leukofiltration may be required.
		METABOLIC	Careful assessment of glucose homeostasis in infants

Table 74.4	American Society of Anesthesiology Physical Status Classification

Class 1: Healthy patient, no systemic disease
Class 2: Mild systemic disease with no functional limitations (mild chronic renal failure, iron-deficiency anemia, mild asthma)
Class 3: Severe systemic disease with functional limitations (hypertension, poorly controlled asthma or diabetes, congenital heart disease, cystic fibrosis)
Class 4: Severe systemic disease that is a constant threat to life (critically and/or acutely ill patients with major systemic disease)
Class 5: Moribund patients not expected to survive 24 hr, with or without surgery
Additional classification: "E"—emergency surgery

Copyright American Society of Anesthesiology, http://www.asahq.org. Used with permission.

Table 74.5	Common Difficult Airway Syndromes

Achondroplasia
Airway tumors, hemangiomas
Apert syndrome
Beckwith-Wiedemann syndrome
Choanal atresia
Cornelia de Lange syndrome
Cystic hygroma/teratoma
DiGeorge syndrome
Fractured mandible
Goldenhar syndrome
Juvenile rheumatoid arthritis
Mucopolysaccharidosis
Pierre Robin syndrome
Smith-Lemli-Opitz syndrome
Treacher-Collins syndrome
Trisomy 21
Turner syndrome

Table 74.6	Guidelines for Preoperative Fasting ("2-4-6-8 Rule")*

TIME BEFORE SURGERY (hr)	ORAL INTAKE
2	Clear, sweet liquids
4	Breast milk
6	Infant formula, fruit juices, gelatin
8	Solid food

*These are general guidelines and may differ among hospitals.

ventriculoperitoneal (VP) shunt insertion to divert cerebrospinal fluid (CSF) and to prevent intracranial hypertension (ICH). Repeated shunt malfunction is common, and these children my present for shunt revision with signs of ICH (vomiting, altered mentation, sundowning). Similarly, shunt patency and function should be ensured preoperatively in children with VP shunts presenting for nonneurosurgical procedures.

Psychological Assessment
Surgery and painful medical procedures are psychologically traumatic events for children and families. Children who require anesthesia may experience fear and anxiety. They may also sense stressful signals from parents and caregivers. Many children undergoing surgery have new-onset negative behavioral changes postoperatively. These maladaptive behavioral responses may include enuresis, separation anxiety, temper tantrums, and nighttime crying, as well as fear of strangers, doctors, and hospitals. Sleep quality may be altered postoperatively, resulting in further behavioral compromise. Risk factors for postoperative behavioral changes include preoperative anxiety and emergence excitation. Need for recurrent procedures is another risk factor. Preoperative psychological preparation programs decrease the incidence of postoperative behavioral changes. **Parental presence during induction (PPI)** has not been shown to improve postoperative behavior (see later). Oral midazolam (0.5 mg/kg) may decrease negative behavioral changes after surgery. Midazolam has the benefit of providing rapid-onset anxiolysis and amnesia.

Genetic Evaluation
Children with genetic conditions may have syndrome-specific anesthetic considerations. For example, children with trisomy 21 may have cardiac anomalies, macroglossia, upper airway obstruction, and hypothyroidism (see Chapter 98.2). Atlantoaxial instability, common in trisomy 21, has been linked to cervical dislocation and spinal cord trauma with neck

extension during intubation. Some anesthesiologists recommend extension and flexion lateral neck films to detect instability before surgery. For children with other known genetic disorders it is essential to review specific anesthetic considerations.

PREOPERATIVE PREPARATION
Preoperative Fasting
Preoperative fasting guidelines have been developed to reduce the incidence of aspiration of gastric contents during anesthesia. Aspiration may lead to laryngospasm, bronchospasm, and postoperative pneumonitis. Aspiration of gastric contents may be a potentially lethal complication in children with chronic lung disease or critical illness. Table 74.6 lists preoperative fasting guidelines (e.g., nothing by mouth, or nil per os [NPO] status). Clear, sweet liquids (e.g., Pedialyte, 5% dextrose in water [D5W]) facilitate gastric emptying, prevent hypoglycemia, and may be given up to 2 hr before anesthesia. Breast milk may be given to infants up to 4 hr before surgery. Solids should be avoided for 6-8 hr before surgery. Many conditions delay gastric emptying and may require prolonged periods of fasting.

The Full Stomach
Gastric emptying may be delayed for up to 96 hr after an acute episode of trauma or surgical illness. Because of the serious complications of aspiration of gastric contents, it is desirable to secure the airway as rapidly as possible during induction of anesthesia in patients at risk for having a full stomach. Under these circumstances, rapid sequence induction of anesthesia is indicated (**rapid sequence induction**; see Chapter 89).

Parental Presence During Induction of Anesthesia
Parents may expect to be with their child during the induction of anesthesia. Removing a fearful child from the comforting arms of a parent is stressful for the child, parents, and caregivers. When parental separation cannot be achieved comfortably with premedication and behavioral modification (patient education and desensitization to the operative environment), there may be a need to defer parent–child separation until general anesthesia is induced. Premedication with the oral benzodiazepine midazolam more frequently provides calm, smooth induction conditions than PPI without pharmacologic preparation. Although PPI in the hands of a confident, competent anesthesia practitioner may replace the need for preoperative medication, it does not reliably predict smooth induction. PPI has not been shown to decrease emergence delirium or postoperative behavioral changes, and it does not appear to be superior to premedication with oral midazolam.

GENERAL ANESTHESIA
Analgesia
Pediatric anesthesiologists are responsible for providing analgesia to children for procedures within operating room (OR) and non-OR settings (Table 74.7). Multimodal techniques exist to provide pain relief during operative procedures for children of all ages, including critically ill infants. Effective analgesia is essential to blunt physiologic responses to painful stimuli (surgery) and modulate the deleterious physiologic and metabolic consequences. The response to painful and stressful

stimuli may provoke **systemic inflammatory response syndrome (SIRS)**, which has been linked to increased catabolism, physiologic instability, and mortality (see Chapter 88).

Hypnosis and Amnesia

The attenuation of both consciousness (**hypnosis**) and conscious recall (**amnesia**) is critical during pediatric anesthesia care. Awareness during procedures may be as physically and psychologically deleterious as the experience of pain. A primary goal of anesthetic management is to minimize fear and anxiety during both painful and nonpainful procedures. Many drugs provide anxiolysis and amnesia for such events (Table 74.8). However, it is important to remember that sedative-hypnotic agents may alter consciousness without producing analgesia; *analgesia* and *hypnosis* are not synonymous. It is also possible to provide analgesia (local, spinal, or epidural) without altering consciousness.

Sedation describes a medically induced state in the continuum between wakefulness and general anesthesia (see Table 74.7). **General anesthesia** is characterized by unconsciousness, amnesia, and reduced physiologic reflexes. Cardiorespiratory reflexes (**airway-protective and vasomotor reflexes**) are reduced with general anesthesia. *Light (minimal) sedation* is anxiolysis with minimally reduced reflexes or airway patency. *Deep sedation* occurs when cardiorespiratory reflexes are obtunded or lost. Respiratory depression and hemodynamic compromise may be profound. As sedation deepens toward general anesthesia, loss of airway patency, loss of airway-protective reflexes, and loss of cardiovascular stability occur. Individuals providing sedation and anesthesia for children must be able to detect and support cardiorespiratory insufficiency.

Akinesia (Immobility or Muscular Relaxation)

Akinesia, the absence of movement, is commonly indicated to ensure safe and adequate operative conditions. Neuromuscular blocking agents (NMBAs) may be used to produce akinesia (see Table 74.8). However, the absence of movement is not indicative of hypnosis, amnesia, or analgesia. Whenever NMBAs are used, *analgesia and sedation must be provided.*

Monitoring

Administration of anesthesia increases the need to monitor and support physiologic integrity and homeostasis due to potentially life-threatening physiologic consequences (see Tables 74.7 and 74.8). Consequently, ASA mandates routine monitoring of oxygenation, ventilation, and circulation during the provision of anesthesia. This includes assessment of continuous pulse oximetry, capnography, electrocardiography, intermittent blood pressure measurements (every 5 min), and temperature when temperature instability is anticipated. The use of advanced invasive or noninvasive monitors varies based on procedural complexity and ASA-PS.

Specific Medications
Inhalational Anesthetics

Inhalational anesthetics are frequently used for the induction and maintenance of general anesthesia in children. Pediatric inhalational anesthetics include sevoflurane, isoflurane, and desflurane. Although halothane is the prototypical pediatric inhalational anesthetic, it has been replaced by sevoflurane and is no longer used in the United States.

The **minimum alveolar concentration (MAC)** of an inhalational anesthetic is the alveolar concentration (expressed as percent at 1 atmosphere) that provides sufficient depth of anesthesia for surgery in 50% of patients. For potent inhalational agents, the alveolar concentration of an anesthetic reflects the arterial concentration of anesthetic in the blood perfusing the brain. Thus the MAC is an indication of anesthetic potency and is analogous to the ED_{50} (effective dose in 50% of recipients)

Table 74.7	Definitions of Anesthesia Care

MONITORED ANESTHESIA CARE

A designated anesthesia service in which an anesthesiologist has been requested to participate in the care of a patient undergoing a diagnostic or therapeutic procedure.

Monitored anesthesia care includes all aspects of anesthesia care: a preprocedure assessment, intraprocedure care, and postprocedure anesthesia management.

During monitored anesthesia care, the anesthesiologist or a member of the anesthesia care team provides a number of specific services, which may include but are not limited to the following:

- Discussing anesthesia care with the family and child, obtaining consent for anesthesia, allaying anxiety and answering questions—family-centered anesthesia care.
- Monitoring of vital signs, maintenance of the patient's airway, and continual evaluation of vital functions.
- Diagnosing and treating clinical problems that occur during the procedure.
- Administering sedatives, analgesics, hypnotics, anesthetic agents, or other medications as necessary to ensure patient safety and comfort.
- Providing other medical services as needed to accomplish the safe completion of the procedure.

Anesthesia care often includes the administration of medications for which the loss of normal protective reflexes or loss of consciousness is likely.

Monitored anesthesia care refers to those clinical situations in which the patient remains able to protect the airway for the majority of the procedure.

If the patient is rendered unconscious and/or loses normal protective reflexes for an extended period, this is considered a general anesthetic.

LIGHT SEDATION

Administration of anxiolysis or analgesia that obtunds consciousness but does not obtund normal protective reflexes (cough, gag, swallow, hemodynamic), or spontaneous ventilation.

DEEP SEDATION

Sedation that obtunds consciousness and normal protective reflexes or possesses a significant risk of blunting normal protective reflexes (cough, gag, swallow, hemodynamic), hemodynamic and respiratory insufficiency may occur.

GENERAL ANESTHESIA

Administration of hypnosis, sedation, and analgesia that results in the loss of normal protective reflexes.

REGIONAL ANESTHESIA

Induction of neural blockade (either central, neuraxial, epidural, or spinal; or peripheral nerve block, e.g., digital nerve block, brachial plexus block), which provides analgesia and is associated with regional motor blockade.

Consciousness is not obtunded.

Special expertise is required.

Frequently, in children, anxiolysis and sedation are also necessary for this technique to be successful.

Regional anesthesia (e.g., caudal epidural blockade) is used to supplement general anesthesia and provide postoperative analgesia.

LOCAL ANESTHESIA

Provision of analgesia by local infiltration of an appropriate anesthetic agent.

Does not require the presence or involvement of an anesthesiologist, although an anesthesiologist may provide local anesthesia services.

NO ANESTHESIOLOGIST

An anesthesiologist will not be involved in the care of the child.

Table 74.8	Selected Drugs Used in Anesthesia
DRUG	**USES AND IMPLICATIONS**
MUSCLE RELAXANTS	
Succinylcholine	A depolarizing neuromuscular blocking agent with rapid onset and offset properties Used to facilitate endotracheal intubation and maintain muscle relaxation in emergency situations; rarely used Associated with the development of malignant hyperthermia in susceptible patients Degraded by plasma cholinesterase, which may be deficient in some individuals; such a deficiency may result in prolonged effect Fasciculations may be associated with immediate increases in intracranial and intraocular pressures as well as postoperative muscle pain.
Vecuronium, rocuronium, cis-atracurium, all aminosteroids	Nondepolarizing neuromuscular blockers Have less rapid onset than succinylcholine but are longer acting Prolonged ICU use may lead to profound muscle weakness. Vecuronium and rocuronium are metabolized by the liver and excreted in bile; they are the most commonly used neuromuscular blocking agents. cis-Atracurium is metabolized by plasma cholinesterase and therefore may be of benefit in patients with hepatic or renal disease.
HYPNOTICS	
Propofol	Rapid-acting hypnotic amnestic agent No analgesic properties Respiratory depressant Increases seizure threshold Antiemetic Propofol infusion syndrome may occur with prolonged intravenous infusion (>24 hr).
Etomidate	Cardiovascular stability on induction Inhibits corticosteroid synthesis Increases ICU mortality after use Associated with myoclonus and pain on injection
Ketamine	Hypnotic analgesic Causes sialorrhea and should be co-administered with an antisialogue, such as atropine or glycopyrrolate Induces endogenous catecholamine release and tachycardia Bronchodilator Increases intracranial and intraocular pressures Decreases the seizure threshold
SEDATIVE-ANXIOLYTICS	
Benzodiazepines	Produce sedation, anxiolysis, amnesia, and hypnosis All agents raise the seizure threshold, are metabolized by the liver, and depress respiration, especially when administered with opioids. Effective as premedication Diazepam may be painful on injection and has active metabolites. Midazolam can be administered by various routes. Lorazepam has no active metabolites. Reversed with flumazenil
Dexmedetomidine	Produces anxiolysis, sedation, sympatholysis, by α_2-receptor stimulation centrally; has mild analgesic properties Side effects include hypertension, hypotension, and bradycardia. Commonly used for procedural and ICU sedation Continuous infusion for ICU sedation
ANALGESIC-SEDATIVES	
Opioids	Gold standard for providing analgesia All cause respiratory depression. Morphine and, to a lesser extent, hydromorphone may cause histamine release. The synthetic opioids fentanyl, sufentanil, and short-acting alfentanil may have a greater propensity to cause chest wall rigidity when administered rapidly or in high doses and are also associated with the rapid development of tolerance. These drugs have particular utility in cardiac surgery because of the hemodynamic stability associated with their use. Remifentanil is an ultrashort-acting synthetic opioid that is metabolized by plasma cholinesterase; it may have particular utility when deep sedation and analgesia are required along with the ability to assess neurologic status intermittently.
INHALATIONAL AGENTS	
Nitrous oxide	Produces amnesia and analgesia at low concentrations Danger of hypoxic gas mixture if the oxygen concentration is not monitored and preventive safety mechanisms are not in place
Potent vapors, sevoflurane, desflurane, isoflurane	"Complete anesthetics"—induce hypnosis, analgesia, and amnesia All are myocardial depressants, and some are vasodilators. May trigger malignant hyperthermia in susceptible individuals Sevoflurane is used for induction of anesthesia in children. All bronchodilate at equipotent concentrations. Isoflurane and desflurane are associated with laryngospasm and should not be used for anesthesia induction.

of a drug. MAC is age dependent. MAC is lower in premature than in full-term infants and decreases from term through infancy to preadolescence. In adolescence, MAC again increases, falling thereafter.

Respiratory Effects. The advantages of inhalational anesthesia are rapid onset and offset with the convenient route of delivery and respiratory excretion. These agents provide profound analgesia and amnesia. Inhalational anesthetic agents are poorly soluble in blood but rapidly equilibrate between alveolar gas and blood. They are airway irritants that may provoke laryngospasm. All inhalational anesthetics depress ventilation in a dose-dependent manner. Thus, expired carbon dioxide (CO_2) and $PaCO_2$ (arterial partial pressure of CO_2) will increase in spontaneously breathing children. Inhalational anesthetics also shift the CO_2 response curve to the right, thus decreasing the normal increase in minute ventilation with increasing $PaCO_2$. Inhalational anesthesia decreases end-expiratory lung volume (functional residual capacity). Small lung volumes are associated with reduced lung compliance, increased pulmonary vascular resistance, and restrictive lung defects. Volatile agents depress normal hypoxic pulmonary vasoconstriction, increasing intrapulmonary arteriovenous shunting and hypoxemia.

Cardiovascular Effects. All volatile anesthetic agents reduce cardiac output and peripheral vascular resistance; hypotension is common. This is accentuated in hypovolemic patients and more pronounced in neonates. Inhalational anesthetics also depress baroreceptor and heart rate responses. The administration of inhalational anesthesia may result in decreased tissue oxygen delivery. Perioperatively, cellular metabolism increases, creating a potential imbalance between oxygen demand and oxygen delivery. Development of intraoperative dysoxia is a sign of this imbalance. All volatile inhalational anesthetic agents cause **cerebrovasodilation** and uncouple cerebral blow flow with cerebral metabolic rate. Although inhalational anesthetics decrease cerebral oxygen consumption, they may also disproportionately increase cerebral oxygen blood flow. Thus, inhalational anesthetics should be used with caution in children who have elevated intracranial pressure (ICP) or impaired cerebral perfusion (i.e., traumatic brain injury).

Sevoflurane

Sevoflurane is the most commonly used inhalational agent for induction and maintenance of general anesthesia in children. Sevoflurane is not a significant airway irritant and is a useful induction agent when co-administered with nitrous oxide. Emergence from sevoflurane anesthesia is rapid; however, there is a significant incidence of **emergence delirium**, especially with inadequate pain control. This effect may be attenuated with adequate analgesia and supplemental hypnotic agents (e.g., midazolam, dexmedetomidine, propofol), although hypnotics may delay recovery from anesthesia. Metabolism of sevoflurane by cytochrome P450 (CYP) yields free fluoride, which may be potentially nephrotoxic. Sevoflurane degradation by desiccated CO_2 absorbents at low fresh gas flows (<2 L/min) may produce the nephrotoxin Compound A. Large-scale studies of sevoflurane-associated renal injury in humans are lacking. However, the U.S. Food and Drug Administration (FDA) has recommended maintenance of fresh gas flow rates >2 L/min for surgical cases lasting >2 MAC hr.

Isoflurane

Isoflurane is a pungent volatile anesthetic and airway irritant, not suitable for induction because of the high incidence of complications, such as laryngospasm. However, maintenance of anesthesia with isoflurane is common after induction with sevoflurane or an intravenous (IV) hypnotic. Emergence from anesthesia with isoflurane is slower than for sevoflurane. Isoflurane administration in the setting of desiccated CO_2 absorbents may yield the production of carbon monoxide.

Desflurane

Desflurane is a potent airway irritant associated with coughing, breath holding, and laryngospasm and is *not* useful for induction. Desflurane has the lowest solubility and potency of all commonly used volatile agents. It is frequently administered for maintenance of anesthesia. Emergence from desflurane anesthesia is rapid due to its low tissue solubility.

Nitrous Oxide

Nitrous oxide (N_2O) is a tasteless, colorless, odorless gas with potent analgesic properties. It produces a state of euphoria (thus its nickname, "laughing gas"). The MAC of N_2O is >100; consequently, it may not be used as a sole agent to maintain anesthesia. N_2O produces little hemodynamic or respiratory depression. N_2O is typically used in combination with volatile and IV anesthetic agents during maintenance of general anesthesia. The deleterious effects of N_2O include postoperative nausea and vomiting and, with long-term use (i.e., days), bone marrow suppression. N_2O diffuses out of blood rapidly and is contraindicated in patients with closed gas-filled body cavities (pneumothorax, lung cysts, bowel injury).

Intravenous Anesthetic Agents

Intravenous anesthetics may be administered for induction and maintenance of anesthesia in bolus form or as continuous infusions. Common IV agents include propofol, opioids, benzodiazepines, ketamine, dexmedetomidine, and barbiturates. For children with vascular access, IV induction should be routine. All IV agents affect cardiorespiratory function.

Propofol

Propofol is the most commonly administered IV induction agent. Administered in doses of 2-5 mg/kg, propofol rapidly produces unconsciousness. Propofol may burn and itch on injection. After induction of anesthesia, propofol is a useful agent for maintaining hypnosis and amnesia and may be used as a sole anesthetic agent for nonpainful procedures (e.g., radiation therapy) and imaging studies. When combined with opioids, propofol provides excellent anesthesia for brief painful procedures, such as lumbar puncture and bone marrow aspiration. Although hemodynamic stability, and even spontaneous respirations, may be maintained during propofol administration, it remains a potent anesthetic that obtunds airway reflexes, respiration, and hemodynamic function, and should not be considered a "sedation agent." Propofol frequently induces both respiratory depression and hypotension. Extrapyramidal symptoms are a rarer complication. Prolonged use may cause hemodynamic collapse, bradycardia, metabolic acidosis, cardiac failure, rhabdomyolysis, hyperlipidemia, profound shock, and death (**propofol infusion syndrome**). Prolonged propofol administration (>24-48 hr) in the ICU in children is not recommended. Propofol is formulated in 10% soy emulsion with egg emulsifiers and was once thought to be contraindicated in patients with soy or egg allergy. According to the American Academy of Allergy, Asthma, and Immunology, however, patients with soy and egg allergies may safely receive propofol for anesthesia.

Etomidate

Etomidate is an imidazole derivative used for the induction of anesthesia, frequently in emergent situations. Its onset of action is slower than propofol. Etomidate lacks significant cardiovascular depressant effects, making it a popular induction agent in patients with hemodynamic compromise, cardiac disease, and septic shock. However, etomidate inhibits 11β-hydroxylase, thereby suppressing mineralocorticoid and glucocorticoid synthesis for up to 72 hr after a single induction dose. Etomidate is associated with increased mortality when used as a sedative in the ICU (for which it is now contraindicated), even with a single induction dose. Any decision to use etomidate must weigh the short-term benefits of hemodynamic stability with the serious risks of adrenal suppression.

Ketamine

Ketamine (1-3 mg/kg IV) produces rapid induction of general anesthesia that lasts for 15-30 min. Ketamine is effective when given intramuscularly, subcutaneously, nasally, or orally. However, the dose must be increased for alternative routes. Ketamine dissociates connections between the cerebral cortex and limbic system (*dissociative anesthesia*) through inhibition of N-methyl-D-aspartate receptors. Ketamine is also an analgesic and may be used as a sole IV agent to provide general anesthesia. It has few side effects and generally preserves blood pressure and cardiac output. However, ketamine increases myocardial oxygen demand and should be used cautiously in patients with impaired myocardial oxygen delivery or ventricular outflow tract obstruction. With low-dose (1-2 mg/kg) ketamine, airway reflexes and spontaneous ventilation may be maintained; at higher doses (3-5 mg/kg), loss of airway reflexes, apnea, and respiratory depression occur. Aspiration of gastric contents remains a risk during deep sedation with ketamine. IV ketamine is a useful general anesthetic agent for short procedures.

Ketamine has been linked to disturbing postanesthetic dreams and hallucinations following emergence from anesthesia. In adults the incidence of this effect is 30–50%; in prepubertal children it may be 5–10%. Benzodiazepines (e.g., midazolam) reduce these sequelae and should be routinely given to children receiving ketamine. Ketamine is also a potent secretagogue, enhancing oral and bronchial secretions. An antisialogue, such as atropine or glycopyrrolate, should also be considered before the administration of ketamine. Ketamine is a bronchodilator and is a useful agent for sedating asthmatic patients in the ICU. Ketamine has been reported to increase ICP and therefore is contraindicated in patients with elevated ICP.

Opioids

Opioids are superb analgesics for painful procedures and postprocedural pain (see Chapter 75). Opioids are respiratory depressants that suppress CO_2 responsiveness and can produce apnea. Importantly, in equianalgesic doses, all opioids are equally potent respiratory depressants. Other inhalational or IV anesthetics generally potentiate opioid-induced respiratory depression.

Morphine is a long-acting opioid analgesic with important age-dependent pharmacokinetics. Large doses of morphine (0.5-2 mg/kg), combined with N_2O provide adequate analgesia for painful procedures. Equivalent doses of morphine per kilogram are associated with higher blood levels in neonates than in older children, with plasma concentrations approximating 3 times those of adults. Morphine exhibits a longer elimination half-life (14 hr) in young children than in adults (2 hr). The immature blood-brain barrier of neonates is more permeable to morphine. Morphine is often associated with hypotension and bronchospasm from histamine release and should be used with caution in children with asthma. Morphine has renally excreted active metabolites and is relatively contraindicated in renal failure. Because of morphine's prolonged duration of action and cardiorespiratory side effects, the fentanyl class of synthetic opioids has increased in popularity for perioperative analgesia.

Fentanyl is a potent synthetic opioid with a shorter duration of action and a more stable hemodynamic profile than morphine. Fentanyl attenuates the hemodynamic response to surgery and provides stable operating conditions. Effective analgesia and anesthesia may be provided with IV fentanyl administered as a 2-3 μg/kg bolus followed by a 1-3 μg/kg/hr continuous infusion. Nitrous-narcotic anesthetic techniques that incorporate fentanyl are effective for maintenance of stable hemodynamics while still providing adequate hypnosis and analgesia. Fentanyl is the most commonly used *synthetic* opioid, but other formulations of varying potency are available (alfentanil < fentanyl < sufentanil). *Sufentanil* is 10 times more potent than fentanyl and is frequently used during pediatric cardiac anesthesia. *Alfentanil* is approximately ¼ as potent as fentanyl. *Remifentanil* has very rapid onset and offset of action. In doses of 0.25 μg/kg/min, surgical anesthesia can be maintained with this agent. Remifentanil is metabolized through nonspecific ester hydrolysis and has a short elimination half-life (<10 min) advantageous for rapid emergence from anesthesia. Unfortunately, this short duration of action has been linked to inadequate postprocedural analgesia and increased need for postprocedural opioid analgesic supplementation, limiting remifentanil's use.

Benzodiazepines

Benzodiazepines induce hypnosis, anxiolysis, sedation, and amnesia and have anticonvulsant properties. In high doses, benzodiazepines cause respiratory depression and are synergistic with opioids and barbiturates in their respiratory depressant effects. Benzodiazepines are γ-aminobutyric acid (GABA) agonists.

Midazolam is the most commonly used benzodiazepine in pediatric anesthesia. Short acting and water soluble, it can be injected without pain. It is a potent hypnotic-anxiolytic-anticonvulsant and is approximately 4 times more potent than diazepam. Midazolam may be administered orally, nasally, rectally, intravenously, or intramuscularly. Midazolam (0.10-0.15 mg/kg IV) has minimal effect on respiratory rate, heart rate, or blood pressure and provides excellent preoperative anxiolysis and amnesia. Premedication with oral midazolam (0.5-1.0 mg/kg) mixed in sweet-flavored syrup induces anxiolysis in approximately 90% of children without hemodynamic or respiratory depressant effects. However, children may experience loss of coordination (head control), blurred vision, and rarely dysphoria. A child sedated with midazolam should not be left unattended. Most children rapidly accept an inhalational anesthetic by face mask after oral midazolam premedication. The widespread use of preoperative oral midazolam has decreased the practice of PPI.

Dexmedetomidine

Dexmedetomidine is a central α_2 adrenergic receptor agonist similar to clonidine. Dexmedetomidine lacks respiratory depressant effects and produces anxiolysis, sedation, mild analgesia, and sympatholysis. Interestingly, rapid bolus administration may produce hypertension and bradycardia, whereas continuous infusions may produce hypotension and bradycardia. Dexmedetomidine is frequently used for sedation in ICU patients as well as for procedures. Dexmedetomidine has become a popular adjuvant for general anesthesia during pediatric cardiac surgery.

Barbiturates

Sodium thiopental is the classic barbiturate IV induction agent, although it is now rarely used. Side effects of thiopental include respiratory depression, apnea, and hypotension. Induction with 3-5 mg/kg of thiopental produces unconsciousness within seconds, lasting 5-10 min. Thiopental is not useful for maintenance of anesthesia, which requires other IV or inhalational anesthetics. Pentobarbital is a barbiturate frequently administered IV for sedation in children during imaging procedures of intermediate duration (e.g., imaging studies) that require akinesia. **Pentobarbital** is a potent respiratory depressant, particularly when combined with opioids and benzodiazepines. Pentobarbital has a prolonged duration of action. Pentobarbital sedation for nonpainful procedures generally results in delayed emergence. **Sodium methohexital** (Brevital) is another IV induction agent, similar to sodium thiopental in respiratory depressant effects. Barbiturates lack analgesic properties, and painful procedures require supplemental analgesia.

Neuromuscular Blocking Agents

Neuromuscular blockade is performed to facilitate endotracheal intubation and akinesia during surgery. NMBAs may be *depolarizing* (e.g., succinylcholine) or *nondepolarizing* (e.g., vecuronium, rocuronium, cisatracurium). **Succinylcholine** has a high-risk profile in children. Its use is associated with postoperative pain from muscle spasms; hyperkalemia; elevated intracranial, intraocular, and intragastric pressures; malignant hyperthermia; myoglobinuria; and renal damage. Consequently, succinylcholine is now rarely used, except to provide rapid relief of laryngospasm. Endotracheal intubation is most often facilitated with nondepolarizing NMBAs. **Rocuronium** is most commonly used for intubation because of its rapid onset of action. For procedures that last >40 min, **vecuronium** and **cisatracurium** are also suitable to induce muscle relaxation for intubation. After intubation, repeat administration of NMBAs may be indicated to maintain muscle relaxation to facilitate surgery. Prolonged use of nondepolarizing NMBAs in critical illness may contribute to myopathy, especially when combined with high-dose corticosteroids.

INDUCTION OF GENERAL ANESTHESIA

The primary goal of induction of general anesthesia is the rapid and safe transition to a state of unconsciousness. Induction in children is usually achieved by inhalational anesthetics, although IV agents are indicated when patients have IV access. Many children will not tolerate the establishment of vascular access before induction of anesthesia, and it is routine to induce anesthesia by face mask with inhaled anesthetics.

Before the induction of anesthesia, monitors applied may include pulse oximetry, ECG, and noninvasive blood pressure cuff. The child is then cautiously introduced to the face mask, which contains a high gas flow (5-7 L/min O_2), frequently mixed with N_2O. Inhalation of N_2O and O_2 for 60-90 sec induces a state of euphoria. Nitrous oxide blunts the airway responses to potent volatile inhalational agents, and sevoflurane may then be safely introduced into the inhaled gas mixture. This leads to unconsciousness within 30-60 sec while the child continues to breathe spontaneously.

Following induction, IV access is obtained, and comprehensive intraoperative monitoring initiated. Thereafter, definitive airway management is performed. Airway management for short procedures (i.e., myringotomy tubes) frequently includes a mask airway and spontaneous ventilation; this is safe when the airway is secure, and patent and aspiration risk is low. Longer procedures (>30-60 min) are not usually performed with mask airways. Definitive artificial airways include laryngeal mask airways and endotracheal tubes. The **laryngeal mask** is a supraglottic airway generally reserved for procedures in spontaneously ventilating patients and does not effectively prevent the aspiration of gastric contents.

For complex surgical procedures, **endotracheal intubation** in required (e.g., intraabdominal, intrathoracic, airway). Although endotracheal intubation may be performed under deep inhalational anesthesia, the depth of anesthesia required to attenuate airway reflexes may produce hemodynamic instability. Therefore, NMBAs are frequently administered to facilitate intubation. The depolarizing NMBA succinylcholine is rarely used, and nondepolarizing NMBAs such as rocuronium and vecuronium are most frequently used (see earlier). After muscle relaxation, direct laryngoscopy and endotracheal intubation can be performed. Correct endotracheal tube (ETT) placement is confirmed by direct laryngoscopy, end-tidal CO_2 measurement, and bilaterally equal breath sounds. Additional confirmatory tests include chest radiograph and fiberoptic bronchoscopy. After endotracheal intubation, controlled mechanical ventilation is required in the setting of neuromuscular blockade (see Chapter 89).

Children with full stomach precautions may require **rapid sequence induction**. Before performing a rapid sequence induction, preoxygenation with 100% oxygen for 2-5 min increases alveolar oxygen content and provides an extra margin of safety if intubation is difficult. Rapid sequence induction involves concurrent administration of hypnotic and NMBAs. Assisted ventilation before or after drug administration is avoided due to the risk of gastric distention, regurgitation, and aspiration. After administering a sedative and NMBA, the Sellick maneuver (cricoid pressure) is performed by applying firm pressure in a posterior direction, against the cricoid cartilage. This displaces the cricoid cartilage into the esophagus, forming an artificial sphincter to prevent reflux of the gastroesophageal contents. Cricoid pressure should be maintained until correct ETT placement is verified by positive end-tidal CO_2 and bilateral breath sounds.

The major risk of rapid sequence induction is intubation failure. In this situation the child is paralyzed without a protected airway, and ventilation may be hazardous or impossible. Only experienced airway specialists should undertake rapid sequence induction. It should be avoided in patients with a history of failed endotracheal intubation or features (micrognathia) associated with difficult intubation. Under these circumstances, bronchoscopic awake intubation may be indicated.

Complications During Induction
During induction of anesthesia the transition between full wakefulness to unconsciousness is fraught with potential complications, including laryngospasm, bronchospasm, vomiting, and aspiration. Concerns for vomiting and aspiration dictate adherence to preanesthetic fasting guidelines and may be an indication for rapid sequence anesthetic induction.

During induction of anesthesia, especially with inhalational anesthetics, a period of excitement may occur. This period is associated with heightened airway reflexes, which can lead to coughing, gagging, laryngospasm, and bronchospasm. **Laryngospasm** is the reflex closure of the larynx, which prevents spontaneous or assisted ventilation. The child may make violent inspiratory efforts against a closed glottis, generating significantly negative intrathoracic pressure. This may affect cardiovascular function and cause postobstructive pulmonary edema. Laryngospasm can be prolonged, and hypoxia may ensue. Laryngospasm occurs in up to 2% of all anesthetic inductions in children <9 yr old and is much less common in older patients. Laryngospasm occurs twice as frequently in children with active or recent upper respiratory tract infection. A history of tobacco exposure increases the likelihood of laryngospasm significantly.

Laryngospasm can be relieved by increasing the depth of anesthesia, either intravenously or through inhalation (although with the glottis closed, further administration of inhalational anesthesia is not possible). Neuromuscular blockade relieves laryngospasm, and an acute situation may be an indication for succinylcholine administration. Continuous positive airway pressure administration may be beneficial in alleviating laryngospasm. Laryngospasm may also occur during emergence from anesthesia because airway tone is increased during the transition to wakefulness.

Bronchospasm may result from increased airway reactivity during the hyperexcitable stage of induction, or secondary to histamine release induced by anesthetic agents. Endotracheal intubation may provoke bronchospasm, especially in asthmatic patients, which may be associated with life-threatening hypoxemia and inability to ventilate. Alternative airway management strategies such as laryngeal mask should be considered when appropriate in children with severe reactive airway disease. The use of histamine-releasing anesthetic agents has been associated with severe bronchospasm, and in rare instances cardiorespiratory failure. Environmental tobacco smoke is another risk factor.

Hypoxemia during induction may be secondary to reduced functional residual capacity, atelectasis, and ventilation-perfusion ($\dot{V}/\dot{Q}$) mismatch. Volatile anesthetics blunt hypoxic pulmonary vasoconstriction further contributing to $\dot{V}/\dot{Q}$ abnormalities. **Hypersecretion** may result in airway obstruction and should managed with antisialogues, such as glycopyrrolate and atropine. The newer inhalation agents are less potent secretagogues, and the routine use of atropine premedication is much less common, but often indicated when ketamine is used.

Hemodynamic complications may also develop during induction of anesthesia. **Hypotension** is common and may be exaggerated patients with hypervolemia, decreased myocardial function, or CHD. Inhalational anesthetics sensitize the myocardium to circulating catecholamines, and induction and excitement are associated with a hypercatecholaminergic state.

MAINTENANCE OF ANESTHESIA
Maintenance of anesthesia is the period between induction and emergence. The child should be unaware of pain, unresponsive to painful stimuli, and physiologically supported. Anesthesia is typically maintained with a volatile anesthetic (e.g., isoflurane, sevoflurane) supplemented with opioid-based analgesia. IV hypnotic agents (e.g., dexmedetomidine, benzodiazepines) may be administered to augment hypnosis and amnesia. Choice of ventilatory strategy (spontaneous, assisted, or controlled) varies according to procedure type and patient condition (see Chapter 89). Surgical trauma may result in hypothermia and hypovolemia due to blood loss and significant fluid shifts (third spacing). Management of these physiologic disturbances is the responsibility of the anesthesiologist during maintenance.

Temperature Management
Thermoregulation is critical during anesthesia. The absence of movement and inhibition of shivering reduce thermogenesis. Mechanisms of heat loss during anesthesia include convection, radiation, evaporation, and conduction. Although temperature sensing may remain normal, the autonomic response to hypothermia is reduced. Anesthetic agents cause vasoparesis, which further impairs thermoregulation and increases heat loss. In newborns, inhalational anesthetics inhibit nonshivering thermogenesis from brown fat, increasing the risk for hypothermia. Humidification and warming of inspired gases is required. Additional warming devices, such as forced-air warming blankets and radiant

warmers, should also be used.

Fluid Management

Most anesthetics produce vasodilation and increase venous capacitance, effectively reducing myocardial preload. Surgical bleeding and insensible/third space fluid losses further contribute to intravascular volume depletion. Volume expansion with isotonic salt-containing solutions (normal saline, lactated Ringer, Plasmalyte) may be required to maintain cardiac output and organ perfusion. Increased renin-angiotensin-aldosterone axis activation and antidiuretic hormone (ADH) secretion further complicate fluid regulation.

Intraoperative fluid management must account for (1) deficits acquired during preoperative fasting, (2) maintenance fluid requirements, (3) surgical blood loss, and (4) insensible fluid loss. Infants should receive glucose-containing isotonic fluid to prevent perioperative hypoglycemia. Table 74.9 is a guideline for determining fluid deficits and maintenance requirements in the OR. For longer procedures, fluid deficits should be replaced with isotonic fluid over the 1st 3 hr of intraoperative management. Deficits are generally calculated as the number of hours of fasting status multiplied by the hourly maintenance rate for the child. Half the deficit is replaced during the 1st hr and half during the subsequent 2 hr. If hypotension or tachycardia persists in the early stages of anesthesia, more rapid replacement of the fluid deficit may be indicated.

Third space interstitial fluid losses should be replaced with isotonic salt solutions. For smaller operations, such as herniorrhaphy, pyloromyotomy, and minor procedures, fluid replacement at 3-5 mL/kg/hr is indicated for insensible losses. Complex abdominal or thoracic procedures with large insensible losses may require an additional 8-10 mL/kg/hr of IV fluid replacement. Crystalloid solution is indicated for blood loss as a 3:1 ratio. Allogenic blood products should be replaced as a 1:1 ratio. Colloid (albumin) administration also decreases the amount of crystalloid replacement needed for blood loss. During large-volume transfusions, active fluid warming should be performed to prevent hypothermia. With major surgery and resultant SIRS, capillary integrity is lost and third space losses are common. Failure to replace fluid loss and restore intravascular volume may lead to shock.

Perioperative **hypoglycemia** may result from preoperative fasting, most often in neonates or in children with metabolic disorders. In neonates, perioperative glucose monitoring is indicated and glucose replacement is frequently required. In older children with normal nutritional status, isotonic salt solutions without glucose are adequate. In patients receiving total parenteral alimentation containing high glucose concentrations (>10%), continuous glucose administration should be ensured to avoid rebound hypoglycemia.

Postprocedural care includes supervision of emergence and recovery from anesthesia and surgery. **Emergence** describes the transition period between the anesthetized state and consciousness. During emergence, patients experience decreased anesthetic effect and increased physiologic and psychological responses to painful stimuli (e.g., reactive autonomic tone, excitement, anxiety). Inhalational anesthetic agents are rapidly excreted during ventilation, and muscle relaxants can be reversed; however, the effects of opioids, benzodiazepines, and IV hypnotics may be prolonged. Normal physiologic functions such as spontaneous ventilation resume, and hemodynamic function improves. Before leaving the OR after routine elective procedures, the child should be conscious with intact airway reflexes and a patent airway. The effects of muscle relaxants should be reversed. Ideally, emergence should be as brief as possible, with maintenance of analgesia and anxiolysis and restoration of cardiorespiratory function. However, critically ill patients scheduled for ICU admission may require postoperative endotracheal intubation and mechanical ventilation. In these patients, deeper levels of sedation and analgesia should be maintained after the procedure.

During emergence, it is essential to assess whether **residual neuromuscular blockade** (NMB) exists. If weakness or respiratory depression is observed in the postoperative phase, prolonged NMB should be considered. *Reversal of residual NMB is standard anesthetic practice.* With the virtual abandonment of succinylcholine, only nondepolarizing NMBAs are routinely used for intubation. The termination of NMB depends on metabolism and elution away from the neuromuscular junction. Classically, nondepolarizing muscle relaxants are reversed by increasing the acetylcholine concentration at the neuromuscular junction with acetylcholine esterase inhibitors (neostigmine, edrophonium), which work through competitive antagonism. Vagolytic agents (e.g., atropine, glycopyrrolate) must be co-administered to prevent bradycardia. This process, even for the shortest-acting muscle relaxant, rocuronium, can take several minutes. An intubating dose of rocuronium to rapidly induce paralysis in emergency situations may not spontaneously reverse for 20 min or longer (compared with about 3 min for succinylcholine). The effects of long-acting, nondepolarizing NMBAs (vecuronium, pancuronium) are invariably reversed. Residual NMB is common despite reversal with these agents. **Sugammadex** is an alternative reversal agent that has a very low rate of residual NMB. Its mechanism of action involves noncompetitive antagonism through encapsulation of neuromuscular agents.

POSTANESTHESIA CARE UNIT

In the postanesthesia care unit (PACU), the child is observed until there is adequate recovery from anesthesia and sedation. Achievement of spontaneous breathing, adequate pulse oximetry saturation (>95%), and hemodynamic stability are key recovery end-points. The child should be arousable, responsive, and oriented before discharge from the PACU. The amount of time spent in the PACU varies based on disposition (transfer to acute care or ICU, transfer to day surgery postrecovery unit, or discharge to home). Parents should be permitted to comfort their children in the PACU. Discharge from the PACU depends on the child's overall functional status—not merely the physiologic end-points, but also the adequate provision of analgesia and control of postoperative nausea and vomiting. Various scoring systems have been used for determining readiness for discharge from the PACU (Table 74.10).

Postanesthetic Complications

Respiratory insufficiency following general anesthesia is common. Prolonged emergence from anesthesia and respiratory depression may be caused by the residual effects of opioids, hypnotic agents, or NMBAs. Pain may also cause significant hypoventilation, especially after thoracic or abdominal surgery. Delayed emergence from anesthesia may result from retention of inhaled anesthetics worsened by hypoventilation. Hypothermia, especially in neonates, delays metabolism and excretion of anesthetics and prolongs NMB. Hypoventilation after surgery is associated with the development of **atelectasis**. Microatelectasis may lead to postoperative infections. When airway obstruction is present, maintenance of airway patency may necessitate oropharyngeal or nasopharyngeal airway placement. In the setting of profound respiratory depression, endotracheal intubation and mechanical ventilation may be indicated.

Opioid reversal with naloxone may be indicated in rare instances when excessive **opioid effect** is suspected. However, naloxone reverses both the respiratory depressant and the analgesic effects of opioids. Following naloxone reversal, a somnolent child with respiratory depression may experience increased pain. Opioid reversal requires bedside attention by the physician to monitor the child's behavioral, hemodynamic, and respiratory status. Importantly, naloxone is shorter-acting than most opioid analgesics, which may result in re-narcotization.

Postoperative stridor occurs in up to 2% of all pediatric patients. The use of appropriately sized ETTs and assurance of an air leak <30 cm

Table 74.9	Intraoperative Pediatric Fluid Replacement
INFUSION RATE	**PATIENT WEIGHT**
4 mL/kg/hr	1-10 kg
2 mL/kg/hr	10-20 kg
1 mL/kg/hr	per kg >20 kg

Example: 22 kg child requires (4 × 10) + (2 × 10) + (1 × 2) = 62 mL/hr

Table 74.10	Postanesthesia Recovery Scores

ALDRETE RECOVERY SCORE	>9 REQUIRED FOR DISCHARGE
ACTIVITY—VOLUNTARILY OR ON COMMAND	
Moves 4 extremities	2
Moves 2 extremities	1
No motion	0
BREATHING	
Deep breath, cough, cry	2
Dyspnea or shallow breathing	1
Apnea	0
BLOOD PRESSURE	
Within 20% of preanesthetic value	2
Within 20–50% of preanesthetic value	1
>50% outside preanesthetic value	0
COLOR	
Pink	2
Pale, blotchy, dusky	1
Cyanotic	0
CONSCIOUSNESS	
Fully aware, responds	2
Arouses to stimulus	1
Unresponsive	0

STEWARD RECOVERY SCORE	6 REQUIRED FOR DISCHARGE
ACTIVITY	
Moves limbs purposefully	2
Nonpurposeful movement	1
Still	0
CONSCIOUSNESS	
Awake	2
Responsive	1
Unresponsive	0
AIRWAY	
Coughing on command or crying	2
Maintaining patent airway	1
Requires airway maintenance	0

H_2O pressure decreases the risk of airway trauma or edema. A history of stridor increases the likelihood of postoperative complications. Stridor may be severe enough after extubation to require reintubation. Racemic epinephrine aerosols and dexamethasone are effective therapies; their use requires prolonged observation because of the potential for rebound stridor. Stridor in infants suggests the need for overnight observation.

Cardiovascular complications are less frequently encountered in the PACU. Volume expansion may be required to maintain adequate cardiac output, peripheral perfusion, and urine output. Large-volume fluid resuscitation (>30 mL/kg) in the postoperative period may be an indication of evolving shock physiology, and sources of hypovolemia (e.g., occult bleeding) or myocardial dysfunction (e.g., tamponade, pneumothorax) should be considered.

Emergence delirium immediately after anesthesia is noted in 5–10% of children and is more common in those 3-9 yr old. Manifestations include restlessness, combativeness, disorientation, and inconsolability. Almost all anesthetic agents have been linked to the development of delirium, especially newer volatile anesthetic agents (e.g., sevoflurane, desflurane). Potential postoperative complications, such as hypoglycemia and hypoxemia, should also be ruled out. Occasionally, it is necessary to provide additional sedation (e.g., propofol, dexmedetomidine, benzodiazepines) although these agents prolong postanesthesia recovery time and may not effectively reduce delirium.

Awareness During Anesthesia

A fundamental aim of anesthesia is to prevent recall by inducing hypnosis and amnesia. In adults, certain anesthetic techniques and surgical procedures have been associated with recall during anesthesia. The long-term sequelae of recall in children are unknown. Continuous cerebral bispectral index (BIS) electroencephalographic monitoring has been used to assess intraoperative awareness. Unfortunately, pediatric studies have not confirmed the usefulness of BIS monitoring as a means of determining anesthetic depth. Existing data do not support the routine use of BIS monitoring during pediatric anesthesia. Volatile anesthetic agents reliably produce dose-dependent hypnotic and amnestic effects and remain a mainstay of general anesthesia.

Postoperative Nausea and Vomiting

Following general anesthesia, 40–50% of children may experience postoperative nausea and vomiting (PONV) that generally lasts for several hours. This complication prolongs recovery room times and requires significant nursing attention. The etiology is not completely understood but is likely multifactorial related to the emetic effects of anesthetics, pain, and surgical stress. Opioid analgesics may provoke nausea and vomiting. Importantly, preoperative fasting does not decrease the incidence of PONV. Indeed, hydration and glucose supplementation appear to be important factors in decreasing PONV. Multimodal analgesia with nonopioid agents (e.g., acetaminophen, ibuprofen, ketorolac) and regional or local anesthesia may decrease PONV. The serotonin antagonist ondansetron is an effective treatment of PONV. Ondansetron prophylaxis is also recommended for patients at increased risk of PONV, such as after eye and otolaryngology surgery. Serotonin antagonists are contraindicated in children taking serotonin reuptake inhibitors for migraine headaches. Dexamethasone may also be used for the treatment of PONV.

Thermoregulation and Malignant Hyperthermia

Following anesthesia, thermoregulation remains abnormal for several hours. **Hypothermia**, especially in neonates, may to cardiorespiratory depression and prolongation of the effect of opioids and NMBAs. Although hypothermia has deleterious effects, active rewarming should be performed cautiously to avoid hyperthermia and cutaneous burns. Postoperative shivering is common and may occur in the absence of hypothermia. **Hyperthermia**, with temperatures in excess of 39°C (102.2°F), is of concern in the postoperative period. When high fevers occur within hours of the use of an inhalational anesthetic, especially if succinylcholine was used, malignant hyperthermia must be ruled out.

Malignant hyperthermia (MH) is a hypermetabolic syndrome triggered by volatile anesthetic agents and succinylcholine. The onset of MH may be acute, fulminant, and lethal without appropriate interventions. The disease is genetically heterogeneous, with >10 genes contributing to susceptibility, but typically displays an autosomal dominant inheritance pattern. A family history of death or febrile reactions during anesthesia should alert the anesthesiologist to its potential. Mutations within the gene encoding for the ryanodine receptor (the calcium channel of the sarcoplasmic reticulum) predispose to MH susceptibility and have been identified in 20–40% of humans with MH. Certain **myopathies** are associated with the risk of MH, including Duchenne muscular dystrophy, central core disease, and King Denborough syndrome.

The pathophysiology of MH involves uncontrolled intracellular calcium release from skeletal muscle sarcolemma, resulting in prolonged muscle contraction, adenosine triphosphate (ATP) depletion, and muscle cell death. Myolysis results in the release of myoglobin, creatine phosphokinase (CPK), and potassium into the blood. The clinical course of MH is characterized by rapid onset of high fever (>38.5°C), muscle rigidity, acidosis (metabolic and respiratory), high end-tidal CO_2, and multiorgan dysfunction. Death may ensue secondary to hemodynamic collapse from shock and cardiac dysrhythmias. Signs of MH generally occur within the 1st 2 hr of anesthesia, but (rarely) can occur up to 24 hr later.

Aggressive therapy involves discontinuation of all inhalational anesthetics, correction of the metabolic acidosis, and treatment with the muscle relaxant dantrolene. IV dantrolene (2.5 mg/kg as initial dose) should be initiated when MH is suspected. The need for repeat doses, up to a maximum of 10 mg/kg, is indicated for persistent fever, muscle rigidity, acidosis, and tachycardia. Once symptoms are controlled, the patient should be observed for at least 24 hr, because recrudescence may occur. The MH mortality rate was once >70% and is now <5% with standardized treatment algorithms. A MH cart with sufficient supplies of dantrolene should be present at every site where pediatric anesthesia is provided.

Certain phenomena suggest an increased risk of MH. Masseter spasm during induction, with rigid clenching of the masseter muscles and an inability to open the mouth, may signal MH susceptibility. Acute myoglobinuria associated with an MH-triggering agent is another clue. The child may not be hypermetabolic or febrile, but may have dark urine, high CPK levels, and risk of myoglobin-induced renal tubular damage. The finding of dark urine after administration of an anesthetic requires further investigation, including measurement electrolytes on CPK. Prevention of MH in susceptible patients requires the avoidance of triggering agents, which include inhalational anesthetics and succinylcholine. IV anesthesia and nitrous-opioid techniques are safe. MH-safe anesthesia machines devoid of trace concentrations of volatile anesthetic vapors should be used. Dantrolene prophylaxis is not recommended because MH is rapidly treatable and the drug causes respiratory depression and muscle weakness. For a child in whom MH is suspected, the MH hotline, 1-800-MHHYPER (1-800-644-9737), should be used to notify the Malignant Hyperthermia Association of the United States (MHAUS). MHAUS registers susceptible patients and provides diagnostic and therapeutic information. Preanesthesia susceptibility testing includes genetic analysis of the ryanodine receptor gene, muscle biopsies, in vitro contraction studies, and possibly measurement of muscle CO_2 production in response to intramuscular caffeine.

Mediastinal Masses

Children with anterior mediastinal masses such as lymphomas, teratomas, and other primary mediastinal tumors are at serious risk for cardiorespiratory failure during anesthesia. Even mild sedation may result in airway compromise, inability to ventilate, cardiac tamponade, vascular obstruction, and circulatory collapse. These patients generally require surgical tissue diagnosis before treatment is initiated. Significant compression of vital structures can occur with seemingly mild symptoms. Tachypnea, orthopnea, wheezing, and avoidance of prone or supine positions are significant indications of serious risk. Echocardiographic or CT evidence of pericardial tamponade, right ventricular compression, or compression of the pulmonary artery suggests severe risk. Biopsy with light sedation under local anesthesia may be indicated. When anesthesia is required, preservation of spontaneous ventilation is critical during induction of anesthesia. Rigid bronchoscopy may be used to assist with ventilation in the setting of external airway compression Provisions to provide mechanical circulatory support (cardiopulmonary bypass) should also be available. In high-risk children, consideration should be given to initiating treatment with corticosteroids, radiation therapy, and chemotherapy before obtaining a tissue diagnosis.

Postoperative Apnea

Neonates and infants are at increased risk for the development of postoperative apnea after exposure to potent hypnotic and analgesic medications. Both central and obstructive apnea may occur. Postanesthetic apnea is most common within the 1st 12 hr, although apnea has been reported in premature infants up to 48 hr later. The risk of apnea is inversely proportional to postconceptual age at surgery and is highest in premature neonates <44 wk postconceptual age. This risk is minimal by the time premature infants have reached 60 wk postconceptual age. Theophyllines do not reliably decrease the incidence of postoperative apnea and are not routinely used. When surgery is required within the 1st mo of life, overnight observation and monitoring are indicated. In term infants >44 wk postconceptual age, management should include observation and monitoring for 6 hr with at least 1 sleep-wake-feed cycle without hypoxia, bradycardia, or supplemental oxygen. Premature infants <56 wk postconceptual age require observation for 12 hr after anesthesia.

POSTOPERATIVE PAIN MANAGEMENT

Postprocedural pain management should ensure adequate analgesia and anxiolysis (see Chapter 76). Preoperative education focusing on pain management through development of skills designed to decrease anticipatory anxiety and participation in treatment planning can be helpful for children and families. Pediatric pain management relies on multimodal therapy, including opioid and nonopioid analgesics. Nonsteroidal antiinflammatory drugs, cyclooxygenase-2 inhibitors, IV acetaminophen, opioids, and regional analgesia all have roles in postoperative pain management. Repeated evaluation is critical to effective pain management. Adjunctive therapy, such as pet therapy, may also decrease the need for potent analgesics postoperatively.

Patient-controlled analgesia (PCA) and **parent/nurse-controlled analgesia (PNCA)** are widely accepted postoperative pain regimens. PCA/PNCA provide a low-dose continuous (basal) infusion of opioid with intermittent (bolus) supplements as needed. The practitioner must determine the basal rate, bolus dose, lockout interval, and acceptable number of bolus doses per hour. PCA/PNCA safety requires appropriate medication dosing and assumes that patients are unlikely to overdose because somnolence will limit repeated self-administration. In young children, use of the *pain button* (for pain relief) may be more difficult to ensure, although children as young as 5 yr have been able to use PNCA successfully. In older children and adolescents, PCA is a standard modality of postoperative pain management.

Regional Anesthesia

Regional anesthesia is the use of anesthetics to block the conduction of afferent neural impulses to the central nervous system. Forms of regional anesthesia include local anesthesia, peripheral nerve blocks, nerve plexus blocks, and neuraxial (epidural and subarachnoid/spinal) blocks. Anesthetics may be administered as a single injection or as a continuous infusion. Regional anesthesia may be used for both intraoperative and postoperative analgesia. It has been linked to shortened recovery times and hospital stays in children. A major benefit of regional anesthesia is lesser central cardiorespiratory depressant effects. Injection of local anesthetics (e.g., lidocaine, bupivacaine) into the affected area may provide procedural analgesia lasting for hours to days. Wound infiltration with local anesthetics at the conclusion of surgery may also decrease early postoperative pain.

Neuraxial (epidural, spinal) analgesia is common in pediatric practice. The epidural space lies between the dura and the pia and arachnoid membranes, an area through which all nerve roots pass. Caudal epidural analgesia is placed through the sacral hiatus, inferior to the distal end of the spinal cord. This site is often used for pelvic and lower-limb anesthesia during urologic and orthopedic surgery in infants and toddlers. A single dose of caudal epidural anesthesia may provide hours of pain relief, and a continuous infusion may provide effective pain relief for hours to days. The epidural injection of opioids can provide analgesia for 12-24 hr and is a potential supplement to postoperative analgesia. Longer-acting local anesthetics (e.g., bupivacaine, ropivacaine) combined with an opioid (e.g., fentanyl, preservative-free morphine) are typically used in single-injection and continuous epidural therapy. It is also possible to provide epidural PCA with a continuous infusion pump and the patient's ability to self-administer analgesia as needed. Epidural analgesia can also provide pain relief in patients with chronic pain or pain caused by advanced malignant conditions.

Complications of neuraxial anesthesia include cephalad spread of blockade with respiratory depression, paralysis of respiratory muscles, and brainstem depression. Common complications of neuraxial analgesia are paresthesias and, if opioids are used, pruritus, nausea, and vomiting. Neuraxial opioid use necessitates antipruritic and antiemetic therapy. Infection and epidural hematoma are extremely rare. Neuraxial opioids, especially when administered intrathecally, may cause respiratory depression and require postoperative monitoring.

Bibliography is available at Expert Consult.

74.1 Anesthetic Neurotoxicity

John P. Scott

Laboratory animal studies have suggested a link between anesthetic exposure at an early age and neurotoxicity in developing brains. Existing nonclinical data implicate *N*-methyl-D-aspartate and γ-aminobutyric acid (GABA) pathways in apoptosis and neuronal cell death. Both histopathologic changes and adverse neurodevelopmental outcomes have been associated with exposure to both inhalational and IV anesthetics, including isoflurane, sevoflurane, ketamine, benzodiazepines, and propofol. Animal studies were initially performed in nonprimates (rodents), and controversy remains concerning experimental design (dose, duration of treatment, species differences). However, work in nonhuman primates has also shown an increased incidence of adverse neurodevelopmental outcomes after prolonged and/or multiple exposures to volatile anesthetics.

Human studies of anesthesia-induced neurotoxicity have yielded conflicting results. Further complicating the situation are other potential triggers for adverse neurodevelopmental outcomes, including comorbidities, surgical trauma, and perioperative cardiorespiratory status. Multiple population-based epidemiologic studies have suggested a potential association between anesthetic exposure and adverse neurodevelopmental outcomes following multiple or prolonged anesthetic exposures. Large-scale European and Canadian cohort studies utilizing national registries have revealed subtle differences in standardized psychometric testing of early school-aged children after exposure to general anesthesia. Interestingly, other studies in children have failed to yield similar results. The Pediatric Anesthesia and Neurodevelopmental Assessment (PANDA), a multicenter matched-sibling control study, revealed no association between brief anesthetic exposure for inguinal hernia repair and aptitude on psychometric testing. Similarly, the General Anaesthesia and Awake-Regional Anaesthesia in Infancy (GAS) study, a prospective multicenter randomized controlled trial comparing general and neuraxial spinal anesthesia in infants for hernia repair, *did not* demonstrate any significant differences in neurodevelopment at 2 yr of age between groups. The primary outcome of the GAS study is neurodevelopment at 5 yr of age, and these results have not yet been made available. Importantly, studies have not shown an association between adverse neurodevelopmental outcomes and anesthetic exposure <3 hr.

Alternatives to general anesthesia for many procedures in young children do not exist. Regional anesthetic techniques and narcotic-based anesthetics may gain popularity. Dexmedetomidine may also have some neuroprotective properties. Currently, there is insufficient data to make conclusions regarding the safety of one anesthetic approach over another. Ultimately, the potential for neurotoxicity must be balanced against the necessity of providing adequate anesthesia for children presenting for surgery.

Bibliography is available at Expert Consult.

Chapter **75**
Procedural Sedation
John P. Scott
第七十五章
操作时的镇静

中文导读

本章主要介绍了操作时的镇静。镇静描述的是清醒状态和全身麻醉之间的连续状态。许多用于诱导全身麻醉的药物也可用于镇静。儿科操作时的镇静需要警惕和常识，以确保安全，并遵循与麻醉照护相同的指南。本章详细阐述了儿童镇静的系统方法，使用合适的语言来帮助患儿处理操作时的镇静的方法，以及父母和健康照护者的推荐语言。

See also Chapters 74 and 76.

Sedation describes the continuum between wakefulness and general anesthesia (see Table 74.7). Many of the same drugs used to induce general anesthesia may be used to provide sedation (see Table 74.8). Analogous to the provision of anesthesia, performance of procedural sedation requires a comprehensive presedation evaluation, intraprocedural monitoring, and postsedation recovery care. The term **conscious sedation** refers to a condition in which a patient is sleepy, comfortable, and cooperative but maintains airway-protective and ventilatory reflexes. Depending on the choice of pharmacotherapy, sedation may not provide analgesia. Sedation that is sufficient to obtund painful responses describes deep sedation. **Deep sedation** is a state of unarousability to voice and is accompanied by suppression of reflex responses.

Pediatric procedural sedation requires vigilance and knowledge to ensure safety and is governed by the same guidelines as anesthesia care (Table 75.1). Adherence to guidelines for appropriate monitoring and management of sedation in children is imperative. Sedative doses that cause minimal sedation in one patient may produce complete unconsciousness and apnea in another. Anxiolysis or light sedation with chloral hydrate, benzodiazepines, and dexmedetomidine is often sufficient for nonpainful procedures. The use of dexmedetomidine for procedural sedation is safe; recovery time can be prolonged and success variable. For painful procedures (e.g., bone marrow aspiration), the combination of hypnosis and analgesia is required. The addition of opioids to sedation regimens increases the risk of respiratory insufficiency. Short-acting anesthetics (e.g., propofol, methohexital, remifentanil) provide effective procedural sedation, but their use carries a higher likelihood of inadvertent induction of general anesthesia. Use of these medications requires the presence of an anesthesiologist and/or specially trained, experienced, credentialed, and qualified physicians.

Many pediatric subspecialists provide sedation and anesthesia care for children. The use of anesthetic agents is not limited to anesthesiologists, but anesthesiology departments are obligated to help develop, manage, and oversee sedation services. Together, hospitals and providers, including anesthesiologists, share responsibility for the oversight and credentialing of individuals administering sedation and anesthesia.

The elements of a safe pediatric procedural sedation system include the following:

- Clearly defined knowledge and skill sets
- Adequate prerequisite training
- Credentialing of providers
- Maintenance of certification
- Ensuring that sedation sites meet recognized standards
- Continuous quality improvement

Table 75.2 provides an approach to proper language to help the child cope with procedural pain.

Bibliography is available at Expert Consult.

Table 75.1	Systematic Approach to Sedation in Children

Comprehensive medical history and organ system assessment, anticipating underlying medical problems that predispose the patient to anesthetic complications
Careful physical examination focused on the cardiorespiratory system and airway
Appropriate fasting
Informed consent
Pediatric drug dosing (mg/kg)
Appropriately sized equipment
Documentation of vital signs and condition on a time-based record
Rapid response ("code") team to respond to emergencies with "crash cart"
Fully equipped and staffed recovery area
Discharge criteria documenting recovery from sedation

Table 75.2	Suggested Language for Parents and Health-Care Providers

LANGUAGE TO AVOID	LANGUAGE TO USE
You will be fine; there is nothing to worry about. (reassurance)	What did you do in school today? (distraction)
This is going to hurt/this won't hurt. (vague; negative focus)	It might feel like a pinch. (sensory information)
The nurse is going to take some blood. (vague information)	First, the nurse will clean your arm, you will feel the cold alcohol pad, and next … (sensory and procedural information)
You are acting like a baby. (criticism)	Let's get your mind off of it; tell me about that film … (distraction)
It will feel like a bee sting. (negative focus)	Tell me how it feels. (information)
The procedure will last as long as … (negative focus)	The procedure will be shorter than … (television program or other familiar time for child) (procedural information; positive focus)
The medicine will burn. (negative focus)	Some children say they feel a warm feeling. (sensory information; positive focus)
Tell me when you are ready. (too much control)	When I count to three, blow the feeling away from your body. (coaching to cope; distraction-limited control)
I am sorry. (apologizing)	You are being very brave. (praise; encouragement)
Don't cry. (negative focus)	That was hard; I am proud of you. (praise)
It is over. (negative focus)	You did a great job doing the deep breathing, holding still … (labeled praise)

Adapted from Krauss BS, Calligaris L, Green SM, Barbi E: Current concepts in management of pain in children in the emergency department, *Lancet* 387:83–92, 2016.

Chapter **76**

Pediatric Pain Management

Lonnie K. Zeltzer, Elliot J. Krane, and Rona L. Levy

第七十六章

疼痛管理

中文导读

本章主要介绍了疼痛的定义和分类，儿童疼痛的评估及治疗。鉴于儿童不同年龄段认知水平存在差异，本章介绍了几种评估方法：数字法、表情法、FLCC量表法等。疼痛治疗则包括药物治疗如非甾体药、阿片类药物、抗抑郁药、镇静药等，以及非药物治疗如介入治疗、按摩疗法、针刺疗法等内容。

Pain is both a sensory and an emotional experience. When unrecognized and undertreated, pain extracts a significant physiologic, biochemical, and psychological toll on both the child and the family. Many disease processes and most interventional diagnostic or treatment procedures in pediatrics are associated with pain. Similarly, traumatic, developmental, cognitive, psychological, and social experiences can also trigger and maintain chronic pain.

DEFINITION AND CATEGORIES OF PAIN

The International Association for the Study of Pain (IASP) defines **pain** as "an unpleasant sensory and emotional experience associated with actual or potential tissue damage or described in terms of such damage." The important elements to emphasize in this definition are (1) pain encompasses both peripheral physiologic and central neural components and (2) pain may or may not be associated with ongoing tissue damage. The experience of pain lies primarily in the strength and patterning of central neural connectivity (Fig. 76.1). While immediate upstream neural activation can originate from inflammatory, structural, or biochemical events, processes not only in the periphery of the body but also in the spinal cord and the brain influence the intensity and duration of pain. Similarly, central neural processes in the brain are associated with the location, intensity, and distress associated with pain. Chronic pain can develop when the upstream neural signaling continues to activate central neural circuits, such as with continued peripheral inflammatory or structural pain-associated processes.

Often, however, pediatricians face the most difficult problems when either acute pain becomes chronic or chronic pain develops and is maintained without a definable infectious, inflammatory, metabolic, or structural cause. When no "cause" can be found, patients are often referred to mental health specialists, or the cause for the pain is labeled as "stress." Children read this message as, "The doctor thinks I am faking pain or am crazy." Parents see their child suffering and often seek care elsewhere, with the child undergoing numerous tests, procedures, medication trials, and visits and many physicians looking for the cause of the pain so it can be "fixed." Meanwhile, the child may be missing school, social, and physical activities and developing poor sleep habits with increasing fatigue.

It is recognized that chronic pain, in the absence of a specific identified structural, biochemical, or inflammatory cause, develops through the initiation, maintenance, and strength of central neural connectivity patterns, the *connectome* of the child's brain (see Chapter 147). That is, what is now called "centrally mediated pain" derives from neural connectivity patterns in the brain that include centers involved in autonomic nervous system control, memory, and other cognitive centers, as well as emotional centers of the brain. In pediatrics, birth history and child development overlay these central patterns that contribute to the development of chronic pain. A child with high-functioning autism spectrum disorder (ASD) may perseverate on a pain symptom (e.g., headache) in the same way the child might perseverate on an idea or point of view (e.g., the parents may never "win" an argument with their child). Parents may understand the concept of a "sticky nervous system" as the perpetuator of the continued pain in such a child. This model of brain connectivity patterns or "top-down" mediators of chronic pain is important, since it explains how psychological and other nonpharmacologic interventions work to reduce pain and suffering. Science has come a long way since the model of pain as "psychological" or "physical." The current model of pain also includes the impact of the gut microbiome in altering central neural processes in relation to the development and maintenance of pain.

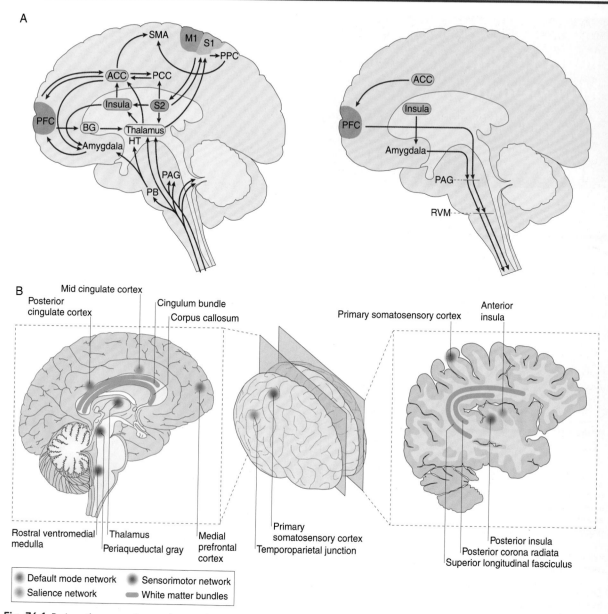

Fig. 76.1 Brain pathways, regions, and networks involved in acute and chronic pain. *ACC,* Anterior cingulate cortex; *PCC,* posterior cingulate cortex; *BG,* basal ganglia; *HT,* hypothalamus; *PAG,* periaqueductal gray; *PB,* parabrachial nuclei; *PFC,* prefrontal cortex; *PPC,* posterior parietal cortex; *SMA,* supplementary motor area; *RVM,* rostral ventromedial medulla. (A, left panel, *From Apkarian AV, Bushnell MC, Treede RD, Zubieta JK: Human brain mechanisms of pain perception and regulation in health and disease, Eur J Pain 9:463–484, 2005; A, right panel, from Schweinhardt P, Bushnell MC: Pain imaging in health and disease—how far have we come? J Clin Invest 120:3788–3797, 2010; B, from Davis KD, Flor H, Greely HT, et al: Brain imaging tests for chronic pain: medical, legal and ethical issues and recommendations, Nat Rev Neurol 13:624–638, 2017.)*

Table 76.1 specifies important pain categories typically treated (somatic, visceral, and neuropathic) and defines the elements and characteristics of **nociception,** the peripheral physiologic aspect of pain perception. Nociception refers to how specialized fibers (largely but not exclusively the small, unmyelinated A-delta and C fibers) in the peripheral nervous system transmit nerve impulses (usually transmitting signals originating from peripheral mechano- and chemoreceptors) through synapses in the spinal cord's dorsal horn through (but not exclusively through) the spinothalamic tracts to the brain's higher centers, where the development of neural connectivity patterns creates the experience of pain.

ASSESSMENT AND MEASUREMENT OF PAIN IN CHILDREN

Assessing pain entails much more than merely quantifying it. Whenever feasible, the physician should ask the patient about the character, location, quality, duration, frequency, and intensity of the pain. Some children may not report pain because of fears (often well founded) of talking to strangers, disappointing or bothering others, receiving an injection if they report pain, returning to the hospital if they admit to pain, and other negative reactions. For infants and nonverbal children, their parents, pediatricians, nurses, and other caregivers are constantly challenged to

Table 76.1	Pain Categories and Characteristics	
PAIN CATEGORY	**DEFINITION AND EXAMPLES**	**CHARACTERISTICS**
Somatic	Pain resulting from injury to or inflammation of tissues (e.g., skin, muscle, tendons, bone, joints, fascia, vasculature) *Examples:* burns, lacerations, fractures, infections, inflammatory conditions	In skin and superficial structures: sharp, pulsatile, well localized In deep somatic structures: dull, aching, pulsatile, not well localized
Visceral	Pain resulting from injury to or inflammation of viscera *Examples:* angina, hepatitic distention, bowel distention or hypermobility, pancreatitis	Aching and cramping; nonpulsatile; poorly localized (e.g., appendiceal pain perceived around umbilicus) or referred to distant locations (e.g., angina perceived in shoulder)
Neuropathic	Pain resulting from injury to, inflammation of, or dysfunction of the peripheral or central nervous system *Examples:* complex regional pain syndrome (CRPS), phantom limb pain, Guillain-Barré syndrome, sciatica	Spontaneous; burning; lancinating or shooting; dysesthesias (pins and needles, electrical sensations); hyperalgesia (amplification of noxious stimuli); hyperpathia (widespread pain in response to a discrete noxious stimulus); allodynia (pain in response to nonpainful stimulation); pain may be perceived distal or proximal to site of injury, usually corresponding to innervation pathways (e.g., sciatica)

interpret whether the child's distressed behaviors represent pain, fear, hunger, or a range of other perceptions or emotions. Similarly, lack of normal interest in play without behavioral distress signals can be manifestations of pain. Therapeutic trials of comfort measures (cuddling, feeding) and analgesic medication may be helpful in clarifying the triggers of the behaviors.

Behavior and physiologic signs are useful but can be misleading. A toddler may scream and grimace during an ear examination because of fear rather than pain. Conversely, children with inadequately relieved persistent pain from cancer, sickle cell disease, trauma, or surgery may withdraw from their surroundings and appear very quiet, leading observers to conclude falsely that these children are comfortable or sedated or, for adolescent patients, are "drug seeking." In these situations, increased dosing of analgesics may make the child become more, not less, interactive and alert. Similarly, neonates and young infants may close their eyes, furrow their brows, and clench their fists in response to pain. Adequate analgesia is often associated with eye opening and increased involvement in surroundings. A child who is experiencing significant chronic pain may play normally as a way to distract attention away from pain. This coping behavior is sometimes misinterpreted as evidence of the child's "faking" or exaggerating pain at other times.

Age-Specific and Developmentally Specific Measures
Because infants, young children, and nonverbal children cannot express the quantity of pain they experience, several pain scales have been devised in an attempt to quantify pain in these populations (Fig. 76.2 and Table 76.2).

The Newborn and Infant
There are several behavioral distress scales for the infant and young child, mostly emphasizing the patient's facial expressions, crying, and body movement. Facial expression measures appear most useful and specific in neonates. Autonomic and vital signs can indicate pain, but because they are nonspecific, they may reflect other processes, including fever, hypoxemia, and cardiac or renal dysfunction (Table 76.3).

The Older Child
Children age 3-7 yr become increasingly articulate in describing the intensity, location, and quality of pain. Pain is occasionally referred to adjacent areas; referral of hip pain to the thigh or area above the knee is common in this age range. Self-report measures for children this age include using drawings, pictures of faces, or graded color intensities. Children ≥8 yr can usually use verbal numerical rating scales or visual analog pain scales (VAS) accurately (Fig. 76.2). Verbal numerical ratings are preferred and considered the gold standard; valid and reliable ratings can be obtained from children ≥8 yr. The numerical rating scale (NRS) consists of numbers from 0-10, in which 0 represents no pain and 10

represents very severe pain. There is debate about the label for the highest pain rating, but the current agreement is *not* to use the phrase "worst pain possible," because children can always imagine a greater pain. In the United States, regularly documented pain assessments are required for hospitalized children and children attending outpatient hospital clinics and emergency departments (EDs). Pain scores do not always correlate with changes in heart rate or blood pressure.

The Cognitively Impaired Child
Measuring pain in cognitively impaired children remains a challenge. Understanding pain expression and experience in this population is important, because behaviors may be misinterpreted as indicating that cognitively impaired children are more insensitive to pain than cognitively competent children. Children with trisomy 21 may express pain less precisely and more slowly than the general population. Pain in children with ASD may be difficult to assess because these children may be both *hyposensitive* and *hypersensitive* to many different types of sensory stimuli, and they may have limited communication abilities. Although self-reports of pain can be elicited from some children who are cognitively impaired, observational measures have better validation among these children. The **Noncommunicating Child's Pain Checklist—Postoperative Version** is recommended for children up to 18 yr. Maladaptive behaviors and reduction in function may also indicate pain. Children with severe cognitive impairments experience pain frequently, mostly not because of accidental injury. Children with the fewest abilities experience the most pain.

CONCEPTUAL FRAMEWORK FOR TREATMENT OF PEDIATRIC PAIN
A number of models have been developed to understand the various factors that influence children's pain. Many of these theories focus on factors that explain the interindividual variability in pain perception and the chronicity and impairment experienced with pain. Central to these models are interrelationships among biologic, cognitive, affective, and social factors that influence children's pain and disability, commonly referred to as "biopsychosocial models" of pain. **Biologic** factors include the child's physical health, central nervous system (CNS) factors (pain processing), sex, pubertal status, and genetic factors. Individual child **cognitive and affective** factors related to perception of pain are anxiety, fear, negative affect, pain behaviors, and functional disability, whereas **social** factors include such areas as culture, socioeconomic status, school environment, social and peer interactions, and parental and family factors. For children, **developmental** factors need to be considered, such as cognitive and motor development, birth history, and epigenetic factors (the interaction in development between genetic and environmental factors).

A framework that considers the interplay of biologic, psychological, and social factors is useful for understanding pediatric pain and to

Behavioral Indicators

Facial grimacing: The Neonatal Facial Coding System* uses several facial actions that may be indicators of pain. Pain is characterized by a bulging brow with tight creases in between; tightly closed eyelids; a deeply furrowed nasolabial groove; a horizontal, wide opened mouth; and a taut tongue that may be quivering along with the chin.

Crying: May be an indicator of pain.

Activity: Withdrawal or immobilization of a limb may be an indicator of pain.

Response to comfort measures: Feeding, swaddling, holding, and ensuring that the infant is neither wet nor cold may help to discriminate between pain and other conditions.

Physiologic indicators: Alterations in heart rate, blood pressure, SpO_2, respiratory rate, or alterations in pattern of respiration may be nonspecific indicators of pain.

Multidimensional Instrument

FLACC[†] Scoring System: May be used in preverbal, mechanically ventilated, or cognitively impaired patients; it is an acronym that includes five indicators, each scored as a 0, 1, or 2 that forms a ten-point composite scale with a range from "0" (no pain) to "10" (worst pain).

FLACC: Score each category between 0 and 2. The total score may be any number from 0 to 10.

Score:	0	1	2
Face	No expression	Occational action	Frequent action
Legs	Normal	Restless or tense	Kicking, legs withdrawn
Activity	Quiet	Shifting or tense	Rigid, arched, jerking
Cry	None	Moan, whimper	Steady crying, screaming, sobbing, or frequent complaints
Consolability	Content	Consolable	Inconsolable

Self-Report of Pain

Categorical description: Toddlers or young children are asked to say if they are having "a little bit," a "middle amount," or "a lot" of pain.

Faces Scales[‡]: Children who do not have an appreciation of ordinal numbering are asked to rate their pain based upon cartoons depicting facial indicators of distress.

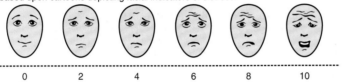

NRS[§]: Older children and teenagers are asked to rate their pain on a scale of "0" (no pain) to "10" (worst pain).

VAS[§]: Children or teenagers are asked to move an indicator along a mechanical slide to depict the level of pain; the clinician reads a number along a 10-cm indicator on the back to determine the numeric score.

Fig. 76.2 **Clinically useful pain assessment tools.** *(Adapted from Burg FD, Ingelfinger JR, Polin RA, et al, editors: Current pediatric therapy, ed 18, Philadelphia, 2006, Saunders/Elsevier, p 16; and Hicks CL, von Baeyer CL, Spafford P, et al: The Faces Pain Scale—revised: toward a common metric in pediatric pain measurement, Pain 93:173–183, 2001.)*

guide pain assessment and the delivery of pain prevention and management. Many simple interventions designed to promote relaxation and patient control can work either alone or synergistically with pain medications for relief of pain and related distress. Moreover, psychological interventions are often coupled with physical therapy interventions to assist in the management of disabling chronic pain.

Pharmacologic Treatment of Pain

The pharmacokinetics and pharmacodynamics of analgesics vary with age; drug responses in infants and young children differ from those in older children and adults. The elimination half-life of most analgesics is prolonged in neonates and young infants because of their immature hepatic enzyme systems and glomerular filtration. Clearance of analgesics may also be variable in young infants and children. Renal blood flow, glomerular filtration, and tubular secretion increase dramatically in the 1st few weeks, approaching adult values by 3-5 mo of age. Renal clearance of analgesics is often greater in toddlers and preschool-aged children than in adults, whereas in premature infants, clearance is reduced. Age-related differences in body composition and protein binding also exist. Total body water as a fraction of body weight is greater in neonates than in children or adults. Tissues with high perfusion, such as the brain and heart, account for a larger proportion of body mass in neonates than do other tissues, such as muscle and fat. Because of decreased serum concentrations of albumin and α_1-acid glycoprotein, neonates have reduced protein binding of some drugs, resulting in higher amounts of free, unbound, pharmacologically active drug.

Acetaminophen, Aspirin, Nonsteroidal Antiinflammatory, and Coxib Drugs

Acetaminophen and nonsteroidal antiinflammatory drugs (NSAIDs) have replaced aspirin as the most commonly used antipyretics and oral, nonopioid analgesics (Table 76.4).

Acetaminophen, a generally safe, nonopioid analgesic and antipyretic, has the advantage of intravenous (IV), rectal, and oral routes of administration. Acetaminophen is not associated with the gastrointestinal (GI) or antiplatelet effects of aspirin and NSAIDs, making it a particularly useful drug in patients with cancer. Unlike aspirin and NSAIDs, acetaminophen has only mild antiinflammatory action.

Acetaminophen toxicity can result from a large single dose or cumulative excessive dosing over days or weeks (see Chapter 77). A single massive overdose overwhelms the normal glucuronidation and sulfation metabolic pathways in the liver, whereas long-term overdosing exhausts supplies of the sulfhydryl donor glutathione, leading to alternative cytochrome P-450 (CYP)–catalyzed oxidative metabolism and the production of the hepatotoxic metabolite *N*-acetyl-*p*-benzoquinone imine (NAPQI). Toxicity manifests as fulminant hepatic necrosis and failure in infants, children, and adults. Drug biotransformation processes are immature in neonates, very active in young children, and somewhat less active in adults. Young children are more resistant to acetaminophen-induced hepatotoxicity than are adults as a result of metabolic differences; sulfation predominates over glucuronidation in young children, leading to a reduction in NAPQI production.

Aspirin is indicated for certain rheumatologic conditions and for inhibition of platelet adhesiveness, as in the treatment of Kawasaki

Table 76.2	Pain Measurement Tools				
NAME	**FEATURES**	**AGE RANGE**	**ADVANTAGES**	**VALIDATION AND USES**	**LIMITATIONS**
Visual Analog Scale (VAS)	Horizontal 10-cm line; subject marks a spot on the line between anchors of "no pain" (or neutral face) and "most pain imaginable" (or sad face)	6-8 yr and older	Good psychometric properties; validated for research purposes	Acute pain Surgical pain Chronic pain	Cannot be used in younger children or in those with cognitive limitations Requires language skills and numerical processing; upper anchor of "most pain" requires an experiential reference point that is lacking in many children.
Likert Scale	Integers from 0-10, inclusive, corresponding to a range from no pain to most pain	6-8 yr and older	Good psychometric properties; validated for research purposes	Acute pain Surgical pain Chronic pain	Same as for VAS.
Faces Scales (e.g., FACES-R, Wong-Baker, Oucher, Bieri, McGrath scales)	Subjects rate their pain by identifying with line drawings of faces, or photos of children	4 yr and older	Can be used at younger ages than VAS and Likert	Acute pain Surgical pain	Choice of "no pain" face affects responses (neutral vs smiling); not culturally universal.
Behavioral or combined behavioral-physiologic scales (e.g., FLACC, N-PASS, CHEOPS, OPS, FACS, NIPS)	Scoring of observed behaviors (e.g., facial expression, limb movement) ± heart rate and blood pressure	Some work for any ages; some work for specific age-groups, including preterm infants	May be used in both infants and nonverbal children	FLACC, N-PASS: Acute pain Surgical pain	Nonspecific; overrates pain in toddlers and preschool children; underrates persistent pain; some measures are convenient, but others require videotaping and complex processing; vital sign changes unrelated to pain can occur and may affect total score.
Autonomic measures (e.g., heart rate, blood pressure, heart rate spectral analyses)	Scores changes in heart rate, blood pressure, or measures of heart rate variability (e.g., "vagal tone")	All ages	Can be used at all ages; useful for patients receiving mechanical ventilation		Nonspecific; vital sign changes unrelated to pain may occur, and may artifactually increase or decrease score.
Hormonal-metabolic measures	Plasma or salivary sampling of "stress" hormones (e.g., cortisol, epinephrine)	All ages	Can be used at all ages		Nonspecific; changes unrelated to pain can occur; inconvenient; cannot provide "real-time" information; standard normal values not available for every age bracket.

Table 76.3	Signs and Symptoms of Pain in Infants and Young Children
PHYSIOLOGIC CHANGES • Increase in heart rate, respiratory rate, blood pressure, muscle tone • Oxygen desaturation • Sweating • Flushing • Pallor **BEHAVIORAL CHANGES** • Change in facial expression (grimacing, furrowing of the	brow, nasal flaring, deep nasolabial groove, curving of the tongue, quivering of the chin) • Finger clenching • Thrashing of limbs • Writhing • Back arching • Head banging • Poor feeding • Sleep disturbance • Pseudoparalysis

From Krauss BS, Calligaris L, Green SM, Barbi E: Current concepts in management of pain in children in the emergency department, *Lancet* 387:83–92, 2016.

disease. Concerns about Reye syndrome have resulted in a substantial decline in pediatric aspirin use.

The **NSAIDs** are used widely to treat pain and fever in children. NSAIDs are nonselective cyclooxygenase (COX) inhibitors, that is, drugs that nonselectively block the activity of both COX-1 (found in gastric mucosa and platelets) and COX-2 (active in inflammatory pathways and cortical renal blood flow regulation) enzymes that synthesize prostaglandins. In children with juvenile idiopathic arthritis, ibuprofen and aspirin are equally effective, but ibuprofen is associated with fewer side effects and better drug adherence. NSAIDs and coxibs used adjunctively in surgical patients reduce opioid requirements (and therefore opioid side effects) by as much as 35–40%. Although NSAIDs can be useful postoperatively, they should be used as an adjunct to, not as a substitute for, opioids in patients with acute, moderate to severe pain.

Ketorolac, an IV NSAID, is useful in treating moderate to severe acute pain in patients who are unable or unwilling to swallow oral NSAIDs. U.S. Food and Drug Administration (FDA) recommendations limit ketorolac to 5 consecutive days of administration. IV ibuprofen (Caldolor) is FDA approved for the management of pain and fever in infants and children >6 mo of age. Adverse effects of NSAIDs are uncommon but may be serious when they occur, including inhibition of bone growth and healing; gastritis with pain and bleeding; decreased

Table 76.4	Commonly Used Nonopioid Medications	
MEDICATION	**DOSAGE**	**COMMENT(S)**
Acetaminophen	10-15 mg/kg PO q4h 10 mg/kg IV q4h 15 mg/kg IV q6h 10 mg/kg IV q6h (<2 yr) 20-30 mg/kg/PR q4h 40 mg/kg/PR q6-8h *Maximum daily dosing:* 90 mg/kg/24 hr (children) 60 mg/kg/24 hr (<2 yr) 30-45 mg/kg/24 hr (neonates)	Minimal antiinflammatory action; no antiplatelet or adverse gastric effects; overdosing can produce fulminant hepatic failure.
Aspirin	10-15 mg/kg PO q4h *Maximum daily dosing:* 120 mg/kg/24 hr (children)	Antiinflammatory; prolonged antiplatelet effects; may cause gastritis; associated with Reye syndrome.
Ibuprofen	8-10 mg/kg PO q6h 10 mg/kg IV q4-6h to maximum of 400 mg *Maximum daily dose:* 2400 mg	Antiinflammatory; transient antiplatelet effects; may cause gastritis; extensive pediatric safety experience.
Naproxen	5-7 mg/kg PO q8-12h	Antiinflammatory; transient antiplatelet effects; may cause gastritis; more prolonged duration than that of ibuprofen.
Ketorolac	Loading dose 0.5 mg/kg, then 0.25-0.3 mg/kg IV q6h to a maximum of 5 days; maximum dose 60 mg loading with maximum dosing of 30 mg q6h	Antiinflammatory; reversible antiplatelet effects; may cause gastritis; useful for short-term situations in which oral dosing is not feasible.
Diclofenac sodium	2-3 mg/kg/day divided in 2 or 3 doses	Antiinflammatory; reversible antiplatelet effects; lower risk of gastritis and ulceration compared with other NSAIDs.
Choline magnesium salicylate	10-20 mg/kg PO q8-12h	Weak antiinflammatory; lower risk of bleeding and gastritis than with conventional NSAIDs.
Celecoxib	3-6 mg/kg PO q12-24h	Antiinflammatory; no or minimal antiplatelet or gastric effects; cross-reactivity with sulfa allergies.
Nortriptyline, amitriptyline, desipramine	0.1-0.5 mg/kg PO qhs Larger doses may be divided bid.	For neuropathic pain; facilitates sleep; may enhance opioid effect; may be useful in sickle cell pain; risk of dysrhythmia in prolonged QTc syndrome; may cause fatal dysrhythmia in overdose; FDA states agents may enhance suicidal ideation; little or no antidepression or antianxiety effects at lower dosages.
Gabapentin	100 mg bid or tid titrated to up to 3600 mg/24 hr	For neuropathic pain; associated with sedation, dizziness, ataxia, headache, and behavioral changes.
Quetiapine, risperidone, chlorpromazine, haloperidol	Quetiapine: 6.25 or 12.5 mg PO qd (hs); may use q6hr prn acute agitation with pain. Escalate dose to 25 mg/dose if needed. Risperidone: useful for PDD spectrum or tic disorder and chronic pain; 0.25-1 mg (in 0.25 mg increments) qd or bid; see PDR for other dosing.	Useful when arousal is amplifying pain; often used when patient first starting SSRI and then weaned after at least 2 wk; check for normal QTc before initiating; side effects include extrapyramidal reactions (diphenhydramine may be used to treat) and sedation; in high doses, can lower the seizure threshold.
Venlafaxine, duloxetine	Venlafaxine: start 37.5 mg daily as the XR formulation and titrate up monthly to effective dose, 2-4 mg/kg. Duloxetine: start 20 mg daily and titrate upward to effective dose, 1-1.5 mg/kg.	SNRIs with both clinically significant antidepression and antianxiety effects as well as analgesic effects.
Fluoxetine	10-20 mg PO qd (usually in morning)	SSRI for children with anxiety disorders in which arousal amplifies sensory signaling; useful in PDD spectrum disorders in very low doses; best to use in conjunction with psychiatric evaluation.
Sucrose solution via pacifier or gloved finger	*Preterm infants (gestational age):* 28 wk: 0.2 mL swabbed into mouth 28-32 wk: 0.2-2 mL, depending on suck/swallow >32 wk: 2 mL *Term infants:* 1.5-2 mL PO over 2 min	Allow 2 min before starting procedure; analgesia may last up to 8 min; the dose may be repeated once.

FDA, U.S. Food and Drug Administration; IV, intravenously; NSAIDs, nonsteroidal antiinflammatory drugs; PDD, pervasive developmental disorder; PDR, *Physicians' Desk Reference*; PO, orally; PR, rectally; QTc, corrected QT interval on an electrocardiogram; SSRI, selective serotonin reuptake inhibitor.

renal blood flow that may reduce glomerular filtration and enhance sodium reabsorption, in some cases leading to tubular necrosis; hepatic dysfunction and liver failure; inhibition of platelet function; and an increased incidence of cardiovascular events in patients predisposed to stroke and myocardial infarction. Although the overall incidence of bleeding is very low, gastric bleeding is the most common cause of mortality related to this class of analgesics. NSAIDs should not be used in the child with a bleeding diathesis or at risk for bleeding or when surgical hemostasis is a concern, such as after tonsillectomy. The drug class is usually not used in the setting of bone healing, except perhaps in the 1st few days after surgery. Renal injury from short-term use of ibuprofen in euvolemic children is quite rare; the risk is increased by hypovolemia or cardiac dysfunction. The safety of both ibuprofen and acetaminophen for short-term use is well established (see Table 76.4).

Coxib drugs available in the United States are limited to oral celecoxib, whereas in Europe and elsewhere parenteral parecoxib and oral rofecoxib are available. Parecoxib was not FDA approved, whereas rofecoxib was approved and withdrawn from marketing due to concern of enhanced risk of heart attack and stroke in high-risk adults, which has subsequently been found to be associated with all the coxibs and all the NSAID drugs as well. The coxib drugs are selective COX-2 enzyme inhibitors; therefore they are effective antiinflammatory and analgesic molecules that generally do not result in platelet inhibition or bleeding, or in gastric inflammation or ulceration, findings that may be seen with the nonselective COX inhibitors in the NSAID class. However, coxib drugs do inhibit regulation of cortical renal blood flow, and therefore carry the same risk of renal toxicity and acute tubular necrosis, particularly in the setting of low cardiac output states or dehydration. Celecoxib is therefore an appropriate primary or adjunctive analgesic to use in children after surgery, children with gastric mucosal pathology, or oncology patients in whom concern for hemostasis contraindicates conventional NSAIDs.

Opioids

Opioids are analgesic substances either derived from the opium poppy (**opiates**) or synthesized to have a similar chemical structure and mechanism of action (**opioids**). The older, pejorative term "narcotics" (narcotic analgesics) should not be used for these agents because it connotes criminality and lacks pharmacologic descriptive specificity. Opioids are administered for moderate and severe pain, such as acute postoperative pain, sickle cell crisis pain, and cancer pain. Opioids can be administered by the oral, rectal, oral transmucosal, transdermal, intranasal, IV, epidural, intrathecal, subcutaneous (SC), or intramuscular (IM) route. Regardless of route of administration, the site of action is at mu (µ) opioid receptors in the peripheral nervous system, spinal cord, brainstem, and higher CNS centers. Historically, infants and young children have been underdosed with opioids because of concern about significant respiratory side effects. Once thought to represent infants' particular sensitivity, the opioids' respiratory depressant effects are now known to result from infants' lower metabolic clearance of opioids and higher blood levels with frequent dosing. With proper understanding of the pharmacokinetic and pharmacodynamics of opioids, children can receive effective relief of pain and suffering with a good margin of safety, regardless of pharmacokinetic maturity, age, or size (Tables 76.5 to 76.8).

Opioids act by mimicking the actions of endogenous opioid peptides, binding to receptors in the brain, brainstem, spinal cord, and to a lesser extent in the peripheral nervous system, and thus leading to inhibition of nociception. Opioids also bind to µ receptors in the pleasure centers of the midbrain, particularly in genetically susceptible individuals, a factor responsible for the euphoric effect in some individuals as well as the predilection to psychological dependence and addictive behavior. Opioids also have dose-dependent respiratory depressant effects when interacting with the µ-opioid receptors in the respiratory centers of the brainstem, depressing ventilator drive and blunting ventilatory responses to both hypoxia and hypercarbia. These respiratory depressant effects are increased with co-administration of other sedating drugs, particularly benzodiazepines or barbiturates.

Optimal use of opioids requires proactive and anticipatory management of side effects (see Table 76.7). Common side effects include sedation, constipation, nausea, vomiting, urinary retention, and pruritus. Tolerance usually develops to the side effect of **nausea**, which typically subsides with long-term dosing, but nausea may require treatment with antiemetics, such as a phenothiazine, butyrophenones, antihistamines, or a serotonin receptor antagonist such as ondansetron or granisetron. Pruritus and other complications during patient-controlled analgesia with opioids may be effectively managed by low-dose IV naloxone.

The most common, troubling, but treatable side effect is **constipation**. Patients who take opioids for chronic pain for long periods predictably develop tolerance to the sedative and analgesic effects of opioids over time, but tolerance to constipation does not occur, and constipation remains a troublesome and distressing problem in almost all patients with long-term opioid administration. Stool softeners and stimulant laxatives should be administered to most patients receiving opioids for

Table 76.5	Practical Aspects of Prescribing Opioids

- Morphine, hydromorphone, or fentanyl is regarded as 1st choice for severe pain.
- Dosing should be titrated and individualized. There is no "right" dose for everyone.
- The right dose is the dose that relieves pain with a good margin of safety.
- Dosing should be more cautious in infants, in patients with coexisting diseases that increase risk or impair drug clearance, and with concomitant administration of sedatives.
- Hydromorphone is metabolized by CYP2D6 and fentanyl by CYP3A4, and to some extent 2D6; drugs that compete for 2D6 enzyme will raise blood levels and increase risk of respiratory depression.
- Morphine is metabolized by glucuronidation to an active metabolite, morphine-6-glucuronide, which accumulates and causes CNS toxicity in renal impairment.
- Anticipate and treat peripheral side effects, including constipation, nausea, and itching.
- Give doses at sufficient frequency to prevent the return of severe pain before the next dose.
- Use a drug delivery method, such as patient-controlled anesthesia or continuous infusions, that avoids the need for "prn" decision-making.
- With opioid dosing for >1 wk, taper gradually to avoid abstinence syndrome.
- When converting between parenteral and oral opioid doses, use appropriate potency ratios (see Table 76.6).
- *Tolerance* refers to decreasing drug effect with continued administration of a drug. Over time a patient will need higher dosing to achieve the same clinical effect; however, tolerance to sedation and respiratory depression develop more rapidly than tolerance to analgesia. Thus, with higher doses, patients do not experience oversedation or respiratory depression.
- *Dependence* refers to the need for continued drug dosing to prevent abstinence syndrome when a drug is abruptly discontinued, or its dose reduced. Abstinence syndrome is characterized by irritability, agitation, autonomic arousal, nasal congestion, piloerection, diarrhea, jitteriness, and yawning; it is produced by administration of potent opioids for >5-7 days.
- *Addiction*, a psychiatric pathology, refers to psychological craving, compulsive drug-seeking behavior, and drug use despite medical harm. Addiction has strong genetic and environmental determinants. Opioid therapy will not lead to addiction in nonsusceptible individuals, and opioid underdosing does not prevent addiction; it may in fact increase drug-seeking behavior for relief of pain (e.g., watching the clock), referred to as "pseudoaddiction."

more than a few days. Osmotic and bulk laxatives are less effective, usually producing more distention and discomfort. A peripherally acting opiate µ-receptor antagonist, **methylnaltrexone,** promptly and effectively reverses opioid-induced constipation in patients with chronic pain who are receiving opioids daily. Methylnaltrexone is approved for use as either an injectable or oral formulation, but only the SC injection is commercially available, which most children will object to receiving. Naldemedine and naloxegol are other agents with actions similar to methylnaltrexone. A novel laxative, **lubiprostone,** is a colonic chloride channel inhibitor that impairs water reabsorption in the colon and is very effective for opioid-induced constipation.

Media and government attention the "opioid epidemic" has reasonably led to scrutiny of the prescription of opioids to children, and recent FDA approval of opioid formulations for children has raised alarm and criticism by some vocal critics of the use of opioids for medical purposes. Thus, one of the potent barriers to effective management of pain with opioids is the fear of addiction held by many prescribing pediatricians and parents alike. Pediatricians should understand the phenomena of tolerance, dependence, withdrawal, and addiction (see Table 76.5). **Opioid addiction** is the result of the complex interplay of genetic predisposition, psychiatric pathology, and social forces, including poverty, joblessness, hopelessness, and despair. The dramatic increase in the

Table 76.6 | Pediatric Dosage Guidelines for Opioid Analgesics

DRUG	EQUI-ANALGESIC DOSES		PARENTERAL DOSING		IV:PO DOSE RATIO	ORAL DOSING		COMMENTS
	IV	Oral	<50 kg	>50 kg		<50 kg	>50 kg	
Fentanyl	10 µg	100 µg	0.5-1 µg/kg q1-2h 0.5-1.5 µg/kg/hr	0.5-1 µg/kg q1-2h 0.5-1.5 µg/kg/hr	Oral transmucosal: 1:10 Transdermal: 1:1	Oral transmucosal: 10 µg/kg Transdermal: 12.5-50 µg/hr	Transdermal patches available; patch reaches steady state at 24 hr and should be changed q72h	70-100 times as potent as morphine with rapid onset and shorter duration. With high doses and rapid administration, can cause chest-wall rigidity. Useful for short procedures; transdermal form should be used only in opioid-tolerant patients with chronic pain.
Hydrocodone	N/A	1.5 mg	N/A	N/A	N/A	0.15 mg/kg	10 mg	Weak opioid; only available in form with acetaminophen.
Hydromorphone	0.2 mg	0.6 mg	0.01 mg q2-4h 0.002 mg/kg/hr	0.01 mg q2-4h 0.002 mg/kg/hr	1:3	0.04-0.08 mg/kg q3-4h	2-4 mg q3-4h	5 times the potency of morphine; no histamine release and fewer adverse events than morphine.
Meperidine	10 mg	30 mg	0.5 mg/kg q2-4h	0.5 mg/kg q2-4h	1:4	2-3 mg/kg q3-4h	100-150 mg q3-4h	Primary use in low doses is for treatment of rigors and shivering after anesthesia or with amphotericin or blood products. Not appropriate for repeated dosing.
Methadone	1 mg	2 mg	0.1 mg/kg q8-24h	0.1 mg/kg q8-24h	1:2	0.2 mg/kg q8-12h PO; available as liquid or tablet	2.5 mg TID	Duration 12-24 hr; useful in certain types of chronic pain; requires additional vigilance because it will accumulate over 72 hr and produce delayed sedation. When patients tolerant of opioids are switched to methadone, they show incomplete cross-tolerance and improved efficacy. Since methadone is associated with prolonged QTc, monitoring is needed for children receiving high and extended dosing.
Morphine	1 mg	3 mg	0.05 mg/kg q2-4h 0.01-0.03 mg/kg/hr	Bolus: 5-8 mg q2-4h	1:3	Immediate release: 0.3 mg/kg q3-4h Sustained release: 20-35 kg: 10-15 mg q8-12h 35-50 kg: 15-30 mg q8-12h	Immediate release: 15-20 mg q3-4h Sustained release: 30-90 mg q8-12h	Potent opioid for moderate/severe pain; may cause histamine release. Sustained-release form must be swallowed whole; if crushed, becomes immediate acting, leading to acute overdose.
Oxycodone	N/A	3 mg	N/A	N/A	N/A	0.1-0.2 mg q3-4h; available in liquid (1 mg/mL)	Immediate release: 5-10 mg q4h Sustained release: 10-120 mg q8-12h	Strong opioid only available as an oral agent in North America; more potent than and preferable to hydrocodone. Sustained-release form must be swallowed whole; if crushed, becomes immediate acting, leading to acute overdose.

N/A, not available.

Table 76.7	Management of Opioid-Induced Adverse Effects
Respiratory depression	*Naloxone:* 0.01-0.02 mg/kg up to a full reversal dose of 0.1 mg/kg. May be given IV, IM, SC, or via ET. The full reversal dose should initially be used for apnea in opioid-naive patients. In opioid-tolerant patients, a reduced dose should be given and titrated up slowly to treat symptoms but prevent acute withdrawal. Ventilation may need to be supported during this process. Dose may be repeated every 2 min to a total of 10 mg. Adult maximum dose is 2 mg/dose. Give with caution to patients who are receiving long-term opioid therapy, as it may precipitate acute withdrawal. Duration of effect is 1-4 hr; therefore close observation for re-narcotization is essential to prevent re-narcotization.
Excessive sedation without evidence of respiratory depression	*Methylphenidate**: 0.3 mg/kg per dose PO (typically 10-20 mg/dose to a teenager) before breakfast and lunch. Do not administer to patients receiving clonidine, because dysrhythmias may develop. *Dextroamphetamine:* 2.5-10 mg on awakening and at noon. Not for use in young children or in patients with cardiovascular disease or hypertension. *Modafinil:* Pediatric dose not established. May be useful in selected patients. Typical adult dose: 50-200 mg/day. Change opioid or decrease the dose.
Nausea and vomiting	*Metoclopramide*†: 0.15 mg/kg IV up to 10 mg/dose q6-12h for 24 hr. *Trimethobenzamide:* PO or PR if weight <15 kg, 100 mg q6h; if >15 kg, 200 mg q6h. (*Note:* Suppository contains benzocaine 2%.) Not for use in newborn infants or premature infants. 5-HT$_3$ receptor blockers: *Ondansetron:* 0.15 mg/kg up to 8 mg IV q6-8h not to exceed 32 mg/day (also available as a sublingual tablet). *Granisetron:* 10 to 20 µg/kg IV q12-24h. *Prochlorperazine** (Compazine): >2 yr or >20 kg, 0.1 mg/kg per dose q8h IM or PO up to 10 mg/dose. Change opioid.
Pruritus	*Hydroxyzine:* 0.5 mg/kg PO q6h. *Nalbuphine:* 0.1 mg/kg IV q6h for pruritus caused by intraaxial opioids, especially fentanyl. Administer slowly over 15-20 min. May cause acute reversal of systemic μ-receptor effects and leave κ-agonism intact. *Naloxone:* 0.003 to 0.1 mg/kg/hr IV infusion (titrate up to decrease pruritus and reduce infusion if pain increases). *Ondansetron:* 0.05 to 0.1 mg/kg IV or PO q8h. *Cyproheptadine*†: 0.1-0.2 mg/kg PO q8-12h. Maximum dose 12 mg. Change opioid.
Constipation	Encourage water consumption, high-fiber diet, and vegetable fiber. *Bulk laxatives:* Metamucil, Maltsupex. *Lubricants:* Mineral oil 15-30 mL PO qd as needed (not for use in infants because of aspiration risk). *Surfactants:* Sodium docusate (Colace): <3 yr: 10 mg PO q8h 3-6 yr: 15 mg PO q8h 6-12 yr: 50 mg PO q8h >12 yr: 100 mg PO q8h *Stimulants:* Bisacodyl suppository (Dulcolax): <2 yr: 5 mg PR qhs >2 yr: 10 mg PR qhs Senna syrup (218 mg/5 mL): >3 yr: 5 mL qhs. *Enema:* Fleet hypertonic phosphate enema (older children; risk of hyperphosphatemia). *Electrolytic/osmotic:* Milk of magnesia; for severe impaction: polyethylene glycol (GoLYTELY, MiraLax). Methylnaltrexone is an opioid antagonist that works in the colon and does not cross the blood-brain barrier to reverse analgesia; given as subcutaneous injection every day or every other day (0.15 mg/kg) and is effective in producing stool in 30-60 min in most patients.
Urinary retention	Straight catheterization, indwelling catheter.

*Avoid in patients taking monoamine oxidase inhibitors.
†May be associated with extrapyramidal side effects, which may be more often seen in children than in adults.
ET, Endotracheal tube; IV, intravenously; IM, intramuscularly; PO, orally; PR, rectally; SC, subcutaneously.
Modified from Burg FD, Ingelfinger JR, Polin RA, et al, editors: *Current pediatric therapy*, ed 18, Philadelphia, 2006, Saunders/Elsevier, p 16.

amount of opioid abuse and overdoses and opioid-related deaths since 2001 has been largely restricted to the adult white population age 30-55 yr, not in children or adolescents. A longitudinal study of children and adolescents treated for medical reasons with opioids found that there was no increased risk of the development of substance abuse, at least until their mid-20s. Other epidemiologic studies have shown a negligible increase in opioid overdoses and deaths in the black and Latino populations, but rather a relationship to the unemployment rate. Thus the rational short- or even long-term use of opioids in children does not lead to a predilection for or risk of addiction in a child not otherwise at risk because of genetic background, race, or social milieu.

It is equally important for pediatricians to realize that even patients with recognized substance abuse diagnoses are entitled to effective analgesic management, which often includes the use of opioids. If legitimate concerns exist about addiction in a patient, safe effective opioid pain management is often best managed by specialists in pain management and addiction medicine. Table 76.9 outlines the U.S. Centers for Disease Control and Prevention (CDC) opioid recommendations for **chronic pain** (primarily in adults).

There is no longer a reason to administer opioids by IM injection. Continuous IV infusion of opioids is an effective option that permits more constant plasma concentrations and clinical effects than intermittent IV bolus dosing, without the pain associated with IM injection. The most common approach in pediatric centers is to administer a low-dose basal opioid infusion, while permitting patients to use a **patient-controlled analgesia (PCA)** device to titrate the dosage above the infusion (Fig. 76.3) (see Chapter 74). Compared with children given intermittent IM morphine, children using PCA reported better pain scores. PCA has several other advantages: (1) dosing can be adjusted to account for individual pharmacokinetic and pharmacodynamic

Table 76.8	Equianalgesic Doses and Half-Life ($T_{1/2\beta}$) of Some Commonly Used Opioids		
OPIOID	**IM/IV DOSE (mg)**	**ORAL DOSE (mg)**	**$T_{1/2\beta}$ (hr)**
Morphine	10	30	2-3
Meperidine	100	400	3-4
Oxycodone	15	20-30	2-3
Fentanyl	0.15-0.2	—	3-5
Alfentanil	0.75-1.5	—	1-2
Sufentanil	0.02	—	2-3
Diamorphine	5	60	0.5*
Methadone	10	10-15	15-40
Hydromorphone	1.5	7.5	3-4
Tramadol†	100	100	5-7
Buprenorphine	0.4	0.8 (sublingual)	3-5
Pentazocine	60	150	3-5
Nalbuphine	10-20	—	2-4
Butorphanol	2	—	2-3

NOTES:
- Published reports vary in the suggested doses considered to be equianalgesic to morphine. Therefore, titration to clinical response in each patient is necessary.
- Suggested doses are the results of single-dose studies only. Therefore, use of the data to calculate total daily dose requirements and repeated or continuous doses may not be appropriate.
- There may be incomplete cross-tolerance between these drugs. In patients who have been receiving one opioid for a prolonged period, it is usually necessary to use a dose lower than the expected equianalgesic dose when changing to another opioid, and to titrate to effect.
*Rapidly hydrolyzed to morphine.
†Only part of its analgesic action results from action on μ-opioid receptors.
Modified from Macintyre PE, Ready LB: *Acute pain management: a practical guide*, ed 2, Philadelphia, 2001, Saunders, p 19.

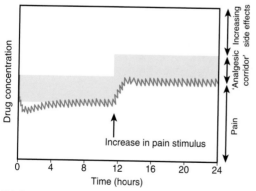

Fig. 76.3 Patient-controlled analgesia is more likely to keep blood concentrations of opioid within the "analgesic corridor" and allows rapid titration if there is an increase in pain stimulus requiring higher blood levels of opioid to maintain the analgesia. (*From Burg FD, Ingelfinger JR, Polin RA, et al, editors:* Current pediatric therapy, *ed 18. Philadelphia, 2006, Saunders/Elsevier, p 16.*)

variation and for changing pain intensity during the day; (2) psychologically the patient is more in control, actively coping with the pain; (3) overall opioid consumption tends to be lower; (4) therefore fewer side effects occur; and (5) patient satisfaction is generally much higher. Children as young as 5-6 yr can effectively use PCA. The device can also be activated by parents or nurses, known as **PCA-by-proxy (PCA-P)**, which produces analgesia in a safe, effective manner for children who cannot activate the PCA demand button themselves because they are too young or intellectually or physically impaired. PCA overdoses have occurred when well-meaning, inadequately instructed parents pushed the PCA button in medically complicated situations, with or without the use of PCA-P, highlighting the need for patient and family education, use of protocols, and adequate nursing supervision.

Because of the high risk of adverse side effects (respiratory depression), the FDA has issued contraindications for the pediatric use of codeine and tramadol (Table 76.10).

Local Anesthetics

Local anesthetics are widely used in children for topical application, cutaneous infiltration, peripheral nerve block, neuraxial blocks (intrathecal or epidural infusions), and IV infusions (Table 76.11) (see Chapter 74). Local anesthetics can be used with excellent safety and effectiveness. Local anesthetics interfere with neural transmission by blocking neuronal sodium channels. Excessive systemic dosing can cause seizures, CNS depression, and (by cardiac and arteriolar sodium channel blockade) hypotension, arrhythmias, cardiac depression, and cardiovascular collapse. Local anesthetics therefore require a strict maximum dosing schedule. Pediatricians should be aware of the need to calculate these doses and adhere to guidelines.

Topical local anesthetic preparations do not generally result in measurable systemic blood levels and can reduce pain in diverse circumstances: suturing of lacerations, placement of peripheral IV catheters, lumbar punctures, and accessing indwelling central venous ports. The application of tetracaine, epinephrine, and cocaine results in good anesthesia for suturing wounds but should not be used on mucous membranes. Combinations of tetracaine with phenylephrine and lidocaine-epinephrine-tetracaine are equally as effective, eliminating the need to use a controlled substance (cocaine). EMLA, a topical eutectic mixture of lidocaine and prilocaine used to anesthetize intact skin, is frequently applied for venipuncture, lumbar puncture, and other needle procedures. A 5% lidocaine cream (Elemax) is also effective as a topical anesthetic.

Lidocaine is the most commonly used local anesthetic for cutaneous infiltration. Maximum safe doses of lidocaine are 5 mg/kg without epinephrine and 7 mg/kg with epinephrine. Although concentrated solutions (2%) are commonly available from hospital pharmacies, more dilute solutions (0.25% and 0.5%) are equally as effective as 1–2% solutions. The diluted solutions cause less burning discomfort on injection and permit use of larger volumes without achieving toxic doses. In the surgical setting, cutaneous infiltration is more often performed with bupivacaine 0.25% or ropivacaine 0.2% because of the much longer duration of effect; maximum dosage of these long-acting amide anesthetics is 2-3 mg/kg and 3-4 mg/kg, respectively.

Neuropathic pain may respond well to the local application of a lidocaine topical patch (Lidoderm) for 12 hr/day (Table 76.12). Peripheral and central neuropathic pain also may respond to IV lidocaine infusions, which may be used in hospital settings for refractory pain, complex regional pain syndromes, and pain associated with malignancies or the therapy of malignancies, such as oral mucositis following bone marrow transplantation. In these patients, 1-2 mg/kg/hr should be administered, and the infusion titrated to achieve a blood lidocaine level in the 2-5 μg/mL range, with use of twice-daily therapeutic blood monitoring. Table 76.13 outlines approaches to central neuropathic pain.

UNCONVENTIONAL MEDICATIONS IN PEDIATRIC PAIN

Unconventional analgesic medication refers to a wide number of drugs developed for other indications but found to have analgesic properties. These drugs include some antidepressants, antiepileptic drugs, and neurotropic drugs.

The unconventional analgesics are generally used to manage neuropathic pain conditions, migraine disorders, fibromyalgia syndrome, and some forms of functional chronic abdominal pain syndromes. These agents also are used as components of multimodal analgesia in the management of surgical, somatic, and musculoskeletal pain. Fig. 76.4

Table 76.9	CDC Recommendations for Prescribing Opioids for Chronic Pain Outside of Active Cancer, Palliative, and End-of-Life Care

Determining When to Initiate or Continue Opioids for Chronic Pain

1. Nonpharmacologic therapy and nonopioid pharmacologic therapy are preferred for chronic pain. Clinicians should consider opioid therapy only if expected benefits for both pain and function are anticipated to outweigh risks to the patient. If opioids are used, they should be combined with nonpharmacologic therapy and nonopioid pharmacologic therapy, as appropriate.
2. Before starting opioid therapy for chronic pain, clinicians should establish treatment goals with all patients, including realistic goals for pain and function, and should consider how therapy will be discontinued if benefits do not outweigh risks. Clinicians should continue opioid therapy only if there is clinically meaningful improvement in pain and function that outweighs risks to patient safety.
3. Before starting and periodically during opioid therapy, clinicians should discuss with patients known risks and realistic benefits of opioid therapy and patient and clinician responsibilities for managing therapy.

Opioid Selection, Dosage, Duration, Follow-Up, and Discontinuation

4. When starting opioid therapy for chronic pain, clinicians should prescribe immediate-release opioids instead of extended-release/long-acting (ER/LA) opioids.
5. When opioids are started, clinicians should prescribe the lowest effective dosage. Clinicians should use caution when prescribing opioids at any dosage, should carefully reassess evidence of individual benefits and risks when increasing dosage to ≥50 morphine milligram equivalents (MME)/day, and should avoid increasing dosage to ≥90 MME/day or carefully justify a decision to titrate dosage to ≥90 MME/day.
6. Long-term opioid use often begins with treatment of acute pain. When opioids are used for acute pain, clinicians should prescribe the lowest effective dose of immediate-release opioids and should prescribe no greater quantity than needed for the expected duration of pain severe enough to require opioids. Three days or less will often be sufficient; more than seven days will rarely be needed.

7. Clinicians should evaluate benefits and harms with patients within 1 to 4 weeks of starting opioid therapy for chronic pain or of dose escalation. Clinicians should evaluate benefits and harms of continued therapy with patients every 3 months or more frequently. If benefits do not outweigh harms of continued opioid therapy, clinicians should optimize other therapies and work with patients to taper opioids to lower dosages or to taper and discontinue opioids.

Assessing Risk and Addressing Harms of Opioid Use

8. Before starting and periodically during continuation of opioid therapy, clinicians should evaluate risk factors for opioid-related harms. Clinicians should incorporate into the management plan strategies to mitigate risk, including considering offering naloxone when factors that increase risk for opioid overdose, such as history of overdose, history of substance use disorder, higher opioid dosages (≥50 MME/day), or concurrent benzodiazepine use, are present.
9. Clinicians should review the patient's history of controlled substance prescriptions using state prescription drug monitoring program (PDMP) data to determine whether the patient is receiving opioid dosages or dangerous combinations that put him or her at high risk for overdose. Clinicians should review PDMP data when starting opioid therapy for chronic pain and periodically during opioid therapy for chronic pain, ranging from every prescription to every 3 months.
10. When prescribing opioids for chronic pain, clinicians should use urine drug testing before starting opioid therapy and consider urine drug testing at least annually to assess for prescribed medications as well as other controlled prescription drugs and illicit drugs.
11. Clinicians should avoid prescribing opioid pain medication and benzodiazepines concurrently whenever possible.
12. Clinicians should offer or arrange evidence-based treatment (usually medication-assisted treatment with buprenorphine or methadone in combination with behavioral therapies) for patients with opioid use disorder.

All recommendations are category A (apply to all patients outside of active cancer treatment, palliative care, and end-of-life care) except recommendation 10 (designated category B, with individual decision making required); see full guideline for evidence ratings.
From Dowell D, Haegerich TM, Chou R: CDC guideline for prescribing opioids for chronic pain—United States, 2016, *MMWR* 65(1):1–49, 2016.

Table 76.10	Summary of FDA Recommendations

- Use of codeine to treat pain or cough in children <12 yr old is contraindicated.
- Use of tramadol to treat pain in children <12 yr old is contraindicated.
- Use of tramadol for treatment of pain after tonsillectomy or adenoidectomy in patients <18 yr old is contraindicated. (Codeine was already contraindicated in such patients).
- Use of codeine or tramadol in children 12-18 yr old who are obese or who have an increased risk of serious breathing problems, such as those with obstructive sleep apnea or severe lung disease, is not recommended.
- Use of codeine or tramadol in breastfeeding women should be avoided.

From The Medical Letter: FDA warns against use of codeine and tramadol in children and breastfeeding women, *Med Lett* 59(1521):86–88, 2017.

presents a decision-making tree to help the physician select the appropriate analgesic category for various types of pain.

Although several unconventional analgesics are FDA approved for analgesic use, none is approved for use in youths with acute or chronic pain. Thus, these drugs should be used with caution, with a focus on mitigating pain to allow a child to participate effectively in therapies and return to normal activity as soon as possible. The use of psychotropic medications should be guided by the principles applied to pharmacologic treatment of any symptom or disease. Target symptoms should be identified, and medication side effects monitored. To determine dosing regimens, the physician should consider the child's weight and the effects that the medical condition and other medications, such as psychotropic drugs, may have on the child's metabolism. When available, therapeutic blood level monitoring should be performed. Side effects should be addressed in detail with both parent and child, and specific instructions given for responding to possible adverse events. Directly addressing concerns about addiction, dependence, and tolerance may be necessary to decrease treatment-related anxiety and improve medication adherence.

Antidepressant Medications

Antidepressants are useful in adults with chronic pain, including neuropathic pain, headaches, and rheumatoid arthritis, independent of their effects on depressive disorders. Antidepressants' analgesic mechanism of action is inhibition of norepinephrine reuptake in the CNS. In children, because clinical trials have been limited, the practitioner should use antidepressants cautiously to treat chronic pain or associated depressive or anxiety symptoms. The FDA has issued a "black box warning," its strongest warning, to inform the public of a small but significant increase in suicidal thoughts and attempts in children and adolescents receiving antidepressants. A meta-analysis of studies

Table 76.11	Topical Pharmacologic Management of Acute Pain in Children	
DRUG	**DOSE**	**NOTES**
INTACT SKIN		
Lidocaine 2·5% and prilocaine 2·5% (EMLA cream)	<3 mo old or <5 kg: 1 g 3–12 mo and >5 kg: 2 g 1–6 yr and >10 kg: 10 g 7–12 yr and >20 kg: 20 g	60 min is needed to achieve maximum effect; cover cream with an occlusive dressing
Lidocaine 70 mg and tetracaine 70 mg (Synera patch)	Age ≥3 yr: apply patch	20–30 min needed to achieve maximum effect
Tetracaine 4% (Ametop)	>1 mo and <5 yr: apply 1 tube of gel (1 g) >5 yr: apply up to 5 tubes of gel (5 g)	30 min before venipuncture 45 min before intravenous cannulation
WOUNDS		
Lidocaine, epinephrine, tetracaine (LET) solution or gel*	Age ≥1 yr: apply to wound	20 min needed for maximum effect

*Also referred to as ALA on the basis of alternative names for the constituents: adrenaline, lignocaine, amethocaine. These mixtures are locally made by hospital formularies, with a common formula being lidocaine 4% plus epinephrine 0·1% plus tetracaine 0·5%. The cocaine-based formulation was historically avoided on wounds of digits, ears, penis, nose, mucous membranes, close to the eye, or deep wounds involving bone, cartilage, tendon, or vessels. The lidocaine-based formulation can be used in such settings.
Adapted from Krauss BS, Calligaris L, Green SM, Barbi E: Current concepts in management of pain in children in the emergency department, *Lancet* 387:83–92, 2016.

Table 76.12	Examples of Neuropathic Pain Syndromes

PERIPHERAL NERVOUS SYSTEM FOCAL AND MULTIFOCAL LESIONS
Postherpetic neuralgia
Cranial neuralgias (e.g., trigeminal neuralgia, glossopharyngeal neuralgia)
Diabetic mononeuropathy
Nerve entrapment syndromes
Plexopathy from malignancy or irradiation
   Phantom limb pain
Posttraumatic neuralgia (e.g., nerve root compression, after thoracotomy)
   Ischemic neuropathy
Complex regional pain syndrome types 1 and 2
Erythromelalgia

PERIPHERAL NERVOUS SYSTEM GENERALIZED POLYNEUROPATHIES
Metabolic/nutritional: Diabetes mellitus, pellagra, beriberi, multiple nutritional deficiency, hypothyroidism
Toxic: Alcohol-, platinum-, or taxane-based chemotherapy, isoniazid, antiretroviral drugs
Infective/autoimmune: HIV, acute inflammatory polyneuropathy (Guillain-Barré syndrome), neuroborreliosis (Bannwarth syndrome)
Hereditary: Fabry disease
Malignancy: Carcinomatosis
Others: Idiopathic small-fiber neuropathy, erythromelalgia

CENTRAL NERVOUS SYSTEM LESIONS
Spinal cord injury
Prolapsed disc
Stroke (brain infarction, spinal infarction)
Multiple sclerosis
Surgical lesions (e.g., rhizotomy, cordotomy)
Complex neuropathic disorders
Complex regional pain syndrome types 1 and 2

Adapted from Freynhagen R, Bennett MI: Diagnosis and management of neuropathic pain, *BMJ* 339:b3002, 2009.

Table 76.13	Treatment Recommendations for Central Neuropathic Pain Adapted From Current Evidence-Based Literature	
MEDICATION CLASS/DRUG	**RECOMMENDED STAGE OF TREATMENT**
ANTIDEPRESSANTS	
Tricyclics (e.g., amitriptyline, nortriptyline)	1st or 2nd
Serotonin and norepinephrine reuptake inhibitors (e.g., duloxetine, venlafaxine)	1st or 2nd
ANTICONVULSANTS	
Pregabalin	1st or 2nd
Gabapentin	1st or 2nd
Lamotrigine	2nd or 3rd (in pain after stroke)
Valproate	3rd
OPIOIDS*	
Levorphanol	
MISCELLANEOUS	
Cannabinoids	2nd (in multiple sclerosis)
Mexiletine	3rd

*2nd or 3rd treatment stage (no specification).
Adapted from Freynhagen R, Bennett MI: Diagnosis and management of neuropathic pain, *BMJ* 339:b3002, 2009.

involving children and adolescents receiving antidepressants indicated that no suicides had been completed. The pediatrician should address this issue with parents of patients being treated with antidepressants and should develop monitoring plans consistent with current FDA recommendations.

Tricyclic antidepressants (TCAs) have been studied most in children with chronic pain and found to be effective in pain relief for symptoms that include neuropathic pain, functional abdominal pain, and migraine.

TCA efficacy may be based on inhibition of the neurochemical pathways involved in norepinephrine and serotonin reuptake and interference with other neurochemicals involved in the perception or neural conduction of pain. Because sedation is the most common side effect, TCAs are also effective in treating the sleep disorders that frequently accompany pediatric pain. Biotransformation of TCAs is extensive in healthy children. Typically, TCAs are administered only at bedtime. Alternatively, the patient can be started on a bedtime dose of a TCA, which may be able to then be titrated to a daily divided dose, with the larger dose given at bedtime. The reader should note that pain symptoms usually remit at lower doses than those recommended or required for the treatment of mood disorders. Most children and adolescents do not require more than 0.25-0.5 mg/kg of amitriptyline or nortriptyline once daily at bedtime.

Attention should also be paid to hepatic microsomal enzyme metabolism, because CYP2D6 inhibitors, such as cimetidine and quinidine, can increase levels of TCAs. Anticholinergic side effects, which are less common in children than adults, may remit over time. Constipation,

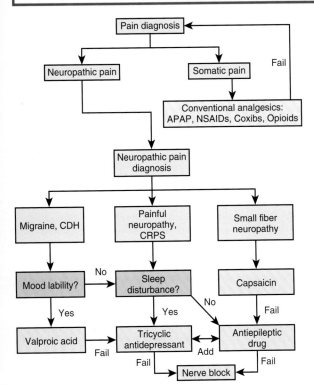

Fig. 76.4 Decision tree for selection of conventional and nonconventional analgesics. APAP, Acetaminophen; CDH, chronic daily headaches; CRPS, complex regional pain syndromes; NSAIDs, nonsteroidal antiinflammatory drugs.

orthostatic hypotension, and dental caries from dry mouth should be addressed by emphasizing the importance of hydration and oral hygiene. Other side effects include weight gain, mild bone marrow suppression, and liver dysfunction. Some practitioners recommend monitoring complete blood count (CBC) and liver function values at baseline and periodically during therapy. TCA blood levels can be obtained as well, but therapeutic blood monitoring generally should occur individually, particularly if adherence, overdose, or sudden change in mental status is an issue.

All TCAs inhibit cardiac conduction pathways and prolong the QT interval. Sudden cardiac death has been reported in children taking TCAs, principally desipramine, probably related to QTc prolongation. There is no general agreement for monitoring the electrophysiologic effects of these drugs, but it is prudent to obtain a careful personal and family history focusing on cardiac arrhythmias, heart disease, and syncope before the initiation of treatment. If personal or family history is positive for any of these conditions, a baseline electrocardiogram (ECG) should be obtained, with care taken to ensure that the QTc is <445 msec. We recommend that if the dose of amitriptyline or nortriptyline is increased beyond 0.25-0.5 mg/kg/day, an ECG should be performed for each dosing increase. With TCAs, as with other antidepressants, physical dependence and a known discontinuation syndrome can occur. The *discontinuation syndrome* includes agitation, sleep disturbances, appetite changes, and GI symptoms. These medications should be tapered slowly to assist in distinguishing among symptoms that indicate rebound, withdrawal, or the need for continuing the medication.

Selective serotonin reuptake inhibitors (SSRIs) have minimal efficacy in the treatment of a variety of pain syndromes in adults. SSRIs are very useful when symptoms of depression or anxiety disorders are present and cannot be addressed adequately by nonpharmacologic means. Escitalopram (Lexapro), fluoxetine (Prozac), and sertraline (Zoloft) have been approved by the FDA for use in children and adolescents. SSRIs

have a significantly milder side effect profile than TCAs (most side effects are transient), and they have no anticholinergic side effects. Chief side effects include GI symptoms, headaches, agitation, insomnia, sexual dysfunction, and anxiety. Rarely, hyponatremia, or the syndrome of inappropriate antidiuretic hormone secretion (SIADH), may occur. Interactions with other medications that have serotonergic effects (tramadol, trazodone, tryptophan, and triptan migraine medication) may also occur in theory. When these medications are used in combination, many sources state there may be increased likelihood that a life-threatening **serotonergic syndrome** may occur, with associated symptoms of myoclonus, hyperreflexia, autonomic instability, muscle rigidity, and delirium (see Chapter 77). In fact, serotonin syndrome has never been reported in adults or children taken with triptans for headache disorder and SSRIs. There is also a **discontinuation syndrome** associated with shorter-acting SSRIs (e.g., paroxetine), which includes dizziness, lethargy, paresthesias, irritability, and vivid dreams. Dosages of medications should be tapered slowly over several weeks.

The **selective serotonin-norepinephrine reuptake inhibitors (SNRIs)** duloxetine and venlafaxine have demonstrated significant efficacy with chronic neuropathic and other pain syndromes because they inhibit both serotonin and norepinephrine reuptake, and they may directly block associated pain receptors as well. Venlafaxine has no pain indication labeling. Duloxetine is FDA approved for managing neuropathic pain (specifically, diabetic neuropathy) and fibromyalgia syndrome and for use in children as young as 7 yr. A significant advantage of SNRIs over TCAs when used for headache prophylaxis or neuropathic pain is that they have therapeutic effects on mood and anxiety at dosages effective for pain control.

Because both SSRIs and SNRIs have fewer anticholinergic side effects than TCAs, adherence to them is better than in psychiatric populations taking TCAs. Side effects of both types of drugs include GI symptoms, hyperhidrosis, dizziness, and agitation, but these effects generally wane over time. Hypertension and orthostatic hypotension may occur; in addition, the patient's blood pressure should be closely followed, and appropriate hydration should be stressed. Note that whereas appetite stimulation and weight gain are associated with all TCAs, duloxetine is often associated with weight loss, frequently a desirable side effect, especially in weight-conscious adolescent females.

All antidepressants, including the TCAs, SSRIs and SNRIs, are thought to have the potential to increase the risk of suicidal ideation and the risk of suicide in patients. The FDA states, "All pediatric patients being treated with antidepressants for any indication should be observed closely for clinical worsening, suicidality, and unusual changes in behavior, especially during the initial few months of a course of drug therapy, or at times of dose changes, either increases or decreases." However, the FDA also notes, "Although there has been a long-standing concern that antidepressants may have a role in inducing worsening of depression and the emergence of suicidality in certain patients, a causal role for antidepressants in inducing such behaviors has not been established. Nevertheless, patients being treated with antidepressants should be observed closely for clinical worsening and suicidality, especially at the beginning of a course of drug therapy, or at the time of dose changes, either increases or decreases."

Antiepileptic Drugs

Anticonvulsants, such as gabapentin, carbamazepine, and valproic acid, are believed to relieve chronic pain by blocking sodium (valproate and the gabapentanoids) or calcium (carbamazepine and oxcarbazepine) channels at the cellular neuronal level, thereby suppressing spontaneous electrical activity and restoring the normal threshold to depolarization of hypersensitive nociceptive neurons, without affecting normal nerve conduction. These medications are particularly useful in patients with mood disorders who have neuropathic pain. In adults, the FDA has approved carbamazepine for trigeminal neuralgia, valproate for migraine prophylaxis, and pregabalin for neuropathic pain complicating diabetes, for zoster, and for management of fibromyalgia. Anticonvulsant medications generally have GI side effects in addition to sedation, anemia, ataxia, rash, and hepatotoxicity. Carbamazepine and oxcarbazepine are also associated with Stevens-Johnson syndrome.

Liver function and CBC should be monitored at the start of therapy and periodically with antiepileptic drugs (AEDs). Carbamazepine and valproic acid have narrow therapeutic windows and variability in therapeutic blood medication levels, as well as many drug-drug interactions, and may cause liver disease and renal impairment. Drug levels should be measured with each dose increase and periodically thereafter. Carbamazepine, in particular, causes autoinduction of hepatic microsomal enzymes, which can further complicate obtaining a therapeutic medication level. Female patients should have pregnancy testing before taking valproate, and those who are sexually active must be cautioned to use effective contraception, because neural tube defects are associated with carbamazepine.

Less toxic AEDs have supplanted the use of valproate and carbamazepine in patients with pain. These newer agents have their own, sometimes troubling, side effect profiles, but they are much less toxic than their predecessors and do not require monitoring of liver or bone marrow function or blood levels. Furthermore, they are also far less lethal in accidental or deliberate overdose.

Gabapentin, the most widely prescribed AED for the management of pain disorders, demonstrates efficacy in treating children with chronic pain, particularly neuropathic pain, and is playing an increasing role in the management of routine surgical pain. Gabapentin has proved effective in treating chronic headache disorders and many neuropathic pain syndromes, including complex regional pain syndromes, chemotherapy-induced neuropathy, postherpetic neuralgia, and diabetic neuropathy in both children and adults. This agent has a relatively benign side effect profile and no drug interactions. Side effects include somnolence, dizziness, and ataxia. Children occasionally demonstrate side effects not reported in adults, such as impulsive or oppositional behavior, agitation, and occasionally depression. These side effects do not seem to be dose related.

Pregabalin works by similar mechanisms as gabapentin but has a better side effect profile. Both gabapentin and pregabalin undergo virtually no hepatic metabolism, with no significant drug-drug interactions, a concern in patients with chronic pain, who frequently take multiple medications—for both the pain and the underlying medical condition associated with the pain. However, because both AEDs depend on renal function for clearance, doses must be adjusted in the presence of renal dysfunction.

Topiramate also demonstrates greater success than traditional anticonvulsants in treating trigeminal neuralgia in adults and in migraine prophylaxis. Topiramate therapy results more frequently in cognitive dysfunction and short-term memory loss than gabapentin or pregabalin, and these neurocognitive effects are particularly problematic for school-aged children. The pediatrician should also be aware that topiramate is associated with weight loss, whereas other anticonvulsants are typically associated with significant weight gain. This side effect is particularly valuable in weight-conscious adolescents, whereas in the anorexic cancer patient, a TCA would be preferable to induce appetite and weight gain.

Benzodiazepines

Children and adolescents with chronic pain may have comorbid psychological conditions, such as depressed mood, sleep disturbances, and anxiety disorders, including generalized anxiety disorder, separation anxiety, posttraumatic stress disorder (PTSD), and panic attacks. Pervasive developmental disorders are common in this population. Psychological factors affect a youth's ability to cope with a pain disorder. A *conditioned response* to pain may be to feel out of control and increase anxiety and pain, and conversely, *anticipatory anxiety* related to pain will inhibit activities and recovery. Feelings of helplessness sensitize the child to increasing amounts of pain, leading the child to perseverate on pain, think catastrophically, and feel hopeless. Changes in children's normal routines, with a negative impact on participation in valued activities, may further promote hopelessness, resulting in increased pain experiences and development of a depressive disorder.

Benzodiazepines are anxiolytic medications that also have muscle relaxant effects. They are particularly appropriate in acute situations as valuable adjuncts to the management of pain in the hospital setting, because they inhibit painful muscle spasms in surgical patients, but

more importantly because they suppress the anxiety that virtually every hospitalized child experiences, anxiety that interferes with restorative sleep and amplifies the child's perception of pain. Benzodiazepines are useful to calm children with anxiety and anticipatory anxiety about planned, painful procedures.

Because dependence, tolerance, and withdrawal may occur with prolonged use, benzodiazepines are generally not recommended for the routine management of *chronic pain*. Further, the risk of respiratory depression when benzodiazepines are combined with opioid therapy has contributed to the increasing number of opioid-related deaths in the United States since 2001. In concert with psychotherapy, however, benzodiazepines help control anxiety symptoms that amplify the perception of pain.

Infrequently, benzodiazepines may cause behavioral disinhibition, psychosis-like behaviors, or, in large doses, respiratory depression. When dosing these medications, the pediatrician should consider that many benzodiazepines are metabolized by the cytochrome P-450 microsomal enzyme system. This issue may be less significant with lorazepam and oxazepam, which undergo first-pass hepatic conjugation. Side effects common to benzodiazepines include sedation, ataxia, anemia, increased bronchial secretions, and depressed mood. If a benzodiazepine is administered for more than several consecutive days, the dosage should be slowly tapered over 2 or more weeks; if therapy is abruptly discontinued, autonomic instability, delirium, agitation, seizures, and profound insomnia may occur. The child psychiatric literature cites concerns that the use of benzodiazepines during hospitalization for serious disease (e.g., organ transplantation, prolonged intensive care unit [ICU] stay) might increase the risk for development of PTSD or increase PTSD symptomatology by reducing orientation used in coping with stress. Thus, other anxiolytics, such as atypical antipsychotics, are often recommended.

Antipsychotics and Major Sedatives

Low doses of antipsychotic medications are often used to address the more severe anxiety, agitation, and behavioral decompensation sometimes associated with severe pain. The use of these medications is controversial because associated adverse events may be severe and irreversible. Typical antipsychotics used in the past, including thioridazine (Mellaril), haloperidol (Haldol), and chlorpromazine (Thorazine), are associated with a decreased seizure threshold, dystonia, agranulocytosis, weight gain, cardiac conduction disturbances, tardive dyskinesia, orthostatic hypotension, hepatic dysfunction, and life-threatening laryngeal dystonia. These side effects are generally less severe with atypical antipsychotics. Because these effects may still occur, the pediatrician should obtain a baseline ECG, liver function values, and CBC analysis, and if possible obtain a child psychiatry consultation. If the pediatrician is using typical antipsychotics, an inventory of movement disturbances, such as the Abnormal Involuntary Movement Scale (AIMS) test, should be performed at baseline and at every follow-up visit, because movement disorders can worsen with abrupt withdrawal of medications or can become irreversible.

Atypical antipsychotics are generally associated with less severe side effect profiles, particularly dyskinesias and dystonias. Use of olanzapine (Zyprexa), which is particularly helpful with insomnia and severe anxiety, requires assessing and monitoring blood levels of glucose, cholesterol, and triglyceride; olanzapine's side effects may include diabetes, hypercholesterolemia, or significant weight gain. The anticholinergic side effects associated with quetiapine (Seroquel) warrant frequent monitoring of blood pressure. Risperidone at doses >6 mg may cause side effects similar to those of typical antipsychotics. Clozapine (Clozaril), which causes increased incidence of life-threatening agranulocytosis, should generally be avoided as a treatment for children and adolescents with chronic pain. Aripiprazole (Abilify) has been used for severe anxiety and/or for treatment-resistant depression. All antipsychotics are associated with the rare, but potentially lethal **neuroleptic malignant syndrome,** which includes severe autonomic instability, muscular rigidity, hyperthermia, catatonia, and altered mental status.

Other Pain Control Medications

Alpha-adrenergic receptor agonists such as clonidine are typically used as antihypertensive agents. However, they are often helpful as both anxiolytics and sleep-onset agents in the anxious hospitalized child. The α-agonists also have central effects on pain reduction. **Clonidine** can be given orally or transdermally, if the child's blood pressure permits. In the ICU, IV **dexmedetomidine**, an α-agonist sedating agent, can be used for the anxious, medically unstable child. Weaning off the dexmedetomidine can often be accomplished with a transition to clonidine. **Propranolol** is a β-blocking agent typically used for the child with autonomic instability and for thalamic storm. There are reports that a β-blocker can enhance depression in a child who already has a major depressive disorder, and discussion with a child psychiatrist can be helpful in decisions about using propranolol if needed. Both clonidine and propranolol have been found useful for the agitated child with ASD. Another α-agonist, **guanfacine**, is more likely to be used during the day for the child with ASD because it is less sedating than clonidine. Despite research on the impact of clonidine on chronic pain, no data are available to determine if guanfacine is as effective in reducing pain. Lastly, **ketamine**, a blocker of N-methyl-D-aspartate (NMDA) receptors, has been used for intractable pain in hospitalized children and in outpatients with severe sickle cell disease–related chronic pain, as well as others in palliative care for whom opioids are not sufficient to reduce pain. Since ketamine can have central hallucinatory effects, such children should be monitored closely.

NONPHARMACOLOGIC TREATMENT OF PAIN

Numerous psychological and physical treatments for relieving pain, fear, and anxiety as well as enhancing functioning have excellent safety profiles and proven effectiveness and should always be considered for incorporation into pediatric pain treatment (Fig. 76.5). In acute and procedural pain, nonpharmacologic strategies have long been used to help reduce distress in children undergoing medical procedures and surgery. Many of these methods aim to help children shift attention from pain and alter pain perception (e.g., distraction, hypnosis, imagery). Similarly, in the treatment of chronic pain, several strategies, often falling under the umbrella category of **cognitive-behavioral therapies (CBTs)**, have been shown to reduce pain and improve functioning and quality of life. CBT was developed with the goal of modifying social/environmental and behavioral factors that may exacerbate the child's experience of pain and pain-related disability. Several decades of research is available on CBTs for pediatric chronic pain. Meta-analyses of randomized controlled trials (RCTs) of CBT interventions have found large positive effects of psychological intervention on reductions in pain and/or its deleterious effects in children with headache, abdominal pain, and fibromyalgia, with relative or comparative effectiveness of different interventions examined in areas such as headache and abdominal pain in children. Biofeedback and relaxation therapies have been found to have superior effects to pharmacologic treatments in reducing headache pain in children and adolescents. Similarly, for recurrent abdominal pain, positive effects for CBT were found relative to attention-control conditions and pharmaceutical, botanical, and dietary interventions (which had very

weak evidence). Positive results have even resulted from very brief (3 sessions) and remotely delivered (telephone or internet) therapies, with outcomes lasting as long as 12 mo after intervention.

When deciding how to incorporate nonpharmacologic techniques to treat pain, the practitioner should (1) conduct a thorough assessment of individual, social, and environmental factors that may be contributing to the patient's pain and functioning limitations; (2) based on this assessment, decide whether nonpharmacologic techniques alone may be sufficient as a beginning to treatment, or if these treatments should be integrated with appropriate analgesics; (3) give children (and family members) developmentally and situationally appropriate information as to the rationale for treatment selection, and what to expect, given the child's medical condition, procedures, and treatments; (4) include patients and their families in decision making to ensure an appropriate treatment choice and to optimize adherence to treatment protocols; and (5) above all, develop a communication plan among the different **care providers**, typically with the pediatrician as the case manager, so that the messages to the child and parent are consistent and the modes of therapy are organized into an integrative team approach. Finally, it is important to recognize that in addition to pain, other psychological disorders (e.g., anxiety disorders, major depression) may impact the presenting pain complaint and may need to be identified and addressed as part of, or separate from, the pain management plan. Individual psychotherapy or psychiatric intervention may be warranted to adequately treat a comorbid disorder.

CBT strategies refer to a range of techniques that teach children (and their caregivers) how to manage pain by learning new ways to think about the pain and how to change behaviors associated with the pain. Strategies focusing on **cognitions** are typically aimed at enhancing parents' and children's confidence and self-efficacy to handle pain and decrease fear of pain. In addition, pain coping skills may shift the child's attentional focus away from pain and painful stimuli.

The goals of those strategies focusing on **behavior** change are to modify (1) contingencies in the child's environment, such as teaching parents how to respond to pain behaviors in ways that encourage wellness, rather than illness behaviors; (2) the ways parents model reactions to pain or discomfort; (3) child and parent coping techniques when psychosocial distress or problems in social relations exist; and (4) the child's behavioral reactions to situations, such as relaxation and exposure to previously avoided activities. Common examples of these strategies are discussed next. Whereas comprehensive CBTs are typically conducted by trained mental health specialists over several sessions, some basic CBT strategies can be briefly and easily introduced by practitioners into most medical settings. If more in-depth CBT treatment is needed, a referral to a qualified mental health specialist with CBT skills would be warranted.

Parent and family education and/or **psychotherapy**, particularly within cognitive-behavioral family approaches, is one treatment modality through which these goals are accomplished, and thus has been shown

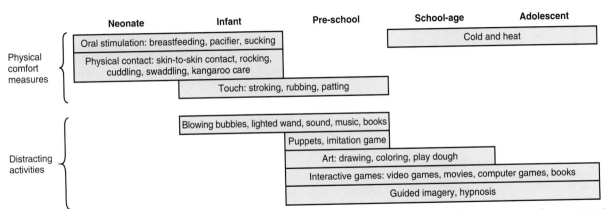

Fig. 76.5 Nonpharmacologic interventions for pediatric pain. *(From Krauss BS, Calligaris L, Green SM, Barbi E: Current concepts in management of pain in children in the emergency department, Lancet 387:83–92, 2016.)*

to be effective for treating chronic pain. Parents can learn to cope with their own distress and to understand pain mechanisms and appropriate treatment of pain. Key components include teaching parents to alter family patterns that may inadvertently exacerbate pain through developing behavior plans. Parents are taught to create plans for the child to manage the child's own symptoms and increase independent functioning. Often, adult caregivers (e.g., parents, teachers) need only guidance on developing a behavioral incentive plan to help the child return to school, gradually increase attendance, and receive tutoring, after a prolonged, pain-related absence. *Suggested sample brief strategy:* Ask caregivers how they react to the child's pain complaints; assess whether they encourage wellness activities or give attention and "rewards" primarily when the child says he or she does not feel well; and suggest that caregivers respond to the child in ways that encourage wellness both when complaining and not complaining.

Relaxation training is often employed to promote muscle relaxation and reduction of anxiety, which often accompanies and increases pain. Relaxation training, along with distraction and biofeedback, are treatments often included in CBT, but also are discussed in the literature without mention of CBT.

Controlled breathing and **progressive muscle relaxation** are commonly used relaxation techniques taught to preschool-age and older children. *Suggested sample brief strategy:* Ask the child (or instruct the caregiver to do so) to practice the following and use if pain is coming on: focus on the breath, and pretend to be blowing up a big balloon, while pursing the lips and exhaling slowly. This is one way to help induce controlled breathing.

Distraction can be used to help a child of any age shift attention away from pain and onto other activities. Common attention sustainers in the environment include bubbles, music, video games, television, the telephone, conversation, school, and play. Asking children to tell stories, asking parents to read to the child, and even mutual storytelling can be helpful distracters. Being involved with social, school, physical, or other activities helps the child in chronic pain to regain function. *Suggested sample brief strategy:* Encourage the child (or instruct the caregiver to do so) to shift attention away from the pain by continuing to engage in other activities and/or think of something else.

Biofeedback involves controlled breathing, relaxation, or hypnotic techniques with a mechanical device that provides visual or auditory feedback to the child when the desired action is approximated. Common targets of actions include muscle tension, peripheral skin temperature through peripheral vasodilation, and anal control through rectal muscle contraction and relaxation. Biofeedback also enhances the child's sense of mastery and control, especially for the child who needs more "proof" of change than that generated through hypnotherapy alone.

Hypnotherapy has also been used in the treatment of chronic pain in children, although the evidence for its effectiveness has not been as extensively studied as CBT. Hypnotherapy helps a child focus on an imaginative experience that is comforting, safe, fun, or intriguing. Hypnotherapy captures the child's attention, alters his or her sensory experiences, reduces distress, reframes pain experiences, creates time distortions, helps the child dissociate from the pain, and enhances feelings of mastery and self-control. Children with chronic pain can use *metaphor,* for example, imagining they have overcome something feared because of pain in real life. As the child increases mastery of imagined experiences, the enhanced sense of control can be used during actual pain rehabilitation. Hypnotherapy is best for children of school age or older.

Nonpharmacologic treatments of pain may also be applied to other treatment needs. A child who learns relaxation to reduce distress from lumbar punctures in cancer treatment may also apply this skill to other stressful medical and nonmedical situations, such as stressors caused by school.

Yoga is intended to achieve balance in mind, body, and spirit. **Therapeutic yoga** can be helpful in treating chronic pain; improving mood, energy, and sleep; and reducing anxiety. Yoga involves a series of *asanas* (body poses) oriented to the specific medical condition or symptoms. Some forms of yoga use poses within a movement flow and format. *Iyengar* yoga is unique in its use of props, such as blankets, bolsters, blocks, and belts, to support the body while the child assumes more healing poses. Yoga promotes a sense of energy, relaxation, strength, balance, and flexibility and, over time, enhances a sense of mastery and control. Within a yoga practice, the child may learn certain types of breathing (*pranayama*) for added benefit. With a focus on body postures or in types of *flow* yoga, the child learns mindfulness or being present and in the moment. By focusing on body and breath, the child can develop strategies to avoid ruminating about the past or worrying about the future.

Mindfulness meditation involves a focus on the present, "in-the-moment" experience using a variety of strategies. Many studies in adults report the value of meditation for chronic pain states as well as for anxiety and depression. These strategies help children learn how to be mindful and in the present, with enhanced parasympathetic control. Many mindfulness smartphone applications are geared to children of different ages, as well as books for parents on how to help their children achieve a mindful state to enhance relaxation (see Susan Kaiser-Greenland's book). Although there are different schools of mindfulness, such as *Vipassana* (insight-oriented meditation often using a focus on the breath) and *transcendental* meditation (in which the child learns the use of a silent mantra to facilitate acquiring a deeper inner calmness), the goal is to help the child learn strategies that enhance self-competence in reducing stress and enhancing a state of well-being.

Massage therapy involves the therapist's touching and applying varied degrees of pressure on the child's muscles. Massage is very useful for children with chronic pain and especially helpful for those with myofascial pain. There are several types of massage, including craniosacral therapy. For young children, it can be helpful to have parents learn and perform brief massage on their children before bedtime. Massage therapy likely will not be helpful to or tolerated by the child with sensory sensitivity and sensory aversion.

Physical therapy can be especially useful for children with chronic, musculoskeletal pain and for those deconditioned from inactivity. Exercise appears specifically to benefit muscle functioning, circulation, and posture, also improving body image, body mechanics, sleep, and mood. The physical therapist and the child can develop a graded exercise plan for enhancing the child's overall function and for the child to continue at home. Recent research indicates that physical therapy affects central neurobiologic mechanisms that enhance "top-down" pain control.

Acupuncture involves the placement of needles at specific acupuncture points along a *meridian*, or energy field, after the acupuncturist has made a diagnosis of excess or deficiency energy in that meridian as the primary cause of the pain. Acupuncture is a feasible, popular part of a pain management plan for children with chronic pain. Acupuncture alleviates chronic nausea, fatigue, and several chronic pain states, including migraine and chronic daily headaches, abdominal pain, and myofascial pain. Acupuncture also has efficacy in adults with myofascial pain, primary dysmenorrhea, sickle cell crisis pain, and sore throat pain. The acupuncturist must relate well to children so that the experience is not traumatic, because added stress would undo the benefits gained.

Transcutaneous electrical nerve stimulation (TENS) is the use of a battery-operated tool worn on the body to send electrical impulses into the body at certain frequencies set by the machine. TENS is believed to be safe and can be tried for many forms of localized pain. Children often find TENS helpful and effective.

Music therapy and **art therapy** can be especially helpful for young and nonverbal children who would otherwise have trouble with traditional talk psychotherapies. Also, many creative children can more easily express fears and negative emotions through creative expression and, with the therapist's help, learn about themselves in the process. There is also increasing research on the impact of art and music therapy on altering central neural circuits that maintain and enhance pain.

Dance, movement, and pet therapies, and **aromatherapy** have also been used and may be helpful, but these have not been as well studied in children for pain control as have other complementary therapies. Often, clinical experience helps guide the pediatrician in the benefits of these therapies with individual patients. For example, pet therapy is gaining favor in hospitals and in stress reduction for sick children. Pets often can become self-regulators for the child with ASD, although the neurobiologic mechanisms are not yet understood.

INVASIVE INTERVENTIONS FOR TREATING PAIN

Interventional neuraxial and peripheral nerve blocks provide intra-operative anesthesia, postoperative analgesia (see Chapter 74), and treatment of acute pain (e.g., long-bone fracture, acute pancreatitis) and contribute to the management of chronic pain such as headache, abdominal pain, complex regional pain syndrome (CRPS), and cancer pain. Interventional procedures are often used in the treatment of nonmalignant chronic pain in children in some centers and are described here so that the pediatrician will understand the different types of procedures available to children but rarely described in pediatric texts. Interventional procedures may be useful in some children who have specific types of chronic pain, but their use in children (as widely practiced in adult pain clinics) generally is not recommended because the pediatric research is insufficient. Therefore the data are largely extrapolated from the adult population. In children with CRPS receiving multiple focal blocks at an adult pain center, the first block may work "wonders," but the pain-free intervals between blocks may become shorter, until the blocks are no longer effective, and the CRPS pain spreads, including to the sites of the blocks. This does not mean that no block should be recommend in children, but that blocks should be used judiciously and in conjunction with other biopsychosocial treatments.

Regional anesthesia provides several benefits. As an alternative to or in augmentation of opioid-based pain control, regional anesthesia minimizes opioid requirements and therefore opioid side effects, such as nausea, vomiting, somnolence, respiratory depression, pruritus, constipation, and physical dependence. It generally provides better-quality pain relief than systemic medication because it interrupts nociceptive pathways and more profoundly inhibits endocrine stress responses. Regional anesthesia also results in earlier ambulation in recovering surgical patients, helps prevent atelectasis in the patient with chest pain, and usually results in earlier discharge from the hospital. Theoretically, the interruption of nociceptive pathways in the periphery by regional anesthetics will prevent, or reverse, the process of amplification of pain signals induced by nociception (e.g., CNS wind-up, glial cell activation). For postoperative pain, effective regional anesthesia reduces the risks of acute pain evolving to chronic pain. Regional anesthesia is considered safe and effective if performed by trained staff with the proper instruments and equipment. Most frequently, nerve blocks are performed by an anesthesiologist or pain management physician; a few are easily performed by a nonanesthesiologist with appropriate training.

Head and Neck Blocks

Primary pain syndromes of the head, such as trigeminal neuralgia, are distinctly unusual in the pediatric population, and few surgical procedures in the head and neck are amenable to regional anesthesia. Pain following tonsillectomies is not amenable to nerve blockade, and neurosurgical incisional pain is usually mitigated by local infiltration of local anesthetic into the wound margins by the surgeon. Headache disorders, very common in the pediatric age-group, often respond well to regional anesthesia of the greater occipital nerve (2nd cervical, C2), which provides sensation to much of the cranial structures, from the upper cervical region, the occiput to the apex of the head, or even to the hairline. The greater occipital nerve can be blocked medial to the occipital artery, which can usually be identified at the occipital ridge midway between the occipital prominence and the mastoid process by palpation, Doppler sound amplification, or visually by high-frequency ultrasound. The short-term and especially long-lasting effects of nerve blocks for chronic headaches in children have not been documented by research. Studies are needed to determine which children with which types of headaches will benefit most from occipital nerve blocks.

Upper-Extremity Blocks

The brachial plexus block controls pain of the upper extremity. This block also protects the extremity from movement, reduces arterial spasm, and blocks sympathetic tone of the upper extremity. The brachial plexus,

responsible for cutaneous and motor innervation of the upper extremity, is an arrangement of nerve fibers originating from spinal nerves C5 through 1st thoracic (T1), extending from the neck into the axilla, arm, and hand. The brachial plexus innervates the entire upper limb, except for the trapezius muscle and an area of skin near the axilla. If pain is located proximal to the elbow, the brachial plexus may be blocked above the clavicle (roots and trunks); if the pain is located distal to the elbow, the brachial plexus may be blocked at the axilla (cords and nerves). The block may be given as a single injection with a long-acting anesthetic (bupivacaine or ropivacaine, sometimes augmented with clonidine or dexamethasone to prolong block duration and intensity) to provide up to 12 hr of analgesia, or by a percutaneous catheter attached to a pump that can provide continuous analgesia over days or even weeks.

Trunk and Abdominal Visceral Blocks

Trunk blocks provide somatic and visceral analgesia and anesthesia for pain or surgery of the thorax and abdominal area. Sympathetic, motor, and sensory blockade may be obtained. These blocks are often used in combination to provide optimal relief. Intercostal and paravertebral blocks may be beneficial in patients for whom a thoracic epidural injection or catheter is contraindicated (e.g., patient with coagulopathy). Respiratory function is maintained, and the side effects of opioid therapy are eliminated.

The intercostal, paravertebral, rectus sheath, and transverse abdominal plane blocks are most useful for pediatric chest and somatic abdominal pain. The celiac plexus and splanchnic nerve block is most useful for abdominal visceral pain, such as caused by malignancy or pancreatitis. These blocks are best performed by an experienced anesthesiologist, pain physician, or interventional radiologist using ultrasound or CT imaging guidance.

The **intercostal block** is used to block the intercostal nerves, the anterior rami of the thoracic nerves from T1 to T11. These nerves lie inferior to each rib, between the inner and innermost intercostal muscles with their corresponding vein and artery, where they can be blocked, generally posterior to the posterior axillary line. Ultrasound imaging of the intercostal nerves helps avoid injury to intercostal vessels or insertion of the needle through the pleura, which may result in pneumothorax.

The **paravertebral block**, an alternative to intercostal nerve block or epidural analgesia, is useful for pain associated with thoracotomy or with unilateral abdominal surgery, such as nephrectomy or splenectomy. Essentially this block results in multiple intercostal blocks with a single injection. The thoracic paravertebral space, lateral to the vertebral column, contains the sympathetic chain, rami communicantes, dorsal and ventral roots of the spinal nerves, and dorsal root ganglion. Because it is a continuous space, local anesthetic injection will provide sensory, motor, and sympathetic blockade to several dermatomes. The paravertebral block may be performed as a single injection or, for a very prolonged effect, as a continuous infusion over several days or weeks via a catheter. This block is best performed by an anesthesiologist or interventional pain physician under ultrasound guidance.

Ilioinguinal and iliohypogastric nerve blocks are indicated with surgery for inguinal hernia repair, hydrocele, or orchiopexy repair, as well as for chronic pain subsequent to these procedures. The 1st lumbar (L1) nerve divides into the iliohypogastric and ilioinguinal nerves, which emerge from the lateral border of the psoas major muscle. The iliohypogastric nerve supplies the suprapubic area as it pierces the transversus abdominis muscle and runs deep to the internal oblique muscle. The ilioinguinal nerve supplies the upper medial thigh and superior inguinal region as it also pierces the transversus abdominis muscle and runs across the inguinal canal. Ultrasound guidance has made this nerve block almost always successful.

The **celiac plexus block** is indicated for surgery or pain of the pancreas and upper abdominal viscera. The celiac plexus, located on each side of the L1 vertebral body, contains 1-5 ganglia. The aorta lies posterior, the pancreas anterior, and the inferior vena cava lateral to these nerves. The celiac plexus receives sympathetic fibers from the greater, lesser, and least splanchnic nerves, as well as from parasympathetic fibers from the vagus nerve. Autonomic fibers from the liver, gallbladder, pancreas, stomach, spleen, kidneys, intestines, and adrenal glands originate from the celiac plexus. This block is best performed with CT guidance to provide direct visualization of the appropriate landmarks, avoid vascular and visceral structures, and confirm correct needle placement. The close proximity of structures such as the aorta and vena cava make this a technical procedure best performed by an anesthesiologist, interventional pain physician, or interventional radiologist.

Lower-Extremity Blocks

Lumbar plexus and sciatic nerve blocks provide pain control for painful conditions or surgical procedures of the lower extremities, with the benefit of providing analgesia to only one extremity while preserving motor and sensory function of the other. The lumbosacral plexus is an arrangement of nerve fibers originating from spinal nerves L2-L4 and S1-S3. The lumbar plexus arises from L2-L4 and forms the lateral femoral cutaneous, femoral, and obturator nerves. These nerves supply the muscles and sensation of the upper leg, with a sensory branch of the femoral nerve (saphenous nerve) extending below the knee to innervate the medial aspect of the foreleg, ankle, and foot. The sacral plexus arises from L4-S3 and divides into the major branches of the sciatic, tibial, and common peroneal nerves. These nerves in turn supply the posterior thigh, lower leg, and foot. Unlike the brachial plexus block, blockade of the entire lower extremity requires >1 injection because the lumbosacral sheath is not accessible. Separate injections are necessary for the posterior (sciatic) and anterior (lumbar plexus) branches, and the injections can be performed at any of several levels during the course of the nerve, as is clinically expedient. The lumbar plexus can be blocked in the back, resulting in analgesia of the femoral, lateral femoral cutaneous, and obturator nerves. Alternatively, any of these 3 nerves can be individually anesthetized, depending on the location of the pain. Similarly, the sciatic nerve can be anesthetized proximally as it emerges from the pelvis or more distally in the posterior thigh, or its major branches (tibial and peroneal nerves) can be individually anesthetized. These nerve blocks are generally best performed by an anesthesiologist, pain physician, or radiologist.

Sympathetic Blocks

Sympathetic blocks were once thought to be useful in the diagnosis and treatment of sympathetically mediated pain, CRPS, and other neuropathic pain conditions, but more recently, large meta-analyses have shown their utility to be minimal. The peripheral sympathetic trunk is formed by the branches of the thoracic and lumbar spinal segments, and it extends from the base of the skull to the coccyx. The sympathetic chain, which consists of separate ganglia containing nerves and autonomic fibers with separate plexuses, can be differentially blocked. These separate plexuses include the stellate ganglion in the lower neck and upper thorax, the celiac plexus in the abdomen, the 2nd lumbar plexus for the lower extremities, and the ganglion impar for the pelvis. When blocks of these plexuses are performed, sympathectomy is obtained without attendant motor or sensory anesthesia.

The **stellate ganglion block** is indicated for pain in the face or upper extremity as well as for CRPS, phantom limb pain, amputation stump pain, or circulatory insufficiency of the upper extremities. The stellate ganglion arises from spinal nerves C7-T1 and lies anterior to the 1st rib. It contains ganglionic fibers to the head and upper extremities. Structures in close proximity include the subclavian and vertebral arteries anteriorly, the recurrent laryngeal nerve, and the phrenic nerve. Chassaignac tubercle, the transverse process of the C6 vertebral body superior to the stellate ganglion, is a useful and easily palpable landmark for the block, but radiographic or ultrasound imaging is used more often than surface anatomy and palpation.

The **lumbar sympathetic block** addresses pain in the lower extremity, CRPS, phantom limb pain, amputation stump pain, and pain from circulatory insufficiency. The lumbar sympathetic chain contains ganglionic fibers to the pelvis and lower extremities. It lies along the anterolateral surface of the lumbar vertebral bodies and is most often injected between the L2 and L4 vertebral bodies.

The analgesia produced by peripheral sympathetic blocks usually outlives the duration of the local anesthetic, often persisting for weeks or indefinitely. If analgesia is transient, the blocks may be performed with catheter insertion for continuous local anesthesia of the sympathetic chain over days or weeks. Because precise, radiographically guided placement of the needle and/or catheter is required for safety and success, sympathetic blocks are generally best performed by an anesthesiologist, interventional pain physician, or interventional radiologist.

Epidural Anesthesia (Thoracic, Lumbar, and Caudal)

Epidural anesthesia and analgesia are indicated for pain below the clavicles, management of regional pain syndromes, cancer pain unresponsive to systemic opioids, and pain limited by opioid side effects.

The 3 layers of the spinal meninges—dura mater (outer), arachnoid mater (middle), and pia mater (inner)—envelop the spinal neural tissue. The subarachnoid space contains cerebrospinal fluid between the arachnoid mater and pia mater. The epidural space extends from the foramen magnum to the sacral hiatus and contains fat, lymphatics, blood vessels, and the spinal nerves as they leave the spinal cord. The epidural space separates the dura mater from the periosteum of the surrounding vertebral bodies. In children the fat in the epidural space is not as dense as in adults, predisposing to greater spread of the local anesthetic from the site of injection.

Epidural local anesthetics block both sensory and sympathetic fibers, and if the local anesthetic is of sufficient concentration, they also block motor fibers. Mild hypotension may occur, although it is unusual in children <8 yr. Epidural local anesthetics high in the thoracic spine may also anesthetize the sympathetic nerves to the heart (the cardiac accelerator fibers), producing bradycardia. In addition to using local anesthetics, it is routine to use opioids and α-agonists as adjunctive medications in the epidural space. Clonidine and opioids have been well studied and shown not to be neurotoxic. Other drugs (neostigmine, ketamine, diazepam) also are analgesic in the epidural space, but neurotoxicity studies have not established their safety. These agents have their primary site of action in the spinal cord, to which they diffuse from their epidural depot. Side effects of epidural opioid administration include delayed respiratory depression, particularly when hydrophilic opioids such as morphine are used. The risk of this effect requires that children receiving epidural opioids by intermittent injection or continuous infusion be monitored by continuous pulse oximetry and nursing observation, particularly during the 1st 24 hr of therapy or after significant dose escalations. Respiratory depression occurring after the 1st 24 hr of epidural opioid administration is distinctly unusual.

Epidural clonidine (an α2-agonist with μ-opioid analgesic properties) is associated with minimal risk and side effects. Although product labeling indicates use only in children with severe cancer pain, clonidine is frequently used for routine postoperative pain as well as pain syndromes such as CRPS. Mild sedation is the most common side effect of epidural clonidine, and it is not associated with respiratory depression.

Because performing epidural blockade is technical and may result in spinal cord injury, it is best done by an anesthesiologist or pain physician skilled in the technique. Caution is advised in the use of epidural anesthesia/analgesia for CRPS in children because no published RCTs have shown these procedures superior to a combination of less invasive physical and psychological therapy with or without neuropathic pain-focused medications.

INTRATHECAL ANALGESIA

Intrathecal catheters infused with opioids, clonidine, ziconotide (derived from a marine neurotoxin produced by the cone snail), and local anesthetics are occasionally applicable in pediatric patients with intractable pain from cancer or other conditions. Typically, intrathecal catheters are attached to an implanted electronic pump containing a drug reservoir sufficient for several months of dosing. The technique is technical and best performed by an experienced pain management physician.

NERVE ABLATION AND DESTRUCTION

In some cases, pain remains refractory despite maximal reliance on oral and IV medications and nerve blockade. In these patients, temporary (pulsed radiofrequency ablation) or permanent (neurolytic) destruction of one or more nerves may be performed. The techniques should be carefully weighed against the consideration of permanent nerve destruction in a growing child with decades of life ahead. On the other hand, when pain is severe in life-limiting disease processes, the long-term considerations are less concerning, and these techniques should be discussed with a skilled pain management specialist.

CONSIDERATIONS FOR SPECIAL PEDIATRIC POPULATIONS

Pain Perception and Effects of Pain on Newborns and Infants

Pain has a number of sources in the newborn period, including acute pain (diagnostic and therapeutic procedures, minor surgery, monitoring), continuous pain (pain from thermal/chemical burns, postsurgical and inflammatory pain), and chronic or disease-related pain (repeated heelsticks, indwelling catheters, necrotizing enterocolitis, nerve injury, chronic conditions, thrombophlebitis). The most common sources of pain in healthy infants are acute procedures, such as heel lances, surgical procedures, and in boys, circumcision.

Many procedures are performed for premature infants in the neonatal intensive care unit (NICU). In the 1st wk of life, approximately 94% of preterm infants <28 wk gestational age are mechanically ventilated. Other procedures are heelsticks (most common) and airway suctioning. Few of these procedures are preceded by any type of analgesia. Repeated handling and acute pain episodes sensitize the neonate to increased reactivity and stress responses to subsequent procedures. Typical stress responses include increases in heart rate, respiratory rate, blood pressure, and intracranial pressure. Cardiac vagal tone, transcutaneous oxygen saturation, carbon dioxide levels, and peripheral blood flow are decreased. Autonomic signs include changes in skin color, vomiting, gagging, hiccupping, diaphoresis, dilated pupils, and palmar and forehead sweating.

Untreated pain in the newborn has serious short- and long-term consequences. There has been a shift in most NICUs to more liberal use of opioids. Nonetheless, **morphine**, the traditional gold standard of analgesia for acute pain, may not be effective and may have adverse long-term consequences. No differences have been found in the incidence of severe intraventricular hemorrhage or in the mortality rate when infants receiving morphine are compared with the placebo group, and there are no changes in assessed pain from tracheal suctioning in ventilated infants receiving morphine compared with those receiving a placebo infusion. Morphine may not alleviate acute pain in ventilated preterm neonates, although there are few data on the effects of morphine and fentanyl in nonventilated newborns. The lack of opioid effects for acute pain in neonates may result from immaturity of opioid receptors; acute pain may cause the uncoupling of μ-opioid receptors in the forebrain. Repetitive acute pain may create central neural changes in the newborn that may have long-term consequences for later pain vulnerability, cognitive effects, and opioid tolerance. Most neonatologists use opioids in painful situations. Sucrose and pacifiers are also being used in the NICU. The effects of **sucrose** (sweet taste) are believed to be opioid mediated because they are reversed with naloxone; stress and pain relief are integrated through the endogenous opioid system. Sucrose, with or without a pacifier, may be effective for acute pain and stress control. Other nonpharmacologic strategies for stress and pain control include infant care by an individual primary nurse, tactile-kinesthetic stimuli (massage), "kangaroo care," and soothing sensorial saturation.

Children With Cancer Pain

The World Health Organization (WHO) proposed an analgesic therapy model for cancer pain known as the *analgesic ladder* (Table 76.14). Designed to guide therapy in the Third World, this ladder consists of a hierarchy of oral pharmacologic interventions intended to treat pain of increasing magnitude. The hierarchy ignores modalities such as the use of nonconventional analgesics and interventional pain procedures, which are within the capability of physicians to prescribe in developed countries. Nevertheless, because oral medications are simple and efficacious, especially for home use, the ladder presents a framework for rationally using them before applying other drugs and techniques of drug administration.

Table 76.14	World Health Organization Analgesic Ladder for Cancer Pain

STEP 1
Patients who present with mild to moderate pain should be treated with a nonopioid.

STEP 2
Patients who present with moderate to severe pain or for whom the step 1 regimen fails should be treated with an oral opioid for moderate pain combined with a nonopioid analgesic.

STEP 3
Patients who present with very severe pain or for whom the step 2 regimen fails should be treated with an opioid used for severe pain, with or without a nonopioid analgesic.

Oral medications are the first line of analgesic treatment. Because NSAIDs affect platelet adhesiveness, they are typically not used. Opioid therapy is the preferred approach for moderate or severe pain. Nonopioid analgesics are used for mild pain, a weak opioid is added for moderate pain, and strong opioids are administered for more severe pain. Adjuvant analgesics can be added, and side effects and comorbid symptoms are actively managed. Determining the type and sources of the pain will help develop an effective analgesic plan. Certain treatments, such as the chemotherapeutic agent vincristine, are associated with neuropathic pain. Such pain might require anticonvulsants or TCAs. Organ-stretching pain from tumor growth within an organ might require strong opioids and/or radiation therapy if the tumor is radiosensitive. Organ obstruction, such as intestinal obstruction, should be diagnosed to relieve or bypass the obstruction.

It is important to consider both pharmacologic and nonpharmacologic strategies (e.g., CBT, family/parent support) to treat pain in children with cancer.

Children With Pain Associated With Advanced Disease

Patients with advanced diseases, including cancer, acquired immunodeficiency syndrome (AIDS), neurodegenerative disorders, and cystic fibrosis, need palliative care approaches that focus on optimal quality of life. Nonpharmacologic and pharmacologic management of pain and other distressing symptoms is a key component. *Palliative care* should be offered to all children with serious diseases, whether or not the diseases are potentially curable or long life expectancy is predicted. Examples include young children diagnosed with acute lymphoblastic leukemia (>90% posttreatment life expectancy) and children undergoing organ transplantation. Palliative care in pediatrics connotes treatment that focuses on symptom reduction, quality of life, and good family and clinical team communication. It is not only for patients in hospice care or those at the end of life. Differences in the progression of underlying illness, associated distressing symptoms, and common emotional responses in these conditions should shape individual treatment plans. For end-of-life care, >90% of children and adolescents with cancer can be made comfortable by standard escalation of opioids according to the WHO protocol. A small subgroup (5%) has enormous opioid dose escalation to >100 times the standard morphine or other opiate infusion rate. Most of these patients have spread of solid tumors to the spinal cord, roots, or plexus, and signs of neuropathic pain are evident. **Methadone** given orally is often used in palliative care, not only end-of-life care, because of its long half-life and its targets at both opioid and NMDA receptors.

The type of pain experienced by the patient (neuropathic, myofascial) should determine the need for adjunctive agents. Complementary measures, such as massage, hypnotherapy, and spiritual care, must also be offered in palliative care. Although the oral route of opioid administration should be encouraged, especially to facilitate care at home if possible, some children are unable to take oral opioids. Transdermal and sublingual routes, as well as IV infusion with PCA, are likely next choices. Small, portable infusion pumps are convenient for home use. If venous access is limited, a useful alternative is to administer opioids (especially morphine or hydromorphone, but not methadone or meperidine) through continuous SC infusion, with or without a bolus option. A small (e.g., 22-gauge) cannula is placed under the skin and secured on the thorax, abdomen, or thigh. Sites may be changed every 3-7 days, as needed. As noted, alternative routes for opioids include the transdermal and oral transmucosal routes. These latter routes are preferred over IV and SC drug delivery when the patient is being treated at home.

CHRONIC AND RECURRENT PAIN SYNDROMES

Chronic pain is defined as recurrent or persistent pain lasting longer than the normal tissue healing time, 3-6 mo. Children may experience pain related to injury (e.g., burns) or to a chronic or underlying disease process (e.g., cancer, arthritis), or pain can also be the chronic condition itself (e.g., CRPS, fibromyalgia, functional abdominal pain) (see Chapter 147). During childhood, abdominal, musculoskeletal, and headache pain are the most frequently occurring conditions. However, definitions of chronic pain do not take into account standard criteria for assessing particular pain symptoms or for evaluating the intensity or impact of pain, and therefore includes individuals with varying symptoms and experiences. Consequently, in epidemiologic surveys, prevalence estimates vary widely. Overall prevalence rates for different childhood pains range from 4–88%. For example, an average of 13.5–31.8% of adolescents in a community sample reported having weekly abdominal, headache, or musculoskeletal pains. Most epidemiologic studies report prevalence and do not report the *severity* or impact of the pain. Research indicates that only a subset of children and adolescents with chronic pain (approximately 5%) experience moderate to severe disability, and this likely better represents the estimated population for whom help is needed to treat pain and associated problems.

Neuropathic Pain Syndromes

Neuropathic pain is caused by abnormal excitability in the peripheral or central nervous system that may persist after an injury heals or inflammation subsides. The pain, which can be acute or chronic, is typically described as burning or stabbing and may be associated with cutaneous hypersensitivity (allodynia), distortion of sensation (dysesthesia), and amplification of noxious sensations (hyperalgesia and hyperpathia). Neuropathic pain conditions may be responsible for >35% of referrals to chronic pain clinics, conditions that typically include posttraumatic and postsurgical peripheral nerve injuries, phantom pain after amputation, pain after spinal cord injury, and pain caused by metabolic neuropathies. Patients with neuropathic pain typically respond poorly to opioids. Evidence supports the efficacy of antidepressants (nortriptyline, amitriptyline, venlafaxine, duloxetine) and anticonvulsants (gabapentin, pregabalin, oxcarbazepine) for treatment of neuropathic pain (see Tables 76.12 and 76.13).

Complex regional pain syndrome, formerly known as "reflex sympathetic dystrophy" (RSD), is well described in the pediatric population. **CRPS type 1** is a syndrome of neuropathic pain that typically follows an antecedent and usually minor injury or surgery to an extremity without identifiable nerve injury. It is often seen in oncology patients as a complication of their malignancy, IV infiltrations in the periphery, or surgery. The syndrome of CRPS type 1 includes severe spontaneous neuropathic pain, hyperpathia, hyperalgesia, severe cutaneous allodynia to touch and cold, changes in blood flow (typically extremity cyanosis), and increased sweating. In more advanced cases, symptoms include dystrophic changes of the hair, nails, and skin, immobility of the extremity (dystonia), and muscle atrophy. In the most advanced cases, symptoms include ankylosis of the joints of the extremity. Specific causal factors in CRPS type 1 in both children and adults remain elusive, although coincidental events may be noted. **CRPS type 2**, formerly referred to as "causalgia," is less common and describes a very similar constellation of symptoms but is associated with a known nerve injury. CRPS type 2 pain may be restricted to the distribution of the injured nerve or too much of the involved limb in a stocking-glove distribution, whereas CRPS type 1 is generally seen in a stocking-glove distribution and by

definition is not limited to a peripheral nerve or dermatomal distribution of signs and symptoms.

Treatment of CRPS in children has been extrapolated from that in adults, with some evidence for efficacy of physical therapy, CBT, nerve blocks, antidepressants, AEDs, and other related drugs. All experts in pediatric pain management agree on the value of aggressive physical therapy. Some centers provide aggressive therapy without the use of pharmacologic agents or interventional nerve blocks. Unfortunately, recurrent episodes of CRPS may be seen in up to 50% of patients, particularly adolescent females. Physical therapy can be extraordinarily painful for children to endure; it is tolerated only by the most stoic and motivated patients. If children have difficulty enduring the pain, there is a well-established role for pharmacologic agents with or without peripheral or central neuraxial nerve blocks to render the affected limb sufficiently analgesic so that physical therapy can be tolerated. Pharmacologic interventions include the use of AEDs such as gabapentin and/or TCAs such as amitriptyline (see Fig. 76.4). Although there is clear evidence of a peripheral inflammatory component of CRPS, with release of cytokines and other inflammatory mediators from the peripheral nervous system in the affected limb, the use of antiinflammatory agents has been disappointing. Common nerve block techniques include IV regional anesthetics, epidural analgesia, and peripheral nerve blocks. In extreme and refractory cases, more invasive strategies have been reported, including surgical sympathectomy and spinal cord stimulation.

Although an array of treatments has some benefit, the mainstay of treatment remains **physical therapy** emphasizing desensitization, strengthening, and functional improvement. Additionally, pharmacologic agents and psychological and complementary therapies are important components of a treatment plan. Invasive techniques, although not curative, can be helpful if they permit the performance of frequent and aggressive physical therapy that cannot be carried out otherwise. A good biopsychosocial evaluation will help determine the orientation of the treatment components. There are insufficient data to indicate the superior value of interventional blocks, such as epidural anesthesia, in children with CRPS over physical and psychological interventions, with or without pharmacologic support.

Myofascial Pain Disorders and Fibromyalgia

Myofascial pain disorders are associated with tender points in the affected muscles as well as with muscle spasms (tight muscles). Treatment is targeted at relaxing the affected muscles through physical therapy, Iyengar yoga, massage, and acupuncture. Rarely are pharmacologic muscle relaxants helpful other than for creating tiredness at night for sleep. Dry needling or injections of local anesthetic into the tender points has been advocated, but the data do not support this as a standard treatment. Similarly, although botulinum toxin injections may be used, no data support this practice in children. Often, poor body postures, repetitive use of a body part not accustomed to that movement, or carrying heavy backpacks initiates pain. When it becomes widespread with multiple tender points, the diagnosis may be made of *juvenile fibromyalgia*, which may or may not continue to subsequently become adult fibromyalgia. Likely there are different subtypes of widespread pain syndromes, and physical therapy is a key component of treatment. Psychological interventions may play an important role to assist the child in resuming normal activities and to manage any psychological comorbidities. Any pain rehabilitation plan should enhance return to full function. Because there is a high incidence of chronic pain in parents of children presenting with a chronic pain condition, especially fibromyalgia, attention to parent and family factors is important. Parent training may entail teaching the parent to model more appropriate pain coping behaviors and to recognize the child's independent attempts to manage pain and function adaptively. Parents may also need referrals to obtain appropriate pain management for their own pain condition.

Pregabalin and duloxetine are FDA approved for management of fibromyalgia in adults, but no clinical studies have confirmed their effectiveness in children and adolescents. One recent large study in adolescents with fibromyalgia found that CBT and physical therapy were superior to typical pharmacologic agents used in adults.

Erythromelalgia

Erythromelalgia in children is generally primary, whereas in adults it may be either primary or secondary to malignancy or other hematologic disorders, such as polycythemia vera. Patients with erythromelalgia exhibit red, warm, hyperperfused distal limbs. The disorder is usually bilateral and may involve either or both the hands and feet. Patients perceive burning pain and typically seek relief by immersing the affected extremities in ice water, sometimes so often and for so long so that skin pathology results. **Primary erythromelalgia** is caused by a genetic mutation (autosomal dominant) in the gene for the NaV1.7 neuronal sodium channel on peripheral C nociceptive fibers, resulting in their spontaneous depolarization, and thus continuous burning pain. The most common mutation identified is in the *SCN9A* gene, although there are several mutations that affect the NaV1.7 channel. Interestingly, another mutation in the NaV1.7 channel results in a rare but devastating genetic condition, the congenital indifference to pain.

It is easy to distinguish erythromelalgia (or related syndromes) from CRPS. The limb afflicted with CRPS is typically cold and cyanotic, the disease is typically unilateral, and children with CRPS have cold allodynia, making immersion in cold water exquisitely painful. In erythromelalgia, ice water immersion is analgesic, the condition is bilateral and symmetric, and it is associated with hyperperfusion of the distal extremity. The evaluation of hyperperfused limbs with burning pain should include genetic testing for **Fabry disease** and screening for hematologic malignancies, with diagnosis of primary erythromelalgia being one of exclusion. At present, few clinical laboratories are Clinical Laboratory Improvement Amendments (CLIA) certified to perform the DNA analysis required to identify the common NaV1.7 mutations.

The definitive treatment of Fabry disease includes enzyme replacement as disease-modifying treatment and administration of neuropathic pain medications such as gabapentin, although the success of antineuropathic pain drugs in small-fiber neuropathies has not been impressive. The treatment of erythromelalgia is much more problematic. Antineuropathic pain medications (AEDs, TCAs) are typically prescribed but rarely helpful (see Fig. 76.4). Although one might predict that sodium channel–blocking AEDs might be effective in this sodium channelopathy, oxcarbazepine has not proved to be a particularly effective modality. The pain responds well to regional anesthetic nerve blocks, but it returns immediately when the effects of the nerve block resolve. In contrast, in other neuropathic syndromes, the analgesia usually (and inexplicably) persists well after the resolution of the pharmacologic nerve block. Aspirin and even nitroprusside infusions have been anecdotally reported to be of benefit with secondary erythromelalgia, but have not been reported to be helpful in children with primary erythromelalgia. Case reports in adults and clinical experience in children suggest that periodic treatment with high-dose **capsaicin cream** is effective in alleviating the burning pain and disability of erythromelalgia. Capsaicin (essence of chili pepper) cream is a vanilloid receptor (TRPV1) agonist that depletes small-fiber peripheral nerve endings of the neurotransmitter substance P, an important neurotransmitter in the generation and transmission of nociceptive impulses. Once depleted, these nerve endings are no longer capable of generating spontaneous pain until the receptors regenerate, a process that takes many months.

Other Chronic Pain Conditions in Children

A variety of genetic and other medical/surgical conditions are often associated with chronic pain. Examples include Fabry disease, Chiari/syringomyelia, epidermolysis bullosa, juvenile idiopathic arthritis, porphyria, mitochondrial disorders, degenerative neurologic diseases, cerebral palsy, ASD, intestinal pseudoobstruction, inflammatory bowel disease, chronic migraine/daily headaches, and irritable bowel disease. In many cases, treating the underlying disease, such as enzyme replacement in Fabry disease and in other lysosomal disorders, will reduce what otherwise might be progression of symptoms, but may not totally reduce pain and suffering, and other modalities will be needed. Finally, pain that persists and is not well treated can lead to central sensitization and widespread pain, such as seen in children with one pain source who develop fibromyalgia.

MANAGING COMPLEX CHRONIC PAIN PROBLEMS

Some patients with chronic pain have a prolonged course of evaluation in attempts to find what is expected as the singular "cause" of the pain and thus also undergo many failed treatments (see Chapter 147). Parents worry that the doctors have not yet discovered the cause that may be serious and life threatening, and children often feel not believed, that they are faking their pain, or are "crazy." There may be no identifiable or diagnosable condition, and families may seek opinions from multiple treatment facilities in an attempt to find help for their suffering child. For some children, what may have begun as an acute injury or infectious event may result in a chronic pain syndrome, with changes in the neurobiology of the pain-signaling system.

In the context of disabling chronic pain, it is very important for the pediatrician to avoid overmedication because this can exacerbate associated disability, maintain an open mind and reassess the diagnosis if the clinical presentation changes, and understand and communicate to the family that pain has a biologic basis (likely related to neural signaling and neurotransmitter dysregulation), and that the pain is naturally distressing to the child and family. All patients and families should receive a simple explanation of pain physiology that helps them understand the importance of (1) functional rehabilitation to normalize pain signaling, (2) the low risk of causing further injury with systematic increases in normal functioning, and (3) the likely failure of treatment if pain is managed as if it were acute. Because it is counterintuitive for most people to move a part of the body that hurts, many patients with chronic pain have atrophy or contractures of a painful extremity from disuse. Associated increases in worry and anxiety may exacerbate pain and leave the body even more vulnerable to further illness, injury, and disability. Pain can have a significant impact on many areas of normal functioning and routines for children, and school absenteeism and related consequences of missed schooling are often significant problems. Appropriate assessment and evaluation of the child with chronic pain and the family is the critical 1st step necessary in developing a treatment plan. For example, a high–academically functioning child might have an acute injury that leads to chronic pain and significant school absenteeism. While many downstream contributors to pain and disability maintenance can accumulate the more school that is missed, often previously unrecognized focal learning disabilities may become the increasing trigger for a downhill cascade of pain, disability, and school absenteeism. Even for the child with outstanding grades, it may be helpful to learn about the amount of time spent on each subject. As certain subjects become more complicated, such as math, the child with a previously unrecognized math learning disability may be spending hours on math homework each night, even with good grades in math. In this case the acute illness or injury becomes the "final straw" that breaks down the child's coping and turns the acute pain into a chronic problem.

Interdisciplinary pediatric pain programs have become the standard of care for treating complex chronic pain problems in youth. Although available in many parts of the United States, Canada, Europe, Australia, and New Zealand, the overall number of programs is still small. Therefore, many children and adolescents with chronic pain will be unable to receive specialized pain treatment in their local communities. In recognition of the severity and complexity of pain and disability for some children, different settings and treatment delivery models for providing pain care have been explored. One option is inpatient and day hospital treatment programs, which often address barriers to access to outpatient treatment and coordination of care. In addition, these programs provide an intensive treatment option for children who do not make adequate progress in outpatient treatment or who are severely disabled by pain. Early programs developed in the 1990s focused on CRPS treatment through intensive inpatient rehabilitation and exercise-based programs. Later programs expanded to other clinical populations and broadened the treatment focus to incorporate a range of rehabilitation and psychological therapies delivered both individually and in groups. The typical length of inpatient admissions for children with chronic pain in such programs is 3-4 wk, and emerging evidence suggests benefit from these programs. A major problem that limits such care for children with complex chronic disabling pain is the long waiting list for entry into these still relatively few programs, as well as obtaining insurance approval. Additional more widespread models of care are needed.

Another intervention delivery option is *remote management,* referring to pain interventions utilized outside the clinic/hospital setting to reach children in their homes or communities. Interventions are typically delivered using some form of technology, such as the internet, or may rely on other media, such as telephone counseling or written self-help materials. Typically, remote management of pain includes monitoring, counseling, and delivery of behavioral and CBT interventions. Internet interventions have received the most research attention to date, with published examples of several different pediatric chronic pain conditions with promising findings for pain reduction. *Telemedicine,* while in widespread use clinically for many pediatric health conditions, has not yet been formally evaluated in pediatric pain. Within any community, the pediatrician will need to locate appropriate referral sources for patients with complex chronic pain. However, while psychological interventions can be delivered through these telemedicine strategies, the pediatrician is still relied on to obtain the needed biopsychosocial history, complete a thorough physical examination, and provide the pharmacologic management as needed. The pediatrician also communicates with the family to help the child and family understand the pain and how the different pharmacologic and nonpharmacologic treatments will enhance function and alter the long-term neural processes underlying pain.

Bibliography is available at Expert Consult.

Chapter **77**

Poisoning

Jillian L. Theobald and Mark A. Kostic

第七十七章

中毒

中文导读

中毒是导致儿童及青少年意外伤害的重要原因之一，可导致严重后果。本章介绍了如何预防中毒，接触、评估和处置中毒患儿的原则及注意事项，以及常见毒物中毒后的表现，建议选用的解毒剂种类和用法用量等。并进一步根据毒物种类不同，介绍了药物中毒、日用品中毒、植物中毒、气体中毒，以及其他可能发生在家中的儿童中毒情形。

Poisoning is the leading cause of injury-related death in the United States, surpassing that from motor vehicle crashes. Most these deaths are unintentional (i.e., not suicide). In adolescents, poisoning is the 3rd leading cause of injury-related death. Of the >2 million human poisoning exposures reported annually to the National Poison Data Systems (NPDS) of the American Association of Poison Control Centers (AAPCC), approximately 50% occur in children <6 yr old, with the highest number of exposures occurring in 1 and 2 yr olds. Almost all these exposures are unintentional and reflect the propensity for young children to put virtually anything in their mouth. Fortunately, children <6 yr old account for <2% of all poisoning fatalities reported to NPDS.

More than 90% of toxic exposures in children occur in the home, and most involve a single substance. Ingestion accounts for the majority of exposures, with a minority occurring by the dermal, inhalational, and ophthalmic routes. Approximately 40% of cases involve nondrug substances, such as cosmetics, personal care items, cleaning solutions, plants, and foreign bodies. Pharmaceutical preparations account for the remainder of exposures, and analgesics, topical preparations, vitamins, and antihistamines are the most commonly reported categories.

The majority of poisoning exposures in children <6 yr old can be managed without direct medical intervention beyond a call to the regional **poison control center (PCC).** This is because the product involved is not inherently toxic or the quantity of the material is not sufficient to produce clinically relevant toxic effects. However, a number of substances can be highly toxic to toddlers in small doses (Table 77.1). In 2015, carbon monoxide (CO), batteries, and analgesics (mainly opioids) were the leading causes of poison-related fatalities in young children (<6 yr). In addition, stimulants/street drugs, cardiovascular (CV) drugs, and aliphatic hydrocarbons were significant causes of mortality.

Poison prevention education should be an integral part of all well-child visits, starting at the 6 mo visit. Counseling parents and other caregivers about potential poisoning risks, poison-proofing a child's environment, and actions in the event of an ingestion diminishes the likelihood of serious morbidity or mortality. Poison prevention education materials

Table 77.1	Common Agents Potentially Toxic to Young Children (<6 yr) in Small Doses*

SUBSTANCE	TOXICITY
Aliphatic hydrocarbons (e.g., gasoline, kerosene, lamp oil)	Acute lung injury
Antimalarials (chloroquine, quinine)	Seizures, dysrhythmias
Benzocaine	Methemoglobinemia
β-Adrenergic receptor blockers[†]	Bradycardia, hypotension
Calcium channel blockers	Bradycardia, hypotension, hyperglycemia
Camphor	Seizures
Caustics (pH <2 or >12)	Airway, esophageal and gastric burns
Clonidine	Lethargy, bradycardia, hypotension
Diphenoxylate and atropine (Lomotil)	CNS depression, respiratory depression
Hypoglycemics, oral (sulfonylureas and meglitinides)	Hypoglycemia, seizures
Laundry detergent packets (pods)	Airway issues, respiratory distress, altered mental status
Lindane	Seizures
Monoamine oxidase inhibitors	Hypertension followed by delayed cardiovascular collapse
Methyl salicylate	Tachypnea, metabolic acidosis, seizures
Opioids (especially methadone, buprenorphine)	CNS depression, respiratory depression
Organophosphate pesticides	Cholinergic crisis
Phenothiazines (especially chlorpromazine, thioridazine)	Seizures, dysrhythmias
Theophylline	Seizures, dysrhythmias
Tricyclic antidepressants	CNS depression, seizures, dysrhythmias, hypotension

*"Small dose" typically implies 1 or 2 pills or 5 mL.
[†]Lipid-soluble β-blockers (e.g., propranolol) are more toxic than water-soluble β-blockers (e.g., atenolol).
CNS, Central nervous system.

are available from the American Academy of Pediatrics (AAP) and regional PCCs. Through a U.S. network of PCCs, anyone at any time can contact a regional poison center by calling the toll-free number **1-800-222-1222**. Parents should be encouraged to share this number with grandparents, relatives, babysitters, and any other caregivers.

Product safety measures, poison prevention education, early recognition of exposures, and around-the-clock access to regionally based PCCs all contribute to the favorable exposure outcomes in young children. Poisoning exposures in children 6-12 yr are much less common, involving only approximately 10% of all reported pediatric exposures. A 2nd peak in pediatric exposures occurs in adolescence. Exposures in the adolescent age-group are primarily intentional (suicide or abuse or misuse of substances) and thus often result in more severe toxicity (see Chapter 140). Families should be informed and given anticipatory guidance that nonprescription and prescription medications, and even household products (e.g., inhalants), are common sources of adolescent exposures. Although adolescents (age 13-19 yr) account for only about 12% of exposures, they constituted a much larger proportion of deaths. Of the 90 poison-related pediatric deaths in 2015 reported to NPDS, 58 were adolescents (5% of all fatalities called in to poison centers). Pediatricians

should be aware of the signs of drug abuse or suicidal ideation in adolescents and should aggressively intervene (see Chapter 40).

PREVENTION
Deaths caused by unintentional poisoning among younger children have decreased dramatically over the past 2 decades, particularly among children <5 yr old. In 1970, when the U.S. Poison Packaging Prevention Act was passed, 226 poisoning deaths of children <5 yr old occurred, compared with only 24 in 2015. Poisoning prevention demonstrates the effectiveness of passive strategies, including the use of child-resistant packaging and limited doses per container. Difficulty using child-resistant containers by adults is an important cause of poisoning in young children today. In 18.5% of households in which poisoning occurred in children <5 yr old, the child-resistant closure was replaced, and 65% of the packaging used did not work properly. Almost 20% of ingestions occur from drugs belonging to grandparents, who have difficulty using traditional child-resistant containers and often put their medications in pill organizers that are not childproof.

Even though there has been success in preventing poisoning in young children, there has been a remarkable rise in adolescent poison-related death over the past 20 years. This has mirrored the increasing rate of antidepressant prescriptions written by healthcare providers and the epidemic increase in opioid-related fatalities.

APPROACH TO THE POISONED PATIENT
The initial approach to the patient with a witnessed or suspected poisoning should be no different than that in any other sick child, starting with stabilization and rapid assessment of the airway, breathing, circulation (pulse, blood pressure), and mental state, including Glasgow Coma Scale score and laryngeal reflexes (see Chapters 80 and 81). In any patient with altered mental status, a serum dextrose concentration should be obtained early, and naloxone administration should be considered. A targeted history and physical examination serves as the foundation for a thoughtful differential diagnosis, which can then be further refined through laboratory testing and other diagnostic studies.

History
Obtaining an accurate problem-oriented history is of paramount importance. *Intentional* poisonings (suicide attempts, drug abuse/misuse) are typically more severe than unintentional, exploratory ingestions. In patients without a witnessed exposure, historical features such as age of the child (toddler or adolescent), acute onset of symptoms without prodrome, multisystem organ dysfunction, or high levels of household stress should suggest a possible diagnosis of poisoning. In patients with a witnessed exposure, determining exactly what the child was exposed to and the circumstances surrounding the exposure is crucial to initiating directed therapy quickly. For household and workplace products, names (brand, generic, chemical) and specific ingredients, along with their concentrations, can often be obtained from the labels. PCC specialists can also help to identify possible ingredients and review the potential toxicities of each component. Poison center specialists can also help identify pills based on markings, shape, and color. If referred to the hospital for evaluation, parents should be instructed to bring the products, pills, and/or containers with them to assist with identifying and quantifying the exposure. If a child is found with an unknown pill, a list of all medications in the child's environment, including medications that grandparents, parents, siblings, caregivers, or other visitors might have brought into the house, must be obtained. In the case of an unknown exposure, clarifying where the child was found (e.g., garage, kitchen, laundry room, bathroom, backyard, workplace) can help to generate a list of potential toxins.

Next, it is important to clarify the *timing* of the ingestion and to obtain some estimate of how much of the substance was ingested. It is better to overestimate the amount ingested to prepare for the worst-case scenario. Counting pills or measuring the remaining volume of a liquid ingested can sometimes be useful in generating estimates. For inhalational, ocular, or dermal exposures, the concentration of the agent and the length of contact time with the material should be determined, if possible.

Symptoms

Obtaining a description of symptoms experienced after ingestion, including their timing of onset relative to the time of ingestion and their progression, can generate a list of potential toxins and help anticipate the severity of the ingestion. Coupled with physical exam findings, reported symptoms assist practitioners in identifying **toxidromes,** or recognized poisoning syndromes, suggestive of toxicity from specific substances or classes of substances (Tables 77.2 to 77.4).

Past Medical and Developmental History

Underlying diseases can make a child more susceptible to the effects of a toxin. Concurrent drug therapy can also increase toxicity because certain drugs may interact with the toxin. A history of psychiatric illness can make patients more prone to substance abuse, misuse, intentional ingestions, and polypharmacy complications. Pregnancy is a common precipitating factor in adolescent suicide attempts and can influence both evaluation of the patient and subsequent treatment. A developmental history is important to ensure that the exposure history provided is appropriate for the child's developmental stage (e.g., report of 6 mo old picking up a large container of laundry detergent and drinking it should indicate urgent need for treatment, or indicate a severe condition, or "red flag").

Social History

Understanding the child's social environment helps to identify potential sources of exposures (caregivers, visitors, grandparents, recent parties or social gatherings) and social circumstances (new baby, parent's illness, financial stress) that might have contributed to the ingestion (suicide or unintentional). Unfortunately, some poisonings occur in the setting of serious neglect or intentional abuse.

Physical Examination

A targeted physical examination is important to identifying the potential toxin and assessing the severity of the exposure. Initial efforts should be directed toward assessing and stabilizing the airway, breathing, circulation, and mental status. Once the airway is secure and the patient is stable from a cardiopulmonary standpoint, a more extensive physical exam can help to identify characteristic findings of specific toxins or classes of toxins.

In the poisoned patient, key features of the physical exam are vital signs, mental status, pupils (size, reactivity), nystagmus, skin, bowel sounds, and muscle tone. These findings might suggest a toxidrome, which can then guide the differential diagnosis and management.

Laboratory Evaluation

A basic chemistry panel (electrolytes, renal function, glucose) is necessary for all poisoned or potentially poisoned patients. Any patient with acidosis (low serum bicarbonate level on serum chemistry panel) must have an anion gap calculated because of the more specific differential diagnoses associated with an elevated **anion gap metabolic acidosis** (Table 77.5). Patients with a known overdose of acetaminophen should have liver transaminases (ALT, AST) assessed, as well as an international normalized ratio (INR). A serum creatinine kinase level is indicated on any patient with a prolonged "down time" to evaluate for **rhabdomyolysis.** Serum osmolality is only helpful as a surrogate marker for a toxic alcohol exposure if a serum concentration of the alcohol cannot be obtained in a reasonable time frame. A urine pregnancy test is mandatory for all postpubertal female patients. Based on the clinical presentation and the presumed poison, additional lab tests may also be helpful. Acetaminophen is a widely available medication and a commonly detected co-ingestant with the potential for severe toxicity. There is an effective antidote to acetaminophen poisoning that is time dependent. Given that patients might initially be asymptomatic and might not report or be aware of acetaminophen ingestion, an acetaminophen level should be checked in all patients who present after an intentional exposure or ingestion.

For select intoxications (e.g., salicylates, some anticonvulsants, acetaminophen, iron, digoxin, methanol, ethanol, lithium, ethylene glycol, theophylline, CO, lead), quantitative **blood concentrations** are integral to confirming the diagnosis and formulating a treatment plan.

However, for most exposures, quantitative measurement is not readily available and is not likely to alter management. All intoxicant levels must be interpreted in conjunction with the history. For example, a methanol level of 20 mg/dL 1 hr after ingestion may be nontoxic, whereas a similar level 24 hr after ingestion implies a significant poisoning. In general, patients with multiple or chronic exposures to a drug or other chemical will be more symptomatic at lower drug levels than those with a single exposure.

Both the rapid urine drug-of-abuse screens and the more comprehensive drug screens vary widely in their ability to detect toxins and generally add little information to the clinical assessment. This is particularly true if the agent is known and the patient's symptoms are consistent with that agent. If a drug screen is ordered, it is important to know that the components screened for, and the lower limits of detection, vary from laboratory to laboratory. In addition, the interpretation of most drug screens is hampered by many false-positive and false-negative results. Many opiate toxicology screens poorly detect hydrocodone, and do not detect the fully synthetic opioids at all (e.g., methadone, buprenorphine, fentanyl). Several common benzodiazepines may not be detected, as may not synthetic cannabinoids or "bath salts." The amphetamine screen, on the other hand, is typically overly sensitive and often is triggered by prescription amphetamines and some over-the-counter cold preparations. As such, the urine drug-of-abuse screen is typically of limited utility for medical clearance, but may serve a useful function for psychiatrists in their evaluation of the adolescent patient. Besides its psychiatric usefulness, urine drug-of-abuse screens are potentially helpful in patients with altered mental status of unknown etiology, persistent unexplained tachycardia, and acute myocardial ischemia or stroke at a young age. These screens can also be useful in the assessment of a neglected or abused child. Consultation with a medical toxicologist can be helpful in interpreting drug screens and directing which specific drug levels or other lab analyses might aid in patient management.

In the case of a neglected or allegedly abused child, a positive toxicology screen can add substantial weight to a claim of abuse or neglect. In these cases and any case with medicolegal implications, any positive screen *must* be confirmed with gas chromatography/mass spectroscopy, which is considered the gold standard measurement for legal purposes.

Additional Diagnostic Testing

An electrocardiogram (ECG) is a quick and noninvasive bedside test that can yield important clues to diagnosis and prognosis. Particular attention should be paid to the ECG intervals (Table 77.6). A widened QRS interval, putting the patient at risk for monomorphic ventricular tachycardia, suggests blockade of fast sodium channels. A widened QTc interval suggests effects at the potassium rectifier channels and portends a risk of torsades de pointes (polymorphic ventricular tachycardia).

Chest radiography may reveal signs of pneumonitis (e.g., hydrocarbon aspiration), noncardiogenic pulmonary edema (e.g., salicylate toxicity), or a foreign body. Abdominal radiography is most helpful in screening for the presence of lead paint chips or other foreign bodies. It may detect a *bezoar* (concretion), demonstrate radiopaque tablets, or reveal drug packets in a "body packer." Further diagnostic testing is based on the differential diagnosis and pattern of presentation.

PRINCIPLES OF MANAGEMENT

The principles of management of the poisoned patient are supportive care, decontamination, directed therapy (antidotes, ILE), and enhanced elimination. Few patients meet criteria for all these interventions, although clinicians should consider each option in every poisoned patient so as not to miss a potentially lifesaving intervention. Antidotes are available for relatively few poisons (Tables 77.7 and 77.8), thus emphasizing the importance of meticulous supportive care and close clinical monitoring.

Poison control center personnel are specifically trained to provide expertise in the management of poisoning exposures. Parents should be instructed to call the poison control center (**1-800-222-1222**) for any concerning exposure. PCC specialists can assist parents in assessing the potential toxicity and severity of the exposure. They can further

Table 77.2	Selected Historical and Physical Findings in Poisoning

SIGN	TOXIN
ODOR	
Bitter almonds	Cyanide
Acetone	Isopropyl alcohol, methanol, paraldehyde, salicylates
Rotten eggs	Hydrogen sulfide, sulfur dioxide, methyl mercaptans (additive to natural gas)
Wintergreen	Methyl salicylate
Garlic	Arsenic, thallium, organophosphates, selenium
OCULAR SIGNS	
Miosis	Opioids (except propoxyphene, meperidine, and pentazocine), organophosphates and other cholinergics, clonidine, phenothiazines, sedative-hypnotics, olanzapine
Mydriasis	Anticholinergics (e.g., antihistamines, TCAs, atropine), sympathomimetics (cocaine, amphetamines, PCP), post–anoxic encephalopathy, opiate withdrawal, cathinones, MDMA
Nystagmus	Anticonvulsants, sedative-hypnotics, alcohols, PCP, ketamine, dextromethorphan
Lacrimation	Organophosphates, irritant gas or vapors
Retinal hyperemia	Methanol
CUTANEOUS SIGNS	
Diaphoresis	Cholinergics (organophosphates), sympathomimetics, withdrawal syndromes
Alopecia	Thallium, arsenic
Erythema	Boric acid, elemental mercury, cyanide, carbon monoxide, disulfiram, scombroid, anticholinergics, vancomycin
Cyanosis (unresponsive to oxygen)	Methemoglobinemia (e.g., benzocaine, dapsone, nitrites, phenazopyridine), amiodarone, silver
ORAL SIGNS	
Salivation	Organophosphates, salicylates, corrosives, ketamine, PCP, strychnine
Oral burns	Corrosives, oxalate-containing plants
Gum lines	Lead, mercury, arsenic, bismuth
GASTROINTESTINAL SIGNS	
Diarrhea	Antimicrobials, arsenic, iron, boric acid, cholinergics, colchicine, opioid withdrawal
Hematemesis	Arsenic, iron, caustics, NSAIDs, salicylates
Constipation	Lead
CARDIAC SIGNS	
Tachycardia	Sympathomimetics, anticholinergics, antidepressants, antipsychotics, methylxanthines (theophylline, caffeine), salicylates, cellular asphyxiants (cyanide, carbon monoxide, hydrogen sulfide), withdrawal (ethanol, sedatives, clonidine, opioids), serotonin syndrome, neuroleptic malignant syndrome, MDMA, cathinones
Bradycardia	β-Blockers, calcium channel blockers, digoxin, clonidine, organophosphates, opioids, sedative-hypnotics
Hypertension	Sympathomimetics, anticholinergics, monoamine oxidase inhibitors, serotonin syndrome, neuroleptic malignant syndrome, clonidine withdrawal
Hypotension	β-Blockers, calcium channel blockers, cyclic antidepressants, iron, antipsychotics, barbiturates, clonidine, opioids, arsenic, amatoxin mushrooms, cellular asphyxiants (cyanide, carbon monoxide, hydrogen sulfide), snake envenomation
RESPIRATORY SIGNS	
Depressed respirations	Opioids, sedative-hypnotics, alcohol, clonidine, barbiturates
Tachypnea	Salicylates, sympathomimetics, caffeine, metabolic acidosis, carbon monoxide, hydrocarbon aspiration
CENTRAL NERVOUS SYSTEM SIGNS	
Ataxia	Alcohols, anticonvulsants, sedative-hypnotics, lithium, dextromethorphan, carbon monoxide, inhalants
Coma	Opioids, sedative-hypnotics, anticonvulsants, antidepressants, antipsychotics, ethanol, anticholinergics, clonidine, GHB, alcohols, salicylates, barbiturates
Seizures	Sympathomimetics, anticholinergics, antidepressants (especially TCAs, bupropion, venlafaxine), cholinergics (organophosphates), isoniazid, camphor, lindane, salicylates, lead, nicotine, tramadol, water hemlock, withdrawal
Delirium/psychosis	Sympathomimetics, anticholinergics, LSD, PCP, hallucinogens, lithium, dextromethorphan, steroids, withdrawal, MDMA, cathinones
Peripheral neuropathy	Lead, arsenic, mercury, organophosphates, nicotine

GHB, γ-Hydroxybutyrate; LSD, lysergic acid diethylamide; MDMA, 3,4-methylenedioxymethamphetamine (Ecstasy); NSAIDs, nonsteroidal antiinflammatory drugs; PCP, phencyclidine; TCAs, tricyclic antidepressants.

determine which children can be safely monitored at home and which children should be referred to the emergency department for further evaluation and care. Although up to one third of calls to PCCs involve hospitalized patients, and 90% of all calls for exposures in children <6 yr old are managed at home. The AAPCC has generated consensus statements for out-of-hospital management of common ingestions (e.g., acetaminophen, iron, calcium channel blockers) that serve to guide poison center recommendations.

Supportive Care

Careful attention is paid first to the "ABCs" of airway, breathing, and circulation; there should be a low threshold to aggressively manage the airway of a poisoned patient because of the patient's propensity to quickly become comatose. In fact, endotracheal intubation is often the only significant intervention needed in many poisoned patients. An important caveat is the tachypneic patient with a clear lung examination and normal oxygen saturation. This should alert the clinician to the likelihood that

Table 77.3 Recognizable Poison Syndromes ("Toxidromes")

TOXIDROME	SIGNS						POSSIBLE TOXINS
	Vital Signs	Mental Status	Pupils	Skin	Bowel Sounds	Other	
Sympathomimetic	Hypertension, tachycardia, hyperthermia	Agitation, psychosis, delirium, violence	Dilated	Diaphoretic	Normal to increased		Amphetamines, cocaine, PCP, bath salts (cathinones), ADHD medication
Anticholinergic	Hypertension, tachycardia, hyperthermia	Agitated, delirium, coma, seizures	Dilated	Dry, hot	Diminished	Ileus urinary retention	Antihistamines, TCAs, atropine, jimsonweed
Cholinergic	Bradycardia, BP, and temp typically normal	Confusion, coma, fasciculations	Small	Diaphoretic	Hyperactive	Diarrhea, urination, bronchorrhea, bronchospasm, emesis, lacrimation, salivation	Organophosphates (insecticides, nerve agents), carbamates (physostigmine, neostigmine, pyridostigmine) Alzheimer medications, myasthenia treatments
Opioids	Respiratory depression bradycardia, hypotension, hypothermia	Depression, coma, euphoria	Pinpoint	Normal	Normal to decreased		Methadone, buprenorphine, morphine, oxycodone, heroin, etc.
Sedative-hypnotics	Respiratory depression, HR normal to decreased, BP normal to decreased, temp normal to decreased	Somnolence, coma	Small or normal	Normal	Normal		Barbiturates, benzodiazepines, ethanol
Serotonin syndrome (similar findings with neuroleptic malignant syndrome)	Hyperthermia, tachycardia, hypertension or hypotension (autonomic instability)	Agitation, confusion, coma	Dilated	Diaphoretic	Increased	Neuromuscular hyperexcitability: clonus, hyperreflexia (lower > upper extremities)	SSRIs, lithium, MAOIs, linezolid, tramadol, meperidine, dextromethorphan
Salicylates	Tachypnea, hyperpnea, tachycardia, hyperthermia	Agitation, confusion, coma	Normal	Diaphoretic	Normal	Nausea, vomiting, tinnitus, ABGs with primary respiratory alkalosis and primary metabolic acidosis; tinnitus or difficulty hearing	Aspirin and aspirin-containing products, methyl salicylate
Withdrawal (sedative-hypnotic)	Tachycardia, tachypnea, hyperthermia	Agitation, tremor, seizure, hallucinosis, delirium tremens	Dilated	Diaphoretic	Increased		Lack of access to ethanol, benzodiazepines, barbiturates, GHB, or excessive use of flumazenil
Withdrawal (opioid)	Tachycardia	Restlessness, anxiety	Dilated	diaphoretic	Hyperactive	Nausea, vomiting, diarrhea	Lack of access to opioids or excessive use of naloxone

ABGs, Arterial blood gases; ADHD, attention-deficit/hyperactivity disorder; BP, blood pressure; GHB, γ-hydroxybutyrate; HR, heart rate; MAOIs, monoamine oxidase inhibitors; PCP, phencyclidine; SSRIs, selective serotonin reuptake inhibitors; temp, temperature; TCAs, tricyclic antidepressants.

Table 77.4	Mini-Toxidromes	
TOXIDROME	**SYMPTOMS AND SIGNS**	**EXAMPLES**
α_1-Adrenergic receptor antagonists	CNS depression, tachycardia, miosis	Chlorpromazine, quetiapine, clozapine, olanzapine, risperidone
α_2-Adrenergic receptor agonist	CNS depression, bradycardia, hypertension (early), hypotension (late), miosis	Clonidine, oxymetazoline, tetrahydrozoline, tizanidine, dexmedetomidine
Clonus/myoclonus	CNS depression, myoclonic jerks, clonus, hyperreflexia	Carisoprodol, lithium, serotonergic agents, bismuth, organic lead, organic mercury, serotonin or neuroleptic malignant syndrome
Sodium channel blockers	CNS toxicity, wide QRS	Cyclic antidepressants and structurally related agents, propoxyphene, quinidine/quinine, amantadine, antihistamines, bupropion, cocaine
Potassium channel blockers	CNS toxicity, long QT interval	Antipsychotics, methadone, phenothiazines
Cathinones, synthetic cannabinoids	Hyperthermia, tachycardia, delirium, agitation, mydriases	See Chapter 140.

CNS, Central nervous system.
From Ruha AM, Levine M: Central nervous system toxicity. *Emerg Med Clin North Am* 32(1):205–221, 2014, p 208.

Table 77.5	Laboratory Clues in Toxicologic Diagnosis

ANION GAP METABOLIC ACIDOSIS (MNEMONIC = MUDPILES CAT)
Methanol, metformin
Uremia
Diabetic ketoacidosis
Propylene glycol
Isoniazid, iron, massive ibuprofen
Lactic acidosis
Ethylene glycol
Salicylates
Cellular asphyxiants (cyanide, carbon monoxide, hydrogen sulfide)
Alcoholic ketoacidosis
Tylenol (clinical significance depends upon presence or absence of liver injury)

ELEVATED OSMOLAR GAP
Alcohols: ethanol, isopropryl, methanol, ethylene glycol

HYPOGLYCEMIA (MNEMONIC = HOBBIES)
Hypoglycemics, oral: sulfonylureas, meglitinides
Other: quinine, unripe ackee fruit
Beta Blockers
Insulin
Ethanol
Salicylates (late)

HYPERGLYCEMIA
Salicylates (early)
Calcium channel blockers
Caffeine

HYPOCALCEMIA
Ethylene glycol
Fluoride

RHABDOMYOLYSIS
Neuroleptic malignant syndrome, serotonin syndrome
Statins
Mushrooms (*Tricholoma equestre*)
Any toxin causing prolonged immobilization (e.g., opioids, antipsychotics) or excessive muscle activity or seizures (e.g., sympathomimetics)

RADIOPAQUE SUBSTANCE ON KUB (MNEMONIC = CHIPPED)
Chloral hydrate, calcium carbonate
Heavy metals (lead, zinc, barium, arsenic, lithium, bismuth)
Iron
Phenothiazines
Play-Doh, potassium chloride
Enteric-coated pills
Dental amalgam, drug packets

KUB, Kidney-ureter-bladder radiograph.

the patient is compensating for an acidemia. Paralyzing such a patient and underventilating might prove fatal. If intubation is absolutely necessary for airway protection or a tiring patient, a good rule of thumb is to match the ventilatory settings to the patient's preintubation minute ventilation.

Hypotensive patients often are not hypovolemic but are poisoned, and aggressive fluid resuscitation may lead to fluid overload. If hypotension persists after 1 or 2 standard boluses of crystalloid, infusion of a direct-acting vasopressor, such as norepinephrine or epinephrine, is preferred. Dysrhythmias are managed in the standard manner, except for those caused by agents that block fast sodium channels of the heart, for which boluses of sodium bicarbonate are given.

Seizures should primarily be managed with agents that potentiate the γ-aminobutyric acid (GABA) complex, such as benzodiazepines or barbiturates. The goal of supportive therapy is to support the patient's vital functions until the patient can eliminate the toxin. Patients with an elevated creatine phosphokinase (CPK) should be aggressively hydrated

with crystalloid, with a goal urine output of 1-2 mL/kg/hr and close monitoring of CPK trend.

Decontamination

The majority of poisonings in children are from ingestion, although exposures can also occur by inhalational, dermal, and ocular routes. The goal of decontamination is to minimize absorption of the toxic substance. The specific method employed depends on the properties of the toxin itself and the route of exposure. Regardless of the decontamination method used, the efficacy of the intervention decreases with increasing time since exposure. *Decontamination should not be routinely employed for every poisoned patient.* Instead, careful decisions regarding the utility of decontamination should be made for each patient and should include consideration of the toxicity and pharmacologic properties of the exposure, route of the exposure, time since the exposure, and risks vs benefits of the decontamination method.

Dermal and ocular decontamination begins with removal of any

Table 77.6	Electrocardiographic Findings in Poisoning

PR INTERVAL PROLONGATION
Digoxin
Lithium

QRS PROLONGATION
Tricyclic antidepressants
Diphenhydramine
Carbamazepine
Cardiac glycosides
Chloroquine, hydroxychloroquine
Cocaine
Lamotrigine
Quinidine, quinine, procainamide, disopyramide
Phenothiazines
Propoxyphene
Propranolol
Bupropion, venlafaxine (rare)

QTC PROLONGATION*
Amiodarone
Antipsychotics (typical and atypical)
Arsenic
Cisapride
Citalopram
Clarithromycin, erythromycin
Disopyramide, dofetilide, ibutilide
Fluconazole, ketoconazole, itraconazole
Methadone
Pentamidine
Phenothiazines
Sotalol

*This is a select list of important toxins, other medications are also associated with QTc prolongation.

contaminated clothing and particulate matter, followed by flushing of the affected area with tepid water or normal saline (NS). Treating clinicians should wear proper protective gear when performing irrigation. Flushing for a minimum of 10-20 min is recommended for most exposures, although some chemicals (e.g., alkaline corrosives) require much longer periods of flushing. Dermal decontamination, especially after exposure to adherent or lipophilic (e.g., organophosphates) agents, should include thorough cleansing with soap and water. Water should *not* be used for decontamination after exposure to highly reactive agents, such as elemental sodium, phosphorus, calcium oxide, and titanium tetrachloride. After an inhalational exposure, decontamination involves moving the patient to fresh air and administering supplemental oxygen if indicated.

Gastrointestinal (GI) decontamination strategies are most likely to be effective in the 1 or 2 hours after an acute ingestion. GI absorption may be delayed after ingestion of agents that slow GI motility (anticholinergic medications, opioids), massive amounts of pills, sustained-release (SR) preparations, and agents that can form pharmacologic bezoars (e.g., enteric-coated salicylates). GI decontamination more than 2 hr after ingestion may be considered in patients who ingest toxic substances with these properties. However, even rapid institution of GI decontamination with activated charcoal will, at best, bind only approximately 30% of the ingested substance. GI decontamination should never supplant excellent supportive care and should not be employed in an unstable or persistently vomiting patient. Described methods of GI decontamination include induced emesis with ipecac, gastric lavage, cathartics, activated charcoal, and whole-bowel irrigation (WBI). *Of these, only activated charcoal and WBI are of potential benefit.*

Syrup of Ipecac
Syrup of ipecac contains 2 emetic alkaloids that work in both the central nervous system (CNS) and locally in the GI tract to produce vomiting. Many studies have failed to document a significant clinical impact from the use of ipecac and have documented multiple adverse events from its use. The AAP, the American Academy of Clinical Toxicology (AACT),

and the AAPCC have all published statements in favor of *abandoning the use of ipecac.*

Gastric Lavage
Gastric lavage involves placing a large tube orally into the stomach to aspirate contents, followed by flushing with aliquots of fluid, usually water or NS. Although gastric lavage was used routinely for many years, objective data do not document or support clinically relevant efficacy. This is particularly true in children, in whom only small-bore tubes can be used. Lavage is time-consuming and painful and can induce bradycardia through a vagal response to tube placement. It can delay administration of more definitive treatment (activated charcoal) and under the best circumstances, only removes a fraction of gastric contents. *Thus, in most clinical scenarios, the use of gastric lavage is no longer recommended.*

Single-Dose Activated Charcoal
Activated charcoal is a potentially useful method of GI decontamination. Charcoal is "activated" by heating to extreme temperatures, creating an extensive network of pores that provides a very large adsorptive surface area that many (but not all) toxins will bind to, preventing absorption from the GI tract. Charged molecules (i.e., heavy metals, lithium, iron) and liquids do not bind well to activated charcoal (Table 77.9). *Charcoal is most likely to be effective when given within 1 hr of ingestion.* Administration should also be avoided after ingestion of a caustic substance, as it can impede subsequent endoscopic evaluation. A repeat dose of activated charcoal may be warranted in the cases of ingestion of an extended-release product or, more frequently, with a significant salicylate poisoning as a result of its delayed and erratic absorption pattern.

The dose of activated charcoal, with or without sorbitol, is 1 g/kg in children or 50-100 g in adolescents and adults. Before administering charcoal, one *must* ensure that the patient's airway is intact or protected and that the patient has a benign abdominal examination. In the awake, uncooperative adolescent or child who refuses to drink the activated charcoal, there is little utility and potential morbidity associated with forcing activated charcoal down a nasogastric (NG) tube, and such practice should be avoided. In young children, practitioners can attempt to improve palatability by adding flavorings (chocolate or cherry syrup) or giving the mixture over ice cream. Approximately 20% of children vomit after receiving a dose of charcoal, emphasizing the importance of an intact airway and avoiding administration of charcoal after ingestion of substances that are particularly toxic when aspirated (e.g., hydrocarbons). If charcoal is given through a gastric tube in an intubated patient, placement of the tube should be carefully confirmed before activated charcoal is given. Instillation of charcoal directly into the lungs can have disastrous effects. Constipation is another common side effect of activated charcoal, and in rare cases, bowel perforation has been reported.

Cathartics (sorbitol, magnesium sulfate, magnesium citrate) have been used in conjunction with activated charcoal to prevent constipation and accelerate evacuation of the charcoal-toxin complex. There are no data demonstrating their value and numerous reports of adverse effects from cathartics, such as dehydration and electrolyte imbalance.

Whole-Bowel Irrigation
Whole-bowel irrigation (WBI) involves instilling large volumes (35 mL/kg/hr in children or 1-2 L/hr in adolescents) of a polyethylene glycol electrolyte solution (e.g., GoLYTELY) to "wash out" the entire GI tract. This technique may have some success for the ingestion of SR preparations, substances not well adsorbed by charcoal (e.g., lithium, iron), transdermal patches, foreign bodies, and drug packets. In children, WBI is most frequently administered to decontaminate the gut of a child whose abdominal radiograph demonstrates multiple lead paint chips. Careful attention should be paid to assessment of the airway and abdominal exam before initiating WBI. WBI should never be given to a patient with signs of obstruction or ileus or with a compromised airway. Given the rate of administration and volume needed to flush the system, WBI is typically administered by NG tube. WBI is continued until the rectal effluent is clear. If the WBI is for a child with ingested

Table 77.7	Common Antidotes for Poisoning			
POISON	**ANTIDOTE**	**DOSAGE**	**ROUTE**	**ADVERSE EFFECTS, WARNINGS, COMMENTS**
Acetaminophen	N-Acetylcysteine (Mucomyst)	140 mg/kg loading, followed by 70 mg/kg q4h	PO	Vomiting (patient-tailored regimens are the norm)
	N-Acetylcysteine (Acetadote)	150 mg/kg over 1 hr, followed by 50 mg/kg over 4 hr, followed by 100 mg/kg over 16 hr	IV	Anaphylactoid reactions (most commonly seen with loading dose) (Higher doses of the infusion are often recommended depending on acetaminophen level or degree of injury)
Anticholinergics	Physostigmine	0.02 mg/kg over 5 min; may repeat q5-10 min to 2 mg max	IV/IM	Bradycardia, seizures, bronchospasm *Note:* Do not use if conduction delays on ECG.
Benzodiazepines	Flumazenil	0.2 mg over 30 sec; if response is inadequate, repeat q1min to 1 mg max	IV	Agitation, seizures from precipitated withdrawal (doses over 1 mg) **Do not use for unknown or polypharmacy ingestions.**
β-Blockers	Glucagon	0.15 mg/kg bolus followed by infusion of 0.05-0.15 mg/kg/hr	IV	Vomiting, relative lack of efficacy
Calcium channel blockers	Insulin	1 unit/kg bolus followed by infusion of 0.5-1 unit/kg/hr	IV	Hypoglycemia Follow serum potassium and glucose closely.
	Calcium salts	Dose depends on the specific calcium salt	IV	
Carbon monoxide	Oxygen	100% FiO_2 by non-rebreather mask (or ET if intubated)	Inhalation	Some patients may benefit from hyperbaric oxygen (see text).
Cyanide	Hydroxocobalamin (Cyanokit)	70 mg/kg (adults: 5 g) given over 15 min	IV	Flushing/erythema, nausea, rash, chromaturia, hypertension, headache
Digitalis	Digoxin-specific Fab antibodies (Digibind, DigiFab)	1 vial binds 0.6 mg of digitalis glycoside; #vials = digitalis level × weight in kg/100	IV	Allergic reactions (rare), return of condition being treated with digitalis glycoside
Ethylene glycol, methanol	Fomepizole	15 mg/kg load; 10 mg/kg q12h × 4 doses; 15 mg/kg q12h until ethylene glycol level is <20 mg/dL	IV	Infuse slowly over 30 min. If fomepizole is not available, can treat with oral ethanol (80 proof)
Iron	Deferoxamine	Infusion of 5-15 mg/kg/hr (max: 6 g/24 hr)	IV	Hypotension (minimized by avoiding rapid infusion rates)
Isoniazid (INH)	Pyridoxine	Empirical dosing: 70 mg/kg (max dose = 5 g) If ingested dose is known: 1 g per gram of INH	IV	May also be used for *Gyromitra* mushroom ingestions
Lead and other heavy metals (e.g., arsenic, inorganic mercury)	BAL (dimercaprol)	3-5 mg/kg/dose q4h, for the 1st day; subsequent dosing depends on the toxin	Deep IM	Local injection site pain and sterile abscess, vomiting, fever, salivation, nephrotoxicity *Caution:* prepared in peanut oil; contraindicated in patients with peanut allergy
	Calcium disodium EDTA	35-50 mg/kg/day × 5 days; may be given as a continuous infusion or 2 divided doses/day	IV	Vomiting, fever, hypertension, arthralgias, allergic reactions, local inflammation, nephrotoxicity (maintain adequate hydration; follow UA and renal function)
	Dimercaptosuccinic acid (succimer, DMSA, Chemet)	10 mg/kg/dose q8h × 5 days, then 10 mg/kg q12h × 14 days	PO	Vomiting, hepatic transaminase elevation, rash
Methemoglobinemia	Methylene blue, 1% solution	0.1-0.2 mL/kg (1-2 mg/kg) over 5-10 min; may be repeated q30-60 min	IV	Vomiting, headache, dizziness, blue discoloration of urine
Opioids	Naloxone	1 mg if patient not likely to be addicted. 0.04-0.4 mg if possibly addicted; repeated as needed; may need continuous infusion	IV, intranasal, IO, IM, nebulized	Acute withdrawal symptoms if given to addicted patients May also be useful for clonidine ingestions (typically at higher doses)

Continued

Table 77.7	Common Antidotes for Poisoning—cont'd			
POISON	**ANTIDOTE**	**DOSAGE**	**ROUTE**	**ADVERSE EFFECTS, WARNINGS, COMMENTS**
Organophosphates	Atropine	0.05-0.1 mg/kg repeated q5-10 min as needed	IV/ET	Tachycardia, dry mouth, blurred vision, urinary retention
	Pralidoxime (2-PAM)	25-50 mg/kg over 5-10 min (max: 200 mg/min); can be repeated after 1-2 hr, then q10-12h as needed	IV/IM	Nausea, dizziness, headache, tachycardia, muscle rigidity, bronchospasm (rapid administration)
Salicylates	Sodium bicarbonate	Bolus 1-2 mEq/kg followed by continuous infusion	IV	Follow potassium closely and replace as necessary. Goal urine pH: 7.5-8.0
Sulfonylureas	Octreotide and dextrose	1-2 µg/kg/dose (adults 50-100 µg) q6-8h	IV/SC	
Tricyclic antidepressants	Sodium bicarbonate	Bolus 1-2 mEq/kg; repeated bolus dosing as needed to keep QRS <110 msec	IV	Indications: QRS widening (≥110 msec), hemodynamic instability; follow potassium.

BAL, British antilewisite; DMSA, dimercaptosuccinic acid; ECG, electrocardiogram; FIO_2, fraction of inspired oxygen; EDTA, ethylenediaminetetraacetic acid; ET, endotracheal tube; IO, intraosseous; max, maximum; UA, urinalysis.

Table 77.8	Other Antidotes
ANTIDOTES	**TOXIN OR POISON**
Latrodectus antivenin	Black widow spider
Botulinum antitoxin	Botulinum toxin
Diphenhydramine and/or benztropine	Dystonic reactions
Calcium salts	Fluoride, calcium channel blockers
Protamine	Heparin
Folinic acid	Methotrexate, trimethoprim, pyrimethamine
Crotalidae-specific Fab antibodies	Rattlesnake envenomation
Sodium bicarbonate	Sodium channel blockade (tricyclic antidepressants, type 1 antiarrhythmics)

Table 77.9	Substances Poorly Adsorbed by Activated Charcoal

Alcohols
Caustics: alkalis and acids
Cyanide
Heavy metals (e.g., lead)
Hydrocarbons
Iron
Lithium

paint chips, the end-point will be clearing of the chips from the bowel based on repeat radiographs. Complications of WBI include vomiting, abdominal pain, and abdominal distention. Bezoar formation might respond to WBI but may also require endoscopy or surgery.

Directed Therapy
Antidotal Therapy
Antidotes are available for relatively few toxins (Tables 77.7 and 77.8), but early and appropriate use of an antidote is a key element in managing the poisoned patient.

Intralipid Emulsion Therapy
Intralipid emulsion (ILE) therapy is a potentially lifesaving intervention. ILE therapy sequesters fat-soluble drugs, decreasing their impact at target organs. It also enhances cardiac function by supplying an alternative energy source to a depressed myocardium and acting on calcium channels in the heart, increasing myocardial calcium and thus cardiac function. Intralipid is most effective as a reversal agent for toxicity from inadvertent intravenous (IV) injection of bupivacaine. Using the same 20% Intralipid used for total parenteral nutrition (TPN), a bolus dose of 1.5 mL/kg is given over 3 min, followed by an infusion of 0.25 mL/kg/min until recovery or until a total of 10 mL/kg has been infused. *Lipophilic drugs,* those in which the logarithm of the coefficient describing the partition between 2 solvents (hydrophobic phase and hydrophilic phase) is >2,

have the most potential to be bound by ILE. These include, but are not limited to, calcium channel blockers (verapamil, diltiazem), bupropion, and tricyclic antidepressants.

Enhanced Elimination
Enhancing elimination results in increased clearance of a poison that has already been absorbed. It is only useful for a few toxins and in these cases is a potentially lifesaving intervention. Methods of enhanced elimination include urinary alkalinization, hemodialysis, and multidose activated charcoal.

Urinary Alkalinization
Urinary alkalinization enhances the elimination of drugs that are weak acids by forming charged molecules, which then become trapped in the renal tubules. Charged molecules, being polar and hydrophilic, do not easily cross cellular membranes, thus they remain in the renal tubules and are excreted. Urinary alkalinization is accomplished by a continuous infusion of sodium bicarbonate–containing IV fluids, with a goal urine pH of 7.5-8. Alkalinization of the urine is most useful in managing salicylate and methotrexate toxicity. Complications of urinary alkalinization include electrolyte derangements (e.g., hypokalemia, hypocalcemia), fluid overload, and excessive serum alkalinization. Serum pH should be closely monitored and not exceed a pH >7.55. Patients typically unable to tolerate the volumes required for alkalinization are those with heart failure, kidney failure, pulmonary edema, or cerebral edema.

Hemodialysis
Few drugs or toxins are removed by dialysis in amounts sufficient to justify the risks and difficulty of dialysis. Toxins amenable to dialysis have the following properties: low volume of distribution (<1 L/kg) with a high degree of water solubility, low molecular weight, and low degree of protein binding. Hemodialysis may be useful for toxicity from

methanol, ethylene glycol, salicylates, theophylline, bromide, lithium, and valproic acid. Hemodialysis is also used to correct severe electrolyte disturbances and acid-base derangements resulting from the ingestion (e.g., severe metformin-associated lactic acidosis).

Multidose Activated Charcoal

Whereas single-dose activated charcoal is used as a method of decontamination, multidose activated charcoal (**MDAC**) can help to enhance the elimination of certain toxins. MDAC is typically given as 0.5 g/kg every 4-6 hr (for 4 doses). MDAC enhances elimination by 2 proposed mechanisms: interruption of enterohepatic recirculation and "GI dialysis." The concept of GI dialysis involves using the intestinal mucosa as a dialysis membrane and pulling toxins from the bloodstream back into the intraluminal space, where they are adsorbed to the charcoal. The AACT/European Association of Poisons Centres and Clinical Toxicologists position statement recommends MDAC in managing significant ingestions of carbamazepine, dapsone, phenobarbital, quinine, and theophylline. As with single-dose activated charcoal, contraindications to use of MDAC include an unprotected airway and a concerning abdominal examination (e.g., ileus, distention, peritoneal signs). Thus the airway and abdominal exam *should be assessed before each dose.* A cathartic (e.g., sorbitol) may be given with the 1st dose, but it should not be used with subsequent doses because of the risk of dehydration and electrolyte derangements. Although MDAC reduces the serum level of an intoxicant quicker than without MDAC, it has not been shown to have a significant impact on outcome.

SELECT COMPOUNDS IN PEDIATRIC POISONING

See other chapters for herbal medicines (Chapter 78), drugs of abuse (Chapter 140), and environmental health hazards (Chapters 735-741).

Pharmaceuticals
Analgesics

Acetaminophen. Acetaminophen (APAP) is the most widely used analgesic and antipyretic in pediatrics, available in multiple formulations, strengths, and combinations. Consequently, APAP is commonly available in the home, where it can be unintentionally ingested by young children, taken in an intentional overdose by adolescents and adults, or inappropriately dosed in all ages. In the United States, APAP toxicity remains the most common cause of acute liver failure and is the leading cause of intentional poisoning death.

Pathophysiology. APAP toxicity results from the formation of a highly reactive intermediate metabolite, N-acetyl-p-benzoquinone imine (NAPQI). In therapeutic use, only a small percentage of a dose (approximately 5%) is metabolized by the hepatic cytochrome P450 enzyme CYP2E1 to NAPQI, which is then immediately joined with glutathione to form a nontoxic mercapturic acid conjugate. In overdose, glutathione stores are overwhelmed, and free NAPQI is able to combine with hepatic macromolecules to produce hepatocellular necrosis. The single acute toxic dose of APAP is generally considered to be >200 mg/kg in children and >7.5-10 g in adolescents and adults. Repeated administration of APAP at supratherapeutic doses (>90 mg/kg/day for consecutive days) can lead to hepatic injury or failure in some children, especially in the setting of fever, dehydration, poor nutrition, and other conditions that serve to reduce glutathione stores.

Any child with a history of acute ingestion of >200 mg/kg (unusual in children <6 yr) or with an acute intentional ingestion of any amount should be referred to a healthcare facility for clinical assessment and measurement of a serum APAP level.

Clinical and Laboratory Manifestations. Classically, 4 general stages of APAP toxicity have been described (Table 77.10). The initial signs are nonspecific (i.e., nausea and vomiting) and may not be present. Thus the diagnosis of APAP toxicity cannot be based on clinical symptoms alone, but instead requires consideration of the combination of the patient's history, symptoms, and laboratory findings.

If a toxic ingestion is suspected, a serum APAP level should be measured 4 hr after the reported time of ingestion. For patients who present to medical care more than 4 hr after ingestion, a stat APAP level should be obtained. *APAP levels obtained <4 hr after ingestion,*

Table 77.10	Classic Stages in Clinical Course of Acetaminophen Toxicity	
STAGE	**TIME AFTER INGESTION**	**CHARACTERISTICS**
I	0.5-24 hr	Anorexia, vomiting, malaise Lab tests typically normal, except for acetaminophen level
II	24-48 hr	Resolution of earlier symptoms; right upper quadrant abdominal pain and tenderness; elevated hepatic transaminases (aspartate > alanine), INR
III	3-5 days	Peak transaminase elevations; development of liver failure, multi organ-system failure, death or recovery begins
IV	4 days to 2 wk	Resolution of liver function abnormalities Clinical recovery precedes histologic recovery

unless "nondetectable," are difficult to interpret and cannot be used to estimate the potential for toxicity. Other important baseline lab tests include hepatic transaminases, renal function tests, and coagulation parameters.

Treatment. When considering the treatment of a patient poisoned or potentially poisoned with APAP, and after assessment of the ABCs, it is helpful to place the patient into one of the following four categories.

1. *Prophylactic.* By definition, these patients have a normal aspartate transaminase (AST). If the APAP level is known and the ingestion is within 24 hr of the level being drawn, treatment decisions are based on where the level falls on the Rumack-Matthew nomogram (Fig. 77.1). Any patient with a serum APAP level in the possible or probable hepatotoxicity range per the nomogram should be treated with N-acetylcysteine (NAC). This nomogram is only intended for use in patients who present within 24 hr of a single *acute* APAP ingestion with a known time of ingestion. If treatment is recommended, they should receive NAC as either oral Mucomyst or IV Acetadote for 24 or 21 hr, respectively. Repeat AST and APAP concentration drawn toward the end of that interval should be obtained. If the AST remains normal and the APAP becomes nondetectable, treatment may be discontinued. If the AST becomes elevated, the patient moves into the next category of treatment (injury). If APAP is still present, treatment should be continued until the level is nondetectable. In the case of a patient with a documented APAP level, normal AST, and an unknown time of ingestion, treatment should ensue until the level is nondetectable, with normal transaminases.

The importance of instituting therapy with either IV or oral NAC *no later than 8 hr from the time of ingestion* cannot be overemphasized. No patient, regardless of the size of the ingestion, who receives NAC within 8 hr of overdose should die from liver failure. The longer from the 8 hr mark the initiation of therapy is delayed, the greater the risk of acute liver failure. Any patient presenting close to or beyond the 8 hr mark after an APAP overdose should be empirically started on NAC pending laboratory results.

2. *Hepatic Injury.* These patients are exhibiting evidence of hepatocellular necrosis, manifested first as elevated liver transaminases (usually AST first, then alanine transaminase [ALT]), followed by a rise in the INR. Any patient in this category requires therapy with NAC (IV or oral). When to discontinue therapy in the clinically well patient remains controversial, but in general the transaminases and INR have peaked and fallen significantly "toward" normal (they do not need to be normal). Most patients' liver enzymes will peak 3 or 4 days after their ingestion.

3. *Acute Liver Failure.* The King's College criteria are used to determine which patients should be referred for consideration of liver transplant. These criteria include acidemia (serum pH <7.3) after adequate fluid resuscitation, coagulopathy (INR >6), renal dysfunction (creatinine

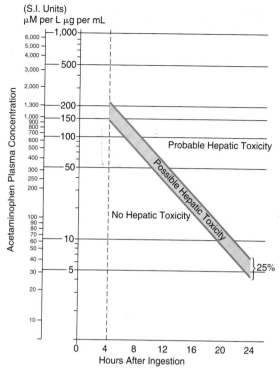

Fig. 77.1 Rumack-Matthew nomogram for acetaminophen poisoning, a semilogarithmic plot of plasma acetaminophen concentrations vs time. *Cautions for the use of this chart:* The time coordinates refer to time after ingestion; serum concentrations obtained before 4 hr are not interpretable; and the graph should be used only in relation to a single acute ingestion with a known time of ingestion. This nomogram is not useful for chronic exposures or unknown time of ingestion and should be used with caution in the setting of co-ingestants that that slow gastrointestinal motility. The *lower solid line* is typically used in the United States to define toxicity and direct treatment, whereas the *upper line* is generally used in Europe. (From Rumack BH, Hess AJ, editors: *Poisindex, Denver, 1995, Micromedix. Adapted from Rumack BH, Matthew H: Acetaminophen poisoning and toxicity, Pediatrics 55:871–876, 1975.)*

>3.4 mg/dL), and grade III or IV hepatic encephalopathy (see Chapter 391). A serum lactic acid >3 mmol/L (after IV fluids) adds to both sensitivity and specificity of the criteria to predict death without liver transplant. The degree of transaminase elevation does not factor in to this decision-making process.

4. Repeated Supratherapeutic Ingestion. APAP is particularly prone to unintentional overdose through the ingestion of multiple medications containing the drug or simply because people assume it to be safe at any dose. Ingestion of amounts significantly greater than the recommended daily dose for several days or more puts one at risk for liver injury. Because the Rumack-Matthew nomogram is not helpful in this scenario, a conservative approach is taken. In the asymptomatic patient, if the AST is normal and the APAP is <10 μg/mL, no therapy is indicated. A normal AST and an elevated APAP warrants NAC dosing for at least long enough for the drug to metabolize while the AST remains normal. An elevated AST puts the patient in the "hepatic injury" category previously described. A patient presenting with symptoms (i.e., right upper quadrant pain, vomiting, jaundice) should be empirically started on NAC pending lab results.

NAC is available in oral and IV forms, and both are considered equally efficacious (see Table 77.7 for the dosing regimens of the oral vs IV form). The IV form is used in patients with intractable vomiting, those with evidence of hepatic failure, and pregnant patients. Oral NAC has an unpleasant taste and smell and can be mixed in soft drink or fruit juice or given by NG tube to improve tolerability of the oral regimen. Administration of IV NAC (as a standard 3% solution to avoid administering excess free water, typically in 5% dextrose), especially the initial loading dose, is associated in some patients with the development of anaphylactoid reactions (non–immunoglobulin E mediated). These reactions are typically managed by stopping the infusion; treating with diphenhydramine, albuterol, and/or epinephrine as indicated; and restarting the infusion at a slower rate once symptoms have resolved. IV NAC is also associated with mild elevation in measured INR (range: 1.2-1.5) because of laboratory interference. IV dosing, however, delivers less medication to the liver compared with the oral regimen. As a result, many toxicologists now recommend higher doses of the IV formulation in patients with large overdoses. Transaminases, synthetic function, and renal function should be followed daily while the patient is being treated with NAC. Patients with worsening hepatic function or clinical status might benefit from more frequent lab monitoring. A patient-tailored approach is now the norm for when to stop NAC therapy, for deciding whom to refer for transplantation evaluation, and often for the dose of IV NAC in patients with either very high APAP levels or signs of injury. Consultation with the regional PCC and medical toxicologist can help streamline the care of these patients, ultimately shortening their length of stay with potentially improved outcomes.

Salicylates. The incidence of salicylate poisoning in young children has declined dramatically since APAP and ibuprofen replaced aspirin as the most commonly used analgesics and antipyretics in pediatrics. However, salicylates remain widely available, not only in aspirin-containing products but also in antidiarrheal medications, topical agents (e.g., keratolytics, sports creams), oil of wintergreen, and some herbal products. Oil of wintergreen contains 5 g of salicylate in 1 teaspoon (5 mL), meaning ingestion of very small volumes of this product has the potential to cause severe toxicity.

Pathophysiology. Salicylates lead to toxicity by interacting with a wide array of physiologic processes, including direct stimulation of the respiratory center, uncoupling of oxidative phosphorylation, inhibition of the tricarboxylic acid cycle, and stimulation of glycolysis and gluconeogenesis. The acute toxic dose of salicylates is generally considered to be >150 mg/kg. More significant toxicity is seen after ingestions of >300 mg/kg, and severe, potentially fatal, toxicity is described after ingestions of >500 mg/kg.

Clinical and Laboratory Manifestations. Salicylate ingestions are classified as acute or chronic, and acute toxicity is much more common in pediatric patients. Early signs of acute salicylism include nausea, vomiting, diaphoresis, and tinnitus. Moderate salicylate toxicity can manifest as tachypnea and hyperpnea, tachycardia, and altered mental status. The tachycardia largely results from marked insensible losses from vomiting, tachypnea, diaphoresis, and uncoupling of oxidative phosphorylation. Thus, careful attention should be paid to volume status and early volume resuscitation in the significantly poisoned patient. Signs of severe salicylate toxicity include mild hyperthermia, coma, and seizures. Chronic salicylism can have a more insidious presentation, and patients can show marked toxicity (e.g. altered mental status, noncardiogenic pulmonary edema, acidemia) at significantly lower salicylate levels than in acute toxicity.

Classically, laboratory values from a patient poisoned with salicylates reveal a primary respiratory alkalosis and a primary, elevated anion gap metabolic acidosis. Early in the course of acute salicylism, respiratory alkalosis dominates and the patient is alkalemic. As the respiratory stimulation diminishes, the patient will move toward acidemia. Hyperglycemia (early) and hypoglycemia (late) have been described. Abnormal coagulation studies and acute kidney injury may be seen but are not common.

Serial serum salicylate levels should be closely monitored (every 2-4 hr initially) until they are consistently downtrending. Salicylate absorption in overdose is unpredictable and erratic, especially with an enteric-coated product, and levels can rapidly increase into the highly toxic range, even many hours after the ingestion. The Done nomogram is of poor value and should not be used. Serum and urine pH and electrolytes should be followed closely. An APAP level should be checked in any patient who intentionally overdoses on salicylates, because APAP is a common co-ingestant, and people often confuse or combine their nonprescription analgesic medications. Salicylate toxicity can cause a noncardiogenic pulmonary edema, especially in chronic overdose; consequently, a chest radiograph is recommended in any patient in respiratory distress.

Treatment. For the patient who presents soon after an acute ingestion, initial treatment should include gastric decontamination with activated charcoal. Salicylate pills occasionally form bezoars, which should be suspected if serum salicylate concentrations continue to rise many hours after ingestion or are persistently elevated despite appropriate management. Gastric decontamination is typically not useful after chronic exposure.

Initial therapy focuses on aggressive volume resuscitation and prompt initiation of sodium bicarbonate therapy in the symptomatic patient, even before obtaining serum salicylate levels. Therapeutic salicylate levels are 10-20 mg/dL, and levels >25 or 30 mg/dL warrant treatment.

The primary mode of therapy for salicylate toxicity is **urinary alkalinization**. Urinary alkalinization enhances the elimination of salicylates by converting salicylate to its ionized form, "trapping" it in the renal tubules, thus enhancing elimination. In addition, maintaining an alkalemic serum pH decreases CNS penetration of salicylates because charged particles are less able to cross the blood-brain barrier. Alkalinization is achieved by administration of a sodium bicarbonate infusion at approximately 2 times maintenance fluid rates. *The goals of therapy include a urine pH of 7.5-8, a serum pH of 7.45-7.55, and decreasing serum salicylate levels.* In general, in the presence of an acidosis, an aspirin-poisoned patient's status can be directly related to the patient's serum pH: the lower the pH, the greater the relative amount of salicylate in the uncharged, nonpolar form and the greater the penetration of the blood-brain barrier by the drug. Careful attention should also be paid to serial potassium levels in any patient on a bicarbonate infusion, since potassium will be driven intracellularly and hypokalemia impairs alkalinization of the urine. For these reasons, potassium is often added to the bicarbonate drip. Repeat doses of charcoal may be beneficial because of the often delayed and erratic absorption of aspirin. Parenteral glucose should be provided to any salicylate-poisoned patients with altered mental status because they may have CNS hypoglycemia (i.e., neuroglycopenia) not seen in a peripheral serum glucose test.

In patients with severe toxicity, hemodialysis may be required. Indications for dialysis include severe acid-base abnormalities (specifically severe acidosis and acidemia), a rising salicylate level (despite adequate decontamination and properly alkalinized urine), pulmonary edema, cerebral edema, seizures, and renal failure. Serum salicylate concentrations alone are not a clear indicator of the need for dialysis and should always be interpreted along with the clinical status of the patient.

Ibuprofen and Other Nonsteroidal Antiinflammatory Drugs (NSAIDs). Ibuprofen and other NSAIDs are often involved in unintentional and intentional overdoses because of their widespread availability and common use as analgesics and antipyretics. Fortunately, serious effects after acute NSAID overdose are rare because of their wide therapeutic index.

Pathophysiology. NSAIDs inhibit prostaglandin synthesis by reversibly inhibiting the activity of cyclooxygenase (COX), the primary enzyme responsible for the biosynthesis of prostaglandins. In therapeutic use, side effects include GI irritation, reduced renal blood flow, and platelet dysfunction. To minimize these side effects, NSAID analogs have been developed that are more specific for the inducible form of COX (the COX-2 isoform) than the constitutive form, COX-1. However, overdose of the more selective COX-2 inhibitors (e.g., celecoxib [Celebrex]) is treated the same as overdose of nonspecific COX inhibitors (e.g., ibuprofen) because at higher doses, COX-2–selective agents lose their COX inhibitory selectivity.

Ibuprofen, the primary NSAID used in pediatrics, is well tolerated, even in overdose. In children, acute doses of <200 mg/kg rarely cause toxicity, but ingestions of >400 mg/kg can produce more serious effects, including altered mental status and metabolic acidosis.

Clinical and Laboratory Manifestations. Symptoms usually develop within 4-6 hr of ingestion and resolve within 24 hr. If toxicity does develop, it is typically manifested as nausea, vomiting, and abdominal pain. Although GI bleeding and ulcers have been described with chronic use, they are rare in the setting of acute ingestion. After massive ingestions, patients can develop marked CNS depression, anion gap metabolic acidosis, renal insufficiency, and (rarely) respiratory depression. Seizures have also been described, especially after overdose of mefenamic acid. Specific drug levels are not readily available, nor do they inform management decisions. Renal function studies, acid-base balance, complete blood count (CBC), and coagulation parameters should be monitored after very large ingestions. Co-ingestants, especially APAP, should be ruled out after any intentional ingestion.

Treatment. Supportive care, including use of antiemetics and acid blockade as indicated, is the primary therapy for NSAID toxicity. Decontamination with activated charcoal should be considered if a patient presents within 1-2 hr of a potentially toxic ingestion. There is no specific antidote for this class of drugs. Given the high degree of protein binding and excretion pattern of NSAIDs, none of the modalities used to enhance elimination is particularly useful in managing these overdoses. Unlike in patients with salicylate toxicity, urinary alkalinization is not helpful for NSAID toxicity. Patients who develop significant clinical signs of toxicity should be admitted to the hospital for ongoing supportive care and monitoring. Patients who remain asymptomatic for 4-6 hr after ingestion may be considered medically cleared.

Prescription Opioids. Opioids are a frequently abused class of medications in both IV and oral forms. The opioid epidemic gripping the United States and other countries is discussed in Chapter 140. Two specific oral opioids, buprenorphine and methadone, merit mention because of potential life-threatening toxicity in toddlers with ingestion of even 1 pill. Both agents are used in managing opioid dependence, although **buprenorphine** is the drug of choice. **Methadone** is also widely used in the treatment of chronic pain, meaning multiday prescriptions can be filled. Both drugs are readily available for illicit purchase and potential abuse. Both drugs are of great potential toxicity to a toddler, especially buprenorphine because of its long half-life and high potency.

Pathophysiology. Methadone is a lipophilic synthetic opioid with potent agonist effects at μ-opioid receptors, leading to both its desired analgesic effects and undesired side effects, including sedation, respiratory depression, and impaired GI motility. Methadone is thought to cause QTc interval prolongation through interactions with the human ether-a-go-go–related gene (hERG)-encoded potassium rectifier channel. Its duration of effect for pain control averages only about 8 hr, whereas the dangerous side effects can occur up to 24 hr from the last dose and longer after overdose. Methadone has an average half-life >25 hr, which may be extended to >50 hr in overdose.

Suboxone is a combination of buprenorphine, a potent opioid with partial agonism at μ-opioid receptors and weak antagonism at κ-opioid receptors, and naloxone. Naloxone has poor oral bioavailability but is included in the formulation to discourage diversion for IV use, during which it can precipitate withdrawal. Suboxone is formulated for buccal or sublingual administration; consequently, toddlers can absorb significant amounts of drug even by sucking on a tablet. Buprenorphine has an average half-life of 37 hr.

Clinical and Laboratory Manifestations. In children, methadone and buprenorphine ingestions can manifest with the classic opioid toxidrome of respiratory depression, sedation, and miosis. Signs of more severe toxicity can include bradycardia, hypotension, and hypothermia. Even in therapeutic use, methadone is associated with a prolonged QTc interval and risk of torsades de pointes. Accordingly, an ECG should be part of the initial evaluation after ingestion of methadone or any unknown opioid. Neither drug is detected on routine urine opiate screens, although some centers have added a separate urine methadone screen. Levels of both drugs can be measured, although this is rarely done clinically and is seldom helpful in the acute setting. An exception may be in the cases involving concerns about neglect or abuse, at which point urine for gas chromatography/mass spectroscopy, the legal gold standard, should be sent to confirm and document the presence of the drug.

Treatment. Patients with significant respiratory depression or CNS depression should be treated with the opioid antidote **naloxone** (see

Table 77.7). In pediatric patients who are not chronically taking opioids, the full reversal dose of 1-2 mg should be used. In contrast, opioid-dependent patients should be treated with smaller initial doses (0.04-0.4 mg), which can then be repeated as needed to achieve the desired clinical response, avoiding abrupt induction of withdrawal. Because the half-life of methadone and buprenorphine is much longer than that of naloxone, patients can require multiple doses of naloxone. These patients may benefit from a continuous infusion of naloxone, typically started at two thirds of the reversal dose per hour and titrated to maintain an adequate respiratory rate and level of consciousness. Patients who have ingested methadone should be placed on a cardiac monitor and have serial ECGs to monitor for the development of a prolonged QTc interval. If a patient does develop a prolonged QTc, management includes close cardiac monitoring, repletion of electrolytes (potassium, calcium, and magnesium), and having a defibrillator readily available should the patient develop torsades de pointes.

Given the potential for clinically significant and prolonged toxicity, any toddler who has ingested opioids, even if asymptomatic, should be admitted to the hospital for at least 24 hr of monitoring. Some experts advocate a similar approach to management of buprenorphine ingestions, even in the asymptomatic patient. All such cases should be discussed with a PCC or medical toxicologist before determining disposition.

Cardiovascular Medications

β-Adrenergic Receptor Blockers. β-Blockers competitively inhibit the action of catecholamines at the β-adrenergic receptor. Therapeutically, β-blockers are used for a variety of conditions, including hypertension, coronary artery disease, tachydysrhythmias, anxiety disorders, migraines, essential tremor, and hyperthyroidism. Because of its lipophilicity and blockade of fast sodium channels, **propranolol** is considered to be the most toxic member of the β-blocker class. Overdoses of water-soluble β-blockers (e.g., atenolol) are associated with milder symptoms.

Pathophysiology. In overdose, β-blockers decrease chronotropy and inotropy in addition to slowing conduction through atrioventricular nodal tissue. Clinically, these effects are manifested as bradycardia, hypotension, and heart block. Patients with reactive airways disease can experience bronchospasm as a result of blockade of β₂-mediated bronchodilation. β₂-Blockers interfere with glycogenolysis and gluconeogenesis, which can sometimes lead to hypoglycemia, especially in patients with poor glycogen stores (e.g., toddlers).

Clinical and Laboratory Manifestations. Toxicity typically develops within 6 hr of ingestion, although it may be delayed after ingestion of sotalol or slow-release (SR) preparations. The most common features of severe poisoning are bradycardia and hypotension. Lipophilic agents, including propranolol, can enter the CNS and cause altered mental status, coma, and seizures. Overdose of β-blockers with membrane-stabilizing properties (e.g., propranolol) can cause QRS interval widening and ventricular dysrhythmias.

Evaluation after β-blocker overdose should include an ECG, frequent reassessments of hemodynamic status, and blood glucose. Serum levels of β-blockers are not readily available for routine clinical use and are not useful in management of the poisoned patient.

Treatment. In addition to supportive care and GI decontamination as indicated, **glucagon** is theoretically the preferred antidote of choice for β-blocker toxicity (see Table 77.7). Glucagon stimulates adenyl cyclase and increases levels of cyclic adenosine monophosphate (cAMP) independent of the β-receptor. Glucagon is typically given as a bolus and, if this is effective, followed by a continuous infusion. In practice, glucagon is often only marginally effective, limited by its proemetic effects, especially at the high doses typically required. Other potentially useful interventions include calcium, vasopressors, and high-dose insulin. Seizures are managed with benzodiazepines, and QRS widening should be treated with sodium bicarbonate. Children who ingest 1 or 2 water-soluble β-blockers are unlikely to develop toxicity and can typically be discharged to home if they remain asymptomatic over a 6 hr observation period. Children who ingest SR products, highly lipid-soluble agents, and sotalol can require longer periods of observation before safe discharge. Any symptomatic child should be admitted for ongoing monitoring and directed therapy.

Calcium Channel Blockers. Calcium channel blockers (CCBs) are used for a variety of therapeutic indications and have the potential to cause severe toxicity, even after exploratory ingestions. Specific agents include verapamil, diltiazem, and the dihydropyridines (e.g., amlodipine, nifedipine). Of these, diltiazem and verapamil are the most dangerous in overdose because of their higher lipophilicity and direct cardiac suppressant effects.

Pathophysiology. CCBs antagonize L-type calcium channels, inhibiting calcium influx into myocardial and vascular smooth muscle cells. Verapamil works primarily by slowing inotropy and chronotropy and has no effect on systemic vascular resistance (SVR). Diltiazem has effects both on the heart and the peripheral vasculature. The dihydropyridines exclusively diminish SVR. Verapamil and diltiazem can significantly diminish myocardial contractility and conduction, with diltiazem also lowering SVR. By contrast, dihydropyridines will decrease the SVR, leading to vasodilation and reflex tachycardia, although this receptor selectivity may be lost after a large overdose. Because the same L-type calcium channels blocked by CCBs are also on the pancreatic islet cells, any patient significantly poisoned with a CCB usually is hyperglycemic.

Clinical and Laboratory Manifestations. The onset of symptoms typically is soon after ingestion, although it may be delayed with ingestions of SR products. Overdoses of CCBs lead to hypotension, accompanied by bradycardia, normal heart rate, or even tachycardia, depending on the agent. A common feature of CCB overdose is the patient exhibiting profound hypotension with preserved consciousness.

Initial evaluation should include an ECG, continuous and careful hemodynamic monitoring, and rapid measurement of serum glucose levels. Both the absolute degree of hyperglycemia and the percentage increase in serum glucose have been correlated with the severity of CCB toxicity in adults. The development of hyperglycemia can even precede the development of hemodynamic instability. Blood levels of CCBs are not readily available and are not useful in guiding therapy.

Treatment. Once initial supportive care has been instituted, GI decontamination should begin with activated charcoal as appropriate. WBI may be beneficial in a stable patient after ingestion of an SR product. Calcium channel blockade in the smooth muscles of the GI tract can lead to greatly diminished motility; thus any form of GI decontamination should be undertaken with careful attention to serial abdominal tests.

Calcium salts, administered through a peripheral IV line as calcium gluconate or a central line as calcium chloride, help to overcome blocked calcium channels. **High-dose insulin euglycemia therapy** is considered the antidote of choice for CCB toxicity. An initial bolus of 1 unit/kg of regular insulin is followed by an infusion at 0.5-1 unit/kg/hr (see Table 77.7). The main mechanism of high-dose insulin euglycemia is to improve the metabolic efficiency of a poisoned heart that is in need of carbohydrates for energy (instead of the usual free fatty acids), but has minimal circulating insulin. Blood glucose levels should be closely monitored, and supplemental glucose may be given to maintain euglycemia, although this is rarely necessary in the severely poisoned patient.

Additional therapies include judicious IV fluid boluses and vasopressors (often in very high doses). Cardiac pacing is rarely of value. Lipid emulsion therapy (discussed earlier) is a potentially lifesaving intervention, especially for patients poisoned with the more lipid-soluble CCBs, verapamil and diltiazem. In extreme cases an intraaortic balloon pump or extracorporeal membrane oxygenation (ECMO) are potential rescue devices. Given the potential for profound and sometimes delayed toxicity in toddlers after ingestion of 1 or 2 CCB tablets, hospital admission and 12-24 hr of monitoring for all of these patients is strongly recommended.

Clonidine. Although originally intended for use as an antihypertensive, the number of clonidine prescriptions in the pediatric population has greatly increased because of its reported efficacy in the management of attention-deficit/hyperactivity disorder (ADHD), tic disorders, and other behavioral disorders. With this increased use has come a significant rise in pediatric ingestions and therapeutic misadventures. Clonidine is available in pill and transdermal patch forms.

Pathophysiology. Clonidine, along with the closely related agent **guanfacine**, is a centrally acting α₂-adrenergic receptor agonist with a very narrow therapeutic index. Agonism at central α_2 receptors decreases sympathetic outflow, producing lethargy, bradycardia, hypotension, and apnea. Toxicity can develop after ingestion of only 1 pill or after sucking on or swallowing a discarded transdermal patch. Even a "used" transdermal patch might contain as much as one-third to one-half the original amount of drug.

Clinical and Laboratory Manifestations. The most common clinical manifestations of clonidine toxicity are lethargy, miosis, and bradycardia. Hypotension, respiratory depression, and apnea may be seen in severe cases. Very early after ingestion, patients may be hypertensive in the setting of agonism at peripheral α-receptors and resulting vasoconstriction. Symptoms develop relatively soon after ingestion and typically resolve within 24 hr. Serum clonidine concentrations are not readily available and are of no clinical value in the acute setting. Although signs of clinical toxicity are common after clonidine overdose, death from clonidine alone is extremely unusual.

Treatment. Given the potential for significant toxicity, most young children warrant referral to a healthcare facility for evaluation after unintentional ingestions of clonidine. Gastric decontamination is usually of minimal value because of the small quantities ingested and the rapid onset of serious symptoms. Aggressive supportive care is imperative and is the cornerstone of management. Naloxone, often in high doses, has shown variable efficacy in treating clonidine toxicity. Other potentially useful therapies include atropine, IV fluid boluses, and vasopressors. Symptomatic children should be admitted to the hospital for close cardiovascular and neurologic monitoring. Also, in a patient receiving chronic clonidine or guanfacine therapy, rapid discontinuation of the drug, or even missing 1 or 2 doses, could lead to potentially dangerous elevations in blood pressure.

Digoxin. Digoxin is a cardiac glycoside extracted from the leaves of *Digitalis lanata*. Other natural sources of cardiac glycosides include *Digitalis purpura* (foxglove), *Nerium oleander* (oleander), *Convallaria majalis* (lily of the valley), Siberian ginseng, and the *Bufo marinus* toad. Therapeutically, digoxin is used in the management of heart failure and some supraventricular tachydysrhythmias. Acute overdose can occur in the setting of dosing errors (especially in younger children), unintentional or intentional medication ingestion, or exposure to plant material containing digitalis glycosides. Regarding exposure to such plants, toxicity is unusual unless the poison is concentrated in the form of a tea. Chronic toxicity can result from alteration of the digoxin dose, alteration in digoxin clearance as a result of renal impairment, or drug interactions.

Pathophysiology. Digoxin blocks the sodium-potassium adenosine triphosphatase (Na^+,K^+-ATPase) pump, leading to intracellular loss of K^+ and gain of Na^+ and calcium (Ca^{2+}). This resulting rise in Ca^{2+} available to the contractile myocardium improves inotropy. An increase in myocardial automaticity leads to subsequent atrial, nodal, and ventricular ectopy. Digoxin also affects nodal conduction, leading to a prolonged refractory period, decreased sinus node firing, and slowed conduction through the atrioventricular node. Impaired Na^+/K^+ exchange results in dangerously high levels of serum K^+. Overall, digoxin overdose manifests as a combination of slowed or blocked conduction and increased ectopy.

Clinical and Laboratory Manifestations. Nausea and vomiting are common initial symptoms of acute digoxin toxicity, manifesting within 6 hr of overdose. Cardiovascular manifestations include bradycardia, heart block, and a wide variety of dysrhythmias. CNS manifestations consist of lethargy, confusion, and weakness. Chronic toxicity is more insidious and may also manifest as altered mental status and visual disturbances (rare).

Initial assessment should include an ECG, serum digoxin level, serum potassium, and kidney function tests. The serum digoxin level should be assessed at least 6 hr after ingestion and carefully interpreted in the setting of clinical symptoms, because the digoxin level alone does not entirely reflect the severity of intoxication. In acute ingestions, serum potassium is an independent marker of morbidity and mortality, with levels >5.5 mEq/L predicting poor outcomes. In chronic toxicity, serum K^+ concentration is less useful as a prognostic marker and may be altered from concomitant use of diuretics.

Digoxin has a very narrow therapeutic index. Therapeutic plasma digoxin concentrations are 0.5-2.0 ng/mL; a level >2 ng/mL is considered toxic and >6 ng/mL is considered potentially fatal (in chronic poisonings). As with all serum levels of intoxicants, one must be careful to interpret the number in the context of the scenario of the poisoning and the status of the patient. An acutely poisoned patient may have a very high serum level and minimal to no symptoms, whereas a patient with a chronic or acute on chronic poisoning will usually be sicker with a lower serum level.

Numerous drug interactions affect plasma digoxin concentrations. Medications known to increase serum digoxin concentrations include the macrolides, erythromycin and clarithromycin, spironolactone, verapamil, amiodarone, and itraconazole.

Treatment. Initial treatment includes good general supportive care and gastric decontamination with activated charcoal if the ingestion was recent. An antidote for digoxin, digoxin-specific antibody fragments (Fab: Digibind or DigiFab) is available (see Table 77.7). Fab fragments bind free digoxin in both the intravascular and the interstitial spaces to form a pharmacologically inactive complex that is subsequently eliminated renally. Indications for Fab fragments include life-threatening dysrhythmias, K^+ value >5-5.5 mEq/L, serum digoxin level >15 ng/mL at any time or >10 ng/mL 6 hr after ingestion, clinically significant hypotension or other CV instability, altered mental state, and renal failure. Atropine is potentially useful in managing symptomatic bradycardia. Although dogma states that patients on digoxin with severe hyperkalemia and QRS widening on the ECG should not receive calcium salts, this has not been supported in the literature. Once stabilized, consultation with a cardiologist is recommended in the management of patients receiving chronic digoxin therapy, because administration of Fab fragments can lead to recurrence of the patient's underlying dysrhythmias or dysfunction.

Iron. Historically, iron was a common cause of childhood poisoning deaths. However, preventive measures such as childproof packaging have significantly decreased the rates of serious iron toxicity in young children. Iron-containing products remain widely available, with the most potentially toxic being adult iron preparations and prenatal vitamins. The severity of an exposure is related to the amount of *elemental iron* ingested. Ferrous sulfate contains 20% elemental iron, ferrous gluconate 12%, and ferrous fumarate 33%. Multivitamin preparations and children's vitamins rarely contain enough elemental iron to cause significant toxicity. Furthermore, nonionic forms of iron, carbonyl iron and iron polysaccharide also do not cause significant toxicity.

Pathophysiology. Iron is directly corrosive to the GI mucosa, leading to hematemesis, melena, ulceration, infarction, and potential perforation. Early iron-induced hypotension is caused by massive volume losses, increased permeability of capillary membranes, and vasodilation mediated by free iron. Iron accumulates in tissues, including the Kupffer cells of the liver and myocardial cells, leading to hepatotoxicity, coagulopathy, and cardiac dysfunction. Metabolic acidosis develops in the setting of hypotension, hypovolemia, and iron's direct interference with oxidative phosphorylation and the Krebs cycle. Pediatric patients who ingest >40 mg/kg of elemental iron should be referred to medical care for evaluation, although moderate to severe toxicity is typically seen with ingestions >60 mg/kg.

Clinical and Laboratory Manifestations. Iron toxicity is described in 5 often-overlapping stages. The **1st stage**, 30 min to 6 hr after ingestion, consists of profuse vomiting and diarrhea (often bloody), abdominal pain, and significant volume losses leading to potential hypovolemic shock. Patients who do not develop GI symptoms within 6 hr of ingestion are unlikely to develop serious toxicity. The **2nd stage**, 6-24 hr after ingestion, is often referred to as the "quiescent phase" since the GI symptoms typically have resolved. However, careful clinical examination can reveal subtle signs of hypoperfusion, including tachycardia, pallor, and fatigue. During the **3rd stage**, 12-36 hr after ingestion, patients develop multisystem organ failure, shock, hepatic and cardiac dysfunction, acute lung injury, and profound metabolic acidosis. Death usually occurs during the 3rd stage. The **4th stage** (hepatic) results in fulminant liver failure and coagulopathy about 2-5 days after ingestion. The **5th stage**, 4-6 wk after ingestion, is marked by formation of strictures and signs of GI obstruction.

Symptomatic patients and patients with a large exposure by history should have serum iron levels drawn 4-6 hr after ingestion. Serum iron concentrations of <500 μg/dL 4-8 hr after ingestion suggest a low risk of significant toxicity, whereas concentrations of >500 μg/dL indicate that significant toxicity is likely. Additional laboratory evaluation in the ill patient should include arterial or venous blood gas, CBC, serum glucose level, liver transaminases, and coagulation parameters. Careful attention should be paid to the patient's hemodynamic status. An abdominal radiograph might reveal the presence of iron tablets, although not all formulations of iron are radiopaque.

Treatment. Close clinical monitoring, combined with aggressive supportive and symptomatic care, is essential to the management of iron poisoning. Activated charcoal does not adsorb iron, and WBI remains the decontamination strategy of choice. **Deferoxamine**, a specific chelator of iron, is the antidote for moderate to severe iron intoxication (see Table 77.7). Indications for deferoxamine treatment include a serum iron concentration >500 μg/dL or moderate to severe symptoms of toxicity (e.g., acidosis), regardless of serum iron concentration. Deferoxamine is preferably given by continuous IV infusion at 15 mg/kg/hr. Hypotension is a common side effect of deferoxamine infusion and is managed by slowing the rate of the infusion and administering fluids and vasopressors as needed. Prolonged deferoxamine infusion (>24 hr) has been associated with pulmonary toxicity (acute respiratory distress syndrome, ARDS) and *Yersinia* sepsis. The deferoxamine-iron complex can color the urine reddish ("vin rosé"), although the degree of this coloration should not guide therapy. Deferoxamine is typically continued until clinical symptoms and acidosis resolve. Consultation with a PCC or medical toxicologist can yield guidelines for discontinuing deferoxamine.

Oral Hypoglycemics

Oral medications used in the management of type 2 diabetes include sulfonylureas, biguanides (e.g., metformin), thiazolidinediones, and meglitinides. Of these, only the sulfonylureas and meglitinides have the potential to cause profound hypoglycemia in both diabetic and nondiabetic patients. These classes of medications are widely prescribed and thus readily available for both unintentional and intentional exposures. In toddlers, ingestion of a single sulfonylurea tablet can lead to significant toxicity.

Pathophysiology. Sulfonylureas work primarily by enhancing endogenous insulin secretion. In binding to the sulfonylurea receptor, these drugs induce closure of K^+ channels, leading to membrane depolarization, opening of Ca^{2+} channels, and stimulation of Ca^{2+}-mediated insulin release. Even in therapeutic use, the duration of hypoglycemic action can last up to 24 hr.

Clinical and Laboratory Manifestations. Hypoglycemia and symptoms associated with hypoglycemia are the primary clinical manifestations of sulfonylurea toxicity. These signs and symptoms can include diaphoresis, tachycardia, lethargy, irritability, coma, seizures, and even focal neurologic findings. As with other hyperinsulinemic states, sulfonylurea overdoses are associated with a nonketotic hypoglycemia. In the majority of patients, hypoglycemia develops within 6 hr of ingestion but can be delayed up to 16-18 hr after ingestion. Toddlers are particularly susceptible to hypoglycemia during an overnight fast.

Treatment. Patients with symptomatic hypoglycemia should be promptly treated with dextrose. In patients with mild symptoms, oral dextrose may be sufficient. However, patients with severe symptoms or profound hypoglycemia should be treated with a bolus of IV dextrose. Continuous dextrose infusions and repeated IV dextrose boluses should be avoided if possible, because this can stimulate further insulin release and lead to recurrent and prolonged hypoglycemia. Instead, the preferred antidote for persistent (i.e., requiring ≥2 doses of IV dextrose) sulfonylurea toxicity is **octreotide** (see Table 77.7). Octreotide is a somatostatin analog that inhibits insulin release. Octreotide is given intravenously (IV) or subcutaneously (SC), typically in doses of 1-2 μg/kg (50-100 μg in teens or adults) every 6-8 hr.

Given the potential for significant hypoglycemia, toddlers with witnessed or suspected sulfonylurea ingestions should be admitted to the hospital for serial glucose measurements for at least 12 hr, including an overnight fast. Patients of any age who develop hypoglycemia are also candidates for admission given the prolonged duration of hypoglycemic activity. Prophylactic IV dextrose infusions are not recommended because they can mask the symptoms of toxicity and stimulate further insulin secretion. Patients who require IV dextrose and/or octreotide should be monitored until they can demonstrate euglycemia for at least 8 hr off all therapy.

With the increasing numbers of adolescents with type 2 diabetes, pediatricians should be familiar with the toxic effects of **metformin** as well. Although metformin does not cause hypoglycemia, its association with lactic acidosis is well documented (metformin-associated lactic acidosis, MALA). This state typically arises after a large overdose in which the agent interferes with the liver's ability to clear lactic acid. Dangerously high serum lactate levels can result, leading to hemodynamic instability. Hemodialysis is usually the best option for patients with severe MALA.

Psychiatric Medications: Antidepressants

Selective serotonin reuptake inhibitors (SSRIs; e.g., fluoxetine, sertraline, paroxetine, citalopram) are the most commonly prescribed class of antidepressants. This trend largely results from their wide therapeutic index and more favorable side effect profile compared with older agents such as tricyclic antidepressants (TCAs; amitriptyline, clomipramine, desipramine, doxepin, nortriptyline, imipramine) and monoamine oxidase inhibitors (MAOIs). Other agents include the serotonin-norepinephrine reuptake inhibitors (SNRIs; e.g., venlafaxine) and atypical antidepressants (e.g., bupropion).

Tricyclic Antidepressants. Although now prescribed less often for depression, TCAs remain in use for a variety of other conditions, including chronic pain syndromes, enuresis, ADHD, and obsessive-compulsive disorder. TCAs can cause significant toxicity in children, even with ingestion of 1 or 2 pills (10-20 mg/kg).

Pathophysiology. TCAs achieve their desired antidepressant effects primarily through blockade of norepinephrine and serotonin reuptake. TCAs have complex interactions with other receptor types. Antagonism at muscarinic acetylcholine receptors leads to clinical features of the anticholinergic toxidrome. Antagonism at peripheral α-receptors leads to hypotension and syncope. Key to the toxicity of TCAs is their ability to block fast sodium channels, leading to impaired cardiac conduction and arrhythmias.

Clinical and Laboratory Manifestations. Cardiovascular and CNS symptoms dominate the clinical presentation of TCA toxicity. Symptoms typically develop within 1-2 hr of ingestion, and serious toxicity usually manifests within 6 hr of ingestion. Patients can have an extremely rapid progression from mild symptoms to life-threatening dysrhythmias. Patients often develop features of the **anticholinergic toxidrome**, including delirium, mydriasis, dry mucous membranes, tachycardia, hyperthermia, urinary retention, and slow GI motility. CNS toxicity can include lethargy, coma, myoclonic jerks, and seizures. Sinus tachycardia is the most common cardiovascular manifestation of toxicity; however, patients can also develop widening of the QRS complex, premature ventricular contractions, and ventricular dysrhythmias. Refractory hypotension is a poor prognostic indicator and is the most common cause of death in TCA overdose.

An ECG is a readily available bedside test that can help determine the diagnosis and prognosis of the TCA-poisoned patient (Fig. 77.2; see Table 77.6). A QRS duration >100 msec identifies patients who are at risk for seizures and cardiac arrhythmias. An R wave in lead aVR of ≥3 mm is also an independent predictor of toxicity. Both ECG parameters are superior to measured serum TCA concentrations for identifying patients at risk for serious toxicity, and obtaining levels is rarely helpful in management of the acutely ill patient.

Treatment. Initial attention should be directed to supporting vital functions, including airway and ventilation as needed. Gastric decontamination can be accomplished with activated charcoal in appropriate patients. Treating clinicians should obtain an ECG as soon as possible and follow serial ECGs to monitor for progression of toxicity. The 4 primary effects described next are seen at the bedside.

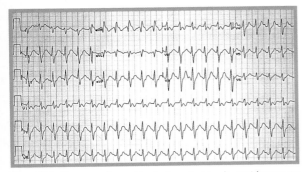

Fig. 77.2 Electrocardiographic findings in tricyclic antidepressant toxicity. Note the tachycardia, widened QRS interval (144 msec), and prominent R wave in lead aVR. These findings are consistent with blockade of fast sodium channels.

Table 77.11	Drugs Associated With the Serotonin Syndrome
DRUG TYPE	**DRUGS**
Selective serotonin reuptake inhibitors	Sertraline, fluoxetine, fluvoxamine, paroxetine, citalopram
Antidepressant drugs	Trazodone, nefazodone, buspirone, clomipramine, venlafaxine
Monoamine oxidase inhibitors	Phenelzine, moclobemide, clorgyline, isocarboxazid
Anticonvulsants	Valproate
Analgesics	Meperidine, fentanyl, tramadol, pentazocine
Antiemetic agents	Ondansetron, granisetron, metoclopramide
Antimigraine drugs	Sumatriptan
Bariatric medications	Sibutramine
Antibiotics	Linezolid (a monoamine oxidase inhibitor), ritonavir (through inhibition of cytochrome P450 enzyme isoform 3A4)
Nonprescription cough and cold remedies	Dextromethorphan
Drugs of abuse	Methylenedioxymethamphetamine (MDMA, "Ecstasy"), lysergic acid diethylamide (LSD), 5-methoxydiisopropyltryptamine ("foxy methoxy"), Syrian rue (contains harmine and harmaline, both monoamine oxidase inhibitors)
Dietary supplements and herbal products	Tryptophan, *Hypericum perforatum* (St. John's wort), *Panax ginseng* (ginseng)
Other	Lithium

From Boyer EW, Shannon M: The serotonin syndrome, *N Engl J Med* 352:1112–1120, 2005.

1. *Altered Mental State.* TCA-poisoned patients can become deeply comatose relatively quickly, so careful and prompt attention to the airway and placement of an endotracheal tube is of paramount importance. The airway should be secured before any GI decontamination efforts.

2. *Widened QRS on ECG.* TCAs, as well as with other agents (e.g., diphenhydramine, cocaine), will block the fast Na^+ channels on the myocardial cells, slowing the upstroke of the QRS complex. Because the effect on Na^+ channels is greatest within the 1st 6 hr, frequent ECGs (i.e., every 20-30 min) during this period are important. As the QRS approaches 160 msec, the risk of the patient developing monomorphic ventricular tachycardia rises to 30%. Sodium, usually in the form of sodium bicarbonate, is the antidote of choice. *Indications for sodium bicarbonate include a QRS duration ≥110 msec, ventricular dysrhythmias, and hypotension.* Multiple bolus doses of sodium bicarbonate, 1-2 mEq/kg each, may be needed to narrow the QRS to <110 msec. Some prefer then to place the patient on an infusion of sodium bicarbonate, but this may not be necessary if the QRS is carefully monitored after the initial doses and repeat bolus dosing is provided as needed during the 1st 6-12 hr. Hypertonic (3%) saline and/or lipid emulsion therapy may be beneficial in refractory cases.

3. *Hypotension.* A direct-acting vasopressor such as norepinephrine or epinephrine is the agent of choice. Boluses of IV crystalloid fluids should be used with caution to prevent fluid overload.

4. *Seizures.* Likely a result of the anticholinergic effects of TCAs, seizures are relatively common, typically brief, and should be treated with agents targeting the GABA-receptor complex in the brain. Benzodiazepines are the agent of choice.

Asymptomatic children should receive appropriate decontamination and have continuous cardiac monitoring and serial ECGs for at least 6 hr after exposure. If any manifestations of toxicity develop, the child should be admitted to a monitored setting. Children who remain completely asymptomatic with normal serial ECGs may be candidates for discharge after that monitoring period.

Selective Serotonin Reuptake Inhibitors. In overdose, SSRIs are considerably less toxic than TCAs. SSRIs are unlikely to cause significant toxicity in exploratory ingestions. Some data suggest that initiating SSRI therapy is associated with an increased risk of suicidal ideation and behavior (see Chapter 40).

Pathophysiology. SSRIs selectively block the reuptake of serotonin in the CNS. In contrast to TCAs and atypical antidepressants, SSRIs do not directly interact with other receptor types.

Clinical and Laboratory Manifestations. In overdose, the principal manifestations of toxicity are sedation and tachycardia. Cardiac conduction abnormalities (primarily QTc prolongation) and seizures have been described in significant overdoses, especially after ingestions of citalopram. An ECG should be part of the initial assessment after SSRI ingestion. Serum creatine kinase (CK) levels are almost always elevated in a patient with clinically significant **serotonin syndrome**. Although seen more often after therapeutic use or overdose of several serotonergic

agents in combination, the serotonin syndrome has also been described in ingestion of SSRIs alone (Table 77.11). Clinically, serotonin syndrome describes a spectrum of altered mental status, autonomic instability, fever, and neuromuscular hyperactivity (hyperreflexia, tremors, clonus in lower extremities > upper extremities). One or all of these signs may be present to varying degrees.

Treatment. Initial management includes a careful assessment for signs and symptoms of serotonin syndrome and an ECG. Most patients simply require supportive care and observation until their mental status improves and tachycardia, if present, resolves. Management of serotonin syndrome is directed by the severity of symptoms; possible therapeutic interventions include benzodiazepines in mild cases and intubation, sedation, and paralysis in patients with severe manifestations (e.g., significant hyperthermia). Because agonism at the 5-HT_{2A} serotonin receptor is thought to be primarily responsible for the development of serotonin syndrome, use of the 5-HT_{2A} receptor antagonist cyproheptadine may also be helpful. Cyproheptadine is only available in an oral form.

Atypical Antidepressants. The atypical antidepressant class includes agents such as venlafaxine and duloxetine (SNRIs), bupropion (dopamine, norepinephrine, and some serotonin reuptake blockade), and trazodone (serotonin reuptake blockade and peripheral α-receptor antagonism). The variable receptor affinities of these agents lead to some distinctions in their clinical manifestations and management.

Clinical and Laboratory Manifestations. In overdose, **venlafaxine** and other SNRIs have been associated with cardiac conduction defects, including QRS and QTc prolongation, and seizures. **Bupropion** warrants special consideration because it is one of the most common etiologies of toxicant-induced seizures in the United States. After ingestion of

SR or extended-release (ER) preparations, seizures can occur as late as 18-20 hr after ingestion. In addition, bupropion can cause tachycardia, agitation, and QRS and QTc prolongation. These cardiac effects are thought to result from a reduction in cardiac intracellular coupling caused by inhibition at gap junctions in the heart. Mortality results from not only status epilepticus but also the cardiac conduction disturbances causing ventricular tachycardia. Bupropion is of growing concern with the rising popularity of the drug, especially in the ER formulation. In addition to sedation and signs of serotonin excess, trazodone overdose may be associated with hypotension from blockade of peripheral α-receptors.

Treatment. Management is directed to clinical signs and symptoms. QRS and QTc interval prolongation after bupropion poisoning is typically resistant to the standard treatments of sodium bicarbonate and magnesium. Seizures are often brief and self-limited but can be treated with benzodiazepines if necessary. A patient poisoned with bupropion who shows unstable hemodynamics with prolonged ECG intervals or persistent seizure activity should receive Intralipid emulsion therapy. Because of the potential for delayed seizures, asymptomatic patients who have ingested an SR preparation of bupropion should be admitted to a monitored setting for at least 20-24 hr. Trazodone-associated hypotension typically responds to fluids, though it can require vasopressors in extreme cases.

Monoamine Oxidase Inhibitors. Although now rarely used therapeutically, MAOIs remain important agents given their potential for serious and delayed toxicity. Ingestions of only 1 or 2 pills (6 mg/kg) are associated with toxicity in children. Clinical manifestations initially include hypertension, hyperthermia, tachycardia, muscle rigidity, and seizures, followed up to 24 hr later by hemodynamic instability and CV collapse. *Any child who ingests a MAOI should be admitted to a monitored setting for at least 24 hr, regardless of symptoms.* Management includes blood pressure control, cooling and benzodiazepines for hyperthermia, serial monitoring of CK and renal function, and fluid and vasopressor therapy for hemodynamic instability.

Psychiatric Medications: Antipsychotics

Clinicians are increasingly prescribing antipsychotic medications in the pediatric population. Antipsychotics are usually classified as either typical or atypical. In general, typical agents are associated with more side effects and toxicity than the atypical agents.

Pathophysiology. Typical or "traditional" antipsychotics (haloperidol, droperidol, thioridazine, chlorpromazine, fluphenazine) are characterized by their antagonism at D_2 dopamine receptors. In therapeutic use, these agents are associated with extrapyramidal symptoms, tardive dyskinesia, and development of the **neuroleptic malignant syndrome (NMS)**. The *atypical* agents (aripiprazole, clozapine, quetiapine, risperidone, ziprasidone) were developed with relatively less dopamine (D_2-receptor) antagonism in the nigrostriatum in an effort to avoid these side effects and improve their efficacy in managing the "negative" symptoms of schizophrenia. Instead, these agents have complex and varied interactions with multiple receptor types, including α-receptors, serotonin receptors, muscarinic acetylcholine receptors, and histamine receptors.

Clinical and Laboratory Manifestations. Typical antipsychotic toxicity usually includes sedation, tachycardia, and QTc prolongation. Patients can present with acute dystonia, akathisia, and NMS, although these are seen less frequently in acute overdoses than in therapeutic use. The phenothiazines (e.g., thioridazine) can cause widening of the QRS interval from blockade of fast sodium channels. Clinically, NMS can be difficult to distinguish from serotonin syndrome.

Although the presentation of atypical antipsychotic toxicity can vary based on the receptor affinities of the specific agent, sedation, tachycardia, and QTc prolongation are common. Peripheral α-receptor blockade (e.g., with quetiapine) is associated with hypotension. In therapeutic use, clozapine is associated with agranulocytosis.

Diagnostic testing should include an ECG. Patients with hyperthermia or muscle rigidity should have a serum CK level sent to monitor for possible rhabdomyolysis. Antipsychotic levels are not readily available and are not helpful in managing acute poisoning.

Management. Initial management involves assessing and supporting vital functions. In some patients, CNS depression may be so profound

as to require intubation for airway control. Acute dystonia is treated with diphenhydramine and benztropine. Management of NMS includes conscientious supportive care, IV fluids, cooling, benzodiazepines, and bromocriptine or dantrolene in severe cases. QTc prolongation is managed with repletion of electrolytes (especially calcium, magnesium, and potassium), continuous cardiac monitoring, prevention of bradycardia (overdrive pacing, isoproterenol, atropine), and defibrillation if the patient develops torsades de pointes. Seizures typically are well controlled with benzodiazepines. Hypotension usually responds to boluses of IV fluids, although vasopressor therapy is necessary in some patients.

Household Products
Caustics

Caustics include acids and alkalis as well as a few common oxidizing agents (see Chapter 353). Strong acids and alkalis can produce severe injury even in small-volume ingestions.

Pathophysiology. **Alkalis** produce a *liquefaction necrosis*, allowing further tissue penetration of the toxin and setting the stage for possible perforation. **Acids** produce a *coagulative necrosis*, which limits further tissue penetration, although perforation can still occur. The severity of the corrosive injury depends on the pH and concentration of the product as well as the length of contact time with the product. Agents with a pH of <2 or >12 are most likely to produce significant injury.

Clinical Manifestations. Ingestion of caustic materials can produce injury to the oral mucosa, posterior pharynx, vocal cords, esophagus, and stomach. Patients can have significant esophageal injury even in the absence of visible oral burns. Symptoms include pain, drooling, vomiting, abdominal pain, and difficulty swallowing or refusal to swallow. Laryngeal injury can manifest as stridor and respiratory distress, necessitating intubation. In the most severe cases, patients can present in shock after perforation of a hollow viscus. Circumferential burns of the esophagus are likely to cause strictures when they heal, which can require repeated dilation or surgical correction and long-term follow-up for neoplastic changes in adulthood. Caustics on the skin or in the eye can cause significant tissue damage.

Treatment. Initial treatment of caustic exposures includes thorough removal of the product from the skin or eye by flushing with water. *Emesis and lavage are contraindicated.* Activated charcoal should not be used because it does not bind these agents and can predispose the patient to vomiting and subsequent aspiration. Stridor or other signs of respiratory distress should alert the provider to the need for a thorough evaluation of the airway for potential intubation or surgical airway management. Endoscopy can be performed within 12-24 hr of ingestion for prognostic and diagnostic purposes in symptomatic patients or those with suspected injury on the basis of history and known characteristics of the ingested product. Endoscopy's role is purely diagnostic. Whether the risks of the procedure are justified is debatable. Expectant management with a period of nothing by mouth (NPO) and proton pump inhibitor therapy is likely appropriate for the majority of patients *without* airway burns or signs of mediastinitis or peritonitis. Endoscopy is contraindicated in such patients, who instead require immediate surgical consultation. Corticosteroids or prophylactic antibiotics are not beneficial.

Pesticides

Cholinesterase-Inhibiting Insecticides. The most commonly used insecticides in agriculture are **organophosphates** and **carbamates**; both are inhibitors of cholinesterase enzymes: acetylcholinesterase (AChE), pseudocholinesterase, and erythrocyte AChE. Most pediatric poisonings occur as the result of unintentional exposure to insecticides in and around the home or farm. The chemical warfare weapons known as "nerve agents" are also organophosphate compounds with a similar mechanism of action but much greater potency.

Pathophysiology. Organophosphates and carbamates produce toxicity by binding to and inhibiting AChE, preventing the degradation of acetylcholine (ACh) and resulting in its accumulation at nerve synapses. If left untreated, organophosphates form an irreversible bond to AChE, permanently inactivating the enzyme. This process, called *aging*, occurs over a variable time period depending on the characteristics of the specific organophosphate. A period of weeks to months is required to regenerate inactivated enzymes. In contrast, carbamates form a temporary bond to the enzymes, typically allowing reactivation of AChE within 24 hr.

Clinical and Laboratory Manifestations. Clinical manifestations of organophosphate and carbamate toxicity relate to ACh accumulation at peripheral nicotinic and muscarinic synapses and in the CNS. Symptoms of carbamate toxicity are usually less severe than those seen with organophosphates. A commonly used mnemonic for the symptoms of cholinergic excess at muscarinic receptors is **DUMBBELS**: diarrhea/defecation, urination, miosis, bronchorrhea/bronchospasm, bradycardia, emesis, lacrimation, and salivation. Nicotinic signs and symptoms include muscle weakness, fasciculation, tremors, hypoventilation (diaphragm weakness), hypertension, tachycardia, and dysrhythmias. Severe manifestations include coma, seizures, shock, arrhythmias, and respiratory failure.

Diagnosis of poisoning is based primarily on history and physical exam findings. Red blood cell cholinesterase and pseudocholinesterase activity levels can be measured in the laboratory. These are only helpful when compared to the patient's known baseline. As such, these assessments are typically limited to farmworkers undergoing ongoing occupational surveillance.

Treatment. Basic decontamination should be performed, including washing all exposed skin with soap and water and immediately removing all exposed clothing. Activated charcoal is unlikely to be of benefit because these are liquids that are rapidly absorbed. Basic supportive care should be provided, including fluid and electrolyte replacement, intubation, and ventilation if necessary. The use of succinylcholine for rapid sequence intubation should be avoided because the same cholinesterase enzymes that are poisoned metabolize this neuromuscular blocking agent, leading to prolonged paralysis.

Two antidotes are useful in treating cholinesterase inhibitor poisoning: atropine and pralidoxime (see Table 77.7). **Atropine**, which antagonizes the muscarinic ACh receptor, is useful for both organophosphate and carbamate intoxication. Often, large doses of atropine must be administered by intermittent bolus or continuous infusion to control symptoms. Atropine dosing is primarily targeted to drying the respiratory secretions. **Pralidoxime** breaks the bond between the organophosphate and the enzyme, reactivating AChE. Pralidoxime is only effective if it is used before the bond ages and becomes permanent. Pralidoxime is not necessary for carbamate poisonings because the bond between the insecticide and the enzyme degrades spontaneously.

Without treatment, symptoms of organophosphate poisoning can persist for weeks, requiring continuous supportive care. Even with treatment, some patients develop a delayed polyneuropathy and a range of chronic neuropsychiatric symptoms.

Pyrethrins and Pyrethroids. Pyrethrins are derived from the chrysanthemum flower and along with pyrethroids, synthetic derivatives, are the most commonly used pesticides in the home. Although >1,000 pyrethrins and pyrethroids exist, <20 are available in the United States, with **permethrin** being the most common. Exposure to these compounds occurs by inhalation, dermal absorption, or ingestion. Ingestion is the predominant route and typically occurs by eating contaminated foods. Permethrin is also a prescribed medication for the treatment of scabies and lice.

Pathophysiology. Pyrethrins and pyrethroids prolong the open state of the voltage-gated Na⁺ channel conduction, which is the main mechanism resulting in its pesticide activity. Pyrethrins have minimal toxicity in mammals because of rapid metabolism, higher affinity for the insect Na⁺ channel, and decreased activity at higher temperatures seen in warm-blooded animals. Since pyrethroids were specifically manufactured to be more stable in the environment, they have a higher likelihood of toxicity.

Clinical and Laboratory Manifestations. Pyrethrin exposures can lead to allergic reactions ranging from dermatitis to urticaria to anaphylaxis. Acute exposure can result in headache, nausea, dizziness, tremors, ataxia, choreoathetosis, loss of consciousness, and seizures. The severity of the symptoms depends on the magnitude of the exposure. Reports of acute lung injury have also occurred after pyrethroid exposures, although this is likely from the other components of the insecticide, such as surfactants and solvents. Paresthesias limited to the cutaneous exposure area can also occur following a dermal exposure. Chronic exposures have not been shown to result in any clinical manifestations. Although one can test for urinary pyrethroid metabolites, this is only useful for monitoring occupational exposure and has no role for the acute exposure.

Treatment. Initial treatment should focus on decontamination, which involves removing all clothing and irrigation of exposed areas. Allergic reactions are treated the same as for antihistamines and corticosteroids. Systemic toxicity should be treated with excellent supportive care, using benzodiazepines for tremors and seizures.

Hydrocarbons

Hydrocarbons include a wide array of chemical substances found in thousands of commercial products. Specific characteristics of each product determine whether exposure will produce systemic toxicity, local toxicity, both, or neither. Nevertheless, aspiration of even small amounts of certain hydrocarbons can lead to serious, potentially life-threatening toxicity.

Pathophysiology. The most important manifestation of hydrocarbon toxicity is *aspiration pneumonitis* through inactivation of the type II pneumocytes and resulting in surfactant deficiency (see Chapter 425). Aspiration usually occurs during coughing and gagging at the time of ingestion or vomiting after the attempted ingestion of an aliphatic hydrocarbon. The propensity of a hydrocarbon to cause aspiration pneumonitis is inversely proportional to its viscosity, and directly proportional to its volatility. Compounds with low viscosity and high volatility, such as mineral spirits, naphtha, kerosene, gasoline, and lamp oil, spread rapidly across surfaces and cover large areas of the lungs when aspirated. Only small quantities (<1 mL) of such chemicals need be aspirated to produce significant injury. Pneumonitis does not result from dermal absorption of hydrocarbons or from ingestion in the absence of aspiration. Gasoline and kerosene are poorly absorbed, but they often cause considerable irritation of the GI mucosa as they pass through the intestines.

Certain hydrocarbons have unique toxicities and can cause symptoms after ingestion, inhalation, or dermal exposures. Several chlorinated solvents, most notably carbon tetrachloride, can produce hepatic toxicity. **Methylene chloride**, found in some paint removers, is metabolized to carbon monoxide. **Benzene** is known to cause cancer, most often acute myelogenous leukemia, after long-term exposure. Nitrobenzene, aniline, and related compounds can produce methemoglobinemia. A number of **volatile** hydrocarbons, including toluene, propellants, refrigerants, and volatile nitrites, are frequently abused by inhalation. Some of these substances, principally the **halogenated** hydrocarbons (which contain a chlorine, bromine, or fluorine), can sensitize the myocardium to the effects of endogenous catecholamines. This can result in dysrhythmias and "sudden sniffing death." Chronic abuse of these agents can lead to cerebral atrophy, neuropsychologic changes, peripheral neuropathy, and kidney disease (see Chapter 140).

Clinical and Laboratory Manifestations. Transient, mild CNS depression is common after hydrocarbon ingestion or inhalation. Aspiration is characterized by coughing, which usually is the 1st clinical finding. Chest radiographs may initially be normal, but they often show abnormalities within 6 hr of exposure in patients who have aspirated. Respiratory symptoms can remain mild or progress rapidly to acute respiratory distress syndrome (ARDS) and respiratory failure. Fever and leukocytosis are common accompanying signs in patients with pneumonitis and do not necessarily imply bacterial superinfection. Chest radiographs can remain abnormal long after the patient is clinically normal. Pneumatoceles can appear on the chest radiograph 2-3 wk after exposure.

After inhalational exposures to halogenated hydrocarbons, patients can present with ventricular dysrhythmias, often refractory to conventional management. Recurrent inhalation of the aromatic hydrocarbon **toluene** can lead to a type IV renal tubular acidosis.

Treatment. *Emesis and lavage are contraindicated given the risk of aspiration.* Activated charcoal is not useful because it does not bind the common hydrocarbons and can also induce vomiting. If hydrocarbon-induced pneumonitis develops, respiratory treatment is supportive (see

Chapter 425). Neither corticosteroids nor prophylactic antibiotics have shown any clear benefit. Standard mechanical ventilation, high-frequency ventilation, and extracorporeal membrane oxygenation (ECMO) have all been used to manage the respiratory failure and ARDS associated with severe hydrocarbon-induced pneumonitis.

Patients with dysrhythmias in the setting of halogenated hydrocarbon inhalation should be treated with β-blockers (usually esmolol) to block the effects of endogenous catecholamines on the sensitized myocardium.

Toxic Alcohols

Methanol is found in windshield washer fluids, deicers, paint removers, fuel additives, liquid fuel canisters, and industrial solvents. **Ethylene glycol** is found in antifreeze. Unintentional ingestion is the most common exposure in children, and small-volume ingestions of concentrated products can theoretically cause toxicity. The pathophysiology, acid-base derangements, and treatment of both chemicals are similar, although they differ in their primary end-organ toxicity. In both cases the metabolites of the parent compounds are responsible for the serious clinical effects that can follow exposure.

Isopropyl alcohol (rubbing alcohol), found in hand sanitizers, causes intoxication similar to that associated with ethanol but can also cause a hemorrhagic gastritis and myocardial depression in massive ingestions. Unlike ethylene glycol and methanol, isopropyl alcohol is metabolized to a ketone and does not cause a metabolic acidosis. Management is similar to that of ethanol ingestions (see Chapter 140) and is not further discussed here.

Methanol

Pathophysiology. Methanol is oxidized in the liver by alcohol dehydrogenase to formaldehyde, which is further oxidized to formic acid by aldehyde dehydrogenase. Toxicity is caused primarily by formic acid, which inhibits mitochondrial respiration.

Clinical and Laboratory Manifestations. Drowsiness, mild inebriation, nausea, and vomiting develop early after methanol ingestion. The onset of serious effects, including profound metabolic acidosis and visual disturbances, is often delayed up to 12-24 hr as the parent methanol undergoes metabolism to its toxic metabolites. This metabolism is further slowed if *ethanol* has also been ingested, since the liver will preferentially metabolize ethanol. Visual disturbances include blurred or cloudy vision, constricted visual fields, decreased acuity, and the "feeling of being in a snowstorm" and appear only after acidosis is well established. These visual defects may be reversible if treated early, but untreated can lead to permanent blindness. On examination, dilated pupils, retinal edema, and optic disc hyperemia may be noted. Initially, patients have an elevated osmolar gap, then develop an anion gap metabolic acidosis as the parent compound is metabolized to formic acid.

In young children, determining if a significant exposure has occurred is usually difficult based on history. Methanol blood levels are available at some laboratories and should be sent after a concerning exposure. If methanol blood levels are not readily available, estimation of an osmolar gap may be used as a surrogate marker, but a normal osmolar gap does not rule out ingestion of any alcohol. Serum osmolality is measured by the freezing-point depression method and compared with a calculated serum osmolarity.

Treatment. Treatment is as discussed for ethylene glycol toxicity.

Ethylene Glycol

Pathophysiology. Ethylene glycol is oxidized by alcohol dehydrogenase in the liver to glycolaldehyde, which is further converted to glycolic acid by aldehyde dehydrogenase. Glycolic acid is responsible for the metabolic acidosis and is further metabolized to glyoxylic and then to oxalic acid. Oxalic acid combines with serum and tissue calcium, forming calcium oxalate crystals that deposit throughout the body, especially in the renal parenchyma, leading to acute tubular necrosis.

Clinical and Laboratory Manifestations. Early symptoms include nausea, vomiting, CNS depression, and inebriation. Delayed manifestations include an anion gap metabolic acidosis, hypocalcemia, and acute kidney injury. Even later, patients can develop cranial nerve palsies.

Both ethylene glycol and methanol can produce profound, life threatening metabolic acidosis and acidemia, with measured serum

bicarbonates that may even be nondetectable. The onset of the acidosis is delayed up to 4-12 hr after ethylene glycol ingestion and may be delayed further with any concomitant ingestion of ethanol. Ethylene glycol blood concentrations are technically difficult to perform and are available only at some larger reference laboratories. In the absence of readily available ethylene glycol concentrations, calculation of the osmolar gap may be helpful as a surrogate marker.

Examination of the urine with a Wood lamp is neither sensitive nor specific for ethylene glycol ingestion. The earliest sign on a urinalysis of ethylene glycol poisoning is usually hematuria. Calcium oxalate crystals can be seen on urine microscopy but might not be evident early after exposure. Electrolytes (including calcium), acid-base status, kidney function, and ECG should be closely monitored in poisoned patients.

Treatment. Because methanol and ethylene glycol are rapidly absorbed, gastric decontamination is generally not of value. The classic antidote for methanol and ethylene glycol poisoning was ethanol, a preferential substrate for alcohol dehydrogenase, thus preventing the metabolism of parent compounds to toxic metabolites. **Fomepizole**, a potent competitive inhibitor of alcohol dehydrogenase, has almost entirely replaced ethanol because of its ease of administration, lack of CNS and metabolic effects, and overall excellent patient tolerability profile (see Table 77.7). A serum concentration must be interpreted along with the time removed from exposure. A patient with a methanol level of 20 mg/dL 24 hr after exposure had a much larger dose than a patient with the same level only 1 hr after ingestion. Classic indications for fomepizole include ethylene glycol or methanol level >20 mg/dL (assuming no ethanol is present), history of potentially toxic ingestion (e.g., any intentional overdose), or history of ingestion with evidence of acidosis. There are few disadvantages to giving the initial dose of fomepizole to patients with a concerning history of ingestion or lab findings, and given the dosing schedule of fomepizole (every 12 hr), this strategy buys the clinician time to confirm or exclude the diagnosis before giving a 2nd dose. Adjunctive therapy includes folate (methanol toxicity), pyridoxine (ethylene glycol toxicity), and sodium bicarbonate infusion for both (if acidemic). If a child has had an unintentional exposure and the alcohol level cannot be obtained, a reasonable approach is to follow serum chemistries every 4 hr until 12 hr after the exposure. If the bicarbonate level on the chemistry panel does not fall in that period, a toxic exposure is unlikely (assuming no ethanol is present).

Hemodialysis effectively removes ethylene glycol, methanol, and their metabolites (except calcium oxalate) and corrects acid-base and electrolyte disturbances. Fomepizole should be given both before and immediately after dialysis. Indications for dialysis include a methanol level >50 mg/dL, acidosis, severe electrolyte disturbances, and renal failure. However, in the absence of acidosis and kidney failure, even massive ethylene glycol ingestions have been managed without dialysis. Methanol, however, because its elimination in the setting of alcohol dehydrogenase inhibition is prolonged, often warrants dialysis to remove the parent compound. Therapy (fomepizole and/or dialysis) should be continued until ethylene glycol and methanol levels are <20 mg/dL. While the visual effects from methanol poisoning are usually permanent, the kidney injury from ethylene glycol injury is not. Patients requiring hemodialysis after ethylene glycol poisoning will almost always recover complete renal function within 2-6 wk. Consultation with a PCC, medical toxicologist, and nephrologist may be helpful in managing toxic alcohol ingestions.

Plants

Exposure to plants, both inside the home and outside in backyards and fields, is one of the most common causes of unintentional poisoning in children. Fortunately, the majority of ingestions of plant parts (leaves, seeds, flowers) result in either no toxicity or mild, self-limiting effects. However, ingestion of certain plants can lead to serious toxicity (Table 77.12).

The potential toxicity of a particular plant is highly variable, depending on the part of the plant involved (flowers are generally less toxic than the root or seed), the time of year, growing conditions, and the route of exposure. Assessment of the potential severity after an exposure is also complicated by the difficulty in properly identifying the plant. Many plants are known by several common names, which can

Table 77.12	Commonly Ingested Plants With Significant Toxic Potential	
PLANT	**SYMPTOMS**	**MANAGEMENT**
Autumn crocus (*Colchicum autumnale*)	Vomiting Diarrhea Initial leukocytosis followed by bone marrow failure Multisystem organ failure	Activated charcoal decontamination Aggressive fluid resuscitation and supportive care
Belladonna alkaloids: jimson weed (*Datura stramonium*) Belladonna ("deadly nightshade"; *Atropa belladonna*)	Anticholinergic toxidrome Seizures	Supportive care, benzodiazepines Consider physostigmine if patient is a threat to self or others; only use if no conduction delays on ECG
Cardiac glycoside–containing plants (foxglove, lily of the valley, oleander, yellow oleander, etc)	Nausea Vomiting Bradycardia Dysrhythmias (AV block, ventricular ectopy) Hyperkalemia	Digoxin-specific Fab fragments
Jequirity bean and other abrin-containing species (e.g., rosary pea, precatory bean)	Oral pain Vomiting Diarrhea Shock Hemolysis Renal failure	Supportive care, including aggressive volume resuscitation and correction of electrolyte abnormalities
Monkshood (*Aconitum* species)	Numbness and tingling of lips/tongue Vomiting Bradycardia	Atropine for bradycardia Supportive care
Oxalate-containing plants: *Philodendron*, *Dieffenbachia*, *Colocasia* ("elephant ear")	Local tissue injury Oral pain Vomiting	Supportive care, pain control
Poison hemlock (*Conium maculatum*)	Vomiting Agitation followed by CNS depression Paralysis Respiratory failure	Supportive care
Pokeweed	Hemorrhagic gastroenteritis Burning of mouth and throat	Supportive care
Rhododendron	Vomiting Diarrhea Bradycardia	Atropine for symptomatic bradycardia Supportive care
Tobacco	Vomiting Agitation Diaphoresis Fasciculations Seizures	Supportive care
Water hemlock (*Cicuta* species)	Abdominal pain Vomiting Delirium Seizures	Supportive care, including benzodiazepines for seizures
Yew (*Taxus* species)	GI symptoms QRS widening Hypotension CV collapse	Supportive care Atropine for bradycardia Sodium bicarbonate does not appear to be effective

AV, Atrioventricular; CNS, central nervous system; CV, cardiovascular; ECG, electrocardiogram; Fab, fragment, antigen binding; GI, gastrointestinal.

vary among communities. Poison control centers have access to professionals who can assist in properly identifying plants. They also are well versed in the common poisonous plants in their service area and the seasons when they are more abundant. For these reasons, consultation with the local PCC may be very helpful in the management of these ingestions.

For potentially toxic plant ingestions, consider decontamination with activated charcoal in patients who present within 1-2 hr of ingestion; otherwise, treatment is primarily supportive and based on symptoms. The most common manifestation of toxicity after plant ingestion is GI upset, which can be managed with antiemetics and fluid and electrolyte support. Table 77.12 outlines management strategies for a few specific toxicities.

Toxic Gases
Carbon Monoxide
Although many industrial and naturally occurring gases pose a health risk by inhalation, the most common gas involved in pediatric exposures is carbon monoxide. CO is a colorless, odorless gas produced during the combustion of any carbon-containing fuel; the less efficient the combustion, the greater the amount of CO produced. Wood-burning stoves, kerosene heaters, old furnaces, hot-water heaters, closed-space fires, and automobiles are a few of the potential sources of CO.

Pathophysiology. CO binds to hemoglobin with an affinity >200 times that of oxygen, forming carboxyhemoglobin (HbCO). In doing so, CO displaces oxygen and creates a conformational change in hemoglobin that impairs the delivery of oxygen to the tissues, leading to tissue hypoxia. HbCO levels are not well correlated with clinical signs of toxicity, likely because CO interacts with multiple proteins in addition to hemoglobin. CO binds to cytochrome oxidase, disrupting cellular respiration. CO displaces nitric oxide (NO) from proteins, allowing NO to bind with free radicals to form the toxic metabolite peroxynitrite, leading to lipid peroxidation and cellular damage. NO is also a potent vasodilator, in part responsible for clinical symptoms such as headache, syncope, and hypotension.

Clinical and Laboratory Manifestations. Early symptoms are nonspecific and include headache, malaise, nausea, and vomiting. These symptoms are often misdiagnosed as indicating flu or food poisoning. At higher exposure levels, patients can develop mental status changes, confusion, ataxia, syncope, tachycardia, and tachypnea. Severe poisoning is manifested by coma, seizures, myocardial ischemia, acidosis, cardiovascular collapse, and potentially death. Physical examination should focus on the cardiovascular and neurologic systems because these are the most detrimentally effected by CO. Emergency department evaluation should include arterial or venous blood gas analysis with HbCO determined by CO-oximetry, CK level in severely poisoned patients, pregnancy test, and ECG in any patient with cardiac symptoms.

Treatment. Prevention of CO poisoning is paramount and should involve educational initiatives and the use of home CO detectors. Treatment of CO poisoning focuses on the administration of 100% oxygen to enhance elimination of CO. In ambient air the average half-life of HbCO is 4-6 hr. This is dramatically reduced to 60-90 min by providing 100% oxygen at normal atmospheric pressures by non-rebreather face mask. Severely poisoned patients might benefit from **hyperbaric oxygen (HBO)**, which decreases the half-life of HbCO to 20-30 min and is thought also to decrease the risk of delayed neurologic sequelae. Although the clinical benefits and referral guidelines for HBO therapy remain controversial, frequently cited indications include syncope, coma, seizure, altered mental status, acute coronary syndrome, HbCO level >25%, abnormal cerebellar examination, and pregnancy. Consultation with a PCC, medical toxicologist, or HBO facility can assist clinicians in determining which patients could benefit from HBO therapy. Sequelae of CO poisoning include persistent and delayed cognitive and cerebellar effects. HBO advocates believe that the risk of such sequelae is minimized through the delivery of 100% oxygen at 3 atm of pressure. Patients typically receive oxygen, by non-rebreather mask or hyperbaric chamber, for 6-24 hr.

Hydrogen Cyanide

Pathophysiology. Cyanide inhibits cytochrome-*c* oxidase, part of the electron transport chain, interrupting cellular respiration and leading to profound tissue hypoxia. Patients may be exposed to hydrogen cyanide (HCN) gas in the workplace (manufacturing of synthetic fibers, nitriles, and plastics) or by smoke inhalation in a closed-space fire.

Clinical and Laboratory Manifestations. Onset of symptoms is rapid after a significant exposure. Clinical manifestations of toxicity include headache, agitation/confusion, sudden loss of consciousness, tachycardia, cardiac dysrhythmias, and metabolic acidosis. Cyanide levels can be measured in whole blood but are not readily available at most institutions. A severe lactic acidosis (lactate >10 mmol/L) in fire victims suggests cyanide toxicity. Impaired oxygen extraction by tissues is implied by elevated mixed-venous oxyhemoglobin saturation, another laboratory finding suggesting cyanide toxicity.

Treatment. Treatment includes removal from the source of exposure, rapid administration of high concentrations of oxygen, and antidotal therapy. The cyanide antidote kit (no longer manufactured) includes nitrites (amyl nitrite and sodium nitrite) used to produce methemoglobin, which then reacts with cyanide to form cyanomethemoglobin. The 3rd part of the kit is sodium thiosulfate, given to hasten the metabolism of cyanomethemoglobin to hemoglobin and the less toxic thiocyanate. In patients for whom induction of methemoglobinemia could produce more risk than benefit, the sodium thiosulfate component of the kit may be given alone.

The U.S. Food and Drug Administration (FDA) has approved **hydroxocobalamin** for use in known or suspected cyanide poisoning (see Table 77.7). This antidote reacts with cyanide to form the nontoxic cyanocobalamin (vitamin B_{12}), which is then excreted in urine. Side effects of hydroxocobalamin include red discoloration of the skin and urine, transient hypertension, and interference with colorimetric lab assays. *Hydroxocobalamin has an overall safety profile that appears superior to that of the cyanide antidote kit and thus is the preferred antidote for cyanide poisoning.*

Miscellaneous Toxic Agents Found in the Home
Nicotine-Containing Products

Nicotine poisoning has become increasingly common with the recent advent of vaporizer ("vaping") and e-cigarette devices. Although there are many nicotine-containing products (patches, gums, snuff, chewing tobacco, sprays, lozenges), tobacco cigarettes remain the main source of exposure. Prescription medications (varenicline and cytisine) are available that are partial nicotine receptor agonists. For children, some of the most concerning exposures are from the bottles of liquid nicotine used to refill vaping and e-cigarette devices. These bottles typically do not have childproof caps and contain a large amount of concentrated nicotine.

Pathophysiology. Nicotine acts on nicotinic ACh receptors in the nervous system, neuromuscular junctions, and adrenal medulla, stimulating neurotransmitter release. Nicotine's effects on the dopaminergic reward pathway play a significant role in its addictive properties. The effects of nicotine are dose dependent; at lower doses it primarily acts on the brain, causing stimulation. At higher doses, nicotine overstimulates receptors, leading to inhibition and resulting in neuromuscular and nervous system blockade.

Clinical and Laboratory Manifestations. Clinical effects of nicotine also depend on the dose. At low doses typically achieved through smoking, nicotine results in cognitive and mood enhancement, increased energy, and appetite suppression. At higher doses, significant toxicity follows a biphasic pattern, where cholinergic stimulation symptoms predominate and are later followed by inhibition. The first signs of nicotine poisoning are nausea, vomiting, diarrhea, and often muscle fasciculations. Tachycardia and hypertension occur initially, although in severe poisoning these progress to bradycardia, hypotension, coma, and respiratory muscle failure, which typically leads to death if not treated. Serum and urinary levels of nicotine and its metabolite cotinine can be obtained, but these rarely are available in real time and therefore have little effect on diagnosis and management.

Treatment. Treatment of nicotine poisoning focuses on maximizing symptomatic and supportive care. Aggressive airway management should be the priority, especially in severe poisonings, because death usually occurs from respiratory muscle paralysis. IV fluids with escalation to vasopressors should be used for hypotension. Seizures should be managed with benzodiazepines, barbiturates, or propofol.

Single-Use Detergent Sacs

Commonly known as laundry "pods" for clothing, these products resemble candy to many children. When bitten into, a relatively large dose of concentrated detergent is expelled under pressure onto the posterior pharynx and vocal cords. This can lead to stridor and other signs of respiratory distress. Occasionally, and for unknown reasons, these children may also develop altered mental status. Supportive care with attention to any airway and breathing issues is warranted. Admission to the hospital is often indicated. Importantly, these are not considered caustic ingestions; the pH of these products is in the neutral zone. As such, upper GI endoscopy is rarely indicated. Curiously, laundry detergent drank from a bottle is rarely of significant concern.

Electric Dishwasher Detergent

Especially when in the form of crystals, these products are highly alkaline (pH >13), and exposure by ingestion can cause significant burns to the vocal cords and GI tract. Admission for expectant management or upper GI endoscopy is usually indicated.

Magnets

Most foreign body ingestions pass through the GI tract once known to have passed into the stomach. However, ingestion of ≥2 magnets (unless very weak refrigerator-style magnets) cause concern for bowel obstruction and perforation. Admission for attempted retrieval by endoscopy or clearance by WBI should be considered.

Batteries

Any disk or button-style battery lodged in the esophagus or airway should be considered a true emergency warranting immediate referral to an endoscopist for removal. These batteries can cause necrosis of the tissues in which they are lodged by continued electrical discharge and leaking of their contents (the former is likely the primary method of injury). Mucosal contact for even 2 hr might induce necrosis. Once past the lower esophageal sphincter, button or even larger batteries (e.g., AA, AAA) can usually be allowed to pass through the GI tract with close follow-up.

Bibliography is available at Expert Consult.

Chapter **78**

Complementary Therapies and Integrative Medicine

Paula M. Gardiner and Caitlin M. Neri

第七十八章
辅助治疗

中文导读

本章介绍了一系列非药物治疗方法，我们将其称为辅助治疗或整合医学治疗，包括膳食补充疗法（如维生素、微量元素）、按摩疗法、身心疗法（如催眠、瑜伽、太极）、针刺疗法和大麻疗法等。同时，特别在膳食补充治疗项下，详细介绍了其安全性和有效性。此外，祈祷和医治仪式虽然也属于辅助治疗范畴，但不在本章讨论。

Integrative medicine focuses on promoting physical, mental, emotional, spiritual, social, and educational well-being in the context of a medical home in a healthy family and community. The foundations of integrative medicine are health-promoting practices such as optimal nutrition and dietary supplements to prevent deficiencies, avoidance of addictive substances (e.g., nicotine, illicit drugs), physical activity, adequate sleep, a healthy environment, and supportive social relationships. Evidence-based **complementary therapies** such as dietary supplements, massage, chiropractic, other forms of bodywork, yoga, meditation practices, hypnosis, guided imagery, biofeedback, and acupuncture may also be used. Although prayer and healing rituals are sometimes included under the rubric of complementary and integrative therapies, they are not covered in this chapter.

Not including multivitamins and mineral supplements such as iron and calcium, an estimated 10–40% of healthy children and >50% of children with chronic conditions use integrative medicine in the United States. The prevalence could be even higher because these treatments usually occur without disclosure to the children's primary care physician.

Common therapies include dietary supplements, deep breathing, guided imagery, mediation, biofeedback, hypnosis, yoga, acupuncture, massage, and aromatherapy.

Use of complementary therapies is most common among youth with chronic, incurable, or recurrent conditions such as cancer, depression and other mental health conditions, asthma, autism, headaches, abdominal pain, and other chronic painful conditions. Children's hospitals and pediatric subspecialty programs are increasingly offering integrative medicine strategies alongside traditional medicine, as part of the care of children in both inpatient and outpatient settings. In a 2014 survey the American Pain Society identified 48 pediatric chronic pain clinics, with most offering some type of integrative medicine or behavioral health strategies with conventional medicine. For example, integrative therapies are increasingly being used in pediatric chronic pain clinics to treat functional bowel disorders. Recent reviews include supplements (e.g., ginger, peppermint oil) and mind-body techniques (e.g., hypnotherapy, biofeedback, acupuncture/acupressure) with traditional medical management for these common pediatric conditions.

DIETARY SUPPLEMENTS

Under the 1994 U.S. Dietary Supplement Health and Education Act, a **dietary supplement** is a product taken by mouth that contains a *dietary ingredient* intended to supplement the diet. These may include vitamins, minerals, herbs or other botanicals, amino acids, and substances such as enzymes, organ tissues, glands, and metabolites. Dietary supplements are the most frequently used complementary therapies for children and adolescents (Table 78.1). Some uses are common and recommended, such as vitamin D supplements for breastfed infants and probiotics to prevent antibiotic-associated diarrhea, whereas other uses are more controversial, such as using herbal products to treat otitis media.

In the United States, dietary supplements do not undergo the same stringent evaluation and postmarketing surveillance as prescription medications. Although they may not claim to prevent or treat specific medical conditions, product labels may make *structure-function* claims. For example, a label may claim that a product "promotes a healthy immune system," but it may not claim to cure the common cold.

According to the 2012 National Health Interview Survey, 5% of U.S. children used non-vitamin/mineral dietary supplements. (e.g., fish oil, melatonin, prebiotics, probiotics) Use of dietary supplements is most common among children whose families have higher income and education and whose parents use supplements, among older children, and among those with chronic conditions.

Despite this widespread use, many patients and their parents who use dietary supplements do not talk with their physician about their use. Several guidelines have called for more complete dietary supplement history taking by healthcare professionals. The Joint Commission recommends that clinicians routinely ask patients about their use of dietary supplements and include this information as part of the medication reconciliation process.

DIETARY SUPPLEMENT SAFETY

Dietary supplements may have safety issues in children, but toxicity is much less common with nonprescription dietary supplements than with prescription medications (Table 78.2). Toxicity depends on dose, use of other therapies, and the child's underlying medical condition. Current use of a dietary supplement (e.g., ephedra for weight loss) may not reflect its traditional use (e.g., ephedra as a component of a traditional Chinese medicine tea in small doses to improve allergic or respiratory symptoms). Moreover, herbs that are apparently safe for most adults may be more hazardous in specific conditions (e.g., newborns, patients with impaired renal or hepatic function), under special circumstances (e.g., after organ transplantation or other surgery), or when combined with prescription medications. Some natural products are toxic in and of themselves. Even when a product is safe when used correctly, it can cause mild or severe toxicity when used incorrectly. For example, although peppermint is a commonly used and usually benign gastrointestinal spasmolytic included in after-dinner mints, it can exacerbate gastro-esophageal reflux.

Although there are good manufacturing practices for dietary supplements in the United States, dietary supplement labels might not accurately reflect the contents or concentrations of ingredients. Because of natural variability, variations of 10–1,000–fold have been reported for several popular herbs, even across lots produced by the same manufacturer. Herbal products may be contaminated with pesticides, microbial agents or products, or the wrong herb misidentified during harvesting. Products from developing countries (e.g., Ayurvedic products from South Asia) might contain toxic levels of mercury, cadmium, arsenic, or lead, either from unintentional contamination during manufacturing or from intentional additions by producers who believe that these metals have therapeutic value. Approximately 30–40% of Asian patent medicines include potent pharmaceuticals, such as analgesics, antibiotics, hypoglycemic agents, or corticosteroids; typically the labels for these products are not written in English and do not note the inclusion of pharmaceutical agents. Even conventional mineral supplements, such as calcium, have been contaminated with lead or had significant problems with product variability.

Many families use supplements concurrently with medications, posing hazards of interactions (Table 78.3). Using the same principles of drug-drug interactions can help determine if a supplement-drug interaction is a concern. For example, St. John's wort induces CYP3A4 activity of the cytochrome P450 enzyme system and thus can enhance elimination of most drugs that use this pathway, including digoxin, cyclosporine, protease inhibitors, oral contraceptives, and numerous antibiotics, leading to subtherapeutic serum levels.

DIETARY SUPPLEMENT EFFICACY

Evidence about the effectiveness of dietary supplements to prevent or treat pediatric problems is mixed, depending on the product used and condition treated. Some herbal products may be helpful adjunctive treatments for common childhood problems; some herbs have proved helpful for colic (fennel and the combination of chamomile, fennel, vervain, licorice, and balm mint), nausea (ginger), irritable bowel syndrome (peppermint), and diarrhea (probiotics).

MASSAGE AND CHIROPRACTIC

Massage is usually provided at home by parents and in clinical settings by professional massage therapists, physical therapists, and nurses. **Infant massage** is routinely provided in many neonatal intensive care units to promote growth and development in preterm infants. Massage also has been demonstrated to be beneficial for pediatric patients with asthma, insomnia, colic, cystic fibrosis, or juvenile arthritis and patients undergoing cancer therapy. **Massage therapy** is generally safe. Professional massage practice is regulated by state government and may be in the form of a license, registration, or certification. More than 40 states license massage therapists, with licensure being the strictest form of

Table 78.1	Commonly Used Dietary Supplements in Pediatrics	
PRODUCT	**USES**
VITAMINS	
B$_2$ (riboflavin)	Migraine headache prophylaxis
B$_6$ (pyridoxine)	Pyridoxine-dependent epilepsy; neuropathy; nausea associated with pregnancy
B$_9$ (folate)	Prevention of neural tube defects
D	Prevention of rickets; treatment of vitamin D deficiencies
Multivitamins	General health promotion
MINERALS	
Iodine (salt)	Prevent goiter and mental retardation
Iron	Prevent and treat iron-deficiency anemia
Magnesium	Constipation, asthma, migraine prevention
Zinc	Diarrhea in nutrient-poor populations
HERBS	
Aloe vera	Mild burns
Chamomile	Mild sedative, dyspepsia
Echinacea	Prevention of upper respiratory infections
Ginger	Nausea
Lavender (aromatherapy)	Mild sedative
Peppermint	Irritable bowel syndrome
Tea tree oil	Antibacterial (acne remedies), pediculicide (lice)
OTHER	
Melatonin	Insomnia
Omega-3 fatty acids	ADHD, allergies, inflammation, anxiety and mood disorders
Probiotics	Antibiotic-associated diarrhea; *Clostridium difficile*–associated diarrhea; constipation; irritable bowel syndrome; pouchitis; inflammatory bowel disorders

ADHD, Attention-deficit/hyperactivity disorder.

Table 78.2	Clinical Toxicity of Selected Herbs		
COMMON NAME	**BOTANICAL NAME**	**THERAPEUTIC USES**	**POTENTIAL TOXICITY**
Aconite (monkshood, wolfsbane)	*Aconitum* spp.	Sedative, analgesic, antihypertensive	Cardiac arrhythmias
Aloe	*Aloe* spp.	Burns, skin diseases	Nephritis, GI upset
Betel nut	*Areca catechu*	Mood elevation	Bronchoconstriction, oral cancers
Bloodroot	*Sanguinaria canadensis*	Emetic, cathartic, eczema	GI upset, vertigo, visual disturbances
Chaparral (greasewood)	*Larrea tridentata*	Aging, free radical scavenging	Hepatitis
Compound Q	*Trichosanthes kirilowii*	Anthelmintic, cathartic	Diarrhea, hypoglycemia, CNS toxicity
Dandelion	*Taraxacum officinale*	Diuretic, heartburn remedy	Anaphylaxis
Figwort (xuan shen)	*Scrophularia* spp.	Antiinflammatory, antibacterial	Cardiac stimulation
Ginseng	*Panax quinquefolium*	Antihypertensive, aphrodisiac, stimulant, mood elevation, digestive aid	Ginseng abuse syndrome
Goldenseal	*Hydrastis canadensis*	Digestive aid, mucolytic, anti-infective	Uterine, cardiac stimulation; GI upset, leukopenia
Hellebore	*Veratrum* spp.	Antihypertensive	Vomiting, bradycardia, hypotension
Hyssop	*Hyssopus officinalis*	Asthma, mucolytic	Seizures
Juniper	*Juniperus communis*	Hallucinogen	GI upset, seizures, renal injury, hypotension, bradycardia
Kava kava	*Piper methysticum*	Sedative	Inebriation
Kombucha		Stimulant	Metabolic acidosis, hepatotoxicity, death
Licorice	*Glycyrrhiza* spp.	Indigestion	Mineralocorticoid effects
Lily of the valley	*Convallaria* spp.	Cardiotonic	GI (nausea, vomiting), cardiac arrhythmias
Linn (willow)	*Salix caprea*	Purgative	Hemolysis with glucose-6-phosphate dehydrogenase deficiency
Lobelia (Indian tobacco)	*Lobelia* spp.	Stimulant	Nicotine intoxication
Ma Huang	*Ephedra sinica*	Stimulant	Sympathetic crisis, especially with monamine oxidase inhibitors
Mandrake	*Mandragora officinarum*	Hallucinogen	Anticholinergic syndrome
Mormon tea	*Ephedra nevadensis*	Stimulant, asthma, antipyretic	Hypertension, sympathomimetic
Nutmeg	*Myristica fragrans*	Hallucinogen, abortifacient	Hallucinations, GI upset
Oleander	*Nerium oleander*	Cardiac stimulant	Cardiac arrhythmias
Passionflower	*Passiflora caeruliea*	Hallucinogen	Hallucinations, seizures, hypotension
Periwinkle	*Vinca* spp.	Antiinflammatory, diabetes	Alopecia, seizures, hepatotoxicity
Pokeweed	*Phytolacca* spp.	Arthritis, chronic pain	GI upset, seizures, death
Sabah	*Sauropus androgynus*	Weight loss, vision	Pulmonary injury
Sage	*Salvia* spp.	CNS stimulant	Seizures
Snakeroot	*Rauwolfia serpentina*	Sedative, antihypertensive	Bradycardia, coma
Squill	*Urginea maritima*	Arthritis, cardiac stimulant	Seizures, arrhythmias, death
Thorn apple (jimsonweed)	*Datura stramonium*	Hallucinations	Anticholinergic
Tonka bean	*Dipteryx odorata*	Anticoagulant	Bleeding diathesis
Valerian root	*Valeriana* spp.	Sedative	Sedation, obtundation
Wild (squirting) cucumber	*Ecballium elaterium*	Constipation, antiinflammatory, rheumatic disease	Airway obstruction
Wormwood (mugwort)	*Artemisia* spp.	Stimulant, hallucinogen	Hallucinations, seizures, uterine stimulation
Yohimbine	*Corynanthe yohimbe*	Aphrodisiac, stimulant	Hypertension, sympathetic crisis

CNS, Central nervous system; GI, gastrointestinal.
From Kingston RL, Foley C: Herbal, traditional, and alternative medicines. In *Haddad and Winchester's clinical management of poisoning and drug overdose*, ed 4, Philadelphia, 2007, Saunders/Elsevier, p 1081.

Table 78.3	Common Herbal Dietary Supplement (HDS)–Drug Interactions	
HDS	**DRUGS**	**POTENTIAL CONSEQUENCES/REACTIONS**
Aloe vera	Glibenclamide (glyburide)	↑ Oral aloe vera gel can cause additive glycemic-lowering effects when taken concurrently with a hypoglycemic agent.
Bitter orange	Phenelzine	↑ Risk of hypertensive crisis
Garlic	Ritonavir Saquinavir	↓ Effect of ritonavir ↓ Effect of saquinavir
Licorice	Warfarin	↑ Risk of bleeding
Grapefruit	Calcium channel blockers	Grapefruit juice has been found to increase bioavailability of certain drugs by inhibition of cytochrome P450 (CYP) 3A4 isozyme in liver and gut wall.
Melatonin	Zolpidem	↑ Sedative effects
Valerian	Alprazolam, phenobarbital	↑ Central nervous system depression
Goldenseal	Inhibition of CYP2D6 and CYP3A4	May affect approximately 50% of common pharmaceutical agents
St. John's wort	Cyclosporine, tacrolimus, warfarin, protease inhibitors, digoxin, theophylline, venlafaxine, oral contraceptives	May decrease drug effectiveness

↓, Decreasing; ↑, increasing.

regulation, making it illegal for any nonlicensed professional to practice massage therapy.

Chiropractic healthcare deals with the diagnosis, treatment, and prevention of disorders of the neuromusculoskeletal system and their effects on general health. Currently, >60,000 chiropractors have licensure in the United States, with licensure in all 50 states. Most medical insurance companies cover chiropractic funding. Children and families seek chiropractic care for common childhood conditions such as asthma, infantile colic, nocturnal enuresis, constipation, and headache. A recent consensus update on chiropractic care in children overall found limited support in a small number of high-quality studies for effectiveness of chiropractic care for such common childhood conditions. With respect to safety, the evidence is also limited; however, published cases of serious adverse events in infants and children receiving chiropractic care are rare. If children and families are seeking chiropractic care, it is appropriately done in collaboration with the child's pediatric primary care provider to ensure patient safety.

MIND-BODY THERAPIES

Mind-body therapies such as slow, deep breathing, meditation, guided imagery, biofeedback, hypnosis, tai chi, and yoga are also frequently used complementary therapies in pediatrics. These practices can be learned informally through books, YouTube videos, compact discs, digital video discs, smartphone apps, or classes, as well as in therapeutic sessions with health professionals, such as psychologists and social workers (Table 78.4). Substantial research suggests that such practices can aid in reducing anxiety, insomnia, and stress-related conditions, including migraine headaches and functional abdominal pain. These therapies can also help patients struggling with chronic pain.

ACUPUNCTURE

Modern acupuncture incorporates treatment traditions from China, Japan, Korea, France, and other countries. In the United States, acupuncturists are licensed to practice in 45 states. Acupuncture can be delivered to pediatric patients in hospital and clinic settings to treat a variety of ailments. Acupuncture is particularly useful for children experiencing pain, and acupuncture services are offered alongside conventional medicine and psychology by >50% of North American academic pediatric chronic pain programs. The technique that has undergone most scientific study involves penetrating the skin with thin, solid, metallic needles manipulated by hand or by electrical stimulation. Variants include rubbing (**shiatsu**), heat (**moxibustion**), lasers, magnets, pressure (**acupressure**), or electrical currents.

Although pediatric patients may be averse to needles, when approached in a developmentally appropriate way by an acupuncturist trained in

Table 78.4	Commonly Used Mind-Body Practices in Pediatrics
PRACTICE	**USES**
Biofeedback	Preventing migraine headaches; reducing stress and anxiety; encopresis/constipation treatment; treatment of stress incontinence; neurofeedback is experimental for ADHD.
Deep breathing	Relaxation; stress management
Guided imagery	Stress management; anxiety reduction; pain relief
Hypnosis	Correcting habit disorders; preventing headaches; managing pain
Meditation	Stress management; improving concentration
Tai chi	Improving balance, coordination, concentration, and discipline
Yoga	Improving balance, coordination, and concentration

ADHD, Attention-deficit/hyperactivity disorder.

pediatrics, children are often amenable to acupuncture and report that it is helpful. Acupuncture can offer significant benefits in the treatment of recurrent headache, anxiety, back and other types of pain, depression, abdominal pain, and nausea. As with any needle therapy, infections and bleeding are rare but can occur, and more serious complications, such as pneumothorax, occur in <1 in 30,000 treatments.

CANNABIS

Because marijuana has been legalized in many states for both recreational (adult) use and medical use, caregivers and families have inquired about the potential health benefits of cannabis for both children and adults. At this time, no pediatric studies support any health benefit of cannabis for children. Furthermore, significant safety concerns remain, since detrimental effects of marijuana on the developing brain have been documented.

It is important to note that in some children with severe refractory **epilepsy**, oral **cannabidiol**, a nonpsychoactive component in marijuana, has provided improvement in seizure control. On a case-by-case basis, this is a reasonable consideration for families facing this rare and difficult challenge, and additional research is required in this area, especially since the purity and regulation of marijuana and its commercially available component products are variable. Most of the recent pediatric literature on cannabis describes an increase in accidental ingestions in young children, presumably in association with the increase in products now available for adult use; this is an additional safety risk for pediatricians to consider.

Internet Resources

American Academy of Pediatrics Section on Integrative Medicine: http://www2.aap.org/sections/chim/default.cfm.

Academic Consortium Integrative Medicine and Health: http://www.imconsortium.org/.

National Institutes of Health, National Center for Complementary and Integrative Health: https://nccih.nih.gov/.

American Pain Society; pediatric chronic pain programs by state: http://americanpainsociety.org/uploads/get-involved/PediatricPainClinicList_Update_2.10.15.pdf.

Bibliography is available at Expert Consult.

Emergency Medicine and Critical Care

急危重症

Chapter 79
Emergency Medical Services for Children

Joseph L. Wright and Steven E. Krug

第七十九章
儿科急诊医疗服务

中文导读

本章主要介绍了初级医疗医师和办公室日常工作的准备、儿科院前急救以及急诊室。初级医疗医师和办公室日常工作的准备具体阐述了人员培训和继续教育、规程、复苏器械及转运；儿科院前急救描述了如何启动急诊医疗服务（EMS）系统、施救者的能力及目的地；急诊室部分介绍了如何进行灾难准备。本章还详细阐述了危重或受伤患儿在院间的转运，其中包括交流和调度中心、医疗总负责医师、转运队伍、救护车和转运飞机、转运生理学、安全、以家庭为中心的护理、涉及医院的责任及宣传教育，还详细阐述了儿科急诊医疗服务的结果和风险调整及适用于发展中国家的原则。

The overwhelming majority of the 27 million children who present annually for emergency care in the United States are seen at community hospital emergency departments (EDs). Visits to children's hospital EDs account for just 10% of initial emergency care encounters. This distribution suggests that the greatest opportunity to optimize care for acutely ill or injured pediatric patients, on a population basis, occurs broadly as part of a systems-based approach to emergency services, an approach that incorporates the unique needs of children at every level. Conceptually, emergency medical services for children are characterized by an integrated, continuum-of-care model (Fig. 79.1). The model is designed such that patient care flows seamlessly from the primary care medical home through transport and on to hospital-based definitive care. It includes the following 5 principal domains of activity:

1. Prevention, primary and secondary
2. Out-of-hospital care, both emergency response and prehospital transport
3. Hospital-based care: ED and inpatient, including critical care
4. Interfacility transport, as necessary, for definitive or pediatric medical and surgical subspecialty care (see Chapter 79.1)
5. Rehabilitation

The federal **Emergency Medical Services for Children (EMSC)** program of the Health Resources and Services Administration's Maternal and Child Health Bureau has stewarded improvements in the care of children in the context of the continuum-of-care model. The programmatic mission of the EMSC program is as follows:

- To ensure state-of-the-art emergency medical care for ill or injured children and adolescents of all ages.
- To ensure that pediatric services are well integrated into an emergency medical services (EMS) system and backed by optimal resources.
- To ensure that the entire spectrum of emergency services—including primary prevention of illness and injury, acute care, and rehabilitation—is provided to infants, children, adolescents, and young adults.

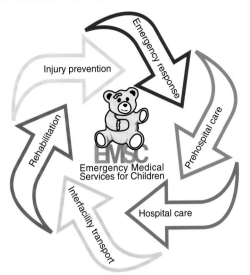

Fig. 79.1 The emergency medical services for children (EMSC) continuum of care. Seriously ill and injured children interface with a large number of healthcare personnel as they move through the EMSC system.

PRIMARY CARE PHYSICIAN AND OFFICE PREPAREDNESS

The primary care physician (PCP) has multiple important roles in the EMS system. Through anticipatory guidance, the PCP can help shape the attitudes, knowledge, and behaviors of parent and child, with the primary goal of preventing acute medical events, such as injury and status asthmaticus. The point-of-care initiation for many acute problems is often the PCP office. From the standpoint of personnel, equipment, training, and protocols, the PCP office setting must be adequately prepared to initially manage acute and emergency exacerbations of common pediatric conditions, such as respiratory distress and seizures. Furthermore, on rare occasion, the PCP office environment may be confronted with a child in clinical extremis who requires resuscitative intervention and stabilization. It is therefore incumbent on the PCP not only to ensure access to EMS, that is, 911 system activation, but also to ensure that there is adequate, on-site psychomotor skill preparation to deal with such an emergency. **Office preparedness** requires training and continuing education for staff members, protocols for emergency intervention, ready availability of appropriate resuscitation drugs and equipment, and knowledge of local EMS resources and ED capabilities. PCPs can also play a pivotal role in informing and advocating for pediatric emergency and disaster readiness in local EMS agencies, schools and childcare programs, and community hospitals; this is particularly important in rural communities.

Staff Training and Continuing Education

It is a reasonable expectation that all office staff, including receptionists and medical assistants, be trained in cardiopulmonary resuscitation (CPR) with their certification maintained annually. Nurses and physicians should also have training in a systematic approach to pediatric resuscitation. Core knowledge may be obtained through standardized courses in **advanced life support (ALS)** offered by national medical associations and professional organizations. Frequent practice and timely recertification is important for knowledge retention and skill maintenance. Examples include the Pediatric Advanced Life Support (PALS) and Pediatric Emergency Assessment, Recognition and Stabilization (PEARS) courses sponsored by the American Heart Association (AHA), the Advanced Pediatric Life Support (APLS) course sponsored by the American Academy of Pediatrics (AAP) and American College of Emergency Physicians (ACEP), and the Emergency Nurses Pediatric Course (ENPC) sponsored by the Emergency Nurses Association (ENA).

Protocols

Standardized protocols for telephone triage of seriously ill or injured children are essential. When a child's clinical status is in question and prehospital care is available, ambulance transport in the care of trained personnel is always preferable to transport by other means (e.g., private vehicle). This obviates the potentially serious medical consequences of relying on unskilled and distraught parents without the ability to provide even **basic life support (BLS)** measures to an unstable child during transport to an ED. Practitioners can work with their local pediatric emergency care resource center (e.g., children's hospital, academic medical center, trauma center) to develop and maintain written protocols for office-based management of a range of conditions, including anaphylaxis, cardiopulmonary arrest, head trauma, ingestions, shock, status asthmaticus, status epilepticus, and upper airway obstruction. Regular practice using mock code scenarios improves office-based practitioner and office staff confidence and self-efficacy in managing these problems.

Resuscitation Equipment

Availability of necessary equipment is a vital part of an emergency response. Every physician's office should have essential resuscitation equipment and medications packaged in a pediatric resuscitation cart or kit (Table 79.1). This cart or kit should be checked on a regular basis and kept in an accessible location known to all office staff. Outdated medication, a laryngoscope with a failed light source, or an empty oxygen tank represents a potential catastrophe in a resuscitation scenario. Such an incident can be easily avoided if an equipment checklist and regular maintenance schedule are implemented. A pediatric kit that includes posters, laminated cards, or a color-coded length-based resuscitation tape specifying emergency drug doses and equipment size are invaluable in avoiding critical therapeutic errors during resuscitation.

To facilitate emergency response when a child needs rapid intervention in the office, all personnel should have designated roles. Organizing a "code team" within the office ensures that necessary equipment is made available to the physician in charge, that an appropriate medical record detailing all interventions and the child's response is generated, and that the 911 call for EMS response or a transport team is made in a timely fashion.

Transport

Once the child has been stabilized, a decision must be made on how best to transport a child to a facility capable of providing definitive care. If a child has required airway or cardiovascular support, has altered mental state or unstable vital signs, or has significant potential to deteriorate en route, it is not appropriate to send the child via privately owned vehicle, regardless of proximity to a hospital. Even when an ambulance is called, it is the PCP's responsibility to initiate essential life support measures and to attempt to stabilize the child before transport.

In metropolitan centers with numerous public and private ambulance agencies, the PCP must be knowledgeable about the level of service provided by each. The availability of BLS vs ALS services, the configuration of the transport team, and pediatric expertise vary greatly among agencies and across jurisdictions. BLS services provide basic support of airway, breathing, and circulation, whereas ALS units are capable of providing resuscitation drugs and procedural interventions as well. Some communities may have only BLS services available, whereas others may have a 2-tiered system, providing both BLS and ALS. It may be appropriate to consider **medical air transport** when definitive or specialized care is not available within an immediate community or when ground transport times are prolonged. In that case, initial transport via ground to an appropriate helicopter landing zone or a local hospital for interval stabilization may be undertaken, pending arrival of the air transport team. Independent of whether a child is to be transported by air or ground, copies of the pertinent medical records and any imaging or laboratory studies should be sent with the patient, and a call made to the physicians at the receiving facility to alert them to the referral and any treatments administered. Such notification is not merely a courtesy; direct physician-to-physician communication is essential to ensure

Table 79.1	Recommended Drugs and Equipment for Pediatric Office Emergencies

DRUGS/EQUIPMENT	PRIORITY
DRUGS	
Oxygen	E
Albuterol for inhalation	E
Epinephrine (1 : 1,000 [1 mg/mL])	E
Activated charcoal	S
Antibiotics	S
Anticonvulsants (diazepam/lorazepam)	S
Corticosteroids (parenteral/oral)	S
Dextrose (25%)	S
Diphenhydramine (parenteral, 50 mg/mL)	S
Epinephrine (1 : 10,000 [0.1 mg/mL])	S
Atropine sulfate (0.1 mg/mL)	S
Naloxone (0.4 mg/mL)	S
Sodium bicarbonate (4.2%)	S
INTRAVENOUS FLUIDS	
Normal saline (0.9 NS) or lactated Ringer solution (500 mL bags)	S
5% dextrose, 0.45 NS (500 mL bags)	S
EQUIPMENT FOR AIRWAY MANAGEMENT	
Oxygen and delivery system	E
Bag-valve-mask (450 mL and 1,000 mL)	E
Clear oxygen masks, breather and non-rebreather, with reservoirs (infant, child, adult)	E
Suction device, tonsil tip, bulb syringe	E
Nebulizer (or metered-dose inhaler with spacer/mask)	E
Oropharyngeal airways (sizes 00-5)	E
Pulse oximeter	E
Nasopharyngeal airways (sizes 12-30F)	S
Magill forceps (pediatric, adult)	S
Suction catheters (sizes 5-16F and Yankauer suction tip)	S
Nasogastric tubes (sizes 6-14F)	S
Laryngoscope handle (pediatric, adult) with extra batteries, bulbs	S
Laryngoscope blades (straight 0-2; curved 2-3)	S
Endotracheal tubes (uncuffed 2.5-5.5; cuffed 6.0-8.0)	S
Stylets (pediatric, adult)	S
Esophageal intubation detector or end-tidal carbon dioxide detector	S
EQUIPMENT FOR VASCULAR ACCESS AND FLUID MANAGEMENT	
Butterfly needles (19-25 gauge)	S
Catheter-over-needle device (14-24 gauge)	S
Arm boards, tape, tourniquet	S
Intraosseous needles (16 and 18 gauge)	S
Intravenous tubing, micro-drip	S
MISCELLANEOUS EQUIPMENT AND SUPPLIES	
Color-coded tape or preprinted drug doses	E
Cardiac arrest board/backboard	E
Sphygmomanometer (infant, child, adult, thigh cuffs)	E
Splints, sterile dressings	E
Automated external defibrillator with pediatric capabilities	S
Spot glucose test	S
Stiff neck collars (small/large)	S
Heating source (overhead warmer/infrared lamp)	S

E, Essential; S, strongly suggested.
From Frush K, American Academy of Pediatrics, Committee on Pediatric Emergency Medicine: Policy statement-preparation for emergencies in the offices of pediatricians and pediatric primary care providers, *Pediatrics* 120:200–212, 2007. Reaffirmed *Pediatrics* 128:e748, 2011.

adequate transmission of patient care information, to allow mobilization of necessary resources in the ED, and to redirect the transport if the emergency physician believes that the child would be more optimally treated at a facility with specialized services.

PEDIATRIC PREHOSPITAL CARE

Prehospital care refers to emergency assistance rendered by trained emergency medical personnel before a child reaches a treating medical facility. The goals of prehospital care are to further minimize systemic insult or injury through a series of well-defined and appropriate interventions and to embrace principles that ensure patient safety. Most U.S. communities have a formalized EMS system; the organizational structure and nature of emergency medical response depend greatly on local demographics and population base. EMS may be provided by volunteers or career professionals working in a fire department–based or independent 3rd service response system. Key points to recognize in negotiation of the juncture between the community physician and the local EMS system include access to the system, provider capability, and destination determination.

Access to the EMS System

Virtually all Americans have access to the 911 telephone service that provides direct access to a dispatcher who coordinates police, fire, and EMS responses. Some communities have an enhanced telephone 911 system, in which the location of the caller is automatically provided to the dispatcher, permitting emergency response even if the caller, such as a young child, cannot give an address. The extent of medical training for these dispatchers varies among communities, as do the protocols by which they assign an emergency response level (BLS vs ALS). In some smaller communities, no coordinated dispatch exists, and emergency medical calls are handled by the local law enforcement agency.

When activating the 911 system, the physician must make clear to the dispatcher the nature of the medical emergency and the condition of the child. In many communities, emergency medical dispatchers are trained to ask a series of questions per protocol that determines the appropriate level of provider to be sent.

Provider Capability

There are many levels of training for prehospital EMS providers, ranging from individuals capable of providing only first aid to those trained and licensed to provide ALS. All EMS personnel, whether basic *emergency medical technicians* (EMTs) or paramedics, receive some training in pediatric emergencies; however, pediatric cases constitute approximately 10% of all EMS transports.

First responders may be law enforcement officers or firefighters, who are dispatched to provide emergency medical assistance, or bystanders. Public safety personnel have a minimum of 40 hr of training in first aid and CPR. Their role is to provide rapid response and stabilization pending the arrival of more highly trained personnel. In some smaller communities, this may be the only prehospital emergency medical response available.

In the United States the bulk of emergency medical response is provided by EMTs, who may be volunteers or paid professionals. Basic EMTs may staff an ambulance after undergoing a training program of approximately 100 hr. They are licensed to provide BLS services but may receive further training in some jurisdictions to expand their scope of practice to include intravenous catheter placement and fluid administration, management of airway adjuncts, and use of an automated external defibrillator (AED).

Paramedics, or EMT-Ps, represent the highest level of EMT response, with medical training and supervised field experience of approximately 1,000 hr. Paramedic skills include advanced airway management, including endotracheal intubation; placement of peripheral, central, or intraosseous lines; intravenous administration of drugs; administration of nebulized aerosols; needle thoracostomy; and cardioversion and defibrillation. These professionals provide ALS services, functioning out of an ambulance equipped as a mobile intensive care unit (ICU). In the joint policy statement *Equipment for Ground Ambulances*, the AAP, ACEP, American College of Surgeons Committee on Trauma, EMSC, ENA, National Association of EMS Physicians, and National Association of EMS Officials have published guideline standards for essential ambulance equipment, medications, and supplies necessary to provide BLS and ALS care across the age spectrum. This essential equipment list represents one of the reference standards that the federal

EMSC program has adopted as a performance measure for state-level operational readiness to care for children in an EMS system.

Both basic EMTs and paramedics function under the delegated licensing authority of a supervisory EMS medical director. This physician oversight of prehospital practice is broadly characterized under the umbrella term *medical control*. **Direct**, or online, **medical control** refers to medical direction either at the scene or in real time via voice or video transmission. **Indirect**, or **offline**, **medical control** refers to the administering of medical direction before and after the provision of care. Offline activities, such as provider education and training, protocol development, and medical leadership of quality assurance/quality improvement programs, represent areas in need of greater pediatric input. As a measure of the degree to which EMSC permanence is being established in state EMS systems, the federal EMSC program has required demonstration of participation in online and offline medical direction activities for pediatric patients and the presence of an EMSC advisory committee at the state level. These advisory bodies are well positioned to support EMS agencies in their pediatric readiness as well as provide a forum for the active engagement of pediatric care experts at a system level.

Destination Determination

The destination to which a pediatric patient is transported may be defined by parental preference, provider preference, or jurisdictional protocol, which is typically predicated on field assessment of anatomic and physiologic criteria and, in the case of trauma, mechanism of injury. In communities served by an organized trauma or regionalized EMS system that incorporates pediatric designation based on objectively verified hospital capabilities, seriously ill or injured children may be triaged by protocol to the highest-level center reachable within a reasonable amount of time. The mantra is to deliver the child to the *right care in the right time*, even if it requires bypassing closer hospitals. An exception is the child in full cardiorespiratory arrest, for whom expeditious transport to the nearest facility is always warranted.

Regionalization in the context of EMS is defined as a geographically organized system of services that ensures access to care at a level appropriate to patient needs while maintaining efficient use of available resources. This system concept is especially germane in the care of children, given the relative scarcity of facilities capable of managing the full range and scope of pediatric conditions (Fig. 79.2). Regionalized systems of care coordinated with emergency medical dispatch, field triage, and EMS transport have demonstrated efficacy in improving outcomes for **pediatric trauma** patients, especially for younger children and for children with isolated head injury. Emerging evidence also suggests a similar benefit conferred to children in **shock** identified in the field who are preferentially transported to hospital EDs with documented pediatric ALS capability. The existence of statewide or regional standardized systems that formally recognize hospitals able to stabilize and/or manage pediatric medical emergencies is another federal EMSC performance measure against which operational capacity to provide optimal pediatric emergency care in the United States is currently being evaluated.

In communities that do not have a hospital with the equipment and personnel resources to provide definitive pediatric inpatient care, **interfacility transport** of a child to a regional center should be undertaken after initial stabilization (see Chapter 79.1).

THE EMERGENCY DEPARTMENT

The ability of hospital EDs to respond to the emergency care of children varies and depends on a number of factors in addition to availability of equipment and supplies. Training, awareness, and experience of the staff as well as access to pediatricians and medical and surgical subspecialists also play a key role. The majority of children who require emergency care are evaluated in community hospitals by physicians, nurses, and other healthcare providers with variable degrees of pediatric training and experience. Although children account for approximately 25% of all ED visits, only a fraction of these encounters represent true emergencies. Because the volume of critical pediatric cases is low, emergency physicians and nurses working in lower-volume community hospital EDs often have limited opportunity to reinforce their knowledge and skills in the assessment of ill or injured children and in pediatric resuscitation. Indeed, 50% of U.S. hospital EDs provide care for <10 children per day. General pediatricians from the community or pediatric hospitalists may be consulted when a seriously ill or injured child presents to the ED, and they should have a structured approach to the initial evaluation and treatment of an unstable child of any age, regardless of the underlying diagnosis. *Early recognition of life-threatening abnormalities in oxygenation, ventilation, perfusion, and central nervous system function and rapid intervention to correct those abnormalities are key to successful resuscitation and stabilization of the pediatric patient.*

The **National Pediatric Readiness Project (NPRP)**, a 2013-2014 survey of pediatric readiness in U.S. EDs, found higher readiness levels (as measured by compliance with published guidelines) in larger-volume EDs and in hospitals with a physician and/or nurse pediatric emergency care coordinator. Further information about the NPRP, including data by state, may be found on the website of the EMSC Innovation and Improvement Center, https://emscimprovement.center/.

Baseline readiness standards must be met by all EDs that care for children, to ensure that children receive the best emergency care possible. Specific recommendations on equipment, supplies, and medications for the ED are listed and updates available on the AAP website. Table 79.2 lists sample policies, procedures, and protocols specifically addressing the needs of children in the ED.

The way the family supports the child during a crisis, and consequently how the family is supported in the ED when caring for the child, are critical to patient recovery, family satisfaction, and mitigation of behavioral and mental health impact. Commitment to patient- and family-centered care in the ED ensures that the patient and family experience guides the practice of culturally sensitive care and promotes patient dignity, comfort, and autonomy. In the ED setting, particular issues, such as family presence, deserve specific attention. Surveys of parents have indicated that most want to be with their child during invasive procedures and even during resuscitation. Allowing their presence has been shown to reduce parental and patient anxiety and does not interfere with procedure performance. Patient- and family-centered care practices are also strongly associated with improved care quality and patient safety.

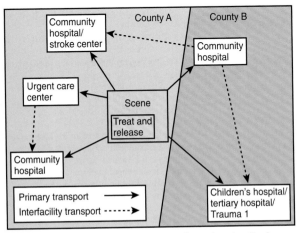

Fig. 79.2 Transport options within a coordinated, regionalized emergency medical services system model. The objective is to ensure access to definitive care at a level appropriate to meet patient needs. *Solid arrows,* Primary transport; *dotted arrows,* interfacility transport. (*Adapted from Institute of Medicine, Committee on the Future of Emergency Care in the U.S. Health System: Hospital-based emergency care: at the breaking point, Washington, DC, 2006, National Academies Press.*)

Disaster Preparedness

Throughout a catastrophic event, natural or human-made, several unique factors place children at disproportionate, increased risk. During an

Table 79.2	Guidelines for Pediatric-Specific Policies, Procedures, and Protocols for the Emergency Department (ED)

Illness and injury triage
Pediatric patient assessment and reassessment
Documentation of pediatric vital signs, abnormal vital signs, and actions to be taken for abnormal vital signs
Immunization assessment and management of the underimmunized patient
Sedation and analgesia for procedures, including medical imaging
Consent (including situations in which a parent is not immediately available)
Social and mental health issues
Physical or chemical restraint of patients
Child maltreatment (physical and sexual abuse, sexual assault, and neglect) mandated reporting criteria, requirements, and processes
Death of the child in the ED
Do-not-resuscitate orders
Family-centered care, including:
1. Involving families in patient care decision-making and in medication safety processes.
2. Family presence during all aspects of emergency care, including resuscitation.
3. Education of the patient, family, and regular caregivers.
4. Discharge planning and instruction.
5. Bereavement counseling.

Communication with patient's medical home or primary healthcare provider
Medical imaging policies that address age- or weight-appropriate dosing for children receiving studies that impart ionizing radiation, consistent with ALARA (as low as reasonably achievable) principles
All-hazard disaster preparedness plan that addresses the following pediatric issues:
  a. Availability of medications, vaccines, equipment, and appropriately trained providers for children in disasters.
  b. Pediatric surge capacity for both injured and noninjured children.
  c. Decontamination, isolation, and quarantine of families and children of all ages.
  d. A plan that minimizes parent-child separation and includes system tracking of pediatric patients, allowing for the timely reunification of separated children with their families.
  e. Access to specific medical and mental health therapies, as well as social services, for children in the event of a disaster.
  f. Disaster drills, which should include a pediatric mass casualty incident at least every 2 yr.
  g. Care of children with special healthcare needs.
  h. A plan that includes evacuation of pediatric units and pediatric specialty units.

Adapted from Gausche-Hill M, Krug SE, American Academy of Pediatrics Committee on Pediatric Emergency Medicine; American College of Emergency Physicians Pediatric Committee; Emergency Nurses Association Pediatric Committee: Joint policy statement—guidelines for care of children in the emergency department, *Pediatrics* 124:1233–1243, 2009. Reaffirmed *Pediatrics* 132:e281, 2013.

average workday, an estimated 69 million U.S. children are separated from their families, in schools and childcare centers, where mass casualty events can easily occur. This separation adds the additional challenge of safe and timely reunification of children with family during or after an incident. Furthermore, in the event of a biologic, chemical, or radionuclear attack, unique anatomic, developmental, and physiologic features make children especially vulnerable to absorption, ingestion, or inhalation of toxic agents and related morbidity and mortality.

Similar to day-to-day emergency readiness for ill and injured children, pediatric disaster preparedness requires advance considerations of the unique vulnerabilities and needs of children within planning, and exercises, at local, state, regional and even national levels. Pediatric planning considerations include training of first responders and other care providers, patient triage, decontamination, surge capacity and capability, medical countermeasures (medications, vaccines, equipment, supplies), evacuation, transport, sheltering, and family reunification. Planning for children should occur at all levels of the healthcare system, including the medical home, urgent care centers, EMS, acute care hospitals, pediatric tertiary hospitals, alternate care facilities, and rehabilitation services. While the NPRP noted meaningful progress in day-to-day emergency readiness, no improvement was found in disaster preparations, with less than half of U.S. hospitals having a disaster plan addressing the needs of children. Beyond acute medical treatment needs, pediatric planning must also consider the typically broad mental and behavioral health impact disasters have on children and families. Pediatric plans must also be in place for locations where children congregate, such as schools and childcare.

At the local, state, or regional level, healthcare coalitions have been identified as an optimal forum for disaster planning; core participants should include local or state public health departments, emergency management authorities, EMS agencies, and hospitals. Many other key stakeholder groups should be involved in coalition planning, such as healthcare professional organizations. To ensure that the needs of children are effectively considered, it has been recommended that disaster planning at all levels include pediatric subject matter experts. Pediatricians are an obvious source for this expertise and are also uniquely positioned to educate families about emergency readiness, particularly families with special needs children. The presence of an intact medical home during a public health emergency, and after a disaster has occurred,

will contribute enormously toward response, recovery, and community resiliency. Lastly, community practice and healthcare system readiness and resiliency begin with *personal readiness planning* engaged by healthcare providers and support staff.

The AAP's Children and Disasters website* contains toolkits, checklists and other resources pertinent to pediatric readiness within the community, schools, the medical home, and hospitals; educational materials are also available for families. Reliable information and excellent disaster readiness resources may also located on the websites of the EMSC Innovation and Improvement Center (https://emscimprovement.center), U.S. Centers for Disease Control and Prevention (https://emergency.cdc.gov), U.S. Department of Health and Human Services (https://www.phe.gov/preparedness/Pages/default.aspx), and U.S. Federal Emergency Management Agency (https://www.fema.gov).

Bibliography is available at Expert Consult.

79.1 Interfacility Transport of the Seriously Ill or Injured Pediatric Patient
Corina Noje and Bruce L. Klein

Patients often seek treatment at facilities that lack sufficient expertise to treat their conditions, necessitating transfer to more appropriate specialty centers. This is especially pronounced in pediatrics. Emergency medical services (EMS) providers or parents usually take children to local emergency departments (EDs) first, where their conditions and physiologic stabilities are assessed. Although bringing a child directly to the local ED may be proper logistically, local EDs can be less than ideal for pediatric emergencies. Children account for 27% of all ED visits, but only 6% of EDs have all the necessary supplies for pediatric emergencies. Also, general EDs are less likely to have pediatric expertise or policies in place for the care of children. Outcomes for critically ill children treated in pediatric intensive care units (PICUs) are better than for those treated in adult ICUs. When pediatric critical care is

*https://www.aap.org/en-us/advocacy-and-policy/aap-health-initiatives/Children-and-Disasters/Pages/default.aspx.

required, transport to a regional PICU is indicated. In addition, often the type of subspecialty care needed (e.g., pediatric orthopedics) is available only at the pediatric center.

Pediatric transport medicine consists of the interfacility transfer of infants, children, and adolescents from community facilities to pediatric centers that can provide the needed level of expertise. Transport is performed by professionals proficient in pediatric transport using age-equipped ground, rotorcraft, or fixed-wing ambulances. Pediatric transport medicine is a multidisciplinary field comprising pediatric critical care and **pediatric emergency medicine** (PEM) physicians (and, sometimes for very young infants, neonatologists); nurses, respiratory therapists, and paramedics with advanced training for pediatric transport; and communications specialists. The goal is to deliver quality pediatric care to the region's children, while optimizing the use of regional resources. For the individual child, the aim is to stabilize and, when appropriate, begin treating as soon as possible—that is, at the local ED and during transport, well before arrival at the referral center.

Models for pediatric transport services vary depending on the needs and available resources in a geographic region, but all should have certain basic components: a network of community hospitals and regional pediatric centers; an established communications and dispatch system that easily facilitates transfer to the pediatric center; ground and/or air ambulances; medical and nursing leadership from pediatric critical care or PEM (or neonatology); experienced pediatric **medical control physicians** (**MCPs**); a multidisciplinary team of pediatric transport professionals specially trained to provide the appropriate level of care required during transport; operational and clinical policies and procedures that guarantee safe, state-of-the-art, and timely pediatric critical care transport; and a database for quality and performance assessment.

COMMUNICATIONS AND DISPATCH CENTER

Communications are one of the most vital components of a regional transport system. Treating a critically ill or injured child is generally an uncommon event for most community physicians. Therefore, they need to know *whom*, *how*, and *when* to call for assistance in the stabilization and transfer of a pediatric patient. The communications and dispatch center provides a single telephone number for such calls.

The communications and dispatch center coordinates communications among the outlying facility, receiving unit, MCP, transport team, and other consultants. This center may be part of a hospital unit (e.g., ED, PICU), self-contained in a single institution (e.g., Emergency Communications and Information Center), or based offsite as a freestanding center coordinating communications and dispatch for multiple transport programs.

Staffing varies depending on the type of center. On-duty nurses or physicians may receive calls at unit-based models with low volumes. In contrast, dedicated communications specialists usually staff self-contained or freestanding centers, which tend to be busier. The communications specialist has numerous responsibilities, including answering the referring physician's call promptly; documenting essential patient demographic information; arranging for immediate consultation with the MCP; dispatching the transport team to the referring facility expeditiously; updating the referring facility with any changes in the arrival time; and coordinating medical control and other necessary transport-related calls. The transport team must be equipped with a cellular telephone or radio for immediate contact with the receiving and referring facilities. Furthermore, with advances in technology and wireless communication systems, **telemedicine**—either *interactive* (synchronous) or *store and forward* (asynchronous)—is being used during pediatric transport; certain programs have incorporated it into their routine transport operations.

MEDICAL CONTROL PHYSICIAN

The MCP is involved in the clinical care and safe transport of the patient from the time of referral through arrival at the receiving hospital unit. The MCP's oversight increases once the transport team arrives at the referring facility. The MCP should have expertise in pediatric critical care or PEM (or sometimes neonatology). Besides having the knowledge required to stabilize a critically ill or injured child, the MCP must be

familiar with the transport environment; the transport team members' resources and capabilities; the program's policies and procedures; and the region's geography, medical resources, and regulations regarding interhospital transport. The MCP must possess good interpersonal and communication skills and must be able to maintain collegiality with the referring hospital's staff during a potentially difficult and stressful situation.

Once a transport call is received, the MCP must be immediately available to confer with the referring physician. Although the MCP may have other responsibilities, these transport responsibilities take priority in order to avoid undue delays when transferring a critically ill child. Often the MCP recommends further testing or therapeutic interventions that can be delivered by the referring hospital before the transport team arrives. The MCP may seek additional guidance from other specialists, as necessary. Because the child's condition may change rapidly, the MCP must remain ready to give additional advice. All conversations and recommendations regarding the care of the patient should be documented. Some centers record these conversations.

After discussion with the referring physician—and when warranted, with the transport staff—the MCP determines the best team composition and vehicle for transport. The MCP usually does not accompany the team but remains available, by phone or radio (and sometimes through telemedicine), to supervise care.

TRANSPORT TEAM

Transport team composition varies among programs—and sometimes within an individual program. The team's composition is based on a variety of factors, including the child's age; the severity of the illness or injury; the distance to the referring facility; the transport vehicle used; the team members' advanced practice scope and abilities; the referrer's (reasonable or unreasonable) insistence that a physician be present; the program's historical professional makeup; and the region's staffing regulations. Team members are generally physicians, nurse practitioners, nurses, respiratory therapists, and paramedics who have expertise in pediatric critical care, PEM, or neonatology (in some cases), as well as advanced education and training in those cognitive and procedural areas important for pediatric critical care transport. There is a lower incidence of transport-related morbidity for critically ill and injured children transported by pediatric specialty teams than for those transported by generalist teams. Nevertheless, in-transit critical events occur in almost 1 in 8 pediatric critical care transports.

Various scoring systems have been developed to predict the need for a physician during transport. It seems that a team member's training, experience, and skill in treating critically ill patients are more important considerations than that team member's professional degree. Team members must understand basic pediatric pathophysiology and collectively must be able to assess and monitor a critically ill or injured child; manage the airway and provide respiratory support; obtain vascular access; perform point-of-care testing; and administer medications typically used in pediatric critical care transport. They must be familiar with the physiologic alterations as well as practical difficulties of the transport environment and, importantly, must be comfortable working in an out-of-hospital setting. Physicians are less often deployed on transport teams in part because of the advanced training that other healthcare professionals on the transport team receive.

The transport team should have a designated team leader who, in addition to the team leader's many other responsibilities, interacts with the MCP during the transport. Once the team arrives at the referring facility, the team should reassess the child's condition, review all of the pertinent diagnostic studies and therapies, and discuss the situation with the referring staff and parents. If the patient's condition has changed significantly, the team leader may need to contact the MCP for additional advice. Otherwise, the team leader should generally notify the MCP before starting to bring the child to the receiving facility. Any care delivered by the team during transport should be documented, and copies of all medical records—including laboratory data, radiographs, and scans—should accompany the child to the pediatric center. The receiving unit must be updated prior to arrival so it can finalize preparations for the patient.

GROUND VS AIR AMBULANCE

Transport vehicle options include ground, rotorcraft, and fixed-wing ambulances. Vehicle selection depends on the child's emergency needs; transport team's capabilities; any out-of-ordinary staffing or equipment requirements (e.g., for extracorporeal membrane oxygenation, inhaled nitric oxide or heliox); referring facility's abilities; distance; terrain; traffic patterns; ground or air ambulance availability; helicopter landing pad or airport access; weather conditions; and expense.

The transport vehicle must be equipped with electrical power, oxygen, and suction and must have sufficient space for the equipment and supplies that the team brings along—stretcher or isolette, monitor, ventilator, oxygen tank(s), medication pack(s), infusion pumps, and more. Compared with helicopters, ambulances are more spacious and able to carry more weight, so they can accommodate larger teams and more equipment. Another advantage of ground ambulance transport is the ability to stop en route if the patient's condition deteriorates; this may facilitate the performance of certain interventions, such as intubation.

An airplane may be able to fly to an area when distance (>150 miles), altitude, or weather precludes helicopter use. However, the use of an airplane necessitates several ambulance transfers, with their attendant delays and potential complications. There also are delays when the plane must fly from a remote base to the program's jurisdiction.

TRANSPORT PHYSIOLOGY

When possible, the transport team tries to provide the same care during transport as the patient would receive in the specialty center. This can be difficult, however, because of limitations in personnel, equipment, and space, as well as other environmental challenges.

The team and child are subjected to variable intensities of background noise and vibration while traveling in the vehicle cabin. **Noise** can impair the team's ability to auscultate breath sounds and heart sounds or accurately measure the blood pressure manually—another reason for monitoring vital signs mechanically and relying on other assessment modalities, such as the level of mentation, skin color, and capillary refill. For rotor transports in particular, the crew and patient should wear helmets or headphones (or another wearable noise attenuator, such as MiniMuffs, Natus Medical, San Carlos, CA) to mitigate noise. **Motion** and **vibration** are additional transport hazards and can lead to increased metabolic rate, shortness of breath, and fatigue in the patient, as well as motion sickness in the patient and staff.

On fixed-wing or certain rotary-wing transports, the patient may suffer adverse physiologic effects from **altitude**. With increasing altitude, the barometric (atmospheric) pressure decreases and gas expands to occupy a greater volume due to decreased pressure exerted on it. Therefore, as barometric pressure drops with altitude, the partial pressures of inspired oxygen (PiO_2) and, consequently, arterial oxygen (PaO_2) decrease, as does the arterial oxygen-hemoglobin saturation (SpO_2). For example, at 8,000 feet—an elevation at which unpressurized airplanes may fly, as well as the effective cabin altitude for many pressurized airplanes flying at 35,000 to 40,000 feet—the barometric pressure, PiO_2, PaO_2, and SpO_2 fall to 565 mm Hg, 118 mm Hg, 61 mm Hg, and 93%, respectively. In comparison, the barometric pressure, PiO_2, PaO_2, and SpO_2 are 760 mm Hg, 159 mm Hg, 95 mm Hg, and 100% at sea level. Although healthy individuals usually tolerate these changes well, patients with respiratory insufficiency, pulmonary hypertension, significant blood loss, or shock may decompensate and should receive supplemental oxygen and/or have the cabin pressured at sea level.

Gases expand 10–15% at the few-thousand feet where helicopters typically fly, and approximately 30% at 8,000 feet. Gases within the body itself also expand as the altitude increases. The degree of gas expansion must be considered during transport via air of any patient with a pneumocephalus, pneumothorax, bowel obstruction, or another condition involving entrapped gas. Before transport, a pneumothorax should be decompressed and a nasogastric tube inserted for ileus.

SAFETY

Safety is of paramount importance and mandates constant vigilance by everyone involved. Accident rates for pediatric air and ground transport are estimated at approximately 1 in 1,000 transports. The team should routinely attend pilot briefs, as well as perform safety inspections of the vehicles and equipment, aided by checklists. When in doubt, the MCP should solicit input from the staff about whether to transport via air or ground ambulance or to employ lights and sirens, decisions that cannot be taken lightly. The pilot's or driver's judgment as to the safety of proceeding during inclement weather or with a mechanical problem must not be overruled.

Organizations such as the Federal Aviation Administration (FAA) and the National Transportation Safety Board (NTSB), play a role in ensuring safe interfacility transport. The **Commission on Accreditation of Medical Transport Systems (CAMTS)** is an independent, peer-review organization established in 1990 in response to the number of air medical accidents in the 1980s. CAMTS, through voluntary participation, audits and accredits fixed-wing, rotary-wing, and ground interfacility medical transport services.

FAMILY-CENTERED CARE

Family-centered care represents a philosophy that respects the important role that family members play in a child's care. It recognizes family members and healthcare providers as partners in caring for the child. Family presence during transport is beneficial because it provides support to children in stressful situations and assists healthcare providers in delivering care to patients with complex and chronic medical problems.

As care is transitioned from the referring hospital, it is the transport team's responsibility to maintain family-centered care. The team meets with family members to explain the transport process, help obtain consent, and discuss anticipated management. When possible, the transport team should attempt to accommodate a family member's presence onboard. However, the family member and child may need to be separated when the child is critically ill and rapid transport is essential, or in case of space or weight limitations in the air or ground ambulance. In these situations, it is important that family members have a clear understanding of how the child will be cared for during the separation.

REFERRING HOSPITAL RESPONSIBILITIES

Transfer of a child to another facility requires written documentation by the referring physician of the need and reasons for transfer, including a statement that the risks and benefits, as well as any alternatives, have been discussed with the parents. Informed consent should be obtained from the parent/legal guardian before transfer.

Federal law under the Emergency Medical Treatment and Active Labor Act (EMTALA), part of the Consolidated Omnibus Budget Reconciliation Act (COBRA), imposes specific requirements that a patient presenting to an ED be given a medical screening examination without regard to ability to pay. If on examination an emergency medical condition is found, the hospital is required to stabilize the patient or to transfer the patient to another facility if unable to stabilize the patient or if requested by the patient. The primary requirement is that the referring physician must certify that the medical risks of transfer are outweighed by its potential benefits. The receiving hospital must agree to accept the patient if it has the space and staff to provide the necessary level of care. The transferring hospital is responsible for arranging for the transfer and ensuring that it is performed by qualified medical personnel with appropriate equipment. The transferring hospital must also send copies of the patient's medical records and test results, even those that become available after the transfer is complete.

Some referring hospitals have entered into transfer agreements with specialty centers to facilitate the smooth and safe transfer of pediatric patients. Having prepared forms for all the above purposes also aids in the transfer process.

Each hospital needs to review its facility's guidelines; if established guidelines do not exist, the Emergency Medical Services for Children National Resource Center in partnership with the Emergency Nurses Association and the Society of Trauma Nurses has developed the "Inter Facility Transfer Tool Kit for the Pediatric Patient" (www.pediatricreadiness.org). This tool kit includes the essentials for comprehensively and safely transferring the pediatric patient to the most appropriate level of care in a timely manner.

EDUCATIONAL OUTREACH

Besides safe and rapid transport, regional pediatric transport programs (and their specialty centers) have an obligation to provide educational opportunities to community healthcare providers so that these providers can acquire the necessary skills to evaluate and stabilize a critically ill or injured child until the transport team arrives. These learning activities may include transport case reviews; lectures on pediatric acute care topics; resuscitation and related programs such as the Pediatric Advanced Life Support (PALS) course, Advanced Pediatric Life Support (APLS) course, Pediatric Education for Prehospital Professionals (PEPP) course, and S.T.A.B.L.E. (sugar and safe care, temperature, airway, blood pressure, lab work, emotional support) program; and rotations through the specialty center's pediatric ED and PICU. These activities also help cement relationships with the referring facility's staff.

Bibliography is available at Expert Consult.

79.2 Outcomes and Risk Adjustment of Pediatric Emergency Medical Services

Robert C. Tasker and Evaline A. Alessandrini

Health services research has documented wide variation in the likelihood that patients receive quality, evidence-based healthcare, and this can negatively impact the health of children and youth (see Chapter 2). The complexities of delivering high-quality healthcare are magnified in the emergency department (ED). Patients are in crisis, EDs are often overcrowded, patient–physician relationships are based on brief interactions, and the varieties of complaints and diagnoses are immense. Practitioners want to know whether the system is working well, and whether local performance is good compared with a recognized benchmark or standard. Physicians can make their practice better only if they can make the appropriate measurements. However, no two places of practice are the same, so besides assessing raw outcomes (e.g., times, mortality, patient satisfaction), practitioners also need to make some adjustment for severity of illness, case mix, or risk of morbidity (e.g., one ED's practice and cases may differ significantly from a theoretical standard being used as a benchmark for "best practice").

OUTCOME MEASURES IN EMERGENCY MEDICAL SERVICES FOR CHILDREN

Pediatric emergency medical systems must support the development of national standards for emergency care performance measurement. The *Donabedian structure-process-outcome model* has set the framework for most contemporary quality measurement and improvement activities. **Structural** elements provide indirect quality-of-care measures related to a physical setting and resources. **Process** indicators provide a measure of the quality of care and services by evaluating the method or process by which care is delivered, including both technical and interpersonal components. **Outcome** elements describe valued results related to lengthening life, relieving pain, reducing disabilities, and satisfying the consumer.

A true *outcome-based* approach describes observable measures such as mortality, risk of organ system failure, and disability. An alternative approach is a *resource-based* outcome measure with a definition related to the level of care required. Children who are more ill, in general, require more resources. Thus, resource use across groups of patients reflects **severity of illness** in the groups, provided clinicians have a similar approach to practice. Examples of resource-based outcomes include need for hospital admission (ED disposition), ED length-of-stay, costs, and diagnostic and therapeutic interventions performed in the ED. This approach, certainly provides a measurement of activity, but child healthcare providers do not really know whether the patient receiving the therapeutic interventions or resources actually needed them (i.e., data may also reflect physician behavior or [lack of] experience). Therefore, some other assessment is needed that incorporates information on *how sick* the patient is, or their specific diagnosis.

Table 79.3	Stakeholder-Endorsed Outcome Measures for Pediatric Emergency Care

- Overall patient satisfaction with ED visit—nurses
- Overall patient satisfaction with ED visit—physicians
- Parent/caregiver understanding of ED discharge instructions
- ED length of stay for patients <18 yr of age
- Percentage of patients <18 yr of age left without being seen (LWBS)
- Effective pediatric procedural sedation
- Acute fracture patients with documented reduction in pain within 90 min of ED arrival
- Improvement in asthma severity score for patients with acute exacerbations
- ED revisit within 48 hr resulting in admission
- Medication error rates
- Global sentinel never events
- Unplanned return visit within 72 hr for the same/related asthma exacerbation
- Failure to achieve seizure control within 30 min of ED arrival
- Return visits within 48 hr resulting in admission for all urgent and emergency patients

Table 79.3 provides a list of outcome measures for pediatric ED care developed by **Emergency Medical Services for Children Innovation and Improvement Cente**r supported by the Health Resources and Services Administration of the U.S. Department of Health and Human Services.

RISK ADJUSTMENT

The purpose of measuring outcomes in the ED is to evaluate **performance** and therefore to offer EDs and other components of the healthcare system the opportunity to make effective improvements over time, using a benchmark within and between units. When making comparisons over time, one must ensure that patient-related attributes (e.g., age, preexisting conditions associated with outcome of interest, severity of illness) has not changed; otherwise one may be looking at changes in demography and case mix rather than any change in performance. The approach is to make some form of *risk adjustment* to *level the playing field*, so that comparison of outcomes is as fair and meaningful as possible. Because children present to EDs with illnesses of varying acuity, severity is inextricably linked to outcomes. Severity typifies the concept of *risk*—the higher the severity, the higher the risk of a given outcome. Without risk adjustment, EDs with sicker patients may appear to have poorer outcomes.

In the population of children admitted to a pediatric intensive care unit (PICU), 2 models, the **Pediatric Risk of Mortality** (PRISM) and **Pediatric Index of Mortality** (PIM),– have been developed and validated against the outcome of death during PICU admission and in, the case of PRISM IV, against functional outcome. These models or prediction algorithms, use a composite of a priori known high- or low-risk diagnoses, as well as acute physiology measurements taken around the time of presentation. In PRISM IV the data collection is from 2 hr before to 4 hr after admission, or the 1st 4 hr of care. The main concept is that deranged physiology reflects underlying severity of illness; the other features of the patient (e.g., age, diagnoses, postintervention status) modify the relationship between physiologic status and risk and enable accurate and reliable estimates of mortality and morbidity risks. Importantly, in the PRISM methodology, physiologic status is not conflated with therapies (e.g., mechanical ventilation) used at presentation (i.e., in the initial window for assessment). Historically, the measure used after the initial window of assessment with its laboratory and clinical evaluation was a period of intervention in the PICU, lasting a median of 2 days, and then discharge survival. However, the mortality rate in many U.S. PICUs is now <2.5%, and thus the need for algorithms that also include development of morbidity, now approximately 5%. The PRISM IV methodology has been validated using a *trichotomous* outcome (i.e., death, new morbidity, no new morbidity) at hospital discharge.

The previous approach is not well suited for the population presenting to the ED. Interventions may have already occurred in the prehospital setting, or physiology may have stabilized. Mortality rate is very low, and the other outcome measures may reflect what happens on the PICU or during hospital ward care. A number of disease-specific acuity scoring systems are available for use in the ED population, predominantly for those involved in trauma (e.g., Injury Severity Score, Trauma Score, Pediatric Trauma Score).

Risk Adjustment Tools in the ED
In the ED the choice of a risk adjustment tool depends on the outcomes of interest. Two general risk adjustment tools have been developed specifically for PEM, the second-generation Pediatric Risk of Admission (PRISA II) score and the Revised Pediatric Emergency Assessment Tool (RePEAT).

Pediatric Risk of Admission II
PRISA II uses components of acute and chronic medical history and physiology to determine the probability of hospitalization. The outcome measure of interest is *mandatory hospital admission* (admissions utilizing therapies best delivered as an inpatient). Table 79.4 lists the patient-related attributes contributing to the PRISA II risk adjustment score. Analytic models, including the PRISA II score, have good **calibration** (how well the probabilities predicted from the model correlated with the observed outcomes in the population) and **discrimination** (the ability to categorize subjects correctly into the categories of interest) with respect to mandatory hospital admission. Construct validity of the PRISA score has been demonstrated by measuring rates of the secondary outcomes: mandatory admission, PICU admission, and mortality. As the probability of hospital admission rises, the proportion of patients with these increasing care requirements also increases. This finding supports the use of the PRISA II score as a measure of severity of illness.

Table 79.4	Elements of the PRISA II Score

- Age <90 days
- Minor injury
- Abdominal pain in an adolescent
- Immunodeficiency
- Indwelling medical device
- Controller asthma medication
- Referral status
- Temperature
- Decreased mental status
- Low systolic blood pressure (<70 neonates and infants; <83 children; <100 adolescents)
- High diastolic blood pressure (>59 neonates and infants; >70 children; >90 adolescents)
- Low serum bicarbonate value (<20 mEq/L)
- High potassium value (>4.9 mEq/L)
- High blood urea nitrogen value (>80 mg/dL)
- High white blood cell count (>20,000/mm³)
- Oxygen therapy other than during inhaled bronchodilator treatments
- Low bicarbonate and high potassium values

Table 79.5	Elements of the RePEAT Score

- Age
- Chief complaint
- Triage category
- Current use of prescription medications
- Arrival via EMS (ground/air)
- Heart rate
- Respiratory rate
- Temperature

PRISA II has also been used to demonstrate racial/ethnic differences in severity-adjusted hospitalization rates. One study demonstrated that teaching hospitals had higher-than-expected severity-adjusted admission rates than nonteaching hospitals.

Revised Pediatric Emergency Assessment Tool
RePEAT uses a limited set of data collected at the time of ED triage to model severity of illness as reflected by the level of care provided in the ED, for example, routine assessment (clinical examination only ± nonprescription medicine) vs specific ED care (ED diagnostics and/or therapeutics) vs hospital admission. It is assumed that patients needing a higher level of care have a higher severity of illness. Table 79.5 lists the patient-related attributes contributing to the RePEAT risk adjustment score. Analytic models such as RePEAT have good calibration and discrimination with respect to predicting ED care and hospital admission. Furthermore, analytic models that compare costs and ED length of stay between EDs are improved by adjustment for severity of illness using the RePEAT score. RePEAT is a reasonable objective marker of severity of illness that could be used in the administrative process comparing outcomes between EDs.

Bibliography is available at Expert Consult.

79.3 Principles Applicable to the Developing World
Victorio R. Tolentino Jr, Jennifer I. Chapman, and David M. Walker

The maturity of **pediatric emergency medicine** (PEM) in any given area depends on the healthcare priorities and resources of that geographic or physical setting. The places in which emergency care takes place range from the community (for those with no access to organized medical care) to state-of-the-art pediatric EDs in populated centers. The scope ranges from care of the individual patient to the management of populations of children involved in large-scale disasters. Barriers to quality care are different in each situation and in each part of the world, with the implication for the astute international PEM practitioner that solutions must be targeted to the local context of healthcare within a given environment.

CONTINUUM-OF-CARE MODEL
This Emergency Medical Services for Children (EMSC) framework can also be applied to discussion of emergency care for children on a global level (see Chapter 79). With medical infrastructures that may not be consistent or well organized, or that have been weakened by civil strife, natural disasters, or economic loss, the focus of child health in the developing world has mostly been on prevention and acute care.

Prevention
Infectious Diseases
International child health has focused mainly on reducing preventable childhood illnesses, primarily through immunizations. Enormous advances have been realized in measles, neonatal tetanus, and polio reduction; wild-type smallpox was eradicated in 1978. Although there are advocates for providing primary care interventions (e.g., vaccinations) in the ED, the role of the PEM practitioner in this area of prevention has been limited.

Injuries
Injuries are a leading cause of childhood morbidity and mortality. Unintentional injuries constitute 90% of injury mortality to children 5-19 yr old and are the cause of 9% of the world's mortality (see Chapter 13). Intentional injuries, which remain underrecognized and underreported, make a smaller but significant contribution. Unintentional injuries cause more than 2,000 childhood deaths daily, or 950,000 annually worldwide. The burden of these deaths is borne disproportionately by children in middle- and lower-income countries, where >95% of all

injury deaths occur. For each of these deaths, many more children are permanently disabled, and an even larger number are treated and released without permanent sequelae.

The World Health Organization (WHO) and United Nations Children's Fund (UNICEF) have outlined several proven injury prevention strategies, of which child health practitioners in the global community must be aware. The top 3 causes of injury mortality are traffic-related injuries, burns, and drowning. There are 7 specific effective strategies for reducing **traffic-related injuries**: a minimum drinking age, appropriate child restraints and seatbelts, helmets for motorcycle and bicycle riders, reduced vehicle speeds around schools and residential areas, running lights on motorcycles, graduated licensing for drivers, and separation of different types of road users. There is insufficient evidence to demonstrate that school-based programs on drunk driving, increased pedestrian visibility, or designated driver programs are effective. Although these strategies have proved effective, the data are based on U.S. research and may not be generalizable to other countries. It may be difficult to reduce vehicle speeds around schools when there is insufficient infrastructure for street signs. Alternatively, lack of separation of car and bus traffic from bicyclists and pedestrians contributes to unsafe and dangerous road conditions. This is more of a problem in lower- and middle-income countries, where bicycles and motorized 2-wheel vehicles are used to carry children as well as goods, while the drivers negotiate among rapidly moving vehicles. With rising income, these countries have seen increases in both the number of cars and the number of 2-wheeled vehicles, with a corresponding increase in the number of related injuries.

For reducing **drowning deaths**, strategies that have proven effective focus on creating barriers between children and water hazards, such as covering wells, buckets, and other standing sources of water, and placing high fences around pools (see Chapter 91). **Burns** have been addressed by advocating for installation of smoke detectors and lowering the temperature of water from water heaters (see Chapter 92).

Out-of-Hospital Care

Out-of-hospital care comprises access to emergency services, prehospital care, and interfacility transport of patients. Morbidity and mortality arise from delayed or limited access to emergency care, lack of prehospital care, transport without proper monitoring or trained personnel, or delayed transport to a higher level of care. *Safe transport of seriously ill children* is a neglected global health issue. An emergency response system must address the following links in the patient's care: a communication system with prompt activation of EMS, the correct assessment and initial treatment of the patient, and the rapid transport to definitive care.

Access to Care

When a child is injured or ill, a parent or caretaker must be able to access help and activate EMS. Many countries worldwide have dedicated emergency numbers to rapidly dispatch medical, police, or fire services. The simple 112 emergency number has been adopted and is being phased in throughout the European Union (EU) member states, to access medical, fire, and police services, in addition to secondary regional emergency access numbers. The universal U.S. emergency number system 911 today covers the large majority of the country (98%) and has enhanced features of automatically linking the phone number to an address. However, there remain limitations to universal access resulting from absence of phones in some households, unclear addresses in rural areas, and insufficient reach of the emergency system.

In the majority of low- and middle-income countries, no such universal emergency numbers have been established, requiring access by direct dialing to an ambulance, if such private services exist. In most low- and middle-income countries, the family must bring the ill or injured child to the health facility for stabilization and treatment. For this to occur, families must overcome financial and geographic barriers, which can result in delayed presentation for care. This delay predictably increases the acuity of the illness or injury and associated complications and decreases the likelihood of full recovery and survival.

Prehospital Care

In regions with maturing EMS systems, there must be adequately trained personnel to stabilize and transport the child to a medical facility. The quality and level of training of such prehospital personnel vary tremendously among countries and within regions of the same country. In urban areas, there is a greater concentration of medical care and therefore a greater opportunity to have strong prehospital training. In most of Asia and sub-Saharan Africa, trained personnel are used primarily to transfer patients between health facilities, not from the initial site of illness or injury. In most high-income countries, medical services are dispatched to the patient.

In the French model, Service d'Aide Médicale Urgente (SAMU), a physician, often an emergency medicine specialist, will review calls for acuity and can dispatch a physician-led team by ambulance to go to the patient's home to assess, stabilize, and initiate treatment. This Franco-German system is used in other countries, including many in Latin America and Europe. There are no clear data on the cost-effectiveness and patient outcomes associated with delivery of patients to the nearest facility vs bringing hospital resources to the patient.

Around the world, the effort to establish standardized approaches to prehospital care exists primarily in the form of courses to educate EMS and hospital personnel in the emergency management of patients. For trauma care, the WHO manuals *Prehospital Trauma Care Systems* and *Guidelines for Essential Trauma Care* both focus on guidelines for prehospital and trauma care systems that are affordable and sustainable. The AAP course Pediatric Education for Prehospital Professionals is a dynamic, modularized teaching tool designed to provide specific pediatric prehospital education that can be adapted to any EMS system. Table 79.6 describes additional prehospital resources.

Although most middle- and high-income countries have a system of trained EMS workers, low-income countries lack this advanced tier of emergency care. In these countries, commercial drivers, volunteers, and willing bystanders provide the first line of care. Training a cadre of first responders can rely on existing networks of aid or can be drawn from specific populations, such as students, soldiers, or public servants. Training needs to emphasize basic lifesaving and limb-saving interventions, including how to stop bleeding and support breathing, access advanced care, and splint broken limbs. In Ghana, for example, taxi drivers participated in a first-aid course that relied heavily on demonstration and practice rather than knowledge transfer through didactic sessions. Taxi drivers were selected because they already provided much of the transport for injured patients, either voluntarily or for pay by the family. Two years after the course, external evaluators favorably rated the quality of their care compared with untrained drivers. In rural areas, such first responders become vital in providing emergency interventions when more definitive care is distant. Thus a system of trained first responders forms the foundation of an effective prehospital system.

Methods of Transport

In many low-income countries, there is no means of transport other than the family's motorized or other type of transport. Health centers may only have 1 vehicle for transport to a higher-level facility. This vehicle may also be used for outreach primary care services, such as offering immunizations and collecting drugs and equipment from a central supply location, and sometimes, improperly for personal reasons by local officials or politicians. In large cities, taxis and auto rickshaws are frequently used because they are rapidly available, well disseminated, and able to pass around traffic jams. Where organized prehospital systems exist, different types of vehicles are adapted for emergency transportation, from fully equipped ambulances to basic transport with trained personnel. The WHO recommends identifying transport vehicles in advance, choosing vehicles that can be repaired and maintained locally, and equipping the vehicles according to recognized standards. Therefore the provision of available and appropriately staffed and equipped transport vehicles is crucial to the realization of recommended emergency care plans.

Hospital-Based Care

Once a child has reached a medical facility for the care of an injury or illness, adequate emergency services must be available. In many countries

Table 79.6	Pediatric Emergency Care Resources

PREHOSPITAL

Advanced Medical Life Support (AMLS)
Newest course developed by the National Association of Emergency Medical Technicians (NAEMT) to provide more clinical teaching and reasoning around emergent medical problems. Course is open to physicians, nurses EMTs and paramedics.
www.naemt.org/education/amls/amls.aspx

Prehospital Trauma Life Support
Available in 33 countries, PHTLS is the leading continuing education program for prehospital emergency trauma care.
www.phtls.org

International Trauma Life Support
Training course for prehospital trauma care.
www.itrauma.org

Pediatric Education for Prehospital Professionals (PEPP)
Curriculum designed specifically to teach prehospital professionals how to assess and manage ill or injured children.
www.peppsite.org

HOSPITAL CARE

Pocket Book of Hospital Care for Children
WHO publication providing guidelines for the management of common illnesses with limited resources; incorporates both the Emergency Triage Assessment and Treatment (ETAT) and Integrated Management of Childhood Illness (IMCI) guidelines.
www.who.int/maternal_child_adolescent/documents/9241546700/en/index.html

AFEM Handbook of Acute and Emergency Care
Management strategies based on available resources. It leads providers through a rapid, systematic, and integrated approach to stabilization and resuscitation of patients stratified to 3 resource levels: where there are no available resources, where there are minimal resources, and where there are full resources.
Available for purchase online.

Where There Is No Doctor: A Village Health Handbook
Healthcare manual for health workers, clinicians, and others involved in primary healthcare delivery and health promotion programs around the world. Available for purchase or as a free download.
www.hesperian.org

International Federation for Emergency Medicine
2012 International Standards of Care for Children in Emergency Departments.
https://www.ifem.cc/wp-content/uploads/2016/07/International-Standards-for-Children-in-Emergency-Departments-V2.0-June-2014-1.pdf

HUMANITARIAN EMERGENCIES

CHILDisaster Network
Registry for those with education and experience in humanitarian emergencies to volunteer their time when needed in a disaster.
www.aap.org/disaster

The Sphere Project
Downloadable modules on disaster preparedness.
www.sphereproject.org

Management of Complex Humanitarian Emergencies: Focus on Children and Families
Training course offered by the Children in Disasters Project, sponsored by the Rainbow Center for Global Child Health (RCGCH) in Cleveland, OH. Held in early June annually.

Manual for the Health Care of Children in Humanitarian Emergencies
WHO publication that provides comprehensive guidance on childcare in emergencies; includes information on care of traumatic injuries and mental health emergencies.
www.who.int/child_adolescent_health/documents/9789241596879/en/index.html

ACCESS TO ACADEMIC PUBLICATIONS RELEVANT TO PEM

PEMdatabase.org
A website devoted to pediatric emergency medicine (PEM). Contains links to conferences, evidence-based medicine reviews, research networks, and professional organizations.
www.pemdatabase.org

HINARI Access to Research Initiative
Program established by WHO and others to enable developing countries to gain access to one of the world's largest collections of biomedical and health literature.
www.who.int/hinari/en

INVOLVEMENT

ACEP Ambassador Program
Provides the names of U.S.-boarded emergency medicine physicians who can provide advice and information on issues pertaining to the progress and status of emergency medicine in their assigned countries.
www.acep.org/content.aspx?id=25138

Section on International Emergency Medicine, American College of Emergency Physicians
This group maintains a list of international organizations and clinical opportunities, many of which involve emergency care of children.
http://www.acep.org/_InternationalSection/International-Emergency-Medicine-Related-Resources/

Section of International Child Health, American Academy of Pediatrics
Lists non-U.S. clinical opportunities, many of which involve emergency care.
http://www2.aap.org/sections/ich/working_overseas.htm

ORGANIZATIONS INVOLVED IN INTERNATIONAL PEM ACTIVITIES

U.S. Agency for International Development (USAID)
Government agency providing U.S. economic and humanitarian assistance worldwide.
www.usaid.gov

World Health Organization (WHO)
Publication catalog, media resources, health articles, and current health news.
www.who.int/topics/child_health/en

United Nations Children's Fund (UNICEF)
Organization dedicated to providing lifesaving assistance to children affected by disasters and to protecting their rights in any circumstances; formerly United Nations International Children's Emergency Fund.
www.unicef.org

Safe Kids Worldwide
The first and only international nonprofit organization dedicated solely to preventing unintentional childhood injury.
www.safekids.org

the ED serves only as a triage area where patients are distinguished by their likely disease process and directed for admission to the corresponding unit within the hospital. Strengthening emergency services includes seeing the ED as a unit where definitive treatment can be provided to the ill and injured child. Critically ill children must receive not only prompt care but also correct care. Such expedience and accuracy are ensured by implementation of an effective triage system, moving the sickest patients to immediate care and standardizing the initial care of emergency conditions.

Triage

Children requiring emergency care frequently are not promptly recognized. Too often, children presenting to EDs are treated on a first-come first-served basis, in an approach that creates long waiting times for critically ill children, a contributor to unnecessary mortality. Medical facilities need to adopt an efficient and effective triage system to respond rapidly to the needs of patients and to assign the appropriate amount of resources. To this end, WHO has developed a course entitled **Emergency Triage Assessment and Treatment (ETAT)**.

This course teaches to triage patients on arrival as having emergency, priority, or nonurgent signs and to provide emergency treatment for life-threatening conditions. ETAT emphasizes the evaluation of a patient's **ABCD status** to identify emergency situations—the patency of the airway (A), the quality of breathing (B), the quality of circulation and presence of coma or convulsions (C), and the presence of severe dehydration (D).

One of the benefits of the ETAT guidelines is that they can be adapted to centers with limited resources and are applicable to areas with high morbidity and mortality from meningitis, dehydration, malaria, respiratory illness, and malnutrition. Another benefit is that the care algorithms are based on limited diagnostic studies, that is, hemoglobin measurement, blood smear for malaria, and bedside blood glucose testing. Widely accepted triage assessment guidelines are teachable to emergency care staff, and their adoption can provide better organization within a healthcare center. At the Queen Elizabeth Central Hospital in Blantyre, Malawi, for example, the institution of triage and rapid treatment in its emergency care center led to a 50% decrease in the mortality of children within 24 hr of presentation to the hospital, with a further 50% decrease as implementation and practice of triaging patients have continued.

Beyond triage, education on overall emergency center organization is a low-resource intervention that can obviate some of the obstacles to quality care delivery. Additionally, the arrangement of short-stay areas (hydration and infusion rooms) can lessen the burden on inpatient units.

Pediatric-Specific Emergency Centers
Anecdotally, most countries have developed at least 1 pediatric-capable center, usually as part of an academic medical center. The emergency services in these centers are variable, but certainly can be a starting point from which to build overall improvement in pediatric emergency care.

Practitioners
Throughout the world, nurses, paramedics, and nonspecialist physicians provide most of the care to acutely ill or injured children. The majority of sick children attend local clinics or district or central hospitals, where financial and human resources are not always matched to the potential acuity of presenting patient complaints. Nominal supervision is provided to staff attending these patients. Pediatric EDs located in tertiary hospitals are often staffed by training physicians with little or no supervision from faculty, who themselves may have limited exposure to or training in PEM. General hospitals lack dedicated pediatric staff; guidelines as to which patients should be moved to a higher level of care are often not standardized and depend on local influences and/or cultural beliefs about health and illness.

Clinical Guidelines
The **Integrated Management of Childhood Illnesses (IMCI)** guidelines were developed by the WHO and UNICEF to provide assistance in the initial triage and management of the presenting signs and symptoms of the major killers of children <5 yr old in first-level health facilities (e.g., clinics, health centers, outpatient departments of hospitals). The flow charts within each chapter of the IMCI manuals allow easy accessibility to materials that can enhance education and outreach to less experienced health workers.

Evaluations in various countries of the implementation of IMCI guidelines have shown improvements in health worker performance and quality of care, as well as decreases in delay in treatment and mortality of the under-5 population. These guidelines also dramatically reduce the cost of healthcare. The WHO website provides all the necessary implementation tools, including course manuals and evaluation tools.

The International Federation of Emergency Medicine developed standards to improve emergency care globally. These standards are not just aimed at dedicated EDs, but at any setting where emergency care takes place, regardless of the providers or the resources available. At the same time, however, the existence of the standards allows sites to advocate for improved resources dedicated to expertise in the various aspects of providing quality emergency care for children. The standards address design of care spaces, child- and family-centered care, assessment of ill and injured children, staff training and competencies, quality and safety, and disaster response.

Trauma
Morbidity and mortality from trauma are among the most prevalent problems for children worldwide. Trauma care presents the challenge of sequential, often simple, interventions that must be performed in a timely manner to limit the severity of the outcome. However, with lack of specific training, signs and symptoms of pediatric trauma may go unrecognized or may be underappreciated. Trauma courses such as Advanced Trauma Life Support (ATLS) are educational tools that can be disseminated to improve the quality of care at emergency centers worldwide. For low-resource settings, WHO has developed the Integrated Management for Emergency and Essential Surgical Care toolkit, which provides clear directions and reasoning for the initial care of injured patients. Not expressly addressed in the ATLS course is specific concern about **child abuse** as the cause of trauma. This is an area of pediatric care that many countries do not yet address comprehensively in their medical training, their law enforcement, or their judicial systems. The epidemiologic need for reliable trauma registries is great, as is the need to identify personnel with trauma management skill sets and dedicated trauma centers to serve as higher-level referral sites.

Equipment
Pediatric emergency equipment guidelines are available for a variety of settings where acutely ill and injured children would present. Although these equipment guidelines may represent minimum supplies to treat the widest variety of pediatric emergencies, the roles of substitution and improvisation often provide for equivalent function of recommended supplies.

Inpatient Services
After the initial stabilization, children requiring ongoing care are admitted to the hospital. The quality of inpatient services varies greatly depending on institutional and provider experience, comfort with pediatric conditions, and the resources available to treat them. WHO has produced the *Pocket Book of Hospital Care for Children*, which is based on IMCI guidelines and focuses on inpatient management of high-morbidity/high-mortality illnesses common in developing countries.

HUMANITARIAN DISASTERS
Children are a vulnerable population who experience disproportionate suffering during humanitarian emergencies, either natural (earthquakes, tsunamis, hurricanes, floods, droughts) or manmade (armed conflicts, terrorist attacks). The under-5 population is especially susceptible to infectious diseases, malnutrition, and trauma following disasters. The **Rainbow Center for Global Child Health** at the Case Western Reserve University School of Medicine offers a training course, *Management of Humanitarian Emergencies: Focus on Children and Families*, to educate and train health professionals, relief workers, and policymakers to recognize and address the unique needs of children affected by manmade and natural disasters worldwide. AAP also maintains a CHILD disaster Network, which acts as an electronic database of child health professionals with education and experience in humanitarian emergencies. Nongovernmental organizations can access the database to solicit practitioners to aid in disaster response.

The WHO *Manual for the Health Care of Children in Humanitarian Emergencies* is based on IMCI guidelines and addresses the emergency care of children in disaster situations where hospital facilities and resources are not immediately available. It goes beyond the IMCI guidelines by discussing initial assessment and management of trauma, burns, and poisonings. Preexisting IMCI guidelines assumed a functioning health system that facilitated the referral of children, which may not be available in all emergency situations. This manual also includes the initial management of severe conditions, such as injuries, burns, neonatal illness, and psychosocial problems, which are considered high priority in acute care settings.

Exchange and Dissemination of Information

The WHO established the **HINARI** (Health InterNetwork Access to Research Initiative) program to allow free or reduced-cost access to more than 6,200 journal publications. This internet access is made available to the 108 countries with gross national income per capita <$3,500. For middle-income countries not meeting the financial eligibility, internet access continues to be a barrier, and resources may be limited to out-of-date textbooks and journals.

Another valuable tool is the website pemdatabase.org. This nonproprietary site was started as an online resource for PEM practitioners. It contains links to PEM abstracts and articles, evidence-based reviews, pediatric resuscitation websites, and relevant journals, as well as PEM conferences and professional organizations.

Bibliography is available at Expert Consult.

Chapter 80

Triage of the Acutely Ill Child

Anna K. Weiss and Frances B. Balamuth

第八十章

危重患儿的分诊

中文导读

　　本章主要介绍了危重患儿生命体征的评估、询问病史、体格检查、管理和处置。生命体征的评估包括体温、心率、呼吸频率和血压；病史包括发热、头痛、腹痛、呕吐等症状及既往用药史；体格检查包括观察孩子对刺激的反应、生命体征及全身各系统的检查；管理包括对潜在的不稳定儿童应从ABC，即气道、呼吸、循环开始评估；处置包括应根据患儿病情轻重决定进一步处理的方法。

Identifying the acutely ill child in the ambulatory setting is a challenge. Children presenting to pediatricians' offices, urgent care practices, and emergency departments (EDs) may have a range of illnesses from simple viral infections to life-threatening emergencies. Although most children in this setting will have a benign course of illness, it is incumbent on the pediatric practitioner to quickly and accurately discern which children are likely to deteriorate from potentially serious or life-threatening disease. When assessing an acutely ill child, practitioners must remember that the early signs of severe illness may be subtle.

ASSESSMENT OF VITAL SIGNS

Assessment of vital signs is critical in all pediatric visits for acute illness, including temperature, heart rate, respiratory rate, and blood pressure. Normal vital signs vary with age. Although there have been increasing efforts to build evidence-based vital sign cutoffs for different age-groups, most institutions use nonempirically derived cutoffs such as those in Pediatric Advanced Life Support (PALS). **Tachycardia** is common in children presenting for acute care and can result from benign (fever, pain, dehydration) to life-threatening (septic shock, hemorrhage) conditions. An abnormal heart rate should prompt a full history and physical examination, as described later, and careful *reassessment* (often multiple times) after the presumed cause is identified and treated. The vast majority of children will improve after initiation of simple interventions such as antipyretics or analgesia. Tachycardia that persists after fever, pain, and dehydration have been treated *must* be evaluated further, particularly if the child appears ill or has deficit in perfusion or altered mental state.

Tachypnea is also common and has many causes, including fever, respiratory conditions (bronchiolitis, asthma, pneumonia), cardiac disease (e.g., heart failure), and metabolic acidosis (shock, poisoning, diabetic ketoacidosis). Similar to tachycardia, tachypnea often resolves with antipyretics in febrile children, and should be reassessed to ensure resolution once fever has been managed. In cases where bronchiolitis and asthma have been ruled out, persistent tachypnea and fever can be a sign of pneumonia, even in the absence of focal lung findings on examination. Consider evaluation for metabolic acidosis in cases of significant tachypnea without apparent pulmonary or cardiac causes. **Apnea** is a sign of respiratory failure and should be *treated emergently with bag-valve-mask ventilation and immediate ED evaluation.*

Hypotension is rare in children, and when present, it is a sign of critical illness. Children with hypotension should be evaluated in an ED. Hypotension is evidence of decompensated circulatory shock and can result from severe dehydration, sepsis, hemorrhage, neurogenic spinal shock, or cardiogenic shock.

Pulse oximetry (oxygen-hemoglobin saturation, SpO_2) should be assessed in children with respiratory or cardiac illness/compromise and also in children with underlying abnormalities of oxygenation. Healthy children have SpO_2 >95%. The practitioner should consider evaluating for any underlying respiratory or cardiac causes in children with SpO_2 <93–95%. For children with underlying abnormalities, the child's baseline SpO_2 should be assessed and alterations from that baseline should be investigated further.

The combination of bradycardia, hypertension, and altered breathing known as **Cushing triad** can be a sign of life-threatening increased intracranial pressure (ICP) and should be evaluated in an ED. Anisocoria and a 6th cranial nerve palsy are other signs of increased ICP. **Toxidromes** should also be considered in children with abnormal combinations of vital signs (see Chapter 77).

HISTORY

A thorough history is paramount to identifying patients whose condition will require prompt intervention. Obtaining an accurate history from young patients is challenging, particularly with preverbal or very anxious children who are unable or unwilling to localize the source of their discomfort. In such instances, parents or caretakers often provide the most important information, and their perceptions of the child's course of illness must be carefully considered. Pediatricians should be guided by the patient's chief complaint to ask *open-ended questions* that help distinguish between benign and potentially life-threatening disease entities. The most common complaints leading to acute care visits among children include fever, headache and altered mental status, trauma, abdominal pain and vomiting, respiratory distress, and chest pain. Table 80.1 describes signs and symptoms that should prompt immediate transfer to an ED or, if already in the ED, initiation of rapid intervention.

Fever is the most common reason for a sick-child visit. Most cases of fever are the result of self-limited viral infection. However, pediatricians need to be aware of the age-dependent potential for serious bacterial infections, such as urinary tract infection (UTI), sepsis, meningitis, pneumonia, acute abdominal infection, and osteoarticular infection.

During the 1st 2 mo of life, the neonate is at risk for sepsis caused by pathogens that are uncommon in older children. These organisms include group B streptococcus, *Escherichia coli*, *Listeria monocytogenes*, and herpes simplex virus (HSV). In neonates, the history must include untreated maternal obstetric information and the patient's birth history. Risk factors for sepsis include untreated maternal group B streptococcus colonization, prematurity, chorioamnionitis, and prolonged rupture of membranes. If there is a maternal history of sexually transmitted infections (STIs) during the pregnancy, the differential diagnosis must be expanded to include those pathogens. Septic infants can present with lethargy, poor feeding, grunting respirations, and cool or mottled extremities, in addition to fever (or hypothermia). Febrile infants in the 1st 1-2 mo of life should be evaluated broadly for infection, including sampling blood, urine, and cerebrospinal fluid (CSF).

When the infant matures beyond 2 mo of age and receives their 1st set of vaccinations, serious bacterial infections become less common. Evaluation to rule out serious infection is an important part of treating the febrile older child. Children with fever should have a full set of vital signs, history, and physical examination to ensure that critical illness is absent and to identify any focal source. Red flags for **septic shock** include hypotension, poor perfusion, altered mental status, or the presence of purpuric or erythrodermic rash. Red flags for **meningitis** include severe headache, meningismus, and altered mental state. The presence of any of these signs should prompt emergency evaluation in the ED or rapid treatment if the patient is already in the ED.

Additional focal findings to consider include evaluation for acute otitis media, pharyngitis, pneumonia, abdominal infections (bacterial enteritis, appendicitis), skin and soft tissue infections, septic arthritis,

Table 80.1	History and Examination Findings That Should Prompt Immediate Intervention and/or Transfer to Emergency Department
HISTORY AND EXAM FINDINGS	**RISK FACTORS**
RED FLAGS FOR RESPIRATORY FAILURE	
Tachycardia	Tracheostomy
Tachypnea	Ventilator dependence
Cyanosis	History of critical airway
Apnea	
Brief resolved unexplained event (BRUE) with cyanosis or change in tone	
Suspected button-battery ingestion	
Foreign body aspiration with respiratory distress	
Respiratory distress with hypoxemia and/or altered mental status	
RED FLAGS FOR CIRCULATORY FAILURE	
Tachycardia	Oncology (or other immunosuppressed) patients
Tachypnea	
Cyanosis	Bone marrow or solid-organ transplants
Apnea	
Petechial or purpuric rashes	Sickle cell (or otherwise asplenic) patients
Erythroderma	
Peritonitis	Infants <56 days old
Bilious emesis	Cardiac patient with change from baseline pulse oximetry
Posttonsillectomy or postadenoidectomy with bleeding	
Extremity trauma with neurovascular deficits	Bleeding disorder with trauma
RED FLAGS FOR NEUROLOGIC FAILURE	
Tachycardia	Ventriculoperitoneal shunt
Bradycardia-hypertension	
Double vision	Diabetes or metabolic disease with altered mental status
Unequal pupils	
Apnea	
Frequent or prolonged seizure(s)	Hypoxic-ischemic encephalopathy
Focal neurologic deficit(s)	
Acute onset of severe headache	Clotting disorder with neurologic change(s)
Suicidal or homicidal ideation, psychosis	

Adapted from Farah MM, Tay Y, Lavelle J. A general approach to ill and injured children. In Shaw KN, Bachur RG, editors: *Fleischer and Ludwig's textbook of pediatric emergency medicine*, Philadelphia, 2015, LWW.

and osteomyelitis. Occult UTI should be considered if 3 of the following risk factors are present: age <1 yr, fever >39°C, fever >48 hr, and no focal source of fever. Pneumonia should be considered in the presence of tachypnea, hypoxia, or focal findings on chest examination. Bacteremia is rare in the post–pneumococcal and *Haemophilus influenzae* vaccine era but should be considered if staphylococcal infection or meningococcemia is suspected, as well as in unvaccinated children or children with signs of septic shock. In addition to infection, inflammatory conditions to consider include juvenile idiopathic arthritis and Kawasaki disease. The diagnosis of **Kawasaki disease** should be considered if the patient meets the diagnostic criteria for this illness although some patients may have an atypical or incomplete presentation (see Chapter 191).

For patients presenting in an **altered mental state**, the pediatrician should inquire about any symptoms, such as fever or headache. Screening questions should explore feeding changes, medications in the household, ill contacts, and the possibility of trauma. Parents will often describe a febrile child as lethargic, but further questioning will reveal a tired-appearing child who interacts appropriately when no longer febrile. The child who appears ill only when febrile must be differentiated from the lethargic patient who presents with suspected sepsis or meningitis, and from the child whose altered behavior is secondary to an intracranial emergency or seizure. Infants with meningitis, sepsis, or cardiac defects may have a history of irritability, being inconsolable, poor feeders, grunting breathing, seizures, poor urine output, and/or color changes such as pallor, mottling, or cyanosis. Patients with poisoning or inborn error of metabolism can also present with lethargy, poor feeding, unusual odors, seizures, and vomiting. Nonaccidental **trauma** should always be considered in a lethargic infant, particularly in the absence of additional signs or symptoms. In infants and young toddlers, rapidly growing head circumference or bulging anterior fontanel may signal increased ICP. Older children may present with altered mental state as a result of meningitis/encephalitis, trauma, or ingestions. School-age children and adolescents with meningitis may have a history of fever and neck pain; other associated symptoms may include rash, headache, photophobia, or vomiting. Children with ingestions can present with other abnormal neurologic symptoms, such as ataxia, slurred speech, and seizures, or with characteristic constellations of vital sign changes and other physical findings consistent with certain toxidromes.

In patients with **headache**, ask questions about the chronicity of the headache and any accompanying symptoms. Headaches that occur on arising in the morning, are worse when lying flat, or are accompanied by vomiting are concerning for increased ICP. Similarly, headache accompanied by focal neurologic deficit should be referred to an ED for urgent head imaging. While migraine headaches in teenagers are similar in presentation to those in adults (unilateral, throbbing, accompanied by an aura), pediatric practitioners should be aware that migraines in prepubertal children may have a nonclassic presentation and may be bilateral and not accompanied by aura, photophobia, or phonophobia.

Parents may interpret a variety of symptoms as **respiratory distress**, and care must be taken to distinguish normal and benign respiratory patterns from true respiratory distress. Tachypnea secondary to fever is a common source of parental anxiety, and parents of newborn infants are sometimes alarmed by the presence of periodic breathing. Parents should be questioned about their child's other symptoms, such as fever, limitation of neck movement, drooling, choking, and the presence of stridor or wheezing. A history of apnea or cyanosis warrants further investigation. Practitioners should also remember that tachypnea in a child without evidence of true respiratory distress may be evidence of compensation for shock or metabolic acidosis, both of which will require rapid treatment. Although wheezing is often secondary to bronchospasm, it can also be caused by cardiac disease or congenital airway anomalies such as vascular rings. Parents may interpret true **stridor** as noisy breathing or wheezing. Stridor is most frequently caused by upper airway obstruction such as croup. However, anatomic abnormalities such as laryngeal webs, laryngomalacia, subglottic stenosis, and paralyzed vocal cords also cause stridor. Toddlers who present with breathing difficulty after a coughing or choking episode should be evaluated for **foreign body aspiration**. In these cases, practitioners must ask about the possibility of button-battery ingestion, as this constitutes a true medical emergency that warrants immediate endoscopic removal or transfer to a facility that can perform the procedure. In toxic-appearing children with stridor, the pediatrician should consider epiglottitis, bacterial tracheitis, or a rapidly expanding retropharyngeal abscess. The incidence of epiglottitis has greatly declined with the advent of the *H. influenzae* type b (Hib) vaccine, but it remains a possibility in the unimmunized or partially immunized patient. Children with retropharyngeal abscesses may also present with drooling and limitation of neck movement (especially hyperextension) after a recent upper respiratory infection or penetrating mouth injury.

Abdominal pain is a very common complaint in the ambulatory setting and can herald either acute intraabdominal or pelvic pathology, or it can be a subtler sign of systemic illness. Both relatively benign (e.g., streptococcal infection, UTI, pneumonia) and severe abdominal (e.g., appendicitis) or systemic (e.g., diabetic ketoacidosis) illness can present with abdominal pain, and questions to the patient and parent should include whether there is an extraabdominal source of discomfort. Questions should include details about pain onset and location; presence of accompanying symptoms, such as fever, abdominal distention; and changes in feeding, urination, and stooling patterns. Care should be taken to elicit a history of peritonitis or obstruction, including worsening pain with abrupt movements and persistent or bilious vomiting.

In neonates, a tender abdomen with or without bilious emesis should raise concern for the presence of a small bowel obstruction (volvulus).

These infants appear ill and may have a history of decreased stooling. Pediatricians should be wary of neonates with abdominal tenderness and bloody stools, because 10% of cases of necrotizing enterocolitis occur in term infants. Infants with milk protein intolerance can also present with bloody stools, but these infants appear well and do not have abdominal tenderness. In older patients the differential diagnosis for emergency causes of abdominal pain expands to include intussusception and appendicitis. Patients with intussusception present in a variety of ways, ranging from colicky abdominal pain but otherwise well between episodes to being lethargic or in shock. The diagnosis of appendicitis in the child younger than 3 yr is extremely difficult because children in this age-group cannot localize pain well. In adolescent females with abdominal pain, practitioners must obtain a menstrual and sexual history, because acute lower abdominal pain may be caused by adnexal pathology, including ovarian torsion or ectopic pregnancy.

For patients with **vomiting**, pediatricians should ask if they have experienced bilious or blood-stained emesis, abdominal distention or constipation, weight changes, and diarrhea or bloody stools. An infant with bilious emesis and abdominal distention may have intestinal obstruction (as with midgut volvulus or Hirschsprung disease), whereas an infant who appears immediately hungry after nonbilious projectile vomiting may have pyloric stenosis. In an older child, vomiting may be caused by peritonitis or obstruction, as well as by systemic illnesses, including diabetic ketoacidosis, ingestion, or trauma. Patients with headache and vomiting raise the concern for increased ICP and should be questioned about neurologic changes, meningismus, and fever.

Practitioners should also obtain a thorough account of the child's **past medical history**. It is important to be aware of any underlying chronic problems that might predispose the child to recurring infections or a serious acute illness. Children with sickle cell anemia, indwelling central venous access devices, or immune compromise are at increased risk for bacteremia and sepsis. Similarly, children with prior surgery, including ventriculoperitoneal shunt placement or intraabdominal procedures, can develop complications from their previous surgeries.

PHYSICAL EXAMINATION

Observation is important when evaluating the acutely ill child. Most observational data that the pediatrician gathers should focus on assessing the child's response to stimuli. Does the child awaken easily? Does the child smile and interact with the parent, or with the examiner? Evaluating these responses requires knowledge of normal child development and an understanding of the manner in which normal responses are elicited, depending on the child's age.

During the physical examination, the pediatric practitioner seeks evidence of illness. The portions of the exam that require the child to be most cooperative are completed first. Initially, it is best to seat the child on the parent's lap; the older child may be seated on the examination table. It is also important to assess the child's willingness to move, as well as ease of movement. It is reassuring to see the child moving about on the parent's lap with ease and without discomfort. *Vital signs are often overlooked but are invaluable in assessing ill children.* The presence of tachycardia out of proportion to fever and the presence of tachypnea and blood pressure abnormalities raise the suspicion for more serious illness. The respiratory evaluation includes determining respiratory rate, noting the presence or absence of hypoxia by SpO_2, and noting any evidence of inspiratory stridor, expiratory wheezing, grunting, coughing, or increased work of breathing (e.g., retractions, nasal flaring, accessory muscle use). The **skin** should be carefully examined for rashes. Frequently, viral infections cause an exanthem, and many of these eruptions are diagnostic, such as the reticulated rash and slapped-cheek appearance of parvovirus infections and the stereotypical appearance of hand-foot-and-mouth disease caused by coxsackieviruses, as well as measles, chickenpox, and roseola. The skin examination may also yield evidence of more serious infections, including petechiae and purpura associated with bacteremia and erythroderma associated with a toxin-producing systemic infection. Cutaneous perfusion should be assessed by warmth and capillary refill time. The extremities may then be evaluated not only for ease of movement but also for the presence of swelling, warmth, tenderness, or alterations in perfusion. Such abnormalities may indicate focal infections (e.g., cellulitis, bone/joint infection) or vascular changes (e.g., arterial or venous thromboembolus).

When an infant is seated and is least perturbed, the examiner should assess the anterior fontanel to determine whether it is depressed, flat, or bulging. While the child is calm and cooperative, the **eyes** should be examined to identify features that might indicate an infectious or neurologic process. Often, viral infections result in watery discharge or redness of the bulbar conjunctivae. Bacterial infection, if superficial, results in purulent drainage; if the infection is more deep-seated, tenderness, swelling, and redness of the tissues surrounding the eye may be present, as well as proptosis, altered visual acuity, and impaired extraocular movement. Abnormalities in pupillary response or extraocular movements may also be indicators of cranial nerve abnormalities and if new, are indications for head imaging.

During this initial portion of the physical examination, when the child is most comfortable (and therefore most likely to be quiet), the **heart and lungs** are auscultated. It is important to assess the adequacy of air entry into the lungs, the equality of breath sounds, and any evidence of adventitial breath sounds, especially wheezes, rales, or rhonchi. The coarse sound of air moving through a congested nasal passage is frequently transmitted to the lungs. The examiner can become attuned to these coarse sounds by placing the stethoscope near the child's nose and then compensating for this sound as the chest is auscultated. The cardiac examination is next; findings such as pericardial friction rubs, loud murmurs, and distant heart sounds may indicate cardiac inflammation or infection. In the neonate, murmurs may herald congenital heart disease, especially in the presence of cyanosis, unequal extremity pulses, or a differential in upper- vs lower-extremity blood pressures. A complete cardiac exam should also look for displacement of the PMI (point of maximal impulse) and the presence of jugular venous distention or facial plethora.

The components of the physical examination that are more bothersome to the child are completed last. This is best done with the patient on the examination table. Initially, the **neck** is examined to assess for areas of swelling, redness, or tenderness, as may be seen in cervical adenitis. Resistance to neck movement should prompt evaluation for signs of meningeal irritation or retropharyngeal abscess. During examination of the **abdomen**, the diaper, if present, is removed. The abdomen is inspected for distention. Auscultation is performed to assess adequacy of bowel sounds, followed by palpation. Every attempt should be made to quiet a fussing child during this part of the exam; if this is not possible, practitioners should note that increased crying as the abdomen is palpated may indicate tenderness, especially if this finding is focally reproducible. In addition to focal tenderness, palpation may elicit involuntary guarding or rebound tenderness (including tenderness to percussion); these findings indicate peritoneal irritation, as seen in appendicitis. During palpation of the abdomen, practitioners should look for signs of hepatomegaly or splenomegaly. When palpating the bottom-most edge of the liver or spleen, examiners should begin in the pelvis and work upward toward the ribs, because severe organomegaly can be missed if the examiner begins palpating in the mid-abdomen. The **inguinal area and genitals** are then examined. One should assess the inguinal area for hernias. Care should be taken to examine the testicles of boys with abdominal pain; testicular trauma, testicular torsion, and epididymitis all may present with abdominal discomfort. A unilateral swollen or painful testicle with an absent cremasteric reflex on the affected side is concerning for testicular torsion and should be referred for emergent ultrasound and urologic consultation. After the genital exam, the child is then placed in the prone position, and abnormalities of the **back** are sought. The spine and costovertebral angle areas are percussed to elicit any tenderness; such findings may be indicative of vertebral osteomyelitis or diskitis and pyelonephritis, respectively.

Examining the **ears and throat** completes the physical examination. These are usually the most bothersome parts of the examination for the child, and parents frequently can be helpful in minimizing head movement. During the oropharyngeal examination, it is important to document the presence of enanthemas; these may be seen in many infectious processes, such as stomatitis caused by herpes or enteroviruses.

This portion of the examination is also important in documenting inflammation or exudates on the tonsils, which may indicate viral or bacterial infection. Findings such as trismus or unilateral tonsillar swelling are concerning for peritonsillar abscess and for infections in the para- and retropharyngeal spaces; such cases should be referred for specialist ear, nose, and throat evaluation and imaging of the neck.

Repeating portions of the assessment may be indicated. If the child cried continuously during the initial clinical evaluation, the examiner may not be certain whether the crying was caused by the high fever, stranger anxiety, or pain, or is indicative of a serious or localizing illness. Constant crying also makes portions of the physical examination, such as auscultation of the chest, more difficult. Before a repeat assessment is performed, efforts to make the child as comfortable as possible are indicated. In young infants, **persistent irritability**, even when the examiner is absent from the room, is concerning for meningitis, encephalitis, or other causes of meningeal irritation (e.g., intracranial injury from nonaccidental trauma). When faced with a truly inconsolable infant, practitioners should have a low threshold to obtain head imaging and/or perform lumbar puncture, as the clinical scenario dictates.

MANAGEMENT

Most patients who present to the pediatrician's office with an acute illness will not require acute stabilization. However, the pediatrician needs to be prepared to evaluate and begin resuscitation for the seriously ill or unstable child. Outpatient pediatric offices and urgent care facilities should be stocked with appropriate equipment necessary to stabilize an acutely ill child. Maintenance of that equipment and ongoing training of the office staff in its use is required, and every effort should be made to ensure that pediatric clinicians are PALS certified (see Chapter 81).

The evaluation of the potentially unstable child must begin with assessment of the ABCs—airway, breathing, and circulation. When assessing the **airway**, chest rise should be evaluated and evidence of increased work of breathing sought. The examiner should ensure that the trachea is midline and should listen carefully for evidence of air exchange at the level of the extrathoracic airway. If the airway is patent and no signs of obstruction are present, the patient is allowed to assume a position of comfort. If the child shows signs of airway obstruction, repositioning of the head with the chin-lift maneuver may alleviate the obstruction. An oral or nasal airway may be necessary in patients in whom airway patency cannot be maintained. These devices are not well tolerated in conscious patients because they may induce gagging or vomiting; instead, they are most often used to facilitate effective bag-valve-mask ventilation in semiconscious or unconscious children. Once airway patency has been established, the adequacy of **breathing** should be evaluated. Slow respiratory rates or cyanosis may signal impending respiratory failure. If the airway is patent but the child's respiratory effort is inadequate, positive pressure ventilation via bag-valve-mask support should be initiated. Oxygen should be administered to all seriously ill or hypoxic children via nasal cannula or face mask. Auscultation of the lung fields should assess for air entry, symmetry of breath sounds, and presence of adventitial breath sounds such as crackles or wheezes. Bronchodilator therapy can be initiated to alleviate bronchospasm. Racemic epinephrine is indicated for stridor at rest in a patient with croup. Once airway and breathing have been addressed, **circulation** must be evaluated. Symptoms of *shock* include tachycardia, cool extremities, delayed capillary refill time, mottled or pale skin, and effortless tachypnea. In children, hypotension is a late finding in shock and indicates that significant decompensation has already taken place. Vascular access is necessary for volume resuscitation in patients with impaired circulation, and an intraosseous line should be considered early if there is any difficulty in obtaining vascular access for a patient requiring resuscitation. Each time an intervention is performed, the clinician should **reassess the patient** to determine whether interventions have been successful and whether additional care is needed.

DISPOSITION

The majority of children evaluated in the office or urgent care setting for an acute illness can be managed as an **outpatient**. These patients should have a reassuring physical examination, stable vital signs, and an adequate follow-up plan before being sent home. A mildly dehydrated patient can be discharged home for a trial of oral rehydration. Patients with respiratory illness who exhibit signs of mild respiratory distress may be monitored at home, with a repeat examination scheduled the next day. Depending on the child's condition, the comfort of the parents, and the relationship of the family with the physician, telephone follow-up may be all that is necessary. When no specific diagnosis has been established at the first outpatient visit, a follow-up examination may yield the diagnosis and can provide reassurance for both the caregiver and the practitioner that a child's severity of illness has not progressed.

However, if it is deemed that the child needs a higher level of care, it is the pediatrician's responsibility to decide what method of transfer is appropriate. Physicians may be reluctant to call for help because of a misperception that emergency 911 services should be activated only for ongoing resuscitation. Emergency medical services (EMS) transport should be initiated for any child who is physiologically unstable (e.g., with severe respiratory distress, hypoxia, signs of shock, or altered mental state). If the family's ability to comply promptly with recommendation for ED evaluation is in question, this patient also should be transported by EMS. Some physicians and families may defer calling EMS because of the perception that a parent can reach the hospital faster by private motor vehicle. Although rapidity of transport should be considered, the need for further interventions during transport and the risk of clinical decompensation are other important factors in the decision to activate EMS. Ultimately, the legal responsibility for choosing an appropriate level of transport for a patient lies with the referring physician, until responsibility of care is officially transferred to another medical provider.

Bibliography is available at Expert Consult.

Chapter **81**
Pediatric Emergencies and Resuscitation

Mary E. Hartman and Ira M. Cheifetz

第八十一章
儿科急症和复苏

中文导读

本章主要介绍了急诊对儿童进行评估的方法、呼吸窘迫和呼吸衰竭的识别与治疗、休克的识别和管理、心动过缓和快速型心律失常的识别、血管通路、非血管的应急处理及复苏后治疗。急诊对儿童进行评估的方法具体描述了一般评估、初级评估、二次评估；呼吸窘迫和呼吸衰竭的识别与治疗包括气道梗阻、气道狭窄、肺实质疾病和高级气道管理技术；心动过缓和快速型心律失常的识别部分具体描述了心动过缓和快速型心律失常；血管通路中具体描述了血管通路、骨髓通路、动脉通路的建立；非血管的应急处理包括胸腔穿刺术和胸腔引流管的放置及心包穿刺术。

Injuries are the leading cause of death in American children and young adults and account for more childhood deaths than all other causes combined (see Chapter 13). Rapid, effective bystander cardiopulmonary resuscitation (CPR) for children is associated with survival rates as high as 70%, with good neurologic outcome. However, bystander CPR is still provided for <50% of children who experience cardiac arrest outside medical settings. This failing has led to long-term survival rates of <40%, often with a poor neurologic outcome.

APPROACH TO THE EMERGENCY EVALUATION OF A CHILD

The first response to a pediatric emergency of any cause is a systematic, rapid **general assessment** of the scene and the child to identify immediate threats to the child, care providers, or others. If an emergency is identified, the emergency response system (emergency medical services, EMS) should be activated immediately. Care providers should then proceed through **primary**, **secondary**, and **tertiary** assessments as allowed by the child's condition, safety of the scene, and resources available. This standardized approach provides organization to what might otherwise be a confusing or chaotic situation and reinforces an organized thought process for care providers. If at any point in these assessments the caregiver identifies a life-threatening problem, the assessment is halted and lifesaving interventions are initiated. Further assessment and intervention should be delayed until other caregivers arrive or the condition is successfully treated or stabilized.

General Assessment

On arrival at the scene of a compromised child, a caregiver's first task is a quick survey of the scene itself. Is the rescuer or child in imminent danger because of circumstances at the scene (e.g., fire, high-voltage electricity)? If so, can the child be safely extricated to a safe location for assessment and treatment? Can the child be safely moved with the appropriate precautions (i.e., cervical spine protection), if indicated? A rescuer is expected to proceed only if these important safety conditions have been met.

Once the caregiver and patient's safety has been ensured, the caregiver performs a rapid **visual survey** of the child, assessing the child's **general appearance** and **cardiopulmonary function**. This action should be only a few seconds and include assessment of (1) general appearance, determining color, tone, alertness, and responsiveness; (2) adequacy of breathing, distinguishing between normal, comfortable respirations and respiratory distress or apnea; and (3) adequacy of circulation, identifying cyanosis, pallor, or mottling. A child found unresponsive from an *unwitnessed* collapse should be approached with a gentle touch and the verbal question, "Are you OK?" If there is no response, the caregiver should immediately shout for help and send someone to activate the emergency response system and locate an **automated external defibrillator (AED)**. Figs. 81.1 and 81.2 present basic life support (BLS) pediatric cardiac arrest algorithms for 1 rescuer and 2 or more rescuers, respectively. The provider should then determine whether the child is breathing and, if not, provide 2 rescue breaths. If the child is breathing adequately, the circulation is quickly assessed. Any child with heart rate <60 beats/min or without a pulse requires immediate CPR. If the caregiver *witnesses* the sudden collapse of a child, the caregiver should have a higher suspicion for a sudden cardiac event. In this case, rapid deployment of an AED is crucial. Any interruptions in care of the child to activate EMS and locate the nearest AED should be very brief. If >1 caregiver is present, someone should always remain with the child and provide initial care or stabilization (see Fig. 81.2).

Primary Assessment

Once the emergency response system has been activated and the child is determined not to need CPR, the caregiver should proceed with a primary assessment that includes a brief, **hands-on assessment** of cardiopulmonary and neurologic function and stability. This assessment includes a limited physical examination, evaluation of vital signs, and measurement of pulse oximetry if available. The American Heart Association, in its Pediatric Advanced Life Support (PALS) curriculum, supports the structured format of **airway, breathing, circulation, disability, exposure (ABCDE)**. The goal of the primary assessment is to obtain a focused, systems-based assessment of the child's injuries or abnormalities, so that resuscitative efforts can be directed to these areas; if the caregiver identifies a life-threatening abnormality, further evaluation is postponed until appropriate corrective action has been taken.

The exam and vital sign data can be interpreted only if the caregiver has a thorough understanding of normal values. In pediatrics, normal respiratory rate, heart rate, and blood pressure have age-specific norms (Table 81.1). These ranges can be difficult to remember, especially if used infrequently. However, several standard principals apply: (1) a child's respiratory rate should not be >60 breaths/min for a sustained period; (2) normal heart rate is 2-3 times normal respiratory rate for age; and (3) a simple guide for pediatric blood pressure is that the lower limit of systolic blood pressure should be ≥60 mm Hg for neonates; ≥70 mm Hg for 1 mo-1 yr olds; ≥70 mm Hg + (2 × age) for 1-10 yr olds; and ≥90 mm Hg for any child older than 10 yr.

Airway and Breathing

The most common precipitating event for cardiac instability in infants and children is respiratory insufficiency. Therefore, rapid assessment of respiratory failure and immediate restoration of adequate ventilation and oxygenation remain the first priority in the resuscitation of a child. Using a systematic approach, the caregiver should first assess whether the child's airway is patent and maintainable. A healthy, **patent** airway is unobstructed, allowing normal respiration without noise or effort. A **maintainable** airway is one that is either already patent or can be made patent with a simple maneuver. To assess airway patency, the provider should look for breathing movements in the child's chest and abdomen, listen for breath sounds, and feel the movement of air at the child's mouth and nose. Abnormal breathing sounds (e.g., snoring or stridor), increased work of breathing, and apnea are all findings potentially consistent with airway obstruction. If there is evidence of airway obstruction, maneuvers to relieve the obstruction should be instituted before the caregiver proceeds to evaluate the child's breathing.

Assessment of breathing includes evaluation of the child's respiratory rate, respiratory effort, abnormal sounds, and pulse oximetry. Normal breathing appears comfortable, is quiet, and occurs at an age-appropriate rate. Abnormal respiratory rates include apnea and rates that are either too slow (bradypnea) or too fast (tachypnea). *Bradypnea and irregular respiratory patterns require urgent attention because they are often signs of impending respiratory failure and/or apnea.* Signs of increased respiratory effort include nasal flaring, grunting, chest or neck muscle retractions, head bobbing, and seesaw respirations. Hemoglobin oxygen desaturation, as measured by pulse oximetry, often accompanies parenchymal lung disease apnea or airway obstruction. However, providers should keep in mind that adequate perfusion is required to produce a reliable oxygen saturation (SO_2) measurement. A child with low SO_2 is a child in distress. **Central cyanosis** is a sign of severe hypoxia and indicates an emergent need for oxygen supplementation and respiratory support.

Circulation

Cardiovascular function is assessed by evaluation of skin color and temperature, heart rate, heart rhythm, pulses, capillary refill time, and blood pressure. In nonhospital settings, much of the important information can be obtained without measuring the blood pressure; lack of blood pressure data should not prevent the provider for determining adequacy of circulation or implementing a lifesaving response. Mottling, pallor, delayed capillary refill, cyanosis, poor pulses, and cool extremities

Table 81.1	Normal Vital Signs According to Age		
AGE	**HEART RATE (beats/min)**	**BLOOD PRESSURE (mm Hg)**	**RESPIRATORY RATE (breaths/min)**
Premature	120-170*	55-75/35-45†	40-70‡
0-3 mo	100-150*	65-85/45-55	35-55
3-6 mo	90-120	70-90/50-65	30-45
6-12 mo	80-120	80-100/55-65	25-40
1-3 yr	70-110	90-105/55-70	20-30
3-6 yr	65-110	95-110/60-75	20-25
6-12 yr	60-95	100-120/60-75	14-22
12+ yr	55-85	110-135/65-85	12-18

*In sleep, infant heart rates may drop significantly lower, but if perfusion is maintained, no intervention is required.

†A blood pressure cuff should cover approximately two thirds of the arm; too small a cuff yields spuriously high pressure readings, and too large a cuff yields spuriously low pressure readings. Values are systolic/diastolic.

‡Many premature infants require mechanical ventilatory support, making their spontaneous respiratory rate less relevant.

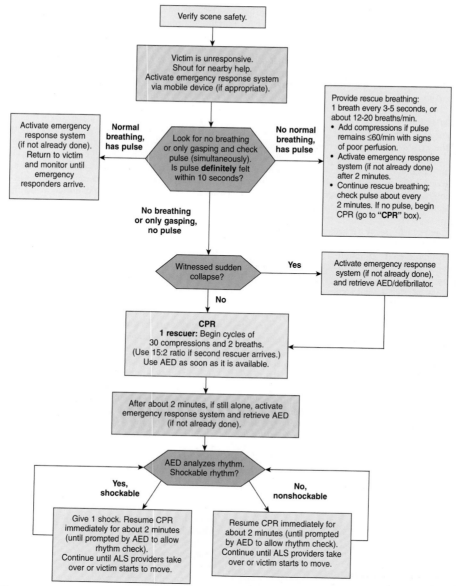

© 2015 American Heart Association

Fig. 81.1 Basic life support (BLS) healthcare provider: pediatric cardiac arrest algorithm for the single rescuer—2015 update. AED, Automated external defibrillator; ALS, advanced life support; CPR, cardiopulmonary resuscitation. (From Atkins DL, Berger S, Duff JP, et al: Part 11. Pediatric basic life support and cardiopulmonary resuscitation quality: 2015 American Heart Association guidelines update for cardiopulmonary resuscitation and emergency cardiovascular care, Circulation 132[Suppl 2]:S519–S525, 2015, Fig 1, p S521.)

are all signs of diminished perfusion and compromised cardiac output. **Tachycardia** is the earliest and most reliable sign of shock but is itself fairly nonspecific and should be correlated with other components of the exam, such as weakness, threadiness, and absence of pulses. An age-specific approach to pulse assessment will yield best results.

Disability

In the setting of a pediatric emergency, *disability* refers to a child's neurologic function in terms of the level of consciousness and cortical function. Standard evaluation of a child's neurologic condition can be done quickly with an assessment of pupillary response to light (if one is available) and use of either of the standard scores used in pediatrics: the Alert, Verbal, Pain, Unresponsive (AVPU) Pediatric Response Scale

and the Glasgow Coma Scale (GCS). The causes of decreased level of consciousness in children are numerous and include conditions as diverse as respiratory failure with hypoxia or hypercarbia, hypoglycemia, poisonings or drug overdose, trauma, seizures, infection, and shock. *Most often, an ill or injured child has an altered level of consciousness because of respiratory compromise, circulatory compromise, or both.* Any child with a depressed level of consciousness should be immediately assessed for abnormalities in cardiorespiratory status.

Alert, Verbal, Pain, Unresponsive Pediatric Response Scale. The AVPU scoring system is used to determine a child's level of consciousness and cerebral cortex function (Table 81.2). Unlike the GCS, the AVPU scale is not developmentally dependent—a child does not have to understand spoken language or follow commands, merely respond to a stimulus.

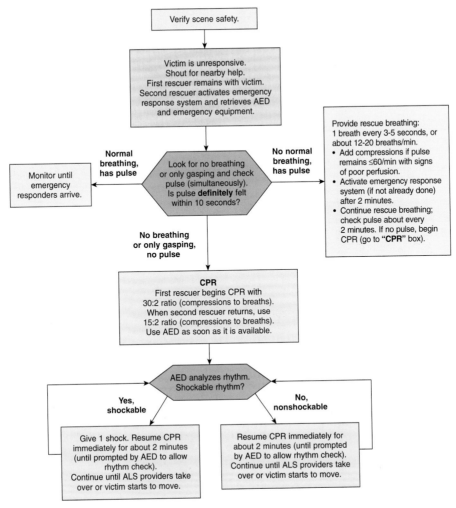

Fig. 81.2 Basic life support (BLS) healthcare provider pediatric cardiac arrest algorithm for 2 or more rescuers—2015 update. AED, Automated external defibrillator; ALS, advanced life support; CPR, cardiopulmonary resuscitation. (*From Atkins DL, Berger S, Duff JP, et al: Part 11. Pediatric basic life support and cardiopulmonary resuscitation quality: 2015 American Heart Association guidelines update for cardiopulmonary resuscitation and emergency cardiovascular care, Circulation 132[Suppl 2]:S519–S525, 2015, Fig 2, p S522.)*

The child is scored according to the amount of stimulus required to obtain a response, from *alert* (no stimulus, the child is already awake and interactive) to *unresponsive* (child does not respond to any stimulus).

Glasgow Coma Scale. Although it has not been systematically validated as a prognostic scoring system for infants and young children as it has in adults, GCS is frequently used in the assessment of pediatric patients with an altered level of consciousness. The GCS is the most widely used method of evaluating a child's neurologic function and has 3 components. Individual scores for eye opening, verbal response, and motor response are added together, with a maximum of 15 points (Table 81.3). Patients with a GCS score ≤8 require aggressive management, generally including stabilization of the airway and breathing with endotracheal intubation and mechanical ventilation, respectively, and if indicated, placement of an intracranial pressure monitoring device. The **Full Outline of Unresponsiveness** (FOUR) score is another useful assessment and monitoring tool (see Table 85.1).

Exposure

Exposure is the final component of the pediatric primary assessment. This component of the exam is reached only after the child's airway, breathing, and circulation have been assessed and determined to be stable or have been stabilized through simple interventions. In this setting, *exposure* stands for the dual responsibility of the provider to both expose the child to assess for previously unidentified injures and consider prolonged exposure in a cold environment as a possible cause of hypothermia and cardiopulmonary instability. The provider should undress the child (as is feasible and reasonable) to perform a focused physical exam, assessing for burns, bruising, bleeding, joint laxity, and fractures. If possible, the provider should assess the child's temperature. All maneuvers should be performed with careful maintenance of cervical spine precautions.

Secondary Assessment

For healthcare providers in community or outpatient settings, transfer of care of a child to emergency or hospital personnel may occur before a full secondary assessment is possible. However, before the child is removed from the scene and separated from witnesses or family, a brief history should be obtained for medical providers at the accepting facility. The components of a secondary assessment include a **focused history** and **focused physical examination**.

Table 81.2 | AVPU Neurologic Assessment

A	The child is awake, alert, and interactive with parents and care providers.
V	The child responds only if the care provider or parents call the child's name or speak loudly.
P	The child responds only to painful stimuli, such as pinching the nail bed of a toe or finger.
U	The child is unresponsive to all stimuli.

A, Alert; V, verbal, P, pain, U, unresponsive.
From Ralston M, Hazinski MF, Zaritsky AL, et al, editors: *Pediatric advanced life support course guide and PALS provider manual: provider manual*, Dallas, 2007, American Heart Association.

Table 81.3 | Glasgow Coma Scale

EYE OPENING (TOTAL POSSIBLE POINTS 4)

Spontaneous	4
To voice	3
To pain	2
None	1

VERBAL RESPONSE (TOTAL POSSIBLE POINTS 5)

Older Children		Infants and Young Children	
Oriented	5	Appropriate words; smiles, fixes, and follows	5
Confused	4	Consolable crying	4
Inappropriate	3	Persistently irritable	3
Incomprehensible	2	Restless, agitated	2
None	1	None	1

MOTOR RESPONSE (TOTAL POSSIBLE POINTS 6)

Obeys	6
Localizes pain	5
Withdraws	4
Flexion	3
Extension	2
None	1

Adapted from Teasdale G, Jennett B: Assessment of coma and impaired consciousness: a practical scale, *Lancet* 2:81–84, 1974.

The history should be targeted to information that could explain cardiorespiratory or neurologic dysfunction and should take the form of a **SAMPLE history**: signs/symptoms, allergies, medications, past medical history, timing of last meal, and events leading to this situation. Medical personnel not engaged in resuscitative efforts can be dispatched to elicit history from witnesses or relatives. The physical examination during the secondary assessment is a thorough head-to-toe exam, although the severity of the child's illness or injury could necessitate curtailing portions of the exam or postponing nonessential elements until a later time.

Tertiary Assessment

The tertiary assessment occurs in a hospital setting, where ancillary laboratory and radiographic assessments contribute to a thorough understanding of the child's condition. A basic blood chemistry profile, complete blood count, liver function tests, coagulation studies, and arterial blood gas analyses give fairly broad (but somewhat nonspecific) estimates of renal function, acid-base balance, cardiorespiratory function, and presence or absence of shock. Chest radiographs can be useful to evaluate both the heart and lungs, although more detailed estimates of heart function and cardiac output can be made with **echocardiography**. Arterial and central venous catheters can be placed to monitor arterial and central venous pressure.

RECOGNITION AND TREATMENT OF RESPIRATORY DISTRESS AND FAILURE

The goals of initial management of respiratory distress or failure are to rapidly stabilize the child's airway and breathing and to identify the cause of the problem so that further therapeutic efforts can be appropriately directed.

Airway Obstruction

Children <5 yr old are particularly susceptible to foreign body aspiration and choking. Liquids are the most common cause of choking in infants, whereas small objects and food (e.g., grapes, nuts, hot dogs, candy) are the most common source of foreign bodies in the airways of toddlers and older children. A history consistent with foreign body aspiration is considered diagnostic. Any child in the proper setting with the sudden onset of choking, stridor, or wheezing has foreign body aspiration until proven otherwise.

Airway obstruction is treated with a sequential approach, starting with the head-tilt/chin-lift maneuver to open and support the airway, followed by inspection for a foreign body, and finger-sweep clearance or suctioning if one is visualized (Fig. 81.3). *Blind suctioning or finger sweeps of the mouth are not recommended.* A nasopharyngeal airway or oropharyngeal airway can be inserted for airway support, if indicated. A conscious child suspected of having a partial foreign body obstruction should be permitted to cough spontaneously until coughing is no longer effective, respiratory distress and stridor increase, or the child becomes unconscious.

If the child becomes unconscious, the child should be gently placed on the ground, supine. The provider should then open the airway with the head-tilt/chin-lift maneuver and attempt mouth-to-mouth ventilation (Figs. 81.4 and 81.5). If ventilation is unsuccessful, the airway is repositioned and ventilation attempted again. If there is still no chest rise, attempts to remove a foreign body are indicated. In an infant <1 yr old, a combination of 5 back blows and 5 chest thrusts is administered (Fig. 81.6). After each cycle of back blows and chest thrusts, the child's mouth should be visually inspected for the presence of the foreign body. If identified within finger's reach, it should be removed with a gentle finger sweep. If no foreign body is visual, ventilation is again attempted. If this is unsuccessful, the head is repositioned and ventilation attempted again. If there is still no chest rise, the series of back blows and chest thrusts is repeated.

For a conscious child >1 yr old, providers should give a series of 5 abdominal thrusts (**Heimlich maneuver**) with the child standing or sitting (Fig. 81.7); this should occur with the child lying down if unconscious (Fig. 81.8). After the abdominal thrusts, the airway is examined for a foreign body, which should be removed if visualized. If no foreign body is seen, the head is repositioned and ventilation attempted. If unsuccessful, the head is repositioned and ventilation attempted again. If these efforts are unsuccessful, the Heimlich sequence is repeated.

Airway Narrowing

Airway obstruction can also be caused by airway narrowing, in both the upper and lower airways. *Upper airway obstruction* refers to narrowing of the extrathoracic portion of the airway, including the oropharynx, larynx, and trachea. In the upper airways, narrowing is most often caused by airway **edema** (e.g., croup or anaphylaxis). Lower airway disease affects all intrathoracic airways, notably the bronchi and bronchioles. In the lower airways, **bronchiolitis** and acute **asthma** exacerbations are the major contributors to intrathoracic airway obstruction in children, causing airway narrowing through a combination of airway swelling, mucus production, and circumferential smooth muscle constriction of smaller airways.

Airway support for these processes is dictated by both the underlying condition and the clinical severity of the problem. In cases of mild upper airway obstruction, the child has minimally elevated work of breathing (evidenced by tachypnea and few to mild retractions). Stridor, if present at all, should be audible with only coughing or activity. Children with these findings can be supported with supplemental oxygen as needed. In cases with moderate obstruction, in which the child has a

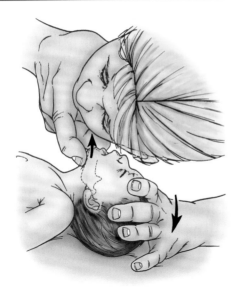

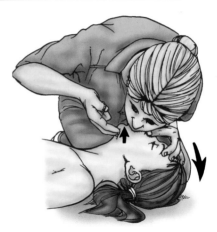

Fig. 81.5 Rescue breathing in a child. The rescuer's mouth covers the child's mouth, creating a mouth-to-mouth seal. One hand maintains the head-tilt; the thumb and forefinger of the same hand are used to pinch the child's nose. *(From Guidelines for cardiopulmonary resuscitation and emergency cardiac care. Emergency Cardiac Care Committee and Subcommittees, American Heart Association. Part V. Pediatric basic life support, JAMA 268:2251–2261, 1992.)*

Fig. 81.3 Opening the airway with the head-tilt/chin-lift maneuver. One hand is used to tilt the head, extending the neck. The index finger of the rescuer's other hand lifts the mandible outward by lifting the chin. Head-tilt should not be performed if a cervical spine injury is suspected. *(From Guidelines for cardiopulmonary resuscitation and emergency cardiac care. Emergency Cardiac Care Committee and Subcommittees, American Heart Association. Part V. Pediatric basic life support, JAMA 268:2251–2261, 1992.)*

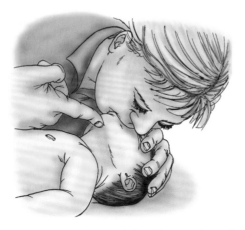

Fig. 81.4 Rescue breathing in an infant. The rescuer's mouth covers the infant's nose and mouth, creating a seal. One hand performs the head-tilt while the other hand lifts the infant's jaw. Avoid head-tilt if the infant has sustained head or neck trauma. *(From Guidelines for cardiopulmonary resuscitation and emergency cardiac care. Emergency Cardiac Care Committee and Subcommittees, American Heart Association. Part V. Pediatric basic life support, JAMA 268:2251–2261, 1992.)*

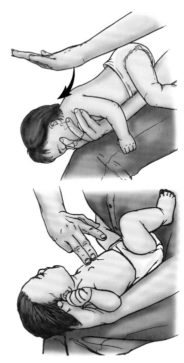

Fig. 81.6 Back blows *(top)* and chest thrusts *(bottom)* to relieve foreign body airway obstruction in the infant. *(From Guidelines for cardiopulmonary resuscitation and emergency cardiac care. Emergency Cardiac Care Committee and Subcommittees, American Heart Association. Part V. Pediatric basic life support, JAMA 268:2251–2261, 1992.)*

higher work of breathing and more pronounced stridor, nebulized racemic **epinephrine** and oral or intravenous (IV) **dexamethasone** can be added. **Heliox** (combined helium-oxygen therapy) administration may also be considered. Children with severe upper airway obstruction have marked intercostal retractions, prominent stridor, and decreased air entry on auscultation of the lung fields. Most children with significant airway obstruction are also hypoxic, and many appear dyspneic and agitated. A child in severe distress needs to be closely observed because the signs of impending respiratory failure may be initially confused

with improvement. Stridor becomes quieter and intercostal retractions less prominent when a child's respiratory effort begins to diminish. The child in respiratory failure can be distinguished from one who is improving by evidence of poor air movement on auscultation and lethargy or decreased level of consciousness from hypercarbia, hypoxia, or both.

When **anaphylaxis** is suspected as the cause for upper airway edema, providers should administer an intramuscular (IM) or IV dose of epinephrine as needed (see Chapter 174). No matter the cause, any child in impending respiratory failure should be prepared for endotracheal intubation and respiratory support. Prompt notification of providers trained in airway management is essential.

In cases of *lower airway obstruction*, therapies are targeted to both

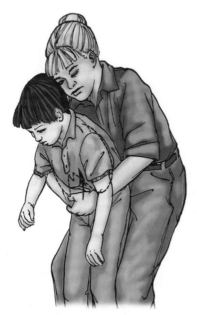

Fig. 81.7 Abdominal thrusts with the victim standing or sitting (conscious). *(From Guidelines for cardiopulmonary resuscitation and emergency cardiac care. Emergency Cardiac Care Committee and Subcommittees, American Heart Association. Part V. Pediatric basic life support, JAMA 268:2251–2261, 1992.)*

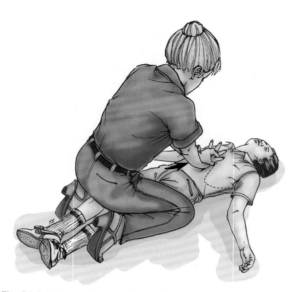

Fig. 81.8 Abdominal thrusts with victim lying (conscious or unconscious). *(From Guidelines for cardiopulmonary resuscitation and emergency cardiac care. Emergency Cardiac Care Committee and Subcommittees, American Heart Association. Part V. Pediatric basic life support, JAMA 268:2251–2261, 1992.)*

relieving the obstruction and reducing the child's work of breathing. Inhaled **bronchodilators**, such as albuterol, augmented by oral or IV corticosteroids, remain the mainstay of therapy in settings of mild to moderate acute distress caused by lower airway obstruction (e.g., **asthma**). Children with more significant obstruction appear dyspneic, with tachypnea, retractions, and easily audible wheezing. In these cases, the addition of an anticholinergic agent, such as nebulized ipratropium bromide, or a smooth muscle relaxant, such as magnesium sulfate, may provide further relief, although the evidence for these measures remains controversial (see Chapter 169). Supplemental oxygen and IV fluid hydration can also be useful adjuncts. As in cases of upper airway obstruction, impending respiratory failure in children with lower airway obstruction can be insidious. When diagnosed early in a school-age child who is cooperative, respiratory failure can be averted through judicious use of noninvasive support, including heated, high-flow nasal cannula (HFNC) therapy, continuous positive airway pressure (CPAP), bilevel positive airway pressure (BiPAP), or heliox therapy. Endotracheal intubation should be performed only by skilled providers, preferably in a hospital setting, because there is a high risk of cardiorespiratory compromise in patients with lower airway obstruction during the procedure.

Parenchymal Lung Disease

Parenchymal lung disease includes a heterogeneous list of conditions, such as pneumonia, acute respiratory distress syndrome (ARDS), pneumonitis, bronchiolitis, bronchopulmonary dysplasia, cystic fibrosis, and pulmonary edema. The commonalities of these conditions are their effects on the small airways and alveoli, including inflammation and exudation leading to consolidation of lung tissue, decreased gas exchange, and increased work of breathing. Clinical management of these conditions includes specific treatment as indicated (e.g., antibiotics for bacterial pneumonia) and supportive care in the form of supplemental oxygen, noninvasive respiratory support (with HFNC, CPAP, or BiPAP), or invasive mechanical ventilation.

Advanced Airway Management Techniques
Bag-Valve-Mask Positive Pressure Ventilation

Rescue breathing with a bag-valve-mask apparatus can be as effective as endotracheal intubation and safer when the provider is inexperienced with intubation. Bag-valve-mask ventilation itself requires training to ensure that the provider is competent to select the correct mask size, open the child's airway, form a tight seal between the mask and the child's face, deliver effective ventilation, and assess the effectiveness of the ventilation. An appropriately sized mask is one that fits over the child's mouth and nose but does not extend below the chin or over the eyes (Fig. 81.9). An adequate seal is best achieved through a combination "C-E" grip on the mask, in which the thumb and index finger form the letter "C" on top of the mask, pressing the mask downward onto the child's face, and the remaining 3 fingers form an "E" grip under the child's mandible, holding the jaw forward and extending the head up toward the mask. Using this method, the care provider can secure the mask to the child's face with one hand and use the other hand to compress the ventilation bag (Fig. 81.10).

The provider may have to move the head and neck through a range of positions to find the one that best maintains airway patency and allows maximal ventilation. In infants and young children, optimal ventilation is often provided when the child's head is in the neutral sniffing position without hyperextension of the head (Fig. 81.11). Poor chest rise and persistently low SO₂ values indicate inadequate ventilation. In this setting the care provider should recheck the mask's seal on the child's face, reposition the child's head, and consider suctioning the airway, if indicated. If these maneuvers do not restore ventilation, the provider should consider noninvasive or invasive respiratory support (i.e., endotracheal intubation) as clinically indicated.

Endotracheal Intubation

A child generally requires intubation when at least one of these conditions exists: (1) the child is unable to maintain airway patency or protect the airway against aspiration (as occurs in settings of neurologic compromise); (2) the child is failing to maintain adequate oxygenation; (3) the child is failing to control blood carbon dioxide levels and maintain safe acid-base balance; (4) sedation and/or paralysis is required for a procedure; and (5) care providers anticipate a deteriorating course that will eventually lead to any of the first 4 conditions. It should be noted that in centers *experienced in noninvasive respiratory support,* a trial of HFNC, CPAP, and/or BiPAP may be indicated based on the specific clinical scenario.

There are few *absolute contraindications* to tracheal intubation, but experts generally agree that in settings of known complete airway obstruction, endotracheal intubation should be avoided, and emergency cricothyroidotomy performed instead. Another important consideration is to ensure that caregivers provide appropriate cervical spine (C-spine) protection during the intubation procedure when neck or spinal cord injury is suspected.

The most important phase of the intubation procedure is the pre-procedural preparation, when the provider ensures all the equipment and staff needed for safe intubation are present and functioning. An easy pneumonic for this is **SOAP MM:** *suction* (Yankauer suction catheter attached to wall suction); *oxygen* (both preoxygenation of the patient and devices needed to deliver oxygen, such as a bag-valve-mask); *airway* (appropriately sized endotracheal tube and laryngoscope); *people* (all those needed during and immediately after the procedure, including respiratory therapists and nurses); *monitor* (SO_2, heart rate, blood pressure, capnography); and *medications* (sedation and often neuromuscular blockade to allow the provider(s) to control the airway). A simple formula for selecting the appropriately sized endotracheal tube (ETT) is:

$$\text{Uncuffed ETT size (in mm)} = \left(\frac{\text{age in years}}{4}\right) + 4$$

Cuffed ETTs should generally be 0.5 mm smaller. Providers should always have a range of ETTs available given the heterogeneity of patients and airway size.

Analgesia is recommended to reduce metabolic stress, discomfort, and anxiety during intubation. Pretreatment with a sedative, an analgesic, and possibly a muscle relaxant is recommended unless the situation is emergent (i.e., apnea, asystole, unresponsiveness) and the administration of drugs would cause an unacceptable delay.

Because many intubations in critically ill children are emergency procedures, caregivers should be prepared for **rapid sequence intubation** (RSI) (Fig. 81.12 and Table 81.4). The goals of RSI are to induce anesthesia and paralysis and to complete intubation quickly. This approach minimizes elevations of intracranial pressure and blood pressure that may accompany intubation in awake or lightly sedated patients. Because the stomach generally cannot be emptied before RSI, the **Sellick maneuver** (downward pressure on the cricoid cartilage to compress the esophagus against the vertebral column) should be used to prevent aspiration of gastric contents.

Once the patient is intubated, proper ETT placement should be assessed by auscultation of breath sounds, evidence of symmetric chest rise, and analysis of exhaled carbon dioxide (CO_2) by a colorimetric device placed within the respiratory tubing near the ETT or a device that directly measures CO_2 elimination (capnogram or capnograph). Chest radiography is necessary to confirm appropriate tube position.

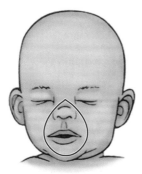

Correct
Covers mouth, nose, and chin but not eyes

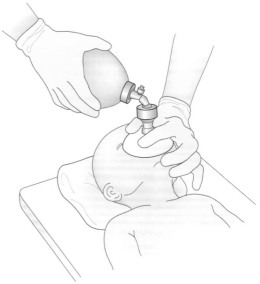

Fig. 81.10 "C-E" grip to secure bag-valve-mask to a child's face with appropriate seal.

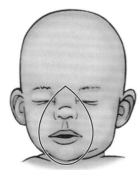

Incorrect
Too large: covers eyes and extends over chin

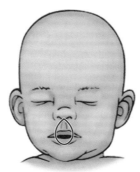

Incorrect
Too small: does not cover nose and mouth well

Fig. 81.9 Appropriate sizing technique for pediatric bag-valve-mask apparatus. *(From American Academy of Pediatrics and the American Heart Association; Kattwinkel J (ed): Textbook of Neonatal Resuscitation, ed 6. Elk Grove, IL: American Academy of Pediatrics, 2011. Fig 3-17.)*

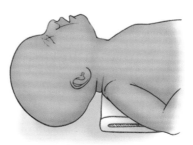

Fig. 81.11 Appropriate head position for bag-valve-mask ventilation. *(From American Academy of Pediatrics and the American Heart Association; Kattwinkel J (ed): Textbook of Neonatal Resuscitation, ed 6. Elk Grove, IL: American Academy of Pediatrics, 2011. Fig 3-19.)*

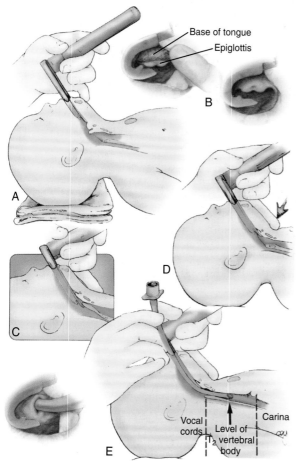

Base of tongue
Epiglottis

B

A

D

C

E

Vocal cords
Level of T₂ vertebral body
Carina

Fig. 81.12 A-E, Intubation technique. *(From Fleisher G, Ludwig S: Textbook of pediatric emergency medicine, Baltimore, 1983, Williams & Wilkins, p. 1250.)*

RECOGNITION AND MANAGEMENT OF SHOCK

In simple terms, shock occurs when oxygen and nutrient delivery to the tissues is inadequate to meet metabolic demands (see Chapter 88). The definition of shock *does not* include hypotension, and it is important for care providers to understand that **shock does not begin when blood pressure drops; it merely worsens and becomes more difficult (refractory) to treat once blood pressure is abnormal.**

Early *compensated* shock, whereby oxygen delivery is mostly preserved through compensatory mechanisms, is defined by the presence of normal blood pressure. When compensatory mechanisms fail, the shock progresses to *decompensated* shock, as defined by hypotension and organ dysfunction. In *irreversible* shock, organ failure progresses and death ensues.

Shock is also often described according to the underlying pathophysiology, which dictates the appropriate therapeutic response. **Hypovolemic shock** is the most common type of shock in children worldwide, usually related to fluid losses from severe diarrhea. Hemorrhage is a cause of hypovolemic shock after trauma or intestinal hemorrhage. When hypovolemia occurs because of third spacing of intravascular fluids into the extravascular compartment, the shock is described as **distributive shock**. The most common causes of distributive shock are sepsis, anaphylaxis, and burn injuries, in which release of inflammatory cytokines causes massive capillary leak of fluid and proteins, leading to low oncotic pressure and intravascular volume. In settings of profound myocardial dysfunction, a child has tissue hypoperfusion from

cardiogenic shock. The most common causes of cardiogenic shock are myocarditis, cardiomyopathy, and congenital heart disease, generally in the postoperative setting. **Obstructive shock** occurs when cardiac output is lowered by obstruction of blood flow to the body, as occurs when a ductus arteriosus closes in a child with ductus-dependent systemic blood flow, pericardial tamponade, tension pneumothorax, or massive pulmonary embolism.

The evaluation of a child in shock should proceed as described in the preceding sections on primary, secondary, and tertiary assessments. If the child presents in a hospital setting, providers should generally place a central venous line to provide secure venous access and an arterial line to permit continuous blood pressure monitoring and a more thorough laboratory assessment of organ systems, including studies of renal and liver function, acid-base balance and presence of lactic acidosis, hypoxemia and/or hypercapnia, and evidence of coagulopathy or disseminated intravascular coagulation. Chest radiography and echocardiography may also be useful. Respiratory and cardiovascular support should be provided as clinically indicated.

The treatment of shock focuses on the modifiable determinants of oxygen delivery while reducing the imbalance between oxygen supply and demand. A multipronged approach is recommended consisting of optimizing the arterial oxygen content of the blood, improving the volume and distribution of cardiac output, correcting metabolic derangements, and reducing oxygen demand. Blood oxygen content is maximized when hemoglobin values are normal and 100% of available hemoglobin is saturated with oxygen. Transfusion may be considered in the presence of hemorrhagic or distributive shock, in which crystalloid volume resuscitation has led to hemodilution and anemia. Appropriate SO_2 may be achieved by simple maneuvers, such as oxygen administration by nasal cannula or face mask; supportive measures (e.g., HFNC, CPAP, BiPAP) or invasive mechanical ventilation may be necessary. Therapies to increase cardiac output should be selected on the basis of the underlying pathophysiology. For hypovolemic and distributive shock, aggressive volume resuscitation, guided by arterial and central venous pressures, is the mainstay of therapy. In obstructive shock, relief of the obstruction is critical. The ductus arteriosus can often be reopened with prostaglandin administration and tamponade physiology relieved with appropriate drainage.

RECOGNITION OF BRADYARRHYTHMIAS AND TACHYARRHYTHMIAS

In the advanced life support (ALS) setting, arrhythmias are most usefully classified according to the observed heart rate (i.e., slow or fast) and its effect on perfusion (i.e., adequate or poor). If, in the primary survey, a caregiver finds a child with an abnormal heart rate plus poor perfusion and/or altered mental status, the rhythm is inadequate no matter its rate. In those settings the child is diagnosed with shock, and further evaluation is generally halted until appropriate resuscitation has been initiated.

Bradyarrhythmias

By definition, a child is *bradycardic* when the heart rate is slower than the normal range for age (see Table 81.1). Sinus bradycardia can be a harmless incidental finding in an otherwise healthy person and not usually associated with cardiac compromise. A relative bradycardia occurs when the heart rate is too slow for a child's activity level or metabolic needs. A clinically significant bradycardia occurs when the heart rate is slow and there are signs of systemic hypoperfusion (i.e., pallor, altered mental status, hypotension, acidosis). Symptomatic bradycardia occurs most often in the setting of hypoxia but can also be caused by hypoglycemia, hypocalcemia, other electrolyte abnormalities, hypothermia, heart block, and intracranial hypertension. Bradyarrhythmias are often the most common *prearrest* rhythms in young children.

Initial management of symptomatic bradycardia includes support or opening of the airway and confirming or establishing adequate SO_2 and ventilation (Fig. 81.13). After breathing has been secured, the child should be reassessed for continued bradycardia and poor perfusion. If

Table 81.4	Rapid Sequence Intubation	
STEP	**PROCEDURE**	**COMMENT/EXPLANATION**
1	Obtain a brief history and perform an assessment.	Rule out drug allergies; examine the airway anatomy (e.g., micrognathia, cleft palate).
2	Assemble equipment, medications, etc.	ETT: select the proper size for the age and weight of the child. Laryngoscope blades: a variety of Miller and the Macintosh blades.
3	Preoxygenate the patient.	With bag/mask, nasal cannula, hood or blow-by.
4	Position the patient.	Patient supine; neck is extended moderately to the "sniffing" position.
5	Premedicate the patient with lidocaine, atropine.	Lidocaine minimizes the ICP rise with intubation and can be applied topically to the airway mucosa for local anesthesia. Atropine helps blunt the bradycardia associated with upper airway manipulation and reduces airway secretions.
6	Perform a Sellick maneuver.	Pressure on the cricoid cartilage, to occlude the esophagus and prevent regurgitation or aspiration.
7	Induce sedation and analgesia.	**Sedatives** *Midazolam* (0.1 mg/kg): onset ~1 min; elimination in 30-40 min. *Ketamine* (2 mg/kg, may repeat as clinically indicated): onset 1-2 min; elimination in 30-40 min. May cause hallucinations if used alone; can cause higher ICP, mucous secretions, increased vital signs, and bronchodilation. **Analgesics** *Fentanyl* (3-5 μg/kg, may repeat as clinically indicated): onset ~1 min; elimination in 20-30 min. Rapid administration risks "tight chest" response, with no effective ventilation. Effects wear off in 20-30 min. *Morphine* (0.05-0.1 mg/kg dose): may last 30-60 min; may lead to hypotension in hypovolemic patients.
8	Administer muscle relaxants.	**Option 1:** Rocuronium (1 mg/kg): rapid onset and short duration. Other nondepolarizing agents include vecuronium and pancuronium, both dosed at 0.1 mg/kg. **Option 2:** Succinylcholine dose is 1-2 mg/kg; causes initial contraction of muscles, then relaxation. This depolarization can, however, increase ICP and blood pressure. Onset of paralysis in 30-40 sec; duration is 5-10 min. Pretreat with a small dose of a nondepolarizing paralytic agent, with intent of diminishing the depolarizing effect of succinylcholine.
9	Perform endotracheal intubation.	Performed by trained personnel.
10	Secure the tube, and verify position with radiograph.	ETT secured with tape to the cheeks and upper lip or to an adhesive patch applied to the skin near the mouth.
11	Begin mechanical ventilation.	Verify tube placement before ventilating with positive pressure; if an ETT is in 1 bronchus, barotraumas may occur.

ETT, Endotracheal tube; ICP, intracranial pressure.

cardiac compromise was solely the result of respiratory insufficiency, support of the child's airway and breathing may have been sufficient to restore normal hemodynamics. If respiratory support does not correct the perfusion abnormalities, further care is based on the quality of perfusion and degree of bradycardia. *A heart rate <60 beats/min with poor perfusion is an indication to begin chest compressions.* If the bradycardia persists, vascular access should be obtained; resuscitative epinephrine should be administered, and it should be repeated every 3-5 min for persistent symptomatic bradycardia. If increased vagal tone (e.g., in the setting of head injury with increased intracranial pressure) or primary atrioventricular block is suspected, atropine can also be given. For cases of refractory bradycardia, cardiac pacing should be considered. During the resuscitation of a child with bradycardia, providers should assess and treat factors known to cause bradycardia, referred to collectively as the **6 Hs**—hypoxia, hypovolemia, hydrogen ions (acidosis), hypokalemia or hyperkalemia, hypoglycemia, and hypothermia—and **5 Ts**—toxins, tamponade, tension pneumothorax, thrombosis (in either the pulmonary or cardiac circulations), and trauma (causing hypovolemia, intracranial hypertension, cardiac compromise or tamponade) (Table 81.5).

Tachyarrhythmias
Tachyarrhythmias represent a wide variety of rhythm disturbances of atrial and ventricular origin (see Chapter 462). Sinus tachycardia is a normal physiologic response to the body's need for increased cardiac output or oxygen delivery, as occurs with fever, exercise, or stress. It can also occur in more pathologic states, such as hypovolemia, anemia,

pain, anxiety, and metabolic stress. Tachyarrhythmias that do not originate in the sinus node are often categorized as *narrow complex rhythms* (i.e., originating in the atrium, such as atrial flutter or supraventricular tachycardia, SVT) and *wide complex rhythms* (i.e., rhythms of ventricular origin, such as ventricular tachycardia).

The initial management of tachycardia includes confirmation that the child has an adequate airway and life-sustaining breathing and circulation (Fig. 81.14). For children with persistent symptoms, further treatment is based on whether the QRS complex of the electrocardiogram (ECG) is narrow (≤0.09 sec) or wide (>0.09 sec). For narrow complex tachycardia, providers must distinguish between sinus tachycardia and SVT. In **sinus tachycardia**, (a) the history and onset are consistent with a known cause of tachycardia, such as fever or dehydration, and (b) P waves are consistently present, are of normal morphology, and occur at a rate that varies somewhat. In **supraventricular tachycardia**, (a) onset is often abrupt without prodrome, and (b) P waves are absent or polymorphic, and when present, their rate is often fairly steady at or above 220 beats/min. For children with SVT and good perfusion, vagal maneuvers can be attempted. When SVT is associated with poor perfusion, providers should rapidly move to convert the child's heart rhythm back to sinus rhythm. If the child already has IV access, adenosine can be given via IV access with rapid push. Adenosine has an extremely short half-life, so a proximal IV line is best, and the adenosine should be set up with a 3-way stopcock so it can be given and immediately flushed into the circulation. If the child does not have IV access, or adenosine does not successfully convert the heart rhythm back to sinus

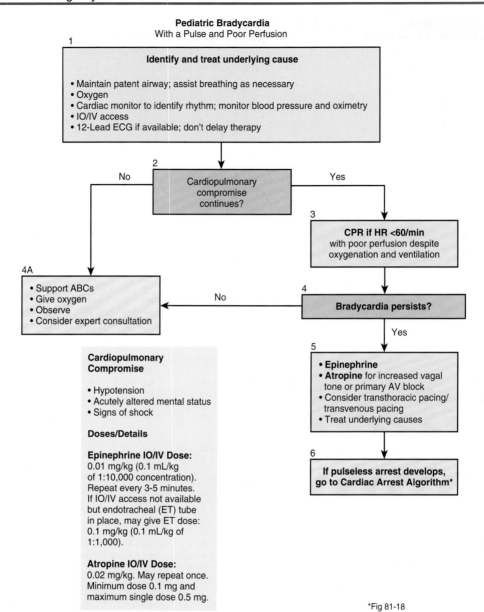

Pediatric Bradycardia
With a Pulse and Poor Perfusion

1
Identify and treat underlying cause

- Maintain patent airway; assist breathing as necessary
- Oxygen
- Cardiac monitor to identify rhythm; monitor blood pressure and oximetry
- IO/IV access
- 12-Lead ECG if available; don't delay therapy

2
Cardiopulmonary compromise continues?
No → Yes

3
CPR if HR <60/min
with poor perfusion despite oxygenation and ventilation

4A
- Support ABCs
- Give oxygen
- Observe
- Consider expert consultation

4
No ← **Bradycardia persists?**
Yes

Cardiopulmonary Compromise

- Hypotension
- Acutely altered mental status
- Signs of shock

Doses/Details

Epinephrine IO/IV Dose:
0.01 mg/kg (0.1 mL/kg of 1:10,000 concentration). Repeat every 3-5 minutes. If IO/IV access not available but endotracheal (ET) tube in place, may give ET dose: 0.1 mg/kg (0.1 mL/kg of 1:1,000).

Atropine IO/IV Dose:
0.02 mg/kg. May repeat once. Minimum dose 0.1 mg and maximum single dose 0.5 mg.

5
- **Epinephrine**
- **Atropine** for increased vagal tone or primary AV block
- Consider transthoracic pacing/ transvenous pacing
- Treat underlying causes

6
If pulseless arrest develops, go to Cardiac Arrest Algorithm*

*Fig 81-18

Fig. 81.13 Pediatric advanced life support bradycardia algorithm. ABCs, Airway, breathing, and circulation; AV, atrioventricular (conductor); ECG, electrocardiogram; HR, heart rate; IO/IV, intraosseous/intravenous. (*From Kleinman ME, Chameides L, Schexnayder SM, et al: 2010 American Heart Association guidelines for cardiopulmonary resuscitation and emergency cardiovascular care, part 14, Circulation 122[Suppl 3]:S876–S908, 2010, Fig. 2, p. S887.*)

rhythm, then **synchronized cardioversion**, using 0.5-1.0 joule (J)/kg, should be performed. In cases of wide complex tachycardia, providers should generally move immediately to cardioversion and increase the dose to 2 J/kg if 1 J/kg is not effective. As with cases of bradycardia, providers should review the 6 Hs and 5 Ts to identify factors that might be contributing to the tachycardia (see Table 81.5).

RECOGNITION AND MANAGEMENT OF CARDIAC ARREST

Cardiac arrest occurs when the heart fails as an effective pump and blood flow ceases. Outwardly, the patient in cardiac arrest presents as unresponsive and apneic with no palpable pulse. Internally, the cessation of nutrient flow causes progressive tissue ischemia and organ dysfunction.

If not rapidly reversed, cardiac arrest leads to progressive deterioration in brain, heart, and other organ function, such that resuscitation and recovery are no longer possible.

Pediatric cardiac arrest is rarely caused by a sudden coronary event or arrhythmia. Instead, cardiac arrest in children is most often the end result of progressive organ and tissue ischemia, caused by tissue hypoxia, acidosis, and nutrient depletion at the end stages of respiratory deterioration, shock, or heart failure. Therefore, **the most important treatment of cardiac arrest is anticipation and prevention. Intervening when a child manifests respiratory distress or early stages of shock can prevent deterioration to full arrest**. When sudden cardiac arrest does occur, it is often associated with an arrhythmia, specifically ventricular fibrillation (VF) or pulseless ventricular tachycardia (VT). In sudden

Table 81.5	Potentially Treatable Conditions Associated With Cardiac Arrest	
CONDITION	**COMMON CLINICAL SETTINGS**	**CORRECTIVE ACTIONS**
Acidosis	Preexisting acidosis, diabetes, diarrhea, drugs and toxins, prolonged resuscitation, renal disease, and shock	Reassess the adequacy of cardiopulmonary resuscitation, oxygenation, and ventilation; reconfirm endotracheal tube placement. Hyperventilate. Consider intravenous bicarbonate if pH <7.2 after above actions have been taken.
Cardiac tamponade	Hemorrhagic diathesis, cancer, pericarditis, trauma, after cardiac surgery, and after myocardial infarction	Administer fluids; obtain bedside echocardiogram, if available. Perform pericardiocentesis; immediate surgical intervention is appropriate if pericardiocentesis is unhelpful but cardiac tamponade is known or highly suspected.
Hypothermia	Alcohol abuse, burns, central nervous system disease, debilitated patient, drowning, drugs and toxins, endocrine disease, history of exposure, homelessness, extensive skin disease, spinal cord disease, and trauma	If hypothermia is severe (temperature <30°C [86°F]), limit initial shocks for ventricular fibrillation or pulseless ventricular tachycardia to 3; initiate active internal rewarming and cardiopulmonary support. If hypothermia is moderate (temperature 30-34°C [86-93.2°F]), proceed with resuscitation (space medications at longer intervals than usual), passively rewarm child, and actively rewarm truncal body areas.
Hypovolemia, hemorrhage, anemia	Major burns, diabetes, gastrointestinal losses, hemorrhage, hemorrhagic diathesis, cancer, pregnancy, shock, and trauma	Administer fluids. Transfuse packed red blood cells if hemorrhage or profound anemia is present. Thoracotomy is appropriate when a patient has cardiac arrest from penetrating trauma and a cardiac rhythm and the duration of cardiopulmonary resuscitation before thoracotomy is <10 min.
Hypoxia	Consider in all patients with cardiac arrest.	Reassess the technical quality of cardiopulmonary resuscitation, oxygenation, and ventilation; reconfirm endotracheal tube placement.
Hypomagnesemia	Alcohol abuse, burns, diabetic ketoacidosis, severe diarrhea, diuretics, and drugs (e.g., cisplatin, cyclosporine, pentamidine)	Administer 1-2 g magnesium sulfate intravenously over 2 min.
Poisoning	Alcohol abuse, bizarre or puzzling behavioral or metabolic presentation, classic toxicologic syndrome, occupational or industrial exposure, and psychiatric disease	Consult a toxicologist for emergency advice on resuscitation and definitive care, including an appropriate antidote. Prolonged resuscitation efforts may be appropriate; immediate cardiopulmonary bypass should be considered, if available.
Hyperkalemia	Metabolic acidosis, excessive administration of potassium, drugs and toxins, vigorous exercise, hemolysis, renal disease, rhabdomyolysis, tumor lysis syndrome, and clinically significant tissue injury	If hyperkalemia is identified or strongly suspected, treat* with all the following: 10% calcium chloride (5-10 mL by slow IV push; do not use if hyperkalemia is secondary to digitalis poisoning), glucose and insulin (50 mL of 50% dextrose in water and 10 units of regular insulin IV), sodium bicarbonate (50 mmol IV; most effective if concomitant metabolic acidosis is present), and albuterol (15-20 mg nebulized or 0.5 mg by IV infusion).
Hypokalemia	Alcohol abuse, diabetes, use of diuretics, drugs and toxins, profound gastrointestinal losses, hypomagnesemia	If profound hypokalemia (<2.0-2.5 mmol of potassium) is accompanied by cardiac arrest, initiate urgent IV replacement (2 mmol/min IV for 10-15 mmol);* then reassess.
Pulmonary embolism	Hospitalized patient, recent surgical procedure, peripartum, known risk factors for venous thromboembolism, history of venous thromboembolism, or prearrest presentation consistent with a diagnosis of acute pulmonary embolism	Administer fluids; augment with vasopressors as necessary. Confirm the diagnosis, if possible; consider immediate cardiopulmonary bypass to maintain patient's viability. Consider definitive care (e.g., thrombolytic therapy, embolectomy by interventional radiology or surgery).
Tension pneumothorax	Placement of a central catheter, mechanical ventilation, pulmonary disease (including asthma, chronic obstructive pulmonary disease, and necrotizing pneumonia), thoracentesis, and trauma	Needle decompression, followed by chest tube insertion.

*Adult dose. Adjust for size of child. See Table 81.6.
From Eisenberg MS, Mengert TJ: Cardiac resuscitation, *N Engl J Med* 344:1304–1313, 2001.

events such as these, the key to successful resuscitation is early recognition of the arrhythmia and prompt treatment with high-quality CPR *and* defibrillation.

The principle behind high-quality CPR is that adequate chest compressions—those that circulate blood around the body with a good pulse pressure—are the most important component of CPR. The caregiver providing chest compressions should **push hard, push fast, allow for complete chest recoil, and minimize interruptions**. Ideally, chest compressions should be interrupted only for a rhythm check or delivery of a defibrillating shock. Providers should refer to the most recent American Heart Association (AHA) guidelines for pediatric BLS and ALS (eccguidelines.heart.org).

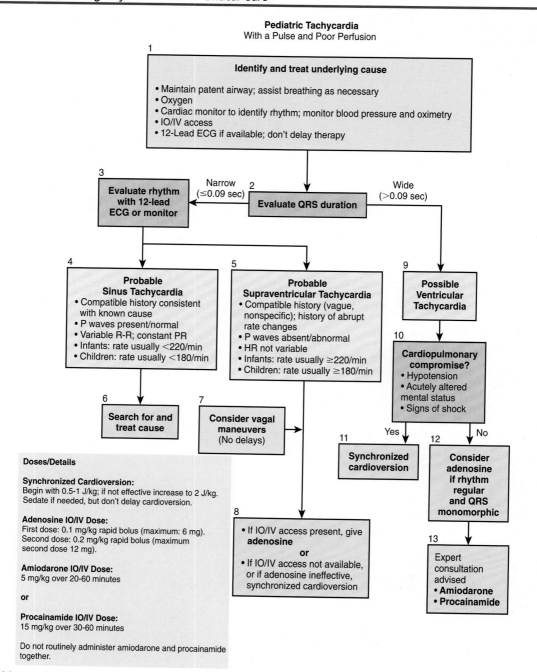

Fig. 81.14 Pediatric advanced life support tachycardia algorithm. AV, Atrioventricular (conductor); ECG, electrocardiogram; HR, heart rate; IO/IV, intraosseous/intravenous. (*From Kleinman ME, Chameides L, Schexnayder SM, et al: 2010 American Heart Association guidelines for cardiopulmonary resuscitation and emergency cardiovascular care. Part 14, Circulation 122[Suppl 3]:S876–S908, 2010, Fig 3, p S888.*)

Cardiac arrest is recognized from general and primary survey findings consistent with a pale or cyanotic child who is unresponsive, apneic, and pulseless. Even experienced providers have a relatively high error rate when asked to determine presence or absence of pulse in a child. Therefore, any child found unresponsive and apneic can be presumed to be in cardiac arrest, and a rescuer should respond accordingly. **A lone rescuer for an *unwitnessed* pediatric cardiac arrest in an outpatient setting should treat the arrest as asphyxial in nature, immediately initiate CPR, and activate the emergency response system via a mobile phone (if available).** If a mobile phone is not immediately available, the rescuer should perform initial rescue breaths and 2 min of chest compressions and ventilations before leaving the child to activate the emergency response system. For an in-hospital arrest, the provider should call for help and have a team member activate the emergency response system while beginning CPR. **A lone rescuer in an outpatient setting who *witnesses* a child's sudden collapse should treat the arrest as a primary arrhythmia, should immediately activate the EMS system, and obtain an AED.** On returning to the child, the rescuer should confirm pulselessness, turn on the AED, place the leads on the child's chest, and follow the defibrillator's voice commands.

The initial step in CPR for a child of any age is to restore ventilation and oxygenation as quickly as possible. On confirmation of unresponsiveness, apnea, and/or pulselessness, resuscitation should follow current AHA Basic Life Support (BLS), (or Advanced Cardiac Life Support, ACLS) guidelines, as appropriate (eccguidelines.heart.org).

If a person is pulseless, chest compressions should be initiated. Chest compressions in infants <1 yr old may be performed by placing 2 thumbs on the midsternum with the hands encircling the thorax or by placing 2 fingers over the midsternum and compressing (Figs. 81.15 and 81.16). For children >1 yr old, the care provider should perform chest compressions over the lower half of the sternum with the heel of 1 hand, or with 2 hands as used for adult resuscitation (Fig. 81.17). In all cases, care should be taken to avoid compression of the xiphoid and the ribs. When feasible, a cardiac resuscitation board should be placed under the child's back to maximize the efficiency of compressions. CPR and rescue breathing should be performed based on current AHA BLS/ACLS guidelines.

The goal of CPR is to reestablish spontaneous circulation at a level that is compatible with survival. If resuscitative efforts do not succeed in reestablishing life-sustaining breathing and circulation, the medical team must decide whether continued efforts are warranted or whether the resuscitation should be stopped. If EMS care is en route, bringing the potential for further escalation in care, such as endotracheal intubation, vascular access, and medications, CPR should be continued as long as possible or deemed reasonable by the rescuers.

In the in-hospital setting, the ECG should dictate further resuscitative efforts. For children without a pulse and in asystole or electromechanical dissociation (**pulseless electrical activity**, PEA), providers should continue rescue breathing and CPR, obtain vascular access, and administer emergency IV epinephrine (Fig. 81.18). For continued asystole or PEA, epinephrine can be repeated every 3-5 min. Patient history, physical exam findings, and laboratory evaluation should be used to elicit correctable causes of arrest (e.g., 6 Hs, 5 Ts; see Table 81.5). CPR should be continued after epinephrine administration, to circulate the drug through the body. After 5 cycles of CPR, providers should reassess the child for the presence of a pulse or a change in the ECG rhythm that would necessitate a different response.

For those children with pulseless VT or VF, emergency defibrillation is indicated (Fig. 81.18). Providers should apply the pads to the child's bare chest and back and follow the verbal instructions given by the AED. For younger children, a defibrillator (if available) set to the dose of 2 J/kg should be used. Ideally, the AED used in a child ≤8 yr of age should be equipped with an attenuated adult dose or should be designed for children; if neither device is available, a standard adult AED should be used. CPR should be immediately restarted after defibrillation. Emergency dose epinephrine can also be administered with another 5 cycles of CPR to ensure its circulation throughout the child's body. If the ECG rhythm continues to show VF or VT, defibrillation can be alternated with epinephrine. For refractory VF or VT, an IV antiarrhythmic, such as lidocaine or amiodarone, can be given (Tables 81.6 and 81.7). Some adult studies have suggested that a combination of epinephrine, vasopressin, and methylprednisolone improves intact survival after CPR.

Traditionally, continuing CPR >20 min in children with in-hospital cardiac arrest has been considered futile. With current practice for CPR, survival for in-hospital cardiac arrest is approximately 40% for CPR duration <15 min, compared with approximately 12% for CPR lasting >35 min. Survivors had a favorable neurologic outcome in 70% with a CPR duration <15 min, compared with 60% for those requiring resuscitation for >35 min.

VASCULAR ACCESS
Venous Access
Veins suitable for cannulation are numerous, but there is considerable anatomic variation from patient to patient. In the upper extremities, the *median antecubital vein*, located in the antecubital fossa, is often the largest and easiest to access (Fig. 81.19). Many veins on the dorsum of the hand are also suitable for cannulation because they are often large and easily located, and their cannulation is generally well tolerated.

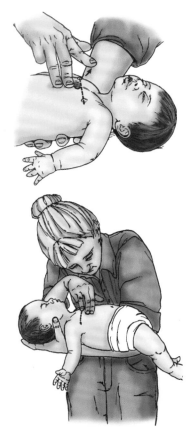

Fig. 81.15 *Cardiac compressions. Top*, The infant is supine on the palm of the rescuer's hand. *Bottom*, Performing CPR while carrying an infant or small child. Note that the head is kept level with the torso. *(From Guidelines for cardiopulmonary resuscitation and emergency cardiac care. Emergency Cardiac Care Committee and Subcommittees, American Heart Association. Part V. Pediatric basic life support, JAMA 268:2251–2261, 1992.)*

The *cephalic vein* is usually cannulated at the wrist, along the forearm, or at the elbow. The *median vein* of the forearm is also suitable as it lies along a flat surface of the forearm. In the lower extremity, the *great saphenous vein*, located just anterior to the medial malleolus, is accessible in most patients. The dorsum of the foot usually has a large vein in the midline, passing across the ankle joint, but catheters are difficult to maintain in this vein because dorsiflexion tends to dislodge them. A 2nd large vein on the lateral side of the foot, running in the horizontal plane, usually 1-2 cm dorsal to the lower margin of the foot, is preferable (Fig. 81.20). The most notable scalp veins are the *superficial temporal* (just anterior to the ear) and *posterior auricular* (just behind the ear).

Deeper and larger central veins can provide more reliable, larger-bore access for medications, nutritive solutions, and blood sampling than peripheral venous lines. They may be reached by percutaneous cannulation or surgical exposure. In infants and young children, the *femoral vein* is often the easiest to access and cannulate, but the *internal jugular* and *subclavian* veins may also be used (Figs. 81.21 and 81.22). Because of its proximity to the median nerve, the brachial vein is not often recommended for cannulation.

Intraosseous Access
Intraosseous (IO) needles (for intramedullary venous plexus access) are special rigid, large-bore needles. IO cannulation is recommended for patients in whom IV access proves difficult or unattainable, even in older children. If venous access is not available within approximately

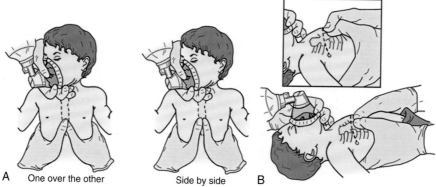

A   One over the other   Side by side   B

Fig. 81.16 Thumb method of chest compressions. **A,** Infant receiving chest compressions with thumb 1 fingerbreadth below the nipple line and hands encircling chest. **B,** Hand position for chest encirclement technique for external chest compressions in neonates. Thumbs are side by side over the lower third of the sternum. In the small newborn, thumbs may need to be superimposed *(inset)*. Gloves should be worn during resuscitation. *(From Fleisher GR, Ludwig S, editors: Textbook of pediatric emergency medicine, Philadelphia, 2010, Wolters Kluwer/Lippincott Williams & Wilkins Health, Fig 2.2.)*

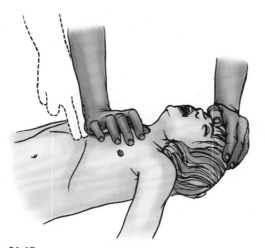

Fig. 81.17 Locating the hand position for chest compression in a child. Note that the rescuer's other hand is used to maintain the head position to facilitate ventilation. *(From Guidelines for cardiopulmonary resuscitation and emergency cardiac care. Emergency Cardiac Care Committee and Subcommittees, American Heart Association. Part V. Pediatric basic life support, JAMA 268:2251–2261, 1992.)*

1 min in a child with cardiopulmonary arrest, an IO needle should be placed in the anterior proximal tibia (with care taken to avoid traversing the epiphyseal plate). The needle should penetrate the anterior layer of compact bone, and its tip is advanced into the spongy interior of the bone (Fig. 81.23). Commercially available IO kits frequently include drills that obviate the complications of needle placement associated with manual placement. All medications, blood products, and fluids may be administered through the IO route, including medications required for emergency resuscitation. Complications are uncommon but may include osteomyelitis with prolonged infusions and tibial fracture.

If IV and IO routes are unavailable in an intubated patient, medication can be given through the ETT (epinephrine, atropine, naloxone, vasopressin).

Arterial Access

Arterial access is indicated when care providers need frequent blood sampling, particularly to assess adequacy of oxygenation, ventilation, or acid-base balance, and/or continuous blood pressure monitoring.

The *radial artery*, the most commonly cannulated artery, lies on the lateral side of the anterior wrist, just medial to the styloid process of the radius (Fig. 81.24). The ulnar artery, just lateral to the tendon of the flexor carpi ulnaris, is used less often because of its proximity to the ulnar nerve. Useful sites in the lower extremity, particularly in neonates and infants, are the *dorsalis pedis artery*, on the dorsum of the foot between the tendons of the tibialis anterior and the extensor hallucis longus, and the *posterior tibial artery*, posterior to the medial malleolus. Arterial catheters require special care for insertion and subsequent management.

NONVASCULAR EMERGENCY PROCEDURES
Thoracentesis and Chest Tube Placement

Thoracentesis is the placement of a needle or catheter into the pleural space to evacuate fluid, blood, or air. Most insertions are performed in one of the intercostal spaces between the 4th and 9th ribs in the plane of the midaxillary line. After appropriate systemic and local anesthesia/sedation is performed as clinically indicated, a skin incision is made, and dissection through the chest wall is accomplished in layers with use of blunt dissection techniques. The needle (and later the chest tube) that enters the pleural space should penetrate the intercostal space by passing over the superior edge of the lower rib, because there are larger vessels along the inferior edge of the rib. Ideally, the chest tube should lie *anterior* in the pleural space for air accumulation and *posterior* for fluid accumulation. A radiograph must be obtained to verify chest tube placement and evacuation of the pleural space.

Pericardiocentesis

When fluid, blood, or gas accumulates in the pericardial sac, the heart may become compressed and may be unable to fill/empty with normal volumes of blood, leading to diminished cardiac output. The cardinal signs of such a restrictive pericardial effusion are tachycardia, hypotension generally with a narrowed pulse pressure, and decreased So_2. Pericardiocentesis includes needle aspiration of the pericardial sac, often followed by the placement of a catheter for continuous drainage. As with thoracentesis, chest radiography should be done to confirm catheter location as well as evaluate for any complications, such as pneumothorax or hemothorax. Pericardiocentesis may be performed with echocardiography.

POSTRESUSCITATION CARE

After successful resuscitation, close observation in an intensive care unit, where the child can receive ongoing multiorgan system assessments and support, is critical. Optimal postresuscitation care includes ongoing support of cardiovascular and respiratory system function as needed and the identification and treatment of other organ system dysfunction

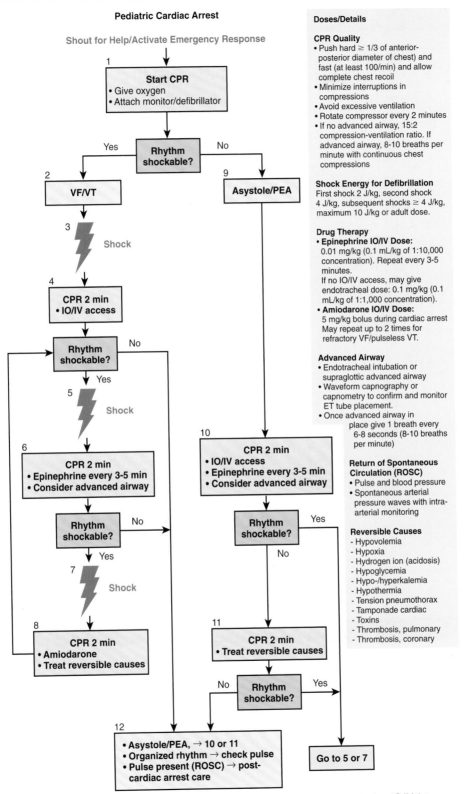

Fig. 81.18 Pediatric advanced life support pulseless arrest algorithm. CPR, Cardiopulmonary resuscitation; IO/IV, intraosseous/intravenous; PEA, pulseless electrical activity; VF/VT, ventricular fibrillation/tachycardia. *(From Kleinman ME, Chameides L, Schexnayder SM, et al: 2010 American Heart Association guidelines for cardiopulmonary resuscitation and emergency cardiovascular care. Part 14, Circulation 122[Suppl 3]:S876–S908, 2010, Fig 1, p S885.)*

Table 81.6	Medications for Pediatric Resuscitation and Arrhythmias	
MEDICATION	**DOSE**	**REMARKS**
Adenosine	0.1 mg/kg (max: 6 mg) Repeat: 0.2 mg/kg (max: 12 mg)	Monitor ECG. Rapid IV/IO bolus.
Amiodarone	5 mg/kg IV/IO; repeat up to 15 mg/kg Max: 300 mg	Monitor ECG and blood pressure. Adjust administration rate to urgency (give more slowly when perfusing rhythm is present). Use caution when administering with other drugs that prolong QT interval (consider expert consultation).

Atropine	0.02 mg/kg IV/IO
	0.03 mg/kg ETT*
	Repeat once if needed
	Minimum dose: 0.1 mg
	Minimum single dose:
	    Child, 0.5 mg
	    Adolescent, 1 mg
		Higher doses may be used with organophosphate poisoning.

Calcium chloride (10%)	20 mg/kg IV/IO (0.2 mL/kg)	Slowly Adult dose: 5-10 mL
Epinephrine	0.01 mg/kg (0.1 mL/kg 1:10,000) IV/IO 0.1 mg/kg (0.1 mL/kg 1:1,000) ETT* Max dose: 1 mg IV/IO; 10 mg ET	May repeat every 3-5 min
Glucose	0.5-1 g/kg IV/IO	D10W: 5-10 mL/kg D25W: 2-4 mL/kg D50W: 1-2 mL/kg
Lidocaine	Bolus: 1 mg/kg IV/IO Max dose: 100 mg Infusion: 20-50 µg/kg/min ETT*: 2-3 mg	
Magnesium sulfate	25-50 mg/kg IV/IO over 10-20 min; faster in torsades de pointes Max dose: 2 g	
Naloxone	<5 yr or ≤20 kg: 0.1 mg/kg IV/IO/ETT* ≥5 yr or >20 kg: 2 mg IV/IO/ETT*	Use lower doses to reverse respiratory depression associated with therapeutic opioid administration (1-15 µg/kg).
Procainamide	15 mg/kg IV/IO over 30-60 min Adult dose: 20 mg/min IV infusion up to total max dose of 17 mg/kg	Monitor EGG and blood pressure. Use caution when administering with other drugs that prolong QT interval (consider expert consultation).
Sodium bicarbonate	1 mEq/kg/dose IV/IO slowly	After adequate ventilation

*Flush with 5 mL of normal saline and follow with 5 ventilations.
ECG, Electrocardiogram; ETT, endotracheal tube; IO, intraosseous; IV, intravenous.
From ECC Committee, Subcommittees and Task Forces of the American Heart Association: 2005 American Heart Association guidelines for cardiopulmonary resuscitation and emergency cardiovascular care, *Circulation* 112:IV1–203, 2005.

Table 81.7	Medications to Maintain Cardiac Output and for Postresuscitation Stabilization*	
MEDICATION	**DOSE RANGE**	**COMMENT**
Inamrinone	0.75-1 mg/kg IV/IO over 5 min; may repeat 2x; then: 2-20 µg/kg/min	Inodilator
Dobutamine	2-20 µg/kg/min IV/IO	Inotrope; vasodilator
Dopamine	2-20 µg/kg/min IV/IO in low doses; pressor in higher doses	Inotrope; chronotrope; renal and splanchnic vasodilator
Epinephrine	0.1-1 µg/kg/min IV/IO	Inotrope; chronotrope; vasodilator in low doses; vasopressor in higher doses
Milrinone	50-75 µg/kg IV/IO over 10-60 min then 0.5-0.75 µg/kg/min	Inodilator
Norepinephrine	0.1-2 µg/kg/min	Inotrope; vasopressor
Sodium nitroprusside	1-8 µg/kg/min	Vasodilator; prepare only in D5W

*Alternative formula for calculating an infusion: Infusion rate (mL/hr) = [weight (kg) × dose (µg/kg/min) × 60 (min/hr)]/concentration µg/mL).
D5W, 5% Dextrose in water; IO, intraosseous; IV, intravenous.
From ECC Committee, Subcommittees and Task Forces of the American Heart Association: 2005 American Heart Association guidelines for cardiopulmonary resuscitation and emergency cardiovascular care, *Circulation* 112:IV1–IV203, 2005.

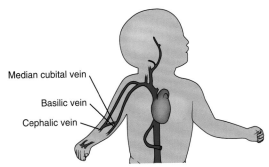

Fig. 81.19 Veins of the upper extremity. *(From Roberts JR, Hedges JR, editors: Clinical procedures in emergency medicine, ed 4, Philadelphia, 2004, Saunders.)*

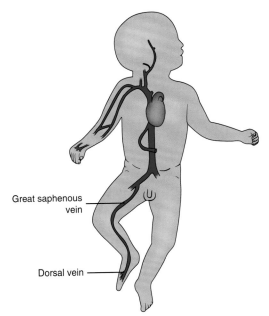

Fig. 81.20 Veins of the lower extremity. *(From Roberts JR, Hedges JR, editors: Clinical procedures in emergency medicine, ed 4, Philadelphia, 2004, Saunders.)*

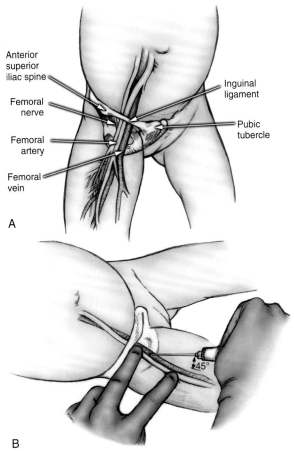

A

B

Fig. 81.21 Femoral vein approach. Remember the mnemonic NAVEL for nerve, artery, vein, empty space, and lymphatics. *(From Putigna F, Solenberger R: Central venous access. http://emedicine.medscape.com/article/940865-overview.)*

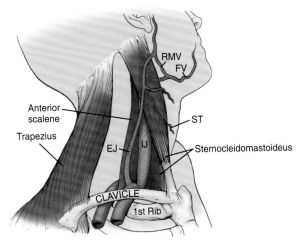

Fig. 81.22 Internal and external jugular veins. EJ, External jugular vein; FV, facial vein; IJ, internal jugular vein; RMV, retromandibular vein; ST, superior thyroid vein. The 2 heads of the sternocleidomastoideus are indicated by the *lines*. *(From Mathers LW, Smith DW, Frankel L: Anatomic considerations in placement of central venous catheters, Clin Anat 5:89, 1992. Reprinted by permission of Wiley-Liss.)*

that may have contributed to (or resulted from) the child's cardiopulmonary instability. Good postresuscitation intensive care also includes supportive services for the child's parents, siblings, family, and friends.

Induced hypothermia (32-34°C [89.6-91.4°F] versus targeted temperature 36.8°C (98.2°F) [range, 36-37.5°C [96.8-99.5°F]]) for about 48 hr) has *not* been shown to improve survival and neurologic function in pediatric survivors of CPR. However, *hyperthermia must be avoided.* **Hypoxic-ischemic encephalopathy** with subsequent development of seizures, intellectual impairment, and spasticity, is a serious and common complication of cardiac arrest. In addition, *hyperglycemia and hypoglycemia should be avoided.*

Postresuscitation management generally has 2 phases. First, the providers must assess the child's airway and breathing and support oxygenation and ventilation as indicated. If the child has ongoing respiratory failure and has been supported with bag-valve-mask ventilation until this time, the providers should now move forward with intubation. Once the child is intubated, mechanical ventilation must be established and respiratory assessments performed, such as chest radiography and arterial blood gas analysis. The child's circulatory system must also be assessed and supported as needed. Continuous arterial

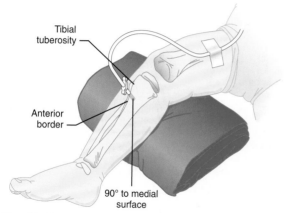

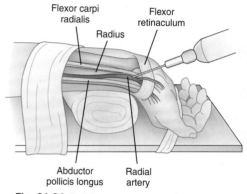

Fig. **81.24** Radial artery anatomy and cannulation.

Fig. **81.23** Intraosseous cannulation technique. (From Zwass MS, Gregory GA: Pediatric and neonatal intensive care. In Miller RD, Eriksson LI, Fleisher LA, et al, editors: Miller's anesthesia, ed 7, Philadelphia, 2009, Churchill Livingstone, Fig 84-1.)

blood pressure monitoring can help the provider determine the need for, and response to, inotropic and chronotropic medications (see Table 81.7). Once the ABCs have been managed, providers can move on to full organ system assessments. A systematic approach should be used, with a full physical exam and laboratory evaluation to reveal the child's respiratory, cardiovascular, neurologic, gastrointestinal, renal, and hematologic system function.

Communication with the patients' family is an essential element of postresuscitation care. The family should be thoroughly briefed on the elements of the resuscitation performed, the child's condition, and ongoing medical concerns, uncertainties, or issues by the *most senior provider available.* This provider should be available to answer the family's questions, clarify information, and provide comfort. Other support staff, including social workers and chaplains, should be contacted, as the family wishes, to provide additional support and comfort. For situations in which the resuscitation is ongoing and the child is not expected to survive, it is recommended that the provider make every effort possible to have the family present at the bedside, if they wish. Family presence during CPR or other emergency resuscitative efforts, even if the child dies, is associated with a more positive medical experience than if they are excluded. In situations where the child is critically ill but stable, the family should be brought to the bedside as soon as the healthcare team deems it safe and appropriate (see Chapter 7).

Bibliography is available at Expert Consult.

Chapter **82**
Acute Care of Multiple Trauma

Cindy Ganis Roskind, Howard I. Pryor II, and Bruce L. Klein

第八十二章
多发性创伤的急救

中文导读

　　本章主要介绍了多发性创伤的流行病学、地域性和创伤急救队伍、初级评估、二次评估及心理和社会支持。在初级评估中，具体描述了气道/颈椎、呼吸、循环、神经功能缺陷的评估及暴露/环境的控制；在二次评估中，具体描述了头部创伤、颈椎创伤、胸部创伤、腹部创伤、骨盆创伤、下泌尿生殖道创伤、四肢创伤及影像学和实验室检查。

EPIDEMIOLOGY

Injury is a leading cause of death and disability in children throughout the world (see Chapter 13). Deaths represent only a small fraction of the total trauma burden. Approximately 140,000 children were treated in U.S. trauma centers in 2016 for serious injury. Many survivors of trauma have permanent or temporary functional limitations. Motor vehicle–related injuries and falls rank among the top 15 causes of disability-adjusted life years in children worldwide.

Trauma is frequently classified according to the number of significantly injured body parts (≥1), the severity of injury (mild, moderate, or severe), and the mechanism of injury (blunt or penetrating). In childhood, blunt trauma predominates, accounting for the majority of injuries. In adolescence, penetrating trauma increases in frequency, accounting for approximately 15% of injuries, and penetrating trauma secondary to a firearm is associated with a high case fatality rate of 11%.

REGIONALIZATION AND TRAUMA TEAMS

Mortality and morbidity rates have decreased in geographic regions with comprehensive, coordinated trauma systems. Treatment at designated trauma centers is associated with decreased mortality. At the scene of injury, paramedics should administer necessary advanced life support and perform **triage** (Fig. 82.1). It is usually preferable to bypass local hospitals and rapidly transport a seriously injured child directly to a pediatric trauma center (or a trauma center with pediatric commitment). *Children have lower mortality rates, lower complication rates, and less operative interventions after severe blunt trauma when they are treated in designated pediatric trauma centers or in hospitals with pediatric intensive care units.*

When the receiving emergency department (ED) is notified before the child's arrival, the trauma team should also be mobilized in advance. Each member has defined tasks. A senior surgeon (surgical coordinator) or, sometimes initially, an emergency physician leads the team. Team compositions vary somewhat from hospital to hospital; Fig. 82.2 shows the model used at The Johns Hopkins Hospital Bloomberg Children's Center (Baltimore, MD). Consultants, especially neurosurgeons and orthopedic surgeons, must be promptly available; and the operating room staff should be alerted.

Physiologic status, anatomic locations, and/or mechanism of injury are used for field triage as well as to determine whether to activate the trauma team. More importance should be placed on physiologic compromise and less on mechanism of injury. Scoring scales such as the Abbreviated Injury Scale (AIS), Injury Severity Score (ISS), Pediatric Trauma Score (Table 82.1), and Revised Trauma Score use these parameters to predict patient outcome. The AIS and ISS are used together. First, the AIS is used numerically to score injuries—as 1 minor, 2 moderate, 3 serious, 4 severe, 5 critical, or 6 probably lethal—in each of 6 ISS body regions: head/neck, face, thorax, abdomen and pelvic contents, extremities and bony pelvis, and external. The ISS is the sum of the squares of the highest 3 AIS region scores.

PRIMARY SURVEY

During the primary survey, the physician quickly assesses and treats any life-threatening injuries. The principal causes of death shortly after trauma are airway obstruction, respiratory insufficiency, shock from hemorrhage, and central nervous system (CNS) injury. The primary survey addresses the **ABCDEs**: Airway, Breathing, Circulation, neurologic Deficit, and Exposure of the patient and control of the Environment.

Airway/Cervical Spine

Optimizing oxygenation and ventilation, while protecting the cervical spine (C-spine) from potential further injury, is of paramount importance. Initially, C-spine injury should be suspected in any child sustaining multiple, blunt trauma. Although C-spine injuries occur less often in children than adults, children are at risk for such injuries because of their relatively large heads in proportion to the rest of their body, which augment flexion-extension forces, and weak neck muscles, which predispose them to ligament injuries. To prevent additional spinal injury, paramedics have traditionally been taught to immobilize the cervical (and thoracic and lumbar) spine in neutral position with a stiff collar, head blocks, tape or cloth placed across the forehead, torso, and thighs to restrain the child, and a rigid backboard.

Airway obstruction manifests as snoring, gurgling, hoarseness, stridor, and/or diminished breath sounds (even with apparently good respiratory effort). Children are more likely than adults to have airway obstruction because of their smaller oral and nasal cavities, proportionately larger tongues and more tonsillar and adenoidal tissue, higher and more anterior glottic opening, and narrower larynx and trachea. Obstruction is common in patients with severe head injuries, partly because of decreased muscle tone, which allows the tongue to fall posteriorly and occlude the airway. With trauma, obstruction can also result from fractures of the mandible or facial bones, secretions such as blood or vomit, crush injuries of the larynx or trachea, and foreign body aspiration.

If it is necessary to open the airway, a jaw thrust without head tilt is recommended. This procedure minimizes cervical spine motion. In an unconscious child, an oropharyngeal airway may be inserted to prevent posterior displacement of the mandibular tissues. A semiconscious child will gag with an oropharyngeal airway but may tolerate a nasopharyngeal airway. A nasopharyngeal airway is contraindicated when there is a possibility of cribriform plate fracture. If these maneuvers plus suctioning do not clear the airway, oral endotracheal intubation is indicated. When endotracheal intubation proves difficult, a laryngeal mask airway can be used as a temporary alternative. A laryngeal mask airway consists of a tube with an inflatable cuff that rests above the larynx and thus does not require placement of the tube into the trachea. Video-assisted laryngoscopy or the use of a bougie can also be helpful in the management of a difficult airway. Emergency cricothyrotomy is needed in <1% of trauma victims.

Breathing

The physician assesses breathing by counting the respiratory rate; visualizing chest wall motion for symmetry, expansion, and accessory muscle use; and auscultating breath sounds in both axillae. Continuous

Table 82.1	Pediatric Trauma Score*		
COMPONENT	**+2**	**+1**	**−1**
Size	≥20 kg	10-20 kg	<10 kg
Airway	Normal	Maintainable	Unmaintainable
Systolic BP	≥90 mm Hg	50-90 mm Hg	<50 mm Hg
CNS	Awake	Obtunded/LOC	Coma/decerebrate
Open wound	None	Minor	Major/penetrating
Skeletal	None	Closed fracture	Open/multiple fractures
Sum total points			

*Children with a Pediatric Trauma Score ≤6 are at increased risk of mortality as well as morbidity.

BP, Blood pressure; CNS, central nervous system; LOC, loss of consciousness.
From Tepas JJ 3rd, Mollitt DL, Talbert JL, et al: The Pediatric Trauma Score as a predictor of injury severity in the injured child, *J Pediatr Surg* 22:14–18, 1987 (Table 1, p 15).

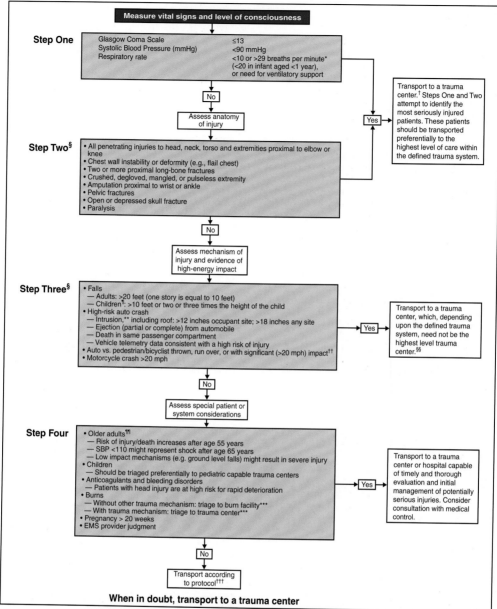

Fig. 82.1 Guidelines for field triage of injured patients—United States, 2011. *(From Guidelines for field triage of injured patients: recommendations of the National Expert Panel on Field Triage, MMWR 61:6, 2012.)*

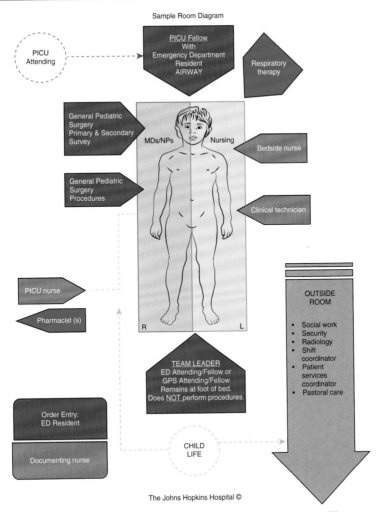

Sample Room Diagram

Fig. 82.2 Staff in the ED trauma bay at The Johns Hopkins Hospital Bloomberg Children's Center. ED, emergency department; NP, nurse practitioner; GPS, general pediatric surgery; PICU, pediatric intensive care unit; PSC, patient services coordinator. *(Courtesy The Johns Hopkins Hospital, Baltimore, Maryland.)*

Table 82.2	Differential Diagnosis of Immediately Life-Threatening Cardiopulmonary Injuries		
	TENSION PNEUMOTHORAX	**MASSIVE HEMOTHORAX**	**CARDIAC TAMPONADE**
Breath sounds	Ipsilaterally decreased more than contralaterally	Ipsilaterally decreased	Normal
Percussion note	Hyperresonant	Dull	Normal
Tracheal location	Contralaterally shifted	Midline or shifted	Midline
Neck veins	Distended	Flat	Distended
Heart tones	Normal	Normal	Muffled

Modified from Cooper A, Foltin GL: Thoracic trauma. In Barkin RM, editor: *Pediatric emergency medicine*, ed 2, St Louis, 1997, Mosby, p 325.

waveform capnography monitoring should also be used as an adjunct; however, it is less reliable in patients with shock. In addition to looking visually for cyanosis, pulse oximetry is standard. If ventilation is inadequate, bag-valve-mask ventilation with 100% oxygen must be initiated immediately, followed by endotracheal intubation. End-expiratory carbon dioxide (CO_2) detectors or capnography help verify accurate tube placement.

Head trauma is the most common cause of respiratory insufficiency. An unconscious child with severe head injury may have a variety of breathing abnormalities, including Cheyne-Stokes respiration, slow irregular breaths, and apnea.

Although less common than a pulmonary contusion, tension pneumothorax and massive hemothorax are immediately life threatening (Tables 82.2 and 82.3). **Tension pneumothorax** occurs when air accumulates under pressure in the pleural space. The adjacent lung is compacted, the mediastinum is pushed toward the opposite hemithorax, and the heart, great vessels, and contralateral lung are compressed or kinked (see Chapter 439). Both ventilation and cardiac output are impaired. Characteristic findings include cyanosis, tachypnea, retractions, asymmetric chest rise, contralateral tracheal deviation, diminished breath sounds on the ipsilateral (more than contralateral) side, and signs of shock. Needle thoracentesis, followed by thoracostomy tube insertion, is diagnostic and lifesaving. **Hemothorax** results from injury to the intercostal vessels, lungs, heart, or great vessels. When ventilation is adequate, fluid resuscitation should begin before evacuation, because a large amount of blood may drain through the chest tube, resulting in shock.

Circulation

Signs of **shock** include tachycardia; weak pulse; delayed capillary refill; cool, mottled, pale skin; and altered mental state (see Chapter 88). The most common type of shock in trauma is *hypovolemic* shock caused by hemorrhage. *Cardiac tamponade*, which is a form of obstructive shock, may be suspected clinically or diagnosed by **focused assessment with sonography in trauma (FAST)** examination or echocardiography. Cardiac tamponade is best managed by thoracotomy or pericardial window,

Table 82.3	Life-Threatening Chest Injuries

TENSION PNEUMOTHORAX

One-way valve leak from the lung parenchyma or tracheobronchial tree

Lung collapse with mediastinal and tracheal shift to the side opposite the leak

Compromises venous return and decreases ventilation of the other lung

Clinically, manifests as respiratory distress, unilateral absence of breath sounds, tracheal deviation, distended neck veins, tympany to percussion of the involved side, and cyanosis

Relieve first with needle aspiration, then with chest tube drainage

OPEN PNEUMOTHORAX (SUCKING CHEST WOUND)

Effect on ventilation depends on size

MAJOR FLAIL CHEST

Usually caused by blunt injury resulting in multiple rib fractures

Loss of bone stability of the thoracic cage

Major disruption of synchronous chest wall motion

Mechanical ventilation and positive end-expiratory pressure required

MASSIVE HEMOTHORAX

Must be drained with a large-bore tube

Initiate drainage only with concurrent vascular volume replacement

CARDIAC TAMPONADE

Beck's triad:
1. Decreased or muffled heart sounds
2. Jugular venous distention
3. Hypotension (with narrow pulse pressure)

Must be drained

Modified from Krug SE: The acutely ill or injured child. In Behrman RE, Kliegman RM, editors: *Nelson essentials of pediatrics*, ed 4, Philadelphia, 2002, Saunders, p 97.

although pericardiocentesis may be necessary as a temporizing maneuver (see Table 82.3).

Early in shock, blood pressure remains normal because of compensatory increases in heart rate and peripheral vascular resistance (Table 82.4). Some individuals can lose up to 30% of blood volume before blood pressure declines. It is important to note that 25% of blood volume equals 20 mL/kg, which is only 200 mL in a 10 kg child. Losses >40% of blood volume cause severe hypotension that, if prolonged, may become irreversible. Direct pressure should be applied to control external hemorrhage. When direct pressure does not control hemorrhage, a tourniquet should be applied to a proximal pressure point. Blind clamping of bleeding vessels, which risks damaging adjacent structures, is not advisable.

Cannulating a larger vein, such as an antecubital vein, is usually the quickest way to achieve intravenous (IV) access. A short, large-bore catheter offers less resistance to flow, allowing for more rapid fluid administration. Ideally, a 2nd catheter should be placed within the first few minutes of resuscitation in a severely injured child. If IV access is not rapidly obtainable, an intraosseous (IO) needle should be inserted; all medications and fluids can be administered intraosseously. Other alternatives are central venous access using the Seldinger technique (e.g., in the femoral vein) and, rarely, surgical cutdown (e.g., in saphenous vein). Ultrasonography should be used to facilitate central venous catheter placement, if possible.

Traditionally, fluids are administered aggressively early in hemorrhagic shock to reverse and prevent further clinical deterioration. Isotonic crystalloid solution, such as lactated Ringer injection or normal saline (20 mL/kg), should be infused rapidly. When necessary, repeated crystalloid boluses may be given. Most children are stabilized with administration of crystalloid solution alone. However, if the patient remains in shock after boluses totaling 40-60 mL/kg of crystalloid, packed red blood cells should be transfused. Massive transfusion protocols (including fresh-frozen plasma) should be initiated early to prevent coagulopathy. When shock persists despite these measures, surgery to stop internal hemorrhage is usually indicated. Although literature is emerging regarding the benefits of permissive hypotension, hemostatic resuscitation, and damage control surgery for adult trauma patients, currently there are no pediatric data.

Neurologic Deficit

Neurologic status is briefly assessed by determining the level of consciousness and evaluating pupil size and reactivity. The level of consciousness can be classified using the mnemonic **AVPU**: Alert, responsive to Verbal commands, responsive to Painful stimuli, or Unresponsive.

At least 75% of pediatric blunt trauma deaths are accounted for by head injuries. Primary direct cerebral injury occurs within seconds of the event and is irreversible. Secondary injury is caused by subsequent anoxia or ischemia. *The goal is to minimize secondary injury by ensuring adequate oxygenation, ventilation, and perfusion, and maintaining normal cerebral perfusion pressure.* A child with severe neurologic impairment—i.e., with a Glasgow Coma Scale (GCS; see Chapter 85) score of ≤8—should undergo endotracheal intubation and supportive mechanical ventilation.

Table 82.4	Systemic Responses to Blood Loss in Pediatric Patients		
SYSTEM	**MILD BLOOD LOSS (<30%)**	**MODERATE BLOOD LOSS (30–45%)**	**SEVERE BLOOD LOSS (>45%)**
Cardiovascular	Increased heart rate; weak, thready peripheral pulses; normal systolic blood pressure; normal pulse pressure	Markedly increased heart rate; weak, thready central pulses; peripheral pulses absent; low normal systolic blood pressure; narrowed pulse pressure	Tachycardia followed by bradycardia; central pulses very weak or absent; peripheral pulses absent; hypotension; narrowed pulse pressure (or undetectable diastolic blood pressure).
Central nervous	Anxiety; irritability; confusion	Lethargy; dulled response to pain	Coma
Skin	Cool, mottled; capillary refill prolonged	Cyanotic; capillary refill markedly prolonged	Pale and cold
Urine output	Low to very low	Minimal	None

Adapted from American College of Surgeons Committee on Trauma: *Advanced trauma life support for doctors: student course manual*, ed 9, Chicago, 2012, American College of Surgeons.

Signs of **increased intracranial pressure** (ICP), including progressive neurologic deterioration and evidence of transtentorial herniation, must be treated immediately (see Chapter 85). Hyperventilation lowers the arterial partial pressure of carbon dioxide (PaCO$_2$), resulting in cerebral vasoconstriction, reduced cerebral blood flow, and decreased ICP. Brief hyperventilation remains an immediate option for patients with acute increases in ICP. Prophylactic hyperventilation, or vigorous or prolonged hyperventilation, is not recommended, because the consequent vasoconstriction may excessively decrease cerebral perfusion and oxygenation. Mannitol lowers ICP and may improve survival. Because mannitol induces an osmotic diuresis, it can exacerbate hypovolemia and must be used cautiously. Hypertonic saline may be a more useful agent for control of increased ICP in patients with severe head injury. Neurosurgical consultation is mandatory. If signs of increased ICP persist, the neurosurgeon must decide whether to operate emergently.

Exposure and Environmental Control
All clothing should be cut away to reveal any injuries. Cutting is quickest and minimizes unnecessary patient movement. Children often arrive in the ED mildly hypothermic because of their higher body surface area-to-mass ratios. They can be warmed with use of radiant heat as well as heated blankets and IV fluids.

SECONDARY SURVEY
During the secondary survey, the physician completes a detailed, head-to-toe physical examination.

Head Trauma
A GCS or Pediatric GCS score (see Chapter 85) should be assigned to every child with significant head trauma. This scale assesses eye opening and motor and verbal responses. In the Pediatric GCS, the verbal score is modified for age. The GCS helps categorize neurologic disability, and serial measurements identify improvement or deterioration over time. Patients with low scores 6-24 hr after injuries have poorer prognosis.

In the ED, cranial CT scanning of the head without a contrast agent has become standard to determine the type of injury in patients with concerning findings. Diffuse cerebral injury with edema is a common

and serious finding on CT scan in severely brain-injured children. Focal hemorrhagic lesions (e.g., epidural hematoma) that can be evacuated occur less often but may require immediate neurosurgical intervention (Fig. 82.3).

Monitoring of ICP should be strongly considered for children with severe brain injury, particularly for those with a GCS score of ≤8 and abnormal head CT findings (see Chapter 85). One advantage of an intraventricular catheter over an intraparenchymal device is that cerebrospinal fluid can be drained to treat acute increases in ICP. Hypoxia, hypercarbia, hypotension, and hyperthermia must be aggressively managed to prevent secondary brain injury. Cerebral perfusion pressure (i.e., the difference between mean arterial blood pressure and mean ICP) should be maintained >40 mm Hg, at least (and an even higher minimum, >50 mm Hg, especially for older children).

A child with a severe brain injury must be treated aggressively in the ED because it is difficult to predict the long-term neurologic outcome.

Cervical Spine Trauma
Cervical spine injuries occur in <3% of children with blunt trauma—with the risk being substantially higher in those with GCS scores ≤8—but they are associated with significant mortality and morbidity. Bony injuries occur mainly from C1 to C4 in children younger than 8 yr. In older children, they occur equally in the upper and lower cervical spine. The mortality rate is significantly higher in patients with upper C-spine injuries. **Spinal cord injury without radiographic abnormalities (SCIWORA)** on plain films or CT may be present. Patients with SCIWORA have neurologic symptoms, and spinal cord abnormalities are nearly always noted on MRI. Approximately 30% of all patients with C-spine injuries have permanent neurologic deficits.

Evaluation begins with a detailed history and neurologic examination. Identifying the mechanism of injury helps in estimating the likelihood of a C-spine injury. Both the patient and the paramedic should be asked whether any neurologic symptoms or signs, such as weakness or abnormal sensation, were present before arrival in the ED. In a child with neurologic symptoms and normal findings on C-spine plain radiographs and CT scan, SCIWORA must be considered.

Whenever the history, physical examination, or mechanism of injury suggests a C-spine injury, radiographs should be obtained after initial resuscitation. The **National Emergency X-Radiography Utilization Study (NEXUS)** cervical spine rule helps identify low-risk patients who may not require radiographs (Table 82.5). The standard series of plain radiographs includes lateral, anteroposterior (AP), and odontoid views. Some centers use cervical spine CT as the primary diagnostic tool, particularly in patients with abnormal GCS scores and/or significant injury mechanisms, recognizing that CT is more sensitive in detecting bony injury than plain radiographs. CT is also helpful if an odontoid fracture is suspected, because young children typically do not cooperate enough to obtain an open-mouth (odontoid) radiographic view. Use of cervical spine CT scan must be balanced with the knowledge that CT exposes thyroid tissue to 90-200 times the amount of radiation from plain films. MRI is indicated in a child with suspected SCIWORA and in the evaluation of children who remain obtunded.

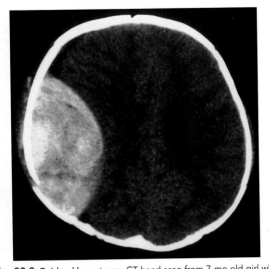

Fig. 82.3 Epidural hematoma. CT head scan from 7 mo old girl who, according to the history provided, did not wake up for her nightly feeding and began vomiting in the morning. The mother's boyfriend reported that the infant had fallen from a chair the previous day. The CT scan shows a large epidural hematoma on the right and marked shift of the midline from right to left. The right lateral ventricle is compressed as a result of the mass effect, and the left lateral ventricle is slightly prominent. The infant underwent emergency surgical evacuation of the epidural hematoma and recovered uneventfully. *(From O'Neill JA Jr: Principles of pediatric surgery, ed 2, St Louis, 2003, Mosby, p 191.)*

Table 82.5	National Emergency X-Radiography Utilization Study (NEXUS) to Rule Out Cervical Spine Injury Following Blunt Trauma

*If **none** of the following is present, the patient is at very low risk for clinically significant cervical spine injury:*
  Midline cervical tenderness
  Evidence of intoxication
  Altered level of alertness
  Focal neurologic deficit
  Distracting painful injury

Data from Hoffman JR, Mower WR, Wolfson AB, et al: Validity of a set of clinical criteria to rule out injury to the cervical spine in patients with blunt trauma, *N Engl J Med* 343:94–99, 2000; and Viccellio P, Simon H, Pressman BD, et al: A prospective multicenter study of cervical spine injury in children, *Pediatrics* 108:e20, 2001.

Table 82.6	Indications for Operation in Thoracic Trauma

THORACOTOMY IMMEDIATELY OR SHORTLY AFTER INJURY
Massive continuing pneumothorax or large air leak from
    tracheobronchial injury (cannot expand lung and ventilate)
Cardiac tamponade
Open pneumothorax
Esophageal injury
Aortic or other vascular injury
Acute rupture of the diaphragm

DELAYED THORACOTOMY
Chronic rupture of the diaphragm
Clotted hemothorax
Persistent chylothorax
Traumatic intracardiac defects
Evacuation of large foreign bodies
Chronic atelectasis from traumatic bronchial stenosis

Modified from O'Neill JA Jr: *Principles of pediatric surgery*, ed 2, St Louis, 2003, Mosby, p 157.

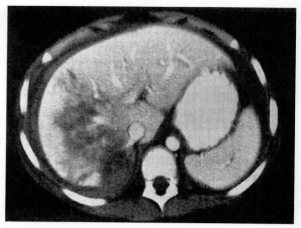

Fig. 82.5 Liver injury. CT scan performed after severe blunt injury of the abdomen shows a bursting injury of the liver. The patient was stable, and no operative intervention was required. The decision to perform surgery should be based on the patient's physiologic stability. *(From O'Neill JA Jr: Principles of pediatric surgery, ed 2, St Louis, 2003, Mosby, p 168.)*

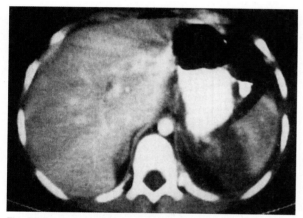

Fig. 82.4 Splenic rupture. CT scan with intravenous and gastrointestinal contrast enhancement shows an isolated splenic rupture that resulted from blunt trauma. This injury responded to nonoperative management, as do most splenic injuries. *(From O'Neill JA Jr: Principles of pediatric surgery, ed 2, St Louis, 2003, Mosby, p 166.)*

Rapid diagnosis of spinal cord injury is essential. Initiating high-dose IV methylprednisolone within 8 hr of spinal cord injury has been reported to improve motor outcome, but this treatment has become controversial.

Thoracic Trauma

Pulmonary contusions occur frequently in young children with blunt chest trauma. A child's chest wall is relatively pliable; therefore, less force is absorbed by the rib cage, and more is transmitted to the lungs. Respiratory distress may be noted initially or may develop during the 1st 24 hr after injury.

Rib fractures result from significant external force. They are noted in patients with more severe injuries and are associated with a higher mortality rate. Flail chest, which is caused by multiple rib fractures, is rare in children. Table 82.6 lists indications for operative management in thoracic trauma. (See Table 82.2 for the differential diagnosis of immediately life-threatening cardiopulmonary injuries.)

Abdominal Trauma

Liver and spleen contusions, hematomas, and lacerations account for the majority of intraabdominal injuries from blunt trauma. The kidneys, pancreas, and duodenum are relatively spared because of their retroperitoneal location. Pancreatic and duodenal injuries are more common after a bicycle handlebar impact or a direct blow to the abdomen.

Although a thorough examination for intraabdominal injuries is

essential, achieving it often proves difficult. Misleading findings can result from gastric distention after crying or in an uncooperative toddler. Calm reassurance, distraction, and gentle, persistent palpation help with the examination. Important findings include distention, bruises, and tenderness. Specific symptoms and signs give insight into the mechanism of injury and the potential for particular injuries. Pain in the left shoulder may signify splenic trauma. A lap belt mark across the abdomen raises concern for bowel or mesentery injury. The presence of certain other injuries, such as lumbar spinal fractures and femur fractures, increases the likelihood of intraabdominal injury.

An abdominal (and pelvic) CT scan with IV contrast medium enhancement rapidly identifies structural abnormalities and is the preferred study in a stable child. Negative abdominal CT scan has been shown to have a negative predictive value (NPV) of 99.6%. It has excellent sensitivity and specificity for splenic (Fig. 82.4), hepatic (Fig. 82.5), and renal injuries, but is less sensitive for diaphragmatic, pancreatic, or intestinal injuries. Small amounts of free fluid or air or a mesenteric hematoma may be the only sign of an intestinal injury. Administration of an oral contrast agent is not routinely recommended for all abdominal CT scans, but it sometimes aids in identifying an intestinal, especially a duodenal, injury.

Although the **FAST** examination helps detect hemoperitoneum, the variably low sensitivity of this test in children suggests that it should not be used alone to exclude intraabdominal injury in patients with a moderate to high pretest probability for injury. A positive FAST exam for hemoperitoneum requires further investigation. Serial FAST exams over time (by a skilled ultrasonographer) may be used to rule out injury in need of intervention. The FAST exam is most clinically useful in patients who have blunt trauma and are hemodynamically unstable or in patients who require operative intervention for nonabdominal injuries, because in these cases the performance of a CT scan may not be feasible.

Nonoperative treatment has become standard for hemodynamically stable children with splenic, hepatic, and renal injuries from blunt trauma. The majority of such children can be treated nonsurgically. In addition to avoiding perioperative complications, nonoperative treatment decreases the need for blood transfusions and shortens hospital stay. When laparotomy is indicated, splenic repair is preferable to splenectomy.

Pelvic Trauma

Pelvic fractures in children are much less common than in adults, occurring in approximately 4% of children with more severe blunt trauma. Pelvic fractures are typically caused by high forces (e.g., high-speed motor vehicle crashes or pedestrian impacts) and are often associated with intraabdominal and/or vascular injuries. The pelvis itself forms a ring, and high-force impacts can lead to disruption of this ring. When the ring is disrupted in >1 location, such as the symphysis pubis and the sacroiliac joint, the ring can become unstable and displaced, potentially injuring large pelvic vessels and leading to massive blood loss. Catheter-directed embolization to control bleeding, performed by an interventional radiologist, may be required.

The pelvis should be assessed for stability by means of compression-distraction maneuvers. If instability is noted, immediate external fixation with a pelvis-stabilizing device or a sheet should be applied and orthopedic consultation sought. A trauma patient with a potential pelvic fracture should receive an AP pelvic radiograph in the trauma bay, or a CT scan, if there is high suspicion of injury. Children *without* a high-risk clinical finding (i.e., GCS <14; abdominal pain or tenderness; pelvic tenderness, laceration, ecchymosis, or abrasion; gross hematuria or >20 red blood cells/high-power field on urinalysis; or femur fracture) or a high-risk mechanism of injury (i.e., unrestrained motor vehicle collision, motor vehicle collision with ejection, motor vehicle collision rollover, auto vs pedestrian, or auto vs bicycle), however, are unlikely to have pelvic fractures.

Lower Genitourinary Trauma

The perineum should be inspected and the stability of the bones of the pelvis assessed. Urethral injuries are more common in males. Findings suggestive of urethral injury include scrotal or labial ecchymosis, blood at the urethral meatus, gross hematuria, and a superiorly positioned prostate on rectal examination (in an adolescent male). Certain pelvic fractures also increase the risk for potential genitourinary injury. Any of these findings is a contraindication to urethral catheter insertion and warrants consultation with a urologist. Retrograde urethrocystogram and CT scan of the pelvis and abdomen are used to determine the extent of injury.

Extremity Trauma

Thorough examination of the extremities is essential because extremity fractures are among the most frequently overlooked injuries in children with multiple trauma. All limbs should be inspected for deformity, swelling, and bruises; palpated for tenderness; and assessed for active and passive range of motion, sensory function, and perfusion.

Before radiographs are obtained, suspected fractures and dislocations should be immobilized and an analgesic administered. Splinting a femur fracture helps alleviate pain and may decrease blood loss. An orthopedic surgeon should be consulted immediately to evaluate children with compartment syndrome, neurovascular compromise, open fracture, or most traumatic amputations.

Radiologic and Laboratory Evaluation

Most authorities recommend ordering multiple laboratory tests (e.g., complete blood cell count, electrolytes, glucose, blood urea nitrogen, creatinine, liver function tests, amylase, lipase, lactate, blood gas, prothrombin and partial thromboplastin times, type and cross-match, urinalysis) and x-ray films (e.g., lateral C-spine, AP chest, AP pelvis) in the ED. One benefit of standardizing the evaluation of patients with major trauma is that fewer decisions need to be made on an individual basis, possibly expediting ED management. Some of these studies have prognostic importance. A large base deficit is associated with a higher mortality rate, and elevated lactate values correlate with poor prognosis.

There are some limitations in standard tests. The lateral cervical spine radiograph can miss clinically significant injuries. Hemoglobin and hematocrit values provide baseline values in the ED, but they may not have yet equilibrated after a hemorrhage. Abnormal liver function test results or elevated serum amylase and lipase values may be noted in patients with significant abdominal trauma, but most patients with significant trauma to the abdomen already have clinical indications for CT scanning or surgery. The majority of previously healthy children have normal coagulation profiles; these may become abnormal after major head trauma. Although routine urinalysis or dipstick urine testing for blood has been recommended for children, other data suggest that this evaluation may be unnecessary in patients without gross hematuria,

Table 82.7	Prediction Rule for Identification of Children at Very Low Risk of Clinically Important Brain Injuries After Head Trauma

*Children <2 yr old are at very low risk of clinically important traumatic brain injury if they have **none** of the following:*
Severe mechanism of injury
History of LOC >5 sec
GCS ≤14 or other signs of altered mental status
Not acting normally per parent
Palpable skull fracture
Occipital/parietal/temporal scalp hematoma
*Children 2-18 yr old are at very low risk of clinically important traumatic brain injury if they have **none** of the following:*
Severe mechanism of injury
History of LOC
History of vomiting
GCS ≤14 or other signs of altered mental status
Severe headache in the ED
Signs of basilar skull fracture

ED, Emergency department; GCS, Glasgow Coma Scale score; LOC, loss of consciousness.

Modified from Kuppermann N, Holmes JF, Dayan PS, et al: Identification of children at very low risk of clinically-important brain injuries after head trauma: a prospective cohort study, *Lancet* 374:1160–1170, 2009.

Table 82.8	Prediction Rule for Identification of Children at Very Low Risk of Clinically Important Intraabdominal Injuries After Blunt Trauma

*If **none** of the following is present, the patient is at very low risk for clinically significant intraabdominal injury:*
Glasgow Coma Scale score <14
Vomiting
Evidence of thoracic wall trauma
Decreased breath sounds
Evidence of abdominal wall trauma or seatbelt sign
Abdominal pain
Abdominal tenderness

Modified from Holmes JF, Lillis K, Monroe D, et al: Identifying children at very low risk of clinically important blunt abdominal injuries, *Ann Emerg Med* 62:107–116, e2, 2013.

hypotension, or other associated abdominal injuries.

Clinical prediction rules that combine patient history with physical examination findings have been developed to identify those at low risk of injury for whom specific radiographic and laboratory studies may not be necessary. The NEXUS C-spine rule is a sensitive, easily applicable rule that was validated for adults and children, although there were fewer young patients studied (see Table 82.5). Several clinical prediction rules have been developed to identify children at low risk of traumatic brain injury (Table 82.7). Another clinical prediction rule has been developed to identify children at very low risk of clinically important intraabdominal injuries following blunt trauma (Table 82.8). Although this rule has an NPV of 99.9%, it needs to be externally validated before widespread implementation.

PSYCHOLOGICAL AND SOCIAL SUPPORT

Serious multisystem trauma may result in significant long-term psychological and social difficulties for the child and family, particularly when there is a major head injury. Like adults, children are at risk for depressive symptoms and posttraumatic stress disorder. Caregivers face persistent stress and have been noted to have more psychological symptoms. Psychological and social support, during the resuscitation period and afterward, is extremely important. Parents often prefer to be offered the choice to be present during resuscitations. A member of the resuscitation team should be made responsible for answering the family's questions and supporting them in the trauma room.

Bibliography is available at Expert Consult.

Chapter 83
Spinal Cord Injuries in Children
Mark R. Proctor

第八十三章
儿童脊髓损伤

中文导读

本章主要介绍了儿童脊髓损伤的临床表现、如何明确儿童颈椎骨折、治疗及预防。其中临床表现包括脊髓休克、矛盾呼吸、短暂的四肢瘫及圆锥综合征等；明确儿童颈椎骨折的方法包括X线片、MRI及CT；治疗首先要维持正常血容量及血压，药物治疗包括大剂量甲泼尼龙（30mg/kg），但此种方法尚有争议，此外还可通过手术治疗解除脊髓压迫；预防措施包括安全驾驶、使用安全带或安全座椅及游泳时遵守"脚先入水"规则等。

See also Chapter 729.

Compared with adults, spine and spinal cord injuries are rare in children, particularly young children, because of both anatomic differences and etiologies of injury. The main mechanisms of injury to the spine are motor vehicle crashes, falls, sports, and violence, which affect young children less often (see Chapter 82).

Several anatomic differences affect the pediatric spine. The head of a young child is larger relative to body mass than in adults, and the neck muscles are still underdeveloped, which places the fulcrum of movement higher in the spine. Therefore, children <9 yr old have a higher percentage of injuries in the upper cervical spine than older children and adults. The spine of a small child also is very mobile, with pliable bones and ligaments, so fractures of the spine are exceedingly rare. However, this increased mobility is not always a positive feature. Transfer of energy leading to spinal distortion may not affect the structural integrity of the bones and ligaments of the spine but can still lead to significant injuries of the spinal cord. This phenomenon of **spinal cord injury without radiographic abnormalities (SCIWORA)** is more common in children than adults. The term is relatively outdated, since almost all injuries are detectable by MRI, but is still clinically useful when referring to spinal cord injuries evaluated by plain radiographs or CT. There seem to be 2 distinct forms of SCIWORA. The **infantile** form involves severe injury of the cervical or thoracic spinal cord; these patients have a poor chance of complete recovery. In older children and adolescents, SCIWORA is more likely to be a less severe injury, with a high likelihood of complete recovery over time. The **adolescent** form, also called *transient neurapraxia*, is assumed to be a spinal cord concussion or mild contusion, as opposed to the severe spinal cord injury related to the mobility of the spine in small children.

Although the mechanisms of spinal cord injury in children include birth trauma, falls, and child abuse, the major cause of morbidity and mortality across all ages remains **motor vehicle injuries**. Adolescents incur spinal cord injuries with epidemiology similar to that of adults, including significant male predominance and a high likelihood of fracture dislocations of the lower cervical spine or thoracolumbar region. In infants and children <5 yr old, fractures and mechanical disruption of spinal elements are more likely to occur in the upper cervical spine between the occiput and C3, for the reasons previously discussed.

CLINICAL MANIFESTATIONS

One in 3 patients with significant trauma to the spine and spinal cord will have a concomitant severe head injury, which makes early diagnosis challenging. For these patients, clinical evaluation may be difficult. Patients with a potential spine injury need to be maintained in a protective environment, such as a collar, until the spine can be cleared by clinical and/or radiographic means. A careful neurologic examination is necessary for infants with suspected spinal cord injuries. Complete spinal cord injury will lead to **spinal shock** with early areflexia (see Chapter 729). Severe cervical spinal cord (C-spine) injuries will usually lead to paradoxical respiration in patients who are breathing spontaneously. **Paradoxical respiration** occurs when the diaphragm, which is innervated by the phrenic nerves with contributions from C3, C4, and C5, is functioning normally, but the intercostal musculature innervated by the thoracic spinal cord is paralyzed. In this situation, inspiration fails to expand of the chest wall but distends the abdomen. Other complications during the acute (2-48 hr) phase include autonomic dysfunction (brady- and tachyarrhythmias, orthostatic hypotension, hypertension), temperature instability, thromboembolism, dysphagia, and bowel/bladder dysfunction.

The *mildest* injury to the spinal cord is **transient quadriparesis** evident for seconds or minutes with complete recovery in 24 hr. This injury follows a concussion of the cord and is most frequently seen in adolescent athletes. If their imaging is normal, these children can generally return to normal activities after a period of rest from days to weeks, depending on the initial severity, similar to cerebral concussion management.

Significant spinal cord injury in the cervical region is characterized by: flaccid quadriparesis, loss of sphincter function, and a sensory level corresponding to the level of injury. An injury at the high cervical level (C1-C2) can cause respiratory arrest and death in the absence of ventilatory support. Injuries in the *thoracic* region are generally the result of fracture dislocations. They may produce paraplegia when at T10 or above, or the **conus medullaris syndrome** if at the T12-L1 level. This includes a loss of urinary and rectal sphincter control, flaccid weakness, and sensory disturbances of the legs. A **central cord lesion** may result from contusion and hemorrhage in the center of the spinal cord. It typically involves the upper extremities to a greater degree than the legs, because the motor fibers to the cervical and thoracic region are more centrally located in the spinal cord. There are lower motor neuron signs in the upper extremities and upper motor neuron signs in the legs, bladder dysfunction, and loss of sensation caudal to the lesion. There may be considerable recovery, particularly in the lower extremities, although sequelae are common (see Chapter 729).

CLEARING THE CERVICAL SPINE IN CHILDREN

The management of children following major trauma is challenging. For older children, the clearance is similar to a lucid adult, and the NEXUS (National Emergency X-Radiography Utilization Study) criteria are appropriate (see Chapter 82, Table 82.5). Clearing the cervical spine in younger and uncooperative children involves similar issues as in adults with an altered level of consciousness. Small children generally have a difficult-to-assess physical examination, and it is difficult to determine if they have cervical pain. Plain radiography remains a mainstay for assessing the spine because it is easy to obtain. There has been increasing emphasis on MRI for evaluation of potential C-spine instability, but in small children MRI requires sedation and in most centers the presence of an anesthesiologist (Fig. 83.1). CT scan is another important study with high sensitivity and specificity, but the risk of radiation exposure must be considered.

TREATMENT

The cervical spine should be immobilized in the field by the emergency medical technicians. In cases of acute spinal cord injury, weak data suggest the acute infusion of a bolus of high-dose (30 mg/kg) methylprednisolone, followed by a 23 hr infusion (5.4 mg/kg/hr). The data for this treatment are controversial and have not been tested specifically in children; *many centers no longer use it routinely.* Maintenance of euvolemia and

normotension are very important, and vasopressors might be needed if the sympathetic nervous system has been compromised.

Surgical management of spinal injuries must be tailored to the patient's age but can be a crucial step in management. Any compression of the spinal cord must be surgically relieved to afford the best chance of a favorable outcome. In addition, spinal cord injury can be worsened by instability, so surgical stabilization can prevent further injury (Fig. 83.2). In general, younger children have a higher healing capacity for bones and ligaments, and external immobilization might be considered for injuries that require surgery in older children and adults. However, some injuries are highly unstable and always require surgery. **Occipitocervical dislocation** is one such highly unstable injury, and early surgery with fusion from the occiput to C2 or C3 should be performed, even in very young children. Fixation of the subaxial spine must be tailored to the size of the pedicles and other osseous structures of the developing axial skeleton.

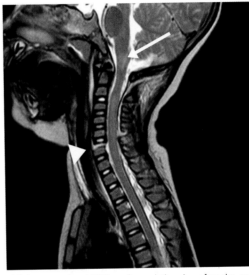

Fig. 83.1 T2-weighted MRI performed the day after the accident showed cervical spinal cord swelling combined with high signal intensity (C1-C3) (*arrow*) and dislocation of C5-C6 (*arrowhead*). (*From Inoue K, Kumada T, Fujii T, Kimura N: Progressive cervical spinal cord atrophy after a traffic accident, J Pediatr 180:287, 2017, Fig 1, p 287.*)

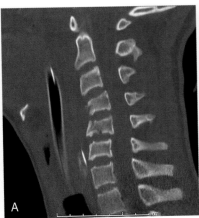 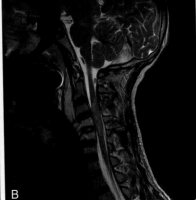 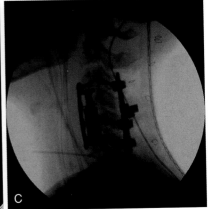

Fig. 83.2 A 15 yr old hockey player suffered acute paraplegia after his head struck the boards during a hockey game. **A,** CT scan shows compression fractures of C4 and C5. **B,** MRI shows severe spinal cord contusion. **C,** Because of the need to decompress the spinal cord and stabilize the spine, anterior and posterior surgery was performed. No meaningful recovery was obtained.

PREVENTION

The most important aspect of the care of spinal cord injuries in children is injury prevention. Use of appropriate child restraints in automobiles is the most important precaution. In older children and adolescents, rules against "spear tackling" in American football and the *Feet First, First Time* aimed at adolescents diving into swimming pools and natural water areas are important ways to help prevent severe cervical spinal cord injuries. Safe driving practices, such as using safety belts, avoiding distracted driving, and following the speed limit, can have substantial beneficial effects on injury rates.

Bibliography is available at Expert Consult.

Chapter **84**

Care of Abrasions and Minor Lacerations

Joanna S. Cohen and Bruce L. Klein

第八十四章
擦伤和轻微撕裂伤的处理

中文导读

本章主要介绍了撕裂伤和切割伤以及擦伤的处理。其中在撕裂伤和切割伤的流行病学部分介绍了撕裂伤在美国的发生率；评估包括询问病史，如损伤机制、损伤程度以及受伤的时间，还包括对伤口的检查，如大小，深度，是否伤及血管、神经、肌腱或其他组织，位置等；治疗的目标是止血，最大限度减少感染风险，修复皮肤和保持组织的完整性，并尽可能恢复功能及美观；擦伤的治疗包括彻底清创，使用不粘连敷料，局部使用抗生素和常规敷料，有指征时应注射破伤风疫苗。

LACERATIONS AND CUTS

Lacerations are tears of the skin caused by blunt or shearing forces. A **cut** (or a *stab*), in contrast, is an injury inflicted by a sharp object. Although distinguishing between the two can be important for forensic purposes, their evaluation and management are similar. In this chapter, lacerations include cuts and stabs.

Epidemiology

More than half of the 12 million wounds treated annually in U.S. emergency departments (EDs) are lacerations. Approximately 30% occur in children younger than 18 yr. Approximately 2% of pediatric office visits are related to wound management.

Evaluation

The history should include the mechanism of injury, the amount of force, and the time the injury occurred. The mechanism helps determine whether there may be foreign material in the wound, which would increase the risk for infection. Particularly in children, it is essential to determine whether the injury was inflicted intentionally. *If nonaccidental trauma is suspected, child protective services should be notified.* The type of force causing the laceration also influences the risk of infection, because a significant crush injury is more likely to become infected than a shearing one. **Blunt injury**, such as bumping the head, is a common cause of lacerations in children and is less likely to become infected. Theoretically, the amount of bacteria in the wound should increase exponentially with the time from injury to repair; however, the length of time that results in a clinically significant increase in wound infection is unclear. Older wounds may require delayed primary closure or healing by secondary intention. The patient or parent should be asked about any special host factors that may predispose to infection or impede healing, such as diabetes, malnutrition, obesity, and corticosteroid therapy, as well as immunization status, with particular attention to tetanus administration.

On examination, the clinician should note the size and depth of the wound, as well as any associated vascular, neurologic, tendon, or other tissue injury. The laceration's location also is important with regard to both the risk for infection and the cosmetic outcome. Compared with lacerations in adults, those in children occur more often on the face and scalp and less often on the upper extremities. Because the face and scalp are more vascular, wounds located there are less likely to become infected. Lacerations overlying joints are more likely to develop wider scars as a result of tension during healing.

Treatment

The goals of treatment are to establish hemostasis, minimize the risk of infection, restore skin and underlying tissue integrity, and produce the most functionally and cosmetically acceptable result possible. Complications of wounds, including infection, hypertrophic scar formation, and functional limitation occur in approximately 8% of children.

Any significant bleeding must be controlled, usually with external pressure, before a thorough evaluation of the wound can occur. If there is a skin flap, it should be returned to its original position before application of pressure. Infrequently, a tourniquet may need to be applied if bleeding cannot be controlled with direct pressure. Clothing over the injury should be removed to minimize wound contamination. Jewelry encircling an injured extremity should be removed to prevent the jewelry from forming a constricting band when the extremity swells.

It is best to administer a **local anesthetic** early, before exploration and more meticulous cleansing of the wound. This anesthetic can be applied topically (e.g., lidocaine, epinephrine, and tetracaine gel) or infiltrated locally or as a regional nerve block (e.g., lidocaine or bupivacaine), depending on the location of the laceration and the complexity of the repair. Buffering the acidic lidocaine with sodium bicarbonate can reduce pain during injection. Sometimes, nonpharmacologic or additional pharmacologic methods of analgesia and anxiolysis are required for a young, frightened, or uncooperative child. The wound should be examined under proper light to enable identification of foreign bodies or damage to vessels, nerves, or tendons.

Many lacerations, especially heavily contaminated ones, benefit from **irrigation**, with either water or sterile saline, to reduce the risk of infection. It is important to recognize that many traumatic lacerations treated in the ED, or office, are only minimally contaminated, containing <10^2 bacterial colonies. In fact, in one of the few human studies on irrigation, irrigation did not decrease the infection rate of *minimally* contaminated scalp or facial lacerations in patients who presented to an ED within 6 hr of injury. Higher-pressure irrigation may actually increase tissue damage, making the wound and adjacent tissue more susceptible to infection and delaying healing. These caveats notwithstanding, irrigation has benefits, although which technique to use—that is, which device, what size syringe, what size needle, which solution, how much volume, how much pressure—remains to be determined. These features may vary for different types of lacerations. In heavily contaminated wounds, the benefit of higher-pressure irrigation likely outweighs the harm of tissue damage. For heavily contaminated lacerations, a typical recommendation is to use a 35-65 mL syringe attached to a plastic splatter shield, or a 19-gauge needle if a splatter shield is unavailable, and to irrigate with approximately 100 mL of solution per centimeter of wound. Conversely, for relatively clean wounds, lower-pressure irrigation minimizes tissue damage, which may be more important for outcome than any decrease in bacterial clearance that may ensue. Debridement of devitalized tissue with higher-pressure irrigation, scrubbing, or surgical excision can also be necessary in certain cases, such as crush injuries.

Most lacerations seen in the pediatric ED or office should be closed primarily. Contraindications exist to **primary closure** (e.g., certain bite wounds; see Chapter 743). Although it is accepted that the time from injury to repair should be as brief as possible to minimize the risk of infection, there is no universally accepted guideline as to what length of time is too long for primary wound closure. Also, this length of time varies for different types of lacerations. A prudent recommendation is that higher-risk wounds should be closed within 6 hr at most after the injury but that some low-risk wounds (e.g., clean facial lacerations) may be closed as late as 12-24 hr.

Many lacerations can be closed with simple, interrupted, 4-0, 5-0, or 6-0, **nonabsorbable sutures**. For certain lacerations, absorbable sutures for external skin closure are not necessarily inferior to nonabsorbable sutures, and may provide cost and time savings, as well as avoiding having to remove them, an unpleasant procedure in a young child. For lacerations under tension, horizontal or vertical mattress sutures, which provide added strength and may evert the wound edges better, can be used instead. For lacerations in cosmetically significant areas, a **running intradermal stitch** may produce a less conspicuous, more aesthetic scar than simple or mattress skin sutures, which can leave unattractive track marks. Deeper lacerations may need repair with an absorbable dermal and/or fascial layer. Other complex lacerations, such as those involving the ear, eyelid, nose, lip, tongue, genitalia, or fingertip, sometimes require more advanced techniques as well as subspecialty consultation.

Staples, topical skin adhesives, and surgical tape are acceptable alternatives to sutures, depending on the laceration's location and the healthcare provider's preference. **Staples** are particularly useful for scalp lacerations, where the scar's appearance tends to be less important. Topical **skin adhesives** (octyl cyanoacrylates or butyl cyanoacrylates) are ideal for linear, relatively superficial lacerations with easily approximated edges that are not under tension. Adhesives are particularly useful for lacerations located in areas where suture track marks are especially undesirable, or in situations where resources are constrained.

Maintaining a warm, moist, wound environment following repair accelerates wound healing without increasing the risk of infection. A topical antimicrobial ointment (e.g., bacitracin or bacitracin, neomycin, and polymyxin B combination) and conventional gauze dressing provide such an environment and reduce the infection rate. Compared with conventional dressings, **occlusive dressings** (hydrocolloids, hydrogels, polyurethane films) may be better at accelerating healing, reducing infection, and decreasing pain but are more expensive. Occlusive dressings that adhere (hydrocolloids or polyurethane films) are impractical for lacerations with protruding sutures. If the laceration overlies or is near a joint, **splinting** helps limit mobility and can speed healing and minimize dehiscence.

For most routine lacerations that are repaired early and meticulously, prophylactic systemic antibiotics are unnecessary because they do not decrease the rate of infection. **Antibiotic prophylaxis** is or may be indicated for human and many animal bites, for open fractures and joints, and for grossly contaminated wounds, as well as for wounds in patients who are immunosuppressed or have prosthetic devices. *Tetanus prophylaxis should be administered, if indicated,* according to U.S. Centers for Disease Control and Prevention guidelines (see Chapter 238).

ABRASIONS

An **abrasion** is a scrape to the epidermis, and sometimes the dermis, that is usually caused by friction of the skin against a rough surface. *Road rash* is a colloquial term for abrasions that result from friction of the skin against pavement. Motor vehicle collisions with pedestrians and cycling accidents are common causes of road rash in children. Road rash can be extensive, involving multiple areas on the body. These abrasions also can be deep, and they often contain embedded debris. A *rug burn* is an abrasion sustained by sliding across a carpet. Some abrasions display specific patterns and are called **imprint abrasions**. *Ligature marks* are a type of imprint abrasion caused by a rope or cord that has been tied around a part of the body and has rubbed against the skin. These injuries should alert the clinician to the likelihood of nonaccidental (including self-inflicted) trauma.

Treatment

All abrasions should be cleansed thoroughly and any debris or foreign material removed. If debris is not removed, abnormal skin pigmentation, known as **posttraumatic tattooing**, can occur and can be difficult to treat. A nonadherent occlusive dressing or a topical antibiotic and conventional dressing should be applied. *Tetanus prophylaxis should be administered, if indicated* (see Chapter 238). Large and/or deep abrasions that have not healed in a few weeks require consultation with a plastic surgeon for more advanced care.

Bibliography is available at Expert Consult.

Chapter 85
Neurologic Emergencies and Stabilization
Patrick M. Kochanek and Michael J. Bell

第八十五章
神经系统急症和稳定

中文导读

　　本章主要介绍了神经系统疾病治疗原则及创伤性颅脑损伤（TBI）。治疗原则是保障对大脑的营养供应。造成TBI的病因，包括车祸伤、跌倒、袭击和虐待性头部创伤；TBI的病理学特点为硬膜外、硬膜下和脑实质出血；TBI的发病机制分为原发性损伤和继发性损伤；重型TBI临床表现为昏迷和颅内压增高；

实验室检查包括头CT和MRI；根据病史和临床表现通常可以诊断重型TBI；治疗原则为防止二次损伤及降颅压，支持治疗包括维持氧饱和度、监测血糖、提倡早期肠内营养、慎重使用糖皮质激素、吸痰前后使用镇痛或镇静药及预防惊厥，预后与颅脑和全身损伤程度有关。

NEUROCRITICAL CARE PRINCIPLES

The brain has high metabolic demands, which are further increased during growth and development. Preservation of nutrient supply to the brain is the mainstay of care for children with evolving brain injuries. *Intracranial dynamics* describes the physics of the interactions of the contents—brain parenchyma, blood (arterial, venous, capillary), and cerebrospinal fluid (CSF)—within the cranium. Normally, brain parenchyma accounts for up to 85% of the contents of the cranial vault, and the remaining portion is divided between CSF and blood. The brain resides in a relatively rigid cranial vault, and cranial compliance decreases with age as the skull ossification centers gradually replace cartilage with bone. The **intracranial pressure (ICP)** is derived from the volume of its components and the bony compliance. The **perfusion pressure** of the brain (cerebral perfusion pressure, CPP) is equal to the pressure of blood entering the cranium (mean arterial pressure, MAP) minus the ICP, in most cases.

Increases in intracranial volume can result from swelling, masses, or increases in blood and CSF volumes. As these volumes increase, compensatory mechanisms decrease ICP by (1) decreasing CSF volume (CSF is displaced into the spinal canal or absorbed by arachnoid villi), (2) decreasing cerebral blood volume (venous blood return to the thorax is augmented), and/or (3) increasing cranial volume (sutures pathologically expand or bone is remodeled). Once compensatory mechanisms are exhausted (the increase in cranial volume is too large), small increases in volume lead to large increases in ICP, or intracranial hypertension (Fig. 85.1). As ICP continues to increase, brain ischemia can occur as CPP falls. Further increases in ICP can ultimately displace the brain downward into the foramen magnum—a process called **cerebral herniation,** which can become irreversible in minutes and may lead to severe disability or death; Fig. 85.2 notes other sites of brain herniation.

Oxygen and glucose are required by brain cells for normal functioning, and these nutrients must be constantly supplied by cerebral blood flow (CBF). Normally, CBF is constant over a wide range of blood pressures (i.e., blood pressure autoregulation of CBF) via actions mainly within the cerebral arterioles. Cerebral arterioles are maximally dilated at lower blood pressures and maximally constricted at higher pressures so that CBF does not vary during normal fluctuations (Fig. 85.3). Above the upper limit of autoregulation, breakthrough dilation occurs, which if severe can produce hypertensive encephalopathy. Acid-base balance of the CSF, often reflected by acute changes in arterial partial pressure of carbon dioxide ($PaCO_2$), body/brain temperature, glucose utilization, blood viscosity, and other vasoactive mediators (i.e., adenosine, nitric oxide), can also affect the cerebral vasculature.

Knowledge of these concepts is instrumental to preventing secondary brain injury. Increases in CSF pH that occur because of inadvertent hyperventilation (which decreases $PaCO_2$) can produce cerebral ischemia. Hyperthermia-mediated increases in cerebral metabolic demands may damage vulnerable brain regions after injury. Hypoglycemia can produce neuronal death when CBF fails to compensate. Prolonged seizures can lead to permanent injuries if hypoxemia occurs from loss of airway control.

Attention to detail and constant reassessment are paramount in managing children with critical neurologic insults. Among the most valuable tools for serial, objective assessment of neurologic condition

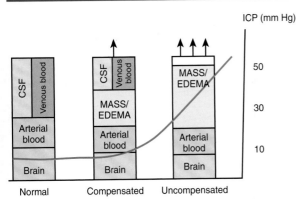

Fig. 85.1 The Munro-Kellie doctrine describes intracranial dynamics in the setting of an expanding mass lesion (i.e., hemorrhage, tumor) or brain edema. In the normal state, the brain parenchyma, arterial blood, cerebrospinal fluid (CSF), and venous blood occupy the cranial vault at a low pressure, generally <10 mm Hg. With an expanding mass lesion or brain edema, initially there is a compensated state as a result of reduced CSF and venous blood volumes, and intracranial pressure (ICP) remains low. Further expansion of the lesion, however, leads to an uncompensated state when compensatory mechanisms are exhausted, and intracranial hypertension results.

is the **Glasgow Coma Scale (GCS)** (see Chapter 81, Table 81.3). Originally developed for use in comatose adults, the GCS is also valuable in pediatrics. Modifications to the GCS have been made for nonverbal children and are available for infants and toddlers. Serial assessments of the GCS score along with a focused neurologic examination are invaluable to detection of injuries before permanent damage occurs in the vulnerable brain. The **full outline of unresponsiveness (FOUR)** score is a modification of the GCS, with eye and motor response, but eliminates the verbal response and adds 2 functional assessments of the brainstem (pupil, corneal, and cough reflexes) and respiratory patterns (Table 85.1).

The most studied monitoring device in clinical practice is the **ICP monitor**. Monitoring is accomplished by inserting a catheter-transducer either into the cerebral ventricle or into brain parenchyma (i.e., externalized ventricular drain and parenchymal transducer, respectively). ICP-directed therapies are standard of care in traumatic brain injury (TBI) and are used in other conditions, such as intracranial hemorrhage, some cases of encephalopathy, meningitis, and encephalitis. Other devices being used include catheters that measure brain tissue oxygen concentration, external probes that noninvasively assess brain oxygenation by absorbance of near-infrared light (i.e., near-infrared spectroscopy), monitors of brain electrical activity (continuous electroencephalography [EEG] or somatosensory, visual, or auditory evoked potentials), and CBF monitors (transcranial Doppler, xenon CT, perfusion MRI, or tissue probes). In the severe TBI guidelines, brain tissue oxygen concentration monitoring received level III support and thus may be considered.

TRAUMATIC BRAIN INJURY
Etiology and Epidemiology
Mechanisms of TBI include motor vehicle crashes, falls, assaults, and abusive head trauma. Most TBIs in children are from closed-head injuries (Fig. 85.4). TBI is an important pediatric public health problem, with approximately 37,000 cases resulting in the death of >7,000 children annually in the United States.

Pathology
Epidural, subdural, and parenchymal intracranial hemorrhages can result. Injury to gray or white matter is also commonly seen and includes focal cerebral contusions, diffuse cerebral swelling, axonal injury, and injury to the cerebellum or brainstem. Patients with severe TBI often have multiple findings; diffuse and potentially delayed cerebral swelling is common.

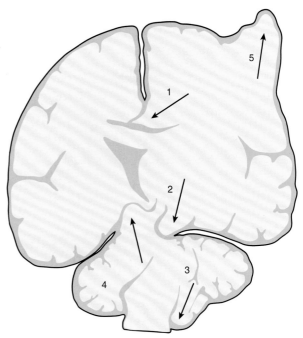

Fig. 85.2 Different forms of brain herniation. *1*, Cingulate. *2*, Uncal. *3*, Cerebellar tonsillar. *4*, Upward cerebellar. *5*, Transcalvarial. *(From Fishman RA: Cerebrospinal fluid in diseases of the nervous system, Philadelphia, 1980, Saunders.)*

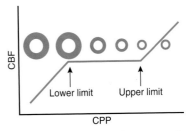

Fig. 85.3 Schematic of the relationship between cerebral blood flow (CBF) and cerebral perfusion pressure (CPP). The diameter of a representative cerebral arteriole is also shown across the center of the y axis to facilitate understanding of the vascular response across CPP that underlies blood pressure autoregulation of CBF. CPP is generally defined as the mean arterial pressure (MAP) minus the intracranial pressure (ICP). At normal values for ICP, this generally represents MAP. Thus, normally, CBF is kept constant between the lower limit and upper limit of autoregulation; in normal adults, these values are approximately 50 mm Hg and 150 mm Hg, respectively. In children, the upper limit of autoregulation is likely proportionally lower than the adult value relative to normal MAP for age. However, according to the work of Vavilala et al. (2003), lower-limit values are surprisingly similar in infants and older children. Thus, infants and young children may have less reserve for adequate CPP.

Pathogenesis
TBI results in primary and secondary injury. Primary injury from the impact produces irreversible tissue disruption. In contrast, 2 types of secondary injury are targets of neurointensive care. First, some of the ultimate damage seen in the injured brain evolves over hours or days, and the underlying mechanisms involved (e.g., edema, apoptosis, secondary axotomy) are therapeutic targets. Second, the injured brain is vulnerable to additional insults because injury disrupts normal autoregulatory defense mechanisms; disruption of autoregulation of CBF can lead to

ischemia from hypotension that would otherwise be tolerated by the uninjured brain.

Clinical Manifestations

The hallmark of **severe TBI** is coma (**GCS score 3-8**). Often, coma is seen immediately after the injury and is sustained. In some cases, such as with an epidural hematoma, a child may be alert on presentation but may deteriorate after a period of hours. A similar picture can be seen in children with diffuse swelling, in whom a "talk-and-die" scenario has been described. Clinicians should also not be lulled into underappreciating the potential for deterioration of a child with **moderate TBI** (**GCS score 9-12**) with a significant contusion, because progressive swelling can potentially lead to devastating complications. In the comatose child with severe TBI, the second key clinical manifestation is the development of *intracranial hypertension*. The development of increased ICP with impending herniation may be heralded by new-onset or worsening headache, depressed level of consciousness, vital sign changes (hypertension, bradycardia, irregular respirations), and signs of 6th (lateral rectus palsy) or 3rd (anisocoria [dilated pupil], ptosis, down-and-out position of globe as a result of rectus muscle palsies) cranial nerve compression. Increased ICP is managed with continuous ICP monitoring, as well as monitoring for clinical signs of increased ICP or impending herniation. The development of brain swelling is progressive. Significantly raised ICP (>20 mm Hg) can occur early after severe TBI, but peak ICP generally is seen at 48-72 hr. Need for ICP-directed therapy may persist for longer than a week. A few children have coma without increased ICP, resulting from axonal injury or brainstem injury. *In addition to head trauma, it is critical to identify potential cervical spine injury* (see Chapter 83).

Laboratory Findings

Cranial CT should be obtained immediately after resuscitation and cardiopulmonary stabilization (Figs. 85.5 to 85.11). In some cases, MRI can be diagnostic (Fig. 85.12). Generally, other laboratory findings are normal in isolated TBI, although occasionally coagulopathy or the development of the syndrome of inappropriate antidiuretic hormone (SIADH) secretion or, rarely, cerebral salt wasting (CSW) is seen. In the setting of TBI with polytrauma, other injuries can result in laboratory and radiographic abnormalities, and a **full trauma survey** is important in all patients with severe TBI (see Chapter 82).

Diagnosis and Differential Diagnosis

In severe TBI the diagnosis is generally obvious from the history and clinical presentation. Occasionally, TBI severity can be overestimated because of concurrent alcohol or drug intoxication. The diagnosis of TBI can be problematic in cases of **abusive head trauma** or following an anoxic event such as drowning or smoke inhalation.

Table 85.1	Commonly Used Coma Scores	
POINTS		**DESCRIPTION**
GLASGOW COMA SCALE (GCS) SCORE		
Eye Opening		
1		Does not open eyes
2		Opens eyes in response to noxious stimuli
3		Opens eyes in response to voice
4		Opens eyes spontaneously
Verbal Output		
1		Makes no sounds
2		Makes incomprehensible sounds
3		Utters inappropriate words
4		Confused and disoriented
5		Speaks normally and oriented
Motor Response (Best)		
1		Makes no movements
2		Extension to painful stimuli
3		Abnormal flexion to painful stimuli
4		Flexion/withdrawal to painful stimuli
5		Localized to painful stimuli
6		Obeys commands
FULL OUTLINE OF UNRESPONSIVENESS (FOUR) SCORE		
Eye Response		
4		Eyelids open or opened, tracking, or blinking to command
3		Eyelids open but not tracking
2		Eyelids closed but open to loud voice
1		Eyelids closed but open to pain
0		Eyelids remain closed with pain
Motor Response		
4		Thumbs-up, fist, or "peace" sign
3		Localizing to pain
2		Flexion response to pain
1		Extension response to pain
0		No response to pain or generalized myoclonus status
Brainstem Reflexes		
4		Pupil and corneal reflexes present
3		One pupil wide and fixed
2		Pupil or corneal reflexes absent
1		Pupil and corneal reflexes absent
0		Absent pupil, corneal, and cough reflex
Respiration		
4		Not intubated, regular breathing pattern
3		Not intubated, Cheyne-Stokes breathing pattern
2		Not intubated, irregular breathing
1		Breathes above ventilatory rate
0		Breathes at ventilator rate or apnea

Adapted from Edlow JA, Rabinstein A, Traub SJ, Wijdicks EFM: Diagnosis of reversible causes of coma, *Lancet* 384:2064-2076, 2014.

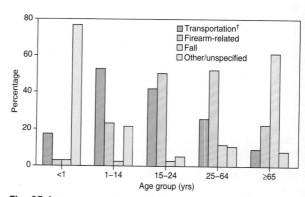

Fig. 85.4 Percentage of traumatic brain injury (TBI)–related deaths* by underlying cause and age group—United States, 2013. *TBI-related deaths were identified using the *International Classification of Diseases, Tenth Revision*, underlying cause of death codes of *U01–*U03, V01–Y36, Y85–Y87, or Y89 with a multiple cause of death code of S01.0–S01.9, S02.0, S02.1, S02.3, S02.7–S02.9, S04.0, S06.0–S06.9, S07.0, S07.1, S07.8, S07.9, S09.7–S09.9, T01.0, T02.0, T04.0, T06.0, T90.1, T90.2, T90.4, T90.5, T90.8, or T90.9, for a total of 54,185 deaths in 2013 for all ages. †Transportation includes all modes, such as motor vehicle, motorcycle, pedal cycle, pedestrian, other land transport, railway, watercraft, and aircraft. The causes of injury that result in TBI-related deaths vary by age-group. In 2013, 77% of the TBI-related deaths among infants <1 yr old were from causes other than transportation, firearms, or falls and primarily resulted from assault and maltreatment. Transportation accounted for 53% of the TBI-related deaths among children 1-14 yr. Firearm-related injuries accounted for 50% and 52% of the TBI-related deaths for persons 15-24 and 25-64 yr, respectively. Most of the firearm-related TBI deaths in these 2 age-groups were suicides (62% and 83%, respectively). The majority (61%) of TBI-related deaths for those aged ≥65 yr resulted from falls. (*From National Vital Statistics System mortality data.* http://www.cdc.gov/nchs/deaths.htm. *Additional information on TBI available at* http://www.cdc.gov/traumaticbraininjury/. *The Lancet: The burden of traumatic brain injury in children, Lancet 391:813, 2018.*)

Treatment

Infants and children with severe or moderate TBI (GCS score 3-8 or 9-12, respectively) receive intensive care unit (ICU) monitoring. Evidence-based guidelines for management of severe TBI have been published (Fig. 85.13). This approach to ICP-directed therapy is also reasonable for other conditions in which ICP is monitored. Care involves a multidisciplinary team comprising pediatric caregivers from neurologic surgery, critical care medicine, surgery, and rehabilitation and is directed at preventing secondary insults and managing increased ICP. Initial stabilization of infants and children with severe TBI includes rapid sequence tracheal intubation with spine precautions along with maintenance of normal extracerebral hemodynamics, including blood gas values (PaO$_2$, PaCO$_2$), MAP, and temperature. Intravenous (IV) fluid boluses may be required to treat hypotension. Euvolemia is the target, and hypotonic fluids must be rigorously avoided; *normal saline is the fluid of choice*. Vasopressors may be needed as guided by monitoring of central venous pressure, with avoidance of both fluid overload and exacerbation of brain edema. A trauma survey should be performed. Once stabilized, the patient should be taken for CT scanning to rule out the need for emergency neurosurgical intervention. If surgery is not required, an ICP monitor should be inserted to guide the treatment of intracranial hypertension.

During stabilization or at any time during the treatment course, patients can present with signs and symptoms of *cerebral herniation* (pupillary dilation, systemic hypertension, bradycardia, extensor posturing). Because herniation and its devastating consequences can sometimes be reversed if promptly addressed, it should be treated as a *medical emergency*, with use of hyperventilation, with a fraction of inspired oxygen of 1.0, and intubating doses of either thiopental or pentobarbital and either mannitol (0.25-1.0 g/kg IV) or hypertonic saline (3% solution, 5-10 mL/kg IV).

Intracranial pressure should be maintained at <20 mm Hg. Age-dependent cerebral perfusion pressure targets are approximately 50 mm Hg for children 2-6 yr old; 55 mm Hg for those 7-10 yr old; and 65 mm Hg for those 11-16 yr old. **First-tier** therapy includes elevation of the head of the bed, ensuring midline positioning of the head, controlled mechanical ventilation, and analgesia and sedation (i.e., narcotics and benzodiazepines). If neuromuscular blockade is needed, it may be desirable to monitor EEG continuously because status epilepticus can

occur; this complication will not be recognized in a paralyzed patient and is associated with increased ICP and unfavorable outcome. If a ventricular rather than parenchymal catheter is used to monitor ICP, therapeutic CSF drainage is available and can be provided either continuously (often targeting an ICP >5 mm Hg) or intermittently in response to ICP spikes, generally >20 mm Hg. Other first-tier therapies include the osmolar agents **hypertonic saline** (often given as a continuous infusion of 3% saline at 0.1-1.0 mL/kg/hr) and **mannitol** (0.25-1.0 g/kg IV over 20 min), given in response to ICP spikes >20 mm Hg or

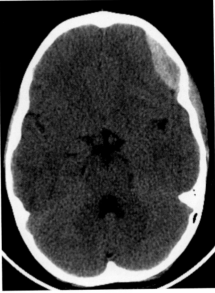

Fig. 85.6 Epidural hematoma. Left frontal epidural hematoma observed on CT imaging in a 12 yr old child who fell off his bike onto concrete surface.

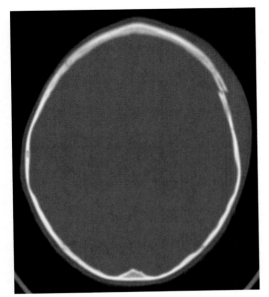

Fig. 85.5 Skull fracture. Mildly displaced skull fracture seen on CT imaging (bone window view) in a 4 yr old child who fell and hit her head on a curb.

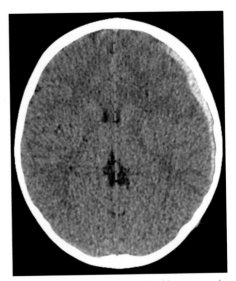

Fig. 85.7 Subdural hematoma. Left subdural hematoma observed on CT imaging in a 10 yr old child after motor vehicle crash. Note effacement of the left lateral ventricle and midline shift (see *dotted line* for midline reference).

with a fixed (every 4-6 hr) dosing interval. Use of hypertonic saline is more common and has stronger literature support than mannitol, although both are used; these 2 agents can be used concurrently. It is recommended to avoid serum osmolality >320 mOsm/L. A Foley urinary catheter should be placed to monitor urine output.

If increased ICP remains refractory to treatment, careful reassessment of the patient is needed to rule out unrecognized hypercarbia, hypoxemia, fever, hypotension, hypoglycemia, pain, and seizures. Repeat imaging should be considered to rule out a surgical lesion. Guidelines-based **second-tier** therapies for refractory raised ICP are available, but evidence favoring a given second-tier therapy is limited. In some centers, surgical decompressive **craniectomy** is used for refractory traumatic intracranial

hypertension. Others use a **pentobarbital infusion**, with a loading dose of 5-10 mg/kg over 30 min followed by 5 mg/kg every hour for 3 doses and then maintenance with an infusion of 1 mg/kg/hr. Careful blood pressure monitoring is required because of the possibility of drug-induced hypotension and the frequent need for support with fluids and pressors. Mild hypothermia (32-34°C [89.6-93.2°F]) in an attempt to control refractory ICP may be induced and maintained by means of surface

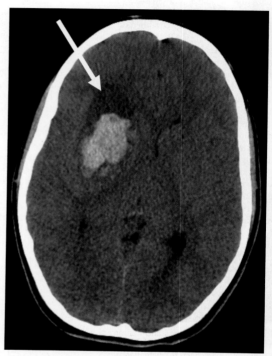

Fig. 85.10 Hemorrhage and edema. In a 16 yr old child who fell from his dirt bike, CT imaging demonstrates intraparenchymal hemorrhage and significant surrounding edema (*arrow*).

Fig. 85.8 Subdural hematoma. Hyperacute right frontal subdural hematoma observed on CT imaging in a 5 yr old child after motor vehicle crash. Note that the hyperacute aspect of the subdural hematoma is dark on CT imaging in the early stage after injury. Also, there is marked midline shift of intracranial contents, with both lateral ventricles displaced into the left side of the skull (*dotted line* for midline reference).

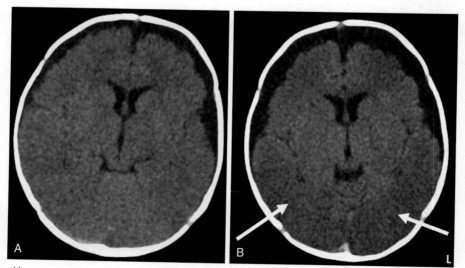

Fig. 85.9 Subdural hematoma. A, In a 3 mo old child who suffered from abusive head trauma, initial CT imaging demonstrates chronic subdural hematoma bilaterally. **B,** Three days after hospitalization, the subdural hematomas are slightly larger, but infarctions are noted in the posterior areas of brain parenchyma (*arrows*).

cooling. Hypothermia for increased ICP after traumatic brain injury remains controversial for pediatric and adult patients. **Hyperthermia** *must* be avoided and if present should be treated aggressively. Sedation and neuromuscular blockade are used to prevent shivering, and rewarming should be slow, no faster than 1°C (1.8°F) every 4-6 hr. Hypotension should be prevented during rewarming. Refractory raised ICP can also be treated with hyperventilation (PaCO$_2$ 25-30 mm Hg). Combinations of these second-tier therapies are often required.

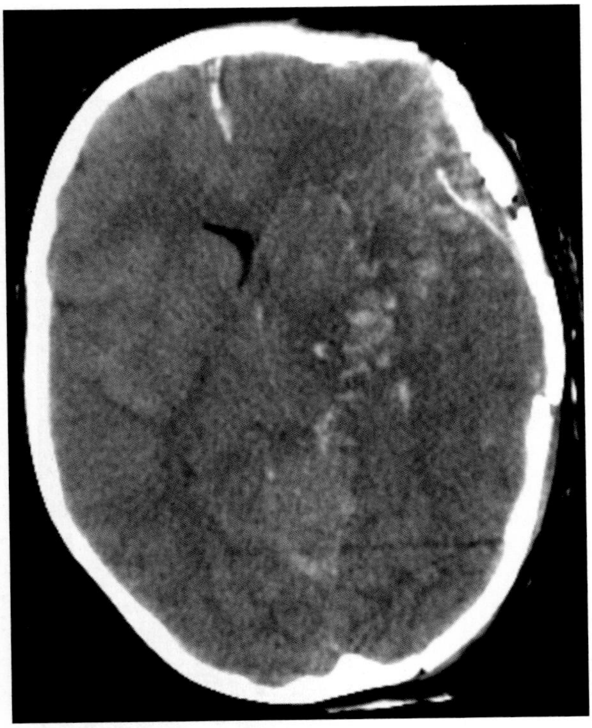

Supportive Care

Euvolemia should be maintained, and isotonic fluids are recommended throughout the ICU stay. SIADH and CSW can develop and are important to differentiate, because management of SIADH is fluid restriction and that of CSW is sodium replacement. Severe hyperglycemia (blood glucose level >200 mg/dL) should be avoided and treated. The blood glucose level should be monitored frequently. Early nutrition with enteral feedings is advocated. Corticosteroids should generally not be used unless adrenal insufficiency is documented. Tracheal suctioning can exacerbate raised ICP. Timing of the use of analgesics or sedatives around suctioning events and use of tracheal or IV lidocaine can be helpful. Seizures are common after severe acute TBI. Early posttraumatic seizures (within 1 wk) will complicate management of TBI and are often difficult to treat. Anticonvulsant prophylaxis with fosphenytoin, carbamazepine, or levetiracetam is a common treatment option. Late posttraumatic seizures (≥7 days after TBI) and, if recurrent, late posttraumatic epilepsy are *not* prevented by prophylactic anticonvulsants, whereas early posttraumatic seizures are prevented by initiating anticonvulsants soon after TBI. Antifibrinolytic agents (tranexamic acid) reduce hemorrhage size, as well as the development of new focal ischemic cerebral lesions, and improve survival in adults with severe TBI.

Prognosis

Mortality rates for children with severe TBI who reach the pediatric ICU range between 10% and 30%. Ability to control ICP is related to patient survival, and the extent of cranial and systemic injuries correlates with quality of life. Motor and cognitive sequelae resulting from severe TBI generally benefit from rehabilitation to minimize long-term disabilities. Recovery from TBI may take months to achieve. Physical therapy, and in some centers methylphenidate or amantadine, helps with motor and behavioral recovery. Pituitary insufficiency may be an uncommon but significant complication of severe TBI.

Bibliography is available at Expert Consult.

Fig. 85.11 Skull fractures and hemorrhage. An 11 yr old child was hit in the head by a horse, and CT imaging demonstrates multiple, comminuted skull fractures with fragments of bone within the brain parenchyma, multifocal areas of intraparenchymal hemorrhage, and obliteration of the left lateral ventricle.

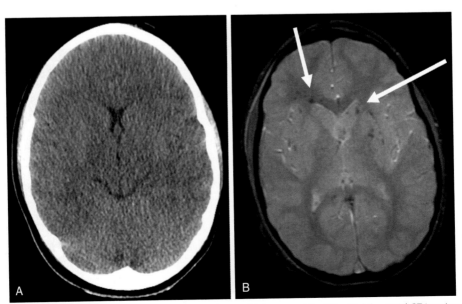

Fig. 85.12 Hemorrhages and axonal injury. A, In a 6 yr old child who was hit by a car while riding his bike, initial CT imaging demonstrated no obvious abnormality. **B,** However, immediate MRI demonstrates multiple areas of punctate hemorrhages (lucencies) consistent with diffuse axonal injury *(arrows)*.

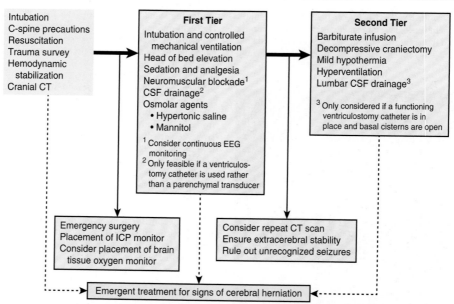

Fig. 85.13 Schematic outlining the approach to management of a child with severe traumatic brain injury (TBI). This schematic is specifically presented for severe TBI, for which the experience with intracranial pressure (ICP)–directed therapy is greatest. Nevertheless, the general approach provided here is relevant to the management of intracranial hypertension in other conditions for which evidence-based data on ICP monitoring and ICP-directed therapy are lacking. The ICP and CPP targets are discussed in the text. (*Based on 2012 guidelines for the management of severe TBI, along with minor modifications from later literature.*)

Chapter **86**

Brain Death

K. Jane Lee and Binod Balakrishnan

第八十六章
脑死亡

中文导读

本章主要介绍了脑死亡的临床表现和诊断。临床表现为原因明确的昏迷、脑干反射消失和无自主呼吸；在美国两次脑死亡判定的间隔时间：妊娠37周至足月30天新生儿间隔24小时，>30天的婴儿和儿童间隔12小时；在临床判定（包括自主呼吸激发试验）不能完全或可靠地完成时，可通过确认试验来协助判定脑死亡，包括脑电图和放射性核素脑血流检测；完整的文档记录也是脑死亡判定的一个重要方面；在脑死亡判定后，还需要一段时间的支持性治疗，帮助家人接受脑死亡的判定。

Brain death is the irreversible cessation of all functions of the entire brain, including the brainstem. It is also known as **death by neurologic criteria** and is legally accepted as death in the United States.

EPIDEMIOLOGY

In children, brain death usually develops after traumatic brain injury (TBI, including brain injury from nonaccidental trauma) or asphyxial injury. Pathogenesis is multifactorial, with the end result being irreversible loss of brain and brainstem function.

CLINICAL MANIFESTATIONS AND DIAGNOSIS

Current guidelines do not apply to preterm infants <37 wk gestational age (Fig. 86.1).

Brain death is determined by clinical assessment. Although ancillary tests such as electroencephalography (EEG) and cerebral blood flow (CBF) studies are sometimes used to assist in making the diagnosis, repeated clinical examination is the standard for diagnosis. The 3 components for determining brain death are demonstration of coexisting **irreversible coma with a known cause**, **absence of brainstem reflexes**, and **apnea**.

Before a determination of brain death may be made, it is of utmost importance that the cause of the coma be determined using the history, any radiology, and laboratory data, to rule out a reversible condition. *Potentially reversible causes of coma* include metabolic disorders, toxins, sedative drugs, paralytic agents, hypothermia, hypoxia, hypotension/shock, recent cardiopulmonary resuscitation (CPR), hypo-/hyperglycemia, hypo-/hypernatremia, hypercalcemia, hypermagnesemia, nonconvulsive status epilepticus, hypothyroidism, hypocortisolism, hypercarbia, liver or renal failure, sepsis, meningitis, encephalitis, subarachnoid hemorrhage, and surgically remediable brainstem lesions. Confounding factors must be corrected before initiation of brain death assessment.

Coma

The state of coma requires that the patient be unresponsive, even to noxious stimuli. Any purposeful motor response, such as localization, does not constitute coma. Likewise, any posturing (decerebrate or decorticate) is not consistent with coma, and therefore not consistent with brain death. The presence of spinal cord reflexes—even complex reflexes—does not preclude the diagnosis of brain death.

Brainstem Reflexes

Brainstem reflexes must be absent. Table 86.1 lists the brainstem reflexes to be tested, the brainstem location of each reflex, and the result of each test that is consistent with a diagnosis of brain death.

Apnea

Apnea is the absence of respiratory effort in response to an adequate stimulus. An arterial partial pressure of carbon dioxide ($PaCO_2$) value ≥60 mm Hg *and* >20 mm Hg above baseline is a sufficient stimulus. Apnea is clinically confirmed through the apnea test. Because the apnea test has the potential to destabilize the patient, it is performed only if the 1st 2 criteria for brain death (irreversible coma and absence of brainstem reflexes) are already confirmed.

The **apnea test** assesses the function of the medulla in driving ventilation. It is performed by first ensuring appropriate hemodynamics and temperature (>35°C) and the absence of apnea-producing drug effects or significant metabolic derangements. The patient is then preoxygenated with 100% oxygen for approximately 10 min, and ventilation is adjusted to achieve a $PaCO_2$ of approximately 40 mm Hg. A baseline arterial blood gas (ABG) result documents the starting values. During the test, oxygenation can be maintained with 100% oxygen via a T-piece attached to the endotracheal tube or via a resuscitation bag such as a Mapleson device. Throughout the test, the child's hemodynamics and pulse oximetry oxygen-hemoglobin saturation (SpO_2) are monitored while the physician observes for respiratory efforts. An ABG sample is obtained approximately 10 min into the test and every 5 min thereafter until the target $PaCO_2$ is surpassed; ventilatory support is resumed at that time. If at any point during the test the patient becomes hypoxic (SpO_2 <85%) or hypotensive, the test is aborted and ventilatory support resumed. Absence of respiratory efforts with a $PaCO_2$ ≥60 mm Hg and >20 mm Hg above baseline is consistent with brain death.

OBSERVATION PERIODS

To determine brain death in the United States, the findings must remain consistent for 2 examinations performed by different attending physicians (apnea testing may be performed by the same physician) separated by an observation period. The 1st exam determines that the child has met the criteria for brain death, whereas the 2nd exam confirms brain death based on an unchanged and irreversible condition. Recommended observation periods are 24 hr for neonates from 37 wk gestation to term infants 30 days old, and 12 hr for infants and children >30 days old. An observation period of 24-48 hr before initiation of brain death assessment is recommended after CPR or severe acute brain injury.

ANCILLARY STUDIES

Ancillary studies are not required for the diagnosis of brain death unless the clinical examination including the apnea test cannot be safely or reliably completed. Examples include cervical spinal cord injury, presence of high therapeutic or supratherapeutic levels of sedative medications, or hemodynamic instability or SpO_2 desaturation during an apnea test. Ancillary studies may also be used to shorten the recommended observation period. In this case, 2 complete clinical examinations, including apnea test, should be carried out and documented along with the ancillary study. Ancillary studies are no substitute for the neurologic examination.

The 2 most widely used ancillary tests are EEG and radionuclide CBF studies. A valid **electroencephalogram** to support suspected brain death must be performed according to the American EEG Society standards and technical requirements, under conditions of normothermia and appropriate hemodynamics, and in the absence of drug levels sufficient to suppress the EEG response. An EEG that demonstrates **electrocerebral silence** over a 30 min recording time under these conditions supports the diagnosis of brain death. Advantages of this study are its wide availability and low risk. Disadvantages include potential confounders, such as artifact in the tracing and the presence of suppressing levels of drugs such as barbiturates.

A **radionuclide cerebral blood flow study** consists of intravenous (IV) injection of a radiopharmaceutical agent followed by imaging of the brain to look for cerebral uptake. As with EEG, nuclear medicine scans are widely available and low risk. Unlike EEG, radionuclide CBF studies are not affected by drug levels. A study that shows absence of uptake in the brain demonstrates absence of CBF and is supportive of brain death. Four-vessel intracranial contrast angiography was previously used as the definitive ancillary test, but practical technical difficulties and risks have led to the use of nuclear medicine scans instead.

Interpretation of both EEG and radionuclide CBF studies should be done by appropriately trained and qualified individuals. If the studies show electrical activity or presence of CBF, brain death cannot be declared. A 24 hr waiting period is recommended before repeating the clinical examination or ancillary study.

DOCUMENTATION

Documentation is an important aspect of diagnosing brain death. Complete documentation should include statements of the following:
1. Etiology and irreversibility of the coma.
2. Absence of confounding factors: hypothermia, hypotension, hypoxia, significant metabolic derangement, and significant drug levels.
3. Absence of motor response to noxious stimulation.
4. Absence of brainstem reflexes: pupillary light reflex, oculocephalic/oculovestibular reflex, corneal reflex, cough reflex, and gag reflex.
5. Absence of respiratory effort in response to an adequate stimulus; ABG values should be documented at the start and end of the apnea test.

SUPPORTIVE CARE

Following a diagnosis of brain death, supportive care may continue for hours to days as the family makes decisions about potential organ donation and comes to terms with the diagnosis. A diagnosis of brain

Checklist for Documentation of Brain Death

Brain Death Examination for Infants and Children[a]		
Age of Patient	**Timing of First Examination**	**Interexamination Interval**
Term newborn 37 weeks gestational age and up to 30 days old	☐ First examination may be performed 24 hours after birth OR following cardiopulmonary resuscitation or other severe brain injury	☐ At least 24 hours ☐ Interval shortened because ancillary study (Section 4) is consistent with brain death
31 days to 18 years old	☐ First examination may be performed 24 hours following cardiopulmonary resuscitation or other severe brain injury	☐ At least 12 hours OR ☐ Interval shortened because ancillary study (Section 4) is consistent with brain death

Section 1. Prerequisites for Brain Death Examination and Apnea Test

A. Irreversible and Identifiable Cause of Coma (please check)

☐ Traumatic brain injury   ☐ Anoxic brain injury   ☐ Known metabolic disorder   ☐ Other (specify) _____

B. Correction of Contributing Factors That Can Interfere with the Neurologic Examination

	Examination 1		Examination 2	
a. Core body temperature is >95°F (35°C)	☐ Yes	☐ No	☐ Yes	☐ No
b. Systolic blood pressure or MAP in acceptable range (Systolic BP not less than 2 standard deviations below age-appropriate norm) based on age	☐ Yes	☐ No	☐ Yes	☐ No
c. Sedative/analgesic drug effect excluded as a contributing factor	☐ Yes	☐ No	☐ Yes	☐ No
d. Metabolic intoxication excluded as a contributing factor	☐ Yes	☐ No	☐ Yes	☐ No
e. Neuromuscular blockade excluded as a contributing factor	☐ Yes	☐ No	☐ Yes	☐ No

☐ If ALL prerequisites are marked YES, then proceed to section 2, OR

☐ _____ confounding variable was present. Ancillary study was therefore performed to document brain death (Section 4).

Section 2. Physical Examination (please check); Note: Spinal Cord Reflexes Are Acceptable

	Examination 1, Date/Time: _____		Examination 2, Date/Time: _____	
a. Flaccid tone, patient unresponsive to deep painful stimuli	☐ Yes	☐ No	☐ Yes	☐ No
b. Pupils are midposition or fully dilated and light reflexes are absent	☐ Yes	☐ No	☐ Yes	☐ No
c. Corneal, cough, gag reflexes are absent	☐ Yes	☐ No	☐ Yes	☐ No
d. Sucking and rooting reflexes are absent (in neonates and infants)	☐ Yes	☐ No	☐ Yes	☐ No
e. Oculovestibular reflexes are absent	☐ Yes	☐ No	☐ Yes	☐ No
f. Spontaneous respiratory effort while on mechanical ventilation is absent	☐ Yes	☐ No	☐ Yes	☐ No

☐ The _____ (specify) element of the examination could not be performed because _____.

Ancillary study (EEG or radionuclide CBF) was therefore performed to document brain death (Section 4).

Section 3. Apnea Test

	Examination 1, Date/Time: _____	Examination 2, Date/Time: _____
No spontaneous respiratory efforts were observed despite final $PaCO_2$ ≥60mmHg and a ≥20mmHg increase above baseline (Examination 1). No spontaneous respiratory efforts were observed despite final $PaCO_2$ Đ≥60mmHg and a ≥20mmHg increase above baseline (Examination 2).	Pretest $PaCO_2$: _____ Apnea duration: _____ min Post-test $PaCO_2$: _____	Pretest $PaCO_2$: _____ Apnea duration: _____ min Post-test $PaCO_2$: _____

Apnea test is contraindicated or could not be performed to completion because _____.

Ancillary study (EEG or radionuclide CBF) was therefore performed to document brain death (Section 4).

Section 4. Ancillary Testing

Ancillary testing is required (1) when any components of the examination or apnea testing cannot be completed; (2) if there is uncertainty about the results of the neurologic examination; or (3) if a medication effect may be present. Ancillary testing can be performed to reduce the interexamination period; however, a second neurologic examination is required. Components of the neurologic examination that can be performed safely should be completed in close proximity to the ancillary test.

Date/Time:_____

☐ EEG report documents electrocerebral silence OR   ☐ Yes   ☐ No

☐ CBF study report documents no cerebral perfusion   ☐ Yes   ☐ No

Section 5. Signatures

Examiner 1

I certify that my examination is consistent with cessation of function of the brain and brainstem. Confirmatory examination to follow.

Printed name _____

Signature _____

Specialty _____

Pager #/license # _____

Date mm/dd/yyyy _____

Time _____

Examiner 2

I certify that my examination ☐ and/or ancillary test report ☐ confirms unchanged and irreversible cessation of function of the brain and brainstem. The patient is declared brain dead at this time.

Date/time of death _____

Printed name _____

Signature _____

Specialty _____

Pager #/license # _____

Date mm/dd/yyyy _____

Time _____

[a]Two physicians must perform independent examinations separated by specified intervals.

BP = blood pressure; CBF = cerebral blood flow; EEG = electroencephalography; MAP = mean arterial pressure.

Fig. 86.1 Checklist for documentation of brain death. (*From Nakagawa TA, Ashwal S, Mathur M, et al. Guidelines for the determination of brain death in infants and children: an update of the 1987 Task Force recommendations—executive summary, Ann Neurol 71:573–585, 2012, Table 2.*).

Table 86.1	Brainstem Reflex Testing to Determine Brain Death		
BRAINSTEM REFLEX	**AREA TESTED**	**HOW TO PERFORM EXAM**	**EXPLANATION OF RESULTS**
Pupillary light reflex	Cranial nerves (CNs) II and III, midbrain	Shine a light into the eyes while closely observing pupillary size.	Midposition (4-6 mm) or fully dilated pupils that are not reactive to light are consistent with brain death. Pinpoint pupils, even if nonreactive, suggest intact function of the Edinger-Westphal nucleus in the midbrain and are therefore *not* consistent with brain death.
Oculocephalic reflex (doll's eyes reflex)	CNs III, VI, and VIII; midbrain; pons	Manually rotate the patient's head side to side and closely watch the position of the eyes. Should not be performed in a patient with a cervical spine injury.	In the intact patient, the eyes remain fixed on a distant spot, as if maintaining eye contact with that spot. In an exam consistent with brain death, the eyes move in concert with the patient's head movement.
Corneal reflex	CNs III, V, and VII; pons	Touch the patient's cornea with a cotton swab.	In the intact patient, the touch results in eyelid closure, and the eye may rotate upward. In an exam consistent with brain death, there is no response.
Oculovestibular reflex	CNs III, IV, VI, and VIII; pons; midbrain	Irrigate the tympanic membrane with iced water or saline and look for eye movement.	Absence of eye movement is consistent with brain death.
Gag and cough reflex	CNs IX and X, medulla	Touch the posterior pharynx with a tongue depressor or a cotton-tipped swab to stimulate a gag. Advance a suction catheter through the endotracheal tube to the carina to stimulate a cough.	Absence of both a cough and a gag is consistent with brain death.

death may not be accepted by the family for personal, religious, or cultural reasons. It is important for care providers to be patient and supportive of the family dealing with this difficult situation.

OBJECTIONS TO THE IDEA OF BRAIN DEATH

Although the concept of brain death is widely accepted and very useful in facilitating organ transplantation, it is not accepted by all. Several countries do not recognize brain death, and some individuals, both medical personnel and laypeople, object to the idea of brain death.

It has been pointed out that some patients who meet brain death criteria continue to show evidence of *integrative functioning*, such as control over free-water homeostasis (absence of diabetes insipidus), control of temperature regulation, capacity for growth and wound healing, and variability of heart rate and blood pressure in response to stimulus. Along with scientific arguments, there are also philosophical arguments about what constitutes death and whether a person who lacks function of the brain, but not of the body, is truly dead.

Bibliography is available at Expert Consult.

Chapter **87**

Syncope

Aarti S. Dalal and George F. Van Hare

第八十七章

晕厥

中文导读

本章主要介绍了晕厥的机制、评估和治疗。引　起晕厥的机制包括心脏的原因，如心律失常、严重的主动脉狭窄、冠状动脉异常、原发性肺动脉高压、艾森伯格综合征等；非心脏的原因，如癫痫、发作性睡病、低血糖和过度换气等。晕厥的评估包括病史、

体格检查和实验室检查，如心电图等；不同原因的晕厥，治疗措施不同；此外，本章还详细阐述了体位性心动过速综合征的临床表现、诊断和治疗。

Syncope is defined as a sudden transient loss of consciousness with inability to maintain postural tone. The most common cause of syncope in the normal pediatric population is **neurocardiogenic syncope** (vasovagal syncope, fainting). **Vasovagal syncope** is classically associated with a prodrome that includes diaphoresis, warmth, pallor, or feeling lightheaded and is often triggered by a specific event or situation such as pain, medical procedures, or emotional distress (Table 87.1). This type of syncope is characterized by hypotension and bradycardia. Approximately 30–50% of children will have had a **fainting** episode before 18 yr of age.

Most patients with a vasovagal syncope episode will have prodromal features followed by loss of motor tone. Once in a horizontal position, consciousness returns rapidly, in 1-2 min; some patients may have 30 sec of tonic-clonic motor activities, which should not be confused with a **seizure** (Table 87.2). Syncope must also be distinguished from **vertigo** and **ataxia** (Table 87.3).

Although this type of syncope is very common in adolescence and has an excellent prognosis, other causes for loss of consciousness are more dangerous; thus syncope may be the first sign of more serious conditions (Table 87.4). Indeed, the occurrence of syncope may well be the pediatrician's best opportunity to diagnose a life-threatening condition before the patient subsequently succumbs. The task of the clinician, therefore, is not only to counsel the family and the patient concerning the common form, but also to rule out a number of important life-threatening cardiac problems.

MECHANISMS
Syncope by whatever mechanism is caused by a lack of adequate cerebral blood flow with loss of consciousness and inability to remain upright.

Primary **cardiac causes** of syncope (Table 87.4) include arrhythmias such as long QT syndrome (LQTS), Wolff-Parkinson-White syndrome (particularly with atrial fibrillation), ventricular tachycardia (VT), and occasionally supraventricular tachycardia (see Chapter 462). VT may be associated with hypertrophic cardiomyopathy (HCM), arrhythmogenic cardiomyopathy, repaired congenital heart disease, or a genetic cause such as catecholaminergic polymorphic ventricular tachycardia (CPVT). Other arrhythmias that may lead to syncope are bradyarrhythmias such as sinus node dysfunction and high-grade second- or third-degree atrioventricular (AV) block. Patients with congenital complete AV block may present with syncope. Syncope may also be caused by cardiac obstructive lesions, such as critical aortic stenosis, or coronary artery anomalies, such as an aberrant left coronary artery arising from the right sinus of Valsalva. Patients with primary pulmonary hypertension or Eisenmenger syndrome may experience syncope. In all the obstructive forms of syncope, exercise increases the likelihood of an episode because the obstruction interferes with the ability of the heart to increased cardiac output in response to exercise.

Noncardiac causes of loss of consciousness include epilepsy, as well as basilar artery migraine, hysterical syncope, and pseudoseizures (see Table 87.1). Occasionally, patients with narcolepsy may present with syncope. Hypoglycemia and hyperventilation may also present as syncope.

EVALUATION
The most important goal in the evaluation of the new patient with syncope is to diagnose life-threatening causes of syncope so that these causes can be managed. Many patients presenting with sudden cardiac arrest caused by conditions such as LQTS will have previously experienced an episode of syncope, so the presentation with syncope is an opportunity to prevent sudden death.

The most important tool in evaluation is a careful **history**. The characteristics of cardiac syncope differ significantly from the prodrome seen in neurocardiogenic syncope (Table 87.5). Several red flags can be identified that should lead the clinician to suspect that the mechanism is a life-threatening cardiac cause rather than simple fainting (Table 87.6). The occurrence during exercise suggests an arrhythmia or coronary obstruction. Injury because of an episode of syncope indicates sudden occurrence with a lack of adequate prodromal symptoms and suggests an arrhythmia. The occurrence of syncope while recumbent would be quite unusual in a patient with neurocardiogenic syncope and therefore suggests a cardiac or neurologic cause. Occasionally, a patient with syncope caused by a tachyarrhythmia will report the sensation of a racing heart before the event, but this is unusual.

A careful family history is essential in evaluation of syncope. Specifically, if there are first-degree relatives with inherited syndromes, such as a LQTS or HCM, this should lead to more specific evaluation of the patient. Also, if relatives died suddenly at a young age without a clear and convincing cause, inherited cardiac arrhythmias or cardiomyopathies should also be suspected.

Patients with a history of heart disease, especially cardiac repair, may have causes that are specific to their repair. Sinus node dysfunction is common after the Senning or Mustard procedure for transposition of the great vessels. VT may be seen after repair of tetralogy of Fallot. A patient with a history of septal defect repair should be evaluated for the late occurrence of AV block, and patients with an implanted pacemaker should be evaluated for pacemaker lead failure.

The physical examination may also offer clues (Table 87.6). Patients with HCM may have a prominent cardiac impulse and/or an ejection murmur, as will patients with aortic stenosis. The patient with primary pulmonary hypertension will have a loud and single second heart sound and may also have an ejection click and the murmur of pulmonary insufficiency. Scars from prior cardiac surgery and pacemaker implantation would be evident.

All patients presenting with a first episode of syncope *must* have an electrocardiogram obtained, looking primarily for QT interval prolongation, preexcitation, ventricular hypertrophy, T-wave abnormalities, and conduction abnormalities. Other tests that may be needed depending on the results of the initial evaluation may include echocardiography, exercise testing, cardiac MRI, or 24 hr Holter monitoring. In patients for whom there is a strong suspicion of a paroxysmal arrhythmia, an implantable loop recorder may be the most effective means of diagnosis. Additional tests to look for anemia, hypoglycemia, drugs of abuse, and other etiologies noted in Table 87.1 will be determined by the history and physical examination.

TREATMENT
Therapy for vasovagal syncope includes avoiding triggering events (if possible), fluid and salt supplementation, and if needed, midodrine (see Chapter 87.1, Table 87.7). Immediately after the event, the patient should remain supine until symptoms abate to avoid recurrence.

Treatment for cardiac causes of syncope will be determined by the diagnosis. If a reentrant tachycardia (AVNRT, AVRT) is found, then a catheter ablation is indicated. If bradycardia from AV block was the cause of the syncope, a pacemaker may be warranted. Patients with syncope from medically refractory malignant arrhythmias, as may be seen in HCM, LQTS, arrhythmogenic cardiomyopathy, or CPVT, require

Table 87.1	Noncardiac Causes of Syncope

Reflex vasodepressor syncope
  Neurocardiogenic (vasovagal)
  Emotion (seeing blood)
  Pain (needle phobia)
Miscellaneous situational reflex
  Tussive
  Sneeze
  Exercise, after exercise
  Swallowing
  Stretching
  Defecation
  Micturition
  Hair grooming
  Valsalva (increased intrathoracic pressure)
  Trumpet playing
  Weightlifting
  Breath-holding spells
Systemic illness
  Hypoglycemia
  Anemia
  Infection
  Hypovolemia, dehydration
  Adrenal insufficiency
  Narcolepsy, cataplexy
  Pulmonary embolism
  Pheochromocytoma
  Mastocytosis
  Ruptured ectopic pregnancy

Central nervous system
  Seizure (atonic, absence, myoclonic-astatic)
  Stroke, transient ischemic attack
  Subarachnoid hemorrhage
Dysautonomia
Myotonic dystrophy
Kearns-Sayre syndrome
Friedreich ataxia
Basilar artery migraine
Drug effects
  β-Blocking agents
  Vasodilating agents
  Opiates
  Sedatives
  Drugs prolonging QT interval
  Diuretics
  Anticonvulsant agents
  Antihistamines
  Antidepressant agents
  Anxiolytic agents
  Drugs of abuse
  Insulin, oral hypoglycemic agents
  Carbon monoxide
Other etiologies
  Carotid sinus sensitivity
  Subclavian steal
  Panic attack, anxiety
  Conversion disorder

Table 87.2	Comparison of Clinical Features of Syncope and Seizures

FEATURES	SYNCOPE	SEIZURES	FEATURES	SYNCOPE	SEIZURES
Relation to posture	Common	No	Injury	Rare	Common (with convulsive seizures)
Time of day	Diurnal	Diurnal or nocturnal	Urinary incontinence	Rare	Common
Precipitating factors	Emotion, injury, pain, crowds, heat, exercise, fear, dehydration, coughing, micturition	Sleep loss, drug/alcohol withdrawal	Tongue biting	No	Can occur with convulsive seizures
Skin color	Pallor	Cyanosis or normal	Postictal confusion	Rare	Common
Diaphoresis	Common	Rare	Postictal headache	No	Common
Aura or premonitory symptoms	Long	Brief	Focal neurologic signs	No	Occasional
Convulsion	Rare, brief	Common	Cardiovascular signs	Common (cardiac syncope)	No
Other abnormal movements	Minor twitching	Rhythmic jerks	Abnormal findings on EEG	Rare (generalized slowing may occur during the event)	Common

From Bruni J: Episodic impairment of consciousness. In Daroff RB, Jankovic JM, Mazziotta JC, Pomeroy SL, editors: *Bradley's neurology in clinical practice*, ed 7, Philadelphia, 2016, Elsevier.

Table 87.3	Syncope and Dizziness

	VERTIGO	PRESYNCOPE	DISEQUILIBRIUM	LIGHTHEADEDNESS
Patient complaint	"My head is spinning." "The room is whirling."	"I feel I might pass out." "I feel faint." "I feel like blacking out."	"I feel unsteady." "My balance is off."	"I feel dizzy." "I feel disconnected, drugged."
Associated features	Motion, swaying, spinning, nystagmus	Syncope: loss of postural tone, brief loss of consciousness Situational	Poor balance No vertigo or ataxia	Anxiety, hyperventilation, paresthesias, respiratory alkalosis, panic attacks
Usual cause	Vestibular disorders	Impaired cerebral perfusion	Sensory and/or central neurologic dysfunction	Anxiety and/or depressive disorders
Key differential diagnoses	Peripheral (labyrinthine-cochlear) vs central neurologic disorder	Neurocardiogenic (vagal) vs cardiac syncope vs neuropsychiatric syncope	Sensory deficit vs central neurologic disease	Anxiety/depression vs hyperventilation vs medication effects

From Cohen G: Syncope and dizziness. In *Nelson pediatric symptom-based diagnosis*, Philadelphia, 2018, Elsevier (Table 6.1, p 84).

Table 87.4	Life-Threatening Cardiac Causes as Risk With Syncope

Long QT syndromes (congenital and drug induced)
Short QT syndromes
Cardiomyopathies
  Hypertrophic cardiomyopathy
  Dilated cardiomyopathy
  Arrhythmogenic right ventricular dysplasia
Brugada syndrome
Catecholaminergic polymorphic ventricular tachycardia
Myocarditis
Lyme myocarditis
Chagas disease
Wolff-Parkinson-White syndrome
Coronary artery anomalies
Late postoperative arrhythmias
Adult congenital heart patients
Congenital or acquired complete atrioventricular block
Aortic, mitral, or pulmonic valve stenosis
Primary pulmonary hypertension
Eisenmenger syndrome
Dissecting aortic aneurysm (Marfan syndrome)
Cardiac tumor
Pacemaker malfunction
Takotsubo cardiomyopathy

an implantable cardioverter-defibrillator. Patients with structural heart disease (valvular disease or coronary artery anomalies) should be referred for surgery.

Bibliography is available at Expert Consult.

87.1 Postural Tachycardia Syndrome
Gisela G. Chelimsky and Thomas C. Chelimsky

Several complex and interrelated mechanisms allow humans to stand despite the pull of gravity on the cerebral circulation. In the supine posture, most blood sits in the thoracic cavity, with 25–30% of total volume in the splanchnic vasculature. When an adult stands up, about 500 mL of blood shifts to the lower extremities and to the splanchnic vasculature. The decrease in hydrostatic pressure in the carotid sinuses produces vasoconstriction in the peripheral vessels mediated by sympathetic outflow, as well as in the splanchnic vasculature. This action is mediated by norepinephrine, adenosine triphosphate (ATP), and neuropeptide Y. The muscles in the legs and gluteal area work as a pump when the individual is upright and during exercise, to help return the blood to the heart.

Understanding postural tachycardia syndrome (**POTS**), or postural orthostatic tachycardia syndrome, requires an understanding of other orthostatic conditions. Many adolescents have lightheadedness or tunnel vision in the first few seconds of assuming the upright posture. This phenomenon, termed **initial orthostatic hypotension (IOH)**, can lead to *syncope*, but usually is very short, perhaps 30-60 sec, and occurs primarily with active standing, not passive upright tilt. Blood pressure (BP) may drop 30% of baseline at 10-20 sec of standing and may be associated with tachycardia. BP returns to baseline in 30-60 sec, whereas heart rate (HR) typically returns to a new, higher value above the baseline when supine. Because of its transient rapidity, IOH escapes detection with standard BP machines and requires beat-to-beat monitoring of BP and HR. The clinical diagnosis requires a careful history. The symptoms usually happen after prolonged recumbence and when the individual stands. The person complains of lightheadedness and "blacking out" or tunnel vision 5-10 sec after standing.

In contrast to IOH, **orthostatic hypotension (OH)** is defined as a *sustained* decrease in the systolic BP of >20 mm Hg or diastolic BP >10 mm Hg in the 1st 3 min of upright tilt. This 2nd type of orthostatic

Table 87.5	Differentiating Features for Causes of Syncope

NEUROCARDIOGENIC
Symptoms after prolonged motionless standing, sudden unexpected pain, fear, or unpleasant sight, sound, or smell; pallor
Syncope in a well-trained athlete *after* exertion (without heart disease)
Situational syncope during or immediately after micturition, cough, swallowing, or defecation
Syncope with throat or facial pain (glossopharyngeal or trigeminal neuralgia)

ORGANIC HEART DISEASE (PRIMARY ARRHYTHMIA, OBSTRUCTIVE HYPERTROPHIC CARDIOMYOPATHY, PULMONARY HYPERTENSION)
Brief sudden loss of consciousness, no prodrome, history of heart disease
Syncope while sitting or supine
Syncope with exertion
History of palpitations
Family history of sudden death

NEUROLOGIC
Seizures: preceding aura, post event symptoms lasting > 5 min (includes postictal state of decreased level of consciousness, confusion, headache or paralysis)
Migraine: syncope associated with antecedent headaches with or without aura

OTHER VASCULAR
Carotid sinus: syncope with head rotation or pressure on the carotid sinus (as in tumors, shaving, tight collars)
Orthostatic hypotension: syncope immediately on standing especially after prolonged bed rest

DRUG INDUCED
Patient is taking a medication that may lead to long QT syndrome, orthostasis, or bradycardia

PSYCHIATRIC ILLNESS
Frequent syncope, somatic complaints, no heart disease

From Cohen G: Syncope and dizziness. In Kliegman RM, Lye PS, Bordini BJ, et al, editors: Nelson pediatric symptom-based diagnosis. Philadelphia, 2018, Elsevier, Table 6.4.

Table 87.6	Red Flags in Evaluation of Patients With Syncope

Syncope with activity or exercise or supine
Syncope not associated with prolonged standing
Syncope precipitated by loud noise or extreme emotion
Absence of presyncope or lightheadedness
Family history of syncope, drowning, sudden death, familial ventricular arrhythmia syndromes,* cardiomyopathy
Syncope requiring CPR
Injury with syncope
Anemia
Other cardiac symptoms
Chest pain
Dyspnea
Palpitations
History of cardiac surgery
History of Kawasaki disease
Implanted pacemaker
Abnormal physical examination
  Murmur
  Gallop rhythm
  Loud and single second heart sound
  Systolic click
  Increased apical impulse (tachycardia)
  Irregular rhythm
  Hypo- or hypertension
  Clubbing
  Cyanosis

*Long QT syndrome, Brugada syndrome, catecholamine polymorphic ventricular tachycardia, arrhythmogenic right ventricular dysplasia.

Table 87.7	First-Line Medications in Treatment of Postural Tachycardia Syndrome (POTS)		
DRUG	**MECHANISM OF ACTION**	**SIDE EFFECTS**	**TREATMENT GUIDELINES**
Fludrocortisone	Low dose: sensitizes α receptors Higher doses: mineralocorticoid effect	Peripheral edema, headache, irritability, hypokalemia, hypomagnesemia, acne	Monitor basic metabolic panel and magnesium.
Midodrine	α_1-Agonist; produces vasoconstriction	Scalp tingling, urinary retention, goose bumps, headache, supine hypertension	Monitor supine blood pressure 30-60 min after dose.
Metoprolol succinate/tartrate	β-Blocker	Worsening of asthma, dizziness, fatigue	Use with caution in asthma. If fatigue is severe, use at bedtime.
Propranolol	Nonselective β-blocker	Bradycardia, gastrointestinal symptoms, lightheadedness, sleepiness, hypotension, syncope	Use with caution in diabetes and asthma.
Pyridostigmine	Peripheral acetylcholinesterase inhibitor that increases synaptic acetylcholine in autonomic ganglia and at peripheral muscarinic receptors	Symptoms of excessive cholinergic activity (diarrhea, urinary incontinence, salivation)	Very useful if patient has POTS and constipation. Use with caution in asthma. Contraindicated in urinary or bowel obstruction.

disorder rarely occurs in children. The patient frequently has no orthostatic symptoms while upright despite very low pressures (Fig. 87.1). This distinguishes OH from POTS, which *requires* symptoms while upright. A 3rd orthostatic disorder, **reflex syncope** (i.e., vasovagal or neurally mediated), is defined as relatively sudden change in autonomic nervous system activity that leads to a sudden decrease in BP, HR, and cerebral perfusion (Fig. 87.2).

In children, POTS is defined as a syndrome characterized by HR increase of >40 beats/min during the 1st 10 min of upright tilt test without associated hypotension, (>30 beats/min if >19 yr old) while replicating orthostatic symptoms that occur when upright (Fig. 87.3). Improvement of symptoms in the supine position is expected. The diagnosis of POTS also requires *daily* orthostatic symptoms. In patients with POTS, the larger decline in cardiac stroke volume appears to be the primary trigger for the tachycardia, which may result from various pathophysiologic mechanisms, such as the following:

- **Neuropathic** POTS, an autonomic neuropathy impairing sympathetic venoconstriction in the lower extremities or splanchnic circulation, decreasing stroke volume, and consequently resulting in a tachycardia
- **Hypovolemic** POTS, a common contributor, often related to decreased aldosterone with reduced renin activity, resulting in a tachycardia caused by decrease blood volume
- **Hyperadrenergic** POTS, with norepinephrine levels rising 3-4–fold in the standing position (norepinephrine normally doubles on standing), which may occur in norepinephrine transporter deficiency or strong stimulation of central baroreflex responses
- **Autoimmune** POTS, typically assumed based on a postviral chronology, but seldom proven; such a form may or may not exist. The antiganglionic antibody is almost never elevated in these patients. Nonetheless, a group of patients report that intravenous immune globulin (IVIG) is helpful to them. Whether they benefit from the increase in intravascular volume or an actual immune effect is unknown.

Some patients have orthostatic symptoms while upright but do not meet criteria for syncope, OH, or POTS. This group has **orthostatic intolerance otherwise not specified (OI-NOS).**

CLINICAL PRESENTATION
The symptoms that intrinsically relate to POTS are those that are replicated during upright tilt testing or standing. Many other symptoms also occur in patients with POTS, fitting the description of comorbid conditions, but not reproduced while upright. A patient may have nausea while upright associated with lightheadedness and has a diagnosis of POTS. Another patient may complain of nausea on awakening and have POTS, but has no nausea while upright. In the former patient the nausea is a symptom of POTS itself, whereas in the latter nausea is an

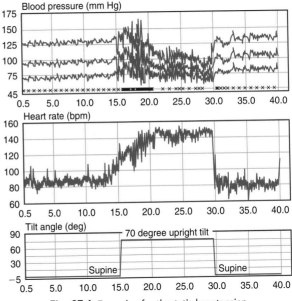

Fig. 87.1 Example of orthostatic hypotension.

associated condition. The symptoms that often directly relate to POTS include lightheadedness, orthostatic nausea, sometimes orthostatic headaches, fatigue, tunnel vision, and brain fog. About 20–30% of pediatric patients with POTS will also have syncope (Fig. 87.4). Other comorbid conditions frequently occur in these patients but are not caused by POTS (i.e., not an orthostatic phenomenon). These comorbidities include (1) sleep issues, usually delayed onset of sleep, frequent awakening, and not feeling refreshed in the morning; (2) aches in different parts of the body; (3) abdominal pain; (4) headaches and migraines; (5) nausea and vomiting; and (6) Raynaud like symptoms and other, less frequent problems (e.g., urinary symptoms).

The association of upper gastrointestinal (GI) symptoms and POTS are well described. Nausea, early satiety, and bloating are described in association with POTS. Such GI symptoms relate mechanistically to POTS only when they occur in the upright position. Many patients with POTS have comorbid GI symptom that are not a consequence of the orthostatic challenge. Therefore, only the GI symptoms replicated during tilt testing will improve with treatment aimed at orthostasis.

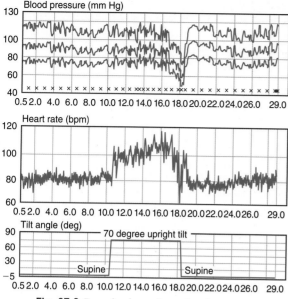

Fig. 87.2 Example of neurally mediated syncope.

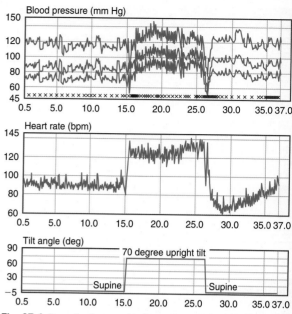

Fig. 87.4 Example of postural tachycardia syndrome (POTS) followed by a neurally mediated syncope.

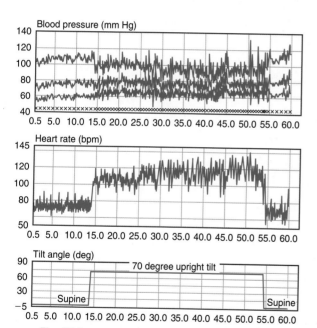

Fig. 87.3 Example of postural tachycardia syndrome.

Patients with POTS have changes in the electrical activity of the stomach while upright, which may explain the upright GI symptoms; they usually do not have delayed gastric emptying. The emptying is either normal or accelerated, implying that the cause of nausea is not gastroparesis.

Patients with **hypermobility Ehlers-Danlos syndrome** (h-EDS) may have POTS. Typically, such individuals have more migraine and syncope. Joint hypermobility itself in *adults* is associated with more autonomic complaints such as syncope, presyncope, palpitations, chest discomfort, fatigue, and heat intolerance. Those with hypermobility have more frequent positive tilt tests than healthy controls. Interestingly, in children, joint hypermobility does not influence the number of comorbidities or

autonomic disorders. Similarly, those with pediatric chronic overlapping pain conditions with or without POTS have the same comorbidities, suggesting that neither POTS nor hypermobility are drivers of the comorbidities or the chronic overlapping pain condition, but rather another associated disorder (Chapter 147).

DIAGNOSIS

Orthostatic intolerance is clinically diagnosed by detailed history attending specifically to symptoms as they relate to body position. Dizziness that begins in the supine position cannot be a manifestation of orthostatic intolerance. Furthermore, those symptoms that do develop while upright should improve or resolve when supine. Importantly, the history should include a detailed description of current physical exercise habits, with frequency, type, and endurance. One should also assess sleep, diet (mainly evaluating intake of salt), fluid intake, and other comorbidities. The physical examination is also important and should include a cardiac and neurologic evaluation with supine and standing BP and HR. Examination of the extremities may provide information about venous pooling, such as mild edema or reddish purple discoloration when sitting or standing. Cold, clammy hands can signify excess sympathetic activity.

To diagnose POTS the patient needs to undergo a *head-up tilt test for at least 10 min*. It is important to have the patient supine for at least 20 min before the tilt test. POTS can also be assessed by a standing test, measuring BP and HR at 1, 3, 5, and 10 min standing, but to have a reliable test similar to the tilt test, the patient needs to be supine for 1 hr before standing. The HR increase with active standing is typically less than with tilt, because the lower-extremity muscle pump is less active in tilt. The diagnosis of POTS requires replication of the day-to-day symptoms while upright, not just the increased HR while upright. A small but significant proportion of healthy teenagers in school will have an increased HR that may be diagnosed as POTS but will not have associated symptoms.

Other tests may include electrocardiogram, echocardiogram, and Holter monitor when there is concern of a primary cardiac cause of tachycardia, or if there is a need to determine if symptoms correlate with tachycardia (see Chapter 87). Supine and standing plasma catecholamines help confirm the diagnosis of POTS, as one expects to see either the normal doubling of norepinephrine levels from supine to standing, or a tripling with hyperadrenergic POTS. Beyond tilt table testing, autonomic testing will also include cardiac response to deep breathing (checking cardiac parasympathetic function), Valsalva maneuver (checking cardiac sympathetic and parasympathetic functions and vasomotor sympathetic function), and quantitative axon reflex sudomotor test (to assess for an autonomic neuropathy and vasomotor sympathetic dysfunction).

Additional studies depend on the clinical symptoms and include morning cortisol (to rule out Addison disease) and hypo- or hyperthyroid studies if the patient has unusually severe fatigue or is not responsive to usual treatment. Serum tryptase and urine methylhistamine are tested if mast cell activation disorder is suspected, based on a history of flushing during the spells. If an autoimmune cause for the POTS is a concern, antibodies such as voltage-gated potassium channel and acetylcholine receptor antibodies could be checked, but this etiology for POTS is being questioned. Patients rarely (<5 in 1000) benefit from IVIG; if this mechanism is really causing POTS, such patients will experience peak benefit at about 10 days after the infusion, rather than immediately, which may simply reflect increasing intravascular volume. If the patient has hypertension, plasma and urine metanephrines should be measured to test for a pheochromocytoma. In addition, if symptoms are associated with perimenstrual timing, an assessment of sex hormone axis is helpful, with occult polycystic ovarian syndrome or low testosterone levels sometimes present.

MANAGEMENT

The core of POTS management is **nonpharmacologic**. Medications will be of little benefit without these measures being undertaken first. The best measure for treating POTS is a regular **aerobic exercise** program. Given the combination of orthostatic symptoms and severe deconditioning found in most patients, the exercise program must be introduced in a slow, progressive manner. Patients with POTS typically have moderate to severe exercise intolerance, and compared with sedentary healthy controls, have decreased peak oxygen uptake. After 3 mo of exercise, POTS patients have an increase in cardiac mass and size, blood volume, and peak oxygen uptake, as reflected in a better exercise performance.

The tachycardia in POTS is caused by a decrease in stroke volume and not an intrinsic circulatory problem. An exercise program should start with water exercises combined with recumbent aerobic activities (recumbent bike or rowing machine). Slowly increase the exercise time to 45 min at least 5 times per week. When tolerance increases, patients can advance to more upright aerobic activities. These aerobic activities need to be combined with light core- and limb-strengthening exercises.

Exercise usually cannot be performed without simultaneous expansion of the intravascular volume. To this end, encourage teenagers to drink >80 oz of fluids daily and to add 2 g of salt to usual diet in both the morning and the early afternoon. **Salt supplementation** increases plasma and blood volume, improves orthostatic tolerance, and decreases baroreflex sensitivity. Salt also reduces nitric oxide production, resulting in less vasodilation. Trial and error of different salt formulation can help to identify the best method for each individual patient. Salt tablets are simple and inexpensive but may make some people nauseous. An alternative is simply to obtain empty capsules on the internet and fill them with table salt. A "0" size capsule contains about 400 mg of salt.

The content of sodium in the body determines the extracellular fluid volume that in turn dictates orthostatic tolerance. Patients with POTS who have lower urinary sodium excretion have more symptoms than those with higher urinary sodium (> 123 mmol/24 hr), and they often respond less well to salt supplementation. Those with severe orthostatic symptoms either in the morning or before sports should drink 16 oz of plain water, which is known to increase sympathetic response mainly in individuals with baroreflex dysregulation. The effect starts soon after drinking the water and lasts for about 1 hr. Compression garments may also be useful. These can be thigh or waist high; the waist-high compression garments may not be tolerated.

Medications can be added when the nonpharmacologic interventions are not insufficient (). Different centers use different strategies, and there is no single correct evidence-based approach. Table 87.3 addresses first-line medications that primary care physicians could use; only the most common side effects are included.

Bibliography is available at Expert Consult.

Chapter **88**
Shock
David A. Turner and Ira M. Cheifetz

第八十八章
休克

中文导读

　　本章主要介绍了休克的流行病学、休克类型、病理生理学、临床表现、诊断、实验室检查、治疗和预后。休克的类型包括低血容量性休克、心源性休克、梗阻性休克、分布性休克和脓毒性休克；其临床表现

最初可能仅表现为心动过速，可伴或不伴有呼吸急促，随着病情进展会出现尿量减少、外周血流灌注不良、呼吸窘迫或衰竭、精神状态改变和低血压；休克的诊断需要通过深入了解病史和体格检查才能做出；

在休克治疗中，主要介绍了初始治疗、其他的早期注　意事项及继续治疗的考虑因素。

Shock is an acute process characterized by the body's inability to deliver adequate oxygen to meet the metabolic demands of vital organs and tissues. Insufficient oxygen at the tissue level is unable to support normal aerobic cellular metabolism, resulting in a shift to less efficient anaerobic metabolism. As shock progresses, increases in tissue oxygen extraction are unable to compensate for this deficiency in oxygen delivery, leading to progressive clinical deterioration and lactic acidosis. If inadequate tissue perfusion persists, adverse vascular, inflammatory, metabolic, cellular, endocrine, and systemic responses worsen physiologic instability.

Compensation for inadequate oxygen delivery involves a complex set of responses that attempt to preserve oxygenation of the vital organs (i.e., brain, heart, kidneys, liver) at the expense of other organs (i.e., skin, gastrointestinal tract, muscles). Of importance, the brain is especially sensitive to periods of poor oxygen supply given its lack of capacity for anaerobic metabolism. Initially, shock is often well compensated, but it may rapidly progress to an *uncompensated* state requiring more aggressive therapies to achieve clinical recovery. The combination of a continued presence of an inciting trigger and the body's exaggerated and potentially harmful neurohumoral, inflammatory, and cellular responses lead to the progression of shock. Irrespective of the underlying cause of shock, the specific pattern of response, pathophysiology, clinical manifestations, and treatment may vary significantly depending on the specific etiology (which may be unknown), the clinical circumstances, and an individual patient's biologic response to the shock state. Untreated shock causes irreversible tissue and organ injury (i.e., *irreversible shock*) and, ultimately, death.

EPIDEMIOLOGY

Shock occurs in approximately 2% of all hospitalized infants, children, and adults in developed countries, and the mortality rate varies substantially depending on the etiology and clinical circumstances. Of patients who do not survive, most do not die in the acute hypotensive phase of shock, but rather as a result of associated complications and **multiple-organ dysfunction syndrome (MODS)**. MODS is defined as any alteration of organ function that requires medical support for maintenance, and the presence of MODS in patients with shock substantially increases the probability of death. In pediatrics, educational efforts and the utilization of standardized management guidelines that emphasize early recognition and intervention along with the rapid transfer of critically ill patients to a pediatric intensive care unit (PICU) have led to decreases in the mortality rate for shock (Figs. 88.1 and 88.2).

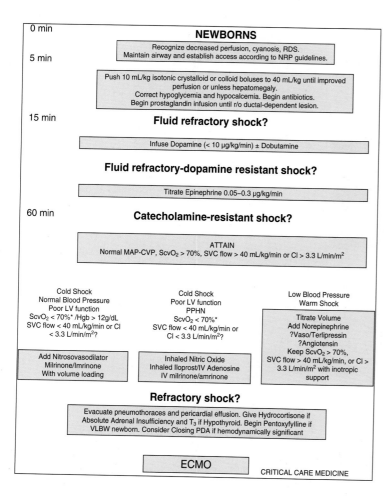

Fig. 88.1 American College of Critical Care Medicine algorithm for time-sensitive, goal-directed stepwise management of hemodynamic support in *newborns*. Proceed to next step if shock persists. (1) First-hour goals—restore and maintain heart rate thresholds, capillary refill ≤ 2 sec, and normal blood pressure in the 1st hr. (2) Subsequent ICU goals—restore normal perfusion pressure (mean arterial pressure – central venous pressure), preductal and postductal oxygen saturation difference < 5%, and either ScvO₂ > 70% (*except congenital heart patients with mixing lesions), superior vena cava flow > 40 mL/min/m² in NICU. (*From Davis AL, Carcillo JA, Aneja RK, et al: American College of Critical Care Medicine clinical practice parameters for hemodynamic support of pediatric and neonatal septic shock, Crit Care Med 45:1061–1093, 2017, Fig 4.)*

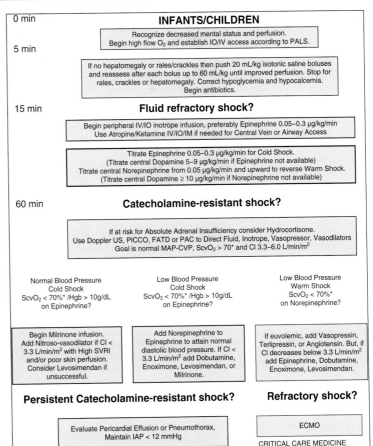

Fig. 88.2 American College of Critical Care Medicine algorithm for time-sensitive, goal-directed stepwise management of hemodynamic support in *infants and children.* Proceed to next step if shock persists. (1) First-hour goals—restore and maintain heart rate thresholds, capillary refill ≤ 2 sec, and normal blood pressure in the 1st hr/emergency department. (2) Subsequent ICU goals—if shock not reversed, proceed to restore and maintain normal perfusion pressure (MAP – CVP) for age, ScvO$_2$ > 70% (*except congenital heart patients with mixing lesions), and cardiac index > 3.3 and < 6.0 L/min/m^2 in PICU. (*From Davis AL, Carcillo JA, Aneja RK, et al: American College of Critical Care Medicine clinical practice parameters for hemodynamic support of pediatric and neonatal septic shock, Crit Care Med 45:1061–1093, 2017, Fig 2.*)

Table 88.1	Types of Shock				
HYPOVOLEMIC	**CARDIOGENIC**	**DISTRIBUTIVE**	**SEPTIC**	**OBSTRUCTIVE**	
Decreased preload secondary to internal or external losses	Cardiac pump failure secondary to poor myocardial function	Abnormalities of vasomotor tone from loss of venous and arterial capacitance	Encompasses multiple forms of shock Hypovolemic: third spacing of fluids into the extracellular, interstitial space Distributive: early shock with decreased afterload Cardiogenic: depression of myocardial function by endotoxins	Decreased cardiac output secondary to direct impediment to right- or left-sided heart outflow or restriction of all cardiac chambers	
POTENTIAL ETIOLOGIES					
Blood loss: hemorrhage Plasma loss: burns, nephrotic syndrome Water/electrolyte loss: vomiting, diarrhea	Congenital heart disease Cardiomyopathies: infectious or acquired, dilated or restrictive Ischemia Arrhythmias	Anaphylaxis Neurologic: loss of sympathetic vascular tone secondary to spinal cord or brainstem injury Drugs	Bacterial Viral Fungal (immunocompromised patients are at increased risk)	Tension pneumothorax Pericardial tamponade Pulmonary embolism Anterior mediastinal masses Critical coarctation of aorta	

TYPES OF SHOCK

Shock classification systems generally define 5 major types of shock: hypovolemic, cardiogenic, distributive, obstructive, and septic (Table 88.1). **Hypovolemic shock,** the most common cause of shock in children worldwide, is most frequently caused by diarrhea, vomiting, or hemorrhage. **Cardiogenic shock** is seen in patients with congenital heart disease (before or after surgery, including heart transplantation) or those with congenital or acquired cardiomyopathies, including acute myocarditis. **Obstructive shock** stems from any lesion that creates a mechanical barrier that impedes adequate cardiac output, which includes pericardial tamponade, tension pneumothorax, pulmonary embolism, and ductus-dependent congenital heart lesions. **Distributive shock** is caused by inadequate vasomotor tone, which leads to capillary leak and maldistribution of fluid into the interstitium. **Septic shock** is often discussed synonymously with distributive shock, but the septic process usually involves a more complex interaction of distributive, hypovolemic, and cardiogenic shock.

PATHOPHYSIOLOGY

An initial insult triggers shock, leading to inadequate oxygen delivery to organs and tissues. Compensatory mechanisms attempt to maintain blood pressure (BP) by increasing cardiac output and systemic vascular resistance (SVR). The body also attempts to optimize oxygen delivery to the tissues by increasing oxygen extraction and redistributing blood flow to the brain, heart, and kidneys at the expense of the skin and gastrointestinal (GI) tract. These responses lead to an initial state of **compensated shock** in which BP is maintained. If treatment is not initiated or is inadequate during this period, **decompensated shock** develops, with hypotension and tissue damage that may lead to **multisystem organ dysfunction** and, ultimately, death (Tables 88.2 and 88.3).

In the early phases of shock, multiple compensatory physiologic mechanisms act to maintain BP and preserve tissue perfusion and oxygen delivery. Cardiovascular effects include increases in heart rate (HR), stroke volume, and vascular smooth muscle tone, which are regulated through sympathetic nervous system activation and neurohormonal responses. Respiratory compensation involves greater carbon dioxide (CO_2) elimination in response to the metabolic acidosis and increased CO_2 production from poor tissue perfusion. Renal excretion of hydrogen ions (H^+) and retention of bicarbonate (HCO_3^-) also increase in an effort to maintain normal body pH (see Chapter 68.7). Maintenance of intravascular volume is facilitated via sodium regulation through the renin-angiotensin-aldosterone and atrial natriuretic factor axes, cortisol and catecholamine synthesis and release, and antidiuretic hormone secretion. Despite these compensatory mechanisms, the underlying shock and host response lead to vascular endothelial cell injury and significant leakage of intravascular fluids into the interstitial extracellular space.

Another important aspect of the initial pathophysiology of shock is the impact on cardiac output. All forms of shock affect cardiac output through several mechanisms, with changes in HR, preload, afterload, and myocardial contractility occurring separately or in combination (Table 88.4). **Hypovolemic shock** is characterized primarily by fluid loss and decreased preload. Tachycardia and an increase in SVR are the initial compensatory responses to maintain cardiac output and systemic BP. Without adequate volume replacement, hypotension develops, followed by tissue ischemia and further clinical deterioration. When there is preexisting low plasma oncotic pressure (caused by nephrotic syndrome, malnutrition, hepatic dysfunction, acute severe burns, etc.), even further volume loss and exacerbation of shock may result from endothelial breakdown and worsening capillary leak.

In contrast, the underlying pathophysiologic mechanism leading to **distributive shock** is a state of abnormal vasodilation and decreased SVR. Sepsis, hypoxia, poisoning, anaphylaxis, spinal cord injury, or mitochondrial dysfunction can cause *vasodilatory shock* (Fig. 88.3). The lowering of SVR is accompanied initially by a maldistribution of blood flow away from vital organs and a compensatory increase in cardiac

Table 88.2	Criteria for Organ Dysfunction
ORGAN SYSTEM	**CRITERIA FOR DYSFUNCTION**
Cardiovascular	Despite administration of isotonic intravenous fluid bolus ≥60 mL/kg in 1 hr: decrease in BP (hypotension) systolic BP <90 mm Hg, mean arterial pressure <70 mm Hg, <5th percentile for age, or systolic BP <2 SD below normal for age *or* Need for vasoactive drug to maintain BP in normal range (dopamine >5 µg/kg/min or dobutamine, epinephrine, or norepinephrine at any dose) *or* Two of the following: Unexplained metabolic acidosis: base deficit >5.0 mEq/L Increased arterial lactate: >1 mmol/L or >2× upper limit of normal Oliguria: urine output <0.5 mL/kg/hr Prolonged capillary refill: >5 sec Core-to-peripheral temperature gap: >3°C (5.4°F)
Respiratory	PaO_2/FIO_2 ratio <300 in absence of cyanotic heart disease or preexisting lung disease *or* $PaCO_2$ >65 torr or 20 mm Hg over baseline $PaCO_2$ *or* Need for >50% FIO_2 to maintain saturation ≥92% *or* Need for nonelective invasive or noninvasive mechanical ventilation
Neurologic	GCS score ≤11 *or* Acute change in mental status with decrease in GCS score ≥3 points from abnormal baseline
Hematologic	Platelet count <100,000/mm³ or decline of 50% in platelet count from highest value recorded over last 3 days (for patients with chronic hematologic or oncologic disorders) *or* INR >1.5 *or* Activated prothrombin time >60 sec
Renal	Serum creatinine >0.5 mg/dL, ≥2× upper limit of normal for age, or 2-fold increase in baseline creatinine value
Hepatic	Total bilirubin ≥4 mg/dL (not applicable for newborn) Alanine transaminase level 2× upper limit of normal for age

BP, Blood pressure; FIO_2, fraction of inspired oxygen; GCS, Glasgow Coma Scale; INR, international normalized ratio; $PaCO_2$, arterial partial pressure of carbon dioxide; PaO_2, partial pressure arterial oxygen; SD, standard deviations.

Table 88.3	Signs of Decreased Perfusion		
ORGAN SYSTEM	**↓ PERFUSION**	**↓↓ PERFUSION**	**↓↓↓ PERFUSION**
Central nervous system	—	Restless, apathetic, anxious	Agitated/confused, stuporous, coma
Respiration	—	↑ Ventilation	↑↑ Ventilation
Metabolism	—	Compensated metabolic acidemia	Uncompensated metabolic acidemia
Gut	—	↓ Motility	Ileus
Kidney	↓ Urine volume ↑ Urinary specific gravity	Oliguria (<0.5 mL/kg/hr)	Oliguria/anuria
Skin	Delayed capillary refill	Cool extremities	Mottled, cyanotic, cold extremities
Cardiovascular system	↑ Heart rate	↑↑ Heart rate ↓ Peripheral pulses	↑↑ Heart rate ↓ Blood pressure, central pulses only

Table 88.4	Pathophysiology of Shock

Extracorporeal Fluid Loss
Hypovolemic shock may be a result of direct blood loss through hemorrhage or abnormal loss of body fluids (diarrhea, vomiting, burns, diabetes mellitus or insipidus, nephrosis).

Lowering Plasma Oncotic Forces
Hypovolemic shock may also result from hypoproteinemia (liver injury, or as a progressive complication of increased capillary permeability).

Abnormal Vasodilation
Distributive shock (neurogenic, anaphylaxis, or septic shock) occurs when there is loss of vascular tone—venous, arterial, or both (sympathetic blockade, local substances affecting permeability, acidosis, drug effects, spinal cord transection).

Increased Vascular Permeability
Sepsis may change the capillary permeability in the absence of any change in capillary hydrostatic pressure (endotoxins from sepsis, excess histamine release in anaphylaxis).

Cardiac Dysfunction
Peripheral hypoperfusion may result from any condition that affects the heart's ability to pump blood efficiently (ischemia, acidosis, drugs, constrictive pericarditis, pancreatitis, sepsis).

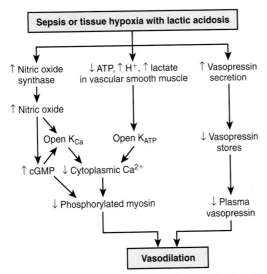

Fig. 88.3 Mechanisms of vasodilatory shock. Septic shock and states of prolonged shock causing tissue hypoxia with lactic acidosis increase nitric oxide synthesis, activate the adenosine triphosphate (ATP)–sensitive and calcium-regulated potassium channels (K_{ATP} and K_{Ca}, respectively) in vascular smooth muscle, and lead to depletion of vasopressin. cGMP, Cyclic guanosine monophosphate. *(From Landry DW, Oliver JA: The pathogenesis of vasodilatory shock, N Engl J Med 345:588.595, 2001.)*

output. This process leads to significant decreases in both preload and afterload. Therapies for distributive shock must address both these problems simultaneously.

Cardiogenic shock may be seen in patients with myocarditis, cardiomyopathy, arrhythmias and congenital heart disease (generally following cardiac surgery) (see Chapter 461). In these patients, myocardial contractility is affected, leading to systolic and/or diastolic dysfunction. The later phases of all forms of shock frequently have a negative impact on the myocardium, leading to development of a cardiogenic component to the initial shock state.

Septic shock is generally a unique combination of distributive, hypovolemic, and cardiogenic shock. Hypovolemia from intravascular fluid losses occurs through capillary leak. Cardiogenic shock results from the myocardial-depressant effects of sepsis, and distributive shock is the result of decreased SVR. The degree to which a patient exhibits each of these responses varies, but there are frequently alterations in preload, afterload, and myocardial contractility.

In septic shock, it is important to distinguish between the inciting infection and the host inflammatory response. Normally, host immunity prevents the development of sepsis through activation of the reticular endothelial system along with the cellular and humoral immune systems. This host immune response produces an *inflammatory cascade* of toxic mediators, including hormones, cytokines, and enzymes. If this inflammatory cascade is uncontrolled, derangement of the microcirculatory system leads to subsequent organ and cellular dysfunction.

The **systemic inflammatory response syndrome** (**SIRS**) is an inflammatory cascade that is initiated by the host response to an infectious or noninfectious trigger (Table 88.5). This inflammatory cascade is triggered when the host defense system does not adequately recognize and/or eliminate the triggering event. The inflammatory cascade initiated by shock can lead to hypovolemia, cardiac and vascular failure, acute respiratory distress syndrome (ARDS), insulin resistance, decreased cytochrome P450 activity (decreased steroid synthesis), coagulopathy, and unresolved or secondary infection. Tumor necrosis factor (TNF) and other inflammatory mediators increase vascular permeability, causing diffuse capillary leak, decreased vascular tone, and an imbalance between perfusion and metabolic demands of the tissues. TNF and interleukin (IL)-1 stimulate the release of proinflammatory and antiinflammatory mediators, causing fever and vasodilation. Proinflammatory mediators include IL-6, IL-12, interferon-γ, and macrophage migration inhibitory factor; antiinflammatory cytokines include IL-10, transforming growth factor-β, and IL-4. Arachidonic acid metabolites lead to the development of fever, tachypnea, ventilation-perfusion abnormalities, and lactic acidosis. Nitric oxide (NO), released from the endothelial or inflammatory cells, is a major contributor to hypotension. Myocardial depression is caused directly by myocardial-depressant factors, TNF, and some interleukins and is further depressed by depleted catecholamines, increased β-endorphin, and production of myocardial NO.

The inflammatory cascade is initiated by toxins or superantigens through macrophage binding or lymphocyte activation (Fig. 88.4). The vascular endothelium is both a target of tissue injury and a source of mediators that may cause further injury. Biochemical responses include the production of arachidonic acid metabolites, release of myocardial-depressant factors and endogenous opiates, activation of the complement system, and production and release of other mediators, which may be proinflammatory or antiinflammatory. The balance among these mediator groups for an individual patient contributes to the progression (and resolution) of disease and affects the prognosis.

CLINICAL MANIFESTATIONS

Table 88.1 shows a classification system for shock. Categorization is important, but there may be significant overlap among these groups, especially in septic shock. The clinical presentation of shock depends in part on the underlying etiology, but if unrecognized and untreated, all forms of shock follow a common and untoward progression of clinical signs and pathophysiologic changes that may ultimately lead to irreversible organ injury and death.

Shock may initially manifest as only tachycardia, with or without tachypnea. Progression leads to decreased urine output, poor peripheral perfusion, respiratory distress or failure, alteration of mental status, and low BP (see Table 88.3). A significant misconception is that shock occurs only with low BP; hypotension is often a late finding and is not a criterion for the diagnosis of shock because of a complex set of compensatory mechanisms that attempt to preserve BP and peripheral perfusion. Hypotension reflects an advanced state of decompensated shock and is associated with increased morbidity and mortality.

Hypovolemic shock often manifests initially as orthostatic hypotension and is associated with dry mucous membranes, dry axillae, poor skin turgor, and decreased urine output. Depending on the degree of dehydration, the patient with hypovolemic shock may present with either normal

| Table 88.5 | Differential Diagnosis of Systemic Inflammatory Response Syndrome (SIRS) |

INFECTION
Bacteremia or meningitis (*Streptococcus pneumoniae, Haemophilus influenzae* type b, *Neisseria meningitidis*, group A streptococcus, *Staphylococcus aureus*)
Viral illness (influenza, enteroviruses, hemorrhagic fever group, herpes simplex virus, respiratory syncytial virus, cytomegalovirus, Epstein-Barr virus)
Encephalitis (arboviruses, enteroviruses, herpes simplex virus)
Rickettsiae (Rocky Mountain spotted fever, *Ehrlichia*, Q fever)
Syphilis
Vaccine reaction (pertussis, influenza, measles)
Toxin-mediated reaction (toxic shock, staphylococcal scalded skin syndrome)

CARDIOPULMONARY
Pneumonia (bacteria, virus, mycobacteria, fungi, allergic reaction)
Pulmonary emboli
Heart failure
Arrhythmia
Pericarditis
Myocarditis

METABOLIC-ENDOCRINE
Adrenal insufficiency (adrenogenital syndrome, Addison disease, corticosteroid withdrawal)
Electrolyte disturbances (hypo- or hypernatremia; hypo- or hypercalcemia)
Diabetes insipidus
Diabetes mellitus
Inborn errors of metabolism (organic acidosis, urea cycle, carnitine deficiency, mitochondrial disorders)
Hypoglycemia
Reye syndrome

GASTROINTESTINAL
Gastroenteritis with dehydration
Volvulus
Intussusception
Appendicitis
Peritonitis (spontaneous, associated with perforation or peritoneal dialysis)
Necrotizing enterocolitis
Hepatitis
Hemorrhage
Pancreatitis

HEMATOLOGIC
Anemia (sickle cell disease, blood loss, nutritional)
Methemoglobinemia
Splenic sequestration crisis
Leukemia or lymphoma
Hemophagocytic syndromes

NEUROLOGIC
Intoxication (drugs, carbon monoxide, intentional or accidental overdose)
Intracranial hemorrhage
Infant botulism
Trauma (child abuse, accidental)
Guillain-Barré syndrome
Myasthenia gravis

OTHER
Anaphylaxis (food, drug, insect sting)
Hemolytic-uremic syndrome
Kawasaki disease
Erythema multiforme
Hemorrhagic shock–encephalopathy syndrome
Poisoning
Toxic envenomation
Macrophage activation syndrome
Idiopathic systemic capillary leak (Clarkson) syndrome

| Table 88.6 | Hemodynamic Variables in Different Shock States |

TYPE OF SHOCK	CARDIAC OUTPUT	SYSTEMIC VASCULAR RESISTANCE	MEAN ARTERIAL PRESSURE	CAPILLARY WEDGE PRESSURE	CENTRAL VENOUS PRESSURE
Hypovolemic	↓	↑	↔ or ↓	↓↓↓	↓↓↓
Cardiogenic*					
Systolic	↓↓	↑↑↑	↔ or ↓	↑↑	↑↑
Diastolic	↔	↑↑	↔	↑↑	↑
Obstructive	↓	↑	↔ or ↓	↑↑↑†	↑↑↑†
Distributive	↑↑	↓↓↓	↔ or ↓	↔ or ↓	↔ or ↓
Septic					
Early	↑↑↑	↓↓↓	↔ or ↓‡	↓	↓
Late	↓↓	↓↓	↓↓	↑	↑ or ↔

*Systolic or diastolic dysfunction.
†Wedge pressure, central venous pressure, and pulmonary artery diastolic pressures are equal.
‡Wide pulse pressure.

or slightly cool distal extremities, and pulses may be normal, decreased, or absent depending on disease severity. The presenting signs of **cardiogenic shock** are tachypnea, cool extremities, delayed capillary filling time, poor peripheral and/or central pulses, declining mental status, and decreased urine output caused by the combination of decreased cardiac output and compensatory peripheral vasoconstriction (see Chapter 469.1). **Obstructive shock** often also manifests as inadequate cardiac output because of a physical restriction of forward blood flow, and the acute presentation may quickly progress to cardiac arrest. **Distributive shock** manifests initially as peripheral vasodilation and

increased but inadequate cardiac output.

Regardless of etiology, uncompensated shock, with hypotension, high SVR, decreased cardiac output, respiratory failure, obtundation, and oliguria, occurs late in the progression of disease. Table 88.6 lists the hemodynamic findings in various shock states. Additional clinical findings in shock include cutaneous lesions such as petechiae, diffuse erythema, ecchymoses, ecthyma gangrenosum, and peripheral gangrene. Jaundice can be present either as a sign of infection or as a result of MODS.

Sepsis is defined as SIRS resulting from a suspected or proven infectious etiology. The clinical spectrum of sepsis begins when a *systemic*

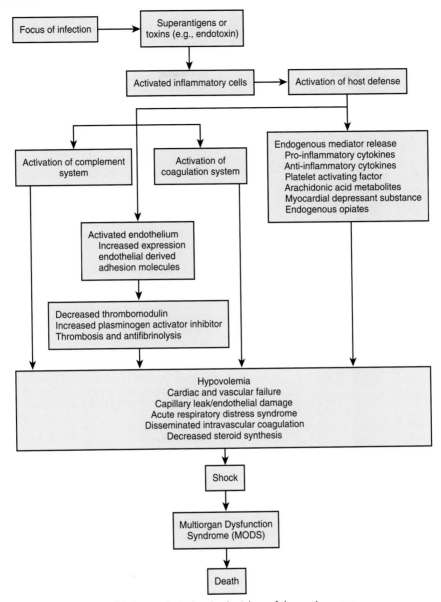

Fig. 88.4 Hypothetical pathophysiology of the septic process.

(e.g., bacteremia, rickettsial disease, fungemia, viremia) or *localized* (e.g., meningitis, pneumonia, pyelonephritis, peritonitis, necrotizing fasciitis) infection progresses from sepsis to **severe sepsis** (i.e., presence of sepsis combined with organ dysfunction). Further clinical deterioration leads to **septic shock** (severe sepsis plus the persistence of hypoperfusion or hypotension despite adequate fluid resuscitation or a requirement for vasoactive agents), MODS, and possibly death (Table 88.7). This is a complex spectrum of clinical problems that is a leading cause of mortality in children worldwide. Mortality can be mitigated and outcomes improved with early recognition and treatment.

Although **septic shock** is primarily distributive in nature, multiple other elements of pathophysiology are represented in this disease process. The initial signs and symptoms of sepsis include alterations in temperature regulation (hyperthermia or hypothermia), tachycardia, and tachypnea. In the early stages (hyperdynamic phase, low SVR, or *warm* shock), cardiac output increases to maintain adequate oxygen delivery and meet the greater metabolic demands of the organs and tissues. As septic shock progresses, cardiac output falls in response to the effects of numerous inflammatory mediators, leading to a compensatory elevation in SVR and the development of *cold* shock.

DIAGNOSIS

Shock is a clinical diagnosis based on a thorough history and physical examination (see Tables 88.2 and 88.3). Septic shock has a specific consensus conference definition (see Table 88.7). In cases of suspected septic shock, an infectious etiology should be sought through culture of clinically appropriate specimens and prompt initiation of empirical antimicrobial therapy based on patient age, underlying disease, and geographic location, recognizing that time is necessary for incubation of cultures, and results often are not positive. Additional evidence for identifying an infectious etiology as the cause of SIRS includes physical examination findings, imaging, presence of white blood cells in normally sterile body fluids,

Table 88.7	International Consensus Definitions for Pediatric Sepsis

Infection
Suspected or proven infection or a clinical syndrome associated with high probability of infection.

Systemic Inflammatory Response Syndrome (SIRS)
Two of 4 criteria, 1 of which must be abnormal temperature or abnormal leukocyte count:
1. Core temperature >38.5°C (101.3°F) or <36°C (96.8°F) (rectal, bladder, oral, or central catheter)
2. Tachycardia:
   Mean heart rate >2 SD above normal for age in absence of external stimuli, chronic drugs or painful stimuli
   or
   Unexplained persistent elevation over 0.5-4 hr
   or
   In children <1 yr old, persistent bradycardia over 0.5 hr (mean heart rate <10th percentile for age in absence of vagal stimuli, β-blocker drugs, or congenital heart disease)
3. Respiratory rate >2 SD above normal for age or acute need for mechanical ventilation not related to neuromuscular disease or general anesthesia
4. Leukocyte count elevated or depressed for age (not secondary to chemotherapy) or >10% immature neutrophils

Sepsis
SIRS plus a suspected or proven infection

Severe Sepsis
Sepsis plus 1 of the following:
1. Cardiovascular organ dysfunction, defined as:
   Despite >40 mL/kg of isotonic intravenous fluid in 1 hr:
   • Hypotension <5th percentile for age or systolic blood pressure <2 SD below normal for age
   or
   • Need for vasoactive drug to maintain blood pressure
   or
   Two of the following:
   • Unexplained metabolic acidosis: base deficit >5 mEq/L
   • Increased arterial lactate: >2 times upper limit of normal
   • Oliguria: urine output <0.5 mL/kg/hr
   • Prolonged capillary refill: >5 sec
   • Core-to-peripheral temperature gap: >3°C (5.4°F)
2. Acute respiratory distress syndrome (ARDS), as defined by the presence of a PaO_2/FIO_2 ratio ≤300 mm Hg, bilateral infiltrates on chest radiograph, and no evidence of left-sided heart failure.
   or
   Sepsis plus ≥2 organ dysfunctions (respiratory, renal, neurologic, hematologic, or hepatic).

Septic Shock
Sepsis plus cardiovascular organ dysfunction as defined above.

Multiple-Organ Dysfunction Syndrome (MODS)
Presence of altered organ function such that homeostasis cannot be maintained without medical intervention.

FIO_2, Fraction of inspired oxygen; PaO_2, partial pressure of arterial oxygen; SD, standard deviations.

and suggestive rashes such as petechiae and purpura. Affected children should be admitted to a PICU or other highly monitored environment as indicated by clinical status and the resources of the medical facility. These patients necessitate continuous monitoring, with a combination of non-invasive (e.g., pulse oximetry, capnography, near-infrared spectroscopy) and invasive (e.g., central venous pressure, arterial BP) techniques as clinically indicated.

LABORATORY FINDINGS

Laboratory findings often include evidence of hematologic abnormalities and electrolyte disturbances. Hematologic abnormalities

may include thrombocytopenia, prolonged prothrombin and partial thromboplastin times, reduced serum fibrinogen level, elevation of fibrin split products, and anemia. Elevated neutrophil counts and increased immature forms (i.e., bands, myelocytes, promyelocytes), vacuolation of neutrophils, toxic granulations, and Döhle bodies can be seen with infection. Neutropenia or leukopenia may be an ominous sign of overwhelming sepsis.

Glucose dysregulation, a common stress response, may manifest as hyperglycemia or hypoglycemia. Other electrolyte abnormalities are hypocalcemia, hypoalbuminemia, and metabolic acidosis. Renal and/ or hepatic function may also be abnormal. Patients with ARDS or pneumonia have impairment of oxygenation (decreased partial pressure of arterial oxygen [PaO_2]) as well as of ventilation (increased arterial partial pressure of carbon dioxide [$PaCO_2$]) in the later stages of lung injury (see Chapter 89).

The hallmark of *uncompensated* shock is an imbalance between oxygen delivery (DO_2) and oxygen consumption (VO_2). Oxygen delivery normally exceeds oxygen consumption by threefold. The oxygen extraction ratio is approximately 25%, thus producing a normal mixed venous oxygen saturation (SvO_2) of approximately 75%. A falling SvO_2 value, as measured by cooximetry, reflects an increasing oxygen extraction ratio and documents a decrease in oxygen delivery relative to consumption. This increase in oxygen extraction by the end organs is an attempt to maintain adequate oxygen delivery at the cellular level. This state is manifested clinically by increased lactic acid production (e.g., high anion gap, metabolic acidosis) caused by anaerobic metabolism and a compensatory increase in tissue oxygen extraction. The gold standard measurement of SvO_2 is from a pulmonary arterial catheter, but measurements from this location are often not clinically feasible. Sites such as the right ventricle, right atrium, superior vena cava ($SvcO_2$), or inferior vena cava can be as surrogate measures of mixed venous blood to follow the adequacy of oxygen delivery and effectiveness of therapeutic interventions. *Elevated blood lactate levels reflect poor tissue oxygen delivery noted in all forms of shock.*

TREATMENT
Initial Management

Early recognition and prompt intervention are extremely important in the management of all forms of shock (Tables 88.8 to 88.12; see Figs. 88.1 and 88.2). *The vital sign targets and dose recommendations in Tables 88.9 to 88.12 should be adjusted to pediatric-size patients.* Baseline mortality is much lower in pediatric shock than in adult shock, and further improvements in mortality are associated with early interventions (see Fig. 81.1). The initial assessment and treatment of the pediatric shock patient should include stabilization of airway, breathing, and circulation as established by the American Heart Association's pediatric advanced life support and neonatal advanced life support guidelines (see Chapter 81). Depending on the severity of shock, further airway intervention, including intubation and mechanical ventilation, may be necessary to lessen the work of breathing and decrease the body's overall metabolic demands.

Given the predominance of sepsis and hypovolemia as the most common causes of shock in the pediatric population, most therapeutic regimens are based on guidelines established in these settings. Immediately following establishment of intravenous (IV) or intraosseous (IO) access, aggressive, early goal-directed therapy should be initiated unless there are significant concerns for cardiogenic shock as an underlying pathophysiology. Rapid IV administration of 20 mL/kg isotonic fluid should be initiated to reverse the shock state. This bolus should be repeated quickly up to 60-80 mL/kg; it is not unusual for severely affected patients to require this volume within the 1st 3 hr of treatment.

Rapid fluid resuscitation totaling 60-80 mL/kg or more is associated with improved survival without an increased incidence of pulmonary edema. Fluid resuscitation in increments of 20 mL/kg should be titrated to normalize HR (according to age-based HRs), urine output (to 1 mL/kg/hr), capillary refill time (to <2 sec), and mental status. If shock remains refractory following 60-80 mL/kg of volume resuscitation, vasopressor therapy (e.g., norepinephrine, epinephrine) should be instituted while additional fluids are administered. Pediatric guidelines for septic

Table 88.8	Goal-Directed Therapy of Organ System Dysfunction in Shock		
SYSTEM	**DISORDERS**	**GOALS**	**THERAPIES**
Respiratory	Acute respiratory distress syndrome Respiratory muscle fatigue Central apnea	Prevent/treat: hypoxia and respiratory acidosis Prevent barotrauma Decrease work of breathing	Oxygen Noninvasive ventilation Early endotracheal intubation and mechanical ventilation Positive end-expiratory pressure (PEEP) Permissive hypercapnia High-frequency ventilation Extracorporeal membrane oxygenation (ECMO)
Renal	Prerenal failure Renal failure	Prevent/treat: hypovolemia, hypervolemia, hyperkalemia, metabolic acidosis, hypernatremia/hyponatremia, and hypertension Monitor serum electrolytes	Judicious fluid resuscitation Establishment of normal urine output and blood pressure for age Furosemide (Lasix) Dialysis, ultrafiltration, hemofiltration
Hematologic	Coagulopathy (disseminated intravascular coagulation) Thrombosis	Prevent/treat: bleeding Prevent/treat: abnormal clotting	Vitamin K Fresh-frozen plasma Platelets Heparinization
Gastrointestinal	Stress ulcers Ileus Bacterial translocation	Prevent/treat: gastric bleeding Avoid aspiration, abdominal distention Avoid mucosal atrophy	Histamine H_2-receptor–blocking agents or proton pump inhibitors Nasogastric tube Early enteral feedings
Endocrine	Adrenal insufficiency, primary or secondary to chronic steroid therapy	Prevent/treat: adrenal crisis	Stress-dose steroids in patients previously given steroids Physiologic dose for presumed primary insufficiency in sepsis
Metabolic	Metabolic acidosis	Correct etiology Normalize pH	Treatment of hypovolemia (fluids), poor cardiac function (fluids, inotropic agents) Improvement of renal acid excretion Low-dose (0.5-2.0 mEq/kg) sodium bicarbonate if patient is not showing response, pH <7.1, and ventilation (CO_2 elimination) is adequate

Table 88.9	Recommendations for Shock: Initial Resuscitation and Infection Issues—Adults

INITIAL RESUSCITATION

1. Protocolized, quantitative resuscitation of patients with sepsis-induced tissue hypoperfusion (defined as hypotension persisting after initial fluid challenge or blood lactate concentration ≥4 mmol/L). Goals during the 1st 6 hr of resuscitation:
   a. Central venous pressure 8-12 mm Hg
   b. Mean arterial pressure (MAP) ≥65 mm Hg
   c. Urine output ≥0.5 mL kg^{-1} hr
   d. Central venous (superior vena cava) or mixed venous oxygen saturation: 70% or 65%, respectively
2. In patients with elevated lactate levels, targeting resuscitation to normalize lactate as rapidly as possible.

SCREENING FOR SEPSIS AND PERFORMANCE IMPROVEMENT

1. Routine screening of potentially infected seriously ill patients for severe sepsis to allow earlier implementation of therapy.
2. Hospital-based performance improvement efforts in severe sepsis.

DIAGNOSIS

1. Cultures as clinically appropriate before antimicrobial therapy if no significant delay (>45 min) in the start of antimicrobial(s). At least 2 sets of blood cultures (both aerobic and anaerobic bottles) should be obtained before antimicrobial therapy with at least 1 drawn percutaneously and 1 drawn through each vascular access device, unless the device was recently (<48 hr) inserted.
2. Use of the 1,3 β-D-glucan assay, mannan and antimannan antibody assays, if available, and invasive candidiasis is in differential diagnosis of cause of infection.
3. Imaging studies performed promptly to confirm a potential source of infection.

ANTIMICROBIAL THERAPY

1. Administration of effective intravenous antimicrobials within the 1st hr of recognition of septic shock and severe sepsis without septic shock as the goal of therapy.
2a. Initial empirical antiinfective therapy of 1 or more drugs that have activity against all likely pathogens (bacterial and/or fungal or viral) and that penetrate in adequate concentrations into tissues presumed to be the source of sepsis.
2b. Antimicrobial regimen should be reassessed daily for potential deescalation.
3. Use of low procalcitonin levels or similar biomarkers to assist the clinician in the discontinuation of empirical antibiotics in patients who initially appeared septic, but have no subsequent evidence of infection.
4a. Combination empirical therapy for neutropenic patients with severe sepsis and for patients with difficult-to-treat, multidrug-resistant bacterial pathogens such as *Acinetobacter* and *Pseudomonas* spp.
   For patients with severe infections associated with respiratory failure and septic shock, combination therapy with an extended-spectrum β-lactam and either an aminoglycoside or a fluoroquinolone for *Pseudomonas aeruginosa* bacteremia. A combination of β-lactam and macrolide for patients with septic shock from bacteremic *Streptococcus pneumoniae* infections.
4b. Empirical combination therapy should not be administered for more than 3-5 days. Deescalation to the most appropriate single therapy should be performed as soon as the susceptibility profile is known.
5. Duration of therapy typically 7-10 days; longer courses may be appropriate in patients who have a slow clinical response,

Continued

Table 88.9	Recommendations for Shock: Initial Resuscitation and Infection Issues—Adults—cont'd

undrainable foci of infection, bacteremia with *Staphylococcus aureus*, some fungal and viral infections, or immunodeficiencies (e.g., neutropenia).
6. Antiviral therapy initiated as early as possible in patients with severe sepsis or septic shock of viral origin.
7. Antimicrobial agents should *not* be used in patients with severe inflammatory states determined to be of noninfectious cause.

SOURCE CONTROL
1. A specific anatomic diagnosis of infection requiring consideration for emergent source control should be sought and diagnosed or excluded as rapidly as possible, and intervention undertaken for source control within the 1st 12 hr after the diagnosis is made, if feasible.
2. When infected peripancreatic necrosis is identified as a potential source of infection, definitive intervention is best delayed until adequate demarcation of viable and nonviable tissues has occurred.

3. When source control in a severely septic patient is required, the effective intervention associated with the least physiologic insult should be used (e.g., percutaneous rather than surgical drainage of an abscess).
4. If intravascular access devices are a possible source of severe sepsis or septic shock, these should be removed promptly after other vascular access has been established.

INFECTION PREVENTION
1a. Selective oral decontamination and selective digestive decontamination should be introduced and investigated as a method to reduce the incidence of ventilator-associated pneumonia; this infection control measure can then be instituted in healthcare settings and regions where this methodology is found to be effective.
1b. Oral chlorhexidine gluconate be used as a form of oropharyngeal decontamination to reduce the risk of ventilator-associated pneumonia in ICU patients with severe sepsis.

Adapted from Dellinger PR, Levy MM, Rhodes A, et al: Surviving sepsis campaign: International guidelines for management of severe sepsis and septic shock: 2012, *Crit Care Med* 41(2):580–637, 2013 (Table 5, p 589).

Table 88.10	Surviving Sepsis Campaign: Care Bundles

To be completed within 3 hr:
1. Measure lactate level.
2. Obtain blood cultures before administration of antibiotics.
3. Administer broad-spectrum antibiotics.
4. Administer 30 mL/kg crystalloid for hypotension or lactate ≥4 mmol/L.
To completed within 6 hr:
5. Apply vasopressors (for hypotension that does not respond to initial fluid resuscitation) to maintain a mean arterial pressure (MAP) ≥65 mm Hg.

6. In the event of persistent arterial hypotension despite volume resuscitation (septic shock) or initial lactate ≥4 mmol/L (36 mg/dL): Measure central venous pressure (CVP).*
Measure central venous oxygen saturation (ScvO₂).*
7. Remeasure lactate if initial lactate was elevated.*

*Targets for quantitative resuscitation included in the guidelines are CVP of ≥8 mm Hg, ScvO₂ of ≥70%, and normalization of lactate.
Adapted from Dellinger PR, Levy MM, Rhodes A, et al: Surviving Sepsis campaign: international guidelines for management of severe sepsis and septic shock: 2012. *Crit Care Med* 41(2):580–637, 2013 (Fig 1, p 591).

Table 88.11	Recommendations for Shock: Hemodynamic Support and Adjunctive Therapy—Adults

FLUID THERAPY OF SEVERE SEPSIS
1. Crystalloids as the initial fluid of choice in the resuscitation of severe sepsis and septic shock.
2. Against the use of hydroxyethyl starches for fluid resuscitation of severe sepsis and septic shock.
3. Albumin in the fluid resuscitation of severe sepsis and septic shock when patients require substantial amounts of crystalloids.
4. Initial fluid challenge in patients with sepsis-induced tissue hypoperfusion with suspicion of hypovolemia, to achieve a minimum of 30 mL/kg of crystalloids (a portion of this may be albumin equivalent). More rapid administration and greater amounts of fluid may be needed in some patients.
5. Fluid challenge technique be applied in which fluid administration is continued as long as there is hemodynamic improvement either based on dynamic (e.g., change in pulse pressure, stroke volume variation) or static (e.g., arterial pressure, heart rate) variables.

VASOPRESSORS
1. Vasopressor therapy initially to target a mean arterial pressure (MAP) of 65 mm Hg.
2. Norepinephrine as the first-choice vasopressor.
3. Epinephrine (added to and potentially substituted for norepinephrine) when an additional agent is needed to maintain adequate blood pressure.
4. Vasopressin 0.03 units/min can be added to norepinephrine (NE) with intent of either raising MAP or decreasing NE dosage.
5. Low-dose vasopressin is not recommended as the single initial vasopressor for treatment of sepsis-induced hypotension, and

vasopressin doses >0.03-0.04 units/min should be reserved for salvage therapy (failure to achieve adequate MAP with other vasopressor agents).
6. Dopamine as an alternative vasopressor agent to NE only in highly selected patients (e.g., with low risk of tachyarrhythmias and absolute or relative bradycardia).
7. Phenylephrine is not recommended in the treatment of septic shock except in circumstances where (a) NE is associated with serious arrhythmias, (b) cardiac output is known to be high and blood pressure persistently low, or (c) as salvage therapy when combined inotrope/vasopressor drugs and low-dose vasopressin have failed to achieve MAP target.
8. Low-dose dopamine should not be used for renal protection.
9. All patients requiring vasopressors have an arterial catheter placed as soon as practical if resources are available.

INOTROPIC THERAPY
1. A trial of dobutamine infusion up to 20 µg/kg/min be administered or added to vasopressor (if in use) in the presence of (a) myocardial dysfunction as suggested by elevated cardiac filling pressures and low cardiac output, or (b) ongoing signs of hypoperfusion, despite achieving adequate intravascular volume and adequate MAP.
2. Not using a strategy to increase cardiac index to predetermined supranormal levels.

CORTICOSTEROIDS
1. Not using intravenous hydrocortisone to treat adult septic shock patients, if adequate fluid resuscitation and vasopressor therapy

Continued

Table 88.11	Recommendations for Shock: Hemodynamic Support and Adjunctive Therapy—Adults—cont'd

are able to restore hemodynamic stability (see goals for Initial Resuscitation). In the event this is not achievable, we suggest IV hydrocortisone alone at a dose of 200 mg/day. 2. Not using the ACTH stimulation test to identify adults with septic shock who should receive hydrocortisone.	3. In treated patients, hydrocortisone tapered when vasopressors are no longer required. 4. Corticosteroids should *not* be administered for the treatment of sepsis in the absence of shock. 5. When hydrocortisone is given, use continuous flow.

Adapted from Dellinger PR, Levy MM, Rhodes A, et al: Surviving Sepsis campaign: international guidelines for management of severe sepsis and septic shock: 2012, *Crit Care Med* 41(2):580–637, 2013 (Table 6, p 596).

Table 88.12	Recommendations for Shock: Special Considerations in Pediatric Patients

INITIAL RESUSCITATION

1. For respiratory distress and hypoxemia, start with face mask oxygen or, if needed and available, high-flow nasal cannula oxygen or nasopharyngeal CPAP (NP CPAP). For improved circulation, peripheral intravenous access or intraosseous access can be used for fluid resuscitation and inotrope infusion when a central line is not available. If mechanical ventilation is required, cardiovascular instability during intubation is less likely after appropriate cardiovascular resuscitation.
2. Initial therapeutic end-points of resuscitation of septic shock: capillary refill of ≤2 sec, normal blood pressure for age, normal pulses with no differential between peripheral and central pulses, warm extremities, urine output >1 mL kg^{-1} hr^{-1}, and normal mental status. ScvO$_2$ saturation ≥70% and cardiac index between 3.3 and 6.0 L/min/m^2 should be targeted thereafter.
3. Follow American College of Critical Care Medicine–Pediatric Advanced Life Support (ACCM-PALS) guidelines for the management of septic shock.
4. Evaluate for and reverse pneumothorax, pericardial tamponade, or endocrine emergencies in patients with refractory shock.

ANTIBIOTICS AND SOURCE CONTROL

1. Empirical antibiotics should be administered within 1 hr of the identification of severe sepsis. Blood cultures should be obtained before administering antibiotics when possible, but this should not delay administration of antibiotics. The empirical drug choice should be changed as epidemic and endemic ecologies dictate (e.g., H1N1, methicillin-resistant *Staphylococcus aureus* [MRSA], chloroquine-resistant malaria, penicillin-resistant pneumococci, recent ICU stay, neutropenia).
2. Clindamycin and antitoxin therapies for toxic shock syndromes with refractory hypotension.
3. Early and aggressive source control.
4. *Clostridium difficile* colitis should be treated with enteral antibiotics if tolerated. Oral vancomycin is preferred for severe disease.

FLUID RESUSCITATION

1. In the industrialized world with access to inotropes and mechanical ventilation, initial resuscitation of hypovolemic shock begins with infusion of isotonic crystalloids or albumin with boluses of up to 20 mL/kg crystalloids (or albumin equivalent) over 5-10 min, titrated to reversing hypotension, increasing urine output, and attaining normal capillary refill, peripheral pulses, and level of consciousness without inducing hepatomegaly or rales. If hepatomegaly or rales present, inotropic support should be implemented, not fluid resuscitation. In nonhypotensive children with severe hemolytic anemia (severe malaria or sickle cell crises), blood transfusion is considered superior to crystalloid or albumin bolus.

INOTROPES, VASOPRESSORS, AND VASODILATORS

1. Begin peripheral inotropic support until central venous access can be attained in children who are not responsive to fluid resuscitation.
2. Patients with low cardiac output and elevated systemic vascular resistance states with normal blood pressure should be given vasodilator therapies in addition to inotropes.

EXTRACORPOREAL MEMBRANE OXYGENATION

1. Consider ECMO for refractory pediatric septic shock and respiratory failure.

CORTICOSTEROIDS

1. Timely hydrocortisone therapy in children with fluid-refractory, catecholamine-resistant shock and suspected or proven absolute (classic) adrenal insufficiency.

PROTEIN C AND ACTIVATED PROTEIN CONCENTRATE

No recommendations (no longer available).

BLOOD PRODUCTS AND PLASMA THERAPIES

1. Similar hemoglobin targets in children as in adults. During resuscitation of low superior vena cava oxygen saturation shock (<70%), hemoglobin levels of 10 g/dL are targeted. After stabilization and recovery from shock and hypoxemia, a lower target (>7.0 g/dL) can be considered reasonable.
2. Similar platelet transfusion targets in children as in adults.
3. Use plasma therapies in children to correct sepsis-induced thrombotic purpura disorders, including progressive disseminated intravascular coagulation, secondary thrombotic microangiopathy, and thrombotic thrombocytopenic purpura.

MECHANICAL VENTILATION

1. Lung-protective strategies during mechanical ventilation.

SEDATION, ANALGESIA, AND DRUG TOXICITIES

1. We recommend use of sedation with a sedation goal in critically ill, mechanically ventilated patients with sepsis.
2. Monitor drug toxicity lab results because drug metabolism is reduced during severe sepsis, putting children at greater risk of adverse drug-related events.

GLYCEMIC CONTROL

1. Control hyperglycemia using a similar target as in adults (≤180 mg/dL). Glucose infusion should accompany insulin therapy in newborns and children because some hyperglycemic children make no insulin whereas others are insulin resistant.

DIURETICS AND RENAL REPLACEMENT THERAPY

1. Use diuretics to reverse fluid overload when shock has resolved, and if unsuccessful, use continuous venovenous hemofiltration (CVVH) or intermittent dialysis to prevent >10% total body weight fluid overload.

DEEP VEIN THROMBOSIS (DVT) PROPHYLAXIS

No recommendation on the use of DVT prophylaxis in prepubertal children with severe sepsis.

STRESS ULCER (SU) PROPHYLAXIS

No recommendation on the use of SU prophylaxis in prepubertal children with severe sepsis.

NUTRITION

1. Enteral nutrition given to children who can be fed enterally, and parenteral feeding in those who cannot (grade 2C).

CPAP, Continuous positive airway pressure.
Adapted from Dellinger PR, Levy MM, Rhodes A, et al: Surviving Sepsis campaign: *International guidelines for management of severe sepsis and septic shock: 2012, Crit Care Med* 41(2):580–637, 2013 (Table 9, p 614).

shock unresponsive to fluid resuscitation suggest epinephrine (Fig. 88.2) or dopamine (Fig. 88.1), whereas adult guidelines recommend norepinephrine.

Fluid resuscitation may sometimes require as much as 200 mL/kg or greater. It must be stressed that hypotension is often a late and ominous finding, and BP normalization alone is not a reliable end-point for assessing the effectiveness of resuscitation. Although the type of fluid (crystalloid vs colloid) is an area of ongoing debate, fluid resuscitation (usually crystalloid) in the 1st hr is unquestionably essential to survival in septic shock, regardless of the fluid type administered.

Additional Early Considerations

In **septic shock** specifically, early (*within 1 hr*) administration of broad-spectrum antimicrobial agents is associated with a reduction in mortality. The choice of antimicrobial agents depends on the predisposing risk factors and the clinical situation. Bacterial resistance patterns in the community and/or hospital should be considered in the selection of optimal antimicrobial therapy. Neonates should be treated with ampicillin plus cefepime and/or gentamicin. Acyclovir should be added if herpes simplex virus is suspected clinically. In infants and children, community-acquired infections with *Neisseria meningitidis* can initially be treated empirically with a third-generation cephalosporin (e.g., ceftriaxone, cefepime), as can *Haemophilus influenzae* infections. The prevalence of resistant *Streptococcus pneumoniae* requires the addition of vancomycin. Suspicion of community- or hospital-acquired, methicillin-resistant *Staphylococcus aureus* (MRSA) infection warrants coverage with vancomycin, depending on local resistance patterns. If an intraabdominal process is suspected, anaerobic coverage should be included with an agent such as metronidazole, clindamycin, or piperacillin-tazobactam.

Nosocomial sepsis should generally be treated with at least a third- or fourth-generation cephalosporin or a penicillin with an extended gram-negative spectrum (e.g., piperacillin-tazobactam). An aminoglycoside should be added as the clinical situation warrants. Vancomycin should be added to the regimen if the patient has an indwelling medical device (see Chapter 206), if gram-positive cocci are isolated from the blood, if MRSA infection is suspected, or as empirical coverage for *S. pneumoniae* in a patient with meningitis. Empirical coverage for fungal infections should be considered for selected immunocompromised patients (see Chapter 205). It should be noted that these are broad, generalized recommendations that must be tailored to the individual clinical scenario and to the local resistance patterns of the community and hospital.

Distributive shock that is not secondary to sepsis is caused by a primary abnormality in vascular tone. Cardiac output in affected patients is usually maintained and may initially be supranormal. These patients may benefit temporarily from volume resuscitation, but the early initiation of a vasoconstrictive agent to increase SVR is an important element of clinical care. Patients with spinal cord injury and spinal shock may benefit from either phenylephrine or vasopressin to increase SVR; epinephrine is the treatment of choice for patients with anaphylaxis (Table 88.13). Epinephrine has peripheral α-adrenergic as well as inotropic effects that may improve the myocardial depression seen with anaphylaxis and its associated inflammatory response (see Chapter 174).

Patients with **cardiogenic shock** have poor cardiac output secondary to systolic and/or diastolic myocardial depression, often with a compensatory elevation in SVR. These patients may show poor response to fluid resuscitation and may decompensate quickly when fluids are administered. Smaller boluses of fluid (5-10 mL/kg) should be given in cardiogenic shock to replace deficits and maintain preload. In any patient with shock whose clinical status deteriorates with fluid resuscitation, a cardiogenic etiology should be considered, and further administration of IV fluids should be provided judiciously. Early initiation of myocardial

Table 88.13	Cardiovascular Drug Treatment of Shock		
DRUG	**EFFECT(S)**	**DOSING RANGE**	**COMMENT(S)**
Dopamine	↑ Cardiac contractility Significant peripheral vasoconstriction at >10 μg/kg/min	3-20 μg/kg/min	↑ Risk of arrhythmias at high doses
Epinephrine	↑ Heart rate and ↑ cardiac contractility Potent vasoconstrictor	0.05-3.0 μg/kg/min	May ↓ renal perfusion at high doses ↑ Myocardial O_2 consumption Risk of arrhythmia at high doses
Dobutamine	↑ Cardiac contractility Peripheral vasodilator	1-10 μg/kg/min	—
Norepinephrine	Potent vasoconstriction No significant effect on cardiac contractility	0.05-1.5 μg/kg/min	↑ Blood pressure secondary to ↑ systemic vascular resistance ↑ Left ventricular afterload
Phenylephrine	Potent vasoconstriction	0.5-2.0 μg/kg/min	Can cause sudden hypertension ↑ O_2 consumption

Table 88.14	Vasodilators/Afterload Reducers in Treatment of Shock		
DRUG	**EFFECT(S)**	**DOSING RANGE**	**COMMENT(S)**
Nitroprusside	Vasodilator (mainly arterial)	0.5-4.0 μg/kg/min	Rapid effect Risk of cyanide toxicity with prolonged use (>96 hr)
Nitroglycerin	Vasodilator (mainly venous)	1-20 μg/kg/min	Rapid effect Risk of increased intracranial pressure
Prostaglandin E_1	Vasodilator Maintains an open ductus arteriosus in the newborn with ductal-dependent congenital heart disease	0.01-0.2 μg/kg/min	Can lead to hypotension Risk of apnea
Milrinone	Increased cardiac contractility Improves cardiac diastolic function Peripheral vasodilation	Load 50 μg/kg over 15 min 0.5-1.0 μg/kg/min	Phosphodiesterase inhibitor—slows cyclic adenosine monophosphate breakdown

support with epinephrine or dopamine to improve cardiac output is important in this context, and early consideration should be given to administration of an inodilator, such as milrinone.

Despite adequate cardiac output with the support of inotropic agents, a high SVR with poor peripheral perfusion and acidosis may persist in cardiogenic shock. Therefore, if not already started, milrinone therapy may improve systolic function and decrease SVR without causing a significant increase in HR. Furthermore, this agent has the added benefit of enhancing diastolic relaxation. Dobutamine or other vasodilating agents, such as nitroprusside, may also be considered in this setting (Table 88.14). Titration of these agents should target clinical end-points, including increased urine output, improved peripheral perfusion, resolution of acidosis, and normalization of mental status. Even though they may be beneficial in other forms of shock, agents that improve BP by increasing SVR, such as norepinephrine and vasopressin, should generally be avoided in patients with cardiogenic shock. These agents may cause further decompensation and potentially precipitate cardiac arrest as a result of the increased afterload and additional work imposed on the myocardium. The combination of inotropic and vasoactive agents must be tailored to the pathophysiology of the individual patient with close and frequent reassessment of the patient's cardiovascular status.

For patients with **obstructive shock**, fluid resuscitation may be briefly temporizing in maintaining cardiac output, but the primary insult must be immediately addressed. Examples of lifesaving therapeutic interventions for such patients are pericardiocentesis for pericardial effusion, pleurocentesis or chest tube placement for pneumothorax, thrombectomy/thrombolysis for pulmonary embolism, and the initiation of a prostaglandin infusion for ductus-dependent cardiac lesions. There is often a *last-drop phenomenon* associated with some obstructive lesions, in that small additional amounts of intravascular volume depletion may lead to a rapid deterioration, including cardiac arrest, if the obstructive lesion is not corrected.

Regardless of the etiology of shock, metabolic status should be meticulously maintained (see Table 88.8). Electrolyte levels should be monitored closely and corrected as needed. Hypoglycemia is common and should be promptly treated. Neonates and infants in particular may have profound glucose dysregulation in association with shock. Glucose levels should be checked routinely and treated appropriately, especially early in the course of illness. Hypocalcemia, which may contribute to myocardial dysfunction, should be treated with a goal of normalizing the ionized calcium concentration. There is no evidence that supranormal calcium levels benefit the myocardium, and hypercalcemia may be associated with increased myocardial toxicity.

Adrenal function is another important consideration in shock, and hydrocortisone replacement may be beneficial. Up to 50% of critically ill patients may have absolute or relative adrenal insufficiency. Patients at risk for adrenal insufficiency include those with congenial adrenal hypoplasia, abnormalities of the hypothalamic-pituitary axis, and recent therapy with corticosteroids (including those with asthma, rheumatic diseases, malignancies, and inflammatory bowel disease). These patients are at high risk for adrenal dysfunction and should receive stress doses of hydrocortisone. *Corticosteroids may also be considered in patients with shock that is unresponsive to fluid resuscitation and catecholamines.* Although a subset of pediatric septic shock patients may benefit from treatment with hydrocortisone, currently available pediatric data do not demonstrate an overall survival benefit in patients with shock treated with hydrocortisone. Determination of baseline cortisol levels before corticosteroid administration may be beneficial in guiding therapy, although this approach remains controversial.

Considerations for Continued Therapy

After the 1st hr of therapy and attempts at early reversal of shock, focus on goal-directed end-points should continue in an intensive care setting (see Figs. 88.1 and 88.2 and Table 88.8). Clinical end-points serve as global markers for organ perfusion and oxygenation. Laboratory parameters such as SvO_2 (or $ScvO_2$), serum lactate concentration, cardiac index, and hemoglobin serve as adjunctive measures of tissue oxygen delivery. Hemoglobin should be generally maintained at 10 g/dL, SvO_2 (or $ScvO_2$) >70%, and cardiac index at 3.3-6.0 $L/min/m^2$ to optimize oxygen delivery in the acute phase of shock. It is important to note that cardiac index is rarely monitored in the clinical setting because of the limited use of pulmonary artery catheters and lack of accurate noninvasive cardiac output monitors for infants and children. Blood lactate levels and calculation of base deficit from arterial blood gas values are very useful markers for the adequacy of oxygen delivery. These traditional markers are indicators of global oxygen utilization and delivery. There is increasing use of measures of local tissue oxygenation, including near-infrared spectroscopy of the cerebrum, flank, or abdomen.

Respiratory support should be used as clinically appropriate. When shock leads to ARDS requiring mechanical ventilation, lung-protective strategies to keep plateau pressure <30 cm H_2O and maintain tidal volume at 6 mL/kg have been shown to improve mortality in adult patients (see Chapter 89). These data are extrapolated to pediatric patients because of the lack of definitive pediatric studies in this area. Additionally, after the initial shock state has been reversed, data demonstrate that judicious fluid administration, renal replacement therapy, and fluid removal may also be useful in children with anuria or oliguria and fluid overload (see Chapter 550). Other interventions include correction of coagulopathy with fresh-frozen plasma or cryoprecipitate and platelet transfusions as necessary, especially in the presence of active bleeding.

If shock remains refractory despite maximal therapeutic interventions, mechanical support with **extracorporeal membrane oxygenation** (ECMO) or a **ventricular assist device** (VAD) may be indicated. ECMO may be lifesaving in cases of refractory shock regardless of underlying etiology. Similarly, a VAD may be indicated for refractory cardiogenic shock in the setting of cardiomyopathy or recent cardiac surgery. Systemic anticoagulation, which is required while patients are receiving mechanical support, may be difficult, given the significant coagulopathy often encountered in refractory shock, especially when the underlying etiology is sepsis. Mechanical support in refractory shock poses substantial risks but can improve survival in specific populations of patients.

PROGNOSIS

In septic shock, mortality rates are as low as 3% in previously healthy children and 6–9% in children with chronic illness (compared with 25–30% in adults). With early recognition and therapy, the mortality rate for pediatric shock continues to improve, but shock and MODS remain one of the leading causes of death in infants and children. The risk of death involves a complex interaction of factors, including the underlying etiology, presence of chronic illness, host immune response, and timing of recognition and therapy.

Bibliography is available at Expert Consult.

Chapter **89**

Respiratory Distress and Failure

Ashok P. Sarnaik, Jeff A. Clark, and Sabrina M. Heidemann

第八十九章
呼吸窘迫和呼吸衰竭

中文导读

　　本章主要介绍了呼吸窘迫、呼吸衰竭、呼吸窘迫和呼吸衰竭儿童监测以及治疗。呼吸窘迫中描述了伴有和不伴有呼吸系统疾病的呼吸窘迫；呼吸衰竭中描述了呼吸衰竭的病理生理学；在呼吸窘迫和呼吸衰竭儿童监测部分介绍了临床检查、血气异常、酸碱紊乱及氧合不足和通气障碍的评估；在治疗中描述了氧疗、人工气道、吸入气体、正压呼吸支持、气管内插管和机械通气以及插管前后即刻短暂的人工通气；详细阐述了机械通气，其中包括呼吸机管理的基本概念、无创机械通气、有创机械通气及附加的通气方式等内容。

The term *respiratory distress* is used to indicate signs and symptoms of abnormal respiratory pattern. A child with nasal flaring, tachypnea, chest wall retractions, stridor, grunting, dyspnea, and wheezing has respiratory distress. Taken together, the magnitude of these findings is used to judge clinical severity. Nasal flaring is nonspecific, but the other signs are useful in localizing the site of pathology (see Chapter 400). *Respiratory failure* is defined as inability of the lungs to provide sufficient oxygen (hypoxic respiratory failure) or remove carbon dioxide (ventilator failure) to meet metabolic demands. Therefore, whereas respiratory distress is determined by a clinical impression, the diagnosis of respiratory failure is indicated by inadequacy of oxygenation or of ventilation, or both. Respiratory distress can occur in patients without respiratory disease, and respiratory failure can occur in patients without respiratory distress.

RESPIRATORY DISTRESS

A careful physical examination must be performed when managing a child in respiratory distress. **Nasal flaring**, although nonspecific, is an extremely important sign of distress in infants. It may indicate discomfort, pain, fatigue, or breathing difficulty. The state of **responsiveness** is another crucial sign. Lethargy, disinterest in surroundings, and poor cry are suggestive of exhaustion, hypercarbia, and impending respiratory failure. Abnormalities of the rate and depth of **breathing** can occur with both pulmonary and nonpulmonary causes of respiratory distress. In diseases of decreased lung compliance, such as pneumonia and pulmonary edema, breathing is characteristically rapid and shallow

(decreased tidal volume). In obstructive airway diseases, such as asthma and laryngotracheitis, breathing is deep with increased tidal volume, but less rapid. Rapid and deep breathing without other respiratory signs should alert the physician to possible nonpulmonary or nonthoracic causes of respiratory distress, such as response to metabolic acidosis (e.g., diabetic ketoacidosis, renal tubular acidosis) or stimulation of the respiratory center (e.g., encephalitis, ingestion of central nervous system stimulants). Chest wall, suprasternal, and subcostal **retractions** are manifestations of increased inspiratory effort, weak chest wall, or both. Inspiratory **stridor** indicates airway obstruction above the thoracic inlet, whereas expiratory wheezing results from airway obstruction below the thoracic inlet. **Grunting** is most commonly heard in diseases with decreased functional residual capacity (e.g., pneumonia, pulmonary edema) and peripheral airway obstruction (e.g., bronchiolitis).

Respiratory Disease Manifesting as Respiratory Distress

Clinical examination is important in localizing the site of pathology (see Chapter 400). Extrathoracic airway obstruction occurs anywhere above the thoracic inlet. Inspiratory stridor, suprasternal, chest wall, and subcostal retractions; and prolongation of inspiration are hallmarks of extrathoracic airway obstruction. By comparison, features of intrathoracic airway obstruction are prolongation of expiration and expiratory wheezing. Typical manifestations of alveolar interstitial pathology are rapid, shallow respirations, chest wall retractions, and grunting. The site of pathology can be localized and the differential diagnosis

Table 89.1	Typical Localizing Signs for Pulmonary Pathology		
SITE OF PATHOLOGY	**RESPIRATORY RATE**	**RETRACTIONS**	**AUDIBLE SOUNDS**
Extrathoracic airway	↑	↑↑↑↑	Stridor
Intrathoracic extrapulmonary	↑	↑↑	Wheezing
Intrathoracic intrapulmonary	↑↑	↑↑	Wheezing
Alveolar interstitial	↑↑↑	↑↑↑	Grunting

established on the basis of the clinical signs and symptoms (Tables 89.1 and 89.2).

Respiratory Distress Without Respiratory Disease

Although respiratory distress most frequently results from diseases of lungs, airways, and chest wall, pathology in other organ systems can manifest as respiratory distress and lead to misdiagnosis and inappropriate management (Table 89.3). Respiratory distress resulting from heart failure or diabetic ketoacidosis may be misdiagnosed as asthma and improperly treated with albuterol, resulting in worsened hemodynamic state or ketoacidosis. Careful history and physical examination provide essential clues in avoiding misdiagnosis.

Cardiovascular Disease Manifesting as Respiratory Distress

A child with cardiovascular pathology may present with respiratory distress caused by either *decreased lung compliance* or *cardiogenic shock* (Table 89.4). Diseases that result in increased pulmonary arterial blood flow (e.g., left-to-right shunts) or increased pulmonary venous pressure (e.g., left ventricular dysfunction from hypertension or myocarditis, obstructed total anomalous pulmonary venous return) cause an increase in pulmonary capillary pressure and transudation of fluid into the pulmonary interstitium and alveoli. The increased pulmonary blood and water content lead to decreased lung compliance and result in rapid shallow breathing.

It is important to recognize that interstitial lung edema cannot only manifest as alveolar fluid, but as small airway obstruction as well. **Wheezing** as a sign of congestive cardiac disease is common in infants and young children and should be recognized. Patients with cardiac lesions, resulting in low cardiac output, often present in shock. For example, obstructive lesions of left side of the heart and acquired or congenital cardiomyopathy result in decreased perfusion and metabolic acidosis, as well as respiratory distress because of chemoreceptor and baroreceptor stimulation. The likelihood of a particular cardiovascular illness manifesting as respiratory distress depends on age at presentation (Table 89.5).

Neurologic Disease Manifesting as Respiratory Distress

Central nervous system (CNS) dysfunction can lead to alterations in respiratory patterns and manifest as respiratory distress. Increased intracranial pressure (ICP) may manifest as respiratory distress. Early rise in intracranial pressure (ICP) results in stimulation of respiratory centers, leading to increases in the rate (**tachypnea**) and depth (**hyperpnea**) of respiration. The resultant decrease in arterial blood partial pressure of carbon dioxide ($PaCO_2$) and elevation of cerebrospinal fluid (CSF) pH lead to cerebral vasoconstriction and amelioration of intracranial hypertension. Stereotypical respiratory patterns are associated with dysfunction at multiple levels of the brain. Cerebral hemisphere and midbrain lesions result in hyperpnea as well as tachypnea. In such situations, arterial blood gas (ABG) measurements typically show respiratory alkalosis without hypoxemia. Pathology affecting the pons and medulla manifests as irregular breathing patterns such as **apneustic breathing** (prolonged inspiration with brief expiratory periods), **Cheyne-Stokes breathing** (alternate periods of rapid and slow breathing), and irregular, ineffective breathing or apnea (Table 89.6). Along with respiratory changes, other manifestations of CNS dysfunction and

Table 89.2	Examples of Anatomic Sites of Lesions Causing Respiratory Failure
LUNG	**RESPIRATORY PUMP**

LUNG	**RESPIRATORY PUMP**
CENTRAL AIRWAY OBSTRUCTION	
Choanal atresia	**THORACIC CAGE**
Tonsilloadenoidal hypertrophy	Kyphoscoliosis
Retropharyngeal/peritonsillar abscess	Diaphragmatic hernia
Laryngomalacia	Flail chest
Epiglottitis	Eventration of diaphragm
Vocal cord paralysis	Asphyxiating thoracic dystrophy
Laryngotracheitis	Prune-belly syndrome
Subglottic stenosis	Dermatomyositis
Vascular ring/pulmonary sling	Abdominal distention
Mediastinal mass	
Foreign body aspiration	
Obstructive sleep apnea	
PERIPHERAL AIRWAY OBSTRUCTION	
Asthma	**BRAINSTEM**
Bronchiolitis	Arnold-Chiari malformation
Foreign body aspiration	Central hypoventilation syndrome
Aspiration pneumonia	CNS depressants
Cystic fibrosis	Trauma
α_1-Antitrypsin deficiency	Increased intracranial pressure
	CNS infections
ALVEOLAR-INTERSTITIAL DISEASE	
Lobar pneumonia	**SPINAL CORD**
ARDS, hyaline membrane disease	Trauma
Interstitial pneumonia	Transverse myelitis
Hydrocarbon pneumonia	Spinal muscular atrophy
Pulmonary hemorrhage/hemosiderosis	Poliomyelitis
	Tumor/abscess
	Acute flaccid myelitis
	NEUROMUSCULAR
	Phrenic nerve injury
	Birth trauma
	Infant botulism
	Guillain-Barré syndrome
	Muscular dystrophy
	Myasthenia gravis
	Organophosphate poisoning

ARDS, Acute respiratory distress syndrome; CNS, central nervous system.

increased ICP may be present, such as focal neurologic signs, pupillary changes, hypertension, and bradycardia (see Chapter 85). Occasionally, severe CNS dysfunction can result in **neurogenic pulmonary edema** and respiratory distress, which may follow excessive sympathetic discharge resulting in increased pulmonary venous hydrostatic pressure as well as increased pulmonary capillary permeability. **Central neurogenic hyperventilation** is characteristically observed in CNS involvement by illnesses such as urea cycle defects and encephalitis. **Bradycardia** and **apnea** may be caused by CNS-depressant medications, poisoning, prolonged hypoxia, trauma, or infection (see Table 89.2).

Table 89.3	Nonpulmonary Causes of Respiratory Distress	
SYSTEM	**EXAMPLE(S)**	**MECHANISM(S)**
Cardiovascular	Left-to-right shunt Congestive heart failure Cardiogenic shock	↑ Pulmonary blood/water content Metabolic acidosis Baroreceptor stimulation
Central nervous	Increased intracranial pressure Encephalitis Neurogenic pulmonary edema Toxic encephalopathy	Stimulation of brainstem respiratory centers
Metabolic	Diabetic ketoacidosis Organic acidemia Hyperammonemia	Stimulation of central and peripheral chemoreceptors
Renal	Renal tubular acidosis Hypertension	Stimulation of central and peripheral chemoreceptors Left ventricular dysfunction → increased pulmonary blood/water content
Sepsis	Toxic shock syndrome Meningococcemia	Cytokine stimulation of respiratory centers Baroreceptor stimulation from shock Metabolic acidosis

Table 89.4	Cardiovascular Pathology Manifesting as Respiratory Distress

I. **Decreased lung compliance**
  A. Left-to-right shunts
    1. Ventricular septal defect, atrial septal defect, patent ductus arteriosus, atrioventricular canal, truncus arteriosus
    2. Cerebral or hepatic arteriovenous fistula
  B. Ventricular failure
    1. Left heart obstructive lesions
      a. Aortic stenosis
      b. Coarctation of the aorta
      c. Mitral stenosis
      d. Interrupted aortic arch
      e. Hypoplastic left heart syndrome
    2. Myocardial infarction
      a. Anomalous left coronary artery arising from the pulmonary artery
    3. Hypertension
      a. Acute glomerulonephritis
    4. Inflammatory/infectious
      a. Myocarditis
      b. Pericardial effusion
    5. Idiopathic
      a. Dilated cardiomyopathy
      b. Hypertrophic obstructive cardiomyopathy
  C. Pulmonary venous obstruction
    1. Total anomalous pulmonary venous return with obstruction
    2. Cor triatriatum
II. **Shock resulting in metabolic acidosis**
  A. Left heart obstructive lesions
  B. Acute ventricular failure
    1. Myocarditis, myocardial infarction

Toxic Metabolic States Manifesting as Respiratory Distress

Direct stimulation of respiratory centers resulting in respiratory alkalosis is encountered in intoxication involving agents such as salicylates and theophylline. Similarly, intoxication with general CNS stimulants, such

Table 89.5	Typical Chronology of Heart Disease Presentation in Children	
AGE	**MECHANISM**	**DISEASE**
Newborn (1–10 days)	↑ Arteriovenous pressure difference Ductal closure	Arteriovenous fistula (brain, liver) Single ventricle lesions or severe ventricular outflow obstruction
	Independent pulmonary and systemic blood flow Pulmonary venous obstruction	Transposition of the great arteries Total anomalous pulmonary venous return (TAPVR)
Young infant (1–6 mo)	↓ Pulmonary vascular resistance ↓ Pulmonary artery pressure	Left-to-right shunt Anomalous left coronary artery to the pulmonary artery
Any age	Rate disturbance Infection Abnormal cardiac myocytes Excess afterload	Tachy- or bradyarrhythmias Myocarditis, pericarditis Cardiomyopathy hypertension

as cocaine and amphetamines, may result in increased respiration. Presence of endogenous and exogenous toxins, such as organic acidemias, ingestion of methanol and ethylene glycol, and late stages of salicylism, cause metabolic acidosis and compensatory hyperventilation, which can manifest as respiratory distress. ABG measurements show decreased pH and compensatory hypocarbia with normal oxygenation. Metabolic disorders causing hyperammonemia, on the other hand, cause respiratory alkalosis (decreased $PaCO_2$ with increased pH) because ammonia stimulates the respiratory centers. Carbon monoxide and cyanide poisoning or methemoglobinemia may produce respiratory distress.

Other Nonpulmonary Entities Manifesting as Respiratory Distress

Sepsis and **septic shock** may cause an acute respiratory distress syndrome (ARDS) with hypovolemic stimulation of baroreceptors, cytokine stimulation of respiratory centers, and lactic acidosis. Other indirect causes of lung injury include systemic inflammatory conditions, trauma, transfusion-related acute lung injury, and pancreatitis. Similarly, renal disease may manifest as respiratory distress by causing metabolic acidosis (e.g., renal tubular acidosis or renal failure) or hypertensive left ventricular failure and fluid overload.

RESPIRATORY FAILURE

Respiratory failure occurs when oxygenation and ventilation are insufficient to meet the metabolic demands of the body. Respiratory failure may result from an abnormality in (1) lung and airways, (2) chest wall and muscles of breathing, or (3) central and peripheral chemoreceptors. Clinical manifestations depend largely on the site of pathology. Although respiratory failure is traditionally defined as respiratory dysfunction resulting in arterial partial pressure of oxygen (PaO_2) <60 mm Hg when breathing room air and $PaCO_2$ >50 mm Hg resulting in acidosis, the patient's general state, respiratory effort, and potential for impending exhaustion are more important indicators than ABG values.

The Berlin definition of ARDS was once used to describe pediatric patients with ARDS, even though the pathophysiology is different between children and adults. The current pediatric definition differs in chest imaging findings, definition of oxygenation, consideration of both noninvasive and invasive mechanical ventilation, and consideration of special populations (Table 89.7 and Fig. 89.1).

Pathophysiology

Respiratory failure can be classified into *hypoxic* respiratory failure (failure of oxygenation) and *hypercarbic* respiratory failure (failure of

Table 89.6	Respiratory Patterns in Neurologic Disease	
INJURY	**PATTERN***	**COMMENTS**

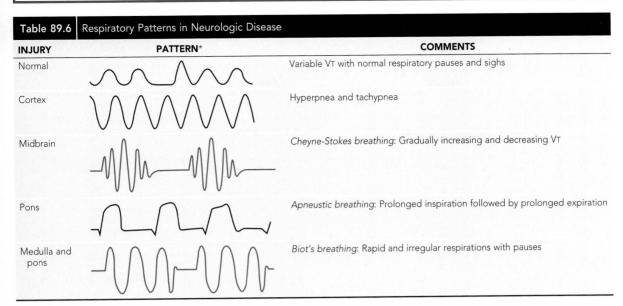

Normal		Variable VT with normal respiratory pauses and sighs
Cortex		Hyperpnea and tachypnea
Midbrain		*Cheyne-Stokes breathing*: Gradually increasing and decreasing VT
Pons		*Apneustic breathing*: Prolonged inspiration followed by prolonged expiration
Medulla and pons		*Biot's breathing*: Rapid and irregular respirations with pauses

*Lung volume vs time.
VT, Tidal volume.

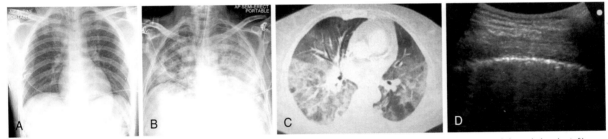

Fig. 89.1 Acute respiratory distress syndrome (ARDS). **A,** Normal chest radiograph. **B,** Chest radiograph demonstrating bilateral alveolar infiltrates consistent with ARDS. (**C,** Chest CT showing bilateral pneumonitis and consolidation with air bronchograms consistent with ARDS, **D,** Lung ultrasonogram illustrating smooth pleural line, absence of horizontal A lines, and presence of vertical B lines suggestive of ARDS. *(Modified from MacSweeney R, McAuley DF: Acute respiratory distress syndrome, Lancet 388:2416–2430, 2016, Fig 3.)*

ventilation). Systemic venous (pulmonary arterial) blood is arterialized after equilibration with alveolar gas in the pulmonary capillaries and is carried back to the heart by pulmonary veins. The ABG is influenced by the composition of inspired gas, effectiveness of alveolar ventilation, pulmonary capillary perfusion, and diffusion capacity of the alveolar capillary membrane. Abnormality in any of these steps can result in respiratory failure. **Hypoxic respiratory failure** results from intrapulmonary shunting and venous admixture or insufficient diffusion of oxygen from alveoli into pulmonary capillaries. This physiology can be caused by small airways obstruction, increased barriers to diffusion (e.g., interstitial edema, fibrosis), and conditions in which alveoli are collapsed or filled with fluid (e.g., ARDS, pneumonia, atelectasis, pulmonary edema). In most cases, hypoxic respiratory failure is associated with decreased functional residual capacity and can be managed by lung volume recruitment with positive pressure ventilation. **Hypercarbic respiratory failure** is caused by decreased minute ventilation (i.e., tidal volume multiplied by respiratory rate). This physiology can result from centrally mediated disorders of respiratory drive, increased dead space ventilation, or obstructive airways disease. *Hypoxic and hypercarbic respiratory failure may coexist as a combined failure of oxygenation and ventilation.*

Ventilation-Perfusion Mismatch

For exchange of O_2 and CO_2 to occur, alveolar gas must be exposed to blood in pulmonary capillaries. Both ventilation and perfusion are lower in nondependent areas of the lung and higher in dependent areas. The difference in perfusion ($\dot{Q}$) is greater than the difference in ventilation ($\dot{V}$). Perfusion in excess of ventilation results in incomplete arterialization of systemic venous (pulmonary arterial) blood and is referred to as **venous admixture**. Perfusion of unventilated areas is referred to as **intrapulmonary shunting** of systemic venous blood to systemic arterial circulation. Conversely, ventilation that is in excess of perfusion is wasted; that is, it does not contribute to gas exchange and is referred to as **dead space ventilation**. Dead space ventilation results in return of greater amounts of atmospheric gas (which has not participated in gas exchange and has negligible CO_2) back to the atmosphere during exhalation. The respiratory dead space is divided into the anatomic dead space and the alveolar dead space. The *anatomic dead space* includes the conducting airways from the nasopharynx to the terminal bronchioles, ends at the alveoli, and has no contact with the pulmonary capillary bed. The *alveolar dead space* refers to areas of the lung where alveoli are ventilated but not perfused. Under normal conditions, this physiology usually occurs in West zone I, where alveolar pressure is greater than pulmonary

Table 89.7	Pediatric Acute Respiratory Distress Syndrome (PARDS) Definition	
	BERLIN DEFINITION	**PARDS**
Age	Adults and children	Excludes patients with perinatal-related lung disease
Timing	Within 1 wk of known clinical insult or new or worsening respiratory symptoms	Within 1 wk of a known clinical insult
Origin of edema	Respiratory failure not fully explained by cardiac failure or fluid overload. Need objective assessment (e.g., echocardiography) to exclude hydrostatic edema, even if no risk factor present.	Respiratory failure not fully explained by cardiac failure or fluid overload
Chest imaging[a]	Bilateral opacities not fully explained by effusions, lobar/lung collapse, or nodules. (Illustrative clinical cases and chest radiographs have been provided.)	Chest imaging findings of new infiltrate(s) consistent with acute pulmonary parenchymal disease

Oxygenation[b]
  Mild
  Moderate
  Severe
	200 mm Hg < PaO_2/FIO_2 ≤300 mm Hg with PEEP, or CPAP ≥5 cm H_2O[c]
	100 mm Hg < PaO_2/FIO_2 ≤200 mm Hg with PEEP ≥5 cm H_2O
	PaO_2/FIO_2 <100 mm Hg with PEEP ≥5 cm H_2O
		Noninvasive mechanical ventilation:
		  PARDS (No severity stratification)
		  Full face-mask bilevel ventilation or CPAP >5 cm H_2O[e]
		  PF ratio <300
		  SF ratio <264[d]
		Invasive mechanical ventilation[f]:
		  Mild: 4 < OI <8, or 5 < OSI <7.5[d]
		  Moderate: 8 < OI <16, or 7.5 < OSI <12.3[d]
		  Severe: OI >16, or OSI >12.3[d]

In addition to the above, the Pediatric Acute Lung Injury Consensus Conference Group added definitions for special populations, including cyanotic heart disease, chronic lung disease, and left ventricular function.

[a]Chest radiograph or CT scan in Berlin criteria only.
[b]If altitude is >1,000 m, the correction factor should be calculated as follows: PaO_2/FIO_2 × Barometric pressure/760.
[c]This may be delivered noninvasively in the mild acute respiratory distress syndrome group.
[d]Use PaO_2-based metric when available. If PaO_2 not available, wean FIO_2 to maintain SpO_2 <97% to calculate OSI or SF ratio.
[e]For nonintubated patients treated with supplemental oxygen or nasal modes of noninvasive ventilation, refer to reference below for "At Risk Criteria."
[f]ARDS severity groups stratified by OI or OSI should not be applied to children with chronic lung disease who normally receive invasive mechanical ventilation or children with cyanotic heart disease.
CPAP, Continuous positive airway pressure; FIO_2, fraction of inspired oxygen; PaO_2, partial pressure of arterial oxygen; PEEP, positive end-expiratory pressure. OI, oxygenation index; OSI, oxygen saturation index.
Adapted from Pediatric Acute Lung Injury Consensus Conference Group, Pediatric Acute Respiratory Distress Syndrome: Consensus recommendations from the Pediatric Acute Lung Injury Consensus Conference, Pediatr Crit Care Med 16;428–439, 2015.

capillary pressure. Under clinical conditions, this physiology may result from dynamic hyperinflation, high levels of positive end-expiratory pressure (PEEP), or large tidal volume in ventilated patients. Additionally, decreased pulmonary artery perfusion from pulmonary embolism or decreased cardiac output and hypovolemia can result in alveolar dead space. The end result is a decrease in mixed expired CO_2 ($PECO_2$) and an increase in the $PaCO_2 - PECO_2$ gradient. Dead space as a fraction of tidal volume (VD/VT) is calculated as:

$$(PaCO_2 - PECO_2) \div PaCO_2$$

Normal VD/VT is approximately 0.33. Venous admixture and intrapulmonary shunting predominantly affect oxygenation, resulting in a alveolar oxygen (PAO_2) to PaO_2 (A-aO_2) gradient without elevation in $PaCO_2$. This physiology is caused by greater ventilation of perfused areas, which is sufficient to normalize $PaCO_2$ but not PaO_2 because of their respective dissociation curves. The relative straight-line relationship of the hemoglobin-CO_2 dissociation allows for averaging of capillary PCO_2 ($PcCO_2$) from hyperventilated and hypoventilated areas. Because the association between oxygen tension and hemoglobin saturation plateaus with increasing PaO_2, the decreased hemoglobin-O_2 saturation in poorly ventilated areas cannot be compensated for by well-ventilated areas where hemoglobin-O_2 saturation has already reached near-maximum. This physiology results in decreased arterial oxyhemoglobin saturation (SaO_2) and PaO_2. Elevation of $PaCO_2$ in such situations is indicative of coincident alveolar hypoventilation. Examples of diseases leading to venous admixture include asthma and aspiration pneumonia, and those of intrapulmonary shunt include lobar pneumonia and ARDS.

Diffusion

Even if ventilation and perfusion are matched, gas exchange requires diffusion across the interstitial space between alveoli and pulmonary

capillaries. Under normal conditions, there is sufficient time for the pulmonary capillary blood to equilibrate with alveolar gas across the interstitial space. When the interstitial space is filled with inflammatory cells or fluid, diffusion is impaired. Because the diffusion capacity of CO_2 is 20 times greater than that of O_2, diffusion defects manifest as hypoxemia rather than hypercarbia. Even with the administration of 100% oxygen, PAO_2 increases to approximately 660 mm Hg from 100 mm Hg at sea level, and the concentration gradient for diffusion of O_2 is increased by only 6.6 times. Therefore, with diffusion defects, lethal hypoxemia will set in before clinically significant CO_2 retention results. In fact, in such situations, $PaCO_2$ is often decreased because of the hyperventilation that accompanies hypoxemia. Presence of hypercarbia in diseases that impair diffusion is indicative of alveolar hypoventilation from coexisting airway obstruction, exhaustion, or CNS depression. Examples of disease that impair diffusion are interstitial pneumonia, ARDS, scleroderma, and pulmonary lymphangiectasia.

MONITORING A CHILD IN RESPIRATORY DISTRESS AND RESPIRATORY FAILURE
Clinical Examination

It cannot be overemphasized that clinical observation is the most important component of monitoring. The presence and magnitude of abnormal clinical findings, their progression with time, and their temporal relation to therapeutic interventions serve as guides to diagnosis and management (see Chapter 400). As much as possible, the child with respiratory distress or failure should be observed in the position of greatest comfort and in the least threatening environment.

Pulse oximetry is the most commonly used technique to monitor oxygenation. Noninvasive and safe, it is the standard of care in bedside monitoring of children during transport, procedural sedation, surgery, and critical illness. It indirectly measures arterial hemoglobin-O_2

saturation by differentiating oxyhemoglobin from deoxygenated hemoglobin using their respective light absorption at wavelengths of 660 nm (red) and 940 nm (infrared). A pulsatile circulation is required to enable detection of oxygenated blood entering the capillary bed. Percentage of arterial oxyhemoglobin is reported as SaO_2; however, the correct description is *oxyhemoglobin saturation as measured by pulse oximetry* (SpO_2). Such precision is needed because SpO_2 may not always reflect SaO_2. It is important to be familiar with the hemoglobin-O_2 dissociation curve (see Chapter 400) to estimate PaO_2 at a given oxyhemoglobin saturation. Because of the shape of the hemoglobin-O_2 dissociation curve, changes in PaO_2 above 70 mm Hg are not readily identified by pulse oximetry. Also, at the same PaO_2, there may be significant change in SpO_2 at a different blood pH value. In most situations, SpO_2 >95% is a reasonable goal, especially in emergency care. In some adult studies of ARDS, the recommended saturation is 94–96% to avoid oxygen toxicity. There are exceptions, such as in patients with single-ventricle cardiac lesions, in whom the pulmonary and systemic circulations are receiving blood flow from the same ventricle (e.g., after Norwood procedure for hypoplastic left heart syndrome), or with large left-to-right shunts (e.g., ventricular septal defect, patent ductus arteriosus). In these types of pathophysiologic situations, a lower SpO_2 is desired to avoid excessive blood flow to the lungs and pulmonary edema from the pulmonary vasodilatory effects of oxygen, in the patient with a single ventricle, diverting blood flow away from the systemic circulation. Because most commercially available pulse oximeters recognize all types of hemoglobin as either oxyhemoglobin or deoxygenated hemoglobin, they provide inaccurate information in the presence of carboxyhemoglobin and methemoglobin. In carbon monoxide poisoning, **carboxyhemoglobin** absorbs light in the same (red) wavelength as oxyhemoglobin, leading to overestimation of oxygen saturation. **Methemoglobin** absorbs light in both the oxygenated and deoxygenated wavelengths, which can cause either an overestimation or underestimation of oxygen saturation. Data suggest that increasing methemoglobin concentrations tend to drive SpO_2 toward 85%, no matter the actual percent of oxyhemoglobin. At lower methemoglobin levels, the pulse oximetry reading is falsely low, whereas high levels lead to a falsely high pulse oximetry reading. Newer pulse oximeters may have the ability to distinguish dyshemoglobinemias and to prevent false readings, but these are not currently in widespread use. It should be recognized that dangerous levels of hypercarbia may exist in patients with ventilatory failure, who have satisfactory SpO_2 if they are receiving supplemental oxygen. Pulse oximetry should not be the only monitoring method in patients with primary ventilatory failure, such as neuromuscular weakness and CNS depression. It is also unreliable in patients with poor perfusion and poor pulsatile flow to the extremities. Despite these limitations, pulse oximetry is a noninvasive, easily applicable, and effective means of evaluating the percentage of oxyhemoglobin in most patients.

Volumetric capnography (end-tidal CO_2 [$PetCO_2$] measurement) is helpful in non-invasively determining the effectiveness of ventilation and pulmonary circulation. The $PetCO_2$ can be used to determine the alveolar dead space fraction and is calculated as follows: [($PaCO_2$ − $PetCO_2$)/$PaCO_2$]. Changes in the alveolar dead space fraction usually correlate well with changes in the gradient of $PaCO_2$ and $PetCO_2$ ($PaCO_2$ − $PetCO_2$). Thus a change in $PaCO_2$ − $PetCO_2$ can be used as an index of changes in alveolar dead space. In healthy children the gradient is smaller than in adults and is usually <3 mm Hg. Diseases resulting in increased alveolar dead space (e.g., dynamic hyperinflation) or decreased pulmonary blood flow (e.g., pulmonary embolism, low cardiac output) lead to decreases in $PetCO_2$ and an increase in $PaCO_2$ − $PetCO_2$. $PetCO_2$ alone may overestimate adequacy of ventilation.

Blood Gas Abnormalities

Arterial blood gas analysis offers valuable assistance in diagnosis, monitoring, and management of a child in respiratory distress and failure. Because of technical difficulties in obtaining an arterial sample in children, a *capillary blood gas* (CBG) sample is most often obtained in emergency situations. A properly arterialized CBG sample obtained by warming the digit and obtaining free-flowing blood is acceptable. The blood sample needs to be processed without delay. CBG provides

a good estimate of $PaCO_2$ and arterial pH, but less so for PaO_2. In patients who mainly require monitoring of ventilation (especially those whose oxygenation is being monitored with pulse oximetry) a *venous blood gas* sample provides reliable estimate of arterial pH and $PaCO_2$ values, provided tissue perfusion is reasonably adequate. Venous PCO_2 ($PvCO_2$) is approximately 6 mm Hg higher and pH approximately 0.03 lower than the arterial values. PvO_2 has a poor correlation with PaO_2. Mixed venous O_2 saturation obtained from a central venous catheter in the right atrium is an excellent marker of the balance between oxygen delivery and oxygen consumption. In patients with a constant arterial O_2 content and O_2 consumption, mixed venous O_2 saturation offers valuable information about cardiac output.

Blood gas analysis is important not only for determining the adequacy of oxygenation and ventilation but also for determining site of respiratory pathology and planning treatment (see Chapter 400). Briefly, in the presence of pure alveolar hypoventilation (e.g., airway obstruction above carina, decreased CO_2 responsiveness, neuromuscular weakness), the blood gas will show respiratory acidosis with an elevated $PaCO_2$ but a relative sparing of oxygenation. $\dot{V}/\dot{Q}$ mismatch (peripheral airway obstruction, bronchopneumonia) will be reflected in increasing hypoxemia and variable levels of $PaCO_2$ (low, normal, high) depending on severity of disease. Intrapulmonary right-to-left shunting and diffusion defects (alveolar-interstitial diseases such as pulmonary edema, ARDS) will be associated with a large A-aO_2 gradient and hypoxemia with relative sparing of CO_2 elimination, unless there is coincident fatigue or CNS depression.

Acid-Base Abnormalities

It is crucial to analyze the magnitude and appropriateness of changes in pH, $PaCO_2$, and bicarbonate concentration ([HCO_3^-]) because they provide useful clues to the underlying pathophysiology and presence of more than 1 disorder. To do so, it is useful to assume baseline values of pH 7.40, $PaCO_2$ 40 mm Hg, and [HCO_3^-] 24 mEq/L. Newborns have lower renal threshold for bicarbonate and therefore have slightly different baseline values of pH 7.38, $PaCO_2$ 35 mm Hg, and [HCO_3^-] 20 mEq/L.

Metabolic Acidosis With Respiratory Compensation

Patients with metabolic acidosis have decreased pH resulting from decreased serum [HCO_3^-]. Chemoreceptor stimulation results in hyperventilation and respiratory compensation that may clinically manifest as respiratory distress. Normal compensation does not completely correct the pH but rather minimizes a change in pH that would otherwise occur without compensation. The adequacy of respiratory compensation is judged by the extent of the decline in $PaCO_2$ in response to the decline in [HCO_3^-] or pH. A normal compensation for metabolic acidosis results in a fall in $PaCO_2$ by 1.2 mm Hg for every 1 mEq/L fall in [HCO_3^-]. The most commonly used method to analyze the adequacy of respiratory compensation is Winter's formula:

$$PaCO_2 = ([HCO_3^-] \times 1.5) + 8 \pm 2$$

A quick method is to look at the last 2 digits of pH (provided it is not <7.10), which should be within 2 mm Hg of $PaCO_2$. For example, pH 7.27, $PaCO_2$ 26 mm Hg, and [HCO_3^-] 12 mEq/L represents metabolic acidosis with a normal respiratory compensation response. On the other hand, pH 7.15, $PaCO_2$ 30 mm Hg, and [HCO_3^-] 10 mEq/L constitutes metabolic acidosis with inadequate respiratory compensation. The reasons for inadequate compensation include decreased CO_2 responsiveness (e.g., narcotic poisoning, cerebral edema), abnormalities of lungs and airways, or neuromuscular weakness. A decrease in $PaCO_2$ that is greater than what could be expected as a normal compensatory response to metabolic acidosis is indicative of a mixed disorder. A pH 7.20, $PaCO_2$ 15 mm Hg, and [HCO_3^-] 7.5 mEq/L represents metabolic acidosis with a concomitant respiratory alkalosis because the decline in $PaCO_2$ is greater than what can be expected as normal compensation. Combination of metabolic acidosis and respiratory alkalosis is often encountered in serious conditions such as cardiogenic shock (e.g., anxiety, stimulation of baroreceptors), sepsis, or toxic-metabolic states (e.g., salicylates, organic acidemia).

Respiratory Acidosis With Metabolic Compensation

Patients with respiratory acidosis have decreased pH as a result of elevated $PaCO_2$. An acute increase in $PaCO_2$ of 10 mm Hg results in a decrease in pH by 0.08. Thus a child with severe status asthmaticus and a $PaCO_2$ of 60 mm Hg will have blood pH of approximately 7.24. Chronically elevated (>3-5 days) $PaCO_2$ is accompanied by renal compensation and increase in serum $[HCO_3^-]$, limiting the fall in pH to 0.03 for every 10 mm Hg rise in $PaCO_2$. Thus an infant with bronchopulmonary dysplasia who has a basal $PaCO_2$ of 60 mm Hg will have blood pH of approximately 7.34. These findings are helpful in distinguishing acute from chronic changes in $PaCO_2$. Also, for a given level of CO_2 accumulation, a decrease in pH that is greater than expected is indicative of concomitant metabolic acidosis, and a decline in pH that is less than expected is caused by accompanying metabolic alkalosis.

Assessment of Oxygenation and Ventilation Deficits

For standardizing management, following clinical progress, and determining prognosis for patients with defects in oxygenation or ventilation, the following indicators have been proposed, each with its strengths and limitations:

A-aO_2 gradient is calculated by the subtraction, $PAO_2 - PaO_2$. For the comparison to be valid, both values must be taken at the same time and with the same fraction of oxygen in the inspired gas (FIO_2).

PaO_2/FiO_2 ratio (P/F) is calculated by dividing PaO_2 by FIO_2. In hypoxic respiratory failure, a PaO_2/FIO_2 value <300 mm Hg is consistent with acute lung injury, and a value <200 mm Hg is consistent with ARDS. Although the intent is to measure $\dot{V}/\dot{Q}$ mismatch, intrapulmonary shunt, and diffusion defect, the status of alveolar hypoventilation could have a significant impact on PaO_2/FIO_2.

SpO_2/FiO_2 ratio is a surrogate measure of oxygenation when PaO_2 is not available. It is calculated by dividing the pulse oximeter saturation by the FIO_2. P/F ratios of 200 mm Hg and 300 mm Hg correlate approximately with S/F ratios of 235 and 315 respectively. This relationship is most valid for SpO_2 values between 80% and 97%.

PaO_2/PAO_2 ratio is determined by dividing PaO_2 by PAO_2. The level of alveolar ventilation is accounted for in the calculation of PAO_2. Therefore, PaO_2/PAO_2 is more indicative of $\dot{V}/\dot{Q}$ mismatch and alveolar capillary integrity.

Oxygenation index (OI) is aimed at standardizing oxygenation to the level of therapeutic interventions, such as mean airway pressure (MAP) and FIO_2 used during mechanical ventilation, which are directed toward improving oxygenation. None of the indicators of oxygenation mentioned above takes into account the degree of positive pressure respiratory support.

$$OI = (MAP \times FIO_2 \times 100) \div PaO_2$$

The limitation of OI is that level of ventilation is not accounted for in the assessment.

Ventilation index (VI) is aimed at standardizing alveolar ventilation to the level of therapeutic interventions, such as peak inspiratory pressure (PIP), positive end-expiratory pressure (PEEP), and ventilator rate ([R] directed toward lowering $PaCO_2$.

$$VI = [R \times (PIP - PEEP) \times PaCO_2] \div 1000$$

MANAGEMENT

The goal of management for respiratory distress and respiratory failure is to ensure a patent airway and provide necessary support for adequate oxygenation of the blood and removal of CO_2. Compared with hypercapnia, **hypoxemia** is a life-threatening condition; therefore initial therapy for respiratory failure should be aimed at ensuring adequate oxygenation.

Oxygen Administration

Supplemental oxygen administration is the least invasive and most easily tolerated therapy for hypoxemic respiratory failure. **Nasal cannula** oxygen provides low levels of oxygen supplementation and is easy to administer. Oxygen is humidified in a bubble humidifier and delivered via nasal prongs inserted in to the nares. In children, a flow rate <5 L/min is most often used because of increasing nasal irritation with higher flow rates. A common formula for an estimation of the FIO_2 during use of a nasal cannula in older children and adults follows:

$$FIO_2 \text{ (as percentage)} = 21\% + [(\text{Nasal cannula flow (L/min)} \times 3)]$$

The typical FIO_2 value (expressed as percentage rather than fraction of 1) using this method is between 23% and 40%, although the FIO_2 varies according to the size of the child, the respiratory rate, and the volume of air moved with each breath. In a young child, because typical nasal cannula flow rates are a greater percentage of total minute ventilation, significantly higher FIO_2 may be provided. Alternately, a **simple mask** may be used, which consists of a mask with open side ports and a valveless oxygen source. Variable amounts of room air are entrained through the ports and around the side of the mask, depending on the fit, size, and minute volume of the child. Oxygen flow rates vary from 5-10 L/min, yielding typical FIO_2 values (expressed as percentage rather than fraction of 1) between 30% and 65%. If more precise delivery of oxygen is desired, other mask devices should be used.

A **Venturi mask** provides preset FIO_2 through a mask and reservoir system by entraining precise flow rates of room air into the reservoir along with high-flow oxygen. The adapter at the end of each mask reservoir determines the flow rate of entrained room air and the subsequent FIO_2. (Adapters provide FIO_2 of 0.30-0.50.) Oxygen flow rates of 5-10 L/min are recommended to achieve the desired FIO_2 and to prevent rebreathing. Partial rebreather and non-rebreather masks use a reservoir bag attached to a mask to provide higher FIO_2. **Partial rebreather masks** have 2 open exhalation ports and contain a valveless oxygen reservoir bag. Some exhaled gas can mix with reservoir gas, although most exhaled gas exits the mask via the exhalation ports. Through these same ports, room air is entrained, and the partial rebreather mask can provide FIO_2 up to 0.60, for as long as oxygen flow is adequate to keep the bag from collapsing (typically 10-15 L/min). As with nasal cannulas, smaller children with smaller tidal volumes entrain less room air, and their FIO_2 values will be higher. **Non-rebreather masks** include 2 one-way valves, 1 between the oxygen reservoir bag and the mask and the other on 1 of the 2 exhalation ports. This arrangement minimizes mixing of exhaled and fresh gas and entrainment of room air during inspiration. The 2nd exhalation port has no valve, a safeguard to allow some room air to enter the mask in the event of disconnection from the oxygen source. A non-rebreather mask can provide FIO_2 up to 0.95. The use of a non-rebreather mask in conjunction with an oxygen blender allows delivery of FIO_2 between 0.50 and 0.95 (Table 89.8). When supplemental oxygen alone is inadequate to improve oxygenation, or when ventilation problems coexist, additional therapies may be necessary.

Airway Adjuncts

Maintenance of a patent airway is a critical step in maintaining adequate oxygenation and ventilation. Artificial pharyngeal airways may be useful in patients with oropharyngeal or nasopharyngeal airway obstruction

Table 89.8	Approximate Oxygen Delivery According to Device and Flow Rates in Infants and Older Children*	
DEVICE	**FLOW (L/min)**	**FiO_2 DELIVERED**
Nasal cannula	0.1-6	0.21-0.4
Simple face mask	5-10	0.4-0.6
Partial rebreather	6-15	0.55-0.7
Non-rebreather	6-15	0.7-0.95
Venturi mask	5-10	0.25-0.5
Hood/tent	7-12	0.21-1.0
High-flow systems	1-40	0.21-1.0

*Individual delivery varies and depends on the patient's size, respiratory rate, and volume moved with every breath.

and in those with neuromuscular weakness in whom inherent extrathoracic airway resistance contributes to respiratory compromise. An **oropharyngeal airway** is a stiff plastic spacer with grooves along each side that can be placed in the mouth to run from the teeth along the tongue to its base just above the vallecula. The spacer prevents the tongue from opposing the posterior pharynx and occluding the airway. Because the tip sits at the base of the tongue, it is usually not tolerated by patients who are awake or whose gag reflex is strong. The **nasopharyngeal airway**, or *nasal trumpet*, is a flexible tube that can be inserted into the nose to run from the nasal opening along the top of the hard and soft palate with the tip ending in the hypopharynx. It is useful in bypassing obstruction from enlarged adenoids or from contact of the soft palate with the posterior nasopharynx. Because it is inserted past the adenoids, a nasopharyngeal airway should be used with caution in patients with bleeding tendencies.

Inhaled Gases

Helium-oxygen mixture (heliox) is useful in overcoming airway obstruction and improving ventilation. Helium is much less dense and slightly more viscous than nitrogen. When substituted for nitrogen, helium helps maintain laminar flow across an obstructed airway, decreases airway resistance, and improves ventilation. It is especially helpful in diseases of large airways obstruction in which turbulent airflow is more common, such as acute laryngotracheobronchitis, subglottic stenosis, and vascular ring. It is also used in patients with severe status asthmaticus. To be effective, helium should be administered in concentrations of at least 60%, so associated hypoxemia may limit its use in patients requiring >40% oxygen.

Inhaled nitric oxide (iNO) is a powerful inhaled pulmonary vasodilator. Its use may improve pulmonary blood flow and $\dot{V}/\dot{Q}$ mismatch in patients with diseases that elevate pulmonary vascular resistance, such as occurs in persistent pulmonary hypertension of the newborn, primary pulmonary hypertension, and secondary pulmonary hypertension as a result of chronic excess pulmonary blood flow (e.g., ventriculoseptal defect) or collagen vascular diseases. iNO is administered in doses ranging from 5 to 20 parts per million of inspired gas. Although administration of iNO to unintubated patients is possible, it is usually administered to patients undergoing mechanical ventilation via an endotracheal tube, because of the need for precision in iNO dosing.

Positive Pressure Respiratory Support

Noninvasive positive pressure respiratory support is useful in treating both hypoxemic and hypoventilatory respiratory failure. Positive airway pressure helps with aeration of partially atelectatic or filled alveoli, prevention of alveolar collapse at end-exhalation, and increase in functional residual capacity (FRC). These actions improve pulmonary compliance and hypoxemia, as well as decrease intrapulmonary shunt. In addition, positive pressure ventilation is useful in preventing collapse of extrathoracic airways by maintaining positive airway pressure during inspiration. Improving compliance and overcoming airway resistance also improves tidal volume and therefore ventilation. A **high-flow nasal cannula** delivers gas flow at 4-16 L/min and up to 60 L/min, with newer systems for older children and adolescents, capable of providing significant **continuous positive airway pressure (CPAP)**. In this setting, the amount of CPAP provided is not quantifiable and varies with each patient, depending on the percentage of total inspiratory flow that is delivered from the cannula, airway anatomy, and degree of mouth breathing. In small children the relative amount of CPAP for a given flow is usually greater than in older children and may provide significant positive pressure. The FIO_2 can be adjusted by provision of gas flow through an oxygen blender. Another benefit of a high-flow nasal cannula system is the washout of CO_2 from the nasopharynx, which decreases rebreathing of CO_2 and dead space ventilation. When delivering high-flow air or oxygen, adequate humidification is essential, by using a separate heated humidification chamber. CPAP can also be provided through snugly fitting nasal prongs or a tight-fitting face mask attached to a mechanical ventilator or other positive pressure device. Noninvasive CPAP is most useful in diseases of mildly decreased lung compliance

and low FRC, such as atelectasis and pneumonia. Patients with diseases of extrathoracic airway obstruction, in which extrathoracic negative airway pressures during inspiration lead to airway narrowing (e.g., laryngotracheitis, obstructive sleep apnea, postextubation airway edema), may also benefit from CPAP. Potential risks include nasal irritation, hyperinflation from excessive CPAP in smaller patients, and abdominal distention from swallowed air.

Noninvasive positive airway pressure ventilation (NIPPV) provides positive airway pressure during exhalation, and bilevel modes can apply additional positive pressure during inspiration (see Chapter 89.1).

Endotracheal Intubation and Mechanical Ventilation

When hypoxemia or significant hypoventilation persists despite the interventions already described, endotracheal intubation and mechanical ventilation are indicated. Additional indications for intubation include maintaining airway patency in patients who have the potential for airway compromise, such as those with actual or potential neurologic deterioration, and in patients with hemodynamic instability.

Proper monitoring is essential to ensuring a safe and successful endotracheal intubation. Pulse oximetry, heart rate, and blood pressure monitoring are mandatory and should be forgone only in situations calling for emergency intubation. All necessary equipment, including bag-mask ventilation device, laryngoscope, endotracheal tube (ETT) with stylet, and suction equipment, must be available and working properly before the procedure of intubation. The proper internal diameter (ID) for the ETT can be estimated using the following formula:

$$ID = (Age [yr]/4) + 4$$

Table 89.9 provides average values for age, size, and depth of insertion for tracheal tubes. Preoxygenation of the patient with high FIO_2 is essential and will allow maximum procedure time before the onset of hypoxemia. Although intubation can be accomplished without sedation and pharmacologic paralysis in selected patients, the physiologic benefits of these measures to the patient as well as to the facilitation of the intubation usually far outweigh the risks. Administration of a sedative and analgesic followed by a paralytic agent is a common pharmacologic regimen for facilitating intubation. In fact, sedation and paralysis with neuromuscular blocking agents should be considered standard unless contraindicated. The particular type and dose of each agent often depends on the underlying disease and clinician preference. Table 89.10 lists commonly used agents. *Dexmedetomidine* has been a standard sedating agent for maintenance during mechanical ventilation. An alternative to this pharmacologic approach is **rapid sequence intubation**, used when

Table 89.9	Average Size and Depth Dimensions for Tracheal Tubes		
PATIENT AGE	**INTERNAL DIAMETER (mm)**	**OROTRACHEAL DEPTH (cm)**	**NASOTRACHEAL DEPTH (cm)**
Premature	2.0-3.0	8-9	9-10
Full-term neonate	3.0-3.5	10	11
6 mo	4.0	11	13
12-24 mo	4.5	13-14	16-17
4 yr	5.0	15	17-18
6 yr	5.5	17	19-20
8 yr	6.0	19	21-22
10 yr	6.5	20	22-23
12 yr	7.0	21	23-24
14 yr	7.5	22	24-25
Adult	8.0-9.0	23-25	25-28

Table 89.10	Medications Commonly Used for Intubation			
DRUG	**DOSE**	**ONSET (min)**	**DURATION (min)**	**COMMENTS**
SEDATIVES/ANESTHETICS				
Midazolam	0.1 mg/kg IV	3-5	60-120	Amnesia Respiratory depression
Lorazepam	0.1 mg/kg IV	3-5	120-240	Amnesia Respiratory depression
Ketamine	1-2 mg/kg IV 4-6 mg/kg IM	2-3	10-15	↑ HR, BP, and ICP Bronchodilation
Propofol	1-3 mg/kg IV	0.5-2	10-15	↓ BP Apnea
Thiopental	4-7 mg/kg IV	0.5-1	5-10	↓ BP Apnea
ANALGESICS				
Fentanyl	2-5 µg/kg IV	3-5	30-90	Respiratory depression Chest wall rigidity
Morphine	0.1 mg/kg IV	5-15	120-240	↓ BP Respiratory depression
NEUROMUSCULAR BLOCKING AGENTS				
Vecuronium	0.1 mg/kg IV	2-3	30-75	↑ HR Renal elimination
Rocuronium	0.6-1.2 mg/kg IV 1 mg/kg IM	5-15	15-60	↑ HR Renal elimination
Cisatracurium	0.1 mg/kg IV	2-3	25-30	Histamine release Nonrenal elimination

BP, Blood pressure; HR, heart rate; ICP, intracranial pressure; IM, intramuscularly; IV, intravenously.

endotracheal intubation is urgent, or the patient is suspected of having a full stomach and at increased risk of aspiration (see Chapter 81).

Once adequate sedation and/or paralysis have been achieved, ventilation should be assisted with a **bag-mask device**. After optimal preoxygenation, intubation can be performed. The clinician uses the dominant hand to open the patient's mouth and insert the laryngoscope blade gently along the tongue to its base. The airway opening can be visualized by applying lift up-and-away from the clinician, along the axis of the laryngoscope handle. When a *straight* (Miller) laryngoscope blade is used to visualize the glottis, the tip of the blade lifts the epiglottis anteriorly. When a *curved* (Macintosh) blade is used to visualize the glottis, the tip of the blade should be advanced into the vallecula and then lifted. Secretions often obscure visualizations at this step and should be suctioned clear. Once clear visualization of the vocal cords is accomplished, the ETT can be placed through the vocal cords. Rapid confirmation of ETT placement is essential and should be assessed by as many of the following steps as possible: presence of PetCO$_2$ determined by a monitor attached in-line with ETT; auscultation of both lung fields as well as the epigastrium for equal breath sounds; and, good air movement and evaluation of the abdomen for increasing distention. Adequate, bilateral chest expansion and misting inside the ETT with each breath confirm proper tube placement. An increasing heart rate, if heart rate has decreased during the attempt, and a rising or normal SpO$_2$ reading are suggestive of successful tube placement. Preoxygenation may significantly delay any drop in SpO$_2$ with improper tube placement, leading to a significant delay in its recognition. Confirmation of exhaled PetCO$_2$ is mandatory, using a disposable colorimetric CO$_2$ detector or with capnography. In situations of very low pulmonary perfusion, such as cardiac arrest, PetCO$_2$ may not be detected. A chest radiograph should also be obtained to confirm proper placement of the ETT, which should lie with the tip about halfway between the glottis and the carina (see Chapter 81).

Transient Manual Ventilation in Immediate Preintubation and Postintubation Periods

Establishment of supportive ventilation via bag-mask or bag-ETT is required before transport of the patient to a setting of continued critical care. The technique of manual ventilation should take into account the underlying pathology. Mechanical ventilation of patients with diseases characterized by low FRC (e.g., pneumonia, pulmonary edema, ARDS) should include the application of PEEP to prevent alveolar derecruitment. Lung volume recruitment can be accomplished with a PEEP valve on a self-inflating ventilation bag or by careful manipulation of exhaust gas using an anesthesia bag. Such diseases are also characterized by a short time constant for lung deflation and therefore are best managed with relatively small tidal volumes and high ventilation rates.

In contrast, diseases characterized by airway obstruction have prolonged deflation time constants and are therefore best managed with relatively slow rates and high tidal volumes.

Bibliography is available at Expert Consult.

89.1 Mechanical Ventilation

Ashok P. Sarnaik, Christian P. Bauerfeld, and Ajit A. Sarnaik

The decision to institute support with mechanical ventilation is based mainly on the need to assist lung function; supporting left ventricular (LV) performance and treating intracranial hypertension are additional indications. Although there are no absolute criteria for derangement of gas exchange, PaO$_2$ <60 mm Hg while breathing >60% oxygen, PaCO$_2$ >60 mm Hg, and pH <7.25 are often reasons to initiate mechanical ventilation. Clinical impressions of fatigue and impending exhaustion are also indications for ventilatory support, even in the presence of adequate gas exchange. Positive pressure ventilation is a powerful means of decreasing LV afterload, and it is used for this purpose in patients with cardiogenic shock resulting from LV dysfunction. Mechanical ventilation is also used in patients whose breathing is unreliable (e.g., unconscious patients, those with neuromuscular dysfunction) and when deliberate hyperventilation is desired, such as in patients with intracranial hypertension.

Mechanical ventilation is not intended to normalize gas exchange, nor is it a cure. The goals are to maintain sufficient oxygenation and ventilation to ensure tissue viability until the disease process that has compromised the patient's lung function has resolved, while minimizing any complications. Thus, PaO$_2$, PaCO$_2$, and pH levels are maintained in ranges that provide a safe environment for the patient, while protecting the lungs from damage caused by oxygen toxicity, pressure (**barotrauma**), tidal volume overdistention (**volutrauma**), **atelectrauma**, and cytokine release (**biotrauma**) (Figs. 89.2 and 89.3).

BASIC CONCEPTS OF VENTILATOR MANAGEMENT
Equation of Motion

A pressure gradient is required for air to move from one place to another. During natural spontaneous ventilation, inspiration results from generation of negative intrapleural pressure from contraction of the diaphragm and intercostal muscles, drawing air from the atmosphere across the airways into the alveoli. During mechanical ventilation, inspiration results from positive pressure created by compressed gases through the ventilator, which pushes air across the airways into alveoli. In both spontaneous and mechanical ventilation, exhalation results from alveolar pressure generated by the elastic recoil of the lung and the chest wall. Pressure necessary to move a given amount of air into the lung is determined by 2 factors: lung and chest wall elastance and airway resistance. Fig. 89.4 describes the relationship in pressure gradient, compliance, and resistance. *Elastance*—defined as the change in pressure (ΔP) divided by the change in volume (ΔV)—refers to the property of a substance to oppose deformation. It is opposite of *compliance* ($\Delta V \div \Delta P$), the property of a substance to allow distention or lengthening when subjected to pressure. Compliance (C) is therefore expressed as 1/elastance.

The pressure needed to overcome tissue elastance is measured in conditions in which there is no flow (at end-inspiration and end-expiration) and is therefore a reflection of static conditions in the lung. It is influenced by tidal volume (VT) and compliance ($P = \Delta V \div C$). It is increased with high VT and low compliance. This pressure gradient is used to calculate the static compliance of the respiratory system (C_{STAT}).

Resistance (R) refers to the opposition to generation of flow. It is measured as the amount of pressure needed to generate a unit of flow ($\Delta P \div \Delta Flow$). Pressure needed to overcome airway resistance is calculated as flow multiplied by resistance. Because this pressure is needed only when the flow is occurring through the airways, it is referred to as the *dynamic component*. Pressure to overcome flow-resistive properties is measured when there is maximum flow and is therefore under dynamic conditions. It is increased in conditions with greater airway resistance and flow rate. Flow rate depends on the time allowed for inspiration and expiration. At higher respiratory rates, there is less time available for each inspiration and expiration, necessitating higher flows; therefore higher pressure is required to overcome flow-resistive properties. The pressure gradient necessary to move air from one place to another is the sum of pressure needed to overcome the elastic and flow-resistive properties of the lung. This pressure gradient is taken into account to calculate the dynamic compliance of the respiratory system (C_{DYN}). The difference in change in pressure between static conditions and dynamic conditions is attributable to airway resistance.

Functional Residual Capacity

During inspiration, oxygen-enriched gas enters alveoli. During exhalation, oxygen continues to be removed by the pulmonary capillary circulation. FRC is the volume of gas left in the alveoli at end-expiration. It is the only source of gas available for gas exchange during exhalation. In diseases with decreased FRC (e.g., ARDS, pulmonary edema), PaO_2 declines sharply throughout expiration, resulting in hypoxemia. Two ventilator strategies used to improve oxygenation in such situations are the application of PEEP and increasing the *inspiratory time* (TI) (Fig. 89.5). PEEP increases FRC, whereas a longer TI allows longer exposure of pulmonary capillary blood to a higher concentration of O_2 during inspiration. (See also Chapter 400.)

Time Constant

At the beginning of inspiration, the atmospheric pressure is higher than the pressure in the alveoli, resulting in movement of air into the alveoli. During mechanical ventilation, the ventilator circuit serves as the patient's

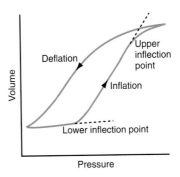

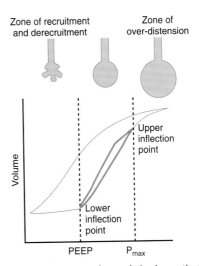

Fig. 89.3 Pulmonary pressure-volume relation in a patient with acute lung injury. **Top,** The lower inflection point is typically 12-18 cm H_2O, and the upper inflection point 26-32 cm H_2O. **Bottom,** Specific protective ventilation strategies require that positive end-expiratory pressure (PEEP) is set just above the lower inflection point and the pressure limit (P_{max}) just below the upper inflection point. Thus the lung is ventilated in the safe zone between the zone of recruitment and derecruitment and the zone of overdistention, and both high-volume and low-volume injuries are avoided. *(From Pinhu L, Whitehead T, Evans T, et al: Ventilator-associated lung injury, Lancet 361:332–340, 2003.)*

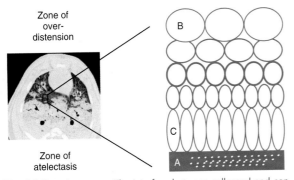

Fig. 89.2 Atelectrauma. The interface between collapsed and consolidated lung *(A)* and overdistended lung units *(B)* is heterogeneous and unstable. Depending on ambient conditions, this region is prone to cyclic recruitment and derecruitment and localized asymmetric stretch of lung units *(C)* immediately apposed to regions of collapsed lung. *(From Pinhu L, Whitehead T, Evans T, et al: Ventilator-associated lung injury, Lancet 361:332–340, 2003.)*

1. Pressure gradient is required to move air from one place to another
2. Movement of air is opposed by flow-resistive and elastic properties of the system

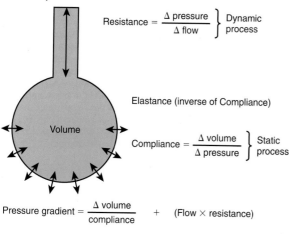

$$\text{Resistance} = \frac{\Delta\ \text{pressure}}{\Delta\ \text{flow}} \left.\right\}\ \begin{array}{l}\text{Dynamic}\\\text{process}\end{array}$$

Elastance (inverse of Compliance)

Volume

$$\text{Compliance} = \frac{\Delta\ \text{volume}}{\Delta\ \text{pressure}} \left.\right\}\ \begin{array}{l}\text{Static}\\\text{process}\end{array}$$

$$\text{Pressure gradient} = \frac{\Delta\ \text{volume}}{\text{compliance}}\ +\ (\text{Flow} \times \text{resistance})$$

Elastic properties   Flow-resistive properties

Fig. 89.4 Equation of motion. A pressure gradient is required to move air from one place to another. In the lungs, the required pressure gradient must overcome the lung and chest wall elastance (static component) and the flow-resistive properties (dynamic component). The static component is increased in alveolar interstitial diseases and stiff chest wall, whereas the dynamic component is increased with airway obstruction.

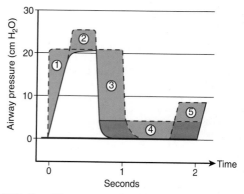

Fig. 89.5 Five different ways to increase mean airway pressure. (1) Increase the respiratory flow rate, producing a square wave inspiratory pattern; (2) increase the peak inspiratory pressure; (3) reverse the inspiratory-expiratory ratio or prolong the inspiratory time without changing the rate; (4) increase positive end-expiratory pressure; and (5) increase the ventilatory rate by reducing the expiratory time without changing the inspiratory time. *(From Harris TR, Wood BR: Physiologic principles. In Goldsmith JP, Karotkin EH, editors: Assisted ventilation of the neonate, ed 3, Philadelphia, 1996, Saunders.)*

atmosphere. As alveoli expand with air, the alveolar pressure rises throughout inspiration until it equilibrates with the ventilator pressure, at which time airflow ceases. Expiration starts when the ventilator pressure falls below the alveolar pressure. Alveolar pressure decreases throughout expiration until it reaches the ventilator pressure, at which time no further egress of air from the alveoli occurs. If inspiration or expiration is terminated before pressure equilibration between alveoli and the ventilator is allowed to occur, alveolar expansion during inspiration or alveolar emptying during expiration is incomplete. Incomplete inspiration results in delivery of decreased VT, whereas incomplete expiration is associated with air trapping and the presence of residual PEEP in the alveoli that is greater than the ventilator pressure, referred to as **auto-PEEP**. Some time is required for pressure equilibration to occur between alveoli and the atmosphere, which is reflected in the *time constant* (TC). It takes 3 TCs for 95% (and 5 TCs for 99%) of pressure equilibration to occur. The TC depends on compliance (C) and resistance (R), and their relationship is depicted in Fig. 89.6. TC is calculated as compliance multiplied by resistance (C × R) and is measured in seconds.

Diseases with decreased compliance (increased elastance) are characterized by high elastic recoil pressure, which results in more rapid equilibration of alveolar and ventilator pressures, thereby decreasing TC. Diseases with increased airway resistance are associated with slower flow rates, require longer time for movement of air from one place to another, and therefore have increased TC. Airways expand during inspiration and narrow during expiration. Therefore, expiratory time constant (TCE) is longer than inspiratory time constant (TCI). In intrathoracic airway obstruction (e.g., asthma, bronchiolitis, aspiration syndromes), airway narrowing is much more pronounced during expiration. Therefore, although both TCE and TCI are prolonged in such diseases, TCE is much more prolonged than TCI. Patients with such diseases therefore are best ventilated with slower rates, higher VT, and longer expiratory time than inspiratory time. In diseases characterized by decreased compliance, both TCE and TCI are short; however, the TCE is closer to TCI than in normal lungs because of the stiffer alveoli recoil with greater force. Patients with these diseases are best ventilated with small

VT to prevent ventilator-induced lung injury and with a relatively longer inspiratory time in each breath to improve oxygenation.

Critical Opening Pressure
Collapsed or atelectatic alveoli require a considerable amount of pressure to open. Once open, the alveoli require relatively less pressure for continued expansion. The process of opening atelectatic alveoli is called **recruitment**. In a normal lung, alveoli remain open at end-expiration, and therefore the lung requires relatively less pressure to receive its VT. In a disease process in which the alveoli collapse at end-expiration (e.g., ARDS), a substantial amount of pressure is required to open the alveoli during inspiration. This pressure causes ventilator-induced lung injury by 2 mechanisms: *barotrauma* at the terminal airway–alveolar junction and *volutrauma* as a result of overdistention of alveoli that are already open (see Figs. 89.2 and 89.3). Although a pulmonary parenchymal disease process is rarely uniform, and each of the millions of alveoli may have its own mechanical characteristics, a composite volume-pressure relationship could be conceptualized for the whole lung (Fig. 89.7).

In these situations, the lower and upper portions of the curve are relatively horizontal, and the middle portion is more vertical. At the beginning of inspiration, atelectatic alveoli are being recruited, requiring high pressure for a relatively small increase in volume. Once they are recruited, further increase in volume requires relatively less pressure. The pressure at which most alveoli are open is called *critical opening pressure*; this point is also referred to as the *lower inflection point* (lower P_FLEX). After the lower P_FLEX, greater volume can be delivered for relatively less pressure until the upper P_FLEX is reached, at which the volume-pressure curve again becomes relatively horizontal. The goal of mechanical ventilation in alveolar interstitial pathology is to deliver a VT between the lower and upper inflection points, the so-called safe zone of ventilation. If VT is delivered with a change in inflation pressure that includes the lower P_FLEX, alveoli are likely to open *and* close during every breath, a process termed **tidal recruitment** that is injurious to the lung, especially at the terminal airway–alveolar junction. If VT is delivered with a change of pressure that includes the upper P_FLEX, overdistention of alveoli is likely to occur, resulting in volutrauma and barotrauma. Keeping tidal ventilation between the upper and lower P_FLEX values is accomplished by maintaining a level of PEEP to produce baseline alveolar recruitment and delivering a relatively small (6 mL/kg) VT. Called "open lung" strategy, this approach has proved to be beneficial in alveolar interstitial diseases such as ARDS.

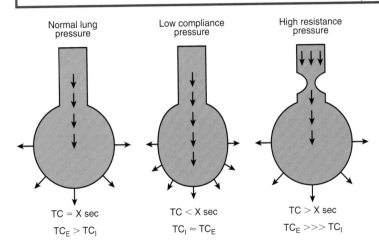

Fig. 89.6 Time constant (TC). A certain amount of time is necessary for pressure equilibration (and therefore completion of delivery of gas) to occur between proximal airway and alveoli. TC, a reflection of time required for pressure equilibration, is a product of compliance and resistance. In diseases of decreased lung compliance, less time is needed for pressure equilibration to occur, whereas in diseases of increased airway resistance, more time is required. Expiratory TC is increased much more than inspiratory TC in obstructive airway diseases, because airway narrowing is exaggerated during expiration.

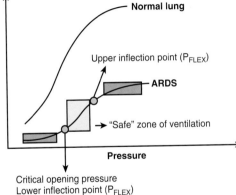

Fig. 89.7 Volume-pressure relationship in normal lung and in acute respiratory distress syndrome. In ARDS, atelectatic alveoli require a considerable amount of pressure to open. Critical opening pressure, also referred to as lower P_{FLEX}, is the airway pressure above which further alveolar expansion occurs with relatively less pressure. Upper P_{FLEX} is the airway pressure above which further increase in pressure results in less alveolar expansion; this is the area of alveolar overdistention. Keeping tidal volume between upper and lower P_{FLEX} values is considered less injurious to the lung.

Mechanical ventilation may be delivered either noninvasively with a patient-machine interface other than an ETT or invasively after endotracheal intubation.

NONINVASIVE MECHANICAL VENTILATION

Delivering positive pressure mechanical respiratory support without the use of endotracheal intubation is called noninvasive positive pressure ventilation (**NIPPV**). This type of respiratory support has been increasingly used in the pediatric intensive care setting.

The most common techniques applied are continuous positive airway pressure (**CPAP**) or biphasic (inspiratory and expiratory) positive airway pressure (**BiPAP**). A variety of devices with increasing sophistication has been developed in recent years, and different interfaces are available, such as nasal prongs, nasal and full-face masks, as well as helmets. Especially in the pediatric population a comfortable interface is critical for the successful application of NIPPV. NIPPV has been successfully used in acute and chronic hypoxic and/or hypercarbic respiratory failure.

Indications range from acute lower airway obstruction such as asthma or acute upper airway obstruction including postextubation airway swelling, to parenchymal lung diseases such as pneumonia and ARDS. Acute and chronic respiratory failure, from neuromuscular weakness and chest wall deformities, has been the classic indication for its use. NIPPV can also be used to help prevent reintubation after prolonged mechanical ventilation.

BiPAP provides positive airway pressure during exhalation and additional positive pressure during inspiration. These pressures can be adjusted independently to suit individual needs and comfort, and a respiratory rate can be delivered. The additional positive pressure during inspiration helps improve alveolar ventilation in low compliance and obstructive lung disease. During exhalation, expiratory positive airway pressure can decrease the effects of airway closure by raising intraluminal pressure and ameliorating intrathoracic airway collapse. During inspiration, inspiratory positive airway pressure can unload inspiratory muscle work.

These mechanics may explain many of the physiological benefits of NIPPV including an increase in lung compliance and FRC, a decrease of dynamic airway narrowing ("stenting" of the airway), augmentation of V_T and alveolar ventilation, and decreased work of breathing. Physiologic benefits of NIPPV in obstructive (e.g., asthma) and restrictive (e.g., ARDS) lung disease are schematically presented in Figs. 89.8 and 89.9. Additional benefits result from improving cardiopulmonary interactions, especially LV afterload reduction, thereby improving cardiac output in patients with acute or chronic LV dysfunction.

NIPPV is usually well tolerated and safer than invasive mechanical ventilation. Airway trauma from endotracheal intubation can be avoided, and less sedation is required. Breaks can be given for the application of oral medications and clearance of respiratory secretions, and selected stable patients can be fed by mouth. The number of nosocomial infections, ventilator-associated pneumonia, and ventilator-induced lung injury is expected to decrease as well. In addition, aerosol therapy driven by NIPPV, appears to be more effective.

Complications of NIPPV may include upper airway mucosal irritation, pulmonary hyperinflation with resulting interstitial emphysema and pneumothorax, abdominal distention, aspiration, and feeding intolerance. Patients initiated on NIPPV need close cardiorespiratory monitoring because the respiratory failure may progress, leading to the need for endotracheal intubation.

Some authorities have suggested independent predictors of NIPPV failure. Patients with more severe respiratory distress and those who do not show improvement of respiratory indices (i.e., respiratory rate, reduction in FiO_2) within 2 hr of initiation are more likely to fail. Underlying severe systemic diseases such as sepsis, multiorgan dysfunction, and malignancies are less likely to respond favorably to NIPPV. Absolute contraindications include loss of airway reflexes, acute severe

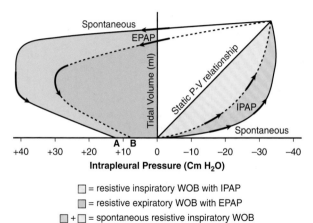

□ = resistive inspiratory WOB with IPAP

□ = resistive expiratory WOB with EPAP

□ + □ = spontaneous resistive inspiratory WOB

□ + □ = spontaneous resistive expiratory WOB

Fig. 89.8 Work of breathing (WOB) in status asthmaticus with and without noninvasive positive pressure ventilation. In the expiratory limb of the respiratory cycle, the equal pressure point is displaced distally, causing airways to begin to close at a higher lung volume (increased closing capacity), leading to dynamic hyperinflation, and auto–positive end-expiratory pressure (auto-PEEP) (A). Application of expiratory positive airway pressure (EPAP) stents the airways, reducing intrathoracic airway collapse, dynamic hyperinflation, auto-PEEP (B), and WOB. In the inspiratory limb, the patient needs to generate less negative pressure to initiate inspiration because of lower auto-PEEP. Inspiratory muscles are further unloaded by inspiratory positive airway pressure (IPAP) throughout inspiration for the given tidal volume. Both expiratory and inspiratory WOB are thus reduced by application of noninvasive positive pressure ventilation. P-V, Pressure-volume. (From Sarnaik AA, Sarnaik AP: Noninvasive ventilation in pediatric status asthmaticus: sound physiologic rationale but is it really safe, effective, and cost-efficient? Pediatr Crit Care Med 13:484–485, 2012.)

Total WOB = WOB/Breath Cycle X Respiratory Rate

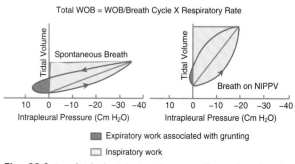

■ Expiratory work associated with grunting

□ Inspiratory work

Fig. 89.9 Beneficial physiologic pulmonary effects of noninvasive positive pressure ventilation (NIPPV) in restrictive lung disease (e.g., ARDS). **Left,** Without NIPPV, the slope of pressure-volume relationship is flatter, resulting in lower tidal volume for a given inflation pressure and necessitating in increased respiratory rate to maintain required minute alveolar ventilation. Start of inspiration is at a lower lung volume, indicating decreased functional residual capacity (FRC). Expiration is active toward the end as a result of grunting aimed at increasing FRC. **Right,** On institution of NIPPV, the slope of pressure-volume relationship is increased, resulting in greater tidal volume for a given inflation pressure, with a subsequent decrease in respiratory rate and inspiratory work of breathing (WOB). FRC is increased because of expiratory positive airway pressure (EPAP), resulting in improved oxygenation and decreased expiratory work associated with grunting.

neurologic insults, cardiorespiratory arrest, and severe hemodynamic instability. Patients with mid-face abnormalities or facial trauma and burns should not be considered as candidates for NIPPV. Other contraindications include the immediate postoperative period after facial

and upper airway surgery, recent gastrointestinal surgery, or patients with bowel obstruction and vomiting. Patients who are severely agitated and confused should not be initiated on NIPPV. NIPPV has been shown to decrease intubation rates, as well as reintubation rates, and is increasingly used to treat acute or chronic respiratory failure in pediatric patients.

INVASIVE MECHANICAL VENTILATION

Mechanical ventilation involves considering the four phases of the respiratory cycle: (1) initiation of respiration and a variable that is controlled, often referred to as *mode*; (2) inspiratory phase characteristics, which determine the duration of inspiration and how the pressure or volume is delivered; (3) termination of inspiration, often referred to as *cycle*; and (4) expiratory phase characteristics. Ideally, mechanical ventilation should not completely take over the work of breathing, but rather should assist the patient's own respiratory effort. In the absence of any patient effort, respiratory muscle deconditioning may occur, making weaning from mechanical ventilation more difficult.

Initiation of Inspiration and the Control Variable (Mode)

The initiation of inspiration may be set to occur at a predetermined rate and interval regardless of patient effort, or it could be timed in response to patient effort. Once inspiration is initiated, the ventilator breath either is controlled entirely by the ventilator (*control mode*) or supports the patient's inspiratory effort to a predetermined inspiratory volume or pressure target (*support mode*). Advances in technology allow for greater patient-ventilator synchrony to occur. The ventilator may be set to be *triggered* by the signal it receives as a result of patient effort. This feature may be in the form of lowering of either pressure (*pressure trigger*) or airflow (*flow trigger*) in the ventilator circuit generated by the patient's inspiratory effort. If no such signal is received because of lack of patient effort, the ventilator delivers a breath at an interval selected by the operator.

Control Modes

Intermittent Mandatory Ventilation Mode. In intermittent mandatory ventilation (**IMV**), the inspiration is initiated at a set frequency with a timing mechanism independent of patient effort. In between machine-delivered breaths, the patient can breathe spontaneously from a fresh source of gas. IMV allows for adjustment of ventilator support according to the patient's needs, making it useful in the weaning process. Lack of synchrony between machine-delivered breaths and patient efforts may result in ineffective ventilation and patient discomfort, especially when IMV is delivered at a high rate. In such cases the patient may require sedation and pharmacologic neuromuscular blockade for efficient delivery of VT. To obviate this problem, **synchronized** IMV (**SIMV**) is used, whereby the machine-delivered breaths are triggered by the patient's inspiratory efforts (Fig. 89.10). In between the machine-delivered breaths, a fresh source of gas is available for spontaneous patient breaths. In the absence of patient effort, the patient receives a backup rate, as in IMV mode. Even with SIMV, ventilator-patient asynchrony can occur, because VT, inflation pressure, and inspiratory time are determined by the ventilator alone.

Assist-Control Mode. In assist-control (AC) mode, every patient breath is triggered by pressure or flow generated by patient inspiratory effort and "assisted" with either preselected inspiratory pressure or volume. The rate of respirations is therefore determined by the patient's inherent rate. A backup total (patient and ventilator) obligatory rate is set to deliver a minimum number of breaths. On AC mode, with a backup rate of 20 breaths/min and a patient's inherent rate of 15 breaths/min; the ventilator will assist all the patient's breaths, and the patient will receive 5 additional breaths/min. On the other hand, a patient with an inherent rate of 25 breaths/min will receive all 25 breaths assisted. Although useful in some patients, the AC mode cannot be used in the weaning process, which involves gradual decrease in ventilator support.

Control Variable

Once initiated, either the VT or the pressure delivered by the machine can be controlled. The machine-delivered breath is thus referred to as either volume controlled or pressure controlled (Table 89.11). With **volume-controlled ventilation (VCV)**, machine-delivered volume is the primary control, and the inflation pressure generated depends on the respiratory system's compliance and resistance. Changes in respiratory system compliance and resistance are therefore easily detected from changes observed in inflation pressure. In **pressure-controlled ventilation (PCV)** the pressure change above the baseline is the primary control, and the Vt delivered to the lungs depends on the respiratory system's C and R. Changes in respiratory system C and R do not affect inflation pressure and may therefore go undetected unless the exhaled Vt is monitored.

VCV and PCV have their own advantages and disadvantages (Table 89.11). Generally speaking, PCV is more efficient than VCV in terms of amount of VT delivered for a given inflation pressure during ventilation of a lung that has nonuniform TC, as in asthma. In VCV, relatively less-obstructed airways are likely to receive more of the machine-delivered volume throughout inspiration than relatively more-obstructed airways with longer TC (Fig. 89.11A). This situation would result in uneven ventilation, higher peak inspiratory pressure (PIP), and a decrease in C_{DYN}. In PCV, because of a constant inflation pressure that is held throughout inspiration, relatively less-obstructed lung units with shorter TC would achieve pressure equilibration earlier during inspiration than the relatively more-obstructed areas. Thus, units with shorter TCs would attain their final volume earlier in inspiration, and those with longer TCs would continue to receive additional volume later in inspiration (Fig. 89.11B). This situation would result in more even distribution of inspired gas, delivery of more VT for the same inflation pressure, and improved C_{DYN} compared with VCV.

Pressure-regulated volume control (PRVC) combines the advantages of VCV and PCV. In this mode, the VT and TI are controlled as primary variables, but the ventilator determines the amount of pressure needed to deliver the desired VT. Inflation pressure is thus adjusted to deliver the prescribed VT over the TI, depending on the patient's respiratory C and R.

Support Modes

Pressure-support ventilation (PSV) and **volume-support ventilation (VSV)** are designed to support the patient's spontaneous respirations. With PSV, initiation of inspiration is triggered by the patient's spontaneous breath, which is then "supported" by a rapid rise in ventilator pressure to a preselected level. The inspiration is continued until the inspiratory flow rate falls to a set level (generally 25% of peak flow rate) as the patient's lungs fill up. Thus, TI is controlled by the patient's own efforts. PSV can be combined with SIMV so that any breath above the SIMV rate is supported by PSV. Allowing the patient to control as much of the rate, VT, and inspiratory time as possible is considered a gentler form of mechanical ventilation than SIMV, in which the VT (or inflation pressure) and TI are preset. PSV as the sole source of mechanical ventilator support is often not adequate for patients with severe lung disease. However, PSV is especially useful in patients being weaned and in those who require mechanical ventilation for relatively minor lung disease or for neuromuscular weakness.

VSV is similar to PSV, in that all the spontaneous breaths are supported. In VSV, inspiratory pressure to support spontaneous breaths is adjusted to guarantee a preset VT. If there is a change in respiratory mechanics or patient effort, the inspiratory pressure to support the breath initiated by patient effort is automatically adjusted to deliver the set VT.

Inspiratory Phase Characteristics

TI, inspiratory flow waveform, and pressure rise time can be adjusted in the inspiratory phase to suit the patient's respiratory mechanics.

In PCV the duration of TI is directly set in seconds. In VCV the TI can be adjusted by adjusting the inspiratory flow (volume/time). The choice of TI value depends on the respiratory rate, which determines the total duration of each breath, and on the estimation of inspiratory and expiratory TCs. Decreasing the flow rate delivery increases TI, and vice versa. With an increase in TI, the pulmonary capillary blood is exposed to a higher level of PAO_2 for a longer time. This feature is

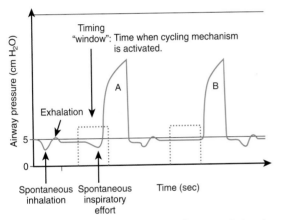

Fig. 89.10 Synchronized intermittent mandatory ventilation. At set intervals, the ventilator's timing circuit becomes activated and a timing "window" appears (*dotted line area*). If the patient initiates a breath in the timing window, the ventilator delivers a mandatory breath (*A*). If no spontaneous effort occurs, the ventilator delivers a mandatory breath at a fixed time after the timing window (*B*). (*From Banner MJ, Gallagher TJ: Respiratory failure in the adult: ventilatory support. In Kirby RR, Smith RA, Desautels DA, editors: Mechanical ventilation, New York, 1985, Churchill Livingstone.*)

Table 89.11	Characteristics of Pressure-Controlled and Volume-Controlled Methods of Ventilation	
	PRESSURE-CONTROLLED VENTILATION	**VOLUME-CONTROLLED VENTILATION**
Control setting(s)	Inflation pressure Inspiratory time Rise time	Tidal volume Flow rate Inspiratory flow pattern (constant vs decelerating)
Machine-delivered volume	Depends on respiratory system compliance and resistance	Constant
Inflation pressure	Constant	Depends on respiratory system compliance and resistance
Endotracheal tube leak	Somewhat compensated	Leaked volume part of tidal volume
Distribution of ventilation	More uniform in lungs with varying time constant units	Less uniform in lungs with varying time constant units
Patient comfort	Possibly compromised	Possibly enhanced
Weaning	Inflation pressure adjustment required to deliver desired tidal volume	Tidal volume remains constant; inflation pressure automatically weaned

Volume control ventilation

Areas with low resistance are preferentially filled throughout inspiration (both early and late) resulting in uneven ventilation especially in obstructive lesions

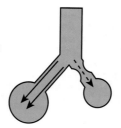

A

Pressure control ventilation

Early inspiration: Areas with short time constants fill up quickly and equilibriate with proximal airway pressure.

Late inspiration: Areas with prolonged time constants receive more volume with slower equilibrium of pressure.

Result: More even gas distribution compared to volume-controlled ventilation especially in obstructive lesions

Early phase
Pressure equilibration
Max volume reached

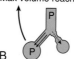

Late phase
Pressure & volume
equilibration still occurring

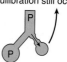

B

Fig. 89.11 A, In volume-controlled ventilation (VCV), tidal volume (VT) is delivered to the less-obstructed areas throughout inspiration. Obstructed areas of the lung therefore receive a lower proportion of VT, resulting in uneven ventilation. **B,** In pressure-controlled ventilation (PCV), less-obstructed areas equilibrate with inflation pressure and therefore receive most of their VT early during inspiration. More-obstructed areas, with prolonged time constants, require longer time for pressure equilibration and therefore continue to receive a portion of their VT later during inspiration. The entire VT is more evenly distributed than with volume-cycled ventilation.

beneficial in diseases with decreased FRC, such as ARDS and pulmonary edema. An increase in TI also increases VT without increasing inflation pressure in PCV if inspiratory flow is still occurring at end-expiration. It must be recognized that at a given ventilator rate, an increase in TI decreases expiratory time (TE). Therefore, any strategy that employs an increase in the inspiratory component of the respiratory cycle should ensure that the decreased TE is still sufficient for complete exhalation.

Inspiratory flow waveform can be adjusted in VCV mode as either a constant flow (square waveform) or a decelerating flow (descending ramp waveform). With a square waveform, flow is held constant throughout inspiration. In a descending ramp waveform, flow is maximal at the start of inspiration and declines throughout its duration. It is debatable which flow pattern is better for a given disease.

In PCV and PSV, the prescribed PIP is reached through delivery of airflow. *Pressure rise time* reflects the time required for the ventilator to reach PIP and can be adjusted by control of flow at the beginning of the inspiratory phase. The inspiratory flow rise time is adjusted to provide comfort for a patient who is awake and also to prevent an extremely rapid rise in inspiratory pressure, which might result in barotrauma.

Termination of Inspiration (Cycle)

The 2 most commonly used inspiratory terminating mechanisms in control modes are time-cycled and volume-cycled. With a **time-cycled** mechanical breath, inspiration is terminated after a preselected TI has elapsed, whereas with **volume-cycled** breath the inspiration ends after a preselected volume has been delivered by the machine into the ventilator circuit. A time-cycled breath is almost always pressure-limited, with the PIP held constant for the duration of inspiration. A volume-cycled breath can be pressure-limited as a safety mechanism to avoid barotrauma. The inspiration-terminating mechanism is set somewhat differently in support modes. In PSV the inspiration is set to end after the inspiratory flow decreases below a certain percentage (usually 25%) of peak inspiratory flow. This happens when the patient no longer desires to receive additional VT. Such a breath can be termed **flow-cycled**. In VSV the inspiration is terminated when the patient has received the desired VT.

Expiratory Phase Maneuvers

The most useful expiratory phase maneuver is the application of PEEP, which is applied to both the control breath and the assisted breath. The most important clinical benefits of PEEP are to recruit atelectatic alveoli and to increase FRC in patients with alveolar-interstitial diseases and thereby improve oxygenation. There is growing recognition that even a brief disconnection from a ventilator, and therefore having zero

end-expiratory pressure (ZEEP), can result in significant alveolar **derecruitment** and decline in oxygenation. In patients with obstructive lesions in which insufficient exhalation results in air trapping and auto-PEEP, extrinsic PEEP (that applied through a mechanical device) can prevent airway closure during expiration and improve ventilation. Other salutary effects of PEEP include redistribution of extravascular lung water away from gas-exchanging areas, improved V̇/Q̇ relationship, and stabilization of the chest wall. The effect of PEEP on lung C is variable, depending on the level of PEEP provided and the patient's pulmonary mechanics. By shifting the VT ventilation to a more favorable part of the pressure-volume curve, PEEP may recruit more alveoli, delay airway closure, and improve lung C. Excessive PEEP, on the other hand, may lead to overdistention of alveoli and reduced C. The effect of PEEP in individual patients can be ascertained by measuring exhaled VT and calculating C_{DYN}. Other deleterious effects of PEEP include decreased venous return, increased pulmonary vascular resistance, and decreased cardiac output.

ADDITIONAL VENTILATORY MODALITIES
Airway Pressure Release Ventilation

Airway pressure release ventilation (**APRV**) improves oxygenation in patients with severe hypoxemic respiratory failure resulting from alveolar-interstitial disease. This modality applies a CPAP, designated $CPAP_{HIGH}$, to recruit and maintain FRC with brief intermittent release phases of $CPAP_{LOW}$ to allow alveolar gas to escape. $CPAP_{HIGH}$ is analogous to PIP, and $CPAP_{LOW}$ is similar to setting PEEP. In contrast to the patient receiving conventional mechanical ventilation, a patient receiving APRV spends the majority of time in the $CPAP_{HIGH}$ phase, which may last as long as 3-5 sec with a brief (0.3-0.5 sec) time in the $CPAP_{LOW}$ phase. These atypically long TIs are tolerated because of a floating expiratory valve in the ventilator circuit that permits spontaneous breathing during $CPAP_{HIGH}$ phase. Therefore, even if the $CPAP_{HIGH}$ phase can be considered "inspiratory" and the $CPAP_{LOW}$ phase "expiratory" in regard to the ventilator, the patient is able to breathe spontaneously during both these phases. The longer ventilator TI recruits lung units, and the ability to breathe spontaneously during this phase allows distribution of gas flow to atelectatic lung regions. The outcome benefit of APRV in pediatric hypoxemic respiratory failure has not been proved.

High-Frequency Ventilation

Mechanical ventilation at supraphysiologic rates and low VT, known as high-frequency ventilation (**HFV**), improves gas exchange in a select group of patients who show no response to traditional ventilatory modalities. The mechanism of alveolar ventilation in HFV is very different from that in conventional ventilation, in that HFV is less dependent on VT and more dependent on asymmetric velocities and convective dispersion of inspired gas. Patients with severe persistent hypoxic failure are most likely to benefit from HFV. HFV is also helpful in patients with bronchopleural fistula and persistent air leaks. The main tenet of HFV is to recruit lung volume with a high MAP and produce smaller fluctuations in alveolar pressure during inspiration and expiration, thus maintaining a satisfactory FRC and reducing alveolar stretch. The 2 most investigated techniques of HFV are HFO and HFJV.

The most commonly used HFV modality is **high-frequency oscillation (HFO)**, which employs a mechanism to generate to-and-fro air movement. Additional air is drawn in (entrained) through a parallel circuit via a Venturi effect. Air is pushed in during inspiration and actively sucked out during expiration. The main determinants of oxygenation are FIO_2 and MAP, whereas ventilation is determined by changes in pressure (amplitude) from the MAP. Commonly used respiratory frequency varies from 5 Hz (300 breaths/min) in adults and older children, to 6-8 Hz (360-480 breaths/min) in young children, 8-10 Hz (480-600 breaths/min) in infants, and 10-12 Hz (600-720 breaths/min) in newborn and premature infants.

In **high-frequency jet ventilation (HFJV)**, a high-frequency interrupter is interposed between a high-pressure gas source and a small cannula that is incorporated in the ETT. The cannula propels tiny amounts of gas (jets) at high velocity and high frequency through the ETT. An additional amount of gas is entrained from a parallel circuit. Unlike in HFO, expiration occurs passively in HFJV as a result of elastic recoil of the lung and the chest wall. PEEP is set through the parallel circuit by a conventional ventilator in line. Respiratory rate is generally set at 420 breaths/min. Major determinants of oxygenation are FIO_2 and PEEP, and the major determinant of ventilation is PIP.

CONVENTIONAL VENTILATOR SETTINGS
Fraction of Inspired Oxygen
The shape of the hemoglobin-O_2 dissociation curve dictates that oxygen content in the blood is not linearly related to PaO_2. A PaO_2 value that results in an oxyhemoglobin saturation of 94% is reasonable in most situations, because a higher PaO_2 would cause minimal increase in arterial oxygen content, and a modest (10 mm Hg) drop in PaO_2 would result in minimal decrease in oxyhemoglobin saturation. In most cases, a PaO_2 value of 70-75 mm Hg is a reasonable goal. FIO_2 values that are higher than those necessary to attain oxyhemoglobin saturations of approximately 95% expose the patient to unnecessary oxygen toxicity. Whenever possible, FIO_2 values should be decreased to a level ≤0.40 as long as oxyhemoglobin saturation remains ≥95%.

Mode
The choice of mode of ventilation depends on how much ventilator-patient interaction is desired and the disease entity that is being treated. SIMV or AC is chosen as the control mode; PCV, VCV, or PRVC as the variable that is to be controlled; and pressure support and volume support are the choices for support modes.

Tidal Volume and Rate
As previously discussed, alveolar ventilation, the chief determinant of $PaCO_2$, is calculated using VT, respiratory rate, and VD. A change in VT results in a corresponding change in alveolar ventilation without affecting VD-ventilation. A change in respiratory rate will affect alveolar ventilation as well as the VD-ventilation. Choice of VT and rate depends on the TC. In a patient with relatively normal lungs, an age-appropriate ventilator rate and a VT of 7-10 mL/kg would be appropriate initial settings. Diseases associated with decreased TC (decreased static compliance; e.g., ARDS, pneumonia, pulmonary edema) are best treated with small (6 mL/kg) VT and relatively rapid rates (e.g., 25-40 breaths/min). Diseases associated with prolonged TCs (increased airway resistance; e.g., asthma, bronchiolitis) are best treated with relatively slow rates and higher (10-12 mL/kg) VT. In PCV the delivered VT depends on the C and R of the patient's respiratory system and needs to be monitored to ensure the appropriate amount for a given situation. An inflation

pressure of 15-35 cm H_2O is sufficient for most patients, but it may need adjustment, depending on the volume of exhaled VT. It should be emphasized that achieving a *normal* $PaCO_2$ value is not a goal of mechanical ventilation. Mild hypercapnia (permissive hypercapnia) should be acceptable, especially when one is attempting to limit injurious inflation pressures or VTs.

Inspiratory Time and Expiratory Time
TI and TE are adjusted by setting inspiratory flow rate in VCV and by setting the precise TI in PCV. Increasing the TI results in increased MAP, improved oxygenation in diseases with decreased FRC, and better distribution of VT in obstructive lung disease. Sufficient expiratory time must be provided to ensure adequate emptying of the alveoli.

Positive End-Expiratory Pressure
The best level of PEEP depends on the disease entity that is being treated, and it may change in the same patient from time to time. Decisions are often based on the PaO_2/FIO_2 ratio and the measurement of C_{DYN}.

PATIENT-VENTILATOR ASYNCHRONY
Patient-ventilator asynchrony occurs when the patient's respiratory pattern does not match that of the ventilator. This can occur during all phases of respiration. Adverse effects of patient-ventilator asynchrony include wasted effort, ineffective delivery of desired VT, excessive generation of intrathoracic pressure resulting in barotrauma and adverse effects on cardiac output, increased work of breathing, and patient discomfort. Although several mechanisms exist to facilitate patient-ventilator asynchrony, a certain amount of asynchrony is inevitable unless the patient is pharmacologically sedated and paralyzed.

Triggering the Ventilator
The patient must be able to trigger the ventilator without excessive effort. Ventilators can be pressure-triggered or flow-triggered. With **pressure triggering**, the inspiratory valve opens and flow is delivered when a set negative pressure is generated within the patient-ventilator circuit during inspiration. The amount of pressure required to trigger an inspiration depends on the pressure trigger sensitivity. In **flow triggering** the ventilator provides a base flow of gas through the ventilator-patient circuit. When a flow sensor on the expiratory limb of the patient-ventilator circuit detects a decrease in flow as a result of the patient's inspiratory effort, the inspiratory valve opens and a ventilator breath is delivered. The degree of change in flow required to trigger an inspiration depends on the flow trigger sensitivity. Flow triggering is considered to be more comfortable, primarily because the patient receives some flow before triggering the ventilator, in contrast to pressure triggering, in which no flow is provided until the ventilator breath is triggered. Increasing the trigger sensitivity by decreasing the change in either pressure or flow needed to trigger an inspiration decreases the work of breathing. However, reducing the required pressure or flow excessively could result in accidental triggering and unwanted breaths by turbulence, caused by condensation in the ventilator circuit, ETT air leaks, or cardiac oscillations.

Selection of Appropriate Inspiratory Time
The duration of TI should match the patient's own inspiratory phase. If TI is too long, the patient's drive to exhale may begin before the ventilator breath has cycled off. When this occurs, exhalation occurs against inspiratory flow and a closed exhalation valve, resulting in increased work of breathing, excessive rise in intrathoracic pressure, and discomfort. If TI is too short, the patient may be still inhaling without respirator support. In general terms, TI is usually initiated at 0.5-0.7 sec for neonates, 0.8-1 sec in older children, and 1-1.2 sec for adolescents and adults. Adjustments need to be made through individual patient observations and according to the type of lung disease present. In patients with severe lung disease (both obstructive and restrictive), unnatural TI and TE values may have to be selected, as discussed earlier. In such situations, adequate analgesia, sedation, and in extreme cases neuromuscular blockade may be needed.

Selection of Inspiratory Flow Pattern

In VCV, inappropriate flow may be another source of patient-ventilator dyssynchrony. After initiation of inspiration, if the set amount of flow is inadequate to meet patient demand, a state of **flow starvation** occurs, resulting in excessive work of breathing and discomfort. Such patients may require a decelerating inspiratory flow pattern, in which a higher flow is provided in the beginning of inspiration and less toward the end as the lungs fill up. On the other hand, such a pattern may be uncomfortable for a patient who desires more gradual alveolar filling. The selection of inspiratory flow pattern should be based on the individual patient's respiratory mechanics. In PCV and PSV, the inspiratory rise time determines the manner in which the airway pressure is raised and VT delivered. Considerations for choosing the appropriate rise time in PCV and PSV are similar to those for choosing the inspiratory flow pattern in VCV.

Use of Support Modes

A conscious patient should be allowed to have spontaneous breaths that are supported by either PSV or VSV. This approach minimizes the mandatory breaths generated by the ventilator that are beyond the patient's control to modulate. Therefore, continued assessments should be made to determine whether the patient is able to maintain ventilatory requirements more in support modes and less in control modes.

Use of Sedation and Pharmacologic Neuromuscular Blockade

Having a conscious but comfortable patient is a desirable goal during mechanical ventilation. Spontaneous breaths with good muscle tone and presence of cough are important for adequate clearance of tracheobronchial secretions. The patient's ability to indicate distress is also important in identifying and preventing potential injurious factors. In certain situations, management of patient-ventilator asynchrony assumes much greater importance when the asynchrony is causing unacceptable derangement of gas exchange and ventilator-induced lung injury. Both alveolar interstitial lung pathology and obstructive airway diseases may necessitate unnatural and uncomfortable settings for respiratory rate, TI, and inflation pressures. In such patients, deep sedation is often necessary; dexmedetomidine, benzodiazepines, and opiates are the agents most commonly used for this purpose. In extreme situations, pharmacologic neuromuscular blockade with a nondepolarizing agent, such as vecuronium, is required to abolish any patient effort and respiratory muscle tone. When such pharmacologic paralysis is used, deep sedation must be ensured so that the patient does not sense pain and discomfort. Pharmacologic sedation and paralysis can ensure total control of the patient's ventilation by mechanical means and may result in lifesaving improvement in gas exchange with reduction in inflation pressures. However, long-term use of such agents may be associated with undesirable consequences and higher morbidity. The risk of inadequate tracheobronchial secretions and atelectasis is potentially greater. Long-term use of pharmacologic sedation may be associated with chemical dependency and withdrawal manifestations, and prolonged neuromuscular blockade is associated with neuromyopathy in critically ill patients. The benefits of sedation and pharmacologic paralysis therefore should be carefully balanced with the risks, and periodic assessments should be made to determine the need for their continuation.

Cardiopulmonary Interactions

Mechanical ventilation can have salutary as well as adverse effects on cardiac performance. By decreasing oxygen consumption necessary for work of breathing, oxygen supply to vital organs is improved. Positive pressure breathing decreases LV afterload, thus enhancing stroke volume and cardiac output in patients with failing myocardium (e.g., myocarditis). On the other hand, the decreased systemic venous return may further compromise stroke volume in hypovolemic patients. Such patients will require intravascular fluid loading. Also, an increase in pulmonary vascular resistance (PVR) caused by positive intrathoracic pressure may result in further decompensation of a poorly performing right ventricle. PVR is at its lowest value at an optimum FRC. When FRC is too low or too high, PVR (and therefore the right ventricular afterload) is increased. Both desirable

Table 89.12	Suggested Mechanical Ventilation Strategies in Various Clinical Situations	
SITUATION	**DISEASE**	**STRATEGY**
Low compliance, normal resistance	ARDS	PCV, APRV, HFO, HFJV
Normal compliance, high resistance	Asthma	PVC, PRVC
Normal compliance, normal resistance, for weaning	Head trauma, drug overdose, subglottic stenosis	VCV

APRV, Airway pressure release ventilation; ARDS, acute respiratory distress syndrome; HFO, high-frequency oscillation; HFJV, high-frequency jet ventilation; PCV, pressure-controlled ventilation; PRVC, pressure-regulated volume control; VCV, volume-controlled ventilation.

and undesirable effects of cardiopulmonary interactions may coexist and require ongoing assessment and necessary interventions (Table 89.12).

MONITORING RESPIRATORY MECHANICS

Exhaled Tidal Volume

Exhaled tidal volume (VTE) is measured by a pneumotachometer in the ventilator circuit during exhalation. In VCV, part of the machine-delivered volume may leak out during inspiration and therefore never reach the patient. Measurement of VTE more accurately describes the VT that is contributing to the patient's alveolar ventilation. In PCV the VTE depends on the patient's respiratory system compliance and resistance and therefore offers valuable diagnostic clues. A decrease in VTE during PCV is indicative of either decrease in compliance or increase in resistance and is helpful in directing the clinician to appropriate investigation and management. An increase in VTE is indicative of improvement and may require weaning of inflation pressures to adjust the VTE.

Peak Inspiratory Pressure

In VCV and PRVC, the PIP is the secondary variable determined by the patient's respiratory system compliance and resistance. An increase in PIP in these modes is indicative of decreased C (e.g., atelectasis, pulmonary edema, pneumothorax) or increased R (e.g., bronchospasm, obstructed ET). During VCV and PRVC, decreasing the respiratory rate or prolonging the TI will result in a lower PIP in patients with prolonged TCs because more time will be available for alveoli to fill. In such patients, a decrease in PIP suggests increased C or decreased R of the respiratory system.

Respiratory System Dynamic Compliance and Static Compliance

The changes in PIP during VCV and PRVC, and in VTE during PCV, are determined by C_{DYN} of the respiratory system (lung and chest wall). C_{DYN} is calculated as follows:

$$C_{DYN} = V_{TE} \div (PIP - PEEP)$$

C_{DYN} takes into account both the flow-resistive and the elastic properties of the respiratory system. Changes in C_{DYN} can be used to assess effects of different levels of PEEP as tidal ventilation is shifted along the slope of the volume-pressure curve (see Fig. 89.7). An increase in PEEP in alveolar-interstitial diseases (increased elastance), resulting in an increase in C_{DYN} suggests alveolar recruitment, whereas a decrease in C_{DYN} may indicate overdistention. Similarly, in obstructive diseases (increased R), adjustment in PEEP levels to ameliorate airway collapse during exhalation can be guided by monitoring C_{DYN}. To assess only the elastic recoil of the lung, measurement of C_{STAT} when there is no airflow is required. This measurement is performed by using an inspiratory hold maneuver with the patient under neuromuscular blockade and observing pressure-time and flow-time waveforms (Fig. 89.12). During this maneuver, inspiratory flow ceases while the expiratory valve continues to remain closed, thus allowing pressure to equilibrate

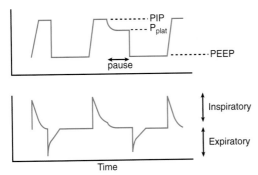

Fig. 89.12 Alveolar pressure is best determined by measurement of plateau pressure (P$_{plat}$). Inspiration is paused for an extended period, and alveolar gas pressure is allowed to equilibrate with the ventilator circuit pressure. Airway pressure at the end of the inspiratory pause is P$_{plat}$. The difference between peak inspiratory pressure (PIP) and P$_{plat}$ is meant to overcome flow-resistive properties of the lung, whereas P$_{plat}$ reflects the pressure needed to overcome elastic properties of lung and chest wall. PEEP, Positive end-expiratory pressure.

throughout the ventilator circuit and the patient's lungs. This pressure, referred to as the *plateau pressure* (P$_{plat}$), reflects alveolar pressure. C$_{STAT}$ is calculated as follows:

$$C_{STAT} = V_{TE} \div (P_{plat} - PEEP)$$

The difference between C$_{DYN}$ and C$_{STAT}$ is attributable to airway resistance. This difference is minimal in alveolar-interstitial diseases but substantial in airway obstruction.

Assessment of Auto-PEEP

Auto-PEEP is assessed with the use of an expiratory pause maneuver in which inspiration is delayed and alveolar pressure is allowed to equilibrate with the airway. In diseases with airway obstruction, insufficient alveolar emptying may occur if exhalation time is not adequate. The alveolar pressure in excess of the set PEEP at the completion of the expiratory pause is measured as auto-PEEP or intrinsic PEEP. Auto-PEEP can have adverse effects on ventilation and hemodynamic status. It can be managed by decreasing the respiratory rate or T$_I$ and thus allowing longer time for exhalation. Auto-PEEP may also be managed by increasing the set PEEP (*extrinsic* PEEP), thereby delaying airway closure during exhalation and improving alveolar emptying.

Assessment of Dead Space Ventilation

Positive pressure ventilation and application of PEEP may result in a decrease in venous return, cardiac output, and therefore pulmonary perfusion as well. Ventilation of poorly perfused alveoli results in dead space ventilation, which does not contribute to gas exchange. The V$_D$/V$_T$ fraction can be calculated (see Chapter 89). Normal V$_D$/V$_T$ is 0.33. Increased V$_D$/V$_T$ is indicative of poorly perfused alveoli. Patients with increased V$_D$/V$_T$ may require intravascular volume infusion or other means of augmenting the cardiac output to improve pulmonary perfusion. The V$_D$/V$_T$ fraction is calculated and displayed by commercially available capnographs, which measure endotracheal PetCO$_2$ continuously.

VENTILATOR-INDUCED LUNG INJURY

As with most medical therapies, mechanical ventilation can be harmful. Pathophysiology of ventilator-induced lung injury can be multifactorial. Large lung volumes and high pressures delivered with increased frequency cause cyclic strain, which may lead to disruption of the tight junctions between the alveolar epithelial and capillary endothelial cells, with intracapillary blebs resulting in alveolar and interstitial edema. This **biotrauma** may cause the release of proinflammatory cytokines that further injure the lung and travel in the blood outside the lung, leading to multiorgan failure. Evidence shows that in patients with ARDS, avoidance of V$_T$ ≥10 mL/kg and P$_{plat}$ ≥30 cm H$_2$O limits diffuse alveolar damage.

Atelectrauma is shear stress on the alveolar walls caused by cyclic opening and closing of the alveoli. PEEP can be used to prevent collapse and keep alveoli open. It is important that alveolar units are neither overdistended nor collapsed. Careful adjustments of PEEP may also permit the clinician to wean a patient from a high FIO$_2$, another potential source of lung injury (**oxytrauma**). Although most patients receive an FIO$_2$ of 1.00 during endotracheal intubation and at the beginning of mechanical ventilation, increasing PEEP to recruit alveoli without overdistention should be quickly instituted to improve oxygenation and permit weaning of the FIO$_2$. Although the FIO$_2$ value below which there is no risk of oxygen toxicity is unknown, most clinicians aim for a value <0.6. Regional mechanics may play a role in lung injury.

Ventilator-Associated Pneumonia

The pathophysiology of ventilator-associated pneumonia (VAP) is multifactorial. Aspiration of oral and/or gastric secretions, colonization of ETTs, and suppression of cough reflexes with sedation all play a role. New-onset fever and leukocytosis accompanied by demonstration of an infiltrative process on chest radiography are consistent with a diagnosis of VAP. This complication can lead to worsened gas exchange, increased duration of ventilation, and even death. Elevation of the head of the bed to 30 degrees after initiation of mechanical ventilation and use of a protocol for oral decontamination during mechanical ventilation are 2 means of reducing the risk for VAP. The most effective strategy to minimize any of the aforementioned complications is regular assessment of extubation readiness and liberation from mechanical ventilation as soon as clinically possible.

Weaning

Weaning from mechanical ventilation should be considered as a patient's respiratory insufficiency begins to improve. Most pediatricians favor gradual weaning from ventilator support. With SIMV, the ventilator rate is slowly reduced, allowing the patient's spontaneous breaths (typically assisted with pressure or volume support) to assume a larger proportion of the minute ventilation. When the ventilator rate is low (<5 breaths/min) such that its contribution to minute ventilation is minimal, assessment of extubation readiness is performed. An alternative method of gradual weaning is transition to PSV. In this mode, no ventilator rate is set, allowing all triggered breaths to be assisted with pressure support. The clinician reduces the pressure support slowly to a low value (<5-10 cm H$_2$O), at which point assessment of extubation readiness is performed. During either technique, weaning should be halted if tachypnea, increased work of breathing, hypoxemia, hypercapnia, acidosis, diaphoresis, tachycardia, or hypotension occurs.

The most objective means of assessing extubation readiness is a **spontaneous breathing trial (SBT)**. Before performance of an SBT, a patient should be awake with intact airway reflexes, capable of handling oropharyngeal secretions, and with stable hemodynamic status. In addition, gas exchange should be adequate, defined as PaO$_2$ >60 mm Hg while receiving FIO$_2$ <0.4 and PEEP ≤5 cm H$_2$O. If these criteria are present, a patient should be started on CPAP with minimal or no pressure support (≤5 cm H$_2$O). If this SBT is tolerated with no episodes of respiratory or cardiovascular decompensation, successful extubation is likely.

Some neonates and small children cannot be calmed or consoled long enough to complete the SBT. In this situation, extubation readiness must be assessed on a low level of ventilator support. Data suggest a low risk of extubation failure if the patient is comfortable and has stable hemodynamic status, with adequate gas exchange and spontaneous V$_T$ >6.5 mL/kg, while receiving <20% of total minute ventilation from the ventilator. Certain patient populations are at increased risk for extubation failure, such as young infants, children mechanically ventilated for >7 days, and patients with chronic respiratory or neurologic conditions. These children often benefit from transition to a noninvasive form of positive pressure ventilation (e.g., high-flow nasal cannula, CPAP, or BiPAP) delivered via nasal prongs or face mask to increase the odds of successful extubation.

The likelihood of **postextubation upper airway obstruction**, the most common cause of extubation failure in children, cannot be predicted on the basis of an SBT result or bedside measurements of physiologic variables. Traumatic endotracheal intubation and subglottic swelling from ETT irritation, especially in patients who exhibit agitation while receiving mechanical ventilation, are common causes of airway narrowing after extubation. Administration of intravenous corticosteroids (dexamethasone, 0.5 mg/kg every 6 hr for 4 doses before extubation) has been shown to minimize the incidence of postextubation airway obstruction. In patients in whom postextubation airway obstruction develops, the need for reintubation may be obviated by administration of nebulized racemic epinephrine and heliox.

Bibliography is available at Expert Consult.

89.2 Long-Term Mechanical Ventilation

See Chapter 446.4.

Chapter 90
Altitude-Associated Illness in Children (Acute Mountain Sickness)
Christian A. Otto
第九十章
儿童高原病（急性高山病）

中文导读

　　本章主要介绍了儿童高原病的病因学、低压缺氧的常见效应、急性高山病、高原性脑水肿、高原性肺水肿及特殊注意事项。低压缺氧的常见效应中描述了环境适应的重要性；急性高山病中介绍了其流行病学和危险因素、病理生理学、预防、诊断、周期性呼吸及治疗；在高原肺水肿中介绍了其流行病学和危险因素、病理生理学、诊断和治疗；在特殊注意事项中介绍了复发性高原肺水肿以及带小婴儿一起旅行时的注意事项。

High-altitude illness represents a spectrum of clinical entities with neurologic and pulmonary manifestations that overlap in their presentations and share common elements of pathophysiology. **Acute mountain sickness (AMS)** is the relatively benign and self-limited presentation, whereas **high-altitude pulmonary edema (HAPE)** and **high-altitude cerebral edema (HACE)** have potentially life-threatening manifestations.

Often overlooked by travelers as high-altitude destinations are cities such as La Paz, Bolivia (3,700 meters, approximately 12,100 feet), Lhasa, Tibet (3,600 m, ~11,800 ft), Cusco, Peru (3,400 m, ~11,200 ft), and Quito, Ecuador (2,850 m, ~9,350 ft), which reside at an elevation where altitude illness is likely to develop. In 2014, >15 million people visited Lhasa, a 6-fold increase over 8 yr since the opening of the Qinghai-Tibet Railway. In the western United States, 35 million people visit alpine resorts each year. Over 40% of those who stay above 3,300 m (~11,000 ft) have been found to suffer from AMS. In Colorado alone, approximately 150,000 children <12 yr old visit the mountains annually on ski holidays with their families. In 2014, AMS symptoms were severe enough to result in 1,350 visits to emergency departments (EDs) throughout Colorado. Because of the increasing family travel to high altitude, thousands of children are likely to develop AMS symptoms.

ETIOLOGY
The altitude threshold where clinical illness may begin to occur is 1,500 m (~4,900 ft). At this altitude a mild impairment in oxygen transport begins, although altitude illness is relatively rare until higher elevations are reached. Children with underlying medical problems that impair oxygen transport may be predisposed to developing altitude illness at these lower levels. At *moderate high altitude*, 2,500-3,500 m (~8,000-11,500

ft), arterial oxygen saturation (SaO$_2$) is generally well maintained; however, mild tissue hypoxia may occur as a result of low arterial oxygen partial pressure (PaO$_2$), and altitude illness becomes common after rapid ascent above 2,500 m (~8,200 ft). This is the altitude range that most people visit and the elevation of many popular U.S. ski resorts and thus the most common range to find the greatest number of altitude illness cases. *Very high altitude,* 3,500-5,500 m (~11,500-18,000 ft), is associated with the most serious altitude illness; SaO$_2$ falls below 90%, on the steep portion of the oxyhemoglobin dissociation curve, and marked desaturation may occur with relatively small increases in altitude. At these heights, severe hypoxemia is seen with sleep, exercise, and illness. HAPE and HACE are most common in this environment. *Extreme high altitude,* above 5,500 m (~18,000 ft), generally results in severe altitude illness during acute ascent without supplemental oxygen. Acclimatization at intermediate altitudes is required to reach extreme altitudes. Complete acclimatization is not possible, and long visits result in progressive deterioration.

GENERAL EFFECTS OF HYPOBARIC HYPOXIA

The partial pressure of oxygen (PO$_2$) in the atmosphere decreases logarithmically as geographic altitude rises, but oxygen remains a constant 20.93% of the barometric pressure. SaO$_2$ falls with increasing altitude, eventually triggering central chemoreceptor responses to produce hyperventilation in an attempt to normalize SaO$_2$; relative hypoventilation exacerbates the hypoxemia of high-altitude exposure. During sleep, periodic breathing associated with high-altitude exposure may result in periods of apnea, causing further arterial oxygen desaturation. Fluid homeostasis often shifts at altitude, resulting in a generalized fluid retention and redistribution into intracellular and interstitial spaces, manifested by peripheral edema, decreased urine output, and impaired gas exchange.

Acclimatization

Gradual ascents allowing for acclimatization over several weeks have allowed successful summiting of many of the world's highest peaks without supplemental oxygen. Without this gradual approach, rapid exposure to extreme altitude results in loss of consciousness and asphyxia in minutes. Children acclimatize as well as, if not better than, adults when comparing heart rate and SaO$_2$ of 7-9 yr olds to their parents during a slow ascent.

Some of the responses to hypoxia are mediated at the molecular level by *hypoxia-inducible factor* (HIF). This transcriptional activator orchestrates the expression of hundreds of genes in response to both acute and chronic hypoxic conditions. Acclimatization begins at the altitude that causes SaO$_2$ to fall below sea-level values. Most healthy, unacclimatized visitors to high altitude will not experience a significant drop in SaO$_2$ (<90%) until they reach elevations above 2,500 m (~8,200 ft). Children with preexisting conditions that reduce oxygen transport may have altitude intolerance and hypoxic stress at lower levels. Of particular importance are both acute and chronic cardiac and respiratory illnesses. An individual's inherent ability to acclimatize is also important. Previous successful acclimatization may be predictive of future responses for adults in similar conditions but may not be the case for children. Some acclimatize easily without developing clinical symptoms; others may transiently develop AMS during acclimatization; and a few have marked reactions to altitude exposure, fail to acclimatize, and develop severe altitude illness.

The most important response to acute hypoxia is an increase in minute ventilation. Peripheral chemoreceptors in the carotid bodies respond to hypoxia by signaling the respiratory control center in the medulla to increase ventilation. This decreases alveolar carbon dioxide partial pressure (PACO$_2$), resulting in a corresponding increase of PAO$_2$ and arterial oxygenation. This increased ventilation, known as the **hypoxic ventilatory response (HVR)**, varies in magnitude among individuals, may be genetically predetermined, and is related to the ability to acclimatize. Changes in the HVR and the onset of AMS with ascent to high altitude have been found to be remarkably similar between children and their fathers. Additional research has demonstrated that familial clustering of AMS accounts for up to 50% of the variability of AMS

onset among children. A low HVR and relative hypoventilation are implicated in the pathogenesis of both AMS and HAPE, whereas a strong HVR enhances acclimatization. As ventilation increases, a respiratory alkalosis occurs, exerting negative feedback on central respiratory control and limiting further ventilation increase. The kidneys excrete bicarbonate in an effort to compensate for the alkalosis. As the pH normalizes, ventilation rises slowly, reaching a maximum after 4-7 days. *This process is enhanced by acetazolamide, which induces a bicarbonate diuresis.*

Increased sympathetic activity and catecholamine release on ascent result in elevation of heart rate, blood pressure, cardiac output, and venous tone. Except at extreme altitudes, acclimatization results in the resting heart rate gradually returning to near sea-level values. *Resting relative tachycardia is evidence of poor acclimatization.*

Hematopoietic acclimatization consists of an increase in hemoglobin (Hb) and red blood cells (RBCs) and in 2,3-diphosphoglycerate (DPG). After acute ascent, an early increase of up to 15% occurs in Hb concentration primarily from fluid shifting into the extravascular space. Acclimatization leads to an increase in plasma volume and total blood volume. Erythropoietin is secreted in a HIF-mediated response to hypoxemia within hours of ascent, stimulating the production of new RBCs, which begin to appear in the circulation in 4 or 5 days. Hypoxemia also increases 2,3-DPG, resulting in a rightward shift of the oxyhemoglobin dissociation curve, favoring release of oxygen from the blood to the tissues. This is counteracted by the leftward shift of the curve caused by the respiratory alkalosis from hyperventilation. The result is a net null change in the oxyhemoglobin dissociation curve and an increase in O$_2$-Hb binding in the lung, raising SaO$_2$. Climbers at extreme altitude respond with marked hyperventilation, alkalosis, and a leftward shift that favors oxygen loading in a hypoxic environment and increases SaO$_2$.

ACUTE MOUNTAIN SICKNESS
Epidemiology and Risk Factors

The incidence of high-altitude illness depends on several variables, including the rate of ascent, previous altitude exposure, and individual genetic susceptibility. Sleeping altitude, final altitude reached, and duration of stay at altitude are also clear risk factors for AMS development. AMS is very common with **rapid ascent**. Climbers around the world who ascend quickly (1 or 2 days) from sea level to altitudes of about 4,300-6100 m (14,000-20,000 ft) have a very high incidence of AMS (27–83%). The rapid ascent profile associated with air travel to high-altitude locations also results in high AMS attack rates. Trekkers who fly into the Khumbu region to explore the Mt. Everest area have a higher incidence of AMS (47%) compared with those who walk (23%). Skiers who visit resorts in the western United States from sea level generally fly or drive to the region but sleep at relatively moderate altitudes (2,000-3,000 m, 6,300-9,700 ft). Among this population, AMS occurs in approximately 25%.

Children have the same incidence of AMS as adults. Individual (genetic) susceptibility for the development of AMS plays a significant role in risk assessment. Most individuals with a previous history of AMS after acute ascent are likely to experience similar symptoms with repeated visits to altitude. Gender does not affect the incidence of AMS.

Pathophysiology

The symptoms of AMS develop several hours after arrival at high altitude, whereas the development of HAPE and HACE generally requires several days of altitude exposure. Because hypoxemia occurs within minutes of arrival, it cannot be the direct cause of high-altitude illness, but rather the initiating factor.

The clinical manifestations of AMS/HACE are primarily the result of central nervous system (CNS) dysfunction caused by hemodynamic mechanical factors and biochemical mediators of permeability. The CNS vasodilatory response to hypoxemia causes an increase in cerebral blood flow and volume. Significant elevation of brain volume is observed in moderate to severe AMS and HACE but has not been demonstrated in mild AMS. Hypoxic alteration of CNS vascular autoregulation and hypertension from exercise may increase pressure transmission to the brain's capillary beds, resulting in transcapillary leakage and vasogenic edema. HIF-mediated vascular endothelial growth factor, the inducible form of nitric oxide synthase, reactive cytokines, and free radical formation may increase permeability. Both mechanical and biochemical activation of the trigeminovascular system have been proposed as the cause of **high-altitude headache**, the primary symptom of AMS. Vasogenic edema has been implicated in severe AMS and HACE, but MRI reveals signal changes in persons with and without clinical AMS. It has been well established that adults can have changes in cognitive function with acute exposure to high altitude. Investigation of cognitive dysfunction in healthy, lowlander European children found significant impairment in verbal short-term memory, episodic memory, and executive functions 24 hr after arrival at 3,450 m (11,400 ft). These impairments were attributed to hypoxia-induced dysfunction of the cerebral white matter. The neuropsychological changes were found to be reversible, since cognitive function returned to baseline on reevaluation 3 mo after returning to sea level.

Many of the responses to hypoxia and altitude exposure occur in both individuals who develop symptoms and those who remain free of AMS. To address the discrepancy in symptomatic illness, the "tight fit" hypothesis was proposed. This theory suggests that the development of AMS/HACE is the result of a lack of intracranial space to accommodate increasing volume from brain swelling and edema that develop at altitude. The adequacy of the intracranial and intraspinal space to buffer changes in brain and cerebrospinal fluid (CSF) volume is the central concept. Buffering occurs as the intracranial CSF is displaced by the foramen magnum into the space available in the spinal canal, followed by increased CSF absorption and decreased CSF production. Individuals with less CSF buffering capacity have less compliance and are hypothesized to become more symptomatic (develop AMS).

Prevention

A comprehensive approach to travel to high altitude with children should focus on 3 phases: planning the ascent and assessment of risk, recognition and management of altitude-associated illness, and follow-up of any illness relative to future travel or diagnostic testing necessary.

Planning for travel to high altitude with children should consider rate of ascent, formulation of an emergency plan for communication and evacuation, and availability of medical care at the high-altitude destination. The availability of medical care and evacuation from altitude will influence the degree of personal preparation necessary. *Slow ascent with time for acclimatization is the best prevention for all forms of altitude illness.* Residing for a few days at moderate altitudes (2,000-3,100 m, 6,600-10,200 ft) followed by graded ascent before arriving at high altitude. One extra night of acclimatization (at the same sleeping altitude) should be taken for every 1,000 m (~3,300 ft) gained. Rapid ascent by air may be avoidable through alternate routes or alternate means of transportation. Exposure to hypobaric hypoxia (reduced barometric pressure with maintained O_2 of 20.9%) decreases end-tidal CO_2 and AMS score, while increasing SaO_2 and exercise endurance on exposure to higher altitude. Staying over in Denver, Colorado, for 1 or 2 days before traveling to higher alpine destinations is an example of such a strategy and has been an effective technique of acclimatization; it has the advantage of reducing the likelihood of developing AMS, HACE, or HAPE. A similar trend in preacclimatization was found with preexposure to *normobaric* hypoxia (maintained barometric pressure with O_2 <20.9%) using commercially available low-O_2 tents or hypoxia breathing masks, although not as effective as preacclimatization with *hypobaric* hypoxia. Slow, gradual ascent is another effective means of acclimatization. The altitude at which someone sleeps is considered more important than the highest altitude reached during waking hours. Guidelines recommend that *above 3,000 m (~9,800 ft), one should not increase sleeping elevation by >500 m (1,600 ft) per day and should include a rest day every 3-4 days with no ascent to a higher sleeping elevation.* Acclimatization and slow ascent are by far the best ways to avoid AMS. The first few days at altitude, individuals should limit their activity and maintain adequate hydration.

Medical risk assessment encompasses consideration of age, previous altitude-associated illness, and possible predisposing circumstances to altitude illness. Very young infants (<4-6 wk) may not have completed the postnatal circulatory transition and may be more vulnerable to altitude-associated desaturation with periodic breathing, right-to-left shunting across the foramen ovale, and hypoxic pulmonary vasoconstriction. Infants who required supplemental oxygen during the neonatal period, especially for pulmonary hypertension, may be at risk for hypoxemia with prolonged altitude exposure. History and physical examination are useful to identify conditions predisposing to HAPE, including recent viral infections, cardiac malformations, or obstructive sleep apnea. Children are known to have greater pulmonary vascular reactivity than adults. Thus, respiratory illnesses such as otitis media, pneumonia, or bronchiolitis that cause release of inflammatory mediators will increase capillary permeability; although normally tolerated at sea level, when superimposed on hypoxia at high elevations, it may predispose children to serious altitude illness. If a child has had a recent upper or lower respiratory infection or otitis media, careful consideration should be given to rapid ascent above 2,000 m (~6,600 ft).

Children with chronic lung disease (e.g., cystic fibrosis, bronchopulmonary dysplasia) and obstructive sleep apnea (OSA) are at increased risk of hypoxia at altitude and development of HAPE. Therefore they should undergo SO_2 monitoring during altitude travel. Similarly, children with cardiac lesions involving an increase in pulmonary blood flow or pulmonary hypertension are at greater risk of developing HAPE. Children with trisomy 21 have increased pulmonary vascular reactivity and a higher risk of pulmonary hypertension, and are also more likely to have OSA and hypoventilation. *Children with sickle cell anemia who live at sea level should reconsider travel to altitude, or else ascend carefully because sickle cell crisis may occur at as low as 1,500 m (~5,000 ft).* Those with sickle cell trait may become symptomatic at altitudes above 2,500 m (~8,200 ft).

Acetazolamide is commonly prescribed as prophylaxis against AMS because of its ability to stimulate respiration and increase alveolar and arterial oxygenation. It acts as a carbonic anhydrase inhibitor that induces a renal bicarbonate diuresis, causing a metabolic acidosis that increases ventilation and arterial oxygenation. However, prophylactic pharmacologic therapy with acetazolamide in children is generally not recommended because preacclimatization with slow ascent achieves the same effect. Exceptions include children with previous susceptibility to AMS and an unavoidably rapid ascent, such as flying to La Paz, Bolivia (3,700 m, 12,100 ft), or Cusco, Peru (3,400 m, 11,200 ft), from sea level. The pediatric dose of acetazolamide is 2.5 mg/kg (maximum, 125 mg/dose) every 12 hr (Table 90.1). In adults, it is recommended that prophylaxis begin 24 hr before arriving at altitude and be continued for 48 hr at altitude, or until the final destination high altitude is reached. The respiratory stimulation caused by acetazolamide also improves sleep by eradicating periodic breathing. Side effects are common and include paresthesias, polyuria, lightheadedness, dry mouth, and metallic taste with carbonated beverages. Acetazolamide is a nonbacteriostatic sulfonamide drug, so a history of anaphylactic reaction to sulfa medications is a contraindication to its use. Acetazolamide should be avoided in breastfeeding mothers and pregnant women. **Dexamethasone** is another agent that has been used for AMS prophylaxis in the adult population. However, it should not be used for prophylaxis in children because of the potential for side effects; pancreatitis, pseudotumor cerebri, and interference with normal growth. Low-risk children should not need medications for prophylaxis and should use gradual ascent to prevent illness.

Diagnosis

AMS is easily identified in older children and adolescents using the **Self-Report Lake Louise AMS Scoring System**. The criteria require that the individual be in the setting of a recent gain in altitude, be at the new altitude for at least several hours, and report a headache *plus* at least 1 of the following symptoms: gastrointestinal (GI) upset (anorexia, nausea, or vomiting), general weakness or fatigue, dizziness or lightheadedness, or difficulty sleeping. Shortness of breath on exertion may also be a part of the clinical picture, although if occurring at rest, the presence of HAPE should be considered in the absence of other causes. The headache may vary from mild to severe; anorexia and nausea, with or without vomiting, are common. Sleep disturbance caused by periodic breathing is common in all visitors to high altitudes but is exacerbated

Table 90.1	Medications for Treatment of Altitude-Associated Illness in Children (No Studies in Children for High-Altitude Indications)			
MEDICATION	**CLASSIFICATION**	**INDICATION**	**DOSE AND ROUTE**	**ADVERSE EFFECTS**
Acetazolamide	Carbonic anhydrase inhibitor	AMS prevention*	2.5 mg/kg PO every 12 hr; max 125 mg/dose	Collateral effects include paresthesias and taste alteration
		AMS treatment	2.5 mg/kg PO every 12 hr; max 250 mg/dose	
Dexamethasone	Steroid	AMS prevention†		Risk of adverse effects precludes prophylactic use
		AMS HACE treatment‡	0.15 mg/kg PO/IM/IV every 6 hr; max 4 mg/dose	Hypertension, gastrointestinal hemorrhage, pancreatitis, growth inhibition
Nifedipine	Calcium channel blocker	HAPE treatment (small children)§	0.5 mg/kg PO every 4-8 hr; max 20 mg/dose	Hypotension
		HAPE treatment (>60 kg)§	30 mg SR PO every 12 hr or 20 mg SR PO every 8 hr	
		Reentry HAPE prevention	Same dose as HAPE treatment	
Sildenafil	Phosphodiesterase-5 inhibitor	HAPE¶	0.5 mg/kg/dose PO every 4-8 hr; max 50 mg/dose every 8 hr	

*AMS prophylaxis is not routinely recommended in children. It is indicated when rapid ascent profile is unavoidable or with previous altitude illness in child about to undergo similar ascent profile. Doses as low as 1.25 mg/kg every 12 hr have been successful in some children.
†Use not warranted due to risk of adverse effects. Use slow, graded ascent or acetazolamide.
‡Oxygen and descent are the treatment of choice for severe AMS. If acetazolamide is not tolerated, dexamethasone may be used. Oxygen, descent, and dexamethasone should be used in HACE.
§In emergency settings where oxygen and descent are not an option, nifedipine is indicated.
¶In emergency settings where oxygen and descent are not an option, if nifedipine is not well tolerated, sildenafil may provide an alternative.
AMS, Acute mountain sickness; HACE, high-altitude cerebral edema; HAPE, high-altitude pulmonary edema, IM, intramuscularly; IV, intravenously; PO, orally; SR, sustained release.

in the setting of AMS. All the symptoms of AMS can range in severity from mild to incapacitating. Symptoms develop within a few hours after ascent and generally reach maximum severity between 24 and 48 hr, followed by gradual resolution. Most adults become symptom free by the 3rd or 4th day. The vague nature of this presentation has resulted in many misdiagnoses and morbidity among adults. In the setting of recent altitude exposure, these symptoms warrant a presumptive diagnosis of AMS and limitation of further ascent. Any evidence of CNS dysfunction, such as mild ataxia or altered mentation, is early evidence of HACE.

In nonverbal young children and infants, recognition of AMS symptoms is more challenging. AMS is often a diagnosis of exclusion and is characterized by nonspecific signs: fussiness, lack of playfulness, anorexia, nausea, vomiting, and disordered sleep. In most cases of AMS in nonverbal young children and infants, all these symptoms are present. *Fussiness* is defined as a state of irritability that is not easily explained by a cause, such as tiredness, wet diaper, hunger, teething, or pain from an injury. Fussy behavior may include crying, restlessness, or muscular tension. Decreased playfulness may be profound. Alterations of appetite may progress to frank vomiting. Sleep disturbance can manifest with either increased or decreased sleep compared to normal patterns. Most often, decreased sleep and the inability to nap are noted.

The **Children's Lake Louise Score (CLLS)** has been successfully tested in preverbal children <4 yr old by parents briefed on the use of the scoring system. The CLLS combines a score for the amount and intensity of unexplained fussiness with a symptom score of how well the child has eaten, played, and slept in the past 24 hr. Evaluating for headache is done by asking if the head hurts or by using a "faces" pain scale. GI symptoms are evaluated by asking children if they are "hungry" rather than trying to evaluate their appetite. A combined score of ≥7 is indicative of AMS (Fig. 90.1). Many of the symptoms manifested by AMS in children may also result from the disruption of normal routine with travel. A change in environment, sleeping accommodation, or eating options can result in a fussy child. The threshold scores for AMS diagnostic criteria are modified to account for these baseline variations. Supplemental oxygen may serve as a diagnostic aid; 2-4 L/min by nasal cannula (27-33% O_2) for 15-20 min should significantly improve headache and other symptoms.

If symptoms occur >2 days after arrival at altitude and headache and dyspnea at rest are absent, and if the child fails to improve with supplemental oxygen, an alternative diagnosis should be sought. It must be emphasized that altered mental status, neurologic abnormalities, breathing difficulty, or cyanosis are *not* part of uncomplicated AMS. **Any of these signs warrants immediate medical attention.** If serious bacterial illness, a surgical condition, or another problem meriting specific intervention is suspected in a child, descent to lower altitude is recommended to eliminate the confounding variable of altitude illness.

Periodic Breathing
Periodic breathing at altitude is common at all ages during sleep, resulting in brief, repeated episodes of oxyhemoglobin desaturation. Prepubertal children (9-12 yr old) have similar nighttime oxygen desaturation as their parents but have somewhat more stable breathing patterns with less periodicity. Periodic breathing is not a sign of AMS, but the exacerbation of hypoxia during sleep plays a role in AMS development. Newborn infants normally have periodicity in their respiratory pattern, which is increased by high-altitude exposure and sleep. SaO_2 of awake neonates born in Colorado at 3,100 m ranges from 88-91%. During sleep with increased periodic breathing, SaO_2 may drop to 81% during the 1st wk of life. The amount and magnitude of respiratory periodicity decrease as the child matures, and SaO_2 during sleep increases to 86% after 2 mo. A stable, mature pattern is usually reached by 6 mo of age. Preterm babies may demonstrate marked periodicity with prolonged desaturation as a result of their immaturity. Acute ascent with a child born preterm is best delayed until maturity, when normal pulmonary function and respiratory drive can be demonstrated. Parents of normal healthy babies may become distressed by the marked periodic breathing pattern in their child after ascent to moderate altitude. Clinicians can reassure parents that this is generally not a precursor of true apnea; however, desaturation can occur with periodic breathing in sleep, especially at higher altitudes.

Management
The management of AMS must include strict adherence to the principle that further ascent to a higher sleeping altitude is contraindicated after the symptoms of altitude illness occur. Halting ascent or activity to allow

AMOUNT OF UNEXPLAINED FUSSINESS

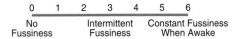

0	1	2	3	4	5	6
No Fussiness		Intermittent Fussiness		Constant Fussiness When Awake		

INTENSITY OF FUSSINESS

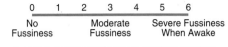

0	1	2	3	4	5	6
No Fussiness		Moderate Fussiness		Severe Fussiness When Awake		

FUSSINESS SCORE **(FS)** = Amount + Intensity

RATE HOW WELL YOUR CHILD HAS **EATEN** TODAY **(E)**

0—Normal
1—Slightly less than normal
2—Much less than normal
3—Vomiting or not eating

RATE HOW **PLAYFUL** YOUR CHILD IS TODAY **(P)**

0—Normal
1—Playing slightly less
2—Playing much less than normal
3—Not playing

RATE ABILITY OF YOUR CHILD TO **SLEEP** TODAY **(S)**

0—Normal
1—Slightly less or more than normal
2—Much less or more than normal
3—Not able to sleep

CLLS = FS + E + P + S

The CLLS must be ≥7 with both the FS ≥4 and E+P+S ≥3 to confirm acute mountain sickness.

Fig. 90.1 Children's Lake Louise Score (CLLS). *Fussiness* is defined as a state of irritability that is not easily explained by a cause, such as tiredness, hunger, teething, or pain from an injury. Fussy behavior may include crying, restlessness, or muscular tension. Please rate your child's typical fussy behavior *during the last 24 hr* without the benefit of your intervention.

further acclimatization may reverse the symptoms. However, the ascent exacerbates the underlying pathologic processes and may lead to disastrous results. Stopping further ascent and waiting for acclimatization treats most AMS in 1-4 days. Mild cases of AMS may be treated without descent if monitoring by a reliable caregiver is available. Conservative treatment may be provided, including rest, analgesics for headache, and antiemetics for nausea. Ibuprofen and acetaminophen are useful for the treatment of high-altitude headache; for nausea and vomiting, ondansetron dissolving tablets may be used.

More moderate symptoms may require acetazolamide and/or oxygen when conservative measures have proved inadequate. Oxygen is effective in the treatment of moderate AMS, titrated to maintain SaO_2 >94%. Although no studies have formally assessed its use in pediatric patients, anecdotal reports have demonstrated efficacy of acetazolamide in treating mild AMS in this population. AMS that becomes worse or does not respond to maintenance of altitude, rest, and pharmacologic intervention after 48 hr mandates descent. Descent (500-1,000 m, ~1,600-3,300 ft) is effective treatment for all forms of altitude illness and should be tailored to the individual response. *The presence of neurologic abnormalities (ataxia or altered mentation) or evidence of pulmonary edema (dyspnea at rest) mandates descent because these signs indicate a progression of AMS to severe altitude illness.*

HIGH-ALTITUDE CEREBRAL EDEMA

The incidence of HACE is very low and practically unheard of below 4,000 m (~13,100 ft), but it is rapidly fatal if unrecognized. Generally seen in adults with prolonged stays above 4,000 m, HACE is usually associated with concurrent AMS or HAPE but can occur on its own.

HACE is regarded as the extreme expression of the same pathophysiology underlying AMS. The etiology is believed to be secondary to increased cerebral blood flow leading to increased intracranial pressure (ICP). Cerebral venous congestion caused by compression and/or elevated central venous pressure may be an underappreciated mechanism of the increased ICP. In patients with HACE, MRI reveals white matter changes consistent with vasogenic edema that correlate with symptoms; evidence of cytotoxic edema has also been described.

HACE is frequently preceded by AMS, but it is differentiated from severe AMS by the presence of **neurologic signs**, most often ataxia and altered mental status, including confusion, progressive decrease in responsiveness, and eventually coma. Less common signs are focal cranial nerve palsies, motor and sensory deficits, and seizures. The CT scan is consistent with edema and increased ICP. MRI shows a high T2 signal in the white matter, specifically in the splenium of the corpus callosum, with diffusion-weighted technique.

Descent remains the most effective treatment for HACE. If available, supplemental oxygen is useful, especially when descent is not possible or delayed. Portable hyperbaric treatment is beneficial, but its use should not delay descent. Dexamethasone should be administered at a dose of 0.15 mg/kg orally every 6 hr. The few children reported with mild cases of HACE have recovered with dexamethasone and descent.

HIGH-ALTITUDE PULMONARY EDEMA
Epidemiology and Risk Factors

HAPE is a **noncardiogenic pulmonary edema** caused by intense pulmonary vasoconstriction and subsequent high capillary pressure, secondary to hypoxia, resulting in altered permeability of the alveolocapillary membrane and the extravasation of intravascular fluid into the extravascular space of the lung. *HAPE is the deadliest of the high-altitude illnesses;* its reported incidence is 0.5%, without an underlying predisposition, and typically requires recent ascent above 3,000 m. The development of HAPE depends on genetic factors typically affecting pulmonary vasoreactivity, rate of ascent, altitude achieved, and time spent at that altitude. Among children, HAPE occurs in 2 distinct settings. **Type I** HAPE (or simply HAPE) occurs in a child who resides at low altitude who travels to high altitude. **Type II** HAPE (also termed **reentry** or **reascent** HAPE) affects children who reside at high altitude but become ill on their return home after descent to lower altitudes. HAPE may also occur in children who develop acute respiratory illnesses that exacerbate hypoxia at high altitude. Fatal outcomes of HAPE in children have been reported. Most mild and moderate cases resolve without difficulty; however, if unrecognized and untreated, rapid progression to death can occur, especially when infection or cardiac conditions complicate the illness.

HAPE affects male and female children more equally than adults, among whom the observed male predominance appears to result from strenuous sport activities and military assignments. The occurrence and even the pathophysiology of HAPE may vary by population and genetic background. Individuals of Tibetan ancestry, resident on the Himalayan plateau and having minimal admixture with other populations, represent the extreme of adaptation to high altitude and rarely experience HAPE. Other native populations residing at high altitude, such as Andeans, do not appear to be protected from HAPE, and certain populations may have genetic polymorphisms associated with pulmonary edema.

A number of conditions may predispose a child to HAPE (Table 90.2). Preexisting viral respiratory infections have been linked to HAPE, especially in children. Cardiorespiratory conditions associated with pulmonary hypertension, such as atrial and ventricular septal defects, pulmonary vein stenosis, congenital absence of a pulmonary artery, and OSA, also predispose to HAPE. Down syndrome is a risk factor for HAPE development, as are previously repaired congenital heart

Table 90.2	Conditions Associated With Increased Risk of High-Altitude Pulmonary Edema (HAPE)

ENVIRONMENTAL

Ascent above 2,500 m (~8,200 ft)
Rapid rate of ascent (generally >1,000 m [~3,300 ft] per day)
Cold exposure

CARDIAC

Anomalies causing increased pulmonary blood flow or increased
   pulmonary artery pressure
Ventricular septal defect, atrial septal defect, patent foramen ovale,
   patent ductus arteriosus
Anomalous pulmonary venous return or pulmonary vein stenosis
Unilateral absent pulmonary artery or isolated pulmonary artery of
   ductal origin
Coarctation of the aorta
Congestive heart failure

PULMONARY

Chronic lung disease
   Bronchopulmonary dysplasia
   Pulmonary hypoplasia
   Supplemental oxygen requirement at sea level
Pulmonary hypertension
Perinatal respiratory distress
   Persistent pulmonary hypertension of the newborn
   Perinatal asphyxia or depression
Sleep apnea

INFECTIOUS

Upper respiratory tract infection
Bronchitis/bronchiolitis
Pneumonitis
Otitis media

PHARMACOLOGIC

Any medication causing central nervous system and respiratory
   depression
Alcohol
Sympathomimetics

SYSTEMIC

Down syndrome (trisomy 21)
History of premature birth or low birthweight

defects and the presence of hypoplastic lungs. Undiagnosed structural cardiopulmonary abnormalities may result in severe hypoxia and/or altitude illness once ascent occurs.

Pathophysiology

Alveolar hypoxia results in vasoconstriction of pulmonary arterioles just proximal to the alveolar capillary bed. Hypoxic pulmonary vasoconstriction is a normal physiologic response to optimize ventilation/perfusion ($\dot{V}/\dot{Q}$) matching by redistributing regional pulmonary blood flow to areas of highest ventilation, thereby optimizing arterial oxygenation. Under conditions that result in widespread alveolar hypoxia, extensive pulmonary vasoconstriction will lead to significant elevations in pulmonary arterial pressure; uneven pulmonary vasoconstriction can result in localized overperfusion, increased capillary pressures, distention, and leakage in the remaining vessels. This explains the patchy and heterogeneous edema that is classically observed in HAPE. The combination of pulmonary hypertension and uneven pulmonary vasoconstriction appears to be necessary in the pathogenesis of HAPE. Children and adolescents acutely exposed to high-altitude hypoxia demonstrated pulmonary hypertension, with increases in pulmonary artery pressure inversely related to age. Once the vascular leak occurs and alveolar fluid accumulates, a defect in transepithelial sodium transport impairs the clearance of alveolar fluid and contributes to HAPE.

Diagnosis

The diagnosis of HAPE is based on clinical findings and their evolution in the context of recent ascent from lower elevation. There is no single diagnostic test or constellation of laboratory findings. Symptoms usually develop within 24-96 hr, with onset of symptoms the 1st or 2nd night at altitude, when hypoxia may be exacerbated during sleep. HAPE generally is not observed beyond 5 days after ascent to altitude (unless additional ascent occurs) because pulmonary vascular remodeling and acclimatization have taken place. The minimum criteria to diagnose HAPE include recent exposure to altitude, dyspnea at rest, radiographic evidence of alveolar infiltrates, and near-complete resolution of both clinical and radiographic signs within 48 hr after descent or institution of oxygen therapy. Portable ultrasound is useful to diagnose HAPE through the finding of *comet tails*, artifacts created by microreflections of the ultrasound beam within interlobular septa thickened by interstitial and alveolar edema.

Frequently, patients first exhibit general malaise that may progress to more specific signs of dyspnea at rest, then cardiopulmonary distress. In preverbal toddlers and infants, HAPE may manifest as worsening respiratory distress over 1-2 days, pallor, depressed consciousness, increased fussiness, decreased playfulness, crying, decreased appetite, poor sleep, and sometimes vomiting. Young children may show agitation and general debility. Older children and adolescents may complain of headache and orthopnea and present with cough, dyspnea not relieved by rest or out of proportion to effort, and production of frothy, rust-colored sputum. Physical exam findings include tachypnea, cyanosis, elevated jugular venous pressure, and diffuse crackles on lung auscultation. Dyspnea at rest, orthopnea, cyanosis, tachycardia, and chest pain herald worsening compromise, which may advance within hours to production of pink-tinged sputum.

Findings on physical examination frequently are less severe than the patient's chest radiograph and hypoxemia on pulse oximetry would predict. Children often appear pale, with or without visible cyanosis. Low-grade fever (<38.5°C [101.3°F]) is common, and respiratory rate is generally increased. Auscultation typically reveals rales, usually greater in the right lung than the left on presentation. Chest radiograph reveals diffuse interstitial changes typical of noncardiogenic pulmonary edema, with central interstitial edema associated with peribronchial cuffing, poorly defined vessels, enlargement of the pulmonary artery silhouette with dilation of more peripheral pulmonary arteries, and patchy air space consolidation; Kerley lines may be present. In severe cases, air space consolidation may become confluent and involve the entire lung (Fig. 90.2). Often the right lung shows more radiographic changes of edema than the left. Cardiomegaly is an uncommon finding, but enlargement of the pulmonary artery is a frequent finding. Significant arterial oxygen desaturation, as measured by pulse oximetry, is a consistent finding, with SpO_2 frequently below 75%. A complete blood count often reveals a leukocytosis with a left shift of the granulocyte series.

The **differential diagnosis** of HAPE includes pneumonia, bronchitis/bronchiolitis, asthma, and other forms of cardiogenic and noncardiogenic pulmonary edema, as well as pulmonary embolism. HAPE is most frequently misdiagnosed as pneumonia or a viral respiratory illness, especially when suspicion of altitude-associated pathology is not appropriately high. The presenting signs of cough, dyspnea, and orthopnea, followed by sputum production, can easily be misinterpreted as pneumonia, an impression reinforced by the frequent low-grade fever. Respiratory viral infections increase the risk of developing HAPE, which may lead to further confusion in diagnosis.

Complications of HAPE in children often relate to underlying, sometimes undiagnosed, cardiopulmonary pathology or coexisting viral infections that potentiate the severity of pulmonary edema and pulmonary hypertension. Acute altitude exposure in such circumstances may lead to severe presentations that progress rapidly to extreme hypoxemia or cardiac failure and death. Children with trisomy 21, with or without structural cardiac anomalies, show increased susceptibility to HAPE and rapid symptom progression. Neonatal respiratory distress with pulmonary hypertension has been linked to exaggerated hypoxic pulmonary vasoreactivity in early adulthood and thereby a theoretical predisposition to HAPE. Other conditions related to pulmonary

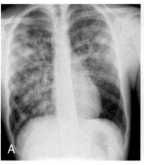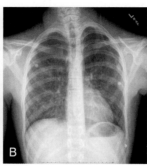

Fig. 90.2 Acute mountain sickness (AMS) and high-altitude pulmonary edema (HAPE). A healthy 15 yr old boy flew from Buffalo, NY, to Denver, CO, and immediately drove with his school group from the airport to a ski resort at 9,300 ft in the Rocky Mountains. The following day he felt dizzy and complained of headache. Symptoms of headache and dizziness continued along with emesis daily for 2 days. A snowboarding coach brought the patient to the local emergency facility the next day because of dyspnea, cough, headache, emesis, and fatigue. Pulse oximetry showed an arterial oxygen saturation of 51%. Chest radiograph showed diffuse pulmonary edema (**A**). The patient was transported to Denver (5,280 ft) by ambulance with 15 L/min oxygen via a non-rebreathing mask. SaO$_2$ improved with descent and was 94% on arrival at the Children's Hospital Colorado emergency department. Breath sounds remained coarse, and the patient was tachycardic and tachypneic. Oxygen flow was weaned to 1 L/min shortly after admission. Two days after presentation, lung exam was improved, without crackles. Repeat chest radiograph showed clearing of edema pattern (**B**). The patient maintained adequate SaO$_2$ without supplemental oxygen and was discharged. (*Courtesy of the Department of Radiology, Children's Hospital of Colorado.*)

overcirculation, small cross-sectional area of the pulmonary vascular bed, obstruction to pulmonary venous return, or left-sided obstruction potentiate HAPE. Inflammatory processes, such as viral infection, predispose to HAPE and may worsen hypoxemia.

Management
Descent with supplemental oxygen is the treatment of choice for HAPE in children. Unlike AMS, HAPE does not respond to rest and oxygen alone. When feasible, or in the absence of medical care, rapid descent of at least 1,000 m (~3,300 ft) usually results in rapid recovery. As with all altitude illness, the magnitude of the descent is tailored to the resolution of symptoms. Those affected should exert themselves as little as possible on descent and prevent exposure to cold, to avoid exacerbation of pulmonary artery pressure and pulmonary edema. Oxygen and bed rest without descent can be safe and effective treatment for mild HAPE in children where careful medical observation is available. Mild HAPE in children and young adults at 3,750 m (~12,300 ft) has been treated with bed rest alone, although clinical recovery may be slower than with supplemental oxygen therapy.

Supplemental oxygen at altitude is administered at 2-6 L/min by nasal cannula for 48-72 hr to maintain an SaO$_2$ of at least 90%. Oxygen flow can be weaned with improvement in symptoms and SaO$_2$; at flow rates <2-4 L/min, children may be sufficiently stable and comfortable to continue treatment at home under family monitoring. Most children experience complete resolution of mild HAPE within 24-72 hr of oxygen therapy when treated at the altitude of symptom onset.

Pharmacotherapy for pediatric HAPE is rarely needed since oxygen and descent are so effective. However, in emergency situations without the option of descent or oxygen, pharmacotherapy should be considered for treatment of HAPE. In adults, nifedipine, a calcium channel blocker, is the preferred drug. Although its use has not been studied in children for treatment of HAPE, **nifedipine** is indicated for treatment of pulmonary hypertension. Extrapolated dosing for children is 0.5 mg/kg orally every 4-8 hr and titrated to response (maximum, 10 mg/dose). Liquid-filled capsules of nifedipine (10 mg/0.34 mL) can be punctured to obtain

doses for children <20 kg. Patients should be monitored for hypotension during nifedipine administration. Alternatively, diltiazem can be given at 0.5-1.0 mg/kg/dose every 8 hr in tablet form or compounded oral suspension (12 mg/mL). Phosphodiesterase-5 inhibitors reduce pulmonary pressure at high altitude in adults through vasodilation and may be used if a calcium channel blocker is not available or poorly tolerated. However, concurrent use of multiple pulmonary vasodilators is not recommended. Pulmonary hypertension guidelines for children cite level I evidence for sildenafil in treatment of pulmonary hypertension.

β-Adrenergic agonists upregulate the clearance of alveolar fluid through transepithelial sodium transport and therefore could have a positive effect on HAPE. A single randomized controlled study in adults susceptible to HAPE exposed to very high altitude found that those receiving inhaled salmeterol had a 50% decreased incidence of HAPE compared to those who received placebo. Prevention of pulmonary edema using salmeterol was not associated with a decrease in pulmonary pressure, underscoring the clearance of alveolar fluid and improved hypoxia, which is believed to have accounted for the improved AMS score in these patients compared with the placebo group.

SPECIAL CONSIDERATIONS
Reentry HAPE
Children residing at high altitude may also experience HAPE of the type termed *reentry* or *reascent* HAPE. Reentry HAPE occurs on reascent to the altitude of residence after a sojourn to low altitude. Most cases occur after several days at lower altitude, and probability of recurrence may justify pharmacologic prophylaxis.

Travel With Young Infants
Newborn infants retain some of the circulatory characteristics of recent fetal life, and these can pose a unique risk for altitude exposure. The fetal circulation has high pulmonary resistance, low pulmonary blood flow, and both intra- and extracardiac shunts that optimize oxygenation through the placenta rather than the fetal lungs. After birth, a transition begins that closes fetal shunts and establishes normal pulmonary circulation and oxygen transport. *Exposure to marked hypoxia (3,000-5,000 m) can result in reversion to fetal shunting patterns despite the absence of a placenta.* Therefore, prolonged exposure to high altitude should be avoided for infants <6 mo old who normally live at low altitude, or whose gestation occurred at low altitude. Normal infants at sea level complete these changes in 4-6 wk, although for infants born at moderate or high altitude, changes may last ≥3 mo. Travel to high altitude with young infants is generally safe after 4-6 wk, when circulatory changes have occurred, breastfeeding is established, and congenital abnormalities may have been detected. Infants between 6 wk and 1 yr of age may have a higher incidence of pulmonary hypertension with hypoxia, patent ductus arteriosus (PDA), and patent foramen ovale (PFO) with prolonged exposure to high altitudes. Hypoxic exposure induces medial hypertrophy of pulmonary arteries and pulmonary arterioles, together with dilation of the pulmonary trunk and impressive hypertrophy and dilation of the right ventricle.

Infants residing at an altitude above 2,400 m (~8,000 ft) are at an increased risk of **sudden infant death syndrome (SIDS)**, possibly from greater hypoxia. Altitude may be an independent risk factor for SIDS. Similar to low altitude, infants should be placed on their backs for sleeping, and parents should be counseled on the potential elevated risk of SIDS at altitude.

Sickle Trait and Sickle Cell Disease
Children with sickle cell disease or sickle trait should avoid travel to altitude, because hypoxemia may trigger sickling and painful crises, including splenic crises. Up to 20% of pediatric patients with sickle cell and sickle-thalassemia disease may experience a vasoocclusive crisis at moderate altitude. Although the majority of children with sickle trait remain asymptomatic, children can experience splenic ischemia or infarction, with severe left upper quadrant pain.

Bibliography is available at Expert Consult.

Chapter **91**

Drowning and Submersion Injury

Anita A. Thomas and Derya Caglar

第九十一章

溺水和淹溺伤害

中文导读

　　本章主要介绍了溺水和淹溺伤害的病因、流行病学、病理生理学、治疗、预后及预防。在流行病学中描述了<1岁儿童、1~4岁儿童、学龄期儿童、青少年溺水的发生率及原因，并描述了基础疾病、服用乙醇、运动和娱乐、全球不同区域特点对溺水发生的影响；病理生理学中主要描述了缺氧缺血性损伤、肺损伤及冷水损伤；在治疗中主要描述了初步评估和复苏、院内评估和治疗、其他治疗问题及低体温的治疗。

Drowning is one of the leading causes of childhood morbidity and mortality in the world. Prevention is the most important step to reducing the impact of drowning injury, followed by early initiation of cardiopulmonary resuscitation (CPR) at the scene.

ETIOLOGY

Children are at risk of drowning when they are exposed to a water hazard in their environment. The World Congress of Drowning definition of drowning is "the process of experiencing respiratory impairment from submersion/immersion in liquid." The term *drowning* does not imply the final outcome—death or survival; the outcome should be denoted as *fatal* or *nonfatal* drowning. Use of this terminology should improve consistency in reporting and research; the use of confusing descriptive terms such as "near," "wet," "dry," "secondary," "silent," "passive," and "active" should be abandoned. The injury following a drowning event is *hypoxia*.

EPIDEMIOLOGY

From 2005 to 2014, an average 3,536 people per year were victims of **fatal drowning**, and an estimated 6,776 persons per year were treated in U.S. hospital emergency departments (EDs) for **nonfatal drowning**. Compared with other types of injuries, drowning has one of the highest rapid case fatality rates and is in the top-10 causes of death related to unintentional injuries for all pediatric age-groups. From 2010 to 2015, the highest drowning death rates were seen in children age 1-4 yr and 15-19 yr (crude rates of 2.56 and 1.2 per 100,000, respectively). In children age 1-4 yr, drowning was the number-one cause of death from *unintentional injury* in the United States in 2014. Pediatric hospitalization rates associated with drowning ranged from 4.7 to 2.4 per 100,000 between 1993 and 2008. Rates of fatal drowning hospitalization declined from 0.5 to 0.3 deaths per 100,000 during the same period. Morbidity following nonfatal drowning is poorly studied.

The risk of drowning and the circumstances leading to it vary by age (Fig. 91.1). Drowning risk also relates to other host factors, including male gender, alcohol use, a history of seizures, and swimming lessons. Environmental risk factors include exposure to water and varying supervision. These factors are embedded in the context of geography, climate, socioeconomic status, and culture.

Children <1 Yr Old

Most (71%) drowning deaths in children younger than 1 yr occur in the **bathtub**, when an infant is left alone or with an older sibling. Infant tub seats or rings may exacerbate the risk by giving caregivers a false sense of security that the child is safe in the tub. The next major risk to children <1 yr is the large (5-gallon) household bucket, implicated in 16% of infant drowning deaths. These buckets are approximately 30 cm (1 ft) tall and designed not to tip over when half-full. The average 9 mo old child tends to be top-heavy and thus can easily fall headfirst into a half-full bucket, become stuck, and drown within minutes.

Children 1-4 Yr Old

Drowning rates are consistently highest in 1-4 yr old children, likely because of their curious but unaware nature, coupled with the rapid progression of their physical capabilities. From 1999 to 2015, U.S. rates are highest in the southern regions, in some areas as high as 3.8 per 100,000. A common factor in many of these deaths is a lapse in adult supervision, often reportedly <5 min. Most U.S. drownings occur in residential **swimming pools**. Usually, the child is in the child's own home, and the caregiver does not expect the child to be near the pool.

In rural areas, children 1-4 yr old often drown in irrigation ditches

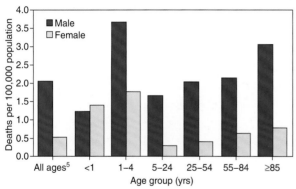

Fig. 91.1 Death rates from unintentional drowning* by age-group and sex—United States,[†] 2011. A total of 3,961 deaths from unintentional drowning were reported in the United States in 2011; the overall death rate for males was 2.05 per 100,000 population, almost 4 times the rate for females (0.52). In each age-group except for infants (i.e., those age <1 yr), the drowning death rate was higher for males. Males age 1-4 yr had the highest rate (3.67); for males and females, death rates increased with age after age 5-24 yr. *Unintentional drowning as the underlying cause of death includes codes for accidental drowning and submersion (W65-74), watercraft causing drowning and submersion (V90), and water-transport–related drowning and submersion without accident to watercraft (V92) in the *International Classification of Diseases, 10th Revision.* [†]U.S. residents only. [§]Includes decedents whose ages were not reported. *(From National Vital Statistics System: Mortality public use data file for 2011. http://www.cdc.gov/nchs/data_access/vitalstatsonline.htm.)*

or nearby ponds and rivers. The circumstances are similar to those noted previously, in a body of water that is near the house. Drowning is one of the leading causes of *farm injury–related deaths* in children.

School-Age Children
School-age children are at increased risk of drowning in natural bodies of water such as lakes, ponds, rivers, and canals. Although swimming pools account for most nonfatal drownings across all ages, **natural waterways** account for a higher death rate in children 10-19 yr old. Unlike for preschool children, swimming or boating activities are important factors in drowning injuries in school-age children.

Adolescents
The 2nd major peak in drowning death rates occurs in older adolescents, age 15-19 yr. Almost 90% drown in open water. In this age-group particularly, striking disparities in drowning deaths exist in gender and race. From 1999 to 2015, adolescent males fatally drowned at a rate of 2.4/100,000 compared to 0.3/100,000 in adolescent females. The gender disparity may likely be related to males' greater risk-taking behavior, greater alcohol use, less perception about risks associated with drowning, and greater confidence in their swimming ability than females.

Dangerous underwater breath-holding behaviors (DUBBs) are often performed by experienced healthy swimmers or fitness enthusiasts (hypoxic training) or when teenagers hold breath-holding contests during horseplay. DUBBs have been primarily reported in regulated swimming facilities. Behaviors include intentional hyperventilation before submersion, static apnea, and extended periods of underwater distance swimming or breathhold intervals. Swimmers are found motionless and submerged; resuscitation is often unsuccessful.

There is also significant racial disparity seen across drowning rates and causes. In 2015, as in previous years, drowning rates for black males age 15-19 yr were double those for white males of the same age. Non-Caucasian children are 4 times more likely to have a nonfatal drowning across all age-groups through 19 yr old. Black children are more likely to drown in unguarded public or apartment pools; white children are more likely to drown in private residential pools. Hispanic and

foreign-born children have lower rates of drowning than their white counterparts. Those with private insurance have lower rates of nonfatal drowning. Other factors include differences in exposure to swimming lessons, cultural attitudes, and fears about swimming, as well as experience around water, all of which may contribute to overall drowning risk.

Underlying Conditions
Several underlying medical conditions are associated with drowning at all ages. A number of studies have found an increased risk, up to 19-fold, in individuals with **epilepsy**. Drowning risk for children with seizures is greatest in bathtubs and swimming pools. Cardiac etiologies, including arrhythmias, myocarditis, and prolonged QT syndromes, have been found in some children who die suddenly in the water, particularly in those with a family history of syncope, cardiac arrest, prior drowning, or QT prolongation. Some children with long QT syndrome are misdiagnosed as having seizures (see Chapter 462.5).

Drowning may also be an **intentional injury**. A history of the event that changes or is inconsistent with the child's developmental stage is the key to recognition of intentional drowning. Physical examination and other physical injuries rarely provide clues. **Child abuse** is more often recognized in bathtub-related drownings. **Suicide** usually occurs in lone swimmers in open water.

Alcohol Use
The use of alcohol and drugs greatly increases the risk of drowning. Of teenagers and adults who die, up to 70% are associated with alcohol use. Alcohol can impair judgment, leading to riskier behavior, decreased balance and coordination, and blunted ability to self-rescue. Furthermore, an intoxicated adult may provide less effective supervision of children around water.

Sports and Recreation
Most U.S. drowning deaths occur during recreational activities. Drowning is the leading cause of *noncardiac sports-related deaths.* Surveys confirm that alcohol use is common during water recreation, as is not using a personal flotation device (PFD) during boating activities. In 2015 the U.S. Coast Guard reported that 85% of those who drowned in boating accidents were not wearing a PFD.

Global Impact of Drowning
Drowning injury is the 3rd leading cause of unintentional death worldwide, with the majority (90%) of fatalities occurring in low- and middle-income countries. More than half of the global drowning occurs in the World Health Organization (WHO) Western Pacific and Southeast Asia regions. Global drowning rates are vastly underestimated, since many drowning deaths in this region go unreported, and many immediate fatalities are unrecognized. In addition, these data exclude any cases of drowning as the result of intentional harm or assault, accidents of watercraft or water transport, and drowning related to forces of nature or cataclysmic storms, which usually claim large numbers of lives per incident; thus, true numbers of fatal drowning are likely much higher.

Some patterns of pediatric drowning are similar in all countries. By most accounts, the highest rates are seen in males and in children 1-4 yr old.

Whereas bathtubs and places of recreation (i.e., pools, spas) are significant locations for drowning in U.S. children, these are virtually unreported locations for drownings in developing countries. Instead, the predominant locations are near or around the home, involving bodies of water used for activities of daily living. These include water-collecting systems, ponds, ditches, creeks, and watering holes. In tropical areas, death rates increase during monsoon season, when ditches and holes rapidly fill with rain, and are highest during daylight hours, when caregivers are busy with daily chores.

Drowning during natural disasters such as **storms** and **floods** is important in all areas of the world. The largest numbers of reported flood-related deaths occur in developing nations; most are drownings that occur during the storm surge. In the United States and much of Europe, advances in weather monitoring and warning systems have reduced such deaths. U.S. flooding incidents, including hurricanes

Katrina and Sandy, showed that drowning caused the most deaths, particularly when people became trapped in their vehicles, were unable or refused to evacuate homes, or attempted to rescue others.

PATHOPHYSIOLOGY

Drowning victims drown silently and do not signal distress or call for help. Vocalization is precluded by efforts to achieve maximal lung volume to keep the head above the water or by aspiration leading to **laryngospasm**. Young children can struggle for only 10-20 sec and adolescents for 30-60 sec before final submersion. A swimmer in distress is vertical in the water, pumping the arms up and down. This splashing or efforts to breathe are often misconstrued by nearby persons as merely playing in the water, until the victim sinks.

Anoxic-Ischemic Injury

After experimental submersion, a conscious animal initially panics, trying to surface. During this stage, small amounts of water enter the hypopharynx, triggering laryngospasm. There is a progressive decrease in arterial blood oxyhemoglobin saturation (SaO_2), and the animal soon loses consciousness from hypoxia. Profound hypoxia and medullary depression lead to terminal apnea. At the same time, the cardiovascular response leads to progressively decreasing cardiac output and oxygen delivery to other organs. By 3-4 min, myocardial hypoxia leads to abrupt circulatory failure. Ineffective cardiac contractions with electrical activity may occur briefly, without effective perfusion (**pulseless electrical activity**). With early initiation of CPR, spontaneous circulation may initially be successfully restored. The extent of the global **hypoxic-ischemic injury** determines the final outcome and becomes more evident over subsequent hours.

With modern intensive care, the cardiorespiratory effects of resuscitated drowning victims are usually manageable and are less often the cause of death than irreversible hypoxic-ischemic central nervous system (CNS) injury (see Chapter 85). CNS injury is the most common cause of mortality and long-term morbidity. Although the duration of anoxia before irreversible CNS injury begins is uncertain, it is probably on the order of 3-5 min. Submersions <5 min are associated with a favorable prognosis, whereas those >25 min are generally fatal.

Several hours after cardiopulmonary arrest, **cerebral edema** may occur, although the mechanism is not entirely clear. Severe cerebral edema can elevate intracranial pressure (ICP), contributing to further ischemia; intracranial hypertension is an ominous sign of profound CNS damage.

All other organs and tissues may exhibit signs of hypoxic-ischemic injury. In the lung, damage to the pulmonary vascular endothelium can lead to **acute respiratory distress syndrome** (see Chapter 89). Aspiration may also compound pulmonary injury. Myocardial dysfunction (so-called stunning), arterial hypotension, decreased cardiac output, arrhythmias, and cardiac infarction may also occur. Acute kidney injury, cortical necrosis, and renal failure are common complications of major hypoxic-ischemic events (see Chapter 550.1). Vascular endothelial injury may initiate disseminated intravascular coagulation, hemolysis, and thrombocytopenia. Many factors contribute to gastrointestinal damage; bloody diarrhea with mucosal sloughing may be seen and often portends a fatal injury. Serum levels of hepatic transaminases and pancreatic enzymes are often acutely increased. Violation of normal mucosal protective barriers predisposes the victim to bacteremia and sepsis.

Pulmonary Injury

Pulmonary aspiration occurs in many drowning victims, but the amount of aspirated fluid is usually small (see Chapter 425). Aspirated water does not obstruct airways and is readily moved into the pulmonary circulation with positive pressure ventilation. More importantly, it can wash out surfactant and cause alveolar instability, ventilation-perfusion mismatch, and intrapulmonary shunting. In humans, aspiration of small amounts (1-3 mL/kg) can lead to marked hypoxemia and a 10–40% reduction in lung compliance. The composition of aspirated material can also affect the patient's clinical course: Gastric contents, pathogenic organisms, toxic chemicals, and other foreign matter can injure the lung or cause airway obstruction. Clinical management is not significantly

different in saltwater and freshwater aspirations, because most victims do not aspirate enough fluid volume to make a clinical difference.

Cold Water Injury

Drowning should be differentiated from cold water **immersion** injuries, in which the victim remains afloat, keeping the head above water without respiratory impairment in cold waters. The definition of cold water varies from <15 to 20°C (<59 to 68°F).

Heat loss through conduction and convection is more efficient in water than in air. Children are at increased risk for **hypothermia** because of their relatively high ratio of body surface area (BSA) to mass, decreased subcutaneous fat, and limited thermogenic capacity. Hypothermia can develop because of prolonged surface contact with cold water during immersion, while the airway is above water, or with submersion. Body temperature may also continue to fall because of cold air, wet clothes, hypoxia, and hospital transport. Hypothermia in pediatric drowning victims may be observed even after drowning in relatively warm water and in warm climates.

Immersion in cold water has immediate respiratory and cardiovascular effects. Victims experience **cold water shock**, a dynamic series of cardiorespiratory physiologic responses that can cause drowning. In adults, immersion in icy water results in intense involuntary reflex hyperventilation and to a decrease in breath-holding ability to <10 sec, which leads to fluid aspiration. Severe bradycardia, the *diving reflex*, occurs in adults but is transient and rapidly followed by supraventricular and ectopic tachycardia and hypertension. There is *no evidence* that the diving reflex has any protective effect.

Even after surviving the chaotic minutes of cold water shock, after an additional 5-10 min of cold water immersion, the victim can become incapacitated. Cooling of large and small muscles disables the victim's ability to grab hold, swim, or perform other self-rescue maneuvers. Depending on water and air temperature, insulation, BSA, thermogenic capacity, physical condition, swimming efforts, or high-water flow rates, heat loss with continued immersion can significantly decrease core temperature to hypothermic levels within 30-60 min.

The symptoms and severity of hypothermia are categorized based on body temperature. The victim with mild hypothermia has a temperature of 34-36°C (93.2-96.8°F) with intact thermogenic mechanisms (shivering and nonshivering thermogenesis, vasoconstriction) and active movements. Compensatory mechanisms usually attempt to restore normothermia at body temperatures >32°C (89.6°F). Lower core temperatures lead to impaired cognition, coordination, and muscle strength and with it, less ability to self-rescue. Thermoregulation may fail and spontaneous rewarming will not occur. With moderate hypothermia (30 to <34°C [86 to <93.2°F]), loss of consciousness leads to water aspiration. Progressive bradycardia, impaired myocardial contractility, and loss of vasomotor tone contribute to inadequate perfusion, hypotension, and possible shock. At body temperatures <28°C (82.4°F), extreme bradycardia is usually present with decreases in cardiac output, and the propensity for spontaneous ventricular fibrillation or asystole is high. Central respiratory center depression with moderate to severe hypothermia results in hypoventilation and eventual apnea. A deep coma, with fixed and dilated pupils and absence of reflexes at very low body temperatures (<25-29°C [77-84.2°F]), may give the false appearance of death.

If the cooling process is quick—and cardiac output lasts long enough for sufficient heat loss to occur before the onset of severe hypoxia—the brain can cool to a level that may be considered in the *neuroprotective* range, approximately 33°C (91.4°F) in controlled, experimental conditions. However, if submersion leading to drowning occurs before development of a neuroprotective level of hypothermia, severe anoxia devastates tissue organs. The theoretical benefits, implications, and consequences of hypothermia in drowning victims are areas of controversy. Known adverse effects are associated with hypothermia, and these must be balanced against the potential benefits observed in experimental data. One should clearly differentiate among **controlled hypothermia**, such as that used in the operating room before the onset of hypoxia or ischemia; **accidental hypothermia**, such as occurs in drowning, which is uncontrolled and variable, with onset during or shortly after hypoxia-ischemia; and **therapeutic hypothermia**, involving the purposeful and controlled lowering and maintenance of body (or brain) temperature after a hypoxic-ischemic event.

In drowning victims with uncontrolled accidental hypothermia associated with icy water submersion, there are a few case reports of good neurologic recovery after prolonged (10-150 min) cardiopulmonary arrest. Almost all these rare survivors have been in freezing water (<5°C [41°F]) and had core body temperatures <30°C (86°F), often much lower. Presumably, very rapid and sufficiently deep hypothermia developed in these fortunate survivors before irreversible hypoxic-ischemic injury occurred.

Most often, hypothermia is a poor prognostic sign, and a neuroprotective effect has not been demonstrated A 2014 study from Washington State found that submersion duration <6 min is most strongly related to good outcome, not water temperature. In another study of comatose drowning patients admitted to pediatric intensive care unit (PICU), 65% of hypothermic patients (body temperature <35°C [95°F]) died, compared with a 27% observed mortality rate in nonhypothermic victims. Similarly, in Finland (where the median water temperature was 16°C [60.9°F]) and in the United States, a beneficial effect of drowning-associated hypothermia was not seen in pediatric submersion victims; submersion duration <10 min was most strongly related to good outcome, not water temperature.

MANAGEMENT

Duration of submersion, speed of the rescue, effectiveness of resuscitative efforts, and clinical course determine the outcome in submersion victims. Two groups may be identified on the basis of responsiveness at the scene. The **first group** consists of children who require minimal resuscitation at the scene and quickly regain spontaneous respiration and consciousness. They have good outcomes and minimal complications. These victims should be transported from the scene to the ED for further evaluation and observation. The **second group** comprises children in cardiac arrest who require aggressive or prolonged resuscitation and have a high risk of multiple–organ system complications, major neurologic morbidity, or death. Compared with cardiac arrest from other causes, cardiac arrest from drowning has a higher survival rate.

Initial management of drowning victims requires coordinated and experienced prehospital care following the ABCs (airway, breathing, circulation) of emergency resuscitation. CPR of drowning victims must include providing ventilation. Children with severe hypoxic injury and symptoms often remain comatose and lack brainstem reflexes despite the restoration of oxygenation and circulation. Subsequent ED and PICU care often involve advanced life support (ALS) strategies and management of multiorgan dysfunction with discussions about end-of-life care.

Initial Evaluation and Resuscitation

See Chapter 81.

Once a submersion has occurred, immediate institution of CPR efforts at the scene is imperative. The goal is to reverse the anoxia from submersion and limit secondary hypoxic injury after submersion. Every minute that passes without the reestablishment of adequate breathing and circulation dramatically decreases the possibility of a good outcome. When safe for the victim and the rescuer, institution of in-water resuscitation for nonbreathing victims by trained personnel may improve the likelihood of survival. Victims usually need to be extricated from the water as quickly as possible so that effective CPR can be provided. Common themes in children who have good recovery are a short duration of event and initiation of CPR as soon as possible, before arrival of emergency medical services.

Initial resuscitation must focus on rapidly restoring oxygenation, ventilation, and adequate circulation. The airway should be clear of vomitus and foreign material, which may cause obstruction or aspiration. Abdominal thrusts should not be used for fluid removal, because many victims have a distended abdomen from swallowed water; abdominal thrusts may increase the risk of regurgitation and aspiration. In cases of suspected airway foreign body, chest compressions or back blows are preferable maneuvers.

The cervical spine should be protected in anyone with potential traumatic

neck injury (see Chapters 82 and 85). Cervical spine injury is a rare concomitant injury in drowning; only approximately 0.5% of submersion victims have C-spine injuries, and history of the event and victim's age should guide suspicion of C-spine injury. Drowning victims with C-spine injury are usually preteens or teenagers whose drowning event involved diving, a motor vehicle crash, a fall from a height, a water sport accident, child abuse, or other clinical signs of serious traumatic injury. In such cases, the neck should be maintained in a neutral position and protected with a well-fitting cervical collar. Patients rescued from unknown circumstances may also warrant C-spine precautions. In low-impact submersions, spinal injuries are exceedingly rare, and routine spinal immobilization is not warranted.

If the victim has ineffective respiration or apnea, ventilatory support must be initiated immediately. Mouth-to-mouth or mouth-to-nose breathing by trained bystanders often restores spontaneous ventilation. As soon as it is available, supplemental oxygen should be administered to all victims. Positive pressure bag-mask ventilation with 100% inspired oxygen should be instituted in patients with respiratory insufficiency. If apnea, cyanosis, hypoventilation, or labored respiration persists, trained personnel should perform endotracheal intubation as soon as possible. Intubation is also indicated to protect the airway in patients with depressed mental status or hemodynamic instability. Hypoxia must be corrected rapidly to optimize the chance of recovery.

Concurrent with securing of airway control, oxygenation, and ventilation, the child's cardiovascular status must be evaluated and treated according to the usual resuscitation guidelines and protocols. Heart rate and rhythm, blood pressure, temperature, and end-organ perfusion require urgent assessment. CPR should be instituted immediately in pulseless, bradycardic, or severely hypotensive victims. Continuous monitoring of the electrocardiogram (ECG) allows appropriate diagnosis and treatment of arrhythmias. Slow capillary refill, cool extremities, and altered mental status are potential indicators of shock (see Chapter 88).

Recognition and treatment of hypothermia are the unique aspects of cardiac resuscitation in the drowning victim. Core temperature must be evaluated, especially in children, because moderate to severe hypothermia can depress myocardial function and cause arrhythmias. Wet clothing should be removed to prevent ongoing heat losses, although in the hemodynamically stable patient, rewarming should be initiated in the controlled environment of the receiving ED or PICU. Unstable patients (i.e., arrhythmias) should be warmed to 34°C (93.2°F), taking care not to overheat. Trials are investigating if therapeutic hypothermia might be helpful, or if avoiding hyperthermia is the key element to long-term neurologic survival.

Often, intravenous (IV) fluids and vasoactive medications are required to improve circulation and perfusion. Vascular access should be established as quickly as possible for the administration of fluids or pressors. Intraosseous catheter placement is a potentially lifesaving vascular access technique that avoids the delay usually associated with multiple attempts to establish IV access in critically ill children. Epinephrine is usually the initial drug of choice in victims with bradyasystolic cardiopulmonary arrest (IV dose is 0.01 mg/kg using the 1:10,000 [0.1 mg/mL] solution given every 3-5 min, as needed). Epinephrine can be given intratracheally (endotracheal tube dose is 0.1-0.2 mg/kg of 1:1,000 [1 mg/mL] solution) if no IV access is available. An intravascular bolus of lactated Ringer solution or 0.9% normal saline (10-20 mL/kg) is often used to augment preload; repeated doses may be necessary. Hypotonic or glucose-containing solutions should not be used for intravascular volume administration of drowning victims.

Hospital-Based Evaluation and Treatment

Most pediatric drowning victims should be observed for at least 6-8 hr, even if they are asymptomatic on presentation to the ED. At a minimum, serial monitoring of vital signs (respiratory rate, heart rate, blood pressure, and temperature) and oxygenation by pulse oximetry, repeated pulmonary examination, and neurologic assessment should be performed in all drowning victims. Other studies may also be warranted, depending on the specific circumstances (possible abuse or neglect, traumatic injuries, or suspected intoxication). Almost half of asymptomatic or minimally symptomatic alert children (those who do not require ALS in the prehospital setting or who have an initial ED **Glasgow Coma Scale [GCS]** score of ≥13) experience some level of respiratory distress or hypoxemia progressing to pulmonary edema, usually during the 1st 4-8 hr after submersion. Most alert children with early respiratory symptoms respond to oxygen and, despite abnormal initial radiographs, become asymptomatic with a return of normal room-air pulse oximetry oxyhemoglobin saturation (SpO$_2$) and pulmonary examination by 4-6 hr. Subsequent delayed respiratory deterioration is extremely unlikely in such children. Selected low-risk patients who are alert and asymptomatic with normal physical findings and oxygenation levels may be considered for discharge after 6-8 hr of observation if appropriate follow-up can be ensured.

Cardiorespiratory Management

For children who are not in cardiac arrest, the level of respiratory support should be appropriate to the patient's condition and is a continuation of prehospital management. Frequent assessments are required to ensure that adequate oxygenation, ventilation, and airway control are maintained (see Chapter 89). Hypercapnia should generally be avoided in potentially brain-injured children. Patients with actual or potential hypoventilation or markedly elevated work of breathing should receive mechanical ventilation to avoid hypercapnia and decrease the energy expenditures of labored respiration.

Measures to stabilize cardiovascular status should also continue. Conditions contributing to myocardial insufficiency include hypoxic-ischemic injury, ongoing hypoxia, hypothermia, acidosis, high airway pressures during mechanical ventilation, alterations of intravascular volume, and electrolyte disorders. Heart failure, shock, arrhythmias, or cardiac arrest may occur. Continuous ECG monitoring is mandatory for recognition and treatment of arrhythmias (see Chapter 462).

The provision of adequate oxygenation and ventilation is a prerequisite to improving myocardial function. Fluid resuscitation and inotropic agents are often necessary to improve heart function and restore tissue perfusion (see Chapter 81). Increasing preload with IV fluids may be beneficial through improvements in stroke volume and cardiac output. Overzealous fluid administration, however, especially in the presence of poor myocardial function, can worsen pulmonary edema.

For patients with persistent cardiopulmonary arrest on arrival in the ED after *non–icy water* drowning, the decision to withhold or stop resuscitative efforts can be addressed by review of the history and the response to treatment. Because there are reports of good outcome following ongoing CPR in the ED, most drowning victims should be treated aggressively on presentation. However, for children who do not show ready response to aggressive resuscitative efforts, the need for prolonged ongoing CPR after non–icy water submersion almost invariably predicts death or persistent vegetative state. Consequently, in most cases, discontinuation of CPR in the ED is probably warranted for victims of non–icy water submersion who do not respond to resuscitation within 25-30 min. Final decisions regarding whether and when to discontinue resuscitative efforts must be individualized, with the understanding that the possibility of good outcome is generally very low with protracted resuscitation efforts.

Neurologic Management

Drowning victims who present to the hospital awake and alert usually have normal neurologic outcomes. In comatose victims, irreversible CNS injury is highly likely. The most critical and effective neurologic intensive care measures after drowning are rapid restoration and maintenance of adequate oxygenation, ventilation, and perfusion. Core body temperature and glucose management may also be important modulators of neurologic injury after hypoxia-ischemia.

Comatose drowning patients are at risk for intracranial hypertension. There is little evidence that ICP monitoring and therapy to reduce intracranial hypertension improve outcomes for drowning victims. Patients with elevated ICP usually have poor outcomes—either death or persistent vegetative state. Children with normal ICP can also have poor outcomes, although less frequently. Conventional neurologic

intensive care therapies, such as fluid restriction, hyperventilation, and administration of muscle relaxants, osmotic agents, diuretics, barbiturates, and corticosteroids, have not been shown to benefit the drowning victim, either individually or in combination. There is some evidence that these therapies may reduce overall mortality but increase the number of survivors with severe neurologic morbidity.

Seizures after hypoxic brain injury are common, although detection is often difficult in the ICU because these patients are frequently sedated, thus masking clinical signs. Continuous electroencephalographic (EEG) monitoring in critically ill patients revealed a 13% incidence of seizures, 92% of which were exclusively nonconvulsive. However, EEG monitoring has only limited value in the management of drowning victims, except to detect seizures or as an adjunct in the clinical evaluation of brain death (see Chapter 86). Seizures should be treated if possible to stabilize cerebral oxygen use, although benefits are inconclusive. Fosphenytoin or phenytoin (loading dose of 10-20 mg of phenytoin equivalents/kg, followed by maintenance dosing with 5-8 mg of phenytoin equivalents/kg/day in 2-3 divided doses; levels should be monitored) may be considered as an anticonvulsant; it may have some neuroprotective effects and may mitigate neurogenic pulmonary edema. Benzodiazepines, barbiturates, and other anticonvulsants may also have some role in seizure therapy, although no conclusive studies have shown improved neurologic outcome.

With optimal management, many initially comatose children can have impressive neurologic improvement, but usually do so within the 1st 24-72 hr. Unfortunately, half of deeply comatose drowning victims admitted to the PICU die of their hypoxic brain injury or survive with severe neurologic damage. Many children become brain dead. Deeply comatose drowning victims who do not show substantial improvement on neurologic examination after 24-72 hr and whose coma cannot be otherwise explained should be seriously considered for limitation or withdrawal of support.

Other Management Issues

A few drowning victims may have traumatic injury (see Chapter 82), especially if their drowning event involved participation in high-energy water sports such as personal watercraft, boating, diving, or surfing. A high index of suspicion for such injury is required. *Spinal precautions should be maintained in victims with altered mental status and suspected traumatic injury.* Significant anemia suggests trauma and internal hemorrhage.

Hypoxic-ischemic injury can have multiple systemic effects, although protracted organ dysfunction is uncommon in the absence of severe CNS injury. Hyperglycemia is associated with a poor outcome in critically ill pediatric drowning victims. Its etiology is unclear, but hyperglycemia is possibly a stress response. Glucose control in patients after drowning should be focused on avoiding hypoglycemia, hyperglycemia, and wide or rapid fluctuations in serum glucose, to prevent further harm.

Manifestations of acute kidney injury may be seen after hypoxic-ischemic injury (see Chapter 550). Diuretics, fluid restriction, and dialysis are occasionally needed to treat fluid overload or electrolyte disturbances; renal function usually normalizes in survivors. **Rhabdomyolysis** after drowning has been reported.

Profuse bloody diarrhea and mucosal sloughing usually portend a grim prognosis; conservative management includes bowel rest, nasogastric suction, and gastric pH neutralization. Nutritional support for most drowning victims is usually not difficult, because the majority of children either die or recover quickly and resume a normal diet within a few days. Enteral tube feeding or parenteral nutrition is occasionally indicated in children who do not recover quickly.

Hyperthermia after drowning or other types of brain injury may increase the risk of mortality and exacerbate hypoxic-ischemic CNS damage. Almost half of drowning victims have a fever during the 1st 48 hr after submersion. Hyperthermia is usually not caused by infection and resolves without antibiotics in approximately 80% of patients. Generally, prophylactic antibiotics are not recommended. However, there is general consensus that fever or hyperthermia (core body temperature >37.5°C [99.5°F]) in comatose drowning victims resuscitated from cardiac arrest should be prevented at all times in the acute recovery period (at least the 1st 24-48 hr).

Psychiatric and psychosocial sequelae in the family of a pediatric drowning victim are common. Grief, guilt, and anger are typical among family members, including siblings. Divorce rates increase within a few years of the injury, and parents often report difficulties with employment or substance abuse. Friends and family may blame the parents for the event. Professional counseling, pastoral care, or social work referral should be initiated for drowning victims and their families.

Hypothermia Management

Attention to core body temperature starts in the field and continues during transport and in the hospital. The goal is to prevent or treat moderate or severe hypothermia. Damp clothing should be removed from all drowning victims. Rewarming measures are generally categorized as passive, active external, or active internal (see Chapter 93). **Passive rewarming measures** can be applied in the prehospital or hospital setting and include the provision of dry blankets, a warm environment, and protection from further heat loss. These should be instituted as soon as possible for hypothermic drowning victims who have not had a cardiac arrest.

Full CPR with chest compressions is indicated for hypothermic victims if no pulse can be found or if narrow complex QRS activity is absent on ECG (see Chapters 81 and 93). When core body temperature is <30°C (86°F), resuscitative efforts should proceed according to the American Heart Association guidelines for CPR, but IV medications may be given at a lower frequency in moderate hypothermia because of decreased drug clearance. When ventricular fibrillation is present in severely hypothermic victims (core temperature <30°C [86°F]), defibrillation should be initiated but may not be effective until the core temperature is ≥30°C (86°F), at which time successful defibrillation may be more likely.

Significant controversy surrounds the discontinuation of prolonged resuscitative efforts in hypothermic drowning victims. Body temperature should be taken into account before resuscitative efforts are terminated. Other considerations include whether the victim may have been immersed before submerged, whether water was icy, or the cooling was very rapid with fast-flowing cold water. Victims with profound hypothermia may appear clinically dead, but full neurologic recovery is possible, although rare. Attempts at lifesaving resuscitation should not be withheld based on initial clinical presentation unless the victim is obviously dead (dependent lividity or rigor mortis). Rewarming efforts should usually be continued until the temperature is 32-34°C (89.6-93.2°F); if the victim continues to have no effective cardiac rhythm and remains unresponsive to aggressive CPR, resuscitative efforts can be discontinued.

Complete rewarming is not indicated for all arrest victims before resuscitative efforts are abandoned. Discontinuing resuscitation in victims of non–icy water submersion who remain asystolic despite 30 min of CPR is probably warranted. Physicians must use their individual clinical judgment about deciding to stop resuscitative efforts, taking into account the unique circumstances of each incident.

Once a drowning victim has undergone successful CPR after a cardiac arrest, temperature management should be carefully considered and body temperature continuously monitored. In victims in whom resuscitation duration was brief and who are awake soon after resuscitation, attempts to restore and maintain normothermia are warranted. Careful monitoring is necessary to prevent unrecognized worsening hypothermia, which can have untoward consequences.

For drowning victims who remain comatose after successful CPR, more contentious issues include rewarming of hypothermic patients and controlled application of therapeutic hypothermia. Although there is no evidence basis or opinion consensus, many investigators cautiously recommend that hypothermic drowning victims who remain unresponsive because of hypoxic-ischemic encephalopathy after restoration of adequate spontaneous circulation should not be actively rewarmed to normal body temperatures. Active rewarming should be limited to victims with core body temperatures <32°C (89.6°F), but temperatures 32-37.5°C (89.6-99.5°F) should be allowed without further rewarming efforts.

More controversial is the **induction of therapeutic hypothermia** in drowning victims who remain comatose because of hypoxic-ischemic encephalopathy after CPR for cardiac arrest. *A specific recommendation for therapeutic hypothermia, especially in children, is not yet generally accepted.* The Advanced Life Support Task Force of the International Liaison Committee on Resuscitation (2002) did not recommend therapeutic hypothermia in drowned children resuscitated after cardiopulmonary arrest, citing insufficient evidence and older studies demonstrating a potential deleterious effect in pediatric drowning victims. Several subsequent studies evaluating extracorporeal membrane circulation, rewarming, and therapeutic hypothermia in pediatric and adult drowning patients have shown no significant improvement in neurologic outcome or mortality.

The Therapeutic Hypothermia After Out-of-Hospital Pediatric Cardiac Arrest (THAPCA) randomized controlled trial (RCT) investigators analyzed post hoc the findings of *targeted temperature management* (TTM) in pediatric comatose survivors of out-of-hospital cardiac arrest due to drowning. Drowning comprised 28% of the landmark pediatric TTM (33°C vs 36.8°C) RCT, and the authors' principal observation is that targeting hypothermia, compared with targeting normothermia, did not result in better survival.

PROGNOSIS

The outcomes for drowning victims are remarkably bimodal: The great majority of victims either have a good outcome (intact or mild neurologic sequelae) or a poor outcome (severe neurologic sequelae, persistent vegetative state, or death), with very few exhibiting intermediate neurologic injury at hospital discharge. Subsequent evaluation of good outcome survivors may identify significant persistent cognitive deficits. Of hospitalized pediatric drowning victims, 15% die and as many as 20% survive with severe permanent neurologic damage.

Strong predictors of outcome are based on the incident and response to treatment at the scene. Intact survival or mild neurologic impairment has been seen in 91% of children with submersion duration <5 min and in 87% with resuscitation duration <10 min. Children with normal sinus rhythm, reactive pupils, or neurologic responsiveness at the scene virtually always had good outcomes (99%). Poor outcome is highly likely in patients with deep coma, apnea, absence of papillary responses, and hyperglycemia in the ED, with submersion durations >10 min, and with failure of response to CPR given for 25 min. In one comprehensive case series, all children with *resuscitation durations* >25 min either died or had severe neurologic morbidity, and all victims with *submersion durations* >25 min died. Long-term health-related quality of life and school performance in those who had received either bystander- or emergency medical service personnel–initiated CPR was high if their submersion duration was <5 min. Higher morbidity, mortality, and lower quality of life were reported in patients with >10 min submersion duration. In several studies of pediatric drowning, submersion duration was the best predictor of outcome, and water temperature was not. However, there are rare case reports of intact recovery following non–icy water drowning with longer submersion or resuscitation duration.

The GCS score has some limited utility in predicting recovery. Children with a score ≥6 on hospital admission generally have a good outcome, whereas those with a score ≤5 have a much higher probability of poor neurologic outcome. Occasionally, children with a GCS score of 3 or 4 in the ED have complete recovery. Improvement in the GCS score during the 1st several hr of hospitalization may indicate a better prognosis. Overall, early GCS assessments fail to adequately distinguish who will survive intact from those with major neurologic injury.

Neurologic examination and progression during the 1st 24-72 hr are the best prognosticators of long-term CNS outcome. Children who regain consciousness within 48-72 hr, even after prolonged resuscitation, are unlikely to have serious neurologic sequelae. On the contrary, several studies have shown that patients with minimal improvement during this initial period rarely show significant subsequent neurologic recovery despite aggressive resuscitation efforts and remain in a persistent vegetative state or die. Laboratory and technologic methods to improve prognostication have not yet proved superior to neurologic examination. Serial neurologic evaluations after CPR should be performed over the ensuing 48-72 hr, with consideration given to limitation or withdrawal of support in patients who do not have significant neurologic recovery, even though this may occur before absolute prognostic certainty is achieved.

PREVENTION

The most effective way to decrease the injury burden of drowning is prevention. Drowning is a multifaceted problem, but several evidence-based preventive strategies are effective. The pediatrician has a prime opportunity to identify and inform families at risk of these strategies through anticipatory guidance. Advocacy should focus on anticipatory guidance regarding the appropriate supervision of children, access to swim lessons, presence of lifeguards, barriers to swimming pools, and use of personal floatation devices (PFDs). A family-centered approach to anticipatory guidance for water safety helps explore and identify the water hazards that each family is exposed to in their environment. The practitioner can then discuss the best tools and strategies for prevention that are relevant for the family. It is important to identify the risk both in and around the home and in other locations they may frequent, often when vacationing, such as vacation or relatives' homes. For some families the focus may be on bathtubs and bucket safety; for others, home pools or hot tubs may be the major hazards. If the family recreates near or on open water, they also need to learn about safety around boats and open water. In a rural environment, water collection systems and natural bodies of water may pose great risk.

Parents must build layers of water protection around their children. Table 91.1 provides an approach to the hazards and preventive strategies relevant to the most common sources of water involved in childhood drowning. A common preventive strategy for exposure to all water types and all ages is ensuring **appropriate supervision**. Pediatricians should define for parents what constitutes appropriate supervision at the various developmental levels of childhood. Many parents either underestimate the importance of adequate supervision or are simply unaware of the risks associated with water. Even parents who say that constant supervision is necessary will often admit to brief lapses while their child is alone near water. Parents also overestimate the supervisory abilities of older siblings; many bathtub drownings occur when an infant or toddler is left with a child <5 yr old.

Supervision of infants and young children means that a responsible adult should be with the child every moment. The caregiver must be alert, must not be consuming alcohol or other drugs or socializing, and must be attentive and focused entirely on watching the child. Even a brief moment of inattention, such as to answer a phone, get a drink, or hold a conversation, can have tragic consequences. If the child does not swim, *touch supervision* is required, meaning that the caregiver should be within arm's reach at all times. Adolescents require active adult supervision and avoidance of alcohol or drug use during water activities.

Learning to swim offers another layer of protection. Children may start swim lessons at an early age that are developmentally appropriate and aimed at the individual child's readiness and skill level. Swim lessons are beneficial and provide some level of protection to young children. A study from Bangladesh, where drowning accounts for 20% of all deaths in children ages 1-4 yr, showed that swim lessons and water safety curricula are cost-effective and led to a decrease in mortality from drowning. As with any other water safety intervention, parents need to know that swimming lessons and acquisition of swim skills cannot be solely relied on to prevent drowning. *No child can be drown-proof.* A supervising caretaker should be aware of where and how to get help and know how to safely rescue a child in trouble. Because only those trained in water rescue can safely attempt it, families should be encouraged to swim in designated areas only when and where a lifeguard is on duty.

Children and adolescents should never swim alone regardless of their swimming abilities. Even as they become more independent and participate in recreational activities without their parents, they should be encouraged to seek areas that are watched by **lifeguards**. In 2015, lifeguards rescued 940,000 Americans from drowning, and they probably prevent millions more drownings through verbal warnings and prompt interventions when needed. It is important to emphasize that even if the child is considered a strong swimmer, the ability to swim in a pool does not translate to being safe in open water, where water temperature, currents, and underwater obstacles can present additional and unfamiliar challenges. For swimmers, supervision by lifeguards reduces drowning risk, because lifeguards monitor risk behaviors and are trained in the difficult and potentially dangerous task of rescuing drowning victims.

Two of the preventive strategies listed in Table 91.1 deserve special mention. The most vigorously evaluated and effective drowning

Table 91.1	Approach to Prevention Strategies for Drowning		
	HOME	**RECREATION**	**NEIGHBORHOOD**
Water hazards	Swimming pools Ponds Bathtubs Large buckets	Playing in water-swimming, wading Playing near water Being on water—boating	Irrigation ditches Watering holes Water drainage
Common risks	Lapse in supervision Unexpected toddler exposure Delayed discovery of child Reliance on water wings or pool toys Reliance on sibling or bath seat for bathing supervision	Lapse in supervision Change in weather Unfamiliarity with or change(s) in water conditions: 　Steep drop-off 　Current/tide 　Low temperature Alcohol use Peer pressure	Lapse in supervision, particularly when caregiver is socializing Risky behavior when with peers
Prevention strategies	Recognize hazards and risks. Provide constant adult supervision around water. Install 4-sided, isolation fencing of pools. Install rescue equipment and phone at poolside. Learn swimming and water survival skills. Avoid bath; instead shower, if a child/teen with seizure disorder. Learn first aid and CPR.	Provide constant adult supervision. Swim in lifeguarded areas. Know when and how to wear U.S. Coast Guard–approved PFDs. Avoid alcohol and other drugs. Learn swimming and water survival skills. Teach children about water safety. Be aware of current weather and water conditions. Learn first aid and CPR.	Identify hazardous bodies of water. Prevent access to water with barriers. Provide fenced-in "safe area" for water recreation. Provide lifeguarded swim sites. Provide access to low-cost swim/water survival lessons.

CPR, Cardiopulmonary resuscitation; PFDs, personal floatation devices.

intervention applies to swimming pools. **Isolation fencing** that surrounds a pool with a secure, self-locking gate could prevent up to 75% of swimming pool–related drowning. Guidelines for appropriate fencing, provided by the U.S. Consumer Product Safety Commission, are very specific; they were developed through testing of active toddlers in a gymnastics program on their ability to climb barriers of different materials and heights, and recent studies show them to be effective in preventing drowning in young children. In families who have a pool on their property, caregivers often erroneously believe that if a child falls into the water, there will be a loud noise or splash to alert them. Unfortunately, these events are usually silent, delaying timely rescue. This finding highlights the need for a fence that separates the pool from the house, not just surrounds the entire property.

The use of U.S. Coast Guard–approved **lifejackets or PFDs** should be advised with all families spending time around open water, not just those who consider themselves boaters. This issue is also particularly important for families who will participate in aquatic activities on a vacation. A PFD should be chosen with respect to the weight of the child and the proposed activity. Young children should wear PFDs that will float their head up. Parents should be urged to wear PFDs as well, since their use of PFDs is associated with greater use by their children. Toys such as water wings and "floaties" should not be relied on as drowning prevention measures.

Effective preventive efforts must also consider **cultural practices**. Different ethnic groups may have certain attitudes, beliefs, dress, or other customs that may affect their water safety. The higher drowning risk of minority children needs to be addressed by community-based prevention programs.

In addition to anticipatory guidance, pediatricians can play an active role in drowning prevention by participating in advocacy efforts to improve legislation for pool fencing, PFD use, and alcohol consumption in various water activities. Several counties in the United States, Australia, and New Zealand have laws requiring isolation fencing for pools. Their effectiveness has been limited by a lack of enforcement. Similarly, all states have boating-under-the-influence laws but, similarly, rarely enforce them. Furthermore, efforts at the community level may be needed to ensure the availability of swimming lessons for underserved populations and lifeguarded swim areas.

Bibliography is available at Expert Consult.

Chapter **92**

Burn Injuries

Alia Y. Antoon

第九十二章

烧伤

中文导读

　　本章主要介绍了烧伤的流行病学、预防、紧急处理、复苏和评估、治疗和电烧伤。在紧急处理、复苏和评估中主要介绍了住院指征、紧急处理措施、急救处理、烧伤分类及烧伤体表面积的评估方法；在治疗中主要介绍了轻度烧伤的门诊治疗、液体复苏、预防感染和烧伤的外科处理、营养支持、局部治疗、吸入性损伤、缓解疼痛和心理调整、整形和康复，以及重返学校和长期预后。

Burns are a leading cause of *unintentional injury* in children, second only to motor vehicle crashes. There has been a decline in the incidence of burn injury requiring medical care that has coincided with a stronger focus on burn treatment and prevention, increased fire and burn prevention education, greater availability of regional treatment centers, widespread use of smoke detectors, greater regulation of consumer products and occupational safety, and societal changes such as reductions in smoking and alcohol abuse.

EPIDEMIOLOGY

Approximately 2 million people in the United States require medical care for burn injuries each year. Approximately 50% of these patients are younger than 5 yr, with an average age of 32 mo. The principal cause of the burn is scald; one of the causes of **scald burn** is heating liquids in the microwave. The leading cause of burn in children 5-14 yr old is **flame injury**. In children 5-10 yr old, burns are usually a result of match play, whereas for older children, it is usually a result of gasoline ignition. **Fires** are a major cause of mortality in children, accounting for up to 34% of fatal injuries in those <16 yr old.

Scald burns account for 85% of total injuries and are most prevalent in children <4 yr old. Although the incidence of hot water scalding has been reduced by legislation requiring new water heaters to be preset at 48.9°C (120°F), scald injury remains the leading cause of hospitalization for burns. *Steam inhalation* used as a home remedy to treat respiratory infections is another potential cause of burns. Flame burns account for 13%; the remaining are electrical and chemical burns. **Clothing ignition** events have declined since passage of the Federal Flammable Fabric Act requiring sleepwear to be flame-retardant; however, the U.S. Consumer Product Safety Commission has voted to relax the existing children's sleepwear flammability standard. *Polyester* is the fabric most resistant to ignition by small flame source. Polyester does burn deeply as it melts, but it self-extinguishes when the flame source is removed. *Cotton*, on the other hand, continues to burn after the flame source has been removed, resulting in large, deep burns. Polyester melts downward, sparing the face and respiratory tract; cotton burns upward toward the face. Pellet stove, glass front stoves, and flat top stoves are becoming frequent sources of hand burns in children. Approximately 18% of burns are the result of **child abuse** (usually scalds), making it important to assess the pattern and site of injury and their consistency with the patient history (see Chapter 16). **Friction burns** from treadmills are also a problem. Hands are the most commonly injured sites, with deep 2nd-degree friction injury sometimes associated with fractures of the fingers. *Anoxia,* not the actual burn, is a major cause of morbidity and mortality in house fires.

Review of the history usually shows a common pattern: scald burns to the side of the face, neck, and arm if liquid is pulled from a table or stove; burns in the pant leg area if clothing ignites; burns in a splash pattern from cooking; and burns on the palm of the hand from contact with a hot stove. However, **glove or stocking burns** of the hands and feet; single-area deep burns on the trunk, buttocks, or back; and small, full-thickness burns (e.g., cigarette burns) in young children should raise the suspicion of child abuse.

Burn care involves a range of activities: prevention, acute care and resuscitation, wound management, pain relief, reconstruction, rehabilitation, and psychosocial adjustment. Children with massive burns require early and appropriate psychological and social support as well as resuscitation. Surgical debridement, wound closure, and rehabilitative efforts should be instituted concurrently to promote optimal rehabilitation. In order to maximize survival, the clinical approach includes aggressive surgical removal of devitalized tissue, infection control, and judicious use of antibiotics; life support with endotracheal intubation and mechanical ventilation; and use of early nutrition. Children who have sustained burn injuries differ in appearance from their peers, necessitating supportive efforts for reentry to school and social and sporting activities.

PREVENTION

The aim of burn prevention is a continuing reduction in the number of serious burn injuries (Table 92.1). Effective first aid and triage can decrease both the extent (area) and the severity (depth) of injuries. The use of flame-retardant clothing and smoke detectors, control of hot water temperature (thermostat settings) to 48.9°C (120°F) within buildings, and prohibition of cigarette smoking have been partially successful in reducing the incidence of burn injuries. Treatment of children with significant burn injuries in dedicated burn centers facilitates medically effective care, improves survival, and leads to greater cost efficiency. Survival of at least 80% of patients with burns of 90% of the body surface area (BSA) is possible; the overall survival rate of children with burns of all sizes is 99%. Death is more likely in children with irreversible anoxic brain injury sustained at the time of the burn. It is well known that burns occur in predictable patterns. Sources of burns include, by season:

Winter:
- Glass front fireplaces/pellet stoves and radiators increase hand burns.
- Treadmill injuries as more people exercise inside—child imitates adults or young child touches belt.

Table 92.1	Burn Prophylaxis

PREVENT FIRES
Install and use smoke detectors.
Control the hot water thermostat; in public buildings, maximum water temperature should be 48.9°C (120°F).
Keep fire, matches, and lighters out of the reach of children.
Avoid cigarette smoking, especially in bed.
Do not leave lit candles unattended.
Use flame retardant–treated clothing.
Use caution when cooking, especially with oil.
Keep cloth items off heaters.

PREVENT INJURY
Roll, but do not run, if clothing catches fire; wrap in a blanket.
Practice escape procedures.
Crawl beneath smoke if a fire occurs indoors.
Use educational materials.*

*National Fire Protection Association pamphlets and videos.

Table 92.2	Indications for Hospitalization for Burns

Burns affecting >10% of BSA
Burns >10–20% of BSA in adolescent/adult
3rd-degree burns
Electrical burns caused by high-tension wires or lightning
Chemical burns
Inhalation injury, regardless of the amount of BSA burned
Inadequate home or social environment
Suspected child abuse or neglect
Burns to the face, hands, feet, perineum, genitals, or major joints
Burns in patients with preexisting medical conditions that may complicate the acute recovery phase
Associated injuries (fractures)
Pregnancy

BSA, Body surface area.

Summer:
- Fireworks, sparkler—temperatures reach 537.8°C (1,000°F).
- Burn contact with hot grill; hand/feet burn from hot embers.
- Lawnmowers

Spring/Fall:
- Burning leaves
- Gasoline burns
- Tap water scalds are essentially preventable through a combination of behavioral and environmental changes.

Pediatricians can play a major role in preventing the most common burns by educating parents and healthcare providers. Simple, effective, efficient, and cost-effective preventive measures include the use of appropriate clothing and smoke detectors and the planning of routes for emergency exit from the home. The National Fire Protection Association (NFPA) recommends replacing smoke detector batteries annually and the smoke detector alarm every 10 yr (or earlier, if indicated on the device). Child neglect and abuse must be seriously considered when the history of the injury and the distribution of the burn do not match.

ACUTE CARE, RESUSCITATION, AND ASSESSMENT
Indications for Admission
Burns covering >10% of total body surface area (BSA), burns associated with smoke inhalation, burns resulting from high-tension (voltage) electrical injuries, and burns associated with suspected child abuse or neglect should be treated as emergencies and the child hospitalized (Table 92.2). Small 1st- and 2nd-degree burns of the hands, feet, face, perineum, and joint surfaces also require admission if close follow-up care is difficult to provide. Children who have been in enclosed-space fires and those who have face and neck burns should be hospitalized for at least 24 hr for observation for signs of central nervous system

(CNS) effects of anoxia from carbon monoxide (CO) poisoning and pulmonary effects from smoke inhalation.

First Aid Measures

Acute care should include the following measures:

1. Extinguish flames by rolling the child on the ground; cover the child with a blanket, coat, or carpet.
2. After determining that the airway is patent, remove smoldering clothing or clothing saturated with hot liquid. Jewelry, particularly rings and bracelets, should be removed or cut away to prevent constriction and vascular compromise during the edema phase in the first 24-72 hr after burn injury.
3. In cases of **chemical injury**, brush off any remaining chemical, if powdered or solid; then use copious irrigation or wash the affected area with water. Call the local poison control center for the neutralizing agent to treat a chemical ingestion.
4. Cover the burned area with clean, dry sheeting and apply cold (not iced) wet compresses to small injuries. Significant large-burn injury (>15% of BSA) decreases body temperature control and contraindicates the use of cold compresses.
5. If the burn is caused by **hot tar**, use mineral oil to remove the tar.
6. Administer analgesic medications.

Emergency Care

Supportive measures are as follows (Table 92.3 and Table 92.4)

1. Rapidly review the cardiovascular and pulmonary status and document preexisting or physiologic lesions (asthma, congenital heart disease, renal or hepatic disease).
2. Ensure and maintain an adequate airway, and provide humidified oxygen by mask or endotracheal intubation (Fig. 92.1). The latter may be needed in children who have facial burns or a burn sustained in an enclosed space, before facial or laryngeal edema becomes evident. If hypoxia or CO poisoning is suspected, 100% oxygen should be used (see Chapters 81 and 89).
3. Children with burns >15% of BSA require intravenous (IV) fluid resuscitation to maintain adequate perfusion. In an emergency situation if IV access is unattainable, an intraosseous line should be placed. When inserting central lines to provide high-volume fluid, special attention should be paid to use a very-small-caliber catheter in small

children to avoid injury to the vascular lining, which may predispose to formation of clots. All inhalation injuries, regardless of the extent of BSA burn, require venous access to control fluid intake. All high-tension and electrical injuries require venous access to ensure forced alkaline diuresis in case of muscle injury to avoid myoglobinuric renal damage. Lactated Ringer solution, 10-20 mL/kg/hr (normal saline may be used if lactated Ringer solution is not available), is initially infused until proper fluid replacement can be calculated. Consultation with a specialized burn unit should be made to coordinate fluid therapy, the type of fluid, the preferred formula for calculation, and preferences for the use of colloid agents, particularly if transfer to a burn center is anticipated.

4. Evaluate the child for associated injuries, which are common in patients with a history of high-tension electrical burn, especially if there has also been a fall from a height. Injuries to the spine, bones, and thoracic or intraabdominal organs may occur (see Chapter 82). Cervical spine precautions should be observed until this injury is ruled out. There is a very high risk of cardiac abnormalities, including ventricular tachycardia and ventricular fibrillation, resulting from conductivity of the high electric voltage. Cardiopulmonary resuscitation (CPR) should be instituted promptly at the scene and cardiac monitoring started on the patient's arrival at the emergency department (ED) (see Chapter 81).
5. Children with burns of >15% of BSA should not receive oral fluids (initially) because gastric distention may develop. These children require insertion of a nasogastric tube in the ED to prevent aspiration.
6. A Foley catheter should be inserted into the bladder to monitor urine output in all children who require IV fluid resuscitation.
7. All wounds should be wrapped with sterile dressings until it is decided whether to treat the patient on an outpatient basis or refer to an appropriate facility.
8. A CO measurement (carboxyhemoglobin [HbCO]) should be obtained for fire victims and 100% oxygen administered until the result is known.
9. Review child immunization. Burns <10% BSA do not require tetanus prevention, whereas burns >10% need tetanus immunization. Use diphtheria, tetanus toxoids, and acellular pertussis (DTaP) for tetanus prophylaxis for children <11 yr old, and use tetanus, diphtheria, and pertussis (TdaP) for children >11 yr old (see Chapter 238).

Classification of Burns

Proper triage and treatment of burn injury require assessment of the extent and depth of the injury (Table 92.5 and Fig. 92.2). **1st-degree burns** involve only the epidermis and are characterized by swelling, erythema, and pain (similar to mild sunburn). Tissue damage is usually minimal, and there is no blistering. Pain resolves in 48-72 hr; in a small percentage of patients, the damaged epithelium peels off, leaving no residual scars.

A **2nd-degree burn** involves injury to the entire epidermis and a variable portion of the dermal layer (vesicle and blister formation are characteristic). A *superficial* 2nd-degree burn is extremely painful because

Table 92.3	Acute Treatment of Burns

First aid, including washing of wounds and removal of devitalized tissue
Fluid resuscitation
Provision of energy requirements
Control of pain
Prevention of infection—early excision and grafting
Prevention of excessive metabolic expenditures
Control of bacterial wound flora
Use of biologic and synthetic dressings to close the wound

Table 92.4	Four Phases of Burn Care, With Physiologic Changes and Objectives	
PHASE AND TIMING	**PHYSIOLOGIC CHANGES**	**OBJECTIVES**
1: Initial evaluation and resuscitation, 0 to 72 hr	Massive capillary leak and burn shock	Accurate fluid resuscitation and thorough evaluation
2: Initial wound excision and biologic closure, days 1-7	Hyperdynamic and catabolic state with high risk of infection	Accurately identify and remove all full-thickness wounds and achieve biologic closure
3: Definitive wound closure, day 7 to week 6	Continued catabolic state and risk of nonwound septic events	Replace temporary with definitive covers, and close small complex wounds
4: Rehabilitation, reconstruction, and reintegration, day 1 through discharge	Waning catabolic state and recovering strength	Initially to maintain range of motion and reduce edema; subsequently to strengthen and facilitate return to home, work, and school

From Sheridan RL: Burns, including inflammation injury. In Vincent JL, Abraham E, Moore FA, et al, editors: *Textbook of critical care*, ed 7, Philadelphia, 2017, Elsevier (Table 168-1, p. 1173).

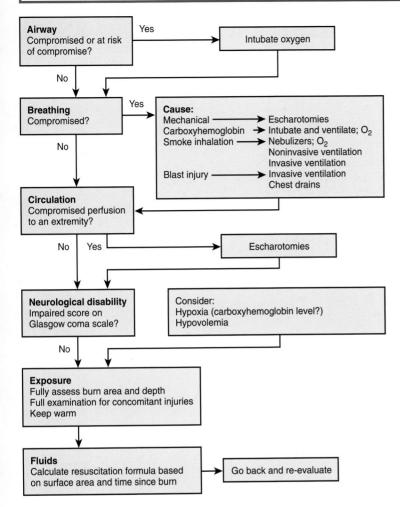

Fig. 92.1 Algorithm for primary survey of a major burn injury. *(From Hettiaratchy S, Papini R: Initial management of a major burn. I. Overview, BMJ 328: 1555–1557, 2004.)*

many remaining viable nerve endings are exposed. Superficial 2nd-degree burns heal in 7-14 days as the epithelium regenerates in the absence of infection. *Mid-level to deep* 2nd-degree burns also heal spontaneously if wounds are kept clean and infection free. Pain is less with these burns than in more superficial burns because fewer nerve endings remain viable. Fluid losses and metabolic effects of deep dermal (2nd-degree) burns are essentially the same as those of 3rd-degree burns.

Full-thickness, or **3rd-degree, burns** involve destruction of the entire epidermis and dermis, leaving no residual epidermal cells to repopulate the damaged area. The wound cannot epithelialize and can heal only by wound contraction or skin grafting. The absence of painful sensation and capillary filling demonstrates the loss of nerve and capillary elements.

Technologies are being used to help accurately determine the depth of burns. Laser *Doppler imaging* can be used from 48 hr to 5 days after the burn. It produces a color map of the affected tissue; *yellow* indicates second-degree burns, reflecting the presence of capillaries, arterioles, and venules, and *blue* reflects very low or absence of blood flow, which indicates third-degree burns. Its accuracy is up to 95%, and with accurate assessment, the proper treatment can be applied without delay. Doppler imaging can be used in both outpatients and inpatients.

Another technology called *reflectance confocal microscopy* (RCM), can be combined with *optical coherence tomography* (OCT) to visualize tissue morphology at the subcellular level. It determines if the cells are damaged and enables detection of skin morphologic changes up to 1 mm in depth. It provides accurate determination of the depth of the burn, allowing for the appropriate treatment.

Estimation of Body Surface Area for a Burn
Appropriate burn charts for different childhood age-groups should be used to accurately estimate the extent of BSA burned. The volume of fluid needed in resuscitation is calculated from the estimation of the extent and depth of burn surface. Mortality and morbidity also depend on the extent and depth of the burn. The variable growth rate of the head and extremities throughout childhood makes it necessary to use BSA charts, such as that modified by Lund and Brower or the chart used at the Shriners Hospital for Children in Boston (Fig. 92.3). The **rule of nines** used in adults may be used only in children >14 yr old or as a rough estimate to institute therapy before transfer to a burn center. In small burns, <10% of BSA, the **rule of palm** may be used, especially in outpatient settings; the area from the wrist crease to the finger crease (the palm) in the child equals 1% of the child's BSA.

TREATMENT
Outpatient Management of Minor Burns
A patient with 1st- and 2nd-degree burns of <10% BSA may be treated on an outpatient basis unless family support is judged inadequate or there are issues of child neglect or abuse. These outpatients do not require a tetanus booster (unless not fully immunized) or prophylactic penicillin therapy. Blisters should be left intact and dressed with *bacitracin* or *silver sulfadiazine* cream (Silvadene). Dressings should be changed once daily, after the wound is washed with lukewarm water to remove any cream left from the previous application. Very small wounds, especially those on the face, may be treated with bacitracin ointment

Table 92.5	Categories of Burn Depth		
	1ST-DEGREE BURN	**2ND-DEGREE, OR PARTIAL-THICKNESS, BURN**	**3RD-DEGREE, OR FULL-THICKNESS, BURN**
Surface appearance	Dry, no blisters Minimal or no edema Erythematous Blanches, bleeds	Moist blebs, blisters Underlying tissue is mottled pink and white, with fair capillary refill Bleeds	Dry, leathery eschar Mixed white, waxy, khaki, mahogany, soot-stained No blanching or bleeding
Pain	Very painful	Very painful	Insensate
Histologic depth	Epidermal layers only	Epidermis, papillary, and reticular layers of dermis May include domes of subcutaneous layers	Down to and may include fat, subcutaneous tissue, fascia, muscle, and bone
Healing time	2-5 days with no scarring	Superficial: 5-21 days with no grafting Deep partial: 21-35 days with no infection; if infected, converts to full-thickness burn	Large areas require grafting, but small areas may heal from the edges after weeks

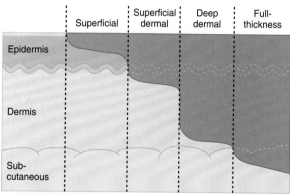

Fig. 92.2 Diagram of different burn depths. (*From Hettiaratchy S, Papini R: Initial management of a major burn. II. Assessment and resuscitation, BMJ 329:101–103, 2004.*)

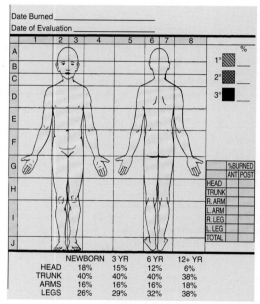

Fig. 92.3 Chart to determine developmentally related percentage of body surface area affected by burn injury. ANT, Anterior; POST, posterior; R., right; L., left. (*Courtesy of Shriners Hospital for Crippled Children, Burn Institute, Boston Unit.*)

and left open. **Debridement** of the devitalized skin is indicated when the blisters rupture. A variety of wound dressings and wound membranes (e.g., AQUACEL Ag dressing [ConvaTec USA, Skillman, NJ] in soft felt-like material impregnated with silver ion) may be applied to 2nd-degree burns and wrapped with a dry sterile dressing. Similar wound membranes provide pain control, prevent wound desiccation, and reduce wound colonization (Table 92.6). These dressings are usually kept on for 7-10 days but are checked twice a week.

Burns to the palm with large blisters usually heal beneath the blisters; they should receive close follow-up on an outpatient basis. The great majority of superficial burns heal in 10-20 days. Deep 2nd-degree burns take longer to heal and may benefit from enzymatic debridement ointment (collagenase) applied daily on the wound, which aids in the removal of the dead tissue. These ointments should not be applied to the face, to avoid the risk of getting into the eyes.

The depth of scald injuries is difficult to assess early; conservative treatment is appropriate initially, with the depth of the area involved determined before grafting is attempted (Fig. 92.4). This approach obviates the risk of anesthesia and unnecessary grafting.

Fluid Resuscitation
Fluid resuscitation should begin soon after the injury has occurred, in the ED before transferring to a burn center. For most children, the *Parkland formula* is an appropriate starting guideline for fluid resuscitation (4 mL lactated Ringer solution/kg/% BSA burned). Half the fluid is given over the 1st 8 hr, calculated from the time of onset of injury; the remaining fluid is given at an even rate over the next 16 hr. The rate of infusion is adjusted according to the patient's response to therapy.

Pulse and blood pressure should return to normal, and an adequate urine output (>1 mL/kg/hr in children; 0.5-1.0 mL/kg/hr in adolescents) should be accomplished by varying the IV infusion rate. Vital signs, acid-base balance, and mental status reflect the adequacy of resuscitation. Because of interstitial edema and sequestration of fluid in muscle cells, patients may gain up to 20% over baseline (preburn) body weight. Patients with burns of 30% BSA require a large venous access (central venous line) to deliver the fluid required over the critical 1st 24 hr. Patients with burns of >60% BSA may require a multilumen central venous catheter; these patients are best cared for in a specialized burn unit. In addition to fluid resuscitation, children should receive standard maintenance fluids (see Chapter 69).

During the 2nd 24 hr after the burn, patients begin to reabsorb edema fluid and to experience diuresis. Half the 1st day's fluid requirement is infused as lactated Ringer solution in 5% dextrose. Children <5 yr old may require the addition of 5% dextrose in the 1st 24 hr of resuscitation. Controversy surrounds whether *colloid* should be provided in the early period of burn resuscitation. One preference is to use colloid replacement concurrently if the burn is >85% of total BSA. Colloid is usually instituted

Table 92.6	Select Common Wound Membranes for Burns
MEMBRANE	**CHARACTERISTIC(S)**
Porcine xenograft	Adheres to coagulum Excellent pain control
Biobrane	Bilaminate Fibrovascular in growth into inner layer
Acticoat	Nonadherent dressing that delivers silver
AQUACEL Ag	Absorptive hydrofiber that delivers silver
Various semipermeable membranes	Provide vapor and bacterial barrier
Various hydrocolloid dressings	Provide vapor and bacterial barrier Absorb exudates
Various impregnated gauzes	Provide barrier while allowing drainage

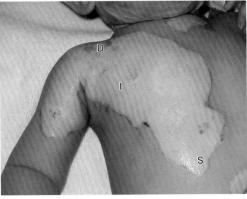

Fig. 92.4 Tea scald over the chest and shoulder of a child showing heterogeneity of burn depth. D, Deep; I, intermediate; S, superficial. *(From Enoch S, Roshan A, Shah M: Emergency and early management of burns and scalds, BMJ 338:937–941, 2009.)*

8-24 hr after the burn injury. In children <12 mo old, sodium tolerance is limited; the volume and sodium concentration of the resuscitation solution should be decreased if the urinary sodium level is rising. The adequacy of resuscitation should be constantly assessed by means of vital signs as well as urine output, blood gas, hematocrit, and serum protein measurements. Some patients require arterial and central venous lines, particularly those undergoing multiple excision and grafting procedures, as needed, for monitoring and replacement purposes. Central venous pressure monitoring may be indicated to assess circulation in patients with hemodynamic or cardiopulmonary instability. Femoral vein cannulation is a safe access for fluid resuscitation, especially in infants and children. Burn patients who require frequent blood gas monitoring benefit from radial or femoral arterial catheterization.

Oral supplementation may start as early as 48 hr after the burn. Milk formula, artificial feedings, homogenized milk, or soy-based products can be given by bolus or constant infusion through a nasogastric or small bowel feeding tube. As oral fluids are tolerated, IV fluids are decreased proportionally in an effort to keep the total fluid intake constant, particularly if pulmonary dysfunction is present.

A **5% albumin infusion** may be used to maintain the serum albumin levels at a desired 2 g/dL. The following rates are effective: for burns of 30–50% of total BSA, 0.3 mL of 5% albumin/kg/% BSA burn is infused over 24 hr; for burns of 50–70% of total BSA, 0.4 mL/kg/% BSA burn is infused over 24 hr; and for burns of 70–100% of total BSA, 0.5 mL/kg/% BSA burn is infused over 24 hr. **Infusion of packed red blood cells** is recommended if the hematocrit falls to <24% (hemoglobin = 8 g/dL). Some authorities recommend treatment for hematocrit <30% or hemoglobin <10 g/dL in patients with systemic infection, hemoglobinopathy, cardiopulmonary disease, anticipated (or ongoing) blood loss, and if repeated excision and grafting of full-thickness burns are needed. **Fresh-frozen plasma** (FFP) is indicated if clinical and laboratory assessment shows a deficiency of clotting factors, a prothrombin level >1.5 times control, or a partial thromboplastin time >1.2 times control in children who are bleeding or are scheduled for an invasive procedure or a grafting procedure that could result in an estimated blood loss of more than half of blood volume. FFP may be used for volume resuscitation within 72 hr of injury in patients <2 yr old with burns >20% BSA and associated inhalation injury.

Sodium supplementation may be required for children with burns of >20% BSA if 0.5% silver nitrate solution is used as the topical antibacterial burn dressing. Sodium losses with silver nitrate therapy are regularly as high as 350 mEq/m^2 burn surface area. Oral sodium chloride supplement of 4 g/m^2 burn area/24 hr is usually well tolerated, divided into 4-6 equal doses to avoid osmotic diarrhea. The aim is to maintain serum sodium levels >130 mEq/L and urinary sodium concentration >30 mEq/L. Young children <5 yr are especially susceptible

to hyponatremic and cerebral edema. IV **potassium supplementation** is supplied to maintain a serum potassium level >3 mEq/dL. Potassium losses may be significantly increased when 0.5% silver nitrate solution is used as the topical antibacterial agent or when aminoglycoside, diuretic, or amphotericin therapy is required.

Prevention of Infection and Surgical Management of the Burn Wound

Controversy surrounds the use of **prophylactic penicillin** for all patients hospitalized with acute burn injury and the periodic **replacement of central venous catheters** to prevent infection. In some units, a 5-day course of penicillin therapy is used for all patients with acute burns; standard-dose crystalline penicillin is given orally or intravenously in 4 divided doses. *Erythromycin* may be used as an alternative in penicillin-allergic children. Other units have discontinued prophylactic use of penicillin therapy without an increase in the infection rate. Similarly, there is conflicting evidence as to whether relocation of the IV catheter every 48-72 hr decreases or increases the incidence of catheter-related sepsis. Some recommend that the central venous catheter be replaced and relocated every 5-7 days, even if the site is not inflamed and there is no suspicion of catheter-related sepsis.

Mortality related to burn injury is associated not with the toxic effect of thermally injured skin, but with the metabolic and bacterial consequences of a large open wound, reduction of the patient's host resistance, and malnutrition. These abnormalities set the stage for life-threatening bacterial infection originating from the burn wound. Wound treatment and prevention of wound infection also promote early healing and improve aesthetic and functional outcomes. Topical treatment of the burn wound with 0.5% silver nitrate solution, silver sulfadiazine cream, or mafenide acetate (Sulfamylon) cream or topical solution at a concentration of 2.5–5% to be used for wounds with multidrug–resistant bacteria aims at prevention of infection (Table 92.7). These 3 agents have tissue-penetrating capacity. Regardless of the choice of topical antimicrobial agent, it is essential that all 3rd-degree burn tissue be fully excised before bacterial colonization occurs, and that the area is grafted as early as possible to prevent deep wound sepsis. Children with a burn of >30% BSA should be housed in a bacteria-controlled nursing unit to prevent cross-contamination and to provide a temperature- and humidity-controlled environment to minimize hypermetabolism.

Deep 3rd-degree burns of >10% BSA benefit from early excision and grafting. To improve outcome, sequential excision and grafting of 3rd-degree and deep 2nd-degree burns is required in children with large burns. Prompt excision with immediate wound closure is achieved with **autografts**, which are often meshed to increase the efficiency of coverings. Alternatives for wound closure, such as allografts, xenografts, and Integra (Integra LifeSciences, York, PA) and other synthetic skin coverings

Table 92.7	Topical Agents Used for Burns		
AGENT	**EFFECTIVENESS**		**EASE OF USE**
Silver sulfadiazine cream (Silvadene)	Good penetration		Changed once daily Residue *must* be washed off with each dressing change
Mafenide acetate cream* (Sulfamylon)	Broad spectrum, including *Pseudomonas* Rapid and deep wound penetration		Closed dressings Changed twice daily Residue *must* be washed off with each dressing changed
0.5% Silver nitrate solution	Bacteriostatic Broad spectrum, including some fungi Superficial penetration		Closed bulky dressing soaked every 2 hr and changed once daily
AQUACEL Ag	Dressing impregnated with silver		Applied directly to 2nd-degree burn; occlusive dressing kept for 10 days

*Mafenide acetate solution at concentrations of 2.5% or 5% for use on heavily colonized, multidrug-resistant organisms to be used for 5 days only.

(bilaminate membrane composed of a porous lattice of crosslinked chondroitin-6-sulfate engineered to induce neovascularization as it is biodegraded), may be important for wound coverage in patients with extensive injury to limit fluid, electrolyte, and protein losses and to reduce pain and minimize temperature loss. Epidermal cultured cells (autologous keratinocytes) are a costly alternative and are not always successful. An experienced burn team can safely perform early-stage or total excision while burn fluid resuscitation continues. Important keys to success are: (1) accurate preoperative and intraoperative determination of burn depth; (2) the choice of excision area and appropriate timing; (3) control of intraoperative blood loss; (4) specific instrumentation; (5) the choice and use of perioperative antibiotics; and (6) the type of wound coverage chosen. This process can accomplish early wound coverage without the use of recombinant human growth hormone.

Nutritional Support
Supporting the increased energy requirements of a patient with a burn is a high priority. The burn injury produces a hypermetabolic response characterized by both protein and fat catabolism. Depending on the time lapse since the burn, children with a burn of 40% of total BSA require basal energy expenditure (oxygen consumption) approximately 50–100% higher than predicted for their age. Early excision and grafting can decrease the energy requirement. Pain, anxiety, and immobilization increase the physiologic demands. Additional energy expenditure is caused by cold stress if environmental humidity and temperature are not controlled; this is especially true in young infants, in whom the large BSA:mass ratio allows proportionately greater heat loss than in adolescents and adults. Providing environmental temperatures of 28-33°C (82.4-91.4°F), adequate covering during transport, and liberal use of analgesics and anxiolytics can decrease caloric demands. Special units to control ambient temperature and humidity may be necessary for children with large surface area burns. Appropriate sleep intervals are necessary and should be part of the regimen. Sepsis increases metabolic rates, and early enteral nutrition, initially with high-carbohydrate, high-protein caloric support (1,800 kcal/m²/24 hr maintenance plus 2,200 kcal/m² of burn/24 hr) reduces metabolic stress.

The objective of **caloric supplementation** programs is to maintain body weight and minimize weight loss by meeting metabolic demands. This reduces the loss of lean body mass. Calories are provided at approximately 1.5 times the basal metabolic rate, with 3-4 g/kg of protein/day. The focus of nutritional therapy is to support and compensate for the metabolic needs. Multivitamins, particularly the B vitamin group, vitamin C, vitamin A, and zinc, are also necessary.

Alimentation should be started as soon as is practical, both enterally and parenterally, to meet all the caloric needs and keep the gastrointestinal (GI) tract active and intact after the resuscitative phase. Patients with burns of >40% of total BSA need a flexible nasogastric or small bowel feeding tube to facilitate continuous delivery of calories without the risk of aspiration. To decrease the risk of infectious complications, parenteral nutrition is discontinued as soon as is practical, after delivery of sufficient enteral calories are established. Continuous GI feeding is

essential, even if feeding is interrupted, causing frequent visits to the operating room, until full grafting takes place. The use of anabolic agents (growth hormone, oxandrolone, low-dose insulin) or anticatabolic agents (propranolol) remains controversial, although β-blocking agents may reduce metabolic stress. Burn centers caring for large burns (>50% BSA, 3rd-degree) in patients who might be malnourished have used the anabolic steroid *oxandrolone*, at a dose of 0.1-0.2 mg/kg/day orally, to promote better protein synthesis while the nutritional support by nasogastric feeding and IV hyperalimentation continues.

Topical Therapy
Topical therapy is widely used and is effective against most burn wound pathogens (see Table 92.7). A number of topical agents are used: 0.5% silver nitrate solution, sulfacetamide acetate cream or solution, silver sulfadiazine cream, and Accuzyme ointment or AQUACEL Ag⁺. Accuzyme is an enzymatic debridement agent and may cause a stinging feeling for 15 min after application. Preferences vary among burn units. Each topical agent has advantages and disadvantages in application, comfort, and bacteriostatic spectrum. *Mafenide acetate* is a very effective broad-spectrum agent with the ability to diffuse through the burn eschar; it is the treatment of choice for injury to cartilaginous surface, such as the ear. Mafenide acetate solution at a concentration of 5% is useful for the treatment of burn wounds that are heavily colonized with multidrug-resistant bacteria (use should be limited to 5 days). The carbonic anhydrase inhibition activity of mafenide acetate may cause acid-base imbalance if large surface areas are treated, and adverse reactions to the sulfur-containing agents may produce transient **leukopenia**. This latter reaction is mostly noted with the use of silver sulfadiazine cream when applied over large surface areas in children <5 yr old. This phenomenon is transient, self-limiting, and reversible. No sulfa-containing agent should be used if the child has a history of sulfa allergies.

Inhalational Injury
Inhalational injury is serious in the infant and child, particularly if preexisting pulmonary conditions are present (see Chapter 89). Inhalation injury should be suspected in a patient confined to a closed space (building), with a history of an explosion or a decreased level of consciousness, or with evidence of carbon deposits in the oropharynx or nose, singed facial hair, and carbonaceous sputum. Mortality estimates vary, depending on the criteria for diagnosis, but are 45–60% in adults; exact figures are not available in children. Evaluation aims at early identification of inhalation airway injuries, which may result from (1) direct heat (greater problems with steam burns); (2) acute asphyxia; (3) CO poisoning; and (4) toxic fumes, including cyanides from combustible plastics. Sulfur and nitrogen oxides and alkalis formed during the combustion of synthetic fabrics produce corrosive chemicals that may erode mucosa and cause significant tissue sloughing. Exposure to smoke may cause degradation of surfactant and decrease its production, resulting in atelectasis. Inhalation injury and burn injury are synergistic, and the combined effect can increase morbidity and mortality.

The pulmonary complications of burns and inhalation can be divided into 3 syndromes that have distinct clinical manifestations and temporal patterns:

1. Early complications include CO and/or cyanide poisoning, airway obstruction, and pulmonary edema.
2. Acute respiratory distress syndrome (ARDS) usually becomes clinically evident later, at 24-48 hr, although it can occur even later (see Chapter 89).
3. Late complications (days to weeks) include pneumonia and pulmonary emboli.

Inhalation injury should be assessed from the evidence of obvious injury (swelling or carbonaceous material in the nasal passages), wheezing, crackles or poor air entry, and laboratory determinations of HbCO and arterial blood gases.

Treatment is initially focused on establishing and maintaining a patent airway through prompt and early nasotracheal or orotracheal intubation and adequate ventilation and oxygenation. **Wheezing** is common, and β-agonist aerosols or inhaled corticosteroids are useful. Aggressive pulmonary toilet and chest physiotherapy are necessary in patients with prolonged nasotracheal intubation or in the rare patient with a tracheotomy. An endotracheal tube can be maintained for months without the need for tracheostomy. If tracheotomy must be performed, it should be delayed until burns at and near the site have healed, and then it should be performed electively, with the child under anesthesia with optimal tracheal positioning and hemostasis. In children with inhalation injury or burns of the face and neck, upper airway obstruction can develop rapidly; endotracheal intubation becomes a lifesaving intervention. Extubation should be delayed until the patient meets the accepted criteria for maintaining the airway.

Signs of CNS injury from hypoxemia caused by asphyxia or **carbon monoxide poisoning** vary from irritability to depression. CO poisoning may be *mild* (<20% HbCO), with slight dyspnea, headache, nausea, and decreased visual acuity and higher cerebral functions; *moderate* (20–40% HbCO), with irritability, agitation, nausea, dimness of vision, impaired judgment, and rapid fatigue; or *severe* (40–60% HbCO), producing confusion, hallucination, ataxia, collapse, acidosis, and coma. Measurement of HbCO is important for diagnosis and treatment. The PaO_2 value may be normal and the HbCO saturation values misleading because HbCO is not detected by the usual tests of oxygen saturation. CO poisoning is assumed until the tests are performed, and it is treated with 100% oxygen. Significant CO poisoning requires hyperbaric oxygen therapy (see Chapter 77). **Cyanide poisoning** should be suspected if a metabolic acidosis persists despite adequate fluid resuscitation, and in environments containing synthetic polymers. Unless specifically suspected, most burn centers do not routinely screen for cyanide poisoning.

Patients with severe inhalation injury or with other causes of respiratory deterioration that lead to ARDS who do not improve with conventional pressure-controlled ventilation (progressive oxygenation failure, as manifested by oxygen saturation <90% while receiving FIO_2 of 0.9-1.0 and positive end-expiratory pressure of at least 12.5 cm H_2O) may benefit from high-frequency ventilation or nitric oxide inhalation treatment. Nitric oxide usually is administered through the ventilator at 5 parts per million (ppm) and increased to 30 ppm. This method of therapy reduces the need for extracorporeal membrane oxygenation (see Chapter 89).

Pain Relief and Psychologic Adjustment
See Chapter 76.

It is important to provide adequate analgesia, anxiolytics, and psychologic support to reduce early metabolic stress, decrease the potential for posttraumatic stress disorder (PTSD), and allow future stabilization as well as physical and psychologic rehabilitation. Patients and family members require team support to work through the grieving process and accept long-term changes in appearance.

Children with burn injury show frequent and wide fluctuations in pain intensity. Appreciation of pain depends on the depth of the burn; the stage of healing; the patient's age, stage of emotional development, and cognition; the experience and efficiency of the treating team; the use of analgesics and other drugs; the patient's pain threshold; and interpersonal and cultural factors. From the onset of treatment, **preemptive pain control** during dressing changes is crucial. The use of a variety of nonpharmacologic interventions as well as pharmacologic agents must be reviewed throughout the treatment period. Opiate analgesia, prescribed in an adequate dose and timed to cover dressing changes, is essential to comfort management. A supportive person who is consistently present and knows the patient profile can integrate and encourage patient participation in burn care. The problem of *undermedication* is most prevalent in adolescents, in whom fear of drug dependence may inappropriately influence treatment. A related problem is that the child's specific pain experience may be misinterpreted; for anxious patients, those who are confused and alone, or those with preexisting emotional disorders, even small wounds may illicit intense pain. Anxiolytic medication added to the analgesic is usually helpful and has more than a synergistic effect. Equal attention is necessary to decrease stress in the intubated patient. Other modalities of pain and anxiety relief (**relaxation techniques**) can decrease the physiologic stress response.

Oral *morphine sulfate* (immediate release) is recommended at a consistent schedule at a dose of 0.3-0.6 mg/kg every 4-6 hr initially and until wound cover is accomplished. Morphine sulfate IV bolus is administered at a dose of 0.05-0.1 mg/kg (maximum, 2-5 mg) every 2 hr. Morphine sulfate rectal suppositories may be useful at a dose of 0.3-0.6 mg/kg every 4 hr when oral administration is not possible. The use of *codeine* preparation should be limited to children >6 yr old because of the ultrarapid metabolizers of codeine into morphine. For anxiety, *lorazepam* is given on a consistent schedule, 0.05-0.1 mg/kg/dose every 6-8 hr. To control pain during a procedure (dressing change or debridement), oral morphine, (0.3-0.6 mg/kg) is given 1-2 hr before the procedure, supplemented by a morphine IV bolus (0.05-0.1 mg/kg) given immediately before the procedure. Lorazepam, 0.04 mg/kg, is given orally or intravenously, if necessary, for anxiety before the procedure. *Midazolam* is also very useful for conscious sedation at a dose of 0.01-0.02 mg/kg for nonintubated patients and 0.05-0.1 mg/kg for intubated patients, as an IV infusion or bolus, and may be repeated in 10 min. During the process of weaning from analgesics, the dose of oral opiates is reduced by 25% over 1-3 days, sometimes with the addition of acetaminophen as opiates are tapered. When weaning off antianxiety medications, the approach involves reducing the dose of benzodiazepines, at 25–50% per dose, daily over 1-3 days. *Risperidone*, up to 2.5 mg/day, is being used in children with severe burns.

For ventilated patients, pain control is accomplished by using morphine sulfate intermittently as an IV bolus at 0.05-0.1 mg/kg every 2 hr. Doses may need to be increased gradually, and some children may need continuous infusion; a starting dose of 0.05 mg/kg/hr as an infusion is increased gradually as the need of the child changes. Naloxone is rarely needed but should be immediately available to reverse the effect of morphine, if necessary; if needed for an airway crisis, it should be given in a dose of 0.1 mg/kg up to a total of 2 mg, either intramuscularly or intravenously. For patients undergoing assisted respiration who require treatment of anxiety, midazolam is used as an intermittent IV bolus (0.04 mg/kg by slow push every 4-6 hr) or as a continuous infusion. For intubated patients, opiates do not need to be discontinued during the process of weaning from the ventilator. Benzodiazepine should be reduced to approximately half the dose over 24-72 hr before extubation; too-rapid weaning from a benzodiazepine can lead to seizures.

There is a growing use of *psychotropic medication* in the care of children with burns, including prescription of selective serotonin reuptake inhibitors as antidepressants, the use of haloperidol as a neuroleptic in the critical care setting, and the treatment of PTSD with benzodiazepines. Conscious sedation using ketamine or propofol may be used for major dressing changes.

Reconstruction and Rehabilitation
To ensure maximum cosmetic and functional outcome, occupational and physical therapy must begin on the day of admission, continue throughout hospitalization, and for some patients, continue after discharge. Physical rehabilitation involves body and limb positioning, splinting, exercises (active and passive movement), assistance with activities of daily living, and gradual ambulation. These measures maintain adequate joint and muscle activity with as normal a range of movement as possible after healing or reconstruction. **Pressure therapy** is necessary to reduce

hypertrophic scar formation; a variety of prefabricated and custom-made garments are available for use in different body areas. These custom-made garments deliver consistent pressure on scarred areas, shorten the time of scar maturation, and decrease scar thickness, redness, and associated itching. Continued adjustments to scarred areas (scar release, grafting, rearrangement) and multiple minor cosmetic surgical procedures are necessary to optimize long-term function and improve appearance. Replacement of areas of alopecia and scarring has been achieved with the use of tissue-expander techniques. The use of ultrapulse laser for reduction of scarring is an adjunct in scar management.

School Reentry and Long-Term Outcome

It is best for the child to return to school immediately after discharge. Occasionally, a child may need to attend a few half-days (because of rehabilitation needs). It is important for the child to return to the normal routine of attending school and being with peers. Planning for a return to home and school often requires a **school reentry program** that is individualized to each child's needs. For a school-age child, planning for the return to school occurs simultaneously with planning for discharge. The hospital schoolteacher contacts the local school and plans the program with the school faculty, nurses, social workers, recreational/child-life therapists, and rehabilitation therapists. This team should work with students and staff to ease anxiety, answer questions, and provide information. Burns and scars evoke fears in those who are not familiar with this type of injury and can result in a tendency to withdraw from or reject the burned child. A school reentry program should be appropriate to a child's development and changing educational needs.

Major advances have made it possible to save the lives of children with massive burns. Although some children have had lingering physical difficulties, most have a satisfactory quality of life. The comprehensive burn care that includes experienced multidisciplinary aftercare plays an important role in recovery. Table 92.8 lists the long-term disabilities and complications of burns.

ELECTRICAL BURNS

There are 3 types of electrical burns: extension cord (minor), high-tension wire, and lightning. **Minor electrical burns** usually occur as a result of biting on an extension cord. These injuries produce localized burns to the mouth, which usually involve the portions of the upper and lower lips that come in contact with the extension cord. The injury may involve or spare the corners of the mouth. Because these are *nonconductive*

injuries (do not extend beyond the site of injury), hospital admission is not necessary, and care is focused on the area of the injury visible in the mouth, ensuring it is low voltage and does not cause entry or exit wounds or cardiac issues. Treatment with topical antibiotic creams is sufficient until the patient is seen in a burn unit outpatient department or by a plastic surgeon.

A more serious category of electrical burn is the **high-tension electrical wire burn**, for which children must be admitted for observation, regardless of the extent of the surface area burn. Deep muscle injury is typical and cannot be readily assessed initially. These injuries result from high voltage (>1,000 V) and occur particularly at high-voltage installations, such as electric power stations or railroads; children climb an electric pole and touch an electric box out of curiosity or accidentally touch a high-tension electrical wire. Such injuries have a mortality rate of 3–15% for children who arrive at the hospital for treatment. Survivors have a high rate of morbidity, including major limb amputations. Points of entry of current through the skin and the exit site show characteristic features consistent with current density and heat. The majority of entrance wounds involve the upper extremity, with small exit wounds in the lower extremity. The electrical path, from entrance to exit, takes the shortest distance between the 2 points and may produce injury in any organ or tissue in the path of the current. Multiple exit wounds in some patients attest to the possibility of several electrical pathways in the body, placing virtually any structure in the body at risk (Table 92.9). Damage to the abdominal viscera, thoracic structures, and the nervous system (confusion, coma, paralysis) in areas remote from obvious extremity injury occurs and must be sought, particularly in injuries with multiple current pathways or those in which the victim falls from a high pole. Sometimes an *ignition* occurs and results in concurrent flame burn and clothing fire. **Cardiac abnormalities**, manifested as ventricular fibrillation or cardiac arrest, are common; patients with high-tension electrical injury need an initial electrocardiogram and cardiac monitoring until they are stable and have been fully assessed. Higher-risk patients have abnormal electrocardiographic findings and a history of loss of consciousness. Renal damage from **deep muscle necrosis** and subsequent myoglobinuria is another complication; such patients need forced alkaline diuresis to minimize renal damage. Soft tissue (muscle) injury of an extremity may produce a **compartment syndrome**. Aggressive removal of all dead and devitalized tissue, even with the risk of functional loss, remains the key to effective management of the electrically damaged extremity. Early debridement facilitates early

Table 92.8	Common Long-Term Complications and Disabilities in Patients With Burn Injuries
COMPLICATIONS AFFECTING THE SKIN AND SOFT TISSUE Hypertrophic scars Susceptibility to minor trauma Dry skin Contractures Itching and neuropathic pain Alopecia Chronic open wounds Skin cancers **ORTHOPEDIC DISABILITIES** Amputations Contractures Heterotopic ossification Temporary reduction in bone density **METABOLIC DISABILITIES** Heat sensitivity Obesity	**PSYCHIATRIC AND NEUROLOGIC DISABILITIES** Sleep disorders Adjustment disorders Posttraumatic stress disorder Depression Body image issues Neuropathy and neuropathic pain Long-term neurologic effects of carbon monoxide poisoning Anoxic brain injury **LONG-TERM COMPLICATIONS OF CRITICAL CARE** Deep vein thrombosis, venous insufficiency, or varicose veins Tracheal stenosis, vocal cord disorders, or swallowing disorders Renal or adrenal dysfunction Hepatobiliary or pancreatic disease Cardiovascular disease Reactive airway disease or bronchial polyposis **PREEXISTING DISABILITIES THAT CONTRIBUTED TO THE INJURIES** Risk-taking behavior Untreated or poorly treated psychiatric disorder

Modified from Sheridan RL, Schultz JT, Ryan CM, et al: Case records of the Massachusetts General Hospital. Weekly clinicopathological exercises. Case 6-2004: a 35-year-old woman with extensive, deep burns from a nightclub fire, *N Engl J Med* 350:810–821, 2004.

Table 92.9	Electrical Injury: Clinical Considerations	
SYSTEM	**CLINICAL MANIFESTATIONS**	**MANAGEMENT**
General	—	Extricate the patient. Perform ABCs of resuscitation; immobilize the spine. Obtain history: voltage, type of current. Obtain complete blood count with platelets, electrolytes, BUN, creatinine, and glucose.
Cardiac	Dysrhythmias: asystole, ventricular fibrillation, sinus tachycardia, sinus bradycardia, premature atrial contractions, premature ventricular contractions, conduction defects, atrial fibrillation, ST-T wave changes	Treat dysrhythmias. Provide cardiac monitor, electrocardiogram, and radiographs with suspected thoracic injury. Perform creatinine phosphokinase with isoenzyme measurements if indicated.
Pulmonary	Respiratory arrest, acute respiratory distress, aspiration syndrome	Protect and maintain the airway. Provide mechanical ventilation if indicated, chest radiograph, and arterial blood gas levels.
Renal	Acute kidney injury, myoglobinuria	Provide aggressive fluid management unless central nervous system injury is present. Maintain adequate urine output, >1 mL/kg/hr. Consider central venous or pulmonary artery pressure monitoring. Measure urine myoglobin; perform urinalysis; measure BUN, creatinine.
Neurologic	Immediate: loss of consciousness, motor paralysis, visual disturbances, amnesia, agitation; intracranial hematoma Secondary: pain, paraplegia, brachial plexus injury, syndrome of inappropriate antidiuretic hormone secretion, autonomic disturbances, cerebral edema Delayed: paralysis, seizures, headache, peripheral neuropathy	Treat seizures. Provide fluid restriction if indicated. Consider spine radiographs and MRI, especially cervical. Perform CT or MRI scan of the brain if indicated.
Cutaneous/oral	Oral commissure burns, tongue and dental injuries; skin burns resulting from ignition of clothes, entrance and exit burns, and arc burns Electrical burns to mouth could include oral commissures and lips; low-voltage electrical burns secondary to high conductivity of saliva	Search for the entrance and exit wounds. Treat cutaneous burns; determine patient's tetanus status. Obtain consultation for plastic surgery of ear, nose, and throat, if indicated. Ensure no entry or exit wounds and no cardiac involvement. Confirm all injuries are localized. Management is observation until eschar sloughs off and granulation tissue fills in. Obtain plastic surgeon evaluation after first healing, usually with scar formation.
Abdominal	Viscus perforation and solid-organ damage; ileus; abdominal injury rare without visible abdominal burns	Place nasogastric tube if patient has airway compromise or ileus. Obtain serum ALT, AST, amylase, BUN, and creatinine measurements and CT scans as indicated.
Musculoskeletal	Compartment syndrome from subcutaneous necrosis limb edema and deep burns Long-bone fractures, spine injuries	Monitor patient for possible compartment syndrome. Obtain radiographs and orthopedic/general surgery consultations as indicated.
Ocular	Visual changes, optic neuritis, cataracts, extraocular muscle paresis	Obtain an ophthalmology consultation as indicated.

AST, Aspartate transaminase; ALT, alanine transaminase; BUN, blood urea nitrogen.
  Adapted from Hall ML, Sills RM: Electrical and lightning injuries. In Barkin RM, editor: *Pediatric emergency medicine*, St Louis, 1997, Mosby, p 484.

closure of the wound. Damaged major vessels must be isolated and buried in a viable muscle to prevent exposure. Survival depends on immediate intensive care; functional result depends on long-term care and delayed reconstructive surgery.

Lightning burns occur when a high-voltage current directly strikes a person (most dangerous) or when the current strikes the ground or an adjacent (in-contact) object. A *step voltage burn* is observed when lightning strikes the ground and travels up one leg and down the other (the path of least resistance). Lightning burns depend on the current path, the type of clothing worn, the presence of metal, and cutaneous moisture. Entry, exit, and path lesions are possible; the prognosis is poorest for lesions of the head or legs. Internal organ injury along the path is common and does not relate to the severity of the cutaneous burn. Linear burns, usually 1st or 2nd degree, are in the locations where

sweat is present. *Feathering*, or an arborescent pattern, is characteristic of lightning injury. Lightning may ignite clothing or produce serious cutaneous burns from heated metal in the clothing. Internal complications of lightning burns include cardiac arrest caused by asystole, transient hypertension, premature ventricular contractions, ventricular fibrillation, and myocardial ischemia. Most severe cardiac complications resolve if the patient is supported with CPR (see Chapter 81). CNS complications include cerebral edema, hemorrhage, seizures, mood changes, depression, and paralysis of the lower extremities. Rhabdomyolysis and myoglobinuria (with possible renal failure) also occur. Ocular manifestations include vitreous hemorrhage, iridocyclitis, retinal tearing, or retinal detachment.

Bibliography is available at Expert Consult.

中文导读

本章主要介绍了冻伤的病理生理学、病因、临床表现及寒冷诱发的脂肪坏死（脂膜炎）。其病因中主要为低体温引起的低体温综合征；在临床表现中主要介绍了冻伤、浸渍足、冻疮、低体温及严重冻疮的临床表现及治疗方法。冻伤表现为面部、耳朵或手足变硬、冰凉、苍白；浸渍足表现为双足冰凉、麻木、苍白、水肿和湿冷；冻疮指皮肤初期的刺痛和疼痛进展到冰冷、发硬、苍白麻木和冻僵；低体温应以预防为主；严重冻疮则表现为红斑、水疱或溃疡。治疗中主要描述了预防为主、保暖、温和的复温、抗炎或止痛药、血管舒张药的使用等措施。

The involvement of children and youth in snowmobiling, mountain climbing, winter hiking, and skiing places them at risk for cold injury. Cold injury may produce either local tissue damage, with the injury pattern depending on exposure to *damp cold* (frostnip, immersion foot, or trench foot), *dry cold* (which leads to local frostbite), or generalized systemic effects (hypothermia).

PATHOPHYSIOLOGY

Ice crystals may form between or within cells, interfering with the sodium pump, and may lead to rupture of cell membranes. Further damage may result from clumping of red blood cells or platelets, causing microembolism or thrombosis. Blood may be shunted away from an affected area by secondary neurovascular responses to the cold injury; this shunting often further damages an injured part while improving perfusion of other tissues. The spectrum of injury ranges from mild to severe and reflects the result of structural and functional disturbance in small blood vessels, nerves, and skin.

ETIOLOGY

Body heat may be lost by *conduction* from wet clothing or contact with metal or other solid conducting objects, *convection* from wind chill, *evaporation,* or *radiation.* Susceptibility to cold injury may be increased by dehydration, alcohol or drug use, impaired consciousness, exhaustion, hunger, anemia, impaired circulation from cardiovascular disease, and sepsis; very young or older persons also are more susceptible. Certain medications may contribute to hypothermia, whereas others may cause reduced metabolism or clearance during hypothermia (Table 93.1).

Hypothermia occurs when the body can no longer sustain normal core temperature by physiologic mechanisms, such as vasoconstriction, shivering, muscle contraction, and nonshivering thermogenesis. When

Table 93.1	Drugs Displaying Reduced Metabolism or Clearance in Hypothermia
Atropine	Procaine
Digoxin	Propranolol
Fentanyl	Sulfanilamide (AVC cream)
Gentamicin	Succinylcholine
Lidocaine	D-Tubocurarine
Phenobarbital	

Adapted from Bope ET, Kellerman RD, editors: *Conn's current therapy 2014,* Philadelphia, 2014, Elsevier/Saunders (Box 3, p 1135).

shivering ceases, the body is unable to maintain its core temperature; when the body core temperature falls to <35°C (95°F), the syndrome of hypothermia occurs. Wind chill, wet or inadequate clothing, and other factors increase local injury and may cause dangerous hypothermia, even in the presence of an ambient temperature that is not <17-20°C (50-60°F).

CLINICAL MANIFESTATIONS
Frostnip

Frostnip results in the presence of firm, cold, white areas on the face, ears, or extremities. Blistering and peeling may occur over the next 24-72 hr, occasionally leaving mildly increased hypersensitivity to cold for days or weeks. Treatment consists of warming the area with an unaffected hand or a warm object before the lesion reaches a stage of stinging or aching and before numbness supervenes. Rewarming in a water bath (40-42.2°C [104-108°F]) is effective.

Immersion Foot (Trench Foot)

Immersion foot occurs in cold weather when the feet remain in damp or wet, poorly ventilated boots. The feet become cold, numb, pale, edematous, and clammy. Tissue maceration and infection are likely, and prolonged autonomic disturbance is common. This autonomic disturbance leads to increased sweating, pain, and hypersensitivity to temperature changes, which may persist for years. Treatment includes drying the foot, gentle rewarming and nonsteroidal antiinflammatory drugs (NSAIDs) for pain. Prevention consists of using well-fitting, insulated, waterproof, nonconstricting footwear. Once damage has occurred, patients must choose clothing and footwear that are more appropriate, dry, and well fitting. The disturbance in skin integrity is managed by keeping the affected area dry and well ventilated and by preventing or treating infection. Only supportive measures are possible for control of autonomic symptoms.

Frostbite

With frostbite, initial stinging or aching of the skin progresses to cold, hard, white anesthetic and numb areas. Clear or hemorrhagic vesicles may develop over the exposed areas. On rewarming, the area becomes blotchy, itchy, and often red, swollen, and painful. The injury spectrum ranges from complete normality to extensive tissue damage, even gangrene, if early relief is not obtained.

Treatment consists of warming the damaged area. It is important not to cause further damage by attempting to rub the area with ice or snow. The area may be warmed against an unaffected hand, the abdomen, or an axilla during transfer of the patient to a facility where more rapid warming with a warm (and not hot) water bath is possible. If the skin becomes painful and swelling occurs, NSAIDs are helpful, and an analgesic agent is necessary. Freeze and rethawing cycles are most likely to cause permanent tissue injury, and it may be necessary to delay definitive warming and apply only mild measures if the patient is required to walk on the damaged feet en route to definitive treatment. In the hospital the affected area should be immersed in warm water (approximately 42°C [107.6°F]), with care taken not to burn the anesthetized skin. Broken vesicles may be debrided, but intact vesicles should be left alone. Vasodilating agents, such as prazosin and phenoxybenzamine, may be helpful. Use of anticoagulants (e.g., heparin, dextran) has had equivocal results; results of chemical and surgical sympathectomy have also been equivocal. Oxygen is of help only at high altitudes. Meticulous local care, prevention of infection, and keeping the rewarmed area dry, open, and sterile provide optimal results.

Recovery can be complete, and prolonged observation with conservative therapy is justified before any excision or amputation of tissue is considered. Analgesia and maintenance of good nutrition are necessary throughout the prolonged waiting period.

Hypothermia

Hypothermia may occur in winter sports when injury, equipment failure, or exhaustion decreases the level of exertion, particularly if sufficient attention is not paid to wind chill. Immersion in frozen bodies of water and wet wind chill rapidly produce hypothermia. As the core temperature of the body falls, insidious onset of extreme lethargy, fatigue, incoordination, and apathy occurs, followed by mental confusion, clumsiness, irritability, hallucinations, and finally, bradycardia. A number of medical conditions, such as cardiac disease, diabetes mellitus, hypoglycemia, sepsis, β-blocking agent overdose, and substance abuse, may need to be considered in a differential diagnosis. The decrease in rectal temperature to <34°C (93°F) is the most helpful diagnostic feature. Hypothermia associated with drowning is discussed in Chapter 91.

Prevention is a high priority. Of extreme importance for those who participate in winter sports is wearing layers of warm clothing, gloves, socks within insulated boots that do not impede circulation, and a warm head covering, as well as application of adequate waterproofing and protection against the wind. Thirty percent of heat loss for infants occurs from the head. Ample food and fluid must be provided during exercise. Those who participate in sports should be alert to the presence of cold or numbing of body parts, particularly the nose, ears, and extremities, and they should review methods to produce local warming

Table 93.2 | Management of Hypothermia

HISTORY AND PHYSICAL EXAMINATION
Gentle handling of the patient to prevent arrhythmias
ABCDE: cardiopulmonary resuscitation for ventricular fibrillation and asystole
Underlying disease diagnosis and treatment
Vital signs, pulse oximetry, electrocardiogram
Wet or cold clothing removed and patient placed in warm environment

LABORATORY TESTS
Arterial blood gas analysis corrected for temperature
Electrolytes, BUN, creatinine, Ca, Mg, P
CBC with differential, PT/PTT, fibrinogen
Glucose, amylase/lipase
Liver function tests
Additional lab tests, if appropriate, such as toxicology screen

PASSIVE REWARMING
≥32°C (89.6°F) in patients who are capable of spontaneous thermogenesis

ACTIVE REWARMING
<32°C (89.6°F), cardiovascular instability, patients at risk for developing hypothermia
Close monitoring for core-temperature afterdrop
Acute: external and/or core rewarming
Chronic (<32°C [89.6°F] for >24 hr): core rewarming
Extracorporeal membrane oxygenation
Availability of rapid deployment

ABCDE, Airway and possibly antibiotics, breathing, circulation, disability or neurologic and possible dextrose, extracorporeal support if all else fails; BUN, blood urea nitrogen; Ca, calcium; CBC, complete blood count; Mg, magnesium; P, phosphorus; PT, prothrombin time; PTT, partial thromboplastin time.
Adapted from Burg FD, Ingelfinger JR, Polin RA, Gershon AA, editors: *Current pediatric therapy*, ed 18, Philadelphia, 2006, Saunders/Elsevier (Table 4, p 174).

and know to seek shelter if they detect symptoms of local cold injury. Application of petrolatum (Vaseline) to the nose and ears helps protect against frostbite.

Treatment at the scene aims at prevention of further heat loss and early transport to adequate shelter (Table 93.2). Dry clothing should be provided as soon as practical, and transport should be undertaken if the victim has a pulse. If no pulse is detected at the initial review, cardiopulmonary resuscitation is indicated (Fig. 93.1) (see Chapter 81). During transfer, jarring and sudden motion should be avoided because of the risk of ventricular arrhythmia. It is often difficult to attain a normal sinus rhythm during hypothermia.

If the patient is conscious, mild muscle activity should be encouraged and a warm drink offered. If the patient is unconscious, external warming should be undertaken initially with use of blankets and a sleeping bag; wrapping the patient in blankets or sleeping bag with a warm companion may increase the efficiency of warming. On arrival at a treatment center, while a warming bath of 45-48°C (113-118°F) water is prepared, the patient should be warmed through inhalation of warm, moist air or oxygen or with heating pads or thermal blankets. Monitoring of serum chemistry values and an electrocardiogram are necessary until the core temperature rises to >35°C (95°F) and can be stabilized. Control of fluid balance, pH, blood pressure, and arterial partial pressure of oxygen (PaO$_2$) is necessary in the early phases of the warming period and resuscitation. In severe hypothermia, there may be a combined respiratory and metabolic acidosis. Hypothermia may falsely elevate pH; nonetheless, most authorities recommend warming the arterial blood gas specimen to 37°C (98.6°F) before analysis and regarding the result as one from a normothermic patient. In patients with marked abnormalities, warming measures, such as gastric or colonic irrigation with warm saline or peritoneal dialysis, may be considered, but the effectiveness of these measures in treating hypothermia is unknown. In accidental *deep hypothermia* (core temperature 28°C [82.4°F]) with circulatory arrest, rewarming with cardiopulmonary bypass may be lifesaving for previously

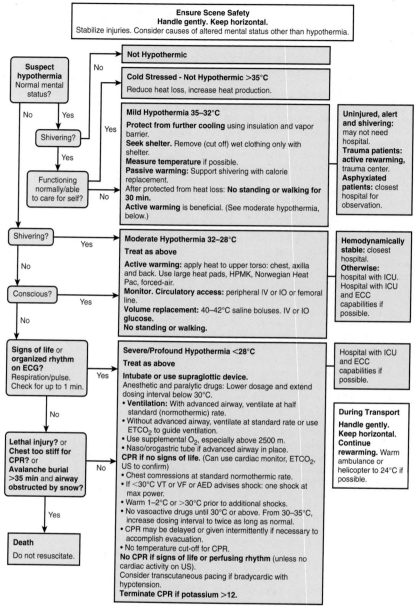

Fig. 93.1 Recommendations for out-of-hospital evaluation and treatment of accidental hypothermia. *AED,* Automatic external defibrillator; *CPR,* cardiopulmonary resuscitation; *ECC,* extracorporeal circulation; *ECG,* electrocardiogram; *ETCO₂,* end-tidal carbon dioxide; *HPMK,* Hypothermia Prevention Management Kit; *ICU,* intensive care unit; *IO,* intraosseous; *IV,* intravenous; *US,* ultrasound; *VF,* ventricular fibrillation; *VT,* ventricular tachycardia. *(From Zafren K, Giesbrecht GG, Danzl DF, et al: Wilderness Medical Society practice guidelines for the out-of-hospital evaluation and treatment of accidental hypothermia: 2014 update,* Wilderness Environ Med *25:S66–S85, 2014, Fig 2.)*

healthy young individuals. If rewarming is not successful despite appropriate measures, one should suspect infection, drug overdose, endocrine disorders, or a futile resuscitation.

Chilblain (Pernio)

Chilblain (pernio) is a form of cold injury in which erythematous, vesicular, or ulcerative lesions occur. The lesions are presumed to be of vascular or vasoconstrictive origin. They are often itchy, may be painful, and result in swelling and scabbing. The lesions are most often found on the ears, the tips of the fingers and toes, and exposed areas of the legs. The lesions last for 1-2 wk but may persist for longer. Treatment

consists of prophylaxis: avoiding prolonged chilling and protecting potentially susceptible areas with a cap, gloves, and stockings. Prazosin and phenoxybenzamine may be helpful in improving circulation if this is a recurrent problem. For significant itching, local corticosteroid preparations may be helpful.

Familial chilblain lupus, an autosomal dominant variant of lupus, is caused by mutations in the *TREX1, SAMHD1,* and *STING* genes. Patients develop cold-induced erythematous peripheral skin lesions and also manifest systemic disease typical of lupus (Chapter 183). In addition, fever and arthralgias may be present. Those with the *STING* mutation may develop a necrotizing acral vasculitis.

COLD-INDUCED FAT NECROSIS (PANNICULITIS)

A common, usually benign injury, cold-induced fat necrosis occurs on exposure to cold air, snow, or ice and manifests in exposed (or less often covered) surfaces as red (or less often purple to blue) macular, papular, or nodular lesions. Treatment is with NSAIDs. The lesions may last 10 days to 3 wk but may persist for longer. Severe coagulopathy may be associated with poor outcome in some severe cold injuries, thus meriting anticoagulation therapy (see Chapter 680.1).

Bibliography is available at Expert Consult.

Chapter 94
Integration of Genetics Into Pediatric Practice

Brendan Lee

第九十四章
遗传学与儿科实践的结合

中文导读

　　本章主要介绍了诊断性检测、预测性检测、倾向性检测和药理学检测。详细阐述了遗传咨询，其中包括与家庭谈话的内容，特定疾病、诊断知识、疾病史、遗传因素与复发风险、产前诊断与预防、治疗和转诊、支持小组、随访、非指导性咨询等内容。详细阐述了遗传病的管理和治疗，其中包括生理疗法和替代疗法。

Genetic testing involves analyzing genetic material to obtain information related to a person's health status using chromosomal (cytogenetic) analysis (see Chapter 98) or DNA-based testing.

DIAGNOSTIC TESTING

Diagnostic genetic testing helps explain a set of signs and symptoms of a disease. The list of disorders for which specific genetic tests are available is extensive. The website http://www.ncbi.nlm.nih.gov/gtr/ provides a database of available tests that is provider driven, so claims are not validated by the site's host, the National Institutes of Health (NIH).

Single-gene disorders can be tested by at least 3 different approaches: linkage analysis (though this is now rarely used), array comparative genomic hybridization (**aCGH**), and direct mutation analysis, usually by DNA sequencing (Table 94.1). Linkage analysis is used if the responsible gene is mapped but not yet identified, or if it is impractical to find specific mutations, usually because of the large size and larger number of different mutations in some genes. Array CGH can be used to detect large, multigene deletions or duplications (**copy number variations**). In addition, with increasing resolution, single-gene or smaller intragenic deletions or duplications can be detected by aCGH, although it is important to note that coverage of each gene may vary from different providers. *Direct DNA mutation analysis is preferred and is possible with the availability of the complete human genome sequence.* An emerging feature is the increasing recognition of oligogenic disease where more than one disease gene contributes to a complex, or "blended," phenotype. The ability to sequence hundreds to thousands of genes at once has provided insight into this added layer of complexity in disease pathogenesis.

Linkage testing involves tracking a genetic trait through a family using closely linked polymorphic markers as a surrogate for the trait (Fig. 94.1). It requires testing an extended family and is vulnerable to several pitfalls, such as genetic recombination, genetic heterogeneity, and incorrect diagnosis in the proband. **Genetic recombination** occurs between any pair of loci, the frequency being proportional to the distance between them. This problem can be ameliorated by using very closely linked markers and, if possible, using markers that flank the specific gene. **Genetic heterogeneity** can be problematic for a linkage-based test if there are multiple distinct genomic loci that can cause the same phenotype, resulting in the risk that the locus tested for is not the one responsible for disease in the family. **Incorrect diagnosis** in the proband also leads to tracking the wrong gene. Linkage testing remains useful for several genetic conditions, but it is increasingly being superseded by the availability of direct DNA sequencing of either single genes or of the whole collection of genes that encode all proteins. It is critically important that genetic counseling be provided to the family to explain the complexities of interpretation of test results.

Array comparative genomic hybridization can detect copy number variation in a patient's DNA by comparing it to a standard control DNA (see Chapter 98). In so doing, aCGH provides a level of genetic resolution

Table 94.1	Approaches for Genetic Testing			
TYPE OF MUTATION TESTING	**RESOLUTION**	**ADVANTAGES**	**DISADVANTAGES**	**SAMPLE REQUIREMENTS**
Linkage analysis	Depends on location of polymorphic markers near putative disease gene	Possible when specific disease-causing genetic mutation is not identifiable or found	Can give only diagnostic probability based on likelihood of genetic recombination between presumed DNA mutation and polymorphic markers	Requires multiple family members with documented mendelian pattern of inheritance within family
Array comparative genomic hybridization (aCGH)	Several hundred base pairs to several hundreds of kilobases	Able to detect small deletion or duplications within 1 or more genes	Can miss small deletions or insertions depending on resolution of the array used	Single patient sample sufficient, but having sample from biological parents can help with interpretation
Direct DNA-based testing (e.g., DNA sequencing)	Single–base-pair changes	High specificity if previously described deleterious mutation is found	Can miss deletion or duplication of a segment of gene	Single patient sample sufficient, but having sample from biological parents can help with interpretation

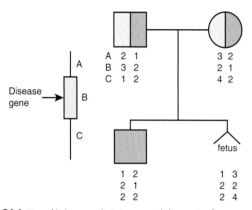

Fig. 94.1 Use of linkage analysis in prenatal diagnosis of an autosomal recessive disorder. Both parents are carriers, and they have 1 affected son. The numbers below the symbols indicate alleles at 3 polymorphic loci: A, B, and C. Locus B resides within the disease gene. The affected son inherited the 1-2-2 chromosome from his father and the 2-1-2 chromosome from his mother. The fetus has inherited the same chromosome from the father, but the 3-2-4 chromosome from the mother and therefore is most likely to be a carrier.

between that available with DNA sequencing and that available with chromosome analysis. Whereas earlier technologies could only identify large deletions or duplications that might encompass multiple genes, aCGH can resolve deletions or duplications of several kilobases within 1 gene. In theory, this approach can detect deletion and duplication mutations that would be missed by either chromosome analysis or direct mutation testing by DNA sequencing. However, because the specific resolution and coverage of different aCGH platforms can vary tremendously for different gene regions, the sensitivity for detecting deletions and duplications can vary for different diseases and laboratories. The highest resolution is what would be detection of on average deletion or duplication at the single exon level.

Direct DNA-based mutation testing avoids the pitfalls of linkage testing by detecting the specific gene mutation (i.e., sequence change). The specific approach used is customized to the biology of the gene being tested. In some disorders, 1 or a few distinct mutations occur in all affected individuals. This is the case in sickle cell anemia, in which the same single-base substitution occurs in everyone with the disorder. In other conditions, many possible mutations may account for the disorder in different individuals. In cystic fibrosis, for example, >1,000 distinct

mutations have been found in the *CFTR* gene. Mutation analysis is challenging because no single technique can detect all possible mutations. However, with the completion of the human genome sequence and high-throughput DNA sequencing technology, the approach of choice is to directly sequence DNA that is generated by **polymerase chain reaction (PCR)** amplification of DNA isolated from peripheral blood white blood cells. The limitation of this approach is that only DNA that is amplified is sequenced, and usually this is restricted to the *coding* or *exonic* regions of a gene. Because mutations sometimes occur in the *noncoding intronic* regions, failure to detect a mutation does not exclude the diagnosis. Whole *genome* sequencing should identify mutations in the noncoding regions. In addition, genes in a deleted region will not be detected. Although DNA sequencing can be highly specific, it is not completely sensitive because of practical limitations of what is commercially available. Gene sequencing techniques may not be able to identify diseases caused by triplet repeat sequences; specific tests are needed.

The most useful development in clinical DNA diagnosis is application of **next-generation sequencing** technology to testing panels of genes that target disease symptoms (e.g., seizures, ataxia syndromes) or the whole exome (**whole exome sequencing [WES]**). Soon, whole genome sequencing (WGS), where both coding and noncoding sequences are identified, will provide even more information, although initial clinical interpretation will still be limited to the coding sequences of the approximately 20,000 human genes, the so-called digital exome, as it is extracted electronically from the whole genome data. The challenge is not so much the generation of DNA sequence, but the interpretation of enormous genetic variation within a single sample. Direct sequencing of tens to hundreds of genes in next-generation sequencing panels offer a potentially higher sensitivity because the "depth" of read is higher without complicating high discovery rate of **variants of unknown sequences (VUS)**. WES and WGS also offer the potential for identifying new disease-gene associations as well as phenotypes caused by more than one disease gene (i.e., oligogenic phenotypes).

An important ethical consideration is the reporting of *incidental findings*, whether medically actionable or not medically actionable in a patient. WES and WGS may identify mutations that cause aminoglycoside-sensitive hearing loss, which would be medically actionable. At the same time, the discovery of apolipoprotein E variants in a child that increase Alzheimer disease risk susceptibility may not be medically actionable. Therefore, counseling for patients undergoing these tests is important so that only wanted results are reported back to the patient. Guidelines are currently evolving for reporting of incidental findings for WES by the American College of Medical Genetics (www.acmg.net). Practice varies among institutions and recommendations vary among international genetic organizations about the approach for revealing incidental findings from WES/WGS to patients; many leave the choice up to the patient and family. Most require revealing to the

Table 94.2	Variants That Are Incidental Findings Are Assigned to 1 of 4 Categories
Childhood onset	Medically actionable*
Childhood onset	Not medically actionable†
Adult onset	Medically actionable*
Adult onset	Not medically actionable†

*"Medically actionable" refers to a variant in a gene in which knowledge of the particular variant will affect medical decision-making, such as initiation of a treatment or family planning.

†"Not medically actionable" refers to variants that increase the individual's risk for a disease in which no treatment is proven to significantly change medical decision-making.

From Bick D, Dimmock D: Whole exome and whole genome sequencing. *Curr Opin Pediatr* 23:594–600, 2011.

patient and/or family significant diseases (actionable) with a specific and successful treatment or prevention strategy (Table 94.2).

Genetic testing is interpreted by 3 factors: analytic validity, clinical validity, and clinical utility. **Analytical validity** is test accuracy: Does the test correctly detect the presence or absence of mutation? Most genetic tests have a very high analytical validity, assuming that human error, such as sample mix-up, has not occurred. Human errors are possible, and unlike most medical tests, a genetic test is unlikely to be repeated, because it is assumed that the result will not change over time. Therefore, human errors can go undetected for long periods of time. However, it may be reinterpreted over time as our knowledge base of what are disease-causing mutations and genes increases over time.

Clinical validity is the degree to which the test correctly predicts presence or absence of disease. False-positive and false-negative test results can occur. **False-positive results** are more likely for predictive tests than for diagnostic tests. An important contributing factor is **nonpenetrance**: an individual with an at-risk genotype might not clinically express the condition. Another factor is the finding of a **genetic variant of unknown significance** (VUS). Detection of a base sequence variation in an affected patient does not prove that it is the cause of the patient's disorder. In WES there may be more than 30,000 VUS; in WGS there may be more than 3,000,000 VUS. Various lines of evidence are used to establish pathogenicity. These include finding the variant only in affected individuals, inferring that the variant alters the function of the gene product, determining whether the amino acid altered by the mutation is conserved in evolution, and determining whether the mutation segregates with disease in the family. In some cases, it is possible to be certain whether the variant is pathogenic or incidental, but in other cases it might be impossible to definitively assign causality with 100% confidence.

False-negative results reflect an inability to detect a mutation in an affected patient. This occurs principally in disorders where genetic heterogeneity—**allelic** (different mutations occur in 1 causative gene) or **locus** (>1 gene can cause a disease) heterogeneity—is the rule. It is difficult to detect all possible mutations within a gene, because mutations can be varied in location within the gene and in the type of mutation. Direct sequencing may miss gene deletions or rearrangements (i.e. structural variants), and mutations may be found within noncoding sequences such as introns or the promoter; a negative DNA test does not necessarily exclude a diagnosis.

Clinical utility is the degree to which the results of a test guide clinical management. For genetic testing, clinical utility includes establishing a diagnosis that obviates the need for additional workup or guiding surveillance or treatment. Test results may also be used as a basis for genetic counseling. For some disorders, genetic testing is possible, but the test results do not add to the clinical assessment. If the diagnosis and genetic implications are already clear, it might not be necessary to pursue genetic testing.

PREDICTIVE TESTING

Predictive genetic testing involves performing a test in a person who is at risk for developing a genetic disorder (**presymptomatic**), usually on the basis of family history, yet who does not manifest signs or symptoms. This is usually done for disorders that display age-dependent penetrance; the likelihood of manifesting signs and symptoms increases with age, as in cancer or Huntington disease.

A major caution with predictive testing is that the presence of a gene mutation does not necessarily mean that the disease will develop. Many of the disorders with age-dependent penetrance display *incomplete penetrance*. A person who inherits a mutation might never develop signs of the disorder. There is concern that a positive DNA test could result in stigmatization of the person and might not provide information that will guide medical management. Stigmatization might include psychological stress, but it could also include discrimination, including denial of health, life, or disability insurance, or employment (see Chapter 95).

It is generally agreed that predictive genetic tests should be performed for children only if the results of the test will benefit the medical management of the child. Otherwise, the test should be deferred until the child has an understanding of the risks and benefits of testing and can provide informed consent. Individual states offer varying degrees of protection from discrimination on the basis of genetic testing. A major milestone in the prevention of genetic discrimination was the passage of the **Genetic Information Nondiscrimination Act** (GINA) in 2008, which is a U.S. federal law that prohibits discrimination in health coverage or employment based on genetic information; *it does not* protect against refusal of life insurance.

PREDISPOSITIONAL TESTING

It is expected that genetic tests will become available that will predict risk of disease. Common disorders are multifactorial in etiology; many different genes may contribute to risk of any specific condition (see Chapter 99). Most of the genetic variants that have been found to correlate with risk of a common disease add small increments of relative risk, probably in most cases too little to guide management. It is possible that further discovery of genes that contribute to common disorders will reveal examples of variants that convey more significant levels of risk. It is also possible that testing several genes together will provide more information about risk than any individual gene variant would confer.

The rationale for predispositional testing is that the results would lead to strategies aimed at risk reduction as part of a *personalized approach* to healthcare maintenance. This might include avoidance of environmental exposures that would increase risk of disease (cigarette smoking and α_1-antitrypsin deficiency), medical surveillance (familial breast cancer and mammography), or in some cases, pharmacologic treatment (statins and hypercholesterolemia). The value of predispositional testing will need to be critically appraised through outcomes studies as these tests are developed.

PHARMACOGENETIC TESTING

Polymorphisms in drug metabolism genes can result in distinctive patterns of drug absorption, metabolism, excretion, or effectiveness (see Chapters 72 and 99). Knowledge of individual genotypes will guide pharmacologic therapy, allowing customization of choice of drug and dosage to avoid toxicity and provide a therapeutic response. An example is testing for polymorphisms within the methylenetetrahydrofolate reductase (*MTHFR*) gene for susceptibility of potentially increased toxicity to methotrexate antimetabolite therapy for acute lymphoblastic leukemia.

94.1 Genetic Counseling

Brendan Lee and Pilar L. Magoulas

Genetic counseling is a communication process in which the genetic contribution to health, specific risks of transmission of a trait, and options to manage the condition are explained to individuals and their family members (Table 94.3). Genetic counselors are specialized healthcare providers trained in the psychosocial aspects of counseling and the science of medical genetics who may serve as members of medical teams in many different specialties. The genetic counselor is expected to present information in a neutral, nondirective manner while

Table 94.3	Indications for Genetic Counseling

Advanced parental age
- Maternal age ≥35 yr
- Paternal age ≥40 yr

Previous child with or family history of:
- Congenital abnormality
- Dysmorphology
- Intellectual disability
- Isolated birth defect
- Metabolic disorder
- Chromosome abnormality
- Single-gene disorder

Adult-onset genetic disease (presymptomatic testing)
- Cancer
- Huntington disease

Pharmacogenomics

Consanguinity

Teratogen exposure (occupational, abuse)

Repeated pregnancy loss or infertility

Pregnancy screening abnormality

- Maternal serum α-fetoprotein

Maternal 1st-trimester screen
- Maternal triple or quad screen or variant of this test
- Fetal ultrasonography

Noninvasive prenatal testing (NIPT)
- Fetal karyotype

Heterozygote screening based on ethnic risk
- Sickle cell anemia
- Tay-Sachs, Canavan, and Gaucher diseases
- Thalassemias

Universal carrier screening panels

Follow-up to abnormal neonatal genetic testing

Prior to whole genome or exome sequencing

Prior to preimplantation genetic testing

providing resources and psychosocial support to the individual and family to cope with decisions that are made.

Genetic counseling has evolved from a model of care that was developed in the context of prenatal diagnosis and pediatrics into a multidisciplinary approach to medicine that factors into all aspects of healthcare (Table 94.3). In the prenatal setting, a common indication for genetic counseling is to assess risk of occurrence or recurrence of having a child with a genetic condition and to discuss management or treatment options that might be available before, during, or after the pregnancy, such as preimplantation genetic diagnosis, prenatal diagnosis or fetal intervention, and perinatal management. In pediatrics and adult genetics practices, the goals of genetic counseling are to help establish a diagnosis in an individual, provide longitudinal care and psychosocial support to the family, and discuss the genetic basis and inheritance of the condition as it relates to immediate and distant family members.

The genetic counseling role has expanded, particularly with advances in understanding the genetics of adult-onset or common and rare disease therapeutics. In the former context, genetic counseling has a major role in risk assessment for cancer, especially breast, ovarian, or colon cancer, for which well-defined risk models and genetic tests are available to assess risk to an individual. In the latter, the genetic counselor may discuss developments in rare disease therapeutics and make appropriate referral for medical therapies.

TALKING TO FAMILIES

The type of information provided to a family depends on the urgency of the situation, the need to make decisions, and the need to collect additional information. There are 4 situations in which genetic counseling plays a particularly important role in this process.

The 1st situation is the **prenatal diagnosis** of a congenital anomaly or genetic disease. The need for information is urgent because a family must often make time-sensitive decisions about treatment and management options, such as fetal intervention or continuation of a pregnancy in the context of fetal anomalies. Risks to the mother must also be considered. The 2nd type of situation occurs when a child is born with a life-threatening **congenital anomaly** or suspected **genetic disease**. Decisions must be made immediately with regard to how much support should be provided for the child and whether certain types of therapy should be attempted. The 3rd situation arises when there are concerns about a **genetic condition** affecting one later in life. For example, this

may occur in an adolescent or young adult with a family history of an adult-onset genetic disorder (e.g., Huntington disease, hereditary breast/ ovarian cancer), in an individual with a suspected yet undiagnosed genetic condition, or if a couple with a personal or family history of a genetic condition (or a carrier) is planning a family. In these situations it is often necessary to have several meetings with a family to discuss possible testing, screening, and management options. Urgency is not as much of an issue as being sure that they have as much information and as many options as are available. The 4th situation is **genetic counseling** before genome sequencing, where the family is given options of what they want reported back to them (actionable/nonactionable incidental findings vs a specific diagnosis).

GENETIC COUNSELING

Providing accurate information to families requires the following:
- Taking a careful family history and constructing a pedigree that lists the patient's relatives (including miscarriages, abortions, stillbirths, deceased persons) with their sex, age, ethnicity, and state of health, up to and including third-degree relatives.
- Gathering information from hospital records about the affected individual and, in some cases, about other family members.
- Documenting prenatal, pregnancy, and delivery histories.
- Reviewing the latest available medical, laboratory, and genetic information concerning the disorder.
- Performing a careful physical examination of the affected individual (photographs, measurements) and of apparently unaffected individuals in the family (this is usually performed by a physician rather than a genetic counselor).
- Establishing or confirming the diagnosis by the diagnostic tests available.
- Giving the family information about support groups and local and national resources.
- Providing new information to the family as it becomes available (a mechanism for updating needs to be established).

Counseling sessions must include the specific condition, knowledge of the diagnosis of the particular condition, natural history of the condition, genetic aspects of the condition and risk of recurrence, prenatal diagnosis and reproductive options, therapies and referrals, support groups, and nondirective counseling.

Specific Condition or Conditions

If a specific diagnosis is made and confirmed, this should be discussed with the family and information provided in writing. Often, however, the disorder fits into a spectrum (e.g., one of many types of arthrogryposis) or the diagnosis is clinical rather than laboratory based. In these situations the family needs to understand the limits of present knowledge, and that additional research will probably lead to better information in the future.

Knowledge of the Diagnosis of the Particular Condition

Although it is not always possible to make an exact diagnosis, having a diagnosis *as accurate as possible* is important. Estimates of recurrence risk for various family members depend on an accurate diagnosis, that considers the likelihood that a particular finding is isolated, associated with a syndrome, or nonsyndromic (e.g., isolated cleft lip and palate). When a specific diagnosis cannot be made (as in many cases of multiple congenital anomalies), the various possibilities in the differential diagnosis should be discussed with the family and empirical information provided. If available, specific diagnostic tests should be discussed. Often, empirical recurrence risks can be given even without a specific laboratory-based diagnosis. At the same time, even negative laboratory testing can further modify this risk.

Natural History of the Condition

It is important to discuss the natural history of the specific genetic disorder in the family. Affected persons and their families have questions regarding the prognosis and potential management or therapy that can be answered only with knowledge of the natural history. If there are other possible diagnoses, their natural history may also be discussed. If the disorder is associated with a spectrum of clinical outcomes or complications, the range of possible outcomes and variability of the condition, as well as treatment and referral to the appropriate specialist, should be addressed.

Genetic Aspects of the Condition and Recurrence Risk

The genetic aspects and risk of recurrence are important because all family members should be informed of their reproductive choices. The genetic basis of the disorder can be explained with visual aids (e.g., diagrams of chromosomes and inheritance patterns). It is important to provide accurate occurrence and recurrence risks for various members of the family, including unaffected individuals. If a definite diagnosis cannot be made, it is necessary to use empirical recurrence risks. Genetic counseling gives patients the necessary information to understand the various options and to make their own informed decisions regarding pregnancy, adoption, artificial insemination, prenatal diagnosis, screening, carrier detection, or termination of pregnancy. It may be necessary to have more than one counseling session.

Prenatal Diagnosis and Prevention

Many different methods of prenatal diagnosis are available, depending on the specific genetic disorder (see Chapter 115). The use of ultrasonography allows prenatal screening of anatomic abnormalities such as congenital heart defects. Amniocentesis and chorionic villus sampling are used to obtain fetal tissue for analysis of chromosomal abnormalities, biochemical disorders, and DNA studies. Maternal blood or serum sampling is used for some types of screening, including noninvasive prenatal screening by direct analysis of fetal DNA fragments found in maternal blood. This has gained widespread use for screening of conditions such as trisomy 21. In addition, this source of cell free fetal DNA has also been used clinically for DNA sequencing for dominant de novo conditions in the fetus that may occur with increased frequency with increasing paternal age. In the research arena, intact fetal cells can also be retrieved from maternal blood (though this is not yet readily available compared to free fetal DNA) for testing, and this may potentially offer higher resolution testing including whole exome or whole genome testing. Importantly, current tests of fetal DNA from maternal blood should be considered screening tests, and invasive testing like amniocentesis or chorionic villus sampling should be considered for confirmatory diagnostic testing.

Therapies and Referral

A number of genetic disorders require the care of multiple specialists. Many genetic conditions now have diagnosis and management guidelines to aid in the treatment and management of these complex patients. Prevention of known complications is a priority, so close follow-up with the necessary specialists involved in the child's care is essential to identify any potentially concerning issues early. The psychological adjustment of the family might also require specific intervention. Some challenges may involve when to discuss the diagnosis of a chronic disease with the patient, siblings, and other family members or friends. The decision to do so should always involve the parents and an assessment of the maturity and capacity of the child or adolescent.

Alternative medicines or nontraditional therapies are often brought to attention by parents after exhaustive internet searches. Such treatments should not necessarily be dismissed out of hand because the physician and genetic counselor should serve as an important resource for helping parents navigate the maze of nonstandard treatments. Instead, the relative merits of treatments should be framed in the context of cost and benefit, scientific rationale, evidence from controlled and observational studies, the placebo effect, safety of the treatment, and the gaps in our own scientific knowledge base.

Support Groups

A large number of community and online lay support groups have been formed to provide information and to fund research on specific genetic and nongenetic conditions. An important part of genetic counseling is to give information about these groups to patients and to suggest a contact person for the families. Many groups have established websites with very helpful information. With the rise of social media and its ability to connect families with rare syndromes from around the world, it is important to stress to families that their individual disease course will be unique.

Follow-up

Families should be encouraged to continue to ask questions and keep up with new information about the specific disorder. New developments often influence the diagnosis and therapy of specific genetic disorders. Lay support groups are a good source of new information.

Nondirective Counseling

Genetic counseling is usually nondirective; choices about reproduction are left to the family to decide what is right for them. The role of the counselor (physician, genetic counselor, nurse, medical geneticist) is to provide information in understandable terms and outline the range of options available.

94.2　Management and Treatment of Genetic Disorders

Brendan Lee and Nicola Brunetti-Pierri

Genetic conditions are often chronic disorders; few are amenable to curative therapies, although there has been a rapid increase in the number available in recent years. All patients and families should be provided information about the disorder, genetic counseling, anticipatory guidance, and appropriate medical surveillance. Surgical management is available for many conditions that are associated with congenital anomalies or predisposition to tumors.

Resources for patients include the National Organization of Rare Disorders (www.rarediseases.org), the Genetic Alliance (www.geneticalliance.org), the National Library of Medicine (www.nlm.nih.gov/medlineplus/geneticdisorders.html), and a large number of disease-specific websites. A current listing of federally and privately funded clinical trials, including many for genetic diseases, is available at www.ClinicalTrials.gov.

Specific medical therapies for genetic disorders can be classified into physiologic and replacement therapies. Another approach corrects protein misfolding induced by missense mutations through use of small molecules that specifically bind to mutant proteins stabilizing their conformation, thereby preventing early degradation and allowing proper cellular trafficking and localization. This strategy has found successful applications for therapy of cystic fibrosis caused by specific *CFTR* mutations, including the F508del (see Chapter 432).

PHYSIOLOGIC THERAPIES

Physiologic therapies attempt to ameliorate the phenotype of a genetic disorder by modifying the physiology of the affected individual. The underlying defect itself is not altered by treatment. Physiologic therapies are used in the treatment of **inborn errors of metabolism** (see Chapter 102). These include dietary manipulation, such as avoiding phenylalanine by persons with phenylketonuria; coenzyme supplementation for some patients with methylmalonic acidemia and mitochondrial diseases; stimulation of alternative pathways to excrete ammonia for those with urea cycle disorders; phototherapy to increase excretion of neurotoxic unconjugated bilirubin in Crigler-Najjar syndrome; bisphosphonate treatment for those with osteogenesis imperfecta to reduce bone fractures; and avoiding cigarette smoking by persons with α_1-antitrypsin deficiency or specific foods and drugs by persons with glucose-6-phosphate dehydrogenase deficiency or acute intermittent porphyria. Physiologic treatments can be highly effective, but they usually need to be maintained for a lifetime because they do not affect the underlying genetic disorder. Many of these treatments are most effective when begun early in life, before irreversible damage has occurred. This is the rationale for comprehensive newborn screening for inborn errors of metabolism.

Many physiologic therapies use small-molecule pharmaceuticals (e.g., to remove ammonia in those with urea cycle disorders). **Pharmacologic treatments** directly target a defective cellular pathway that is altered by an abnormal or a missing gene product. However, there are relatively few such therapies. One example is the inhibition of an enzyme reaction that is upstream of the deficient enzyme, to prevent accumulation of the toxic metabolites, such as the nitisinone (NTBC) for therapy of tyrosinemia type I. A similar approach focuses on partially reducing the synthesis of the substrate of the mutant enzyme or its precursors in lysosomal storage disorders (see Chapter 104.4).

REPLACEMENT THERAPIES

Replacement therapies include replacement of a missing metabolite, an enzyme, an organ, or even a specific gene.

Enzyme Replacement

Enzyme replacement therapy is a component of the treatment of cystic fibrosis to manage intestinal malabsorption. Pancreatic enzymes are easily administered orally, because they must be delivered to the gastrointestinal tract. Recombinant alkaline phosphatase coupled to bone targeting motif is available for intravenous therapy of hypophosphatasia, a skeletal disorder caused by alkaline-phosphatase deficiency.

Enzyme replacement strategies are effective for several lysosomal storage disorders. Enzymes are targeted for the lysosome by modification with mannose-6-phosphate, which binds to a specific receptor. This receptor is also present on the cell surface, so lysosomal enzymes with exposed mannose-6-phosphate residues can be infused into the blood and are taken into cells and transported to lysosomes. Enzyme replacement therapies are available for Gaucher disease and Fabry disease, some mucopolysaccharidoses (MPS I, II, IVA, VI), acid lipase deficiency, and Pompe disease, and are being tested for MPS IIIA, MPS VII, metachromatic leukodystrophy, α-mannosidosis, Niemann-Pick disease type B, and neuronal ceroid lipofuscinosis, late infantile (CLN2). Other examples include enzyme replacement therapy for hypophosphatasia.

One complication of enzyme replacement therapy is antibody response to the infused recombinant enzyme. The magnitude of this response is not always predictable and varies depending on the enzyme preparation and the disease. In most cases, the patient's antibody response does not affect the treatment's efficacy (e.g., Gaucher disease), but in other situations it may be a significant hurdle (e.g., Pompe disease and phenylketonuria).

Transplantation

Cell transplantation and **organ transplantation** are potentially effective approaches to replacement of a defective gene. Aside from transplantation to replace damaged tissues, transplantation of stem cells, liver, or bone marrow is also used for several diseases, mainly inborn errors of metabolism, and hematologic or immunologic disorders. A successful transplant is essentially curative, although there may be significant risks and side effects (see Chapters 161-165). Cell and tissue transplantation is effective in many clinical scenarios, but there is always short-term morbidity, often associated with either surgical (liver) or preparative (bone marrow) regimens, and long-term morbidity related to chronic immunosuppression and graft failure. Bone marrow transplantation is the best example of stem cell therapy, but much effort also is focused on identifying, characterizing, expanding, and using other tissue stem cells for regenerative therapies.

Alternatively, research has focused on replacing a defective gene (**gene therapy**). In theory, if one can target the specific tissue that has a deficiency in the gene or gene product, this can offer a less invasive means of achieving a cure for a genetic disorder. Ultimately, gene therapy depends on the unique interaction of the disease pathophysiology, which is specific to the patient, and the gene delivery vehicle.

Gene-transfer vehicles include viral and nonviral vectors administered through ex vivo or in vivo approaches. In ex vivo approaches the patient's cells are removed and after gene correction are infused into the patient. An example of this is the FDA approved CAR-T cell therapy for non-Hodgkin lymphoma. In the in vivo approaches the gene therapy vector is directly injected into the body by either systemic (e.g., intravenous) or localized (e.g., intramuscular, intracerebral, intraocular) injections. Most human clinical trials have used viral vectors because of their efficiency of tissue transduction. In some diseases, such as X-linked and adenosine deaminase–deficient severe combined immunodeficiency, chronic granulomatous disease, and Wiskott-Aldrich syndrome, clinical gene therapy is a viable and effective option (see Chapter 152.1). Ex vivo gene transfer of hematopoietic stem cells can now be considered at least as effective to allogenic hematopoietic stem cells transplantation in presymptomatic patients with X-linked adrenoleukodystrophy and metachromatic leukodystrophy. In vivo gene therapy is also promising for Leber congenital amaurosis by intraocular delivery, lipoprotein lipase deficiency by intramuscular injections, and hemophilia B by systemic intravenous injection. The first ever human in vivo gene therapy was recently approved in the United States by the FDA for treatment of a specific RPE65-deficient form of retinitis pigmentosa using adenoassociated virus (AAV)-mediated expression of the normal RPE65 gene via intraretinal injection.

Gene editing with direct correction of a pathologic mutation is a possible approach to genetic therapy. **CRISPR/Cas9** (clustered regularly interspaced short palindromic repeats/CRISPR-associated system) is a mechanism that permits permanent gene modification of genes in cells. CRISPR genes are bacterial DNA sequences used as a defense mechanism to destroy DNA from viral infections. Combined with related Cas nuclease proteins, the foreign RNA or DNA is recognized, excised, and digested. In gene editing, a complex of the nuclease enzyme and a complementary RNA sequence recognizes the base sequence in the mutated gene. Once bound to the targeted sequence, the nuclease excises both strands and inserts the corrected (nonmutated) sequence. The CRISPR system has corrected the gene defect in a mouse model of Duchenne muscular dystrophy and reduced the tumor burden in explanted human prostate cancer cells in mice. CRISPR-edited T cells can be modified to target and kill tumor cells. CRISPR/Cas9 has been employed to correct the mutation in *MYBPC3* (hypertrophic cardiomyopathy) in an experimental human embryo model. Clinical trials are now in progress applying this approach in somatic tissue. Currently, germline and/or embryonic gene editing studies in humans have not been approved.

Prevention of genetic disease has been accomplished by **preimplantation genetic diagnosis**. This procedure requires in vitro fertilization and single–embryo cell genetic testing of the known families' mutation and is performed with PCR amplification of the affected gene. To avoid recurrent disease, only the unaffected embryos are used for implantation.

In addition, mitochondrial DNA mutations may be avoided by using **mitochondrial replacement therapies**. In one technique the mutation carrier mother's nuclear DNA is removed from the unfertilized oocyte and transferred to the unaffected mitochondrial donor oocyte (minus that cell's nuclear DNA). In another approach the pronucleus from the mutation-carrier mother's fertilized oocyte is transferred to the unaffected mitochondrial donor's fertilized oocyte (minus the pronucleus).

These different and promising methodologies have many technical and ethical considerations that are being discussed by medical, ethical, legal, and policymaking organizations.

Bibliography is available at Expert Consult.

Chapter 95

The Genetic Approach in Pediatric Medicine

Daryl A. Scott and Brendan Lee

第九十五章

儿科医学中的遗传学研究方法

中文导读

　　本章主要介绍了儿童期的遗传病负担、遗传学在医学应用中的范式的改变和伦理问题。具体描述了儿童期的遗传病负担的单基因病和基因组病的负担；遗传学在医学应用中的范式的改变中描述了植入前遗传学诊断、先天性代谢缺陷以及溶酶体贮积病；伦理问题中详细阐述了一般性建议、诊断性检测、新生儿筛查、携带者筛查、预测性基因检测、组织相容性检测、收养、基因公开、直接对消费者的检测等内容。

Since the completion of the Human Genome Project, we have seen an unprecedented expansion in our understanding of how human health is impacted by variations in genomic sequence and **epigenetic**, non-sequence-based, changes that affect gene expression. This period has also seen the development and implementation of new clinical tests that have made it easier for physicians to detect such changes. In addition, there has been a dramatic increase in the availability of information about the genetic aspects of pediatric diseases, particularly on the internet (Table 95.1).

THE BURDEN OF GENETIC DISORDERS IN CHILDHOOD

Medical problems associated with genetic disorders can appear at any age, with the most obvious and serious problems typically manifesting in childhood. It has been estimated that 53/1,000 children and young adults can be expected to have diseases with an important genetic component. If congenital anomalies are included, the rate increases to 79/1,000. In 1978 it was estimated that just over half of admissions to pediatric hospitals were for a genetically determined condition. By 1996, because of changes in healthcare delivery and a greater understanding of the genetic basis of many disorders, that percentage rose to 71%, in one large pediatric hospital in the United States, with 96% of chronic disorders leading to admission having an obvious genetic component or being influenced by genetic susceptibility.

Major categories of genetic disorders include single-gene, genomic, chromosomal, and multifactorial conditions.

Individually, each **single-gene disorder** is rare, but collectively they represent an important contribution to childhood disease. The hallmark of a single-gene disorder is that the phenotype is overwhelmingly determined by changes that affect an individual gene. The phenotypes associated with single-gene disorders can vary from one patient to another

based on the severity of the change affecting the gene and additional modifications caused by genetic, environmental, and stochastic factors. This feature of genetic disease is termed **variable expressivity**. Common single-gene disorders include sickle cell anemia and cystic fibrosis. Some identifiable syndromes and diseases can be caused by more than one gene (e.g., Noonan syndrome by *RAF1, NF1, NRAS, PTPN11, SOS1, SOS2, KRAS, BRAF, SOC2, LZTR1,* and *RIT1*). In addition, mutations affecting a single gene may produce different phenotypes (e.g., *SCN5A* and Brugada syndrome, long QT syndrome 3, dilated cardiomyopathy, familial atrial fibrillation, and congenital sick sinus syndrome).

Single-gene disorders tend to occur when changes in a gene have a profound effect on the *quantity* of the gene product produced, either too much or too little, or the *function* of the gene product, either a loss of function or a harmful gain of function. Single-gene disorders can be caused by de novo sequence changes that are not found in the unaffected parents of the affected individual, or they may be caused by inherited changes. When a single-gene disorder is known to be caused by changes in only 1 gene, or a small number of individual genes, searching for deleterious changes is most often performed by directly sequencing that gene and, in some cases, looking for small deletions and/or duplications. When multiple genes can cause a particular disorder, it is sometimes more efficient and cost-effective to screen large numbers of disease-causing genes using a disease-specific panel that takes advantage of next-generation sequencing technology than to screen genes individually. When such panels are not available, or when the diagnosis is in question, physicians may consider screening the protein-coding regions of all genes by **whole exome sequencing (WES)** on a clinical basis. In many circumstances, WES is less expensive than sequencing multiple individual genes. In the future, **whole genome sequencing**, in which an individual's entire genome is sequenced, may become a valid clinical option as the cost of such tests fall and our ability to interpret

Table 95.1	Useful Internet Genetic Reference Sites	
RESOURCE		**WEB ADDRESS**
National Center for Biotechnology Information. A general reference maintained by the National Library of Medicine.		www.ncbi.nlm.nih.gov
Online Mendelian Inheritance in Man. A useful resource for clinicians containing information on all known mendelian disorders and >12,000 genes. Information focuses on the relationship between phenotype and genotype.		www.ncbi.nlm.nih.gov/omim
Genetic Testing Registry. A resource that provides information on individual genes, genetic tests, clinical laboratories, and medical conditions. This resource also provides access to GeneReviews, a collection of expert-authored reviews on a variety of genetic disorders.		www.ncbi.nlm.nih.gov/gtr/
Genetics Home Reference. A resource that provides consumer-friendly information about the effects of genetic variations on human health.		www.ghr.nlm.nih.gov
National Human Genome Research Institute. A resource for information about human genetics and ethical issues.		www.genome.gov
Human Gene Mutation Database. A searchable index of all described mutations in human genes with phenotypes and references.		www.hgmd.cf.ac.uk
DECIPHER. A database designed to aid physicians in determining the potential consequences of chromosomal deletions and duplications.		http://decipher.sanger.ac.uk
Database of Genomic Variants. A database of chromosomal alterations seen in normal controls.		http://dgv.tcag.ca/dgv/app/home
Gene Letter. An online magazine of genetics.		www.geneletter.com
American Society of Human Genetics		www.ashg.org
American College of Medical Genetics		www.acmg.net

the clinical consequences of the thousands of changes identified in such tests improves (see Chapter 94).

The risk of having a child with a particular single-gene disorder can vary from one population to another. In some cases, this is the result of a **founder effect**, in which a specific change affecting a disease-causing gene becomes relatively common in a population derived from a small number of founders. This high frequency is maintained when there is relatively little interbreeding with persons outside that population because of social, religious, or physical barriers. This is the case for Tay-Sachs disease in Ashkenazi Jews and French Canadians. Other changes may be subject to **positive selection** when found in the heterozygous carrier state. In this case, individuals who carry a single copy of a genetic change (**heterozygotes**) have a survival advantage over noncarriers. This can occur even when individuals who inherit 2 copies of the change (**homozygotes**) have severe medical problems. This type of positive selection is evident among individuals in sub-Saharan Africa who carry a single copy of a hemoglobin mutation that confers relative resistance to malaria but causes sickle cell anemia in homozygotes.

Genomic disorders are a group of diseases caused by alterations in the genome, including **deletions** (copy number loss), **duplications** (copy number gain), **inversions** (altered orientation of a genomic region), and **chromosomal rearrangements** (altered location of a genomic region). **Contiguous gene disorders** are caused by changes that affect 2 or more genes that contribute to the clinical phenotype and are located near one other on a chromosome. DiGeorge syndrome, which is caused by deletions of genes located on chromosome 22q11, is a common example. Some genomic disorders are associated with distinctive phenotypes whose pattern can be recognized clinically. Other genomic disorders do not have a distinctive pattern of anomalies but can cause developmental delay, cognitive impairment, structural birth defects, abnormal growth patterns, and changes in physical appearance. **Fluorescent in situ hybridization (FISH)** can provide information about the copy number and location of a specific genomic region. **Array-based copy number detection assays** can be used to screen for chromosomal deletions (large and small) and duplications across the genome, but do not provide information about the orientation or location of genomic regions. A **chromosome analysis (karyotype)** can detect relatively large chromosomal deletions and duplications and can also be useful in identifying inversions and chromosomal rearrangements even when they are **copy number neutral**

changes that do not result in a deletion or duplication of genomic material.

Deletions, duplications, and chromosomal rearrangements that affect whole chromosomes, or large portions of a chromosome, are typically referred to as **chromosomal disorders**. One of the most common chromosomal disorders is Down syndrome, most often associated with the presence of an extra copy, or **trisomy**, of an entire chromosome 21. When all or a part of a chromosome is missing, the disorder is referred to as **monosomy**. **Translocations** are a type of chromosomal rearrangement in which a genomic region from one chromosome is transferred to a different location on the same chromosome or on a different (nonhomologous) chromosome. Translocations can be *balanced,* meaning that no genetic material has been lost or gained, or they can be *unbalanced,* in which some genetic material has been deleted or duplicated.

In some cases, only a portion of cells that make up a person's body are affected by a single-gene defect, a genomic disorder, or a chromosomal defect. This is referred to as **mosaicism** and indicates that the individual's body is made up of 2 or more distinct cell populations.

Polygenic disorders are caused by the cumulative effects of changes or variations in more than 1 gene. **Multifactorial** disorders are caused by the cumulative effects of changes or variations in multiple genes and/or the combined effects of both genetic and environmental factors. Spina bifida and isolated cleft lip or palate are common birth defects that display multifactorial inheritance patterns. Multifactorial inheritance is seen in many common pediatric disorders, such as asthma and diabetes mellitus. These traits can cluster in families but do not have a mendelian pattern of inheritance (see Chapter 97). In these cases the genetic changes or variations that are contributing to a particular disorder are often unknown, and genetic counseling is based on empirical data.

THE CHANGING PARADIGM OF GENETICS IN MEDICINE

Genetic testing is increasingly available for a wide variety of both rare and relatively common genetic disorders. Genetic testing is typically used in pediatric medicine to resolve uncertainty regarding the underlying etiology of a child's medical problems and provides a basis for improved genetic counseling and possibly a specific therapy. Even in cases where a specific treatment is not available, identifying a genetic cause can aid physicians in providing individuals and family with accurate prognostic and recurrence risk information and usually helps to relieve unfounded feelings of guilt and stem the tide of misdirected blame.

Genetic tests will ultimately come to underlie a high proportion of medical decisions and will be seamlessly incorporated into routine medical care. Although most genetic testing is presently aimed at identifying or confirming a diagnosis, in the future, genetic testing may find wider application as a means of determining if an individual is predisposed to develop a particular disease. Another area in which genetic testing could make a significant impact is on individualized drug treatment. It has long been known that genetic variation in the enzymes involved in drug metabolism underlies differences in the therapeutic effect and toxicity of some drugs. As the genetic changes that underlie these variations are identified, new genetic tests are being developed that allow physicians to tailor treatments based on individual variations in drug metabolism, responsiveness, and susceptibility to toxicity (see Chapter 72). It is likely that the expansion of such testing will depend, at least in part, on the extent to which such tests can be linked to strategies to prevent disease or improve outcome (see Chapter 94). As such links are made, we will enter into a new era of personalized medical treatment.

Long-standing and highly successful carrier screening programs have existed for disorders such as Tay-Sachs disease and many other rare, single-gene disorders that are prevalent in specific populations. Couples are usually offered screening for a variety of conditions, in part based on ancestry (Tay-Sachs disease, hemoglobinopathies, cystic fibrosis). Couples found to be at increased risk for such disorders can be offered preconception or prenatal testing aimed at detecting specific disease-causing mutations.

Prenatal screening is routinely offered for chromosomal disorders such as trisomy 13, trisomy 18, and Down syndrome. An increasing number of pregnancies affected by these and other genetic disorders are being recognized by noninvasive screening tests targeting fetal cell-free DNA in maternal blood and by fetal ultrasound. When genetic disorders are suspected, chorionic villus sampling at 10-12 wk of gestation or amniocentesis at 16-18 wk of gestation can provide material for genetic testing. When a couple are at risk for a specific genetic defect, **preimplantation genetic diagnosis** can sometimes be used to select unaffected early embryos, which are then implanted as part of an in vitro fertilization procedure.

Although prenatally obtained genetic material can be used to identify single-gene disorders, genomic disorders, and chromosomal anomalies, the information obtained on any pregnancy depends on the tests that are ordered. It is important that physicians select the most appropriate prenatal tests, and that couples understand the limitations of these tests. No amount of genetic testing can guarantee the birth of a healthy child.

Specific treatments are not available for the majority of genetic disorders, although some important exceptions exist (Chapter 94). **Inborn errors of metabolism** were the first genetic disorders to be recognized, and many are amenable to treatment by dietary manipulation (see Chapter 102). These conditions result from genetically determined deficiency of specific enzymes, leading to the buildup of toxic substrates and/or deficiency of critical end products.

Individual metabolic disorders tend to be very rare, but their combined impact on the pediatric population is significant. Tandem mass spectrometry has made it relatively inexpensive to screen for a large number of these disorders in the newborn period. Use of this technology not only dramatically increases the number of metabolic disorders identified within a population, but also allows treatment to be initiated at a much earlier stage in development.

Another area showing progress in genetic therapies is the treatment of **lysosomal storage disorders** (see Chapter 104.4). These metabolic diseases are caused by defects in lysosomal function. *Lysosomes* are cellular organelles that contain specific digestive enzymes. Some of these disorders that were characterized by early lethal or intractable chronic illness can now be treated using specially modified enzymes administered by intravenous infusion. These enzymes are taken up by cells and incorporated into lysosomes. Conditions such as Gaucher disease and Fabry disease are routinely treated using **enzyme replacement**, and similar therapies are being developed for other lysosomal disorders.

Therapeutic advances are also being made in the treatment of nonmetabolic genetic disorders. Improvements in surgical techniques and intensive care medicine are extending the survival of children with life-threatening birth defects such as congenital diaphragmatic hernia and severe cardiac defects. In many cases the life expectancy of children with debilitating genetic disorders is also increasing. For example, in cystic fibrosis, improvements in nutrition and the management of chronic pulmonary disease allow an increasing percentage of affected patients to survive into adulthood, creating a need to transition care from pediatric to adult providers.

Gene replacement therapies have long been anticipated and are starting to show some benefit (see Chapter 94). Stem cell–based therapies have also been touted as a potential treatment for a number of intractable disorders, but clear evidence that such therapies are effective has yet to materialize.

ETHICS ISSUES

As with all medical care, genetic testing, diagnosis, and treatment should be performed *confidentially*. Nothing is as personal as one's genetic information, and all efforts should be made to avoid any stigma for the patient. Many people worry that results of genetic testing will put them, or their child, at risk for genetic discrimination. **Genetic discrimination** occurs when people are treated unfairly because of a difference in their DNA that suggests they have a genetic disorder or they are at an increased risk of developing a certain disease. In the United States the Genetic Information Nondiscrimination Act of 2008 protects individuals from genetic discrimination at the hands of health insurers and employers, but does not extend protection against discrimination from providers of life, disability, or long-term care insurance.

As in all medical decision-making, the decisions about genetic testing should be based on a careful evaluation of the potential benefits and risks. In the pediatric setting, these decisions may be more difficult because physicians and parents are often called on to make decisions for a child who cannot directly participate in discussions about testing. Molecular diagnostic tests are often used to diagnose malformation syndromes, cognitive delay, or other disabilities in which there is a clear benefit to the child. In other cases, such as genetic testing for susceptibility to adult-onset diseases, it is appropriate to wait until the child or adolescent is mature enough to weigh the potential risks and benefits and make his or her own decisions about genetic testing.

Policies regarding genetic testing of children have been developed collaboratively by the American Academy of Pediatrics (AAP) and the American College of Medical Genetics and Genomics (ACMG; *Pediatrics* 131[3]:620–622, 2013). These recommendations are outlined next.

General Recommendations

1. Decisions about whether to offer genetic testing and screening should be driven by the best interest of the child.
2. Genetic testing is best offered in the context of genetic counseling. Genetic counseling can be performed by clinical geneticists, genetic counselors, or any other health care provider with appropriate training and expertise. AAP and ACMG support the expansion of educational opportunities in human genomics and genetics for medical students, residents, and practicing pediatric primary care providers.

Diagnostic Testing

3. In a child with symptoms of a genetic condition, the rationale for genetic testing is similar to that of other medical diagnostic evaluations. Parents or guardians should be informed about the risks and benefits of testing, and their permission should be obtained. Ideally, and when appropriate, the assent of the child should be obtained.
4. When performed for therapeutic purposes, pharmacogenetic testing of children is acceptable, with permission of parents or guardians and, when appropriate, the child's assent. If a pharmacogenetic test result carries implications beyond drug targeting or dose responsiveness, the broader implications should be discussed before testing.

Newborn Screening

5. AAP and ACMG support the mandatory offering of newborn screening for all children. After education and counseling about the substantial benefits of newborn screening, its remote risks, and

the next steps in the event of a positive screening result, parents should have the option of refusing the procedure, and an informed refusal should be respected.

Carrier Testing

6. AAP and ACMG do not support routine carrier testing in minors when such testing does not provide health benefits in childhood. The AAP and ACMG advise against school-based testing or screening programs, because the school environment is unlikely to be conducive to voluntary participation, thoughtful consent, privacy, confidentiality, or appropriate counseling about test results.

7. For pregnant adolescents or for adolescents considering reproduction, genetic testing and screening should be offered as clinically indicated, and the risks and benefits should be explained clearly.

Predictive Genetic Testing

8. Parents or guardians may authorize predictive genetic testing for asymptomatic children at risk of childhood-onset conditions. Ideally, the assent of the child should be obtained.

9. Predictive genetic testing for adult-onset conditions generally should be deferred unless an intervention initiated in childhood may reduce morbidity or mortality. An exception might be made for families for whom diagnostic uncertainty poses a significant psychosocial burden, particularly when an adolescent and the parents concur in their interest in predictive testing.

10. For ethical and legal reasons, healthcare providers should be cautious about providing predictive genetic testing to minors without the involvement of their parents or guardians, even if a minor is mature. Results of such tests may have significant medical, psychological, and social implications, not only for the minor but also for other family members.

Histocompatibility Testing

11. Tissue compatibility testing of minors of all ages is permissible to benefit immediate family members but should be conducted only after thorough exploration of the psychosocial, emotional, and physical implications of the minor serving as a potential stem cell donor. A donor advocate or similar mechanism should be in place from the outset to avert coercion and safeguard the interests of the child.

Adoption

12. The rationale for genetic testing of children in biological families should apply for adopted children and children awaiting placement for adoption. If a child has a known genetic risk, prospective adoptive parents must be made aware of this possibility. In rare cases, it may be in a child's best interest to undergo predictive genetic testing for a known risk before adoption, to ensure the child's placement with a family capable of and willing to accept the child's potential medical and developmental challenges. In the absence of such indications, genetic testing should not be performed as a condition of adoption.

Disclosure

13. At the time of genetic testing, parents or guardians should be encouraged to inform their child of the test results at an appropriate age. Parents or guardians should be advised that, under most circumstances, a request by a mature adolescent for test results should be honored.

14. Results from genetic testing of a child may have implications for the parents and other family members. Healthcare providers have an obligation to inform parents and the child, when appropriate, about these potential implications. Healthcare providers should encourage patients and families to share this information and offer to help explain the results to the extended family or refer them for genetic counseling.

15. Misattributed paternity, use of donor gametes, adoption, or other questions about family relationships may be uncovered "incidentally" whenever genetic testing is performed, particularly when testing multiple family members. This risk should be discussed, and a plan about disclosure or nondisclosure should be in place before testing.

Direct-to-Consumer Testing

16. AAP and ACMG strongly discourage the use of direct-to-consumer and home-kit genetic testing of children because of the lack of oversight on test content, accuracy, and interpretation.

Bibliography is available at Expert Consult.

Chapter 96
The Human Genome
Daryl A. Scott and Brendan Lee

第九十六章
人类基因组

中文导读

　　本章主要介绍了分子遗传学基础、遗传变异、遗传病的基因型–表型相关性以及人类基因组计划。具体描述了分子遗传学基础中的双螺旋结构、DNA聚合酶、信使RNA、核糖体RNA等概念；具体描述了遗传变异中的替换、插入以及缺失等变异类型和功能丧失性突变以及功能获得性突变；具体描述了遗传病的基因型–表型相关性中的长QT综合征、马方综合征以及囊性纤维化。

The human genome has approximately 20,000 genes that encode the wide variety of proteins found in the human body. Reproductive or germline cells contain 1 copy (N) of this genetic complement and are **haploid**, whereas somatic (nongermline) cells contain 2 complete copies (2N) and are **diploid**. Genes are organized into long segments of deoxyribonucleic acid (**DNA**), which, during cell division, are compacted into intricate structures together with proteins to form chromosomes. Each somatic cell has 46 chromosomes: 22 pairs of **autosomes**, or nonsex chromosomes, and 1 pair of **sex chromosomes** (XY in a male, XX in a female). Germ cells (ova or sperm) contain 22 autosomes and 1 sex chromosome, for a total of 23. At fertilization, the full diploid chromosome complement of 46 is again realized in the embryo.

Most of the genetic material is contained in the cell's nucleus. The mitochondria (the cell's energy-producing organelles) contain their own unique genome. The **mitochondrial chromosome** consists of a double-stranded circular piece of DNA, which contains 16,568 base pairs (bp) of DNA and is present in multiple copies per cell. The proteins that occupy the mitochondria are produced either in the mitochondria, using information contained in the mitochondrial genome, or are produced outside of the mitochondria, using information contained in the nuclear genome, and then transported into the organelle. Sperm do not usually contribute mitochondria to the developing embryo, so all mitochondria are maternally derived, and a child's mitochondrial genetic makeup derives exclusively from the child's biological mother (see Chapter 106).

FUNDAMENTALS OF MOLECULAR GENETICS
DNA consists of a pair of chains of a sugar-phosphate backbone linked by pyrimidine and purine bases to form a **double helix** (Fig. 96.1). The sugar in DNA is deoxyribose. The pyrimidines are cytosine (C) and thymine (T); the purines are guanine (G) and adenine (A). The bases are linked by hydrogen bonds such that A always pairs with T and G with C. Each strand of the double helix has polarity, with a free phosphate at one end (5′) and an unbonded hydroxyl on the sugar at

the other end (3′). The 2 strands are oriented in opposite polarity in the double helix.

The replication of DNA follows the pairing of bases in the parent DNA strand. The original 2 strands unwind by breaking the hydrogen bonds between base pairs. Free nucleotides, consisting of a base attached to a sugar-phosphate chain, form new hydrogen bonds with their complementary bases on the parent strand; new phosphodiester bonds are created by enzymes called **DNA polymerases.** Replication of chromosomes begins simultaneously at multiple sites, forming replication bubbles that expand bidirectionally until the entire DNA molecule (chromosome) is replicated. Errors in DNA replication, or mutations induced by environmental mutagens such as irradiation or chemicals, are detected and potentially corrected by DNA repair systems.

The central tenet of molecular genetics is that information encoded in DNA, predominantly located in the cell nucleus, is transcribed into **messenger** ribonucleic acid (**mRNA**), which is then transported to the cytoplasm, where it is translated into protein. A prototypical gene consists of a regulatory region, segments called **exons** that encode the amino acid sequence of a protein, and intervening segments called **introns** (Fig. 96.2).

Transcription is initiated by attachment of ribonucleic acid (**RNA**) polymerase to the promoter site upstream of the beginning of the coding sequence. Specific proteins bind to the region to repress or activate transcription by opening up the **chromatin**, which is a complex of DNA and histone proteins. It is the action of these regulatory proteins (**transcription factors**) that determines, in large part, when a gene is turned on or off. Some genes are also turned on and off by methylation of cytosine bases that are adjacent to guanine bases (**cytosine-phosphate-guanine bases, CpGs**). Methylation is an example of an **epigenetic** change, meaning a change that can affect gene expression, and possibly the characteristics of a cell or organism, but that *does not* involve a change in the underlying genetic sequence. Gene regulation is flexible and responsive, with genes being turned on or off during development and in response to internal and external environmental conditions and stimuli.

Transcription proceeds through the entire length of the gene in a 5′ to 3′ direction to form an mRNA transcript whose sequence is complementary to that of one of the DNA strands. RNA, like DNA, is a sugar-phosphate chain with pyrimidines and purines. In RNA the sugar is ribose, and uracil replaces the thymine found in DNA. A "cap" consisting of 7-methylguanosine is added to the 5′ end of the RNA in a 5′-5′ bond, and for most transcripts, several hundred adenine bases are enzymatically added to the 3′ end after transcription.

mRNA processing occurs in the nucleus and consists of excision of the introns and splicing together of the exons. Specific sequences at the start and end of introns mark the sites where the splicing machinery will act on the transcript. In some cases, there may be tissue-specific patterns to splicing, so that the same primary transcript can produce multiple distinct proteins.

The processed transcript is next exported to the cytoplasm, where it binds to ribosomes, which are complexes of protein and **ribosomal RNA** (**rRNA**). The genetic code is then read in triplets of bases, each triplet corresponding with a specific amino acid or providing a signal that terminates **translation**. The triplet codons are recognized by **transfer RNAs** (**tRNAs**) that include complementary anticodons and bind the corresponding amino acid, delivering it to the growing peptide. New amino acids are enzymatically attached to the peptide. Each time an amino acid is added, the ribosome moves 1 triplet codon step along the mRNA. Eventually a **stop codon** is reached, at which point translation ends and the peptide is released. In some proteins, there are **post-translational modifications**, such as attachment of sugars (**glycosylation**); the protein is then delivered to its destination within or outside the cell by trafficking mechanisms that recognize portions of the peptide.

Another mechanism of genetic regulation is **noncoding** RNAs, which are RNAs transcribed from DNA but not translated into proteins. Noncoding RNAs function in mediating splicing, the processing of coding RNAs in the nucleus, and the translation of coding mRNAs in ribosomes. The roles of *large* noncoding RNAs (>200 bp) and *short* noncoding RNAs (<200 bp) extend beyond these processes to impact

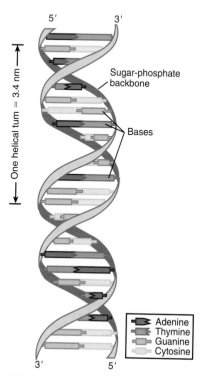

← One helical turn = 3.4 nm →

5′   3′

Sugar-phosphate backbone

Bases

■▶ Adenine
■▶ Thymine
■▶ Guanine
■▶ Cytosine

3′   5′

Fig. 96.1 DNA double helix, with sugar-phosphate backbone and nitrogenous bases. *(From Jorde LB, Carey JC, Bamshad MJ, et al, editors: Medical genetics, ed 2, St Louis, 1999, Mosby, p 8.)*

a diverse set of biologic functions, including the regulation of gene expression. For example, **microRNAs (miRNAs)** are a class of small RNAs that control gene expression in the cell by directly targeting specific sets of coding RNAs by direct RNA–RNA binding. This RNA–RNA interaction can lead to degradation of the target-coding RNA or inhibition of translation of the protein specified by that coding RNA. miRNAs, in general, target and regulate several hundred mRNAs.

GENETIC VARIATION

The process of producing protein from a gene is subject to disruption at multiple levels because of alterations in the coding sequence (Fig. 96.3). Changes in the regulatory region can lead to altered gene expression, including increased or decreased rates of transcription, failure of gene activation, or activation of the gene at inappropriate times or in inappropriate cells. Changes in the coding sequence can lead to **substitution** of one amino acid for another (**missense variant** or **nonsynonymous variant**) or creation of a stop codon in the place of an amino acid codon. Overall, missense or nonsense variants are the most common (56% of variants); small deletions or insertions represent approximately 24% of variants (Table 96.1). Some single-base changes do not affect the amino acid (**silent**, **wobble**, or **synonymous variants**), because there may be several triplet codons that correspond to a single amino acid. Amino acid substitutions can have a profound effect on protein function if the chemical properties of the substituted amino acid are markedly different from the usual one. Other substitutions can have a subtle or no effect on protein function, particularly if the substituted amino acid is chemically similar to the original one.

Genetic changes can also include **insertions** or **deletions**. Insertions or deletions of a nonintegral multiple of 3 bases into the coding sequence leads to a **frameshift**, altering the grouping of bases into triplets. This leads to translation of an incorrect amino acid sequence and often a premature stop to translation. Insertion or deletion of an integral multiple of 3 bases into the coding sequence will insert or delete a corresponding number of amino acids from the protein, leading to **in-frame** alterations that maintain the amino acid sequence outside the deleted or duplicated amino acids. Larger-scale insertions or deletions can disrupt a coding sequence or result in complete deletion of an entire gene or group of genes.

Pathogenic variants usually can be classified as causing a loss of function or a gain of function. **Loss-of-function variants** cause a reduction in the level of protein function as a result of decreased expression or production of a protein that does not work as efficiently. In some cases, loss of protein function from 1 gene is sufficient to cause disease. **Haploinsufficiency** describes the situation in which maintenance of a normal phenotype requires the proteins produced by both copies of a gene, and a 50% decrease in gene function results in an abnormal phenotype. Thus, haploinsufficient phenotypes are, by definition, dominantly inherited. Loss-of-function variants can also have a dominant negative effect when the abnormal protein product actively interferes with the function of the normal protein product. Both these situations lead to diseases inherited in a dominant fashion. In other cases, loss-of-function variants must be present in both copies of a gene before an abnormal phenotype results. This situation typically results in diseases inherited in a recessive fashion (see Chapter 97).

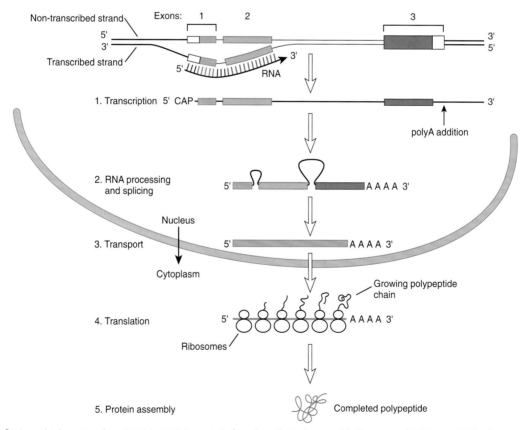

Fig. 96.2 Flow of information from DNA to RNA to protein for a hypothetical gene with 3 exons and 2 introns. Within the exons, *colored regions* indicate coding sequences. Steps include transcription, RNA processing and splicing, RNA transport from the nucleus to the cytoplasm, translation, and protein assembly. (*From Nussbaum RL, McInnis RR, Willard HF, Hamosh A, editors:* Thompson & Thompson genetics in medicine, *ed 7, Philadelphia, 2007, Saunders/Elsevier, p 31.*)

Gain-of-function variants typically cause dominantly inherited diseases. These variants can result in production of a protein molecule with an increased ability to perform a normal function or can confer a novel property on the protein. The gain-of-function variant in **achondroplasia**, the most common of the disproportionate, short-limbed short stature disorders, exemplifies the enhanced function of a normal protein. Achondroplasia results from a mutation in the fibroblast growth factor (FGF) receptor 3 gene (*FGFR3*), which leads to activation of the receptor, even in the absence of FGF. In **sickle cell disease** an amino acid is substituted into the hemoglobin molecule and has little effect on the ability of the protein to transport oxygen. However, sickle hemoglobin chains have a novel property. Unlike normal hemoglobin,

sickle hemoglobin chains aggregate under conditions of deoxygenation, forming fibers that deform the red cells.

Other gain-of-function mutations result in overexpression or inappropriate expression of a gene product. Many cancer-causing genes (**oncogenes**) are normal regulators of cellular proliferation during development. However, expression of these genes in adult life and/or in cells in which they usually are not expressed can result in neoplasia.

In some cases, changes in gene expression are caused by changes in the number of copies of a gene that are present in the genome (Fig. 96.4). Although some **copy number variations** are common and do not appear to cause or predispose to disease, others are clearly disease causing. **Charcot-Marie-Tooth disease type 1A**, the most common

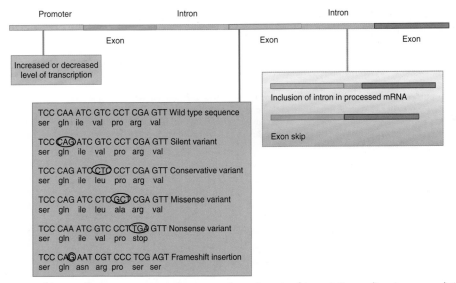

Fig. 96.3 Various types of intragenic sequence variants. Promoter variants alter rate of transcription or disrupt gene regulation. Base changes within exons can have various effects, as shown. Variants within introns can lead to inclusion of some intronic sequence in the final processed mRNA, or it can lead to exon skipping.

Table 96.1	Main Classes, Groups, and Types of Sequence Variants and Their Effects on Protein Products		
CLASS	**GROUP**	**TYPE**	**EFFECT ON PROTEIN PRODUCT**
Substitution	Synonymous	Silent*	Same amino acid
	Nonsynonymous	Missense*	Altered amino acid—may affect protein function or stability
		Nonsense*	Stop codon—loss of function or expression from degradation of mRNA
		Splice site	Aberrant splicing—exon skipping or intron retention
		Promoter	Altered gene expression
Deletion	Multiple of 3 (codon)		In-frame deletion of 1 or more amino acid(s)—may affect protein function or stability
	Not multiple of 3	Frameshift	Likely to result in premature termination with loss of function or expression
	Large deletion	Partial gene deletion	May result in premature termination with loss of function or expression
		Whole gene deletion	Loss of expression
Insertion	Multiple of 3 (codon)		In-frame insertion of 1 or more amino acid(s)—may affect protein function or stability
	Not multiple of 3	Frameshift	Likely to result in premature termination with loss of function or expression
	Large insertion	Partial gene duplication	May result in premature termination with loss of function or expression
		Whole gene duplication	May have an effect because of increased gene dosage
	Expansion of trinucleotide repeat	Dynamic mutation	Altered gene expression or altered protein stability or function

*Some have been shown to cause aberrant splicing.
From Turnpenny P, Ellard S (Editors): *Emery's elements of medical genetics*, ed 14, Philadelphia, 2012, Elsevier/Churchill Livingstone, p 23.

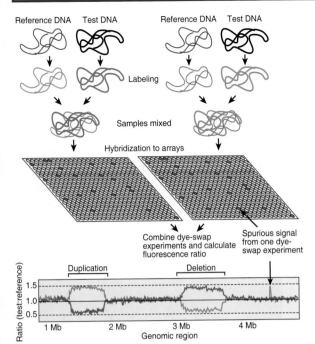

Fig. 96.4 Array comparative genomic hybridization. Test and reference DNA samples are differentially labeled, mixed, and passed over a target array of probes (e.g., bacterial artificial chromosome clones or oligonucleotides) containing DNA fragments from across the whole human genome. The experiment is often repeated with reversal of the test and reference dyes to detect dye effects or identify spurious signals. DNA samples hybridize with their corresponding probe, and the ratio of fluorescence from each probe (test:reference) is used to detect regions that vary in copy number between the test and the reference sample (*red line*, original hybridization; *blue line*, dye-swapped hybridization). Equal copy number for both the test and the reference DNA is identified by equal binding, resulting in a ratio of 1:1. Duplication in a genomic region of the test sample is identified by an increased ratio, and a deletion is identified by a decreased ratio, but a deletion in the test sample is indistinguishable from a duplication in the reference sample. These ratios are usually converted to log2 scale for further analysis. (*Adapted from Feuk L, Carson AR, Scherer SW: Structural variation in the human genome, Nat Rev Genet 7:85–97, 2006, with permission from Nature Reviews Genetics.*)

inherited form of chronic peripheral neuropathy of childhood, is caused by duplications of the gene for peripheral myelin protein 22, resulting in overexpression as a result of the existence of 3 active copies of this gene (see Chapter 631.1). Deletions of this same gene leaving only 1 active copy are responsible for a different disorder, hereditary neuropathy with liability to pressure palsies.

Deletions and duplications can vary in their extent and can involve several genes, even when they are not visible on a traditional chromosome analysis. Such changes are commonly called **microdeletions** and **microduplications**. When deletion or duplication of 2 or more genes in the same chromosomal region each play a role in the resulting clinical features, the condition can also be referred to as a **contiguous gene disorder**.

In some cases the recognition of a specific constellation of features leads the clinician to suspect a specific microdeletion or microduplication syndrome. Examples of such disorders include Smith-Magenis, DiGeorge, and Williams syndromes. In other cases the clinician may be alerted to this possibility by an unusually diverse array of clinical features in one patient or the presence of unusual features in a person with a known condition. Because of the close physical proximity of a series of genes, different deletions involving the short arm of the X chromosome can produce individuals with various combinations of ichthyosis, Kallmann

syndrome, ocular albinism, intellectual disability, chondrodysplasia punctata, and short stature.

DNA rearrangements can also take place in **somatic cells** (cells that do not go on to produce ova or sperm). Rearrangements that occur in **lymphoid** cells are required for the formation of functional immunoglobulin in B cells and antigen-recognizing receptors on T cells. Large segments of DNA, which code for the variable and the constant regions of either immunoglobulin or the T-cell receptor (TCR), are physically joined at a specific stage in the development of an immunocompetent lymphocyte. These rearrangements take place during development of the lymphoid cell lineage in humans and result in the extensive diversity of immunoglobulin and TCR molecules. Because of this postgermline DNA rearrangement, no 2 individuals, not even identical twins, are really identical, because mature lymphocytes from each will have undergone random DNA rearrangements at these loci.

Studies of the human genome sequence reveal that any 2 individuals differ in about 1 base in 1,000. Some of these differences are silent; some result in changes that explain phenotypic differences (hair or eye color, physical appearance); some have medical significance, causing single-gene disorders such as sickle cell anemia or explaining susceptibility to common pediatric disorders such as asthma. Genetic variants in a single gene that occur at a frequency of >1% in a population are often referred to as **polymorphisms**. These variations may be silent or subtle or may have significant phenotypic effects.

GENOTYPE-PHENOTYPE CORRELATIONS IN GENETIC DISEASE

The term **genotype** is used to signify the internally coded, heritable information of an individual and can also be used to refer to which particular alternative version (**allele**) of a gene is present at a specific location (**locus**) on a chromosome. A **phenotype** is the observed structural, biochemical, and physiologic characteristics of an individual, determined by the genotype, and can also refer to the observed structural and functional effects of a variant allele at a specific locus. Many sequence variants result in predictable phenotypes. In these cases, physicians can predict clinical outcomes and plan appropriate treatment strategies based on a patient's genotype. Increasingly, there is phenotypic expansion where multiple alleles (variants) within a gene can be associated with often diverse and distinct clinical presentations.

The **long QT syndrome** exemplifies a disorder with predictable associations between a patient's genotype and his or her phenotype (see Chapter 462.5). Long QT syndrome is genetically heterogeneous, meaning that pathogenic variants in several different genes can cause the same disorder. The risk for cardiac events (syncope, aborted cardiac arrest, or sudden death) is higher in patients with long QT syndrome involving the *KCNQ1* gene (63%) or *KCNH2* (46%) than in those with pathogenic variants in *SCN5A* (18%). In addition, those with *KCNQ1* variants experience most of their episodes during exercise and rarely during rest or sleep. In contrast, individuals with pathogenic variants in *KCNH2* and *SCN5A* are more likely to have episodes during sleep or rest and rarely during exercise. Therefore, variants in specific genes (genotype) are correlated with specific manifestations (phenotype) of long QT syndrome. These types of relationships are commonly referred to as *genotype-phenotype correlations*.

Pathogenic variants in the fibrillin-1 gene associated with **Marfan syndrome** represent another example of predictable genotype-phenotype correlations (see Chapter 722). Marfan syndrome is characterized by the combination of skeletal, ocular, and aortic manifestations, with the most devastating outcome being aortic root dissection and sudden death. The fibrillin-1 gene consists of 65 exons, and mutations have been found in almost all these. The location of the mutation within the gene (genotype) might play a significant role in determining the severity of the condition (phenotype). Neonatal Marfan syndrome is caused by mutations in exons 24-27 and in exons 31 and 32, whereas milder forms are caused by mutations in exons 59-65 and in exons 37 and 41.

Genotype-phenotype correlations have also been observed in some complications of **cystic fibrosis** (CF; see Chapter 432). Although pulmonary disease is the major cause of morbidity and mortality, CF is a multisystem disorder that affects not only the epithelia of the respiratory tract but also the exocrine pancreas, intestine, male genital tract, hepatobiliary system, and exocrine sweat glands. CF is caused by pathologic variants in the CF transmembrane conductance regulator (*CFTR*) gene; >1,600 different pathogenic variants have been identified. The most common is a deletion of 3 nucleotides that removes the amino acid phenylalanine (F) at the 508th position on the protein (ΔF508 variant), which accounts for approximately 70% of all pathogenic CF variants and is associated with severe disease. The best genotype-phenotype correlations in CF are seen in the context of pancreatic function, with most common mutations being classified as either *pancreatic sufficient* or *pancreatic insufficient*. Persons with pancreatic sufficiency usually have either 1 or 2 pancreatic-sufficient alleles, indicating that pancreatic-sufficient alleles are dominant. In contrast, the genotype-phenotype correlation in pulmonary disease is much weaker, and persons with identical genotypes have wide variations in the severity of their pulmonary disease. This finding may be accounted for in part by genetic modifiers or environmental factors.

In many disorders the effects of variants on phenotype can be modified by changes in the other allele of the same gene, by changes in specific **modifier genes**, and/or by variations in a number of unspecified genes (**genetic background**). When sickle cell anemia is co-inherited with the gene for hereditary persistence of fetal hemoglobin, the sickle cell phenotypic expression is less severe. Modifier genes in CF can influence the development of congenital meconium ileus, or colonization with *Pseudomonas aeruginosa*. Modifier genes can also affect the manifestations of Hirschsprung disease, neurofibromatosis type 2, craniosynostosis, and congenital adrenal hyperplasia. The combination of genetic variants producing glucose-6-phosphate dehydrogenase deficiency and longer versions of the TATAA element in the uridine diphosphate–glucuronosyltransferase gene promoter exacerbates neonatal physiologic hyperbilirubinemia.

HUMAN GENOME PROJECT

A rudimentary genetic map can be made using genetic linkage, which is based on the principle that alleles at 2 genetic loci that are located near each other segregate together in a family unless they are separated by genetic **recombination**. The frequency of recombination between the loci can be used to estimate the physical distance between points. Some of the first maps of the human genome were linkage maps based on a set of polymorphic genetic loci located along the entire human genome. Linkage analysis is still used to map the location of genetic changes responsible for phenotypic traits and genetic disorders that are inherited in a mendelian fashion.

In contrast to linkage maps, which are based on recombination frequencies, physical maps rely on overlapping DNA fragments to determine the location of loci with respect to one another. Several strategies can be used to create physical maps of a chromosomal region. In one strategy, segments of the region of interest with lengths from hundreds or thousands to a few million base pairs are isolated and placed in microorganisms such as bacteria or yeast. Common regions contained in different organisms can then be identified and this information used to piece together a map composed of overlapping DNA pieces, each contained in a different microorganism. The pieces contained in each organism can then be sequenced to obtain the DNA sequence of the entire region. An alternative strategy involves breaking the entire genome into random fragments, sequencing the fragments, and then using a computer to order the fragments based on overlapping segments. This whole genome approach in combination with new next-generation sequencing technologies has resulted in a dramatic reduction in the cost of sequencing an individual's entire genome.

Analysis of the human genome has produced some surprising results. The number of genes appears to be about 20,000. This is fewer than had been expected and is in the same range as many simpler organisms. *The number of protein products encoded by the genome is greater than the number of genes.* This is a result of the presence of alternative promoter regions, alternative splicing, and posttranslational modifications, which can allow a single gene to encode a number of protein products.

It is also apparent that most of the human genome does not encode protein, with <5% being transcribed and translated, although a much

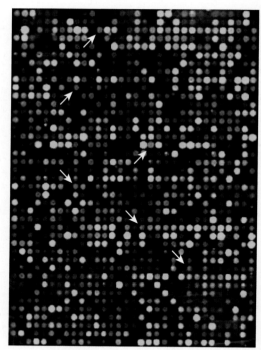

Fig. 96.5 Microarray containing 36,000 oligonucleotides. The microarray was exposed to RNA from normal fibroblasts (labeled in *red*; see *arrows*) and fibroblasts from a patient with Niemann-Pick disease, type C (labeled *green*). *Arrows* point to regions in which there was a strong hybridization signal with either normal or disease RNA. This microarray was used to search for genes that are highly expressed in the fibroblasts of patients. (*From Jorde LB, Carey JC, Bamshad MJ, et al, editors: Medical genetics, ed 3, St Louis, 2006, Mosby, p 116.*)

larger percentage may be transcribed without translation. Many transcribed sequences are not translated but represent genes that encode RNAs that serve a regulatory role. A large fraction of the genome consists of repeated sequences that are interspersed among the genes. Some of these are transposable genetic elements that can move from place to place in the genome. Others are static elements that were expanded and dispersed in the past during human evolution. Other repeated sequences might play a structural role. There are also regions of genomic duplications. Such duplications are substrate for evolution, allowing genetic motifs to be copied and modified to serve new roles in the cell. Duplications can also play a role in chromosomal rearrangement, permitting nonhomologous chromosome segments to pair during meiosis and exchange material. This is another source of evolutionary change and a potential source of chromosomal instability leading to congenital anomalies or cancer. Low copy repeats also play an important role in causing genomic disorders. When low copy repeats flank unique genomic segments, these regions can be duplicated or deleted through a process known as *nonallelic homologous recombination*.

Availability of the entire human genomic sequence permits the study of large groups of genes, looking for patterns of gene expression or genome alteration. Microarrays permit the expression of thousands of genes to be analyzed on a small glass chip. Increasingly, studies of gene expression are being performed using next generation sequencing techniques to obtain information about all of the RNA transcripts in a tissue sample. In some cases the patterns of gene expression provide signatures for particular disease states, such as cancer, or change in response to therapy (Fig. 96.5).

Bibliography is available at Expert Consult.

Chapter **97**
Patterns of Genetic Transmission

Daryl A. Scott and Brendan Lee

第九十七章
遗传传递的模式

中文导读

本章主要介绍了家族史和系谱、孟德尔遗传、Y连锁遗传、与假常染色体区域相关的遗传、双基因遗传、假性遗传与家族聚集、非传统遗传以及多因素和多基因遗传。具体描述了家族史和系谱中家系、先证者以及一级亲属的概念；具体描述了孟德尔遗传的常染色体显性遗传、常染色体隐性遗传、假显性遗传以及X连锁遗传；具体描述了非传统遗传的线粒体遗传、三联体重复疾病以及遗传印记。

FAMILY HISTORY AND PEDIGREE NOTATION

The family history remains the most important screening tool for pediatricians in identifying a patient's risk for developing a wide range of diseases, from multifactorial conditions such as diabetes and attention-deficit/hyperactivity disorder, to single-gene disorders such as sickle cell anemia and cystic fibrosis. Through a detailed family history, the physician can often ascertain the mode of genetic transmission and the risks to family members. Because not all familial clustering of disease is caused by genetic factors, a family history can also identify common environmental and behavioral factors that influence the occurrence of disease. The main goal of the family history is to identify genetic susceptibility, and the cornerstone of the family history is a systematic and standardized pedigree.

A **pedigree** provides a graphic depiction of a family's structure and medical history. It is important when taking a pedigree to be systematic and use standard symbols and configurations so that anyone can read and understand the information (Figs. 97.1 to 97.4). In the pediatric setting, the **proband** is typically the child or adolescent who is being evaluated. The proband is designated in the pedigree by an arrow.

A 3 to 4–generation pedigree should be obtained for every new patient as an initial screen for genetic disorders segregating within the family. The pedigree can provide clues to the inheritance pattern of these disorders and can aid the clinician in determining the risk to the proband and other family members. The closer the relationship of the proband to the person in the family with the genetic disorder, the greater is the shared genetic complement. **First-degree** relatives, such as a parent, full sibling, or child, share one-half their genetic information on average; first cousins share one-eighth. Sometimes the person providing the family history may mention a distant relative who is affected with a genetic disorder. In such cases a more extensive pedigree may be needed to identify the risk to other family members. For example, a history of a distant maternally related cousin with intellectual disability caused by fragile X syndrome can still place a male proband at an elevated risk for this disorder.

MENDELIAN INHERITANCE

There are 3 classic forms of genetic inheritance: **autosomal dominant, autosomal recessive**, and **X-linked**. These are referred to as **mendelian inheritance** forms, after Gregor Mendel, the 19th-century monk whose experiments led to the laws of **segregation of characteristics, dominance, and independent assortment**. These remain the foundation of single-gene inheritance.

Autosomal Dominant Inheritance

Autosomal dominant inheritance is determined by the presence of one abnormal gene on one of the **autosomes** (chromosomes 1-22). Autosomal genes exist in pairs, with each parent contributing 1 copy. In an autosomal dominant trait, a change in 1 of the paired genes affects the phenotype of an individual, even though the other copy of the gene is functioning correctly. A **phenotype** can refer to a physical manifestation, a behavioral characteristic, or a difference detectable only through laboratory tests.

The pedigree for autosomal dominant disorders demonstrates certain characteristics. These disorders show a **vertical transmission** (parent-to-child) pattern and can appear in multiple generations. In Fig. 97.5, this is illustrated by individual I.1 passing on the changed gene to II.2 and II.5. An affected individual has a 50% (1 in 2) chance of passing on the deleterious gene in *each* pregnancy and, therefore, of having a child affected by the disorder. This is referred to as the **recurrence risk** for the disorder. Unaffected individuals (family members who do not manifest the trait and do not harbor a copy of the deleterious gene) do not pass the disorder to their children. Males and females are equally affected.

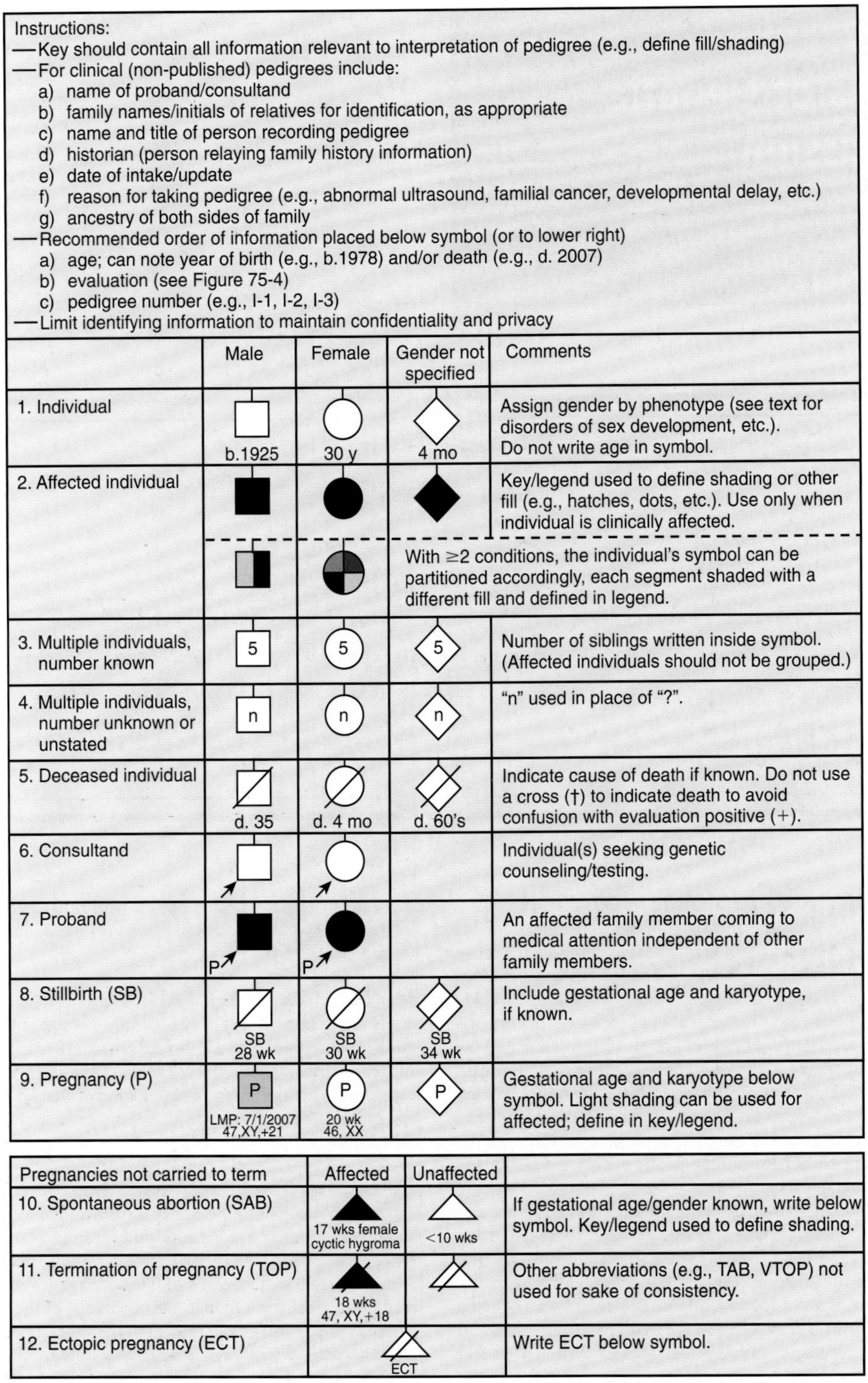

Instructions:
— Key should contain all information relevant to interpretation of pedigree (e.g., define fill/shading)
— For clinical (non-published) pedigrees include:
  a) name of proband/consultand
  b) family names/initials of relatives for identification, as appropriate
  c) name and title of person recording pedigree
  d) historian (person relaying family history information)
  e) date of intake/update
  f) reason for taking pedigree (e.g., abnormal ultrasound, familial cancer, developmental delay, etc.)
  g) ancestry of both sides of family
— Recommended order of information placed below symbol (or to lower right)
  a) age; can note year of birth (e.g., b.1978) and/or death (e.g., d. 2007)
  b) evaluation (see Figure 75-4)
  c) pedigree number (e.g., I-1, I-2, I-3)
— Limit identifying information to maintain confidentiality and privacy

	Male	Female	Gender not specified	Comments
1. Individual	b.1925	30 y	4 mo	Assign gender by phenotype (see text for disorders of sex development, etc.). Do not write age in symbol.
2. Affected individual	■	●	◆	Key/legend used to define shading or other fill (e.g., hatches, dots, etc.). Use only when individual is clinically affected.
				With ≥2 conditions, the individual's symbol can be partitioned accordingly, each segment shaded with a different fill and defined in legend.
3. Multiple individuals, number known	5	5	5	Number of siblings written inside symbol. (Affected individuals should not be grouped.)
4. Multiple individuals, number unknown or unstated	n	n	n	"n" used in place of "?".
5. Deceased individual	d. 35	d. 4 mo	d. 60's	Indicate cause of death if known. Do not use a cross (†) to indicate death to avoid confusion with evaluation positive (+).
6. Consultand				Individual(s) seeking genetic counseling/testing.
7. Proband	P■	P●		An affected family member coming to medical attention independent of other family members.
8. Stillbirth (SB)	SB 28 wk	SB 30 wk	SB 34 wk	Include gestational age and karyotype, if known.
9. Pregnancy (P)	P LMP: 7/1/2007 47,XY,+21	P 20 wk 46,XX	P	Gestational age and karyotype below symbol. Light shading can be used for affected; define in key/legend.

Pregnancies not carried to term	Affected	Unaffected	
10. Spontaneous abortion (SAB)	17 wks female cyctic hygroma	<10 wks	If gestational age/gender known, write below symbol. Key/legend used to define shading.
11. Termination of pregnancy (TOP)	18 wks 47, XY,+18		Other abbreviations (e.g., TAB, VTOP) not used for sake of consistency.
12. Ectopic pregnancy (ECT)		ECT	Write ECT below symbol.

Fig. 97.1 Common pedigree symbols, definitions, and abbreviations. (*From Bennett RL, French KS, Resta RG, et al: Standardized human pedigree nomenclature: update and assessment of the recommendations of the National Society of Genetic Counselors, J Genet Couns 17:424–433, 2008.*)

Although not a characteristic per se, the finding of male-to-male transmission essentially confirms autosomal dominant inheritance. Vertical transmission can also be seen with X-linked traits. However, because a father passes on his Y chromosome to a son, male-to-male transmission cannot be seen with an X-linked trait. Therefore, male-to-male transmission eliminates X-linked inheritance as a possible explanation. Although male-to-male transmission can occur with Y-linked genes as well, there are very few **Y-linked** disorders, compared with thousands having the autosomal dominant inheritance pattern.

Although parent-to-child transmission is a characteristic of autosomal dominant inheritance, many patients with an autosomal dominant disorder have no history of an affected family member, for several

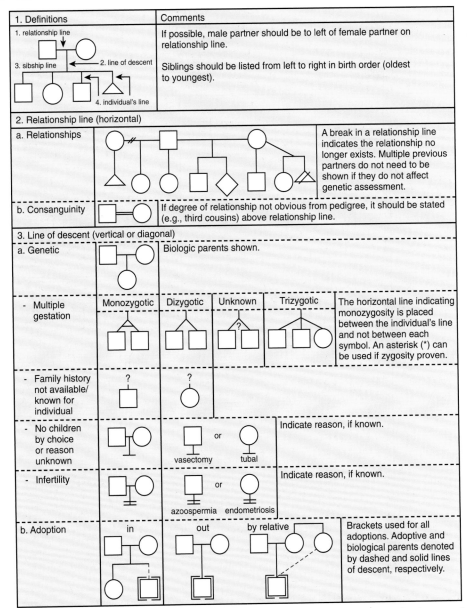

Fig. 97.2 Pedigree line definitions. *(From Bennett RL, French KS, Resta RG, et al: Standardized human pedigree nomenclature: update and assessment of the recommendations of the National Society of Genetic Counselors, J Genet Couns 17:424–433, 2008.)*

possible reasons. First, the patient may have the disorder due to a **de novo** (new) mutation that occurred in the DNA of the egg or sperm that formed that individual. Second, many autosomal dominant conditions demonstrate **incomplete penetrance**, meaning that not all individuals who carry the mutation have phenotypic manifestations. In a pedigree this can appear as a **skipped generation**, in which an unaffected individual links 2 affected persons (Fig. 97.6). There are many potential reasons that a disorder might exhibit incomplete penetrance, including the effect of modifier genes, environmental factors, gender, and age. Third, individuals with the same autosomal dominant variant can manifest the disorder to different degrees. This is termed **variable expression** and is a characteristic of many autosomal dominant disorders. Fourth, some spontaneous genetic mutations occur not in the egg or sperm that forms a child, but rather in a *cell* in the developing embryo. Such events are referred to as **somatic mutations**, and because not all cells

are affected, the change is said to be **mosaic**. The phenotype caused by a somatic mutation can vary but is usually milder than if all cells were affected by the mutation. In **germline mosaicism** the mutation occurs in cells that populate the germline that produces eggs or sperm. An individual who is germline mosaic might not have any manifestations of the disorder but may produce multiple eggs or sperm that are affected by the mutation.

Autosomal Recessive Inheritance

Autosomal recessive inheritance requires deleterious variants in both copies of a gene to cause disease. Examples include cystic fibrosis and sickle cell disease. Autosomal recessive disorders are characterized by **horizontal transmission**, the observation of multiple affected members of a kindred in the same generation, but no affected family members in other generations (Fig. 97.7). They are associated with a recurrence

Instructions:
— D represents egg or sperm donor
— S represents surrogate (gestational carrier)
— If the woman is both the ovum donor and a surrogate, in the interest of genetic assessment, she will only be referred to as a donor (e.g., 4 and 5); the pregnancy symbol and its line of descent are positioned below the woman who is carrying the pregnancy
— Available family history should be noted on the gamete donor and/or gestational carrier

Possible Reproductive Scenarios		Comments
1. Sperm donor	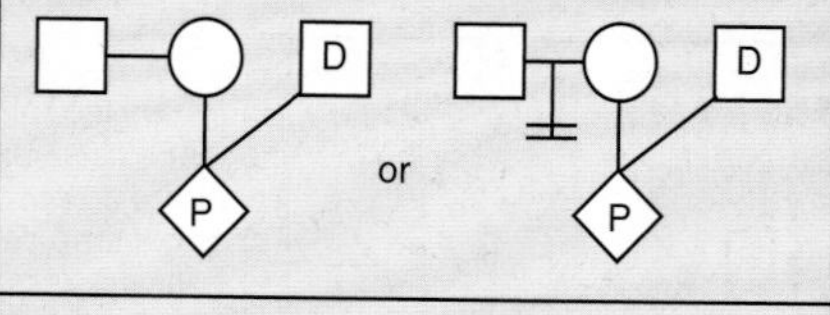	Couple in which woman is carrying pregnancy using donor sperm. No relationship line is shown between the woman carrying the pregnancy and the sperm donor.
2. Ovum donor	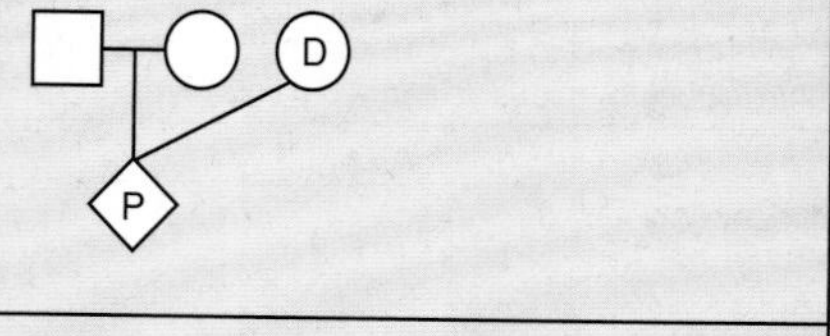	Couple in which woman is carrying pregnancy using a donor egg and partner's sperm. The line of descent from the birth mother is solid because there is a biologic relationship that may affect the fetus (e.g., teratogens).
3. Surrogate only	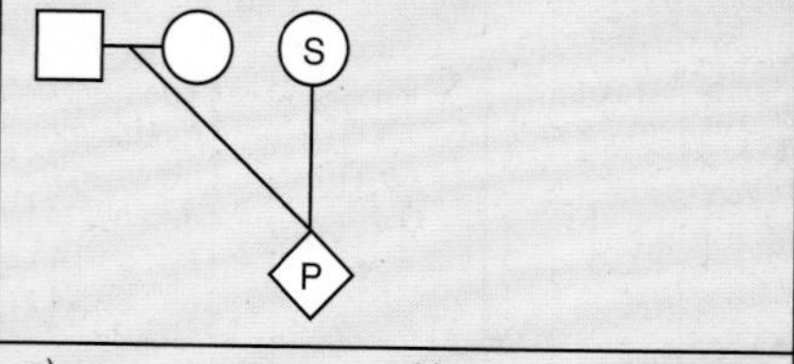	Couple whose gametes are used to impregnate a woman (surrogate) who carries the pregnancy. The line of descent from the surrogate is solid because there is a biological relationship that may affect the fetus (e.g., teratogens).
4. Surrogate ovum donor	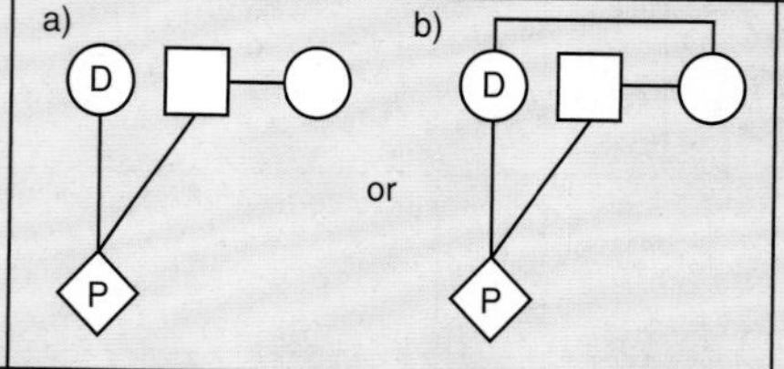	Couple in which male partner's sperm is used to inseminate (a) an unrelated woman or (b) a sister who is carrying the pregnancy for the couple.
5. Planned adoption	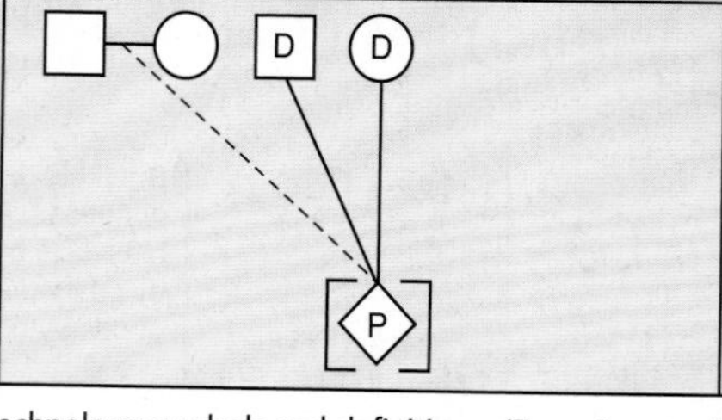	Couple contracts with a woman to carry a pregnancy using ovum of the woman carrying the pregnancy and donor sperm.

Fig. 97.3 Assisted reproductive technology symbols and definitions. (From Bennett RL, French KS, Resta RG, et al: Standardized human pedigree nomenclature: update and assessment of the recommendations of the National Society of Genetic Counselors, J Genet Couns 17:424–433, 2008.)

risk of 25% for carrier parents who have had a previous affected child. Male and female offspring are equally likely to be affected, although some traits exhibit differential expression between sexes. The offspring of consanguineous parents are at increased risk for rare, autosomal recessive traits due to the increased chance that that both parents may carry a gene affected by a deleterious mutation that they inherited from a common ancestor. **Consanguinity** between parents of a child with a suspected genetic disorder implies, but certainly does not prove, autosomal recessive inheritance. Although consanguineous unions are uncommon in Western society, in other parts of the world (southern India, Japan, and the Middle East) as high as 50% of all children may be conceived in consanguineous unions. The risk of a genetic disorder for the offspring of a first-cousin union (6–8%) is about double the risk in the general population (3–4%).

Every individual probably has several rare, deleterious recessive pathogenic sequence variants. Because most pathogenic variants carried in the general population occur at a very low frequency, it does not make economic sense to screen the entire population in order to identify the small number of persons who carry these variants. As a result, these variants typically remain undetected unless an affected child is born to a couple who both carry pathogenic variants affecting the same gene.

However, in some **genetic isolates** (small populations isolated by geography, religion, culture, or language), certain rare recessive pathogenic variants are much more common than in the general population. Even though there may be no known consanguinity, couples from these genetic isolates have a greater chance of sharing pathogenic alleles inherited from a common ancestor. Screening programs have been developed among some such groups to detect persons who carry common disease-causing variants and therefore are at increased risk for having affected children. A variety of autosomal recessive conditions are more common among Ashkenazi Jews than in the general population. Couples of Ashkenazi Jewish ancestry should be offered prenatal or preconception screening

Instructions:
— E is used for evaluation to represent clinical and/or test information on the pedigree
    a. E is to be defined in key/legend
    b. If more than one evaluation, use subscript (E_1, E_2, E_3) and define in key
    c. Test results should be put in parentheses or defined in key/legend
— A symbol is shaded only when an individual is clinically symptomatic
— For linkage studies, haplotype information is written below the individual. The haplotype of interest should be on left and appropriately highlighted
    Repetitive sequences, trinucleotides, and expansion numbers are written with affected allele first and placed in parentheses
— If mutation known, identify in parentheses

Definition	Symbol	Scenario
1. Documented evaluation (*) Use only if examined/evaluated by you or your research/clinical team or if the outside evaluation has been reviewed and verified.	◯*	Woman with negative echocardiogram. E− (echo)
2. Carrier—not likely to manifest disease regardless of inheritance pattern	⊡ (dot)	Male carrier of Tay-Sachs disease by patient report (* not used because results not verified).
3. Asymptomatic/presymptomatic carrier—clinically unaffected at this time but could later exhibit symptoms	◯ (vertical line)	Woman age 25 with negative mammogram and positive BRCA1 DNA test. 25 y E_1− (mammogram) E_2+ (5385insC BRCA1)
4. Uninformative study (u)	☐ Eu	Man age 25 with normal physical exam and uninformative DNA test for Huntington disease (E_2). 25 y E_1− (physical exam) E_2u (36n/18n)
5. Affected individual with positive evaluation (E+)	■ E+	Individual with cystic fibrosis and positive mutation study; only one mutation has currently been identified. E+(ΔF508) Eu E+(ΔF508/u) --- 10 week male fetus with a trisomy 18 karyotype. P 10 wk E+(CVS) 47,XY,+18

Fig. 97.4 Pedigree symbols of genetic evaluation and testing information. *(From Bennett RL, French KS, Resta RG, et al: Standardized human pedigree nomenclature: update and assessment of the recommendations of the National Society of Genetic Counselors, J Genet Couns 17:424–433, 2008.)*

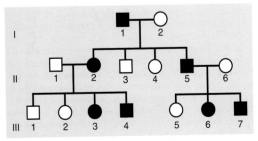

Fig. 97.5 Autosomal dominant pedigree. Pedigree showing typical inheritance of a form of achondroplasia *(FGFR3)* inherited as an autosomal dominant trait. *Black,* Affected patients.

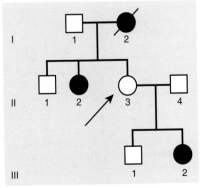

Fig. 97.6 Incomplete penetrance. This family segregates a familial cancer syndrome, familial adenomatous polyposis. Individual II.3 is an obligate carrier, but there are no findings to suggest the disorder. This disorder is nonpenetrant in this individual. *Black,* Affected patients.

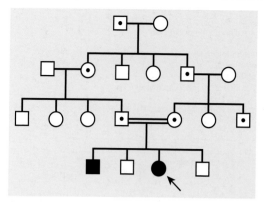

Fig. 97.7 Autosomal recessive pedigree with parental consanguinity. *Central dot,* Carriers; *Black,* Affected patients.

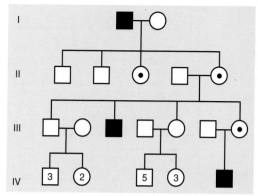

Fig. 97.9 Pedigree demonstrating X-linked recessive inheritance. *Central dot,* Carriers; *Black,* Affected patients.

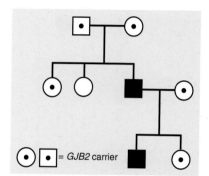

Fig. 97.8 Pseudodominant inheritance. *Black,* Affected (deaf); *central dot* shows carrier who is asymptomatic (unaffected).

for Gaucher disease type 1 (carrier rate 1:14), cystic fibrosis (1:25), Tay-Sachs disease (1:25), familial dysautonomia (1:30), Canavan disease (1:40), glycogen storage disease type 1A (1:71), maple syrup urine disease (1:81), Fanconi anemia type C (1:89), Niemann-Pick disease type A (1:90), Bloom syndrome (1:100), mucolipidosis IV (1:120), and possibly neonatal familial hyperinsulinemic hypoglycemia.

The prevalence of carriers of certain autosomal recessive variants in some larger populations is unusually high. In such cases, **heterozygote advantage** is postulated. The carrier frequencies of sickle cell disease in the African population and of cystic fibrosis in the northern European population are much higher than would be expected from the rate of new mutations. In these populations, heterozygous carriers may have had an advantage in terms of survival and reproduction over noncarriers. In sickle cell disease the carrier state is thought to confer some resistance to malaria; in cystic fibrosis the carrier state has been postulated to confer resistance to cholera or enteropathogenic *Escherichia coli* infections. Population-based **carrier screening** for cystic fibrosis is recommended for persons of northern European and Ashkenazi Jewish ancestry; population-based screening for sickle cell disease is recommended for persons of African ancestry.

If the frequency of an autosomal recessive disease is known, the frequency of the heterozygote or carrier state can be calculated from the **Hardy-Weinberg formula:**

$$p^2 + 2pq + q^2 = 1$$

where *p* is the frequency of one of a pair of alleles and *q* is the frequency of the other. For example, if the frequency of cystic fibrosis among white Americans is 1 in 2,500 (p^2), then the frequency of the heterozygote

(2pq) can be calculated: If $p^2 = 1/2,500$, then p = 1/50 and q = 49/50; 2pq = 2 × (1/50) × (49/50) = 98/2500, or 3.92%.

Pseudodominant Inheritance

Pseudodominant inheritance refers to the observation of apparent dominant (parent to child) transmission of a known autosomal recessive disorder (Fig. 97.8). This occurs when a homozygous affected individual has a partner who is a heterozygous carrier. This is most likely to occur for relatively common recessive traits within a population, such as sickle cell anemia or nonsyndromic autosomal recessive hearing loss caused by deleterious mutations in the *GJB2*, the gene that encodes connexin 26.

X-Linked Inheritance

X-linked inheritance describes the inheritance pattern of most disorders caused by deleterious changes in genes located on the X chromosome (Fig. 97.9). In X-liked disorders, males are more commonly affected than females. Female carriers of these disorders are generally unaffected, or if affected, they are affected more mildly than males. In each pregnancy, female carriers have a 25% chance of having an affected son, a 25% chance of having a carrier daughter, and a 50% chance of having a child that does not inherit the mutated X-linked gene. Since affected males pass their X chromosome to all their daughters and their Y chromosome to all their sons, they have a 50% chance of having an unaffected son that does not carry the disease gene and a 50% chance of having a daughter who is a carrier. Male-to-male transmission excludes X-linked inheritance but is seen with autosomal dominant and Y-linked inheritance.

A female occasionally exhibits signs of an X-linked trait similar to a male. This occurs rarely from homozygosity for an X-linked trait or the presence of a sex chromosome abnormality (45,X or 46,XY female) or skewed or nonrandom X-inactivation. **X chromosome inactivation** occurs early in development and involves the random and irreversible inactivation of most genes on one X chromosome in female cells (Fig. 97.10). In some cases, a preponderance of cells inactivates the same X chromosome, resulting in phenotypic expression of an X-linked pathogenic variant if it resides on the active chromosome. This can occur because of chance, selection against cells that have inactivated the X chromosome carrying the normal gene, or an X chromosome abnormality that results in inactivation of the X chromosome carrying the normal gene.

In some X-linked disorders, both **hemizygous** males and heterozygous females who carry an affected X-linked gene have similar phenotypic manifestations. In these cases, an affected male will have a 50% chance of having an affected daughter and a 50% chance of having an unaffected son in each pregnancy, whereas half the male and female offspring of an affected woman will be affected (Fig. 97.11). Some X-linked conditions are lethal in a high percentage of males, such as **incontinentia pigmenti** (see Chapter 614.7). In such cases the pedigree typically shows only

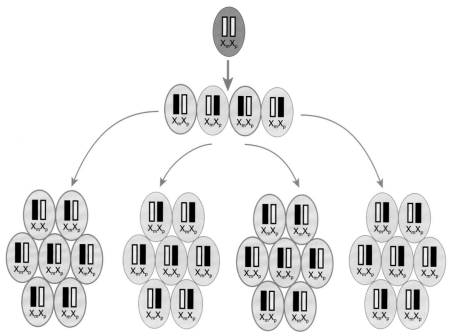

Fig. 97.10 X-inactivation. *Black* marks the active X chromosome. Color of the cell represents its active X chromosome is paternally (X_p, *blue*) or maternally (X_m, *pink*) derived.

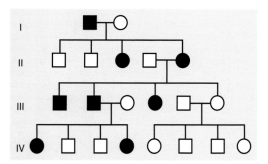

Fig. 97.11 Pedigree pattern demonstrating X-linked dominant inheritance. *Black,* Affected patients. Note there is no father-to-son transmission in this situation, and hemizygosity (i.e., X-linked gene in a male) is not lethal. In some X-linked dominant conditions, X-linked males have a more severe phenotype and might not survive. In that case, only females manifest the disease (see Fig. 97.12).

affected females and an overall female/male ratio of $2:1$, with an increased number of miscarriages (Fig. 97.12).

Y-LINKED INHERITANCE

There are few Y-linked traits. These demonstrate *only* male-to-male transmission, and only males are affected (Fig. 97.13). Most Y-linked genes are related to male sex determination and reproduction and are associated with infertility. Therefore, it is rare to see familial transmission of a Y-linked disorder. However, advances in assisted reproductive technologies might make it possible to have familial transmission of male infertility.

INHERITANCE ASSOCIATED WITH PSEUDOAUTOSOMAL REGIONS

Of special note are the pseudoautosomal regions on the X and Y chromosomes. Since these regions are made up of homologous sequences

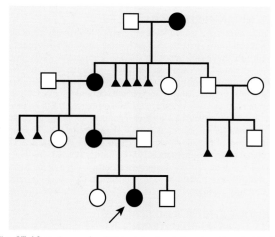

Fig. 97.12 Pedigree of an X-linked dominant disorder with male lethality, such as incontinentia pigmenti. *Black,* Affected patients.

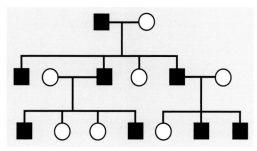

Fig. 97.13 Y-linked inheritance. *Black,* Affected patients.

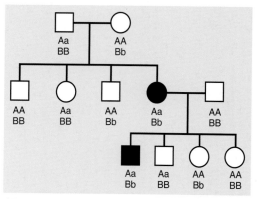

Fig. 97.14 Digenic pedigree. Here, the disease alleles are *a* and *b* and they reside on distinct genetic loci or genes. For a person to have the disease, heterozygosity for mutant alleles in both genes (A/a; B/b) is required. *Black*, Affected patients.

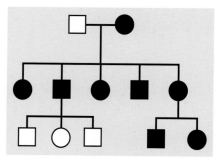

Fig. 97.15 Pedigree of a mitochondrial disorder, exhibiting maternal inheritance. *Black*, Affected patients.

of nucleotides, genes that are located in these regions are present in equal numbers among both males and females. *SHOX* is one of the best-characterized disease genes located in these regions. Heterozygous *SHOX* mutations cause **Leri-Weil dyschondrosteosis**, a rare skeletal dysplasia that involves bilateral bowing of the forearms with dislocations of the ulna at the wrist and generalized short stature. Homozygous *SHOX* mutations cause the much more severe **Langer mesomelic dwarfism**.

DIGENIC INHERITANCE

Digenic inheritance explains the occurrence of **retinitis pigmentosa (RP)** in children of parents who each carry a pathogenic variant in a different RP-associated gene (Fig. 97.14). Both parents have normal vision, as would be expected, but their offspring who are **double heterozygotes**—having inherited both mutations—develop RP. Digenic pedigrees can exhibit characteristics of both autosomal dominant (vertical transmission) and autosomal recessive inheritance (1 in 4 recurrence risk). A couple in which the 2 unaffected partners are carriers for mutation in 2 different RP-associated genes that show digenic inheritance have a 1 in 4 risk of having an affected child, similar to what is seen in autosomal recessive inheritance. However, their affected children, and affected children in subsequent generations, have a 1 in 4 risk of transmitting both mutations to their offspring, who would be affected (vertical transmission).

PSEUDOGENETIC INHERITANCE AND FAMILIAL CLUSTERING

Sometimes nongenetic reasons for the occurrence of a particular disease in multiple family members can produce a pattern that mimics genetic transmission. These nongenetic factors can include identifiable environmental factors, teratogenic exposures, or as yet undetermined or undefined factors. Examples of identifiable factors might include multiple siblings in a family having asthma because of exposure to cigarette smoke from their parents or having failure to thrive, developmental delay, and unusual facial appearance caused by exposure to alcohol during pregnancy.

In some cases the disease is sufficiently common in the general population that some familial clustering occurs simply by chance. Breast cancer affects 11% of all women, and it is possible that several women in a family will develop breast cancer even in the absence of a genetic predisposition. However, hereditary breast cancer associated with mutations in *BRCA1* and *BRCA2* should be suspected in any individual who has a personal history of breast cancer with onset before age 50, early-onset breast and ovarian cancer at any age, bilateral or multifocal breast cancer, a family history of breast cancer or breast and ovarian

cancer consistent with autosomal dominant inheritance, or a personal or family history of male breast cancer.

Nonetheless, such clustering within families may be caused by as yet undefined genetic factors or unidentified pathogenic sequence variants (nuclear or mitochondrial).

NONTRADITIONAL INHERITANCE

Some genetic disorders are inherited in a manner that does not follow classical mendelian patterns. Nontraditional inheritance is seen in mitochondrial disorders, triplet repeat expansion diseases, and imprinting defects.

Mitochondrial Inheritance

An individual's mitochondrial genome is entirely derived from the mother because sperm contain relatively few mitochondria, and these are degraded after fertilization. It follows that **mitochondrial inheritance is essentially maternal inheritance**. A woman with a mitochondrial genetic disorder can have affected offspring of either sex, but an affected father cannot pass on the disease to his offspring (Fig. 97.15). Mitochondrial DNA mutations are often deletions or point mutations; overall, 1 person in 400 has a maternally inherited pathogenic mitochondrial DNA mutation (see Chapter 106). In individual families, mitochondrial inheritance may be difficult to distinguish from autosomal dominant or X-linked inheritance, but in many cases, the sex of the transmitting and nontransmitting parents can suggest a mitochondrial basis (Table 97.1).

The mitochondria are the cell's suppliers of energy, and it is not surprising that the organs that are most affected by the presence of abnormal mitochondria are those that have the greatest energy requirements, such as the brain, muscle, heart, and liver (see Chapters 105.4, 388, 616.2, and 629.4) (Fig. 97.16). Common manifestations include developmental delay, seizures, cardiac dysfunction, decreased muscle strength and tone, and hearing and vision problems.

Mitochondrial diseases can be highly variable in clinical manifestation. This is partly because cells can contain multiple mitochondria, each bearing several copies of the mitochondrial genome. Thus a cell can have a mixture of normal and abnormal mitochondrial genomes, which is referred to as **heteroplasmy**. In contrast, **homoplasmy** refers a state in which all copies of the mitochondrial genome carry the same sequence variant. Unequal segregation of mitochondria carrying normal and abnormal genomes and replicative advantage can result in varying degrees of heteroplasmy in the cells of an affected individual, including the individual ova of an affected female. Because of this, a mother may be asymptomatic yet have children who are severely affected. The level of heteroplasmy at which disease symptoms typically appear can also vary based on the type of mitochondrial variant. Detection of mitochondrial genome variants can require sampling of the affected tissue for DNA analysis. In some tissues, such as blood, testing for mitochondrial DNA variants may be inadequate because the variant may be found primarily in affected tissues such as muscle (Fig. 97.17).

Growth and differentiation factor 15 (GDF-15) and blood lactate levels are screening tests for mitochondrial disorders.

Table 97.1	Representative Examples of Disorders Caused by Mutations in Mitochondrial DNA and Their Inheritance			
DISEASE	**PHENOTYPE**	**MOST FREQUENT MUTATION IN mtDNA MOLECULE**	**HOMOPLASMY vs HETEROPLASMY**	**INHERITANCE**
Leber hereditary optic neuropathy	Rapid optic nerve atrophy, leading to blindness in young adult life; sex bias approximately 50% males with visual loss, only 10% females	Substitution p.Arg340His in *ND1* gene of complex I of electron transport chain; other complex I missense mutations	Homoplasmic (usually)	Maternal
NARP, Leigh disease	Neuropathy, ataxia, retinitis pigmentosa, developmental delay, intellectual disability lactic academia	Point mutations in ATPase subunit 6 gene	Heteroplasmic	Maternal
MELAS	*Mitochondrial encephalomyopathy, lactic acidosis, and strokelike episodes;* may manifest only as diabetes mellitus or deafness	Point mutation in tRNA^{Leu}	Heteroplasmic	Maternal
MERRF	*Myoclonic epilepsy, ragged red fibers in* muscle, ataxia, sensorineural deafness	Point mutation in tRNA^{Lys}	Heteroplasmic	Maternal
Deafness	Progressive sensorineural deafness, often induced by aminoglycoside antibiotics	m.1555A>G mutation in 12S rRNA	Homoplasmic	Maternal
	Nonsyndromic sensorineural deafness	m.7445A>G mutation in 12S rRNA	Homoplasmic	Maternal
Chronic progressive external ophthalmoplegia (CPEO)	Progressive weakness of extraocular muscles, cardiomyopathy, ptosis, heart block, ataxia, retinal pigmentation, diabetes	The common MELAS point mutation in tRNA^{Lys}; large deletions similar to KSS	Heteroplasmic	Maternal if point mutations
Pearson syndrome	Pancreatic insufficiency, pancytopenia, lactic acidosis	Large deletions	Heteroplasmic	Sporadic, somatic mutations
Kearns-Sayre syndrome (KSS)	PEO of early onset with heart block, retinal pigmentation	5-kb large deletion	Heteroplasmic	Sporadic, somatic mutations

mtDNA, Mitochondrial DNA; rRNA, ribosomal RNA; tRNA, transfer RNA.
From Nussbaum RL, McInnes RR, Willard HF, editors: *Thompson & Thompson genetics in medicine*, ed 6, Philadelphia, 2001, Saunders, p 246.

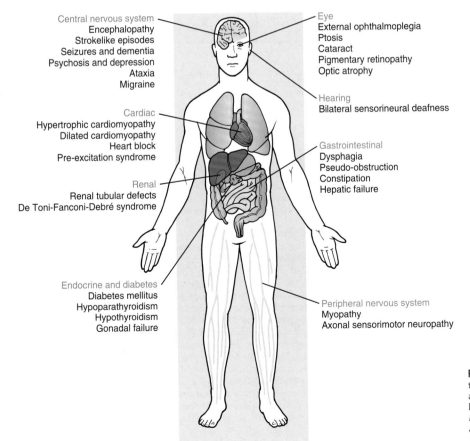

Central nervous system
Encephalopathy
Strokelike episodes
Seizures and dementia
Psychosis and depression
Ataxia
Migraine

Eye
External ophthalmoplegia
Ptosis
Cataract
Pigmentary retinopathy
Optic atrophy

Hearing
Bilateral sensorineural deafness

Cardiac
Hypertrophic cardiomyopathy
Dilated cardiomyopathy
Heart block
Pre-excitation syndrome

Gastrointestinal
Dysphagia
Pseudo-obstruction
Constipation
Hepatic failure

Renal
Renal tubular defects
De Toni-Fanconi-Debré syndrome

Endocrine and diabetes
Diabetes mellitus
Hypoparathyroidism
Hypothyroidism
Gonadal failure

Peripheral nervous system
Myopathy
Axonal sensorimotor neuropathy

Fig. 97.16 The range of affected tissues and clinical phenotypes associated with mutations in mitochondrial DNA (mtDNA). (*Modified from Chinnery PF, Turnbull DM: Mitochondrial DNA and disease, Lancet 345:SI17–SI21, 1999.*)

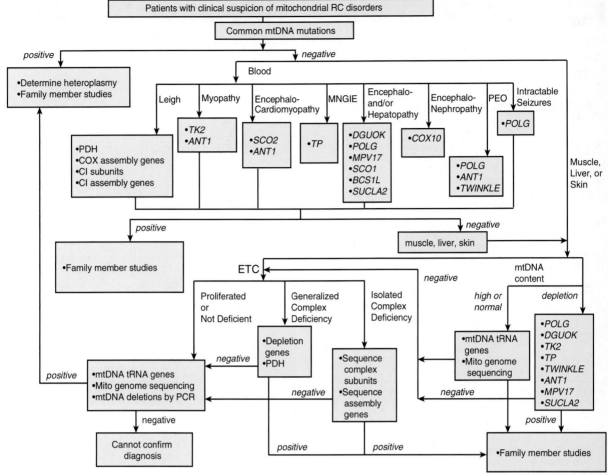

Fig. 97.17 Clinical algorithm for genetic diagnostic testing of mitochondrial DNA (mtDNA) and nuclear DNA (nDNA) genes in patients suspected of mitochondrial disorders (Baylor College of Medicine, Mitochondrial Diagnostics Laboratory). RC, Respiratory chain; MNGIE, mitochondrial neurogastrointestinal encephalopathy; PEO, progressive external ophthalmoplegia; PDH, pyruvate dehydrogenase; CI, respiratory complex I; ETC, electron transport chain; PCR, polymerase chain reaction. *(From Haas RH, Parikh S, Falk MJ, et al: The in-depth evaluation of suspected mitochondrial disease,* Mol Genet Metab *94:16–37, 2008.)*

Triplet Repeat Expansion Disorders

Triplet repeat expansion disorders are distinguished by the special dynamic nature of the disease-causing variant. Triplet repeat expansion disorders include fragile X syndrome, myotonic dystrophy, Huntington disease, and spinocerebellar ataxias (Table 97.2 and Fig. 97.18). These disorders are caused by expansion in the number of 3-bp repeats. The fragile X gene, *FMR1*, normally has 5-40 CGG triplets. An error in replication can result in expansion of that number to a level in the gray zone between 41 and 58 repeats, or to a level referred to as **premutation**, which comprises 59-200 repeats. Some premutation carriers, more often males, develop fragile X–associated tremor/ataxia syndrome (FXTAS) as adults. Female premutation carriers are at risk for fragile X–associated primary ovarian insufficiency (*FXPOI*). Persons with a premutation are also at risk for having the repeat expand further in subsequent meiosis, thus crossing into the range of a **full mutation** (>200 repeats) in offspring. With this number of repeats, the *FMR1* gene becomes hypermethylated, and protein production is lost.

Some triplet expansions associated with other genes can cause disease through a mechanism other than decreased protein production. In Huntington disease the expansion causes the gene product to have a new, toxic effect on the neurons of the basal ganglia. For most triplet repeat disorders, there is a clinical correlation to the size of the expansion,

with a greater expansion causing more severe symptoms and having an earlier age of disease onset. The observation of increasing severity of disease and early age at onset in subsequent generations is termed **genetic anticipation** and is a defining characteristic of many triplet repeat expansion disorders (Fig. 97.19).

Genetic Imprinting

The 2 copies of most autosomal genes are functionally equivalent. However, in some cases, only 1 copy of a gene is transcribed and the 2nd copy is silenced. This gene silencing is typically associated with methylation of DNA, which is an **epigenetic** modification, meaning it does not change the nucleotide sequence of the DNA (Fig. 97.20). In **imprinting**, gene expression depends on the parent of origin of the chromosome (see Chapter 98.8). Imprinting disorders result from an imbalance of active copies of a given gene, which can occur for several reasons. Prader-Willi and Angelman syndromes, two distinct disorders associated with developmental impairment, are illustrative. Both can be caused by microdeletions of chromosome 15q11-12. The microdeletion in **Prader-Willi syndrome** is always on the paternally derived chromosome 15, whereas in **Angelman syndrome** it is on the maternal copy. *UBE3A* is the gene responsible for Angelman syndrome. The paternal copy of *UBE3A* is transcriptionally silenced in the brain, and the maternal

| Table 97.2 | Diseases Associated With Polynucleotide Repeat Expansions |

DISEASE	DESCRIPTION	REPEAT SEQUENCE	NORMAL RANGE	ABNORMAL RANGE	PARENT IN WHOM EXPANSION USUALLY OCCURS	LOCATION OF EXPANSION
CATEGORY 1						
Huntington disease	Loss of motor control, dementia, affective disorder	CAG	6-34	36-100 or more	More often through father	Exon
Spinal and bulbar muscular atrophy	Adult-onset motor-neuron disease associated with androgen insensitivity	CAG	11-34	40-62	More often through father	Exon
Spinocerebellar ataxia type 1	Progressive ataxia, dysarthria, dysmetria	CAG	6-39	41-81	More often through father	Exon
Spinocerebellar ataxia type 2	Progressive ataxia, dysarthria	CAG	15-29	35-59	—	Exon
Spinocerebellar ataxia type 3 (Machado-Joseph disease)	Dystonia, distal muscular atrophy, ataxia, external ophthalmoplegia	CAG	13-36	68-79	More often through father	Exon
Spinocerebellar ataxia type 6	Progressive ataxia, dysarthria, nystagmus	CAG	4-16	21-27	—	Exon
Spinocerebellar ataxia type 7	Progressive ataxia, dysarthria, retinal degeneration	CAG	7-35	38-200	More often through father	—
Spinocerebellar ataxia type 17	Progressive ataxia, dementia, bradykinesia, dysmetria	CAG	29-42	47-55	—	Exon
Dentatorubral-pallidoluysian atrophy/Haw River syndrome	Cerebellar atrophy, ataxia, myoclonic epilepsy, choreoathetosis, dementia	CAG	7-25	49-88	More often through father	Exon
CATEGORY 2						
Pseudoachondroplasia, multiple epiphyseal dysplasia	Short stature, joint laxity, degenerative joint disease	GAC	5	6-7	—	Exon
Oculopharyngeal muscular dystrophy	Proximal limb weakness, dysphagia, ptosis	GCG	6	7-13	—	Exon
Cleidocranial dysplasia	Short stature, open skull sutures with bulging calvaria, clavicular hypoplasia, shortened fingers, dental anomalies	GCG, GCT, GCA	17	27 (expansion observed in 1 family)	—	Exon
Synpolydactyly	Polydactyly and syndactyly	GCG, GCT, GCA	15	22-25	—	Exon
CATEGORY 3						
Myotonic dystrophy (DM1; chromosome 19)	Muscle loss, cardiac arrhythmia, cataracts, frontal balding	CTG	5-37	100 to several thousand	Either parent, but expansion to congenital form through mother	3′ untranslated region
Myotonic dystrophy (DM2; chromosome 3)	Muscle loss, cardiac arrhythmia, cataracts, frontal balding	CCTG	<75	75-11,000	—	3′ untranslated region
Friedreich ataxia	Progressive limb ataxia, dysarthria, hypertrophic cardiomyopathy, pyramidal weakness in legs	GAA	7-2	200-900 or more	Autosomal recessive inheritance, so disease alleles are inherited from both parents	Intron
Fragile X syndrome (FRAXA)	Intellectual impairment, large ears and jaws, macroorchidism in males	CGG	6-52	200-2,000 or more	Exclusively through mother	5′ untranslated region
Fragile site (FRAXE)	Mild intellectual impairment	GCC	6-35	>200	More often through mother	5′ untranslated region
Spinocerebellar ataxia type 8	Adult-onset ataxia, dysarthria, nystagmus	CTG	16-37	107-127	More often through mother	3′ untranslated region
Spinocerebellar ataxia type 10	Ataxia and seizures	ATTCT	12-16	800-4,500	More often through father	Intron
Spinocerebellar ataxia type 12	Ataxia, eye movement disorders; variable age at onset	CAG	7-28	66-78	—	5′ untranslated region
Progressive myoclonic epilepsy type 1	Juvenile-onset convulsions, myoclonus, dementia	12-bp repeat motif	2-3	30-75	Autosomal recessive inheritance, so transmitted by both parents	5′ untranslated region

From Jorde LB, Carey JC, Bamshad MJ, et al: *Medical genetics*, ed 3, St Louis, 2006, Mosby, p 82.

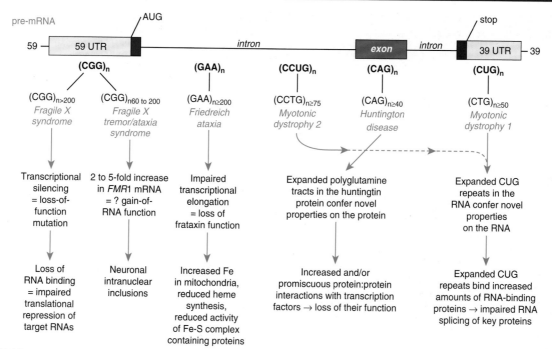

Fig. 97.18 The locations of the trinucleotide repeat expansions and the sequence of each trinucleotide in 5 representative trinucleotide repeat diseases, shown on a schematic of a generic pre–messenger RNA (mRNA). The minimal number of repeats in the DNA sequence of the affected gene associated with the disease is also indicated, as well as the effect of the expansion on the mutant RNA or protein. *(From Nussbaum RL, McInnes RR, Willard HF, editors: Thompson & Thompson genetics in medicine, ed 8, Philadelphia, 2016, Elsevier; based partly on an unpublished figure of John A. Phillips III, Vanderbilt University.)*

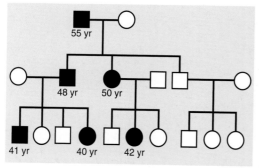

Fig. 97.19 Myotonic dystrophy pedigree illustrating genetic anticipation. In this case the age at onset for family members affected with an autosomal dominant disease is lower in more recent generations. *Black,* Affected patients.

copy continues to be transcribed. If an individual has a maternal deletion, an insufficient amount of UBE3A protein is produced in the brain, resulting in the neurologic deficits seen in Angelman syndrome.

Uniparental disomy (UPD), the rare occurrence of a child inheriting both copies of a chromosome from the same parent, is another genetic mechanism that can cause Prader-Willi and Angelman syndromes. Inheriting both chromosomes 15 from the mother is functionally the same as deletion of the paternal 15q12 and results in Prader-Willi syndrome. Approximately 30% of cases of Prader-Willi syndrome are caused by maternal UPD15, whereas paternal UPD15 accounts for only 3% of Angelman syndrome (see Chapter 98.8).

A mutation in an imprinted gene is another cause. Pathologic variants in *UBE3A* account for almost 11% of patients with Angelman syndrome and also result in familial transmission. The most uncommon cause is a mutation in the imprinting center, which results in an inability to

correctly imprint *UBE3A*. In a woman, inability to reset the imprinting on her paternally inherited chromosome 15 imprint results in a 50% risk of passing on an incorrectly methylated copy of *UBE3A* to a child, who would then develop Angelman syndrome.

Besides 15q12, other imprinted regions of clinical interest include the short arm of chromosome 11, where the genes for Beckwith-Wiedemann syndrome and nesidioblastosis map, and the long arm of chromosome 7 with maternal UPD of 7q, which has been associated with some cases of idiopathic short stature and Russell-Silver syndrome.

Imprinting of a gene can occur during gametogenesis or early embryonic development (reprogramming). Genes can become inactive or active by various mechanisms including DNA methylation or demethylation or histone acetylation or deacetylation, with different patterns of (de)methylation noted on paternal or maternal imprintable chromosome regions. Some genes demonstrate tissue-specific imprinting (see Fig. 97.20). Several studies suggest a small but significantly increased incidence of imprinting disorders, specifically Beckwith-Wiedemann and Angelman syndrome, associated with assisted reproductive technologies such as in vitro fertilization and intracytoplasmic sperm injection. However, the overall incidence of these disorders in children conceived using assisted reproductive technologies is likely to be <1%.

MULTIFACTORIAL AND POLYGENIC INHERITANCE

Multifactorial inheritance refers to traits that are caused by a combination of inherited, environmental, and stochastic factors (Fig. 97.21). Multifactorial traits differ from **polygenic inheritance**, which refers to traits that result from the additive effects of multiple genes. Multifactorial traits segregate within families but do not exhibit a consistent or recognizable inheritance pattern. Characteristics include the following:

◆ There is a similar rate of recurrence among all first-degree relatives (parents, siblings, offspring of affected child). It is unusual to find a substantial increase in risk for relatives related more distantly than second degree to the index case.
◆ The risk of recurrence is related to the incidence of the disease.

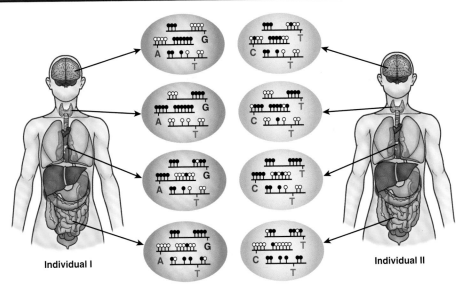

Fig. 97.20 Tissue-specific DNA methylation and epigenetic heterogeneity among individuals. A subset of the DNA methylation patterns within a cell is characteristic of that cell type. Cell type–specific and tissue-specific DNA methylation patterns are illustrated by organ-to-organ variations in the clusters of methylated CpGs (cytosine-phosphate-guanine bases) within the same individual. Despite overall consistency in tissue-specific DNA methylation patterns, variations in these patterns exist among different individuals. Methylated CpGs are indicated by a *filled circle* and unmethylated CpGs by an *open circle*. Single nucleotide polymorphisms (SNPs) are indicated by the corresponding base. *(Redrawn from Brena RM, Huang THM, Plass C: Toward a human epigenome, Nat Genet 38:1359–1360, 2006.)*

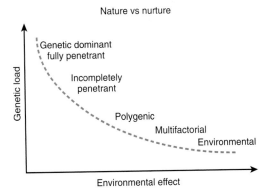

Fig. 97.21 The progressive decrease in the genetic load contributing to the development of a disease creates a smooth transition in the distribution of illnesses on an etiologic diagram. In theory, no diseases are completely free from the influence of both genetic and environmental factors. *(From Bomprezzi R, Kovanen PE, Martin R: New approaches to investigating heterogeneity in complex traits, J Med Genet 40:553–559, 2003. Reproduced with permission from the BMJ Publishing Group.)*

◆ Some disorders have a sex predilection, as indicated by an unequal male:female incidence. Pyloric stenosis, for example, is more common in males, whereas congenital dislocation of the hips is more common in females. With an altered sex ratio, the risk is higher for the relatives of an index case whose gender is less often affected than relatives of an index case of the more frequently affected gender. For example, the risk to the son of an affected female with infantile pyloric stenosis is 18%, compared with the 5% risk for the son of an affected male. An affected female presumably has a greater genetic susceptibility, which she can then pass on to her offspring.

◆ The likelihood that both identical twins will be affected with the same malformation is <100% but much greater than the chance that both members of a nonidentical twin pair will be affected. This contrasts with the pattern seen in mendelian inheritance, in which identical twins almost always share fully penetrant genetic disorders.

◆ The risk of recurrence is increased when multiple family members are affected. A simple example is that the risk of recurrence for unilateral cleft lip and palate is 4% for a couple with 1 affected child and increases to 9% with 2 affected children. It is sometimes difficult to distinguish between a multifactorial and mendelian etiology in families with multiple affected individuals.

◆ The risk of recurrence may be greater when the disorder is more severe. For example, an infant who has long-segment Hirschsprung disease has a greater chance of having an affected sibling than the infant who has short-segment Hirschsprung disease.

There are two types of multifactorial traits. One exhibits continuous variation, with "normal" individuals falling within a statistical range—often defined as having a value 2 standard deviations (SDs) above and/or below the mean—and "abnormals" falling outside that range. Examples include such traits as intelligence, blood pressure, height, and head circumference. For many of these traits, offspring values can be estimated based on a modified average of their parental values, with nutritional and environmental factors playing an important role.

With other multifactorial traits, the distinction between normal and abnormal is based on the presence or absence of a particular trait. Examples include pyloric stenosis, neural tube defects, congenital heart defects, and cleft lip and cleft palate. Such traits follow a **threshold model** (see Fig. 97.15). A distribution of liability because of genetic and nongenetic factors is postulated in the population. Individuals who exceed a threshold liability develop the trait, and those below the threshold do not.

The balance between genetic and environmental factors is demonstrated by neural tube defects. Genetic factors are implicated by the increased recurrence risk for parents of an affected child compared with the general population, yet the recurrence risk is about 3%, less than what would be expected if the trait was caused by a single, fully penetrant mutation. The role of nongenetic environmental factors is shown by the recurrence risk decreasing up to 87% if the mother-to-be takes 4 mg of folic acid daily starting 3 mo before conception.

Many adult-onset diseases behave as if caused by multifactorial inheritance. Diabetes, coronary artery disease, and schizophrenia are examples.

Bibliography is available at Expert Consult.

Chapter **98**

Cytogenetics

Carlos A. Bacino and Brendan Lee

第九十八章

细胞遗传学

中文导读

本章主要介绍了染色体分析方法、唐氏综合征及其他染色体数目异常、染色体结构异常、性染色体非整倍体、染色体易断裂位点、嵌合体、染色体不稳定综合征以及单亲二倍体和印记。具体描述了染色体结构异常的易位、倒位、缺失和重复、插入、等臂染色体以及标记染色体和环状染色体；具体描述了性染色体非整倍体的特纳综合征、克林费尔特综合征以及47,XYY；具体描述了嵌合体的PALLISTER-KILLIAN综合征和伊藤黑素过少症。

Clinical cytogenetics is the study of chromosomes: their structure, function, inheritance, and abnormalities. Chromosome abnormalities are very common and occur in approximately 1–2% of live births, 5% of stillbirths, and 50% of early fetal losses in the 1st trimester of pregnancy (Table 98.1). Chromosome abnormalities are more common among individuals with intellectual disability and play a significant role in the development of some neoplasias.

Chromosome analyses are indicated in persons presenting with multiple congenital anomalies, dysmorphic features, and/or intellectual disability. The specific indications for studies include advanced maternal age (>35 yr), multiple abnormalities on fetal ultrasound (prenatal testing), multiple congenital anomalies, unexplained growth restriction in the fetus, postnatal problems in growth and development, ambiguous genitalia, unexplained intellectual disability with or without associated anatomic abnormalities, primary amenorrhea or infertility, recurrent miscarriages (≥3) or prior history of stillbirths and neonatal deaths, a first-degree relative with a known or suspected structural chromosome abnormality, clinical findings consistent with a known anomaly, some malignancies, and chromosome breakage syndromes (e.g., Bloom syndrome, Fanconi anemia).

98.1 Methods of Chromosome Analysis

Carlos A. Bacino and Brendan Lee

Cytogenetic studies are usually performed on peripheral blood lymphocytes, although cultured fibroblasts obtained from a skin biopsy may also be used. Prenatal (fetal) chromosome studies are performed with cells obtained from the amniotic fluid (amniocytes), chorionic villus tissue, and fetal blood or, in the case of preimplantation diagnosis,

by analysis of a *blastomere* (cleavage stage) biopsy, polar body biopsy, or blastocyst biopsy. Cytogenetic studies of bone marrow have an important role in tumor surveillance, particularly among patients with leukemia. These are useful to determine induction of remission and success of therapy or in some cases the occurrence of relapses.

Chromosome anomalies include abnormalities of number and structure and are the result of errors during cell division. There are 2 types of cell division: mitosis, which occurs in most somatic cells, and meiosis, which is limited to the germ cells. In **mitosis,** 2 genetically identical daughter cells are produced from a single parent cell. DNA duplication has already occurred during **interphase** in the S phase of the cell cycle (DNA synthesis). Therefore, at the beginning of mitosis the chromosomes consist of 2 double DNA strands joined together at the centromere, known as *sister chromatids.* Mitosis can be divided into 4 stages: prophase, metaphase, anaphase, and telophase. **Prophase** is characterized by condensation of the DNA. Also during prophase, the nuclear membrane and the nucleolus disappear and the mitotic spindle forms. In **metaphase** the chromosomes are maximally compacted and are clearly visible as distinct structures. The chromosomes align at the center of the cell, and spindle fibers connect to the centromere of each chromosome and extend to centrioles at the 2 poles of the mitotic figure. In **anaphase** the chromosomes divide along their longitudinal axes to form 2 daughter chromatids, which then migrate to opposite poles of the cell. **Telophase** is characterized by formation of 2 new nuclear membranes and nucleoli, duplication of the centrioles, and cytoplasmic cleavage to form the 2 daughter cells.

Meiosis begins in the female oocyte during fetal life and is completed years to decades later. In males it begins in a particular spermatogonial cell sometime between adolescence and adult life and is completed in a few days. Meiosis is preceded by DNA replication so that at the outset, each of the 46 chromosomes consists of 2 chromatids. In meiosis, a

Table 98.1	Incidence of Chromosomal Abnormalities in Newborn Surveys	
TYPE OF ABNORMALITY	**NUMBER**	**APPROXIMATE INCIDENCE**
SEX CHROMOSOME ANEUPLOIDY		
Males (43,612 newborns)		
47,XXY	45	1/1,000*
47,XYY	45	1/1,000
Other X or Y aneuploidy	32	1/1,350
Total	122	1/360 male births
Females (24,547 newborns)		
45,X	6	1/4,000
47,XXX	27	1/900
Other X aneuploidy	9	1/2,700
Total	42	1/580 female births
AUTOSOMAL ANEUPLOIDY (68,159 NEWBORNS)		
Trisomy 21	82	1/830
Trisomy 18	9	1/7,500
Trisomy 13	3	1/22,700
Other aneuploidy	2	1/34,000
Total	96	1/700 live births
STRUCTURAL ABNORMALITIES (68,159 NEWBORNS)		
Balanced Rearrangements		
Robertsonian	62	1/1,100
Other	77	1/885
Unbalanced Rearrangements		
Robertsonian	5	1/13,600
Other	38	1/1,800
Total	182	1/375 live births
All chromosome abnormalities	442	1/154 live births

*Recent studies show the prevalence is currently 1:580.
  Data from Hsu LYF: Prenatal diagnosis of chromosomal abnormalities through amniocentesis. In Milunsky A, editor: *Genetic disorders and the fetus*, ed 4, Baltimore, 1998, Johns Hopkins University Press, pp 179–248.

diploid cell (2n = 46 chromosomes) divides to form **4 haploid cells** (n = 23 chromosomes). Meiosis consists of 2 major rounds of cell division. In **meiosis I**, each of the homologous chromosomes pair precisely so that **genetic recombination**, involving exchange between 2 DNA strands (**crossing over**), can occur. This results in reshuffling of the genetic information for the recombined chromosomes and allows further genetic diversity. Each daughter cell then receives 1 of each of the 23 homologous chromosomes. In oogenesis, one of the daughter cells receives most of the cytoplasm and becomes the egg, whereas the other smaller cell becomes the first polar body. **Meiosis II** is similar to a mitotic division but without a preceding round of DNA duplication (replication). Each of the 23 chromosomes divides longitudinally, and the homologous chromatids migrate to opposite poles of the cell. This produces 4 spermatogonia in males, or an egg cell and a 2nd polar body in females, each with a haploid (n = 23) set of chromosomes. Consequently, meiosis fulfills 2 crucial roles: It reduces the chromosome number from diploid (46) to haploid (23) so that on fertilization a diploid number is restored, and it allows genetic recombination.

Two common errors of cell division may occur during meiosis or mitosis, and either can result in an abnormal number of chromosomes. The 1st error is **nondisjunction**, in which 2 chromosomes fail to separate during meiosis and thus migrate together into one of the new cells, producing 1 cell with 2 copies of the chromosome and another with no copy. The 2nd error is **anaphase lag**, in which a chromatid or chromosome is lost during mitosis because it fails to move quickly enough during anaphase to become incorporated into 1 of the new daughter cells (Fig. 98.1).

For chromosome analysis, cells are cultured (for varying periods depending on cell type), with or without stimulation, and then artificially arrested in mitosis during metaphase (or prometaphase), later subjected to a hypotonic solution to allow disruption of the nuclear cell membrane

and proper dispersion of the chromosomes for analysis, fixed, banded, and finally stained. The most commonly used banding and staining method is the **GTG banding** (G-bands trypsin Giemsa), also known as **G banding**, which produces a unique combination of dark (G-positive) and light (G-negative) bands that permits recognition of all individual 23 chromosome pairs for analysis.

Metaphase chromosome spreads are first evaluated microscopically, and then their images are photographed or captured by a video camera and stored on a computer for later analysis. Humans have 46 chromosomes or 23 pairs, which are classified as *autosomes* for chromosomes 1-22, and the *sex chromosomes*, often referred as *sex complement*: XX for females and XY for males. The homologous chromosomes from a metaphase spread can then be paired and arranged systematically to assemble a karyotype according to well-defined standard conventions such as those established by International System for Human Cytogenetic Nomenclature (ISCN), with chromosome 1 being the largest and 22 the smallest. According to nomenclature, the description of the karyotype includes the total number of chromosomes followed by the sex chromosome constitution. A normal karyotype is 46,XX for females and 46,XY for males (Fig. 98.2). Abnormalities are noted after the sex chromosome complement.

Although the internationally accepted system for human chromosome classification relies largely on the length and banding pattern of each chromosome, the position of the centromere relative to the ends of the chromosome also is a useful distinguishing feature (Fig. 98.3). The centromere divides the chromosome in 2, with the short arm designated the **p arm** and the long arm designated the **q arm**. A plus or minus sign before the number of a chromosome indicates that there is an extra or missing chromosome, respectively. Table 98.2 lists some of the abbreviations used for the descriptions of chromosomes and their abnormalities. A metaphase chromosome spread usually shows 450-550 bands. Prophase and prometaphase chromosomes are longer, are less condensed, and often show 550-850 bands. High-resolution analysis may detect small chromosome abnormalities although has been mostly replaced by chromosome microarray studies (array CGH or aCGH).

Molecular techniques (e.g., FISH, CMA, aCGH) have filled a significant void for the diagnosing cryptic chromosomal abnormalities. These techniques identify subtle abnormalities that are often below the resolution of standard cytogenetic studies. **Fluorescence in situ hybridization (FISH)** is used to identify the presence, absence, or rearrangement of *specific* DNA segments and is performed with gene- or region-specific DNA probes. Several FISH probes are used in the clinical setting: unique sequence or single-copy probes, repetitive-sequence probes (alpha satellites in the pericentromeric regions), and multiple-copy probes (chromosome specific or painting) (Fig. 98.4A and B). FISH involves using a unique, known DNA sequence or probe labeled with a fluorescent dye that is complementary to the studied region of disease interest. The labeled probe is exposed to the DNA on a microscope slide, typically metaphase or interphase chromosomal DNA. When the probe pairs with its complementary DNA sequence, it can then be visualized by fluorescence microscopy (Fig. 98.5). In metaphase chromosome spreads, the exact chromosomal location of each probe copy can be documented, and often the *number of copies* (deletions, duplications) of the DNA sequence as well. When the interrogated segments (as in genomic duplications) are close together, only interphase cells can accurately determine the presence of 2 or more copies or signals since in metaphase cells, some duplications might falsely appear as a single signal.

Chromosome rearrangements <5 million bp (5 Mbp) cannot be detected by conventional cytogenetic techniques. FISH was initially used to detect deletions as small as 50-200 kb of DNA and facilitated the early clinical characterization of a number of **microdeletion syndromes**. Some FISH probes hybridize to repetitive sequences located in the pericentromeric regions. Pericentromeric probes are still widely used for the rapid identification of certain trisomies in interphase cells of blood smears, or even in the rapid analysis of prenatal samples from cells obtained through amniocentesis. Such probes are available for chromosomes 13, 18, and 21 and for the sex pair X and Y (see Fig. 98.4C and D). With regard to the detection of genomic disorders, FISH is no longer the first line of testing, and its role has also mostly changed

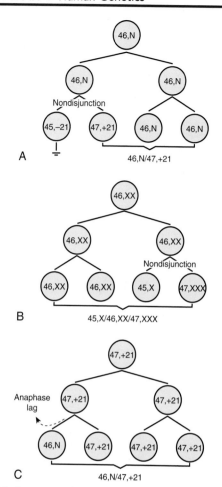

A, Postzygotic nondisjunction in an initially normal conceptus.

B, Postzygotic nondisjunction in an initially 46,XX conceptus.

C, Postzygotic anaphase lag in an initially 47,+21 conceptus.

Fig. 98.1 Generation of mosaicism. **A,** Postzygotic nondisjunction in an initially normal conceptus. In this example, 1 cell line (monosomic 21) is subsequently lost, with the final karyotype 46,N/47,+21. **B,** Postzygotic nondisjunction in an initially 46,XX conceptus, resulting in 45,X/46,XX/47,XXX mosaicism. **C,** Postzygotic anaphase lag in an initially 47,+21 conceptus. (*From Gardner RJM, Sutherland GR. Chromosome abnormalities and genetic counseling, ed 3 New York, 2003, Oxford University Press, p 33, Figure 43.1. By permission of Oxford University Press, Inc, www.oup.com.*)

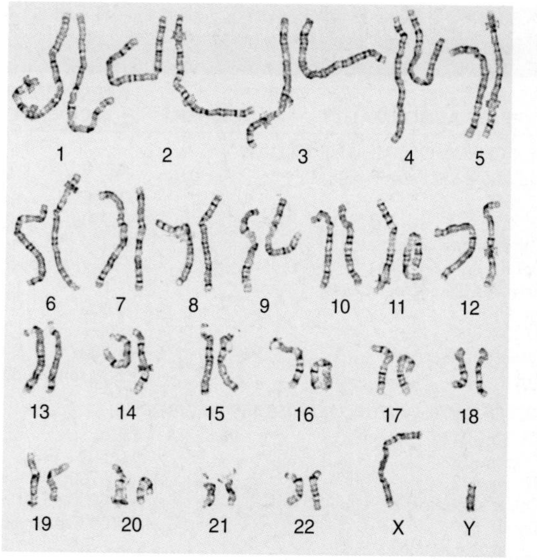

Fig. 98.2 Karyotype of a normal male at the 550-600 band level. The longer the chromosomes are captured at metaphase or sometimes prometaphase, the more bands that can be visualized.

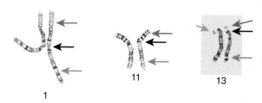

Fig. 98.3 Example of different chromosome types according to the position of the centromere. On the *left* is a chromosome 1 pair with the centromere equidistant from the short and long arm (also known as *metacentric*). In the center is a chromosome 11 pair that is submetacentric. On the *right* is a chromosome 13 pair that is an example of an acrocentric chromosome. Acrocentric chromosomes contain a very small short arm, stalks, and satellite DNA. The *black arrow* indicates the position of the centromere. The *blue arrow* shows the long arm of a chromosome. The *red arrow* shows the short arm of a chromosome. The *green arrow* highlights the satellite region, which is made of DNA repeats. The *light area* between the short arm and the satellite is known as the *stalk*.

to the confirmation of microarray findings. In summary, FISH is reserved for (1) confirmation studies of abnormalities detected by CMA, (2) rapid prenatal screening on interphase amniotic fluid cells, and (3) interphase blood smear for sex assignment of newborns who present with ambiguous genitalia.

Array comparative genomic hybridization (aCGH) and **chromosomal microarray (CMA)** are molecular-based techniques that involve differentially labeling the patient's DNA with a fluorescent dye (green fluorophore) and a normal reference DNA with a red fluorophore (Fig. 98.6). Oligonucleotides (short DNA segments) encompassing the entire genome are spotted onto a slide or **microarray** grid. Equal amounts of the 2-label DNA samples are mixed, and the green:red fluorescence ratio is measured along each tested area. Regions of amplification of the patient's DNA display an excess of green fluorescence, and regions of loss show excess red fluorescence. If the patient's and the control DNA are equally represented, the green:red ratio is 1:1, and the tested regions appear yellow (see Chapter 96, Fig. 96.5). The detection is

currently possible at the single-exon resolution level, depending on the arrays used. In the near future, copy number detections may further evolve to be detected by next generation sequencing in the context of whole *genome* sequencing.

The many advantages of aCGH include its ability to test all critical disease-causing regions in the genome at once, detect duplications and deletions not currently recognized as recurrent disease-causing regions probed by FISH, and detect single-gene and contiguous gene deletion syndromes. Also, aCGH does not always require cell culture to generate sufficient DNA, which may be important in the context of prenatal testing because of timing. Limitations of aCGH are that it does not detect balanced translocations or inversions and may not detect low levels of chromosomal mosaicism. Among different types of aCGH, some are more targeted than others. **Targeted aCGH** can be an efficient way to detect clinically known cryptic chromosomal aberrations, which are typically associated with known disease phenotypes. **Whole genome arrays** target the entire genome and allow better and denser coverage

ABBREV	MEANING	EXAMPLE	CONDITION
Table 98.2	Some Abbreviations Used for Description of Chromosomes and Their Abnormalities		
XX	Female	46,XX	Normal female karyotype
XY	Male	46,XY	Normal male karyotype
[##]	Number [#] of cells	46,XY[12]/47,XXY[10]	Number of cells in each clone, typically inside brackets Mosaicism in Klinefelter syndrome with 12 normal cells and 10 cells with an extra X chromosome
cen	Centromere		
del	Deletion	46,XY,del(5p)	Male with deletion of chromosome 5 short arm
der	Derivative	46,XX,der(2),t(2p12;7q13)	Female with a structurally rearranged chromosome 2 that resulted from a translocation between chromosomes 2 (short arm) and 7 (long arm)
dup	Duplication	46,XY,dup(15)(q11-q13)	Male with interstitial duplication in the long arm of chromosome 15 in the Prader-Willi/Angelman syndrome region
ins	Insertion	46,XY,ins(3)(p13q21q26)	Male with an insertion within chromosome 3 A piece between q21q26 has reinserted on p13
inv	Inversion	46,XY,inv(2)(p21q31)	Male with pericentric inversion of chromosome 2 with breakpoints at bands p21 and q31
ish	Metaphase FISH	46,XX.ish del(7)(q11.23q11.23)	Female with deletion in the Williams syndrome region detected by in situ hybridization
nuc ish	Interphase FISH	nuc ish(DXZ1 × 3)	Interphase in situ hybridization showing 3 signals for the X chromosome centromeric region
mar	Marker	47,XY,+mar	Male with extra, unidentified chromosome material
mos	Mosaic	mos 45,X[14]/46,XX[16]	Turner syndrome mosaicism (analysis of 30 cells showed that 14 cells were 45,X and 16 cells were 46,XX)
p	Short arm	46,XY,del(5)(p12)	Male with a deletion on the short arm of chromosome 5, band p12 (short nomenclature)
q	Long arm	46,XY,del(5)(q14)	Male with a deletion on the long arm of chromosome 5, band 14
r	Ring chromosome	46,X,r(X)(p21q27)	Female with 1 normal X chromosome and a ring X chromosome
t	Translocation	t(2;8)(q33;q24.1)	Interchange of material between chromosomes 2 and 8 with breakpoints at bands 2q33 and 8q24.1
ter	Terminal	46,XY,del(5)(p12-pter)	Male with a deletion of chromosome 5 between p12 and the end of the short arm (long nomenclature)
/	Slash	45,X/46,XY	Separate lines or clones Mosaicism for monosomy X and a male cell line
+	Gain of	47,XX,+21	Female with trisomy 21
−	Loss of	45,XY,−21	Male with monosomy 21

in evenly spaced genomic regions. Its disadvantage is that interpretation of deletions or duplications may be difficult if it involves areas not previously known to be involved in disease.

A frequently used array in the clinical setting is the **single nucleotide polymorphism (SNP)**. SNPs are polymorphic variations between 2 nucleotides, and when analyzed in massive parallel fashion, they can provide valuable clinical information. Several million SNPs normally occur in the human genome. SNP arrays can help with the detection of **uniparental disomies** (i.e., genetic information derived from only 1 parent), as well as consanguinity in the family. Many arrays currently used in clinical practice combine the use of oligonucleotides for the detection of **copy number variations** in conjunction with SNPs. There are many copy number variations causing deletion or duplication in the human genome. Thus, most detected genetic abnormalities, unless associated with well-known clinical phenotypes, require *parental investigations* because a detected copy number variation that is inherited could be benign or an incidental polymorphic variant. A **de novo** abnormality (i.e., one found only in the child and not the parents) is often more significant if it is associated with an abnormal phenotype found only in the child, and if it involves genes with important functions.

aCGH is a very valuable technology alone or when combined with FISH and conventional chromosome studies (Fig. 98.7).

Bibliography is available at Expert Consult.

98.2 Down Syndrome and Other Abnormalities of Chromosome Number

Brendan Lee

ANEUPLOIDY AND POLYPLOIDY

Human cells contain a multiple of 23 chromosomes (n = 23). A haploid cell (n) has 23 chromosomes (typically in the ovum or sperm). If a cell's chromosomes are an exact multiple of 23 (46, 69, 92 in humans), those cells are referred to as **euploid**. **Polyploid** cells are euploid cells with more than the normal **diploid** number of 46 (2n) chromosomes: 3n, 4n. Polyploidy conceptions are usually not viable, but the presence of mosaicism with a karyotypically normal cell line can allow survival. **Mosaicism** is an abnormality defined as the presence of 2 or more cell

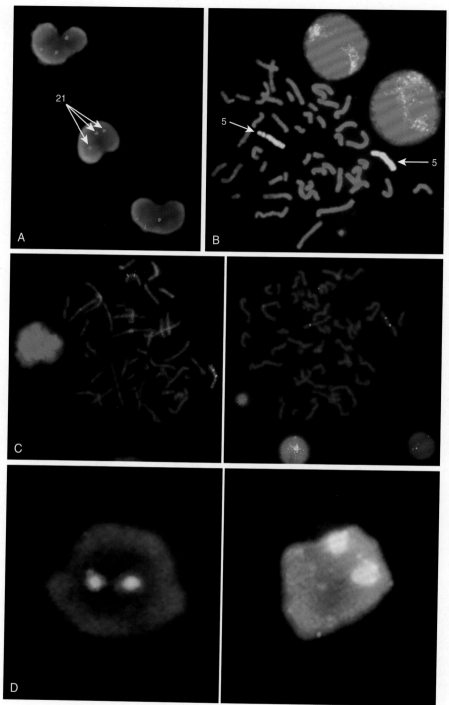

Fig. 98.4 A, FISH analysis of interphase peripheral blood cells from a patient with Down syndrome using a chromosome 21–specific probe. The 3 red signals mark the presence of 3 chromosomes 21. **B,** FISH analysis of a metaphase chromosome spread from a clinically normal individual using a whole chromosome paint specific for chromosome 5. Both chromosomes 5 are completely labeled (*yellow*) along their entire length. **C,** FISH on metaphase cells using a unique sequence probe that hybridizes to the elastin gene on chromosome 7q11.23, inside the Williams syndrome critical region. The elastin probe is labeled in *red,* and a control probe on chromosome 7 is labeled in *green.* The *left* image shows normal hybridization to chromosome 7, with 2 signals for the elastin region and 2 for the control probe. The *right* image shows a normal chromosome on the right with control and elastin signals, and a deleted chromosome 7 on the left, evidenced by a single signal for the control probe. This image corresponds to a patient with a Williams syndrome region deletion. **D,** FISH in interphase cells using DNA probes that hybridize to repetitive α-satellite sequences in the pericentromeric region for the sex chromosomes. *Left,* interphase cells with 2 signals, 1 labeled in *red* for the X chromosome and *green* for the Y chromosome, consistent with a normal male chromosome complement. *Right,* interphase cell showing 2 *red* signals for the X chromosome, compatible with a normal female chromosome complement.

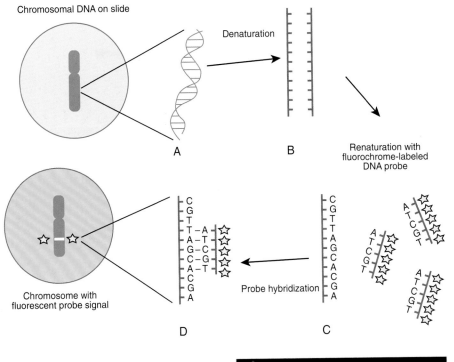

Fig. 98.5 FISH involves denaturation of double-stranded DNA as present in metaphase chromosomes or interphase nuclei on cytogenetic slide preparations (**A**) into single-stranded DNA (**B**). The slide-bound (in situ) DNA is then renatured or reannealed in the presence of excess copies of a single-stranded, fluorochrome-labeled DNA base-pair sequence or probe (**C**). The probe anneals or "hybridizes" to sites of complementary DNA sequence (**D**) within the chromosomal genome. Probe signal is visualized and imaged on the chromosome by fluorescent microscopy. *(From Lin RL, Cherry AM, Bangs CD, et al: FISHing for answers: the use of molecular cytogenetic techniques in adolescent medicine practice. In Hyme HE, Greydanus D, editors: Genetic disorders in adolescents: state of the art reviews. Adolescent medicine, Philadelphia, 2002, Hanley and Belfus, pp. 305–313.)*

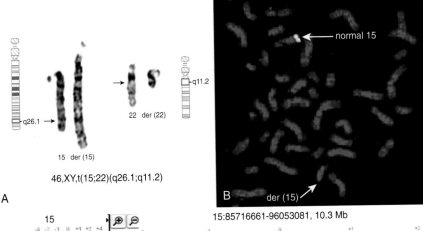

Fig. 98.6 Example of a cryptic microdeletion at a translocation breakpoint of an apparently balanced translocation in a patient with developmental delay (dd) and growth defect. **A,** Partial karyotype shows t(15;22)(q26.1;q11.2). **B,** FISH with clones 2O19 *(green)* and 354M14 *(red)* at 15q26.1; arrows indicate signals only present on the normal chromosome 15, suggesting a deletion on the der(15). **C,** Two-color aCGH with dye swap with 244 K oligo probes; *arrowhead* indicates a 3.3-Mbp deletion at chromosome 15q26.1-q26.2, *arrow* points to the close-up view of the deletion. *(From Li MM, Andersson HC: Clinical application of microarray-based molecular cytogenetics: an emerging new era of genomic medicine, J Pediatr 155:311–317, 2009, with permission of the authors and publisher.)*

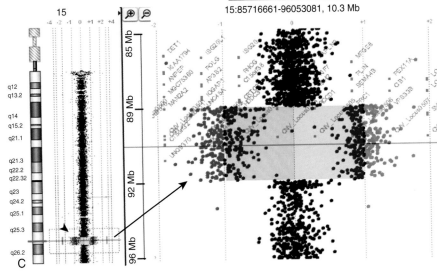

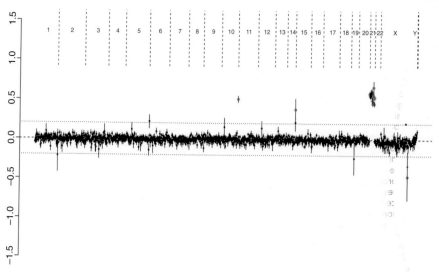

Fig. 98.7 aCGH in a female patient with Down syndrome. Each *black dot* represents a piece of DNA segment specific for different chromosome location. Most of the dots displayed between the 0.0 and 0.2 axis are considered within normal range. Exceptions are often a result of polymorphic variations. A group of dots colored in *green* clusters on chromosome 21 and above 0.5. These represent a *gain* in copy number of DNA segments for chromosome 21, as seen in Down syndrome and consistent with trisomy 21.

lines in a single individual. **Polyploidy** is a common abnormality seen in 1st-trimester pregnancy losses. **Triploid cells** are those with 3 haploid sets of chromosomes (3n) and are only viable in a mosaic form. Triploid infants can be liveborn but do not survive long. Triploidy is often the result of fertilization of an egg by 2 sperm (dispermy). Failure of 1 of the meiotic divisions, resulting in a diploid egg or sperm, can also result in triploidy. The phenotype of a triploid conception depends on the origin of the extra chromosome set. If the extra set is of **paternal** origin, it results in a partial *hydatidiform mole* (excessive placental growth) with poor embryonic development, but triploid conceptions that have an extra set of **maternal** chromosomes results in severe embryonic restriction with a small, fibrotic placenta (insufficient placental development) that is typically spontaneously aborted.

Abnormal cells that do not contain a multiple of haploid number of chromosomes are termed **aneuploid** cells. **Aneuploidy** is the most common and clinically significant type of human chromosome abnormality, occurring in at least 3–4% of all clinically recognized pregnancies. **Monosomies** occur when only 1, instead of the normal 2, of a given chromosome is present in an otherwise diploid cell. In humans, most autosomal monosomies appear to be lethal early in development, and survival is possible in **mosaic forms** or by means of chromosome rescue (restoration of the normal number by duplication of single monosomic chromosome). An exception to this rule is monosomy for the X chromosome (45,X), seen in Turner syndrome; the majority of 45,X conceptuses are believed to be lost early in pregnancy for as yet unexplained reasons.

The most common cause of aneuploidy is **nondisjunction**, the failure of chromosomes to disjoin normally during meiosis (see Fig. 98.1). Nondisjunction can occur during meiosis I or II or during mitosis, although maternal meiosis I is the most common nondisjunction in aneuploidies (e.g., Down syndrome, trisomy 18). After meiotic nondisjunction, the resulting gamete either lacks a chromosome or has 2 copies instead of 1 normal copy, resulting in a monosomic or trisomic zygote, respectively.

Trisomy is characterized by the presence of 3 chromosomes, instead of the normal 2, of any particular chromosome. Trisomy is the most common form of aneuploidy. Trisomy can occur in all cells or it may be mosaic. Most individuals with a trisomy exhibit a consistent and specific phenotype depending on the chromosome involved.

FISH is a technique that can be used for rapid diagnosis in the prenatal detection of common fetal aneuploidies, including chromosomes 13,

18, and 21, as well as sex chromosomes (see Fig. 98.4C and D). Direct detection of fetal cell-free DNA from maternal plasma for fetal trisomy is a safe and highly effective screening test for fetal aneuploidy. The most common numerical abnormalities in liveborn children include trisomy 21 (Down syndrome), trisomy 18 (Edwards syndrome), trisomy 13 (Patau syndrome), and sex chromosomal aneuploidies: Turner syndrome (usually 45,X), Klinefelter syndrome (47,XXY), 47,XXX, and 47,XYY. By far the most common type of trisomy in liveborn infants is trisomy 21 (47,XX,+21 or 47,XY,+21) (see Table 98.1). Trisomy 18 and trisomy 13 are relatively less common and are associated with a characteristic set of congenital anomalies and severe intellectual disability (Table 98.3). The occurrence of trisomy 21 and other trisomies increases with advanced maternal age (≥35 yr). Because of this increased risk, women who are ≥35 yr old at delivery should be offered genetic counseling and prenatal diagnosis (including serum screening, ultrasonography, and cell-free fetal DNA detection, amniocentesis, or chorionic villus sampling; see Chapter 115).

DOWN SYNDROME

Trisomy 21 is the most common genetic etiology of moderate intellectual disability. The incidence of Down syndrome in live births is approximately 1 in 733; the incidence at conception is more than twice that rate; the difference is accounted for by early pregnancy losses. In addition to cognitive impairment, Down syndrome is associated with congenital anomalies and characteristic dysmorphic features (Figs. 98.8 and 98.9 and Table 98.4). Although there is variability in the clinical features, the constellation of phenotypic features is fairly consistent and permits clinical recognition of trisomy 21. Affected individuals are more prone to congenital heart defects (50%) such as atrioventricular septal defects, ventricular septal defects, isolated secundum atrial septal defects, patent ductus arteriosus, and tetralogy of Fallot. Pulmonary complications include recurrent respiratory infections, sleep-disordered breathing, laryngo- and tracheobronchochomalacia, tracheal bronchus, pulmonary hypertension, and asthma. Congenital and acquired gastrointestinal anomalies (celiac disease) and hypothyroidism are common (Table 98.5). Other abnormalities include megakaryoblastic leukemia, immune dysfunction, diabetes mellitus, seizures, alopecia, juvenile idiopathic arthritis, and problems with hearing and vision. Alzheimer disease–like dementia is a known complication that occurs as early as the 4th decade and has an incidence 2-3 times higher than sporadic Alzheimer disease.

Most males with Down syndrome are sterile, but some females have been able to reproduce, with a 50% chance of having trisomy 21 pregnancies. Two genes (*DYRK1A, DSCR1*) in the putative critical region of chromosome 21 may be targets for therapy.

Developmental delay is universal (Tables 98.6 and 98.7 and Fig. 98.10). Cognitive impairment does not uniformly affect all areas of development. Social development is often relatively spared, but autism spectrum disorder can occur. Children with Down syndrome have considerable difficulty using expressive language. Understanding the individual developmental strengths and challenges is necessary to maximize the educational process. Persons with Down syndrome often benefit from programs aimed at cognitive training, stimulation, development, and education. Children with Down syndrome also benefit from anticipatory guidance, which establishes the protocol for screening, evaluation, and care for patients with genetic syndromes and chronic disorders (Table 98.8). Up to 15% of children with Down syndrome have misalignment of the 1st cervical vertebra (C1), which places them at risk for spinal cord injury with neck hyperextension or extreme flexion. Special Olympics recommends sports participation and training but requires x-ray examination (full extension and flexion views) of the neck before participation in sports that may result in hyperextension or radical flexion or pressure on the neck or upper spine. Such sports include diving starts in swimming, butterfly stroke, diving, pentathlon, high jump, equestrian sports, gymnastics, football, soccer, alpine skinning, and warm-up exercises placing stress on the head and neck. If atlantoaxial instability is diagnosed, Special Olympics will permit participation if the parents or guardians request so and only after obtaining written certification from a physician and acknowledgment of the risks by the parent or guardian.

Compared with the general population, children with Down syndrome are at increased risk for behavior problems; psychiatric comorbidity is an estimated 18–38% in this population. Common behavioral difficulties that occur in children with Down syndrome include inattentiveness, stubbornness, and a need for routine and sameness. Aggression and self-injurious behavior are less common in this population than other children with similar degrees of intellectual disability from other etiologies. All these behaviors can respond to educational, behavioral, or pharmacologic interventions.

The life expectancy for children with Down syndrome is reduced and is approximately 50-55 yr. Little prospective information about the secondary medical problems of adults with Down syndrome is known. Retrospective studies have shown premature aging and an increased risk of Alzheimer disease in adults with Down syndrome. These studies have also shown unexpected negative (protective) associations between

Table 98.3	Chromosomal Trisomies and Their Clinical Findings	
SYNDROME	**INCIDENCE**	**CLINICAL MANIFESTATIONS**
Trisomy 13, Patau syndrome	1/10,000 births	Cleft lip often midline; flexed fingers with postaxial polydactyly; ocular hypotelorism, bulbous nose; low-set, malformed ears; microcephaly; cerebral malformation, especially holoprosencephaly; microphthalmia, cardiac malformations; scalp defects; hypoplastic or absent ribs; visceral and genital anomalies Early lethality in most cases, with a median survival of 12 days; ~80% die by 1 year; 10-year survival ~13%. Survivors have significant neurodevelopmental delay.
Trisomy 18, Edwards syndrome	1/6,000 births	Low birthweight, closed fists with index finger overlapping the 3rd digit and the 5th digit overlapping the 4th, narrow hips with limited abduction, short sternum, rocker-bottom feet, microcephaly, prominent occiput, micrognathia, cardiac and renal malformations, intellectual disability ~88% of children die in the 1st year; 10-year survival ~10%. Survivors have significant neurodevelopmental delay.
Trisomy 8, mosaicism	1/20,000 births	Long face; high, prominent forehead; wide, upturned nose, thick, everted lower lip; microretrognathia; low-set ears; high-arched, sometimes cleft, palate; osteoarticular anomalies common (camptodactyly of 2nd-5th digits, small patella); deep plantar and palmar creases; moderate intellectual disability

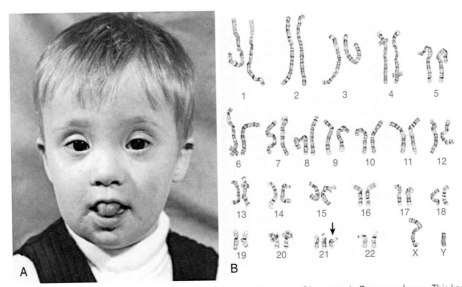

Fig. 98.8 A, Face of a child with Down syndrome. **B,** Karyotype of a male with trisomy 21 as seen in Down syndrome. This karyotype reveals 47 chromosomes instead of 46, with an extra chromosome in pair 21.

Down syndrome and comorbidities. Persons with Down syndrome have fewer-than-expected deaths caused by solid tumors and ischemic heart disease. This same study reported increased risk of adult deaths from congenital heart disease, seizures, and leukemia. In one large study, leukemias accounted for 60% of all cancers in people with Down syndrome and 97% of all cancers in children with Down syndrome. There was decreased risk of solid tumors in all age-groups with Down syndrome, including neuroblastomas and nephroblastomas in children and epithelial tumors in adults.

Most adults with Down syndrome are able to perform activities of daily living. However, most have difficulty with complex financial, legal, or medical decisions, and a guardian may be appointed.

The risk of having a child with trisomy 21 is highest in women who conceive after age 35 yr. Even though younger women have a lower risk, they represent half of all mothers with babies with Down syndrome because of their higher overall birth rate. *All women should be offered screening for Down syndrome* in their 2nd trimester by means of 4 maternal serum tests (free β-human chorionic gonadotropin [β-hCG], unconjugated estriol, inhibin, and α-fetoprotein). This is known as the *quad screen;* it can detect up to 80% of Down syndrome pregnancies

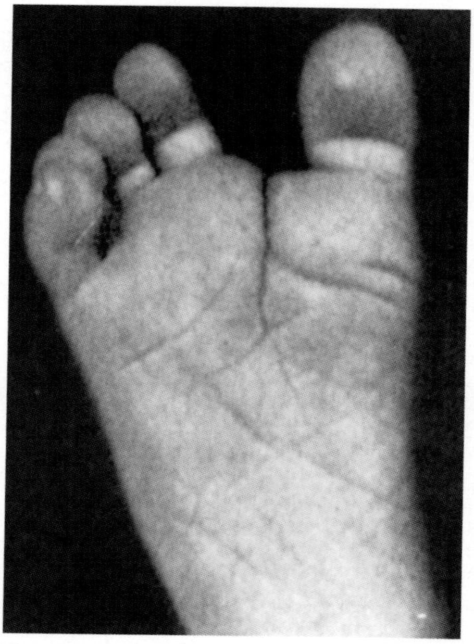

Fig. 98.9 Prehensile foot in a 1 mo old child with Down syndrome. *(From Wiedemann HR, Kunze J, Dibbern H:* Atlas of clinical syndromes: a visual guide to diagnosis, *ed 3, St Louis, 1989, Mosby.)*

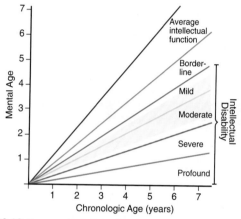

Fig. 98.10 The area shaded in *yellow* denotes the range of intellectual function of the majority of children with Down syndrome. *(From Levine MD, Carey WB, Crocker AC, editors:* Developmental-behavioral pediatrics, *ed 2, Philadelphia, 1992, Saunders, p 226.)*

Table 98.4 | Clinical Features of Down Syndrome in the Neonatal Period

CENTRAL NERVOUS SYSTEM
Hypotonia*
Developmental delay
Poor Moro reflex*

CRANIOFACIAL
Brachycephaly with flat occiput
Flat face*
Upward slanted palpebral fissures*
Epicanthal folds
Speckled irises (Brushfield spots)
Three fontanels
Delayed fontanel closure
Frontal sinus and midfacial hypoplasia
Mild microcephaly
Short, hard palate
Small nose, flat nasal bridge
Protruding tongue, open mouth
Small dysplastic ears*

CARDIOVASCULAR
Endocardial Cushing defects
Ventricular septal defect
Atrial septal defect
Patent ductus arteriosus
Aberrant subclavian artery
Pulmonary hypertension

MUSCULOSKELETAL
Joint hyperflexibility*
Short neck, redundant skin*
Short metacarpals and phalanges
Short 5th digit with clinodactyly*
Single transverse palmar creases*
Wide gap between 1st and 2nd toes
Pelvic dysplasia*
Short sternum
Two sternal manubrium ossification centers

GASTROINTESTINAL
Duodenal atresia
Annular pancreas
Tracheoesophageal fistula
Hirschsprung disease
Imperforate anus
Neonatal cholestasis

CUTANEOUS
Cutis marmorata

*Hall's criteria to aid in diagnosis.

| Table 98.5 | Additional Features of Down Syndrome That Can Develop or Become Symptomatic With Time |

NEUROPSYCHIATRIC
Developmental delay
Seizures
Autism spectrum disorders
Behavioral disorders (disruptive)
Depression
Alzheimer disease

SENSORY
Congenital or acquired hearing loss
Serous otitis media
Refractive errors (myopia)
Congenital or acquired cataracts
Nystagmus
Strabismus
Glaucoma
Blocked tear ducts

CARDIOPULMONARY
Acquired mitral, tricuspid, or aortic valve regurgitation
Endocarditis
Obstructive sleep apnea

MUSCULOSKELETAL
Atlantoaxial instability
Hip dysplasia
Slipped capital femoral epiphyses
Avascular hip necrosis
Recurrent joint dislocations (shoulder, knee, elbow, thumb)

ENDOCRINE
Congenital or acquired hypothyroidism
Diabetes mellitus
Infertility
Obesity
Hyperthyroidism

HEMATOLOGIC
Transient myeloproliferative syndrome
Acute lymphocytic leukemia
Acute myelogenous leukemia

GASTROINTESTINAL
Celiac disease
Delayed tooth eruption
Respiratory
Obstructed sleep apnea
Frequent infections (sinusitis, nasopharyngitis, pneumonia)

CUTANEOUS
Hyperkeratosis
Seborrhea
Xerosis
Perigenital folliculitis

| Table 98.6 | Developmental Milestones |

	CHILDREN WITH DOWN SYNDROME		UNAFFECTED CHILDREN	
Milestone	Average (mo)	Range (mo)	Average (mo)	Range (mo)
Smiling	2	1.5-3	1	1.5-3
Rolling over	6	2-12	5	2-10
Sitting	9	6-18	7	5-9
Crawling	11	7-21	8	6-11
Creeping	13	8-25	10	7-13
Standing	10	10-32	11	8-16
Walking	20	12-45	13	8-18
Talking, words	14	9-30	10	6-14
Talking, sentences	24	18-46	21	14-32

From Levine MD, Carey WB, Crocker AC, editors: *Developmental-behavioral pediatrics*, ed 2, Philadelphia, 1992, Saunders.

| Table 98.7 | Self-Help Skills |

	DOWN SYNDROME CHILDREN		UNAFFECTED CHILDREN	
Skill	Average (mo)	Range (mo)	Average (mo)	Range (mo)
EATING				
Finger feeding	12	8-28	8	6-16
Using spoon/fork	20	12-40	13	8-20
TOILET TRAINING				
Bladder	48	20-95	32	18-60
Bowel	42	28-90	29	16-48
DRESSING				
Undressing	40	29-72	32	22-42
Putting clothes on	58	38-98	47	34-58

From Levine MD, Carey WB, Crocker AC, editors: *Developmental-behavioral pediatrics*, ed 2, Philadelphia, 1992, Saunders.

vs 70% in the triple screen. Both tests have a 5% false-positive rate. There is a method of screening during the 1st trimester using fetal nuchal translucency (NT) thickness that can be done alone or in conjunction with maternal serum β-hCG and pregnancy-associated plasma protein-A (PAPP-A). In the 1st trimester, NT alone can detect ≤70% of Down syndrome pregnancies, but with β-hCG and PAPP-A, the detection rate increases to 87%. If both 1st- and 2nd-trimester screens are combined using NT and biochemical profiles (integrated screen), the detection rate increases to 95%. If only 1st-trimester quad screening is done, maternal serum α-fetoprotein (which is decreased in affected pregnancies) is recommended as a 2nd-trimester follow-up.

Detection of cell-free fetal DNA in maternal plasma is also diagnostic and replacing conventional 1st- and 2nd-trimester screens. The non-invasive detection of fetal trisomy 21 by analyzing cell-free fetal DNA in maternal serum is an important advance in prenatal diagnosis of Down syndrome. Next-generation DNA sequencing has reduced the cost of this procedure, which has a high degree of accuracy (98% detection rate) and applicability. The prenatal screens are also useful for other trisomies, although the detection rates may be different from those given for Down syndrome. Current tests can detect microdeletions including 22q11.2 deletion syndrome, Angelman syndrome, Prader Willi syndrome deletion, cri du chat syndrome, Williams syndrome, and 1p36.3 deletion syndrome. Importantly, especially for microdeletions, cell-free noninvasive prenatal testing (NIPT) should be considered

Table 98.8	Health Supervision for Children With Down Syndrome	
CONDITION	**TIME TO SCREEN**	**COMMENT**
Congenital heart disease	Birth; by pediatric cardiologist Young adult for acquired valve disease	50% risk of congenital heart disease; increased risk for pulmonary hypertension
Strabismus, cataracts, nystagmus	Birth or by 6 mo; by pediatric ophthalmologist **Check vision annually**	Cataracts occur in 15%, refractive errors in 50%
Hearing impairment or loss	Birth or by 3 mo with auditory brainstem response or otoacoustic emission testing; check hearing q6mo up to 3 yr if tympanic membrane is not visualized; **annually thereafter**	Risk for congenital hearing loss plus 50–70% risk of serous otitis media
Constipation	Birth	Increased risk for Hirschsprung disease
Celiac disease	At 2 yr or with symptoms	Screen with IgA and tissue transglutaminase antibodies
Hematologic disease	At birth and in adolescence or if symptoms develop	Increased risk for neonatal polycythemia (18%), leukemoid reaction, leukemia (<1%)
Hypothyroidism	Birth; repeat at 6-12 mo and **annually**	Congenital (1%) and acquired (5%)
Growth and development	At each visit Use Down syndrome growth curves	Discuss school placement options Proper diet to avoid obesity
Obstructive sleep apnea	Start at ~1 yr and at each visit	Monitor for snoring, restless sleep
Atlantoaxial subluxation or instability (incidence 10–30%)	At each visit by history and physical exam Radiographs at 3-5 yr or when planning to participate in contact sports Radiographs indicated wherever neurologic symptoms are present even if transient (neck pain, torticollis, gait disturbances, weakness) Many are asymptomatic	Special Olympics recommendations are to screen for high-risk sports, e.g., diving, swimming, contact sports
Gynecologic care	Adolescent girls	Menstruation and contraception issues
Recurrent infections	When present	Check IgG subclass and IgA levels
Psychiatric, behavioral disorders	At each visit	Depression, anxiety, obsessive-compulsive disorder, schizophrenia seem in 10–17% Autism spectrum disorder in 5–10% Early-onset Alzheimer disease

IgA, Immunoglobulin A; IgG, immunoglobulin G.
Data from Committee on Genetics: Health supervision for children with Down syndrome, *Pediatrics* 107:442–449, 2001; and Baum RA, Spader M, Nash PL, et al: Primary care of children and adolescents with Down syndrome: an update, *Curr Probl Pediatr Adolesc Health Care* 38:235–268, 2008.

primarily for screening tests and follow-up invasive testing (e.g., amniocentesis) pursued for definitive diagnosis.

In approximately 95% of the cases of Down syndrome, there are 3 copies of chromosome 21. The origin of the supernumerary chromosome 21 is maternal in 97% of the cases as a result of errors in meiosis. The majority of these occur in maternal meiosis I (90%). Approximately 1% of persons with trisomy 21 are mosaics, with some cells having 46 chromosomes, and another 4% have a **translocation** that involves chromosome 21. The majority of translocations in Down syndrome are fusions at the centromere between chromosomes 13, 14, 15, 21, and 22, known as *robertsonian translocations*. The translocations can be de novo or inherited. Very rarely is Down syndrome diagnosed in a patient with only a part of the long arm of chromosome 21 in triplicate (**partial trisomy**). Isochromosomes and ring chromosomes are other rarer causes of trisomy 21. Down syndrome patients without a visible chromosome abnormality are the least common. It is not possible to distinguish the phenotypes of persons with full trisomy 21 and those with a translocation. Representative genes on chromosome 21 and their potential effects on development are noted in Table 98.9. Patients who are mosaic tend to have a milder phenotype.

Chromosome analysis is indicated in every person suspected of having Down syndrome. If a translocation is identified, parental chromosome studies must be performed to determine whether one of the parents is a translocation carrier, which carries a high recurrence risk for having another affected child. That parent might also have other family members at risk. Translocation (21;21) carriers have a 100% recurrence risk for a chromosomally abnormal child, and other robertsonian translocations,

such as t(14;21), have a 5–7% recurrence risk when transmitted by females. Genomic dosage imbalance contributes through direct and indirect pathways to the Down syndrome phenotype and its phenotypic variation.

Tables 98.10 and 98.11 provide more information on other aneuploidies and partial autosomal aneuploidies (Figs. 98.11 to 98.14).

Bibliography is available at Expert Consult.

98.3 Abnormalities of Chromosome Structure

Carlos A. Bacino and Brendan Lee

TRANSLOCATIONS

Translocations, which involve the transfer of material from one chromosome to another, occur with a frequency of 1 in 500 liveborn human infants. They may be inherited from a carrier parent or appear de novo, with no other affected family member. Translocations are usually reciprocal or robertsonian, involving 2 chromosomes (Fig. 98.15).

Reciprocal translocations are the result of breaks in nonhomologous chromosomes, with reciprocal exchange of the broken segments. Carriers of a reciprocal translocation are usually phenotypically normal but are at an increased risk for miscarriage caused by transmission of unbalanced reciprocal translocations and for bearing chromosomally abnormal offspring. Unbalanced translocations are the result of abnormalities in

Table 98.9	Genes Localized to Chromosome 21 That May Affect Brain Development, Neuronal Loss, and Alzheimer-Type Neuropathology		
SYMBOL	**NAME**	**POSSIBLE EFFECT IN DOWN SYNDROME**	**FUNCTION**
SIM2	Single-minded homolog 2	Brain development	Required for synchronized cell division and establishment of proper cell lineage
DYRK1A	Dual-specificity tyrosine-(Y)-phosphorylation regulated kinase 1A	Brain development	Expressed during neuroblast proliferation Believed important homolog in regulating cell-cycle kinetics during cell division
GART	Phosphoribosylglycinamide formyltransferase Phosphoribosylglycinamide synthetase Phosphoribosylaminoimidazole synthetase	Brain development	Expressed during prenatal development of the cerebellum
PCP4	Purkinje cell protein 4	Brain development	Function unknown but found exclusively in the brain and most abundantly in the cerebellum
DSCAM	Down syndrome cell adhesion molecule	Brain development and possible candidate gene for congenital heart disease	Expressed in all molecule regions of the brain and believed to have a role in axonal outgrowth during development of the nervous system
GRIK1	Glutamate receptor, ionotropic kainite1	Neuronal loss	Function unknown, found in the cortex in fetal and early postnatal life and in adult primates, most concentrated in pyramidal cells in the cortex
APP	Amyloid beta (A4) precursor protein (protease nexin-II, Alzheimer disease)	Alzheimer type neuropathy	Seems to be involved in plasticity, neurite outgrowth, and neuroprotection
S100B	S100 calcium binding protein β (neural)	Alzheimer type neuropathy	Stimulates glial formation
SOD1	Superoxide dismutase 1, soluble (amyotrophic lateral sclerosis, adult)	Accelerated aging?	Scavenges free superoxide molecules in the cell and might accelerate aging by producing hydrogen peroxide and oxygen

Table 98.10	Other Rare Aneuploidies and Partial Autosomal Aneuploidies	
DISORDER	**KARYOTYPE**	**CLINICAL MANIFESTATIONS**
Trisomy 8	47,XX/XY,+8	Growth and mental deficiency are variable. The majority of patients are mosaics. Deep palmar and plantar furrows are characteristic. Joint contractures
Trisomy 9	47,XX/XY,+9	The majority of patients are mosaics. Clinical features include craniofacial (high forehead, microphthalmia, low-set malformed ears, bulbous nose) and skeletal (joint contractures) malformations and heart defects (60%).
Trisomy 16	47,XX/XY,+16	The most commonly observed autosomal aneuploidy in spontaneous abortion; the recurrence risk is negligible.
Tetrasomy 12p	46,XX[12]/46,XX, +i(12p)[8] (mosaicism for an isochromosome 12p)	Known as Pallister-Killian syndrome Sparse anterior scalp hair (more so temporal region), eyebrows, and eyelashes; prominent forehead; chubby cheeks; long philtrum with thin upper lip and cupid-bow configuration; polydactyly; streaks of hyper- and hypopigmentation

Table 98.11	Findings That May Be Present in Trisomy 13 and Trisomy 18
TRISOMY 13	**TRISOMY 18**

TRISOMY 13

HEAD AND FACE
Scalp defects (e.g., cutis aplasia)
Microphthalmia, corneal abnormalities
Cleft lip and palate in 60–80% of cases
Microcephaly
Microphthalmia
Sloping forehead
Holoprosencephaly (arrhinencephaly)
Capillary hemangiomas
Deafness

TRISOMY 18

Small and premature appearance
Tight palpebral fissures
Narrow nose and hypoplastic nasal alae
Narrow bifrontal diameter
Prominent occiput
Micrognathia
Cleft lip or palate
Microcephaly

CHEST
Congenital heart disease (e.g., VSD, PDA, ASD) in 80% of cases
Thin posterior ribs (missing ribs)

Congenital heart disease (e.g., VSD, PDA, ASD)
Short sternum, small nipples

Continued

Table 98.11	Findings That May Be Present in Trisomy 13 and Trisomy 18—cont'd
TRISOMY 13	**TRISOMY 18**
EXTREMITIES	
Overlapping of fingers and toes (clinodactyly) Polydactyly Hypoplastic nails, hyperconvex nails	Limited hip abduction Clinodactyly and overlapping fingers; index over 3rd, 5th over 4th; closed fist Rocker-bottom feet Hypoplastic nails
GENERAL	
Severe developmental delays and prenatal and postnatal growth restriction Renal abnormalities Survival (see Table 98.3)	Severe developmental delays and prenatal and postnatal growth restriction Premature birth, polyhydramnios Inguinal or abdominal hernias Survival (see Table 98.3)

ASD, Atrial septal defect; PDA, patent ductus arteriosus; VSD, ventricular septal defect.
From Behrman RE, Kliegman RM: *Nelson essentials of pediatrics*, ed 4, Philadelphia, 2002, Saunders, p 142.

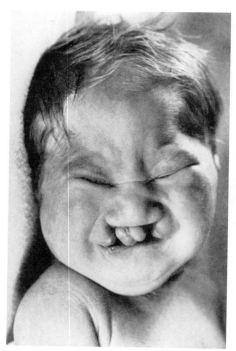

Fig. 98.11 Facial appearance of a child with trisomy 13. *(From Wiedemann HR, Kunze J, Dibbern H: Atlas of clinical syndromes: a visual guide to diagnosis, ed 3, St Louis, 1989, Mosby.)*

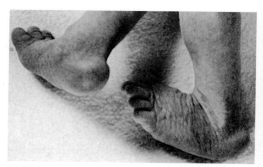

Fig. 98.13 Trisomy 18: rocker-bottom feet (protruding calcanei). *(From Wiedemann HR, Kunze J, Dibbern H: Atlas of clinical syndromes: a visual guide to diagnosis, ed 3, St Louis, 1989, Mosby.)*

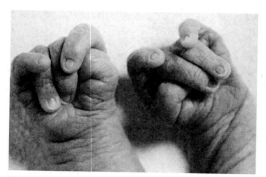

Fig. 98.12 Trisomy 18: overlapping fingers and hypoplastic nails. *(From Wiedemann HR, Kunze J, Dibbern H: Atlas of clinical syndromes: a visual guide to diagnosis, ed 3, St Louis, 1989, Mosby.)*

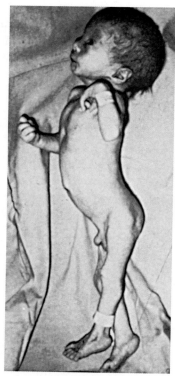

Fig. 98.14 Male infant with trisomy 18 at age 4 days. Note prominent occiput, micrognathia, low-set ears, short sternum, narrow pelvis, prominent calcaneus, and flexion abnormalities of the fingers.

the segregation or crossover of the translocation carrier chromosomes in the germ cells.

Robertsonian translocations involve 2 acrocentric chromosomes (chromosomes 13, 14, 15, 21, and 22) that fuse near the centromeric region with a subsequent loss of the short arms. Because the short arms of all 5 pairs of acrocentric chromosomes have multiple copies of genes encoding for ribosomal RNA, loss of the short arm of 2 acrocentric chromosomes has no deleterious effect. The resulting karyotype has only 45 chromosomes, including the translocated chromosome, which consists of the long arms of the 2 fused chromosomes. Carriers of robertsonian translocations are usually phenotypically normal. However, they are at increased risk for miscarriage and unbalanced translocations in phenotypically abnormal offspring.

In some rare instances, translocations can involve 3 or more chromosomes, as seen in complex rearrangements. Another, less common type is the insertional translocation. **Insertional translocations** result from a piece of chromosome material that breaks away and later is reinserted inside the same chromosome at a different site or inserted in another chromosome.

INVERSIONS

An inversion requires that a single chromosome break at 2 points; the broken piece is then inverted and joined into the same chromosome. Inversions occur in 1 in 100 live births. There are 2 types of inversions: pericentric and paracentric. In **pericentric inversions** the breaks are in the 2 opposite arms of the chromosome and include the centromere. They are usually discovered because they change the position of the centromere. The breaks in **paracentric inversions** occur in only 1 arm. Carriers of inversions are usually phenotypically normal, but they are at increased risk for miscarriages, typically in paracentric inversions, and chromosomally abnormal offspring in pericentric inversions.

DELETIONS AND DUPLICATIONS

Deletions involve loss of chromosome material and, depending on their location, can be classified as **terminal** (at the end of chromosomes) or **interstitial** (within the arms of a chromosome). They may be isolated or may occur along with a duplication of another chromosome segment. The latter typically occurs in unbalanced reciprocal chromosomal translocation secondary to abnormal crossover or segregation in a translocation or inversion carrier.

A carrier of a deletion is monosomic for the genetic information of the missing segment. Deletions are usually associated with intellectual disability and malformations. The most commonly observed deletions in routine chromosome preparations include 1p–, 4p–, 5p–, 9p–, 11p–, 13q–, 18p–, 18q–, and 21q– (Table 98.12 and Fig. 98.16), all distal or terminal deletions of the short or the long arms of chromosomes. Deletions may be observed in routine chromosome preparations, and deletions and translocations larger than 5-10 Mbp are usually visible microscopically.

High-resolution banding techniques, FISH, and molecular studies such as aCGH can reveal deletions that are too small to be seen in ordinary or routine chromosome spreads (see Fig. 98.7). **Microdeletions** involve loss of small chromosome regions, the largest of which are detectable only with prophase chromosome studies and molecular methods. For submicroscopic deletions, the missing piece can only be detected using molecular methodologies such as DNA-based studies (e.g., aCGH, FISH). The presence of extra genetic material from the same chromosome is referred to as **duplication**. Duplications can also be sporadic or result from abnormal segregation in translocation or inversion carriers.

Microdeletions and microduplications usually involve regions that include several genes, so the affected individuals can have a distinctive phenotype depending on the number of genes involved. When such a deletion involves more than a single gene, the condition is referred to as a **contiguous gene deletion syndrome** (Table 98.13). With the advent of clinically available aCGH, a large number of duplications, most of them microduplications, have been uncovered. Many of those **microduplication syndromes** are the reciprocal duplications of the known deletions or microdeletion counterparts and have distinctive clinical features (Table 98.14).

Subtelomeric regions are often involved in chromosome rearrangements that cannot be visualized using routine cytogenetics. *Telomeres,* which are the distal ends of the chromosomes, are gene-rich regions. The distal structure of the telomeres is essentially common to all chromosomes, but proximal to these are unique regions known as *subtelomeres,* which typically are involved in deletions and other chromosome rearrangements. Small subtelomeric deletions, duplications, or rearrangements (translocations, inversions) may be relatively common in children with nonspecific intellectual disability and minor anomalies. Subtelomeric rearrangements have been found in 3–7% of children with moderate to severe intellectual disability and 0.5% of those with mild intellectual disability and can be detected by aCGH studies.

Telomere mutations and length abnormalities have also been associated with dyskeratosis congenita and other aplastic anemia syndromes, as well as pulmonary or hepatic fibrosis. Both the subtelomeric rearrangements and the microdeletion and microduplication syndromes are typically diagnosed by molecular techniques such as aCGH and multiple ligation-dependent primer amplification studies. Recent studies show that aCGH can detect 14–18% of abnormalities in patients who previously had normal chromosome studies.

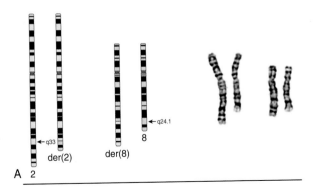

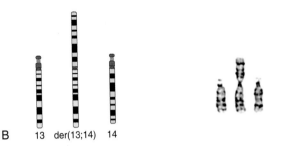

Fig. 98.15 A, Schematic diagram *(left)* and partial G-banded karyotype *(right)* of a reciprocal translocation between chromosome 2 *(blue)* and chromosome 8 *(pink)*. The breakpoints are on the long *(q)* arm of both chromosomes at bands 2q33 and 8q24.1, with the reciprocal exchange of material between the derivative *(der)* chromosomes 2 and 8. This translocation is balanced, with no net gain or loss of material. The nomenclature for this exchange is t(2;8)(q33:q24.1). **B,** Schematic diagram *(left)* and partial G-banded karyotype *(right)* of a robertsonian translocation between chromosomes 13 *(blue)* and 14 *(pink)*. The breakpoints are at the centromere (band q10) of both chromosomes, with fusion of the long arms into a single derivative chromosome and loss of the short *(p)* arm material. The nomenclature for this exchange is der(13;14) (q10;q10).

INSERTIONS

Insertions occur when a piece of a chromosome broken at 2 points is incorporated into a break in another part of a chromosome. A total of 3 breakpoints are then required, and they can occur between 2 or within

Table 98.12	Common Deletions and Their Clinical Manifestations
DELETION	**CLINICAL ABNORMALITIES**
4p–	Wolf-Hirschhorn syndrome. The main features are a typical "Greek helmet" facies secondary to ocular hypertelorism, prominent glabella, and frontal bossing; microcephaly, dolichocephaly, hypoplasia of the orbits, ptosis, strabismus, nystagmus, bilateral epicanthic folds, cleft lip and palate, beaked nose with prominent bridge, hypospadias, cardiac malformations, and intellectual disability.
5p–	Cri du chat syndrome. The main features are hypotonia, short stature, characteristic shrill cry in the first few weeks of life (also called cat's cry syndrome), microcephaly with protruding metopic suture, hypertelorism, bilateral epicanthic folds, high arched palate, wide and flat nasal bridge, and intellectual disability.
9p–	The main features are craniofacial dysmorphic features with trigonocephaly, slanted palpebral fissures, discrete exophthalmos secondary to supraorbital hypoplasia, arched eyebrows, flat and wide nasal bridge, short neck with low hairline, genital anomalies, long fingers and toes with extra flexion creases, cardiac malformations, and intellectual disability.
13q–	The main features are low birthweight, failure to thrive, microcephaly, and severe intellectual disability. Facial features include high, wide nasal bridge; hypertelorism; ptosis; and micrognathia. Ocular malformations are common (retinoblastoma). The hands have hypoplastic or absent thumbs and syndactyly.
18p–	A few patients (15%) are severely affected and have cephalic and ocular malformations: holoprosencephaly, cleft lip and palate, ptosis, epicanthal folds, and varying degrees of intellectual disability. Most (80%) have only minor malformations and mild intellectual disability.
18q–	The main features are growth deficiency and hypotonia with a "froglike" position with the legs flexed, externally rotated, and in hyperabduction. The face is characteristic, with depressed midface and apparent protrusion of the mandible, deep-set eyes, short upper lip, and everted lower lip ("carplike" mouth); antihelix of the ears is very prominent. Varying degrees of intellectual disability and belligerent personality are present. Myelination abnormalities occur in the central nervous system.

Table 98.13	Microdeletion and Contiguous Gene Syndromes and Their Clinical Manifestations	
DELETION	**SYNDROME**	**CLINICAL MANIFESTATIONS**
1p36	1p deletion	Growth restriction, dysmorphic features with midface hypoplasia, straight thin eyebrows, pointy chin, sensorineural hearing loss, progressive cardiomyopathy, hypothyroidism, seizures, intellectual disability
5q35	Sotos (50% are deletions of *NSD1* gene in Asians but only 6% in whites)	Overgrowth, macrocephaly, prominent forehead, prominence of extraaxial fluid spaces on brain imaging, large hands and feet, hypotonia, clumsiness, mental disabilities
6p25	Axenfeld-Rieger	Axenfeld-Rieger malformation, hearing loss, congenital heart defects, dental anomalies, developmental delays, facial dysmorphism
7q11.23	Williams	Round face with full cheeks and lips, long philtrum, stellate pattern in iris, strabismus, supravalvular aortic stenosis and other cardiac malformations, varying degrees of intellectual disability, friendly personality
8p11	8p11	Kallmann syndrome type 2 (hypogonadotropic hypogonadism and anosmia), spherocytosis (deletions of ankyrin 1), multiple congenital anomalies, intellectual disability
8q24.1-q24.13	Langer-Giedion or trichorhinophalangeal type II	Sparse hair, multiple cone-shaped epiphyses, multiple cartilaginous exostoses, bulbous nasal tip, thickened alar cartilage, upturned nares, prominent philtrum, large protruding ears, mild intellectual disability
9q22	Gorlin	Multiple basal cell carcinomas, odontogenic keratocysts, palmoplantar pits, calcification falx cerebri
9q34	9q34 deletion	Distinct face with synophrys, anteverted nares, tented upper lip, protruding tongue, midface hypoplasia, conotruncal heart defects, intellectual disability
10p12-p13	DiGeorge type 2	Many of the DiGeorge type 1 and velocardiofacial type 1 features (conotruncal defects, immunodeficiency, hypoparathyroidism, dysmorphic features)
11p11.2	Potocki-Shaffer	Multiple exostoses, parietal foramina, craniosynostosis, facial dysmorphism, syndactyly, intellectual disability
11p13	WAGR	Hypernephroma (*Wilms* tumor), aniridia, male genital hypoplasia of varying degrees, gonadoblastoma, long face, upward-slanting palpebral fissures, ptosis, beaked nose, low-set poorly formed auricles, intellectual disability (retardation)
11q24.1-11qter	Jacobsen	Growth restriction, intellectual disability, cardiac and digit anomalies, thrombocytopenia
15q11-q13 (paternal)	Prader-Willi	Severe hypotonia and feeding difficulties at birth, voracious appetite and obesity in infancy, short stature (responsive to growth hormone), small hands and feet, hypogonadism, intellectual disability
15q11-q13 (maternal)	Angelman	Hypotonia, feeding difficulties, gastroesophageal reflux, fair hair and skin, midface hypoplasia, prognathism, seizures, tremors, ataxia, sleep disturbances, inappropriate laughter, poor or absent speech, severe intellectual disability

Continued

Table 98.13	Microdeletion and Contiguous Gene Syndromes and Their Clinical Manifestations—cont'd	
DELETION	**SYNDROME**	**CLINICAL MANIFESTATIONS**
16p13.3	Rubinstein-Taybi	Microcephaly, ptosis, beaked nose with low-lying philtrum, broad thumbs and large toes, intellectual disability
17p11.2	Smith-Magenis	Brachycephaly, midfacial hypoplasia, prognathism, myopia, cleft palate, short stature, severe behavioral problems, intellectual disability
17p13.3	Miller-Dieker	Microcephaly, lissencephaly, pachygyria, narrow forehead, hypoplastic male external genitals, growth restriction, seizures, profound intellectual disability
20p12	Alagille	Bile duct paucity with cholestasis; heart defects, particularly pulmonary artery stenosis; ocular abnormalities (posterior embryotoxon); skeletal defects such as butterfly vertebrae; long nose
22q11.2	Velocardiofacial-DiGeorge	Conotruncal cardiac anomalies, cleft palate, velopharyngeal incompetence, hypoplasia or agenesis of thymus and parathyroid glands, hypocalcemia, hypoplasia of auricle, learning disabilities, psychiatric disorders
22q13.3 deletion		Hypotonia, developmental delay, normal or accelerated growth, severe expressive language deficits, autistic behavior
Xp21.2-p21.3		Duchenne muscular dystrophy, retinitis pigmentosa, adrenal hypoplasia, intellectual disability, glycerol kinase deficiency
Xp22.2-p22.3		Ichthyosis, Kallmann syndrome, intellectual disability, chondrodysplasia punctata
Xp22.3	MLS	*Microphthalmia, linear skin defects, poikiloderma, congenital heart defects, seizures, intellectual disability*

Table 98.14	Microduplications and Their Clinical Manifestations	
DUPLICATION CHROMOSOME REGION	**DISEASE REGION**	**CLINICAL FEATURES**
1q21.1		Macrocephaly, DD, learning disabilities
3q29		Mild to moderate MR, microcephaly
7q11.23	Williams syndrome	DD and severe expressive language disorder, autistic features, subtle dysmorphisms
15q13.3	Prader-Willi/Angelman syndrome	DD, MR, autistic features in duplications of maternal origin
15q24		Growth restriction, DD, microcephaly, digital anomalies, hypospadias, connective tissue abnormalities
16p11.2		FTT, severe DD, short stature, GH deficiency, dysmorphic features
17p11.2	Potocki-Lupski syndrome	Hypotonia, cardiovascular anomalies, FTT, DD, verbal apraxia, autism, anxiety
17q21.31		Severe DD, microcephaly, short and broad digits, dysmorphic features
22q11.2	Velocardiofacial-DiGeorge syndrome	Cardiovascular defects, velopharyngeal insufficiency
Xq28	*MECP2* gene (Rett syndrome)	In males: infantile hypotonia, immune deficiency, dysmorphic features, DD, speech delay, autistic behavior, regression in childhood

DD, Developmental delay; ID, intellectual disability; FTT, failure to thrive; GH, growth hormone; MR, mental retardation.

1 chromosome. A form of nonreciprocal translocation, insertions are rare. Insertion carriers are at risk of having offspring with deletions or duplications of the inserted segment.

ISOCHROMOSOMES

Isochromosomes consist of 2 copies of the same chromosome arm joined through a single centromere and forming mirror images of one another. The most commonly reported autosomal isochromosomes tend to involve chromosomes with small arms. Some of the more common chromosome arms involved in this formation include 5p, 8p, 9p, 12p, 18p, and 18q. There is also a common isochromosome abnormality seen in long arm of the X chromosome and associated with Turner syndrome. Individuals who have 1 isochromosome X within 46 chromosomes are monosomic for genes in the lost short arm and trisomic for the genes present in the long arm of the X chromosome.

MARKER AND RING CHROMOSOMES

Marker chromosomes are rare and are usually chromosome fragments that are too small to be identified by conventional cytogenetics; they usually occur in addition to the normal 46 chromosomes. Most are sporadic (70%); mosaicism is often (50%) noted because of the mitotic instability of the marker chromosome. The incidence in newborn infants is 1 in 3,300, and the incidence in persons with intellectual disability is 1 in 300. The associated phenotype ranges from normal to severely abnormal, depending on the amount of chromosome material and number of genes included in the fragment.

Ring chromosomes, which are found for all human chromosomes, are rare. A ring chromosome is formed when both ends of a chromosome are deleted and the ends are then joined to form a ring. Depending on the amount of chromosome material that is lacking or in excess (if the ring is in addition to the normal chromosomes),

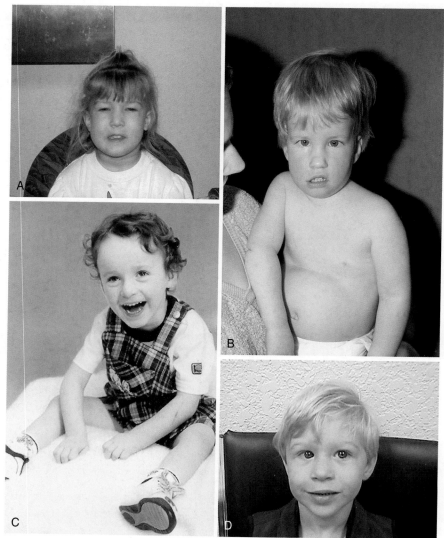

Fig. 98.16 A, Child with velocardiofacial syndrome (deletion 22q11.2). **B,** Child with Prader-Willi syndrome (deletion 15q11-13). **C,** Child with Angelman syndrome (deletion 15q11-13). **D,** Child with Williams syndrome (deletion 7q11.23). *(From Lin RL, Cherry AM, Bangs CD, et al: FISHing for answers: the use of molecular cytogenetic techniques in adolescent medicine practice. In Hyme HE, Greydanus D, editors: Genetic disorders in adolescents: state of the art reviews. Adolescent medicine, Philadelphia, 2002, Hanley and Belfus, pp 305–313.)*

a patient with a ring chromosome can appear normal or nearly normal or can have intellectual disability and multiple congenital anomalies.

Marker and ring chromosomes can be found in the cells of solid tumors of children the cells of whose organs do not contain this additional chromosomal material.

Bibliography is available at Expert Consult.

98.4 Sex Chromosome Aneuploidy

Carlos A. Bacino and Brendan Lee

About 1 in 400 males and 1 in 650 females have some form of sex chromosome abnormality. Considered together, sex chromosome abnormalities are the most common chromosome abnormalities seen in liveborn infants, children, and adults. Sex chromosome abnormalities can be either structural or numerical and can be present in all cells or in a mosaic form. Those affected with these abnormalities might have few or no physical or developmental problems (Table 98.15).

TURNER SYNDROME

Turner syndrome is a condition characterized by complete or partial monosomy of the X chromosome and defined by a combination of phenotypic features (Table 98.16). Half the patients with Turner syndrome have a 45,X chromosome complement. The other half exhibit mosaicism and varied structural abnormalities of the X or Y chromosome. Maternal age is not a predisposing factor for children with 45,X. Turner syndrome occurs in approximately 1 in 5,000 female live births. In 75% of patients, the lost sex chromosome is of paternal origin (whether an X or a Y). 45,X is one of the chromosome abnormalities most often associated with spontaneous abortion. It has been estimated that 95–99% of 45,X conceptions are miscarried.

Table 98.15	Sex Chromosome Abnormalities	
DISORDER	**KARYOTYPE**	**APPROXIMATE INCIDENCE**
Klinefelter syndrome	47,XXY 48,XXXY Other (48,XXYY; 49,XXXYY; mosaics)	1/580 males 1/50,000-1/80,000 male births
XYY syndrome	47,XYY	1/800-1,000 males
Other X or Y chromosome abnormalities		1/1,500 males
XX males	46,XX	1/20,000 males
Turner syndrome	45,X Variants and mosaics	1/2,500-1/5,000 females
Trisomy X	47,XXX 48,XXXX and 49,XXXXX	1/1,000 females Rare
Other X chromosome abnormalities		1/3,000 females
XY females	46,XY	1/20,000 females

Table 98.16	Signs Associated With Turner Syndrome

Short stature
Congenital lymphedema
Horseshoe kidneys
Patella dislocation
Increased carrying angle of elbow (cubitus valgus)
Madelung deformity (chondrodysplasia of distal radial epiphysis)
Congenital hip dislocation
Scoliosis
Widespread nipples
Shield chest
Redundant nuchal skin (in utero cystic hygroma)
Low posterior hairline
Coarctation of aorta
Bicuspid aortic valve
Cardiac conduction abnormalities
Hypoplastic left heart syndrome and other left-sided heart abnormalities
Gonadal dysgenesis (infertility, primary amenorrhea)
Gonadoblastoma (increased risk if Y chromosome material is present)
Learning disabilities (nonverbal perceptual motor and visuospatial skills) (in 70%)
Developmental delay (in 10%)
Social awkwardness
Hypothyroidism (acquired in 15–30%)
Type 2 diabetes mellitus (insulin resistance)
Strabismus
Cataracts
Red-green color blindness (as in males)
Recurrent otitis media
Sensorineural hearing loss
Inflammatory bowel disease
Celiac disease (increased incidence)

Clinical findings in the newborns can include small size for gestational age, webbing of the neck, protruding ears, and lymphedema of the hands and feet, although many newborns are phenotypically normal (Fig. 98.17). Older children and adults have short stature and exhibit variable dysmorphic features. Congenital heart defects (40%) and structural renal anomalies (60%) are common. The most common heart defects are bicuspid aortic valves, coarctation of the aorta, aortic stenosis,

and mitral valve prolapse. The gonads are generally streaks of fibrous tissue (**gonadal dysgenesis**). There is primary amenorrhea and lack of secondary sex characteristics. These children should receive regular endocrinologic testing (see Chapter 604). Most patients tend to be of normal intelligence, but intellectual disability is seen in up to 6% of affected children. They are also at increased risk for behavioral problems and deficiencies in spatial and motor perception. Guidelines for health supervision for children with Turner syndrome are published by the American Academy of Pediatrics (AAP) and include pubertal induction, as well as treatment with growth hormone and oxandrolone.

Patients with **45,X/46,XY mosaicism** can have Turner syndrome, although this form of mosaicism can also be associated with male pseudohermaphroditism, male or female genitalia in association with mixed gonadal dysgenesis, or a normal male phenotype. This variant is estimated to represent approximately 6% of patients with mosaic Turner syndrome. Some of the patients with Turner syndrome phenotype and a Y cell line exhibit masculinization. Phenotypic females with 45,X/46,XY mosaicism have a 15–30% risk of developing **gonadoblastoma**. The risk for the patients with a male phenotype and external testes is not so high, but tumor surveillance is nevertheless recommended. AAP has recommended the use of FISH analysis to look for Y chromosome mosaicism in all 45,X patients. If Y chromosome material is identified, laparoscopic gonadectomy is recommended.

Noonan syndrome shares many clinical features with Turner syndrome and was formerly called *pseudo-Turner syndrome*, although it is an autosomal dominant disorder resulting from mutations in several genes involved in the RAS-MAPK (mitogen-activated protein kinase) pathway. The most common of these is *PTPN11* (50%), which encodes a protein-tyrosine phosphatase (SHP-2) on chromosome 12q24.1. Other genes include *SOS1* in 10–13%, *RAF1* in 3–17%, *RITI* in 5%, *KRAS* <5%, *BRAF* <2%, *MAP2K* <2%, and *NRAS* (only few reported families). Overlapping phenotypes are seen in LEOPARD (lentigines, electrocardiographic abnormalities, ocular hypertelorism, pulmonary stenosis, abnormalities of genitalia, retardation of growth, deafness) syndrome, cardiofaciocutaneous (CFC) syndrome, and Costello syndrome; these are Noonan-related disorders. Features common to Noonan syndrome include short stature, low posterior hairline, shield chest, congenital heart disease, and a short or webbed neck (Table 98.17). In contrast to Turner syndrome, Noonan syndrome affects both sexes and has a different pattern of congenital heart disease, typically involving right-sided lesions.

KLINEFELTER SYNDROME

Persons with Klinefelter syndrome are phenotypically male; this syndrome is the most common cause of hypogonadism and infertility in males and the most common sex chromosome aneuploidy in humans (see Chapter 601). Eighty percent of children with Klinefelter syndrome have a male karyotype with an extra chromosome X-47,XXY. The remaining 20% have multiple sex chromosome aneuploidies (48,XXXY; 48,XXYY; 49,XXXXY), mosaicism (46,XY/47,XXY), or structurally abnormal X chromosomes; the greater the aneuploidy, the more severe the mental impairment and dysmorphism. Early studies showed a birth prevalence of approximately 1 in 1,000 males, but more recent studies suggest that the prevalence of 47,XXY appears has increased to approximately 1 in 580 liveborn males; the reasons for this are still unknown but hypothesized to be the result of environmental factors acting in spermatogenesis. Errors in paternal nondisjunction in meiosis I account for half the cases.

Puberty commences at the normal age, but the testes remain small. Patients develop secondary sex characters late, and 50% ultimately develop gynecomastia. They have taller stature. Because many patients with Klinefelter syndrome are phenotypically normal until puberty, the syndrome often goes undiagnosed until they reach adulthood, when their infertility leads to identification. Patients with 46,XY/47,XXY have a better prognosis for testicular function. Their intelligence shows variability and ranges from above to below average. Persons with Klinefelter syndrome can show behavioral problems, learning disabilities, and deficits in language. Problems with self-esteem often occur in adolescents and adults. Substance abuse, depression, and anxiety have

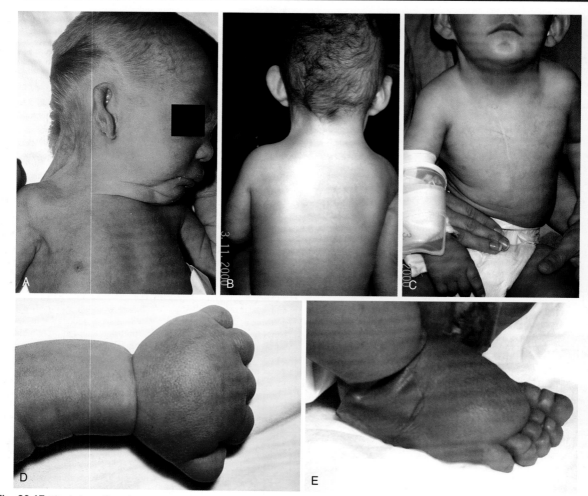

Fig. 98.17 Physical manifestations associated with turner syndrome. **A,** This newborn shows a webbed neck with low hairline, shield chest with widespread nipples, abnormal ears, and micrognathia. **B,** The low-set posterior hairline can be better appreciated in this older child, who also has protruding ears. **C,** In this frontal view, mild webbing of the neck and small, widely spaced nipples are evident, along with a midline scar from prior cardiac surgery. The ears are low set and prominent, protruding forward. **D** and **E,** The newborn shown in **A** also has prominent lymphedema of the hands and feet. *(From Madan-Khetarpal S, Arnold G: Genetic disorders and dysmorphic conditions. In Zitelli BJ, McIntire SC, Nowalk AJ, editors: Zitelli and Davis' atlas of pediatric physical diagnosis, ed 6, Philadelphia, 2012, Elsevier, Fig 1.25.)*

Table 98.17	Signs Associated With Noonan Syndrome
Short stature Failure to thrive (best to use Noonan growth curve) Tall forehead Epicanthal folds Ptosis Blue-green irises Hypertelorism Low nasal bridge, upturned nose Downward-slanting palpebral fissures Myopia Nystagmus Low-set and posteriorly rotated auricles Dental malocclusion Low posterior hairline Short, webbed neck (excessive nuchal skin), cystic hygroma Shield chest	Pectus carinatum superiorly Scoliosis Pigmented villonodular synovitis (polyarticular) Cubitus valgus Pulmonary valve stenosis (dysplastic valve) Hypertrophic cardiomyopathy Atrial septal defect, ventricular septal defect Lymphedema Nevi, lentigines, café au lait spots Cryptorchidism Small penis Delayed puberty Bleeding disorders, including thrombocytopenia and coagulation factor deficiencies Leukemia, myeloproliferative disorders, other malignancies Cognitive delay (*KRAS* mutation)

been reported in adolescents with Klinefelter syndrome. Those who have higher X chromosome counts show impaired cognition. It has been estimated that each additional X chromosome reduces the IQ by 10-15 points, when comparing these individuals with typical siblings. The main effect is seen in language skills and social domains.

47,XYY

The incidence of 47,XYY is approximately 1 in 800-1,000 males, with many cases remaining undiagnosed, because most affected individuals have a normal appearance and normal fertility. The extra Y is the result of nondisjunction at paternal meiosis II. Those with this abnormality have normal intelligence but are at risk for learning disabilities. Behavioral abnormalities, including hyperactive behavior, pervasive developmental disorder, and aggressive behavior, have been reported. Early reports that assigned stigmata of criminality to this disorder have long been disproved.

Bibliography is available at Expert Consult.

98.5 Fragile Chromosome Sites
Carlos A. Bacino and Brendan Lee

Fragile sites are regions of chromosomes that show a tendency for separation, breakage, or attenuation under particular growth conditions. They visually appear as a gap in the staining in chromosome studies. At least 120 chromosomal loci, many of them heritable, have been identified as fragile sites in the human genome (see Table 97.2).

A clinically significant fragile site is on the distal long arm of chromosome Xq27.3 associated with the **fragile X syndrome**. Fragile X syndrome accounts for 3% of males with intellectual disability. There is another fragile site on the X chromosome (FRAXE on Xq28) that has also been implicated in mild intellectual disability. The FRA11B (11q23.3) breakpoints are associated with **Jacobsen syndrome** (condition caused by deletion of the distal long arm of chromosome 11). Fragile sites can also play a role in tumorigenesis. In fragile X syndrome the CGG repeat expansion silences the gene producing **fragile X mental retardation protein (FMRP)** that regulates the translation of multiple mRNAs to specific proteins, thus affecting synaptic function. FMRP

deficiency upregulates the metabotropic glutamate receptor (mGluR) 5 pathway. FMRP deficiency also alters the expression of matrix metalloproteinase (MMP) 9.

The main clinical manifestations of fragile X syndrome in affected males are intellectual disability, autistic behavior, postpubertal macroorchidism, hyperextensible finger joints, and characteristic facial features (Table 98.18). The facial features, which include a long face, large ears, and a prominent square jaw, become more obvious with age. Females affected with fragile X show varying degrees of intellectual disability and/or learning disabilities. Diagnosis of fragile X syndrome is possible by DNA testing that shows an expansion of a triplet DNA repeat inside the *FMR1* gene on the X chromosome >200 repeats. The expansion involves an area of the gene that contains a variable number of trinucleotide (CGG) repeats (typically <50 in unaffected individuals). The larger the triplet repeat expansion, the more significant is the intellectual disability. In cases where the expansion is large, females can also manifest different degrees of intellectual disability. Males with premutation triple repeat expansions (55-200 repeats) have been found to have a adult, late-onset, progressive neurodegenerative disorder known as **fragile X–associated tremor/ataxia syndrome**. Females with premutation triple repeat expansions are at high risk for developing premature ovarian failure (POF).

Table 98.19 outlines therapy of the diverse neuropsychiatric manifestations associated with fragile X syndrome. Inhibitors of mGluR (overexpressed in fragile X) are undergoing clinical trials. In preliminary trials, minocycline (lowers MMP-9) has resulted in short-term improvements in anxiety, mood, and the clinical Global Impression Scale.

Bibliography is available at Expert Consult.

98.6 Mosaicism
Carlos A. Bacino and Brendan Lee

Mosaicism describes an individual or tissue that contains ≥2 different cell lines typically derived from a single zygote and the result of mitotic nondisjunction (see Fig. 98.1). Study of placental tissue from chorionic villus samples collected at or before the 10th wk of gestation has shown that ≥2% of all conceptions are mosaic for a chromosome abnormality.

Table 98.18	Clinical Features of Full and Premutation *FMR1* Alleles			
	PHENOTYPE			
DISORDER	**Cognitive or Behavioral**	**Clinical and Imaging Signs**	**ONSET**	**PENETRANCE**
FULL MUTATION (>200 REPEATS)				
FXS	Developmental delay: mean IQ = 42 in M; IQ is higher if significant residual FMRP is produced (e.g., females and mosaic males or unmethylated full mutations) Autism 20–30% ADHD 80% Anxiety 70–100%	Hypothalamic dysfunction: macroorchidism, 40%* Facial features, 60%,* large cupped ears, elongated face, high arched palate Connective tissue abnormalities: mitral valve prolapse, scoliosis, joint laxity, flat feet Others: seizures (20%), recurrent otitis media (60%), strabismus (8–30%)	Neonate	M 100%
PREMUTATION (55-200 REPEATS)				
Female reproductive symptoms		POF (<40 yr) Early menopause (<45 yr)	Adult/childhood	F 20%[†] F 30%[†]
FXTAS	Cognitive decline, dementia, apathy, disinhibition, irritability, depression	Gait ataxia, intention tremor, parkinsonism, neuropathy, autonomic dysfunction	>50 yr	M 33%[‡] F unknown
Neurodevelopmental disorder	ADHD, autism, or developmental delay	Mild features of FXS	Childhood	8% (1/13)*

*Frequency of those signs in prepubertal boys; one third of boys with FXS are without classic facial features. Macroorchidism is present in 90% of men.
[†]Maximum penetrance reported for allele size approximately 80-90 CGG repeats.
[‡]Penetrance is correlated with age and repeat size.
ADHD, Attention-deficit/hyperactivity disorder; F, female; FMRP, fragile X mental retardation protein; FXS, fragile X syndrome; FXTAS, fragile X–associated tremor/ataxia syndrome; M, male; POF, premature ovarian failure.
From Jacquemont S, Hagerman RJ, Hagerman PJ, et al: Fragile-X syndrome and fragile X-associated tremor/ataxia syndrome: two faces of FMRI, *Lancet Neurol* 6:45–55, 2007, Table 1.

Table 98.19	Therapy for *FMR1*-Related Disorders		
DISORDER	**SYMPTOM**	**THERAPY AND INTERVENTIONS**	**FUTURE POTENTIAL THERAPY**
FULL MUTATION			
FXS*	ADHD	Stimulants	mGluR5 antagonists
	Anxiety, hyperarousal, aggressive outbursts	SSRIs, atypical antipsychotics, occupational therapy, behavioral therapy, counseling	mGluR5 antagonists
	Seizures	Carbamazepine, valproic acid	mGluR5 antagonists
	Cognitive deficit	Occupational therapy, speech therapy, special education support	mGluR5 antagonists
PREMUTATION			
POF	Premature ovarian failure	Reproductive counseling, egg donation Hormone replacement therapy	Cryopreservation of ovarian tissue
FXTAS†	Intention tremor	β-Blockers	
	Parkinsonism	Carbidopa/levodopa	
	Cognitive decline, dementia	Acetylcholinesterase inhibitors	
	Anxiety, apathy, disinhibition, irritability, depression	Venlafaxine, SSRIs	
	Neuropathic pain	Gabapentin	

*These data are based on a survey in 2 large referral centers. Drugs for anxiety were more frequently prescribed than those for neurologic signs.
†There have been no controlled studies to assess drugs for FXTAS. These data were collected through a questionnaire study (n = 56).
ADHD, Attention-deficit/hyperactivity disorder; FXS, fragile-X syndrome; FXTAS, fragile X–associated tremor/ataxia syndrome; POF, premature ovarian failure; SSRIs, selective serotonin reuptake inhibitors.
From Jacquemont S, Hagerman RJ, Hagerman PJ, et al: Fragile-X syndrome and fragile X-associated tremor/ataxia syndrome: two faces of FMRl, *Lancet Neurol* 2006:45–55, 2007, Table 2.

With the exception of chromosomes 13, 18, and 21, complete autosomal trisomies are usually nonviable; the presence of a normal cell line might allow these other trisomic conceptions to survive to term. Depending on the point at which the new cell line arises during early embryogenesis, mosaicism may be present in some tissues but not in others. **Germline mosaicism**, which refers to the presence of mosaicism in the germ cells of the gonad, may be associated with an increased risk for recurrence of an affected child if the germ cells are affected with a chromosomal abnormality or with a specific gene mutation.

PALLISTER-KILLIAN SYNDROME
Pallister-Killian syndrome is characterized by coarse facies (prominent full cheeks), abnormal ear lobes, localized alopecia (sparse hair in the temporal regions), pigmentary skin anomalies, diaphragmatic hernia, cardiovascular anomalies, supernumerary nipples, seizures, and profound intellectual disability. The syndrome is caused by mosaicism for an isochromosome 12p. The presence of the isochromosome 12p in cells gives 4 functional copies for the short arm of chromosome 12 in the affected cells. The isochromosome 12p is preferentially cultured from fibroblasts that can be readily obtained from a skin punch biopsy and is seldom present in lymphocytes. The abnormalities seen in affected persons probably reflect the presence of abnormal cells during early embryogenesis.

HYPOMELANOSIS OF ITO
Hypomelanosis of Ito is characterized by unilateral or bilateral macular hypo- or hyperpigmented whorls, streaks, and patches (see Chapter 672). Sometimes these pigmentary defects follow the lines of Blaschko. Hair and tooth anomalies are common. Abnormalities of the eyes, musculoskeletal system (growth asymmetry, syndactyly, polydactyly, clinodactyly), and central nervous system (microcephaly, seizures, intellectual disability) may also be present. Patients with hypomelanosis of Ito might have two genetically distinct cell lines. The mosaic chromosome anomalies that have been observed involve both autosomes and sex chromosomes and have been demonstrated in about 50% of clinically affected patients. The mosaicism might not be visible in lymphocyte-derived chromosome studies; it is more likely to be found when chromosomes are analyzed from skin fibroblasts. The distinct cell lines might not always be caused by observable chromosomal anomalies but might result from single-gene mutations or other mechanisms.

98.7 Chromosome Instability Syndromes
Carlos A. Bacino and Brendan Lee

Chromosome instability syndromes, formerly known as *chromosome breakage syndromes*, are characterized by an increased risk of malignancy and specific phenotypes. They display autosomal recessive inheritance and have an increased frequency of chromosome breakage and/or rearrangement, either spontaneous or induced. Chromosome instability syndromes result from specific defects in DNA repair, cell cycle control, and apoptosis. The resulting chromosomal instability leads to the increased risk of developing neoplasms. The classic chromosome instability syndromes are Fanconi anemia, ataxia telangiectasia, Nijmegen syndrome, ICF (immunodeficiency, centromere instability, facial anomalies) syndrome, Roberts syndrome, Werner syndrome, and Bloom syndrome.

98.8 Uniparental Disomy and Imprinting
Carlos A. Bacino and Brendan Lee

UNIPARENTAL DISOMY
Uniparental disomy (**UPD**) occurs when both chromosomes of a pair or areas from one chromosome in any individual have been inherited from a single parent. UPD can be of 2 types: uniparental isodisomy or uniparental heterodisomy. **Uniparental isodisomy** means that both chromosomes or chromosomal regions are identical (typically the result of monosomy rescue by duplication). **Uniparental heterodisomy** means that the 2 chromosomes are different members of a pair, both of which were still inherited from 1 parent. This results from a trisomy that is later reduced to disomy, leaving 2 copies from 1 parent. The phenotypic result of UPD varies according to the chromosome involved, the parent who contributed the chromosomes, and whether it is isodisomy or heterodisomy. Three types of phenotypic effects are seen in UPD: those related to imprinted genes (i.e., the absence of a gene that is normally expressed only when inherited from a parent of a specific sex), those related to the uncovering of autosomal recessive disorders, and those related to a vestigial aneuploidy producing mosaicism (see Chapter 97).

In uniparental isodisomy, both chromosomes or regions (and thus the genes) in the pair are identical. This is particularly important when the parent is a carrier of an autosomal recessive disorder. If the offspring of a carrier parent has UPD with isodisomy for a chromosome that carries an abnormal gene, the abnormal gene will be present in 2 copies, and the phenotype will be that of the autosomal recessive disorder; the child has an autosomal recessive disorder even though only 1 parent is a carrier of that recessive disorder. It is estimated that all humans carry approximately 20 abnormal autosomal recessive genes. Some autosomal recessive disorders, such as spinal muscular atrophy, cystic fibrosis, cartilage-hair hypoplasia, α- and β-thalassemias, and Bloom syndrome, have been reported in cases of UPD. The possibility of uniparental isodisomy should also be considered when a person is affected with >1 recessive disorder because the abnormal genes for both disorders could be carried on the same isodisomic chromosome. Uniparental isodisomy is a *rare* cause of recessively inherited disorders. Uniparental isodisomies can also be detected by SNP microarrays.

Maternal UPD involving chromosomes 2, 7, 14, and 15 and **paternal UPD** involving chromosomes 6, 11, 15, and 20 are associated with phenotypic abnormalities of growth and behavior. UPD of maternal chromosome 7 is associated with a phenotype similar to Russell-Silver syndrome with intrauterine growth restriction. These phenotypic effects may be related to imprinting (see later) (Fig. 98.18).

UPD for chromosome 15 is seen in some cases of Prader-Willi syndrome and Angelman syndrome. In **Prader-Willi syndrome**, approximately 25–29% of cases have maternal UPD (missing the paternal chromosome 15) (Fig. 98.19). In **Angelman syndrome**, paternal UPD of chromosome 15 is rarer and is observed in approximately 5% of the cases (missing the maternal chromosome 15). The phenotype for Prader-Willi syndrome and Angelman syndrome in cases of UPD is thought to result from the lack of the functional contribution from a particular parent of chromosome 15. In Prader-Willi syndrome the paternal contribution is missing, and the maternal contribution is missing in Angelman syndrome. Prader-Willi syndrome may be caused by

paternal deficiency of HB11-85 small nucleolar RNAs (snoRNAs). These findings suggest that there are differences in function of certain regions of chromosome 15, depending on whether it is inherited from the mother or from the father. Angelman syndrome is caused by absence of a maternally contributed gene known as *UBE3A* and can be the result of maternal deletion, maternal *UBE3A* mutation, paternal UPD, and abnormalities in the maternal imprinting center on chromosome 15q11-13 region.

UPD most frequently arises when a pregnancy starts off as a **trisomic conception** followed by **trisomy rescue**. Because most trisomies are lethal, the fetus can only survive if a cell line loses 1 of the extra chromosomes to revert to the disomic state. One third of the time, the disomic cell line is uniparental. This is the typical mechanism for Prader-Willi syndrome, and it is often associated with advanced maternal age. The embryo starts off as trisomy 15 secondary to maternal meiosis I nondisjunction, followed by random loss of the paternal chromosome. In this case the disomic cell line becomes the more viable one and outgrows the trisomic cell line. When mosaic trisomy is found at prenatal diagnosis, care should be taken to determine whether UPD has resulted and whether the chromosome involved is one of the disomies known to be associated with phenotypic abnormalities. There must always be concern that some residual cells that are trisomic are present in some tissues, leading to malformations or dysfunction. The presence of aggregates of trisomic cells might account for the spectrum of abnormalities seen in persons with UPD.

IMPRINTING

Traditional genetics for many years has suggested that most genes are equally expressed when inherited from maternal vs paternal lineages. The only exception to this rule were genes on the X chromosome that are subject to inactivation, and the immunoglobulin genes subject to allelic exclusion, a phenomenon that results in monoallelic expression

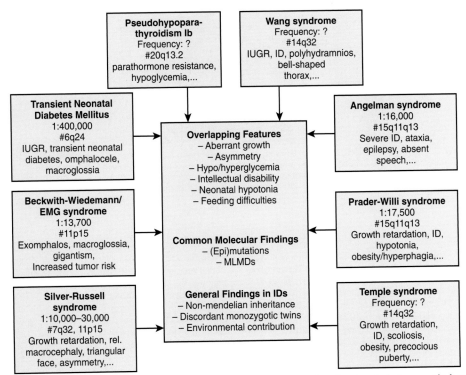

Fig. 98.18 Overview of the common clinical and molecular findings in the 8 known imprinting disorders, including specific features, frequencies, and major chromosomal localization. *#6q24*, Chromosome 6q24; *EMG*, exomphalos-macroglossia-gigantism; *IUGR*, intrauterine growth restriction; *ID*, intellectual disability; *MLMDs*, multilocus methylation defects. (*From Eggermann T, Elbracht M, Schröder C, et al: Congenital imprinting disorders: a novel mechanism linking seemingly unrelated disorders, J Pediatr 163:1204, 2013*).

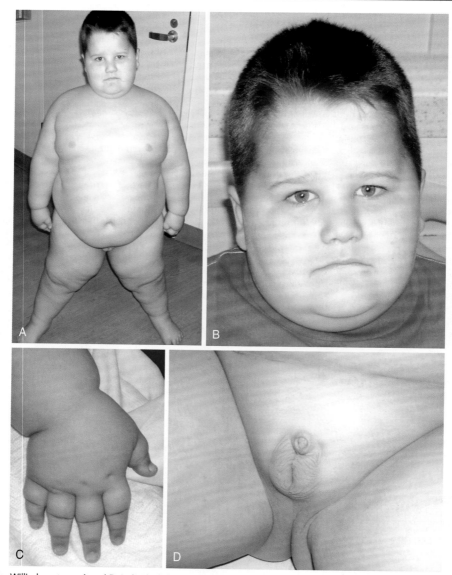

Fig. 98.19 Prader-Willi phenotype. **A** and **B,** Individual showing morbid obesity with facial features as shown. **C,** Upper extremities are notable for small hands relative to body size. **D,** External genitalia after laparoscopic orchiopexy at 13 mo. Parental informed consent, as approved by the Baylor College of Medicine Institutional Review Board, was obtained to publish the photographs. *(From Sahoo T, del Gaudio D, German JR, et al: Prader-Willi phenotype caused by paternal deficiency for the HBII-85 C/D box small nucleolar RNA cluster, Nat Genet 40:719–721, 2008.)*

of a particular immunoglobulin chain by switching expression of parental alleles on and off. Genomic imprinting occurs when the phenotypic expression of a gene depends on the parent of origin for certain genes or in some cases entire chromosome regions. Whether the genetic material is expressed or not depends on the sex of the parent from whom it was derived. Genomic imprinting can be suspected in some cases on the basis of a pedigree. In these pedigrees the disease is always transmitted from one sex and could be passed on silently for several generations by the opposite sex (Figs. 98.20 and 98.21). Imprinting probably occurs in many different parts of the human genome and is thought to be particularly important in gene expression related to development, growth, cancer, and even behavior; >60 genes have been classified as imprintable. Imprinting disorders may arise from UPD, deletions or duplications, epigenetic aberrant methylation patterns, or point mutations in a specific gene.

A classic example of imprinting disorder is seen in Prader-Willi syndrome and Angelman syndrome, 2 very different clinical conditions. These syndromes are usually associated with deletion of the same region in the proximal long arm of chromosome 15. A deletion on the paternally derived chromosome causes Prader-Willi syndrome, in which the maternally derived copy is still intact, but some of the imprinted genes within this region normally remain silent. Prader-Willi syndrome can be diagnosed clinically (Table 98.20) and confirmed with genetic testing. Additional clinical features and issues of weight gain are noted in Table 98.21. The weight gain is difficult to control, but treatment with growth hormone has resulted in improvements in height, lean body mass, decreased adipose tissue, and improvement in cognitive function.

A maternal deletion of the same region as in Prader-Willi syndrome causes Angelman syndrome, leaving intact the paternal copy that in

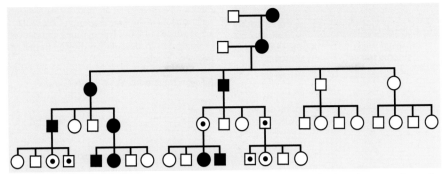

Fig. 98.20 In this hypothetical pedigree suggestive of imprinting, phenotypic effects occur only when the mutated gene is transmitted from the mother, but not when it is transmitted from the father, that is, maternal deficiency. Equal numbers of males and females can be affected and not affected phenotypically in each generation. A nonmanifesting transmitter gives a clue to the sex of the parent who passes the expressed genetic information; that is, in maternal deficiency disorders (also termed *paternal imprinting*), there are "skipped" nonmanifesting females. This is theoretical, because in most clinical scenarios of maternal deficiency, such as Angelman syndrome, affected persons do not reproduce.

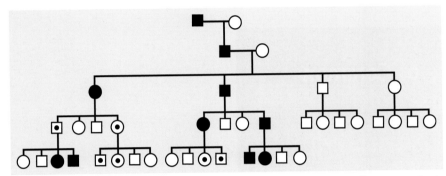

Fig. 98.21 In theoretical pedigrees suggestive of paternal deficiency (maternal imprinting), phenotypic effects occur only when the mutated gene is transmitted from the father, but not when transmitted from the mother. Equal numbers of males and females can be affected and not affected phenotypically in each generation. In a theoretical situation, a nonmanifesting transmitter gives a clue to the sex of the parent who passes on the expressed genetic information; that is, in paternal deficiency (also known as *maternal imprinting*), there are "skipped" nonmanifesting males. In real-life clinical cases of Prader-Willi syndrome, affected persons do not reproduce.

Table 98.20	Consensus Diagnostic Criteria for Prader-Willi Syndrome	
	MAJOR CRITERIA (1 point each)	**MINOR CRITERIA (1/2 point each)**
1	Neonatal/infantile hypotonia	Decreased fetal movement and infantile lethargy
2	Feeding problems and failure to thrive as an infant	Typical behavior problems
3	Weight gain at 1-6 yr; obesity; hyperphagia	Sleep apnea
4	Characteristic dysmorphic facial features	Short stature for family by 15 yr
5	Small genitalia; pubertal delay and insufficiency	Hypopigmentation for the family
6	Developmental delay/intellectual disability	Small hands and feet for height
7		Narrow hands, straight ulnar border
8		Esotropia, myopia
9		Thick, viscous saliva
10		Speech articulation defects
11		Skin picking

Data from Cassidy SB, Schwartz S, Miller JL, Driscoll DJ: Prader-Willi syndrome, *Genet Med* 14(1):15, 2012, Table 2.

Table 98.21	Nutritional Phases in Prader-Willi Syndrome	
PHASE	**MEDIAN AGES**	**CLINICAL CHARACTERISTICS**
0	Prenatal to birth	Decreased fetal movements and lower birthweight than siblings
1a	0-9 mo	Hypotonia with difficulty feeding and decreased appetite
1b	9-25 mo	Improved feeding and appetite and growing appropriately
2a	2.1-4.5 yr	Weight increasing without appetite increase or excess calories
2b	4.5-8 yr	Increased appetite and calories, but can feel full
3	8 yr to adulthood	Hyperphagic, rarely feels full
4	Adulthood	Appetite is no longer insatiable

Modified from Miller JL, Lynn CH, Driscoll DC, et al. Nutritional phases in Prader-Willi syndrome. *Am J Med Genet A* 155A:1040–1049, 2011.

Table 98.22	Molecular Mechanisms Causing Prader-Willi and Angelman Syndromes	
	PRADER-WILLI SYNDROME	**ANGELMAN SYNDROME**
15q11-q13 deletion	~70% (paternal)	~70% (maternal)
Uniparental disomy	~30% (maternal)	~5% (paternal)
Single-gene mutation	None detected	E6-AP ubiquitin-protein ligase (11% of total but mostly in familial cases)
Imprinting center mutation	5%	1%
Unidentified	<1%	10–15%

Data from Nicholls RD, Knepper JL: Genome organization, function and imprinting in Prader-Willi and Angelman syndromes, *Annu Rev Genomics Hum Genet* 2:153–175, 2001; and Horsthemke B, Buiting K: Imprinting defects on human chromosome 15, *Cytogenet Genome Res* 113:292–299, 2006.

Chapter 99
Genetics of Common Disorders

Bret L. Bostwick and Brendan Lee

第九十九章
常见疾病的遗传学

中文导读

本章主要介绍了常见儿科疾病的主要遗传学研究方法。介绍了遗传流行病学、家族性、遗传度、连锁定位、关联研究、单核苷酸多态性、表型、二分性状、数量性状、位点异质性、等位基因异质性、拟表型、等位基因、外显率以及基因–环境相互作用等概念。描述了连锁定位和遗传关联。具体介绍了连锁定位中微卫星和核型的概念；具体介绍了遗传关联中直接关联、间接关联以及连锁不平衡的概念。

---

this case has genes that are also normally silent. In other situations, UPD can lead to the same diagnosis (Table 98.22). Many other disorders are associated with this type of parent-of-origin effect, as in some cases of Beckwith-Wiedemann syndrome, Russell-Silver syndrome, and neonatal diabetes.

Bibliography is available at Expert Consult.

Common pediatric diseases are usually multifactorial. The combination of many genes and environmental factors contribute to a complex sequence of events leading to disease. The complexity of the combination of contributing factors increases the challenge of finding genetic variants that cause disease. Genetic tools include the completed human genome sequence, public databases of genetic variants, and the human haplotype map. In addition to public genetic databases, dramatic reduction in the cost of genotyping and DNA sequencing has allowed very large numbers of genetic variants to be efficiently tested in large numbers of patients. Most of these studies focus on common variants (those with frequencies >5%). Technologies for DNA sequencing are allowing whole exome sequencing in many individuals at very low cost. This technology is being used to investigate the role of rare coding sequence variants in common diseases. The incorporation of these tools into large, well-designed population studies is the field of **genetic epidemiology**. Many new methods for analyzing genetic data have been developed, stimulating a renaissance in applied population genetics.

99.1 Major Genetic Approaches to the Study of Common Pediatric Disorders

Bret L. Bostwick and Brendan Lee

Millions of genetic variants are present in every person. Many of these variants have no impact on health, while others have a measureable influence. Sometimes, single-gene mutations consistently cause a disease, as with cystic fibrosis and sickle cell anemia. Other types of genetic variation, however, can contribute much less to the emergence of specific medical conditions, and these are best conceptualized as *modifiers* of disease risk. Fig. 99.1 demonstrates the relationship between variant frequency and the relative medical impact of the allele. The spectrum of variant impact is logarithmic, ranging widely from a slightly increased risk of illness to predetermined fully expressed disease. Studies aimed at discovering rare variants with outsized health effects only require small sample populations to achieve statistical significance, while those studying common variants require much larger sample sizes because of the small anticipated impact of each variant.

The cumulative risk of many common variants determines genetic susceptibility. For common conditions, the genetic predisposition alone is not sufficient to cause disease. Everyone inherits a different degree of disease vulnerability, which is then augmented by exposure to certain environmental factors. Fig. 99.2 shows a model for the contribution of common genetic variants to individual health. One of the goals in medical genetics is to identify the genes that contribute to initial genetic susceptibility and to help prevent the occurrence of disease, either by avoiding inciting environmental factors or by instituting interventions that reduce risk. For persons who cross the threshold of disease, the goal is to better understand the pathogenesis in the hope that this will suggest better approaches to treatment. Common genetic variation can also influence response to medications and the risk of adverse drug reactions (see Chapter 72) and augment the health impacts of environmental toxins.

Complex traits may be inherently difficult to study if the precision of clinical diagnosis (phenotype) is problematic, as often occurs with neurobehavioral traits. A starting point in the genetic analysis of a complex trait is to obtain evidence in support of a genetic contribution and to estimate the relative strength of genetic and environmental factors. Complex traits typically exhibit familial clustering but are not transmitted in a regular pattern as is autosomal dominant or recessive inheritance. Complex traits often show variation among different ethnic or racial groups, possibly reflecting the differences in gene variants among these groups.

Assessing the potential genetic contribution begins by determining whether the trait is seen among related individuals more often than in the general population. A common measure of **familiality** is the first-degree relative risk (usually designated by the symbol λ_s), which is equal to the ratio of the prevalence rate in siblings and/or parents to the prevalence rate in the general population. The λ_s for type 1 diabetes is about 15. The relative strength of genetic and nongenetic risk factors can be estimated by variance components analysis. The **heritability** of a trait is the estimate of the fraction of the total variance contributed by genetic factors (Fig. 99.3).

A minority of cases of common diseases such as diabetes may be caused by single-gene mutations (mendelian inheritance), chromosomal disorders, and other genomic disorders. These *less common* causes of the disease can often provide important insight into the most important molecular pathways involved. Chromosomal regions with genes that might contribute to disease susceptibility could theoretically be located with **linkage mapping**, which locates regions of DNA that are inherited in families with the specific disease. In practical terms, however, this has become quite difficult for most complex traits either because of a dearth of families or because the effect of individual genetic loci is weak.

Genetic **association studies** are more powerful in identifying common gene variants (>5% in the population) that confer increased risk of disease, but they fail if the disease-causing gene variants are relatively rare. Detection of the modest effect of each variant and interactions with environmental factors requires well-powered studies that often include thousands of individuals. A number of parallel approaches for analyzing the aggregate effects of rare variants in genes have also been developed. Such rare variant association methods also seem to require large sample sizes because the gene effects have also proved to be relatively weak.

Linkage mapping and association studies require markers along the DNA that can be ascertained, or **genotyped**, with large-scale, high-throughput laboratory techniques. Markers that are typically used are in the forms of microsatellites and **single nucleotide polymorphisms** (**SNPs**; Fig. 99.4). A sample of the same region of genome from 50 people will reveal that approximately 1 in every 200 bases varies from

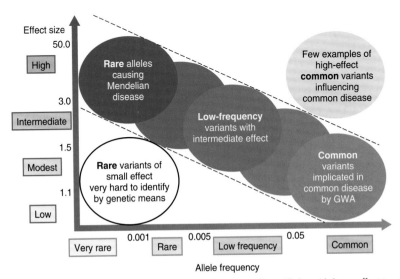

Fig. 99.1 Relationship between allele frequency and relative strength of genetic effect. Alleles with large effect tend to be very rare but can be studied with a small sample size because of the relative ease of allele detection when medical impact is high. Common variants tend to have a modest or low effect on health, requiring large datasets to visualize statistically small effects. The vast majority of disease-associated alleles identified to date have the characteristics shown within the *diagonal dotted lines*. *GWA*, Genome-wide association. (*Adapted from McCarthy MI, Abecasis GR, Cardon LR, et al: Genome-wide association studies for complex traits: consensus, uncertainty and challenges, Nat Rev Genet 9:356–369, 2008.*)

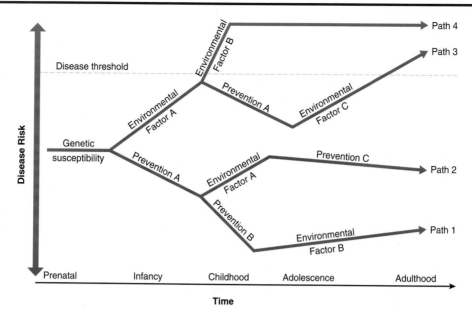

Fig. 99.2 Model for the influence of gene-environment interaction on genetic susceptibility to common diseases. Everyone inherits common variants that determine initial genetic liability for disease risk. For multifactorial disorders, the initial genetic susceptibility is insufficient to produce disease on its own. Over time, exposure to environmental factors increases the likelihood of a disease state. Identifying the gene variants responsible for risk can lead to prevention strategies or treatments.

Phenotypic variance	Genetic variance	Environmental variance	Measurement variance
V_P	$= V_G$	$+ V_E$	$+ V_M$

$$h^2 = V_G / V_P$$
Heritability

Fig. 99.3 Heritability concept. The phenotypic variance of a particular trait can be partitioned between the contributions of the genetic variance, environmental variance, and measurement variance. This is usually empirically determined. Heritability is defined by the proportion of the phenotypic variance that is accounted for by the genetic variance. One can estimate the heritability from correlation of a quantitative trait between relatives.

the more common form. Although most SNPs lack any obvious function, a few alter the amino acid sequence of the protein or affect regulation of gene expression. Some of these functional alterations directly affect susceptibility to disease. A complex clinical **phenotype** can be defined by the presence or absence of a disease as a **dichotomous trait**, or by selection of a clinically meaningful variable such as serum glucose in type 2 diabetes, which is a continuous or **quantitative trait**.

Although it might not be possible to define subgroups of patients in advance based on common disease mechanisms, the more uniform the phenotype, the more likely that a genetic study will be successful. **Locus heterogeneity** refers to the situation in which a trait results from the independent action of more than 1 gene. **Allelic heterogeneity** indicates that more than 1 variant in a particular gene can contribute to disease risk. The development of a trait or disease from a nongenetic mechanism results in a **phenocopy**. These 3 factors often contribute to the difficulty in identifying individual disease susceptibility genes, because they reduce the effective size of the study population.

A person bearing any variant or **allele** (inherited unit, DNA segment, or chromosome) in a gene has a certain probability of being affected with a specific gene variant–associated disease. This is called the **penetrance**. Some diseases manifest signs only later in life (age-related

penetrance), which could lead to misclassifying children who actually have the disease-producing gene as unaffected. Single-gene disorders are typically caused by mutations with relatively high penetrance, but some common variants have very low penetrance because their overall contribution to the disease is small. Many such common variants can contribute to disease risk for a complex trait. Normal human height is influenced by >400 genes.

Ideally, important environmental exposures should be measured and accounted for in a population because there may be a dependent interaction between the environmental factor and specific genetic variant. An example is the likely requirement for a viral infection preceding onset of type 1 diabetes. Although **gene-environment interactions** are strongly suspected to play an important role in common diseases, it is difficult to identify and measure them. Very large studies with uniform collection of information about environmental exposures are rare. Methods, such as genome-wide analysis of DNA methylation, may show evidence of environmental effects—so-called developmental programming (see Chapter 100). This information might be used to discover and validate gene-environment interactions.

LINKAGE MAPPING
Linkage studies were used in the past to isolate genes that cause rare genetic syndromes; modified methods have been used to identify chromosomal regions linked to more common diseases. Linkage studies involve tagging segments of a person's genome with markers that allow identification of segments that have been inherited through the family along with disease. The markers are typically **microsatellites** or SNPs that define and help to distinguish which type of an allele any person carries. **Genotype** refers to the combination of alleles at a locus in a diploid organism. Linkage analyses of common diseases have shown inconsistent results. Factors such as heterogeneity, pleiotropy, variable expressivity, and reduced penetrance, in addition to variability in environmental exposures, weaken the power of linkage studies in complex traits.

GENETIC ASSOCIATION
For multifactorial common diseases, association analyses may be used to identify causally important genes. There are two types of association

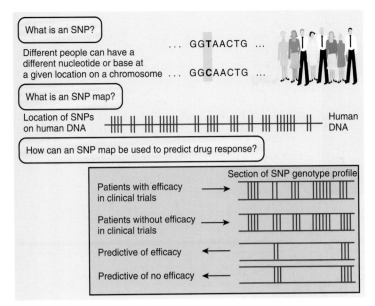

What is an SNP?

Different people can have a different nucleotide or base at a given location on a chromosome

... GGTAACTG ...

... GGCAACTG ...

What is an SNP map?

Location of SNPs on human DNA

Human DNA

How can an SNP map be used to predict drug response?

Section of SNP genotype profile

Patients with efficacy in clinical trials →

Patients without efficacy in clinical trials →

Predictive of efficacy ←

Predictive of no efficacy ←

Fig. 99.4 Different combinations of SNPs are found in different individuals. The locations of these SNPs can be pinpointed on maps of human genes. Subsequently, they can be used to create profiles that are associated with difference in response to a drug, such as efficacy and nonefficacy. (*Adapted from Roses A: Pharmacogenetics and the practice of medicine, Nature 405:857–865, 2000. Copyright 2000. Reprinted by permission of Macmillan Publishers Ltd.*)

study: **direct association**, in which the causal variant itself is tested to see whether its presence correlates with disease, and **indirect association**, in which markers that are physically close to the biologically important variant are used as proxies. The correlation of markers with other genetic variants in a small region of the genome is called **linkage disequilibrium**. Indirect association is enabled by the construction of a detailed genetic map in 3 reference populations (Europeans, Asians, West Africans) through the International HapMap Project. SNPs that tag most of the genome have been identified and can be genotyped at low cost using specially designed microarrays.

Three basic study designs are used for association testing. In a case control design, the frequency of an allele in the affected group is compared with the unaffected group. In a family-based control design, parents or siblings of an affected individual are used as the controls. In a cohort design, large numbers of people are ascertained and then followed for the onset of any number of diseases. The cohort analysis is very expensive, and there are few true cohort studies.

Family-based control study designs are somewhat attractive for pediatric diseases because it is usually possible to enroll parents. These studies solve a major problem in testing for association because the parents are perfectly matched for genetic background. When parents are collected, the statistical test used for these studies is called the **transmission disequilibrium test**. TDT compares the transmitted genotype with the inferred nontransmitted genotype. The success of all association analysis depends on the design of a well-powered study and an accurately measured trait to avoid phenotypic misclassification. In large, population-based studies, confounding by ethnicity or **population stratification** could distort results. Some genetic variants are more common in people from a particular ethnic group, which could cause an apparent association of a variant with a disease, when the disease rate happens to be higher in that group. This association would not be a true association between an allele and a disease, because the association

would be confounded by genetic background. The family-based tests using the TDT are immune to population stratification. However, TDT and related study designs are inherently less efficient than case control studies. Newer methods for measuring subtle mismatching between cases and controls using many thousands of markers routinely genotyped in genome-wide association studies allow researchers to account for this effect.

Association studies should be a powerful tool to find genetic variation that confers risk to an individual; the effect of any 1 genetic variant will be a very small contribution to the complex disease pathway. Genetic variants have been found that implicate a novel gene in a process, motivating more in-depth research into systems that will affect disease outcome. Associations such as the *APOEε4* variant with an increased risk of Alzheimer disease are noted by many studies. Many published association results are not reproducible; insufficient power and stratification might account for the inconsistencies. As of late 2016, 2,650 studies and 29,954 unique SNP-trait associations have been catalogued (https://www.ebi.ac.uk/gwas/).

Low-cost methods for sequencing the complete exomes *and* genomes of individuals will allow a more comprehensive evaluation of the full range of genetic variants involved in common diseases. Rare genetic variants, including small insertions or deletions, could turn out to be extremely important in explaining the impact of genetic factors in important pediatric diseases such as autism, cardiovascular malformations, and other birth defects. Common traits such as obesity, diabetes, and autoimmune diseases might also be affected by rare variants. In common severe disorders such as intellectual disability and complex heart malformations, de novo mutations (i.e., mutations not present in either parent) are known to play an important role.

Bibliography is available at Expert Consult.

Chapter **100**

Epigenome-Wide Association Studies and Disease

John M. Greally

第一百章

表观基因组关联研究和疾病

中文导读

　　本章主要介绍了疾病的表观遗传机制：活黄鼠模型、表观遗传学与基因表达调控、涉及表观遗传过程的儿科疾病、表观基因组相关研究：DNA甲基化、细胞命运可变性可作为表观遗传学和疾病的模型以及表观遗传病与治疗干预。具体描述了表观遗传学与基因表达调控中的"表观遗传学"一词的演变。并介绍了表观遗传、DNA甲基化、印迹、X失活、剂量补偿等概念。

Pediatricians are asked to consider the possibility that certain conditions involve epigenetic mechanisms. The assumption is that **epigenetic** processes, generally defined as regulatory control of gene expression, are capable of overriding information encoded in the DNA sequence to increase or decrease the risk of a disease. Despite powerful genomic assays to test these regulators of gene expression, it has proved difficult to provide clear answers about how epigenetic mechanistic insights could improve patient care. Clarifying the fundamental concepts and definitions that underlie proposed epigenetic contributions to phenotypes should lead to valuable insights into their role in human health.

EPIGENETIC MECHANISMS OF DISEASE: VIABLE YELLOW MOUSE MODEL

The back-translated meaning of **epigenetics** (*epi*, above, upon; *genetic*, DNA sequence) implies that information encoded in the DNA sequence may be modifiable in some way by higher-order information that regulates the levels of activity of specific genes. Such a concept is attractive when trying to understand why monozygotic twins, who have identical DNA sequences, are sometimes discordant for certain heritable diseases, such as Alzheimer disease and type 1 diabetes mellitus. Genetic predisposition that fails to account fully for the development of a disease (or other) phenotype has been called "missing heritability," a gap that epigenetic regulatory processes have been proposed to fill. Furthermore, because the environment influences the risk of certain disorders by modifying an underlying genetic predisposition, environmental stimuli may act through epigenetic regulatory processes of gene expression.

The most compelling evidence for the epigenetic, higher-level regulation of genes and predisposition to disease was the viable yellow mouse model (Fig. 100.1). This mouse was found to have a mutation involving an endogenous retrovirus, a component of the genome that can replicate itself and move to a new location. In the case of the viable yellow mouse, the endogenous retrovirus was the type called an **intracisternal A particle (IAP)**, which inserted upstream from a gene called *a* (*nonagouti*). The *nonagouti* gene encodes agouti-signaling protein precursor, which binds to and has a negative effect on melanocortin receptors. When it stimulates melanocytes in hair follicles, it causes the production of the yellow pheomelanin pigment rather than black eumelanin. Without the upstream IAP element, *nonagouti* would normally switch on for a very short burst of activity and stimulate a limited amount of yellow pigment production. The presence of the active IAP element upstream was found to create a new, constitutively active start site for the *nonagouti* gene, leading to the hair being produced with pheomelanin throughout its length, and a distinctive yellow fur phenotype. Because the agouti-signaling protein precursor is also expressed in other cell types, the extra activity of the *nonagouti* gene driven by the IAP element caused the yellow mice to become obese (due to actions on adipocytes), creating a syndrome comparable to human type 2 diabetes mellitus in these animals.

These mice became an intriguing model of a potential epigenetic role in disease risk because of the unexpected observation that pups from the same litter, all containing the same IAP insertion mutation, differed strikingly in their amount of yellow fur and associated adult obesity. Some of the mice had so little yellow fur that they had no visible evidence of having a mutation at all. The IAP element in these littermates was active in the cells of the yellow mice, as expected, but had undergone **silencing** in the mice with the brown fur. The inactive IAP element was distinctive for having acquired **DNA methylation**, the modification of cytosines located immediately before guanines (CG

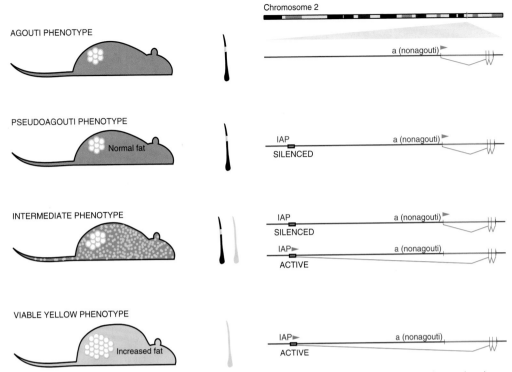

Fig. 100.1 The viable yellow mouse model of epigenetic modification of disease risk. The wild-type strain is depicted at the *top*; the brown coat color is caused by a band of yellow pheomelanin within the shaft of the otherwise black hair, resulting from a pulse of expression during hair growth from the *a* (*nonagouti*) gene on chromosome 2. The lower examples represent what happens when the intracisternal A particle (IAP) transposable element inserts upstream from the *nonagouti* gene. These mice can be indistinguishable from wild-type mice when the IAP element is completely silenced (pseudoagouti phenotype), or the IAP element can be active in every cell (*bottom*), driving continuous transcription of the *nonagouti* gene and causing pheomelanin to be expressed throughout the growth of the hair, causing the yellow color of the fur (viable yellow phenotype). These mice are also obese because of the effect of agouti-signaling protein on adipocytes. When some cells express and others silence the IAP element, an intermediate fur phenotype, often described as "mottled," is generated, accompanied by a less pronounced obesity. This demonstrates how the same genetic mutation (the IAP insertion) is variable in its association with a phenotype, depending on differences in transcriptional regulation at a specific locus in the genome.

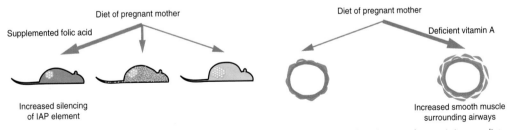

Fig. 100.2 Modification of adult disease risk by maternal diet during pregnancy. On the *left* is the pseudoagouti, intermediate, and viable yellow phenotypes associated with differences in silencing of the IAP element inserted upstream from the *nonagouti* gene. Increasing the amount of folic acid in the mother's diet during pregnancy is associated with an increased proportion of pups born with pseudoagouti and intermediate phenotypes, as well as less obesity during adulthood. On the *right* is the effect of vitamin A deficiency in the pregnant mother's diet during lung formation in the offspring. The lack of vitamin A during development is associated with the accumulation of smooth muscle (brown) around the airways and increased airway resistance during adulthood. The vitamin A deficiency results in a lack of retinoic acid in the developing embryos, leading to changes in gene expression regulation that alter cell fates and cause more smooth muscle cells to form. Both examples represent how dietary influences during pregnancy alter decisions made by cells during development, acting through regulation of gene expression, and predispose to adult diseases.

or CpG dinucleotides) to 5-methylcytosine. Methylation of cytosines at CG dinucleotides is the default state throughout the genome, but it is usually absent at the sites regulating expression of nearby genes, so its acquisition at these sites indicates that the gene has undergone silencing. This suggested that an influence on how genes are expressed overrode innate genetic susceptibility, modifying the risk of acquiring a disease. Further, researchers modified the diets of mothers pregnant with a litter of pups with the IAP insertion by supplementing **folic acid**, a single-carbon donor that increased the availability of a cofactor needed for DNA methylation. The outcome was a higher proportion of pups born with DNA methylation and inactivation of the IAP mutation (Fig. 100.2).

Therefore, a reason for the variability in whether the mice developed the yellow fur and obesity could be influences during pregnancy, such as maternal diet. This supported suggestions that intrauterine stresses were associated with increased risks of certain adult conditions, such as cardiovascular, renal, and metabolic diseases. This field of study is often known as the **Developmental Origins of Health and Disease (DOHaD)**, which asks how someone's cells remember an intrauterine stress years or decades later. The viable yellow mouse model suggested that such memory could be mediated by regulators of gene expression and influenced by environmental factors such as maternal diet during pregnancy.

EPIGENETICS AND REGULATION OF GENE EXPRESSION

Two examples of gene regulation provide a model for locking in a regulatory pattern early in development and maintaining it indefinitely thereafter. The first is **X chromosome inactivation**. Because males have only 1 X chromosome, it does not undergo inactivation. However, a person with 2 X chromosomes will inactivate 1, a person with trisomy for the X chromosome will inactivate 2, and so on. The result is that males and females have 1 active X chromosome per cell, despite starting with different numbers of X chromosomes, a process referred to as **dosage compensation**.

X chromosome inactivation is generally a random event, choosing the maternal X for inactivation in half the cells of the body and the paternal X in the other half. The inactivation occurs very early during development, when the blastocyst is implanting itself into the uterine wall. However, once established in this small number of pluripotent cells, the inactivation persists in all the cells of the individual throughout life.

The other relevant model of gene regulation is **genomic imprinting** (see Chapter 97). Gene activation in a specific cell type usually switches on the copies present on both the paternal and the maternal chromosomes. However, an **imprinted locus** is distinctive because only the copy on the *paternal* chromosome is switched on for some imprinted genes, while other imprinted genes are distinctive for only switching on the maternal copy. The timing of this inactivation event is even earlier than X chromosome inactivation, occurring during the formation of the male or female gametes. Again, these patterns of inactivation persist throughout life into old age.

Evolution of the Term "Epigenetics"

Because the 2 previous examples both involved a gene regulation event (silencing) that occurred early in development and was maintained into adulthood, they were described as "epigenetic," emphasizing how a cell retains a memory of past regulatory processes. This highlights that epigenetics has long been held to have a 2nd property, mediating cellular memory.

In the 1950s, Nanney interpreted the epigenetic landscape to define epigenetics as the property of a cell to remember past events. In the 1970s, Riggs and Holliday both noted that DNA methylation patterns could be propagated from parent to daughter cells, potentially providing a molecular mechanism of cellular memory, and described this as an "epigenetic property." When DNA methylation was found to be a feature of the alleles silenced during X chromosome inactivation and genomic imprinting, this appeared to confirm the idea of a "heritable molecular mark" being involved in remembering a past silencing event during development, leading DNA methylation to be described as an "epigenetic regulator." When the active and silenced alleles at X inactivated or imprinted loci were further studied, differences in chromatin states and long noncoding RNAs were found to distinguish the chromosomes, suggesting that they helped to mediate the long-term silencing at these loci.

There have been attempts to test whether chromatin states are heritable through cell division in the same way as DNA methylation. Despite the evidence for their heritability being less compelling, the field has tended to be *inclusive* rather than exclusive in labeling transcriptional regulators as epigenetic, but needed to redefine epigenetics as *epi* (above, upon) and *genetics* (DNA sequence), the back-translated definition. This definition is not only dissociated from the original ideas of cell fates and cellular memory, but now also encompasses all transcriptional regulatory processes. Because of the broadened definition of epigenetics, an experiment testing for differences in cellular memory is no different in design from an experiment testing for differences in transcriptional regulation, which may or may not mediate cellular memory.

PEDIATRIC DISEASES INVOLVING EPIGENETIC PROCESSES

Prime examples of epigenetics are those involving imprinted loci, exemplified by the Prader-Willi and Angelman syndromes (see Chapter 97). Each of these syndromes may be caused by the same deletion on chromosome 15, distinguished by the deletion occurring on the *paternal* chromosome 15 causing **Prader-Willi syndrome** and the *maternal* chromosome 15 causing **Angelman syndrome**. There are imprinted genes located within the 15q11-q13 region, some of which are expressed only on the paternal chromosome, some only on the maternal chromosome. When an individual is missing the region on the paternally inherited chromosome, the person still has a copy of the gene on the remaining maternal chromosome, but if it is silenced by imprinting, the individual effectively has *no functional copy* of the gene, leading to the Prader-Willi phenotype. The converse happens for Angelman syndrome; a deletion of the maternal chromosome leaves a silenced copy of the gene on the paternal chromosome.

Although deletions cause these syndromes in the majority of affected individuals, a subset results from **uniparental disomy (UPD)**, in which there are 2 intact chromosomes 15, but both are inherited from *1 parent*. Maternal UPD has the same effect as a paternal deletion in that there is no contribution of a paternally inherited chromosome, causing Prader-Willi syndrome, with paternal UPD causing Angelman syndrome. UPD is thought to start with trisomy for that chromosome, with a 2nd event occurring early in development in which 1 of the 3 chromosomes is lost, occasionally leaving 2 chromosomes derived from the same parent. In a further, very small proportion of individuals, mutations within the 15q11-q13 region seem to affect the imprinted domain as a whole.

Prader-Willi and Angelman syndromes occur because of **genetic mutations**: large deletions, nondisjunction events leading to whole chromosomal gains or losses, or smaller DNA mutations. These mutations reveal the underlying pattern of genomic imprinting, a distinctive organization of gene regulation at chromosome 15q11-q13 that reflects a memory of the gamete of origin of each chromosome, described as epigenetic. What is *not* occurring in these individuals is an alteration of the normal epigenetic regulation of the locus, as exemplified by the yellow agouti mouse. To find examples of altered epigenetic regulation associated with disease, researchers take advantage of assays that studied DNA methylation patterns throughout the genome. If we had never known about the IAP element insertion in the yellow agouti mice, for example, the locus would have revealed itself by having distinctive DNA methylation in the yellow, obese animals compared with the brown, lean, genetically identical littermates. This approach, referred to as an **epigenome-wide association study (EWAS)**, was initially applied to study individuals who had intrauterine perturbations, environmental exposures, or various types of cancer, to look for cellular reprogramming events.

EPIGENOME-WIDE ASSOCIATION STUDIES: DNA METHYLATION

Because of the availability of genome-wide assays and its demonstrated heritability through mitosis, DNA methylation has been the primary focus for studies attempting to link altered epigenetic regulation with disease phenotypes. The *genome-wide association study* (GWAS) template was used for EWAS, but instead of linking variability in DNA sequences, the EWAS links variability in DNA methylation with the presence of a phenotype.

Interpretation of EWAS is more complex than foreseen partly because DNA methylation in a sample of cells reflects not only its reprogramming in these cells but also other influences. For example, if a sample of cells contains more than 1 subtype (each subtype of cells in the body has distinctive DNA methylation patterns), a change in proportion of *cell subtypes* between individuals will cause a change in the pattern of DNA methylation, at the loci where differences in DNA methylation distinguish the cell subtypes. In this way, DNA methylation changes can be found in an EWAS without any individual cells having altered their DNA methylation.

Another major influence, accounting for an estimated 22–80% of DNA methylation variation between individuals, is DNA sequence variability. Epigenetic regulation is defined as a level of information above that of DNA sequence, but the reciprocal influence of DNA sequence *variation* on DNA methylation is substantial. The typical EWAS to date has not taken genetic variation into account when interpreting its results, again suggesting misinterpretation of DNA methylation changes as reflective of reprogramming of cells, when in fact the differences in DNA methylation may reflect *sequence differences* in the individuals studied.

The typical design of an EWAS is cross-sectional: comparing a group of individuals with a condition against a group without the condition; by the time these people are studied, they have already developed the disorder of interest. This makes the study vulnerable to the effects of *reverse causation*, in which the condition studied alters DNA methylation, rather than reprogramming of DNA methylation causing the condition. This has been shown to occur in peripheral blood leukocytes in individuals with high body mass index. The results of all EWAS to date therefore should be interpreted with caution.

CELL FATE VARIABILITY AS MODEL FOR EPIGENETICS AND DISEASE

A universally held belief is that 1 or more cell types in the body undergo a change in the regulation of gene expression, a type of cellular reprogramming that alters the properties of the cell to contribute to the disease. However, another model to consider is a reprogramming occurring earlier, during cell fate decision-making, and changing the repertoire of cells in the organ in such a way that it predisposes to disease.

Studies are guided by a mouse model characterized by maternal **vitamin A deficiency** during pregnancy. Vitamin A is the dietary precursor of **retinoic acid**, which binds to a retinoic acid receptor that then finds its way to specific locations in the genome to regulate the expression

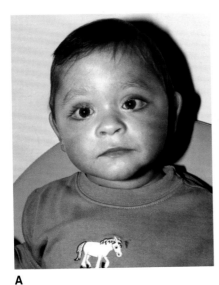
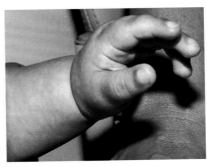

B

A

Fig. 100.3 Kabuki syndrome in 18 mo old boy. **A,** Long palpebral fissures and eversion of lateral portion of lower eyelids. **B,** Prominent fingertip pads. *(From Jones, KL, Jones MC, Del Campo, M, editors: Smith's recognizable patterns of human malformation, ed 7, Philadelphia, 2013, Elsevier, p 158.)*

Table 100.1	Clinical Manifestations of Kabuki Syndrome	

FACIAL	**EXTREMITY/SKELETAL**
Long palpebral tissues and eversions of lateral third of lower eyelids	Short, incurved 5th finger
Ptosis	Brachydactyly
Broad, arched eyebrows with sparse hair on lateral third	Kyphosis
Long eyelashes	Joint hyperextensibility
Blue sclerae	Persistent fetal fingertip pads
Protuberant ears	Hypoplastic finger nails
Short nasal columella (depressed nasal tip)	
	CARDIOVASCULAR
NEURODEVELOPMENTAL	Multiple forms of congenital heart disease
Hypotonia	
Developmental delay (IQ about 60; >80 in 10%)	**OTHER**
Low birthweight	Nonimmune hydrops
Postnatal growth deficiency	Hypothyroidism
Microcephaly	Precocious puberty
Seizures	Delayed puberty
Autism	Lymphatic malformations
	Feeding difficulties

of groups of genes. When vitamin A was restricted in the diet of pregnant female mice from embryonic days 9.5-14.5, the period when most lung formation occurs, the mice were born with increased amounts of smooth muscle around the airways, later in their lives shown to be associated with increased airway resistance. The mice were thus showing a component of the reactive airways disease (asthma) phenotype caused solely by a micronutrient deficiency during fetal life (see Fig. 100.2). The change in a cell fate decision to alter the proportion of 1 or more cell types in the mature organ is a strikingly attractive mechanism for DOHaD and highly consistent with the original definition of epigenetic events based on cell fate decisions, but it is not considered the outcome of interest in current EWAS.

The same model can be considered for the epigenetic response to toxins, in particular **endocrine disruptors**, defined by their interaction with the endocrine system, for which links with epigenetic regulatory processes have been frequently sought. One interesting class of endocrine-disrupting chemical is the *organotins,* biocides used in different types of manufacturing. The organotin tributyltin was found to cause obesity and to direct tissue stem cells preferentially toward the production of adipocytes, signaling through a transcriptional pathway involving PPAR gamma. Again, this is not an outcome generally sought in a typical EWAS at present, but it represents a perturbation acting to change cell fate through transcriptional regulatory mechanisms and leading to an altered repertoire of cells in the exposed individual.

EPIGENETIC DISEASE AND THERAPEUTIC INTERVENTIONS

The question arises whether interventions can ameliorate or reverse a disease phenotype when it is caused by epigenetic processes. In cancer, involving somatic mutations that can target various mediators of transcriptional regulation, numerous therapeutic avenues have emerged that show promise. An interesting noncancer example is the genetic condition called **Kabuki syndrome**, which is caused by mutations in either a histone methyltransferase (*KMT2D*) or a histone demethylase (*KDM6A*) gene, each of which has a role in creating accessible chromatin to allow genes to be expressed appropriately (Fig. 100.3 and Table 100.1). With the idea that increasing the amount of histone acetylation could help to compensate for the inappropriate histone methylation, mice with Kabuki syndrome were placed on a ketogenic diet, which increases the amount of β-hydroxybutyrate, an endogenous inhibitor of histone deacetylases. Mice on this diet showed improved neurogenesis and memory, suggesting that such an intervention in children with Kabuki syndrome may also have beneficial effects.

Bibliography is available at Expert Consult.

Chapter **101**

Genetic Approaches to Rare and Undiagnosed Diseases

William A. Gahl, David R. Adams, Thomas C. Markello, Camilo Toro, and Cynthia J. Tifft

第一百零一章
罕见和未确诊疾病的遗传学研究方法

中文导读

　　本章主要介绍了遗传病范围、临床评估、单核苷酸多态性阵列、外显子组测序、基因功能研究、儿科问题以及诊断谱。具体描述了NIH未确诊疾病计划、商业化遗传学检测以及对未确诊儿童家庭的思考，这些思考包括我的孩子有什么病（诊断）？为什么会这样（病因/遗传模式）？未来会发生什么（自然史、预后）？有治疗方法吗（治疗）？其他家庭成员也会发生同样的事情吗（再发风险）？

Rare and novel disorders often present in childhood and represent a diagnostic challenge that can be addressed using advanced genetic techniques. In the United States, **rare disorders** are defined as those affecting <200,000 people (about 1 in 1,500 persons), but no single definition has been agreed on internationally.

SCOPE OF GENETIC DISEASE

An estimated 8000 rare disorders are recognized, and the existence of approximately 23,000 human genes suggests that many more genetic diseases will be discovered in the future. Potential reasons patients may remain undiagnosed despite extensive prior investigation include:

- The genetic variant had not previously been associated with the disease phenotype.
- There is genetic *pleiotropy* (same gene but different variant producing a different phenotype).
- There is genetic *heterogeneity* (different genes producing similar phenotype).
- Presentation is known but atypical features for a known disease.
- Multiple diseases are contributing to the presenting set of disease features.
- Somatic mosaicism

NIH Undiagnosed Diseases Program

One approach toward investigating undiagnosed diseases was taken by the National Institutes of Health (NIH) Undiagnosed Diseases Program (**UDP**), which was expanded to a nationwide Undiagnosed Diseases Network (UDN). For the >4,000 patient applications to the UDP, prior investigations are recounted in a summary letter from the referring clinician and documented with medical records that include photos, videos, imaging, and histologic slides of biopsy material. Specialty consultants review the records, and the UDP directors determine the next steps. Accepted patients come to the NIH Clinical Center for a week-long inpatient admission. Approximately half the patients with undiagnosed diseases have neurologic disease; cardiovascular, rheumatology, immunology, and pulmonary problems are also common. Approximately 40% of accepted patients are children, who often have congenital anomalies and neurologic disorders.

CLINICAL EVALUATION

Patients remain without a definitive diagnosis after an extensive workup in part because every individual has a unique genetic and environmental background, and diseases have variable expression. Undiagnosed conditions include those never before seen, unusual presentations of otherwise recognizable conditions, and combinations of conditions that obfuscate each other's identities. A thorough clinical investigation allows the clinician to broaden the differential diagnosis through research, consultation, and clinical testing. Extensive phenotyping, imaging, and other tests provide better documentation of the presentation and allow for association with diseases not yet discovered, genetic variants, and patient cohorts.

A complete history anchors the data and includes prenatal and neonatal findings, developmental milestones, growth pattern, onset and progression of symptoms and signs, precipitating influences, response to medications, and a pedigree to determine which family members are possibly affected. Pertinent physical findings include dysmorphisms, organomegaly, neurologic impairment, bone involvement, and dermatologic findings. Because many rare and novel disorders are *multisystemic,* consultants play a critical role in every diagnostic evaluation. Typical studies performed to address possible diagnoses are listed in Table 101.1; neurodevelopmental or neurodegenerative phenotypes require even more extensive studies (Table 101.2).

An inpatient admission allows for close interaction among experts in different fields, informs the evaluation of complex cases, and often leads to new disease discovery. In the last situation, other family members require evaluation to ascertain whether they are affected with the disorder.

Commercial Genetic Studies

Once **phenotyping** is complete, a list of candidate genetic disorders can be compiled. Laboratory testing is available for an increasingly large

Table 101.1	Initial Studies to Generate New Diagnostic Hypotheses
TEST	**RELATED DISORDERS/ DISORDER GROUPS**
Electrolytes, lactate, pyruvate	Energy metabolism defects, including mitochondrial disorders
Plasma amino acids	Renal disorders, amino acid disorders
Urine organic acids	Renal disorders, organic acid disorders, energy metabolism disorders, vitamin deficiencies
Aldolase, creatine phosphokinase	Muscle disorders
Carnitine (free, total, acyl, panel)	Fatty acid oxidation disorders, carnitine metabolism disorders
Cerebrospinal fluid (CSF) analysis	Neurotransmitter disorders, inborn errors of metabolism, select disorders that may present only in the CSF
Brain MRI/magnetic resonance spectroscopy	Structural and morphologic clues to disorders affecting central nervous system
Mass spectrometry to detect N- and O-linked proteoglycan abnormalities	Congenital disorders of glycosylation
Lysosomal enzyme testing	Lysosomal storage diseases
White cell and skin electron microscopy	Lysosomal storage diseases; neuronal lipofuscinoses
Pathologic evaluation of affected tissues with special stains, DNA hybridization	Any
Echocardiogram, electrocardiogram	Structural and functional abnormalities of the heart
Nerve conduction velocity, electromyogram	Dysfunction of anterior horn cells, nerves, neuromuscular junction, or muscle
Fibroblast cell line	Any
Single nucleotide polymorphism, exome/genome/karyotype	Any
Erythrocyte sedimentation rate, C-reactive protein	Inflammatory disorders

number of molecular disorders. Examples of genetic panels include those for X-linked cognitive impairment, hereditary spastic paraplegia, spastic paraplegia and gait disorders, spinocerebellar ataxias, dystonias, and mitochondrial disorders. Some of these are expensive and may exceed the cost of **exome sequencing**. On the other hand, exome and genome sequencing are not useful for detecting diseases caused by many types of genetic disorder, including from DNA repeats. In addition, exome sequencing may provide less certainty for excluding genetic diseases than a disease-specific test panel.

SINGLE NUCLEOTIDE POLYMORPHISM ARRAYS

Single nucleotide polymorphism (**SNP**) arrays and next-generation sequencing (NGS) provide valuable genome-wide structural information. The human genome's 3.2 billion bases include many that are **polymorphic,** customarily defined as differing between any 2 people >1% of the time. In most human populations, about 4 million differences exist between any 2 unrelated individuals (about 1 polymorphism for every 1,000 bases in the genome on average). Within a single ethnic population, about 1 common SNP occurs per 3,000-7,000 bases, where *common* means a >10% chance that the base will differ between 2 unrelated

Table 101.2	Diagnostic Evaluation of the Neurologically Impaired Child

CONSULTATIONS
Genetics/genetic counseling
Neurology
Ophthalmology
Endocrinology
Immunology
Rheumatology
Dermatology
Cardiology
Neuropsychology
Nutrition
Rehabilitative medicine
    Physical therapy
    Occupational therapy
    Speech therapy

PROCEDURES
Swallow study for aspiration
Abdominal ultrasound (hepatosplenomegaly)
Skeletal survey (dysostosis)
Bone density scan (nonambulatory or growth failure patients)
Bone age
Electroencephalogram, evoked responses, electroretinogram (ERG)
Muscle biopsy for electron transport chain function, histology,
    immunohistochemistry
Neuropsychometric testing
Nerve biopsy

LABORATORY EVALUATIONS
Complete blood count with differential and peripheral smear
Comprehensive metabolic panel
Prothrombin time/partial thromboplastin time (for anesthesia
    sedation)
Thyroid-stimulating hormone, thyroxine
Vitamins A and E, 1,25-dihydroxyvitamin D
Lactate, pyruvate
Ammonia
Amino acids (plasma and urine)
Organic acids (urine)
Acylcarnitine profile
Total and free carnitine
Lysosomal enzyme analysis in leukocytes/fibroblasts
White blood cell coenzyme Q
Purines and pyrimidines (urine)
α-Glucosidase (plasma and urine)
Peroxisomal panel

Oxysterols
Methylmalonic acid and homocysteine (plasma)
Copper/ceruloplasmin
Transferrin isoelectric focusing
N- and O-glycans (plasma)
Oligosaccharides and free glycans (urine)
Glycosaminoglycans (urine)

ADDITIONAL TESTING IF CLINICALLY INDICATED
Electron microscopy of white blood cell buffy coat for inclusion
    bodies
Electron microscopy of skin biopsy for evidence of storage
Stool for ova and parasites, occult blood, fecal fat, or fecal
    calprotectin
Autoimmune antibodies
Vaccine response titers
C3/C4
Quantitative immunoglobulins
T-cell subsets
Conjunctival or salivary gland biopsy

RESEARCH SPECIMENS
Cerebrospinal fluid
Serum
Plasma
Skin biopsy for fibroblasts and/or melanocytes
Isolated DNA/RNA
Urine

STUDIES UNDER SEDATION
3T MRI/magnetic resonance spectroscopy of brain (and spine if
    indicated)
Skin biopsy
Ophthalmologic exam
Brainstem auditory evoked response
Electroretinogram
Lumbar puncture for biopterin, neopterin, neurotransmitters, folate,
    and inflammatory markers
Dental exam
Large blood draws
Catheterization for urine
Any part of the physical exam difficult to do in an awake child,
    including dysmorphology measurements and genital and rectal
    exam
Electromyography and nerve conduction studies   .

people. Approximately 1 million of these common SNPs can be included on a DNA hybridization array and examined simultaneously, revealing copy number variants, mosaicism, and regions of identity by descent. These results complement NGS results; one example is the pairing of sequence variants detected by exome or genome sequencing with *trans*-oriented deletions detected by SNP assay.

EXOME SEQUENCING

Technical advances have allowed for massive, inexpensive DNA sequencing, making it feasible to determine the sequence of the coding regions of almost all the human genes. Because this involves 1.9% of the 3.2 billion bases in the human genome, exome sequences comprise approximately 60,000,000 bases. Using current technology, clinical exome sequencing adequately sequences >80% of known genes and >90% of genes that have been associated with human disease. The average exome sequencing produces about 35,000 bases (0.06%) that differ from the "reference" sequence and from any other unrelated human sequence of the same ethnic group. These variants include some laboratory and computational errors. In practice, most variants are inconsequential polymorphisms and minor polynucleotide repeats that occur near intron/exon boundaries. However, each of the 35,000 variants of unknown significance is a *potential* disease-causing variant, yet only 1 (or 2 for

compound heterozygous recessive cases) is *the* disease-causing mutation for a monogenic disorder (with perhaps 2 or 3 additional loci modifying severity). The clinician and bioinformatician must reduce the number of candidate variants to a tractable number, which is challenging. For instance, a variant causing an adult-onset disease may look just as damaging as a different variant causing congenital-onset disease. However, the likelihood of the presence of the associated diseases is much different in an adult vs a child.

Certain rules are used to separate *likely-interesting variants* from likely-uninteresting variants. For example, variants that segregate in a family consistent with a given inheritance model (e.g., dominant or recessive) are retained, while those that segregate in an inconsistent manner are set aside. This segregation filter requires careful clinical data collection and experimental design, since it depends on correct assignment of affected vs unaffected statuses in the family and collection of sequencing data for family members besides the proband.

A 2nd technique used to evaluate sequence variants is **pathogenicity assessment**. Bioinformaticians estimate the likelihood that a given DNA sequence variant will have biologic consequences (e.g., change protein function or gene expression). Factors such as nucleotide conservation and differences in coded amino acids are used to create a pathogenicity estimate, or score. Various software programs take different, often overlapping, approaches. PolyPhen-2, SIFT, and MutationTaster rate the pathogenicity of amino acid changes. Computer modeling programs such as CADD, Eigen, and M-CAP, trained on model genetic changes that are already validated, predict effects on gene expression of noncoding variants. These filters are very powerful because of large population datasets that are publically available, including the 1000Genomes project, ExAC, and the UK's 10K genome project. In the next 1 or 2 yr, datasets with genome populations in the 100,000 to 1 million range (e.g., GnomAD database) will further improve these filters and provide better subpopulation frequencies. Ultimately, a multiethnic, graph theory-based alignment should allow successful filtering of variants in currently incomplete genomic regions such as the HLA region. Overall, computational pathogenicity assessment has false-positive and false-negative rates of 10–20%.

Some filters compare variants to databases that contain previously measured or asserted properties of variants found in human populations, such as population frequency information (e.g., ExAC), or curated evidence for association with human disease (e.g., CLINVAR). The latter, while potentially useful, is quite incomplete for many genes, but this is improving. One common pitfall of database-derived filters is an inaccurate designation of certain variants as rare. This typically happens when the database is missing information from human populations in whom the variant is seen more often than in the included populations.

Several points need to be considered when employing genome-scale sequencing for clinical diagnostics. **Positive predictive value** gives the likelihood that a positive test is a true positive. This is higher in a population in whom a disease is common and lower in a population in whom the disease is rare. A person being tested with exome sequencing will show no clinical signs or symptoms of most of the genetic diseases for which the exome sequencing tests. Therefore, many apparently positive findings will be *false positives,* variants associated with phenotypes that do not match the person being tested.

Individual vs family studies are relevant because family data allow for the proband's variants to be substantially filtered. This advantage must be weighed against the financial costs of studying families vs individuals. Furthermore, family studies are useless if an affected person is called unaffected, or vice versa. Therefore, *phenotyping family members is critical.* For later-onset conditions, younger siblings may not be suitable for inclusion in an exome sequencing study unless their affected status can be determined unambiguously. Datasets with large numbers of young individuals may have many pathologic variants that cause disease in elderly persons and are inappropriate for filtering variants in late-onset adult diseases or for prenatal counseling about late-onset disease inheritance risks.

Data revisiting policies must be addressed. Genome-scale sequencing generates data for many genes besides those involved in the current diagnostic effort; these data may be useful in the future care of the patient. Some unreported mutated genes, not currently associated with disease, may be implicated in the future as disease risk factors or even as protective factors. In the current testing environment, time-limited data reuse policies and storage and reuse fees are increasingly common. In fact, the storage of data is now becoming more expensive than the cost of re-generating the data.

Early discussion with a genetic specialist is critical. Genetic counseling should be sought before an exome sequencing study is sent. Proper consent for exome sequencing studies is an involved process, including discussions of disease risk factors, unrelated medical conditions, carrier states, and cancer susceptibility. Consented individuals should be asked which types of results they would like to receive.

Anticipating findings that are difficult to use clinically is an important part of counseling. Variants of unknown significance (VUS) are problematic, and genome-scale sequencing amplifies the problem by including variable numbers of results that are difficult to use for medical decision-making. Discussing such variants with families can be challenging; counseling families about the likelihood of receiving this type of result before testing is performed can help the family to cope when the report is returned (see Chapter 94).

When used as a gene panel, exome sequencing rules *in* but does not rule *out*. An exome study is a cost-effective way to test many genes simultaneously, but coverage of any given exon varies. Therefore, exome studies cannot always exclude **variants** in a panel of genes. With careful analysis involving laboratory validation performed on many similarly processed individuals, the exome coverage of any given gene can be assessed. However, commercial/clinical testing facilities may be unwilling to perform such an analysis when a large set of genes needs to be considered. Therefore, a gene panel can be useful when the index of suspicion is high for a disorder caused by a large group of genes. Cerebellar ataxia and hereditary spastic paraplegia are examples (see Chapters 615.1 and 631).

Providing information to the testing facility improves the chance of diagnosis. Exome sequencing interpretation benefits substantially from the incorporation of an accurate and detailed phenotype. The more clinical information provided to the testing lab, the more specific and useful will be the clinical report.

The role of whole *genome* sequencing (WGS) is not yet defined in clinical practice but remains a consideration when *exome* sequencing yields no diagnosis. The fundamental issue is whether the VUS findings in an exome will be more meaningful than any additional variants discovered by WGS, rather than a clinical conclusion that there is no germline genetic/molecular cause for the undiagnosed patient. WGS tools have less confidence because of net lower coverage, take more time to process, and generate variants in noncoding regions of the genome that are much more difficult to filter and interpret.

GENE FUNCTION STUDIES

Despite filtering for frequency and predicted deleteriousness, a variant identified by exome or genome sequencing cannot be interpreted as the cause of an individual's disease unless it has been previously demonstrated to cause a disease with a similar phenotype. To prove causality, medical genetics relies on **association** (the recurrence of mutations within a gene among individuals with a similar phenotype). For rare diseases, there may be too few affected patients to demonstrate a statistically significant association, and other evidence from phenotype ontologies, metabolomics, glycomics, proteomics, and lipidomics may be required. In addition, models (e.g., mice, zebrafish, fruit flies, yeast, cultured cells) can be developed to recapitulate the disease. The variant in question can also be linked to a biologic process or pathway that is known to cause a similar phenotype when disturbed. Finally, standardized and correlated phenotypic and genomic data are deposited into a database to identify other individuals with a similar phenotype and mutations in the same gene.

Physicians may apply their past biases to a group of variants that could be disease causing, but this is often misleading. A standardized computational approach is preferable. For example, the Human Phenotype Ontology standardizes the description of a disease and, because the descriptors have been mapped to other human diseases and to mutant model organisms, identifies possible candidate genes and genetic networks for causing the disease. Similarly, untargeted laboratory screening tests provide an unbiased survey of patient cellular biology and physiology and a more informed prioritization of candidate variants.

The ultimate proof of causality is to ameliorate the disease process by correcting the genetic defect; this might be demonstrable in a model system that recapitulates the human disease. Alternatively, a search for other patients with a similar phenotype and mutations in the same gene can be performed using public databases established using strict statistical and biologic standards.

PEDIATRIC ISSUES

Of the UDP's 1st 500 pediatric applications, >10% had more than 1 family member (usually a sibling) similarly affected. The age distribution had peaks at 4-5 yr (reflecting patients with congenital disorders) and at 16-18 yr (representing disorders with symptom onset at early school age). Most applicants had been on a diagnostic odyssey for >5 yr. Of the 200 pediatric cases accepted, 25% received a diagnosis; half were obtained using conventional diagnostic methods, including clinical suspicion, biochemical testing with molecular confirmation, or radiographic interpretation. Otherwise, SNP analysis and NGS yielded the diagnosis; all involved rare diseases.

Pediatric medical records require attention to what has and what has not been completed previously. The electronic medical record is an important tool, but "copy forward" functions can perpetuate errors, such as reports of normal testing when in fact the test was recommended or ordered but not performed. Repetitive copying also fosters sloppiness in critical thinking, failure to take an adequate history, and missing the nuances of symptom progression. A history and physical examination should be performed anew and all prior testing results confirmed through copies of original laboratory reports.

Prolonged and painful procedures should be performed under sedation, but the risks associated with sedation must be weighed against the value of information and samples obtained.

Considerations for Families of Undiagnosed Children

When a child comes to a genetics clinic for evaluation, the parents ask these questions:

- What does my child have? (diagnosis)
- Why did it happen? (etiology/inheritance)
- What will happen in the future? (natural history; prognosis)
- Is there a treatment? (therapy)
- Could the same thing happen to other family members? (recurrence risk)

The answers all require an accurate diagnosis. The lack of a diagnosis makes both the family and the physician uncomfortable, raises suspicion among relatives and acquaintances, and creates feelings of guilt about not having worked hard enough to obtain a diagnosis. Families often consult more and more specialists, becoming frustrated with the lack of coordination among providers. Families should save copies of every test and every visit from each institution in a binder for travel among institutions. A 2- to 3-page narrative summarizing the child's history, medications, list of healthcare providers with contact information, main medical issues, level of functioning on well days and sick days, and interventions that worked in the past can be invaluable in an emergency room setting. An electronic copy is easily updated. Parents can always be the best advocates for their child, particularly an undiagnosed child.

Recommendations to parents of an undiagnosed child are similar to those that apply to any child with chronic illness:

- Organize copies of all records, especially original reports from "send-out" laboratories.
- Carry an updated emergency letter.
- Establish a medical home even if you obtain many second opinions.
- Find a physiatrist (rehabilitation medicine physician) to coordinate rehabilitative care.
- Strongly advocate with the school system for needed services (see Chapter 48), using a legal advocate if necessary;
- Explore parent support groups for unknown disorders (Syndromes Without a Name, National Organization for Rare Disorders).
- Periodically check with providers (especially geneticists) for new diagnoses reported in the medical literature.
- Carve out time for yourselves as caregivers by engaging extended family members or respite care services.
- Work at supporting and being attentive to well children in the family.
- For the dying child, consider an autopsy to establish a diagnosis, especially when there is a possibility of future pregnancies.

THE DIAGNOSTIC SPECTRUM

Rare and new genetic disorders can present at any age; a gene's "severe" mutations may manifest early in life while "mild" mutations present later. Diagnoses of known disorders can have very different bases, such as the extent of recognition of a clinical entity, a molecular confirmation, or biochemical evidence. Some variants identified by SNP and exome sequencing analyses may represent new diseases.

One example of the use of these technologies to discover a new diagnosis involves 2 brothers whose parents were first cousins. The brothers had an early-onset spastic ataxia-neuropathy syndrome, with lower-extremity spasticity, peripheral neuropathy, ptosis, oculomotor apraxia, dystonia, cerebellar atrophy, and progressive myoclonic epilepsy. A homozygous missense mutation (c.1847G>A; p.Y616C) in *AFG3L2*, which encodes a subunit of a mitochondrial protease, was identified by exome sequencing. The AFG3L2 protein can bind to another AFG3L2 molecule or to paraplegin. UDP collaborators in Germany used a yeast model system to demonstrate that the patients' mutation affects the specific amino acid involved in the formation of both these complexes. As a result, the brothers exhibited the signs and symptoms of a known AFG3L2 defect, autosomal dominant spinocerebellar ataxia type 28 (SCA28), and also deficits attributable to a paraplegin defect, hereditary spastic paraplegia type 7 (SPG7). Other features of a mitochondrial disorder (oculomotor apraxia, extrapyramidal dysfunction, myoclonic epilepsy) were also present. The 2 brothers represent the 1st such cases in the world and expand the phenotype of AFG3L2 disease.

A 2nd example involves 2 siblings ages 5 and 10 yr with hypotonia, developmental delays, facial dysmorphisms, hearing loss, nystagmus, seizures, and atrophy on brain MRI. In this case the leading clue was biochemical in nature, and genetic analysis confirmed the diagnosis. Urine thin-layer chromatography for oligosaccharides identified a strong band determined by mass spectrometry to consist of a tetrasaccharide containing 3 glucoses and 1 mannose. This suggested a defect of glucosidase I, the 1st enzyme involved in endoplasmic reticulum trimming of *N*-linked glycoproteins from a high-mannose to a complex form. Mutation analysis confirmed compound heterozygous variants in the glucosidase I gene, establishing the diagnosis of congenital disorder of glycosylation IIb. The 2 siblings were the 2nd and 3rd patients in the world with this disorder.

Occasionally an autosomal dominant disorder, typically presenting in adulthood, can manifest as a completely different and more severe disorder when pathologic variants in the same gene are inherited from each parent; the child is a *compound heterozygote*. This was the case in a 3 yr old child who inherited 2 variants in *GARS*, the gene causing autosomal dominant Charcot-Marie-Tooth disease (CMT) 2D. The child had severe intrauterine and postnatal growth retardation, microcephaly, developmental delay, optic nerve atrophy and retinal pigment changes, as well as an atrial septal defect. Neither parent was symptomatic at the time the child was evaluated; the parents had normal electromyography and nerve conduction studies. This case emphasizes the need to consent families before any genetic testing as to the possibility of receiving unexpected results in additional family members. In this case, genetic counseling was expanded to include possible CMT2D in the parents.

Bibliography is available at Expert Consult.

Metabolic Disorders
代谢性疾病

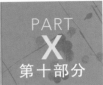

Chapter **102**

An Approach to Inborn Errors of Metabolism

Oleg A. Shchelochkov and
Charles P. Venditti

第一百零二章
遗传代谢病诊疗思路

中文导读

本章主要介绍了新生儿筛查、遗传代谢病的临床表现及诊治。首先介绍了美国医学遗传学会推荐的应纳入新生儿筛查的主要疾病；继而以多个表格的形式总结了主要遗传代谢病的新生儿神经系统及实验室表现，临床表现疑似遗传代谢疾病的足月新生儿的诊断流程，表现有新生儿低血糖、肝功能障碍、心肌病、特征畸形、胎儿水肿、特殊气味的遗传代谢病，高氨血症的鉴别诊断，遗传代谢病相关的病理组织学临床发现以及提示应该进行遗传代谢检测的临床表现、实验室检查结果；简要介绍了遗传代谢病治疗包括的主要方法，如特殊饮食、血液透析、液体疗法等。

Many childhood conditions are caused by single-gene mutations that encode specific proteins. These mutations can change primary protein structure or the amount of protein synthesized. The function of a protein, whether it is an enzyme, receptor, transport vehicle, membrane component, transcriptional co-regulator, or structural element, may be compromised or abolished. Hereditary diseases that disrupt normal biochemical processes are termed **inborn errors of metabolism** or **inherited metabolic diseases**.

Most genetic changes are clinically inconsequential and represent *benign* variants. However, pathogenic variants produce diseases that range in severity of presentation and time of onset. Severe metabolic disorders usually become clinically apparent in the newborn period or shortly thereafter, whereas milder forms may present later in childhood and even in adulthood. With some exceptions, the presenting symptoms of most metabolic conditions lack the specificity to enable a definitive diagnosis without further evaluation. The combination of *low specificity* of presenting symptoms and *low prevalence* of metabolic disorders makes determination of the diagnosis difficult. Progressive symptoms, the lack of plausible non-genetic diagnosis after detailed evaluation, history of overlapping symptoms in patient's relatives, or consanguinity should alert a pediatrician to seek a consultation with a geneticist and consider metabolic testing early in the evaluation.

Correct diagnosis is often only the beginning of a long medical journey for most families affected by metabolic conditions (see Chapter 95). Although each inherited metabolic disorder is individually rare, improved diagnosis and increasing survival of patients with metabolic conditions virtually ensure that a pediatrician will encounter and provide care to affected patients. Pediatricians can play a critical role in establishing the continuity of care, managing some aspects of treatment, fostering adherence, and delivering routine pediatric interventions such as immunizations, referrals to specialists, and elements of genetic counseling (see Chapter 94.1).

The greater awareness of metabolic conditions, wider availability of biochemical laboratories, global metabolomic analysis, and routine application of exome sequencing dramatically increased the detection rate of the known disorders and contributed to the discovery of new metabolic disorders. Nonetheless, collection and analysis of family history remains a critical screening test that a healthcare provider can use to identify an infant or child at risk for a metabolic disorder. The identification of consanguinity or a particular ethnic background with an unusually high incidence of inborn errors of metabolism can be important to direct further studies. For example, tyrosinemia type 1 is more common among French-Canadians of Quebec, maple syrup urine disease is seen with higher frequency in the U.S. Amish population, and Canavan disease in patients of the Ashkenazi Jewish ancestry.

NEWBORN SCREENING

The individual rarity of inborn errors of metabolism, the importance of early diagnosis, and the ensuing genetic counseling ramifications make a strong argument for the universal screening all newborn infants. **Tandem mass spectrometry** of metabolites and **digital microfluidics analysis** of enzyme activities form the foundation of newborn screening today. Both methods require a few drops of blood to be placed on a filter paper and delivered to a central laboratory for assay. Many genetic conditions can be identified by these methods, and the list of disorders continues to grow (Tables 102.1 and 102.2). Pediatricians need to be aware of the general screening procedure and limitations of screening. As a screening method, a positive result may require a repeat newborn screen or confirmatory testing to secure the diagnosis. Time required to return the results vary from country to country and even within states in the same country. Some metabolic conditions can be severe enough to cause clinical manifestations before the results of the newborn screening become available. Conversely, diagnostic metabolites in milder forms of screened disorders may not reach a set threshold to trigger secondary studies, thus leading to a negative newborn screen results and delayed diagnosis. *Therefore, negative newborn screening in a patient with symptoms suggestive of a metabolic disorder warrants a referral to genetics center for further evaluation.*

Table 102.1	Disorders Recommended by the American College of Medical Genetics Task Force for Inclusion in Newborn Screening ("Primary Disorders")*

DISORDERS OF ORGANIC ACID METABOLISM	DISORDERS OF AMINO ACID METABOLISM
Isovaleric acidemia	Phenylketonuria
Glutaric aciduria type I	Maple syrup urine disease
3-Hydroxy-3-methylglutaric aciduria	Homocystinuria
Multiple carboxylase deficiency	Citrullinemia type 1
Methylmalonic acidemia (methylmalonyl-CoA mutase deficiency)	Argininosuccinic acidemia
Methylmalonic acidemia (*cbl*A and *cbl*B defects)	Tyrosinemia type I
Propionic acidemia	
3-Methylcrotonyl-CoA carboxylase deficiency	**HEMOGLOBINOPATHIES**
β-Ketothiolase deficiency	Sickle cell anemia (hemoglobin SS disease)
	Hemoglobin S/β-thalassemia
DISORDERS OF FATTY ACID METABOLISM	Hemoglobin S/C disease
Medium-chain acyl-CoA dehydrogenase deficiency	
Very-long-chain acyl-CoA dehydrogenase deficiency	**OTHER DISORDERS**
Long-chain 3-hydroxy-acyl-CoA dehydrogenase deficiency	Congenital hypothyroidism
Trifunctional protein deficiency	Biotinidase deficiency
Carnitine uptake defect	Congenital adrenal hyperplasia
	Galactosemia
	Hearing loss
	Cystic fibrosis
	Severe combined immunodeficiency (SCID)†
	Critical congenital heart disease†

*As of November 2014, there is state-to-state variation in newborn screening; a list of the disorders that are screened for by each state is available at http://genes-r-us.uthscsa.edu/sites/genes-r-us/files/nbsdisorders.pdf.
†The inclusion of SCID and critical congenital heart disease received support of the American College of Medical Genetics and Genomics.
*cbl*A, Cobalamin A defect; *cbl*B, cobalamin B defect; CoA, coenzyme A.

Table 102.2	Secondary Conditions Recommended by American College of Medical Genetics* Task Force for Inclusion in Newborn Screening

ORGANIC ACID METABOLISM DISORDERS	AMINO ACID METABOLISM DISORDERS
Methylmalonic acidemia (*cbl*C and *cbl*D defects)	Hyperphenylalaninemia, benign (not classic phenylketonuria)
Malonic acidemia	Tyrosinemia type II
2-Methyl-3-hydroxybutyric aciduria	Tyrosinemia type III
Isobutyryl-CoA dehydrogenase deficiency	Defects of biopterin cofactor biosynthesis
2-Methylbutyryl-CoA dehydrogenase deficiency	Defects of biopterin cofactor regeneration
3-Methylglutaconic aciduria	Argininemia
	Hypermethioninemia
FATTY ACID OXIDATION DISORDERS	Citrullinemia type II (citrin deficiency)
Short-chain acyl-CoA dehydrogenase deficiency	
Glutaric acidemia type 2	**HEMOGLOBINOPATHIES**
Medium/short-chain 3-hydroxy-acyl-CoA dehydrogenase deficiency	Hemoglobin variants (including hemoglobin E)
Medium-chain ketoacyl-CoA thiolase deficiency	
Carnitine palmitoyltransferase IA deficiency	**OTHERS**
Carnitine palmitoyltransferase II deficiency	Galactose epimerase deficiency
Carnitine:acylcarnitine translocase deficiency	Galactokinase deficiency
Dienoyl-CoA reductase deficiency	

*The American College of Medical Genetics Newborn Screening Expert Group (May 2006) recommended reporting, in addition to the primary disorders, 25 disorders ("secondary targets") that can be detected through screening but that do not meet the criteria for primary disorders (https://www.acmg.net/resources/policies/nbs/NBS_Main_Report_01.pdf).
*cbl*C, Cobalamin C defect; *cbl*D, cobalamin D defect; CoA, coenzyme A.

Universal newborn screening may also identify mild forms of inherited metabolic conditions, some of which may never cause clinical manifestations in the lifetime of the individual. For example, short-chain acyl-CoA dehydrogenase deficiency has been identified with unexpectedly high frequency in screening programs using tandem mass spectrometry, but most of these children have remained asymptomatic. This highlights the need for an ongoing evaluation of metabolite cutoff values and approaches to confirmatory testing to maximize the diagnostic yield and minimize potential psychosocial and economic implications of such findings. Premature infants represent a special patient population in whom the incidence of false-positive or false-negative test results can be especially high.

With the advent of genetic therapy for spinal muscular atrophy (SMA) and enzyme replacement therapy for some lysosomal storage diseases (e.g., Pompe disease, Fabry disease, Gaucher disease, and mucopolysaccharidosis type 1), pilot newborn screening programs have demonstrated initial success in identifying SMA or lysosomal storage disorders, often before severe symptoms develop.

CLINICAL MANIFESTATIONS OF GENETIC METABOLIC DISEASES

Physicians and other healthcare providers who care for children should familiarize themselves with early manifestations of genetic metabolic disorders, because (1) severe forms of some of these conditions may cause symptoms before the results of screening studies become available, and (2) the current screening methods, although quite extensive, identify a small number of all inherited metabolic conditions. In the newborn period, the clinical findings are usually nonspecific and similar to those seen in infants with sepsis. A genetic disorder of metabolism should be considered in the differential diagnosis of a severely ill newborn infant, and special studies should be undertaken if the index of suspicion is high (Fig. 102.1).

Signs and symptoms such as lethargy, hypotonia, hypothermia, convulsions (Table 102.3), poor feeding, and vomiting may develop as early as a few hours after birth. Occasionally, vomiting may be severe enough to suggest the diagnosis of pyloric stenosis, which is usually not present, although it may occur simultaneously in such infants. Lethargy, poor feeding, seizures, and coma may also be seen in infants

with hypoglycemia (Table 102.4) (see Chapters 111 and 127), hypocalcemia (Chapters 64 and 589), and hyperammonemia (Table 102.5) (Chapter 103). Measurements of blood concentrations of glucose and calcium and response to intravenous injection of glucose or calcium help establish these diagnoses. Every organ system can be affected by metabolic disorders. However, *physical examination* usually reveals nonspecific findings; most signs are related to the central nervous system such as opisthotonus in the case of maple syrup urine disease (MSUD). Hepatomegaly is a common finding in a variety of inborn errors of metabolism (Table 102.6). Cardiomyopathy (Table 102.7), dysmorphology (Table 102.8), and fetal hydrops (Table 102.9) are additional potential manifestations of a metabolic disorder (Table 102.10). Occasionally, a peculiar odor may offer an invaluable aid to the diagnosis (Table 102.11).

In an increasing number of patients, a metabolic condition may be recognized months or years after birth. This is more typical in patients carrying milder autosomal recessive pathogenic variants, in mitochondrial disorders, in females affected by X-linked recessive conditions, and specific metabolic conditions that usually present later in life. *Clinical manifestations,* such as intellectual disability, motor deficits, developmental regression, seizures, psychosis, cardiomyopathy, myopathy, organomegaly, and recurrent emesis, in patients beyond the neonatal period should suggest an inherited metabolic disease (Table 102.12). There may be an episodic or intermittent pattern, with episodes of acute clinical manifestations separated by periods of seemingly disease-free states. The episodes are usually triggered by stress or nonspecific catabolic stress such as an infection. The child may die during one of these acute attacks. An inborn error of metabolism should be considered in any child with 1 or more of the following manifestations: unexplained developmental delay; intellectual disability; developmental regression; motor deficits or adventitious movements (e.g., dystonia, choreoathetosis, ataxia); seizures; catatonia; unusual odor (particularly during an acute illness); intermittent episodes of unexplained vomiting, acidosis, mental deterioration, psychosis, or coma; hepatomegaly; renal stones; renal dysfunction, especially Fanconi syndrome or renal tubular acidosis; muscle weakness; and cardiomyopathy (Table 102.12).

Diagnosis usually requires a variety of specific *laboratory studies.* Plasma amino acid analysis, plasma acylcarnitine profile, total and free

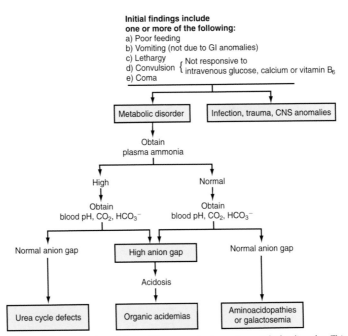

Fig. 102.1 Initial clinical approach to a full-term newborn infant with a suspected genetic metabolic disorder. This schema is a guide to elucidate some of the metabolic disorders in newborn infants. Although some exceptions to this schema exist, it is appropriate for most cases affected by disorders or intermediate metabolism. CNS, Central nervous system; GI, gastrointestinal; HCO_3^-, bicarbonate.

Table 102.3	Select Inborn Errors of Metabolism Associated With Neurologic and Laboratory Manifestations in Neonates

DETERIORATION IN CONSCIOUSNESS
Metabolic Acidosis
Organic acidemias
Disorders of pyruvate metabolism
Fatty acid oxidation defects
Fructose-1,6-bisphosphatase deficiency
Glycogen storage diseases
Mitochondrial respiratory chain defects
Disorders of ketone metabolism
Hypoglycemia*
Fatty acid oxidation defects
Disorders of gluconeogenesis
Disorders of fructose and galactose metabolism
Glycogen storage diseases

Disorders of ketogenesis
Organic acidemias
Hyperinsulinemic hypoglycemias
Mitochondrial respiratory chain defects
Neonatal intrahepatic cholestasis caused by citrin deficiency
Pyruvate carboxylase deficiency
Carbonic anhydrase VA deficiency
Hyperammonemia**
Urea cycle disorders
Organic acidemias
Fatty acid oxidation disorders
Disorders of pyruvate metabolism
GLUD1-related hyperinsulinemic hypoglycemia
Carbonic anhydrase VA deficiency

SEIZURES AND HYPOTONIA

Antiquitin deficiency (pyridoxine-dependent epilepsy)

Pyridoxamine 5′-phosphate oxidase (PNPO) deficiency (pyridoxal phosphate-responsive epilepsy)

Folate metabolism disorders
Multiple carboxylase deficiency (holocarboxylase synthetase deficiency and biotinidase deficiency)
Urea cycle disorders
Organic acidemias
Fatty acid oxidation disorders
Disorders of creatine biosynthesis and transport
Disorders of neurotransmitter metabolism
Molybdenum cofactor deficiency and sulfite oxidase deficiency
Serine deficiency disorders
Glycine encephalopathy

Asparagine synthetase deficiency
Mitochondrial respiratory chain defects
Zellweger spectrum disorders
Congenital disorders of glycosylation
Purine and pyrimidine metabolism defects

NEONATAL APNEA
Glycine encephalopathy
Asparagine synthetase deficiency
Urea cycle disorders
Organic acidemias
Disorders of pyruvate metabolism
Fatty acid oxidation defects
Mitochondrial respiratory chain defects

*Refer to Table 102.4 for more details on the metabolic disorders associated with neonatal hypoglycemia.
**Refer to Table 102.5 for more details on the differential diagnosis of neonatal and infantile hyperammonemia.
Modified from El-Hattab AW: Inborn errors of metabolism, Clin Perinatol 42:413-439, 2015 (Box 1, p 415).

Table 102.4	Select Inborn Errors of Metabolism Associated With Neonatal Hypoglycemia

CATEGORY OF DISORDERS	DISORDERS	CATEGORY OF DISORDERS	DISORDERS
Fatty acid oxidation disorders	Carnitine-acylcarnitine translocase deficiency Carnitine palmitoyltransferase Ia deficiency Carnitine palmitoyltransferase II deficiency Long-chain 3-hydroxyacyl-CoA dehydrogenase deficiency/trifunctional protein deficiency Medium-chain acyl-CoA dehydrogenase deficiency Very-long-chain acyl-CoA dehydrogenase deficiency Multiple acyl-CoA dehydrogenase deficiency	Disorders of ketogenesis	3-Hydroxy-3-methylglutaryl-CoA lyase deficiency Mitochondrial 3-hydroxy-3-methylglutaryl-CoA synthase deficiency
		Organic acidemias	Propionic acidemia Methylmalonic acidemia Isovaleric acidemia Maple syrup urine disease Multiple carboxylase deficiency (holocarboxylase synthetase deficiency and biotinidase deficiency)
Disorders of gluconeogenesis	Fructose-1,6-diphosphatase deficiency Phosphoenolpyruvate carboxykinase deficiency	Hyperinsulinemic hypoglycemia	*HADH*-related disorder (3-alpha-hydroxyacyl-CoA dehydrogenase deficiency) *GLUD1*-related disorder (hyperammonemia-hyperinsulinism syndrome, HIHA)
Disorders of fructose and galactose metabolism	Hereditary fructose intolerance Classic galactosemia		
Glycogen storage diseases (GSD)	GSD type Ia (glucose-6-phosphatase deficiency) GSD type Ib (impaired glucose-6-phosphate exchanger) GSD type III (glycogen debrancher enzyme deficiency) GSD type VI (liver glycogen phosphorylase deficiency) GSD type IX (phosphorylase kinase deficiencies)	Other	Mitochondrial respiratory chain defects Neonatal intrahepatic cholestasis caused by citrin deficiency Pyruvate carboxylase deficiency Carbonic anhydrase VA deficiency

Modified from Zinn AB: Inborn errors of metabolism. In *Fanaroff & Martin's neonatal-perinatal medicine: diseases of the fetus and infant*, ed 10, vol 2, Philadelphia, 2015, Elsevier (Table 99.17, p 1605).

| Table 102.5 | Differential Diagnosis of Hyperammonemia |

INBORN ERRORS OF METABOLISM
Urea Cycle Enzyme Defects
N-acetylglutamate synthase (NAGS) deficiency
Carbamoyl phosphate synthetase 1 (CPS1) deficiency
Ornithine transcarbamylase (OTC) deficiency
Argininosuccinate synthetase (ASS) deficiency (citrullinemia type 1)
Argininosuccinate lyase (ASL) deficiency (argininosuccinic aciduria)
Arginase 1 deficiency
Transport and Synthesis Defects of Urea Cycle Intermediates
Hyperornithinemia-hyperammonemia-homocitrullinemia (HHH syndrome)
Citrullinemia type 2 caused by citrin deficiency
Lysinuric protein intolerance
Ornithine aminotransferase deficiency
Carbonic anhydrase VA deficiency
Organic Acidemias
Propionic acidemia
MUT-related methylmalonic acidemia and cobalamin metabolism disorders
Isovaleric acidemia
Fatty Acid Oxidation Disorders
Long-chain fatty acid oxidation defects
Systemic primary carnitine deficiency
Other
Pyruvate carboxylase deficiency
GLUD1-related hyperinsulinemic hypoglycemia
Neonatal iron overload disorders (e.g. hereditary hemochromatoses)

ACQUIRED DISORDERS
Transient Hyperammonemia of the Newborn
Diseases of the Liver and Biliary Tract
Liver failure
Biliary atresia
Severe Systemic Neonatal Illness
Neonates sepsis
Heart failure
Medications
Valproic acid
Cyclophosphamide
5-Pentanoic acid
Asparaginase
Other
Reye syndrome

ANATOMIC VARIANTS
Vascular bypass of the liver (e.g. a portosystemic anastomosis)

TECHNICAL
Inappropriate sample collection (e.g., capillary blood or prolonged placement of a tourniquet)
Sample not immediately analyzed

Modified from El-Hattab AW: Inborn errors of metabolism, Clin Perinatol 42:413-439, 2015 (Box 8, p 428).

carnitine profile, and urine organic acid assay, while not exhaustive in their diagnostic scope, are useful as initial screening tests to evaluate for a suspected inborn error of metabolism. Measurements of plasma ammonia, lactate, bicarbonate, and pH are readily available in hospitals and very helpful initially in differentiating major causes of genetic metabolic disorders (Table 102.13; see Fig. 102.1). Elevation of blood ammonia is usually caused by defects of urea cycle enzymes, organic acidemias, and disorders of fatty acid oxidation. Infants with elevated blood ammonia levels from urea cycle defects tend to have normal serum pH and bicarbonate values; without measurement of blood ammonia, they may remain undiagnosed and succumb to their disease. In organic acidemias, elevated plasma ammonia is accompanied by severe acidosis caused by accumulation of organic acids, ketone bodies, and lactate in body fluids.

When blood ammonia, pH, and bicarbonate values are normal, other aminoacidopathies (e.g. hyperglycinemia) or galactosemia should be considered. Galactosemic infants may also manifest cataracts, hepatomegaly, ascites, and jaundice.

TREATMENT

The majority of patients with genetic disorders of metabolism respond to one or more of the following treatments:
1. Special diets play an important role in the treatment of affected children. Dietary changes should be tailored to the pathophysiology of the condition and vary greatly among disorders.
2. Hemodialysis for expeditious removal of accumulated noxious compounds. This is a very effective modality for treatment of the acute phase of the condition.
3. Catabolic states in patients at risk for metabolic crisis can be treated with fluids containing dextrose and electrolytes.
4. Administration of the deficient metabolite.
5. Administration of the cofactor or coenzyme to maximize the residual enzyme activity.
6. Activation of alternate pathways to reduce the noxious compounds accumulated because of the genetic mutation.
7. Administration of the deficient enzyme.
8. Bone marrow transplantation.
9. Liver and kidney transplantation.

The organ transplantation modalities may offer the best treatment modality to stabilize a metabolic patient and improve quality of life. To date, replacement of the mutant gene with a normal copy using gene therapy has been successful in only a few diseases.

Treatment of genetic disorders of metabolism is complex and requires medical and technical expertise. The therapeutic regimen often needs to be tailored to the individual patient because of large phenotypic variations in the severity of the disease, even within a single family. Providing education and support for the family is the key to successful long-term therapy. Even in patients with poor prognoses, every effort should be made to establish correct diagnoses premortem. Effective treatment is best achieved by a team of specialists—metabolic genetics specialist, nutritionist, neurologist, and psychologist—in a major medical center.

Bibliography is available at Expert Consult.

Table 102.6	Select Metabolic Disorders Associated With Hepatic Dysfunction

CATEGORY OF DISORDERS	DISORDERS
Disorders of amino acid metabolism	Tyrosinemia type I Citrullinemia type II caused by citrin deficiency Disorders of methionine metabolism Urea cycle disorders
Biliary tract disorders and disorder of bile acid synthesis	See Chapter 383
Disorders of fructose and galactose metabolism	Hereditary fructose intolerance Classic galactosemia Epimerase deficiency galactosemia
Congenital disorders of glycosylation	Multiple types
Fatty acid oxidation disorders	Carnitine-acylcarnitine translocase deficiency Carnitine palmitoyltransferase Ia deficiency Carnitine palmitoyltransferase II deficiency Long-chain 3-hydroxyacyl-CoA dehydrogenase deficiency/trifunctional protein deficiency Very-long-chain acyl-CoA dehydrogenase deficiency Multiple acyl-CoA dehydrogenase deficiency
Glycogen storage disorders (GSD)	GSD type III (glycogen debrancher enzyme deficiency) GSD type IV (glycogen branching enzyme deficiency) GSD type VI (liver glycogen phosphorylase deficiency)
Peroxisomal disorders	Zellweger spectrum disorders Disorders of peroxisomal β-oxidation
Mitochondrial respiratory chain (RC) defects	*Mitochondrial DNA (mtDNA) or nuclear DNA (nDNA) defects* Specific single nucleotide pathogenic variants in mtDNA Large-scale mtDNA re-arrangements (Pearson syndrome) Disorders of mitochondrial translation (e.g., tRNA^{Glu}) Disorder of protein synthesis of RC complexes Disorders affected the assembly or stabilization of RC complexes (e.g., *BCS1L*) Disorders of cofactor biosynthesis (e.g. coenzyme Q10) Disorders of mitochondrial transport and dynamics mtDNA depletion syndromes (e.g., *DGUOK, MPV17, POLG, SUCLG1*)
Lysosomal storage disorders	Niemann-Pick disease type C
Other	α$_1$-Antitrypsin deficiency

Modified from Zinn AB: Inborn errors of metabolism. In Fanaroff & Martin's neonatal-perinatal medicine: diseases of the fetus and infant, ed 10, vol 2, Philadelphia, 2015, Elsevier (Table 99.5, p 1579).

Table 102.7	Select Metabolic Disorders Associated With Cardiomyopathy

CATEGORY OF DISORDERS	DISORDERS
Organic acidemias	Propionic acidemia Cobalamin C deficiency 3-methylglutaconic acidurias (e.g., Barth syndrome and DCMA syndrome)
Lysosomal storage disorders	Sphingolipidoses (e.g., Fabry disease) Oligosaccharidoses and mucolipidoses (e.g., I-cell disease) Mucopolysaccharidoses
Glycogen storage disorders (GSD)	GSD type II (Pompe disease) GSD type III (glycogen debrancher enzyme deficiency) *PRKAG2*-related disorders (includes lethal congenital glycogen storage disease of heart)
Congenital disorders of glycosylation	Multiple types
Fatty acid oxidation disorders	Carnitine-acylcarnitine translocase deficiency Carnitine palmitoyltransferase II deficiency Long-chain 3-hydroxyacyl-CoA dehydrogenase deficiency/trifunctional protein deficiency *ACAD9*-related disorder (mitochondrial acyl-CoA dehydrogenase deficiency) Multiple acyl-CoA dehydrogenase deficiency (includes glutaric aciduria type 2) Very-long-chain acyl-CoA dehydrogenase deficiency Systemic primary carnitine deficiency
Mitochondrial respiratory chain (RC) defects	*Mitochondrial DNA (mtDNA) or nuclear DNA (nDNA) defects* Specific single nucleotide pathogenic variants in mtDNA Large-scale mtDNA deletions Disorders of mitochondrial translation (e.g., tRNA^{Leu}) Disorders of protein synthesis of RC complexes (e.g., *MT-ATP6, MT-ATP8, NDUFS2, NDUFV2, SDHA, SCO2, COX10, COX15*) Disorders affecting the assembly or stabilization of RC complexes (e.g., *TMEM70*) Disorders of cofactor biosynthesis (e.g. coenzyme Q10) Disorders of mitochondrial transport and dynamics (e.g., *SLC25A3*) mtDNA depletion syndromes (e.g., *SUCLG1*)
Other	Danon disease

Modified from Zinn AB: Inborn errors of metabolism. In Fanaroff & Martin's neonatal-perinatal medicine: diseases of the fetus and infant, ed 10, vol 2, Philadelphia, 2015, Elsevier (Table 99.4, p 1576).

Table 102.8	Select Inborn Errors of Metabolism Associated With Dysmorphic Features		
CATEGORY OF DISORDERS	**DISORDERS**	**CATEGORY OF DISORDERS**	**DISORDERS**
Congenital disorders of glycosylation	N-Glycosylation disorders (e.g., PMM2-CDG and ALG3-CDG) O-Glycosylation disorders (e.g., Walker-Warburg syndrome)	Lysosomal storage disorders	Sphingolipidoses Oligosaccharidoses and mucolipidoses Mucopolysaccharidoses
Disorders of cholesterol biosynthesis	Smith-Lemli-Opitz syndrome Desmosterolosis Lathosterolosis *EBP*-related disorder (includes Conradi-Hunermann syndrome)	Organic acidurias	Multiple acyl-CoA dehydrogenase deficiency (includes glutaric aciduria type 2) Mevalonic aciduria*
		Peroxisomal disorders	Zellweger spectrum disorders Disorders of peroxisomal β-oxidation
		Other	Pyruvate dehydrogenase complex deficiency

*Mevalonic aciduria has been classified as an organic acidemia based on the method used for its diagnosis, but it can also be classified as a peroxisomal single-enzyme disorder or as a defect in cholesterol biosynthesis because of its intracellular location and function, respectively.
Modified from Zinn AB: Inborn errors of metabolism. In Fanaroff & Martin's neonatal-perinatal medicine: diseases of the fetus and infant, ed 10, vol 2, Philadelphia, 2015, Elsevier (Table 99.8, p 1583).

Table 102.9	Select Inborn Errors of Metabolism Associated With Hydrops Fetalis

Lysosomal storage disorders
  Mucopolysaccharidoses types I, IVA, and VII
  Sphingolipidoses (e.g., Gaucher disease, Farber disease, Niemann-Pick disease A, GM$_1$ gangliosidosis, multiple sulfatase deficiency)
  Lipid storage diseases (Wolman and Niemann-Pick disease C)
  Oligosaccharidoses (e.g., sialidosis type I)
  Mucolipidoses (e.g., I-cell disease)
	Zellweger spectrum disorders
	Glycogen storage disease type IV
	Congenital disorders of glycosylation
	Mitochondrial respiratory chain defects
	Transaldolase deficiency

Modified and adapted from El-Hattab AW: Inborn errors of metabolism, Clin Perinatol 42:413-439, 2015 (Box 6, p 417).

Table 102.10	Pathognomonic Clinical Findings Associated With Inborn Errors of Metabolism (Select Examples)		
FINDINGS	**DISORDERS**	**FINDINGS**	**DISORDERS**
Hepatomegaly	Disorders of fructose and galactose metabolism (e.g., classic galactosemia and hereditary fructose intolerance) Glycogen storage diseases Disorders of gluconeogenesis Disorders of fatty acid oxidation and transport Mitochondrial respiratory chain defects Tyrosinemia type 1 Urea cycle disorders Zellweger spectrum disorders Niemann-Pick disease type C Congenital disorders of glycosylation	Dystonia or extrapyramidal signs	Gaucher disease type 2 Glutaric acidemia type 1 Methylmalonic acidemia Propionic acidemia Krabbe disease Crigler–Najjar syndrome Disorders of neurotransmitter metabolism Pyruvate dehydrogenase complex deficiency
		Macular "cherry-red spot"	GM$_1$ gangliosidosis Tay-Sachs disease (GM$_2$ gangliosidosis) Farber disease (acid ceramidase deficiency) Galactosialidosis Niemann-Pick disease type A Sialidosis Multiple sulfatase deficiency
Hepatosplenomegaly	Mucopolysaccharidoses Niemann-Pick disease types A, B, and C Sphingolipidoses (e.g., GM$_1$ gangliosidosis or Gaucher disease) Wolman disease Farber disease (acid ceramidase deficiency)		
		"Bull eye" maculopathy	*cbl*C deficiency (combined methylmalonic acidemia and homocystinuria, type C)
Macrocephaly	Glutaric acidemia type 1 Canavan disease	Retinitis pigmentosa	Mitochondrial respiratory chain defects Peroxisomal disorders Abetalipoproteinemia
Microcephaly	Mitochondrial respiratory chain defects Disorders of intracellular cobalamin metabolism (e.g., *cbl*C deficiency)	Optic nerve atrophy or hypoplasia	Pyruvate dehydrogenase complex deficiency Mitochondrial respiratory chain defects Peroxisomal disorders Propionic acidemia *MUT*-related methylmalonic acidemia and cobalamin metabolism disorders
Coarse facial features	Mucopolysaccharidoses Oligosaccharidoses and mucolipidoses (e.g., α-mannosidosis) Sphingolipidoses (e.g., GM$_1$ gangliosidosis) Galactosialidosis		
		Corneal clouding or opacities	Mucolipidoses Mucopolysaccharidoses Steroid sulfatase deficiency Tyrosinemia type II Cystinosis
Macroglossia	Glycogen storage disease type II (Pompe disease) Mucopolysaccharidoses Oligosaccharidoses and mucolipidoses Sphingolipidoses Galactosialidosis		

Continued

Table 102.10 | Pathognomonic Clinical Findings Associated With Inborn Errors of Metabolism (Select Examples)—cont'd

FINDINGS	DISORDERS	FINDINGS	DISORDERS
Cataracts	Disorders of galactose metabolism (e.g., classic galactosemia) Congenital disorders of glycosylation Mitochondrial respiratory chain (RC) defects Peroxisomal disorders Lowe oculocerebrorenal syndrome	Ichthyosis	Gaucher disease type 2 Steroid sulfatase deficiency Refsum disease ELOVL4-related disorder Serine deficiency disorders
Dislocated lens	Cystathionine β-synthase deficiency Molybdenum cofactor deficiency and sulfite oxidase deficiency	Alopecia	Multiple carboxylase deficiency (holocarboxylase synthetase deficiency and biotinidase deficiency)
Skeletal dysplasias and dysostosis multiplex	Oligosaccharidoses and mucolipidoses Mucopolysaccharidoses Sphingolipidoses Galactosialidosis Peroxisomal disorders Disorders of cholesterol biosynthesis Congenital disorders of glycosylation	Steely or kinky hair	Menkes disease
		Trichorrhexis nodosa	Argininosuccinic aciduria (ASL deficiency)
Thick skin	Oligosaccharidoses and mucolipidoses Mucopolysaccharidoses Sphingolipidoses	Persistent diarrhea	Glucose-galactose malabsorption Congenital lactase deficiency Congenital chloride diarrhea Sucrase-isomaltase deficiency Acrodermatitis enteropathica Abetalipoproteinemia Congenital folate malabsorption Wolman disease Lysinuric protein intolerance Classic galactosemia
Desquamating, eczematous, or vesiculobullous skin lesions	Acrodermatitis enteropathica Essential amino acid deficiencies in organic acidemias Hartnup disorder Multiple carboxylase deficiency (holocarboxylase synthetase deficiency and biotinidase deficiency) Porphyrias		

Modified from Cederbaum S: Introduction to metabolic and biochemical genetic diseases. In Gleason CA, Juul SE, editors: Avery's diseases of the newborn, ed 10, Philadelphia, 2018, Elsevier (Table 21.1, p 227).

Table 102.11 | Inborn Errors of Amino Acid Metabolism Associated With Peculiar Odor

INBORN ERROR OF METABOLISM	URINE ODOR	INBORN ERROR OF METABOLISM	URINE ODOR
Isovaleric acidemia Glutaric acidemia (type II)	Sweaty feet, acrid	Trimethylaminuria Dimethylglycine dehydrogenase deficiency	Rotten fish
Maple syrup urine disease	Maple syrup, burnt sugar	Tyrosinemia type 1	Boiled cabbage, rancid butter
Multiple carboxylase deficiency 3-Methylcrotonyl-CoA carboxylase deficiency 3-Hydroxy-3-methylglutaric aciduria	Cat urine	Hypermethioninemia	Boiled cabbage
		Cystinuria Tyrosinemia type I	Sulfur
Phenylketonuria	Mousey or musty	Hawkinsinuria	"Swimming pool"
		Oasthouse urine disease	Hops-like

Table 102.12 | Clinical Findings That Should Prompt a Metabolic Workup

Family history	Sibling(s) who died from unexplained causes or exhibit overlapping symptoms Ethnic groups with high prevalence of metabolic disorders Consanguinity	Cardiovascular system	Cardiac failure with or without cardiomyopathy, arrhythmia
		Musculoskeletal system	Rhabdomyolysis, myopathy Osteopenia, early-onset osteoporosis, skeletal dysplasia, epiphyseal abnormalities, bone crises
Perinatal history	Intrauterine growth retardation, sepsis-like presentation in the neonatal period, nonimmune fetal hydrops		
		Eye	Retinitis pigmentosa, macular dystrophy, cataracts, corneal opacities, nystagmus, cherry-red spot
Growth	Postnatal failure to thrive, microcephaly, macrocephaly, short stature		
Central and peripheral nervous systems	Progressive encephalopathy, lethargy, coma, intractable seizures, developmental delay, developmental regression, intellectual disability, autism spectrum disorder, hypotonia, spasticity, dystonia, strokes, ataxia, psychosis, intracranial calcifications, white matter disease, peripheral neuropathy	Hearing	Sensorineural hearing loss
		Gastrointestinal system	Hepatomegaly, splenomegaly, liver failure, Reye syndrome, cholestasis, cirrhosis, chronic diarrhea, vomiting, acute pancreatitis
		Kidney	Renal dysfunction, renal stones
		Hematological system	Anemia, leukopenia, thrombocytopenia, pancytopenia, hemolytic-uremic syndrome
Respiratory system	Hyperventilation, apnea	Skin	Hair abnormality, alopecia, lipodystrophy, recalcitrant eczema

Table 102.13	Laboratory Findings That Should Prompt a Metabolic Workup
Hyperammonemia Metabolic acidosis Lactic acidosis Ketosis	Hypoglycemia Liver dysfunction Pancytopenia

Chapter 103
Defects in Metabolism of Amino Acids

第一百零三章
氨基酸代谢病

中文导读

本章详细阐述了苯丙氨酸、酪氨酸、甲硫氨酸、半胱氨酸及胱氨酸、色氨酸、异亮氨酸、亮氨酸、缬氨酸及相关有机酸血症、甘氨酸、丝氨酸代谢障碍（丝氨酸合成及转运障碍）、脯氨酸、谷氨酸、遗传性神经递质病、尿素循环障碍（精氨酸、瓜氨酸、鸟氨酸）、组氨酸、赖氨酸及N-乙酰天冬氨酸（Canavan病）等疾病的病因、临床表现、诊断、治疗和预后等内容。

103.1 Phenylalanine

Oleg A. Shchelochkov and Charles P. Venditti

Phenylalanine is an essential amino acid. Dietary phenylalanine not utilized for protein synthesis is normally degraded by way of the tyrosine pathway (Fig. 103.1). Deficiency of the enzyme **phenylalanine hydroxylase (PAH)** or of its cofactor **tetrahydrobiopterin (BH₄)** causes accumulation of phenylalanine in body fluids and in the brain.

Elevations of phenylalanine in the plasma depend on the degree of enzyme deficiency. In patients with **severe PAH deficiency** (previously referred to as *classic phenylketonuria*), plasma phenylalanine levels on unrestricted diet usually exceed 20 mg/dL (>1,200 μmol/L). Patients with milder PAH pathogenic variants have plasma phenylalanine levels between 10 mg/dL (600 μmol/L) and 20 mg/dL (1,200 μmol/L). Levels between 2 and 10 mg/dL (120-600 μmol/L) on unrestricted diet are observed in patients with **mild hyperphenylalaninemia**. In affected infants with plasma concentrations >20 mg/dL, excess phenylalanine is metabolized to phenylketones (phenylpyruvate and phenylacetate; see Fig. 103.1) that are excreted in the urine, giving rise to the term *phenylketonuria* (PKU).

These metabolites have no known role in pathogenesis of central nervous system (CNS) damage in PKU patients; their presence in the body fluids simply signifies the severity of the condition. The **brain** is the main organ damaged by PKU, but the exact mechanism of injury remains elusive. Both toxic levels of phenylalanine and insufficient tyrosine may play a role. Phenylalanine hydroxylase converts phenylalanine to **tyrosine**, which is necessary for the production of neurotransmitters such as epinephrine, norepinephrine, and dopamine (Fig. 103.2). If the degree of enzymatic block is severe, tyrosine becomes an essential amino acid and may be deficient if intake is not adequate. On the other hand, observations that lower concentration of phenylalanine in plasma and brain tissue are associated with improved neurobehavioral outcomes support the view that toxic levels of phenylalanine are key to the mechanisms of the disease. High blood levels of phenylalanine can saturate the transport system across the blood-brain barrier and cause inhibition of the cerebral uptake of other large neutral amino acids such as branched-chain amino acids, tyrosine, and tryptophan, impairing brain protein synthesis.

SEVERE PHENYLALANINE HYDROXYLASE DEFICIENCY (CLASSIC PHENYLKETONURIA)

Elevations of plasma phenylalanine >20 mg/dL (>1,200 μmol/L), if untreated, invariably result in the development of signs and symptoms of classic PKU, except in uncommon and unpredictable cases.

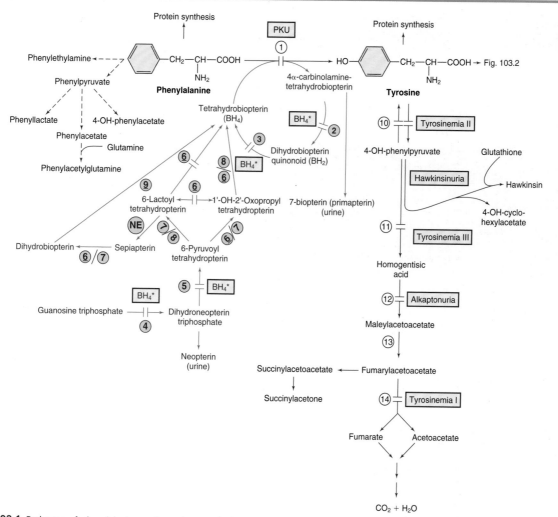

Fig. 103.1 Pathways of phenylalanine and tyrosine metabolism. Enzyme defects causing genetic conditions are depicted as *horizontal bars* crossing the reaction arrow(s). Pathways for synthesis of cofactor BH₄ are shown in *purple*. BH₄* refers to defects of BH₄ metabolism that affect the phenylalanine, tyrosine, and tryptophan hydroxylases (see Figs. 103.2 and 103.5). PKU, Phenylketonuria; NE, nonenzymatic. **Enzymes:** (1) Phenylalanine hydroxylase, (2) pterin-carbinolamine dehydratase, (3) dihydrobiopterin reductase, (4) guanosine triphosphate (GTP) cyclohydrolase, (5) 6-pyruvoyltetrahydropterin synthase, (6) sepiapterin reductase, (7) carbonyl reductase, (8) aldolase reductase, (9) dihydrofolate reductase, (10) tyrosine aminotransferase, (11) 4-hydroxyphenylpyruvate dioxygenase, (12) homogentisic acid dioxygenase, (13) maleylacetoacetate isomerase, (14) fumarylacetoacetate hydrolase.

Clinical Manifestations

The affected infant appears normal at birth. Profound intellectual disability develops gradually if the infant remains untreated. Cognitive delay may not be evident for the 1st few months. In untreated patients, 50–70% will have an IQ below 35, and 88–90% will have an IQ below 65. Only 2–5% of untreated patients may have normal intelligence. Vomiting, sometimes severe enough to be misdiagnosed as pyloric stenosis, may be an early symptom. Older untreated children become hyperactive with autistic behaviors, including purposeless hand movements, rhythmic rocking, and athetosis.

Untreated and undertreated infants are lighter in their complexion than unaffected siblings. Some may have a seborrheic or eczematoid rash, which is usually mild and disappears as the child grows older. These children have an odor of phenylacetic acid, which has been described as musty or "mousey." Neurologic signs include seizures (approximately 25%), spasticity, hyperreflexia, and tremors; >50% have electroencephalographic (EEG) abnormalities. Microcephaly, prominent maxillae with widely spaced teeth, enamel hypoplasia, and growth

retardation are other common findings in untreated children. Low bone mineral density and osteopenia have been reported in affected individuals of all ages. Although inadequate intake of natural proteins seems to be the major culprit, the exact pathogenesis of this sequela remains unclear. Long-term care of patients with PKU is best achieved by a team of experienced professionals (metabolic specialist, nutritionist, and psychologist) in a regional treatment center. The clinical manifestations of classic PKU are rarely seen in countries where neonatal screening programs for the detection of PKU are in effect.

Non-PKU Hyperphenylalaninemia

In any screening program for PKU, a group of infants will be identified in whom initial plasma concentrations of phenylalanine are above normal (i.e., >2 mg/dL, or 120 μmol/L) but <20 mg/dL (1,200 μmol/L). These infants typically do not excrete phenylketones. Patients with non-PKU hyperphenylalaninemia may still require dietary therapy, depending on their untreated plasma phenylalanine level. Attempts have been made to classify these patients in different subgroups depending on the degree of

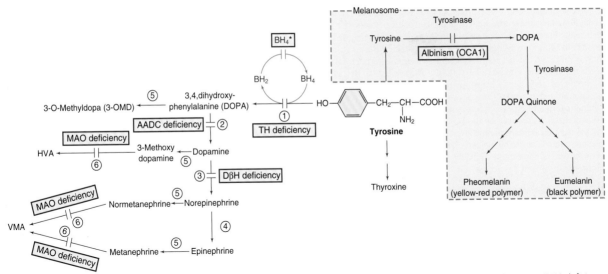

Fig. 103.2 Other pathways involving tyrosine metabolism. BH₄* indicates hyperphenylalaninemia caused by tetrahydrobiopterin (BH₄) deficiency (see Fig. 103.1). HVA, Homovanillic acid; VMA, vanillylmandelic acid. **Enzymes:** *(1)* Tyrosine hydroxylase (TH), *(2)* aromatic L-amino acid decarboxylase (AADC), *(3)* dopamine β-hydroxylase (DβH), *(4)* phenylethanolamine-N-methyltransferase (PNMT), *(5)* catechol O-methyltransferase (COMT), *(6)* monoamine oxidase (MAO).

hyperphenylalaninemia, but such a practice has little clinical or therapeutic advantage. The possibility of deficiency of BH₄ should be investigated in all infants with the milder forms of hyperphenylalaninemia.

Diagnosis
Because of the gradual and nonspecific nature of early clinical symptoms such as vomiting, developmental delay, or eczematoid rash, hyperphenylalaninemia is usually diagnosed through newborn screening in all developed countries. In infants with positive screening results, diagnosis should be confirmed by quantitative measurement of plasma phenylalanine concentration. Identification and measurement of phenylketones in the urine has no place in any screening program. In countries and places where such programs are not in effect, identification of phenylketones in the urine by ferric chloride may offer a simple test for diagnosis of infants with developmental and neurologic abnormalities. Once the diagnosis of hyperphenylalaninemia is established, additional studies for BH₄ metabolism should be performed to rule out BH₄ deficiency as the cause of hyperphenylalaninemia.

Neonatal Screening for Hyperphenylalaninemia
Effective and relatively inexpensive methods for mass screening of newborn infants are used in the United States and many other countries. A few drops of blood, which are placed on a filter paper and mailed to a central laboratory, are used for assay. The screening method of choice uses **tandem mass spectrometry**, which identifies all forms of hyperphenylalaninemia with a low false-positive rate and excellent accuracy and precision. The addition of the phenylalanine:tyrosine molar ratio has further reduced the number of false-positive results. Diagnosis must be confirmed by measurement of plasma phenylalanine concentration. Blood phenylalanine in affected infants with PKU may rise to diagnostic levels as early as 4 hr after birth, even in the absence of protein feeding. It is recommended that the blood for screening be obtained in the 1st 24-48 hr of life after feeding protein to reduce the possibility of false-negative results, especially in the milder forms of the condition.

Treatment
The mainstay of treatment of PKU is a *low-phenylalanine diet.* The general consensus is to start diet treatment immediately in patients with blood phenylalanine levels >10 mg/dL (600 μmol/L). It is generally accepted that infants with persistent (more than a few days) plasma levels of phenylalanine ≥6 mg/dL (360 μmol/L) should also be treated with a phenylalanine-restricted diet similar to that in classic PKU. The goal of therapy is to reduce phenylalanine levels in the plasma and brain. Formulas free of, or low in, phenylalanine are commercially available. The diet should be started as soon as the diagnosis is established. Because phenylalanine is not synthesized endogenously, the diet should provide phenylalanine to prevent phenylalanine deficiency. Dietary phenylalanine tolerance is determined based on age and severity of the PAH deficiency. **Phenylalanine deficiency** is manifested by lethargy, failure to thrive, anorexia, anemia, rashes, diarrhea, and even death. Further, tyrosine becomes an essential amino acid in this disorder, and its adequate intake must be ensured. Special food items low in phenylalanine are commercially available for dietary treatment of affected children and adults.

There is no firm consensus concerning optimal levels of blood phenylalanine in affected patients either across different countries or among treatment centers in the United States. The current recommendation is to maintain blood phenylalanine levels between 2 and 6 mg/dL (120-360 μmol/L) throughout life. Discontinuation of therapy, even in adulthood, may cause deterioration of IQ and cognitive performance. Lifelong adherence to a low-phenylalanine diet is extremely difficult. Patients who maintain good control as children but discontinue the phenylalanine-restricted diet as teenagers or adults may experience significant difficulties with executive function, concentration, emotional liability, and depression. Executive dysfunction may also occur in early-treated children despite diet treatment.

Given the difficulty of maintaining a strict low-phenylalanine diet, there are continuing attempts to find other modalities for treatment of these patients. Administration of **large neutral amino acids** (LNAAs) is another approach to dietary therapy. LNAAs (tyrosine, tryptophan, leucine, isoleucine, valine, methionine, histidine, and phenylalanine) share the same transporter protein (LNAA type 1 or LAT-1) for transit through the intestinal cell membrane and blood-brain barrier (BBB). Binding of LNAAs to the transporter protein is a competitive process. The rationale for use of LNAA is that these molecules compete with phenylalanine for transport across the BBB; therefore, large concentrations of other LNAAs in the intestinal lumen and in the blood reduce the uptake of phenylalanine into bloodstream and the brain. Large, controlled clinical trials are necessary to establish the efficacy of this treatment.

Oral administration of BH$_4$, the cofactor for PAH, may result in reduction of plasma levels of phenylalanine in some patients with PAH deficiency. Plasma levels of phenylalanine in these patients may decrease enough to allow for considerable modification of their dietary restriction. In very rare cases the diet may be discontinued because the phenylalanine levels remain under 6 mg/dL (360 µmol/L). The response to BH$_4$ cannot be predicted consistently based on the genotype alone, especially in compound heterozygous patients. **Sapropterin dihydrochloride**, a synthetic form of BH$_4$, which acts as a cofactor in patients with residual PAH activity, is approved by the U.S. Food and Drug Administration (FDA) to reduce phenylalanine levels in PKU. A sustained decrease of plasma phenylalanine by at least 30% is consistent with sapropterin responsiveness. Injectable PEGylated recombinant phenylalanine ammonia lyase is in development.

Pregnancy in Women With PAH Deficiency (Maternal Phenylketonuria)
Pregnant women with PAH deficiency who are not on a phenylalanine-restricted diet have a very high risk of having offspring with intellectual disability, microcephaly, growth retardation, congenital malformations, and congenital heart disease. These complications are directly correlated with elevated maternal blood phenylalanine levels during pregnancy. Prospective mothers who have been treated for PAH deficiency should be maintained on a phenylalanine-restricted diet before and during pregnancy. The best observed outcomes occur when strict control of maternal blood phenylalanine concentration is instituted before pregnancy. Plasma phenylalanine levels >6 mg/dL (360 µmol/L) after conception are associated with increased incidence of intrauterine growth restriction and congenital malformations, as well as lower IQ. However, there is strong evidence that phenylalanine control instituted after conception results in improved outcomes. The currently recommended phenylalanine concentration is 2-6 mg/dL (120-360 µmol/L) throughout the pregnancy, although some expert groups advocate plasma phenylalanine levels <4 mg/dL (<240 µmol/L). All women with PAH deficiency who are of childbearing age should be counseled properly regarding the risk of congenital anomalies in their offspring.

HYPERPHENYLALANINEMIA CAUSED BY DEFICIENCY OF THE COFACTOR TETRAHYDROBIOPTERIN
In 1-3% of infants with hyperphenylalaninemia, the defect resides in one of the enzymes necessary for production or recycling of the cofactor BH$_4$ (see Fig. 103.1). If these infants are misdiagnosed as having PKU, they may deteriorate neurologically despite adequate control of plasma phenylalanine. BH$_4$ is synthesized from guanosine triphosphate (GTP) through several enzymatic reactions (see Fig. 103.1). In addition to acting as a cofactor for PAH, BH$_4$ is also a cofactor for tyrosine hydroxylase and tryptophan hydroxylase, which are involved in the biosynthesis of dopamine (see Fig. 103.2) and serotonin (see Fig. 103.5), respectively. Therefore, patients with hyperphenylalaninemia resulting from BH$_4$ deficiency also manifest neurologic findings related to deficiencies of these neurotransmitters. Four enzyme deficiencies leading to defective BH$_4$ formation cause hyperphenylalaninemia with concomitant deficiencies of dopamine and serotonin: autosomal recessive GTP cyclohydrolase I deficiency, 6-pyruvoyl-tetrahydropterin synthase deficiency, dihydropteridine reductase deficiency, and pterin-4-α-carbinolamine dehydratase deficiency. More than half the reported patients have had a deficiency of 6-pyruvoyl-tetrahydropterin synthase. Autosomal dominant forms of GTP cyclohydrolase I deficiency and sepiapterin reductase deficiency result in deficiencies of neurotransmitters without hyperphenylalaninemia (see Chapter 103.11).

Clinical Manifestations
Infants with cofactor BH$_4$ deficiency are identified during screening programs for PKU because of evidence of hyperphenylalaninemia. Plasma phenylalanine levels may be as high as those in classic PKU or may be in the milder range. However, the clinical manifestations of the neurotransmitter disorders differ greatly from those of PKU. Neurologic symptoms of the neurotransmitter disorders often manifest in the 1st few months of life and include extrapyramidal signs (choreoathetotic or dystonic limb movements, axial and truncal hypotonia, hypokinesia), feeding difficulties, and autonomic abnormalities. Intellectual disability, seizures, hypersalivation, and swallowing difficulties are also seen. The symptoms are usually progressive and often have a marked diurnal fluctuation. Prognosis and outcome strongly depend on the age at diagnosis and at introduction of treatment, but also on the specific nature of the pathogenic variant and resulting enzyme defect.

Diagnosis
Despite the low incidence of BH$_4$ synthesis defects, all newborns with hyperphenylalaninemia detected through newborn screening *must* be screened for BH$_4$ synthesis defects. BH$_4$ deficiency and the responsible enzyme defect may be diagnosed by several studies.

Measurement of Neopterin and Biopterin. Neopterin (oxidative product of dihydroneopterin triphosphate) and biopterin (oxidative product of dihydrobiopterin and BH$_4$) are measured in body fluids, especially urine (see Fig. 103.1). In patients with GTP cyclohydrolase I deficiency, urinary excretion of both neopterin and biopterin is very low. In patients with 6-pyruvoyl-tetrahydropterin synthase deficiency, there is a marked elevation of neopterin excretion and a concomitant decrease in biopterin excretion. In patients with dihydropteridine reductase deficiency, the excretion of neopterin and biopterin is elevated. Excretion of biopterin increases in this enzyme deficiency because the quinonoid dihydrobiopterin cannot be recycled back to BH$_4$. Patients with pterin-4-α-carbinolamine dehydratase deficiency excrete 7-biopterin (an unusual isomer of biopterin) in their urine.

Cerebrospinal Fluid Studies. Examination of cerebrospinal fluid (CSF) may reveal decreased levels of dopamine and serotonin metabolites (see Chapter 103.11).

BH$_4$ Loading Test. An oral dose of BH$_4$ (20 mg/kg) normalizes plasma phenylalanine and phenylalanine:tyrosine ratio in patients with BH$_4$ deficiency within 4-12 hr. The blood phenylalanine should be elevated (>400 µmol/L) to enable interpretation of the results. This may be achieved by discontinuing diet therapy for 2 days before the test or by administering a loading dose of phenylalanine (100 mg/kg) 3 hr before the test. In BH$_4$-responsive PKU caused by PAH deficiency, blood phenylalanine levels may decrease during the BH$_4$ loading test, but increase later even with BH$_4$ supplementation. Patients who demonstrate phenylalanine levels within normal range over at least 1 wk without a phenylalanine-restricted diet can continue BH$_4$ supplementation as the sole treatment for the hyperphenylalaninemia. However, it is imperative that plasma phenylalanine levels be monitored prospectively to ensure that phenylalanine levels remain within the normal range.

Molecular Testing. Sequencing and deletion/duplication analysis are clinically available and play an increasingly more important role in confirming the biochemical diagnosis.

Enzyme Assay. The activity of dihydropteridine reductase can be measured in the dry blood spots on the filter paper used for screening purposes. 6-Pyruvoyl-tetrahydropterin synthase activity can be measured in the liver, fibroblasts, and erythrocytes. Pterin-4-α-carbinolamine dehydratase activity can be measured in the liver and fibroblasts. GTP cyclohydrolase I activity can be measured in the liver and in cytokine (interferon-γ)–stimulated mononuclear cells or fibroblasts (the enzyme activity is normally very low in unstimulated cells).

Treatment
The goals of therapy are to correct hyperphenylalaninemia and to restore neurotransmitter deficiencies in the CNS. The control of hyperphenylalaninemia is important in patients with cofactor deficiency, because high levels of phenylalanine cause intellectual disability and interfere with the transport of neurotransmitter precursors (tyrosine and tryptophan) into the brain. Plasma phenylalanine should be maintained as close to normal as possible (<6 mg/dL or <360 µmol/L). This can be achieved by oral supplementation of BH$_4$ (5-20 mg/kg/day). Sapropterin dihydrochloride, the synthetic form of BH$_4$, is commercially available but expensive.

Lifelong supplementation with neurotransmitter precursors such as

L-dopa and 5-hydroxytryptophan, along with carbidopa to inhibit degradation of L-dopa before it enters the CNS, is necessary in most of these patients even when treatment with BH_4 normalizes plasma levels of phenylalanine. BH_4 does not readily enter the brain to restore neurotransmitter production. To minimize untoward side effects (especially L-dopa–induced dyskinesia), the treatment should be started with low doses of L-dopa/carbidopa and 5-hydroxytryptophan and should be gradually adjusted based on response to therapy and clinical improvement for each individual patient. Supplementation with folinic acid is also recommended in patients with dihydropteridine reductase deficiency. Unfortunately, attempting to normalize neurotransmitter levels using neurotransmitter precursors usually does not fully resolve the neurologic symptoms, because of the inability to attain normal levels of BH_4 in the brain. Patients often demonstrate intellectual disability, fluctuating abnormalities of tone, eye movement abnormalities, poor balance and coordination, decreased ability to ambulate, and seizures despite supplementation with neurotransmitter precursors.

Hyperprolactinemia occurs in patients with BH_4 deficiency and may be the result of hypothalamic dopamine deficiency. Measurement of serum prolactin levels may be a convenient method for monitoring adequacy of neurotransmitter replacement in affected patients.

Some drugs, such as trimethoprim/sulfamethoxazole, methotrexate, and other antileukemic agents, are known to inhibit dihydropteridine reductase enzyme activity and should be used with great caution in patients with BH_4 deficiency.

Genetics and Prevalence
All defects causing hyperphenylalaninemia are inherited as autosomal recessive traits. The prevalence of PKU in the United States is estimated at 1 in 14,000 to 1 in 20,000 live births. The prevalence of non-PKU hyperphenylalaninemia is estimated at 1 in 50,000 live births. The condition is more common in whites and Native Americans and less prevalent in blacks, Hispanics, and Asians.

The gene for PAH is located on chromosome 12q23.2, and many disease-causing mutations have been identified in different families. Most patients are compound heterozygotes for 2 different mutant alleles. The gene for 6-pyruvoyl-tetrahydropterin synthase (PTS), the most common cause of BH_4 deficiency, resides on chromosome 11q23.1, the gene for dihydropteridine reductase (QDPR) is located on chromosome 4p15.32, and those of pterin-4-α-carbinolamine dehydratase (PCBD1) and GTP cyclohydrolase I (GCH1) are on 10q22.1 and 14q22.2, respectively. Prenatal diagnosis is possible if causative mutations are known.

TETRAHYDROBIOPTERIN DEFECTS WITHOUT HYPERPHENYLALANINEMIA
See Chapter 103.11.

Bibliography is available at Expert Consult.

103.2 Tyrosine
Oleg A. Shchelochkov and Charles P. Venditti

Tyrosine is derived from ingested proteins or is synthesized endogenously from phenylalanine. It is used for protein synthesis and is a precursor of dopamine, norepinephrine, epinephrine, melanin, and thyroxine. Excess tyrosine is metabolized to carbon dioxide and water (see Fig. 103.1). Hereditary causes of hypertyrosinemia include deficiencies of the enzymes fumarylacetoacetate hydrolase (**FAH**), tyrosine aminotransferase, and 4-hydroxyphenylpyruvate dioxygenase (**4-HPPD**). **Acquired hypertyrosinemia** may occur in severe hepatocellular dysfunction (liver failure), scurvy (vitamin C is the cofactor for 4-HPPD), and hyperthyroidism. Hypertyrosinemia is common in blood samples obtained soon after eating and in premature infants.

TYROSINEMIA TYPE I (FUMARYLACETOACETATE HYDROLASE DEFICIENCY, HEPATORENAL TYROSINEMIA)

Tyrosinemia type I is a severe multisystemic disease caused by FAH deficiency. Liver, kidney, and nerve damage is likely caused by metabolites of tyrosine degradation, especially fumarylacetoacetate and succinylacetone.

Clinical Manifestations and Natural History
Without treatment, affected infants appear normal at birth and develop symptoms in the 1st yr of life. Most patients present between 2 and 6 mo of age but rarely may become symptomatic in the 1st mo or appear healthy beyond the 1st yr of life. Earlier presentation confers poorer prognosis. The 1-yr mortality of untreated children, which is approximately 60% in infants developing symptoms before 2 mo of age, decreases to 4% in infants who become symptomatic after 6 mo.

An acute **hepatic crisis** typically heralds the onset of the disease and is usually precipitated by an intercurrent illness that produces a catabolic state. Fever, irritability, vomiting, hemorrhage, hepatomegaly, jaundice, elevated levels of serum transaminases, hypoglycemia, and neuropathy are common. An odor resembling boiled cabbage may be present, resulting from increased methionine metabolites. Hepatic crises may progress to liver failure and death. Between the crises, varying degrees of failure to thrive, hepatomegaly, and coagulation abnormalities often persist. Cirrhosis and eventually hepatocellular carcinoma occur with increasing age.

Episodes of acute **peripheral neuropathy** resembling acute porphyria occur in approximately 40% of affected children. These crises, often triggered by a minor infection, are characterized by severe pain, often in the legs, associated with extensor hypertonia of the neck and trunk, vomiting, paralytic ileus, and occasionally self-induced injuries of the tongue or buccal mucosa. Marked weakness occurs in about 30% of episodes, which may lead to respiratory failure requiring mechanical ventilation. Crises typically last 1-7 days, but recuperation from paralytic crises can require weeks to months.

Renal involvement is manifested as a Fanconi-like syndrome with hyperphosphaturia, hypophosphatemia, normal–anion gap metabolic acidosis, and vitamin D–resistant rickets. Nephromegaly and nephrocalcinosis may be present on ultrasound examination. Glomerular failure may occur in adolescents and older patients.

Hypertrophic cardiomyopathy and hyperinsulinism are seen in some infants.

Laboratory Findings
Elevated levels of succinylacetone in serum and urine are diagnostic for tyrosinemia type I (see Fig. 103.1). Succinylacetone levels may fall below the diagnostic threshold in patients treated with nitisinone. In untreated patients, the blood level of α-fetoprotein is increased, often greatly, and liver-synthesized coagulation factors are decreased in most patients. Increased levels of α-fetoprotein are present in the cord blood of affected infants, indicating intrauterine liver damage. Serum transaminase levels are often increased, with marked increases possible during acute hepatic episodes. Serum concentration of bilirubin is usually normal but can be increased with liver failure. Plasma tyrosine levels are usually elevated at diagnosis, but this is a nonspecific finding and depends on dietary intake. Plasma levels of other amino acids, particularly methionine, may also be elevated in patients with liver damage. Hyperphosphaturia, hypophosphatemia, and generalized aminoaciduria may occur. The urinary level of 5-aminolevulinic acid (also known as delta aminolevulinic acid) is elevated because of inhibition of 5-aminolevulinate dehydratase by succinylacetone (see Fig. 110.1).

Diagnosis is usually established by demonstration of elevated levels of succinylacetone in urine or blood. Neonatal screening for hypertyrosinemia using tyrosine alone detects only a fraction of patients with tyrosinemia type I. Succinylacetone, which is assayed by many neonatal screening programs, has higher sensitivity and specificity than tyrosine and is the preferred metabolite for screening. Tyrosinemia type I should be differentiated from other causes of hepatitis and hepatic failure in infants, including galactosemia, hereditary fructose intolerance, neonatal iron storage disease, giant cell hepatitis, and citrullinemia type II (see Chapter 103.12).

Treatment and Outcome

A diet low in phenylalanine and tyrosine can slow but does not halt the progression of the condition. The treatment of choice is **nitisinone** (NTBC), which inhibits 4-HPPD and reduces the flux of tyrosine metabolites to FAH, thus decreasing the production of the offending compounds, fumarylacetoacetate and succinylacetone (see Fig. 103.1). The dose of nitisinone is titrated to the lowest, most effective dose (usually targeting the blood range of 20-40 μmol/L) to suppress production of succinylacetone while maintaining plasma tyrosine level <400 μmol/L (7.2 mg/dL). This treatment prevents acute hepatic and neurologic crises. Although nitisinone greatly slows disease progression, some pretreatment liver damage is not reversible. Therefore, patients must be followed for development of *cirrhosis* or *hepatocellular carcinoma*. On imaging, the presence of even a single liver nodule usually indicates underlying cirrhosis. Most liver nodules in tyrosinemic patients are benign, but current imaging techniques do not accurately distinguish all malignant nodules. For patients with severe liver failure not responding to nitisinone, liver transplantation is an effective therapy, which can also alleviate the risk of hepatocellular carcinoma. The impact of nitisinone treatment on the need for liver transplantation is still under study, but the greatest effect is in patients treated early, such as children detected by neonatal screening, prior to developing clinical symptoms. In early-treated patients, nitisinone has greatly reduced the need for liver transplantation. Because nitisinone treatment increases plasma tyrosine, a low-tyrosine, low-phenylalanine diet is recommended. Rarely, nitisinone-treated patients develop corneal crystals, presumably of tyrosine, which are reversible by strict dietary compliance. This finding, combined with observations of developmental delay in some patients with tyrosinemia type II who chronically have elevated tyrosine levels, suggest that a diet low in phenylalanine and tyrosine should be continued in patients treated with nitisinone. The dietary treatment of patients with tyrosine and phenylalanine restriction necessitates surveillance of growth and development by ensuring adequate intakes of amino acids and other nutrients.

Genetics and Prevalence

Tyrosinemia type I is inherited as an autosomal recessive trait. The *FAH* gene maps to chromosome 15q25.1. DNA analysis is useful for molecular prenatal diagnosis if the familial pathogenic variants are known and for carrier testing in groups at risk for specific mutations, such as French-Canadians from the Saguenay-Lac Saint-Jean region of Quebec. The prevalence of the condition is estimated to be 1 in 1,846 live births in the Saguenay-Lac Saint-Jean region and approximately 1 in 100,000 live births worldwide. Prenatal screening can be performed by measurement of succinylacetone in amniotic fluid. Prenatal diagnosis is possible using DNA analysis of amniocytes or of chorionic villi, if the familial pathogenic variants are known.

TYROSINEMIA TYPE II (TYROSINE AMINOTRANSFERASE DEFICIENCY, RICHNER-HANHART SYNDROME, OCULOCUTANEOUS TYROSINEMIA)

Tyrosinemia type II is a rare autosomal recessive disorder caused by deficiency of cytosolic tyrosine aminotransferase and results in palmar and plantar hyperkeratosis, herpetiform corneal ulcers, and intellectual disability (see Fig. 103.1). *Ocular manifestations*, which may occur as early as 6 mo of age, include excessive tearing, redness, pain, and photophobia. Corneal lesions are presumed to be caused by tyrosine deposition. In contrast to herpetic ulcers, corneal lesions in tyrosinemia type II stain poorly with fluorescein and often are bilateral. *Skin lesions*, which may develop later in life, include painful, nonpruritic hyperkeratotic plaques on the soles, palms, and fingertips. Intellectual disability, which occurs in approximately 50% of patients, is usually mild to moderate. The contribution of consanguinity in this rare disorder is incompletely understood.

The principal **laboratory finding** in untreated patients is marked

hypertyrosinemia, >500 μmol/L and may reach 1,100-2,750 μmol/L. Surprisingly, 4-hydroxyphenylpyruvic acid and its metabolites are also elevated in urine despite being downstream from the metabolic block (see Fig. 103.1). This is hypothesized to occur via the action of other transaminases in the presence of high tyrosine concentrations, producing 4-hydroxyphenylpyruvic acid in mitochondria, where it cannot be further degraded. In contrast to tyrosinemia type I, liver and kidney function are normal, as are serum concentrations of other amino acids and succinylacetone. Tyrosinemia type II is caused by tyrosine aminotransferase (*TAT*) gene pathogenic variants, causing deficiency of cytosolic TAT activity in liver. *TAT* maps to chromosome 16q22.

Diagnosis of type II tyrosinemia is established by assay of plasma tyrosine concentration in patients with suggestive findings. Molecular diagnosis is possible. Assay of liver TAT requires a liver biopsy and is rarely indicated.

Treatment with a diet low in tyrosine and phenylalanine aiming to achieve plasma tyrosine levels <500 μmol/L improves skin and eye manifestations. The claim that intellectual disability may be prevented by early diet therapy is reasonable and is consistent with some case reports.

TYROSINEMIA TYPE III (PRIMARY DEFICIENCY OF 4-HYDROXYPHENYLPYRUVATE DIOXYGENASE)

Only a few patients with tyrosinemia type III have been reported. Most were detected by amino acid chromatography performed for various neurologic findings; therefore ascertainment bias likely confounds our current understanding of this disorder. Apparently, asymptomatic infants with 4-HPPD deficiency have been identified by neonatal screening for hypertyrosinemia. Age at presentation has been from 1-17 mo. In symptomatic patients, developmental delay, seizures, intermittent ataxia, and self-injurious behavior have been reported. Liver and renal abnormalities are absent.

The role of 4-HPPD deficiency in the disease mechanisms needs further study. The **diagnosis** is suspected in children with sustained moderate increases in plasma levels of tyrosine (typically 350-700 μmol/L on a normal diet) and the presence of 4-hydroxyphenylpyruvic acid and its metabolites 4-hydroxyphenyllactic and 4-hydroxyphenylacetic acids in urine. Diagnosis may be refined by demonstrating the presence of pathogenic variants in the *HPD* gene encoding 4-HPPD, or rarely by demonstrating a low activity of 4-HPPD enzyme; the latter requires a liver biopsy and is not usually indicated.

Given the possible association with neurologic abnormalities, dietary reduction of plasma tyrosine levels is prudent. It is also logical to attempt a trial of vitamin C, the cofactor for 4-HPPD. The condition is inherited as an autosomal recessive trait.

HAWKINSINURIA

A missense variant c.722A>G (p.Asn241Ser) in *HPD* encoding 4-HPPD results in the uncoupling of normal oxidization of 4-hydroxyphenylpyruvate to homogentisic acid and premature release of quinolacetic acid. The abnormal enzyme, incapable of normally oxidizing 4-hydroxyphenylpyruvate to homogentisic acid, forms an intermediate that reacts with glutathione to form the unusual organic acid **hawkinsin** ([2-L-cystein-S-yl-1,4-dihydroxycyclohex-5-en-1-yl] acetic acid), named after the first affected family (see Fig. 103.1). As a result, secondary glutathione deficiency may ensue. Hawkinsinuria is inherited as an autosomal dominant trait. In one patient, compound heterozygosity for hawkinsinuria and tyrosinemia type III alleles produced only biochemical features of hawkinsinuria.

The clinical course of this rare disorder is incompletely understood. Individuals with hawkinsinuria may be symptomatic only during infancy. The symptoms usually appear in the 1st few months of life, typically after weaning from breastfeeding and with the introduction of a high-protein diet. Severe metabolic acidosis, ketosis, failure to thrive, anemia, mild hepatomegaly, renal tubular acidosis, and an unusual odor are reported manifestations of this disorder. Neurocognitive development is usually normal.

Symptomatic infants and asymptomatic affected children and adults excrete hawkinsin, 4-hydroxyphenylpyruvic acid, and its metabolites (4-hydroxyphenyllactic and 4-hydroxyphenylacetic acids), 4-hydroxycyclohexylacetic acid and 5-oxoproline (from secondary glutathione deficiency) in their urine. The plasma tyrosine level, which is moderately elevated in the symptomatic infants, may become normal in the asymptomatic affected individuals.

Treatment consists of a low-protein diet during infancy. Breastfeeding is encouraged. Avoidance of protein overrestriction is important because some patients may present with failure to thrive. Successful long-term use of N-acetyl-L-cysteine to treat secondary glutathione deficiency has been reported. A trial with vitamin C is recommended. The abnormal enzyme is susceptible to inhibition by nitisinone. Clinical studies showing the efficacy of this agent in symptomatic infants are lacking at this time, and the indications for its use are not known.

TRANSIENT TYROSINEMIA OF THE NEWBORN

In a small number of newborn infants, plasma tyrosine may be as high as 3,300 μmol/L during the 1st 2 wk of life. Most affected infants are premature and are receiving a high-protein diet. Transient tyrosinemia is thought to result from delayed maturation of 4-HPPD (see Fig. 103.1). Lethargy, poor feeding, and decreased motor activity are noted in some patients. Most are asymptomatic and are identified by a high blood phenylalanine or tyrosine level on routine screening. Laboratory findings include marked elevation of plasma tyrosine with a moderate increase in plasma phenylalanine. The finding of hypertyrosinemia differentiates this condition from PKU. 4-Hydroxyphenylpyruvic acid and its metabolites are present in the urine. Hypertyrosinemia usually resolves spontaneously in the 1st 2 mo of life. It can be corrected by reducing dietary protein to below 2 g/kg/24 hr and by administering vitamin C. Mild intellectual deficits have been reported in some infants who had this condition, but the causal relationship to hypertyrosinemia is not conclusively established.

ALKAPTONURIA

Alkaptonuria is a rare (approximately 1 in 250,000 live births) autosomal recessive disorder caused by a deficiency of homogentisate 1,2-dioxygenase. Large amounts of homogentisic acid are formed (see Fig. 103.1), which are excreted in urine or deposited in tissues.

The main **clinical manifestations** of alkaptonuria consist of ochronosis and arthritis in adulthood. The only sign in children is blackening of the urine on standing, caused by oxidation and polymerization of homogentisic acid. A history of gray- or black-stained diapers should suggest the diagnosis. This sign may never be noted; thus diagnosis is often delayed until adulthood. *Ochronosis*, which is seen clinically as dark spots on the sclera or ear cartilage, results from the accumulation of the black polymer of homogentisic acid. *Arthritis* is another result of this deposition and can be disabling with advancing age. It involves the spine and large joints (shoulders, hips, and knees) and is usually more severe in males. As with rheumatoid arthritis, the alkaptonuric arthritis has acute exacerbations, but the radiologic findings are typical of osteoarthritis, with characteristic narrowing of the joint spaces and calcification of the intervertebral disks. High incidence of heart disease (mitral and aortic valvulitis, calcification of heart valves, myocardial infarction) has been reported.

The **diagnosis** is confirmed by finding massive excretion of homogentisic acid on urine organic acid testing. Tyrosine levels are normal. The enzyme is expressed only in the liver and kidneys.

Treatment of the arthritis is symptomatic. Nitisinone efficiently reduces homogentisic acid production in alkaptonuria. If presymptomatic individuals are detected, treatment with nitisinone, combined with a phenylalanine- and tyrosine-restricted diet, seems reasonable, although no experience is available regarding long-term efficacy.

The gene for homogentisate 1,2-dioxygenase (HGD) maps to chromosome 3q13.3. Alkaptonuria is most common in the Dominican Republic and Slovakia.

TYROSINE HYDROXYLASE DEFICIENCY

See Chapter 103.11.

ALBINISM

See also Chapters 640 and 672.

Albinism is caused by deficiency of **melanin**, the main pigment of the skin and eye (Table 103.1). Melanin is synthesized by melanocytes from tyrosine in a membrane-bound intracellular organelle, the melanosome. Melanocytes originate from the embryonic neural crest and migrate to the skin, eyes (choroid and iris), hair follicles, and inner ear. The melanin in the eye is confined to the iris stromal and retinal pigment epithelia, whereas in skin and hair follicles, it is secreted into the epidermis and hair shaft. Albinism can be caused by deficiencies of melanin synthesis, by some hereditary defects of melanosomes, or by disorders of melanocyte migration. Neither the biosynthetic pathway of melanin nor many facets of melanocyte cell biology are completely elucidated (see Fig. 103.2). The end products are 2 pigments: *pheomelanin*, which is a yellow-red pigment, and *eumelanin*, a brown-black pigment.

Clinically, primary albinism can be *generalized* or *localized*. Primary generalized albinism can be *ocular* or *oculocutaneous*. Some syndromes feature albinism in association with platelet, immunologic, or neurologic dysfunction. In generalized oculocutaneous albinism, hypopigmentation can be either complete or partial. Individuals with complete albinism do not develop either generalized (tanning) or localized (pigmented nevi) skin pigmentation.

The **diagnosis** of albinism is usually evident, but for some white children whose families are particularly light-skinned, normal variation may be a diagnostic consideration. Unlike patients with albinism, normal fair-skinned children progressively develop pigmentation with age, do not exhibit the eye manifestations of albinism, and have pigmentary development similar to other family members. The clinical diagnosis of oculocutaneous albinism, as opposed to other types of cutaneous hypopigmentation, requires the presence of characteristic eye findings.

The **ocular manifestations** of albinism include hypopigmentation of iris and retina with foveal hypoplasia, along with reduced visual acuity, refractive errors, nystagmus, alternating strabismus, and iris transillumination (diffuse reddish hue of iris produced during ophthalmoscopic or slit-lamp examination of eye). There is also an abnormality in routing of the optic fibers at the chiasm. Unlike in pigmented individuals, in patients with albinism the majority of the nerve fibers from the temporal side of the retina cross to the contralateral hemisphere of the brain. This results in lack of binocular (stereoscopic) vision and depth perception and in repeated switching of vision from eye to eye, causing alternating strabismus. This abnormality also causes a characteristic pattern of visual evoked potentials. These findings are highly specific for albinism and can be used to enable the clinical diagnosis. Regular ophthalmologic follow-up is recommended for patients with oculocutaneous albinism. Correction of refractive errors can maximize visual

Table 103.1	Classification of Major Causes of Albinism	
TYPE	**GENE**	**CHROMOSOME**
OCULOCUTANEOUS ALBINISM (OCA)		
OCA1 (tyrosinase deficient)	*TYR*	11q14-q21
OCA1A (severe deficiency)	*TYR*	11q14-q21
OCA1B (mild deficiency)*	*TYR*	11q14-q21
OCA2 (tyrosinase positive)†	*OCA2*	15q12-q13
OCA3 (Rufous, red OCA)	*TYRP1‡*	9p23
OCA4	*SLC45A2*	5p13.3
Hermansky-Pudlak syndrome	*HPS1-9*	Different chromosomes
Chédiak-Higashi syndrome	*LYST*	1q42.1
OCULAR ALBINISM (OA)		
OA1 (Nettleship-Falls type)	*OA*	Xp22.3
LOCALIZED ALBINISM		
Piebaldism	*KIT*	4q12
Waardenburg syndrome (WS1-WS4)	See text	See text

*This includes Amish, minimal pigment, yellow albinism, and platinum and temperature-sensitive variants.
†Includes brown OCA.
‡Tyrosinase-related protein 1.

function. Usually, the alternating strabismus does not result in amblyopia and does not require surgery.

Patients with albinism should be counseled to avoid ultraviolet (UV) radiation by wearing protective long-sleeved clothing and by using sunscreens with a sun protection factor (SPF) rating >30. Melanin is also present in the cochlea. Albino individuals may be more susceptible to ototoxic agents such as gentamicin.

Oculocutaneous albinism is inherited as autosomal recessive trait. Many clinical forms of albinism have been identified. Some of the seemingly distinct clinical forms are caused by different pathogenic variants of the same gene. Several genes located on different chromosomes are involved in melanogenesis (see Table 103.1). Attempts to differentiate types of albinism based on the mode of inheritance, tyrosinase activity, or extent of hypopigmentation have failed to yield a comprehensive classification. The classification outlined next is based on the distribution of albinism in the body and the affected genes.

Genetic analysis is clinically available for most albinism genes (see Table 103.1). Molecular diagnosis is of little use therapeutically in isolated albinism but can be helpful for precise genetic counseling of families.

Oculocutaneous (Generalized) Albinism

Lack of pigment is generalized, affecting skin, hair, and eyes. At least 4 genetically distinct forms of oculocutaneous albinism (**OCA**) have been identified: OCA_1, OCA_2, OCA_3, and OCA_4. The lack of pigment is complete in patients with OCA_1 A; the other types may not be clinically distinguishable from one another. All affected individuals have ocular manifestations of albinism. All forms are inherited as autosomal recessive traits.

OCA_1 (Tyrosinase-Deficient Albinism)

The defect in patients with OCA_1 resides in the tyrosinase gene, *TYR*, located on chromosome 11q14.3. Many mutant alleles have been identified. Most affected individuals are compound heterozygotes. A clinical clue to the diagnosis of OCA_1 is complete lack of pigment at birth. The condition can be subdivided to OCA_1 A and OCA_1 B, based on enzyme activity and difference in clinical manifestations as a function of age.

OCA_1 A (Tyrosinase-Negative OCA)

In patients with OCA_1 A, the most severe form of OCA, both *TYR* alleles have pathogenic variants that completely inactivate tyrosinase. Clinically, lack of pigment in the skin (milky white), hair (white hair), and eyes (red-gray irides) is evident at birth and remains unchanged throughout life. They do not tan and do not develop pigmented nevi or freckles.

OCA_1 B

Patients with OCA_1 B have *TYR* gene pathogenic variants that preserve some residual activity. Clinically, they completely lack pigment at birth, but with age become light blond with light-blue or hazel eyes. They develop pigmented nevi and freckles, and they may tan. OCA_1 B patients, depending on the degree of pigmentation, were once subdivided into different groups and thought to be genetically distinct.

OCA_2 (Tyrosinase-Positive OCA)

OCA_2 is the *most common form of generalized OCA*, particularly in patients of African ancestry. Clinically, the phenotype is highly variable; most patients demonstrate some pigmentation of the skin and eyes at birth and continue to accumulate pigment throughout life. The hair is yellow at birth and may darken with age. They have pigmented nevi and freckles, and some may tan. They may be clinically indistinguishable from OCA_1 B patients. Individuals with OCA_2, however, have normal tyrosinase activity in hair bulbs. The defect is in the *OCA2* gene, which is an orthologue of the *p* (pink-eyed dilution) gene in the mouse. This gene produces the P protein, a melanosome membrane protein. Patients with **Prader-Willi** and **Angelman** syndromes caused by microdeletion of chromosome 15q12 that includes the *OCA2* gene have mild pigmentary deficiency (see Chapter 98.8).

OCA_3 (Rufous Albinism)

This form has been identified predominantly in Africans, African-Americans, and natives of New Guinea. Patients with OCA_3 can make pheomelanin but not eumelanin. Patients have reddish hair and reddish brown skin as adults. The skin color is peculiar to this form. In young persons the coloration may resemble that of OCA_2. The pathogenic variant is in the tyrosinase-related protein 1 (*TYRP1*) gene (located on chromosome 9p23), the function of which is not well-understood.

OCA_4

Similar manifestations to OCA_2 (both in the skin and the eyes) have been observed in OCA_4 patients (mostly from Japan) with pathogenic variants in the *SLC45A2* (previously called *MATP*) gene (located on chromosome 5p13.2).

Ocular Albinism

Patients with ocular albinism (**OA**) present in the 1st months of life with nystagmus, hypopigmentation of iris and fundus, foveal hypoplasia, and decreased visual acuity. Electron microscopy demonstrates characteristic macromelanosomes in skin biopsies or hair root specimens. Most patients affected by ocular albinism have ocular albinism type 1 (**OA₁**), an X-linked disorder caused by pathogenic variants in the *GPR143* gene. A rare form of OA with late-onset sensorineural deafness and apparent autosomal dominant inheritance has also been reported.

Ocular Albinism Type 1 (Nettleship-Falls Ocular Albinism)

OA_1 is an X-linked disorder characterized by congenital nystagmus, reduced pigmentation of ocular structures, and visual impairment in affected males. Heterozygous females may present with segments of abnormal retinal pigmentations. Infrequently, depending on the pattern of X chromosome inactivation, heterozygous females may also present with severe manifestations, including nystagmus, iris and foveal hypopigmentation, foveal hypoplasia, and reduced visual acuity. In families with darker skin complexion, mild skin hypopigmentation can be seen. The diagnosis of OA_1 is suspected in males with features of albinism in the eye, normal to mildly reduced skin pigmentation, and a family history suggestive of an X-linked transmission. It is a nonprogressive disorder, and the eye findings often improve with age. In patients who are the first of their families to be affected, genetic analysis of the *GPR143* gene (Xp22.2) helps confirm the diagnosis.

Syndromic Forms of Generalized Albinism
Hermansky-Pudlak Syndrome

This group of autosomal recessive disorders is caused by pathogenic variants of 1 of 9 different genes located on different chromosomes, *HPS1* to *HPS9*. Hermansky-Pudlak syndrome (**HPS**) is suspected in patients with albinism and a bleeding diathesis with inflammatory bowel disease (IBD) or pulmonary fibrosis. Disease subtype can be established with molecular studies (see Chapter 511).

The *HPS* genes are necessary for normal structure and function of lysosome-derived organelles, including melanosomes and platelet dense bodies. Patients have a tyrosinase-positive OCA of variable severity associated with platelet dysfunction (caused by the absence of platelet dense bodies). A ceroid-like material accumulates in tissues. HPS is panethnic. However, taking into account patients' ancestry can help develop a cost-effective testing strategy. HPS is prevalent in two regions of Puerto Rico (**type 1** in the northwest and **type 3** in the central regions as a result of different founder effects). The cutaneous and ocular symptoms of albinism are present. Patients can develop epistaxis, postsurgical bleeding, or abundant menses. Bleeding time is prolonged, but platelet count is normal. Major complications include progressive pulmonary fibrosis in young adults and Crohn-like IBD in adolescents and young adults. Kidney failure and cardiomyopathy have been reported. Neutropenia has been described in HPS **type 2**. Treatment is symptomatic.

Chédiak-Higashi Syndrome

Patients with this rare autosomal recessive condition have OCA of variable severity and susceptibility to infection (see Chapter 156). Bacterial infections of skin and upper respiratory tract are common. Giant peroxidase-positive lysosomal granules can be seen in granulocytes in a blood smear. Patients have a reduced number of melanosomes, which are abnormally large (macromelanosomes). The bleeding tendency is typically mild. If treatment is not successful, children can reach a stage of the disease known as the **accelerated phase**, which is a major, life-threatening complication of Chédiak-Higashi syndrome. It is caused by macrophage activation resulting in hemophagocytic lymphohistiocytosis, and systemic manifestations include fever, lymphadenopathy, hepatosplenomegaly, cytopenia, and elevated plasma ferritin level. Patients surviving childhood may develop cerebellar atrophy, peripheral neuropathy, and cognitive delay. Pathogenic variants in the *LYST* gene on chromosome 1q42.3 are the only known cause of this syndrome. Hematopoietic stem cell transplantation offers an effective approach to control immunodeficiency and hematologic abnormalities as well as prevent development of the accelerated phase.

Other Disorders Featuring Generalized Albinism

Hypopigmentation is a feature of other syndromes, some with abnormalities of lysosomal biogenesis or melanosome biology. **Griscelli syndrome** patients have silver-gray hair, pigmentary dilution of skin, and melanosomal clumping in hair shafts and the center of melanocytes, with intellectual disability or macrophage activation with hemophagocytosis in different subtypes. **Vici syndrome** patients have combined immunodeficiency, intellectual disability, agenesis of the corpus callosum, cataracts, and cleft lip/palate. Patients with **MAPBP-interacting protein deficiency** have short stature, recurrent infections, neutropenia.

Localized Albinism

Localized albinism refers to localized patches of hypopigmentation of skin and hair, which may be evident at birth or develop with time. These conditions are caused by abnormal migration of melanocytes during embryonic development.

Piebaldism

Piebaldism is an autosomal dominant inherited condition in which the individual is usually born with a white forelock. The underlying skin is depigmented and devoid of melanocytes. In addition, there are usually white macules on the face, trunk, and extremities. Pathogenic variants in the *KIT* and *SNAI2* genes have been shown in affected patients.

Waardenburg Syndrome

In Waardenburg syndrome, a white forelock is often associated with lateral displacement of inner canthi of the eyes, broad nasal bridge, heterochromia of irides, and sensorineural deafness. This condition is inherited as an autosomal dominant trait; 4 major types have been identified. Patients with Waardenburg syndrome type 1 (**WS1**, the *most common form*) have all the previous clinical findings, including lateral displacement of inner canthi. The condition is caused by pathogenic variants (>90%) in the *PAX3* gene. Patients with Waardenburg syndrome type 2 (**WS2**) have the clinical findings of WS1 except for the lateral displacement of inner canthi. Genetically, this is a heterogeneous condition caused by pathogenic variants in several genes, including *MITF*, *SOX10*, and *SNAI2*. Patients with Waardenburg syndrome type 3 (**WS3**) have all the findings seen in individuals with WS1 plus hypoplasia and contractures of the upper limbs. It is caused by heterozygous or homozygous pathogenic variants of *PAX3* gene. Waardenburg syndrome type 4 (**WS4**), associated with **Hirschsprung disease**, is genetically heterogeneous; pathogenic variants in different genes (*EDN3*, *EDNRB*, or *SOX10*) have been identified in different patients.

Other causes of **localized hypopigmentation** include vitiligo and hypomelanosis of Ito (see Chapter 672).

Bibliography is available at Expert Consult.

103.3 Methionine

Oleg A. Shchelochkov and Charles P. Venditti

The usual pathway for catabolism of methionine, an essential amino acid, produces S-*adenosylmethionine*, which serves as a methyl group donor for methylation of a variety of compounds in the body, and *cysteine*, which is formed through a series of reactions collectively called *trans-sulfuration* (Fig. 103.3).

HOMOCYSTINURIA (HOMOCYSTINEMIA)

Normally, most *homocysteine*, an intermediate compound of methionine degradation, is remethylated to methionine. This methionine-sparing reaction is catalyzed by the enzyme methionine synthase, which requires a metabolite of folic acid (5-methyltetrahydrofolate) as a methyl donor and a metabolite of vitamin B_{12} (methylcobalamin) as a cofactor (see Fig. 103.3). In healthy individuals, most plasma homocysteine is either protein-bound or exists as disulfides. Three major forms of homocystinemia and homocystinuria have been identified.

Homocystinuria Caused by Cystathionine β-Synthase Deficiency (Classic Homocystinuria)

This is the most common inborn error of methionine metabolism. Approximately 40% of affected patients respond to high doses of vitamin B_6 and usually have milder clinical manifestations than those who are unresponsive to vitamin B_6 therapy. These patients possess some residual enzyme activity.

Infants with classic homocystinuria appear normal at birth. **Clinical manifestations** during infancy are nonspecific and may include failure to thrive and developmental delay. Without newborn screening, the diagnosis can be delayed and is usually made after 3 yr of age, when subluxation of the ocular lens (*ectopia lentis*) occurs. This causes severe myopia and iridodonesis (quivering of the iris). Astigmatism, glaucoma, staphyloma, cataracts, retinal detachment, and optic atrophy may develop later in life. Progressive intellectual disability is common. Normal intelligence has been reported. In an international survey of >600 patients, IQ scores ranged from 10-135. Higher IQ scores are seen in vitamin B_6–responsive patients. Psychiatric and behavioral disorders have been observed in more than 50% of affected patients. Seizures are seen in approximately 20% of untreated patients. Affected individuals with homocystinuria manifest skeletal abnormalities resembling those of Marfan syndrome (see Chapter 722): tall with elongated limbs and arachnodactyly. Scoliosis, pectus excavatum or pectus carinatum, genu valgum, pes cavus, high-arched palate, and crowding of the teeth are typically seen. These children usually have fair complexions, blue eyes, and a peculiar malar flush. Generalized osteoporosis, especially of the spine, is the main x-ray finding. Thromboembolic episodes involving both large and small vessels, especially those of the brain, are common and may occur at any age. Optic atrophy, paralysis, cor pulmonale, and severe hypertension (from renal infarcts) are among the serious consequences of thromboembolism, which is likely caused by elevated homocysteine levels leading to abnormal angiogenesis and inhibition of fibrinolytic activity. The risk of thromboembolism increases after surgical procedures. Spontaneous pneumothorax and acute pancreatitis are rare complications.

Elevations of both methionine and homocystine (or homocysteine) in body fluids are the diagnostic **laboratory findings**. Freshly voided urine should be tested for homocystine because this compound is unstable and may disappear after prolonged storage. Cysteine is low or absent in plasma. Total plasma homocysteine is the preferred analyte for management of classic homocystinuria. Free plasma homocysteine may normalize or remain normal when total plasma homocysteine is lowered. The diagnosis may be established by molecular analysis of cystathionine β-synthase (*CBS*) or by assay of the enzyme in cultured fibroblasts, phytohemagglutinin-stimulated lymphocytes, or liver biopsy specimens.

Treatment with high doses of vitamin B_6 (100-500 mg/24 hr) causes dramatic improvement in patients who are responsive to this therapy. The degree of response to vitamin B_6 treatment may vary across families. Some patients may not respond because of folate depletion; a patient

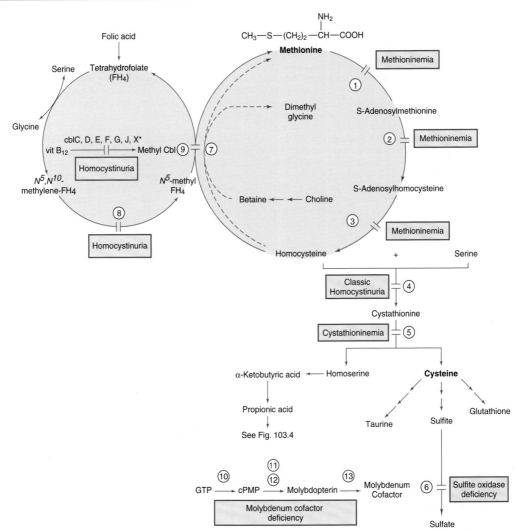

Fig. 103.3 Pathways in the metabolism of sulfur-containing amino acids. **Enzymes:** *(1)* Methionine adenosyltransferase (MAT I/III), *(2)* glycine N-methyltransferase, *(3)* S-adenosylhomocysteine hydrolase, *(4)* cystathionine synthase, *(5)* cystathionase, *(6)* sulfite oxidase, *(7)* betaine homocysteine methyltransferase, *(8)* methylene tetrahydrofolate reductase, *(9)* methionine synthase (cblG), *(10)* molybdenum cofactor biosynthesis protein 1, *(11)* molybdopterin synthase, *(12)* adenylyltransferase and sulfurtransferase (*MOCS3*), *(13)* gephyrin. GTP, Guanosine triphosphate; cPMP, cyclic pyranopterin monophosphate. *Defects in cblC, D, F, J, X result in methylmalonic acidemia and homocystinuria.

should not be considered unresponsive to vitamin B₆ until folic acid (1-5 mg/24 hr) has been added to the treatment regimen. For patients who are unresponsive to vitamin B₆, restriction of methionine intake in conjunction with cysteine supplementation is also recommended. The need for dietary restriction and its extent remains controversial in patients with vitamin B₆–responsive form. In some patients with this form, addition of betaine may obviate the need for any dietary restriction. *Betaine* (trimethylglycine, 6 g/24 hr for adults or 200-250 mg/kg/day for children) lowers homocysteine levels in body fluids by remethylating homocysteine to methionine (see Fig. 103.3), which may result in elevation of plasma methionine levels. This treatment has produced clinical improvement (preventing vascular events) in patients who are unresponsive to vitamin B₆ therapy. Cerebral edema has occurred in a patient with vitamin B₆–nonresponsive homocystinuria and dietary noncompliance during betaine therapy.

More than 100 pregnancies in women with classic homocystinuria have been reported with favorable outcomes for both mothers and infants. The majority of infants were full-term and normal. Postpartum thromboembolic events occurred in a few mothers.

The screening of newborn infants for classic homocystinuria has been performed worldwide, with an estimated prevalence of 1 in 200,000 to 1 in 350,000 live births, although it can be more common in some parts of the world (e.g., 1:1,800 in Qatar). Early treatment of patients identified by screening has produced favorable results. The mean IQ of patients with vitamin B₆–unresponsive form treated in early infancy was in the normal range. Dislocation of the lens seemed to be prevented in some patients.

Classic homocystinuria is inherited as an autosomal recessive trait. The gene for cystathionine β-synthase (*CBS*) is located on chromosome 21q22.3. Prenatal diagnosis is feasible by DNA analysis or by performing an enzyme assay of cultured amniotic cells. Most affected patients are compound heterozygotes for 2 different alleles. Heterozygous carriers are asymptomatic.

Homocystinuria Caused by Defects in Methylcobalamin Formation
Methylcobalamin is the cofactor for the enzyme methionine synthase, which catalyzes remethylation of homocysteine to methionine. At least

7 distinct defects in the intracellular metabolism of cobalamin may interfere with the formation of methylcobalamin. (To better understand the metabolism of cobalamin, see Methylmalonic Acidemia in Chapter 103.6 and Figs. 103.3 and 103.4.) The 7 defects are designated as *cbl*C, *cbl*D (including *cbl*D variant 1), *cbl*E (methionine synthase reductase), *cbl*G (methionine synthase), *cbl*F, *cbl*J, and *cbl*X. Patients with *cbl*C, *cbl*D, *cbl*F, *cbl*J, and *cbl*X defects have **methylmalonic acidemia** in

addition to homocystinuria, because the formation of both adenosyl-cobalamin and methylcobalamin is impaired.

Patients with *cbl*E, *cbl*G, and *cbl*D variant 1 defects are unable to form methylcobalamin and develop homocystinuria without methylmalonic acidemia (Fig. 103.4). The clinical manifestations are similar in patients with these 3 defects. Nonspecific symptoms such as vomiting, poor feeding, failure to thrive, lethargy, hypotonia, seizures, and

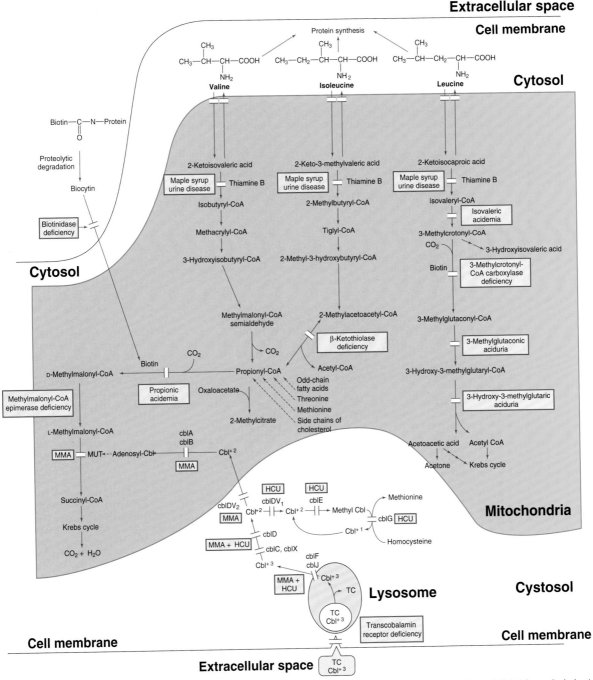

Fig. 103.4 Pathways in the metabolism of the branched-chain amino acids, biotin, and vitamin B$_{12}$ (cobalamin). Adenosyl Cbl, Adenosylcobalamin; Cbl, cobalamin; *cbl*, defect in metabolism of cobalamin; *cbl*DV1, *cbl*D variant 1; *cbl*DV2, *cbl*D variant 2; HCU, homocystinuria; methyl Cbl, methylcobalamin; MMA, methylmalonic acidemia; MUT, mutase; OHCbl, hydroxycobalamin; TC, transcobalamin; TCR, transcobalamin receptor. See text for the name of the enzymes.

developmental delay may occur in the 1st few months of life. Late-onset forms of these disorders may present with neurocognitive defects, psychosis, and peripheral neuropathy. **Laboratory findings** include megaloblastic anemia, hyperhomocysteinemia, homocystinuria, and hypomethioninemia. The absence of hypermethioninemia differentiates these conditions from cystathionine β-synthase deficiency (see earlier). Renal artery thrombosis, hemolytic uremic syndrome, pulmonary hypertension, and optic nerve atrophy have been reported in some patients with these defects.

Diagnosis is established by DNA testing or by complementation studies performed in cultured fibroblasts. Prenatal diagnosis has been accomplished by studies in amniotic cell cultures. *cbl*E, *cbl*G, and *cbl*D variant 1 deficiencies are inherited as autosomal recessive traits. The gene for *cbl*E is *MTRR*, encoding methionine synthase reductase (located on chromosome 5p15.31). The gene for *cbl*G is *MTR*, encoding methionine synthase (located on chromosome 1q43). The *cbl*D variant 1 deficiency is caused by pathogenic variants affecting the C-terminal of the *MMADHC* gene (located on chromosome 2q23.2).

Treatment with vitamin B_{12} in the form of high-dose hydroxycobalamin helps improve the clinical and biochemical findings. Results vary among both diseases and sibships.

Homocystinuria Caused by Deficiency of Methylenetetrahydrofolate Reductase (MTHFR Deficiency)

This enzyme reduces 5,10-methylenetetrahydrofolate to form 5-methyltetrahydrofolate, which provides the methyl group needed for remethylation of homocysteine to methionine (see Fig. 103.3). The severity of the enzyme defect and the clinical manifestations vary considerably in different families. **Clinical findings** vary from apnea, seizure, microcephaly, coma, and death to developmental delay, ataxia, motor abnormalities, peripheral neuropathy, and psychiatric manifestations. Thromboembolism has also been observed. Exposure to the anesthetic nitrous oxide (which inhibits methionine synthase) in patients with MTHFR deficiency may result in neurologic deterioration and death.

Laboratory findings include moderate homocystinemia and homocystinuria. The methionine concentration is low or low-normal. This finding helps differentiate this condition from classic homocystinuria caused by cystathionine β-synthase deficiency. The diagnosis may be confirmed by molecular analysis of *MTHFR* or by the enzyme assay in cultured fibroblasts or leukocytes.

MTHFR deficiency should be differentiated from **mild hyperhomocysteinemia** due to two common polymorphisms in the *MTHFR* gene. Two "thermolabile" polymorphisms have been extensively studied, c.665C>T (p.Ala222Val, previously referred to as c.677C>T) and c.1286A>C (p.Glu429Ala, formerly referred to as c.1298A>C). These polymorphisms may minimally affect levels of plasma total homocysteine in some patients and are often confounded by dietary folate deficiency. Both polymorphisms have been studied as possible risk factors for a wide variety of medical conditions, including birth defects, autism, vascular disease, stroke, pregnancy loss, cancer, and response to chemotherapy. Population-based studies revealed a surprisingly high prevalence of homozygosity for these polymorphisms in the general population: up to 10–15% of the North American Caucasians and >25% in some Hispanics. It is hypothesized that fortification of flour with folate may have decreased the strength of associations observed in the past. To date, the best data support a role for the c.665C>T polymorphism (formerly c. 677C>T) as a risk factor for neural tube defects. Although a clinical test for this polymorphism is widely available, recent meta-analyses have not supported the association between the *MTHFR* polymorphism and risk for venous thromboembolism or between mild hyperhomocysteinemia and an increased risk for coronary heart disease.

The condition is inherited as an autosomal recessive trait. The **diagnosis** can be confirmed by *MTHFR* gene analysis. Prenatal diagnosis can be achieved by molecular analysis of *MTHFR* of the known familial pathogenic variants or by measuring MTHFR enzyme activity in cultured chorionic villus cells or amniocytes.

Treatment of MTHFR deficiency with a combination of folic acid,

vitamin B_6, vitamin B_{12}, methionine supplementation, and betaine has been tried. Of these, early treatment with betaine appears to have the most beneficial effect.

HYPERMETHIONINEMIA
Primary (Genetic) Hypermethioninemia

Elevation of plasma level of methionine occurs in several genetic conditions.

Classic Homocystinuria. See earlier discussion.

Hepatic Methionine Adenosyltransferase (MAT I/MAT III) Deficiency (Mudd Disease). This enzyme, which has 2 isoforms, MAT I (tetrameric) and MAT III (dimeric), is encoded by a single gene (*MAT1A* on chromosome 10q22.3) and is involved in the 1st step of methionine catabolism (see Fig. 103.3). Another structurally similar enzyme, MAT II, is encoded by a different gene (*MAT2A* on chromosome 2p11.2) and is expressed predominantly in nonhepatic tissues (kidney, brain, lymphocytes). Deficiency of MAT I/MAT III causes hypermethioninemia. In severe deficiency, total plasma homocysteine can also be elevated. The majority of these patients have been diagnosed in the neonatal period through screening for homocystinuria. Most affected individuals have residual enzyme activity and remain asymptomatic throughout life despite persistent hypermethioninemia. Some complain of an unusual odor to their breath, likely caused by accumulation of dimethylsulfide. A few patients with complete enzyme deficiency have had neurologic abnormalities related to demyelination (intellectual disability, dystonia, dyspraxia).

Laboratory studies reveal markedly elevated levels of plasma methionine with a normal or low level of S-adenosylmethionine and normal concentrations of S-adenosylhomocysteine and homocysteine. These findings help differentiate MAT I/MAT III deficiency from other causes of hypermethioninemia.

No uniformly accepted therapeutic regimen has yet emerged. Although no specific treatment is used in most patients, long-term follow-up to monitor for neurologic and liver abnormalities should be considered. Diets low in methionine result in lowering of plasma methionine, but the advisability of such diets has been questioned since lowering the plasma methionine level causes further lowering of S-adenosylmethionine in the body. Supplementation with S-adenosylmethionine in conjunction with a low-methionine diet seems prudent, but no large clinical experience is yet available. Normal pregnancies producing normal offspring have been reported in mothers with MAT I/MAT III (*MAT1A*) deficiency. The condition is inherited as an autosomal recessive trait, although pathogenic variant p.R264H in *MAT1A* appears to disrupt protein dimerization and may result in mild hypermethioninemia even in heterozygous patients.

Glycine N-Methyltransferase Deficiency. Glycine N-methyltransferase mediates catabolism of S-adenosylmethionine to S-adenosylhomocysteine (see Fig. 103.3). A few patients with deficiency of this enzyme have been reported to date. Clinically, patients were asymptomatic except for mild hepatomegaly and elevated serum levels of transaminases. Other laboratory findings included hypermethioninemia and very high levels of serum S-adenosylmethionine. No specific treatment has yet been identified. The condition is inherited as an autosomal recessive trait; the gene *GNMT* is on chromosome 6p21.1.

S-Adenosylhomocysteine Hydrolase (SAHH) Deficiency. Deficiency of SAHH (see Fig. 103.3) has been described infrequently. Intellectual disability, severe hypotonia, and progressive liver dysfunction were common clinical findings. Laboratory studies included elevated levels of serum creatine kinase, hypoalbuminemia (associated with fetal hydrops in one family), hypoprothrombinemia and greatly elevated levels of serum S-adenosylhomocysteine with moderate elevations of plasma methionine and S-adenosylmethionine. Marked elevation in S-adenosylhomocysteine has been thought to cause inhibition of methyltransferases, including those involved in the synthesis of creatine (see Fig. 103.10) and choline, resulting in their deficiencies. MRI of the brain can reveal delayed myelination of the white matter. The diagnosis can be achieved by the *AHCY* gene analysis (chromosome 20q11.22) or by biochemical assay of red blood cells, cultured skin fibroblasts, or liver biopsy. Treatment with a low-methionine diet has been used, but its long-term effectiveness has not been established.

Tyrosinemia Type I. See Chapter 103.2.

Citrin Deficiency. See Chapter 103.12.

Acquired (Nongenetic) Hypermethioninemia

Hypermethioninemia occurs in premature and some full-term infants receiving high-protein diets, in whom it may represent delayed maturation of the enzyme MAT. Lowering the protein intake usually resolves the abnormality. It is also commonly found in patients with various forms of liver disease.

PRIMARY CYSTATHIONINEMIA (CYSTATHIONINURIA)

Cystathionase (cystathionine γ-lyase) deficiency results in massive cystathioninuria and mild to moderate cystathioninemia. Deficiency of this enzyme is inherited as an autosomal recessive trait, with an estimated prevalence of 1 in 14,000 live births. A wide variety of clinical manifestations have been reported. Lack of a consistent clinical picture and the presence of cystathioninuria in a number of individuals free of clinical findings suggest that cystathionase deficiency may be of no clinical significance. Many reported cases are responsive to oral administration of large doses of vitamin B_6 (≥100 mg/24 hr). When cystathioninuria is discovered in a patient, vitamin B_6 treatment can be tried, but its beneficial effect has not been established. The gene encoding for cystathionase (*CTH*) is located on chromosome 1p31.1. The disorder is inherited as an autosomal recessive trait.

Primary cystathioninuria needs to be differentiated from secondary cystathioninuria, which can occur in patients with vitamin B_6 or B_{12} deficiency, liver disease (particularly damage caused by galactosemia), thyrotoxicosis, hepatoblastoma, neuroblastoma, ganglioblastoma, or defects in remethylation of homocysteine.

Bibliography is available at Expert Consult.

103.4 Cysteine and Cystine
Oleg A. Shchelochkov and Charles P. Venditti

Cysteine is a sulfur-containing amino acid that is synthesized from methionine (see Fig. 103.3). Oxidation of cysteine forms *cystine*, a poorly soluble dimer. The most common genetic disorders of cysteine and cystine metabolism are cystinuria (see Chapter 562) and cystinosis (see Chapter 547.3).

SULFITE OXIDASE DEFICIENCY AND MOLYBDENUM COFACTOR DEFICIENCY

In the last step in cysteine metabolism, sulfite is oxidized to sulfate by sulfite oxidase, and the sulfate is excreted in the urine (see Fig. 103.3). Sulfite oxidase is encoded by *SUOX* (located on chromosome 12q13.2). This enzyme requires a molybdenum-pterin complex termed *molybdenum cofactor*. This cofactor is also necessary for the function of 2 other enzymes in humans: xanthine dehydrogenase (which oxidizes xanthine and hypoxanthine to uric acid) and aldehyde oxidase (involved in oxidizing a number of natural compounds and drugs). Three enzymes, encoded by 3 different genes (*MOCS1, MOCS2,* and *GPHN,* mapped to chromosomes 6p21.2, 5q11.2, and 14q23.3, respectively), are involved in the synthesis of the cofactor. Deficiency of any of the 3 enzymes causes cofactor deficiency with similar phenotypes. Most patients, who were originally diagnosed as having **sulfite oxidase deficiency**, have been shown to have **molybdenum cofactor deficiency**. Sulfite oxidase deficiency and molybdenum cofactor deficiency are inherited as autosomal recessive traits.

The enzyme and cofactor deficiencies produce overlapping **clinical manifestations**. Refusal to feed, vomiting, an exaggerated startle reaction, severe intractable seizures (tonic, clonic, myoclonic), cortical atrophy with subcortical multicystic lesions, and severe developmental delay may develop within a few weeks after birth. The biochemical diagnosis should be considered in infants presenting with neonatal seizures and

neonates with symptoms reminiscent of hypoxic-ischemic encephalopathy. Bilateral dislocation of ocular lenses is a common finding in patients who survive the neonatal period. The intractable seizures seen in this condition are in part a consequence of secondary vitamin B_6 dependency. The accumulation of sulfites in body fluids in this condition causes the inhibition of *antiquitin* enzyme, which is necessary for conversion of α-amino adipic semialdehyde to α-aminoadipic acid; the resultant accumulation of α-aminoadipic semialdehyde and its cyclic form, P6C, causes the inactivation of pyridoxal-5-phosphate (active form of vitamin B_6) and thus the vitamin B_6–dependent epilepsy (see also Chapter 103.14).

Affected children excrete large amounts of sulfite, thiosulfate, S-sulfocysteine, xanthine, and hypoxanthine in the urine. Urinary and serum levels of uric acid and urinary concentration of sulfate are diminished. Fresh urine should be used for screening purposes and for quantitative measurements of sulfite, because oxidation of sulfite to sulfate at room temperature may produce false-negative results. Increased concentrations of α-aminoadipic semialdehyde and P6C are present in the cerebrospinal fluid, plasma, and urine.

Diagnosis is confirmed by measurement of sulfite oxidase and molybdenum cofactor in fibroblasts and liver biopsies, respectively or by DNA studies. Prenatal diagnosis is possible by performing an assay of sulfite oxidase activity in cultured amniotic cells, in samples of chorionic villi or by DNA studies. The prevalence of these deficiencies in the general population is not known, but likely is very low.

No effective treatment is available. Large doses of vitamin B_6 (5-100 mg/kg) result in alleviation of seizures but do not seem to alter the devastating neurologic outcome. Most children die in the 1st 2 yr of life. Patients with molybdenum cofactor deficiency caused by pathogenic variants in *MOCS1* have benefited from supplementation using intravenous **cyclic pyranopterin monophosphate** (cPMP), which is undergoing a multicenter clinical trial.

Bibliography is available at Expert Consult.

103.5 Tryptophan
Oleg A. Shchelochkov and Charles P. Venditti

Tryptophan is an essential amino acid and a precursor for nicotinic acid (niacin) and serotonin (Fig. 103.5). The genetic disorders of metabolism of serotonin, one of the major neurotransmitters, are discussed in Chapter 103.11.

HARTNUP DISORDER

In the autosomal recessive Hartnup disorder, named after the 1st affected family, a defect occurs in the transport of monoamino-monocarboxylic amino acids (neutral amino acids), including tryptophan, by the intestinal mucosa and renal tubules. The transporter protein for these amino acids (B^0AT1) is encoded by the *SLC6A19* gene (located on chromosome 5p15.33). Most children with Hartnup defect remain asymptomatic. Patients show significant variability in presentation, likely related to the nutritional factors, environment, and genetic heterogeneity (e.g., 2 proteins, TMEM27 and ACE2, that interact with B^0AT1). Decreased intestinal absorption of tryptophan in conjunction with its increased renal loss can lead to reduced availability of tryptophan for niacin synthesis. **Tryptophan deficiency** can be accentuated by malabsorption such as celiac disease. The major clinical manifestation in the rare symptomatic patient is **cutaneous photosensitivity**. The skin becomes rough and red after moderate exposure to the sun, and with greater exposure, a *pellagra-like rash* may develop. The rash may be pruritic, and a chronic eczema may develop. The skin changes have been reported in affected infants as young as 10 days of age. Some patients may have intermittent ataxia manifested as an unsteady, wide-based gait. The ataxia may last a few days and can respond to niacin supplementation. Cognitive development is usually normal. Episodic psychiatric manifestations such as irritability, emotional instability, depression, and suicidal tendencies, have been observed; these changes are usually associated

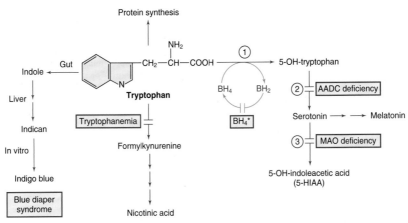

Fig. 103.5 Pathways in the metabolism of tryptophan. BH₄* indicates hyperphenylalaninemia caused by tetrahydrobiopterin deficiency (see Fig. 103.1). **Enzymes:** *(1)* Tryptophan hydroxylase, *(2)* aromatic L-amino acid decarboxylase (AADC), *(3)* monoamine oxidase (MAO).

with bouts of ataxia. Short stature and atrophic glossitis are seen in some patients.

Most children diagnosed with Hartnup disorder by neonatal screening have remained asymptomatic. This indicates that other factors are also involved in pathogenesis of the clinical condition.

The main laboratory finding is **aminoaciduria**, which is restricted to neutral amino acids (alanine, serine, threonine, valine, leucine, isoleucine, phenylalanine, tyrosine, tryptophan, histidine). Urinary excretion of proline, hydroxyproline, and arginine remains normal. This finding helps differentiate Hartnup disorder from other causes of generalized aminoaciduria, such as Fanconi syndrome. Plasma concentrations of neutral amino acids are normal or mildly decreased. This seemingly unexpected finding reflects compensatory mechanisms required to maintain normal transport and utilization of amino acids. The indole derivatives (especially indican) may be found in large amounts in some patients, resulting from bacterial breakdown of unabsorbed tryptophan in the intestines.

Diagnosis of Hartnup disorder is established by the intermittent nature of symptoms and characteristic findings on the urine amino acid analysis. If necessary, the diagnosis can be confirmed molecularly by *SLC6A19* gene analysis.

Treatment with nicotinic acid or nicotinamide (50-300 mg/24 hr) and a high-protein diet results in a favorable response in symptomatic patients with Hartnup disorder. Because of the intermittent nature of the clinical manifestations, the efficacy of these treatments is difficult to evaluate. The prevalence of Hartnup disorder is estimated to be 1 in 20,000 to 1 in 55,000 live births. Normal outcome for both mother and fetus has been reported in several affected women.

Bibliography is available at Expert Consult.

103.6 Isoleucine, Leucine, Valine, and Related Organic Acidemias

Oleg A. Shchelochkov, Irini Manoli, and Charles P. Venditti

The early steps in the degradation of the branched-chain amino acids (BCAAs)—isoleucine, leucine, and valine—are similar (see Fig. 103.4). Under catabolic conditions, BCAAs in the muscle tissue undergo a reversible reaction of transamination catalyzed by BCAA transaminase. α-Ketoacids formed by this reaction then undergo an oxidative decarboxylation step mediated by branched-chain α-ketoacid dehydrogenase (**BCKDH**) complex. The deficiency of BCKDH results in maple syrup urine disease, whereas the deficiency of enzymes mediating more distal

steps results in accumulation of enzyme-specific organic acids excreted in the urine, thus giving those inborn errors of metabolism the eponyms **organic acidemias** and **organic acidurias**. These disorders typically cause metabolic acidosis, which usually occurs in the 1st few days of life. Although most of the clinical findings are nonspecific, some manifestations may provide important clues to the nature of the enzyme deficiency. Fig. 103.6 presents an approach to infants suspected of having an organic acidemia. The diagnosis is usually established by identifying and measuring specific organic acids in body fluids (blood, urine), identifying pathogenic variants in a respective gene, and enzyme assay.

Organic acidemias are *not* limited to defects in the catabolic pathways of BCAAs. Disorders causing accumulation of other organic acids include those derived from lysine (see Chapter 103.14), disorders of γ-glutamyl cycle (see Chapter 103.11), those associated with lactic acid (see Chapter 105), and dicarboxylic acidemias associated with defective fatty acid degradation (see Chapter 104.1).

MAPLE SYRUP URINE DISEASE

Decarboxylation of leucine, isoleucine, and valine is accomplished by a complex enzyme system (BCKDH) using thiamine (vitamin B₁) pyrophosphate as a coenzyme. This mitochondrial enzyme consists of 4 subunits: $E_{1\alpha}$, $E_{1\beta}$, E_2, and E_3. The E_3 subunit is shared with 2 other dehydrogenases, pyruvate dehydrogenase and α-ketoglutarate dehydrogenase. Deficiency of any of these subunits causes maple syrup urine disease (**MSUD**) (see Fig. 103.4), a disorder named after the sweet odor of maple syrup found in body fluids, especially urine. Clinical conditions caused by defects in $E_{1\alpha}$, $E_{1\beta}$, E_2 and E_3 are designated as MSUD type IA, type IB, type 2 and type 3, respectively. This classification, however, is not very helpful clinically because the severity of clinical manifestations does not correlate with, or correspond specifically to, any single enzyme subunit. An affected infant with type 1A defect can have clinical manifestations ranging from relatively mild to very severe. A more useful classification, based on clinical findings and response to thiamine administration, delineates 5 phenotypes of MSUD.

Classic Maple Syrup Urine Disease

Classic MSUD has the **most severe** clinical manifestations. The BCKDH complex activity in this group varies between 0% and 2% of controls. Patients with uncontrolled or poorly controlled disease develop signs of acute encephalopathy. The mechanisms underlying this life-threatening complication are complex, but leucine and its derivative, α-ketoisocaproic acid, appear to be the key factors underlying acute encephalopathy. Elevated leucine competitively inhibits the uptake of other amino acids by the large neutral amino acid (LNAA) transporter. Once taken up by the brain tissue, leucine is metabolized by BCAA aminotransferase to α-ketoisocaproic acid, which leads to the disrupted metabolism of

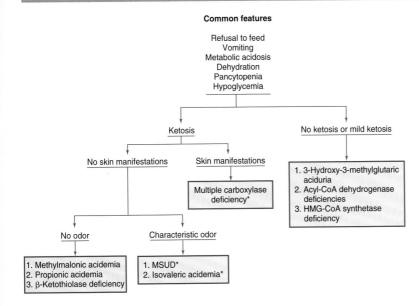

Common features

Refusal to feed
Vomiting
Metabolic acidosis
Dehydration
Pancytopenia
Hypoglycemia

Ketosis — No ketosis or mild ketosis

No skin manifestations — Skin manifestations

Multiple carboxylase deficiency*

1. 3-Hydroxy-3-methylglutaric aciduria
2. Acyl-CoA dehydrogenase deficiencies
3. HMG-CoA synthetase deficiency

No odor — Characteristic odor

1. Methylmalonic acidemia
2. Propionic acidemia
3. β-Ketothiolase deficiency

1. MSUD*
2. Isovaleric acidemia*

Fig. 103.6 Clinical approach to infants with organic acidemia. *Asterisks* indicate disorders in which patients have a characteristic odor (see text and Table 103.2). MSUD, Maple syrup urine disease.

neurotransmitters and amino acids (glutamate, GABA, glutamine, alanine, and aspartate). α-Ketoisocaproic acid can reversibly inhibit oxidative phosphorylation and result in cerebral lactic acidosis. Collectively, these processes are detrimental to the normal function of neurons and glia, clinically manifesting as encephalopathy and brain edema and referred to as **leucinosis**. Affected infants who appear healthy at birth develop poor feeding and vomiting in the 1st days of life. Lethargy and coma may ensue within a few days. Physical examination reveals hypertonicity and muscular rigidity with severe opisthotonos. Periods of hypertonicity may alternate with bouts of flaccidity manifested as repetitive movements of the extremities ("boxing" and "bicycling"). Neurologic findings are often mistakenly thought to be caused by generalized sepsis and meningitis. Cerebral edema may be present; convulsions occur in most infants, and hypoglycemia is common. In contrast to most hypoglycemic states, correction of the blood glucose concentration does not improve the clinical condition. Aside from the blood glucose, routine laboratory findings are usually unremarkable, except for varying degrees of ketoacidosis. If left untreated, death can occur in the 1st few weeks or months of life.

Diagnosis is often suspected because of the peculiar odor of maple syrup in urine, sweat, and cerumen. It is usually confirmed by amino acid analysis showing marked elevations in plasma levels of leucine, isoleucine, valine, and alloisoleucine (a stereoisomer of isoleucine not normally found in blood) and depressed level of alanine. Leucine levels are usually higher than those of the other 3 amino acids. Urine contains high levels of leucine, isoleucine, and valine and their respective ketoacids. These ketoacids may be detected qualitatively by adding a few drops of 2,4-dinitrophenylhydrazine reagent (0.1% in 0.1N HCl) to the urine; a yellow precipitate of 2,4-dinitrophenylhydrazone is formed in a positive test. Neuroimaging during the acute state may show cerebral edema, which is most prominent in the cerebellum, dorsal brainstem, cerebral peduncle, and internal capsule. After recovery from the acute state and with advancing age, hypomyelination and cerebral atrophy may be seen in neuroimaging of the brain.

Treatment of the acute state is aimed at hydration and rapid removal of the BCAAs and their metabolites from the tissues and body fluids. Uptake of leucine by the brain and accumulation of the downstream metabolite, α-ketoisocaproic acid, appear to be the key metabolic events underlying MSUD encephalopathy. Therefore, strategies of MSUD management focus on decreasing plasma leucine to control acute and chronic manifestations of the disease.

Because renal clearance of leucine is poor, hydration alone may not produce a rapid improvement. *Hemodialysis* is the most effective mode of therapy in critically ill infants and should be instituted promptly; significant decreases in plasma levels of leucine, isoleucine, and valine are usually seen within 24 hr. Sufficient calories and nutrients should be provided intravenously or orally as soon as possible to reverse patient's catabolic state. Cerebral edema, if present, may require treatment with mannitol, diuretics (e.g., furosemide), or hypertonic saline. Counterintuitively, supplementation with isoleucine and valine is also needed to control plasma leucine level in MSUD patients. Judiciously administered isoleucine and valine will compete with leucine for the LNAA transporter at the blood-brain barrier and thus decrease leucine entry into the central nervous system (CNS) and help in the prevention and treatment of leucine encephalopathy.

Treatment after recovery from the acute state requires a diet low in BCAAs. Synthetic formulas devoid of leucine, isoleucine, and valine are available commercially. Because these amino acids cannot be synthesized endogenously, age-appropriate amounts of BCAAs should be provided in the diet in the form of complete protein. To avoid essential amino acid deficiencies, the amount should be titrated carefully by performing frequent analyses of the plasma amino acids, with close attention to plasma isoleucine, leucine, and valine levels. A clinical condition resembling **acrodermatitis enteropathica** (see Chapter 691) occurs in affected infants whose plasma isoleucine or valine become *very low*; addition of isoleucine or valine, respectively, to the diet will hasten the recovery of skin rash. Patients with MSUD need to remain on the diet for the rest of their lives. Liver transplantation has been performed in patients with classic MSUD, with promising results.

The long-term prognosis of affected children remains guarded. Severe ketoacidosis, cerebral edema, and death may occur during any stressful situation such as infection or surgery, especially in mid-childhood. Cognitive and other neurologic deficits are common sequelae.

Intermediate (Mild) Maple Syrup Urine Disease
Children with intermediate MSUD develop milder disease after the neonatal period. Clinical manifestations are insidious and limited to the CNS. Patients have mild to moderate intellectual disability with or without seizures. They have the odor of maple syrup and excrete moderate amounts of the BCAAs and their ketoacid derivatives in the urine. Plasma concentrations of leucine, isoleucine, and valine are moderately increased whereas those of lactate and pyruvate tend to be normal. These children are commonly diagnosed during an intercurrent illness, when signs and symptoms of classic MSUD may occur. The dehydrogenase activity is 3–40% of controls. Because patients with thiamine-responsive MSUD usually have manifestations similar to the mild form,

a trial of thiamine therapy is recommended. Diet therapy, similar to that of classic MSUD, is needed.

Intermittent Maple Syrup Urine Disease

In intermittent MSUD, seemingly normal children develop vomiting, odor of maple syrup, ataxia, lethargy, and coma during any stress or catabolic state such as infection or surgery. During these attacks, laboratory findings are indistinguishable from those of the classic form, and death may occur. Treatment of the acute attack of intermittent MSUD is similar to that of the classic form. After recovery, although a normal diet can be tolerated, a low-BCAA diet is recommended. The BCKDH activity in patients with the intermittent form is higher than in the classic form and may reach 40% of the control activity.

Thiamine-Responsive Maple Syrup Urine Disease

Some children with mild or intermediate forms of MSUD who are treated with high doses of thiamine have dramatic clinical and biochemical improvement. Although some respond to treatment with thiamine at 10 mg/24 hr, others may require as much as 100 mg/24 hr for at least 3 wk before a favorable response is observed. These patients also require BCAA-restricted diets. The enzymatic activity in these patients can be up to 40% of normal.

Maple Syrup Urine Disease Caused by Deficiency of E₃ Subunit (MSUD Type 3)

Although sometimes referred to as "maple syrup urine disease type 3," this very rare disorder leads to clinical and biochemical abnormalities that encompass a wide range of mitochondrial reactions. E_3 subunit, dihydrolipoamide dehydrogenase, is a component of the BCKDH complex, pyruvate dehydrogenase complex, and α-ketoglutarate dehydrogenase complex. Pathogenic variants in dihydrolipoamide dehydrogenase cause lactic acidosis, elevated pyruvate, as well as signs and symptoms similar to intermediate MSUD. Progressive neurologic impairment manifested by hypotonia and developmental delay occurs after 2 mo of age. Abnormal movements progress to ataxia or Leigh syndrome. Death may occur in early childhood.

Laboratory findings include persistent lactic acidosis with high levels of plasma pyruvate and alanine. Plasma BCAA concentrations are moderately increased. Patients excrete large amounts of lactate, pyruvate, α-ketoglutarate, and the 3 branched-chain ketoacids in their urine.

No effective treatment is available. BCAA-restricted diets and treatment with high doses of thiamine, biotin, and lipoic acid have been ineffective.

Genetics and Prevalence of Maple Syrup Urine Disease

All forms of MSUD are inherited as an autosomal recessive trait. The gene for each subunit resides on different chromosomes. The gene for $E_{1\alpha}$ (*BCKDHA*) is on chromosome 19q13.2; that for $E_{1\beta}$ (*BCKDHB*) is on chromosome 6q14.1; the gene for E_2 (*DBT*) is on chromosome 1p21.2; and that for E_3 (*DLD*) is on chromosome 7q31.1. Genotype-phenotype correlations are difficult to establish and are usually imprecise. The exception is thiamine-responsive MSUD, shown to be caused by pathogenic variants in *DBT*. Most patients are compound heterozygotes inheriting 2 different pathogenic alleles. Pathogenic variants in *BCKDHA* (45%) and *BCKDHB* (35%) account for approximately 80% of cases. Pathogenic variants in *DBT* are responsible for 20% of MSUD cases.

The prevalence is estimated at 1 in 185,000 live births. Classic MSUD is more prevalent in the Old Order Mennonites in the United States, at an estimated 1 in 380 live births. Affected patients in this population are homozygous for a specific pathogenic variant (c.1312T>A) in *BCKDHA*-encoding $E_{1\alpha}$ subunit.

Early detection of MSUD is feasible by universal newborn screening. In most cases, however, especially those with classic MSUD, the infant may be quite sick by the time screening results become available (see Chapter 102). Prenatal diagnosis has been accomplished by enzyme assay of the cultured amniocytes, cultured chorionic villus tissue, or direct assay of samples of the chorionic villi and by identification of the known pathogenic variants in the affected gene.

Several successful pregnancies have occurred in women with different forms of MSUD. The teratogenic potential of leucine during pregnancy is unknown. Tight control of isoleucine, leucine, and valine before and during the pregnancy is important to minimize the risk of metabolic decompensation and to optimize fetal nutrition. Mothers affected by MSUD require close monitoring and meticulous management of nutrition, electrolytes, and fluids in the postpartum period.

BRANCHED-CHAIN α-KETOACID DEHYDROGENASE KINASE DEFICIENCY

A defect in the regulation of branched-chain α-ketoacid dehydrogenase (BCKDH) by BCKDH kinase (BCKDK), the enzyme responsible for the phosphorylation-mediated inactivation of the BCKDH complex, causes the *reverse* biochemical phenotype of MSUD. Pathogenic variants in *BCKDK* decrease the negative regulation by the kinase, resulting in uncontrolled degradation and depletion of isoleucine, leucine, and valine in plasma and brain. Patients with BCKDK deficiency present with low plasma concentrations of isoleucine, leucine, and valine associated with autism, intellectual impairment, fine motor coordination problems, and seizures.

BRANCHED-CHAIN AMINO ACID TRANSPORTER DEFICIENCY

Isoleucine, leucine, and valine are transported across the BBB mainly by the heterodimeric LNAA transporter LAT1 encoded by *SLC7A5*. A defect in LAT1 caused by pathogenic variants in *SLC7A5* results in low brain concentrations of isoleucine, leucine, and valine. Patients with this defect may present clinically similar to BCKDK-deficient patients, with autism, microcephaly, gross motor delays, and in some cases, seizures.

ISOVALERIC ACIDEMIA

Isovaleric acidemia (**IVA**) is caused by deficiency of isovaleryl–coenzyme A (CoA) dehydrogenase (see Fig. 103.4). Decreased or lost activity of isovaleryl-CoA dehydrogenase results in impaired leucine degradation. Accumulating derivatives of isovaleric acid, isovalerylcarnitine, isovalerylglycine, and 3-hydroxyisovaleric acid can be detected in body fluids and thus enable the biochemical diagnosis and screening. Clinically, the course of IVA is highly variable, ranging from essentially asymptomatic to severe. Introduction of newborn screening and proactive management of IVA changed its outlook and the clinical course. Older siblings of symptomatic newborn infants have been reported with identical genotype and biochemical abnormalities but without clinical manifestations, suggesting that presymptomatic detection of affected patients on the newborn screen can improve clinical outcomes.

Patients with severe IVA can present with vomiting, severe acidosis, hyperammonemia, hypoglycemia, hypocalcemia, and bone marrow suppression in the infantile period. Lethargy, convulsions, and coma may ensue, and death may occur if proper therapy is not initiated. Vomiting may be severe enough to suggest pyloric stenosis. The characteristic odor of *sweaty feet* or *rancid-cheese* may be present. Infants who survive this acute episode are at risk to develop episodes of metabolic decompensation later in life. In the mild form without treatment, typical clinical manifestations of severe IVA (vomiting, lethargy, acidosis or coma) may not appear until the child is a few months or a few years old. Acute episodes of metabolic decompensation may occur during a catabolic state, such as infection, dehydration, surgery, or high-protein intake. Acute episodes may be mistaken for diabetic ketoacidosis. Some patients may experience acute and recurrent episodes of pancreatitis.

Laboratory findings during the acute attacks include ketoacidosis, neutropenia, thrombocytopenia, and occasionally pancytopenia. Hypocalcemia, hypoglycemia, and moderate to severe hyperammonemia may be present in some patients. Increases in plasma ammonia may suggest a defect in the urea cycle (see Chapter 103.12). In urea cycle defects, however, the infant usually shows no significant ketoacidosis (see Fig. 103.6).

Diagnosis is established by demonstrating marked elevations of isovaleric acid metabolites (isovalerylglycine, 3-hydroxyisovaleric acid) in body fluids, especially urine. The main compound in plasma is isovalerylcarnitine (C5-carnitine). C5-carnitine can be measured in dried blood spots, thus enabling universal newborn screen using tandem mass spectrometry. The diagnosis can be confirmed by molecular analysis of the *IVD* gene. In some patients with equivocal results, measurement of the enzyme activity in cultured skin fibroblasts may be necessary.

Treatment of the acute attack is aimed at hydration, reversal of the catabolic state (by providing adequate calories orally or intravenously), correction of metabolic acidosis, and facilitation of the isovaleric acid excretion. L-Carnitine (100 mg/kg/24 hr orally) also increases removal of isovaleric acid by forming isovalerylcarnitine, which is excreted in the urine. Because isovalerylglycine has a high urinary clearance, some centers recommend glycine supplementation (250 mg/kg/24 hr) to enhance the formation of isovalerylglycine. Temporary restriction of protein intake (<24 hr) may be beneficial in some cases. In patients with significant hyperammonemia (blood ammonia >200 μmol/L), measures that reduce blood ammonia should be employed (see Chapter 103.12). Renal replacement therapy may be needed if the previously described measures fail to produce significant clinical and biochemical improvement. Long-term management of IVA patients requires restriction of protein according to age-appropriate intake (recommended dietary allowance of protein). Patients benefit from carnitine supplementation with or without glycine. Normal development can be achieved with early and proper treatment.

Prenatal diagnosis can be accomplished by enzyme assay in cultured amniocytes, or if causative mutations are known, by the *IVD* gene analysis. Successful pregnancies with favorable outcomes have been reported. Universal newborn screening of IVA is used in the United States and other countries (see Chapter 102). IVA is caused by autosomal recessive pathogenic variants in *IVD*. The prevalence of IVA is estimated from 1 in 62,500 (in parts of Germany) to 1 in 250,000 live births (in the United States).

MULTIPLE CARBOXYLASE DEFICIENCIES (DEFECTS OF BIOTIN CYCLE)

Biotin is a water-soluble vitamin that is a cofactor for all 4 carboxylase enzymes in humans: pyruvate carboxylase, acetyl-CoA carboxylase, propionyl-CoA carboxylase, and 3-methylcrotonyl-CoA carboxylase. The latter 2 are involved in the catabolic pathways of leucine, isoleucine, and valine (see Fig. 103.4).

Most of the dietary biotin is bound to proteins. Free biotin is generated in the intestine by the action of digestive enzymes, by intestinal bacteria, and perhaps by biotinidase. **Biotinidase**, which is found in serum and most tissues, is also essential for the recycling of biotin in the body by releasing it from the apoenzymes (carboxylases; see Fig. 103.4). Free biotin must form a covalent bond with the apocarboxylases to produce the activated enzyme (holocarboxylase). This binding is catalyzed by holocarboxylase synthetase. Deficiencies in this enzyme activity or in biotinidase result in malfunction of all the carboxylases and in organic acidemias.

Holocarboxylase Synthetase Deficiency

Infants with this rare autosomal recessive disorder become symptomatic in the 1st few weeks of life. Symptoms may appear as early as a few hours after birth to as late as 8 yr of age. Clinically, shortly after birth, the affected infant develops breathing difficulties (tachypnea and apnea). Feeding problems, vomiting, and hypotonia are also usually present. If the condition remains untreated, *generalized erythematous rash with exfoliation and alopecia*, failure to thrive, irritability, seizures, lethargy, and even coma may occur. Developmental delay is common. Immune deficiency manifests with susceptibility to infection. Urine may have a peculiar odor, which has been described "tomcat urine." The rash, when present, helps differentiate this condition from other organic acidemias (see Fig. 103.6).

Laboratory findings include metabolic acidosis, ketosis, hyperammonemia, and the presence of a variety of organic acids (lactic acid, 3-methylcrotonic acid, 3-methylcrotonylglycine, tiglylglycine, 3-OH-propionic acid, methylcitric acid, and 3-hydroxyisovaleric acid) in body fluids. **Diagnosis** is confirmed by identification of pathogenic variants in *HLCS* or by the enzyme assay in lymphocytes or cultured

fibroblasts. Most pathogenic variants cause the enzyme to have an increased K_m (Michaelis-Menten dissociation constant) for biotin; the enzyme activity in such patients can be restored by the administration of large doses of biotin. Newborn screening can identify holocarboxylase synthetase–deficient infants by detecting elevated C5-OH-carnitine on tandem mass spectrometry. In these infants, biotinidase enzymatic assay would be normal.

Treatment with biotin (10-20 mg/day orally) usually results in an improvement in clinical manifestations and biochemical abnormalities. Early diagnosis and treatment are critical to prevent irreversible neurologic damage. In some patients, however, complete resolution may not be achieved even with large doses (up to 60 mg/day) of biotin.

The gene for holocarboxylase synthetase *(HLCS)* is located on chromosome 21q22.13. **Prenatal diagnosis** can be accomplished by prenatal molecular analysis of the known pathogenic variants in *HLCS* or by assaying enzyme activity in cultured amniotic cells. Pregnant mothers who had previous offspring with holocarboxylase synthetase deficiency have been treated with biotin late in pregnancy. Affected infants were normal at birth, but the efficacy of prenatal treatment remains unclear.

Biotinidase Deficiency

Impaired biotinidase activity results in biotin deficiency. Affected infants may develop clinical manifestations similar to those seen in infants with holocarboxylase synthetase deficiency. Unlike the latter, however, symptoms tend to appear later, when the child is several months or years old. The delay in onset of symptoms presumably results from the presence of free biotin derived from the mother or the diet. Clinical manifestations are mostly confined to skin and the nervous system. Atopic or seborrheic dermatitis, candidiasis, alopecia, ataxia, seizures (usually myoclonic), hypotonia, developmental delay, optic nerve atrophy, sensorineural hearing loss, and immunodeficiency resulting from impaired T-cell function may occur. A small number of children with *intractable seborrheic dermatitis* and *partial* (15–30% activity) biotinidase deficiency, in whom the dermatitis resolved with biotin therapy, have been reported; these children were otherwise asymptomatic. Asymptomatic children and adults with this enzyme deficiency have been identified in screening programs. Most of these individuals have been shown to have partial biotinidase deficiency. With universal newborn screening leading to early identification and treatment of the affected patients, the clinical disease is predicted to become extinct.

Laboratory findings and the pattern of organic acids in body fluids resemble those associated with holocarboxylase synthetase deficiency (see above). **Diagnosis** can be established by measurement of the enzyme activity in the serum or by the identification of the mutant gene. **Treatment** with free biotin (5-20 mg/day) results in a dramatic clinical and biochemical improvement. Treatment with biotin is also suggested for individuals with partial biotinidase deficiency. The prevalence of this autosomal recessive trait is estimated at 1 in 60,000 live births. The gene for biotinidase *(BTD)* is located on chromosome 3p25.1. **Prenatal diagnosis** is possible by identification of the known pathogenic variants in *BTD*, or less frequently by the measurement of the enzyme activity in the amniotic cells, although in practice, a prenatal approach is rarely used.

Multiple Carboxylase Deficiency Caused by Acquired Biotin Deficiency

Acquired deficiency of biotin may occur in infants receiving total parenteral nutrition without added biotin, in patients with prolonged use of antiepileptic drugs (phenobarbital, phenytoin, primidone, carbamazepine), and in children with short bowel syndrome or chronic diarrhea who are receiving formulas low in biotin. Excessive ingestion of raw eggs may also cause biotin deficiency because the protein avidin in egg white binds biotin, decreasing its absorption. Infants with biotin deficiency may develop dermatitis, alopecia, and candidal skin infections. This condition readily responds to treatment with oral biotin.

3-METHYLCROTONYL-CoA CARBOXYLASE DEFICIENCY

This enzyme is 1 of the 4 carboxylases requiring biotin as a cofactor (see Fig. 103.4). An isolated deficiency of this enzyme must be differentiated from disorders of biotin metabolism (multiple carboxylase deficiency), which causes diminished activity of all 4 carboxylases (see earlier). 3-Methylcrotonyl-CoA carboxylase (3-MCC) is a heteromeric enzyme consisting of α (biotin containing) and β subunits, encoded by genes *MCCC1* and *MCCC2*, respectively. 3-MCC deficiency can be detected in the newborn period by identifying elevated 3-hydroxyisovalerylcarnitine (C5-OH) in dried blood spots. Universal newborn screening using tandem mass spectrometry has identified an unexpectedly high number of infants with 3-MCC deficiency, with prevalence ranging from 1:2,400 to 1:68,000.

Clinical manifestations are highly variable, ranging from completely asymptomatic adults (including mothers of affected newborn infants), to children presenting with developmental delay without episodes of metabolic decompensation, to patients with seizures, hyperammonemia, and metabolic acidosis. In severe 3-MCC deficiency the affected infant who has been seemingly normal develops an acute episode of vomiting, hypotonia, lethargy, and convulsions after a minor infection, in some cases progressing to life-threatening complications (e.g., Reye syndrome, coma). In patients prone to developing these symptoms, the onset is usually between 3 wk and 3 yr of age. Among infants identified through newborn screening, 85–90% of children remain apparently asymptomatic. The reason for differences in outcomes is unknown. None of the symptoms reported so far could be clearly attributed to the degree of enzyme deficiency.

Laboratory findings during acute episodes include mild to moderate metabolic acidosis, ketosis, hypoglycemia, hyperammonemia, and elevated serum transaminase levels. Large amounts of 3-hydroxyisovaleric acid and 3-methylcrotonylglycine are found in the urine. Urinary excretion of 3-methylcrotonic acid is not usually increased in this condition because the accumulated 3-methylcrotonyl-CoA is converted to 3-hydroxyisovaleric acid. Plasma acylcarnitine profile shows elevated 3-hydroxyisovalerylcarnitine (C5-OH). Severe secondary carnitine deficiency is common. 3-MCC deficiency should be differentiated biochemically from multiple carboxylase deficiency (see earlier), in which, in addition to 3-hydroxyisovaleric acid, lactic acid and metabolites of propionic acid are also present. **Diagnosis** may be confirmed by molecular analysis or by measurement of the enzyme activity in cultured fibroblasts. Documentation of normal activities of other carboxylases is necessary to rule out multiple carboxylase deficiency.

Treatment of acute episodes is similar to that of isovaleric acidemia (see earlier). Hydration and measures to correct hypoglycemia and severe metabolic acidosis by infusing glucose and sodium bicarbonate should be instituted promptly. Secondary carnitine deficiency, seen in up to 50% of patients, can be corrected with L-carnitine supplementation. For symptomatic patients, some centers recommend keeping protein intake at the recommended dietary allowance in conjunction with the oral administration of L-carnitine and the proactive management of catabolic states. Normal growth and development are expected in most patients.

3-MCC deficiency is an autosomal recessive condition. The gene for α-subunit (*MCCC1*) is located on chromosome 3q27.1, and that for the β-subunit (*MCCC2*) is mapped to chromosome 5q13.2. Pathogenic variants in either of these genes result in the enzyme deficiency with overlapping clinical features.

3-METHYLGLUTACONIC ACIDURIAS

The 3-methylglutaconic acidurias are a heterogeneous group of metabolic disorders characterized by excessive excretion of 3-methylglutaconic acid in the urine (Table 103.2). Other metabolites found in 3-methylglutaconic aciduria patients may include 3-methylglutaric acid and 3-hydroxyisovaleric acid. Current classification distinguishes primary and secondary forms. **Primary** 3-methylglutaconic aciduria is caused by the deficiency of mitochondrial 3-methylglutaconyl-CoA hydratase (see Fig. 103.4), formerly *3-methylglutaconic aciduria type I*. **Secondary** 3-methylglutaconic aciduria can be further classified based on the underlying mechanism (e.g., defective phospholipid remodeling vs dysfunction of mitochondrial membrane) or the known molecular cause. Known secondary 3-methylglutaconic aciduria includes *TAZ*-related syndrome (**Barth syndrome**), *OPA3*-related 3-methylglutaconic aciduria (**Costeff syndrome**), *SERAC1*-related syndrome (**MEGDEL syndrome**), *TMEM70*-related syndrome, and *DNAJC19*-related syndrome (**DCMA syndrome**).

Significant and persistent 3-methylglutaconic aciduria with negative molecular evaluation for known genetic causes represents a heterogeneous group called 3-methylglutaconic aciduria **not otherwise specified**

Table 103.2	3-Methylglutaconic Acidurias				
GROUP	**DISORDER**	**GENE (CHROMOSOME)**	**PREVIOUS CLASSIFICATION**	**DISEASE MECHANISM**	**CLINICAL DESCRIPTION**
Primary 3-methylglutaconic aciduria	3-Methylglutaconyl-CoA hydratase deficiency	*AUH* (9q22.31)	Type I	Enzyme deficiency in the leucine degradation pathway	Depending on age, variable presentation is seen ranging from younger asymptomatic patients to older patients with progressive leukoencephalopathy
Secondary 3-methylglutaconic acidurias	Barth syndrome	*TAZ* (Xq28)	Type II	Defective phospholipid remodeling	X-linked inheritance, cardiomyopathy, endocardial fibroelastosis, proximal myopathy, failure to thrive, neutropenia, dysmorphic findings
	Costeff syndrome	*OPA3* (19q13.32)	Type III	Mitochondrial membrane dysfunction	Progressive optic nerve atrophy, chorea, spastic paraparesis, cognitive impairment
	MEGDEL syndrome	*SERAC1* (6q25.3)	Type IV	Defective phospholipid remodeling	Progressive deafness, dystonia, spasticity, basal ganglia changes
	TMEM70-related disorder	*TMEM70* (8q21.11)	Type IV	Mitochondrial membrane dysfunction	Developmental delay, failure to thrive, metabolic decompensations, microcephaly, cardiomyopathy, dysmorphic findings
	3-Methylglutaconic aciduria, not otherwise specified	Unknown	Type IV	Unknown	Variable presentation
	DCMA syndrome	*DNAJC19* (3q26.33)	Type V	Mitochondrial membrane dysfunction	Cardiomyopathy, ataxia, optic nerve atrophy, failure to thrive

awaiting further molecular characterization. Primary and secondary 3-methylglutaconic aciduria should be distinguished from mild and transient urinary elevations of 3-methylglutaconic acid seen in patients affected by other metabolic disorders, such as mitochondrial disorders of diverse etiology.

3-Methylglutaconyl-CoA Hydratase Deficiency

Two main clinical forms of 3-methylglutaconyl-CoA hydratase deficiency have been described (see Fig. 103.4). In the **childhood** form, nonspecific neurodevelopmental findings such as speech delay or regression, choreoathetoid movements, optic nerve atrophy, and mild psychomotor delay may be present. Metabolic acidosis may occur during a catabolic state. In the **adulthood** form, affected individuals may remain asymptomatic until the 2nd or 3rd decade of life, when a clinical picture of *slowly progressing leukoencephalopathy* with optic nerve atrophy, dysarthria, ataxia, spasticity, and dementia occurs. Brain MRI typically shows white matter abnormalities, which may precede the appearance of clinical symptoms by years. Asymptomatic pediatric and adult patients have also been reported. Patients excrete large amounts of 3-methylglutaconic acid and moderate amounts of 3-hydroxyisovaleric and 3-methylglutaric acids in urine. **Treatment** with L-carnitine may help some patients. The effectiveness of a low-leucine diet has not been established. The condition is inherited as an autosomal recessive trait. The gene for the hydratase enzyme *(AUH)* is mapped to chromosome 9q22.31.

Barth Syndrome (*TAZ*-Related Disorder)

This X-linked condition is caused by deficiency of *tafazzin,* a mitochondrial protein, encoded by *TAZ* gene. This enzyme is necessary for remodeling of immature cardiolipin into its mature form. *Cardiolipin,* a mitochondrial phospholipid, is critical for the integrity of inner mitochondrial membrane. **Clinical manifestations** of Barth syndrome, which usually occur in the 1st yr of life in a male infant, include cardiomyopathy, hypotonia, growth retardation, hypoglycemia, and mild to severe neutropenia. The onset of clinical manifestations may be as late as adulthood, but most affected individuals become symptomatic by adolescence. If patients survive infancy, relative improvement may occur with advancing age. Cognitive development is usually normal, although delayed motor function and learning disabilities are possible.

Laboratory findings include mild to moderate increases in urinary excretion of 3-methylglutaconic, 3-methylglutaric, and 2-ethylhydracrylic acids. Unlike primary 3-methylglutaconic aciduria (type I), urinary excretion of 3-hydroxyisovaleric acid is not elevated. The activity of the enzyme 3-methylglutaconyl-CoA hydratase is normal. *Neutropenia is a common finding.* Lactic acidosis, hypoglycemia, low serum cholesterol concentration, low prealbumin, and abnormal mitochondrial ultrastructure have been shown in some patients. Total cardiolipin and subclasses of cardiolipin are very low in skin fibroblast cultures from these patients. The monolysocardiolipin/cardiolipin ratio in cultured fibroblast may be useful for establishing the diagnosis in patients with negative or equivocal molecular results. Because of its nonspecific presentation, the condition could be underdiagnosed and underreported.

The condition is inherited as an *X-linked* recessive trait. The gene *(TAZ)* has been mapped to chromosome Xq28. The modest 3-methylglutaconic aciduria seen in Barth syndrome is thought to be related to the defect in mitochondrial membrane, causing the leakage of this organic acid. *Specific treatment is not available.* Patients with an unsatisfactory response to medical management of cardiomyopathy may benefit from cardiac transplantation. Daily aspirin to reduce the risk of strokes has been described.

OPA3-Related 3-Methylglutaconic Aciduria (Costeff Syndrome)

Clinical manifestations in patients with Costeff syndrome include early-onset optic nerve atrophy and later development of choreoathetoid movements, spasticity, ataxia, dysarthria, and cognitive impairment. Patients excrete moderate amounts of 3-methylglutaconic and 3-methylglutaric acids. Activity of the enzyme 3-methylglutaconyl-CoA hydratase is normal. The condition is inherited as an autosomal recessive

trait. The gene for this condition *(OPA3)* is mapped to chromosome 19q13.32. Pathogenic variants in *OPA3* are thought to cause electron transport chain dysfunction. Treatment is supportive.

Disorders Formerly Described as 3-Methylglutaconic Aciduria Type IV

3-Methylglutaconic aciduria type IV represents a group of disorders with diverse genetic etiology. Two disorders in this group have been linked to specific molecular etiology, while other conditions are still awaiting the discovery of their underlying molecular defect.

MEGDEL syndrome (3-*me*thylglutaconic aciduria with *deafness,* encephalopathy and *Leigh*-like) is an autosomal recessive disorder caused by deleterious mutations in *SERAC1* on chromosome 6q25.3. Affected patients experience progressive deafness, dystonia, spasticity and basal ganglia injury similar to patients with Leigh syndrome. Treatment is symptomatic.

***TMEM70*-related disorder** is also inherited in an autosomal recessive fashion. Pathogenic variants in *TMEM70* result in the mitochondrial complex V deficiency, although the exact mechanism of disease is unknown. Clinical manifestations include developmental delay, developmental regression, Reye syndrome–like episodes, intellectual disability, failure to thrive, microcephaly, cardiomyopathy, and dysmorphic findings. Patients are prone to metabolic decompensation, characterized by hyperammonemia (up to 900 μmol/L) and lactic acidosis, which are more common in the 1st yr of life. **Acute hyperammonemic** episodes are treated with intravenous glucose, lipid emulsion, ammonia-scavenging drugs, and occasionally require hemodialysis. Long-term therapy that has been described includes L-carnitine, coenzyme Q_{10}, and bicarbonate substitution (e.g., citric acid/sodium citrate). Patients require interval echocardiographic and electrocardiographic (ECG) monitoring to enable early diagnosis and management of cardiomyopathy.

DCMA Syndrome (*DNAJC19*-Related Syndrome, 3-Methylglutaconic Aciduria Type V)

DCMA syndrome (dilated *c*ardio*m*yopathy with *a*taxia) is a novel autosomal recessive disorder identified in patients of the Canadian Dariusleut Hutterite ancestry living in The Great Plains of North America. As the disorder's abbreviated name suggests, affected individuals present with dilated cardiomyopathy, long QTc interval, and CNS involvement. Neurologic symptoms include intellectual disability, cerebellar involvement, and optic atrophy. Growth is affected in all patients. Intrauterine growth restriction is seen in up to 50% of patients. Cryptorchidism and hypospadias are frequent findings in affected boys. Urine organic acid assay reveals increased 3-methylglutaconic acid and 3-methylglutaric acid. Pathogenic variants in *DNAJC19* (3q26.33) are the underlying cause of DCMA syndrome. Treatment is symptomatic. Interval echocardiography and ECG can prospectively identify patients requiring treatment of cardiomyopathy and long QTc interval.

β-KETOTHIOLASE (3-OXOTHIOLASE) DEFICIENCY (MITOCHONDRIAL ACETOACETYL-CoA THIOLASE [T_2] DEFICIENCY)

This reversible mitochondrial enzyme is involved in the final steps of isoleucine catabolism and in ketolysis. In the isoleucine catabolic pathway, the enzyme cleaves 2-methylacetoacetyl-CoA into propionyl-CoA and acetyl-CoA (see Fig. 103.4). In the fatty acid oxidation pathway, the enzyme generates 2 moles of acetyl-CoA from 1 mole of acetoacetyl-CoA (Fig. 103.7). The same enzyme synthesizes 2-methyacetoacetate-CoA and acetoacetyl-CoA in the reverse direction. The hallmark of this disorder is **ketoacidosis**, often triggered by infections, prolonged fasting, and large protein load. The mechanism of ketosis in this condition is incompletely understood, because in this enzyme deficiency one expects impaired ketone formation (Fig. 103.7). It is postulated that excess acetoacetyl-CoA produced from other sources can be used as a substrate for 3-hydroxy-3-methylglutaryl-CoA synthesis in the liver.

Clinical manifestations are quite variable, ranging from mild cases showing normal development to severe episodes of acidosis starting in the 1st yr of life causing severe cognitive impairment. Unless identified on the newborn screening, affected children present with intermittent

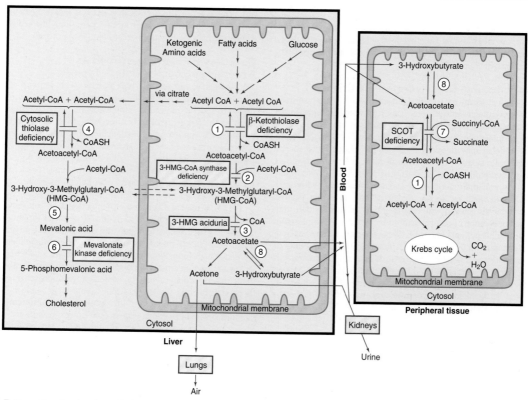

Fig. 103.7 Formation (liver) and metabolism (peripheral tissues) of ketone bodies and cholesterol synthesis. **Enzymes:** *(1)* Mitochondrial acetoacetyl CoA thiolase, *(2)* HMG-CoA synthase, *(3)* HMG-CoA lyase, *(4)* cytosolic acetoacetyl-CoA thiolase, *(5)* HMG-CoA reductase, *(6)* mevalonic kinase, *(7)* succinyl CoA:3-ketoacid CoA transferase (SCOT), *(8)* 3-hydroxybutyrate dehydrogenase.

episodes of unexplained ketoacidosis. These episodes usually occur after an intercurrent infection and typically respond promptly to intravenous fluids and bicarbonate therapy. Mild to moderate hyperammonemia may also be present during attacks. Both hypoglycemia and hyperglycemia have been reported in isolated cases. The child may be completely asymptomatic between episodes and may tolerate a normal protein diet. Cognitive development is normal in most children. The episodes may be misdiagnosed as salicylate poisoning because of the similarity of the clinical findings and the interference of elevated blood levels of acetoacetate with the colorimetric assay for salicylate.

Laboratory findings during the acute attack include ketoacidosis, and hyperammonemia. Findings of ketones in the urine and hyperglycemia may be interpreted as diabetic ketoacidosis, and the high index of suspicion is needed to identify this metabolic disorder. Urine organic acid assay can provide clues leading to correct diagnosis. Urine contains large amounts of 2-methylacetoacetate and its decarboxylated products butanone, 2-methyl-3-hydroxybutyrate, and tiglylglycine. Lower concentrations of urinary metabolites are stable. Mild hyperglycinemia may also be present. Plasma acylcarnitine profile show elevations of C5:1 and C5-OH carnitines, although these metabolites can normalize in between catabolic episodes. Minimal elevations of C5:1 and C5-OH carnitines can result in false-negative results on the newborn screening of affected infants who were clinically well at the time of blood collection. The clinical and biochemical findings should be differentiated from those seen with propionic and methylmalonic acidemias (see later).

Treatment of acute episodes includes hydration. Recalcitrant metabolic acidosis can be severe enough to require infusion of bicarbonate. A 10% glucose solution with the appropriate electrolytes is used to suppress protein catabolism, lipolysis, and ketogenesis. Restriction of protein intake to age-appropriate physiologic requirements is recommended for long-term therapy. Oral L-carnitine (50-100 mg/kg/24 hr) is also recommended to prevent possible secondary carnitine deficiency. Long-term prognosis for achieving normal quality of life seems very favorable. Successful pregnancy with a normal outcome has been reported.

β-Ketothiolase deficiency is inherited as an autosomal recessive trait and may be more prevalent than previously appreciated. The gene *(ACAT1)* for this enzyme is located on chromosome 11q22.3. **Diagnosis** may be confirmed by molecular analysis of the *ACAT1* gene or using enzyme assay of leukocytes or cultured fibroblasts.

CYTOSOLIC ACETOACETYL-CoA THIOLASE DEFICIENCY

This enzyme catalyzes the cytosolic production of acetoacetyl-CoA from two moles of acetyl-CoA (see Fig. 103.7). Cytosolic acetoacetyl-CoA is the precursor of hepatic cholesterol synthesis. Cytosolic acetoacetyl-CoA thiolase should be differentiated from the mitochondrial thiolase (see earlier and Fig. 103.4). Clinical manifestations in patients with this very rare enzyme deficiency have been incompletely characterized. Patients may present with severe progressive developmental delay, hypotonia, and choreoathetoid movements in the 1st few months of life. Laboratory findings are nonspecific; elevated levels of lactate, pyruvate, acetoacetate, and 3-hydroxybutyrate may be found in blood and urine. One patient had normal levels of acetoacetate and 3-hydroxybutyrate. Diagnosis can be aided by demonstrating a deficiency in cytosolic thiolase activity in liver biopsy or in cultured fibroblasts or by DNA analysis. No effective treatment has been described, although a low-fat diet helped to diminish ketosis in one patient.

MITOCHONDRIAL 3-HYDROXY-3-METHYLGLUTARYL-CoA SYNTHASE DEFICIENCY

This enzyme catalyzes synthesis of 3-hydroxy-3-methylglutaryl (HMG)-CoA from acetoacetyl-CoA and acetyl-CoA in the mitochondria. This is a critical step in ketone body synthesis in the liver (see Fig. 103.7). A few patients with deficiency of this enzyme have been reported. The principal clinical syndrome is hypoketotic hypoglycemia triggered by physiologic stress, such as infections or fasting. Age at presentation has ranged from infancy to 6 yr. Children tend to be asymptomatic before these episodes and with appropriate management can remain stable after the recovery (except for mild hepatomegaly with fatty infiltration). Future episodes can be prevented by avoiding prolonged fasting during ensuing intercurrent illnesses. Hepatomegaly is a consistent physical finding in these patients. **Laboratory findings** include hypoglycemia, acidosis with mild or no ketosis, elevated levels in liver function tests, and massive dicarboxylic aciduria. The clinical and laboratory findings may be confused with fatty acid metabolism defects (see Chapter 104.1). In contrast to the latter, in patients with HMG-CoA synthase deficiency the blood concentrations of acylcarnitine conjugates are negative for acylcarnitine findings characteristic of fatty acid oxidation disorders. Treatment of the secondary carnitine deficiency with L-carnitine supplementation can result in elevated plasma acetylcarnitine (C2-carnitine), likely reflecting intracellular accumulation of acetyl-CoA. A controlled fasting study can produce the clinical and biochemical abnormalities.

Treatment consists of provision of adequate calories and avoidance of prolonged periods of fasting. No dietary protein restriction was needed.

The condition is inherited as an autosomal recessive trait. The gene *(HMGCS2)* for this enzyme is located on chromosome 1p12. The condition should be considered in any child with fasting hypoketotic hypoglycemia and may be more common than appreciated.

3-HYDROXY-3-METHYLGLUTARYL-CoA LYASE DEFICIENCY (3-HYDROXY-3-METHYLGLUTARIC ACIDURIA)

3-HMG-CoA lyase (see Fig. 103.4) catalyzes the conversion of 3-HMG-CoA to acetoacetate and is a rate-limiting enzyme for ketogenesis (see Fig. 103.7). The deficiency of this enzyme is a rare disorder seen with increased frequency in Saudi Arabia, the Iberian Peninsula, and in Brazil in patients of Portuguese ancestry. Clinically, approximately 30% develop symptoms in the 1st few days of life, and >60% of patients become symptomatic between 3 and 11 mo of age. Infrequently, patients may remain asymptomatic until adolescence. With the addition of 3-HMG-CoA lyase deficiency to the newborn screening using C5-OH-carnitine, many infants are identified presymptomatically in the newborn period. Similar to 3-HMG-CoA synthase deficiency, patients affected by 3-HMG-CoA lyase deficiency may present with acute hypoketotic hypoglycemia. Episodes of vomiting, severe hypoglycemia, hypotonia, acidosis with mild or no ketosis, and dehydration may rapidly lead to lethargy, ataxia, and coma. These episodes often occur during a catabolic state such as prolonged fasting or an intercurrent infection. Hepatomegaly is common. These manifestations may be mistaken for Reye syndrome or fatty acid oxidation defects such as medium-chain acyl-CoA dehydrogenase deficiency. Long-term complications can include dilated cardiomyopathy, hepatic steatosis, and pancreatitis. Development can be normal, but intellectual disability and seizures with abnormalities in the white matter seen on MRI have been observed in patients after prolonged episodes of hypoglycemia.

Laboratory findings include hypoglycemia, moderate to severe hyperammonemia, and acidosis. There is mild or no ketosis (see Fig. 103.7). Urinary excretion of 3-hydroxy-3-methylglutaric acid and other proximal intermediate metabolites of leucine catabolism (3-methylglutaric acid, 3-methylglutaconic acid, and 3-hydroxyisovaleric acid) is markedly increased, causing the urine to smell like *cat urine*. Glutaric and dicarboxylic acids may also be increased in urine during acute attacks. Secondary carnitine deficiency is common. The condition is inherited as an autosomal recessive trait. 3-HMG-CoA lyase is encoded by gene *HMGCL*. **Diagnosis** may be confirmed by molecular analysis of *HMGCL* or by enzyme assay in cultured fibroblasts, leukocytes, or liver specimens.

Prenatal diagnosis is possible by molecular DNA analysis if the familial pathogenic variants are known or by enzymatic assay of the cultured amniocytes or a chorionic villi biopsy.

Treatment of acute episodes includes hydration, infusion of glucose to control hypoglycemia, provision of adequate calories, and administration of bicarbonate to correct acidosis. Hyperammonemia should be treated promptly (see Chapter 103.12). Renal replacement therapy may be required in patients with severe recalcitrant hyperammonemia. Restriction of protein and fat intake is recommended for long-term management. Oral administration of L-carnitine (50-100 mg/kg/24 hr) prevents secondary carnitine deficiency. Prolonged fasting should be avoided.

SUCCINYL-CoA:3-OXOACID-CoA TRANSFERASE DEFICIENCY

Succinyl-CoA:3-oxoacid-CoA transferase (**SCOT**) deficiency and β-ketothiolase deficiency collectively are referred to as **ketone utilization disorders.** SCOT participates in the conversion of ketone bodies (acetoacetate and 3-hydroxybutyrate) generated in liver mitochondria into *acetoacetyl-CoA in the nonhepatic tissues* (see Fig. 103.7). A deficiency of this enzyme results in the accumulation of ketone bodies, ketoacidosis, increased utilization of glucose, and hypoglycemia. During fasting, patients tend to have a proportional elevation of plasma free fatty acids. More than 30 patients with SCOT deficiency have been reported to date. The condition may not be rare because many cases may be mild and may remain undiagnosed. SCOT deficiency can be distinguished from β-ketothiolase deficiency by the absence of 2-methylacetoacetate, 2-methyl-3-hydroxybutyrate, and tiglylglycine, characteristic of the latter disorder. Plasma acylcarnitine profile tends to show no specific abnormalities.

A common clinical presentation is an acute episode of severe ketoacidosis in an infant who had been growing and developing normally. About half the patients become symptomatic in the 1st wk of life, and practically all become symptomatic before 2 yr of age. The acute episode is often precipitated by a catabolic state triggered by an infection or prolonged fasting. Without treatment, the ketoacidotic episode can result in death. A chronic subclinical ketosis may persist between the attacks. Development is usually normal, although severe and recurrent episodes of ketoacidosis and hypoglycemia can predispose patients to neurocognitive impairment.

Laboratory findings during the acute episode are nonspecific and include metabolic acidosis and ketonuria with high levels of acetoacetate and 3-hydroxybutyrate in blood and urine. No other organic acids are found in the blood or in the urine. Blood glucose levels are usually normal, but hypoglycemia has been reported in some affected newborn infants with severe ketoacidosis. Plasma amino acids and plasma acylcarnitine profile are usually normal. Severe SCOT deficiency can be accompanied by ketosis even when patients are clinically stable. This condition should be considered in any infant with unexplained bouts of ketoacidosis. **Diagnosis** can be established by molecular analysis of *OXCT1* or by demonstrating a deficiency of enzyme activity in cultured fibroblasts. The condition is inherited as an autosomal recessive trait.

Treatment of acute episodes consists of rehydration with solutions containing dextrose, correction of acidosis, and the provision of a diet adequate in calories. Long-term treatment should include high-carbohydrate diet and avoidance of prolonged fasting and administration of dextrose before anticipated or during established catabolic states.

MEVALONATE KINASE DEFICIENCY

Mevalonic acid, an intermediate metabolite of cholesterol synthesis, is converted to 5-phosphomevalonic acid by the action of the enzyme mevalonate kinase (MVK) (see Fig. 103.7). Based on clinical manifestations and degree of enzyme deficiency, 2 conditions have been recognized: mevalonic aciduria and hyperimmunoglobulinemia D syndrome. Both disorders are accompanied by recurrent fever, gastrointestinal symptoms, mucocutaneous manifestations, and lymphadenopathy. Patients with mevalonic aciduria also show growth retardation and nervous system involvement. In practice, the 2 disorders represent the 2 ends of the spectrum.

Mevalonic Aciduria

Clinical manifestations include failure to thrive, growth retardation, intellectual disability, hypotonia, ataxia, myopathy, hepatosplenomegaly, cataracts, and facial dysmorphisms (dolichocephaly, frontal bossing, low-set ears, downward slanting of eyes, long eyelashes). Most patients experience recurrent crises characterized by fever, vomiting, diarrhea, hepatosplenomegaly, arthralgia, lymphadenopathy, edema, and morbilliform rash. These episodes typically last 2-7 days and recur up to 25 times a year. Death may occur during these crises.

Laboratory findings include marked elevation of mevalonic acid in urine; the concentration of urinary mevalonic acid ranges between 500 and 56,000 mmol/mol of creatinine (normal: <0.3 mmol/mol of creatinine). Plasma levels of mevalonic acid are also greatly increased (as high as 540 μmol/L; normal: <0.04 μmol/L). Mevalonic acid levels tend to correlate with the severity of the condition and increase during crises. Serum cholesterol concentration is normal or mildly decreased. Serum concentration of creatine kinase can be greatly increased. Inflammatory markers are elevated during the crises. Brain MRI may reveal progressive atrophy of the cerebellum.

Diagnosis may be confirmed by DNA analysis or by assaying the MVK activity in lymphocytes or cultured fibroblasts. The enzyme activity in this form of the condition is below the detection level. **Treatment** with high doses of prednisone helps in the acute crises, but due to side effects, it is not routinely used long term. *Etanercept* (tumor necrosis factor inhibitor) and *anakinra* (interleukin-1 receptor antagonist) have shown to be effective in bringing significant clinical improvement. The condition is inherited as an autosomal recessive trait. **Prenatal diagnosis** is possible by identifying known familiar pathogenic variants in *MVK*, by measurement of mevalonic acid in the amniotic fluid, or by assaying the enzyme activity in cultured amniocytes or chorionic villi samples. The gene (*MVK*) for the enzyme is on chromosome 12q24.11.

Hyperimmunoglobulinemia D Syndrome (Hyperimmunoglobulinemia D and Periodic Fever Syndrome)

Some pathogenic variants of mevalonic kinase gene (*MVK*) cause milder enzyme deficiency and produce the clinical picture of periodic fever with hyperimmunoglobulinemia D. These patients have periodic bouts of fever associated with abdominal pain, vomiting, diarrhea, arthralgia, arthritis, hepatosplenomegaly, lymphadenopathy, and morbilliform rash (even petechiae and purpura), which usually start before 1 yr of age. The attacks can be triggered by vaccination, minor trauma, or stress and can occur every 1-2 mo, lasting 2-7 days. Patients are free of symptoms between acute attacks. The diagnostic laboratory finding is elevation of serum immunoglobulin D (IgD). IgA is also elevated in 80% of patients. During acute attacks, leukocytosis, increased C-reactive protein, and mild mevalonic aciduria may be present. High concentrations of serum IgD help differentiate this condition from familial Mediterranean fever. See Chapter 188 for treatment recommendations.

PROPIONIC ACIDEMIA (PROPIONYL-CoA CARBOXYLASE DEFICIENCY)

Propionic acid is an intermediate metabolite of isoleucine, valine, threonine, methionine, odd-chain fatty acids, and side chains of cholesterol. Normally, propionic acid in the form of propionyl-CoA undergoes carboxylation to D-methylmalonyl-CoA, catalyzed by the mitochondrial enzyme propionyl-CoA carboxylase. This enzyme requires biotin as a cofactor; thus the disorders of biotin metabolism, among other findings, can also result in elevation of propionic acid metabolites (see Fig. 103.4). Propionyl-CoA carboxylase is a multimeric enzyme composed of 2 nonidentical subunits, α and β, encoded by 2 genes, *PCCA* and *PCCB*, respectively. Pathogenic variants in propionyl-CoA carboxylase result in the disorder called propionic acidemia.

Clinical findings of propionic acidemia are not specific to this disorder only. In the severe form, patients develop symptoms in the 1st few days of life. Poor feeding, vomiting, hypotonia, lethargy, dehydration, a sepsislike picture, and clinical signs of severe ketoacidosis progress rapidly

to coma and death. Seizures occur in approximately 30% of affected infants. If an infant survives the first attack, similar episodes of metabolic decompensation may occur during an intercurrent infection, trauma, surgery, prolonged fasting, severe constipation, or after ingestion of a high-protein diet. Moderate to severe intellectual disability and neurologic manifestations reflective of extrapyramidal (dystonia, choreoathetosis, tremor) and pyramidal (paraplegia) dysfunction are common sequelae in the survivors. Neuroimaging shows that these abnormalities, which often occur after an episode of metabolic decompensation, are the result of damage to the basal ganglia, especially to the globus pallidus. This phenomenon has been referred to as **metabolic stroke**. This is the main cause of neurologic sequelae seen in the surviving affected children. Additional long-term complications include failure to thrive, optic nerve atrophy, pancreatitis, cardiomyopathy, and osteopenia.

In the *milder* form, episodes of metabolic decompensation are less frequent, but these children are still at risk to develop intellectual disability, seizures, long QTc interval, and severe cardiomyopathy. Universal newborn screening can identify propionic acidemia by detecting elevated propionylcarnitine (C3) in dried blood spots. However, in patients with the mild form of propionic acidemia, propionylcarnitine could remain below the cutoff value set by the screening laboratory, resulting in a false-negative result. Therefore, physicians should maintain a high index of suspicion for this disorder and follow up with a biochemical evaluation of infants and children presenting with unexplained ketosis or metabolic acidosis.

Laboratory findings during the acute attack include various degrees of metabolic acidosis, often with a large anion gap, ketosis, ketonuria, hypoglycemia, anemia, neutropenia, and thrombocytopenia. Moderate to severe hyperammonemia is common; plasma ammonia concentrations usually correlate with the severity of the disease. In contrast to other causes of hyperammonemia, plasma concentration of glutamine tends to be within normal limits or decreased. Presence of severe metabolic acidosis and normal to reduced plasma glutamine help differentiate propionic academia from hyperammonemia caused by urea cycle defects. Measurement of plasma ammonia is especially helpful in planning therapeutic strategy during episodes of exacerbation in a patient whose diagnosis has been established. Mechanisms of hyperammonemia in propionic acidemia are not well understood but are likely related to the perturbed biochemical and pH environment of the mitochondrial matrix, where the proximal part of urea cycle resides. **Glycine** concentration can be elevated in all body fluids (blood, urine, CSF) and possibly are the result of the inhibited glycine cleavage system in the hepatic mitochondria (Fig. 103.8). Glycine elevation has also been observed in patients with methylmalonic acidemia. These disorders were collectively referred to as *ketotic hyperglycinemia* in the past before the specific enzyme deficiencies were elucidated. Mild to moderate increase in blood lactate and lysine may also be present in these patients. Concentrations of propionylcarnitine, 3-hydroxypropionic acid, and methylcitric acid (presumably formed through condensation of propionyl-CoA with oxaloacetic acid) are greatly elevated in the plasma and urine of infants with propionic acidemia. Propionylglycine and other intermediate metabolites of branched-chain amino acid catabolism, such as tiglylglycine, can also be found in urine. Moderate elevations in blood levels of glycine, and previously mentioned organic acids can persist between the acute attacks. Brain imaging may reveal cerebral atrophy, delayed myelination, and abnormalities in the globus pallidus and other parts of the basal ganglia.

The **diagnosis** of propionic acidemia should be differentiated from multiple carboxylase deficiencies (see earlier and Fig. 103.6). In addition to propionic acid metabolites, infants with the latter condition excrete large amounts of lactic acid, 3-methylcrotonylglycine, and 3-hydroxyisovaleric acid. The presence of hyperammonemia may suggest a genetic defect in the urea cycle enzymes. Infants with defects in the urea cycle are usually *not* acidotic (see Fig. 103.1) and have elevated levels of plasma glutamine. The definitive diagnosis of propionic acidemia can be established through molecular analysis of *PCCA* and *PCCB* or by measuring the enzyme activity in leukocytes or cultured fibroblasts.

Treatment of acute episodes of metabolic decompensation includes hydration with solutions containing glucose, correction of acidosis, and

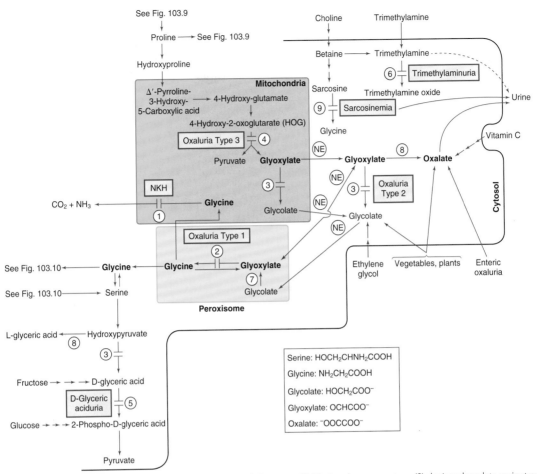

Fig. 103.8 Pathways in the metabolism of glycine and glyoxylic acid. **Enzymes:** *(1)* Glycine cleavage system, *(2)* alanine:glyoxylate aminotransferase, *(3)* glyoxylic reductase/hydroxypyruvate reductase (GR/HRP), *(4)* hydroxyoxoglutarate aldolase 1 (HOGA1), *(5)* glycerate kinase, *(6)* trimethylamine oxidase, *(7)* glycolate oxidase (D-amino acid oxidase), *(8)* lactate dehydrogenase, *(9)* sarcosine dehydrogenase. NE, Nonenzymatic; NKH, nonketotic hyperglycinemia.

amelioration of the catabolic state by provision of adequate calories through enteral or parenteral hyperalimentation. A brief restriction of protein intake, no more than 24 hr, is often necessary. Depending on the clinical status, gradual reintroduction of protein is recommended. If enteral feedings cannot be tolerated after 48 hours of protein restriction, parenteral nutrition should be instituted to achieve the age-specific recommended dietary protein intake. Patients unable to tolerate the recommended dietary allowance of protein can receive specialized medical foods free of isoleucine, valine, threonine, and methionine. The composition and the amount of protein vary among patients. The metabolic diet composition can be adjusted by monitoring growth and plasma amino acids drawn 3-4 hr after the typical feeding. Some patients may benefit from the suppression of propionogenic gut microflora. This can be achieved by oral antibiotics such as oral neomycin or metronidazole. Prolonged use of metronidazole should be avoided because it has been associated with reversible peripheral neuropathy and increased QTc interval. The risk of QTc prolongation can be problematic in propionic acidemia patients, who are at risk for cardiomyopathy and long QT interval. Baseline and interval electrocardiograms (ECGs) are recommended before and after initiation of the metronidazole therapy. Patients may benefit from management of constipation.

Patients with propionic acidemia often develop secondary carnitine deficiency, presumably as a result of the urinary loss of propionylcarnitine. Administration of L-carnitine (50-100 mg/kg/24 hr orally or intravenously) helps restore free carnitine in blood. In patients with concomitant hyperammonemia, measures to reduce blood ammonia should be employed (see Chapter 103.12). Very ill patients with severe acidosis and hyperammonemia require hemodialysis to remove ammonia and other toxic compounds rapidly and efficiently. *N*-carbamoylglutamate (carglumic acid) and nitrogen scavengers (sodium benzoate, sodium phenylacetate, sodium phenylbutyrate) can aid in the treatment of acute hyperammonemia. Although no infant with propionic acidemia has been found to be responsive to biotin, this compound should be administered (10 mg/24 hr orally) to all infants during the first attack and until the diagnosis is established and multiple carboxylase deficiency ruled out.

Long-term treatment consists of a low-protein diet meeting age-specific recommended dietary allowance and administration of L-carnitine (50-100 mg/kg/24 hr orally). Some centers manage mild cases of propionic acidemia without medical foods, opting for only restricting the protein intake to recommended dietary allowance. Patients unable to tolerate the recommended dietary intake of protein may require medical foods free of propionate precursors (isoleucine, valine, methionine, and threonine). Excessive use of medical foods while restricting natural-source protein may cause a deficiency of the essential amino acids, especially isoleucine and valine, which may cause a condition resembling **acrodermatitis enteropathica** (see Chapter 691). Overrestriction of methionine, especially in the 1st years of life, may contribute to the reduced brain growth and microcephaly. To avoid this problem, natural proteins should comprise most of the dietary protein. Some patients may require bicarbonate substitution (e.g., citric acid/sodium citrate) to correct chronic acidosis. The concentration of plasma ammonia usually normalizes between attacks, although some patients may experience mild chronic hyperammonemia. Acute attacks triggered by infections, fasting, trauma, stress, constipation, or dietary indiscretions should be treated promptly and aggressively. Close monitoring of plasma ammonia, plasma amino acids obtained 3-4 hr after the last typical meal (especially isoleucine, leucine, valine, threonine, and methionine), and growth parameters is necessary to ensure the diet is appropriate. Orthotopic liver transplantation is used in clinically unstable patients experiencing recurrent hyperammonemia, frequent metabolic decompensations, and poor growth. Liver transplantation does not cure propionic acidemia, and lifelong dietary management and proactive management during periods of significant metabolic stress are recommended.

Long-term **prognosis** is guarded. Death may occur during an acute attack. Normal psychomotor development is possible in the mild form identified through newborn screening. Children identified clinically may manifest some degree of permanent neurodevelopmental deficit, such as tremor, dystonia, chorea, and spasticity despite adequate therapy. These neurologic findings may be the sequelae of a metabolic stroke occurring during an acute decompensation. Long QTc interval as well as cardiomyopathy with potential progression to heart failure, fatal arrhythmias, and death may develop in older affected children despite adequate metabolic control. Acute pancreatitis is a common and severe complication in propionic acidemia. Osteoporosis can predispose to fractures, which can occur even after minimal mechanical stress.

Prenatal diagnosis can be achieved by identification of the known familial pathogenic variants in *PCCA* or *PCCB* or by measuring the enzyme activity in cultured amniotic cells or in samples of uncultured chorionic villi.

Propionic acidemia is inherited as an autosomal recessive trait and has a worldwide prevalence of 1:105,000 to 1:250,000 live births. It is more prevalent in Greenlandic Inuits (1:1,000) and in some Saudi Arabian tribes (1:2,000 to 1:5,000 live births). The gene for the α-subunit (*PCCA*) is located on chromosome 13q32.3 and that of the β-subunit (*PCCB*) is mapped to chromosome 3q22.3. Pathogenic variants in either gene result in similar clinical and biochemical manifestations. Although pregnancies with normal outcomes have been reported, the perinatal period poses special risks to females with propionic acidemia because of hyperemesis gravidarum, worsening cardiomyopathy, changing protein requirements, and risk of metabolic decompensation.

ISOLATED METHYLMALONIC ACIDEMIAS

Methylmalonic acidemias are a group of metabolic disorders of diverse etiology characterized by impaired conversion of methylmalonyl-CoA into succinyl-CoA. Propionyl-CoA derived from catabolism of isoleucine, valine, threonine, methionine, side chain of cholesterol, and odd-chain fatty acids is catalyzed by propionyl-CoA carboxylase to form D-methylmalonyl-CoA. Methylmalonyl-CoA epimerase then converts D-methylmalonyl-CoA to its enantiomer L-methylmalonyl-CoA. **Methylmalonyl-CoA epimerase deficiency** is a rare disorder associated with persistent elevations of propionate-related metabolites and methylmalonic acid. It may present with metabolic acidosis, ketosis, but known patients appear more clinically stable than those with severe forms of methylmalonic acidemia.

In the next biochemical step, L-methylmalonyl-CoA is converted to succinyl-CoA by methylmalonyl-CoA mutase (see Fig. 103.4). The latter enzyme requires adenosylcobalamin, a metabolite of vitamin B_{12}, as a coenzyme. Deficiency of either the mutase or its coenzyme results in the accumulation of methylmalonic acid and its precursors in body fluids. Two biochemical forms of methylmalonyl-CoA mutase deficiencies have been identified. These are designated *mut⁰*, referring to no detectable enzyme activity, and *mut⁻*, indicating residual, although insufficient, mutase activity. Patients with methylmalonic acidemia due to deficiency of the mutase apoenzyme (*mut⁰*) are not responsive to hydroxocobalamin

therapy.

In the remaining methylmalonic acidemia patients, the defect resides in the formation of adenosylcobalamin from dietary vitamin B_{12}. The absorption of dietary vitamin B_{12} in the terminal ileum requires *intrinsic factor,* a glycoprotein secreted by the gastric parietal cells. It is transported in the blood by haptocorrin and transcobalamin II. The transcobalamin II–cobalamin complex (TCII-Cbl) is recognized by a specific receptor on the cell membrane (transcobalamin receptor encoded by *CD320*) and enters the cell by endocytosis. In the lysosome, TCII-Cbl is hydrolyzed, and, with the participation of LMBRD1 (*cblF*) and ABCD4 (*cblJ*), free cobalamin is released into the cytosol (see Fig. 103.4). Pathogenic variants in either *LMBRD1* or *ABCD4* genes result in impaired release of cobalamin from lysosomes. In the cytoplasm, cobalamin binds to the MMACHC protein (see *cblC* later), which removes a moiety attached to cobalt in the cobalamin molecule and reduces the cobalt from oxidation state +3 (cob[III]alamin) to +2 (cob[II]alamin). It then enters the mitochondria, where it is catalyzed by MMAB (*cblB*) and MMAA (*cblA*) to form adenosylcobalamin, a coenzyme for methylmalonyl-CoA mutase. The other arm of the pathway directs cytosolic cobalamin toward methionine synthase reductase (*cblE*), which forms methylcobalamin, acting as a coenzyme for methionine synthase (*cblG*, see Fig. 103.3). The MMADHC protein (see *cblD*) appears to play a role in determining whether cobalamin enters the mitochondria or remains in the cytoplasm.

The uptake of TCII-Cbl by cells is impaired in individuals with pathogenic variants affecting transcobalamin receptor (*CD320*), which is located on the cell surface. Individuals homozygous for pathogenic variants in the *CD320* gene encoding the transcobalamin receptor may have mild elevations of methylmalonic acid in blood and urine. These patients can be identified by the newborn screen based on the elevated propionylcarnitine (C3). In **transcobalamin receptor deficiency**, methylmalonic acid levels and plasma propionylcarnitine tend to normalize in the 1st yr of life. It is not clear whether there is a long-term clinical phenotype associated with this defect.

Nine different defects in the intracellular metabolism of cobalamin have been identified. These are designated *cblA* through *cblG*, *cblJ*, and *cblX*, where *cbl* stands for a defect in any step of cobalamin metabolism. The *cblA*, *cblB*, and *cblD* variant 2 defects cause methylmalonic acidemia *alone*. In patients with *cblC*, classic *cblD*, *cblF*, *cblJ*, and *cblX* defects, synthesis of both adenosylcobalamin and methylcobalamin is impaired, resulting in *combined* methylmalonic acidemia and homocystinuria. The *cblD* variant 1, *cblE*, and the *cblG* defects affect only the synthesis of methylcobalamin, resulting in homocystinuria without methylmalonic aciduria (see Chapter 103.3).

Biochemical manifestations of patients with isolated methylmalonic acidemia caused by *mut⁰*, *mut⁻*, *cblA*, *cblB*, and *cblD* variant 2 overlap. The wide variations in severity of clinical course range from very sick newborn infants to apparently asymptomatic adults. In **severe** forms, lethargy, feeding problems, vomiting, a sepsis-like picture, tachypnea (from metabolic ketoacidosis), and hypotonia may develop in the 1st few days of life and may progress to hyperammonemic encephalopathy, coma, and death if left untreated. Infants who survive the first attack may go on to develop similar acute metabolic episodes during a catabolic state such as infection or prolonged fasting or after ingestion of a high-protein diet. In certain situations, such acute events can cause a sudden injury of the basal ganglia (movement centers in CNS), a metabolic stroke, resulting in a debilitating movement disorder. Between the acute attacks, the patient usually continues to exhibit hypotonia and feeding problems with failure to thrive, while other complications of the disease occur with age, including recurrent episodes of pancreatitis, bone marrow suppression, osteopenia, and optic nerve atrophy. Chronic renal failure and tubulointerstitial nephritis necessitating renal transplant have been reported in older patients. Renal complications are more severe in patients with the *mut⁰* and severe *cblB* forms of methylmalonic acidemia. In milder forms, patients may present later in life with hypotonia, failure to thrive, and developmental delay. Neurocognitive development of patients with mild methylmalonic acidemia may remain within the normal range.

The episodic nature of the condition and its biochemical abnormalities in some patients may be confused with those of *ethylene glycol* (antifreeze) ingestion. The peak of propionate in a blood sample from an infant with methylmalonic acidemia has been mistaken for ethylene glycol when the sample was assayed by gas chromatography without mass spectrometry.

Laboratory findings include ketosis, metabolic acidosis, hyperglycinemia, hyperammonemia, hypoglycemia, anemia, neutropenia, thrombocytopenia, and the presence of large quantities of methylmalonic acid in body fluids (see Fig. 103.6). Metabolites of propionic acid (3-hydroxypropionate and methylcitrate) are also found in the urine. Plasma acylcarnitine profile reveals elevated propionylcarnitine (C3) and methylmalonylcarnitine (C4DC). Hyperammonemia in methylmalonic acidemia may be confused with a urea cycle disorder. However, patients with defects in urea cycle enzymes are typically not acidotic and tend to have high plasma glutamine (see Fig. 103.12). The reason for hyperammonemia is not well understood, but it is likely related to the inhibition of proximal urea cycle in the mitochondrial matrix.

Diagnosis can be confirmed by identifying pathogenic variants in the causal gene, by measuring propionate incorporation with complementation analysis in cultured fibroblasts, and by measuring the specific activity of the mutase enzyme in biopsies or cell extracts.

Treatment of acute attacks is similar to propionic acidemia. Long-term treatment consists of administration of a low-protein diet limited to the recommended dietary allowance, L-carnitine (50-100 mg/kg/24 hr orally). Patients with severe forms of methylmalonic acidemia may require protein diet modifications similar to those prescribed for patients with propionic acidemia. Patients with isolated methylmalonic acidemia caused by defects in the intracellular metabolism of cobalamin (*cbl*A, *cbl*D variant 2, and some patients with *cbl*B) respond to parenteral hydroxocobalamin. Chronic bicarbonate replacement therapy is usually required to correct chronic acidosis. Plasma ammonia tends to normalize between the attacks, and chronic treatment of hyperammonemia is rarely needed. Stressful situations that may trigger acute attacks (infection, prolonged fasting, trauma, surgeries, high-protein meals) should be treated promptly.

Inadequate oral intake secondary to poor appetite, protein overrestriction, or essential amino acid deficiencies are common complications in long-term management of these patients. Consequently, enteral feeding through gastrostomy is often recommended early in the course of treatment. Close monitoring of blood pH, essential amino acid levels, blood and urinary concentrations of methylmalonate, and growth parameters is required to ensure the nutritional prescription meets patient's metabolic demands. In addition, frequent monitoring of kidney function, vision, hearing, and bone mineral density are necessary for early recognition and management of chronic complications. Glutathione deficiency responsive to treatment with ascorbate has been described.

Liver, kidney, and combined liver-kidney transplantations have been attempted in an increasing number of affected patients. Liver and liver-kidney transplantation can alleviate but not eliminate the metabolic abnormalities. Liver and liver-kidney transplants do not provide complete protection against the occurrence of metabolic stroke. Kidney transplantation alone can restore the renal function but results in only minor improvement of the clinical stability of patients.

Prognosis depends on the severity of symptoms and the occurrence of complications. In general, patients with complete deficiency of mutase apoenzyme (*mut⁰*) and severe forms of *cbl*B deficiency have the least favorable prognosis, and those with *mut⁻* and *cbl*A defects have a better outcome.

Methylmalonic acidemia can be identified on the universal newborn screening by measuring propionylcarnitine (C3) using tandem mass spectrometry. The prevalence of all forms of methylmalonic aciduria is estimated at 1:50,000 to 1:100,000 live births. All defects causing isolated methylmalonic acidemia are inherited as autosomal recessive traits. The gene for the mutase (*MUT*) is on the short arm of chromosome 6p12.3. Neonates with methylmalonic acidemia and severe diabetes caused by β-cell agenesis, who have paternal uniparental isodisomy of chromosome 6, have been reported. Pathogenic variants in the genes for *cbl*A (*MMAA,* on chromosome 4q31.21), *cbl*B (*MMAB,* on

chromosome 12q24.11), and all forms of *cbl*D (*MMADHC,* on chromosome 2q23.2) have been identified in affected patients. The previously described *cbl*H group is identical to *cbl*D variant 2.

COMBINED METHYLMALONIC ACIDURIA AND HOMOCYSTINURIA (*cbl*C, *cbl*D, *cbl*F, *cbl*J, AND *cbl*X DEFECTS)

Combined methylmalonic acidemia and homocystinuria caused by *cbl*C deficiency is the most common type of intracellular cobalamin (vitamin B₁₂) biosynthesis defects. Deficiency of *cbl*C is as common as methylmalonyl-CoA mutase deficiency. The other disorders (*cbl*D, *cbl*F, *cbl*J, *cbl*X) are much rarer (see Figs. 103.3 and 103.4). Neurologic findings are prominent in patients with *cbl*C, *cbl*D and *cbl*X defects. Most patients with the *cbl*C defect present in the 1st mo of life because of failure to thrive, lethargy, poor feeding, developmental delay, nystagmus and seizures. Hyperammonemia may be seen infrequently, while hyperglycinemia is not present, unlike in isolated *mut*-type methylmalonic acidemia. Intrauterine growth restriction and microcephaly suggest that *cbl*C can manifest prenatally in some affected infants. Late-onset patients with sudden development of dementia and myelopathy have been reported, even with presentation in adulthood. Megaloblastic anemia is a common finding in patients with *cbl*C defect. Mild to moderate increases in concentrations of methylmalonic acid and significant elevations in total plasma homocysteine are found in blood. Unlike classic homocystinuria, in untreated *cbl*C patients plasma methionine is low to normal. Retinal abnormalities (e.g., bull's eye maculopathy) resulting in severe progressive vision loss are common and can be seen as early as 3 mo of age, even in prospectively identified and well-treated patients. **Thrombotic microangiopathy** can present as hemolytic uremic syndrome, pulmonary hypertension, and cor pulmonale. Hydrocephalus, and non-compaction cardiomyopathy have been reported as complications in patients with *cbl*C defect.

Similar to *cbl*C patients, males with *cbl*X have elevations of both total plasma homocysteine and methylmalonic acid, but they tend to have milder elevations of these metabolites. Unlike *cbl*C-deficient patients, who tend to respond to treatment, *cbl*X-deficient patients experience failure to thrive, severe developmental delay, and intractable epilepsy despite aggressive treatment.

Clinical findings in *cbl*F deficiency are quite variable. Patients may present with poor feeding, growth and developmental delay, and persistent stomatitis manifesting in the 1st mo of life. Delay in diagnosis and treatment can be accompanied by hyperpigmentation of skin, developmental delay, intellectual disability, and short stature. Vitamin B₁₂ malabsorption and low plasma vitamin B₁₂ has been noted in patients with *cbl*F defect. Clinical manifestations of *cbl*J defect show significant overlap with those of the *cbl*F deficiency. Dysmorphic features and congenital heart disease have been reported in some patients with *cbl*F and *cbl*J defects.

Experience with **treatment** of patients with *cbl*C, *cbl*D, *cbl*F, *cbl*J, and *cbl*X defects is limited. Large doses of hydroxocobalamin (up to 0.3 mg/kg/day) in conjunction with betaine (up to 250 mg/kg/day) produce biochemical improvement with variable clinical effect. Patients with *cbl*F and *cbl*J deficiency typically show favorable biochemical and clinical response to smaller hydroxocobalamin doses (1 mg once weekly to 1 mg daily parenterally). Folic or folinic acid supplementation is recommended. Dietary methionine deficiency should be avoided.

The *cbl*C disorder is caused by pathogenic variants in the *MMACHC* gene (on chromosome 1p34.1). A frameshift variant (c.271dupA) is seen in up to 40% of *MMACHC* alleles and is associated with a less favorable clinical outcome. The *cbl*D disorder is caused by pathogenic variants in the *MMADHC* gene (on chromosome 2q23.2). Pathogenic variants resulting in *cbl*D variant 1 (causing only homocystinuria) affect the C-terminal domain of the gene product; those resulting in *cbl*D variant 2 (causing only methylmalonic aciduria) affect the N-terminus. Patients with classic *cbl*D, with both homocystinuria and methylmalonic acidemia, have pathogenic variants resulting in decreased protein expression. The *cbl*F disorder is caused by pathogenic variants in the *LMBRD1* gene (on chromosome 6q13) encoding a lysosomal membrane protein. The *cbl*J disorder is associated with pathogenic variants in the

ABCD4 gene (on chromosome 14q24.3), encoding an adenosine triphosphate–binding cassette protein localized to the lysosomal membrane. The *cbl*X disorder is caused by pathogenic variants in the *HCFC1* gene on the X chromosome (Xq28), which encodes a transcription factor that appears to be essential for expression of the *MMACHC* gene. This is the only X-linked disorder in the B_{12} intracellular metabolism pathway.

ISOLATED HOMOCYSTINURIA
Patients with *cbl*D variant 1, *cbl*E, and *cbl*G deficiency present with isolated homocystinuria without methylmalonic acidemia (see Chapter 103.3, Homocystinuria Caused by Defects in Methylcobalamin Formation).

COMBINED MALONIC AND METHYLMALONIC ACIDURIA (*ACSF3*-RELATED DISORDER)
Combined *m*alonic and *methylm*alonic *a*ciduria (**CMAMMA**) is a rare autosomal recessive disorder resulting from pathogenic variants in *ACSF3*. ACSF3 is a putative acyl-CoA synthetase required for the conversion of malonic and methylmalonic acids to their CoA derivatives in the mitochondrial matrix. The disorder can be suspected based on the presence of elevated malonic and methylmalonic acids in urine and plasma. It is distinguished from malonyl-CoA decarboxylase, because methylmalonic acid is about 5-fold greater than malonic acid in the urine. Plasma propionylcarnitine (C3-carnitine) in CMAMMA patients is normal, so universal newborn screening programs using C3-carnitine in blood spots to screen for methylmalonic acidemia would not detect this condition. The clinical phenotype is incompletely understood. Young patients identified prospectively in infancy through urine-based newborn screening were reported to be asymptomatic, but the long-term outcome in this cohort awaits further characterization. Older patients ascertained clinically have highly variable presentations, including metabolic crises, failure to thrive, seizures, memory problems, optic nerve or spinal cord atrophy, and progressive neurodegeneration. Treatment of CMAMMA is supportive and includes avoidance of an excessively high-protein diet. Vitamin B_{12} supplementation does not appear to lower malonic and methylmalonic metabolites in body fluids.

Bibliography is available at Expert Consult.

103.7 Glycine
Oleg A. Shchelochkov and Charles P. Venditti

Glycine is a nonessential amino acid synthesized mainly from serine and threonine. Structurally, it is the simplest amino acid. Glycine is involved in many reactions in the body, especially in the nervous system, where it functions as a neurotransmitter (excitatory in the cortex, inhibitory in the brainstem and the spinal cord; see Chapter 103.11). Its main catabolic pathway requires the *glycine cleavage system,* a pyridoxal phosphate–dependent, mitochondrial enzyme complex that converts glycine to carbon dioxide and ammonia and transfers α-carbon to tetrahydrofolate (see Fig. 103.8). The glycine cleavage system is composed of 4 proteins: P protein (glycine decarboxylase), H protein, T protein, and L protein, which are encoded by 4 different genes.

HYPOGLYCINEMIA
Defects in the biosynthetic pathway of serine (see Chapter 103.8) cause deficiency of glycine in addition to that of serine in body fluids, especially in the cerebrospinal fluid (CSF). Isolated primary deficiency of glycine has not been reported.

HYPERGLYCINEMIA
Elevated levels of glycine in body fluids occur in propionic acidemia, methylmalonic acidemia, isovaleric acidemia, and β-ketothiolase deficiency, which are collectively referred to as *ketotic hyperglycinemia* because of the coexistence of acidosis and ketosis. The pathogenesis of hyperglycinemia in these disorders is not fully understood, but inhibition of the glycine cleavage enzyme system by the various organic acids has been shown to occur in some of these patients. The term **nonketotic hyperglycinemia (NKH)** is reserved for the clinical condition caused by the genetic deficiency of the glycine cleavage enzyme system (see Fig. 103.8). In this condition, hyperglycinemia is present without ketosis.

NONKETOTIC HYPERGLYCINEMIA (GLYCINE ENCEPHALOPATHY)
Four forms of NKH have been identified: neonatal, infantile, late onset, and transient.

Neonatal Nonketotic Hyperglycinemia
This is the most common form of NKH. Clinical manifestations develop in the 1st few days of life (between 6 hr and 8 days after birth). Poor feeding, failure to suck, lethargy, and profound hypotonia may progress rapidly to a deep coma, apnea, and death. Convulsions, especially myoclonic seizures and hiccups, are common.

Laboratory findings reveal moderate to severe hyperglycinemia (as high as 8 times normal) and hyperglycinuria. The unequivocal elevation of glycine concentration in CSF (15-30 times normal) and the high ratio of glycine concentration in CSF to that in plasma (a value >0.08, normal <0.02) are diagnostic of NKH. Affected patients' blood pH is usually normal, and urine assay is negative for organic acids. CSF serine levels can be low.

Approximately 30% of NKH infants die despite supportive therapy. Those who survive develop profound psychomotor retardation and intractable seizure disorders (myoclonic and/or grand mal seizures). Hydrocephalus, requiring shunting, and pulmonary hypertension have been noted in some survivors. In some patients the hyperglycemia is transient.

Infantile Nonketotic Hyperglycinemia
These previously normal infants develop signs and symptoms of neonatal NKH after 6 mo of age. Seizures and hypotonia are the common presenting signs. Infantile NKH appears to be a milder form of neonatal NKH; infants usually survive, and intellectual disability is not as profound as in the neonatal form.

Laboratory findings in patients with infantile NKH are identical to those seen in neonatal NKH.

Late-Onset Nonketotic Hyperglycinemia
Clinical manifestations of this atypical form of NKH include progressive spastic diplegia, optic nerve atrophy, and choreoathetotic movements. Age of onset has been between 2 and 33 yr. Symptoms of delirium, chorea, and vertical gaze palsy may occur episodically in some patients during an intercurrent infection. Mental development is usually normal, but mild cognitive impairment and infrequent seizures have been reported in some patients.

Laboratory findings in late-onset NKH are similar but not as pronounced as in neonatal NKH.

All forms of NKH should be differentiated from *ketotic* hyperglycinemia, pyridox(am)ine phosphate oxidase (PNPO) deficiency, ingestion of valproic acid, and transient glycine encephalopathy. Valproic acid can moderately increase blood, CSF, and urinary concentrations of glycine. Repeat assays after discontinuation of the drug will help establish the diagnosis.

Transient Nonketotic Hyperglycinemia
Most clinical and laboratory manifestations of transient NKH are indistinguishable from those of the neonatal form. By 2-8 wk of age, however, a complete clinical recovery may occur, and the elevated glycine levels in plasma and CSF normalize after the patient stops a glycine-lowering medication. Some of these patients develop normally with no neurologic sequelae, but intellectual disability has been noted in others. The etiology of this condition is not known, but it is thought to be a consequence of immaturity of the enzyme system.

Diagnosis and Treatment
Diagnosis of NKH can be suspected based on the findings of elevated glycine in plasma or CSF and the abnormal CSF/plasma ratio of glycine.

The diagnosis is confirmed using molecular analysis of the NKH-related genes. Rarely, assay of the enzyme in liver or brain specimens is necessary to establish the diagnosis. Enzyme activity in the neonatal form is close to zero, whereas in the other forms, some residual activity is present. In most patients with neonatal NKH, the enzyme defect resides in the P protein (75%); defects in the T protein account for approximately 20% of cases, whereas <1% are caused by pathogenic variants in the H protein.

No effective treatment is known. Exchange transfusion, dietary restriction of glycine, and administration of sodium benzoate or folate have not altered the neurologic outcome in severe forms of NKH. Patients with attenuated NKH may experience clinical improvement from enteral sodium benzoate. Drugs that counteract the effect of glycine on neuronal cells, such as dextromethorphan and felbamate, have shown some beneficial effects in patients with the mild forms of the condition.

NKH is inherited as an autosomal recessive trait. The prevalence is not known, but high frequency of the disorder has been noted in northern Finland (1 in 12,000 live births) suggesting that this disorder is likely underdiagnosed. The gene for P protein (*GLDC*) is on chromosome 9p24.1. The gene encoding T protein (*AMT*) is on chromosome 3p21.31 and that for H protein (*GCSH*) is mapped to chromosome 16q23.2. The L protein gene (*DLD*) on chromosome 7q31.7 encodes dihydrolipoamide dehydrogenase, the E3 component of α-ketoacid dehydrogenase complexes and is discussed in Chapter 103.6 (Valine, Leucine, Isoleucine, and Related Organic Acidemias). **Prenatal diagnosis** has been accomplished by identification of the known familial pathogenic variants in the affected gene or by performing an assay of the enzyme activity in chorionic villus biopsy specimens.

SARCOSINEMIA

Increased concentrations of sarcosine (*N*-methylglycine) are observed in both blood and urine, but no consistent clinical picture has been attributed to sarcosinemia. This autosomal recessive metabolic condition is caused by a defect in sarcosine dehydrogenase, the enzyme that converts sarcosine to glycine (see Fig. 103.8). The gene for this enzyme (*SARDH*) is on chromosome 9q34.2.

PRIMARY TRIMETHYLAMINURIA

Trimethylamine is normally produced in the intestine from the breakdown of dietary choline and trimethylamine oxide by bacteria. Egg yolk and liver are the main sources of choline, and fish is the major source of trimethylamine oxide. Trimethylamine is absorbed and oxidized in the liver by trimethylamine oxidase (flavin-containing monooxygenases) to trimethylamine oxide, which is odorless and excreted in the urine (see Fig. 103.8). Deficiency of this enzyme results in massive excretion of trimethylamine in urine. There is a body odor that resembles that of a fish, which may have significant social and psychosocial ramifications. Transient symptomatic trimethylaminuria can occur in normal individuals following ingestion of large quantities of the above mentioned foods. **Treatment** with oral activated charcoal, short courses of oral metronidazole, neomycin, or lactulose cause temporary reduction in the body odor. Restriction of fish, eggs, liver, and other sources of choline (e.g., nuts, grains) in the diet significantly reduces the odor. Topical use of acidic soaps (pH 5.5) can also help control the odor. The gene for trimethylamine oxidase (*FMO3*) has been mapped to chromosome 1q24.3.

HYPEROXALURIA AND OXALOSIS

Normally, oxalic acid is derived mostly from oxidation of glyoxylic acid and, to a lesser degree, from oxidation of ascorbic acid (see Fig. 103.8). Glyoxylic acid is formed from oxidation of glycolic acid and glycine in the peroxisomes, and catabolism of **hydroxyproline** in the mitochondria (Fig. 103.9). Vegetables and foods containing oxalic acid, such as spinach, rhubarb, and almond milk, are the main *exogenous* sources of glycolic and oxalic acids; most of glyoxylic and oxalic acids are produced endogenously. Normally, a major portion of glyoxylate produced in the body is shuttled to peroxisomes, where it is converted to glycine by the action of the enzyme alanine:glyoxylate transaminase. Deficiency of this enzyme causes hyperoxaluria **type 1.** Most of the remaining glyoxylate in the cytosol is reduced to glycolate by the action of the enzyme glyoxylate reductase/hydroxypyruvate reductase. Deficiency of this enzyme causes hyperoxaluria **type 2.** These 2 pathways protect the body from excessive production of oxalic acid (see Fig. 103.8). Any glyoxylate that cannot be disposed of through these pathways is readily converted to oxalic acid by the action of the enzyme lactate dehydrogenase (LDH). Oxalic acid cannot be further metabolized in humans and is excreted in the urine as oxalates. Calcium oxalate is relatively insoluble in water and precipitates in tissues (kidneys and joints) if its concentration increases in the body.

Secondary hyperoxaluria has been observed in pyridoxine deficiency (cofactor for alanine:glyoxylate transaminase), in patients with inflammatory bowel disease, extensive resection of small bowel, or jejunoileal bypass (*enteric hyperoxaluria*), after ingestion of ethylene glycol or high doses of vitamin C, and after administration of the anesthetic agent methoxyflurane (which oxidizes directly to oxalic acid). Acute, fatal hyperoxaluria may develop after ingestion of plants with high oxalic acid content (e.g., sorrel) or intentional ingestion of oxalic acid.

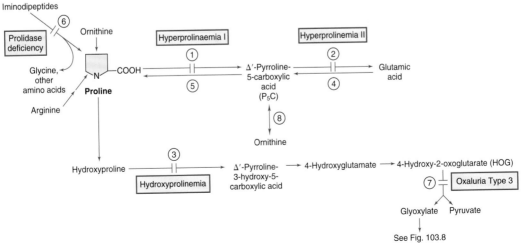

Fig. 103.9 Pathways in the metabolism of proline. **Enzymes:** *(1)* Proline oxidase (dehydrogenase), *(2)* Δ¹-pyrroline-5-carboxylic acid (P5C) dehydrogenase, *(3)* hydroxyproline oxidase, *(4)* Δ¹-pyrroline-5-carboxylic acid (P5C) synthase, *(5)* Δ¹-pyrroline-5-carboxylic acid (P5C) reductase, *(6)* prolidase, *(7)* 4-hydroxyoxoglutarate aldolase 1 (HOGA1), *(8)* ornithine aminotransferase.

Precipitation of calcium oxalate in tissues causes hypocalcemia, liver necrosis, renal failure, cardiac arrhythmia, and death. The lethal dose of oxalic acid is estimated at 5-30 g.

Primary hyperoxaluria is a group of disorders in which large amounts of oxalates accumulate in the body. Three types of primary hyperoxaluria have been identified to date. The term **oxalosis** refers to deposition of calcium oxalate in parenchymal tissues.

Primary Hyperoxaluria Type 1

This rare condition (prevalence of 1 : 120,000 live births in Europe) is the most common form of primary hyperoxaluria. It is caused by deficiency of the peroxisomal enzyme alanine:glyoxylate transaminase, which is expressed only in the liver peroxisomes and requires pyridoxine (vitamin B_6) as a cofactor. In the absence of this enzyme, glyoxylic acid, which cannot be converted to glycine, is transferred to the cytosol, where it is oxidized to oxalic acid (see earlier and Fig. 103.8).

The age of presentation varies widely, from neonatal period to late adulthood. The majority of patients become symptomatic in late childhood or early adolescence. In about 20% of cases, symptoms develop before 1 yr of age. The initial clinical manifestations are related to renal stones and nephrocalcinosis. Renal colic and asymptomatic hematuria lead to a gradual deterioration of renal function, manifested by growth retardation and uremia. If the disorder is left untreated, most patients die before 20 yr of age from renal failure. Other frequent manifestations of the disease include failure to thrive, short stature, arterial calcifications, arrhythmia, heart failure, hypothyroidism, and skin nodules. Acute arthritis is a rare manifestation and may be misdiagnosed as gout because uric acid is usually elevated in patients with type 1 hyperoxaluria. Crystalline retinopathy and optic neuropathy causing visual loss have occurred in a few patients.

A marked increase in urinary excretion of oxalate (normal excretion: 10-50 mg/24 hr) is the most important laboratory finding. The presence of oxalate crystals in urinary sediment is rarely helpful for diagnosis because such crystals can also be seen in normal individuals. Urinary excretion of glycolic acid and glyoxylic acid is increased in most but not all patients. Diagnosis can be confirmed by identification of pathogenic variants in the *AGXT* gene or by performing an enzymatic assay in liver specimens.

Treatment focuses on the reduction of oxalic acid production and on increasing calcium oxalate disposal. Patients with primary hyperoxaluria type 1 should receive a 3-mo trial of pyridoxine treatment to establish pyridoxine responsiveness. In up to 30% of patients (e.g., homozygous for pathogenic variant c.508G>A in *AGXT*), administration of large doses of pyridoxine reduces plasma level and urinary excretion of oxalate. To increase calcium oxalate disposal and prevent nephrolithiasis, high oral fluid intake (2-3 L/m²/24 hr while controlling for fluid balance), urine alkalinization, phosphate supplementation, monitoring of vitamin C and vitamin D intake, and avoidance of drugs that increase urinary calcium excretion (e.g., loop diuretics) are recommended. Urinary stones should be managed by experienced urologists because excessive surgical trauma may contribute to renal dysfunction. Renal function replacement strategies (e.g., hemodialysis) are used in some patients (e.g., to bridge patients to transplant or when transplant is not a viable option).

Organ **transplantation** has emerged as the most definitive treatment. The decision to undergo kidney, liver, or liver-kidney transplant is complex and may vary from one medical center to another. Except for older patients with pyridoxine-responsive form of disease, renal transplantation for patients in renal failure may not improve the outcome, because oxalosis will recur in the transplanted kidney. Combined liver-kidney transplants have resulted in a significant decrease in plasma and urinary oxalate and thus may be the most effective treatment strategy in this disorder, particularly in children.

The condition is inherited as an autosomal recessive trait. The gene for this enzyme (*AGXT*) is mapped to chromosome 2q37.3. The most common pathogenic variant in patients with high residual enzyme activity (c.508G>A, p.Gly170Arg) results in mistargeting of the enzyme to the mitochondria instead of the peroxisomes and loss of in vivo function. **Prenatal diagnosis** has been achieved by DNA analysis of chorionic villus samples or by the measurement of fetal hepatic enzyme

activity obtained by needle biopsy.

Primary Hyperoxaluria Type 2 (L-Glyceric Aciduria)

This rare condition is caused by a deficiency of the glyoxylate reductase–hydroxypyruvate reductase enzyme complex (see Fig. 103.8). A deficiency in the activity of this complex results in an accumulation of two intermediate metabolites, hydroxypyruvate (the ketoacid derivative of serine) and glyoxylic acid. Both these compounds are further metabolized by LDH to L-glyceric acid and oxalic acid, respectively. A high prevalence of this disorder is reported in the Saulteaux-Ojibway Indians of Manitoba.

Primary hyperoxaluria type 2 results in the deposition of calcium oxalate in the renal parenchyma and urinary tract. Renal stones presenting with renal colic and hematuria may develop before age 2 yr. Renal failure is less common in this condition than in primary hyperoxaluria type 1.

Urinary testing reveals large amounts of L-glyceric acid in addition to high levels of oxalate. Urinary L-glyceric acid is considered a pathognomonic finding in primary hyperoxaluria type 2. Urinary excretion of glycolic acid and glyoxylic acid is not increased. The presence of L-glyceric acid without increased levels of glycolic and glyoxylic acids in urine differentiates this type from type 1 hyperoxaluria. Diagnosis can be confirmed by molecular analysis of *GRHPR* (9p13.2) or by the enzyme assay in liver biopsy.

Principles of therapy are similar to those in primary hyperoxaluria type 1. Renal transplant is used in some patients; no experience with kidney-liver transplantation is available at this time.

Primary Hyperoxaluria Type 3

Approximately 10% of patients with primary hyperoxaluria have deficiency of 4-hydroxy-2-oxoglutarate aldolase 1 (HOGA1), the underlying cause of hyperoxaluria type 3. The enzyme is encoded by *HOGA1* mapped to chromosome 10q24.2. This mitochondrial enzyme catalyzes the final step in the metabolic pathway of hydroxyproline generating pyruvate and glyoxylate from 4-hydroxy-2-oxoglutarate (HOG; see Figs. 103.8 and 103.9). In vitro studies show inhibition of glyoxylate reductase–hydroxypyruvate reductase enzyme activity by high concentration of HOG that accumulates in patients with hyperoxaluria type 3. This inhibition results in a biochemical phenotype similar to hyperoxaluria type 2 (see Fig. 103.8).

Patients with primary hyperoxaluria type 3 usually presented with calcium oxalate kidney stones in early childhood, but asymptomatic older siblings were also identified. Gradually, renal function may decline, infrequently resulting in end-stage renal disease. Increased levels of HOG in urine, serum, and liver biopsy samples of these patients is the distinguishing feature of this disorder. **Treatment** involves high oral fluid intake, management of oral citrate or phosphate intake to prevent calcium oxalate renal stone formation, and avoidance of dehydration to prevent acute kidney injury. In severe forms of this disorder, dialysis and transplantation may be required to address the end-stage renal disease.

Creatine Deficiency Disorders

Creatine is synthesized mainly in the liver, pancreas, and kidneys and to a lesser degree in the brain from arginine and glycine and is transported to muscles and the brain, where there is high activity of the enzyme creatine kinase (Fig. 103.10). Phosphorylation and dephosphorylation of creatine in conjunction with adenosine triphosphate and diphosphate provide high-energy phosphate transfer reactions in these organs. Creatine is nonenzymatically metabolized to creatinine at a constant daily rate and is excreted in the urine. Three genetic conditions are known to cause creatine deficiency in the brain and other tissues. Two enzymes, arginine:glycine amidinotransferase (**AGAT**) and guanidinoacetate methyltransferase (**GAMT**; Fig. 103.10), are involved in the biosynthesis of creatine. Both conditions may respond to creatine supplementation, especially when the treatment is started in early age. The 3rd condition, an X-linked inherited defect, is caused by deficiency of the creatinine transporter (CRTR) protein mediating uptake of creatine by brain and muscle.

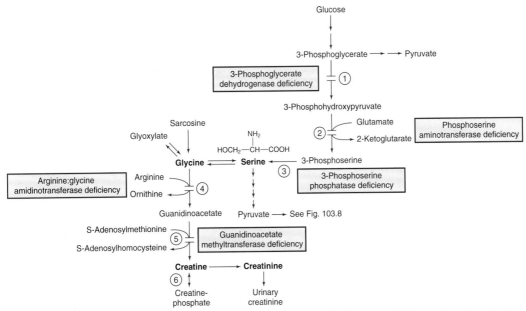

Fig. 103.10 Biosynthesis of serine and creatine. **Enzymes:** *(1)* 3-Phosphoglycerate dehydrogenase, *(2)* 3-phosphoserine aminotransferase, *(3)* 3-phosphoserine phosphatase, *(4)* arginine:glycine amidinotransferase (AGAT), *(5)* guanidinoacetate methyltransferase (GAMT), *(6)* creatine kinase.

Clinical manifestations of the 3 defects overlap, relate to the brain and muscle, and may appear in the 1st few wk or mo of life. Developmental delay, intellectual disability, speech delay, psychiatric symptoms (autism and psychosis), hypotonia, ataxia, and seizures are common findings. Dystonic movements have been documented in GAMT and CRTR deficiency.

Laboratory findings include decreased creatine in plasma in patients with AGAT and GAMT defects. Plasma creatinine level alone is insufficient to diagnose these disorders. Secondary to impaired reabsorption of creatine in kidneys, the urinary ratio of creatine to creatinine is increased in male patients with a CRTR defect but can also be mildly elevated in female carriers. Marked elevations of guanidinoacetate in blood, urine, and especially in CSF, are diagnostic of GAMT defects. In contrast, low levels of guanidinoacetate can be found in body fluids in the AGAT defect. Absence of creatine and creatine phosphate (in all 3 defects) and high levels of guanidinoacetate (in GAMT defect) can be demonstrated in the brain by magnetic resonance spectroscopy (MRS). Brain MRI may show signal hyperintensity in the globus pallidus. Diagnosis of AGAT deficiency or GAMT deficiency may be confirmed by DNA analysis or by measuring of enzymatic activity in cultured fibroblasts (GAMT) or lymphoblasts (AGAT). Diagnosis of CRTR deficiency can be confirmed by DNA analysis or a creatine uptake assay in fibroblasts.

The outcomes of **treatment** are age-dependent and best with treatment started in the neonatal period or presymptomatically. In AGAT-deficient patients, oral creatine monohydrate (up to 400-800 mg/kg/24 hr) may improve muscle weakness in most and neurocognitive outcomes in some patients. In GAMT-deficient patients, supplementation with oral creatine monohydrate (up to 400-800 mg/kg/24 hr), ornithine (up to 400-800 mg/kg/24 hr), and dietary arginine restriction may result in improved muscle tone and neurocognitive development and may alleviate seizures. In CRTR-deficient patients, administration of creatine and its precursors (arginine and glycine) does not restore creatine in the brain, but some patients may experience improvements of seizures and neurocognitive outcomes.

AGAT and GAMT defects are inherited as autosomal recessive traits. The gene for AGAT *(GATM)* is on chromosome 15q21.1 and that for GAMT *(GAMT)* is on chromosome 19p13.3. CRTR is an X-linked disorder and the gene *(SLC6A8)* is on Xq28. CRTR defect is the most common cause of creatine deficiency, accounting for up to 1–2% of males with intellectual disability of unknown cause.

Bibliography is available at Expert Consult.

103.8 Serine Deficiency Disorders (Serine Biosynthesis and Transport Defects)
Oleg A. Shchelochkov and Charles P. Venditti

Serine is a nonessential amino acid supplied through dietary sources and through its endogenous synthesis, mainly from glucose and glycine. The endogenous production of serine comprises an important portion of the daily requirement of this amino acid, especially in the synaptic junctions where it contributes to the metabolism of phospholipids as well as D-serine and glycine, both involved in neurotransmission (see Chapter 103.11). Consequently, deficiency of any of the enzymes involved in the biosynthesis of serine or its transport causes neurologic manifestations. The clinical spectrum of serine deficiency disorders is wide and varies from Neu-Laxova syndrome on the severe end of spectrum to epilepsy and developmental delay on the milder end. Affected patients respond favorably to oral supplementation with serine and glycine provided that the treatment is initiated very early in life. Figs. 103.8 and 103.10 show the metabolic pathway for synthesis and catabolism of serine.

3-PHOSPHOGLYCERATE DEHYDROGENASE DEFICIENCY
3-Phosphoglycerate dehydrogenase (**PHGDH**) deficiency has a broad range of symptoms and ages of presentation. **Neu-Laxova syndrome type 1** is the most severe manifestation and presents prenatally with intrauterine growth restriction and congenital anomalies, including dysmorphic facial features, microcephaly, CNS malformations, limb deformities, and ichthyosis. Most patients with this form are stillborn or have early neonatal mortality. Infantile-onset PHGDH deficiency presents with feeding problems, failure to thrive, vomiting, irritability, intractable seizures, severe developmental delay, and hypertonia progressing to spastic quadriplegia. Nystagmus, cataracts, hypogonadism, and megaloblastic anemia have been observed in some affected infants.

Patients with a milder form of this disorder experience cognitive impairment, behavioral problems, sensorineural polyneuropathy, and childhood-onset seizures.

Laboratory findings include low fasting levels of serine and glycine in plasma and very low levels of serine and glycine in CSF. No abnormal organic acid metabolite is found in the urine. MRI of the brain shows cerebral atrophy with enlarged ventricles, significant attenuation of white matter, and impaired myelination. **Diagnosis** can be confirmed by DNA analysis or by measurement of the enzyme activity in cultured fibroblasts. **Treatment** with high doses of serine (200-700 mg/kg/24 hr orally) and glycine (200-300 mg/kg/24 hr) normalizes the serine levels in the blood and CSF. When started postnatally, this treatment may improve seizures, spasticity, and brain myelination. One case report suggests that developmental delay may be prevented if the treatment commences in the 1st days of life or prenatally.

The condition is inherited as an autosomal recessive trait. The gene for 3-phosphoglycerate dehydrogenase enzyme *(PHGDH)* has been mapped to chromosome 1p12. If familial pathogenic variants are known, molecular **prenatal diagnosis** is possible. Administration of serine to the mother carrying an affected fetus was associated with stabilization of the fetal head circumference, as evidenced by ultrasound. Treatment with supplemental serine has continued postnatally; the patient remained normal neurologically at 4 yr of age. The favorable response of this condition to a relatively straightforward treatment makes this diagnosis an important consideration in any child with microcephaly and neurologic defects such as psychomotor delay or a seizure disorder. Measurements of serine and glycine in the CSF are critical for diagnosis because mild decreases of these amino acids in the plasma can be easily overlooked.

PHOSPHOSERINE AMINOTRANSFERASE DEFICIENCY

Phosphoserine aminotransferase 1 **(PSAT1)** catalyzes conversion of 3-phosphohydroxypyruvate to 3-phosphoserine (see Fig. 103.10). Deficiency of this enzyme may present in the neonatal period with poor feeding, cyanotic episodes, and irritability and may progress to intractable, multifocal seizures and microcephaly. Brain imaging may reveal generalized cerebral and cerebellar atrophy. Laboratory studies done on postprandial plasma samples may reveal normal or mildly decreased levels of serine and glycine. Serine and glycine levels are usually more depressed on the CSF amino acid analysis. **Treatment** with serine and glycine as outlined earlier may result in clinical improvement. The condition is inherited as an autosomal recessive trait, and the gene *(PSAT1)* is mapped to chromosome 9q21.2.

3-PHOSPHOSERINE PHOSPHATASE DEFICIENCY

3-Phosphoserine phosphatase catalyzes the final step in the L-serine synthesis converting 3-phosphoserine to L-serine. Deficiency of this enzyme results in a rare disorder with clinical and biochemical findings indistinguishable from the PHGDH and PSAT1 deficiencies. The disorder is caused by autosomal recessive pathogenic variants in *PSPH* mapped to chromosome 7p11.2.

Bibliography is available at Expert Consult.

103.9 Proline

Oleg A. Shchelochkov and Charles P. Venditti

Proline is a nonessential amino acid synthesized endogenously from glutamic acid, ornithine, and arginine (see Fig. 103.9). Proline and hydroxyproline are found in high concentrations in collagen. Normally, neither of these amino acids is found in large quantities in urine. Excretion of proline and hydroxyproline as *iminopeptides* (dipeptides and tripeptides containing proline or hydroxyproline) is increased in disorders of accelerated collagen turnover, such as rickets or hyperparathyroidism. Proline is also found in synapses, where it can interact with glycine and glutamate receptors (see Chapter 103.11). The catabolic pathway of proline and hydroxyproline produces glyoxylic acid, which can be further

metabolized to glycine or oxalic acid (see Fig. 103.8).

Accumulation of proline in tissues is associated with disorders of hyperprolinemia type 1 and hyperprolinemia type 2. Reduced de novo synthesis of proline causes syndromes manifesting with **cutis laxa** (see Fig. 678.8) with **progeroid features** or **spastic paraplegia**. Two types of primary hyperprolinemia have been described.

HYPERPROLINEMIA TYPE I

This rare autosomal recessive condition is caused by deficiency of proline oxidase (proline dehydrogenase; see Fig. 103.9). Most patients with hyperprolinemia type 1 appear asymptomatic, although some may present with intellectual disability, seizures, and behavioral problems. Hyperprolinemia may also be a risk factor for autism spectrum disorders and schizophrenia. The nature of such wide phenotypic range in this biochemical condition has not been elucidated. The gene encoding proline oxidase *(PRODH)* is mapped to 22q11.2 and is located within the critical region for the **velocardiofacial syndrome**. Laboratory studies reveal high concentrations of proline in plasma, urine, and CSF. Increased urinary excretion of hydroxyproline and glycine is also present, which could be related to saturation of the shared tubular reabsorption mechanism due to massive prolinuria.

No effective treatment has yet emerged. Restriction of dietary proline causes modest improvement in plasma proline with no proven clinical benefit.

HYPERPROLINEMIA TYPE II

This is a rare autosomal recessive condition caused by the deficiency of Δ^1-pyrroline-5-carboxylate dehydrogenase (aldehyde dehydrogenase 4; see Fig. 103.9). Intellectual disability and seizures (usually precipitated by an intercurrent infection) have been reported in affected children, but asymptomatic patients have also been described. The cause for such disparate clinical outcomes is incompletely understood. The gene encoding P5C dehydrogenase *(ALDH4A1)* is mapped to chromosome 1p36.13.

Laboratory studies reveal increased concentrations of proline and Δ^1-pyrroline-5-carboxylic acid (P5C) in blood, urine, and CSF. The presence of P5C differentiates this condition from hyperprolinemia type I. Increased level of P5C in body fluids, especially in the CNS, appears to antagonize vitamin B_6 and lead to vitamin B_6 dependency (see Chapter 103.14). Vitamin B_6 dependency may be the main cause of seizures and neurologic findings in this condition and may explain the variability in clinical manifestations in different patients. **Treatment** with high doses of vitamin B_6 is recommended.

PROLIDASE DEFICIENCY

During collagen degradation, imidodipeptides are formed and are normally cleaved by tissue prolidase. Deficiency of prolidase, which is inherited as an autosomal recessive trait, results in the accumulation of imidodipeptides in body fluids. Age at onset varies from 6 mo to the 3rd decade of life.

The **clinical manifestations** of this rare condition also vary and include recurrent, severe, and painful skin ulcers, which are typically on hands and legs. Other skin lesions that may precede ulcers by several years may include a scaly erythematous maculopapular rash, purpura, and telangiectasia. Most ulcers become infected. Healing of the ulcers may take months. Other findings include developmental delays, intellectual disability, organomegaly, anemia, thrombocytopenia, and immune dysfunction resulting in increased susceptibility to infections (recurrent otitis media, sinusitis, respiratory infection, splenomegaly). Some patients may have craniofacial abnormalities such as ptosis, ocular proptosis, hypertelorism, small beaked nose, and prominent cranial sutures. Asymptomatic cases have also been reported. Increased incidence of systemic lupus erythematosus has been noted in children. High levels of urinary excretion of imidodipeptides are diagnostic. The gene for prolidase *(PEPD)* has been mapped to chromosome 19q13.11. The diagnosis can be confirmed using DNA analysis. Enzyme assay may be performed in erythrocytes or cultured skin fibroblasts.

Treatment of prolidase deficiency is supportive. Infectious complications can be fatal and warrant close and proactive antibiotic management.

Oral supplementation with proline, ascorbic acid, and manganese and topical proline and glycine have not been found to be consistently effective in all patients.

DISORDERS OF DE NOVO PROLINE SYNTHESIS

De novo synthesis of proline and ornithine from glutamate appears to be critical in the normal biology of connective tissue and to maintain urea cycle in a repleted state. Correspondingly, clinical manifestations of these disorders encompass connective tissue abnormalities, nervous system abnormalities, and variable biochemical abnormalities reflecting urea cycle dysfunction. This section summarizes clinical and laboratory findings associated with the deficient function of Δ^1-pyrroline-5-carboxylate (P5C) synthase (see Fig. 103.9) encoded by *ALDH18A1* (mapped to 10q24.1) and PSC reductase encoded by *PYCR1* (mapped to 17q25.3).

Deficient activity of P5C synthase has been associated with several phenotypes, including **de Barsy syndrome**, characterized by cataracts, growth retardation, intellectual disability, a prematurely aged appearance (progeroid features), and cutis laxa. Some patients may show pyramidal signs. Skin biopsy may reveal decreased size of elastic fibers and collagen abnormalities. Brain imaging studies show cortical atrophy, ventriculomegaly, and reduced creatine. Laboratory findings include reduced levels of proline, ornithine, citrulline, and arginine as well as mild fasting hyperammonemia. Patients may show only intermittent abnormalities of plasma amino acids, likely related to the time of blood sampling in relation to the last meal. Interestingly, both autosomal recessive and autosomal dominant forms of inheritance have been described. The diagnosis can be suspected in a patient presenting with cutis laxa, developmental delay, mild hyperammonemia, and amino acid abnormalities. The diagnosis can be confirmed using molecular DNA analysis or using the glutamine loading test on skin fibroblasts. Treatment is supportive, although supplementation with citrulline or arginine to address hyperammonemia and cerebral creatine depletion have been proposed.

Deleterious mutations in *PYCR1* result in the abnormal function of the mitochondrial Δ^1-pyrroline-5-carboxylate reductase, which catalyzes the last step in the synthesis of proline from P5C. The most consistent finding in patients carrying proven pathogenic variants in *PYCR1* include triangular facies, cutis laxa (**de Barsy–like syndrome**), joint hypermobility, wrinkled skin, gerodermia osteodysplastica, and progeroid features. Skin biopsy reveals reduction of the elastic fibers and infiltration with inflammatory cells. Some patients may have epilepsy, developmental delays, intellectual disability, cataracts, osteopenia, and failure to thrive. However, many of the affected families are consanguineous, thus confounding the phenotype. Of note, plasma amino acid analysis typically reveals no specific abnormalities. The diagnosis depends on the recognition of the skin findings and can be confirmed using molecular DNA analysis. Available pedigrees of families affected by *PYCR1*-related disorder supports the autosomal recessive mode of inheritance.

Bibliography is available at Expert Consult.

103.10 Glutamic Acid
Oleg A. Shchelochkov and Charles P. Venditti

Glutamic acid and its amide derivative glutamine have a wide range of functions in the body. *Glutamate* plays numerous biologic roles, functioning as a neurotransmitter, an intermediate compound in many fundamental biochemical reactions, and a precursor of an inhibitory neurotransmitter γ-aminobutyric acid (GABA) (see Chapter 103.11). Another major product of glutamate is *glutathione* (γ-glutamylcysteinylglycine). This ubiquitous tripeptide, with its function as the major antioxidant in the body, is synthesized and degraded through a complex cycle called the γ-glutamyl cycle (Fig. 103.11). Because of its free sulfhydryl (–SH) group and its abundance in the cell, glutathione protects other sulfhydryl-containing compounds (e.g., enzymes, coenzyme

A) from oxidation. It is also involved in the detoxification of peroxides, including hydrogen peroxide, and in keeping the intracellular milieu in a reduced state. In addition, glutathione participates in amino acid transport across the cell membrane through the γ-glutamyl cycle.

One of the biochemical manifestations of γ-glutamyl cycle deficiency is increased urinary excretion of 5-oxoproline, which could be the result of both genetic and non-genetic causes. 5-Oxoprolinemia should be routinely considered in the differential diagnosis of **high–anion gap metabolic acidosis** (HAGMA). Two metabolic disorders can present with massive 5-oxoprolinuria: **glutathione synthetase deficiency** and **5-oxoprolinase deficiency** (Fig. 103.11). However, a more common clinical scenario is a transient and mild urinary elevation of 5-oxoproline in urine that can be seen in a variety of metabolic and acquired conditions, such as exposure to acetaminophen and some hydrolyzed-protein formulas, severe burns, Stevens-Johnson syndrome, homocystinuria, urea cycle defects, and tyrosinemia type I.

GLUTATHIONE SYNTHETASE DEFICIENCY

Three forms of this rare condition have been reported. In the **mild form**, enzyme deficiency causes glutathione deficiency only in erythrocytes. These patients present with hemolytic anemia without chronic metabolic acidosis and demonstrate high residual activity of glutathione synthetase on enzymatic testing. A **moderate form** has also been observed in which the hemolytic anemia is associated with variable degrees of metabolic acidosis and 5-oxoprolinuria. Its **severe form** is distinguished by presence of hemolytic anemia accompanied by severe acidosis, massive 5-oxoprolinuria, and neurologic manifestations.

Glutathione Synthetase Deficiency, Severe and Moderate Forms

Affected newborn infants with this rare condition usually develop acute symptoms of metabolic acidosis, jaundice, and mild to moderate hemolytic anemia in the 1st few days of life. Chronic acidosis continues after recovery. Similar episodes of life-threatening acidosis may occur during an infection (e.g., gastroenteritis) or after a surgical procedure. Progressive neurologic damage develops with age, manifested by intellectual disability, spastic tetraparesis, ataxia, tremor, dysarthria, and seizures. Susceptibility to infections, presumably because of granulocyte dysfunction, is observed in some patients. Patients with the moderate form of glutathione synthetase deficiency have milder acidosis and less 5-oxoprolinuria than is seen in the severe form, with no neurologic manifestations.

Laboratory findings include metabolic acidosis, mild to moderate degrees of hemolytic anemia, and 5-oxoprolinuria. High concentrations of 5-oxoproline are also found in blood. The urinary and blood levels of 5-oxoproline is less pronounced in patients with moderate form of the condition. The glutathione content of erythrocytes is markedly decreased. Increased synthesis of 5-oxoproline in this disorder is thought to be the result of the conversion of γ-glutamylcysteine to 5-oxoproline by the enzyme γ-glutamyl cyclotransferase (see Fig. 103.11). γ-Glutamylcysteine production increases greatly because the normal inhibitory effect of glutathione on the γ-glutamylcysteine synthetase enzyme is removed.

Treatment of acute attack includes hydration, correction of acidosis (by infusion of sodium bicarbonate), and measures to correct anemia and hyperbilirubinemia. Chronic administration of alkali is usually needed indefinitely. Supplementation with vitamin C, vitamin E, and selenium is recommended. Drugs and oxidants known to cause hemolysis and stressful catabolic states should be avoided. Oral administration of glutathione analogs has been tried with variable success.

Prenatal diagnosis can be achieved by the measurement of 5-oxoproline in amniotic fluid, by enzyme analysis in cultured amniocytes or chronic villus samples, or by DNA analysis. Successful pregnancy in an affected female (moderate form) has been reported, with favorable outcomes for both mother and infant.

Glutathione Synthetase Deficiency, Mild Form

The mild form has been reported in only a few patients. Mild to moderate hemolytic anemia has been the only clinical finding. Splenomegaly has been reported in some patients. Cognitive development is normal.

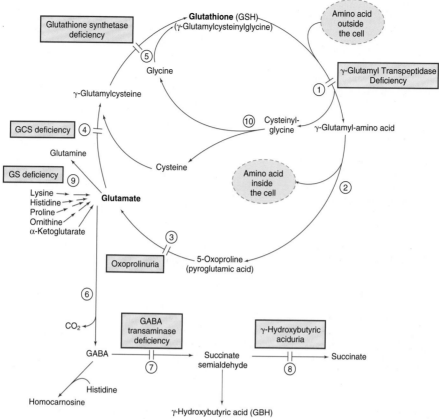

Fig. 103.11 The γ-glutamyl cycle and related pathways. Defects of the glutathione (GSH) synthesis and degradation are noted. **Enzymes:** *(1)* γ-Glutamyl transpeptidase (GGT), *(2)* γ-glutamyl cyclotransferase, *(3)* 5-oxoprolinase, *(4)* γ-glutamyl-cysteine synthetase, *(5)* glutathione synthetase, *(6)* glutamate decarboxylase, *(7)* γ-aminobutyric acid (GABA) transaminase, *(8)* succinate-semialdehyde dehydrogenase, *(9)* glutamine synthetase, *(10)* dipeptidase.

Chronic metabolic acidosis typically is not seen. Some patients can have increased concentrations of 5-oxoproline in the urine. Pathogenic variants in the gene for this enzyme *(GSSD)* appear to decrease the half-life of the enzyme, which causes an increased rate of protein turnover without affecting its catalytic function. The expedited rate of enzyme turnover caused by these pathogenic variants is of little or no consequence for tissues with protein synthetic capability. However, inability of mature erythrocytes to synthesize protein results in glutathione deficiency in the erythrocytes. **Treatment** is that of hemolytic anemia and avoidance of drugs and oxidants that can trigger the hemolytic process.

All forms of glutathione synthetase deficiency are inherited as an autosomal recessive trait. *GSSD* is located on chromosome 20q11.22. **Diagnosis** can be confirmed by DNA analysis or enzyme activity in erythrocytes or skin fibroblasts.

5-Oxoprolinase Deficiency

More than 20 patients with 5-oxoprolinuria (4-10 g/day) caused by 5-oxoprolinase (see Fig. 103.11) deficiency have been described. No specific clinical picture has yet emerged; completely asymptomatic affected individuals have also been identified. It is therefore not clear whether 5-oxoprolinase deficiency is of any clinical consequence. *No treatment is currently recommended.* The gene for the enzyme *(OPLAH)* is on chromosome 8q24.3.

γ-Glutamylcysteine Synthetase Deficiency (Glutamate-Cysteine Ligase Deficiency)

Only a few patients with this enzyme deficiency have been reported. The most consistent clinical manifestation has been mild chronic

hemolytic anemia. Acute attacks of hemolysis have occurred after exposure to sulfonamides. Peripheral neuropathy and progressive spinocerebellar degeneration have been noted in 2 siblings in adulthood. Laboratory findings of chronic hemolytic anemia were present in all patients. Generalized aminoaciduria is also present because the γ-glutamyl cycle is involved in amino acid transport in cells (see Fig. 103.11). **Treatment** should focus on the management of hemolytic anemia and avoidance of drugs and oxidants that may trigger the hemolytic process. The condition is inherited as an autosomal recessive trait; the gene *(GCLC)* is mapped to chromosome 6p12.1.

γ-GLUTAMYL TRANSPEPTIDASE DEFICIENCY (GLUTATHIONEMIA)

γ-Glutamyl transpeptidase (GGT) is present in any cell that has secretory or absorptive functions. It is especially abundant in the kidneys, pancreas, intestines, and liver. The enzyme is also present in the bile. Measurement of GGT in the blood is frequently performed to evaluate liver and bile duct diseases.

GGT deficiency causes elevation in glutathione concentrations in body fluids, but the cellular levels remain normal (see Fig. 103.11). Because only a few patients with GGT deficiency have been reported, the scope of clinical manifestations has not yet been defined. Mild to moderate intellectual disability and severe behavioral problems were observed in 3 patients. However, 1 of 2 sisters with this condition had normal intelligence as an adult, and the other had Prader-Willi syndrome.

Laboratory findings include marked elevations in urinary concentrations of glutathione (up to 1 g/day), γ-glutamylcysteine, and cysteine. None of the reported patients has had generalized aminoaciduria, a finding that would have been expected to occur in this enzyme deficiency (see Fig. 103.11).

Diagnosis can be confirmed by measurement of the enzyme activity in leukocytes or cultured skin fibroblasts. *No effective treatment has been proposed.* The condition is inherited as an apparent autosomal recessive trait. γ-Glutamyl transpeptidases represent a large family of enzymes encoded by at least 7 genes.

GENETIC DISORDERS OF METABOLISM OF γ-AMINOBUTYRIC ACID
See Chapter 103.11.

Bibliography is available at Expert Consult.

103.11 Genetic Disorders of Neurotransmitters
Oleg A. Shchelochkov and Charles P. Venditti

Neurotransmitters are chemical substances released from the axonal end of excited neurons at the synaptic junctions; they mediate initiation and amplification or inhibition of neural impulses. A number of amino acids and their metabolites comprise the bulk of neurotransmitters. Pathogenic variants in genes responsible for the synthesis, transport, or degradation of these substances may cause conditions that manifest neurologic and/or psychiatric abnormalities (Table 103.3). Previously, children affected by disorders of neurotransmitters have been given syndromic diagnoses such as cerebral palsy, epilepsy, parkinsonism, dystonia, or autism. Diagnosis, in most cases, requires specialized laboratory studies of the cerebrospinal fluid (CSF), because some of the neurotransmitters generated in the central nervous system (CNS), dopamine and serotonin, do not cross the blood-brain barrier, and their abnormal concentrations are not detected in the serum or urine.

Table 103.3	Genetic Disorders of Neurotransmitters in Children		
TRANSMITTER	**SYNTHESIS DEFECTS**		**DEGRADATION DEFECTS**
MONOAMINES			
Dopamine	TH deficiency		MAO deficiency
Serotonin and dopamine	AADC deficiency BH₄ deficiency With and without hyperphenylalaninemia		MAO deficiency
Norepinephrine	DβH deficiency		MAO deficiency
GABA	?		GABA transaminase deficiency GHB aciduria
Histamine	HDC deficiency		?
TRANSPORTER PROTEINS			
Dopamine transporter	DAT deficiency		?
Vesicular monoamine transporter	VMAT2 deficiency		?
AMINO ACIDS			
Proline	?		Hyperprolinemia
Serine	3-PGD, PSAT, PSPH deficiencies		?
Glycine	3-PDG, PSAT deficiencies		NKH

AADC, Aromatic L-amino acid decarboxylase; BH₄, tetrahydrobiopterin; DAT, dopamine transporter; DβH, dopamine β-hydroxylase; GABA, γ-aminobutyric acid; GHB, γ-hydroxybutyric acid; HDC, histidine decarboxylase; hyperphe, hyperphenylalaninemia; MAO, monoamine oxidase; NKH, nonketotic hyperglycinemia; 3-PGD, 3-phosphoglycerate dehydrogenase; PSAT, phosphoserine aminotransferase; PSPH, 3-Phosphoserine Phosphatase Deficiency; TH, tyrosine hydroxylase; VMAT2, vesicular monoamine transporter 2.

A growing number of these conditions are being identified; diseases once thought to be rare are now diagnosed with increasing frequency.

TYROSINE HYDROXYLASE DEFICIENCY (INFANTILE PARKINSONISM, AUTOSOMAL RECESSIVE DOPA-RESPONSIVE DYSTONIA, AUTOSOMAL RECESSIVE SEGAWA SYNDROME)
Tyrosine hydroxylase catalyzes the formation of L-dopa from tyrosine. Deficiency of this enzyme results in deficiencies of dopamine and norepinephrine (see Fig. 103.2). The differential diagnosis includes a wide range of inherited dystonias, including autosomal dominant dystonia caused by GTP cyclohydrolase 1 deficiency.

Clinical manifestations range from mild to very severe. In general, 2 phenotypes have been recognized. In the **mild** form (dopa-responsive dystonia, or **type A**), symptoms of unilateral limb dystonia causing gait incoordination and postural tremor occur in childhood and worsen with age if the condition remains untreated. Diurnal variation of symptoms (worse at the end of the day) may be present. Cognitive development is usually normal.

In the **severe** form of tyrosine hydroxylase deficiency (infantile parkinsonism, infantile encephalopathy, or **type B**), the clinical manifestations occur at birth or shortly thereafter and include microcephaly, developmental delay, involuntary movements of the limbs with spasticity, dystonia, ptosis, expressionless face, oculogyric crises (upward eye-rolling movements), and autonomic dysfunction (temperature instability, excessive sweating, hypoglycemia, salivation, tremor, gastrointestinal reflux, constipation). Brisk reflexes, myoclonus, athetosis, and distal chorea may be present. The patient with the severe form usually shows incomplete response to treatment with L-dopa and is prone to developing L-dopa–induced dyskinesia as a side effect.

Laboratory findings include reduced levels of dopamine and its metabolite homovanillic acid (HVA) and normal concentrations of tetrahydrobiopterin (BH₄), neopterin, and 5-hydroxyindoleacetic acid (5-HIAA, a metabolite of serotonin) in the CSF. Serum prolactin levels are usually elevated. These findings are not diagnostic of the condition; diagnosis should be established by molecular gene analysis.

Treatment with L-dopa/carbidopa results in significant clinical improvement in most patients, but the severe forms are invariably associated with L-dopa–induced dyskinesias. To minimize the side effects of therapy, the treatment should be started with a low dose and increased very slowly, if needed. Other therapeutic interventions include anticholinergics, serotonergic agents, and monoamine oxidase (MAO) B inhibitors, including amantadine, biperiden, and selegiline. Bilateral subthalamic nucleus deep brain stimulation has shown clinical efficacy in one case. Tyrosine hydroxylase deficiency is inherited as an autosomal-recessive trait. Molecular testing for pathogenic variants in the *TH* gene is available clinically.

AROMATIC L-AMINO ACID DECARBOXYLASE DEFICIENCY
Aromatic L-amino acid decarboxylase (AADC) is a vitamin B₆–dependent enzyme that catalyzes the decarboxylation of both 5-hydroxytryptophan to form serotonin (see Fig. 103.5) and L-dopa to generate dopamine, (see Fig. 103.2). **Clinical manifestations** are related to reduced availability of dopamine and serotonin. Poor feeding, lethargy, hypotension, hypothermia, oculogyric crises, and ptosis have been observed in affected neonates. Clinical findings in infants and older children include developmental delay, truncal hypotonia with hypertonia of limbs, oculogyric crises, extrapyramidal movements (choreoathetosis, dystonia, myoclonus), and autonomic abnormalities (sweating, salivation, irritability, temperature instability, hypotension). Symptoms may have a diurnal variation, becoming worse by the end of the day.

Laboratory findings include decreased concentrations of dopamine and serotonin and their metabolites (HVA, 5-HIAA, norepinephrine, vanillylmandelic acid [VMA]) and increased levels of 5-hydroxytryptophan, L-dopa, and its metabolite (3-O-methyldopa) in body fluids, especially in CSF. Elevated serum concentrations of prolactin (a result of dopamine deficiency) have also been observed. MRI of the brain reveals cerebral atrophy with degenerative changes in the white matter. A urine screening program, focused on 3-*O*-methyl-dopa and VMA, has demonstrated diagnostic promise in high-disease prevalence populations.

Treatment with neurotransmitter precursors has produced limited clinical improvement. Dopamine and serotonin have no therapeutic value because of their inability to cross the blood-brain barrier. Dopamine agonists (L-dopa/carbidopa, bromocriptine), MAO inhibitors (tranylcypromine), serotonergic agents and high doses of pyridoxine, a cofactor for AADC enzyme, have been tried. Pyridoxine supplementation in patients harboring the p.S250F variant in AADC may be beneficial. The recent demonstration of CNS-directed gene therapy with an adeno-associated viral vector has shown benefit in some patients. Preimplantation genetic diagnosis after in vitro fertilization has been achieved in the high-prevalence Taiwanese population. The gene encoding AADC (*DDC*) is on chromosome 7p12.1. The condition is inherited as an autosomal recessive trait.

TETRAHYDROBIOPTERIN DEFICIENCY
See Chapter 103.1.

BH$_4$ is the cofactor for phenylalanine hydroxylase (see Fig. 103.1), tyrosine hydroxylase (see Fig. 103.2), tryptophan hydroxylase (see Fig. 103.5), and nitric oxide synthase. It is synthesized from GTP in many tissues (see Fig. 103.1). Deficiencies of enzymes involved in the biosynthesis of BH$_4$ result in inadequate production of this cofactor, which causes deficiencies of monoamine neurotransmitters with or without concomitant hyperphenylalaninemia.

Tetrahydrobiopterin Deficiency With Hyperphenylalaninemia
See Chapter 103.1.

Tetrahydrobiopterin Deficiency Without Hyperphenylalaninemia
GTP Cyclohydrolase 1 Deficiency (Hereditary Progressive Dystonia, Autosomal Dominant Dopa-Responsive Dystonia, Autosomal Dominant Segawa Syndrome)
This form of dystonia, caused by guanosine triphosphate (GTP) cyclohydrolase 1 deficiency, is inherited as an autosomal dominant trait and is more common in females than males (4 : 1 ratio) (see Chapter 615.4). **Clinical manifestations** usually start in early childhood with tremor and dystonia of the lower limbs (**toe gait**), which may spread to all extremities within a few years. Torticollis, dystonia of the arms, and poor coordination may precede dystonia of the lower limbs. Early development is generally normal. Symptoms have an impressive diurnal variation, becoming worse by the end of the day and improving with sleep. Autonomic instability is not uncommon. Parkinsonism may also be present or develop with advancing age. Late presentation in adult life has also been reported, associated with **action dystonia** ("writer's cramp"), torticollis, or generalized rigid hypertonia with tremor but without postural dystonia. Additionally, limited data on adults suggest symptoms related to serotonin deficiency (sleep disturbance, cognitive impairment, impulsivity).

Laboratory findings show reduced levels of BH$_4$ and neopterin in the CSF without hyperphenylalaninemia (see Chapter 103.1). Dopamine and its metabolite (HVA) may also be reduced in CSF. The serotonergic pathway is less affected by this enzyme deficiency; thus concentrations of serotonin and its metabolites are usually normal. Plasma phenylalanine is normal, but an oral phenylalanine loading test (100 mg/kg) produces an abnormally high plasma phenylalanine level with an elevated phenylalanine/tyrosine ratio. The ratio, obtained at the 2-3 hr after the load, in combination with urine neopterin level, has optimal diagnostic specificity and sensitivity. The existence of asymptomatic carriers indicates that other factors or genes may play a role in pathogenesis. The asymptomatic carrier may be identified by the phenylalanine loading test. **Diagnosis** may be confirmed by reduced levels of BH$_4$ and neopterin in CSF, measurement of the enzyme activity, and molecular genetic analysis (see Chapter 103.1). Clinically, the condition should be differentiated from other causes of dystonias and childhood parkinsonism, especially tyrosine hydroxylase, sepiapterin reductase, and aromatic

amino acid decarboxylase deficiencies.

Treatment with L-dopa/carbidopa usually produces dramatic clinical improvement. Oral administration of BH$_4$ is also effective but is rarely used. The gene for GTP cyclohydroxylase 1 (*GCH1*) is located on chromosome 14q22.2.

Sepiapterin Reductase Deficiency
Sepiapterin reductase is involved in conversion of 6-pyruvoyl-tetrahydropterin to BH$_4$. It also participates in the salvage pathway of BH$_4$ synthesis (see Fig. 103.1). Sepiapterin reductase deficiency results in accumulation of 6-lactoyl-tetrahydropterin, which can be converted to sepiapterin nonenzymatically. The majority of sepiapterin is metabolized to BH$_4$ through the salvage pathway in peripheral tissues (see Fig. 103.1), but because of the low activity of dihydrofolate reductase in brain, the amount of BH$_4$ remains insufficient for proper synthesis of dopamine and serotonin. This explains the absence of hyperphenylalaninemia and the often-delayed diagnosis.

Clinical manifestations usually appear within a few months of life. Cardinal manifestations include paroxysmal stiffening, oculogyric crises, and hypotonia. Additional findings include motor and language delays, weakness, limb hypertonia, dystonia, hyperreflexia, and early-onset parkinsonism. The symptoms usually have a diurnal variation. Misdiagnosis as cerebral palsy is common and a wide variability of symptoms have been reported. **Diagnosis** is established by measurement of CSF neurotransmitters and pterin metabolites, which reveal decreased dopamine, HVA, norepinephrine, and 5-HIAA and marked elevations of sepiapterin and dihydrobiopterin. The serum concentration of prolactin may be elevated. The phenylalanine loading test may have diagnostic utility. Diagnosis may be confirmed by molecular genetic analysis or enzyme assay in fibroblasts. **Treatment** with slowly increasing doses of L-dopa/carbidopa and 5-hydroxytryptophan usually produces dramatic clinical improvement. The condition is inherited as an autosomal recessive trait; the gene *SPR* encoding sepiapterin reductase is located on chromosome 2p13.2.

DOPAMINE β-HYDROXYLASE DEFICIENCY
Dopamine β-hydroxylase catalyzes the conversion of dopamine to norepinephrine (see Fig. 103.2). The deficiency of this enzyme results in reduced or absent synthesis of norepinephrine, leading to dysregulation of the sympathetic function. Infants and children may present with difficulty opening eyes, ptosis, hypotension, hypothermia, hypoglycemia, and nasal stuffiness. Adult patients may present with profound deficits of autonomic regulation, resulting in severe orthostatic hypotension, and sexual dysfunction in males. Presyncopal symptomatology includes dizziness, blurred vision, dyspnea, nuchal discomfort, and chest pain; olfactory function remains relatively intact. The **diagnosis** can be aided by performing autonomic function testing (measurement of the sinus arrhythmia ratio, blood pressure studies during controlled hyperventilation, Valsalva maneuver, cold pressor, handgrip exercise). **Laboratory findings** include decreased or absent norepinephrine and epinephrine and their metabolites, with elevated levels of dopamine and its metabolite (HVA), in plasma, CSF, and urine. Elevated plasma dopamine may be pathognomonic for this disease. MRI of the brain shows decreased brain volume, consistent with the neurotrophic role of norepinephrine. **Treatment** with L-dihydroxyphenylserine, which is converted to norepinephrine directly in vivo by the action of AADC, leads to significant improvement in orthostatic hypotension and normalizes noradrenaline and its metabolites. The condition is inherited as an autosomal recessive trait; the gene (*DBH*) encoding dopamine β-hydroxylase resides on chromosome 9q34.2.

MONOAMINE OXIDASE A DEFICIENCY
Human genome encodes 2 monoamine oxidase (MAO) isoenzymes: MAO A and MAO B. Both enzymes catalyze oxidative deamination of most biogenic amines in the body, including serotonin (see Fig. 103.5), norepinephrine, epinephrine, and dopamine (see Fig. 103.2). The genes for both isoenzymes are on the X chromosome (Xp11.3), residing in close proximity. A deletion of both genes can also encompass a neighboring gene, *NDP*, resulting in a contiguous deletion syndrome, which can

present as an atypical **Norrie disease** (see Chapter 640). Male patients with MAO A deficiency manifest borderline intellectual deficiency and impaired impulse control. The consequences of the isolated MAO B deficiency are incompletely understood. Combined MAO A and B deficiency causes severe intellectual disability and behavioral problems and can be associated with pronounced laboratory abnormalities (e.g., 4-6–fold serotonin elevation in physiologic fluids, elevated *O*-methylated amine metabolites, and reduced deamination products [VMA, HVA]). Dietary intervention (low tyramine, phenylethylamine, and L-dopa/dopamine intake) did not improve patients' blood serotonin levels. Inheritance of MAO deficiency is X-linked. **Treatment** of MAO A deficiency is supportive.

DISORDERS OF γ-AMINOBUTYRIC ACID (GABA) METABOLISM
GABA is the main inhibitory neurotransmitter synthesized in the synapses through decarboxylation of glutamic acid by glutamate decarboxylase (GAD). The same pathway is responsible for production of GABA in other organs, especially the kidneys and the β-cells of the pancreas. GAD enzyme requires pyridoxine (vitamin B_6) as cofactor. Two GAD enzymes, GAD1 (GAD_{67}) and GAD2 (GAD_{65}) have been identified. **GAD1** is the main enzyme in the brain, and **GAD2** is the major enzyme in the β-cells. Antibodies against GAD_{65} and GAD_{67} have been implicated in the development of type 1 diabetes and **stiff-person syndrome**, respectively. GABA is catabolized to succinic acid by 2 enzymes, GABA transaminase and succinic semialdehyde dehydrogenase (SSADH) (see Fig. 103.11).

γ-Aminobutyric Acid Transaminase Deficiency
Clinical manifestations in the 2 index infant siblings included severe psychomotor retardation, hypotonia, hyperreflexia, lethargy, refractory seizures, and increased linear growth likely related to GABA-mediated increased secretion of growth hormone. Increased concentrations of GABA and β-alanine were found in CSF (see Fig. 103.11). Evidence of leukodystrophy was noted in the postmortem examination of the brain. A 3rd patient showed severe psychomotor retardation, recurrent episodic lethargy, and intractable seizures with comparable CSF metabolite abnormalities to those of the index probands. GABA transaminase deficiency is demonstrated in brain and lymphocytes. **Treatment** is symptomatic. Intervention with vitamin B_6, the cofactor for the enzyme, was without therapeutic benefit. The gene *(ABAT)*, maps to chromosome 16p13.2; the condition is inherited as an autosomal recessive trait.

Succinic Semialdehyde Dehydrogenase Deficiency (γ-Hydroxybutyric Aciduria)
Clinical manifestations of SSADH deficiency usually begin in infancy with developmental delays with a disproportionate deficit in expressive language, hypotonia, and ataxia; seizures occur in approximately 50% of patients (see Fig. 103.11). Many patients also carry the diagnosis of **autism spectrum disorder**. Neuropsychiatric comorbidity (especially oppositional defiance, obsession-compulsion, and hyperactivity) can be disabling, particularly in adolescents and adults. Abnormal EEG findings include background slowing and generalized spike-wave paroxysms, with variable lateralization in hemispheric onset and voltage predominance. Photosensitivity and electrographic status epilepticus of sleep have been reported in combination with difficulties in sleep maintenance and excessive daytime somnolence. MRI of the brain shows an increased T2-weighted hyperintensity involving the globus pallidi, cerebellar dentate nuclei, and subthalamic nuclei, usually in a bilaterally symmetric distribution.

The biochemical hallmark, γ-hydroxybutyric acid (GHB), is elevated in physiologic fluids (CSF, plasma, urine) in all patients. Increased concentrations of GABA are also found in CSF. Heightened diagnostic suspicion evolves through documentation of elevated urinary GHB, and confirmation is achieved by molecular genetic testing.

Treatment remains elusive; vigabatrin (GABA-transaminase inhibitor) has been employed empirically, with mixed outcomes, and there is

concern with its use as it further elevates CNS GABA in an already hyper-GABAergic disorder. Additionally, vigabatrin can cause constriction of the visual field and long-term use is contraindicated.

The gene for SSADH *(ALDH5A1)* is located on chromosome 6p22, and inheritance follows an autosomal-recessive pattern. **Prenatal diagnosis** has been achieved by measurement of GHB in the amniotic fluid, assay of the enzyme activity in the amniocytes, chorionic villus sampling, or DNA analysis.

DEFECTS IN NEUROTRANSMITTER TRANSPORTER PROTEINS
More than 20 different proteins are involved in transporting different neurotransmitters across the neuronal membranes. The main function of most of these transporters is to remove the excess neurotransmitters from the synaptic junction back into the presynaptic neurons (reuptake). This recycling process not only regulates the precise effect of neurotransmitters at the synaptic junction, but also resupplies the presynaptic neurons with neurotransmitters for future use. A few transporter proteins are involved in shuttling neurotransmitters from the neuronal cytoplasm across the membrane of synaptic vesicles for storage (vesicular transporters). On neuronal stimulation, these vesicles release a bolus of neurotransmitters through exocytosis. As expected, pathogenic variants in transporter proteins interfere with the proper reuptake and storage of neurotransmitters and may result in clinical manifestations similar to those seen in deficiencies of neurotransmitters metabolism. Several conditions caused by pathogenic variants of neurotransmitter protein transporters have been described, including dopamine transporter protein deficiency and dopamine-serotonin vesicular transporter disease.

Dopamine Transporter Protein Deficiency
This transporter protein is involved in reuptake of dopamine by the presynaptic neurons, and its deficiency causes depletion of dopamine and thus a dopamine deficiency state. Dopamine transporter protein (DAT) is encoded by *SLC6A3* gene on chromosome 5p15.33. Pathogenic variants of this gene has been reported in 13 children. These children presented with symptoms of infantile **parkinsonism-dystonia syndrome**. Irritability and feeding difficulties started shortly after birth and progressed to hypotonia, lack of head control, parkinsonism, dystonia, and global developmental delay by early infancy. Brain MRI usually shows no abnormalities.

CSF examination revealed elevation of HVA and normal level of 5-HIAAs. The urinary level of HVA and serum concentration of prolactin were increased. Diagnosis was established by demonstrating the loss-of-function mutation in the *SLC6A3* gene. *No effective treatment* has been identified; L-dopa/carbidopa did not result in improvements in clinical or biochemical parameters.

Dopamine-Serotonin Vesicular Transporter Disease (Vesicular Monoamine Transporter Deficiency)
This autosomal recessive condition, described in 8 children from a consanguineous Saudi Arabian family, is caused by a pathogenic variant in the *SLC18A2* gene. This gene encodes the vesicular monoamine transporter 2 (VMAT2), which is involved in transporting dopamine and serotonin from the cytoplasm into the synaptic storage vesicles located in the axonal terminals of the presynaptic neurons. Most affected children presented in the 1st yr of life with symptoms consistent with deficiencies of dopamine (hypotonia progressing into dystonia, parkinsonism, oculogyric crises), serotonin (sleep and psychiatric disturbances), and norepinephrine-epinephrine (excessive sweating, tremors, temperature instability, postural hypotension, ptosis). Neurocognitive delays become apparent in the 1st yr of life. No diurnal variation of the symptoms was noted. Brain imaging studies were within normal limits. Changes in the levels of CNS neurotransmitters and their metabolites have been inconsistent.

The phenotype resembles that seen in AADC and BH_4 deficiencies (see earlier). Diagnosis requires molecular analysis of *SLC18A2* (located on chromosome 10q25.3). **Treatment** with L-dopa/carbidopa caused exacerbation of symptoms, whereas pramipexole, a dopamine receptor agonist, resulted in a promising clinical response.

HISTIDINE DECARBOXYLASE DEFICIENCY

Decarboxylation of histidine by histidine decarboxylase produces histamine, which functions as a neurotransmitter in the brain. Deficiency of this enzyme (expressed mainly in the posterior hypothalamus) results in deficiency of histamine in the CNS and in one family caused an autosomal dominant form of Tourette syndrome (see Chapter 103.13).

HYPERPROLINEMIA

Intellectual disability and seizures are common findings in most patients with hyperprolinemia types I and II. Patients with **type I** hyperprolinemia typically show a benign clinical course but could have an increased risk of developing schizophrenia. The contribution of increased concentration of proline to the mechanisms of schizophrenia, however, remains unclear. The neurologic abnormalities observed in hyperprolinemia **type II** are mainly caused by development of vitamin B_6 dependency in this condition (see Chapter 103.9). Dietary intervention in hyperprolinemias type I and II is neither feasible nor recommended.

3-PHOSPHOGLYCERATE DEHYDROGENASE DEFICIENCY

See Chapter 103.8.

PHOSPHOSERINE AMINOTRANSFERASE DEFICIENCY

See Chapter 103.8.

NONKETOTIC HYPERGLYCINEMIA

See Chapter 103.7.

Bibliography is available at Expert Consult.

103.12 Urea Cycle and Hyperammonemia (Arginine, Citrulline, Ornithine)

Oleg A. Shchelochkov and Charles P. Venditti

Catabolism of amino acids results in the production of free ammonia, which in high concentration is toxic to the CNS. Mammals detoxify ammonia to urea through a series of reactions known as the **urea cycle** (Fig. 103.12), which is composed of 5 enzymes: carbamoyl phosphate synthetase 1 (**CPS1**), ornithine transcarbamylase (**OTC**), argininosuccinate synthetase (**ASS**), argininosuccinate lyase (**ASL**), and arginase 1. A 6th enzyme, *N*-acetylglutamate (NAG) synthetase (**NAGS**), catalyzes synthesis of NAG, which is an obligatory activator (effector) of the CPS1 enzyme. Individual deficiencies of these enzymes have been observed and, with an overall estimated prevalence of 1 in 35,000 live births, they are the most common genetic causes of hyperammonemia in infants.

GENETIC CAUSES OF HYPERAMMONEMIA

Hyperammonemia, sometimes severe, occurs in inborn errors of metabolism other than the urea cycle defects (Table 103.4; see also Table 102.5). The mechanisms of hyperammonemia in some of these conditions are diverse and include accumulation of toxic metabolites (e.g., organic acids), impaired transport of urea cycle intermediates (e.g., HHH syndrome), or depletion of urea cycle intermediates (e.g., lysinuric protein intolerance), leading to compromised function of the urea cycle.

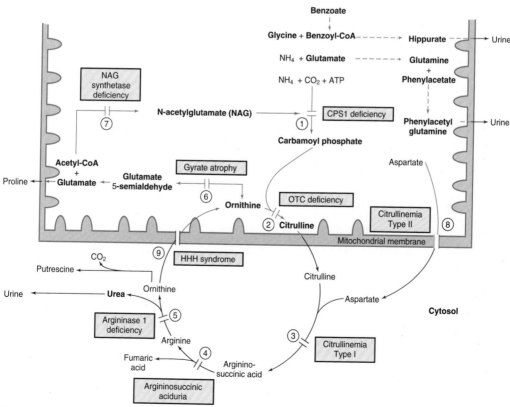

Fig. 103.12 Urea cycle: pathways for ammonia disposal and ornithine metabolism. Reactions occurring in the mitochondria are depicted in *purple*. Reactions shown with *interrupted arrows* are the alternate pathways for the disposal of ammonia. **Enzymes:** *(1)* Carbamyol phosphate synthetase type 1 (CPS1), *(2)* ornithine transcarbamylase (OTC), *(3)* argininosuccinate synthetase (ASS), *(4)* Argininosuccinate lyase (ASL), *(5)* arginase 1, *(6)* ornithine aminotransferase, *(7) N*-acetylglutamate (NAG) synthetase, *(8)* citrin, *(9)* ornithine transporter (ORNT1). HHH syndrome, Hyperammonemia-hyperornithinemia-homocitrullinemia.

Table 103.4	Inborn Errors of Metabolism Causing Hyperammonemia

Deficiencies of the urea cycle enzymes
  Carbamyl phosphate synthetase 1
  Ornithine transcarbamylase
  Argininosuccinate synthetase
  Argininosuccinate lyase
  Arginase 1
  N-acetylglutamate synthetase
Organic acidemias
  Propionic acidemia
  Methylmalonic acidemia
  Isovaleric acidemia
  β-Ketothiolase deficiency
  Multiple carboxylase deficiencies
  Medium-chain fatty acid acyl-CoA dehydrogenase deficiency
  Glutaric acidemia type I
  3-Hydroxy-3-methylglutaric aciduria
Lysinuric protein intolerance
Hyperammonemia-hyperornithinemia-homocitrullinemia syndrome
Transient hyperammonemia of the newborn
Congenital hyperinsulinism with hyperammonemia

CLINICAL MANIFESTATIONS OF HYPERAMMONEMIA

In the **neonatal period**, symptoms and signs are mostly related to brain dysfunction and are similar regardless of the cause of the hyperammonemia. The affected infant appears normal at birth but becomes symptomatic following the introduction of dietary protein. Refusal to eat, vomiting, tachypnea, and lethargy can quickly progress to a deep coma. Seizures are common. Physical examination may reveal hepatomegaly in addition to obtundation. Hyperammonemia can trigger increased intracranial pressure that may be manifested by a bulging fontanelle and dilated pupils.

In **infants and older children**, acute hyperammonemia is manifested by vomiting and neurologic abnormalities such as ataxia, confusion, agitation, irritability, combativeness, and psychosis. These manifestations may alternate with periods of lethargy and somnolence that may progress to coma.

Routine laboratory studies show no specific findings when hyperammonemia is caused by defects of the urea cycle enzymes. Blood urea nitrogen is usually low in these patients. Some patients may initially present with unexplained elevated serum alanine transaminase (ALT) and aspartate transaminase (AST) and even meet the criteria for acute liver failure. In infants with organic acidemias, hyperammonemia is commonly associated with severe *acidosis* as well as *ketonuria*. Newborn infants with hyperammonemia are often misdiagnosed as having sepsis; they may succumb without a correct diagnosis. Neuroimaging may reveal cerebral edema. Autopsy may reveal microvesicular steatosis, mild cholestasis, and fibrosis of the liver. Thus, because of the nonspecific presentation or urea cycle disorders, it is imperative to measure plasma ammonia levels in any ill infant with severe sepsis, unexplained liver dysfunction, recurrent emesis, or progressive encephalopathy.

DIAGNOSIS

The main criterion for diagnosis is hyperammonemia. Each clinical laboratory should establish its own normal values for blood ammonia. Normal newborn values are higher than those of the older child or adult. Levels as high as 100 μmol/L can occur in healthy term infants. An ill infant usually manifests a blood ammonia level >150 μmol/L. Fig. 103.13 illustrates an approach to the differential diagnosis of hyperammonemia in the newborn infant. Careful inspection of individual plasma amino acids usually reveals abnormalities that may help the diagnosis. In patients with deficiencies of CPS1, OTC, or NAGS, frequent findings include elevations in plasma glutamine and alanine with concurrent decrements in citrulline and arginine. These disorders cannot be differentiated from

one another by the plasma amino acid levels alone. A marked increase in urinary orotic acid in patients with OTC deficiency helps differentiate this defect from CPS1 deficiency. Differentiation between the CPS1 deficiency and the NAGS deficiency may require an assay of the respective enzymes or molecular analysis of the relevant genes. Clinical improvement occurring after oral administration of carbamylglutamate, however, may suggest NAGS deficiency. Patients with a deficiency of ASS, ASL, or arginase 1 have marked increases in the plasma levels of citrulline, argininosuccinic acid, or arginine, respectively. The combination of hyperammonemia and marked hypercitrullinemia or argininosuccinic acidemia is virtually pathognomonic for these disorders. Children with urea cycle defects often self-select a low-protein, high-carbohydrate diet, especially those with late-onset disease or symptomatic females with partial OTC deficiency.

Mass screening of newborn infants identifies patients with ASS, ASL, and arginase 1 deficiencies.

TREATMENT OF ACUTE HYPERAMMONEMIA

Clinical outcome depends mainly on the severity and the duration of hyperammonemia. Serious neurologic sequelae are likely in newborns with severe elevations in blood ammonia (>300 μmol/L) for more than 12 hr. Thus, acute hyperammonemia should be treated promptly and vigorously. The goal of therapy is to lower the concentration of ammonia. This is accomplished by (1) removal of ammonia from the body in a form other than urea and (2) minimizing endogenous protein breakdown and favoring endogenous protein synthesis by providing adequate calories and essential amino acids (Table 103.5). Fluid, electrolytes, glucose (10–15%), and lipids (1-2 g/kg/24 hr) should be infused intravenously, together with minimal amounts of protein (0.25 g/kg/24 hr), preferably including essential amino acids. Oral feeding with a low-protein formula (0.5-1.0 g/kg/24 hr) through a nasogastric tube should be started as soon as sufficient improvement is seen.

Because the kidneys clear ammonia poorly, its removal from the body must be expedited by formation of compounds with a high renal clearance. An important advance in the treatment of hyperammonemia has been the introduction of **acylation therapy** by using an exogenous organic acid that is acylated endogenously with nonessential amino acids to form a nontoxic compound with high renal clearance. The main organic acids used for this purpose are sodium salts of benzoic acid and phenylacetic acid. **Benzoate** forms hippurate with endogenous glycine in the liver (see Fig. 103.12). Each mole of benzoate removes 1 mole of ammonia as glycine. **Phenylacetate** conjugates with glutamine to form phenylacetylglutamine, which is readily excreted in the urine. One mole of phenylacetate removes 2 moles of ammonia as glutamine from the body (see Fig. 103.12). Sodium phenylbutyrate, metabolized to phenylacetate, is the primary oral formulation. For intravenous (IV) use, a combined formulation of benzoate and phenylacetate (Ammonul) is commercially available.

Another valuable therapeutic adjunct is IV infusion of **arginine**, which is effective in all patients (except those with arginase deficiency). Arginine administration supplies the urea cycle with ornithine (see Fig. 103.12). In patients with citrullinemia, 1 mole of arginine reacts with 1 mole of ammonia (as carbamoyl phosphate) to form citrulline. In patients with argininosuccinic acidemia, 2 moles of ammonia (as carbamoyl phosphate and aspartate) react with arginine to form argininosuccinic acid. Citrulline and argininosuccinate are less toxic than ammonia and more readily excreted by the kidneys. In patients with CPS1 or OTC deficiencies arginine administration is indicated because this amino acid is not produced in sufficient amounts to enable endogenous protein synthesis. For enteral therapy, patients with OTC deficiency benefit from supplementation with *citrulline* (200 mg/kg/24 hr) because 1 mole of citrulline reacts with 1 mole of ammonia (through aspartic acid) to form arginine. Administration of arginine or citrulline is contraindicated in patients with **arginase deficiency**, a rare condition in which the usual presenting clinical picture is spastic diplegia rather than hyperammonemia. Arginine therapy is of no benefit if hyperammonemia is secondary to an organic acidemia. In a newborn infant with an initial episode of hyperammonemia, arginine should be used until the diagnosis is established (see Table 103.5).

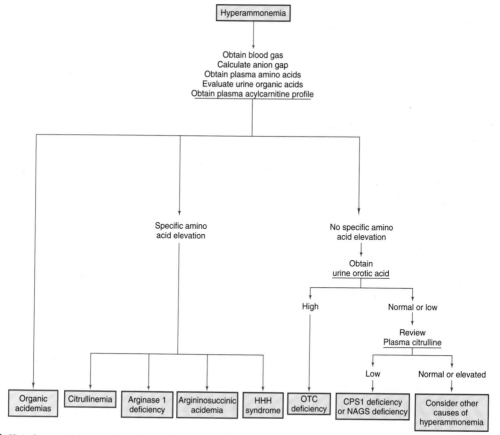

Fig. 103.13 Clinical approach to a newborn infant with symptomatic hyperammonemia. CPS1, Carbamoyl phosphate synthetase 1; HHH syndrome, hyperornithinemia-hyperammonemia-homocitrullinemia; NAGS, N-acetylglutamate synthetase; OTC, ornithine carbamoyltransferase.

Benzoate, phenylacetate, and arginine may be administered together for maximal therapeutic effect. A priming dose of these compounds is followed by continuous infusion until recovery from the acute state occurs. Both benzoate and phenylacetate are usually supplied as concentrated solutions and should be properly diluted (1–2% solution) for IV use. The recommended therapeutic doses of both compounds deliver a substantial amount of sodium to the patient; this amount should be included in calculation of the daily sodiumn requirement. Benzoate and phenylacetate (or the combined formulation, Ammonul) should be used with caution in newborn infants with hyperbilirubinemia because they may displace bilirubin from albumin; however, there are no documented cases of kernicterus (see Chapter 123.4) reported in neonates with hyperammonemia who have received such therapies. In infants at risk, it is advisable to reduce bilirubin to a safe level while considering IV administration of benzoate or phenylacetate.

If the initial ammonia level is <500 μmol/L, and if the foregoing therapies fail within 4-6 hr to produce any appreciable change in the blood ammonia level, **hemodialysis** should be used. For patients presenting with an ammonia level >500 μmol/L, extracorporeal detoxification is the initial method of ammonia removal. Exchange transfusion has little effect on reducing total body ammonia. It should be used only if dialysis cannot be employed promptly or when the patient is a newborn infant with hyperbilirubinemia (see earlier). Hemodialysis dramatically lowers blood ammonia within a few hours, but if it is unavailable or technically unfeasible, peritoneal dialysis may be used as an alternative. When hyperammonemia is caused by an organic acidemia and hemodialysis is not available, peritoneal dialysis can be used to remove both the offending organic acid and ammonia.

Table 103.5	Treatment of Acute Hyperammonemia in an Infant

1. Provide adequate calories, fluid, and electrolytes intravenously (10% glucose, NaCl* and intravenous lipids 1 g/kg/24 hr). Add minimal amounts of protein preferably as a mixture of essential amino acids (0.25 g/kg/24 hr) during the 1st 24 hr of therapy.
2. Give priming doses of the following compounds:
   (To be added to 20 mL/kg of 10% glucose and infused within 1-2 hr)
   • Sodium benzoate 250 mg/kg[†]
   • Sodium phenylacetate 250 mg/kg[†]
   • Arginine hydrochloride 200-600 mg/kg as a 10% solution
3. Continue infusion of sodium benzoate[†] (250-500 mg/kg/24 hr), sodium phenylacetate[†] (250-500 mg/kg/24 hr), and arginine (200-600 mg/kg/24 hr[‡]) following the above priming doses. These compounds should be added to the daily intravenous fluid.
4. Initiate peritoneal dialysis or hemodialysis if above treatment fails to produce an appreciable decrease in plasma ammonia.

*The concentration of sodium chloride should be calculated to be 0.45–0.9%, including the amount of the sodium in the drugs.
[†]Sodium from these drugs should be included as part of the daily sodium requirement.
[‡]The higher dose is recommended in the treatment of patients with citrullinemia and argininosuccinic aciduria. Arginine is not recommended in patients with arginase deficiency and in those whose hyperammonemia is secondary to organic acidemia. Sodium benzoate and sodium phenylacetate should be used with caution in patients with organic acidemias.

Oral administration of **neomycin** limits growth of intestinal bacteria that can produce ammonia. However, this modality is of limited use in patients (e.g., affected neonates) in whom reduction of hyperammonemia is an urgent priority. Oral **lactulose** acidifies the intestinal lumen, thereby reducing the diffusion of ammonia across the intestinal epithelium. This agent is of limited applicability in newborns, who have a high risk of acidemia and dehydration.

There has been interest in the use of **cooling** as a therapeutic adjunct in newborn infants with metabolic encephalopathy such as that caused by hyperammonemia. Clinical studies are in progress to evaluate the efficacy of this approach. There may be considerable lag between the normalization of ammonia level and an improvement in the patient's neurologic status. Several days may be needed before the infant becomes fully alert.

Long-Term Therapy

Once the infant is alert, therapy should be tailored to the underlying cause of the hyperammonemia. In general, all patients, regardless of the enzymatic defect, require protein restriction limited to age-adjusted recommended dietary allowance (RDA). In pediatric patients with defects in the urea cycle, chronic administration of sodium benzoate (250 mg/kg/24 hr), sodium phenylbutyrate (250-500 mg/kg/24 hr), and arginine (200-400 mg/kg/24 hr) or citrulline (in patients with OTC deficiency, 200-400 mg/kg/24 hr) is effective in maintaining blood ammonia levels within the normal range (shown doses are for patients who weigh <20 kg). Arginine and citrulline are contraindicated in patients with argininemia. Patients who have difficulty taking sodium phenylbutyrate can receive a trial of glycerol phenylbutyrate. This compound conceals the offensive odor of sodium phenylbutyrate and may help with patient adherence. Glycerol phenylbutyrate is not yet approved for use in children <2 months of age. Benzoate and phenylacetate may lower carnitine levels, but clinical signs of carnitine deficiency or benefit from carnitine supplementation have not yet been demonstrated. These compounds have been used during pregnancy without obvious teratogenic effect. However, experience is still limited, and appropriate caution should be exercised.

Growth parameters, especially head circumference, and nutritional indices (blood albumin, prealbumin, pH, electrolytes, amino acids, zinc, selenium) should be followed closely. Long-term care of these patients is best achieved by a team of experienced professionals (pediatrician, nutritionist, child neurologist, metabolic geneticist). Skin lesions resembling **acrodermatitis enteropathica** (see Chapter 691) have been noted in a few patients with different types of urea cycle defects, presumably from deficiency of essential amino acids, caused by overzealous dietary protein restriction. Catabolic states (infections, fasting) that may trigger hyperammonemia should be avoided. They must be treated vigorously if they occur. It is important that all children with urea cycle defects avoid valproic acid because this drug can elevate blood ammonia even in some healthy individuals. In patients with CPS1, OTC, or ASS deficiency, acute hyperammonemic attacks may be precipitated by valproate administration.

CARBAMOYL PHOSPHATE SYNTHETASE 1 AND N-ACETYLGLUTAMATE SYNTHASE DEFICIENCIES

Deficiencies of these 2 enzymes produce similar clinical and biochemical manifestations (see Figs. 103.12 and 103.13). There is a wide variation in severity of symptoms and in the age at presentation. In near-complete enzymatic deficiency, symptoms appear during the 1st few days or even hours of life with signs and symptoms of hyperammonemia (refusal to eat, vomiting, lethargy, convulsion, coma). Increased intracranial pressure is frequent. Late forms (as late as the 4th decade of life) may present as an acute bout of hyperammonemia (lethargy, headache, seizures, psychosis) in a seemingly normal individual. Coma and death may occur during these episodes (a previously asymptomatic 26-yr-old female died from hyperammonemia during childbirth). Diagnostic confusion with migraine is common. Intermediate forms with intellectual disability and chronic subclinical hyperammonemia interspersed with bouts of acute hyperammonemia have also been observed.

Laboratory findings include hyperammonemia. The plasma amino acid analysis typically shows a marked increase of glutamine and alanine with relatively low levels of citrulline and arginine. These are nondiagnostic changes that occur in hyperammonemia of diverse cause. Urinary orotic acid is usually low or may be absent (see Fig. 103.13).

Treatment of acute hyperammonemic attacks and the long-term therapy of the condition are previously outlined (see Table 103.5). Patients with NAGS deficiency benefit from oral administration of carbamylglutamate. It is therefore important to differentiate between CPS1 and NAGS deficiencies by gene sequencing. Deficiency of NAGS is rare in North America.

CPS1 and NAGS deficiencies are inherited as an autosomal recessive trait; the CPS1 enzyme is normally present in liver and intestine. The gene *(CPS1)* is mapped to chromosome 2q34. The prevalence of the condition is approximately 1 : 1,300,000. The gene for NAG synthetase *(NAGS)* is located on chromosome 17q21.31. Neither of these conditions is identified by the mass screening of the newborn infants.

ORNITHINE TRANSCARBAMYLASE DEFICIENCY

In this X-linked disorder, the hemizygous males are more severely affected than heterozygous females (see Figs. 103.12 and 103.13). The heterozygous females may have a mild form of the disease, but the majority (approximately 75%) remain asymptomatic, although investigations indicate subtle neurologic defects even in women without a frank history of hyperammonemia. Ornithine transcarbamylase (OTC) deficiency is the most common form of all the urea cycle disorders, comprising approximately 40% of cases of urea cycle disorders.

Clinical manifestations in a male newborn are usually those of **severe** hyperammonemia (see earlier) occurring in the 1st few days of life. **Mild forms**, such as in some heterozygous females, characteristically have episodic manifestations, which may occur at any age (usually after infancy). Episodes of hyperammonemia, manifested by vomiting and neurologic abnormalities (e.g., ataxia, mental confusion, agitation, combativeness, frank psychosis), are separated by periods of wellness. These episodes usually occur after ingestion of a high-protein diet or as a result of a catabolic state such as infection. Hyperammonemic coma, cerebral edema, and death may occur during one of these attacks. Cognitive development may proceed normally. Mild to moderate intellectual disability, however, is common. Gallstones have been seen in the survivors; the mechanism remains unclear.

The major **laboratory finding** during the acute attack is hyperammonemia accompanied by marked elevations of plasma concentrations of glutamine and alanine with low levels of citrulline and arginine. The blood level of urea is usually low. A marked increase in the urinary excretion of orotic acid differentiates this condition from CPS1 deficiency (see Fig. 103.13). Orotate may precipitate in urine as pink-colored gravel or stones. In the **mild form**, these laboratory abnormalities may revert to normal between attacks. This form should be differentiated from all the episodic conditions of childhood. In particular, patients with lysinuric protein intolerance (see Chapter 103.14) may demonstrate some features of OTC deficiency, but the former can be differentiated by increased urinary excretion of lysine, ornithine, and arginine and elevated blood concentrations of citrulline.

The **diagnosis** is most conveniently confirmed by gene analysis. As many as 20% of affected patients demonstrate a normal sequence, perhaps because the pathogenic variant involves copy number variants and pathogenic variants involving introns or a promoter region. Copy number variants can be evaluated using a chromosomal microarray, and if positive, a contiguous gene deletion should be considered. If the molecular diagnostic approach is negative, a liver biopsy may be indicated. Prenatal diagnosis is feasible by analysis of DNA in amniocytes or chorionic villus samples. Increase in urinary excretion of orotidine after an allopurinol loading test can identify female carriers. Mild cerebral dysfunction may be present in asymptomatic female carriers. The importance of a detailed family history should be emphasized. A history of migraine or protein aversion is common in maternal female relatives of the proband. Indeed, careful scrutiny of the family history may reveal a pattern of unexplained deaths in male newborns in the maternal lineage.

Treatment of acute hyperammonemic attacks and the long-term therapy of the condition are previously outlined. For enteral use, citrulline is used in place of arginine in patients with OTC deficiency. Liver transplantation is a successful treatment for patients with severe OTC deficiency.

The gene for OTC has been mapped to the X chromosome (Xp21.1). Many disease-causing pathogenic variants (>300) have been identified. The prevalence of OTC deficiency is $1:56,000$-$1:77,000$ live births. Genotype and the resulting degree of enzyme deficiency determine severity of the phenotype in most cases. Mothers of affected infants are expected to be carriers of the mutant gene unless a de novo pathogenic variant has occurred. A mother who gave birth to 2 affected male offspring was found to have a normal genotype, suggesting that gonadal mosaicism can be seen in some families. This condition is not identified by the mass screening of newborn infants.

CITRULLINEMIA

Two clinically and genetically distinct forms of citrullinemia have been identified. The classic form (**type I**) is caused by the deficiency of the ASS enzyme. Citrullinemia **type II** is caused by the deficiency of a mitochondrial transport protein named *citrin*. (See Figs. 103.12 and 103.13.)

Citrullinemia Type I (Argininosuccinate Synthetase Deficiency, Classic Citrullinemia)

This condition is caused by the deficiency of ASS (see Fig. 103.12) and has variable clinical manifestations depending on the degree of the enzyme deficiency. Two major forms of the condition have been identified. The **severe** or **neonatal form**, which is most common, appears in the 1st few days of life with signs and symptoms of hyperammonemia (see earlier). In the **subacute or mild form**, clinical findings such as failure to thrive, frequent vomiting, developmental delay, and dry, brittle hair appear gradually after 1 yr of age. Acute hyperammonemia, triggered by an intercurrent catabolic state, may bring the diagnosis to light.

Laboratory findings are similar to those found in patients with OTC deficiency, except that the plasma citrulline concentration is greatly elevated (50-100 times normal) (see Fig. 103.13). Urinary excretion of orotic acid is moderately increased; crystalluria may also occur as a result of precipitation of orotates. The diagnosis is confirmed by DNA analysis or less frequently by assay of enzyme activity in cultured fibroblasts. Prenatal diagnosis is feasible with enzyme assay in cultured amniotic cells or by DNA analysis of cells obtained from chorionic villus biopsy.

Treatment of acute hyperammonemic attacks and long-term therapy are outlined earlier (see Table 103.5). Plasma concentration of citrulline remains elevated at all times and may increase further after administration of arginine. Patients can do well on a protein-restricted diet in conjunction with sodium benzoate, phenylbutyrate, and arginine therapy. Mild to moderate cognitive impairment is a common sequela, even in a well-treated patient.

Citrullinemia is inherited as an autosomal recessive trait. The gene (*ASS1*) is located on chromosome 9q34.11. The majority of patients are compound heterozygotes for 2 different alleles. The prevalence of the condition is $1:250,000$ live births. The recent introduction of neonatal screening for urea cycle defects has shown that some affected patients are ostensibly asymptomatic even with ingestion of a regular diet. Long-term follow-up is needed to be certain that these individuals do not sustain neurologic sequelae.

Citrin Deficiency (Citrullinemia Type II)

Citrin (aspartate-glutamate carrier protein) is a mitochondrial transporter encoded by a gene (*SLC25A13*) located on chromosome 7q21.3. One of this protein's functions is to transport aspartate from mitochondria into cytoplasm and replenish the cytosolic aspartate pool required for converting citrulline to argininosuccinic acid (see Fig. 103.12). If aspartate is unavailable to the cytoplasmic component of the urea cycle, urea will not be formed at a normal rate, and citrulline will accumulate. ASS activity is diminished in the liver of these patients, but no pathogenic variant in the *ASS1* gene has been found. It is postulated that citrin deficiency interferes with translation of messenger RNA for ASS enzyme

in the liver. The condition initially was reported in Japan, but non-Japanese patients have also been identified. Two clinical forms of citrin deficiency have been described.

Neonatal Intrahepatic Cholestasis (Citrullinemia Type II, Neonatal Form)

Clinical and laboratory manifestations, which usually start before 1 yr of age, include cholestatic jaundice with mild to moderate direct (conjugated) hyperbilirubinemia, marked hypoproteinemia, clotting dysfunction (increased prothrombin time and partial thromboplastin time), and increased serum γ-glutamyltransferase and alkaline phosphatase activities; liver transaminases are usually normal. Plasma concentrations of ammonia and citrulline are usually normal, but moderate elevations have been reported. There may be increases in plasma concentrations of methionine, tyrosine, alanine, and threonine. Elevated levels of serum galactose have been found, even though the enzymes of galactose metabolism are normal. The reason for hypergalactosemia is not known. Marked elevation in the serum level of α-fetoprotein is also present. These findings resemble those of tyrosinemia type I, but unlike the latter condition, urinary excretion of succinylacetone is not elevated (see Chapter 103.2). Liver biopsy shows fatty infiltration, cholestasis with dilated canaliculi, and a moderate degree of fibrosis. The condition is usually self-limiting, and the majority of infants recover spontaneously by 1 yr of age with supportive and symptomatic treatment. Hepatic failure requiring liver transplantation has occurred in a few cases. Although the condition is commonly seen in Japan, the diagnosis should be considered in any case of unexplained neonatal hepatitis with cholestasis. Data on the long-term prognosis and the natural history of the condition are limited; development into the adult form of the condition after several years of seemingly asymptomatic hiatus has been observed.

Citrullinemia Type II, Adult Form (Adult-Onset Citrullinemia; Citrullinemia Type II, Mild Form)

This form of citrullinemia type II starts acutely in a previously apparently normal individual and manifests with neuropsychiatric symptoms such as disorientation, delirium, delusion, aberrant behavior, tremors, and frank psychosis. Moderate degrees of hyperammonemia and hypercitrullinemia are present. The age at onset is usually between 20 and 40 yr (range: 11 to >100 yr). Patients who recover from the 1st episode may have recurrent attacks. Pancreatitis, hyperlipidemia, and hepatoma are major complications among the survivors. Medical **treatment** has been mostly ineffective for prevention of future attacks. Diet enriched for protein and lipids helps restore cytosolic aspartate pool and stimulate ureagenesis. Indeed, some have speculated that the administration of large amounts of glucose might even prove deleterious, because the citrin transporter is important to the glycolytic pathway. Although liver transplantation appears to be effective in preventing future episodes of hyperammonemia, enteral supplementation with arginine, pyruvate, and medium-chain triglycerides can be tried first to improve hyperammonemic episodes and growth.

Several disease-causing mutations of the gene have been identified in affected Japanese and non-Japanese families. Although the frequency of homozygosity is relatively high in Japan ($1:20,000$ people), the clinical condition has a frequency of only $1:100,000$ to $1:230,000$. This indicates that a substantial number of homozygous individuals remain asymptomatic.

ARGININOSUCCINATE LYASE DEFICIENCY (ARGININOSUCCINIC ACIDURIA)

The severity of the clinical and biochemical manifestations varies considerably (see Figs. 103.12 and 103.13). In severe form of ASL deficiency, signs and symptoms of severe hyperammonemia (see earlier) develop in the 1st few days of life, and without treatment, mortality can be high. Clinical course of ASL deficiency in patients who survive the initial acute episode can be characterized by intellectual disability, failure to thrive, hypertension, gallstones, liver fibrosis, and hepatomegaly. A common finding in untreated patients is dry and brittle hair (**trichorrhexis nodosa**). Acute attacks of severe hyperammonemia may occur during a catabolic state.

Laboratory findings include hyperammonemia, moderate elevations in liver enzymes, nonspecific increases in plasma levels of glutamine and alanine, a moderate increase in plasma levels of citrulline (less than in citrullinemia), and marked increase in the concentration of argininosuccinic acid in plasma, urine, and CSF. The CSF levels are usually higher than those in plasma. The enzyme is normally present in erythrocytes, the liver, and cultured fibroblasts. **Prenatal diagnosis** is possible by measurement of the enzyme activity in cultured amniotic cells or by identification of pathogenic variants in the *ASL* gene. Argininosuccinic acid is also elevated in the amniotic fluid of affected fetuses.

Treatment of acute hyperammonemic attacks and the long-term therapy of the condition are outlined earlier in this chapter. Intellectual disability, persistent hepatomegaly with mild increases in liver enzymes, and bleeding tendencies as a result of abnormal clotting factors are common sequelae. This deficiency is inherited as an autosomal recessive trait with a prevalence of about 1 in 220,000 live births. The gene *(ASL)* is located on chromosome 7q11.21. Early detection is achieved through mass screening of newborn infants.

ARGINASE 1 DEFICIENCY (HYPERARGININEMIA)

This defect is inherited as an autosomal recessive trait (see Figs. 103.12 and 103.13). There are 2 genetically distinct arginases in humans. One is cytosolic (ARG1) and is expressed in the liver and erythrocytes, and the other (ARG2) is found in renal and brain mitochondria. The gene for ARG1, the enzyme that is deficient in patients with arginase 1 deficiency, is mapped to chromosome 6q23.2. The role of the mitochondrial enzyme is not well understood; its activity increases in patients with argininemia but has no protective effect.

Clinical manifestations of this rare distal urea cycle enzyme defects are somewhat different from those of other urea cycle enzyme defects, although acute neonatal form with intractable seizures, cerebral edema, and death has also been reported. The onset arginase 1 deficiency often is insidious; the infant can remain asymptomatic in the 1st few mo or yr of life. A **progressive spastic diplegia** with scissoring of the lower extremities, choreoathetotic movements, loss of developmental milestones, and failure to thrive in a previously normal infant may suggest a degenerative disease of the CNS. Some children were treated for years as cases of cerebral palsy before their arginase 1 deficiency was confirmed. Intellectual disability is progressive; seizures are common, but episodes of severe hyperammonemia are not as frequent as in the more proximal urea cycle defects. Hepatomegaly may be present.

Laboratory findings include marked elevations of arginine in plasma and CSF (see Fig. 103.13). Urinary orotic acid can be increased. Determination of amino acids in plasma is a critical step in the diagnosis of argininemia. The guanidino compounds (α-keto-guanidinovaleric acid and α-keto-argininic acid) are markedly increased in urine. The diagnosis is confirmed by assaying arginase activity in erythrocytes or by the identification of the mutant gene.

Treatment consists of a low-protein diet providing the RDA. The composition of the diet and the daily intake of protein should be monitored by frequent plasma amino acid determinations. Sodium benzoate or sodium phenylbutyrate are also effective in controlling hyperammonemia and lowering plasma arginine levels. Intellectual disability is a common sequela of the condition. One patient developed type 1 diabetes by 9 yr of age while his argininemia was under good control. Liver transplantation has produced promising results, but experience with long-term outcome is limited. Early detection is feasible through mass screening of newborn infants.

TRANSIENT HYPERAMMONEMIA OF THE NEWBORN

The blood concentration of ammonia in full-term infants may be as high as 100 µmol/L, or 2-3 times greater than that of the older child or adult. Blood levels approach the adult normal values after a few weeks of life (see Fig. 103.13).

Severe transient hyperammonemia is observed in some newborn infants. The majority of affected infants are premature and have mild respiratory distress syndrome. Hyperammonemic coma may develop within 2-3 days of life, and the infant may succumb to the disease if treatment is not started immediately. Laboratory studies reveal marked hyperammonemia (plasma ammonia as high as 4,000 µmol/L) with moderate increases in plasma levels of glutamine and alanine. Plasma concentrations of urea cycle intermediate amino acids are usually normal except for citrulline, which may be moderately elevated. The cause of the disorder is unknown. Urea cycle enzyme activities are normal. **Treatment** of hyperammonemia should be initiated promptly and continued vigorously. Recovery without sequelae is common, and hyperammonemia does not recur even with a normal protein diet.

DISORDERS OF ORNITHINE METABOLISM

Ornithine, a key intermediate of the urea cycle, is not incorporated into natural proteins. Rather, it is generated in the cytosol from arginine and must be transported into mitochondria, where it becomes a substrate for the reaction catalyzed by OTC that forms citrulline. Excess ornithine is catabolized by 2 enzymes, ornithine aminotransferase, which is a mitochondrial enzyme converting ornithine to a proline precursor, and ornithine decarboxylase, which resides in the cytosol and converts ornithine to putrescine (see Fig. 103.12). Two genetic disorders feature **hyperornithinemia**: gyrate atrophy of the retina and hyperammonemia-hyperornithinemia-homocitrullinemia syndrome.

Gyrate Atrophy of the Retina and Choroid

This rare, autosomal recessive disorder is caused by deficiency of ornithine aminotransferase (see Fig. 103.12). Approximately 30% of the reported cases are from Finland. Clinical manifestations may include hyperammonemia in the 1st mo of life in some patients. Findings that define the phenotype of ornithine aminotransferase deficiency include night blindness, myopia, loss of peripheral vision, and posterior subcapsular cataracts. These eye changes start between 5 and 10 yr of age and progress to complete blindness by the 4th decade of life. Atrophic lesions in the retina resemble cerebral gyri. These patients usually have normal intelligence. Besides the characteristic 10-20–fold increase in plasma levels of ornithine (400-1,400 µmol/L), plasma levels of glutamate, glutamine, lysine, creatine, and creatinine can be moderately decreased. Some patients respond partially to high doses of pyridoxine. An arginine-restricted diet in conjunction with supplemental lysine, proline, and creatine has been successful in reducing plasma ornithine concentration and has produced some clinical improvement. The gene for ornithine aminotransferase *(OAT)* is mapped to chromosome 10q26.13. Many (at least 60) pathogenic variants have been identified in different families.

Hyperammonemia-Hyperornithinemia-Homocitrullinemia Syndrome

In this rare autosomal recessive disorder the defect is in the transport system of ornithine from the cytosol into the mitochondria, resulting in accumulation of ornithine in the cytosol and a depletion of this amino acid in mitochondria. The former causes hyperornithinemia, and the latter results in disruption of the urea cycle and hyperammonemia (see Fig. 103.12). Homocitrulline is presumably formed from the reaction of mitochondrial carbamoyl phosphate with lysine, which can become a substrate for the OTC reaction when ornithine is deficient. Clinical manifestations of hyperammonemia may develop shortly after birth or may be delayed until adulthood. Acute episodes of hyperammonemia manifest as refusal to feed, vomiting, and lethargy; coma may occur during infancy. Progressive neurologic signs, such as lower limb weakness, increased deep tendon reflexes, spasticity, clonus, seizures, and varying degrees of psychomotor retardation may develop if the condition remains undiagnosed. No clinical ocular findings have been observed in these patients. Laboratory findings reveal marked increases in plasma levels of ornithine and homocitrulline in addition to hyperammonemia (see Fig. 103.13). Acute episodes of hyperammonemia should be treated promptly (see earlier). Restriction of protein intake improves hyperammonemia. Oral supplementation with arginine (or citrulline) has produced clinical improvement in some patients. The gene for this disorder *(SLC25A15)* is located on chromosome 13q14.11.

CONGENITAL GLUTAMINE DEFICIENCY

Glutamine is synthesized endogenously from glutamate and ammonia by a ubiquitous enzyme, glutamine synthetase (see Fig. 103.11). Glutamine is known to be involved in several important functions, including detoxification of ammonia. Deficiency of this enzyme, resulting in glutamine deficiency, has been reported in 3 infants from 3 unrelated families. All affected infants manifested multiorgan involvement, including significant brain malformations (abnormal gyrations, hypomyelination), facial abnormalities (broad nasal root, low-set ears), hypotonia and seizures at birth. Two of the patients died from multiorgan failure (respiratory and heart failure) in the neonatal period. One child was alive at 3 yr of age with severe developmental delay. Glutamine was absent in plasma, urine, and CSF, but plasma levels of glutamic acid were normal. Genetic defects of this enzyme underline the critical role of glutamine in embryogenesis, especially for normal brain development. The condition is inherited as an autosomal recessive trait; the gene for glutamine synthetase (GLUL) is mapped to chromosome 1q25.3.

Bibliography is available at Expert Consult.

103.13　Histidine

Oleg A. Shchelochkov and Charles P. Venditti

Histidine is degraded through the urocanic acid pathway to glutamic acid. Several genetic biochemical aberrations involving the degradative pathway of histidine have been reported, but the clinical significance of elevated histidine levels has not been established.

Decarboxylation of histidine by histidine decarboxylase produces histamine. Deficiency of this enzyme has been implicated in the familial form of **Tourette syndrome** (see Chapter 103.11).

Bibliography is available at Expert Consult.

103.14　Lysine

Oleg A. Shchelochkov and Charles P. Venditti

Lysine is catabolized through 2 pathways. In the 1st pathway, lysine is condensed with α-ketoglutaric acid to form saccharopine. Saccharopine is then catabolized to α-aminoadipic semialdehyde and glutamic acid. These 1st 2 steps are catalyzed by α-aminoadipic semialdehyde synthase, which has 2 activities: lysine-ketoglutarate reductase and saccharopine dehydrogenase (Fig. 103.14). In the 2nd pathway, lysine is first transaminated and then condensed to its cyclic forms, pipecolic acid and piperideine-6-carboxylic acid (**P6C**). P6C and its linear form, α-aminoadipic semialdehyde, are oxidized to α-aminoadipic acid by the enzyme **antiquitin**. This is the major pathway for D-lysine in the body and for the L-lysine in the brain.

Hyperlysinemia-saccharopinuria and **α-aminoadipic-α-ketoadipic acidemia** are biochemical conditions caused by inborn errors of lysine degradation. Individuals with these conditions are usually asymptomatic.

PYRIDOXINE (VITAMIN B₆)–DEPENDENT EPILEPSY

Pyridoxal 5′-phosphate (**P5P**), the active form of pyridoxine, is the cofactor for many enzymes including those involved in the metabolism of neurotransmitters. Intracellular P5P deficiency in the brain may result in a seizure disorder that is refractory to common anticonvulsant agents but is responsive to high doses of pyridoxine. These pyridoxine-responsive phenotypes are seen in the following genetic metabolic conditions:

Antiquitin (α-Aminoadipic Semialdehyde Dehydrogenase) Deficiency

This is the most common cause of pyridoxine-dependent epilepsy. Deficiency of antiquitin results in accumulation of P6C in brain tissue (see Fig. 103.14); P6C reacts with P5P and renders it inactive. Large doses of pyridoxine are therefore needed to overcome this inactivation. The condition is inherited as an autosomal recessive trait; the gene for antiquitin (ALDH7A1) is on chromosome 5q31.

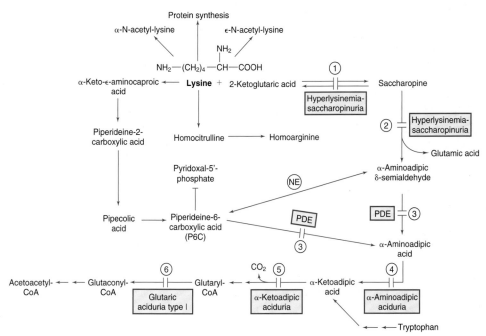

Fig. 103.14 Pathways in the metabolism of lysine. **Enzymes:** *(1)* Lysine ketoglutarate reductase, *(2)* saccharopine dehydrogenase, *(3)* α-aminoadipic semialdehyde/piperidine-6-carboxylic acid (P6C) dehydrogenase (antiquitin), *(4)* α-aminoadipic acid transferase, *(5)* α-ketoadipic acid dehydrogenase, *(6)* glutaryl-CoA-dehydrogenase. NE, Nonenzymatic; PDE, pyridoxine-dependent epilepsy.

Pyridox(am)ine 5′-Phosphate Oxidase (PNPO) Deficiency

PNPO deficiency clinically overlaps with antiquitin deficiency. PNPO-deficient patients often present with neonatal-onset seizures, developmental delays, spastic tetraplegia, and nonspecific findings on brain imaging (delayed myelination, cerebral atrophy, and abnormal signals in basal ganglia). Developmental regression, optic disc pallor, and retinopathy have been reported infrequently. Plasma and CSF amino acid analysis may reveal elevated glycine, prompting evaluation for nonketotic hyperglycinemia (see Chapter 103.7) and lead to a delay in initiating treatment with P5P. CSF neurotransmitter assay revealed inconsistent changes in the levels of 3-O-methyldopa, homovanillic acid, and 5-hydroxyindoleacetic acid. Normal CSF level of P5P was reported in one patient, suggesting that a therapeutic trial with P5P and molecular analysis may be a prudent strategy in some patients irrespective of the CSF studies. The lowest effective dose of P5P should be used to avoid toxicity. The disorder is caused by autosomal recessive pathogenic variants in *PNPO*.

Sulfite Oxidase Deficiency and Molybdenum Cofactor Deficiency

In this rare condition (see Chapter 103.4), accumulation of sulfites causes inhibition of enzymatic activity of antiquitin and accumulation of P6C, which in turn causes inactivation of P5P and vitamin B_6 dependency.

Hyperprolinemia Type II

In this condition, accumulation of Δ1-pyrroline-5-carboxylate (P5C) in brain tissue causes inactivation of P5P, leading to pyridoxine dependency (see Chapter 103.9 and Fig. 103.9).

Hypophosphatasia

Pyridoxal-5′-phosphate is the main circulating form of pyridoxine. Alkaline phosphatase (ALP) is required for dephosphorylation of P5P to generate free pyridoxine, which is the only form of vitamin B_6 that can cross the blood-brain barrier and enter the brain cells. Pyridoxine is rephosphorylated intracellularly to form P5P. In the infantile form of hypophosphatasia, P5P cannot be dephosphorylated to free pyridoxine because of marked deficiency of tissue-nonspecific ALP. This results in deficiency of pyridoxine in the brain and pyridoxine-dependent epilepsy (see Chapters 611 and 724).

The main **clinical manifestation** of pyridoxine-dependent epilepsy caused by antiquitin deficiency is generalized seizures, which usually occur in the first days of life and are unresponsive to conventional anticonvulsant therapies. Some mothers of affected fetuses report abnormal intrauterine fluttering movements. The seizures are usually tonic-clonic in nature but can be almost any type. Other manifestations such as dystonia, respiratory distress, and abdominal distention with vomiting, hepatomegaly, hypoglycemia and hypothermia may be present. Learning problems and speech delay are common sequelae. Late-onset forms of the condition (as late as 5 years of age) have been reported. Consequently, a trial with vitamin B_6 is recommended in any infant with intractable convulsions (see Chapters 611.04 and 611.06).

Laboratory findings show increased concentrations of α-aminoadipic semialdehyde and pipecolic acid in the CSF, plasma, and urine. EEG abnormalities may normalize after treatment. Neuroimaging may be normal but cerebellar and cerebral atrophy, periventricular hyperintensity, intracerebral hemorrhage, and hydrocephalus have been reported.

Treatment with vitamin B_6 (50-100 mg/day) usually results in a dramatic improvement of both seizures and the EEG abnormalities. High doses of pyridoxine can result in peripheral neuropathy, and doses >500 mg/day should be avoided. The pyridoxine dependency and thus the therapy are lifelong. The therapeutic benefit of a lysine-restricted diet is being evaluated.

GLUTARIC ACIDURIA TYPE 1 (GLUTARYL-CoA DEHYDROGENASE DEFICIENCY)

Glutaric acid is an intermediate in the degradation of lysine (see Fig. 103.14), hydroxylysine, and tryptophan. Glutaric aciduria **type 1**, a

disorder caused by a deficiency of glutaryl-CoA dehydrogenase, should be differentiated from glutaric aciduria **type 2**, a distinct clinical and biochemical disorder caused by defects in the mitochondrial electron transport chain (see Chapter 104.1).

Clinical Manifestations

Macrocephaly is a common but nonspecific finding in patients with glutaric aciduria type 1. It develops in the 1st yr of life but can also be present at birth and precede the onset of neurologic manifestations. Some affected infants may also show subtle neurologic symptoms, such as delayed onset of motor milestones, irritability, and feeding problems, during this seemingly asymptomatic period. The onset of the condition is usually heralded by **acute encephalopathic findings**, such as loss of normal developmental milestones (head control, rolling over, or sitting), seizures, generalized rigidity, opisthotonos, choreoathetosis, and dystonia caused by acute striatal injury. These symptoms may occur suddenly in an apparently normal infant after a minor infection. Brain imaging reveals increased extraaxial (particularly frontal) fluid with stretched bridging veins, striatal lesions, dilated lateral ventricles, cortical atrophy (mainly in frontotemporal region), and fibrosis. Recovery from the 1st attack usually occurs slowly, but some residual neurologic abnormalities may persist, especially dystonia and choreoathetosis. Without treatment, additional acute attacks resembling the first can occur during subsequent episodes of intercurrent infections or catabolic states. In some patients these signs and symptoms may develop gradually in the 1st few yr of life. Hypotonia and choreoathetosis may gradually progress into rigidity and dystonia (**insidious form**). Acute episodes of metabolic decompensation with vomiting, ketosis, seizures, and coma also occur in this form after infection and other catabolic states. Without treatment, death may occur in the 1st decade of life during one of these episodes. Affected infants are prone to development of subdural hematoma and retinal hemorrhage following minor falls and head traumas. This can be misdiagnosed as child abuse. The intellectual abilities usually remain relatively normal in most patients.

Laboratory Findings

During acute episodes, mild to moderate metabolic acidosis and ketosis may occur. Hypoglycemia, hyperammonemia, and elevations of serum transaminases are seen in some patients. High concentrations of glutaric acid are usually found in urine, blood, and CSF. 3-Hydroxyglutaric acid may also be present in the body fluids. Acylcarnitine profile shows elevated glutarylcarnitine (C5-DC) in blood and urine. Plasma concentrations of amino acids are usually within normal limits. Laboratory findings may be unremarkable between attacks. Glutaric aciduria type 1 can be identified on the newborn screen by measuring glutarylcarnitine levels in blood spots. The sensitivity of this screening method depends on the cutoff value used by a newborn screen program, and some patients can be missed. For example, it can happen in a subset of patients with glutaric aciduria type 1 who may present with normal plasma and urinary levels of glutaric acid and variably elevated plasma glutarylcarnitine. This type of glutaric aciduria type 1 referred to as a "low-excretor" phenotype carries the same risk of developing brain injury as in a "high-excretor" phenotype. In some low-excreting patients, glutaric acid is elevated only in CSF. Urinary glutarylcarnitine appears to be a more sensitive screening method to identify affected low-excreting patients. In any child with progressive dystonia and dyskinesia, activity of the enzyme glutaryl-CoA dehydrogenase and molecular analysis of *GCDH* should be performed.

Treatment

Patients require lysine- and tryptophan-restricted diet while meeting physiologic requirements for protein, micronutrients, and vitamins. Increased dietary arginine may decrease cellular uptake of lysine and decrease the endogenous formation of glutaryl-CoA. Patients should be routinely evaluated for lysine and tryptophan deficiency by monitoring plasma amino acids and growth. L-Carnitine supplementation (50-100 mg/kg/24 hr orally) is recommended in all cases. Emergency treatment during acute illness, including temporary cessation of protein intake for 24 hr, replacement of lost calories using carbohydrates or lipids, IV L-carnitine, IV dextrose, prompt treatment of infection, and control of fever, is critical to decreasing the risk of striatal injury. All patients should be provided with an emergency letter describing the underlying diagnosis, recommended evaluation, and treatment. Early diagnosis through newborn screening with prevention and aggressive treatment of intercurrent catabolic states (infections) can help minimize striatal injury and ensure a more favorable prognosis. Patients with movement disorder and spasticity may require treatment with baclofen, diazepam, trihexyphenidyl, and injectable botulinum toxin A.

Glutaric aciduria type 1 is inherited as an autosomal recessive trait. The prevalence is estimated at 1:100,000 live births worldwide. The condition is more prevalent in some ethnic populations (Canadian Oji-Cree Indians, Irish Travelers, black South Africans, Swedes, and the Old Order Amish population in the United States). The gene for glutaryl-CoA dehydrogenase (GCDH) is located on chromosome 19p13.2. Molecular analysis of GCDH can aid in identifying patients with a low-excretor phenotype associated with specific pathogenic variants (e.g., p.M405V, p.V400M, p.R227P). High prevalence of known pathogenic variants in specific ethnic populations can enable a cost-effective molecular evaluation and counseling.

Prenatal diagnosis can be accomplished by demonstrating increased concentrations of glutaric acid in amniotic fluid, by assay of the enzyme activity in amniocytes or chorionic villus samples, or by identification of the known pathogenic variants in GCDH.

LYSINURIC PROTEIN INTOLERANCE (FAMILIAL PROTEIN INTOLERANCE)

This rare autosomal recessive disorder is caused by a defect in the transport of the cationic amino acids lysine, ornithine, and arginine in both intestine and kidneys. Deficiency of the transporter protein (Y+L amino acid transporter 1) in this condition causes multisystem manifestations, which start initially with gastrointestinal (GI) symptoms. The transport defect in this condition resides in the basolateral (antiluminal) membrane of enterocytes and renal tubular epithelia. This explains the observation that cationic amino acids are unable to cross these cells even when administered as dipeptides. Lysine in the form of dipeptide crosses the luminal membrane of the enterocytes but hydrolyzes to free lysine molecules in the cytoplasm. Free lysine, unable to cross the basolateral membrane of the cells, diffuses back into the lumen.

Refusal to feed, nausea, aversion to protein, vomiting, and mild diarrhea, which may result in failure to thrive, wasting, and hypotonia, may be seen shortly after birth. Breastfed infants usually remain asymptomatic until soon after weaning, possibly because of the low-protein content of breast milk. Episodes of hyperammonemia may occur after ingestion of a high-protein meal. Mild to moderate hepatosplenomegaly, osteoporosis, sparse brittle hair, thin extremities with moderate centripetal adiposity, and growth retardation are common physical findings in patients whose condition has remained undiagnosed. Neurocognitive status is usually normal, but moderate intellectual disability has been observed in some patients.

Progressive interstitial pneumonitis with bouts of acute exacerbation often occurs in these patients. This usually progresses to severe alveolar proteinosis. Clinical manifestations include progressive exertional dyspnea, fatigue, cough, diminished breath sound, and inspiratory rales; cyanosis may develop in older patients. Some patients have remained undiagnosed until the appearance of pulmonary manifestations. Radiographic evidence of pulmonary fibrosis has been observed in up to 65% of patients without clinical manifestations of pulmonary involvement.

Renal involvement is manifested initially by proteinuria, hematuria, and elevation of serum creatinine, which may progress to end-stage renal failure. Renal tubular involvement with laboratory findings of renal Fanconi syndrome may also be present. Renal biopsy reveals pathologic findings consistent with glomerulonephritis and tubulointerstitial nephritis. Hematologic findings of anemia, leukopenia, thrombocytopenia, and elevated ferritin may also be present. A condition resembling hemophagocytic lymphohistiocytosis/macrophage activation syndrome has also been reported. Immunologic abnormalities (impaired

lymphocyte function, abnormalities in immune globulins, hypocomplementemia) and acute pancreatitis are frequent features of lysinuric protein intolerance.

Laboratory findings may reveal hyperammonemia and an elevated concentration of urinary orotic acid, which develop after high-protein feeding. Plasma concentrations of lysine, arginine, and ornithine are usually mildly decreased, but urinary levels of these amino acids, especially lysine, are greatly increased. The pathogenesis of hyperammonemia is likely related to the depletion of urea cycle intermediates caused by poor absorption and the increased renal loss of ornithine and arginine. Plasma concentrations of alanine, glutamine, serine, glycine, and proline are usually increased. Anemia, increased serum levels of ferritin, lactate dehydrogenase (LDH), thyroxine-binding globulin, hypercholesterolemia, and hypertriglyceridemia are common findings. This condition should be differentiated from hyperammonemia caused by urea cycle defects (see Chapter 103.12), especially in heterozygous females with OTC deficiency, in whom increased urinary excretion of lysine, ornithine, and arginine is not seen.

Treatment with a low-protein diet providing the RDA of protein and supplemented with oral citrulline (50-100 mg/kg/day) can produce biochemical and clinical improvements. Episodes of hyperammonemia should be treated promptly (see Chapter 103.12). Supplementation with lysine (10-30 mg/kg/day) given in small and frequent doses helps improve plasma levels. The dose of lysine should be titrated down if patients develop abdominal pain and diarrhea. Treatment with high doses of prednisone has been effective in the management of acute pulmonary complications in some patients. **Bronchopulmonary lavage** is the treatment of choice for patients with alveolar proteinosis. The condition is more prevalent in Finland and Japan, where the prevalence is 1:60,000 and 1:57,000 live births, respectively.

The gene for lysinuric protein intolerance (SLC7A7) is mapped to chromosome 14q11.2. Pregnancies in affected mothers have been complicated by anemia, thrombocytopenia, toxemia, and bleeding, but offspring have been normal.

Bibliography is available at Expert Consult.

103.15 N-Acetylaspartic Acid (Canavan Disease)

Reuben K. Matalon and Joseph M. Trapasso

N-Acetylaspartic acid (**NAA**), a derivative of aspartic acid, is synthesized in the brain and is found in a high concentration similar to glutamic acid. Studies suggest that NAA has multiple functions, such as serving as an acetate reservoir for myelin synthesis and being an organic osmolyte that helps regulate cerebral osmolality. However, the complete function of NAA is not yet fully understood. **Aspartoacylase** cleaves the N-acetyl group from NAA. Deficiency of aspartoacylase leads to **Canavan disease**, a severe **leukodystrophy** characterized by excessive excretion of NAA and spongy degeneration of the white matter of the brain. Canavan disease is an autosomal recessive disorder and is more prevalent in individuals of Ashkenazi Jewish descent than in other ethnic groups. The defective gene for Canavan disease (ASPA) is located on chromosome 17, and genetic testing can be offered for patients, family members, and at-risk populations.

ETIOLOGY AND PATHOLOGY

The deficiency of the enzyme aspartoacylase leads to NAA accumulation in the brain, especially in white matter, and massive urinary excretion of this compound. Excessive amounts of NAA are also present in the blood and CSF. Brain biopsies of patients with Canavan disease show spongy degeneration of the myelin fibers, astrocytic swelling, and elongated mitochondria. There is striking vacuolization and astrocytic swelling in white matter. Electron microscopy reveals distorted mitochondria. As the disease progresses, the ventricles enlarge because of cerebral atrophy.

CLINICAL MANIFESTATIONS

The severity of Canavan disease covers a wide spectrum. Infants usually appear normal at birth and may not manifest symptoms of the disease until 3-6 mo of age, when they develop **progressive macrocephaly**, severe hypotonia, persistent head lag, and delayed milestones. As the disease progresses, there is spasticity, joint stiffness, and contractures. Optic atrophy and seizures develop. Feeding difficulties, poor weight gain, and gastroesophageal reflux may occur in the 1st yr of life; swallowing deteriorates, and nasogastric feeding or permanent gastrostomy may be required. In the past, most patients died in the 1st decade of life, but with the advances in medical technology and improved supportive care, now they often survive to the 2nd or 3rd decade.

ATYPICAL CANAVAN DISEASE

Juvenile or **mild** Canavan disease is less common than **infantile** Canavan disease and is most prevalent in non-Ashkenazi Jews. Affected patients with juvenile Canavan disease usually present with mild speech and motor delay and may have **retinitis pigmentosa**. The other typical features of Canavan disease are usually not present. These children have moderately increased urinary excretion of NAA, which suggests Canavan disease. Brain MRI demonstrates increased signal intensity in the basal ganglia rather than global white matter disease, sometimes leading to confusion with mitochondrial disease.

DIAGNOSIS

In a typical patient with Canavan disease, CT scan and MRI reveal diffuse white matter degeneration, primarily in the cerebral hemispheres, with less involvement of the cerebellum and brainstem (Fig. 103.15). Repeated evaluations may be required. MRS performed at the time of MRI can be done to show the high peak of NAA, suggesting Canavan disease. The diagnosis can also be established by finding elevated amounts of NAA in the urine or blood. NAA is found only in trace amounts (24 ±16 μmol/mmol creatinine) in the urine of unaffected individuals, whereas in patients with Canavan disease its concentration is in the range of 1,440 ±873 μmol/mmol creatinine. High levels of NAA can also be detected in plasma, CSF, and brain tissue. Aspartoacylase in fibroblasts is often used to confirm the diagnosis but is not necessary. The activity of aspartoacylase in the fibroblasts of obligate carriers is half or less the activity found in normal individuals. Genotyping of patients with Canavan disease should always be done and will show mutations of *ASPA*. The differential diagnosis of Canavan disease should include **Alexander disease**, which is another leukodystrophy associated with macrocephaly. Alexander disease is caused by a defect in the synthesis of glial fibrillary acidic protein, and the diagnosis can be ruled out by molecular diagnosis on blood lymphocytes.

There are 2 predominant pathogenic variants leading to Canavan disease in the Ashkenazi Jewish population. The first is an amino acid substitution (E285A) in which glutamic acid is substituted for alanine. This mutation is the most frequent and encompasses 83% of 100 mutant alleles examined in Ashkenazi Jewish patients. The 2nd common pathogenic variant is a change from tyrosine to a nonsense mutation, leading to a stop in the coding sequence (Y231X). This accounts for 13% of mutant alleles. In the non-Jewish population, more diverse pathogenic variants have been observed, and the 2 variants common in Jewish people are rare. A different mutation (A305E), the substitution of alanine for glutamic acid, accounts for 40% of 62 mutant alleles in non-Jewish patients. More than 50 pathogenic variants are described in the non-Jewish population. With Canavan disease, it is important to obtain a molecular diagnosis because this will lead to accurate counseling and prenatal guidance for the family. If the mutations are not known, **prenatal diagnosis** relies on the NAA level in the amniotic fluid. In Ashkenazi Jewish patients, the carrier frequency can be as high as 1:40, which is close to that of Tay-Sachs disease. Carrier screening for Canavan disease is available for Jewish individuals. Genotype phenotype correlation and aspartoacylase expression show that expression studies may aid in understanding the disease.

Patients with juvenile or mild forms of Canavan disease have been compound heterozygotes with a mild pathogenic variant on one allele and a severe variant on the other allele. Mild variants include p.Tyr288Cys and p.Arg71His.

TREATMENT AND PREVENTION

No specific treatment is currently available. Recent studies of gene therapy using recombinant adeno-associated viruses (**rAAVs**) have shown some positive results in rescuing knockout mice but have yet to be tested in humans. Feeding problems and seizures should be treated on an individual basis. Genetic counseling, carrier testing, and prenatal diagnosis are the only methods of prevention. Gene therapy attempts in children with Canavan disease have shown lack of long-term adverse events, some decrease in the brain elevation of *N*-acetylaspartic acid, improved seizure frequency, and stabilization of overall clinical status.

Bibliography is available at Expert Consult.

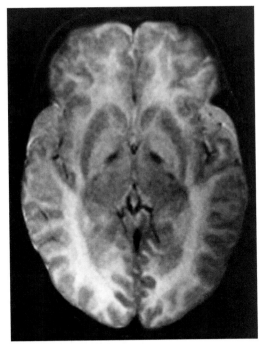

Fig. 103.15 Axial T-weighted MRI of a 2 yr old patient with Canavan disease. Extensive thickening of the white matter is seen.

Chapter 104

Defects in Metabolism of Lipids

第一百零四章
脂肪代谢病

中文导读

　　本章详细阐述了线粒体脂肪酸β－氧化障碍，其中包括β－氧化循环障碍、肉碱循环障碍、电子传递通路障碍、酮体合成通路障碍及酮体利用障碍；详细阐述了极长链脂肪酸代谢障碍及其他过氧化物酶体功能障碍，其中包括过氧化物酶体病及肾上腺脑白质营养不良；详细阐述了脂蛋白代谢及转运障碍，其中包括血脂及心血管疾病流行病学、血脂及动脉粥样硬化形成、血浆脂蛋白代谢及转运和高脂蛋白血症；详细阐述了脂质贮积症（溶酶体贮积症）及黏脂贮积症等内容。

104.1 Disorders of Mitochondrial Fatty Acid β-Oxidation

Charles A. Stanley and Michael J. Bennett

Mitochondrial β-oxidation of fatty acids is an essential energy-producing pathway. It is particularly important during prolonged periods of starvation and during periods of reduced caloric intake caused by gastrointestinal illness or increased energy expenditure during febrile illness. Under these conditions, the body switches from using predominantly *carbohydrate* to predominantly *fat* as its major fuel. Fatty acids are also important fuels for exercising skeletal muscle and are the preferred substrate for normal cardiac metabolism. In these tissues, fatty acids are completely oxidized to carbon dioxide and water. The end products of hepatic fatty acid oxidation are the ketone bodies β-*hydroxybutyrate* and *acetoacetate*. These cannot be oxidized by the liver but are exported to serve as important fuels in peripheral tissues, particularly the brain, where ketone bodies can partially substitute for glucose during periods of fasting.

Genetic defects have been identified in almost all the known steps in the fatty acid oxidation pathway; all are recessively inherited (Table 104.1).

Clinical manifestations characteristically involve tissues with a high β-oxidation flux, including liver, skeletal, and cardiac muscle. The most common presentation is an acute episode of life-threatening coma, hepatic encephalopathy, and hypoglycemia induced by a period of fasting resulting from defective hepatic ketogenesis. Other manifestations may include chronic cardiomyopathy and muscle weakness or exercise-induced acute rhabdomyolysis. The fatty acid oxidation defects can often be asymptomatic during periods when there is no fasting stress or increased energy demand. Acutely presenting disease may be misdiagnosed as **Reye syndrome** or, if fatal, as **sudden unexpected infant death**. Fatty acid oxidation disorders are easily overlooked because the only specific clue to the diagnosis may be the finding of inappropriately low concentrations of plasma or urinary ketones in an infant who has hypoglycemia, unless specialized metabolic testing is performed. Genetic defects in ketone body utilization may also be overlooked because ketonemia is an expected finding with fasting hypoglycemia. In some circumstances, clinical manifestations appear to arise from toxic effects of fatty acid metabolites rather than inadequate energy production. These circumstances include certain long-chain fatty acid oxidation disorders (deficiencies of long-chain 3-hydroxyacyl dehydrogenase [LCHAD], carnitine palmitoyltransferase-IA [CPT-IA], or mitochondrial trifunctional protein [MTP; also known as TFP]) in which the presence of a homozygous affected fetus increases the risk of a life-threatening illness in the heterozygote mother, resulting in **acute fatty liver of pregnancy** (AFLP) or **preeclampsia with HELLP** (hemolysis, elevated liver enzymes, low platelets) syndrome. The mechanism of these obstetric complications is likely accumulation of toxic intermediates. Malformations of the brain and kidneys have been described in severe deficiencies of electron transfer flavoprotein (**ETF**), ETF dehydrogenase (**ETF-DH**), and carnitine palmitoyltransferase-II (**CPT-II**), which might reflect in utero toxicity of fatty acid metabolites or a developmental role for these enzymes. Progressive retinal degeneration, peripheral neuropathy, and chronic progressive liver disease have been identified in LCHAD and MTP deficiency. Newborn screening programs using tandem mass spectrometry detect characteristic plasma acylcarnitine profiles in most of these disorders, allowing early and presymptomatic diagnosis. Screening programs have demonstrated that all the fatty acid oxidation disorders combined are among the most common inborn errors of metabolism,

Table 104.1	Mitochondrial Fatty Acid Oxidation Disorders—Clinical and Biochemical Features		
ENZYME DEFICIENCY	**GENE**	**CLINICAL PHENOTYPE**	**LABORATORY FINDINGS**
Carnitine transporter	OCTN2 SLC22A5	Cardiomyopathy, skeletal myopathy, liver disease, sudden death, endocardial fibroelastosis, prenatal and newborn screening diagnosis reported	↓ Total and free carnitine, normal acylcarnitines, acylglycine, and organic acids
Long-chain fatty acid transporter	FATP1-6	Rare, acute liver failure in childhood requiring liver transplantation	↓ intracellular C_{14}-C_{18} fatty acids, ↓ fatty acid oxidation
Carnitine palmitoyl transferase-I	CPT-IA	Liver failure, renal tubulopathy, and sudden death. Prenatal and newborn screening diagnosis reported, maternal preeclampsia, HELLP syndrome association described in a few patients.	Normal or ↑ free carnitine, normal acylcarnitines, acylglycine, and organic acids
Carnitine acylcarnitine translocase	CACT SLC25A20	Chronic progressive liver failure, persistent ↑ NH_3, hypertrophic cardiomyopathy. Newborn screening diagnosis reported.	Normal or ↓ free carnitine, abnormal acylcarnitine profile
Carnitine palmitoyl transferase-II	CPT-II	Early and late onset types. Liver failure, encephalopathy, skeletal myopathy, cardiomyopathy, renal cystic changes, newborn screening diagnosis reported. Adult form with acute rhabdomyolysis, myoglobinuria.	Normal or ↓ free carnitine, abnormal acylcarnitine profile
Short-chain acyl-CoA dehydrogenase	SCAD ACADS	Clinical phenotype unclear. Many individuals appear to be normal. Others have a variety of inconsistent signs and symptoms. Subset may have severe manifestations of unclear relationship to biochemical defects. Newborn screening diagnosis reported; significance being questioned.	Normal or ↓ free carnitine, elevated urine ethylmalonic acid, inconsistently abnormal acylcarnitine profile
Medium-chain acyl-CoA dehydrogenase	MCAD ACADM	Hypoglycemia, hepatic encephalopathy, sudden death. Newborn screening diagnosis possible, maternal preeclampsia, HELLP syndrome association described rarely, possible long Qt interval.	Normal or ↓ free carnitine, ↑ plasma acylglycine, plasma C_6-C_{10} free fatty acids, ↑ C_8-C_{10} acyl-carnitine
Very long-chain acyl-CoA dehydrogenase	VLCAD ACADVL	Dilated cardiomyopathy, arrhythmias, hypoglycemia, and hepatic steatosis. Late-onset, stress-induced rhabdomyolysis, episodic myopathy. Prenatal and newborn screening diagnosis possible.	Normal or ↓ free carnitine, ↑ plasma $C_{14:1}$, C_{14} acylcarnitine, ↑ plasma C_{10}-C_{16} free fatty acids
ETF dehydrogenase*	ETF-DH	Nonketotic fasting hypoglycemia, congenital anomalies, milder forms of liver disease, cardiomyopathy, and skeletal myopathy. Newborn screening diagnosis reported.	Normal or ↓ free carnitine, increased ratio of acyl:free carnitine, ↑ acylcarnitine, urine organic acid and acylglycines
ETF-α*	α-ETF	Nonketotic fasting hypoglycemia, congenital anomalies, liver disease, cardiomyopathy, and skeletal myopathy also described. Newborn screening diagnosis reported.	Normal or ↓ free carnitine, increased ratio of acyl:free carnitine, ↑ acylcarnitine, urine organic acid and acylglycines
ETF-β*	β-ETF	Fasting hypoglycemia, congenital anomalies, liver disease, cardiomyopathy, and skeletal myopathy also described. Newborn screening diagnosis reported.	Normal or ↓ free carnitine, increased ratio of acyl:free carnitine, ↑ acylcarnitine, urine organic acid and acylglycines
Short-chain L-3-hydroxyacyl-CoA dehydrogenase	SCHAD HAD1	Hyperinsulinemic hypoglycemia, cardiomyopathy, myopathy. Newborn screening diagnosis reported.	Normal or ↓ free carnitine, elevated free fatty acids, inconsistently abnormal urine organic acid, ↑ 3-OH glutarate, ↑ plasma C_4-OH acylcarnitine
Long-chain L-3-hydroxyacyl-CoA dehydrogenase	LCHAD HADH-A	Newborn screening diagnosis reported, maternal preeclampsia, HELLP syndrome, and AFLP association described frequently. See also MTP below for clinical manifestations.	Normal or ↓ free carnitine, increased ratio of acyl:free carnitine, ↑ free fatty acids, ↑ C_{16}-OH and C_{18}-OH carnitines
MTP	HADH-A, HADH-B	Severe cardiac and skeletal myopathy, hypoglycemia, acidosis, hyper NH_3, sudden death, elevated liver enzymes, retinopathy. Maternal preeclampsia, HELLP syndrome, and AFLP association described frequently.	Normal or ↓ free carnitine, increased ratio of acyl:free carnitine, ↑ free fatty acids, ↑ C_{16}-OH and C_{18}-OH carnitines
Long-chain 3-ketoacyl-CoA thiolase	LKAT HADH-B	Severe neonatal presentation, hypoglycemia, acidosis, ↑ creatine kinase, cardiomyopathy, neuropathy, and early death	Normal or ↓ free carnitine, increased ratio of acyl:free carnitine, ↑ free fatty acids, ↑ 2-trans, 4-cis-decadienoylcarnitine
Short-chain 2,3-enoyl-CoA hydratase	ECHS1	Leigh disease, lactic acidosis, seizures, cystic degeneration of white matter, microcephaly, metabolic acidosis, extrapyramidal dystonia, dilated cardiomyopathy	Abnormal organic acids, 2-methacrylglycine, 2-methyl-2,3 dihydroxybutyrate, also S-(2-carboxypropyl)cysteine, S-(2-carboxyethyl) cysteamine. Acylcarnitine shows ↑ C4OH (inconsistently).

Continued

Table 104.1	Mitochondrial Fatty Acid Oxidation Disorders—Clinical and Biochemical Features—cont'd		
ENZYME DEFICIENCY	**GENE**	**CLINICAL PHENOTYPE**	**LABORATORY FINDINGS**
2,4-Dienoyl-CoA reductase	DECR1	Only 1 patient described, hypotonia in the newborn, mainly severe skeletal myopathy and respiratory failure. Hypoglycemia rare.	Normal or ↓ free carnitine, ↑ acyl:free carnitine ratio, normal urine organic acids and acylglycines
HMG CoA synthetase	HMGCS2	Hypoketosis and hypoglycemia, rarely myopathy	↑ total plasma fatty acids, enzyme studies in biopsied liver may be diagnostic, genetic testing preferred
HMG CoA lyase	HMGCL	Hypoketosis and hypoglycemia, rarely myopathy	Normal free carnitine, ↑ C_5-OH, and methylglutaryl-carnitine, enzymes studies in fibroblasts may be diagnostic
Monocarboxylate transporter 1 (MCT1)	SLC16A1	Severe fasting induced ketoacidosis, rarely hypoglycemia	Profound ketoacidosis; no specific biomarkers yet identified

*Also known as glutaric acidemia type II or multiple acyl-CoA dehydrogenase defect (MADD).

AFLP, Acute fatty liver of pregnancy; CoA, coenzyme A; ETF, electron transport flavoprotein; HELLP, hemolysis, elevated liver enzymes, low platelets; MTP, mitochondrial trifunctional protein; NH_3, ammonia.

From Shekhawat PS, Matern D, Strauss AW: Fetal fatty oxidation disorders, their effect on maternal health and neonatal outcome: impact of expanded newborn screening on their diagnosis and management, *Pediatr Res* 57:78R–84R, 2005.

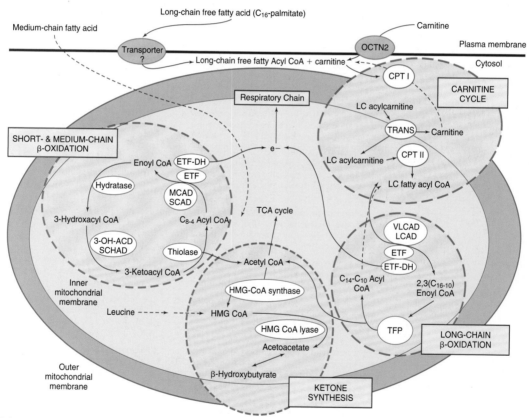

Fig. 104.1 Mitochondrial fatty acid oxidation. Carnitine enters the cell through the action of the organic cation/carnitine transporter (OCTN2). Palmitate, a typical 16-carbon long-chain fatty acid, is transported across the plasma membrane and can be activated to form a long-chain (LC) fatty acyl coenzyme A (CoA). It then enters into the carnitine cycle, where it is transesterified by carnitine palmitoyltransferase-I (CPT-I), translocated across the inner mitochondrial membrane by carnitine/acylcarnitine translocase (TRANS), and then reconverted into a long-chain fatty acyl-CoA by carnitine palmitoyltransferase-II (CPT-II) to undergo β-oxidation. Very-long-chain acyl-CoA dehydrogenase (VLCAD/LCAD) leads to the production of (C_{16}-C_{10}) 2,3-enoyl CoA. Mitochondrial trifunctional protein (MTP) contains the activities of enoyl CoA hydratase (hydratase), 3-OH-hydroxyacyl-CoA dehydrogenase (3-OH-ACD), and β-ketothiolase (thiolase). Acetyl-CoA, reduced form of flavin adenine dinucleotide (FADH), and reduced form of nicotinamide adenine dinucleotide (NADH) are produced. Medium- and short-chain fatty acids (C8-4) can enter the mitochondrial matrix independent of the carnitine cycle. Medium-chain acyl-CoA dehydrogenase (MCAD), short-chain acyl-CoA dehydrogenase (SCAD), and short-chain hydroxy acyl-CoA dehydrogenase (SCHAD) are required. Acetyl-CoA can then enter the Krebs (TCA) cycle. Electrons are transported from FADH to the respiratory chain via the electron transfer flavoprotein (ETF) and the electron transfer flavoprotein dehydrogenase (ETF-DH). NADH enters the electron transport chain through complex I. In liver, acetyl-CoA can be converted into hydroxymethylglutaryl (HMG) CoA by β-hydroxy-β-methylglutaryl-CoA synthase (HMG CoA synthase) and then the ketone body acetoacetate by the action of β-hydroxy-β-methylglutaryl-CoA lyase (HMG-CoA lyase).

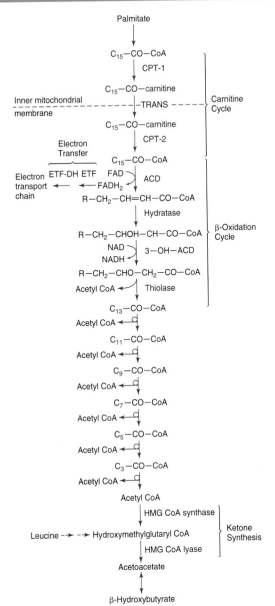

Fig. 104.2 Pathway of mitochondrial oxidation of palmitate, a typical 16-carbon long-chain fatty acid. Enzyme steps include carnitine palmitoyltransferase (CPT) 1 and 2, carnitine/acylcarnitine translocase (TRANS), electron transfer flavoprotein (ETF), ETF dehydrogenase (ETF-DH), acyl-CoA dehydrogenase (ACD), enoyl CoA hydratase (hydratase), 3-hydroxy-acyl-CoA dehydrogenase (3-OH-ACD), β-ketothiolase (thiolase), β-hydroxy-β-methylglutaryl-CoA (HMG-CoA) synthase, and lyase.

at least in predominantly Caucasian populations.

Figs. 104.1 and 104.2 outline the steps involved in the oxidation of a typical long-chain fatty acid. In the *carnitine cycle*, long-chain fatty acids are transported across the barrier of the inner mitochondrial membrane as acylcarnitine esters. (Medium-chain fatty acids, which are commonly provided as medium-chain triglyceride supplementation in infants who are failing to thrive, can bypass the carnitine cycle and enter the mitochondrial β-oxidation cycle directly.) Within the mitochondria, successive turns of the 4-step β-*oxidation cycle* convert the **coenzyme A (CoA)**–activated fatty acids to acetyl-CoA units. Two or

3 different specific isoenzymes are needed for each of these β-oxidation steps to accommodate the different chain-length fatty acyl-CoA species. The electrons generated in the first β-oxidation step (acyl-CoA dehydrogenase) are carried by the *electron transfer pathway* to the *electron transport chain* at the level of coenzyme Q for adenosine triphosphate production; while electrons generated from the 3rd step (3-hydroxyacyl-CoA dehydrogenase) enter the *electron transport chain* at the level of complex 1. Most of the acetyl-CoA generated from fatty acid β-oxidation in the liver flows through the *pathway of ketogenesis* to form β-hydroxybutyrate and acetoacetate, whereas in muscle and heart the fatty acids are completely oxidized to CO_2 and water.

DEFECTS IN THE β-OXIDATION CYCLE
Medium-Chain Acyl-CoA Dehydrogenase Deficiency
Medium-chain acyl-CoA dehydrogenase (**MCAD**) deficiency is the most common fatty acid oxidation disorder. The disorder shows a strong founder effect; most patients have a northwestern European ancestry, and the majority of these patients are homozygous for a single common MCAD missense mutation, an A-G transition at cDNA position 985 (c.985A>G) that changes a lysine to glutamic acid at residue 329 (p.K329E).

Clinical Manifestations
Previously undiagnosed affected patients usually present in the 1st 3 mo to 5 yr of life with episodes of acute illness triggered by prolonged fasting (>12-16 hr). Signs and symptoms include vomiting and lethargy, which rapidly progress to coma or seizures and cardiorespiratory collapse. Sudden unexpected infant death may occur. The liver may be slightly enlarged with fat deposition. Attacks are rare until the infant is beyond the 1st few mo of life, presumably because of more frequent feedings at a younger age. Affected older infants are at higher risk of illness as they begin to fast through the night or are exposed to fasting stress during an intercurrent childhood illness. Presentation in the 1st days of life with neonatal hypoglycemia has been reported in newborns who were fasted inadvertently or were being breastfed. Diagnosis of MCAD has occasionally been documented in previously healthy teenage and adult individuals, indicating that even patients who have been asymptomatic in infancy are still at risk for metabolic decompensation if exposed to sufficient periods of fasting. An unknown number of patients may remain asymptomatic. Prior to routine newborn screening testing, as many as 25% of MCAD-deficient patients died or suffered severe brain damage from their first episode. Most patients are now diagnosed in the newborn period by **blood spot acylcarnitine screening**, allowing the initiation of early treatment and prevention of many of the severe signs and symptoms. In some reports, newborns with MCAD deficiency presented acutely before newborn screening results were obtained; neonates who are exclusively breastfed are at higher risk because of early poor caloric intake.

Laboratory Findings
During acute episodes, hypoglycemia is usually present. Plasma and urinary ketone concentrations are inappropriately low (**hypoketotic hypoglycemia**). Because of the hypoketonemia, there is little or no metabolic acidosis, which is expected to be present in many children with hypoglycemia. Liver function tests (LFTs) are abnormal, with elevations of liver enzymes (alanine transaminase, aspartate transaminase), elevated blood ammonia, and prolonged prothrombin and partial thromboplastin times. Liver biopsy at times of acute illness shows microvesicular or macrovesicular steatosis from triglyceride accumulation. During fasting stress or acute illness, urinary organic acid profiles by gas chromatography/mass spectrometry show inappropriately low concentrations of ketones and elevated levels of medium-chain dicarboxylic acids (adipic, suberic, and sebacic acids) that derive from microsomal and peroxisomal omega oxidation of accumulated medium-chain fatty acids. Plasma and tissue concentrations of total carnitine are reduced to 25–50% of normal, and the fraction of total esterified carnitine is increased. This pattern of **secondary carnitine deficiency** is seen in most fatty acid oxidation defects and reflects competition between increased acylcarnitine levels and free carnitine for transport

at the renal tubular plasma membrane. Significant exceptions to this rule are the plasma membrane carnitine transporter, CPT-IA, and β-hydroxy-β-methylglutaryl-CoA (HMG-CoA) synthase deficiencies, which do not manifest secondary carnitine deficiency.

Diagnostic metabolite patterns for MCAD deficiency include increased plasma $C_{6:0}$, $C_{8:0}$, $C_{10:0}$, and $C_{10:1}$ acylcarnitine species and increased urinary acylglycines, including hexanoylglycine, suberylglycine, and 3-phenylpropionylglycine. Newborn screening, which almost all babies born in the United States receive, can detect presymptomatic MCAD deficiency based on these abnormal acylcarnitines in filter paper blood spots. The diagnosis can be confirmed by finding the common A985G mutation or sequencing the *MCAD* gene. A 2nd common variant, T199C, has been detected in infants identified by newborn screening. Interestingly, this allele has not been seen to date in symptomatic MCAD patients; it may represent a milder mutation.

Treatment
Acute illnesses should be promptly treated with intravenous (IV) fluids containing 10% dextrose to correct or prevent hypoglycemia and to suppress lipolysis as rapidly as possible (see Chapter 111). Chronic therapy consists of avoiding fasting. This usually requires simply adjusting the diet to ensure that overnight fasting periods are limited to <10-12 hr. Restricting dietary fat or treatment with carnitine is controversial. The need for active therapeutic intervention for individuals with the T199C variant has not yet been established.

Prognosis
Up to 25% of unrecognized patients may die during their first attack of illness. There is frequently a history of a previous sibling death that is presumed to be from an unrecognized MCAD deficiency. Some patients may sustain permanent brain injury during an attack of profound hypoglycemia. For survivors without brain damage, the prognosis is excellent because progressive cognitive impairment or cardiomyopathy does not occur in MCAD deficiency. Fasting tolerance improves with age, and the risk of illness decreases. Because as many as 35% of affected patients have never had an episode, testing of siblings of affected patients is important to detect asymptomatic family members.

Very-Long-Chain Acyl-CoA Dehydrogenase Deficiency
Very-long-chain acyl-CoA dehydrogenase (**VLCAD**) deficiency is the second most commonly diagnosed disorder of fatty acid oxidation. It was originally termed "long-chain acyl-CoA dehydrogenase deficiency" before the existence of the inner mitochondrial membrane-bound VLCAD was known. *All patients previously diagnosed as having long-chain acyl-CoA dehydrogenase deficiency have VLCAD gene defects.* Patients with VLCAD deficiency have no ability to oxidize physiologic long-chain fatty acids and are usually more severely affected than those with MCAD deficiency, who have a milder oxidative defect. VLCAD deficiency presents earlier in infancy and has more chronic problems with muscle weakness or episodes of muscle pain and rhabdomyolysis. Cardiomyopathy may be present during acute attacks provoked by fasting. The left ventricle may be hypertrophic or dilated and may show poor contractility on echocardiography. Sudden unexpected death has occurred in several patients, but most who survive the initial episode show improvement, including normalization of cardiac function. Other physical and routine laboratory features are similar to those of MCAD deficiency, including secondary carnitine deficiency. The urinary organic acid profile shows a nonketotic dicarboxylic-aciduria with increased levels of C_{6-12} dicarboxylic acids. Diagnosis may be suggested by an abnormal acylcarnitine profile with plasma or blood spot $C_{14:0, \, 14:1, \, 14:2}$ acylcarnitine species. However, the specific diagnosis requires mutational analysis of the *VLCAD* gene. Treatment is based primarily on avoidance of fasts for >10-12 hr. Continuous intragastric feeding is useful in some patients.

Short-Chain Acyl-CoA Dehydrogenase Deficiency
A small number of patients with 2 null mutations in the short-chain acyl-CoA dehydrogenase (*SCAD*) gene have been described with variable phenotype. Most individuals classified as being SCAD deficient actually have polymorphic DNA changes in the *SCAD* gene; for example, 2 common polymorphisms are G185S and R147W, which are homozygously present in 7% of the population. Some investigators argue that these variants may be susceptibility factors, which require a 2nd, as yet unknown, genetic mutation to express a clinical phenotype; many other investigators believe that SCAD deficiency is a harmless biochemical condition. This autosomal recessive disorder presents with neonatal hypoglycemia and may have normal levels of ketone bodies. The diagnosis is indicated by elevated levels of butyrylcarnitine (C4-carnitine) on newborn blood spots or plasma and increased excretion of urinary ethylmalonic acid and butyrylglycine. These metabolic abnormalities are most pronounced in patients with null mutations and are variably present in patients who are homozygous for the common polymorphisms.

The need for treatment in SCAD deficiency has not yet been established. It has been proposed that long-term evaluation of asymptomatic individuals is necessary to determine whether this is or is not a real disease. Most individuals with SCAD deficiency remain asymptomatic throughout life, but there may be a subset of individuals with **severe manifestations**, including dysmorphic facial features, feeding difficulties/failure to thrive, metabolic acidosis, ketotic hypoglycemia, lethargy, developmental delay, seizures, hypotonia, dystonia, and myopathy.

Long-Chain 3-Hydroxyacyl-CoA Dehydrogenase/ Mitochondrial Trifunctional Protein Deficiency
The LCHAD enzyme is part of the MTP, which also contains 2 other steps in β-oxidation: long-chain 2,3-enoyl CoA hydratase and long-chain β-ketothiolase. MTP is a hetero-octameric protein composed of 4 α and 4 β chains derived from distinct contiguous genes sharing a common promoter region. In some patients, only the LCHAD activity of the MTP is affected (**LCHAD deficiency**), whereas others have deficiencies of all 3 activities (**MTP deficiency**).

Clinical manifestations include attacks of acute hypoketotic hypoglycemia similar to MCAD deficiency; however, patients often show evidence of more severe disease, including cardiomyopathy, muscle cramps and weakness, and abnormal liver function (cholestasis). Toxic effects of fatty acid metabolites may produce pigmented retinopathy leading to blindness, progressive liver failure, peripheral neuropathy, and rhabdomyolysis. Life-threatening obstetric complications (AFLP, HELLP syndrome) have been observed in heterozygous mothers carrying homozygous fetuses affected with LCHAD/MTP deficiency. Sudden unexpected infant death may occur. The **diagnosis** is indicated by elevated levels of blood spot or plasma 3-hydroxy acylcarnitines of chain lengths C_{16}-C_{18}. Urinary organic acid profile in patients may show increased levels of 3-hydroxydicarboxylic acids of chain lengths C_6-C_{14}. Secondary carnitine deficiency is common. A common mutation in the α subunit, E474Q, is seen in more than 60% of LCHAD-deficient patients. This mutation in the fetus is especially associated with the obstetric complications, but other mutations in either subunit may also be linked to maternal illness.

Treatment is similar to that for MCAD or VLCAD deficiency; that is, avoiding fasting stress. Some investigators have suggested that dietary supplements with medium-chain triglyceride oil to bypass the defect in long-chain fatty acid oxidation and docosahexaenoic acid (for protection against the retinal changes) may be useful. Liver transplantation has been attempted in patients with severe liver failure, but does not ameliorate the metabolic abnormalities or prevent the myopathic or retinal complications.

Short-Chain 3-Hydroxyacyl-CoA Dehydrogenase Deficiency
Only 14 patients with proven mutations of short-chain 3-hydroxyacyl-CoA dehydrogenase (**SCHAD**) have been reported. Most cases with recessive mutations of the *SCHAD* gene have presented with episodes of hypoketotic hypoglycemia that was caused by hyperinsulinism. In contrast to those with other forms of fatty acid oxidation disorders, these patients required specific therapy with diazoxide for hyperinsulinism to avoid recurrent hypoglycemia. A single patient with compound heterozygous mutations presented with fulminant hepatic failure at age

10 mo. The SCHAD protein has a nonenzymatic function in which it directly interacts with glutamate dehydrogenase (GDH) to inhibit its activity. In the absence of SCHAD protein, this inhibition is removed, leading to upregulation of GDH enzyme activity, a recognized cause of hyperinsulinism usually from activating mutations of the *GDH* gene. Severe deficiency of SCHAD protein often presents predominantly as protein-sensitive hypoglycemia rather than as fasting hypoglycemia. It appears that if SCHAD protein is present, inhibition of GDH is maintained even when there is no SCHAD enzyme activity; these patients may present with a more traditional fatty acid oxidation defect. Specific metabolic markers for SCHAD deficiency include elevated plasma C4-hydroxy acylcarnitine and urine 3-hydroxyglutaric acid. Successful newborn screening for SCHAD deficiency has been recorded, but the sensitivity of the process has not yet been established.

Treatment of SCHAD-deficient patients with hyperinsulinism is with diazoxide. There is insufficient experience with the nonhyperinsulinemic form of SCHAD deficiency at present to recommend treatment modalities, but prevention of fasting seems advisable.

Short-Chain 2,3-Enoyl-CoA Hydratase Deficiency

This disorder, resulting from mutations in the *ECHS1* gene, has only recently been defined. Many patients were identified through exome sequencing, and currently there are approximately 20 cases in the literature. The disorder affects a shared pathway of short-chain fatty acid and valine metabolism. The clinical phenotypes are more characteristic of mitochondrial disorders of pyruvate metabolism with predominantly a Leigh-like disease (see Chapter 616.2) with profound and often-fatal lactic acidosis. Currently, no treatment modalities or specific biomarkers have been established. Several patients were found to excrete increased levels of methacrylylglycine, a highly reactive and potentially toxic intermediate; 2-methyl-2.3 dihydroxybutyrate; *S*-(2-carboxypropyl) cysteine; and *S*-(2-carboxpropyl) cysteamine.

DEFECTS IN THE CARNITINE CYCLE
Plasma Membrane Carnitine Transport Defect (Primary Carnitine Deficiency)

Primary carnitine deficiency is the only genetic defect in which carnitine deficiency is the cause, rather than the consequence, of impaired fatty acid oxidation. The most common presentation is progressive **cardiomyopathy** with or without **skeletal muscle weakness** beginning at age 1-4 yr. A smaller number of patients may present with fasting hypoketotic hypoglycemia in the 1st yr of life, before the cardiomyopathy becomes symptomatic. The underlying defect involves the plasma membrane sodium gradient–dependent carnitine transporter that is present in heart, muscle, and kidney. This transporter is responsible both for maintaining intracellular carnitine concentrations 20-50-fold higher than plasma concentrations and for renal conservation of carnitine.

Diagnosis of the carnitine transporter defect is aided by patients having extremely reduced carnitine levels in plasma and muscle (1–2% of normal). Heterozygote parents have plasma carnitine levels approximately 50% of normal. Fasting ketogenesis may be normal because liver carnitine transport is normal, but it may become impaired if dietary carnitine intake is interrupted. The fasting urinary organic acid profile may show a hypoketotic dicarboxylic aciduria pattern if hepatic fatty acid oxidation is impaired, but is otherwise unremarkable. The defect in carnitine transport can be demonstrated clinically by the severe reduction in renal carnitine threshold or by in vitro assay of carnitine uptake using cultured fibroblasts or lymphoblasts. Mutations in the organic cation/carnitine transporter *(OCTN2)* underlie this disorder. **Treatment** with pharmacologic doses of oral carnitine (100-200 mg/kg/day) is highly effective in correcting the cardiomyopathy and muscle weakness, as well as any impairment in fasting ketogenesis. Muscle total carnitine concentrations remain <5% of normal on treatment.

Carnitine Palmitoyltransferase-IA Deficiency

Several dozen infants and children have been described with a deficiency of the liver and kidney CPT-I isozyme (CPT-IA). **Clinical manifestations** include fasting-induced hypoketotic hypoglycemia, occasionally with extremely abnormal LFTs and rarely with renal tubular acidosis. The heart and skeletal muscle are not involved because the muscle isozyme is unaffected. Fasting urinary organic acid profiles sometimes show a hypoketotic C_6–C_{12} dicarboxylic aciduria but may be normal. Plasma acylcarnitine analysis demonstrates mostly free carnitine with very little acylated carnitine. This observation has been used to identify CPT-IA deficiency on newborn screening by tandem mass spectrometry. CPT-IA deficiency is the only fatty acid oxidation disorder in which plasma total carnitine levels may be elevated, often to 150–200% of normal. This phenomenon is explained by the absence of inhibitory effects of long-chain acylcarnitines on the renal tubular carnitine transporter in CPT-IA deficiency. The enzyme defect can be demonstrated in cultured fibroblasts or lymphoblasts. CPT-IA deficiency in the fetus has been associated in a single case report with AFLP in the mother. A common variant in the *CPTIA* gene (c.1436C>t, p.P479L) has been identified in individuals of Inuit background in the United States, Canada, and Greenland. This variant is associated with an increased risk for sudden infant death syndrome (SIDS) in the Inuit population. The variant can be detected by newborn screening; enzyme activity is reduced by 80%, and regulation by malonyl-CoA is lost. It has not been established whether CPT-IA (c.1436C>t, p.P479L) is a pathologic enzyme variant or an adaptation to ancient Inuit high-fat diets. **Treatment** for the severe form of CPT-IA deficiency that is found in non-Inuit populations is similar to that for MCAD deficiency, with avoidance of situations where fasting ketogenesis is necessary. The need for treatment of the Inuit variant has not yet been determined.

Carnitine:Acylcarnitine Translocase Deficiency

This defect of the inner mitochondrial membrane carrier protein for long-chain acylcarnitines blocks the entry of long-chain fatty acids into the mitochondria for oxidation. The clinical phenotype of this disorder is characterized by a severe and generalized impairment of fatty acid oxidation. Most newborn patients present with attacks of fasting-induced hypoglycemia, hyperammonemia, and cardiorespiratory collapse. All symptomatic newborns have had evidence of cardiomyopathy and muscle weakness. Several patients with a partial translocase deficiency and milder disease without cardiac involvement have also been identified. No distinctive urinary or plasma organic acids are noted, although increased levels of plasma long-chain acylcarnitines of chain lengths C_{16}–C_{18} are reported. **Diagnosis** can be confirmed using genetic analysis. Functional carnitine:acylcarnitine translocase activity can be measured in cultured fibroblasts or lymphoblasts. **Treatment** is similar to that of other long-chain fatty acid oxidation disorders.

Carnitine Palmitoyltransferase-II Deficiency

Three forms of CPT-II deficiency have been described. A **severe neonatal lethal** presentation associated with a profound enzyme deficiency and early death has been reported in several newborns in association with dysplastic kidneys, cerebral malformations, and mild facial anomalies. A milder defect is associated with an **adult presentation** of episodic rhabdomyolysis. The first episode usually does not occur until late childhood or early adulthood. Attacks are frequently precipitated by prolonged exercise. There is aching muscle pain and myoglobinuria that may be severe enough to cause renal failure. Serum levels of creatine kinase are elevated to 5,000-100,000 units/L. Hypoglycemia has not been described, but fasting may contribute to attacks of myoglobinuria. Muscle biopsy shows increased deposition of neutral fat. This adult myopathic presentation of CPT-II deficiency is associated with a common mutation, c.338C>T, p.S113L. This mutation produces a heat-labile protein that is unstable to increased muscle temperature during exercise resulting in the myopathic presentation. The 3rd, **intermediate form** of CPT-II deficiency presents in infancy or early childhood with fasting-induced hepatic failure, cardiomyopathy, and skeletal myopathy with hypoketotic hypoglycemia, but is not associated with the severe developmental changes seen in the neonatal lethal presentation. This pattern of illness is similar to that seen in VLCAD deficiency, and management is identical.

Diagnosis of all forms of CPT-II deficiency can be made by a combination of molecular genetic analysis and demonstrating deficient enzyme activity in muscle or other tissues and in cultured fibroblasts.

DEFECTS IN THE ELECTRON TRANSFER PATHWAY
Electron Transfer Flavoprotein and Electron Transfer Flavoprotein Dehydrogenase Deficiencies (Glutaric Acidemia Type 2, Multiple Acyl-CoA Dehydrogenation Defects)

ETF and ETF-DH function to transfer electrons into the mitochondrial electron transport chain from dehydrogenation reactions catalyzed by VLCAD, MCAD, and SCAD, as well as by glutaryl-CoA dehydrogenase and 4 enzymes involved in branched-chain amino acid (BCAA) oxidation. Deficiencies of ETF or ETF-DH produce illness that combines the features of impaired fatty acid oxidation and impaired oxidation of several amino acids. Complete deficiencies of either protein are associated with severe illness in the newborn period, characterized by acidosis, hypoketotic hypoglycemia, coma, hypotonia, cardiomyopathy, and an unusual odor of sweaty feet caused by isovaleryl-CoA dehydrogenase inhibition. Some affected neonates have had congenital facial dysmorphism and polycystic kidneys similar to that seen in severe CPT-II deficiency, which suggests that toxic effects of accumulated metabolites may occur in utero.

Diagnosis can be made from the newborn blood spot acylcarnitine profile and urinary organic acids; both tests show abnormalities corresponding to blocks in the oxidation of fatty acids (ethylmalonate and C_6-C_{10} dicarboxylic acids), lysine (glutarate), and BCAAs (isovaleryl-, isobutyryl-, and α-methylbutyryl-glycine). The diagnosis can be confirmed by genetic testing for ETF (2 genes, A and B) and ETF dehydrogenase. Most severely affected infants do not survive the neonatal period.

Partial deficiencies of ETF and ETF-DH produce a disorder that may mimic MCAD deficiency or other milder fatty acid oxidation defects. These patients have attacks of fasting hypoketotic coma. The urinary organic acid profile reveals primarily elevations of dicarboxylic acids and ethylmalonate, derived from short-chain fatty acid intermediates. Secondary carnitine deficiency is present. Some patients with mild forms of ETF/ETF-DH deficiency may benefit from treatment with high doses of *riboflavin*, a precursor of the various flavoproteins involved in electron transfer.

DEFECTS IN THE KETONE SYNTHESIS PATHWAY

The final steps in production of ketones from mitochondrial fatty acid β-oxidation convert acetyl-CoA to acetoacetate through 2 enzymes of the HMG-CoA pathway (Fig. 104.2).

β-Hydroxy-β-Methylglutaryl-CoA Synthase Deficiency
See Chapter 103.6.

HMG-CoA synthase is the rate-limiting step in the conversion of acetyl-CoA derived from fatty acid β-oxidation in the liver to ketones. Several patients with this defect have been identified. The presentation is one of fasting hypoketotic hypoglycemia without evidence of impaired cardiac or skeletal muscle function. Urinary organic acid profile shows only a nonspecific hypoketotic dicarboxylic aciduria. Plasma and tissue carnitine levels are normal, in contrast to all the other disorders of fatty acid oxidation. A separate synthase enzyme, present in cytosol for cholesterol biosynthesis, is not affected. The HMG-CoA synthase defect is expressed only in the liver (and kidney) and cannot be demonstrated in cultured fibroblasts. The diagnosis can be made by genetic mutation analysis. *Avoiding fasting is usually a successful treatment.*

β-Hydroxy-β-Methylglutaryl-CoA Lyase Deficiency (3 Hydroxy-3-Methylgutaric Aciduria)
See Chapter 103.6.

DEFECTS IN KETONE BODY UTILIZATION

The ketone bodies, β-hydroxybutyrate and acetoacetate, are the end products of hepatic fatty acid oxidation and are important metabolic fuels for the brain during fasting. Three defects in utilization of ketones in brain and other peripheral tissues present as episodes of **hyperketotic coma**, with or without hypoglycemia.

Monocarboxylate Transporter-1 Deficiency
About 10 patients have been described with recurrent episodes of potentially lethal ketoacidosis, with or without hypoglycemia, caused by deficiency of monocarboxylate transporter 1 (MCT1), a plasma membrane carrier encoded by *SLC16A1* that is required to transport ketones into tissues from plasma. Although the first cases identified were homozygous for inactivating mutations of *MCT1*, heterozygous carriers can also be affected. Affected patients developed severe ketoacidosis provoked by fasting or infections in their 1st years of life; hypoglycemia was not always present. The differential includes ketotic hypoglycemia associated with milder forms of glycogen storage disease, such as phosphorylase or phosphorylase kinase deficiency (see Chapter 105). **Treatment** for acute episodes includes IV dextrose to suppress lipolysis and inhibit ongoing ketogenesis. Long-term treatment includes avoidance of prolonged fasting stress. The **diagnosis** can be suspected by unusually severe ketosis and delayed suppression of ketones after starting treatment with dextrose. There are no specific metabolic markers or newborn screening methods. The diagnosis can be established by genetic sequencing of *SLC16A1*.

Succinyl-CoA:3-Ketoacid-CoA Transferase Deficiency
See Chapter 103.6.

Several patients with succinyl-CoA:3-ketoacid-CoA transferase (**SCOT**) deficiency have been reported. The characteristic presentation is an infant with recurrent episodes of severe ketoacidosis induced by fasting. Plasma acylcarnitine and urine organic acid abnormalities do not distinguish SCOT deficiency from other causes of ketoacidosis. **Treatment** of episodes requires infusion of glucose and large amounts of bicarbonate until metabolically stable. Patients usually exhibit inappropriate hyperketonemia even between episodes of illness. SCOT is responsible for activating acetoacetate in peripheral tissues, using succinyl CoA as a donor to form acetoacetyl-CoA. Deficient enzyme activity can be demonstrated in the brain, muscle, and fibroblasts from affected patients. The gene has been cloned, and numerous mutations have been characterized.

β-Ketothiolase Deficiency
See Chapter 103.6.

Bibliography is available at Expert Consult.

104.2 Disorders of Very-Long-Chain Fatty Acids and Other Peroxisomal Functions
Michael F. Wangler and Gerald V. Raymond

PEROXISOMAL DISORDERS

Disorders of very-long-chain fatty acids (VLCFAs) fall within the broader group of peroxisomal diseases. The **peroxisomal diseases** are genetically determined disorders caused either by the failure to form or maintain the peroxisome or by a defect in the function of a single protein that is normally located in this organelle. These disorders cause serious disability in childhood and occur more frequently and present a wider range of phenotypes than recognized in the past. Many, but not all, peroxisomal disorders are associated with elevations of VLCFAs. This discussion addresses the broader group of peroxisomal disorders with a focus on pediatric presentations.

Etiology
Peroxisomal disorders are subdivided into two major categories (Table 104.2). In the **peroxisomal biogenesis disorders (PBDs)** the basic defect is the failure to import 1 or more proteins into the organelle. In the other group, defects affect a single peroxisomal protein (**single-enzyme defects**). The *peroxisome* is present in all cells except mature erythrocytes and is a subcellular organelle surrounded by a single membrane; >50 peroxisomal enzymes are identified. Some enzymes are involved in production and decomposition of hydrogen peroxide and others in lipid and amino acid metabolism. Most peroxisomal enzymes are first

synthesized in their mature form on free polyribosomes and enter the cytoplasm. Proteins that are destined for the peroxisome contain specific **peroxisome targeting sequences** (PTSs). Most peroxisomal matrix proteins contain **PTS1**, a 3-amino acid sequence at the carboxyl terminus. **PTS2** is an aminoterminal sequence that is critical for the import of enzymes involved in plasmalogen and branched-chain fatty acid metabolism. Import of proteins involves a complex series of reactions that involves at least 23 distinct proteins. These proteins, referred to as *peroxins,* are encoded by *PEX* genes.

Epidemiology

Except for X-linked **adrenoleukodystrophy (ALD)**, all the peroxisomal disorders listed in Table 104.2 are **autosomal recessive diseases**. ALD is the most common peroxisomal disorder, with an estimated incidence of 1 in 17,000 live births. The combined incidence of the other peroxisomal disorders is estimated to be 1 in 50,000 live births, although with broader newborn screening it is expected that the actual incidences of all of the disorders of very-long-chain fatty acids will be more accurately established.

Pathology

Absence or reduction in the number of peroxisomes is pathognomonic for disorders of peroxisome biogenesis. In most disorders, membranous sacs contain peroxisomal integral membrane proteins, which lack the normal complement of matrix proteins; these are peroxisome "ghosts." Pathologic changes are observed in most organs and include profound and characteristic defects in neuronal migration, micronodular cirrhosis of the liver, renal cysts, chondrodysplasia punctata, sensorineural hearing loss, retinopathy, congenital heart disease, and dysmorphic features.

Pathogenesis

All pathologic changes likely are secondary to the peroxisome defect. Multiple peroxisomal enzymes fail to function in the PBDs (Table 104.3). The enzymes that are diminished or absent are synthesized but are degraded abnormally fast because they may be unprotected outside the peroxisome. It is not clear how defective peroxisome functions lead to the widespread pathologic manifestations.

Table 104.2	Classification of Peroxisomal Disorders
PEROXISOMAL BIOGENESIS DISORDERS	**SINGLE-ENZYME DEFECTS**
Zellweger spectrum disorder	X-linked adrenoleukodystrophy
Zellweger syndrome	Acyl-CoA oxidase deficiency
Neonatal	Bifunctional enzyme deficiency
adrenoleukodystrophy (ALD)	2-Methylacyl-CoA racemase
Infantile Refsum disease	deficiency
Rhizomelic chondrodysplasia	DHAP acyltransferase deficiency
punctata (RCDP) and other	Alkyl-DHAP synthase deficiency
PEX7 conditions	Adult Refsum disease

Table 104.3	Abnormal Laboratory Findings Common to Zellweger Spectrum Disorders

Peroxisomes absent to reduced in number
Catalase in cytosol
Deficient synthesis and reduced tissue levels of plasmalogens
Defective oxidation and abnormal accumulation of very-long-chain fatty acids
Deficient oxidation and age-dependent accumulation of phytanic acid
Defects in certain steps of bile acid formation and accumulation of bile acid intermediates
Defects in oxidation and accumulation of L-pipecolic acid
Increased urinary excretion of dicarboxylic acids

Mutations in 12 different *PEX* genes have been identified in PBDs. The pattern and severity of pathologic features vary with the nature of the import defects and the degree of import impairment. These gene defects lead to disorders that were named before their relationship to the peroxisome was recognized, namely, Zellweger syndrome, neonatal ALD, infantile Refsum disease, and rhizomelic chondrodysplasia punctata (**RCDP**). The first 3 disorders are considered to form a *clinical continuum*, with Zellweger syndrome the most severe, infantile Refsum disease the least severe, and neonatal ALD intermediate. They can be caused by mutations in any of the 11 genes involved in peroxisome assembly. The specific gene defects cannot be distinguished by clinical features. The clinical severity varies with the degree to which protein import is impaired. Mutations that abolish import completely are often associated with the Zellweger syndrome phenotype, whereas a missense mutation, in which some degree of import function is retained, leads to the somewhat milder phenotypes. A defect in *PEX7*, which involves the import of proteins that utilize PTS2, is associated with RCDP. *PEX7* defects that leave import partially intact are associated with milder phenotypes, some of which resemble classic (adult) Refsum disease.

The genetic disorders that involve single peroxisomal enzymes usually have clinical manifestations that are more restricted and relate to the single biochemical defect. The primary adrenal insufficiency of ALD is caused by accumulation of VLCFAs in the adrenal cortex, and the peripheral neuropathy in adult Refsum disease is caused by the accumulation of phytanic acid in Schwann cells and myelin.

Zellweger Spectrum Disorder

Newborn infants with **Zellweger syndrome** show striking and consistent recognizable abnormalities. Of central diagnostic importance are the typical facial appearance (high forehead, unslanting palpebral fissures, hypoplastic supraorbital ridges, and epicanthal folds; Fig. 104.3), severe weakness and hypotonia, neonatal seizures, and eye abnormalities. Because of the hypotonia and craniofacial appearance, Down syndrome may be suspected. Infants with Zellweger syndrome rarely live more than a few months. More than 90% show postnatal growth failure. Table 104.4 lists the main clinical abnormalities.

Patients with **neonatal ALD** show fewer, less prominent craniofacial features. Neonatal seizures occur frequently. Some degree of psychomotor developmental delay is present; function remains in the range of severe intellectual disability, and development may regress after 3-5 yr of age, probably from a progressive leukodystrophy. Hepatomegaly, impaired liver function, pigmentary degeneration of the retina, and severely impaired hearing are invariably present. Adrenocortical function is usually impaired and may require adrenal hormone replacement. Chondrodysplasia punctata and renal cysts are absent.

Patients with **infantile Refsum disease** have survived to adulthood. They can walk, although gait may be ataxic and broad based. Cognitive function is generally impaired, but accurate assessment is limited, usually by the presence of both vision and hearing impairment. Almost all have some degree of sensorineural hearing loss and pigmentary degeneration of the retina. They have moderately dysmorphic features that may include epicanthal folds, a flat nose bridge, and low-set ears. Early hypotonia and hepatomegaly with impaired function are common. Levels of plasma cholesterol and high-density and low-density lipoprotein are often moderately reduced. Chondrodysplasia punctata and renal cortical cysts are absent. Postmortem study in infantile Refsum disease reveals micronodular liver cirrhosis and small, hypoplastic adrenals. The brain shows no malformations, except for severe hypoplasia of the cerebellar granule layer and ectopic locations of the Purkinje cells in the molecular layer. The mode of inheritance is autosomal recessive.

Some patients with PBDs have milder and atypical phenotypes. They may present with peripheral neuropathy or with retinopathy, impaired vision, or cataracts in childhood, adolescence, or adulthood and have been diagnosed to have **Charcot-Marie-Tooth disease** or **Usher syndrome**. Some patients have survived to the fifth decade. Defects in *PEX7*, which most frequently lead to the RCDP phenotype, may also lead to a milder phenotype with clinical manifestations similar to those of adult Refsum disease.

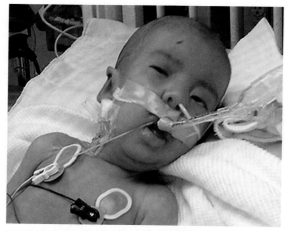

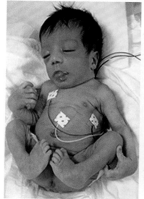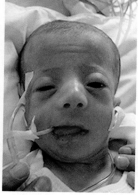

Fig. 104.3 Zellweger syndrome. Three affected neonates. Note the hypotonia, high forehead with shallow supraorbital ridges, anteverted nares, and mild micrognathia, as well as the talipes equinovarus and contractures at the knees. *(From Shaheen R, Al-Dirbashi OY, Al-Hassnan ZN, et al: Clinical, biochemical and molecular characterization of peroxisomal diseases in Arabs, Clin Genet 79(1):60–70, 2011.)*

Table 104.4	Main Clinical Abnormalities in Zellweger Syndrome	
	PATIENTS IN WHOM THE FEATURE WAS PRESENT	
ABNORMAL FEATURE	Number	%
High forehead	58	97
Flat occiput	13	81
Large fontanelle(s), wide sutures	55	96
Shallow orbital ridges	33	100
Low/broad nasal bridge	23	100
Epicanthus	33	92
High-arched palate	35	95
External ear deformity	39	97
Micrognathia	18	100
Redundant skin fold of neck	13	100
Brushfield spots	5	83
Cataract/cloudy cornea	30	86
Glaucoma	7	58
Abnormal retinal pigmentation	6	40
Optic disc pallor	17	74
Severe hypotonia	94	99
Abnormal Moro response	26	100
Hyporeflexia or areflexia	56	98
Poor sucking	74	96
Gavage feeding	26	100
Epileptic seizures	56	92
Psychomotor retardation	45	100
Impaired hearing	9	40
Nystagmus	30	81

From Heymans HAS: Cerebro-hepato-renal (Zellweger) syndrome: clinical and biochemical consequences of peroxisomal dysfunctions, Thesis, University of Amsterdam, 1984.

Rhizomelic Chondrodysplasia Punctata

RCDP is characterized by the presence of stippled foci of calcification within the hyaline cartilage and is associated with dwarfing, cataracts (72%), and multiple malformations caused by contractures. Vertebral bodies have a coronal cleft filled by cartilage that is a result of an embryonic arrest. Disproportionate short stature affects the proximal parts of the extremities (Fig. 104.4*A*). Radiologic abnormalities consist of shortening of the proximal limb bones, metaphyseal cupping, and disturbed ossification (Fig. 104.4*B*). Height, weight, and head circumference are less than the 3rd percentile, and these children have a severe intellectual disability. Skin changes such as those observed in **ichthyosiform erythroderma** are present in approximately 25% of patients.

Isolated Defects of Peroxisomal Fatty Acid Oxidation

In the group of single-enzyme defects, acyl-CoA oxidase and bifunctional enzyme deficiency involve a single enzymatic step in peroxisomal fatty acid oxidation. **Defects of bifunctional enzyme** are common and are found in approximately 15% of patients who are initially suspected of having Zellweger spectrum disorder. Patients with isolated **acyl-CoA oxidase deficiency** have a somewhat milder phenotype that resembles, and comes to attention because of the development of, an early childhood leukodystrophy.

Isolated Defects of Plasmalogen Synthesis

Plasmalogens are lipids in which the first carbon of glycerol is linked to an alcohol rather than a fatty acid. They are synthesized through a complex series of reactions, the first 2 steps of which are catalyzed by the peroxisomal enzymes dihydroxyacetone phosphate alkyl transferase (DHAPT) and synthase. Deficiency of either of these enzymes leads to a phenotype that is clinically indistinguishable from the peroxisomal import disorder RCDP. This latter disorder is caused by a defect in *PEX7*, the receptor for PTS2. RCDP shares the severe deficiency of plasmalogens with these single-enzyme disorders but also has defects of phytanic oxidation. The fact that these single genetic disorders are associated with the full phenotype of RCDP suggests that a deficiency of plasmalogens is sufficient to produce it.

Adult (Classic) Refsum Disease

The defective enzyme (phytanoyl-CoA hydroxylase) is localized to the peroxisome. The manifestation of Refsum disease includes impaired vision from retinitis pigmentosa, anosmia, ichthyosis, peripheral neuropathy, ataxia, and occasionally cardiac arrhythmias. In contrast to infantile Refsum disease, cognitive function is normal, and there are no congenital malformations. Refsum disease often does not manifest until young adulthood, but visual disturbances such as night blindness,

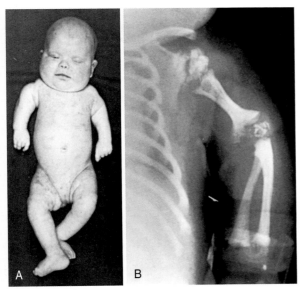

Fig. 104.4 A, Newborn infant with rhizomelic chondrodysplasia punctata. Note the severe shortening of the proximal limbs, the depressed bridge of the nose, hypertelorism, and widespread scaling skin lesions. **B,** Note the marked shortening of the humerus and epiphyseal stippling at the shoulder and elbow joints. *(Courtesy of John P. Dorst, MD.)*

ichthyosis, and peripheral neuropathy may already be present in childhood and adolescence. Early diagnosis is important because institution of a phytanic acid–restricted diet can reverse the peripheral neuropathy and prevent the progression of the visual and central nervous system (CNS) manifestations. The adult Refsum disease phenotype may also be caused by defects in *PEX7*.

2-Methylacyl-CoA Racemase Deficiency (AMACR)

This disorder is caused by an enzyme defect that leads to the accumulation of the branched-chain fatty acids (phytanic and pristanic acid) and bile acids. Individuals present with typically an adult-onset peripheral neuropathy and may also have pigmentary degeneration of the retina.

Laboratory Findings

Diagnosis of a peroxisomal disorder often follows from a biochemical determination of an abnormality and then is confirmed through further genetic testing.

The biochemical characterization of peroxisomal disorders uses the generally available testing listed in Table 104.5. Measurement of plasma

VLCFA levels is the most common assay. It must be emphasized that although plasma VLCFA levels are elevated in many patients with peroxisomal disorders, this is not always the case. The most important exception is RCDP, in which VLCFA levels are normal, but plasma phytanic acid levels are increased and red blood cell (RBC) plasmalogen levels are reduced. In other peroxisomal disorders, the biochemical abnormalities are still more restricted. Therefore, a panel of tests is recommended and includes plasma levels of VLCFAs and phytanic, pristanic, and pipecolic acids and RBC levels of plasmalogens. Tandem mass spectrometry techniques also permit convenient quantitation of bile acids in plasma and urine. This panel of tests can be performed on very small amounts of venous blood and permits detection of most peroxisomal disorders. Furthermore, normal results make the presence of the typical peroxisomal disorder unlikely. Biochemical findings combined with the clinical presentation are often sufficient to arrive at a clinical diagnosis. *Methods using dried blood spots of filter paper have been developed and are being incorporated into newborn screening assays.*

The next step in diagnosis is generally to proceed to molecular DNA diagnosis, and many clinical laboratories provide a peroxisomal panel using next-generation technology. In some circumstances the diagnosis has been revealed through whole exome sequencing and the pathogenic nature of the alteration then confirmed through biochemical means.

Definition of the molecular defect in the *proband* is essential for carrier detection and speeds **prenatal diagnosis**. Characterization of the mutation may be of prognostic value in patients with *PEX1* defects. This defect is present in approximately 60% of PBD patients, and about half the *PEX1* defects have the G843D allele, which is associated with a significantly milder phenotype than found in other mutations.

Diagnosis

Several noninvasive laboratory tests permit precise and early diagnosis of peroxisomal disorders (see Table 104.5). The challenge in PBDs is to differentiate them from the large variety of other conditions that can cause hypotonia, seizures, failure to thrive, or dysmorphic features. Experienced clinicians readily recognize classic Zellweger syndrome by its clinical manifestations. However, more mildly affected PBD patients often do not show the full clinical spectrum of disease and may be identifiable only by laboratory assays. Clinical features that warrant diagnostic assay include intellectual disability; weakness and hypotonia; dysmorphic features; neonatal seizures; retinopathy, glaucoma, or cataracts; hearing deficits; enlarged liver and impaired liver function; and chondrodysplasia punctata. The presence of 1 or more of these abnormalities increases the likelihood of this diagnosis. Atypical milder forms presenting as peripheral neuropathy have also been described.

Some patients with the isolated defects of peroxisomal fatty acid oxidation resemble those with Zellweger spectrum disorder and can be detected by the demonstration of abnormally high levels of VLCFAs.

Patients with RCDP must be distinguished from patients with other causes of chondrodysplasia punctata. RCDP is suspected clinically

Table 104.5	Diagnostic Biochemical Abnormalities in Peroxisomal Disorders			
DISORDER	**VLCFA**	**PHYTANIC ACID**	**PRISTANIC ACID**	**PLASMALOGENS**
ZSD	↑↑	↑*	↑*	↓
RCDP	NI	↑	NI	↓↓
ALD	↑	NI	NI	NI
ACoX	↑	NI	NI	NI
Bifunctional enzyme deficiency	↑	↑	↑	NI
AMACR	NI	↑	↑	NI
Refsum disease	NI	↑	↑	NI

*Phytanic acid and pristanic acid accumulation is age dependent, and normal (NI) levels may be seen in infants and young children.
VLCFA, Very-long-chain fatty acids; ZSD, Zellweger spectrum disorder; RCDP, rhizomelic chondroplasia punctata; ALD, adrenoleukodystrophy; ACoX, acyl-CoA oxidase deficiency; AMACR, 2-methylacyl-CoA racemase deficiency.

because of the shortness of limbs, developmental delays, and ichthyosis. The most decisive laboratory test is the demonstration of abnormally low plasmalogen levels in RBCs and an alteration in *PEX7*.

Complications

Patients with Zellweger syndrome have multiple disabilities involving muscle tone, swallowing, cardiac abnormalities, liver disease, and seizures. These conditions are treated symptomatically, but the prognosis is poor, and most patients succumb in the 1st yr of life. Similarly, individuals with RCDP have multiple systemic and neurologic issues. In addition, they may develop quadriparesis from compression at the base of the brain.

Treatment

The most effective therapy is the dietary treatment of adult Refsum disease with a phytanic acid–restricted diet. However, this only applies to this specific condition.

For patients with the somewhat milder variants of the peroxisome import disorders, success has been achieved with multidisciplinary early intervention, including physical and occupational therapy, hearing aids or cochlear implants, augmentative and alternative communication, nutrition, and support for the families. Although most patients continue to function in the impaired range, some make significant gains in self-help skills, and several are in stable condition in their teens or even early 20s.

Attempts to mitigate some of the secondary biochemical abnormalities include the oral administration of docosahexaenoic acid (DHA). DHA level is greatly reduced in patients with disorders of peroxisome biogenesis, and this therapy normalizes DHA plasma levels. Although there were anecdotal reports of clinical improvement with DHA therapy, a randomized placebo-controlled study failed to find benefit.

Genetic Counseling

All the discussed peroxisomal disorders can be diagnosed prenatally. Prenatal testing using chorionic villi sampling or amniocentesis will usually rely on genetic testing when the alteration is known, but biochemical measurements may be made using the same tests as described for postnatal diagnosis (see Table 104.5). Because of the 25% recurrence risk, couples with an affected child should be advised about the availability of prenatal diagnosis.

ADRENOLEUKODYSTROPHY

ALD is an X-linked disorder associated with the accumulation of saturated VLCFAs and a progressive dysfunction of the adrenal cortex and nervous system. It is the most common peroxisomal disorder.

Etiology

The key biochemical abnormality in ALD is the tissue accumulation of saturated VLCFAs, with a carbon chain length of 24 or more. Excess hexacosanoic acid ($C_{26:0}$) is the most striking and characteristic feature. This accumulation of fatty acids is caused by genetically deficient peroxisomal degradation of fatty acid. The defective gene (*ABCD1*) codes for a peroxisomal membrane protein (ALDP, the ALD protein). Many alterations in *ABCD1* have been determined to be pathogenic, with over half these being private or unique to the kindred. A curated database of mutations is maintained (www.x-ald.nl). The mechanism by which the ALDP defect leads to VLCFA accumulation appears to be a disruption of transport of saturated fatty acids into the peroxisome, with resultant continued elongation of progressively longer fatty acids.

Epidemiology

The minimum incidence of ALD in males is 1 in 21,000, and the combined incidence of ALD males and heterozygous females in the general population is estimated to be 1 in 17,000. All races are affected. The various phenotypes often occur in members of the same kindred. Increased implementation of newborn screening in the United States and other countries is expected to improve the accuracy of these incidence estimates.

Pathology

Characteristic lamellar cytoplasmic inclusions can be demonstrated on electron microscopy in adrenocortical cells, testicular Leydig cells, and nervous system macrophages. These inclusions probably consist of cholesterol esterified with VLCFA. They are most prominent in cells of the zona fasciculata of the adrenal cortex, which at first are distended with lipid and later atrophy.

The nervous system displays 2 types of ALD lesions. In the severe cerebral form, demyelination is associated with an inflammatory response manifested by the accumulation of perivascular lymphocytes that is most intense in the involved region. In the slowly progressive adult form, **adrenomyeloneuropathy**, the main finding is a distal axonopathy that affects the long tracts in the spinal cord. In this form the inflammatory response is mild or absent.

Pathogenesis

The adrenal dysfunction is probably a direct consequence of the accumulation of VLCFAs. The cells in the adrenal zona fasciculata are distended with abnormal lipids. Cholesterol esterified with VLCFA is relatively resistant to adrenocorticotropic hormone (ACTH)–stimulated cholesterol ester hydrolases, and this limits the capacity to convert cholesterol to active steroids. In addition, $C_{26:0}$ excess increases the viscosity of the plasma membrane, which may interfere with receptor and other cellular functions.

There is no correlation between the neurologic phenotype and the nature of the mutation or the severity of the biochemical defect as assessed by plasma VLCFA levels or between the degree of adrenal involvement and nervous system involvement. The severity of the illness and rate of progression correlate with the intensity of the **inflammatory response**. The inflammatory response may be partially cytokine mediated and may involve an autoimmune response triggered in an unknown way by the excess of VLCFAs. Mitochondrial damage and oxidative stress also appear to contribute. Approximately half the patients do not experience the inflammatory response; this difference is not understood.

Clinical Manifestations

There are 5 relatively distinct ALD phenotypes, 3 of which are present in childhood with symptoms and signs. In all the phenotypes, development is usually normal in the 1st 3-4 yr of life.

In the **childhood cerebral form** of ALD, symptoms most often are first noted between ages 4 and 8 yr. The most common initial manifestations are hyperactivity, inattention, and worsening school performance in a child who had previously been a good student. *Auditory discrimination* is often impaired, although tone perception is preserved. This may be evidenced by difficulty in using the telephone and greatly impaired performance on intelligence tests in items that are presented verbally. Spatial orientation is often impaired. Other initial symptoms are disturbances of vision, ataxia, poor handwriting, seizures, and strabismus. Visual disturbances are often caused by involvement of the parietooccipital cortex rather than eye or optic tract abnormalities, which leads to variable and seemingly inconsistent visual capacity. Seizures occur in nearly all patients and may represent the first manifestation of the disease. Some patients present with increased intracranial pressure. Impaired cortisol response to ACTH stimulation is present in 85% of patients, and mild hyperpigmentation is noted. In most patients with this phenotype, adrenal dysfunction is recognized only after the condition is diagnosed because of the cerebral symptoms. Cerebral childhood ALD tends to progress rapidly with increasing spasticity and paralysis, visual and hearing loss, and loss of ability to speak or swallow. The mean interval between the first neurologic symptom and an apparently vegetative state is 1.9 yr. Patients may continue in this apparently vegetative state for ≥10 yr.

Adolescent ALD designates patients who experience neurologic symptoms between ages 10 and 21 yr. The manifestations resemble those of childhood cerebral ALD except that progression is slower. Approximately 10% of patients present acutely with status epilepticus, adrenal crisis, acute encephalopathy, or coma.

Adrenomyeloneuropathy first manifests in late adolescence or adulthood as a progressive paraparesis caused by long tract degeneration in the spinal cord. Approximately half the affected men also have involvement of the cerebral white matter.

The **Addison-only** phenotype is an important condition. Of male patients with Addison disease, 25% may have the biochemical defect of ALD. Many of these patients have intact neurologic systems, whereas others have subtle neurologic signs. Many acquire adrenomyeloneuropathy in adulthood.

The term **asymptomatic ALD** is applied to persons who have the biochemical defect of ALD but are free of neurologic or endocrinal disturbances. Almost all persons with the gene defect eventually become neurologically symptomatic.

Approximately 50% of female heterozygotes acquire a syndrome that resembles adrenomyeloneuropathy but is milder and of later onset. Adrenal insufficiency and cerebral disease are rare.

Cases of typical ALD have occurred in relatives of those with adrenomyeloneuropathy. One of the most difficult problems in the management of ALD is the common observation that affected individuals in the same family may have quite different clinical courses. For example, in one family, an affected boy may have severe classic ALD culminating in death by age 10 yr, and another brother will have the later-onset adrenomyeloneuropathy.

Laboratory and Radiographic Findings

The most specific and important laboratory finding is the demonstration of abnormally high levels of VLCFAs in plasma, RBCs, or cultured skin fibroblasts. Positive results are obtained in all male patients with ALD and in approximately 85% of female carriers of ALD. Mutation analysis is the most reliable method for the identification of carriers. Simply finding a variation in *ABCD1* is not adequate for making the diagnosis of ALD. It must be shown to segregate with elevated VLCFA levels.

Neuroimaging

Patients with childhood cerebral or adolescent ALD have characteristic white matter lesions on MRI. In 80% of patients the lesions are symmetric and involve the splenium of the corpus callosum and periventricular white matter in the posterior parietal and occipital lobes. Many will show a garland of contrast enhancement adjacent and anterior to the posterior hypodense lesions (Fig. 104.5). This zone corresponds to the zones of intense perivascular lymphocytic infiltration where the blood-brain barrier breaks down. In 10–15% of patients, the initial lesions are frontal. Unilateral lesions that produce a mass effect suggestive of a brain tumor may occur rarely. MRI provides a clearer delineation of normal and abnormal white matter than does CT and is the preferred imaging modality.

Impaired Adrenal Function

More than 85% of patients with the childhood form of ALD have elevated levels of ACTH in plasma and a subnormal rise of cortisol levels in plasma after IV injection of 250 µg of ACTH (Cortrosyn).

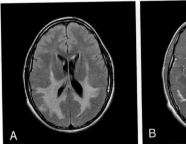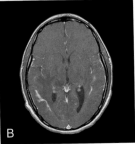

Fig. 104.5 Characteristic MRI findings in cerebral adrenoleukodystrophy. **A,** Symmetric T2-weighted MRI abnormalities involve the posterior white matter, including the corpus callosum. **B,** Contrast administration reveals a garland of enhancement.

Diagnosis and Differential Diagnosis

Diagnosis of asymptomatic males has become available by newborn screening that has been added to the recommended uniform screening panel. After diagnosis, confirmatory testing and genetic counseling should be provided. Males then enter a program of surveillance for adrenal insufficiency and early detection of potential cerebral disease. Females identified through these programs should also have confirmatory testing, genetic counseling for the family, and screening of other at-risk males. Females do not generally require any other monitoring in childhood.

The earliest manifestations of childhood cerebral ALD are difficult to distinguish from the more common attention-deficit disorders or learning disabilities of school-age children. Rapid progression, signs of dementia, or difficulty in auditory discrimination suggest ALD. Even in early stages, neuroimaging shows abnormal changes. Other leukodystrophies or multiple sclerosis may sometimes mimic these radiographic findings, although early ALD has more of a predilection for the posterior brain than its mimics. Definitive diagnosis depends on demonstration of VLCFA excess, which occurs only in ALD and the other peroxisomal disorders.

Cerebral forms of ALD, especially if asymmetric, may be misdiagnosed as gliomas or other mass lesion. Individuals have received brain biopsy and rarely other therapies before the correct diagnosis was made. Measurement of VLCFAs in plasma is the most reliable differentiating test.

Adolescent or adult cerebral ALD can be confused with psychiatric disorders, dementing disorders, multiple sclerosis, or epilepsy. The first clue to the diagnosis of ALD may be the demonstration of characteristic white matter lesions by neuroimaging; VLCFA assays are confirmatory.

ALD *cannot* be distinguished clinically from other forms of Addison disease; it is recommended that assays of VLCFA levels be performed in all male patients with Addison disease. ALD patients *do not* usually have antibodies to adrenal tissue in their plasma.

Complications

An avoidable complication is the occurrence of **adrenal insufficiency**. The most difficult neurologic problems are those related to bed rest, contracture, coma, and swallowing disturbances. Other complications involve behavioral disturbances and injuries associated with defects of spatial orientation, impaired vision and hearing, and seizures.

Treatment

Corticosteroid replacement for adrenal insufficiency or adrenocortical hypofunction is effective. It may be lifesaving and may increase general strength and well-being, but it does not alter the course of the neurologic disability.

Bone Marrow Transplantation

Bone marrow transplantation (BMT) or hematopoietic stem cell therapy benefits patients who show early evidence of the inflammatory demyelination characteristic of the rapidly progressive neurologic disability in boys and adolescents with the cerebral ALD phenotype. BMT carries risk, and patients must be evaluated and selected with care. The mechanism of the beneficial effect is incompletely understood. Bone marrow–derived cells do express ALDP, the protein that is deficient in ALD; approximately 50% of brain microglial cells are bone marrow derived. The favorable effect may be caused by modification of the brain inflammatory response. Follow-up of boys and adolescents who had early cerebral involvement has shown stabilization. On the other hand, BMT does not arrest the course in those who already had severe brain involvement and may accelerate disease progression under these circumstances. The ALD MRI score and the use of performance measures on IQ testing have shown some predictive ability for boys likely to benefit from this procedure. Transplant is not recommended in patients with performance IQ significantly <80. Unfortunately, in more than half the patients who are diagnosed because of neurologic symptoms, the illness is so advanced at diagnosis that they are not candidates for transplant.

Consideration of BMT is most relevant in neurologically asymptomatic or mildly involved patients. Screening at-risk relatives of symptomatic patients identifies these patients most frequently. Screening by measurement of plasma VLCFA levels in patients with Addison disease may also identify candidates for BMT. Because of its risk (10–20% mortality) and because up to 50% of untreated patients with ALD do not develop inflammatory brain demyelination, transplant is not recommended in patients who are free of demonstrable brain involvement on MRI. MRI is also of key importance for the crucial decision of whether transplant should be performed. MRI abnormalities precede clinically evident neurologic or neuropsychologic abnormalities. The brain MRI should be monitored at 6 mo intervals in neurologically asymptomatic boys and adolescents age 3-15 yr. If the MRI is normal, BMT is not indicated. If brain MRI abnormalities develop, the boy should be evaluated by a center familiar with transplant for ALD. This should include MRI, neurologic, and neuropsychologic evaluations. It is not known whether BMT has a favorable effect on the noninflammatory spinal cord involvement in adults with the adrenomyeloneuropathy phenotype.

Lorenzo's Oil Therapy

Lorenzo's oil (4:1 mixture of glyceryl trioleate and glyceryl trierucate) combined with a dietary regimen has been under investigation to prevent the development of various aspects of ALD. The compound does lower plasma levels of VLCFAs, but despite early enthusiasm, clinical trials have been equivocal. Lorenzo's oil has not been shown to alter disease progression in males with cerebral disease. Whether it or another agent that lowers VLCFA levels has disease-modifying effects is as yet uncertain.

Supportive Therapy

The progressive behavioral and neurologic disturbances associated with the childhood form of ALD are extremely difficult for the family. ALD patients require the establishment of a comprehensive management program and partnership among the family, physician, visiting nursing staff, school authorities, and counselors. In addition, parent support groups (e.g., United Leukodystrophy Foundation) are often helpful. Communication with school authorities is important because under the provisions of Public Law 94-142, children with ALD qualify for special services as "other health impaired" or "multi-handicapped." Depending on the rate of progression of the disease, special needs might range from relatively low-level resource services within a regular school program to home- and hospital-based teaching programs for children who are not mobile.

Management challenges vary with the stage of the illness. The early stages are characterized by subtle changes in affect, behavior, and attention span. Counseling and communication with school authorities are of prime importance. Changes in the sleep–wake cycle can be benefited by the judicious use of nighttime sleep medications.

As the leukodystrophy progresses, the modulation of muscle tone and support of bulbar muscular function are major concerns. **Baclofen** in gradually increasing doses (5 mg twice a day to 25 mg 4 times a day) is an effective pharmacologic agent for the treatment of acute episodic painful muscle spasms. Other agents may also be used, with care taken to monitor the occurrence of side effects and drug interactions. As the leukodystrophy progresses, bulbar muscular control is lost. Although initially this can be managed by changing the diet to soft and pureed foods, most patients eventually require a gastrostomy tube. At least 30% of patients have focal or generalized seizures that usually readily respond to standard anticonvulsant medications.

Genetic Counseling and Prevention

Genetic counseling and appropriate monitoring are of crucial importance. Extended-family screening should be offered to all at-risk relatives of symptomatic patients; one program led to the identification of >250 asymptomatic affected males and 1,200 women heterozygous for ALD. The plasma assay permits reliable identification of affected males in whom plasma VLCFA levels are increased already on the day of birth. Identification of asymptomatic males permits institution of steroid replacement therapy when appropriate and prevents adrenal crisis, which

may be fatal. Monitoring of brain MRI also permits identification of patients who are candidates for BMT at a stage when this procedure has the greatest chance of success. Plasma VLCFA assay is recommended in all male patients with Addison disease. ALD has been shown to be the cause of adrenal insufficiency in >25% of boys with Addison disease of unknown cause. Identification of women heterozygous for ALD is more difficult than that of affected males. Plasma VLCFA levels are normal in 15–20% of heterozygous women, and failure to note this has led to serious errors in genetic counseling. DNA analysis permits accurate identification of carriers, provided that the mutation has been defined in a family member, and this is the procedure recommended for the identification of heterozygous women.

Prenatal diagnosis of affected male fetuses can be achieved by determination of the known mutation or by the measurement of VLCFA levels in cultured amniocytes or chorionic villus cells. Whenever a new patient with ALD is identified, a detailed pedigree should be constructed and efforts made to identify all at-risk female carriers and affected males. These investigations should be accompanied by careful and sympathetic attention to social, emotional, and ethical issues during counseling.

Bibliography is available at Expert Consult.

104.3 Disorders of Lipoprotein Metabolism and Transport

Lee A. Pyles and William A. Neal

EPIDEMIOLOGY OF BLOOD LIPIDS AND CARDIOVASCULAR DISEASE

There is a strong association between average intake of saturated fats, plasma cholesterol, and mortality from coronary heart disease (CHD). Of all common chronic diseases, none is so clearly influenced by both environmental *and* genetic factors as CHD. This multifactorial disorder is strongly associated with increasing age and male gender, although it is increasingly apparent that heart disease is underrecognized in women. Tobacco use confers a 2-fold higher lifetime risk. Sedentary activity and high intake of processed sugars leading to adiposity increase risk through differences in the plasma levels of atherogenic lipoproteins. Family history reflects the combined influence of lifestyle and genetic predisposition to early heart disease. Risk of premature heart disease associated with positive family history is 1.7 times higher than in families with no such history.

Atherosclerosis begins during childhood. The Johns Hopkins Precursors Study demonstrated that white male medical students with blood cholesterol levels in the lowest quartile showed only a 10% incidence of CHD 3 decades later, whereas those in the highest quartile had a 40% incidence. The Pathobiological Determinants of Atherosclerosis in Youth Study demonstrated a significant relationship between the weight of the abdominal fat pad and the extent of atherosclerosis found at autopsy on individuals 15-34 yr of age. The Bogalusa Heart Study of more than 3,000 black and white children and adolescents has provided the most comprehensive longitudinal data relating the presence and severity of CHD risk factors with semiquantifiable severity of atherosclerosis. Coronary atherosclerosis was present in 8.5% of military autopsies performed following combat or unintentional injuries.

The *fetal origins hypothesis* is based on the observation that infants born with low birthweight have a higher incidence of heart disease as adults. Epidemiologic studies support the idea that prenatal and early postnatal conditions may affect adult health status. Children who are large for gestational age at birth and exposed to an intrauterine environment of either diabetes or maternal obesity are at increased risk of eventually developing the **metabolic syndrome** (insulin resistance, type II diabetes, obesity, CHD). Breastfeeding preterm infants confers a long-term cardioprotective benefit 13-16 yr later. Those adolescents who were breastfed as infants had lower C-reactive protein (CRP) concentrations and a 14% lower low-density lipoprotein (LDL)/high-density lipoprotein (HDL) ratio than formula-fed infants. The impact of early nutrition and other lifestyle variables on gene expression, *epigenetics*, is one mechanism by which adult metabolism and body composition may be determined.

Secondary causes of hyperlipidemia may be the result of drugs (cyclosporine, corticosteroids, isotretinoin, protease inhibitors, alcohol, thiazide diuretics, β-blocking agents, valproate); or various diseases (nephrotic syndrome, hypothyroidism, Cushing syndrome, anorexia nervosa, obstructive jaundice). Psychotropic medications, including second-generation antipsychotics such as olanzapine, are associated with dyslipidemia, obesity, and insulin resistance.

BLOOD LIPIDS AND ATHEROGENESIS

Numerous epidemiologic studies demonstrate the association of hypercholesterolemia, referring to elevated total and LDL blood cholesterol, with atherosclerotic disease. The ability to measure subcomponents within classes of lipid particles, as well as markers of inflammation, have further elucidated the process of atherogenesis and plaque rupture leading to acute coronary syndromes. Atherosclerosis affects primarily the coronary arteries but may also involve the aorta, arteries of the lower extremities, and carotid arteries.

The early stage of development of atherosclerosis is thought to begin with vascular endothelial dysfunction and intima-media thickness, which has been shown to occur in preadolescent children with risk factors such as obesity or familial hypercholesterolemia. The complex process of penetrating the intimal lining of the vessel may result from a variety of insults, including the presence of highly toxic oxidized LDL particles. Lymphocytes and monocytes penetrate the damaged endothelial lining, where they become macrophages laden with LDL lipids and then become foam cells. Such accumulation is counterbalanced by HDL particles capable of removing lipid deposits from the vessel wall. Fundamental to plaque formation is an inflammatory process (elevated CRP) involving macrophages and the arterial wall. The deposition of lipid within the subendothelial lining of the arterial wall appears macroscopically as fatty streaks, which may to some degree be reversible. A later stage of plaque development involves disruption of arterial smooth muscle cells stimulated by the release of tissue cytokines and growth factors. The *atheroma* is composed of a core of fatty substance separated from the lumen by collagen and smooth muscle (Fig. 104.6). Growth of the atherosclerotic plaque may result in ischemia of the tissue supplied by the artery. Chronic inflammation within the atheroma results in plaque instability and subsequent rupture. Platelet adherence leads to clot formation at the site of rupture, resulting in myocardial infarction (MI) or a cerebrovascular accident (CVA), depending on the site of thrombosis or thromboembolism.

PLASMA LIPOPROTEIN METABOLISM AND TRANSPORT

Abnormalities of lipoprotein metabolism are associated with diabetes mellitus and premature atherosclerosis. *Lipoproteins* are soluble complexes of lipids and proteins that effect transport of fat absorbed from the diet, or synthesis by the liver and adipose tissues, for utilization and storage. Dietary fat is transported from the small intestine as chylomicrons. Lipids synthesized by the liver as very-low-density lipoproteins (VLDLs) are catabolized to intermediate-density lipoproteins (IDLs) and LDLs. HDL is fundamentally involved in VLDL and chylomicron metabolism and cholesterol transport. Nonesterified free fatty acids are metabolically active lipids derived from lipolysis of triglycerides stored in adipose tissue and bound to albumin for circulation in the plasma (Fig. 104.7).

Lipoproteins consist of a central core of triglycerides and cholesteryl esters surrounded by phospholipids, cholesterol, and proteins (Fig. 104.8). The density of the several classes of lipoproteins is inversely proportional to the ratio of lipid to protein, which is generally denser (Fig. 104.9). Lipoproteins consist of a central core of triglycerides and cholesteryl esters surrounded by phospholipids, cholesterol, and proteins.

Constituent proteins known as *apolipoproteins* are responsible for a variety of metabolic functions in addition to their structural role, including as cofactors or inhibitors of enzymatic pathways and mediators of lipoprotein binding to cell surface receptors (Table 104.6). **ApoA** is the major apolipoprotein (Apo) of HDL. **ApoB** is present in LDL, VLDL, IDL, and chylomicrons. ApoB-100 is derived from the liver, whereas apoB-48 comes from the small intestine. ApoC-I, C-II, and C-III are small peptides important in triglyceride metabolism. Loss of function and disruptive mutations of the *APOC3* gene are associated with low levels of triglycerides and a reduced risk of ischemic CHD. Likewise, **apoE**, which is present in VLDL, HDL, chylomicrons, and chylomicron remnants, plays an important role in the clearance of triglycerides.

Transport of Exogenous (Dietary) Lipids

All dietary fat except medium-chain triglycerides is efficiently carried into the circulation by way of lymphatic drainage from the intestinal mucosa. Triglyceride and cholesteryl esters combine with apoA and apoB-48 in the intestinal mucosa to form chylomicrons, which are carried into the peripheral circulation via the lymphatic system. HDL particles contribute apoC-II to the chylomicrons, required for the activation of *lipoprotein lipase* (LPL) within the capillary endothelium of adipose, heart, and skeletal muscle tissue. Free fatty acids are oxidized, esterified for storage as triglycerides, or released into the circulation

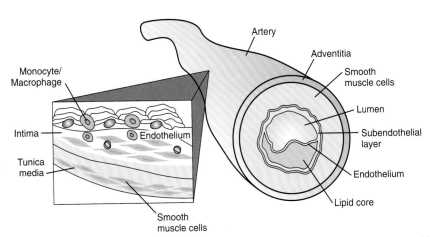

Fig. 104.6 The early stage of development of atherosclerosis begins with penetration of the intimal lining of the vessel by inflammatory cells. Deposition of lipid within the subendothelial lining of the arterial wall eventually leads to disruption of smooth muscle cells to form an atheromatous lipid core that impinges on the lumen. Chronic inflammation leads to plaque instability, setting the stage for plaque rupture and complete occlusion of the vessel lumen by clot formation.

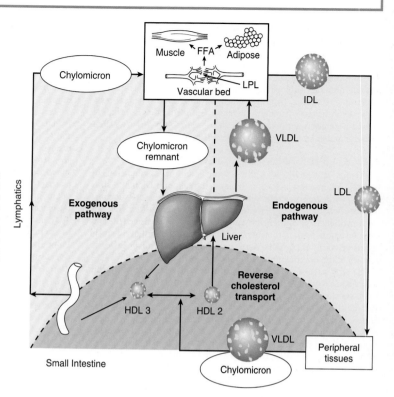

Fig. 104.7 The exogenous, endogenous, and reverse cholesterol pathways. The exogenous pathway transports dietary fat from the small intestine as chylomicrons to the periphery and the liver. The endogenous pathway denotes the secretion of very-low-density lipoprotein (VLDL) from the liver and its catabolism to intermediate-density lipoprotein (IDL) and low-density lipoprotein (LDL). Triglycerides are hydrolyzed from the VLDL particle by the action of lipoprotein lipase (LPL) in the vascular bed, yielding free fatty acids (FFA) for utilization and storage in muscle and adipose tissue. High-density lipoprotein (HDL) metabolism is responsible for the transport of excess cholesterol from the peripheral tissues back to the liver for excretion in the bile. Nascent HDL-3 particles derived from the liver and small intestine are esterified to more mature HDL-2 particles by enzyme-mediated movement of chylomicron and VLDL into the HDL core, which is removed from the circulation by endocytosis.

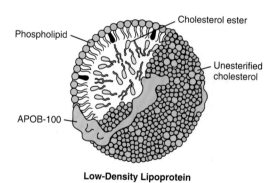

Fig. 104.8 Schematic of low-density lipoprotein. Lipoprotein consists of a central core of cholesteryl esters, surrounded by phospholipids, cholesterol, and protein.

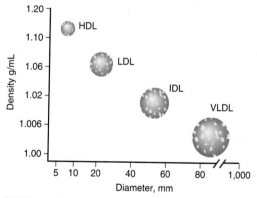

Fig. 104.9 The density of the several classes of lipoprotein is inversely proportional to the ratio of lipid to protein. As lipid is less dense than protein, the more lipid contained in the particle increases its size and decreases its density. HDL, High-density lipoprotein; LDL, low-density lipoprotein; IDL, intermediate-density lipoprotein; VLDL, very-low-density lipoprotein.

bound to albumin for transport to the liver. After hydrolysis of the triglyceride core from the chylomicron, apoC particles are recirculated back to HDL. The subsequent contribution of apoE from HDL to the remnant chylomicron facilitates binding of the particle to hepatic LDL receptor (LDL-R). Within the hepatocyte, the chylomicron remnant may be incorporated into membranes, resecreted as lipoprotein back into the circulation, or secreted as bile acids. Normally, all dietary fat is disposed of within 8 hr after the last meal, an exception being individuals with a disorder of chylomicron metabolism. **Postprandial hyperlipidemia** is a risk factor for atherosclerosis. Abnormal transport of chylomicrons and their remnants may result in their absorption into the blood vessel wall as foam cells, caused by the ingestion of cholesteryl esters by macrophages, the earliest stage in the development of fatty streaks.

Transport of Endogenous Lipids From the Liver
The formation and secretion of VLDL from the liver and its catabolism to IDL and LDL particles describe the endogenous lipoprotein pathway. Fatty acids used in the hepatic formation of VLDL are derived primarily by uptake from the circulation. VLDL appears to be transported from the liver as rapidly as it is synthesized, and it consists of triglycerides, cholesteryl esters, phospholipids, and apoB-100. Nascent particles of VLDL secreted into the circulation combine with apoC and apoE. The size of the VLDL particle is determined by the amount of triglyceride present, progressively shrinking in size as triglyceride is hydrolyzed by

Table 104.6 | Characteristics of the Major Lipoproteins

LIPOPROTEIN	SOURCE	SIZE (nm)	DENSITY (g/mL)	COMPOSITION Protein (%)	Lipid (%)	Apolipoproteins
Chylomicrons	Intestine	80–1,200	<0.95	1–2	98–99	C-I, C-II, C-III, E, A-I, A-II, A-IV, B-48
Chylomicron remnants	Chylomicrons	40–150	<1.0006	6–8	92–94	B-48, E
VLDL	Liver, intestine	30–80	0.95–1.006	7–10	90–93	B-100, C-I, C-II, C-III
IDL	VLDL	25–35	1.006–1.019	11	89	B-100, E
LDL	VLDL	18–25	1.019–1.063	21	79	B-100
HDL	Liver, intestine VLDL, chylomicrons	5–20	1.125–1.210	32–57	43–68	A-I, A-II, A-IV C-I, C-II, C-III D, E

HDL, High-density lipoproteins; IDL, intermediate-density lipoproteins; LDL, low-density lipoproteins; VLDL, very-low-density lipoproteins.

Table 104.7 | Hyperlipoproteinemias

DISORDER	LIPOPROTEINS ELEVATED	CLINICAL FINDINGS	GENETICS	ESTIMATED INCIDENCE
Familial hypercholesterolemia	LDL	Tendon xanthomas, CHD	AD	1 in 500
Familial defective ApoB-100	LDL	Tendon xanthomas, CHD	AD	1 in 1,000
Autosomal recessive hypercholesterolemia	LDL	Tendon xanthomas, CHD	AR	<1 in 1,000,000
Sitosterolemia	LDL	Tendon xanthomas, CHD	AR	<1 in 1,000,000
Polygenic hypercholesterolemia	LDL	CHD		1 in 30?
Familial combined hyperlipidemia	LDL, TG	CHD	AD	1 in 200
Familial dysbetalipoproteinemia	LDL, TG	Tuberoeruptive xanthomas, peripheral vascular disease	AD	1 in 10,000
Familial chylomicronemia (Frederickson type I)	TG ↑↑	Eruptive xanthomas, hepatosplenomegaly, pancreatitis	AR	1 in 1,000,000
Familial hypertriglyceridemia (Frederickson type IV)	TG ↑	±CHD	AD	1 in 500
Familial hypertriglyceridemia (Frederickson type V)	TG ↑↑	Xanthomas ± CHD	AD	—
Familial hepatic lipase deficiency	VLDL	CHD	AR	<1 in 1,000,000

AD, Autosomal dominant; AR, autosomal recessive; CHD, coronary heart disease; LDL, low-density lipoproteins, TG, triglycerides; VLDL, very-low-density lipoproteins.

the action of LPL, yielding free fatty acids for utilization or storage in muscle and adipose tissue. Hydrolysis of approximately 80% of the triglyceride present in VLDL particles produces IDL particles containing an equal amount of cholesterol and triglyceride. The remaining remnant IDL is converted to LDL for delivery to peripheral tissues or to the liver. ApoE is attached to the remnant IDL particle to allow binding to the cell and subsequent incorporation into the lysosome. Individuals with deficiency of either apoE2 or hepatic triglyceride lipase accumulate IDL in the plasma.

LDL particles account for approximately 70% of the plasma cholesterol in normal individuals. LDL receptors are present on the surfaces of nearly all cells. Most LDL is taken up by the liver, and the rest is transported to peripheral tissues such as the adrenal glands and gonads for steroid synthesis. Dyslipidemia is greatly influenced by LDL-R activity. The efficiency with which VLDL is converted into LDL is also important in lipid homeostasis. The normal newborn LDL level of 50 mg/dL is probably adequate for steroid synthesis throughout the life cycle.

High-Density Lipoprotein and Reverse Cholesterol Transport

Because hepatic secretion of lipid particles into the bile is the only mechanism by which cholesterol can be removed from the body, transport of excess cholesterol from the peripheral cells is a vitally important function of HDL. HDL is heavily laden with apoA-I–containing lipoproteins, which is nonatherogenic, in contrast to B lipoproteins.

Cholesterol-poor nascent HDL particles secreted by the liver and small intestine are esterified to more mature HDL-2 particles by the action of the enzyme lecithin-cholesterol acyltransferase (**LCAT**), which facilitates movement of chylomicrons and VLDL into the HDL core. HDL-2 may transfer cholesteryl esters back to apoB lipoproteins mediated by cholesteryl ester transfer protein (CETP), or the cholesterol-rich particle may be removed from the plasma by endocytosis, completing reverse cholesterol transport. Low HDL may be genetic (deficiency of apoA-I) or secondary to increased plasma triglyceride.

LCAT deficiency results in diminished maturation of HDL particles, affecting their ability to do reverse cholesterol transport. This reduces its protective effect on atherosclerosis. There are rare reports, however, of less-than-expected severity of atherosclerosis despite low HDL secondary to LCAT deficiency, suggesting that the relationship may, for unknown reasons, be variable.

HYPERLIPOPROTEINEMIAS
Hypercholesterolemia
See Table 104.7.

Familial Hypercholesterolemia
Familial hypercholesterolemia (FH) is a monogenic autosomal co-dominant disorder characterized by strikingly elevated LDL cholesterol (LDL-C), premature cardiovascular disease (CVD), and tendon xanthomas. In the past, FH referred to defects of LDL-R activity. The etiology

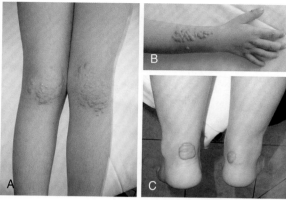

Fig. 104.10 Homozygous familial hypercholesterolemia. Tendon xanthomas in a 5 yr old male with homozygous FH noted at the knee (**A**), wrist (**B**), and Achilles (**C**). *(Modified from Macchiaiolo M, Gagliardi MG, Toscano A, et al: Homozygous familial hypercholesterolaemia, Lancet 379:1330, 2012.)*

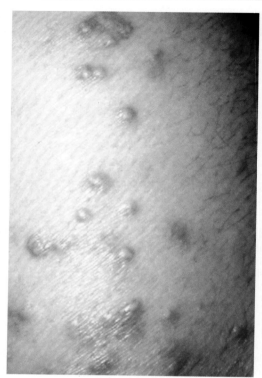

Fig. 104.12 Eruptive xanthomata on extensor surface of forearm. *(From Durrington P: Dyslipidaemia, Lancet 362:717–731, 2003.)*

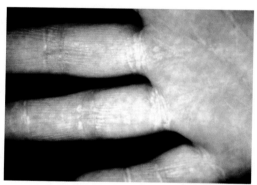

Fig. 104.11 Striate palmar xanthomata. *(From Durrington P: Dyslipidaemia, Lancet 362:717–731, 2003.)*

of this lipoprotein abnormality also includes defects in the genes for apoB (as well as PCSK-9). Of the almost 1200 mutations described, some result in failure of synthesis of the LDL-R (receptor negative), and others cause defective binding or release at the lipoprotein-receptor interface. Receptor-negative mutations result in more severe phenotypes than receptor-defective mutations.

Homozygous Familial Hypercholesterolemia
FH homozygotes inherit 2 abnormal LDL receptor genes, resulting in markedly elevated plasma cholesterol levels ranging between 500 and 1,200 mg/dL. Triglyceride levels are normal to mildly elevated, and HDL levels may be slightly decreased. The condition occurs in 1 in 500,000 persons. Receptor-negative patients have <2% normal LDL-R activity, whereas those who are receptor defective may have as much as 25% normal activity and a better prognosis.

The prognosis is poor regardless of the specific LDL-R aberration. Severe atherosclerosis involving the aortic root and coronary arteries is present by early to middle childhood. These children usually present with **xanthomas**, which may cause thickening of the Achilles tendon or extensor tendons of the hands, or cutaneous lesions on the hands, elbows, knees, or buttocks (Figs. 104.10 to 104.12). Corneal arcus may be present. Family history is informative because premature heart disease is strongly prevalent among relatives of both parents. The diagnosis may be confirmed genetically or by measuring LDL-R activity in cultured skin fibroblasts. Phenotypic expression of the disease may also be assessed

by measuring receptor activity on the surface of lymphocytes by using cell-sorting techniques.

Untreated homozygous patients rarely survive to adulthood. Symptoms of coronary insufficiency may occur; sudden death is common. LDL apheresis to remove LDL particles selectively from the circulation is recommended for many children because it slows the progression of atherosclerosis. Liver transplantation is also successful in decreasing LDL-C levels, but complications related to immunosuppression are common. HMG-CoA reductase inhibitors may be modestly effective depending on the specific class of LDL-R defect present. Combination therapy with *ezetimibe,* selectively blocking cholesterol adsorption in the gut, usually results in further decline in LDL levels; it has largely replaced the use of bile acid sequestrants. Early clinical trials using microsomal triglyceride transfer protein inhibition with *lomitapide* (oral agent) resulted in a significant reduction in all apoB lipoproteins, including LDL, but hepatic fat deposition as a side effect limits consideration of this pharmacologic approach. *Mipomersen* (subcutaneous injection), an antisense oligonucleotide that binds to the sequence that encodes apolipoprotein B, reduces the synthesis of apoB and thus also VLDL and LDL; LDL cholesterol levels may decline approximately 25% with this treatment. Adverse effects include flulike symptoms, hepatic steatosis, and cirrhosis.

Heterozygous Familial Hypercholesterolemia
Heterozygous FH is the most common single-gene mutations associated with acute coronary syndromes and atherosclerotic CHD in adults. Its prevalence is approximately 1 in 250 individuals worldwide, but the frequency may be greater in select populations, such as French Canadians, Afrikaners, and Christian Lebanese, as a result of the founder effect of unique new mutations. The founder effect noted in Ashkenazi Jews can be traced through gene disequilibrium analysis to an initial mutation in Lithuania in the 1400s.

Heart disease accounts for more than half of all deaths in Western society. The pathogenesis of CHD is both environmental and genetic, and the complex interrelationship determines the phenotypic expression of disease.

Because heterozygous FH is a co-dominant condition with nearly full penetrance, 50% of first-degree relatives of affected individuals will have the disease, as will 25% of second-degree relatives. An estimated 20 million people have FH worldwide. Symptoms of CHD usually occur at the mean age of 45-48 yr in males and a decade later in females. Genetic testing of individuals who fulfill clinical criteria for the diagnosis of heterozygous FH is variably positive dependent on the population under investigation, including pediatric vs adult participants.

The World Health Organization (WHO) has targeted FH for individualized intervention strategies because of its large effect on morbidity and mortality. A relatively small percentage of the population accounts for a disproportionately high share of the burden of CVD. The clinical expression of the disease is straightforward, and treatment is effective.

One cannot overemphasize the importance of family history for suspecting the possibility of FH, especially given the 3% cholesterol screening rate for children in primary care offices. American Academy of Pediatrics (AAP) and National Heart, Lung, and Blood Institute (NHLBI) guidelines advocate for universal screening for cholesterol in childhood, but with poor acceptance and disagreement. There is an increased interest in genetic testing for persons with suspected FH because of variability in phenotype based on genotype. In fact, the risk of CHD in individuals with FH can be up to 20 times greater than in the general population.

Plasma levels of LDL-C do not allow unequivocal diagnosis of FH heterozygotes, but values are generally twice normal for age because of 1 absent or dysfunctional allele. The U.S. MED-PED (*Make Early Diagnosis–Prevent Early Death*) Program has formulated diagnostic criteria. Similar criteria with minor variations exist in the United Kingdom (Simon Broome criteria) and Holland (Dutch Lipid Clinic Network criteria). Within well-defined FH families, the diagnosis is reliably established according to LDL cutoff points. More stringent criteria are required to establish the diagnosis in previously undiagnosed families, requiring strong evidence of an autosomal inheritance pattern and higher LDL cutoff points. At a total cholesterol level of 310 mg/

dL, only 4% of adults in the general population would have FH, whereas 95% of adults who were first-degree relatives of known cases would have the disease. The mathematical probability of FH in MED-PED, verified by molecular genetics, is derived from a U.S. population cohort and may not be applicable to other countries.

Very high cholesterol levels in children should prompt extensive screening of adult first- and second-degree relatives ("reverse cascade" cholesterol screening). In the general population, a child younger than age 18 yr with total plasma cholesterol of 270 mg/dL and/or LDL-C of 200 mg/dL has an 88% chance of having FH (Table 104.8). *Formal clinical diagnosis of FH is based on the presence of 2 or more family members having elevated LDL-C levels* (the 95th percentile LDL-C level cutoff points for children vary with age and are lower than for adults; see Table 104.9). Thus the criteria for probable FH in a child whose first-degree relative has known FH require only modest elevation of total cholesterol to 220 mg/dL (LDL-C 160 mg/dL; Table 104.8). The challenge of childhood FH diagnosis is heightened by the lack of clinical stigmata such as xanthomata that are employed in the Simon Broome and Dutch Lipid Clinic Network schema and highlights the shift toward genetic diagnosis.

Treatment of children with FH should begin with a rather rigorous low-fat diet. Diet alone is rarely sufficient for decreasing blood cholesterol levels to acceptable levels (LDL-C <130 mg/dL). Ezetimibe blocks cholesterol adsorption in the gastrointestinal (GI) tract and has a low risk of side effects. Data suggest that ezetimibe will lower total cholesterol by 20-30 mg/dL. *HMG-CoA reductase inhibitors (statins) are the drug of choice for treatment of FH because of their remarkable effectiveness and acceptable risk profile.* There is sufficient clinical experience with this class of drugs in children over age 10 yr to document that they are as effective in children as in adults, and the risks of elevated hepatic enzymes and myositis are no greater than in adults. Another class of drugs, the proprotein convertase subtilisin/kexin type 9 (**PCSK-9**) inhibitors, are monoclonal antibodies (mAbs) that block the action of PCSK-9 to downregulate the LDL-R. These agents boost LDL-R levels and result in a marked decrease in plasma LDL-C levels. PCSK-9 inhibitors have a role in adults intolerant of statins and those with subtherapeutic statin effect. Use in children is experimental.

Table 104.8	Percentage of Youths Younger than Age 18 Yr Expected to Have Familial Hypercholesterolemia (FH) According to Cholesterol Levels and Closest Relative With FH				
		PERCENTAGE WITH FH AT THAT LEVEL			
		Degree of Relative			
TOTAL CHOL (mg/dL)	**LDL CHOL (mg/dL)**	**First**	**Second**	**Third**	**General Population**
180	122	7.2	2.4	0.9	0.01
190	130	13.5	5.0	2.2	0.03
200	138	26.4	10.7	4.9	0.07
210	147	48.1	23.6	11.7	0.19
220	155	73.1	47.5	27.9	0.54
230	164	90.0	75.0	56.2	1.8
240	172	97.1	93.7	82.8	6.3
250	181	99.3	97.6	95.3	22.2
260	190	99.9	99.5	99.0	57.6
270	200	100.0	99.9	99.8	88.0
280	210	100.0	100.0	100.0	97.8
290	220	100.0	100.0	100.0	99.6
300	230	100.0	100.0	100.0	99.9
310	240	100.0	100.0	100.0	100.0

Chol, Cholesterol; LDL, low-density lipoprotein.
From Williams RR, Hunt SC, Schumacher MC, et al: Diagnosing heterozygous familial hypercholesterolemia using new practical criteria validated by molecular genetics, *Am J Cardiol* 72:171–176, 1993.

Table 104.9 | Plasma Cholesterol and Triglyceride Levels in Childhood and Adolescence: Means and Percentiles

	TOTAL TRIGLYCERIDE (mg/dL)					TOTAL CHOLESTEROL (mg/dL)					LDL CHOLESTEROL (mg/dL)					HDL CHOLESTEROL (mg/dL)*				
	5th	Mean	75th	90th	95th	5th	Mean	75th	90th	95th	5th	Mean	75th	90th	95th	5th	10th	25th	Mean	95th
Cord	14	34	—	—	84	42	68	—	—	103	17	29	—	—	50	13	—	—	35	60
1-4 YR																				
Male	29	56	68	85	99	114	155	170	190	203	—	—	—	—	—	—	—	—	—	—
Female	34	64	74	95	112	112	156	173	188	200	—	—	—	—	—	—	—	—	—	—
5-9 YR																				
Male	28	52	58	70	85	125	155	168	183	189	63	93	103	117	129	38	42	49	56	74
Female	32	64	74	103	126	131	164	176	190	197	68	100	115	125	140	36	38	47	53	73
10-14 YR																				
Male	33	63	74	94	111	124	160	173	188	202	64	97	109	122	132	37	40	46	55	74
Female	39	72	85	104	120	125	160	171	191	205	68	97	110	126	136	37	40	45	52	70
15-19 YR																				
Male	38	78	88	125	143	118	153	168	183	191	62	94	109	123	130	30	34	39	46	63
Female	36	73	85	112	126	118	159	176	198	207	59	96	111	29	137	35	38	43	52	74

*Note that different percentiles are listed for high-density lipoprotein (HDL) cholesterol. LDL, Low-density lipoprotein.

Data for cord blood from Strong W: Atherosclerosis: its pediatric roots. In Kaplan N, Stamler J, editors: *Prevention of coronary heart disease*, Philadelphia, 1983, Saunders. Data for children 1-4 yr from Tables 6, 7, 20, and 21, and all other data from Tables 24, 25, 32, 33, 36, and 37 in *Lipid research clinics population studies data book*, Vol 1, "The prevalence study," NIH Pub No 80-1527, Washington, DC, 1980, National Institutes of Health.

Familial Defective ApoB-100

Familial defective apoB-100 is an autosomal dominant condition that is indistinguishable from heterozygous FH. LDL cholesterol levels are increased, triglycerides are normal, adults often develop tendon xanthomas, and premature CHD occurs. Familial defective apoB-100 is caused by mutation in the receptor-binding region of apoB-100, the ligand of the LDL receptor, with an estimated frequency of 1 in 700 people in Western cultures. It is usually caused by substitution of glutamine for arginine in position 3500 in apoB-100, which results in reduced ability of the LDL-R to bind LDL-C, thus impairing its removal from the circulation. Specialized laboratory testing can distinguish familial defective apoB-100 from FH, but this is not necessary, except in research settings, because treatment is the same.

Autosomal Recessive Hypercholesterolemia

This rare condition, caused by a defect in LDL-R–mediated endocytosis in the liver, clinically presents with severe hypercholesterolemia at levels intermediate between those found in homozygous and heterozygous FH. It is disproportionately present among Sardinians and is modestly responsive to treatment with HMG-CoA reductase inhibitors.

Sitosterolemia

A rare autosomal recessive condition characterized by excessive intestinal adsorption of plant sterols, sitosterolemia is caused by mutations in the adenosine triphosphate (ATP)–binding cassette transporter system (*ABCG5* or *ABCG8*), which is responsible for limiting adsorption of plant sterols in the small intestine and promotes biliary excretion of the small amounts adsorbed. Plasma cholesterol levels may be severely elevated, resulting in tendon xanthomas and premature atherosclerosis. Other features include hemolytic anemia, macrothrombocytopenia (large platelets, reduced number), and hemorrhage. Diagnosis can be confirmed by measuring elevated plasma sitosterol levels. Treatment with HMG-CoA reductase inhibitors is not effective, but cholesterol adsorption inhibitors, such as ezetimibe, and bile acid sequestrants are effective.

Polygenic Hypercholesterolemia

Primary elevation in LDL-C among children and adults is most often polygenic; the small effects of many genes are impacted by environmental influences (diet). Plasma cholesterol levels are modestly elevated; triglyceride levels are normal. Polygenic hypercholesterolemia aggregates in families sharing a common lifestyle but does not follow predictable hereditary patterns found in single-gene lipoprotein defects. Treatment of children with polygenic hypercholesterolemia is directed toward adoption of a healthy lifestyle: reduced total and saturated fat consumption and at least 1 hr of physical activity daily. Cholesterol-lowering medication is rarely necessary.

Hypercholesterolemia With Hypertriglyceridemia
Familial Combined Hyperlipidemia

This autosomal dominant condition is characterized by moderate elevation in plasma LDL-C and triglycerides and reduced plasma HDL-C. Familial combined hyperlipidemia (FCHL) is the most common primary lipid disorder, affecting approximately 1 in 200 people. Family history of premature heart disease is typically positive; the formal diagnosis requires that at least 2 first-degree relatives have evidence of 1 of 3 variants of dyslipidemia: (1) >90th percentile plasma LDL-C; (2) >90th percentile LDL-C and triglycerides; and (3) >90th percentile triglycerides. Individuals switch from one phenotype to another. Xanthomas are not a feature of FCHL. Elevated plasma apoB levels with increased small, dense LDL particles support the diagnosis.

Children and adults with FCHL have coexisting adiposity, hypertension, and hyperinsulinemia, suggesting the presence of the **metabolic syndrome**. Formal diagnosis in adults, as defined by the National Cholesterol Education Program (**NCEP**) Adult Treatment Panel III, identifies 6 major components: abdominal obesity, atherogenic dyslipidemia, hypertension, insulin resistance with or without impaired glucose tolerance, evidence of vascular inflammation, and prothrombotic state. An estimated 30% of overweight adults fulfill criteria for the diagnosis of metabolic syndrome, including 65% of those with FCHL. Hispanics

and South Asians from the Indian subcontinent are especially susceptible. *There is no official definition of metabolic syndrome for children.* Absolute cutoffs for diagnosis in children do not account for continuous variables in aging, sexual maturation, and race/ethnicity.

FCHL and type 2 diabetes share many features of the metabolic syndrome, suggesting that they are less distinct entities than originally conceptualized. Genetic association studies reveal evidence for a common genetic background. The resultant metabolic overlap is associated with ectopic fat accumulation and insulin resistance. The mechanisms associating visceral adiposity with the metabolic syndrome and type 2 diabetes are not fully understood. A plausible unifying principle is that obesity causes endoplasmic reticulum stress, leading to suppression of insulin receptor signaling and thus insulin resistance and heightened inflammatory response. How this relates to atherogenesis is unclear. It is assumed that hypercholesterolemia and, with less certainty, hypertriglyceridemia confer risk for CVD in patients with FCHL. When features of the metabolic syndrome are included in logistic models, shared etiologic features such as increased visceral adiposity become apparent. Visceral adiposity increases with age, and its importance in children as a risk factor for heart disease and diabetes is limited by the relative paucity of data. Although longitudinal measurement of waist circumference and the presence of intraabdominal fat as determined by MRI is being conducted in the research setting, body mass index (BMI) remains the surrogate for adiposity in the pediatric clinical setting.

The metabolic syndrome is a dramatic illustration of the interaction of genetics and the environment. Genetic susceptibility is essential as an explanation for premature heart disease in individuals with FCHL. Unhealthy lifestyle, poor diet, and physical inactivity contribute to obesity and attendant features of the metabolic syndrome.

The cornerstone of management is lifestyle modification. This includes a diet low in saturated fats, *trans* fats, and cholesterol, as well as reduced consumption of processed sugars. Increased dietary intake of fruits and vegetables is important, as is 1 hr of moderate physical activity daily. Compliance among children and their parents is often a problem, but small incremental steps are more likely to succeed than aggressive weight loss strategies. It is very important that the child's caregivers participate in the process. Plasma triglyceride levels are usually quite responsive to dietary restriction, especially reduction in the amount of sweetened drinks consumed. Blood cholesterol levels may decrease by 10–15%, but if LDL-C remains >160 mg/dL, drug therapy should be considered.

Familial Dysbetalipoproteinemia (Type III Hyperlipoproteinemia)

Familial dysbetalipoproteinemia (FDBL) is caused by mutations in the gene for apoE, which when exposed to environmental influences (e.g., high-fat high-caloric diet, excessive alcohol intake) results in a mixed type of hyperlipidemia. Patients tend to have elevated plasma cholesterol and triglycerides to a relatively similar degree. HDL-C is typically normal, in contrast to other causes of hypertriglyceridemia associated with low HDL. This rare disorder affects approximately 1 in 10,000 persons. ApoE mediates removal of chylomicron and VLDL remnants from the circulation by binding to hepatic surface receptors. The polymorphic *APOE* gene expresses in 3 isoforms: *apoE3, apoE2,* and *apoE4*. E4 is the "normal" allele present in the majority of the population. The *apoE2* isoform has lower affinity for the LDL receptor, and its frequency is approximately 7%. Approximately 1% of the population is homozygous for *apoE2/E2,* the most common mutation associated with FDBL, but only a minority expresses the disease. Expression requires precipitating illnesses such as diabetes, obesity, renal disease, or hypothyroidism. Individuals homozygous for *apoE4/E4* are at risk for late-onset Alzheimer disease and dementia from repeated sports-related head injuries.

Most patients with FDBL present in adulthood with distinctive xanthomas. Tuberoeruptive xanthomas resemble small, grapelike clusters on the knees, buttocks, and elbows. Prominent orange-yellow discoloration of the creases of the hands (palmar xanthomas) is also typically present. Atherosclerosis, often presenting with peripheral vascular disease, usually occurs in the 4th or 5th decade. Children may present with a less distinctive rash and generally have precipitating illnesses.

The diagnosis of FDBL is established by lipoprotein electrophoresis, which demonstrates a broad beta band containing remnant lipoproteins. Direct measurement of VLDL by ultracentrifugation can be performed in specialized lipid laboratories. A VLDL/total triglyceride ratio >0.30 supports the diagnosis. *APOE* genotyping for *apoE2* homozygosity can be performed, confirming the diagnosis in the presence of the distinctive physical findings. A negative result does not necessarily rule out the disease as other mutations in *APOE* may cause even more serious manifestations.

Pharmacologic treatment of FDBL is necessary to decrease the likelihood of symptomatic atherosclerosis in adults. HMG-CoA reductase inhibitors, nicotinic acid, and fibrates are all effective. FDBL is quite responsive to recommended dietary restriction.

Hypertriglyceridemias

The familial disorders of triglyceride-rich lipoproteins include both common and rare variants of the **Frederickson classification** system. These include familial chylomicronemia (type I), familial hypertriglyceridemia (type IV), and the more severe combined hypertriglyceridemia and chylomicronemia (type V). Hepatic lipase deficiency also results in a similar combined hyperlipidemia.

Familial Chylomicronemia (Type I Hyperlipidemia)

This rare single-gene defect, like FH, is caused by mutations affecting clearance of apoB-containing lipoproteins. Deficiency or absence of LPL or its cofactor apoC-II, which facilitates lipolysis by LPL, causes severe elevation of triglyceride-rich plasma chylomicrons. HDL-C levels are decreased. Clearance of these particles is greatly delayed, so the plasma is noted to have a turbid appearance even after prolonged fasting (Fig. 104.13). Chylomicronemia caused by LPL deficiency is associated with modest elevation in triglycerides, whereas this is not the case when the cause is deficient or absent apoC-II. Both are autosomal recessive conditions with a frequency of approximately 1 in 1 million population. The disease usually presents during childhood with acute pancreatitis.

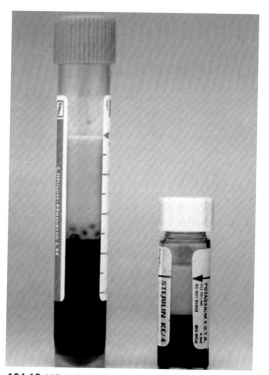

Fig. 104.13 Milky plasma from patient with acute abdominal pain. (*From Durrington P: Dyslipidaemia, Lancet 362:717–731, 2003.*)

Eruptive xanthomas on the arms, knees, and buttocks may be present, and there may be hepatosplenomegaly. The diagnosis is established by assaying triglyceride lipolytic activity. **Treatment** of chylomicronemia is by vigorous dietary fat restriction supplemented by fat-soluble vitamins. Medium-chain triglycerides that are adsorbed into the portal venous system may augment total fat intake, and administration of fish oils may also be beneficial.

Familial Hypertriglyceridemia (Type IV Hyperlipidemia)

Familial hypertriglyceridemia (FHTG) is an autosomal dominant disorder of unknown etiology that occurs in approximately 1 in 500 individuals. It is characterized by elevation of plasma triglycerides >90th percentile (250-1,000 mg/dL range), often accompanied by slight elevation in plasma cholesterol and low HDL. FHTG does not usually manifest until adulthood, although it is expressed in approximately 20% of affected children. In contrast to FCHL, FHTG is not thought to be highly atherogenic. It is most likely caused by defective breakdown of VLDL, or less often by overproduction of this class of lipoproteins.

The diagnosis should include the presence of at least 1 first-degree relative with hypertriglyceridemia. FHTG should be distinguished from FCHL and FDBL, which require more vigorous treatment to prevent coronary or peripheral vascular disease. The differentiation is usually possible on clinical grounds, in that lower LDL-C levels accompany FHTG, but measurement of normal apoB levels in FHTG may be helpful in ambiguous situations.

A more severe hypertriglyceridemia characterized by increased levels of chylomicrons as well as VLDL particles (Frederickson **type V**) may occasionally be encountered. Triglyceride levels are often >1,000 mg/dL. The disease is rarely seen in children. In contrast to chylomicronemia (Frederickson **type I**), LPL or apoC-II deficiency is not present. These patients often develop eruptive xanthomas in adulthood, whereas **type IV** hypertriglyceridemia individuals do not. Acute pancreatitis may be the presenting illness. As with other hypertriglyceridemias, excessive alcohol consumption and estrogen therapy can exacerbate the disease.

Secondary causes of *transient hypertriglyceridemia* should be ruled out before making a diagnosis of FHTG. A diet high in simple sugars and carbohydrates or excessive alcohol consumption, as well as estrogen therapy, may exacerbate hypertriglyceridemia. Adolescents and adults should be questioned about excessive consumption of soda and other sweetened drinks, as it is common to encounter people who drink supersized drinks or multiple 12 oz cans of sweetened drinks daily. Cessation of this practice often results in dramatic fall in triglyceride levels as well as weight among those who are obese. HDL-C levels will tend to rise as BMI stabilizes.

Pediatric diseases associated with hyperlipidemia include hypothyroidism, nephrotic syndrome, biliary atresia, glycogen storage disease, Niemann-Pick disease, Tay-Sachs disease, systemic lupus erythematosus, hepatitis, and anorexia nervosa (Table 104.10). Certain medications exacerbate hyperlipidemia, including isotretinoin (Accutane), thiazide diuretics, second-generation antipsychotic agents, oral contraceptives, corticosteroids, β blockers, immunosuppressants, and protease inhibitors used in HIV treatment.

Treatment of hypertriglyceridemia in children rarely requires medication unless levels >1,000 mg/dL persist after dietary restriction of fats, sugars, and carbohydrates, accompanied by increased physical activity. In such patients the aim is to prevent episodes of pancreatitis. The common use of fibrates (fenofibric acid) and niacin in adults with hypertriglyceridemia is not recommended in children. HMG-CoA reductase inhibitors are variably effective in lowering triglyceride levels, and there is considerably more experience documenting the safety and efficacy of this class of lipid-lowering medications in children. In adults, the U.S. Food and Drug Administration (FDA) has approved prescription (Lovaza, Vascepa) and nonprescription fish oils as adjuncts to diet in the treatment of severe hypertriglyceridemias.

Hepatic Lipase Deficiency

Hepatic lipase deficiency is a very rare autosomal recessive condition causing elevation in both plasma cholesterol and triglycerides. Hepatic

Table 104.10	Secondary Causes of Hyperlipidemia

HYPERCHOLESTEROLEMIA
Hypothyroidism
Nephrotic syndrome
Cholestasis
Anorexia nervosa
Drugs: progesterone, thiazides, carbamazepine (Tegretol),
   cyclosporine

HYPERTRIGLYCERIDEMIA
Obesity
Type 2 diabetes
Alcohol
Renal failure
Sepsis
Stress
Cushing syndrome
Pregnancy
Hepatitis
AIDS, protease inhibitors
Drugs: anabolic steroids, β-blockers, estrogen, thiazides

REDUCED HIGH-DENSITY LIPOPROTEIN
Smoking
Obesity
Type 2 diabetes
Malnutrition
Drugs: β-blockers, anabolic steroids

lipase hydrolyzes triglycerides and phospholipids in VLDL remnants and IDL, preventing their conversion to LDL. HDL-C levels tend to be increased rather than decreased, suggesting the diagnosis. Laboratory confirmation is established by measuring hepatic lipase activity in heparinized plasma.

Disorders of High-Density Lipoprotein Metabolism
Primary Hypoalphalipoproteinemia
Isolated low HDL cholesterol is a familial condition that often follows a pattern suggestive of autosomal dominant inheritance but may occur independent of family history. It is the most common disorder of HDL metabolism. It is defined as HDL-C <10th percentile for gender and age with normal plasma triglycerides and LDL-C. Whether it is associated with more rapid atherosclerosis is uncertain. Primary hypoalphalipoproteinemia appears to be related to a reduction in apoA-I synthesis and increased catabolism of HDL. Secondary causes of low HDL-C, such as the metabolic syndrome, and rare diseases such as LCAT deficiency and Tangier disease must be ruled out.

Familial Hyperalphalipoproteinemia
This is an unusual condition conferring decreased risk for CHD among family members. Plasma levels of HDL-C exceed 80 mg/dL.

Familial Apolipoprotein A-I Deficiency
Mutations in the *apoA-I* gene may result in complete absence of plasma HDL. Nascent HDL is produced in the liver and small intestine. Free cholesterol from peripheral cells is esterified by LCAT, enabling formation of mature HDL particles. ApoA-I is required for normal enzymatic functioning of LCAT. The resultant accumulation of free cholesterol in the circulation eventually leads to corneal opacities, planar xanthomas, and premature atherosclerosis. Some patients, however, may have mutations of *apoA-I* that result in very rapid catabolism of the protein not associated with atherogenesis, despite HDL-C levels in the 15-30 mg/dL range.

Tangier Disease
This autosomal co-dominant disease is associated with HDL-C levels <5 mg/dL. It is caused by mutations in ABCA1, a protein that facilitates the binding of cellular cholesterol to apoA-I. This results in free cholesterol accumulation in the reticuloendothelial system, manifested by tonsillar hypertrophy of a distinctive orange color and hepatosplenomegaly. Intermittent peripheral neuropathy may occur from cholesterol accumulation in Schwann cells. Diagnosis should be suspected in children with enlarged orange tonsils and extremely low HDL-C levels.

Familial Lecithin–Cholesterol Acyltransferase (LCAT) Deficiency
Mutations affecting LCAT interfere with the esterification of cholesterol, thereby preventing formation of mature HDL particles. This is associated with rapid catabolism of apoA-I. Free circulating cholesterol in the plasma is greatly increased, which leads to corneal opacities and HDL-C levels <10 mg/dL. Partial LCAT deficiency is known as "fish-eye" disease. Complete deficiency causes hemolytic anemia and progressive renal insufficiency early in adulthood. This rare disease is not thought to cause premature atherosclerosis. Laboratory confirmation is based on demonstration of decreased cholesterol esterification in the plasma.

Cholesteryl Ester Transfer Protein Deficiency
Mutations involving the *CETP* gene are localized to chromosome 16y21. Cholesteryl ester transfer protein (CETP) facilitates the transfer of lipoproteins from mature HDL to and from VLDL and chylomicron particles, thus ultimately regulating the rate of cholesterol transport to the liver for excretion in the bile. About half of mature HDL-2 particles are directly removed from the circulation by HDL receptors on the surface of the liver. The other half of cholesteryl esters in the core of HDL exchange with triglycerides in the core of apoB lipoproteins (VLDL, IDL, LDL) for transport to the liver. Homozygous deficiency of CETP has been observed in subsets of the Japanese population with extremely high HDL-C levels (>150 mg/dL).

Conditions Associated With Low Cholesterol
Disorders of apoB-containing lipoproteins and intracellular cholesterol metabolism are associated with low plasma cholesterol.

Abetalipoproteinemia
This rare autosomal recessive disease is caused by mutations in the gene encoding microsomal triglyceride transfer protein necessary for the transfer of lipids to nascent chylomicrons in the small intestine and VLDL in the liver. This results in absence of chylomicrons, VLDL, LDL, and apoB and very low levels of plasma cholesterol and triglycerides. Fat malabsorption, diarrhea, and failure to thrive present in early childhood. Spinocerebellar degeneration, secondary to vitamin E deficiency, manifests in loss of deep tendon reflexes progressing to ataxia and lower-extremity spasticity by adulthood. Patients with abetalipoproteinemia also acquire a progressive pigmented retinopathy associated with decreased night and color vision and eventual blindness. The neurologic symptoms and retinopathy may be mistaken for **Friedreich ataxia**. Differentiation from Friedreich ataxia is suggested by the presence of malabsorption and acanthocytosis on peripheral blood smear in abetalipoproteinemia. Many of the clinical manifestations of the disease are a result of malabsorption of fat-soluble vitamins, such as vitamins E, A, and K. *Early treatment with supplemental vitamins, especially E, may significantly slow the development of neurologic sequelae.* Vitamin E is normally transported from the small intestine to the liver by chylomicrons, where it is dependent on the endogenous VLDL pathway for delivery into the circulation and peripheral tissues. Parents of children with abetalipoproteinemia have normal blood lipid and apoB levels.

Familial Hypobetalipoproteinemia
Familial homozygous hypobetalipoproteinemia is associated with symptoms very similar to those of abetalipoproteinemia, but the inheritance pattern is autosomal co-dominant. The disease is caused by mutations in the gene encoding apoB-100 synthesis. It is distinguishable from abetalipoproteinemia in that heterozygous parents of probands have plasma LDL-C and apoB levels less than half normal. There are no symptoms or sequelae associated with the heterozygous condition.

Table 104.11	Major Clinical Characteristics of Smith-Lemli-Opitz Syndrome: Frequent Anomalies (>50% of Patients)

CRANIOFACIAL
Microcephaly
Blepharoptosis
Anteverted nares
Retromicrognathia
Low-set, posteriorly rotated ears
Midline cleft palate
Broad maxillary alveolar ridges
Cataracts (<50%)

SKELETAL ANOMALIES
Syndactyly of toes II/III
Postaxial polydactyly (<50%)
Equinovarus deformity (<50%)

GENITAL ANOMALIES
Hypospadias
Cryptorchidism
Sexual ambiguity (<50%)

DEVELOPMENT
Prenatal and postnatal growth retardation
Feeding problems
Mental impairment
Behavioral abnormalities

From Haas D, Kelley RI, Hoffmann GF: Inherited disorders of cholesterol biosynthesis, *Neuropediatrics* 32:113–122, 2001.

Table 104.12	Characteristic Malformations of Internal Organs in Severely Affected Smith-Lemli-Opitz Patients

CENTRAL NERVOUS SYSTEM
Frontal lobe hypoplasia
Enlarged ventricles
Agenesis of corpus callosum
Cerebellar hypoplasia
Holoprosencephaly

CARDIOVASCULAR
Atrioventricular canal
Secundum atrial septal defect
Patent ductus arteriosus
Membranous ventricular septal defect

URINARY TRACT
Renal hypoplasia or aplasia
Renal cortical cysts
Hydronephrosis
Ureteral duplication

GASTROINTESTINAL
Hirschsprung disease
Pyloric stenosis
Refractory dysmotility
Cholestatic and noncholestatic progressive liver disease

PULMONARY
Pulmonary hypoplasia
Abnormal lobation

ENDOCRINE
Adrenal insufficiency

From Haas D, Kelley RI, Hoffmann GF: Inherited disorders of cholesterol biosynthesis, *Neuropediatrics* 32:113–122, 2001.

The selective inability to secrete apoB-48 from the small intestine results in a condition resembling abetalipoproteinemia or homozygous hypobetalipoproteinemia. Sometimes referred to as **Anderson disease**, the failure of chylomicron absorption causes steatorrhea and fat-soluble vitamin deficiency. The blood level of apoB-100, derived from normal hepatocyte secretion, is normal in this condition.

Smith-Lemli-Opitz Syndrome

Patients with Smith-Lemli-Opitz syndrome (**SLOS**) often have multiple congenital anomalies and developmental delay caused by low plasma cholesterol and accumulated precursors (Tables 104.11 and 104.12) (see Chapter 606.2). Family pedigree analysis has revealed its autosomal recessive inheritance pattern. Mutations in the *DHCR7* (7-dehydrocholesterol-Δ7 reductase) gene result in deficiency of the microsomal enzyme DHCR7, which is necessary to complete the final step in cholesterol synthesis. It is not known why defects in cholesterol synthesis result in congenital malformations, but since cholesterol is a major component of myelin and a contributor to signal transduction in the developing nervous system, neurodevelopment is severely impaired. The incidence of SLOS is estimated to be 1 in 20,000-60,000 births among whites, with a somewhat higher frequency in Hispanics and lower incidence in individuals of African descent.

Spontaneous abortion of SLOS fetuses may occur. **Type II** SLOS often leads to death by the end of the neonatal period. Survival is unlikely when the plasma cholesterol level is <20 mg/dL. Laboratory measurement should be performed by gas chromatography, because standard techniques for lipoprotein assay include measurement of cholesterol precursors, which may yield a false-positive result. Milder cases may not present until late childhood. Phenotypic variance ranges from microcephaly, cardiac and brain malformation, and multiorgan system failure to only subtle dysmorphic features and mild developmental delay. **Treatment** includes supplemental dietary cholesterol (egg yolk) and HMG-CoA reductase inhibition to prevent the synthesis of toxic precursors proximal to the enzymatic block.

Disorders of Intracellular Cholesterol Metabolism
Cerebrotendinous Xanthomatosis

This autosomal recessive disorder presents clinically in late adolescence with tendon xanthomas, cataracts, and progressive neurodegeneration. It is caused by tissue accumulation of bile acid intermediates shunted into cholestanol, resulting from mutations in the gene for sterol 27-hydroxylase. This enzyme is necessary for normal mitochondrial synthesis of bile acids in the liver. Early treatment with chenodeoxycholic acid reduces cholesterol levels and prevents the development of symptoms.

Wolman Disease and Cholesterol Ester Storage Disease

These autosomal recessive disorders are caused by lack of lysosomal acid lipase. After LDL cholesterol is incorporated into the cell by endocytosis, it is delivered to lysosomes, where it is hydrolyzed by lysosomal lipase. Failure of hydrolysis because of complete absence of the enzyme causes accumulation of cholesteryl esters within the cells. Hepatosplenomegaly, steatorrhea, and failure to thrive occur during early infancy, leading to death by age 1 yr. In cholesterol ester storage disease, a less severe form than Wolman disease, there is low but detectable acid lipase activity (see Chapter 104.4).

Niemann-Pick Disease Type C

This disorder of intracellular cholesterol transport is characterized by accumulation of cholesterol and sphingomyelin in the CNS and reticuloendothelial system. Death from this autosomal recessive neurologic disease usually occurs by adolescence (see Chapter 104.4).

Lipoprotein Patterns in Children and Adolescents

Derived primarily from the Lipid Research Clinics Population Studies, Table 104.9 shows the distribution of lipoprotein levels in American youth at various ages. Total plasma cholesterol rises rapidly from a mean of 68 mg/dL at birth to a level approximately twice that by the end of the neonatal period. A very gradual rise in total cholesterol level occurs until puberty, when the mean level reaches 160 mg/dL. Total cholesterol falls transiently during puberty, in males because of a small decrease in HDL-C, and in females secondary to a slight fall in LDL-C. Blood cholesterol levels track reasonably well as individuals age.

High blood cholesterol tends to aggregate in families, a reflection of genetic and environmental influences.

Acceptable total cholesterol among children and adolescents is <170 mg/dL; borderline is 170-199 mg/dL; and high >200 mg/dL. Acceptable LDL-C is <110 mg/dL; borderline 110-129 mg/dL; and high >130 mg/dL. HDL-C should be >40 mg/dL.

Blood Cholesterol Screening

The AAP began recommending a universal approach for cholesterol screening to all children in 2011. *A lipid profile should be checked for all children between ages 9 and 11 yr and then another between ages 17 and 21 yr*, because cholesterol levels may vary after puberty. However, if a child would have met the selective criteria from the previous risk-based guidelines (premature coronary artery disease in parent or grandparent, parent with cholesterol >240 mg/dL), screening can occur as early as 2 yr. Data also suggest that obtaining a *nonfasting* lipid profile can be just as useful in detecting severe genetic dyslipidemias as a fasting lipid profile, and thus can be used as first-line screening in children. Fasting lipid profiles may also be used depending on parental, child, and clinician preference, especially if there is concern for hypertriglyceridemia, since triglycerides are affected more by fasting status. Abnormal lipid panels should be repeated, and especially when the concern is the triglycerides, the 2nd panel should be obtained ≥2 wk later in the fasted state. Treatment other than lifestyle modification is not initiated based on a single lipid panel determination.

Risk Assessment and Treatment of Hyperlipidemia

The NCEP recommends a population-based approach toward healthy lifestyle applicable to all children, and an individualized approach directed at those children at high risk (Fig. 104.14). The important focus on maintenance of a healthy lifestyle rather than aggressive weight reduction is recommended by the AAP.

All children with dyslipidemias are stratified according to the presence of high-level or moderate-level risk factors to determine their ultimate treatment. **High-level risk factors** are defined as hypertension requiring drug therapy (blood pressure ≥99th percentile + 5 mm Hg), current cigarette smoker, BMI at the ≥97th percentile, presence of type 1 or type 2 diabetes mellitus, chronic kidney disease, postorthoptic heart transplant, and/or Kawasaki disease with current aneurysms. **Moderate-level risk factors** are defined as hypertension that does not require drug therapy, BMI at the ≥95th percentile but <97th percentile, HDL-C <40 mg/dL, Kawasaki disease with regressed coronary aneurysms, chronic inflammatory disease, HIV infection, and/or presence of nephrotic syndrome.

The initial treatment for dyslipidemia in a child always begins with a 6-mo trial of lifestyle modification, namely, improvements in dietary and physical activity patterns. Being overweight confers special risk of CVD because of the strong association with the insulin resistance syndrome (metabolic syndrome). Although there is no standardized definition of metabolic syndrome defined for youth, it is likely that half of all severely obese children are insulin resistant. Data from the CARDIAC project noted that 49% of 5th grade children with the hyperpigmented rash, acanthosis nigricans, had 3 or more factors for the insulin resistance syndrome when using the definition classically used for adults, including evidence of insulin resistance, hypertension, HDL-C <40 mg/dL, and triglycerides >150 mg/dL, in addition to obesity.

The Cardiovascular Health Integrated Lifestyle Diet-1 (**CHILD-1**) diet is the first level of dietary change to be recommended for all children with dyslipidemias. The CHILD-1 diet is specially designed for children with risk factors for coronary artery disease and focuses on limiting dietary cholesterol to 300 mg/day, limiting sugary drink consumption, using reduced-fat/skim milk, avoiding foods high in *trans*-type fats,

limiting foods high in sodium, and encouraging consumption of foods high in fiber. Specific recommendations depend on the child's age.

The use of the Cardiovascular Health Integrated Lifestyle Diet-2 (**CHILD-2**) diet is recommended if the CHILD-1 diet alone is unsuccessful. Although similar in many aspects to the CHILD-1 diet, the CHILD-2 diet is geared toward a specific dyslipidemia type; the **CHILD-2 LDL** diet is recommended for children with elevated LDL levels and the **CHILD-2 TG** diet for those presenting with elevated triglycerides. The basic recommendations of calorie consumption for the CHILD-2 diet are as follows: only 25–30% of calories from fat, ≤7% of calories from saturated fat, 10% of calories from monounsaturated fat, and <200 mg/day of cholesterol. If the CHILD-2 LDL diet is recommended, the use of plant sterols and water-soluble fiber is emphasized. If the CHILD-2 TG diet is recommended, the increasing consumption of omega-3 fatty acids and complex rather than simple carbohydrates is emphasized.

If followed, these dietary recommendations will provide adequate calories for optimal growth and development without promoting obesity. Compliance on the part of children and their caregivers is challenging. Children learn eating habits from their parents. Successful adoption of a healthier lifestyle is much more likely to occur if meals and snacks in the home are applicable to the entire family rather than an individual child. A regular time for meals together as a family is desirable. Grandparents and other nonparental caregivers sometimes need to be reminded not to indulge the child who is on a restricted diet. Additionally, the rise in obesity is prompting some school districts to restrict sweetened drink availability and offer more nutritious cafeteria selections.

Changes in physical activity habits are also an important part of the initial lifestyle modification. The National Association for Sport and Physical Education recommends that children should accumulate at least 60 min of age-appropriate physical activity on most days of the week. Extended periods (≥2 hr) of daytime inactivity are discouraged, as is >2 hr of television and other forms of screen time.

Pharmacologic Therapy. See Tables 104.13 and 104.14.

Pharmacologic therapy with cholesterol-lowering medication is the cornerstone of therapy for children who fail to respond to 6 mo of rigorous lifestyle modification. Drug therapy should be considered when 1 of the following conditions are met (also shown in Fig. 104.14):

◆ LDL cholesterol remains >190 mg/dL
◆ LDL cholesterol remains >160 mg/dL with presence of 1 high-level risk factor *and/or* at least 2 moderate-level risk factors
◆ LDL cholesterol remains >130 mg/dL with presence of at least 2 high-level risk factors, 1 high-level risk factor, *and* at least 2 moderate-level risk factors, *or* evidence of coronary artery disease (CAD)

HMG-CoA reductase inhibitors, also known as "statins" are remarkably effective in lowering LDL cholesterol levels and reducing plaque inflammation, thereby reducing the likelihood of a sudden coronary event in an at-risk adult within weeks of starting the medication. As a class, they work by blocking the intrahepatic biosynthesis of cholesterol, thereby stimulating the production of more LDL receptors on the cell surface and facilitating the uptake of LDL-C from the bloodstream. The NCEP Adult Treatment Panel advocates aggressive lowering of LDL to <70 mg/dL in individuals with known CAD. This information is relevant because a child who fulfills criteria for consideration of cholesterol-lowering medication will almost always have inherited the condition from one of the child's parents. Not infrequently, when providing care for the child, questions arise about screening and treatment of parents or grandparents. Statins are equally effective in children, capable of lowering LDL-C levels by 50% when necessary. They are considered first-line therapy for children who meet criteria for pharmacologic therapy. They also will affect a modest reduction in triglycerides and an inconsistent increase in HDL-C. Their side effect profile, mainly liver dysfunction and rarely rhabdomyolysis with secondary renal failure, should be taken into consideration before prescribing the drug. However, there has been no evidence that complications are any more frequent in children than adults, and skeletal muscle discomfort seems to be somewhat less of a problem. Drug interactions may occur as well, so careful attention should be paid to a child's active prescriptions to avoid potentiation of the side effects. Children should have liver enzymes

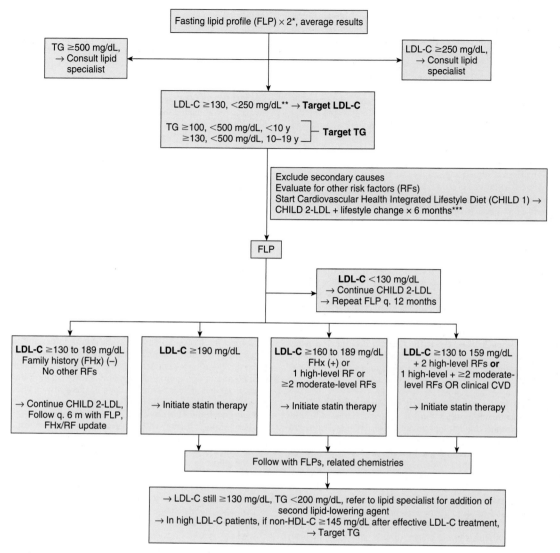

Fig. 104.14 Dyslipidemia treatment algorithm: Target LDL-C (low-density lipoprotein cholesterol). Note: Values given are in mg/dL. To convert to SI units, divide results for total cholesterol (TC), low-density lipoprotein cholesterol (LDL-C), high-density lipoprotein cholesterol (HDL-C), and non-HDL-C by 38.6; for triglycerides (TG), divide by 88.6. (*From US Department of Health and Human Services, National Institutes of Health, National Heart, Lung, and Blood Institute: Expert Panel on Integrated Guidelines for Cardiovascular Health and Risk Reduction in Children and Adolescents. NIH Publication No. 12-7486A, Oct 2012, Fig 9-1.*)

monitored regularly, and creatine phosphokinase measured if muscle aches or weakness occurs. Liver (muscle) enzymes may be allowed to rise 3-fold before discontinuing the drug. There is a suggested link between the use of statins and increased risk of developing type 2 diabetes mellitus in adults, but these results have not been replicated in children. Sex hormones have been measured in children receiving statins and are unchanged. It should be reemphasized that children with modest elevations in cholesterol, such as that seen in polygenic hypercholesterolemia, are not, as a rule, candidates for statins because of their side effect profile and the childhood response to lifestyle modifications. Statins should be started at the lowest effective dose and allowed at least 8 wk to achieve their peak effect. If LDL levels are not at goal, which in children who are treated is generally established to be <130 mg,

the medication may be titrated upward with careful monitoring of side effects.

Other cholesterol-lowering medications, such as nicotinic acid and fibrates, have been used far less often in children than bile acid sequestrants and statins. Nicotinic acid and fibrates have been used selectively in children with marked hypertriglyceridemia (>500 mg/dL) at risk for acute pancreatitis, though dietary restriction of complex sugars (stressing elimination of sugar-sweetened beverages) and carbohydrates will usually result in significant lowering of triglyceride levels. Current guidelines recommend treatment of LDL-C as the initial priority and after LDL levels are at goal, then if triglycerides remain between 200 and 499 mg/dL and non-HDL cholesterol ≥145 mg/dL, pharmacologic treatment to reduce triglyceride levels is indicated. Omega-3 fatty acid supplementa-

Table 104.13	Drugs Used for the Treatment of Hyperlipidemia		
DRUG	**MECHANISM OF ACTION**	**INDICATION**	**STARTING DOSE**
HMG-CoA reductase inhibitors (statins)	↓ Cholesterol and VLDL synthesis ↑ Hepatic LDL receptors	Elevated LDL	5-80 mg every night at bedtime
Bile acid sequestrants: Cholestyramine Colestipol	↑ Bile and excretion	Elevated LDL	4-32 g daily 5-40 g daily
Nicotinic acid	↓ Hepatic VLDL synthesis	Elevated LDL Elevated TG	100-2,000 mg 3 times daily
Fibric acid derivatives: Gemfibrozil	↑ LPL ↓ VLDL	Elevated TG	600 mg twice daily
Fish oils	↓ VLDL production	Elevated TG	3-10 g daily
Cholesterol absorption inhibitors: Ezetimibe	↓ Intestinal absorption cholesterol	Elevated LDL	10 mg daily

LDL, Low-density lipoprotein(s); LPL, lipoprotein lipase; TG, triglycerides; VLDL, very-low-density lipoprotein.

tion, available in both over-the-counter and prescription form, is a safe and useful treatment thought to reduce triglyceride levels by decreasing the hepatic synthesis of triglycerides. LDL-C levels in adults of about 70 mg/dL were recently associated with coronary artery atheromatous plaque reduction and reversal of CAD. Knowledge in this area will continue to evolve.

Ezetimibe has proved to be useful in the pediatric population because of its efficacy and low side effect profile. Ezetimibe reduces plasma LDL-C by blocking sterol absorption in enterocytes. The drug is marketed as an adjunct to statins when adults are not achieving sufficient blood lipid lowering with statins alone. Sufficient reports documenting its effectiveness without side effects support recommending ezetimibe instead of a statin when moderate hypercholesterolemia is encountered, or apprehension from parents makes using a statin difficult.

Bibliography

Austin MA, Hutter CH, Zimmern RL, et al: Familial hypercholesterolemia and coronary heart disease: a huge association review, *Am J Epidemiol* 160:421–429, 2004.

Bhatnagar D, Soran H, Durrington PN: Hypercholesterolaemia and its management, *BMJ* 337:503–508, 2008.

Bremer AA, Mietus-Snyder M, Lustig RH: Toward a unifying hypothesis of metabolic syndrome, *Pediatrics* 129:557–570, 2012.

Brunzell JD: Hypertriglyceridemia, *N Engl J Med* 357:1009–1016, 2007.

Buonuomo PS, Malamisura M, Macchiaiolo M, et al: Eruptive xanthomas in pipoprotein lipase deficiency, *J Pediatr* 187:330, 2017.

Centers for Disease Control and Prevention: Prevalence of abnormal lipid levels among youths—United States, 1999–2006, *MMWR Morb Mortal Wkly Rep* 59:29–33, 2010.

Chan YM, Merkens LS, Connor WB, et al: Effects of dietary cholesterol and simvastatin on cholesterol synthesis in Smith-Lemli-Opitz syndrome, *Pediatr Res* 65:681–685, 2009.

Cuchel M, Meagher EA, du Toit Theron H, et al: Efficacy and safety of a microsomal triglyceride transfer protein inhibitor in patients with homozygous familial hypercholesterolaemia: a single-arm, open-label, phase 3 study, *Lancet* 381:40–46, 2013.

Daniels SR, Greer FR, et al: Lipid screening and cardiovascular health in childhood, *Pediatrics* 122:198–208, 2008.

Expert Panel on Integrated Guidelines for cardiovascular health and risk reduction in children and adolescents: summary report, *Pediatrics* 128:S1–S44, 2011.

Ford ES, Li C, Zhao G, et al: Concentrations of low-density lipoprotein cholesterol and total cholesterol among children and adolescents in the United States, *Circulation* 119:1108–1115, 2009.

Gillman MW, Daniels SR: Is universal pediatric lipid screening justified?, *JAMA* 307:259–260, 2012.

Grundy SM, Hansen B, Smith SC, et al: Clinical management of metabolic syndrome: report of the American Heart Association/National Heart, Lung, Blood Institute/American Diabetes Association Conference on Scientific Issues Related to Management, *Circulation* 109:551–556, 2004.

Table 104.14	Adverse Effects of Cholesterol-Lowering Drugs

STATINS
Myalgia, myositis, transaminase elevations, hepatic dysfunction, increased risk of diabetes mellitus
Rare: Rhabdomyolysis, hemorrhagic stroke

EZETIMIBE
Diarrhea, arthralgia, rhabdomyolysis, hepatitis, pancreatitis, thrombocytopenia

PCSK9 INHIBITORS
Nasopharyngitis, upper respiratory tract infection, influenza, back pain, injection site reactions, rash, allergic skin reactions, cognitive effects, antidrug antibodies

BILE ACID SEQUESTRANTS
Constipation, heartburn, nausea, eructation, bloating
Adverse effects are more common with colestipol and cholestyramine and may diminish over time.

FIBRIC ACID DERIVATIVES
Gastrointestinal (GI) disturbances, cholelithiasis, hepatitis, myositis

NIACIN
Skin flushing, pruritus, GI disturbances, blurred vision, fatigue, glucose intolerance, hyperuricemia, hepatic toxicity, exacerbation of peptic ulcers
Adverse effects, especially flushing, occur more frequently with immediate-release products.
Rare: Dry eyes, hyperpigmentation

FISH OIL
Eructation, dyspepsia, unpleasant aftertaste

From *The Medical Letter:* Lipid-lowering drugs, *Med Lett* 58:133-140, 2016 (Table 2, p 136).

Jørgensen AB, Frikke-Schmidt R, Nordestgaard BG, et al: Loss-of-function mutations in *APOC3* and risk of ischemic vascular disease, *N Engl J Med* 371:32–40, 2014.

Kastelein JJP, Besseling J, Shah S, et al: Anacetrapib as lipid-modifying therapy in patients with heterozygous familial hypercholesterolaemia (REALIZE): a randomized, double-blind, placebo-controlled, phase 3 study, *Lancet* 385:2153–2160, 2015.

Kavey REW, Mietus-Snyder M: Beyond cholesterol: the atherogenic consequences of combined dyslipidemia, *J Pediatr* 161:977–979, 2012.

Khera AV, et al: Diagnostic yield and clinical utility of sequencing familial hypercho-lesterolemia genes in patients with severe hypercholesterolemia, *J Am Coll Cardiol* 67(22):2578–2589, 2016.

Klancar G, et al: Universal screening for familial hypercholesterolemia in children, *J Am Coll Cardiol* 66(11):1250–1257, 2015.

Kumanyika SK, Obarzanek E: Population-based prevention of obesity: the need for comprehensive practices of healthful eating, physical activity and energy balance. A scientific statement from American Heart Association Council on Epidemiology and Prevention, *Circulation* 118:428–464, 2008.

Kusters DM, Caceres M, Coll M, et al: Efficacy and safety of ezetimibe monotherapy in children with heterozygous familial or nonfamilial hypercholesterolemia, *J Pediatr* 166:1377–1384, 2015.

Lebenthal Y, Horvath A, Dziechciarz P, et al: Are treatment targets for hyperchole-sterolemia evidence-based? Systematic review and meta-analysis of randomized controlled trials, *Arch Dis Child* 95:673–680, 2010.

Lozano P, Henrikson NB, Dunn J, et al: Lipid screening in childhood and adolescence for detection of familial hypercholesterolemia: evidence report and systematic review for the US Preventive Services Task Force, *JAMA* 316(6):645–655, 2016.

Lozano P, Henrikson NB, Morrison CC, et al: Lipid screening in childhood and adolescence for detection of multifactorial dyslipidemia: evidence report and systematic review for the US Preventive Services Task Force, *JAMA* 316(6):634–644, 2016.

Lufti R, Huang J, Wong HR: Plasmapheresis to treat hypertriglyceridemia in a child with diabetic ketoacidosis and pancreatitis, *Pediatrics* 129:e195–e198, 2012.

Macchiaiolo M, Gagliardi MG, Toscano A, et al: Homozygous familial hyperchole-sterolaemia, *Lancet* 379:1330, 2012.

Magnussen CG, Raitakari OT, Thomson R, et al: Utility of currently recommended pediatric dyslipidemia classifications in predicting dyslipidemia in adulthood, *Circulation* 117:32–42, 2008.

Manlhiot C, Larsson P, Gurofsky R, et al: Spectrum and management of hypertri-glyceridemia among children in clinical practice, *Pediatrics* 123:458–465, 2009.

Marks D, et al: A review on the diagnosis, natural history, and treatment of familial hypercholesterolaemia, *Atherosclerosis* 168(1):1–14, 2003.

McCrindle BW, Gidding SS: What should be the screening strategy for familial hypercholesterolaemia?, *N Engl J Med* 375(17):1685–1686, 2016.

The Medical Letter: Lipid-lowering drugs, *Med Lett Drugs Ther* 58:133–140, 2016.

The Medical Letter: Fenofibric acid (Trilipix), *Med Lett Drugs Ther* 51:33–34, 2009.

The Medical Letter: Icosapent ethyl (Vascepa) for severe hypertriglyceridemia, *Med Lett Drugs Ther* 55:33–34, 2013.

The Medical Letter: Drugs for hypertriglyceridemia, *Med Lett Drugs Ther* 55:17–20, 2013.

The Medical Letter: Two new drugs for homozygous familial hypercholesterolemia, *Med Lett Drugs Ther* 55:25–26, 2013.

Merkens LS, Connor WE, Linck LM, et al: Effects of dietary cholesterol on plasma lipoproteins in Smith-Lemli-Opitz syndrome, *Pediatr Res* 56:726–732, 2004.

Othman RA, Myrie SB, Mymin D, et al: Ezetimibe reduces plant sterol accumulation and favorably increases platelet count in sitosterolemia, *J Pediatr* 166:125–131, 2015.

Psaty BM, Rivara FP: Universal screening and drug treatment of dyslipidemia in children and adolescents, *JAMA* 307:257–258, 2012.

Raal FJ: Lomitapide for homozygous familial hypercholesterolaemia, *Lancet* 381:7–8, 2013.

Raitakari OT: Arterial abnormalities in children with familial hypercholesteremia, *Lancet* 363:342–343, 2004.

Roth EM, McKenney JM, Hanotin C, et al: Atorvastatin with or without an anti-body to PCSK9 in primary hypercholesterolemia, *N Engl J Med* 367:1891–1900, 2012.

Silverstein J, Haller M: Coronary artery disease in youth: present markers, future hope?, *J Pediatr* 157(4):523–524, 2010.

Stein EA, Raal FJ: Polygenic familial hypercholesterolaemia: does it matter?, *Lancet* 381:1255–1258, 2013.

Steiner MJ, Skinner AC, Perrin EM: Fasting might not be necessary before lipid screening: a nationally representative cross-sectional study, *Pediatrics* 128(3):463–470, 2011.

The SEARCH Collaborative Group: SLCO1B1 variants and statin-induced myopathy—a genomewide study, *N Engl J Med* 359:789–799, 2008.

The TG and HDL Working Group of the Exome Sequencing Project, National Heart, Lung, and Blood Institute: Loss-of-function mutations in APOC3 triglycerides, and coronary disease, *N Engl J Med* 371:22–30, 2014.

Urbina EM, de Ferranti SD: Lipid screening in children and adolescents, *JAMA* 316(6):589–591, 2016.

US Preventive Services Task Force: Screening for lipid disorders in children and adolescents, *JAMA* 316(6):625–632, 2016.

Vinci S, et al: Cholesterol testing among children and adolescents during health visits, *JAMA* 311(17):1804–1806, 2014.

Wald DS, Bestwick JP, Morris JK, et al: Child-parent familial hypercholesterolemia screening in primary care, *N Engl J Med* 375(17):1628–1636, 2016.

Wald DS, Kasturiratne A, Godoy A, et al: Child-parent screening for familial hyper-cholesterolaemia, *J Pediatr* 159:865–867, 2011.

Webber BJ, Seguin PG, Burnett DG, et al: Prevalence of and risk factors for autopsy-determined atherosclerosis among US service members, *JAMA* 308:2577–2582, 2012.

104.4 Lipidoses (Lysosomal Storage Disorders)

Margaret M. McGovern and Robert J. Desnick

The lysosomal lipid storage diseases are diverse disorders, each caused by an inherited deficiency of a specific lysosomal hydrolase leading to the intralysosomal accumulation of the enzyme's particular substrate (Tables 104.15 and 104.16). Except for Wolman disease and cholesterol ester storage disease, the lipid substrates share a common structure that includes a ceramide backbone (2-*N*-acylsphingosine) from which the various sphingolipids are derived by substitution of hexoses, phosphor-ylcholine, or 1 or more sialic acid residues on the terminal hydroxyl group of the ceramide molecule. The pathway of sphingolipid metabolism in nervous tissue (Fig. 104.15) and in visceral organs (Fig. 104.16) is known; each catabolic step, with the exception of the catabolism of lactosylceramide, has a genetically determined metabolic defect and a resultant disease. Because **sphingolipids** are essential components of all cell membranes, the inability to degrade these substances and their subsequent accumulation results in the physiologic and morpho-logic alterations and characteristic clinical manifestations of the lipid storage disorders (Table 104.15). Progressive lysosomal accumulation of glycosphingolipids in the CNS leads to neurodegeneration, whereas storage in visceral cells can lead to organomegaly, skeletal abnormali-ties, pulmonary infiltration, and other manifestations. The storage of a substrate in a specific tissue depends on its normal distribution in the body.

Diagnostic assays for the identification of affected individuals rely on the measurement of the specific enzymatic activity, typically in isolated leukocytes. Fig. 104.17 shows an approach to differentiating these disorders. For most, carrier identification and prenatal diagnosis are available; a specific diagnosis is essential to permit genetic counseling. Neonatal screening using dried blood spots and performing enzyme assays and mutational analysis for Gaucher, Pompe, Fabry, and Niemann-Pick diseases are undergoing pilot studies, and the FDA has approved the *Seeker System* for detection of Gaucher and Fabry diseases. The characterization of the genes that encode the specific enzymes required for sphingolipid metabolism permit the development of therapeutic options, such as recombinant enzyme replacement therapy, as well as the potential of cell or gene therapy. Identification of specific disease-causing mutations improves diagnosis, prenatal detection, and carrier identification. For several disorders (Gaucher, Fabry, Niemann-Pick types A and B), it has been possible to make genotype-phenotype correlations that predict disease severity and allow more precise genetic counseling. Inheritance is autosomal recessive except for X-linked Fabry disease.

GM₁ GANGLIOSIDOSIS

GM_1 gangliosidosis most frequently presents in early infancy but has been described in patients with juvenile- and adult-onset subtypes. Inherited as an autosomal recessive trait, each subtype results from a different gene mutation that leads to the deficient activity of β-galactosidase, a lysosomal enzyme encoded by a gene on chromosome 3 (3p21.33). Although the disorder is characterized by the pathologic accumulation of GM_1 gangliosides in the lysosomes of both neural and visceral cells, GM_1 ganglioside accumulation is most marked in the brain. In addition, keratin sulfate, a mucopolysaccharide, accumulates in liver and is excreted in the urine of patients with GM_1 gangliosidosis. The β-galactosidase gene has been isolated and sequenced; mutations causing the disease subtypes have been identified.

The clinical manifestations of the **infantile** form of GM_1 gangliosidosis may be evident in the newborn as hepatosplenomegaly, edema, and skin eruptions (**angiokeratoma**). It most frequently presents in the 1st

6 mo of life with developmental delay followed by progressive psychomotor retardation and the onset of tonic-clonic seizures. Typical facies is characterized by low-set ears, frontal bossing, a depressed nasal bridge, and an abnormally long philtrum. Up to 50% of patients have a macular cherry-red spot. Hepatosplenomegaly and skeletal abnormalities are present, such as those of the mucopolysaccharidoses, including anterior beaking of the vertebrae, enlargement of the sella turcica, and thickening of the calvarium. By the end of the 1st yr of life, most patients are blind and deaf, with severe neurologic impairment characterized by decerebrate rigidity. Death usually occurs by 3-4 yr of age. The **juvenile-onset** form of GM$_1$ gangliosidosis is clinically distinct, with a variable age at onset. Affected patients present primarily with neurologic symptoms, including ataxia, dysarthria, intellectual disability, and spasticity. Deterioration is slow; patients may survive through the 4th decade of life. These patients lack the visceral involvement, facial abnormalities, and skeletal features seen in type 1 disease. Adult-onset patients have been described who present with gait and speech abnormalities, dystonia and mild skeletal abnormalities. *There is no specific treatment* for either form of GM$_1$ gangliosidosis.

The diagnosis of GM$_1$ gangliosidosis should be suspected in infants with typical clinical features and is confirmed by the demonstration of the deficiency of β-galactosidase activity in peripheral leukocytes. Other disorders that share some of the features of the GM$_1$ gangliosidoses include Hurler disease (mucopolysaccharidosis type I), I-cell disease, and Niemann-Pick disease type A, each of which can be distinguished by the demonstration of their specific enzymatic deficiencies. Carriers of the disorder are detected by the measurement of the enzymatic activity

in peripheral leukocytes or by identifying the specific gene mutations; prenatal diagnosis is accomplished by determination of the enzymatic activity in cultured amniocytes or chorionic villi or identification of the specific disease-causing mutations. Only supportive therapy is available for patients with GM$_1$ gangliosidosis. However, studies in mice with GM$_1$ gangliosidosis have demonstrated that oral *N*-octyl-4-epi-β-valienamine (NOEV), which stabilizes the mutant enzyme protein produced by the affected animals, crossed the brain and improved neurologic deterioration, suggesting that this approach may be useful in human study.

THE GM$_2$ GANGLIOSIDOSES

The GM$_2$ gangliosidoses include Tay-Sachs disease and Sandhoff disease; each results from deficiency of β-hexosaminidase activity and lysosomal accumulation of GM$_2$ gangliosides, particularly in the CNS. Both disorders have been classified into infantile-, juvenile-, and adult-onset forms based on the age at onset and clinical features. β-Hexosaminidase occurs as 2 isozymes: β-hexosaminidase A, which is composed of 1 α and 1 β subunit, and β-hexosaminidase B, which has 2 β subunits. B-Hexosaminidase A deficiency results from mutations in the α subunit and causes Tay-Sachs disease, whereas mutations in the β subunit result in the deficiency of both β-hexosaminidases A and B and cause Sandhoff disease. Both are autosomal recessive traits, with Tay-Sachs disease being more common in the Ashkenazi Jewish population, in whom the carrier frequency is approximately 1 in 25.

More than 50 mutations have been identified; most are associated with the infantile forms of disease. Three mutations account for >98%

Text continued on p. 828

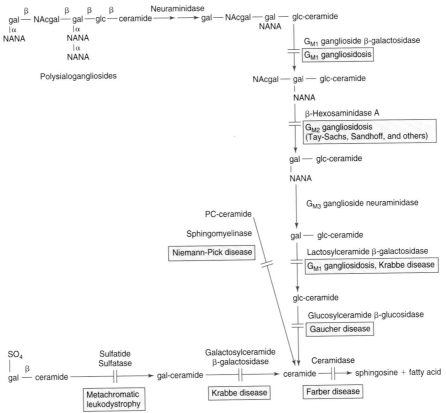

Fig. 104.15 Pathways in the metabolism of sphingolipids found in nervous tissues. The name of the enzyme catalyzing each reaction is given with the name of the substrate that it hydrolyzes. Inborn errors are depicted as *bars* crossing the reaction arrows, and the name of the associated defect or defects is given in the nearest *box*. The gangliosides are named according to the nomenclature of Svennerholm. Anomeric configurations are given only at the largest starting compound. Gal, Galactose; glc, glucose; NAcgal, *N*-acetylgalactosamine; NANA, *N*-acetylneuraminic acid; PC, phosphorylcholine.

Table 104.15 | Clinical Findings in Lysosomal Storage Diseases

NOMENCLATURE	ENZYME DEFECT	HYDROPS FETALIS	COARSE FACIAL FEATURES DYSOSTOSIS MULTIPLEX	HEPATOSPLENOMEGALY
MUCOLIPIDOSES				
Mucolipidoses II, I-cell disease	N-Acetylglucosaminylphosphotransferase	(+)	++	+
Mucolipidosis III, pseudo-Hurler	N-Acetylglucosaminylphosphotransferase	–	+	(+)
Mucolipidosis IV	Unknown	–	–	+
SPHINGOLIPIDOSES				
Fabry disease	α-Galactosidase	–	–	–
Farber disease	Acid ceramidase	–	–	(+)
Galactosialidosis	β-Galactosidase and sialidase	(+)	++	++
GM$_1$ gangliosidosis	β-Galactosidase	(+)	++	+
GM$_2$ gangliosidosis (Tay-Sachs, Sandhoff disease)	β-Hexosaminidases A and B	–	–	(+)
Gaucher type I	Glucocerebrosidase	–	–	++
Gaucher type II	Glucocerebrosidase	(+)	–	++
Gaucher type III	Glucocerebrosidase	(+)	–	+
Niemann-Pick type A	Acid Sphingomyelinase	(+)	–	++
Niemann-Pick type B	Acid Sphingomyelinase	–	–	++
Metachromatic leukodystrophy	Arylsulfatase A	–	–	–
Krabbe disease	β-Galactocerebrosidase	–	–	–
LIPID STORAGE DISORDERS				
Niemann-Pick type C	Intracellular cholesterol transport	–	–	(+)
Wolman disease	Lysosomal acid lipase	(+)	–	+
Ceroid lipofuscinosis, infantile (Santavuori-Haltia)	Palmitoyl-protein thioesterase (CLN1)	–	–	–
Ceroid lipofuscinosis, late infantile (Jansky-Bielschowsky)	Pepstatin-insensitive peptidase (CLN2); variants in Finland (CLN5), Turkey (CLN7), and Italy (CLN6)	–	–	–
Ceroid lipofuscinosis, juvenile (Spielmeyer-Vogt)	CLN3, membrane protein	–	–	–
Ceroid lipofuscinosis, adult (Kufs, Parry)	CLN4, probably heterogeneous	(+)	–	–
OLIGOSACCHARIDOSES				
Aspartylglucosaminuria	Aspartylglucosylaminase	–	+	(+)
Fucosidosis	α-Fucosidase	–	++	(+)
α-Mannosidosis	α-Mannosidase	–	++	+
β-Mannosidosis	β-Mannosidase	–	+	(+)
Schindler disease	α-N-Acetylgalactosaminidase	–	–	–
Sialidosis I	Sialidase	(+)	–	–
Sialidosis II	Sialidase	(+)	++	+

++, Prominent; +, often present; (+), inconstant or occurring later in the disease course; –, not present.
Modified from Hoffmann GF, Nyhan WL, Zschoke J, et al: *Storage disorders in inherited metabolic diseases*, Philadelphia, 2002, Lippincott Williams & Wilkins, pp 346–351.

CARDIAC INVOLVEMENT CARDIAC FAILURE	MENTAL DETERIORATION	MYOCLONUS	SPASTICITY	PERIPHERAL NEUROPATHY	CHERRY-RED SPOT	CORNEAL CLOUDING	ANGIOKERATOMATA
++	++	−	−	−	−	(+)	−
−	(+)	−	−	−	−	+	−
−	(+)	−	−	−	−	−	−
+	−	−	−	−	−	+	++
++	+	−	−	+	(+)	−	−
+	++	(+)	+	−	+	+	+
(+)	++	−	(+)	−	(+)	+	+
−	++	+	+	−	++	−	−
−	−	−	−	−	−	−	−
−	++	+	+	−	−	−	−
−	+	(+)	(+)	−	−	−	−
−	+	(+)	−	(+)	(++)	−	−
−	−	−	−	(+)	(+)	−	−
−	++	−	+	++	(+)	−	−
−	++	−	+	++	(+)	−	−
−	+	−	−	−	(+)	−	−
(+)	−	−	−	−	(+)	−	−
−	+	+	+	−	−	−	−
−	+	+	+	−	−	−	−
−	+	−	(+)	−	−	−	−
−	+	−	−	−	−	−	−
(+)	+	−	−	−	−	(+)	(+)
+	++	+	+	−	−	−	(+)
−	++	−	(+)	−	−	++	(+)
−	+	−	+	+	−	−	(+)
−	+	+	+	−	−	−	−
−	−	++	+	+	++	(+)	−
+	++	(+)	−	−	++	−	+

Table 104.16 | Lysosomal Storage Disorders in the Newborn Period: Genetic and Clinical Characteristics of Neonatal Presentation

DISORDER	ONSET	FACIES	NEUROLOGIC FINDINGS	DISTINCTIVE FEATURES	EYE FINDINGS	DEFECT	GENE LOCATION/ MOLECULAR FINDINGS	ETHNIC PREDILECTION
Niemann–Pick A disease	Early infancy	Frontal bossing	Difficulty feeding, apathy, deafness, blindness, hypotonia	Brownish-yellow skin, xanthomas	Cherry-red spot (50%)	Sphingomyelinase deficiency	*SMPD1* gene at 11p15.4; three of 18 mutations account for approximately 92% of mutant alleles in the Ashkenazi population	1:40,000 in Ashkenazi Jews with carrier frequency of 1:60
Niemann–Pick C disease	Birth–3 months	Normal	Developmental delay, vertical gaze paralysis, hypotonia, later spasticity	—	—	Abnormal cholesterol esterification	*NPC1* gene at 18q11 accounts for >95% of cases; *HE1* gene mutations may account for remaining cases	Increased in French Canadians of Nova Scotia and Spanish Americans in the southwest United States
Gaucher disease type 2	In utero–6 months	Normal	Poor suck and swallow, weak cry, squint, trismus, strabismus, opsoclonus, hypertonic, later flaccidity	Congenital ichthyosis, collodion skin	—	Glucocerebrosidase deficiency	1q21; large number of mutations known; five mutations account for approximately 97% of mutant alleles in the Ashkenazi population but approximately 75% in the non-Jewish population	Panethnic
Krabbe disease	3–6 months	Normal	Irritability, tonic spasms with light or noise stimulation, seizures, hypertonia, later flaccidity	Increased CSF protein level	Optic atrophy	Galactocerebrosidase deficiency	14q 24.3-q32.1; >60 mutations with some common mutations in specific populations	Increased in Scandinavian countries and in a large Druze kindred in Israel
GM1 gangliosidosis	Birth	Coarse	Poor suck, weak cry, lethargy, exaggerated startle, blindness, hypotonia, later spasticity	Gingival hypertrophy, edema, rashes	Cherry-red spot (50%)	β-Galactosidase deficiency	3pter-3p21; heterogeneous mutations; common mutations in specific populations	Panethnic
Farber disease type I	2 weeks–4 months	Normal	Progressive psychomotor impairment, seizures, decreased reflexes, hypotonia	Joint swelling with nodules, hoarseness, lung disease, contractures, fever, granulomas, dysphagia, vomiting, increased CSF protein level	Grayish opacification surrounding retina in some patients, subtle cherry-red spot	Lysosomal acid ceramidase	8p21.3-22; nine disease-causing mutations identified	Panethnic

Continued

Farber disease types II and III	Birth–9 months (≤20 months)	Normal	—	Joint swelling with nodules, hoarseness	Normal macula, corneal opacities	—	8p21.3-p22	Panethnic
Farber disease type IV (neonatal)	Birth	Normal	Nodules not consistent findings	Corneal opacities (1/3)	—	—	Unknown	Panethnic
Congenital sialidosis	In utero–birth	Cognitive, edema	Intellectual impairment, hypotonia	Neonatal ascites, inguinal hernias, renal disease	Corneal clouding	Neuraminidase deficiency	NEU1 gene (sialidase) at 6p21	Panethnic
Galactosialidosis	In utero–birth	Coarse	Intellectual impairment, occasional deafness, hypotonia	Ascites, edema, inguinal hernias, renal disease, telangiectasias	Cherry-red spot, corneal clouding	Absence of a protective protein that safeguards neuraminidase and β-galactosidase from premature degradation	20q13.1	Panethnic
Wolman disease	First weeks of life	Normal	Cognitive deterioration	Vomiting, diarrhea, steatorrhea, abdominal distention, failure to thrive, anemia, adrenal calcifications	—	Lysosomal acid lipase deficiency	10q23.2-q23.3; variety of mutations identified	Increased in Iranian Jews and in non-Jewish and Arab populations of Galilee
Infantile sialic acid storage disease	In utero–birth	Coarse, dysmorphic	Intellectual impairment, hypotonia	Ascites, anemia, diarrhea, failure to thrive	—	Defective transport of sialic acid out of the lysosome	SLC17A5 gene at 6q	Panethnic
I-cell disease	In utero–birth	Coarse	Intellectual impairment, deafness	Gingival hyperplasia, restricted joint mobility, hernias	Corneal clouding	Lysosomal enzymes lack mannose 6-phosphate recognition marker and fail to enter the lysosome (phosphotransferase deficiency, 3-subunit complex [α2 β2 γ2])	Enzyme encoded by two genes; α and β subunits encoded by gene at 12p; γ subunit encoded by gene at 16p	Panethnic
Mucolipidosis type IV	Birth–3 months	Normal	Intellectual impairment, hypotonia	—	Severe corneal clouding, retinal degeneration, blindness	Unknown; some patients with partial deficiency of ganglioside sialidase	MCOLN1 gene at 19p13.2-13.3 encoding mucolipin 1; two founder mutations accounting for 95% of mutant alleles in the Ashkenazi population	Increased in Ashkenazi Jews
Mucopolysaccharidosis type VII	In utero–childhood	Variable coarseness	Mild to severe intellectual impairment	Hernias	Variable corneal clouding	β-Glucuronidase deficiency	GUSB gene at 7q21.2-q22; heterogeneous mutations	Panethnic

Modified from Thomas JA, Lam C, Berry GT: Lysosomal storage, peroxisomal, and glycosylation disorders and Smith-Lemli-Opitz syndrome presenting in the neonate. In Gleason CA, Juul SE, editors: Avery's diseases of the newborn, ed 10, Philadelphia, 2018, Elsevier, Table 23.1.

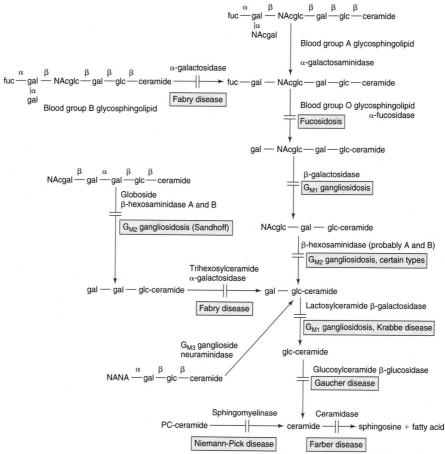

Fig. 104.16 Pathways in the degradation of sphingolipids found in visceral organs and red or white blood cells. See also the legend for Fig. 104.15. Fuc, Fucose; NAcglc, *N*-acetylglucosamine.

of mutant alleles among Ashkenazi Jewish carriers of Tay-Sachs disease, including one allele associated with the adult-onset form. Mutations that cause the subacute or adult-onset forms result in enzyme proteins with residual enzymatic activities, the levels of which correlate with the severity of the disease.

Patients with the infantile form of **Tay-Sachs disease** have clinical manifestations in infancy such as loss of motor skills, increased startle reaction, and macular pallor and retinal cherry-red spots (see Table 104.15). Affected infants usually develop normally until 4-5 mo of age, when decreased eye contact and an exaggerated startle response to noise (**hyperacusis**) are noted. **Macrocephaly**, not associated with hydrocephalus, may develop. In the 2nd yr of life, seizures develop, which may be refractory to anticonvulsant therapy. Neurodegeneration is relentless, with death occurring by age 4 or 5 yr. The juvenile- and later-onset forms initially present with ataxia and dysarthria and may not be associated with a macular cherry-red spot.

The clinical manifestations of **Sandhoff disease** are similar to those of Tay-Sachs disease. Infants with Sandhoff disease have hepatosplenomegaly, cardiac involvement, and mild bony abnormalities. The **juvenile** form of this disorder presents as ataxia, dysarthria, and mental deterioration, but without visceral enlargement or a macular cherry-red spot. *No treatment is available* for Tay-Sachs disease or Sandhoff disease, although experimental approaches are being evaluated.

The diagnosis of **infantile** Tay-Sachs disease and Sandhoff disease is usually suspected in an infant with neurologic features and a cherry-red spot. Definitive diagnosis is made by determination of β-hexosaminidase A and B activities in peripheral leukocytes. The 2 disorders are distinguished by the enzymatic assay, because in Tay-Sachs disease only the β-hexosaminidase A isozyme is deficient, whereas in Sandhoff disease both the β-hexosaminidase A and B isozymes are deficient. At-risk pregnancies for both disorders can be prenatally diagnosed by determining the enzyme levels in fetal cells obtained by amniocentesis or chorionic villus sampling. Identification of carriers in families is also possible by β-hexosaminidases A and B determination. Indeed, for Tay-Sachs disease, carrier screening of all couples in which at least 1 member is of Ashkenazi Jewish descent is recommended before the initiation of pregnancy to identify couples at risk. These studies can be conducted by the determination of the level of β-hexosaminidase A activity in peripheral leukocytes or plasma. Molecular studies to identify the exact molecular defect in enzymatically identified carriers should also be performed to permit more specific identification of carriers in the family and to allow prenatal diagnosis in at-risk couples by both enzymatic and genotype determinations. The incidence of Tay-Sachs disease has been greatly reduced since the introduction of carrier screening programs in the Ashkenazi Jewish population. Newborn screening may be possible by measuring specific glycosphingolipid markers or the relevant enzymatic activities in dried blood spots.

GAUCHER DISEASE

Gaucher disease is a multisystemic lipidosis characterized by hematologic abnormalities, organomegaly, and skeletal involvement, the latter usually manifesting as bone pain and pathologic fractures (see Table 104.15). It is one of the most common lysosomal storage diseases and the most prevalent genetic defect among Ashkenazi Jews. There are 3 clinical

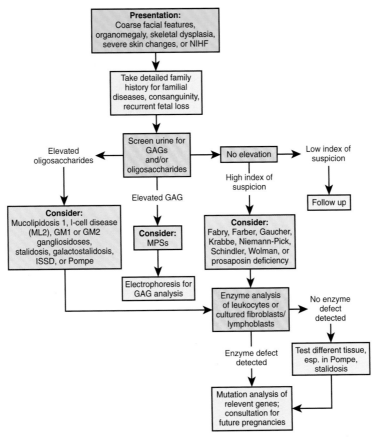

Fig. 104.17 Algorithm of the clinical evaluation recommended for an infant with a suspected lysosomal storage disease. GAGs, Glycosaminoglycans; ISSD, infantile sialic acid storage disease; NIHF, nonimmune hydrops fetalis. *(From Staretz-Chacham O, Lang TC, LaMarca ME, et al: Lysosomal storage disorders in the newborn,* Pediatrics *123:1191–1207, 2009.)*

subtypes, delineated by the absence or presence and progression of neurologic manifestations: **type 1**, or the adult, nonneuronopathic form; **type 2**, the infantile or acute neuronopathic form; and **type 3**, the juvenile or subacute neuronopathic form. All are autosomal recessive traits. Type 1, which accounts for 99% of cases, has a striking predilection for Ashkenazi Jews, with an incidence of approximately 1 in 1,000 live births and a carrier frequency of approximately 1 in 18 adults.

Gaucher disease results from the deficient activity of the lysosomal hydrolase, acid β-glucosidase, which is encoded by a gene located on chromosome 1q21-q31. The enzymatic defect results in the accumulation of undegraded glycolipid substrates, particularly glucosylceramide, in cells of the reticuloendothelial system (RES). This progressive deposition results in infiltration of the bone marrow, progressive hepatosplenomegaly, and skeletal complications. Four mutations—N370S, L444P, 84insG, and IVS2+2—account for approximately 95% of mutant alleles among Ashkenazi Jewish patients, permitting screening for this disorder in this population. Genotype-phenotype correlations have been noted, providing the molecular basis for the clinical heterogeneity seen in Gaucher disease type 1. Patients who are homozygous for the N370S mutation tend to have a later onset of clinical manifestations, with a more indolent course than patients with 1 copy of N370S and another common allele.

Clinical manifestations of **type 1 Gaucher disease** have a variable age at onset, from early childhood to late adulthood, with most symptomatic patients presenting by adolescence. At presentation, patients may have bruising from thrombocytopenia, chronic fatigue secondary to anemia, hepatomegaly with or without elevated LFT results,

splenomegaly, and bone pain. Occasional patients have pulmonary involvement at presentation. Patients presenting in the 1st decade frequently are not Jewish and have growth retardation and a more malignant course. Other patients may be discovered fortuitously during evaluation for other conditions or as part of routine examinations; these patients may have a milder or even a benign course. In symptomatic patients, splenomegaly is progressive and can become massive. Most patients develop radiologic evidence of skeletal involvement, including an Erlenmeyer flask deformity of the distal femur. Clinically apparent bony involvement, which occurs in most patients, can present as bone pain, a pseudoosteomyelitis pattern, or pathologic fractures. Lytic lesions can develop in the long bones, including the femur, ribs, and pelvis; osteosclerosis may be evident at an early age. Bone crises with severe pain and swelling can occur. Bleeding secondary to thrombocytopenia may manifest as epistaxis or bruising and is frequently overlooked until other symptoms become apparent. With the exception of the severely growth-retarded child, who may experience developmental delay secondary to the effects of chronic disease, development and intelligence are normal.

The pathologic hallmark of Gaucher disease is the Gaucher cell in the RES, particularly in the bone marrow (Fig. 104.18). These cells, which are 20-100 μm in diameter, have a characteristic wrinkled-paper appearance resulting from the presence of intracytoplasmic substrate inclusions. The cytoplasm of the Gaucher cell reacts strongly positive with the periodic acid–Schiff (PAS) stain. The presence of this cell in bone marrow and tissue specimens is highly suggestive of Gaucher disease, although it also may be found in patients with granulocytic

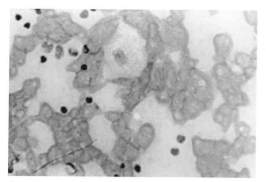

Fig. 104.18 Cells from the spleen of a patient with Gaucher disease. A characteristic spleen cell is shown engorged with glucocerebroside.

leukemia and myeloma.

Gaucher disease type 2 is a rare form and does not have an ethnic predilection. It is characterized by a rapid neurodegenerative course with extensive visceral involvement and death early in life. It presents in infancy with increased tone, strabismus, and organomegaly. Failure to thrive and stridor caused by laryngospasm are typical. After a several-year period of psychomotor regression, death typically occurs secondary to respiratory compromise. **Gaucher disease type 3** presents with clinical manifestations that are intermediate to those seen in types 1 and 2, with presentation in childhood and death by age 10-15 yr. It has a predilection for the Swedish Norrbottnian population, in whom the incidence is approximately 1 in 50,000. Neurologic involvement is present. Type 3 disease is further classified as types 3a and 3b based on the extent of neurologic involvement and whether there is progressive myotonia and dementia (**type 3a**) or isolated supranuclear gaze palsy (**type 3b**).

Gaucher disease should be considered in the differential diagnosis of patients with unexplained organomegaly, who bruise easily, who have bone pain, or who have a combination of these conditions. Bone marrow examination usually reveals the presence of Gaucher cells. All suspected diagnoses should be confirmed by determination of the acid β-glucosidase activity in isolated leukocytes or cultured fibroblasts, as well as by identification of their specific acid β-glucosidase gene mutations. In Ashkenazi Jewish individuals the identification of carriers can be achieved best by molecular testing for the common Ashkenazi mutations. Testing should be offered to all family members, keeping in mind that heterogeneity, even among members of the same kindred, can be so great that nonsymptomatic affected individuals may be diagnosed. **Prenatal diagnosis** is available by determination of enzyme activity and/or the specific family mutations in chorionic villi or cultured amniotic fluid cells.

Treatment of patients with Gaucher disease type 1 includes enzyme replacement therapy (ERT). The efficacy of ERT with mannose-terminated recombinant human acid β-glucosidase (*imiglucerase* [Cerezyme, Genzyme]), *velaglucerase alfa* [VPRIV, Shire HGT]), or *taliglucerase alfa* (Uplyso, Protalix Biotherapeutics) is the standard of care for the treatment of patients with type 1 disease. Most symptoms (organomegaly, hematologic indices, bone pain) are reversed by ERT (60 IU/kg) administered by IV infusion every other week, and the bone involvement can be stabilized or improved. Although ERT does not alter the neurologic progression of patients with Gaucher disease types 2 and 3, it has been used in selected patients as a palliative measure, particularly in type 3 patients with severe visceral involvement. Alternative treatment with oral substrate reduction agents designed to decrease the synthesis of glucosylceramide by chemical inhibition of glucosylceramide synthase include *miglustat* (Zavesca, Actelion), although its efficacy on hematologic parameters is not as great as ERT. A 2nd, more effective substrate inhibitor, *eliglustat* (Cerdelga, Sanofi-Genzyme), has demonstrated significant efficacy versus placebo and is not inferior to imiglucerase

making this an alternative first-line oral treatment for patients with type 1 disease. A small number of patients have undergone bone marrow transplantation (BMT), which is curative but is associated with significant morbidity and mortality from the procedure, limiting the selection of appropriate candidates.

NIEMANN-PICK DISEASE

The original description of Niemann-Pick disease (NPD) was what is now known as **type A** NPD, a fatal disorder of infancy characterized by failure to thrive, hepatosplenomegaly, and a rapidly progressive neurodegenerative course that leads to death by 2-3 yr of age. **Type B** disease is a nonneuronopathic form observed in children and adults. **Type C** disease is a neuronopathic form that results from defective cholesterol transport. All subtypes are inherited as autosomal recessive traits and display variable clinical features (see Table 104.15).

NPD types A and B result from the deficient activity of **acid sphingomyelinase (ASM)**, a lysosomal enzyme encoded by a gene on chromosome 11 (11p15.1-p15.4). The enzymatic defect results in the pathologic accumulation of *sphingomyelin,* a ceramide phospholipid, and other lipids in the monocyte-macrophage system, the primary pathologic site. The progressive deposition of sphingomyelin in the CNS results in the neurodegenerative course seen in type A and in nonneural tissue in the systemic disease manifestations of type B, including progressive lung disease in some patients. A variety of mutations in the acid sphingomyelinase gene that cause types A and B NPD have been identified.

The **clinical manifestations** and course of type A NPD are uniform and characterized by a normal appearance at birth followed by hepatosplenomegaly, moderate lymphadenopathy, and psychomotor retardation evident by 6 mo of age. Over time, the loss of motor function and the deterioration of intellectual capabilities are progressively debilitating; spasticity and rigidity develop; and death occurs by 3 yr of age. In contrast to the stereotyped type A phenotype, the clinical presentation and course of patients with type B disease are more variable. Most are diagnosed in infancy or childhood when enlargement of the liver or spleen, or both, is detected during a routine physical examination. At diagnosis, type B NPD patients usually have evidence of mild pulmonary involvement, usually detected as a diffuse reticular or finely nodular infiltration on the chest radiograph. Pulmonary symptoms may present in adults. In most patients, hepatosplenomegaly is particularly prominent in childhood, but with increasing linear growth, the abdominal protuberance decreases and becomes less conspicuous. In mildly affected patients the splenomegaly may not be noted until adulthood, and disease manifestations may be minimal.

Severely affected patients may have liver involvement leading to life-threatening cirrhosis, portal hypertension, and ascites. Clinically significant pancytopenia caused by secondary hypersplenism may require partial or complete splenectomy; this should be avoided if possible because splenectomy frequently causes progression of pulmonary disease, which can be life threatening. In general, type B patients do not have neurologic involvement and have a normal IQ. Some patients with type B disease have cherry-red maculae or haloes and subtle neurologic symptoms (peripheral neuropathy). In some type B patients, decreased pulmonary diffusion caused by alveolar infiltration becomes evident in late childhood or early adulthood and progresses with age. Severely affected individuals may experience significant pulmonary compromise by 15-20 yr of age. Such patients have low oxygen tension (PO_2) values and dyspnea on exertion. Life-threatening bronchopneumonia may occur, and cor pulmonale has been described.

Type C NPD patients often present with prolonged neonatal jaundice, appear normal for 1-2 yr, and then experience a slowly progressive and variable neurodegenerative course. Their hepatosplenomegaly is less severe than that of patients with types A or B NPD, and they may survive into adulthood. The underlying biochemical defect in type C patients is an abnormality in cholesterol transport, leading to the accumulation of sphingomyelin and cholesterol in their lysosomes and a secondary partial reduction in ASM activity (see Chapter 104.3).

In type B NPD patients, splenomegaly is usually the first manifestation detected. The splenic enlargement is noted in early childhood; in very mild disease the enlargement may be subtle and detection delayed until adolescence or adulthood. The presence of the characteristic NPD cells in bone marrow aspirates supports the diagnosis of type B NPD. Patients with type C NPD, however, also have extensive infiltration of NPD cells in the bone marrow, and thus all suspected cases should be evaluated enzymatically to confirm the clinical diagnosis by measuring the ASM activity level in peripheral leukocytes. Patients with types A and B NPD have greatly decreased ASM levels (1–10%), whereas patients with type C NPD have normal or somewhat decreased ASM activities. The enzymatic identification of NPD carriers is problematic. For families in whom the specific molecular lesion has been identified, however, family members can be accurately tested for heterozygote status by DNA analysis. **Prenatal diagnosis** of types A and B NPD can be made reliably by the measurement of ASM activity in cultured amniocytes or chorionic villi; molecular analysis of fetal cells to identify the specific *ASM* mutations can provide the specific diagnosis or serve as a confirmatory test. The clinical diagnosis of type C NPD can be supported by filipin stain positivity in cultured fibroblasts and identification of a specific mutation in the *NPC1* or *NPC2* gene.

There is no specific treatment for NPD. Orthotopic liver transplantation in an infant with type A disease and cord blood transplantation in several type B NPD patients have been attempted with little or no success. BMT in a small number of type B NPD patients has been successful in reducing the spleen and liver volumes, the sphingomyelin content of the liver, the number of Niemann-Pick cells in the marrow, and radiologically detected infiltration of the lungs. In one patient, liver biopsies taken up to 33 mo after transplant showed only a moderate reduction in stored sphingomyelin. ERT with recombinant human ASM is currently in clinical trials for the treatment of type B patients. A 26-wk phase 1b study in adult patients with NPD type B established initial proof of concept in this patient group, and a phase 1/2 clinical trial in pediatric patients and a phase 2/3 trial in adult patients with ASM deficiency are ongoing. Clinical trials of miglustat have been performed, and the drug has been approved in Europe for the treatment of type C disease. Treatment of type A disease by BMT has not been successful, presumably because of the severe neurologic involvement.

FABRY DISEASE

Fabry disease is an X-linked inborn error of glycosphingolipid metabolism caused by the absent or extremely deficient activity of α-galactosidase A (α-gal A). There are 2 major phenotypes. Affected males with the **classic** phenotype present in childhood with angiokeratomas (telangiectatic skin lesions), hypohidrosis, corneal and lenticular opacities, and painful acroparesthesias. With advancing age, they develop kidney failure, heart disease, and stroke (see Table 104.15). This classic phenotype is caused by the absent activity of the α-gal A and has an estimated

prevalence of approximately 1 in 40,000 males. The **later-onset** phenotype occurs in affected males with residual α-gal A activity and presents in the 4th to 8th decades with cardiac disease and renal failure. This phenotype is more prevalent than the classic phenotype. Heterozygous females for the classic phenotype can be asymptomatic or as severely affected as the males, the variability a result of random X-chromosomal inactivation. The enzyme deficiency results from mutations in the α-gal A gene located on the long arm of the X chromosome (Xq22). The enzymatic defect leads to the systemic accumulation of neutral glycosphingolipids, primarily globotriaosylceramide, particularly in the plasma and lysosomes of vascular endothelial and smooth muscle cells, cardiac myocytes, and renal podocytes. The progressive vascular glycosphingolipid deposition in classically affected males results in small-vessel occlusion and ischemia, leading to the major disease manifestations. The complementary DNA (cDNA) and genomic sequences encoding α-gal A have been characterized, and >900 different mutations in the α-gal A gene are responsible for this lysosomal storage disease.

The **angiokeratomas** usually occur in childhood and may lead to early diagnosis (Fig. 104.19). They increase in size and number with age and range from barely visible to several millimeters in diameter. The lesions are punctate, dark red to blue-black, and flat or slightly raised. They do not blanch with pressure, and the larger ones may show a slight hyperkeratosis. Characteristically, the lesions are densest between the umbilicus and knees, in the "bathing trunk area," but may occur anywhere, including the oral mucosa. The hips, thighs, buttocks, umbilicus, lower abdomen, scrotum, and glans penis are common sites, and there is a tendency toward symmetry. Variants without skin lesions have been described. Sweating is usually decreased or absent. Corneal opacities and characteristic lenticular lesions, observed under slit-lamp examination, are present in affected males, as well as in approximately 90% of heterozygotes from families with the classic phenotype. Conjunctival and retinal vascular tortuosity is common and results from the systemic vascular involvement.

Pain is the most debilitating symptom in childhood and adolescence. **Fabry crises,** lasting from hours to several days, consist of agonizing, burning pain in the hands, feet, and proximal extremities and are usually associated with exercise, fatigue, fever, or a combination of these factors. These painful acroparesthesias usually become less frequent in the 3rd and 4th decades, although in some men these may become more frequent and severe. Attacks of abdominal or flank pain may simulate appendicitis or renal colic. Pain may suggest other diagnoses (Table 104.17).

The major morbid symptoms in classically affected males result from the progressive involvement of the vascular system. Early in the course of the classic phenotype, casts, RBCs, and lipid inclusions with characteristic birefringent "Maltese crosses" appear in the urinary sediment. Proteinuria, isosthenuria, and gradual deterioration of renal function and development of azotemia occur in the 2nd to 4th decades in the classic phenotype and in the 4th to 8th decades in the later-onset

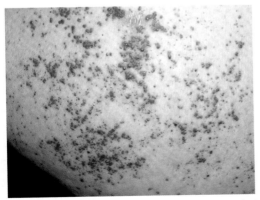

Fig. 104.19 Typical angiokeratomas. Angiokeratomas are quite large and easily recognizable, but if only a few lesions exist or they are restricted only to the genitalia or umbilical regions, they can be easily missed. *(From Zarate VA, Hopkin RJ: Fabry's disease,* Lancet *372:1427, 2008.)*

Table 104.17	Common Misdiagnoses for Fabry Disease	
Growing pains	Polyphyria	Erythromelalgia
Chronic overlapping pain syndrome	Guillain-Barre syndrome	Meniere disease
Irritable bowel syndrome	Hereditary neuropathy	Coronary heart disease
Malingering	Uremic neuropathy	Complex regional pain syndromes
Systemic lupus erythematous	Diabetic neuropathy	Multiple sclerosis
Rheumatic fever	Polyneuropathy	Osler disease
Fibromyalgia	C1 esterase deficiency	Appendicitis
Dermatomyositis	TNF receptor-associated periodic syndrome (TRAPS)	Metabolic bone disease (rickets, uremia, scurvy)
Raynaud phenomenon	Joint and recurrent fever syndromes (juvenile idiopathic arthritis, familial Mediterranean fever)	
Raynaud syndrome		

Adapted from Sivley MD: Fabry disease: a review of ophthalmic and systemic manifestations. Optometry Vision Sci 90(2)e63-e78, 2013 (Table 2, p e71).

form. Cardiovascular findings may include arrhythmias, hypertrophic cardiomyopathy, and heart failure. Mitral insufficiency is the most common valvular lesion. Cerebrovascular manifestations, including transient ischemic attack (TIA) and stroke (CVA), result secondary to cardiac arrhythmias as well as multifocal small-vessel involvement, other features may include chronic bronchitis and dyspnea, lymphedema of the legs without hypoproteinemia, episodic diarrhea, osteoporosis, impaired growth, and delayed puberty. Death most often results from renal failure, cardiac disease, or stroke. Before hemodialysis or renal transplantation, the mean age at death for affected men was about 40 yr. Patients with the later-onset phenotype with residual α-gal A activity have cardiac and/or renal disease. The cardiac manifestations include hypertrophy of the left ventricular wall and interventricular septum, and electrocardiographic abnormalities consistent with cardiomyopathy. Hypertrophic cardiomyopathy may lead to ventricular tachycardia as a cause of death.

The **diagnosis** of Fabry disease in classically affected males is most readily made from the history of painful acroparesthesias, hypohidrosis, the presence of the characteristic skin lesions, and the observation of the corneal opacities and lenticular lesions. The disorder is often misdiagnosed as rheumatic fever, erythromelalgia, or neurosis. The skin lesions must be differentiated from the benign angiokeratomas of the scrotum (**Fordyce disease**) or from angiokeratoma circumscriptum. Angiokeratomas identical to those of Fabry disease have been reported in fucosidosis, aspartylglycosaminuria, late-onset GM$_1$ gangliosidosis, galactosialidosis, α-N-acetylgalactosaminidase deficiency, and sialidosis. Later-onset patients have been identified among patients on hemodialysis and patients with hypertrophic cardiomyopathy or who had cryptogenic strokes. Later-onset patients lack the early classic manifestations previously described. The diagnosis of classic and later-onset Fabry disease is confirmed biochemically by the demonstration of greatly decreased α-gal A activity in plasma, isolated leukocytes, or cultured fibroblasts or lymphoblasts. The specific α-gal A mutation can be determined by gene sequencing.

Heterozygous females from classic families may have corneal opacities, isolated skin lesions, and intermediate activities of α-gal A in plasma or cells. Rare female heterozygotes may have manifestations as severe as those in affected males. Asymptomatic at-risk females in classic and later-onset families affected by Fabry disease, however, should be optimally diagnosed by the direct analysis of their family's specific mutation. Prenatal detection of affected males can be accomplished by demonstrating deficient α-gal A activity and the family's specific gene mutation in chorionic villi obtained in the 1st trimester or in cultured amniocytes obtained by amniocentesis in the 2nd trimester of pregnancy. Fabry disease can be detected by newborn screening, and pilot studies have been conducted in Europe, Asia, and North America.

Treatment for Fabry disease may include the use of phenytoin and carbamazepine to decrease the frequency and severity of the chronic acroparesthesias and the periodic crises of excruciating pain. Renal transplantation and long-term hemodialysis are lifesaving procedures for patients with renal failure.

Enzyme replacement therapy (ERT) for Fabry patients using recombinant human α-gal A preparations produced in Chinese hamster ovary cells (*agalsidase beta*, Fabrazyme, Genzyme) and in human fibrosarcoma cells (*agalsidase alfa*, Replagal, Shire HGT) is available. Both Fabrazyme and Replagal were approved by the European Medicines Agency in the European Union, but only Fabrazyme is approved by the U.S. FDA. The effectiveness of ERT with Fabrazyme has been demonstrated in stabilization of renal disease, regression of hypertrophic cardiomyopathy, reduction of pain, and improvement in quality of life. Because most classically affected males produce no enzyme protein, these patients can produce immunoglobulin G (IgG) antibodies in response to the infused enzyme, which does not reduce the effectiveness of substrate clearance unless the antibody titer is very high. Treatment of classically affected males should begin in childhood.

FUCOSIDOSIS

Fucosidosis is a rare autosomal recessive disorder caused by the deficient activity of α-fucosidase and the accumulation of fucose-containing glycosphingolipids, glycoproteins, and oligosaccharides in the lysosomes of the liver, brain, and other organs (see Table 104.15). The α-fucosidase gene is on chromosome 1 (1p24), and specific mutations are known. Although the disorder is panethnic, most reported patients are from Italy and the United States. There is wide variability in the clinical phenotype, with the most severely affected patients presenting in the 1st yr of life with developmental delay and somatic features similar to those of the mucopolysaccharidoses. These features include frontal bossing, hepatosplenomegaly, coarse facial features, and macroglossia. The CNS storage results in a relentless neurodegenerative course, with death in childhood. Patients with milder disease have angiokeratomas and longer survival. *No specific therapy exists for fucosidosis.* The disorder can be diagnosed by the demonstration of deficient α-fucosidase activity in peripheral leukocytes or cultured fibroblasts. Carrier identification and prenatal diagnosis are possible by determination of the enzymatic activity or the specific family mutations.

SCHINDLER DISEASE

This autosomal recessive neurodegenerative disorder results from the deficient activity of α-N-acetylgalactosaminidase and the accumulation of asialoglycopeptides and sialyloligosaccharides (see Table 104.15). The gene for the enzyme is located on chromosome 22 (22q11). Schindler disease is clinically heterogeneous, and 2 major phenotypes have been identified. **Type I** disease is an infantile-onset neuroaxonal dystrophy. Affected infants have normal development for the 1st 9-15 mo of life followed by a rapid neurodegenerative course that results in severe psychomotor retardation, cortical blindness, and frequent myoclonic seizures. **Type II** disease is characterized by a variable age at onset, mild intellectual disability, and angiokeratomas. *There is no specific therapy* for either form of the disorder. The diagnosis is by demonstration of the enzymatic deficiency in leukocytes or cultured skin fibroblasts or specific gene mutations.

METACHROMATIC LEUKODYSTROPHY

This autosomal recessive white matter disease is caused by a deficiency of **arylsulfatase A (ASA)**, which is required for the hydrolysis of sulfated glycosphingolipids. Another form of metachromatic leukodystrophy (**MLD**) is caused by a deficiency of a sphingolipid activator protein (SAP1), which is required for the formation of the substrate-enzyme complex. The deficiency of this enzymatic activity results in the white matter storage of sulfated glycosphingolipids, which leads to demyelination and a neurodegenerative course. The *ASA* gene is on chromosome 22 (22q13.31qter); specific mutations tend to fall into 2 groups that correlate with disease severity.

The **clinical manifestations** of the **late-infantile** form of MLD, which is most common, usually present between 12 and 18 mo of age as irritability, inability to walk, and hyperextension of the knee, causing genu recurvatum. The clinical progression of the disease relates to the pathologic involvement of both central and peripheral nervous systems, giving a mixture of upper and lower motor neuron and cognitive and psychiatric signs. Deep tendon reflexes are diminished or absent. Gradual muscle wasting, weakness, and hypotonia become evident and lead to a debilitated state. As the disease progresses, nystagmus, myoclonic seizures, optic atrophy, and quadriparesis appear, with death in the 1st decade of life (see Table 104.15). The **juvenile** form of MLD has a more indolent course, with onset that may occur as late as 20 yr of age. This form of the disease presents with gait disturbances, mental deterioration, urinary incontinence, and emotional difficulties. The **adult** form, which presents after the 2nd decade, is similar to the juvenile form in its clinical manifestations, although emotional difficulties and psychosis are more prominent features. Dementia, seizures, diminished reflexes, and optic atrophy also occur in both juvenile and adult forms. The pathologic hallmark of MLD is the *deposition of metachromatic bodies*, which stain strongly positive with PAS and Alcian blue, in the white matter of the brain. Neuronal inclusions may be seen in the midbrain, pons, medulla, retina, and spinal cord; demyelination occurs in the peripheral nervous system. The **diagnosis** of MLD should be suspected in patients with the clinical features of leukodystrophy. Decreased nerve conduction velocities, increased cerebrospinal fluid protein, metachromatic deposits in sampled segments of sural nerve, and metachromatic granules in urinary sediment are all suggestive of MLD. Confirmation of the diagnosis is based on the demonstration of the reduced activity of ASA in leukocytes or cultured skin fibroblasts. SAP deficiency is diagnosed by measuring the concentration of SAP1 in cultured fibroblasts using a specific antibody to the protein. The diagnosis, identification of carriers, and prenatal diagnosis are available for both forms of MLD by detection of the causative mutations in the *ASA* or *SAP* genes.

Unrelated-donor umbilical cord blood transplantation has been undertaken in some pediatric patients with MLD. A longitudinal study of 6 patients with late-infantile onset and 14 with juvenile onset revealed that motor deficits present at the time of transplant did not improve, and that neurologic symptoms continued to progress in those with late-infantile presentation. In contrast, in juvenile patients the brainstem auditory evoked responses, visual evoked potentials, electroencephalogram, and/or peripheral nerve conduction velocities stabilized or improved. Therefore, consideration of umbilical cord blood transplantation for children with presymptomatic late-infantile MLD or minimally symptomatic juvenile MLD may be indicated. Clinical trials of a recombinant human arylsulfatase A (rhARSA) enzyme (Metazym, Shire HGT) demonstrated its safety in children with late-infantile MLD, but a lack of efficacy. A multicenter phase I/II clinical trial to evaluate the safety and efficacy of rhARSA administered intrathecally is ongoing.

MULTIPLE-SULFATASE DEFICIENCY
This autosomal recessive disorder results from the enzymatic deficiency of at least 9 sulfatases, including arylsulfatases A, B, and C and iduronate-2-sulfatase. The specific defect is an enzyme in the C-α-formylglycine–generating system (the gene for which is located at 3p26), which introduces a common posttranslational modification in all the affected sulfatases and explains the occurrence of these multiple enzyme defects. Because of the deficiency of these enzymes, sulfatides, mucopolysaccharides, steroid sulfates, and gangliosides accumulate in the cerebral cortex and visceral tissues, resulting in a clinical phenotype with features of a **leukodystrophy** as well as those of the **mucopolysaccharidoses**. Severe ichthyosis may also occur. Carrier testing and prenatal diagnosis can be done by measurement of the enzymatic activities or the specific gene defects. *There is no specific treatment for multiple sulfatase deficiency* other than supportive care.

KRABBE DISEASE
Also called *globoid cell leukodystrophy,* Krabbe disease is an autosomal recessive fatal disorder of infancy. It results from the deficient activity of **galactocerebrosidase** and the white matter accumulation of **galactosylceramide**, which is normally found almost exclusively in the myelin sheath. Both peripheral and central myelin is affected, resulting in spasticity and cognitive impairment coupled with deceptively normal or even absent deep tendon reflexes. The galactocerebrosidase gene is on chromosome 14 (14q31), and specific disease-causing mutations are known. The **infantile** form of Krabbe disease is rapidly progressive, and patients present in early infancy with irritability, seizures, and hypertonia (see Table 104.15). Optic atrophy is evident in the 1st yr of life, and mental development is severely impaired. As the disease progresses, optic atrophy and severe developmental delay become apparent; affected children exhibit opisthotonos and die before 3 yr of age. A **late-infantile** form of Krabbe presents after age 2 yr. Affected individuals have a course similar to that of the early-infantile form.

The **diagnosis** of Krabbe disease relies on the demonstration of the specific enzymatic deficiency in white blood cells or cultured skin fibroblasts. Causative gene mutations have been identified. Carrier identification and prenatal diagnosis are available. The development of methods to measure galactocerebrosidase activity on dried blood spots has led to the inclusion of Krabbe disease in the newborn screening programs of some states. **Treatment** of infants with Krabbe disease with umbilical cord blood transplantation has been reported in prenatally identified asymptomatic newborns and symptomatic infants. Transplanted infants appear to develop neurologic manifestations at a slower rate

but succumb to a neurologic demise.

FARBER DISEASE
This rare autosomal recessive disorder results from the deficiency of the lysosomal enzyme acid ceramidase and the accumulation of ceramide in various tissues, especially the joints. Symptoms can begin in the 1st yr of life with painful joint swelling and nodule formation (Fig. 104.20), which is sometimes diagnosed as **rheumatoid arthritis**. As the disease progresses, nodule or granulomatous formation on the vocal cords can lead to hoarseness and breathing difficulties; failure to thrive is common. In some patients, moderate CNS dysfunction is present (see Table 104.15). Patients may die of recurrent pneumonias in their teens. *There is currently no specific therapy.* The **diagnosis** of Farber disease should be suspected in patients who have nodule formation over the joints but no other findings of rheumatoid arthritis. In such patients, acid ceramidase activity should be determined in cultured skin fibroblasts or peripheral leukocytes. Various disease-causing mutations have been identified in the acid ceramidase gene. Carrier detection and prenatal diagnosis are available.

WOLMAN DISEASE AND CHOLESTEROL ESTER STORAGE DISEASE
These autosomal recessive lysosomal storage diseases result from deficiency of **lysosomal acid lipase (LAL)** and accumulation of cholesterol esters and triglycerides in histiocytic foam cells of most visceral organs. The *LAL* gene is on chromosome 10 (10q24-q25). **Wolman disease** is the more severe clinical phenotype and is a fatal disorder of infancy. Clinical features become apparent in the 1st weeks of life and include failure to thrive, relentless vomiting, abdominal distention, steatorrhea, and hepatosplenomegaly (see Table 104.15). There usually is hyperlipidemia. Hepatic dysfunction and fibrosis may occur. **Calcification of the adrenal glands** occurs in about 50% of patients. Death usually occurs within the 1st 6 mo of life.

Cholesterol ester storage disease is less severe than Wolman disease and may not be diagnosed until adulthood. Hepatomegaly can be the only detectable abnormality, but affected individuals are at significant risk for premature cirrhosis and atherosclerosis. Adrenal calcification can occur in patients with severe early onset.

Diagnosis and carrier identification are based on measuring LAL activity in peripheral leukocytes or cultured skin fibroblasts. Disease-causing mutations have been identified in the *LAL* gene. Prenatal diagnosis depends on measuring decreased enzyme levels or identifying

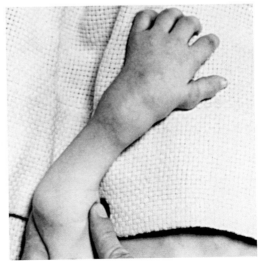

Fig. 104.20 Forearm of an 18 mo old girl with Farber disease. Note the painful joint swelling and the nodule formation. The infant was suspected of having rheumatoid arthritis.

specific mutations in cultured chorionic villi or amniocytes. Pharmacologic agents to suppress cholesterol synthesis, in combination with cholestyramine and diet modification, have been used in patients, but with little to no clinical benefit. *Sebelipase alfa* (Kanuma, Alexion) is a recombinant form of LAL approved by the FDA in 2015. In a clinical study, 67% of infants with LAL deficiency survived beyond 12 mo of age, compared with 0% of untreated infants in a historical cohort, all of whom died by 8 mo. In a study of 66 pediatric and adult patients with cholesteryl ester storage disease, those treated with Kanuma had demonstrated significant reductions in serum alanine transaminase (ALT) levels and liver fat and improvements in LDL-C, triglycerides, and HDL-C, compared to placebo-treated patients (see Chapter 104.3).

Bibliography is available at Expert Consult.

104.5 Mucolipidoses
Margaret M. McGovern and Robert J. Desnick

I-cell disease (mucolipidosis II [ML-II]) and **pseudo-Hurler polydystrophy (mucolipidosis III [ML-III])** are rare autosomal recessive disorders that share some clinical features with Hurler syndrome (see Chapter 107). These diseases result from the abnormal targeting of newly synthesized lysosomal enzymes that normally have phosphorylated mannose residues for binding to the mannose-6-phosphate receptors that transport the enzymes to the lysosomes. These mannose-6-phosphate residues are synthesized in a 2-step reaction that occurs in the Golgi apparatus and is mediated by 2 enzymatic activities. The enzyme that catalyzes the first step, the lysosomal enzyme *N*-acetylglucosamine-1-phosphotransferase, is defective in both ML-II and ML-III, which are allelic disorders resulting from mutations in the GlcNAc-phosphotransferase α/β-subunits precursor gene (*GNPTAB*). This enzyme deficiency results in abnormal targeting of the lysosomal enzymes, which are consequently secreted into the extracellular matrix. Because the lysosomal enzymes require the acidic environment of the lysosome to function, patients with this defect accumulate a variety of different substrates because of the intracellular deficiency of most lysosomal enzymes. The **diagnosis** of ML-II and ML-III can be made by the determination of the serum lysosomal enzymatic activities, which are markedly elevated, or by the demonstration of their reduced enzymatic activity levels in cultured skin fibroblasts. Direct measurement of the phosphotransferase activity is possible as well. **Prenatal diagnosis** is available for both disorders by measurement of lysosomal enzymatic activities in amniocytes or chorionic villus cells. Carrier identification is available for both disorders by measurement of enzymatic activities using cultured skin fibroblasts or by mutation analysis of the causative gene. Neonatal screening by tandem mass spectroscopy may detect I-cell disease.

I-CELL DISEASE
I-cell disease, or ML-II, shares many of the clinical manifestations of Hurler syndrome (see Chapter 107), although there is no mucopolysacchariduria, and the presentation is earlier (see Table 104.15). Some patients have clinical features evident at birth, including coarse facial features, craniofacial abnormalities, restricted joint movement, and hypotonia. Nonimmune hydrops may be present in the fetus. The remainder of patients present in the 1st yr with severe psychomotor retardation, coarse facial features, and skeletal manifestations that include kyphoscoliosis and a lumbar gibbus. Patients may also have congenital dislocation of the hips, inguinal hernias, and gingival hypertrophy. Progressive, severe psychomotor impairment leads to death in early childhood. *No treatment is available for I-cell disease.*

PSEUDO-HURLER POLYDYSTROPHY
Pseudo-Hurler polydystrophy, or ML-III, is a less severe disorder than I-cell disease, with later onset and survival to adulthood reported. Affected children may present around age 4 or 5 yr with joint stiffness and short stature. Progressive destruction of the hip joints and moderate dysostosis multiplex are evident. Radiographic evidence of low iliac wings, flattening of the proximal femoral epiphyses with valgus deformity of the femoral head, and hypoplasia of the anterior third of the lumbar vertebrae are characteristic findings. Ophthalmic findings include corneal clouding, retinopathy, and astigmatism; visual complaints are uncommon (see Table 104.15). Some patients have learning disabilities or intellectual disability. **Treatment**, which should include orthopedic care, is symptomatic.

Bibliography is available at Expert Consult.

Chapter **105**
Defects in Metabolism of Carbohydrates
Priya S. Kishnani and Yuan-Tsong Chen
第一百零五章
碳水化合物代谢病

中文导读

本章详细阐述了糖原累积症，包括肝脏糖原生　　成和肌肉糖原生成障碍；半乳糖代谢障碍，包括半乳糖–1–磷酸尿苷酰转移酶缺乏性半乳糖血症、半乳糖激酶缺乏症及尿苷二磷酸–半乳糖–4–差向异构酶缺乏症；果糖代谢障碍，包括果糖激酶缺乏症（特发性或良性果糖尿）及果糖1,6–二磷酸醛缩酶缺乏症；戊糖代谢障碍，包括特发性戊糖尿症、一过性醛酸转移酶缺乏症及5–磷酸核糖异构酶缺乏症；先天性糖基化障碍，包括先天性蛋白N–糖基化障碍、先天性蛋白O–糖基化障碍、脂质糖基化及糖基磷脂酰肌醇锚蛋白生物合成障碍、多种糖基化路径障碍及磷酸多萜醇生物合成等其他路径障碍、先天性去糖基化障碍。

Carbohydrate synthesis and degradation provide the energy required for most metabolic processes. The important carbohydrates include 3 monosaccharides—glucose, galactose, and fructose—and a polysaccharide, glycogen. Fig. 105.1 shows the relevant biochemical pathways of these carbohydrates. **Glucose** is the principal substrate of energy metabolism, continuously available through dietary intake, gluconeogenesis (glucose made de novo from amino acids, primarily alanine), and glycogenolysis (breakdown of glycogen). Metabolism of glucose generates adenosine triphosphate (ATP) via glycolysis (conversion of glucose or glycogen to pyruvate), mitochondrial oxidative phosphorylation (conversion of pyruvate to carbon dioxide and water), or both. Dietary sources of glucose come from polysaccharides, primarily starch, and the disaccharides lactose, maltose, and sucrose. However, oral intake of glucose is intermittent and unreliable. Gluconeogenesis contributes to maintaining euglycemia (normal levels of glucose in the blood), but this process requires time. Hepatic glycogenolysis provides the rapid release of glucose, and is the most significant factor in maintaining euglycemia. **Glycogen** is also the primary stored energy source in muscle, providing glucose for muscle activity during exercise. Galactose and fructose are monosaccharides that provide fuel for cellular metabolism, though their role is less significant than that of glucose. **Galactose** is derived from lactose (galactose + glucose), which is found in milk and milk products. Galactose is an important energy source in infants, but it is first metabolized to glucose. Galactose (exogenous or endogenously synthesized from glucose) is also an important component of certain glycolipids, glycoproteins, and glycosaminoglycans. The dietary sources of **fructose** are sucrose (fructose + glucose, sorbitol) and fructose itself, which is found in fruits, vegetables, and honey.

Defects in glycogen metabolism typically cause an accumulation of glycogen in the tissues, thus the name **glycogen storage disease** (Table 105.1). Defects in gluconeogenesis or the glycolytic pathway, including galactose and fructose metabolism, do not result in an accumulation of glycogen (Table 105.1). The defects in pyruvate metabolism in the pathway of the conversion of pyruvate to carbon dioxide and water via mitochondrial oxidative phosphorylation are more often associated with **lactic acidosis** and some tissue glycogen accumulation.

105.1 Glycogen Storage Diseases

Priya S. Kishnani and Yuan-Tsong Chen

The disorders of glycogen metabolism, the glycogen storage diseases (**GSDs**), result from deficiencies of various enzymes or transport proteins in the pathways of glycogen metabolism (see Fig. 105.1). Glycogen found in these disorders is abnormal in quantity, quality, or both. GSDs are categorized by numerical type in accordance with the chronological order in which these enzymatic defects were identified. This numerical classification is still widely used, at least up to number VII. The GSDs can also be classified by organ involvement into liver and muscle glycogenoses (see Table 105.1).

There are more than 12 forms of GSDs. Glucose-6-phosphatase deficiency (type I), lysosomal acid α-glucosidase deficiency (type II), debrancher deficiency (type III), and liver phosphorylase kinase deficiency

(type IX) are the most common of those that typically present in early childhood; myophosphorylase deficiency (type V, McArdle disease) is the most common in adolescents and adults. The cumulative frequency of all forms of GSD is approximately 1 in 20,000 live births.

LIVER GLYCOGENOSES

The GSDs that principally affect the liver include glucose-6-phosphatase deficiency (**type I**), debranching enzyme deficiency (**type III**), branching enzyme deficiency (**type IV**), liver phosphorylase deficiency (**type VI**), phosphorylase kinase deficiency (**type IX**, formerly GSD VIa), glycogen synthase deficiency (**type 0**), and glucose transporter-2 defect. Because hepatic carbohydrate metabolism is responsible for plasma glucose homeostasis, this group of disorders typically causes fasting hypoglycemia and hepatomegaly. Some (types III, IV, IX) can be associated with liver cirrhosis. Other organs can also be involved and may manifest as renal dysfunction in type I, myopathy (skeletal and/or cardiomyopathy) in types III and IV, as well as in some rare forms of phosphorylase kinase deficiency, and neurologic involvement in types III (peripheral nerves) and IV (diffuse central and peripheral nervous system dysfunction).

Type I Glycogen Storage Disease (Glucose-6-Phosphatase or Translocase Deficiency, Von Gierke Disease)

Type I GSD is caused by the absence or deficiency of **glucose-6-phosphatase** activity in the liver, kidney, and intestinal mucosa. It has 2 subtypes: **type Ia**, in which the defective enzyme is glucose-6-phosphatase, and **type Ib**, in which the defective enzyme is a **translocase** that transports glucose-6-phosphate across the microsomal membrane. Deficiency of the enzymes in both type Ia and type Ib lead to inadequate hepatic conversion of glucose-6-phosphate to glucose through normal glycogenolysis and gluconeogenesis, resulting in fasting hypoglycemia.

Type I GSD is an autosomal recessive disorder. The gene for glucose-6-phosphatase (*G6PC*) is located on chromosome 17q21; the gene for translocase (*SLC37A4*) is on chromosome 11q23. Common pathogenic variants have been identified. Carrier detection and prenatal diagnosis are possible with DNA-based methodologies.

Clinical Manifestations

Patients with type I GSD may present in the neonatal period with hypoglycemia and lactic acidosis but more often present at 3-4 mo of age with hepatomegaly, hypoglycemic seizures, or both. Affected children often have a **doll-like face** with fat cheeks, relatively thin extremities, short stature, and a protuberant abdomen that is a consequence of massive hepatomegaly. The kidneys are also enlarged, whereas the spleen and heart are not involved.

The biochemical characteristics of type I GSD are *hypoglycemia, lactic acidosis, hyperuricemia,* and *hyperlipidemia.* Hypoglycemia and lactic acidosis can develop after a short fast. Hyperuricemia is present in young children; it rarely progresses to symptomatic gout before puberty. Despite marked hepatomegaly, the liver transaminase levels are usually normal or only slightly elevated. Intermittent diarrhea may occur in GSD I. In patients with GSD Ib, the loss of mucosal barrier function as a result of inflammation, which is likely related

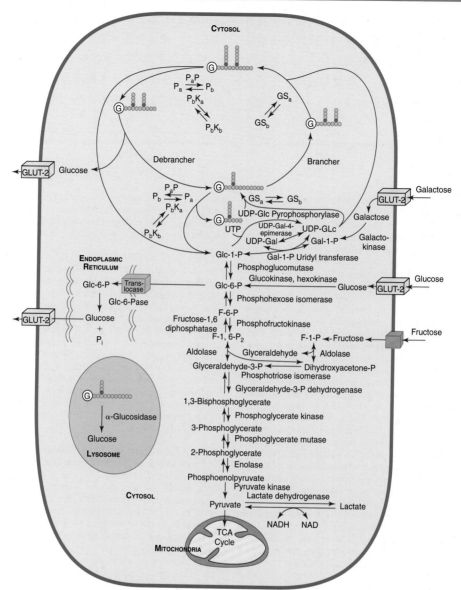

Fig. 105.1 Pathway related to glycogen storage diseases and galactose and fructose disorders. G, Glycogen, the primer for glycogen synthesis; GLUT-2, glucose transporter 2; GSa, active glycogen synthase; GSb, inactive glycogen synthase; NAD/NADH, nicotinamide adenine dinucleotide; Pa, active phosphorylase; PaP, phosphorylase a phosphatase; Pb, inactive phosphorylase; PbKa, active phosphorylase b kinase; PbKb, inactive phosphorylase b kinase; UDP, uridine diphosphate. *(Adapted from Beaudet AR: Glycogen storage disease. In Harrison TR, Isselbacher KJ, editors: Harrison's principles of internal medicine, ed 13, New York, 1994, McGraw-Hill. Reproduced with permission of The McGraw-Hill Companies.)*

to the disturbed neutrophil function, seems to be the main cause of diarrhea. Easy bruising and epistaxis are common and are associated with a **prolonged bleeding time** as a result of impaired platelet aggregation and adhesion.

The plasma may be "milky" in appearance due to strikingly elevated triglyceride levels. Cholesterol and phospholipids are also elevated, but less prominently. The lipid abnormality resembles type IV hyperlipidemia and is characterized by increased levels of very-low-density lipoprotein, low-density lipoprotein, and a unique apolipoprotein profile consisting of increased levels of apolipoproteins B, C, and E, with relatively normal or reduced levels of apolipoproteins A and D. The histologic appearance of the liver is characterized by a universal distention of hepatocytes by glycogen and fat. The lipid vacuoles are particularly large and prominent. There is no associated liver fibrosis.

Although type I GSD affects mainly the liver, multiple organ systems are involved. **Delayed puberty** is often seen. Females can have ultrasound findings consistent with **polycystic ovaries** even though other features of polycystic ovary syndrome (acne, hirsutism) are not seen. Nonetheless, fertility appears to be normal, as evidenced in several reports of successful pregnancy in women with GSD I. Increased bleeding during menstrual cycles, including life-threatening menorrhagia, has been reported and could be related to the impaired platelet aggregation. Symptoms of gout usually start around puberty from long-term hyperuricemia. There is an increased risk of **pancreatitis,** secondary to the lipid abnormalities. The dyslipidemia, together with elevated erythrocyte aggregation, could predispose these patients to atherosclerosis, but premature atherosclerosis has not yet been clearly documented except for rare cases. Impaired platelet aggregation and increased antioxidative defense to prevent lipid

Table 105.1	Features of the Disorders of Carbohydrate Metabolism		
DISORDERS	**BASIC DEFECTS**	**CLINICAL PRESENTATION**	**COMMENTS**
LIVER GLYCOGENOSES *Type/Common Name*			
Ia/Von Gierke	Glucose-6-phosphatase	Growth retardation, hepatomegaly, hypoglycemia; elevated blood lactate, cholesterol, triglyceride, and uric acid levels	Common, severe hypoglycemia Adulthood: hepatic adenomas and carcinoma, osteoporosis, pulmonary hypertension, and renal failure
Ib	Glucose-6-phosphate translocase	Same as type Ia, with additional findings of neutropenia, periodontal disease, inflammatory bowel disease	10% of type Ia
IIIa/Cori or Forbes	Liver and muscle debrancher deficiency (amylo-1,6-glucosidase)	Childhood: hepatomegaly, growth retardation, muscle weakness, hypoglycemia, hyperlipidemia, elevated transaminase levels Adult form: muscle atrophy and weakness, peripheral neuropathy, liver cirrhosis and failure, risk for hepatocellular carcinoma	Common, intermediate severity of hypoglycemia Muscle weakness may progress to need for ambulation assistance such as wheelchair.
IIIb	Liver debrancher deficiency; normal muscle enzyme activity	Liver symptoms same as in type IIIa; no muscle symptoms	15% of type III
IV/Andersen	Branching enzyme	Childhood: failure to thrive, hypotonia, hepatomegaly, splenomegaly, progressive cirrhosis (death usually before 5th yr), elevated transaminase levels; a subset does not have progression of liver disease Adult form: isolated myopathy, central and peripheral nervous system involvement	Rare neuromuscular variants exist
VI/Hers	Liver phosphorylase	Hepatomegaly, typically mild hypoglycemia, hyperlipidemia, and ketosis	Often underdiagnosed, severe presentation also known
IX/phosphorylase kinase (PhK) deficiency			Common, X-linked, typically less severe than autosomal forms; clinical variability within and between subtypes; severe cases being recognized across different subtypes
IX (*PHKA2* variant)	Liver PhK	Hypoglycemia, hyperketosis hepatomegaly, chronic liver disease, hyperlipidemia, elevated liver enzymes, growth retardation	X-linked
IX (*PHKB* variant)	Liver and muscle PhK	Hepatomegaly, growth retardation	Autosomal recessive
IX (*PHKG2* variant)	Liver PhK	More severe than IXa; marked hepatomegaly, recurrent hypoglycemia, liver cirrhosis	Autosomal recessive
Glycogen synthase deficiency	Glycogen synthase	Early morning drowsiness and fatigue, fasting hypoglycemia, and ketosis, no hepatomegaly	Decreased liver glycogen store
XI/Fanconi-Bickel syndrome	Glucose transporter 2 (GLUT-2)	Failure to thrive, rickets, hepatorenomegaly, proximal renal tubular dysfunction, impaired glucose and galactose utilization	GLUT-2 expressed in liver, kidney, pancreas, and intestine
MUSCLE GLYCOGENOSES *Type/Common Name*			
IX (*PHKA1* variant)	Muscle PhK	Exercise intolerance, cramps, myalgia, myoglobinuria; no hepatomegaly	X-linked or autosomal recessive
II/Pompe infantile	Acid α-glucosidase (acid maltase)	Cardiomegaly, hypotonia, hepatomegaly; onset: birth to 6 mo	Common, cardiorespiratory failure leading to death by age 1-2 yr; minimal to no residual enzyme activity
II/Late-onset Pompe (juvenile and adult)	Acid α-glucosidase (acid maltase)	Myopathy, variable cardiomyopathy, respiratory insufficiency; onset: childhood to adulthood	Residual enzyme activity
Danon disease	Lysosome-associated membrane protein 2 (LAMP2)	Hypertrophic cardiomyopathy, heart failure	Rare, X-linked
PRKAG2 deficiency	Adenosine monophosphate (AMP)–activated protein kinase γ	Hypertrophic cardiomyopathy. Congenital fetal form is rapidly fatal; myopathy, myalgia, seizures	Autosomal dominant
V/McArdle	Myophosphorylase	Exercise intolerance, muscle cramps, myoglobinuria, "second wind" phenomenon	Common, male predominance

Continued

Table 105.1	Features of the Disorders of Carbohydrate Metabolism—cont'd		
DISORDERS	**BASIC DEFECTS**	**CLINICAL PRESENTATION**	**COMMENTS**
VII/Tarui	Phosphofructokinase	Exercise intolerance, muscle cramps, compensatory hemolytic anemia, myoglobinuria	Prevalent in Japanese and Ashkenazi Jews
Late-onset polyglucosan body myopathy	Glycogenin-1	Adult-onset proximal muscle weakness, nervous system involvement uncommon	Autosomal recessive, rare
Phosphoglycerate kinase deficiency	Phosphoglycerate kinase	As with type V	Rare, X-linked
Phosphoglycerate mutase deficiency	M subunit of phosphoglycerate mutase	As with type V	Rare, majority of patients are African American
Lactate dehydrogenase deficiency	M subunit of lactate dehydrogenase	As with type V	Rare
GALACTOSE DISORDERS			
Galactosemia with transferase deficiency	Galactose-1-phosphate uridyltransferase	Vomiting, hepatomegaly, cataracts, aminoaciduria, failure to thrive	Black patients tend to have milder symptoms
Galactokinase deficiency	Galactokinase	Cataracts	Benign
Generalized uridine diphosphate galactose-4-epimerase deficiency	Uridine diphosphate galactose-4-epimerase	Similar to transferase deficiency with additional findings of hypotonia and nerve deafness	A benign variant also exists
FRUCTOSE DISORDERS			
Essential fructosuria	Fructokinase	Urine reducing substance	Benign
Hereditary fructose intolerance	Fructose-1-phosphate aldolase	Acute: vomiting, sweating, lethargy Chronic: failure to thrive, hepatic failure	Prognosis good with fructose restriction
DISORDERS OF GLUCONEOGENESIS			
Fructose-1,6-diphosphatase deficiency	Fructose-1,6-diphosphatase	Episodic hypoglycemia, apnea, acidosis	Good prognosis, avoid fasting
Phosphoenolpyruvate carboxykinase deficiency	Phosphoenolpyruvate carboxykinase	Hypoglycemia, hepatomegaly, hypotonia, failure to thrive	Rare
DISORDERS OF PYRUVATE METABOLISM			
Pyruvate dehydrogenase complex defect	Pyruvate dehydrogenase	Severe fatal neonatal to mild late onset, lactic acidosis, psychomotor retardation, failure to thrive	Most commonly caused by $E_{1\alpha}$ subunit, defect X-linked
Pyruvate carboxylase deficiency	Pyruvate carboxylase	Same as above	Rare, autosomal recessive
Respiratory chain defects (oxidative phosphorylation disease)	Complexes I-V, many mitochondrial DNA mutations	Heterogeneous with multisystem involvement	Mitochondrial inheritance
DISORDERS IN PENTOSE METABOLISM			
Pentosuria	L-Xylulose reductase	Urine-reducing substance	Benign
Transaldolase deficiency	Transaldolase	Liver cirrhosis and failure, cardiomyopathy	Autosomal recessive
Ribose-5-phosphate isomerase deficiency	Ribose-5-phosphate isomerase	Progressive leukoencephalopathy and peripheral neuropathy	

peroxidation may function as a protective mechanism to help reduce the risk of atherosclerosis. Frequent fractures and radiographic evidence of **osteopenia** are common; bone mineral content is reduced, even in prepubertal patients.

By the 2nd or 3rd decade of life, some patients with type I GSD develop **hepatic adenomas** that can hemorrhage and turn malignant in some cases. **Pulmonary hypertension** has been seen in some long-term survivors of the disease. Iron-refractory anemia and an increased prevalence of thyroid autoimmunity are also being recognized.

Renal disease is another late complication, and most patients with type I GSD >20 yr of age have proteinuria. Many also have hypertension, renal stones, nephrocalcinosis, and altered creatinine clearance. Glomerular hyperfiltration, increased renal plasma flow, and microalbuminuria are often found in the early stages of renal dysfunction and can occur before the onset of proteinuria. In younger patients, hyperfiltration and hyperperfusion may be the only signs of renal abnormalities. With the advancement of renal disease, focal segmental glomerulosclerosis and interstitial fibrosis become evident. In some patients, renal function has deteriorated and progressed to failure, requiring dialysis and transplantation. Other renal abnormalities include amyloidosis, a Fanconi-like syndrome, hypocitraturia, hypercalciuria, and a distal renal tubular acidification defect.

Patients with GSD Ib can have additional features of recurrent bacterial infections from **neutropenia** and impaired neutrophil function. Oral involvement including recurrent mucosal ulceration, gingivitis, and rapidly progressive periodontal disease may occur in type Ib. Intestinal mucosa ulceration culminating in GSD enterocolitis is also common. Type 1b is also associated with a chronic inflammatory bowel disease (IBD)–like picture involving the colon that may be associated with neutropenia and/or neutrophil dysfunction; it may resemble ulcerative colitis or Crohn disease.

Diagnosis

The clinical presentation and laboratory findings of hypoglycemia, lactic acidosis, hyperuricemia, and hyperlipidemia lead to a suspected diagnosis of type I GSD. Neutropenia is noted in GSD Ib patients, typically before 1 yr of age. Neutropenia has also been noted in some patients with GSD Ia, especially those with the p.G188A variant. Administration of glucagon or epinephrine leads to a negligible increase, if any, in blood glucose levels, but the lactate level rises significantly. Before the availability of genetic testing, a definitive diagnosis required a liver biopsy. Gene-based variant analysis by single-gene sequencing or gene panels provides a noninvasive way to diagnose most patients with GSD types Ia and Ib.

Treatment

Treatment focuses on maintaining normal blood glucose levels and is achieved by continuous nasogastric (NG) infusion of glucose or oral administration of uncooked cornstarch. In infancy, overnight NG drip feeding may be needed to maintain normoglycemia. NG feedings can consist of an elemental enteral formula or only glucose or a glucose polymer to provide sufficient glucose to maintain euglycemia. During the day, frequent feedings with high-carbohydrate content are typically sufficient.

Uncooked cornstarch acts as a slow-release form of glucose and can be introduced at a dose of 1.6 g/kg every 4 hr for children <2 yr of age. The response of young children is variable. For older children, the cornstarch regimen can be changed to every 6 hr at a dose of 1.6-2.5 g/kg body weight and can be given orally as a liquid. Newer starch products, such as extended-release waxy maize starch, are thought to be longer acting, better tolerated, and more palatable. Medium-chain triglyceride (MCT) supplementation improves metabolic control, leading to improved growth in children. Since fructose and galactose cannot be converted directly to glucose in GSD type I, these sugars should be restricted in the diet. Sucrose (table sugar, cane sugar, other ingredients), fructose (fruit, juice, high-fructose corn syrup), lactose (dairy foods), and sorbitol should be avoided or limited. As a result of these dietary restrictions, vitamins and minerals such as calcium and vitamin D may be deficient, and supplementation is required to prevent nutritional deficiencies.

Dietary therapy improves hyperuricemia, hyperlipidemia, and renal function, slowing the development of renal failure. This therapy fails, however, to normalize blood uric acid and lipid levels completely in some individuals, despite good metabolic control, especially after puberty. The control of hyperuricemia can be further augmented by the use of allopurinol, a xanthine oxidase inhibitor. The hyperlipidemia can be reduced with lipid-lowering drugs such as β-hydroxy-β-methylglutaryl-coenzyme A (HMG-CoA) reductase inhibitors and fibrate (see Chapter 104). **Microalbuminuria**, an early indicator of renal dysfunction in type I disease, is treated with angiotensin-converting enzyme (ACE) inhibitors. Citrate supplements can be beneficial for patients with hypocitraturia by preventing or ameliorating nephrocalcinosis and development of urinary calculi. Thiazide diuretics increase renal reabsorption of filtered calcium and decrease urinary calcium excretion, thereby preventing hypercalciuria and nephrocalcinosis. Growth hormone (GH) should be used with extreme caution and limited to only those with a documented GH deficiency. Even in those patients, there should be close monitoring of metabolic parameters and for the presence of adenomas.

In patients with type Ib GSD, granulocyte and granulocyte-macrophage colony-stimulating factors are successful in correcting the neutropenia, decreasing the number and severity of bacterial infections, and improving the chronic IBD. The minimum effective dose should be used because side effects are noted on these agents, including splenomegaly, hypersplenism, and bone pain. Bone marrow transplantation has been reported to correct the neutropenia of type Ib GSD.

Orthotopic liver transplantation is a potential cure of type I GSD, especially for patients with liver malignancy, multiple liver adenomas, metabolic derangements refractory to medical management, and liver failure. However, this should be considered as a last resort because of the inherent short- and long-term complications. Large adenomas (>2 cm) that are rapidly increasing in size and/or number may necessitate partial hepatic resection. Smaller adenomas (<2 cm) may be treated with percutaneous ethanol injection or transcatheter arterial embolization. Recurrence of liver adenomas is a challenge and may potentiate malignant transformation in these patients, ultimately requiring a liver transplant.

Before any surgical procedure, the bleeding status must be evaluated and good metabolic control established. Prolonged bleeding times can be normalized by the use of intensive intravenous (IV) glucose infusion for 24-48 hr before surgery. DDAVP (1-deamino-8-D-arginine vasopressin) can reduce bleeding complications, but it should be used with caution because of the risk of fluid overload and hyponatremia when administered as an IV infusion. Lactated Ringer solution should be avoided because it contains lactate and no glucose. Glucose levels should be maintained in the normal range throughout surgery with the use of 10% dextrose. Overall, metabolic control is assessed by growth, improvement, and correction of the metabolic abnormalities, such as elevated lactate, glucose, triglyceride, cholesterol, and uric acid levels.

Prognosis

Previously, type I GSD was associated with a high mortality at a young age, and even for those who survived, the prognosis was guarded. Inadequate metabolic control during childhood can lead to long-term complications in adults. Clinical outcomes have improved dramatically with early diagnosis and effective treatment. However, serious complications such as renal disease and formation of hepatic adenomas with potential risk for malignant transformation persist. The ability to identify transformation to hepatocellular carcinoma in the liver adenomas remains a challenge: α-fetoprotein (AFP) and carcinoembryonic antigen (CEA) levels often remain normal in the setting of hepatocellular carcinoma.

Type III Glycogen Storage Disease (Debrancher Deficiency, Limit Dextrinosis)

Type III GSD is caused by deficient activity of the **glycogen debranching enzyme**. Debranching enzyme, together with phosphorylase, is responsible for complete degradation of glycogen. When debranching enzyme is defective, glycogen breakdown is incomplete, resulting in the accumulation of an abnormal glycogen with short outer-branch chains, which resemble *limit dextrin*. Symptoms of glycogen debranching enzyme deficiency include hepatomegaly, hypoglycemia, short stature, variable skeletal myopathy, and variable cardiomyopathy. GSD **type IIIa** usually involves both liver and muscle, whereas in **type IIIb**, seen in approximately 15% of patients, the disease appears to involve only liver.

Type III GSD is an autosomal recessive disease that has been reported in many different ethnic groups. The frequency is relatively high in Sephardic Jews from North Africa, inhabitants of the Faroe Islands, and in Inuits. The gene for debranching enzyme *(AGL)* is located on chromosome 1p21. More than 130 different pathogenic variants have been identified; 2 pathogenic variants in exon 3, c.18_19delGA (previously described as c.17_18delAG) and p.Gln6X, are specifically associated with glycogenosis IIIb. Carrier detection and prenatal diagnosis are possible using DNA-based methodologies.

Clinical Manifestations

In infancy and childhood, GSD type III may be indistinguishable from type I GSD because of overlapping features such as hepatomegaly, hypoglycemia, hyperlipidemia, and growth retardation (Fig. 105.2). Splenomegaly may be present, but the kidneys are typically not affected. Hepatomegaly in most patients with type III GSD improves with age; however, liver fibrosis, cirrhosis progressing to liver failure, and hepatocellular carcinoma (HCC) are noted in many in late adulthood. Hepatic adenomas occur less often in individuals with GSD III than those with GSD I. The relationship between hepatic adenomas and malignancy in GSD III remains unclear. AFP and CEA levels are not good predictors of the presence of hepatocellular adenomas or malignant transformation. A single case of malignant transformation at the site of adenomas has been noted.

In patients with GSD type IIIa, the **muscle weakness** is slowly progressive and associated with wasting. The weakness is less remarkable in childhood but can become severe after the 3rd or 4th decade of life. Low bone mineral density in patients with GSD III put them at an increased risk of potential fractures. Myopathy does not follow any particular pattern of involvement; both proximal and distal muscles are involved. Electromyography reveals a widespread myopathy; nerve conduction studies are often abnormal.

Although overt cardiac dysfunction is rare, ventricular hypertrophy

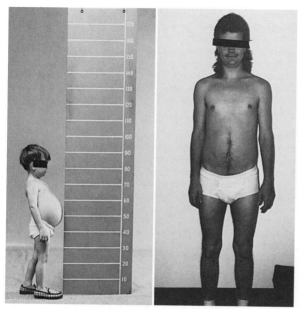

Fig. 105.2 Growth and development in a patient with type IIIb glycogen storage disease. The patient has debrancher deficiency in the liver but normal activity in muscle. As a child, he had hepatomegaly, hypoglycemia, and growth retardation. After puberty, he no longer had hepatomegaly or hypoglycemia, and his final adult height is normal. He had no muscle weakness or atrophy; this is in contrast to type IIIa patients, in whom a progressive myopathy is seen in adulthood.

is a frequent finding. **Cardiac pathology** has shown diffuse involvement of various cardiac structures, including vacuolation of myocytes, atrioventricular conduction, and hyperplasia of smooth muscles. Life-threatening arrhythmia and the need for heart transplant have been reported in some GSD III patients. Hepatic symptoms in some patients may be so mild that the diagnosis is not made until adulthood, when the patients show symptoms and signs of neuromuscular disease.

The initial diagnosis has been confused with Charcot-Marie-Tooth disease (see Chapter 631.1). Polycystic ovaries are noted; some patients can develop hirsutism, irregular menstrual cycles, and other features of polycystic ovarian syndrome. Fertility does not appear to be affected; successful pregnancies have been reported.

Hypoglycemia and hyperlipidemia are common. In contrast to type I GSD, elevation of liver transaminase levels and fasting ketosis are prominent, but blood lactate and uric acid concentrations are usually normal. Glucagon administration 2 hr after a carbohydrate meal provokes a normal increase in blood glucose; after an overnight fast, however, glucagon may provoke no change in blood glucose level. Serum creatine kinase levels can be useful to identify patients with muscle involvement, although normal levels do not rule out muscle enzyme deficiency.

Diagnosis

The histologic appearance of the liver is characterized by a universal distention of hepatocytes by glycogen and the presence of fibrous septa. The fibrosis and the paucity of fat distinguish type III glycogenosis from type I. The fibrosis, which ranges from minimal periportal fibrosis to micronodular cirrhosis, appears in most cases to be nonprogressive. Overt cirrhosis has been seen in some patients with GSD III.

Patients with myopathy and liver symptoms have a generalized enzyme defect (type IIIa). The deficient enzyme activity can be demonstrated not only in liver and muscle, but also in other tissues such as heart, erythrocytes, and cultured fibroblasts. Patients with hepatic symptoms without clinical or laboratory evidence of myopathy have debranching enzyme deficiency only in the liver, with enzyme activity retained in

the muscle (type IIIb). Before the availability of genetic testing, a definitive diagnosis required enzyme assay in liver, muscle, or both. Gene sequencing now allows for diagnosis and subtype assignment in the majority of patients.

Treatment

The mainstay of treatment of GSD III is dietary management, as in GSD I, although it is less demanding. Patients do not need to restrict dietary intake of fructose and galactose, although simple sugars should be avoided to prevent sudden spikes in blood glucose levels. Hypoglycemia is treated with small, frequent meals high in complex carbohydrates, such as cornstarch supplements or nocturnal gastric drip feedings. Additionally, a high-protein diet during the daytime as well as overnight protein enteral infusion is effective in preventing hypoglycemia. The exogenous protein can be used as a substrate for gluconeogenesis which helps to meet energy needs and prevent endogenous protein breakdown. Protein in the diet also reduces the overall starch requirement. Overtreatment with cornstarch should be avoided as it can result in excessive glycogen buildup, which is detrimental and can lead to excessive weight gain. MCT supplementation is being considered as an alternative source of energy. There is no satisfactory treatment for the progressive myopathy other than recommending a high-protein diet and a submaximal exercise program. Close monitoring with abdominal MRI is needed to detect progression of liver fibrosis to cirrhosis and further to HCC. Liver transplantation has been performed in GSD III patients with progressive cirrhosis and/or HCC. There are reports of cardiac transplant in GSD III patients with end stage cardiac disease.

Type IV Glycogen Storage Disease (Branching Enzyme Deficiency, Amylopectinosis, Polyglucosan Disease, or Andersen Disease)

Type IV GSD is caused by the deficiency of **branching enzyme** activity, which results in the accumulation of an abnormal glycogen with poor solubility. The disease is also known as *amylopectinosis* because the abnormal glycogen has fewer branch points, more α 1-4 linked glucose units, and longer outer chains, resulting in a structure resembling amylopectin. Accumulation of polyglucosan, which is positive on periodic acid–Schiff (PAS) and partially resistant to diastase digestion, is seen in all tissues of patients, but to different degrees.

Type IV GSD is an autosomal recessive disorder. The glycogen branching enzyme *(GBE)* gene is located on chromosome 3p21. More than 20 pathogenic variants responsible for type IV GSD have been identified, and their characterization in individual patients can be useful in predicting clinical outcome. The nearly complete absence of GBE activity with null variants has been associated with perinatal death and fatal neonatal hypotonia. Residual GBE enzyme activity >5% and presence of at least 1 missense variant are associated with a nonlethal hepatic cirrhosis phenotype and, in some situations, a lack of progressive liver disease.

Clinical Manifestations

There is a high degree of clinical variability associated with type IV GSD. The most common and classic form is characterized by progressive cirrhosis of the liver and manifests in the 1st 18 mo of life as hepatosplenomegaly and failure to thrive. Cirrhosis may present with portal hypertension, ascites, and esophageal varices and may progress to liver failure, usually leading to death by 5 yr of age. Rare patients survive without progression of liver disease; they have a milder hepatic form and do not require a liver transplant. Extrahepatic involvement in some patients with GSD IV consists of musculoskeletal involvement, particularly cardiac and skeletal muscles, as well as central nervous system (CNS) involvement.

A **neuromuscular** form of type IV GSD has been reported, with 4 main variants recognized based on age at presentation. The **perinatal** form is characterized by a *fetal akinesia deformation sequence* (FADS) and death in the perinatal period. The **congenital** form presents at birth with severe hypotonia, muscle atrophy, and neuronal involvement, with death in the neonatal period; some patients have cardiomyopathy. The

childhood form presents primarily with myopathy or cardiomyopathy. The **adult** form, *adult polyglucosan body disease* (APBD), presents as an isolated myopathy or with diffuse CNS and peripheral nervous system dysfunction, accompanied by accumulation of polyglucosan material in the nervous system. Symptoms of neuronal involvement include peripheral neuropathy, neurogenic bladder, and leukodystrophy, as well as mild cognitive decline in some patients. For APBD, a leukocyte or nerve biopsy is needed to establish the diagnosis because branching enzyme deficiency is limited to those tissues.

Diagnosis

Deposition of amylopectin-like materials can be demonstrated in liver, heart, muscle, skin, intestine, brain, spinal cord, and peripheral nerve in type IV GSD. Liver histology shows micronodular cirrhosis and faintly stained basophilic inclusions in the hepatocytes. The inclusions are composed of coarsely clumped, stored material that is PAS positive and partially resistant to diastase digestion. Electron microscopy (EM) shows, in addition to the conventional α and β glycogen particles, accumulation of the fibrillar aggregations that are typical of amylopectin. The distinct staining properties of the cytoplasmic inclusions, as well as EM findings, could be diagnostic. However, polysaccharides with histologic features reminiscent of type IV disease, but without enzymatic correlation, have been observed. The definitive diagnosis rests on the demonstration of the deficient branching enzyme activity in liver, muscle, cultured skin fibroblasts, or leukocytes, or on the identification of pathogenic variants in the *GBE* gene. Prenatal diagnosis is possible by measuring enzyme activity in cultured amniocytes, chorionic villi, or DNA-based methodologies.

Treatment

There is no specific treatment for type IV GSD. Nervous system involvement, such as gait problems and bladder involvement, requires supportive, symptomatic management. Unlike patients with the other liver GSDs (I, III, VI, IX), those with GSD IV do not have hypoglycemia, which is only seen when there is overt liver cirrhosis. Liver transplantation has been performed for patients with progressive liver disease, but patients must be carefully selected as this is a multisystem disease, and in some patients, extrahepatic involvement may manifest after transplant. The long-term success of liver transplantation is unknown. Individuals with significant diffuse reticuloendothelial involvement may have greater risk for morbidity and mortality, which may impact the success rate for liver transplant.

Type VI Glycogen Storage Disease (Liver Phosphorylase Deficiency, Hers Disease)

Type VI GSD is caused by deficiency of **liver glycogen phosphorylase**. Relatively few patients are documented, likely because of underreporting of this disease. Patients usually present with hepatomegaly and growth retardation in early childhood. Hypoglycemia, hyperlipidemia, and hyperketosis are of variable severity. Ketotic hypoglycemia may present after overnight or prolonged fasting. Lactic acid and uric acid levels are normal. Type VI GSD presents within a broad spectrum of involvement, some with a more severe clinical presentation. Patients with severe hepatomegaly, recurrent severe hypoglycemia, hyperketosis, and postprandial lactic acidosis have been reported. Focal nodular hyperplasia of liver and hepatocellular adenoma with malignant transformation into carcinoma is reported in some patients. While cardiac muscle was thought to be unaffected, recently mild cardiomyopathy has been reported in a patient with GSD VI.

Treatment is symptomatic and aims to prevent hypoglycemia while ensuring adequate nutrition. A high-carbohydrate, high-protein diet and frequent feeding are effective in preventing hypoglycemia. Blood glucose and ketones should be monitored routinely, especially during periods of increased activity/illness. Long-term follow-up of these patients is needed to expand the understanding of the natural history of this disorder.

GSD VI is an autosomal recessive disease. **Diagnosis** can be confirmed through molecular testing of the liver phosphorylase gene *(PYGL)*, which is found on chromosome 14q21-22 and has 20 exons. Many pathogenic

variants are known in this gene; a splice-site variant in intron 13 has been identified in the Mennonite population. A liver biopsy showing elevated glycogen content and decreased hepatic phosphorylase enzyme activity can also be used to make a diagnosis. However, with the availability of DNA analysis and next-generation sequencing panels, liver biopsies are considered unnecessary.

Type IX Glycogen Storage Disease (Phosphorylase Kinase Deficiency)

Type IX GSD represents a heterogeneous group of glycogenoses. It results from deficiency of the enzyme **phosphorylase kinase** (PhK), which is involved in the rate-limiting step of glycogenolysis. This enzyme has 4 subunits (α, β, γ, δ), each encoded by different genes on different chromosomes and differentially expressed in various tissues. Pathogenic variants in the *PHKA1* gene cause muscle PhK deficiency; pathogenic variants in the *PHKA2* and *PHKG2* genes cause liver PhK deficiency; pathogenic variants in the *PHKB* gene cause PhK deficiency in liver and muscle. Pathogenic variants in the *PHKG1* gene have not been identified. Defects in subunits α, β, and γ are responsible for liver presentation.

Clinical manifestations of liver PhK deficiency are usually recognizable within the 1st 2 yr of life and include short stature and abdominal distention from moderate to marked hepatomegaly. The clinical severity of liver PhK deficiency varies considerably. Hyperketotic hypoglycemia, if present, can be mild but may be severe in some cases. Ketosis may occur even without glucose levels are normal. Some children may have mild delays in gross motor development and hypotonia. It is becoming increasingly clear that GSD IX is not a benign condition. Severe phenotypes are reported, with liver fibrosis progressing to cirrhosis and HCC, particularly in patients with *PHKG2* variants. Progressive splenomegaly and portal hypertension are reported secondary to cirrhosis. Mild cardiomyopathy has been reported in a patient with GSD IX *(PHKB variant)*. Cognitive and speech delays have been reported in a few individuals, but it is not clear whether these delays are caused by PhK deficiency or coincidental. Renal tubular acidosis has been reported in rare cases. Unlike in GSD I, lactic acidosis, bleeding tendency, and loose bowel movements are not characteristic. Although growth is retarded during childhood, normal height and complete sexual development are eventually achieved. As with debrancher deficiency, abdominal distention and hepatomegaly usually decrease with age and may disappear by adolescence. Most adults with liver PhK deficiency are asymptomatic, although further long-term studies are needed to fully assess the impact of this disorder in adults.

Phenotypic variability within each subtype is being uncovered with the availability of molecular testing. The incidence of all subtypes of PhK deficiency is approximately 1 : 100,000 live births.

X-Linked Liver Phosphorylase Kinase Deficiency (From *PHKA2* Variants)

X-linked liver PhK deficiency is one of the most common forms of liver glycogenosis in males. In addition to liver, enzyme activity can also be deficient in erythrocytes, leukocytes, and fibroblasts; it is normal in muscle. Typically, a 1-5 yr old boy presents with growth retardation, an incidental finding of hepatomegaly, and a slight delay in motor development. Cholesterol, triglycerides, and liver enzymes are mildly elevated. Ketosis may occur after fasting. Lactate and uric acid levels are normal. Hypoglycemia is typically mild, if present, but can be severe. The response in blood glucose to glucagon is normal. Hepatomegaly and abnormal blood chemistries gradually improve and can normalize with age. Most adults achieve a normal final height and are usually asymptomatic despite a persistent PhK deficiency. It is increasingly being recognized that this disorder is not benign as previously thought, and there are patients with severe disease and long-term hepatic sequelae. In rare cases, liver fibrosis can occur and progress to cirrhosis.

Liver histology shows glycogen-distended hepatocytes, steatosis, and potentially mild periportal fibrosis. The accumulated glycogen (β particles, rosette form) has a frayed or burst appearance and is less compact than the glycogen seen in type I or III GSD. Fibrous septal formation and low-grade inflammatory changes may be seen.

The gene for the common liver isoform of the PhK α subunit, *PHKA2*, is located on the X chromosome (αL at Xp22.2). Mutations in the *PHKA2* gene account for 75% of all PhK cases. X-linked liver PhK deficiency is further subdivided into 2 biochemical subtypes: XLG1, with measurable deficiency of PhK activity in both blood cells and liver, and XLG2, with normal in vitro PhK activity in blood cells and variable activity in liver. It is suspected that XLG2 may be caused by missense variants that affect enzyme regulation, whereas nonsense variants affecting the amount of protein result in XLG1. Female carriers are unaffected.

Autosomal Liver and Muscle Phosphorylase Kinase Deficiency (From *PHKB* Variants)

PhK deficiency in liver and blood cells with an autosomal recessive mode of inheritance has been reported. Similar to the X-linked form, chief symptoms in early childhood include hepatomegaly and growth retardation. Some patients also exhibit muscle hypotonia. In a few cases where enzyme activity has been measured, reduced PhK activity has been demonstrated in muscle. Mutations are found in *PHKB* (chromosome 16q12-q13), which encodes the β subunit, and result in liver and muscle PhK deficiency. Several nonsense variants, a single-base insertion, a splice-site mutation, and a large intragenic mutation have been identified. In addition, a missense variant was discovered in an atypical patient with normal blood cell PhK activity.

Autosomal Liver Phosphorylase Kinase Deficiency (From *PHKG2* Variants)

This form of PhK deficiency is caused by pathogenic variants in the testis/liver isoform (TL) of the γ subunit gene *(PHKG2)*. In contrast to X-linked PhK deficiency, patients with variants in *PHKG2* typically have more severe phenotypes, with recurrent hypoglycemia, prominent hepatomegaly, significant liver fibrosis, and progressive cirrhosis. Liver involvement may present with cholestasis, bile duct proliferation, esophageal varices, and splenomegaly. Other reported presentations include delayed motor milestones, muscle weakness, and renal tubular damage. The spectrum of involvement continues to evolve as more cases are recognized. *PHKG2* maps to chromosome 16p12.1-p11.2; many pathogenic variants are known for this gene.

Phosphorylase Kinase Deficiency Limited to Heart

These patients have been reported with **cardiomyopathy** in infancy and rapidly progress to heart failure and death. Recent studies have shown that this is not a case of cardiac-specific primary PhK deficiency as suspected previously, but rather linked to the γ₂ subunit of adenosine monophosphate (AMP)–activated protein kinase (see later). The γ₂ subunit is encoded by the *PRKAG2* gene.

Diagnosis

PhK deficiency may be diagnosed by demonstration of the enzymatic defect in affected tissues. PhK can be measured in leukocytes and erythrocytes, but because the enzyme has many isozymes, the diagnosis can be easily missed without studies of liver, muscle, or heart. Individuals with liver PhK deficiency also usually have elevated transaminases, mildly elevated triglycerides and cholesterol, normal uric acid and lactic acid concentrations, and normal glucagon responses. Gene sequencing is used for diagnostic confirmation and subtyping of GSD IX.

The *PHKA2* gene encoding the α subunit is most frequently involved, followed by the *PHKB* gene encoding the β subunit. Variants in the *PHKG2* gene underlying γ-subunit deficiency are typically associated with severe liver involvement with recurrent hypoglycemia and liver fibrosis.

Treatment and Prognosis

The treatment for liver PhK deficiency is symptomatic. It includes a diet high in complex carbohydrates and proteins and small, frequent feedings to prevent hypoglycemia. Cornstarch can be administered with symptom-dependent dosage and timing (0.6-2.5 g/kg every 6 hr). Oral intake of glucose, if tolerated, should be used to treat hypoglycemia. If not, IV glucose should be given.

Prognosis for the X-linked and certain autosomal forms is typically good; however, long term complications are being recognized. Patients with mutations in the γ subunit typically have a more severe clinical course with progressive liver disease. Liver involvement needs to be monitored in all patients with GSD IX by periodic imaging (abdominal ultrasound or MRI every 6-12 mo) and serial hepatic function tests.

Liver Glycogen Synthase Deficiency

Liver glycogen synthase deficiency type 0 (**GSD 0**) is caused by deficiency of **hepatic glycogen synthase** (GYS2) activity, leading to a marked decrease of glycogen stored in the liver. The gene *GYS2* is located at 12p12.2. Several pathogenic variants have been identified in patients with GSD 0. The disease appears to be rare in humans, and in the true sense, this is not a type of GSD because the deficiency of the enzyme leads to decreased glycogen stores. Patients present in infancy with early-morning (prebreakfast) drowsiness, pallor, emesis, and fatigue and sometimes convulsions associated with hypoglycemia and hyperketonemia. Blood lactate and alanine levels are low, and there is no hyperlipidemia or hepatomegaly. Prolonged *hyperglycemia*, glycosuria, lactic acidosis, and hyperalaninemia, with normal insulin levels after administration of glucose or a meal, suggest a deficiency of glycogen synthase. Definitive diagnosis may be by a liver biopsy to measure the enzyme activity or identification of pathogenic variants in *GYS2*.

Treatment consists of frequent meals, rich in protein and nighttime supplementation with uncooked cornstarch to prevent hypoglycemia and hyperketonemia. Most children with GSD 0 are cognitively and developmentally normal. Short stature and osteopenia are common features. The **prognosis** seems good for patients who survive to adulthood, including resolution of hypoglycemia, except during pregnancy.

Hepatic Glycogenosis With Renal Fanconi Syndrome (Fanconi-Bickel Syndrome)

Fanconi-Bickel Syndrome is a rare autosomal recessive disorder is caused by defects in the facilitative glucose transporter 2 (GLUT-2), which transports glucose in and out of hepatocytes, pancreatic β cells, and the basolateral membranes of intestinal and renal epithelial cells. The disease is characterized by proximal renal tubular dysfunction, impaired glucose and galactose utilization, and accumulation of glycogen in liver and kidney.

The affected child typically presents in the 1st yr of life with failure to thrive, rickets, and a protuberant abdomen from hepatomegaly and nephromegaly. The disease may be confused with GSD I because a Fanconi-like syndrome can also develop in type I patients. Adults typically present with short stature, dwarfism, and excess fat in the abdomen and shoulders. Patients are more susceptible to fractures because of early-onset generalized osteopenia. In addition, intestinal malabsorption and diarrhea may occur.

Laboratory findings include glucosuria, phosphaturia, generalized aminoaciduria, bicarbonate wasting, hypophosphatemia, increased serum alkaline phosphatase levels, and radiologic findings of rickets. Mild fasting hypoglycemia and hyperlipidemia may be present. Liver transaminase, plasma lactate, and uric acid levels are usually normal. Oral galactose or glucose tolerance tests show intolerance, which could be explained by the functional loss of GLUT-2 preventing liver uptake of these sugars. Tissue biopsy results show marked accumulation of glycogen in hepatocytes and proximal renal tubular cells, presumably from the altered glucose transport out of these organs. Diffuse glomerular mesangial expansion along with glomerular hyperfiltration and microalbuminuria similar to nephropathy in GSD Ia and diabetes have been reported.

This condition is rare, and 70% of patients with Fanconi-Bickel syndrome have consanguineous parents. Most patients have homozygous pathogenic variants; some patients are compound heterozygotes. The majority of variants detected thus far predict a premature termination of translation. The resulting loss of the C-terminal end of the GLUT-2 protein predicts a nonfunctioning glucose transporter with an inward-facing substrate-binding site.

There is no specific treatment. Symptom-dependent treatment with phosphate and bicarbonate can result in growth improvement. Growth may also improve with symptomatic replacement of water, electrolytes, and vitamin D; restriction of galactose intake; and a diet similar to that used for diabetes mellitus, with small, frequent meals and adequate caloric intake.

MUSCLE GLYCOGENOSES

The role of glycogen in muscle is to provide substrates for the generation of ATP for muscle contraction. The muscle GSDs are broadly divided into 2 groups. The first group is characterized by hypertrophic cardiomyopathy, progressive skeletal muscle weakness and atrophy, or both, and includes deficiencies of **acid α-glucosidase**, a lysosomal glycogen-degrading enzyme (**type II** GSD), lysosomal-associated membrane protein 2 (**LAMP2**), and AMP-activated protein kinase γ_2 (**PRKAG2**). The 2nd group comprises muscle energy disorders characterized by muscle pain, exercise intolerance, myoglobinuria, and susceptibility to fatigue. This group includes myophosphorylase deficiency (McArdle disease, **type V** GSD) and deficiencies of phosphofructokinase (**type VII**), phosphoglycerate kinase, phosphoglycerate mutase, lactate dehydrogenase, and muscle-specific phosphorylase kinase. Some of these latter enzyme deficiencies can also be associated with *compensated hemolysis*, suggesting a more generalized defect in glucose metabolism.

Type II Glycogen Storage Disease (Lysosomal Acid α-1,4-Glucosidase Deficiency, Pompe Disease)

Pompe disease, also referred to as GSD type II or **acid maltase deficiency**, is caused by a deficiency of acid α-1,4-glucosidase (acid maltase), an enzyme responsible for the degradation of glycogen in lysosomes. This enzyme defect results in lysosomal glycogen accumulation in multiple tissues and cell types, predominantly affecting cardiac, skeletal, and smooth muscle cells. In Pompe disease, glycogen typically accumulates within lysosomes, as opposed to its accumulation in cytoplasm in the other glycogenoses. However, as the disease progresses, lysosomal rupture and leakage lead to the presence of cytoplasmic glycogen as well.

Pompe disease is an autosomal recessive disorder. The incidence was thought to be approximately 1 in 40,000 live births in Caucasians and 1 in 18,000 live births in Han Chinese. Newborn screening for Pompe disease in the United States suggests that the prevalence is much higher than previously thought (between 1 in 9,132 and 1 in 24,188). The gene for acid α-glucosidase (*GAA*) is on chromosome 17q25.2. More than 500 pathogenic variants have been identified that could be helpful in delineating the phenotypes. A splice-site variant (IVS1-13T→G; c.-32-13T>G) is commonly seen in late-onset Caucasian patients.

Clinical Manifestations

Pompe disease is broadly classified into infantile and late-onset forms. **Infantile Pompe disease** (IPD) is uniformly lethal without enzyme replacement therapy (ERT) with *alglucosidase alfa*. Affected infants present in the 1st day to weeks of life with hypotonia, generalized muscle weakness with a *floppy infant* appearance, neuropathic bulbar weakness, feeding difficulties, macroglossia, hepatomegaly, and hypertrophic cardiomyopathy, which if untreated leads to death from cardiorespiratory failure or respiratory infection, usually by 1 yr of age.

Late-onset Pompe disease (LOPD; juvenile-, childhood-, and adult-onset disease) is characterized by proximal limb girdle muscle weakness and early involvement of respiratory muscles, especially the diaphragm. Cardiac involvement ranges from cardiac rhythm disturbances to cardiomyopathy and a less severe, short-term prognosis. Symptoms related to progressive dysfunction of skeletal muscles can start as early as within 1 yr of age to as late as the 6th decade of life. The clinical picture is dominated by slowly progressive proximal muscle weakness with truncal involvement and greater involvement of the lower limbs than the upper limbs. The pelvic girdle, paraspinal muscles, and diaphragm are the muscle groups most seriously affected in patients with LOPD. Other symptoms may include lingual weakness, ptosis, and dilation of blood vessels (e.g., basilar artery, ascending aorta). With disease progression, patients become confined to a wheelchair and

require artificial ventilation. The initial symptoms in some patients may be respiratory insufficiency manifested by somnolence, morning headache, orthopnea, and exertional dyspnea, which eventually lead to sleep-disordered breathing and respiratory failure. Respiratory failure is the cause of significant morbidity and mortality in LOPD. Basilar artery aneurysms with rupture also contribute to mortality in some cases. Small-fiber neuropathy presenting as painful paresthesia has been identified in some LOPD patients. Gastrointestinal disturbances such as postprandial bloating, dysphagia, early satiety, diarrhea, chronic constipation, and irritable bowel disease have been reported. Genitourinary tract involvement is not uncommon and may present as bladder and bowel incontinence, weak urine stream or dribbling. If untreated, the age of death varies from early childhood to late adulthood, depending on the rate of disease progression and the extent of respiratory muscle involvement. With the advent of ERT, a new natural history is emerging for both survivors of infantile and LOPD.

Laboratory Findings

These include elevated levels of serum creatine kinase (CK), aspartate transaminase (AST), alanine transaminase (ALT), and lactate dehydrogenase (LDH). Urine glucose tetrasaccharide, a glycogen breakdown metabolite, is a reliable biomarker for disease severity and treatment response. In the infantile form a chest x-ray film showing massive cardiomegaly is frequently the first symptom detected. **Electrocardiographic findings** include a high-voltage QRS complex, Wolff-Parkinson-White (WPW) syndrome, and a shortened PR interval. Echocardiography reveals thickening of both ventricles and/or the intraventricular septum and/or left ventricular outflow tract obstruction. Muscle biopsy shows the presence of vacuoles that stain positively for glycogen; acid phosphatase is increased, presumably from a compensatory increase of lysosomal enzymes. EM reveals glycogen accumulation within a membranous sac and in the cytoplasm. Electromyography reveals myopathic features with excessive electrical irritability of muscle fibers and pseudomyotonic discharges. Serum CK is not always elevated in adult patients. Depending on the muscle sampled or tested, the muscle histologic appearance and electromyography may not be abnormal.

Some patients with infantile Pompe disease who had peripheral nerve biopsies demonstrated glycogen accumulation in the neurons and Schwann cells.

Diagnosis

Diagnosis of Pompe disease can be made by enzyme assay in dried blood spots, leukocytes, blood mononuclear cells, muscle, or cultured skin fibroblasts demonstrating deficient acid α-glucosidase activity. Gene sequencing showing 2 pathogenic variants in the *GAA* gene is confirmatory. The enzyme assay should be done in a laboratory with experience using maltose, glycogen, or 4-methylumbelliferyl-α-D-glucopyranoside (4MUG) as a substrate. The infantile form has a more severe enzyme deficiency than the late-onset forms. Detection of percent residual enzyme activity is captured in skin fibroblasts and muscle. Blood-based assays, especially dried blood spots, have the advantage of a rapid turnaround time and are being increasingly used as the first-line tissue to make a diagnosis. A muscle biopsy is often done with suspected muscle disease and a broad differential; it yields faster results and provides additional information about glycogen content and site of glycogen storage within and outside the lysosomes of muscle cells. However, a normal muscle biopsy *does not* exclude a diagnosis of Pompe disease. Late-onset patients show variability in glycogen accumulation in different muscles and within muscle fibers; muscle histology and glycogen content can vary depending on the site of muscle biopsy. There is also a high risk from anesthesia in infantile patients. An electrocardiogram can be helpful in making the diagnosis in suspected cases of the infantile form and should be done for patients suspected of having Pompe disease before any procedure requiring anesthesia, including muscle biopsy, is performed. Urinary glucose tetrasaccharides can be elevated in the urine of affected patients, and levels are extremely high in infantile patients. Availability of next-generation sequencing panels and whole exome sequencing allows for identification of additional patients with

Pompe disease, especially when the diagnosis is ambiguous. **Prenatal diagnosis** using amniocytes or chorionic villi is available.

Treatment

Enzyme replacement therapy with recombinant human acid α-glucosidase (alglucosidase alfa) is available for treatment of Pompe disease. Recombinant acid α-glucosidase is capable of preventing deterioration or reversing abnormal cardiac and skeletal muscle functions (Fig. 105.3). ERT should be initiated as soon as possible across the disease spectrum, especially for babies with the infantile form, because the disease is rapidly progressive. Infants who are negative for cross-reacting immunologic material (CRIM) develop a high-titer antibody against the infused enzyme and respond to the ERT less favorably. Treatment using immunomodulating agents such as methotrexate, rituximab, and intravenous immune globulin (IVIG) have demonstrated efficacy in preventing the development of an immune response to ERT and immune tolerance. Nocturnal ventilatory support, when indicated, should be used; it has been shown to improve the quality of life and is particularly beneficial during a period of respiratory decompensation.

In addition to ERT, other adjunctive therapies have demonstrated benefit in Pompe patients. For patients with the late-onset disease, a high-protein diet may be beneficial. Respiratory muscle strength training has demonstrated improvements in respiratory parameters when combined with ERT. Submaximal exercise regimens are of assistance to improve muscle strength, pain, and fatigue. Other approaches are under clinical development to improve the safety and efficacy of enzyme delivery to affected tissues. These include use of chaperone molecules to enhance rhGAA delivery, and neoGAA, which is a second-generation ERT with a high number of mannose-6-phosphate (M6P) tags that enhances M6P receptor targeting and enzyme uptake. Gene therapy studies to correct the endogenous enzyme production pathways have shown promise.

Early diagnosis and treatment are necessary for optimal outcomes.

Newborn screening using blood-based assays in Taiwan has resulted in early identification of Pompe cases and thus improved disease outcomes through the early initiation of ERT.

Glycogen Storage Diseases Mimicking Hypertrophic Cardiomyopathy (Danon Disease)

Danon disease is caused by pathogenic variants in the *LAMP2* gene, which leads to a deficiency of **lysosomal-associated membrane protein 2** (LAMP2). This leads to accumulation of glycogen in the heart and skeletal muscle, which presents primarily with hypertrophic cardiomyopathy and skeletal muscle weakness. Danon disease can be distinguished from the usual causes of hypertrophic cardiomyopathy (defects in sarcomere-protein genes) by their electrophysiologic abnormalities, particularly ventricular preexcitation and conduction defects. Patients present with cardiac symptoms, including chest pain, palpitations, syncope, and cardiac arrest, usually between ages 8 and 15 yr. Other clinical manifestations in Danon disease include peripheral pigmentary retinopathy, lens changes, and abnormal electroretinograms. This disorder is inherited in an X-linked dominant pattern. Diagnosis can be done by genetic testing for the *LAMP2* gene. The prognosis for LAMP2 deficiency is poor, with progressive end-stage heart failure early in adulthood. **Treatment** is directed toward management of symptoms in affected individuals, including management of cardiomyopathy, correction of arrhythmias, and physical therapy for muscle weakness. Cardiac transplantation has been tried successfully in some patients.

Adenosine Monophosphate–Activated Protein Kinase γ₂ Deficiency (PRKAG2 Deficiency)

AMP-activated protein kinase γ₂ (PRKAG2) deficiency is caused by pathogenic variants in the *PRKAG2* gene mapped to chromosome 7q36. *PRKAG2* is required for the synthesis of the enzyme AMP-activated protein kinase (AMPK), which regulates cellular pathways involved in

Pre-treatment   **Post-treatment**

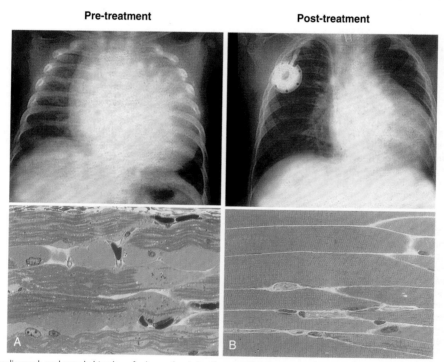

Fig. 105.3 Chest radiograph and muscle histology findings of an infantile-onset Pompe disease patient before (**A**) and after (**B**) enzyme replacement therapy. Note the decrease in heart size and muscle glycogen with the therapy. (*Modified from Amalfitano A, Bengur AR, Morse RP, et al: Recombinant human acid alpha-glucosidase enzyme therapy for infantile glycogen storage disease type II: results of a phase I/II clinical trial, Genet Med 3:132–138, 2001.*)

ATP metabolism. Common presentations include hypertrophic cardiomyopathy and electrophysiologic abnormalities such as WPW syndrome, atrial fibrillation, and progressive atrioventricular block. Cardiac involvement is variable and includes supraventricular tachycardia, sinus bradycardia, left ventricular dysfunction, and even sudden cardiac death in some cases. In addition to cardiac involvement, there is a broad spectrum of phenotypic presentations including myalgia, myopathy, and seizures. Cardiomyopathy caused by *PRKAG2* variants usually allows for long-term survival, although a rare congenital form presenting in early infancy is associated with a rapidly fatal course. Cardiomyopathy in PRKAG2 syndrome often mimics that in other conditions, especially Pompe disease, and should be considered as a differential diagnosis in infants presenting with severe hypertrophic cardiomyopathy. **Treatment** is primarily symptomatic, including management of cardiac failure and correction of conduction defects.

Muscle Glycogen Synthase Deficiency

This GSD results from muscle glycogen synthase (**glycogen synthase I**, GYS1) deficiency. The gene GYS1 has been localized to chromosome 19q13.3. In the true sense, this is not a type of GSD because the deficiency of the enzyme leads to decreased glycogen stores. The disease is extremely rare and has been reported in 3 children of consanguineous parents of Syrian origin. Muscle biopsies showed lack of glycogen, predominantly oxidative fibers, and mitochondrial proliferation. Glucose tolerance was normal. Molecular study revealed a homozygous stop mutation (R462→ter) in the muscle glycogen synthase gene. The phenotype was variable in the 3 siblings and ranged from sudden cardiac arrest, muscle fatigability, hypertrophic cardiomyopathy, an abnormal heart rate, and hypotension while exercising, to mildly impaired cardiac function at rest.

Late-Onset Polyglucosan Body Myopathy (From GYG1 Variants)

Late-onset polyglucosan body myopathy is an autosomal recessive, slowly progressive skeletal myopathy caused by pathogenic variants in the *GYG1* gene blocking **glycogenin-1** biosynthesis. There is a reduced or complete absence of glycogenin-1, which is a precursor necessary for glycogen formation. Polyglucosan accumulation in skeletal muscles causes adult-onset proximal muscle weakness, prominently affecting hip and shoulder girdles. Cardiac involvement is not seen. Compared with GSD IV–APBD, nervous system involvement is uncommon, although polyglucosan deposition is seen in both disorders. *GYG1* is mapped to chromosome 3q24. Muscle biopsies show PAS-positive storage material in 30–40% of muscle fibers. EM reveals the typical polyglucosan structure, consisting of ovoid form composed of partly filamentous material.

Type V Glycogen Storage Disease (Muscle Phosphorylase Deficiency, McArdle Disease)

GSD type V is caused by deficiency of **myophosphorylase** activity. Lack of this enzyme limits muscle ATP generation by glycogenolysis, resulting in muscle glycogen accumulation, and is the prototype of muscle energy disorders. A deficiency of myophosphorylase impairs the cleavage of glucosyl molecules from the straight chain of glycogen.

Clinical Manifestations

Symptoms usually first develop in late childhood or in the 2nd decade of life. Clinical heterogeneity is uncommon, but cases suggesting otherwise have been documented. Studies have shown that McArdle disease can manifest in individuals as old as 74, as well as in infancy in a fatal, early-onset form characterized by hypotonia, generalized muscle weakness, and respiratory complication. Symptoms are generally characterized by exercise intolerance with muscle cramps and pain. Symptoms are precipitated by 2 types of activity: brief, high-intensity exercise, such as sprinting or carrying heavy loads, and less intense but sustained activity, such as climbing stairs or walking uphill. Most patients can perform moderate exercise, such as walking on level ground, for long periods. Many patients experience a characteristic "second wind" phenomenon, with relief of muscle pain and fatigue after a brief period of rest. As a result of the underlying myopathy, these patients may be at

risk for statin-induced myopathy and rhabdomyolysis. While patients typically experience episodic muscle pain and cramping from exercise, 35% of patients with McArdle disease report permanent pain that has a serious impact on sleep and other activities. Studies also suggest that there may also be a link between GSD V and variable cognitive impairment.

Approximately 50% of patients report burgundy-colored urine after exercise as a result of exercise-induced **myoglobinuria** secondary to **rhabdomyolysis**. Excessive myoglobinuria after intense exercise may precipitate acute renal failure.

Lab findings show elevated levels of serum CK at rest, which further increases after exercise. Exercise also elevates the levels of blood ammonia, inosine, hypoxanthine, and uric acid, which may be attributed to accelerated recycling of muscle purine nucleotides caused by insufficient ATP production. Type V GSD is an autosomal recessive disorder. The gene for muscle phosphorylase *(PYGM)* has been mapped to chromosome 11q13.

Diagnosis

The standard diagnosis for GSD V includes a muscle biopsy to measure glycogen content as well as enzyme and sequencing of *PYGM*. An ischemic exercise test offers a rapid diagnostic screening for patients with a metabolic myopathy. Lack of an increase in blood lactate levels and exaggerated blood ammonia elevations indicate muscle glycogenosis and suggest a defect in the conversion of muscle glycogen or glucose to lactate. The abnormal ischemic exercise response is *not limited* to type V GSD. Other muscle defects in glycogenolysis or glycolysis produce similar results (deficiencies of muscle phosphofructokinase, phosphoglycerate kinase, phosphoglycerate mutase, or LDH). An ischemic exercise test was once used to be a rapid diagnostic screening for suspected patients but was associated with severe complications and false-positive results. A nonischemic forearm exercise test with high sensitivity that is easy to perform and cost-effective has been determined to be indicative of muscle glycogenosis. However, as with the ischemic test, it cannot differentiate between abnormal exercise responses due to type V disease versus other defects in glycogenolysis or glycolysis or debranching enzyme (noted when the test is done after fasting).

The diagnosis is confirmed by molecular genetic testing of PYGM. A common nonsense variant, p.R49X in exon 1, is found in 90% of Caucasian patients, and a deletion of a single codon in exon 17 is found in 61% of Japanese patients. The p.R49X variant represents 55% of alleles in Spanish patients, whereas the p.W797R variant represents 14% and the p.G204S 9% of pathogenic alleles in the Spanish population. There seems to be an association between clinical severity of GSD V and presence of the D allele of the ACE insertion/deletion polymorphism. This may help explain the spectrum of phenotypic variability manifested in this disorder.

Treatment

Avoidance of strenuous exercise prevents the symptoms; regular and moderate exercise is recommended to improve exercise capacity. Glucose or sucrose given before exercise or injection of glucagon can greatly improve tolerance in these patients. A high-protein diet may increase muscle endurance, and low-dose creatine supplement has been shown to improve muscle function in some patients. The clinical response to creatine is dose dependent; muscle pain may increase on high doses of creatine supplementation. Vitamin B_6 supplementation reduces exercise intolerance and muscle cramps. Longevity is not generally affected.

Type VII Glycogen Storage Disease (Muscle Phosphofructokinase Deficiency, Tarui Disease)

Type VII GSD is caused by pathogenic variants in the *PFKM* gene, located on chromosome 12q13.1, which results in a deficiency of **muscle phosphofructokinase** enzyme. This enzyme is a key regulatory enzyme of glycolysis and is necessary for the ATP-dependent conversion of fructose-6-phosphate to fructose-1,6-diphosphate. Phosphofructokinase is composed of 3 isoenzyme subunits according to the tissue type and are encoded by different genes: (*PFKM* [M: muscle], *PFKL* [L: liver], and *PFKP* [P: platelet]). Skeletal muscle has only the M subunit, whereas red blood cells (RBCs) express a hybrid of L and M forms. In type VII GSD the M isoenzyme is defective, resulting in complete deficiency of enzyme activity in muscle and a partial deficiency in RBCs.

Type VII GSD is an autosomal recessive disorder with increased prevalence in individuals of Japanese ancestry and Ashkenazi Jews. A splicing defect and a nucleotide deletion in *PFKM* account for 95% of pathogenic variants in Ashkenazi Jews. Diagnosis based on molecular testing for the common variants is thus possible in this population.

Clinical Manifestations

Although the clinical picture is similar to that of type V GSD, the following features of type VII GSD are distinctive:

1. Exercise intolerance, which usually commences in childhood, is more severe than in type V disease and may be associated with nausea, vomiting, and severe muscle pain; vigorous exercise causes severe muscle cramps and myoglobinuria.
2. Compensatory hemolysis occurs, as indicated by an increased level of serum bilirubin and an elevated reticulocyte count.
3. Hyperuricemia is common and exaggerated by muscle exercise to a greater degree than that observed in type V or III GSD.
4. An abnormal polysaccharide is present in muscle fibers; it is PAS positive but resistant to diastase digestion.
5. Exercise intolerance is especially worse after carbohydrate-rich meals because the ingested glucose prevents lipolysis, thereby depriving muscle of fatty acid and ketone substrates. This is in contrast to patients with type V disease, who can metabolize blood borne glucose derived from either endogenous liver glycogenolysis or exogenous glucose; indeed, glucose infusion improves exercise tolerance in type V patients.
6. The "second wind" phenomenon is absent because of the inability to break down blood glucose.

Several rare type VII variants occur. One variant presents in infancy with hypotonia and limb weakness and proceeds to a rapidly progressive myopathy that leads to death by 4 yr of age. A 2nd variant occurs in infancy and results in congenital myopathy and arthrogryposis with a fatal outcome. A 3rd variant presents in infancy with hypotonia, mild developmental delay, and seizures. An additional presentation is *hereditary nonspherocytic hemolytic anemia*. Although these patients do not experience muscle symptoms, it remains unclear whether these symptoms will develop later in life. One variant presents in adults and is characterized by a slowly progressive, fixed muscle weakness rather than cramps and myoglobinuria. It may also cause mitral valve thickening from glycogen buildup.

Diagnosis

To establish a diagnosis, a biochemical or histochemical demonstration of the enzymatic defect in the muscle is required. The absence of the M isoenzyme of phosphofructokinase can also be demonstrated in muscle, blood cells, and fibroblasts. Gene sequencing can identify pathogenic variants for the phosphofructokinase gene.

Treatment

There is no specific treatment. Strenuous exercise should be avoided to prevent acute episodes of muscle cramps and myoglobinuria. Consuming simple carbohydrates before strenuous exercise may benefit by improving exercise tolerance. A ketogenic diet has been reported to show clinical improvement in a patient with infantile GSD VII. Drugs such as statins should be avoided. Precautionary measures should be taken to avoid hyperthermia while undergoing anesthesia. Carbohydrate meals and glucose infusions have demonstrated worsening symptoms because of the body's inability to utilize glucose. The administered glucose tends to lower the levels of fatty acids in the blood, a primary source of muscle fuel.

Muscle-Specific Phosphorylase Kinase Deficiency (From *PHKA1* Variants)

A few cases of PhK deficiency restricted to muscle are known. Patients, both male and female, present either with muscle cramps and

myoglobinuria with exercise or with progressive muscle weakness and atrophy. PhK activity is decreased in muscle but normal in liver and blood cells. There is no hepatomegaly or cardiomegaly. This is inherited in an X-linked or autosomal recessive manner. The gene for the muscle-specific form α subunit (αM) is located at Xq12. Pathogenic variants of the gene have been found in some male patients with this disorder. The gene for muscle γ subunit (γM, *PHKG1*) is on chromosome 7p12. No pathogenic variants in this gene have been reported so far.

Other Muscle Glycogenoses With Muscle Energy Impairment

Six additional defects in enzymes—phosphoglycerate kinase, phosphoglycerate mutase, lactate dehydrogenase, fructose-1,6-bisphosphate aldolase A, muscle pyruvate kinase, and β-enolase in the pathway of the terminal glycolysis—cause symptoms and signs of muscle energy impairment similar to those of types V and VII GSD. The failure of blood lactate to increase in response to exercise is a useful diagnostic test and can be used to differentiate muscle glycogenoses from disorders of lipid metabolism, such as carnitine palmitoyltransferase II deficiency and very-long-chain acyl-CoA dehydrogenase deficiency, which also cause muscle cramps and myoglobinuria. Muscle glycogen levels can be normal in the disorders affecting terminal glycolysis, and assaying the muscle enzyme activity is needed to make a definitive diagnosis. There is no specific treatment (see preceding Treatment section).

Bibliography is available at Expert Consult.

105.2 Defects in Galactose Metabolism
Priya S. Kishnani and Yuan-Tsong Chen

Milk and dairy products contain **lactose**, the major dietary source of galactose. The metabolism of galactose produces fuel for cellular metabolism through its conversion to glucose-1-phosphate (see Table 105.1). Galactose also plays an important role in the formation of galactosides, which include glycoproteins, glycolipids, and glycosaminoglycans. **Galactosemia** denotes the elevated level of galactose in the blood and is found in 3 distinct inborn errors of galactose metabolism in 1 of the following enzymes: galactose-1-phosphate uridyl transferase, galactokinase, and uridine diphosphate galactose-4-epimerase. The term galactosemia, although adequate for the deficiencies in any of these disorders, generally designates the *transferase* deficiency.

GALACTOSE-1-PHOSPHATE URIDYL TRANSFERASE DEFICIENCY GALACTOSEMIA

Two forms of the deficiency exist: infants with complete or near-complete deficiency of the enzyme (classic galactosemia) and those with partial transferase deficiency. **Classic galactosemia** is a serious disease with onset of symptoms typically by the 2nd half of the 1st wk of life. The incidence is predicted to be 1 in 60,000 live births. The newborn infant receives high amounts of lactose (up to 40% in breast milk and certain formulas), which consists of equal parts of glucose and galactose. Without the transferase enzyme, the infant is unable to metabolize galactose-1-phosphate, the accumulation of which results in injury to kidney, liver, and brain. This injury may begin prenatally in the affected fetus by transplacental galactose derived from the diet of the heterozygous mother or by endogenous production of galactose in the fetus.

Clinical Manifestations

The diagnosis of uridyl transferase deficiency should be considered in newborn or young infants with any of the following features within a few days or weeks after birth: jaundice, hepatomegaly, vomiting, hypoglycemia, seizures, lethargy, feeding difficulties, poor weight gain or failure to regain birthweight, and aminoaciduria. Untreated children may show nuclear cataracts, vitreous hemorrhage, hepatic failure, cirrhosis, ascites, splenomegaly, or intellectual disability. Patients with galactosemia are at increased risk for *Escherichia coli* neonatal sepsis; the onset of sepsis often precedes the diagnosis of galactosemia. Pseudotumor cerebri can occur and cause a bulging fontanel. Complete withdrawal of lactose from the diet results in improvement of the acute symptoms. If untreated, death from liver and kidney failure and sepsis may follow within days. When the diagnosis is not made at birth, damage to the liver (cirrhosis) and brain (intellectual disability) becomes increasingly severe and irreversible.

Partial transferase deficiency is generally asymptomatic. It is more common than classic galactosemia and is diagnosed in newborn screening because of moderately elevated blood galactose and/or low transferase activity. Galactosemia should be considered for the newborn or young infant who is not thriving or who has any of the preceding findings. Light and electron microscopy of hepatic tissue reveals fatty infiltration, the formation of pseudoacini, and eventual macronodular cirrhosis. These changes are consistent with a metabolic disease but do not indicate the precise enzymatic defect.

Diagnosis

The *initial* diagnosis of galactosemia is done by demonstration of a **reducing substance** in several urine specimens collected while the patient is on a diet containing human milk, cow's milk, or any other formula containing lactose. The reducing substance detected in urine by Clinitest (e.g., glucose, galactose) can be identified by chromatography or an enzymatic test specific for galactose. Galactose can be detected in urine, provided the milk feeding was within the last few hours and the child is not vomiting excessively. Clinistix urine test results are usually negative because the test relies on the action of glucose oxidase, which is specific for glucose but is nonreactive with galactose. Amino acids may be detected in urine since they are excreted together with glucose because of a proximal renal tubular syndrome. Since galactose is injurious to persons with galactosemia, diagnostic challenge tests dependent on administering galactose orally or intravenously should not be used. *Direct enzyme assay using erythrocytes establishes the diagnosis.* The clinician needs to confirm that the patient did not receive a blood transfusion before the collection of the blood sample, because a diagnosis could be missed. A novel method utilizes nonradioactive ultraviolet (UV) light and high-performance liquid chromatography (HPLC) to accurately detect levels of galactose-1-phosphate uridyl transferase in erythrocytes.

Genetics

Transferase deficiency is an autosomal recessive disorder. Based on newborn screening in the United States, the frequency of the disease is approximately 1 in 47,000 live births. There are several enzymatic variants of galactosemia. The *Duarte variant,* a single–amino acid substitution (p.N314D), has diminished RBC enzyme activity (50% of normal), but usually is of no clinical significance. This variant is the most common, with a carrier frequency of 12% in the general population. Those who are heterozygous for the Duarte variant of galactosemia typically have 25% of normal galactose activity, few symptoms, elevated metabolites, and no need for intervention. Other similar variants expressing little enzyme activity typically require no intervention. Some black patients have milder symptoms despite the absence of measurable transferase activity in erythrocytes; these patients retain 10% enzyme activity in liver and intestinal mucosa, whereas most white patients have no detectable activity in any of these tissues. More than 230 identifiable pathogenic variants have been associated with transferase deficiency. In blacks, 62% of alleles are represented by the p.S135L variant, a variant that is responsible for a milder disease course. In the white population, 70% of alleles are represented by the p.Q188R and p.K285N missense variants and are associated with severe disease. Carrier testing and prenatal diagnosis can be performed by direct enzyme analysis of amniocytes or chorionic villi; testing can also be DNA based.

Treatment and Prognosis

With the availability of newborn screening for galactosemia, it is possible to identify and treat patients earlier than before. All galactose-containing foods should be removed from the diet on initial suspicion of galactosemia. Various non–lactose-containing milk substitutes are available (casein hydrolysates, soybean-based formula). Elimination of galactose from the diet along with adequate calcium supplementation reverses growth failure and renal and hepatic dysfunction. Cataracts regress, and most patients have no impairment of vision. Early diagnosis and treatment have improved the prognosis of galactosemia. On long-term follow-up, however, patients still manifest ovarian failure with primary or secondary amenorrhea, decreased bone mineral density, developmental delay, and learning disabilities that increase in severity with age. *Hypergonadotropic hypogonadism* is reported in 80% to >90% of female patients with classic galactosemia. Although most women with classic galactosemia are infertile when they reach childbearing age, a small number have given birth. Most patients manifest speech disorders, whereas a smaller number demonstrate poor growth and impaired motor function and balance (with or without overt ataxia). The relative control of galactose-1-phosphate levels does not always correlate with long-term outcome, leading to the belief that other factors, such as elevated galactitol, decreased uridine diphosphate galactose (a donor for galactolipids and proteins), and endogenous galactose production may be responsible.

GALACTOKINASE DEFICIENCY

The deficient enzyme is **galactokinase**, which normally catalyzes the phosphorylation of galactose. The principal metabolites accumulated are galactose and galactitol. Two genes are reported to encode galactokinase: *GK1* on chromosome 17q24 and *GK2* on chromosome 15. **Cataracts** are usually the sole manifestation of galactokinase deficiency; pseudotumor cerebri is a rare complication. The affected infant is otherwise asymptomatic. Heterozygous carriers may be at risk for presenile cataracts. Lab findings show an increased concentration of blood galactose levels, provided the infant has been fed a lactose-containing formula. The diagnosis is made by demonstrating an absence of galactokinase activity in erythrocytes or fibroblasts. Transferase activity is normal. Treatment is dietary restriction of galactose.

URIDINE DIPHOSPHATE GALACTOSE-4-EPIMERASE DEFICIENCY

There are 2 distinct forms of **epimerase** deficiency. The first is a **benign** form that is diagnosed incidentally through newborn screening programs. Affected individuals are asymptomatic because the enzyme deficiency is limited to leukocytes and erythrocytes. This form does not require treatment. The second variety is **severe** because the epimerase deficiency is more generalized. Clinical manifestations resemble transferase deficiency, with the additional symptoms of hypotonia and nerve deafness. Clinical symptoms improve with restriction of galactose in diet. Although the severe form of galactosemia is rare, it must be considered in a symptomatic patient with measurable galactose-1-phosphate who has normal transferase activity. The abnormally accumulated metabolites are similar to those in transferase deficiency; however, there is also an increase in cellular uridine diphosphate (UDP) galactose. Diagnosis is confirmed by the assay of epimerase in erythrocytes.

Patients with the severe form of epimerase deficiency cannot synthesize UDP galactose from UDP glucose and are galactose dependent. Because galactose is an essential component of many nervous system structural proteins, patients are placed on a galactose-restricted diet rather than a galactose-free diet.

Infants with the mild form of epimerase deficiency have not required treatment. It is advisable to follow urine specimens for reducing substances and exclude aminoaciduria within a few weeks of diagnosis while the infant is still on lactose-containing formula.

The gene for UDP galactose-4-epimerase *(GALE)* is located on chromosome 1 at 1p36. Carrier detection is possible by measurement of epimerase activity in the erythrocytes. **Prenatal diagnosis** for the severe form of epimerase deficiency can be done using an enzyme assay of cultured amniotic fluid cells.

Bibliography is available at Expert Consult.

105.3 Defects in Fructose Metabolism
Priya S. Kishnani and Yuan-Tsong Chen

Two inborn errors are known in the specialized pathway of fructose metabolism: benign or essential fructosuria and hereditary fructose intolerance. Fructose-1,6-bisphosphatase deficiency, although strictly speaking not a defect of the specialized fructose pathway, is discussed in Chapter 105.4.

DEFICIENCY OF FRUCTOKINASE (ESSENTIAL OR BENIGN FRUCTOSURIA)
Deficiency of fructokinase is not associated with any clinical manifestations. **Fructosuria** is an accidental finding usually made because the asymptomatic patient's urine contains a reducing substance. No treatment is necessary, and the prognosis is excellent. Inheritance is autosomal recessive with an incidence of 1 in 120,000 live births. The gene encoding fructokinase (*KHK*) is located on chromosome 2p23.3.

Fructokinase catalyzes the first step of metabolism of dietary fructose: conversion of fructose to fructose-1-phosphate (see Fig. 105.1). Without this enzyme, ingested fructose is not metabolized; its level is increased in the blood, and it is excreted in urine because practically no renal threshold exists for fructose. Clinitest results reveal the urinary reducing substance, which can be identified as fructose by chromatography.

DEFICIENCY OF FRUCTOSE-1,6-BISPHOSPHATE ALDOLASE (ALDOLASE B, HEREDITARY FRUCTOSE INTOLERANCE)
Deficiency of fructose-1,6-bisphosphate aldolase (**aldolase-B**) is a severe condition of infants caused by a deficiency of aldolase B activity in the liver, kidney, and intestine. This enzyme catalyzes the hydrolysis of fructose-1,6-bisphosphate into triose phosphate and glyceraldehyde phosphate. The same enzyme also hydrolyzes fructose-1-phosphate. In the absence of enzyme activity, there is a rapid accumulation of fructose-1-phosphate, which presents with severe symptoms when fructose-containing food is ingested.

Epidemiology and Genetics
The exact incidence of **hereditary fructose intolerance (HFI)** is unknown but is estimated to be as high as 1 in every 26,000 live births. HFI is inherited in an autosomal recessive manner. The *ALDOB* gene is mapped to chromosome 9q22.3. At least 40 pathogenic variants causing HFI are known. The most common pathogenic variant identified in northern Europeans is a single missense variant, a G→C transversion in exon 5 resulting in the normal alanine at position 149 being replaced by proline. This variant, along with 2 other missense variants (p.A174D and p.N334K), account for 80–85% of HFI in Europe and the United States. Diagnosis of HFI can be made by direct DNA analysis for the common variants and phosphorus magnetic resonance spectroscopy.

Clinical Manifestations
Affected individuals remain asymptomatic until fructose or sucrose (table sugar) is introduced in diet (usually from fruit, fruit juice, or sweetened cereal). Signs and symptoms typically manifest in infancy when foods or formulas containing these sugars are introduced. Certain patients are very sensitive to fructose, whereas others can tolerate moderate intakes (up to 250 mg/kg/day). The average intake of fructose in Western societies is 1-2 g/kg/day. Early clinical manifestations resemble galactosemia and include jaundice, hepatomegaly, vomiting, lethargy, irritability, and convulsions. There may also be a higher incidence of *celiac disease* in HFI patients (>10%) than in the general population (1–3%). As they grow older, patients usually develop an aversion to fructose-containing foods due to associated symptoms of nausea, vomiting, and abdominal pain.

Characteristic lab findings include lactic acidosis, hypophosphatemia, hyperuricemia, and hypermagnesemia. A prolonged clotting time, hypoalbuminemia, elevation of bilirubin and transaminase levels, and proximal tubular dysfunction are also seen. Acute fructose ingestion produces symptomatic hypoglycemia; the higher the intake, the more severe the clinical picture. Chronic ingestion results in failure to thrive and hepatic disease. If the intake of fructose persists, hypoglycemic episodes recur, leading to progressive renal and hepatic failure and eventually death.

Diagnosis
The presence of a reducing substance in urine during an acute episode raises the possibility of HFI. Oral fructose challenge is *no longer* considered a diagnostic approach because of high risk to the patient, who can become acutely ill after the test. Definitive diagnosis is made by demonstration of 2 pathogenic variants in *ALDOB* on molecular genetic testing. A common pathogenic variant (substitution of *Pro* for *Ala* at position 149) accounts for 53% of HFI alleles worldwide. An alternative is to show deficient hepatic fructose 1-phosphate aldolase (aldolase B) activity on liver biopsy.

Treatment
Acute episodes are managed symptomatically by correcting hypoglycemia with IV glucose (dextrose) administration, providing supportive treatment of hepatic insufficiency, and correcting metabolic acidosis. Complete elimination of fructose usually rapidly reverses symptoms and results in normalization of related metabolic disturbances. The cornerstone of long-term treatment is the complete restriction of all sources of sucrose, fructose, and sorbitol from the diet. It may be difficult because these sugars are widely used additives, found even in most medicinal preparations. With treatment, liver and kidney dysfunction improves, and catch-up in growth is common. Intellectual development is usually unimpaired. As the patient matures, symptoms become milder even after fructose ingestion; the long-term prognosis is good. Because of voluntary dietary avoidance of sucrose, affected patients have few dental caries. Care should be taken to avoid fructose-containing IV fluids during hospitalizations.

Bibliography is available at Expert Consult.

105.4 Defects in Intermediary Carbohydrate Metabolism Associated With Lactic Acidosis
Priya S. Kishnani and Yuan-Tsong Chen

Lactic acidosis (**type B3**) occurs with defects of carbohydrate metabolism that interfere with the conversion of pyruvate to glucose via the pathway of gluconeogenesis or to carbon dioxide and water via the mitochondrial enzymes of the Krebs cycle. Fig. 105.4 depicts the relevant metabolic pathways. Type I GSD, fructose-1,6-diphosphatase deficiency, and phosphoenolpyruvate carboxylase deficiency are disorders of gluconeogenesis associated with lactic acidosis. Pyruvate dehydrogenase complex deficiency, respiratory chain defects, and pyruvate carboxylase deficiency are disorders in the pathway of pyruvate metabolism causing lactic acidosis. Lactic acidosis (type B3) can also occur in defects of fatty acid oxidation, organic acidurias (see Chapters 103.6, 103.10, and 104.1), or biotin utilization diseases (type B3) (Table 105.2). These disorders are easily distinguishable by the presence of abnormal acyl carnitine profiles, amino acids in the blood, and unusual organic acids in the urine. Blood lactate, pyruvate, and acyl carnitine profiles, and the presence of these unusual urine organic acids should be determined in infants and children with unexplained acidosis, especially if there is an increase of anion gap.

Lactic acidosis unrelated to an enzymatic defect occurs in hypoxemia (**type A** lactic acidosis). In this case, as well as in defects in the respiratory chain, the serum pyruvate concentration may remain normal (<1.0 mg/dL, with increased lactate:pyruvate ratio), whereas pyruvate is usually increased when lactic acidosis results from an enzymatic defect in gluconeogenesis or pyruvate dehydrogenase complex (both lactate and pyruvate are increased, and the ratio is normal). Lactate and pyruvate should be measured in the same blood specimen and on multiple blood specimens obtained when the patient is symptomatic because lactic acidosis can be intermittent. Fig. 105.5 is an algorithm for the differential diagnosis of lactic acidosis. Lactic acidosis is also noted with various underlying diseases (**type B1**) and drugs or toxins (**type B2**) (Table 105.2).

DISORDERS OF GLUCONEOGENESIS
Deficiency of Glucose-6-Phosphatase (Type I Glycogen Storage Disease)
Type I GSD is the only glycogenosis associated with significant **lactic acidosis**. The chronic metabolic acidosis predisposes these patients to osteopenia; after prolonged fasting, the acidosis associated with hypoglycemia is a life-threatening condition (see Chapter 105.1).

Fructose-1,6-Diphosphatase Deficiency
Fructose-1,6-diphosphatase deficiency impairs the formation of glucose from all gluconeogenic precursors, including dietary fructose. Hypoglycemia occurs when glycogen reserves are limited or exhausted. The **clinical manifestations** are characterized by life-threatening episodes of acidosis, hypoglycemia, hyperventilation, convulsions, and coma. In about half the cases, the deficiency presents in the 1st wk of life. In infants and small children, episodes are triggered by febrile infections and gastroenteritis if oral food intake decreases. The frequency of the attacks decreases with age. Laboratory findings include low blood glucose, high lactate and uric acid levels, and metabolic acidosis. In contrast to

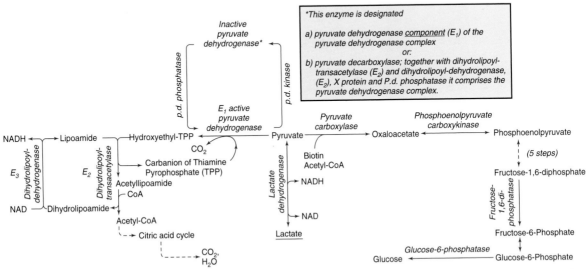

Fig. 105.4 Enzymatic reactions of carbohydrate metabolism, deficiencies of which can give rise to lactic acidosis, pyruvate elevations, or hypoglycemia. The pyruvate dehydrogenase complex comprises, in addition to E_1, E_2, and E_3, an extra lipoate-containing protein (not shown), called protein X, and pyruvate dehydrogenase phosphatase.

Table 105.2	Causes of Type B Lactic Acidosis

TYPE B1—UNDERLYING DISEASES Renal failure Hepatic failure Diabetes mellitus Malignancy Systemic inflammatory response syndrome Human immunodeficiency virus **TYPE B2—DRUGS AND TOXINS** Acetaminophen Alcohols—ethanol, methanol, diethylene glycol, isopropanol, and propylene glycol Antiretroviral nucleoside analogs—zidovudine, didanosine, and lamivudine β-Adrenergic agonists—epinephrine, ritodrine, and terbutaline Biguanides—phenformin and metformin Cocaine, methamphetamine Cyanogenic compounds—cyanide, aliphatic nitriles, and nitroprusside Diethyl ether Fluorouracil Halothane Iron Isoniazid Linezolid Nalidixic acid Niacin	Propopol Salicylates Strychnine Sugars and sugar alcohols—fructose, sorbitol, and xylitol Sulfasalazine Total parenteral nutrition Valproic acid Vitamin deficiencies—thiamine and biotin **TYPE B3—INBORN ERRORS OF METABOLISM** Glucose-6-phosphatase deficiency (von Gierke disease) Fructose-1,6-diphosphatase deficiency Phosphoenolpyruvate carboxykinase deficiency Pyruvate carboxylase deficiency Pyruvate dehydrogenase complex (PDHC) deficiency Krebs cycle defects Methylmalonic aciduria and other organic acidemias Kearns-Sayre syndrome Pearson syndrome Barth syndrome Mitochondrial DNA depletion syndromes Nuclear DNA respiratory chain defects Mitochondrial DNA respiratory defects Mitochondrial encephalomyopathy, lactic acidosis, and stroke-like episodes (MELAS) Myoclonic epilepsy with ragged red fibers (MERRF)

Adapted from Vernon C, LeTourneau JL: Lactic acidosis: recognition, kinetics, and associated prognosis, Crit Care Clin 26:255–283, 2010 (Box 1, p 264).

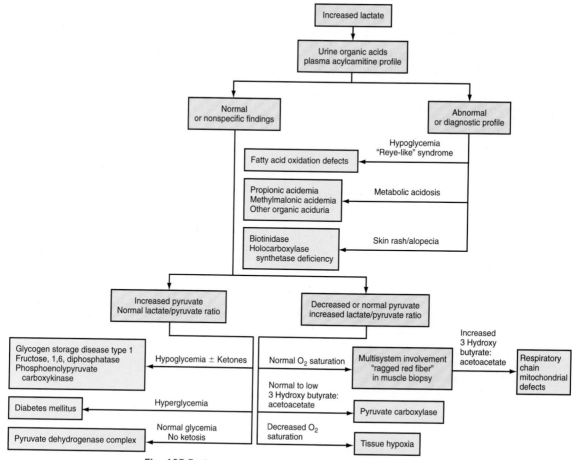

Fig. 105.5 Algorithm of the differential diagnosis of lactic acidosis.

HFI, there is usually no aversion to sweets; renal tubular and liver function is normal.

The **diagnosis** is established by demonstrating an enzyme deficiency in either liver or intestinal biopsy. The enzyme defect can also be demonstrated in leukocytes in some cases. The gene coding for fructose-1,6-diphosphatase *(FBP1)* is located on chromosome 9q22; pathogenic variants are characterized, making carrier detection and prenatal diagnosis possible. **Treatment** of acute attacks consists of correction of hypoglycemia and acidosis by IV glucose infusion; the response is usually rapid. Avoidance of fasting, aggressive management of infections, and restriction of fructose and sucrose from the diet can prevent further episodes. For long-term prevention of hypoglycemia, a slowly released carbohydrate such as cornstarch is useful. Patients who survive childhood develop normally.

Phosphoenolpyruvate Carboxykinase Deficiency
Phosphoenolpyruvate carboxykinase (**PEPCK**) is a key enzyme in gluconeogenesis. It catalyzes the conversion of oxaloacetate to phosphoenolpyruvate (see Fig. 105.4). PEPCK deficiency is both a mitochondrial enzyme deficiency and a cytosolic enzyme deficiency, encoded by 2 distinct genes.

PEPCK deficiency has been reported in only a few cases. The clinical features are heterogeneous, with hypoglycemia, lactic acidemia, hepatomegaly, hypotonia, developmental delay, and failure to thrive as the major manifestations. There may be multisystem involvement, with neuromuscular deficits, hepatocellular damage, renal dysfunction, and cardiomyopathy. The **diagnosis** is based on the reduced

activity of PEPCK in liver, fibroblasts, or lymphocytes. Fibroblasts and lymphocytes are not suitable for diagnosing the cytosolic form of PEPCK deficiency because these tissues possess only mitochondrial PEPCK. To avoid hypoglycemia, patients should receive **treatment** with slow-release carbohydrates such as cornstarch, and fasting should be avoided.

DISORDERS OF PYRUVATE METABOLISM
Pyruvate is formed from glucose and other monosaccharides, from lactate, and from alanine. It is metabolized through 4 main enzyme systems: lactate dehydrogenase, alanine transaminase, pyruvate carboxylase, and pyruvate dehydrogenase complex. Deficiency of the M subunit of LDH causes exercise intolerance and myoglobinuria (see Chapter 105.1).

Pyruvate Dehydrogenase Complex Deficiency
After entering the mitochondria, pyruvate is converted into acetyl-CoA by the pyruvate dehydrogenase complex (**PDHC**), which catalyzes the oxidation of pyruvate to acetyl-CoA, which then enters the tricarboxylic acid cycle for ATP production. The complex comprises 5 components: E_1, an α-ketoacid decarboxylase; E_2, a dihydrolipoyl transacylase; E_3, a dihydrolipoyl dehydrogenase; **protein X**, an extra lipoate-containing protein; and pyruvate dehydrogenase phosphatase. The most common is a defect in the E_1 (see Fig. 105.4).

Deficiency of the PDHC is the most common of the disorders leading to lactic acidemia and CNS dysfunction. The CNS dysfunction occurs because the brain obtains its energy primarily from oxidation of glucose. Brain acetyl-CoA is synthesized almost exclusively from pyruvate.

The E_1 defects are caused by pathogenic variants in the gene coding for E_1 α subunit, which is X-linked dominant. Although X-linked, its deficiency is a problem in both male and female patients, despite only one E_1 α allele in females carrying a variant.

Clinical Manifestations

PDHC deficiency has a wide spectrum of presentations, from the most severe neonatal presentation to a mild late-onset form. The **neonatal onset** is associated with lethal lactic acidosis, white matter cystic lesions, agenesis of the corpus callosum, and the most severe enzyme deficiency. **Infantile onset** can be lethal or associated with psychomotor delay and chronic lactic acidosis, cystic lesions in the brainstem and basal ganglia, and pathologic features resembling **Leigh disease** (see later and Chapter 616.2). Neurologic symptoms in PDHC can be categorized into 2 groups: abnormal brain development, seen in both males and females, and brain lesions and epilepsy, seen in male patients only. Older children, usually boys, may have less acidosis, have greater enzyme activity, and manifest ataxia with high-carbohydrate diets. Intelligence may be normal. Patients of all ages may have facial dysmorphology, features similar to those of fetal alcohol syndrome.

The E_2 and **protein X–lipoate** defects are rare and result in severe psychomotor retardation. The E_3 **lipoamide dehydrogenase** defect leads to deficient activity not only in the PDHC, but also in the α-ketoglutarate and branched-chain ketoacid dehydrogenase complexes. This deficiency is more common in the Ashkenazi Jewish population. The reactive oxygen species generated by the pathogenic variants responsible for lipoamide dehydrogenase deficiency may in fact explain certain disease characteristics and suggest the utility of antioxidant therapy. **Pyruvate dehydrogenase phosphatase** deficiency has also been reported. These other PDHC defects have clinical manifestations within the variable spectrum associated with PDHC deficiency caused by E_1 deficiency.

Treatment

The general prognosis is poor, except in rare patients in whom variants are associated with altered affinity for thiamine pyrophosphate, who may respond to thiamine supplementation. Because carbohydrates can aggravate lactic acidosis, a ketogenic diet is recommended. The diet has been found to lower the blood lactate level; the long-term benefit to patient outcome is unclear. A potential treatment strategy is to maintain any residual PDHC in its active form by oral administration of **dichloroacetate**, an inhibitor of E_1 kinase. Beneficial effects of controlling postprandial lactic acidosis have been shown in some patients. Young children with congenital acidosis generally tolerate dichloroacetate well, but continued exposure is associated with peripheral neuropathy, a condition that could be attributable to the drug or the disease.

Deficiency of Pyruvate Carboxylase

Pyruvate carboxylase is a mitochondrial, biotin-containing enzyme essential in the process of gluconeogenesis; it catalyzes the conversion of pyruvate to oxaloacetate. The enzyme is also essential for Krebs cycle function as a provider of oxaloacetate and is involved in lipogenesis and formation of nonessential amino acids. **Clinical manifestations** of this deficiency have varied from neonatal severe lactic acidosis accompanied by hyperammonemia, citrullinemia, and hyperlysinemia (**type B**) to late-onset mild to moderate lactic acidosis and developmental delay (**type A**). In both types, patients who survived usually had severe psychomotor retardation with seizures, spasticity, and microcephaly. Some patients have pathologic changes in the brainstem and basal ganglia that resemble **Leigh disease**. The clinical severity appears to correlate with the level of the residual enzyme activity. A "benign" form of pyruvate carboxylase deficiency has also been described, characterized by recurrent attacks of lactic acidosis and mild neurologic deficits (**type C**). Laboratory findings are characterized by elevated levels of blood lactate, pyruvate, alanine, and ketonuria. In the case of type B, blood ammonia, citrulline, and lysine levels are also elevated, which might suggest a primary defect of the urea cycle. The mechanism is likely

caused by depletion of oxaloacetate, which leads to reduced levels of aspartate, a substrate for argininosuccinate synthase in the urea cycle (see Chapter 103.12). The gene for pyruvate carboxylase (*PC*) is located on chromosome 11q13.4-q13.5, and about 15 pathogenic variants have been identified.

Treatment consists of avoidance of fasting and eating a carbohydrate meal before bedtime. During acute episodes of lactic acidosis, patients should receive continuous IV glucose. Aspartate and citrate supplements restore the metabolic abnormalities; whether this treatment can prevent the neurologic deficits is not known. Liver transplantation has been attempted; its benefit remains unknown. **Diagnosis** of pyruvate carboxylase deficiency is made by the measurement of enzyme activity in liver or cultured skin fibroblasts and must be differentiated from holocarboxylase synthase or biotinidase deficiency.

Deficiency of Pyruvate Carboxylase Secondary to Deficiency of Holocarboxylase Synthase or Biotinidase

Deficiency of either holocarboxylase synthase (**HCS**) or biotinidase, which are enzymes of biotin metabolism, result in multiple-carboxylase deficiency (pyruvate carboxylase and other biotin-requiring carboxylases and metabolic reactions) and in **clinical manifestations** associated with the respective deficiencies, as well as rash, lactic acidosis, and alopecia (see Chapter 103.6). The course of HCS or biotinidase deficiency can be protracted, with intermittent exacerbation of chronic lactic acidosis, failure to thrive, seizures, and hypotonia leading to spasticity, lethargy, coma, and death. Auditory and optic nerve dysfunction can lead to deafness and blindness, respectively. Late-onset milder forms have also been reported. Laboratory findings include metabolic acidosis and abnormal organic acids in the urine. In HCS deficiency, biotin concentrations in plasma and urine are normal. **Diagnosis** can be made in skin fibroblasts or lymphocytes by assay for HCS activity, and in the case of biotinidase, in the serum by a screening blood spot.

Treatment consists of biotin supplementation, 5-20 mg/day, and is generally effective if treatment is started before the development of brain damage. Patients identified through newborn screening and treated with biotin have remained asymptomatic.

Both enzyme deficiencies are autosomal recessive disorders. The incidence of HCS deficiency is approximately 1 in 87,000 live births. *HCS* and biotinidase (*BTD*) are located on chromosome 21q22 and 3p25, respectively. Ethnic-specific pathogenic variants in the *HCS* gene have been identified. Two common pathogenic variants (del7/ins3 and p.R538C) in the *BTD* account for 52% of all pathogenic alleles in symptomatic patients with biotinidase deficiency.

Mitochondrial Respiratory Chain Defects (Oxidative Phosphorylation Disease)

The mitochondrial respiratory chain catalyzes the oxidation of fuel molecules and transfers the electrons to molecular oxygen with concomitant energy transduction into adenosine triphosphate (**oxidative phosphorylation**) (see Chapter 106). The respiratory chain produces ATP from adenosine diphosphate and inorganic phosphate utilizing the energy from electrons transferred from nicotinamide adenine dinucleotide (NADH) or flavin adenine dinucleotide and includes 5 specific complexes (I: NADH–coenzyme Q reductase; II: succinate–coenzyme Q reductase; III: coenzyme QH_2 cytochrome-*c* reductase; IV: cytochrome-*c* oxidase; V: ATP synthase). Each complex is composed of 4-35 individual proteins and, with the exception of complex II (which is encoded solely by nuclear genes), is encoded by nuclear or mitochondrial DNA (inherited only from the mother by mitochondrial inheritance). Defects in any of these complexes or assembly systems produce chronic lactic acidosis, presumably because of a change of the reduction-oxidation state with increased concentrations of NADH (see Table 105.3).

In contrast to PDHC or pyruvate carboxylase deficiency, skeletal muscle and heart are usually involved in the respiratory chain disorders. On muscle biopsy, **ragged red fibers** indicating mitochondrial proliferation are very suggestive when present (see Fig. 105.5). Because of the ubiquitous nature of oxidative phosphorylation, a defect of the

Table 105.3 | Clinical and Genetic Heterogeneity of Disorders Related to Mutations in Mitochondrial DNA*

SYMPTOMS, SIGNS, AND FINDINGS	LARGE DELETIONS IN MITOCHONDRIAL DNA			MUTATION IN TRANSFER RNA		MUTATION IN RIBOSOMAL RNA	MUTATION IN MESSENGER RNA		
	KSS	PEO	PS	MERRF	MELAS	AID	NARP	MILS	LHON
CENTRAL NERVOUS SYSTEM									
Seizures	−	−	−	+++	+		−	+	−
Ataxia	+	−	−	+	+		+	±	−
Myoclonus	−	−	−	+	±		−	−	−
Psychomotor retardation	−	−	−	−	−		−	+	−
Psychomotor regression	+	−	−	±	+		−	+	−
Hemiparesis and hemianopia	−	−	−	−	+++		−	−	−
Cortical blindness	−	−	−	−	+		−	−	−
Migraine-like headaches	−	−	−	−	+		−	−	−
Dystonia	−	−	−	−	+		−	+	±
PERIPHERAL NERVOUS SYSTEM									
Peripheral neuropathy	±	−	−	±	±		+	−	−
MUSCLE									
Weakness and exercise intolerance	+	+++	−	+	+		+	+	−
Ophthalmoplegia	+	+	±	−	−		−	−	−
Ptosis	−	+	−	−	−		−	−	−
EYE									
Pigmentary retinopathy	+	−	−	−	−		+	±	−
Optic atrophy	−	−	−	−	−		±	±	−
BLOOD									
Sideroblastic anemia	±	−	+	−	−		−	−	−
ENDOCRINE SYSTEM									
Diabetes mellitus	±	−	−	−	±		−	−	−
Short stature	+	−	−	+	+		−	−	−
Hypoparathyroidism	±	−	−	−	−		−	−	−
HEART									
Conduction disorder	+	−	−	−	±		−	−	±
Cardiomyopathy	±	−	−	−	±	+	−	±	−
GASTROINTESTINAL SYSTEM									
Exocrine pancreatic dysfunction	±	−	+	−	−		−	−	−
Intestinal pseudoobstruction	−	−	−	−	+		−	−	−
EAR, NOSE, AND THROAT									
Sensorineural hearing loss	±	−	−	+	+	+	±	−	−
KIDNEY									
Fanconi syndrome		−	±	−	±		−	−	−
LABORATORY FINDINGS									
Lactic acidosis	+	±	+	+	+	±	±	±	−
Ragged-red fibers on muscle biopsy	+	+	±	+	+	−	−	−	−
MODE OF INHERITANCE									
Maternal	−	−	−	+	+	−	+	+	+
Sporadic	+	+	+	−	−	−	−	−	−

*Characteristic constellations of symptoms and signs are in **bold**.

+, Presence of a symptom, sign, or finding; −, absence of a symptom, sign, or finding; ±, possible presence of a symptom, sign, or finding; AID, aminoglycoside-induced deafness; KSS, Kearns-Sayre syndrome; LHON, Leber hereditary optic neuropathy; MELAS, mitochondrial encephalomyopathy, lactic acidosis, and stroke-like episodes; MERRF, myoclonic epilepsy with ragged-red fibers; MILS, maternally inherited Leigh syndrome; NARP, neuropathy, ataxia, and retinitis pigmentosa; PEO, progressive external ophthalmoplegia; PS, Pearson syndrome.

From DiMauro S, Schon EA: Mitochondrial respiratory-chain diseases, *N Engl J Med* 348:2656–2668, 2003. Copyright 2003 Massachusetts Medical Society. All rights reserved.

mitochondrial respiratory chain accounts for a vast array of clinical manifestations and should be considered in patients in all age-groups presenting with multisystem involvement. Some deficiencies resemble **Leigh disease**, whereas others cause infantile myopathies such as **MELAS** (mitochondrial encephalopathy, lactic acidosis, and stroke-like episodes), **MERRF** (myoclonic epilepsy and ragged red fibers), and **Kearns-Sayre syndrome** (external ophthalmoplegia, acidosis, retinal degeneration, heart block, myopathy, and high cerebrospinal fluid protein) (Table 105.3) (see Chapters 616.2 and 629.4). There is a higher incidence of psychiatric disorders in adults with a primary oxidative phosphorylation

disease than in the general population. Elevated serum growth and differentiation factor (GDF)-15 levels help screen for mitochondrial disorders.

Diagnosis requires demonstration of abnormalities of oxidative phosphorylation enzyme complex activities in tissues or of mitochondrial DNA or a nuclear gene coding for mitochondrial functions, or both (Fig. 105.6). Muscle histology, including EM, can detect ragged red fibers and other abnormalities typical of mitochondrial myopathies. Analysis of oxidative phosphorylation complexes I-IV from intact mitochondria isolated from fresh skeletal muscle is the most sensitive

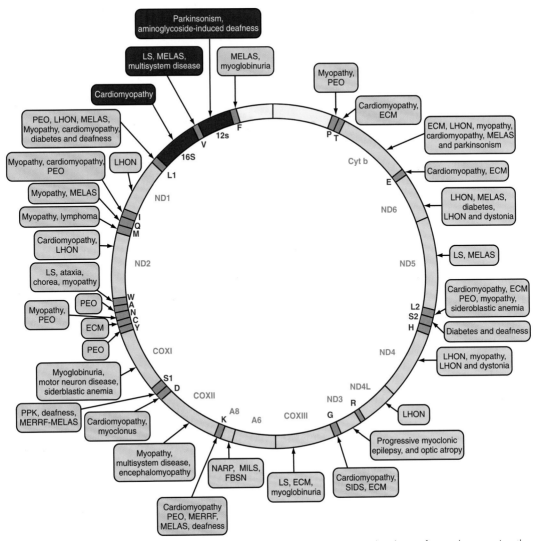

Fig. 105.6 Mutations in the human mitochondrial genome that are known to cause disease. Disorders that are frequently or prominently associated with mutations in a particular gene are shown in **bold**. Diseases caused by mutations that impair mitochondrial protein synthesis are shown in *blue*. Diseases caused by mutations in protein-coding genes are shown in *red*. ECM, Encephalomyopathy; FBSN, familial bilateral striatal necrosis; LHON, Leber hereditary optic neuropathy; LS, Leigh syndrome; MELAS, mitochondrial encephalomyopathy, lactic acidosis, and stroke-like episodes; MERRF, myoclonic epilepsy with ragged red fibers; MILS, maternally inherited Leigh syndrome; NARP, neuropathy, ataxia, and retinitis pigmentosa; PEO, progressive external ophthalmoplegia; PPK, palmoplantar keratoderma; SIDS, sudden infant death syndrome. *(From DiMauro S, Schon EA: Mitochondrial respiratory-chain diseases, N Engl J Med 348:2656–2668, 2003. Copyright 2003 Massachusetts Medical Society. All rights reserved.)*

assay for mitochondrial disorders; however, electron transport chain testing of flash-frozen muscle provides an alternative approach when fresh muscle testing is not available. Next-generation sequencing of mitochondrial DNA and panels of nuclear genes provides a noninvasive alternative to diagnosis. Specific criteria may assist in making a diagnosis (Table 105.4). Table 105.5 lists clues to the diagnosis of mitochondrial diseases.

The majority of mitochondrial disorders are caused by nuclear genes involved in mitochondrial function, and >300 genes have been included in nuclear gene panels for mitochondrial disorder diagnosis. However, pathogenic variants can be identified in 50% or fewer of patients diagnosed clinically with a mitochondrial disorder. An important consideration is that many genetic and multifactorial conditions have been associated with defects in 1 or more of the 4 complexes assayed in mitochondrial oxidative phosphorylation testing. These latter conditions

feature so-called secondary mitochondrial dysfunction, because the conditions are not considered to be mitochondrial disorders per se.

Treatment remains largely symptomatic and does not significantly alter the outcome of disease. Some patients appear to respond to cofactor supplements, typically coenzyme Q_{10} ± L-carnitine at pharmacologic doses. The addition of creatine monohydrate and α-lipoic acid supplementation may add a significant benefit. EPI-743 is a parobenzoquinone like agent that has protective activity against oxidative injury; it is a promising agent in the treatment of mitochondrial disorders, including Leigh syndrome.

Leigh Disease (Subacute Necrotizing Encephalomyelopathy)

Leigh disease is a heterogeneous neurologic disease characterized by demyelination, gliosis, necrosis, relative neuronal sparing, and capillary

Table 105.4	Mitochondrial Disease Criteria (Simplified Version for Bedside Use)*			
I. CLINICAL SIGNS AND SYMPTOMS, 1 POINT/SYMPTOM (max. 4 points)				
A. Muscular Presentation (max. 2 points)	**B. CNS Presentation (max. 2 points)**	**C. Multisystem Disease (max. 3 points)**	**II. Metabolic/Imaging Studies (max. 4 points)**	**III. Morphology (max. 4 points)**
Ophthalmoplegia[†]	Developmental delay	Hematology	Elevated lactate[†]	Ragged red/blue fibers[‡]
Facies myopathica	Loss of skills	GI tract	Elevated L/P ratio	COX-negative fibers[‡]
Exercise intolerance	Stroke-like episode	Endocrine/growth	Elevated alanine[†]	Reduced COX staining[‡]
Muscle weakness	Migraine	Heart	Elevated CSF lactate[†]	Reduced SDH staining
Rhabdomyolysis	Seizures	Kidney	Elevated CSF protein	SDH positive blood vessels[†]
Abnormal EMG	Myoclonus	Vision	Elevated CSF alanine[†]	Abnormal mitochondria/EM[†]
	Cortical blindness	Hearing	Urinary TA excretion[†]	
	Pyramidal signs	Neuropathy	Ethylmalonic aciduria	
	Extrapyramidal signs	Recurrent/familial	Stroke-like picture/MRI	
	Brainstem involvement		Leigh syndrome/MRI[†]	
			Elevated lactate/MRS	

*Score 1: mitochondrial disorder unlikely; score 2 to 4: possible mitochondrial disorder; score 5 to 7: probable mitochondrial disorder; score 8 to 12: definite mitochondrial disorder.
[†]This specific symptom scores 2 points.
[‡]This symptom in a higher percentage scores 4 points.
GI, gastrointestinal; L/P, lactate/pyruvate; COX, cytochrome C oxidase; SDH, succinate dehydrogenase; EM, electron microscopy; EMG, electromyography; TA, tricarbon acid.
From Morava E, van den Heuvel L, Hol F, et al: Mitochondrial disease criteria – diagnostic applications in children. Neurology 67:1823-1826, 2006, p 1824.

proliferation in specific brain regions (see Chapter 616.2). Patients with Leigh disease frequently present with feeding and swallowing problems, failure to thrive, and developmental delay. The presentation is highly variable and may include seizures, altered consciousness, pericardial effusion, and dilated cardiomyopathy. **Diagnosis** is usually confirmed by radiologic or pathologic evidence of symmetric lesions affecting the basal ganglia, brainstem, and subthalamic nuclei. Patients with Leigh disease have defects in several enzyme complexes. Dysfunction in cytochrome-c oxidase (complex IV) is the most commonly reported defect, followed by NADH–coenzyme Q reductase (complex I), PDHC, and pyruvate carboxylase (see Chapter 106). Pathogenic variants in the nuclear *SURF1* gene, which encodes a factor involved in the biogenesis of cytochrome-c oxidase and mitochondrial DNA variants in the adenosine triphosphatase 6 coding region, have been reported in patients with Leigh disease in association with complex IV deficiency. The most common mitochondrial DNA variant in Leigh disease is the T8993G variant in *MT-ATP6*. The **prognosis** for Leigh syndrome is poor. In a study of 14 cases, there were 7 fatalities before age 1.5 yr.

Lactic acidosis, hypoglycemia, and encephalopathy have also been reported in patients with thiamine transporter deficiency and with pyridoxine-dependent epilepsy. Both disorders should improve by the provision of thiamine and pyridoxine, respectively.

Bibliography is available at Expert Consult.

105.5 Defects in Pentose Metabolism
Priya S. Kishnani and Yuan-Tsong Chen

Approximately 90% of glucose metabolism in the body is via the glycolytic pathway, with the remaining 10% via the hexose monophosphate pathway. The hexose monophosphate shunt leads to formation of pentoses, as well as providing NADH. One of the metabolites is ribose-5-phosphate, which is used in the biosynthesis of ribonucleotides and deoxyribonucleotides. Through the transketolase and transaldolase reactions, the pentose phosphates can be converted back to fructose-6-phosphate and glucose-6-phosphate.

ESSENTIAL PENTOSURIA
Essential pentosuria is a benign disorder encountered principally in Ashkenazi Jews and is an autosomal recessive trait. The urine contains L-xylulose, which is excreted in increased amounts because of a block in the conversion of L-xylulose to xylitol as a result of **xylitol dehydrogenase deficiency**. The condition is usually discovered accidentally in a urine test for reducing substances. No treatment is required.

TRANSALDOLASE DEFICIENCY
Few patients have reported symptoms that include liver cirrhosis, hepatosplenomegaly, severe neonatal hepatopathy, and cardiomyopathy. Biochemical abnormalities revealed elevated levels of arabitol, ribitol, and erythritol in the urine. Erythronic acid has been identified by urine nuclear magnetic resonance spectroscopy as another hallmark metabolite. Enzyme assay in the lymphoblasts and fibroblasts demonstrated low transaldolase activity, which was confirmed by pathogenic variants in the transaldolase gene. In addition, measurement of transaldolase activity in fibroblasts, lymphoblasts, or liver tissue, as well as assessing urinary concentrations of polyols, also can be used to confirm the diagnosis.

RIBOSE-5-PHOSPHATE ISOMERASE DEFICIENCY
Only one case of this disorder has been reported. The affected male had psychomotor delay from early in life and developed epilepsy at 4 yr of age. Thereafter, a slow neurologic regression developed, with prominent cerebellar ataxia, some spasticity, optic atrophy, and a mild sensorimotor neuropathy. MRI of the brain at ages 11 and 14 yr showed extensive abnormalities of the cerebral white matter. Proton magnetic resonance spectroscopy (MRS) of the brain revealed elevated levels of ribitol and D-arabitol. These pentitols were also increased in urine and plasma similar to the patient found in transaldolase deficiency. Enzyme assays in cultured fibroblasts showed deficient **ribose-5-phosphate isomerase** activity, which was confirmed by a molecular study. These results, combined with a study of ribose-5-phosphate isomerase–deficient mice, demonstrated that the specific genetic pairing of a null allele with an allele coding for a form of the enzyme that is only partly active, allowing for cell type–dependent expression deficits, is a contributing factor to the rarity of the disease. Ribose-5-phosphate isomerase deficiency may represent an example of a single-gene disease that appears seldom because of its complex molecular etiology.

Bibliography is available at Expert Consult.

Table 105.5	Clues to the Diagnosis of Mitochondrial Disease

NEUROLOGIC
Cerebral stroke-like lesions in a nonvascular pattern
Basal ganglia disease
Encephalopathy: recurrent or with low/moderate dosing of
valproate
Neurodegeneration
Epilepsia partialis continua
Myoclonus
Ataxia
MRI findings consistent with Leigh disease
Characteristic MRS peaks
Lactate peak at 1.3 ppm TE (time to echo) at 35 and 135
Succinate peak at 2.4 ppm

CARDIOVASCULAR
Hypertrophic cardiomyopathy with rhythm disturbance
Unexplained heart block in a child
Cardiomyopathy with lactic acidosis (>5 mM)
Dilated cardiomyopathy with muscle weakness
Wolff-Parkinson-White arrhythmia

OPHTHALMOLOGIC
Retinal degeneration with signs of night blindness, color vision
deficits, decreased visual acuity, or pigmentary retinopathy
Ophthalmoplegia/paresis
Fluctuating, dysconjugate eye movements
Ptosis
Sudden- or insidious-onset optic neuropathy/atrophy

GASTROENTEROLOGIC
Unexplained or valproate-induced liver failure
Severe dysmotility
Pseudoobstructive episodes

OTHER
A newborn, infant, or young child with unexplained hypotonia,
weakness, failure to thrive, and a metabolic acidosis (particularly
lactic acidosis)
Exercise intolerance that is not in proportion to weakness
Hypersensitivity to general anesthesia
Episodes of acute rhabdomyolysis
Elevated GDF-15 level

MRI, Magnetic resonance imaging, MRS, magnetic resonance spectroscopy; GDF, growth and differentiation factor.
From Haas RH, Parikh S, Falk MJ, et al: Mitochondrial disease: a practical approach for primary care physicians, *Pediatrics* 120:1326–1333, 2007 (Table 1, p 1327).

105.6 Disorders of Glycoprotein Degradation and Structure

Margaret M. McGovern and Robert J. Desnick

The disorders of glycoprotein degradation and structure include several lysosomal storage diseases that result from defects in glycoprotein degradation, and the congenital disorders of glycosylation (see Chapter 105.7). *Glycoproteins* are macromolecules composed of oligosaccharide chains linked to a peptide backbone. They are synthesized by 2 pathways: the glycosyltransferase pathway, which synthesizes oligosaccharides linked *O*-glycosidically to serine or threonine residues; and the dolichol, lipid-linked pathway, which synthesizes oligosaccharides linked *N*-glycosidically to asparagine.

The **glycoprotein lysosomal storage diseases** result from the deficiency of the enzymes that normally participate in the degradation of oligosaccharides and include sialidosis, galactosialidosis, aspartylglucosaminuria, and α-mannosidosis. In some instances the underlying abnormality that leads to glycoprotein accumulation also results in abnormal degradation of other classes of macromolecules that contain similar

oligosaccharide linkages, such as certain glycolipids and proteoglycans. In these cases the underlying enzymatic deficiency results in the accumulation of both glycoproteins and *glycolipids*. The classification of these types of disorders as *lipidoses* or *glycoproteinoses* depends on the nature of the predominantly stored substance. In general, the glycoprotein disorders are characterized by autosomal recessive inheritance and a progressive disease course with clinical features that resemble those seen in the mucopolysaccharidoses.

SIALIDOSIS AND GALACTOSIALIDOSIS

Sialidosis is an autosomal recessive disorder that results from the primary deficiency of neuraminidase because of mutations in the gene (*NEU1*) that encodes this protein, located on chromosome 6p21.33. In contrast, **galactosialidosis** is caused by the deficiency of 2 lysosomal enzymes—neuraminidase and β-galactosidase. The loss of these enzymatic activities results from mutations in a single gene, *CTSA*, located on chromosome 20q13.12, that encodes the protective protein cathepsin A, which functions to stabilize these enzymatic activities. Neuraminidase normally cleaves terminal sialyl linkages of several oligosaccharides and glycoproteins. Its deficiency results in the accumulation of oligosaccharides, and the urinary excretion of sialic acid terminal oligosaccharides and sialylglycopeptides. Examination of tissues from affected individuals reveals pathologic storage of substrate in many tissues, including liver, bone marrow, and brain.

The clinical phenotype associated with neuraminidase deficiency is variable and includes **type I** sialidosis, which usually presents in the 2nd decade of life with myoclonus and cherry-red spots in the macula. These patients typically present secondary to gait disturbances, myoclonus, or visual complaints. In contrast, **type II** sialidosis occurs at several ages of onset (congenital, infantile, and juvenile), depending on the severity of the gene mutation. The **congenital** and **infantile** forms result from isolated neuraminidase deficiency, whereas the **juvenile** form results from both neuraminidase and β-galactosidase deficiency. The congenital type II disease is characterized by hydrops fetalis, neonatal ascites, hepatosplenomegaly, stippling of the epiphyses, periosteal cloaking, and stillbirth or death in infancy. The type II infantile form presents in the 1st yr of life with dysostosis multiplex, moderate global developmental delays, visceromegaly, corneal clouding, cherry-red maculae, and seizures. The juvenile type II form of sialidosis, which is sometimes designated *galactosialidosis*, has a variable age of onset ranging from infancy to adulthood. In infancy, the phenotype is similar to that of GM₁ gangliosidosis, with edema, ascites, skeletal dysplasia, and cherry-red spots. Patients with later-onset disease have dysostosis multiplex, visceromegaly, intellectual disability, dysmorphism, corneal clouding, progressive neurologic deterioration, and cherry-red spots.

No specific therapy exists for any form of the disease, although studies in animal models have demonstrated improvement in the phenotype after bone marrow transplantation. The **diagnosis** of sialidosis and galactosialidosis is achieved by the demonstration of the specific enzymatic deficiency or by mutations in the responsible gene. **Prenatal diagnosis** using cultured amniotic cells or chorionic villi is available by demonstrating the enzyme defect and/or specific gene mutations.

ASPARTYLGLUCOSAMINURIA

This is a rare autosomal recessive lysosomal storage disorder, except in Finland, where the carrier frequency is estimated at 1 in 36 adults, the high frequency due to a *founder* gene. The disorder results from the deficient activity of **aspartylglycosaminidase** and the subsequent accumulation of aspartylglycosamine, particularly in the liver, spleen, and thyroid. The gene for the enzyme (*AGA*) has been localized to chromosome 4q32-33, and the DNA and gene have been isolated and sequenced. In the Finnish population, a single *AGA* mutation encoding p.C163S accounts for most mutant alleles, whereas outside of Finland, a large number of private mutations have been described.

Affected individuals with aspartylglucosaminuria typically present in the 1st yr of life with recurrent infections, diarrhea, and umbilical hernias. Coarsening of the facies and short stature usually develop later. Other features include joint laxity, macroglossia, hoarse voice, crystal-like lens opacities, hypotonia, and spasticity. Psychomotor development is usually near normal until age 5 yr, when a decline is noted. Behavioral abnormalities are typically seen, and IQ values in affected adults are usually<40 (severe intellectual disability). Survival to adulthood is common, with most early deaths attributable to pneumonia or other pulmonary causes. Definitive **diagnosis** requires demonstration of markedly deficient aspartylglucosaminidase in peripheral blood leukocytes, and/or the specific *AGA* mutation(s). Several patients have undergone allogeneic bone marrow transplants, but this approach has not proved effective, and *no specific treatment is available*. **Prenatal diagnosis** is available by the determination of aspartylglucosaminidase deficiency and/or the specific *AGA* mutations in cultured amniocytes or chorionic villi.

α-MANNOSIDOSIS

This autosomal recessive disorder results from the deficient activity of **α-mannosidase** and the accumulation of mannose-rich compounds. The gene *MAN2B1* encoding the enzyme has been localized to chromosome 19p13.2-q12, and the cDNA and gene sequence have been determined. To date >140 gene mutations have been reported. Affected patients display clinical heterogeneity. There is a severe infantile form, or **type I** disease, and a milder juvenile variant, **type II** disease. All patients have psychomotor retardation, facial coarsening, and dysostosis multiplex. The **infantile** form of the disorder, however, is characterized by more rapid cognitive deterioration, with death occurring between ages 3 and 10 yr. Patients with the infantile form also have more severe skeletal involvement and hepatosplenomegaly. The **juvenile** disorder is characterized by onset of symptoms in early childhood or adolescence, with milder somatic features and survival to adulthood. Hearing loss, destructive synovitis, pancytopenia, and spastic paraplegia have been reported in type II patients. The **diagnosis** is made by the demonstration of the marked deficiency of α-mannosidase activity in white blood cells

or cultured fibroblasts. Clinical trials of ERT with recombinant human α-mannosidase are underway. **Prenatal diagnosis** can be made by demonstrating the enzyme defect and/or the specific gene mutations in cultured amniocytes or chorionic villi.

Bibliography is available at Expert Consult.

105.7 Congenital Disorders of Glycosylation
Eva Morava and Peter Witters

Glycosylation is the complex multistep metabolic process of adding (oligo) saccharides to proteins and lipids. The classification of **disorders of hypoglycosylation** is based on biochemical structures: (1) defects in protein *N*-linked glycosylation, (2) defects in protein *O*-linked glycosylation, (3) defects in glycosphingolipid and in glycosylphosphatidylinositol-anchor glycosylation, and (4) defects in multiple glycosylation pathways and in other pathways (Fig. 105.7). No disorders are known to result from abnormal *C*-linked glycosylation. Congenital disorders of glycosylation are labeled based on their genetic defect *(CDG)*.

Protein glycosylation is an essential pathway. Most functional proteins are glycosylated, including serum proteins (e.g., transferrin, ceruloplasmin, TBG), hormones (e.g., TSH, FSH, FH, ACTH, IGFBP3), and clotting and anticoagulation factors (e.g., factors IX and XI, antithrombin). Membrane proteins are also highly glycosylated. Important intracellular glycoproteins include enzymes such as glycosyltransferases or lysosomal enzymes.

N-glycans are linked to the amide group of asparagine. They are synthetized in a complicated process throughout the cytoplasm, endoplasmic reticulum (ER), and Golgi complex, starting with sugar activation and nucleotide sugar synthesis, then oligosaccharide assembly, and finally glycan processing (Fig. 105.8). The majority of the pediatric disorders are *N*-glycosylation disorders. **O-glycans** are linked to the

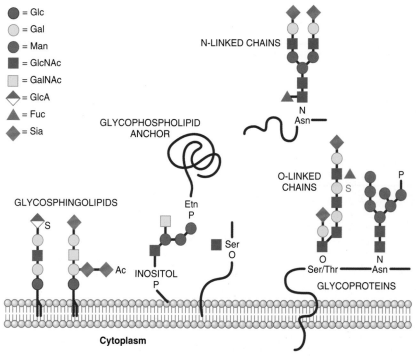

Fig. 105.7 Schematic of different types of glycosylation. *Left to right,* Glycosphingolipids, glycophospholipid anchor (GPI anchor), *O*-linked membrane protein glycosylation, *N*-linked membrane glycosylation, and secretory *N*-linked glycan.

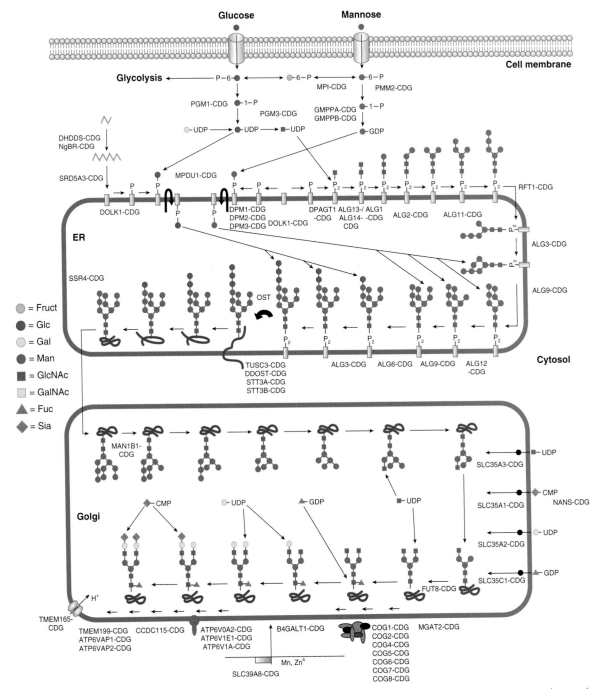

Fig. 105.8 Overview of different cell compartments involved in *N*-linked protein glycosylation. Activation of nucleotide sugars in the cytoplasm is followed by step-by-step dolichol-linked synthesis of glycans associated with the endoplasmic reticulum. Transfer of the glycan from the lipid arm to the protein is followed by transport to the Golgi for further modifications.

hydroxyl group of serine or threonine. These diverse glycoproteins are mostly formed in the Golgi complex; their defects can involve xylosylation, fucosylation, mannosylation, or other modifications. An important focus is *O*-mannosylation defects because of their relevance for dystroglycanopathies.

Lipid glycosylation is an essential process for the synthesis of ceramide and ganglioside synthesis. **Glycosylphosphatidylinositols** (GPIs) are very special glycolipids that link various proteins to the

plasma membrane, as complex lipid-sugar anchors (GPI anchors, see Fig. 105.7).

Congenital disorders of glycosylation (CDG) are predominantly multisystem diseases, caused by >140 different genetic defects in glycoprotein and glycolipid glycan synthesis. This rapidly growing group is one of the newest and largest metabolic disorder groups. Most patients described with CDG have *N*-glycosylation defects, followed by the fastest-growing group of CDGs, involving multiple glycosylation pathways and dolicholphosphate synthesis. Smaller groups are *O*-glycosylation disorders and disorders of glycosylphosphatidylinositol. The "oldest" CDG is PMM2-CDG, in which the genetic defect leads to the loss of **phosphomannomutase 2** (PMM2), the enzyme that catalyzes the conversion of mannose-6-phosphate into mannose-1-phosphate. The majority of CDGs have an autosomal recessive inheritance. Only 2 *N*-linked CDGs are autosomal dominant, GANAB-CDG and PRKCSH-CDG. The dominantly inherited *O*-linked CDGs include EXT1/EXT2-CDG, POFUT1-CDG, and POGLUT1-CDG. X-linked CDGs include ALG13-CDG, SSR4-CDG, PIGA-CDG, SLC35A2-CDG, ATP6AP2-CDG and ATP6AP1-CDG.

Some CDGs are lethal; 20% of PMM2-CDG patients die in the 1st 2 yr of life. Some patients, however, stabilize throughout young adulthood. Almost any clinical phenotype can be present in a patient with CDG. It can affect any organ or organ system and most often includes the central nervous system (CNS). The most common clinical features include developmental and speech delay, seizures, ataxia, spasticity, peripheral neuropathy, hypotonia, strabismus, abnormal fat distribution, visual loss, cardiomyopathy, feeding difficulties, liver dysfunction, endocrine abnormalities, bleeding diathesis, and thrombosis (Fig. 105.9 and Table 105.6). Single-organ presentations are rare in CDGs (e.g., TUSC3-CDG and ST3GAL3-CDG: brain; DHDDS-CDG: retina; ALG14-CDG: neuromuscular junction; POFUT1-CDG and POGLUT1-

CDG: skin; SEC23B-CDG: red cell lineage; EXT1/EXT2-CDG: cartilage; TMEM199-CDG: liver). Many CDGs are recognizable syndromes. CDG should be considered in any patient with a developmental disability or an unexplained clinical condition, especially in multisystem disease with neurologic involvement.

There are also **congenital disorders of deglycosylation**, including known lysosomal disorders and a severe neurologic condition caused by defective *N*-glycanase function (*NGLY1* defect).

Laboratory evaluations in most *N*-linked CDGs rely on a primary screening method called serum **transferrin isoelectric focusing (TIEF)**. Transferrin isoforms, which are hyposialylated (missing terminal sialic acid residues), show different cathodal shifts depending on either missing glycan chains or truncated glycans. A **type 1 pattern** suggests an early metabolic defect in the cytosolic-ER–related glycan synthesis and assembly. A **type 2 pattern** suggests Golgi-related glycan-processing defects (Fig. 105.10).

Isoelectric focusing of apolipoprotein C-III (**IEF apoC-III**), a serum mucine type *O*-glycosylated protein, can detect some *O*-glycosylation disorders (combined *N*- and *O*-linked glycosylation defects). Mass spectrometry in serum for type 1 defects is highly sensitive for mild glycosylation abnormalities. Glycomics by matrix-assisted laser desorption/ionization time of flight (**MALDI-TOF**) can be diagnostic in specific types of CDG (mostly Golgi related with a type 2 pattern). Dolichol-linked

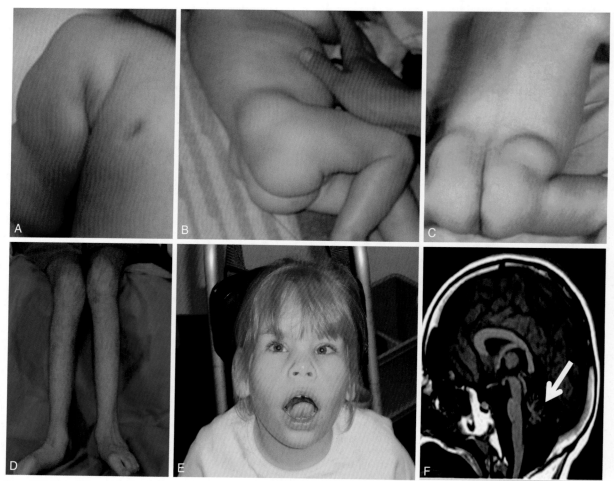

Fig. 105.9 Patients with phosphomannomutase-2 deficiency (PMM2-CDG) and recognizable clinical features. **A,** Inverted nipples. **B** and **C,** Abnormal fat distribution. **D,** Muscle atrophy caused by peripheral neuropathy after puberty. **E,** Characteristic facial features with strabismus, short nose, anteverted nares, long philtrum, and large ears. **F,** MRI of brain with T1-weighted sagittal image showing cerebellar vermis hypoplasia (*arrow*) and brain atrophy.

Table 105.6	Clinical and Laboratory Features in Common Congenital Disorders of Glycosylation (CDGs), with Clinically Recognizable Phenotype and Abnormal Glycosylation, Detectable by Serum Transferrin Isoform Analysis (TIEF)			
DEFECTIVE GENE	**MOST FREQUENT CLINICAL FEATURES**	**SUGGESTIVE FEATURES**	**LABORATORY ABNORMALITIES**	**OTHER BIOCHEMICAL ANOMALIES**
PMM2	Strabismus, nystagmus, smooth philtrum, large ears, vomiting, diarrhea, FTT, axial hypotonia, cerebellar vermis hypoplasia, ataxia, psychomotor disability, seizures, spasticity, neuropathy, pigmentary retinitis	Inverted nipples and/or abnormal fat pads, stroke-like episodes	Elevated serum transaminases, hypoalbuminemia, decreased factor IX, XI and AT activity, low serum ceruloplasmin and TBG levels	Type 1 serum TIEF, decreased PMM activity in leukocytes and fibroblasts
PMI	Cholestasis, hepatomegaly, feeding difficulties, recurrent vomiting, chronic diarrhea, ascites, recurrent thrombosis, gastrointestinal bleeding	Hyperinsulinism, protein losing enteropathy Normal intelligence and absence of neurologic features	Elevated transaminases, hypoalbuminemia, hypoglycemia, decreased factor IX, XI, and AT-III activity	Type 1 serum TIEF, decreased PMI activity in leukocytes and fibroblasts
ALG6	Hypotonia, muscle weakness, seizures, ataxia, intellectual disability, behavioral abnormalities	(Distal limb malformations)	Elevated serum transaminases; hypoalbuminemia; decreased factor IX, XI, and AT activity; low serum IgG level	Type 1 serum TIEF, abnormal LLO results in fibroblasts
DPAGT1	Microcephaly, brain malformations, hypotonia, severe psychomotor disability, seizures, spasticity, proximal weakness, failure to thrive, joint contractures	Congenital myasthenia phenotype In multisystem phenotype: cataract	Decreased AT, protein C, and protein S activity; increased creatine kinase; hypoalbuminemia; normal creatine kinase in myasthenia	Type 1 serum TIEF
SRD5A3	Developmental delay, hypotonia, ataxia, cerebellar vermis hypoplasia, intellectual disability, speech delay, visual loss	Congenital cataract, retinal and iridic coloboma, glaucoma, optic nerve dysplasia, ichthyosis	Low anticoagulation factors (AT, protein C, and protein S activity), increased serum transaminases	Type 1 serum TIEF *but reported false-negative TIEF*
ATP6V0A2	Generalized cutis laxa, hypotonia, strabismus, characteristic facial features, joint laxity, seizures, motor and language developmental delay, spontaneous improvement of cutis laxa by aging	Cobblestone-like brain dysgenesis	Mild coagulation abnormalities, increased serum transaminase levels	Type 2 serum TIEF *but reported false-negative TIEF*
ATP6V1A and ATP6V1E1		Cardiovascular anomalies	Mild coagulation abnormalities and increased serum transaminase levels, hypercholesterolemia	Abnormal apoC-III IEF, characteristic MALDI TOF profile (Note abnormal skin histology)
PGM1	Pierre Robin sequence, cholestasis, short stature, dilated cardiomyopathy,	Cleft palate, hyperinsulinism, normal intelligence	Hypoglycemia, increased serum transaminase levels, decreased AT	Mixed type 1/2 serum TIEF, decreased fibroblast PGM1 activity
MAN1B1	Developmental delay, speech delay, intellectual disability, muscle weakness	Obesity, autistic features, inverted nipples, characteristic face	Increased serum transaminase levels, low AT	Type 2 serum TIEF, abnormal apoC-III IEF, diagnostic MALDI TOF profile
TMEM199	Cholestasis, hepatomegaly, liver steatosis, liver fibrosis, liver failure, spontaneous bleedings, motor developmental delay	Normal intelligence	Decreased serum ceruloplasmin, increased serum transaminase levels, hypercholesterolemia, high AP	Type 2 serum TIEF, abnormal apoC-III IEF, characteristic MALDI TOF profile
CCDC115		Hepatomegaly		
ATP6AP1 and ATP6AP2		Immune deficiency		
SLC39A8	Seizures, hypsarrhythmia, hypotonia, developmental and speech delay, FTT	Dwarfism, craniosynostosis, rhizomelia, Leigh disease	Decreased serum manganese, high serum transaminases, abnormal coagulation	Type 2 serum TIEF, abnormal apoC-III, characteristic MALDI TOF profile

AP, Alkaline phosphatase; AT, antithrombin; apoC-III: apolipoprotein C-III; FTT, failure to thrive; LLO, lipid-linked oligosaccharides; MALDI-TOF, matrix-assisted laser desorption/ionization time of flight; TBG, thyroxine-binding globulin; TIEF, transferrin isoelectric focusing.

glycan or lipid-linked oligosaccharide (LLO) analysis is a complicated but sensitive method to detect ER-related N-glycan assembly (CDG type 1) defects in patient fibroblasts. GPI-anchor defects can be suspected based on *recurrent elevation of alkaline phosphatase levels* in blood.

Dystroglycanopathies can be confirmed based on abnormal immunohistochemistry in muscle biopsy. Fluorescence-activated cell sorting (**FACS**) analysis of the membrane-anchored markers CD16 and CD24 in leukocytes is highly suggestive for a GPI-anchor abnormality, especially when alkaline phosphatase in blood is significantly elevated. Enzyme analysis in blood is only available for a few, more common CDGs (PMM2-CDG, MPI-CDG, PGM1-CDG); it is more reliable in fibroblasts.

With an abnormal TIEF pattern result or clinical suspicion of any type of CDG, most metabolic centers use a direct *CDG* gene panel analysis or next-generation sequencing (NGS; whole exome sequencing) (see Fig. 105.10).

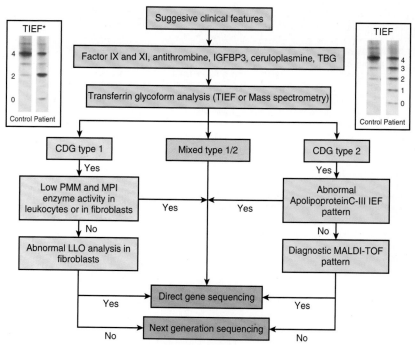

Fig. 105.10 Diagnostic flow chart of glycosylation disorders affecting N-linked glycosylation. *Instead of TIEF, mass spectrometry methods can be used as well. IGFBP3, Insulin-like growth factor–binding protein 3; TBG, thyroxine-binding globulin; CDG, congenital disorders of glycosylation; PMM, phosphomannomutase; MPI, mannosephosphoisomerase; LLO, lipid-linked oligosaccharides; TIEF, transferrin isoelectric focusing; IEF, isoelectric focusing; MALDI-TOF, matrix-assisted laser desorption/ionization time of flight.

CONGENITAL DISORDERS OF PROTEIN N-GLYCOSYLATION
Phosphomannomutase-2 Deficiency (PMM2-CDG)
Clinical Manifestations
PMM2-CDG is the most common and easily recognizable CDG. Most patients have alternating strabismus, characteristic facial features (short nose, long philtrum, large ears) (Fig. 105.9E), inverted nipples and/or abnormal fat pads (Fig. 105.9A-C), feeding difficulties, axial hypotonia, and decreased reflexes, already in the 1st few mo of life. Nystagmus (caused by pontocerebellar and vermis hypoplasia; Fig. 105.9F) is also common. Psychomotor disability is present in most patients, but normal intellectual development has been described in a few patients. Most patients develop a multisystem disease, and <25% show an isolated neurologic phenotype without other organ involvement, normal endocrine regulation, and no coagulopathy. The neurologic involvement is quite diverse, with ataxia, seizures, spasticity, and peripheral neuropathy (Fig. 105.9D) the most common features. Dystonia, stroke-like episodes, and proximal myopathy can also occur. PMM2-CDG is not a progressive disease, but certain features, when present, typically appear at different ages during the disease. From birth, pericardial fluid collection, cardiomyopathy, or chronic vomiting/diarrhea can occur; after 7 yr, retinitis pigmentosa and cataract; and after puberty, scoliosis, neuropathy, and recurrent thrombotic events. Liver function anomalies are mild, and only a few patients develop cholestasis or liver fibrosis. Most patients have a hypergonadotropic hypogonadism; no successful pregnancies have been reported. Intellectual disability can be mild to severe; speech development is frequently delayed and can even be absent. Autistic behavior is common, although patients usually have a cheerful personality.

Pathophysiology
Phosphomannomutase 2 catalyzes the conversion of mannose-6-phosphate to mannose-1-phosphate, essential for the formation of activated mannose units used in the synthesis of the growing glycan chain in the ER. Hypoglycosylation leads to abnormal function affecting many essential glycoproteins, such as coagulation and anticoagulation factors, endocrine regulation, transport proteins, liver function, and immune, membrane, and receptor proteins.

Diagnosis
The primary screening method for PMM2-CDG is serum transferrin glycoform analysis, which is most frequently performed by TIEF. Intact transferrin has 4 negatively charged sialic acid residues (tetrasialotransferrin). Transferrin glycoforms, missing terminal sialic acid residues, show different cathodal shifts, less abundant tetrasialotransferrin, increased disialotransferrin, and some a-sialotransferrin (see Fig. 105.10). This is the so-called type 1 pattern, suggestive of a defect in glycan assembly in the cytosol-ER. Transferrin isoforms are also detectable by mass spectrometry. Certain other disorders can cause a *false-positive* transferrin isoform pattern, including galactosemia, hereditary fructose intolerance, and excessive alcohol use. PMM enzyme analysis is available in leukocytes and fibroblasts.

The presence of elevated serum transaminases, hypoalbuminemia, decreased factor IX and XI and antithrombin activity, or low ceruloplasmin or thyroxine-binding globulin (TBG) level is highly suggestive of CDG, including the most common type, PMM2-CDG.

PMM2-CDG is autosomal recessive. Genetic testing is mostly performed by direct sequencing. The most frequent pathogenic variant (c.422G>A; R141H) is present in 75% of patients of Caucasian origin. The exact incidence of PMM2-CDG is not known, but it is estimated to be as high as 1 in 40,000-80,000 in Europe. Prenatal diagnosis is only reliable by genetic testing.

Treatment
The therapy in PMM2-CDG relies on supportive treatment. Even with the best treatment, mortality is about 20% in the 1st 2 yr of life, mostly

from cardiac or kidney involvement and severe infections. Current recommended therapy includes adequate nutrition, diet or tube feeding if needed, cardiac support, hormone supplements, physical and occupational therapy, speech therapy, seizure management, and strabismus surgery. Therapeutic developments include targeted mannose-phosphate treatment, and chaperone therapy; these are only in preclinical trial phases.

Mannosephosphoisomerase Deficiency (MPI-CDG)
Clinical Manifestations
MPI deficiency is a recognizable and treatable CDG. Most patients show early symptoms of liver disease (cholestasis, elevated transaminases) and feeding difficulties, with recurrent vomiting and chronic diarrhea, most frequently with protein-losing enteropathy. Life-threatening episodes might appear as early as the 1st few mo of life with recurrent thrombosis and severe gastrointestinal bleeding because of severe coagulation abnormalities. Hypoglycemia is usually caused by hyperinsulinism. Hypoalbuminemia can be severe; patients might develop visible abdominal distention from a combination of ascites and hepatomegaly. Patients with MPI-CDG have no other organ involvement, and the CNS is not affected. There are no dysmorphic features. The liver disease frequently progresses to fibrosis or cirrhosis.

Pathophysiology
Mannosephosphoisomerase (MPI) catalyzes the conversion of fructose-6-phosphate to mannose-6-phosphate, 1 step before PMM2, therefore blocking the formation of activated mannose units (GDP mannose) for oligosaccharide synthesis. Hypoglycosylation leads to abnormal glycoprotein function the same as in PMM2-CDG, especially coagulation and anticoagulation factors, liver function, and hormone receptors.

Diagnosis
The primary screening method in a suspected MPI-CDG patient is serum transferrin isoform analysis by TIEF (see Fig. 105.10) or MS analysis. MPI deficiency leads to a type 1 pattern, as seen in PMM2 deficiency. MPI enzyme analysis is available in leukocytes and fibroblasts. The presence of elevated serum transaminases, hypoalbuminemia, decreased factor IX and XI and antithrombin activity, hyperinsulinism, and nonketotic hypoglycemia are highly suggestive for MPI-CDG.

MPI-CDG is autosomal recessive. Genetic testing is mostly performed by direct sequencing. The exact incidence of MPI-CDG is not known, but it is estimated at 1 : 800 000 in Europe. Prenatal diagnosis is only reliable by genetic testing. Although this is a rare CDG, early diagnosis is imperative because it is treatable.

Treatment
MPI-CDG is the first CDG type treatable by dietary therapy. Mannose therapy is clinically effective by both IV and oral supplementation of 1 g/kg/day divided into 3-4 doses. A known side effect is hemolysis. The treatment uses an alternative pathway: mannose can be phosphorylated by hexokinases to mannose 6-phosphate, bypassing the MPI defect. The clinical symptoms improve rapidly, but liver function might further deteriorate. Liver fibrosis and cirrhosis might necessitate liver transplantation, which will resolve the metabolic disease. The oldest patient known with MPI-CDG has survived into her late 30s.

Glucosyltransferase-1 Deficiency (ALG6-CDG)
Clinical Manifestations
ALG6-CDG is the 2nd most common CDG. Most patients have hypotonia, muscle weakness, seizures, and ataxia. To date, no patient with ALG6-CDG has normal intelligence. Speech delay and nystagmus are common neurologic signs. Brachydactyly, skeletal abnormalities, and transverse limb defects have been observed. Strabismus and characteristic facial dysmorphism are rare (hypertelorism, oval face, short nose). Inverted nipples and/or abnormal fat pads are exceptional in ALG6-CDG.

The most severe ALG6-CDG patients show a multisystem phenotype in the 1st few mo of life, including severe infections, protein-losing enteropathy, hypoalbuminemia, anemia, and failure to thrive. Autistic behavior and mood changes have been observed in several patients. The oldest patient to date is almost 45 yr.

Pathophysiology
The metabolic problem is caused by defective binding of the 1st of 3 glucoses to the lipid-linked oligosaccharide in the ER. This glucose binding is essential for attachment of the oligosaccharyltransferase enzyme complex to the newly built oligosaccharide chain and the ability to transfer it to the protein. This leads to protein hypoglycosylation and abnormal glycoprotein function similar to PMM2-CDG and MPI-CDG. Laboratory abnormalities are also similar, including abnormalities in coagulation and anticoagulation factors, liver function, thyroid hormones, and immunoglobulins (IgG).

Diagnosis
The primary screening method in a suspected ALG6-CDG patient is serum transferrin glycoform analysis by TIEF or MS analysis. ALG6 deficiency leads to a type 1 pattern (see Fig. 105.10), as seen in PMM2 and MPI deficiency. There is no available enzyme analysis, although lipid-linked oligosaccharides could be evaluated in patient fibroblasts.

ALG6-CDG is autosomal recessive. Genetic testing is mostly performed by direct sequencing. The most common mutations are p.A333V and p.I299Del. Prenatal diagnosis is only reliable by genetic testing. The exact incidence of ALG6-CDG is not known.

Treatment
The current therapy in ALG6-CDG relies on supportive treatment. Mortality is about 10% in the 1st years of life, mostly from protein-losing enteropathy and severe infections.

UDP-GlcNAc:Dol-P-GlcNAc-P Transferase Deficiency (DPAGT1-CDG)
Clinical Manifestations
DPAGT1 deficiency is a recognizable and potentially treatable CDG. About one third of patients show the **congenital myasthenia** phenotype, indistinguishable from other genetic congenital myasthenias. Creatine kinase (CK) levels are normal. These patients have a relatively good prognosis, especially with early myasthenia therapy. The other patients show a multisystem phenotype with microcephaly, brain malformations, hypotonia, severe psychomotor disability, seizures, spasticity, failure to thrive, joint contractures, and cataracts.

Pathophysiology
DPAGT1 defect leads to very early arrest of glycan synthesis outside the ER membrane, by slowing down the addition of the 2nd GlcNAc sugar to the phosphorylated dolichol arm. Abnormal receptor glycosylation in the *neuromuscular junction* leads to myasthenia. Hypoglycosylation in the multisystem type leads to abnormal glycoprotein function similar to that in PMM2-CDG, especially involving the anticoagulation factors, and interestingly leading to high serum CK (in contrast to the congenital myasthenia phenotype) and hypoalbuminemia.

Diagnosis
The primary screening method is serum transferrin glycoform analysis or MS analysis. Most patients show a type 1 pattern (see Fig. 105.10), but patients with the congenital myasthenia phenotype can show normal screening. There is no clinically available enzyme analysis.

DPAGT1-CDG is autosomal recessive. Genetic testing is mostly performed by direct sequencing. The exact incidence is not known. Prenatal diagnosis is only reliable by genetic testing. Because of the false-negative TIEF results in several patients with the myasthenic phenotype, congenital myasthenia panel testing is suggested in suspected cases, especially for determining the potential therapy.

Treatment
The congenital myasthenia phenotype is frequently treatable by high-dose pyridostigmine, eventually enhanced with salbutamol. In the multisystem phenotype of DPAGT1-CDG, treatment is supportive.

CONGENITAL DISORDERS OF PROTEIN O-GLYCOSYLATION
Cerebro-Ocular Dysplasia–Muscular Dystrophy and Muscle-Eye-Brain Disease Spectrum (POMT1-CDG, POMT2-CDG, POMGNT1-CDG)

From isolated muscular dystrophy to **Walker Warburg syndrome**, this group of O-linked glycosylation disorders presents with severe muscle weakness, congenital eye malformations, and neuronal migration defects. Pachygyria, cobblestone dysgenesis, hydrocephalus, polymicrogyria, heterotopias, and corpus callosum agenesis are variably present. Eye malformations include anophthalmia, microphthalmia, congenital cataract, or colobomas. **Congenital muscular dystrophy** is associated with significant CK level elevations. There is severe psychomotor disability.

The underlying metabolic defect is the abnormal synthesis of the O-mannosylglycan core, which is essential for the proper glycosylation of α-dystroglycan. The α-dystroglycan is heavily O-glycosylated with mannose residues and is expressed in both muscle and brain. Defective mannosylation of α-dystroglycan leads to muscle degeneration and migration defects. Muscle biopsy shows abnormal α-dystroglycan staining on immunohistochemistry.

Transferrin isoelectric focusing is normal in patients with isolated O-mannosylation defects. There is also no clinically available enzyme analysis. **Diagnosis** is based on histology (muscle biopsy) and genetic analysis.

POMT1-CDG, POMT2-CDG, POMGNT1-CDG are the most common autosomal recessive α-dystroglycanopathies. Additional gene defects occur in the pathway; POMK, FKTN, FKRP, LARGE, B4GAT1, TMEM5, and ISPD have been described in association with human disease. The exact incidence of α-dystroglycanopathies is not known.

In α-dystroglycanopathies the **treatment** is supportive.

DEFECTS IN LIPID GLYCOSYLATION AND IN GLYCOSYLPHOSPHATIDYLINOSITOL ANCHOR BIOSYNTHESIS
Hyperphosphatasia–Intellectual Disability Syndromes: PIGA Deficiency (PIGA-CDG)

This clinically recognizable syndrome is an epilepsy syndrome with intellectual disability, hypotonia, dysmorphic facial features, skin anomalies, congenital brain malformations, and behavioral abnormalities, including autism. Other organ malformations, including cardiac and renal defects, have also been reported. (Note that *somatic* mutations with *PIGA* defect can also lead to paroxysmal nocturnal hemoglobinuria.)

N-acetylglucosamine (GlcNAc) cannot be efficiently transferred to phosphatidylinositol for glycophosphatidylinositol synthesis. Abnormal anchoring of alkaline phosphatase leads to hyperphosphatasemia in blood and loss of specific surface antigens on blood cells.

Transferrin isoform analysis is normal in GPI-anchor defects. FACS analysis of the membrane-anchored markers CD16 and CD24 in leukocytes is highly suggestive for a GPI-anchor abnormality, especially in association with increased levels of serum alkaline phosphatase. Mutation analysis confirms the defect.

PIGA-CDG is X-linked. The exact incidence is not known. A similar phenotype has been described in *PIGO, PIGV, PIGY, PIG, PGAP2,* and *PGAP3* defects.

In PIGA-CDG the **treatment** is supportive.

DEFECTS IN MULTIPLE GLYCOSYLATION PATHWAYS AND IN OTHER PATHWAYS, INCLUDING DOLICHOLPHOSPHATE BIOSYNTHESIS DEFECTS
Steroid 5α-Reductase Deficiency (SRD5A3-CDG)
Clinical Manifestations

SRD5A3 deficiency is a clinically recognizable CDG, originally described as a multiple–congenital malformation syndrome. About 20 patients have been diagnosed at different ages, including one at 45 yr. Patients have hypotonia, ataxia, and eye abnormalities, including congenital cataract, retinal and iridic colobomas, glaucoma, optic nerve dysplasia,

and visual loss. Cerebellar vermis hypoplasia can be variable. Intellectual disability has been described in all affected patients thus far. About one third of patients have severe *congenital ichthyosis*. Hypertrichosis and dysmorphic facial features are common, including squared face, high forehead, large ears, and coarsening. Some children with SRD5A3-CDG have a severe autism spectrum disorder. Skeletal abnormalities (scoliosis) and cardiac malformations are less common.

Pathophysiology

SRD5A3 deficiency leads to abnormal dolichol synthesis affecting early glycan synthesis outside the ER membrane and affects O-mannosylation and GPI-anchor synthesis. Hypoglycosylation affects anticoagulation factors and leads to increased serum transaminases.

Diagnosis

The primary screening method in a suspected SRD5A3-CDG patient is serum transferrin glycoform analysis or MS analysis. Most patients show a type 1 pattern (see Fig. 105.10), but several false-negative cases have been described. There is no clinically available enzyme analysis.

SRD5A3-CDG is autosomal recessive. Genetic testing is mostly performed by direct sequencing. The exact incidence is not known.

Treatment

In SRD5A3-CDG the treatment is supportive.

Autosomal Recessive Cutis Laxa Type 2 (ARCL-2A or ATP6V0A2-CDG, ATP6V1A-CDG and ATP6V1E1-CDG)
Clinical Manifestations

ATP6V02-CDG is a multiple-malformation syndrome originally described as *cutis laxa syndrome* and recently discovered to be a combined N- and O-linked glycosylation disorder. Patients show generalized cutis laxa with inelastic, sagging skin at birth, hypotonia, strabismus, myopia, characteristic facial features, and joint laxity. The facial features include hypertelorism, short nose, long philtrum, down-slanting palpebral fissures with sagging eyelids, and sagging cheeks. Cardiovascular involvement is rare, and there is variable CNS involvement. Seizures and motor and language developmental disability are common, but normal intelligence has been described as well. Sensorineural hearing loss is sometimes observed. Some patients have vermis hypoplasia, and several children have been described with cobblestone like dysgenesis and partial pachygyria on brain MRI. Skeletal abnormalities and short stature are common, as well as late-closing fontanels, and/or brachydactyly and scoliosis. There is frequently enamel dysplasia. The skin features spontaneously improve with age. **ATP6V1A-CDG** and **ATP6V1E1-CDG** show a highly overlapping phenotype with associated cardiovascular symptoms and hypercholesterolemia.

Pathophysiology

ATP6V0A2 is a membrane subunit of the proton pump of the vesicular adenosine triphosphatase (V-ATPase) complex. Abnormal function of the V-ATPase complex alters the pH gradient in the secretory pathway and affects the maturation and transport of several glycosyltransferases and elastic fibers (e.g., elastin). ATP6V1A and ATP6V1E1 are other complex subunits affecting ATP6V0A2 function and cause secondary ATPase deficiency. Both N- and O-linked glycosylation are affected. There are mild coagulation abnormalities and high serum transaminase levels in some patients.

Diagnosis

The primary screening method in a suspected ATP6V0A2-CDG patient is serum transferrin glycoform analysis or MS analysis. Most patients show a type 2 pattern (see Fig. 105.10), but false-negative cases have been described before age 6 wk. Apolipoprotein III-C (apoC-III) is a mucin-type secretory glycoprotein that is only O-glycosylated. ApoC-III IEF shows a hypoglycosylation pattern in patients, even when the TIEF is falsely negative. Skin biopsy in patients show classic histologic changes of cutis laxa with diminished, short, abnormal, and fuzzy elastic fibers.

ATP6V0A2-CDG is autosomal recessive. Genetic testing is mostly performed by direct sequencing. The exact incidence is not known. *ATP6V1A* and *ATP6V1E1* defects have been recently described.

Treatment

In autosomal recessive cutis laxa type 2, the treatment is supportive. There is continuous and spontaneous improvement of skin symptoms throughout the disease course, especially in ATP6V0A2-CDG.

Golgi-α$_{1-2}$ Mannosidase-1 Deficiency (MAN1B1-CDG)
Clinical Manifestations

MAN1B1 defect was originally described as an intellectual disability syndrome in association with dysmorphic features. Additional patients were recognized with psychomotor disability, muscle hypotonia, and inverted nipples in association with truncal obesity. The degree of intellectual disability is quite variable. Autistic behaviors, eating disorders, and aggressive behavior are frequent features. More than 30 patients have been reported.

Pathophysiology

MAN1B1 codes for a Golgi mannosidase, which is essential for the final "trimming" of mannose units during the glycan processing in the Golgi. Hypermannosylation leads to abnormal, truncated glycans and CDG-II. The glycosylation abnormality in serum is relatively mild. Increased serum transaminases and abnormal coagulation are uncommon.

Diagnosis

Most patients show a mild type 2 pattern by TIEF, but false-negative cases have been described. MALDI-TOF analysis shows characteristic, hybrid glycans in serum. In suspected cases, direct sequence analysis is recommended, even if the TIEF is normal.

MAN1B1-CDG is autosomal recessive. The exact incidence is unknown; several adult patients are known.

Treatment

Only supportive treatment is available.

Phosphoglucomutase-1 Deficiency (PGM1-CDG)
Clinical Manifestations

PGM1-CDG is a disorder presenting with midline malformations (cleft palate, Pierre Robin sequence, bifid uvula), liver dysfunction, hypoglycemia, and short stature in almost all patients. *Hypoglycemia* is usually caused by hyperinsulinism in the 1st years of life. It can resolve with aging; ketotic hypoglycemia has also been observed. Cholestasis, liver fibrosis, and even cirrhosis have been described in a few patients. About one third of patients also show proximal muscle weakness and dilated cardiomyopathy; the latter led to mortality in at least 7 reported cases. Other malformations, including cardiac and skeletal anomalies, have also been described. Wound healing is frequently abnormal, and there is a very high risk for bleeding during surgery. Intelligence is normal.

Pathophysiology

Phosphoglucomutase 1 (PGM1) is an essential enzyme for glycogenolysis and glycolysis. It also provides substrates for nucleotide sugars needed for normal glycosylation. PGM1 regulates the bidirectional conversion of glucose-1-phosphate and glucose-6-phosphate. During fasting it leads to a glycogenosis-like phenotype (also called GSD XIV, MIM 614921). PGM1-CDG affects both the ER- and Golgi-related glycosylation and causes a mixed type 1/type 2 hypoglycosylation pattern. Abnormal serum proteins include coagulation and anticoagulation factors, insulin-like growth factor–binding protein 3 (IGFBP3), TBG, and thyroid-stimulating hormone (TSH), in addition to serum transaminases, hypoglycemia, and elevated CK.

Diagnosis

The primary screening method in a suspected PGM1-CDG is serum transferrin glycoform analysis or MS analysis. Patients show a mixed type 1/type 2 pattern.

PGM1-CDG is autosomal recessive. It is among the relatively common CDGs; >40 patients have been described. Enzyme testing is possible in blood, but is more reliable in fibroblasts. Direct sequencing is available for testing.

Treatment

PGM1-CDG seems to be the 2nd treatable CDG besides MPI-CDG. D-Galactose is hypothesized to restore the balance in the availability of different nucleotide sugars. Adding 1 g/kg/day D-galactose for a few weeks to the diet improves glycosylation significantly, although the TIEF pattern does not fully normalize. This treatment improves liver transaminases and antithrombin levels and in some patients the hormonal status. The effect of D-galactose on hypoglycemic episodes and the myopathy is not yet clear. Larger, long-term dietary trials are ongoing.

Disorders of Golgi Homeostasis: TMEM199-, CCDC115-, ATP6AP2-CDG, and ATP6AP1-CDG
Clinical Manifestations

These 4 disorders are clinically and biochemically indistinguishable. They have been described with liver function anomalies, cholestasis, fibrosis, and cirrhosis with liver failure, necessitating liver transplantation in a few patients. The phenotype resembles **Wilson disease**, especially because of low serum ceruloplasmin and copper levels, but there is no Kayser-Fleischer ring. In CCDC115-CDG there are frequently also neurologic features. The intellectual outcome is variable. Additional abnormalities include hypercholesterolemia and elevated alkaline phosphatase. In ATP6AP1-CDG there is also immunologic involvement.

Pathophysiology

TMEM199-, CCDC115-, ATP6AP1-CDG, and ATP6AP2-CDG are important for Golgi homeostasis. The exact pathologic mechanism is not yet known, but it is hypothesized that the secondary Golgi dysfunction affects and delays the normal glycosylation process.

Diagnosis

The primary screening method in a patient with suspected PGM1-CDG is serum transferrin glycoform analysis or MS analysis. Patients show a type 2 pattern (see Fig. 105.10). ApoC-III IEF is abnormal. Glycomics results by MALDI-TOF analysis are characteristic but cannot discriminate between the 3 defects. Final diagnosis requires mutation analysis.

TMEM199-CDG and CCDC115-CDG are autosomal recessive, whereas ATP6AP1-CDG, and ATP6AP2-CDG are X-linked.

Treatment

Treatment is supportive; 2 patients successfully underwent liver transplantation.

Manganese Transporter Defect: SLC39A8-CDG
Clinical Manifestations

This intriguing disorder was originally described as a neurologic disease with hypotonia, seizures (hypsarrhythmia), and developmental disability. Some of the later-described patients had severe *skeletal dysplasia* with rhizomelic chondrodysplasia, craniosynostosis, and dwarfism. Mitochondrial dysfunction (Leigh disease, cerebral lactic acidemia, dystonia) may also be present.

Pathophysiology

SLC39A8 is a membrane transporter, responsible for the manganese (Mn) transmembrane transport. SLC39A8 deficiency affects all Mn-dependent enzymes and therefore different parts of the metabolism. Since several glycosyltransferases (e.g. β-1,4-galactosyltransferase) are Mn dependent, a secondary Golgi glycosylation occurs with a type 2 glycosylation defect. Low serum Mn levels are suggestive but not always present in patients.

Diagnosis

The primary screening method in a suspected SLC39A8-CDG is serum transferrin glycoform analysis or MS analysis. Patients show a type 2 pattern (see Fig. 105.10). MALDI-TOF analysis is suggestive, but not discriminative. Final diagnosis requires mutation analysis.

SLC39A8-CDG is an autosomal recessive disease. Its incidence is unknown.

Treatment

Besides supportive treatment, a few patients showed biochemical and clinical improvement (better seizure control) with oral D-galactose (1-3 g/kg/day) therapy.

CONGENITAL DISORDERS OF DEGLYCOSYLATION
N-Glycanase 1 Deficiency (*NGLY1* Defect)
Clinical Manifestations

Patients with NGLY1 deficiency do have a glycosylation disorder, but not from the deficient synthesis; rather, it is caused by deficient breakdown of glycoproteins. The phenotype comprises severe CNS involvement, microcephaly, intellectual disability, seizures, neuropathy, movement disorders, and hypotonia. The presence of *alacrimia*, hypolacrimia, or chalazion is highly suggestive for the diagnosis, but not all patients have problems with tearing. Other features include failure to thrive, intrauterine growth restriction, and liver involvement. Some patients have a recognizable oval face with a short nose, flat profile, and hypertelorism. Masklike face also occurs, imitating the phenotype of mitochondrial disorders, especially when serum lactic acid levels are also elevated.

Pathophysiology

N-glycanase is responsible for the deglycosylation of misfolded *N*-linked glycoproteins. The enzyme is essential for cutting off the glycans before the proteins are degraded in the ER. The increased abundance of misfolded *N*-glycans increases ER stress, which has been suggested as a possible reason for lactate elevation in several patients. Serum transaminase and α-fetoprotein levels are also frequently increased.

Diagnosis

Serum transferrin isoform analysis shows a normal pattern. Final diagnosis requires mutation analysis.

NGLY1-CDG is an autosomal recessive disease. The most common mutation is c.1201A>T/p.R401X. The exact incidence of the condition is unknown, but >20 patients have been reported in a few years since the discovery of the disease.

Treatment

Only supportive treatment is available for the patient with NGLY1 deficiency.

THERAPEUTIC SUMMARY

Most CDGs are only treatable with supportive therapy. The initially discovered oral mannose treatment in MPI-CDG (1 g/kg/day) has proved to be efficient for coagulation problems and protein-losing enteropathy but cannot prevent liver fibrosis in all patients. Liver transplantation in MPI-CDG has been successful in a few patients. Oral D-galactose in PGM1-CDG (1g/kg/day) improves serum transaminases and coagulation, and has a positive effect on endocrine function, but cannot restore glycosylation fully. Seizure frequency improved in patients with SLC39A8-CDG receiving oral D-galactose treatment (1 g/kg/day) and oral Mn intake. The congenital myasthenic syndrome in DPAGT1-CDG, GFPT1-CDG and GMPPB-CDG has been successfully treated with high dose of cholinesterase inhibitors. Several CDG have been positively controlled by transplantation; including DOLK-CDG (DK1-CDG; heart transplantation) PGM3-CDG (hematopoietic stem cell transplantation), CCDC155-CDG (liver transplantation).

Additional CDG treatment options are available for disorders not described in this chapter. Patients with CAD-CDG show significant clinical improvement on receiving oral uridine therapy, especially with seizure control. Two children with SLC35C1-CDG–defective immune function improved on oral fucose therapy. GNE-CDG patients showed significant improvement in muscle strength on *N*-acetylmannoseamin therapy. Several dietary trials are currently ongoing in different CDG.

Bibliography is available at expert consult.

Chapter **106**

Mitochondrial Disease Diagnosis

Marni J. Falk

第一百零六章
线粒体病诊断

中文导读

　　本章主要介绍了线粒体病概述、何时疑诊线粒体病、线粒体病遗传、线粒体病诊断性检测及线粒体病治疗原则。强调了线粒体疾病是多系统能量衰竭状态，具有高度的临床和遗传异质性。原发性线粒体疾病是由氧化磷酸化功能障碍导致的，这可能是由编码氧化磷酸化亚单位、装配因子或辅因子、线粒体DNA代谢和维持以及在线粒体内进行的许多其他基本代谢过程的基因突变所导致的。并且以图表形式清晰地归纳了线粒体基因的主要分子分类，线粒体病患者的所　有症状及其出现频率以及疑似线粒体病的诊断流程。

See also Chapter 105.4.

OVERVIEW OF MITOCHONDRIAL DISEASE

Mitochondrial diseases are multisystemic energy failure states with extensive clinical and genetic heterogeneity. Their common basis is best understood through recognition that mitochondria function as biologic "fuel cells," or "batteries," producing chemical energy in the form of adenosine triphosphate (ATP) by aerobic metabolism of nutrient-derived reducing equivalents, through the integrated function of the 5-complex mitochondrial **respiratory chain (RC)** (Fig. 106.1). Mitochondria also play other essential roles that can be variably disrupted in disease states, such as regulating calcium homeostasis, diverse aspects of intermediary nutrient metabolism, nucleotide metabolism, and oxidative stress. Primary mitochondrial disease results from deficient RC function, which can be caused by mutations in genes that encode RC subunits, assembly factors or cofactors, components of mitochondrial DNA (mtDNA)

metabolism and maintenance, or a host of other basic metabolic processes ongoing within mitochondria. Approximately 1,500 proteins exist within the mitochondrial proteome of different tissues, with variants in more than 350 unique genes across both the nuclear and the mitochondrial genomes already implicated as causal in human mitochondrial disease.

Collectively recognized as the most common group of inherited metabolic diseases, **primary** (genetic-based) mitochondrial disease has a combined minimal prevalence of 1 in 4,300 individuals across all ages. In addition, **secondary** mitochondrial dysfunction is broadly implicated in the pathogenesis of a host of complex diseases, ranging from metabolic syndrome to ischemia-reperfusion injury after stroke, to neurodegenerative diseases. Failure of high-energy demand organs in mitochondrial diseases may clinically present as severe neurodevelopmental, cardiac, myopathic, renal, hepatic, endocrine, immune, gastrointestinal, hearing, and vision disabilities, as well as global metabolic instability with lactic acidosis (Fig. 106.2) (see Tables 105.2 and 105.3).

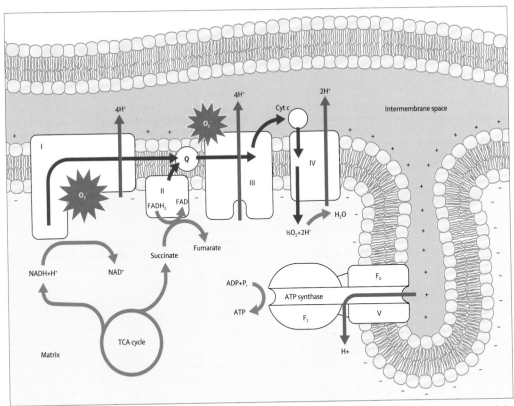

Fig. 106.1 Electron transport chain. The electron transport chain consists of 4 protein complexes (I-IV) coupled to a 5th (V), unlinked complex, ATP synthase. Together, these 5 complexes are known as the respiratory chain and are the site where oxidative phosporylation (OXPHOS) occurs to generate energy. The transport chain accepts electrons from NADH (complex I) or FADH₂ (complex II) that have been produced by glycolysis, the formation of acetyl–coenzyme A, and the TCA cycle (green arrows). Electrons flow from one complex to another (red arrows) because of the redox potential of each complex and lose a small amount of energy as they move through the chain. Three of the 4 complexes act as pumps, driven by electron flow, moving H⁺ ions from the matrix to the intermembrane space (blue arrows). This pumping builds a concentration gradient and creates an electrochemical force that is used by ATP synthase to produce ATP. Under normal conditions, this machinery provides almost all (90%) of the ATP in a cell. However, a small proportion of electrons escape the electron transport chain even under normal conditions and can react with oxygen and complexes I and III to form superoxide (O₂⁻). ADP, Adenosine diphosphate; ATP, adenosine triphosphate; Cyt c, cytochrome c; Q, coenzyme Q; NADH, nicotinamide dinucleotide; Pi, inorganic phosphate; TCA, tricarboxylic acid cycle; FADH2, 1,5-dihydro-flavin adenine dinucleotide. (Adapted from Hagberg H, Mallard C, Rousset CI, Thornton C: Mitochondria: hub of injury responses in the developing brain, Lancet Neurol 13(2):217–232, 2014.)

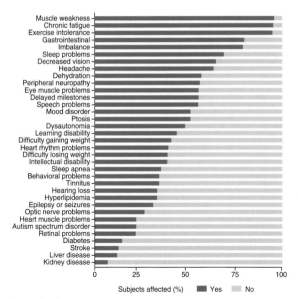

Fig. 106.2 Mitochondrial disease subject cohort, experienced symptoms. Frequency of experienced symptoms as reported by the RDCRN self-reported cohort revealed muscle weakness, chronic fatigue, exercise intolerance, imbalance, and gastrointestinal problems to be the top 5 common symptoms. *(Modified from Zolkipli-Cunningham Z, Xiao R, Stoddart A, et al: Mitochondrial disease patient motivations and barriers to participate in clinical trials. PLoS ONE 13(5):e0197513 [Fig. 2].)*

In most mitochondrial disorders, the phenotype may vary depending on the patient's age or the specific gene or genetic variant. Particularly common mitochondrial disease clinical syndromes that present in children include Leigh syndrome (for which there are more than 90 causal genes), mtDNA depletion syndrome (MDS, for which there are dozens of causal genes), mtDNA deletion syndromes (Pearson, Kearns Sayre), primary lactic acidosis, and pyruvate dehydrogenase deficiency. Common clinical features in children present in at least 90 percent of patients include fatigue, exercise intolerance, weakness, gastrointestinal problems, ataxia, and developmental delay. Thus, mitochondrial diseases present to and must be considered by clinicians across every medical specialty.

Patients with suspected mitochondrial disease may frequently experience a *diagnostic odyssey*, both clinically and genetically. Their extensive phenotypic heterogeneity without a common biomarker (GDF-15 may be one screening test that may be elevated in some mitochondrial myopathies particularly involving mtDNA deletions or depletion, along with lactic acidosis) presents a challenge to the readily available and accurate **clinical diagnosis** of mitochondrial disorders in many medical settings. Similarly, their extensive genetic heterogeneity involving known etiologies in >300 nuclear genes and all 37 mitochondrial DNA (mtDNA) genes, with likely dozens to hundreds more causative nuclear disease genes awaiting discovery, can make the accurate **genetic diagnosis** of an individual patient challenging. The diagnostic uncertainty can be further compounded by poor genotype-phenotype correlations and variable clinical presentations of individual gene disorders, high locus heterogeneity (i.e., multiple different causal disease genes) for similar clinical phenotypes, incomplete penetrance for some gene disorders, variable life stressors or environmental exposures that may exacerbate a given child's disease, and the unique biologic aspects of maternal inheritance for the subset of mitochondrial diseases caused by mtDNA gene mutations.

WHEN TO SUSPECT MITOCHONDRIAL DISEASE

Because of failure in the ability to generate cellular energy, mitochondrial diseases can involve any organ system at any age (see Fig. 106.2).

Mitochondrial disease should be suspected when classic symptoms are present or if unexplained symptoms occur in 3 or more apparently unrelated organs. Individuals may present with a vast array of symptoms, including fatigue, muscle weakness, exercise intolerance, metabolic strokes, seizures, cardiomyopathy, arrhythmias, developmental or cognitive disabilities, autism, diabetes mellitus, other endocrinopathies (adrenal, thyroid), dysautonomia, and autoimmune disorders, as well as impairment of hearing, vision, growth, liver, gastrointestinal (GI), or kidney function. Although individuals may have just one or a few symptoms and a fluctuating disease course in terms of symptom severity, most patients with primary mitochondrial disease tend to develop *progressive* symptoms over time. A study of patients with mitochondrial diseases showed an average of 16 different clinically significant symptoms per patient, with a range of 7-35. When considering the diagnosis, it is helpful to recognize that most symptoms of mitochondrial disease involve *functional*, rather than structural, problems.

When mitochondrial disease is considered in the differential diagnosis, it is often helpful to obtain several **laboratory screening** studies for common biochemical features of mitochondrial disease and overlapping disorders, both at baseline and if unrevealing, during an acute illness or period of decompensation. Blood-based metabolic screening studies include comprehensive chemistry panel, complete blood count with differential, plasma amino acid quantitative analysis, carnitine analysis (total, free, acyl-carnitine profile), ammonia, creatine kinase, and testing for common secondary manifestations of mitochondrial disease (e.g., thyroid screen, lipoprotein profile, hemoglobin A_{1c}). Urine-based metabolic screening studies include urinalysis, urine organic acid quantitative analysis, and urine amino acid quantitative analysis. Consideration should also be given for screening for congenital disorders of glycosylation or vitamin deficiencies, which may have overlapping clinical features in some cases with mitochondrial disease. Lactic acidemia is neither highly sensitive nor specific for primary mitochondrial disease, but laboratory findings suggestive of primary mitochondrial disease include elevations of blood lactate, pyruvate, lactate:pyruvate ratio, alanine, ratios of alanine to lysine (>3) and alanine to sum of phenylalanine and tyrosine (>4), and anion gap. Biochemical alterations further suggestive of mitochondrial disease may include secondary impairment of fatty acid oxidation with elevation of dicarboxylic acids on acyl-carnitine profile, increased branched-chain amino acids and proline on plasma amino acid analysis, increased tricarboxylic acid cycle intermediates and lactate excretion on urine organic acid analysis, and generalized aminoaciduria on urine amino acid analysis. Growth and differentiation factor 15 (**GDF-15**) may be a useful screening test for mitochondrial depletion based myopathies.

Similarly, when mitochondrial disease is considered in the differential diagnosis, obtaining additional **clinical evaluations** to carefully phenotype the patient for prevalent or highly morbid and potentially modifiable features of mitochondrial disease is important. Because many individuals with mitochondrial disease develop problems with their *vision* (reduced visual acuity not correctable with glasses, photophobia or nyctalopia with reduced peripheral vision associated with retinal disease or optic atrophy, ophthalmoplegia, ptosis), *hearing* (high-frequency sensorineural hearing loss), and *heart* (arrhythmia, conduction block, cardiomyopathy), carefully evaluating for involvement of these high-energy systems is indicated. **Neurologic** evaluation is essential because many mitochondrial disease patients experience a range of *central* (metabolic stroke in cortical or deep gray matter including basal ganglia, midbrain, and/or brainstem, white matter changes, seizures, ataxia, movement disorder, migraine, cognitive changes), *peripheral* (axonal sensorimotor neuropathy), or *autonomic* nervous system dysfunction; brain imaging (MRI), spectroscopy (MRS), and on occasion electromyogram or nerve conduction velocity (EMG/NCV) studies can be helpful to support the diagnosis. Formal **exercise physiology** evaluation can also be useful to quantify and advise patients on their exercise capacity and safety, with some specific features (e.g., reduced $\dot{V}O_2$ maximal capacity) suggestive of quantifiable mitochondrial dysfunction. **Sleep** study may be useful for individuals with sleep dysfunction because sleep disorders may mimic mitochondrial disease symptoms, and sleep problems are common and potentially treatable in mitochondrial disease. **Gastrointestinal** symptoms are common and underrecognized in mitochondrial disease patients, usually involving dysmotility of any portion of the GI tract with reflux, swallowing dysfunction, delayed gastric emptying, feeding and/or growth problems, pseudoobstruction, malabsorption, and constipation. **Endocrine** abnormalities are also common but underappreciated in many patients, including pituitary, adrenal, thyroid, and pancreatic dysfunction. Such careful phenotyping of patients with suspected mitochondrial disease can thus provide reassurance that the common, and potentially treatable, clinical aspects of mitochondrial disease are not present although they may develop over time, or conversely if identified, increase diagnostic suspicion and direct further diagnostic evaluation.

MITOCHONDRIAL DISEASE INHERITANCE

Primary mitochondrial disease may result from variants in either nuclear genes or mtDNA genes, which may be inherited from a parent or occur de novo in an affected individual. Thus, all *mendelian* (autosomal recessive, autosomal dominant, X-linked) or *maternal* (mtDNA) inheritance patterns can be consistent with mitochondrial diseases (Table 106.1). Obtaining a detailed, three-generation pedigree is important to potentially highlight the specific inheritance pattern in a given family. Individuals with inherited mtDNA disorders may report family members related through their maternal lineage (both males and females may be affected, but only affected individuals will be connected through the female germline), with a range of functional problems in different organs, such as migraines, fatigue, exercise intolerance, stroke, diabetes mellitus, thyroid dysfunction, irritable bowel spectrum, mood disorder, or vision and hearing problems. Inherited X-linked disorders typically present with symptoms only, or more severely, in males related through unaffected or minimally affected females. **Autosomal recessive** disorders are common in pediatric mitochondrial disease, particularly in consanguineous pedigrees, where a rare variant in the general population becomes enriched and passed down through both maternal and paternal lineages to become homozygous in the affected proband and also affect multiple individuals in a given generation without having affected individuals in earlier generations. **Autosomal dominant** variants may occur de novo or are passed on from either parent to their child, although many disorders may have reduced penetrance, which may make the genetic disorder appear to skip a generation. Identifying a likely inheritance pattern through pedigree analysis can inform accurate interpretation of large-scale genetic diagnostic evaluations, such as multigene sequencing and deletion/duplication analysis panels and exome or genome sequencing. Establishing a correct genetic diagnosis for mitochondrial disease in an affected individual is essential to enable reliable recurrence risk

counseling and testing options in a given family, whether in a future pregnancy by chorionic villus sampling (CVS, typically performed at 10-12 weeks' gestation) or amniocentesis (typically performed at 16-20 weeks' gestation) or in the in vitro fertilization (IVF) setting with preimplantation genetic diagnosis (PGD) for a specific disease-causing variant.

Special mention is warranted to consider the unique aspects of *maternal inheritance* that typify mtDNA disorders. More than 300 disease-causing mtDNA variants have been identified, with extensive variation in disease manifestations and features. Most disease-causing variants are present in only a portion of an individual's mtDNA genomes, a concept known as **heteroplasmy**. For heteroplasmic mtDNA variants, the precise mutation level (percent) can vary between an individual's different tissues and can change over time, with symptom severity corresponding to different threshold mutation levels that can be difficult to define and that typically vary between organs. An individual's mtDNA genome background set of fixed sequence variants, known as a **haplogroup**, can also influence the penetrance or severity of a mtDNA disease. When a novel or rare mtDNA variant is identified in a given individual, it may be useful to use highly sensitive sequencing methods to test the levels of that mutation (which may be accurate to detect 1% mutation levels) in their tissues (blood, urine, buccal, skin cells, muscle), as well as tissues from their mother or maternal relatives, to accurately determine whether it may be causal of disease in that family. Research-based functional testing may also be necessary to characterize fully the effects of a newly recognized mtDNA variant. When it is not known whether an mtDNA variant is maternally inherited or occurs de novo, the recurrence risk to future offspring of their asymptomatic parent is empirically estimated at 1 in 25 (4%), although the empirical recurrence risk rises to 1 in 2 (50%) when the mother is symptomatic.

DIAGNOSTIC TESTING FOR MITOCHONDRIAL DISEASE

The diagnosis of mitochondrial disease relies foremost on genetic testing (genomic analysis), with biochemical screens useful in blood or urine and invasive tissue testing often seen as secondary, or sometimes not required at all (Fig. 106.3).

When the clinical evaluation—medical history; detailed review of systems; careful physical, neurologic, and dysmorphic examinations; pedigree-, blood-, and urine-based biochemical screening studies; and additional phenotyping clinical evaluations—is suggestive of mitochondrial disease, a range of clinical diagnostic testing options can be pursued. Absent a known molecular etiology in an affected family member,

Table 106.1	Major Molecular Categories of Mitochondrial Genes			
COMPONENT	**CAUSAL GENOME**	**GENE MUTATION EFFECTS**		**DISEASE EXAMPLES**
Electron transport chain enzyme subunits	Nuclear or mtDNA	Decreased functioning of electron transport chain complex		Complex I deficiency Complex II deficiency
Electron transport chain assembly factors	Nuclear	Decreased assembly of electron transport chain enzyme complex		Complex III deficiency Complex IV deficiency Complex V deficiency
Electron transport chain cofactors	Nuclear	Decreased functioning of electron transport chain		Coenzyme Q10 deficiency Iron sulfur cluster defect Lipoyltransferase deficiency
mtDNA translation	Nuclear or mtDNA	Decreased translation of protein-coding mitochondrial DNA genes leading to decreased functioning of electron transport chain enzymes		Combined oxidative phosphorylation complexes deficiency
mtDNA maintenance	Nuclear	Increased errors in mitochondrial DNA leading to increased presence of point mutations and deletions, resulting in decreased translation of electron transport chain subunits		Mitochondrial DNA depletion syndromes Mitochondrial DNA multiple deletion disorders
Mitochondrial membrane fission and fusion	Nuclear	Increased mtDNA point mutations and deletions; clumped and fragmented mitochondria		*OPA1*-related conditions *MFN2*-related conditions

From McCormick EM, Muraresku CC, Falk MJ: Mitochondrial genomics: a complex field now coming of age. *Curr Genet Med Rep* 6:52–61, 2018 (Table 1, p. 57).

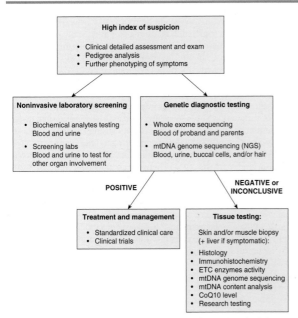

Fig. 106.3 Diagnostic algorithm for suspected mitochondrial disease. *(From Murareshu CC, McCormick EM, Flak MJ: Mitochondrial disease: advances in clinical diagnosis, management, therapeutic development, and preventative strategies. Curr Genet Med Rep 6:62–72, 2018.)*

first-line genetic diagnostic testing may involve a focused panel of hundreds to thousands of known nuclear genes and the mtDNA genome using **next-generation sequencing** (NGS) methodologies that will detect both single-nucleotide variants and larger-scale gene deletions and duplications. If such testing is unrevealing, clinically based **whole exome sequencing** (WES) may be pursued. The standard of care is moving to pursue initial diagnostic testing by WES, which is more comprehensive for genes known not only to cause mitochondrial disease, but also to cause all human genetic diseases. The rationale for this evolution in diagnostic testing approach includes the following factors:

1. An increasingly similar cost and turnaround-time for panel-based and WES-based massively parallel NGS studies.
2. The common genetic diagnostic laboratory practice of generating WES data for all tests ordered, but only evaluating and reporting variants in specific gene subsets when panel-based testing is requested, leaving the remaining genes uninterpreted.
3. The mtDNA genome sequence is often included at no extra cost when clinical WES is ordered in blood, but may need to be repeated in a symptomatic tissue (e.g., muscle, liver) to detect heteroplasmic mtDNA variants that may not be present in blood.
4. The utility of performing concurrent proband and both parental sample sequencing *(trio-based testing)*, as usually pursued with WES but not panel-based testing, thereby allowing concurrent segregation analysis of a suspected pathogenic variants as well as ready identification of de novo dominant variants in the proband.
5. The improved diagnostic yield of exome relative to panel-based testing increasingly being reported by clinical diagnostic laboratories, given the highly heterogeneous nature of mitochondrial disease, rapid rate of change in the recognition of *new* gene diagnoses making prior established gene panels obsolete, and the extensive phenotypic overlap with non-mitochondrial diseases.
6. The ability to utilize WES raw data (either on a research basis or for reanalysis at a later date by the clinical diagnostic laboratory) to highlight and/or identify "novel" gene disorders not previously recognized or associated with human disease.

A mitochondrial disease community resource to centrally curate all mitochondrial disease, gene, and variant knowledge across both genomes

is publicly accessible at www.mseqdr.org. Exome sequencing including mtDNA is estimated to identify the definitive genetic etiology for mitochondrial disease in at least 60% of patients in whom it is strongly suspected, reducing the diagnostic odyssey in many patients from decades or years to months.

Tissue-based diagnostic testing has decreased in frequency as a front-line test in all patients with suspected mitochondrial disease, although it still has clinical utility in some cases. These include (1) in the setting of rapidly deteriorating clinical status when genetic testing results may not be available in a timely fashion; (2) when a variant of uncertain significance identified on genomic testing has unclear biochemical consequences; and (3) when uninformative genomic sequencing in blood in an individual with myopathy or muscle symptoms raises concern for other disease processes that may be evident on histology, electron microscopy, immunohistochemistry or enzymatic tissue testing. In addition, some mitochondrial diseases are only evident by tissue-based diagnostic testing. These include mtDNA deletion disorders (typically involving several-thousand nucleotides) not present in blood that cause chronic **progressive external ophthalmoplegia** (CPEO) or **Kearns-Sayre syndrome** (KSS) spectrum disorder, as well as different tissue (muscle or liver)-specific mtDNA depletion disorders (e.g., reduced mtDNA tissue content) that confirm a mitochondrial pathophysiology in a given patient and highlight a likely underlying nuclear gene cause for their disease, since mtDNA maintenance requires a host of nuclear-encoded proteins. Muscle analysis for integrated RC oxidative phosphorylation capacity assessment requires analysis of a fresh muscle biopsy only available at a very limited number of sites worldwide, whereas **electron transport chain enzyme** activity analyses are the accepted gold standard to evaluate for mitochondrial dysfunction in a previously frozen tissue sample, often shipped elsewhere for diagnostic analysis. Skin biopsies are useful to establish fibroblast cell lines in which these same studies of mitochondrial function can be clinically performed. If detected, abnormalities can be revealing of a specific type of mitochondrial disorder, although not all mitochondrial diseases may be expressed or detectable in skin analysis. Thus, if fibroblast testing is unrevealing, more invasive tissue studies may subsequently need to be pursued. Fibroblast cell lines, and occasionally blood-based lymphoblastoid cell lines, also provide a minimally invasive cell source to allow other clinical enzymatic analyses to be performed, as well as novel disease gene validation and research-based therapeutic modeling.

TREATMENT PRINCIPLES FOR MITOCHONDRIAL DISEASE

Effective therapies for both primary and secondary mitochondrial diseases are lacking, because little has been known about the biochemical and physiologic abnormalities that contribute to their diverse clinical manifestations. Clinical complexity and imprecisely defined or understood biochemical phenotypes of different mitochondrial disease subtypes have made it difficult for clinicians to effectively apply or monitor targeted therapies for RC disease. *Mitochondrial cocktails* of vitamins and supplements variably include vitamins (B_1, B_2, C), antioxidants (CoQ_{10}, lipoic acid, vitamin E), and metabolic modifiers (creatine, L-carnitine, L-arginine, folinic acid). Although the efficacy, toxicity, and optimal dose of these drugs are not known and have not been objectively assessed in human RC disease patients, they continue to be empirically prescribed in hopes of enhancing residual RC enzymatic function or quenching toxic metabolites theorized to accumulate in RC dysfunction, and because of patient-based reports of improved well-being. However, provision of these therapies has often adopted a one-size-fits-all approach, ignoring the inherent variation in primary mitochondrial disease subtypes, the tissue-specific manifestations, and the major pathogenic factors, such as the predominant downstream metabolic and signaling alterations that occur in different disease subclasses.

Although no cure or U.S. Food and Drug Administration (FDA)–approved therapy yet exists for any mitochondrial disease, improved molecular delineation has enabled selected therapies to advance from the theoretical, empirical, and largely ineffective stage to a promising horizon of rational, personalized, and effective interventions. An increasing number of mitochondrial disease diagnoses have interventions involving the initiation or avoidance of specific medications (corticosteroids, valproic acid, phenytoin, barbiturates, propofol for prolonged duration beyond 30-60 min, certain anesthetics, statins, β-blocking agents, amiodarone, nucleoside reverse transcriptase inhibitors), provision of cofactors or diets, and screening regimens for progressive clinical involvement of modifiable manifestations. General therapies for **Leigh syndrome** such as L-arginine and citrulline may prevent or reverse neurodevelopmental sequelae from a metabolic stroke. Nutritional therapies in these disorders are tailored to specific disease genes, such as thiamine and biotin for *SLC19A3* disease, ubiquinol for *PDSS2* (CoQ$_{10}$ deficiency) disease, and thiamine and the ketogenic diet for *PDHA1* (pyruvate dehydrogenase) deficiency. Establishing the precise molecular diagnosis can further be lifesaving by avoiding fasting and mitochondrial-toxic medicines or general anesthetics in specific mitochondrial disease

subsets, improving recurrence risk counseling and prevention, enabling targeted screening for reported medical complications, and in some cases providing necessary cofactors or vitamins that may not otherwise have been considered. In addition, reproductive methodologies emerging in some countries for mitochondrial disease prevention, such as **mitochondrial replacement technologies** (MRTs), are only appropriate to consider in the setting of known pathogenic, inherited mtDNA variants. Finally, the ability to molecularly identify primary mitochondrial disease patients has enabled the design of an increasing number of clinical treatment trials now being planned or underway for a diverse range of symptoms that occur in primary mitochondrial diseases (see www.clinicaltrials.gov).

Bibliography is available at Expert Consult.

Chapter **107**
Mucopolysaccharidoses
Jürgen W. Spranger

第一百零七章
黏多糖贮积症

中文导读

　　本章主要介绍了黏多糖贮积症疾病实体、诊断和鉴别诊断以及治疗。具体描述了黏多糖贮积症 I 型、黏多糖贮积症 II 型、黏多糖贮积症 III 型、黏多糖贮积症 IV 型、黏多糖贮积症 VI 型、黏多糖贮积症 VII 型，黏多糖贮积症 IX 型以及黏多糖贮积症附加综合征。

Mucopolysaccharidoses are hereditary, progressive diseases caused by mutations of genes coding for lysosomal enzymes needed to degrade glycosaminoglycans (acid mucopolysaccharides). *Glycosaminoglycans* (GAGs) are long-chain complex carbohydrates composed of uronic acids, amino sugars, and neutral sugars. The major GAGs are chondroitin-4-sulfate, chondroitin-6-sulfate, heparan sulfate, dermatan sulfate, keratan sulfate, and hyaluronan. These substances are synthesized and, with the exception of hyaluronan, linked to proteins to form *proteoglycans*, major constituents of the ground substance of connective tissue and of nuclear and cell membranes. Degradation of proteoglycans starts with the proteolytic removal of the protein core, followed by the stepwise degradation of the GAG moiety. Failure of this degradation because of absent or grossly reduced activity of mutated lysosomal enzymes results in the intralysosomal accumulation of GAG fragments (Fig. 107.1). Distended lysosomes accumulate in the cell, interfere with cell function, and lead to characteristic patterns of clinical, radiologic, and biochemical abnormalities (Table 107.1 and Fig. 107.2). Within these patterns, specific

diseases can be recognized that evolve from the intracellular accumulation of different degradation products (Table 107.2). As a general rule, the impaired degradation of heparan sulfate is more closely associated with **mental deficiency**, and that of dermatan, chondroitin, and keratan sulfate with **mesenchymal abnormalities**. Variable expression within a given entity results from allelic mutations and varying residual activity of mutated enzymes. For instance, allelic mutations of the gene encoding L-iduronidase may result in severe **Hurler disease** (Hurler syndrome) with early death or in mild **Scheie disease** (Scheie syndrome) manifesting only with limited joint mobility, mild skeletal abnormalities, and corneal opacities.

Mucopolysaccharidoses are autosomal recessive disorders, with the exception of **Hunter disease** (Hunter syndrome), which is X-linked recessive. Their birth prevalence varies between 1.2 per 100,000 births (United States) and 16.9 per 100,000 births (Saudi Arabia). In the United States the most common subtype is MPS-III, followed by MPS-I and MPS-II.

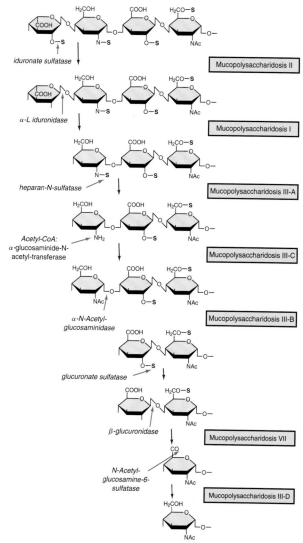

Fig. 107.1 Degradation of heparan sulfate and mucopolysaccharidoses resulting from the deficiency of individual enzymes. Some of the enzymes are also involved in the degradation of other glycosaminoglycans (not shown).

| Table 107.1 | Recognition Pattern of Mucopolysaccharidoses |

MANIFESTATIONS	MUCOPOLYSACCHARIDOSIS (MPS) TYPE						
	I-H	I-S	II	III	IV	VI	VII
Intellectual disability	+	−	±	+	−	−	±
Coarse facial features	+	(+)	+	+	−	+	±
Corneal clouding	+	+	−	−	(+)	+	±
Visceromegaly	+	(+)	+	(+)	−	+	+
Short stature	+	(+)	+	−	+	+	+
Joint contractures	+	+	+	−	+	+	+
Dysostosis multiplex	+	(+)	+	(+)	+	+	+
Leucocyte inclusions	+	(+)	+	+	−	+	+
Mucopolysacchariduria	+	+	+	+	+	+	+

I-H, Hurler syndrome; I-S, Scheie syndrome; II, Hunter syndrome; III, Sanfilippo syndrome; IV, Morquio syndrome; VI, Maroteaux-Lamy syndrome; VII, Sly syndrome.

+, Presence of manifestation, −, absence of manifestation; ±, possible presence of manifestation; (+), mild manifestation.

Hurler Syndrome

The Hurler form of MPS-I (**MPS I-H**) is a severe, progressive disorder with involvement of multiple organs and tissues that results in premature death, usually by 10 yr of age. An infant with Hurler syndrome appears normal at birth, but inguinal hernias and failed neonatal hearing tests may be early signs. Diagnosis is usually made at 6-24 mo, with evidence of hepatosplenomegaly, coarse facial features, corneal clouding, large tongue, enlarged head circumference, joint stiffness, short stature, and skeletal dysplasia. Acute cardiomyopathy has been found in some infants <1 yr. Most patients have recurrent upper respiratory tract and ear infections, noisy breathing, and persistent copious nasal discharge. Valvular heart disease, notably with incompetence of the mitral and aortic valves, regularly develops, and narrowing of the coronary arteries occurs. Obstructive airway disease, especially during sleep, may necessitate tracheotomy. Obstructive airway disease, respiratory infection, and cardiac complications are the common causes of death (Table 107.3).

Most children with Hurler syndrome acquire only limited language skills because of intellectual disability, combined conductive and neurosensory hearing loss, and an enlarged tongue. Progressive ventricular enlargement with increased intracranial pressure caused by communicating hydrocephalus also occurs. Corneal clouding, glaucoma, and retinal degeneration are common. Radiographs show a characteristic skeletal dysplasia known as **dysostosis multiplex** (Figs. 107.3 and 107.4). The earliest radiographic signs are thick ribs and ovoid vertebral bodies. Skeletal abnormalities (in addition to those shown in the figures) include enlarged, coarsely trabeculated diaphyses of the long bones with irregular metaphyses and epiphyses. With disease progression, macrocephaly develops with thickened calvarium, premature closure of lambdoid and sagittal sutures, shallow orbits, enlarged J-shaped sella, and abnormal spacing of teeth with dentigerous cysts.

Hurler-Scheie Syndrome

The clinical phenotype of the Hurler-Scheie form of MPS-I (**MPS I-H/S**) is *intermediate* between Hurler and Scheie syndromes and is characterized by progressive somatic involvement, including dysostosis multiplex with little or no intellectual dysfunction. The onset of symptoms is usually observed between 3 and 8 yr of age. Survival to adulthood is common. Cardiac involvement and upper airway obstruction contribute to clinical morbidity. Some patients have spondylolisthesis, which may cause cord compression.

Scheie Syndrome

The Scheie form of MPS-I (**MPS I-S**) is a comparatively mild disorder

DISEASE ENTITIES
Mucopolysaccharidosis I

Mucopolysaccharidosis I (MPS-I) is caused by mutations of the *IUA* gene on chromosome 4p16.3 encoding α-L-iduronidase. Mutation analysis has revealed 2 major alleles, W402X and Q70X, which account for more than half the MPS-I alleles in the white population. The mutations that introduce stop codons with ensuing absence of functional enzyme (null alleles), and in homozygosity or compound heterozygosity, give rise to Hurler syndrome. Other mutations occur in only one or a few individuals.

Deficiency of α-L-iduronidase results in a wide range of clinical involvement, from severe Hurler syndrome to mild Scheie syndrome, which are ends of a broad clinical spectrum. Homozygous nonsense mutations result in severe forms of MPS-I, whereas missense mutations are more likely to preserve some residual enzyme activity associated with a milder form of the syndrome.

characterized by joint stiffness, aortic valve disease, corneal clouding, and mild dysostosis multiplex. Onset of significant symptoms is usually after age 5 yr, with diagnosis made between 10 and 20 yr. Patients with Scheie syndrome have normal intelligence and stature but have significant joint and ocular involvement. A carpal tunnel syndrome often develops. Ophthalmic features include corneal clouding, glaucoma, and retinal degeneration. Obstructive airway disease, causing sleep apnea, develops in some patients, necessitating tracheotomy. Aortic valve disease is common and has required valve replacement in some patients.

Mucopolysaccharidosis II

Hunter syndrome (MPS-II) is an X-linked disorder caused by the deficiency of iduronate 2-sulfatase. The *IDS* gene is mapped to Xq28. Point mutations of *IDS* have been detected in about 80% of patients with MPS-II. Major deletions or rearrangements of *IDS* have been found in the rest, and these are usually associated with a more severe clinical phenotype. As an X-linked recessive disorder, Hunter syndrome manifests almost exclusively in males. However, it has been observed in females, because of skewed inactivation of the X-chromosome carrying the normal gene.

Marked molecular heterogeneity explains the wide clinical spectrum of Hunter syndrome. Patients with severe MPS-II have features similar to those of Hurler syndrome, except for the lack of corneal clouding and the somewhat slower progression of somatic and central nervous system (CNS) deterioration. Coarse facial features, short stature, dysostosis multiplex, joint stiffness, and intellectual disability manifest between 2 and 4 yr of age. Grouped skin papules are present in some patients. Extensive mongolian spots have been observed in African and Asian patients and may be an early marker of the disease. Gastrointestinal (GI) storage may produce chronic diarrhea. Communicating hydrocephalus and spastic paraplegia may result from thickened meninges. In severely affected patients, extensive, slowly progressive neurologic involvement precedes death, which usually occurs at age 10-15 yr.

Patients with the mild form have a near-normal or normal life span, minimal CNS involvement, and slow progression of somatic deterioration with preservation of cognitive function in adult life. Survival to ages 65 and 87 yr has been reported, and some patients have had children. Somatic features are Hurler-like but milder with a greatly reduced rate of progression. Adult height may exceed 150 cm (60 inches). Airway involvement, valvular cardiac disease, hearing impairment, carpal tunnel

syndrome, and joint stiffness are common and can result in significant loss of function in both the mild and severe forms.

Mucopolysaccharidosis III

Sanfilippo syndrome (MPS-III) is a genetically heterogeneous but clinically similar group of 4 recognized types (IIIA-IIID). Each type is caused by a different enzyme deficiency involved in the degradation of heparan sulfate (see Fig. 107.1). Genes encoding these enzymes are listed in Table 107.2.

Sanfilippo syndrome is characterized by slowly progressive, severe CNS degeneration with mild somatic disease. Onset of clinical features usually occurs at age 2–6 yr in a child who previously appeared normal. Presenting features include delayed cognitive development, hyperactivity with aggressive behavior, coarse hair, hirsutism, sleep disorders, and mild hepatosplenomegaly. Delay in diagnosis of MPS-III is common because of the mild physical features, hyperactivity, and slowly progressive neurologic disease. Severe neurologic deterioration occurs in most patients by age 6-10 yr, accompanied by rapid deterioration of social and adaptive skills. Severe behavior problems are common, such as sleep disturbance, uncontrolled hyperactivity, temper tantrums, destructive behavior, and physical aggression. Profound intellectual disability and behavior problems often occur in patients with normal physical strength, making management particularly difficult.

Mucopolysaccharidosis IV

Morquio syndrome (MPS-IV) is caused by a deficiency of N-acetylgalactosamine-6-sulfatase **(MPS-IVA)** or of β-galactosidase **(MPS-IVB)**. Both result in the defective degradation of keratan sulfate. The gene encoding N-acetylgalactosamine-6-sulfatase is *GALNS* on chromosome 16q24.3, and the gene encoding β-galactosidase is *GLB1* on chromosome 3p21.33. β-Galactosidase catalyzes GM$_1$ ganglioside in addition to endohydrolysis of keratan sulfate, and most mutations of *GLB1* result in generalized **gangliosidosis**, a spectrum of neurodegenerative disorders associated with dysostosis multiplex. A W273L mutation of the *GLB1* gene, either in the homozygous state or as part of compound heterozygosity, usually results in Morquio B syndrome.

Both types of Morquio syndrome are characterized by short-trunk dwarfism, a skeletal dysplasia that is distinct from other mucopolysaccharidoses, and preservation of intelligence. MPS-IVA is usually more severe than MPS-IVB, with adult height of <125 cm (50 inches)

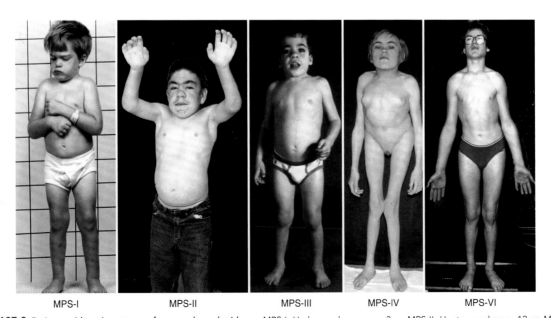

Fig. 107.2 Patients with various types of mucopolysaccharidoses. MPS-I: Hurler syndrome, age 3 yr; MPS-II: Hunter syndrome, 12 yr; MPS-III: Sanfilippo syndrome, 4 yr; MPS-IV: Morquio syndrome, 10 yr; MPS-VI: Maroteaux-Lamy syndrome, 15 yr.

| Table 107.2 | | Mucopolysaccharidoses: Clinical, Molecular, and Biochemical Aspects | | | | | |

MPS TYPE	EPONYM	INHERITANCE	GENE CHROMOSOME	MAIN CLINICAL FEATURES	DEFECTIVE ENZYME	ASSAY	MIM NUMBER
I-H	(Pfaundler-) Hurler	AR	IDUA 4p16.3	Severe Hurler phenotype, mental deficiency, corneal clouding, death usually before age 14 yr	α-L-iduronidase	L, F, Ac, Cv	252800 607014
I-S	Scheie	AR	IDUA 4p16.4	Stiff joints, corneal clouding, aortic valve disease, normal intelligence, survive to adulthood	α-L-iduronidase	L, F, Ac, Cv	607016
I-HS	Hurler-Scheie	AR	IDUA 4p16.4	Phenotype intermediate between I-H and I-S	α-L-iduronidase	L, F, Ac, Cv	607015
II	Hunter	XLR	IDS Xq27.3-28	Severe course: similar to I-H but clear corneas Mild course: less pronounced features, later manifestation, survival to adulthood with mild or without mental deficiency	Iduronate sulfate sulfatase	S, F, Af, Ac, Cv	309900
IIIA	Sanfilippo A	AR	SGSH 17q25.3	Behavioral problems, sleeping disorder, aggression, progressive dementia, mild dysmorphism, coarse hair, clear corneas Survival to adulthood possible	Heparan-S-sulfamidase	L, F, Ac, Cv	252900 605270
IIIB	Sanfilippo B	AR	NAGLU 17q21		N-Acetyl-α-D-glucosaminidase	S, F, Ac, Cv	252920
IIIC	Sanfilippo C	AR	HGSNAT 8p11.21		Acetyl-CoA-glucosaminide N-acetyltransferase	F, Ac	252930
IIID	Sanfilippo D	AR	GNS 12q14		N-Acetylglucosamine–6-sulfate sulfatase	F, Ac	252940 607664
IVA	Morquio A	AR	GALNS 16q24.3	Short-trunk dwarfism, fine corneal opacities, characteristic bone dysplasia; final height <125 cm	N-Acetylgalactosamine-6-sulfate sulfatase	L, F, Ac	253000
IVB	Morquio B	AR	GLB1 3p21.33	Same as IVA, but milder; adult height >120 cm	β-Galactosidase	L, F, Ac, Cv	253010 230500
VI	Maroteaux-Lamy	AR	ARSB 5q11-q13	Hurler phenotype with marked corneal clouding but normal intelligence; mild, moderate, and severe expression in different families	N-Acetylgalactosamine-α-4-sulfate sulfatase (arylsulfatase B)	L, F, Ac	253200
VII	Sly	AR	GUSB 7q21.11	Varying from fetal hydrops to mild dysmorphism; dense inclusions in granulocytes	β-Glucuronidase	S, F, Ac, Cv	253220
IX	Hyaluronidase deficiency	AR	HYAL1 3p21.3	Periarticular masses, no Hurler phenotype	Hyaluronidase 1	S	601492
MPSPS	MPS plus syndrome	AR	VPS33A	Mild Hurler phenotype, cognitive deficiency, organomegaly, skeletal dysplasia, pancytopenia, renal insufficiency, optic atrophy, early death	No lysosomal enzyme deficiency		617303

AR, Autosomal recessive; XLR, X-linked recessive; L, Leukocytes; S, serum; F, cultured fibroblasts; Ac, cultured amniotic cells; Af, amniotic fluid; Cv, chorionic villus sampling; MIM, Mendelian Inheritance in Man Catalogue.

and >150 cm, respectively. However, there is considerable variability of expression in both subtypes. The appearance of genu valgum, kyphosis, growth retardation with short trunk and neck, and waddling gait with a tendency to fall are early symptoms of MPS-IV. Extraskeletal manifestations include mild corneal clouding, small teeth with abnormally thin enamel, frequent caries formation, and occasionally hepatomegaly and cardiac valvular lesions. Instability of the odontoid process and ligamentous laxity are invariably present and can result in life-threatening atlantoaxial instability and dislocation. Thickened anterior extradural tissue contributes to spinal cord compression. Regular neurologic assessment and radiologic imaging are imperative. Surgery to stabilize the upper cervical spine, usually by posterior

spinal fusion, before the development of cervical myelopathy, can be lifesaving.

Mucopolysaccharidosis VI

Maroteaux-Lamy syndrome (MPS-VI) is caused by mutations of the *ARSB* gene on chromosome 5q11-13 encoding N-acetylgalactosamine-4-sulfatase (arylsulfatase B). It is characterized by severe to mild somatic involvement, as seen in MPS-I, but with preservation of intelligence. The somatic involvement of the severe form of MPS-IV is characterized by corneal clouding, coarse facial features, joint stiffness, valvular heart disease, communicating hydrocephalus, and dysostosis multiplex. In the severe form, growth can be normal for the 1st few years of life but

Table 107.3	Analysis of Symptom Frequency in Patients With MPS-I ≤2 Yr of Age

SYMPTOMS/COMPLICATIONS	PERCENTAGE OF PATIENTS WITH SYMPTOM
Coarse facies	98
Valvular disease	95
Corneal clouding	90
Hepatomegaly	84
Upper airway obstruction → OSA	82
Kyphosis gibbus	75
Joint contractures	72
Hernia	70
Dysostosis multiplex	70
Cognitive impairment	60
Enlarged tongue	60
Splenomegaly	60
Eustachian tube obstruction → otitis media	55
Hip dysplasia	42
Genu valgum	38
Reactive airway disease	37
Scoliosis	35
Carpal tunnel syndrome	25
Pes cavus	18
Glaucoma	10
Heart failure	3
Cor pulmonale	2

OSA, Obstructive sleep apnea.
From Clarke LA, Atherton AM, Burton BK, et al: Mucopolysaccharidosis type I newborn screening: best practices for diagnosis and management, *J Pediatr* 182:363–370, 2017 (Table 1, p 364).

seems to virtually stop after age 6-8 yr. The mild to intermediate forms of Maroteaux-Lamy syndrome can be easily confused with Scheie syndrome. Spinal cord compression from thickening of the dura in the upper cervical canal with resultant myelopathy is common in patients with MPS-VI.

Mucopolysaccharidosis VII
Sly syndrome (MPS-VII) is caused by mutations of the *GUSB* gene located on chromosome 7q21.11. Mutations result in a deficiency of ß-glucuronidase, intracellular storage of GAG fragments, and extensive clinical involvement. The most severe form presents as lethal **nonimmune fetal hydrops** and may be detected in utero by ultrasound. Some severely affected newborns survive for months and have, or develop, signs of lysosomal storage disease, including thick skin, visceromegaly, and dysostosis multiplex. Less severe forms of MPS-VII present during the 1st years of life with features of MPS-I but slower progression. Corneal clouding varies. Patients with manifestation after 4 yr of life have skeletal abnormalities of dysostosis multiplex but normal intelligence and usually clear corneas. They may be found incidentally on the basis of a blood smear that shows coarse granulocytic inclusions.

Mucopolysaccharidosis IX
MPS-IX is caused by a mutation in the *HYAL1* gene on chromosome 3p21.2-21.2 encoding 1 of 3 hyaluronidases. Clinical findings in the only known patient, a 14 yr old girl, were bilateral nodular soft tissue periarticular masses, lysosomal storage of GAGs in histiocytes, mildly

dysmorphic craniofacial features, short stature, normal joint movement, and normal intelligence. Small erosions in both acetabula were the only radiographic findings.

Mucopolysaccharidosis Plus Syndrome
Coarse facial features, organomegaly, joint contractures, dysostosis multiplex, cognitive deficiency, increased mucopolysacchariduria, and massive intracellular accumulation of heparin sulfate were found in 13 children in Northeastern Siberia and 2 Turkish children. Further findings were optic atrophy, intracerebral calcifications, pancytopenia, and renal insufficiency. Most children died within the 1st 2 yr of life from cardiorespiratory failure.

Lysosomal enzyme activities were normal in children with MPS plus syndrome. This autosomal recessive multisystem disorder is caused by homozygous mutations of *VPS33A* encoding a protein involved in lysosomal fusion processes.

DIAGNOSIS AND DIFFERENTIAL DIAGNOSIS
Clinical suspicion of a MPS justifies a skeletal survey. Radiographs of chest, spine, pelvis, and hands may show signs of dysostosis multiplex. The next diagnostic step is to assay the urinary excretion of GAGs. Semiquantitative spot tests for increased urinary GAG excretion are quick, inexpensive, and useful for initial evaluation but are subject to both false-positive and false-negative results. Quantitative analysis of single GAG and/or oligosaccharides by mass spectrometry detection tests reveals type-specific profiles in urine, serum, plasma, and dried blood spots.

Any individual with a suspected MPS disorder based on clinical features, radiographic results, or urinary GAG screening tests should have a definitive diagnosis established by **enzyme assay**. Serum, leukocytes, or cultured fibroblasts are used as the tissue source for measuring lysosomal enzymes (see Table 107.2).

Molecular analysis is typically performed using appropriate gene panels. In many cases the type and location of the mutation are related to the future course of the disease and thus have a predictive value. The specific mutation is also needed if **prenatal diagnosis** on fetal cells from a subsequent pregnancy is considered. Carrier testing in Hunter syndrome, an X-linked disorder, requires analysis of *IDS* once the specific mutation or chromosome arrangement in the family is known. Prenatal molecular analysis must be offered in a male fetus of a proven female carrier of the *IDS* gene. His risk to be affected is 50%. In a female fetus the risk is small, but not zero, as a result of skewed maternal X-chromosome inactivation.

Newborn screening for mucopolysaccharidoses is available from dried blood spots and is essential for their early detection and therapeutic intervention.

Mucolipidoses and **oligosaccharidoses** manifest with the same clinical and radiographic features as mucopolysaccharidoses. In these conditions the urinary excretion of GAGs is not elevated. Hurler-like facial features, joint contractures, dysostosis multiplex, and elevated urinary GAG excretion differentiate the mucopolysaccharidoses from other neurodegenerative and dwarfing conditions.

TREATMENT
Hematopoietic stem cell transplantation has resulted in significant clinical improvement of somatic disease in patients with MPS I, II, and VI (Table 107.4). Clinical effects are increased life expectancy with resolution or improvement of growth, hepatosplenomegaly, joint stiffness, facial appearance, skin changes, obstructive sleep apnea, heart disease, communicating hydrocephalus, and hearing loss. Enzyme activity in serum and urinary GAG excretion normalize. This is true for MPS I-H, II, and III. Patients with MPS-I who have undergone transplantation before 9 mo of age may show normal cognitive development. Transplantation before 24 mo and with a baseline mental development index >70 have improved long-term outcome. Transplantation does not significantly improve the neuropsychological outcome of MPS patients with impaired cognition at transplantation. Early transplantation in the MPS-II patient may have the same effect. Transplantation in the MPS-VI patient stabilizes or improves cardiac manifestations, posture, and joint mobility. Stem cell transplantation does not correct skeletal or ocular

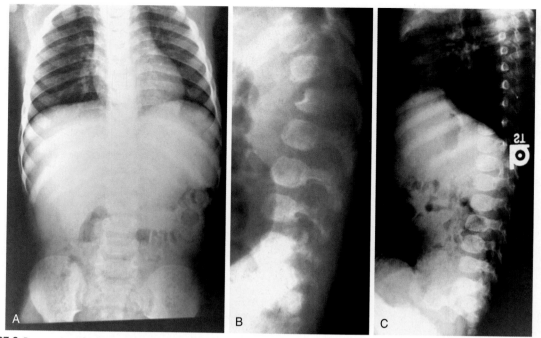

Fig. 107.3 Dysostosis multiplex. **A,** Sanfilippo syndrome, patient age 4 yr; the ribs are wide. **B,** Sanfilippo syndrome, age 4 yr; immature, ovoid configuration of the vertebral bodies. **C,** Hurler syndrome, age 18 mo; anterosuperior hypoplasia of 1st lumbar vertebra (L1) resulting in hook-shaped appearance.

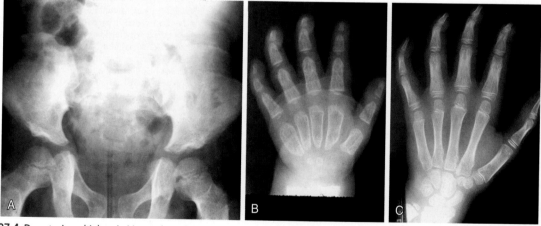

Fig. 107.4 Dysostosis multiplex. **A,** Mucopolysaccharidosis I-H, patient age 10 yr. The inferior portions of the ilia are hypoplastic, with resulting iliac flare and shallow acetabular fossae. The femoral necks are in valgus position. **B,** MPS I-H, age 4 yr. Metacarpals and phalanges are abnormally short, wide, and deformed with proximal pointing of the metacarpals and bullet-shaped phalanges. Bone trabeculation is coarse, and the cortices are thin. **C,** MPS I-S, age 13 yr. The carpal bones are small, leading to a **V**-shaped configuration of the digits. The short, tubular bones are well modeled. Flexion of the middle and distal phalanges II-V is caused by joint contractures.

anomalies.

Enzyme replacement therapy (ERT) using recombinant α-L-iduronidase has been approved for patients with MPS-I (Table 107.4). It reduces organomegaly and ameliorates rate of growth, improves joint mobility, and reduces the number of episodes of sleep apnea and urinary GAG excretion. The enzyme does not cross the blood-brain barrier and does not prevent deterioration of neurocognitive function. Consequently, ERT is appropriate for patients with mild CNS involvement or to stabilize extraneural manifestations in young patients before stem cell transplantation. Recombinant iduronate-2-sulfatase is the treatment of choice for MPS-II to ameliorate nonneural manifestations.

ERT with recombinant human *GALNS* improves physical endurance, respiratory function, and daily living activity of patients with MPS-IV. Similar effects produce recombinant *N*-acetylgalactosamine-4-sulfatase in patients with MPS-VI.

Symptomatic therapy focuses on respiratory and cardiovascular complications, hearing loss, carpal tunnel syndrome, spinal cord compression, hydrocephalus, and other problems (Table 107.5). The multisystem involvement and progressive nature of MPS syndromes usually requires the complex care provided by medical centers.

Bibliography is available at Expert Consult.

Table 107.4		Therapies Aimed at Proximate Causes of Mucopolysaccharidoses	
MPS TYPE	**HEMATOPOIETIC STEM CELL TRANSPLANTATION**	**ENZYME REPLACEMENT THERAPY**	**REMARKS**
I	Yes	Laronidase (Aldurazyme)	Developmental trajectory dependent on time of transplantation. Little effect on connective tissue manifestations. Enzyme replacement immediately after diagnosis.
II	Yes	Idursulfase (Elaprase)	
III	No	No	Experimental intrathecal application of recombinant heparin-N-sulfatase in MPS-IIIA.
IV	Yes	Elosulfase (Vimizim)	Improved daily activities. No effect on growth or skeletal dysplasia.
VI	Yes	Galsulfase (Naglazyme)	Improved daily activities. Improved growth. No effect on skeletal dysplasia.
VII	Yes	rhGUS	Phase 3 study by Ultragenyx, 2016. Limited experience because of rarity of condition.

Table 107.5		Symptomatic Management of Mucopolysaccharidoses	
PROBLEM		**PREDOMINANTLY IN**	**MANAGEMENT**
NEUROLOGIC			
Hydrocephalus		MPS I, II, VI, VII	Funduscopy, CT scan
Chronic headaches		All	Ventriculoperitoneal shunting
Behavioral disturbance		MPS-III	Behavioral medication, sometimes CT scan, ventriculoperitoneal shunting
Disturbed sleep–wake cycle		MPS-III	Melatonin
Seizures		MPS I, II, III	EEG, anticonvulsants
Atlantoaxial instability		MPS IV	Cervical MRI, upper cervical fusion
Spinal cord compression		All	Laminectomy, dural excision
OPHTHALMOLOGIC			
Corneal opacity		MPS I, VI, VII	Corneal transplant
Glaucoma		MPS I, VI, VII	Medication, surgery
Retinal degeneration		MPS I, II	Night-light
EARS, AIRWAYS			
Recurrent otitis media		MPS I, II, VI, VII	Ventilating tubes
Impaired hearing		All except MPS-IV	Audiometry, hearing aids
Obstruction		All except MPS-III	Adenotomy, tonsillectomy, bronchodilator therapy, CPAP at night, laser excision of tracheal lesions, tracheotomy
CARDIAC			
Cardiac valve disease		MPS I, II, VI, VII	Endocarditis prevention, valve replacement
Coronary insufficiency		MPS I, II, VI, VII	Medical therapy
Arrhythmias		MPS I, II, VI, VII	Antiarrhythmic medication, pacemaker
ORAL, GASTROINTESTINAL			
Hypertrophic gums, poor teeth		MPS I, II, VI, VII	Dental care
Chronic diarrhea		MPS-II	Diet modification, loperamide
MUSCULOSKELETAL			
Joint stiffness		All except MPS IV	Physical therapy
Weakness		All	Physical therapy, wheelchair
Gross long-bone malalignment		All	Corrective osteotomies
Carpal tunnel syndrome		MPS I, II, VI, VII	Electromyography, surgical decompression
ANESTHESIA		All except III	Avoid atlantoaxial dislocation; use angulated video intubation laryngoscope and small endotracheal tubes.

CT, Computed tomography; CPAP, continuous positive airway pressure; EEG, electroencephalogram; MRI, magnetic resonance imaging.

Chapter 108

Disorders of Purine and Pyrimidine Metabolism

James C. Harris

第一百零八章

嘌呤和嘧啶代谢障碍

中文导读

本章主要介绍了痛风、嘌呤补救异常、嘌呤核苷酸合成相关障碍、嘌呤分解代谢异常所致疾病以及嘧啶代谢障碍。包括痛风的遗传学及治疗；次黄嘌呤-鸟嘌呤-磷酸核糖转移酶（HPRT）缺乏症及腺嘌呤磷酸核糖转移酶缺乏症；磷酸核糖焦磷酸合成酶活性过强或缺乏症、腺苷酸琥珀酸裂解酶缺乏症及氨基咪唑羧酰胺核苷酸转甲酰基酶/肌苷一磷酸环化水解酶

缺乏症；肌腺苷酸脱氨酶缺乏症、腺苷酸脱氨酶缺乏症、嘌呤核苷酸磷酸化酶缺乏症及黄嘌呤氧化还原酶缺乏症；尿苷单磷酸合成酶缺乏症I型、二氢乳清酸脱氢酶缺乏症、二氢嘧啶脱氢酶缺乏症、二氢嘧啶酶缺乏症、β-脲基丙酸酶缺乏症、嘧啶5'-核苷酸酶缺乏症、胞质5'-核苷酸酶活性过强、胸腺嘧啶磷酸酶缺乏症以及胸腺嘧啶激酶2缺乏症等。

The inherited disorders of purine and pyrimidine metabolism cover a broad spectrum of illnesses with various presentations. These include hyperuricemia, acute renal failure, renal stones, gout, unexplained neurologic deficits (seizures, muscle weakness, choreoathetoid and dystonic movements), intellectual and developmental disabilities, acrofacial dysostosis, compulsive self-injury and aggression, autistic-like behavior, unexplained anemia, failure to thrive, susceptibility to recurrent infection (immune deficiency), and deafness. When identified, all family members should be screened.

Purines and pyrimidines form the basis of *nucleotides* and *nucleic acids* (DNA and RNA) and thus are involved in all biologic processes. Metabolically active nucleotides are formed from heterocyclic nitrogen-containing purine bases (guanine and adenine) and pyrimidine bases (cytosine, uridine, and thymine): all cells require a balanced supply of nucleotides for growth and survival. Purines provide the primary source of cellular energy through adenosine triphosphate (ATP) and the basic coenzymes (nicotinamide adenine dinucleotide and its reduced form) for metabolic regulation and play a major role in signal transduction (guanosine triphosphate [GTP], cyclic adenosine monophosphate, cyclic guanosine monophosphate). Fig. 108.1 shows the early steps in the biosynthesis of the purine ring. Purines are primarily produced from endogenous sources, and in usual circumstances, dietary purines have a small role. The end product of purine metabolism in humans is uric acid (2,6,8-trioxypurine).

Uric acid is not a specific disease marker, so the cause of its elevation must be determined. The serum level of uric acid present at any time

depends on the size of the purine nucleotide pool, which is derived from de novo purine synthesis, catabolism of tissue nucleic acids, and increased turnover of preformed purines. Uric acid is poorly soluble and must be excreted continuously to avoid toxic accumulation in the body. Baseline serum uric acid is established by the balancing of activity between secretory and absorptive urate transporters in both kidney and intestine. Urate secretion and absorption are mediated by separate, opposing groups of transporters. The majority of the genes involved in the variation in uric acid blood level encode urate transporters or associated regulatory proteins.

Thus the fraction of uric acid excreted by the kidney is the result of a complex interplay between secretion and reabsorption by specific and nonspecific uric acid transporters in the proximal tubule, and this sets the level of uric acid in the plasma. Because renal tubule excretion is greater in children than in adults, serum uric acid levels are a less reliable indicator of uric acid production in children than in adults, and therefore measurement of the level in urine may be required to determine excessive production. Clearance of a smaller portion of uric acid is through the gastrointestinal (GI) tract (biliary and intestinal secretion). Because of poor solubility of uric acid under normal circumstances, uric acid is near the maximal tolerable limits, and small alterations in production or solubility or changes in secretion may lead to hyperuricemia and can result in precipitation monosodium urate crystals in extremities (e.g., fingers or toes), which defines **clinical gout**. In renal insufficiency, urate excretion is increased by residual nephrons and the GI tract. Increased production of uric acid is found in malignancy,

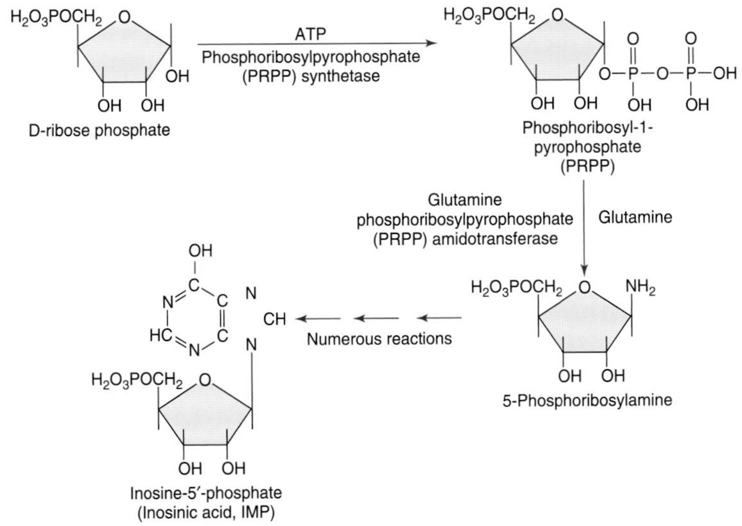

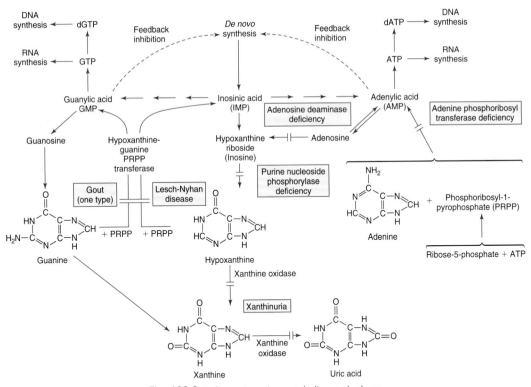

Fig. 108.1 Early steps in the biosynthesis of the purine ring.

Fig. 108.2 Pathways in purine metabolism and salvage.

Reye syndrome, Down syndrome, psoriasis, sickle cell anemia, cyanotic congenital heart disease, pancreatic enzyme replacement, glycogen storage disease (types I, III, IV, and V), hereditary fructose intolerance, and acyl-coenzyme A dehydrogenase deficiency.

The metabolism of both purines and pyrimidines can be divided into biosynthetic, salvage, and catabolic pathways. The first, the de novo pathway, involves a multistep biosynthesis of phosphorylated ring structures from precursors such as CO_2, glycine, and glutamine. Purine and pyrimidine nucleotides are produced from ribose-5-phosphate or carbamyl phosphate, respectively. The second, a single-step salvage pathway, recovers purine bases and pyrimidine nucleosides derived from either dietary intake or the catabolic pathway (Figs. 108.2 and 108.3). In the de novo pathway, the nucleosides guanosine, adenosine, cytidine, uridine, and thymidine are formed by the addition of ribose-1-phosphate to the purine bases guanine or adenine and to the pyrimidine bases cytosine, uracil, and thymine, respectively. The phosphorylation of these nucleosides produces monophosphate, diphosphate, and triphosphate nucleotides, as well as the deoxy-nucleotides that are utilized

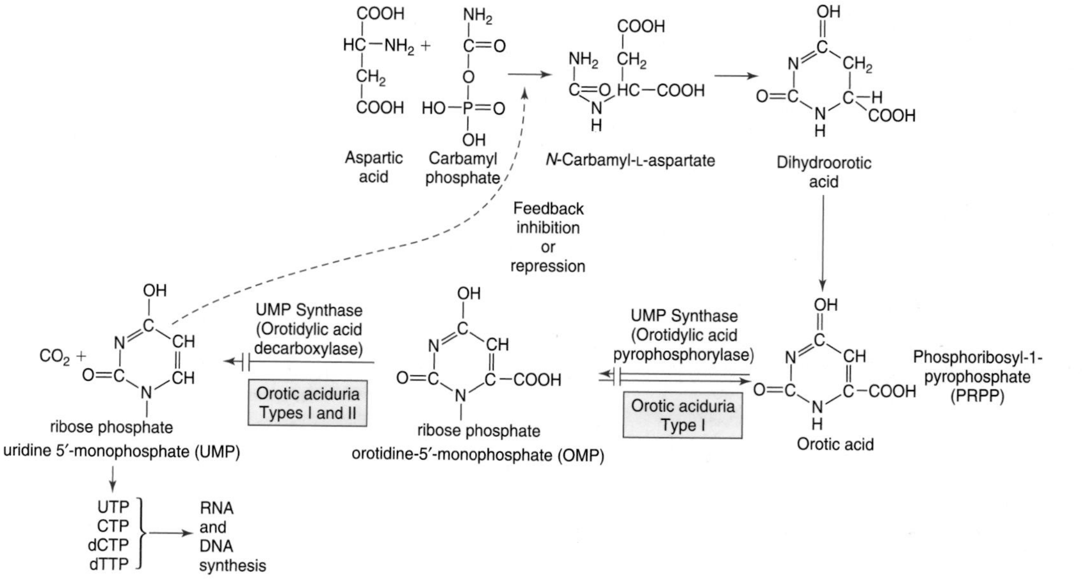

Fig. 108.3 Pathways in pyrimidine biosynthesis.

for DNA formation. Under usual circumstances, the salvage pathway predominates over the biosynthetic pathway because nucleotide salvage saves energy for cells. Only a small fraction of the nucleotides turned over by the body each day are degraded and excreted. Synthesis of nucleotides is most active in tissues with high rates of cellular turnover, such as gut epithelium, skin, and bone marrow. The third pathway is catabolism. The end product of the catabolic pathway of the purines in humans is uric acid, whereas catabolism of pyrimidines produces citric acid cycle intermediates.

Inborn errors in the **synthesis of purine nucleotides** comprise the phosphoribosylpyrophosphate synthetase spectrum of disorders, including deficiency and superactivity, adenylosuccinate lyase deficiency, and 5-amino-4-imizolecarboxamide (AICA) riboside deficiency (AICA-ribosiduria). Disorders resulting from abnormalities in **purine catabolism** comprise muscle adenosine monophosphate (AMP) deaminase deficiency, adenosine deaminase deficiency, purine nucleoside phosphorylase deficiency, and xanthine oxidoreductase deficiency. Disorders resulting from the **purine salvage** pathway include hypoxanthine-guanine phosphoribosyltransferase (HPRT) deficiency and adenine phosphoribosyltransferase (APRT) deficiency.

Hereditary orotic aciduria (uridine monophosphate synthase deficiency) is an inborn error of **pyrimidine synthesis** that leads to an excessive excretion of orotic acid in urine. Dihydrorotate dehydrogenase deficiency (Miller syndrome), also a disorder of de novo pyrimidine synthesis, paradoxically may lead to orotic aciduria. Other pyrimidine disorders lead to abnormalities in **pyrimidine catabolism**, including dihydropyrimidine dehydrogenase (DPD) deficiency, dihydropyrimidinase (DPH) deficiency, β-ureidopropionase deficiency, pyrimidine 5′-nucleotidase deficiency, and thymidine phosphorylase deficiency. A disorder resulting from the **pyrimidine salvage** is thymidine kinase-2 deficiency.

GOUT

Gout presents with hyperuricemia, uric acid nephrolithiasis, and acute inflammatory arthritis. **Gouty arthritis** is caused by monosodium urate crystal deposits that result in inflammation in joints and surrounding tissues. The presentation is most commonly monoarticular, typically in the metatarsophalangeal joint of the big toe. *Tophi*, deposits of monosodium urate crystals, may occur over points of insertion of tendons at the elbows, knees, and feet or over the helix of the ears. **Primary**

gout usually occurs in middle-aged males and results mainly from decreased renal excretion of uric acid, or purine overconsumption, or high intake of alcohol or fructose, or a combination of these factors. Gout occurs in any condition that leads to reduced clearance of uric acid: during therapy for malignancy or with dehydration, lactic acidosis, ketoacidosis, starvation, diuretic therapy, and renal failure. Excessive purine, alcohol, or fructose ingestion may increase uric acid levels. The biochemical etiology of gout is unknown for most patients, and it is considered to have a basis in genetic polymorphisms, predominantly in uric acid transporters. Purine overproduction is a rare cause of primary gout and is associated with several genetic disorders discussed later. **Secondary gout** is either the result of another disorder with rapid tissue breakdown or cellular turnover, leading to increased production or decreased excretion of uric acid, or the result of some types of drug treatment; for example, diuretics cause plasma volume reduction and can precipitate a gouty attack.

Gout resulting from **endogenous purine overproduction** is associated with hereditary disorders of 3 different enzymes that result in hyperuricemia. These include the HPRT deficiency spectrum (ranging from severe deficiency or Lesch-Nyhan syndrome to partial HPRT deficiency), 2 forms of superactivity of PP-ribose-P synthetase, and glycogen storage disease type I (glucose-6-phosphatase deficiency). In the first 2 disorders, the basis of hyperuricemia is purine nucleotide and uric acid overproduction, whereas in the 3rd disorder it is both excessive uric acid production and diminished renal excretion of urate. Glycogen storage disease types III, V, and VII are associated with exercise-induced hyperuricemia, the consequence of rapid ATP utilization and failure to regenerate it effectively during exercise (see Chapter 105.1).

Juvenile gout results from purine underexcretion. The earlier terminology *juvenile hyperuricemic nephropathy* has been replaced by the newer term (autosomal dominant) *tubulointerstitial kidney disease* (ADTKD). The term **ADTKD-UMOD** (*uromodulin-associated kidney disease*) is used for medullary cystic kidney disease type 2 and maps to chromosome 16p11.2. It results from uromodulin mutations. Other genes classified as forms of familial juvenile hyperuricemic nephropathy include those for renin and hepatic nuclear factor-1β. Unlike the 3 inherited purine disorders that are X-linked and the recessively inherited glycogen storage disease, these are autosomal dominant conditions. Familial juvenile hyperuricemic nephropathy is associated with a reduced fractional excretion of uric acid. Although it typically presents from puberty up to the 3rd decade, it has been reported in early childhood. It is characterized by early onset, hyperuricemia, gout, familial renal disease, and low urate clearance relative to glomerular filtration rate. It occurs in both males and females and is frequently associated with a rapid decline in renal function that may lead to death unless diagnosed and treated early. Once familial juvenile hyperuricemic nephropathy is recognized, presymptomatic detection is of critical importance to identify asymptomatic family members with hyperuricemia and to begin treatment, when indicated, to prevent nephropathy.

Genetics

Familial juvenile hyperuricemic nephropathy-2 (HNFJ2; 613092) is caused by mutation in the renin gene (*REN*; 179820) on chromosome 1q32. HNFJ3 (614227) has been mapped to chromosome 2p22.1-p21. ADTKD involves mutations of the mucin (*MUC1*) gene. The mutation of uromodulin has been traced to chromosome 16.

Treatment

Treatment of hyperuricemia involves the combination of allopurinol or febuxostat (xanthine oxidase inhibitors) to decrease uric acid production, probenecid to increase uric acid clearance in those with normal renal function, and increased fluid intake to reduce the concentration of uric acid. A low-purine diet, weight reduction, and reduced alcohol and fructose intake (fructose both reduces urate clearance and accelerates ATP breakdown to uric acid) are recommended.

ABNORMALITIES IN PURINE SALVAGE
Hypoxanthine-Guanine Phosphoribosyltransferase (HPRT) Deficiency

Lesch-Nyhan disease (LND) is a rare X-linked disorder of purine metabolism that results from HPRT deficiency. This enzyme is normally present in each cell in the body, but its highest concentration is in the brain, especially in the basal ganglia. Clinical manifestations include hyperuricemia, intellectual disability, dystonic movement disorder that may be accompanied by choreoathetosis and spasticity, dysarthric speech, and compulsive self-biting, usually beginning with the eruption of teeth.

There is a spectrum of severity for the clinical presentations. HPRT levels are related to the extent of motor symptoms, to the presence or absence of self-injury, and possibly to the level of cognitive function. Purine overproduction is present. The majority of individuals with classic LND have low or undetectable levels of the HPRT enzyme. Partial deficiency in HPRT (**Kelley-Seegmiller syndrome**) with >1.5–2.0% enzyme is associated with purine overproduction and variable neurologic dysfunction (neurologic HPRT deficiency). HPRT deficiency with activity levels >8% of normal still shows purine (and uric acid) overproduction but apparently normal cerebral functioning (HPRT-related hyperuricemia), although cognitive deficits may occur. Qualitatively similar cognitive deficit profiles have been reported in both LND and variant cases. Variants produced scores intermediate between those of patients with LND and normal controls on almost every neuropsychological measure tested.

Genetics

The *HPRT* gene has been localized to the long arm of the X chromosome (q26-q27). The complete amino acid sequence for HPRT is known and is encoded by the *HPRT1* gene (approximately 44 kb; 9 exons). The disorder appears in males; occurrence in females is extremely rare and ascribed to nonrandom inactivation of the normal X chromosome. Absence of HPRT activity results in a failure to salvage hypoxanthine, which is degraded to uric acid. Failure to consume phosphoribosyl-pyrophosphate in the salvage reaction results in an increase in this metabolite, which drives de novo purine synthesis, leading to the overproduction of uric acid. Excessive uric acid production manifests as gout, necessitating specific drug treatment (allopurinol). Because of the enzyme deficiency, hypoxanthine accumulates in the cerebrospinal fluid (CSF), but uric acid does not; uric acid is not produced in the brain and does not cross the blood-brain barrier. The behavior disorder is not caused by hyperuricemia or excess hypoxanthine because patients with partial HPRT deficiency, the variants with hyperuricemia, do not

self-injure, and infants with isolated hyperuricemia from birth do not develop self-injurious behavior.

The prevalence of the classic LND has been estimated at 1 in 100,000 to 1 in 380,000 persons based on the number of known cases in the United States. The incidence of partial variants is not known. Those with the classic syndrome rarely survive the 3rd decade because of renal or respiratory compromise. The life span may be normal for patients with partial HPRT deficiency without severe renal involvement.

Pathology

No specific brain abnormality is documented after detailed histopathology and electron microscopy of affected brain regions. MRI has documented reductions in the volume of basal ganglia nuclei. Abnormalities in neurotransmitter metabolism have been identified in 3 autopsied cases. All 3 patients had very low HPRT levels (<1% in striatal tissue and 1–2% of control in thalamus cortex). There was a functional loss of 65–90% of the nigrostriatal and mesolimbic dopamine terminals, although the cells of origin in the substantia nigra did not show dopamine reduction. The brain regions primarily involved were the caudate nucleus, putamen, and nucleus accumbens. It is proposed that the neurochemical changes may be linked to functional abnormalities, possibly resulting from a diminution of arborization or branching of dendrites rather than cell loss. A neurotransmitter abnormality is demonstrated by changes in CSF neurotransmitters and their metabolites and is confirmed by positron emission tomography (PET) scans of dopamine function. In vivo reductions in the presynaptic dopamine transporter have been documented in the caudate and putamen of 6 individuals.

The mechanism whereby HPRT leads to the neurologic and behavioral symptoms is unknown. However, both hypoxanthine and guanine metabolism are affected, and GTP and adenosine have substantial effects on neural tissues. The functional link between purine nucleotides and the dopamine system is through salvage of guanine by HPRT to form GTP; this is essential for GTP cyclohydrolase activity, the first step in the synthesis of pterins and dopamine. In a controlled study that sought correlations between HPRT and GPRT and behavior, GPRT was more highly correlated than HPRT on 13 of 14 measures of the clinical phenotype; these included severity of dystonia, cognitive impairment, and behavioral abnormalities. These findings suggest that loss of guanine recycling might be more closely linked to the LND/LNV phenotype than loss of hypoxanthine recycling. Moreover, patients with inherited GTP cyclohydrolase deficiency show clinical features in common with LND.

Dopamine reduction in brain is documented in HPRT-deficient strains of mutant mice. Dopamine binding to its receptor results in either an activation (D1 receptor) or an inhibition (D2 receptor) of adenylcyclase. Both receptor effects are mediated by G proteins (GTP-binding proteins) dependent on guanine diphosphate in the guanine diphosphate/GTP exchange for cellular activation. Dopamine and adenosine systems are also linked through the role of adenosine as a neuroprotective agent in preventing neurotoxicity. Adenosine derives from AMP, which depends on hypoxanthine salvage in the brain by HPRT. Adenosine agonists mimic the biochemical and behavioral actions of dopamine antagonists, whereas adenosine receptor antagonists act as functional dopamine agonists. LND can thus be seen as arising ultimately from nucleotide depletion specifically in the brain, which relies on the HPRT salvage pathway, leading to dopamine and adenosine depletions.

Clinical Manifestations

At birth, infants with LND have no apparent neurologic dysfunction. After several months, developmental delay and neurologic signs become apparent. Before age 4 mo, hypotonic, recurrent vomiting, and difficulty with secretions may be noted. By 8-12 mo, extrapyramidal signs appear, primarily dystonic movements. In some patients, spasticity may become apparent at this time; in others it becomes apparent later in life.

Cognitive function is usually reported to be in the mild to moderate range of intellectual disability, although some individuals test in the low-normal range. Because test scores may be influenced by difficulty in testing caused by movement disorder and dysarthric speech, overall intelligence may be underestimated.

The age of onset of self-injury may be as early as 1 yr and occasionally as late as the teens. Self-injury occurs, although all sensory modalities, including pain, are intact. The **self-injurious behavior** (SIB) usually begins with self-biting, although other SIB patterns emerge with time. Most characteristically, the fingers, mouth, and buccal mucosa are mutilated. Self-biting is intense and causes tissue damage and may result in the amputation of fingers and substantial loss of tissue around the lips. Extraction of primary teeth may be required. The biting pattern can be asymmetric, with preferential mutilation of the left or right side of the body. The type of behavior is different from that seen in other intellectual disability syndromes involving self-injury. Self-hitting and head-banging are the most common initial presentations in *other* syndromes. The intensity of SIB generally requires that the patient be restrained. When restraints are removed, the patient with LND may appear terrified, and stereotypically place a finger in the mouth. The patient may ask for restraints to prevent elbow movement; when the restraints are placed, or replaced, he may appear relaxed and cheerful. Dysarthric speech may cause interpersonal communication problems; however, the higher-functioning children can express themselves fully and participate in verbal therapy.

The self-mutilation presents as a compulsive behavior that the child tries to control but frequently is unable to resist. Older individuals may enlist the help of others and notify them when they are comfortable enough to have restraints removed. In some cases the behavior may lead to deliberate self-harm. The LND patient may also show compulsive aggression and inflict injury to others through pinching, grabbing, or hitting or by using verbal forms of aggression. Afterward he may apologize, stating that this behavior was out of his control. Other maladaptive behaviors include head- or limb-banging, eye-poking, and psychogenic vomiting.

Diagnosis

The presence of **dystonia** along with self-mutilation of the mouth and fingers suggests LND. With partial HPRT deficiency, recognition is linked to either hyperuricemia alone or hyperuricemia and a dystonic movement disorder. Serum levels of uric acid that exceed 4-5 mg uric acid/dL and a urine uric acid:creatinine ratio of ≥3-4:1 are highly suggestive of HPRT deficiency, particularly when associated with neurologic symptoms. The definitive diagnosis requires an analysis of the HPRT enzyme. This is assayed in an erythrocyte lysate. Individuals with classic LND have near 0% enzyme activity, and those with partial variants show values between 1.5% and 60%. The intact cell HPRT assay in skin fibroblasts offers a good correlation between enzyme activity and severity of disease. Molecular techniques are used for gene sequencing and identification of carriers.

Differential diagnosis includes other causes of infantile hypotonia and dystonia. Children with LND are often initially *incorrectly* diagnosed as having athetoid cerebral palsy. When a diagnosis of cerebral palsy is suspected in an infant with a normal prenatal, perinatal, and postnatal course, LND should be considered. Partial HPRT deficiency may be associated with acute renal failure in infancy; therefore clinical awareness of partial HPRT deficiency is of particular importance. The simplest test to exclude LND or partial deficiency is the urinary uric acid:creatinine ratio.

An understanding of the molecular disorder has led to effective drug treatment for uric acid accumulation and arthritic tophi, renal stones, and neuropathy. However, reduction in uric acid alone does not influence the neurologic and behavioral aspects of LND. Despite treatment from birth for uric acid elevation, behavioral and neurologic symptoms are unaffected. The most significant complications of LND are renal failure and self-mutilation.

Treatment

Medical management of LND focuses on prevention of renal failure by pharmacologic treatment of hyperuricemia, with high fluid intake along with alkalization and allopurinol (or more often febuxostat). A low-purine diet and reduced fructose intake are desirable.

Allopurinol treatment must be monitored because urinary oxypurine excretion with all overproduction disorders is sensitive to allopurinol, resulting in an increased urine concentration of xanthine, which

is extremely insoluble. Self-mutilation is reduced through behavior management and the use of restraints and/or removal of teeth. Pharmacologic approaches to decrease anxiety and spasticity with medication have mixed results. Drug therapy focuses on symptomatic management of anticipatory anxiety, mood stabilization, and reduction of self-injurious behavior. Although there is no standard drug treatment, diazepam may be helpful for anxiety symptoms, risperidone for aggressive behavior, and carbamazepine or gabapentin for mood stabilization. Each of these medications may reduce SIB by helping to reduce anxiety and stabilize mood. S-adenosylmethionine (**SAMe**), which is thought to act by countering nucleotide depletion in the brain, has been reported specifically to reduce the rate of self-injury in some cases. Animal studies have suggested that D1-dopamine receptor antagonists such as ecopipam may suppress SIB. Despite limited data, the drug appears to reduce SIB in most patients, suggesting further study to establish an appropriate dosing regimen and assess toxicity.

Several patients have received **bone marrow transplantation** (BMT), based on the hypothesis that the central nervous system (CNS) damage is produced by a circulating toxin. There is no evidence that BMT is a beneficial treatment approach; it remains an experimental and potentially dangerous therapy. Two patients received partial exchange transfusions every 2 mo for 3-4 yr. Erythrocyte HPRT activity was 10–70% of normal during this period, but no reduction of neurologic or behavioral symptoms was apparent. Successful preimplantation genetic diagnosis and in vitro fertilization for LND has been reported with the birth of an unaffected male infant.

Both the motivation for self-injury and its biologic basis must be addressed in treatment programs. However, behavioral techniques alone, using operant conditioning approaches, have not proved to be an adequate general treatment. Although **behavioral procedures** have had some selective success in reducing self-injury, difficulty with generalization outside the experimental setting limits this approach, and patients under stress may revert to their previous SIB. Behavioral approaches may also focus on reducing SIB through treatment of phobic anxiety associated with being unrestrained. The most common techniques are systematic desensitization, extinction, and differential reinforcement of other (competing) behavior. Stress management has been recommended to assist patients to develop more effective coping mechanisms. Individuals with LND do not respond to contingent electric shock or similar aversive behavioral measures. An increase in self-injury may be observed when aversive methods are used.

Restraint (day and night) and dental procedures are common means to prevent self-injury. The time in restraints is linked to the age of onset of self-injury. Children with LND can participate in making decisions regarding restraints and the type of restraints. The time in restraints may potentially be reduced with systematic behavior treatment programs. Many patients have teeth extracted to prevent self-injury. Others use a protective mouth guard designed by a dentist. Most parents suggest that stress reduction and awareness of the patient's needs are the most effective in reducing self-injury. Positive behavioral techniques of reinforcing appropriate behavior are rated effective by almost half the families.

Deep brain stimulation to the anteroventral internal globus pallidus is a procedure that has successfully treated self-injury and lessened dystonia in several case reports.

Adenine Phosphoribosyltransferase Deficiency (Dihydroxyadeninuria)

APRT, a purine salvage enzyme, catalyzes the synthesis of AMP from adenine and 5-phosphoribosyl-1-pyrophosphate (PP-ribose-P). The absence of this enzyme results in the cellular accumulation of adenine and it being oxidized as an alternative substrate by xanthine dehydrogenase to form **2,8-dihydroxyadenine**, which is extremely insoluble. APRT deficiency is present from birth, becoming apparent as early as 5 mo and as late as the 7th decade.

Genetics

The disorder is an autosomal recessive trait with considerable clinical heterogeneity. The *APRT* gene is located on chromosome 16q (16q24.3) and encompasses 2.8 kb of genomic DNA.

Clinical Manifestations

These include urinary calculus formation with crystalluria, urinary tract infections, hematuria, renal colic, dysuria, and acute renal failure. Brownish spots on the infant's diaper or yellow-brown crystals in the urine suggest the diagnosis. The 2,8-dihydroxyadenine is cleared efficiently by the kidneys and so does not accumulate in plasma, but precipitates readily in the renal lumen.

Laboratory Findings

Urinary levels of adenine, 8-hydroxyadenine, and 2,8-dihydroxyadenine are elevated, whereas plasma uric acid is normal. The deficiency may be complete (**type I**) or partial (**type II**); the partial deficiency is reported in Japan. The diagnosis is made based on the level of residual enzyme in erythrocyte lysates. The renal calculi, composed of 2,8-dihydroxyadenine, are radiolucent, soft, and easily crushed. These stones are not distinguishable from uric acid stones by routine tests but require high-performance liquid chromatography (HPLC), ultraviolet (UV) light, infrared light, mass spectrometry, x-ray crystallography, or capillary electrophoresis for diagnosis, particularly to distinguish from stones in HPRT deficiency.

Treatment

Treatment includes high fluid intake, dietary purine restriction, and allopurinol, which inhibits the conversion of adenine to its metabolites and prevents further stone formation. Alkalinization of the urine is to be avoided, because unlike that of uric acid, the solubility of 2,8-dihydroxyadenine does not increase up to pH 9. **Shock wave lithotripsy** has been reported to be successful. The **prognosis** depends on renal function at diagnosis. Early treatment is critical in the prevention of stones because severe renal insufficiency may accompany late recognition.

DISORDERS LINKED TO PURINE NUCLEOTIDE SYNTHESIS
Phosphoribosylpyrophosphate Synthetase Superactivity and Deficiency

Phosphoribosylpyrophosphate (**PRPP**) is a substrate involved in the synthesis of essentially all nucleotides and important in the regulation of the de novo pathways of purine and pyrimidine nucleotide synthesis. The synthetase enzyme (**PRPS**) produces PRPP from ribose-5-phosphate and ATP (see Figs. 108.1 and 108.2). PRPP is the first intermediary compound in the de novo synthesis of purine nucleotides that lead to the formation of inosine monophosphate, then to ATP and GTP.

Genetic disorders of this enzyme affect only the PRPS-1 isoform; PRPS-2 mutations have not been described. PRPS-1 disorders are all X-linked and are divided into "superactivity," which occurs as 2 phenotypes (infantile or early childhood onset, and a milder form with late-juvenile or early-adult onset), and "deficiency," which is a spectrum disorder that is distinguished clinically according to severity as 3 disorders: Arts syndrome, Charcot-Marie-Tooth disease X-linked-5, and X-linked deafness-2.

Superactivity of the enzyme results in an increased generation of PRPP in dividing cells. Because PRPP aminotransferase, the first enzyme of the purine de novo pathway, is not physiologically saturated by PRPP, the synthesis of purine nucleotides increases, and consequently the production of uric acid is increased. PRPP synthetase superactivity is one of the few hereditary disorders in which the activity of an enzyme is enhanced. The infantile or early childhood form of PRPS-1 superactivity has severe neurologic consequences accompanied by uric acid overproduction, whereas individuals with the late-juvenile or early-adult presentation are neurologically normal but still have uric acid overproduction.

Deficiency of PRPS-1 produces depleted purine nucleotide synthesis in tissues dependent on PRPS-1, which includes brain as well as other neural tissues and lung.

Genetics

Three distinct complementary DNAs for PRPS have been cloned and sequenced. Two forms, PRPS-1 and PRPS-2, are X-linked to Xq22-q24 and Xp22.2-p.22.3 (escapes X inactivation), respectively, and are widely expressed. The 3rd locus maps to human chromosome 7 and appears to be transcribed only in the testes. PRPS-1 defects are thus inherited as X-linked traits and present with varying degrees of severity. The **late-onset** form of superactivity arises from increased transcription of normal messenger RNA; the cause of this has not been discovered. The **early-onset** form of superactivity arises from mutations affecting allosteric regulation of the protein that controls feedback inhibition by inorganic phosphate and dinucleotides. At the same time, these mutations destabilize the protein, so that in slow or nonreplicating cells, such as neurons and red blood cells (RBCs), the enzyme becomes inactive. In contrast, the deficiency phenotypes of PRPS-1 are produced by mutations directly affecting enzyme function, usually in the substrate binding site. Even though the defect is X-linked, it should be considered in a child or young adult of either sex with hyperuricemia and/or hyperuricosuria and normal HPRT activity in lysed RBCs.

Clinical Manifestations

Affected hemizygous males with early-onset superactivity show signs of uric acid overproduction that are apparent in infancy or early childhood, as well as psychomotor delay and sensorineural deafness. Hypotonia, ataxia, and autistic-like behavior have been described. Heterozygous female carriers may also develop gout and hearing impairment. The late-onset type is found in males who show only hyperuricemia and hyperuricosuria, but no neurologic signs. The mildest form of PRPS-1 deficiency manifests as progressive postlingual hearing loss in **X-linked deafness-2 (DFN2)**. More severe mutations constitute the **Charcot-Marie-Tooth disease X-linked-5** phenotype, which includes peripheral neuropathy, hearing impairment, and optic atrophy. The most severe PRPS-1 mutations occur in patients with **Arts syndrome**, who also have central neuropathy and an impaired immune system. Females appear to be unaffected, but hemizygous males have usually not survived beyond the 1st decade, typically succumbing to lung disease. SAMe therapy has prolonged survival, although the neurologic deficits, including the deafness, do not appear to be responsive.

A mechanism for the neurologic symptoms is not yet known, but it can be hypothesized that nucleotide depletion is present in neural tissues, including the brain. Abnormalities of hearing and vision are typical of PRPS-1 deficiency, where the absence of this enzyme presumably compromises these highly energy-dependent neural functions. The high transcript level of PRPS-1 in lung and bone marrow also suggests that its absence may be causal for the recurrent lung infections that characterize Arts syndrome.

Laboratory Findings

For PRPS-1 "superactivity" (both juvenile and adult presentations), serum uric acid may be grossly raised and the urinary excretion of uric acid increased. For PRPS "deficiency," uric acid is normal, not low, probably because PRPS-2 provides the major uric acid–forming activity in liver and other major organs. Diagnosis requires that PRPS-1 activity be measured in erythrocytes and cultured fibroblasts. The adult superactivity disorder must be differentiated from partial HPRT deficiency involving the salvage pathway, which also presents with mild or absent neurologic traits accompanied by hyperuricemia.

Treatment

Treatment of PRPS deficiency, specifically Arts syndrome, has involved mainly experimental therapy with SAMe, as a dietary supplement to correct the depletion of purines. Dietary purines are usually not absorbed into the body but are degraded to uric acid by the gut. SAMe supplementation (beginning at 20 mg/kg/day orally) has been effective in greatly reducing the acute hospitalization episodes of 2 brothers with Arts syndrome, over a period of 10 yr. Treatment of PRPS superactivity is aimed at controlling the hyperuricemia with allopurinol, which inhibits xanthine oxidase, the last enzyme of the purine catabolic pathway. Uric acid production is reduced and is replaced by hypoxanthine, which is more soluble, and xanthine. The initial dose of allopurinol is 10-20 mg/kg/24 hr in children and is adjusted to maintain normal uric acid levels in plasma. The risk of xanthine stone formation is similar to that described for LND. A low-purine diet (free of organ meats, dried beans, and sardines), high fluid intake, and alkalinization of the urine to establish a urinary pH of 6.0-6.5 are necessary. These measures control the hyperuricemia and urate nephropathy but do not affect the neurologic symptoms. There is no known treatment for the neurologic complications.

Adenylosuccinase Lyase Deficiency (Succinylpurinuria)

Adenylosuccinase lyase deficiency is an inherited deficiency of de novo purine synthesis in humans. Adenylosuccinase lyase is an enzyme that catalyzes 2 pathways in de novo synthesis and purine nucleotide recycling. These are the conversion of succinylaminoimidazole carboxamide ribotide (SAICAr) into aminoimidazole carboxamide ribotide (AICAR) in the de novo synthesis of purine nucleotides and the conversion of adenylosuccinate (S-AMP) into AMP, the 2nd step in the conversion of inosine monophosphate (IMP) into AMP, in the purine nucleotide cycle. Adenylosuccinase lyase deficiency results in the accumulation in urine, CSF, and to a smaller extent in plasma, of SAICAr and succinyladenosine (S-Ado), the dephosphorylated derivatives of SAICAr and S-AMP, respectively.

Genetics

Succinylpurinuria is an autosomal recessive disorder; the gene has been mapped to chromosome 22q13.1-q13.2, and approximately 50 gene mutations have been identified. Laboratory investigations show grossly raised succinylpurines in urine and CSF, which are normally undetectable.

Clinical Manifestations

The fatal **neonatal** form presents with lethal encephalopathy. Clinical manifestations include varying degrees of psychomotor retardation, generally accompanied by a seizure disorder and autistic-like behaviors (poor eye contact and repetitive behaviors). Neonatal seizures and a severe infantile epileptic encephalopathy are often the first manifestations of this disorder. Others demonstrate moderate to severe intellectual disability, sometimes associated with growth retardation and muscle hypotonia. One female tested in the mild range of intellectual disability. The form of adenylosuccinase lyase deficiency with profound intellectual disability has been designated **type I** and the variant case with mild intellectual disability **type II**. Other patients have an intermediate clinical symptom pattern with moderately delayed psychomotor development, seizures, stereotypies, and agitation.

Pathology

CT and MRI of the brain may show hypotrophy or hypoplasia of the cerebellum, particularly the vermis. It is proposed that rather than being caused by purine nucleotide depletion, the symptoms are from the neurotoxic effects of accumulating succinylpurines. The S-Ado: SAICAr ratio has been linked to phenotype severity, suggesting that SAICAr is the more toxic compound and that S-Ado might be neuroprotective.

The laboratory diagnosis is based on the presence in urine and CSF of SAICAr and S-Ado, both normally undetectable.

Treatment

No successful treatment has been demonstrated for adenylosuccinase lyase deficiency. SAMe supplementation therapy was tested for 6 mo for an infant diagnosed in the early postnatal period, but no amelioration of symptoms was noted, providing further evidence that the disorder arises from nucleotide toxicity rather than depletion. Prenatal diagnosis has been reported. Systematic screening is suggested in infants and children with unexplained psychomotor retardation or seizure disorder.

Aminoimidazole Carboxamide Ribotide (AICAR) Transformylase/Inosine Monophosphate (IMP) Cyclohydrolase Deficiency

AICA riboside is the dephosphorylated product of AICAR, also termed *ZMP*. Along with its di- and triphosphates, ZMP accumulates in RBCs and fibrocytes in inherited deficiency of the bifunctional enzyme AICAR transformylase/IMP cyclohydrolase (**ATIC**), which catalyzes the conversion of AICAR to formyl-AICAR.

Genetics

This inborn error of purine biosynthesis is caused by a mutation of the *ATIC* gene effecting AICAR transformylase activity. In a single reported case, AICAR transformylase was profoundly deficient, whereas the IMP cyclohydrolase level was 40% of normal.

Clinical Features

The disorder is described in a female infant with profound intellectual disability, epilepsy, dysmorphic features (prominent forehead and metopic suture, brachycephaly, wide mouth with thin upper lip, low-set ears, and prominent clitoris because of fused labia minora), and congenital blindness.

Laboratory Findings

Urinary screening with the Bratton-Marshall test to detect AICA resulted in the identification of this disorder. The transformylase was found to be deficient in fibroblasts, confirming diagnosis of ATIC deficiency.

Treatment

No successful treatment is described.

DISORDERS RESULTING FROM ABNORMALITIES IN PURINE CATABOLISM
Myoadenylate Deaminase Deficiency (Muscle Adenosine Monophosphate Deaminase Deficiency)

Myoadenylate deaminase is a muscle-specific isoenzyme of AMP deaminase that is active in skeletal muscle. During exercise, the deamination of AMP leads to increased levels of IMP and ammonia in proportion to the work performed by the muscle. Two forms of myoadenylate deaminase deficiency are known: an inherited (**primary**) form that may be asymptomatic or associated with cramps or myalgia with exercise, and a **secondary** form that may be associated with other neuromuscular or rheumatologic disorders.

Clinical Manifestations

Clinical manifestations are typically isolated muscle weakness, fatigue, myalgias following moderate to vigorous exercise, or cramps. Myalgia may be associated with an increased serum creatine kinase level and detectable electromyelographic abnormalities. Muscle wasting or histologic changes on biopsy are absent. The age of onset may be as early 8 mo, with approximately 25% of cases recognized between 2 and 12 yr. The enzyme defect has been identified in asymptomatic family members. Secondary forms of muscle AMP deaminase deficiency have been identified in Werdnig-Hoffmann disease, Kugelberg-Welander syndrome, polyneuropathies, and amyotrophic lateral sclerosis (see Chapter 630.2). The metabolic disorder involves the purine nucleotide cycle. As shown in Fig. 108.2, the enzymes involved in this cycle are AMP deaminase, S-AMP synthetase, and S-AMP lyase. It is proposed that muscle dysfunction in AMP deaminase deficiency results from impaired energy production during muscle contraction. It is unclear how individuals may carry the deficit and be asymptomatic. In addition to muscle dysfunction, a mutation of liver AMP deaminase has been proposed as a cause of primary gout, leading to overproduction of uric acid.

Genetics

The inherited form of the disorder is an autosomal recessive trait. *AMPD1*, the gene responsible for encoding muscle AMP deaminase, is located on the short arm of chromosome 1 (1p13-21). Population studies reveal that a mutant allele is found at high frequency in white populations, but alternative splicing of the gene can result in removal of the mutation and normal enzyme function. As a result, the disorder is usually screened by performing the forearm ischemic exercise test. The elevation of venous plasma ammonia following exercise that is seen in unaffected individuals is *absent* in AMP deaminase deficiency.

Laboratory Findings

The final diagnosis is made by histochemical or biochemical assays of a muscle biopsy. The primary form is distinguished by the finding of enzyme levels <2% with little or no immunoprecipitable enzyme. Affected individuals are advised to exercise with caution to prevent rhabdomyolysis and myoglobinuria.

Treatment

Although there are no documented fully effective treatments for myoadenylate deaminase deficiency, it has been proposed that enhancing the rate of replenishment of the ATP pool might be beneficial. Using this rationale, treatment with **ribose** (2-60 g/24 hr orally in divided doses) or **xylitol**, which is converted to ribose, has been reported to improve endurance and muscle strength in some patients, but is ineffective in others. Genetic approaches may be feasible in the future for inherited cases, whereas treatment of the underlying condition is essential in secondary cases.

Adenosine Deaminase Deficiency

See Chapter 152.1.

Purine Nucleoside Phosphorylase Deficiency

See Chapter 152.2.

Xanthine Oxidoreductase Deficiency (Hereditary Xanthinuria/Molybdenum Cofactor Deficiency)

Xanthine oxidoreductase (XOR) is the catalytic enzyme in the final step of the purine catabolic pathway and oxidizes hypoxanthine to xanthine and xanthine to uric acid. Because XOR exists in 2 forms, xanthine dehydrogenase and xanthine oxidase, the deficiency is also referred to as **xanthine dehydrogenase/xanthine oxidase deficiency**. Xanthine, the immediate precursor of uric acid, is less soluble than uric acid in urine, and deficiency of the enzyme results in xanthinuria. XOR deficiency may occur in isolated form (**xanthinuria type 1**), in a combined form involving XOR and aldehyde oxidase deficiencies (**xanthinuria type II**), or multiple deficiencies of XOR, aldehyde oxidase, and sulfite oxidase (**molybdenum cofactor deficiency**). All 3 forms result in an almost total replacement of uric acid by hypoxanthine and xanthine in urine, while plasma uric acid is very low or undetectable.

Patients with the isolated form can be asymptomatic or can have mild symptoms; renal stones, often not visible on radiography, are a risk for renal damage and may appear at any age, when patients may present with loin pain or renal insufficiency. For type II xanthinuria the clinical presentation is similar to type I, but patients also have aldehyde oxidase deficiency, which has no known clinical attributes. Molybdenum cofactor deficiency arises from inherited deficiency of molybdenum cofactor synthase, which affects all 3 molybdoenzymes; as with isolated sulfite oxidase deficiency, it usually presents with neonatal feeding problems, neonatal seizures, increased or decreased muscle tone, ocular lens dislocation, severe intellectual disability, and death in early childhood. Milder cases have presented with lens dislocation only.

Genetics

The inheritance of all 3 types of xanthinuria is complex and autosomal recessive. Type I results from mutations in the human *XDH* gene located on chromosome 2p22. Type II xanthinuria arises from mutations in the molybdenum cofactor sulfurase gene located on chromosome 18q12.2; this enzyme completes the synthesis of the molybdenum cofactor, which is essential for the activity of both XOR and aldehyde oxidase. Type III xanthinuria (XOR, aldehyde oxidase, and sulfite oxidase deficiencies) can arise from functional mutations in any of 3 genes: *MOCS1* (encoding 2 enzymes for synthesis of the precursor via a bicistronic transcript), *MOCS2* (encoding molybdopterin synthase), or *GPHN* (encoding gephyrin), located at 6p21.2, 5q11.2, and 14q23.3, respectively.

Laboratory Findings

Diagnosis is made initially by measuring plasma and/or urinary concentrations of uric acid. Plasma uric acid is very low or absent (<1 mg/dL). Urinary uric acid is reduced, being replaced by xanthine and hypoxanthine. Type II patients can be distinguished by the absence in urine of methyl-2-pyridone-carboxamide, the product of nicotinamide (niacin) breakdown by aldehyde oxidase. Alternately, type II patients can

be distinguished from type I by their inability to oxidize a test dose of allopurinol to oxypurinol via aldehyde oxidase. Molybdenum cofactor deficiency is distinguished by an additional excessive urinary excretion of sulfite and other sulfur-containing metabolites such as sulfocysteine.

Enzyme assay of XOR is not usually offered because it requires jejunal or liver biopsy, because these are the only human tissues that contain appreciable amounts of the enzyme. Sulfite oxidase and the molybdenum cofactor synthase can be measured in liver and fibroblasts. Molecular genetic analysis can be used to confirm diagnosis by searching for functional mutations among the 3 groups of genes.

Treatment

Although isolated deficiency is generally benign, treatment with a diet of low purines and low fructose (which reduces ATP breakdown to xanthine) with increased fluid intake is recommended. Allopurinol is not recommended. The prognosis for molybdenum cofactor deficiency has previously been very poor, but trials of cyclic pyranopterin monophosphate are promising in patients with a defect in the *MOCS1* gene.

DISORDERS OF PYRIMIDINE METABOLISM

The pyrimidines are the building blocks of DNA and RNA and involved in the formation of active intermediates in carbohydrate and phospholipid metabolism (e.g., uridine diphosphate glucose, cytidine diphosphate choline), glucuronidation in detoxification processes (uridine diphosphate), and glycosylation of proteins and lipids.

The essential precursor for pyrimidine biosynthesis is carbamylphosphate, which is shared with the urea cycle. Consequently, proximal blockages of the urea cycle results in carbamyl-phosphate overflowing into the pyrimidine pathway. Pyrimidine synthesis differs from that of purines in that the single pyrimidine ring is first assembled to form orotic acid and then linked to ribose phosphate to form the central pyrimidine nucleotide *uridine monophosphate* (UMP). The pyrimidine bases, uracil and thymine, are catabolized in 4 steps (see Fig. 108.3). Eight disorders of pyrimidine metabolism are reviewed. Purine catabolism has an easily measurable end-point in uric acid; however, there is no equivalent compound in pyrimidine catabolism. Disorders of de novo pyrimidine synthesis include hereditary **orotic aciduria** and dihydroorotate dehydrogenase deficiency (**Miller syndrome**). **Thymidine kinase deficiency** is part of pyrimidine salvage, and the other disorders involve overactivity (in one syndrome) or defects in the pyrimidine degradation pathway. Pyrimidine disorders may present as anemia, neuropathologies, acrofacial dysostosis, or multisystem mitochondrial disorders. The first 3 steps of the degradation pathways for thymine and uracil, respectively, make use of the same enzymes (DPD, DPH, and UP). These 3 steps result in the conversion of uracil into β-alanine. There is increasing evidence that pyrimidines play an important role in the regulation of the nervous system. Reduced production of the neurotransmitter function of β-alanine is hypothesized to produce clinical symptoms. Clinically, pyrimidine disorders may be overlooked because they are rare and their symptoms are not highly specific; however, they should be considered as possible causes of anemia and neurologic disease and are a contraindication for treatment of cancer patients with certain pyrimidine analogs.

Uridine Monophosphate Synthase Type 1 Deficiency (Hereditary Orotic Aciduria)

Hereditary orotic aciduria is a disorder of pyrimidine synthesis associated with deficient activity of the last 2 steps of the de novo pyrimidine synthetic pathway: orotate phosphoribosyltransferase and orotidine-5'-monophosphate decarboxylase (ODC). The activities of these 2 steps reside in separate domains of a bifunctional protein, UMP synthase. This catalyzes the 2-step conversion of orotic acid to UMP via orotidine monophosphate. Hereditary orotic aciduria (UMP synthase deficiency) results in the excessive accumulation of orotic acid.

Genetics

UMP synthase deficiency is inherited as an autosomal recessive disorder, with both functional domains encoded on a single gene, *UMPS*, located on the long arm of chromosome 3 (3q13). Theoretically, random mutations in the gene should have equal chances of producing either orotate phosphoribosyltransferase or ODC deficiency, but there has been only a single case of ODC deficiency reported. Genetic metabolic defects that involve 4 of the 6 enzymes associated with the urea cycle may also result in orotic aciduria, secondary to PPRP depletion resulting from a substantial increased flux through the pyrimidine synthesis pathway.

Clinical Manifestations

Patients with hereditary orotic aciduria (UMP synthase type 1 deficiency) have a macrocytic hypochromic megaloblastic anemia unresponsive to usual therapy (iron, folic acid, vitamin B_{12}) and may develop leukopenia. Onset is usually in 1st months of life. Untreated, this disorder can lead to intellectual disability, failure to thrive, cardiac disease, strabismus, crystalluria, and occasional ureteric obstruction. Renal function is generally normal. Heterozygotes may have mild orotic aciduria but are not otherwise affected. The clinical features are thought to be related to pyrimidine nucleotide depletion. Metabolites derived from several pharmacologic agents (e.g., 5-azauridine, allopurinol) can produce secondary orotic aciduria and orotidinuria by specifically inhibiting the ODC step of UMP synthase. Orotic aciduria may also occur in association with parenteral nutrition, essential amino acid deficiency, and Reye syndrome.

Laboratory Findings

The enzymatic defect may be demonstrated in liver, lymphoblasts, erythrocytes, leukocytes, and cultured skin fibroblasts. A carrier detection test is available, as is prenatal diagnosis.

Treatment

The administration of **uridine** in doses of 50-300 mg/kg/day has led to clinical improvement and reduction in orotic acid excretion in UMP synthase type 1 deficiency. Lifelong treatment is required. Uracil is ineffective because, unlike purines, pyrimidine salvage occurs at the nucleoside (uridine) level. The long-term prognosis in uncomplicated cases is good; however, congenital malformations and other associated features may adversely affect outcome.

Dihydroorotate Dehydrogenase Deficiency (Miller Syndrome)

Miller syndrome was the first mendelian disorder whose molecular basis was identified by whole exome sequencing and shown to correlate with mutations in dihydroorotate dehydrogenase *(DHODH)*. The enzyme DHODH is associated with the mitochondrial electron transport chain and is required for de novo pyrimidine synthesis, catalyzing the oxidation of DHO to orotic acid.

Clinical Manifestations

Miller syndrome is a recognizable **acrofacial dysostosis syndrome** with a combination of craniofacial and limb anomalies. It includes micrognathia, orofacial clefts, malar hypoplasia, aplasia of the medial lower-lid eyelashes, cleft lip/palate, coloboma of the lower eyelid, and cup-shaped ears, combined with postaxial limb deformities, hypoplasia of the limbs with or without ulnar and fibular hypoplasia, and supernumerary nipples. Many of these features are similar to **Treacher Collins syndrome** (see Chapter 337).

Laboratory Findings

Assays of disease-associated *DHODH* alleles predict affected individuals have a deficiency of de novo pyrimidine synthesis, but with significant residual function.

Treatment

Theoretically, dietary supplementation with orotic acid or uridine should bypass the metabolic block. However, because the main effects occur in utero, it is unlikely that the phenotypic abnormality could be corrected.

Dihydropyrimidine Dehydrogenase Deficiency (Thymine-Uraciluria, Pyrimidinuria)

DPD catalyzes the initial and rate-limiting step in the degradation of the pyrimidine bases uracil and thymine. DPD has been identified in most tissues, with the highest activity being in lymphocytes.

Genetics

DPD deficiency is an autosomal recessive disorder, with the *DPYD* gene mapping to chromosome 1p22, with at least 32 polymorphisms detected. It is estimated that the frequency of heterozygosity may be as high as 3%.

Clinical Manifestations

Children may have seizure disorder, intellectual disability and motor delay. Less common features are growth retardation, microcephaly, autistic-like behavior, and ocular anomalies. Others may have milder neurologic symptoms and language disorder. Unaffected individuals have been reported, suggesting possible secondary gene effects. Most patients have an initial period of normal psychomotor development, followed by subsequent developmental delays. Symptoms may be linked to altered uracil, thymine, or β-alanine homeostasis. Because β-alanine is a structural analog of γ-aminobutyric acid and glycine, it has been proposed that it may affect inhibitory neurotransmission. DPD is the initial and rate-limiting enzyme in the inactivation of the antineoplastic drug 5-fluorouracil (5-FU), being responsible for 80% of its catabolism. Patients with partial DPD deficiency are at risk for developing a severe 5-FU–associated toxicity. In adult patients, neurotoxicity (headache, somnolence, visual illusions, memory impairment) linked to pyrimidinemia after 5-FU treatment for cancer is reported in previously healthy individuals.

Laboratory Findings

DPD deficiency is characterized by a variable phenotype and diagnosed by the gross accumulation of thymine and uracil in urine (**thymine-uraciluria**), plasma, and CSF. Uric acid levels have been reported to be normal. Prenatal diagnosis has been reported.

Treatment

There is no established treatment for this disorder, although patients with seizures do respond to anticonvulsant medications. *DPYD* genetic variants associated with partial or complete DPD activity and occurring with relatively high frequency in populations are potentially useful predictive markers of patient response to 5-FU chemotherapy.

Dihydropyrimidinase Deficiency (Dihydropyrimidinuria)

DPH is the 2nd enzyme in the 3-step degradation pathway of uracil and thymine. DPH deficiency is characterized by increased urinary excretion of dihydrouracil and dihydrothymine (**dihydropyrimidinuria**), as well as uracil and thymine. Similar to DPD deficiency, there is a variable clinical phenotype.

Genetics

This is an autosomal recessive disorder, with the *DPYS* gene mapped to chromosome 8q22. One study found no significant difference in residual activity between mutations observed in symptomatic and asymptomatic individuals, again similar to DPD deficiency. Population prevalence in a Japanese sample was 0.1%.

Clinical Manifestations

Clinical manifestations are similar to DPD deficiency, which is evidence that defects in these sequential steps produce a common disorder. Symptoms in 3 unrelated affected cases included seizures with dysmorphic features and developmental delay in 2 patients. However, 3 unrelated infants and 2 adult asymptomatic cases were identified in a screening program for pyrimidine degradation disorders in Japan and were asymptomatic despite the accumulation of pyrimidine degradation products in body fluids.

Laboratory Findings

Organic acid screening may identify increased amounts of uracil and thymine in urine. Oral loading tests with uracil, dihydrouracil, thymine, and dihydrothymine have been used to detect carriers of DPH deficiency.

In symptomatic cases, treatment with β-alanine has been attempted with equivocal results. A single case of increased sensitivity to 5-FU has been reported.

Deficiency of β-Ureidopropionase (N-Carbamyl-β-Amino Aciduria)

The pyrimidine bases uracil and thymine are degraded via the consecutive action of 3 enzymes to β-alanine and β-aminoisobutyric acid, respectively. The 3rd enzyme in the pathway is **ureidopropionase (UP)**, and its deficiency leads to N-carbamyl-β-amino aciduria. 3-Ureidopropionic acid (3-UPA) acts as an endogenous neurotoxin through inhibition of mitochondrial energy metabolism, resulting in the initiation of secondary, energy-dependent excitotoxic mechanisms.

Genetics
Fluorescence in situ hybridization (FISH) localized the human β-ureidopropionase gene, UPB1, to 22q11.2.

Clinical Manifestations
These include muscular hypotonia, dystonic movements, seizures, and severe developmental delay. Some individuals with UP deficiency and no neurologic problems have been reported.

Laboratory Findings
Neuropathology involves both gray and white matter. UP deficiency leads to pathologic accumulation of 3-UPA in body fluids. Urinary analysis in a reported case showed elevated levels of N-carbamyl-β-alanine and N-carbamyl-β-aminoisobutyric acid (ureidoisobutyric acid). The enzyme is expressed only in the liver, and no activity of β-ureidopropionase is detected in a liver biopsy.

Treatment
There is no known treatment for UP deficiency.

Pyrimidine 5′-Nucleotidase Deficiency

Erythrocyte maturation is accompanied by RNA degradation and the release of mononucleotides. Pyrimidine 5′-nucleotidase is the first degradative enzyme of the pyrimidine salvage cycle and catalyzes the hydrolysis of pyrimidine 5′-nucleotides to the corresponding nucleosides. Enzyme deficiency results in the accumulation of high levels of cytidine and uridine nucleotides in the erythrocytes, which in turn results in hemolysis. Deficiency of pyrimidine 5′-nucleotidase may be at least in part compensated in vivo by other nucleotidases or perhaps other nucleotide metabolic pathways.

Genetics
This is an autosomal recessive disorder involving the gene NT5C3A on chromosome 7 (7p15).

Clinical Manifestations
Affected patients with pyrimidine 5′-nucleotidase deficiency clinically present with a defect restricted to erythrocytes and characterized by nonspherocytic hemolytic anemia with basophilic stippling. Other characteristic features include splenomegaly, increased indirect bilirubin, and hemoglobinuria. **Lead** is a powerful inhibitor of pyrimidine 5′-nucleotidase, and assessment of lead levels should be included whenever hemolytic anemia, pyrimidine 5′-nucleotidase deficiency, and basophilic stippling are found together.

Laboratory Findings
Diagnosis requires assay of erythrocyte UMP hydrolysis to form uridine and inorganic phosphate. The enzyme defect should be suspected in patients with nonspherocytic hemolytic anemia with basophilic stippling. The anemia is usually moderate, and transfusions are rarely necessary.

Treatment
There is no specific treatment. Splenectomy has not proved to be effective. Lead-induced acquired pyrimidine 5′ nucleotidase deficiency is treatable,

unlike the congenital deficiency.

Overactive Cytosolic 5′-Nucleotidase (Pyrimidine Nucleotide Depletion)

Pyrimidine nucleotide depletion and overactive cytosolic 5′-nucleotidase, may lead to a neurodevelopmental disorder. Four unrelated patients showed 6-10–fold elevation in the activity of pyrimidine 5′-nucleotidase in fibroblasts with both purine and pyrimidine substrates. Investigation in cultured fibroblasts derived from these patients showed normal incorporation of purine bases into nucleotides but decreased incorporation of uridine and orotic acid.

Clinical Manifestations
These include developmental delay, seizures, ataxia, recurrent infections, severe language deficit, hyperactivity, short attention span, and aggressive behavior appearing within the 1st few years of life. Affected patients show electroencephalogram abnormalities. Metabolic testing is normal except for persistent hypouricosuria. It is proposed that increased catabolic activity and decreased pyrimidine salvage cause a deficiency of pyrimidine nucleotides.

Treatment
Treatment is with oral uridine based on compensating for the increased nucleotide catabolism. All reported patients treated with uridine showed improved speech and behavior, decreased seizure activity with discontinuation of seizure medications, and decreased infections.

Thymidine Phosphorylase Deficiency (Mitochondrial Neurogastrointestinal Encephalomyopathy)

Thymidine phosphorylase catalyzes the catabolism of thymidine to thymine. This enzyme is also known as *platelet-derived endothelial cell growth factor* because of its angiogenic properties, or *gliostatin*, indicating its inhibitory effects on glial cell proliferation. It has been implicated in mitochondrial nucleoside metabolism. Plasma thymidine level is increased more than 20-fold in patients compared to controls. Loss of function of thymidine phosphorylase causes **mitochondrial neurogastrointestinal encephalomyopathy (MNGIE)**, which is inherited as a single autosomal recessive disorder, causing mitochondrial DNA depletion and instability. In MNGIE, loss of thymidine phosphorylase activity causes toxic accumulations of the nucleosides thymidine and deoxyuridine, which are phosphorylated to the corresponding nucleoside triphosphate in the mitochondrion, leading to mitochondrial deoxynucleoside triphosphate pool imbalances and aberrant mitochondrial DNA replication.

Genetics
The TYMP gene encoding thymidine phosphorylase has been identified as the MNGIE gene and is mapped to chromosome 22q13.32-qter, but the protein is imported into mitochondria.

Clinical Manifestations
Clinical manifestations of MNGIE usually begin in adolescence and young adulthood and include ptosis, progressive external ophthalmoparesis, GI dysmotility (pseudoobstruction) and malabsorption, cachexia, peripheral neuropathy, skeletal muscle myopathy, and leukoencephalopathy.

Laboratory Findings
Muscle biopsies typically reveal mitochondrial abnormalities. Screening is performed by detection of grossly raised thymidine and deoxyuridine in urine and plasma, which are normally absent. Confirmation of the diagnosis can be made by assay of thymidine phosphorylase activity in peripheral leukocytes. Molecular genetic analysis will show functional mutations in the TYMP gene. Increased thymidine and/or deoxyuridine nucleotides may cause mitochondrial nucleotide pool imbalance, resulting in mitochondrial DNA alterations, in particular DNA depletion.

Treatment
Supportive treatment is indicated. There is no established therapy for

MNGIE; bone marrow transplantation has been performed on several patients, but no improvement in symptoms or disease progression has been reported. Allogeneic hematopoietic stem cell transplantation to restore thymidine phosphorylase activity and eliminate toxic metabolites is a potential therapy for MNGIE.

Thymidine Kinase 2 Deficiency
Thymidine kinase 2 (TK2) is a key enzyme for the pyrimidine salvage pathway to provide precursor nucleotide for mitochondrial DNA. TK2 deficiency causes tissue-specific depletion of mitochondrial DNA. TK2 normally phosphorylates thymidine and deoxycytidine.

Genetics
The TK2 gene is located on chromosome 16q 22; the deficiency is inherited in an autosomal recessive manner.

Clinical Manifestations
Affected individuals with TK2 deficiency have severe myopathy and depletion of muscular mitochondrial DNA in infancy.

Treatment
No specific treatment is available. Supportive treatment is indicated.

Bibliography is available at Expert Consult.

Chapter **109**

Hutchinson-Gilford Progeria Syndrome (Progeria)

Leslie B. Gordon

第一百零九章
Hutchinson-Gilford早老综合征

中文导读

　　本章主要介绍了Hutchinson-Gilford早老综合征的临床特征、实验室检查、分子发病机制、诊断与鉴别诊断、治疗及预后以及患者资源。在临床特征中描述了该疾病的皮肤改变、生长迟缓、眼部异常、颅面及牙齿表型、骨骼肌及软骨异常、听力、心血管疾病、脑血管动脉病变及卒中、性发育以及机体功能维持系统等内容。

Hutchinson-Gilford progeria syndrome (HGPS), or progeria, is a rare, fatal, autosomal dominant segmental premature aging disease. With an estimated incidence of 1 in 4 million live births and prevalence of 1 in 20 million living individuals, there are an estimated total of 400 children living with progeria in 2018 worldwide. There is no gender, ethnic, or regional bias.

Progeria is caused by a single-base mutation in the *LMNA* gene, which results in the production of a mutant lamin A protein called **progerin**. Lamin A is an intermediate filament inner nuclear membrane protein found in most differentiated cells of the body. Without progerin-specific treatment, children with progeria develop **premature progressive atherosclerosis** and die of heart failure, usually between ages 5 and 20 yr. Progerin is found in increased concentration in skin and the vascular wall of normal older individuals compared to younger individuals, suggesting a role in normal aging.

CLINICAL MANIFESTATIONS
Children develop the appearance of accelerated aging, but both clinical and biologic overlaps with aging are segmental, or partial. Physical appearance changes dramatically each year that they age (Fig. 109.1). The descriptions discussed next are roughly in order of clinical appearance.

Dermatologic Changes
Skin findings are often apparent as initial signs of progeria. These are variable in severity and include areas of discoloration, stippled pigmentation, tightened areas that can restrict movement, and areas of the trunk or legs where small (1-2 cm), soft, bulging skin is present. Although usually born with normal hair presence, cranial hair is lost within the first few years, leaving soft, downy, sparse immature hair on the scalp, no eyebrows, and scant eyelashes. Nail dystrophy occurs later in life.

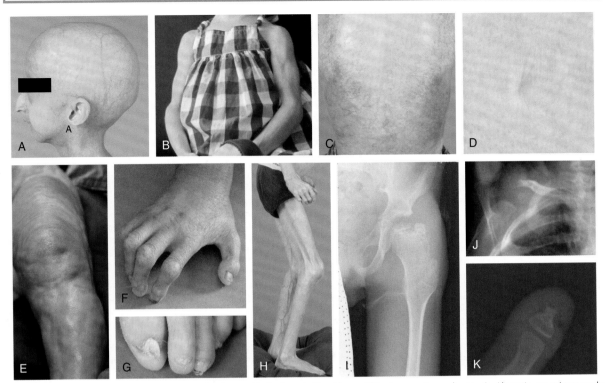

Fig. 109.1 Distinguishing clinical features and radiographic findings in Hutchinson-Gilford progeria syndrome. **A,** Alopecia, prominent scalp veins, narrowed nasal bridge, retrognathia; **B,** generalized lipoatrophy leaves muscular prominence; **C,** skin tightening and mottling; **D,** flat umbilicus with scarred-over appearance; **E,** skin bulging; **F,** digital joint contractures; **G,** nail dystrophy with spooning; **H,** knee joint contractures, lipodystrophy; **I,** coxa valga of the hip; **J,** clavicular osteolysis; **K,** acroosteolysis in a thumb. *(Photos courtesy of The Progeria Research Foundation and Boston Children's Hospital.)*

Failure to Thrive

Children with progeria experience apparently normal fetal and early postnatal development. Between several months and 1 yr of age, abnormalities in growth and body composition are readily apparent. Severe failure to thrive ensues, heralding generalized lipoatrophy, with apparent wasting of limbs, circumoral cyanosis, and prominent veins around the scalp, neck, and trunk. The mean weight percentile is usually normal at birth, but decreases to below the 3rd percentile despite adequate caloric intake for normal growth and normal resting energy expenditure. A review of 35 children showed an average weight increase of only 0.44 kg/yr, beginning at 24 mo of age and persisting through life. There is interpatient variation in weight gain, but the projected weight gain over time in individual patients is constant, linear, and very predictable; this sharply contrasts with the parabolic growth pattern for normal age- and gender-matched children. Children reach an average final height of approximately 1 meter and weight of approximately 15 kg. Head circumference is normal. The weight deficit is more pronounced than the height deficit and, associated with the loss of subcutaneous fat, results in the emaciated appearance characteristic of progeria. Clinical problems caused by the lack of subcutaneous fat include sensitivity to cold temperatures and foot discomfort caused by lack of fat cushioning. Overt diabetes is very unusual in progeria, but about 30–40% of children have insulin resistance.

Ocular Abnormalities

Ophthalmic signs and symptoms are caused in part by tightened skin and a paucity of subcutaneous fat around the eyes. Children often experience hyperopia and signs of ocular surface disease from nocturnal lagophthalmos and exposure keratopathy, which in turn may lead to corneal ulceration and scarring. Some degree of photophobia is common.

Most patients have relatively good acuity; however, advanced ophthalmic disease can be associated with reduced acuity. *Children with progeria should have an ophthalmic evaluation at diagnosis and at least yearly thereafter.* Aggressive ocular surface lubrication is recommended, including the use of tape tarsorrhaphy at night.

Craniofacial and Dental Phenotypes

Children develop craniofacial disproportion, with micrognathia and retrognathia caused by mandibular hypoplasia. Typical oral and dental manifestations include hypodontia, delayed tooth eruption, severe dental crowding, ogival palatal arch, ankyloglossia, presence of median sagittal palatal fissure, and generalized gingival recession. Eruption may be delayed for many months, and primary teeth may persist for the duration of life. Secondary teeth are present but may or may not erupt. They sometimes erupt on the lingual and palatal surfaces of the mandibular and maxillary alveolar ridges, rather than in place of the primary incisors. In some, but not all cases, extracting primary teeth promotes movement of secondary teeth into place.

Bone and Cartilaginous Abnormalities

Development of bone structure and bone density represents a unique skeletal dysplasia that is not based in malnutrition. Acroosteolysis of the distal phalanges, distal clavicular resorption, and thin, tapered ribs are early signs of progeria (as early as 3 mo of age). *Facial disproportion a narrowed nasal bridge and retrognathia makes intubation extremely difficult, and fiberoptic intubation is recommended.* A pyriform chest structure and small clavicles can lead to reducible glenohumeral joint instability. Growth of the spine and bony pelvis are normal. However, dysplastic growth of the femoral head and neck axis result in coxa valgus (i.e., straightening of the femoral head-neck axis >125 degrees) and coxa magna, where the diameter of the femoral head is disproportionately large for the acetabulum, resulting in hip instability. The resulting hip dysplasia can be progressive and may result in osteoarthritis, avascular necrosis, hip dislocation, and inability to bear weight. Other changes to the appendicular skeleton include flaring of the humeral and femoral metaphyses and constriction of the radial neck. Growth plate morphology is generally normal but can be variable within a single radiograph. The appearance of ossification centers used to define bone age is normal. Bone structure assessed by peripheral quantitative computed tomography (pQCT) of the radius demonstrates distinct and severe abnormalities in bone structural geometry, consistent with progeria representing a *skeletal dysplasia*. Areal bone mineral density (aBMD) z scores measured by dual-energy X-ray absorptiometry (DXA) adjusted for height-age, and true (volumetric) BMD assessed by pQCT are normal to mildly reduced, refuting the assumption that patients with progeria are osteoporotic. Fracture rates in progeria are normal and not associated with fragility fractures observed in other pediatric metabolic bone diseases, such as osteogenesis imperfecta.

Contractures in multiple joints (e.g., fingers, elbows, hips, knees, ankles) may be present at birth and may progress with age because of changes in the laxity of the surrounding soft tissue structures (joint capsule, ligament, skin). Along with irregularities in the congruency of articulating joint surfaces, these changes serve to limit joint motion and affect the pattern of gait. Physical therapy is recommended routinely and throughout life to maximize joint function.

Hearing

Low-tone conductive hearing loss is pervasive in progeria and indicative of a stiff tympanic membrane and/or deficits in the middle ear bony and ligamentous structures. Overall, this does not affect ability to hear the usual spoken tones, but preferential classroom seating is recommended, with annual hearing examinations.

Cardiovascular Disease

Approximately 80% of progeria deaths are caused by heart failure, possibly precipitated by events such as superimposed respiratory infection or surgical intervention. Progeria is a **primary vasculopathy** characterized by pervasive accelerated vascular stiffening, followed by large- and small-vessel occlusive disease from atherosclerotic plaque formation, with valvular and cardiac insufficiency in later years. Hypertension, angina, cardiomegaly, metabolic syndrome, and congestive heart failure are common end-stage events.

A study of transthoracic echocardiography in treatment-naïve patients revealed diastolic left ventricular dysfunction associated with age-related decline in lateral and septal early (E′) diastolic tissue Doppler velocity z scores and an increase in the ratio of mitral inflow (E) to lateral and septal E' velocity z scores. Other echocardiographic findings included left ventricular hypertrophy, left ventricular systolic dysfunction, and mitral or aortic valve disease. These tend to appear later in life. Routine carotid ultrasound for plaque monitoring, carotid-femoral pulse wave velocity (PWV_{cf}) measures for vascular stiffening, and echocardiography are recommended.

Cerebrovascular Arteriopathy and Stroke

Cerebral infarction may occur while the child exhibits a normal electrocardiogram. The earliest incidence of stroke occurred at age 0.4 yr. More often strokes occur in the later years. Over the life span, MRI evidence of infarction can be found in 60% of progeria patients, with half of these clinically silent. Both large- and small-vessel disease is found; collateral vessel formation is extensive. Carotid artery blockages are well documented, but infarction can occur even in their absence. A propensity for strokes and an underlying stiff vasculature make maintaining adequate blood pressure through hydration (habitually drinking well) a priority in progeria patients; special care should be taken when considering maintenance of consistent blood pressure during general anesthesia, airplane trips, and hot weather. In addition, 15% of deaths in children with progeria occur from head injury or trauma, including subdural hematoma. This implies an underlying susceptibility to subdural hematoma.

Sexual Development

Females with progeria can develop Tanner Stage II secondary sexual characteristics, including signs of early breast development and sparse pubic hair. They do not achieve Tanner Stage III. Despite minimal to no physical signs of pubertal development and minimal body fat, over half of females experience spontaneous menarche at a median age of 14 yr. Those experiencing menarche vs nonmenstruating females have similar body mass indices, percentage body fat, and serum leptin levels, all of which are vastly below the healthy adolescent population. If bleeding becomes severe, the complete blood count may be decreased, and an oral contraceptive may be used to decrease bleeding severity. Secondary sexual characteristics in males have not been studied. There are no documented cases of reproductive capacity in females or males with progeria.

Normally Functioning Systems

Liver, kidney, thyroid, immune, gastrointestinal, and neurologic systems (other than stroke related) remain intact. Intellect is normal for age, possibly in part from downregulation of progerin expression in the brain by a brain-specific micro-RNA, miRNA-9.

LABORATORY FINDINGS

The most consistent laboratory findings are low serum leptin below detectable levels (>90%) and insulin resistance (60%). Platelet count is often moderately high. High-density lipoprotein (HDL) cholesterol and adiponectin concentrations decrease with increasing age to values significantly below normal. Otherwise, lipid panels, high-sensitivity C-reactive protein, blood chemistries, liver and kidney function tests, endocrine test, and coagulation tests are generally normal.

MOLECULAR PATHOGENESIS

Mutations in the *LMNA* gene cause progeria. The normal *LMNA/C* gene encodes the proteins lamins A and C, of which only lamin A is associated with human diseases. The lamin proteins are the principal proteins of the nuclear lamina, a complex molecular interface located between the inner membrane of the nuclear envelope and chromatin. The integrity of the lamina is central to many cellular functions, creating and maintaining structural integrity of the nuclear scaffold, DNA replication, RNA transcription, organization of the nucleus, nuclear pore assembly, chromatin function, cell cycling, senescence, and apoptosis.

Progeria is almost always a sporadic autosomal dominant disease. There are 2 documented sibling occurrences, both presumably stemming from parental mosaicism, where 1 phenotypically normal parent has germline mosaicism. It is caused by the accelerated use of an alternative, internal splice site that results in the deletion of 150 base pairs in the 3′ portion of exon 11 of the *LMNA* gene. In about 90% of cases, this results from a single C to T transition at nucleotide 1824 that is silent (Gly608Gly) but optimizes an internal splice site within exon 11. The remaining 10% of cases possess 1 of several single-base mutations within the intron 11 splice donor site, thus reducing specificity for this site and altering the splicing balance in favor of the internal splice. Subsequent to all these mutations, translation followed by posttranslational processing of the altered mRNA produces progerin, a shortened abnormal lamin A protein with a 50–amino acid deletion near its C-terminal end. An understanding of the posttranslational processing pathway and how it is altered to create progerin has led to a number of treatment prospects for the disease (Fig. 109.2).

Both lamin A and progerin possess a methylated farnesyl side group attached during posttranslational processing. This is a lipophilic moiety that facilitates intercalation of proteins into the inner nuclear membrane, where most of the lamin and progerin functions are performed. For normal lamin A, loss of the methylated farnesyl anchor releases prelamin from the nuclear membrane, rendering it soluble for autophagic degradation. However, progerin retains its farnesyl moiety. It remains anchored to the membrane, binding other proteins, causing blebbing of the nucleus, disrupting mitosis, and altering gene expression. Progerin also retains a methyl moiety.

Disease in progeria is produced by a dominant negative mechanism; *the action of progerin,* not the diminution of lamin A, causes the disease phenotype. The severity of disease is determined in part by progerin levels, which are regulated by the particular mutation, tissue type, or other factors influencing use of the internal splice site.

DIAGNOSIS AND DIFFERENTIAL DIAGNOSIS

Overall, the constellation of small body habitus, bone, hair, subcutaneous fat, and skin changes results in the marked physical resemblance among patients with progeria (Fig. 109.3). For this reason, clinical diagnosis can be achieved or excluded with relative confidence even at young ages, even though there have been a few cases of low–progerin-expressing patients with extremely mild signs. Clinical suspicion should be followed by *LMNA* genetic sequence testing. The disorders that resemble progeria are those grouped as the senile-like syndromes and include Wiedmann-Rautenstrauch syndrome, Werner syndrome, Cockayne syndrome, Rothmund-Thomson syndrome, restrictive dermopathy, and Nestor-Guillermo progeria syndrome (Table 109.1). Patients often fall under none of these diagnoses and represent ultra-rare, unnamed progeroid laminopathies that carry either non–progerin-producing mutations in *LMNA* or the lamin-associated enzyme *(ZMPSTE24)*, or progeroid syndromes without lamin-associated mutations.

TREATMENT AND PROGNOSIS

Children with progeria develop a severe premature form of atherosclerosis. Prior to death, cardiac decline with left-sided hypertrophy, valvular insufficiency, and pulmonary edema develop; neurovascular decline with transient ischemic attacks (TIAs), strokes, and occasionally seizures can result in significant morbidity. Death occurs generally between ages 5 and 20 yr, with a median life span of 14.5 yr, resulting from heart failure, sometimes with superimposed respiratory infection (approximately 80%); from head injury or trauma, including subdural hematoma (approximately 15%); and rarely from stroke (1–3%) or complications from anesthesia during surgery (1–3%).

Growth hormone, 0.05 mg/kg/day subcutaneously, has resulted in increased rate of weight gain and overall size, but still well below that seen in normal children. Low-dose aspirin therapy is recommended at 2 mg/kg/day, as an extension of what is known about decreasing cardiovascular risk in the general at-risk adult population. It is not known whether growth hormone or low-dose aspirin has any effect on morbidity or mortality.

Several clinical treatment trials have been based on medications that target the posttranslational pathway of progerin (see Fig. 109.2). Inhibiting posttranslational progerin farnesylation is aimed at preventing this disease-causing protein from anchoring to the nuclear membrane, where it carries out much of its damage. A prospective single-arm clinical trial was conducted with the farnesyltransferase inhibitor **lonafarnib** (NCT00425607). Lonafarnib was well tolerated; the most common side effects were diarrhea, nausea, and loss of appetite, which generally improved with time. Subgroups of patients experienced increased rate of weight gain, decreased vascular stiffness measured by decreased PWV_{cf} and carotid artery echodensity, improved left ventricular diastolic function, increased radial bone structural rigidity, improved sensorineural hearing, and early evidence of decreased headache, TIA, and stroke rates. Dermatologic, dental, joint contracture, insulin resistance, lipodystrophy, BMD, and joint contractures were unaffected by drug treatment. A lonafarnib extension study was initiated, which added 30 children to the study. Children treated with lonafarnib demonstrated an increase in estimated survival over untreated children with progeria.

A clinical trial that added *pravastatin* (FDA approved to lower cholesterol) and *zoledronate* (FDA approved for osteoporosis) to the

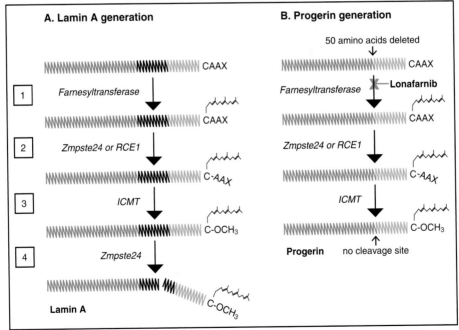

Fig. 109.2 Posttranslational processing pathways producing lamin A and progerin, including the target site for lonafarnib. **A,** Prelamin A polypeptide chain, showing its central α-helical rod domain and C-terminal –CAAX box, representing cysteine (C), aliphatic amino acids (AA), and any amino acid (X). The α-helical rod domain is divided into segments that assist in displaying the progerin defect. Posttranslational processing consists of 4 steps: *1,* a farnesyl group is attached to the cysteine residue of the –CAAX box by farnesyltransferase; *2,* the last 3 residues are proteolytically cleaved by the zinc metalloprotease Zmpste24 or Ras-converting enzyme (RCE1); *3,* carboxy-methylation by isoprenyl-cysteine carboxyl methyltransferase (ICMT); and *4,* the terminal 15 C-terminal residues, including the farnesylated and carboxymethylated cysteine, are cleaved off by Zmpste24. **B,** A 50–amino acid deletion in prelamin A (represented by black segment of the lamin A rod) is the result of a mutation that activates a cryptic splice site within exon 11 of the *LMNA* gene. This deletion leaves progerin without an attachment site for the last processing step—cleavage of the farnesylation and carboxymethylated terminal 15 amino acid residues. Thus, progerin remains farnesylated and intercalated within the inner nuclear membrane, where it causes much of its cellular damage.

lonafarnib regimen was similarly aimed at inhibiting progerin farnesylation (NCT00916747), but results showed no detected improvements in clinical status over lonafarnib monotherapy. An ongoing clinical trial adding *everolimus* (FDA-approved mTOR inhibitor) to the lonafarnib regimen is aimed at accelerating autophagy of progerin, thus theoretically reducing its accumulation and cellular damage (NCT02579044). Results of this study are forthcoming.

PATIENT RESOURCES

The **Progeria Research Foundation** (www.progeriaresearch.org) maintains an international progeria patient registry, provides a diagnostics program and complete patient care manual, and coordinates clinical treatment trials. It funds preclinical and clinical research to define the molecular basis of the disorder and to discover treatments and a cure. The Foundation website is an excellent source of current information on progeria for families of children with the disorder, their physicians, and interested scientists. Additional resources include the National Human Genome Research Institute (www.genome.gov/11007255/), National Center for Biotechnology Information Genereviews (www.ncbi.nlm.nih.gov/books/NBK1121/), and National Center for Advancing Translational Sciences (www.rarediseases.info.nih.gov/diseases/7467/progeria).

Bibliography is available at Expert Consult.

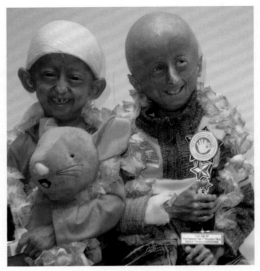

Fig. 109.3 Unrelated 7 yr old female and 10 yr old male with progeria. Appearance is remarkably similar between patients. *(Photograph courtesy of The Progeria Research Foundation)*

| Table 109.1 | Features of Hutchinson-Gilford Progeria Syndrome and Other Disorders With Overlapping Features |

	HUTCHINSON-GILFORD PROGERIA SYNDROME	WIEDEMANN-RAUTENSTRAUCH SYNDROME	WERNER SYNDROME	COCKAYNE SYNDROME	ROTHMUND-THOMPSON SYNDROME	RESTRICTIVE DERMOPATHY
Causative gene(s)	*LMNA*	Unknown	*WRN, LMNA*	*CSA (ERCC8)* *CSB (ERCC6)*	*RECQL4*	*ZMPSTE24, LMNA*
Inheritance	Autosomal Dominant	Unknown, likely recessive	Recessive	Recessive	Recessive	Recessive
Onset	Infancy	Newborn	Young adult	Newborn/infancy	Infancy	Newborn
Growth retardation	Postnatal	Intrauterine	Onset after puberty	Postnatal	Postnatal	Intrauterine
Hair loss	+ Total	+ Scalp patchy	+ Scalp, sparse, graying	−	+ Diffuse	+ Diffuse
Skin abnormalities	+	+	+	+	+	+
Subcutaneous fat loss	+	+	+	+	−	−
Skin calcification	+ Rarely	−	+	−	−	−
Short stature	+	+	+	+	+	+
Coxa valga	+	−	−	−	−	−
Acroosteolysis	+	+	+	−	−	−
Mandibular dysplasia	+	+	−	−	−	+
Osteopenia	+ Mild	+	+	−	+	+
Vasculopathy	+	−	+	+	−	−
Heart failure	+	−	+	−	−	−
Strokes	+	−	−	−	−	−
Insulin Resistance	+	−	+ Rarely	−	−	−
Diabetes	−	−	+	−	−	−
Hypogonadism	+	−	+	+	+	−
Dental abnormality	+	+	+	+	+	+
Voice abnormality	+	−	+	−	−	−
Hearing loss	+	−	−	+	−	−
Joint contractures	+	−	−	−	−	+

Continued

Table 109.1	Features of Hutchinson-Gilford Progeria Syndrome and Other Disorders With Overlapping Features—cont'd					
	HUTCHINSON-GILFORD PROGERIA SYNDROME	WIEDEMANN-RAUTENSTRAUCH SYNDROME	WERNER SYNDROME	COCKAYNE SYNDROME	ROTHMUND-THOMPSON SYNDROME	RESTRICTIVE DERMOPATHY
Hyperkeratosis	−	−	+	−	+	−
Cataracts	−	−	+	+	+	−
Tumor predisposition	−	−	+	−	+	−
Intellectual disability	−	+	−	+	−	−
Neurologic disorder	−	+	+ Mild	+	−	−

Adapted from Hegele RA: Drawing the line in Progeria syndromes, *Lancet* 362;416–417, 2003.

Chapter 110
The Porphyrias

Manisha Balwani, Robert J. Desnick, and Karl E. Anderson

第一百一十章
卟啉病

中文导读

　　本章主要介绍了血红素生物合成途径、卟啉病分类及诊断、δ–氨基乙酰丙酸脱氢酶缺乏性卟啉病、急性间歇性卟啉病、先天性红细胞生成卟啉病、迟发皮肤型卟啉病、肝红细胞生成性卟啉病、遗传性粪卟啉病、变异性卟啉病、红细胞生成性原卟啉病及X连锁原卟啉病、双重卟啉病以及肿瘤所致卟啉病。具体描述了卟啉病分类及诊断的一线实验室诊断检查、二线检查及亚临床卟啉病相关检查；具体描述了各具体疾病的病因、病理及发病机制、临床表现、实验室发现、诊断与鉴别诊断、并发症、治疗、预后以及遗传咨询等内容。

Porphyrias are metabolic diseases resulting from altered activities of specific enzymes of the heme biosynthetic pathway. These enzymes are most active in bone marrow and liver. **Erythropoietic porphyrias**, in which overproduction of heme pathway intermediates occurs primarily in bone marrow erythroid cells, usually present at birth or in early childhood with *cutaneous photosensitivity,* or in the case of congenital erythropoietic porphyria, even in utero as nonimmune hydrops. Erythropoietic protoporphyria is the most common porphyria in children and of most interest to pediatricians. Most porphyrias are *hepatic*, with overproduction and initial accumulation of porphyrin precursors or porphyrins in the liver. Activation of hepatic porphyrias is very rare during childhood, reflecting the distinct hepatic regulatory mechanisms for heme biosynthesis that are influenced by pubertal development.

Homozygous forms of the hepatic porphyrias may manifest clinically before puberty. Children who are heterozygous for inherited hepatic porphyrias may present with nonspecific and unrelated symptoms, and parents often request advice about long-term prognosis and express concerns about drugs that may exacerbate these conditions.

The DNA sequences and chromosomal locations are established for the genes of the enzymes in this pathway, and multiple disease-related mutations have been found for each porphyria. However, benign variants identified by gene sequencing can be misleading. The inherited porphyrias display autosomal dominant, autosomal recessive, or X-linked inheritance. Although initial diagnosis of porphyria by biochemical methods remains essential, it is especially important to confirm the diagnosis by demonstrating a specific pathogenic gene mutation(s).

THE HEME BIOSYNTHETIC PATHWAY

Heme is required for a variety of hemoproteins, such as hemoglobin, myoglobin, respiratory cytochromes, and cytochrome P450 enzymes (CYPs). It is believed that the 8 enzymes in the pathway for heme biosynthesis are active in all tissues. Hemoglobin synthesis in erythroid precursor cells accounts for approximately 85% of daily heme synthesis in humans. Hepatocytes account for most of the rest, primarily for synthesis of CYPs, which are especially abundant in the liver endoplasmic reticulum, and turn over more rapidly than many other hemoproteins, such as the mitochondrial respiratory cytochromes. Pathway intermediates are the porphyrin precursors **δ-aminolevulinic acid** (**ALA**, also known as 5-aminolevulinic acid) and **porphobilinogen** (**PBG**), as well as porphyrins (mostly in their reduced forms, known as **porphyrinogens**) (Fig. 110.1). These intermediates do not accumulate in significant amounts under normal conditions or have important physiologic functions.

Altered activity of each enzyme in the pathway has been associated with a specific type of porphyria (Table 110.1). The first enzyme, ALA synthase (ALAS), occurs in 2 forms. An erythroid specific form, ALAS2, is deficient in X-linked sideroblastic anemia, as a result of mutations of the *ALAS2* gene on chromosome Xp11.2. Gain-of-function mutations of *ALAS2* caused by deletions in the last exon cause X-linked protoporphyria (**XLP**), which is phenotypically identical to erythropoietic protoporphyria.

Regulation of heme synthesis differs in the 2 major heme-forming tissues. Liver heme biosynthesis is primary controlled by the ubiquitous form of ALAS (ALAS1). Synthesis of ALAS1 in liver is regulated by a "free" heme pool (see Fig. 110.1), which can be augmented by newly synthesized heme or by existing heme released from hemoproteins and destined for breakdown to biliverdin by heme oxygenase.

In the erythron, novel regulatory mechanisms allow for the production of the very large amounts of heme needed for hemoglobin synthesis. The response to stimuli for hemoglobin synthesis occurs during cell differentiation, leading to an increase in cell number. Also, unlike the liver, heme has a stimulatory role in hemoglobin formation, and the stimulation of heme synthesis in erythroid cells is accompanied by increases not only in ALAS2, but also by sequential induction of other heme biosynthetic enzymes. Separate erythroid-specific and nonerythroid or "housekeeping" transcripts are known for the first 4 enzymes in the pathway. The separate forms of ALAS are encoded by genes on different chromosomes, but for each of the other three, erythroid and nonerythroid transcripts are transcribed by alternative promoters in the same gene. Heme also regulates the rate of its synthesis in erythroid cells by controlling the transport of iron into reticulocytes.

Intermediates of the heme biosynthetic pathway are efficiently converted to heme and, normally, only small amounts of the intermediates are excreted. Some may undergo chemical modifications before excretion. Whereas the porphyrin precursors ALA and PBG are colorless, nonfluorescent, and largely excreted unchanged in urine, PBG may degrade to colored products such as the brownish pigment called *porphobilin* or spontaneously polymerize to uroporphyrins. Porphyrins are red in color and display bright-red fluorescence when exposed to long-wavelength ultraviolet (UV) light. Porphyrinogens are the reduced form of porphyrins, and are colorless and nonfluorescent, but are readily autoxidized to the corresponding porphyrins when they accumulate or are outside the cell. Only the type III isomers of uroporphyrinogen and coproporphyrinogen are converted to heme (see Fig. 110.1).

ALA and PBG are excreted in urine. Excretion of porphyrins and porphyrinogens in urine or bile is determined by the number of carboxyl groups. Those with many carboxyl groups, such as *uroporphyrin* (octacarboxyl porphyrin) and *heptacarboxyl porphyrin,* are water soluble and readily excreted in urine. Those with fewer carboxyl groups, such as *protoporphyrin* (dicarboxyl porphyrin), are not water soluble and are excreted in bile and feces. *Coproporphyrin* (tetracarboxyl porphyrin) is excreted partly in urine and partly in bile. Because coproporphyrin I is more readily excreted in bile than coproporphyrin III, impaired hepatobiliary function may increase total urinary coproporphyrin excretion and the ratio of these isomers.

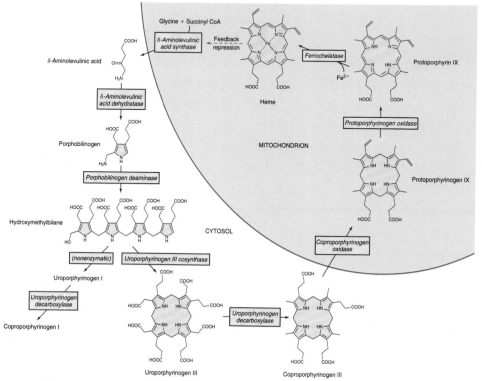

Fig. 110.1 Enzymes and intermediates of the heme biosynthetic pathway. The pathway is regulated in the liver by the end product, heme, mainly by feedback repression (*dashed arrow*).

Table 110.1 | The Human Porphyrias: Mutations, Time of Presentation, and Tissue- and Symptom-Based Classifications

DISEASE	ENZYME	INHERITANCE	PRESENTATION	H	E	A/N	C
X-Linked protoporphyria (XLP)	δ-Aminolevulinate synthase 2 (ALAS2)	X-linked	Childhood		X		X
δ-Aminolevulinic acid dehydratase porphyria (ADP)	δ-Aminolevulinic acid dehydratase (ALAD)	Autosomal recessive	Mostly post puberty	X	X*	X	
Acute intermittent porphyria (AIP)	Porphobilinogen deaminase (PBGD)	Autosomal dominant	Post puberty	X		X	
Homozygous AIP		Homozygous dominant	Childhood	X	X	X	
Congenital erythropoietic porphyria (CEP)	Uroporphyrinogen III synthase (UROS)	Autosomal recessive	In utero or infancy		X		X
Porphyria cutanea tarda (PCT) type 1	Uroporphyrinogen decarboxylase (UROD)	Sporadic	Adults	X			X
PCT type 2†		Autosomal dominant	Adults	X			X
PCT type 3		Unknown	Adults	X			X
Hepatoerythropoietic porphyria (HEP)		Homozygous dominant	Childhood	X	X*		X
Hereditary coproporphyria (HCP)	Coproporphyrinogen oxidase (CPOX)	Autosomal dominant	Post puberty	X		X	X
Homozygous HCP		Homozygous dominant	Childhood	X	X	X	X
Variegate porphyria (VP)	Protoporphyrinogen oxidase (PPOX)	Autosomal dominant	Post puberty	X		X	X
Homozygous VP		Homozygous dominant	Childhood	X	X	X	X
Erythropoietic protoporphyria (EPP)	Ferrochelatase (FECH)	Autosomal recessive (most commonly heteroallelic with hypomorphic allele)	Childhood		X		X

ADP and HEP are considered primarily hepatic porphyrias, but substantial increases in erythrocyte zinc protoporphyrin suggest an erythropoietic component.
*Classification abbreviations: H, Hepatic; E, Erythropoietic; A/N, Acute/Neurologic; C, Cutaneous.
†PCT is a result of inhibition of hepatic UROD. Autosomal dominant inheritance of a partial deficiency of UROD is a predisposing factor in cases defined as familial (type 2) PCT.

Table 110.2 | Three Most Common Human Porphyrias and Major Features

	PRESENTING SYMPTOMS	EXACERBATING FACTORS	MOST IMPORTANT SCREENING TESTS	TREATMENT
Acute intermittent porphyria	Neurologic, adult onset	Drugs (mostly P450 inducers), progesterone, dietary restriction	Urinary porphobilinogen	Hemin, glucose
Porphyria cutanea tarda	Skin blistering and fragility (chronic), adult onset	Iron, alcohol, smoking, estrogens, hepatitis C, HIV, halogenated hydrocarbons	Plasma (or urine) porphyrins	Phlebotomy, low-dose hydroxychloroquine
Erythropoietic protoporphyria	Phototoxic pain and swelling (mostly acute), childhood onset		Total erythrocyte protoporphyrin with metal-free and zinc protoporphyrin	Sun protection

CLASSIFICATION AND DIAGNOSIS OF PORPHYRIAS

Two useful classification schemes reflect either the underlying pathophysiology or the clinical features of porphyrias (see Table 110.1). In **hepatic porphyrias** and **erythropoietic porphyrias** the source of excess production of porphyrin precursors and porphyrins is the liver and bone marrow, respectively. **Acute porphyrias** cause neurologic symptoms that are associated with increases of one or both of the porphyrin precursors, ALA and PBG. In the **cutaneous porphyrias**, photosensitivity results from transport of porphyrins in blood from the liver or bone marrow to the skin. **Dual porphyria** refers to the very rare cases of porphyria with deficiencies of 2 different heme pathway enzymes.

Porphyria cutanea tarda (**PCT**), acute intermittent porphyria (**AIP**), and erythropoietic protoporphyria (**EPP**) are the 3 most common porphyrias, in that order, considering all age-groups, and are very different in clinical presentation, precipitating factors, methods of diagnosis, and effective therapy (Table 110.2). Two less common acute porphyrias, hereditary coproporphyria (**HCP**) and variegate porphyria (**VP**), can also cause blistering photosensitivity (see Table 110.1). Congenital erythropoietic porphyria (**CEP**) causes more severe blistering lesions, often with secondary infection and mutilation. EPP and XLP have the same phenotype and are distinct from the other cutaneous porphyrias in causing nonblistering photosensitivity that occurs acutely after sun exposure. EPP is also the most common porphyria to become manifest before puberty.

First-Line Laboratory Diagnostic Testing

A few sensitive and specific first-line laboratory tests should be obtained whenever symptoms or signs suggest the diagnosis of porphyria. If a first-line or screening test is significantly abnormal, more comprehensive testing should follow to establish the type of porphyria. Overuse of lab tests for screening can lead to unnecessary expense and even delay in diagnosis. In patients who present with a past diagnosis of porphyria, lab reports that were the basis for the original diagnosis must be reviewed, and if these were inadequate, further testing considered.

Acute porphyria should be suspected in patients with neurovisceral symptoms such as abdominal pain after puberty, when initial clinical evaluation does not suggest another cause. *Urinary PBG* and *total porphyrins* should be measured. Urinary PBG is virtually always increased during acute attacks of AIP, HCP, and VP and is not substantially increased in any other medical conditions. Therefore this measurement is both sensitive and specific. Results from spot (single void) urine specimens are highly informative because very substantial increases are expected during acute attacks of porphyria. A 24 hr collection can unnecessarily delay diagnosis. The same spot urine specimen should be saved for quantitative determination of PBG and total porphyrins (both expressed relative to creatinine) to confirm the qualitative PBG result. ALA is often measured as well, but is usually less elevated than PBG in AIP, HCP, and VP. In ALA dehydratase porphyria, urinary ALA and porphyrins, but not PBG, are greatly elevated. Urinary porphyrins may remain increased longer than porphyrin precursors in some cases of HCP and VP. Measurement of urinary porphyrins alone should be avoided for screening, however, because they are often increased in many disorders other than porphyrias, such as liver diseases, and misdiagnoses of porphyria can result from minimal increases in urinary porphyrins that have no diagnostic significance.

Blistering Cutaneous Porphyrias

Blistering skin lesions caused by porphyria are virtually always accompanied by increases in *total plasma* and *urinary porphyrins*. Porphyrins in plasma in VP are mostly covalently linked to plasma proteins and readily detected by a diagnostic peak in a fluorescence scanning method. The normal range for plasma porphyrins is somewhat increased in patients with end-stage renal disease.

Nonblistering Cutaneous Porphyria

Measurement of total erythrocyte protoporphyrin and, if the total amount is elevated, fractionation of protoporphyrin into its metal-free and zinc-chelated forms, is essential for diagnosis of EPP and XLP. Unfortunately, this is not offered by some major commercial laboratories. Results of zinc protoporphyrin measurements are often recorded (even in the same report) as both *protoporphyrin* and *free erythrocyte protoporphyrin*, with each calculated differently, based on past practices for screening for lead poisoning (which only increases zinc protoporphyrin). Thus the obsolete term *free protoporphyrin* does not mean metal-free protoporphyrin, because it was defined as iron-free protoporphyrin, and dates from before it was known that (except in protoporphyrias) protoporphyrin in erythrocytes is mostly zinc chelated. This unnecessary confusion makes diagnosis and reliable exclusion of protoporphyrias difficult. Total plasma porphyrins are elevated in most but not all cases of protoporphyria, so a normal level should not be relied on to exclude protoporphyria when total erythrocyte protoporphyrin is elevated.

Increases in erythrocyte total and zinc-chelated protoporphyrin occur in many other conditions, including iron deficiency, lead poisoning, hemolysis, anemia of chronic disease, and other erythrocyte disorders. Therefore the diagnosis of EPP must be confirmed by showing a predominant increase in metal-free protoporphyrin. In XLP, both free and zinc protoporphyrin are elevated.

Second-Line Testing

More extensive testing is well justified when a first-line test is positive. For example, a substantial increase in PBG may be caused by AIP, HCP, or VP, and these can be distinguished by measuring erythrocyte porphobilinogen deaminase, urinary porphyrins (using the same spot urine sample), fecal porphyrins, and plasma porphyrins. The various porphyrins that cause blistering skin lesions are differentiated by measuring porphyrins in urine, feces, and plasma. Confirmation at the gene level is important once the diagnosis is established by biochemical testing.

Testing for Subclinical Porphyria

It is often difficult to diagnose or rule out porphyria in patients who had suggestive symptoms months or years in the past, and in relatives of patients with acute porphyrias, because porphyrin precursors and porphyrins may be normal. More extensive testing and consultation with a specialist laboratory and physician may be needed. Before evaluating relatives, the diagnosis of porphyria should be firmly established in an index case, and the lab results reviewed to guide the choice of tests for the family members. The index case or another family member with confirmed porphyria should be retested if necessary. Identification of a disease-causing mutation in an index case greatly facilitates detection of additional gene carriers, because biochemical tests in latent carriers may be normal.

δ-AMINOLEVULINIC ACID DEHYDRATASE DEFICIENT PORPHYRIA

ALA dehydratase deficient porphyria (**ADP**) is sometimes termed *Doss porphyria* after the investigator who described the first cases. The term *plumboporphyria* emphasizes the similarity of this condition to lead poisoning, but incorrectly implies that it is caused by lead exposure.

Etiology

This porphyria results from a deficiency of ALA dehydratase (ALAD), which is inherited as an autosomal recessive trait. Only six cases have been confirmed by mutation analysis. The prevalence of heterozygous ALAD deficiency was estimated to be <1% in Germany and approximately 2% in Sweden.

Pathology and Pathogenesis

ALAD catalyzes the condensation of 2 molecules of ALA to form the pyrrole PBG (see Fig. 110.1). The enzyme is subject to inhibition by a number of exogenous and endogenous chemicals. ALAD is the principal lead-binding protein in erythrocytes, and lead can displace the zinc atoms of the enzyme. Inhibition of erythrocyte ALAD activity is a sensitive index of lead exposure.

Eleven abnormal ALAD alleles, most with point mutations, have been identified, some expressing partial activity, such that heme synthesis is partially preserved. The amount of residual enzyme activity may predict the phenotypic severity of this disease.

ADP is often classified as a hepatic porphyria, although the site of overproduction of ALA is not established. A patient with severe, early-onset disease underwent liver transplantation, without significant clinical or biochemical improvement, which might suggest that the excess intermediates did not originate in the liver. Excess urinary coproporphyrin III in ADP might originate from metabolism of ALA to porphyrinogens in a tissue other than the site of ALA overproduction. Administration of large doses of ALA to normal individuals also leads to substantial coproporphyrinuria. Increased erythrocyte protoporphyrin, as in all other homozygous porphyrias, may be explained by accumulation of earlier pathway intermediates in bone marrow erythroid cells during hemoglobin synthesis, followed by their transformation to protoporphyrin after hemoglobin synthesis is complete. Neurologic symptoms are attributed to neurotoxic effects of ALA, but this is unproven.

Clinical Manifestations

In most cases, symptoms resemble other acute porphyrias, including acute attacks of abdominal pain and peripheral neuropathy. Precipitating factors, such as exposure to harmful drugs, have not been evident in most cases. Four of the reported cases were adolescent males. A Swedish infant had more severe disease, with neurologic impairment and failure to thrive. A 63 yr old man in Belgium developed an acute motor polyneuropathy concurrently with a myeloproliferative disorder.

Laboratory Findings

Urinary ALA, coproporphyrin III, and erythrocyte zinc protoporphyrin are substantially increased. Urinary PBG is normal or slightly increased. Erythrocyte ALAD activity is markedly reduced, and both parents have approximately half-normal activity of this enzyme and normal urinary ALA.

Diagnosis and Differential Diagnosis

The other 3 acute porphyrias are characterized by substantial increases in both ALA and PBG. In contrast, ALA but not PBG is substantially increased in ADP. A marked deficiency of erythrocyte ALAD and half-normal activity in the parents support the diagnosis. Other causes of ALAD deficiency, such as **lead poisoning**, must be excluded. Succinylacetone accumulates in hereditary tyrosinemia type 1 and is structurally similar to ALA, inhibits ALAD, and can cause increased urinary excretion of ALA and clinical manifestations that resemble acute porphyria. Idiopathic acquired ALAD deficiency has been reported. Unlike lead poisoning, the deficient ALAD activity in ADP is not restored by the in vitro addition of sulfhydryl reagents such as dithiothreitol. Even if no other cause of ALAD deficiency is found, it is essential to confirm the diagnosis of ADP by molecular studies.

Treatment

Treatment experience with ADP is limited but is similar to other acute porphyrias. Glucose seems to have minimal effectiveness but may be tried for mild symptoms. **Hemin therapy** was apparently effective for acute attacks in male adolescents, and weekly infusions prevented attacks in 2 of these patients. Hemin was not effective either biochemically or clinically in the Swedish child with severe disease, and it produced a biochemical response but no clinical improvement in the Belgian man with a late-onset form, who had a peripheral neuropathy but no acute attacks. Hemin is also effective in treating porphyria-like symptoms associated with hereditary tyrosinemia and can significantly reduce urinary ALA and coproporphyrin in lead poisoning. Avoidance of drugs that are harmful in other acute porphyrias is advisable. Liver transplantation was not effective in the child with severe disease.

Prognosis

The outlook is generally good in typical ADP cases, although recurrent attacks may occur. The course was unfavorable in the Swedish child with more severe disease and is uncertain in adults with late-onset disease associated with myeloproliferative disorders.

Prevention and Genetic Counseling

Heterozygous parents should be aware that subsequent children are at risk for ADP, as in any autosomal recessive disorder. Prenatal diagnosis is possible but has not been reported.

ACUTE INTERMITTENT PORPHYRIA

AIP is also termed *pyrroloporphyria, Swedish porphyria,* and *intermittent acute porphyria* and is the most common type of acute porphyria in most countries.

Etiology

AIP results from the deficient activity of the housekeeping form of **porphobilinogen deaminase (PBGD)**. This enzyme is also known as hydroxymethylbilane (HMB) synthase (the prior term, uroporphyrinogen I synthase, is obsolete). PBGD catalyzes the deamination and head-to-tail condensation of 4 PBG molecules to form the linear tetrapyrrole, HMB (also known as preuroporphyrinogen; see Fig. 110.1). A unique dipyrromethane cofactor binds the pyrrole intermediates at the catalytic site until 6 pyrroles (including the dipyrrole cofactor) are assembled in a linear fashion, after which the tetrapyrrole HMB is released. The apodeaminase generates the dipyrrole cofactor to form the holodeaminase, and this occurs more readily from HMB than from PBG. Indeed, high concentrations of PBG may inhibit formation of the holodeaminase. The product HMB can cyclize nonenzymatically to form nonphysiologic uroporphyrinogen I, but in the presence of the next enzyme in the pathway is more rapidly cyclized to form uroporphyrinogen III.

Erythroid and housekeeping forms of the enzyme are encoded by a single gene on human chromosome 11 (11q24.1→q24.2), which contains 15 exons. The 2 isoenzymes are both monomeric proteins and differ only slightly in molecular weight (approximately 40 and 42 kDa), and result from alternative splicing of 2 distinct messenger RNA (mRNA) transcripts arising from 2 promoters. The housekeeping promoter functions in all cell types, including erythroid cells.

The pattern of inheritance of AIP is autosomal dominant, with very rare homozygous cases that present in childhood. More than 400 *PBGD* mutations, including missense, nonsense, and splicing mutations, and insertions and deletions have been identified in AIP and in many population groups, including blacks. Most mutations are found in only one or a few families. Because of founder effects, however, some are more common in certain geographic areas, such as northern Sweden (W198X), Holland (R116W), Argentina (G116R), Nova Scotia (R173W), and Switzerland (W283X). De novo mutations may be found in approximately 3% of cases. The nature of the *PBGD* mutation does not account for the severity of the clinical presentation, which varies greatly within families. **Chester porphyria** was initially described as a variant form of acute porphyria in a large English family but was found to be caused by a *PBGD* mutation.

Most mutations lead to approximately half-normal activity of the housekeeping and erythroid isozymes and half-normal amounts of their respective enzyme proteins in all tissues of heterozygotes. In approximately 5% of unrelated AIP patients, the housekeeping isozyme is deficient, but the erythroid-specific isozyme is normal. Mutations causing this variant are usually found within exon 1 or its 5′ splice donor site or initiation of translation codon.

Pathology and Pathogenesis

Induction of the rate-limiting hepatic enzyme ALAS1 is thought to underlie acute exacerbations of this and the other acute porphyrias. AIP remains latent (or asymptomatic) in the great majority of those who are heterozygous carriers of *PBGD* mutations, and this is almost always the case before puberty. In those with no history of acute symptoms, porphyrin precursor excretion is usually normal, suggesting that half-normal hepatic PBGD activity is sufficient unless hepatic ALAS1 activity is increased. Patients can also be asymptomatic with elevated levels of porphyrin precursors and are classified as *asymptomatic high excretors*. These patients may have a remote history of symptoms. Many factors that lead to clinical expression of AIP, including certain drugs and steroid hormones, have the capacity to induce hepatic ALAS1 and CYPs. When hepatic heme synthesis is increased, half-normal PBGD activity may become limiting, and ALA, PBG, and other heme pathway intermediates may accumulate. In addition, heme synthesis becomes impaired, and heme-mediated repression of hepatic ALAS1 is less effective.

It is not proved, however, that hepatic PBGD remains constant at approximately 50% of normal activity during exacerbations and remission of AIP, as in erythrocytes. An early report suggested that the enzyme activity is considerably less than half-normal in the liver during an acute attack. Hepatic PBGD activity might be reduced further once AIP becomes activated if, as suggested, excess PBG interferes with assembly of the dipyrromethane cofactor for this enzyme. It also seems likely that currently unknown genetic factors play a contributing role in, for example, patients who continue to have attacks even when known precipitants are avoided.

AIP is almost always latent before puberty and becomes active mostly in adult women, which suggests that endocrine factors, and especially adult levels of female steroid hormones, are important for clinical expression. Premenstrual attacks are probably the result of endogenous progesterone. Acute porphyrias are sometimes exacerbated by exogenous steroids, including oral contraceptive preparations containing progestins. Surprisingly, pregnancy is usually well tolerated, suggesting that beneficial metabolic changes may ameliorate the effects of high levels of progesterone.

Drugs that are unsafe in acute porphyrias (Table 110.3) include those having the capacity to induce hepatic ALAS1, which is closely associated with induction of CYPs. Some chemicals (e.g., griseofulvin) can increase heme turnover by promoting the destruction of specific CYPs to form an inhibitor (e.g., *N*-methyl protoporphyrin) of ferrochelatase (FECH, the final enzyme in the pathway). Sulfonamide antibiotics are harmful but apparently not inducers of hepatic heme synthesis. Ethanol and other alcohols are inducers of ALAS1 and some CYPs.

Nutritional factors, principally reduced intake of calories and carbohydrates, as may occur with illness or attempts to lose weight, can increase porphyrin precursor excretion and induce attacks of porphyria.

Table 110.3	Drugs Regarded as Unsafe and Safe in Acute Porphyrias

UNSAFE	SAFE
Barbiturates (all)	Narcotic analgesics
Sulfonamide antibiotics*	Aspirin
Meprobamate* (also mebutamate,* tybutamate*)	Acetaminophen (paracetamol)
Carisoprodol*	Phenothiazines
Glutethimide*	Penicillin and derivatives
Methyprylon	Streptomycin
Ethchlorvynol*	Glucocorticoids
Mephenytoin	Bromides
Phenytoin*	Insulin
Succinimides	Atropine
Carbamazepine*	Cimetidine
Clonazepam‡	Ranitidine†
Primidone*	Acetazolamide
Valproic acid*	Allopurinol
Pyrazolones (aminopyrine, antipyrine)	Amiloride
Griseofulvin*	Bethanidine
Ergots	Bumetanide
Metoclopramide*‡	Coumarins
Rifampin*	Fluoxetine
Pyrazinamide*‡	Gabapentin
Diclofenac*‡	Gentamicin
Fluconazole*	Guanethidine
Oral contraceptives	Ofloxacin
Progesterone and synthetic progestins*	Propranolol
Danazol*	Succinylcholine
Alcohol	Tetracycline
ACEIs (especially enalapril)‡	
Spironolactone	
CCBs (especially nifedipine)‡	
Ketoconazole	
Ketamine*	

This partial listing does not include all available information about drug safety in acute porphyrias. Other sources should be consulted for drugs not listed here.

*Porphyria has been listed as a contraindication, warning, precaution, or adverse effect in U.S. labeling for these drugs. Estrogens are also listed as harmful in porphyria but have been implicated as harmful in acute porphyrias, mostly based only on experience with estrogen-progestin combinations. Although estrogens can exacerbate porphyria cutanea tarda, there is little evidence they are harmful in the acute porphyrias.

†Porphyria has been listed as a precaution in U.S. labeling for this drug. However, this drug is regarded as safe by other sources.

‡These drugs have been classified as probably safe by some sources, but this is controversial, and they should be avoided.

ACEIs, Angiotensin-converting enzyme inhibitors; CCBs, calcium channel blockers.

Increased carbohydrate intake may ameliorate attacks. Hepatic ALAS1 is modulated by the peroxisome proliferator-activated receptor-γ coactivator-1α, which is an important link between nutritional status and exacerbations of acute porphyria.

Other factors have been implicated. Chemicals in cigarette smoke, such as polycyclic aromatic hydrocarbons, can induce hepatic CYPs and heme synthesis. A survey of AIP patients found an association between **smoking** and repeated porphyric attacks. Attacks may result from metabolic stress and impaired nutrition associated with major illness, infection, or surgery. Clinical observations suggest an additive effect of multiple predisposing factors, including drugs, endogenous hormones, nutritional factors, and smoking, are common.

Neurologic Mechanisms

The mechanism of neural damage in acute porphyrias is poorly understood. The most favored hypothesis at present is that 1 or more heme precursors, or perhaps a derivative, are neurotoxic. Increased ALA in AIP, HCP, VP, ADP, plumbism, and hereditary tyrosinemia type 1, which have similar neurologic manifestations, suggests that this substance or a derivative may be neuropathic. Porphyrins derived from ALA after its uptake into cells may have toxic potential. ALA can also interact with γ-aminobutyric acid (GABA) receptors. Severe AIP greatly improves after allogeneic liver transplantation. This experience and the demonstration that recipients of AIP livers develop porphyria support the hypothesis that heme precursors from the liver cause the neurologic manifestations.

Epidemiology

AIP occurs in all races and is the most common acute porphyria, with an estimated prevalence in most countries of 5 in 100,000. In Sweden, prevalence was estimated to be 7.7 in 100,000, including latent cases with normal porphyrin precursors. A much higher prevalence of 60-100 in 100,000 in northern Sweden is the result of a founder effect. The combined prevalence of AIP and VP in Finland is approximately 3.4 in 100,000. A survey of chronic psychiatric patients in the United States using an erythrocyte PBGD determination found a high prevalence (210 in 100,000) of PBGD deficiency, but a study in Mexico found a similar prevalence in psychiatric patients and controls. Population screening by erythrocyte PBGD activity or DNA analysis revealed a prevalence of 200 heterozygotes per 100,000 people in Finland, and 1 in approximately 1,675 (60 in 100,000) in France. Studies using exomic/genomic databases show that the estimated frequency of pathogenic mutations in the *HMBS* gene is 0.00056 (56 in 100,000) suggesting that the penetrance of this disorder may be as low as 1%, and that carriers of *PBGD* mutations that can cause AIP are much more common than previously believed.

Clinical Manifestations

Neurovisceral manifestations of acute porphyrias may appear any time after puberty, but rarely before (Table 110.4). Symptomatic childhood cases have been reported, but most were not adequately documented biochemically and confirmed by genetic testing. Abdominal pain is the most common presenting symptom in such cases, but seizures are common and may precede the diagnosis of AIP. Other manifestations reported in children include peripheral neuropathy, myalgias, hypertension, irritability, lethargy, and behavioral abnormalities. A population-based study in Sweden indicated that symptoms suggestive of porphyria may occur in heterozygotes during childhood, even, in contrast to adults, when urinary porphyria precursors are not elevated. This study did not compare the frequency of such nonspecific symptoms in a control group of children. Very rare cases of homozygous AIP present differently, with severe neurologic manifestations early in childhood.

Acute attacks in adults are characterized by a constellation of non-specific symptoms, which may become severe and life threatening. **Abdominal pain** occurs in 85–95% of AIP patients; is usually severe, steady, and poorly localized, but is sometimes cramping; and accompanied by signs of ileus, including abdominal distention and decreased bowel sounds. Nausea, vomiting, and constipation are common, but increased bowel sounds and diarrhea may occur. Bladder dysfunction may cause hesitancy and dysuria. **Tachycardia**, the most common physical sign, occurs in up to 80% of attacks. This is often accompanied by **hypertension**, restlessness, coarse or fine tremors, and excess sweating, which are attributed to sympathetic overactivity and increased catecholamines. Other common manifestations include mental symptoms; pain in the extremities, head, neck, or chest; muscle weakness; and sensory loss.

Table 110.4 | Common Presenting Symptoms and Signs of Acute Porphyria

SYMPTOMS AND SIGNS	FREQUENCY (%)	COMMENT
GASTROINTESTINAL		
Abdominal pain	85–95	Usually unremitting (for hours or longer) and poorly localized but can be cramping.
Vomiting	43–88	Neurologic in origin and rarely accompanied by peritoneal signs, fever, or leukocytosis.
Constipation	48–84	Nausea and vomiting often accompany abdominal pain. May be accompanied by bladder paresis.
Diarrhea	5–12	
NEUROLOGIC		
Pain in extremities, back	50–70	Pain may begin in the chest or back and move to the abdomen. Extremity pain chest, neck, or head indicates involvement of sensory nerves; objective sensory loss reported in 10–40% of cases.
Paresis	42–68	May occur early or late during a severe attack. Muscle weakness usually begins proximally rather than distally and more often in the upper than lower extremities.
Respiratory paralysis	9–20	Preceded by progressive peripheral motor neuropathy and paresis.
Mental symptoms	40–58	May range from minor behavioral changes to agitation, confusion, hallucinations, and depression.
Convulsions	10–20	A central neurologic manifestation of porphyria or caused by hyponatremia, which often results from syndrome of inappropriate antidiuretic hormone secretion or sodium depletion.
CARDIOVASCULAR		
Tachycardia	64–85	May warrant treatment to control rate, if symptomatic
Systemic arterial hypertension	36–55	May require treatment during acute attacks, and sometimes becomes chronic.

From Anderson KE, Bloomer JR, Bonkovsky HL, et al: Desnick recommendations for the diagnosis and treatment of the acute porphyrias, *Ann Intern Med* 142(6):439–450, 2005.

Because all these manifestations are neurologic rather than inflammatory, there is little or no abdominal tenderness, fever, or leukocytosis.

Porphyric neuropathy is primarily motor and appears to result from axonal degeneration rather than demyelinization. Sensory involvement is indicated by pain in the extremities, which may be described as muscle or bone pain, and by numbness, paresthesias, and dysesthesias. Paresis may occur early in an attack but is more often a late manifestation in an attack that is not recognized and adequately treated. Rarely, severe neuropathy develops when there is little or no abdominal pain. Motor weakness most commonly begins in the proximal muscles of the upper extremities and then progresses to the lower extremities and the periphery. It is usually symmetric, but occasionally asymmetric or focal. Initially, tendon reflexes may be little affected or hyperactive and become decreased or absent. Cranial nerves, most often X and VII, may be affected, and blindness from involvement of the optic nerves or occipital lobes has been reported. More common central nervous system (CNS) manifestations include seizures, anxiety, insomnia, depression, disorientation, hallucinations, and paranoia. Seizures may result from hyponatremia, porphyria itself, or an unrelated cause. Chronic depression and other mental symptoms occur in some patients, but attribution to porphyria is often difficult.

Hyponatremia is common during acute attacks. Inappropriate antidiuretic hormone (ADH) secretion is often the most likely mechanism, but salt depletion from excess renal sodium loss, gastrointestinal (GI) loss, and poor intake have been suggested as causes of hyponatremia in some patients. Unexplained reductions in total blood and red blood cell volumes are sometimes found and increased ADH secretion might then be an appropriate physiologic response. Other electrolyte abnormalities may include hypomagnesemia and hypercalcemia.

The attack usually resolves within several days, unless treatment is delayed. Abdominal pain may resolve within a few hours and paresis within a few days. Even severe motor neuropathy can improve over months or several years, but may leave some residual weakness. Progression of neuropathy to respiratory paralysis and death seldom occurs with appropriate treatment and removal of harmful drugs. Sudden death may result from cardiac arrhythmia.

Laboratory Findings
Levels of ALA and PBG are substantially increased during acute attacks. These levels may decrease after an attack but usually remain increased unless the disease becomes asymptomatic for a prolonged period.

Porphyrins are also markedly increased, which accounts for reddish urine in AIP. These are predominantly uroporphyrins, which can form nonenzymatically from PBG. Because the increased urinary porphyrins in AIP are predominantly isomer III, however, their formation is likely to be largely enzymatic, which might occur if excess ALA produced in the liver enters cells in other tissues and is then converted to porphyrins by the heme biosynthetic pathway. Porphobilin, a degradation product of PBG, and dipyrrylmethenes appear to account for brownish urinary discoloration. Total fecal porphyrins and plasma porphyrins are normal or slightly increased in AIP. Erythrocyte protoporphyrin may be somewhat increased in patients with manifest AIP.

Erythrocyte PBGD activity is approximately half-normal in most patients with AIP. The normal range is wide and overlaps with the range for AIP heterozygotes. Some *PBGD* gene mutations cause the enzyme to be deficient only in nonerythroid tissues. PBGD activity is also highly dependent on erythrocyte age, and an increase in erythropoiesis from concurrent illness in an AIP patient may raise the activity into the normal range. Thus, PBGD activity alone is insufficient to make the diagnosis of AIP.

Diagnosis and Differential Diagnosis
An increased urinary PBG level establishes that a patient has 1 of the 3 most common acute porphyrias (see Table 110.2). Measuring PBG in serum is preferred when there is coexistent severe renal disease but is less sensitive when renal function is normal. Measurement of urinary ALA is less sensitive than PBG and also less specific, but will detect ADP, the 4th type of acute porphyria. Erythrocyte PBGD activity is decreased in most AIP patients and helps confirm the diagnosis in a patient with high PBG. A normal enzyme activity in erythrocytes does not exclude AIP.

Knowledge of the *PBGD* mutation in a family enables reliable identification of other gene carriers. Prenatal diagnosis can be performed by amniocentesis or chorionic villus sampling (CVP) in a fetus with a known *PBGD* mutation in the family. Prenatal diagnosis is typically not performed due to the low penetrance of the disorder and favorable prognosis with treatment.

Complications
AIP and other acute porphyrias are typically associated with mild abnormalities in liver function tests; some patients develop chronic

liver disease. The risk of hepatocellular carcinoma is also increased, perhaps 60-70–fold after age 50, even in asymptomatic individuals who have increased porphyrins or porphyrin precursors. Few patients who developed this neoplasm had increases in serum α-fetoprotein. Patients with acute porphyrias, especially >50 yr old, should be screened at least yearly by ultrasound or an alternative imaging method.

The risk of chronic hypertension and impaired renal function is increased in these patients, most often with evidence of interstitial nephritis. A nephrotoxic effect of ALA may contribute. This may progress to severe renal failure and require renal transplantation.

Patients with recurrent attacks may develop **chronic neuropathic pain**, although this has not been well characterized. Referral to a neurologist is recommended for any patient with ongoing or residual neurologic symptoms. In addition, depression and anxiety are common in these patients.

Treatment
Hemin
Intravenous (IV) hemin is the treatment of choice for most *acute* attacks of porphyria. There is a favorable biochemical and clinical response to early treatment with hemin, but less rapid clinical improvement if treatment is delayed. It is no longer recommended that therapy with hemin for a severe attack be started only after an unsuccessful trial of IV glucose for several days. Mild attacks without severe manifestations, such as paresis, seizures, hyponatremia, or pain requiring opioids, may be treated with IV glucose. After IV administration, hemin binds to hemopexin and albumin in plasma and is taken up primarily in hepatocytes, where it augments the regulatory heme pool in hepatocytes, represses the synthesis of hepatic ALAS1, and dramatically reduces porphyrin precursor overproduction.

Hemin* is available for IV administration in the United States as *lyophilized hematin* (Panhematin, Recordati). Degradation products begin to form as soon as the lyophilized product is reconstituted with sterile water, and these are responsible for phlebitis at the site of infusion and a transient anticoagulant effect. Loss of venous access due to phlebitis is common after repeated administration. Stabilization of lyophilized hematin by reconstitution with 30% human albumin can prevent these adverse effects; this is recommended especially if a peripheral vein is used for the infusion. Uncommon side effects of hemin include fever, aching, malaise, hemolysis, anaphylaxis, and circulatory collapse. Heme arginate, a more stable hemin preparation, is available in Europe and South Africa.

Hemin treatment should be instituted only after a diagnosis of acute porphyria has been initially confirmed by a marked increase in urinary PBG. When prior documentation of the diagnosis is available for review, it is not essential to confirm an increase in PBG with every recurrent attack, if other causes of the symptoms are excluded clinically. The standard regimen of hemin for treatment of acute porphyric attacks is 3-4 mg/kg/day for 4 days. Lower doses have less effect on porphyrin precursor excretion and probably less clinical benefit.

General and Supportive Measures
Drugs that may exacerbate porphyrias (see Table 110.3) should be discontinued whenever possible, and other precipitating factors identified. Hospitalization is warranted, except for mild attacks; for treatment of severe pain, nausea, and vomiting; for administration of hemin and fluids; and for monitoring vital capacity, nutritional status, neurologic function, and electrolytes. Pain usually requires an opioid; there is low risk for addiction after recovery from the acute attack. Ondansetron or a phenothiazine such as chlorpromazine is needed for nausea, vomiting, anxiety, and restlessness. Low doses of short-acting benzodiazepines can be given for restlessness or insomnia. β-Adrenergic blocking agents may be useful during acute attacks to control tachycardia and

hypertension but may be hazardous in patients with hypovolemia and incipient cardiac failure.

Carbohydrate Loading
The effects of carbohydrates on repressing hepatic ALAS1 and reducing porphyrin precursor excretion are weak compared to those of hemin. Therefore, carbohydrate loading is seldom beneficial except in mild attacks. Glucose polymer solutions by mouth are sometimes tolerated. At least 300 g of IV glucose, usually given as a 10% solution, has been recommended for adults hospitalized with attacks of porphyria. Amounts up to 500 g daily may be more effective, but large volumes may favor development of hyponatremia.

Other Therapies
Liver transplantation was effective in several patients with severe AIP. A group from the United Kingdom reported their experience with liver transplantation in 10 AIP patients with significantly impaired quality of life and recurrent attacks refractory to medical management. Patients had a complete biochemical and symptomatic resolution after transplantation; 2 patients succumbed to multiorgan failure. Liver transplantation was also successful in a U.S. patient with AIP and intractable symptoms who became unresponsive to hemin therapy; liver transplantation normalized porphyrin precursor excretion, and symptoms resolved. However, liver transplantation is a high-risk procedure and should be considered only as a last resort. Hepatocyte-targeted RNA interference (**RNAi**) therapy is being developed to reverse directly the extremely elevated hepatic ALAS1 mRNA in this disease. Preliminary results from clinical trials are promising.

Seizures and Other Complications
Seizures caused by hyponatremia or other electrolyte imbalances may not require prolonged treatment with anticonvulsant drugs, most of which have at least some potential for exacerbating acute porphyrias. Bromides, gabapentin, and probably vigabatrin are safe. Clonazepam may be less harmful than phenytoin or barbiturates. Control of hypertension is important and may help prevent chronic renal impairment, which can progress and require renal transplantation.

Safe and Unsafe Drugs
Patients often do well with avoidance of harmful drugs. Table 110.3 lists some drugs known or strongly suspected to be harmful or safe in the acute porphyrias. More extensive listings are available from the **European Porphyria Network** (www.porphyria-europe.com) and **American Porphyria Foundation** (www.porphyriafoundation.com), but some listings are controversial. Information regarding safety is lacking for many drugs, especially for those recently introduced.

Exogenous progestins, usually in combination with estrogens, can induce attacks of porphyria. Estrogens are seldom reported to be harmful when given alone. Synthetic steroids with an ethynyl substituent can cause a mechanism-based destruction of hepatic CYPs and should probably be avoided in patients with acute porphyria. Danazol is especially contraindicated.

Other Situations
Major surgery can be carried out safely in patients with acute porphyria, especially if barbiturates are avoided. Halothane has been recommended as an inhalation agent and propofol and midazolam as IV induction agents.

Pregnancy is usually well tolerated, which is surprising, because levels of progesterone, a potent inducer of hepatic ALAS1, are considerably increased during pregnancy. Some women do experience continuing attacks during pregnancy. This has sometimes been attributed to reduced caloric intake or metoclopramide, a drug sometimes used to treat hyperemesis gravidarum and considered harmful in acute porphyrias.

Diabetes mellitus and other endocrine conditions are not known to precipitate attacks of porphyria. In fact, the onset of diabetes mellitus and resulting high circulating glucose levels may decrease the frequency of attacks and lower porphyrin precursor levels in AIP.

---

*Hemin is the generic name for all heme preparations used for intravenous administration. Hemin is also a chemical term that refers to the oxidized (ferric) form of heme (iron protoporphyrin IX) and is usually isolated as hemin chloride. In alkaline solution, the chloride is replaced by the hydroxyl ion, forming hydroxyheme, or hematin.

Prognosis

The outlook for patients with acute porphyrias has improved greatly in the past several decades. In Finland, for example, 74% of patients with AIP or VP reported that they led normal lives, and <30% had recurrent attacks during several years of follow-up. In those presenting with acute symptoms, recurrent attacks were most likely within the next 1-3 yr. Moreover, only 6% of gene carriers who had never had attacks developed symptoms. The improved outlook may result from earlier detection, better treatment of acute attacks, and replacement of harmful drugs such as barbiturates and sulfonamides with safer drugs. However, some patients continue to have recurrent attacks, chronic pain, and other symptoms, even after avoiding known exacerbating factors.

Prevention

For prevention of attacks, it is important to identify multiple inciting factors and remove as many as possible. Drugs for concurrent medical conditions should be reviewed. Because dietary factors are often unapparent, consultation with a dietitian may be useful. A well-balanced diet that is somewhat high in carbohydrate (60–70% of total calories) and sufficient to maintain weight is recommended. There is little evidence that additional dietary carbohydrate helps further in preventing attacks, and it may lead to weight gain. Patients who wish to lose excess weight should do so gradually and when they are clinically stable. Rapid weight loss after bariatric surgery may exacerbate acute porphyrias. Iron deficiency, which can be detected by a low serum ferritin level, should be corrected.

Gonadotropin-releasing hormone (GnRH) analogs, which reversibly suppress ovulation, can be dramatically effective for preventing frequently recurring luteal phase attacks, but baseline and continuing gynecologic evaluation and bone mineral density measurements are important; transdermal estrogen or a bisphosphonate may be added to prevent bone loss. Hemin administered once or twice weekly can prevent frequent, noncyclic attacks of porphyria in some patients. Alternatively, single-dose hemin can be administered "on demand" at an outpatient infusion center to abort an attack and prevent hospitalization, if a patient can recognize early "prodromal" symptoms. Inpatient management is warranted, however, if advanced manifestations such as vomiting, paresis, or other neuropsychiatric symptoms have developed.

Genetic Counseling

A mutation identified in the index case can be sought in the child. Counseling should emphasize that the great majority of those who inherit a *PBGD* mutation never develop symptoms, and the prognosis of those who do is favorable. Therefore a normal, healthy life is expected, especially with avoidance of harmful drugs and other factors and prompt recognition and treatment of symptoms should they occur. Given the favorable outlook for most mutation carriers, even during pregnancy, having children is not precluded, and prenatal diagnosis of acute porphyrias is less important than it is for many other inherited diseases.

CONGENITAL ERYTHROPOIETIC PORPHYRIA

Also termed *Günther disease,* this rare disease usually presents with photosensitivity shortly after birth or in utero as nonimmune hydrops.

Etiology

CEP is an autosomal recessive disease caused by a marked deficiency of uroporphyrinogen III synthase (UROS). Many *UROS* mutations have been identified among CEP families. Later-onset disease in adults is likely to be associated with myeloproliferative disorders and expansion of a clone of erythroblasts that carry a *UROS* mutation.

Pathology and Pathogenesis

UROS, which is extremely deficient in CEP, catalyzes inversion of pyrrole ring D of HMB and rapid cyclization of the linear tetrapyrrole to form uroporphyrinogen III. This enzyme is also termed *uroporphyrinogen III cosynthase.* The human enzyme is a monomer. The gene for the enzyme is found on chromosome 10q25.3→q26.3 and contains 10 exons. Erythroid and housekeeping transcripts are generated by alternative promoters but encode the same enzyme.

In CEP, HMB accumulates in erythroid cells during hemoglobin synthesis and cyclizes nonenzymatically to form uroporphyrinogen I, which is auto-oxidized to uroporphyrin I. Some of the uroporphyrinogen I that accumulates is metabolized to coproporphyrinogen I, which accumulates because it is not a substrate for coproporphyrinogen oxidase. Thus, both uroporphyrin I and coproporphyrin I accumulate in the bone marrow and are then found in circulating erythrocytes, plasma, urine, and feces.

A variety of *UROS* mutations have been identified in CEP, including missense and nonsense mutations, large and small deletions and insertions, splicing defects, and intronic branch point mutations. At least 4 mutations have been identified in the erythroid-specific promoter. Many patients inherited a different mutation from each parent, and most mutations have been detected in only one or a few families. An exception is a common mutation, C73R, which is at a mutational hot spot and was found in approximately 33% of alleles. One child with CEP had a *GATA1* mutation, with no *UROS* mutation. The CEP phenotype may be modulated by gain of function *ALAS2* mutations, which were first identified as causing XLP.

Genotype–phenotype correlations have been based on the in vitro expression of various CEP mutations and the severity of associated phenotypic manifestations. The C73R allele, which is associated with a severe phenotype in homozygotes or in patients heteroallelic for C73R and another mutation expressing little residual activity, resulted in <1% of normal enzyme activity. Patients with the C73R allele and heteroallelic for other mutations expressing more residual activity have milder disease.

Hemolysis is a common feature of CEP. Excess porphyrins in circulating erythrocytes cause cell damage, perhaps by a phototoxic mechanism, leading to both intravascular hemolysis and increased splenic clearance of erythrocytes. Also important is ineffective erythropoiesis, with intramedullary destruction of porphyrin-laden erythroid cells and breakdown of heme. Expansion of the bone marrow as a result of erythroid hyperplasia may contribute, along with vitamin D deficiency, to bone loss. Nutrient deficiencies sometimes cause erythroid hypoplasia. Despite the marked deficiency of UROS, heme production in the bone marrow is increased because of hemolysis and a compensatory increase in hemoglobin production. This occurs, however, at the expense of marked accumulation of HMB, which is converted to porphyrinogens and porphyrins.

Clinical Manifestations

In severe cases, CEP can cause fetal loss or may be recognized in utero as causing intrauterine hemolytic anemia and **nonimmune hydrops fetalis.** CEP may be associated with neonatal hyperbilirubinemia, and *phototherapy may unintentionally induce severe photosensitivity and scarring.*

The most characteristic presentation is reddish urine or pink staining of diapers by urine or meconium shortly after birth (Fig. 110.2). With sun exposure, severe blistering lesions appear on exposed areas of skin on the face and hands and have been termed *hydroa estivale* because they are more severe with greater sunlight exposure during summer (Fig. 110.3). Vesicles and bullae, as well as friability, hypertrichosis, scarring, thickening, and areas of hypopigmentation and hyperpigmentation are very similar to those seen in PCT but usually much more severe. Infection and scarring sometimes cause loss of facial features and fingers and damage to the cornea, ears, and nails. Porphyrins are deposited in dentin and bone in utero. Reddish brown teeth in normal light, an appearance termed **erythrodontia,** display reddish fluorescence under long-wave UV light (Fig. 110.4). Unaffected children born to a mother with CEP may have erythrodontia. Hemolysis and splenomegaly are common in CEP. Bone marrow compensation may be adequate, especially in milder cases. Patients with severe phenotypes, however, are often transfusion dependent. Splenomegaly may contribute to the anemia and cause leukopenia and thrombocytopenia, which may be

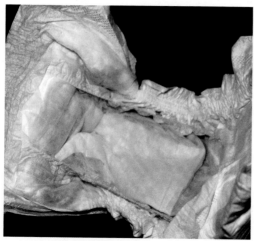

Fig. 110.2 Congenital erythropoietic porphyria (CEP). The diaper of a baby with CEP demonstrates the red color of urine. *(From Paller AS, Macini AJ: Hurwitz clinical pediatric dermatology, ed 3, Philadelphia, 2006, Elsevier Saunders, p 517.)*

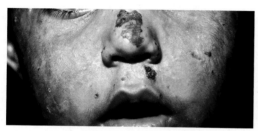

Fig. 110.3 Congenital erythropoietic porphyria. Vesicles, bullae, and crusts on sun-exposed areas. *(From Paller AS, Macini AJ: Hurwitz clinical pediatric dermatology, ed 3, Philadelphia, 2006, Elsevier Saunders, p 517.)*

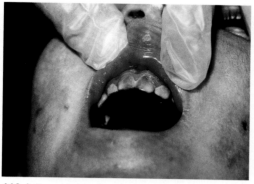

Fig. 110.4 Congenital erythropoietic porphyria. Brownish teeth that fluoresce under Wood lamp examination. *(From Paller AS, Macini AJ: Hurwitz clinical pediatric dermatology, ed 3, Philadelphia, 2006, Elsevier Saunders, p 517.)*

complicated by significant bleeding. Neuropathic symptoms are absent, and there is no sensitivity to drugs, hormones, or carbohydrate restriction. The liver may be damaged by iron overload or viral hepatitis acquired from blood transfusions.

Milder cases of CEP with onset of symptoms in adult life and without erythrodontia may mimic PCT. These late-onset cases are likely to be associated with myeloproliferative disorders and expansion of a clone of cells carrying a *UROS* mutation.

Laboratory Findings
Urinary porphyrin excretion and circulating porphyrin levels in CEP are much higher than in almost all other porphyrias. Urinary porphyrin excretion can be as high as 50-100 mg daily and consists mostly of uroporphyrin I and coproporphyrin I. ALA and PBG are normal. Fecal porphyrins are greatly increased, with a predominance of coproporphyrin I.

Marked increases in erythrocyte porphyrins in CEP also consist mostly of uroporphyrin I and coproporphyrin I. These porphyrins are also increased in bone marrow, spleen, plasma, and to a lesser extent, liver. The porphyrin pattern in erythrocytes is influenced by rates of erythropoiesis and erythroid maturation. A predominance of protoporphyrin has been noted in some CEP patients, and in 1 such patient, uroporphyrin and coproporphyrin increased when erythropoiesis was stimulated by blood removal.

Diagnosis and Differential Diagnosis
The diagnosis of CEP should be documented by full characterization of porphyrin patterns and identification of the underlying mutations. In later-onset cases, an underlying myeloproliferative disorder and a *UROS* somatic mutation should be suspected and studied in detail.

The clinical picture in hepatoerythropoietic porphyria (HEP) may be very similar, but the porphyrin patterns in urine and feces in HEP resemble PCT. A predominant increase in erythrocyte protoporphyrin is unusual in CEP but is characteristic of HEP as well as rare homozygous cases of AIP, HCP, and VP. EPP and XLP are also distinguished by normal urinary porphyrins and by increases in erythrocyte metal-free protoporphyrin, whereas the increased protoporphyrin in other conditions is mostly complexed with zinc.

CEP should be suspected as a cause of nonimmune hydrops or hemolytic anemia in utero. With recognition of the disease at this stage, intrauterine transfusion can be considered, avoiding severe, scarring photosensitivity from phototherapy for hyperbilirubinemia after birth. Prenatal diagnosis is feasible by finding red-brown discoloration and increased porphyrins in amniotic fluid and measuring porphyrins in fetal erythrocytes and plasma. UROS activity can be measured in cultured amniotic fluid cells, or *UROS* mutations identified in chorionic villi or cultured amniotic cells.

Treatment
Protection from sunlight exposure, minimizing skin trauma, and prompt treatment of any cutaneous infections are essential in managing CEP. Sunscreen lotions and beta-carotene are sometimes beneficial. Transfusions to achieve a level of hemoglobin sufficient to suppress erythropoiesis significantly can be quite effective in reducing porphyrin levels and photosensitivity. Concurrent deferoxamine to reduce iron overload and hydroxyurea to suppress erythropoiesis further may provide additional benefit. Splenectomy reduces hemolysis and transfusion requirements in some patients. Oral charcoal may increase fecal loss of porphyrins but may contribute little in more severe cases. IV hemin may be somewhat effective but has not been extensively studied and seems unlikely to provide long-term benefit.

The most effective treatment is marrow stem cell transplantation in early childhood, which has greatly reduced porphyrin levels and photosensitivity and increased long-term survival.

Prognosis
The outlook is favorable in milder cases and in patients with more severe disease, especially after successful bone marrow or stem cell transplantation. Otherwise, prognosis relates to adherence to sunlight avoidance.

Prevention and Genetic Counseling
Genetic counseling is important for affected families because CEP can be recognized before birth, and a severe phenotype can often be predicted by identifying the nature of the *UROS* mutations.

PORPHYRIA CUTANEA TARDA

Porphyria cutanea tarda is the most common and readily treated human porphyria (see Table 110.2). It occurs in mid or late adult life and is rare in children. Previous terms include *symptomatic porphyria*, *PCT symptomatica,* and *idiosyncratic porphyria.* The underlying cause is a liver-specific, acquired deficiency of uroporphyrinogen decarboxylase (UROD) with contributions by several types of genetic and acquired susceptibility factors, including heterozygous *UROD* mutations in familial PCT. HEP, the homozygous form of familial PCT, usually has a more severe presentation in childhood, resembling CEP clinically.

Etiology

PCT is caused by a reduction of hepatic UROD activity to ≤20% of normal activity. An inhibitor of hepatic UROD has been characterized as a *uroporphomethene*, which is derived from partial oxidation of the enzyme substrate uroporphyrinogen. CYPs, such as CYP1A2, as well as iron, are involved in its formation (Fig. 110.5). Although enzyme activity is inhibited, the amount of hepatic enzyme protein measured immunochemically remains at its genetically determined level.

UROD catalyzes the decarboxylation of the 4 acetic acid side chains of uroporphyrinogen (an octacarboxyl porphyrinogen) to form copro-porphyrinogen (a tetracarboxyl porphyrinogen). The enzyme reaction occurs in a sequential, clockwise fashion, with the intermediate formation of hepta-, hexa-, and pentacarboxyl porphyrinogens. Uroporphyrinogen III, as compared with other uroporphyrinogen isomers, is the preferred substrate. Human UROD is a dimer with the 2 active site clefts juxtaposed. The UROD gene is on chromosome 1p34 and contains 10 exons, with only 1 promoter. Therefore the gene is transcribed as a single mRNA in all tissues.

The majority of PCT patients (80%) have no *UROD* mutations and have sporadic (**type 1**) disease. Some are heterozygous for *UROD* mutations and have familial (**type 2**) PCT. Described mutations include missense, nonsense, and splice-site mutations; several small and large deletions; and small insertions, with only a few identified in more than 1 family. A few of these mutations may be located near the active site cleft, but most appear to involve regions with important structural roles. Being heterozygous for a *UROD* mutation is insufficient to cause PCT. Individuals with type 2 PCT are born with 50% of normal UROD activity, and later in life other susceptibility factors (as in type 1) lead to production of the uroporphomethene inhibitor and further reduction on hepatic UROD activity to <20% of normal. Because penetrance of the genetic trait is low, many patients with familial PCT have no family history of the disease.

Induction of hepatic ALAS1 is not a prominent feature in PCT, although alcohol may increase this enzyme slightly. Iron and estrogens are not potent inducers of ALAS1, and drugs that are potent inducers of ALAS1 and CYPs are much less frequently implicated in PCT than in acute porphyrias.

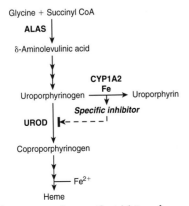

Fig. 110.5 Formation of a specific inhibitor of uroporphyrinogen decarboxylase in the liver in porphyria cutanea tarda. ALAS, δ-Aminolevulinic acid synthase; CYP1A2, cytochrome P450 1A2; UROD, uroporphyrinogen decarboxylase.

Blistering skin lesions result from porphyrins that are released from the liver. Sunlight exposure leads to generation of reactive oxygen species (ROS) in the skin, complement activation, and lysosomal damage.

Epidemiology

Differences in prevalence probably relate to geographic variations in susceptibility factors such as hepatitis C and ethanol use. The yearly incidence in the United Kingdom was estimated at 2-5 in 1 million in the general population, and the prevalence in the United States and Czechoslovakia was estimated at 1 in 25,000 and 1 in 5,000 in the general population, respectively. The disease was reported to be prevalent in the Bantus of South Africa in association with iron overload. PCT is more common in males, possibly because of greater alcohol intake, and in women it is usually associated with estrogen use.

A massive outbreak of PCT occurred in eastern Turkey in the 1950s. Wheat intended for planting and treated with hexachlorobenzene as a fungicide was consumed by many at a time of food shortage. Cases and small outbreaks of PCT after exposure to other chemicals including di- and trichlorophenols and 2,3,7,8-tetrachlorodibenzo-*p*-dioxin (TCDD, dioxin) have been reported. The manifestations improved in most cases when the exposure was stopped. There are reported cases of delayed onset many years after chemical exposure.

Pathology and Pathogenesis

Porphyria cutanea tarda is classified into 3 clinically similar types. Generation of a UROD inhibitor in the liver plays an important role in all 3 types. The 80% of patients with type 1 (**sporadic**) PCT have no *UROD* mutations, and UROD activity is normal in nonhepatic tissues such as erythrocytes. In type 2 (**familial**) PCT, a heterozygous *UROD* mutation results in a partial (approximately 50%) deficiency of UROD in all tissues from birth, and the disease becomes active in some heterozygotes after further reduction of hepatic UROD activity to ≤20% of normal. HEP results from inheritance of a *UROD* mutation from each parent and typically causes severe photosensitivity resembling CEP starting in early childhood. Some compound heterozygotes have developed symptoms in childhood more typical of PCT. **Type 3** is rare and describes PCT without a *UROD* mutation occurring in more than 1 family member. Another genetic basis, such as *HFE* mutations, may be identified in type 3.

CYPs, especially CYP1A2, can catalyze the oxidation of uroporphyrinogen to uroporphyrin. This uroporphyrinogen oxidase activity is enhanced by iron and leads to formation of a UROD inhibitor (see Fig. 110.5). CYP1a2 seems essential for development of uroporphyria in rodents, because experimental uroporphyria does not develop in *CYP1a2* knockout mice.

Susceptibility Factors

The following factors are implicated in the development of PCT, and these occur in various combinations in individual patients.

Iron

A normal or increased amount of iron in the liver is essential for developing PCT, and treatment by phlebotomy to reduce hepatic iron leads to remission. Serum ferritin levels are usually in the upper part of the normal range or moderately increased, and liver histology commonly shows increased iron staining. Prevalence of the C282Y mutation of the *HFE* gene, which is the major cause of hemochromatosis in people of northern European ancestry, is increased in both type 1 and type 2 PCT, and approximately 10% of patients are C282Y homozygotes. In southern Europe the H63D mutation is more prevalent. PCT may develop in patients with secondary iron overload. Reduced hepatic expression of the hormone hepcidin occurs in hemochromatosis and also in PCT, regardless of *HFE* genotype, which may explain hepatic siderosis in this condition.

Hepatitis C

Hepatitis C virus (HCV) infection is highly prevalent in PCT in most geographic locations; in the United States, for example, HCV is present in 56-74% of cases, which is similar to rates in southern Europe.

Prevalence of hepatitis C in PCT is lower in northern Europe (<20%). Steatosis and oxidative stress in HCV infection may favor iron-mediated generation of ROS and a UROD inhibitor. Dysregulation of hepcidin occurs in hepatitis C and may lead to increased iron absorption.

Human Immunodeficiency Virus
Many reports suggest that HIV infection can contribute to the development of PCT, although less frequently than HCV.

Ethanol
The long-recognized association between alcohol and PCT may be explained by the generation of ROS, which may cause oxidative damage, mitochondrial injury, depletion of reduced glutathione and other antioxidant defenses, increased production of endotoxin, and activation of Kupffer cells. Also, alcohol may contribute to iron overload by impairing hepcidin production.

Smoking and Cytochrome P450 Enzymes
Smoking has not been extensively studied as a susceptibility factor but is often associated with alcohol use in PCT. It may act to induce hepatic CYPs and oxidative stress. Hepatic CYPs are thought to be important in oxidizing uroporphyrinogen and generating a UROD inhibitor (see Fig. 110.5). Genetic polymorphisms of *CYP1A2* and *CYP1A1* have been implicated in human PCT. The frequency of an inducible *CYP1A2* genotype was more common in PCT patients than in controls in several studies.

Antioxidant Status
Ascorbic acid deficiency contributes to uroporphyria in laboratory models and perhaps in human PCT. In one series, plasma ascorbate levels were substantially reduced in 84% of patients with PCT. Low levels of serum carotenoids were also described, further suggesting that oxidant stress in hepatocytes is important in PCT.

Estrogens
Use of estrogen-containing oral contraceptives (OCs) or postmenopausal estrogen replacement therapy is frequently associated with PCT (type 1 or 2) in women. PCT sometimes occurs during pregnancy, although it is not clear whether the risk is increased.

Clinical Manifestations
Cutaneous Manifestations
PCT is readily recognized by blistering and crusted skin lesions on the backs of the hands, which are the most sun-exposed areas of the body, and somewhat less often on the forearms, face, ears, neck, legs, and feet (Fig. 110.6). The fluid-filled vesicles usually rupture and become crusted or denuded areas, heal slowly, and are subject to infection. The skin on the backs of the hands is characteristically friable, and minor trauma may cause blisters or denudation of skin. Small white plaques, termed *milia*, may precede or follow vesicle formation. Facial hypertrichosis and hyperpigmentation are also common. Severe scarring and thickening of sun-exposed skin may resemble scleroderma. Skin biopsy findings include subepidermal blistering and deposition of periodic acid–Schiff-(PAS)–positive material around blood vessels and fine fibrillar material at the dermoepithelial junction, which may be related to excessive skin fragility. IgG, other immunoglobulins, and complement are also deposited at the dermoepithelial junction and around dermal blood vessels. The skin lesions and histologic changes are not specific for PCT. The same findings occur in VP and HCP and resemble those of CEP and HEP, but are usually less severe. PCT usually develops in mid or late adult life. Onset in early adult life may be seen in those with *UROD* or *HFE* mutations. Childhood onset is rare and may be associated with cancer chemotherapy and *UROD* mutations.

Liver Abnormalities
PCT is almost always associated with nonspecific liver abnormalities, especially increased serum transaminases and γ-glutamyltranspeptidase, even in the absence of heavy alcohol intake or hepatitis C. Most histologic findings, such as necrosis, inflammation, increased iron, and increased

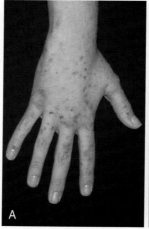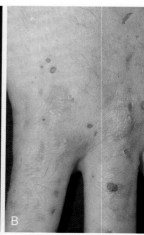

Fig. 110.6 Porphyria cutanea tarda (PCT). **A,** Right hand of a patient with PCT, revealing numerous erosions and erythematous patches. **B,** Close-up of right hand. *(From Horner ME, Alikhan A, Tintle S, et al: Cutaneous porphyrias. Part 1. Epidemiology, pathogenesis, presentation, diagnosis, and histopathology, Int J Dermatol 52:1464–1480, 2013, Fig 2, p 1470.)*

fat, are nonspecific. Specific findings include red fluorescence of liver tissue, and fluorescent, birefringent, needle-like inclusions presumably consisting of porphyrins. Electron microscopy shows these inclusions are in lysosomes, and paracrystalline inclusions are found in mitochondria. Distorted lobular architecture and cirrhosis are more common with long-standing disease.

The risk of developing hepatocellular carcinoma is increased, with reported incidences ranging from 4–47% in PCT. These tumors seldom contain large amounts of porphyrins.

Other Features and Associations
Mild or moderate erythrocytosis in some adult patients is not well understood, but chronic lung disease from smoking may contribute. An earlier onset of symptoms may be noted in patients with genetic predisposing factors, such as an inherited partial deficiency of UROD or the C282Y/C282Y *HFE* genotype. Iron overload secondary to conditions such as myelofibrosis and end-stage renal disease (ESRD) may be associated with PCT. The disease can be especially severe in patients with ESRD because the lack of urinary excretion leads to much higher concentrations of porphyrins in plasma, and the excess porphyrins are poorly dialyzable. PCT occurs more frequently in patients with systemic lupus erythematosus and other immunologic disorders than would be expected by chance.

Laboratory Findings
Porphyrins accumulate in the liver mostly as the oxidized porphyrins rather than porphyrinogens in PCT, as indicated by the immediate *red fluorescence* observed in liver tissue. This develops over weeks or months before porphyrins appear in plasma and are transported to the skin, causing photosensitivity. In contrast to the acute hepatic porphyrias, only a very small increase in synthesis of heme pathway intermediates and little or no increase in hepatic ALAS1 are required to account for the excess porphyrins excreted in PCT.

Hepatic UROD deficiency leads to a complex pattern of excess porphyrins, which initially accumulate as porphyrinogens and then undergo nonenzymatic oxidation to the corresponding porphyrins (uro-, hepta-, hexa-, and pentacarboxyl porphyrins, and isocoproporphyrins). Uroporphyrin and heptacarboxyl porphyrin predominate in urine, with lesser amounts of coproporphyrin and penta- and hexacarboxyl porphyrin. A normally minor pathway is accentuated by UROD deficiency, whereby pentacarboxyl porphyrinogen is oxidized by coproporphyrinogen oxidase (CPOX; the next enzyme in the pathway), forming isocopro-porphyrinogen, an atypical tetracarboxyl porphyrinogen. Relative to normal values, urinary porphyrins are increased to a greater extent than fecal porphyrins. However, the total amount of porphyrins excreted in feces in PCT exceeds that in urine, and total excretion of type III isomers (including isocoproporphyrins, which are mostly derived from the type III series) exceeds that of type I isomers. Perhaps because uroporphyrinogen III is the preferred substrate for UROD, more uroporphyrinogen I than III accumulates and is excreted as uroporphyrin I in PCT. Hepta- and hexacarboxyl porphyrin are mostly isomer III; and pentacarboxyl porphyrin and coproporphyrin are approximately equal mixtures of isomers I and III.

Diagnosis and Differential Diagnosis

Plasma porphyrins are always increased in clinically manifest PCT, and a total plasma porphyrin determination is useful for screening. A normal value rules out PCT and other porphyrias that produce blistering skin lesions. If increased, it is useful to determine the plasma fluorescence emission maximum at neutral pH, because a maximum near 619 nm is characteristic of PCT (as well as CEP and HCP) and importantly, excludes VP, which has a distinctly different fluorescence maximum. Increased urinary or plasma porphyrins, with a predominance of uroporphyrin and heptacarboxyl porphyrin, is confirmatory. Urine porphyrins are less useful for initial screening because nonspecific increases, especially of coproporphyrin, occur in liver disease and other medical conditions. Urinary ALA may be increased slightly, and PBG is normal. Mild cases of CEP can mimic PCT clinically, and this possibility is ruled out by finding normal or only mildly increased levels of erythrocyte porphyrins.

Familial (type 2) can be distinguished from sporadic (type 1) PCT by finding decreased erythrocyte UROD activity (in type 2), or more reliably by finding a disease-related *UROD* mutation. Type 3 is distinguished from type 1 only by occurrence of PCT in a relative. Biochemical findings in HEP are similar to those in PCT, but with an additional marked increase in erythrocyte zinc protoporphyrin.

Pseudoporphyria (also known as pseudo-PCT) presents with skin lesions that closely resemble PCT, but without significant increases in plasma porphyrins. A photosensitizing agent such as a nonsteroidal antiinflammatory drug (NSAID) is sometimes implicated. Both PCT and pseudoporphyria may occur in patients with ESRD.

Complications

Cutaneous blisters may rupture and become infected, sometimes leading to cellulitis. In more-severe disease in patients with ESRD, repeated infections can be mutilating, as in CEP. **Pseudoscleroderma**, with scarring, contraction, and calcification of skin and subcutaneous tissue, is a rare complication. Other complications include advanced liver disease and hepatocellular carcinoma.

Treatment

Two specific and effective forms of treatment, phlebotomy and low-dose hydroxychloroquine, are available. Susceptibility factors should be removed when possible. The diagnosis of PCT must be firmly established because conditions that produce identical cutaneous lesions do not respond to these treatments. Treatment can usually be started after demonstrating an increase in plasma total porphyrins and excluding VP by analysis of the fluorescence spectrum at neutral pH, while urine and fecal studies are still pending. Use of alcohol, estrogens (in women), and smoking should be stopped and patients tested for HCV, HIV, and *HFE* mutations. Susceptibility factors and degree of iron overload, as assessed by the serum ferritin concentration, can influence the choice of treatment.

Phlebotomy is considered standard therapy and is effective in both children and adults with PCT because it reduces hepatic iron content. Treatment is guided by plasma (or serum) ferritin and porphyrin levels. Hemoglobin or hematocrit levels should be followed to prevent symptomatic anemia. For adults, a unit of blood (450 mL) is removed at about 2 wk intervals until a target serum ferritin near the lower limit of normal (15 ng/mL) is achieved. A total of 6-8 phlebotomies is often

sufficient in adults. After this, plasma porphyrin concentrations continue to fall from pretreatment levels (generally 10-25 µg/dL) to below the upper limit of normal (1 µg/dL), usually after several more weeks. This is followed by gradual clearing of skin lesions, sometimes including pseudoscleroderma. Liver function abnormalities may improve, and hepatic siderosis, needle-like inclusions, and red fluorescence of liver tissue will disappear. Although remission usually persists even if ferritin levels later return to normal, it is advisable to follow porphyrin levels and reinstitute phlebotomies if porphyrins begin to increase. Infusions of deferoxamine, an iron chelator, may be used when phlebotomy is contraindicated.

An alternative when phlebotomy is contraindicated or poorly tolerated is a low-dose regimen of **hydroxychloroquine** (or chloroquine). Normal doses of these 4-aminoquinoline antimalarials in PCT increase plasma and urinary porphyrin levels and increase photosensitivity, reflecting an outpouring of porphyrins from the liver. This is accompanied by acute hepatocellular damage, with fever, malaise, nausea, and increased serum transaminases, but is followed by complete remission of the porphyria. These adverse consequences of normal doses are largely avoided by a low-dose regimen (for adults, hydroxychloroquine 100 mg or chloroquine 125 mg, i.e., half a normal tablet, twice weekly), which can be continued until plasma or urine porphyrins are normalized. In young children, half the adult dose is recommended. There is at least some risk of retinopathy, which may be lower with hydroxychloroquine. The mechanism of action of 4-aminoquinolines in PCT is not known but is quite specific, because these drugs are not useful in other porphyrias. Recent studies indicate that low-dose hydroxychloroquine is as safe and effective as phlebotomy in adults with PCT.

In patients with PCT and hepatitis C, PCT should be treated first because this condition is more symptomatic and can be treated more quickly and effectively. Treatment of PCT by phlebotomy may not be possible once interferon-ribavirin treatment is complicated by anemia. Moreover, treatment of hepatitis C may be more effective after iron reduction. Whether direct-acting antiviral agents should be used initially for treating both hepatitis C and PCT is under investigation.

PCT in patients with ESRD is often more severe and difficult to treat. However, erythropoietin administration can correct anemia, mobilize iron, and support phlebotomy in many cases. Improvement after renal transplantation may be partly from resumption of endogenous erythropoietic production.

Liver imaging and a serum α-fetoprotein determination may be advisable in all PCT patients, perhaps at 6-12 mo intervals, for early detection of hepatocellular carcinoma. Finding low-erythrocyte UROD activity or a *UROD* mutation identifies those with an underlying genetic predisposition, which does not alter treatment but is useful for genetic counseling.

Prognosis

Porphyria cutanea tarda is the most readily treated form of porphyria, and complete remission is expected with treatment either by phlebotomy or low-dose hydroxychloroquine. There is little information on rates of recurrence and long-term outlook. Risk for hepatocellular carcinoma is increased, and some susceptibility factors such as hepatitis C can lead to complications even after PCT is in remission.

Prevention and Genetic Counseling

A heritable *UROD* mutation can usually be detected or excluded by measuring erythrocyte UROD activity, although DNA studies are more sensitive. Relatives of patients with *UROD* mutations have an increased risk for developing PCT and may have increased motivation to avoid adverse behaviors such as ethanol and tobacco use and exposures to HCV and HIV (although such counseling would be given to anyone). The finding of *HFE* mutations, and especially C282Y, should prompt screening of relatives, some of whom may be C282Y homozygotes and warrant lifelong monitoring of serum ferritin.

HEPATOERYTHROPOIETIC PORPHYRIA

HEP is the homozygous form of familial (type 2) PCT; it resembles CEP clinically. Excess porphyrins originate mostly from liver, with a pattern consistent with severe UROD deficiency. This rare disorder has no particular racial predominance.

Etiology

HEP is an autosomal recessive disorder, and most patients have inherited a different mutation from unrelated parents. In contrast to most mutations in familial PCT, most causing HEP are associated with expression of some residual enzyme activity. At least 1 genotype is associated with the predominant excretion of pentacarboxyl porphyrin.

Pathology and Pathogenesis

Excess porphyrins originate primarily from the liver in HEP, although the substantial increase in erythrocyte zinc protoporphyrin indicates that the heme biosynthetic pathway is also impaired in bone marrow erythroid cells. Apparently, porphyrinogens accumulate in the marrow while hemoglobin synthesis is most active and are metabolized to protoporphyrin after hemoglobin synthesis is complete. The cutaneous lesions are a result of photoactivation of porphyrins in skin, as in other cutaneous porphyrias.

Clinical Manifestations

As in CEP, this disease usually presents with blistering skin lesions, hypertrichosis, scarring, and red urine in infancy or childhood. *Sclerodermoid* skin changes are sometimes prominent. Unusually mild cases have been described. Concurrent conditions that affect liver function can alter disease severity; the disease manifested because of hepatitis A in a 2 yr old child and then improved with recovery of liver function.

Laboratory Findings

Biochemical findings resemble those in PCT, with accumulation and excretion of uroporphyrin, heptacarboxyl porphyrin, and isocoproporphyrin. In addition, erythrocyte zinc protoporphyrin is substantially increased.

Diagnosis and Differential Diagnosis

HEP is distinguished from CEP by increases in both uroporphyrin and heptacarboxyl porphyrin, and isocoproporphyrins. In CEP, the excess erythrocyte porphyrins are predominantly uroporphyrin I and coproporphyrin I rather than protoporphyrin. Blistering skin lesions are unusual in EPP, the excess erythrocyte protoporphyrin in that disease is metal free and not complexed with zinc, and urinary porphyrins are normal.

Treatment and Prognosis

Avoiding sunlight exposure is most important in managing HEP, as in CEP. Oral charcoal was helpful in a severe case associated with dyserythropoiesis. Phlebotomy has shown little or no benefit. The outlook depends on the severity of the enzyme deficiency and may be favorable if sunlight can be avoided.

Prevention and Genetic Counseling

As part of genetic counseling in affected families, it is feasible to diagnose HEP in utero, either by analysis of porphyrins in amniotic fluid or DNA studies.

HEREDITARY COPROPORPHYRIA

This autosomal dominant hepatic porphyria is caused by a deficiency of coproporphyrinogen oxidase (CPOX). The disease presents with acute attacks, as in AIP. Cutaneous photosensitivity may occur, but much less often than in VP. Rare homozygous cases present in childhood.

Etiology

A partial (50%) deficiency in CPOX activity has been found in all cells studied from patients with HCP. A much more profound deficiency is found in homozygous cases. Human CPOX is a homodimer composed of 39 kDa subunits and contains no metals or prosthetic groups. The enzyme requires molecular oxygen and is localized in the mitochondrial intermembrane space. A single active site on the enzyme catalyzes the oxidative decarboxylation of 2 of the 4 propionic acid groups of coproporphyrinogen III to form the 2 vinyl groups at positions 2 and 4, on rings A and B, respectively, of protoporphyrinogen IX. Most of the intermediate tricarboxyl porphyrinogen, termed *harderoporphyrinogen*, is not released before undergoing the 2nd decarboxylation to protoporphyrinogen IX. Coproporphyrinogen I is not a substrate for this enzyme.

The human CPOX gene contains 7 exons and is located on chromosome 3q12.1. A single promoter contains elements for both housekeeping and erythroid-specific expression. A variety of CPOX mutations have been described in HCP, with a predominance of missense mutations and no genotype-phenotype correlations. **Harderoporphyria**, an autosomal recessive biochemical variant form of HCP, is caused by CPOX mutations that impair substrate binding, leading to premature release of harderoporphyrinogen.

Epidemiology

HCP is less common than AIP and VP, but its prevalence has not been carefully estimated. There is no obvious racial predominance. Homozygous HCP is rare and presents during childhood. Harderoporphyria, a biochemically distinguishable variant of HCP, has been recognized in heteroallelic and homoallelic forms.

Pathology and Pathogenesis

Increased ALA and PBG during acute attacks of HCP may be explained by induction of ALAS1 and by the normally relatively low activity of PBGD in the liver. Hepatic ALAS1 is increased during acute attacks but is normal when the disease is latent and porphyrin precursor excretion is normal. Because coproporphyrinogen III concentration in the liver is probably less than the K_m for CPOX, the reaction rate is likely to be determined in part by substrate concentration. The substrate coproporphyrinogen appears to be lost more readily from the liver cell than, for example, uroporphyrinogen, especially when heme synthesis is stimulated. Coproporphyrin and coproporphyrinogen are both transported into bile and excreted in urine, and do not appear to accumulate in the liver in HCP.

Clinical Manifestations

Symptoms are identical to those of AIP except that attacks are generally milder, and cutaneous lesions that resemble those in PCT develop occasionally. Severe motor neuropathy and respiratory paralysis can occur. As in other acute porphyrias, HCP is almost always latent before puberty, and symptoms are most common in adult women. Attacks are precipitated by the same factors that cause attacks in AIP, including fasting, OCs, and hormone increases during the luteal phase of the menstrual cycle. Concomitant liver diseases may increase porphyrin retention and photosensitivity. The risk of hepatocellular carcinoma is increased, as in other acute porphyrias.

The clinical features of homozygous HCP or harderoporphyria begin in early childhood and include jaundice, hemolytic anemia, hepatosplenomegaly, and skin photosensitivity. These symptoms are generally quite distinct from those seen in heterozygotes. Hematologic features are particularly characteristic in harderoporphyria.

Laboratory Findings

The porphyrin precursors ALA and PBG are increased during acute attacks in HCP but may decrease more rapidly than in AIP. Marked increases in coproporphyrin III in urine and feces are more persistent in HCP. In homozygous cases, porphyrin excretion may be more increased and is accompanied by substantial increases in erythrocyte zinc protoporphyrin. Harderoporphyria is characterized by a marked increase in fecal excretion of harderoporphyrin (tricarboxyl porphyrin) as well as coproporphyrin. Plasma porphyrins are usually normal or only slightly increased.

Diagnosis and Differential Diagnosis

The diagnosis of HCP is readily established in patients with clinically manifest disease, although urinary ALA, PBG, and uroporphyrin may revert to normal more quickly than in AIP. Urinary coproporphyrin III is increased. Urinary porphyrins, especially coproporphyrin, can be increased in many medical conditions (e.g., liver disease), and small increases that are not diagnostically significant may lead to an incorrect diagnosis of HCP. Fecal porphyrins are mostly coproporphyrin (isomer III) in HCP, whereas in VP, coproporphyrin III and protoporphyrin are often increased approximately equally. Plasma porphyrins are usually normal in HCP and increased in VP.

The ratio of fecal coproporphyrin III to coproporphyrin I is especially sensitive for detecting latent heterozygotes (especially adults). Assays for CPOX, a mitochondrial enzyme, require cells such as lymphocytes and are not widely available. Identification of a *CPOX* mutation in an index case greatly facilitates screening family members.

Treatment and Prognosis

Acute attacks of HCP are treated as in AIP, which includes IV hemin and identifying and avoiding precipitating factors. Cholestyramine may be of some value for photosensitivity occurring with liver dysfunction. Phlebotomy and chloroquine are not effective. GnRH hormone analogs can be effective for prevention of cyclic attacks. The prognosis is generally better than in AIP.

Prevention and genetic counseling are the same as in other acute porphyrias.

VARIEGATE PORPHYRIA

This hepatic porphyria is caused by a deficiency of protoporphyrinogen oxidase (PPOX), which is inherited as an autosomal dominant trait. The disorder is termed *variegate* because it can present with neurologic or cutaneous manifestations, or both. Other terms have included *porphyria variegata, protocoproporphyria,* and *South African genetic porphyria.* Rare cases of homozygous VP are symptomatic in childhood.

Etiology

PPOX is approximately half normal in all cells studied in patients with VP. The enzyme is more markedly deficient in rare cases of homozygous VP, with approximately half-normal enzyme activity in parents.

Human PPOX is a homodimer that contains flavin adenine dinucleotide and is localized to the cytosolic side of the inner mitochondrial membrane. Membrane-binding domains may be docked onto human FECH, the next enzyme in the pathway, which is embedded in the opposite side of the membrane. PPOX catalyzes the oxidation of protoporphyrinogen IX to protoporphyrin IX by the removal of 6 hydrogen atoms. The enzyme requires molecular oxygen. The substrate is readily oxidized nonenzymatically to protoporphyrin under aerobic conditions, or if exported into the cytosol. PPOX is highly specific for protoporphyrinogen IX and is inhibited by tetrapyrroles such as heme, biliverdin, and bilirubin and by certain herbicides that cause protoporphyrin to accumulate and induce phototoxicity in plants. Inhibition by bilirubin may account for decreased PPOX activity in Gilbert disease.

The human *PPOX* gene on chromosome 1q22-q23 consists of 1 noncoding and 12 coding exons. A single PPOX transcript is produced in a variety of tissues, but putative transcriptional element binding sequences may allow for erythroid-specific expression. Many *PPOX* mutations have been reported in VP families. A missense mutation, R59W, is prevalent in South Africa. No convincing genotype-phenotype correlations have been identified. Mutations in homozygous cases of VP are more likely to encode enzyme proteins with residual activity.

Epidemiology

VP is less common than AIP in most countries. The R59W mutation is highly prevalent in South African whites (3 in 1,000 in this population). This example of "genetic drift" or founder effect has been traced to a man or his wife who emigrated from Holland to South Africa in 1688. In Finland, prevalence is 1.3 in 100,000 people and is about as common as AIP.

Pathology and Pathogenesis

Acute attacks develop in a minority (approximately 25%) of heterozygotes for PPOX deficiency and are often attributable to drugs, steroids, and nutritional factors that play a role in other acute porphyrias. Protoporphyrinogen IX accumulates and undergoes autoxidation to protoporphyrin IX. Coproporphyrinogen III accumulates, perhaps as the result of a close functional association between PPOX in the inner mitochondrial membrane and CPOX in the intermembrane space. Liver porphyrin content is not increased. The increased porphyrin content in plasma consists of porphyrin-peptide conjugates, which may be formed from protoporphyrinogen. Increased ALA and PBG during acute attacks may be explained, as in HCP, by induction of ALAS1 by exacerbating factors, and by the normally relatively low activity of PBGD in liver. Furthermore, PBGD is inhibited by protoporphyrinogen, the substrate for PPOX.

Clinical Manifestations

Symptoms develop in some heterozygotes after puberty. Neurovisceral symptoms occurring as acute attacks are identical to AIP but are generally milder and less often fatal. Drugs, steroids, and nutritional alterations such as fasting, which are harmful in AIP, can also induce attacks of VP. Attacks occur equally in males and females, at least in South Africa. Cutaneous fragility, vesicles, bullae, hyperpigmentation, and hypertrichosis of sun-exposed areas are much more common than in HCP. They are likely to occur apart from and to be longer lasting than the neurovisceral symptoms. OCs can precipitate cutaneous manifestations. Acute attacks have become less common, and skin manifestations are more frequently the initial presentation; this may result from earlier diagnosis and counseling. The risk of hepatocellular carcinoma is increased.

Symptoms of homozygous VP begin in infancy or childhood. These children generally have severe photosensitivity, neurologic symptoms, seizures, developmental disturbances, and sometimes growth retardation, but they do not have acute attacks.

Laboratory Findings

Urinary ALA, PBG, and uroporphyrin are increased during acute attacks, but often less so than in AIP, and may be normal or only slightly increased during remission. Plasma porphyrins, urinary coproporphyrin III, and fecal coproporphyrin III and protoporphyrin are more persistently increased between attacks. Erythrocyte zinc protoporphyrin levels are greatly increased in homozygous VP and may be modestly increased in heterozygous cases.

Diagnosis and Differential Diagnosis

VP is readily distinguished biochemically from AIP and HCP, which also present with acute attacks and increases in PBG. Plasma porphyrin analysis is especially useful because the plasma porphyrins in VP are tightly protein bound, resulting in a characteristic fluorescence emission spectrum at neutral pH. Fecal porphyrins are increased, with approximately equal amounts of coproporphyrin III and protoporphyrin. Fluorometric detection of plasma porphyrins is more sensitive than stool porphyrin analysis in asymptomatic VP. PPOX assays using cells that contain mitochondria, such as lymphocytes, are sensitive for identifying asymptomatic carriers but are not widely available. Knowing the *PPOX* mutation in an index case enables the identification of relatives who carry the same mutation.

Treatment

Acute attacks are treated as in AIP. Hemin is beneficial for acute attacks but not for cutaneous symptoms. Light protection is important in patients with skin manifestations, using long-sleeved clothing, gloves, a broad-brimmed hat, and opaque sunscreen preparations. Exposure to short-wavelength UV light, which does not excite porphyrins, may increase skin pigmentation and provide some protection. Phlebotomy and chloroquine are not effective. Surprisingly, oral activated charcoal was reported to increase porphyrin levels and worsen skin manifestations.

Prognosis and Prevention

The outlook of patients with VP has improved, which may be attributed to improved treatment, earlier diagnosis, and detection of latent cases. Cyclic acute attacks in women can be prevented with a GnRH analog, as in AIP. A diagnosis of VP or any other acute porphyria should not lead to difficulty obtaining insurance, because the prognosis is usually good once the diagnosis is established.

Genetic counseling is the same as in other acute porphyrias.

ERYTHROPOIETIC PROTOPORPHYRIA AND X-LINKED PROTOPORPHYRIA

These forms of protoporphyria are genetically distinct but have essentially the same phenotype. In EPP, an autosomal recessive disorder, protoporphyrin accumulates as the result of a marked deficiency of FECH, the last enzyme in the heme biosynthetic pathway, because of *FECH* mutations. EPP is sometimes termed *erythrohepatic protoporphyria*, although the liver does not contribute substantially to production of excess protoporphyrin in uncomplicated cases. XLP is the most recently described porphyria, in which gain-of-function *ALAS2* mutations leads to overproduction of ALA in the marrow, where it is metabolized to excess amounts of protoporphyrin.

Etiology

Ferrochelatase (FECH), the enzyme that is deficient in EPP, catalyzes the final step in heme synthesis, which is insertion of ferrous iron (Fe^{2+}) into protoporphyrin IX (see Fig. 110.1). The enzyme is also termed *heme synthetase* or *protoheme ferrolyase*. The human enzyme is a dimer, and each homodimer contains a [2Fe-2S] cluster, which may have a role in bridging homodimers. FECH is found in the mitochondrial inner membrane, where its active site faces the mitochondrial matrix. It may be associated with complex I of the mitochondrial electron transport chain, and the ferrous iron substrate may be produced on nicotinamide adenine dinucleotide oxidation. FECH is specific for the reduced form of iron but can utilize other metals, such as Zn^{2+} and Co^{2+}, and other dicarboxyl porphyrins. Accumulation of free protoporphyrin rather than zinc protoporphyrin in EPP indicates that formation of the latter is dependent on FECH activity in vivo.

The human *FECH* gene is located on chromosome 18q21.3, has a single promoter sequence, and contains 11 exons. Two mRNAs of 1.6 and 2.5 kb were described, which may be explained by the use of 2 alternative polyadenylation signals. The larger transcript is more abundant in murine erythroid cells, suggesting erythroid-specific regulation of FECH. A variety of *FECH* mutations have been reported in EPP, including missense, nonsense, and splicing mutations; small and large deletions; and an insertion.

The inheritance of 2 alleles associated with reduced FECH activity is required for disease expression. This is consistent with FECH activities as low as 15–25% of normal in EPP patients. In most patients, a pathogenic mutation on 1 *FECH* allele is combined with a common variant affecting the other allele. This common variant *FECH* allele (IVS3-48T>C) produces less-than-normal amounts of enzyme because it expresses an aberrantly spliced mRNA that is degraded by a nonsense-mediated RNA decay mechanism. The IVS3-48T > C *FECH* variant by itself does not cause disease, even when homozygous. In a few families, 2 severe *FECH* mutations have been found, without the IVS3-48T> C allele.

EPP with autosomal recessive inheritance occurs naturally in cattle and in mouse models.

XLP is associated with gain-of-function deletions in the last exon of *ALAS2*. These lesions delete the last 10-20 amino acids of the ALAS2 polypeptide and apparently make the enzyme more stable. Metal-free protoporphyrin predominates in erythrocytes in these cases, but because FECH activity is normal, the proportion of zinc protoporphyrin is greater than in classic EPP. XLP accounts for approximately 2% of cases with the EPP phenotype in Europe and approximately 10% of cases in North America.

EPP is sometimes associated with **myelodysplastic syndromes** and expansion of a clone of hematopoietic cells with deletion of 1 *FECH* allele or with other *FECH* mutations. In such cases there is late onset of the disease.

Epidemiology

EPP is the most common porphyria to cause symptoms in children but is often not diagnosed until adult life. Overall it is the 3rd most common

porphyria, although its prevalence is not precisely known (see Table 110.2). It is described mostly in white people but occurs in other races. The IVS3-48T>C splice variant is common in whites and Japanese but rare in Africans, which explains lower disease prevalence in populations of African origin.

Pathology and Pathogenesis

FECH is deficient in all tissues in EPP, but bone marrow reticulocytes are thought to be the primary source of the excess protoporphyrin, some of which enters plasma and circulates to the skin. Circulating erythrocytes are no longer synthesizing heme and hemoglobin, but they contain excess free protoporphyrin, which also contributes. In XLP caused by terminal deletions in exon 11 of *ALAS2*, all intermediates of the heme pathway are overproduced and ultimately accumulate in bone marrow erythroblasts as protoporphyrin. FECH is not deficient in XLP, so this enzyme chelates some of the excess protoporphyrin with zinc. An aberrantly spliced mitoferrin transcript, which limits iron transport into mitochondria, has also been described in XLP. The liver functions as an excretory organ rather than a major source for excess protoporphyrin. FECH deficiency in the skin and liver may be important, however, because tissue transplantation studies in mice suggest that skin photosensitivity and liver damage occur only when FECH is deficient in these tissues.

Patients with EPP and XLP are maximally sensitive to light in the 400 nm range, which corresponds to the so-called Soret band, the narrow peak absorption maximum that is characteristic for protoporphyrin and other porphyrins. Having absorbed light, porphyrins enter an excited energy state and release energy as fluorescence, singlet oxygen, and other ROS. Resulting tissue damage is accompanied by lipid peroxidation, oxidation of amino acids, cross linking of proteins in cell membranes, and damage to capillary endothelial cells. Such damage may be mediated by photoactivation of the complement system and release of histamine, kinins, and chemotactic factors. Repeated acute damage leads to thickening of the vessel walls and perivascular deposits from accumulation of serum components. Deposition of amorphous material containing immunoglobulin, complement components, glycoproteins, acid glycosaminoglycans, and lipids occurs around blood vessels in the upper dermis.

There is little evidence for impaired erythropoiesis or hemolysis in EPP. However, mild anemia with microcytosis, hypochromia, and reticulocytosis is common. Iron accumulation in erythroblasts and ring sideroblasts has been noted in bone marrow in some patients. Decreased transferrin saturation and low or low-normal serum ferritin suggest iron deficiency. Iron status should be carefully evaluated in EPP patients, keeping in mind that iron deficiency may lead to further increases in protoporphyrin and increase the risk for cholestasis. Poor response to oral iron supplements is described in EPP and is unexplained. Some patients report increased photosensitivity when given iron supplements, but whether this is from transient increases in porphyrins when iron deficiency is corrected and erythropoiesis increases is not known. Case reports suggest that iron supplementation decreases protoporphyrin and improves anemia, especially in patients with XLP.

Liver damage develops in a small proportion of EPP and XLP patients and is attributed to excess protoporphyrin, which is insoluble in water and excreted only by hepatic uptake, and biliary excretion is cholestatic. Some may be reabsorbed by the intestine and undergo enterohepatic circulation. With cholestasis the excess protoporphyrin that accumulates in the liver can form crystalline structures in hepatocytes and impair mitochondrial function.

Clinical Manifestations

Symptoms of cutaneous photosensitivity begin in childhood and consist of acute pain and itching often occurring within minutes of sunlight exposure and followed by redness and swelling with continued exposure (Fig. 110.7). Petechiae and purpuric lesions may be seen, but blisters are rare. Swelling may resemble angioneurotic edema and *solar urticaria*. Symptoms are usually worse in the spring and summer. Chronic changes may include lichenification, leathery pseudovesicles, labial grooving, and nail changes, but changes in pigmentation and pronounced scarring

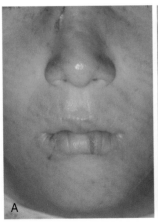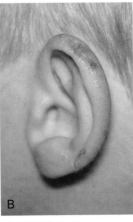

Fig. 110.7 Erythropoietic protoporphyria (EPP). **A,** Linear erosions of the lateral nasal bridge and lower lip in a patient with EPP. **B,** Erosions with crusting on the left helix of a patient with EPP. *(From Horner ME, Alikhan A, Tintle S, et al: Cutaneous porphyrias. Part 1. epidemiology, pathogenesis, presentation, diagnosis, and histopathology, Int J Dermatol 52:1464–1480, 2013, Figs 7 and 8, p 1473.)*

are unusual. Although physical findings in EPP and XLP may not be impressive, the symptoms significantly impair quality of life to a greater extent than in PCT or VP. An association between EPP caused by mutations affecting both FECH alleles and seasonal palmar keratoderma is unexplained. Neuropathy develops only in some patients with severe hepatic decompensation. XLP males have a more severe phenotype with higher protoporphyrin levels than most EPP patients. XLP females have a variable clinical presentation—some with no symptoms or mild symptoms and others with severe symptoms similar to XLP males. This variability in females is likely the result of random X-chromosome inactivation.

Unless hepatic or other complications develop, protoporphyrin levels and symptoms of photosensitivity remain remarkably stable for many years in most patients. Factors that exacerbate hepatic porphyrias play little or no role in EPP or XLP. Erythrocyte protoporphyrin levels may decrease and sunlight tolerance may improve during pregnancy, which is unexplained.

Laboratory Findings
Protoporphyrin is substantially increased in circulating erythrocytes in EPP and consists almost entirely of free protoporphyrin. In XLP, both zinc protoporphyrin and free protoporphyrin are increased, although the latter still predominates. Protoporphyrin is also increased in bone marrow, plasma, bile, and feces. Other porphyrins and porphyrin precursors are normal in uncomplicated EPP and XLP.

Diagnosis and Differential Diagnosis
A diagnosis of EPP is confirmed biochemically by finding a substantially elevated concentration of total erythrocyte protoporphyrin, which is predominantly (at least 85%) metal free and not complexed with zinc. In XLP, both free and zinc-complexed protoporphyrins are elevated. Erythrocyte total protoporphyrin levels are on average higher in XLP and more variable between individuals with EPP, possible reflecting differences in severity of the many reported FECH mutations. Erythrocyte zinc protoporphyrin concentration is increased with little increase in metal-free protoporphyrin in homozygous porphyrias (except CEP), iron deficiency, lead poisoning, anemia of chronic disease, hemolytic conditions, and many other erythrocytic disorders. Measurement of FECH activity requires cells containing mitochondria and is not widely available.

Plasma total porphyrin concentration is often less increased in EPP than in other cutaneous porphyrias and may be normal. Great care must be taken to avoid light exposure during sample processing, because

plasma porphyrins in EPP are particularly subject to photodegradation. Urinary porphyrin precursors and porphyrins are not increased.

DNA studies are strongly recommended for confirming FECH or ALAS2 mutations and for genetic counseling.

Life-threatening **protoporphyric hepatopathy** is characterized by greater increases in erythrocyte and plasma protoporphyrin levels, increased photosensitivity and either chronically abnormal liver function tests or rapidly progressive hepatic failure. Presumably this is heralded by increases above the patient's baseline erythrocyte and plasma porphyrin levels, but this has not been documented, because most such patients have not had adequate baseline determinations of porphyrin values. Increases in urinary porphyrins, especially coproporphyrin, in this setting are attributable to liver dysfunction.

Complications
There is an increased risk of biliary stones, which contain protoporphyrin and are sometimes symptomatic, requiring cholecystectomy. Protoporphyric hepatopathy occurs in <5% of protoporphyria patients, including children, and may be chronic or progress rapidly to death from liver failure. This liver disease is sometimes the major presenting feature of EPP. In XLP, liver disease may be more frequent, and in one report of 8 families, 17% of patients had overt liver dysfunction. Protoporphyric hepatopathy can cause acute upper abdominal pain suggesting biliary obstruction, and unnecessary laparotomy to exclude this possibility can be detrimental. Concurrent conditions that impair liver function, such as viral hepatitis, alcohol- or drug-induced liver disease, or OCs may contribute. Whether iron deficiency may contribute is unclear. Liver histology shows marked deposition of protoporphyrin as inclusions in liver cells and bile canaliculi. Patients with protoporphyric liver failure most often have FECH "null mutations" and the IVS3–48T>C hypoexpression allele, but some may have 2 severe mutant FECH alleles or XLP caused by ALAS2 exon 11 deletions. The bone marrow is probably the major source of protoporphyrin, even in EPP patients with hepatic failure.

Treatment
Exposure to sunlight should be avoided, which is aided by wearing closely woven clothing. A systematic review of treatment options, including beta-carotene, oral cysteine, and vitamin C, showed no proven efficacy of these treatments. One report suggested that high doses of cimetidine were effective in reducing symptoms in 3 children with EPP, but no objective clinical evidence of efficacy was presented.

Measures to darken the skin may also be helpful. This may be accomplished by narrow-band UV-B phototherapy. Double-blind, placebo-controlled studies in the United States and Europe of **afamelanotide,** a synthetic analog of melanocyte-stimulating hormone, showed an increase in pain-free sun exposure and improved quality of life in patients with protoporphyria. This drug is approved for adult use in Europe and is pending U.S. Food and Drug Administration (FDA) approval, and studies in children are anticipated.

Drugs or hormone preparations that impair hepatic excretory function should be avoided, particularly in patients with liver dysfunction, and iron deficiency should be corrected if present, especially in XLP. Vitamin D supplementation and hepatitis A and B vaccination are recommended.

Treatment of protoporphyric hepatopathy must be individualized, and results are unpredictable. Ursodeoxycholic acid may be of some value in early stages. Cholestyramine or activated charcoal may interrupt the enterohepatic circulation of protoporphyrin, promote its fecal excretion, and reduce liver protoporphyrin content. Spontaneous resolution may occur, especially if another reversible cause of liver dysfunction, such as viral hepatitis or alcohol abuse, is contributing. In patients with severe hepatic decompensation, combined treatment with plasmapheresis, transfusion to correct anemia and suppress erythropoiesis, IV hemin to suppress erythroid and possibly hepatic protoporphyrin production, ursodeoxycholic acid, vitamin E, and cholestyramine may be beneficial and bridge patients for liver transplantation.

Motor neuropathy resembling that seen in acute porphyrias sometimes develops in protoporphyria patients with liver disease before or after transfusion or liver transplantation and is sometimes reversible. Artificial lights, such as operating room lights during liver transplantation or other surgery, may cause severe photosensitivity, with extensive burns of the skin and peritoneum and damage to circulating erythrocytes.

Although liver disease may recur in the transplanted liver as a result of continued bone marrow production of excess protoporphyrin, outcomes are comparable to transplantation for other types of liver disease. Bone marrow transplantation should also be considered after liver transplantation if a suitable donor is available.

Prognosis

Typical EPP patients have lifelong photosensitivity but can otherwise expect normal longevity. Protoporphyric liver disease is often life-threatening; however, the incidence is low.

Prevention and Genetic Counseling

Symptoms can be prevented by avoiding sunlight. Avoiding agents that may cause liver damage may help prevent liver complications. Opinions vary on the value of iron replacement, and this is currently under study.

DNA studies to identify *FECH* mutations, the common IVS3–48T>C *FECH* hypoexpression allele, or *ALAS2* exon 11 deletions are important for genetic counseling. When EPP is caused by a severe *FECH* mutation and the common IVS3–48T>C *FECH* allele, DNA studies in the spouse to determine the presence, or more likely the absence, of the hypoexpression allele can predict whether offspring are at risk for EPP. EPP may improve during pregnancy.

DUAL PORPHYRIA

An unusual pattern of porphyrin precursors and porphyrins may suggest mutations of 2 heme pathway enzymes, as documented in 2 patients. One presented with acute porphyria and had heterozygous mutations of both *CPOX* and *ALAD*. The other had symptoms of AIP and PCT and was reported to have both *HMBS* and *UROD* mutations. In other reported cases, 1 or both enzyme deficiencies were based on enzyme measurements.

PORPHYRIA RESULTING FROM TUMORS

Very rarely, hepatocellular tumors contain and presumably produce excess porphyrins, but such cases have not been studied carefully. Hepatocellular carcinomas complicating PCT and acute hepatic porphyrias usually are not described as containing large amounts of porphyrins. Erythropoietic porphyrias can develop late in life from clonal expansion of erythroid cells containing a specific enzyme deficiency in patients who have developed myelodysplastic or myeloproliferative syndromes.

Bibliography is available at Expert Consult.

Chapter **111**

Hypoglycemia

Mark A. Sperling

第一百一十一章
低血糖症

中文导读

　　本章主要介绍了低血糖症的定义、重要意义及后遗症、维持葡萄糖稳态的底物和酶及激素、临床表现、婴儿及儿童低血糖症分类、诊断与鉴别诊断、治疗以及预后。具体描述了维持葡萄糖稳态的底物和酶及激素分别在新生儿期、婴儿及儿童期的不同；婴儿及儿童低血糖症分类中具体描述了新生儿和暂时性及小于胎龄儿及早产儿、糖尿病母亲婴儿、婴儿及儿童持续性或反复性低糖血症、内分泌缺乏症、底物限制性病因、糖原累积症、糖异生障碍、其他酶缺陷、葡萄糖转运缺陷以及系统性疾病等内容。

Glucose has a central role in fuel economy and is a source of energy storage in the form of glycogen, fat, and protein (see Chapter 105). As an immediate source of energy, glucose provides 38 mol of adenosine triphosphate (ATP) per mole of glucose oxidized. Glucose is essential for energy metabolism in the brain, where it is usually the preferred substrate and where its utilization accounts for nearly all the brain's oxygen consumption. Cerebral transport of glucose is a GLUT-1, carrier-mediated, facilitated diffusion process that is dependent on blood glucose concentration and not regulated by insulin. Therefore, low concentrations of blood glucose result in cerebral glucopenia. Deficiency of brain glucose transporters can result in seizures because of low cerebral and cerebrospinal fluid (CSF) glucose concentrations *(hypoglycorrhachia)* despite normal blood glucose levels. To maintain the blood glucose concentration and prevent it from falling precipitously to levels that impair brain function, an elaborate regulatory system has evolved.

The defense against hypoglycemia includes the autonomic nervous system and hormones that act in concert to enhance glucose production through enzymatic modulation of glycogenolysis and gluconeogenesis, while simultaneously limiting peripheral glucose utilization, which conserves glucose for cerebral metabolism. Hypoglycemia represents a defect in one or several of the complex interactions that normally integrate glucose homeostasis during feeding and fasting. This process is particularly important for neonates, in whom there is an abrupt transition from intrauterine life, characterized by dependence on transplacental glucose supply, to extrauterine life, characterized ultimately by the autonomic ability to maintain euglycemia. Because prematurity or placental insufficiency may limit tissue nutrient deposits, and genetic abnormalities in enzymes or hormones may become evident in the neonate, hypoglycemia is common in the neonatal period.

DEFINITION

In neonates, there is not always an obvious correlation between blood glucose concentration and the classic clinical manifestations of hypoglycemia. The absence of symptoms does not indicate that glucose concentration is normal and has not fallen to less than some optimal level for maintaining brain metabolism. There is evidence that hypoxemia and ischemia may potentiate the role of hypoglycemia in causing permanent brain sequelae. Consequently, the lower limit of accepted normality of the blood glucose level in newborn infants with associated illness that already impairs cerebral metabolism has not been determined (see Chapter 127). Because of concern for possible neurologic, intellectual, or psychologic sequelae in later life, most authorities recommend that any value of blood glucose <55 mg/dL in neonates be viewed with suspicion, investigated, and vigorously treated if there are symptoms or it persists or recurs after a meal. This is particularly applicable after the initial 2-3 hr of life, when glucose normally has reached its nadir; subsequently, blood glucose levels begin to rise and achieve values of 55-65 mg/dL or higher after 12-24 hr. By day 3 of life in normal full-term newborns, blood glucose averages approximately 65 mg/dL (range 65-100). Therefore, in otherwise normal, full-term infants after day 3 of life and in older infants and children, a whole blood glucose concentration <55 mg/dL (10-15% higher for serum or plasma) represents hypoglycemia, because counter-regulatory mechanisms are activated at these glucose concentrations. In older children an idealized definition of hypoglycemia is based on "Whipple's Triad"; a plasma glucose concentration less than 60 mg/dL, together with concurrent CNS- or catecholamine-based symptoms, and resolution of symptoms when glucose concentration is restored to normal by treatment with glucose.

SIGNIFICANCE AND SEQUELAE

Most of the endogenous hepatic glucose production in infants and young children, which occurs several hours after feeding and during fasting, can be accounted for by brain metabolism.

Because the brain grows most rapidly in the 1st yr of life, and the larger proportion of glucose turnover is used for brain metabolism, sustained or repetitive hypoglycemia in infants and children can retard brain development and function. *Transient isolated and asymptomatic hypoglycemia of short duration does not appear to be associated with these severe sequelae.* In the rapidly growing brain, glucose may also be

a source of membrane lipids and, together with protein synthesis, can provide structural proteins and myelination important for normal brain maturation. Under conditions of severe and sustained hypoglycemia, these cerebral structural substrates may become degraded to energy-usable intermediates such as lactate, pyruvate, amino acids, and ketoacids, which can support brain metabolism at the expense of brain growth. The capacity of the newborn brain to take up and oxidize ketone bodies is about 5-fold greater than that of the adult brain. However, the capacity of the liver to produce ketone bodies is limited in the immediate newborn period, especially in the presence of **hyperinsulinism**, which acutely inhibits hepatic glucose output, lipolysis, and ketogenesis, thereby depriving the brain of any alternate fuel sources. Although the brain may metabolize ketones, these alternate fuels cannot completely replace glucose as an essential central nervous system (CNS) fuel. The deprivation of the brain's major energy source during hypoglycemia and particularly the limited availability of alternate fuel sources during hyperinsulinism have predictable adverse consequences on brain metabolism and growth: decreased brain oxygen consumption and increased breakdown of endogenous structural components, with destruction of functional membrane integrity.

The major long-term sequelae of **severe, prolonged hypoglycemia** are cognitive impairment, recurrent seizure activity, cerebral palsy, and autonomic dysregulation. Subtle effects on personality are also possible but have not been clearly defined. Permanent neurologic sequelae are present in 25-50% of patients <6 mo old with severe recurrent symptomatic hypoglycemia. These sequelae may be reflected in pathologic changes characterized by reduced myelination in cerebral white matter and atrophy of the cerebral cortex, reflected in enlargement of the sulci and thinning of the gyri of the brain. These sequelae also are more likely when alternative fuel sources are limited, as occurs with hyperinsulinism, when the episodes of hypoglycemia are repetitive or prolonged, or when they are compounded by hypoxia. There is no precise knowledge relating the duration or severity of hypoglycemia to subsequent neurologic development of children in a predictable manner. Although less common, hypoglycemia in older children may also produce long-term neurologic defects through neuronal death mediated, in part, by cerebral excitotoxins released during hypoglycemia.

SUBSTRATE, ENZYME, AND HORMONAL INTEGRATION OF GLUCOSE HOMEOSTASIS
In the Newborn

Under nonstressed conditions, fetal glucose is derived entirely from the mother through placental transfer. Therefore, fetal glucose concentration usually reflects, but is slightly lower than, maternal glucose levels. Catecholamine release, which occurs with fetal stress such as hypoxia, mobilizes fetal glucose and free fatty acids (FFAs) through β-adrenergic mechanisms, reflecting β-adrenergic activity in fetal liver and adipose tissue. Catecholamines may also inhibit fetal insulin and stimulate glucagon release.

The acute interruption of maternal glucose transfer to the fetus at delivery imposes an immediate need to mobilize endogenous glucose. Three related events facilitate this transition: changes in hormones, changes in their receptors, and changes in key enzyme activity. There is a 3-5–fold abrupt increase in glucagon concentration within minutes to hours of birth. The insulin level usually falls initially and remains in the basal range for several days, without demonstrating the usual brisk response to physiologic stimuli such as glucose. A dramatic surge in spontaneous catecholamine secretion is also characteristic. Epinephrine can also augment growth hormone (GH) secretion by α-adrenergic mechanisms; GH levels are markedly elevated at birth. In addition, cortisol levels are higher in the immediate newborn period in infants born vaginally than by cesarean birth, in part reflecting the stress of labor on fetal cortisol secretion. Acting in concert, these hormonal changes at birth mobilize glucose by glycogenolysis and gluconeogenesis, activate lipolysis, and promote ketogenesis. As a result of these processes, plasma glucose concentration stabilizes after a transient decrease immediately after birth; liver glycogen stores become rapidly depleted within hours of birth; and gluconeogenesis from alanine, a major gluconeogenic amino acid, can account for approximately 10% of glucose turnover in the human newborn infant by several hours of age. FFA concentrations also increase sharply in concert with the surges in glucagon and epinephrine, followed later by rises in ketone bodies. Glucose is thus partially spared for brain utilization while FFAs and ketones provide alternative fuel sources for muscle as well as essential gluconeogenic factors such as acetyl-coenzyme A (CoA) and the reduced form of nicotinamide adenine dinucleotide from hepatic fatty acid oxidation, which is required to drive gluconeogenesis.

In the early postnatal period, responses of the endocrine pancreas favor glucagon secretion so that blood glucose concentration can be maintained. These adaptive changes in hormone secretion are paralleled by similarly striking adaptive changes in hormone receptors. Key enzymes involved in glucose production also change dramatically in the perinatal period. Thus, there is a rapid fall in glycogen synthase activity and a sharp rise in phosphorylase activity after delivery. Similarly, the activity of the rate-limiting enzyme for gluconeogenesis, phosphoenolpyruvate carboxykinase, rises dramatically after birth, activated in part by the surge in glucagon and the fall in insulin. This framework can explain several causes of neonatal hypoglycemia based on inappropriate changes in hormone secretion and unavailability of adequate reserves of **substrates** in the form of hepatic glycogen, **muscle** as a source of amino acids for gluconeogenesis, and **lipid** stores for the release of fatty acids. In addition, appropriate activities of key enzymes governing glucose homeostasis are required (see Fig. 105.1).

In Older Infants and Children

Hypoglycemia in older infants and children is analogous to that of adults, in whom glucose homeostasis is maintained by glycogenolysis in the immediate postfeeding period and by gluconeogenesis several hours after meals. The liver of a 10 kg child contains 20-25 g of glycogen, which is sufficient to meet normal glucose requirements of 4-6 mg/kg/min for only 6-12 hr. Beyond this period, hepatic gluconeogenesis must be activated. Both glycogenolysis and gluconeogenesis depend on the metabolic pathway summarized in Fig. 105.1. Defects in glycogenolysis or gluconeogenesis may not be manifested in infants until the frequent feeding at 3-4 hr intervals ceases and infants sleep through the night, a situation usually present by 3-6 mo of age. The source of gluconeogenic precursors is derived primarily from muscle protein. The muscle bulk of infants and small children is substantially smaller relative to body mass than that of adults, whereas glucose requirements per unit of body mass are greater in children. Therefore the ability to compensate for glucose deprivation by gluconeogenesis is more limited in infants and young children, as is the ability to withstand fasting for prolonged periods. The ability of muscle to generate *alanine*, the principal gluconeogenic amino acid, may also be limited. Thus, in normal young children, the blood glucose level falls after 24 hr of fasting, insulin concentrations fall appropriately to levels of <5 μU/mL, lipolysis and ketogenesis are activated, and ketones may appear in the urine.

The switch from glycogen synthesis during and immediately after meals to glycogen breakdown and later gluconeogenesis is governed by hormones, with insulin of central importance. After a meal, plasma insulin concentrations increase to peak levels of 5-10–fold greater than their normal baseline concentration of approximately 5-10 μU/mL, which serves to lower the blood glucose concentration through the activation of glycogen synthesis, enhancement of peripheral glucose uptake, and inhibition of glucose production. In addition, lipogenesis is stimulated, whereas lipolysis and ketogenesis are curtailed. During fasting, plasma insulin concentrations fall to ≤5 μU/mL, and together with the rise of counter-regulatory hormones, this fall in insulin results in activation of gluconeogenic pathways (see Fig. 105.1). Fasting glucose concentrations are maintained through the activation of glycogenolysis and gluconeogenesis, inhibition of glycogen synthesis, and activation of lipolysis and ketogenesis. It should be emphasized that a plasma insulin concentration of >5 μU/mL, in association with a blood glucose concentration of ≤55 mg/dL (2.8-3.0 mM), is abnormal, indicating a state of excessive insulin action, termed *hyperinsulinism,* caused by failure of the mechanisms that normally result in suppression of insulin secretion during fasting or hypoglycemia.

The hypoglycemic effects of insulin are opposed by the actions of several hormones whose concentration in plasma increases as blood glucose falls. These counter-regulatory hormones—glucagon, growth hormone, cortisol, and epinephrine—act synergistically and in concert to increase blood glucose concentrations by activating glycogenolytic enzymes (glucagon, epinephrine); inducing gluconeogenic enzymes (glucagon, cortisol); inhibiting glucose uptake by muscle (epinephrine, growth hormone, cortisol); mobilizing amino acids from muscle for gluconeogenesis (cortisol); activating lipolysis and thereby providing glycerol for gluconeogenesis and fatty acids for ketogenesis (epinephrine, cortisol, GH, glucagon); and inhibiting insulin release and promoting GH and glucagon secretion (epinephrine).

Congenital or acquired deficiency of any one of these hormones is uncommon but will result in hypoglycemia, which occurs when endogenous glucose production cannot be mobilized to meet energy needs in the postabsorptive state, that is, 4-6 hr in the newborn and 8-12 hr after meals or during fasting in an infant or child. Concurrent deficiency of several hormones (**hypopituitarism-ACTH-cortisol deficiency combined with GH deficiency**) may result in hypoglycemia that is more severe or appears earlier during fasting than that seen with isolated hormone deficiencies. Most of the causes of hypoglycemia in neonates, infants, and children reflect inappropriate adaptation to fasting as a result of (1) excess insulin action, (2) inadequate counter-regulatory hormone response primarily of cortisol and GH, (3) enzymatic defects in the mechanisms for glycogen storage and release, or (4) defects in gluconeogenesis.

CLINICAL MANIFESTATIONS
See Chapter 127.

Clinical features of hypoglycemia generally fall into 2 categories: (1) symptoms associated with the activation of the autonomic nervous system and epinephrine release, usually seen with a rapid decline in blood glucose concentration and (2) symptoms caused by decreased cerebral glucose utilization (**cerebral glucopenia**), usually associated with a slow decline in blood glucose level or prolonged hypoglycemia (Table 111.1). Although these classic symptoms occur in older children, the symptoms of hypoglycemia in newborns and infants may be subtler and include cyanosis, apnea, hypothermia, hypotonia, poor feeding, lethargy, and seizures, all reflecting the deprivation of glucose for normal brain activity. Some of these symptoms may be so mild that they are missed. Occasionally, hypoglycemia may be asymptomatic in the immediate newborn period. Newborns with hyperinsulinism are often large for gestational age (LGA), mimicking the features of the infant born to a mother with poorly controlled diabetes. Older infants with hyperinsulinism may eat excessively because of chronic hypoglycemia and become obese. In childhood, hypoglycemia may present as behavior problems, inattention, ravenous appetite, or seizures. It may be misdiagnosed as epilepsy, inebriation, personality disorders, headache, hysteria, and developmental delay. A blood glucose determination should always be performed in sick neonates, who should be vigorously treated if concentrations are <55 mg/dL. At any age, hypoglycemia should be considered a cause of an initial episode of convulsions or a sudden deterioration in psychobehavioral functioning or level of consciousness.

Many neonates have asymptomatic (chemical) hypoglycemia. The incidence of symptomatic hypoglycemia is highest in small-for-gestational-age (SGA) infants (Fig. 111.1). The exact incidence of symptomatic hypoglycemia has been difficult to establish because many of the symptoms in neonates occur together with other conditions, such as infections, especially sepsis and meningitis; CNS anomalies, hemorrhage, or edema; hypocalcemia and hypomagnesemia; asphyxia; drug withdrawal; apnea of prematurity; congenital heart disease; or polycythemia.

The onset of symptoms in neonates varies from a few hours to a week after birth. In approximate order of frequency, symptoms include jitteriness or tremors, apathy, episodes of cyanosis, seizures, intermittent apneic spells or tachypnea, weak or high-pitched cry, limpness or lethargy, difficulty feeding (latching on), and eye rolling. Episodes of sweating, sudden pallor, hypothermia, and cardiac arrest and failure may also occur. Frequently, a clustering of episodic symptoms may be noted.

Table 111.1	Manifestations of Hypoglycemia in Childhood

FEATURES ASSOCIATED WITH ACTIVATION OF AUTONOMIC NERVOUS SYSTEM AND EPINEPHRINE RELEASE*
Anxiety[†]
Perspiration[†]
Palpitation (tachycardia)[†]
Pallor[†]
Tremulousness[‡]
Weakness
Hunger
Nausea
Emesis

FEATURES ASSOCIATED WITH CEREBRAL GLUCOPENIA
Headache[†]
Mental confusion[†]
Visual disturbances (↓ acuity, diplopia)[†]
Organic personality changes[†]
Inability to concentrate[†]
Dysarthria
Staring
Paresthesias
Dizziness
Amnesia
Ataxia, incoordination
Refusal to feed[‡]
Somnolence, lethargy[‡]
Seizures[‡]
Coma
Stroke, hemiplegia, aphasia
Decerebrate or decorticate posture

*Some of these features will be attenuated if the patient is receiving β-adrenergic blocking agents.
[†]Common.
[‡]Most common manifestations in the newborn.

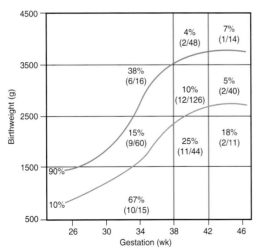

Fig. 111.1 Incidence of hypoglycemia by birthweight, gestational age, and intrauterine growth. *(From Lubchenco LO, Bard H: Incidence of hypoglycemia in newborn infants classified by birthweight and gestational age, Pediatrics 47:831–838, 1971.)*

Because these clinical manifestations may result from various causes, it is critical to measure serum glucose levels and determine whether symptoms disappear with the administration of sufficient glucose to raise the blood glucose to normal levels; if they do not, other diagnoses must be considered.

CLASSIFICATION OF HYPOGLYCEMIA IN INFANTS AND CHILDREN

Classification is based on knowledge of the control of glucose homeostasis in infants and children (Table 111.2).

Neonatal, Transient, Small-for-Gestational-Age, and Premature Infants

The estimated incidence of symptomatic hypoglycemia in newborns is 1-3 in 1,000 live births. This incidence is increased several fold in certain high-risk neonatal groups (see Table 111.2 and Fig. 111.1). Premature and SGA infants are vulnerable to the development of hypoglycemia. The factors responsible for the high frequency of hypoglycemia in this group, as well as in other groups outlined in Table 111.2, are related to the inadequate stores of liver glycogen, muscle protein, and body fat needed to sustain the substrates required to meet energy needs. These infants are small by virtue of prematurity or impaired placental transfer of nutrients. Their enzyme systems for gluconeogenesis may not be fully developed. **Transient hyperinsulinism** responsive to diazoxide has also been reported as contributing to hypoglycemia in asphyxiated, SGA, and premature newborn infants. This form of hyperinsulinism, associated with perinatal asphyxia, intrauterine growth restriction, maternal toxemia, and other perinatal stressors, is probably the most common cause of hyperinsulinemic hypoglycemia in neonates and may be quite severe. In most patients the condition resolves quickly, but it may persist to 7 mo of life or longer.

In contrast to deficiency of substrates or enzymes, the hormonal system appears to be functioning normally at birth in most low-risk neonates. Despite hypoglycemia, plasma concentrations of alanine, lactate, and pyruvate are higher, implying their diminished rate of utilization as substrates for gluconeogenesis. Infusion of alanine elicits further glucagon secretion but causes no significant rise in glucose. During the initial 24 hr of life, plasma concentrations of acetoacetate and β-hydroxybutyrate are lower in SGA infants than in full-term infants, implying diminished lipid stores, diminished fatty acid mobilization, impaired ketogenesis, or a combination of these conditions. Diminished lipid stores most likely occur because fat (triglyceride) feeding of newborns results in elevated plasma levels of glucose, ketones such as β-hydroxybutyrate, and FFAs. For infants with perinatal asphyxia and SGA newborns who have transient hyperinsulinism, the combination of hypoglycemia together with diminished concentrations of β-hydroxybutyrate and FFAs are the diagnostic hallmarks of hyperinsulinism.

The role of FFAs and their oxidation in stimulating neonatal gluconeogenesis is essential. The provision of FFAs as triglyceride feedings from formula or human milk together with gluconeogenic precursors may prevent the hypoglycemia that usually ensues after neonatal fasting. For these and other reasons, milk feedings are introduced early (at birth or within 2-4 hr) after delivery. In the hospital setting, when feeding is precluded by virtue of respiratory distress or other illness, or when feedings alone cannot maintain blood glucose concentrations at levels >55 mg/dL, intravenous (IV) glucose at a rate that supplies 4-8 mg/kg/min should be started. Infants with transient neonatal hypoglycemia can usually maintain the blood glucose level spontaneously after 2-3 days of life, but some require longer periods of support. In these latter infants, insulin values >5 μU/mL at the time of hypoglycemia should be treated with diazoxide.

Infants Born to Diabetic Mothers

See Chapter 127.1.

Of the transient hyperinsulinemic states, infants born to diabetic mothers are the most common. Gestational diabetes affects approximately 2% of pregnant women, and 1 in 1,000 pregnant women have insulin-dependent diabetes. At birth, infants born to these mothers may be large and plethoric, and their body stores of glycogen, protein, and fat are replete.

Hypoglycemia in infants of diabetic mothers is mostly related to hyperinsulinemia and partly related to diminished glucagon secretion. Hypertrophy and hyperplasia of the islets is present, as is a brisk, biphasic, and typically mature insulin response to glucose; this brisk insulin response is absent in normal infants. Infants born to diabetic

Table 111.2	Classification of Hypoglycemia in Infants and Children

NEONATAL TRANSITIONAL (ADAPTIVE) HYPOGLYCEMIA
Associated With Inadequate Substrate or Immature Enzyme Function in Otherwise Normal Neonates
Prematurity
Small for gestational age
Normal newborn

Transient Neonatal Hyperinsulinism
Infant of diabetic mother
Small for gestational age
Discordant twin
Birth asphyxia
Infant of toxemic mother

NEONATAL, INFANTILE, OR CHILDHOOD PERSISTENT HYPOGLYCEMIA
Hyperinsulinism
Recessive K_{ATP} channel HI
Recessive HADH (hydroxyl acyl-CoA dehydrogenase) mutation HI
Recessive UCP2 (mitochondrial uncoupling protein 2) mutation HI
Focal K_{ATP} channel HI
Dominant K_{ATP} channel HI
Atypical congenital hyperinsulinemia (no mutations in *ABCC8* or *KCN11* genes)
Dominant glucokinase HI
Dominant glutamate dehydrogenase HI (hyperinsulinism-hyperammonemia syndrome)
Dominant mutations in HNF-4A and HNF-1A (hepatocyte nuclear factors 4α and 1α) HI with monogenic diabetes of youth later in life
Dominant mutation in SLC16A1 (the pyruvate transporter)—exercise-induced hypoglycemia
Activating mutations in the calcium channel CACNA1D (permit calcium influx and thus unregulated insulin secretion)
Acquired or familial islet adenoma associated with mutations in *MEN1* gene
Beckwith-Wiedemann syndrome
Kabuki syndrome
Insulin administration (Munchausen syndrome by proxy)
Oral sulfonylurea drugs
Congenital disorders of glycosylation

Counter-Regulatory Hormone Deficiency
Panhypopituitarism
Isolated growth hormone deficiency
Adrenocorticotropic hormone deficiency
Addison disease (including congenital adrenal hypoplasia, adrenal leukodystrophy, triple A syndrome, ACTH receptor deficiency, and autoimmune disease complex)
Epinephrine deficiency

Glycogenolysis and Gluconeogenesis Disorders
Glucose-6-phosphatase deficiency (GSD Ia)
Glucose-6-phosphate translocase deficiency (GSD Ib)
Amylo-1,6-glucosidase (debranching enzyme) deficiency (GSD III)
Liver phosphorylase deficiency (GSD VI)
Phosphorylase kinase deficiency (GSD IX)
Glycogen synthetase deficiency (GSD 0)
Fructose-1,6-diphosphatase deficiency
Pyruvate carboxylase deficiency
Galactosemia
Hereditary fructose intolerance

Lipolysis Disorders
Fatty Acid Oxidation Disorders
Carnitine transporter deficiency (primary carnitine deficiency)
Carnitine palmitoyltransferase-1 deficiency
Carnitine translocase deficiency
Carnitine palmitoyltransferase-2 deficiency
Secondary carnitine deficiencies
Very-long-, long-, medium-, short-chain acyl-CoA dehydrogenase deficiency

OTHER ETIOLOGIES
Substrate-Limited Causes
Ketotic hypoglycemia
Poisoning—drugs
Salicylates
Alcohol
Oral hypoglycemic agents
Insulin
Propranolol
Pentamidine
Quinine
Disopyramide
Ackee fruit (unripe)—hypoglycin
Litchi – associated toxin (toxic hypoglycemic syndrome).
Vacor (rat poison)
Trimethoprim-sulfamethoxazole (with renal failure)
L-Asparaginase and other antileukemic drugs

Liver Disease
Reye syndrome
Hepatitis
Cirrhosis
Hepatoma

AMINO ACID AND ORGANIC ACID DISORDERS
Maple syrup urine disease
Propionic acidemia
Methylmalonic acidemia
Tyrosinosis
Glutaric aciduria
3-Hydroxy-3-methylglutaric aciduria

SYSTEMIC DISORDERS
Sepsis
Carcinoma/sarcoma (secreting—insulin-like growth factor II)
Heart failure
Malnutrition
Malabsorption
Antiinsulin receptor antibodies
Antiinsulin antibodies
Neonatal hyperviscosity
Renal failure
Diarrhea
Burns
Shock
Chiari malformation
Postsurgical complication
Pseudohypoglycemia (leukocytosis, polycythemia)
Excessive insulin therapy of insulin-dependent diabetes mellitus
Factitious disorder
Nissen fundoplication (dumping syndrome)
Falciparum malaria

GSD, Glycogen storage disease; HI, hyperinsulinemia; K_{ATP}, regulated potassium channel.

mothers also have a subnormal surge in plasma glucagon immediately after birth, subnormal glucagon secretion in response to stimuli, and initially, excessive sympathetic activity that may lead to adrenomedullary exhaustion, as reflected by decreased urinary excretion of epinephrine. The normal plasma hormonal pattern of low insulin, high glucagon, and high catecholamines is reversed to a pattern of high insulin, low glucagon,

and low epinephrine. As a consequence of this abnormal hormonal profile, endogenous glucose production is significantly inhibited compared with that in normal infants, thus predisposing them to hypoglycemia.

Mothers whose diabetes has been well controlled during pregnancy, labor, and delivery generally have infants near normal size who are less likely to develop neonatal hypoglycemia and other complications formerly considered typical of such infants. In supplying exogenous glucose to these hypoglycemic infants, it is important to avoid hyperglycemia that evokes a prompt exuberant insulin release, which may result in **rebound hypoglycemia**. When needed, glucose should be provided at continuous infusion rates of 4-8 mg/kg/min, but the appropriate dose for each patient must be individually adjusted. During labor and delivery, maternal hyperglycemia should be avoided because it results in fetal hyperglycemia, which predisposes to hypoglycemia when the glucose supply is interrupted at birth. Hypoglycemia persisting beyond day 3 after birth or initially occurring after 1 wk of life requires an evaluation for the causes listed in Table 111.2.

Infants born with **erythroblastosis fetalis** may also have hyperinsulinemia and share many physical features, such as large body size, with infants born to diabetic mothers. The cause of the hyperinsulinemia in infants with erythroblastosis is not clear.

Persistent or Recurrent Hypoglycemia in Infants and Children
Hyperinsulinism
Most children with hyperinsulinism that causes hypoglycemia present in the neonatal period or later in infancy. Hyperinsulinism is the most common cause of persistent hypoglycemia in early infancy. Infants who have hyperinsulinism may be macrosomic at birth, reflecting the anabolic effects of insulin in utero. There is no history or biochemical evidence of maternal diabetes. The onset of symptoms is from birth to 18 mo of age, but occasionally it only becomes evident in older children.

Insulin concentrations are inappropriately elevated at the time of documented hypoglycemia; with nonhyperinsulinemic hypoglycemia, plasma insulin concentrations should be <5 µU/mL. In affected infants, plasma insulin concentrations at the time of hypoglycemia are usually >5 µU/mL. Some authorities set more stringent criteria, arguing that any value of insulin >2 µU/mL with hypoglycemia is abnormal. The insulin (µU/mL):glucose (mg/dL) ratio is typically >0.4; plasma insulin-like growth factor binding protein-1 (IGFBP-1), β-hydroxybutyrate, and FFA levels are low with hyperinsulinism. Rare instances of activating mutations in the insulin receptor signaling pathway have been reported where the clinical and biochemical features are similar to states of excessive insulin secretion, yet insulin concentrations are low to the point of being undetectable. Therefore, the preferred term is *hyperinsulinism*, to describe a state of increased insulin action. Macrosomic infants may present with hypoglycemia from the 1st days of life. Infants with lesser degrees of hyperinsulinism may manifest hypoglycemia only after the 1st few wk to mo, when the frequency of feedings has been decreased to permit the infant to sleep through the night, and hyperinsulinism prevents the mobilization of endogenous glucose. Increasing appetite and demands for feeding, wilting spells, jitteriness, and frank seizures are the most common presenting features.

Additional clues include the rapid development of fasting hypoglycemia within 4-8 hr of food deprivation, compared with other causes of hypoglycemia (Tables 111.3 and 111.4); the need for high rates of exogenous glucose to prevent hypoglycemia, often at rates >10-15 mg/kg/min; the absence of ketonemia or acidosis; and elevated C-peptide or proinsulin levels at the time of hypoglycemia. The latter insulin-related products are absent in **factitious hypoglycemia** from exogenous administration of insulin as a form of child abuse (see Chapter 16.2). Hypoglycemia is invariably provoked by withholding feedings for several hours, permitting simultaneous measurement of glucose, insulin, ketones, and FFAs in the same sample at the time of clinically manifested hypoglycemia. This is termed the *critical sample*. The glycemic response to glucagon at the time of hypoglycemia reveals a brisk increment in glucose concentration of at least 40 mg/dL, which implies that glucose mobilization has been restrained by insulin but that glycogenolytic mechanisms are intact (Tables 111.5 to 111.7).

The measurement of serum IGFBP-1 concentration may help diagnose hyperinsulinism. The secretion of IGFBP-1 is acutely inhibited by insulin action; IGFBP-1 concentrations are low during hyperinsulinism-induced hypoglycemia. In patients with spontaneous or fasting-induced hypoglycemia with a low insulin level (ketotic hypoglycemia, normal fasting), IGFBP-1 concentrations are significantly higher.

The differential diagnosis of endogenous hyperinsulinism includes **diffuse β-cell hyperplasia** or **focal β-cell microadenoma**. The distinction between these 2 major entities is important because the diffuse hyperplasia, if unresponsive to medical therapy, requires near-total pancreatectomy, despite which hypoglycemia may persist or diabetes mellitus may ensue later. Some, but not all, affected infants may respond to sirolimus. By contrast, focal adenomas diagnosed preoperatively or intraoperatively permit localized curative resection with subsequent normal glucose metabolism. Approximately 50% of the autosomal recessive or sporadic forms of neonatal/infantile hyperinsulinism are caused by focal microadenomas, which may be distinguished from the diffuse form by the pattern of insulin response to selective insulin secretagogues infused into an arterial branch supplying the pancreas, with sampling by the hepatic vein. However, these invasive and technically difficult procedures have been largely abandoned in favor of positron emission tomography (PET) using 18-fluoro-L-dopa. This technique can distinguish the diffuse form (uniform fluorescence throughout the pancreas) from the focal form (focal uptake of 18-fluoro-L-dopa and localized fluorescence) with an extremely high degree of reliability, success, specificity, and sensitivity (see Fig. 111.3).

Insulin-secreting **macroadenomas** are rare in childhood and may be diagnosed preoperatively by CT or MRI. The plasma levels of insulin alone, however, cannot distinguish the aforementioned entities. The diffuse or microadenomatous forms of islet cell hyperplasia represent a variety of genetic defects responsible for abnormalities in the endocrine pancreas, characterized by autonomous insulin secretion that is not appropriately reduced when blood glucose declines spontaneously or in response to provocative maneuvers such as fasting (see Tables 111.4, 111.7, and 111.8). Clinical, biochemical, and molecular genetic approaches permit classification of congenital hyperinsulinism, formerly termed *nesidioblastosis,* into distinct entities.

Persistent hyperinsulinemic hypoglycemia of infancy (PHHI) may be inherited or sporadic, is severe, and is caused by mutations that affect the regulation of the potassium channel intimately involved in insulin secretion by the pancreatic β cell (Fig. 111.2). Normally, glucose entry into the β cell is enabled by the non–insulin-responsive glucose transporter GLUT-2. On entry, glucose is phosphorylated to glucose-6-phosphate by the enzyme glucokinase, enabling glucose metabolism to generate ATP. The rise in the molar ratio of ATP relative to adenosine diphosphate (ADP) closes the ATP-sensitive potassium channel in the cell membrane (K$_{ATP}$ channel). This channel is composed of 2 subunits, the K$_{IR}$ 6.2 channel, part of the family of inward-rectifier potassium channels, and a regulatory component in intimate association with K$_{IR}$ 6.2 known as the *sulfonylurea receptor* (SUR1). Together, K$_{IR}$ 6.2 and SUR1 constitute the potassium-sensitive ATP channel K$_{ATP}$. Normally, the K$_{ATP}$ is open, but with the rise in ATP and closure of the channel, potassium accumulates intracellularly, causing depolarization of the membrane, opening of voltage-gated calcium channels, influx of calcium into the cytoplasm, and secretion of insulin by exocytosis. The genes for both SUR1 and K$_{IR}$ 6.2 are located close together on the short arm of chromosome 11, the site of the insulin gene.

Inactivating mutations in the gene for SUR1 or, less often, K$_{IR}$ 6.2 prevent the potassium channel from opening; it remains variably closed with constant depolarization and therefore constant inward flux of calcium. Thus, insulin secretion is continuous and not governed by the glucose concentration. A milder autosomal dominant form of these defects is also reported. Similarly, an **activating** mutation in the gene for glucokinase or for glutamate dehydrogenase enzyme activity increases substrate metabolism and results in closure of the potassium channel through overproduction of ATP, which causes hyperinsulinism. Genetic defects in fatty acid metabolism, in the insulin transcription factors HNF-4α and HNF-1α, and in the uncoupling protein UCP-2 of the mitochondrial gene complex also have been involved in hyperinsulinemic hypoglycemia. Most recently, an activating mutation in the calcium channel has been reported to permit flux of calcium into the β cell, resulting in excessive, dysregulated insulin secretion and hypoglycemia that responds to diazoxide. **Inactivating** mutations of the glucokinase gene or **activating** mutations of the ATP-regulated potassium channel, which prevent or limit closure of the channel, are

Table 111.3	Hypoglycemia in Infants and Children: Clinical and Laboratory Features			
GROUP	**AGE AT DIAGNOSIS (mo)**	**GLUCOSE* (mg/dL)**	**INSULIN (µU/mL)**	**FASTING TIME TO HYPOGLYCEMIA (hr)**
HYPERINSULINEMIA (N = 12)				
Mean	7.4	23.1	22.4	2.1[†]
SEM	2.0	2.7	3.2	0.6
NONHYPERINSULINEMIA (N = 16)				
Mean	41.8	36.1	5.8	18.2
SEM	7.3	2.4	0.9	2.9

*In hypoglycemia caused by hyperinsulinism β-hydroxybutyrate and free fatty acids are low compared with normal at same duration of fasting.
[†]Milder forms of hyperinsulinism may require up to 18 hr of fasting to provoke hypoglycemia.
SEM, Standard error of mean.
Adapted from Antunes JD, Geffner ME, Lippe BM, et al: Childhood hypoglycemia: differentiating hyperinsulinemic from nonhyperinsulinemic causes, *J Pediatr* 116:105–108, 1990.

responsible for inadequate insulin secretion and form the basis of some forms of maturity-onset diabetes of youth and neonatal diabetes mellitus (see Chapter 607).

The familial forms of PHHI are more common in certain populations, notably Arabic and Ashkenazi Jewish communities, where it may reach an incidence of approximately 1 in 2,500, compared with the sporadic rates in the general population of 1 in 50,000. These **autosomal recessive forms** of PHHI typically present in the immediate newborn period as macrosomic newborns with a weight frequently >4.0 kg and severe recurrent or persistent hypoglycemia manifesting in the initial hours or days of life. Glucose infusions as high as 15-20 mg/kg/min and frequent feedings fail to maintain euglycemia. **Diazoxide**, which acts by opening K_{ATP} channels, fails to control hypoglycemia adequately. Somatostatin (**octreotide**), which also opens K_{ATP} channels and inhibits calcium flux, may be partially effective in 50% of patients (see Fig. 111.2). Calcium channel–blocking agents have had inconsistent effects. When affected patients are unresponsive to these measures, **pancreatectomy** is strongly recommended to avoid the long-term neurologic sequelae of hypoglycemia. If surgery is undertaken, preoperative CT or MRI rarely reveals an isolated adenoma, which would then permit local resection. Intraoperative ultrasonography may identify a small impalpable adenoma, permitting local resection. Adenomas often present in late infancy or early childhood.

Distinguishing between **focal** and **diffuse** cases of **persistent hyperinsulinism** has been attempted in several ways. Preoperatively, transhepatic portal vein catheterization and selective pancreatic venous sampling to measure insulin may localize a focal lesion from the step-up in insulin concentration at a specific site. Selective catheterization of arterial branches supplying the pancreas, followed by infusion of a secretagogue such as calcium and portal vein sampling for insulin concentration (arterial stimulation–venous sampling) may localize a lesion. Both approaches are highly invasive, restricted to specialized centers, and not uniformly successful in distinguishing the focal from the diffuse forms. Thus these techniques are not recommended and have largely been abandoned. Fluorine 18 (^{18}F)–labeled L-dopa combined with PET scanning is a highly promising means to distinguish the focal from the diffuse lesions of hyperinsulinism unresponsive to medical management (Fig. 111.3). The gold standard remains intraoperative **histologic** characterization. Diffuse hyperinsulinism is characterized by large β cells with abnormally large nuclei, whereas focal adenomatous lesions display small and normal β-cell nuclei. Although *SUR1* mutations are present in both types, the focal lesions arise by a random loss of a maternally imprinted growth-inhibitory gene on maternal chromosome 11p, in association with paternal transmission of a mutated *SUR1* or K_{IR} 6.2 paternal chromosome 11p, expressing the insulin-like growth factor 2 (*IGF2*) gene. Thus the focal form represents a double hit–loss of maternal repressor and transmission of a paternal mutation that contains a growth-promoting gene. This is similar to what occurs in children with the hyperinsulinemic hypoglycemia seen in Beckwith-Wiedemann syndrome, as discussed later.

Local excision of the focal adenomatous islet cell hyperplasia results in a cure with little or no recurrence. For the diffuse form, near-total

resection of 85–90% of the pancreas is recommended. The near-total pancreatectomy required for the diffuse hyperplastic lesions, however, is often associated with persistent hypoglycemia or later development of hyperglycemia or frank, insulin-dependent diabetes mellitus.

Further resection of the remaining pancreas may occasionally be necessary if hypoglycemia recurs and cannot be controlled by medical measures, such as the use of octreotide or diazoxide.

Experienced pediatric surgeons in medical centers equipped to provide the necessary preoperative and postoperative care, diagnostic evaluation, and management should perform surgery. In some patients who have been managed medically, hyperinsulinism and hypoglycemia regress over months. If hypoglycemia first manifests at 3 and 6 mo of age or later, a therapeutic trial using medical approaches with diazoxide, octreotide, and frequent feedings can be attempted for up to 2-4 wk. Failure to maintain euglycemia without undesirable side effects from the drugs may prompt the need for surgery. Some success in suppressing insulin release and correcting hypoglycemia in patients with PHHI has been reported with the use of the long-acting somatostatin analog octreotide. Most cases of neonatal PHHI are sporadic; familial forms permit genetic counseling on the basis of anticipated autosomal recessive inheritance.

A 2nd form of familial PHHI suggests **autosomal dominant inheritance**. The clinical features tend to be less severe, and onset of hypoglycemia is most likely, but not exclusively, to occur beyond the immediate newborn period and usually beyond the period of weaning, at an average age at onset of 1 yr. At birth, macrosomia is rarely observed, and response to diazoxide is almost uniform. The initial presentation may be delayed and rarely may occur as late as 30 yr, unless provoked by fasting. The genetic basis for this autosomal dominant form has not been delineated; it is not always linked to K_{IR} 6.2/*SUR1*. The activating mutation in glucokinase is transmitted in an autosomal dominant manner. If a family history is present, genetic counseling for a 50% recurrence rate can be given for future offspring.

A 3rd form of persistent PHHI is associated with mild and asymptomatic **hyperammonemia**, usually as a sporadic occurrence, although dominant inheritance occurs. Presentation is more like the autosomal dominant form than the autosomal recessive form. Diet and diazoxide control symptoms, but pancreatectomy may be necessary in some patients. The association of hyperinsulinism and hyperammonemia is caused by an inherited or de novo gain-of-function mutation in the enzyme glutamate dehydrogenase. The resulting increase in glutamate oxidation in the pancreatic β cell raises the ATP concentration and thus the ATP/ADP ratio, which closes K_{ATP}, leading to membrane depolarization, calcium influx, and insulin secretion (see Fig. 111.2). In the liver the excessive oxidation of glutamate to β-ketoglutarate may generate ammonia and divert glutamate from being processed to *N*-acetylglutamate, an essential cofactor for removal of ammonia through the urea cycle by activation of the enzyme carbamoyl phosphate synthetase. The hyperammonemia is mild, with concentrations of 100-200 µM/L, and produces no CNS symptoms or consequences, as seen in other hyperammonemic states. Leucine, a potent amino acid for stimulating insulin secretion and implicated in **leucine-sensitive hypoglycemia**,

| Table 111.4 | Correlation of Clinical Features With Molecular Defects in Persistent Hyperinsulinemic Hypoglycemia in Infancy |

TYPE	MACROSOMIA	HYPOGLYCEMIA/ HYPERINSULINEMIA	FAMILY HISTORY	MOLECULAR DEFECTS	ASSOCIATED CLINICAL, BIOCHEMICAL, OR MOLECULAR FEATURES	RESPONSE TO MEDICAL MANAGEMENT	RECOMMENDED SURGICAL APPROACH	PROGNOSIS
Sporadic	Present at birth	Moderate/severe in 1st days to weeks of life	Negative	? $SUR1/K_{IR}$ 6.2 mutations not always identified in diffuse hyperplasia	Loss of heterozygosity in microadenomatous tissue	Generally poor; may respond better to somatostatin than to diazoxide	Partial pancreatectomy if frozen section shows β-cell crowding with small nuclei—suggests microadenoma Subtotal >95% pancreatectomy if frozen section shows giant nuclei in β-cells—suggests diffuse hyperplasia	Excellent if focal adenoma is removed, thereby curing hypoglycemia and retaining sufficient pancreas to avoid diabetes Guarded if subtotal (>95%) pancreatectomy is performed because diabetes develops, and hypoglycemia persists
Autosomal recessive	Present at birth	Severe in 1st days to weeks of life	Positive	SUR/K_{IR} 6.2	Consanguinity a feature in some populations	Poor	Subtotal pancreatectomy	Guarded
Autosomal dominant	Unusual	Moderate onset usually >6 mo of age	Positive	Glucokinase (activating) Some cases gene unknown	None	Very good to excellent	Surgery usually not required Partial pancreatectomy only if medical management fails	Excellent
Autosomal dominant	Unusual	Moderate onset usually >6 mo of age	Positive	Glutamate dehydrogenase (activating)	Modest hyperammonemia	Very good to excellent	Surgery usually not required	Excellent
Beckwith-Wiedemann syndrome	Present at birth	Moderate, spontaneously resolves >6 mo of age	Negative	Duplicating/ imprinting in chromosome 11p15.1	Macroglossia, omphalocele, hemihypertrophy	Good	Not recommended	Excellent for hypoglycemia; guarded for possible development of embryonal tumors (Wilms hepatoblastoma)
Congenital disorders of glycosylation	Not usual	Moderate/onset >3 mo of age	Negative	Phosphomannose isomerase deficiency	Hepatomegaly, vomiting, intractable diarrhea	Good with mannose supplement	Not recommended	Fair

acts by allosterically stimulating glutamate dehydrogenase. Thus, leucine-sensitive hypoglycemia may be a form of the hyperinsulinemia-hyperammonemia syndrome or a potentiation of mild disorders of the K_{ATP} channel; it need not always be associated with a modest increase in serum ammonia.

Table 111.5	Analysis of Critical Blood Sample During Hypoglycemia and 30 Min After Glucagon*

SUBSTRATES
Glucose
Free fatty acids
Ketones
Lactate
Uric acid
Ammonia

HORMONES
Insulin
Cortisol
Growth hormone
Thyroxine, thyroid-stimulating hormone
Insulin-like growth factor binding protein-1[†]

*Glucagon 0.5 mg with maximum of 1 mg IV or IM.
[†]Measure once only before or after glucagon administration. Rise in glucose of ≥40 mg/dL after glucagon given at the time of hypoglycemia strongly suggests a hyperinsulinemic state with adequate hepatic glycogen stores and intact glycogenolytic enzymes. If ammonia is elevated to 100-200 μM, consider activating mutation of glutamate dehydrogenase.

Hypoglycemia associated with hyperinsulinemia is also seen in approximately 50% of patients with **Beckwith-Wiedemann syndrome** (see Chapter 576). This syndrome is caused by an imprinting disorder (see Chapter 98.8) and characterized by omphalocele, gigantism, macroglossia, microcephaly, and visceromegaly (Fig. 111.4). Distinctive lateral earlobe fissures and facial nevus flammeus are present; hemihypertrophy occurs in many of these infants. Diffuse islet cell hyperplasia occurs in infants with hypoglycemia. The diagnostic and therapeutic approaches are the same as those discussed previously, although microcephaly and slowing of brain development may occur independent of hypoglycemia. Patients with Beckwith-Wiedemann syndrome may acquire tumors, including Wilms tumor, hepatoblastoma, adrenal

Table 111.6	Criteria for Diagnosing Hyperinsulinism Based on "Critical" Samples (Drawn at a Time of Fasting Hypoglycemia: Plasma Glucose <50 mg/dL)

1. Hyperinsulinemia (plasma insulin >2 μU/mL)*
2. Hypofatty acidemia (plasma free fatty acids <1.5 mmol/L)
3. Hypoketonemia (plasma β-hydroxybutyrate <2.0 mmol/L)
4. Inappropriate glycemic response to glucagon, 1 mg IV (change in glucose >40 mg/dL)

*Depends on sensitivity of insulin assay.
From Stanley CA, Thomson PS, Finegold DN, et al: Hypoglycemia in infants and neonates. In Sperling MA, editor: *Pediatric endocrinology*, ed 2, Philadelphia, 2002, Saunders, pp 135–159.

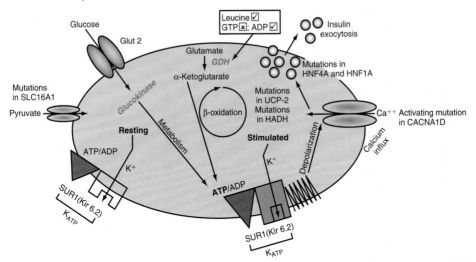

Fig. 111.2 Schematic of the pancreatic cell with some important steps in insulin secretion. The membrane-spanning, adenosine triphosphate (ATP)–sensitive potassium (K^+) channel (K_{ATP}) consists of 2 subunits: the sulfonylurea receptor (SUR) and the inward rectifying K channel (K_{IR} 6.2). In the resting state, the ratio of ATP to adenosine diphosphate (ADP) maintains K_{ATP} in an open state, permitting efflux of intracellular K^+. When blood glucose concentration rises, its entry into the β cell is facilitated by the Glut-2 glucose transporter, a process not regulated by insulin. Within the β cell, glucose is converted to glucose-6-phosphate by the enzyme glucokinase and then undergoes metabolism to generate energy. The resultant increase in ATP relative to ADP closes K_{ATP}, preventing efflux of K^+, and the rise of intracellular K^+ depolarizes the cell membrane and opens a calcium (Ca^{2+}) channel. The intracellular rise in Ca^{2+} triggers insulin secretion via exocytosis. Sulfonylureas trigger insulin secretion by reacting with their receptor (SUR) to close K_{ATP}; diazoxide inhibits this process, whereas somatostatin, or its analog octreotide, inhibits insulin secretion by interfering with calcium influx. Genetic mutations in SUR1 or K_{IR} 6.2 that prevent K_{ATP} from being open tonically maintain inappropriate insulin secretion and are responsible for autosomal recessive forms of persistent hyperinsulinemic hypoglycemia of infancy (PHHI). One form of autosomal dominant PHHI is caused by an activating mutation in glucokinase. The amino acid leucine also triggers insulin secretion by closure of K_{ATP}. Metabolism of leucine is facilitated by the enzyme glutamate dehydrogenase (GDH), and overactivity of this enzyme in the pancreas leads to hyperinsulinemia with hypoglycemia, associated with hyperammonemia from overactivity of GDH in the liver. Mutations in the pyruvate channel SLC16A1 can cause ectopic expression in the β cell and permit pyruvate, accumulated during exercise, to induce insulin secretion and thus exercise-induced hypoglycemia. Mutations in the mitochondrial uncoupling protein 2 (UCP2) and hydroxyl acyl-CoA dehydrogenase (HADH) are associated with hyperinsulinism (HI) by mechanisms yet to be defined. Mutations in the transcription factors hepatocyte nuclear factors (HNF) 4α and 1α can be associated with neonatal macrosomia and HI, but progress to monogenic diabetes of youth (MODY) later in life. Activating mutations in the calcium channel CACNA1D permit calcium influx and hence unregulated insulin secretion at membrane voltages which normally exclude calcium flux. √, Stimulation; GTP, guanosine triphosphate; X, inhibition.

Table 111.7	Diagnosis of Acute Hypoglycemia in Infants and Children

ACUTE SYMPTOMS PRESENT

1. Obtain blood sample before and 30 min after glucagon administration.
2. Obtain urine as soon as possible. Examine for ketones; if not present and hypoglycemia confirmed, suspect hyperinsulinemia or fatty acid oxidation defect; if present, suspect ketotic, hormone deficiency, inborn error of glycogen metabolism, or defective gluconeogenesis.
3. Measure glucose in the original blood sample. If hypoglycemia is confirmed, proceed with substrate-hormone measurement as in Table 111.5.
4. If glycemic increment after glucagon exceeds 40 mg/dL above basal, suspect hyperinsulinemia.
5. If insulin level at time of confirmed hypoglycemia is >5 μU/mL, suspect endogenous hyperinsulinemia; if >100 μU/mL, suspect factitious hyperinsulinemia (exogenous insulin injection). Admit to hospital for supervised fast.
6. If cortisol is <10 μg/dL or growth hormone is <5 ng/mL, or both, suspect adrenal insufficiency or pituitary disease, or both. Admit to hospital for hormonal testing and neuroimaging.

HISTORY SUGGESTIVE: ACUTE SYMPTOMS NOT PRESENT

1. Careful history for relation of symptoms to time and type of food intake, considering age of patient. Exclude possibility of alcohol or drug ingestion. Assess possibility of insulin injection, salt craving, growth velocity, or intracranial pathology.
2. Careful examination for hepatomegaly (glycogen storage disease; defect in gluconeogenesis); pigmentation (adrenal failure); stature and neurologic status (pituitary disease).
3. Admit to hospital for provocative testing:
   a. 24 hr fast under careful observation; when symptoms provoked, proceed with steps 1-4 as when acute symptoms present.
   b. Pituitary-adrenal function using arginine-insulin stimulation test if indicated.
4. Consider molecular diagnostic test before liver biopsy for histologic and enzyme determinations.
5. Oral glucose tolerance test (1.75 g/kg; max 75 g) if reactive hypoglycemia suspected (e.g., dumping syndrome).

carcinoma, gonadoblastoma, and rhabdomyosarcoma. This overgrowth syndrome is caused by mutations in the chromosome 11p15.5 region close to the genes for insulin, *SUR1*, K_{IR} 6.2, and *IGF2*. Duplications in this region and genetic imprinting from a defective or absent copy of the maternally derived gene are involved in the variable features and patterns of transmission. Hypoglycemia may resolve in weeks to months of medical therapy. Pancreatic resection may rarely be needed.

Kabuki syndrome, caused by mutations in a methyltransferase or demethylase, is the 2nd most common syndromic form of hyperinsulinemic hypoglycemia of infancy (HHI) after Beckwith-Wiedemann Syndrome. Neonatal hypoglycemia with congenital hyperinsulinism occurs in about 70% of children with this syndrome; most are diazoxide responsive. Congenital hyperinsulinemia also is reported to occur in **Turner syndrome**. Activating mutations in *AKT2* and in PI3-kinase of the insulin signaling cascade have been reported in association with hypoketotic hypoglycemia and other metabolic features indicative of excessive insulin action, but insulin concentrations are subnormal as a result of negative feedback from the activated insulin receptor signal.

HHI is reported as a manifestation of 1 form of **congenital disorder of glycosylation**. Disorders of protein glycosylation usually present with neurologic symptoms but may also include liver dysfunction with hepatomegaly, intractable diarrhea, protein-losing enteropathy, and hypoglycemia (see Chapter 105.6). These disorders are often underdiagnosed. One entity associated with HHI is caused by phosphomannose isomerase deficiency, and clinical improvement followed supplemental treatment with oral mannose, 0.17 g/kg 6 times per day.

After the 1st 12 mo of life, hyperinsulinemic states are uncommon until islet cell adenomas reappear as a cause after the patient is several years of age. Hyperinsulinemia as a result of **islet cell adenoma** should be considered in any child ≥5 yr who presents with hypoglycemia. Islet cell adenomas do not "light up" during scanning with ^{18}F-labeled L-dopa. An islet cell adenoma in a child should arouse suspicion of the possibility of **multiple endocrine neoplasia type I** (Wermer syndrome), which involves mutations in the menin gene and may be associated with hyperparathyroidism and pituitary tumors. Tables 111.7 and 111.8 outline the diagnostic approach. In a newborn, fasting for only 6-8 hr (1 missed meal in a 3-4 hr feeding schedule) may be sufficient to provoke

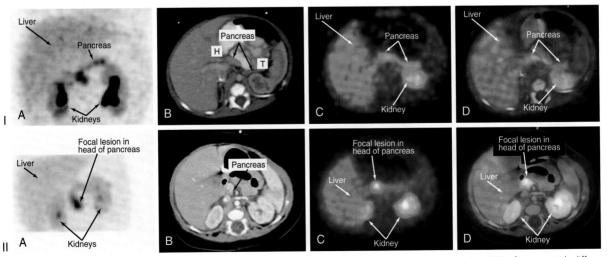

Fig. 111.3 Congenital hyperinsulinism. I Panels (*diffuse*): Fluorine 18 (^{18}F)-L-dopa positron emission tomography (PET) of patient with diffuse form of congenital hyperinsulinism. **A,** Diffuse uptake of ^{18}F-L-dopa is visualized throughout the pancreas. Transverse views show **B,** normal pancreatic tissue on abdominal CT; **C,** diffuse uptake of ^{18}F-L-dopa in pancreas; and **D,** confirmation of pancreatic uptake of ^{18}F-L-dopa with co-registration. H, Head of pancreas; T, tail of pancreas. **II** Panels (*focal*): ^{18}F-L-dopa PET of patient with focal form of congenital hyperinsulinism. **A,** Discrete area of increased ^{18}F-L-dopa uptake is visualized in the head of the pancreas. The intensity of this area is greater than that observed in the liver and neighboring normal pancreatic tissue. Transverse views show **B,** normal pancreatic tissue on abdominal CT; **C,** focal uptake of ^{18}F-L-dopa in pancreatic head; and **D,** confirmation of ^{18}F-L-dopa uptake in the pancreatic head with co-registration. (*Courtesy of Dr. Olga Hardy, Children's Hospital of Philadelphia.*)

hypoglycemia, and this maneuver should be performed to exclude persistent forms of hypoglycemia before discharge from a neonatal unit. In older infants and children, fasting for up to 24-36 hr usually provokes hypoglycemia; coexisting hyperinsulinemia confirms the diagnosis, provided that factitious administration of insulin by the parents is excluded. Occasionally, provocative tests may be required. Exogenously administered insulin can be distinguished from endogenous insulin by simultaneous measurement of C-peptide concentration. If C-peptide levels are elevated, endogenous insulin secretion is responsible for the hypoglycemia; if C-peptide levels are low but insulin values are high, exogenous insulin has been administered, perhaps as a form of child abuse (see Chapter 16.2). Islet cell adenomas at this age are treated by surgical excision. Antibodies to insulin or the insulin receptor (**insulin mimetic action**) are also rarely associated with hypoglycemia. Some **tumors** produce IGFs, thereby provoking hypoglycemia by interacting with the insulin receptor. The astute clinician must also consider the possibility of deliberate or accidental ingestion of drugs such as a sulfonylurea or related compound that stimulates insulin secretion. In such cases, both insulin and C-peptide concentrations in blood will be elevated. Inadvertent substitution of an insulin secretagogue by a dispensing error should be considered in those taking medications who suddenly develop documented hypoglycemia.

A rare form of hyperinsulinemic hypoglycemia has been reported after exercise. Whereas glucose and insulin remain unchanged in most people after moderate, short-term exercise, rare patients manifest severe hypoglycemia with hyperinsulinemia 15-50 min after the same standardized exercise. This form of **exercise-induced hyperinsulinism** is caused by abnormal responsiveness of β-cell insulin release to pyruvate generated during exercise. The gene responsible for this syndrome, *SLC16A1*, regulates a transporter (MCT1R) that controls the entry of pyruvate into cells. Dominant mutations in *SLC16A1* that increase the ectopic expression of MCTR1 in pancreatic β cells permit excessive entry of pyruvate into β cells and act to increase insulin secretion, with resultant hypoglycemia during exercise.

Hypoglycemia with so-called nesidioblastosis has also rarely been reported after **bariatric surgery** for obesity. The mechanism for this form of hyperinsulinemic hypoglycemia remains to be defined.

Infants and children with **Nissen fundoplication**, a relatively common procedure used to ameliorate gastroesophageal reflux, frequently have an associated "dumping" syndrome with hypoglycemia. Characteristic features include significant hyperglycemia of 200 mg/dL and up to 500 mg/dL 30 min postprandially, and severe hypoglycemia (average 32 mg/dL in one series) 1.5-3.0 hr later. The early hyperglycemia phase is associated with brisk and excessive insulin release that causes the rebound hypoglycemia. A role for exaggerated GLP1 secretion has been proposed and glucagon responses have been reported to be inappropriately low in some cases. However, the physiologic mechanisms are not always clearly understood, and attempted treatments not always effective; **acarbose**, an inhibitor of glucose absorption, was reported to be successful in one small series.

Endocrine Deficiencies

Hypoglycemia associated with endocrine deficiency is usually caused by adrenal cortisol insufficiency with or without associated growth hormone deficiency (see Chapters 573 and 593). In **panhypopituitarism**, isolated adrenocorticotropic hormone (ACTH) or GH deficiency, or combined ACTH and GH deficiency, the incidence of hypoglycemia is as high as 20%. In the newborn period, hypoglycemia may be the presenting feature of hypopituitarism; in males, a microphallus may provide a clue to a coexisting deficiency of gonadotropin. Newborns with hypopituitarism often have a form of hepatitis associated with **cholestatic jaundice** and hypoglycemia. The combination of hypoglycemia and cholestatic jaundice requires exclusion of hypopituitarism as a cause, as the jaundice resolves with replacement treatment of GH, cortisol, and thyroid as required. This constellation is often associated with the syndrome of **septooptic dysplasia**. When adrenal disease is severe, as in congenital adrenal hyperplasia caused by enzyme defects in cortisol synthesis, adrenal hemorrhage, or congenital adrenal hypoplasia, serum electrolyte disturbances with hyponatremia and hyperkalemia or disordered genital development may provide diagnostic clues (see Chapter 576). In older children, failure of growth should suggest GH deficiency. Hyperpigmentation, weakness, or salt craving may provide the clue to primary adrenal insufficiency (**Addison disease**), characterized by greatly increased ACTH levels or adrenal unresponsiveness to exogenous ACTH caused by a defect in the adrenal receptor for ACTH, congenital adrenal hypoplasia, adrenoleukodystrophy, or the Allgrove triple A syndrome. The frequent association of Addison disease in childhood with hypoparathyroidism (hypocalcemia), chronic mucocutaneous candidiasis, and other endocrinopathies that constitute the autoimmune polyendocrinopathy syndrome type 1 should be considered. Adrenoleukodystrophy and congenital adrenal hypoplasia are sex-linked conditions and should be considered in the differential diagnosis of primary Addison disease in male children (see Chapter 104.2).

Hypoglycemia in cortisol-GH deficiency may be caused by decreased gluconeogenic enzymes with cortisol deficiency, increased glucose utilization because of a lack of the antagonistic effects of GH on insulin action, or failure to supply endogenous gluconeogenic substrate in the form of alanine and lactate with compensatory breakdown of fat and generation of ketones. Deficiency of these hormones results in reduced gluconeogenic substrate, which resembles the syndrome of ketotic hypoglycemia. Investigation of a child with hypoglycemia therefore requires exclusion of ACTH-cortisol or GH deficiency and, if diagnosed, its appropriate replacement with cortisol or GH.

Epinephrine deficiency could theoretically be responsible for hypoglycemia. Urinary excretion of epinephrine has been decreased in some patients with spontaneous or insulin-induced hypoglycemia in whom absence of pallor and tachycardia were also noted. This suggests that failure of catecholamine release, as the result of a defect anywhere along the hypothalamic-autonomic-adrenomedullary axis, might be responsible for the hypoglycemia. This possibility has been challenged, however, because of the rarity of hypoglycemia in patients

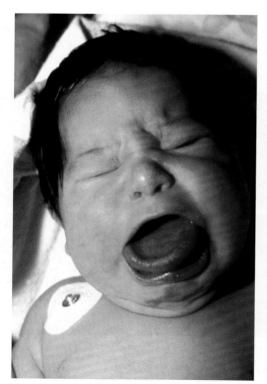

Fig. 111.4 Beckwith-Wiedemann syndrome. *(Courtesy of Dr. Michael Cohen, Dalhousie University, Halifax, Nova Scotia. From Jones KL: Smith's recognizable patterns of human malformation, ed 6, Philadelphia, 2006, Saunders.)*

Table 111.8 | Clinical Manifestations and Differential Diagnosis in Childhood Hypoglycemia

CONDITION	HYPOGLYCEMIA	URINARY KETONES OR REDUCING SUGARS	HEPATOMEGALY	SERUM Lipids	SERUM Uric Acid	EFFECT OF 24-36 HR FAST ON PLASMA Glucose	Insulin	Ketones	Alanine	Lactate	GLYCEMIC RESPONSE TO GLUCAGON Fed	Fasted	GLYCEMIC RESPONSE TO INFUSION OF Alanine	Glycerol
Normal	0	0	0	Normal	Normal	↓	↓	↑	↓	Normal	↑	↓	↑	Not indicated
Hyperinsulinemia	Recurrent severe	0	0	Normal or ↑	Normal	↓↓	↑↑	↓↓	Normal	Normal	↑	↑	↑	Not indicated
Ketotic hypoglycemia	Severe with missed meals	Ketonuria +++	0	Normal	Normal	↓↓	↓	↑↑	↓↓	Normal	↑	↓↓	↑	Not indicated
Fatty acid oxidation disorder	Severe with missed meals	Absent	0 to + Abnormal liver function test results	Abnormal	↑		Contraindicated				↑	↓	↑	Not indicated
Hypopituitarism	Moderate with missed meals	Ketonuria ++	0	Normal	Normal	↓↓	↓	↑↑	↓↓	Normal	↑	↓↓	↑	↑
Adrenal insufficiency	Severe with missed meals	Ketonuria ++	0	Normal	Normal	↓↓	↓	↑↑	↓↓	Normal	↑	↓↓	↑	↑
Type 1 glycogen storage disease[1]	Severe with missed meals	Ketonuria +++[2]	+++	↑↑	↑↑	↓↓	↓	↑↑	↑↑	↑↑	0	0-↓↓	0	0
Glycogen debrancher	Moderate with fasting	++	++	Normal	Normal	↓↓	↓	↑↑	↓↓	Normal	↑	0-↓↓	↑	↑
Glycogen phosphorylase	Mild-moderate	Ketonuria ++	+	Normal	Normal	↓	↓	↑↑	↓↓	Normal	0-↑	0-↓↓	↑	↑
Fructose-1,6-diphosphatase	Severe with fasting	Ketonuria +++	+++	↑↑	↑↑	↓↓	↓	↑↑	↑↑	↑↑	↑	0-↓↓	↓	↓
Galactosemia	After milk or milk products	0 Ketones;(s) +	+++	Normal	Normal	↓	↓	↑	↓	Normal	↑	0-↓↓	↑	↑
Fructose intolerance	After fructose	0 Ketones;(s) +	+++	Normal	Normal	↓	↓	↑	↓	Normal	↑	0-↓↓	↑	↑

Details of each condition are discussed in the text.
0 absence of ketonuria or hepatomegaly; + mildly detected ketonuria or hepatomegaly; ++ moderately increased; +++ markedly increased; 0, Absence; ↑ or ↓ indicates, respectively, small increase or decrease; ↑↑ or ↓↓ indicates, respectively, large increase or decrease.
[1]Glucose-6-phosphatase deficiency.
[2]Hepatomegaly may not be present in the newborn.

with bilateral adrenalectomy, provided that they receive adequate glucocorticoid replacement, and because diminished epinephrine excretion is found in normal patients with repeated insulin-induced hypoglycemia. Many of the patients described as having hypoglycemia with failure of epinephrine excretion fit the criteria for ketotic hypoglycemia (see next). Also, repetitive hypoglycemia leads to diminished cortisol plus epinephrine responses, as seen most often in insulin-treated diabetes mellitus and the syndrome of hypoglycemia unawareness, associated with autonomic failure.

Glucagon deficiency in infants or children may theoretically be associated with hypoglycemia but has never been documented.

Substrate-Limited Etiologies
Ketotic Hypoglycemia

Idiopathic ketotic hypoglycemia is the most common form of *childhood* hypoglycemia. This condition usually presents between ages 18 mo and 5 yr and remits spontaneously by 8-9 yr. Hypoglycemic episodes typically occur during periods of intercurrent illness when food intake is limited. The classic history is of a child who eats poorly or completely avoids the evening meal, is difficult to arouse from sleep the following morning and thus eats poorly again, and may have a seizure or may be comatose by mid-morning. Another common presentation occurs when parents sleep late, and the affected child is unable to eat breakfast, thus prolonging the overnight fast.

At the time of documented hypoglycemia, there is associated marked ketonuria and ketonemia; plasma insulin concentrations are appropriately low, ≤5 μU/mL, thus excluding hyperinsulinemia. A ketogenic-provocative diet, formerly a diagnostic test, is no longer used to establish the diagnosis because fasting alone provokes a hypoglycemic episode with ketonemia and ketonuria within 12-18 hr in susceptible individuals. Normal children of similar age can withstand fasting without hypoglycemia developing during the same period, although even normal children may acquire these features by 36 hr of fasting.

Children with ketotic hypoglycemia have plasma alanine concentrations that are markedly reduced in the basal state after an overnight fast and decline even further with prolonged fasting. **Alanine**, produced in muscle, is a major gluconeogenic precursor. Alanine is the only amino acid that is significantly lower in these children, and infusions of alanine (250 mg/kg) produce a rapid rise in plasma glucose without causing significant changes in blood lactate or pyruvate levels, indicating that the entire gluconeogenic pathway from the level of pyruvate is intact, but that there is a deficiency of substrate. Glycogenolytic pathways are also intact because glucagon induces a normal glycemic response in affected children in the fed state. The levels of hormones that counter hypoglycemia are appropriately elevated, and insulin is appropriately low.

The etiology of ketotic hypoglycemia may be a defect in any of the complex steps involved in protein catabolism, oxidative deamination of amino acids, transamination, alanine synthesis, or alanine efflux from muscle. Children with ketotic hypoglycemia are frequently smaller than age-matched controls and often have a history of transient neonatal hypoglycemia. Any decrease in muscle mass may compromise the supply of gluconeogenic substrate at a time when glucose demands per unit of body weight are already relatively high, thus predisposing the patient to the rapid development of hypoglycemia, with ketosis representing the attempt to switch to an alternative fuel supply. Children with ketotic hypoglycemia may represent the low end of the spectrum of children's capacity to tolerate fasting. Similar relative intolerance to fasting is present in normal children, who cannot maintain blood glucose after 30-36 hr of fasting, compared with the adult's capacity for prolonged fasting. Although the defect may be present at birth, it may not be evident until the child is stressed by more prolonged periods of calorie restriction. Moreover, the spontaneous remission observed in children at age 8-9 yr might be explained by the increase in muscle bulk with its resultant increase in supply of endogenous substrate and the relative decrease in glucose requirement per unit of body mass with increasing age.

In anticipation of spontaneous resolution of this syndrome, **treatment** of ketotic hypoglycemia consists of frequent feedings of a high-protein,

high-carbohydrate diet. During intercurrent illnesses, parents should be taught to test the child's urine for the presence of ketones, the appearance of which precedes hypoglycemia by several hours. In the presence of ketonuria, liquids of high carbohydrate content should be offered to the child. If these cannot be tolerated, the child should be treated with IV glucose administration in a hospital.

Branched-Chain Ketonuria (Maple Syrup Urine Disease)

See Chapter 103.6.

The hypoglycemic episodes were once attributed to high levels of leucine, but evidence indicates that interference with the production of alanine and its availability as a gluconeogenic substrate during calorie deprivation is responsible for hypoglycemia.

Glycogen Storage Disease

See Chapter 105.1.

Glucose-6-Phosphatase Deficiency (Type I Glycogen Storage Disease)

Affected children usually display a remarkable tolerance to their chronic hypoglycemia; blood glucose values in the range of 20-50 mg/dL are not associated with the classic symptoms of hypoglycemia, possibly reflecting the adaptation of the CNS to ketone bodies and lactate as alternative fuels. Hepatomegaly and poor growth are consistent physical features. Hypoglycemia is associated with acidosis (HCO_3^- <18 mEq/L) and increased β-hydroxybutyrate and lactate; hyperuricemia also is frequently seen. Management is discussed in detail in Chapter 105.1.

Amylo-1,6-Glucosidase Deficiency (Debrancher Enzyme Deficiency; Type III Glycogen Storage Disease)

See Chapter 105.1.

Liver Phosphorylase Deficiency (Type VI Glycogen Storage Disease)

Low hepatic phosphorylase activity may result from a defect in any of the steps of activation; a variety of defects have been described. Hepatomegaly, excessive deposition of glycogen in liver, growth retardation, and occasional symptomatic hypoglycemia occur. A diet high in protein and reduced in carbohydrate usually prevents hypoglycemia.

Glycogen Synthetase Deficiency

The inability to synthesize glycogen is rare. Hypoglycemia and hyperketonemia occur after fasting because glycogen reserves are greatly decreased or absent. After feeding, however, hyperglycemia with glucosuria may occur because of the inability to assimilate some of the glucose load into glycogen. During fasting hypoglycemia, levels of the counter-regulatory hormones, including catecholamines, are appropriately elevated or normal, and insulin levels are appropriately low. The liver is not enlarged. Protein-rich feedings at frequent intervals result in dramatic clinical improvement, including growth velocity. Glycogen synthetase deficiency mimics the syndrome of **ketotic hypoglycemia** and should be considered in the differential diagnosis of that syndrome.

Disorders of Gluconeogenesis
Fructose-1,6-Diphosphatase Deficiency

See Chapter 105.3.

A deficiency of this enzyme results in a block of gluconeogenesis from all possible precursors below the level of fructose-1,6-diphosphate. Infusion of these gluconeogenic precursors results in lactic acidosis without a rise in glucose; acute hypoglycemia may be provoked by inhibition of glycogenolysis. Glycogenolysis remains intact, and glucagon elicits a normal glycemic response in the fed, but not in the fasted, state. Accordingly, affected individuals have hypoglycemia only during caloric deprivation, as in fasting, or during intercurrent illness. As long as glycogen stores remain normal, hypoglycemia does not develop. In affected families, there may be a history of siblings with known hepatomegaly who died in infancy with unexplained metabolic acidosis.

Defects in Fatty Acid Oxidation
See Chapter 104.1.

The important role of fatty acid oxidation in maintaining gluconeogenesis is underscored by examples of congenital or drug-induced defects in fatty acid metabolism that may be associated with fasting hypoglycemia.

Various congenital enzymatic deficiencies cause defective carnitine or fatty acid metabolism. A severe and relatively common form of fasting hypoglycemia with hepatomegaly, cardiomyopathy, and hypotonia occurs with long- and medium-chain fatty acid CoA dehydrogenase deficiency. Plasma carnitine levels are low, ketones are not present, but dicarboxylic aciduria is present in urine. Clinically, patients with **acyl-CoA dehydrogenase deficiency** present with a Reye-like syndrome (see Chapter 388), recurrent episodes of severe fasting hypoglycemic coma, and cardiorespiratory arrest (sudden infant death syndrome–like events). Severe hypoglycemia and metabolic acidosis without ketosis also occur in patients with multiple acyl-CoA dehydrogenase disorders. Hypotonia, seizures, and acrid odor are other clinical clues. Survival depends on whether the defects are severe or mild; diagnosis is established from studies of enzyme activity in liver biopsy tissue or in cultured fibroblasts from affected patients. Tandem mass spectrometry can be employed for blood samples, even those on filter paper, for screening of congenital inborn errors. Molecular diagnosis also is available for most entities. The frequency of acyl-CoA dehydrogenase deficiency is at least 1 in 10,000-15,000 births. Avoidance of fasting and supplementation with carnitine may be lifesaving in these patients, who generally present in infancy.

Interference with fatty acid metabolism also underlies the fasting hypoglycemia associated with Jamaican vomiting sickness, with atractyloside, and with the drug valproate. In **Jamaican vomiting sickness** the unripe ackee fruit contains a water-soluble toxin, *hypoglycin*, which produces vomiting, CNS depression, and severe hypoglycemia. The hypoglycemic activity of hypoglycin derives from its inhibition of gluconeogenesis secondary to its interference with the acyl-CoA and carnitine metabolism essential for the oxidation of long-chain fatty acids. The disease is almost totally confined to Jamaica, where ackee forms a staple of the diet for the poor population. The ripe ackee fruit no longer contains this toxin.

Atractyloside is a reagent that inhibits oxidative phosphorylation in mitochondria by preventing the translocation of adenine nucleotides, such as ATP, across the mitochondrial membrane. Atractyloside is a perhydrophenanthrenic glycoside derived from *Atractylis gummifera*. This plant is found in the Mediterranean basin; ingestion of this "thistle" is associated with hypoglycemia and a syndrome similar to Jamaican vomiting sickness. A similar illness noted in India, the **acute toxic encephalopathy-hypoglycemic syndrome**, may be caused by litchi consumption. Litchi contains hypoglycin A and/or methylenecyclopropylglycine, which may inhibit fatty acid oxidation or gluconeogenesis.

The anticonvulsant drug **valproate** is associated with side effects, predominantly in young infants, which include a Reye-like syndrome, low serum carnitine levels, and the potential for fasting hypoglycemia.

In all these conditions, hypoglycemia *is not associated with ketonemia and ketonuria.*

Acute Alcohol Intoxication
The liver metabolizes alcohol as a preferred fuel, and generation of reducing equivalents during the oxidation of ethanol alters the reduced form of nicotinamide adenine dinucleotide:nicotinamide adenine dinucleotide ratio, which is essential for certain gluconeogenic steps. As a result, gluconeogenesis is impaired and hypoglycemia may ensue if glycogen stores are depleted by starvation or by preexisting abnormalities in glycogen metabolism. In toddlers who have been unfed for some time, even the consumption of small quantities of alcohol can precipitate these events. The hypoglycemia promptly responds to IV glucose, which should always be considered in a child who presents initially with coma or seizure, after taking a blood sample to determine glucose concentration. The possibility that child ingested alcoholic drinks must also be considered if there was a preceding evening party. A careful history allows the diagnosis to be made and may avoid needless and expensive hospitalization and investigation.

Salicylate Intoxication
See Chapter 77.

Both hyperglycemia and hypoglycemia occur in children with salicylate intoxication. Accelerated utilization of glucose, resulting from augmentation of insulin secretion by salicylates, and possible interference with gluconeogenesis may contribute to hypoglycemia. Infants are more susceptible than older children. Monitoring of blood glucose levels with appropriate glucose infusion in the event of hypoglycemia should form part of the therapeutic approach to salicylate intoxication in childhood. Ketosis may occur.

Phosphoenolpyruvate Carboxykinase Deficiency
Deficiency of the rate-limiting gluconeogenic enzyme phosphoenolpyruvate carboxykinase is associated with severe fasting hypoglycemia and variable onset after birth. Hypoglycemia may occur within 24 hr after birth, and defective gluconeogenesis from alanine can be documented in vivo. Liver, kidney, and myocardium demonstrate fatty infiltration, and atrophy of the optic nerve and visual cortex may occur. Hypoglycemia may be profound. Lactate and pyruvate levels in plasma have been normal, but a mild metabolic acidosis may be present. The fatty infiltration of various organs is caused by increased formation of acetyl-CoA, which becomes available for fatty acid synthesis. Diagnosis of this rare entity can be made with certainty only through appropriate enzymatic determinations in liver biopsy material or molecular diagnosis. Avoidance of periods of fasting through frequent feedings rich in carbohydrate should be helpful because glycogen synthesis and breakdown are intact.

Pyruvate Carboxylase Deficiency
See Chapter 105.4.

Other Enzyme Defects
Galactosemia (Galactose-1-Phosphate Uridyl Transferase Deficiency)
See Chapter 105.2.

Fructose Intolerance (Fructose-1-Phosphate Aldolase Deficiency)
See Chapter 105.3.

Acute hypoglycemia is caused by fructose-1-phosphate aldolase deficiency, which inhibits glycogenolysis via the phosphorylase system and of gluconeogenesis at the level of fructose-1,6-diphosphate aldolase. Affected individuals usually learn spontaneously to eliminate fructose from their diet.

Defects in Glucose Transporters
GLUT-1 Deficiency
Rarely, infants with a seizure disorder are found to have low CSF glucose concentrations despite normal plasma glucose. Lactate concentrations in CSF are low, suggesting decreased glycolysis rather than bacterial infection, which causes low CSF glucose with high lactate. The erythrocyte glucose transporter (GLUT-1) is defective, suggesting a similar defect in the brain glucose transporter responsible for the clinical features. A ketogenic diet reduces the severity of seizures by supplying an alternate source of brain fuel that bypassed the defect in glucose transport.

GLUT-2 Deficiency
Children with hepatomegaly, galactose intolerance, and renal tubular dysfunction (**Fanconi-Bickel syndrome**) have a deficiency of GLUT-2 of plasma membranes. In addition to liver and kidney tubules, GLUT-2 is also expressed in pancreatic β cells. Thus the clinical manifestations reflect impaired glucose release from liver and defective tubular reabsorption of glucose plus phosphaturia and aminoaciduria.

Systemic Disorders
Several systemic disorders are associated with hypoglycemia in infants and children. **Neonatal sepsis** is often associated with hypoglycemia, possibly as a result of diminished caloric intake with impaired gluconeogenesis. Similar mechanisms may apply to the hypoglycemia found in severely malnourished infants or those with severe malabsorption. **Hyperviscosity**

with a central hematocrit >65% is associated with hypoglycemia in at least 10–15% of affected infants. **Falciparum malaria** is associated with hyperinsulinemia and hypoglycemia. Heart and renal failure are also associated with hypoglycemia, but the mechanism is obscure.

DIAGNOSIS AND DIFFERENTIAL DIAGNOSIS

Table 111.8 and Fig. 111.5 list the pertinent clinical and biochemical findings in the common childhood disorders associated with hypoglycemia. A careful and detailed history is essential in every suspected or documented case of hypoglycemia (see Table 111.7). Specific points to note include age at onset, temporal relation to meals or caloric deprivation, and a family history of prior infants known to have had hypoglycemia or of unexplained infant deaths.

In the 1st week of life, most infants have the transient form of neonatal hypoglycemia either as a result of prematurity/intrauterine growth restriction or by virtue of being born to diabetic mothers. The absence of a history of maternal diabetes, but the presence of macrosomia and the characteristic large plethoric appearance of an infant of a diabetic mother, should arouse the possibility of hyperinsulinemic hypoglycemia of infancy, probably resulting from a K_{ATP} channel defect that is familial (autosomal recessive) or sporadic. Decreased β-hydroxybutyrate, low FFAs, and plasma insulin concentration >5 µU/mL or C-peptide >0.5 ng/mL in the presence of documented hypoglycemia confirm this diagnosis. The presence of hepatomegaly should arouse suspicion of an enzyme deficiency such as glucose-6-phosphatase in glycogen storage disease (GSD) I or other GSDs; if a non–glucose-reducing sugar is present in the urine (e.g., Clinitest positive but Clinistix negative), galactosemia is most likely. In males, the presence of a microphallus suggests the possibility of hypopituitarism, which also may be associated with cholestatic jaundice in both sexes; evidence of a midline facial defect such as cleft palate also suggests possible hypopituitarism as the cause of hypoglycemia from deficiency in GH and/or cortisol. A high index of suspicion and awareness of hypoglycemia as the cause for unusual behavior of any sick newborn should prompt a **bedside glucose determination**. However, because glucose meters have an accuracy of only ±20%, any blood glucose value <60 mg/dL *must be confirmed* by a formal laboratory measurement that is performed without delay on a blood sample preserved in a tube that prevents glycolysis, which can cause spurious low values.

After the newborn period, clues to the cause of persistent or recurrent hypoglycemia may be obtained through a careful history, physical examination, and initial laboratory findings. The temporal relation of the hypoglycemia to food intake may suggest that the defect is one of gluconeogenesis, if symptoms occur 6 hr or more after meals. If hypoglycemia occurs shortly after meals, **hyperinsulinism** should be suspected and confirmed or excluded via measurement of β-hydroxybutyrate, insulin, C-peptide, and FFAs in a sample in which blood glucose is <55 mg/dL. The autosomal dominant forms of hyperinsulinemic hypoglycemia need to be considered, with measurement of glucose, insulin, and ammonia and careful history for other affected family members of any age. Measurement of IGFBP-1 may be useful; it is low in states of hyperinsulinism and high in other forms of hypoglycemia. The presence of hepatomegaly suggests one of the **enzyme deficiencies** in glycogen breakdown or in gluconeogenesis, as outlined in Table 111.8. The absence of ketonemia or ketonuria at the initial presentation strongly suggests hyperinsulinism or a defect in fatty acid oxidation. In most other causes of hypoglycemia, with the exception of galactosemia and fructose intolerance, ketonemia and ketonuria are present at the time of fasting hypoglycemia. During hypoglycemia, serum should be obtained for determination of substrates, especially glucose, β-hydroxybutyrate, lactate, and FFAs, as well as hormones, especially insulin, C-peptide, cortisol, ACTH, and GH, followed by repeated measurement of glucose after an intramuscular or IV injection of glucagon, as outlined in Table 111.7. Table 111.8 summarizes the interpretation of the findings. Hypoglycemia with ketonuria in children between ages 18 mo and 5 yr is most likely to be **ketotic hypoglycemia**, especially if hepatomegaly is absent. The ingestion of a toxin, including alcohol or salicylate, can usually be excluded rapidly by the history. Inadvertent or deliberate drug ingestion and errors in dispensing medicines should also be considered. Factitious disorder

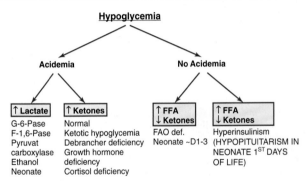

Fig. 111.5 Algorithm for diagnosis of hypoglycemia based on fasting fuel responses. FFA, Free fatty acids; F-1,6-Pase, fructose-1,6-diphosphatase; G-6-Pase, glucose-6-phosphatase; FAO def., fatty acid oxidation defects; D1-3, Days 1-3 of life.

(Munchausen) by proxy should be considered when parents or other caregivers have access to insulin or insulin secretagogues—high insulin concentrations in the sample with low concentrations of C-peptide confirm exogenous insulin administration. Deliberate or accidental ingestion of drugs that stimulate endogenous insulin secretion will result in both high insulin and C-peptide concentrations and may require specialized laboratory methods that identify the offending substance.

When the history is suggestive, but acute symptoms are not present, a 24 hr supervised fast can usually provoke hypoglycemia and resolve the question of hyperinsulinism or other conditions (see Table 111.8). Such a fast rarely needs to be extended to 36 hr, and only in older children. Such a fast is contraindicated if a fatty acid oxidation defect is suspected; other approaches such as mass tandem spectrometry or molecular diagnosis, or both, should be considered. Because adrenal insufficiency may mimic ketotic hypoglycemia, plasma cortisol and ACTH levels should be determined at the time of documented hypoglycemia; increased buccal or skin pigmentation may provide the clue to primary adrenal insufficiency with elevated ACTH (melanocyte-stimulating hormone) activity. Short stature or a decrease in the growth rate may provide the clue to pituitary insufficiency involving GH as well as ACTH. Definitive tests of pituitary-adrenal function, such as the arginine-insulin stimulation test for GH, IGF-1, IGFBP-1, and cortisol release, may be necessary.

In the presence of hepatomegaly and hypoglycemia, a presumptive diagnosis of the enzyme defect can often be made through the clinical manifestations, presence of hyperlipidemia, acidosis, hyperuricemia, response to glucagon in the fed and fasted states, and response to infusion of various appropriate precursors (see Table 111.7). Table 111.8 summarizes these clinical findings and investigative approaches. Definitive diagnosis of the GSD may require molecular diagnosis (see Chapter 105.1). Occasional patients with all the manifestations of GSD are found to have normal enzyme activity. These definitive studies require special expertise available only in certain institutions.

TREATMENT

The prevention of hypoglycemia and its resultant effects on CNS development are critically important in the newborn period. For neonates with hyperinsulinism not associated with maternal diabetes, subtotal or focal pancreatectomy may be needed, unless hypoglycemia can be readily controlled with long-term diazoxide, with somatostatin analogs (e.g., octreotide), or with sirolimus. Other novel approaches for treating hyperinsulinemic hypoglycemia are being investigated.

Treatment of **acute symptomatic** neonatal or infant hypoglycemia includes IV administration of 2 mL/kg of 10% dextrose in water (D10W), followed by a continuous infusion of glucose at 6-8 mg/kg/min, adjusting the rate to maintain blood glucose levels in the normal range. If hypoglycemic seizures are present, some recommend a 4 mL/kg bolus of D10W.

Treatment of asymptomatic hypoglycemia in at-risk infants usually includes enteral feedings rather than parenteral glucose. If symptoms develop or the hypoglycemia persists despite enteral feedings, IV glucose is indicated. Dextrose gel (40% at 400 mg/kg) administered into the mouth may be an alternative to enteral feedings if breast milk or if formula is not available.

The management of **persistent** neonatal or infantile hypoglycemia includes increasing the rate of IV glucose infusion to 10-15 mg/kg/min or more, if needed. This may require a central venous or umbilical venous catheter to administer a hypertonic 15–25% glucose solution. If hyperinsulinism is present, it should be medically managed initially with diazoxide and then somatostatin analogs. If hypoglycemia is unresponsive to IV glucose plus diazoxide (maximal doses up to 15 mg/kg/day) and somatostatin analogs, partial or near-total pancreatectomy should be considered. Such surgery should be performed in centers with the requisite facilities and trained staff experienced in the procedures. If possible, surgery should be preceded by ^{18}F-L-DOPA scanning to localize a lesion which can then provide guidance to the surgeon for curative resection before the operation is undertaken.

Oral **diazoxide**, 5-15 mg/kg/24 hr in divided doses twice daily, may reverse hyperinsulinemic hypoglycemia but may also produce hirsutism, edema, nausea, hyperuricemia, electrolyte disturbances, advanced bone age, IgG deficiency, and rarely, hypertension with prolonged use. The long-acting somatostatin analog **octreotide** may be helpful in controlling hyperinsulinism causing hypoglycemia in patients with islet cell disorders, including genetic mutations in K_{ATP} channel and islet cell adenoma. In neonates and young infants, **glucagon** given by continuous IV infusion at 5 μg/kg/hr, together with octreotide, 20-50 μg/kg/day subcutaneously every 6-12 hr, may maintain blood glucose, but generally these agents are used as a temporizing measure before partial or more complete pancreatectomy. Potential but unusual complications of octreotide include poor growth because of impaired GH release, pain at the injection site, vomiting, diarrhea, and hepatic dysfunction (hepatitis, cholelithiasis), and necrotizing enterocolitis; tachyphylaxis to the drug's effects is more common. Octreotide may be particularly useful for the treatment of refractory hypoglycemia despite subtotal pancreatectomy.

Total pancreatectomy is not optimal therapy because of the risks of surgery, permanent diabetes mellitus, and exocrine pancreatic insufficiency. Continued prolonged medical therapy without pancreatic resection, if hypoglycemia is controllable, is worthwhile because over time some children have a spontaneous resolution of the hyperinsulinism-induced hypoglycemia. This should be balanced against the risk of hypoglycemia-induced CNS injury and the toxicity of drugs.

PROGNOSIS

The prognosis is good in asymptomatic neonates with hypoglycemia of short duration. Hypoglycemia recurs in 10–15% of infants after adequate treatment. Recurrence is more common if IV fluids are extravasated or discontinued too rapidly before oral feedings are well tolerated. Children who had transient neonatal hypoglycemia have an increased incidence of ketotic hypoglycemia later in life.

The prognosis for normal intellectual function must be guarded because prolonged, recurrent, and severe symptomatic hypoglycemia is associated with neurologic sequelae. Symptomatic infants with hypoglycemia, particularly low-birthweight infants, those with persistent hyperinsulinemic hypoglycemia, and severely hypoglycemic infants born to poorly controlled diabetic mothers, have a poorer prognosis for subsequent normal intellectual development than asymptomatic infants.

Bibliography is available at Expert Consult.

The Fetus and the Neonatal Infant
胎儿及新生儿

Chapter 112
Overview of Morbidity and Mortality
James M. Greenberg

第一百一十二章
死亡率和患病率概述

中文导读

本章主要从公共卫生的角度介绍了目前新生儿死亡率的流行病学资料，并专门介绍了美国新生儿死亡率在全球的大致排名情况，以及近几年来全球新生儿死亡率的变化趋势。同时，本章介绍了新生儿及婴儿死亡的主要原因，特别是不同人种新生儿和婴儿死亡率的差别、先天畸形的患病情况，以及与睡眠相关的新生儿死亡发生状况（包括SUID,SIDS）。另外，本章还采用较多的图标和数据介绍了近年来美国本土早产儿、近足月早产儿、胎龄中等的早产儿、低出生体重儿、宫内生长发育受限的新生儿以及小于胎龄儿的死亡率降低的情况。

INFANT MORTALITY

The **infant mortality rate** is a metric used by public health agencies, policymakers, and governments to gauge the overall quality of pediatric and population health among a given population residing within geographically defined boundaries. The rate is stated as the number of infant deaths per 1,000 live births. Specific definitions support each variable. In the United States, an *infant death* is defined as mortality taking place from the time after delivery at any gestational age, up to the 1st birthday. No age correction is made to account for a premature birth. Each infant death is assigned to a geographic entity (e.g., county, state, country) on the basis of the mother's home address at the time of death. The definition of a *live birth* is typically based on the complete expulsion of the productions of conception from the uterus and 1 of 3 criteria: detection of cardiac activity (by auscultation or palpation of the umbilical cord stump), definite movement generated by voluntary muscle contraction, or any respiratory effort. It is important to note that this definition does not incorporate any gestational age cutoff.

The risk of mortality and major morbidity is particularly high around the time of birth (Fig. 112.1). Therefore, within the spectrum of infant mortality, certain subcategories are used in maternal and child health practice to focus on specific periods of high risk. The **perinatal period** is typically defined as the time from the 28th wk of pregnancy through the 7th postpartum day. The **neonatal period** spans the 1st 28 days of life and can be further subdivided into *early neonatal* (1st 7 days) and *late neonatal* (days 8-28) (Fig. 112.2). The primary causes of mortality shift as infancy progresses: during the perinatal and neonatal periods, **preterm birth** (Fig. 112.3) and **congenital malformations** predominate, whereas **unsafe sleep practices** accounts for the majority of deaths during the remainder of infancy. In developing countries with limited resources, preterm birth remains a concern, but other causes, such as infection, birth asphyxia, and complications of labor and delivery, add an additional burden (see Fig. 112.2).

Rankings and Trends

Over the past century, infant mortality rates have declined in the United

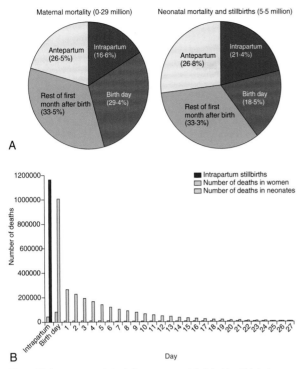

Fig. 112.1 A, Timing of death for women and their babies (third-trimester stillbirths and neonatal deaths) during pregnancy, birth, and the postnatal period. Includes all deaths of mothers and their babies from 28 wk of gestation up to 28 days of life. **B,** Number of deaths during labor and the 1st month after birth of women and their babies (intrapartum stillbirths and neonates). Insufficient data were available to accurately assign the day of death for the 1.4 million antepartum stillbirths and 63,000 maternal deaths occurring during the last trimester of pregnancy (before the onset of labor). *(From Lawn JE, Blencowe H, Oza S, et al: Every newborn: progress, priorities, and potential beyond survival. Lancet 384:189–202, 2014, Fig 5.)*

Table 112.1	Infant Mortality Rate per 1,000 Live Births (IMR) for Select Developed Countries, 2010		
COUNTRY	**IMR**	**COUNTRY**	**IMR**
Finland	2.3	United Kingdom	4.2
Japan	2.3	United States	6.1
Greece	3.8		

Data from the National Center for Health Statistics: *Natl Vital Stat Rep* 63(5):1, 2014 (Fig 1). https://www.cdc.gov/nchs/data/nvsr/nvsr63/nvsr63_05.pdf.

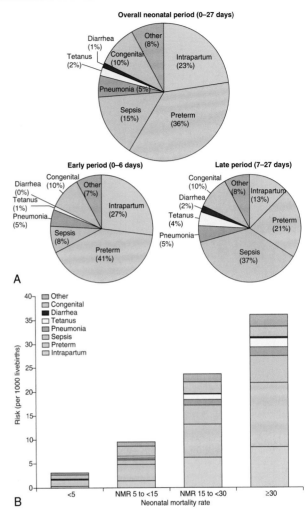

Fig. 112.2 A, Cause of death distribution for the neonatal period, and by the early (<7 days) and late (7–28 days) neonatal periods, for 194 countries in 2012. **B,** Variation in cause-specific neonatal mortality rates (NMRs) by level of NMR in 2012, showing risk difference by cause of death compared with the lowest mortality group (NMR <5). Data from Child Health Epidemiology Reference Group and World Health Organization (WHO) estimates for 194 countries for 2012. Estimates are based on multicause statistical models. In 2012, an additional estimated 196,000 deaths occurred in the postneonatal period from neonatal conditions (preterm birth, intrapartum related) and an estimated further 309,000 from term, small for gestational age. *(From Lawn JE, Blencowe H, Oza S, et al: Every newborn: progress, priorities, and potential beyond survival, Lancet 384:189–202, 2014, Fig 6.)*

States and across most of the world. However, rates continue to differ worldwide. In general, the highest rates are observed in low-resource, developing countries. However, the United States remains an anomaly among nations in the developed world. Table 112.1 shows infant mortality rates from a representative sample of developed countries. The rates are adjusted to exclude deaths before 24 wk gestation to account for potential variation in definitions of live births that might occur at the threshold of viability, to ensure comparability. Beginning in the 1980s, U.S. rates began to consistently exceed other developed nations; in 2015, U.S. infant mortality rates were >2-fold higher than in many developed countries. A wide range of infant mortality rates is also observed, with the highest rates in the Southeast United

States and lower rates in the Upper Midwest, the Northeast, and the West Coast.

MAJOR CAUSES OF INFANT DEATH

In the United States and Europe, most infant deaths fall into 1 of 3 major categories of causation: preterm birth, congenital malformations, and sleep related (e.g., SIDS). Infections, trauma, birth asphyxia, and injuries account for the remainder. The pattern differs in the developing world, where infections and asphyxia predominate. When considered based on the classification of infant cause of death by the *International Classification of Diseases, Tenth Revision,* congenital malformations are the leading cause, followed by disorders related to prematurity and low

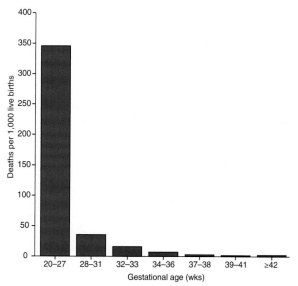

* Deaths in children aged <12 months per 1,000 live births.

Fig. 112.3 Infant mortality rates by gestational age—United States, 2013. Deaths in children age <12 mo per 1,000 live births. *(From Shapiro-Mendoza CK, Barfield WD, Henderson Z, et al: CDC Grand Rounds: Public health strategies to prevent preterm birth, MMWR 65(32):826–830, 2016, p 827.)*

birthweight. Nonetheless, preterm birth rather than congenital malformations accounts for the majority of infant deaths in the United States, when deaths from unique complications of prematurity are included.

The U.S. preterm birth rate is substantially higher than in other developed countries and best explains elevated U.S. infant mortality rates. Worldwide, preterm birth rates display a tight concordance with infant mortality rates, providing further evidence for the importance of this linkage (Fig. 112.4). In the era of modern neonatal intensive care, most preterm birth deaths occur among the earliest gestational ages (<28 wk), and within the 1st few days of life, because of profound respiratory immaturity and insufficiency. The remaining preterm birth deaths result from morbidities associated with prematurity. Late preterm birth (35-36 wk gestation) is not a significant contributor to infant mortality.

International variation in live-birth registration practices may explain the elevated U.S. infant mortality. Although these technical explanations deserve further investigation, they should not be used to justify high U.S. infant mortality. In the United States, where live-birth registration practices are consistent, substantial variation in infant mortality and preterm birth rates implies *systemic* rather than technical explanations.

Racial Disparity and Infant Mortality

There is a significant disparity between infant mortality rates among U.S.-born white and black (African American) infants. This difference persists, even when socioeconomic status (SES) and educational levels are considered. The disparity is restricted to blacks; Hispanic populations in the United States tend to have infant mortality rates in line with the white population. Understanding this *Hispanic paradox* may provide insight into mechanisms driving the African American disparity. Interestingly, South Asian (Indian) populations in the United States may also have elevated infant mortality driven by low birthweight. Preterm birth and low birthweight are the key drivers of the black infant mortality disparity. Black preterm births rates are twice that of other U.S. racial and ethnic groups (Fig. 112.5), a gap that has persisted for decades. This is especially true for preterm birth rates at very low gestational ages, <28 wk, where mortality risks are high, even with the availability of modern neonatal intensive care units (NICUs). Racial

disparities of mortality are not present among those receiving NICU care. Mechanistic explanations for the racial disparity remain elusive. Theories based on concepts of lifetime stress from experiences of racism or adverse life events are compelling (Chapter 2.1) However, studies focusing on stress and pregnancy outcomes fail to demonstrate clear mechanistic links.

Congenital Malformations

Infant deaths from congenital malformations are the 2nd leading cause of infant death after premature birth. Many disorders reside in this category, with **congenital heart disease** the leading etiology. From a public health perspective, specific interventions can reduce the potential for certain congenital malformations, most notably periconceptional folic acid intake and appropriate vaccination programs to prevent diseases such as rubella during pregnancy. However, the mechanism of most congenital malformations remains poorly understood and therefore not yet amenable to population-based prevention strategies. In contrast to preterm birth, there is no discernible racial disparity for mortality caused by congenital malformations in the United States.

Sleep-Related Deaths (SUID, SIDS)

Sudden unexpected infant death (SUID) is a sudden and unexpected death during infancy. Following a thorough investigation of the death, SUID may be explained through mechanisms such as cosleeping and suffocation, or airway obstruction caused by soft objects or excessive bedding. **Sudden infant death syndrome (SIDS)** is a subcategory of SUID assigned to SUIDS that cannot be explained after a thorough investigation, including postmortem examination (see Chapter 402). SIDS represents a small fraction of all sleep-related deaths. With the advent of effective public health messaging, rates of sleep-related deaths in the United States have declined. However, a wide variation of rates is still observed across different geographic jurisdictions. SUID rates also display a racial disparity. The leading cause of infant death beyond the neonatal period is **unsafe infant sleep practices**.

INFANT MORTALITY REDUCTION

Reduction of U.S. infant mortality is a challenging but attainable goal. Decreasing the preterm birth rate, especially extreme prematurity before 28 wk gestation, is an imperative. Improving our understanding of the biologic factors that control gestational duration and initiation of labor and delivery is key. Studies of intramuscular (but not vaginal) progesterone treatment during pregnancy for women known to be at elevated risk for a preterm birth have proved promising. However, the mechanism of action is not well understood, and the public health impact appears limited except perhaps for women with a previous preterm birth. Improving our understanding of how social determinants of health and health behavior influence birth outcomes is also important. **Smoking** during pregnancy is known to drive low birthweight, preterm birth, and elevated mortality. Improving interventions to eliminate smoking during pregnancy should reduce infant mortality. Understanding mechanistic links between the biology of parturition and the social and behavioral determinants of health is imperative.

Preterm Birth

Preterm birth is defined as a live birth occurring before the 37th wk of gestation. Comparison of preterm births between countries or other jurisdictions can be compromised by methods used to calculate gestational age. Three approaches are currently in use: **last menstrual period** (LMP), **obstetric estimate** (OE), and a **combined estimate**. The last defers to the LMP *unless* the value is missing from the vital record information or is extremely inconsistent with the recorded birthweight. In this circumstance (0.4% of record in 2013) the combined method uses the OE value. From a public health perspective, the OE offers superior validity. Since 2014 reports by federal agencies and stakeholder organizations (e.g., March of Dimes) use the OE to state preterm birth rates. The OE is typically a 1–2% lower preterm birth rate than the LMP or combined method. In 2016 the national preterm birth rate based on OE was 9.84%, compared to an 11.40% rate using the combined method.

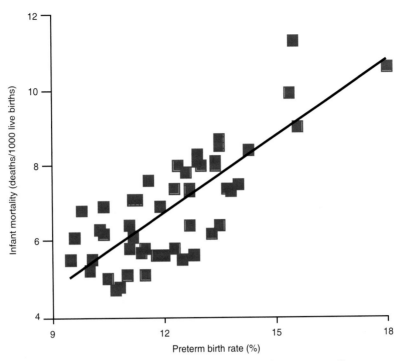

Fig. 112.4 Preterm birth as a function of infant mortality rates for 40 countries. *(Data courtesy of L. Muglia, MD, PhD, Cincinnati Children's Research Foundation.)*

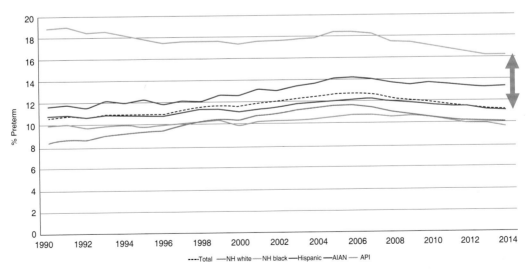

‐‐‐‐Total ——NH white——NH black——Hispanic ——AIAN —— API

Fig. 112.5 The gap between black and white preterm birth rates in the United States has persisted for >3 decades. NH, Non-Hispanic; AIAN, American Indian/Alaskan Native; API, Asian/Pacific Islander. *(Data from the National Center for Health Statistics.)*

Table 112.2	Major Morbidities of the Neonate and Associated Etiologic Conditions
MORBIDITIES	**EXAMPLES OF ETIOLOGY**
CENTRAL NERVOUS SYSTEM	
Spastic diplegic/quadriplegic cerebral palsy	HIE, periventricular leukomalacia, undetermined factors
Choreoathetotic cerebral palsy	Kernicterus/bilirubin encephalopathy
Microcephaly	Intrauterine infections
Hydrocephalus	IVH, HIE, meningitis
Seizures	HIE, encephalopathies, hypoglycemia
Learning disorders, developmental delay	Prematurity, HIE, hypoglycemia, IVH
SENSATION—PERIPHERAL NEUROPATHIES	
Visual impairments	Retinopathy of prematurity, congenital viral infection
Strabismus	Opioid exposure, undetermined
Hearing impairment	HIE, bilirubin toxicity, drug toxicity (loop diuretics, aminoglycosides)
Speech delay	Prematurity, prolonged endotracheal intubation, hearing loss
Paralysis, paresis	Birth trauma (usually affected: phrenic nerve, brachial plexus, spinal cord)
RESPIRATORY SYSTEM	
Bronchopulmonary dysplasia	Prematurity, positive pressure ventilation, oxygen exposure
Subglottic stenosis	Prolonged endotracheal intubation
Sudden unexpected infant death	Prematurity, unsafe sleep conditions
Choanal stenosis, nasal septum injury	Prolonged nasotracheal intubation, nasal CPAP
CARDIOVASCULAR SYSTEM	
Cyanosis	Pulmonary hypertension, cor pulmonale, severe BPD
Heart failure	PDA, congenital heart defects with left-to-right shunting
GASTROINTESTINAL SYSTEM	
Short gut syndrome	NEC, malrotation with mid-gut volvulus, bowel atresia
Cholestatic liver disease	Injury from prolonged parenteral nutrition, sepsis, short gut syndrome
Failure to thrive	Short gut syndrome, BPD, cyanotic heart disease
Inguinal hernia	Preterm birth, male gender, positive pressure ventilation
MISCELLANEOUS	
Cutaneous scarring	Cutis aplasia, chest tube placement
Hypertension	Renal thrombi, prolonged umbilical artery catheterization, unknown

BPD, Bronchopulmonary dysplasia; CPAP, continuous positive airway pressure; HIE, hypoxia-ischemic encephalopathy; IVH, intraventricular hemorrhage; NEC, necrotizing colitis; PDA, patent ductus arteriosus.

The mortality and morbidity challenges encountered by a newborn delivered at 36 wk differ in severity from delivery at 25 wk. Subcategories of preterm birth corresponding to late (35-36 wk), moderate (32-34 wk), and early (<32 wk) acknowledge important differences in morbidity and mortality risk. From an infant mortality perspective, an additional subcategory of the early preterm population, *extreme preterm* births (<28 wk) has substantial importance, because >50% of all infant deaths occur in this population.

In addition to socioeconomic and racial factors, genetic variables may be associated with pregnancy duration and risk for preterm birth. Variants in *EBF1, EEFSEC, AGTR2, WNT4, ADCY5,* and *RAP2C* are reported to be associated with pregnancy length, whereas variants in *EBF1, EEFSEC,* and *AGTR2* loci are associated with preterm birth. In addition, 7 unrelated free RNA transcripts in maternal blood cells have been found to predict preterm delivery. These results are preliminary but may add specific targets for prevention of prematurity.

The Late Preterm Neonate
There is an important appreciation for the significance of late preterm delivery. Often these infants seem similar to their term counterparts, but epidemiologic data demonstrate that they are at significantly higher risk for apneic episodes, disorders of thermoregulation (e.g., hypothermia), hypoglycemia, respiratory distress, feeding difficulties, dehydration, and suspected sepsis. They are more likely to require NICU admission and experience an extended hospital stay. Late preterm neonates also appear to have a higher risk for longer-term neurologic problems, such as attention-deficit disorders and learning disabilities.

Late preterm deliveries may result from complications of pregnancy (e.g., chorioamnionitis, premature rupture of membranes) or maternal conditions (e.g., preeclampsia). Many are caused by elective delivery through induction of labor or scheduled cesarean birth during the late

preterm period. As appreciation grew for an elevated morbidity and mortality risk in late preterm infants, a movement to eliminate elective deliveries before 39 wk gained national traction. The Ohio Perinatal Quality Collaborative initiated a statewide quality improvement initiative to eliminate elective deliveries before 39 wk of gestation through establishment of a multihospital learning network. Their work led to a material and sustained reduction of elective deliveries, with attendant reductions in neonatal morbidity and hospital length of stay.

The Moderate and Early Preterm Neonate
As gestational age at delivery declines, morbidity and mortality risks increase. With modern neonatal intensive care, the potential for survival at a given gestational age has improved. With that, the *threshold* gestational age for offering comprehensive neonatal intensive care has correspondingly declined. However, assigning a specific gestational age for threshold of viability remains a challenging problem. Current published data suggest minimal life-sustaining impact for neonatal intensive care offered before 22-23 wk gestation. However, covariables such as birthweight and perhaps exposure to antenatal steroids must be considered. Neonates born at extremely early gestational ages are at very high risk for morbidities carrying lifelong consequences. Major morbidities of prematurity contribute to infant mortality after the early neonatal period (e.g., BPD, IVH, NEC, PDA). All are more common in extremely premature infants, and when present, each can prolong NICU length of stay or may be listed as an immediate cause of death. Therefore, multidisciplinary decision-making with direct family participation is essential.

Preterm neonates at moderate and early gestational ages are at elevated risk for all the complications of late prematurity. Additional categories of morbidity that are absent or extremely rare in the late preterm and term populations also become much more common at earlier gestational ages (Table 112.2). These include adverse **neurodevelopmental** sequelae such as cerebral palsy, periventricular leukomalacia, intraventricular hemorrhage, hydrocephalus, visual impairment, and hearing impairment. Problems affecting other major organ systems include bronchopulmonary dysplasia, necrotizing enterocolitis, and patent ductus arteriosus. Early preterm infants are at the highest risk for these complications, which also tend to be more severe.

Intraventricular hemorrhage (IVH) occurs when the very fragile capillaries of the periventricular white matter and choroid plexus rupture. The typical pathophysiology is accumulation of blood in the lateral ventricles, which can lead to obstruction of cerebrospinal fluid circulation and ultimately hydrocephalus.

Bronchopulmonary dysplasia (BPD) is a complication of respiratory distress syndrome and prematurity leading to reactive airway disease, alveolar insufficiency, and in severe cases, pulmonary hypertension and death. BPD remains the most common morbidity of prematurity among NICU survivors. The most powerful predictor of BPD is gestational age: as gestational age decreases, the risk of BPD increases. Oxygen exposure and treatment with positive pressure ventilation also increase the risk of developing BPD at any gestational age.

Necrotizing enterocolitis (NEC) is a devastating inflammatory process that can occur anywhere in the lower gastrointestinal tract, most often at the distal ilium and ascending colon. In approximately 40% of patients, surgical exploration and resection of necrotic bowel is required, increasing potential for failure to thrive, malabsorption, and short bowel syndrome. Those at the lowest gestational ages are at the highest risk. Interestingly, preterm infants at the earliest gestational ages tend to develop NEC later in their hospital course than moderate or late preterm infants, suggesting a developmental window of susceptibility.

Patent ductus arteriosus (PDA) is a common finding in preterm neonates born before 28 wk. The ductus arteriosus must be patent during intrauterine life to sustain fetal circulation. Under normal physiologic conditions, the ductus undergoes functional closure within a few minutes of parturition. However, under conditions of marginal oxygenation and ventilation, ductal closure in preterm infants may be delayed. If ductal patency persists, it can promote pulmonary overcirculation, complicating the management of respiratory disease.

Low Birthweight, Intrauterine Growth Restriction, and Small for Gestational Age

Low birthweight (LBW) is classified as any live birth <2,500 g. The **very-low-birthweight (VLBW)** subcategory corresponds to <1,500 g. In general, LBW and VLBW infants are also preterm, although other intrauterine conditions discussed below also contribute. **Intrauterine growth restriction (IUGR)** refers to deficiency of fetal growth and an abnormal fetal growth trajectory. Etiologies of IUGR include certain congenital infections (e.g., rubella, cytomegalovirus), placental insufficiency, environmental factors (e.g., maternal smoking), and certain congenital conditions (e.g., aneuploidy). In contrast, **small-for-gestational-age (SGA)** neonates are constitutionally normal, without known genetic abnormalities or pathologic conditions. SGA and IUGR may occur at any gestational age. Birthweight and gestational age combine to predict mortality and morbidity risk at any gestational age. Healthcare providers can use an online mortality calculator developed by the National Institute of Child Health and Human Development (NICHD) Neonatal Research Network that incorporates gestational age and birthweight to assist with prenatal counseling for families anticipating a preterm delivery.

Bibliography is available at Expert Consult.

Chapter **113**
The Newborn Infant
Neera K. Goyal

第一百一十三章
新生儿

中文导读

　　本章的内容与第二十一章的相关内容相互呼应补充。本章主要介绍了新生儿医学的发展史、新生婴儿的体格检查、新生儿的常规看护和护理、新生儿包皮环切、新生儿与其母亲的母子亲情5个方面的内容。其中新生婴儿的体格检查部分按照从头到脚的顺序，分别介绍了皮肤、颅骨、面部、颈部、胸、肺、心脏、腹、外生殖器、肛门、四肢的体格检查特点和意义。关于新生

儿神经系统体格检查的相关内容请参阅第二十章。关于新生儿的常规护理，本章介绍了如何维持新生儿的正常体温、新生儿皮肤护理和脐带消毒的方法和意义，以及新生儿筛查3个方面的内容。比较有特色的是，本章还专门介绍了新生儿与其母亲的母子亲情，包括母婴同室、新生儿住院期间的家长陪住、母亲用药期间的母乳喂养注意事项、母乳喂养的禁忌证等。

See also Chapter 21.

Although the neonatal period is a highly vulnerable time as infants complete the many physiologic adjustments required for extrauterine existence, this transition is uneventful for most full-term infants. Management of the newborn should focus on parental anticipatory guidance and early detection of conditions or complications that carry risk of morbidity or even death.

113.1 History in Neonatal Pediatrics
Neera K. Goyal

Assessment of the newborn should begin with a review of the maternal and family history, the pregnancy, and the delivery. Details of this history should include the following information, which will guide further evaluation and management in the newborn period:

- Demographic and social data (socioeconomic status, age, race, prenatal care utilization, substance use). Newborns whose mothers are young (<18 yr old) or who have concerns regarding housing, food insecurity, or access to healthcare may warrant evaluation by a social worker or case manager. Newborns exposed in utero to substances such as alcohol, cocaine, nicotine, caffeine, and opioids should be evaluated for associated symptoms (see Chapter 126).
- Maternal medical conditions (cardiopulmonary disorders, infectious diseases, genetic disorders, anemia, diabetes mellitus, current medications). Newborns of diabetic mothers warrant screening within the 1st 24 hr of life for severe hypoglycemia (see Chapter 127.1).
- Past medical illnesses in the mother and family, including previous siblings with a history of jaundice (see Chapter 123.3).
- Previous maternal reproductive problems: stillbirth, prematurity, blood group sensitization (see Chapter 124).
- Events occurring in the present pregnancy (prenatal laboratory and imaging results, preterm labor, fetal assessments, vaginal bleeding, acute illness, duration of rupture of membranes). Such information may prompt additional newborn testing, such as rapid plasma reagin (RPR) testing in the case of a positive maternal syphilis screen, or renal ultrasound imaging if fetal pyelectasis was detected prenatally.
- Description of the labor (duration, fetal presentation, fetal distress, fever) and delivery (cesarean section, anesthesia or sedation, use of forceps, Apgar scores, need for resuscitation). This information, combined with clinical assessment of the newborn, will determine risk for clinical deterioration and need for further monitoring and intervention.

113.2 Physical Examination of the Newborn Infant
Neera K. Goyal

Many physical and behavioral characteristics of a normal newborn infant are described in Chapter 21.

The **initial examination** of a newborn infant should be performed as soon as possible after delivery. Temperature, pulse, respiratory rate, color, signs of respiratory distress, tone, activity, and level of consciousness of infants should be monitored frequently until stabilization. For high-risk deliveries, this examination should take place in the delivery room and should focus on congenital anomalies, maturation and growth, and pathophysiologic problems that may interfere with normal cardiopulmonary and metabolic adaptation to extrauterine life. Congenital anomalies of varying degrees of severity may be present in 3–5% of infants. After a stable delivery room course, a second and more detailed examination should be performed within 24 hr of birth.

If an infant remains in the hospital longer than 48 hr, repeat assessments should be performed throughout the hospital stay including a discharge examination within 24 hr of discharge. For a healthy infant, the mother should be present during this examination; even minor,

seemingly insignificant anatomic variations may worry the parents and should be explained. The explanation must be careful and skillful so that otherwise unworried parents are not unduly alarmed. Infants should not be discharged from the hospital without a final examination because certain abnormalities, particularly cyanosis and heart murmurs, often appear or disappear in the immediate neonatal period; in addition, evidence of disease that has just been acquired may be noted. The pulse (normal: 120-160 beats/min), respiratory rate (normal: 30-60 breaths/min), temperature, weight, length, head circumference, and dimensions of any visible or palpable structural abnormality should be assessed. Blood pressure is determined if a neonate appears ill or has a heart murmur. Pulse oximetry should be performed to screen for critical congenital heart disease and is part of the routine screening for newborn infants.

Examining a newborn requires patience, gentleness, and procedural flexibility. Thus, if the infant is quiet and relaxed at the beginning of the examination, palpation of the abdomen or auscultation of the heart should be performed first, before other, more intrusive manipulations are attempted.

GENERAL APPEARANCE
Physical activity may be decreased by the effects of illness or drugs; an infant may be either lying with the extremities motionless, to conserve energy for the effort of difficult breathing, or vigorously crying, with accompanying activity of the arms and legs. Both active and passive muscle tone and any unusual posture should be noted. Coarse, tremulous movements with ankle or jaw **myoclonus** are more common and less significant in newborn infants than at any other age. Such movements tend to occur when an infant is active, whereas convulsive twitching usually occurs in a quiet state. **Edema** may produce a superficial appearance of good nutrition. Pitting after applied pressure may or may not be noted, but the skin of the fingers and toes lacks the normal fine wrinkles when filled with fluid. Edema of the eyelids commonly results from irritation caused by the administration of silver nitrate. Generalized edema may occur with prematurity, hypoproteinemia secondary to severe erythroblastosis fetalis, nonimmune hydrops, congenital nephrosis, Hurler syndrome, and from unknown causes. Localized edema suggests a congenital malformation of the lymphatic system; when confined to one or more extremities of a female infant, it may be the initial sign of Turner syndrome (see Chapters 98 and 604).

SKIN
Vasomotor instability and peripheral circulatory sluggishness are revealed by deep redness or purple lividity in a crying infant, whose color may darken profoundly with closure of the glottis preceding a vigorous cry, and by harmless cyanosis (**acrocyanosis**) of the hands and feet, especially when they are cool. Mottling, another example of general circulatory instability, may be associated with serious illness or related to a transient fluctuation in skin temperature. An extraordinary division of the body from the forehead to the pubis into red and pale halves is known as *harlequin color change*, a transient and harmless condition. Significant **cyanosis** may be masked by the pallor of circulatory failure or anemia; alternatively, the relatively high hemoglobin content of the 1st few days and the thin skin may combine to produce an appearance of cyanosis at a higher partial pressure of arterial oxygen (PaO_2) than in older children. Localized cyanosis is differentiated from *ecchymosis* by the momentary blanching pallor (with cyanosis) that occurs after pressure. The same maneuver also helps in demonstrating icterus. **Pallor** may be caused by anemia, asphyxia, shock, or edema. Early recognition of anemia may lead to a diagnosis of fetomaternal blood transfusion, erythroblastosis fetalis, subcapsular hematoma of the liver or spleen, subdural hemorrhage, or fetal-maternal or twin-twin transfusion. Without being anemic, postmature infants tend to have paler and thicker skin than term or premature infants. The ruddy appearance of plethora is seen with polycythemia.

The vernix and common transitory macular capillary hemangiomas of the eyelids and neck are described in Chapter 669. Cavernous hemangiomas are deeper, blue masses that, if large, may trap platelets and produce disseminated intravascular coagulation or interfere with local organ function. Scattered petechiae may be seen on the presenting

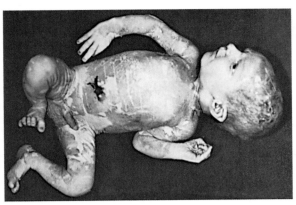

Fig. 113.1 Infant with intrauterine growth restriction as a result of placental insufficiency. Note the long, thin appearance with peeling, parchment-like dry skin, alert expression, meconium staining of the skin, and long nails. (*From Clifford S: Advances in pediatrics, vol 9, Chicago, 1962, Year Book.*)

Table 113.1	Disorders Associated with a Large Anterior Fontanel

Hypothyroidism
Achondroplasia
Apert syndrome
Cleidocranial dysostosis
Congenital rubella syndrome
Hallermann-Streiff syndrome
Hydrocephaly
Hypophosphatasia
Intrauterine growth restriction
Kenny syndrome
Osteogenesis imperfecta
Prematurity
Pyknodysostosis
Russell-Silver syndrome
Trisomies 13, 18, and 21
Vitamin D deficiency rickets

part (usually the scalp or face) after a difficult delivery. Slate-blue, well-demarcated areas of pigmentation called **mongolian spots** are seen over the buttocks, back, and sometimes other parts of the body in more than 50% of black, Native American, and Asian infants, and occasionally in white infants. These benign patches have no known anthropologic significance despite their name; they tend to disappear within the 1st year. The vernix, skin, and especially the cord may be stained brownish yellow if the amniotic fluid has been colored by the passage of meconium during or before birth.

The skin of premature infants is thin and delicate and tends to be deep red; in extremely premature infants, the skin appears almost gelatinous and translucent. Fine, soft, immature hair called **lanugo** frequently covers the scalp and brow and may also cover the face of premature infants. Lanugo has usually been lost or replaced by vellus hair in term infants. **Tufts of hair** over the lumbosacral spine suggest an underlying abnormality, such as occult spina bifida, a sinus tract, or a tumor. The nails are rudimentary in very premature infants, but they may protrude beyond the fingertips in infants born past term. Postterm infants may have a peeling, parchment-like skin (Fig. 113.1), a severe degree of which may mimic **ichthyosis congenita** (see Chapter 677).

In many neonates, small, white papules on an erythematous base develop 1-3 days after birth. This benign rash, **erythema toxicum**, persists for as long as 1 wk, contains eosinophils, and is usually distributed on the face, trunk, and extremities (see Chapter 666). **Pustular melanosis**, a benign lesion seen predominantly in black neonates, contains neutrophils and is present at birth as a vesiculopustular eruption around the chin, neck, back, extremities, and palms or soles; it lasts 2-3 days. Both lesions need to be distinguished from more dangerous vesicular eruptions such as herpes simplex (see Chapter 279) and staphylococcal disease of the skin (Chapter 208.1).

Amniotic bands may disrupt the skin, extremities (amputation, ring constriction, syndactyly), face (clefts), or trunk (abdominal or thoracic wall defects). Their cause is uncertain but may be related to amniotic membrane rupture or vascular compromise with fibrous band formation. Excessive skin fragility and extensibility with joint hypermobility suggest Ehlers-Danlos syndrome (see Chapter 679), Marfan syndrome (Chapter 722), congenital contractural arachnodactyly, and other disorders of collagen synthesis.

SKULL

The skull may be molded, particularly if the infant is the first-born and if the head has been engaged in the pelvic canal for a considerable time. **Caput succedaneum**, caused by scalp pressure from the uterus, cervix, or pelvis, appears as a circular boggy area of edema with indistinct borders and often with overlying ecchymosis. A **cephalohematoma** presents as a well-circumscribed fluid-filled mass that does not cross suture lines. Unlike caput succedaneum, cephalohematoma is often not present at delivery but develops over the 1st few hr of life. Both cephalohematoma and caput succedaneum must be distinguished from a **subgaleal hemorrhage**, which is not restricted by the boundaries of the sutures and therefore is larger and more diffuse. Subgaleal hemorrhage requires prompt recognition because extensive bleeding may result in hypovolemic shock, with estimated mortality up to 20%. The head circumference of all newborns should be plotted on a growth chart to identify an excessively small head (**microcephaly**) or excessively large head (**megalencephaly**). The diagnostic differential for microcephaly is broad and includes underlying genetic disorders, congenital infection, and intrauterine drug exposure (see Chapter 609). Megalencephaly can suggest hydrocephaly, storage disease, achondroplasia, cerebral gigantism, neurocutaneous syndromes, or inborn errors of metabolism, or it may be familial. The suture lines and the size and fullness of the anterior and posterior fontanels should be determined digitally by palpation. The parietal bones tend to override the occipital and frontal bones. Premature fusion of sutures (**cranial synostosis**) is identified as a hard nonmovable ridge over the suture and an abnormally shaped skull. Great variation in the size of the **fontanels** exists at birth; if small, the anterior fontanel usually tends to enlarge during the 1st few mo after birth. The persistence of excessively large anterior (normal: 20 ±10 mm) and posterior fontanels has been associated with several disorders (Table 113.1). Persistently small fontanels suggest microcephaly, craniosynostosis, congenital hyperthyroidism, or wormian bones; presence of a 3rd fontanel suggests trisomy 21 but is seen in preterm infants. Soft areas (**craniotabes**) are occasionally found in the parietal bones at the vertex near the sagittal suture; they are more common in preterm infants and in infants who have been exposed to uterine compression. Although such soft areas are usually insignificant, their possible pathologic cause should be investigated if they persist. Soft areas in the occipital region suggest the irregular calcification and wormian bone formation associated with osteogenesis imperfecta, cleidocranial dysostosis, lacunar skull, cretinism, and occasionally Down syndrome.

Atrophic or alopecic scalp areas may represent **aplasia cutis congenita**, which may be sporadic, or autosomal dominant, or associated with trisomy 13, chromosome 4 deletion, or Johanson-Blizzard syndrome. **Deformational plagiocephaly** may be the result of in utero positioning forces on the skull and manifests as an asymmetric skull and face with ear malalignment (see Chapter 610). It is associated with torticollis and vertex positioning. Depression of the skull (indentation, fracture, Ping-Pong ball deformity) is usually of prenatal onset and a result of prolonged focal pressure by the maternal pelvic bone.

FACE

The general appearance of the face should be noted with regard to **dysmorphic features**, such as epicanthal folds, widely or narrowly spaced eyes, microphthalmos, asymmetry, long philtrum, and low-set ears, which are often associated with congenital syndromes. The face may be asymmetric as a result of a 7th nerve palsy, hypoplasia of the depressor muscle at the angle of the mouth, or an abnormal fetal posture (see Chapter 128); when the jaw has been held against a shoulder or an extremity during the intrauterine period, the mandible may deviate strikingly from the midline. Symmetric facial palsy suggests absence or hypoplasia of the 7th nerve nucleus (**Möbius syndrome**).

Eyes

The eyes often open spontaneously if the infant is held up and tipped gently forward and backward. This maneuver, a result of labyrinthine and neck reflexes, is more successful for inspecting the eyes than is forcing the lids apart. Conjunctival and retinal hemorrhages are usually benign. Retinal hemorrhages are more common with vacuum- or forceps-assisted deliveries than spontaneous vaginal delivery and least common after cesarean section. They are usually bilateral, intraretinal, and in the posterior pole. They resolve in most infants by 2 wk of age (85%) and in all infants by 4 wk. **Pupillary reflexes** are present after 28-30 wk of gestation. The iris should be inspected for colobomas and heterochromia. A cornea >1 cm in diameter in a term infant (with photophobia and tearing) or corneal clouding suggests congenital glaucoma and requires prompt ophthalmologic consultation. The presence of bilateral red reflexes suggests the absence of cataracts and intraocular pathology (see Chapter 637). **Leukokoria** (white pupillary reflex) suggests cataracts, tumor, chorioretinitis, retinopathy of prematurity, or a persistent hyperplastic primary vitreous and warrants an immediate ophthalmologic consultation (see Chapter 640).

Ears

Deformities of the pinnae are occasionally seen. Unilateral or bilateral preauricular skin tags occur frequently; if pedunculated, they can be tightly ligated at the base, resulting in dry gangrene and sloughing. The tympanic membrane, easily seen otoscopically through the short and straight external auditory canal, normally appears dull gray.

Nose

The nose may be slightly obstructed by mucus accumulated in the narrow nostrils. The nares should be symmetric and patent. Dislocation of the nasal cartilage from the vomerian groove results in asymmetric nares. Anatomic obstruction of the nasal passages secondary to unilateral or bilateral choanal atresia results in respiratory distress.

Mouth

A normal mouth may rarely have precocious dentition, with natal (present at birth) or neonatal (eruption after birth) teeth in the lower incisor position or aberrantly placed; these teeth are shed before the deciduous ones erupt (see Chapter 333). Alternatively, such teeth occur in Ellis–van Creveld, Hallermann-Streiff, and other syndromes. Extraction is not usually indicated. Premature eruption of deciduous teeth is even more unusual. The soft and hard palate should be inspected and palpated for a complete or submucosal cleft, and the contour noted if the arch is excessively high or the uvula is bifid. On the hard palate on either side of the raphe, there may be temporary accumulations of epithelial cells called **Epstein pearls**. Retention cysts of similar appearance may also be seen on the gums. Both disappear spontaneously, usually within a few weeks of birth. Clusters of small, white or yellow follicles or ulcers on erythematous bases may be found on the anterior tonsillar pillars, most frequently on the 2nd or 3rd day of life. Of unknown cause, they clear without treatment in 2-4 days.

Neonates do not have active salivation. The tongue appears relatively large; the frenulum may be short, but its shortness (**tongue-tie** or **ankyloglossia**) is rarely a reason for cutting it. If there are problems with feedings (breast or bottle) and the frenulum is short, frenulectomy (**frenotomy**) may be indicated. Frenotomy may reduce maternal nipple pain and improve breastfeeding scores more rapidly than no treatment, but over time, neonates not treated with frenotomy also have successful feeding. The sublingual mucous membrane occasionally forms a prominent fold. The cheeks have fullness on both the buccal and the external aspects as a result of the accumulation of fat in the sucking pads. These pads, as well as the labial tubercle on the upper lip (**sucking callus**), disappear when suckling ceases. A marble-sized buccal mass is usually caused by benign idiopathic fat necrosis.

The throat of a newborn infant is difficult to see because of the low arch of the palate; it should be clearly viewed because posterior palatal or uvular clefts are easy to miss. The tonsils are small.

NECK

The neck appears relatively short. Abnormalities are not common but include goiter, cystic hygroma, branchial cleft cysts, teratoma, hemangioma, and lesions of the sternocleidomastoid muscle that are presumably traumatic or caused by a fixed positioning in utero that produces either a hematoma or fibrosis, respectively. Congenital **torticollis** causes the head to turn toward and the face to turn away from the affected side (see Chapter 700.1). Plagiocephaly, facial asymmetry, and hemihypoplasia may develop if it is untreated (see Chapter 610). Redundant skin or webbing in a female infant suggests intrauterine lymphedema and Turner syndrome (see Chapters 98 and 604). Both clavicles should be palpated for fractures.

CHEST

Breast hypertrophy is common, and milk may be present (but should not be expressed). Asymmetry, erythema, induration, and tenderness suggest mastitis or a breast abscess. Supernumerary nipples, inverted nipples, or widely spaced nipples with a shield-shaped chest may be seen; the last finding suggests Turner syndrome.

LUNGS

Much can be learned by observing breathing. Normal variations in rate and rhythm are characteristic and fluctuate according to the infant's physical activity, the state of wakefulness, or the presence of crying. Because fluctuations are rapid, the **respiratory rate** should be counted for a full minute with the infant in the resting state, preferably asleep. Under these circumstances, the usual rate for normal term infants is 30-60 breaths/min; in premature infants the rate is higher and fluctuates more widely. A rate consistently >60 breaths/min during periods of regular breathing that persists for >1 hr after birth is an indication to rule out pulmonary, cardiac, or metabolic disease (acidosis) etiologies. Preterm infants may breathe with a Cheyne-Stokes rhythm, known as **periodic respiration**, or with complete irregularity. Irregular gasping, sometimes accompanied by spasmodic movements of the mouth and chin, strongly indicates serious impairment of the respiratory centers.

The breathing of newborn infants at rest is almost entirely *diaphragmatic,* so during inspiration, the soft front of the thorax is usually drawn inward while the abdomen protrudes. If the baby is quiet, relaxed, and with good color, this "paradoxical movement" does not necessarily signify insufficient ventilation. On the other hand, labored respiration with retractions is important evidence of respiratory distress syndrome, pneumonia, anomalies, or mechanical disturbance of the lungs. A weak, persistent or intermittent groaning, whining cry, or **grunting** during expiration can signify potentially serious cardiopulmonary disease or sepsis and warrants immediate attention. When benign, the grunting resolves 30-60 min after birth. Flaring of the alae nasi and retraction of the intercostal muscles and sternum are common signs of pulmonary pathology.

Normally, the breath sounds are *bronchovesicular.* Suspicion of pulmonary pathology because of diminished breath sounds, rhonchi, retractions, or cyanosis should always be verified with a chest radiograph.

HEART

Normal variation in the size and shape of the chest makes it difficult to estimate the size of the heart. The location of the heart should be determined to detect **dextrocardia**. The pulse is usually 110-140 beats/min at rest but may vary normally from 90 beats/min in relaxed sleep to 180 beats/min during activity. The still higher rate of supraventricular tachycardia (>220 beats/min) may be determined better with a cardiac monitor or electrocardiogram (ECG) than by auscultation. Preterm

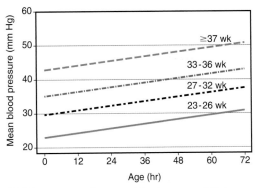

Fig. 113.2 Nomogram for mean blood pressure (BP) in neonates with gestational ages of 23-43 wk. Derived from continuous arterial BP measurements obtained from 103 infants admitted to the neonatal intensive care unit. The graph shows the predicted mean BP of neonates of different gestational ages during the 1st 72 hr of life. Each line represents the lower limit of the 80% confidence interval (2-tail) of the mean BP for each gestational age-group; 90% of infants for each gestational age-group will be expected to have a mean BP value equal to or above the value indicated by the corresponding line, the lower limit of the confidence interval. *(From Nuntnarumit P, Yang W, Bada-Ellzey SB: Blood pressure measurements in the newborn, ClinPerinatol 26: 976–996, 1999.)*

infants usually have a higher resting heart rate, up to about 160 beats/min, but may have a sudden onset of sinus bradycardia secondary to apnea. On both admission to and discharge from the nursery, the infant's pulses should be palpated in the upper and lower extremities to detect **coarctation of the aorta.** Transitory murmurs usually represent a closing ductus arteriosus. Although congenital heart disease (CHD) may not initially produce a murmur, a substantial portion of infants in whom persistent murmurs are detected during routine neonatal examination have underlying malformation. Routine screening for critical CHD using pulse oximetry is performed between 24 and 48 hr of life, which overall yields a sensitivity approaching 80% and specificity >99%. Pulse oximetry screening with SO_2 of ≥95% in the right hand or either foot and <3% difference between the right hand and foot is considered a normal screening test. Those with SO_2 <95% should be referred for evaluation and possible echocardiogram (see Chapter 452). Blood pressure (BP) measurements are indicated in the evaluation of ill-appearing infants and those in whom CHD is suspected. The oscillometric method is the easiest and most accurate noninvasive method available. Mean BP values vary by gestational age, however for all neonates, BP is expected to rise in the 1st 72 hr after birth (Fig. 113.2).

ABDOMEN

The liver is usually palpable, sometimes as much as 2 cm below the rib margin. Less often, the tip of the spleen may be felt. The approximate size and location of each kidney can usually be determined on deep palpation. At no other period of life does the amount of air in the gastrointestinal tract vary so much, nor is it usually so great under normal circumstances. The intestinal tract is gasless at birth. Gas is swallowed soon after birth, and gas should normally be present in the rectum on radiograph by 24 hr of age. The abdominal wall is normally weak (especially in premature infants), and diastasis recti and umbilical hernias are common, particularly among black infants.

Unusual masses should be investigated immediately with ultrasonography. Renal pathology is the cause of most neonatal abdominal masses. **Cystic abdominal masses** include hydronephrosis, multicystic-dysplastic kidneys, adrenal hemorrhage, hydrometrocolpos, intestinal duplication, and choledochal, ovarian, omental, or pancreatic cysts. **Solid masses** include neuroblastoma, congenital mesoblastic nephroma, hepatoblastoma, and teratoma. A solid flank mass may be caused by **renal vein thrombosis,** which becomes clinically apparent with hematuria, hypertension, and thrombocytopenia. Renal vein thrombosis in

infants is associated with polycythemia, dehydration, maternal diabetes, asphyxia, sepsis, nephrosis, and hypercoagulable states such as antithrombin III and protein C deficiency.

Abdominal distention at birth or shortly afterward suggests either obstruction or perforation of the gastrointestinal tract, often as a result of meconium ileus; later distention suggests lower bowel obstruction, sepsis, or peritonitis. A scaphoid abdomen in a newborn suggests diaphragmatic hernia. Abdominal wall defects produce an **omphalocele** when they occur through the umbilicus and gastroschisis when they occur lateral to the midline (see Chapter 125). Omphaloceles are associated with other anomalies and syndromes, such as Beckwith-Wiedemann, conjoined twins, trisomy 18, meningomyelocele, and imperforate anus. **Omphalitis** is an acute local inflammation of the periumbilical tissue that may extend to the abdominal wall, the peritoneum, the umbilical vein or portal vessels, or the liver and may result in later portal hypertension. The umbilical cord should have 2 arteries and 1 vein. A single umbilical artery is associated with an increased risk for an occult renal anomaly.

GENITALS

The genitals and mammary glands normally respond to transplacentally acquired maternal hormones to produce enlargement and secretion of the breasts in both sexes and prominence of the genitals in females, often with considerable nonpurulent discharge. These transitory manifestations require no intervention.

An imperforate hymen or other causes of vaginal obstruction may result in **hydrometrocolpos** and a lower abdominal mass. A normal scrotum at term is relatively large; its size may be increased by the trauma of breech delivery or by a transitory **hydrocele,** which is distinguished from a hernia by palpation and transillumination. The testes should be in the scrotum or should be palpable in the canals in term infants. Black male infants usually have dark pigmentation of the scrotum before the rest of the skin assumes its permanent color. The scrotum may be ecchymotic from breech presentation or a retroperitoneal hemorrhage; it may contain meconium particles associated with meconium peritonitis.

The prepuce or foreskin of a newborn infant is normally tight and adherent to the penile glans at birth and cannot be retracted. The foreskin should separate naturally over several months. Severe **hypospadias** or **epispadias** should always suggest either that abnormal sex chromosomes are present (see Chapter 98) or that the infant is actually a masculinized female with an enlarged clitoris, because this finding may be the first evidence of adrenogenital syndrome (see Chapter 594). Erection of the penis is common and has no significance. Urine is usually passed during or immediately after birth; a period without voiding may normally follow. Most neonates void by 12 hr, and approximately 95% of preterm and term infants void within 24 hr.

ANUS

Some passage of **meconium** usually occurs within the 1st 12 hr after birth; 99% of term infants and 95% of premature infants pass meconium within 48 hr of birth. Physical examination is usually sufficient for diagnosis of **imperforate anus,** if the anal opening is absent or incorrectly located. However, if there is a fistula to the skin, urethra or vagina, a newborn can pass meconium; in such cases, unless a careful exam is done, imperforate anus may not be suspected. Abdominal radiographs are used to confirm distal obstruction and to determine how low the rectum is. In females with imperforate anus, careful examination of the vestibule must be made to ensure separate openings of the urethra and vagina. All newborns with anorectal malformations warrant evaluation for possible associated cardiac, renal and spine anomalies.

The dimple or irregularity in skin fold often normally present in the sacrococcygeal midline may be mistaken for an actual or potential neurocutaneous sinus.

EXTREMITIES

During examination of the extremities, the effects of fetal posture (see Chapter 692) should be noted so that their cause and usual transitory nature can be explained to the mother. Such explanations are particularly important after breech presentations. A fracture or nerve injury associated with delivery can be detected more frequently by observation of the extremities in spontaneous or stimulated activity than by any other means. The hands and feet should be examined for polydactyly, syndactyly, and abnormal dermatoglyphic patterns such as a simian crease.

The hips of all infants should be examined with specific maneuvers to rule out congenital dislocation (see Chapter 698.1).

NEUROLOGIC EXAMINATION
See Chapter 21.

In utero neuromuscular diseases associated with limited fetal motion produce a constellation of signs and symptoms that are independent of the specific disease. Severe positional deformations and contractures produce **arthrogryposis**. Other manifestations of fetal neuromuscular disease include breech presentation, polyhydramnios, failure to breathe at birth, pulmonary hypoplasia, dislocated hips, undescended testes, thin ribs, and clubfoot. Many congenital disorders manifest as hypotonia, hypertonia, or seizures.

Bibliography is available at Expert Consult.

113.3 Routine Newborn Care
Neera K. Goyal

The initial steps of management for all newborns after delivery are to provide warmth, drying, and tactile stimulation, while simultaneously evaluating respiratory effort, heart rate, and color. Full-term, vigorous infants may initially be placed on the mother's abdomen after delivery, during which time **delayed clamping** of the umbilical cord (30-60 sec) is recommended to improve transitional circulation and increase neonatal red blood cell (RBC) volume. Clearing the mouth of secretions with gentle suction with a bulb syringe or soft catheter is indicated if there is an excessive (copious) amount of fluid in the mouth or nares. In resource-poor countries, gentle wiping of the face, nose, and mouth with a soft cloth may be equally effective as a bulb syringe. Spontaneously breathing neonates without distress require no assisted method to clear their airway.

The **Apgar score** is a practical method of systematically evaluating infants immediately after birth and is assessed at 1 and 5 min of life (Table 113.2). Most healthy infants who appear to be in satisfactory condition may remain in skin-to-skin contact with their mothers for immediate bonding and nursing. However, infants who fail to initiate or sustain respiratory effort after stimulation, those with a heart rate <100 beats/min, and those with persistent central cyanosis should be placed under warmers for prompt resuscitation and monitoring (see Chapter 121). Apgar scores should not be used to determine need for resuscitation or to guide steps of resuscitation. However, changes in Apgar scores at sequential time points after birth can reflect how well the infant is responding to resuscitation. If the 5 min score remains <7,

additional scores should be assigned every 5 min for up to 20 min. In addition to fetal distress, a number of factors, including prematurity and drugs given to the mother during labor, can result in low Apgar scores (Table 113.3).

MAINTENANCE OF BODY HEAT
Newborn infants are at risk for heat loss and hypothermia for several reasons. Relative to body weight, the body surface area (BSA) of a newborn infant is approximately 3 times that of an adult. Generation of body heat depends in large part on body weight, but heat loss depends on BSA. In low-birthweight and preterm infants, the insulating layer of subcutaneous fat is thin. The estimated rate of heat loss in a newborn is approximately 4 times that of an adult. Under the usual delivery room conditions (20-25°C [68-77°F]), an infant's skin temperature falls approximately 0.3°C (0.54°F)/min, and deep body temperature decreases approximately 0.1°C (0.18°F)/min during the period immediately after delivery; these rates generally result in a cumulative loss of 2-3°C (3.6-5.4°F) in deep body temperature (corresponding to a heat loss of approximately 200 kcal/kg). The heat loss occurs by 4 mechanisms: **convection** of heat energy to the cooler surrounding air, **conduction** of heat to the colder materials touching the infant, **heat radiation** from the infant to other nearby cooler objects, and **evaporation** from skin and lungs.

Metabolic acidosis, hypoxemia, hypoglycemia, and increased renal excretion of water and solutes may develop in term infants exposed to cold after birth because of their effort to compensate for heat loss. Heat

Table 113.3	Factors Affecting the Apgar Score*

FALSE-POSITIVE RESULT[†]
Prematurity
Analgesics, narcotics, sedatives
Magnesium sulfate
Acute cerebral trauma
Precipitous delivery
Congenital myopathy
Congenital neuropathy
Spinal cord trauma
Central nervous system anomaly
Lung anomaly (diaphragmatic hernia)
Airway obstruction (choanal atresia)
Congenital pneumonia and sepsis
Previous episodes of fetal asphyxia (recovered)
Hemorrhage-hypovolemia

FALSE-NEGATIVE RESULT[‡]
Maternal acidosis
High fetal catecholamine levels
Some full-term infants

*Regardless of the etiology, a low Apgar score because of fetal asphyxia, immaturity, central nervous system depression, or airway obstruction identifies an infant needing immediate resuscitation.
[†]No fetal acidosis or hypoxia; low Apgar score.
[‡]Acidosis; normal Apgar score.

Table 113.2	Apgar Evaluation of Newborn Infants*			
SIGN		**0**	**1**	**2**
Heart rate		Absent	Below 100	Over 100
Respiratory effort		Absent	Slow, irregular	Good, crying
Muscle tone		Limp	Some flexion of extremities	Active motion
Response to catheter in nostril (tested after oropharynx is clear)		No response	Grimace	Cough or sneeze
Color		Blue, pale	Body pink, extremities blue	Completely pink

*At 60 sec after complete birth of the infant (disregarding the cord and placenta), the 5 objective signs listed here are evaluated, and each is given a score of 0, 1, or 2. A total score of 10 indicates an infant in the best possible condition. An infant with a score of 0-3 requires immediate resuscitation.
Adapted from Apgar V: A proposal for a new method of evaluation of the newborn infant, *Curr Res Anesth Analg* 32:260–267, 1953.

production is augmented by increasing the metabolic rate and oxygen consumption in part by releasing **norepinephrine**, which results in nonshivering thermogenesis through oxidation of fat, particularly brown fat. In addition, muscular activity may increase. Hypoglycemic or hypoxic infants cannot increase their oxygen consumption when exposed to a cold environment, and their central temperature decreases. After labor and vaginal delivery, many newborn infants have mild to moderate metabolic acidosis, for which they may compensate by hyperventilating, a response that is more difficult for infants with central nervous system (CNS) depression (asphyxia, drugs) and infants exposed to cold stress in the delivery room. Therefore, to reduce heat loss, it is desirable to ensure that infants are dried and either wrapped in blankets or placed with the mother or under radiant warmers. **Skin-to-skin contact** with the mother is the optimal method of maintaining temperature in the stable newborn. Because carrying out resuscitative measures on a covered infant or one enclosed in an incubator is difficult, a radiant heat source should be used to warm the baby during resuscitation.

ANTISEPTIC SKIN AND CORD CARE

Nursery personnel should use alcohol-based solutions or chlorhexidine or iodophor-containing antiseptic soaps for routine handwashing before caring for each infant. Rigid enforcement of hand-to-elbow washing for 2 min in the initial wash and 15-30 sec in subsequent washes is essential for staff and visitors entering the nursery. Careful removal of the amniotic fluid and blood from the skin shortly after birth may reduce the risk of infection with bloodborne agents. For the infant's first bath, the entire skin and cord should be cleansed with warm water or a mild nonmedicated soap solution and rinsed with water to reduce the incidence of skin and periumbilical colonization with pathogenic bacteria and subsequent infectious complications. Based on World Health Organization (WHO) recommendations, this should be delayed until 24 hr of life to allow full transition to extrauterine life with emphasis on maternal–infant bonding and early breastfeeding. To avoid heat loss, the infant should then be dried and wrapped in clean blankets.

Staphylococcus aureus remains the most frequent pathogenic bacteria to colonize the umbilical cord, although other common pathogens include group A and group B streptococci and gram-negative bacilli. Pathogenic bacteria may derive from the mother's birth canal or various bacterial sources, including the nonsterile hands of personnel attending the delivery. Topical chlorhexidine to the umbilical cord is recommended for infants born outside of birthing centers or hospital settings, and for those born in low-resource communities with high neonatal mortality rates. However, in high-resource countries the incidence of omphalitis is very low and the severity is mild, so **dry cord care** is recommended without the application of topical substances such as alcohol or chlorhexidine. Dry cord care involves leaving the umbilical cord exposed to air or loosely covered, cleaning it with soap and water if it becomes soiled. Colonization and infection of newborns from potentially pathogenic organisms can also be reduced through continuous rooming-in with their mother, which creates an environment conducive for colonization from less pathogenic bacteria acquired from the mother's flora.

Vernix is spontaneously shed within 2-3 days, much of it adhering to the clothing, which should be completely changed daily. The diaper should be checked before and after feeding and when the baby cries; it should be changed when wet or soiled. The perineal area can be cleaned with baby wipes or with mild soap and warm water. Meconium or feces should be cleansed from the buttocks with sterile cotton moistened with sterile water. The foreskin of a male infant should not be retracted.

NEWBORN PROPHYLAXIS AND SCREENING

Newborn assessment and vital sign monitoring may vary by hospital but generally decreases in frequency after the 1st 1-2 hr after birth. For well-appearing newborns, a reasonable interval between assessments is 4 hr during the 1st 2-3 days of life and 8 hr thereafter. The infant's temperature should be taken by axillary measurement, with a normal range of 36.5-37.4°C (97.7-99.3°F). Weighing at birth and daily thereafter is sufficient.

The eyes of all infants, including those of cesarean birth, must be protected against **gonococcal ophthalmia neonatorum** by application of a 1 cm ribbon of erythromycin (0.5%) or tetracycline (1.0%) sterile ophthalmic ointments in each lower conjunctival sac. This procedure may be delayed during the initial short-alert period after birth to promote bonding, but once applied, drops should not be rinsed out (see Chapters 219 and 253.3). A 1% silver nitrate solution is an acceptable alternative but leads to a transient chemical conjunctivitis in 10–20% of cases.

Although hemorrhage in newborn infants can be a result of factors other than vitamin K deficiency, an intramuscular (IM) injection of 0.5-1 mg of water-soluble vitamin K₁ (phytonadione) should be given to all infants shortly after birth to prevent **hemorrhagic disease of the newborn** (see Chapter 124.4). Oral vitamin K is *not* as effective as the parenteral dosage.

Hepatitis B immunization before discharge from the nursery is recommended for newborns with weight >2 kg, irrespective of maternal hepatitis status.

Neonatal screening is available for various genetic, metabolic, hematologic, and endocrine disorders. All states in the United States have adopted the recommendations of the **Advisory Committee on Heritable Disorders in Newborns and Children**, although the specific tests performed vary by state based in part to disease prevalence, detection rates, and costs (see Chapter 102). The most commonly identified disorders (and their rates) include hypothyroidism (52/100,000 births), cystic fibrosis (30/100,000), hemoglobinopathies (26/100,000), medium-chain acyl–coenzyme A dehydrogenase deficiency (6/100,000), galactosemia (5/100,000), phenylketonuria (5/100,000), and adrenal hyperplasia (5/100,000). To be effective in the timely identification and prompt management of treatable diseases, screening programs must include not only high-quality laboratory tests but also follow-up of infants with abnormal test results; education, counseling, and psychologic support for families; and prompt referral of the identified neonate for accurate diagnosis and appropriate treatment.

Hearing impairment, a serious morbidity that affects speech and language development, may be severe in 2/1,000 births and overall affects 5/1,000 births. Universal screening of infants is recommended to ensure early detection of hearing loss and appropriate, timely intervention. Parents of infants who fail screening should be counseled on the importance of screening results, reinforcing the need for prompt audiologic confirmation and emphasizing the potential for normal language development with prompt intervention.

Universal screening with pulse oximetry provides early detection of ductal dependent cyanotic congenital heart disease (see Chapter 452).

Universal screening for hyperbilirubinemia should include risk assessment in all infants with measurement of serum or transcutaneous bilirubin levels before hospital discharge (see Chapter 123.4, Kernicterus).

Universal screening for congenital hip dysplasia with physical examination with the **Ortolani test** (sensation of the dislocated hip reducing) and **Barlow test** (unstable hip dislocating from the acetabulum) is recommended, but routine hip ultrasound is not indicated.

Screening for hypoglycemia is risk based and should be performed in infants who are small for gestational age, large for gestational age, born to mothers who have diabetes, preterm, or symptomatic (see Chapter 127.1).

For infants with suspected maternal chorioamnionitis, current clinical guidelines recommend laboratory screening for sepsis, including a blood culture, and at least 48 hr of broad-spectrum antibiotic therapy. However, evidence suggests a low incidence of sepsis among well-appearing, term neonates, and that frequent, reliable observation to detect early signs of sepsis, with or without laboratory studies, may be appropriate. (see Chapter 129).

Table 113.4 lists minimum criteria to be met before newborn discharge. A shortened hospital stay (<48 hr after delivery) may be reasonable for healthy, term newborns but is not always appropriate. Early discharge requires careful ambulatory follow-up at home (by a visiting nurse) or in the office within 48 hr of discharge.

Bibliography is available at Expert Consult.

Table 113.4	Criteria for Discharge of Healthy Term Newborns*

GENERAL

Normal vital signs including respiratory rate <60 breaths/min; axillary temperature 36.5°C-37.4°C (97.7°-99.3°F) in open crib

Physical examination reveals no abnormalities requiring continued hospitalization

Regular urination; stool × 1

At least 2 uneventful, successful feedings

No excessive bleeding 2 hr after circumcision

LABORATORY AND OTHER SCREENS

Maternal syphilis, hepatitis B surface antigen, and HIV status

Newborn hepatitis B vaccine administered or appointment for vaccination confirmed

Maternal tetanus toxoid, reduced diphtheria toxoid, and acellular pertussis, adsorbed (Tdap) vaccination

Maternal influenza vaccination during flu season

Evaluation and monitoring for sepsis based on maternal risk factors including GBS colonization

Umbilical or newborn direct Coombs test and blood type if clinically indicated

Expanded newborn metabolic screening

Hearing screening

Screening for hypoglycemia based on infant risk factors

Pulse oximetry screening

Screening for hyperbilirubinemia, with management and follow-up as recommended based on level of jaundice

SOCIAL

Evidence of parental knowledge, ability, and confidence to care for the baby at home:
  Feeding
  Normal stool and urine output
  Cord, skin, and genital care
  Recognition of illness (jaundice, poor feeding, lethargy, fever, etc.)
  Infant safety (car seat, supine sleep position, etc.)

Availability of family and physician support (physician follow-up)

Assessment of family, environmental, and social risk factors:
  Substance abuse
  History of child abuse
  Domestic violence
  Mental illness
  Teen mother
  Homelessness
  Barriers to follow-up

Source of continuing medical care is identified.

*Refers to infants born between 37 and 42 wk of gestation after uncomplicated pregnancy, labor, and delivery.

From American Academy of Pediatrics Committee on Fetus and Newborn: Hospital stay for healthy term newborn infants, *Pediatrics* 135:948–953, 2015.

113.4 Circumcision

Neera K. Goyal

Male circumcision consists of the surgical removal of some, or all, of the foreskin from the penis, and is one of the most common procedures performed worldwide. Circumcision performed during the newborn period has considerably lower complication rates than when performed later in life. The procedure should only be performed in healthy newborns whose condition is stable. Those providing circumcision should be adequately trained in both sterile techniques and effective pain management to reduce risk of complications. The surgery includes dilation of the preputial orifice to visualize the glans, freeing the preputial epithelium from the epithelium of the glans, placement of the circumcision device (Gomco clamp, Plastibell, or Mogen clamp) to enhance hemostasis, and removal of foreskin. For pain management, topical 4% lidocaine (i.e., LMX4 cream), a dorsal penile nerve block, and a subcutaneous ring block are all effective options. Topical anesthetic creams may cause a higher incidence of skin irritation in

low-birthweight infants; therefore penile nerve block techniques should be chosen for this group. Usually, the dorsal penile nerve block consists of injections of 0.4 mL of 1% lidocaine *without* epinephrine on both sides of the base of the penis. The subcutaneous **circumferential ring block** involves 0.8 mL of 1% lidocaine *without* epinephrine injected at the base or midshaft of the penis and may provide the most effective analgesia compared with other techniques. Nonpharmacologic techniques, such as positioning on a padded environment and use of sucrose pacifiers, are useful adjuncts to improve infant comfort during the procedure but are insufficient as sole therapies to prevent procedural and postprocedural pain.

Contraindications to this procedure include critically ill infants, those with blood dyscrasias, individuals who have a family history of bleeding disorders, and those who have congenital abnormalities (e.g., hypospadias), congenital chordee, or deficient shaft skin (e.g., penoscrotal fusion, congenital buried penis). In addition, it should be confirmed before the procedure that the newborn received IM vitamin K in accordance with standard practice of newborn care. Premature infants may undergo circumcision before discharge.

Preventive health benefits of elective circumcision for male newborns include significant reductions in the risk of urinary tract infection in the 1st year of life, heterosexual acquisition of HIV and transmission of other sexually transmitted infections (human papillomavirus, herpes simplex virus type 2, and syphilis), and penile cancer. Acute complications from circumcision in the United States and other high-resource countries are rare, including bleeding (0.08–0.18%), infection (0.06%), and penile injury (0.04%). More catastrophic injuries, including glans or penile amputation, are extremely rare and published as case reports only. Later complications can include excessive residual skin (incomplete circumcision), excessive skin removal, adhesions (natural and vascularized skin bridges), meatal stenosis, phimosis, and epithelial inclusion cysts.

Current evidence indicates while health benefits outweigh the risks of male circumcision, health benefits are not great enough to recommend routine circumcision for all male newborns. Therefore, physicians who counsel families about this decision should explain the potential benefits and risks, in a nonbiased manner, and ensure that parents understand that circumcision is an elective procedure. Ultimately, parents should decide whether circumcision is in the best interests of their male child, weighing the medical information in context of their own religious, ethical, and cultural beliefs and practices.

Regardless of whether or not the newborn is circumcised, parents should be instructed in the care of the penis at discharge from the newborn hospital stay. The circumcised penis should be washed gently each day with soap and water. As part of normal healing, the glans may appear raw or yellowish for 7-10 days. Gauze with petroleum jelly can be used to cover the area and should be changed with each urine and stool until the glans heals.

Bibliography is available at Expert Consult.

113.5 Parent–Infant Bonding

Neera K. Goyal

See also Chapter 21.

Normal infant development depends partly on a series of affectionate responses exchanged between a mother and her newborn infant that binds them psychologically and physiologically. This bonding is facilitated and reinforced by the emotional support of a loving family. The attachment process may be important in enabling some mothers to provide loving care during the neonatal period and subsequently during childhood. The power of this attachment is so great that it enables the mother and the father to make unusual sacrifices necessary for the day-to-day care of the infant, care night after night, giving feedings 24 hr a day, attending to crying, and so on. The sacrifices continue for many years as parents dedicate much of their lives to their children.

Parent–infant bonding is initiated before birth with the planning and confirmation of the pregnancy. Subsequently, there is a growing awareness of the baby as an individual, starting usually with the remarkably powerful event of quickening or sensation of fetal movements. After delivery and during the ensuing weeks, sensory (visual, auditory, olfactory) and physical contact between the mother and baby triggers various mutually rewarding and pleasurable interactions, such as the mother touching the infant's extremities and face with her fingertips and encompassing and gently massaging the infant's trunk with her hands. Touching an infant's cheek elicits responsive turning toward the mother's face or toward the breast with nuzzling and licking of the nipple, a powerful stimulus for prolactin secretion. An infant's initial quiet alert state provides the opportunity for eye-to-eye contact, which is particularly important in stimulating the loving and possessive feelings of many parents for their babies. An infant's crying elicits the maternal response of touching the infant and speaking in a soft, soothing, higher-toned voice.

Initial contact between the mother and infant should take place in the delivery room, and opportunities for extended intimate contact and breastfeeding should be provided within the 1st hours after birth. Delayed or abnormal maternal–infant bonding, as occurs because of prematurity, infant or maternal illness, birth defects, or family stress, may harm infant development and maternal caretaking ability. Hospital routines should be designed to encourage parent–infant contact. Rooming-in arrangements, care by parents, and family-centered care increase the opportunities for better parent–infant interaction.

ROOMING-IN AND BREASTFEEDING

See Chapter 56 for full discussions of breastfeeding and formula feeding.

Ample evidence indicates that there are infant and maternal benefits to breastfeeding. One important hospital practice to encourage successful breastfeeding is rooming-in of newborns with their mothers. Therefore, it should be encouraged that term, healthy infants remain continuously in the mother's room whenever possible. To reduce the risk of **sudden infant death syndrome**, infants should be placed to sleep supine in a bassinet, preferably of clear plastic to allow for easy visibility and care. All professional care should be given to the infant in the bassinet, including the physical examination, clothing changes, temperature taking, skin cleansing, and other procedures that, if performed elsewhere, would establish a common contact point and possibly provide a channel for cross-infection. The clothing and bedding should be minimal, only enough needed for an infant's comfort; the room temperature should be kept at approximately 22-26°C (72-78°F).

Additional practices that encourage successful breastfeeding include antepartum education and encouragement, immediate postpartum mother–infant contact with suckling, demand feeding, inclusion of maternal partners in breastfeeding education, and support from experienced women. Nursing at first for least 5 min at each breast is reasonable, allows a baby to obtain most of the available breast contents, and provides effective stimulation for increasing the milk supply. Nursing episodes should then be extended according to the comfort and desire of the mother and infant. A confident and relaxed mother, supported by an encouraging home and hospital environment, is likely to nurse well. The **Baby-Friendly Hospital Initiative**, a global effort sponsored by WHO and the UN Children's Fund to promote breastfeeding, recommends 10 steps to successful breastfeeding (Table 113.5). When instituted together as a complete bundle, these practices can improve multiple outcomes, including breastfeeding initiation, duration of exclusive breastfeeding, and duration of overall breastfeeding. In the United States, however, the vast majority of newborns are still not delivered in Baby-Friendly hospitals that have implemented all 10 steps. Educating mothers during pregnancy and showing mothers how to breastfeed are the most widely implemented strategies, while establishment of written breastfeeding policies, restriction of formula access, and establishment of breastfeeding support groups after discharge are among the most challenging to implement.

Drugs and Breastfeeding

Ideally, drugs of any type should be avoided in breastfeeding women, unless prescribed for specific medical conditions. Many mothers are

Table 113.5	Ten Steps to Successful Breastfeeding

Every facility providing maternity services and care for newborn infants should accomplish the following:
1. Have a written feeding policy that is routinely communicated to staff and patients, comply with WHO restrictions on marketing of breast milk substitutes, and establish ongoing monitoring and data-management systems.
2. Ensure that staff have sufficient knowledge, competence, and skills to support breastfeeding.
3. Discuss the importance and management of breastfeeding with pregnant women and their families.
4. Facilitate immediate and uninterrupted skin-to-skin contact and help initiate breastfeeding as soon as possible after birth.
5. Support mothers to initiate and maintain breastfeeding and manage common difficulties.
6. Give newborn infants no food or drink other than breast milk unless *medically* indicated.
7. Practice rooming-in (allow mothers and infants to remain together) 24 hr a day.
8. Support mothers to recognize and respond to their infants' feeding cues.
9. Counsel mothers on the use and risks of feeding bottles, teats, and pacifiers.
10. Coordinate discharge to ensure timely access to ongoing support and care.

Adapted from Guideline: Protecting, promoting and supporting breastfeeding in facilities providing maternity and newborn services. Geneva, 2017, World Health Organization.

advised to discontinue breastfeeding or avoid taking essential medications due to fears of adverse infant effects. However, such an approach may be inappropriate in many cases, as only a small proportion of medications are contraindicated when breastfeeding. When weighing risks and benefits, healthcare providers should consider the following factors in discussion with the family: maternal need for the medication, potential effects on lactation, extent of excretion into human milk, extent of oral absorption by the breastfeeding infant, potential adverse infant effects, proportion of feedings comprised of breast milk, and age of the infant. Although previous editions of this text sought to list medications potentially used during lactation and to describe their potential for infant harm, revisions to this text can no longer keep pace with rapidly changing information available via the internet, published studies, and new drug approvals. For up-to-date information on drug levels in human milk and infant serum, possible adverse effects on infant health and lactation, and recommendations for possible medication alternatives, providers should refer to LactMed (http://toxnet.nlm.nih.gov).

Among US women of childbearing age, illicit drug use and legal substance use or abuse is common, with >5% of pregnant women reporting active illicit drugs, >9% alcohol use, and >15% cigarette use. Multiple drug use is also common. For mothers desiring to breastfeed with a history of current or past illegal drug abuse or legal drug use or abuse, healthcare providers must carefully and thoughtfully weigh the documented benefits of human milk and breastfeeding against the risks associated with the substance that the infant may be exposed to during lactation. Most illicit drugs are found in human milk with varying degrees of oral bioavailability, and breastfeeding is generally contraindicated (Table 113.6). However, mothers with substance use disorders should be encouraged to breastfeed under the following circumstances: established engagement in substance abuse treatment (e.g., methadone or buprenorphine maintenance therapy) that includes counseling and social support; abstinence from drug use for 90 days before delivery, with maternal urine toxicology testing at delivery negative other than prescribed substances, ability to maintain sobriety demonstrated in an outpatient setting, and engagement and compliance with care.

Contraindications to Breastfeeding

Medical contraindications to breastfeeding in the United States include infants with galactosemia, maple syrup urine disease, and

Table 113.6	Drugs of Abuse and Adverse Infant Effects

CONTRAINDICATED

Amphetamines	Aspirin (salicylates)
Antineoplastic agents	Atropine
Bromocriptine	β-Adrenergic blocking agents
Chloramphenicol	Benzodiazepines
Clozapine	Birth control pills
Cocaine	Bromides
Cyclophosphamide	Cascara
Doxorubicin	Codeine
Ecstasy (MDMA)	Dicumarol
Ergots	Dihydrotachysterol
Gold salts	Domperidone
Heroin	Estrogens
Immunosuppressants	Hydrocodone
Methamphetamine	Lithium
Phencyclidine (PCP)	Marijuana
Radiopharmaceuticals	Metoclopramide
Thiouracil	Meperidine
	Oxycodone
USE WITH CAUTION	Phenobarbital*
Alcohol	Primidone
Amiodarone	Reserpine
Anthraquinones (laxatives)	Salicylazosulfapyridine
	(sulfasalazine)

*Watch for sedation.

phenylketonuria. Maternal conditions that contraindicate breastfeeding include infection with human T-cell lymphotropic virus types 1 and 2, active tuberculosis (until appropriately treated ≥2 wk and not considered contagious), herpesvirus infection on breast, use of or dependence on certain illicit drugs, and maternal treatment with some radioactive compounds (Table 113.7). Because clean water and affordable replacement feeding are available in the United States, it is recommended that HIV-infected mothers not breastfeed their infants regardless of maternal viral load and antiretroviral therapy. However, in resource-limited countries where diarrhea and pneumonia are significant causes of infant and child mortality, breastfeeding may not be contraindicated for HIV-positive mothers receiving antiretroviral therapy. Donor human milk, particularly that purchased online, may be contaminated with potential pathogens. Contamination is much less of a concern with pasteurized human milk obtained from a milk bank.

Bibliography is available at Expert Consult.

Table 113.7	Summary of Infectious Agents Detected in Milk and Newborn Disease

INFECTIOUS AGENT	DETECTED IN BREAST MILK?	BREAST MILK REPORTED AS CAUSE OF NEWBORN DISEASE?	MATERNAL INFECTION CONTRAINDICATION TO BREASTFEEDING?
BACTERIA			
Mastitis/*Staphylococcus aureus*	Yes	No	No, unless breast abscess present
Mycobacterium tuberculosis:			
Active disease	Yes	No	Yes, because of aerosol spread, or tuberculosis mastitis
Purified protein derivative skin test result positive, chest radiograph findings negative	No	No	No
Escherichia coli, other gram-negative rods	Yes, stored	Yes, stored	—
Group B streptococci	Yes	Yes	No*
Listeria monocytogenes	Yes	Yes	No*
Coxiella burnetii	Yes	Yes	No*
Syphilis	No	No	No†
VIRUSES			
HIV	Yes	Yes	Yes, developed countries
Cytomegalovirus:			
Term infant	Yes	Yes	No
Preterm infant	Yes	Yes	Evaluate on an individual basis
Hepatitis B virus	Yes, surface antigen	No	No, developed countries‡
Hepatitis C virus	Yes	No	No§
Hepatitis E virus	Yes	No	No
Human T-cell leukemia virus (HTLV)-1	Yes	Yes	Yes, developed countries
HTLV-2	Yes	Uncertain	Yes, developed countries
Herpes simplex virus	Yes	Yes	No, unless breast vesicles present
Rubella			
Wild type	Yes	Yes, rare	No
Vaccine	Yes	No	No
Varicella-zoster virus	Yes	No	No, cover active lesions¶
Epstein-Barr virus	Yes	No	No
Human herpesvirus (HHV)-6	No	No	No
HHV-7	Yes	No	No
West Nile virus	Possible	Possible	Unknown
Zika virus	Yes	No	No
PARASITES			
Toxoplasma gondii	Yes	Yes, 1 case	No

*Provided that the mother and child are taking appropriate antibiotics.
†Treat mother and child if active disease.
‡Immunize and immune globulin at birth.
§Provided that the mother is HIV seronegative. Mothers should be counseled that breast milk transmission of hepatitis C virus has not been documented, but is theoretically possible.
¶Provide appropriate antivaricella therapy or prophylaxis to newborn.
Adapted from Jones CA: Maternal transmission of infectious pathogens in breast milk, *J Paediatr Child Health* 37:576–582, 2001.

Chapter **114**
High-Risk Pregnancies
Kristen R. Suhrie and Sammy M. Tabbah

第一百一十四章
高危妊娠

中文导读

本章主要介绍了高危妊娠、高危妊娠的相关因素和高危妊娠的分娩方式。相关因素方面具体介绍了遗传因素和母亲因素如孕妇年龄、产妇合并症、感染等具有因果关系的直接因素，以及羊水过多或过少等可提示高危妊娠的间接因素。后者详细描述了妊娠期羊水量的变化、羊水量的测量、羊水量过少或过多与先天性异常的关系、羊水量过少或过多可能带来的胎儿并发症；分娩方式的选择方面，剖宫产新生儿与经阴道产新生儿的风险比较，并描述了剖宫产时麻醉阵痛的选择。

The care of high-risk pregnancies should be coordinated with an experienced maternal-fetal medicine specialist.

In general, high-risk pregnancies are those that increase the likelihood of maternal complications, miscarriage, fetal death, preterm delivery, intrauterine growth restriction (IUGR), poor cardiopulmonary or metabolic transitioning at birth, fetal or neonatal disease, congenital malformations, or intellectual impairment and other handicaps (Table 114.1). There is no accepted comprehensive definition of what constitutes a *high-risk pregnancy*, therefore, specific epidemiologic data regarding the incidence/prevalence cannot be reliably reported. Some factors, such as ingestion of a teratogenic drug in the first trimester, are causally related to the risk, while others, such as polyhydramnios, are associations that alert a physician to determine the etiology and avoid the inherent risks associated with excessive amniotic fluid. Although assessing antepartum risk is important in reducing perinatal mortality and morbidity, some pregnancies become high risk only during labor and delivery; therefore careful monitoring is critical throughout the intrapartum course.

Identifying high-risk pregnancies is important not only because it is the first step toward prevention but also because critical steps may often be taken to reduce the risks to the fetus or neonate if the physician is alerted to the specific condition early in pregnancy.

GENETIC FACTORS
The occurrence of chromosomal abnormalities, congenital anomalies, inborn errors of metabolism, cognitive delay, or any familial disease in blood relatives increases the risk of the same condition in the infant. Because many parents recognize only obvious clinical manifestations of genetically determined diseases, specific inquiry should be made about any disease affecting one or more blood relatives. A high index of suspicion should be maintained to the possibility of autosomal recessive disorders in offspring of couples who are closely related (i.e., consanguinity).

MATERNAL FACTORS
The lowest neonatal mortality rate occurs in infants of mothers who receive adequate prenatal care and who are 20-30 yr of age. Pregnancies in both teenagers and women older than 40, particularly primiparous women, are at increased risk for IUGR, fetal distress, preeclampsia, and stillbirth. Advanced maternal age increases the risk of both chromosomal and nonchromosomal fetal malformations (Fig. 114.1).

Maternal illness (Table 114.2), multiple pregnancies (particularly those involving monochorionic twins), infections (Table 114.3), and certain drugs (see Chapter 115.4) increase the risk for the fetus. The use of assisted reproductive technology (e.g., ovulation induction, in vitro fertilization, intracytoplasmic sperm injection) increases the risk of prematurity, perinatal mortality, infant morbidity, low and very-low birthweight, imprinting disorders, and cerebral palsy. These risks are largely because of the increase in *multiple gestations* with such technology and the association with *prematurity*. The risks for *birth defects* are also increased with assisted reproductive technology, in part because of epigenetic effects on gene expression.

Preterm birth is common in high-risk pregnancies (see Chapter 117). Factors associated with prematurity (see Table 114.1) include multiple gestations as well as biologic markers such as cervical shortening, genital infection, presence of fetal fibronectin in cervicovaginal secretions, serum α-fetoprotein (AFP), and premature rupture of membranes (PROM). PROM occurs in 3% of all pregnancies in the United States and is a leading identifiable cause of prematurity.

The presence of **polyhydramnios** or **oligohydramnios** indicates high-risk pregnancies. Amniotic fluid volume is variable throughout pregnancy and progressively increases from 10 to 30 wk of gestation. On average, volume is typically <10 mL at 8 wk and increases to 630 and 770 mL at 22 and 28 wk, respectively. After 30 wk, the rate of increase slows and the volume remains fairly constant until 36-38 wk gestation. This is followed by a progressive decline, with an average volume of

Table 114.1	Factors Associated With High-Risk Pregnancy

ECONOMIC
Poverty
Unemployment
Uninsured, underinsured
Poor access to prenatal care

CULTURAL/BEHAVIORAL
Low educational status
Poor healthcare attitudes
No care or inadequate prenatal care
Cigarette, alcohol, or illicit drug use
Age <20 or >40 yr
Unmarried
Short interpregnancy interval (<18 mo between pregnancies)
Lack of support group (husband, family, religion)
Stress (physical, psychologic)
Black race (preterm birth rates are 48% higher than for other women)

BIOLOGIC/GENETIC
Previous low-birthweight or preterm infant
Low weight for height
Poor weight gain during pregnancy
Short stature
Poor nutrition
Consanguinity
Intergenerational effects
Low maternal birthweight
Maternal obesity
Hereditary diseases (inborn error of metabolism)

REPRODUCTIVE
Previous cesarean birth
Previous infertility
Conception by reproductive technology
Prolonged gestation (>40 wk)
Prolonged labor
Previous infant with cerebral palsy, intellectual impairment, birth trauma, or congenital anomalies
Abnormal lie (breech)
Multiple gestations
Premature rupture of membranes
Infection (systemic, amniotic, extra-amniotic, cervical)
Preeclampsia or eclampsia
Uterine bleeding (abruptio placentae, placenta previa)
Parity (0 or >5 previous deliveries)
Uterine or cervical anomalies
Fetal disease
Abnormal fetal growth
Idiopathic premature labor
Iatrogenic prematurity
High or low levels of maternal serum α-fetoprotein

MEDICAL
Diabetes mellitus
Hypertension
Congenital heart disease
Autoimmune disease
Sickle cell anemia
Intercurrent surgery or trauma
Sexually transmitted infection
Maternal hypercoagulable states
Exposure to prescription medications
TORCH (toxoplasmosis, other agents, rubella, cytomegalovirus, herpes simplex) infection

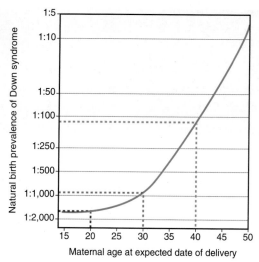

Fig. 114.1 Natural birth prevalence of Down syndrome according to maternal age. *(From Wald NJ, Leck I:* Antenatal and neonatal screening, *ed 2, Oxford, 2000, Oxford University Press.)*

515 mL at 41 wk of gestation. Polyhydramnios complicates 1–3%, and oligohydramnios 1–5%, of pregnancies; although the true incidence of amniotic fluid disorders is confounded by the lack of a uniform approach to diagnosis. The ultrasound (US) criteria for these diagnoses are based on either the *amniotic fluid index* (AFI) or a *deepest vertical pocket* (DVP). The AFI is determined by measuring the vertical dimension of amniotic fluid pockets in 4 quadrants and reporting the sum of these values. An index >24 cm suggests polyhydramnios, whereas an index <5 cm suggests oligohydramnios. The DVP method reports the deepest pocket of fluid identified with a value of 2-8 cm is considered normal.

Polyhydramnios is associated with preterm labor, abruptio placentae, maternal diabetes, multiple congenital anomalies, aneuploidy, and fetal neuromuscular dysfunction or obstruction of the gastrointestinal tract that interferes with reabsorption of the amniotic fluid that is normally swallowed by the fetus (Table 114.4). Increased fetal urination, as with congenital nephrotic syndrome, or edema formation, such as hydrops fetalis, is also associated with excessive amniotic fluid volume. US demonstrates the increased amniotic fluid surrounding the fetus and detects associated fetal anomalies, hydrops, pleural effusions, and ascites. **Idiopathic** polyhydramnios is the most common cause, affecting approximately 40% of patients. About 25% of these cases will demonstrate an abnormality in the postnatal period. Otherwise, approximately 33% of prenatally detected cases have an associated anomaly, and 25% are associated with maternal diabetes. Severe and symptomatic polyhydramnios may be managed by serial reduction amniocenteses. Treatment is indicated for acute maternal respiratory discomfort and threatened preterm labor, or to provide time for the administration of corticosteroids to enhance fetal lung maturity.

Oligohydramnios is associated with congenital anomalies; IUGR; severe renal, bladder, or urethral anomalies; and drugs that interfere with fetal urination (see Table 114.4). Oligohydramnios becomes most evident after 16-20 wk of gestation, when fetal urination is the major source of amniotic fluid. PROM is a common cause of oligohydramnios and must be ruled out if present, especially if a normal-sized bladder and kidneys are seen on fetal US. Oligohydramnios causes fetal compression abnormalities such as fetal distress/stillbirth from umbilical cord compression, clubfoot, spadelike hands, and a flattened nasal bridge. The most serious complication of chronic oligohydramnios is **pulmonary hypoplasia**, especially if present during the canalicular stage of fetal lung development, which occurs between 16 and 24 wk of gestation. The risk of umbilical cord compression during labor and delivery is increased in pregnancies complicated by oligohydramnios and may be alleviated by saline amnioinfusion via a transcervical intrauterine pressure catheter, which has been demonstrated to reduce the need for cesarean section and improve Apgar scores.

A pregnancy should be considered high risk when the uterus is inappropriately large or small. A uterus large for the estimated stage of gestation suggests the presence of multiple fetuses, polyhydramnios, or

Table 114.2	Maternal Conditions Affecting the Fetus or Neonate	
DISORDER	**EFFECT(S)**	**MECHANISM(S)**
Assisted reproductive technology	Beckwith-Wiedemann, Silver-Russel, Angelman syndromes	Altered imprinting
Autoantibody against folate receptors	Neural tube defects	Blockage of cellular uptake of folate
Cervical neoplasia	Preterm premature rupture of membranes, preterm birth	Associated with loop electrosurgical excision procedure or cone therapy
Cholestasis	Preterm delivery, intrauterine fetal demise	Unknown, possibly bile acid–induced fetal arrhythmia
Cyanotic heart disease	IUGR	Low fetal oxygen delivery
Diabetes mellitus:		
Mild	LGA, hypoglycemia	Fetal hyperglycemia: produces hyperinsulinemia; insulin promotes growth
Severe	Growth restriction	Vascular disease, placental insufficiency
Drug addiction	IUGR, neonatal withdrawal	Direct drug effect plus poor nutrition
Endemic goiter	Hypothyroidism	Iodine deficiency
Graves' disease	Transient neonatal thyrotoxicosis	Transplacental passage of IgG thyroid-stimulating antibody
Herpes gestationis (noninfectious)	Bullous rash, intrauterine fetal demise	Autoantibody similar to that in bullous pemphigoid
Hyperparathyroidism	Neonatal hypocalcemia	Maternal calcium crosses to fetus and suppresses fetal parathyroid gland
Hypertension	IUGR, intrauterine fetal demise	Placental insufficiency, fetal hypoxia
Idiopathic thrombocytopenic purpura	Thrombocytopenia	Nonspecific maternal platelet antibodies cross placenta
Isoimmune neutropenia or thrombocytopenia	Neutropenia or thrombocytopenia	Specific antifetus neutrophil or platelet antibody crosses placenta after sensitization of mother
Malignant melanoma	Placental or fetal tumor	Placental metastasis
Myasthenia gravis	Transient neonatal myasthenia	IgG antibody to acetylcholine receptor crosses placenta
Myotonic dystrophy	Neonatal myotonic dystrophy, congenital contractures, respiratory insufficiency	Genetic anticipation
NMDAR antibody encephalitis	Cortical dysplasia	Transplacental antibody
Obesity	LGA or IUGR, hypoglycemia	Unknown, similarities to diabetes
Phenylketonuria	Microcephaly, retardation	Elevated fetal phenylalanine values
Poor nutrition	IUGR, adult insulin resistance	Reduced fetal nutrients, nutritional programming
Preeclampsia, eclampsia	IUGR, thrombocytopenia, neutropenia, fetal demise	Uteroplacental insufficiency, fetal hypoxia, vasoconstriction
Renal transplantation	IUGR	Uteroplacental insufficiency
Rhesus or other blood group sensitization	Fetal anemia, hypoalbuminemia, hydrops, neonatal jaundice	IgG crosses placenta and is directed to fetal cells with antigen
Sickle cell anemia	Preterm birth, IUGR, stillbirth	Placental insufficiency via maternal sickling, producing fetal hypoxia
Systemic lupus erythematosus	Congenital heart block, rash, anemia, thrombocytopenia, neutropenia	Antibody directed to fetal heart, red and white blood cells, and platelets

IgG, Immunoglobulin G; LGA, large for gestational age; NMDAR, antibody to N-methyl-D-aspartate receptor; IUGR, intrauterine growth restriction.

an excessively large infant. An inappropriately small uterus suggests oligohydramnios or poor fetal growth.

Mode of delivery is influenced by a complex interplay between maternal-fetal factors. Spontaneous vaginal delivery is always preferred when not otherwise contraindicated. Operative vaginal delivery with vacuum or forceps is a safe alternative to cesarean delivery in appropriately selected patients. The absolute rate of significant newborn injury from these procedures is low, with rates ranging from 1 in 650-850 for **intracranial hemorrhage** and 1 in 220-385 for **neurologic complications**. With some of these injuries, the *indication* for operative vaginal delivery is more likely to be associated with the injury than the procedure itself, and could not have been prevented with a cesarean birth.

Cesarean delivery is indicated for a wide variety of circumstances. Cesarean-born infants present problems that are often related to the unfavorable obstetric circumstance that necessitated the operation. In normal term pregnancies without indication of fetal distress, cesarean delivery carries a greater neonatal risk than delivery through the birth canal. Even when accounting for gestational age, any malformations, birthweight, and multiple gestations, infants born ≥34 wk of gestation via elective cesarean section have 2 times the mortality rate of babies born following a planned vaginal birth, even if cesarean delivery was ultimately required. They also are 1.4 times as likely to require neonatal intensive care unit (NICU) admission and 1.8 times as likely to require breathing support for >30 min after birth. Cesarean-born infants are

Table 114.3	Maternal Infections Affecting the Fetus or Newborn	
INFECTION	**MODE(S) OF TRANSMISSION**	**NEONATAL OUTCOME**
BACTERIA		
Group B streptococcus	Ascending cervical	Sepsis, pneumonia
Escherichia coli	Ascending cervical	Sepsis, pneumonia
Listeria monocytogenes	Transplacental	Sepsis, pneumonia
Mycoplasma hominis	Ascending cervical	Pneumonia
Chlamydia trachomatis	Vaginal passage	Conjunctivitis, pneumonia
Syphilis	Transplacental, vaginal passage	Congenital syphilis
Neisseria gonorrhoeae	Vaginal passage	Ophthalmia (conjunctivitis), sepsis, meningitis
Mycobacterium tuberculosis	Transplacental	Prematurity, fetal demise, congenital tuberculosis
VIRUS		
Rubella	Transplacental	Congenital rubella
Cytomegalovirus	Transplacental, breast milk (rare)	Congenital cytomegalovirus or asymptomatic
HIV	Transplacental, vaginal passage, breast milk	Congenital or acquired immunodeficiency syndrome
Hepatitis B	Vaginal passage, transplacental, breast milk	Neonatal hepatitis, chronic hepatitis B surface antigen carrier state
Hepatitis C	Transplacental and vaginal passage	Rarely neonatal hepatitis, ~5% chronic carrier state possible
Herpes simplex type 2 or 1	Intrapartum exposure	Neonatal herpes simplex virus
		Neonatal encephalitis; disseminated viremia, or cutaneous infection
Varicella-zoster	Transplacental:	
	Early	Congenital anomalies
	Late	Neonatal varicella
Parvovirus	Transplacental	Fetal anemia, hydrops
Coxsackievirus B	Fecal-oral	Myocarditis, meningitis, hepatitis
Rubeola	Transplacental	Abortion, fetal measles
West Nile	Transplacental (rare)	Uncertain, possible rash, encephalitis
	Possible perinatal	
Zika	Transplacental	Congenital microcephaly, intracranial calcifications, brain abnormalities, retinal lesions
Chikungunya	Transplacental (rare), perinatal	Neonatal encephalitis
Dengue	Transplacental, perinatal	Neonatal sepsis-like symptoms
PARASITES		
Toxoplasmosis	Transplacental	Congenital toxoplasmosis
Malaria	Transplacental	Abortion, prematurity, intrauterine growth restriction
FUNGI		
Candida	Ascending, cervical	Sepsis, pneumonia, rash

Table 114.4	Conditions Associated With Disorders of Amniotic Fluid Volume
OLIGOHYDRAMNIOS	*Syndromes*
Amniotic fluid leak/rupture of membranes	Achondroplasia
Intrauterine growth restriction	Klippel-Feil
Fetal anomalies (particularly GU abnormalities)	Trisomy 18
Twin-twin transfusion (donor)	Trisomy 21
Fetal akinesia syndrome	TORCH*
Prune-belly syndrome	Hydrops fetalis
Pulmonary hypoplasia	Multiple congenital anomalies
Amnion nodosum	Bartter
Indomethacin	*Other*
Angiotensin-converting enzyme inhibitors or receptor antagonists	Diabetes mellitus
POLYHYDRAMNIOS	Twin-twin transfusion (recipient)
Congenital Anomalies	Fetal anemia
CNS abnormalities	Fetal heart failure
Tracheoesophageal fistula	Polyuric renal disease (congenital nephrotic syndrome)
Intestinal atresia	Neuromuscular diseases
Spina bifida	Nonimmune hydrops
Cleft lip or palate	Chylothorax
Cystic adenomatoid lung malformation	Teratoma
Diaphragmatic hernia	Idiopathic

*Toxoplasmosis, other agents, rubella, cytomegalovirus, and herpes simplex.
 CNS, Central nervous system; GU, genitourinary.

also at increased risk for persistent **pulmonary hypertension of the newborn**. An elective cesarean birth should be delayed until ≥39 wk of gestation, assuming there is no indication for delivery earlier.

Obstetric anesthesia is a vital component of care on the labor and delivery unit. The most common form of anesthesia in this patient population is *regional* (i.e., epidural or spinal). From the fetal/neonatal standpoint, the most significant complication encountered with this procedure is acute maternal hypotension, which can significantly impair uteroplacental perfusion. Fetal heart rate (FHR) abnormalities are common in this circumstance and, rarely, require emergent cesarean delivery if not amenable to standard in utero resuscitative efforts. *Opioid analgesia* is sometimes used in women who are not candidates for

regional anesthesia. This form of pain relief is best avoided as delivery approaches, to minimize risk of neonatal depression. To this end, when opioid use is necessary, it is best to prescribe regimens that have a very short half-life. It is essential that the pediatric team is present at the birth in women receiving opioid analgesia. Furthermore, the pediatricians must be alerted to the specific type of opioid used, because all these drugs cross the placenta and have varying neonatal pharmacokinetics. Some of the common regimens used and their respective neonatal half-life are listed in the referenced American College of Obstetricians and Gynecologists (ACOG) practice bulletin on obstetric anesthesia.

Bibliography is available at Expert Consult.

Chapter **115**
The Fetus
Kristen R. Suhrie and Sammy M. Tabbah

第一百一十五章
胎儿

中文导读

本章主要介绍了胎儿生长发育和成熟度、胎儿宫内窘迫、孕母疾病与胎儿、药物暴露致畸、放射线对胎儿的影响以及胎儿疾病的治疗与预防。具体描述了对胎儿生长发育的评估，胎儿成熟度与胎龄的评估；产前胎儿窘迫的原因、胎儿窘迫监测及评估的方法；母亲疾病对胎儿的影响，包括母亲感染性疾病如CMV对胎儿新生儿的影响，非感染性疾病如母亲糖尿病、未控制的母亲甲状腺功能减退症或甲状腺功能亢进症、母亲免疫性疾病、未经治疗的代谢性疾病对胎儿

新生儿的影响；孕妇服用某些药物可能会对胎儿和新生儿的结构或功能产生影响；孕妇暴露于辐射中胎儿发生先天缺陷或恶性肿瘤的概率高；对胎儿疾病进行宫内诊断的方式及应用规范；阐述了一些常见胎儿疾病的治疗与预防，包括母亲预防性应用Rh（D）免疫球蛋白降低Rh溶血病的发生、产前应用糖皮质激素促胎儿肺成熟、应用大剂量维生素治疗某些遗传代谢病、叶酸的补充预防神经管畸形。

The major emphasis in fetal medicine involves (1) assessment of fetal growth and maturity, (2) evaluation of fetal well-being or distress, (3) assessment of the effects of maternal disease on the fetus, (4) evaluation of the effects of drugs administered to the mother on the fetus, and (5) identification and when possible treatment of fetal disease or anomalies.

One of the most important tools used to access fetal well-being is ultrasonography (ultrasound, US); it is both safe and reasonably accurate.

Indications for antenatal US include estimation of gestational age (unknown dates, discrepancy between uterine size and dates, or suspected growth restriction), assessment of amniotic fluid volume, estimation of fetal weight and growth, determination of the location of the placenta and the number and position of fetuses, and identification of congenital anomalies. Fetal MRI is a more advanced imaging method that is thought to be safe to the fetus and neonate and is used for more advanced diagnostic and therapeutic planning (Fig. 115.1).

115.1 Fetal Growth and Maturity

Kristen R. Suhrie and Sammy M. Tabbah

Fetal growth can be assessed by US as early as 6-8 wk of gestation by measurement of the crown-rump length. Accurate determination of

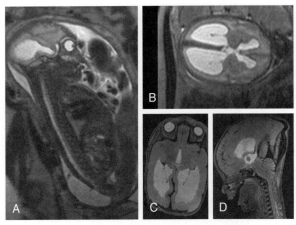

Fig. 115.1 MRI of fetal pathology. **A,** Fetus with sacral myelomeningocele at 30 wk gestation. **B,** Ventriculomegaly in the same fetus as in **A. C,** MRI can also be used for postmortem examination, here in a 33 wk old fetus, demonstrating ventriculomegaly with heterotopic foci in the ventricular walls. **D,** Chiari II malformation of the brainstem. *(Courtesy of Filip Claus, Aalst, Belgium.)*

gestational age can be achieved through the 1st half of pregnancy; however, first-trimester assessment by crown-rump length measurement is the most effective method of pregnancy dating. In the second trimester and beyond, a combination of biometric measures (i.e., biparietal diameter, head and abdominal circumference, femoral diaphysis length) is used for gestational age and growth assessment (Fig. 115.2). If a single US examination is performed, the most information can be obtained with a scan at 18-20 wk, when both gestational age and fetal anatomy can be evaluated. Serial scans assessing fetal growth are performed when risk factors for **fetal growth restriction (FGR)** are present. Two patterns of FGR have been identified: *symmetric* FGR, typically present early in pregnancy, and *asymmetric* FGR, typically occurring later in gestation. The most widely accepted definition of FGR in the United States is an **estimated fetal weight (EFW)** of less than the 10th percentile (Fig. 115.3). Some aspects of human fetal growth and development are summarized in Chapter 20.

Fetal maturity and dating are usually assessed by last menstrual period (LMP), assisted reproductive technology (ART)–derived gestational age, or US assessments. Dating by LMP assumes an accurate recall of the 1st day of LMP, a menstrual cycle that lasted 28 days, and ovulation occurring on the 14th day of the cycle, which would place the **estimated delivery date (EDD)** 280 days after LMP. Inaccuracies with any of these parameters can lead to an incorrectly assigned gestational age if the LMP is used for dating. Dating by ART is the most accurate method for assigning gestational age with EDD occurring 266 days after conception (when egg is fertilized by sperm). When US is used for dating, the most accurate assessment of gestational age is by first-trimester (≤13⁵⁄₇ wk) US measurement of crown-rump length, which is accurate to within 5-7 days. In contrast, US dating in the second trimester is accurate to 10-14 days, and third trimester is only accurate to 21-30 days. Dating of a pregnancy is critical to determine when delivery should occur, if growth is appropriate during

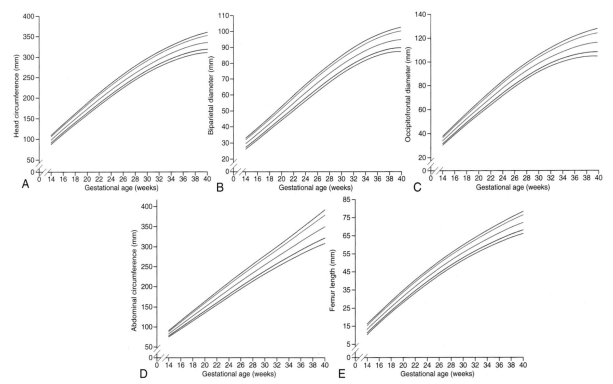

Fig. 115.2 Fetal measurements: 3rd, 10th, 50th, 90th, and 97th smoothed centile curves. **A,** Fetal head circumference; **B,** fetal biparietal diameter; **C,** fetal occipitofrontal diameter; **D,** fetal abdominal circumference; and **E,** fetal femur length measured by ultrasound (US) according to gestational age. *(From Papageorghiou AT, Ohyma EO, Altman DG, et al: International standards for fetal growth based on serial US measurements: the Fetal Growth Longitudinal Study of the INTERGROWTH-21st Project, Lancet 384:869–878, 2014, Fig 3.)*

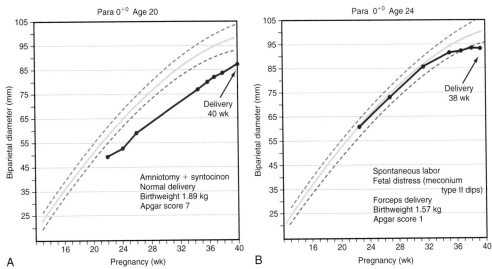

Para 0^{+0} Age 20

Para 0^{+0} Age 24

A Amniotomy + syntocinon
Normal delivery
Birthweight 1.89 kg
Apgar score 7

Delivery
40 wk

B Spontaneous labor
Fetal distress (meconium
type II dips)
Forceps delivery
Birthweight 1.57 kg
Apgar score 1

Delivery
38 wk

Fig. 115.3 A, Example of a "low-profile" growth restriction pattern in an uneventful pregnancy and labor. The baby cried at 1 min, and hypoglycemia did not develop. Birthweight was below the 5th percentile for gestational age. **B,** Example of a "late-flattening" growth restriction pattern. The mother had a typical history of preeclampsia, and the infant had intrapartum fetal distress, a low Apgar score, and postnatal hypoglycemia. Birthweight was below the 5th percentile for gestational age. *(From Campbell S: Fetal growth,* Clin Obstet Gynecol 1:41–65, 1974.)

the pregnancy, and when testing and interventions should be offered. The earliest assessment of pregnancy dating should be used throughout the pregnancy unless methodologies used later in pregnancy are significantly different.

Bibliography is available at Expert Consult.

115.2 Fetal Distress

Kristen R. Suhrie and Sammy M. Tabbah

Fetal compromise may occur during the antepartum or intrapartum period. It may be asymptomatic in the antenatal period but is often suspected by maternal perception of decreased fetal movement. **Antepartum fetal surveillance** is warranted for women at increased risk for fetal death, including those with a history of stillbirth, intrauterine growth restriction (IUGR), oligohydramnios or polyhydramnios, multiple gestation, rhesus sensitization, hypertensive disorders, diabetes mellitus or other chronic maternal disease, decreased fetal movement, preterm labor, preterm rupture of membranes (PROM), and postterm pregnancy. The predominant cause of antepartum fetal distress is uteroplacental insufficiency, which may manifest clinically as IUGR, fetal hypoxia, increased vascular resistance in fetal blood vessels (Figs. 115.4 and 115.5), and, when severe, mixed respiratory and metabolic (lactic) acidosis. The goal of antepartum fetal surveillance is to identify the fetus at risk of stillbirth such that appropriate interventions (i.e., delivery vs optimization of underlying maternal medical condition) can be implemented to allow for a healthy live-born infant. Table 115.1 lists methods for assessing fetal well-being.

The most common noninvasive tests are the nonstress test (**NST**) and the biophysical profile (**BPP**). The NST monitors the presence of fetal heart rate (**FHR**) accelerations that follow fetal movement. A reactive (normal) NST result demonstrates 2 FHR accelerations of at least 15 beats/min above the baseline FHR lasting 15 sec during 20 min of monitoring. A nonreactive NST result suggests possible fetal compromise and requires further assessment with a BPP. Although the NST has a low false-negative rate, it does have a high false-positive rate, which is often remedied by the BPP. The full BPP assesses fetal breathing, body movement, tone, NST, and amniotic fluid volume. It effectively combines

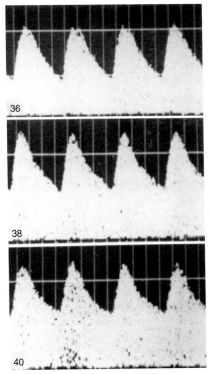

36

38

40

Fig. 115.4 Normal doppler velocity in sequential studies of fetal umbilical artery flow velocity waveforms from one normal pregnancy. Note the systolic peak flow with lower but constant heart flow during diastole. The systolic/diastolic ratio can be determined and, in normal pregnancies, is <3 after the 30th wk of gestation. The *numbers* indicate the weeks of gestation. *(From Trudinger B: Doppler US assessment of blood flow. In Creasy RK, Resnik R, editors:* Maternal-fetal medicine: principles and practice, *ed 5, Philadelphia, 2004, Saunders.)*

acute and chronic indicators of fetal well-being, which improves the predictive value of abnormal testing (Table 115.2). A score of 2 or 0 is given for each observation. A total score of 8-10 is reassuring; a score of 6 is equivocal, and retesting should be done in 12-24 hr; and a score of 4 or less warrants immediate evaluation and possible delivery. The BPP has good negative predictive value. The modified BPP consists of

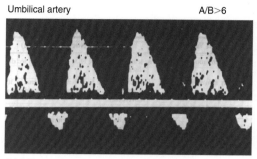

Umbilical artery A/B>6

Fig. 115.5 Abnormal umbilical artery Doppler in which the diastolic component shows flow in a reverse direction. This finding occurs in severe intrauterine hypoxia and intrauterine growth restriction. (*From Trudinger C: Doppler US assessment of blood flow. In Creasy RK, Resnik R, editors: Maternal-fetal medicine: principles and practice, ed 5, Philadelphia, 2004, Saunders.*)

the combination of an US estimate of amniotic fluid volume (the amniotic fluid index) and the NST. When results of both are normal, fetal compromise is very unlikely. Signs of progressive compromise seen on Doppler US include reduced, absent, or reversed diastolic waveform velocity in the fetal aorta or umbilical artery (see Fig. 115.5 and Table 115.1). The umbilical vein and ductus venosus waveforms are also used to assess the degree of fetal compromise. Fetuses at highest risk of stillbirth often have combinations of abnormalities, such as growth restriction, oligohydramnios, reversed diastolic Doppler umbilical artery blood flow velocity, and a low BPP.

Fetal compromise *during labor* may be detected by monitoring the FHR, uterine pressure, and fetal scalp blood pH (Fig. 115.6). **Continuous fetal heart rate monitoring** detects abnormal cardiac patterns by instruments that compute the beat-to-beat FHR from a fetal electrocardiographic signal. Signals are derived either from an electrode attached to the fetal presenting part, from an ultrasonic transducer placed on the maternal abdominal wall to detect continuous ultrasonic waves reflected from the contractions of the fetal heart, or from a phonotransducer placed on the mother's abdomen. Uterine contractions are recorded from an intrauterine pressure catheter or from an external tocotransducer applied to the maternal abdominal wall overlying the uterus. FHR patterns show various characteristics, some of which suggest fetal compromise. The baseline FHR is determined over 10 min devoid of accelerations or decelerations. Over the course of pregnancy, the normal baseline FHR gradually decreases from approximately 155 beats/min in early pregnancy to 135 beats/min at term. The normal range throughout

Table 115.1	Fetal Diagnosis and Assessment
METHOD	**COMMENT(S) AND INDICATION(S)**
IMAGING	
Ultrasound (real-time)	Biometry (growth), anomaly detection, number of fetuses, sites of calcification
	Biophysical profile
	Amniotic fluid volume, hydrops
Ultrasound (Doppler)	Velocimetry (blood flow velocity)
	Detection of increased vascular resistance in the umbilical artery secondary to placental insufficiency
	Detection of fetal anemia (MCA Doppler)
MRI	Defining of lesions before fetal surgery
	Better delineation of fetal CNS anatomy
FLUID ANALYSIS	
Amniocentesis	Karyotype or microarray (cytogenetics), biochemical enzyme analysis, molecular genetic DNA diagnosis, or α-fetoprotein determination
	Bacterial culture, pathogen antigen, or genome detection (PCR)
Cordocentesis (percutaneous umbilical blood sampling)	Detection of blood type, anemia, hemoglobinopathies, thrombocytopenia, polycythemia, acidosis, hypoxia, thrombocytopenia, IgM antibody response to infection
	Rapid karyotyping and molecular DNA genetic diagnosis
	Fetal therapy (see Table 115.5)
FETAL TISSUE ANALYSIS	
Chorionic villus biopsy	Cytogenetic and molecular DNA analysis, enzyme assays
Circulating fetal DNA	Noninvasive molecular DNA genetic analysis including microarray analysis and chromosome number (screening method)
MATERNAL SERUM α-FETOPROTEIN CONCENTRATION	
Elevated	Twins, neural tube defects (anencephaly, spina bifida), intestinal atresia, hepatitis, nephrosis, fetal demise, incorrect gestational age
Reduced	Trisomies, aneuploidy
MATERNAL CERVIX	
Fetal fibronectin	Indicates possible risk of preterm birth
Transvaginal cervical length	Short length suggests possible risk of preterm birth
Bacterial culture	Identifies risk of neonatal infection (group B streptococcus, *Neisseria gonorrhoeae*, *Chlamydia trachomatis*)
Amniotic fluid	Determination of premature rupture of membranes (PROM)
ANTEPARTUM BIOPHYSICAL MONITORING	
Nonstress test	Fetal distress; hypoxia
Biophysical profile and modified biophysical profile	Fetal distress; hypoxia
Intrapartum fetal heart rate monitoring	See Fig. 115.6

Table 115.2	Biophysical Profile Scoring: Technique and Interpretation	
BIOPHYSICAL VARIABLE	**NORMAL SCORE (2)**	**ABNORMAL SCORE (0)**
Fetal breathing movements (FBMs)	At least 1 episode of FBM of at least 30 sec duration in 30 min observation	Absence of FBM or no episode ≥30 sec in 30 min
Gross body movement	At least 3 discrete body/limb movements in 30 min (episodes of active continuous movement considered a single movement)	2 or fewer episodes of body/limb movements in 30 min
Fetal tone	At least 1 episode of active extension with return to flexion of fetal limb(s) or trunk Opening and closing of hand considered evidence of normal tone	Either slow extension with return to partial flexion or movement of limb in full extension or absence of fetal movement with the hand held in complete or partial deflection
Reactive fetal heart rate (FHR)	At least 2 episodes of FHR acceleration of ≥15 beats/min and at least 15 sec in duration associated with fetal movement in 30 min	Less than 2 episodes of acceleration of FHR or acceleration of <15 beats/min in 30 min
Quantitative amniotic fluid (AF) volume*	At least 1 pocket of AF that measures at least 2 cm in 2 perpendicular planes	Either no AF pockets or a pocket <2 cm in 2 perpendicular planes

*Modification of the criteria for reduced amniotic fluid from <1 cm to <2 cm would seem reasonable. Ultrasound is used for biophysical assessment of the fetus.
From Creasy RK, Resnik R, Iams JD, editors: *Maternal-fetal medicine: principles and practice*, ed 5, Philadelphia, 2004, Saunders.

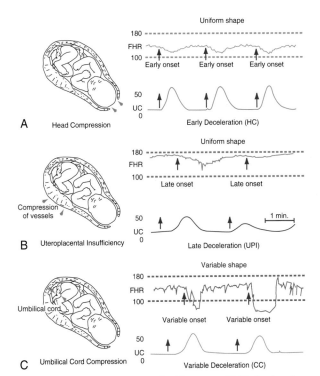

Fig. 115.6 Patterns of periodic fetal heart rate (FHR) deceleration. The tracing in **A** shows early deceleration occurring during the peak of uterine contractions as a result of pressure on the fetal head. **B,** Late deceleration caused by uteroplacental insufficiency. **C,** Variable deceleration as a result of umbilical cord compression. *Arrows* denote the time relationship between the onset of FHR changes and uterine contractions. *(From Hon EH: An atlas of fetal heart rate patterns, New Haven, CT, 1968, Harty Press.)*

Table 115.3	Characteristics of Decelerations of Fetal Heart Rate (FHR)

LATE DECELERATION
Visually apparent, usually symmetric *gradual* decrease and return of the FHR associated with a uterine contraction.
A *gradual* FHR decrease is defined as duration of ≥30 sec from the onset to the nadir of the FHR.
The decrease in FHR is calculated from the onset to the nadir of the deceleration.
The deceleration is delayed in timing, with the nadir of the deceleration occurring after the peak of the contraction.
In most cases, the onset, nadir, and recovery of the deceleration occur after the beginning, peak, and ending of the contraction, respectively.

EARLY DECELERATION
Visually apparent, usually symmetric *gradual* decrease and return of the FHR associated with a uterine contraction.
A *gradual* FHR decrease is defined as duration of ≥30 sec from the onset to the FHR nadir.
The decrease in FHR is calculated from the onset to the nadir of the deceleration.
The nadir of the deceleration occurs at the same time as the peak of the contraction.
In most cases, the onset, nadir, and recovery of the deceleration are coincident with the beginning, peak, and ending of the contraction, respectively.

VARIABLE DECELERATION
Visually apparent, *abrupt* decrease in FHR.
An *abrupt* FHR decrease is defined as duration <30 sec from the onset of the deceleration to the beginning of the FHR nadir of the deceleration.
The decrease in FHR is calculated from the onset to the nadir of the deceleration.
The decrease in FHR is ≥15 beats/min, lasting ≥15 sec, and <2 min in duration.
When variable decelerations are associated with uterine contractions, their onset, depth, and duration commonly vary with successive uterine contractions.

From Macones GA, Hankins GDV, Spong CY, et al: The 2008 National Institute of Child Health and Human Development workshop report on electronic fetal monitoring: update on definitions, interpretation, and research guidelines, *Obstet Gynecol* 112:661–666, 2008.

Table 115.4	Three-Tier Fetal Heart Rate (FHR) Interpretation System

CATEGORY I

Category I FHR tracings include all the following:
- Baseline rate: 110-160 beats/min
- Baseline FHR variability: moderate
- Late or variable decelerations: absent
- Early decelerations: present or absent
- Accelerations: present or absent

CATEGORY II

Category II FHR tracings include all FHR tracings not categorized as category I or category III. Category II tracings may represent an appreciable fraction of those encountered in clinical care. Examples of category II FHR tracings include any of the following:

Baseline Rate
- Bradycardia not accompanied by absence of baseline variability
- Tachycardia

Baseline FHR Variability
- Minimal baseline variability
- Absence of baseline variability not accompanied by recurrent decelerations
- Marked baseline variability

Accelerations
- Absence of induced accelerations after fetal stimulation

Periodic or Episodic Decelerations
- Recurrent variable decelerations accompanied by minimal or moderate baseline variability
- Prolonged deceleration, ≥2 min but <10 min
- Recurrent late decelerations with moderate baseline variability
- Variable decelerations with other characteristics, such as slow return to baseline, "overshoots," and "shoulders"

CATEGORY III

Category III FHR tracings include either:
- Absence of baseline FHR variability
    - or
Any of the following:
- Recurrent late decelerations
- Recurrent variable decelerations
- Bradycardia
- Sinusoidal pattern

Adapted from Macones GA, Hankins GDV, Spong CY, et al: The 2008 National Institute of Child Health and Human Development workshop report on electronic fetal monitoring: update on definitions, interpretation, and research guidelines, *Obstet Gynecol* 112:661–666, 2008.

pregnancy is 110-160 beats/min. **Tachycardia** (>160 beats/min) is associated with early fetal hypoxia, maternal fever, maternal hyperthyroidism, maternal β-sympathomimetic drug or atropine therapy, fetal anemia, infection, and some fetal arrhythmias. Arrhythmias do not generally occur with congenital heart disease and may resolve spontaneously at birth. **Fetal bradycardia** (<110 beats/min) may be normal (e.g., 105-110 beats/min) but may occur with fetal hypoxia, placental transfer of local anesthetic agents and β-adrenergic blocking agents, and occasionally, heart block with or without congenital heart disease.

Normally, the baseline FHR is variable as a result of opposing forces from the fetal sympathetic and parasympathetic nervous systems. **Variability** is classified as follows: *absence of variability,* if an amplitude change is undetectable; *minimal* variability, if amplitude range is ≤5 beats/min; *moderate* variability, if amplitude range is 6-25 beats/min; and *marked* variability, if amplitude range is >25 beats/min. Variability may be decreased or lost with fetal hypoxia or the placental transfer of drugs such as atropine, diazepam, promethazine, magnesium sulfate, and most sedative and narcotic agents. Prematurity, the sleep state, and fetal tachycardia may also diminish beat-to-beat variability.

Accelerations or decelerations of the FHR in response to or independent of uterine contractions may also be monitored (see Fig. 115.6). An **acceleration** is an abrupt increase in FHR of ≥15 beats/min in ≥15 sec. The presence of accelerations or moderate variability reliably predicts the absence of fetal metabolic acidemia. However, their absence does not reliably predict fetal acidemia or hypoxemia. **Early decelerations** are a physiologic vagal response to uterine contractions, with resultant fetal head compression, and represent a repetitive pattern of gradual decrease and return of the FHR that is coincidental with the uterine contraction (Table 115.3). **Variable decelerations** are associated with umbilical cord compression and are characterized by a **V** or **U** shaped pattern, are abrupt in onset and resolution, and may occur with or without uterine contractions.

Late decelerations are associated with fetal hypoxemia and are characterized by onset after a uterine contraction is well established and persists into the interval following resolution of the contraction. The late deceleration pattern is usually associated with maternal hypotension or excessive uterine activity, but it may be a response to any maternal, placental, umbilical cord, or fetal factor that limits effective oxygenation of the fetus. The significance of late decelerations varies according to the underlying clinical context. They are most likely to be associated with true fetal hypoxemia/acidemia when they are recurrent and occur in conjunction with decreased or absent variability. Late decelerations represent a compensatory, chemoreceptor-mediated response to fetal hypoxemia. The transient decrease in FHR serves to increase ventricular preload during the peak of hypoxemia (i.e., at the crest of a uterine contraction). If fetal acidemia progresses, late decelerations may become less pronounced or absent, indicating severe hypoxic depression of myocardial function. Prompt delivery is indicated if late decelerations are unresponsive to oxygen supplementation, hydration, discontinuation of labor stimulation, and position changes. Approximately 10–15% of term fetuses have *terminal* (just before delivery) FHR decelerations that are usually benign if they last <10 min before delivery.

A 3-tier system has been developed by a panel of experts for interpretation of FHR tracings (Table 115.4). **Category I tracings** are normal and are strongly predictive of normal fetal acid-base status at the time of the observation. **Category II tracings** are not predictive of abnormal fetal status, but there is insufficient evidence to categorize them as category I or III; therefore further evaluation, surveillance, and reevaluation are indicated. **Category III tracings** are abnormal and predictive of abnormal fetal acid-base status at the time of observation. Category III tracings require prompt evaluation and efforts to resolve expeditiously the abnormal FHR as previously discussed for late decelerations.

Umbilical cord blood samples obtained at delivery are useful to document fetal acid-base status. Although the exact cord blood pH value that defines significant fetal acidemia is unknown, an umbilical artery pH <7.0 has been associated with greater need for resuscitation and a higher incidence of respiratory, gastrointestinal, cardiovascular, and neurologic complications. Nonetheless, in many cases, even when a low pH is detected, newborn infants are neurologically normal.

Bibliography is available at Expert Consult.

115.3 Maternal Disease and the Fetus
Kristen R. Suhrie and Sammy M. Tabbah

INFECTIOUS DISEASES

See Table 114.3 in Chapter 114 for a list of common maternal infectious diseases that impact the fetus and newborn.

Almost any maternal infection with severe systemic manifestations may result in miscarriage, stillbirth, or premature labor. Whether these results are a consequence of infection of the fetus or are secondary to maternal illness is not always clear. Another important factor to consider when dealing with infectious diseases in pregnancy is the timing of infection. In general, infections that occur earlier in the pregnancy (first or second trimester) are more likely to result in miscarriage or problems with organogenesis, such as the neuromigrational abnormalities seen in newborns with congenital CMV infections.

Cytomegalovirus (CMV) is the most common congenital infection, affecting 0.2–2.2% of all neonates (see Chapter 282). Perinatal transmission can occur at any time during the pregnancy; however, the most devastating sequelae occur with first-trimester infection. After a primary infection, 12–18% of neonates will have signs and symptoms at birth, and as many as 25% can develop long-term complications. The most common complication is **congenital hearing loss**. Severely affected infants have an associated 30% mortality, and 65–80% of survivors develop severe neurologic morbidity. A mother with a history of CMV may experience reactivation of the disease or may be infected with a different strain of the virus and transmit the infection to the fetus. Currently, there are no well-studied or validated antenatal therapies targeted toward decreasing disease severity or preventing congenital infection in the setting of primary maternal CMV infection. Preliminary data from some studies have demonstrated promise with drugs such as valganciclovir and CMV-specific hyperimmune globulin, but confirmatory data are lacking. For this reason, the American College of Obstetricians and Gynecologists (ACOG) does not recommend antenatal therapy for congenital CMV infection outside of an established research protocol.

NONINFECTIOUS DISEASES (see Table 114.2)

Maternal diabetes increases the risk for neonatal hypoglycemia, hypocalcemia, respiratory distress syndrome and other respiratory problems, feeding difficulties, polycythemia, macrosomia, growth restriction, myocardial dysfunction, jaundice, and congenital malformations (see Chapter 127.1). There is an increased risk of uteroplacental insufficiency, polyhydramnios, and fetal demise in poorly controlled diabetic mothers. **Preeclampsia-eclampsia**, **chronic hypertension**, and **chronic renal disease** can result in IUGR, prematurity, and fetal death, all probably caused by diminished uteroplacental perfusion.

Uncontrolled maternal **hypothyroidism** or **hyperthyroidism** is responsible for relative infertility, spontaneous abortion, premature labor, and fetal death. Hypothyroidism in pregnant women (even if mild or asymptomatic) can adversely affect neurodevelopment of the child, especially if the newborn is found to have congenital hypothyroidism.

Maternal **immunologic diseases** such as idiopathic thrombocytopenic purpura, systemic lupus erythematosus, myasthenia gravis, and Graves disease, all of which are mediated by immunoglobulin G autoantibodies that can cross the placenta, frequently cause transient illness in the newborn. Maternal autoantibodies to the folate receptor are associated with neural tube defects (**NTDs**), whereas maternal immunologic sensitization to fetal antigens may be associated with neonatal alloimmune hepatitis and neonatal alloimmune thrombocytopenia (**NAIT**).

Untreated metabolic disorders such as maternal **phenylketonuria** (PKU) results in miscarriage, congenital cardiac malformations, and injury to the brain of a nonphenylketonuric heterozygous fetus. Women whose PKU is well controlled before conception can avoid these complications and have a normal newborn.

Bibliography is available at Expert Consult.

115.4 Medication and Teratogen Exposure

Kristen R. Suhrie and Sammy M. Tabbah

When an infant or child has a congenital malformation or is developmentally delayed, the parents often wrongly blame themselves and attribute the child's problems to events that occurred during pregnancy. Because benign infections occur, and several nonteratogenic drugs are often taken during many pregnancies, the pediatrician must evaluate the presumed viral infections and the drugs ingested to help parents understand their child's birth defect. The causes of approximately 40% of congenital malformations are unknown. Although only relatively few agents are recognized to be teratogenic in humans, new agents continue to be identified. An excellent internet-based resource known as **Reprotox** (reprotox.org) provides comprehensive and routinely updated summaries on drugs and other potentially teratogenic agents in pregnancy. Overall, only 10% of anomalies are caused by recognizable teratogens (see Chapter 128). The time of exposure that is most likely to cause injury is usually during organogenesis at <60 days of gestation. Specific agents produce predictable lesions. Some agents have a dose or *threshold* effect, below which no alterations in growth, function, or

Table 115.5	Agents Acting on Pregnant Women That May Adversely Affect the Structure or Function of the Fetus and Newborn
DRUG	**EFFECT ON FETUS**
Accutane (isotretinoin)	Facial-ear anomalies, heart disease, CNS anomalies
Alcohol	Congenital cardiac, CNS, limb anomalies; IUGR; developmental delay; attention deficits; autism
Aminopterin	Abortion, malformations
Amphetamines	Congenital heart disease, IUGR, withdrawal
ACE inhibitors, angiotensin receptor antagonists	Oligohydramnios, IUGR, renal failure, Potter-like syndrome
Azathioprine	Abortion
Busulfan (Myleran)	Stunted growth; corneal opacities; cleft palate; hypoplasia of ovaries, thyroid, and parathyroids
Carbamazepine	Spina bifida, possible neurodevelopmental delay
Carbimazole	Scalp defects, choanal atresia, esophageal atresia, developmental delay
Carbon monoxide	Cerebral atrophy, microcephaly, seizures
Chloroquine	Deafness
Chorionic villus sampling	Probably no effect, possibly limb reduction
Cigarette smoking	LBW for gestational age
Cocaine/crack	Microcephaly, LBW, IUGR, behavioral disturbances
Cyclophosphamide	Multiple malformations
Danazol	Virilization

Continued

Table 115.5	Agents Acting on Pregnant Women That May Adversely Affect the Structure or Function of the Fetus and Newborn—cont'd
DRUG	**EFFECT ON FETUS**
17α-Ethinyl testosterone (Progestoral)	Masculinization of female fetus
Hyperthermia	Spina bifida
Infliximab	Possible increased risk of live vaccine associated disease in infant; neutropenia
Lithium	Ebstein anomaly, macrosomia
Lopinavir-ritonavir	Transient adrenal dysfunction
6-Mercaptopurine	Abortion
Methyl mercury	Minamata disease, microcephaly, deafness, blindness, mental retardation
Methyltestosterone	Masculinization of female fetus
Misoprostol	Arthrogryposis, cranial neuropathies (Möbius syndrome), equinovarus
Mycophenolate mofetil	Craniofacial, limb, cardiovascular, CNS anomalies
Norethindrone	Masculinization of female fetus
Penicillamine	Cutis laxa syndrome
Phenytoin	Congenital anomalies, IUGR, neuroblastoma, bleeding (vitamin K deficiency)
Polychlorinated biphenyls	Skin discoloration—thickening, desquamation, LBW, acne, developmental delay
Prednisone	Oral clefts
Progesterone	Masculinization of female fetus
Quinine	Abortion, thrombocytopenia, deafness
Selective serotonin reuptake inhibitors	Small increased risk of congenital anomalies, persistent pulmonary hypertension of newborn
Statins	IUGR, limb deficiencies, VACTERAL
Stilbestrol (diethylstilbestrol [DES])	Vaginal adenocarcinoma in adolescence
Streptomycin	Deafness
Tetracycline	Retarded skeletal growth, pigmentation of teeth, hypoplasia of enamel, cataract, limb malformations
Thalidomide	Phocomelia, deafness, other malformations
Toluene (solvent abuse)	Craniofacial abnormalities, prematurity, withdrawal symptoms, hypertonia
Topiramate	Cleft lip
Trimethadione and paramethadione	Abortion, multiple malformations, mental retardation
Valproate	CNS (spina bifida), facial and cardiac anomalies, limb defects, impaired neurologic function, autism spectrum disorder
Vitamin D	Supravalvular aortic stenosis, hypercalcemia
Warfarin (Coumadin)	Fetal bleeding and death, hypoplastic nasal structures

ACE, Angiotensin-converting enzyme; CNS, central nervous system; IUGR, intrauterine growth restriction; LBW, low birthweight; VACTERAL, vertebral, anal, cardiac, tracheoesophageal fistula, renal, arterial, limb.

structure occur. Genetic variables such as the presence of specific enzymes may metabolize a benign agent into a more toxic, teratogenic form (e.g., phenytoin conversion to its epoxide). In many circumstances the same agent and dose may not consistently produce the lesion.

Reduced enzyme activity of the folate methylation pathway, particularly the formation of 5-methyltetrahydrofolate, may be responsible for NTDs or other birth defects. The common thermolabile mutation of 5,10-methylene tetrahydrofolate reductase may be one of the enzymes responsible. Folate supplementation for all pregnant women (by direct fortification of cereal grains, which is mandatory in the United States), and oral folic acid tablets taken during organogenesis may overcome this genetic enzyme defect, thus reducing the incidence of NTDs and perhaps birth defects.

The U.S. Food and Drug Administration (FDA) classifies drugs into 5 pregnancy risk categories. **Category A** drugs pose no risk on the basis of evidence from controlled human studies. For **category B** drugs, either no risk has been shown in animal studies but no adequate studies have been done in humans, *or* some risk has been shown in animal studies but these results are not confirmed by human studies. For **category C** drugs, either definite risk has been shown in animal studies but no adequate human studies have been performed, *or* no data are available from either animal or human studies. **Category D** includes drugs with some risk but with a benefit that may exceed that risk for the treated life-threatening condition, such as streptomycin for tuberculosis. **Category X** is for drugs that are contraindicated in pregnancy on the basis of animal and human evidence and for which the risk exceeds the benefits.

The use of medications or herbal remedies during pregnancy is potentially harmful to the fetus. Consumption of medications occurs during the majority of pregnancies. The average mother has taken 4 drugs other than vitamins or iron during pregnancy. Almost 40% of pregnant women receive a drug for which human safety during pregnancy has not been established (category C pregnancy risk). Moreover, many women are exposed to potential reproductive toxins, such as occupational, environmental, or household chemicals, including solvents, pesticides, and hair products. The effects of drugs taken by the mother vary

Table 115.6	Agents Acting on Pregnant Women That May Adversely Affect the Newborn Infant*

Acebutolol—IUGR, hypotension, bradycardia
Acetazolamide—metabolic acidosis
Amiodarone—bradycardia, hypothyroidism
Anesthetic agents (volatile)—CNS depression
Adrenal corticosteroids—adrenocortical failure (rare)
Ammonium chloride—acidosis (clinically inapparent)
Aspirin—neonatal bleeding, prolonged gestation
Atenolol—IUGR, hypoglycemia
Baclofen—withdrawal
Blue cohosh herbal tea—neonatal heart failure
Bromides—rash, CNS depression, IUGR
Captopril, enalapril—transient anuric renal failure, oligohydramnios
Caudal-paracervical anesthesia with mepivacaine (accidental introduction of anesthetic into scalp of baby)—bradypnea, apnea, bradycardia, convulsions
Cholinergic agents (edrophonium, pyridostigmine)—transient muscle weakness
CNS depressants (narcotics, barbiturates, benzodiazepines) during labor—CNS depression, hypotonia
Cephalothin—positive direct Coombs test reaction
Dexamethasone—periventricular leukomalacia
Fluoxetine and other SSRIs—transient neonatal withdrawal, hypertonicity, minor anomalies, preterm birth, prolonged QT interval
Haloperidol—withdrawal
Hexamethonium bromide—paralytic ileus
Ibuprofen—oligohydramnios, pulmonary hypertension
Imipramine—withdrawal
Indomethacin—oliguria, oligohydramnios, intestinal perforation, pulmonary hypertension
Intravenous fluids during labor (e.g., salt-free solutions)—electrolyte disturbances, hyponatremia, hypoglycemia
Iodide (radioactive)—goiter
Iodides—goiter
Lead—reduced intellectual function
Magnesium sulfate—respiratory depression, meconium plug, hypotonia
Methimazole—goiter, hypothyroidism
Morphine and its derivatives (addiction)—withdrawal symptoms (poor feeding, vomiting, diarrhea, restlessness, yawning and stretching, dyspnea and cyanosis, fever and sweating, pallor, tremors, convulsions)
Naphthalene—hemolytic anemia (in G6PD-deficient infants)
Nitrofurantoin—hemolytic anemia (in G6PD-deficient infants)
Oxytocin—hyperbilirubinemia, hyponatremia
Phenobarbital—bleeding diathesis (vitamin K deficiency), possible long-term reduction in IQ, sedation
Primaquine—hemolytic anemia (in G6PD-deficient infants)
Propranolol—hypoglycemia, bradycardia, apnea
Propylthiouracil—goiter, hypothyroidism
Pyridoxine—seizures
Reserpine—drowsiness, nasal congestion, poor temperature stability
Sulfonamides—interfere with protein binding of bilirubin; kernicterus at low levels of serum bilirubin, hemolysis with G6PD deficiency
Sulfonylurea agents—refractory hypoglycemia
Sympathomimetic (tocolytic β-agonist) agents—tachycardia
Thiazides—neonatal thrombocytopenia (rare)
Tumor necrosis factor blocking agents—neutropenia, possible increased risk of infection during 1st yr of life
Valproate—developmental delay
Zolpidem (Ambien)—low birthweight

*See also Table 115.5.
CNS, Central nervous system; G6PD, glucose-6-phosphate dehydrogenase; IUGR, intrauterine growth restriction; SSRI, selective serotonin reuptake inhibitor.

considerably, especially in relation to the time in pregnancy when they are taken and the fetal genotype for drug-metabolizing enzymes.

Miscarriage or **congenital malformations** result from the maternal ingestion of teratogenic drugs during the period of organogenesis. Maternal medications taken later, particularly during the last few weeks of gestation or during labor, tend to affect the function of specific organs or enzyme systems, and these adversely affect the neonate rather than the fetus (Tables 115.5 and 115.6). The effects of drugs may be evident immediately in the delivery room or later in the neonatal period, or they may be delayed even longer. The administration of diethylstilbestrol during pregnancy, for instance, increased the risk for vaginal adenocarcinoma in female offspring in the 2nd or 3rd decade of life.

Often the risk of controlling maternal disease must be balanced with the risk of possible complications in the fetus. Most women with epilepsy have normal fetuses. Nonetheless, several commonly used **antiepileptic drugs** are associated with congenital malformations. Infants exposed to valproic acid may have multiple anomalies, including NTDs, hypospadias, facial anomalies, cardiac anomalies, and limb defects. In addition,

they have lower developmental index scores than unexposed infants and infants exposed to other common antiepileptic drugs.

Moderate or high alcohol intake (≥7 drinks/wk or ≥3 drinks on multiple occasions) is a risk for **fetal alcohol syndrome**. The exposed fetuses are at risk for growth failure, central nervous system abnormalities, cognitive defects, and behavioral problems. It must be emphasized, however, that there is no known dose-response threshold for fetal alcohol exposure; therefore pregnant women should be counseled toward complete abstinence. **Smoking** during pregnancy is associated with IUGR and facial clefts.

Chronic **heroin (opioid)** use throughout pregnancy is associated with an increased risk of fetal growth restriction, placental abruption, stillbirth, preterm birth, and intrauterine passage of meconium. Opiates readily cross the placenta; therefore these effects are postulated to be related to cyclic fetal opiate withdrawal. Furthermore, the lifestyle issues surrounding opioid abuse, including lack of or late entry into prenatal care, place the mother at higher risk of adverse pregnancy outcome. Therefore, opioid maintenance therapy with either methadone or buprenorphine is recommended for opioid-dependent pregnant women to prevent complications of illicit opioid use and narcotic withdrawal, encourage prenatal care and drug treatment, reduce criminal activity, and avoid risks to the patient of associating with a drug culture.

Neonatal abstinence syndrome (NAS) occurs in the setting of opioid maintenance treatment or illicit drug use; thus opiate maintenance therapy is not preventive in this regard. **Methadone** is considered first-line therapy for treatment of opioid dependence in pregnancy; **buprenorphine** is an acceptable alternative in the appropriately selected patient. There is no established, dose-response relationship between methadone or buprenorphine and risk/severity of NAS, so the lowest effective dose to eliminate maternal cravings/withdrawal is recommended. Methadone is associated with a lower birthweight than buprenorphine. Both medications have a similar rate of NAS requiring treatment (approximately 50%); however, the use of antenatal buprenorphine has been associated with significantly lower dosages of morphine to treat NAS and significantly shorter NAS-related hospital stays than methadone. For these reasons, buprenorphine may be preferred under certain circumstances.

The specific mechanism of action is known or postulated for very few teratogens. **Warfarin**, a vitamin K antagonist used for anticoagulation, prevents the carboxylation of γ-carboxyglutamic acid, which is a component of osteocalcin and other vitamin K–dependent bone proteins. The teratogenic effect of warfarin on developing cartilage, especially nasal cartilage, appears to be avoided if the pregnant woman's anticoagulation treatment is switched from warfarin to heparin for the period between weeks 6 and 12 of gestation. However, the risk of intracranial hemorrhage is maintained with exposure throughout pregnancy. For these reasons, **low-molecular-weight heparin** is the preferred anticoagulant when treating pregnant women.

Hypothyroidism in the fetus may be caused by maternal ingestion of an excessive amount of iodide or propylthiouracil; each interferes with the conversion of inorganic to organic iodides. Furthermore, there is an interaction between genetic factors and susceptibility to certain drugs or environmental toxins. Phenytoin teratogenesis, for example, may be mediated by genetic differences in the enzymatic production of epoxide metabolites. Polymorphisms of genes encoding enzymes that metabolize the polycyclic aromatic hydrocarbons in cigarette smoke influence the growth-restricting effects of smoking on the fetus.

Recognition of teratogenic potential from a variety of sources offers the opportunity to prevent related birth defects. If a pregnant woman is informed of the potentially harmful effects of alcohol, tobacco, and illicit drugs on her unborn infant, she may be motivated to avoid consumption of these substances during pregnancy. A woman with insulin-dependent diabetes mellitus may significantly decrease her risk for having a child with birth defects by achieving good control of her disease before conception. Lastly, in view of the limits of current knowledge regarding the fetal effects of maternal medication use, drugs and herbal agents should only be prescribed during pregnancy after carefully weighing the maternal benefit against the risk of fetal harm.

Bibliography is available at Expert Consult.

115.5 Radiation
Kristen R. Suhrie and Sammy M. Tabbah

See also Chapter 736.

Accidental exposure of a pregnant woman to radiation is a common cause of anxiety about whether her fetus will have genetic abnormalities or birth defects. It is unlikely that exposure to diagnostic radiation will cause gene mutations; no increase in genetic abnormalities has been identified in the offspring exposed as unborn fetuses to the atomic bomb explosions in Japan in 1945.

A more realistic concern is whether the exposed human fetus will show birth defects or a higher incidence of malignancy. The background fetal radiation exposure in a given pregnancy is approximately 0.1 rad. The estimated radiation dose for most radiographs is <0.1 rad and for most CT scans <5 rad (maximum recommended radiation exposure

in pregnancy). Imaging studies with high radiation exposure (e.g., CT scans) can be modified to ensure that radiation doses are kept as low as possible. Thus, single diagnostic studies do not result in radiation doses high enough to affect the embryo or fetus. Pregnancy termination should not be recommended only on the basis of diagnostic radiation exposure. Most of the evidence suggests that usual fetal radiation exposure does not increase the risk of childhood leukemia and other cancers; although some sources suggest that a 1-2 rad fetal radiation exposure may confer a 1.5-2–fold increased risk of childhood leukemia, which has a background risk of 1 in 3,000. Before implantation (0-2 wk postconception), radiation doses of 5-10 rad may result in miscarriage. At 2-8 wk gestation, doses in excess of 20 rad have been associated with congenital anomalies and fetal growth restriction. Severe intellectual disabilities can occur with exposures of ≥25 rad before 25 wk gestation. The available data suggest no harmful fetal effect of diagnostic MRI or US, which do not involve radiation.

Bibliography is available at Expert Consult.

115.6 Intrauterine Diagnosis of Fetal Disease
Kristen R. Suhrie and Sammy M. Tabbah

See Table 115.1 and Chapter 115.2.

Diagnostic procedures are used to identify fetal diseases when direct fetal treatment is possible, to better direct neonatal care, when a decision is made to deliver a viable but premature infant to avoid intrauterine fetal demise, or when pregnancy termination is being considered. Fetal assessment is also indicated in a broader context when the family, medical, or reproductive history of the mother suggests the presence of a high-risk pregnancy or a high-risk fetus (see Chapters 114 and 115.3).

Various methods are used for identifying fetal disease (see Table 115.1). Fetal US imaging may detect fetal growth abnormalities (by previously outlined biometric measurements) or fetal malformations (Fig. 115.7). Serial determinations of growth velocity and the head-to-abdomen circumference ratio enhance the ability to detect IUGR. Real-time US may identify placental abnormalities (abruptio placentae, placenta previa) and fetal anomalies such as hydrocephalus, NTDs, duodenal atresia, diaphragmatic hernia, renal agenesis, bladder outlet obstruction, congenital heart disease, limb abnormalities, sacrococcygeal teratoma, cystic hygroma, omphalocele, gastroschisis, and hydrops (Table 115.7).

Real-time US also facilitates performance of needle-guided procedures (i.e. cordocentesis) and the BPP by imaging fetal breathing, body movements, tone, and amniotic fluid volume (see Table 115.2). Doppler velocimetry assesses fetal arterial blood flow (vascular resistance) (see Figs. 115.4 and 115.5). Fetal MRI is used to better define abnormalities detected on US and to help with prognostication (see Fig. 115.1).

Amniocentesis, the transabdominal withdrawal of amniotic fluid during pregnancy for diagnostic purposes (see Table 115.1), is a common obstetric procedure. It is frequently performed to evaluate for infection. It is also done for genetic indications, usually between the 15th and 20th wk of gestation, with results available as soon as 24-48 hr for fluorescence in situ hybridization (FISH) testing and 2-3 wk for microarray testing. The most common indication for genetic amniocentesis is **advanced maternal age**; the risk for chromosome abnormality at term at age 21 yr is 1:525, vs 1:6 at age 49 yr. ACOG recommends that all pregnant women be offered amniocentesis to evaluate further for an underlying genetic condition such as Down syndrome. Analysis of amniotic fluid may also help in identifying NTDs (elevation of α-fetoprotein [AFP] and presence of acetylcholinesterase). Additionally, families with a known genetic syndrome may be offered prenatal genetic testing from amniotic fluid or amniocytes obtained via amniocentesis or CVS.

Chorionic villus sampling (CVS) is performed in the first trimester, either transvaginally or transabdominally. The sample obtained is placental in origin, which can sometimes be problematic because aneuploidy may be present in the placenta and not the fetus, a condition known as **confined placental mosaicism**, which can give a false-positive rate as high as 3%. Furthermore, CVS may be associated with a slightly higher risk of fetal loss than amniocentesis.

Amniocentesis can be carried out with little discomfort to the mother. Procedure-related complications are relatively rare, and many can be avoided by using a US-guided approach. These risks include direct damage to the fetus, placental puncture and bleeding with secondary damage to the fetus, stimulation of uterine contraction and premature labor, chorioamnionitis, maternal sensitization to fetal blood, and pregnancy loss. Best available data indicate that the pregnancy loss rate associated with amniocentesis is 1:500-900 procedures. Amniocentesis is not recommended before 14 wk of gestation because this has been associated with a higher risk of pregnancy loss, ruptured membranes, and clubfoot.

Cordocentesis, or percutaneous umbilical blood sampling (PUBS), is used to diagnose fetal hematologic abnormalities, genetic disorders, infections, and fetal acidosis (see Table 115.1). Under direct US visualization, a long needle is passed into the umbilical vein at its entrance to the placenta or in a free loop of cord. Transfusion or administration of drugs can be performed through the umbilical vein (Table 115.8). The predominant indication for this procedure is for confirmation of fetal anemia (in Rh isoimmunization) or thrombocytopenia (NAIT), with subsequent transfusion of packed red blood cells or platelets into the umbilical venous circulation.

Aneuploidy screening is offered to pregnant women in the first trimester or at midgestation to evaluate the risk for common aneuploidies such as Down syndrome (trisomy 21), trisomy 18, trisomy 13, and congenital malformations (e.g., abdominal wall or neural tube defects) known to cause elevations of various markers. A combination of these biochemical markers (including AFP, inhibin A, estriol, pregnancy-associated plasma protein A, β–human chorionic gonadotropin [hCG]) and US increases the positive predictive value (PPV) of these screening tests. Fetal DNA in maternal plasma and fetal cells circulating in maternal blood are potential noninvasive sources of material for prenatal genetic testing. This testing, however, is not diagnostic, and a positive test requires either amniocentesis or postnatal analysis to confirm the diagnosis. Nonetheless, fetal karyotyping by analysis of fetal DNA in maternal plasma is another screening test that is very sensitive for the detection of Down syndrome, with a higher PPV than any other prenatal screening test for Down syndrome. Currently, however, the use of this technology is only advocated in pregnancies deemed at high risk for aneuploidy.

Bibliography is available at Expert Consult.

115.7 Treatment and Prevention of Fetal Disease

Kristen R. Suhrie and Sammy M. Tabbah

See also Chapter 116.

Management of a fetal disease depends on coordinated advances in diagnostic accuracy and knowledge of the disease's natural history; an understanding of fetal nutrition, pharmacology, immunology, and pathophysiology; the availability of specific active drugs that cross the placenta; and therapeutic procedures. Progress in providing specific treatments for accurately diagnosed diseases has improved with the advent of real-time ultrasonography, amniocentesis, and cordocentesis (see Tables 115.1 and 115.8).

The incidence of sensitization of Rh-negative women by Rh-positive fetuses has been reduced by prophylactic administration of Rh(D) immunoglobulin to mothers early in pregnancy and after each delivery or abortion, thus reducing the frequency of hemolytic disease in their subsequent offspring. **Fetal erythroblastosis** (see Chapter 124.2) may be accurately detected by fetal Doppler assessment of the peak systolic velocity of the middle cerebral artery and treated with intrauterine transfusions of packed Rh-negative blood cells via the intraperitoneal or, more often, intraumbilical vein approach.

Pharmacologic approaches to fetal immaturity mostly revolve around the administration of antenatal corticosteroids to the mother to promote fetal production of surfactant with a resultant decrease in the incidence of **respiratory distress syndrome** (see Chapter 122.3). Tocolytic agents have been demonstrated to prolong pregnancy to allow the administration of antenatal corticosteroids (48 hr); however, there is no proven benefit beyond this timeframe. Maternal administration

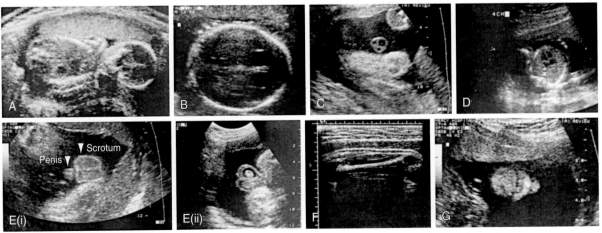

Fig. 115.7 Assessment of fetal anatomy. A, Overall view of the uterus at 24 wk showing a longitudinal section of the fetus and an anterior placenta. **B,** Transverse section at the level of the lateral ventricle at 18 wk showing (*on the right*) prominent anterior horns of the lateral ventricles on either side of the midline echo of the falx. **C,** Cross section of the umbilical cord showing that the lumen of the umbilical vein is much wider than that of the 2 umbilical arteries. **D,** Four-chambered view of the heart at 18 wk with equal-sized atria. **E(i),** Normal male genitals near term. **E(ii),** Hydrocele outlining a testicle within the scrotum projecting into a normal-size pocket of amniotic fluid at 38 wk. Approximately 2% of male infants after birth have clinical evidence of a hydrocele that is often bilateral, not to be confused with subcutaneous edema occurring during vaginal breech birth. **F,** Section of a thigh near term showing thick subcutaneous tissue (4.6 mm between *markers*) above the femur of a fetus with macrosomia. **G,** Fetal face viewed from below, showing (*from right to left*) the nose, alveolar margin, and chin at 20 wk. (*From Special investigative procedures. In Beischer NA, Mackay EV, Colditz PB, editors:* Obstetrics and the newborn, *ed 3, Philadelphia, 1997, Saunders.*)

Table 115.7	Significance of Fetal Ultrasonographic Anatomic Findings			
PRENATAL OBSERVATION	**DEFINITION**	**DIFFERENTIAL DIAGNOSIS**	**SIGNIFICANCE**	**POSTNATAL EVALUATION**
Dilated cerebral ventricles	Ventriculomegaly ≥10 mm	Hydrocephalus Hydranencephaly Dandy-Walker cyst Agenesis of corpus callosum Volume loss	Transient isolated ventriculomegaly is common and usually benign. Persistent or progressive ventriculomegaly is more worrisome. Identify associated cranial and extracranial anomalies.	Serial head US or MRI Evaluate for extracranial anomalies.
Choroid plexus cysts	Size ~10 mm: unilateral or bilateral 1–3% incidence	Abnormal karyotype (trisomy 18, 21) Increased risk if AMA	Often isolated, benign; resolves by 24-28 wk. Fetus should be examined for other organ anomalies; if additional anomalies present, amniocentesis should be performed for karyotype.	Head US Examine for extracranial anomalies; karyotype if indicated.
Nuchal fold thickening	≥6 mm at 15-20 wk	Cystic hygroma trisomy 21, 18 Turner syndrome (XO) Other genetic syndromes Normal (~25%)	~50% of affected fetuses have chromosome abnormalities. Amniocentesis for karyotype needed.	Evaluate for multiple organ malformations; karyotype if indicated.
Dilated renal pelvis	Pyelectasis ≥4 to 10 mm 0.6–1% incidence	Normal variant Uteropelvic junction obstruction Vesicoureteral reflux Posterior ureteral valves Entopic ureterocele Large-volume nonobstruction	Often "physiologic" and transient Reflux is common. If dilation is >10 mm or associated with caliectasis, pathologic cause should be considered. If large bladder present, posterior urethral valves and megacystis–microcolon hypoperistalsis syndrome should be considered.	Repeat ultrasonography on day 5 and at 1 mo; voiding cystourethrogram, prophylactic antibiotics
Echogenic bowel	0.6% incidence	CF, meconium peritonitis, trisomy 21 or 18, other chromosomal abnormalities cytomegalovirus, toxoplasmosis, GI obstruction, intrauterine bleeding (fetal swallowing of blood)	Often normal Consider CF, aneuploidy, and TORCH.	Sweat chloride and DNA testing Karyotype Surgery for obstruction Evaluation for TORCH
Stomach appearance	Small or absent or with double bubble	Upper GI obstruction (esophageal atresia) Double bubble signifies duodenal atresia Aneuploidy Polyhydramnios Stomach in chest signifies diaphragmatic hernia	Must also consider neurologic disorders that reduce swallowing. >30% with double bubble have trisomy 21.	Chromosomes; kidney, ureter, and bladder radiograph if indicated; upper GI series; neurologic evaluation

CF, Cystic fibrosis; CMV, cytomegalovirus; GI, gastrointestinal; TORCH, toxoplasmosis, other agents, rubella, CMV, herpes simplex syndrome; US, ultrasound.

of magnesium sulfate for fetal/neonatal neuroprotection is recommended in pregnancies deemed to be at risk of imminent delivery before 32 wk gestation in light of evidence demonstrating a reduction in frequency of cerebral palsy compared to those who did not receive this treatment.

Management of definitively diagnosed fetal genetic disease or congenital anomalies consists of multidisciplinary parental counseling. Rarely, high-dose **vitamin therapy** for a responsive inborn error of metabolism (e.g., biotin-dependent disorders) or fetal transfusion (with red blood cells or platelets) may be indicated. **Fetal surgery** is well-established treatment for certain conditions but remains a largely experimental approach to therapy for other conditions and is available only in a few, highly specialized perinatal centers (see Table 115.8 and Chapter 116). The nature of the defect and its consequences must be considered, as well as ethical implications for the fetus and the parents. **Termination of pregnancy** is also an option that should be discussed during the initial phases of counseling.

Folic acid supplementation decreases the incidence and recurrence of NTDs. Because the neural tube closes within the 1st 28 days of conception, periconceptional supplementation is needed for prevention. It is recommended that women without a prior history of a NTD ingest 400 µg/day of folic acid throughout their reproductive years. Women with a history of a prior pregnancy complicated by an NTD or a first-degree relative with an NTD should have preconceptional counseling and should ingest 4 mg/day of supplemental folic acid beginning at least 1 mo before conception. Fortification of cereal grain flour with folic acid is established policy in the United States and some other countries. The optimal concentration of folic acid in enriched grains is somewhat controversial. The incidence of NTD in the United States and other countries has decreased significantly since these public health initiatives were implemented. Use of some antiepileptic drugs (valproate, carbamazepine) during pregnancy is associated with an increased risk of NTD. Women taking these medications should ingest 1-5 mg of folic acid daily in the preconception period.

Bibliography is available at Expert Consult.

Table 115.8	Fetal Therapy

DISORDER	POSSIBLE TREATMENT
HEMATOLOGIC	
Anemia with hydrops (erythroblastosis fetalis)	Cordocentesis of umbilical vein with packed red blood cell transfusion
Isoimmune thrombocytopenia	Umbilical vein platelet transfusion, maternal IVIG
Autoimmune thrombocytopenia (ITP)	Maternal steroids and IVIG
METABOLIC/ENDOCRINE	
Maternal phenylketonuria (PKU)	Phenylalanine restriction
Fetal galactosemia	Galactose-free diet (?)
Multiple carboxylase deficiency	Biotin if responsive
Methylmalonic acidemia	Vitamin B_{12} if responsive
21-Hydroxylase deficiency	Dexamethasone if female fetus
Maternal diabetes mellitus	Tight insulin control during pregnancy, labor, and delivery
Fetal goiter	Maternal hyperthyroidism—maternal propylthiouracil
	Fetal hypothyroidism—intraamniotic thyroxine
Bartter syndrome	Maternal indomethacin may prevent nephrocalcinosis and postnatal sodium losses
FETAL DISTRESS	
Hypoxia	Maternal oxygen, position changes
Intrauterine growth restriction	Improve macronutrients and micronutrients if deficient, smoking cessation, treatment of maternal disease, antenatal fetal surveillance
Oligohydramnios, premature rupture of membranes with variable deceleration	Antenatal fetal surveillance
	Approach dependent on etiology
	Amnioinfusion (intrapartum)
Polyhydramnios	Antenatal fetal surveillance
	Approach dependent on etiology
	Amnioreduction if indicated,
Supraventricular tachycardia	Maternal digoxin,* flecainide, procainamide, amiodarone, quinidine
Lupus anticoagulant	Maternal aspirin and heparin
Meconium-stained fluid	Amnioinfusion
Congenital heart block	Dexamethasone, pacemaker (with hydrops)
Premature labor	Magnesium sulfate, nifedipine, indomethacin with antenatal corticosteroids (betamethasone)
RESPIRATORY	
Pulmonary immaturity	Betamethasone
Bilateral chylothorax—pleural effusions	Thoracentesis, pleuroamniotic shunt
CONGENITAL ABNORMALITIES†	
Neural tube defects	Folate, vitamins (prevention); fetal surgery‡
Posterior urethral valves, urethral atresia (lower urinary tract obstruction)	Percutaneous vesicoamniotic shunt
Cystic adenomatoid malformation (with hydrops)	Pleuroamniotic shunt or resection‡
Fetal neck masses	Secure an airway with EXIT procedure‡
INFECTIOUS DISEASE	
Group B streptococcus colonization	Ampicillin, penicillin
Chorioamnionitis	Antibiotics and delivery
Toxoplasmosis	Spiramycin, pyrimethamine, sulfadiazine, folic acid
Syphilis	Penicillin
Tuberculosis	Antituberculosis drugs
Lyme disease	Penicillin, ceftriaxone
Parvovirus	Intrauterine red blood cell transfusion for hydrops, severe anemia
Chlamydia trachomatis	Azithromycin
HIV-AIDS	Maternal and neonatal antiretroviral therapy (see Chapter 302)
Cytomegalovirus	No approved prenatal treatments
OTHER	
Nonimmune hydrops (anemia)	Umbilical vein packed red blood cell transfusion
Narcotic abstinence (withdrawal)	Maternal methadone maintenance
Sacrococcygeal teratoma (with hydrops)	In utero resection or catheter-directed vessel obliteration
Cardiac rhabdomyoma	Maternal sirolimus
Intrapericardial teratoma	Fetal surgery
CRISPR-Cas9 gene editing	Proof of concept in previable in vitro fertilized human embryos
Twin-twin transfusion syndrome	Repeated amniocentesis, yttrium-aluminum-garnet (YAG) laser photocoagulation of shared vessels
Twin reversed arterial perfusion (TRAP) syndrome	Cord occlusion, radiofrequency ablation
Multifetal gestation	Selective reduction
Neonatal hemochromatosis	Maternal IVIG
Aortic stenosis	In utero valvuloplasty

*Drug of choice (may require percutaneous umbilical cord sampling and umbilical vein administration if hydrops is present). Most drug therapy is given to the mother, with subsequent placental passage to the fetus.
†Detailed fetal ultrasonography is needed to detect other anomalies; karyotype is also indicated.
‡EXIT permits surgery and other procedures.
EXIT, Ex utero intrapartum treatment; IVIG, intravenous immune globulin; (?), possible but not proved efficacy.

Chapter 116
Fetal Intervention and Surgery

Paul S. Kingma

第一百一十六章
宫内胎儿手术干预

中文导读

　　本章主要介绍了宫内胎儿手术的相关伦理问题，这个是目前较为有争议的学术焦点。本章同时介绍了宫内胎儿疾病的诊断评估与治疗，以及对胎儿、胎盘、脐带或胎膜进行宫内手术的适应证和依据。关于宫内胎儿手术的特殊疾病及其具体操作方面，本章详细描述了梗阻性尿路疾病、非梗阻性肾病、先天性膈

疝、先天性肺导气管畸形、脊髓脊膜膨出等疾病的概念、发病率、病理生理、预后、手术干预的意义、不同手术方式的优劣选择，以及其他可用于手术干预的相关疾病，如对心脏缺陷的产前干预、激光疗法，以及胎儿中心成立的意义，包括对受严重影响的胎儿的护理计划表。

Numerous diagnoses have been evaluated for the possibility of fetal intervention (Tables 116.1 and 116.2). Some have proved beneficial to the developing infant, some have been abandoned, and some are still under investigation.

FETAL THERAPY ETHICS

With the development of advanced fetal ultrasound (US), fetal MRI, and fetal echocardiography, the ability to accurately diagnose fetal disease has improved substantially over the past 3 decades. There have also been advances in maternal anesthesia and tocolysis, reduction in maternal morbidity, development of fetal surgery–specific equipment, improved clinical expertise of the fetal care team, and construction of state-of-the-art fetal treatment centers. Fetal surgery remains controversial, however, and every discussion of fetal surgery must include a careful consideration of the ethical conflicts inherit to these procedures.

Unlike most surgical procedures, fetal surgery must consider 2 patients simultaneously, balancing the potential risks and benefits to the fetus with those to the mother during the current and future pregnancies. The **International Fetal Medicine and Surgery Society** (IFMSS) established a consensus statement on fetal surgery, as follows:

1. A fetal surgery candidate should be a singleton with no other abnormalities observed on level II ultrasound, karyotype (by amniocentesis), α-fetoprotein (AFP) level or viral cultures.
2. The disease process must not be so severe that the fetus cannot be saved and also not so mild that the infant will do well with postnatal therapy.

3. The family must be fully counseled and understand the risks and benefits of fetal surgery, and they must agree to long-term follow-up to track efficacy of the fetal intervention.
4. A multidisciplinary team must concur that the disease process is fatal without intervention, that the family understands the risks and benefits, and that the fetal intervention is appropriate.

OBSTRUCTIVE UROPATHY

Obstructive uropathy is most frequently caused by **posterior urethral valves** (PUV) but can be caused by a variety of other defects, including urethral atresia, persistent cloaca, caudal regression, and megacystis–microcolon–intestinal hypoperistalsis syndrome (see Chapters 555 and 556). Obstructive uropathy usually presents on fetal US with an enlarged bladder, bilateral hydroureteronephrosis, and oligohydramnios. Mild forms of obstructive uropathy may lead to minimal short- or long-term clinical sequelae. However, the lack of fetal urine output and resulting oligohydramnios or anhydramnios in more severe forms can cause significant **pulmonary hypoplasia**, which is associated with death shortly after delivery in >80% of infants. Pulmonary survivors are still subject to high mortality and chronic morbidity resulting from renal dysplasia, renal failure, and the need for chronic renal replacement therapy.

The primary objective of fetal intervention in fetuses with obstructive uropathy is *restoration of amniotic fluid volume to prevent pulmonary hypoplasia*. Although prevention of ongoing renal injury is also desired, the efficacy of fetal intervention in achieving this goal is uncertain. Several studies have attempted to use fetal urine evaluation to predict

Table 116.1	Fetal Diagnoses Evaluated and Treated in Fetal Centers

Amniotic band syndrome (ABS)	Gastroschisis
Anomalies in monochorionic twins	Hydrocephalus
Aortic stenosis	Hydronephrosis
Arachnoid cyst	Hypoplastic left heart syndrome (HLHS)
Bladder exstrophy	Imperforate anus
Bladder outlet obstruction	Intraabdominal cyst
Bronchopulmonary sequestration (BPS)	Lymphangioma
Cervical teratoma	Mediastinal teratoma
Cloaca	Myelomeningocele, spina bifida
Cloaca exstrophy	Neuroblastoma
Complete heart block	Obstructive uropathy
Congenital pulmonary airway malformation (CPAM)	Omphalocele
Congenital diaphragmatic hernia (CDH)	Pentalogy of Cantrell
Congenital high airway obstruction syndrome (CHAOS)	Pericardial teratoma
EXIT to airway procedure for CHAOS	Pleural effusions
Conjoined twins	Pulmonary agenesis
Dandy-Walker malformation	Pulmonary atresia with intact ventricular septum
Duodenal atresia	Sacrococcygeal teratoma (SCT)
Encephalocele	Twin reversed arterial perfusion (TRAP) sequence
Enteric duplicational atresia	Twin-twin transfusion syndrome (TTTS)
Esophageal atresia	Vein of Galen aneurysm

EXIT, Ex utero intrapartum treatment.

Table 116.2	Indications and Rationales for in Utero Surgery on the Fetus, Placenta, Cord, or Membranes

FETAL SURGERY	PATHOPHYSIOLOGY	RATIONALE FOR IN UTERO INTERVENTION
SURGERY ON THE FETUS		
1. Congenital diaphragmatic hernia	Pulmonary hypoplasia and anatomic substrate for pulmonary hypertension	Reversal of pulmonary hypoplasia and reduced degree of pulmonary hypertension; repair of actual defect delayed until after birth
2. Lower urinary tract obstruction	Progressive renal damage due to obstructive uropathy Pulmonary hypoplasia due to oligohydramnios	Prevention of renal failure and pulmonary hypoplasia by anatomic correction or urinary deviation
3. Sacrococcygeal teratoma	High-output cardiac failure due to AV shunting and/or bleeding Direct anatomic effects of the tumoral mass Polyhydramnios-related preterm labor	Reduction of functional impact of tumor by ablation of tumor or (part of) its vasculature Reduction of anatomic effects by drainage of cysts or bladder Amnioreduction preventing obstetric complications
4. Thoracic space-occupying lesions	Pulmonary hypoplasia (space-occupying mass) Hydrops due to impaired venous return (mediastinal compression)	Creation of space for lung development Reversal of the process of cardiac failure
5. Neural tube defects	Damage to exposed neural tube Chronic CSF leak, leading to Arnold-Chiari malformation and hydrocephalus	Prevention of exposure of the spinal cord to amniotic fluid; restoration of CSF pressure correcting Arnold-Chiari malformation
6. Cardiac malformations	Critical lesions causing irreversible hypoplasia or damage to developing heart	Reversal of process by anatomic correction of restrictive pathology
SURGERY ON THE PLACENTA, CORD, OR MEMBRANES		
7. Chorioangioma	High-output cardiac failure due to AV shunting Effects of polyhydramnios	Reversal of process of cardiac failure and hydrops fetoplacentalis by ablation or reduction of flow
8. Amniotic bands	Progressive constrictions causing irreversible neurologic or vascular damage	Prevention of amniotic band syndrome leading to deformities and function loss
9. Abnormal monochorionic twinning: twin-to-twin transfusion; fetus acardiacus, and discordant anomalies	Intertwin transfusion leading to oligopolyhydramnios sequence, hemodynamic changes; preterm labor, and rupture of membranes; in utero damage to brain, heart, or other organs In utero fetal death may cause damage to co-twin. Cardiac failure of pump twin and consequences of polyhydramnios Serious anomaly raising the question of termination of pregnancy Selective fetocide	Arrest of intertwin transfusion; prevention/reversal of cardiac failure and/or neurologic damage, including at in utero death; prolongation of gestation Selective fetocide to arrest parasitic relationship, to prevent consequences of in utero fetal death, and to avoid termination of entire pregnancy

AV, Arteriovenous; CSF, cerebrospinal fluid.
From Deprest J, Hodges R, Gratacos E, Lewi L: Invasive fetal therapy. In Creasy RK, Resnick R, Iams JD, et al, editors: *Creasy & Resnik's maternal-fetal medicine*, ed 7, Philadelphia, 2014, Elsevier (Table 35-1).

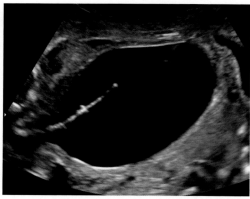

Fig. 116.1 Ultrasound image showing fetoscopic placement of a transurethral vesicoamniotic shunt in a patient with posterior urethral valves. *(Courtesy of Dr. Foong Lim, Cincinnati Fetal Center at Cincinnati Children's Hospital Medical Center.)*

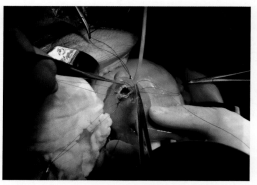

Fig. 116.2 Creation of a fetal vesicostomy. The uterine opening is stapled to prevent bleeding, and a catheter is inserted to replace amniotic fluid and maintain uterine volume. The fetus is positioned with the legs to the lower part of the field and the umbilical cord to the upper part of the field. A vesicostomy is created through the bladder and the abdominal wall to allow drainage of the obstructed bladder and restoration of amniotic fluid volume. *(Courtesy of Dr. Foong Lim, Cincinnati Fetal Center at Cincinnati Children's Hospital Medical Center.)*

renal outcome in these patients, but the reliability of these markers has been disappointing due to the influence of gestational age on many of these markers. Therefore, fetal intervention for obstructive uropathy is currently limited to fetuses in whom the obstruction is sufficient to cause oligohydramnios or anhydramnios.

For fetuses who still have adequate renal function and are capable of producing urine, treatment options include vesicoamniotic shunting, valve ablation via cystoscopy, and vesicostomy. **Vesicoamniotic shunting** is the most common and involves percutaneous, US-guided placement of a double-pigtailed shunt from the fetal bladder to the amniotic space, allowing decompression of the obstructed bladder and restoration of the amniotic fluid volume (Fig. 116.1). Although simple in concept, bladder decompression may not always occur, and many catheters will become dislodged as the fetus develops; a fetus typically requires 3 catheter replacements before completion of pregnancy. Vesicoamniotic shunting may improve perinatal survival, but at the expense of poor long-term renal function.

Fetal cystoscopy is more technically challenging than vesicoamniotic shunt placement, more invasive, and requires more sedation, but this option holds some important advantages. Cystoscopy allows for direct visualization of the obstruction and does not require amnioinfusion. Moreover, when the obstruction is visualized and the diagnosis of PUV confirmed, the valves can be treated, restoring urine flow to the amniotic space and eliminating the need for repeated fetal interventions in most patients. Creation of a **vesicostomy** (direct opening from bladder through fetal abdominal wall) by open fetal surgery has improved perinatal survival (Fig. 116.2). However, the current dataset evaluating this approach is still limited, and direct comparisons to shunting suggest no significant difference between these interventions.

NONOBSTRUCTIVE RENAL DISEASE
Nonobstructive fetal renal disease can result from renal hypoplasia/ dysplasia and from genetic disease such as autosomal recessive polycystic kidney disease. Similar to obstructive uropathy, fetal therapy is focused on restoring amniotic fluid volume in patients with oligohydramnios or anhydramnios. However, restoration of amniotic fluid volume in nonobstructive renal disease requires external sources of amniotic fluid. Current treatment options include serial percutaneous amnioinfusion and infusion of fluid by amnioport. **Serial amnioinfusions** are less invasive as a single procedure, but most pregnancies will require weekly infusions to maintain adequate amniotic fluid volume. Amnioinfusion through an **amnioport** involves open surgical placement of a catheter into the amniotic space that is connected to an ex utero subcutaneous port. This allows repeated fluid infusion into the amniotic space. The amnioport is more challenging and invasive as an individual procedure but provides more reliable access to the amniotic space for the duration of the pregnancy. Small studies suggest both these procedures improve

pulmonary outcomes and perinatal survival in infants with renal disease, but these infants will require dialysis and then renal transplant when the infant is large enough (2-3 yr of age).

CONGENITAL DIAPHRAGMATIC HERNIA
Congenital diaphragmatic hernia (**CDH**) is a defect in the fetal diaphragm causing herniation of the abdominal contents into the thorax and inhibition of fetal lung growth (see Chapter 122.10). CDH occurs in 1 in 3,000 births and can range from mild to severe. In mild cases of CDH, surgical repair of the diaphragm is typically performed in the 1st few days of life. Lungs in these infants are smaller than normal at birth, but as they grow, these patients can lead normal, active lives. In the severe cases of CDH infants experience severe pulmonary hypoplasia and pulmonary hypertension, requiring extracorporeal membrane oxygenation (ECMO) in the perinatal period. Mortality is high in severely affected infants, and survivors often have long-term respiratory, feeding, and neurodevelopmental problems.

Early attempts at fetal intervention for CDH used **in utero** surgical correction of the diaphragm defect in severe CDH infants. Survival rates were poor, with most infants dying during or shortly after the fetal surgery. Since significant complications during this procedure involved reduction of the incarcerated liver, a follow-up study compared **postnatal** repair to in utero repair that was limited to infants without liver herniation in the chest. The fetal repair group had more premature delivery (32 vs 38 wk gestation) without an improvement in survival (75% fetal repair vs 86% postnatal repair). Therefore, attempts at in utero repair of CDH have been abandoned.

Occlusion of the fetal trachea causes lung growth, and this approach was capable of dramatically improving lung growth in animal models of pulmonary hypoplasia. Several groups explored the use of fetal tracheal occlusion in CDH. The fetal surgical team in Philadelphia evaluated both open fetal tracheal ligation and endoscopic tracheal occlusion with an inflatable balloon. Open fetal tracheal ligation was quickly abandoned, with most patients dying from either complications associated with the procedure or shortly after delivery from respiratory failure caused by the lack of alveolar type II cell maturation and surfactant production in the hyperexpanded lungs. Endoscopic balloon tracheal occlusion was eventually evaluated in a larger trial. Survival was better than open fetal tracheal ligation but still not improved over control patients. Development of **fetoscopic balloon tracheal occlusion** in CDH led to the multicenter prospective randomized Tracheal Occlusion to Accelerate Lung Growth (**TOTAL**) study. In this trial the balloon was inserted at 27-30 wk and removed at 34 wk. This timing is based on the hypothesis that tracheal occlusion will promote lung expansion while removal of the balloon before delivery will promote alveolar type

II cell maturation. Initial data suggest that this approach is associated with a high incidence of preterm delivery but a significant increase in survival. The use of fetoscopic tracheal occlusion in CDH therapy is gaining popularity, but this approach in both severe and moderate CDH is still under investigation.

CONGENITAL PULMONARY AIRWAY MALFORMATION

Congenital pulmonary airway malformation (**CPAM**), previously referred to as *congenital cystic adenomatoid malformation* (CCAM), is caused by abnormal branching and hamartomatous growth of the terminal respiratory structures that results in cystic and adenomatoid malformations (see Chapter 423). Although rare, these remain the most common congenital lung lesion. CPAMs usually arise between 5 and 22 wk of gestation and continue to increase in size until around the 26th wk of pregnancy. If large enough, CPAM can cause significant pulmonary hypoplasia and in severe cases, hydrops fetalis. The size of the CPAM is tracked by CPAM volume ratio (**CVR**), an index that compares the volume of the CPAM to the fetal head circumference. Most studies indicate >95% survival in CPAM patients with no hydrops and CVR <1.6, with a much lower survival and greater risk for hydrops in patients with a CVR >1.6. Without intervention, CPAM with hydrops is uniformly fatal.

Open fetal **resection** of CPAM was considered one of the first clearly beneficial fetal surgeries. A less invasive option in fetal patients with CPAM composed of a large, dominant cyst is the insertion of a thoracoamniotic shunt into the dominant cyst. This decreases CPAM size, allowing lung growth and reducing risk of hydrops. An alternative surgical approach involving resection of the CPAM at delivery while the infant remains on placental support via an **ex utero intrapartum therapy (EXIT)** procedure has also demonstrated improved survival in a select group of patients.

Patients (in utero) receiving corticosteroids experience improved survival compared with those receiving open fetal resection. Survival rates approach 100% in high-risk CPAM (CVR >1.6) treated with steroids before the onset of hydrops and 50% in patients who have developed hydrops. Therefore the current approach to fetal therapy for CPAM has been away from open fetal resection and toward single or multiple courses of antenatal corticosteroids in fetuses with CVR >1.6.

MYELOMENINGOCELE

Before the introduction of fetal repair of **myelomeningocele (MMC)**, fetal surgery was limited to diagnoses considered fatal for the fetus or infant without intervention. However, a growing body of data suggests that the neurologic outcome in MMC is directly related to progressive injury from ongoing damage to the exposed spinal cord during pregnancy (see Chapter 609.3). Controversy remained as to whether the maternal and fetal risks of fetal repair should be accepted when the goal was to reduce postnatal morbidity rather than to improve survival.

The observation in early studies that patients receiving open fetal MMC repair were less likely to require **ventriculoperitoneal (VP) shunt** prompted the prospective randomized trial of prenatal vs postnatal MMC management (MOMS) (Fig. 116.3). The study was closed to enrollment in 2010 after 183 patients were randomized and the data safety monitoring board determined a clear advantage for prenatal surgery. The MOMS trial demonstrated a significant reduction in the need for VP shunt in the fetal repair group (40% vs 82% in postnatal repair group). The fetal repair group had an improved composite score for mental development and motor function at 30 mo, but also an increased risk of preterm delivery and uterine dehiscence. The average gestational age at delivery in the fetal repair group was 34 wk, with 10% delivering at <30 wk, compared to 37 wk and no infants <30 wk in the postnatal repair group.

Open fetal repair of MMC has been an important advance but the risk of prematurity significantly decreases the benefit of this procedure. In theory, the less invasive fetoscopic MMC repair approach, which is being developed at a limited number of centers, should reduce maternal morbidity and prematurity rates associated with open fetal MMC repair (Video 116.1).

OTHER INDICATIONS

Antenatal intervention for cardiac defects, such as aortic stenosis, pulmonic stenosis, and hypoplastic left heart syndrome (HLHS), have been used to dilate, with balloon valvuloplasty, stenotic valves (aortic stenosis) to prevent further development of HLHS (creating biventricular physiology) (Fig. 116.4) (see Chapter 458.10).

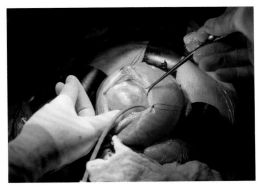

Fig. 116.3 Fetus during open repair of myelomeningocele. The uterine opening is stapled to prevent bleeding, and a catheter is inserted to replace amniotic fluid and maintain uterine volume. The myelomeningocele is exposed through the uterine opening and repaired. (*Courtesy of Dr. Foong Lim, Cincinnati Fetal Center at Cincinnati Children's Hospital Medical Center.*)

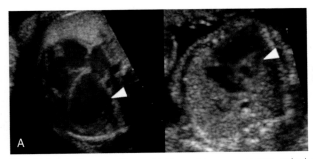
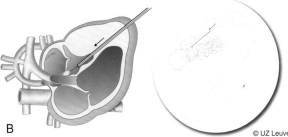

Fig. 116.4 A, Ultrasound image (*right panel*) is a cross section at the level of the fetal chest, demonstrating the 4-chamber view in a fetus with aortic stenosis. Notice that the left ventricle (*arrowhead*) is dilated. Dilation occurs before the development of hypoplasia, which can be seen (*arrowhead*) in another fetus (*left panel*). **B,** Schematic representation of percutaneous valvuloplasty, in this case of the left ventricular outlet tract. (**A,** *From van Mieghem T, Baud D, Devlieger R, et al: Minimally invasive fetal therapy, Best Pract Res Clin Obstet Gynaecol 26:711–725, 2012;* **B,** *copyright © UZ Leuven, Leuven, Belgium.*)

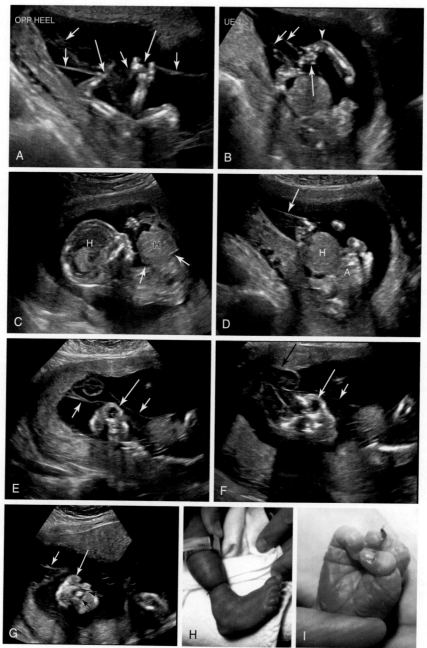

Fig. 116.5 Amniotic band sequence in two different fetuses. **A** and **B,** Effects on the extremities. Images of the limbs of a fetus with amniotic band sequence show multiple amniotic bands (*short arrows,* **A** and **B**), amputation of fingers and toes (*long arrows,* **A** and **B**), and a fixed deformity of the hand at the wrist (*arrowhead,* **B**). **C** and **D,** Effects on the thorax and abdomen of the same fetus as in **A** and **B.** Sagittal image (**C**) shows a thoracoabdominal wall defect (*arrows*) with a large amount of herniated abdominal and thoracic contents (*black H*) outside the body. *White H,* Head. **D,** Axial image of the fetal abdomen (*A*) confirms the presence of a large ventral abdominal hernia (**H**), in the setting of amniotic bands (*arrow*). **E** to **G,** Effects on craniofacial structures in a different fetus. **E,** Coronal image of face shows multiple amniotic bands (*short arrows*) and nonvisualization of the calvarium. This results in a craniofacial appearance that resembles anencephaly (*long arrow*). **F,** A large encephalocele (*black arrow*) is seen above the level of the orbits (*long white arrow*) in a different scan plane. An amniotic band (*short white arrow*) is also seen. **G,** Coronal image of anterior portion of face shows facial clefts (*black arrows*) due to amniotic bands. *Short white arrow,* Amniotic band; *long white arrow,* orbits. **H,** Band constricting the ankle, leading to deformational defects. **I,** Pseudosyndactyly, amputation and disruption of finger morphogenesis. (**A-G,** From Hertzberg BS, Middleton WD: Ultrasound: the requisites, ed 3, Philadelphia, 2016, Elsevier, Fig 19-22; **H** and **I,** From Jones KL, Smith DW, Hall BD, et al. A pattern of craniofacial and limb defects secondary to aberrant tissue bands. J Pediatr 84:90–95:1974.)

Table 116.3	Selection of Patients for Fetal Repair

LEVEL OF CERTAINTY	DIAGNOSIS
DIAGNOSTIC CERTAINTY/PROGNOSTIC CERTAINTY	
Genetic problems	Trisomy 13, 15, or 18
	Triploidy
Central nervous system abnormalities	Anencephaly/acrania
	Holoprosencephaly
	Large encephaloceles
Heart problems	Acardia
	Inoperable heart anomalies
Kidney problems	Potter syndrome/renal agenesis
	Multicystic/dysplastic kidneys
	Polycystic kidney disease
DIAGNOSTIC UNCERTAINTY/PROGNOSTIC CERTAINTY	
Genetic problems	Thanatophoric dwarfism or lethal forms of osteogenesis imperfecta
Early oligo/anhydramnios and pulmonary hypoplasia	Potter syndrome with unknown etiology
Central nervous system abnormalities	Hydranencephaly
	Congenital severe hydrocephalus with absent or minimal brain growth
Prematurity	<23 wk gestation
PROGNOSTIC UNCERTAINTY/BEST INTEREST	
Genetic problems	Errors of metabolism that are expected to be lethal even with available therapy
Mid oligo/anhydramnios	Renal failure requiring dialysis
Central nervous system abnormalities	Complex or severe cases of meningomyelocele
	Neurodegenerative diseases, such as spinal muscular atrophy
Heart problems	Some cases of hypoplastic left heart syndrome
	Pentalogy of Cantrell (ectopia cordis)
Other structural anomalies	Some cases of giant omphalocele
	Severe congenital diaphragmatic hernia with hypoplastic lungs
	Idiopathic nonimmune hydrops
	Inoperable conjoined twins
	Multiple severe anomalies
Prematurity	23-24 wk gestation

From Leuthner SR: Fetal palliative care, *Clin Perinatol* 31:649–665, 2004 (Table 1, p 652).

Laser therapy has been used to treat twin-twin transfusions syndrome (Chapter 117.1) and amniotic bands (Fig. 116.5).

FETAL CENTERS

The value of fetal centers extends beyond fetal surgery. Often, families will present to a fetal center with a newly discovered diagnosis and little understanding of what the diagnosis means for their baby. **Prenatal counseling** by the fetal team can provide comfort to the family by helping them understand the diagnosis and treatment options and by developing a management plan that may include fetal surgery. Some plans may call for enhanced monitoring of the fetus and mother, followed by complex deliveries involving multidisciplinary delivery teams and specialized equipment, as required for EXIT to ECMO, EXIT to airway, EXIT to tumor resection, delivery to cardiac catheterization, and procedures on placental support. Other plans may focus on postnatal therapy.

Not all severely affected fetuses have available therapies in utero or after birth. In these lethal situations, fetal care planning will provide support for the family and a plan for delivery room or nursery palliative care (Table 116.3) (see Chapter 7).

Bibliography is available at Expert Consult.

Chapter **117**

The High-Risk Infant

Jennifer M. Brady, Maria E. Barnes-Davis,
and Brenda B. Poindexter

第一百一十七章

高危婴儿

中文导读

　　高危婴儿是一个笼统的概念，涉及所有的有可能出现临床危险状况的婴儿。本章主要介绍了高危婴儿的概念、导致高危婴儿的因素，以及以下4类高危婴儿的具体临床概念：早产儿、有特殊保健需求或依赖技术的婴儿、因家庭问题有危险的婴儿和预期早亡的婴儿。另外，本章详细介绍了早产儿的定义及发病率，以及妊娠年龄、胎龄、出生体重和性别对新生儿死亡率的影响，同时分节阐述了多胎妊娠、超早产和极早产、近足月早产儿、足月儿和过期产儿的评估和治疗，以及高危儿的出院后随访流程和注意事项。

　　多胎妊娠主要介绍了有关多胎妊娠的流行病学、病因、非典型表现、并发症、诊断、检测、治疗等。具体描述了同卵双生和异卵双生的区别及胎盘检测，详细介绍了多胎妊娠的发生率以及包括种族、辅助生殖技术等导致差异的原因。病因阐述了经典的裂变理论和融合理论。非典型双胎中介绍了连体双胞胎、寄生双胞胎、超级受精等。列举了常见并发症如羊水过多、妊娠剧吐、子痫前期、胎膜早破等，并就双侧动脉灌注反转综合征及双胎输血综合征进行了详细阐述。诊断主要包括常规产前诊断和超声检查。多胎妊娠的预后风险主要包括母亲妊娠期并发症和胎儿围产期死亡率较高等内容。治疗方面包括选择单胚胎移植、择期分娩、儿科医护对新生儿的严密监护等（见原文117.1）。

　　由于超早产儿和极早产儿的整体发育极不成熟，救治成功率低且极易出现远期神经系统后遗症，因此，是考量新生儿重症监护室（NICU）综合实力的典型病例。超早产儿和极早产儿主要介绍了超早产和极早产的概念、发病率、危险因素、胎龄评估、新生儿护理等，具体描述了早产儿药物代谢不成熟以及与早产相关的新生儿疾病等问题。新生儿护理中详细阐述了温度控制、氧疗、营养供给、预防感染；其中营养供给又具体说明了早期肠外营养、母乳的优点、肠内营养以及对出院进行的营养过渡。列表介绍了用于早产儿可能导致不良反应的药物，以及与早产相关可导致发病率及死亡率增高的新生儿疾病（见原文117.2）。

　　近足月早产儿主要介绍了中期早产儿及晚期早产儿的概念和相关风险及研究建议。中度早产婴儿疾病包括且不限于喂养不良、体重减轻、呼吸窘迫综合征、NEC风险和体温调节困难。晚期早产儿出生后需要复苏的风险增加，低血糖、呼吸窘迫、呼吸暂停、进食困难和黄疸的发生率增加，再住院率高，生长后期学习困难风险高。本节的亮点是对于妊娠34~36周、有早产风险的孕妇，建议同样常规使用皮质激素，以减少这部分近足月早产儿出生后的患病风险，同时建议妊娠期无并发症、一般情况良好的孕妇，需在妊娠第39周后才进行无医疗指征的选择性分娩（见原文117.3）。

　　足月儿和过期产儿主要介绍了足月儿中小于胎龄儿、大于胎龄儿、过期产儿的概念、危险因素及相关风险。具体描述了小于胎龄儿与宫内生长限制的区别、可能导致宫内生长限制的因素、对称与不对称生长的区别以及可能带来的问题。大于胎龄儿常由于糖尿病及肥胖导致，其出生损伤、低血糖和红细胞增多症的风险以及先天性异常发病率增高。过期产儿死亡率明显增高，伴有特定的体征，良好的产科管理可帮助解决相关问题（见原文117.4）。

　　高危儿的出院后随访主要介绍了高危儿出院标准、出院后医学随访和长期发育监测。具体描述了包括脱离生命危险、肠内营养获取且体重增加稳定、良好的体温调节、无明显呼吸暂停、相关疾病检测、筛查和预防，以及父母培训、远期随访的出院标准。具体描述了早产儿的常见后遗症，说明医学随访的必要性。详细阐述了长期发育评估的重要性及评估内容和要求以及相关争议，以脑瘫为例说明发育评估可早期发现相关风险，并且建议进行早期干预（见原文117.5）。

The term *high-risk infant* designates an infant at greater risk for neonatal morbidity and mortality; many factors can contribute to an infant being high risk (Table 117.1). High-risk infants are categorized into 4 main groups: the preterm infant, infants with special health care needs or dependence on technology, infants at risk because of family issues, and infants with anticipated early death.

All high-risk infants require closer evaluation and/or treatment by experienced physicians and nurses. This often starts at delivery and continues through a neonatal intensive care unit (NICU) stay (see Chapter 121). Regionalized care for infants is based on the acuity of care that can be provided at hospitals with different levels of care and whether transport should be undertaken (see Chapter 118). It is important to note that additional care does not stop at time of NICU discharge, and that many high-risk infants also benefit from additional resources and follow-up after discharge from the hospital (see Chapter 117.5).

Approximately 15 million infants are born preterm (before 37 wk gestational age) each year worldwide, accounting for approximately 1 in every 10 babies born, and the overwhelming majority of high-risk infants. The World Health Organization (WHO) defines infants born before 28 wk gestational age as *extremely preterm* infants, infants born between 28 and 31⁶⁄₇ wk as *very preterm*, and infants born between 32 and 36⁶⁄₇ weeks as *moderate to late preterm* infants. Risk of both morbidity and mortality increases with earlier gestational age. Gestational age, birthweight, and gender are all important factors that impact neonatal mortality (Fig. 117.1). The **highest risk** of neonatal and infant mortality occurs in infants with birthweight <1,000 g and/or with gestational age <28 wk. The **lowest risk** of neonatal mortality occurs in infants with birthweight of 3,000-4,000 g and a gestational age of 39-41 wk. As birthweight increases from 400 to 3,000 g and gestational age increases from 23 to 39 wk, a logarithmic decrease in neonatal mortality occurs. Once birthweight exceeds 4000 g and/or gestational age exceeds 42 wk, the incidence of neonatal morbidities and mortality increases.

117.1 Multiple-Gestation Pregnancies

Maria E. Barnes-Davis, Jennifer M. Brady, and Brenda B. Poindexter

MONOZYGOTIC VS DIZYGOTIC TWINS

Identifying twins as **monozygotic** or **dizygotic** is useful in determining the relative influence of heredity and environment on human development and disease. The previous assumption that twins not of the same sex are dizygotic can no longer be held as true. Sex discordance, placentation, and determination of amnionicity and chorionicity are not reliable ways of determining zygosity. Detailed blood typing, gene analysis, or tissue (human leukocyte antigen) typing can be used for zygosity testing (an exception being blood typing in cases of **chimeric** twins, where one or both twins contain distinct cell lines from multiple zygotes). Physical and cognitive differences may still exist between monozygotic twins because of other factors. The in utero environment may have been different. Additionally, differences may exist in the mitochondrial genome, in posttranslational gene product modification, and in the epigenetic modification of nuclear genes in response to environmental factors.

Examination of the Placenta

If the placentas are separate, twins are **dichorionic**, but not necessarily dizygotic. One third of monozygotic twins are **dichorionic** and **diamnionic**. An apparently single placenta may be present with either monozygotic or dizygotic twins, but inspection of a dizygotic placenta usually reveals that each twin has a separate chorion that crosses the placenta between the attachments of the cords and 2 amnions. Separate or fused dichorionic placentas may be disproportionate in size. The fetus attached to the smaller placenta or the smaller portion of the placenta is usually smaller than its twin or is malformed. **Monochorionic** twins are usually **diamnionic**, and the placenta is usually a single mass.

INCIDENCE

The incidence of **spontaneous twinning** is highest among blacks and East Indians, followed by northern European whites, and is lowest in the Asian races. Differences in the incidence of twins worldwide mainly involve dizygotic twins. The incidence of monozygotic twins (3-5 per 1,000) is unaffected by racial or familial factors. Until recently, monozygotic twinning rates remained stable across continents and cultures. In 2014 the U.S. final natality report recorded a twin rate of 33.9 per 1,000 live births, which was a new high for the nation. Increases in monozygotic and dizygotic twinning have been associated with advanced maternal age (AMA) and the use of assisted reproductive technologies (ART). The rate of triplets and higher-order multiple births is 113.5 per 100,000 live births in the United States and continues to decline. The use of single-embryo transfer in ART has decreased the numbers of triplet births and higher-order multiples. However, a doubling of **monozygotic** twinning and an increase in atypical twinning have been reported. The incidence of **dizygotic** multifetal gestation is also increasing, attributed to treatment of infertility with ovarian stimulants (clomiphene, gonadotropins).

ETIOLOGY

Polyovular pregnancies are more frequent beyond the 2nd pregnancy, in older women, and in families with a history of dizygotic twins. They may result from simultaneous maturation of multiple ovarian follicles, but follicles containing 2 ova have also been described as a genetic trait leading to twin pregnancies. Twin-prone women have higher levels of gonadotropin. Polyovular pregnancies occur in many women treated for infertility.

The occurrence of monozygotic twins appears to be independent of heritable factors. The etiology of monozygotic twinning is unknown, but there are 2 prevailing theories. In the classic **fission theory**, twinning results from the splitting of a single conceptus, with the timing of splitting resulting in differing amnionicity and chorionicity (i.e., the

Table 117.1	Factors in Considering Infants as High Risk for Morbidity or Mortality in the Neonatal Period

MATERNAL DEMOGRAPHIC/SOCIAL FACTORS
Maternal age <16 yr or >40 yr
Illicit drug, alcohol, cigarette use
Poverty
Unmarried
Emotional or physical stress

MATERNAL MEDICAL HISTORY
Genetic disorders
Diabetes mellitus
Hypertension
Asymptomatic bacteriuria
Rheumatologic illness (systemic lupus erythematosus)
Immune-mediated diseases (IgG crossing placenta)
Long-term medication (see Chapters 115.4 and 115.5)

PREVIOUS PREGNANCY
Intrauterine fetal demise
Neonatal death
Prematurity
Intrauterine growth restriction
Congenital malformation
Incompetent cervix
Blood group sensitization, neonatal jaundice
Neonatal thrombocytopenia
Hydrops
Inborn errors of metabolism

PRESENT PREGNANCY
Vaginal bleeding (abruptio placentae, placenta previa)
Sexually transmitted infections (colonization: herpes simplex, group B streptococcus, chlamydia, syphilis, hepatitis B, HIV)
Multiple gestation
Preeclampsia
Premature rupture of membranes
Short interpregnancy time
Poly-/oligohydramnios
Acute medical or surgical illness
Inadequate prenatal care
Familial or acquired hypercoagulable states
Abnormal fetal ultrasonographic findings
Treatment of infertility

LABOR AND DELIVERY
Premature labor (<37 wk)
Postdates pregnancy (≥42 wk)
Fetal distress
Immature lecithin/sphingomyelin ratio; absence of phosphatidylglycerol
Breech presentation
Meconium-stained fluid
Nuchal cord
Cesarean delivery
Forceps delivery
Apgar score <4 at 5 min

NEONATE
Birthweight <2,500 g or >4,000 g
Birth <37 wk or ≥42 wk of gestation
Small or large for gestational age
Respiratory distress, cyanosis
Congenital malformation
Pallor, plethora, petechiae

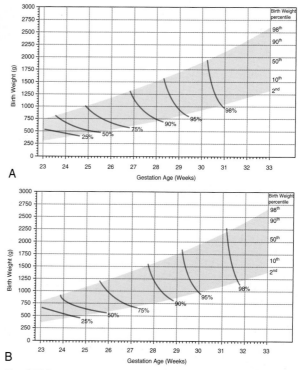

Fig. 117.1 Contour plot of predicted survival according to gestational age, birthweight, and gender. **A,** Female. **B,** Male. The contour lines join combinations of gestational age and birthweight of equal estimated probability of survival. Birthweight percentiles are shown for information. Data based on singleton infants born in the United Kingdom between January 2008 and December 2010 who survived to NICU admission. (*From Manktelow BN, Seaton SE, Fields DJ, et al: Population-based estimates of in-unit survival for very preterm infants, Pediatrics 131:e425–e432, 2013, Fig 2.*)

inner cell masses of trophectoderm fuse after the initial 2-cell splitting stage (Fig. 117.3).

ATYPICAL TWINNING

Conjoined twins (1 in 50,000 pregnancies and 1 in 250,000 live births) are obligate **monozygotes**. Theoretically, they result from later fission of a single zygote (10-14 days) or from fusion of 2 zygotes (as proposed for asymmetrically attached conjoined twins). The majority of conjoined twins are female. The prognosis for symmetrically conjoined twins depends on the possibility of surgical separation, which in turn depends on the extent to which vital organs are shared. The site of connections varies: thoracoomphalopagus (28% of conjoined twins), thoracopagus (18%), omphalopagus (10%), craniopagus (6%), and incomplete duplication (10%). The term *parasitic twin* has historically been used to describe the smaller and less completely developed member of a pair of conjoined twins; this *parasitic* twin has typically had embryonic demise but remains vascularized by the surviving *independent* twin (the **autocyte**). For asymmetrically attached conjoined twins in whom one twin is dependent on the cardiovascular system of the intact autocyte (**exoparasitic twins,** 1 in 1 million live births) survival of the autocyte depends on the feasibility of excising the *exoparasitic* twin. For **endoparasitic twins** (*fetus in fetu,* 1 in 500,000 live births) in whom one (or more) fetus exists as a benign mass in the autocyte, survival of the autocyte is unaffected.

Superfecundation, or fertilization of an ovum by an insemination that takes place after one ovum has already been fertilized, and **superfetation,** or fertilization and subsequent development of an embryo when a fetus is already present in the uterus, have been proposed as explanations for differences in size and appearance of certain twins at birth.

earlier the fission occurs, the more likely the twins are to be diamniotic dichorionic) (Fig. 117.2). However, this theory fails to account for several forms of atypical twinning, including the occurrence of **diamniotic dichorionic monozygotic** twinning after single-embryo transfer in the late blastocyst state, phenotypically-discordant monozygotic twins, and asymmetrically attached conjoined twins. An alternate **fusion theory** of twinning has been proposed to account for this discrepancy, in which the

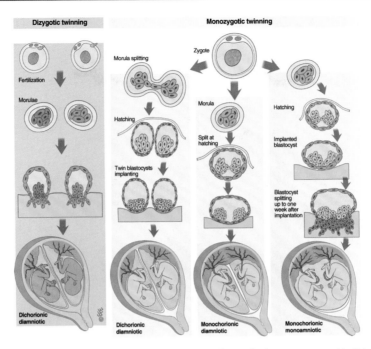

Fig. 117.2 *Classical fission theory of twinning. Dizygotic twins* result from 2 distinct fertilization events, with dichorionic diamniotic twins each developing to become a genetically distinct individual. *Monozygotic twins* result from postzygotic splitting of the product of a single fertilization event. Splitting on days 1-3 (up to the morula stage) results in dichorionic diamniotic twins, on days 3-8 (during which blastocyst hatching occurs) in monochorionic diamniotic twins, on days 8-13 in monochorionic monoamniotic twins. *(Illustration copyright © LeventEfe, CMI. www.leventefe.com.au.)*

COMPLICATIONS

Problems of twin gestation include polyhydramnios, hyperemesis gravidarum, preeclampsia, premature rupture of membranes (PROM), vasa previa, velamentous insertion of the umbilical cord, abnormal presentation (breech), and premature labor. **Monoamniotic** twins have a high fatality rate because of obstruction of the circulation secondary to intertwining of the umbilical cords.

Compared with the 1st-born twin, the 2nd twin is at increased risk for respiratory distress syndrome and asphyxia. Twins are at risk for intrauterine growth restriction, twin-twin transfusion syndrome, and congenital anomalies, which occur predominantly in **monozygotic** twins. Anomalies are a result of compression *deformation* of the uterus from crowding (hip dislocation), vascular communication with embolization (ileal atresia, porencephaly, cutis aplasia) or without embolization (acardiac twin), and unknown factors (conjoined twins, anencephaly, meningomyelocele).

TWIN SYNDROMES (TRAP, TTTS)

Placental vascular anastomoses occur with high frequency in **monochorionic** twins. In monochorionic placentas, the fetal vasculature is usually joined, sometimes in a very complex manner. They are usually balanced so that neither twin suffers. Artery-to-artery communications cross over placental veins, and when anastomoses are present, blood can readily be stroked from one fetal vascular bed to the other. Vein-to-vein communications are similarly recognized but are less common. A combination of artery-to-artery and vein-to-vein anastomoses is associated with the condition of **acardiac fetus**. This rare lethal anomaly (1 in 35,000) is secondary to the **twin reversed arterial perfusion (TRAP) syndrome**. In utero radiofrequency or laser ablation of the anastomosis or cord occlusion can be used to treat heart failure in the surviving twin. However, death of the autocyte is reported in up to 75% of cases. In rare cases, one umbilical cord may arise from the other

after leaving the placenta, and the twin attached to the secondary cord usually is malformed or dies in utero.

In **twin-twin transfusion syndrome (TTTS)**, an artery from one twin acutely or chronically delivers blood that is drained into the vein of the other. The latter develops polyhydramnios, plethoric and large for dates, and the former has oligohydramnios, anemic and small (Fig. 117.4). TTTS is more common in monozygotic twins and affects up to 30% of monochorionic twins. Maternal polyhydramnios in a twin pregnancy suggests TTTS. Anticipating this possibility by preparing to transfuse the donor twin or bleed the recipient twin may be lifesaving. Death of the donor twin in utero may result in generalized fibrin thrombi in the smaller arterioles of the recipient twin, possibly as the result of transfusion of thromboplastin-rich blood from the macerating donor fetus. Disseminated intravascular coagulation (DIC) may develop in the surviving twin. Table 117.2 lists the more frequent changes associated with a large shunt. **Treatment** of this highly lethal problem includes maternal digoxin, aggressive amnioreduction for polyhydramnios, selective twin termination, and more often, laser or fetoscopic ablation of anastomosis (Fig. 117.5).

DIAGNOSIS

A prenatal diagnosis of pregnancy with twins is suggested by a uterine size that is greater than that expected for gestational age, auscultation of 2 fetal hearts, and elevated maternal serum α-fetoprotein (AFP) or human chorionic gonadotropin (hCG) levels. It is confirmed by ultrasonography. Physical examination of twins is necessary but not sufficient to determine zygosity of twins. In the event that congenital anomalies are present or there are transfusion or transplantation considerations, genetic testing of zygosity should be performed. While noninvasive prenatal testing (NIPT) is becoming more common, the results should be interpreted with caution in multiple-gestation pregnancies until more findings are better established.

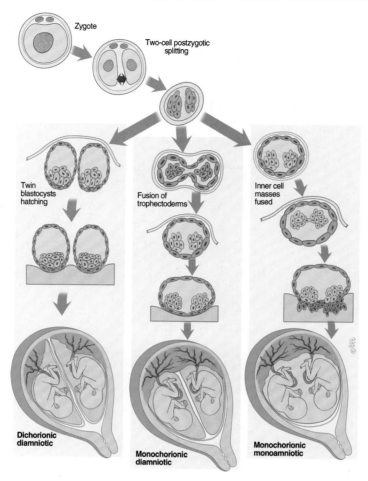

Fig. 117.3 Fusion theory of monozygotic twinning. Splitting occurs at the postzygotic 2-cell stage, with each cell forming a distinct individual. If twin blastocysts hatch from the zona pellucida together, dichorionic diamniotic twins will result. If the 2 trophectoderms fuse before hatching and the inner cells masses are separated within the shared trophectoderm, monochorionic diamniotic twins will result. If the inner cell masses are fused and separated later, monochorionic monoamniotic twins will result. *(Illustration copyright © LeventEfe, CMI. www.leventefe.com.au.)*

PROGNOSIS

Most twins are born prematurely, and maternal complications of pregnancy are more common than with single pregnancies. The risk for twins is most often associated with twin-twin transfusion, ART, and early-onset discordant growth. Because most twins are premature, their overall mortality is higher than that of single-birth infants. The perinatal mortality of twins is about 4 times that of singletons, with **monochorionic** twins being particularly at risk. **Monoamnionic** twins have an increased likelihood of cord entanglement, which may lead to asphyxia. Twins are at greater risk for congenital malformations, with up to 25% of monozygotic twins being affected. Theoretically, the 2nd twin is more subject to anoxia than the 1st because the placenta may separate after birth of the 1st twin and before birth of the 2nd. In addition, delivery of the 2nd twin may be difficult because it may be in an abnormal presentation (breech, entangled), uterine tone may be decreased, or the cervix may begin to close after the 1st twin's birth.

Triplet or higher-order births are associated with an increased risk of death or neurodevelopmental impairment compared with extremely-low-birthweight (ELBW) singleton and twin infants after controlling for gestational age. The mortality for multiple gestations with ≥4 fetuses is excessively high for each fetus. Because of this poor prognosis, selective fetal reduction has been offered as a treatment option. **Monozygotic**

Table 117.2	Characteristic Changes in Monochorionic Twins With Uncompensated Placental Arteriovenous Shunts
TWIN ON:	
Arterial Side—Donor	**Venous Side—Recipient**
Prematurity	Prematurity
Oligohydramnios	Polyhydramnios
Small premature	Hydrops
Malnourished	Large premature
Pale	Well nourished
Anemic	Plethoric
Hypovolemic	Polycythemic
Hypoglycemic	Hypervolemic
Microcardia	Cardiac hypertrophy
Glomeruli small or normal	Myocardial dysfunction
Arterioles thin walled	Tricuspid valve regurgitation
	Right ventricular outflow obstruction
	Glomeruli large
	Arterioles thick walled

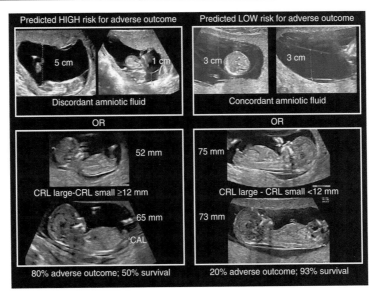

Fig. 117.4 Representation of first-trimester risk assessment for the development of discordant growth, twin-twin transfusion syndrome (TTTS), or intrauterine demise. Discordant amniotic fluid in the first trimester generally corresponded with deepest vertical pockets ≤3 cm in one sac and ≥6.5 cm in the other. Discordance in crown-rump length (CRL) was present if the difference was ≥12 mm. *(From Lewi L, Gucciardo L, Van Mieghem T, et al: Monochorionic diamniotic twin pregnancies: natural history and risk stratification, Fetal Diagn Ther 27:121–133, 2010.)*

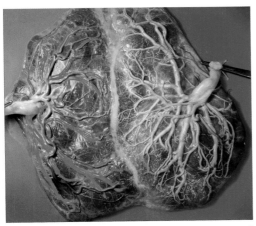

Fig. 117.5 Color-dye-stained twin-to-twin transfusion syndrome placenta that was treated using the Solomon technique. *Blue* and *green* dye used to stain the arteries, and *pink* and *yellow* dye used to stain the veins. After identification and coagulation of each individual anastomosis, the complete vascular equator is coagulated from one placental margin to the other. *(From Slaghekke F, Lopriore E, Lewi L, et al: Fetoscopic laser coagulation of the vascular equator versus selective coagulation for twin-to-twin transfusion syndrome: an open-label randomized controlled trial, Lancet 383:2144–2150, 2014, Fig 3.)*

twins have an increased risk of one twin dying in utero. The surviving twin has a greater risk for cerebral palsy and other neurodevelopmental sequelae.

TREATMENT
Prenatal diagnosis enables the obstetrician and pediatrician to anticipate the birth of infants who are at high risk because of twinning. The risk of multiple-gestation pregnancies using ART may be reduced by elective single-embryo transfers. In addition, elective delivery of twins at 37 wk (or earlier for **monochorionic, monoamniotic** twins) reduces the complication rate for the fetuses and the mother. Furthermore, in twin pregnancies between 32 and 39 wk of gestation, planned vaginal delivery is preferred if the 1st twin is in the cephalic presentation. Close observation and attendance by a pediatric team are indicated in the immediate neonatal period so that prompt treatment of asphyxia or fetal transfusion syndrome can be initiated. The decision to perform an immediate blood transfusion in a severely anemic "donor twin" or a partial exchange transfusion of a "recipient twin" must be based on clinical judgment.

Bibliography is available at Expert Consult.

117.2 Extremely and Very Preterm Infants
Jennifer M. Brady and Brenda B. Poindexter

Traditionally, a delivery date is determined 280 days after the last menstrual period (LMP). However, only 4% of pregnant women actually deliver at 280 days, and only 70% deliver within 10 days of the estimated delivery date.

Infants born before 37 wk from the 1st day of the LMP are termed *premature* by WHO. Infants born before 28 wk gestation are **extremely preterm,** also referred to as **extremely low gestational age newborns (ELGANs)**; whereas infants born between 28 and 31⁶⁄₇ are **very preterm**. Moderate and late preterm infants (born between 32 and 36⁶⁄₇ wk gestation) are discussed in Chapter 117.3.

In addition to classification by gestational age, classification is also based on birthweight. **Extremely low birthweight (ELBW)** is used to describe infants with a birthweight <1000 g, **very low birthweight (VLBW)** describes infants <1500 g, and **low birthweight (LBW)** describes infants <2500 g at birth. Birthweight in general is a proxy for gestational age, but in the cases of intrauterine growth restriction (IUGR) and small-for-gestational-age (SGA) infants, birthweight can sometimes be misleading for true gestational age (see Chapter 117.4).

INCIDENCE
Preterm birth, or birth before 37 wk of gestation, is fairly common. Worldwide, approximately 15 million preterm births occur annually.

In the United States, approximately 10% of all births are preterm. After a prolonged period of increasing rates of preterm birth, preterm births in the United States peaked at 10.44% in 2007. From 2007 until 2014, a slow but steady decline occurred in preterm births, to 9.57% in 2014. Preliminary data show that preterm births have slightly increased since 2014, with 9.84% of all U.S. births being preterm in 2016 and a disproportionate increase in late preterm births (Fig. 117.6). Of preterm births in 2016, the majority were late preterm infants, approximately 72% of preterm births, with the remaining 28% being extremely or early preterm.

ETIOLOGY

Despite the frequency of preterm birth, it is often difficult to determine a specific cause. The etiology of preterm birth is multifactorial and involves complex interactions between fetal, placental, uterine, and maternal factors. In the setting of maternal or fetal conditions that prompt early delivery, as well as placental and uterine pathology, causes of preterm birth can sometimes be identified (Table 117.3).

However, most preterm births are *spontaneous* without an identifiable cause. Older maternal age, poorer maternal health, history of previous preterm delivery, short interpregnancy interval, and lower socioeconomic status (SES) have all been associated with preterm birth. Racial disparities also exist, which seem to persist when taking into account SES. Large population studies have also found associations between maternal genetics and preterm birth. Gestational duration and actual preterm birth have been noted with genetic variants in the maternal genome. Many of these genes have roles in regulation of the estrogen receptor, uterine development, maternal nutrition, or vascular reactivity. In addition, cell free RNA transcripts in maternal blood may also be of value in predicting preterm birth.

ASSESSMENT OF GESTATIONAL AGE

With insufficient prenatal care or discrepancies between birthweight and predicted gestational age at birth, it is often helpful to be able to assess infants at birth for an estimated gestational age. Examination and assessment is needed to distinguish SGA and IUGR infants from preterm infants. Compared with a premature infant of appropriate weight, an infant with IUGR has a reduced birthweight and may appear to have a disproportionately larger head relative to body size; infants in both groups lack subcutaneous fat. Neurologic maturity (nerve conduction velocity) in the absence of asphyxia correlates with gestational age despite reduced fetal weight. Physical signs may be useful in estimating gestational age at birth. The commonly used **Ballard scoring system** is accurate to within 2 wk of actual gestational age (Figs. 117.7 to 117.9).

NURSERY CARE

At birth, the general measures needed to clear the airway, initiate breathing, care for the umbilical cord and eyes, and administer vitamin K are the same for premature infants as for those of normal weight and maturity (see Chapter 121). Additional considerations are the need for (1) thermal control and monitoring of the heart rate and respiration, (2) oxygen therapy, and (3) special attention to the details of fluid requirements and nutrition. Safeguards against infection can never be relaxed. Routine procedures that disturb these infants may result in hypoxia. The need for regular and active participation by the parents in the infant's care in the nursery and the question of prognosis for later growth and development require special consideration.

Thermal Control

Neonatal temperature regulation decreases the risk of morbidity and mortality in ELBW and VLBW infants. Neonates in general, and ELBW and VLBW infants to an even greater extent, are at increased risk of heat loss compared with older children due to an increased body surface/weight ratio, decreased epidermal and dermal skin thickness, minimal subcutaneous fat, and an immature nervous system.

Preterm infants should be kept in a **neutral thermal environment**. This environment is a set of thermal conditions, including air and radiating surface temperatures, relative humidity, and airflow, at which heat production (measured experimentally as oxygen consumption) is minimal and the infant's core temperature is within the normal range. The neutral

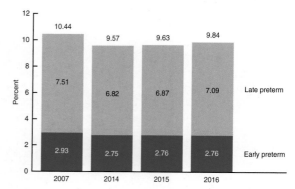

NOTES: Gestational age is measured in completed weeks based on the obstetric estimate. Early preterm is births before 32 weeks; late preterm is births at 34–36 weeks. Figures may not add to totals due to rounding.
SOURCE: NCHS, National Vital Statistics System.

Fig. 117.6 Preterm birth rates in the United States in 2007, 2014, 2015, and 2016 (provisional). There was a recent rise in preterm birth rate from 2014 to 2016. Preterm birth rate further divided into early preterm birth (birth <32 wk) and late preterm birth (birth at 34–36⅞ wk). (*From Hamilton BE, Martin JA, Osterman MJK, et al: Births: provisional data for 2016, Vital Statistics Rapid Release 2017; 1–21, Fig 4.*)

Table 117.3	Identifiable Risk Factors for Preterm Birth

FETAL
Fetal distress
Multiple gestation
Erythroblastosis
Nonimmune hydrops

PLACENTAL
Placental dysfunction
Placenta previa
Placental abruption

UTERINE
Bicornuate uterus
Incompetent cervix (premature dilation)

MATERNAL
Previous preterm birth
Preeclampsia
Black race
Chronic medical illness (cyanotic heart disease, renal disease, thyroid disease)
Short interpregnancy interval
Infection (*Listeria monocytogenes*, group B streptococcus, urinary tract infection, bacterial vaginosis, chorioamnionitis)
Obesity
Drug abuse (cocaine)
Young or advanced maternal age

OTHER
Premature rupture of membranes
Polyhydramnios
Iatrogenic
Assisted reproductive technology
Trauma

thermal environment is a function of the size and postnatal age of an infant; larger, older infants require lower environmental temperatures than smaller, younger infants. Incubators or radiant warmers can be used to maintain body temperature. Body heat is conserved through provision of a warm environment and humidity. The optimal environmental temperature for minimal heat loss and oxygen consumption for an

Physical maturity

	-1	0	1	2	3	4	5
Skin	Sticky, friable, transparent	Gelatinous, red, translucent	Smooth, pink, visible veins	Superficial peeling and/or rash, few veins	Cracking, pale areas, rare veins	Parchment, deep cracking, no vessels	Leathery, cracked, wrinkled
Lanugo	None	Sparse	Abundant	Thinning	Bald areas	Mostly bald	
Plantar surface	Heel-toe 40-50 mm:-1 <40 mm: -2	>50 mm, no crease	Faint red marks	Anterior transverse crease only	Creases on ant. 2/3	Creases over entire sole	
Breast	Impercep- tible	Barely perceptible	Flat areola- no bud	Stripped areola, 1-2 mm bud	Raised areola, 3-4 mm bud	Full areola, 5-10 mm bud	
Eye/ear	Lids fused loosely (-1), tightly (-2)	Lids open, pinna flat, stays folded	Slightly curved pinna; soft; slow recoil	Well-curved pinna, soft but ready recoil	Formed and firm, instant recoil	Thick cartilage, ear stiff	
Genitals, male	Scrotum flat, smooth	Scrotum empty, faint rugae	Testes in upper canal, rare rugae	Testes descending, few rugae	Testes down, good rugae	Testes pendulous, deep rugae	
Genitals, female	Clitoris prominent, labia flat	Prominent clitoris, small labia minora	Prominent clitoris, enlarging minora	Majora and minora equally prominent	Majora large, minora small	Majora cover clitoris and minora	

Fig. 117.7 Physical criteria for maturity. The expanded New Ballard score includes extremely premature infants and has been refined to improve accuracy in more mature infants. *(From Ballard JL, Khoury JC, Wedig K, et al: New Ballard score, expanded to include extremely premature infants, J Pediatr 119:417–423, 1991.)*

Maturity Rating

Score	Weeks
-10	20
-5	22
0	24
5	26
10	28
15	30
20	32
25	34
30	36
35	38
40	40
45	42
50	44

Fig. 117.9 Maturity rating. The physical and neurologic scores are added to calculate gestational age. *(From Ballard JL, Khoury JC, Wedig K, et al: New Ballard score, expanded to include extremely premature infants, J Pediatr 119:417–423, 1991.)*

Neuromuscular maturity

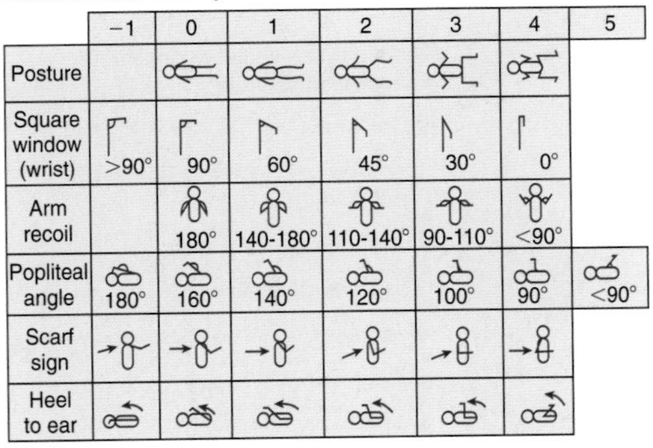

	-1	0	1	2	3	4	5
Posture							
Square window (wrist)	>90°	90°	60°	45°	30°	0°	
Arm recoil		180°	140-180°	110-140°	90-110°	<90°	
Popliteal angle	180°	160°	140°	120°	100°	90°	<90°
Scarf sign							
Heel to ear							

Fig. 117.8 Neuromuscular criteria for maturity. The expanded New Ballard score includes extremely premature infants and has been refined to improve accuracy in more mature infants. *(From Ballard JL, Khoury JC, Wedig K, et al: New Ballard score, expanded to include extremely premature infants, J Pediatr 119:417–423, 1991.)*

unclothed infant is one that maintains the infant's core temperature at 36.5-37.0°C (97.7-98.6°F). The smaller and more immature the infant, the higher is the environmental temperature required. Infant warmth can be maintained by heating the air to a desired temperature or by servo-control. Continuous monitoring of the infant's temperature is required to maintain optimal body temperature. **Kangaroo care** with direct skin-to-skin contact between infant and parent, with a hat and blanket covering the infant, is to be encouraged, without untoward effects on thermoregulation.

Maintaining a relative humidity of 40-60% aids in stabilizing body temperature by reducing heat loss at lower environmental temperatures; by preventing drying and irritation of the lining of respiratory passages, especially during the administration of oxygen and after or during endotracheal intubation; and by thinning viscid secretions and reducing

insensible water loss. An infant should be weaned and then removed from the incubator or radiant warmer only when the gradual change to the atmosphere of the nursery does not result in a significant change in the infant's temperature, color, activity, or vital signs.

Oxygen Administration

Administering oxygen to reduce the risk of injury from hypoxia and circulatory insufficiency (risk of cerebral palsy, death) must be balanced against the risk of hyperoxia to the eyes (**retinopathy of prematurity, ROP**) and oxygen injury to the lungs (**bronchopulmonary dysplasia, BPD**). For ELBW infants at birth, guidelines should be followed to determine need for oxygen during resuscitation to maintain goal O_2 saturation limits (see Chapter 121).

After the initial resuscitation period, ideal target O_2 saturation limits for ELBW infants should be within the range of 90–95% for most infants.

Nutrition for the High-Risk Infant

Extreme prematurity must be considered a nutritional emergency. In the absence of early parenteral and enteral nutritional support, deficits in protein and energy will quickly accrue, placing the infant at risk for poor growth and neurodevelopmental outcomes. The goals of early nutritional support for extremely premature infants include approximating the rate and composition of growth for a normal fetus at the same postmenstrual age. Achieving this goal requires an understanding of the intrauterine growth rate to be targeted as well as the unique nutrient requirements of premature infants. Strategies to prevent growth faltering include a combined approach of early parenteral and enteral nutrition, fortification of human milk, and the use of standardized feeding guidelines. In addition, careful monitoring of not only weight gain but also length and head circumference using appropriate intrauterine growth curves, as well as consultation with an experienced neonatal dietitian, is important to achieve optimal growth outcomes.

Early Parenteral Nutrition

In the absence of intravenous amino acids, extremely premature infants lose 1-2% of body protein stores per day. IV amino acids and dextrose should be started immediately after birth. Many units use a *starter* or *stock* solution of amino acids and dextrose to accomplish this goal in infants weighing <1,500 g. A minimum of 2 g/kg of amino acids should be given in the 1st 24 hr after birth, with the goal of supplying at least 3.5 g/kg within 24-48 hr after birth. To meet total energy requirements, IV lipids will also be needed.

Benefits of Human Milk

Maternal milk is the preferred source of enteral nutrition for premature infants and is associated with decreased in-hospital morbidity, including lower rates of **necrotizing enterocolitis (NEC)**, late-onset sepsis, BPD, and severe ROP. Maternal milk feeding is also associated with superior neurodevelopmental outcomes at 18 and 30 mo corrected age compared to infants fed premature formula. Donor human milk is increasingly being used when maternal milk is not available, but is typically lower in protein and energy content than preterm maternal milk and may result in suboptimal growth unless adequately fortified. Although donor human milk has been associated with a reduction in NEC, the impact of donor human milk on neurodevelopmental outcomes remains unclear.

Enteral Nutrition

Early enteral feedings are recommended in ELBW and VLBW infants, typically beginning between 6 and 48 hr with some period of trophic/minimal enteral feeding volume. Feedings are typically advanced slowly (15-30 mL/kg/day) with a target goal of delivering approximately 110-135 kcal/kg/day and 3.5-4.5 g protein/kg/day. To accomplish these goals, human milk must be fortified, or a premature formula can be given.

Standardized Feeding Guidelines

Standardized feeding guidelines should be developed incorporating evidence-based strategies for the provision of parenteral and enteral nutrition in ELBW and VLBW infants, including a plan to manage feeding intolerance. Regardless of the specific protocol, having a feeding guideline leads to improved outcomes (e.g., time to regain birthweight, time to reach full enteral nutrition), decreased rates of late-onset sepsis and NEC, improved growth at 36 wk postmenstrual age, and reduced length of hospital stay.

Transitioning to Discharge Nutrition

The earlier an infant is born before expected, the greater the likelihood that not all nutritional deficits will be resolved before hospital discharge. Regardless of weight gain during the initial hospital stay, there is strong evidence for improved bone mineralization with the use of higher concentrations of calcium and phosphorus after discharge. Fortified human milk or preterm formula with higher protein, minerals, and trace elements is often recommended after discharge. An individualized approach to postdischarge nutrition should be developed to transition from the NICU.

Prevention of Infection

Extremely preterm infants have an increased susceptibility to infection, and thus meticulous attention to infection control is required. Prevention strategies include strict compliance with handwashing and universal precautions, minimizing the risk of catheter contamination and duration, meticulous skin care, encouraging early appropriate advancement of enteral feeding, education and feedback to staff, and surveillance of nosocomial infection rates in the nursery. Although no one with an active infection should be permitted in the nursery, the risks of infection must be balanced against the disadvantages of limiting the infant's contact with the family. Early and frequent participation by parents in the nursery care of their infant does not increase the risk of infection when preventive precautions are maintained.

Preventing transmission of infection from infant to infant is difficult because often neither term nor premature newborn infants have clear clinical evidence of an infection early in its course. When epidemics occur within a nursery, cohort nursing and isolation rooms should be used. **Hand hygiene** is of upmost importance. Because premature infants have immature immune function, some will develop nosocomial infection even when all precautions are followed.

Routine **immunizations** should be given on the regular schedule based on chronological age at standard doses.

IMMATURITY OF DRUG METABOLISM

Great care must be taken when prescribing and dosing medications for premature infants (Table 117.4). Renal clearance of almost all substances excreted in the urine is diminished in newborn infants, and to even a greater extent in premature infants. The glomerular filtration rate rises with increasing gestational age; therefore, drug dosing recommendations vary with age. For drugs primarily excreted by the kidneys, longer intervals between dosages are often needed with increasing degree of prematurity. Drugs that are detoxified in the liver or require chemical conjugation before renal excretion should also be given with caution and in doses smaller than usual.

Table 117.4	Potential Adverse Reactions to Drugs Administered to Premature Infants
DRUG	**REACTION(S)**
Oxygen	Retinopathy of prematurity, bronchopulmonary dysplasia
Sulfisoxazole	Kernicterus
Chloramphenicol	Gray baby syndrome—shock, bone marrow suppression
Vitamin K analogs	Jaundice
Novobiocin	Jaundice
Hexachlorophene	Encephalopathy
Benzyl alcohol	Acidosis, collapse, intraventricular bleeding
Intravenous vitamin E	Ascites, shock
Phenolic detergents	Jaundice
NaHCO$_3$	Intraventricular hemorrhage
Amphotericin	Anuric renal failure, hypokalemia, hypomagnesemia
Reserpine	Nasal stuffiness
Indomethacin	Oliguria, hyponatremia, intestinal perforation
Cisapride	Prolonged QTc interval
Tetracycline	Enamel hypoplasia
Tolazoline	Hypotension, gastrointestinal bleeding
Calcium salts	Subcutaneous necrosis
Aminoglycosides	Deafness, renal toxicity
Enteric gentamicin	Resistant bacteria
Prostaglandins	Seizures, diarrhea, apnea, hyperostosis, pyloric stenosis
Phenobarbital	Altered state, drowsiness
Morphine	Hypotension, urine retention, withdrawal
Pancuronium	Edema, hypovolemia, hypotension, tachycardia, vecuronium contractions, prolonged hypotonia
Iodine antiseptics	Hypothyroidism, goiter
Fentanyl	Seizures, chest wall rigidity, withdrawal
Dexamethasone	Gastrointestinal bleeding, hypertension, infection, hyperglycemia, cardiomyopathy, reduced growth
Furosemide	Deafness, hyponatremia, hypokalemia, hypochloremia, nephrocalcinosis, biliary stones
Heparin (*not* low-dose prophylactic use)	Bleeding, intraventricular hemorrhage, thrombocytopenia
Erythromycin	Pyloric stenosis

Many drugs apparently safe for adults on the basis of toxicity studies may be harmful to newborns, especially premature infants. Oxygen and a number of drugs have proved toxic to premature infants in amounts not harmful to term infants. Thus, administering any drug, particularly in high doses, that has not undergone pharmacologic testing in premature infants should be undertaken carefully after risks have been weighed against benefits.

MORBIDITY AND MORTALITY

Rates of neonatal morbidity and mortality are high in extremely preterm infants, and risks increase with decreasing gestational age and lower birthweight (Table 117.5). Data on extremely preterm infants born between 2003 and 2007 found that 42% of VLBW infants developed BPD, 12% developed ROP requiring treatment, 11% NEC, 36% late-onset sepsis, 16% grade III or IV **intraventricular hemorrhage (IVH)**, and 3% **periventricular leukomalacia (PVL)**. Morality increased with lower gestational age, with a 94% mortality in infants born at 22 wk and 8% mortality at 28 wk. As a whole, the group of extremely preterm infants had a 28% mortality rate, with 37% surviving without a significant neonatal morbidity.

Table 117.5 Neonatal Morbidities Associated With Prematurity

RESPIRATORY
Respiratory distress syndrome (hyaline membrane disease)
Bronchopulmonary dysplasia*
Pneumothorax, pneumomediastinum; interstitial emphysema
Congenital pneumonia
Apnea

CARDIOVASCULAR
Patent ductus arteriosus
Hypotension
Bradycardia (with apnea)

HEMATOLOGIC
Anemia (early or late onset)

GASTROINTESTINAL
Poor gastrointestinal function—poor motility
Necrotizing enterocolitis*
Hyperbilirubinemia—direct and indirect
Spontaneous gastrointestinal isolated perforation

METABOLIC-ENDOCRINE
Hypocalcemia
Hypoglycemia
Hyperglycemia
Metabolic acidosis
Hypothermia
Euthyroid but low thyroxine status
Osteopenia

CENTRAL NERVOUS SYSTEM
Intraventricular hemorrhage*
Periventricular leukomalacia*
Seizures
Retinopathy of prematurity*
Deafness
Hypotonia

RENAL
Hyponatremia
Hypernatremia
Hyperkalemia
Renal tubular acidosis
Renal glycosuria
Edema

OTHER
Infections* (congenital, perinatal, nosocomial: bacterial, viral, fungal, protozoal)

*Major neonatal morbidities.

Another study found that morbidity and mortality among VLBW infants decreased between 2000 and 2009. This study was limited to live-born infants with birthweight of 500-1500 g. For infants born in 2009, this study found a 12.4% mortality rate; 28% of infants developed BPD, 7% severe ROP, 5% NEC, 15% late-onset sepsis, 6% grade III or IV IVH, and 3% PVL; 51% survived without significant neonatal morbidity.

Outcomes may be slightly improving with time; survival among infants born 22-24 wk gestation increased from 30% in 2000–2003 to 36% in 2008–2011. The percentage surviving without neurodevelopmental impairment increased from 16% to 20% over this same period. However, extreme prematurity is still associated with significant risk of both mortality and major neonatal morbidities. For infants who survive to discharge, prematurity, as well as neonatal morbidities, put them at increased risk for developmental delays and impairment as they age (see Chapter 117.5).

Bibliography is available at Expert Consult.

117.3 Moderate and Late Preterm Infants

Jennifer M. Brady and Brenda B. Poindexter

WHO defines **moderate to late preterm** birth as infants born between 32 and $36\frac{6}{7}$ wk postmenstrual age (PMA). The American College of Obstetricians and Gynecologists (ACOG) further defines **late preterm** infants as those born between 34 and $36\frac{6}{7}$ wk PMA. Therefore, most define **moderate preterm** infants as those born between 32 and $33\frac{6}{7}$ wk PMA.

MODERATE PRETERM INFANT

Moderate preterm infants are still at risk for most postnatal morbidities, although to a lesser extent than very preterm infants are at risk. These morbidities include but are not limited to poor feeding, weight loss, respiratory distress syndrome, risk of NEC, and difficulty with thermoregulation. Moderate preterm infants with birthweight >1,500 g and a fairly unremarkable NICU course are thought to be at fairly minimal risk for IVH and do not routinely need a head ultrasound. Little research has examined moderate preterm infants as an isolated group; more often these infants are grouped with very preterm infants when assessing complications and outcomes. A cohort of approximately 7,000 infants born between 29 and 33 wk gestational age were found in a recent study to have a mean hospital stay of 33.3 days. Compared with term counterparts, these infants had an increased incidence of many morbidities, including BPD, early- and late-onset sepsis, NEC, and PVL.

LATE PRETERM INFANT

Late preterm infants account for approximately 8–9% of all births and almost three fourths of all preterm births in the United States. Historically, late preterm infants were referred to as *near-term infants,* and the approach to their care was similar to that of term infants. It has been increasingly recognized that late preterm infants have significantly increased morbidity, as well as mortality, compared with their term counterparts. There is an increased incidence of congenital anomalies in preterm infants, but even when these infants are excluded, late preterm infants continue to have significantly more morbidities. Immediately after birth, late preterm infants have an increased risk of requiring resuscitation, as well as increased incidence of hypoglycemia, respiratory distress, apnea, feeding difficulties, and jaundice. They also have a higher rehospitalization rate compared to their term peers.

Antenatal corticosteroids were traditionally only recommended for pregnant women between 24 and 34 wk gestation at risk of preterm delivery within the next 7 days, to reduce the incidence of death and respiratory distress syndrome. A randomized controlled trial of women at 34–$36\frac{6}{7}$ wk gestation at risk of preterm labor found a decreased rate of respiratory complications in the newborns whose mothers received antenatal corticosteroids. An increased rate of neonatal hypoglycemia was seen in the steroid group as well, but no other significant differences were found. Based on these findings, ACOG recommends a single course of antenatal corticosteroids for pregnant women between 34 and 36⅞ wk gestation at risk for preterm birth within 7 days, who have not received a previous course of antenatal corticosteroids.

Between 34 and 36⅞ wk gestation is regarded as a critical period for growth and development. In the past, elective deliveries without medical indications often occurred as early as 35 wk. *ACOG recommends elective delivery without medical indications only after 39 wk gestation in well-dated pregnancies.* Some studies suggest a higher risk of lower school readiness at kindergarten and increased risk of academic difficulties in childhood when comparing late preterm infants with term peers.

Bibliography is available at Expert Consult.

117.4 Term and Postterm Infants
Jennifer M. Brady and Brenda B. Poindexter

ACOG further divides term infants into subgroups: **early term** (37–38⅞ wk), **full term** (39–40⅞ wk), and **late term** (41–41⅞ wk). Many risk factors for term infants put them at higher risk for complications, such as meconium aspiration syndrome (see Chapter 122.8), hemolytic disease of the newborn (Chapter 124.2), infant of a diabetic mother (Chapter 127.1), and neonatal abstinence syndrome (Chapter 126.1). Both small for gestational age (SGA) and large for gestational age (LGA) are associated with increased morbidities.

SMALL FOR GESTATIONAL AGE AND IUGR
There is an important distinction between the terms **small for gestational age (SGA)** and **intrauterine growth restriction (IUGR)**. SGA is based on physical evaluation of an infant at birth, usually by a pediatrician or neonatologist. If the infant's weight is <10th percentile, the infant is SGA. The diagnosis of SGA does not differentiate between normal biologic growth potential and a pathologic or growth-restricted state in utero. In contrast, IUGR is a prenatal diagnosis to describe a fetus who fails to reach in utero growth potential, often diagnosed by the obstetrician. Therefore, not all infants with IUGR are SGA, and similarly, not all infants who are SGA have IUGR.

Although it is important to understand the difference between SGA and IUGR, due to difficulty standardizing a classification of IUGR, many studies evaluate postnatal outcomes based on a diagnosis of either SGA or IUGR.

IUGR is associated with medical conditions that interfere with the circulation and efficiency of the placenta, with the development or growth of the fetus, or with the general health and nutrition of the mother (Table 117.6). Many factors are common to both prematurely born and LBW infants with IUGR. IUGR is associated with decreased insulin production or insulin-like growth factor (IGF) action at the receptor level. Infants with IGF-1 receptor defects, pancreatic hypoplasia, or transient neonatal diabetes have IUGR. Genetic mutations affecting the glucose-sensing mechanisms of the pancreatic islet cells result in decreased insulin release (loss of function of the glucose-sensing glucokinase gene) and give rise to IUGR.

IUGR may be a normal fetal response to nutritional or oxygen deprivation; therefore the issue is not the IUGR but rather the ongoing risk of fetal malnutrition or hypoxia. IUGR is often classified as *reduced growth* that is *symmetric* (head circumference, length, and weight equally affected) or *asymmetric* (with relative sparing of head growth). **Symmetric IUGR** often has an earlier onset in the first trimester of pregnancy and is associated with diseases that seriously affect fetal cell number, such as conditions with chromosomal, genetic, malformation, teratogenic, infectious, or severe maternal hypertensive etiologies. It is important to assess gestational age carefully in infants suspected to have symmetric IUGR because incorrect overestimation of gestational age may lead to the diagnosis of symmetric IUGR. **Asymmetric IUGR** is often of late onset in the 2nd half of pregnancy, demonstrates preservation of Doppler waveform velocity to the carotid vessels, and is associated with poor

maternal nutrition or with late onset or exacerbation of maternal vascular disease (preeclampsia, chronic hypertension).

Table 117.7 lists common problems of infants with IUGR. In addition, in both preterm and term infants, SGA has been shown to be associated with an increased risk of neurodevelopmental impairment.

Table 117.6	Factors Often Associated With Intrauterine Growth Restriction

FETAL
Chromosomal disorders
Chronic fetal infections (cytomegalic inclusion disease, congenital rubella, syphilis)
Congenital anomalies—syndrome complexes
Irradiation
Multiple gestation
Pancreatic hypoplasia
Insulin deficiency (production or action of insulin)
Insulin-like growth factor type I deficiency

PLACENTAL
Decreased placental weight, cellularity, or both
Decrease in surface area
Villous placentitis (bacterial, viral, parasitic)
Infarction
Tumor (chorioangioma, hydatidiform mole)
Placental separation
Twin transfusion syndrome

MATERNAL/PATERNAL
Toxemia
Hypertension or renal disease, or both
Hypoxemia (high altitude, cyanotic cardiac or pulmonary disease)
Malnutrition (micronutrient or macronutrient deficiencies)
Chronic illness
Sickle cell anemia
Drugs (narcotics, alcohol, cigarettes, cocaine, antimetabolites)

IGF2 mutation (paternal)

Table 117.7	Problems of Infants Small for Gestational Age or With Intrauterine Growth Restriction*

PROBLEM	PATHOGENESIS
Intrauterine fetal demise	Hypoxia, acidosis, infection, lethal anomaly
Perinatal asphyxia	↓ Uteroplacental perfusion during labor ± chronic fetal hypoxia-acidosis; meconium aspiration syndrome
Hypoglycemia	↓ Tissue glycogen stores, ↓ gluconeogenesis, hyperinsulinism, ↑ glucose needs of hypoxia, hypothermia, large brain
Polycythemia-hyperviscosity	Fetal hypoxia with ↑ erythropoietin production
Reduced oxygen consumption/hypothermia	Hypoxia, hypoglycemia, starvation effect, poor subcutaneous fat stores
Dysmorphology	Syndrome anomalads, chromosomal-genetic disorders, oligohydramnios-induced deformation, TORCH†

*Other problems include pulmonary hemorrhage and those common to the gestational age–related risks of prematurity if born at <37 wk.
†Toxoplasmosis, other agents, rubella, cytomegalovirus, herpes simplex infection.
↓, Decreased; ↑, increased.

LARGE-FOR-GESTATIONAL-AGE INFANTS

Infants with birthweight >90th percentile for gestational age are called **large for gestational age (LGA)**. Neonatal mortality rates decrease with increasing birthweight until approximately 4,000 g, after which they increase. These oversized infants are usually born at term, but preterm infants with weights high for gestational age also have a significantly higher mortality than infants of the same size born at term; maternal diabetes and obesity are predisposing factors. Some infants are constitutionally large because of large parental size. LGA infants, regardless of their gestational age, have a higher incidence of birth injuries, such as cervical and brachial plexus injuries, phrenic nerve damage with paralysis of the diaphragm, fractured clavicles, cephalohematomas, subdural hematomas, and ecchymoses of the head and face. LGA infants are also at increased risk for hypoglycemia and polycythemia.

The incidence of congenital anomalies, particularly congenital heart disease, is also higher in LGA infants than in term infants of normal weight.

POSTTERM INFANTS

Postterm infants are those born after 42 completed wk of gestation, as calculated from the mother's LMP. Historically, approximately 12% of pregnancies resulted in delivery after 42 wk. However, with current evidence suggesting that both morbidity and mortality increase significantly after 42 wk gestation, obstetric interventions to induce labor often occur before 42 wk, resulting in a decreasing rate of postterm births. The cause of postterm birth or postmaturity is unknown. Postterm infants often have normal length and head circumference but may have decreased weight if there is placental insufficiency. Infants born postterm in association with presumed placental insufficiency may have various physical signs. Desquamation, long nails, abundant hair, pale skin, alert faces, and loose skin, especially around the thighs and buttocks, give them the appearance of having recently lost weight; meconium-stained nails, skin, vernix, umbilical cord, and placental membranes may also be noted. Common complications of postmaturity include perinatal depression, meconium aspiration syndrome, persistent pulmonary hypertension, hypoglycemia, hypocalcemia, and polycythemia.

Infants born at ≥42 wk gestational age experience approximately 3 times the mortality of infants born at term. Mortality has been greatly reduced through improved obstetric management. Data suggest that elective delivery during the 39th wk of gestation for both nulliparous and multiparous women is associated with decreased maternal and neonatal complications compared with those who were expectantly managed.

Careful obstetric monitoring, including nonstress testing (NST), biophysical profile (BPP), or Doppler velocimetry, usually provides a rational basis for choosing 1 of 3 courses: nonintervention, induction of labor, or cesarean delivery. Induction of labor or cesarean birth may be indicated in older primigravidas >2-wk beyond term, particularly if evidence of fetal distress is present. Medical problems in the newborn are treated if they arise.

Bibliography is available at Expert Consult.

117.5 Follow-Up of High-Risk Infants After Discharge

Jennifer M. Brady and Brenda B. Poindexter

DISCHARGE FROM THE HOSPITAL

Numerous criteria need to be met before a high-risk infant is ready for discharge from the hospital (Table 117.8). Before discharge, infants should be taking most or all nutrition by nipple, either bottle or breast. Some medically fragile infants may be discharged home while receiving gavage feedings after the parents have received appropriate training and education. Growth should be occurring at steady increments, with a goal weight gain of approximately 30 g/day. Temperature should be stable and normal in an open crib. Infants should have had no recent episodes of apnea or bradycardia requiring intervention for at least 5-7 days prior to discharge. Stable infants recovering from BPD may be discharged on a regimen of home oxygen given by nasal cannula as long as careful follow-up is arranged with home pulse oximetry monitoring and outpatient visits. All infants with birthweight <1,500 g or gestational age <30 wk at birth should undergo an eye examination to screen for ROP. If born preterm, hemoglobin or hematocrit should be determined to evaluate for possible anemia of prematurity. Every infant should have a hearing test before discharge. Routine vaccinations should be given based on chronological age before discharge. In addition, palivizumab (Synagis) should be given to eligible infants during **respiratory syncytial virus (RSV)** season immediately before discharge for prophylaxis against RSV, with continued monthly doses arranged as an outpatient as appropriate.

If all major medical problems have resolved and the home setting is adequate, premature infants may then be discharged when their weight approaches 1,800-2,000 g, they are >34-35 wk PMA, and all the above criteria are met. Parental education, close follow-up, and healthcare provider accessibility are all essential for early discharge protocols. Ideally, the primary caregivers for the infant have a chance to provide infant care in the hospital with nursing supervision and help before discharge home. All high-risk infants should follow-up with their primary care provider within a few days of discharge.

Table 117.8	Readiness for Discharge of High-Risk Infants Criteria

Resolution of acute life-threatening illnesses
Ongoing follow-up for chronic but stable problems:
  Bronchopulmonary dysplasia
  Intraventricular hemorrhage
  Necrotizing enterocolitis after surgery or recovery
  Ventricular septal defect, other cardiac lesions
  Anemia
  Retinopathy of prematurity
  Hearing problems
  Apnea
  Cholestasis
Stable temperature regulation
Gain of weight with enteral feedings:
  Breastfeeding
  Bottle feeding
  Gastric tube feeding
Free of significant apnea
Appropriate immunizations and planning for respiratory syncytial virus prophylaxis if indicated
Hearing screenings
Ophthalmologic examination if <30 wk of gestation or <1,500 g at birth
Parental knowledge, skill, and confidence documented in:
  Administration of medications (diuretics, methylxanthines, aerosols, etc.)
  Use of oxygen, apnea monitors, oximeters
Nutritional support:
  Timing
  Volume
  Mixing concentrated formulas
Recognition of illness and deterioration
Basic cardiopulmonary resuscitation
Infant safety
Scheduling of referrals:
  Primary care provider
  Neonatal follow-up clinic
  Occupational therapy/physical therapy
Imaging (head ultrasound)
Assessment of and solution to social risks

Data from American Academy of Pediatrics, American College of Obstetricians: *Guidelines for perinatal care*, ed 7, Elk Grove Village, IL, 2013, American Academy of Pediatrics.

POSTDISCHARGE FOLLOW-UP
Medical Follow-Up

Even after discharge from the hospital, high-risk infants need very close medical follow-up. They continued to be at increased risk for poor weight gain and failure to thrive. In the setting of viral illness, premature infants are at increased risk for significant respiratory distress. Infants who are sent home on oxygen need very close medical follow-up with frequent visits and assessments, often with pulmonology. Table 117.9 lists common sequelae of prematurity.

Medically complex infants can go home with a multitude of subspecialty appointments to help manage existing morbidities secondary to prematurity. For example, cardiology for management of a patent ductus arteriosus or pulmonary hypertension, pulmonary for BPD, nephrology for hypertension, ophthalmology for ROP, neurosurgery for hydrocephalus, and neurology for history of seizures. The extensive follow-up requirements can be overwhelming and daunting for families. It is very important that these infants have a primary care provider who serves as their "medical home" to help coordinate and assimilate the care from all these providers for families.

Developmental Follow-Up

It is well known that premature infants are at greater risk for **developmental delays** than their term counterparts; the more preterm, the greater the risk of delay. In addition, certain postnatal morbidities (severe BPD, grade III or IV intraventricular hemorrhage, severe ROP) are associated with significantly increased risk of developmental delays. It is very important that preterm infants are followed and assessed for developmental delay, so that if delays are detected, interventions can be instituted early.

It is recommended that developmental follow-up be available for infants born <32 wk PMA, or at a minimum <28 wk PMA and/or <1 kg birthweight. Developmental follow-up in the United States is most often provided in a **neonatal follow-up program** for the 1st 2-3 yr of life, and in some cases, until school age. Assessments focus on 5 main developmental domains: cognitive development, language development, fine and gross motor skills, social development, and emotional development. Although many assessments exist, the most widely used assessment in the United States is the *Bayley Scales of Infant and Toddler Development, Third Edition.*

It is important to note that for at least the 1st 2 yr of life, a child's **corrected age** should be used in determining if a delay exists. Corrected age is calculated by subtracting the weeks born premature from a child's chronological age. In doing so, a corrected age accounts for a child's prematurity. Some debate surrounds whether corrected age should continue to be used after age 2 yr.

If it is determined that a delay exists, a child should be referred for appropriate therapy to help minimize the delay as the child ages. Federal law under the Individuals with Disabilities Act requires states to provide *early intervention* services to children <3 yr old with developmental delay. States vary greatly in how delay is defined and what services are offered. Early intervention is associated with improved cognitive outcomes in infancy and preschool age, but not lasting into school age. Motor outcomes are improved in infancy for children who receive early intervention, but this has not been shown to be a lasting effect into preschool and school age.

Premature infants, especially those with a history of grade III or IV intraventricular hemorrhage or PVL seen on head imaging, are also at increased risk of motor impairments. **Cerebral palsy** is *nonprogressive* but *permanent* disorder of movement and posture caused by disturbance to the developing immature brain. Historically, cerebral palsy had not been diagnosed until 18-24 mo of age, but current tests such as the **General Movements Assessment** (GMA) and **Hammersmith Infant Neurological Examination** (HINE) are helping to identify children at high risk for cerebral palsy within the 1st few mo to yr of life. This enables these children to access early intervention services and therapy at an earlier age, as well as undergo more frequent surveillance as needed.

Children with a history of prematurity who do not show significant developmental delays in the 1st few yr of life are still at risk of later developing learning disabilities, attention problems, and decreased school achievement. Continued screening by their primary care provider may be needed as these children age.

Bibliography is available at Expert Consult.

Table 117.9	Sequelae of Prematurity
IMMEDIATE	**LATE**
Hypoxia, ischemia	Intellectual disability, spastic diplegia, microcephaly, seizures, poor school performance
Intraventricular hemorrhage	Intellectual disability, spasticity, seizures, post hemorrhagic hydrocephalus
Sensorineural injury	Hearing and visual impairment, retinopathy of prematurity, strabismus, myopia
Respiratory failure	Bronchopulmonary dysplasia, pulmonary hypertension, bronchospasm, malnutrition, subglottic stenosis
Necrotizing enterocolitis	Short-bowel syndrome, malabsorption, malnutrition
Cholestatic liver disease	Cirrhosis, hepatic failure, malnutrition
Nutrient deficiency	Osteopenia, fractures, anemia, growth failure
Social stress	Child abuse or neglect, failure to thrive, divorce
Other sequelae	Sudden infant death syndrome, infections, inguinal hernia, cutaneous scars (chest tube, patent ductus arteriosus ligation, intravenous infiltration), gastroesophageal reflux, hypertension, craniosynostosis, cholelithiasis, nephrocalcinosis, cutaneous hemangiomas

Chapter **118**

Transport of the Critically Ill Newborn

Jennifer M. Brady and Brenda B. Poindexter

第一百一十八章

危重新生儿转运

中文导读

本章主要介绍新生儿分级管理中区域化护理以及危重新生儿转运的相关内容。美国儿科学会制定了一级、二级、三级和四级新生儿护理标准。具体说明当新生儿生后需要更高级别护理时，实施危重新生儿转运的具体流程，包括：①新生儿转运团队的组成、转运人员的技能要求，转运所需的设备以及转运方式；②转运前需要进行风险评估并征得父母的同意；③在整个转运过程中，与转运团队和接收医院之间沟通。为有利于医疗资源的合理利用，当婴儿病情稳定后，可转回至下级医疗机构进一步诊治。

REGIONALIZED CARE OF NEWBORNS

The concept of **regionalized care** for neonates was first introduced in the 1976 March of Dimes Report *Toward Improving the Outcome of Pregnancy.* This report and future revisions stress the importance of providing regionalized care for infants in facilities with adequate personnel and equipment for an infant's severity of illness. Ideally, mothers deliver infants at a facility with the appropriate level of expertise and resources to care for the degree of prematurity and illness of the infant. Many studies have shown that very-low-birthweight (VLBW) infants, or infants <1,500 g at birth, have decreased morbidity and mortality when delivered at an appropriate level of care center (**Level III** hospitals). In a meta-analysis, neonatal or predischarge death occurred in 38% of VLBW infants receiving care at a non–Level III hospital and 23% of those receiving care at a Level III hospital. A main objective of *Healthy People 2020* addresses this issue, with a goal of increasing the proportion of VLBW infants born at Level III hospitals or subspecialty perinatal centers to 83.7%. Where this is not possible, the infant should be transported to an appropriate level of care hospital after birth.

LEVELS OF NEONATAL CARE

Although a formal national definition of levels of neonatal care does not exist, the American Academy of Pediatrics (AAP) and March of Dimes have standardized definitions for levels I, II, III, and IV. One must understand the levels of care available before being able to arrange transport to an appropriate facility.

A **Level I** facility must be able to provide *basic neonatal care.* Appropriate equipment and staff must be available to perform neonatal resuscitation and care for healthy term and late preterm infants. In addition, Level I facilities must have the capacity to work to stabilize ill or preterm infants before transport to a higher level of care. A Level I nursery is the minimum requirement for a hospital providing inpatient maternity care. Providers at Level I facilities usually include pediatricians, family physicians, and nurse practitioners.

In addition to the care provided at a Level I facility, **Level II** nurseries must also be capable of providing care to moderately ill term infants with problems expected to resolve quickly. Level II centers also care for infants born ≥32 wk gestational age and >1,500 g at birth, and therefore must be comfortable with treating conditions common in this population, such as difficulty with oral feeds, apnea of prematurity, respiratory distress requiring continuous positive airway pressure (CPAP), and temperature regulation. These centers must also be capable of stabilizing infants born <32 wk gestation and <1,500 g until transfer to a higher-level facility is feasible, including the ability to intubate and provide mechanical ventilation for a brief duration if necessary. In addition to providers in Level I facilities, Level II facilities also typically have pediatric hospitalists, neonatologists, and neonatal nurse practitioners.

Level III neonatal intensive care units (NICUs) are equipped to care for the extremely preterm and critically ill neonates in addition to those infants cared for at Level I and II units. Level III units must have continuously available personnel and equipment to treat conditions commonly seen in this population, such as respiratory distress syndrome, pulmonary hypertension, and need for total parenteral nutrition. Resources should be available to obtain and interpret urgent imaging needed (e.g., CT, echocardiography). Pediatric subspecialists and pediatric surgeons should be available either on site or through prearranged consultative agreements.

In addition to the care available at Level III NICUs, **Level IV** NICUs are also capable of continuously available pediatric subspecialty consultation and pediatric surgical intervention. Many Level IV sites are located at regional children's hospitals and serve to provide outreach education.

TRANSPORT OF THE CRITICALLY ILL NEONATE

In the event that a neonate requires a higher level of care after birth, transport must be arranged to a unit with the appropriate level of care available. Additional decisions that need to be made before transport include composition of the transport team, equipment required for transport, and mode of transportation.

The composition of the **transport team** varies depending on personnel available and the needs of the infant being transported. The transport team often comprises at least 2 individuals, whether 2 registered nurses (RNs), an RN and a respiratory therapist, or an RN and a paramedic. In addition, occasionally a neonatologist, neonatology fellow, or neonatal nurse practitioner will accompany the transport team for critically ill neonates. A designated **medical control physician** is available and in communication with the transport team throughout the transport as needed.

Transport staff must be competent in the treatment of common neonatal conditions and complications, as well as neonatal procedures. Many Level IV facilities have specialized teams available for neonatal transport. A Cochrane review found no evidence to support or to refute improved infant morbidity or mortality when transport occurred with a specialized team. Depending on the volume of neonatal transports and composition of the team, staff may have limited exposure to neonatal transports and procedures. **Simulation-based learning** is recommended by the AAP Section on Transport Medicine (SOTM) as a method to help achieve and retain competency in rarely experienced procedures, as well as improve team interactions for transport teams.

The **transport vehicle** should be equipped with appropriate medicines, intravenous (IV) fluids, oxygen tanks, catheters, chest tubes, endotracheal tubes (ETTs), laryngoscopes, bag-valve-mask, and infant warming device. It should be well illuminated and have ample room for emergency procedures and monitoring equipment. Additional needs for the specific transport should be anticipated (e.g., nitric oxide).

Common **modes of transport** include ground transport by ambulance and air transport by helicopter or fixed-wing aircraft. The stability of the infant, travel distance, traffic, and weather must all be taken into account when deciding the most appropriate mode of transportation.

Steps should be taken to **stabilize infants** as able in a timely fashion prior to transport. Securing an airway, providing oxygen, assisting with infant ventilation, providing antimicrobial therapy, maintaining the circulation, providing a warmed environment, checking a glucose level, and placing IV or arterial lines or chest tubes should be initiated, if indicated, before transport. Appropriate placement of lines and ETT should be evaluated before transport.

Risks of transport and transportation **consent** should be reviewed and obtained from parents before transport. Although transport teams attempt to anticipate and prepare for possible complications that could occur during transport, there is an inherent risk of complications, including death, in the event of a decompensation during transport resulting from the limited resources and personnel available. Parents should be made aware of these risks. If the infant's condition allows, efforts should be made to allow parents to see their baby briefly before transport.

Communication with the transport team as well as the receiving facility is paramount throughout the transport process. Available prenatal history, information on the infant's resuscitation and hospital course, lab data, and radiographic images should be sent with the transport team to the receiving hospital to aid in future care.

Reverse transport of an infant back to a lower level of care should be considered when infants are stabilized after transport and no longer require the higher level care available at the receiving hospital. Transport back to the birth hospital aids in appropriate utilization of resources, decreases costs of care, and may further promote parent–infant bonding because of proximity to the mother's home.

Bibliography is available at Expert Consult.

Chapter 119

Clinical Manifestations of Diseases in the Newborn Period

Elizabeth Enlow and James M. Greenberg

第一百一十九章
新生儿疾病的临床表现

中文导读

由于新生儿不能自主表达，且在大多数情况下，大部分疾病早期的临床表现不典型，因此，本章重点介绍了新生儿患病时的特殊临床表现,包括新生儿某些特殊的异常的动作、如何判断新生儿的精神状态改变、新生儿呼吸暂停、先天发育异常、发绀、胃肠功能异常、低血压、黄疸、疼痛，以及可导致上述情况的相关疾病，其中的新生儿原发性呼吸暂停、新生儿黄疸是新生儿期的特殊临床表现，既可以是独立的疾病诊断，也可以是其他临床疾病的症状之一，还可以是其他临床疾病的体征之一。本章同时针对新生儿发热及低体温、水肿、低钙血症、高镁血症进行病因分析。通过对非特异性临床体征和症状的评估认识新生儿疾病。

A variety of conditions that affect the newborn originate in utero, during birth, or in the immediate postnatal period. These disorders can be caused by prematurity, congenital malformations, disruption of chromosome structure, or acquired diseases and injuries. Recognizing disease in newborn infants requires knowledge of relevant pathophysiology and evaluation of nonspecific clinical signs and symptoms.

ABNORMAL MOVEMENTS

Neonatal seizures usually suggest a central nervous system (CNS) disorder, such as hypoxic-ischemic encephalopathy (HIE), intracranial hemorrhage, stroke, cerebral anomaly, subdural effusion, or meningitis (see Chapter 611.7). In the neonate, seizures can also be secondary to hypocalcemia, hypoglycemia, benign familial seizures, or rarely, pyridoxine dependence, hyponatremia, hypernatremia, inborn errors of metabolism, or drug withdrawal.

Seizures in premature infants are often subtle and associated with abnormal eye movement (fluttering, tonic horizontal deviation, sustained eye opening with ocular fixation) or facial movement (chewing, tongue thrusting); the motor component is often that of tonic extension of the limbs, neck, and trunk. Autonomic phenomena include hypertension and tachycardia. Term infants may have focal or multifocal, clonic or myoclonic movements, but they may also have subtler manifestations of seizure activity. **Apnea** may be the 1st manifestation of seizure activity, particularly in a premature infant. Seizures may adversely affect the subsequent neurodevelopmental outcome and may even predispose an infant to seizures outside the neonatal period. Electroencephalographic evidence of seizures can occur without clinical manifestations, particularly in preterm infants. If seizures are suspected, continuous amplitude integrated EEG (aEEG), or more accurately, long-term video EEG monitoring, will improve detection of both subtle and electrographic but clinically silent seizures. Many medications used to treat seizures have important side effects and limited efficacy, but current evidence suggests that the benefits of treating seizures outweigh the risks.

Seizures should be distinguished from the **jitteriness**, defined as *recurrent tremors*, that may be present in normal newborns, in infants of diabetic mothers, in those who experienced birth asphyxia or drug withdrawal, and in polycythemic neonates. An examiner may stop the tremors by holding the infant's extremity; jitteriness often depends on sensory stimuli and occurs when the infant is active, and it is not associated with abnormal eye movements. Tremors are often more rapid with a smaller amplitude than those of tonic-clonic seizures.

After severe birth asphyxia, infants may exhibit **motor automatisms** characterized by recurrent oral-buccal-lingual movements, rotary limb activities (rowing, pedaling, swimming), tonic posturing, or myoclonus. These motor activities are not usually accompanied by time-synchronized EEG discharges, may not signify cortical epileptic activity, respond poorly to anticonvulsant therapy, and are associated with a poor prognosis. Such automatisms may represent cortical depression that produces a brainstem release phenomenon or subcortical seizures.

Failure to move an extremity (**pseudoparalysis**) suggests fracture, dislocation, or nerve injury, often following a traumatic delivery. It is also seen in septic arthritis, osteomyelitis, and other infections that cause pain on movement of the affected part.

ALTERED MENTAL STATUS

Lethargy may be a manifestation of infection, asphyxia, hypoglycemia, hypercapnia, sedation from maternal analgesia or anesthesia, a cerebral defect, or, indeed, almost any severe disease, including an inborn error of metabolism. Shortly after birth, lethargy is most likely caused by maternal medications (opioids, magnesium, general anesthesia) or severe HIE. Lethargy appearing after the 2nd day should suggest infection or an inborn error of metabolism manifesting with hyperammonemia, acidosis, or hypoglycemia. Lethargy with emesis suggests increased intracranial pressure or an inborn error of metabolism.

Irritability may be a sign of discomfort accompanying intraabdominal conditions, meningeal irritation, drug withdrawal, infections, congenital glaucoma, trauma (birth, abuse), or any condition producing pain. It must be distinguished from normal crying behavior associated with hunger or benign environmental stimuli. **Hyperactivity**, especially in a premature infant, may be a sign of hypoxia, pneumothorax, emphysema, hypoglycemia, hypocalcemia, CNS damage, drug withdrawal, neonatal thyrotoxicosis, bronchospasm, esophageal reflux, or discomfort from a cold environment.

Failure to feed is an important sign of the sick newborn infants and should prompt a careful search for infection, a CNS (brain or spine) or peripheral nervous system disorder, inborn error of metabolism, intestinal obstruction, and other abnormal conditions.

APNEA

Periods of apnea, particularly in premature infants, can be attributed to many different underlying causes (see Chapter 122.2). When apnea recurs, or when the intervals are >20 sec or associated with cyanosis or bradycardia, an immediate diagnostic evaluation for the underlying cause is imperative.

CONGENITAL ANOMALIES

Congenital anomalies are a major cause of stillbirths and in the United States and other developed countries are one of the main causes of neonatal mortality. In addition, congenital anomalies are a major cause of acute illness and long-term morbidity. Anomalies are discussed in general in Chapters 98 and 128 and specifically in the chapters on the various systems of the body. Early recognition of anomalies during fetal life is important to plan for delivery room management and subsequent neonatal care. Some malformations, including congenital heart disease, tracheoesophageal fistula, diaphragmatic hernia, choanal atresia, and intestinal obstruction, require immediate medical/surgical therapy for postnatal survival (Table 119.1). Parents are likely to feel anxious and guilty on learning of the existence of a congenital anomaly and require thoughtful, sensitive counseling.

CYANOSIS

Central cyanosis generates a broad differential diagnosis encompassing respiratory, cardiac, CNS, infectious, hematologic, and metabolic etiologies (Table 119.2). Typically, 5 g/dL of deoxyhemoglobin must be present in the blood for central cyanosis to be clinically apparent. If respiratory insufficiency is caused by pulmonary conditions, respirations tend to be rapid with increased work of breathing. If caused by CNS depression, respirations tend to be irregular and weak and are often slow. Cyanosis unaccompanied by obvious signs of respiratory difficulty suggests cyanotic congenital heart disease or methemoglobinemia. Cyanosis resulting from congenital heart disease may, however, be difficult to distinguish clinically from cyanosis caused by respiratory disease. Episodes of cyanosis may also be the initial sign of hypoglycemia, bacteremia, meningitis, shock, or pulmonary hypertension. **Peripheral acrocyanosis** is common

Table 119.1	Common Life-Threatening Congenital Anomalies
ANOMALY	**MANIFESTATIONS**
Choanal atresia	Respiratory distress in delivery room; nasogastric tube cannot be passed through nares. Suspect CHARGE (coloboma of eye, heart anomaly, choanal atresia, retardation, genital and ear anomalies) syndrome.
Pierre Robin syndrome, Stickler syndrome	Micrognathia, cleft palate, airway obstruction
Diaphragmatic hernia	Scaphoid abdomen, bowel sounds present in chest, respiratory distress
Tracheoesophageal fistula	Polyhydramnios, aspiration pneumonia, excessive salivation; nasogastric tube cannot be placed in stomach. Suspect VATER (vertebral defects, imperforate anus, tracheoesophageal fistula, radial and renal dysplasia) syndrome.
Intestinal obstruction: volvulus, duodenal atresia, ileal atresia	Polyhydramnios, bile-stained emesis, abdominal distention Suspect trisomy 21, cystic fibrosis, or cocaine use.
Gastroschisis, omphalocele	Polyhydramnios, intestinal obstruction
Renal agenesis, Potter syndrome	Oligohydramnios, anuria, pulmonary hypoplasia, pneumothorax
Neural tube defects: anencephalus, meningomyelocele	Polyhydramnios, elevated α-fetoprotein, decreased fetal activity
Ductus-dependent congenital heart disease	Cyanosis, hypotension, murmur

Table 119.2	Differential Diagnosis of Cyanosis in the Newborn

CENTRAL OR PERIPHERAL NERVOUS SYSTEM HYPOVENTILATION	*Obstructed Pulmonary Blood Flow (Pulmonary Blood Flow Decreased)*
Birth asphyxia	Pulmonic atresia with intact ventricular septum
Intracranial hypertension, hemorrhage	Tetralogy of Fallot
Oversedation (direct or through maternal route)	Critical pulmonic stenosis with patent foramen ovale or atrial septal defect
Diaphragm palsy	Tricuspid atresia
Neuromuscular diseases	Single ventricle with pulmonic stenosis
Seizures	Ebstein malformation of tricuspid valve
	Persistent fetal circulation (persistent pulmonary hypertension of newborn)
RESPIRATORY DISEASE	
Airway	**METHEMOGLOBINEMIA**
Choanal atresia/stenosis	Congenital (hemoglobin M, methemoglobin reductase deficiency)
Pierre Robin syndrome	Acquired (nitrates, nitrites)
Intrinsic airway obstruction (laryngeal/bronchial/tracheal stenosis)	Inadequate ambient O_2 or less O_2 delivered than expected (rare)
Extrinsic airway obstruction (bronchogenic cyst, duplication cyst, vascular compression)	Disconnection of O_2 supply to nasal cannula, head hood
Lung	Connection of air, rather than O_2, to a mechanical ventilator
Respiratory distress syndrome	
Transient tachypnea	**SPURIOUS/ARTIFACTUAL**
Meconium aspiration	Oximeter artifact (poor contact between probe and skin, poor pulse searching)
Pneumonia (sepsis)	Arterial blood gas artifact (contamination with venous blood)
Pneumothorax	
Congenital diaphragmatic hernia	
Pulmonary hypoplasia	
CARDIAC RIGHT-TO-LEFT SHUNT	**OTHER**
Abnormal Connections (Pulmonary Blood Flow Normal or Increased)	Hypoglycemia
Transposition of great vessels	Adrenogenital syndrome
Total anomalous pulmonary venous return	Polycythemia
Truncus arteriosus	Blood loss
Hypoplastic left heart syndrome	
Single ventricle or tricuspid atresia with large ventricular septal defect but without pulmonic stenosis	

From Smith F: Cyanosis. In Kliegman RM: *Practical strategies in pediatric diagnosis and therapy*, Philadelphia, 1996, Saunders.

in neonates and thought to represent peripheral venous congestion associated with immature control of peripheral vascular tone. It does not usually warrant concern unless poor perfusion is suspected.

GASTROINTESTINAL DISTURBANCES

Vomiting during the 1st day of life can suggest obstruction in the upper digestive tract, metabolic disease, or increased intracranial pressure and must be distinguished from benign reflux. **Abdominal distention** with emesis, usually a sign of intestinal obstruction or an intraabdominal mass,

may also be seen in infants with enteritis, necrotizing enterocolitis (NEC), isolated intestinal perforation, ileus accompanying sepsis, respiratory distress, ascites, or hypokalemia. Imaging studies are indicated when obstruction is suspected; proximal intestinal obstruction often occurs with a normal physical examination, whereas distal obstruction will likely be accompanied by distention. Vomiting may also be a nonspecific symptom of an illness such as septicemia with associated abdominal distention and ileus. It is a common manifestation of overfeeding, inexperienced feeding technique, or normal reflux. Rarely, vomiting is

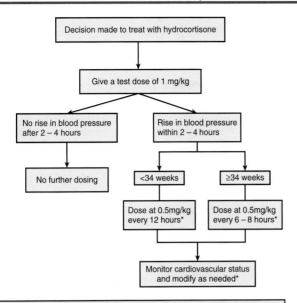

Fig. 119.1 Suggested treatment algorithm for hydrocortisone dosing in the newborn. *(From Watterberg KL: Hydrocortisone dosing for hypotension in newborn infants: less is more, J Pediatr 174:23–26, 2016, p 26.e1.)*

Table 119.3	Pain in the Neonate: General Considerations

- Pain in newborns is often unrecognized and/or undertreated.
- If a procedure is painful in adults, it should be considered painful in newborns.
- Healthcare institutions should develop and implement patient care policies to assess, prevent, and manage pain in neonates.
- Pharmacologic agents with known pharmacokinetic and pharmacodynamic properties and demonstrated efficacy in neonates should be used. Agents known to compromise cardiorespiratory function should be administered only by persons experienced in neonatal airway management and in settings with the capacity for continuous monitoring.
- Educational programs to increase the skills of healthcare professionals in the assessment and management of stress and pain in neonates should be provided.
- Further research is needed to develop and validate neonatal pain assessment tools that are useful in the clinical setting; to determine optimal behavioral and pharmacologic interventions; and to study long-term effects of pain and pain management.

Data from American Academy of Pediatrics Committee on Fetus and Newborn, Committee on Drugs, Section on Anesthesiology, Section on Surgery; Canadian Paediatric Society, Fetus and Newborn Committee: Prevention and management of pain and stress in the neonate, *Pediatrics* 105:454–461, 2000; and from Anand KJS; International Evidence-Based Group for Neonatal Pain: Consensus statement for the prevention and management of pain in the newborn, *Arch Pediatr Adolesc Med* 155:173–180, 2001.

caused by pyloric stenosis, milk allergy, duodenal ulcer, stress ulcer, an inborn error of metabolism (hyperammonemia, metabolic acidosis), or adrenal insufficiency. Vomitus containing dark blood is usually a sign of a serious illness; but the benign possibility of swallowed maternal blood associated with the delivery process should also be considered. Tests for maternal vs fetal hemoglobin can help discriminate between these possibilities. Bilious emesis strongly suggests obstruction below the ampulla of Vater and warrants urgent contrast-enhanced radiography.

Diarrhea may be a symptom of overfeeding (especially high–caloric density formula), acute gastroenteritis, congenital diarrhea syndromes, or malabsorption, or it may be a nonspecific symptom of infection. Diarrhea should be differentiated from the normal loose, seedy, yellow stool seen typically in breastfed infants. Diarrhea may occur in conditions accompanied by compromised circulation of part of the intestinal or genital tract, such as mesenteric thrombosis, NEC, strangulated hernia, intussusception, and torsion of the ovary or testis.

HYPOTENSION

Hypotension in term infants implies hypovolemic shock (hemorrhage, dehydration), a systemic inflammatory response syndrome (bacterial sepsis, intrauterine infection, NEC), cardiac dysfunction (left heart obstructive lesions: hypoplastic left heart syndrome, myocarditis, asphyxia-induced myocardial stunning, anomalous coronary artery), pneumothorax, pneumopericardium, pericardial effusion, or metabolic disorders (hypoglycemia, adrenal insufficiency).

Hypotension is a common problem in sick preterm infants and may also be caused by any of the problems noted in a term infant. Some extremely low gestational age infants do not respond to fluids or inotropic agents but may improve with administration of intravenous hydrocortisone (Fig. 119.1). Sudden onset of hypotension in a very-low-birthweight (VLBW) infant suggests pneumothorax, intraventricular hemorrhage, or subcapsular hepatic hematoma. Strategies used to support blood pressure include volume expansion (normal saline or <5% albumin), vasopressors (dopamine, dobutamine, epinephrine, norepinephrine, vasopressin), or corticosteroids (hydrocortisone) (see Chapter 121).

JAUNDICE

Jaundice during the 1st 24 hr of life warrants diagnostic evaluation and should be considered pathologic until proved otherwise. Septicemia and intrauterine or perinatal infections, such as syphilis, cytomegalovirus, and toxoplasmosis, as well as neonatal hemochromatosis, should also be considered, especially in infants with an increase in *direct* bilirubin value. Immediate evaluation includes obtaining total and direct bilirubin, and confirmation as abnormally elevated indicates albumin level, infant blood type and Coombs status, complete blood cell count (CBC), and reticulocyte count. In the case of Coombs-positive hemolysis, strong consideration should be made to giving intravenous immune globulin (IVIG) if there is no response to intensive phototherapy.

Jaundice beyond the 1st 24 hr may be *physiologic* or may be caused by a wide range of conditions, including septicemia, hemolytic anemia, galactosemia, hepatitis, congenital atresia of the bile ducts, inspissated bile syndrome after erythroblastosis fetalis, syphilis, herpes simplex other congenital infections, or other conditions (see Chapter 123.3).

PAIN

Pain in neonates may be unrecognized and/or undertreated. The intensive care of neonates may involve several painful procedures, including blood sampling (heelstick, venous or arterial puncture), endotracheal intubation and suctioning, mechanical ventilation, and insertion of chest tubes and intravascular catheters. Pain in neonates results in obvious distress and acute physiologic stress responses, which may have developmental implications for pain in later life. Moreover, knowing that infants may experience pain contributes to parental stress.

Pain and discomfort are potentially avoidable problems during the treatment of sick infants. The most common causes of painful stimuli include circumcision pain and that associated with phlebotomy for metabolic screening tests. **Oral sucrose solutions** are well tolerated by most infants and have proven efficacy for procedural pain. For NICU infants, the most frequently used drugs are intermittent or continuous doses of opioids (morphine, fentanyl) and benzodiazepines (midazolam, lorazepam). Although the long-term effects of opioids and sedatives are not well established, the first concern should be the treatment and/or prevention of acute pain. Continuous opiate infusions should be used with caution. Some minor but painful procedures performed in well neonates can be managed with oral sucrose solutions (Table 119.3).

Bibliography is available at Expert Consult.

119.1 Hyperthermia

Elizabeth Enlow and James M. Greenberg

Serious infection (pneumonia, bacteremia, meningitis, and viral infections, particularly herpes simplex or enteroviruses) may cause **fever** and must be considered, although such infections often occur without provoking a febrile response in newborn infants (see Chapters 201 and 202). Providers should consider evaluation for bacterial infection in infants <28 days old with a rectal temperature ≥38°C (100.5°F), including blood culture, urine culture, and lumbar puncture (LP), although stepwise approaches to identify low-risk patients and limiting LP to a subset of higher-risk infants are gaining favor. Fever immediately after birth may be caused by radiant warmers, maternal fever, or maternal epidural analgesia. Fever may also be caused by elevated environmental temperatures because of weather, overheated nurseries, incubators, or radiant warmers, or excessive clothing. It has also been attributed to dehydration, although *dehydration fever* is a diagnosis of exclusion in newborn infants.

Bibliography is available at Expert Consult.

119.2 Hypothermia and Cold Stress

Elizabeth Enlow and James M. Greenberg

Unexplained **hypothermia** may accompany infection or other serious disturbances of the circulation or CNS. A sudden servo-controlled increase in incubator ambient temperature to maintain body temperature is a sign of temperature instability and may be associated with sepsis or any of the conditions already mentioned.

Cold stress can lead to profound decompensation, including apnea, bradycardia, respiratory distress, hypoglycemia, and poor feeding. For this reason, it is paramount for the neonate to maintain normothermia in the delivery room and afterward, especially low-birthweight and premature infants. For VLBW infants, a combination of occlusive plastic wrap, radiant warmers, and thermal mattresses to maintain normothermia can be used to reduce cold stress.

Bibliography is available at Expert Consult.

119.3 Edema

Elizabeth Enlow and James M. Greenberg

Generalized edema in a neonate can be caused by hydrops fetalis secondary to several underlying causes (see Chapter 124.2), excessive fluid administration, respiratory disease, sepsis, NEC, and hepatic, renal, or cardiac dysfunction. An infant with suspected hydrops in utero should be delivered at a specialty perinatal center with capacity for neonatal intubation, thoracentesis, paracentesis, and pericardiocentesis in the delivery room.

Bibliography is available at Expert Consult.

119.4 Hypocalcemia

Elizabeth Enlow and James M. Greenberg

Hypocalcemia in a neonate can manifest as irritability, jitteriness, clonus, or seizures. Electrocardiography can show a prolonged QT interval. The cause may simply represent an exaggerated physiologic decrease in serum calcium levels within the 1st 24 hr of life or pathologic conditions such as genetic disorders (22q deletions), prematurity, growth restriction, perinatal hypoxia, hypomagnesemia, or maternal diabetes. Hypocalcemia is more common in term infants receiving formula than in those exclusively receiving breast milk. Most infants remain asymptomatic and can be managed conservatively with early nutrition and close monitoring, whereas symptomatic neonates should receive IV or oral calcium replacement.

Bibliography is available at Expert Consult.

119.5 Hypermagnesemia

Elizabeth Enlow and James M. Greenberg

Hypermagnesemia is most often caused by maternal administration of magnesium in the perinatal period for treatment of conditions such as preeclampsia and preterm labor, and as prophylaxis to mitigate brain injury associated with preterm birth. Infants are usually present with signs at birth and improve over the next 24-48 hr. Symptoms include respiratory depression, hypotonia, lethargy, and feeding intolerance. No treatment is indicated other than supportive measures.

Chapter **120**
Nervous System Disorders

Stephanie L. Merhar and
Cameron W. Thomas

第一百二十章
神经系统疾病

中文导读

本章主要介绍了与分娩相关的颅骨损伤、颅内出血、脑室内出血和脑室周围白质软化、缺氧缺血性脑病及脊柱脊髓和外周神经损伤的临床表现和治疗，这类疾病既与产科助娩技术相关，也与患儿自身患病状况相关，是最容易引起产科新儿科纠纷的一类疾病。本章同时对缺氧缺血性脑病和脑室内出血和脑室周围白质软化的病因、流行病学、发病机制、诊断和预后也作了详细阐述。

Central nervous system (CNS) disorders are important causes of neonatal mortality and both short-term and long-term morbidity. The CNS can be injured as a result of asphyxia, hemorrhage, trauma, hypoglycemia, or direct cytotoxicity. The etiology of CNS injury is often multifactorial and includes perinatal complications, postnatal hemodynamic instability, and developmental abnormalities that may be genetic and/or environmental. Predisposing factors for brain injury include chronic and acute maternal illness resulting in uteroplacental dysfunction, intrauterine infection, macrosomia/dystocia, malpresentation, prematurity, and intrauterine growth restriction. Acute and often unavoidable emergencies during the delivery process may result in mechanical and hypoxic-ischemic brain injury.

120.1 The Cranium

Stephanie L. Merhar and Cameron W. Thomas

Erythema, abrasions, ecchymoses, and subcutaneous fat necrosis of facial or scalp soft tissues may be noted after a normal delivery or after forceps or vacuum-assisted deliveries. The location depends on the area of contact with the pelvic bones or application of the forceps. Traumatic hemorrhage may involve any layer of the scalp as well as intracranial contents (Fig. 120.1).

Caput succedaneum is a diffuse, sometimes ecchymotic, edematous swelling of the soft tissues of the scalp involving the area presenting during vertex delivery. It may extend across the midline and across suture lines. The edema disappears within the 1st few days of life. Molding of the head and overriding of the parietal bones are frequently associated with caput succedaneum and become more evident after the caput has receded; they disappear during the 1st few weeks of life. Rarely, a hemorrhagic caput may result in shock and require blood transfusion. Analogous swelling, discoloration, and distortion of the face are seen in face presentations. No specific treatment is needed, but if extensive ecchymoses are present, hyperbilirubinemia may develop.

Cephalohematoma is a subperiosteal hemorrhage and thus always limited to the *surface* of one cranial bone (Fig. 120.2). Cephalohematomas occur in 1–2% of live births. No discoloration of the overlying scalp occurs, and swelling is not usually visible for several hours after birth because subperiosteal bleeding is a slow process. The lesion becomes a firm, tense mass with a palpable rim localized over one area of the skull. Most cephalohematomas are resorbed within 2 wk to 3 mo, depending on their size. They may begin to calcify by the end of the 2nd wk. A few remain for years as bony protuberances and are detectable on radiographs as widening of the diploic space; cystlike defects may persist for months or years. An underlying skull fracture, usually linear and not depressed, may be associated with 10–25% of cases. A sensation of central depression suggesting but not indicative of an underlying fracture or bony defect is usually encountered on palpation of the organized rim of a cephalohematoma. Cephalohematomas require no treatment, although phototherapy may be necessary to treat hyperbilirubinemia. Infection of the hematoma is a very rare complication.

A **subgaleal hemorrhage** is a collection of blood beneath the aponeurosis that covers the scalp and serves as the insertion for the occipitofrontalis muscle (see Fig. 120.1). Bleeding can be very extensive into this large potential space and may even dissect into subcutaneous tissues of the neck. There is often an association with vacuum-assisted delivery. The mechanism of injury is most likely secondary to rupture of emissary veins connecting the dural sinuses within the skull and the superficial veins of the scalp. Subgaleal hemorrhages are sometimes associated with skull fractures, suture diastasis, and fragmentation of

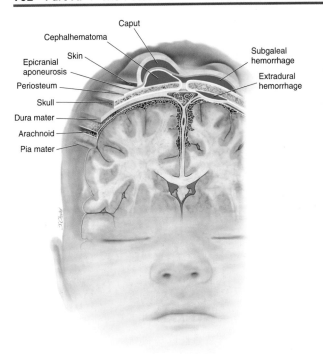

Fig. 120.1 Sites of extracranial (and extradural) hemorrhages in the newborn. Schematic diagram of important tissue planes from skin to dura. *(From Volpe JJ: Injuries of extracranial, cranial, intracranial, spinal cord, and peripheral nervous system structures. In Volpe's neurology of the newborn, ed 6, Philadelphia, 2018, Elsevier, Fig 36-1.)*

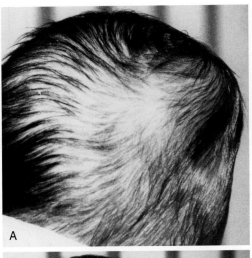

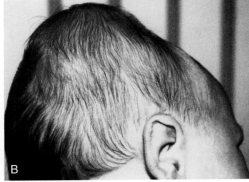

Fig. 120.2 Parietal cephalhematoma. Clinical appearance of 10 day old infant delivered with the aid of mid-forceps. **A,** Posterior view. **B,** Right lateral view. Note prominent swelling that extends medially to the sagittal suture, posteriorly to the lambdoid suture, and laterally to the squamosal suture. *(From Volpe JJ: Injuries of extracranial, cranial, intracranial, spinal cord, and peripheral nervous system structures. In Volpe's neurology of the newborn, ed 6, Philadelphia, 2018, Elsevier, Fig 36-3.)*

the superior margin of the parietal bone. Extensive subgaleal bleeding is occasionally secondary to a hereditary coagulopathy (**hemophilia**). A subgaleal hemorrhage manifests as a fluctuant mass that straddles cranial sutures or fontanels that increases in size after birth. Some patients have a consumptive coagulopathy from massive blood loss. Patients should be monitored for hypotension, anemia, and hyperbilirubinemia. These lesions typically resolve over 2-3 wk.

Fractures of the skull may be caused by pressure from forceps or the maternal pelvis or by accidental falls after birth. *Linear fractures,* the most common, cause no symptoms and require no treatment. Linear fractures should be followed up to demonstrate healing and to detect the possible complication of a leptomeningeal cyst. *Depressed fractures* indent the calvaria similar to dents in a Ping-Pong ball. They are generally a complication of forceps delivery or fetal compression. Affected infants may be asymptomatic unless they have associated intracranial injury; it is advisable to elevate severe depressions to prevent cortical injury from sustained pressure. Although some may elevate spontaneously, some require treatment. Use of a breast pump or vacuum extractor may obviate the need for neurosurgical intervention. Suspected skull fractures should be evaluated with CT (3D reconstruction may be helpful) to confirm fracture and rule out associated intracranial injury.

Subconjunctival and **retinal hemorrhages** are frequent; petechiae of the skin of the head and neck are also common. All are probably secondary to a sudden increase in intrathoracic pressure during passage of the chest through the birth canal. Parents should be assured that these hemorrhages are temporary and the result of normal events of delivery. The lesions resolve rapidly within the 1st 2 wk of life.

120.2 Traumatic, Epidural, Subdural, and Subarachnoid Hemorrhage

Stephanie L. Merhar and Cameron W. Thomas

Traumatic epidural, subdural, or subarachnoid hemorrhage is especially likely when the fetal head is large in proportion to the size of the mother's pelvic outlet, with prolonged labor, in breech or precipitous deliveries, or as a result of mechanical assistance with delivery. Massive **subdural hemorrhage**, often associated with tears in the tentorium cerebelli or less frequently in the falx cerebri, is rare but is encountered more often in full-term than in premature infants. Patients with massive hemorrhage caused by tears of the tentorium or falx cerebri rapidly deteriorate and may die soon after birth. Most subdural and epidural hemorrhages resolve without intervention. Consultation with a neurosurgeon is recommended. Asymptomatic subdural hemorrhage may be noted within 48 hr of birth after vaginal or cesarean delivery. These are typically small hemorrhages, especially common in the posterior fossa, discovered incidentally in term infants imaged in the neonatal period and usually of no clinical significance. The diagnosis of large subdural hemorrhage may be delayed until the chronic subdural fluid volume expands and produces macrocephaly, frontal bossing, a bulging fontanel, anemia, and sometimes seizures. CT scan and MRI are useful imaging techniques to confirm these diagnoses. Symptomatic subdural hemorrhage in term infants can be treated by a neurosurgical evacuation of the subdural fluid collection by a needle placed through the lateral margin of the anterior fontanel. In addition to birth trauma, **child abuse** must be suspected in all infants with subdural effusion after the immediate neonatal period. Most asymptomatic subdural hemorrhages following labor should resolve by 4 wk of age.

Subarachnoid hemorrhage is often clinically silent in the neonate. Anastomoses between the penetrating leptomeningeal arteries or the bridging veins are the most likely source of the bleeding. Most affected infants have no clinical symptoms, but the subarachnoid hemorrhage may be detected because of an elevated number of red blood cells in a lumbar puncture sample. Some infants experience short, benign seizures, which tend to occur on the 2nd day of life. Rarely, an infant has a catastrophic hemorrhage and dies. There are usually no neurologic abnormalities during the acute episode or on follow-up. Significant neurologic findings should suggest an arteriovenous malformation, which can best be detected on CT or MRI.

120.3 Intracranial-Intraventricular Hemorrhage and Periventricular Leukomalacia

Stephanie L. Merhar and Cameron W. Thomas

ETIOLOGY

Intracranial hemorrhage in preterm infants usually develops spontaneously. Less frequently, it may be caused by trauma or asphyxia, and rarely, it occurs from a primary hemorrhagic disturbance or congenital cerebrovascular anomaly. Intracranial hemorrhage often involves the ventricles (**intraventricular hemorrhage, IVH**) of premature infants delivered spontaneously without apparent trauma. The IVH in premature infants is usually not present at birth but may develop during the 1st week of life. Primary hemorrhagic disturbances and vascular malformations are rare and usually give rise to subarachnoid or intracerebral hemorrhage. In utero hemorrhage associated with maternal idiopathic or, more often, fetal alloimmune thrombocytopenia may appear as severe cerebral hemorrhage or as a porencephalic cyst after resolution of a fetal cortical hemorrhage. Intracranial bleeding may be associated with disseminated intravascular coagulation, isoimmune thrombocytopenia, and neonatal vitamin K deficiency, especially in infants born to mothers receiving phenobarbital or phenytoin.

EPIDEMIOLOGY

The overall incidence of IVH has decreased over the past decades as a result of improved perinatal care, increased use of antenatal corticosteroids, surfactant to treat respiratory distress syndrome (RDS), and possibly prophylactic indomethacin. It continues to be an important cause of morbidity in preterm infants, as approximately 30% of premature infants <1,500 g have IVH. The risk is inversely related to gestational age and birthweight; 7% of infants weighing 1,001-1,500 g have a severe IVH (grade III or IV), compared to 14% of infants weighing 751-1,000 g and 24% of infants ≤750 g. In 3% of infants <1,000 g, **periventricular leukomalacia (PVL)** develops.

PATHOGENESIS

The major neuropathologic lesions associated with very-low-birthweight (VLBW) infants are IVH and PVL. IVH in premature infants occurs in the gelatinous subependymal **germinal matrix**. This periventricular area is the site of origin for embryonal neurons and fetal glial cells, which migrate outwardly to the cortex. Immature blood vessels in this highly vascular region of the developing brain combined with poor tissue vascular support predispose premature infants to hemorrhage. The germinal matrix involutes as the infant approaches full-term gestation, and the tissue's vascular integrity improves; therefore IVH is much less common in the term infant. The cerebellum also contains a germinal matrix and is susceptible to hemorrhagic injury. **Periventricular**

hemorrhagic infarction, previously known as **grade IV intraventricular hemorrhage**, often develops after a large IVH because of venous congestion. Predisposing factors for IVH include prematurity, RDS, hypoxia-ischemia, exaggerated fluctuations in cerebral blood flow (hypotensive injury, hypervolemia, hypertension), reperfusion injury of damaged vessels, reduced vascular integrity, increased venous pressure (pneumothorax, venous thrombus), or thrombocytopenia.

Understanding of the pathogenesis of PVL is evolving, and it appears to involve both intrauterine and postnatal events. A complex interaction exists between the development of the cerebral vasculature and the regulation of cerebral blood flow (both of which depend on gestational age), disturbances in the oligodendrocyte precursors required for myelination, and maternal/fetal infection and inflammation. Postnatal hypoxia or hypotension, necrotizing enterocolitis (NEC) with its resultant inflammation, and severe neonatal infection may all result in white matter injury. PVL is characterized by focal necrotic lesions in the periventricular white matter and/or more diffuse white matter damage. Destructive focal necrotic lesions resulting from massive cell death are less common in the modern era. Instead, diffuse injury leading to abnormal maturation of neurons and glia is more frequently seen. The risk for PVL increases in infants with severe IVH or ventriculomegaly. Infants with PVL are at higher risk of cerebral palsy because of injury to the corticospinal tracts that descend through the periventricular white matter.

CLINICAL MANIFESTATIONS

Most infants with **IVH**, including some with moderate to severe hemorrhages, have no initial clinical signs (**silent** IVH). Some premature infants in whom severe IVH develops may have acute deterioration on the 2nd or 3rd day of life (**catastrophic** presentation). Hypotension, apnea, pallor, stupor or coma, seizures, decreased muscle tone, metabolic acidosis, shock, and decreased hematocrit (or failure of hematocrit to increase after transfusion) may be the first clinical indications. A saltatory progression may evolve over several hours to days and manifest as intermittent or progressive alterations of levels of consciousness, abnormalities of tone and movement, respiratory signs, and eventually other features of the acute catastrophic IVH. Rarely, IVH may manifest at birth or even prenatally; 50% of cases are diagnosed within the 1st day of life, and up to 75% within the 1st 3 days. A small percentage of infants have late hemorrhage, between days 14 and 30. IVH as a primary event is rare after the 1st mo of life.

PVL is usually clinically asymptomatic until the neurologic sequelae of white matter damage become apparent in later infancy as spasticity and/or motor deficits. PVL may be present at birth but usually occurs later, when the echodense phase is seen on ultrasound (3-10 days of life), followed by the typical echolucent/cystic phase (14-20 days).

The severity of hemorrhage is defined by the location and degree of bleeding and ventricular dilation on cranial imaging. In a **grade I** hemorrhage, bleeding is isolated to the subependymal area. In **grade II** hemorrhage, there is bleeding within the ventricle without evidence of ventricular dilation. **Grade III** hemorrhage is IVH with ventricular dilation. In **grade IV** hemorrhage, there is intraventricular and parenchymal hemorrhage (Fig. 120.3). Another grading system describes 3 levels of increasing severity of IVH detected on ultrasound: In **grade I**, bleeding is confined to the germinal matrix–subependymal region or to <10% of the ventricle (approximately 35% of IVH cases); **grade II** is defined as intraventricular bleeding with 10–50% filling of the ventricle (40% of IVH cases); and in **grade III**, >50% of the ventricle is involved, with dilated ventricles (Fig. 120.3). **Ventriculomegaly** is defined as mild (0.5-1 cm dilation), moderate (1.0-1.5 cm dilation), or severe (>1.5 cm dilation).

DIAGNOSIS

Intracranial hemorrhage is suspected on the basis of history, clinical manifestations, and knowledge of the birthweight-specific risks for **IVH**. Associated clinical signs of IVH are typically nonspecific or absent; therefore, it is recommended that premature infants <32 wk of gestation be evaluated with routine real-time cranial ultrasonography (US) through the anterior fontanel to screen for IVH. Infants <1,000 g are at highest risk and should undergo cranial US within the 1st 3-7 days of age, when approximately 75% of lesions will be detectable. US is the preferred imaging technique for screening because it is noninvasive, portable, reproducible, and sensitive and specific for detection of IVH. All at-risk infants should undergo follow-up US at 36-40 wk postmenstrual age to evaluate adequately for PVL, as cystic changes related to perinatal injury may not be visible for up to 1 mo. In one study, 29% of low-birthweight (LBW) infants who later experienced cerebral palsy did not have radiographic evidence of PVL until after 28 days of age. US also detects the precystic and cystic symmetric lesions of PVL and the asymmetric intraparenchymal echogenic lesions of cortical hemorrhagic infarction (Fig. 120.4). Cranial US may be useful in monitoring delayed development of cortical atrophy, porencephaly, and the severity, progression, or regression of posthemorrhagic hydrocephalus.

Approximately 3–5% of VLBW infants develop **posthemorrhagic hydrocephalus (PHH)**. If the initial US findings are abnormal, additional interval US studies are indicated to monitor for the development of hydrocephalus and potential need for ventriculoperitoneal shunt insertion.

IVH represents only 1 facet of brain injury in the term or preterm infant. MRI is a more sensitive tool for evaluation of white matter abnormalities and cerebellar injury and may be more predictive of adverse long-term outcome.

PROGNOSIS

The degree of **IVH** and presence of **PVL** are strongly linked to survival and neurodevelopmental impairment (Tables 120.1 and 120.2). For infants with birthweight <1,000 g, the incidence of severe neurologic impairment (defined as Bayley Scales of Infant Development II mental developmental index <70, psychomotor development index <70, cerebral palsy, blindness, or deafness) after IVH is highest with grade IV hemorrhage and lower birthweight. PVL, cystic PVL, and progressive hydrocephalus requiring shunt insertion are each independently associated with a poorer prognosis (Table 120.3). Current data suggest that outcomes for infants with grade III/IV intraventricular hemorrhage may be improving, with rates of cerebral palsy and neurodevelopmental impairment closer to 30–40% at age 2 yr.

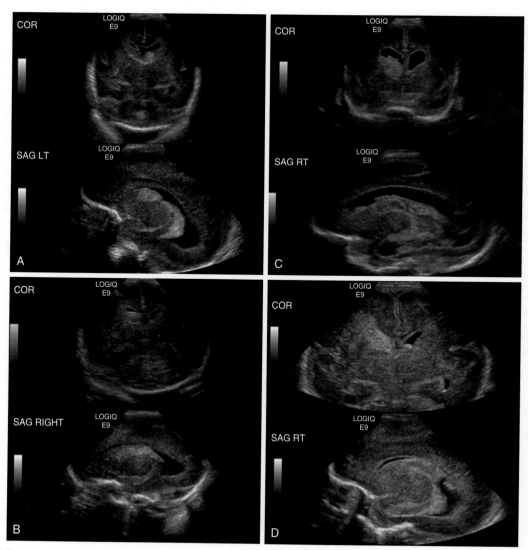

Fig. 120.3 Grading of the severity of germinal matrix–intraventricular hemorrhage (IVH): coronal (cor) and parasagittal (sag) ultrasound scans. **A,** Germinal matrix hemorrhage, grade I. **B,** IVH (filling <50% of ventricular area), grade II. **C,** IVH with ventricular dilatation, grade III. **D,** Large IVH with associated parenchymal echogenicity (hemorrhagic infarct), grade IV. *(From Inder TE, Perlman JM, Volpe JJ: Preterm intraventricular hemorrhage/posthemorrhagic hydrocephalus. In Volpe's neurology of the newborn, ed 6, Philadelphia, 2018, Elsevier, Fig 24-2.)*

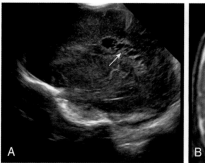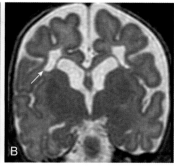

Fig. 120.4 Severe cystic periventricular leukomalacia. **A,** Parasagittal ultrasound image showing numerous large cysts superolateral to the lateral ventricle *(arrow).* **B,** Coronal T_2-weighted MR image in which cysts are present superolateral to the lateral ventricles *(arrow). (From Neil JJ, Volpe JJ: Encephalopathy of prematurity: clinical-neurological features, diagnosis, imaging, prognosis, therapy.* In Volpe's neurology of the newborn, *ed 6, Philadelphia, 2018, Elsevier, Fig 16-1.)*

Table 120.1	Short-Term Outcome of Germinal Matrix–Intraventricular Hemorrhage as a Function of Severity of Hemorrhage and Birthweight*			
	DEATHS IN FIRST 14 DAYS[c]		**PVD (SURVIVORS >14 DAYS)**	
SEVERITY OF HEMORRHAGE	**<750 g (n = 75)**	**751-1500 g (n = 173)**	**<750 g (n = 56)**	**751-1500 g (n = 165)**
Grade I	3/24 (12)	0/80 (0)	1/21 (5)	3/80 (4)
Grade II	5/21 (24)	1/44 (2)	1/16 (6)	6/43 (14)
Grade III	6/19 (32)	2/26 (8)	10/13 (77)	18/24 (75)
Grade III and apparent PHI	5/11 (45)	5/23 (22)	5/6 (83)	12/18 (66)

*Values are n (%). Deaths occurring later in the neonatal period are not shown; the total mortality rates (early and late deaths) are approximately 50–100% greater for each grade of hemorrhage and birthweight than those shown in the table for early deaths alone.

PHI, Periventricular hemorrhagic infarction; PVD, progressive ventricular dilation.

Data from Murphy BP, Inder TE, Rooks V, Taylor GA, et al. Posthemorrhagic ventricular dilatation in the premature infant: natural history and predictors of outcome, *Arch Dis Child Fetal Neonatal Ed* 87:F37–F41, 2002.

Adapted from Inder TE, Perlman JM, Volpe JJ: Preterm intraventricular hemorrhage/posthemorrhagic hydrocephalus. In *Volpe's neurology of the newborn,* ed 6, Philadelphia, 2018, Elsevier (Table 24-15).

Most infants with IVH and acute ventricular distention do not have **PHH**. Only 10–15% of LBW neonates with IVH develop PHH, which may initially present without clinical signs (enlarging head circumference, lethargy, a bulging fontanel or widely split sutures, apnea, and bradycardia). In infants in whom symptomatic hydrocephalus develops, clinical signs may be delayed 2-4 wk despite progressive ventricular distention and compression and thinning of the cerebral cortex. Many infants with PHH have spontaneous regression; only 3–5% of VLBW infants with PHH ultimately require shunt insertion. Those infants who require shunt insertion for PHH have lower cognitive and psychomotor performance at 18-22 mo.

PREVENTION

Improved perinatal care is imperative to minimize traumatic brain injury and decrease the risk of preterm delivery. The incidence of traumatic intracranial hemorrhage may be reduced by judicious management of cephalopelvic disproportion and operative (forceps, vacuum) delivery. Fetal or neonatal hemorrhage caused by maternal idiopathic thrombocytopenic purpura or alloimmune thrombocytopenia may be reduced by maternal treatment with corticosteroids, intravenous immune globulin (IVIG), fetal platelet transfusion, or cesarean birth. Meticulous care of the LBW infant's respiratory status and fluid-electrolyte management—avoidance of acidosis, hypocarbia, hypoxia, hypotension, wide fluctuations in neonatal blood pressure or PCO_2 (and secondarily fluctuation in cerebral perfusion pressure), and pneumothorax—are important factors that may affect the risk for development of IVH and PVL.

A single course of antenatal corticosteroids is recommended in pregnancies 24-37 wk of gestation that are at risk for preterm delivery.

Table 120.2	Long-Term Outcome: Neurologic Sequelae in Survivors With Germinal Matrix–Intraventricular Hemorrhage as a Function of Severity of Hemorrhage*
SEVERITY OF HEMORRHAGE[b]	**INCIDENCE OF DEFINITE NEUROLOGIC SEQUELAE[†] (%)**
Grade I	15
Grade II	25
Grade III	50
Grade III and apparent PVI	75

*Data are derived from reports published since 2002 and include personal published and unpublished cases. Mean values (to nearest 5%); considerable variability among studies was apparent, especially for the severe lesions.

[†]Definite neurologic sequelae included principally cerebral palsy or mental retardation, or both.

PVI, Periventricular hemorrhagic infarction.

Adapted From Inder TE, Perlman JM, Volpe JJ: Preterm intraventricular hemorrhage/posthemorrhagic hydrocephalus. In *Volpe's neurology of the newborn,* ed 6, Philadelphia, 2018, Elsevier (Table 24-16).

Antenatal steroids decrease the risk of death, grades III and IV intraventricular hemorrhage, and PVL in the neonate. The prophylactic administration of low-dose indomethacin (0.1 mg/kg/day for 3 days) to VLBW preterm infants reduces the incidence of severe IVH.

Table 120.3	Ultrasonographic (US) Diagnosis of Periventricular Leukomalacia	
US APPEARANCE	**TEMPORAL FEATURES**	**NEUROPATHOLOGIC CORRELATION**
Echogenic foci, bilateral, posterior > anterior	1st wk	Necrosis with congestion and/or hemorrhage (size >1 cm)
Echolucent foci ("cysts")	1-3 wk	Cyst formation secondary to tissue dissolution (size >3 mm)
Ventricular enlargement, often with disappearance of "cysts"	≥2-3 mo	Deficient myelin formation; gliosis, often with collapse of cyst

From Neil JJ, Volpe JJ: Encephalopathy of prematurity: clinical-neurological features, diagnosis, imaging, prognosis, therapy. In *Volpe's neurology of the newborn*, ed 6, Philadelphia, 2018, Elsevier (Table 16-6).

TREATMENT

Although no treatment is available for **IVH** that has occurred, it may be associated with other complications that require therapy. Seizures should be treated with anticonvulsant drugs. Anemia and coagulopathy require transfusion with packed red blood cells or fresh-frozen plasma. Shock and acidosis are treated with fluid resuscitation.

Insertion of a **ventriculoperitoneal shunt** is the preferred method to treat progressive and symptomatic **PHH**. Some infants require temporary cerebrospinal fluid diversion before a permanent shunt can be safely inserted. Diuretics and acetazolamide are not effective. Ventricular taps or reservoirs and externalized ventricular drains are potential temporizing interventions, although there is an associated risk of infection and *puncture porencephaly* from injury to the surrounding parenchyma. A **ventriculosubgaleal shunt** inserted from the ventricle into a surgically created subgaleal pocket provides a closed system for constant ventricular decompression without these additional risk factors. Decompression is regulated by the pressure gradient between the ventricle and the subgaleal pocket.

Bibliography is available at Expert Consult.

120.4 Hypoxic-Ischemic Encephalopathy

Cameron W. Thomas and Stephanie L. Merhar

Hypoxemia, a decreased arterial concentration of oxygen, frequently results in **hypoxia**, or decreased oxygenation to cells or organs. **Ischemia** refers to blood flow to cells or organs that is inadequate to maintain physiologic function. **Hypoxic-ischemic encephalopathy (HIE)** is a leading cause of neonatal brain injury, morbidity, and mortality globally. In the developed world, incidence is estimated at 1-8 per 1,000 live births, and in the developing world, estimates are as high as 26 per 1,000.

Approximately 20–30% of infants with HIE (depending on the severity) die in the neonatal period, and 33–50% of survivors are left with permanent neurodevelopmental abnormalities (cerebral palsy, decreased IQ, learning/cognitive impairment). The greatest risk of adverse outcome is seen in infants with severe fetal acidosis (pH <6.7) (90% death/impairment) and a base deficit >25 mmol/L (72% mortality). Multiorgan failure and insult can occur (Table 120.4).

ETIOLOGY

Most neonatal encephalopathy and seizure, in the absence of major congenital malformations or metabolic or genetic syndromes, appear to be caused by perinatal events. Brain MRI or autopsy findings in full-term neonates with encephalopathy demonstrate that 80% have acute injuries, <1% have prenatal injuries, and 3% have non–hypoxic-ischemic diagnoses. Fetal hypoxia may be caused by various disorders in the mother, including: (1) inadequate oxygenation of maternal blood from hypoventilation during anesthesia, cyanotic heart disease, respiratory failure, or carbon monoxide poisoning; (2) low maternal blood pressure from acute blood loss, spinal anesthesia, or compression of the vena cava and aorta by the gravid uterus; (3) inadequate relaxation of the uterus to permit placental filling as a result of uterine tetany caused by

Table 120.4	Multiorgan Systemic Effects of Asphyxia
SYSTEM	**EFFECTS**
Central nervous	Hypoxic-ischemic encephalopathy, infarction, intracranial hemorrhage, seizures, cerebral edema, hypotonia, hypertonia
Cardiovascular	Myocardial ischemia, poor contractility, cardiac stunning, tricuspid insufficiency, hypotension
Pulmonary	Pulmonary hypertension, pulmonary hemorrhage, respiratory distress syndrome
Renal	Acute tubular or cortical necrosis
Adrenal	Adrenal hemorrhage
Gastrointestinal	Perforation, ulceration with hemorrhage, necrosis
Metabolic	Inappropriate secretion of antidiuretic hormone, hyponatremia, hypoglycemia, hypocalcemia, myoglobinuria
Integumentary	Subcutaneous fat necrosis
Hematologic	Disseminated intravascular coagulation

the administration of excessive oxytocin; (4) premature separation of the placenta; (5) impedance to the circulation of blood through the umbilical cord as a result of compression or knotting of the cord; and (6) placental insufficiency from maternal infections, exposures, diabetes, toxemia or postmaturity.

Placental insufficiency often remains undetected on clinical assessment. Intrauterine growth restriction may develop in chronically hypoxic fetuses without the traditional signs of fetal distress. Doppler umbilical waveform velocimetry (demonstrating increased fetal vascular resistance) and cordocentesis (demonstrating fetal hypoxia and lactic acidosis) identify a chronically hypoxic infant (see Chapter 115). Uterine contractions may further reduce umbilical oxygenation, depressing the fetal cardiovascular system and CNS and resulting in low Apgar scores and respiratory depression at birth.

After birth, hypoxia may be caused by (1) failure of oxygenation as a result of severe forms of cyanotic congenital heart disease or severe pulmonary disease; (2) severe anemia (severe hemorrhage, hemolytic disease); (3) shock severe enough to interfere with the transport of oxygen to vital organs from overwhelming sepsis, massive blood loss, and intracranial or adrenal hemorrhage; or (4) failure to breathe after birth because of in utero CNS injury or drug-induced suppression.

PATHOPHYSIOLOGY AND PATHOLOGY

The topography of cerebral injury typically correlates with areas of decreased cerebral blood flow and areas of relatively higher metabolic demand, although regional vulnerabilities are impacted by gestational age and severity of insult (Table 120.5). After an episode of hypoxia and ischemia, anaerobic metabolism occurs and generates increased amounts of lactate and inorganic phosphates. Excitatory and toxic amino acids,

Table 120.5	Topography of Brain Injury in Term Infants With Hypoxic-Ischemic Encephalopathy and Clinical Correlates		
AREA OF INJURY	**LOCATION OF INJURY**	**CLINICAL CORRELATES**	**LONG-TERM SEQUELAE**
Selective neuronal necrosis	Entire neuraxis, deep cortical area, brainstem and pontosubicular	Stupor or coma Seizures Hypotonia Oculomotor abnormalities Suck/swallow abnormalities	Cognitive delay Cerebral palsy Dystonia Seizure disorder Ataxia Bulbar and pseudobulbar palsy
Parasagittal injury	Cortex and subcortical white matter Parasagittal regions, especially posterior	Proximal-limb weakness Upper extremities affected > lower extremities	Spastic quadriparesis Cognitive delay Visual and auditory processing difficulty
Focal ischemic necrosis	Cortex and subcortical white matter Vascular injury (usually middle cerebral artery distribution)	Unilateral findings Seizures common and typically focal	Hemiparesis Seizures Cognitive delays
Periventricular injury	Injury to motor tracts, especially lower extremity	Bilateral and symmetric weakness in lower extremities More common in preterm infants	Spastic diplegia

Adapted from Volpe JJ, editor: *Neurology of the newborn*, ed 4, Philadelphia, 2001, Saunders.

particularly glutamate, accumulate in the damaged tissue. prompting overactivation of *N*-methyl-D-aspartate (NMDA), amino-3-hydroxy-5-methyl-4-isoxazole propionate (AMPA), and kainate receptors. This receptor overactivation increases cellular permeability to sodium and calcium ions. Because of inadequate intracellular energy, normal sodium and calcium homeostasis is lost, and intracellular accumulation of these ions results in cytotoxic edema and neuronal death. Intracellular calcium accumulation may also result in apoptotic cell death. Concurrent with the excitotoxic cascade, there is also increased production of damaging free radicals and nitric oxide in these tissues. The initial circulatory response of the fetus is increased shunting through the ductus venosus, ductus arteriosus, and foramen ovale, with transient maintenance of perfusion of the brain, heart, and adrenals in preference to the lungs, liver, kidneys, and intestine. Thus, serum laboratory evidence of injury to these organs may be present in more severe cases.

The pathology of hypoxia-ischemia outside the CNS depends on the affected organ and the severity of the injury. Early congestion, fluid leak from increased capillary permeability, and endothelial cell swelling may lead to signs of coagulation necrosis and cell death. Congestion and petechiae are seen in the pericardium, pleura, thymus, heart, adrenals, and meninges. Prolonged intrauterine hypoxia may result in inadequate perfusion of the periventricular white matter, resulting in PVL. Pulmonary arteriole smooth muscle hyperplasia may develop, which predisposes the infant to pulmonary hypertension (see Chapter 122.9). If fetal distress produces gasping, amniotic fluid contents (meconium, squames, lanugo) may be aspirated into the trachea or lungs with subsequent complications, including pulmonary hypertension and pneumothoraces.

CLINICAL MANIFESTATIONS

Intrauterine growth restriction with increased vascular resistance may be an indication of chronic fetal hypoxia before the peripartum period. During labor, the fetal heart rate slows and beat-to-beat variability declines. Continuous heart rate recording may reveal a variable or late deceleration pattern (see Chapter 115, Fig. 115.4). Particularly in infants near term, these signs should lead to the administration of high concentrations of oxygen to the mother and consideration of immediate delivery to avoid fetal death and CNS damage.

At delivery, the presence of meconium-stained amniotic fluid indicates that fetal distress may have occurred. At birth, affected infants may have neurologic impairment and may fail to breathe spontaneously. Pallor, cyanosis, apnea, a slow heart rate, and unresponsiveness to stimulation are also nonspecific initial signs of potential HIE. During the ensuing hours, infants may be hypotonic, may change from a hypotonic to a hypertonic state, or their tone may appear normal (Tables 120.6 and

Table 120.6	Poor Predictive Variables for Death/Disability After Hypoxic-Ischemic Encephalopathy

- Low (0–3) 10 min Apgar score
- Need for CPR in the delivery room
- Delayed onset (≥20 min) of spontaneous breathing
- Severe neurologic signs (coma, hypotonia, hypertonia)
- Seizures onset ≤12 hr or difficult to treat
- Severe, prolonged (~7 days) EEG findings including burst suppression pattern
- Prominent MRI basal ganglia/thalamic lesions
- Oliguria/anuria >24 hr
- Abnormal neurologic exam ≥14 days

120.7). Cerebral edema may develop during the next 24 hr and result in profound brainstem depression. During this time, seizure activity may occur; it may be severe and refractory to typical doses of anticonvulsants. Although most often a result of the HIE, seizures in asphyxiated newborns may also be caused by vascular events (hemorrhage, arterial ischemic stroke, or sinus venous thrombosis), metabolic derangements (hypocalcemia, hypoglycemia), CNS infection, and cerebral dysgenesis or genetic disorders (nonketotic hyperglycinemia, vitamin-dependent epilepsies, channelopathies). Conditions that result in neuromuscular weakness and poor respiratory effort may also result secondarily in neonatal hypoxic brain injury and seizure. Such conditions might include congenital myopathies, congenital myotonic dystrophy, or spinal muscular atrophy.

In addition to CNS dysfunction, systemic organ dysfunction is noted in up to 80% of affected neonates. Myocardial dysfunction and cardiogenic shock, persistent pulmonary hypertension, RDS, gastrointestinal perforation, and acute kidney and liver injury are associated with perinatal asphyxia secondary to inadequate perfusion (see Table 120.4).

The severity of neonatal encephalopathy depends on the duration and timing of injury. A clinical grading score first proposed by Sarnat continues to be a useful tool. Symptoms develop over days, making it important to perform serial neurologic examinations (see Tables 120.6 and 120.7). During the initial hours after an insult, infants have a depressed level of consciousness. Periodic breathing with apnea or bradycardia is present, but cranial nerve functions are often spared, with intact pupillary response and spontaneous eye movement. Seizures are common with extensive injury. Hypotonia is also common as an early manifestation of HIE, but it should be distinguished from other causes by history and serial examination.

Table 120.7	Hypoxic-Ischemic Encephalopathy in Term Infants		
SIGNS	**STAGE 1**	**STAGE 2**	**STAGE 3**
Level of consciousness	Hyperalert	Lethargic	Stuporous, coma
Muscle tone	Normal	Hypotonic	Flaccid
Posture	Normal	Flexion	Decerebrate
Tendon reflexes/clonus	Hyperactive	Hyperactive	Absent
Myoclonus	Present	Present	Absent
Moro reflex	Strong	Weak	Absent
Pupils	Mydriasis	Miosis	Unequal, poor light reflex
Seizures	None	Common	Decerebration
Electroencephalographic findings	Normal	Low voltage changing to seizure activity	Burst suppression to isoelectric
Duration	<24 hr if progresses; otherwise, may remain normal	24 hr to 14 days	Days to weeks
Outcome	Good	Variable	Death, severe deficits

Adapted from Sarnat HB, Sarnat MS: Neonatal encephalopathy following fetal distress: a clinical and electroencephalographic study, *Arch Neurol* 33:696–705, 1976. Copyright 1976, American Medical Association.

DIAGNOSIS

MRI is the most sensitive imaging modality for detecting hypoxic brain injury in the neonate. Although such injury can be detected at various times and with varying pulse sequences, diffusion-weighted sequences obtained in the 1st 3-5 days following a presumed sentinel event are optimal for identifying acute injury. (Figs. 120.5 to 120.8 and Table 120.8). Where MRI is unavailable or prevented by clinical instability, CT scans may be helpful in ruling out focal hemorrhagic lesions or large arterial ischemic strokes. Loss of gray-white differentiation and injury to the basal ganglia in more severe HIE can be detected on CT by experienced readers, but CT often misses subtler forms of neonatal hypoxic brain injury. US has limited utility in evaluation of hypoxic injury in the term infant, but it too can be useful for excluding hemorrhagic lesions. Because of factors of size and clinical stability, US is the initial preferred (and sometimes only feasible) modality in evaluation of the preterm infant.

Amplitude-integrated electroencephalography (aEEG) may help to determine which infants are at highest risk for developmental sequelae of neonatal brain injury (Tables 120.9 and 120.10). The aEEG background voltage ranges, signal patterns, and rates of normalization, as assessed at various points in the 1st hours and days of life, can provide valuable prognostic information, with positive predictive value of 85% and negative predictive value of 91–96% for infants who will have adverse neurodevelopmental outcome. Unfortunately, even with recent improvements in technology, aEEG still has difficulty detecting seizures, particularly those that are brief or originate far from the electrodes. Sensitivity of aEEG for seizure detection, when used by a typical reader, is <50%. For this reason, *conventional EEG montage with concurrent video of the patient are preferred for seizure monitoring.*

TREATMENT

Therapeutic hypothermia, whether head cooling or systemic cooling (by servo-control to a core rectal or esophageal temperature of 33.5°C [92.3°F] within the 1st 6 hr after birth and maintained for 72 hr), has been shown in various trials to reduce mortality and major neurodevelopmental impairment at 18 mo of age. Infants treated with systemic hypothermia have a lower incidence of cortical neuronal injury on MRI, suggesting systemic hypothermia may result in more uniform cooling of the brain and deeper CNS structures than selective head cooling. The therapeutic effect of hypothermia likely results from decreased secondary neuronal injury achieved by reducing rates of apoptosis and production of mediators known to be neurotoxic, including extracellular glutamate, free radicals, nitric oxide, and lactate. There is also benefit in seizure reduction. The therapeutic benefit of

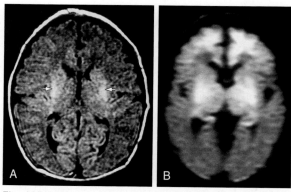

Fig. 120.5 MR images of selective neuronal injury. The infant experienced intrapartum asphyxia and had seizures on the 1st postnatal day. MRI was performed on the 5th postnatal day. **A,** Axial, fluid-attenuated, inversion recovery image shows increased signal in the putamen bilaterally *(arrows)* but no definite abnormality in the cerebral cortex. **B,** By contrast, a diffusion-weighted image shows striking increased signal intensity (i.e., decreased diffusion) in the frontal cortex (in addition to a more pronounced basal ganglia abnormality). *(From Volpe JJ, editor: Neurology of the newborn, ed 5, Philadelphia, 2008, Saunders/Elsevier, p 420.)*

hypothermia noted at 18-22 mo of age is maintained later in childhood. Once established, hypothermia may not alter the prognostic findings on MRI.

Numerous studies seeking ways to extend the benefits of therapeutic hypothermia have been attempted. Assessment of deeper or longer cooling failed to show benefit in short-term outcomes, although longer-term developmental outcomes of that trial are not yet published. Investigations into extending the therapeutic time window of hypothermia initiation beyond 6 hr or offering hypothermia to preterm infants are ongoing.

In addition to extending the benefit of therapeutic hypothermia, there is great interest in augmenting its benefit through other means. High-dose **erythropoietin** given as an adjunct to therapeutic hypothermia shows some promise in decreasing MRI indicators of brain injury and short-term motor outcomes. Further study as well as longitudinal follow-up of the study cohort is warranted to confirm these findings.

Complications of induced hypothermia include thrombocytopenia

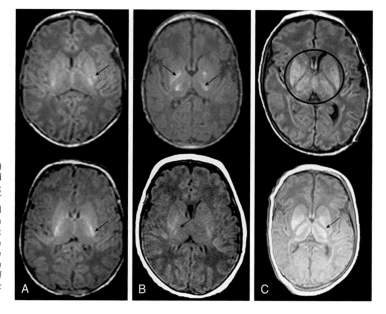

Fig. 120.6 MR images of basal ganglia/thalamic (BG/T) injury and signal intensity. *Top row,* Axial T1-weighted MR images showing **A,** mild BG/T lesions *(arrow);* **B,** moderate BG/T injury *(arrows);* and **C,** severe BG/T abnormalities *(circled). Bottom row,* Axial T1-weighted MR images showing **A,** normal signal intensity (SI) in the posterior limb of the internal capsule (PLIC) *(arrow);* **B,** equivocal, asymmetric, and slightly reduced SI in the PLIC *(arrow);* and **C,** abnormal, absent SI in the PLIC *(arrow). (From Martinez-Biarge M, Diez-Sebastian J, Rutherford MA, Cowan FM. Outcomes after central grey matter injury in term perinatal hypoxic-ischaemic encephalopathy, Early Hum Dev 86:675–682, 2010.)*

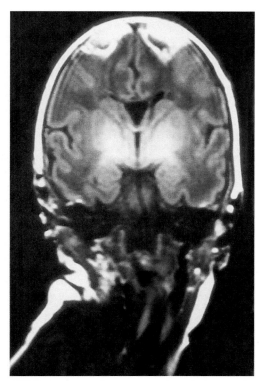

Fig. 120.7 MR image of a parasagittal cerebral injury. Coronal T1-weighted image, obtained on the 5th postnatal day in an asphyxiated term infant, shows striking triangular lesions in the parasagittal areas bilaterally; increased signal intensity is also apparent in the basal ganglia and thalamus bilaterally. *(From Volpe JJ, editor: Neurology of the newborn, ed 5, Philadelphia, 2008, Saunders/Elsevier, p 421.)*

Table 120.8	Major Aspects of MRI in Diagnosis of Hypoxic-Ischemic Encephalopathy in the Term Infant

MAJOR CONVENTIONAL MR FINDINGS IN 1ST WEEK

Cerebral cortical gray-white differentiation lost (on T1W or T2W)

Cerebral cortical high signal (T1W and FLAIR), especially in parasagittal perirolandic cortex

Basal ganglia/thalamus, high signal (T1W and FLAIR), usually associated with the cerebral cortical changes but possibly alone with increased signal in brainstem tegmentum in cases of acute severe insult

Parasagittal cerebral cortex, subcortical white matter, high signal (T1W and FLAIR)

Periventricular white matter, decreased signal (T1W) or increased signal (T2W)

Posterior limb of internal capsule, decreased signal (T1W or FLAIR)

Cerebrum in a vascular distribution, decreased signal (T1W), but much better visualized as decreased diffusion (increased signal) on diffusion-weighted MRI

Diffusion-weighted MRI more sensitive than conventional MRI, especially in 1st days after birth, when former shows decreased diffusion (increased signal) in injured areas

FLAIR, Fluid-attenuated inversion recovery; MRI, magnetic resonance imaging; T1W and T2W, T1- and T2-weighted images.
From Volpe JJ, editor: *Neurology of the newborn,* ed 5, Philadelphia, 2008, Elsevier (Table 9-16).

interval, and affect the interpretation of blood gases. In clinical practice, these concerns have not been observed.

For treating seizures associated with HIE, **phenobarbital**, the historical first-line drug for neonatal seizures, continues to be used in many instances. It is typically given by intravenous loading dose (20 mg/kg). Additional doses of 5-10 mg/kg (up to 40-50 mg/kg total) may be needed. Phenobarbital levels should be monitored 24 hr after the loading dose has been given and maintenance therapy (5 mg/kg/24 hr) begun. Therapeutic phenobarbital levels are 20-40 µg/mL. Animal models demonstrate decreased neurodevelopmental impact of hypoxic brain injury in animals that received a high-dose prophylactic injection of phenobarbital before onset of therapeutic hypothermia. Whether this benefit translates to humans is controversial.

For refractory seizures, there is a high degree of variability regarding choice of 2nd agent. Historically, phenytoin (20 mg/kg loading dose)

(usually without bleeding), reduced heart rate, and subcutaneous fat necrosis (sometimes with associated hypercalcemia) as well as the potential for overcooling and the cold injury syndrome. The latter is usually avoided with a servo-controlled cooling system. Therapeutic hypothermia may theoretically alter drug metabolism, prolong the QT

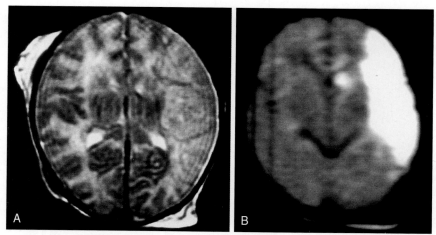

Fig. 120.8 MR images of focal ischemic cerebral injury. MRI was performed on the 3rd postnatal day. **A,** Axial T2-weighted mage shows a lesion in the distribution of the main branch of the left middle cerebral artery. **B,** Diffusion-weighted image demonstrates the lesion more strikingly. *(From Volpe JJ, editor: Neurology of the newborn, ed 5, Philadelphia, 2008, Saunders/Elsevier, p 422.)*

Table 120.9	Value of Electroencephalography in Assessment of Asphyxiated Term Infants

Detection of severe abnormalities (i.e., CLV, FT, BSP) in 1st hours of life has a positive predictive value of an unfavorable outcome of 80–90%.
Severe abnormalities may improve within 24 hr (~50% of BSP and 10% of CLV/FT).
Rapid recovery of severe abnormalities is associated with a favorable outcome in 60% of cases.
The *combination* of early neonatal neurologic examination and early aEEG enhances the positive predictive value and specificity.

aEEG, Amplitude-integrated encephalography; BSP, burst-suppression pattern; CLV, continuous low voltage; FT, flat trace.
From Inder TE, Volpe JJ: Hypoxic-ischemic injury in the term infant: clinical-neurological features, diagnosis, imaging, prognosis, therapy. In *Volpe's neurology of the newborn, ed 6, Philadelphia, 2018, Elsevier (Table 20-28).*

Table 120.10	Electroencephalographic Patterns of Prognostic Significance in Asphyxiated Term Infants*

ASSOCIATED WITH FAVORABLE OUTCOME
Mild depression (or less) on day 1
Normal background by day 7

ASSOCIATED WITH UNFAVORABLE OUTCOME
Predominant interburst interval >20 sec on any day
Burst-suppression pattern on any day
Isoelectric tracing on any day
Mild (or greater) depression after day 12

*Associations with favorable or unfavorable outcome are generally ≥90%, but the clinical context must be considered.
From Inder TE, Volpe JJ: Hypoxic-ischemic injury in the term infant: clinical-neurological features, diagnosis, imaging, prognosis, therapy. In *Volpe's neurology of the newborn, ed 6, Philadelphia, 2018, Elsevier (Table 20-26).*

or lorazepam (0.1 mg/kg) have been preferred, currently the use of **levetiracetam** is preferred (at times even as a first-line agent) as the most used second-line agent. Early reports of administration of levetiracetam in the neonate used low doses, but subsequent pharmacokinetic data suggest that due to the higher volume of distribution created by higher relative body water content in neonates, loading doses should be higher than in older children or adults. Suggested appropriate loading doses may be closer to 60 mg/kg. In addition to levetiracetam and

phenytoin, other second- or third-line agents commonly used include midazolam, topiramate, and lidocaine. Pyridoxine should also be attempted, particularly in ongoing refractory seizures with highly abnormal EEG background.

Status epilepticus, multifocal seizures, and multiple anticonvulsant medications during therapeutic hypothermia are associated with a poor prognosis.

Additional therapy for infants with HIE includes supportive care directed at management of organ system dysfunction. Hyperthermia has been associated with impaired neurodevelopment and should be prevented, particularly in the interval between initial resuscitation and initiation of hypothermia. Careful attention to ventilatory status and adequate oxygenation, blood pressure, hemodynamic status, acid-base balance, and possible infection is important. Secondary hypoxia or hypotension from complications of HIE must be prevented. Aggressive treatment of seizures is critical and may necessitate continuous EEG monitoring. In addition, hyperoxia, hypocarbia, and hypoglycemia are associated with poor outcomes, so careful attention to resuscitation, ventilation, and blood glucose homeostasis is essential.

PROGNOSIS

The outcome of HIE, which correlates with the timing and severity of the insult, ranges from complete recovery to death. The prognosis varies depending on the severity of the insult and the treatment. Infants with initial cord or initial blood pH <6.7 have a 90% risk for death or severe neurodevelopmental impairment at 18 mo of age. In addition, infants with Apgar scores of 0-3 at 5 min, high base deficit (>20-25 mmol/L), decerebrate posture, severe basal ganglia/thalamic (BG/T) lesions (Fig. 120.9; see also Fig. 120.6), persistence of severe HIE by clinical examination at 72 hr, and lack of spontaneous activity are also at increased risk for death or impairment. These predictor variables can be combined to determine a score that helps with prognosis (see Table 120.6). Infants with the highest risk are likely to die or have severe disability despite aggressive treatment, including hypothermia. Those with intermediate scores are likely to benefit from treatment. In general, severe encephalopathy, characterized by flaccid coma, apnea, absence of oculocephalic reflexes, and refractory seizures, is associated with a poor prognosis (see Table 120.7). Apgar scores alone can also be associated with subsequent risk of neurodevelopmental impairment. At 10 min, each point decrease in Apgar score increases odds of death or disability by 45%. Death or disability occurs in 76–82% of infants with Apgar scores of 0-2 at 10 min. Absence of spontaneous respirations at 20 min of age and persistence of abnormal neurologic signs at 2 wk of age also predict death or severe cognitive and motor deficits.

The combined use of early conventional EEG or aEEG and MRI

offers additional insight in predicting outcome in term infants with HIE (see Table 120.10). EEG or aEEG background characteristics such as pattern, voltage, reactivity, state change, and evolution after acute injury are important predictors of outcome. MRI markers include location of injury, identification of injury by certain pulse sequences, measurement of diffusivity and/or fractional anisotropy, and presence of abnormal metabolite ratios on MR spectroscopy, and all have shown correlation with outcome. There is also growing interest in quantitative measures (volumetric analysis, diffusion tensor imaging) of MRI as potential predictors of outcome. Severe BG/T lesions with abnormal signal in the posterior limb of the internal capsule is highly predictive of the poorest cognitive and motor prognosis (see Fig. 120.9). Normal MRI and EEG findings are associated with a good recovery.

Microcephaly and poor head growth during the 1st year of life also correlate with injury to the basal ganglia and white matter and adverse developmental outcome at 12 mo. All survivors of moderate to severe encephalopathy require comprehensive high-risk medical and developmental follow-up. Early identification of neurodevelopmental problems allows prompt referral for developmental, rehabilitative, and neurologic early intervention services so that the best possible outcomes can be achieved.

Brain death after neonatal HIE is diagnosed from the clinical findings of coma unresponsive to pain, auditory, or visual stimulation; apnea with PCO_2 rising from 40 to >60 mm Hg without ventilatory support; and absence of brainstem reflexes (pupillary, oculocephalic, oculovestibular, corneal, gag, sucking) (see Chapter 86). These findings must occur in the absence of hypothermia, hypotension, and elevations of depressant drugs (phenobarbital), which may take days to weeks to be metabolized and cleared completely from the blood. An absence of cerebral blood flow on radionuclide scans and of electrical activity on EEG (electrocerebral silence) is inconsistently observed in clinically brain-dead neonatal infants. Persistence of the clinical criteria for 24 hr in term infants predicts brain death in most asphyxiated newborns. There is no agreement on brain death criteria in preterm infants. Because of inconsistencies and difficulties in applying standard criteria, *no universal agreement has been reached regarding the definition of neonatal brain death.* Consideration of withdrawal of life support should include discussions with the family, the healthcare team, and, if there is disagreement, an ethics committee. The best interest of the infant involves judgments about the benefits and harm of continuing therapy or avoiding ongoing futile therapy.

Bibliography is available at Expert Consult.

120.5 Spine and Spinal Cord
Cameron W. Thomas and Stephanie L. Merhar

See also Chapter 729.

Injury to the spine/spinal cord during birth is rare but can be devastating. Strong traction exerted when the spine is hyperextended or when the direction of pull is lateral, or forceful longitudinal traction on the trunk while the head is still firmly engaged in the pelvis, especially when combined with flexion and torsion of the vertical axis, may produce fracture and separation of the vertebrae. Such injuries are most likely to occur when difficulty is encountered in delivering the shoulders in cephalic presentations and the head in breech presentations. The injury occurs most often at the level of the 4th cervical vertebra with cephalic presentations and the lower cervical–upper thoracic vertebrae with breech presentations. Transection of the cord may occur *with or without* vertebral fractures; hemorrhage and edema may produce neurologic signs that are indistinguishable from those of transection, except that they may not be permanent. Areflexia, loss of sensation, and complete paralysis of voluntary motion occur below the level of injury, although the persistence of a withdrawal reflex mediated through spinal centers distal to the area of injury is frequently misinterpreted as representing voluntary motion.

If the injury is severe, the infant, who from birth may be in poor condition because of respiratory depression, shock, or hypothermia, may deteriorate rapidly to death within several hours before any neurologic signs are obvious. Alternatively, the course may be protracted, with symptoms and signs appearing at birth or later in the 1st wk; Horner syndrome, immobility, flaccidity, and associated brachial plexus injuries may not be recognized for several days. Constipation may also be present. Some infants survive for prolonged periods, their initial flaccidity, immobility, and areflexia being replaced after several weeks or months by rigid flexion of the extremities, increased muscle tone, and spasms. Apnea on day 1 and poor motor recovery by 3 mo are poor prognostic signs.

The **differential diagnosis** of neonatal spine/spinal cord injury includes amyotonia congenita and myelodysplasia associated with spina bifida occulta, spinal muscular atrophy (type 0), spinal vascular malformations

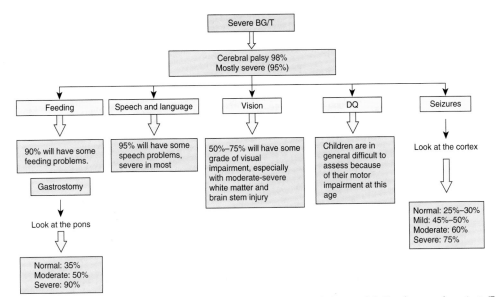

Fig. 120.9 Flow chart showing patterns of outcome with severe basal ganglia/thalamic (BG/T) injury. *DQ,* Developmental quotient. (*From Martinez-Biarge M, Diez-Sebastian J, Rutherford MA, Cowan FM: Outcomes after central grey matter injury in term perinatal hypoxic-ischaemic encephalopathy,* Early Hum Dev 86:675–682, 2010.)

(e.g., arteriovenous malformation causing hemorrhage or stroke), and congenital structural anomalies (syringomyelia, hemangioblastoma). US or MRI confirms the diagnosis. Treatment of the survivors is supportive, including home ventilation; patients often remain permanently disabled. When a fracture or dislocation is causing spinal compression, the prognosis is related to the time elapsed before the compression is relieved.

Bibliography is available at Expert Consult.

120.6 Peripheral Nerve Injuries

Cameron W. Thomas and Stephanie L. Merhar

See also Chapter 731.

BRACHIAL PALSY

Brachial plexus injury is a common problem, with an incidence of 0.6-4.6 per 1,000 live births. Injury to the brachial plexus may cause paralysis of the upper part of the arm with or without paralysis of the forearm or hand or, more often, paralysis of the entire arm. These injuries occur in macrosomic infants and when lateral traction is exerted on the head and neck during delivery of the shoulder in a vertex presentation, when the arms are extended over the head in a breech presentation, or when excessive traction is placed on the shoulders. Approximately 45% of brachial plexus injuries are associated with shoulder dystocia.

In **Erb-Duchenne paralysis** the injury is limited to the 5th and 6th cervical nerves. The infant loses the power to abduct the arm from the shoulder, rotate the arm externally, and supinate the forearm. The

characteristic position consists of adduction and internal rotation of the arm with pronation of the forearm. Power to extend the forearm is retained, but the biceps reflex is absent; the Moro reflex is absent on the affected side (Fig. 120.10). The outer aspect of the arm may have some sensory impairment. Power in the forearm and hand grasps is preserved unless the lower part of the plexus is also injured; the presence of hand grasp is a favorable prognostic sign. When the injury includes the phrenic nerve, alteration in diaphragmatic excursion may be observed with US, fluoroscopy, or as asymmetric elevation of the diaphragm on chest radiograph.

Klumpke paralysis is a rare form of brachial palsy in which injury to the 7th and 8th cervical nerves and the 1st thoracic nerve produces a paralyzed hand and ipsilateral ptosis and miosis (**Horner syndrome**) if the sympathetic fibers of the 1st thoracic root are also injured. Mild cases may not be detected immediately after birth. Differentiation must be made from cerebral injury; from fracture, dislocation, or epiphyseal separation of the humerus; and from fracture of the clavicle. MRI demonstrates nerve root rupture or avulsion.

Most patients have full recovery. If the paralysis was a result of edema and hemorrhage around the nerve fibers, function should return within a few months; if it resulted from laceration, permanent damage may result. Involvement of the deltoid is usually the most serious problem and may result in **shoulder drop** secondary to muscle atrophy. In general, paralysis of the upper part of the arm has a better prognosis than paralysis of the lower part.

Treatment consists of initial conservative management with monthly follow-up and a decision for surgical intervention by 3 mo if function has not improved. Partial immobilization and appropriate positioning are used to prevent the development of contractures. In upper arm paralysis, the arm should be abducted 90 degrees with external rotation

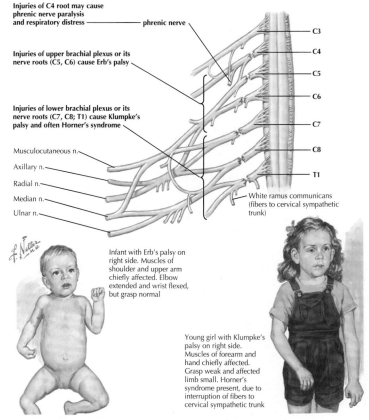

Injuries of C4 root may cause phrenic nerve paralysis and respiratory distress —— phrenic nerve

Injuries of upper brachial plexus or its nerve roots (C5, C6) cause Erb's palsy

Injuries of lower brachial plexus or its nerve roots (C7, C8; T1) cause Klumpke's palsy and often Horner's syndrome

Musculocutaneous n.
Axillary n.
Radial n.
Median n.
Ulnar n.

C3
C4
C5
C6
C7
C8
T1

White ramus communicans (fibers to cervical sympathetic trunk)

Infant with Erb's palsy on right side. Muscles of shoulder and upper arm chiefly affected. Elbow extended and wrist flexed, but grasp normal

Young girl with Klumpke's palsy on right side. Muscles of forearm and hand chiefly affected. Grasp weak and affected limb small. Horner's syndrome present, due to interruption of fibers to cervical sympathetic trunk

Fig. 120.10 Schematic representation of the brachial plexus with its terminal branches. The major sites of brachial plexus injury are shown. *(Courtesy of Netter Images, Image ID 19943. www.netterimages.com.)*

at the shoulder, full supination of the forearm, and slight extension at the wrist with the palm turned toward the face. This position may be achieved with a brace or splint during the 1st 1-2 wk. Immobilization should be intermittent throughout the day while the infant is asleep and between feedings. In lower arm or hand paralysis, the wrist should be splinted in a neutral position and padding placed in the fist. When the entire arm is paralyzed, the same treatment principles should be followed. Gentle massage and range-of-motion exercises may be started by 7-10 days of age. Infants should be closely monitored with active and passive corrective exercises. If the paralysis persists without improvement for 3 mo, neuroplasty, neurolysis, end-to-end anastomosis, and nerve grafting offer hope for partial recovery.

The type of treatment and the prognosis depend on the mechanism of injury and the number of nerve roots involved. The mildest injury to a peripheral nerve (**neurapraxia**) is caused by edema and heals spontaneously within a few weeks. **Axonotmesis** is more severe and is a consequence of nerve fiber disruption with an intact myelin sheath; function usually returns in a few months. Total disruption of nerves (**neurotmesis**) or root avulsion is the most severe, especially if it involves C5-T1; microsurgical repair may be indicated. Fortunately, most (75%) injuries are at the root level C5-C6, involve neurapraxia and axonotmesis, and should heal spontaneously. Botulism toxin may be used to treat biceps-triceps co-contractions.

PHRENIC NERVE PARALYSIS

Phrenic nerve injury (3rd, 4th, 5th cervical nerves) with diaphragmatic paralysis must be considered when cyanosis and irregular and labored respirations develop. Such injuries, usually unilateral, are associated with ipsilateral upper brachial plexus palsies in 75% of cases. Because breathing is thoracic in type, the abdomen does not bulge with inspiration. Breath sounds are diminished on the affected side. The thrust of the diaphragm, which may often be felt just under the costal margin on the normal side, is absent on the affected side. The diagnosis is established by US or fluoroscopic examination, which reveals elevation of the diaphragm on the paralyzed side and seesaw movements of the 2 sides of the diaphragm during respiration. It may also be apparent on chest or abdominal radiograph.

Infants with phrenic nerve injury should be placed on the involved side and given oxygen if necessary. Some may benefit from pressure introduced by continuous positive airway pressure (CPAP) to expand the paralyzed hemidiaphragm. In extreme cases, mechanical ventilation cannot be avoided. Initially, intravenous feedings may be needed; later, progressive gavage or oral feeding may be started, depending on the infant's condition. Pulmonary infections are a serious complication. If the infant fails to demonstrate spontaneous recovery in 1-2 mo, surgical plication of the diaphragm may be indicated.

FACIAL NERVE PALSY

Facial palsy is usually a peripheral paralysis that results from pressure over the facial nerve in utero, during labor, or from forceps use during delivery. Rarely, it may result from nuclear agenesis of the facial nerve.

Peripheral facial paralysis is flaccid and, when complete, involves the entire side of the face, including the forehead. When the infant cries, movement occurs only on the nonparalyzed side of the face, and the mouth is drawn to that side. On the affected side the forehead is smooth, the eye cannot be closed, the nasolabial fold is absent, and the corner of the mouth droops. **Central facial paralysis** spares the forehead (e.g., forehead wrinkles will still be apparent on the affected side) because the nucleus that innervates the upper face has overlapping dual innervation by corticobulbar fibers originating in bilateral cerebral hemispheres. The infant with central facial paralysis usually has other manifestations of intracranial injury, most often 6th nerve palsy from the proximity of the 6th and 7th cranial nerve nuclei in the brainstem. Prognosis depends on whether the nerve was injured by pressure or the nerve fibers were torn; improvement occurs within a few weeks in the former case. Care of the exposed eye is essential. Neuroplasty may be indicated when the paralysis is persistent. Facial palsy may be confused with absence of the depressor muscles of the mouth, which is a benign problem or with variants of Möbius syndrome.

Other peripheral nerves are seldom injured in utero or at birth except when they are involved in fractures or hemorrhage.

Bibliography is available at Expert Consult.

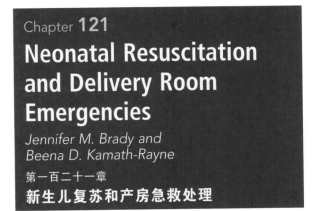

Chapter **121**

Neonatal Resuscitation and Delivery Room Emergencies

Jennifer M. Brady and Beena D. Kamath-Rayne

第一百二十一章
新生儿复苏和产房急救处理

中文导读

本章结合最新版的新生儿复苏教程详细介绍了　　新生儿分娩现场的复苏流程和产房急救处理、早产儿复苏中的特殊关注点。特别是详细介绍了特殊情况下的新生儿复苏及产房急救处理的注意事项以及远期预后，包括：羊水粪染、胎盘早剥、新生儿脑病、气道梗阻、呼吸窘迫、腹壁缺损及神经管缺陷。本章同时介绍了新生儿复苏后，发现合并产伤，例如，头颅损伤（颅内、颅外）、骨折、臂丛损伤时的处理建议。关于复苏后的监护和治疗，本章也进行了详细的阐述。

Most infants complete the transition to extrauterine life without difficulty; however, a small proportion require resuscitation after birth (Fig. 121.1). For a newborn infant, the need for resuscitation is often caused by a problem with respiration leading to inadequate ventilation. This is in contrast to an adult cardiac arrest, which is usually caused by inadequate circulation. The goals of neonatal resuscitation are to reestablish adequate spontaneous respirations, obtain adequate cardiac output, and prevent the morbidity and mortality associated with hypoxic-ischemic tissue (brain, heart, kidney) injury. High-risk situations should be *anticipated* from pregnancy history and labor. Improved perinatal care and prenatal diagnosis of fetal anomalies allow for appropriate maternal transports for high-risk deliveries. Infants who are born limp, cyanotic, apneic, or pulseless require immediate resuscitation before assignment of the 1 min Apgar score. Rapid and appropriate resuscitative efforts improve the likelihood of preventing brain damage and achieving a successful outcome.

NEONATAL RESUSCITATION

See also Chapter 81.

Guidelines for the **Neonatal Resuscitation Program (NRP)** are based on recommendations from the International Liaison Committee on Resuscitation Consensus on Treatment Recommendations. These recommendations propose an *integrated* assessment/response approach for the initial evaluation of an infant, consisting of simultaneous assessment of infant general appearance and risk factors. The fundamental principles include evaluation of the airway and establishing effective respirations and adequate circulation. The guidelines also highlight the assessment and response to the neonatal heart rate.

Before the birth of a baby, sufficient preparation for the birth should occur. At least 1 individual capable of neonatal resuscitation should be present at the delivery, and if advanced resuscitation is anticipated, more individuals should be available to help. Necessary equipment should be available, which routinely includes: a warmer bed, blankets, infant hat, stethoscope, bulb suction, suction catheter with wall suction, bag-mask device, oxygen source with blender, pulse oximeter, laryngoscope with blade, and endotracheal tubes (ETTs). Based on the specific details of the pregnancy, further equipment that may be needed should be anticipated and readily available. The equipment should be checked to make sure it is functioning appropriately. Team members should introduce themselves, define a team leader, assign roles for the resuscitation, and discuss what actions they will take during the resuscitation. For complex resuscitations, there may be 1 individual whose sole job is to keep track of time and record what interventions are taken, both to ensure the correct steps are performed in a timely manner and to review during debriefing later.

Immediately after birth, all term infants should be dried, warmed, and stimulated. If the infant does not need resuscitation, these steps can occur on the mother's abdomen while delayed cord clamping is taking place. Simultaneously, the infant's tone, respiratory effort, and heart rate should be assessed (Fig. 121.2).

Failure to initiate or sustain respiratory effort is fairly common at birth, with 5–10% of births requiring some intervention. Infants with **primary apnea** respond to stimulation by establishing normal breathing. Infants with **secondary apnea** require some ventilatory assistance in order to establish spontaneous respiratory effort. Secondary apnea usually originates in the central nervous system (CNS) as a result of asphyxia

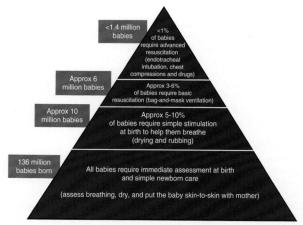

Fig. 121.1 Estimates of infants requiring resuscitation at birth. *(From Wall SN, Lee ACC, Niermeyer S, et al: Neonatal resuscitation in low-resource settings: what, who, and how to overcome challenges to scale up? Int J Gynaecol Obstet 107:S47–S64, 2009, Fig 1.)*

or peripherally because of neuromuscular disorders. The lungs in infants affected by conditions such as pulmonary hypoplasia and prematurity may be noncompliant, and initial efforts to begin respirations may be inadequate to initiate sufficient ventilation.

The steps in neonatal resuscitation follow the ABCs: **A,** anticipate and establish a patent **airway** by positioning the baby with the head slightly extended, sniffing position, and suctioning if secretions are blocking the airway; **B,** initiate **breathing** first by using tactile stimulation, followed by positive pressure ventilation (PPV) with a bag-mask device and ETT insertion should the baby remain apneic or PPV is not achieving effective ventilation; and **C,** maintain the **circulation** with chest compressions and medications, if needed. Fig. 121.2 outlines the steps to follow for immediate neonatal evaluation and resuscitation.

In term infants after stimulation, if no respirations are noted, or if the heart rate is <100 beats/min, PPV should be given through a tightly fitted and appropriately sized bag-mask device. PPV should be initiated at pressures of approximately 20 cm H_2O at a rate of 40-60 breaths/min initially with 21% fraction of inspired oxygen (FIO_2) for full-term infants.

At the same time PPV is initiated, a pulse oximeter should be placed on the right hand (preductal) and cardiac leads placed on the chest. In the past the recommended inspired gas for neonatal resuscitation had been 100% oxygen. However, resuscitation with room air in *term infants* is equally effective and may reduce the risk of hyperoxia, which is associated with decreased cerebral blood flow and generation of oxygen free radicals. Room air is the preferred *initial gas* for neonatal resuscitation in term infants. O_2 concentration administered should then be titrated as needed to obtain expected O_2 saturations in a term infant after birth, as defined by normal reference range by minute of life (see Fig. 121.2).

Successful and effective ventilation is signified by adequate chest rise, symmetric breath sounds, improved pink color, heart rate >100 beats/

Neonatal Resuscitation Algorithm

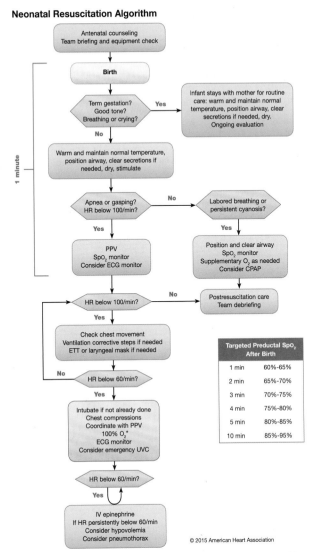

Fig. 121.2 Newborn resuscitation algorithm. *CPAP*, Continuous positive airway pressure; *ETT*, endotracheal tube; *HR*, heart rate; *IV*, intravenous; *PPV*, positive pressure ventilation; *UVC*, umbilical venous catheter. *At this point in resuscitation 100% oxygen is instituted. *(From Wyckoff MH, Aziz K, Escobedo MB, et al. Part 13. Neonatal resuscitation: 2015 American Heart Association guidelines update for cardiopulmonary resuscitation and emergency cardiovascular care, Circulation 132(Suppl 2):S542–S560, 2015, Fig 1.)*

airway obstruction, insufficient pressure, pleural effusions, pneumothorax, excessive air in the stomach leading to abdominal competition, asystole, hypovolemia, diaphragmatic hernia, or prolonged intrauterine asphyxia. Various devices to detect exhaled CO_2 and to confirm accurate ETT placement are available. A laryngeal mask airway may also be an effective tool to establish an airway, especially if PPV is ineffective and intubation attempts are unsuccessful.

The underlying cause for the vast majority of infants having a low heart rate is not a primary cardiac cause, but instead the result of **ineffective ventilation**. Therefore, if the heart rate remains <60 beats/min after 60 sec of PPV with corrective MRSOPA steps, the infant should be intubated (if not already done) to achieve effective ventilation. *Once the infant is intubated, if the heart rate remains <60 beats/min, chest compressions should be initiated with continued ventilation, and FIO_2 increased to 100%.* Chest compressions should be initiated over the lower third of the sternum at a rate of 90/min. The ratio of compressions to ventilation is 3:1 (90 compressions:30 breaths). A provider, separate from the person providing ventilation, is needed to administer chest compressions. Two different techniques exist for performing chest compressions: the thumb technique and the 2-finger technique. For the *thumb technique* the tips of both thumbs are used to depress the sternum, with the fingers on each side encircling the chest; this is the preferred method to administer chest compressions, because it has been shown to achieve a higher blood pressure, increase coronary perfusion, and result in less fatigue. The *2-finger technique* involves depressing the sternum with the tips of the middle finger and index finger while supporting the back with the palm of the other hand. In infants, regardless of whether an alternative airway has been secured, chest compressions are always coordinated with PPV. Chest compressions should continue uninterrupted for 45-60 sec before reassessing heart rate to determine next steps.

Medications are rarely required, but **epinephrine** should be administered when the heart rate is <60 beats/min after 60 sec of combined ventilation and chest compressions or during asystole. Persistent **bradycardia** in neonates is usually attributable to hypoxia resulting from respiratory arrest and often responds rapidly to effective ventilation alone. Persistent bradycardia despite what appears to be adequate resuscitation suggests inadequate ventilation or more severe cardiac compromise.

The umbilical vein can generally be readily cannulated and is the preferred method for administration of medications and volume expanders during neonatal resuscitation (Fig. 121.3). The ETT may be used for the administration of epinephrine if intravenous access is not yet available. Epinephrine (1:10,000 solution at 0.1-0.3 mL/kg *intravenously* or 0.5-1 mL/kg *intratracheally*) is given for asystole or for continued heart rate <60 beats/min after 60 sec of combined resuscitation. The dose may be repeated every 3-5 min. If adequate resuscitation continues for 10 min without a detectable heart rate, it is reasonable to stop resuscitative efforts.

RESUSCITATION OF THE PRETERM INFANT

Resuscitation of the preterm infant should follow the same steps as a term infant, with some special considerations. Whereas resuscitation of term infants should start with room air, resuscitation of most preterm infants can be initiated with slightly higher FIO_2, 21–30%. Pulse oximetry of the preductal (right) hand should be used to titrate O_2 concentrations for targeted saturations per the NRP algorithm (see Fig. 121.2).

Special attention should be paid to *keeping the preterm infant warm in the delivery room.* Quality improvement projects have initiated bundles to improve admission temperatures of preterm infants to the neonatal intensive care unit (NICU) and have included such interventions as higher ambient temperatures in the delivery room, immediate placement of preterm infants into a plastic bag or under plastic wrap rather than drying, and exothermic mattress for resuscitation and transport of the preterm infant.

Delayed cord clamping for 1-3 min can be performed in both preterm and term infants but is especially recommended for preterm infants. Benefits to term infants include higher hemoglobin levels at birth with

min, increasing O_2 saturation, spontaneous respirations, and improved tone. *If after 30 sec of providing PPV there are no signs of effective ventilation, corrective steps should be performed to improve ventilation.* The 6 ventilation corrective steps can be remembered with the mnemonic **MRSOPA**: *m*ask readjustment, *r*eposition the head, *s*uction mouth and nose, *o*pen the mouth, *p*ressure increase, and *a*lternative airway).

In infants with severe respiratory depression who do not respond to PPV by bag-mask, after corrective steps have been taken, endotracheal intubation should be performed. For infants with an otherwise normal airway weighing <1,000 g, ETT size is usually 2.5 mm; for infants 1,000-2,000 g, 3 mm; and for infants >2,000 g, 3.5 mm. A general rule for depth of insertion from upper lip in centimeters is 6 plus infant's weight in kilograms. Poor response to ventilation may be a result of a loosely fitted mask, poor positioning of the ETT, esophageal intubation,

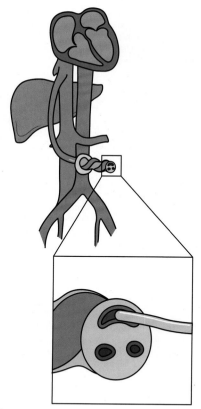

Fig. 121.3 Emergently placed umbilical venous catheter suitable for neonatal resuscitation.

improved iron stores in the 1st several mo of life. Additional benefits for preterm infants include improved hemodynamic stability, decreased need for inotropic support, decreased need for transfusions, and decreased risk of necrotizing enterocolitis and intraventricular hemorrhage. The American College of Obstetricians and Gynecologists (ACOG) recommends at least 30-60 sec of delayed cord clamping after birth for vigorous term and preterm infants. It is unclear, however, whether delayed cord clamping should be continued when an infant requires resuscitation. Studies are investigating whether the onset of respirations before delayed cord clamping is beneficial for both hemodynamic stability and decreased neonatal mortality.

SPECIAL CIRCUMSTANCES IN THE DELIVERY ROOM
Meconium
Meconium staining of the amniotic fluid may be an indication of fetal stress. Previously, the presence of meconium-stained amniotic fluid in a *nonvigorous* infant required tracheal intubation to attempt to aspirate meconium below the cords; NRP recommendations (7th edition) no longer support this practice. If an infant is born through meconium-stained amniotic fluid, it does not matter whether they are vigorous or nonvigorous; the infant should receive the same initial steps of basic resuscitation and should be assessed as any other infant. Tracheal intubation may delay the initiation of effective PPV, which will help the baby to breathe and achieve effective gas exchange.

Placental Abruption
Placental abruption (abruptio placentae) at birth can lead to massive fetal blood loss and a hypovolemic, anemic infant at delivery. Infants can present pale and apneic with poor tone, decreased perfusion, and

bradycardia. In addition to performing routine neonatal resuscitation, when an infant is suspected to be symptomatic from a placental abruption, an emergency low-lying umbilical venous catheter (UVC) should be placed and emergent type O Rh-negative blood should be obtained. In acute blood loss, the blood should be administered as quickly as possible in 10 mL/kg aliquots in the delivery room. Adequate communication between obstetrics and pediatrics regarding suspected abruption is crucial to early recognition and treatment of the infant.

Neonatal Encephalopathy
Infants with neonatal encephalopathy are born with abnormal neurologic function, including level of consciousness, muscle tone, and reflexes. Although there are many possible etiologies, when symptoms are accompanied by a defined perinatal event such as cord prolapse or placental abruption, **hypoxic-ischemic brain injury** is the presumed cause. These infants are often born with impaired respiratory drive. In addition to routine neonatal resuscitation, term infants with concern for neonatal encephalopathy should be passively cooled in the delivery room by not turning on the warmer bed. After initial resuscitation and stabilization, a more thorough neurologic examination can be performed to assess if the infant meets formal criteria for moderate to severe encephalopathy in order to proceed with whole body cooling (see Chapter 120.4).

Airway Obstruction
Hypoplasia of the mandible with posterior displacement of the tongue may result in upper airway obstruction (Pierre Robin, Stickler, DiGeorge, and other syndromes; see Chapter 337). Symptoms may sometimes be temporarily relieved by pulling the tongue or mandible forward or placing the infant in the prone position. Other rare causes of upper airway obstruction at birth include laryngeal atresia or stenosis, teratomas, hygromas, and oral tumors. Critical fetal and then neonatal airway obstruction represents an emergency in the delivery room. High-risk perinatal care has led to the more frequent prenatal diagnosis of these disorders. When diagnosed prenatally, planning can identify the location of delivery and interventions available at delivery. The **ex utero intrapartum treatment (EXIT)** procedure allows time to secure the airway in an infant known prenatally to have critical airway obstruction, before the infant is separated from the placenta (Fig. 121.4). Uteroplacental gas exchange is maintained throughout the procedure.

Respiratory Distress
Both congenital abnormalities and iatrogenic causes secondary to required resuscitation can contribute to respiratory distress in the neonate. A **scaphoid abdomen** suggests a diaphragmatic hernia, as does asymmetry in contour or movement of the chest. An infant with a known diaphragmatic hernia should be immediately intubated in the delivery room and an orogastric tube placed to avoid gaseous distention of the bowel from crying or PPV. The infant should then be transferred to a tertiary referral center for surgical evaluation and treatment (see Chapter 122.1).

In infants with a prenatal diagnosis of hydrops, pleural effusions may be present at delivery, preventing adequate lung expansion and gas exchange. Similarly, infants requiring PPV in the delivery room are at risk for developing a **pneumothorax**. Infants with pulmonary hypoplasia or meconium-stained fluid are at increased risk of this complication. Clinically, infants with a pleural effusion or pneumothorax present with respiratory distress and hypoxia, with *diminished* breath sounds on the affected side. Transillumination may be helpful to confirm the diagnosis. Emergency evacuation of a pneumothorax or pleural effusion without radiographic confirmation is indicated in an infant who is unresponsive to resuscitation efforts and has asymmetric breath sounds, bradycardia, and cyanosis. An angiocatheter attached to a stopcock and syringe should be used for evacuation. For a pneumothorax, an angiocatheter should be inserted perpendicular to the chest wall above the rib in the 2nd intercostal space in the midclavicular line and air evacuated. For a pleural effusion, with the infant in the supine position, the angiocatheter should be inserted in the 4th or 5th intercostal space in the anterior axillary line and directed posteriorly to evacuate the fluid (see Chapter 122).

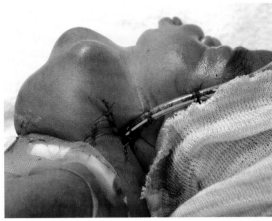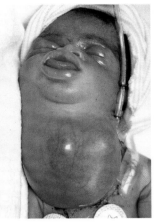

Fig. 121.4 EXIT procedure. Baby with teratoma and critical high airway obstruction syndrome. Trachea is displaced to the lateral neck. *(Courtesy of Dr. Mark Wulkan, Pediatric Surgery, Emory University.)*

Abdominal Wall and Neural Tube Defects

Appropriate management of patients with abdominal wall defects (omphalocele, gastroschisis) in the delivery room prevents excessive fluid loss and minimizes the risk for injury to the exposed viscera. **Gastroschisis** is the more common defect, and typically the intestines are not covered by a membrane. The exposed intestines should be gently placed in a sterile clear plastic bag after delivery. A membrane often covers an **omphalocele**, and care should be taken to prevent its rupture. A nasogastric tube should be placed and the infant transferred to a tertiary referral center for surgical consultation and evaluation for associated anomalies (see Chapter 125).

Similarly, infants born with neural tube defects such as a **myelomeningocele** need special care at delivery to protect the exposed neural tube tissue from trauma and infection; infants should be placed on their side or abdomen for resuscitation. The site of the neural tube defect should be covered with a moist sterile dressing to prevent drying and infection. The infant should then be transferred to a tertiary referral center for surgical evaluation and treatment.

INJURY DURING DELIVERY
Central Nervous System

Both extracranial and intracranial birth injuries can be seen in infants after birth. **Extracranial** lesions include cephalohematoma, caput succedaneum, and subgaleal hemorrhage. **Intracranial** birth injuries include subdural hemorrhage, subarachnoid hemorrhage, and epidural hematoma. The most common intracranial injury experienced at birth is **subdural hemorrhage**, with increasing incidence seen with instrument-assisted vaginal deliveries (see Chapters 120.1 and 120.2).

Fractures

The clavicle is the most frequently fractured bone during labor and delivery. It is particularly vulnerable to injury with difficult delivery of the shoulder in the setting of **shoulder dystocia**, as well as with extended arms in breech deliveries. In the treatment of shoulder dystocia, the obstetrician may intentionally fracture the clavicle so that delivery can proceed. Symptoms of a clavicular fracture include an infant not moving the arm freely on the affected side, palpable crepitus or bony irregularity, and asymmetric or absent Moro reflex on the affected side. The prognosis for this fracture is excellent. Often, no specific treatment is needed, although in some cases the arm and shoulder on the affected side are immobilized for comfort.

Fractures of the long bones are fairly rare. Injuries often present with absent spontaneous movement of the extremity. Associated nerve involvement may also occur. Treatment involves immobilization of the affected extremity with a splint and orthopedic follow-up.

Brachial Plexus Injuries

Brachial plexus injuries result from stretching and tearing of the brachial plexus (spinal roots C5-T1) at delivery. Although shoulder dystocia is associated with an increased risk of brachial plexus injury, it can also occur during a routine delivery (see Chapter 120.6).

ONGOING CARE AFTER RESUSCITATION

The "golden hour" after a baby's birth should emphasize effective neonatal resuscitation, postresuscitation care, prevention of hypothermia, immediate breastfeeding if able, prevention of hypoglycemia, and therapeutic hypothermia for cases of moderate to severe neonatal encephalopathy (birth asphyxia). After supportive measures have stabilized the infant's condition, a specific diagnosis should be established and appropriate continuing treatment instituted.

After initial resuscitation and stabilization, an infant with a significant metabolic acidosis may potentially require further treatment with sodium bicarbonate and/or 10 mL/kg of volume expander. If infection is suspected, appropriate antibiotics should be started as soon as possible. Severe neonatal encephalopathy may also depress myocardial function and cause cardiogenic shock despite the recovery of heart and respiratory rates. Fluids and dopamine or epinephrine as a continuous infusion should be started after initial resuscitation efforts, to improve cardiac output in an infant with poor peripheral perfusion, weak pulses, hypotension, tachycardia, or poor urine output. Regardless of the severity of neonatal encephalopathy or the response to resuscitation, asphyxiated infants should be monitored closely for signs of multiorgan hypoxic-ischemic tissue injury (see Chapter 120.4).

Bibliography is available at Expert Consult.

Chapter 122
Respiratory Tract Disorders

Shawn K. Ahlfeld

第一百二十二章
呼吸系统疾病

中文导读

本章介绍了新生儿分娩脱离母体后其自主呼吸建立的病理生理特点，以及新生儿自身呼吸节律的特点，对早产儿呼吸暂停、呼吸窘迫综合征、支气管肺发育不良、动脉导管未闭等几种特殊疾病的病因、临床特点、诊断和处理分别进行了阐述，并介绍了新生儿持续肺动脉高压、新生儿湿肺、吸入性肺炎、胎粪吸入、肺出血的诊断和鉴别诊断方法，对先天性膈疝、莫尔加尼孔疝、食管旁疝的病因、临床表现及治疗作了详细描述。

Respiratory disorders are the most frequent cause of admission for neonatal intensive care in both term and preterm infants. Signs and symptoms of respiratory distress include cyanosis, expiratory grunting, nasal flaring, retractions, tachypnea, decreased breath sounds with or without rales and/or rhonchi, and pallor. A wide variety of pathologic lesions may be responsible for respiratory disturbances, including pulmonary, airway, cardiovascular, central nervous system, infectious, and other disorders (Fig. 122.1).

It is occasionally difficult to distinguish respiratory from nonrespiratory etiologies on the basis of clinical signs alone. Signs of respiratory distress are an indication for a physical examination and diagnostic evaluation, including determination of ventilation by arterial blood gases and oxygenation by pulse oximetry, and assessment of lung fields with chest radiography. Timely and appropriate therapy is essential to improve outcome.

122.1 Transition to Pulmonary Respiration
Shawn K. Ahlfeld

Successful establishment of adequate lung function at birth depends on airway patency, functional lung development, and maturity of respiratory control. *Fetal lung fluid* must be removed and replaced with gas. This process begins before birth as active sodium transport across the pulmonary epithelium drives liquid from the lung lumen into the interstitium with subsequent absorption into the vasculature. Increased levels of circulating catecholamines, vasopressin, prolactin, and glucocorticoids enhance lung fluid adsorption and trigger the change in lung epithelia from chloride secretion to sodium reabsorption. **Functional residual capacity (FRC)** must be established and maintained to develop a ventilation-perfusion relationship that will provide optimal exchange of oxygen and carbon dioxide between alveoli and blood.

THE FIRST BREATH

Initiation of the first breath is caused by a decline in arterial oxygen tension (PaO_2) and pH and a rise in arterial carbon dioxide partial tension ($PaCO_2$) as a result of interruption of the placental circulation, redistribution of cardiac output, decrease in body temperature, and various tactile and sensory inputs. The relative contributions of these stimuli to the onset of respiration are uncertain.

Although spontaneously breathing infants do not need to generate an opening pressure to create airflow, infants requiring **positive pressure ventilation (PPV)** at birth need an opening pressure of 13-32 cm H_2O and are more likely to establish FRC if they generate a spontaneous, negative pressure breath. Expiratory esophageal pressures associated with the 1st few spontaneous breaths in term newborns range from 45-90 cm H_2O. This high pressure, caused by expiration against a partially closed glottis, may aid in the establishment of FRC but would be difficult to mimic safely with artificial ventilation. The higher pressures needed to initiate respiration are required to overcome the opposing forces of surface tension (particularly in small airways) and the viscosity of liquid remaining in the airways, as well as to introduce about 50 mL/kg of air into the lungs, 20-30 mL/kg of which remains after the first breath to establish FRC. **Surfactant** lining the alveoli enhances the aeration of gas-free lungs by reducing surface tension, thereby lowering the pressure required to open alveoli. Air entry into the lungs displaces fluid, decreases hydrostatic pressure in the pulmonary vasculature, and increases pulmonary blood flow. The greater blood flow in turn increases the blood volume of the lung and the effective vascular surface

Neonate with acute respiratory distress

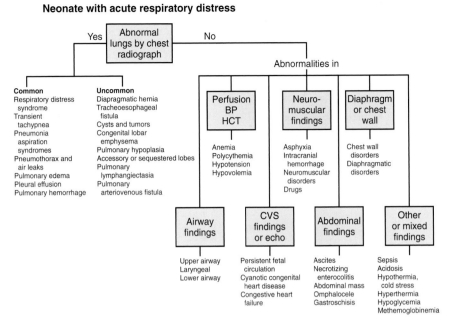

Fig. 122.1 Neonate with acute respiratory distress. BP, Blood pressure; CVS, cardiovascular system; HCT, hematocrit. *(From Battista MA, Carlo WA: Differential diagnosis of acute respiratory distress in the neonate. In Frantz ID, editor:* Tufts University of School of Medicine and Floating Hospital for Children reports on neonatal respiratory diseases, *vol 2, issue 3, Newtown, PA, 1992, Associates in Medical Marketing Co.)*

area available for fluid uptake. The remaining fluid is removed by the pulmonary lymphatics, upper airway, mediastinum, and pleural space. Fluid removal may be impaired after cesarean birth or as a result of surfactant deficiency, endothelial cell damage, hypoalbuminemia, high pulmonary venous pressure, or neonatal sedation.

Compared with term infants, preterm infants have a very compliant chest wall and may be at a disadvantage in establishing FRC. Abnormalities in ventilation-perfusion ratio are greater and persist for longer periods in preterm infants and may lead to hypoxemia and hypercarbia as a result of atelectasis, intrapulmonary shunting, hypoventilation, and gas trapping. The smallest immature infants have the most profound disturbances as a consequence of **respiratory distress syndrome (RDS)**. However, even in healthy term infants, oxygenation is impaired immediately after birth, and oxygen saturation (SO_2) gradually increases and exceeds 90% only at about 5 min. In addition, because of the relatively high pulmonary arterial pressure present in the fetal lung, right-to-left shunting across the ductus arteriosus is common soon after birth. If pulse oximetry is performed soon after birth, the recommendation is to measure preductal SO_2 in the right upper extremity.

BREATHING PATTERNS IN NEWBORNS

During sleep in the 1st few mo after birth, normal full-term infants (and more frequently preterm infants) may have episodes when regular breathing is interrupted by short pauses. This **periodic breathing** pattern is characterized by brief episodes of respiratory pauses lasting 5-10 sec, followed by a burst of rapid respirations at a rate of 50-60 breaths/min for 10-15 sec. The brief interruptions in respiration are not associated with change in color or heart rate. Periodic breathing is a normal characteristic of neonatal respiration and has no prognostic significance.

122.2 Apnea

Shawn K. Ahlfeld

Apnea is a prolonged cessation of respiration and must be distinguished from **periodic breathing** because apnea is often associated with serious

illness. Although there is no universal agreement, apnea is usually defined as cessation of breathing for a period of ≥20 sec, or a period <20 sec that is associated with a change in tone, pallor, cyanosis, or bradycardia (<80-100 beats/min). Based on the absence of respiratory effort and/or airflow, apnea can be obstructive, central, or mixed. **Obstructive apnea** (pharyngeal instability, neck flexion) is characterized by absence of airflow but persistent chest wall motion. Pharyngeal collapse may follow the negative airway pressures generated during inspiration, or it may result from incoordination of the tongue and other upper airway muscles involved in maintaining airway patency. **Central apnea,** which is caused by decreased central nervous system (CNS) stimuli to respiratory muscles, results in both airflow and chest wall motion being absent. Gestational age is the most important determinant of respiratory control, with the frequency of central apnea being inversely related to gestational age. The immaturity of the brainstem respiratory centers is manifest by an attenuated response to CO_2 and a paradoxical response to hypoxia that results in central apnea rather than hyperventilation. **Mixed apnea** is most often observed in **apnea of prematurity** (50–75% of cases), with obstructive apnea preceding central apnea. Short episodes of apnea are usually central, whereas prolonged ones are often mixed. Apnea depends on the sleep state; its frequency increases during active (rapid eye movement) sleep.

Although apnea is usually observed in preterm infants as a result of immature respiratory control or an associated illness, apnea in term infants is uncommon, often associated with serious pathology, and demands prompt diagnostic evaluation. Apnea accompanies many primary diseases that affect neonates (Table 122.1). These disorders produce apnea by direct depression of CNS control of respiration (hypoglycemia, meningitis, drugs, intracranial hemorrhage, seizures), disturbances in oxygen delivery (shock, sepsis, anemia), or ventilation defects (obstruction of the airway, pneumonia, muscle weakness).*The term neonate with apnea should receive continuous cardiorespiratory monitoring while performing an assessment for bacterial or viral sepsis/meningitis, intracranial hemorrhage, seizures, and airway instability.* Supportive care and close monitoring are essential while the underlying etiology is ascertained and appropriately treated.

Table 122.1	Potential Causes of Neonatal Apnea and Bradycardia
Central nervous system	Intraventricular hemorrhage, drugs, seizures, hypoxic injury, herniation, neuromuscular disorders, Leigh syndrome, brainstem infarction or anomalies (e.g., olivopontocerebellar atrophy), spinal cord injury after general anesthesia
Respiratory	Pneumonia, obstructive airway lesions, upper airway collapse, atelectasis, extreme prematurity, laryngeal reflex, phrenic nerve paralysis, pneumothorax, hypoxia
Infectious	Sepsis, meningitis (bacterial, fungal, viral), respiratory syncytial virus, pertussis
Gastrointestinal	Oral feeding, bowel movement, necrotizing enterocolitis, intestinal perforation
Metabolic	↓ Glucose, ↓ calcium, ↓/↑ sodium, ↑ ammonia, ↑ organic acids, ↑ ambient temperature, hypothermia
Cardiovascular	Hypotension, hypertension, heart failure, anemia, hypovolemia, vagal tone
Other	Immaturity of respiratory center, sleep state Sudden unexpected postnatal collapse

APNEA OF PREMATURITY

Apnea of prematurity results from immature respiratory control, most frequently occurs in infants <34 wk of gestational age (GA), and occurs in the absence of identifiable predisposing diseases. The incidence of idiopathic apnea of prematurity varies inversely with GA. Apnea of prematurity is almost universal in infants born at <28 wk GA, and the incidence rapidly decreases from 85% of infants <30 wk GA to 20% of infants <34 wk GA. The onset of apnea of prematurity can be during the initial days to weeks of age but is often delayed if there is RDS or other causes of respiratory distress. In premature infants without respiratory disease, apneic episodes can occur throughout the 1st 7 postnatal days with equal frequency.

Apnea in preterm infants is defined as cessation of breathing for ≥20 sec or for any duration if accompanied by cyanosis and bradycardia (<80-100 beats/min). The incidence of associated bradycardia increases with the length of the preceding apnea and correlates with the severity of hypoxia. Short apnea episodes (10 sec) are rarely associated with bradycardia, whereas longer episodes (>20 sec) have a higher incidence of bradycardia. **Bradycardia** follows the apnea by 1-2 sec in >95% of cases and is most often sinus, but on occasion it can be nodal. Vagal responses and rarely heart block are causes of bradycardia *without* apnea. Short, self-resolving oxygen desaturation episodes noted with continuous monitoring in neonates, and treatment is not necessary.

Preterm infants born at <35 wk GA are at risk for apnea of prematurity and therefore should receive cardiorespiratory monitoring. Apnea that occurs in the absence of other clinical signs of illness in the 1st 2 wk in a preterm infant is likely apnea of prematurity, and therefore additional evaluation for other etiologies is often unwarranted. However, the onset of apnea in a previously well preterm neonate after the 2nd wk of life (or, as previously, in a term infant at any time) is a critical event that may be associated with serious underlying pathology. Prompt investigation for medication side effects, metabolic derangements, structural CNS anomalies, intracranial hemorrhage, seizures, or sepsis/meningitis is warranted.

TREATMENT

Gentle tactile stimulation or provision of flow and/or supplemental oxygen by nasal cannula is often adequate therapy for mild and intermittent episodes. **Nasal continuous positive airway pressure** (nCPAP, 3-5 cm H_2O) and **heated humidified high-flow nasal cannula** (HHHFNC, 1-4 L/min) are appropriate therapies for mixed or obstructive

apnea. The efficacy of both nCPAP and HHHFNC is related to their ability to splint the upper airway to prevent airway obstruction. Both are used widely, but nCPAP may be preferred in extremely preterm infants because of its proven efficacy and safety.

Recurrent or persistent apnea of prematurity is effectively treated with **methylxanthines**. Methylxanthines increase central respiratory drive by lowering the threshold of response to hypercapnia as well as enhancing contractility of the diaphragm and preventing diaphragmatic fatigue. Caffeine and theophylline are similarly effective methylxanthines, but caffeine is preferred because of its longer half-life and lower potential for side effects (less tachycardia and feeding intolerance). In preterm infants, caffeine reduces the incidence and severity of apnea of prematurity, facilitates successful extubation from mechanical ventilation, reduces the rate of **bronchopulmonary dysplasia (BPD)**, and improves neurodevelopmental outcomes. Caffeine therapy can be safely administered orally (PO) or intravenously (IV) with an initial loading dose of 20 mg/kg of caffeine citrate followed 24 hr later by once-daily maintenance doses of 5 mg/kg (increased to 10 mg/kg daily as needed for persistent apnea). Because the therapeutic window is wide (therapeutic level: 8-20 μg/mL) and serious side effects associated with caffeine are rare, monitoring of serum drug concentrations are usually unnecessary. Monitoring is primarily through observation of vital signs (tachycardia) and clinical response. Higher doses of caffeine may be more effective without serious adverse events, but additional studies are needed to ensure safety. Retrospective cohort studies suggest that initiation of caffeine in the 1st 3 days of age in extremely preterm infants (<28 wk GA) may improve outcomes. However, it is reasonable to delay caffeine therapy until apnea occurs. Caffeine therapy is usually continued until an infant is free of clinically significant apnea or bradycardia for 5-7 days without positive pressure respiratory support, or at 34 wk postmenstrual age (PMA).

In an infant with significant anemia, transfusion of packed red blood cells (RBCs) increases blood O_2-carrying capacity, improves tissue oxygenation, and is associated with a short-term reduction in apnea. However, a long-term benefit in regard to apnea appears unlikely. **Gastroesophageal reflux (GER)** is common in neonates, but despite being associated with apnea anecdotally, data *do not* support a causal relationship between GER and apneic events. In preterm infants, medications that inhibit gastric acid production have potentially harmful side effects (increased incidence of sepsis, necrotizing enterocolitis, death) and may actually increase the incidence of apnea and bradycardia. Therefore the routine use of medications that inhibit gastric acid synthesis or promote gastrointestinal motility to reduce the frequency of apnea in preterm infants should be discouraged.

PROGNOSIS

In 92% of infants by 37 wk PMA and in 98% of infants by 40 wk PMA, apnea of prematurity resolves spontaneously. However, infants born well before 28 wk GA may experience apnea and bradycardic events until 44 wk PMA. Beyond 44 wk PMA, extreme events (apnea >30 sec and/or bradycardia <60 beats/min for >10 sec) are very rare. The period that an infant should be observed to ensure resolution of apnea and bradycardia is not defined and among institutions is highly variable. However, many experts would recommend that an infant demonstrate an event-free period of 5-7 days before discharge. Although the nature and severity of events should dictate the length of observation, sufficiently large retrospective cohort studies suggest that a 1-3 day (infants born at ≥30 wk GA), 9-10 day (27-28 wk GA), or 13-14 day (<26 wk GA) event-free period predicts resolution of apnea in up to 95% of infants successfully. Brief, isolated bradycardic episodes associated with oral feeding are common in preterm infants and are generally not considered significant during the event-free period. While not recommended routinely for preterm infants with apnea of prematurity, in *rare* cases an infant with persistent, prolonged apnea may be discharged with home cardiorespiratory monitoring. In the absence of significant events, home monitoring can be safely discontinued at 44 wk PMA. There is no evidence that home monitoring prevents death.

Despite its high frequency in preterm infants, the harm associated with apnea of prematurity is unknown. However, apnea of prematurity does not appear to alter an infant's prognosis unless it is severe, recurrent, and refractory to therapy. Prompt, effective therapy and careful monitoring are vital to avoid prolonged, severe hypoxia, which may increase the risk of death and neurodevelopmental impairment.

APNEA OF PREMATURITY AND SUDDEN INFANT DEATH SYNDROME

Although preterm infants are at higher risk for sudden infant death syndrome (SIDS), apnea of prematurity does not further increase that risk. The peak incidence of SIDS occurs earlier in infants born at 24-28 wk GA (47.1 wk PMA vs 53.5 wk PMA). The epidemiologic evidence that placing babies supine during sleep reduces the rate of SIDS deaths by >50% suggests that positioning, and not prematurity, primarily influences the incidence of SIDS. Supine positioning on a firm sleep surface separate from the parents' bed, promotion of breastfeeding, and pacifier use during sleep reduce the incidence of SIDS. Avoidance of cigarette smoke exposure and no parental use of alcohol or illicit drugs during pregnancy and after birth are also important in the prevention of SIDS.

Bibliography is available at Expert Consult.

122.3 Respiratory Distress Syndrome (Hyaline Membrane Disease)
Shawn K. Ahlfeld

INCIDENCE
Respiratory distress syndrome (RDS) occurs primarily in premature infants; its incidence is inversely related to gestational age and birthweight. It occurs in 60–80% of infants <28 wk GA, in 15–30% of those between 32 and 36 wk GA, and rarely in those >37 wk GA. The risk for development of RDS increases with maternal diabetes, multiple births, cesarean delivery, precipitous delivery, asphyxia, cold stress, and a maternal history of previously affected infants. The risk of RDS is reduced in pregnancies with chronic or pregnancy-associated hypertension, maternal heroin use, prolonged rupture of membranes, and antenatal corticosteroid prophylaxis.

ETIOLOGY AND PATHOPHYSIOLOGY
Surfactant deficiency (decreased production and secretion) is the primary cause of RDS. In the absence of pulmonary surfactant, significantly increased alveolar surface tension leads to atelectasis, and the ability to attain an adequate FRC is impaired. As a consequence of progressive injury to epithelial and endothelial cells from atelectasis (atelectrauma), volutrauma, ischemic injury, and oxygen toxicity, effusion of proteinaceous material and cellular debris into the alveolar spaces (forming the classic *hyaline membranes*) further impairs oxygenation. Alveolar atelectasis, hyaline membrane formation, and interstitial edema make the lungs less compliant in RDS, so greater pressure is required to expand the alveoli and small airways. Additionally, compared with the mature infant, the highly compliant chest wall of the preterm infant offers less resistance to the natural tendency of the lungs to collapse. Thus, at end-expiration, the volume of the thorax and lungs tends to approach residual volume. Although surfactant is present in high concentrations in fetal lung homogenates by 20 wk of gestation, it does not reach the surface of the lungs until later. It appears in amniotic fluid between 28 and 32 wk. Mature levels of pulmonary surfactant are present usually after 35 wk of gestation.

The major constituents of surfactant are dipalmitoyl phosphatidylcholine (lecithin), phosphatidylglycerol, apoproteins (surfactant proteins SP-A, SP-B, SP-C, and SP-D), and cholesterol (Fig. 122.2). With advancing GA, increasing amounts of phospholipids are synthesized and stored in type II alveolar cells (Fig. 122.3). These surface-active agents are released into the alveoli, where they reduce surface tension and help maintain alveolar stability at end-expiration. Synthesis of surfactant depends in part on normal pH, temperature, and perfusion. Asphyxia, hypoxemia, and pulmonary ischemia, particularly in association with hypovolemia, hypotension, and cold stress, may suppress surfactant synthesis. The epithelial lining of the lungs may also be injured by high

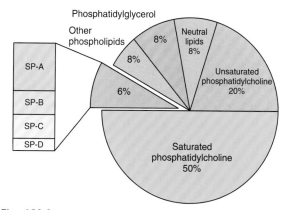

Fig. 122.2 Composition of surfactant. SP-A, Surfactant-associated protein A; SP-B, surfactant-associated protein B; SP-C, surfactant-associated protein C; SP-D, surfactant-associated protein D. *(From Jobe AH, Ikegami M: Biology of surfactant, Clin Perinatol 28:655–669, 2001.)*

O_2 concentrations and mechanical ventilation, thereby further reducing secretion of surfactant.

Atelectasis results in perfused but not ventilated alveoli, causing hypoxia. Decreased lung compliance, small tidal volumes, increased physiologic dead space, and insufficient alveolar ventilation eventually result in hypercapnia. The combination of hypercapnia, hypoxia, and acidosis produces pulmonary arterial vasoconstriction with increased right-to-left shunting through the foramen ovale and ductus arteriosus and within the lung itself. Progressive injury to epithelial and endothelial cells and formation of hyaline membranes further impairs oxygenation, leading to a vicious cycle of diminished surfactant production, worsening atelectasis, lung injury, and severe hypoxia (Fig. 122.4).

CLINICAL MANIFESTATIONS
Signs of RDS usually appear within minutes of birth, although they may not be recognized for several hours in larger premature infants, until rapid, shallow respirations become more obvious. A later onset of tachypnea should suggest other conditions. Some patients require resuscitation at birth because of intrapartum asphyxia or initial severe respiratory distress (especially with birthweight <1,000 g). Characteristically, tachypnea, prominent (often audible) expiratory grunting, intercostal and subcostal retractions, nasal flaring, and cyanosis are noted. Breath sounds may be normal or diminished with a harsh tubular quality, and on deep inspiration, fine crackles may be heard. The natural course of untreated RDS is characterized by progressive worsening of cyanosis and dyspnea. If the condition is inadequately treated, blood pressure may fall; cyanosis and pallor increase, and grunting decreases or disappears, as the condition worsens. *Apnea and irregular respirations are ominous signs requiring immediate intervention.* Untreated patients may also have a mixed respiratory-metabolic acidosis, edema, ileus, and oliguria. Respiratory failure may occur in infants with rapid progression of the disease. In most cases the signs reach a peak within 3 days, after which improvement is gradual. Improvement is often heralded by spontaneous diuresis and improved blood gas values at lower inspired O_2 levels and/or lower ventilator support. Death can result from severe impairment of gas exchange, alveolar air leaks (pulmonary interstitial emphysema, pneumothorax), pulmonary hemorrhage, or intraventricular hemorrhage (IVH).

DIAGNOSIS
The clinical course, chest x-ray findings, and blood gas values help establish the clinical diagnosis. On chest radiograph, the lungs may have a characteristic but not pathognomonic appearance that includes low lung volumes, a diffuse, fine reticular granularity of the parenchyma (ground-glass appearance), and air bronchograms (Fig. 122.5). The initial x-ray appearance is occasionally normal, with the typical pattern

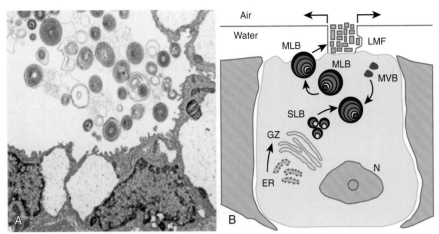

Fig. 122.3 A, Fetal rat lung (low magnification), day 20 (term: day 22) showing developing type II cells, stored glycogen (*pale areas*), secreted lamellar bodies, and tubular myelin. **B,** Possible pathway for transport, secretion, and reuptake of surfactant. ER, Endoplasmic reticulum; GZ, Golgi zone; LMF, lattice (tubular) myelin figure; MLB, mature lamellar body; MVB, multivesicular body; N, nucleus; SLB, small lamellar body. (**A,** *Courtesy of Mary Williams, MD, University of California, San Francisco;* **B,** *from Hansen T, Corbet A: Lung development and function. In Taeusch HW, Ballard RA, Avery MA, editors:* Schaffer and Avery's diseases of the newborn, *ed 6, Philadelphia, 1991, Saunders.*)

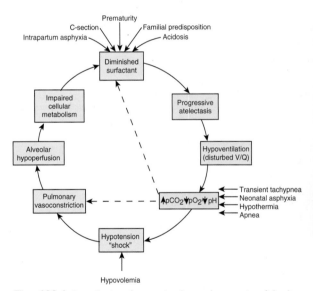

Fig. 122.4 Contributing factors in the pathogenesis of hyaline membrane disease. The potential "vicious circle" perpetuates hypoxia and pulmonary insufficiency. V/Q, Ventilation-perfusion ratio. (*From Farrell P, Zachman R: Pulmonary surfactant and the respiratory distress syndrome. In Quilligan EJ, Kretchmer N, editors: Fetal and maternal medicine, New York, 1980, Wiley. Reprinted by permission of John Wiley and Sons, Inc.*)

Fig. 122.5 Infant with respiratory distress syndrome. Note the granular lungs, air bronchogram, and air-filled esophagus. **A,** Anteroposterior, and **B,** lateral, radiographs are needed to distinguish the umbilical artery from the vein catheter and to determine the appropriate level of insertion. The lateral view clearly shows that the catheter has been inserted into an umbilical vein and is lying in the portal system of the liver. A indicates endotracheal tube; B indicates the umbilical venous catheter at the junction of the umbilical vein, ductus venosus, and portal vein; C indicates the umbilical artery catheter passed up the aorta to T12. (*Courtesy of Walter E. Berdon, Babies Hospital, New York City.*)

developing during the 1st day. Considerable variation in radiographic findings may be seen, especially in infants who have already received treatment with surfactant replacement and/or positive pressure respiratory support; this variation often results in poor correlation between radiographic findings and the clinical course. Blood gas findings are characterized initially by hypoxemia and later by progressive hypoxemia, hypercapnia, and variable metabolic acidosis.

In the differential diagnosis, early-onset sepsis may be indistinguishable from RDS. In neonates with pneumonia, the chest radiograph may be identical to that for RDS. Clinical factors such as maternal group B streptococcal colonization with inadequate intrapartum antibiotic prophylaxis, maternal fever (>38.6°C) or chorioamnionitis, or prolonged rupture of membranes (>12 hr) are associated with an increased risk of early-onset sepsis. Although complete blood counts are neither sensitive nor specific in the diagnosis of early-onset sepsis, the presence of marked neutropenia has been associated with increased risk. Cyanotic congenital heart disease (in particular, total anomalous pulmonary venous return) can also mimic RDS both clinically and radiographically. Echocardiography with color-flow imaging should be performed in infants who show no response to surfactant replacement, to rule out cyanotic congenital heart disease as well as ascertain patency of the ductus arteriosus and assess pulmonary vascular resistance (PVR).

Persistent pulmonary hypertension, aspiration (meconium, amniotic fluid) syndromes, spontaneous pneumothorax, pleural effusions, and congenital anomalies (pulmonary congenital airway malformations, pulmonary lymphangiectasia, diaphragmatic hernia, lobar emphysema) must be considered in patients with an atypical clinical course but can generally be differentiated from RDS through radiographic and other evaluations. Transient tachypnea may be distinguished by its shorter and milder clinical course and is characterized by low or no need for O_2 supplementation.

Although rare, genetic disorders may contribute to respiratory distress. Abnormalities in surfactant protein B and C genes as well as a gene responsible for transporting surfactant across membranes, ABC transporter 3 (*ABCA3*), are associated with severe and often lethal familial respiratory disease. **Congenital alveolar proteinosis** (congenital surfactant protein B deficiency) is a rare familial disease that manifests as severe and lethal RDS in predominantly term and near-term infants (see Chapter 434). In atypical cases of RDS, a lung profile (lecithin:sphingomyelin ratio and phosphatidylglycerol determination) performed on a tracheal aspirate can be helpful in establishing a diagnosis of surfactant deficiency. Other familial causes of neonatal respiratory distress (not RDS) include mucopolysaccharidosis, acinar dysplasia, pulmonary lymphangiectasia, and alveolocapillary dysplasia.

PREVENTION

Avoidance of unnecessary or poorly timed early (<39 wk GA) cesarean delivery or induction of labor, appropriate management of high-risk pregnancy and labor (including administration of antenatal corticosteroids), and prediction of pulmonary immaturity with possible in utero acceleration of maturation (see Chapter 119) are important preventive strategies. Antenatal and intrapartum fetal monitoring may decrease the risk of fetal asphyxia; asphyxia is associated with an increased incidence and severity of RDS.

Administration of antenatal corticosteroids to women before 37 wk gestation significantly reduces the incidence and mortality of RDS as well as overall neonatal mortality. Antenatal steroids also reduce (1) overall mortality, (2) admission to the neonatal intensive care unit (NICU) and need for/duration of ventilatory support, and (3) incidence of severe IVH, necrotizing enterocolitis (NEC), and neurodevelopmental impairment. Postnatal growth is not adversely affected. Antenatal corticosteroids do not increase the risk of maternal death, chorioamnionitis, or puerperal sepsis. **Betamethasone** and **dexamethasone** have both been used antenatally. Betamethasone may reduce neonatal death to a greater extent than dexamethasone.

Although classically, antenatal corticosteroids were reserved for preterm birth before 34 wk gestation, the administration of betamethasone before late preterm birth (34^{+0} to 36^{+6} wk gestation) significantly reduces the need for respiratory support and the incidence of severe respiratory complications. Therefore the American College of Obstetricians and Gynecologists (ACOG) recommends that for all women between 24 and 36 wk gestation who present in preterm labor and are likely to deliver a fetus within 1 wk, antenatal corticosteroid administration should be considered.

TREATMENT

The basic defect requiring treatment in RDS is inadequate pulmonary O_2-CO_2 exchange. Basic supportive care (thermoregulatory, circulatory, fluid, electrolyte, and respiratory) is essential while FRC is established and maintained. Careful and frequent monitoring of heart and respiratory rates, SaO_2, PaO_2, $PaCO_2$, pH, electrolytes, glucose, hematocrit, blood pressure, and temperature are essential. Arterial catheterization is frequently necessary. Because most cases of RDS are self-limited, the goal of treatment is to minimize abnormal physiologic variations and superimposed iatrogenic problems. Treatment of infants with RDS is best carried out in the NICU.

Periodic monitoring of PaO_2, $PaCO_2$, and pH is an important part of the management and is used to provide supportive care; if assisted ventilation is being used, such monitoring is essential. Oxygenation (SO_2) should be assessed by continuous pulse oximetry. Capillary blood samples are of limited value for determining PO_2 but may be useful for PCO_2 and pH monitoring. Monitoring of blood gas parameters and mean arterial blood pressure through an umbilical or peripheral arterial catheter is useful in managing the shock-like state that may occur during the initial hours in premature infants who have been asphyxiated or have severe RDS (see Fig. 121.3). The position of a radiopaque umbilical catheter should be checked radiographically after insertion (see Fig. 122.5). The tip of an umbilical artery catheter should lie at L3-L5 just above the bifurcation of the aorta or at T6-T10. The placement and supervision should be carried out by skilled and experienced personnel. Catheters should be removed as soon as patients no longer have any indication for their continued use—usually when an infant is stable and the fraction of inspired oxygen (FIO_2) is <40%.

Nasal Continuous Positive Airway Pressure

Warm, humidified oxygen should be provided at a concentration sufficient to keep PaO_2 between 50 and 70 mm Hg (91–95% SaO_2) to maintain normal tissue oxygenation while minimizing the risk of O_2 toxicity. If there is significant respiratory distress (severe retractions and expiratory grunting) or if SaO_2 cannot be kept >90% at FIO_2 of ≥40–70%, applying nCPAP at 5-10 cm H_2O is indicated and usually produces a rapid improvement in oxygenation. Nasal CPAP reduces collapse of surfactant-deficient alveoli and improves both FRC and ventilation-perfusion matching. *Early use of nCPAP for stabilization of at-risk preterm infants beginning early (in the delivery room) reduces the need for mechanical ventilation.*

Recognizing the benefits of surfactant replacement therapy, in addition to the potential protective effects of prophylactic nCPAP, some experts recommend intubation for prophylactic or early rescue surfactant replacement therapy, followed by extubation back to nCPAP immediately once the infant is stable (usually within minutes to <1 hr). The aforementioned method is commonly referred to as **intubate surfactant and extubate** (INSURE). A variation of the INSURE method has evolved known as MIST (**minimally invasive surfactant therapy**) or LISA (**less invasive surfactant administration**), in which a small feeding tube, rather than an endotracheal tube (ETT), is used to deliver intratracheal surfactant to a spontaneously breathing infant on nCPAP. The combination of early rescue surfactant by the INSURE, MIST, or LISA method with nCPAP has been associated with the reduced need for mechanical ventilation, and emerging evidence suggests modest benefits in terms of preventing BPD. The amount of nCPAP required usually decreases after approximately 72 hr of age, and most infants can be weaned from nCPAP shortly thereafter. *Assisted ventilation and surfactant are indicated for infants with RDS who cannot keep oxygen saturation >90% while breathing 40–70% oxygen and receiving nCPAP.*

In an effort to minimize ventilator-associated lung injury and prevent long-term pulmonary complications, the use of nCPAP as the initial respiratory support for extremely preterm infants is preferred. The decreased need for ventilator support with the use of nCPAP may allow lung inflation to be maintained while preventing lung injury. Early nCPAP is beneficial compared to intubation and prophylactic surfactant, because avoidance of mechanical ventilation is associated with a reduction in death and/or BPD. Infants at the extremes of GA (<24 wk) and those that were not exposed to antenatal corticosteroids may still benefit from intubation and surfactant prophylaxis.

Mechanical Ventilation

Infants with respiratory failure or persistent apnea require assisted mechanical ventilation. Strict definitions for respiratory failure in extremely preterm infants with RDS are not agreed on universally, but reasonable measures of respiratory failure are (1) arterial blood pH <7.20, (2) $PaCO_2$ ≥60 mm Hg, (3) SaO_2 <90% at O_2 concentration of 40–70% and nCPAP of 5-10 cm H_2O, and (4) persistent or severe apnea. The goal of mechanical ventilation is to improve oxygenation and ventilation without causing pulmonary injury or oxygen toxicity. Acceptable ranges of ABG values vary significantly among institutions but generally range from PaO_2 50-70 mm Hg, $PaCO_2$ 45-65 mm Hg (and higher after the 1st few days when risk of IVH is less), and pH 7.20-7.35. During mechanical ventilation, oxygenation is improved by increasing either FIO_2 or the mean airway pressure. The mean airway pressure can be increased by raising the peak inspiratory pressure (PIP), inspiratory time, ventilator rate, or positive end-expiratory pressure (PEEP). Adjustment in pressure is usually most effective. However, excessive PEEP may impede venous return, thereby reducing cardiac output and O_2 delivery. Assisted ventilation for infants with RDS should always include appropriate PEEP (see Chapter 89.1). PEEP levels of 4-6 cm H_2O are usually safe and effective. CO_2 elimination is determined by the minute ventilation, which is a product of the tidal volume (dependent on the inspiratory time and PIP) and ventilator rate. Because of the homogeneous nature of the lung pathology associated with RDS, a high rate (≥60/min), low tidal volume (4-6 mL/kg) strategy is generally effective. Meta-analyses comparing high (>60 breaths/min) and low (usually 30-40 breaths/min) rates (and presumed low vs high tidal volumes, respectively) revealed that the high ventilatory rate strategy led to fewer air leaks and a trend for increased survival. With use of high ventilatory rates, sufficient expiratory time should be allowed to avoid air-trapping and inadvertent PEEP.

Modes of Mechanical Ventilation

Synchronized intermittent mechanical ventilation (SIMV) delivered by time-cycled, pressure-limited, continuous flow ventilators is a common method of conventional ventilation for newborns. With pressure-limited SIMV, a set PIP is delivered in synchrony with the patient's own breaths for a specified rate per minute. For breaths above the set rate, pressure support breaths (8-10 cm H_2O above PEEP) are provided to help overcome the resistance associated with spontaneous breathing through the ETT. In *pressure-limited ventilation* the delivered tidal volume is directly proportional to the respiratory compliance. Rapid changes in compliance occur with surfactant replacement therapy, requiring careful attention to tidal volumes and appropriate adjustments in PIP. Advances in ventilator technology have allowed the delivery of very small (<10 mL) tidal volume breaths consistently. In *volume-targeted ventilation* a specific tidal volume is set, and the PIP required to deliver it varies inversely with the respiratory compliance. Other modes of volume-targeted ventilation calculate the lowest effective PIP to deliver the set tidal volume. Evidence suggests that volume-targeted ventilation results in fewer air leaks and may improve survival without BPD.

High-frequency ventilation (HFV) achieves desired alveolar ventilation by using smaller tidal volumes and higher rates (300-1,200 breaths/min or 5-20 Hz). HFV may improve elimination of CO_2 and improve oxygenation in patients who show no response to conventional ventilators, as well as those who have severe RDS, interstitial emphysema, recurrent pneumothoraces, or meconium aspiration pneumonia. **High-frequency oscillatory ventilation** (HFOV) and **high-frequency jet ventilation** (HFJV) are the most frequently used methods. HFOV may reduce BPD but the effect size is likely small. In severe respiratory failure unresponsive to conventional mechanical ventilation, HFOV strategies that promote lung recruitment, combined with surfactant therapy, may improve gas exchange. HFJV is particularly useful to facilitate resolution of air leaks. Elective use of either HFV method, in comparison with conventional ventilation, generally does not offer advantages when used as the initial ventilation strategy to treat infants with RDS.

Permissive Hypercapnia and Avoidance of Hyperoxia

Permissive hypercapnia is a strategy for management of patients receiving ventilatory support in whom priority is given to limiting ventilator-associated lung injury by tolerating relatively high levels of $PaCO_2$ (>60-70 mm Hg). Permissive hypercapnia can be implemented during nCPAP and mechanical ventilation but has not been shown to significantly impact outcomes. **Hyperoxia** may also contribute to lung injury in preterm infants. However, a lower target range of oxygenation (85–89%) compared with a higher range (91–95%) increases mortality and does not alter rates of BPD, BPD/death, blindness, or neurodevelopmental impairment. *Therefore the currently recommended range of oxygen saturation targets is 91–95%.*

Discontinuation of Mechanical Ventilation

Strategies for weaning infants from ventilators vary widely and are influenced by lung mechanics as well as the availability of ventilatory

modes. Extubation to nCPAP prevents postextubation atelectasis and reduces the need for reintubation. Synchronized **nasal intermittent positive pressure ventilation** (NIPPV) also decreases the need for reintubation in premature infants, but ventilators capable of synchronization with nasal ventilation are not widely available. HHHFNC (1-8 L/min) oxygen is typically used to support term and near-term infants following extubation. It is not clear whether nCPAP, NIPPV, or HHHFNC is more efficacious for promoting normal lung development and preventing BPD, but there is more evidence associated with nCPAP in extremely preterm infants. Preloading with methylxanthines enhances the success of extubation.

Surfactant Replacement Therapy

Surfactant deficiency is the primary pathophysiology of RDS. Immediate effects of surfactant replacement therapy include improved alveolar-arterial oxygen gradients, reduced ventilatory support, increased pulmonary compliance, and improved chest radiograph appearance. In the past, intratracheal surfactant replacement for symptomatic premature infants immediately after birth (prophylactic) or during the 1st few hr of life (early rescue) showed reduced air leak and mortality from RDS. However, substantial evidence supports the feasibility and efficacy of prophylactic nCPAP as the *primary* means of respiratory support for preterm infants with RDS. CPAP started at birth is as effective as prophylactic or early surfactant and is associated with a reduction in BPD. *Prophylactic nCPAP is therefore the approach of choice for the delivery room management of a preterm neonate at risk for RDS.*

In neonates with RDS who fail nCPAP and require intubation and mechanical ventilation, treatment with endotracheal surfactant should be initiated immediately to avoid lung injury. Repeated dosing is given every 6-12 hr for a total of 2-4 doses, depending on the preparation. Exogenous surfactant should be given by a physician who is qualified in neonatal resuscitation and respiratory management. Additional required onsite staff support includes nurses and respiratory therapists experienced in the ventilatory management of preterm infants. Appropriate monitoring equipment (radiology, blood gas laboratory, pulse oximetry) must also be available. Complications of surfactant replacement therapy include transient hypoxia, hypercapnia, bradycardia and hypotension, blockage of ETT, and pulmonary hemorrhage.

A number of surfactant preparations are available, including synthetic surfactants and natural surfactants derived from animal sources. There do not appear to be significant, consistent benefits to one preparation over another. Infants requiring ventilator support after 1 wk of age may experience transient episodes of surfactant dysfunction temporally associated with episodes of infection and respiratory deterioration. Surfactant treatment may be beneficial in these infants.

Other Pharmacologic Therapies

There are no pharmacologic therapies superior or equal to the efficacy of maintaining FRC (through noninvasive respiratory support and mechanical ventilation when necessary) and providing surfactant replacement therapy in the treatment of RDS. Systemic corticosteroids (predominantly dexamethasone), although effective in improving respiratory mechanics and preventing BPD and death, are associated with increased risk of cerebral palsy and neurodevelopmental impairment when used indiscriminately. Thus, routine use of systemic corticosteroids for the prevention or treatment of BPD is not recommended by the Consensus Group of the American Academy of Pediatrics and the Canadian Pediatric Society. Early (1st 10 days of life), low-dose administration (1 mg/kg/day hydrocortisone twice daily for 7 days; 0.5 mg/kg/day for 3 days) may reduce the risk of BPD in neonates <28 wk GA. In general, administration of inhaled corticosteroids to ventilated preterm infants during the 1st 2 wk after birth has not proved to be consistently advantageous.

Inhaled nitric oxide (iNO) has been evaluated in preterm infants following the observation of its effectiveness in term and near-term infants with hypoxemic respiratory failure. Although iNO improves oxygenation in term and near-term infants with hypoxic respiratory failure or persistent pulmonary hypertension of the neonate, trials in preterm infants have not shown significant benefit. The most current data do not support the routine administration of iNO in preterm infants with hypoxemic respiratory failure.

Hypotension and low flow in the superior vena cava have been associated with higher rates of CNS morbidity and mortality and should be treated with cautious administration of crystalloid (if volume depletion due to hemorrhage or excessive insensible fluid losses is suspected) and early use of vasopressors. Dopamine is more effective in raising blood pressure than dobutamine. Hypotension that is refractory to vasopressor therapy, especially in neonates <1,000 g, may be caused by transient adrenal insufficiency. Administration of intravenous hydrocortisone at 1-2 mg/kg/dose every 6-12 hr may improve blood pressure and allow weaning of vasopressors.

Because of the difficulty in distinguishing group B streptococcal or other bacterial infections from RDS, empirical antibiotic therapy may be indicated until the results of blood cultures are available. Penicillin or ampicillin with an aminoglycoside is suggested, although the choice of antibiotics should be based on the recent pattern of bacterial sensitivity in the hospital where the infant is being treated (see Chapter 129).

COMPLICATIONS

Early provision of intensive observation and care of high-risk newborn infants can significantly reduce the morbidity and mortality associated with RDS and other acute neonatal illnesses. Antenatal corticosteroids, postnatal surfactant use, and improved modes of ventilation have resulted in low mortality from RDS (approximately 10%). Mortality increases with decreasing gestational age. Optimal results depend on the availability of experienced and skilled personnel, care in specially designed and organized regional hospital units, proper equipment, and lack of complications such as severe asphyxia, intracranial hemorrhage, or irremediable congenital malformation.

The most serious complications of endotracheal intubation are **pulmonary air leaks**, asphyxia from obstruction or dislodgment of the tube, bradycardia during intubation or suctioning, and the subsequent development of **subglottic stenosis**. Other complications include bleeding from trauma during intubation, posterior pharyngeal pseudodiverticula, need for tracheostomy, ulceration of the nares caused by pressure from the tube, permanent narrowing of the nostril as a result of tissue damage and scarring from irritation or infection around the tube, erosion of the palate, avulsion of a vocal cord, laryngeal ulcer, papilloma of a vocal cord, and persistent hoarseness, stridor, or edema of the larynx.

Measures to reduce the incidence of these complications include skillful intubation, adequate securing of the tube, use of polyvinyl ETTs, use of the smallest tube that will provide effective ventilation in order to reduce local pressure necrosis and ischemia, avoidance of frequent changes and motion of the tube in situ, avoidance of too frequent or too vigorous suctioning, and prevention of infection through meticulous cleanliness and frequent sterilization of all apparatus attached to or passed through the tube. The personnel inserting and caring for the ETT should be experienced and skilled in such care.

Extrapulmonary air leaks (pneumothorax, pneumomediastinum, pulmonary interstitial emphysema) are observed in 3–9% of extremely preterm infants with RDS (see Chapter 122.12). PPV with excessive inspiratory pressures (and therefore excessive tidal volumes), either during resuscitation at delivery or in the initial hours of mechanical ventilation, is a common risk factor, but air leaks can also occur in infants breathing spontaneously. Although the risk of air leak was increased in infants receiving a higher level of nCPAP (up to 8 cm H_2O) in the CPAP or Intubation at Birth (COIN) trial, subsequent trials have not demonstrated a similar effect.

Risks associated with **umbilical arterial catheterization** include vascular embolization, thrombosis, spasm, and vascular perforation; ischemic or chemical necrosis of abdominal viscera; infection; accidental hemorrhage; hypertension; and impairment of circulation to a leg with subsequent gangrene. Aortography has demonstrated that clots form in or about the tips of 95% of catheters placed in an umbilical artery. Aortic ultrasonography can also be used to investigate for the presence of thrombosis. **Renovascular hypertension** may occur days to weeks after umbilical arterial catheterization in a small proportion of

neonates. Transient blanching of the leg may occur during catheterization of the umbilical artery. It is usually caused by reflex arterial spasm, the incidence of which is lessened by using the smallest available catheter, particularly in very small infants. The catheter should be removed immediately; catheterization of the other artery may then be attempted. **Umbilical vein catheterization** is associated with many of the same risks as umbilical artery catheterization. Additional risks are cardiac perforation and pericardial tamponade; improperly placed catheters in the portal vein can lead to thrombosis. The risk of a serious clinical complication resulting from umbilical catheterization is probably 2–5%.

Bibliography is available at Expert Consult.

122.4 Bronchopulmonary Dysplasia
Shawn K. Ahlfeld

INCIDENCE

Bronchopulmonary dysplasia (**BPD**, also known as **chronic lung disease of prematurity**) is a clinical pulmonary syndrome that develops in the majority of extremely preterm infants and is defined by a prolonged need for respiratory support and supplemental oxygen. Almost 60% of infants born at ≤28 wk gestation will develop BPD, and the incidence of BPD increases inversely with gestational age. For infants born at the extreme of viability (22-24 wk), essentially 100% will develop BPD, the majority of whom will have moderate to severe disease. As neonatal care has improved and use of antenatal corticosteroids has become the standard of care, survival of infants born at the extreme of viability has improved, and BPD is encountered with increased prevalence. In the United States, an additional 10,000-15,000 new cases occur annually. Despite decades of experience, the incidence of BPD remains largely unchanged.

ETIOLOGY AND PATHOPHYSIOLOGY

BPD develops following preterm birth and the necessary life-supporting interventions (particularly mechanical ventilation and supplemental oxygen) that cause neonatal lung injury. As the limit of viability has been lowered by advances in neonatal care, the clinical syndrome associated with BPD has evolved. The clinical, radiographic, and lung histology of classic BPD described in 1967, before widespread use of antenatal corticosteroids and postnatal surfactant, was that of a disease of preterm infants who were more mature. During that era, infants born ≤30-32 wk gestation rarely survived. Infants who developed BPD demonstrated classic RDS initially, but the injurious mechanical ventilation and excessive supplemental oxygen required to support them resulted in a progressive, severe fibroproliferative lung disease. Improvements in respiratory care, as well as the introduction of surfactant and antenatal steroids, have allowed for gentle respiratory support strategies, and the need for excessive ventilator support and high percentages of inspired supplemental oxygen has decreased.

Despite a reduction in the fibroproliferative disease described previously, infants born in the modern era of neonatal care continued to require supplemental oxygen for prolonged periods. The *new* BPD is a disease primarily of infants with birthweight <1,000 g who were born at <28 wk gestation, some of whom have little or no lung disease at birth but over the 1st weeks of age experience progressive respiratory failure. Infants with the new BPD are born at a more immature stage of distal lung development, and lung histology demonstrates variable saccular wall fibrosis, minimal airway disease, abnormal pulmonary microvasculature development, and alveolar simplification. Although the etiology remains incompletely understood, the histopathology of BPD indicates interference with normal alveolar septation and microvascular maturation.

The pathogenesis of BPD is likely multifactorial, but pulmonary inflammation and lung injury are consistently observed. Alveolar collapse (**atelectrauma**) as a consequence of surfactant deficiency, together with ventilator-induced phasic overdistension of the lung (**volutrauma**), promotes lung inflammation and injury. Supplemental oxygen produces free radicals that cannot be metabolized by the immature antioxidant systems of very-low-birthweight (VLBW) neonates and further contributes to the injury. Pulmonary inflammation evidenced by infiltration of neutrophils and macrophages in alveolar fluid, as well as a host of proinflammatory cytokines, contributes to the progression of lung injury. Pre- and postnatal infection, excessive pulmonary blood flow via the patent ductus arteriosus (PDA), excessive administration of intravenous fluid, and pre- and postnatal growth failure are also significantly associated with the development of BPD. While the mechanisms are unclear, all likely promote lung injury by necessitating increased or prolonged respiratory support or interfering with lung repair. Regardless, the result is an interference with normal development of the alveolar-capillary unit and interference with normal gas exchange.

CLINICAL MANIFESTATIONS

Over the 1st several wk of age, infants developing BPD demonstrate persistent, often progressive respiratory distress and the need for respiratory support and supplemental oxygen. In extremely-low-birthweight (ELBW) infants at risk for BPD, the need for supplemental oxygen over the 1st 2 wk of age follows 1 of 3 distinct patterns. Infants that follow the natural course of RDS, and by the 3-4 days of age require minimal (FIO₂ <0.25) supplemental oxygen, have a low (<20%) risk of developing BPD. Infants who initially have a low O₂ requirement (FIO₂ <0.25) during the 1st wk, but then experience early pulmonary deterioration and increased O₂ requirement (FIO₂ >0.25) during the 2nd wk, have a modest risk (approximately 50%) of developing BPD. Infants that have an early, persistently high (FIO₂ >0.25) need for supplemental oxygen have a significantly high (70%) risk of developing BPD.

Respiratory distress, commonly characterized by tachypnea and retractions, persists or worsens and is associated with hypercapnia, hypoxia, and oxygen dependence. The chest radiograph evolves from that of RDS to relative hyperinflation and fine, diffuse interstitial opacities. Wandering atelectasis is common. In the most severe cases, usually associated with prolonged mechanical ventilation and chronically high supplemental oxygen needs, frank cystic changes and/or pneumatoceles are observed (Fig. 122.6). Infants with severe BPD often demonstrate airway obstruction. Excessive airway mucus and edema, airway instability caused by acquired tracheobronchomalacia, and bronchospasm are proposed etiologies. Acute airway obstruction is manifest clinically by abrupt hypoxemia and bradycardia and is often referred to as *BPD spells*. Acute, intermittent right-to-left intracardiac or intrapulmonary shunting caused by abrupt elevations in pulmonary artery pressure may also contribute. Spells are notoriously difficult to control, but occasionally will respond to bronchodilators and sedation acutely.

A common, increasingly recognized complication of BPD is **pulmonary hypertension**. Prospective surveillance indicates that in approximately 15% of all infants born at <1,000 g and <28 wk GA, echocardiographic signs of pulmonary hypertension will develop. Prenatal growth restriction, prolonged duration of mechanical ventilation and supplemental oxygen,

and increasing severity of BPD are all associated with an increased risk. Pulmonary hypertension has been reported in as many as 40% of infants with the most severe BPD and can progress to right-sided heart failure. Consistently, pulmonary hypertension complicating BPD has been associated with increased mortality.

DIAGNOSIS

BPD is diagnosed when a preterm infant requires supplemental oxygen for the 1st 28 postnatal days, and it is further classified at 36 wk PMA according to the degree of O₂ supplementation (Table 122.2). Neonates receiving positive pressure support or ≥30% supplemental O₂ at 36 wk PMA or at discharge (whichever occurs first) are diagnosed as having **severe** BPD; those requiring 22–29% supplemental O₂ have **moderate** BPD; and those who previously required O₂ supplementation for at least 28 days but are currently breathing room air have **mild** BPD. Infants receiving <30% supplemental O₂ should undergo a stepwise 2% reduction in supplemental O₂ to room air while under continuous observation and with SO₂ monitoring to determine whether they can be weaned off oxygen (physiologic definition of BPD). This test is highly reliable and correlated with discharge home on oxygen, length of hospital stay, and hospital readmissions in the 1st yr of life. The risk of neurodevelopmental impairment and pulmonary morbidity and the severity of BPD are directly correlated.

Despite its simplicity, the current severity-based definition of BPD has limitations. Because of incomplete or inaccurate data related to hospital transfer or early discharge, in a significant number of infants the diagnosis of BPD is either not documented or misapplied. Additionally, those infants requiring O₂ support at relatively high flow (>2 L/min) or very low (<0.25 L/min) are not well characterized. Calculation of *effective oxygen* may be helpful but is cumbersome and not well validated. Many clinical trials have simply relied on the need for supplemental O₂ at 36 wk PMA to define BPD. While this definition can diagnose BPD in the highest percentage of infants, it cannot discriminate between infants with milder BPD from those with most severe forms of BPD. In general, any definition of BPD striving to identify infants who benefit from long-term follow up and therapy has been disappointing. Therefore an improved yet feasible definition of BPD is required that accurately evaluates the utility of investigational therapies, predicts long-term outcomes, and directs clinical care.

PREVENTION

In general, there remains a lack of effective interventions that prevent BPD. Avoidance of mechanical ventilation with the early use of **nCPAP** and early, selective **surfactant** replacement therapy with rapid extubation decrease the incidence of BPD modestly. The avoidance of mechanical ventilation achieved by the combination of early rescue surfactant by the INSURE, MIST, or LISA method with nCPAP has been associated with a modest reduction in BPD. Gentle ventilation strategies, including volume-targeted ventilation and HFOV, have also been associated with small, inconsistent reductions in BPD. **Caffeine** therapy for apnea of

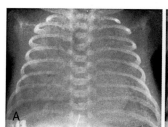 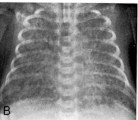 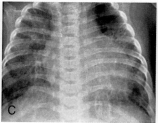 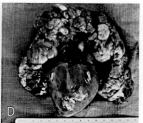

Fig. 122.6 Pulmonary changes in infants treated with prolonged, intermittent positive pressure breathing with air containing 80–100% oxygen in the immediate postnatal period for the clinical syndrome of hyaline membrane disease. **A,** A 5 day old infant with nearly complete opacification of the lungs. **B,** A 13 day old infant with "bubbly lungs" simulating the radiographic appearance of the Wilson-Mikity syndrome. **C,** A 7 mo old infant with irregular, dense strands in both lungs, hyperinflation, and cardiomegaly suggestive of chronic lung disease. **D,** Large right ventricle and a cobbly, irregular aerated lung of an infant who died at 11 mo of age. This infant also had a patent ductus arteriosus. *(From Northway WH Jr, Rosan RC, Porter DY: Pulmonary disease following respiratory therapy of hyaline-membrane disease, N Engl J Med 276:357–368, 1967.)*

Table 122.2	Definition of Bronchopulmonary Dysplasia (BPD): Diagnostic Criteria*	
	GESTATIONAL AGE	
	<32 Wk	**≥32 Wk**
Time point of assessment	36 wk PMA or discharge home, whichever comes first Treatment with >21% oxygen for at least 28 days **plus**:	>28 days but <56 days postnatal age or discharge home, whichever comes first Treatment with >21% oxygen for at least 28 days **plus**:
Mild BPD	Breathing room air at 36 wk PMA or discharge home, whichever comes first	Breathing room air by 56 days postnatal age or discharge home, whichever comes first
Moderate BPD	Need[†] for <30% oxygen at 36 wk PMA or discharge home, whichever comes first	Need[†] for <30% oxygen at 56 days postnatal age or discharge home, whichever comes first
Severe BPD	Need[†] for ≥30% oxygen and/or positive pressure (PPV or NCPAP) at 36 wk PMA or discharge home, whichever comes first	Need[†] for ≥30% oxygen and/or positive pressure (PPV or NCPAP) at 56 days postnatal age or discharge home, whichever comes first

*BPD usually develops in neonates being treated with oxygen and PPV for respiratory failure, most frequently respiratory distress syndrome (RDS). Persistence of the clinical features of respiratory disease (tachypnea, retractions, crackles) is considered common to the broad description of BPD and has not been included in the diagnostic criteria describing the severity of BPD. Infants treated with >21% oxygen and/or PPV for nonrespiratory disease (e.g., central apnea or diaphragmatic paralysis) do not have BPD unless parenchymal lung disease also develops and they have clinical features of respiratory distress. A day of treatment with >21% oxygen means that the infant received >21% oxygen for >12 hr on that day. Treatment with >21% oxygen and/or PPV at 36 wk PMA or at 56 days postnatal age or discharge should not reflect an "acute" event, but should rather reflect the infant's usual daily therapy for several days preceding and after 36 wk PMA, 56 days postnatal age, or discharge.

[†]A physiologic test confirming that the oxygen requirement at the assessment time point remains to be defined. This assessment may include a pulse oximetry saturation range.

NCPAP, Nasal continuous positive airway pressure; PMA, postmenstrual age; PPV, positive pressure ventilation.

From Jobe AH, Bancalari E: Bronchopulmonary dysplasia, *Am J Respir Crit Care Med* 163:1723–1729, 2001.

prematurity has also been associated with a decreased risk of BPD. Although the mechanisms are unknown, caffeine likely supports effective spontaneous respiration and decreases the likelihood that an infant will need invasive mechanical ventilation.

Animal models of BPD have consistently demonstrated that **vitamin A** supplementation promotes distal alveolar development. Previously, provision of intramuscular (IM) vitamin A (5,000 IU 3 times/wk for 4 wk) to VLBW infants was shown to reduce the risk of BPD (1 case prevented for every 14-15 infants treated). However, with the widespread use of early nCPAP, it is unclear if a significant benefit remains, and therefore the use of vitamin A has been inconsistent. Despite promising preclinical data in animal models, the use of prophylactic iNO does not consistently prevent BPD, and its routine use is not recommended.

Systemic corticosteroids (dexamethasone) given either early (<7 days of age to ventilated infants at risk of BPD) or late (>7 days of age to infants with progressing lung disease) prevent both mortality and BPD significantly, but because of the increased risk of **cerebral palsy (CP)** and **neurodevelopmental impairment**, their routine use is not recommended. The risk of neurodevelopmental impairment related to systemic corticosteroid use may be offset by the risk associated with BPD. A systematic review suggested that systemic corticosteroid therapy, when directed to infants with a ≥65% risk of developing BPD, may actually reduce the risk of neurodevelopmental impairment and CP. Although predictive models that use clinical characteristics have been described with promising accuracy, randomized trials using them to guide corticosteroid therapy have not been performed. Systemic hydrocortisone given early to extremely preterm infants at risk for BPD, especially those exposed to chorioamnionitis, may prevent BPD without neurodevelopmental impairment. However, at this time there is insufficient data on safety to support its routine use. **Inhaled corticosteroids** administered to VLBW infants requiring mechanical ventilation at 7-14 days of age did not prevent BPD significantly. However, early, prolonged administration to mechanically ventilated extremely preterm infants until they no longer require oxygen or positive pressure support has been shown to reduce the risk of BPD, but with a concerning trend toward increased mortality. Experience with local delivery of corticosteroids by spiking surfactant with **budesonide** is emerging, and early data suggest that **endotracheal** administration of corticosteroids may reduce pulmonary inflammation and the risk of BPD and death. However, additional evidence is needed before widespread use is implemented. The routine use of antibiotics, inhaled bronchodilators, or diuretics has not been shown to prevent BPD.

TREATMENT

Treatment of evolving and established BPD is supportive, and evidence-based therapies are lacking. The basic tenets of therapy should include appropriate support of ventilation and aggressive nutritional support to optimize linear growth and encourage normal lung repair and development. Despite a lack of support from investigational studies in the current era of BPD, numerous medical interventions are employed. Available evidence suggests short-term benefits (improved pulmonary mechanics, modest reductions in respiratory support parameters) without an indication of impact on clinically relevant outcomes (survival, need for long-term respiratory support, recurrent hospitalization). Currently, available evidence does not support the routine use of any pharmacologic agents in infants with evolving or established BPD. Treatment decisions must weigh the perceived benefit against the potential harm, since data on not only efficacy, but more importantly safety, remain inadequate.

Diuretics and Fluid Restriction

Infants with BPD often have excessive pulmonary interstitial fluid that compromises lung function and increases work of breathing. Diuretic therapy (usually with furosemide or chlorothiazide) has been associated with short-term, temporary improvements in pulmonary compliance and the ability to wean respiratory support. **Furosemide** (1 mg/kg/dose IV or 2 mg/kg/dose PO every 12-24 hr) has been demonstrated to decrease pulmonary interstitial emphysema and PVR, improve pulmonary function, and facilitate weaning from mechanical ventilation and oxygen. Adverse effects of long-term furosemide therapy are common and include hyponatremia, hypokalemia, alkalosis, azotemia, hypocalcemia, hypercalciuria, cholelithiasis, renal stones, nephrocalcinosis, and ototoxicity. Potassium chloride supplementation is often necessary. Thiazide diuretics (e.g., chlorothiazide, 5-10 mg/kg/dose every 12 hr) have been used as an alternative to avoid hypercalciuria, limit nephrocalcinosis, and preserve bone development. Although avoidance of excessive fluid administration in the 1st few wk of age is associated with a reduced risk of BPD, there is no evidence that fluid restriction (130-140 mL/kg/day) in established BPD has any impact. Whether using diuretics or fluid restriction, careful attention to maintaining appropriate electrolyte levels as well as providing adequate caloric intake (often >120-130 kcal/kg/day) is paramount to avoid negatively impacting nutrition.

Bronchodilators

Inhaled bronchodilators improve lung mechanics by decreasing airway resistance. **Albuterol** is a specific β_2-agonist used to treat bronchospasm in infants with BPD. Albuterol may improve lung compliance by decreasing airway resistance secondary to smooth muscle cell relaxation. Changes in pulmonary mechanics may last as long as 4-6 hr. Hypertension and tachycardia are common adverse effects. **Ipratropium bromide** is a muscarinic antagonist related to atropine, but the bronchodilator effect is more potent. Use of ipratropium bromide in BPD has been associated with improved pulmonary mechanics. Compared to either agent used alone, combined use of albuterol and ipratropium bromide may be more effective. Few adverse effects have been noted. With current aerosol administration strategies, exactly how much medication is delivered to the airways and lungs of infants with BPD, especially if they are ventilator dependent, is unclear.

Corticosteroids

In addition to their use at an early age (<7 days) to prevent BPD, **systemic corticosteroids** have also been used to treat evolving and established BPD. In mechanically ventilated infants, systemic corticosteroids improve pulmonary mechanics, allow weaning of ventilator support and supplemental O_2, and facilitate extubation. When given at >7 days of age, long-term benefits include a reduced need for O_2 at 36 wk PMA, improved survival, and decreased need for home O_2. Short-term adverse effects include hyperglycemia, hypertension, and transient hypertrophic obstructive cardiomyopathy. Long-term adverse effects include osteopenia, severe retinopathy of prematurity (ROP), abnormal neurological examination, poor brain growth, neurodevelopmental impairment, and CP. Although meta-analyses suggest that the long-term detrimental effects on neurodevelopment might be mitigated by later postnatal use, open-label use of corticosteroids in control groups makes analysis of safety unreliable. A strategy that utilizes a low cumulative dose (0.89 mg/kg given over 10-day taper) in preterm infants who remain ventilator dependent after 7 days of age (and therefore have a high risk of developing BPD) facilitates weaning of ventilator and oxygen support and promotes successful extubation without an impact on long-term outcomes, including the incidence of BPD or neurodevelopmental impairment. However, randomized controlled trials (RCTs) with appropriate power to assess safety are lacking. The controversy concerning the appropriate use of systemic corticosteroids to prevent and/or treat BPD is ongoing, and until additional evidence is available, their use remains limited to infants with severe respiratory failure (ventilator dependent at >7-14 days of age with significant respiratory and oxygen support needs) at high risk for imminent death.

In an effort to avoid the detrimental effects of systemic corticosteroids, **inhaled corticosteroids** (budesonide, fluticasone, and beclomethasone) have been described as an alternative antiinflammatory therapy in evolving or established BPD. Small RCTs and case reports in infants with established moderate-severe BPD have not shown a significant benefit for pulmonary mechanics or reduction in the need for ventilator or oxygen support.

Pulmonary Vasodilators

Many infants with evolving or established moderate and severe BPD demonstrate pulmonary vascular resistance caused by pulmonary microvascular maldevelopment and abnormal vasoreactivity. In infants with BPD with pulmonary hypertension, acute exposure to even modest levels of hypoxemia can cause pulmonary artery pressure (PAP) to increase abruptly. Maintaining infants with established BPD and pulmonary hypertension at higher SO_2 targets (92-96%) can lower PAP effectively. For infants in whom appropriate O_2 supplementation and support of ventilation are ineffective, the use of low-dose **inhaled NO** may improve oxygenation anecdotally. Despite its frequent use, there is no evidence to support the use of iNO to improve lung function, cardiac function, or oxygenation in evolving BPD. Several case series have reported on the use of the phosphodiesterase-5 inhibitor **sildenafil** in treating pulmonary hypertension in established moderate to severe BPD. Despite its widespread use, no RCTs are evaluating the safety and efficacy of sildenafil in preterm infants with BPD. However, many experts would recommend a trial of low-dose sildenafil (1 mg/kg/dose every 8 hr) for infants with evidence of pulmonary hypertension and persistent respiratory instability despite appropriate oxygen and ventilator support.

Chronic Respiratory Support

Evidence is lacking to guide respiratory management in evolving and established BPD. Experience suggests that maintaining FRC with appropriate positive pressure support (with noninvasive support whenever possible) promotes optimal lung growth and development. Provision of nCPAP until respiratory status improves and oxygen dependence resolves, with subsequent transition directly to room air, may be beneficial but is not based on evidence. Continuation of caffeine therapy may facilitate spontaneous breathing and weaning from support. Established severe BPD with cystic, heterogeneous lung disease requires prolonged mechanical ventilation. A long inspiratory time is required to adequately ventilate diseased lung units, and appropriate expiratory time is required to allow exhalation. The use of a low rate (<20-30 breaths/min), long inspiratory time (≥0.6 sec) strategy is usually required. To attain appropriate minute ventilation, larger tidal volumes (10-12 mL/kg) are necessary. Higher PEEP (often >6-8 cm) may be needed to attain adequate expansion and minimize gas-trapping caused by dynamic airway collapse. Gradual weaning of ventilator settings should be attempted as the infant grows and lung disease improves, but the incidence of death or tracheostomy placement for chronic ventilation may be as high as 20%. By 2-3 yr of age, the majority of infants who undergo tracheostomy for severe BPD are successfully liberated from mechanical ventilation.

PROGNOSIS

Compared with extremely preterm infants without BPD, infants with BPD have higher rates of neurodevelopmental impairment, lung diffusion impairment, wheezing and airflow obstruction, rehospitalization, and mortality. The risk of these complications increases with BPD severity. Prolonged mechanical ventilation, IVH, pulmonary hypertension, cor pulmonale, and oxygen dependence beyond 1 yr of life are poor prognostic signs. Mortality in infants with BPD ranges from 10-25% and is highest in infants who remain ventilator dependent for >6 mo. Cardiorespiratory failure associated with cor pulmonale and acquired infection (respiratory syncytial virus) are common causes of death. Infants are at risk for severe RSV infections and must receive prophylactic therapy (see Chapter 287).

Pulmonary function slowly improves in most survivors because of ongoing lung repair and the natural period of lung growth and alveolarization. *Rehospitalization* for impaired pulmonary function is most common during the 1st 3 yr of life and is much more common in infants requiring respiratory support at discharge. The incidence of physician-diagnosed asthma, use of bronchodilators, and wheezing is elevated. Despite a gradual decrease in symptom frequency, persistence of respiratory symptoms and abnormal pulmonary function test results are measurable in children, adolescence, and young adults. Although not always clinically apparent, pulmonary function testing consistently reveals impaired exercise capacity, reduced pulmonary diffusing capacity, and persistent expiratory flow obstruction. High-resolution chest CT scanning or MRI studies in children and adults with a history of BPD reveal lung abnormalities that correlate directly with the degree of pulmonary function abnormality. The ultimate long-term pulmonary health of survivors of BPD is unknown. As trajectories of developing lung function remain abnormal in survivors of BPD, concerns have been raised highlighting the potential for pulmonary emphysema, chronic obstructive pulmonary disease, and pulmonary vascular disease resulting in early debilitating lung dysfunction.

Other complications of BPD include growth failure, neurodevelopmental impairment, and parental stress, as well as sequelae of therapy, such as nephrolithiasis, osteopenia, and electrolyte imbalance. Airway problems such as vocal cord paralysis, subglottic stenosis, and tracheomalacia are common and may aggravate or cause pulmonary hypertension. Subglottic stenosis may require tracheotomy or an anterior cricoid split procedure to relieve upper airway obstruction. Cardiac complications of BPD include pulmonary hypertension, cor pulmonale, systemic hypertension, left ventricular hypertrophy, and development of aorto-pulmonary collateral vessels, which, if large, may cause heart failure.

Bibliography is available at Expert Consult.

122.5 Patent Ductus Arteriosus
Shawn K. Ahlfeld

INCIDENCE AND PATHOPHYSIOLOGY
Some neonates with RDS may have clinically significant shunting through a patent ductus arteriosus (**PDA**). Although ductal closure occurs by 72 hr after birth in almost all term infants, at the same age in 65% of preterm infants born at <30 wk GA, the ductus remains patent. Risk factors for delayed closure of the PDA include hypoxia, acidosis, increased pulmonary pressure secondary to vasoconstriction, systemic hypotension, immaturity, and local release of prostaglandins (which dilate the ductus). Shunting through the PDA may initially be bidirectional or right to left. As respiratory distress syndrome (RDS) resolves, pulmonary vascular resistance (PVR) decreases, and left-to-right shunting may occur, leading to left ventricular (LV) volume overload and pulmonary edema.

CLINICAL MANIFESTATIONS
Manifestations of PDA may include (1) a hyperdynamic precordium, bounding peripheral pulses, wide pulse pressure, and a machine-like continuous or systolic murmur; (2) radiographic evidence of cardio-megaly and increased pulmonary vascular markings; (3) hepatomegaly; (4) increasing oxygen dependence; (5) carbon dioxide retention; and (6) renal failure. Infants with a hemodynamically significant PDA often require escalation of ventilator and oxygen support. The diag-nosis is confirmed by echocardiographic visualization of a PDA with Doppler flow imaging that demonstrates left-to-right or bidirectional shunting.

TREATMENT
Management of the PDA is controversial, and evidence to guide treatment is limited. Prophylactic closure before signs of a PDA, closure of the asymptomatic but clinically detected PDA, and closure of the symptomatic PDA are 3 management strategies. Interventions to encourage ductal closure include fluid restriction, cyclooxygenase (COX) inhibitors (indomethacin or ibuprofen), and surgical ligation. Short-term benefits of any therapy have to be balanced against adverse effects, such as transient renal dysfunction and fluid imbalances associated with indomethacin.

By the time of discharge in the majority of extremely preterm infants (>90%), the PDA will close spontaneously. Spontaneous ductal closure may be facilitated by general supportive measures, including early (<7 days of age) avoidance of excessive fluid administration and judicious use of diuretics to manage pulmonary edema. However, within the 1st week of age, in 30% of infants with birthweight <1,500 g and 70% of infants <1,000 g, the PDA persists. Although many preterm infants with persistent PDA will remain clinically stable while awaiting spontane-ous closure, approximately 60% of infants <1,000 g will develop significant clinical instability (hypotension, renal failure, worsening respiratory failure secondary to pulmonary edema). Pharmacologic and surgical ductal closure may be indicated in the premature infant with a moderate to large, hemodynamically significant PDA when there is a delay in clinical improvement or deterioration.

Pharmacologic Closure
Pharmacologic closure of the PDA has been described using COX inhibitors that inhibit prostaglandin production, with equivalent efficacy and safety profiles described for ibuprofen and indomethacin. The efficacy of pharmacological therapy is inversely proportional to the gestational and postnatal age, and closure is more likely when medication is administered before 14-21 days of age. However, successful closure has been reported up to 8 wk of age. Whether indomethacin or ibuprofen is used, 20–40% of infants demonstrate treatment failure, and of those infants, 10–20% require eventual surgical ligation. Rates of recurrence following successful pharmacologic closure in general are low (<15%). Neither therapy significantly impacts the rate of NEC, BPD, or mortal-ity. **General contraindications** to both indomethacin and ibuprofen include thrombocytopenia (<50,000 platelets/mm^3), active hemorrhage (including severe IVH), NEC or isolated intestinal perforation, elevated plasma creatinine (>1.8 mg/dL), or oliguria (urine output <1 mL/kg/hr). Importantly, the concomitant use of hydrocortisone and indomethacin in extremely preterm infants must be avoided, because the combination is associated with a dramatic increase in spontaneous intestinal perforation. Despite that indomethacin reduces mesenteric blood flow, mounting experience suggests that low-volume trophic enteral feeding during administration is safe.

Prophylactic **indomethacin** given over the 1st 72 hr of age to preterm infants with birthweight <1,000 g reduces the incidence of severe IVH (grade III/IV), pulmonary hemorrhage, symptomatic PDA, and need for surgical PDA ligation. Although often implicated in spontaneous intestinal perforation and NEC, RCTs have failed to demonstrate that indomethacin increases their risk significantly. Short-term side effects include reductions in cerebral, mesenteric, and renal blood flow. Oliguria unresponsive to diuretic therapy is observed frequently. Dosing regimens for indomethacin vary considerably, but it usually is administered as a slow IV infusion (0.1-0.2 mg/kg/dose over 30 min) every 12-24 hr for 3 doses. A repeat course can be attempted if the duct fails to close or reopens, but additional (>2) courses do not appear to be efficacious. Longer courses (5-7 days) of indomethacin are not recommended because of to an increased risk of NEC in one trial.

Ibuprofen is as effective as indomethacin in closing a PDA, but ibuprofen is associated with reduced rates of oliguria and a small but significant reduction in the length of mechanical ventilation. Although higher doses may improve closure rates in the most immature infants, the typical IV or enteral dosing regimen for ibuprofen is 10 mg/kg for 1 dose, followed by 2 doses of 5 mg/kg every 24 hr. As with indomethacin, a repeat course may be considered, but additional courses of ibuprofen are not efficacious and not recommended. Risk of NEC is not increased with indomethacin, but ibuprofen reduces the relative risk of NEC comparatively. Unlike indomethacin, ibuprofen has not been shown to reduce the risk of severe IVH. Compared to the IV route, enteral ibuprofen may be more efficacious. Whether ibuprofen used in combina-tion with hydrocortisone results in increased risk of spontaneous intestinal perforation is unknown.

Preliminary studies suggest that **acetaminophen** may be an effective drug to close a PDA, with fewer side effects than existing agents.

Surgical Ligation
The infant whose symptomatic PDA fails to close with pharmacologic interventions or who has contraindications to COX inhibitors is a candidate for surgical closure. Although the long-term benefits are unclear, surgical ligation in infants born at <28 wk GA and <1,250 g is associated with improved survival. Surgical mortality is very low even in ELBW infants. However, **postligation cardiac syndrome**, a significant drop in blood pressure 6-12 hr after ductal ligation, is experienced by up to 50% of LBW infants. The hypotension has been attributed to increased systemic vascular resistance along with decreased pulmonary venous return, resulting in impaired preload and LV function. Fluid resuscitation, inotropic support (with dobu-tamine or milrinone), and hydrocortisone are usually effective. Other complications of surgery include hemorrhage, pneumothorax, chylo-thorax, Horner syndrome, and injury to the recurrent laryngeal nerve resulting in vocal cord dysfunction. Inadvertent ligation of the left pul-monary artery or the transverse aortic arch has rarely been reported. Increased rates of neurodevelopmental impairment have been reported following surgical ligation, although a causal relationship remains uncertain.

Bibliography is available at Expert Consult.

122.6 Transient Tachypnea of the Newborn
Shawn K. Ahlfeld

Transient tachypnea of the newborn (**TTN**) is a clinical syndrome of self-limited tachypnea associated with delayed clearance of fetal lung fluid. Although the actual incidence is likely underreported, it is estimated at 3-6 per 1,000 term infant births, making TTN the most common etiology of tachypnea in the newborn. Twin gestation, maternal asthma, late prematurity, precipitous delivery, gestational diabetes, and cesarean delivery without labor are common associated risk factors. Clearance of fetal lung fluid occurs through increased expression of epithelial sodium channels (ENaC) and sodium-potassium adenosine triphosphatase (Na^+,K^+-ATPase) that drive active sodium (and thereby fluid) reabsorption. TTN is believed to result from ineffective expression or activity of ENaC and Na^+,K^+-ATPase, which slows absorption of fetal lung fluid and results in decreased pulmonary compliance and impeded gas exchange.

TTN is characterized by the early onset of tachypnea (>60 breaths/min), sometimes with retractions or expiratory grunting and occasionally with cyanosis that is relieved by minimal O_2 supplementation (<40%). The chest generally sounds clear without crackles or wheeze, and the chest radiograph shows prominent perihilar pulmonary vascular markings, fluid in the intralobar fissures, and rarely small pleural effusions. Hypercapnia and acidosis are uncommon. Respiratory failure requiring positive pressure support (either with nCPAP or mechanical ventilation) also is uncommon, but when it occurs usually resolves rapidly (<12-24 hr). Most infants recover with supportive care alone, and over the first 24-72 hours the tachypnea and O_2 requirements slowly resolve. Distinguishing TTN from RDS and other respiratory disorders (e.g., pneumonia) may be difficult, and transient tachypnea is frequently a diagnosis of exclusion. The distinctive features of TTN are rapid recovery of the infant and the absence of radiographic findings for RDS (low lung volumes, diffuse reticulogranular pattern, air bronchograms) and other lung disorders.

Treatment for TTN is supportive. There is no evidence supporting the use of oral furosemide or nebulized racemic epinephrine in this disorder. Inhaled β_2-agonists such as albuterol (salbutamol) increase expression and activation of ENaC and Na^+,K^+-ATPase and facilitate fluid clearance. Emerging evidence suggests that when given early in the course of TTN, albuterol may improve oxygenation, shorten the duration of supplemental O_2 therapy, and expedite recovery.

Bibliography is available at Expert Consult.

122.7 Aspiration of Foreign Material (Fetal Aspiration Syndrome, Aspiration Pneumonia)
Shawn K. Ahlfeld

With fetal distress, infants often initiate vigorous respiratory movements in utero because of interference with the supply of oxygen through the placenta. Under such circumstances, the infant may aspirate amniotic fluid containing vernix caseosa, epithelial cells, meconium, blood, or material from the birth canal, which may block the smallest airways and interfere with alveolar exchange of O_2 and CO_2. Pathogenic bacteria may accompany the aspirated material, and pneumonia may ensue, but even in noninfected cases, respiratory distress accompanied by radiographic evidence of aspiration is seen (Fig. 122.7).

Postnatal pulmonary aspiration may also occur in newborn infants as a result of prematurity, tracheoesophageal fistula, esophageal and duodenal obstruction, gastroesophageal reflux, improper feeding practices, and administration of depressant medicines. To avoid aspiration of gastric contents, the stomach should be aspirated using a soft catheter just before surgery or other major procedures that require anesthesia or conscious sedation. The treatment of **aspiration pneumonia** is symptomatic and may include respiratory support and systemic antibiot-

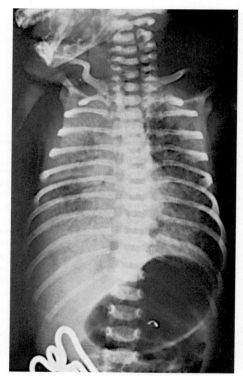

Fig. 122.7 Fetal aspiration syndrome (aspiration pneumonia). Note the coarse granular pattern with irregular aeration typical of fetal distress from the aspiration of material contained in amniotic fluid, such as vernix caseosa, epithelial cells, and meconium. *(From Goodwin SR, Grave SA, Haberkern CM: Aspiration in intubated premature infants, Pediatrics 75:85–88, 1985.)*

ics. Gradual improvement generally occurs over 3-4 days.

122.8 Meconium Aspiration
Shawn K. Ahlfeld

Meconium-stained amniotic fluid is found in 10–15% of births and usually occurs in term or postterm infants. **Meconium aspiration syndrome (MAS)** develops in 5% of such infants; 30% require mechanical ventilation, and 3–5% die. Usually, but not invariably, fetal distress and hypoxia occur before the passage of meconium into amniotic fluid. The infants are meconium stained and may be depressed and require resuscitation at birth. Fig. 122.8 shows the pathophysiology of the MAS. Infants with MAS are at increased risk of **persistent pulmonary hypertension** (see Chapter 122.9).

CLINICAL MANIFESTATIONS
Either in utero or with the first breath, thick, particulate meconium is aspirated into the lungs. The resulting small airway obstruction may produce respiratory distress within the 1st hours, with tachypnea, retractions, grunting, and cyanosis observed in severely affected infants. Partial obstruction of some airways may lead to pneumomediastinum, pneumothorax, or both. Overdistention of the chest may be prominent. The condition usually improves within 72 hr, but when its course requires assisted ventilation, it may be severe with a high risk for mortality. Tachypnea may persist for many days or even several weeks. The typical chest radiograph is characterized by patchy infiltrates, coarse streaking of both lung fields, increased anteroposterior diameter, and flattening of the diaphragm. A normal chest radiograph in an infant with severe

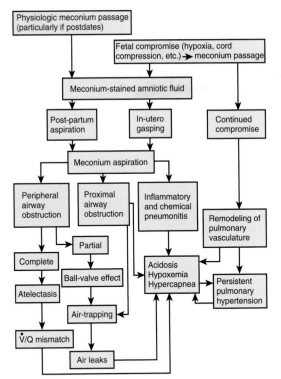

Fig. 122.8 Pathophysiology of meconium passage and the meconium aspiration syndrome. V̇/Q̇, Ventilation-perfusion ratio. *(From Wiswell TE, Bent RC: Meconium staining and the meconium aspiration syndrome: unresolved issues, Pediatr Clin North Am 40:955–981, 1993.)*

hypoxemia and no cardiac malformation suggests the diagnosis of pulmonary hypertension.

PREVENTION

The risk of meconium aspiration may be decreased by rapid identification of fetal distress and initiation of prompt delivery in the presence of late fetal heart rate deceleration or poor beat-to-beat FHR variability. Despite initial enthusiasm for amnioinfusion, it does not reduce the risk of MAS, cesarean delivery, or other major indicators of maternal or neonatal morbidity. Intrapartum nasopharyngeal suctioning in infants with meconium-stained amniotic fluid does not reduce the risk for MAS. Routine intubation and aspiration of depressed infants (those with hypotonia, bradycardia, or decreased respiratory effort) born through meconium-stained fluid is not effective in reducing the MAS or other major adverse outcomes and is not recommended for neonatal resuscitation.

TREATMENT

Treatment of the MAS includes supportive care and standard management for respiratory distress. The beneficial effect of mean airway pressure on oxygenation must be weighed against the risk of pneumothorax. Administration of exogenous surfactant and/or iNO to infants with MAS and hypoxemic respiratory failure, or pulmonary hypertension requiring mechanical ventilation, decreases the need for extracorporeal membrane oxygenation (ECMO), which is required by the most severely affected infants who show no response to therapy. In infants with MAS who demonstrate no other signs of sepsis, there is no role for routine antibiotic therapy. Severe meconium aspiration may be complicated by persistent pulmonary hypertension. Patients with MAS refractory to conventional mechanical ventilation may benefit from HFV or ECMO (see Chapter 122.9).

PROGNOSIS

The mortality rate of meconium-stained infants is considerably higher than that of nonstained infants. The decline in neonatal deaths caused by MAS in recent decades is related to improvements in obstetric and neonatal care. Residual lung problems are rare but include symptomatic cough, wheezing, and persistent hyperinflation for up to 5-10 yr. The ultimate prognosis depends on the extent of CNS injury from asphyxia and the presence of associated problems such as pulmonary hypertension.

Bibliography is available at Expert Consult.

122.9 Persistent Pulmonary Hypertension of the Newborn (Persistent Fetal Circulation)
Shawn K. Ahlfeld

Persistent pulmonary hypertension of the newborn (**PPHN**) occurs in term and postterm infants most often. Predisposing factors include birth asphyxia, MAS, early-onset sepsis, RDS, hypoglycemia, polycythemia, maternal use of nonsteroidal antiinflammatory drugs with in utero constriction of the ductus arteriosus, maternal late trimester use of selective serotonin reuptake inhibitors, and pulmonary hypoplasia caused by diaphragmatic hernia, amniotic fluid leak, oligohydramnios, or pleural effusions. PPHN is often idiopathic. Some patients with PPHN have low plasma arginine and NO metabolite concentrations and polymorphisms of the carbamoyl phosphate synthase gene, findings suggestive of a possible subtle defect in NO production. The incidence is 1 in 500-1,500 live births, with a wide variation among clinical centers. Regardless of etiology of PPHN, profound hypoxemia from right-to-left shunting and normal or elevated $PaCO_2$ are present (Fig. 122.9).

PATHOPHYSIOLOGY

Persistence of the fetal circulatory pattern of right-to-left shunting through the PDA and foramen ovale after birth is a result of excessively high pulmonary vascular resistance (PVR). Fetal PVR is usually elevated relative to fetal systemic or postnatal pulmonary pressure. This fetal state normally permits shunting of oxygenated umbilical venous blood to the left atrium (and brain) through the foramen ovale, from which it bypasses the lungs through the ductus arteriosus and passes to the descending aorta. After birth, PVR normally declines rapidly as a consequence of vasodilation secondary to lung inflation, a rise in postnatal PaO_2, a reduction in $PaCO_2$, increased pH, and release of vasoactive substances. Increased neonatal PVR may be (1) **maladaptive** from an acute injury (not demonstrating normal vasodilation in response to increased O_2 and other changes after birth); (2) the result of increased pulmonary artery medial muscle thickness and extension of smooth muscle layers into the usually nonmuscular, more peripheral pulmonary arterioles in response to chronic fetal hypoxia; (3) a consequence of **pulmonary hypoplasia** (diaphragmatic hernia, Potter syndrome); or (4) **obstructive** as a result of polycythemia, total anomalous pulmonary venous return (TAPVR), or congenital diffuse development disorders of acinar lung development.

CLINICAL MANIFESTATIONS

PPHN usually manifests in the delivery room or within the 1st 12 hr after birth. Idiopathic PPHN or PPHN related to polycythemia, hypoglycemia, hypothermia, or asphyxia may result in severe cyanosis and respiratory distress. In some cases, however, initial signs of respiratory distress may be minimal. Infants who have PPHN associated with meconium aspiration, group B streptococcal pneumonia, diaphragmatic hernia, or pulmonary hypoplasia usually exhibit cyanosis, grunting, flaring, retractions, tachycardia, and shock. Multiorgan involvement may be present (see Table 119.2). Myocardial ischemia, papillary muscle dysfunction with mitral and tricuspid regurgitation, and biventricular dysfunction produce cardiogenic shock with decreases in pulmonary

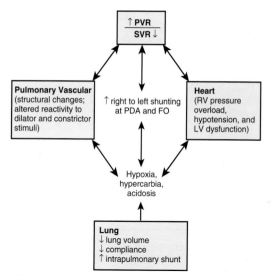

Fig. 122.9 Cardiopulmonary interactions in persistent pulmonary hypertension of the newborn (PPHN). FO, Foramen ovale; LV, left ventricular; PDA, patent ductus arteriosus; PVR, pulmonary vascular resistance; RV, right ventricular; SVR, systemic vascular resistance. *(From Kinsella JP, Abman SH: Recent developments in the pathophysiology and treatment of persistent pulmonary hypertension of the newborn, J Pediatr 126:853–864, 1995.)*

blood flow, tissue perfusion, and O_2 delivery.

Hypoxemia is often labile and out of proportion to the findings on chest radiographs. In asphyxia-associated and idiopathic PPHN, chest x-ray findings are often normal, whereas in PPHN associated with **pneumonia** and **diaphragmatic hernia**, parenchymal opacification and bowel/liver in the chest, respectively, are seen.

DIAGNOSIS
Independent of the prenatal history, PPHN should be suspected in all term infants who have cyanosis. Hypoxemia is universal and intermittently unresponsive to 100% O_2 given by oxygen hood. A transient improvement may occur in response to hyperoxic hyperventilation administered by positive pressure ventilation. A PaO_2 or SaO_2 gradient between a preductal (right radial artery) and a postductal (umbilical artery) site of blood sampling suggests right-to-left shunting through the ductus arteriosus. Intracardiac shunting through the patent foramen ovale does not lead to a PaO_2 or SaO_2 gradient.

Real-time echocardiography combined with Doppler flow imaging is very helpful in evaluating PPHN. Systolic flattening of the interventricular septum as the right ventricular systolic pressure approaches the left ventricular systolic pressure can be used to estimate the degree of pulmonary hypertension. The peak velocity of the tricuspid valve regurgitation jet, when present, yields a quantitative estimate of the right ventricular systolic pressure. Likewise, the direction and velocity of a shunt across the PDA provides a quantitative comparison between the aortic and pulmonary artery pressures. In advanced cases, right-to-left or bidirectional shunting across a PDA and a patent foramen ovale can be observed.

The differential diagnosis of PPHN includes cyanotic heart disease (especially obstructed TAPVR), idiopathic pulmonary vein stenosis, congenital surfactant deficiency syndromes, pulmonary artery thrombosis, and congenital diffuse development disorders of acinar lung development (acinar dysplasia, congenital alveolar dysplasia, and alveolar capillary dysplasia with misalignment of the pulmonary veins).

Alveolocapillary dysplasia (ACD) is a rare, highly lethal autosomal recessive disorder of distal lung development characterized by immature lobular development and reduced capillary density. Infants with ACD present with idiopathic PPHN, demonstrating little or no parenchymal lung disease and profound hypoxemia. Over 60% of infants with ACD manifest hypoxemia and respiratory failure within 48 hr of birth, while some with milder disease present beyond 6 mo of age. The diagnosis is made on autopsy in 90% of cases, and the constellation of findings include thickened alveolar septa, increased muscularization of the pulmonary arterioles, a reduced number of capillaries, with the remaining capillaries demonstrating abnormal apposition to the air interface, and misalignment of the intrapulmonary veins. In up to 80% of cases, extrapulmonary malformations of the genitourinary, gastrointestinal, or cardiovascular system are present. Mutations in the transcription factor gene *FOXFI* have been identified in up to 40% of cases, but the diagnosis continues to rest on clinical and histopathologic features. ACD is uniformly lethal and should be suspected in infants with idiopathic PPHN who fail to respond to maximal medical therapy, or when symptoms recur after successful weaning from ECMO. In a United Kingdom ECMO report, up to 14% of infants who failed ECMO ultimately were diagnosed with ACD. Regardless of the timing of presentation, ACD is uniformly fatal, and lung transplantation remains the sole, experimental therapy.

TREATMENT
Therapy for PPHN is directed toward correcting any predisposing condition (e.g., hypoglycemia, polycythemia) and improving poor tissue oxygenation. The response to therapy is often unpredictable, transient, and complicated by the adverse effects of drugs or mechanical ventilation. Initial management includes O_2 administration and correction of acidosis, hypotension, and hypercapnia. Persistent hypoxemia should be managed with intubation and mechanical ventilation.

Infants with PPHN are usually managed without hyperventilation or alkalization. Gentle ventilation with normocarbia or permissive hypercarbia and avoidance of hypoxemia result in excellent outcomes and a low incidence of chronic lung disease and ECMO use.

Because of their instability and ability to fight the ventilator, newborns with PPHN usually require **sedation**. The use of paralytic agents is controversial and reserved for the newborn who cannot be treated with sedatives alone. Muscle relaxants may promote atelectasis of dependent lung regions and ventilation-perfusion mismatch and may be associated with an increased risk of death.

Inotropic therapy is frequently needed to support blood pressure and perfusion. Whereas dopamine is frequently used as a first-line agent, other agents, such as dobutamine, epinephrine, and milrinone, may be helpful when myocardial contractility is poor. Some of the sickest newborns with PPHN demonstrate hypotension refractory to vasopressor administration. This results from desensitization of the cardiovascular system to catecholamines by overwhelming illness and relative adrenal insufficiency. Hydrocortisone rapidly upregulates cardiovascular adrenergic receptor expression and serves as a hormone substitute in cases of adrenal insufficiency.

Inhaled NO is an endothelium-derived signaling molecule that relaxes vascular smooth muscle and can be delivered to the lung by inhalation. *Use of iNO reduces the need for ECMO support by approximately 40%.* The optimal starting dose is 20 ppm. Higher doses have not been shown to be more effective and are associated with side effects, including methemoglobinemia and increased levels of nitrogen dioxide, a pulmonary irritant. Most newborns require iNO for <5 days. Although NO has been used as long-term therapy in children and adults with primary pulmonary hypertension, prolonged dependency is rare in neonates and suggests the presence of lung hypoplasia, congenital heart disease, or ACD. The maximal safe duration of iNO therapy is unknown. The infant can be weaned to 5 ppm after 6-24 hr of therapy. The dose can then be reduced slowly and discontinued when FIO_2 is <0.6 and the iNO dose is 1 ppm. Abrupt discontinuation should be avoided because it may cause rebound pulmonary hypertension. iNO should be used only at institutions that offer ECMO support or have the capability of transporting an infant on iNO therapy if a referral for ECMO is necessary. Some infants with PPHN do not respond adequately to iNO. Therapy with continuous inhaled or IV prostacyclin (prostaglandin I_2) has improved oxygenation and outcome in infants with PPHN. The safety and efficacy of sildenafil (type 5 phosphodiesterase inhibitor) in newborns with PPHN is under investigation; initial results are promising.

In 5–10% of patients with PPHN, the response to 100% O_2, mechanical ventilation, and drugs is poor, and many of these infants benefit from ECMO. In such patients, 2 parameters have been used to predict mortality: the alveolar-arterial oxygen gradient (PA-aO_2), and the oxygenation index (OI), calculated as FIO_2 (as %) × MAP/PaO_2. A PA-aO_2 >620 for 8-12 hr and OI >40 unresponsive to iNO predict a high mortality rate (>80%) and are indications for ECMO. In carefully selected, severely ill infants with hypoxemic respiratory failure caused by RDS, meconium aspiration pneumonia, congenital diaphragmatic hernia, PPHN, or sepsis, ECMO significantly improves survival.

ECMO is a form of cardiopulmonary bypass that augments systemic perfusion and provides gas exchange. Most experience has been with *venoarterial bypass*, which requires carotid artery ligation and the placement of large catheters in the right internal jugular vein and carotid artery. *Venovenous bypass* avoids carotid artery ligation and provides gas exchange, but it does not support cardiac output. Blood is initially pumped through the ECMO circuit at a rate that approximates 80% of the estimated cardiac output, 150-200 mL/kg/min. Venous return passes through a membrane oxygenator, is rewarmed, and returns to the aortic arch in venoarterial ECMO and to the right atrium in venovenous ECMO. Venous O_2 saturation values are used to monitor tissue O_2 delivery and subsequent extraction for infants undergoing venoarterial ECMO, whereas arterial O_2 saturation values are used to monitor oxygenation for infants receiving venovenous ECMO.

Because ECMO requires complete heparinization to prevent clotting in the circuit, its use is generally avoided in patients with existing intracranial hemorrhage or who are at high risk of developing IVH (weight <2 kg, gestational age <34 wk). In addition, infants being considered for ECMO should have reversible lung disease, no signs of systemic bleeding, and no severe asphyxia or lethal malformations, and they should have been ventilated for <10 days. Complications of ECMO include thromboembolism, air embolism, bleeding, stroke, seizures, atelectasis, cholestatic jaundice, thrombocytopenia, neutropenia, hemolysis, infectious complications of blood transfusions, edema formation, and systemic hypertension.

PROGNOSIS
Survival in patients with PPHN varies with the underlying diagnosis. The long-term outcome for infants with PPHN is related to the associated **hypoxic-ischemic encephalopathy** and the ability to reduce PVR. The long-term prognosis for infants who have PPHN and who survive after treatment with hyperventilation is comparable to that for infants who have underlying illnesses of equivalent severity (e.g., birth asphyxia, hypoglycemia, polycythemia). The outcome for infants with PPHN who are treated with ECMO is also favorable; >80–90% survive, and 60–75% of survivors appear normal at 1-3.5 yr of age.

Bibliography is available at Expert Consult.

122.10 Diaphragmatic Hernia
Shawn K. Ahlfeld

A *diaphragmatic hernia* is defined as a communication between the abdominal and thoracic cavities with or without abdominal contents in the thorax (Fig. 122.10). The etiology is rarely traumatic and usually congenital. The symptoms and prognosis depend on the location of the defect and associated anomalies. The defect may be at the esophageal hiatus (**hiatal hernia**); paraesophageal, adjacent to the hiatus (**paraesophageal hernia**; Chapter 122.12); retrosternal (**foramen of Morgagni hernia**; Chapter 122.11); or at the posterolateral portion of the diaphragm (**Bochdalek hernia**). In **congenital diaphragmatic hernia (CDH)** the Bochdalek hernia accounts for up to 90% of the hernias seen, with 80–90% occurring on the left side. The Morgagni hernia accounts for 2–6% of CDH. The size of the defect is highly

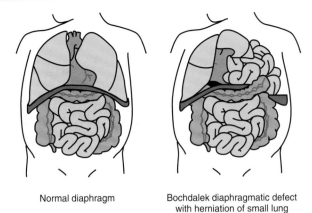

A — Normal diaphragm

B — Bochdalek diaphragmatic defect with herniation of small lung

Fig. 122.10 A, A normal diaphragm separating the abdominal and thoracic cavity. **B,** Diaphragmatic hernia with a small lung and abdominal contents in the thoracic cavity.

variable, ranging from a small hole to complete agenesis of this area of the diaphragm. These lesions may cause significant respiratory distress at birth, can be associated with other congenital anomalies, and have significant mortality and long-term morbidity. The overall survival from the CDH Study Group is approximately 70%, but survival is >80% at many centers.

CONGENITAL DIAPHRAGMATIC HERNIA (BOCHDALEK)
Pathology and Etiology
Although CDH is characterized by a structural diaphragmatic defect, a major limiting factor for survival is the associated **pulmonary hypoplasia**. Lung hypoplasia was initially thought to be solely caused by the compression of the lung from the herniated abdominal contents, which impaired lung growth. However, emerging evidence indicates that pulmonary hypoplasia, at least in some cases, may precede the development of the diaphragmatic defect.

Pulmonary hypoplasia is characterized by a reduction in pulmonary mass and the number of bronchial divisions, respiratory bronchioles, and alveoli. The pathology of pulmonary hypoplasia and CDH includes abnormal septa in the terminal saccules, thickened alveoli, and thickened pulmonary arterioles. Biochemical abnormalities include relative surfactant deficiencies, increased glycogen in the alveoli, and decreased levels of phosphatidylcholine, total DNA, and total lung protein, all of which contribute to limited gas exchange.

Epidemiology
The incidence of CDH is between 1 in 2,000 and 1 in 5,000 live births, with females affected twice as often as males. Defects are more common on the left (85%) and are occasionally bilateral (<5%). Pulmonary hypoplasia and malrotation of the intestine are part of the lesion, not associated anomalies. Most cases of CDH are sporadic, but familial cases have been reported. Associated anomalies have been reported in up to 30% of cases, including CNS lesions, esophageal atresia, omphalocele, and cardiovascular lesions. CDH is recognized as part of several chromosomal syndromes: trisomies 21, 13, and 18 and Fryns, Brachmann–de Lange, Pallister-Killian, and Turner syndromes.

Diagnosis and Clinical Presentation
In >50% of cases, CDH can be diagnosed on prenatal ultrasonography (US) between 16 and 24 wk of gestation. High-speed fetal MRI can further define the lesion. US findings may include polyhydramnios, chest mass, mediastinal shift, gastric bubble or a liver in the thoracic cavity, and fetal hydrops. Certain imaging features may predict outcome;

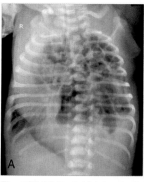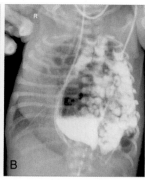

Fig. 122.11 Bochdalek hernia. **A,** Chest radiograph showing herniated bowel loops in the left hemithorax, displacement of the mediastinum to the contralateral side, severely reduced lung space, and unclear lung fields bilaterally. **B,** Upper gastrointestinal tract radiograph showing the stomach and bowel loops stained with contrast in the left hemithorax. *(From Hu X, Liu B: Bochdalek hernia,* Lancet *392:60, 2018.)*

these include liver position in the chest, observed-to-expected total lung volume (TLV), and observed-to-expected lung-to-head ratio (LHR). Nonetheless, no definitive characteristic reliably predicts outcome. After delivery, a chest radiograph is needed to confirm the diagnosis (Fig. 122.11). In some infants with an echogenic chest mass, further imaging is required. The differential diagnosis may include other diaphragm disorders, such as eventration or a cystic lung lesion (pulmonary sequestration, cystic adenomatoid malformation).

Arriving at the diagnosis early in pregnancy allows for prenatal counseling, possible fetal interventions, and planning for postnatal care. A referral to a center providing high-risk obstetrics, pediatric surgery, and tertiary care neonatology is advised. Careful evaluation for other anomalies should include echocardiography and amniocentesis. To avoid unnecessary pregnancy termination and unrealistic expectations, an experienced multidisciplinary group must carefully counsel the parents of a child diagnosed with a diaphragmatic hernia.

Respiratory distress is a cardinal sign in babies with CDH. It may occur immediately after birth, or there may be a "honeymoon" period of up to 48 hr during which the baby is relatively stable. Early respiratory distress, within 6 hr after birth, is thought to be a poor prognostic sign. Respiratory distress is characterized clinically by tachypnea, grunting, use of accessory muscles, and cyanosis. Children with CDH may also have a scaphoid abdomen and increased chest wall diameter. Bowel sounds may also be heard in the chest with decreased breath sounds bilaterally. The point of maximal cardiac impulse may be displaced away from the side of the hernia if mediastinal shift has occurred. A chest radiograph and passage of a nasal gastric tube are usually sufficient to confirm the diagnosis.

A small group of infants with CDH present beyond the neonatal period. Patients with a delayed presentation may experience vomiting as a result of intestinal obstruction or mild respiratory symptoms. Occasionally, incarceration of the intestine proceeds to ischemia with sepsis and shock. Unrecognized diaphragmatic hernia is a rare cause of sudden death in infants and toddlers. Group B streptococcal sepsis has been associated with delayed onset of symptoms and a CDH (often right side).

Treatment
Initial Management
Delivery at a tertiary center with experience in the management of CDH is required to provide early, appropriate respiratory support. In the delivery room, infants with respiratory distress should be rapidly stabilized with endotracheal intubation. *Prolonged mask ventilation in the delivery room, which enlarges the stomach and small bowel and thus makes oxygenation more difficult, must be avoided and a naso- or orogastric tube placed immediately for decompression.* Arterial (preductal and postductal) and central venous (umbilical) lines are mandated, as are a urinary catheter and nasogastric tube. A preductal arterial oxygen saturation (SpO$_2$) value ≥85% should be the minimum goal. Volutrauma is a significant problem. *Gentle ventilation with permissive hypercapnia* reduces lung injury, need for ECMO, and mortality. Factors that contribute to pulmonary hypertension (hypoxia, acidosis, hypothermia) should be avoided. Echocardiography is important to guide therapeutic decisions by measuring pulmonary and system vascular pressures and defining the presence of cardiac dysfunction. Routine use of inotropes is indicated in the presence of left ventricular dysfunction. Babies with CDH may be surfactant deficient. Although surfactant is frequently used, no study has proved that it is beneficial in treatment of CDH, and it may precipitate decompensation. In infants with severe respiratory failure and hypoxemia, sedation and paralysis may be required.

Ventilation Strategies
Conventional mechanical ventilation, high-frequency oscillatory ventilation (HFOV), and ECMO are the 3 main strategies to support respiratory failure in the newborn with CDH. The goal is to maintain oxygenation and CO$_2$ elimination without inducing volutrauma. Conventional ventilation using a gentle, lung protective strategy (PIP <25, PEEP 3-5 cm H$_2$O) that allows for permissive hypercapnia (PaCO$_2$ <65-70 mm Hg) is recommended. Permissive hypercapnia (as opposed to hyperventilation with high PIP) has reduced lung injury and improved survival. HFOV as a rescue therapy is indicated if a PIP >25 is required to maintain appropriate ventilation or if hypoxemia persists.

Inhaled NO is a selective pulmonary vasodilator. Its use reduces ductal shunting and pulmonary pressures and results in improved oxygenation. Although iNO has been helpful in PPHN, randomized trials have not demonstrated improved survival or reduced need for ECMO when iNO is used in newborns with CDH. Nonetheless, iNO is used in patients with CDH as a bridge to ECMO.

Extracorporeal Membrane Oxygenation
The availability of ECMO and the utility of preoperative stabilization has improved survival of babies with CDH. ECMO is the therapeutic option for children in whom conventional ventilation or HFOV fails. ECMO is most often used before repair of the defect. Several objective criteria for ECMO have been developed. Birthweight and the 5 min Apgar score may be the best predictors of outcome in patients treated with ECMO. There is no strict lower weight limit for ECMO, but generally, vessels in infants <1,800-2,000 g are too small to cannulate.

The duration of ECMO for neonates with diaphragmatic hernia is longer (7-14 days) than for those with PPHN (persistent fetal circulation) or meconium aspiration and may last up to 2-4 wk. Timing of repair of the diaphragm while the infant receives ECMO is controversial; some experts prefer early repair to allow a greater duration of ECMO after the repair, whereas many defer repair until the infant has demonstrated the ability to tolerate weaning from ECMO. The recurrence of pulmonary hypertension is associated with high mortality and weaning from ECMO support should be cautious. If the patient cannot be weaned from ECMO after repair of CDH, options include discontinuing support and, in rare cases, lung transplantation.

Novel Strategies for Infants With Congenital Diaphragmatic Hernia
The most reliable prenatal predictors of outcome in children with CDH studied is fetal US. A prospective study of US at 24-26 wk compared fetal LHR with mortality. There were no survivors with LHR <1, but all babies with LHR >1.4 survived. A 2nd important consideration was the presence of liver in the thoracic cavity, which is a poor prognostic feature. Human studies have shown no benefit for in utero repair of CDH. In another single-center study, a late gestation (32-34 wk) fetal MRI-derived TLV >40 mL was associated with >90% survival and only 10% need for ECMO, while TLV <20 mL was associated with <35% survival and >85% need for ECMO.

Based on the observation that hydrostatic pressure exerted by fetal lung fluid plays a critical role in lung growth and maturity, a promising experimental therapy is **in utero tracheal occlusion**. Although initial studies in affected fetuses did not demonstrate success, emerging preliminary reports in those with severe CDH (LHR <1 and intrathoracic liver) suggest that fetoscopic tracheal occlusion is associated with significantly reduced mortality and need for ECMO (see Chapter 116).

Surgical Repair

The ideal time to repair the diaphragmatic defect is under debate. Most experts wait at least 48 hr after stabilization and resolution of the pulmonary hypertension. Good relative indicators of stability are the requirement for conventional ventilation only, a low peak inspiratory pressure, and FIO_2 <50. If the newborn is receiving ECMO, an ability to be weaned from this support should be a consideration before surgical repair. In some centers the repair is done with the cannulas in place; in other centers the cannulas are removed. A subcostal approach is most frequently used (Fig. 122.12). This allows for good visualization of the defect, and if the abdominal cavity cannot accommodate the herniated contents, a polymeric silicone (Silastic) patch can be placed. Both laparoscopic and thoracoscopic repairs have been reported, but these should be reserved for only the most stable infants.

The defect size and amount of native diaphragm present are variable. Whenever possible, a primary repair using native tissue is performed. If the defect is too large, a porous polytetrafluoroethylene (Gore-Tex) patch is used. There is a higher recurrence rate of CDH in children with patches (the patch does not grow as the child grows) than in those with native tissue repairs. A loosely fitted patch may reduce the recurrence rates.

Following surgical repair, the infant must be carefully monitored for worsening pulmonary hypertension. In some patients, a postoperative course of ECMO is needed. Other recognized complications include bleeding, chylothorax, and bowel obstruction.

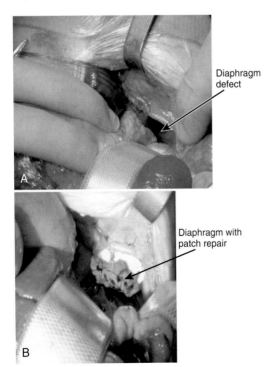

Fig. 122.12 A, Intraoperative photo of congenital diaphragmatic hernia (CDH) before repair. **B,** Intraoperative photo of patch repair of CDH.

Outcome and Long-Term Survival

Overall survival of liveborn infants with CDH is 71%. Relative predictors of a poor prognosis include an associated major anomaly, symptoms before 24 hr of age, severe pulmonary hypoplasia, herniation to the contralateral lung, and the need for ECMO. The size of the defect appears to be the strongest predictor of morbidity.

Pulmonary problems continue to be a source of morbidity for long-term survivors of CDH. Children receiving CDH repair who were studied at 6-11 yr of age demonstrated significant decreases in forced expiratory flow at 50% of vital capacity and decreased peak expiratory flow. Both obstructive and restrictive patterns can occur. Those without severe pulmonary hypertension and barotrauma do the best. Those at highest risk include children who required ECMO and patch repair, but the data clearly show that CDH survivors who did not require ECMO also need frequent attention to pulmonary issues. At discharge, up to 20% of infants require oxygen, but only 1–2% require oxygen past 1 yr old. BPD is frequently documented radiographically but will improve as more alveoli develop and the child ages.

Gastroesophageal reflux disease (GERD) is reported in >50% of children with CDH. GERD is more common in children whose diaphragmatic defect involves the esophageal hiatus. **Intestinal obstruction** is reported in up to 20% of children and may result from a midgut volvulus, adhesions, or a recurrent hernia that became incarcerated. **Recurrent diaphragmatic hernia** is reported in 5–20% in most series. Children with patch repairs are at highest risk.

Children with CDH typically have delayed growth in the 1st 2 yr of life. Contributing factors include poor intake, GERD, and a caloric requirement that may be higher because of the energy required to breathe. Many children normalize and "catch up" in growth by the time they are 2 yr old.

Neurocognitive defects are common and may result from the disease or the interventions. The incidence of neurologic abnormalities is higher in infants who require ECMO (67% vs 24% of those who do not). The abnormalities are similar to those seen in neonates treated with ECMO for other diagnoses and include transient and permanent developmental delay, abnormal hearing or vision, and seizures. Serious hearing loss may occur in up to 28% of children who underwent ECMO. The majority of neurologic abnormalities are classified as mild to moderate.

Other long-term problems include pectus excavatum and scoliosis. Survivors of CDH repair, particularly those requiring ECMO support, have a variety of long-term abnormalities that appear to improve with time but require close monitoring and multidisciplinary support.

Bibliography is available at Expert Consult.

122.11 Foramen of Morgagni Hernia
Shawn K. Ahlfeld

Failure of the sternal and crural portions of the diaphragm to meet and fuse produces the foramen of Morgagni hernia. These defects are usually small, with a greater transverse than anteroposterior diameter, and are more often right sided (90%) but may be bilateral. The transverse colon, small intestine, or liver is usually contained in the hernial sac. Most children with these defects are asymptomatic and are diagnosed beyond the neonatal period, often by chest radiograph performed for evaluation of another condition. The anterolateral radiograph shows a structure behind the heart, and a lateral film localizes the mass to the retrosternal area. Chest CT or MRI confirms the diagnosis. When symptoms occur, they can include recurrent respiratory infections, cough, vomiting, or reflux; in rare cases, incarceration may occur. Repair is recommended for all patients, in view of the risk of bowel strangulation, and can be accomplished laparoscopically. Prosthetic material is rarely required.

122.12 Paraesophageal Hernia

Shawn K. Ahlfeld

Paraesophageal hernia is differentiated from the hiatal hernia in that the gastroesophageal junction is in the normal location. The herniation of the stomach alongside or adjacent to the gastroesophageal junction is prone to incarceration with strangulation and perforation. A previous Nissen fundoplication and other diaphragmatic procedures are risk factors. This unusual diaphragmatic hernia should be repaired promptly after identification.

122.13 Eventration

Shawn K. Ahlfeld

Eventration of the diaphragm is an abnormal elevation consisting of a thinned diaphragmatic muscle that causes elevation of the entire hemidiaphragm or more often the anterior aspect of the hemidiaphragm. This elevation produces a paradoxical motion of the affected hemidiaphragm. Most eventrations are asymptomatic and do not require repair. A congenital form is the result of either incomplete development of the muscular portion or central tendon or abnormal development of the phrenic nerves. Congenital eventration may affect lung development, but it has not been associated with pulmonary hypoplasia. The differential diagnosis includes diaphragmatic paralysis, diaphragmatic hernia, traction injury, and iatrogenic injury after heart surgery. Eventration is also associated with pulmonary sequestration, congenital heart disease, spinal muscular atrophy with respiratory distress, and chromosomal trisomies. Most eventrations are asymptomatic and do not require repair. The indications for surgery include continued need for mechanical ventilation, recurrent infections, and failure to thrive. Large or symptomatic eventrations can be repaired by plication through an abdominal or thoracic approach that is minimally invasive.

Bibliography is available at Expert Consult.

122.14 Extrapulmonary Air Leaks: Pneumothorax, Pneumomediastinum, Pulmonary Interstitial Emphysema, Pneumopericardium

Shawn K. Ahlfeld

Asymptomatic pneumothorax, usually unilateral, is estimated to occur in 1–2% of all newborn infants; symptomatic pneumothorax and pneumomediastinum are less common (see Chapter 113). The incidence of pneumothorax is increased in infants with lung diseases such as meconium aspiration and RDS; in those who receive assisted ventilation, especially if high-frequency ventilation (HFV) support is necessary; and in infants with urinary tract anomalies or oligohydramnios.

ETIOLOGY AND PATHOPHYSIOLOGY

The most common cause of pneumothorax is overdistention resulting in alveolar rupture. Alveolar overdistention can occur with positive pressure ventilation during neonatal resuscitation, or it may occur in association with the "ball-valve" phenomenon that results from aspiration (classically meconium) and bronchial/bronchiolar obstruction. Although **spontaneous rupture** of an underlying pulmonary malformation (e.g., lobar emphysema, congenital lung cyst, pneumatocele) occurs, it is usually in an otherwise normal lung, and no etiology is identified.

Pneumothorax associated with **pulmonary hypoplasia** is common, tends to occur during the 1st few hr after birth, and is caused by reduced alveolar surface area and poorly compliant lungs. It is associated with disorders of decreased amniotic fluid volume (Potter

syndrome, renal agenesis, renal dysplasia, chronic amniotic fluid leak), decreased fetal breathing movement (oligohydramnios, neuromuscular disease), pulmonary space-occupying lesions (diaphragmatic hernia, pleural effusion, chylothorax), and thoracic abnormalities (thoracic dystrophies).

Gas from a ruptured alveolus escapes into the interstitial spaces of the lung, where it tracks along small conducting airways and dissects along the peribronchial and perivascular connective tissue sheaths to the hilum of the lung (pulmonary interstitial emphysema). If the volume of escaped air is great enough, it may collect in the mediastinal space (**pneumomediastinum**) or rupture into the pleural space (**pneumothorax**), subcutaneous tissue (**subcutaneous emphysema**), peritoneal cavity (**pneumoperitoneum**), and/or pericardial sac (**pneumopericardium**). Rarely, increased mediastinal pressure may compress the pulmonary veins at the hilum and thereby interfere with pulmonary venous return to the heart and cardiac output. On occasion, air may embolize into the circulation (pulmonary air embolism) and cause cutaneous blanching, air in intravascular catheters, an air-filled heart and vessels on chest radiographs, and death.

Tension pneumothorax occurs if an accumulation of air within the pleural space is sufficient to elevate intrapleural pressure above atmospheric pressure. Unilateral tension pneumothorax results in impaired ventilation not only in the ipsilateral lung but also in the contralateral lung because of a shift in the mediastinum toward the contralateral side. Compression of the vena cava and torsion of the great vessels may interfere with venous return.

CLINICAL MANIFESTATIONS

The physical findings of a clinically asymptomatic pneumothorax are hyperresonance and diminished ipsilateral breath sounds with or without tachypnea. Symptomatic pneumothorax is characterized by respiratory distress, which varies from merely high respiratory rate to severe dyspnea, tachypnea, and cyanosis. Irritability and restlessness or apnea may be the earliest signs. The onset is usually sudden but may be gradual; an infant may rapidly become critically ill. Physical exam findings include chest asymmetry with an increased anteroposterior diameter, hyperresonance, and diminished or absent breath sounds. The heart is displaced toward the contralateral side, resulting in displacement of the cardiac apex and point of maximal impulse. The diaphragm is displaced downward, as is the liver with right-sided pneumothorax, and may result in abdominal distention. Because pneumothorax may be bilateral in approximately 10% of patients, symmetry of findings does not rule it out. In tension pneumothorax, signs of shock are typical.

Pneumomediastinum can occur in patients with pneumothorax and is usually asymptomatic. The degree of respiratory distress depends on the amount of trapped gas; if great, bulging of the midthoracic area is observed, the neck veins are distended, and blood pressure is low. The last 2 findings are a result of tamponade of the systemic and pulmonary veins. Although often asymptomatic, subcutaneous emphysema in newborn infants is almost pathognomonic of pneumomediastinum.

Pulmonary interstitial emphysema (PIE) may precede the development of a pneumothorax or may occur independently and lead to increasing respiratory distress as a result of decreased compliance, hypercapnia, and hypoxemia. Hypoxemia is caused by an increased $PA\text{-}aO_2$ and intrapulmonary shunting. Progressive enlargement of blebs of gas may result in cystic dilation and respiratory deterioration resembling pneumothorax. In severe cases, pulmonary interstitial emphysema precedes the development of BPD. Avoidance of high inspiratory or mean airway pressures may prevent the development of pulmonary interstitial emphysema. Treatment may include bronchoscopy in patients with evidence of mucous plugging, selective intubation and ventilation of the uninvolved bronchus, oxygen, general respiratory care, and HFV.

DIAGNOSIS

Pneumothorax and other air leaks should be suspected in newborn infants who show signs of respiratory distress, are restless or irritable, or have a sudden change in condition. The diagnosis of **pneumothorax** is established by chest radiography, with the edge of the collapsed lung standing out in relief against the pneumothorax (Fig. 122.13). **Pneumomediastinum** is signified by hyperlucency around the heart border and between the sternum and the heart border (Fig. 122.14). *Transillumination* of the thorax is often helpful in the emergency diagnosis of pneumothorax; the affected side transmits excessive light. Associated renal anomalies are identified by US. **Pulmonary hypoplasia** is suggested by signs of uterine compression (extremity contractures), a small thorax on chest radiographs, severe hypoxia with hypercapnia, and signs of the primary disease (hypotonia, diaphragmatic hernia, Potter syndrome).

Pneumopericardium may be asymptomatic, requiring only general supportive treatment, but it usually manifests as sudden shock with tachycardia, muffled heart sounds, and poor pulses suggesting tamponade. **Pneumoperitoneum** from air dissecting through the diaphragmatic apertures during mechanical ventilation may be confused with intestinal perforation. Abdominal paracentesis can be helpful in differentiating the 2 conditions. The presence of organisms on Gram stain of intestinal contents suggests the latter. Occasionally, pneumoperitoneum can result in an abdominal compartment syndrome requiring decompression.

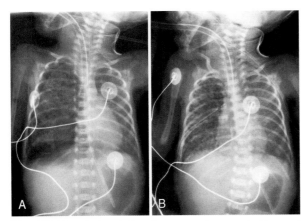

Fig. 122.13 A, Right-sided tension pneumothorax and widespread right lung pulmonary interstitial emphysema in a preterm infant receiving intensive care. **B,** Resolution of pneumothorax with a chest tube in place. Pulmonary interstitial emphysema (PIE) persists. *(From Meerstadt PWD, Gyll C: Manual of neonatal emergency x-ray interpretation, Philadelphia, 1994, Saunders, p 73.)*

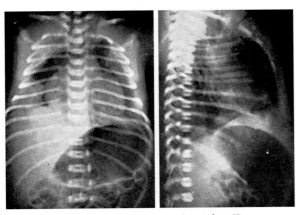

Fig. 122.14 Pneumomediastinum in newborn infant. The anteroposterior view (*left*) demonstrates compression of the lungs, and the lateral view (*right*) shows bulging of the sternum, each resulting from distention of the mediastinum by trapped air.

TREATMENT

Without a continued air leak, asymptomatic and mildly symptomatic, small pneumothoraces require only close observation. Conservative management of a pneumothorax is effective even in selected infants requiring ventilatory support. Frequent small feedings may prevent gastric dilation and minimize crying, which can further compromise ventilation and worsen the pneumothorax. Breathing 100% oxygen in term infants may accelerate the resorption of free pleural air into blood by reducing the nitrogen tension in blood and producing a resultant nitrogen pressure gradient from the trapped gas in the blood; the clinical effectiveness is not proved, however, and the benefit must be weighed against the risks of O_2 toxicity. With severe respiratory or circulatory embarrassment, emergency decompression by *needle thoracentesis* using a soft, small catheter is indicated. Either immediately or after catheter aspiration, a **chest tube** should be inserted and attached to underwater seal drainage (see Fig. 122.13). If the air leak is ongoing, continuous suction (−5 to −20 cm H_2O) may be needed to evacuate the pneumothorax completely. A pneumopericardium requires prompt evacuation of entrapped air. Severe localized PIE may respond to selective bronchial intubation. Surfactant therapy for RDS reduces the incidence of pneumothorax.

Bibliography is available at Expert Consult.

122.15 Pulmonary Hemorrhage
Shawn K. Ahlfeld

Massive pulmonary hemorrhage is a relatively uncommon, but catastrophic complication with a high risk of morbidity and mortality. Some degree of pulmonary hemorrhage occurs in about 10% of extremely preterm infants. However, massive pulmonary hemorrhage is less common and can be fatal. Autopsy demonstrates massive pulmonary hemorrhage in 15% of neonates who die in the 1st 2 wk of life. The reported incidence at autopsy varies from 1-4 per 1,000 live births. Approximately 75% of affected patients weigh <2,500 g at birth. Prophylactic indomethacin in ELBW infants reduces the incidence of pulmonary hemorrhage.

Most infants with pulmonary hemorrhage have had symptoms of respiratory distress that are indistinguishable from those of RDS. The onset may occur at birth or may be delayed several days. **Hemorrhagic pulmonary edema** is the source of blood in many cases and is associated with significant ductal shunting and high pulmonary blood flow or severe left-sided heart failure resulting from hypoxia. In severe cases, sudden cardiovascular collapse, poor lung compliance, profound cyanosis, and hypercapnia may be present. Radiographic findings are varied and nonspecific, ranging from minor streaking or patchy infiltrates to massive consolidation.

The risk of pulmonary hemorrhage is increased in association with acute pulmonary infection, severe asphyxia, RDS, assisted ventilation, PDA, congenital heart disease, erythroblastosis fetalis, hemorrhagic disease of the newborn, thrombocytopenia, inborn errors of ammonia metabolism, and cold injury. Pulmonary hemorrhage is the only severe complication in which the rate is *increased* with surfactant treatment. Pulmonary hemorrhage is seen with all surfactants; the incidence ranges from 1–5% of treated infants and is higher with natural surfactant. Bleeding is predominantly alveolar in approximately 65% of cases and interstitial in the rest. Bleeding into other organs is observed at autopsy of severely ill neonates, suggesting an additional bleeding diathesis, such as disseminated intravascular coagulation. Acute pulmonary hemorrhage may rarely occur in previously healthy full-term infants. The cause is unknown. Pulmonary hemorrhage may manifest as hemoptysis or blood in the nasopharynx or airway with no evidence of upper respiratory or gastrointestinal bleeding. Patients present with acute, severe respiratory failure requiring mechanical ventilation. Chest radiographs usually demonstrate bilateral alveolar infiltrates. The condition usually responds to intensive supportive treatment (see Chapter 436).

Treatment of pulmonary hemorrhage includes blood replacement, suctioning to clear the airway, intratracheal administration of epinephrine, and tamponade with increased mean airway pressure (often requiring HFV). Although surfactant treatment has been associated with the development of pulmonary hemorrhage, administration of exogenous surfactant after the bleeding has occurred can improve lung compliance, because the presence of intraalveolar blood and protein can inactivate surfactant.

Bibliography is available at Expert Consult.

Chapter **123**
Digestive System Disorders
第一百二十三章
消化系统疾病

中文导读

本章将新生儿黄疸及高胆红素血症这种既可以是独立诊断，也可以是疾病症状，又可以是疾病体征的疾病包括在内，详细介绍了新生儿黄疸的病因、临床表现、鉴别诊断；新生儿生理性黄疸、病理性高胆红素血症、母乳性黄疸、新生儿胆汁淤积及先天性胆道闭锁、核黄疸的临床表现、发病率、预后、预防及高胆红素血症的治疗等内容。新生儿在胃肠道功能建立的过程中，可能发生较为严重的消化系统严重疾病，本章主要介绍了胎粪性腹膜炎、肠梗阻、坏死性小肠结肠炎这几种新生儿严重外科疾病，具体描述了坏死性小肠结肠炎的病理生理学、临床表现、诊断、治疗、预后及预防。

123.1 Meconium Ileus, Peritonitis, and Intestinal Obstruction

Juan P. Gurria and Rebeccah L. Brown

Meconium consists of bile salts, bile acids, and debris shed from the intestinal mucosa in the intrauterine period. More than 90% of full-term newborn infants and 80% of very-low-birthweight (VLBW) infants pass meconium within the 1st 24 hr. The possibility of intestinal obstruction should be considered in any infant who does not pass meconium by 24-36 hr.

MECONIUM PLUGS

Meconium plugs syndrome refers to intestinal obstruction, usually in the distal colon, rectum, and anal canal, caused by meconium plugs (Fig. 123.1). Resulting from a disproportionately low amount of water in the intestinal lumen, meconium plugs are a rare cause of intrauterine intestinal obstruction and meconium peritonitis unrelated to cystic fibrosis (CF). **Anorectal plugs** may also cause mucosal ulceration from bowel wall erosion and subsequent intestinal perforation. **Meconium plugs** are associated with small left colon syndrome in infants of diabetic mothers, CF (40%), Hirschsprung disease (40%), maternal opiate use, magnesium sulfate therapy for preeclampsia, and tocolysis. Up to 30% of patients can have spontaneous resolution. Initial treatment may include administration of a glycerin suppository or rectal irrigation with isotonic saline. In up to 95% of patients, a Gastrografin enema (meglumine diatrizoate, a hyperosmolar, water-soluble, radiopaque solution containing 0.1% polysorbate 80 [Tween 80] and 37% organically bound iodine) will be both diagnostic and therapeutic, inducing passage of the plug, presumably because the high osmolarity (1,900 mOsm/L) of the solution draws fluid rapidly into the intestinal lumen and loosens the inspissated material. Such rapid loss of fluid into the bowel may result in acute fluid shifts with dehydration and shock, so it is advisable to dilute the contrast material with an equal amount of water and provide intravenous (IV) fluids, during and for several hours after the procedure, sufficient to maintain normal vital signs, urine output, and electrolytes. After removal of a meconium plug, the infant should be observed closely and consideration given to performing diagnostic testing to identify **Hirschsprung disease** (congenital aganglionic megacolon; see Chapter 358.4) and CF (see Chapter 432).

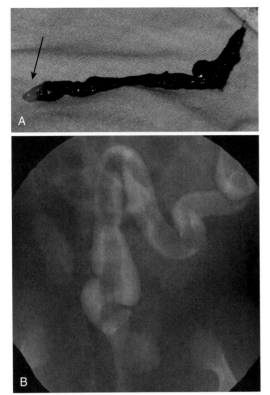

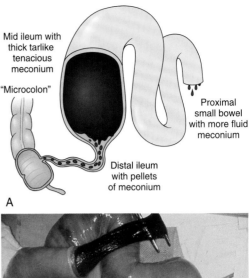

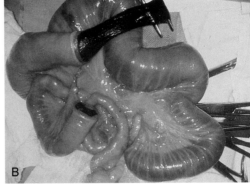

Fig. 123.1 Meconium plug. **A,** Meconium plug evacuated after a diagnostic contrast enema demonstrated the distinctive white tip *(arrow).* **B,** Image from a contrast enema in a term neonate with vomiting and bowel distension demonstrates the long filling defect characteristic of meconium plug syndrome. The child was relieved of the obstruction after evacuation of the plug, without recurrence of symptoms. *(From Hernanz-Schulman M: Congenital and neonatal disorders. In Coley BD, editor:* Caffey's pediatric diagnostic imaging, *ed 12, Philadelphia, 2013, Elsevier, Fig 106-14.)*

Fig. 123.2 Meconium ileus. **A,** Schematic drawing of uncomplicated meconium ileus. Pellets of inspissated meconium fill the terminal ileum proximal to a microcolon. Several loops of more proximal ileum contain thick, tenacious meconium. **B,** Enterotomy of proximal bowel and the nature of the thick and tenacious meconium. Note the dilated proximal loops of bowel filled with meconium and the progressively small caliber of the distal bowel leading to the microcolon. (**A,** *From Leonidas JC, Berdon WE, et al: Meconium ileus and its complications: a reappraisal of plain film roentgen diagnostic criteria, Am J Roentgenol Radium Ther Nucl Med 108[3]:598–609, 1970;* **B,** *courtesy of Dr. Wallace W. Neblett III, Nashville, Ten)*

MECONIUM ILEUS

Meconium ileus, or impaction of inspissated meconium in the distal small bowel, accounts for up to 30% of cases of neonatal intestinal obstruction. It is common in patients with CF in whom the lack of fetal pancreatic enzymes inhibits digestive mechanisms, and meconium becomes viscid and mucilaginous. Clinically, neonates present with intestinal obstruction with or without perforation. Abdominal distention is prominent, and vomiting, often bilious, becomes persistent, although occasionally inspissated meconium stools may be passed shortly after birth. Meconium ileus can present as early as in utero, in which the fetus develops acute intestinal obstruction resulting in volvulus or perforation, peritoneal ascites, meconium peritonitis, and hydrops; if untreated, fetal loss may occur.

Meconium ileus is primarily associated with cystic fibrosis transmembrane regulator (CFTR) mutations F508del, G542X, W1282X, R553X, and G551D. Patients with two copies of the F508del mutation have a 25% chance of presenting with meconium ileus. F508del plus any other CF mutation confers 17% risk, and two other CF mutations confer a 12% risk of meconium ileus. In addition, non-CFTR genetic modifier genes influence meconium ileus. In families who already have at least one child with CF complicated by meconium ileus, there is a 39% risk for meconium ileus in subsequent children, which is more than the rates expected with autosomal recessive inheritance. In a twin study, 82% of monozygotic twins showed concordance for meconium ileus, whereas only 22% of dizygotic and 24% of two affected siblings

showed concordance. Positive newborn screening for CF should prompt sweat testing when the infant weighs >2 kg and is at least 36 wk of corrected gestational age. Genetic testing confirms the diagnosis of CF (see Chapter 432).

The differential diagnosis involves other causes of intestinal obstruction, including intestinal pseudoobstruction, and other causes of pancreatic insufficiency (see Chapter 377). Prenatal diagnosis is readily achieved by ultrasound with identification of enlarged bowel loops or a mass with distention of the proximal small bowel. Clinically the diagnosis can be made with a history of CF in a sibling, by palpation of doughy or cordlike masses of intestines through the abdominal wall, and from the radiographic appearance. Plain radiographs reveal small bowel obstruction. Air-fluid levels may not be apparent because of the thickened meconium.

In contrast to the generally evenly distended intestinal loops above an atresia, the loops may vary in width and are not as evenly filled with gas. At points of heaviest meconium concentration, the infiltrated gas may create a bubbly, granular appearance (Figs. 123.2 and 123.3).

Treatment for simple meconium ileus is a high-osmolarity Gastrografin enema, as described for meconium plugs. If the procedure is unsuccessful or perforation of the bowel wall is suspected, a laparotomy is performed and the ileum opened at the point of largest diameter of the impaction. Approximately 50% of these infants have associated intestinal atresia, stenosis, or volvulus that requires surgery. The inspissated meconium is removed by gentle and patient irrigation with warm isotonic sodium chloride or *N*-acetylcysteine (Mucomyst) solution through a catheter passed between the impaction and the bowel wall. Some patients will require bowel resection with a temporary double-barrel enterostomy followed by serial irrigations and distal refeeding, or primary anastomosis at the initial operation. Most infants with meconium ileus survive the neonatal period. If meconium ileus is associated with CF, the long-term prognosis depends on the severity of the underlying disease (see Chapter 432).

MECONIUM PERITONITIS

Perforation of the intestine may occur in utero or shortly after birth. Frequently, the intestinal perforation seals naturally with relatively little meconium leakage into the peritoneal cavity. Perforations occur most often as a complication of meconium ileus in infants with CF but occasionally result from a meconium plug or in utero intestinal obstruction of another cause.

Cases at the most severe end of the spectrum may be diagnosed on prenatal ultrasound with fetal ascites, polyhydramnios, bowel dilation, intraabdominal calcifications, and hydrops fetalis (Fig. 123.4). At the other end are cases in which an intestinal perforation may seal spontaneously and patients remain asymptomatic, except when meconium becomes calcified and is later discovered on radiographs. Alternatively, the clinical picture may be dominated by signs of intestinal obstruction (as in meconium ileus) with abdominal distention, vomiting, and absence of stools or chemical peritonitis presenting with sepsis. Treatment consists primarily of elimination of the intestinal obstruction and drainage of the peritoneal cavity with a timely surgical intervention proved to result in high survival rate and favorable outcome even in complicated meconium peritonitis.

Bibliography is available at Expert Consult.

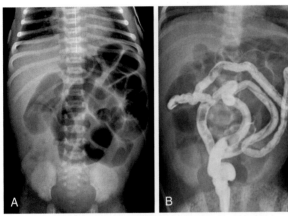

Fig. 123.3 Uncomplicated meconium ileus. **A,** Abdominal radiograph in 3 day old infant with abdominal distention and bilious aspirates shows dilation of multiple loops of bowel. No calcifications are seen on the radiograph to suggest complicated meconium ileus. Orogastric tube near the gastroesophageal junction was subsequently advanced. **B,** Contrast enema demonstrates a microcolon, with multiple meconium plugs, consistent with the diagnosis of meconium ileus. *(From Hernanz-Schulman M: Congenital and neonatal disorders. In Coley BD, editor: Caffey's pediatric diagnostic imaging, ed 13, Philadelphia, 2019, Elsevier, Fig 102-36).*

123.2 Necrotizing Enterocolitis

Rebeccah L. Brown

Necrotizing enterocolitis (NEC) is the most common life-threatening emergency of the gastrointestinal (GI) tract in the newborn period. The disease is characterized by various degrees of mucosal or transmural necrosis of the intestine. The cause of NEC remains unclear but is most likely multifactorial. The incidence of NEC is 5–10% among infants with birthweight <1500 g, with mortality rates of 20–30% and approaching 50% in infants who require surgery. Both incidence and case fatality rates increase with decreasing birthweight and gestational age.

PATHOLOGY AND PATHOGENESIS

Many factors contribute to the development of the pathologic findings of NEC, including mucosal ischemia and subsequent necrosis, gas accumulation in the submucosa of the bowel wall (pneumatosis intestinalis), and progression of the necrosis to perforation, peritonitis, sepsis, and death. The distal part of the ileum and the proximal segment of colon are involved most frequently; in fatal cases, gangrene may extend from the stomach to the rectum (NEC totalis). The pathogenesis of NEC remains to be completely elucidated, but 3 major risk factors have

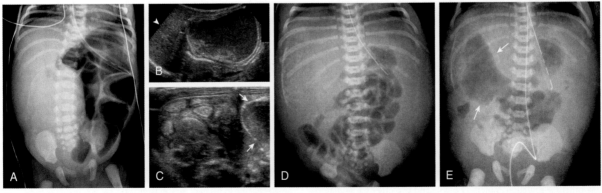

Fig. 123.4 Complicated meconium ileus. **A,** Abdominal radiograph in 2 day old girl with abdominal distention and bilious aspirates shows absence of bowel gas in the right abdomen with a partly calcified mass displacing gas-filled dilated loops of bowel to the left. **B,** Ultrasound image demonstrates the subhepatic, partly calcified mass with internal debris and fluid-fluid level. **C,** Additional ultrasound image shows a portion of the cyst wall *(arrows)* and multiple, abnormal, hyperechoic loops of bowel. **D,** Abdominal radiograph in different 1 day old infant shows a calcified mass in right upper quadrant, shown at sonography to represent a loculated complex meconium collection. **E,** Radiograph a few hours later of the same infant shown in **D** shows a persistent perforation with gas entering into the right upper quadrant collection. *(From Hernanz-Schulman M: Congenital and neonatal disorders. In Coley BD, editor: Caffey's pediatric diagnostic imaging, ed 13, Philadelphia, 2019, Elsevier, Fig 102-37).*

been implicated: prematurity, bacterial colonization of the gut, and formula feeding. NEC develops primarily in premature infants with exposure to metabolic substrate in the context of immature intestinal immunity, microbial dysbiosis, and mucosal ischemia. An underlying genetic predisposition is being recognized with variants in genes regulating immunomodulation and inflammation (e.g., Toll-like receptor-4, IL-6), apoptosis and cellular repair (e.g., platelet-activating factor), and oxidant stress (e.g., vascular endothelial growth factor, arginine, nitric oxide). *The greatest risk factor for NEC is prematurity.* NEC rarely occurs before the initiation of enteral feeding and is much less common in infants fed human milk. Aggressive enteral feeding may predispose to the development of NEC.

Although nearly 90% of all cases of NEC occur in preterm infants, the disease can occur in full-term neonates. NEC in term infants is often a secondary disease, seen more frequently in infants with history of birth asphyxia, Down syndrome, congenital heart disease, rotavirus infections, gastroschisis, and Hirschsprung disease.

CLINICAL MANIFESTATIONS

Infants with NEC have a variety of signs and symptoms and may have an insidious or sudden catastrophic onset (Table 123.1). The onset of NEC is usually in the 2nd or 3rd week of life but can be as late as 3 mo in VLBW infants. Age of onset is inversely related to gestational age. The first signs of impending disease may be nonspecific, including lethargy and temperature instability, or related to GI pathology, such as abdominal distention, feeding intolerance, and bloody stools. Because of nonspecific signs, sepsis may be suspected before NEC. The spectrum of illness is broad, ranging from mild disease with only guaiac-positive stools to severe illness with bowel perforation, peritonitis, systemic inflammatory response syndrome, shock, and death. Laboratory derangements may include neutropenia, anemia, thrombocytopenia, coagulopathy, and metabolic acidosis. Hypotension and respiratory failure are common. Progression may be rapid, but it is unusual for the disease to progress from mild to severe after 72 hr.

DIAGNOSIS

A very high index of suspicion in treating preterm at-risk infants is crucial. Plain abdominal radiographs are essential to make a diagnosis of NEC. The finding of **pneumatosis intestinalis** (air in the bowel wall) confirms the clinical suspicion of NEC and is diagnostic; 50–75% of patients have pneumatosis when treatment is started (Fig. 123.5). Portal

venous gas is a sign of severe disease, and **pneumoperitoneum** indicates a perforation (Figs. 123.6 and 123.7). Ultrasound with Doppler flow assessment may be useful to evaluate for free fluid, abscess, and bowel wall thickness, peristalsis, and perfusion.

The differential diagnosis of NEC includes specific infections (systemic or intestinal), GI obstruction, volvulus, and isolated intestinal perforation. **Idiopathic focal intestinal perforation** can occur spontaneously or after the early use of postnatal corticosteroids and indomethacin. Pneumoperitoneum develops in such patients, but they are usually less ill than those with NEC.

TREATMENT

Rapid initiation of therapy is required for infants with suspected as well as proven NEC. There is no definitive treatment for established NEC, so therapy is directed at providing supportive care and preventing further injury with cessation of feeding, nasogastric decompression, and administration of IV fluids. Careful attention to respiratory status, coagulation profile, and acid-base and electrolyte balances are important. Once blood has been drawn for culture, systemic antibiotics (with broad coverage based on the antibiotic sensitivity patterns of the gram-positive, gram-negative, and anaerobic organisms in the particular neonatal ICU) should be started immediately. If present, umbilical catheters should be removed, but good IV access needs to be maintained. Ventilation should be assisted in the presence of apnea or if abdominal distention is contributing to hypoxia and hypercapnia. Intravascular volume replacement with crystalloid or blood products, cardiovascular support with fluid boluses and/or inotropes, and correction of hematologic, metabolic, and electrolyte abnormalities are essential to stabilize the infant with NEC.

The patient's course should be monitored closely by means of frequent physical assessments; sequential anteroposterior and cross-table lateral or lateral decubitus abdominal radiographs to detect intestinal perforation; and serial determinations of hematologic, electrolyte, and acid-base status. Gown and glove isolation and grouping of infants at similar increased risks into cohorts separate from other infants should be instituted to contain an epidemic.

A surgeon should be consulted early in the course of treatment. The only absolute indication for surgery is evidence of perforation on abdominal radiograph (pneumoperitoneum) present in less than half of infants with perforation or necrosis at operative exploration. Progressive clinical deterioration despite maximum medical management, a single fixed bowel loop on serial radiographs, and abdominal wall erythema are relative indications for exploratory laparotomy. Ideally, surgery should be performed after intestinal necrosis develops but before perforation and peritonitis occur. The optimal surgical approach, however, remains controversial. The options for surgical treatment include **primary peritoneal drainage (PPD)** or exploratory laparotomy with resection of the necrotic intestine and usually stoma creation. Two randomized clinical trials in the mid-2000s comparing these approaches failed to demonstrate significant differences in survival, nutritional outcomes, or length of stay. A Cochrane analysis combining the results of both trials concluded that there were no significant benefits or harms of PPD over exploratory laparotomy. A 3rd randomized clinical trial (Necrotizing Enterocolitis Surgery Trial, NCT01029353) compares the 2 surgical approaches, with the primary outcome being death or neurodevelopmental outcomes at 18-22 mo adjusted age. A large, multicenter cohort study of 8,935 patients demonstrated that laparotomy was the initial therapy in two thirds of VLBW infants with surgical NEC, even in those <1,000 g. Mortality was about 30% in both the laparotomy group and the PPD-converted-to-laparotomy group (46% of PPD group eventually required laparotomy). PPD was found to be an independent risk factor for death (50% mortality), likely from its preferential use in the more seriously ill, unstable patients; however, 27% of patients undergoing PPD survived without further surgery. *The surgical approach depends on surgeon preference and physiologic status of the patient.*

PROGNOSIS

Medical management fails in approximately 20–40% of patients with pneumatosis intestinalis at diagnosis; of these, 20–50% die. Early

Table 123.1	Signs and Symptoms Associated With Necrotizing Enterocolitis

GASTROINTESTINAL
Abdominal distention
Abdominal tenderness
Feeding intolerance
Delayed gastric emptying
Vomiting
Occult/gross blood in stool
Change in stool pattern/diarrhea
Abdominal mass
Erythema of abdominal wall

SYSTEMIC
Lethargy
Apnea/respiratory distress
Temperature instability
"Not right"
Acidosis (metabolic and/or respiratory)
Glucose instability
Poor perfusion/shock
Disseminated intravascular coagulopathy
Positive results of blood cultures

From Kanto WP Jr, Hunter JE, Stoll BJ: Recognition and medical management of necrotizing enterocolitis, *Clin Perinatol* 21:335–346, 1994.

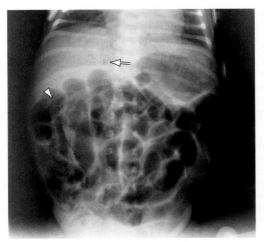

Fig. 123.5 Necrotizing enterocolitis (NEC). Kidney-ureter-bladder film demonstrates abdominal distention, hepatic portal venous gas *(arrow)*, and a bubbly appearance of pneumatosis intestinalis *(arrowhead;* right lower quadrant). The latter 2 signs are thought to be pathognomonic for neonatal NEC.

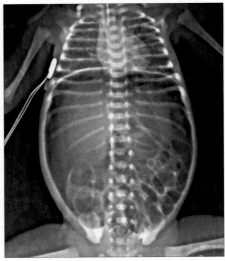

Fig. 123.7 Necrotizing enterocolitis (NEC). Plain abdominal x-ray film of an infant with perforated NEC showing pneumoperitoneum. *(From Tam PKH, Chung PHY, St Peter SD, et al: Advances in paediatric gastroenterology. Lancet 390:1072–1082, 2017, Fig 4).*

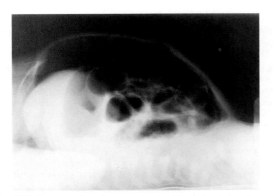

Fig. 123.6 Intestinal perforation. Cross-table abdominal radiograph in patient with neonatal NEC demonstrates marked distention and massive pneumoperitoneum, as evidenced by the free air below the anterior abdominal wall.

probiotics to prevent NEC, there is no clear consensus on the safest, most effective formulation, timing of administration, or length of therapy. Other preventive strategies using **prebiotics** and **synbiotics** have also been studied, with variable outcomes. Inhibitors of gastric acid secretion (H_2-receptor blockers, proton pump inhibitors) or prolonged empirical antibiotics in the early neonatal period have been associated with increased risk of NEC and should be avoided.

Because early detection and treatment may prevent late deleterious consequences of NEC, considerable research is focused on identification of **biomarkers** for early identification of NEC, including C-reactive protein (CRP), urinary intestinal fatty acid–binding protein (I-FABP), claudin-3 (a tight junction protein), fecal calprotectin, acylcarnitine, IL-6, IL-8, and the heart rate characteristics (HRC) index. Near-infrared spectroscopy (NIRS) may be a promising predictive diagnostic modality for NEC.

Bibliography is available at Expert Consult.

postoperative complications include wound infection, dehiscence, and stomal problems (prolapse, necrosis). Later complications include **intestinal strictures**, which occur in approximately 10% of surgically or medically managed patients. After massive intestinal resection, complications from postoperative NEC include **short bowel syndrome** (malabsorption, growth failure, malnutrition), complications related to central venous catheters (sepsis, thrombosis), and cholestatic jaundice. Preterm infants with NEC who require surgical intervention are at increased risk for adverse growth and neurodevelopmental outcomes.

PREVENTION
The most effective preventive strategy for NEC is the use of **human milk**. It is well documented that newborns exclusively breastfed have a reduced risk of NEC. However, because human milk does not provide complete nutritional support, fortification is essential for preterm infants. Some studies have suggested that an "exclusive human milk diet" using human rather than bovine fortifiers may further reduce the risk of NEC. Despite concerns about increased risk of NEC with early and aggressive feeding regimens in VLBW infants, a safe protocol remains unknown. While extensive data and meta-analyses would support the use of

123.3 Jaundice and Hyperbilirubinemia in the Newborn
Erin E. Shaughnessy and Neera K. Goyal

Hyperbilirubinemia is a common and, in most cases, benign problem in neonates. **Jaundice** is observed during the 1st wk after birth in approximately 60% of term infants and 80% of preterm infants. The yellow color usually results from the accumulation of unconjugated, nonpolar, lipid-soluble bilirubin pigment in the skin. This unconjugated bilirubin (designated **indirect-acting** by nature of the van den Bergh reaction) is an end product of heme-protein catabolism from a series of enzymatic reactions by heme-oxygenase and biliverdin reductase and nonenzymatic reducing agents in the reticuloendothelial cells. It may also be partly caused by deposition of pigment from conjugated bilirubin, the end product from indirect, unconjugated bilirubin that has undergone conjugation in the liver cell microsome by the enzyme uridine diphosphoglucuronic acid (UDP)–glucuronyl transferase to form the polar, water-soluble glucuronide of bilirubin (**direct-reacting**). Although bilirubin may have a physiologic role as an antioxidant, elevations of indirect, unconjugated bilirubin are potentially neurotoxic. Even though the conjugated form is not neurotoxic, direct hyperbilirubinemia indicates potentially serious hepatic disorders or a systemic illness.

ETIOLOGY

During the neonatal period, metabolism of bilirubin is in transition from the *fetal stage,* during which the placenta is the principal route of elimination of the lipid-soluble, unconjugated bilirubin, to the *adult stage,* during which the water-soluble conjugated form is excreted from hepatic cells into the biliary system and gastrointestinal tract. **Unconjugated hyperbilirubinemia** may be caused or increased by any factor that (a) increases the load of bilirubin to be metabolized by the liver (hemolytic anemias, polycythemia, bruising or internal hemorrhage, shortened red blood cell [RBC] life as a result of immaturity or transfusion of cells, increased enterohepatic circulation, infection); (b) damages or reduces the activity of the transferase enzyme or other related enzymes (genetic deficiency, hypoxia, infection, thyroid deficiency); (c) competes for or blocks the transferase enzyme (drugs and other substances requiring glucuronic acid conjugation); or (d) leads to an absence or decreased amounts of the enzyme or to reduction of bilirubin uptake by liver cells (genetic defect, prematurity). Gene polymorphisms in the hepatic uridine diphosphate glucuronosyltransferase isoenzyme 1A1 (*UGT1A1*) and the solute carrier organic anion transporter 1B1 (*SLCO1B1*), alone or in combination, influence the incidence of neonatal hyperbilirubinemia.

The toxic effects of elevated serum concentrations of unconjugated bilirubin are increased by factors that reduce the retention of bilirubin in the circulation (hypoproteinemia, displacement of bilirubin from its binding sites on albumin by competitive binding of drugs such as sulfisoxazole and moxalactam, acidosis, and increased free fatty acid concentration secondary to hypoglycemia, starvation, or hypothermia). Neurotoxic effects are directly related not only to the permeability of the blood-brain barrier and nerve cell membranes but also to neuronal susceptibility to injury, all of which are adversely influenced by asphyxia, prematurity, hyperosmolality, and infection. Early and frequent feeding decreases, whereas breastfeeding and dehydration increase, serum levels of bilirubin. Delay in passage of meconium, which contains 1 mg bilirubin/dL, may contribute to jaundice by enterohepatic recirculation after deconjugation by intestinal glucuronidase (Fig. 123.8). Drugs such as oxytocin (in the mother) and chemicals used in the nursery such as phenolic detergents may also produce unconjugated hyperbilirubinemia.

CLINICAL MANIFESTATIONS

Jaundice usually appears during the early neonatal period, depending on etiology. Whereas jaundice from deposition of indirect bilirubin in the skin tends to appear bright yellow or orange, jaundice of the obstructive type (direct bilirubin) has a greenish or muddy yellow cast. Jaundice usually becomes apparent in a cephalocaudal progression, starting on the face and progressing to the abdomen and then the feet, as serum levels increase. Dermal pressure may reveal the anatomic progression of jaundice (face, approximately 5 mg/dL; mid-abdomen, 15 mg/dL; soles, 20 mg/dL), but clinical examination cannot reliably estimate serum levels. Noninvasive techniques for transcutaneous measurement of bilirubin that correlate with serum levels may be used to *screen* infants, but determination of serum bilirubin level is indicated in patients with elevated age-specific transcutaneous bilirubin measurement, progressing jaundice, or risk for hemolysis or sepsis. Infants with severe hyperbilirubinemia may present with lethargy and poor feeding and, without treatment, can progress to acute bilirubin encephalopathy (kernicterus) (see Chapter 123.4).

DIFFERENTIAL DIAGNOSIS

The distinction between *physiologic* and *pathologic* jaundice relates to the timing, rate of rise, and extent of hyperbilirubinemia, because some of the same causes of physiologic jaundice (e.g., large RBC mass, decreased capacity for bilirubin conjugation, increased enterohepatic circulation) can also result in pathologic jaundice. Evaluation should be determined on the basis of risk factors, clinical appearance, and severity of the hyperbilirubinemia (Tables 123.2 to 123.4). Jaundice that is present at birth or appears within the 1st 24 hr after birth should be considered **pathologic** and requires immediate attention. Potential diagnoses would

include erythroblastosis fetalis, concealed hemorrhage, sepsis, or congenital infections, including syphilis, cytomegalovirus (CMV), rubella, and toxoplasmosis. Hemolysis is suggested by a rapid rise in serum bilirubin concentration (>0.5 mg/dL/hr), anemia, pallor, reticulocytosis, hepatosplenomegaly, and a positive family history. An unusually high proportion of direct-reacting bilirubin may characterize jaundice in infants who have received intrauterine transfusions for erythroblastosis fetalis. Jaundice that first appears on the 2nd or 3rd day is usually **physiologic** but may represent a more severe form. Familial nonhemolytic icterus (**Crigler-Najjar syndrome**) and early-onset breastfeeding jaundice are seen initially on the 2nd or 3rd day. Jaundice appearing after the 3rd day and within the 1st week suggests bacterial sepsis or urinary tract infection; it may also be caused by other infections, notably syphilis, toxoplasmosis, CMV, and enterovirus. Jaundice secondary to extensive ecchymosis or blood extravasation may occur during the 1st day or later, especially in premature infants. Polycythemia may also lead to early jaundice.

There is a long differential diagnosis for jaundice first recognized *after* the 1st week of life, including breast milk jaundice, septicemia, congenital atresia or paucity of the bile ducts, hepatitis, galactosemia, hypothyroidism, CF, and congenital hemolytic anemia crises related to RBC morphology and enzyme deficiencies (Fig. 123.9). The differential diagnosis for persistent jaundice during the 1st mo of life includes hyperalimentation-associated cholestasis, hepatitis, cytomegalic inclusion disease, syphilis, toxoplasmosis, familial nonhemolytic icterus, congenital atresia of the bile ducts, galactosemia, and inspissated bile syndrome following hemolytic disease of the newborn. Rarely, physiologic jaundice may be prolonged for several weeks, as in infants with hypothyroidism or pyloric stenosis.

Regardless of gestation or time of appearance of jaundice, patients with *significant* hyperbilirubinemia *and* those with symptoms or signs require a complete diagnostic evaluation, which includes determination of direct and indirect bilirubin fractions, hemoglobin, reticulocyte count,

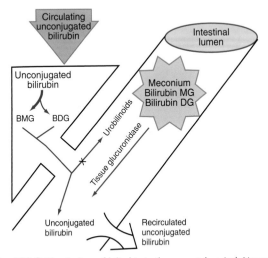

Fig. 123.8 Metabolism of bilirubin in the neonatal period. Neonatal production rate of bilirubin is 6-8 mg/kg/24 hr (in contrast to 3-4 mg/kg/24 hr in adults). Water-insoluble bilirubin is bound to albumin. At the plasma-hepatocyte interface, a liver membrane carrier (bilitranslocase) transports bilirubin to a cytosolic binding protein (ligandin or Y protein, now known to be glutathione *S*-transferase), which prevents back-absorption to plasma. Bilirubin is converted to bilirubin monoglucuronide (BMG). Neonates excrete more BMG than adults. In the fetus, conjugated lipid-insoluble BMG and bilirubin diglucuronide (BDG) must be deconjugated by tissue β-glucuronidases to facilitate placental transfer of lipid-soluble unconjugated bilirubin across the placental lipid membranes. After birth, intestinal or milk-containing glucuronidases contribute to the enterohepatic recirculation of bilirubin and possibly to the development of hyperbilirubinemia.

blood type, Coombs test, and examination of a peripheral blood smear. Indirect hyperbilirubinemia, reticulocytosis, and a smear with evidence of RBC destruction suggest hemolysis (see Table 123.3). In the absence of blood group incompatibility, non–immunologically induced hemolysis should be considered. If the reticulocyte count, Coombs test result, and direct hyperbilirubinemia value are normal, physiologic or pathologic indirect hyperbilirubinemia may be present (see Fig. 123.9). If direct hyperbilirubinemia is present, diagnostic possibilities include hepatitis, congenital bile duct disorders (biliary atresia, paucity of bile ducts, Byler disease), cholestasis, inborn errors of metabolism, CF, congenital hemosiderosis, and sepsis.

PHYSIOLOGIC JAUNDICE (ICTERUS NEONATORUM)

Under normal circumstances, the level of indirect bilirubin in umbilical cord serum is 1-3 mg/dL and rises at a rate of <5 mg/dL/24 hr; thus, jaundice becomes visible on the 2nd or 3rd day, usually peaking between the 2nd and 4th days at 5-6 mg/dL and decreasing to <2 mg/dL between the 5th and 7th days after birth. Jaundice associated with these changes is designated *physiologic* and is believed to be the result of increased bilirubin production from the breakdown of fetal RBCs combined with transient limitation in the conjugation of bilirubin by the immature neonatal liver.

Overall, 6–7% of full-term infants have indirect bilirubin levels >13 mg/dL, and <3% have levels >15 mg/dL. Risk factors for elevated indirect bilirubin include maternal age, race (Chinese, Japanese, Korean, Native American), maternal diabetes, prematurity, drugs (vitamin K_3, novobiocin), altitude, polycythemia, male sex, trisomy 21, cutaneous bruising, blood extravasation (cephalohematoma), oxytocin induction, breastfeeding, weight loss (dehydration or caloric deprivation), delayed bowel

movement, and a family history of, or a sibling who had, physiologic jaundice (see Table 123.2). In infants without these variables, indirect bilirubin levels rarely rise >12 mg/dL, whereas infants with several risk factors are more likely to have higher bilirubin levels. A combination of breastfeeding, variant-glucuronosyltransferase activity (1A1), and alterations of the organic anion transporter-2 gene increases the risk of hyperbilirubinemia. Predicting which neonates are at risk for exaggerated physiologic jaundice can be based on *hour-specific* bilirubin levels in the 1st 24-72 hr of life (Fig. 123.10). Transcutaneous measurements of bilirubin are linearly correlated with serum levels and can be used for screening. Indirect bilirubin levels in full-term infants decline to adult levels (1 mg/dL) by 10-14 days of life. Persistent indirect hyperbilirubinemia beyond 2 wk suggests hemolysis, hereditary glucuronyl transferase deficiency, breast milk jaundice, hypothyroidism, or intestinal obstruction. Jaundice associated with pyloric stenosis may be the result of caloric deprivation, relative deficiency of hepatic UDP–glucuronyltransferase, or an increase in the enterohepatic circulation of bilirubin from the ileus. In premature infants, the rise in serum bilirubin tends to be the same or somewhat slower but of longer duration than in term infants. Peak levels of 8-12 mg/dL are not usually reached until the 4th-7th day, and jaundice is infrequently observed after the 10th day, corresponding to the maturation of mechanisms for bilirubin metabolism and excretion.

The diagnosis of physiologic jaundice in term or preterm infants can be established only by excluding known causes of jaundice on the basis of the history, clinical findings, and laboratory data (see Table 123.4). In general, a search to determine the cause of jaundice should be made if (1) it appears in the 1st 24-36 hr after birth, (2) serum bilirubin is rising at a rate faster than 5 mg/dL/24 hr, (3) serum bilirubin is >12 mg/dL in a full-term infant (especially in the absence of risk factors) or 10-14 mg/dL in a preterm infant, (4) jaundice persists after 10-14 days after birth, or (5) direct bilirubin fraction is >2 mg/dL at any time. Other factors suggesting a pathologic cause of jaundice are family history of hemolytic disease, pallor, hepatomegaly, splenomegaly, failure of phototherapy to lower the bilirubin level, vomiting, lethargy, poor feeding, excessive weight loss, apnea, bradycardia, abnormal vital signs (including hypothermia), light-colored stools, dark urine positive for bilirubin, bleeding disorder, and signs of kernicterus (see Chapter 123.4).

Table 123.2	Risk Factors for Development of Severe Hyperbilirubinemia*

MAJOR RISK FACTORS
Predischarge TSB or TcB level in the high-risk zone (see Fig. 123.10)
Jaundice observed in the 1st 24 hr
Blood group incompatibility with positive direct antiglobulin test, other known hemolytic disease (G6PD deficiency), elevated end-tidal CO concentration
Gestational age 35-36 wk
Previous sibling received phototherapy
Cephalohematoma or significant bruising
Exclusive breastfeeding, particularly if nursing is not going well and weight loss is excessive
East Asian race[†]

MINOR RISK FACTORS
Predischarge TSB or TcB level in the high intermediate-risk zone
Gestational age 37-38 wk
Jaundice observed before discharge
Previous sibling with jaundice
Macrosomic infant of a diabetic mother
Maternal age ≥25 yr
Male gender

DECREASED RISK[‡]
TSB or TcB level in the low-risk zone (see Fig. 123.10)
Gestational age ≥41 wk
Exclusive bottle feeding
Black race
Discharge from hospital after 72 hr

*In infants ≥35 wk of gestation; factors in approximate order of importance.
[†]Race as defined by mother's description.
[‡]These factors are associated with decreased risk of significant jaundice, listed in order of decreasing importance.
G6PD, Glucose-6-phosphate dehydrogenase; TcB, transcutaneous bilirubin; TSB, total serum bilirubin.
Adapted from American Academy of Pediatrics Subcommittee on Hyperbilirubinemia: Management of hyperbilirubinemia in the newborn infant 35 or more weeks of gestation, *Pediatrics* 114:297–316, 2004.

Table 123.3	Evaluation of the Neonate With Significant Jaundice

CONCERN	POSSIBLE DIAGNOSIS	INITIAL LABORATORY TESTS
Jaundice on day 1	Hemolysis[++] TORCH/sepsis Hepatic failure syndromes* Internal hemorrhage	CBC, smear Total and direct bilirubin Blood type and Coombs test
Jaundice requiring phototherapy	Hemolysis[++] TORCH/sepsis	As above
Direct/conjugated hyperbilirubinemia	TORCH/sepsis Biliary atresia Other causes of cholestasis[+] Hepatic failure syndromes*	Hepatic enzymes, INR, check newborn screen for metabolic disease, blood glucose, blood ammonia and lactate, urine and blood cultures, CMV and HSV PCR

[+]See Chapter 383.
[++]Hemolysis may be immune or nonimmune (RBC membrane or enzyme defects).
CMV, Cytomegalovirus; CBC, complete blood count; HSV, herpes simplex virus; PCR, polymerase chain reaction; INR, international normalized ratio; TORCH, toxoplasmosis, other, rubella, CMV, herpes; *Hepatic failure syndromes: HSV, CMV, gestational alloimmune liver disease, mitochondrial liver disease, familial hemophagocytic syndrome; RBC, red blood cell.

Table 123.4	Diagnostic Features of the Various Types of Neonatal Jaundice						
DIAGNOSIS	**NATURE OF VAN DEN BERGH REACTION**	**JAUNDICE**		**PEAK BILIRUBIN CONCENTRATION**		**BILIRUBIN RATE OF ACCUMULATION (mg/dL/day)**	**COMMENTS**
		Appears	**Disappears**	**mg/dL**	**Age in Days**		
"Physiologic jaundice":							Usually relates to degree of maturity
Full-term	Indirect	2-3 days	4-5 days	10-12	2-3	<5	
Premature	Indirect	3-4 days	7-9 days	15	6-8	<5	
Hyperbilirubinemia caused by metabolic factors:							Metabolic factors: hypoxia, respiratory distress, lack of carbohydrate
Full-term	Indirect	2-3 days	Variable	>12	1st wk	<5	Hormonal influences: cretinism, hormones, Gilbert syndrome
Premature	Indirect	3-4 days	Variable	>15	1st wk	<5	Genetic factors: Crigler-Najjar syndrome, Gilbert syndrome
Drugs: vitamin K, novobiocin
Hemolytic states and hematoma	Indirect	May appear in 1st 24 hr	Variable	Unlimited	Variable	Usually >5	Erythroblastosis: Rh, ABO, Kell congenital hemolytic states: spherocytic, nonspherocytic
Infantile pyknocytosis
Drug: vitamin K
Enclosed hemorrhage—hematoma
Mixed hemolytic and hepatotoxic factors	Indirect and direct	May appear in 1st 24 hr	Variable	Unlimited	Variable	Usually >5	Infection: bacterial sepsis, pyelonephritis, hepatitis, toxoplasmosis, cytomegalic inclusion disease, rubella, syphilis
Drug: vitamin K
Hepatocellular damage	Indirect and direct	Usually 2-3 days; may appear by 2nd wk	Variable	Unlimited	Variable	Variable, can be >5	Biliary atresia; paucity of bile ducts, familial cholestasis, galactosemia; hepatitis, infection

From Brown AK: Neonatal jaundice, *Pediatr Clin North Am* 9:575–603, 1962.

PATHOLOGIC HYPERBILIRUBINEMIA

Jaundice and its underlying hyperbilirubinemia are considered pathologic if the time of appearance, duration, or pattern varies significantly from that of physiologic jaundice, or if the course is compatible with physiologic jaundice but other reasons exist to suspect that the infant is at special risk for neurotoxicity. It may not be possible to determine the precise cause of an abnormal elevation of unconjugated bilirubin, but many infants with this finding have associated risk factors such as Asian race, prematurity, breastfeeding, and weight loss. Frequently, the terms *exaggerated physiologic jaundice* and *hyperbilirubinemia of the newborn* are used in infants whose primary problem is probably a deficiency or inactivity of bilirubin glucuronyl transferase (**Gilbert syndrome**) rather than an excessive load of bilirubin for excretion (see Table 123.2). The combination of glucose-6-phosphate dehydrogenase (G6PD) deficiency and a mutation of the promoter region of UDP-glucuronyl transferase-1 produces indirect hyperbilirubinemia in the absence of signs of hemolysis. Nonphysiologic hyperbilirubinemia may also be caused by mutations in the gene for bilirubin UDP–glucuronyl transferase.

The greatest risk associated with indirect hyperbilirubinemia is the development of bilirubin-induced neurologic dysfunction, which typically occurs with high indirect bilirubin levels (see Chapter 123.4). The development of kernicterus (bilirubin encephalopathy) depends on the level of indirect bilirubin, duration of exposure to bilirubin elevation, the cause of jaundice, and the infant's well-being. Neurologic injury including kernicterus may occur at lower bilirubin levels in preterm infants and in the presence of asphyxia, intraventricular hemorrhage, hemolysis, or drugs that displace bilirubin from albumin. The exact serum indirect bilirubin level that is harmful for VLBW infants is unclear.

JAUNDICE ASSOCIATED WITH BREASTFEEDING

Significant elevation in unconjugated bilirubin (**breast milk jaundice**) develops in an estimated 2% of breastfed term infants after the 7th day, with maximal concentrations as high as 10-30 mg/dL reached during the 2nd-3rd wk. If breastfeeding is continued, the bilirubin gradually decreases but may persist for 3-10 wk at lower levels. If nursing is discontinued, the serum bilirubin level falls rapidly, reaching normal range within a few days. With resumption of breastfeeding, bilirubin seldom returns to previously high levels. Phototherapy may be of benefit (see Chapter 123.4). Although uncommon, kernicterus can occur in patients with breast milk jaundice. The etiology of breast milk jaundice is not entirely clear, although β-glucuronidase resulting in deconjugation of bilirubin and increased enterohepatic circulation and other factors in breast milk that might interfere with bilirubin conjugation (e.g., pregnanediol, free fatty acids) have been implicated.

The late jaundice associated with breast milk should be distinguished from an *early onset*, accentuated unconjugated hyperbilirubinemia known as **breastfeeding jaundice**, which occurs in the 1st week after birth in breastfed infants, who normally have higher bilirubin levels than formula-fed infants (Fig. 123.11). Lower milk intake before breast milk production is established can result in dehydration, which hemoconcentrates bilirubin, while also causing fewer bowel movements, which in turn increases the enterohepatic circulation of bilirubin. Prophylactic

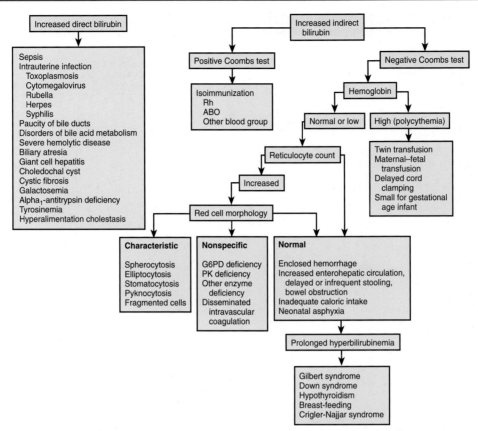

Fig. 123.9 Schematic approach to the diagnosis of neonatal jaundice. *G6PD,* Glucose-6-phosphate dehydrogenase; *PK,* pyruvate kinase. (*From Oski FA: Differential diagnosis of jaundice. In Taeusch HW, Ballard RA, Avery MA, editors: Schaffer and Avery's diseases of the newborn, ed 6, Philadelphia, 1991, Saunders.*)

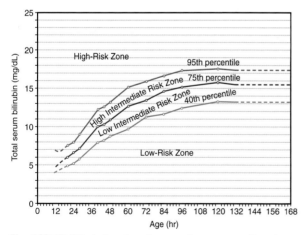

Fig. 123.10 Risk designation of term and near-term well newborns based on their hour-specific serum bilirubin values. The high-risk zone is subdivided by the 95th percentile track. The intermediate -risk zone is subdivided into upper and lower risk zones by the 75th percentile track. The low-risk zone has been electively and statistically defined by the 40th percentile track. (*From Bhutani VK, Johnson L, Sivieri EM: Predictive ability of a predischarge hour-specific serum bilirubin for subsequent significant hyperbilirubinemia in healthy term and near-term newborns, Pediatrics 103:6–14, 1999.*)

supplements of glucose water to breastfed infants are associated with higher bilirubin levels, in part because of reduced intake of the higher–caloric density breast milk, and are *not* indicated. Frequent breastfeeding (>10 in 24 hr), rooming-in with night feeding, and ongoing lactation support may reduce the incidence of early breastfeeding jaundice. In addition, supplementation with formula or expressed breast milk is appropriate if the intake seems inadequate, weight loss is excessive, or the infant appears dehydrated.

NEONATAL CHOLESTASIS
See Chapter 383.1.

CONGENITAL ATRESIA OF THE BILE DUCTS
See Chapter 383.1.

Jaundice persisting for >2 wk or associated with acholic stools and dark urine suggests biliary atresia. All infants with such findings require immediate diagnostic evaluation, including determination of direct bilirubin.

Bibliography is available at Expert Consult.

123.4 Kernicterus
Erin E. Shaughnessy and Neera K. Goyal

Kernicterus, or **bilirubin encephalopathy**, is a neurologic syndrome resulting from the deposition of unconjugated (indirect) bilirubin in the basal ganglia and brainstem nuclei. The pathogenesis of kernicterus is multifactorial and involves an interaction between unconjugated bilirubin levels, albumin binding and unbound bilirubin levels, passage across the blood-brain barrier (BBB), and neuronal susceptibility to injury. Disruption of the BBB by disease, asphyxia, and other factors and maturational changes in BBB permeability affect risk.

The precise blood level above which indirect-reacting bilirubin or free bilirubin will be toxic for an individual infant is unpredictable. In a large series, however, kernicterus occurred only in infants with a bilirubin >20 mg/dL, 90% of whom were previously healthy, predominantly breastfed, term and near-term infants. The duration of exposure to high bilirubin levels needed to produce toxic effects are unknown; the more immature the infant, the greater the susceptibility to kernicterus. Chapter 123.3 discusses the factors that potentiate the movement of bilirubin across the BBB and into brain cells.

CLINICAL MANIFESTATIONS

Signs and symptoms of kernicterus usually appear 2-5 days after birth in term infants and as late as the 7th day in preterm infants, but hyperbilirubinemia may lead to encephalopathy at any time during the neonatal period. The early signs may be subtle and indistinguishable from those of sepsis, asphyxia, hypoglycemia, intracranial hemorrhage, and other acute systemic illnesses in a neonate. Lethargy, poor feeding, and loss of the Moro reflex are common initial signs. Subsequently, the infant may appear gravely ill and prostrate, with diminished tendon reflexes and respiratory distress. Opisthotonos with a bulging fontanel, twitching of the face or limbs, and a shrill, high-pitched cry may follow. In advanced cases, convulsions and spasm occur, with affected infants stiffly extending their arms in an inward rotation with the fists clenched (Table 123.5). Rigidity is rare at this late stage.

Many infants who progress to these severe neurologic signs die; the survivors are usually seriously damaged but may appear to recover and for 2-3 mo show few abnormalities. Later in the 1st yr, opisthotonos, muscle rigidity, irregular movements, and convulsions tend to recur. In the 2nd yr the opisthotonos and seizures abate, but irregular, involuntary movements, muscle rigidity, or, in some infants, hypotonia increase steadily. By 3 yr of age, the complete neurologic syndrome is often apparent: bilateral choreoathetosis with involuntary muscle spasms, extrapyramidal signs, seizures, mental deficiency, dysarthric speech, high-frequency hearing loss, squinting, and defective upward eye movements. Pyramidal signs, hypotonia, and ataxia occur in a few infants. In mildly affected infants, the syndrome may be characterized only by mild to moderate neuromuscular incoordination, partial deafness, or "minimal brain dysfunction," occurring singly or in combination; these problems may be unapparent until the child enters school (see Table 123.5).

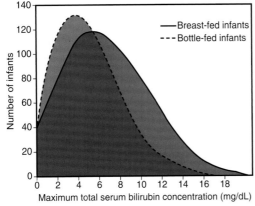

Fig. 123.11 Distribution of maximal bilirubin levels during the 1st wk of life in breastfed and formula-fed white infants weighing >2,500 g. *(From Maisels MJ, Gifford K: Normal serum bilirubin levels in the newborn and the effect of breast-feeding, Pediatrics 78:837–843, 1986.)*

INCIDENCE AND PROGNOSIS

By pathologic criteria, kernicterus develops in 30% of infants (all gestational ages) with untreated hemolytic disease and bilirubin levels >25-30 mg/dL. The incidence at autopsy in hyperbilirubinemic preterm infants is 2–16% and is related to the risk factors discussed in Chapter 123.3. Reliable estimates of the frequency of the clinical syndrome are not available because of the wide spectrum of manifestations. Overt neurologic signs carry a grave prognosis; >75% of infants die, and 80% of affected survivors have bilateral choreoathetosis with involuntary muscle spasms. Developmental delay, deafness, and spastic quadriplegia are common.

PREVENTION

Although kernicterus has been thought to be a disease of the past, there are reports of neurotoxic effects of bilirubin in term and near-term infants who were discharged as healthy newborns. Effective prevention requires ongoing vigilance and a practical, system-based approach to distinguish infants with benign newborn jaundice from those whose course may be less predictable and potentially harmful. Experts recommend predischarge universal screening for hyperbilirubinemia and assessment of clinical risk factors for severe jaundice and bilirubin-induced neurologic dysfunction. Either total serum bilirubin or transcutaneous bilirubin measurement (interchangeably) is recommended for initial screening, although transcutaneous instruments may be less accurate at higher bilirubin levels (>15 mg/dL) or for infants with darker skin. If transcutaneous levels are documented as ≥15 mg/dL or rising rapidly, confirmation with a total serum bilirubin is recommended. Serum values should also be measured once infants begin phototherapy, because transcutaneous measurement may falsely underestimate total bilirubin in this setting.

Protocols using the hour-specific bilirubin nomogram (see Fig. 123.10), physical examination, and clinical risk factors have been successful in identifying patients at risk for hyperbilirubinemia and candidates for targeted management. Potentially preventable causes of kernicterus include (1) early discharge (<48 hr) with no early follow-up (within 48 hr of discharge); this problem is particularly important in near-term infants (35-37 wk of gestation); (2) failure to check the bilirubin level in an infant noted to be jaundiced in the 1st 24 hr; (3) failure to recognize the presence of risk factors for hyperbilirubinemia; (4) underestimation of the severity of jaundice by clinical (visual) assessment; (5) lack of concern regarding the presence of jaundice; (6) delay in measuring the serum bilirubin level despite marked jaundice or delay in initiating phototherapy in the presence of elevated bilirubin levels; and (7) failure to respond to parental concern regarding jaundice, poor feeding, or lethargy. Fig. 123.12 provides an evidence-based management algorithm for infants. In addition, it is recommended to determine before discharge each infant's risk factors from established protocols (see Table 123.2).

The following approach is further recommended: (1) any infant who is jaundiced before 24 hr requires measurement of total *and* direct serum bilirubin levels and, if it is elevated, evaluation for possible hemolytic

Table 123.5	Clinical Features of Kernicterus

ACUTE FORM

Phase 1 (1st 1-2 days): poor suck, stupor, hypotonia, seizures
Phase 2 (middle of 1st wk): hypertonia of extensor muscles, opisthotonos, retrocollis, fever
Phase 3 (after the 1st wk): hypertonia

CHRONIC FORM

1st yr: hypotonia, active deep tendon reflexes, obligatory tonic neck reflexes, delayed motor skills
After 1st yr: movement disorders (choreoathetosis, ballismus, tremor), upward gaze, sensorineural hearing loss

From Dennery PA, Seidman DS, Stevenson DK: Neonatal hyperbilirubinemia, *N Engl J Med* 344:581–590, 2001.

disease, and (2) follow-up should be provided within 2-3 days of discharge to all neonates discharged earlier than 48 hr after birth. Early follow-up is particularly important for infants <38 wk of gestation. The timing of follow-up depends on the age at discharge and the presence of risk factors. In some cases, follow-up within 24 hr is necessary. Postdischarge follow-up is essential for early recognition of problems related to hyperbilirubinemia and disease progression. Parental communication with regard to concerns about the infant's skin color and behavioral activities should be addressed early and frequently, including education about potential risks and neurotoxicity. Ongoing lactation promotion, education, support, and follow-up services are essential throughout the neonatal period. Mothers should be advised to nurse their infants every 2-3 hr and to avoid routine supplementation with water or glucose water to ensure adequate hydration and caloric intake.

TREATMENT OF HYPERBILIRUBINEMIA

Regardless of the cause, the goal of therapy is to prevent neurotoxicity related to indirect-reacting bilirubin while not causing undue harm. Phototherapy and, if it is unsuccessful, exchange transfusion remain the primary treatment modalities used to keep the maximal total serum bilirubin below pathologic levels (Table 123.6 and Figs. 123.13 and 123.14). The risk of injury to the central nervous system from bilirubin must be balanced against the potential risk of treatment. There is lack of consensus regarding the exact bilirubin level at which to initiate phototherapy. Because phototherapy may require 6-12 hr to have a measurable effect, it must be started at bilirubin levels below those indicated for exchange transfusion. When identified, underlying medical causes of elevated bilirubin and physiologic factors that contribute to neuronal susceptibility should be treated, with antibiotics for septicemia and correction of acidosis (Table 123.7).

Phototherapy

Clinical jaundice and indirect hyperbilirubinemia are reduced by exposure to high-intensity light in the visible spectrum. Bilirubin absorbs light maximally in the blue range (420-470 nm). Broad-spectrum white, blue, and special narrow-spectrum (super) blue lights have been effective in reducing bilirubin levels. Bilirubin in the skin absorbs light energy, causing several photochemical reactions. One major product from phototherapy is a result of a reversible photoisomerization reaction converting the toxic native unconjugated 4Z,15Z-bilirubin into an unconjugated configurational isomer, 4Z,15E-bilirubin, which can then be excreted in bile without conjugation. The other major product from phototherapy is lumirubin, which is an irreversible structural isomer converted from native bilirubin that can be excreted by the kidneys in the unconjugated state.

The therapeutic effect of phototherapy depends on the light energy emitted in the effective range of wavelengths, the distance between the lights and the infant, and the surface area of exposed skin, as well as the rate of hemolysis and in vivo metabolism and excretion of bilirubin. Available commercial phototherapy units vary considerably in spectral output and the intensity of radiance emitted; therefore the wattage can be accurately measured only at the patient's skin surface. Dark skin does not reduce the efficacy of phototherapy. Maximal intensive phototherapy should be used when indirect bilirubin levels approach those noted in Fig. 123.13 and Table 123.7. Such therapy includes using "special blue" fluorescent tubes, placing the lamps within 15-20 cm (6-8 inches) of the infant, and putting a fiberoptic phototherapy blanket under the infant's back to increase the exposed surface area.

The use of phototherapy has decreased the need for exchange transfusion in term and preterm infants with hemolytic and nonhemolytic jaundice. When indications for exchange transfusion are present,

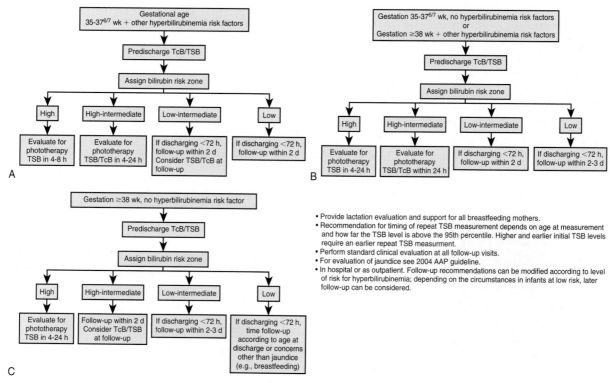

Fig. 123.12 Treatment of hyperbilirubinemia. Algorithm providing recommendations for management and follow-up according to predischarge bilirubin measurements, gestation, and risk factors for subsequent hyperbilirubinemia. TcB, Transcutaneous bilirubin; TSB, total serum bilirubin. (Data from Maisels MJ, Bhutani VK, Bogen D, et al: Hyperbilirubinemia in the newborn infant ≥35 weeks' gestation: an update with clarifications, Pediatrics 124:1193–1198, 2009.)

phototherapy should not be used as a substitute; however, phototherapy may reduce the need for repeated exchange transfusions in infants with hemolysis. Conventional phototherapy is applied continuously, and the infant is turned frequently for maximal skin surface area exposure. It should be discontinued as soon as the indirect bilirubin concentration has reduced to levels considered safe with respect to the infant's age and condition. Serum bilirubin levels and hematocrit should be monitored every 4-8 hr in infants with hemolytic disease and those with bilirubin levels near toxic range for the individual infant. Others, particularly older neonates, may be monitored less frequently. Serum bilirubin monitoring should continue for at least 24 hr after cessation of phototherapy in patients with hemolytic disease, because unexpected rises in bilirubin may occur, requiring further treatment. Skin color cannot be relied on for evaluating the effectiveness of phototherapy; the skin of babies exposed to light may appear to be almost without jaundice in the presence of marked hyperbilirubinemia. Although not necessary for all affected infants, intravenous fluid supplementation added to oral feedings may be beneficial in dehydrated patients or infants with bilirubin levels nearing those requiring exchange transfusion.

Complications associated with phototherapy include loose stools, erythematous macular rash, purpuric rash associated with transient porphyrinemia, overheating, dehydration (increased insensible water loss, diarrhea), hypothermia from exposure, and a benign condition called "bronze baby syndrome," which occurs in the presence of direct hyperbilirubinemia. Phototherapy is contraindicated in the presence of porphyria. Before phototherapy is initiated, the infant's eyes should be closed and adequately covered to prevent light exposure and corneal damage. Body temperature should be monitored, and the infant should be shielded from bulb breakage. Irradiance should be measured directly. In infants with hemolytic disease, care must be taken to monitor for the development of anemia, which may require transfusion. *Anemia may develop despite lowering of bilirubin levels.* Clinical experience suggests that long-term adverse biologic effects of phototherapy are absent, minimal, or unrecognized.

The term **bronze baby syndrome** refers to a dark, grayish brown skin discoloration sometimes noted in infants undergoing phototherapy. Almost all infants observed with this syndrome have had significant elevation of direct-reacting bilirubin and other evidence of obstructive liver disease. The discoloration may result from photo-induced modification of porphyrins, which are often present during cholestatic jaundice and may last for many months. Despite the bronze baby syndrome, phototherapy can continue if needed.

Intravenous Immune Globulin

The administration of intravenous immunoglobulin (IVIG) is an adjunctive treatment for hyperbilirubinemia caused by *isoimmune hemolytic disease.* Its use is recommended when serum bilirubin is approaching exchange levels despite maximal interventions, including phototherapy. IVIG (0.5-1.0 g/kg/dose; repeat in 12 hr) reduces the need for exchange transfusion in both ABO and Rh hemolytic disease, presumably by reducing hemolysis.

Metalloporphyrins

A possible adjunct therapy is the use of metalloporphyrins for hyperbilirubinemia. The metalloporphyrin Sn-mesoporphyrin (SnMP) offers promise as a drug candidate. The proposed mechanism of action is competitive enzymatic inhibition of the rate-limiting conversion of heme-protein to biliverdin (an intermediate metabolite in the production of unconjugated bilirubin) by heme-oxygenase. A single intramuscular dose on the 1st day of life may reduce the need for subsequent phototherapy. Such therapy may be beneficial when jaundice is anticipated, particularly in patients with ABO incompatibility or G6PD deficiency, or when blood products are objected to, as with Jehovah's Witness patients. Complications from metalloporphyrins include transient erythema if the infant is receiving phototherapy. Administration of SnMP may reduce bilirubin levels and decrease both the need for phototherapy and the duration of hospital stay; however, it remains unclear whether treatment with metalloporphyrins for unconjugated

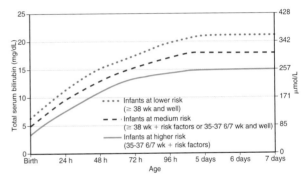

- Use total bilirubin. Do not subtract direct reacting or conjugated bilirubin.
- Risk factors = isoimmune hemolytic disease, G6PD deficiency, asphyxia, significant lethargy, temperature instability, sepsis, acidosis, or albumin < 3.0 g/dL (if measured).
- For well infants 35-37 6/7 wk can adjust TSB levels for intervention around the medium risk line. It is an option to intervene at lower TSB levels for infants closer to 35 wks and at higher TSB levels for those closer to 37 6/7 wk.
- It is an option to provide conventional phototherapy in hospital or at home at TSB levels 2-3 mg/dL (35-50 mmol/L) below those shown, but home phototherapy should not be used in any infant with risk factors.

Fig. 123.13 Guidelines for phototherapy in hospitalized infants of ≥35 wk of gestation. *Note:* These guidelines are based on limited evidence, and the levels shown are approximations. The guidelines refer to the use of intensive phototherapy, which should be used when the total serum bilirubin (TSB) exceeds the line indicated for each category. Infants are designated as "higher risk" because of the potential negative effects of the conditions listed on albumin binding of bilirubin, the blood-brain barrier, and the susceptibility of the brain cells to damage by bilirubin. "Intensive phototherapy" implies irradiance in the blue-green spectrum (wavelengths approximately 430-490 nm) of at least 30 μW/cm²/nm (measured at the infant's skin directly below the center of the phototherapy unit) and delivered to as much of the infant's skin surface area as possible. Note that irradiance measured below the center of the light source is much greater than that measured at the periphery. Measurements should be made with a radiometer specified by the manufacturer of the phototherapy system. If TSB levels approach or exceed the exchange transfusion line (see Fig. 123.14), the sides of the bassinette, incubator, or warmer should be lined with aluminum foil or white material, to increase both the surface area of the infant exposed and the efficacy of phototherapy. The presence of hemolysis is strongly suggested if the TSB does not decrease or continues to rise in an infant who is receiving intensive phototherapy. Infants who receive phototherapy and have an elevated direct-reacting or conjugated bilirubin value (cholestatic jaundice) may inconsistently have the bronze baby syndrome. G6PD, Glucose-6-phosphate dehydrogenase. (*From American Academy of Pediatrics Subcommittee on Hyperbilirubinemia: Management of hyperbilirubinemia in the newborn infant 35 or more weeks of gestation,* Pediatrics 114:297–316, 2004.)

Table 123.6	Suggested Maximal Indirect Serum Bilirubin Concentrations (mg/dL) in Preterm Infants	
BIRTHWEIGHT (g)	**UNCOMPLICATED***	**COMPLICATED***
<1,000	12-13	10-12
1,000-1,250	12-14	10-12
1,251-1,499	14-16	12-14
1,500-1,999	16-20	15-17
2,000-2,500	20-22	18-20

*Complications include perinatal asphyxia, acidosis, hypoxia, hypothermia, hypoalbuminemia, meningitis, intraventricular hemorrhage, hemolysis, hypoglycemia, or signs of kernicterus. Phototherapy is usually started at 50-70% of the maximal indirect level. If values greatly exceed this level, if phototherapy is unsuccessful in reducing the maximal bilirubin level, or if signs of kernicterus are evident, exchange transfusion is indicated.

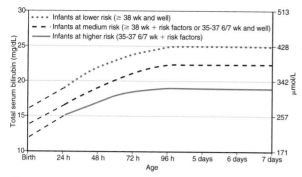

- The dashed lines for the first 24 hours indicate uncertainty due to a wide range of clinical circumstances and a range of responses to phototherapy.
- Immediate exchange transfusion is recommended if infant shows signs of acute bilirubin encephalopathy (hypertonia, arching, retrocollis, opisthotonos, fever, high pitched cry) or if TSB is ≥ 5 mg/dL (85 μmol/L) above these lines.
- Risk factors = isoimmune hemolytic disease, G6PD deficiency, asphyxia, significant lethargy, temperature instability, sepsis, acidosis.
- Measure serum albumin and calculate B/A ratio (see legend).
- Use total bilirubin. Do not subtract direct reacting or conjugated bilirubin.
- If infant is well and 35-37 6/7 wk (median risk), can individualize TSB levels for exchange based on actual gestational age.

Fig. 123.14 Guidelines for exchange transfusion in hospitalized infants of ≥35 wk of gestation. *Note:* These suggested levels represent a consensus of most of the committee but are based on limited evidence, and the levels shown are approximations. During birth hospitalization, exchange transfusion is recommended if the total serum bilirubin (TSB) rises to these levels despite intensive phototherapy. In a readmitted infant, if the TSB level is above the exchange level, TSB measurement should be repeated every 2-3 hr; exchange transfusion should be considered if the TSB remains above the levels indicated after intensive phototherapy for 6 hr. The following B:A (bilirubin:albumin) ratios can be used together with, but not instead of, the TSB level as an additional factor in determining the need for exchange transfusion. G6PD, Glucose-6-phosphate dehydrogenase. *(From American Academy of Pediatrics Subcommittee on Hyperbilirubinemia: Management of hyperbilirubinemia in the newborn infant 35 or more weeks of gestation, Pediatrics 114: 297–316, 2004.)*

hyperbilirubinemia will alter the risk of kernicterus or long-term neurodevelopment impairment. Data on efficacy, toxicity, and long-term benefit are still being evaluated.

Exchange Transfusion

Double-volume exchange transfusion is performed if intensive phototherapy has failed to reduce bilirubin levels to a safe range and the risk of kernicterus exceeds the procedural risk. Potential complications from exchange transfusion are not trivial and include metabolic acidosis, electrolyte abnormalities, hypoglycemia, hypocalcemia, thrombocytopenia, volume overload, arrhythmias, NEC, infection, graft-versus-host disease, and death. This widely accepted treatment is repeated if necessary to keep indirect bilirubin levels in a safe range (see Fig. 123.14 and Table 123.7).

Various factors may influence the decision to perform a double-volume exchange transfusion in an individual patient. The appearance of clinical signs suggesting kernicterus is an indication for exchange transfusion at any level of serum bilirubin. A healthy full-term infant with physiologic or breast milk jaundice may tolerate a concentration slightly higher than 25 mg/dL with no apparent ill effect, whereas kernicterus may develop in a sick premature infant at a significantly lower level. A level approaching that considered critical for the individual infant may be

Table 123.7	Example of a Clinical Pathway for Management of the Newborn Infant Readmitted for Phototherapy or Exchange Transfusion

TREATMENT
Use intensive phototherapy and/or exchange transfusion as indicated in Figs. 123.13 and 123.14.

LABORATORY TESTS
TSB and direct bilirubin levels
Blood type (ABO, Rh)
Direct antibody test (Coombs)
Serum albumin
Complete blood cell count with differential and smear for red cell morphology
Reticulocyte count
End-tidal CO concentration (if available)
Glucose-6-phosphate dehydrogenase if suggested by ethnic or geographic origin or if poor response to phototherapy
Urine for reducing substances
If history and/or presentation suggest sepsis, perform blood culture, urine culture, and cerebrospinal fluid for protein, glucose, cell count, and culture.

INTERVENTIONS
If TSB ≥25 mg/dL (428 μmol/L) or ≥20 mg/dL (342 μmol/L) in a sick infant or infant <38 wk gestation, obtain a type and crossmatch, and request blood in case an exchange transfusion is necessary.
In infants with isoimmune hemolytic disease and TSB level rising in spite of intensive phototherapy or within 2-3 mg/dL (34-51 μmol/L) of exchange level (see Fig. 123.14), administer intravenous immune globulin 0.5-1 g/kg over 2 hr and repeat in 12 hr if necessary.
If infant's weight loss from birth is >12% or there is clinical or biochemical evidence of dehydration, recommend formula or expressed breast milk. If oral intake is in question, give intravenous fluids.

FOR INFANTS RECEIVING INTENSIVE PHOTOTHERAPY:
Breastfeed or bottle-feed (formula or expressed breast milk) every 2-3 hr.
If TSB ≥25 mg/dL (428 μmol/L), repeat TSB within 2-3 hr.
If TSB 20-25 mg/dL (342-428 μmol/L), repeat within 3-4 hr. If TSB <20 mg/dL (342 μmol/L), repeat in 4-6 hr. If TSB continues to fall, repeat in 8-12 hr.
If TSB is not decreasing or is moving closer to level for exchange transfusion, or if the TSB/albumin ratio exceeds levels shown in Fig. 123.14, consider exchange transfusion (see Fig. 123.14 for exchange transfusion recommendations).
When TSB is <13-14 mg/dL (239 μmol/L), discontinue phototherapy. Depending on the cause of the hyperbilirubinemia, it is an option to measure TSB 24 hr after discharge to check for rebound.

TSB, Total serum bilirubin.
From American Academy of Pediatrics Subcommittee on Hyperbilirubinemia: Management of hyperbilirubinemia in the newborn infant 35 or more weeks of gestation, *Pediatrics* 114:297–316, 2004.

an indication for exchange transfusion during the 1st or 2nd day after birth, when a further rise is anticipated, but not typically after the 4th day in a term infant or after the 7th day in a preterm infant, because an imminent fall may be anticipated as the hepatic conjugating mechanism becomes more effective.

Bibliography is available at Expert Consult.

Chapter **124**
Blood Disorders
第一百二十四章
血液系统疾病

中文导读

本章主要介绍了新生儿贫血、胎儿及新生儿溶血性疾病、新生儿红细胞增多症、新生儿出血症、非免疫性水肿。由于新生儿出生前较长时间处于宫内环境中，因此新生儿的血细胞特点与其他年龄阶段完全不同，本章具体描述了正常新生儿红细胞比容及血红蛋白浓度、贫血分类、诊断评估，以及如何正确掌控新生儿贫血的治疗决策。对于新生儿因母子血型不合导致的溶血，本章详细就新生儿Rh系统血型不合溶血病、ABO系统血型不合溶血病及其他类型溶血病的病因、诊断、治疗等进行了阐述。本章还详细介绍了维生素K缺乏性出血症、弥散性血管内凝血病和新生儿血小板减少症等的临床诊治。

124.1 Anemia in the Newborn Infant

Patrick T. McGann and Russell E. Ware

Anemia is a common laboratory and clinical finding in the newborn period and carries a broad differential diagnosis. Anemia in the newborn may be acute or chronic, and its clinical manifestations range from an asymptomatic laboratory finding to life-threatening signs and symptoms. The diagnosis and interpretation of anemia in the newborn infant are therefore complex and require careful consideration of the gestational age and general health of the infant, details of the perinatal course and delivery, and information regarding the general health of the mother both during pregnancy and through delivery into the postpartum period.

Before interpreting hemoglobin and hematocrit values for infants, it is important to understand the pathophysiology of hemoglobin-oxygen binding and delivery, both before and after birth. Because of the hypoxic environment in utero and the lack of direct gas exchange with the ambient atmosphere, fetal hemoglobin (HbF) predominates throughout late gestation because of its increased affinity to bind and transport oxygen compared to the mother's adult hemoglobin. Despite the predominance of HbF, the in utero environment remains hypoxic, such that the normal hemoglobin concentration is relatively high at birth.

NORMAL HEMATOCRIT AND HEMOGLOBIN CONCENTRATIONS IN NEWBORN INFANTS

The diagnostic approach to anemia in the newborn infant begins comparing laboratory results with reference ranges for both gestational age and postnatal age. Although significant variability exists in suggested reference ranges, data collected from more than 25,000 preterm and term infants through the 1st 28 days of life have provided robust data-driven reference ranges. These data, illustrated in Fig. 124.1, demonstrate

a near-linear increase in hemoglobin and hematocrit between 22 and 40 wk of gestation. Notably, the mean corpuscular volume (MCV) in neonates is strikingly higher than toddlers and older children, with normal values ranging from about 100-115 fL at birth. An MCV <100 fL at birth should prompt consideration of underlying α-thalassemia trait or maternal iron deficiency.

Over the first days and weeks of postnatal life, increased oxygen in the environment reduces the erythropoietic drive, and this normal developmental and physiologic process results in a slow decrease in hematocrit and hemoglobin concentration. Fig. 124.2 demonstrates the expected decrease in hematocrit and hemoglobin concentration according to postnatal age for both term/postterm (Fig. 124.2*A* and *B*) and preterm (29-34 wk gestation) infants. The *lower dashed lines* in Fig. 124.2 represent the 5th percentile, below which a diagnosis of neonatal anemia should be defined. Eventually, oxygen delivery becomes limiting enough to stimulate new active erythropoiesis, and the hemoglobin concentration begins to rise. This **physiologic nadir** usually occurs between 6 and 10 wk of life for term infants, with a typical low hemoglobin value of 9-11 g/dL, while preterm infants reach their nadir earlier, at 4-8 wk of age with a hemoglobin concentration of 7-9 g/dL.

CLASSIFICATION OF ANEMIA AND DIAGNOSTIC EVALUATION

As with any diagnostic approach to anemia, low hemoglobin concentration in the newborn period can be classified into 3 broad categories: blood loss; erythrocyte destruction; or underproduction of erythrocytes. Table 124.1 summarizes the most common causes of neonatal anemia according to these categories.

Prior to laboratory testing, a complete medical history, including careful review of the pregnancy and perinatal course, and a careful physical examination are important because they often suggest a specific diagnosis more effectively than extensive laboratory testing. A simple

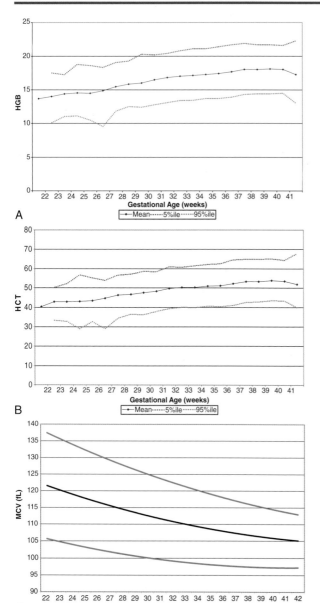

Fig. 124.1 Reference range for hematocrit and hemoglobin concentration according to gestational age. **A** and **B,** Reference ranges (5th percentile, mean, and 95th percentile) are shown for blood hemoglobin (**A**) and hematocrit (**B**). Concentrations were obtained during the 1st 6 hr after birth, among patients 22-42 wk gestation. Values were excluded if the diagnosis included abruption, placenta previa, or known fetal anemia, or if a blood transfusion was given before the first hemoglobin was measured. **C,** References ranges for mean corpuscular volume (MCV) in neonates on 1st day after birth. The *lower line* shows the 5th percentile values, the *middle line* shows the mean values, and the *upper line* shows the 95th percentile values. *(From Christensen RD, Jopling HE, Jopling J, Wiedemeier SE: The CBC: reference ranges for neonates, Semin Perinatol 33(1):3–11, 2009.)*

and efficient laboratory workup is critical to the timely diagnosis and associated treatment of neonatal anemia. In addition to a complete blood count (CBC), additional laboratory tests on the infant include the reticulocyte count, direct antiglobulin test, serum bilirubin, infant

and maternal blood ABO group, and Rh type. The mother should also be screened with an indirect (serum) antiglobulin test for erythrocyte alloantibodies, and the Kleihauer-Betke test can identify fetal erythrocytes in the maternal circulation (Fig. 124.3). Fig. 124.4 shows a proposed diagnostic approach to anemia in newborn infants. Hemolytic anemia is usually associated with difficult-to-treat **hyperbilirubinemia** (Fig. 124.5), whereas **congenital aregenerative anemias** (e.g., Diamond-Blackfan anemia) usually do not manifest jaundice but have other features (Table 124.2).

Review of the peripheral blood smear is an essential component of the evaluation of neonatal anemia. The presence of reticulocytes and nucleated red blood cells (RBCs) indicate chronic anemia with compensatory active erythropoiesis, while distinct erythrocyte morphologies (e.g., elliptocytes, acanthocytes) suggest a congenital intrinsic hemolytic anemia. The presence of spherocytes (often **microspherocytes**) is consistent with immune-mediated hemolysis but can also indicate **hereditary spherocytosis**; the direct antiglobulin test (DAT, formerly the direct Coombs test) is needed to distinguish these 2 important diagnoses (Fig. 124.6). Neonatal blood smears often include atypical erythrocyte morphology with macrocytosis, poikilocytosis, and anisocytosis that reflect normal fetal erythropoiesis, and an experienced hematologist or pathologist may be required to identify a pathologic feature (Table 124.3) (see Chapter 474).

Red Blood Cell Loss

Blood loss is the most common cause of neonatal anemia. Repeated or frequent phlebotomy for routine laboratory tests, especially from premature or acutely ill neonates, is one of the most common causes of anemia. Several reports have documented large volumes of blood removed for laboratory testing among children in neonatal intensive care units (NICUs), with weekly phlebotomy volumes ranging from 15–30% of the infant's total blood volume (11-22 mL/kg/wk). Most other causes of blood loss occur just before or during delivery, such as placental abruption, and fetal hemorrhage is more common in emergent or traumatic deliveries (see Table 124.1).

Fetomaternal hemorrhage (FMH) is caused by bleeding from the fetal into the maternal circulation, either before or during delivery. Such bleeding occurs to some extent in most pregnancies, although the volume lost is typically small. Estimates suggest that more substantial FMH, defined as >30 mL of fetal blood, occurs in 3 per 1,000 births, with *large* (>80 mL) or *massive* (>150 mL) FMH occurring in 0.9 and 0.2 per 1,000 births, respectively. Blood loss during gestation can be slow and well compensated by the fetus in terms of both blood volume and oxygen delivery, but faster or larger bleeds will not be fully compensated. Therefore the presentation of FMH is variable, but *decreased or absent fetal movement* is the most common antenatal presentation and should be associated with a high degree of clinical suspicion. After delivery, infant pallor, hypotension, and poor perfusion will indicate severe anemia. To diagnose FMH, the classic *Kleihauer-Betke test,* which identifies fetal erythrocytes containing HbF resistant to acid elution, is technically the gold standard but is labor intensive, highly dependent on the skills of the technician, and often not available as a rapid or point-of-care test (see Fig. 124.3). Some advanced laboratories offer a more precise test using flow cytometry to quantify fetal cells in the maternal circulation.

Red Blood Cell Destruction

RBC destruction is an important cause of neonatal anemia and most frequently reflects elimination of erythrocytes by immune-mediated mechanisms, which result from RBC antigen incompatibilities between the infant and mother. **Hemolytic disease of the fetus and newborn (HDFN)** is a broad term used to describe any fetus or infant who develops alloimmune hemolysis caused by the presence of maternal antibodies against RBC antigens within the circulation of the child (see Chapter 124.2). HDFN caused by anti-RhD antibodies, occurring in RhD-positive infants born to RhD-negative mothers, is the most severe form because of the highly immunogenic nature of the RhD antigen. ABO incompatibility, most often a mismatch between group O mothers and their non–group O infants, affects approximately 15% of pregnancies but is usually less severe than Rh disease, with only 4% of incompatible

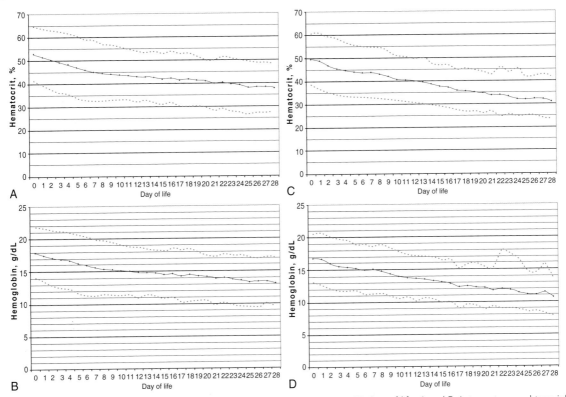

Fig. 124.2 Reference range for hematocrit and hemoglobin concentration during 1st 28 days of life. **A** and **B,** Late preterm and term infants (35-42 wk gestation). **C** and **D,** Preterm infants (29-34 wk gestation). The reference ranges are shown for hematocrit (**A** and **C**) (41,957 patients) and blood hemoglobin (**B** and **D**) (39,559 patients) during the 28 days after birth. Values were divided into 2 groups (**A/B** and **C/D**) on the basis of gestational age at delivery. Patients were excluded when their diagnosis included abruption, placenta previa, or fetal anemia, or when a blood transfusion was given. Analysis was not possible for patients <29 wk gestation because virtually all these had repeated phlebotomy and erythrocyte transfusions. (*From Jopling J, Henry E, Wiedmeier SE, Christensin RD: Reference ranges for hematocrit and blood hemoglobin concentration during the neonatal period: data from a multihospital health care system,* Pediatrics *123(2):e333–e337, 2009.*)

Table 124.1	Differential Diagnosis of Neonatal Anemia

BLOOD LOSS	**↑ RBC DESTRUCTION**	**↓ RBC PRODUCTION**
Iatrogenic blood loss (phlebotomy)	*Immune-Mediated Hemolysis*	Physiologic anemia and anemia of prematurity
Placental hemorrhage	Rh incompatibility	Infection (rubella, CMV, parvovirus B19)
Placental previa	ABO incompatibility	Bone marrow suppression (acute stress in perinatal period)
Injury of umbilical or placental vessels	Minor antigen incompatibility	Hemoglobinopathy (γ-globin mutation, unstable
Fetomaternal transfusion		β-hemoglobinopathy, α-thalassemia major)
Fetoplacental transfusion	*RBC Membrane Disorders*	Bone marrow suppression (CMV, EBV)
Twin-twin transfusion	Hereditary spherocytosis	Diamond Blackfan anemia
Acute perinatal hemorrhage (e.g., cesarean	Hereditary elliptocytosis	Schwachman-Diamond syndrome
birth, other obstetric trauma)	Hereditary pyropoikilocytosis	Congenital dyserythropoietic anemia
Chronic in utero blood loss	Hereditary stomatocytosis	Fanconi anemia
		Pearson syndrome
	RBC Enzyme Disorders	Congenital leukemia
	G6PD deficiency	
	Pyruvate kinase deficiency	

CMV, Cytomegalovirus, EBV, Epstein-Barr virus; G6PD, glucose-6-phosphate dehydrogenase; RBC, red blood cell.

pregnancies resulting in neonatal hemolytic disease. Unlike Rh disease, in which sensitization usually occurs in the first pregnancy and HDFN occurs in subsequent pregnancies, ABO incompatibility can occur during a woman's first pregnancy, since group O mothers have naturally occurring anti-A and anti-B antibodies. A positive DAT on the infant's blood and a positive indirect antiglobulin test (IAT; also known as the antibody screen) in the mother provide diagnostic evidence of HDFN.

In addition to immune-mediated mechanisms of erythrocyte

destruction, **congenital RBC enzyme and membrane disorders** also can result in hemolytic anemia and jaundice within the neonatal period. The erythrocyte membrane is a complex structure with numerous critical proteins and lipids that result in a durable, flexible, circulating biconcave disc shape. Genetic deficiencies or abnormalities in RBC membrane proteins (e.g., ankyrin, band 3, α-spectrin, β-spectrin, protein 4.2) result in instability of the RBC membrane, decreased cellular deformability, and shape changes; the abnormal erythrocytes undergo splenic

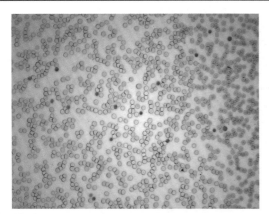

Fig. 124.3 Acid elution technique of Kleithauer (Kleihauer-Betke test). Fetal red blood cells stain with eosin and appear *dark*. Adult RBCs do not stain and appear as "ghosts." *(From Liley HG, Gardener G, Lopriore E, Smits-Wintjens V: Immune hemolytic disease. In Orkin SH, Nathan DG, Ginsburg D, et al, editors: Nathan and Oski's hematology and oncology of infancy and childhood, ed 8, Philadelphia, 2015, Elsevier, Fig 3-2.)*

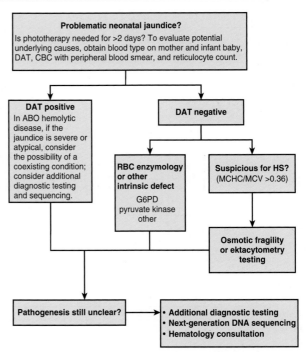

Fig. 124.5 Evaluation of neonate with problematic jaundice of unclear cause. Not all neonates who receive phototherapy for 2 days or more have hemolytic jaundice. However, if hemolytic jaundice is suspected, this algorithm for stepwise evaluation of the cause might be useful. CBC, Complete blood count; DAT, direct antiglobulin test; EMA, eosin 5-maleimide; G6PD, glucose 6-phosphate dehydrogenase; HS, hereditary spherocytosis; MCHC, mean corpuscular hemoglobin concentration; MCV, mean corpuscular volume; RBC, red blood cell. *(From Christensen RD: Neonatal erythrocyte disorders. In Gleason CA, Juul SE, editors: Avery's diseases of the newborn, ed 10, Philadelphia, 2018, Elsevier, Fig 81-15.)*

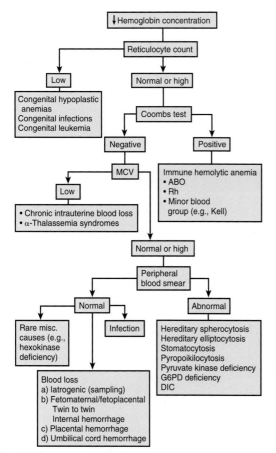

Fig. 124.4 Diagnostic algorithm showing the approach to anemia in newborn infants. DIC, Disseminated intravascular coagulation; G6PD, glucose-6-phosphate dehydrogenase; MCV, mean corpuscular volume. *(Modified from Blanchette VS, Zipursky A: Assessment of anemia in newborn infants, Clin Perinatol 11:489–510, 1984.)*

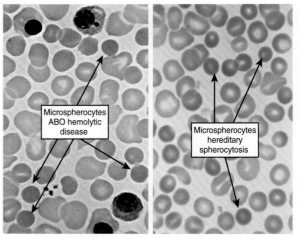

Fig. 124.6 Microspherocytes. *Left*, Neonate with ABO hemolytic disease. *Right*, Neonate with hereditary spherocytosis *(right)*. *(From Christensen RD: Neonatal erythrocyte disorders. In Gleason CA, Juul SE, editors: Avery's diseases of the newborn, ed 10, Philadelphia, 2018, Elsevier, Fig 81-8.)*

Table 124.2	Syndromes Associated With Congenital Hyporegenerative Anemia	
SYNDROME	**PHENOTYPIC FEATURES**	**GENOTYPIC FEATURES**
Adenosine deaminase deficiency	Autoimmune hemolytic anemia, reduced erythrocyte adenosine deaminase activity	AR, 20q13.11
Congenital dyserythropoietic anemias	Type I (rare): megaloblastoid erythroid hyperplasia and nuclear chromatin bridges between nuclei Type II (most common): hereditary erythroblastic multinuclearity with positive acidified serum test result, increased lysis to anti-i antibodies Type III: erythroblastic multinuclearity ("gigantoblasts"), macrocytosis	Type I: 15q15.1-q15.3 Type II: 20q11.2 Type III: 15q21
Diamond-Blackfan syndrome	Steroid-responsive hypoplastic anemia, often macrocytic after 5 mo of age	AR; sporadic mutations and AD inheritance described; 19q13.2, 8p23.3-p22
Dyskeratosis congenita	Hypoproliferative anemia usually presenting between 5 and 15 yr of age	X-linked recessive, locus on Xq28; some cases with AD inheritance
Fanconi syndrome	Steroid-responsive hypoplastic anemia, reticulocytopenia, some macrocytic RBCs, shortened RBC life span Cells are hypersensitive to DNA cross-linking agents.	AR, multiple genes: complementation; group A 16q24.3; group B Xp22.3; group C 9q22.3; group D2 3p25.3; group E 6p22-p21; group F 11p15; group G 9p13
Osler hemorrhagic telangiectasia syndrome	Hemorrhagic anemia	AD, 9q34.1
Osteopetrosis	Hypoplastic anemia from marrow compression; extramedullary erythropoiesis	AR, 16p13, 11q13.4-q13.5; AD, 1p21; lethal, reduced levels of osteoclasts
Pearson syndrome	Hypoplastic sideroblastic anemia, marrow cell vacuolization	Pleioplasmatic rearrangement of mitochondrial DNA; X-linked or AR
Peutz-Jeghers syndrome	Iron-deficiency anemia from chronic blood loss	AD, 19p13.3
ATR-X and ATR-16 syndromes	ATR-X: hypochromic, microcytic anemia; mild form of hemoglobin H disease ATR-16: more significant hemoglobin H disease and anemia are present.	ATR-16, 16p13.3, deletions of α-globin locus

AD, Autosomal dominant; AR, autosomal recessive; ATR-16, chromosome 16–related α-thalassemia/mental retardation; ATR-X, X-linked α-thalassemia/mental retardation; RBC, red blood cell.
From Christensen RD: Neonatal erythrocyte disorders. In Gleason CA, Juul SE, editors: *Avery's diseases of the newborn*, ed 10, Philadelphia, 2018, Elsevier (Table 81-2).

Table 124.3	Morphologic Abnormalities of Erythrocytes From Neonates With Jaundice		
ABNORMAL ERYTHROCYTE MORPHOLOGY	**MOST LIKELY CAUSES**	**SUGGESTED LABORATORY TESTING/FINDINGS**	**OTHER FEATURES**
Microspherocytes	Hereditary spherocytosis	DAT (–) EMA flow (+) Persistent spherocytosis Reticulocytosis	MCHC/MCV elevated (>36, likely >40)
	ABO hemolytic disease	DAT (+) Transient spherocytosis Reticulocytosis	MCHC/MCV normal (<36, likely <34)
Elliptocytes	Hereditary elliptocytosis	DAT (–)	MCHC normal MCV normal
Bite and blister cells	G6PD deficiency Unstable hemoglobin	G6PD enzyme activity Heinz body preparation	Typically affects males, but rarely females are also affected Ethnicity of equatorial origin
Echinocytes	PK deficiency Other glycolytic enzyme deficiency	PK enzyme activity Quantify activity of other glycolytic enzymes	Autosomal recessive, likely to have no family history
Schistocytes	DIC and/or perinatal asphyxia Heinz body HA	Low levels of FV and FVIII, elevated levels of D-dimers Positive result of Heinz body preparation	Low or falling platelet count Normal to high IPF Normal to high MPV DIC, perinatal asphyxia
	ADAMTS-13 deficiency (TTP)	Severely decreased ADAMTS-13 activity (<0.1 U/mL) high levels of LDH	ADAMTS-13 deficiency, early neonatal HUS, and giant hemangiomas all involve
	Neonatal hemolytic-uremic syndrome	Acute renal failure	platelet consumption from endothelial injury and all have
	Homozygous protein C deficiency	Severely decreased functional protein C activity (<1%)	a similar neonatal presentation
	Giant hemangioma	May be internal or external	

DAT, Direct antiglobulin test; DIC, disseminated intravascular coagulation; EMA, eosin 5-maleimide; FV, factor V; FVIII, factor VIII; G6PD, glucose-6-phosphate dehydrogenase; HA, hemolytic anemia; HUS, hemolytic uremic syndrome; IPF, immature platelet fraction; LDH, lactic dehydrogenase; MCHC, mean corpuscular hemoglobin concentration; MCV, mean corpuscular volume; MPV, mean platelet volume; PK, pyruvate kinase; TTP, thrombotic thrombocytopenic purpura.
From Christensen RD, Yaish HM: Hemolytic disorders causing severe neonatal hyperbilirubinemia, *Clin Perinatol* 42:515–527, 2015 (Table 3).

entrapment and removal by macrophages. **Hereditary spherocytosis (HS)**, an autosomal dominant condition characterized by spherical erythrocytes, is the most common RBC membrane disorder, affecting 1 in 2,500-5,000 individuals of European descent. Nearly half of infants born with HS will develop jaundice early in the newborn period.

Hereditary elliptocytosis (HE), another autosomal dominant inherited erythrocyte membranopathy, characterized by elliptical-shaped erythrocytes, is a less common and less severe RBC membrane disorder. In contrast, **hereditary pyropoikilocytosis (HPP)** is an autosomal recessive RBC membrane disorder resulting in striking morphologic shape changes (poikilocytosis) noted on the peripheral blood smear, some of which resemble thermally damaged erythrocytes. HPP is most common in infants of African descent and can be associated with severe anemia and hemolysis in the newborn period. There is substantial clinical and genetic overlap between HPP and HE, because infants with HPP often have a family history of HE and may develop a milder condition resembling HE later in childhood. Clinical suspicion for a RBC membranopathy begins with a positive family history of hemolytic anemia, especially in an infant who develops early jaundice in the 1st 24 hr of life. The diagnostic evaluation should include a negative DAT, indirect hyperbilirubinemia, and hallmark features noted on the peripheral blood smear. The degree of anemia is variable, and reticulocytosis may also be present.

Erythrocyte enzymopathies are another important, but less common, etiology of neonatal anemia. Circulating RBCs lack a nucleus, mitochondria, or other essential organelles and thus rely solely on critical metabolic pathways to allow for their function in the transport and delivery of oxygen. Several enzymes are especially important to RBC metabolism and may result in hemolytic anemia when deficient. **Glucose-6-phosphate dehydrogenase (G6PD) deficiency** is the most common of these RBC enzymopathies. G6PD deficiency is a common X-linked disorder affecting >400 million people worldwide. There are several classes of G6PD deficiency with varying degrees of clinical severity, but most affected persons are asymptomatic. In the setting of oxidative stress (drugs, infection, certain foods), however, some persons with G6PD deficiency may develop acute hemolytic anemia. There is a several-fold increase in the incidence of neonatal jaundice in G6PD-deficient infants, with jaundice typically occurring on day 2-3 of life. Severe anemia with reticulocytosis is not common, but hyperbilirubinemia in the setting of G6PD deficiency can be severe and prolonged. Clinical testing measuring G6PD activity can be performed (<1–2% suggests G6PD deficiency), but the testing will not be accurate in the setting of acute hemolysis or an elevated reticulocyte count, because reticulocytes have higher enzyme activity. **Pyruvate kinase (PK) deficiency** is the 2nd most common RBC enzymopathy and may also be associated with neonatal jaundice and bizarre morphology featuring acanthocytes.

Red Blood Cell Production

RBC underproduction is also common in the neonate, particularly among preterm infants. Because of relative polycythemia and the physiologic right shift in the oxyhemoglobin dissociation curve, there is typically sufficient oxygen delivery to the tissues during the 1st weeks of postuterine life. The erythropoietic drive is thus limited, and active erythropoiesis does not commence until the 2nd mo of life. This physiologic underproduction of erythrocytes appears to be prolonged in preterm infants and results in a steeper physiologic nadir referred to as **anemia of prematurity**. Anemia of prematurity is exacerbated by acute illness, frequent phlebotomy, and other comorbidities observed in premature infants.

In addition to physiologic underproduction of erythrocytes, several acquired and congenital conditions may further suppress bone marrow production (see Table 124.2). Both bacterial and viral infections may result in suppression of erythropoiesis and contribute to neonatal anemia; infectious etiologies are numerous but TORCH infections and parvovirus B19 are the most common. Tables 124.1 and 124.2 list congenital causes of neonatal anemia, including congenital leukemia, bone marrow failure syndromes (Fanconi anemia, Schwachman-Diamond syndrome), Diamond-Blackfan anemia), and variants in γ-globin, β-globin, or α-globin. Notably, common β-hemoglobinopathies such as sickle cell disease and thalassemia do not present in the neonatal period, as a result of the protective effect of high levels of HbF in the first few months of life.

TREATMENT OPTIONS FOR NEONATAL ANEMIA
Packed Red Blood Cell Transfusions

Treatment of neonatal anemia by blood transfusion depends on the severity of symptoms, the hemoglobin concentration, and the presence of comorbidities (e.g., bronchopulmonary dysplasia, cyanotic congenital heart disease, respiratory distress syndrome) that interfere with oxygen delivery. The benefits of blood transfusion should be balanced against its risks, which include hemolytic and nonhemolytic reactions; exposure to blood product preservatives and toxins; volume overload; possible increased risk of retinopathy of prematurity and necrotizing enterocolitis; graft-versus-host reaction; and transfusion-acquired infections such as cytomegalovirus (CMV), HIV, parvovirus, and hepatitis B and C (see Chapter 501). The frequency of transfusion for neonates in the NICU is high, particularly among premature and very-low-birthweight (VLBW) infants.

Few studies have evaluated the efficacy or safety of specific hemoglobin/hematocrit thresholds, but a Cochrane review summarized the available evidence and proposed guidelines for transfusion of VLBW infants. The review identified 4 trials comparing *restrictive* (lower) to *liberal* (higher) hemoglobin thresholds. There were no statistically significant differences in death or serious morbidity, and the restrictive thresholds modestly reduced exposure to blood products. Evidence was inconclusive, however, regarding the effectiveness of either threshold in optimizing long-term neurocognitive outcomes. The proposed guideline for the transfusion of neonates was based primarily on postnatal age and the presence or absence of respiratory support (Table 124.4). In addition to these factors, transfusion should be considered for infants with acute blood loss (>20%) or significant hemolysis, as well as before surgery. With no similar evidence-based guidelines for term infants, transfusion should be based on hemodynamic stability, respiratory status, overall clinical condition, and laboratory values.

When the decision to transfuse has been made, the appropriate blood product should be selected and a safe volume of blood should be transfused at a safe rate. It is important to transfuse packed erythrocytes (PRBCs) to all neonates in the form of **leukocyte-reduced** or **CMV-seronegative** PRBCs, to reduce the risk of CMV transmission. **Irradiation** of PRBCs removes the risk of transfusion-associated graft-versus-host disease (GVHD) *but does not eliminate* the risk of CMV transmission. The volume of transfusion should achieve the intended therapeutic goal while limiting blood product exposure. Typical transfusion protocols choose a transfusion volume ranging from 10-20 mL/kg. There are no clear data to favor a specific amount, but lower volumes exposure infants to risks unnecessarily while higher volumes may cause fluid overload. One logical goal is to target a specific goal hemoglobin (Hb) concentration. The following commonly used shorthand equation can provide a good estimate of required blood volume, which usually results in a transfusion volume within the 10-20 mL/kg range:

$$\text{PRBC transfusion volume} = (\text{Desired Hb}\,[\text{g/dL}] - \text{Actual Hb}) \times \text{Weight}\,(\text{kg}) \times 3$$

Transfusion of PRBCs is typically delivered at a rate of 3-5 mL/kg/hr, with a slower rate preferred for very small, acutely ill infants with

Table 124.4	Suggested Transfusion Thresholds	
	PRESENCE OF RESPIRATORY SUPPORT	**ABSENCE OF RESPIRATORY SUPPORT**
POSTNATAL AGE	**Hemoglobin Concentration, g/dL (Hematocrit %)**	
Week 1	11.5 (35%)	10.0 (30%)
Week 2	10.0 (30%)	8.5 (25%)
Week 3	8.5 (25%)	7.5 (23%)

a tenuous fluid status. Each transfusion should be completed within 4 hours.

Erythropoietin

Because of the low physiologic levels of erythropoietin in neonates, the role of recombinant human erythropoietin (**rhEPO**) has been investigated for the treatment of anemia in neonates, particularly VLBW infants. A Cochrane review documented that rhEPO is associated with a significant reduction in the number of blood transfusions per infant, but also a significantly increased risk of retinopathy of prematurity. There were no differences in mortality or other neonatal morbidities among infants who did or did not receive rhEPO. Because of these limited benefits and potential serious risks of early rhEPO therapy, there is currently no strong indication for the routine use of rhEPO in infants with anemia, although it should be considered in individual settings.

Bibliography is available at Expert Consult.

124.2 Hemolytic Disease of the Fetus and Newborn
Omar Niss and Russell E. Ware

Hemolytic disease of the fetus and newborn (**HDFN**), also known as **erythroblastosis fetalis**, is caused by the transplacental passage of maternal antibodies directed against paternally derived red blood cell (RBC) antigens, which causes increased RBC destruction (hemolysis) in the infant. HDFN is an important cause of anemia and jaundice in newborn infants, and early recognition and diagnosis are crucial for proper management. Although more than 60 different RBC antigens are capable of eliciting a maternal antibody response, clinically significant disease is associated primarily with incompatibility of **ABO blood groups** and the **RhD antigen**. Less frequently, hemolytic disease may be caused by differences in other antigens of the Rh system or by other RBC antigens such as C^W, C^X, D^U, K (**Kell**), M, Duffy, S, P, MNS, Xg, Lutheran, Diego, and Kidd. Notably, anti-Lewis maternal antibodies rarely cause HDFN.

HEMOLYTIC DISEASE CAUSED BY RH INCOMPATIBILITY

The Rh antigenic determinants are genetically transmitted from each parent and determine the Rh blood type by directing the production of Rh proteins (C, c, D, E, and e) on the RBC surface. **RhD** is responsible for 90% of HDFN cases involving the Rh antigen system, but other Rh antigens (especially E and c) also can be etiologic.

Pathogenesis

Alloimmune hemolytic disease from RhD antigen incompatibility is approximately 3 times more common among whites than among blacks, because of differences in Rh allele frequency. Approximately 85% of Caucasians express RhD antigen (**Rh-positive**), whereas 99% of persons from Africa or Asia are Rh-positive. When Rh-positive blood is infused into an unsensitized Rh-negative woman, antibody formation against the mismatched Rh antigen is induced in the recipient. This can occur through transfusion, but the typical scenario is when small quantities (usually >1 mL) of Rh-positive fetal blood, inherited from an Rh-positive father, enter the maternal circulation during pregnancy, through spontaneous or induced abortion, or at delivery. Once sensitization has occurred, considerably smaller doses of antigen can stimulate an increase in antibody titer. Initially, a rise in immunoglobulin (Ig) M antibody occurs, which is later replaced by IgG antibody. Unlike IgM antibodies, IgG readily crosses the placenta to cause hemolytic manifestations.

HDFN requires Rh-antigen mismatch between the infant and the mother, with prior maternal exposure to RBCs expressing the cognate antigen. Hemolytic disease rarely occurs during a first pregnancy because transfusion of Rh-positive fetal blood into an Rh-negative mother usually occurs near the time of delivery, which is too late for the mother to become sensitized and transmit antibody to that infant before delivery.

However, fetal-to-maternal transfusion is thought to occur in only 50% of pregnancies, so Rh incompatibility does not always lead to Rh sensitization. Another important factor is the allele frequency of the RhD antigen because homozygous Rh-positive fathers must transmit the antigen to the fetus, whereas heterozygous fathers have only a 50% chance of having Rh-positive offspring. A smaller family size also reduces the risk of sensitization.

The outcome for Rh-incompatible fetuses varies greatly, depending on the characteristics of both the RBC antigen and the maternal antibodies. Not all maternal-fetal antigen incompatibility leads to alloimmunization and hemolysis. Factors that affect the outcome of antigen-positive fetuses include differential immunogenicity of blood group antigens (RhD antigen being the most immunogenic), a threshold effect of fetomaternal transfusions (a certain amount of the immunizing blood cell antigen is required to induce the maternal immune response), the type of antibody response (IgG antibodies are more efficiently transferred across the placenta to the fetus), and differences in the maternal immune response, presumably related to differences in the efficiency of antigen presentation by various major histocompatibility complex (MHC) loci.

Notably, when the mother and fetus are also ABO incompatible, the Rh-negative mother is partially protected against sensitization due to rapid removal of the fetal Rh-positive cells by maternal isohemagglutinins (preexisting IgM anti-A or anti-B antibodies that do not cross the placenta). Once a mother has been sensitized, all subsequent infants expressing that cognate antigen on RBCs are at risk for HDFN. The severity of Rh illness typically worsens with successive pregnancies because of repeated immune stimulation. The likelihood that Rh sensitization affects a mother's childbearing potential argues urgently for the prevention of sensitization. The injection of anti-Rh immune globulin (RhoGAM) into the Rh-negative mother, both during pregnancy and immediately after the delivery of each Rh-positive infant, reduces HDFN caused by RhD alloimmunization.

Clinical Manifestations

The severity of HDFN is variable, ranging from only laboratory evidence of mild hemolysis to severe anemia with compensatory hyperplasia of erythropoietic tissues, leading to massive enlargement of the liver and spleen. When hemolysis exceeds the compensatory capacity of the hematopoietic system, profound anemia occurs and results in pallor, signs of cardiac decompensation (cardiomegaly, respiratory distress), massive anasarca, and circulatory collapse. This clinical picture of excessive abnormal fluid in 2 or more fetal compartments (skin, pleura, pericardium, placenta, peritoneum, amniotic fluid), termed **hydrops fetalis**, frequently results in death in utero or shortly after birth.

The severity of hydrops is related to the level of anemia and the degree of edema caused by a reduction in serum albumin (oncotic pressure), which is partly a result of hepatic congestion and hepatic dysfunction. Alternatively, heart failure may increase right-sided heart pressure, with the subsequent development of edema and ascites. Failure to initiate spontaneous effective ventilation because of pulmonary edema or bilateral pleural effusions results in birth asphyxia. After successful resuscitation, severe respiratory distress may develop. Petechiae, purpura, and thrombocytopenia may also be present in severe cases, as a result of decreased platelet production or the presence of concurrent disseminated intravascular coagulation (DIC). Fortunately, with the routine use of RhoGAM to prevent Rh sensitization, *hydrops caused by HDFN has become rare and is more frequently encountered in nonhemolytic conditions.*

Jaundice may be absent at birth because of effective placental clearance of lipid-soluble unconjugated bilirubin, but in severe cases, bilirubin pigments can stain the amniotic fluid, cord, and vernix caseosa. *Jaundice is generally evident in the initial 24 hr of life, which is always pathologic,* because the infant's bilirubin-conjugating and excretory systems are unable to cope with the load resulting from massive hemolysis. Indirect-reacting bilirubin accumulates postnatally and may rapidly reach extremely high levels and present a significant risk of bilirubin encephalopathy (kernicterus). The risk of development of kernicterus from HDFN is greater than from comparable nonhemolytic hyperbilirubinemia, although the risk in an individual patient may be affected by other complications such as hypoxia or acidosis. **Hypoglycemia** also occurs in infants with severe HDFN and may be related to hyperinsulinism and hypertrophy of the pancreatic islet cells in these infants.

Infants with signs of severe disease in utero (hydrops, severe fetal anemia) may benefit from **intrauterine transfusion**, given either directly into the peritoneum or through the umbilical cord. Such infants usually have very high (but extremely variable) cord levels of bilirubin, reflecting the severity of the hemolysis and its effects on hepatic function. Infants treated with transfusions in utero may also have a benign postnatal course if the anemia and hydrops resolve before birth. Ongoing hemolysis can be masked by the previous intrauterine transfusion.

Laboratory Data
Before treatment, the direct antiglobulin test (DAT), or Coombs test, is positive, and anemia is generally present. The cord blood hemoglobin content varies and is usually proportional to the severity of the disease. In cases of hydrops fetalis, the hemoglobin concentration may be as low as 3-4 g/dL. Alternatively, despite hemolysis, hemoglobin may be within the normal range because of compensatory bone marrow and extramedullary hematopoiesis. The initial *reticulocyte count* is increased, another abnormal finding at birth, and the peripheral blood smear typically shows polychromasia with a marked increase in nucleated RBCs. The white blood cell count is usually normal but may be elevated, and thrombocytopenia develops in severe cases. Cord bilirubin levels are generally between 3 and 5 mg/dL; the *direct-reacting (conjugated) bilirubin* content may also be elevated (from cholestasis), especially if there was a previous intrauterine transfusion. Indirect-reacting bilirubin content rises rapidly to high levels in the 1st 6-12 hr of life.

After intrauterine transfusions, cord blood may show a normal hemoglobin concentration, *negative* DAT result, predominantly Rh-negative adult RBCs, low/normal reticulocyte count, and relatively normal blood smear findings.

Diagnosis
Definitive diagnosis of HDFN requires demonstration of blood group incompatibility between mother and infant and corresponding maternal antibody bound to the infant's RBCs.

Antenatal Diagnosis
Without proof of immunoglobulin prophylaxis, any Rh-negative women with previous pregnancy or abortion, prior exposure to transfused blood, or receipt of an organ transplant should be considered at risk for Rh sensitization. During pregnancy, the expectant parents should have blood tested for potential incompatibility, particularly for ABO and Rh antigens. If RhD incompatible, the maternal titer of IgG antibodies to the RhD antigen should be measured early in pregnancy. Paternal blood can be tested to determine the fetal risk of inheriting the cognate antigen, typically either 50% or 100% depending on whether the father is heterozygous or homozygous for the antigen. However, paternal serologic testing alone is not fully accurate to predict the zygosity of RhD antigen, and molecular genotyping is recommended for both parents in this setting.

Fetal RBC genotyping provides an accurate prediction for the development of HDFN in sensitized mothers. Fetal Rh status is available by isolating fetal cells or fetal DNA (plasma) from the maternal circulation, which is replacing the more invasive and risky fetal amniocyte testing by amniocentesis and chorionic villus sampling methods. The presence of elevated antibody titers or rising titers increases the risk of the baby developing severe HDFN.

Although maternal antibody titers are often used to predict the risk of HDFN, there is a poor correlation between the anti-D titer level and the severity of the disease, especially in subsequent pregnancies. If an Rh-negative mother is found to have RhD antibody titers of ≥1:16 (15 IU/mL in Europe) at any time during a subsequent pregnancy, the severity of fetal anemia should be monitored by Doppler ultrasonography (US) of the middle cerebral artery (MCA) and then percutaneous umbilical blood sampling (PUBS) if indicated (Fig. 124.7). If the mother has a history of a previously affected infant or a stillbirth, an Rh-positive infant is usually equally or more severely affected than the previous

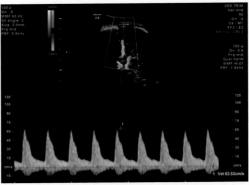

Fig. 124.7 Middle cerebral artery (MCA) Doppler study of elevated peak systolic velocity (PSV). MCA-PSV can predict fetal anemia with sufficient accuracy to determine management, including the need for intrauterine transfusion or, in the mid- to late third trimester, early delivery. Fetal hemoglobin is typically measured at the start and end of intravascular transfusion to validate the prediction from MCA-PSV results. The reliability of MCA-PSV can decrease after intrauterine transfusion because of the altered rheostatic characteristics of transfused adult blood. This is now the method of choice for detecting fetal anemia. *(From Liley HG, Gardener G, Lopriore E, Smits-Wintjens V: Immune hemolytic disease. In Orkin SH, Nathan DG, Ginsburg D, et al, editors:* Nathan and Oski's hematology and oncology of infancy and childhood, *ed 8, Philadelphia, 2015, Elsevier, Fig 3-6.)*

infant, and the severity of disease in the fetus should be monitored starting at 16-24 wk of gestation.

Pregnancies at risk for HDFN should be managed by maternal-fetal specialists. Assessment of the fetus includes US and PUBS. Real-time US is used to detect signs of hydrops (skin or scalp edema, pleural or pericardial effusions, and ascites) and fetal heart rate monitoring. Early US signs of hydrops include organomegaly (liver, spleen, heart), the double–bowel wall sign (bowel edema), and placental thickening. Progression to polyhydramnios, ascites, pleural or pericardial effusions, and skin or scalp edema may then follow. Extramedullary hematopoiesis and hepatic congestion compress the intrahepatic vessels and produce venous stasis with portal hypertension, hepatocellular dysfunction, and decreased albumin synthesis. *Hydrops is typically present when fetal hemoglobin level is <5 g/dL.* Hydrops is also frequently seen with a fetal hemoglobin level <7 g/dL, and in some cases between 7 and 9 g/dL.

Doppler US assesses fetal distress by demonstrating increased vascular resistance in fetal arteries, especially in the infant MCA (see Fig. 124.7). In fetuses without hydrops, moderate to severe anemia can be detected noninvasively by demonstration of an increase in the peak velocity of systolic blood flow in the MCA. The velocity of blood flow correlates with the severity of the anemia and therefore can be used as a noninvasive surrogate marker that can be followed. In pregnancies with moderate-severe fetal anemia (demonstrated by high cerebral velocities) or US evidence of hemolysis (hepatosplenomegaly), early or late hydrops, or fetal distress, further and more direct assessment of fetal hemolysis should be performed.

Amniocentesis was the classic method for assessing fetal hemolysis, by measuring changes in optical density of the amniotic fluid with serial determination of bilirubin levels. However, amniocentesis is an invasive procedure with risks to both the fetus and the mother, including fetal death, bleeding, bradycardia, worsening of alloimmunization, premature rupture of membranes, preterm labor, and chorioamnionitis. Doppler measurement of the peak velocity of systolic blood flow in the MCA has essentially replaced invasive testing in the management of HDFN.

PUBS is the standard approach to the assessment of the fetus if Doppler and real-time US findings suggest that the fetus has moderate to severe anemia. PUBS is performed to determine fetal hemoglobin levels and to transfuse packed RBCs into fetuses with serious fetal anemia (hematocrit <30%) who are immature and not suitable for delivery.

Postnatal Diagnosis

Immediately after the birth of an infant to an Rh-negative woman, or any infant with the appearance of hydrops, blood from the umbilical cord or the infant should be tested for ABO blood group, Rh type, hematocrit and hemoglobin, reticulocyte count, serum bilirubin, and the DAT. A positive DAT result indicates the presence of maternal antibody on the infant RBC, and the incompatible RBC antigen must be identified. The infant's cells can be investigated, but maternal serum should also be screened for RBC antibodies using commercially available panels. These tests not only help establish the diagnosis, but also enable selection of compatible blood for exchange transfusion of the infant, if necessary. The DAT is usually strongly positive in clinically affected infants and may remain so for weeks or even several months.

Treatment

The main goals of therapy for HDFN are (1) to prevent intrauterine or extrauterine death from severe anemia and hypoxia, (2) to prevent neurodevelopmental damage in affected children, and (3) to avoid neurotoxicity from hyperbilirubinemia.

Treatment of the Unborn Fetus

Survival of severely affected fetuses has improved with the advent of fetal US to assess the need for in utero transfusion. Intravascular (umbilical vein) transfusion of packed erythrocytes (PRBCs) is the preferred treatment of choice for fetal anemia, although intrauterine transfusion into the fetal peritoneal cavity is also effective. Hydrops or fetal anemia (hematocrit <30%) is an indication for umbilical vein transfusion in infants with pulmonary immaturity.

Fetal transfusion is facilitated by maternal and hence fetal sedation. PRBCs are slowly infused after being cross-matched against the mother's serum. The erythrocytes should be selected from a donor who is group O, negative for the mismatched antigen (e.g., RhD-negative), and CMV-negative. The blood should also be leukocyte-reduced to reduce the risk of allergic and nonhemolytic reactions and irradiated to avoid transfusion-associated GVHD. Some centers use extended group matching (e.g., RhCE, Kell) to decrease the risk of additional maternal antibody formation. Transfusions should achieve a posttransfusion hematocrit of 45–55% and can be repeated every 3-5 wk.

Intrauterine transfusions ameliorate neurologic complications in many fetuses; however, those with severe hydrops are at risk for cerebral palsy, developmental delay, and deafness. The overall survival rate after intrauterine transfusions is 89%, and the complication rate is 1–3%. In contrast, the outcome after cordocentesis and intrauterine transfusions performed earlier, such as the second trimester, is poor. Complications include rupture of the membranes and preterm delivery, infection, fetal distress requiring emergency cesarean delivery, and perinatal death. Maternal plasma exchange and intravenous immune globulin (IVIG) have been used as adjunctive therapies in women with prior severe HDFN, but there is limited evidence to support their routine use. Indications for early delivery include pulmonary maturity, fetal distress, complications of PUBS, and 35-37 wk of gestation. Careful antenatal care, including intrauterine transfusions, has decreased the need for postdelivery exchange transfusion.

Treatment of the Liveborn Infant

The birth should be attended by a physician skilled in neonatal resuscitation. Fresh, leukoreduced, and irradiated group O and Rh-negative blood, which has been cross-matched against maternal serum, should be immediately available. If clinical signs of **severe hemolytic anemia** (pallor, hepatosplenomegaly, edema, petechiae, ascites) are evident at birth, immediate resuscitation and supportive therapy, temperature stabilization, and monitoring before proceeding with exchange transfusion may save severely affected infants. Such therapy should include a small transfusion of compatible PRBCs to correct anemia; volume expansion for hypotension, especially in those with hydrops; correction of acidosis with 1-2 mEq/kg of sodium bicarbonate; and assisted ventilation for respiratory failure. Infants with HDFN should be closely monitored with frequent hemoglobin and bilirubin testing to determine their need for phototherapy, simple transfusion, or exchange transfusion.

Exchange Transfusion

The decision to proceed with an immediate full or partial exchange transfusion should be based on the infant's clinical condition at birth, with a judgment specifically regarding the likelihood of the infant rapidly developing a dangerous degree of anemia or hyperbilirubinemia. Cord hemoglobin value of ≤10 g/dL or bilirubin concentration ≥5 mg/dL suggest severe hemolysis, but neither consistently predicts the need for exchange transfusion. Some physicians consider previous kernicterus or severe HDFN in a sibling, reticulocyte counts >15%, and prematurity to be additional factors supporting a decision for early exchange transfusion (see Chapters 123.3 and 123.4).

The hemoglobin concentration and serum bilirubin level should be measured at 4-6 hr intervals initially, with extension to longer intervals as the rate of change diminishes. The decision to perform an exchange transfusion is often based on the likelihood that the bilirubin levels, which can be plotted against postnatal hours of life, will reach dangerous levels (see Fig. 123.14 and Table 123.7 in Chapter 123). *Term infants with bilirubin levels ≥20 mg/dL have an increased risk of kernicterus.* Simple transfusions of ABO-compatible, Rh-negative, leukoreduced, and irradiated RBCs may be necessary to correct anemia up to 6-8 wk of age, after which the infant's own erythropoiesis can be expected to overcome any lingering hemolysis. Weekly determinations of hemoglobin values should be performed until the physiologic nadir is passed and a spontaneous rise has been demonstrated.

Careful monitoring of the serum bilirubin level is essential until a decline has been documented in the absence of phototherapy (see Chapter 123.3). Even then, an occasional infant, particularly if premature, may experience a significant rebound in serum bilirubin as late as the 7th day of life. Attempts to predict dangerously high levels of bilirubin based on levels exceeding 6 mg/dL in the 1st 6 hr of life, or 10 mg/dL in the 2nd 6 hr of life, or on increasing rates exceeding 0.5-1.0 mg/dL/hr, are often quoted but not necessarily reliable.

Procedure

The actual exchange transfusion can be performed most easily through an umbilical vein catheter or through peripheral arterial (remove) and venous (return) lines. The exchange should be carried out over 45-60 min and involves serial removal of 15-20 mL aliquots of infant blood (term infant), alternating with infusion of an equivalent volume of donor blood. Smaller, 5-10 mL aliquots may be better tolerated by sick or premature infants. The goal should be an isovolemic exchange of approximately 2 blood volumes of the infant (2×100 mL/kg) to achieve 90% replacement of fetal RBCs and 50% removal of bilirubin.

Blood for exchange transfusion should be as fresh as possible. Standard anticoagulants and preservatives such as citrate-phosphate-dextrose-adenine solution can be used. Blood selection is similar to that of intrauterine transfusions, typically leukoreduced and irradiated erythrocytes from a group O and Rh-negative donor. Although the blood should be negative for the mismatched Rh antigen, a complete crossmatch should be performed before transfusion. Packed erythrocytes should be reconstituted with fresh-frozen plasma to a hematocrit of about 40% before the procedure. Blood should be gradually warmed and maintained at a temperature between 35°C and 37°C throughout the exchange transfusion. It should be kept well mixed by gentle squeezing or agitation of the bag to avoid sedimentation. The infant's stomach should be emptied before transfusion to prevent aspiration, and body temperature should be maintained and vital signs monitored. A competent assistant should be present to help monitor, tally the volume of blood exchanged, and perform emergency procedures.

Infants with acidosis and hypoxia from respiratory distress, sepsis, or shock may be further compromised by the significant exposure to citrate, which provides both an acute acid load (pH 7.0-7.2) and calcium binding. The subsequent metabolism of citrate may later result in metabolic alkalosis. Fresh heparinized blood avoids this problem but is not readily available in most settings. During the exchange transfusion, blood pH and PaO_2 should be serially monitored to avoid acidosis and hypoxia. Symptomatic hypoglycemia may occur before, during, or after an exchange transfusion in moderately to severely affected infants.

Additional acute complications, noted in 5–10% of infants, include transient bradycardia with or without calcium infusion, cyanosis, transient vasospasm, thrombosis, thrombocytopenia, apnea with bradycardia requiring resuscitation, and death. Infectious risks include CMV, HIV, and hepatitis. Necrotizing enterocolitis is a rare complication of exchange transfusion for HDFN.

There is a risk of death from an exchange transfusion, even when performed by an experienced physician team, estimated at 3 per 1,000 procedures. With the fortunate decline of this procedure because of phototherapy and prevention of sensitization, experience with such procedures and physician competence are diminishing, and exchange should be performed only at experienced neonatal referral centers.

After exchange transfusion, the bilirubin level must be measured at frequent intervals (every 4-8 hr) because the serum value may rebound 40–50% because of reequilibration and ongoing production. Repeated exchange transfusions are occasionally necessary, with the primary aim of keeping the indirect bilirubin fraction from exceeding dangerous levels indicated in Table 123.7 (see Chapter 123) for preterm infants and 20 mg/dL for term infants. Signs and symptoms suggestive of kernicterus are mandatory indications for exchange transfusion at any time.

Intravenous Immune Globulin

Because of its ability to interfere with immune-mediated clearance of antibody-sensitized RBCs, early administration of IVIG may be an effective therapeutic intervention for HDFN. IVIG can prevent immune hemolysis, lower peak serum bilirubin levels, shorten the duration of phototherapy, and reduce both length of hospitalization and need for exchange transfusion. However, IVIG does not effectively prevent anemia, which results from both immune-mediated RBC destruction and inadequate erythropoiesis. Consequently, simple transfusions are usually needed as an adjunct to IVIG therapy. An IVIG dose of 0.5-1 g/kg is typically used, but optimal dosing has not been established. Treated infants with blood groups A or B should be monitored for worsening hemolysis caused by anti-A or anti-B antibodies present in IVIG.

Late Complications

Infants with HDFN, including those who have had an intrauterine or postnatal exchange transfusion, must be observed carefully for the development of late anemia and cholestasis.

Late anemia, operationally defined as occurring after the 1st 4-6 wk of life, can result from either persistent hemolysis caused by circulating maternal alloantibodies or from effects on the bone marrow. **Late hyporegenerative anemia** in HDFN results from suppression of erythropoiesis, in part from the higher hemoglobin concentration provided through an intrauterine or exchange transfusion. Late hyporegenerative anemia can be distinguished from hemolytic anemia by a low or absent reticulocyte count and a normal bilirubin level. Infants should be monitored for symptoms and signs of anemia, including poor feeding, sleepiness, and poor growth. Hemoglobin and reticulocyte counts should be monitored weekly to determine the need for transfusion, until the marrow spontaneously recovers after several weeks to months. Neutropenia can also be observed during recovery from HDFN or in association with the late hyporegenerative anemia. In addition to transfusion, treatment with supplemental iron or erythropoietin may be helpful to accelerate marrow recovery.

Inspissated bile syndrome refers to the rare occurrence of persistent icterus in association with significant elevations in both direct and indirect bilirubin levels in infants with hemolytic disease. The cause is unclear, but jaundice clears spontaneously within a few weeks or months with conservative management. **Portal vein thrombosis** and portal hypertension may occur in children who have been subjected to exchange transfusion as newborn infants. It is probably associated with prolonged, traumatic, or septic umbilical vein catheterization.

Prevention of Rh Sensitization

The risk of initial sensitization of Rh-negative mothers has been reduced to less than 0.1% by the routine administration of Rh-immunoglobulin (RhoGAM) to all mothers at risk for Rh alloimmunization. The Rh-immunoglobulin product is administered to Rh-negative mothers as an intramuscular injection of 300 μg (1 mL) of human anti-D globulin within 72 hr of delivery of an Rh-positive infant. Additional clinical indications for RhoGAM administration include ectopic pregnancy, abdominal trauma during pregnancy, amniocentesis, chorionic villus biopsy, or abortion. This quantity of antibody is sufficient to eliminate approximately 10 mL of potentially antigenic fetal Rh-positive cells within the maternal circulation. Larger fetal-to-maternal transfers of blood will require proportionately more human anti-D globulin. RhoGAM administration provided at 28-32 wk of gestation and again at birth is more effective than a single dose.

It is also critical to use appropriately matched blood for all transfusions to Rh-negative girls and young women of childbearing years, including the use of group O, Rh-negative blood during emergencies, as a primary measure to prevent Rh antigen exposure. This approach, coupled with the use of anti-D immunoglobulin during/after pregnancy, plus improved methods of detecting maternal sensitization and measuring the extent of fetal-to-maternal transfusion, have dramatically decreased the incidence and severity of HDFN in developed countries. In addition, the use of fewer obstetric procedures that increase the risk of fetal-to-maternal bleeding should further reduce the incidence of this disorder. However, because serologic testing does not always accurately predict RhD type, since there are now well-recognized weak and partial RhD antigens, the use of fetal RhD genotyping will better guide appropriate use of Rh-immunoglobulin therapy in Rh-negative women.

HEMOLYTIC DISEASE CAUSED BY BLOOD GROUP A AND B INCOMPATIBILITY

Although ABO incompatibility is the most common cause of HDFN, this form is usually much milder than Rh disease and rarely requires aggressive clinical management or therapeutic intervention. Approximately 20% of live births are at theoretical risk for immune-mediated hemolysis based on ABO mismatch, most often the mother being group O and the infant either group A or B. Less often, the mother will be group A and the infant group B, or vice versa.

However, clinical manifestations of hemolysis develop in only 1–10% of at-risk infants, primarily because naturally occurring maternal antibodies against ABO blood group antigens are almost exclusively IgM and therefore do not cross the placenta. Some group O mothers will produce IgG antibodies against blood group A or B antigens, and these can cross the placenta and cause immune-mediated hemolysis. For example, an A-O incompatibility can cause hemolysis even in a firstborn infant, if the mother (group O) produces some anti-A IgG antibodies. A 2nd factor that accounts for the lower-than-predicted incidence of severe ABO hemolytic disease is the relatively low antigen frequency and expression on the RBC of the fetus and newborn infant. With few strong binding sites available for the maternal antibodies to bind, there is less hemolysis.

Clinical Manifestations

Most cases of ABO incompatibility are mild, with jaundice the only clinical manifestation. The infant is not generally affected at birth but will develop jaundice in the 1st 24 hr, which is always abnormal. Pallor and hepatosplenomegaly are not present, and the development of hydrops fetalis or kernicterus is extremely rare.

Diagnosis

A presumptive diagnosis is based on the presence of serologic ABO incompatibility between the mother and infant, plus a weakly to moderately positive DAT result. Hyperbilirubinemia is often the main laboratory abnormality. In 10–20% of affected infants, the unconjugated serum bilirubin level may reach 20 mg/dL or more unless phototherapy is administered. Usually the infant has mild anemia and reticulocytosis; the peripheral blood smear may show polychromasia, nucleated RBCs, and spherocytes. However, the persistence of hemolytic anemia or spherocytosis beyond 2 wk should suggest an alternative diagnosis, such as hereditary (congenital) spherocytosis (see Fig. 124.6).

Treatment

Phototherapy may be effective in lowering serum bilirubin levels (see

Table 124.5	Hemolytic Disease of the Fetus and Newborn		
	Rh	**ABO**	**KELL**
BLOOD GROUPS			
Mother	Rh-negative	O (occasionally B)	K1-negative
Infant	Rh-positive (D is most common)	A (sometimes B)	K1-positive
CLINICAL FEATURES			
Occurrence in firstborn	5%	40–50%	Rare
Severity in subsequent pregnancies:	Predictable	Difficult to predict	Somewhat predictable
Stillbirth/hydrops	Frequent (less with Rh-immunoglobulin use)	Rare	10%
Severe anemia	Frequent	Rare	Frequent
Jaundice	Prominent, severe	Mild-moderate	Mild
LABORATORY TESTS			
Direct antiglobulin test (infant)	Positive	Positive or negative	Positive or negative
Reticulocyte count	Elevated	Elevated	Variable
Red blood cell (RBC) antibodies (mother)	Usually detectable	May not be detectable	Usually detectable
	Antibody titers may help predict severity of fetal disease.	Antibody titers may not correlate with fetal disease.	Antibody titers may not correlate with fetal disease; fetus can be affected at titers lower than for Rh-mediated hemolysis.

Chapter 123.4). In severe cases, IVIG administration can be helpful by reducing the rate of hemolysis and the need for exchange transfusion. Exchange transfusions with group O and Rh-compatible blood type may be needed in some cases to correct dangerous degrees of anemia or hyperbilirubinemia. Indications for this procedure are similar to those previously described for hemolytic disease caused by Rh incompatibility. Some infants with ABO hemolytic disease may require transfusion of PRBC at several weeks of age because of hyporegenerative or slowly progressive anemia. *Postdischarge monitoring of hemoglobin or hematocrit is essential in newborns with ABO hemolytic disease.*

OTHER FORMS OF HEMOLYTIC DISEASE

Blood group incompatibilities other than Rh or ABO account for <5% of HDFN. The pathogenesis of hemolytic disease in this setting is similar, because of other RBC antigens that are mismatched between mother and infant. The likelihood of encountering mismatches for minor antigen mismatches relates to their frequency in the population, their density on the RBC surface, their immunogenicity in the mother, and the index of suspicion. Minor RBC antigen mismatch (especially on Kell group) is emerging as a common cause of HDFN in the developed countries where anti-D immunoglobulin is routinely used. In all cases, the maternal serum should have RBC alloantibodies identified that react against the infant (and paternal) erythrocytes. In addition, the infant's DAT result is invariably positive, and elution techniques can identify the antigen specificity.

Common RBC antigens that can lead to clinically relevant incompatibility include those in the Kell, Duffy, and MNS blood groups. Notably, maternal anti-Lewis antibodies do not lead to HDFN because they are IgM and do not cross the placenta, and Lewis antigens are poorly expressed on fetal erythrocytes. **Kell** is a particularly dangerous incompatibility because the severity of the hemolytic anemia is difficult to predict based on previous obstetric history, amniotic fluid bilirubin determinants, or maternal antibody titer. Kell-alloimmunized infants often have inappropriately low numbers of circulating reticulocytes caused by erythroid suppression, and even low maternal titers of anti-Kell antibodies may cause significant hypoproliferative anemia. Table 124.5 summarizes the clinical characteristics of hemolytic disease caused by Rh, ABO, and Kell antigen systems. There are no specific pharmacologic therapies available to prevent sensitization caused by any blood group other than RhD. As with cases of Rh and ABO incompatibility, exchange transfusion may be indicated for severe hyperbilirubinemia or severe anemia in infants with HDFN caused by minor antigen incompatibility.

Bibliography is available at Expert Consult.

124.3 Neonatal Polycythemia
Omar Niss and Russell E. Ware

Neonatal polycythemia is defined as a central hemoglobin or hematocrit (Hct) exceeding 2 standard deviations (SD) above the normal value for gestational and postnatal age. A full-term infant is therefore considered to have polycythemia when the hemoglobin concentration is ≥22 g/dL or Hct is ≥65%. Measuring the *central hemoglobin* using an automated blood counter is important because both peripheral (heelstick) and capillary tube microcentrifugation yield higher Hct values than central values, by up to 15%. Timing is also important; because of fluid shifts in the newborn period, Hct peaks during the 1st 2-3 hr of life. The frequency of neonatal polycythemia is also increased for births at higher altitudes (5% at high altitude vs 1–2% at sea level). Polycythemia predisposes to **hyperviscosity** (not clinically measurable), which may be the primary issue. When Hct is >65%, hyperviscosity may rapidly increase.

Etiologies of neonatal polycythemia are numerous but can be grouped into two broad categories based on passive RBC transfusion into the fetus and increased intrauterine erythropoiesis. Causes of passive fetal RBC transfusion include delayed clamping of the umbilical cord (most common cause in term infants), twin-twin transfusion for the recipient, and rarely, maternal-fetal transfusions. In contrast, neonatal polycythemia secondary to increased fetal erythropoiesis has many causes, including postmaturity (3%) vs term (1–2%) infants; small-for-gestational-age (8%) or large-for-gestational-age (3%) vs average-for-gestational-age (1–2%) infants; infants of diabetic mothers; infants with trisomy 13, 18, or 21; adrenogenital syndrome; neonatal Graves disease; hypothyroidism; infants of hypertensive mothers or those taking propranolol; and Beckwith-Wiedemann syndrome. Although the pathogenesis of increased erythropoiesis is not always fully understood, infants of diabetic or hypertensive mothers and those with growth restriction may have been exposed to chronic fetal hypoxia, which stimulates erythropoietin production and increases RBC production.

Signs and symptoms of polycythemia can result from hyperviscosity (sluggish blood flow causing decreased tissue perfusion) or metabolic disturbances, or both. Most polycythemic infants are asymptomatic. Symptoms often appear in the 1st few hr of life but can be delayed by up to 2-3 days. Symptoms include irritability, lethargy, tachypnea, respiratory distress, cyanosis, feeding disturbances, hyperbilirubinemia, hypoglycemia, and thrombocytopenia. Severe complications include seizures, stroke, pulmonary hypertension, necrotizing enterocolitis (NEC), renal vein thrombosis, and renal failure. Because most infants are asymptomatic and these symptoms overlap with many neonatal conditions, other respiratory, cardiovascular, and neurologic diseases should be ruled out. Dehydration should also always be considered as a cause. Whether these symptoms are truly caused by, or just associated with, polycythemia is undetermined. Hyperviscosity in infancy may be accentuated because neonatal RBCs are large and have decreased deformability, which together predispose to stasis in the microcirculation.

The **treatment** of polycythemia varies among centers and is often based primarily on local expert opinion. A capillary Hct >65% should always be confirmed with a venous sample and dehydration should be treated. All polycythemic infants should be closely monitored for intake and output, and blood glucose and bilirubin levels should be closely followed. Asymptomatic infants whose central Hct is 60–70% can be monitored closely and hydrated with adequate enteral intake or administration of intravenous (IV) fluids. Treatment of symptomatic polycythemic newborns is not well defined. A partial exchange transfusion (with normal saline) can be used in infants with severe polycythemia and symptoms of hyperviscosity and should be considered if the Hct is ≥70–75% and symptoms worsen despite aggressive IV hydration. Partial exchange transfusion lowers Hct and viscosity acutely and improves acute symptoms but may not affect long-term outcome in polycythemic infants.

Polycythemic infants treated with partial exchange transfusion may be at increased risk of NEC, and their long-term prognosis is unclear. Reported adverse outcomes include speech deficits, abnormal fine motor control, reduced IQ, school problems, and other neurologic abnormalities. The underlying etiology (**chronic intrauterine hypoxia**) is likely the determinant of these outcomes rather than polycythemia itself. Most asymptomatic infants develop normally.

Bibliography is available at Expert Consult.

124.4 Hemorrhage in the Newborn Infant
Cristina Tarango and Russell E. Ware

Neonates have a unique hemostatic system that places them at high risk for hemorrhagic complications, especially in the presence of illness or other stress. Plasma levels of the vitamin K–dependent coagulation factors (II, VII, IX, X, protein C, protein S) and antithrombin are low at birth and do not reach adult ranges until approximately 6 mo of age. Thrombin generation and platelet function are also altered in normal newborns. Consequently, both congenital and acquired bleeding disorders that affect primary or secondary hemostasis can manifest in the newborn period. In general, hemorrhage in a *healthy* neonate suggests an inherited coagulation defect or immune-mediated thrombocytopenia, whereas bleeding symptoms in a *sick* neonate are more likely to reflect underproduction or consumption of coagulation factors and/or platelets. *Congenital hemorrhagic disorders such as hemophilia can present with bleeding in the newborn period.* Common acquired hemorrhagic disorders include vitamin K deficiency bleeding, disseminated intravascular coagulation (see Chapter 510), and immune-mediated thrombocytopenia (Chapter 511.9).

VITAMIN K DEFICIENCY BLEEDING
Vitamin K deficiency bleeding, previously referred to as **hemorrhagic disease of the newborn**, results from transient but severe deficiencies in the vitamin K–dependent factors and is characterized by hemorrhage that is most frequently gastrointestinal, nasal, subgaleal, intracranial, or postcircumcision. Prodromal or warning signs (mild bleeding) may occur before serious intracranial hemorrhage. Laboratory testing reveals that both the prothrombin time (PT) and partial thromboplastin time are prolonged, and plasma levels of prothrombin (II) and factors VII, IX, and X are substantially decreased. The pathophysiology of this acquired hemorrhagic disorder results because vitamin K facilitates posttranscriptional carboxylation of factors II, VII, IX, and X, which is necessary for its full coagulation effects. In the absence of carboxylation, such factors form **PIVKA** (proteins induced in vitamin K absence), which have greatly reduced function; these can be measured and represent a sensitive marker for vitamin K status. In contrast, factors V and VIII, fibrinogen, bleeding time, clot retraction, and platelet count and function are normal for maturity.

Classically, *vitamin K deficiency bleeding occurs early in the newborn period,* typically between day 2 and 7 of life, and most often in exclusively breastfeeding infants who did not receive vitamin K prophylaxis at birth. Severe vitamin K deficiency is also more common in premature infants. This pathogenesis occurs from a lack of free vitamin K from the mother, coupled with absence of bacterial intestinal flora normally responsible for the synthesis of vitamin K. Breast milk is a poor source of vitamin K, which explains why hemorrhagic complications are more frequent in exclusively breastfed than in mixed-fed or formula-fed infants. This classic form of hemorrhagic disease of the newborn, which is responsive to (and entirely prevented by) exogenous vitamin K therapy, should be distinguished from rare congenital deficiencies of clotting factors that are unresponsive to vitamin K, which can occur in otherwise

Table 124.6	Vitamin K Deficiency Bleeding (Hemorrhagic Disease of the Newborn)		
	EARLY-ONSET DISEASE	**CLASSIC DISEASE**	**LATE-ONSET DISEASE**
Age	0-24 hr	2-7 days	1-6 mo
Potential sites of hemorrhage	Cephalohematoma Subgaleal Intracranial Gastrointestinal Umbilicus Intraabdominal	Gastrointestinal Ear-nose-throat-mucosal Intracranial Post-circumcision Cutaneous Injection sites	Intracranial Gastrointestinal Cutaneous Ear-nose-throat-mucosal Injection sites Thoracic
Etiology/risks	Maternal drugs (phenobarbital, phenytoin, warfarin, rifampin, isoniazid) that interfere with vitamin K levels or absorption Inherited coagulopathy	Vitamin K deficiency Exclusive breastfeeding	Cholestasis: malabsorption of vitamin K (biliary atresia, cystic fibrosis, hepatitis) Abetalipoprotein deficiency Idiopathic in Asian breastfed infants Warfarin ingestion
Prevention	Avoidance of high-risk medications Possibly antenatal vitamin K to treatment of mother (20 mg) before birth and postnatal administration to infant soon after birth	Prevented by parenteral vitamin K at birth Oral vitamin K regimens require repeated dosing.	Prevented by parenteral and high-dose oral vitamin K during periods of malabsorption or cholestasis
Incidence	Very rare	~2% if infant not given vitamin K soon after birth	Dependent on primary disease

well-appearing infants (see Chapter 503).

Early-onset vitamin K deficiency bleeding (after birth but in 1st 24 hr) occurs if the mother has been treated chronically with certain drugs (e.g., anticoagulant warfarin, anticonvulsant phenytoin or phenobarbital, cholesterol-lowering medication) that interfere with vitamin K absorption or function. These infants can have severe bleeding, which is usually corrected promptly by vitamin K administration, although some have a poor or delayed response. If a mother is known to be receiving such drugs late in gestation, an infant PT should be measured using cord blood, and *the infant immediately given 1-2 mg of vitamin K intravenously.* If PT is greatly prolonged and fails to improve, or in the presence of significant hemorrhage, *10-15 mL/kg of fresh-frozen plasma should be administered.* In contrast, **late-onset** vitamin K deficiency bleeding (after 2 wk of life) is usually associated with conditions that feature malabsorption of the fat-soluble vitamin K, such as cystic fibrosis, neonatal hepatitis, or biliary atresia, and bleeding can be severe (Table 124.6).

Intramuscular (IM) administration of 1 mg of vitamin K (typically **phytonadione**, or vitamin K_1, the only form of vitamin K available in the United States) soon after birth prevents the pathologic decrease in vitamin K–dependent factors in full-term infants. However, such vitamin K prophylaxis is not uniformly effective to prevent all hemorrhagic disease of the newborn, particularly in exclusively breastfed and premature infants. When an infant presents with hemorrhage, a slow IV infusion of 1-5 mg of vitamin K_1 is effective treatment and leads to improvement in coagulation defects and cessation of bleeding within a few hours. Serious bleeding, particularly in premature infants or those with liver disease, may require transfusion of fresh-frozen plasma or even whole blood. With prompt recognition and treatment, the mortality rate is low.

Decades of experience have demonstrated that the routine use of IM vitamin K for prophylaxis in the United States is safe, and specifically is *not* associated with an increased risk of childhood cancer or leukemia. Although multiple doses of oral vitamin K (1-2 mg at birth, again at discharge, and again at 3-4 wk of life) has been suggested as an alternative, *oral vitamin K is less effective* in preventing late-onset vitamin K deficiency bleeding and thus cannot be recommended for routine therapy. The IM route of vitamin K prophylaxis remains the method of choice.

Other forms of neonatal bleeding may be clinically indistinguishable from hemorrhagic disease of the newborn due to vitamin K deficiency, but they are neither prevented nor successfully treated with vitamin K. For example, an identical clinical presentation may also result from any congenital defect in blood coagulation factors (see Chapters 503 and 504). Hematomas, melena, and postcircumcision and umbilical cord bleeding may be present; up to 70% cases of hemophilia (factor VIII or IX deficiency) are clinically apparent in the newborn period. Treatment of these congenital deficiencies of coagulation factors requires specific factor replacement or fresh-frozen plasma if factor concentrate is not available.

DISSEMINATED INTRAVASCULAR COAGULOPATHY

Disseminated intravascular coagulation (**DIC**) in newborn infants results from consumption of circulating coagulation factors and platelets and therefore can present with either bleeding or thrombosis and usually with evidence of end-organ damage and increased mortality. Affected infants are often premature; their clinical course is frequently characterized by asphyxia, hypoxia, acidosis, shock, hemangiomas, or infection. Since DIC is a secondary event, the most effective treatment is directed at correcting the primary clinical problem, such as infection, to interrupt consumption of clotting factors and allow time to replace them (see Chapter 510). *Infants with DIC who have central nervous system hemorrhage, or other bleeding posing an immediate threat to life, should receive fresh-frozen plasma, vitamin K, and blood* if needed. However, treatment should always be preceded by specific testing for coagulation studies, as well as measurement of the platelet count.

NEONATAL THROMBOCYTOPENIA

See Chapter 511.

Bibliography is available at Expert Consult.

Table 124.7	Conditions Associated With Nonimmune Hydrops

CARDIOVASCULAR	**HEMATOLOGIC**
Malformation	α-Thalassemia
Left heart hypoplasia	Fetomaternal transfusion
Atrioventricular canal defect	Parvovirus B19 infection
Right heart hypoplasia	In utero hemorrhage
Closure of foramen ovale	G6PD deficiency
Single ventricle	Red cell enzyme deficiencies
Transposition of the great vessels	**THORACIC**
Ventral septal defect	Congenital cystic adenomatoid malformation of lung
Atrial septal defect	Diaphragmatic hernia
Tetralogy of Fallot	Intrathoracic mass
Ebstein anomaly	Pulmonary sequestration
Premature closure of ductus	Chylothorax
Truncus arteriosus	Airway obstruction
Tachyarrhythmia	Pulmonary lymphangiectasia
Atrial flutter	Pulmonary neoplasia
Paroxysmal atrial tachycardia	Bronchogenic cyst
Wolff-Parkinson-White syndrome	
Supraventricular tachycardia	**INFECTIONS**
Bradyarrhythmia	Cytomegalovirus
Other arrhythmias	Toxoplasmosis
High-output failure	Parvovirus B19 (fifth disease)
Neuroblastoma	Syphilis
Sacrococcygeal teratoma	Herpes
Large fetal angioma	Rubella
Placental chorioangioma	
Umbilical cord hemangioma	**MALFORMATION SEQUENCES**
Cardiac rhabdomyoma	Noonan syndrome
Other cardiac neoplasia	Arthrogryposis
Cardiomyopathy	Multiple pterygia
	Neu-Laxova syndrome
CHROMOSOMAL	Pena-Shokeir syndrome
45,X	Myotonic dystrophy
Trisomy 21	Saldino-Noonan syndrome
Trisomy 18	
Trisomy 13	**METABOLIC**
18q+	Gaucher disease
13q–	GM_1 gangliosidosis
45,X/46,XX	Sialidosis
Triploidy	Mucopolysaccharide disorders
Other	
	URINARY
CHONDRODYSPLASIAS	Urethral stenosis or atresia
Thanatophoric dwarfism	Posterior urethral valves
Short rib polydactyly	Congenital nephrosis (Finnish)
Hypophosphatasia	Prune-belly syndrome
Osteogenesis imperfecta	
Achondrogenesis	**GASTROINTESTINAL**
	Midgut volvulus
TWIN PREGNANCY	Malrotation of the intestines
Twin-twin transfusion syndrome	Duplication of the intestinal tract
Acardiac twin	Meconium peritonitis
	Hepatic fibrosis
OTHER	Cholestasis
Familial hemophagocytic lymphohistiocytosis	Biliary atresia
Fetal akinesia syndromes	Hepatic vascular malformations
Congenital leukemia	
Infantile arterial calcification syndrome	
Maternal diabetes	
Lymphatic disorders	
IPEX	
Idiopathic	

IPEX, Immune dysregulation polyendocrinopathy enteropathy, X-linked.
Adapted from Wilkins I: Nonimmune hydrops. In Creasy RK, Resnick R, Iams JD, et al, editors: *Creasy & Resnik's maternal-fetal medicine,* ed 7, Philadelphia, 2014, Elsevier (Box 37-1).

124.5 Nonimmune Hydrops

Cristina Tarango and Russell E. Ware

Because of the success in preventing Rh alloimmune fetal hemolysis, nonimmune and often nonhematologic hydrops fetalis is the most common cause of fetal hydrops. **Hydrops** is defined by ≥2 abnormal

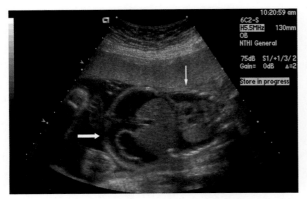

Fig. 124.8 Hydrops fetalis. Longitudinal sonographic image of the fetus, with ascitic fluid outlining the liver *(large arrow)*. The *small arrow* shows pleural effusion above the diaphragm. *(From Wilkins I: Nonimmune hydrops. In Creasy RK, Resnick R, Iams JD, et al, editors: Creasy & Resnik's maternal-fetal medicine, ed 7, Philadelphia, 2014, Elsevier, Fig 37-2.)*

fetal fluid collections, such as ascites, pleural, pericardial, or cutaneous edema (>5 mm) (Fig. 124.8). In addition, there may be associated placental edema (>6 mm), polyhydramnios (50%), and the rare occurrence of the **mirror syndrome**, in which the mother becomes edematous.

The incidence of nonimmune hydrops is approximately 1 in 3,000 births, many of whom are premature. The etiologies are broad; cardiac (structural and SVT) and chromosome disorders are the most common identifiable etiologies (Table 124.7). The etiology is unknown in 10–20%. The mechanisms for the development of nonimmune hydrops are not well established (Fig. 124.9).

In utero treatment has been successful for fetal supraventricular tachycardia (SVT), twin-twin transfusion syndrome, nonimmune fetal anemias, and some surgically treatable fetal conditions. Postnatal therapy includes a team approach to the delivery room management that often requires immediate endotracheal tube intubation and packed RBC transfusion in the presence of anemias. In premature infants, endotracheal surfactant is indicated; drainage of large pleural or pericardial effusions may also be needed. Once the infant is stabilized, diagnostic testing will direct further therapy based on the etiology. For patients with no obvious etiology, lymphangiography, whole exome (or genome) sequencing, and microarray duplication/deletion studies are recommended to establish a diagnosis.

Mortality is approximately 50% and is highest in the most premature infants, those with aneuploidy, and those with fetal anasarca.

Bibliography is available at Expert Consult.

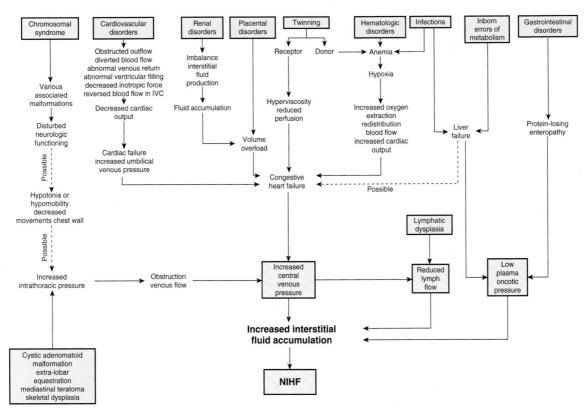

Fig. 124.9 Impact of various etiologies for nonimmune hydrops on fluid homeostasis. *IVC,* Inferior vena cava; *NIHF,* nonimmune hydrops fetalis. *(Adapted from Bellini C, Hennekam RCM: Non-immune hydrops fetalis: a short review of etiology and pathophysiology, Am J Med Genet 158A:597–605, 2012.)*

Chapter **125**
The Umbilicus
Amy T. Nathan

第一百二十五章
脐部

中文导读

脐带是新生儿特殊的解剖结构，在宫内通过脐带与母体相连，靠脐带维系胎儿生存，出生时需要断脐，断脐后则从胎儿血液循环转变为新生儿的自主体肺循环，新生儿靠自身脏器存活。本章主要介绍了脐带、脐带出血、脐肉芽、脐部感染、脐疝、脐膨出及脐部肿瘤等脐带的各种生理病理状况，具体描述了脐带正常结构、断脐后脐部生理改变及常见脐部畸形如卵黄管退化异常、脐尿管，简单描述了脐部出血的原因和造成出血的相关疾病，并简单描述了脐肉芽形成的病理过程和转归、脐部感染性疾病（包括脐炎、脐蜂窝织炎和坏死性筋膜炎）及其预防治疗，介绍了新生儿出生后发生脐疝的病因、好发人群、疝囊组成及其转归。部分新生儿出生后，会出现较严重的脐膨出，本章具体描述了脐膨出的病理生理特点、处理原则及转归，同时简单罗列了常见的脐部肿物以期与脐膨出相鉴别。

UMBILICAL CORD

The umbilical cord typically consists of 2 umbilical arteries, the umbilical vein, and a gelatinous substance called Wharton's jelly, all contained within a sheath derived from the amnion and coiled into a helical shape. The muscular umbilical arteries carry deoxygenated blood from the fetus to the placenta and are contiguous with the fetal internal iliac arteries. The umbilical vein carries oxygenated blood from the placenta back to the fetus, where it flows into the inferior vena cava by way of the ductus venosus. The umbilical cord itself contains an estimated 20 mL/kg of blood, and current recommendations are to delay clamping of the cord at delivery for 30-60 sec, to facilitate placental transfusion. At term, a normal umbilical cord is approximately 55 cm long. Abnormally short cords are associated with conditions causing decreased fetal movement, including fetal hypotonia, oligohydramnios, and uterine constraint, and lead to increased risk for complications during labor and delivery for both mother and infant. Long cords (>70 cm) increase the risk for true knots, wrapping around the fetus, and/or prolapse. Straight uncoiled cords are associated with anomalies, fetal distress, and intrauterine fetal demise.

When the cord is cut after birth, portions of these structures remain in the base but gradually become obliterated. The blood vessels are functionally closed but anatomically patent for 10-20 days. The umbilical arteries become the lateral umbilical ligaments; the umbilical vein, the ligamentum teres; and the ductus venosus, the ligamentum venosum. The umbilical cord stump usually sloughs within 2 wk. Delayed separation of the cord, after more than 1 mo, has been associated with neutrophil chemotactic defects and overwhelming bacterial infection (see Chapter 153).

A single umbilical artery is present in approximately 5-10/1,000 births; the frequency is higher (35-70/1,000) in twin births. It is estimated that 30% of infants with a single umbilical artery have other (and often multiple) congenital structural abnormalities. The presence of multiple anomalies is suggestive of an abnormal karyotype, including trisomies. Infants with isolated single umbilical artery are not thought to be at increased risk of having a chromosomal anomaly, and no specific evaluation is indicated for these infants aside from a thorough physical examination.

The **omphalomesenteric duct (OMD)** is an embryonic connection between the developing midgut and the primitive yolk sac. It typically involutes at 8-9 wk gestation, but failure of this process can leave an abnormal connection between the umbilical cord and the gastrointestinal (GI) tract. The most common remnant of the OMD is a **Meckel diverticulum** (see Chapter 357), whereas abnormalities that would become symptomatic in the neonatal period include a **sinus** or **fistula** that would drain mucus or intestinal contents through the umbilicus. An umbilical **polyp** is one of the least common OMD remnants and represents exposed GI mucosa at the umbilical stump. The tissue of the polyp is bright red, firm, and has a mucoid secretion. Therapy for all OMD remnants is surgical excision of the anomaly.

A **persistent urachus** (urachal cyst, sinus, patent urachus, or diverticulum) is a result of failure of closure of the allantoic duct and may be associated with bladder outlet obstruction. Patency should be suspected if a clear, light-yellow, urine-like fluid is being discharged from the umbilicus. Symptoms include drainage, a mass or cyst, abdominal pain, local erythema, and infection. Urachal anomalies should be investigated by ultrasonography and a cystogram. Therapy for a persistent urachus is surgical excision of the anomaly and correction of any bladder outlet obstruction if present.

HEMORRHAGE

Hemorrhage from the umbilical cord may be the result of trauma, inadequate ligation of the cord, or failure of normal thrombus formation. It may also indicate hemorrhagic disease of the newborn or other coagulopathies (especially factor XIII deficiency), septicemia, or local infection. The infant should be observed frequently during the first few days of life so that if hemorrhage does occur, it will be detected promptly.

GRANULOMA

The umbilical cord stump usually dries and separates within 1-2 wk after birth. The raw surface becomes covered by a thin layer of skin; scar tissue forms, and the wound is usually healed within 12-15 days. The presence of saprophytic organisms delays separation of the cord and increases the possibility of invasion by pathogenic organisms. Mild infection or incomplete epithelialization may result in a moist, granulating area at the base of the cord with a slight mucoid or mucopurulent discharge. Good results are usually obtained by cleansing with alcohol several times daily.

Persistence of granulation tissue at the base of the umbilicus is common. The tissue is soft, 3-10 mm in size, vascular and granular, colored dull red or pink, and may have a seropurulent discharge. Granulation tissue is treated by cauterization with silver nitrate, repeated at intervals of several days until the base is dry.

INFECTIONS

The devitalized umbilical cord provides an ideal medium for bacterial growth and a potential portal of entry for microbes. The term **omphalitis** refers to infection of the umbilical cord stump, navel, or the surrounding abdominal wall. The presence of cellulitis is associated with a high incidence of bacteremia, and complicated omphalitis may spread to the peritoneum, the umbilical or portal vessels, or the liver. **Necrotizing fasciitis** (which is often polymicrobial) is associated with a high mortality rate. Treatment of omphalitis includes prompt antibiotic therapy with agents effective against *Staphylococcus aureus* and *Escherichia coli*, such as an antistaphylococcal penicillin or vancomycin in combination with an aminoglycoside. If abscess formation has occurred, surgical incision and drainage may be required.

In community and primary care settings in developing countries, topical application of chlorhexidine to the umbilical cord has been shown to reduce omphalitis and neonatal mortality. However, the ideal approach to postnatal cord care in hospital settings in developed countries is still debated. There is no convincing evidence that application of antiseptics (including triple dye, alcohol, or chlorhexidine) is superior to dry cord care in minimizing the risk of omphalitis for infants in these settings, although these treatments do reduce bacterial colonization. The American Academy of Pediatrics does not currently recommend any particular method of cord care as superior in the prevention of infection.

UMBILICAL HERNIA

Often associated with **diastasis recti**, an umbilical hernia is caused by incomplete closure or weakness of the muscular umbilical ring. Predisposing factors include black race and low birthweight. The hernia appears as a soft swelling covered by skin that protrudes during crying, coughing, or straining and can be reduced easily through the fibrous ring at the umbilicus. The hernia consists of omentum or portions of the small intestine. The size of the defect varies from <1 cm in diameter to as much as 5 cm (2 inches), but large defects are rare. Most umbilical hernias that appear before age 6 mo disappear spontaneously by 1 yr. Even large hernias (5-6 cm in all dimensions) have been known to disappear spontaneously by 5-6 yr. **Strangulation** of intestinal contents is extremely rare. Surgery is not advised unless the hernia persists to age 4-5 yr, causes symptoms, becomes strangulated, or becomes progressively larger after age 1-2 yr. Defects exceeding 2 cm are less likely to close spontaneously.

CONGENITAL OMPHALOCELE

An **omphalocele** is a herniation or protrusion of the abdominal contents into the base of the umbilical cord (Fig. 125.1). In contrast to the more common umbilical hernia, the sac is covered with peritoneum without

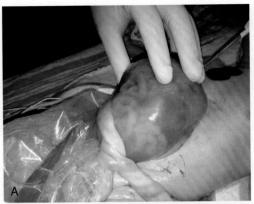
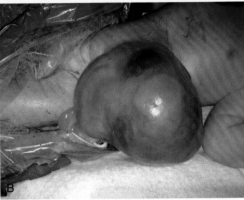

Fig. 125.1 **A,** Omphalocele with umbilical cord insertion into the sac and intestine visible. **B,** Omphalocele with sac containing liver. *(Courtesy of Dr. Foong Lim, Cincinnati Fetal Center at Cincinnati Children's Hospital Medical Center.)*

overlying skin, and the insertion of the distal umbilical cord into the sac itself distinguishes this condition from other abdominal wall defects such as gastroschisis. The size of the sac that lies outside the abdominal cavity depends on its contents. **Herniation** of intestines into the cord occurs in approximately 1/5,000 births, and herniation of liver and intestines in 1/10,000 births. The abdominal cavity may be proportionately small because of the lack of space-occupying viscera. Treatment for an omphalocele consists of covering the sac with moist, sterile dressings, then initiating prompt surgical repair if the abdomen is able to accommodate the eviscerated organs. If the omphalocele is too large to allow immediate repair, continued dressings may temporize and encourage epithelialization of the sac. Occasionally, mesh or similar synthetic material may be used to cover the viscera if the sac has ruptured or if excessive mobilization of the tissues would be necessary to cover the mass and its intact sac.

Many infants with omphalocele (50–70%) have associated malformations, and about 30% have chromosomal abnormalities. The likelihood of an abnormal karyotype is increased when the liver is *intracorporeal* (not within the sac). Omphalocele can be part of well-defined syndromes, including **Beckwith-Wiedemann syndrome**, characterized by omphalocele, macrosomia, and hypoglycemia. The survival rate for affected infants is largely determined by the presence of associated malformations or chromosomal abnormalities. For patients with isolated omphalocele, the survival rate is >90%.

TUMORS

Tumors of the umbilicus are rare and include angioma, enteroteratoma, dermoid cyst, myxosarcoma, and cysts of urachal or OMD remnants.

Bibliography is available at Expert Consult.

Chapter **126**
Abstinence Syndromes
第一百二十六章
戒断综合征

中文导读

　　新生儿的戒断综合征与母亲孕期、特别是孕晚期的不当用药史密切相关。本章主要介绍了新生儿戒断综合征、母孕期选择性5-羟色胺再吸收抑制剂与新生儿行为异常综合征及胎儿酒精综合征，具体描述了新生儿戒断综合征的病因、临床表现、病情程度的评估及其临床干预治疗措施。同时，本章简单描述了母孕期选择性5-羟色胺再吸收抑制剂与新生儿行为异常综合征、持续性肺动脉高压的关系及其治疗，具体介绍了胎儿酒精综合征的流行病学特点、诊断标准、临床特点、干预治疗措施、结局及儿科医师的职责。

126.1 Neonatal Abstinence (Withdrawal)
Scott L. Wexelblatt

Neonatal abstinence syndrome (NAS) is the clinical diagnosis given to infants who experience withdrawal signs after in utero exposure to opioids. Withdrawal signs develop in 55–94% of opioid-exposed infants, 30–65% of whom need pharmacologic treatment for severe withdrawal. The incidence of NAS has been increasing yearly since 2004 and was 5 times more prevalent in 2013 than 2004. This increase in NAS is caused by increased use of prescription medication by pregnant women, an increase in **medication-assisted treatment (MAT)** for opioid addiction, an increase in illicit use of prescription medications, and increased use of heroin. In 2011, 1.1% of pregnant women in the United States abused pain relievers and heroin, and up to 12.9–28% of women were prescribed an opioid at some point during their pregnancy. Many factors affect the severity and duration of withdrawal, including tobacco use during pregnancy, breastfeeding after delivery, rooming-in and parental involvement, genetic makeup, and polysubstance use.

The clinical signs of NAS result from central nervous system (CNS) hyperexcitability and autonomic instability (Fig. 126.1). NAS signs can begin within 24 hr of birth after heroin exposure, within 48 hr after short-acting opioids, and 72-96 hr after exposure to long-acting opioids such as methadone and buprenorphine. Tremors, poor feeding, excessive crying, poor sleeping, and hyperirritability are the most prominent signs of NAS. Other signs include sneezing, yawning, hiccups, myoclonic jerks, skin breakdown and abrasions, vomiting, loose stools, nasal stuffiness, and seizures in the most severe cases.

Identifying which infants are at risk for NAS before discharge is important because of the late onset of signs. Universal maternal screening for drug use is recommended by the American College of Obstetricians and Gynecologists (ACOG), and maternal consent should be obtained if drug testing is indicated. Universal maternal drug testing has been shown to improve identification of infants at risk for NAS but is more expensive and may not be helpful in states with punitive legislation. Maternal testing is preferred over infant testing because results are available promptly, typically by the time the infant is delivered. Testing mothers on admission to the hospital can also exclude iatrogenic exposure. Infant urine, meconium and umbilical cord testing are also used to help identify infants at risk for withdrawal and identify more distant use by the mother. Timing of these results and special collection methods makes routine use of these tests more difficult. Detectability in the neonatal urine specimen is typically 2-3 days for methadone (up to 6 days for methadone metabolites) and buprenorphine and 1-2 days for heroin.

MAT has been shown to be useful for pregnant women with an opioid substance use disorder. Mothers receiving MAT have a decreased mortality, reduced illicit drug use, reduced seroconversion of HIV, and decreased criminal activity. The most common medications in MAT are methadone or buprenorphine. Methadone is a full μ-opioid agonist with a half-life of 24-36 hr, given once daily in methadone clinics because of the potential for overdose. Buprenorphine is a partial μ-opioid agonist with a half-life of 36-48 hr, prescribed monthly as home therapy because a ceiling effect protects against overdosages.

TREATMENT
The first line of treatment for all opioid-exposed infants is **nonpharmacologic support**, which includes swaddling, placing the infant in a dark and quiet environment (e.g., dimmed lights, muted televisions), holding and Kangaroo care, reducing stimulation, and breastfeeding. Illicit (if continued) drug use is a contraindication to breastfeeding infants with NAS. Maternal methadone or buprenorphine use and hepatitis C are not contraindications to breastfeeding. Standardization of nonpharmacologic care with increased emphasis on clinical assessment(i.e., is the infant feeding well, sleeping well, and easily consoled?) over formal scoring

NEONATAL ABSTINENCE SCORE

Date: _____　　　　　　　　Weight: _____

System	Signs & Symptoms	Score	Time AM								PM										Comments
Central Nervous System Disturbances	Excessive High Pitched Cry	2																			
	Continuous High Pitched Cry	3																			
	Sleeps < 1 Hour After Feeding	3																			
	Sleeps < 2 Hours After Feeding	2																			
	Sleeps < 3 Hours After Feeding	1																			
	Hyperactive Moro Reflex	2																			
	Markedly Hyperactive Moro Reflex	3																			
	Mild Tremors Disturbed	1																			
	Moderate - Severe Tremors Disturbed	2																			
	Mild Tremors Undisturbed	3																			
	Moderate - Severe Tremors Undisturbed	4																			
	Increased Muscle Tone	2																			
	Excoriation (Specific Area)	1																			
	Myoclonic Jerks	3																			
	Generalized Convulsions	5																			
Metabolic / Vasomotor / Respiratory Disturbances	Sweating	1																			
	Fever < 101° F (37.2° - 38.2° C)	1																			
	Fever ≥ 101.1° F (≥38.4° C)	2																			
	Frequent Yawning (> 3 - 4 Times/Interval)	1																			
	Mottling	1																			
	Nasal Stuffiness	1																			
	Sneezing (> 3 - 4 Times/Interval)	1																			
	Nasal Flaring	2																			
	Respiratory Rate - 60/min	1																			
	Respiratory Rate - 60/min with Retractions	2																			
Gastrointestinal Disturbances	Excessive Sucking	1																			
	Poor Feeding	2																			
	Regurgitation	2																			
	Projectile Vomiting	3																			
	Loose Stools	2																			
	Watery Stools	3																			
	TOTAL SCORE																				
	Initials of Scorer																				

Fig. 126.1 Neonatal abstinence score used for the assessment of infants displaying neonatal abstinence syndrome. Evaluator should check sign or symptom observed at various time intervals. Add scores for total at each evaluation. (Adapted from Finnegan LP, Kaltenbach K. The assessment and management of neonatal abstinence syndrome. In Hoekelman RA et al, editors: Primary pediatric care, ed 3, St Louis, 1992, Mosby, p 1367.)

tools, which typically require disturbing the infant, was associated with significantly less opioid use among infants with in utero methadone exposure.

The decision for pharmacologic treatment has been traditionally based on the nursing scoring assessment tool. The most widely used tools are the Finnegan and Modified Finnegan (Fig. 126.1). Other scoring tools include the Lipsitz, Neonatal Narcotic Withdrawal Index, Neonatal Withdrawal Inventory, and MOTHER NAS Scale. The main objectives when initiating pharmacologic treatment are to improve signs and comfort of the infant and to prevent worsening withdrawal that could lead to seizures.

Pharmacologic treatment for NAS, when necessary, is typically morphine or methadone (Table 126.1). **Morphine** is a short-acting opioid given every 3-4 hr as a weight-based or symptom-based regimen. **Methadone** is long-acting opioid that can be given twice a day after loading doses, and a pharmacokinetic weight-based weaning protocol is available. Sublingual **buprenorphine** has been proposed as an alternate treatment. Buprenorphine and some methadone formulations contain high ethanol levels, which may be deleterious to the infant. Following a stringent NAS protocol with guidelines on initiation and weaning has

been shown to decrease both length of stay and number of opioid treatment days and may be as important as which primary opioid is used for first-line treatment.

Adjuvant therapy is initiated when the primary opioid is not effective in controlling the signs of NAS. The 2 most common medications used as adjuvant therapy are **phenobarbital** and **clonidine**. Infants with NAS may also expend additional energy. Therefore, the infant should be weighted regularly and strategies to increase caloric intake implemented if weight loss beyond that expected in the 1st week of life occurs.

The long-term prognosis for infants with NAS is multifactorial and not fully known. Close follow-up needs to be initiated to monitor growth and development, visual disturbances, and behavioral/learning problems.

Phenobarbital and benzodiazepine withdrawal may occur in infants of mothers addicted to these drugs, but signs are self-limiting and do not require pharmacologic treatment. Signs may be late onset and begin at a median age of 7 days (range: 2-14 days). Infants may have a brief acute stage consisting of irritability, constant crying, sleeplessness, hiccups, and mouthing movements, followed by a prolonged stage consisting of increased appetite, frequent spit-ups and gagging, irritability, sweating, and a disturbed sleep pattern, all of which may last for weeks.

Table 126.1	Medications Used in Pharmacologic Treatment of Neonatal Abstinence Syndrome (NAS)			
DRUG	**INITIAL DOSING**	**DOSING INCREASES**	**WEANING SCHEDULE**	**ADD ADJUVANT THERAPY**
Morphine	0.05 mg/kg/dose q3h	Increase dose 10–20%	10% of stabilizing dose q24h	>1 mg/kg/day of morphine Unable to wean for 2 days
Methadone	0.1 mg/kg/dose q6h for 4 doses	Increase to q4h if unable to capture	0.7 mg/kg/dose q12h × 2 doses, then 0.05 mg/kg/dose q12h × 2; 0.04 mg/kg/dose q12h × 2; 0.03 mg/kg/dose q12h × 2; 0.02 mg/kg/dose q12h × 2; 0.01 mg/kg/dose q12h × 2; 0.01 mg/kg/dose q24h × 1	Unable to wean for 2 days
Buprenorphine	4 µg/kg q8h	2 µg/kg until maximum of 15 µg/kg	3 µg/kg/dose q8h × 3 doses; 2 µg/kg/dose q8h × 3; 2 µg/kg/dose q8h × 2; 2 µg/kg/dose q24h × 1	Unable to wean for 2 days
Phenobarbital	20 mg/kg	—	5 mg/kg daily	N/A
Clonidine	1.5 µg/kg/dose q3h	25% dose escalation q24hr	10% every day	N/A

N/A, Not available; q24h, every 24 hours.

Cocaine and methamphetamine abuse in pregnant women is less common than opioid abuse, and acute withdrawal in these infants is unusual. However, labor complications can be severe with both drugs and may include preterm labor, placental abruption, intrauterine growth restriction, and fetal asphyxia. Detection in neonatal urine is 6-8 hr for cocaine and 1-2 days for methamphetamine. Early on, exposed infants may have abnormal sleep patterns, poor feeding, tremors, and hypertonia. Long-term outcomes include impaired auditory information processing, developmental delay, and learning disabilities. At age 4 yr, children exposed prenatally to cocaine demonstrate cognitive impairments and are less likely to have an IQ above the normative mean.

Bibliography is available at Expert Consult.

126.2 Maternal Selective Serotonin Reuptake Inhibitors and Neonatal Behavioral Syndromes
Jennifer McAllister

Approximately 18% of women have depression during pregnancy. When pharmacologic treatment is required, selective serotonin reuptake inhibitors (SSRIs; fluoxetine, paroxetine, sertraline, citalopram, fluvoxamine) are most frequently prescribed. Additionally, serotonin norepinephrine reuptake inhibitors (SNRIs; venlafaxine, duloxetine) and tricyclic antidepressants (TCAs) have been used to treat pregnant women with depression or anxiety disorders. About 3.5% of all pregnant women in the Western world use psychotropic medications during their pregnancy, and all these agents cross the placenta. Exposure to these medications in utero may lead to a higher risk of congenital malformations, **poor neonatal adaptation syndrome** (PNAS), and **persistent pulmonary hypertension** (PPHN).

Studies are conflicted on the risk of major birth defects, specifically cardiac defects, and antidepressant use in pregnancy. Use of paroxetine and fluoxetine are thought to have the highest risk of birth defects. Some reported defects include anencephaly, atrial septal defect, right ventricular outflow tract obstruction, omphalocele, and gastroschisis. Although the relative risk may be increased, the occurrence of birth defects is low.

PNAS symptoms usually appear within the 1st 8 hr after birth and often persist for the 1st 2-6 days of life. If symptoms do not develop within 48 hr, the infant is not likely to experience PNAS. PNAS affects the neurologic, autonomic, respiratory, and gastrointestinal systems. Symptoms include a weak suck reflex, irritability, tremors, hypertonia and hypotonia, hyperthermia, weak or absent cry, sleep disturbances,

hypoglycemia, respiratory problems, vomiting and diarrhea, and seizures. Most symptoms are mild, and severe symptoms are rare. No deaths have been reported. Many researchers believe that the etiology of PNAS results from both toxicity and withdrawal from the antidepressant medications, and the symptoms of both toxicity and withdrawal are similar. Symptoms related to toxicity often occur *immediately after birth* when medication levels in the infant are high, whereas symptoms related to withdrawal often occur *8-48 hr after birth* when drug concentrations in the infants are low.

Most studies have reported incidence of PNAS with SSRI exposure to be approximately 30%. Exposure to SNRIs has a similar risk as SSRIs. Infants exposed to TCAs have a 20–50% risk of PNAS.

PPHN is often observed immediately after delivery, but symptoms can be variable in intensity, from mild respiratory insufficiency to severe respiratory failure. SSRI exposure later in pregnancy has been associated with a higher risk of PPHN.

Treatment consists of supportive measures, and most cases are mild, of short duration, and self-limiting. Small, frequent, on-demand feedings; swaddling; and skin-to-skin contact are beneficial to support infants through this process. Breastfeeding is protective against developing PNAS and should be encouraged because many antidepressant medications are safe with breastfeeding. Infants can be observed on the maternity ward with their mothers unless specific symptoms warrant further evaluation and treatment. Infants should be observed for a minimum of 48 hr to ensure they do not develop significant symptoms of PNAS. There have been no reported differences in IQ or development in infants with PNAS. Further research is needed to examine long-term effects of in utero antidepressant exposure.

Bibliography is available at Expert Consult.

126.3 Fetal Alcohol Exposure
Carol Weitzman

EPIDEMIOLOGY
Approximately 1 in 10 pregnant women report consuming alcohol within the past 30 days, and 1 in 33 report binge drinking. When pregnant women report binge drinking, they report an average of 4.6 binge-drinking episodes. Of nonpregnant women of childbearing age, approximately 50% report consuming alcohol within the last 30 days, with about 1 in 5 reporting binge drinking. Because almost 50% of pregnancies in the United States are unplanned, unintentional **prenatal alcohol exposure** (PAE) can occur before a woman knows she is pregnant.

Alcohol is a known teratogen that can cause irreversible CNS damage leading to CNS dysfunction that can range from relatively mild to severe. PAE affects all stages of brain development from neurogenesis to myelination, through mechanisms that include disrupted cell-cell interactions, altered gene expression, and oxidative stress leading to abnormalities such as reduced brain volume in the frontal lobe, striatum and caudate nucleus, thalamus, and cerebellum; thinning of the corpus callosum; and abnormal functioning of the amygdala.

Fetal alcohol spectrum disorders (FASDs) are the most common causes of preventable developmental delay and intellectual disability. Prevalence rates vary for several reasons. First, the method of ascertainment and the specific diagnostic definitions used can influence rates. Further, it is often difficult to obtain accurate information regarding PAE because mothers often deny the extent of alcohol use due to fear of child protective services and removal of their child from the home, shame and guilt associated with alcohol use during pregnancy, and fear of judgment. Lastly, mothers are often not asked in enough detail during or after pregnancy about alcohol consumption during pregnancy to accurately assess the extent of PAE. The U.S. Centers for Disease Control and Prevention (CDC) Fetal Alcohol Syndrome (FAS) Surveillance Network used medical records in several states and identified 0.3 children with FAS per 1,000 children age 7-9 yr. This prevalence rate is much lower than that obtained by active case ascertainment studies in the United States and Western Europe, which have estimated prevalence rates of 2–5%. Another study reported similar rates, 24-48 cases per 1,000 children (2.4–4.8%) for all FASDs, and 6-9 cases per 1,000 (0.6–0.9%) for FAS specifically. Studies that have examined PAE by anonymous meconium testing demonstrate 4.26 times greater identification of alcohol use during pregnancy compared with maternal self-report. Rates of FASDs have been reported to be higher in children living in poverty, in American Indian populations, and in children living in foster care. They often go undetected in these children, and as many as 86.5% of foster and adopted youth with FASDs go undiagnosed or are diagnosed incorrectly within the FAS spectrum.

DIAGNOSTIC CRITERIA

Updated clinical guidelines for diagnosing FASDs in the United States were published in 2016, as were updated Canadian guidelines, which overlap U.S. guidelines but also have important distinctions. PAE can result in a child having 1 of the FASDs, a nondiagnostic umbrella term in the United States. Diagnoses are determined based on the presence or absence of (1) the characteristic facial features; (2) prenatal/postnatal growth deficiency; (3) deficient brain growth, abnormal morphogenesis, or abnormal neurophysiology; (4) neurobehavioral impairment; and (5) maternal alcohol consumption during pregnancy.

FASDs include **fetal alcohol syndrome** (FAS), **partial fetal alcohol syndrome** (pFAS), **alcohol-related neurodevelopmental disorder** (ARND), **alcohol-related birth defect** (ARBD), and **neurobehavioral disorder associated with prenatal alcohol exposure** (ND-PAE), a term introduced in the *Diagnostic and Statistical Manual of Mental Disorders, Fifth Edition* (DSM-5). Table 126.2 describes specific diagnostic features of each of the FASDs. The diagnosis of **FAS** and **pFAS** are the only FASDs that can be diagnosed in the absence of a confirmed maternal history of PAE. The key facial dysmorphologic features include short palpebral fissures, a thin vermilion border of the upper lip, and a smooth philtrum (Fig. 126.2). The differential diagnosis for FAS includes Williams syndrome, Dubowitz syndrome, fetal valproate syndrome, maternal phenylketonuria (PKU) effects, and other prenatal toxin exposures, and when there is unconfirmed PAE, a genetics evaluation may be warranted. **ND-PAE** is included in the DSM-5 as a "condition for further study" and is also provided as an example under "Other Specified Neurodevelopmental Disorder." Although the diagnosis of ND-PAE overlaps with **ARND**, ND-PAE aims to describe the behavioral and mental health effects on an individual with PAE. Unlike ARND, a diagnosis of ND-PAE can be given in addition to FAS or pFAS. ND-PAE has organized the deficits seen into 3 areas: neurocognitive impairment, impaired self-regulation, and impairment in adaptive functioning. In the updated Canadian guidelines, "fetal alcohol spectrum disorder" is considered a diagnostic term with 2 categories: FASD with sentinel facial features

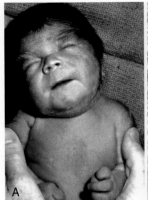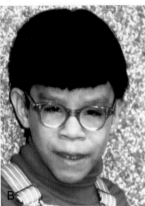

Fig. 126.2 Characteristics of fetal alcohol syndrome. At birth (**A**) and at 4 yr of age (**B**). Note the short palpebral fissures; long, smooth philtrum with vermilion border; and hirsutism in the newborn. *(From Jones KL, Smith DW: Recognition of the fetal alcohol syndrome in early infancy, Lancet 2:999–1001, 1973.)*

and FASD without sentinel facial features. These guidelines have also eliminated *growth restriction* as a diagnostic criterion and have included an at-risk category for children with confirmed PAE who were too young to meet the criteria for neurodevelopmental deficits, or in whom assessment was incomplete, and for children with cardinal facial features without documentation or evidence of severe impairment in neurodevelopmental domains.

A safe threshold or pattern of alcohol consumption has not been identified, and any PAE is believed to present a risk to a developing fetus. Significant alcohol exposure has been carefully defined in the updated guidelines, and information can be obtained from a variety of sources, including, in addition to the birth mother, family members, foster or adoptive parents, social service agencies who observed maternal alcohol consumption during pregnancy, or medical records that document PAE, alcohol treatment, or social, legal, or medical problems related to drinking during pregnancy. PAE in the first trimester leads to the classic *facial dysmorphia* associated with FAS and other structural defects. PAE can have other deleterious effects (e.g., spontaneous abortion, growth defect) on the fetus throughout the pregnancy. Several well-validated screens are used to identify alcohol use in pregnant and nonpregnant women of childbearing years, including the T-ACE (Tolerance, Annoyance, Cut Down, Eye-Opener), CAGE (Cut Back, Annoyed, Guilty, Eye-Opener), CRAFFT, Audit-C (Alcohol Use Disorders Identification Test), and TWEAK (Tolerance, Worried, Eye opener, Amnesia, Kut Down). There are no well-validated screens designed to ask about past consumption of alcohol. Pediatricians can ask the following 2 questions to determine the likelihood of significant PAE: "In the 3 months before you knew you were pregnant, how many times did you have 4 or more alcohol drinks in a day?" and "During your pregnancy, how many times did you have any alcohol?" If a positive response is given to either question, the clinician can follow up to determine the level of PAE by asking, (1) "During your pregnancy, on average, how many days per week did you have any alcohol?" (2) "During your pregnancy, on a typical day when you had an alcoholic beverage, how many drinks did you have?" and (3) "During your pregnancy, what was the maximum number of drinks that you had in a day?"

CLINICAL FEATURES

There is tremendous variability in the presentation of the neurobehavioral and neurocognitive features of children with FASD due to the timing and amount of PAE and unique characteristics of the birth mother and the child. Presentation can range from relatively mild developmental delays to severe intellectual disability, although approximately 75% of individuals with an FASD do not have intellectual disability. In infants, the symptoms can be nonspecific and may include irritability, poor

Table 126.2	Diagnostic Features of Fetal Alcohol Spectrum Disorders (FASDs)

TYPE OF FASD	FACIAL DYSMORPHOLOGY	GROWTH		DEFICIENT BRAIN GROWTH, ABNORMAL MORPHOGENESIS, OR ABNORMAL NEUROPHYSIOLOGY	NEUROBEHAVIORAL FEATURES	PRENATAL ALCOHOL EXPOSURE (PAE)*
Fetal alcohol syndrome (FAS)	≥2 of the following: Short palpebral fissures (≤10th centile) Thin vermilion border of upper lip Smooth philtrum	Height and/or weight ≤10th centile	OR	Head circumference ≤10th centile Structural brain anomalies Recurrent nonfebrile seizures	*With cognitive impairment:* Evidence of global impairment (general conceptual ability ≥1.5 SD below the mean *or* Cognitive deficit in at least 2 neurobehavioral domains ≥1.5 SD below the mean *With behavioral impairment without cognitive impairment:* Evidence of behavioral deficit in at least 2 domains ≥1.5 SD below the mean	Documented PAE not required
Partial FAS (pFAS)	≥2 of the following: Short palpebral fissures (≤10th centile) Thin vermilion border of upper lip Smooth philtrum	Height and/or weight ≤10th centile	OR	Head circumference ≤10th centile Structural brain anomalies Recurrent nonfebrile seizures	*With cognitive impairment:* Evidence of global impairment (general conceptual ability ≥1.5 SD below the mean *or* Cognitive deficit in at least 2 neurobehavioral domains ≥1.5 SD below the mean *With behavioral impairment without cognitive impairment:* Evidence of behavioral deficit in at least 2 domains ≥1.5 SD below the mean	If confirmed PAE, only need facial dysmorphology and neurobehavioral features
Alcohol-related neurodevelopmental disorder (ARND)	—	—		—	*With cognitive impairment:* Evidence of global impairment (general conceptual ability ≥1.5 SD below the mean *or* Cognitive deficit in at least 2 neurobehavioral domains ≥1.5 SD below the mean *With behavioral impairment without cognitive impairment:* Evidence of behavioral deficit in at least 2 domains ≥1.5 SD below the mean	Confirmed PAE required
Alcohol-related birth defect (ARBD)	—	—		One or more specific major malformations demonstrated in animal models and human studies to be the result of prenatal alcohol exposure	—	Confirmed PAE required

Continued

Table 126.2	Diagnostic Features of Fetal Alcohol Spectrum Disorders (FASDs)—cont'd				
TYPE OF FASD	FACIAL DYSMORPHOLOGY	GROWTH	DEFICIENT BRAIN GROWTH, ABNORMAL MORPHOGENESIS, OR ABNORMAL NEUROPHYSIOLOGY	NEUROBEHAVIORAL FEATURES	PRENATAL ALCOHOL EXPOSURE (PAE)*

Neurobehavioral disorder associated with prenatal alcohol exposure (ND-PAE)	—	—	—	Neurocognitive impairment (1)
				  Global intellect
				  Executive functioning
				  Learning
				  Memory
				  Visual-spatial reasoning
				Impaired self-regulation (1)
				  Mood or behavior
				  Attention
				  Impulse control
				Impairments in adaptive functioning (2)
				  Language
				  Social communication and interaction
				  Daily living skills
				  Motor skills
					If no characteristic dysmorphic facial features, confirmed PAE required.

*Documented prenatal alcohol exposure:
   ≥6 drinks/wk for ≥2 wk during pregnancy.
   ≥3 drinks per occasion on ≥2 occasions during pregnancy.
   Documentation of alcohol-related social or legal problems in proximity to (before or during) the index pregnancy (e.g., driving while intoxicated or history of treatment of an alcohol-related condition).
   Documentation of intoxication during pregnancy by blood, breath, or urine alcohol content testing.
   Increased prenatal risk associated with drinking during pregnancy as assessed by a validated screening tool.

feeding, sleep difficulties, a tendency to become easily overstimulated, or difficulty forming attachments with caregivers. Young children may demonstrate developmental delays, inattention, impulsivity, internalizing and externalizing problems, social impairments and difficulty with peers, and behavioral difficulties such as mood lability, frequent tantrums or aggression. The neurocognitive profile of children with an FASD that emerges in elementary or middle school includes challenges with processing speed, memory, visual-spatial reasoning, math, auditory comprehension, use of pragmatic language, and executive functioning skills. Learning strengths often include decoding, reading, and speech. In adolescents, difficulties with abstract reasoning, time and money management, and social and adaptive skills may become more pronounced.

The most common comorbid mental health condition seen in children with an FASD is attention-deficit/hyperactivity disorder (see Chapter 49), which occurs in >50% of children. Individuals with FASD may present with problems of self-regulation, impulse control, and adaptive functioning. Additional mental health disorders typically seen in children and adolescents with an FASD include oppositional defiant and conduct disorder, anxiety disorder, adjustment disorder, sleep disorder, mood disorders (e.g., depression, bipolar disorder), and disinhibited social engagement disorder. FASD may increase the severity or complexity of these conditions.

INTERVENTIONS AND TREATMENT

Given the heterogeneity of presenting problems associated with the FASDs, interventions need to be tailored to address each individual child or adolescent's profile of strengths and difficulties. Although the evidence base examining interventions for children and adolescents with an FASD is limited, with most studies having small sample sizes, there is emerging evidence for effective programs and treatments specifically designed for children with an FASD. Studies support that the most successful interventions begin early and continue across the life span, include a preventive focus, are intensive and individualized, address multiple domains of functioning, include parent education and training,

and are coordinated across systems of care. Children with an FASD often need support and intervention in the areas of learning, executive functioning, adaptive skills, social skills and peer relations, and mental health. To enhance generalizability of skills and to ensure they are encoded into memory, children with an FASD require consistent and predictable interventions, simplified directions, repeated instructions, and reduced distractions. Many children are treated with psychotropic medications, with stimulants most frequently prescribed. Children with an FASD are often treated with a higher number of drugs and at higher doses, likely because of atypical or less favorable responses.

OUTCOMES

Children with an FASD are at higher risk for **victimization and bullying**, often due to poor social judgment. Children and adolescents who are not identified early and aggressively treated are significantly more likely to have secondary disabilities, including encounters with juvenile justice and incarceration, substance abuse problems, severe mental health problems, sexual promiscuity and other inappropriate sexual behaviors, high rates of school failure, dropout and under- or unemployment, and health problems. Children and adolescents with an FASD have a 95% lifetime likelihood of having a mental health diagnosis and are at higher risk for **suicide**. Although an FASD cannot be cured, the long-term negative effects of the brain damage caused by PAE can be reduced through aggressive, sustained intervention initiated early. The estimated lifetime cost of caring for a child with FAS is $1.4 million, with average medical expenditures 9 times higher than expenses for children without FAS. These numbers increase significantly when the costs of caring for all children with any FASD are included.

THE PEDIATRICIAN'S ROLE

Pediatricians play an important role in identifying children and adolescents with an FASD, by asking parents about PAE and counseling mothers to abstain from alcohol consumption if they are planning to have additional children. Pediatricians need to screen all mothers for PAE and reduce the stigma associated with asking. They need to consider an FASD in a child who presents with complex neurodevelopmental and neurobehavioral problems, structural abnormalities, growth deficits, and facial dysmorphology. It is important that pediatricians remember that despite the increased risk in certain groups, FASDs occur across all economic, racial, and ethnic groups. Pediatricians need to document findings related to PAE and establish a **medical home** for the child with an FASD that includes a network of professionals who can help and support the child and family. The American Academy of Pediatrics has developed an FASD toolkit (www.aap.org/fasd) to assist primary care providers in identifying children with an FASD and managing their challenges in an effort to reduce the lifelong adverse consequences.

Bibliography is available at Expert Consult.

Chapter **127**
The Endocrine System
Nicole M. Sheanon and Louis J. Muglia

第一百二十七章
内分泌系统

中文导读

　　本章主要介绍新生儿期内分泌疾病，新生儿出生后体内的各种激素水平，既受母体激素水平的影响，也受自身内分泌组织器官功能的影响，新生儿的暂时性内分泌紊乱现象和永久性内分泌疾病，在新生儿出生后短期内可能具有同样的临床表现和实验室检查结果。本章介绍了生长激素缺乏侏儒症（垂体性侏儒症）、先天性甲状腺功能减退症、短暂性低甲状腺素血症、短暂性甲状旁腺功能减退症、高钙血症、急性肾上腺出血与肾上腺功能衰竭、先天性肾上腺皮质增生症、性发育障碍、短暂性新生儿糖尿病等这几种新生儿最常见的、与新生儿近期远期预后密切相关的内分泌系统疾病，并具体描述了糖尿病母亲婴儿的病理生理学、临床表现、治疗和预后。

Endocrine emergencies in the newborn period are uncommon, but prompt identification and proper treatment are vital to reduce morbidity and mortality.

Pituitary dwarfism (growth hormone deficiency) is not usually apparent at birth, although male infants with **panhypopituitarism** may have neonatal hypoglycemia, hyperbilirubinemia, and micropenis. Conversely, **primordial dwarfism** manifests as in utero growth failure that continues postnatally, with length and weight suggestive of prematurity when born after a normal gestational period; otherwise, physical appearance is normal.

Congenital hypothyroidism is one of the most common preventable causes of developmental disability. Congenital screening followed by thyroid hormone replacement treatment started within 30 days after birth can normalize cognitive development in children with congenital hypothyroidism. Congenital hypothyroidism occurs in approximately 1/2,000 infants worldwide (see Chapter 581). Because most infants with congenital hypothyroidism are asymptomatic at birth, all states screen for it. Even though screening is standard in many countries, millions of infants born throughout the world are not screened for congenital hypothyroidism. Thyroid deficiency may also be apparent at birth in genetically determined cretinism and infants of mothers with hyperthyroidism during pregnancy treated with antithyroid medications (PTU). Infants with trisomy 21 have a higher incidence of congenital hypothyroidism and should be screened in the newborn period. Constipation, prolonged jaundice, goiter, lethargy, umbilical hernia, macroglossia, hypotonia with delayed reflexes, mottled skin, or cold extremities should suggest severe chronic hypothyroidism. **Levothyroxine** is the treatment of choice, with the goal of rapid normalization of thyroid-stimulating hormone (TSH, thyrotropin) and free thyroxine (T_4) to achieve the best outcome. Thyroid hormone treatment is aimed to maintain total thyroxine or free thyroxine in the upper half of the normal range during the 1st 3 yr after birth. Early diagnosis and treatment of congenital thyroid hormone deficiency improve intellectual outcome and are facilitated by screening of all newborn infants for this deficiency. Newborn screening, with early referral to a pediatric endocrinologist for abnormal results, has improved early diagnosis and treatment of congenital hypothyroidism and improved intellectual outcome.

Transient hypothyroxinemia of prematurity is most common in ill and very premature infants. These infants have low thyroxine levels but normal levels of serum thyrotropin and other tests of the pituitary-hypothalamic axis indicating that they are probably chemically euthyroid. Trials of thyroid hormone replacement have reported no difference in developmental outcomes or other morbidities. Current practice is to follow thyroxine until levels normalize. **Transient hyperthyroidism** may occur at birth in infants of mothers with established or cured hyperthyroidism (e.g., Graves disease with positive TSH receptor–stimulating antibodies). See Chapter 584 for details on diagnosis and treatment.

Transient hypoparathyroidism may manifest as tetany or seizure of the newborn due to hypocalcemia and is associated with low levels of parathyroid hormone and hyperphosphatemia. Testing for DiGeorge syndrome should be considered. (see Chapter 589).

Subcutaneous fat necrosis can cause **hypercalcemia** and can occur after a traumatic birth. On examination, firm purple nodules can be appreciated on the trunk or extremities. An infant with hypercalcemia presents with irritability, vomiting, increased tone, poor weight gain, and constipation. Other causes of hypercalcemia in the newborn period are iatrogenic (excess calcium or vitamin D), maternal hypoparathyroidism, Williams syndrome, parathyroid hyperplasia, and idiopathic.

The adrenal glands are subject to numerous disturbances, which may become apparent and require lifesaving treatment during the neonatal period. Acute **adrenal hemorrhage** and adrenal failure are uncommon in the neonatal period. Risk factors include vaginal delivery, macrosomia, and fetal acidemia. The clinical presentation is often mild, with spontaneous regression. In neonates with bilateral adrenal hemorrhage, an evaluation of cortisol production is required (high-dose ACTH stimulation test), and, if insufficient, treatment with glucocorticoids and mineralocorticoids is indicated. Differentiation of unilateral adrenal hemorrhage from neuroblastoma is important. All patients should have sonographic and clinical follow-up to ensure resolution.

Congenital adrenal hyperplasia (CAH) is suggested by vomiting, diarrhea, dehydration, hyperkalemia, hyponatremia, shock, ambiguous genitalia, or clitoral enlargement. Some infants have ambiguous genitalia and hypertension. In an infant with ambiguous genitalia, both pelvic and adrenal ultrasound can be performed to aid in diagnosis. An adrenal ultrasound showing bilateral, enlarged, coiled or cerebriform pattern is specific for CAH. Diagnosis is confirmed with an elevated 17-hydroxyprogesterone level for gestational age. Because the condition is genetically determined, newborn siblings of patients with the salt-losing variety of adrenocortical hyperplasia should be closely observed for manifestations of adrenal insufficiency. Newborn screening and early diagnosis and therapy for this disorder may prevent severe salt wasting and adverse outcomes. Congenitally hypoplastic adrenal glands may also give rise to adrenal insufficiency during the 1st few wk of life (*DAX1* mutation).

Disorders of sexual development can present in the newborn period with ambiguous or atypical genitalia, including bilateral cryptorchidism, hypospadias, micropenis, hypoplastic scrotum, or clitoromegaly. More than 20 genes have been associated with disorders of sexual development. The initial management should involve a multidisciplinary team (endocrinology, urology, genetics, and neonatology) and open communication with the family. Sex assignment and naming of the infant should be delayed until appropriate testing is completed. For more about disorders of sexual development, see Chapter 606.

Female infants with webbing of the neck, lymphedema, hypoplasia of the nipples, cutis laxa, low hairline at the nape of the neck, low-set ears, high-arched palate, deformities of the nails, cubitus valgus, and other anomalies should be suspected of having **Turner syndrome**. Lymphedema of the hands or lower extremities can sometimes be the only indication. A karyotype can confirm diagnosis (see Chapter 604.1).

Transient neonatal diabetes mellitus (TNDM) is rare and typically presents on day 1 of life (see Chapter 607). It usually manifests as polyuria, dehydration, loss of weight, or acidosis in infants who are small for gestational age. The most common cause (70%) is a disruption of the imprinted locus at chromosome 6q24. A select group of patients with TNDM are at risk for recurrence of diabetes later in life.

Bibliography is available at Expert Consult.

127.1 Infants of Diabetic Mothers

Nicole M. Sheanon and Louis J. Muglia

Diabetes (type 1, type 2, or gestational) in pregnancy increases the risk of complications and adverse outcomes in the mother and the baby. Complications related to diabetes are milder in gestational vs pregestational (preexisting type 1 or type 2) diabetes. Pregnancy outcomes are correlated with onset, duration, and severity of maternal hyperglycemia. Prepregnancy planning and tight glycemic control (hemoglobin A_{1c} [HbA_{1c}] <6.5%) is crucial in **pregestational diabetes** in order to achieve the best outcomes for the mother and the baby. The risk of **diabetic embryopathy** (neural tube defects, cardiac defects, caudal regression syndrome) and spontaneous abortions is highest in those with pregestational diabetes who have poor control (HbA_{1c} >7%) in the first trimester. The risk of congenital malformations in **gestational diabetes** is only slightly increased compared to the general population, since the duration of diabetes is less and hyperglycemia occurs later in gestation (typically >25 wk).

Mothers with pregestational and gestational diabetes have a high incidence of complications during the pregnancy. Polyhydramnios, preeclampsia, preterm labor (induced and spontaneous), and chronic hypertension occur more frequently in mothers with diabetes. Accelerated fetal growth is also common, and 36–45% of **infants of diabetic mothers (IDMs)** are born large for gestational age (LGA). Restricted fetal growth is seen in mothers with pregestational diabetes and vascular disease, but it is less common. Fetal mortality rate is greater in both pregestational and gestational diabetic mothers than in nondiabetic mothers, but the rates have dropped precipitously over the years. Fetal loss throughout pregnancy is associated with poorly controlled maternal diabetes, especially **diabetic ketoacidosis**. The neonatal mortality rate of IDMs is >5 times that of infants of nondiabetic mothers and is higher at all gestational ages and in every birthweight for gestational age category. The rate is higher in women with pregestational diabetes, smoking, obesity, hypertension, and poor prenatal care.

PATHOPHYSIOLOGY

The probable pathogenic sequence is that maternal hyperglycemia causes fetal **hyperglycemia**, and the fetal pancreatic response leads to fetal **hyperinsulinemia**, or **hyperinsulinism**. It is important to recognize that while maternal glucose crosses the placenta, maternal and exogenous insulin dose not. Fetal hyperinsulinemia and hyperglycemia then cause increased hepatic glucose uptake and glycogen synthesis, accelerated lipogenesis, and augmented protein synthesis (Fig. 127.1). Related pathologic findings are hypertrophy and hyperplasia of the pancreatic β cells, increased weight of the placenta and infant organs (except the brain), myocardial hypertrophy, increased amount of cytoplasm in liver cells, and extramedullary hematopoiesis. Hyperinsulinism and hyperglycemia produce fetal acidosis, which may result in an increased rate of stillbirth. Separation of the placenta at birth suddenly interrupts glucose infusion into the neonate without a proportional effect on hyperinsulinism, leading to hypoglycemia during the 1st few hr after birth. The risk of rebound hypoglycemia can be diminished by tight blood glucose control during labor and delivery.

Hyperinsulinemia has been documented in infants of mothers with pregestational and gestational diabetes. The infants of mothers with *pregestational* diabetes have significantly higher fasting plasma insulin levels than normal newborns, despite similar glucose levels, and respond to glucose with an abnormally prompt elevation in plasma insulin. After arginine administration, they also have an enhanced insulin response and increased disappearance rates of glucose compared with normal infants. In contrast, fasting glucose production and utilization rates are diminished in infants of mothers with *gestational* diabetes. Although hyperinsulinism is probably the main cause of hypoglycemia, the diminished epinephrine and glucagon responses that occur may be contributing factors. Infants of mothers with pregestational and gestational diabetes are at risk for neonatal hypoglycemia in the 1st hours of life, with an increased risk in both large- and small-for-gestational-age infants. Aggressive screening and treatment is recommended as outlined later.

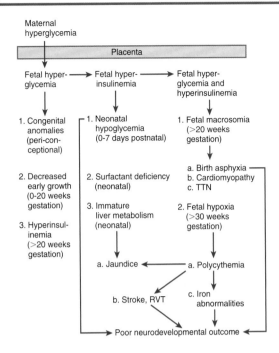

Maternal
hyperglycemia

Placenta

Fetal hyper-glycemia → Fetal hyper-insulinemia → Fetal hyper-glycemia and hyperinsulinemia

1. Congenital anomalies (peri-con-ceptional)

2. Decreased early growth (0-20 weeks gestation)

3. Hyperinsul-inemia (>20 weeks gestation)

1. Neonatal hypoglycemia (0-7 days postnatal)

2. Surfactant deficiency (neonatal)

3. Immature liver metabolism (neonatal)

a. Jaundice

1. Fetal macrosomia (>20 weeks gestation)

a. Birth asphyxia
b. Cardiomyopathy
c. TTN

2. Fetal hypoxia (>30 weeks gestation)

a. Polycythemia

b. Stroke, RVT

c. Iron abnormalities

Poor neurodevelopmental outcome

Fig. 127.1 The fetal and neonatal events attributable to fetal hyper-glycemia *(column 1)*, fetal hyperinsulinemia *(column 2)*, or both in synergy *(column 3)*. Time of risk is denoted in parentheses. RVT, Renal vein thrombosis; TTN, transient tachypnea of the newborn. *(From Nold JL, Georgieff MK: Infants of diabetic mothers, Pediatr Clin North Am 51:619–637, 2004.)*

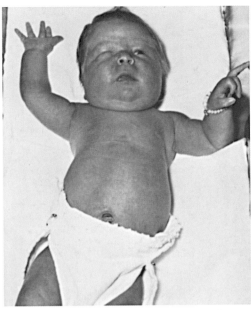

Fig. 127.2 Large, plump, plethoric infant of a mother with gestational diabetes. The baby was born at 38 wk of gestation but weighed 9 lb, 11 oz (4,408 g). Mild respiratory distress was the only symptom other than appearance.

Table 127.1	Morbidity in Infants of Diabetic Mothers

- Congenital anomalies
- Heart failure and septal hypertrophy of heart
- Surfactant deficiency, respiratory distress syndrome, transient tachypnea of the newborn, persistent pulmonary hypertension
- Hyperbilirubinemia
- Hypoglycemia, hypocalcemia, hypomagnesemia
- Macrosomia, nerve injury related to birth trauma
- Renal vein thrombosis
- Small left colon
- Unexplained intrauterine demise
- Polycythemia
- Visceromegaly
- Predisposition to later-life obesity, insulin resistance, and diabetes

From Devaskar SU, Garg M: Disorders of carbohydrate metabolism in the neonate. In Martin RJ, Fanaroff AA, Walsh MC, editors: *Fanaroff & Martin's neonatal-perinatal medicine*, ed 10, Philadelphia, 2015, Elsevier (Box 95-3).

CLINICAL MANIFESTATIONS

Infants of mothers with pregestational diabetes and those of mothers with gestational diabetes often bear a surprising resemblance to each other (Fig. 127.2). They tend to be large and plump as a result of increased body fat and enlarged viscera, with puffy, plethoric facies resembling that of patients who have been receiving corticosteroids. These infants may also be of normal birthweight if diabetes is well controlled; or low birthweight if they are delivered before term or if their mothers have associated diabetic vascular disease. Infants that are macrosomic or LGA are at high risk of birth trauma (brachial plexus injury) and birth asphyxia because of not only their large size but also their decreased ability to tolerate stress, especially if they have cardiomyopathy and other effects of fetal hyperinsulinemia (Table 127.1).

Hypoglycemia develops in approximately 25–50% of infants of mothers with pregestational diabetes and 15–25% of infants of mothers with gestational diabetes, but only a small percentage of these infants become symptomatic. The probability that hypoglycemia will develop in such infants increases with higher cord or maternal fasting blood glucose levels. The nadir in an infant's blood glucose concentration is usually reached between 1 and 3 hr of age. Hypoglycemia can persist for 72 hr and in rare cases last up to 7 days. Frequent feedings can be used to treat the hypoglycemia, but some infants require intravenous (IV) dextrose.

The infants tend to be jittery, tremulous, and hyperexcitable during the 1st 3 days after birth, although hypotonia, lethargy, and poor sucking may also occur. Early appearance of these signs is more likely to be related to hypoglycemia but can also be caused by hypocalcemia and hypomagnesemia, which also occur in the 1st 24-72 hr of life due to delayed response of the parathormone system. Perinatal asphyxia is associated with increased irritability and also increases the risk of hypoglycemia, hypomagnesemia, and hypocalcemia.

Tachypnea develops in many IDMs during the 1st 2 days after birth and may be a manifestation of hypoglycemia, hypothermia, polycythemia, cardiac failure, transient tachypnea, or cerebral edema from birth trauma or asphyxia. IDMs have a higher incidence of **respiratory distress syndrome** (RDS) than do infants of nondiabetic mothers born at comparable gestational age. The greater incidence is possibly related to an antagonistic effect of insulin on stimulation of surfactant synthesis by cortisol, leading to a delay in lung maturation. Polycythemia often occurs with RDS as they are both a result of fetal hyperinsulinism.

Cardiomegaly is common (30%), and heart failure occurs in 5-10% of IDMs. Interventricular septal hypertrophy may occur and may manifest as transient idiopathic hypertrophic subaortic stenosis. This is thought to result from chronic hyperglycemia and chronic hyperinsulinism leading to glycogen loading in the heart. Inotropic agents worsen the obstruction and are contraindicated. β-Adrenergic blockers have been shown to relieve the obstruction, but ultimately the condition resolves

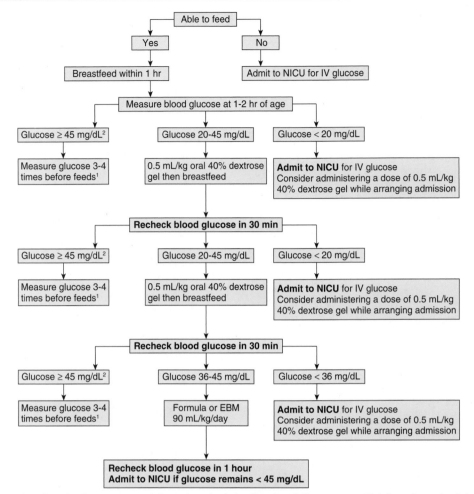

Fig. 127.3 Screening algorithm for *asymptomatic* hypoglycemia during first day of life among at-risk infants. Screening is indicated for late preterm infants, those who are small for gestational age/intrauterine growth restriction, and infants of obese or diabetic mothers.
[1]Continue monitoring blood glucose concentrations until 3 consecutive blood glucose concentrations have been ≥45-50 mg/dL.
[2]There is no consensus for a threshold definition for neonatal hypoglycemia in the first day of life. Nonetheless, if the blood glucose is less than 45-50 mg/dL **AND** symptoms compatible with hypoglycemia are present (see text), treatment must be initiated with an IV minibolus of 10% glucose at 200 mg/kg **followed** by a continuous IV infusion of glucose at a starting rate of 5-8 mg/kg/min.
IV, Intravenous; EBM, expressed breast milk. *(Modified from Newborn Services Clinical Guidelines for the Management of Hypoglycaemia http://www.adhb.govt.nz/newborn/Guidelines/Nutrition/HypoglycaemiaManagement.htm.)*

spontaneously over time.

Acute neurologic abnormalities (lethargy, irritability, poor feeding) can be seen immediately after birth and the cause elucidated by the timing of symptoms, as previously discussed (hypoglycemia, hypocalcemia, hypomagnesemia, or birth asphyxia). The symptoms will resolve with treatment of the underlying cause but may persist for weeks if caused by birth asphyxia. Neurologic development and ossification centers tend to be immature and to correlate with brain size (which is not increased) and gestational age rather than total body weight in infants of mothers with gestational and pregestational diabetes. In addition, IDMs have an increased incidence of hyperbilirubinemia, polycythemia, iron deficiency, and renal vein thrombosis. Renal vein thrombosis should be suspected in the infant with a flank mass, hematuria, and thrombocytopenia.

There is a 4-fold increase in **congenital anomalies** in infants of mothers with pregestational diabetes, and the risk varies with HbA_{1c} during the first trimester when organogenesis occurs. The recommended

goal for periconceptual HbA_{1c} is <6.5%. Although the risk of congenital malformations increases with increasing HbA_{1c} levels, there may still be an increased risk in the therapeutic goal range. Congenital anomalies of the central nervous system and cardiovascular system are most common, including failure of neural tube closure (encephalocele, meningomyelocele, and anencephaly), transposition of great vessels, ventricular septal defect (VSD), atrial septal defect (ASD), hypoplastic left heart, aortic stenosis, and coarctation of the aorta. Other, less common anomalies include caudal regression syndrome, intestinal atresia, renal agenesis, hydronephrosis, and cystic kidneys. **Small left colon syndrome** is a rare anomaly that develops in the second and third trimester because of rapid fluctuations in maternal and therefore fetal glucose, leading to impaired intestinal motility and subsequent intestinal growth. Prenatal ultrasound and a thorough newborn physical examination will identify most of these anomalies. High clinical suspicion and a good prenatal history will help identify needed screening for subtle anomalies.

TREATMENT

Preventive treatment of IDMs should be initiated before birth by means of preconception and frequent prenatal evaluations of all women with preexisting diabetes and pregnant women with gestational diabetes. This involves evaluation of fetal maturity, biophysical profile, Doppler velocimetry, and planning of the delivery of IDMs in hospitals where expert obstetric and pediatric care is continuously available. Preconception glucose control reduces the risk of anomalies and other adverse outcomes in women with pregestational diabetes, and glucose control during labor reduces the incidence of neonatal hypoglycemia. Women with type 1 diabetes who have tight glucose control during pregnancy (average daily glucose levels <95 mg/dL) deliver infants with birthweight and anthropomorphic features similar to those of infants of nondiabetic mothers. Treatment of gestational diabetes (diet, glucose monitoring, metformin, and insulin therapy as needed) decreases the rate of serious perinatal outcomes (death, shoulder dystocia, bone fracture, or nerve palsy). Women with gestational diabetes may also be treated successfully with **glyburide**, which may not cross the placenta. In these mothers, the incidence of macrosomia and neonatal hypoglycemia is similar to that in mothers with insulin-treated gestational diabetes. Women with diabetes can begin to express breast milk before the birth of the baby (≥36 wk gestational age); this will provide an immediate supply of milk to prevent hypoglycemia.

Regardless of size, IDMs should initially receive close observation and care (Fig. 127.3). Infants should initiate feedings within 1 hr after birth. A screening glucose test should be performed within 30 min of the first feed. Transient **hypoglycemia** is common during the 1st 1-3 hr after birth and may be part of normal adaptation to extrauterine life. The target plasma glucose concentration is ≥40 mg/dL before feeds in the 1st 48 hr of life. Clinicians need to assess the overall metabolic and physiologic status, considering these in the management of hypoglycemia. Treatment is indicated if the plasma glucose is <47 mg/dL. Feeding is the initial treatment for *asymptomatic* hypoglycemia. Oral or gavage feeding with breast milk or formula can be given. An alternative is prophylactic use of **dextrose** gel, although early feedings may be equally effective. Recurrent hypoglycemia can be treated with repeat feedings or IV glucose as needed. Infants with *persistent* (and unresponsive to oral therapy) glucose levels <25 mg/dL during the 1st 4 hr after birth and <35 mg/dL at 4-24 hr after birth should be treated with IV glucose, especially if symptomatic. A small bolus of 200 mg/kg of dextrose (2 mL/kg of 10% dextrose) should be administered to infants with plasma glucose below these limits. The small bolus should be followed by a continuous IV glucose infusion to avoid hypoglycemia. If question arises about an infant's ability to tolerate oral feeding, a continuous peripheral IV infusion at a rate of 4-8 mg/kg/min should be given. Neurologic symptoms of hypoglycemia *must* be treated with IV glucose. Bolus injections of hypertonic (25%) glucose should be avoided because they may cause further hyperinsulinemia and potentially produce rebound hypoglycemia (see Chapter 111). For treatment of hypocalcemia and hypomagnesemia, see Chapters 119.4 and 119.5; for RDS treatment, see Chapter 122.3; and for treatment of polycythemia, see Chapter 124.3.

PROGNOSIS

The subsequent incidence of diabetes mellitus in IDMs is higher than that in the general population because of genetic susceptibility in all types of diabetes. Infants of mothers with either pregestational diabetes or gestational diabetes are at risk for obesity and impaired glucose metabolism in later life as a result of intrauterine exposure to hyperglycemia. Disagreement persists about whether IDMs have a slightly increased risk of impaired intellectual development because of the many confounding factors (e.g., parental education, maternal age, neonatal complications). In general, the outcomes have improved over the last several decades due to increased awareness, screening, and improved prenatal care for pregnant women with diabetes.

Bibliography is available at Expert Consult.

Chapter **128**

Dysmorphology

Anne M. Slavotinek

第一百二十八章
外观畸形

中文导读

　　新生儿的结构性畸形对远期生存质量的影响可轻可重，一部分与遗传背景有关，一部分则与宫内感染有关，还有一部分原因不明。本章主要介绍了出生缺陷的分类、畸形的分子机制、识别畸形儿童的方法、本类疾病的发病率及流行病学。出生缺陷分类中分别介绍了畸形和发育不良、变形、破坏、畸形综合征及序列征。分子机制方面详细阐述了先天性基因编码错误、细胞遗传学异常与染色体不平衡两种机制。详细阐述了识别畸形儿童的途径，内容包括病史、体格检查、影像学检查、临床诊断、实验室和基因检测。

并对本类疾病的发病率和流行病学概况进行了介绍。

Dysmorphology is the study of differences in human form and the mechanisms that cause them. It has been estimated that 1 in 40 newborns, or 2.5%, have a recognizable birth defect or pattern of malformations at birth; approximately half these newborns have a single, isolated malformation, whereas in the other half, multiple malformations are present. From 20–30% of infant deaths and 30–50% of deaths after the neonatal period are caused by congenital abnormalities (http://www.marchofdimes.com/peristats/). In 2001, birth defects accounted for 1 in 5 infant deaths in the United States, with a rate of 137.6 deaths per 100,000 live births, which was higher than other causes of mortality, such as preterm/low birthweight (109.5/100,000), sudden infant death syndrome (55.5/100,000), maternal complications of pregnancy (37.3/100,000), and respiratory distress syndrome (25.3/100,000).

CLASSIFICATION OF BIRTH DEFECTS

Birth defects can be subdivided into isolated (single) defects or multiple congenital anomalies (multiple defects) in one individual. An isolated primary defect can be classified, according to the nature of the presumed cause of the defect, as a malformation, dysplasia, deformation, or disruption (Table 128.1 and Fig. 128.1). Most birth defects are malformations. A **malformation** is a structural defect arising from a localized error in morphogenesis that results in the abnormal formation of a tissue or organ. **Dysplasia** refers to the abnormal organization of cells into tissues. Malformations and dysplasias can both affect intrinsic structure. In contrast, a **deformation** is an alteration in shape or structure of a structure or organ that has developed, or differentiated, normally. A **disruption** is a defect resulting from the destruction of a structure that had formed

Table 128.1	Mechanisms, Terminology, and Definitions of Dysmorphology	
TERMINOLOGY	**DEFINITION**	**EXAMPLE**
Sequence	Single error in morphogenesis that results in a series of subsequent defects	Pierre-Robin sequence, in which a small jaw results in glossoptosis and cleft palate DiGeorge sequence of primary 4th brachial arch and 3rd and 4th pharyngeal pouch defects, leading to aplasia or hypoplasia of the thymus and parathyroid glands, aortic arch anomalies, and micrognathia
Deformation sequence	Mechanical (uterine) force that alters structure of intrinsically normal tissue	Oligohydramnios produces deformations by in utero compression of limbs (e.g., dislocated hips, equinovarus foot deformity), crumpled ears, or small thorax
Disruption sequence	In utero tissue destruction after a period of normal morphogenesis	Amnionic membrane rupture sequence, leading to amputation of fingers/toes, tissue fibrosis, and tissue bands
Dysplasia sequence	Atypical organization of cells into tissues or organs	Neurocutaneous melanosis sequence, with atypical migration of melanocyte precursor cells from the neural crest to the periphery, manifesting as melanocytic hamartomas of skin and meninges
Malformation syndrome	Appearance of multiple malformations in unrelated tissues that have a known, unifying cause	Trisomy 21 Teratogens Numerous multiple congenital anomaly syndromes as described above

From Kliegman RM, Greenbaum LA, Lye PS: *Practical strategies in pediatric diagnosis and therapy*, ed 2, Philadelphia, 2004, Elsevier Saunders.

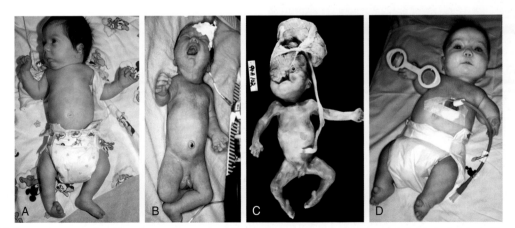

Fig. 128.1 Four major types of problems in morphogenesis: malformation, deformation, disruption, and dysplasia. **A,** Infant with camptomelic dysplasia syndrome, which results in a multiple malformation syndrome caused by a mutation in *SOX9*. **B,** Infant with oligohydramnios deformation sequence caused by premature rupture of membranes from 17 wk gestation until birth at 36 wk; the infant was delivered from persistent transverse lie. **C,** Fetus with early amnion rupture sequence with attachment of the placenta to the head and resultant disruption of craniofacial structures with distal limb contractures. **D,** Infant with diastrophic dysplasia caused by inherited autosomal recessive mutations in a sulfate transporter protein. *(From Graham Jr JM: Smith's recognizable patterns of human deformation, ed 3, Philadelphia, 2007, Saunders, Fig 1-1, p 4.)*

normally before the insult.

Most inherited human disorders with altered morphogenesis display multiple malformations rather than isolated birth defects. When several malformations coexist in a single individual, they can be classified as a syndrome, sequence, or an association. A **syndrome** is defined as a pattern of multiple abnormalities that are related by pathophysiology, resulting from a single, defined etiology. **Sequences** consist of multiple malformations that are caused by a single event, although the sequence itself can have different etiologies. An **association** refers to a nonrandom grouping of malformations in which there is an unclear, or unknown, relationship among the malformations, such that they do not fit the criteria for a syndrome or sequence.

Malformations and Dysplasias

Human malformations and dysplasias can be caused by gene mutations, chromosome aberrations and copy number variants, environmental factors, or interactions between genetic and environmental factors (Table 128.2). Some malformations are caused by deleterious sequence variants in single genes, whereas other malformations arise because of deleterious sequence variants in multiple genes acting in combination (*digenic* or *oligogenic* inheritance). In 1996 it was thought that malformations were caused by monogenic defects in 7.5% of patients; chromosomal anomalies in 6%; multigenic defects in 20%; and known environmental factors, such as maternal diseases, infections, and teratogens, in 6–7% (Table 128.3). In the remaining 60–70% of patients, malformations were classified as caused by unknown etiologies. Currently, the percentages have increased for all categories of known causes of malformations, the result of improved cytogenetic and molecular genetic methods for detecting small chromosomal abnormalities and next-generation sequencing studies that can screen multiple genes simultaneously and identify novel genes and deleterious sequence variants.

Many developmental abnormalities that are caused by deleterious sequence variants (mutations)in a single gene display characteristic, mendelian patterns of inheritance (autosomal dominant, autosomal recessive, and X-linked inheritance). Genes that cause birth defects or multiple congenital anomaly syndromes are often transcription factors, part of evolutionarily conserved signal transduction pathways, or regulatory proteins required for key developmental events (Figs. 128.2 and 128.3). Examples include spondylocostal dysostosis syndromes, Smith-Lemli-Opitz syndrome, Rubinstein-Taybi syndrome, and X-linked lissencephaly ("smooth brain") syndrome (see Table 128.2).

Patients with **spondylocostal dysostosis (SCD)** display a characteristic pattern of vertebral segmentation defects associated with a number of other malformations, such as neural tube defects. The **SCD syndromes** are etiologically heterogeneous and are often caused by mutations in

Table 128.2	Examples of Malformations with Distinct Causes, Clinical Features, and Pathogenesis		
DISORDER	**CAUSE/INHERITANCE**	**SELECTED CLINICAL FEATURES**	**PATHOGENESIS**
Spondylocostal dysostosis syndrome	Mendelian; autosomal recessive	Abnormal vertebral and rib segmentation	Deleterious sequence variants in *DLL3* and other genes
Rubinstein-Taybi syndrome	Autosomal dominant	Intellectual disability Broad thumbs and halluces; valgus deviation of these digits Hypoplastic maxillae Prominent nose and columella Congenital heart disease	Deleterious sequence variants in *CBP* and *EP300*
X-linked lissencephaly	X-linked	Male: severe intellectual disability, seizures Female: variable	Deleterious sequence variants in *DCX*
Aniridia	Autosomal dominant	Absent iris or iris/foveal hypoplasia	Deleterious sequence variants in *PAX6*
Waardenburg syndrome, type I	Autosomal dominant	Deafness White forelock Wide-spaced eyes Iris heterochromia and/or pale skin pigmentation	Deleterious sequence variants in *PAX3*
Holoprosencephaly	Loss of function or heterozygosity for multiple genes	Microcephaly Cyclopia Single central incisor	*SHH*, multiple other genes
Velocardiofacial syndrome	Microdeletion 22q11.2	Congenital heart disease, including conotruncal defects Cleft palate T-cell defects Facial anomalies	*TBX1* haploinsufficiency/mutations; haploinsufficiency for other genes in the deleted interval also contributes to the phenotype.
Down syndrome	Additional copy of chromosome 21 (trisomy 21)	Intellectual disability Characteristic dysmorphic features Congenital heart disease Increased risk of leukemia Alzheimer disease	Increase in dosage of an estimated 250 genes on chromosome 21
Neural tube defects	Multifactorial	Meningomyelocele	Defects in folate sensitive enzymes or folic acid uptake
Fetal alcohol syndrome	Teratogenic	Microcephaly Developmental delay Facial abnormalities Behavioral abnormalities	Ethanol toxicity to developing brain
Retinoic acid embryopathy	Teratogenic	Microtia Congenital heart disease	Isotretinoin effects on neural crest and branchial arch development

Table 128.3	Causes of Congenital Malformations

MONOGENIC
X-linked hydrocephalus
Achondroplasia
Ectodermal dysplasia
Apert syndrome
Treacher Collins syndrome

CHROMOSOMAL ABERRATIONS and COPY NUMBER VARIANTS
Trisomy 21, 18, 13
XO, XXY
Deletions 4p–, 5p–, 7q–, 13q–, 18p–, 18q–, 22q–
Prader-Willi syndrome (70% of affected patients have deletion of
    chromosome 15 q11.2-q13)

MATERNAL INFECTION
Intrauterine infections (e.g., herpes simplex virus, cytomegalovirus,
    varicella-zoster virus, rubella virus, Zika virus, toxoplasmosis)

MATERNAL ILLNESS
Diabetes mellitus
Phenylketonuria
Hyperthermia

UTERINE ENVIRONMENT
Deformation
Uterine pressure, oligohydramnios: clubfoot, torticollis, congenital
    hip dislocation, pulmonary hypoplasia, 7th nerve palsy
Disruption
Amniotic bands, congenital amputations, gastroschisis,
    porencephaly, intestinal atresia
Twinning

ENVIRONMENTAL AGENTS
Polychlorinated biphenyls
Herbicides
Mercury
Alcohol

MEDICATIONS
Thalidomide
Diethylstilbestrol
Phenytoin
Warfarin
Cytotoxic drugs
Paroxetine
Angiotensin-converting enzyme inhibitors
Isotretinoin (vitamin A)
D-Penicillamine
Valproic acid
Mycophenolate mofetil

UNKNOWN ETIOLOGIES
Neural tube defects, such as anencephaly and spina bifida
Cleft lip/palate
Pyloric stenosis

SPORADIC SEQUENCE COMPLEXES
VATER/VACTERL sequence (vertebral defects, anal atresia, cardiac
    defects, tracheoesophageal fistula with esophageal atresia, radial
    and renal anomalies)
Pierre Robin sequence

NUTRITIONAL
Neural tube defects due to low folic acid

From Behrman RE, Kliegman RM, editors: *Nelson's essentials of pediatrics*,
ed 4, Philadelphia, 2002, Saunders.

the gene coding for delta-like 3 (*DLL3*), a ligand of the Notch receptors. The Notch/delta pathway is conserved throughout evolution and regulates a number of developmental events. **Smith-Lemli-Opitz syndrome (SLOS)** results from mutations in the sterol delta-7-dehydrocholesterol reductase (*DHCR7*) gene, an enzyme critical for normal cholesterol biosynthesis. Patients with SLOS (see Fig. 128.2) display syndactyly (fusion of the fingers and toes), in particular affecting the 2nd and 3rd

toes; postaxial polydactyly (extra digits); anteverted (upturned) nose; ptosis; cryptorchidism; and holoprosencephaly (failure of separation of the 2 cerebral hemispheres). Many of the features in SLOS are shared with those arising from deleterious sequence variants in the *SHH* genes, and these mutations link cholesterol biosynthesis pathogenically to the sonic hedgehog (SHH) pathway, because SHH is posttranslationally modified by cholesterol (see Chapter 97). **Rubinstein-Taybi syndrome** (see Fig. 128.2) typically results from heterozygous, loss-of-function deleterious sequence variants in a gene coding for a broadly acting transcriptional coactivator called *CREB-binding protein* (CBP) and from deleterious sequence variants in the *EP300* gene. The CBP coactivator regulates the transcription of a number of genes, which is why patients with deleterious sequence variants in *CBP* have a pleiotropic phenotype that includes developmental delays and intellectual disability, broad and angulated thumbs and halluces (1st toes), and congenital heart disease. One of the transcription factors that binds to CBP is *GLI3*, a member of the SHH pathway (see Fig. 128.2). **X-linked lissencephaly** is a severe neuronal migration defect that causes a smooth brain with reduction or absence of gyri and sulci in males and that gives rise to a variable pattern of intellectual disability and seizures in females. X-linked lissencephaly is caused by deleterious sequence variants in *DCX*. The DCX protein regulates the activity of dynein motors that contribute to movement of the cell nucleus during neuronal migration.

Malformation syndromes can also be caused by chromosomal aberrations or copy number variants and teratogens (see Tables 128.2 and 128.3). **Down syndrome** typically results from an extra copy of an entire chromosome 21 or, less frequently, an extra copy of the Down syndrome critical region on chromosome 21. Chromosome 21 is a small chromosome that contains an estimated 250 genes, and thus individuals with Down syndrome typically have an increased dosage of the numerous genes encoded by this chromosome that causes their physical differences (see Chapter 98.2).

Neural tube defects (NTDs) are an example of a birth defect that displays multifactorial inheritance in most cases. NTDs and a number of other congenital malformations, such as cleft lip and palate, can recur in families, but inheritance for the majority of affected individuals does not occur in a straightforward, mendelian inheritance pattern, and in this situation, multiple genes and environmental factors together likely contribute to the pathogenesis (see Table 128.2). Many of the genes involved in NTDs are unknown, so one cannot predict with certainty the mode of inheritance or a precise recurrence risk in the individual case. Empirical recurrence risks can be provided on the basis of population studies and the presence of single or multiple family members with the same malformation. However, one important gene/environment interaction has been identified for NTDs (see Chapter 609.1). **Folic acid deficiency** is associated with NTDs and can result from a combination of dietary factors and increased utilization during pregnancy. A common variant in the gene for an enzyme in the folate recycling pathway, 5,10-methylene-tetrahydrofolate reductase (*MTHFR*), that makes this enzyme less stable, may also be important in folic acid status. Several teratogenic causes of birth defects have been described (see Tables 128.2 and 128.3). **Ethanol** causes a recognizable malformation syndrome that is variably called fetal alcohol syndrome (FAS), fetal alcohol spectrum disorder (FASD), or fetal alcohol effects (FAE) (see Chapter 126.3). Children who were exposed to ethanol during the pregnancy can display microcephaly, developmental delays, hyperactivity, and facial dysmorphic features. Ethanol, which is toxic to the developing central nervous system (CNS), causes cell death in developing neurons.

Deformations

Many deformations involve the musculoskeletal system (Fig. 128.4). Fetal movement is required for the proper development of the musculoskeletal system, and restriction of fetal movement can cause musculoskeletal deformations such as clubfoot (talipes). Two major intrinsic causes of deformations are primary neuromuscular disorders and **oligohydramnios**, or decreased amniotic fluid, which can be caused by fetal renal defects. The major extrinsic causes of deformation are those that result in fetal crowding and restriction of fetal movement. Examples of extrinsic causes include oligohydramnios resulting from

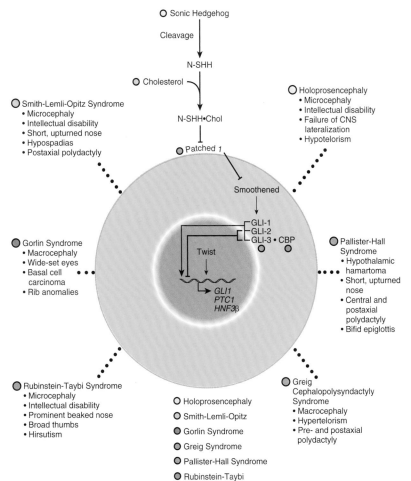

Fig. 128.2 Deleterious sequence variants in genes that function together in a developmental pathway typically have overlapping clinical manifestations. Several components of the sonic hedgehog (SHH) pathway have been identified, and their relationships elucidated (see text for further details). Mutations in several members of this pathway result in phenotypes with facial dysmorphism, as seen in holoprosencephaly, Smith-Lemli-Opitz syndrome, Gorlin syndrome, Greig cephalopolysyndactyly syndrome, Pallister-Hall syndrome, and Rubinstein-Taybi syndrome. CNS, Central nervous system.

chronic leakage of amniotic fluid and abnormal shape of the amniotic cavity. When a fetus is in the breech position (Fig. 128.5), the incidence of deformations is increased 10-fold. The shape of the amniotic cavity also has a profound effect on the shape of the fetus and is influenced by many factors, including uterine shape, volume of amniotic fluid, and the size and shape of the fetus (Fig. 128.6).

It is important to determine whether deformations result from intrinsic or extrinsic causes. Most children with deformations from *extrinsic* causes are otherwise completely normal, and their prognosis is usually excellent. Correction typically occurs spontaneously. Deformations caused by *intrinsic* factors, such as multiple joint contractures resulting from CNS or peripheral nervous system defects, have a different prognosis and may be much more significant for the child (Fig. 128.7).

Disruptions

Disruptions are caused by destruction of a previously normally formed organ or body part. At least 2 mechanisms are known to produce disruptions. One involves entanglement, followed by tearing apart or amputation, of a normally developed structure, usually a digit or limb, by strands of amnion floating within amniotic fluid (amniotic bands) (Fig. 128.8). The other mechanism involves interruption to the blood supply to a developing part, which can lead to infarction, necrosis, and resorption of structures distal to the insult. If interruption to the blood supply occurs early in gestation, the disruptive defect typically involves **atresia,** or absence of a body part. Genetic factors were previously considered to play a minor role in the pathogenesis of disruptions; most occur as sporadic events in otherwise healthy individuals. The prognosis for a

disruptive defect is determined entirely by the extent and location of the tissue loss.

Multiple Anomalies: Syndromes and Sequences

The pattern of multiple anomalies that occurs when a single primary defect in early development produces multiple abnormalities because of a cascade of secondary and tertiary developmental anomalies is called a *sequence* (see Fig. 128.9). When evaluating a child with multiple congenital anomalies, the physician must differentiate between multiple anomalies that are caused by a single localized error in morphogenesis (a sequence) from syndromes with multiple malformations. In the former, recurrence risk counseling for the multiple anomalies depends entirely on the risk of recurrence for the single, localized malformation. **Pierre-Robin sequence** is a pattern of multiple anomalies produced by mandibular hypoplasia. Because the tongue is relatively large for the oral cavity, it drops back (glossoptosis), blocking closure of the posterior palatal shelves and causing a U-shaped cleft palate. There are numerous causes of mandibular hypoplasia, all of which can result in characteristic features of Pierre-Robin sequence.

MOLECULAR MECHANISMS OF MALFORMATIONS
Inborn Errors of Development

Genes that cause malformation syndromes (as well as genes whose expression is disrupted by environmental agents or teratogens) can be part of numerous cellular processes, including evolutionarily conserved signal transduction pathways, transcription factors, or regulatory proteins required for key developmental events. When malformations are

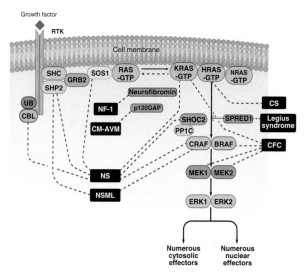

Fig. 128.3 The RAS/MAPK signal transduction pathway. The MAPK signaling pathway of protein kinases is critically involved in cellular proliferation, differentiation, motility, apoptosis, and senescence. The RASopathies are medical genetic syndromes caused by mutations in genes that encode components or regulators of the Ras/MAPK pathway (indicated by *dashed lines*). These disorders include neurofibromatosis type 1 (NF1), Noonan syndrome (NS), Noonan syndrome with multiple lentigines (NSML), capillary malformation–arteriovenous malformation syndrome (CM-AVM), Costello syndrome (CS), cardiofaciocutaneous syndrome (CFC), and Legius syndrome. RAS/MAPK, RAS protein family/mitogen-activated protein kinase. *(From Rauen KA: The RASopathies, Annu Rev Genom Hum Genet 14:355–369, 2013.)*

considered as alterations resulting from disturbances to important developmental pathways, this provides a molecular framework for understanding the birth defects.

Sonic Hedgehog Pathway As Model

The SHH pathway is developmentally important during embryogenesis to induce controlled proliferation in a tissue-specific manner; disruption of specific steps in this pathway results in a variety of related developmental disorders and malformations (see Fig. 128.2). Activation of this pathway in the adult leads to abnormal proliferation and cancer. The SHH pathway transduces an external signal, in the form of a *ligand*, into changes in gene transcription by binding of the ligand to specific cellular receptors. SHH is a ligand expressed in the embryo in regions important for development of the brain, face, limbs, and the gut.

Deleterious sequence variants in *SHH* can cause **holoprosencephaly** (see Fig. 128.2), a variably severe, midline defect associated with clinical effects ranging from cyclopia to a single maxillary incisor with hypotelorism or close spacing of the ocular orbits. The SHH protein is processed by proteolytic cleavage to an active N-terminal form, which is then further modified by the addition of cholesterol. Defects in cholesterol biosynthesis, in particular the sterol, delta-7-dehydrocholesterol reductase gene, result in **SLOS**, which is also associated with holoprosencephaly. The modified and active form of SHH binds to its transmembrane receptor Patched (PTCH1). SHH binding to PTCH1 inhibits the activity of the transmembrane protein Smoothened (SMO). SMO act to suppress downstream targets of the SHH pathway, the GLI family of transcription factors, so inhibition of SMO by PTCH1 results in activation of GLI1, GLI2, and GLI3, resulting in alteration of transcription of GLI targets. *PTCH1* and its orthologue, *PTCH2*, can act as tumor suppressors, and somatic, inactivating sequence variants can be associated with loss of tumor suppressor function, whereas activating mutations in *SMO* can also be oncogenic, particularly in basal cell carcinomas and medulloblastomas. Germline, inactivating mutations in *PTCH1* result in **Gorlin syndrome** (see Fig. 128.4), an

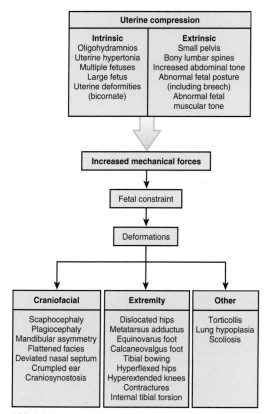

Fig. 128.4 Deformation abnormalities resulting from uterine compression. *(From Kliegman RM, Jenson HB, Marcdante KJ, et al, editors: Nelson essentials of pediatrics, ed 5, Philadelphia, 2005, Saunders.)*

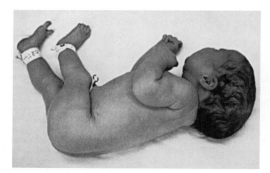

Fig. 128.5 Breech deformation sequence.

autosomal dominant disorder characterized by dysmorphic features (broad face, dental anomalies, rib defects, short metacarpals), basal cell nevi that can undergo malignant transformation, and an increased risk of cancers, including medulloblastomas and rhabdomyosarcomas. *GLI1* amplification has been found in several human tumors, including glioblastoma, osteosarcoma, rhabdomyosarcoma, and B cell lymphomas; mutations or alterations in *GLI3* have been found in **Greig cephalopolysyndactyly syndrome** (GCPS), **Pallister-Hall syndrome** (PHS), postaxial polydactyly type A (and A/B), and preaxial polydactyly type IV (see Fig. 128.2). GCPS consists of hypertelorism (wide-spaced eyes), syndactyly, preaxial polydactyly, and broad thumbs and halluces. PHS is an autosomal dominant disorder characterized by postaxial polydactyly, syndactyly, hypothalamic hamartomas, imperforate anus, and occasionally

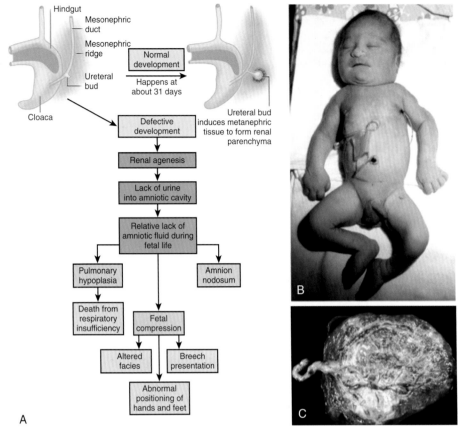

Fig. 128.6 **A,** Consequences of renal agenesis. **B,** Multiple deformational defects. **C,** Defects in amnion nodosum; brown-yellow granules from vernix have been ribbed into defects of the amniotic surface. *(From Jones KL, Jones MC, Del Campo M, editors: Smith's recognizable patterns of human malformation, ed 7, Philadelphia, 2013, Elsevier, p 821.)*

holoprosencephaly. GLI3 binds to CBP, the protein that is haploinsufficient in **Rubinstein-Taybi syndrome**.

Disorders that are caused by mutations in genes that function together in a developmental pathway typically have overlapping clinical manifestations. In this case, the overlapping features result from the expression domains of SHH that are important for development of the brain, face, limbs, and gut. Brain defects are found in holoprosencephaly (Fig. 128.9), SLOS, and PHS. Facial abnormalities are found in holoprosencephaly, SLOS, Gorlin syndrome, GCPS, and PHS. Limb defects are found in SLOS, Gorlin syndrome, GCPS, PHS, and the polydactyly syndromes. Overexpression, or activating mutations, affecting the SHH pathway results in cancer, including basal cell carcinomas, medulloblastomas, glioblastomas, and rhabdomyosarcomas.

The SHH pathway interaction with the primary cilium is critical to transduce the SHH extracellular signal through to the nuclear machinery. A number of disorders, including Bardet-Biedl syndrome, oral-facial-digital (OFD) syndrome type I, and Joubert syndrome, are caused by mutations in genes that function in the primary cilium. These disorders, called **ciliopathies**, overlap clinically with some of the phenotypic features described previously, again demonstrating that perturbations of conserved developmental pathways can cause overlapping presentations (Table 128.4).

Cytogenetic Aberrations and Chromosomal Imbalance

Cytogenetic imbalances resulting from an additional copy of a whole human chromosome can result in characteristic and recognizable syndromes. An additional copy of chromosome 21 results in **Down syndrome** (see Chapter 98.2); loss of one of the X chromosomes results in **Turner syndrome** (see Chapter 98 for discussion of syndromes with whole chromosomal imbalances). With the advent of high-resolution cytogenetic techniques, such as fluorescence in situ hybridization (FISH), array comparative genomic hybridization (array CGH), and single nucleotide polymorphism (SNP) arrays, it has become possible to identify **submicroscopic chromosome deletions and duplications**. A number of recurrent deletions and duplications have been identified that cause characteristic and recognizable syndromes, including **Williams syndrome** (deletion of chromosome 7q11.23), **Miller-Dieker syndrome** (deletion of chromosome 17p13.3), **Smith-Magenis syndrome** (deletion of chromosome 17p11.2), and 22q11 deletion syndrome (deletion of chromosome 22q11.2, also known as **velocardiofacial/DiGeorge syndrome**). Array CGH and SNP arrays have also made it possible to uncover rarer microdeletions and microduplications associated with birth defects, intellectual disability, and neuropsychiatric disorders. The sensitivity and specificity chromosome microarrays have made this the technique of choice for the initial evaluation of a child with multiple congenital anomalies and/or intellectual disability, although it is important to note that all individuals may carry numerous small microdeletions and microduplications as normal or familial variation. Therefore, it is important to compare copy number variants in these children with birth defects with their parents' chromosome analyses and with databases of normal variants detected in individuals without such birth defects.

APPROACH TO THE DYSMORPHIC CHILD

One approach to the dysmorphic child is the *pattern recognition* approach, which compares the manifestations in the patient against a broad and

Table 128.4	Childhood Diseases and Syndromes Associated with Motile and Sensory Ciliopathies	
PEDIATRIC CILIOPATHY	**CLINICAL MANIFESTATIONS**	**SELECTED GENE(S)**
MOTOR		
Primary ciliary dyskinesia	Chronic bronchitis, rhinosinusitis, otitis media, laterality defects, infertility, CHD	*DNAI1, DNAH5, DNAH11, DNAI2, KTU, TXNDC3, LRRC50, RSPH9, RSPH4A, CCDC40, CCDC39*
SENSORY		
Autosomal recessive polycystic kidney disease	RFD, CHF	*PKHD1*
Nephronophthisis	RFD, interstitial nephritis, CHF, RP	*NPHP1-8, ALMS1, CEP290*
Bardet-Biedl syndrome	Obesity, polydactyly, ID, RP, renal anomalies, anosmia, CHD	*BBS1-12, MKS1, MKS3, CEP290*
Meckel-Gruber syndrome	RFD, polydactyly, ID, CNS anomalies, CHD, cleft lip, cleft palate	*MKS1-6, CC2D2A, CEP290, TMEM216*
Joubert syndrome	CNS anomalies, ID, ataxia, RP, polydactyly, cleft lip, cleft palate	*NPHP1, JBTS1, JBTS3, JBTS4, CORS2, AHI1, CEP290, TMEM216*
Alstrom syndrome	Obesity, RP, DM, hypothyroidism, hypogonadism, skeletal dysplasia, cardiomyopathy, pulmonary fibrosis	*ALMS1*
Orofaciodigital syndrome type I	Polydactyly, syndactyly, cleft lip, cleft palate, CNS anomalies, ID, RFD	*OFD1*
Ellis van Creveld syndrome	Chondrodystrophy, polydactyly, ectodermal dysplasia, CHD	*EVC, EVC2*
Jeune asphyxiating thoracic dystrophy	Narrow thorax, RFD, RP, dwarfism, polydactyly	*IFT80*
Sensenbrenner syndrome	Dolichocephaly, ectodermal dysplasia, dental dysplasia, narrow thorax, RFD, CHD	*IFT122, IFT43, WDR35*
Short rib–polydactyly syndromes	Narrow thorax, short limb dwarfism, polydactyly, renal dysplasia	*WDR35, DYNC2H1, NEK1*

CHD, Congenital heart disease; CHF, congenital hepatic fibrosis; CNS, central nervous system; DM, diabetes mellitus; ID, intellectual disabilities; RFD, renal fibrocystic disease; RP, retinitis pigmentosa.
From Ferkol TW, Leigh MW: Ciliopathies: the central role of cilia in a spectrum of pediatric disorders, *J Pediatr* 160:366–371, 2012.

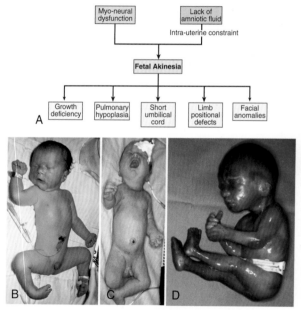

Fig. 128.7 **A,** Diagram demonstrates the etiologically heterogeneous phenotype that results from fetal akinesia. **B,** Infant born with myotonic dystrophy to a mother with the same condition. He had multiple joint contractures with thin bones and respiratory insufficiency. **C,** Infant immobilized in a transverse lie after amnion rupture at 26 wk. **D,** Fetus with bilateral renal agenesis resulting in oligohydramnios. *(From Graham JL. Smith's recognizable patterns of human malformation, ed 3, Philadelphia, 2007, Elsevier, Fig 47-2.)*

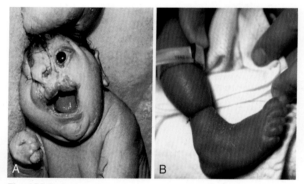

Fig. 128.8 **A,** Amniotic band disruption sequence. **B,** Bands constricting the ankle leading to deformational defects and amputations. *(From Jones KJ: Smith's recognizable patterns of human malformation, ed 6, Philadelphia, 2006, Saunders.)*

memorized (or computerized) knowledge of human pleiotropic disorders. Although this approach can be appropriate for a small number of experienced dysmorphologists, a systematic *genetic mechanism* approach can also be effective for clinicians who are not dysmorphology experts. By gathering and analyzing the clinical data, the general pediatrician can diagnose the patient in a straightforward case or initiate a referral to an appropriate specialist.

Medical History

The history for a patient with birth defects includes a number of elements related to etiologic factors. The *pedigree* or family history is necessary to assess the inheritance pattern, or lack thereof, for the disorder. For disorders that have a simple mendelian inheritance pattern, its recognition can be critical for narrowing the differential diagnosis, then prioritizing common genes with the appropriate inheritance pattern causing the patient's clinical features. A number of common birth defects have a complex or multifactorial genetic etiology, such as isolated cleft palate and spina bifida. The recognition of a close relative affected with a birth defect that is similar to that in the proband can be useful. Typically, a 3-generation pedigree is sufficient for this purpose (see Chapter 97).

The perinatal history is also an essential component of the history. It includes the pregnancy history of the mother (useful for recognition of recurrent miscarriages that may be indicative of a chromosomal disorder), factors that may relate to deformations or disruptions (oligohydramnios),

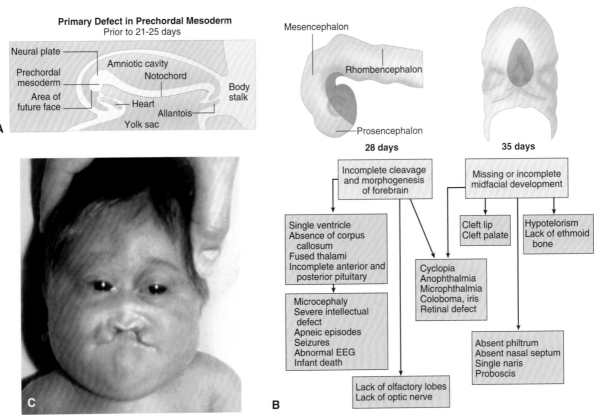

Fig. 128.9 Holoprosencephaly sequence. **A,** Schematic longitudinal section of 21-day embryo. **B,** Developmental pathogenesis of the sequence. **C,** Affected individual. (From Jones KL, Jones MC, Del Campo M, editors: Smith's recognizable patterns of human malformation, ed 7, Philadelphia, 2013 Elsevier, pp 802–803.)

and maternal exposures to teratogenic drugs or chemicals (isotretinoin and ethanol are potential causes of microcephaly).

Another component of the history that is often useful is the natural history of the **phenotype**. Malformation syndromes caused by chromosomal aberrations and single-gene disorders are frequently *static*, meaning that, although the patients can experience new complications over time, the phenotype is typically not progressive. In contrast, disorders that cause dysmorphic features because of metabolic perturbations (e.g., Hunter or Sanfilippo syndrome) can be mild or may not be apparent at birth, but they can progress relentlessly, causing deterioration of patient status over time.

Physical Examination

The physical examination is very important for the diagnosis of a dysmorphic syndrome. The essential element of the physical evaluation is an objective assessment of the patient's clinical findings. The clinician needs to perform an organized evaluation of the size and formation of various body structures. Familiarity with the nomenclature of dysmorphic signs is helpful (Table 128.5). The size and shape of the head is relevant; for example, many children with Down syndrome have mild microcephaly and brachycephaly (shortened anteroposterior dimension of skull). Eye position and shape are useful signs for many disorders. Reference standards are available with which physical measurements (e.g., interpupillary distance) can also be compared. It is also useful to categorize abnormalities as "major" or "minor" birth defects. Major defects either cause significant dysfunction (e.g., absence of a digit) or require surgical correction (e.g., polydactyly), and minor defects neither cause significant dysfunction nor require surgical correction (e.g., mild clinodactyly) (Table 128.6 and Fig. 128.10). By cataloging physical parameters, the clinician may be able to recognize the diagnosis.

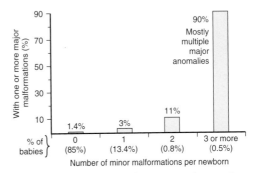

Fig. 128.10 Frequency of major malformations in relation to the number of minor anomalies detected in a given newborn baby. (From Jones KJ: Smith's recognizable patterns of human malformation, ed 6, Philadelphia, 2006, Saunders.)

Imaging Studies

Imaging studies can be critical in diagnosing an underlying genetic etiology. If short stature or disproportionate stature (e.g., long trunk and short limbs) is noted, a full skeletal survey with radiographs should be performed. The skeletal survey can detect anomalies in bone number or structure that can be used to narrow the differential diagnosis. When there are abnormal neurologic signs or symptoms, such as microcephaly or hypotonia, brain imaging can be indicated. Other studies, such as echocardiography and renal ultrasonography, can also be useful to identify additional major or minor malformations that may serve as diagnostic clues.

Table 128.5	Definitions of Common Clinical Signs of Dysmorphic Syndromes
SIGN	**DEFINITION**
Brachycephaly	A condition in which head shape is shortened from front to back along the sagittal plane; typically the back of the skull (occiput) and face are flatter than normal.
Brachydactyly	Short digits.
Brushfield spots	Speckled white spots or rings about two thirds of the distance to the periphery of the iris of the eye.
Camptodactyly	Permanent flexion of 1 or more fingers that can be associated with missing interphalangeal crease.
Clinodactyly	A medial or lateral curving of the fingers or toes; usually refers to incurving of the 5th finger.
Hypoplastic or small nail	A small nail on a digit.
Low-set ears	This designation is made when the helix meets the cranium at a level below a horizontal plane that is an extension of a line through both inner canthi.
Melia	A suffix meaning "limb" (e.g., amelia—missing limb; brachymelia—short limb).
Ocular hypertelorism or wide-set eyes	Increased distance between the center of the pupils of the 2 eyes; also known as *increased interpupillary distance* (IPD).
Plagiocephaly	A condition in which head shape is asymmetric in the sagittal or coronal plane; can result from asymmetry in cranial suture closure, asymmetry of brain growth, or deformation of the skull.
Posterior hair whorl	A single hair whorl occurs to the right or left of midline and is within 2 cm anterior to the posterior fontanel in 95% of cases.
Postaxial polydactyly	Extra finger or toe present on the lateral side of the hand or foot.
Preaxial polydactyly	Extra finger or toe present on the medial side of the hand or foot.
Prominent lateral palatine ridges	Relative overgrowth of the lateral palatine ridges that can be caused by a deficit of tongue thrust into the hard palate.
Scaphocephaly	A condition in which the head is elongated from front to back in the sagittal plane; most normal skulls are scaphocephalic; also termed *dolichocephaly*.
Shawl scrotum	The scrotal skin joins around the superior aspect of the penis and represents a mild deficit in full migration of the labial-scrotal folds.
Short palpebral fissures	Decreased horizontal distance of the eyelid folds based on measurements from the inner canthus to the outer canthus.
Syndactyly	Incomplete separation of the fingers or toes. It most commonly occurs between the 3rd and 4th fingers and between the 2nd and 3rd toes.
Synophrys	Eyebrows that meet in the midline.
Telecanthus	Lateral displacement of the inner canthi. The inner canthal distance (ICD) is increased, but the interpupillary distance (IPD) is normal.
Widow's peak	**V**-shaped midline, downward projection of the scalp hair in the frontal region. It represents an upper forehead intersection of the bilateral fields of periocular hair growth suppression. It usually occurs because the fields are widely spaced, as in ocular hypertelorism.

Diagnosis

The examining physician should gather data on the patient's pedigree and perinatal and pediatric (for older children) history and should have an appreciation for the natural history of the clinical findings. At this point, the physician has examined the child, identified atypical physical features, and obtained appropriate imaging studies.

The clinician should now attempt to organize the findings to elucidate potential developmental processes. An assessment based on **specificity** can be helpful for this process. If a child has multiple findings, such as a patent ductus arteriosus (PDA), mild growth restriction, mild microcephaly, and holoprosencephaly, micropenis, and ptosis, a selection of the rarer or pathognomonic findings may be prioritized. The PDA, ptosis, mild growth restriction, and mild microcephaly are considered to be largely *nonspecific findings* (present in many disorders or often present as isolated features that are not part of a syndrome), whereas holoprosencephaly and micropenis are present in fewer syndromes and are not considered part of normal variation. The clinician can therefore search for disorders that include both holoprosencephaly and micropenis. The search can be performed manually using the features index of a textbook such as *Smith's Recognizable Patterns of Human Malformation*

or a computerized database such as Online Mendelian Inheritance in Man (OMIM). Searching for both holoprosencephaly and micropenis returns a list of diagnostic possibilities, and the physician can then return to the patient to examine for additional features of the leading possible candidate disorders. Appropriate genetic testing can then be undertaken to confirm the clinician's hypothesis and verify the diagnosis.

Laboratory Studies and Genetic Testing

The laboratory evaluation of the dysmorphic child can be critical to reach or confirm the correct diagnosis. Cytogenetic studies with Giemsa-banded (G-banded) chromosome analysis, or karyotyping, was the gold standard previously performed in the evaluation of a dysmorphic patient. Array CGH and SNP arrays enable copy number variant detection and, in the case of SNP arrays, evaluation of loss of heterozygosity. Chromosome deletion syndromes may also be identified with specific and sensitive FISH analysis (Table 128.7). These tests are the most sensitive methods for the detection of cytogenetic alterations associated with birth defects and multiple congenital anomalies.

Molecular testing for deleterious sequence variants that cause pleiotropic malformation syndromes is also available for many disorders

Table 128.6	Minor Anomalies and Phenotype Variants*

CRANIOFACIAL
Large anterior fontanel
Flat or low nasal bridge
Anteverted (upturned) nose
Mild micrognathia
Cutis aplasia of scalp

EYE
Epicanthus
Telecanthus
Slanting of the palpebral fissures
Hypertelorism (widely spaced eyes)
Brushfield spots

EAR
Lack of helical folds
Posteriorly rotated pinna
Small pinnae
Auricular or preauricular pit
Atypical folding of helices
Crushed (crumpled) ear
Asymmetric ear sizes
Low-set ears

SKIN
Skin dimpling over bones
Capillary hemangioma (face, posterior neck)
Dermal melanosis (African Americans, Asians)
Sacral dimple
Pigmented nevi
Redundant skin
Cutis marmorata

HAND
Single palmar creases
Bridged palmar creases
Clinodactyly of 5th digits
Hyperextensibility of thumbs
Mild partial cutaneous syndactyly
Polydactyly
Short, broad thumb
Narrow, hyperconvex nails
Small nails
Camptodactyly
Shortened 4th digit

FOOT
Partial syndactyly of 2nd and 3rd toes
Asymmetric toe length
Clinodactyly of 2nd toe
Overlapping toes
Small nails
Wide gap between hallux and 2nd toe (wide sandal gap)
Deep plantar crease between hallux and 2nd toe

OTHER
Hydrocele
Shawl scrotum
Hypospadias
Hypoplasia of labia majora

*Approximately 15% of newborns have 1 minor anomaly, 0.8% have 2 minor anomalies, and 0.5% have 3. If 2 minor anomalies are present, the probability of an underlying syndrome or a major anomaly (congenital heart disease, renal, central nervous system, limbic) is 5-fold that in the general population. If 3 minor anomalies are present, there is a 20–30% probability of a major anomaly.
From Kliegman RM, Greenbaum LA, Lye PS: *Practical strategies in pediatric diagnosis and therapy*, ed 2, Philadelphia, 2004, Elsevier Saunders.

Table 128.7	Chromosomal Deletion Syndromes	
CONDITION	**BRIEF DESCRIPTION**	**PROBE**
Williams syndrome	Proportionate short stature, mild-moderate to severe intellectual disability, "cocktail patter" for conversation, stellate pattern of iris pigmentation, supravalvular aortic stenosis, recessed nasal bridge, and wide mouth with full lips	7q11
WAGR syndrome	Wilms tumor, aniridia, growth delay, intellectual disability, and genitourinary anomalies	11p13
Prader-Willi syndrome Angelman syndrome	Distinct syndromes with common or overlapping areas of deletion; phenotype depends on gender of the parent of origin of the deletion. Prader-Willi syndrome: hypotonia in infancy, short stature, obesity, mild-moderate and occasionally severe intellectual disability, small hands and feet (caused by paternal deletion of 15q11-13 or maternal uniparental disomy for chromosome 15) Angelman syndrome: severe intellectual disability, absence of speech, ataxia, tremulous movements, large mouth, frequent drooling (caused by maternal deletion of chromosome 15q11-13 or paternal uniparental disomy)	15q11
Smith-Magenis syndrome	Brachycephaly, prognathism, self-destructive behavior, wrist biting, pulling out nails, head banging, indifference to pain, severe intellectual disability, hyperactivity, social behavior problems	17p11.2
Miller-Dieker syndrome	Microcephaly, narrow temples, hypotonia/hypertonia, abnormal posturing, seizures, severe to profound intellectual disability, poor growth, lissencephaly and other brain abnormalities on CT or MRI	17p13
Velocardiofacial (VCF) syndrome (overlaps with DiGeorge syndrome)	VCF: cleft palate, congenital heart disease, learning/behavior problems, long face, prominent nose, limb hypotonia, slender hands with tapering fingers DiGeorge syndrome: T-cell deficiency, immunoglobulin deficiency	22q11

CT, Computed tomography; MRI, magnetic resonance imaging; WAGR, Wilms tumor, aniridia, genitourinary anomalies, and mental retardation.
From Kliegman RM, Lye PS, et al, editors: *Nelson pediatric symptom-based diagnosis*, Philadelphia, 2018, Elsevier (Table 25-10).

as clinical or research testing. In most cases, however, such testing should not be performed indiscriminately, but instead should be ordered thoughtfully after the differential diagnosis has been considered. The introduction of **next-generation sequencing** has led to the identification of innumerable novel genes and revolutionized the testing that is now available for patients and families with intellectual disability, birth defects, or other suspected genetic diseases. A strong suspicion of a genetic diagnosis warrants consideration of testing to confirm the diagnosis, facilitate patient treatment and anticipatory guidance, clarify recurrence risks, and enable carrier testing for relevant inheritance patterns. Single nucleotide variants, exons, or genes are tested by *Sanger sequencing* targeting single or multiple exons. However, for diagnoses that have substantial genetic heterogeneity (e.g., hearing loss), *panel testing*, in which multiple relevant genes can be interrogated for single nucleotide variants, gene deletions, and gene duplications, is more expeditious than Sanger sequencing. Panel tests also frequently have the advantage of providing high coverage for the genes on the panel, compared to coverage for the same genes obtained by exome sequencing. However, in situations with diagnostic uncertainty, such as the investigation of a child with intellectual disability and dysmorphic features, for which there is no clinically recognizable pattern, exome sequencing may be most useful as a broad testing approach. **Whole exome sequencing** (WES) examines approximately 200,000 exons, or the 1–2% of the DNA that comprises the coding regions of the genome. WES is typically performed with a *trio* approach, in which the patient and both biological parents are tested simultaneously, so that the inheritance pattern, or segregation, of deleterious sequence variants can be determined, thus simplifying analysis. Trio sequencing has resulted in higher diagnostic yields than proband-only sequencing and can approach 30–40% for indications such as intellectual disability. In contrast, **whole genome sequencing** (WGS) examines all the DNA content, including noncoding regions, and includes analysis for cytogenetic rearrangements in addition to copy number loss or gain. WES and WGS are applicable to a wide range of birth defects and genetic diseases and can discover causative variants in known or novel genes associated with a particular condition.

Management and Counseling

Management of the affected patient and genetic counseling are essential aspects of the approach to the dysmorphic patient. Children with Down syndrome have a high incidence of hypothyroidism, and children with achondroplasia have a high incidence of cervicomedullary junction abnormalities. One of the many benefits of an early and accurate diagnosis is that **anticipatory guidance and medical monitoring** of patients for syndrome-specific medical risks can prolong and improve their quality of life. When a diagnosis is made, the treating physicians can access published information on the natural history and management of the disorder through published papers, genetics reference texts, and databases.

The 2nd major benefit of an accurate diagnosis is that it provides data for appropriate **recurrence risk** estimates. Genetic disorders may have direct effects on only 1 member of the family, but the diagnosis of the condition can have implications for the entire family. One or both parents may be carriers; siblings may be carriers or may want to know their genetic status when they reach their reproductive years. Recurrence risk provision is an important component of genetic counseling and should be included in all evaluations for families affected with birth defects or other inherited disorders (see Chapter 94).

Bibliography is available at Expert Consult.

Chapter **129**
Epidemiology of Infections
David B. Haslam

第一百二十九章
感染的流行病学

中文导读

　　本章主要介绍了新生儿感染的流行病学，按照新生儿感染发生时间的先后顺序分别介绍了新生儿先天性感染、围产期感染、新生儿早发型和晚发型感染的定义、病因、发病机制及主要感染病原，同时详细介绍了新生儿常见的感染性疾病如细菌性败血症、全身炎症反应综合征、发热或低体温、结膜炎、皮肤软组织感染、脐炎及破伤风等的临床表现，详细阐述了新生儿感染时的实验室检查特点及各感染性疾病的预防和治疗方案。

Infections in the newborn are often classified by their timing relative to birth and include congenital, perinatal, early-onset, and late-onset disease. These are clinically useful designations because the mechanisms of infection, etiologies, and outcomes are distinct at each stage. **Congenital infection** denotes infection acquired in utero. Such infections are generally caused by viral or other non-bacterial organisms and are often associated with injury to developing organs (see Chapter 131). **Perinatal infection** indicates acquisition around the time of delivery. Perinatally acquired organisms include both bacteria and viruses, some of which are the same as those causing congenital infection but often manifest with different features. **Early-onset infection** occurs in the 1st wk of life and is generally the consequence of infection caused by organisms acquired during the perinatal period. **Late-onset infection** occurs between 7 and 30 days of life and may include bacteria, viruses, or other organisms that are typically acquired in the postnatal period. **Hospital-acquired infections** typically occur beyond the 1st wk of life (see Chapter 130).

Neonates are uniquely prone to invasive disease because of their lack of fully responsive innate immunity (Fig. 129.1). Attenuated immune responses often result in minimal or nonspecific clinical manifestations, and effective treatment requires attention to subtle signs of infection. Compared to older infants, newborns are often treated empirically while awaiting results of laboratory investigations. Preterm infants are particularly susceptible to infection because of their decreased innate immune and barrier defenses and their prolonged stay in hospital settings.

INCIDENCE AND EPIDEMIOLOGY

Despite advances in maternal and neonatal care, infections remain a frequent and important cause of neonatal and infant morbidity and mortality. Up to 10% of infants have infections in the 1st mo of life. Newborn infection is more common in areas with limited access to healthcare than in areas with well-established healthcare infrastructure. The overall incidence of neonatal sepsis ranges from 1 to 5 cases per 1,000 live births. Estimated incidence rates vary based on the case definition and the population studied. Globally, neonatal sepsis and other severe infections were responsible for an estimated 430,000 neonatal deaths in 2013, accounting for approximately 15% of all neonatal deaths.

A number of bacterial and nonbacterial agents may infect newborns in the intrapartum or postpartum period (Table 129.1). Although herpes simplex virus (HSV), human immunodeficiency virus (HIV), hepatitis B virus (HBV), hepatitis C virus (HCV), and tuberculosis (TB) can each result in transplacental infection, the most common mode of transmission for these agents is **intrapartum**, during labor and delivery with passage through an infected birth canal (HIV, HSV, HBV), or **postpartum**, from contact with an infected mother or caretaker (TB) or with infected breast milk (HIV) (Fig. 129.2 and Table 129.2). Any microorganism inhabiting the genitourinary or lower gastrointestinal tract may cause intrapartum and postpartum infection. The most common bacteria are group B streptococcus (GBS), *Escherichia coli*, and *Klebsiella* spp. *Salmonella* spp. are common causes of gram-negative sepsis in developing countries; less common causes of bacterial infection in the United States include

Citrobacter, enterococci, gonococci, *Listeria monocytogenes*, *Streptococcus pneumoniae*, and *Haemophilus influenzae*. The more common viruses are cytomegalovirus (CMV), HSV, enteroviruses, and HIV (Table 129.2).

Microorganisms causing pneumonia acquired during labor and delivery include GBS, gram-negative enteric aerobes, *L. monocytogenes*, genital *Mycoplasma*, *Chlamydia trachomatis*, CMV, HSV, and *Candida* spp. (Table 129.3).

The most common bacterial causes of **neonatal meningitis** are GBS, *E. coli*, and *L. monocytogenes*. *S. pneumoniae*, other streptococci, nontypable *H. influenzae*, both coagulase-positive and coagulase-negative staphylococci, *Klebsiella*, *Enterobacter*, *Pseudomonas*, *Treponema pallidum*, and *Mycobacterium tuberculosis* infection involving the central nervous system (CNS) may also result in meningitis.

Early- and Late-Onset Neonatal Infections

The terms *early-onset infection* and *late-onset infection* refer to the different ages at onset of infection in the neonatal period. **Early-onset sepsis** is defined as the onset of symptoms before 7 days of age, although some experts limit the definition to infections occurring within the 1st 72 hr of life. **Late-onset sepsis** is generally defined as the onset of symptoms at ≥7 days of age. Similar to early-onset sepsis, there is variability in the definition, ranging from an onset at >72 hr of life to ≥7 days of age. Early-onset infections are acquired before or during delivery (**vertical** mother-to-child transmission). Late-onset infections develop after delivery from organisms acquired in the hospital or the community. The age at onset depends on the timing of exposure and virulence of the infecting organism. **Very-late-onset infections** (onset after age 1 mo) may also occur, particularly in very-low-birthweight (VLBW) preterm infants or term infants requiring prolonged neonatal intensive care.

The incidence of neonatal bacterial sepsis varies from 1-4 per 1,000 live births, with geographic variation and changes over time. Studies suggest that term male infants have a higher incidence of sepsis than term females. This sex difference is less clear in preterm low-birthweight (LBW) infants. Attack rates of neonatal sepsis increase significantly in LBW infants in the presence of maternal chorioamnionitis, congenital immune defects, mutations of genes involved in the innate immune system, asplenia, galactosemia (*E. coli*), and malformations leading to high inocula of bacteria (e.g., obstructive uropathy).

Data from the Eunice Kennedy Shriver National Institute of Child Health and Human Development (NICHD) Neonatal Research Network documented rates of early-onset sepsis among almost 400,000 live births at Network centers. The overall rate of early-onset sepsis was 0.98 cases per 1,000 live births, with rates inversely related to birthweight: 401-1,500 g, 10.96 per 1,000 births; 1,501-2,500 g, 1.38/1,000; and >2,500 g, 0.57/1,000 (Table 129.4).

The incidence of meningitis is 0.2-0.4 per 1,000 live births in newborn infants and is higher in preterm infants. Bacterial meningitis may be associated with sepsis or may occur as a local meningeal infection. *Up to one third of VLBW infants with late-onset meningitis have negative blood culture results.* The discordance between results of blood and cerebrospinal fluid (CSF) cultures suggests that meningitis may be underdiagnosed among VLBW infants and emphasizes the need for culture of CSF in VLBW infants when *late-onset sepsis* is suspected and in all infants who have positive blood culture results. Most neonates with sepsis presenting in the 1st day of life have a positive blood culture; analysis of CSF is usually deferred until the unstable cardiorespiratory status (shock, respiratory failure) has stabilized.

PATHOGENESIS
Early-Onset Infections

In most cases, the fetus or neonate is not exposed to potentially pathogenic bacteria until the membranes rupture and the infant passes through the birth canal and/or enters the extrauterine environment. The human birth canal is colonized with aerobic and anaerobic organisms that may result in ascending amniotic infection and/or colonization of the neonate at birth. Vertical transmission of bacterial agents that infect the amniotic fluid and vaginal canal may occur in utero or, more often, during labor and delivery (Fig. 129.3).

Table 129.1	Nonbacterial Causes of Systemic Neonatal Infections
VIRUSES	**MYCOPLASMA**
Adenovirus	*Mycoplasma hominis*
Cytomegalovirus (CMV)	*Ureaplasma urealyticum*
Enteroviruses	
Parechoviruses	**FUNGI**
Hepatitis B and C viruses	*Candida* spp.
Herpes simplex virus (HSV)	*Malassezia* spp.
Human immunodeficiency virus (HIV)	**PROTOZOA**
Parvovirus	Plasmodia
Rubella virus	*Toxoplasma gondii*
Varicella-zoster virus (VZV)	*Trypanosoma cruzi*

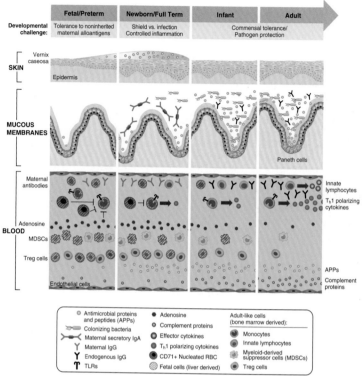

Fig. 129.1 Ontogeny of skin, soluble, and cellular innate defense systems. Host-protective barrier functions include physical, chemical, and functional components of the skin and mucous membrane epithelia of the fetus, neonate (birth to 28 days of age), and infant (1 mo to 1 yr of age). Skin: while physical and chemical barriers are impaired in early in life, especially in the preterm newborn, the vernix caseosa and skin epithelia of full-term newborns robustly express antimicrobial proteins and peptides (APPs). Mucous membranes: in parallel with and induced by an increasingly complex microbiota, the newborn intestinal mucosal epithelium rapidly changes structurally, with an increase in the population of crypts and crypt-based Paneth cells, as well as functionally with increasing APP expression. Blood: the composition of neonatal blood is distinct, with relatively low concentrations of complement components and APPs and high concentrations of the immunosuppressive purine metabolite adenosine. Plasma also contains maternal antibodies that are transferred beginning midgestation and supplemented by postnatal factors derived from breast milk. Innate immunity is detectable from the end of the 1st mo of gestation, with changes driven largely by the increasing exposure to environmental microbes. Neonatal antigen-presenting cells such as blood monocytes express pattern recognition receptors (e.g., Toll-like receptors, TLRs) with distinct functional responses, including limited Th1-polarizing cytokine production, to most stimuli. Adaptive immunity develops from 4 wk of gestation onward, with changes driven by an evolving chimerism reflecting fetal (liver-derived, *shaded cells*) regulatory T (Treg)-cell–rich lymphocytes, and more adultlike (bone marrow derived, *unshaded cells*) lymphocytes with distinct, epigenetically encoded functional programs. Ig, Immunoglobulin; RBC, red blood cell. (*Modified from Kollmann TR, Kampmann B, Mazmanian SK, et al: Protecting the newborn and young infant from infectious diseases: lessons from immune ontogeny.* Immunity *2007;46:350–363.*)

Chorioamnionitis results from microbial invasion of amniotic fluid, often as a result of prolonged rupture of the chorioamniotic membrane. Amniotic infection may also occur with apparently intact membranes or with a relatively brief duration of membrane rupture. The term *chorioamnionitis* refers to the clinical syndrome of intrauterine infection, which includes maternal fever, with or without local or systemic signs of chorioamnionitis (uterine tenderness, foul-smelling vaginal discharge/amniotic fluid, maternal leukocytosis, maternal and/or fetal tachycardia). Chorioamnionitis may also be asymptomatic, diagnosed only by amniotic fluid analysis or pathologic examination of the placenta. The rate of histologic chorioamnionitis is inversely related to gestational age at birth (Fig. 129.4) and directly related to duration of membrane rupture.

Chorioamnionitis was thought to result from infection of the amniotic fluid but is now better defined by the term **intrauterine inflammation or infection at birth (Triple I)**. This is defined by fetal tachycardia, maternal leukocytosis (>15,000 cells in the absence of corticosteroids), purulent fluid from the cervical os, biochemical or microbiologic amniotic fluid changes consistent with infection, and fever (≥39.0°C/10.2°F) (see Chapter 131.2).

Rupture of membranes for >24 hr was once considered prolonged because microscopic evidence of inflammation of the membranes is uniformly present when the duration of rupture exceeds 24 hr. At 18 hr of membrane rupture, however, the incidence of early-onset disease with group B streptococcus (GBS) increases significantly; 18 hr is the appropriate cutoff for increased risk of neonatal infection (see Chapter 211).

Bacterial colonization does not always result in disease. Factors influencing which colonized infant will experience disease are not well understood but include prematurity, underlying illness, invasive procedures, inoculum size, virulence of the infecting organism, genetic predisposition, the innate immune system, host response, and transplacental maternal antibodies (Fig. 129.5). Aspiration or ingestion of bacteria in amniotic fluid may lead to congenital pneumonia or systemic infection, with manifestations becoming apparent before delivery (fetal distress, tachycardia), at delivery (failure to breathe, respiratory distress, shock), or after a latent period of a few hours (respiratory distress, shock). Aspiration or ingestion of bacteria during the birth process may lead to infection after an interval of 1-2 days.

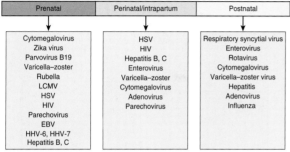

Fig. 129.2 Relative importance of neonatal viral infections related to the timing of acquisition of infection. Viruses are listed in declining order of importance relative to prenatal, perinatal (intrapartum), and postnatal timing of typical infection. Some neonatal virus infections (e.g., cytomegalovirus) can be substantial causes of disease whether acquired during gestation or acquired postpartum, whereas others (e.g., respiratory syncytial virus) are typically acquired in the postnatal period. EBV, Epstein-Barr virus; HHV, human herpesvirus; HIV, human immunodeficiency virus; HSV, herpes simplex virus; LCMV, lymphocytic choriomeningitis virus. (*From Schleiss MR, Marsh KJ: Viral infections of the fetus and newborn. In Gleason CA, Juul SE, editors:* Avery's diseases of the newborn, *ed 10, Philadelphia, 2018, Elsevier, Fig 37-1.*)

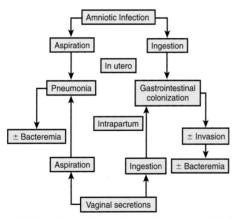

Fig. 129.3 Pathways of ascending or intrapartum infection.

Table 129.2	Period of Transmission of Selected Viruses to the Fetus or Newborn Infant		
VIRUSES	**CONGENITAL**	**NATAL**	**POSTNATAL**
Adenovirus	+	+	+
Chikungunya	++	+	−
Cytomegalovirus	++	++	++
Dengue	++	−	−
Ebola virus	++	+	+
Echoviruses	+	+	+
Epstein-Barr	+	−	+
Hepatitis A	−	++	+
Hepatitis B	+	++	+
Hepatitis C	+	++	−
Herpes simplex	+	++	+
Herpesvirus-6	+	−	+
Human immunodeficiency virus	+	++	+
Human parvovirus B19	+	−	−
Influenza	(+)	−	+
Lymphocytic choriomeningitis virus	++	−	−
Measles	+	−	+
Mumps	+	−	−
Parechovirus	−	+	+
Polioviruses	+	+	+
Rubella	++	−	−
Smallpox	+	+	+
St. Louis encephalitis	(+)	−	(+)
Type B coxsackieviruses	+	+	+
Vaccinia	+	+	+
Varicella-zoster virus	++	+	+
West Nile virus	+	−	+
Western equine encephalitis	+	−	+
Zika virus	++	?	(+)

++, Major demonstrated route; +, minor demonstrated route; (+), suggested route, few supporting data; −, route not demonstrated.
 From Harrison GJ: Approach to infections in the fetus and newborn. In Cherry JD, Demmler-Harrison GJ, Kaplan SL, et al, editors: *Feigin and Cherry's textbook of pediatric infectious diseases*, ed 7, Philadelphia, 2014, Elsevier (Table 66.1, p 878).

Resuscitation at birth, particularly if it involves endotracheal intubation, insertion of an umbilical vessel catheter, or both, is associated with an increased risk of bacterial infection. Explanations include the presence of infection at the time of birth or acquisition of infection during the invasive procedures associated with resuscitation.

Late-Onset Infections
After birth, neonates are exposed to infectious agents in the neonatal intensive care unit (NICU), the nursery, or in the community (including family). Postnatal infections may be transmitted by direct contact with hospital personnel, the mother, or other family members; from breast milk (HIV, CMV); or from inanimate sources such as contaminated equipment. The most common source of postnatal infections in hospitalized newborns is *hand contamination* of healthcare personnel, underscoring the importance of handwashing.

Most cases of meningitis result from hematogenous dissemination. Less often, meningitis results from contiguous spread as a result of contamination of open neural tube defects, congenital sinus tracts, or penetrating wounds from fetal scalp sampling or internal fetal electrocardiographic monitors. Cerebral abscess formation, ventriculitis, septic infarcts, hydrocephalus, and subdural effusions are complications of meningitis that occur more often in newborn infants than in older children. Metabolic factors, including hypoxia, acidosis, hypothermia, and inherited metabolic disorders (e.g., galactosemia), are likely to contribute to risk for and severity of neonatal sepsis

Infection in Premature Infants
The most important neonatal factor predisposing to infection is prematurity or LBW. Preterm LBW infants have a 3- to 10-fold higher incidence of infection than full-term normal-birthweight infants. Possible explanations include (1) maternal genital tract infection is considered to be an important cause of preterm labor, with an increased risk of vertical transmission to the newborn; (2) the frequency of intraamniotic infection is inversely related to gestational age (see Figs. 129.1 and 129.5); (3) premature infants have documented immune dysfunction;

Table 129.3	Etiologic Agents of Neonatal Pneumonia According to Timing of Acquisition

TRANSPLACENTAL	POSTNATAL
Cytomegalovirus (CMV)	Adenovirus
Herpes simplex virus (HSV)	Candida spp.*
Mycobacterium tuberculosis	Coagulase-negative
Rubella virus	staphylococci
Treponema pallidum	CMV
Varicella-zoster virus (VZV)	Enteric bacteria*
Listeria monocytogenes	Enteroviruses
	Influenza viruses A, B
PERINATAL	Parainfluenza
Anaerobic bacteria	Pseudomonas*
Chlamydia	Respiratory syncytial virus (RSV)
CMV	Staphylococcus aureus
Enteric bacteria	Mycobacterium tuberculosis
Group B streptococci	Legionella
Haemophilus influenzae	
HSV	
Listeria monocytogenes	
Mycoplasma	

*More likely with mechanical ventilation or indwelling catheters, or after abdominal surgery.

Table 129.4	Rates of Early-Onset Sepsis Per 1,000 Live Births*

	BIRTHWEIGHT (g)			
	401-1,500	1,501-2,500	>2,500	All
All	10.96	1.38	0.57	0.98
Group B streptococci	2.08	0.38	0.35	0.41
Escherichia coli	5.09	0.54	0.07	0.28

*NICHD Neonatal Research Network/CDC Surveillance Study of Early-Onset Sepsis.

Adapted from Stoll BJ, Hansen NI, Sanchez PJ, et al: Early onset neonatal sepsis: the burden of group B streptococcal and E. coli disease continues, Pediatrics 127(5):817–826, 2011.

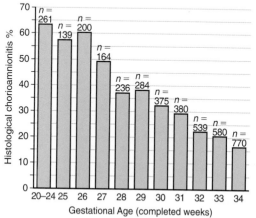

Fig. 129.4 Histologic chorioamnionitis in liveborn preterm babies by gestational age (n = 3,928 babies). (From Lahra MM, Jeffery HE: A fetal response to chorioamnionitis is associated with early survival after preterm birth, Am J Obstet Gynecol 190:147–151, 2004.)

and (4) premature infants often require prolonged intravenous access, endotracheal intubation, or other invasive procedures that provide a portal of entry or impair barrier and clearance mechanisms, putting them at continued risk for hospital-acquired infections.

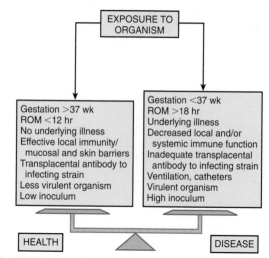

Fig. 129.5 Factors influencing the balance between health and disease in neonates exposed to a potential pathogen. ROM, Rupture of membranes. (Adapted from Baker CJ: Group B streptococcal infections, Clin Perinatol 24:59–70, 1997.)

CLINICAL MANIFESTATIONS

The maternal history provides important information about maternal exposures to infectious diseases, bacterial colonization, immunity (natural and acquired), and obstetric risk factors (prematurity, prolonged ruptured membranes, maternal chorioamnionitis). Signs and symptoms in the neonate are often subtle and nonspecific. Temperature instability, tachypnea, lethargy, and poor feeding are common initial signs and should raise suspicion for systemic or focal infection (Table 129.5).

Bacterial Sepsis

Neonates with bacterial sepsis may have either nonspecific manifestations or focal signs of infection (Table 129.5), including temperature instability, hypotension, poor perfusion with pallor and mottled skin, metabolic acidosis, tachycardia or bradycardia, apnea, respiratory distress, grunting, cyanosis, irritability, lethargy, feeding intolerance, abdominal distention, jaundice, petechiae, purpura, and bleeding. Table 129.6 lists World Health Organization *international criteria* for bacterial sepsis. The initial manifestation may involve only limited symptomatology and only one system, such as apnea alone or tachypnea with retractions, or tachycardia, or the infant may present with an acute catastrophic manifestation with multiorgan dysfunction and shock. Infants should be reevaluated over time to determine whether the symptoms have progressed from mild to severe. Later complications of sepsis include respiratory failure, pulmonary hypertension, cardiac failure, shock, renal failure, liver dysfunction, cerebral edema or thrombosis, adrenal hemorrhage and/or insufficiency, bone marrow dysfunction (neutropenia, thrombocytopenia, anemia), and disseminated intravascular coagulopathy (DIC).

A variety of noninfectious conditions can occur together with neonatal infection or can make the diagnosis of infection more difficult. Respiratory distress syndrome (RDS) secondary to surfactant deficiency can coexist with bacterial pneumonia. Because bacterial sepsis can be rapidly progressive, the physician must be alert to the signs and symptoms of possible infection and must initiate diagnostic evaluation and empirical therapy in a timely manner. The differential diagnosis of many of the signs and symptoms that suggest infection is extensive; noninfectious disorders must also be considered (Table 129.7).

Systemic Inflammatory Response Syndrome

The clinical manifestations of infection depend on the virulence of the infecting organism and the body's inflammatory response. The term *systemic inflammatory response syndrome* (SIRS) is most frequently used

Table 129.5	Initial Signs and Symptoms of Infection in Newborn Infants

GENERAL	CARDIOVASCULAR SYSTEM
Fever, temperature instability	Pallor; mottling; cold, clammy
"Not doing well"	skin
Poor feeding	Tachycardia
Edema	Hypotension
	Bradycardia
GASTROINTESTINAL SYSTEM	
Abdominal distention	**CENTRAL NERVOUS SYSTEM**
Vomiting	Irritability, lethargy
Diarrhea	Tremors, seizures
Hepatomegaly	Hyporeflexia, hypotonia
	Abnormal Moro reflex
RESPIRATORY SYSTEM	Irregular respirations
Apnea, dyspnea	Full fontanel
Tachypnea, retractions	High-pitched cry
Flaring, grunting	
Cyanosis	**HEMATOLOGIC SYSTEM**
	Jaundice
RENAL SYSTEM	Splenomegaly
Oliguria	Pallor
	Petechiae, purpura
	Bleeding

Table 129.6	Clinical Criteria for the Diagnosis of Sepsis in the International Setting

IMCI AND WHO CRITERIA FOR SEVERE INFECTIONS IN CHILDREN

Neurologic: convulsions, drowsy or unconscious, decreased activity, bulging fontanel
Respiratory: respiratory rate >60 breaths/min, grunting, severe chest indrawing, central cyanosis
Cardiac: poor perfusion, rapid and weak pulse
Gastrointestinal: jaundice, poor feeding, abdominal distention
Dermatologic: skin pustules, periumbilical erythema or purulence
Musculoskeletal: edema or erythema overlying bones or joints
Other: temperature >37.7°C (99.9°F; or feels hot) or <35.5°C (95.9°F; or feels cold)

IMCI, Integrated Management of Childhood Illness; WHO, World Health Organization.
Adapted from WHO: *Pocket book of hospital care for children: guidelines for the management of common childhood illnesses*, ed 2, Geneva, 2013, WHO, pp 45–69. http://www.who.int/maternal_child_adolescent/documents/child_hospital_care/en/.

Table 129.7	Serious Systemic Illness in Newborns: Differential Diagnosis of Neonatal Sepsis

CARDIAC
Congenital: hypoplastic left heart syndrome, other structural disease, persistent pulmonary hypertension of the newborn (PPHN)
Acquired: myocarditis, hypovolemic or cardiogenic shock, PPHN

GASTROINTESTINAL
Necrotizing enterocolitis
Spontaneous gastrointestinal perforation
Midgut volvulus
Hepatic failure (inborn errors of metabolism, neonatal iron storage disease)

HEMATOLOGIC
Neonatal purpura fulminans
Immune-mediated thrombocytopenia
Immune-mediated neutropenia
Severe anemia
Malignancies (congenital leukemia)
Langerhans cell histiocytosis
Hereditary clotting disorders
Familial hemophagocytosis syndrome

METABOLIC
Hypoglycemia
Adrenal disorders: adrenal hemorrhage, adrenal insufficiency, congenital adrenal hyperplasia
Inborn errors of metabolism: organic acidurias, lactic acidoses, urea cycle disorders, galactosemia

NEUROLOGIC
Intracranial hemorrhage: spontaneous, caused by child abuse
Hypoxic-ischemic encephalopathy
Neonatal seizures
Infant botulism

RESPIRATORY
Respiratory distress syndrome
Aspiration pneumonia: amniotic fluid, meconium, or gastric contents
Lung hypoplasia
Tracheoesophageal fistula
Transient tachypnea of the newborn

to describe this unique process of infection and the subsequent systemic response (see Chapters 88). In addition to infection, SIRS may result from trauma, hemorrhagic shock, other causes of ischemia, necrotizing enterocolitis, and pancreatitis.

Patients with SIRS have a spectrum of clinical symptoms that represent progressive stages of the pathologic process. In adults, SIRS is defined by the presence of 2 or more of the following: (1) fever or hypothermia, (2) tachycardia, (3) tachypnea, and (4) abnormal white blood cell (WBC) count or an increase in immature forms. In neonates and pediatric patients, SIRS manifests as temperature instability, respiratory dysfunction (altered gas exchange, hypoxemia, acute respiratory distress syndrome), cardiac dysfunction (tachycardia, delayed capillary refill, hypotension), and perfusion abnormalities (oliguria, metabolic acidosis) (Table 129.8). Increased vascular permeability results in capillary leak into peripheral tissues and the lungs, with resultant peripheral and pulmonary edema. DIC results in the more severely affected cases. The cascade of escalating tissue injury may lead to multisystem organ failure and death.

Temperature Instability

Fever or hypothermia may be the only initial manifestation of serious infection in newborns. However, only approximately 50% of infected newborn infants have a temperature >37.8°C (100°F) (axillary) (see Chapter 202). Fever in newborn infants does not always signify infection; it may be caused by increased ambient temperature, isolette or radiant warmer malfunction, dehydration, CNS disorders, hyperthyroidism, familial dysautonomia, or ectodermal dysplasia. A single temperature elevation is infrequently associated with infection; fever sustained over 1 hr is more likely to be caused by infection. Most febrile infected infants have additional signs compatible with infection, although a focus of infection is not always apparent. Acute febrile illnesses occurring later in the neonatal period may be caused by urinary tract infection, meningitis, pneumonia, osteomyelitis, or gastroenteritis, in addition to sepsis, thus underscoring the importance of a diagnostic evaluation that includes blood culture, urine culture, lumbar puncture (LP), and other studies as indicated. Many agents may cause these late infections, including HSV, enteroviruses, respiratory syncytial virus (RSV), and bacterial pathogens. In premature infants, hypothermia or temperature instability requiring increasing ambient (isolette, warmer) temperatures is more likely to accompany infection.

Respiratory and Cardiovascular Symptoms

Early signs and symptoms of **pneumonia** may be nonspecific, including poor feeding, lethargy, irritability, cyanosis, temperature instability, and the overall impression that the infant is not well. Respiratory symptoms of increasing severity are grunting, tachypnea, retractions, flaring of the alae nasi, cyanosis, apnea, and progressive respiratory failure. If the infant is premature, signs of progressive respiratory distress may be

Table 129.8	Definitions of Systemic Inflammatory Respiratory Response Syndrome (SIRS) and Sepsis in Pediatric Patients

SIRS: the systemic inflammatory response to a variety of clinical insults, manifested by 2 or more of the following conditions:
Temperature instability <35°C (95°F) or >38.5°C (101.3°F)
Respiratory dysfunction:
  Tachypnea >2 SD above the mean for age
  Hypoxemia (PaO$_2$<70 mm Hg on room air)
Cardiac dysfunction:
  Tachycardia >2 SD above the mean for age
  Delayed capillary refill >3 sec
  Hypotension >2 SD below the mean for age
Perfusion abnormalities:
  Oliguria (urine output <0.5 mL/kg/hr)
  Lactic acidosis (elevated plasma lactate and/or arterial pH <7.25)
  Altered mental status
Sepsis: the systemic inflammatory response to an infectious process

From Adams-Chapman I, Stoll BJ: Systemic inflammatory response syndrome, *Semin Pediatr Infect Dis* 12:5–16, 2001.

superimposed on RDS or bronchopulmonary dysplasia (BPD). For infants on mechanical ventilation, the need to increase ventilator support may indicate infection. Although a common finding in neonatal sepsis, tachycardia is nonspecific. Bradycardia may also occur. Poor perfusion and hypotension are more sensitive indicators of sepsis but tend to be late findings. In a prospective national surveillance study, 40% of neonates with sepsis required volume expansion, and 29% required vasopressor support.

Signs of pneumonia on physical examination, such as dullness to percussion, change in breath sounds, and the presence of rales or rhonchi, are very difficult to appreciate in a neonate. Radiographs of the chest may reveal new infiltrates or an effusion, but if the neonate has underlying RDS or BPD, it is very difficult to determine whether the radiographic changes represent a new process or worsening of the underlying disease.

The progression of neonatal pneumonia can be variable. Fulminant infection is most frequently associated with pyogenic organisms such as GBS (see Chapter 211). Onset may occur during the 1st hours or days of life, with the infant often manifesting rapidly progressive circulatory collapse and respiratory failure. With early-onset pneumonia in premature infants, the clinical course and chest radiographs may be indistinguishable from those with severe RDS.

In contrast to the rapid progression of pneumonia caused by pyogenic organisms, an indolent course may be seen in nonbacterial infection. The onset can be preceded by upper respiratory tract symptoms or conjunctivitis. The infant may demonstrate a nonproductive cough, and the degree of respiratory compromise is variable. Fever is usually absent or low grade, and radiographic examination of the chest shows focal or diffuse interstitial pneumonitis or hyperinflation. Infection is generally caused by *C. trachomatis*, CMV, *Ureaplasma urealyticum,* or one of the respiratory viruses. Rhinovirus has been reported to cause severe respiratory compromise in infants, particularly those who are preterm. Although *Pneumocystis (carinii) jiroveci* was implicated in the past, its etiologic role is now in doubt, except in newborns infected with HIV.

Conjunctivitis

Conjunctival infection is relatively common and may be caused by a variety of organisms. The presentation includes periorbital swelling, conjunctival injection, and purulent conjunctival drainage. *C. trachomatis* and *Neisseria gonorrhea* are common causes; other gram-positive and gram-negative organisms are occasionally involved. *Pseudomonas aeruginosa* is an important pathogen in hospitalized VLBW infants and may be a precursor to invasive disease. Viral infections (e.g., HSV, adenovirus) are occasionally seen. Recognition of HSV infection is important to prevent corneal injury and dissemination to systemic sites.

Skin and Soft Tissue Infection

Cutaneous manifestations of infection include omphalitis, cellulitis, mastitis, and subcutaneous abscesses. Pustules likely indicate the presence of staphylococcal infection but must be distinguished from the vesicular rash of HSV infection. Staphylococcal pustulosis results in larger, pus-filled lesions 1 mm in diameter and often scattered around the umbilicus, whereas HSV infection often appears as tiny vesicles in crops, often on the scalp. **Ecthyma gangrenosum** indicates infection with *Pseudomonas* spp. and is rare except in VLBW infants. The presence of small, salmon-pink papules suggests *L. monocytogenes* infection. Mucocutaneous lesions suggest *Candida* spp. (see Chapter 261.1). Petechiae and purpura may be the result of systemic viral or bacterial infection.

Omphalitis

Omphalitis is a neonatal infection resulting from unhygienic care of the umbilical cord, which continues to be a problem, particularly in developing countries. The umbilical stump is colonized by bacteria from the maternal genital tract and the environment (see Chapter 125). The necrotic tissue of the umbilical cord is an excellent medium for bacterial growth. Omphalitis may remain a localized infection or may spread to the abdominal wall, the peritoneum, the umbilical or portal vessels, and the liver. Abdominal wall cellulitis or **necrotizing fasciitis**, with associated sepsis and a high mortality rate, may develop in infants with omphalitis. Prompt diagnosis and treatment are necessary to avoid serious complications. *Staphylococcus aureus* and gram-negative organisms are common pathogens involved.

Tetanus

Neonatal tetanus remains a serious infection in resource-limited countries (see Chapter 238). It results from unclean delivery and unhygienic management of the umbilical cord in an infant born to a mother who has not been immunized against tetanus. The surveillance case definition of neonatal tetanus requires the ability of a newborn to suck at birth and for the 1st few days of life, followed by an inability to suck. Neonatal tetanus typically occurs in infants 5-7 days after birth (range: 3-24 days), difficulty swallowing, spasms, stiffness, seizures, and death. **Broncho-pneumonia**, presumably resulting from aspiration, is a common complication and cause of death. Neonatal tetanus can be prevented by immunizing mothers before or during pregnancy and by ensuring a clean delivery, sterile cutting of the umbilical cord and proper cord care after birth.

LABORATORY FINDINGS

Maternal history and infant signs should guide diagnostic evaluation (Table 129.9). Additionally, signs of systemic infection in newborn infants may be unrevealing, so laboratory investigation plays a particularly important role in diagnosis. Cultures and cell counts are obtained from blood and urine. CSF should be sent for Gram stain, routine culture, cell count with differential, and protein/glucose concentrations. Surface swabs, blood, and CSF are often obtained for HSV testing. Except for culture and directed pathogen testing, no single laboratory test is completely reliable for diagnosis of invasive infection in the newborn. Complete blood count may demonstrate elevated or decreased WBC count, often with a shift toward more immature forms. Thrombocytopenia can be seen in systemic bacterial or viral infection. Hyponatremia, acidosis, and other electrolyte abnormalities can be seen. Hyperbilirubinemia is nonspecific but may be an indication of systemic infection. Elevated serum transaminases may be a clue to systemic HSV or enterovirus infection.

Various serum biomarkers have been investigated for their ability to identify infants with **serious bacterial infection** (SBI). An immature-to-total phagocyte count (I/T ratio) (≥0.2) has the best sensitivity of the neutrophil indices for predicting neonatal sepsis. After the newborn period, serum C-reactive protein (CRP) and procalcitonin have demonstrated reasonable sensitivity and specificity for SBI. CRP may be monitored in newborn infants to assess response to therapy. Their value in the initial diagnosis of sepsis in the newborn period has yet to be clarified, as does the value of these biomarkers in determining optimal length of empirical therapy in infants with negative cultures. Cytokines

Table 129.9	Evaluation of a Newborn for Infection or Sepsis

HISTORY (SPECIFIC RISK FACTORS)

Maternal infection during gestation or at parturition (type and duration of antimicrobial therapy):
  Urinary tract infection
  Chorioamnionitis
Maternal colonization with group B streptococci, *Neisseria gonorrhoeae*, herpes simplex
Low gestational age/birthweight
Multiple birth
Duration of membrane rupture
Complicated delivery
Fetal tachycardia (distress)
Age at onset (in utero, birth, early postnatal, late)
Location at onset (hospital, community)
Medical intervention:
  Vascular access
  Endotracheal intubation
  Parenteral nutrition
  Surgery

EVIDENCE OF OTHER DISEASES*

Congenital malformations (heart disease, neural tube defect)
Respiratory tract disease (respiratory distress syndrome, aspiration)
Necrotizing enterocolitis
Metabolic disease (e.g., galactosemia)

EVIDENCE OF FOCAL OR SYSTEMIC DISEASE

General appearance, neurologic status
Abnormal vital signs
Organ system disease
Feeding, stools, urine output, extremity movement

LABORATORY STUDIES

Evidence of Infection

Culture from a normally sterile site (blood, CSF, other)
Demonstration of a microorganism in tissue or fluid
Molecular detection (blood, urine, CSF) by specific PCR and/or 16S ribosomal DNA
Maternal or neonatal serology (syphilis, toxoplasmosis)

Evidence of Inflammation

Leukocytosis, increased immature/total neutrophil count ratio
Acute-phase reactants: C-reactive protein, erythrocyte sedimentation rate, procalcitonin
Cytokines: interleukin-6, interleukin-B, tumor necrosis factor
Pleocytosis in CSF or synovial or pleural fluid
Disseminated intravascular coagulation: fibrin degradation products, D-dimer

Evidence of Multiorgan System Disease

Metabolic acidosis: pH, PCO_2
Pulmonary function: PO_2, PCO_2
Renal function: blood urea nitrogen, creatinine
Hepatic injury/function: bilirubin, alanine transaminase, aspartate transaminase, ammonia, prothrombin time, partial thromboplastin time
Bone marrow function: neutropenia, anemia, thrombocytopenia

*Diseases that increase the risk of infection or may overlap with signs of sepsis.
CSF, Cerebrospinal fluid; PCR, polymerase chain reaction.

(both proinflammatory cytokines such as interleukin (IL)-6 and tumor necrosis factor-α and antiinflammatory cytokines such as IL-4 and IL-10), chemokines, and other biomarkers are increased in infected infants. Elevations of serum amyloid A and the cell surface antigen CD64 also have high sensitivity for identifying infants with sepsis. Chest radiography is generally not indicated in infants without signs of respiratory infection.

Table 129.9 and 129.10 list clinical features and laboratory parameters that are useful in the diagnosis of neonatal infection or sepsis.

GENERAL APPROACH TO MANAGEMENT

In the absence of specific signs of focal infection, therapy for presumed infection in the neonate is often empirical and initiated on the basis of fever or hypothermia, listlessness, irritability, or apneic episodes. Antibiotics are chosen to cover the organisms typically causing neonatal sepsis, including GBS, gram-negative organisms, *Listeria*, and *Enterococcus*. Since the latter 2 organisms are intrinsically resistant to cephalosporins, ampicillin is generally included in the empirical treatment of infants with presumed neonatal infection (Table 129.11).

An empirical regimen for suspected early-onset sepsis in a term or late preterm infant is **ampicillin**, 150 mg/kg/dose intravenously (IV) every 12 hr, and **gentamicin**, 4 mg/kg/dose IV every 24 hr. This has long been a standard regimen for early-onset sepsis and provides coverage for the most prevalent organisms, predominantly GBS and gram-negative ones. Ampicillin plus **cefotaxime** (if available) or **cefepime** may be substituted if the patient presents with infection after discharge from the nursery, or when infection with ampicillin-resistant *E. coli* is suspected. **Ceftriaxone** may be substituted if premature infants are ≥41 wk postconception age; it may be used in term infants if they are not receiving intravenous calcium or do not have hyperbilirubinemia. There is concern this regimen may be associated with higher rates of mortality in NICU patients compared to ampicillin and gentamicin. Alterations to the standard regimen may be appropriate in some circumstances, such as suspected infection with *S. aureus*, in which case **vancomycin** may be substituted for ampicillin, and in environments where infections from antibiotic-resistant bacteria are prevalent.

Herpes simplex virus infection may present without cutaneous signs, in the absence of maternal history of infection, and in mothers receiving suppressive antiviral therapy. Therefore, management of the ill newborn requires a high index of suspicion for HSV infection. Surface swabs, blood, and CSF are obtained for HSV culture or PCR, and empirical acyclovir is often recommended while the results of these studies are pending (see Chapters 202 and 279).

Systemic infection caused by *Candida* spp. is a concern in hospitalized infants, particularly VLBW infants with central venous access catheters and prior antibiotic use. Empirical therapy for fungal infection is generally not recommended unless the patient fails to respond to broad-spectrum antibiotic therapy.

Definitive therapy is based on identification and susceptibility of the offending organism. In almost all circumstances, the *least broad* antibiotic with activity against the organism is chosen. Duration of therapy depends on the organism and the site of infection. In neonates with culture-proven sepsis, the usual course of therapy is 10 days. Longer treatment courses may be warranted if a specific focus of infection is identified (e.g., meningitis, osteomyelitis, septic arthritis). Antimicrobial therapy should be altered based on the susceptibility profile of the pathogen isolated. In infants with a negative blood culture but a clinical status that remains concerning for a systemic infection, antibiotic therapy can be extended for as long as a total of 5 to 10 days. Sepsis is unlikely in these infants if they remain well and the blood culture is sterile at 48 hr. Empirical antibiotic therapy should be discontinued after 48 hr in these neonates.

PREVENTION

Intrapartum antibiotics are used to reduce vertical transmission of GBS (Table 129.12), as well as to lessen neonatal morbidity associated with preterm labor and preterm premature rupture of membranes (see Figs. 211.2 and 211.3 in Chapter 211). With introduction of selective intrapartum antibiotic prophylaxis to prevent perinatal transmission of GBS, rates of early-onset neonatal GBS infection in the United States declined from 1.7/1,000 live births to 0.25/1,000. Intrapartum chemoprophylaxis does *not* reduce the rates of late-onset GBS disease and has no effect on the rates of infection with non-GBS pathogens (see Chapter 211). Of concern is a possible increase in gram-negative infections (especially *E. coli*) in VLBW and possibly term infants despite a reduction in early GBS sepsis by intrapartum antibiotics.

Aggressive management of suspected maternal chorioamnionitis with antibiotic therapy during labor, along with rapid delivery of the infant, reduces the risk of early-onset neonatal sepsis. Vertical transmission

Table 129.10	Culture-Based and Non–Culture-Based Diagnostics for Neonatal Sepsis		
CATEGORY	**PARAMETER**	**OPTIMAL TIMING, VOLUME OF SPECIMEN, ROUTINE/INVESTIGATIONAL***	**APPLICABILITY FOR NEONATAL SEPSIS**
CULTURE BASED			
Blood	Culture	>1 mL of whole blood, from 2 sites	Gold standard for bacteremia
CSF	Culture	When clinically feasible	Optimize antimicrobial therapy
Urine	Culture	>72 hr of life	Not useful for EOS; potential benefits for LOS
Tracheal aspirate	Culture	Neonates with endotracheal tube in place and signs of progressive respiratory distress	Usually reflects colonization
NON–CULTURE BASED			
Immune function	MHC II	Investigational	Both decreased in chorioamnionitis and sepsis
	TNF-α	Investigational	
Neutrophil indices	Neutropenia	After 12 hr of life	Neutropenia better predictor for sepsis than leukocytosis
	Absolute neutrophil count	Consider GA, delivery mode, altitude, arterial versus venous sampling, time since birth	
	Absolute immature neutrophil count		
Neutrophil markers	CD64	Elevated for 24 hr after infection	Cut points between 2.38 and 3.62 optimal sensitivity, specificity, and NPV for EOS
		Requires 50 μL blood	
		Results within hours	
		Investigational	
Platelet count	Thrombocytopenia and thrombocytosis	Late findings; slow to respond	Thrombocytopenia associated with fungal infection
CSF cell count	CSF WBC	Uninfected neonates: mean 10 cells/mm³; range up to 20 cells/mm³	Does not predict culture-proven meningitis
CSF chemistries	CSF protein	Term <100 mg/dL	Elevated in fungal meningitis
	CSF glucose	Preterm higher; 70–80% of serum glucose	Low glucose specific for bacterial meningitis
Acute phase reactants	CRP	8–24 hr after infection	Good NPV
	Procalcitonin	2–12 hr after infection	Better sensitivity but less specificity than CRP
Sepsis panels/scores		After 24 hr of life	Most useful for NPV and discontinuation of antimicrobial therapy
		Investigational	

*Investigational refers to an assay or parameter that is undergoing evaluation for clinical use and applicability.

CRP, C-reactive protein; CSF, cerebrospinal fluid; EOS, early-onset sepsis; GA, gestational age; LOS, late-onset sepsis; MHC II, major histocompatibility complex class II; NPV, negative predictive value; TNF, tumor necrosis factor; WBC, white blood cell count.

From Shane AL, Stoll BJ. Recent developments and current issues in the epidemiology, diagnosis, and management of bacterial and fungal neonatal sepsis, *Am J Perinatol* 30(2):131–141, 2013.

of GBS and early-onset GBS disease is significantly reduced by selective intrapartum chemoprophylaxis (see Fig. 211.4). A number of candidate GBS vaccines are currently being studied. Neonatal infection with *Chlamydia* can be prevented by identification and treatment of infected pregnant women (see Chapter 253). Mother-to-child transmission of HIV is significantly reduced by maternal antiretroviral therapy during pregnancy, labor, and delivery, by cesarean delivery before rupture of membranes, and by antiretroviral treatment of the infant after birth (see Chapter 302).

Prevention of congenital and perinatal infections predominantly focuses on maternal health. The Centers for Disease Control and Prevention (CDC) recommends the following screening tests and treatment when indicated:

1. All pregnant women should be offered voluntary and confidential HIV testing at the first prenatal visit, as early in pregnancy as possible. HIV screening should be part of routine prenatal testing, unless the mother declines testing (opt-out screening). For women at high risk of infection during pregnancy (multiple sexual partners or STIs during pregnancy, intravenous drug use, HIV-infected partners), repeat testing in the third trimester is recommended. Rapid HIV screening is indicated for any women who presents in labor with an undocumented HIV status, unless she declines testing.

2. A serologic test for syphilis should be performed on all pregnant women at the first prenatal visit. Repeat screenings early in the third trimester and again at delivery are recommended for women in whom syphilis test results in the first trimester were positive and for those at high risk for infection during pregnancy. Infants should not be discharged from the hospital unless the syphilis status of the mother has been determined at least once during pregnancy and preferably again at delivery.

3. Serologic testing for hepatitis B surface antigen (HBsAg) should be performed at the first prenatal visit, even if the woman has been previously vaccinated or tested. Women who were not screened prenatally, those who are at high risk for infection (multiple sexual partners, intravenous drug use, HBsAg-positive sex partner) and those with clinical hepatitis should be retested at the time of delivery.

4. A maternal genital culture for *C. trachomatis* should be performed at the first prenatal visit. Young women (<25 yr) and those at increased risk for infection (new or multiple partners during pregnancy) should be retested during the third trimester.

5. A maternal culture for *Neisseria gonorrhoeae* should be performed at the first prenatal visit. Those at high risk for infection should be retested in the third trimester.

6. All pregnant women at high risk for hepatitis C infection (intravenous drug use, blood transfusion or organ transplantation before 1992) should be screened for hepatitis C antibodies at the first prenatal visit.

7. Evidence does not support routine testing for bacterial vaginosis in pregnancy. For asymptomatic women at high risk for preterm delivery, testing may be considered. Symptomatic women should be tested and treated.

8. The CDC recommends universal screening for rectovaginal GBS colonization of all pregnant women at 35-37 wk gestation, and a screening-based approach to selective intrapartum antibiotic prophylaxis against GBS (Table 129.12) (see Figs. 211.2 and 211.3). Fig. 211.4 shows the approach to the infant born after intrapartum prophylaxis (see Chapter 211).

Bibliography is available at Expert Consult.

Table 129.11	Management and Prevention of Neonatal Sepsis	
CONDITION	**THERAPY**	**ADDITIONAL CONSIDERATIONS**
EMPIRICAL MANAGEMENT		
Early-onset sepsis	Ampicillin + aminoglycoside 10 days for bacteremia; 14 days for GBS and uncomplicated meningitis; extend to 21-28 days for complicated infections	Consider a third-generation cephalosporin (cefotaxime preferred) or carbapenem for meningitis. Tailor therapy to pathogen. Consider discontinuation of therapy if pathogen not isolated.
Late-onset sepsis	Vancomycin + aminoglycoside Duration dependent on pathogen and site	Alternatives to vancomycin may be considered based on local epidemiology and clinical presentation. Aminoglycoside-based regimen preferred to cephalosporin given reduced risk of resistance. Consider cephalosporin if meningitis suspected. Consider a carbapenem if third-generation cephalosporin recently received. Consider amphotericin for fungal etiologies. Tailor therapy to pathogen. Consider discontinuation of therapy if pathogen not isolated.
NONANTIMICROBIAL TREATMENT STRATEGIES		
Recombinant G-CSF Recombinant GM-CSF	Enhance neutrophil number and function, but no reduction in infection when administered as prophylaxis or improvement in survival when administered as therapy.	Insufficient evidence to support the clinical use of G-CSF or GM-CSF either as treatment or prophylaxis to prevent systemic infections.
IVIG	Augments antibody-dependent cytotoxicity and improves neutrophilic function, *but* no evidence that IVIG in suspected or proven sepsis reduces death.	Insufficient evidence from 10 RCTs or quasi-RCTs to support use in neonates with confirmed or suspected sepsis.
PREVENTION STRATEGIES		
IAP	Administration of penicillin or ampicillin 4 hr before parturition	Successfully reduces rates of EOS caused by GBS No effect on LOS GBS
Fluconazole prophylaxis	Administration of weight-based dosing to neonates <1,500 g	Most beneficial in NICUs with high baseline rates of invasive candidiasis
BLF supplementation with a probiotic, *Lactobacillus rhamnosus* (GG)	BLF is a human milk glycoprotein with a role in innate immune response. LGG enhances the activity of lactoferrin.	BLF supplementation with and without LGG reduced the incidence of 1st LOS in 472 VLBW neonates in large randomized, double-blind RCT. Additional confirmatory studies warranted.

BLF, Bovine lactoferrin supplementation; EOS, early-onset sepsis; GBS, group B streptococcus; G-CSF, granulocyte colony-stimulating factor; GM-CSF, granulocyte-macrophage colony-stimulating factor; IAP, intrapartum antimicrobial prophylaxis; IVIG, intravenous immune globulin, LGG, *Lactobacillus rhamnosus* GG; LOS, late-onset sepsis; NICUs, neonatal intensive care units; RCTs, randomized controlled trials; VLBW, very-low-birthweight.
    Created with data from Carr R, Modi N, Doré C: G-CSF and GM-CSF for treating or preventing neonatal infections, *Cochrane Database Syst Rev* (3):CD003066, 2003; Brocklehurst P, Farrell B, King A, et al; INIS Collaborative Group: Treatment of neonatal sepsis with intravenous immune globulin, *N Engl J Med* 365:1201–1211, 2011; and Manzoni P, Decembrino L, Stolfi I, et al; Italian Task Force for the Study and Prevention of Neonatal Fungal Infections; Italian Society of Neonatology: Lactoferrin and prevention of late-onset sepsis in the pre-term neonates, *Early Hum Dev* 86(Suppl 1):59–61, 2010.
    Used with permission from Shane AL, Stoll BJ. Recent developments and current issues in the epidemiology, diagnosis, and management of bacterial and fungal neonatal sepsis. *Am J Perinatol* 30(2):131–141, 2013.

Table 129.12	Indications for Intrapartum Antibiotic Prophylaxis to Prevent Early-Onset GBS Disease
INTRAPARTUM GBS PROPHYLAXIS INDICATED	**INTRAPARTUM GBS PROPHYLAXIS NOT INDICATED**
Previous infant with invasive GBS disease	Colonization with GBS during a previous pregnancy (unless an indication for GBS prophylaxis is present for current pregnancy)
GBS bacteriuria during any trimester of the current pregnancy	GBS bacteriuria during previous pregnancy (unless another indication for GBS prophylaxis is present for current pregnancy)
Positive GBS screening culture during current pregnancy (unless a cesarean delivery is performed before onset of labor or amniotic membrane rupture)	Cesarean delivery before onset of labor or amniotic membrane rupture, regardless of GBS colonization status or gestational age
Unknown GBS status at the onset of labor (culture not done, incomplete, or results unknown) and any of the following: Delivery at <37 weeks' gestation* Amniotic membrane rupture ≥18 hr Intrapartum temperature ≥38.0°C (100.4°F)[†] Intrapartum NAAT[‡] positive for GBS	Negative vaginal and rectal GBS screening culture in late gestation during the current pregnancy, regardless of intrapartum risk factors

*Recommendations for the use of intrapartum antibiotics for prevention of early-onset GBS disease in the setting of threatened preterm delivery are presented in Chapter 211.
    [†]If amnionitis is suspected, broad-spectrum antibiotic therapy that includes an agent known to be active against GBS should replace GBS prophylaxis.
    [‡]If intrapartum NAAT is negative for GBS but any other intrapartum risk factor (delivery at <37 wk gestation, amniotic membrane rupture ≥18 hr, or temperature ≥38.0°C/100.4°F) is present, intrapartum antibiotic prophylaxis is indicated.
    GBS, Group B streptococcus; NAAT, nucleic acid amplification test.
    From Verani J, McGee L, Schrag S: Prevention of perinatal group B streptococcal disease—revised guidelines from CDC, 2010, *MMWR Recomm Rep* 59(RR-10): 1–36, 2010.

Chapter **130**
Healthcare-Acquired Infections

David B. Haslam

第一百三十章
医院获得性感染

中文导读

本章主要介绍了新生儿的医院获得性感染，早产儿及低出生体重儿因免疫系统发育不完善、留置导管及气管内插管等侵入性操作时间长等原因，更易发生医院获得性感染。医院获得性感染可以导致患儿住院时间的延长、治疗费用的增加以及死亡率增加。本章

介绍了院内感染的发病率、流行病学及发病机制，详细介绍了各类型医院获得性感染，如与中心静脉相关的血流感染、医院获得性肺炎、皮肤软组织感染、侵袭性真菌感染和病毒感染的临床特点及预防策略。

Premature and very-low-birthweight (VLBW) infants often have prolonged hospitalizations and are particularly prone to healthcare-acquired infection (**HAI**) because of their inefficient innate immunity, deficient skin barriers, presence of indwelling catheters and other devices, and prolonged endotracheal intubation (Table 130.1). HAIs are associated with increased length of hospitalization, increased cost of care, and significant morbidity and mortality.

INCIDENCE

The most common HAIs in the neonatal intensive care unit (NICU) are bloodstream infections, predominantly central line–associated bloodstream infections. Ventilator-associated pneumonia (VAP) is the next most common, followed by surgical site infection and catheter-associated urinary tract infection.

Approximately 11% of NICU patients develop nosocomial infection during their hospitalization; up to 25% of VLBW infants will have blood culture–proven sepsis during their hospitalization. Infection rates are highest among the most premature infants. Ventilator-associated pneumonia accounts for approximately 25% of HAIs.

EPIDEMIOLOGY

HAIs in the NICU are predominantly caused by gram-positive organisms. The largest fraction of **bloodstream infections (BSIs)** in the NICU are caused by coagulase-negative staphylococci (Table 130.2). Other agents that often cause HAIs in the newborn include *Staphylococcus aureus*, enterococci, gram-negative bacilli (*Escherichia coli, Klebsiella pneumoniae, Enterobacter* spp., *Pseudomonas aeruginosa*), and *Candida*. Viruses contributing to HAIs in the neonate include rotavirus, enteroviruses, hepatitis A virus (HAV), adenoviruses, influenza, respiratory syncytial virus (RSV), rhinovirus, parainfluenza, and herpes simplex virus (HSV).

Bacteria responsible for most cases of nosocomial **pneumonia** typically include staphylococcal species, gram-negative enteric aerobes, and occasionally, *P. aeruginosa*. Fungi are responsible for an increasing number of systemic infections, usually acquired during prolonged hospitalization of preterm neonates. Respiratory viruses cause isolated cases and outbreaks of nosocomial pneumonia. These viruses, usually endemic during the winter months and acquired from infected hospital staff or visitors to the nursery, include RSV, parainfluenza virus, influenza viruses, and adenovirus.

PATHOGENESIS

Colonization of the skin, oropharynx, or gastrointestinal (GI) tract is an important precursor to infection in hospitalized infants. Premature infants may first be exposed to pathogenic organisms from a parent or more frequently from the hospital environment. Hospitalized infants are more likely to be colonized with *Staphylococcus aureus*, pathogenic gram-negative bacteria, and *Candida* than are infants in the community setting. Antibiotic exposure, indwelling devices, and frequent contact with contaminated medical equipment or healthcare providers all likely contribute to high rates of pathogen colonization. Following colonization, organisms may gain access to the bloodstream directly through damaged skin or central venous catheters. Recent evidence suggests the intestine is an important reservoir for invasive organisms, which may transit directly from the gut to the bloodstream. Oropharyngeal colonization with subsequent aspiration into the lower respiratory tract is thought to be the major route of infection in infants with ventilator-associated pneumonia.

Gestational age and birthweight are the most important risk factors for HAI. Prolonged use of central venous or umbilical catheters, exposure to broad-spectrum antibiotics, parenteral nutrition, and high nurse-to-

Table 130.1	Definitions of Healthcare-Acquired Infections for Patients <12 Mo Old*

NOSOCOMIAL BLOODSTREAM INFECTIONS

Laboratory-Confirmed Bloodstream Infection (LCBI)

Must meet 1 of the following definitions:

- Recognized pathogen in 1 or more blood specimens (culture-based or non–culture-based microbiologic methods), performed for clinical diagnostic or therapeutic purposes *and* not related to infection at another site.
- Commensal organism (e.g., coagulase-negative staphylococci, diphtheroids, bacillus, viridans streptococci, aerococcus, micrococcus, propionibacterium), identified from 2 or more blood specimens obtained on separate instances (culture- or non–culture-based microbiologic methods), performed for clinical diagnostic or therapeutic purposes *and* not related to infection at another site *and* at least 1 of the following signs: (1) fever (temperature >38.0°C), (2) hypothermia (temperature <36.0°C), or (3) apnea or bradycardia.

Central Line–Associated Bloodstream Infection (CLABSI)

- LCBI (as defined above) *and*
- Central line or umbilical catheter in place for >2 days *and*
- Central line in place on day of or day before CLABSI diagnosis.

Pneumonia

- Two or more serial chest radiographs with new/progressive and persistent infiltrate, cavitation, consolidation, or pneumatoceles for patients with underlying pulmonary or cardiac disease (respiratory distress syndrome, bronchopulmonary dysplasia, pulmonary edema) *or* 1 chest radiograph with the aforementioned abnormalities for patients without underlying pulmonary or cardiac disease *and*
- Worsening gas exchange *and*
- At least 3 of the following; (1) temperature instability; (2) white blood cell count <4,000/μL or >15,000/μL with 10% or more bands, (3) new-onset purulent sputum, change in character of sputum, increased respiratory secretions, or increased suctioning requirements; (4) physical examination findings consistent with increased work of breathing or apnea, wheezing, rales, or rhonchi; (5) cough; (6) bradycardia (<100 beats/min), and (7) tachycardia (>170 beats/min).

Ventilator-Associated Pneumonia (VAP)

- Pneumonia (as defined above) *and*
- Patient on ventilator for >2 days *and*
- Ventilator in place on day of or day before VAP diagnosis

URINARY TRACT INFECTION

Symptomatic Urinary Tract Infection (SUTI)

- At least 1 of the following symptoms: (1) fever (temperature >38.0°C), (2) hypothermia (temperature <36.0°C), (3) apnea, (4) bradycardia, (5) lethargy, (6) vomiting, or (7) suprapubic tenderness *and*
- Urine culture with no more than 2 species identified, at least 1 of which is present at >10⁵ CFU/mL.

Asymptomatic Bacteremic Urinary Tract Infection (ABUTI)

- Urine culture with no more than 2 species identified, at least 1 of which is present at >10⁵ CFU/mL *and*
- Bacteria identified in blood (culture-based or nonculture-based microbiologic method) that matches at least one of the bacteria present at more than 10⁵ CFU/mL in urine.

Catheter–Associated Urinary Tract Infection:

- Urinary tract infection (as defined above, either SUTI or ABUTI) *and*
- Indwelling urinary catheter for >2 days *and*
- Urinary catheter in place on day of or day before urinary tract infection diagnosis.

*Centers for Disease Control and Prevention/National Healthcare Safety Network.
CFU, Colony-forming units.
Adapted from Horan TC, Andrus M, Dudeck MA. CDC/NHSN surveillance definition of health care–associated infection and criteria for specific types of infections in the acute care setting, *Am J Infect Control* 36:309–332, 2008.

Table 130.2	Distribution of Organisms Responsible for Late-Onset Sepsis		
	VLBW INFANTS: NICHD NRN (%)		
ORGANISM	**1991–1993**	**1998–2000**	**2002–2008**
Incidence of late-onset sepsis	25	21	25
GRAM POSITIVE			
Staphylococcus, coagulase-negative	55	48	53
Staphylococcus aureus	9	8	11
Enterococcus/group D streptococcus	5	3	4
Group B streptococcus	2	2	2
Other	2	9	7
GRAM NEGATIVE			
Enterobacter	4	3	3
Escherichia coli	4	5	5
Klebsiella	4	4	4
Pseudomonas	2	3	2
Other	4	1	2
Fungi			
Candida albicans	5	6	5
Candida parapsilosis			
Other	2	2	1

VLBW, Very-low-birthweight (≤1,500 g); NICHD NRN, National Institutes of Child Health and Human Development Neonatal Research Network.
Data from (1) 1991–1993: Stoll BJ, Gordon T, Korones SB, et al: Late-onset sepsis in very low birth weight neonates: a report from the NICHD NRN, *J Pediatr* 129:63–71, 1996; (2) 1998–2000: Stoll BJ, Hansen N, Fanaroff AA, et al: Late-onset sepsis in very low birth weight neonates: the experience of the NICHD NRN, *Pediatrics* 110:285–291, 2002; (3) 2002–2008: Boghossian NS, Page GP, Bell EF, et al: Late-onset sepsis in very low birth weight infants from singleton and multiple gestation births, J Pediatr 162:1120–1120, 2015.
Adapted from Ramasethu J. Prevention and treatment of neonatal nosocomial infections, *Matern Health Neonatol Perinatol* 3(5), 2017.

patient ratios are other documented risk factors. These factors may alter the patient's endogenous microbial community, placing the infant at risk for colonization with pathogenic organisms.

TYPES OF INFECTION

Central Line–Associated Bloodstream Infection

Central venous catheters have become an essential component of the care of critically ill newborns. Presence of a percutaneous or umbilical catheter introduces risk for infection and thrombosis. Central line–associated bloodstream infection (**CLABSI**) is the most common HAI in NICUs, imposing significant burden on the affected infant and on healthcare systems. Each episode has an attributable mortality of 4–20%. Infants with CLABSI subsequently have increased requirement for NICU stay, mechanical ventilation, and increased rates of bronchopulmonary dysplasia and necrotizing enterocolitis. The median estimated additional cost per CLABSI episode is $42,609, and hospitalization is prolonged for a median of 24 days.

Coagulase-negative staphylococci (CoNS) are the most common cause of CLABSI, accounting for approximately half of cases. CoNS are much more likely to cause clinically evident sepsis in VLBW infants than in term infants of comparable postnatal age, despite the organism's low pathogenic potential. Isolation of the organism from blood culture may represent contamination from the infant's or healthcare worker's skin, and blood cultures should be obtained from both peripheral and central venous sites. If both yield CoNS, the likelihood of true infection is high, whereas a single positive is considered questionable. In practice, often a single culture is obtained, and antibiotics are initiated before availability of a 2nd culture. In this circumstance, clinical judgment is often used to assess the need for targeted therapy. *S. aureus, Enterococcus* spp., and gram-negative rods account for most of the remaining CLABSIs during the 1st mo of hospitalization. Thereafter, *Candida* spp. become more prevalent, caused at least in part by their enrichment after broad-spectrum antibiotic exposure.

CLABSIs are generally thought to result from contamination of the central venous catheter, predominantly at the connecting hub or the skin entry site. An association has been shown between density of hub colonization and risk for CLABSI. Prevention of CLABSI is aimed at reducing contamination of these sites. BSI may also result from direct transit from the GI tract or other cutaneous or mucosal surfaces, analogous to recently defined **mucosal barrier injury–associated** BSIs. The contribution of mucosal sites to direct invasive infection remains to be clarified but has implications for infection prevention.

Healthcare-Associated Pneumonia

Ventilator-associated pneumonia (VAP) is overall the 2nd most common HAI in neonatal units, although reported VAP rates vary widely (0.2-1.6 per 1,000 ventilator days). There is also variability in diagnosis of VAP, which consists of clinical, radiographic, and laboratory criteria, some of which are subjective or may be seen in noninfectious circumstances. The National Healthcare Safety Network and Centers for Disease Control and Prevention (CDC) definition of VAP requires at least 48 hr of mechanical ventilation accompanied by new and persistent radiographic infiltrates after the initiation of mechanical ventilation. In addition to these criteria, infants <1 yr old must exhibit worsening gas exchange and at least 3 of the following: (1) temperature instability with no other recognized cause; (2) leukopenia (white blood cell count <4,000/mm^3); (3) change in the character of sputum of increased respiratory secretions or suctioning requirements; (4) apnea, tachypnea, nasal flaring, or grunting; (5) wheezing, rales, rhonchi, or cough; or (6) bradycardia (<100 beats/min) or tachycardia (>170 beats/min). In practice, the diagnosis is often made on the basis of increased need for supplemental oxygen or new infiltrates on chest radiograph; either of which may be caused by factors other than infection. Further complicating the diagnosis of VAP, secretions aspirated from the airways of mechanically ventilated children often yield multiple organisms in culture, whether or not they have signs of infection. The most commonly reported organisms associated with VAP are gram-negative rods (including *Pseudomonas*), *S. aureus*, and *Enterococcus*. The source of infecting organisms is generally thought to be the infant's oropharynx, although contaminated respiratory equipment and tracheal suction catheters are occasionally implicated.

Skin and Soft Tissue Infection

Cutaneous infections are relatively common among hospitalized premature infants. Simple abrasions of frail skin, frequent vascular access, and surgical procedures predispose the skin to infection. *Staphylococcus aureus* is the most frequently isolated organism. **Methicillin-susceptible S. aureus (MSSA)** predominates despite increases in **methicillin-resistant S. aureus (MRSA)** infection rates during the last 2 decades. Gram-negative organisms and *Candida* spp. may occasionally be seen, particularly after intraabdominal surgery.

Invasive Fungal Infection

Up to 3% of extremely-low-birthweight (ELBW) and 20% of extremely-low-birthweight (ELBW) infants will develop invasive fungal infection, with a cumulative incidence of 1–4% of all NICU admissions (see Chapter 261.1). Colonization, a requisite for subsequent infection is common after the 1st wk of hospitalization and is seen in >60% of infants at 1 mo in the NICU. *Candida albicans* accounts for most cases of colonization and infection, although *C. parapsilosis* and *C. glabrata* are prevalent in some NICUs. As with other BSIs, invasive candidiasis is often central venous catheter associated. In addition to gestational age and birthweight, risk factors include exposure to ≥2 antibiotics, receipt of H$_2$ blockers, parenteral nutrition (especially use of lipid emulsifiers), lack of enteral feeding, and GI surgery. Invasive candidiasis is associated with greater morbidity and mortality than invasive bacterial infection, with mortality rates >20% and long term developmental abnormalities seen in >50% of surviving infants.

Viral Infection

Nosocomially acquired viral infections receive less attention than invasive bacterial or fungal infections but can account for significant morbidity.

Approximately 10% of reported episodes in NICUs are caused by viruses. The most common viral agent is **rotavirus**, followed by RSV, enterovirus, HAV, adenovirus, and influenza. Consistent with the viral etiology, GI illness is the most frequently reported virus-associated condition. In most cases of viral infection in the NICU, the source cannot be identified, making it difficult to focus preventive efforts. Response to viral outbreaks in the NICU can include enhanced patient surveillance, patient cohorting, and occasionally, closure of the affected patient care area.

PREVENTION
Hand Hygiene

Hand hygiene is the single most important intervention proven to prevent nosocomial infections, whereas *lack* of hand hygiene is one of the strongest correlates of HAI. Colonization with pathogenic organisms is known to increase with longer time spent performing patient interactions. The CDC and the World Health Organization have published guidelines on timing and choice of sanitizing agent during patient care (Table 130.3). Alcohol-based hand sanitizers are at least as effective as chlorhexidine-containing soaps in decreasing bacterial burden but have poor activity against certain important pathogens, including *Clostridium difficile*, HAV, rotavirus, enterovirus, and adenovirus. Time constraints and workload are considered important barriers to adequate hand care, and recent evidence suggests that shortening the application time of alcohol-based sanitizers to 15 sec may improve frequency of use without impacting antimicrobial efficacy. Observational studies suggest that monitoring with personal or group-level feedback is among the most effective means to improve hand hygiene compliance.

Central Line–Associated Bloodstream Infection

Hand hygiene is the most important intervention to prevent CLABSI in the NICU. "Care bundles" have been studied in numerous neonatal populations and found to reduce catheter-related infection. **Insertion bundles** include a combination of barrier precaution, hand hygiene standards, skin disinfection, dedicated teams and equipment, catheter site evaluation, checklists, and empowerment to stop the procedure. **Maintenance bundles** include recommendations for aseptic technique when accessing the line, dressing change protocols, and prompt removal when the line is no longer required (Table 130.4).

Ventilator-Associated Pneumonia

VAP prevention bundles have been applied to adult patients but are not readily adapted to premature infants. Thus far, few studies have demonstrated efficacy of infection control measures in preventing VAP in NICUs. A number of measures are believed to be helpful, including caregiver education, hand hygiene, donning of gloves when in contact with secretions, minimizing days of ventilation to the extent possible, suctioning the oropharynx, and removing condensate from the ventilator circuit.

Early Feeding and Human Milk

Several studies have demonstrated benefit to feeding infants maternal milk. Enteral feeding of human milk within 2-3 days of life is associated with decreased rates of necrotizing enterocolitis and nosocomial infection. Human milk contains a number of factors thought to contribute to beneficial effects, including secretory antibody, lactoferrin, phagocytes, and oligosaccharides that shape the neonatal microbial community. Interestingly, the benefits of human milk are not as evident when the milk comes from a donor other than the infant's mother, suggesting important compositional differences in maternal milk.

Antifungal Prophylaxis

Prophylactic administration of **fluconazole** during the 1st 6 wk of life reduces fungal colonization and invasive fungal infection in ELBW infants (<1000 g). In addition to the individual benefit afforded by prophylaxis for VLBW neonates, fluconazole prophylaxis may have a community impact by decreasing the overall fungal burden of a NICU. Results from more than 14 trials at multiple institutions with 3,100 neonates suggests that fluconazole prophylaxis decreases colonization of the urine, GI tract, and integument, without promoting the

Table 130.3	U.S. Centers for Disease Control and Prevention (CDC) Guidelines for Hand Hygiene

- When hands are visibly dirty or contaminated with proteinaceous material or are visibly soiled with blood or other body fluids, wash hands with either a nonantimicrobial soap and water or an antimicrobial soap and water (categorization of recommendation: IA)
- If hands are not visibly soiled, use an alcohol-based hand rub for routinely decontaminating hands in all other clinical situations described below (categorization of recommendation: IA). Alternatively, wash hands with an antimicrobial soap and water in all clinical situations described below (categorization of recommendation: IB).
- Decontaminate hands before having direct contact with patients (categorization of recommendation: IB).
- Decontaminate hands before donning sterile gloves when inserting an intravascular catheter (categorization of recommendation: IB).
- Decontaminate hands before inserting indwelling urinary catheters, peripheral vascular catheters, or other invasive devices that do not require a surgical procedure (categorization of recommendation: IB).
- Decontaminate hands after contact with a patient's intact skin (categorization of recommendation: IB).
- Decontaminate hands after contact with body fluids or excretions, mucous membranes, nonintact skin, and wound dressings if hands are not visibly soiled (categorization of recommendation: IB).
- Decontaminate hands if moving from a contaminated body site to a clean body site during patient care (categorization of recommendation: II).
- Decontaminate hands after contact with inanimate objects (including medical equipment) in the immediate vicinity of the patient (categorization of recommendation: II).
- Decontaminate hands after removing gloves (categorization of recommendation: IB).
- Before eating and after using a restroom, wash hands with a nonantimicrobial soap and water or with antimicrobial soap and water (categorization of recommendation: IB).
- Antimicrobial-impregnated wipes may be considered as an alternative to washing hands with nonantimicrobial soap and water. Because they are not as effective as alcohol-based hand rubs or washing hands with an antimicrobial soap and water for reducing bacterial counts on the hands of healthcare workers, they are not a substitute for hand antisepsis (categorization of recommendation: IB).
- Wash hands with nonantimicrobial soap and water or with antimicrobial soap and water if exposure to *Bacillus anthracis* is suspected or proven (categorization of recommendation: II).
- No recommendation can be made regarding the routine use of non–alcohol-based hand rubs for hand hygiene in healthcare settings. Unresolved issue.

CDC/Healthcare Infection Control Practices Advisory Committee System for Categorizing Recommendations

Category IA: Strongly recommended for implementation and strongly supported by well-designed experimental, clinical, or epidemiologic studies.

Category IB: Strongly recommended for implementation and supported by certain experimental, clinical, or epidemiologic studies and using theoretical rationale.

Category IC: Required for implementation, as mandated by federal or state regulation or standard.

Category II: Suggested for implementation and supported by suggestive clinical or epidemiologic studies or a theoretic rationale.

No recommendation; Unresolved issue: Practices for which insufficient evidence or no consensus regarding efficacy exists.

Adapted from Boyce JM, Pittet D; Healthcare Infection Control Practices Advisory Committee: Guideline for hand hygiene in health-care settings: recommendations of the Healthcare Infection Control Practices Advisory Committee and the HIPAC/SHEA/APIC/IDSA Hand Hygiene Task Force, *Am J Infect Control* 30(8):S1–S46, 2002.

Table 130.4	Interventions to Prevent Catheter-Related Infections

- Perform effective hand hygiene before and after any interaction with the catheter.
- Use sterile gowns, gloves, drapes, cap, and mask during catheter insertion.
- Disinfect skin with appropriate agent (chlorhexidine is most often used in United States; other disinfectants may be as effective).
- Use a transparent, semipermeable dressing to cover catheter site.
- Change the dressing when soiled or loose.
- Scrub access point with alcoholic chlorhexidine for at least 15 sec.
- Use aseptic nontouch technique to access the catheter.
- Change administration sets no more frequently than 96 hr unless required by the infused product.
- Avoid use of systemic prophylactic antibiotics for catheter insertion.
- Evaluate daily, and remove central venous catheter when no longer required.
- Ensure all healthcare professionals who interact with the patient are educated on central line management.

Adapted from Taylor JE, McDonald SJ, Tan K: Prevention of central venous catheter–related infection in the neonatal unit: a literature review, *J Matern Fetal Neonatal Med* 28(10):1224–1230, 2015.

development of resistance and without adverse effects. Based on an annual U.S. preterm birth cohort of approximately 30,000 VLBW infants, fluconazole prophylaxis could prevent an estimated 2,000-3,000 cases of invasive candidiasis, 200-300 deaths, and the adverse neurodevelopmental outcomes of invasive candidiasis in 400-500 infants per year. Differing baseline rates of fungal infections, practices related to central venous catheter removal, severity of illness, and administration practices for broad-spectra antimicrobials make universal recommendations regarding prophylaxis challenging. A meta-analysis using patient-level data found that fluconazole prophylaxis was effective at preventing colonization and invasive *Candida* infection and was not associated with adverse drug reactions or increased rates of fluconazole resistance.

Neonatal practices that may reduce the risks of invasive candidiasis include limited use of broad-spectrum antimicrobials, use of an aminoglycoside instead of a cephalosporin for empirical therapy when meningitis or antimicrobial resistance is not suspected, limitation of postnatal corticosteroid use in VLBW infants, early enteral feeding, and establishment of the neonatal gut microbiome with human milk feeding.

Nasal Decolonization

Staphylococcus aureus is the 2nd most common cause of HAI in neonatal units. MSSA generally causes more invasive infections than MRSA, but most prevention efforts have been focused on MRSA. Several studies have documented MRSA transmission within the NICU and have identified nasal colonization as an important risk factor for subsequent invasive infection. Various measures have been implemented in attempt to decrease transmission and invasive infection, including contact precautions, cohorting and isolation, and **nasal decolonization** with **mupirocin**. Contact precautions have been associated with decreased rates of MRSA infection in NICU patients. Studies in other patient populations (predominantly adults undergoing peritoneal dialysis) found increased rates of gram-negative infection in those receiving mupirocin treatment. However, a recent multicenter study of mupirocin use in the NICU found a 64% decrease in gram-positive infections, with no change in gram-negative infection rates, among 384 treated infants.

Bibliography is available at Expert Consult.

Chapter **131**

Congenital and Perinatal Infections

Felicia A. Scaggs Huang
and Rebecca C. Brady

第一百三十一章
先天性和围生期感染

中文导读

感染是导致新生儿发病率和死亡率增加的常见和重要原因，先天性或宫内感染（即通过胎盘传播的感染）和围产期感染（即在分娩过程中从母亲传播给胎儿或新生儿的感染）是新生儿感染的两大途径。这涉及产科和新生儿科两大学科的内容。本章从产前管理、到出生时产房处理、到出生后早期即围产期的感染管理角度，分别详细介绍了几项主要的新生儿先天性或宫内感染及围产期感染的病因、发病机制、临床表现以及诊断策略。

Infections are a frequent and important cause of neonatal morbidity and mortality. **Congenital** or **intrauterine** infections (i.e., those transmitted across the placenta) and **perinatal** infections (i.e., those transmitted from the mother to the fetus or newborn infant during the birth process) represent 2 major routes of neonatal infection.

131.1 Congenital Infections

Felicia A. Scaggs Huang and Rebecca C. Brady

As many as 2% of fetuses are infected in utero; disease can be acquired prenatally from a wide variety of etiologic agents, including bacteria, viruses, fungi, and protozoa. Clinical manifestations can range from asymptomatic or subclinical to life-threatening disease. History and physical examination findings provide insight into the best approach for this immunologically immature population. (See Fig. 129.2 and Table 129.2 in Chapter 129.)

GENERAL APPROACH

Infectious as well as noninfectious processes, such as underlying congenital heart disease, genetic disorders, and inborn errors of metabolism, should be considered in the differential diagnosis of congenital and perinatal infections. Because maternal infection is a prerequisite for infection in the fetus, a thorough history is essential to assess the mother for her symptoms, travel, diet, medication use, occupational exposures, and any **sexually transmitted infections (STIs)** during pregnancy. Clinical manifestations are varied and overlap for many of the pathogens causing intrauterine infection. Laboratory testing and/or radiologic imaging is often required to confirm the diagnosis. Treatment depends on the specific pathogen and can range from symptomatic management with close follow-up for long-term sequelae to targeted antimicrobial therapy.

PATHOGENESIS

The route and timing of infection can provide helpful clues as to the potential infectious etiology (Fig. 131.1 and Table 131.1). First-trimester infection may alter embryogenesis and result in malformations of the heart and eyes, as seen in congenital rubella syndrome. Third-trimester infection (e.g., congenital toxoplasmosis) can result in active infection with signs of hepatomegaly, splenomegaly, and generalized lymphadenopathy at birth. Infections that occur late in gestation (e.g., congenital syphilis) may lead to a delay in clinical manifestations until weeks to years after birth.

Intrauterine infection from cytomegalovirus (CMV), *Treponema pallidum*, *Toxoplasma gondii*, rubella virus, varicella-zoster virus (VZV), and human parvovirus B19 may cause minimal or no symptoms in the mother but still may be transmitted across the placenta to the fetus. The presence of maternal antibodies to rubella prevents infection, but transmission of CMV can occur despite preexisting antibodies. Regardless of the mother's immune status, the placenta may act as a barrier, and the fetus may or may not be infected. If infection occurs, signs may or may not be noted in the fetus during pregnancy. Infection can result in spontaneous abortion, congenital malformation, intrauterine growth restriction (IUGR), premature birth, stillbirth, acute or delayed disease in the neonate, or asymptomatic persistent infection with sequelae later in life.

CLINICAL MANIFESTATIONS

The clinical manifestations of intrauterine infections can range from asymptomatic to severe multiorgan system complications. For some agents (e.g., CMV, *T. pallidum*), ongoing injury after birth leads to late sequelae. The specific clinical signs in the newborn period are usually not sufficient to make a definitive diagnosis but are useful to guide more specific laboratory testing. Symptomatic congenital infections often affect the central nervous system (CNS; brain and eyes) and the reticuloendothelial system (RES; bone marrow, liver, and spleen). Table 131.2 presents the clinical manifestations of some specific congenital infections. Congenital Zika virus infection has features that are rarely seen with other congenital infections (Table 131.3). No hematologic or hepatic laboratory abnormalities have been documented in infants with congenital Zika virus infection. Table 131.4 provides late sequelae of some congenital infections.

DIAGNOSIS
During Pregnancy

The presence of IUGR or a physical abnormality on a prenatal fetal ultrasound raises concern for a congenital infection. The well-known acronym **TORCH**—***Toxoplasma gondii***, **O**ther (*Treponema pallidum*, human parvovirus B19, HIV, Zika virus, others), **R**ubella, **C**ytomegalovirus, and **H**erpes simplex virus (HSV)—is a useful mnemonic. However, the routine ordering of TORCH serology panels is *not* recommended because the presence of a TORCH agent IgG antibody in the mother indicates past infection but does not establish if the infection occurred during pregnancy. Maternal IgM titers to *specific* pathogens are only moderately sensitive, and a negative result cannot be used to exclude infection.

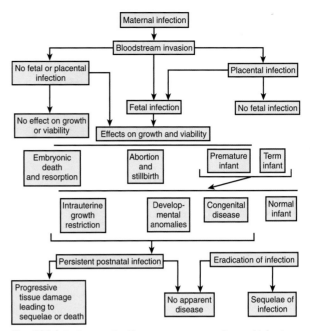

Fig. 131.1 Pathogenesis of hematogenous transplacental infections. *(Adapted from Klein JO, Remington JS: Current concepts of infections of the fetus and newborn infant. In Remington JS, Klein JO, editors: Infectious diseases of the fetus and newborn infant, ed 5, Philadelphia, 2002, Saunders.)*

Table 131.1	Specific Agents in Effects of Transplacental Fetal Infection on the Fetus and Newborn Infant

| | | DISEASE | | | |
ORGANISM	Prematurity	Intrauterine Growth Restriction/Low Birthweight	Developmental Anomalies	Congenital Disease	Persistent Postnatal Infection
Viruses	CMV HSV Rubeola Smallpox HBV HIV*	CMV Rubella VZV* HIV*	CMV Rubella VZV Coxsackievirus B* HIV* Zika	CMV Rubella VZV HSV Mumps* Rubeola Vaccinia Smallpox Coxsackievirus B Poliovirus HBV HIV LCV Parvovirus	CMV Rubella VZV HSV HBV HIV Zika
Bacteria	Treponema pallidum Mycobacterium tuberculosis Listeria monocytogenes Campylobacter fetus Salmonella typhi			T. pallidum M. tuberculosis L. monocytogenes C. fetus S. typhi Borrelia burgdorferi	T. pallidum M. tuberculosis
Protozoa	Toxoplasma gondii Plasmodium* Trypanosoma cruzi	T. gondii Plasmodium T. cruzi		T. gondii Plasmodium T. cruzi	T. gondii Plasmodium

*Association of effect with infection has been suggested and is under consideration.

CMV, Cytomegalovirus; *HBV*, hepatitis B virus; *HIV*, human immunodeficiency virus; *HSV*, herpes simplex virus; *LCV*, lymphocytic choriomeningitis virus; *VZV*, varicella-zoster virus.

From Maldonado YA, Nizet V, Klein JO, et al: Current concepts of infections of the fetus and newborn infant. In Wilson CB, Nizet V, Maldonado Y, et al, editors: *Remington and Klein's infectious diseases of the fetus and newborn*, ed 8, Philadelphia, 2016, Elsevier (Table 1-5).

| Table 131.2 | Clinical Manifestations of Specific Neonatal Infections Acquired in Utero or at Delivery |

Rubella Virus	Cytomegalovirus	*Toxoplasma gondii*	Herpes Simplex Virus	*Treponema pallidum*	Enteroviruses
Hepatosplenomegaly	Hepatosplenomegaly	Hepatosplenomegaly	Hepatosplenomegaly	Hepatosplenomegaly	Hepatosplenomegaly
Jaundice	Jaundice	Jaundice	Jaundice	Jaundice	Jaundice
Pneumonitis	Pneumonitis	Pneumonitis	Pneumonitis	Pneumonitis	Pneumonitis
Petechiae *or* purpura	Petechiae *or* purpura	Petechiae *or* purpura	Petechiae *or* purpura	Petechiae *or* purpura	Petechiae *or* purpura
Meningoencephalitis	Meningoencephalitis	Meningoencephalitis	Meningoencephalitis	Meningoencephalitis	Meningoencephalitis
Hydrocephalus	Hydrocephalus	Hydrocephalus*	Hydrocephalus	Adenopathy	Adenopathy
Adenopathy	Microcephaly*	Microcephaly	Microcephaly	Maculopapular	Maculopapular
Hearing deficits	Intracranial	Maculopapular	Maculopapular	exanthems*	exanthems
Myocarditis	calcifications*	exanthems	exanthems	Bone lesions*	Paralysis*
Congenital defects*	Hearing deficits	Intracranial	Vesicles*	Glaucoma	Myocarditis*
Bone lesions*	Chorioretinitis or	calcifications*	Myocarditis	Chorioretinitis or	Conjunctivitis or
Glaucoma*	retinopathy	Myocarditis	Chorioretinitis or	retinopathy	keratoconjunctivitis
Chorioretinitis or	Optic atrophy	Bone lesions	retinopathy	Uveitis	
retinopathy*		Chorioretinitis or	Cataracts		
Cataracts*		retinopathy*	Conjunctivitis or		
Microphthalmia		Cataracts	keratoconjunctivitis*		
		Optic atrophy			
		Microphthalmia			
		Uveitis			

*Has special diagnostic significance for this infection
From Maldonado YA, Nizet V, Klein JO, et al: Current concepts of infections of the fetus and newborn infant. In Wilson CB, Nizet V, Maldonado Y, et al, editors: *Remington and Klein's infectious diseases of the fetus and newborn*, ed 8, Philadelphia, 2016, Elsevier (Table 1-6).

In certain cases, a fetal blood sample with cordocentesis can be obtained and tested for total and pathogen-specific IgM assays, polymerase chain reaction assays (PCRs), or cultures. A total IgM concentration is a helpful screening test because a normal fetal IgM is <5 mg/dL, so any elevation in total IgM may indicate an underlying infection. A positive *pathogen-specific* IgM test is strongly suggestive of infection, but a negative test does not rule out the organism as the cause of the fetopathy. Amniotic fluid can also be obtained and sent for PCR or culture. The presence of CMV, *T. gondii*, or human parvovirus B19 in amniotic fluid indicates the fetus likely is infected but cannot establish the severity of disease. Although HSV is included in the TORCH acronym, it is rarely isolated from amniotic fluid and is rarely transmitted across the placenta from mother to fetus. Fetal blood can be collected to test for human parvovirus B19 IgM and PCR.

Newborn Infant

When a congenital infection is suspected because clinical signs are present, a complete blood count with differential and platelet count along with measurements of transaminases and total/direct bilirubin are routinely performed. Additional evaluations may include a dilated funduscopic examination, auditory brainstem response (ABR) for those failing the newborn hearing screen, and CNS imaging. If available, pathologic examination of the placenta may be informative. Infectious diseases consultation is valuable in guiding the evaluation.

Neonatal antibody titers for specific pathogens are often difficult to interpret because IgG is acquired from the mother by transplacental passage, and a positive result may reflect the mother's past infection and *not* infection of the newborn. Neonatal IgM antibody titers to specific pathogens have high specificity and only moderate sensitivity; a negative result cannot be used to exclude infection. Paired maternal and fetal-neonatal IgG antibody titers showing higher or rising infant IgG antibodies can diagnose some congenital infections (e.g., syphilis). Total cord blood IgM and IgA are not actively transported across the placenta to the fetus and are not specific for intrauterine infection.

Although viral culture has long been considered the standard for CMV and other viral infections, PCR is sensitive, specific, and now widely accepted. The Palo Alto Medical Foundation Toxoplasma Serology Laboratory (PAMF-TSL; Palo Alto, CA: www.pamf.org/serology/; telephone: (650) 853-4828; e-mail: toxolab@pamf.org) offers specialized tests and physician experts to aid in the diagnosis of congenital toxoplasmosis. If there is concern for congenital Zika virus infection,

| Table 131.3 | Syndromes in the Neonate Caused by Other Congenital Infections |

ORGANISM	SIGNS
VZV	Limb hypoplasia, cicatricial skin lesions, ocular abnormalities, cortical atrophy
Parvovirus B19	Nonimmune hydrops fetalis
HIV	Severe thrush, failure to thrive, recurrent bacterial infections, calcification of basal ganglia
Zika virus	Microcephaly, lissencephaly, cerebellar hypoplasia, akinesia syndrome, macular scarring, retinal mottling, subcortical calcifications, hypertonia

HIV, Human immunodeficiency virus; *VZV,* varicella-zoster virus.
From Maldonado YA, Nizet V, Klein JO, et al: Current concepts of infections of the fetus and newborn infant. In Wilson CB, Nizet V, Maldonado Y, et al, editors: *Remington and Klein's infectious diseases of the fetus and newborn,* ed 8, Philadelphia, 2016, Elsevier (Table 1-7).

healthcare providers should refer to the Centers for Disease Control and Prevention (CDC) Guidance for US Laboratories Testing for Zika Virus Infection (www.cdc.gov/zika/laboratorie/lab-guidance.html) to assist in collecting and sending appropriate laboratory tests from the mother, newborn infant, placenta, and umbilical cord. Currently, testing for Zika virus with real-time reverse-transcription PCR (rRT-PCR) and IgM enzyme-linked immunosorbent assay (ELISA) from neonatal urine and serum specimens is recommended. However, the most reliable method of testing has not been established. In endemic areas, this workup should be done within 2 days of delivery because it is difficult to distinguish congenital from postnatal infection if testing is done later.

SPECIFIC INFECTIOUS AGENTS

Important congenital infections include more than the TORCH agents. The following is a list of pathogens that may be transmitted across the placenta and the respective chapters where they are discussed in more detail, including treatment.

Bacteria

Listeria monocytogenes (Chapter 215)
Syphilis (*Treponema pallidum*) (Chapter 245)

Table 131.4	Late Sequelae of Intrauterine Infections.			
	INFECTION			
CLINICAL SIGN	**Cytomegalovirus**	**Rubella Virus**	**Toxoplasma gondii**	**Treponema pallidum**
Deafness	+	+	+	+
Dental/skeletal problems	+	+	(−)	+
Mental retardation	+	+	+	+
Seizures	+	+	+	+

+, Present; (−), rare or absent.

Viruses

Cytomegalovirus (Chapter 282)
Hepatitis B (Chapter 385)
Hepatitis C (Chapter 385)
Herpes simplex virus (Chapter 279)
Human immunodeficiency virus (Chapter 302)
Human parvovirus B19 (Chapter 278)
Lymphocytic choriomeningitis virus (Chapter 298)
Rubella (Chapter 274)
Varicella-zoster virus (Chapter 280)
Zika virus (Chapter 294.12)

Parasite

Toxoplasmosis (*Toxoplasma gondii*) (Chapter 316)

131.2 Perinatal Infections

Felicia A. Scaggs Huang and Rebecca C. Brady

Perinatal infections are defined as those that are transmitted from the mother to the fetus or newborn infant during the birth process. Despite recommended universal screening of pregnant women for *Chlamydia trachomatis* and gonorrhea, transmission to the newborn still occurs. In addition to these STIs, other bacteria, viruses, and *Candida* spp. may cause perinatal infections. Similar to congenital infections, their presentation can range from asymptomatic to a sepsis-like syndrome.

GENERAL APPROACH

The general approach is similar to that for congenital infections and includes a detailed maternal history and a careful examination of the newborn (see Chapter 129). Many clinical syndromes overlap, and therefore laboratory testing is usually required to establish a specific microbiologic etiology and guide management decisions.

PATHOGENESIS

The human birth canal is colonized with aerobic and anaerobic bacteria. **Ascending amniotic infection** may occur with either apparently intact membranes or relatively brief duration of membrane rupture. Infectious agents can also be acquired as the newborn infant passes through the vaginal canal. This acquisition may result in either colonization or disease. Factors influencing which colonized infants will experience disease are not well understood but include prematurity, underlying illness, invasive procedures, inoculum size, virulence of the infecting organism, genetic predisposition, the innate immune system, host response, and transplacental maternal antibodies.

Chorioamnionitis has been historically used to refer to microbial invasion of the amniotic fluid, often as a result of prolonged rupture of the chorioamniotic membrane for >18 hr. The term *chorioamnionitis* is confusing because it does not convey the spectrum of inflammatory or infectious diseases, it leaves out other intrauterine components that can be involved (e.g., decidua), and it results in significant variability in clinical practice, with the potential for a significant number of well newborns being exposed to antimicrobial agents. The term **intrauterine**

Table 131.5	Classification of Triple I and Isolated Maternal Fever
TERMINOLOGY	**FEATURES**
Isolated maternal fever	Maternal oral temperature ≥39°C is considered a "documented fever." If the oral temperature is ≥38°C but ≤39°C, repeat the measurement in 30 min. If the repeat value is ≥38°C, it is considered a "documented fever."
Suspected Triple I	Fever without a clear source with *any* of the following: 1. Baseline fetal tachycardia (>160 beats/min for 10 min) 2. Maternal WBC >15,000/mm³ 3. Purulent fluid from the cervical os
Confirmed Triple I	All the above (from suspected Triple I) with *any* of the following: 1. Amniocentesis-proven infection through positive Gram stain 2. Low glucose of amniotic fluid or positive amniotic fluid culture 3. Placental pathology consistent with infection

Triple I, Intrauterine inflammation or infection at birth; WBC, white blood cell count.
Adapted from Higgins RD, Saade G; Chorioamnionitis Workshop participants: Evaluation and management of women and newborns with a maternal diagnosis of chorioamnionitis: summary of a workshop, *Obstet Gynecol* 127(3):426–436, 2016.

inflammation or infection at birth, abbreviated as **Triple I**, has become more accepted because of the heterogeneous nature of conditions that can affect the mother and neonate (Table 131.5). Regardless of the definition used, prematurity (<37 wk) is associated with a greater risk of early-onset sepsis, especially with group B streptococcus.

Aspiration or ingestion of bacteria in amniotic fluid may lead to congenital pneumonia or systemic infection, with manifestations becoming apparent before delivery (fetal distress, tachycardia), at delivery (failure to breathe, respiratory distress, shock), or after a latent period of a few hours (respiratory distress, shock). Aspiration or ingestion of bacteria during the birth process may lead to infection after an interval of 1-2 days.

CLINICAL MANIFESTATIONS

Most perinatal infections present clinically during the 1st mo of life. Initial signs and symptoms may be either nonspecific or focal (see Chapter 129). Additional information on specific infectious agents and their management are reviewed in the chapters indicated below.

SPECIFIC INFECTIOUS AGENTS
Bacteria
Chlamydia trachomatis (Chapter 253)
Escherichia coli (Chapter 227)
Genital mycoplasmas (Chapter 251)
Group B streptococci (Chapter 211)
Neisseria gonorrhoeae (Chapter 219)
Syphilis (*Treponema pallidum*) (Chapter 245)

Viruses

Cytomegalovirus (Chapter 282)
Enteroviruses (Chapter 277)
Hepatitis B (Chapter 385)
Herpes simplex virus (Chapter 279)
Human immunodeficiency virus (Chapter 302)

Fungi

Candida spp. (Chapter 261)

DIAGNOSIS

The maternal history provides important information about maternal exposures to infectious diseases, bacterial colonization, immunity (natural and acquired), and obstetric risk factors (prematurity, prolonged ruptured membranes, chorioamnionitis). STIs acquired by a pregnant woman, including syphilis, *N. gonorrhoeae,* and *C. trachomatis,* have the potential for perinatal transmission.

Neonates with perinatal infections often present with nonspecific symptoms and signs; therefore the general diagnostic evaluation for the ill neonate as discussed in Chapter 202 should be followed. Table 131.6 provides a summary of laboratory tests that are useful to diagnose specific perinatal infections.

Bibliography is available at Expert Consult.

Table 131.6	Laboratory Tests in the Diagnosis of Specific Perinatal Infections	
INFECTIOUS AGENT	**ACCEPTABLE SPECIMEN(S) FROM INFANT UNLESS OTHERWISE INDICATED**	**LABORATORY TEST**
Chlamydia trachomatis	Conjunctiva, nasopharyngeal swab, tracheal aspirate	Culture using special transport media Nucleic acid amplification tests (NAATs) are not FDA-approved for specimens from neonates.*
Genital mycoplasmas (*Mycoplasma hominis, M. genitalium, Ureaplasma urealyticum*)	Tracheal aspirate, blood, or cerebrospinal fluid (CSF)	Culture using special transport media Real-time polymerase chain reactions (PCRs)
Neisseria gonorrhoeae	Conjunctiva, blood, CSF, or synovial fluid	Finding gram-negative intracellular diplococci on Gram stain is suggestive. Culture on special media establishes the diagnosis.
Syphilis (*Treponema pallidum*)	Serum (mother) Serum CSF	Rapid plasma reagin (RPR) and if reactive, a specific treponemal test† RPR Venereal Disease Research Laboratories (VDRL)
Cytomegalovirus	Urine, saliva, blood, or CSF	PCR for detection of CMV DNA Obtain within 2-4 wk of birth.
Enteroviruses	Blood, nasopharyngeal swab, throat swab, conjunctival swab, tracheal aspirate, urine, stool, rectal swab, or CSF	PCR Cell culture (sensitivity depends on serotype and cell lines used)
Hepatitis B	Serum (mother) Serum	Hepatitis B surface antigen (HBsAg) If mother's HBsAg is positive, at age 9 mo, test the infant for HBsAg and hepatitis B surface antibody.
Herpes simplex viruses 1 and 2	Conjunctiva, skin vesicle scraping, whole blood, or mouth vesicles CSF "Surface cultures" (mouth, nasopharynx, conjunctiva, and anus)	PCR or cell culture PCR PCR or cell culture
Human immunodeficiency virus (HIV)	Serum (mother) Whole blood	Fourth-generation HIV antigen/antibody test HIV DNA PCR
Candida species	Blood, skin biopsy, or CSF	Culture
Zika virus	Blood, urine, CSF	NAT and serum IgM NAT may be falsely negative IgG antibodies may reflect maternal exposure Antibodies may cross react with other flaviviruses

*Published evaluations of NAATs for these indications are limited, but sensitivity and specificity is expected to be at least as high as those for culture. FDA, U.S. Food and Drug Administration.

†Treponemal tests include the *T. pallidum* particle agglutination (TP-PA) test, *T. pallidum* enzyme immunoassay (TP-EIA), *T. pallidum* chemiluminescent assay (TP-CIA), and fluorescent treponemal antibody absorption (FTA-ABS) test.

Adolescent Medicine
青少年（青春期）医学

Chapter **132**

Adolescent Physical and Social Development

Cynthia M. Holland-Hall

第一百三十二章
青少年身体和社会适应能力的发育

中文导读

　　本章从生物–心理–社会视角探讨了青少年的保健问题，主要介绍了青春期阶段由激素驱动引起的青少年在体格、生理、心理和社会适应力的变化特点、规律以及在男女性别间的变化差异；通过探讨青少年各个阶段神经系统的发育特点，揭示了青少年认知形成的过程；并从环境和文化的角度分析影响青少年性格、心理发展的因素；提出青少年在面临社会环境变化带来的挑战时，父母和社会应给予鼓励和帮助。

See also Part XV and Chapters 577 and 578.

During the preteen, teenage, and young adult years, young people undergo not only dramatic changes in physical appearance, but also rapid changes in physiologic, psychological, and social functioning. Hormonally driven physiologic changes and ongoing neurologic development occur in the setting of social structures that foster the transition from childhood to adulthood. This period of development comprises **adolescence**, which is divided into 3 phases—early, middle, and late adolescence—each marked by a characteristic set of biologic, cognitive, and psychosocial milestones (Table 132.1). Although individual variations in the timing and pace of development undoubtedly exist, these changes follow a fairly predictable pattern of occurrence. Gender and culture profoundly affect the developmental course, as do physical, social, and environmental influences. Given the interaction of these domains, a biopsychosocial perspective is best suited to approach the healthcare of the adolescent.

PHYSICAL DEVELOPMENT

Puberty is the biologic transition from childhood to adulthood. Pubertal changes include the appearance of the secondary sexual characteristics, increase in height, change in body composition, and development of reproductive capacity. Adrenal production of androgen, mainly dehydroepiandrosterone sulfate (DHEAS), may occur as early as 6 yr of age,

with development of underarm odor and faint genital hair (**adrenarche**). Maturation of the gonadotropin-releasing hormone (GnRH) pulse generator is among the earliest neuroendocrine changes associated with the onset of puberty. Under the influence of GnRH, the pituitary gland secretes luteinizing hormone (LH) and follicle-stimulating hormone (FSH); initially this occurs in a pulsatile fashion primarily during sleep, but this diurnal variation diminishes throughout puberty. LH and FSH stimulate corresponding increases in gonadal androgens and estrogens. The triggers for these changes are incompletely understood but may be mediated in part by the hormone leptin, high concentrations of which are associated with increased body fat and earlier onset of puberty. Both genetic and environmental (epigenetic) contributions to the regulation of pubertal timing are likely.

Sexual Development

The progression of the development of the secondary sex characteristics may be described using the **sexual maturity rating (SMR)** scale (ranging from 1, preadolescence, to 5, sexual maturity), or **Tanner stages**. Figs. 132.1 and 132.2 depict the physical findings of breast and pubic hair maturation at each SMR (Tables 132.2 and 132.3). Although the ages at which individual pubertal changes occur may vary, the timing and sequence of these changes relative to one another is predictable (Figs. 132.3 and 132.4). The wide range of normal progress through sexual

Table 132.1	Milestones in Early, Middle, and Late Adolescent Development		
VARIABLE	**EARLY ADOLESCENCE**	**MIDDLE ADOLESCENCE**	**LATE ADOLESCENCE**
Approximate age range	10-13 yr	14-17 yr	18-21 yr
Sexual maturity rating*	1-2	3-5	5
Physical	Females: secondary sex characteristics (breast, pubic, axillary hair), start of growth spurt Males: testicular enlargement, start of genital growth	Females: peak growth velocity, menarche (if not already attained) Males: growth spurt, secondary sex characteristics, nocturnal emissions, facial and body hair, voice changes Change in body composition Acne	Physical maturation slows Increased lean muscle mass in males
Cognitive and moral	Concrete operations Egocentricity Unable to perceive long-term outcome of current decisions Follow rules to avoid punishment	Emergence of abstract thought (formal operations) May perceive future implications, but may not apply in decision-making Strong emotions may drive decision-making Sense of invulnerability Growing ability to see others' perspectives	Future-oriented with sense of perspective Idealism Able to think things through independently Improved impulse control Improved assessment of risk vs reward Able to distinguish law from morality
Self-concept/identity formation	Preoccupied with changing body Self-consciousness about appearance and attractiveness	Concern with attractiveness Increasing introspection	More stable body image Attractiveness may still be of concern Consolidation of identity
Family	Increased need for privacy Exploration of boundaries of dependence vs independence	Conflicts over control and independence Struggle for greater autonomy Increased separation from parents	Emotional and physical separation from family Increased autonomy Reestablishment of "adult" relationship with parents
Peers	Same-sex peer affiliations	Intense peer group involvement Preoccupation with peer culture Conformity	Peer group and values recede in importance
Sexual	Increased interest in sexual anatomy Anxieties and questions about pubertal changes Limited capacity for intimacy	Testing ability to attract partner Initiation of relationships and sexual activity Exploration of sexual identity	Consolidation of sexual identity Focus on intimacy and formation of stable relationships Planning for future and commitment

*See text and Figs. 132.1 and 132.2.

Table 132.2	Sexual Maturity Rating (SMR) Stages in Females	
SMR STAGE	**PUBIC HAIR**	**BREASTS**
1	Preadolescent	Preadolescent
2	Sparse, lightly pigmented, straight, medial border of labia	Breast and papilla elevated as small mound; diameter of areola increased
3	Darker, beginning to curl, increased amount	Breast and areola enlarged, no contour separation
4	Coarse, curly, abundant, but less than in adult	Areola and papilla form secondary mound
5	Adult feminine triangle, spread to medial surface of thighs	Mature, nipple projects, areola part of general breast contour

From Tanner JM: *Growth at adolescence*, ed 2, Oxford, England, 1962, Blackwell Scientific.

Table 132.3	Sexual Maturity Rating (SMR) Stages in Males		
SMR STAGE	**PUBIC HAIR**	**PENIS**	**TESTES**
1	None	Preadolescent	Preadolescent
2	Scant, long, slightly pigmented	Minimal change/enlargement	Enlarged scrotum, pink, texture altered
3	Darker, starting to curl, small amount	Lengthens	Larger
4	Resembles adult type, but less quantity; coarse, curly	Larger; glans and breadth increase in size	Larger, scrotum dark
5	Adult distribution, spread to medial surface of thighs	Adult size	Adult size

From Tanner JM: *Growth at adolescence*, ed 2, Oxford, England, 1962, Blackwell Scientific.

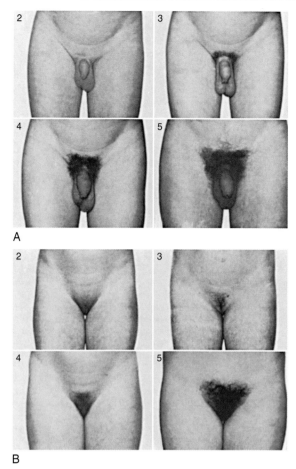

Fig. 132.1 Sexual maturity ratings (2-5) of pubic hair changes in adolescent males (**A**) and females (**B**) (see Tables 132.2 and 132.3). *(Courtesy of J.M. Tanner, MD, Institute of Child Health, Department for Growth and Development, University of London.)*

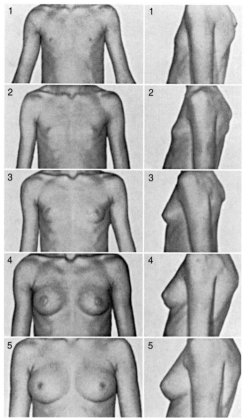

Fig. 132.2 Sexual maturity ratings (1-5) of breast changes in adolescent females. *(Courtesy of J.M. Tanner, MD, Institute of Child Health, Department for Growth and Development, University of London.)*

maturation is affected by genetics, the psychosocial environment, nutrition, and overall health status. Environmental exposures may play a role as well.

In **males** the first visible sign of puberty and the hallmark of SMR 2 is testicular enlargement, beginning as early as 9.5 yr, followed by the development of pubic hair. This is followed by penile growth during SMR 3. Peak growth occurs when testis volumes reach approximately 9-10 cm^3 during SMR 4. Under the influence of LH and testosterone, the seminiferous tubules, epididymis, seminal vesicles, and prostate enlarge. Sperm may be found in the urine by SMR 3; nocturnal emissions may be noted at this time as well. Some degree of breast tissue growth, typically bilateral, occurs in 40–65% of males during SMR 2-4 as a presumed consequence of a relative excess of estrogenic stimulation. This usually resolves with ongoing maturation.

In **females**, typically the first visible sign of puberty and the hallmark of SMR 2 is the appearance of breast buds (**thelarche**), between 7 and 12 yr of age. A significant minority of females develops pubic hair (**pubarche**) prior to thelarche. Less visible changes include enlargement of the ovaries, uterus, labia, and clitoris and thickening of the endometrium and vaginal mucosa. A clear vaginal discharge may be present before menarche (physiologic leukorrhea). Menses typically begins within 3 yr of thelarche, during SMR 3-4 (average age 12.5 yr; normal range 9-15 yr) (see Fig. 132.4). The timing of **menarche** is determined largely by genetics; contributing factors likely include adiposity, chronic

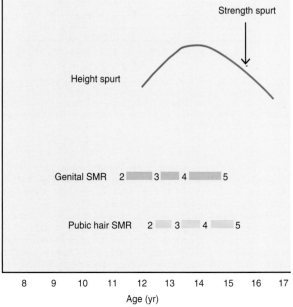

Fig. 132.3 Sequence of pubertal events in males. Although the age of onset of puberty is variable, the sequence of events relative to one another is predictable. SMR, Sexual maturity rating.

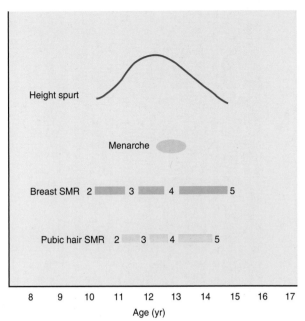

Fig. 132.4 Sequence of pubertal events in females. Although the age of onset of puberty is variable, the sequence of events relative to one another is predictable. SMR, Sexual maturity rating.

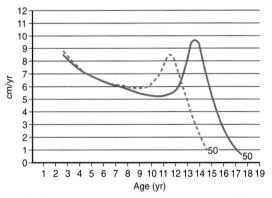

Fig. 132.5 Height velocity curves for American males *(solid line)* and females *(dashed line)* who have their peak height velocity at the average age (i.e., average growth tempo). *(From Tanner JM, Davies PSW: Clinical longitudinal standards for height and height velocity for North American children, J Pediatr 107:317, 1985.)*

illness, nutritional status, and the physical and psychosocial environment. Early menstrual cycles often are anovulatory and thus somewhat irregular, but typically occur every 21-45 days and include 3-7 days of bleeding, even during the 1st year following menarche.

The **onset of puberty** and menarche appear to be occurring at earlier ages than previously reported in the United States. Several studies from 1948–1981 identified the average age for the onset of breast development as ranging from 10.6-11.2 yr of age. Multiple reports since 1997 suggest a significantly earlier average age of onset, ranging from 8.9-9.5 yr in black females to 10.0-10.4 yr in white females. Almost 25% of black females and 10% of white females initiate breast development by 7 yr of age. Early breast development may be associated with a slower tempo of puberty (i.e., longer time to menarche). There also appears to be a trend toward decreasing ages for the onset of pubic hair development and menarche. Data from the National Health and Nutrition Examination

Survey (NHANES), a nationally representative, longitudinal survey in the United States, show a decline in the average age of menarche of 4.9 mo between the 1960s and 2002. Changes in the timing of menarche *within* ethnic groups, however, were significantly smaller. The larger change seen in the population as a whole may be partially explained by changes in the ethnic makeup of the sample. The reasons for the larger decrease in age for breast development have been postulated to include the epidemic of childhood obesity as well as exposure to estrogen-like environmental toxins (endocrine disruptors), but further research in this area is needed.

Although fewer data are available on changes in the timing of puberty in males, they appear to be experiencing a similar trend. Although the method of assessing the onset of puberty (i.e., inspection vs. palpation of the testes) varies between studies, it appears that the average age for the onset of genital and pubic hair development may have decreased by 1-2 yr over the past several decades in many industrialized countries. Evidence for an association of obesity with the timing of puberty in males has been inconsistent.

Somatic Growth

Linear growth acceleration begins in early adolescence for both genders, with 15–20% of adult height accrued during puberty. Females attain a **peak height velocity (PHV)** of 8-9 cm/yr at SMR 2-3, approximately 6 mo before menarche. Males typically begin their growth acceleration at a later SMR stage, achieve a PHV of 9-10 cm/yr later in the course of puberty (SMR 3-4), and continue their linear growth for approximately 2-3 yr after females have stopped growing (Fig. 132.5). The growth spurt begins distally, with enlargement of the hands and feet, followed by the arms and legs, and finally the trunk and chest. This growth pattern imparts a characteristic "awkward" appearance to some early adolescents. Body composition changes as well, after attainment of PHV. Males undergo an increase in lean body mass ("strength spurt"), whereas females develop a higher proportion of body fat. Scoliosis, if present, may progress with rapid axial skeleton growth (see Chapter 699.1). From 50–65% of total body calcium is laid down during puberty. Bone growth precedes increases in bone mineralization and bone density, which may increase the adolescent's risk of fracture during times of rapid growth. Since skeletal growth precedes muscle growth, sprains and strains may be more common during this time as well.

Cardiovascular changes in middle adolescence include increased heart size, higher blood pressure, and increases in blood volume and hematocrit, particularly in males. Coupled with an increase in lung vital capacity, these changes lead to greater aerobic capacity. Androgenic stimulation of sebaceous and apocrine glands may result in acne and body odor. Rapid enlargement of the larynx, pharynx, and lungs leads to changes in vocal quality in males, typically preceded by vocal instability (voice cracking). Elongation of the optic globe may result in the development of myopia (see Chapter 638). Dental changes include jaw growth, loss of the final deciduous teeth, and eruption of the permanent cuspids, premolars, and finally, molars (see Chapter 333). Orthodontic appliances may be needed, secondary to growth exacerbations of bite disturbances. Physiologic changes in sleep patterns and increased sleep requirements occur, causing many adolescents to delay sleep onset at night, with subsequent difficulty awakening for early school start times in the morning (see Chapter 31).

NEUROLOGIC, COGNITIVE, AND MORAL DEVELOPMENT

As children progress through adolescence, they develop and refine their ability to use formal operational thought processes. Abstract, symbolic, and hypothetical thinking replaces the need to manipulate concrete objects. Middle and late adolescents develop the ability to consider multiple options and to assess the long-term consequences of their actions. The capacity for verbal expression is enhanced. Since adolescents' decision-making and subsequent behaviors are the primary determinants of their mortality and morbidity, understanding these cognitive processes is of critical importance.

Both structural and functional brain development continue throughout adolescence. Cortical gray matter volume peaks in preadolescence, then decreases because of selective "pruning" of rarely used synaptic connections. Cerebral white matter volume increases until mid-to-late adolescence, reflecting increasing myelination and subsequent facilitation of integrated brain activity and more efficient transmission of information between different regions of the brain, enhancing the "signal-to-noise" ratio. Although the frontal lobes and prefrontal cortex, regions of the brain associated with executive function, have been considered to be among the last regions to mature, other cortical regions show similarly prolonged trajectories of maturation. Without question, adolescents are capable of the complex cognitive processes attributed to frontal lobe function. *Cognitive control*, however, continues to improve into adulthood, with progressive maturation and *integration* of component processes such as working memory, inhibition and impulse control, performance monitoring, and motivational circuitry.

The behavioral correlates of adolescent neurodevelopment remain speculative but are increasingly supported by a rapidly expanding body of research. Adolescents appear to demonstrate a unique sensitivity to the effects of dopamine on reward-relevant subcortical structures such as the ventral striatum, with some studies demonstrating increased activation in this region when receiving rewards, relative to children or adults. Other studies show reduced responsiveness to aversive stimuli in adolescents. This altered responsiveness to risk vs reward may underlie the increased risk taking and novelty seeking seen in adolescents. Early maturation and distinct patterns of neural reactivity in the amygdala and other limbic structures may explain the strong role that social and emotional stimuli play in adolescents, overwhelming the frontal executive function systems that facilitate the interpretation and regulation of those social and emotional experiences. This may explain why adolescents are more likely to make poor decisions in highly emotionally charged situations, relative to mature adults. These "hot cognition" processes may result in the adolescent making a different decision in the context of a strong affective experience than he or she would in a less emotional state ("cool cognition"). These 2 types of cognitive processes may not develop at the same rate; the adolescent may be able to use higher brain structures and functions more effectively when in states of lower emotional arousal.

Early adolescents often continue to employ the concrete operational cognitive processes of childhood. Although formal operational cognition is developing, it may be applied inconsistently across different domains. A young adolescent may be able to use abstract thought when completing schoolwork, but not when working through a personal dilemma. Early adolescence also is characterized by egocentricity—the belief of some adolescents that they are the center of everyone's attention. Despite being largely imagined, this perception of always being "on stage" can be stressful for adolescents, who may feel that others are constantly judging or evaluating them. Early adolescents express a greater need for privacy than they did in childhood and begin to appreciate the privacy of their own thoughts. With ongoing cognitive development, **middle** adolescents are more able to consider the needs and feelings of other people. Their creativity and intellectual abilities are enhanced. Because of their increased capacity for abstract thought in combination with a persistent perception of uniqueness, middle adolescents may feel a sense of immortality and immunity to the consequences of risky behaviors. **Late** adolescents are more future oriented and able to delay gratification. They can think more independently, consider others' views, and compromise. They have a stronger sense of self and more stable interests. Under times of stress, adolescents may temporarily revert back to the cognitive processes and coping strategies used at younger ages.

Moral development generally accompanies cognitive development. Preadolescents, concrete and individualistic, follow rules in order to please authority figures and avoid punishment. As they move into early adolescence, they develop a stronger sense of right and wrong but are likely to perceive these as absolute and unquestionable. Middle and late adolescents may establish a sense of morality driven by their desire to be seen as a good person, to behave in a manner according to their perceived place in society, or by their sense of obligation to care for others. Moral decision-making, however, still may be highly subject to emotional context. Late adolescents may develop a rational conscience and an independent system of values, although these often are largely consistent with parental values. While going through this complex developmental process, religious or political organizations that promote simple answers to complex social or moral questions may hold great appeal to the adolescent.

PSYCHOSOCIAL DEVELOPMENT

In contrast to cognitive development, psychosocial development correlates more strongly with pubertal status and physical maturation than with chronologic age. Whereas cognitive development is more biologically determined, psychosocial development is subject to greater environmental and cultural influences. Indeed, cultural variation can be dramatic. Some late adolescents move immediately from high school into marriage, childbearing, working, and financial independence; others remain dependent on the parents while pursuing their own education for several more years, in a period sometimes referred to as *emerging adulthood*. Psychosocial development also may be nonlinear, with different domains of growth progressing along different timelines. An overriding theme of psychosocial development is the concept of identity formation and consolidation as the adolescent moves away from the nurturing protection of the family, develops an increased affiliation with the peer group(s), and ultimately defines himself or herself as an individual.

Separation from the parents is a hallmark of adolescent development. Early adolescents start to seek out more privacy at home, spending less time with the parents. They begin to reject parental advice and involvement in their decision-making as they explore the boundaries of their dependence on, and independence from, their parents. With evolving cognitive skills, an adolescent can conceive of an ideal parent and contrast this ideal with his or her own parents. Adolescents may seek out alternative adult role models, such as teachers, coaches, or parents of friends. Parent–child conflict often peaks during middle adolescence, with disagreements over privileges, independence, and other limits set by the parents. Adolescents may appear intermittently to seek and reject parental acceptance. It is theorized that perhaps the adolescent *needs* to conceive of the parents as "wrong" in order to ameliorate the pain of separating from them. Throughout this time, however, the parents remain a critical source of nurturing and support for the adolescent and continue to exert significant influence over the adolescent's decision-making. Paradoxically, frequent arguments and conflict may coexist with strong emotional bonds and closeness. The late adolescent may reestablish a more "adult–adult" type of relationship with the parents, once again seeking out and considering parental advice and guidance as they enter adulthood.

Increasing importance of the **peer group** also may buffer the emotional trauma of separating from the parents. Early adolescents tend to socialize largely with same-sex peers, both in their individual friendships and larger groups. Females' peer groups tend to be more relationship oriented, whereas males' peer groups are more likely to be centered around a particular interest or activity. In both cases, group cohesion and a sense of belonging become important. Peers become increasingly important in middle adolescence, during which time the adolescent may experiment with being a part of different groups and "try on" different identities. These groups may include both sexes. Peer groups may arise from organized activities, such as sports or clubs, or may simply be friendship based. Gang membership is another form of peer acceptance. **Conformity** with the peers in manners of dress, speech, and behavior is a normal part of this process, and should not necessarily be viewed negatively. Similarly, **peer pressure** may exist, but its influence over the adolescent's decision-making may be positive, negative, or negligible. Acceptance and successful navigation of peer groups during adolescence may give the individual more confidence to move into and out of various social, academic, and professional groups in the future. Late adolescents are less vulnerable to peer group influence, having moved closer to establishing their own stable identity. Their cognitive skills allow them to choose selectively among different peer groups, endorsing and adopting individual values and behaviors that best reflect who they are becoming.

Early adolescents have increased **sexual awareness and interest**, which may manifest as sexual talk and gossip, and often is focused on

| Table 132.4 | Recommended Action Bundles* for Adolescent and Young Adult Health Problems and Risks |

PROBLEM/ RISK AREA	STRUCTURAL	SOCIAL MARKETING	COMMUNITY INTERVENTIONS INCLUDING FAMILY	ELECTRONIC HEALTH, MOBILE HEALTH	SCHOOLS	HEALTH SERVICE SECTOR
Sexual and reproductive health, including HIV	Legislation *18 years as the minimum age of marriage Allow provision of contraception to legal minors Legalize abortion*	*Promote community support for sexual and reproductive health, and HIV health access for adolescents*	Cash transfer programs, with payments linked to staying in school *Positive youth development Peer education*	*Target knowledge, attitudes, and risk behaviors*	Quality secondary education Comprehensive sexuality education Safe schools with clean toilets and facilities for menstrual care School-based health services with condoms and modern contraceptives	Condoms and affordable modern contraception including long-acting reversible contraception Early HIV and STI diagnosis and treatment Male circumcision Antenatal, delivery, and postnatal care *Transition to adult care for HIV*
Undernutrition	Fortification of foods (e.g., iron, folate)		Micronutrient supplements (particularly in pregnancy) Protein-energy supplementation Deworming *Cash transfer program Nutrition education*		Micronutrient supplements Healthy school meals	Screening and micronutrient supplementation
Infectious diseases			Deworming *Bednet distribution*	HPV vaccination *Deworming*		Early identification and treatment Adolescent vaccinations (HPV, childhood catch-up) *Deworming Bednet distribution Seasonal malaria chemoprevention*
Violence	Gun control *Legalize homosexuality and protect women from violence and sexual coercion Youth justice reforms to promote second chances and diversion from custody 16 years as the minimum age for criminal responsibility*	*Promote knowledge of the effects of violence and available services*	*Promote parent skills and parent–child communication Positive youth development Promote gender equality Economic empowerment Group training for awareness, knowledge, and skills*		Multicomponent interventions that target violent behavior and substance use	Trauma care
Unintentional injury	Graduated licensing Mandatory helmet wearing Multicomponent traffic injury control	*Promote knowledge of risks*	*Police enforcement of traffic injury control*			Trauma care, including first responders (e.g., ambulances)
Alcohol and illicit drugs	Limit alcohol sales to underage adolescents Taxation on alcohol Drink-driving legislation Restrict illicit alcohol Interventions in licensed premises Diversion from youth justice and custody *Graduated drinking*	Advertising restrictions *Campaigns to build community awareness*	*Promote parent–child communication and parenting skills Needle-syringe exchange access Mentoring*	*Target knowledge, attitudes, and risk behaviors*	Alcohol-free policies	*Risk screening and motivational interviewing*

Continued

Table 132.4	Recommended Action Bundles* for Adolescent and Young Adult Health Problems and Risks—cont'd					
PROBLEM/ RISK AREA	**STRUCTURAL**	**SOCIAL MARKETING**	**COMMUNITY INTERVENTIONS INCLUDING FAMILY**	**ELECTRONIC HEALTH, MOBILE HEALTH**	**SCHOOLS**	**HEALTH SERVICE SECTOR**
Tobacco	**Tobacco control including taxation, pricing, and advertising control** Youth access restrictions Legislation for smoke-free air	Anti-tobacco campaigns	*Interventions to promote parent skills and parent–child communication*	*Text messaging adjunct to quitting*	*Smoke-free policies* Multicomponent	*Routine screening and motivation interviewing to promote cessation*
Mental disorders and suicide	**Restriction of access to means**	*Promote adolescent mental health literacy*	Gatekeeper training	*Electronic mental health interventions*	Educational interventions Gatekeeper training School-based mental health services	**Practitioner training in depression recognition and treatment** *Routine assessment of mental health, including self-harm and suicide risk*
Chronic physical disorders			*Peer support initiatives*		School-based health services	*Promote self-management* *Promote transition to adult health care*
Overweight and obesity	**Taxation of high-sugar, high-salt, and high-fat foods** *Front-of-pack nutrition labels* *Restriction of fast food advertising*	*Promote physical activity*	*Create opportunities for maintenance of physical activity in daily life*	*Interactive or personalized feedback interventions*	*Multicomponent interventions, involving education about healthy diet and increasing opportunities for physical education*	**Manage comorbidities of obesity**

*Actions in **bold** have an evidence base, and actions in *italics* are promising but without yet a strong evidence base, in adolescents and young adults.
HIV, Human immunodeficiency virus; HPV, human papillomavirus; STI, sexually transmitted infection.
From Patton GC, Sawyer SM, Santelli JS, et al: Our future: a Lancet commission on adolescent health and wellbeing, Lancet 387:2458, 2016.

sexual anatomy. Masturbation and other sexual exploration, sometimes with same-sex peers, are common. The prevalence of other forms of sexual behavior varies by culture; in general, these behaviors are less common in early adolescents. Romantic relationships, if they exist at all, lack emotional depth. Sexual curiosity, experimentation, and activity become more common among middle adolescents. Same-sex attraction is common; sexual orientation may become clear to some adolescents, but still may be evolving in others during this time. Dating behaviors may be seen, but this is culture dependent and may not be a popular construct for all adolescents. Individual relationships often continue to emphasize sexual attraction over emotional intimacy; the latter may not be seen until late adolescence. At that time, relationships increasingly involve love and commitment and demonstrate greater stability.

Body image may affect (and be affected by) adolescents' psychosocial development as well. Early and middle adolescence are usually the ages at which poor or distorted body image and eating disorders develop. Early adolescents undergo rapid physical changes and may experience uncertainty about whether all these anatomic and physiologic changes are progressing normally. Reassurance from adults, including their healthcare providers, may be comforting. As puberty comes to an end and these changes slow, the middle adolescent's preoccupation may shift to whether the adolescent is attractive to others. A strong emphasis on physical appearance during this time is normal. Although this focus on physical appearance may continue into adulthood, late adolescence generally is characterized by a shifting balance toward introspection, with somewhat less emphasis placed on external characteristics.

The **timing of pubertal changes** also can affect psychosocial development and well-being. The progression of pubertal changes in males is generally associated with a positive self-image. Females may initially perceive these changes in their physical appearance more negatively. This appears to be especially true for early-maturing females, some of whom experience greater decreases in self-esteem, engage in more disruptive behaviors, and have more conflict with their parents than do on-time or late-maturing females. Perhaps because they are more comfortable associating with older peers, early-maturing females are vulnerable to making poor decisions when exposed to high-risk situations, still lacking the cognitive skills to effectively navigate these situations. Early-maturing males tend to have greater self-confidence, social, and academic success, while later-maturing males are at risk for more internalizing behaviors and diminished self-esteem. Many other factors influence how adolescents experience puberty, and supportive peers and adults can have a positive impact on psychosocial development. With successful navigation of these domains, emerging adults move into the world with a strong sense of personal identity and their place in society. They are able to work toward a vocation and financial independence and to manage the responsibilities of adulthood.

IMPLICATIONS FOR PROVIDERS, PARENTS, AND POLICYMAKERS

Providers can help parents approach their child's adolescent years by reframing some of the "challenges" of adolescence as normal developmental milestones that should be anticipated and accepted. Puberty and emerging sexuality should be approached as positive and health-affirming life changes, rather than focusing discussions only on the negative reproductive risks and outcomes. Even good-natured teasing about bodily changes can be detrimental to the adolescent's self-image. Early-maturing females and late-maturing males should be supported, recognizing their potential increased risk for psychosocial challenges.

Emerging positive coping strategies should be promoted in all youth, particularly those with chronic illness or other challenges. Providers need to determine the young adolescent's cognitive development and capacity for abstract thought and tailor their communication and counseling style accordingly. Physical examinations should be performed in private with the parent outside the exam room (provided the adolescent is comfortable with this), which also affords the adolescent and provider an opportunity to discuss confidential issues. Reassurance of normal development should be provided.

As adolescents develop more independence and parent–child conflict peaks, providers should remind parents that this is typical, and that arguing does not mean the adolescent does not value the parents' input and perspectives. Although some may rebel initially, most adolescents ultimately adopt a value system very similar to that of their parents. Even if discussions feel ineffective to parents, they should continue to demonstrate and model these values to their child. Similarly, rather than categorically dismissing their child's "negative" interests, such as playing a violent video game, parents should be encouraged to use these opportunities to model critical thinking about the impact of such an activity. Potentially negative peer groups may be approached the same way, while fostering the development of positive peer networks. **Authoritative parenting**, in which clear and appropriate negotiated limits are set in the context of a caring and mutually respectful parent–child relationship, is most strongly associated with positive psychosocial development. Parental connectedness and close supervision or monitoring of the youth's activities and peer group can be protective against early onset of sexual activity and involvement in other risk-taking behaviors and can foster positive youth development. Parents should also assume an active role in their adolescent's transition to adulthood to ensure that their child receives appropriate preventive health services.

Parents and providers may each work with adolescents to foster good decision-making. In addition to providing adolescents with accurate and complete health information, the adolescent's cognitive ability to use this information in various contexts must be considered. Adolescents may find themselves needing to make important decisions in highly charged situations where they may be unable to manage their emotions and use their higher cognitive functions to examine the consequences of their decision. For example, a couple in a sexual situation with high emotional arousal may make the decision to proceed with unprotected intercourse. By anticipating this situation ahead of time, under conditions of lower emotional arousal, and making a plan to deal with this, they may make a different decision (e.g., stick with their prior decision never to have sex without protection), when the time comes. Parents and healthcare providers are in a position to encourage and foster this anticipation and planning under conditions of "cool cognition."

Providers may need to help parents distinguish normal adolescent development and risk-taking behaviors from possible signs of a more serious mental health or conduct problem. Bids for **autonomy**, such as avoiding family activities, demanding privacy, and increasing argumentativeness, are normal; extreme **withdrawal** or **antagonism** may be dysfunctional, signaling a mental health or substance use concern. Bewilderment and dysphoria at the start of middle school are normal; continued failure to adapt several months later suggests a more serious problem. Although some degree of risk taking is normal, progressive escalation of risk-taking behaviors is problematic. In general, when the adolescent's behaviors cause significant dysfunction in the domains of home life, academics, or peer relationships, they should be addressed by the parents and healthcare provider, and referral to a mental health provider may be considered. In most cases, parents can be reassured that although adolescence can pose unique challenges, their adolescent, like most adolescents, will come through it to become a successful and happy adult.

At national and international levels, adolescents are at risk for environmental, health, behavioral, and societal challenges. Table 132.4 provides suggestions to address these issues.

Bibliography is available at Expert Consult.

Chapter **133**

Gender and Sexual Identity

Walter O. Bockting

第一百三十三章
性和性别角色的认同

中文导读

　　本章分别从生物性别、性别认同、性别表达和性取向四个方面介绍了儿童和青少年中的性发育和性心理特点；从基因、激素和环境方面分析了影响生物性别和性认知发展的因素。围绕生物性别与性别认同不一致引起的性别焦虑和认知障碍，本章详细介绍了其病因学、流行病学和临床特征，并提出了以合理引导、避免伤害为导向的预防和干预措施。

TERMS AND DEFINITIONS
Sex and Sexual Identity
Sex is multifaceted, with at least 9 components: chromosomal sex, gonadal sex, fetal hormonal sex (prenatal hormones produced by the gonads), internal morphologic sex (internal genitalia), external morphologic sex (external genitalia), hypothalamic sex (sex of the brain), sex of assignment and rearing, pubertal hormonal sex, and gender identity and role. **Sexual identity** is a self-perceived identification distilled from any or all aspects of sexuality and has at least 4 components: sex assigned at birth, gender identity, gender expression, and sexual orientation.

Sex Assigned at Birth
A newborn is assigned a sex before (typically through ultrasound) or at birth based on the external genitalia (natal sex). In case of a *disorder of sex development (intersex)*, these genitalia may appear ambiguous, and additional components of sex (e.g., chromosomal, gonadal, hormonal sex) are assessed. In consultation with specialists, parents assign the child a sex that they believe is most likely to be consistent with gender identity, which cannot be assessed until later in life (see Chapter 606).

Gender Terms
Gender identity refers to a person's basic sense of being a boy/man, girl/woman, or other gender (e.g., transgender, genderqueer, nonbinary, gender fluid). **Gender role** refers to one's role in society, typically the male or female role. Gender identity needs to be distinguished from **gender expression**, which refers to characteristics in personality, appearance, and behavior that are, in a given culture and time, considered masculine or feminine. Gender role is about one's presentation as a boy/man or girl/woman, whereas gender expression is about the masculine and/or feminine characteristics one exhibits in a given gender role. Both boys/men, girls/women, and transgender, genderqueer, or nonbinary persons can be masculine and/or feminine to varying degrees; gender identity and gender expression are not necessarily congruent. A child or adolescent might be **gender nonconforming**, that is, a predominantly feminine boy or a predominantly masculine girl.

Sexual Orientation and Behavior
Sexual orientation refers to attractions, behaviors, fantasies, and emotional attachments toward men, women, or both. **Sexual behavior** refers to any sensual activity to pleasure oneself or another person sexually.

Transgender
Transgender people are a diverse group of individuals whose gender identity differs from their sex assigned at birth. They include **transsexuals** (usually referred to as transgender) (who typically live in the other gender role and seek hormonal and/or surgical interventions to modify primary or secondary sex characteristics); **cross-dressers** (who wear clothing and adopt behaviors associated with the other sex for emotional or sexual gratification and may spend part of the time in the other gender role); **drag queens** and **kings** (female and male impersonators); and individuals identifying as **genderqueer** (differently gendered), **nonbinary** (neither male nor female, both, or in-between), or **gender fluid** (not fixed but changing). Transgender individuals may be attracted to men, women, or other transgender persons.

FACTORS THAT INFLUENCE SEXUAL IDENTITY DEVELOPMENT
During prenatal sexual development, a gene located on the Y chromosome (*XRY*) induces the development of testes. The hormones produced by the testes direct sexual differentiation in the male direction resulting in the development of male internal and external genitalia. In the absence of this gene in XX chromosomal females, ovaries develop and sexual differentiation proceeds in the female direction, resulting in female internal and external genitalia. These hormones may also play a role in sexual differentiation of the brain. In disorders of sex development, chromosomal and prenatal hormonal sex varies from this typical developmental pattern and may result in ambiguous genitalia at birth.

Gender identity develops early in life and is typically fixed by 2-3 yr of age. Children first learn to identify their own and others' sex (**gender labeling**), then learn that gender is most often stable over time (**gender constancy**), and finally learn that gender is typically permanent (**gender consistency**). What determines gender identity remains largely unknown, but it is thought to be an interaction of biologic, environmental, and sociocultural factors.

Some evidence shows the impact of biologic and environmental factors on gender expression, whereas their impact on gender identity remains less clear. Animal research shows the influence of prenatal hormones on sexual differentiation of the brain. In humans, prenatal exposure to unusually high levels of androgens in girls with **congenital adrenal hyperplasia** is associated with more masculine gender expression, transgender identity, and same-sex sexual orientation, but cannot account for all the variance found (see Chapter 594). Research on environmental factors has focused on the influence of sex-typed socialization. Gender-based stereotypes develop early in life. Until later in adolescence, boys and girls are typically socially segregated by gender, reinforcing sex-typed characteristics such as boys' focus on "rough-and-tumble play" and asserting dominance, and girls focus on verbal communication and creating relationships. Parents, other adults, teachers, peers, and the media serve as gender-socializing role models and agents by treating boys and girls differently.

For information on the development of sexual orientation, see Chapter 134.

NONCONFORMITY IN GENDER EXPRESSION AMONG CHILDREN AND ADOLESCENTS
Prevalence
Nonconformity in gender expression needs to be distinguished from a transgender identity. The former operates on the level of personality, appearance, and behavior (masculinity, femininity), whereas the latter is about self-perceived, core gender identity. Nonconformity in gender expression is more common among girls (7%) than boys (5%), but boys are referred more often than girls for concerns regarding gender identity and expression. This is likely a result of parents, teachers, and peers being less tolerant of gender nonconformity in boys than in girls.

Nonconformity in gender expression as part of exploring one's gender identity and role is part of normal sexual development. Gender nonconformity in childhood may or may not persist into adolescence. Marked gender nonconformity in adolescence often persists into adulthood. Only a minority of gender-nonconforming children develop an adult transgender identity; most develop a gay or lesbian identity, and some, a heterosexual identity.

Etiology of Gender-Nonconforming Behavior
Prenatal hormones play a role in the development of nonconformity in gender expression, but cannot completely account for all the variance. A heritable component of gender-nonconforming behavior likely exists, but twin studies indicate that genetic factors also do not account for all of the variance. Family-of-origin factors hypothesized to play a role in the development of gender nonconformity lack empirical support. Maternal psychopathology and emotional absence of the father are the only possible factors associated with gender nonconformity, yet it is unclear whether these factors are cause or effect.

Stigma, Stigma Management, and Advocacy
Gender nonconforming children are subject to **ostracism** and **bullying** (see Chapter 14.1) from peers, which may negatively impact their psychosocial adjustment and lead to social isolation, loneliness, low self-esteem, depression, suicide, and behavioral problems. To assist children and families, individual stigma management strategies, as well as interventions to change the environment, can be offered. **Stigma management** might involve consultation with a health professional to provide support and education, normalizing gender-nonconforming

behavior and encouraging the child and family to build on the child's strengths and interests to foster self-esteem. It might also involve making choices about certain preferences (e.g., a boy who likes to wear feminine attire) to limit these to times and environments that are more accepting. *Most health professionals agree that too much focus on curtailing gender-nonconforming behavior leads to increased shame and undermines the child's self-esteem.*

The health professional and family can also assist the child or adolescent to find others with similar interests (within and beyond the gender-related interests) to strengthen positive peer support. Equally important are interventions in school and society to raise awareness and promote accepting and positive attitudes, take a stand against bullying and abuse, and implement antibullying policies and initiatives. *Gay, lesbian, bisexual, transgender, and straight alliance groups are helpful in providing a haven for gender-nonconforming youth, as well as recognizing them as part of diversity to be respected and embraced within the school system.* Healthcare system level approaches are outlined in Table 133.1.

TRANSGENDER AND GENDER-NONCONFORMING IDENTITIES AMONG CHILDREN AND ADOLESCENTS
Prevalence
Approximately 1% of parents of 4-11 yr old boys report that their son wished to be of the other sex, with 3.5% for 4-11 yr old girls. Only a minority of children's gender identity concerns persist into adolescence (20% in one study of boys). Persistence of gender identity concerns from adolescence into adulthood is higher; the majority identify as transgender in adulthood and may pursue **gender-affirming medical interventions** (i.e., hormone therapy, surgery). The prevalence of transgender adults in the United States is estimated at 1:200.

Etiology of Transgender or Gender-Nonconforming Identities
The etiology of transgender and gender-nonconforming identities remains unknown. Environmental and biologic factors are hypothesized to play a role in the development of a transgender or gender-nonconforming identity. Gender-nonconforming children seem to have more trouble than other children with basic cognitive concepts concerning their gender. They may experience emotional distance from their father. Whether these factors are cause or effect remains unclear.

Prenatal and perinatal hormones may influence sexual differentiation of the brain. Some girls with congenital adrenal hyperplasia develop a male gender identity, but most do not. The size of the sex-dimorphic central part of the bed nucleus of the stria terminalis in the hypothalamus of transgender women is smaller than in males and within the range of nontransgender women; the opposite is true for transgender men. This structure is regulated by hormones in animals, but in humans no evidence yet exists of a direct relationship between prenatal and perinatal hormones and the sexually dimorphic nature of this nucleus. In addition, differences have been shown between transgender men and women and nontransgender controls in white matter microstructure of the brain.

Clinical Presentation
Children and adolescents with a gender-nonconforming identity may experience 2 sources of stress: internal distress inherent to the incongruence between sex assigned at birth and gender identity (gender dysphoria) or distress associated with social stigma. The 1st source of distress is reflected in discomfort with the developing primary and secondary sex characteristics and the gender role assigned at birth. The 2nd source of distress relates to feeling different, not fitting in, peer ostracism, and social isolation, and may result in shame, low self-esteem, anxiety, or depression.

Table 133.1	Systems-Level Principles Underlying Lesbian, Gay, Bisexual, Transgender, Questioning (LGBTQ) Youth-Friendly Services	
PRINCIPLE	**DEFINITION**	**EXAMPLES**
Availability	The presence of healthcare providers with knowledge, competence, and experience working with young people and with people with current or possibly developing LGBTQ identities, feelings, and/or behavior	Providers from various disciplines (e.g., physicians, nonphysician healthcare professionals) provide care sensitive to the needs of LGBTQ youth. Quality of care is high, with LGBTQ youth (and when appropriate, their caregivers) universally receiving recommended screening and anticipatory guidance.
Accessibility	The relative ease with which LGBTQ youth can obtain care from an available provider	Clinical services are located near where LGBTQ youth live, study, work, or otherwise spend time. Clinical services are easily obtained, with expanded hours during evenings and weekends, same-day urgent bookings, drop-in visits, and allowances for late appointments. Technology (e.g., online patient portals, email, telemedicine) is increasingly used to improve access for youth.
Acceptability	The extent to which clinical services are culturally competent and developmentally appropriate for LGBTQ youth, and to which confidentiality is ensured and protected	The clinic has a policy affirming its inclusive services for LGBTQ, and the clinical environment has signs, stickers, and other statements showing it is LGBT-friendly. Health brochures and other reading materials are tailored to the needs of LGBTQ youth. Confidentiality is ensured and protected in every patient encounter, and healthcare providers spend time one-on-one with patients to elicit sensitive information.
Equity	The degree to which clinical care is friendly to *all* LGBTQ youth, regardless of race, ethnicity, language, ability to pay, housing status, and insurance status, among other factors	High-quality care is provided to all youth, regardless of whether they are lesbian, gay, bisexual, or transgender. Culturally competent care is provided to LGBTQ youth of color, and services are available for patients who are not native English speaking. Services are provided free-of-charge for uninsured LGBTQ youth.

Adapted from Tylee A, Haller DM, Graham T, et al. Youth-friendly primary-care services: how are we doing and what more needs to be done? *Lancet* 369(9572):1565–1573, 2007; and Department of Maternal Newborn Child and Adolescent Health. Making health services adolescent friendly—developing national quality standards for adolescent friendly health services, Geneva, 2012, World Health Organization.

Boys with a gender-nonconforming identity may at an early age identify as a girl, expect to grow up female, or express the wish to do so. They may experience distress about being a boy and/or having a male body, prefer to urinate in a sitting position, and express a specific dislike of their male genitals and even want to cut off their genitals. They may dress up in girls' clothes as part of playing dress up or in private. Girls may identify as a boy and expect or wish to grow up male. They may experience distress about being a girl and/or having a female body, pretend to have a penis, or expect to grow one. Girls may express a dislike of feminine clothing and hairstyles. In early childhood, children may spontaneously express these concerns, but depending on the response of the social environment, these feelings may go underground and may be kept more private. The distress may intensify by the onset of puberty; the physical changes of puberty are described by many transgender adolescents and adults as "traumatic." Boys and girls may also identify outside of the gender binary (e.g., as boygirl, girlboy, genderqueer, gender fluid) and describe their identity as neither male nor female, both male and female, in-between, or some other alternative gender different from their sex assigned at birth. Adopting a **nonbinary identity** may be part of identity exploration or constitute a gender identification that persists over time.

Gender-nonconforming children and transgender adolescents may struggle with a number of general behavior problems. Both boys and girls predominantly internalize (anxious and depressed) rather than externalize behavioral difficulties. Boys are more prone to anxiety, have more negative emotions and a higher stress response, and are rated lower in self-worth, social competence, and psychological well-being. Gender-nonconforming children have more peer relationship difficulties than controls. Both femininity in boys and masculinity in girls are

socially stigmatized, although the former seems to carry a higher level of stigma. Boys have been shown to be teased more than girls; teasing for boys increases with age. *Poor peer relations* is the strongest predictor of behavior problems in both boys and girls.

Transgender adolescents may struggle with a number of adjustment problems as a result of social stigma and lack of access to gender-affirming healthcare. Transgender youth, especially those of ethnic/racial minority groups, are vulnerable to verbal and physical abuse, academic difficulties, school dropout, illicit hormone and silicone use, substance use, difficulty finding employment, homelessness, sex work, forced sex, incarceration, HIV/sexually transmitted infections (STIs), and suicide. Parental support can buffer against psychological distress, but many parents react negatively to their child's gender nonconformity, although mothers tend to be more supportive than fathers.

The Diagnosis of Gender Dysphoria: Criteria and Critique

Gender dysphoria (or **gender incongruence**) is classified as a mental disorder in the *Diagnostic and Statistical Manual of Mental Disorders* (DSM) and *International Classification of Diseases* (ICD), which, particularly for children, is controversial (Table 133.2). Critics have argued that the distress children experience is mainly the result of social stigma rather than being inherent to gender nonconformity and thus should not be considered a mental disorder. Critics have also expressed concern about children with normal variation in gender role being labeled with a mental disorder perpetuating social stigma, yet there is a tendency of clinicians to underdiagnose rather than overdiagnose children whose gender nonconformity goes beyond behavior and who report gender dysphoria. These children may benefit from the diagnosis to receive

Table 133.2	Summary of DSM-5 Diagnostic Criteria for Gender Dysphoria

GENDER DYSPHORIA IN CHILDREN (302.6) (F64.2)

A. A marked incongruence between one's experienced/expressed gender and assigned gender, of at least 6 mo duration, as manifested by at least 6 of the following (1 of which must be criterion A1):
1. A strong desire to be of the other gender or an insistence that one is the other gender (or some alternative gender different from one's assigned gender).
2. In boys (assigned gender), a strong preference for cross-dressing or simulating female attire; or in girls (assigned gender), a strong preference for wearing only typical masculine clothing and a strong resistance to the wearing of typical feminine clothing.
3. A strong preferences for cross-gender roles in make-believe play or fantasy play.
4. A strong preference for the toys, games, or activities stereotypically used or engaged in by the other gender.
5. A strong preference for playmates of the other gender.
6. In boys (assigned gender), a strong rejection of typically masculine toys, games, and activities and a strong avoidance of rough-and-tumble play; or in girls (assigned gender), a strong rejection of typically feminine toys, games, and activities.
7. A strong dislike of one's sexual anatomy.
8. A strong desire for the primary and/or secondary sex characteristics that match one's experienced gender.

B. The condition is associated with clinically significant distress or impairment in social, school, or other important areas of functioning.

SPECIFY IF WITH A DISORDER OF SEX DEVELOPMENT (E.G., CONGENITAL ADRENAL HYPERPLASIA OR ANDROGEN INSENSITIVITY SYNDROME)

GENDER DYSPHORIA IN ADOLESCENTS OR ADULTS

A. A marked incongruence between one's experienced/expressed gender and assigned gender, of at least 6 mo duration, as manifested by at least 2 of the following:

1. A marked incongruence between one's experienced/expressed gender and primary and/or secondary sex characteristics (or in young adolescents, the anticipated secondary sex characteristics).
2. A strong desire to be rid of one's primary and/or secondary sex characteristics because of a marked incongruence with one's experienced/expressed gender (or in young adolescents, a desire to prevent the development of the anticipated secondary sex characteristics).
3. A strong desire for the primary and/or secondary sex characteristics of the other gender.
4. A strong desire to be of the other gender (or some alternative gender different from one's assigned gender).
5. A strong desire to be treated as the other gender (or some alternative gender different from one's assigned gender).
6. A strong conviction that one has the typical feelings and reactions of the other gender (or some alternative gender different from one's assigned gender).

B. The condition is associated with clinically significant distress or impairment in social, occupational, or other important areas of functioning.

SPECIFY IF WITH A DISORDER OF SEX DEVELOPMENT (E.G., CONGENITAL ADRENAL HYPERPLASIA OR ANDROGEN INSENSITIVITY SYNDROME)

SPECIFY IF POSTTRANSITION: The individual has transitioned to full-time living in the desired gender (with or without legalization of gender change) and has undergone (or is preparing to have) at least one cross-sex medical procedure or treatment regimen, namely, regular cross-sex hormone treatment or gender reassignment surgery confirming the desired gender (e.g., penectomy, vaginoplasty in a natal male; mastectomy or phalloplasty in a natal female).

early treatment in the form of support, education, advocacy, and, in case of clinically significant distress, changes in gender role, **puberty suppression, and/or feminizing or masculinizing hormone therapy in adolescence**.

Transgender Identity Development

A stages model of coming out might be helpful to understand the experience and potential challenges transgender youth might face. In the **pre–coming out** stage, the child or adolescent is aware that their gender identity is different from that of most boys and girls. In addition to a gender identity that varies from sex assigned at birth, some of these children are also nonconforming in gender expression while others are not. Those who are also nonconforming in gender expression cannot hide their transgender identity, are noticed for who they are, and may face teasing, ridicule, abuse, and rejection. They must learn to cope with these challenges at an early age and usually proceed quickly to the next stage of **coming out**. Children who are not visibly nonconforming in gender expression are able to avoid stigma and rejection by hiding their transgender feelings. They often experience a split between their gender identity cherished in private and expressed in fantasy and a false self presented outwardly to fit in and meet gendered expectations. These children and adolescents often proceed to coming out later in adolescence or adulthood.

Coming out involves acknowledging one's transgender identity to self and others (parents, other caregivers, trusted health providers, peers). An open and accepting attitude is essential; rejection can perpetuate stigma and its negative emotional consequences. By accessing transgender community resources, including peer support (either online or offline), transgender youth can then proceed to the **exploration** stage. This is a time of learning as much as possible about being transgender, getting to know similar others, and experimenting with various options for gender expression. Changes in gender role are carefully considered, as are medical interventions to delay puberty and/or feminize or masculinize the body to alleviate dysphoria. Successful resolution of this stage is a sense of pride in being transgender and comfort with gender role and expression.

Once gender dysphoria has been alleviated, youth can proceed with other human development tasks, including dating and relationships in the **intimacy** stage. As a result of social stigma and rejection, transgender youth may struggle with feeling unlovable. Sexual development has often been compromised by gender and genital dysphoria. Now that greater comfort has been achieved with gender identity and gender expression, dating and sexual intimacy have a greater chance of succeeding. Finally, in the **integration** stage, transgender is no longer the most important signifier of identity, but one of several important parts of overall identity.

Interventions and Treatment

Health providers can assist gender-nonconforming children, transgender adolescents, and their families by directing them to resources and by helping them to make informed decisions about changes in gender role and the available medical interventions to reduce intense and persistent gender dysphoria. To alleviate socially induced distress, interventions focus on stigma management and stigma reduction. It might be in the child's best interest to set reasonable limits on gender expression contributing to teasing and ridicule. The main goal of these interventions is not to change the child's gender-nonconforming behavior but to assist families, schools, and the wider community to create a supportive environment where the child can thrive and safely explore his or her gender identity and expression. Decisions to change gender roles, particularly in school, are not to be taken lightly and are best carefully anticipated and planned in consultation with parents, child, teachers, school counselor, and other providers involved in the adolescent's care. Medical interventions are available as early as Tanner Stage 2. Such treatment is guided by the Standards of Care set forth by the **World Professional Association for Transgender Health** (WPATH). Although some controversy still exists about the appropriateness of early medical intervention, follow-up studies of adolescents treated in accordance with these guidelines show its effectiveness in alleviating intense and persistent gender dysphoria.

Pubertal suppression with gonadotrophin-releasing hormone analogues (usually begun in early puberty) that delay puberty are helpful before gender-affirmation hormone therapies. Certain features of puberty are difficult to reverse (e.g., male facies, Adam's apple), so pubertal suppression avoids these physical features. Pubertal suppression may also reduce gender dysphoria. Gender-affirming hormones can then be initiated; testosterone for masculinizing and estrogen plus an adrogen inhibitor for feminization. Gender-affirming surgery (most commonly "top" surgery) to create a male-typical chest is usually delayed until adulthood.

Pediatricians who encounter transgender youth in their practice should be careful not to make assumptions about gender and sexual identity, but rather ask youth how they would describe themselves. This includes asking if they like being a boy or girl, have ever questioned this, wished they were born the other sex, or define their gender identity in a nonbinary or otherwise different way; and if they have a preferred nickname or pronoun (*he/him, she/her,* or *they/them;* if not sure, avoid pronouns). It also includes asking how they feel about their maturing body and sex characteristics, and what they would change about that if they could. Extra caution should be exercised during physical and genital exams because transgender youth may be particularly uncomfortable with their anatomy. When considering contraceptive options for female-to-male transgender youth, alternatives to feminizing agents should be explored. *For gender-affirming medical interventions, transgender youth should be referred to specialists in the treatment of gender dysphoria* (see www.wpath.org). For other health concerns, ensure referral to transgender or lesbian, gay, bisexual, transgender (LGBT)-friendly providers, especially in the case of gender-segregated treatment facilities. **Gender Spectrum** (www.genderspectrum.org), **Advocates for Youth** (www.advocatesforyouth.org), and **Parents, Families and Friends of Lesbians and Gays** (www.pflag.org) offer excellent support resources for transgender youth and their families.

Bibliography is available at Expert Consult.

Chapter **134**
Gay, Lesbian, and Bisexual Adolescents
Stewart L. Adelson and Mark A. Schuster
第一百三十四章
男同性恋、女同性恋和双性恋青少年

中 文 导 读

本章首先介绍了青少年群体中同性恋和双性恋的流行水平，儿童期和青春期性取向的发展过程及特点；其次，探讨了不同社会、种族和宗教背景下人们对同性恋和双性恋的污名和接受程度；第三，通过介绍同性恋和双性恋青少年遇到的健康问题（抑郁症和自杀倾向、性传播疾病、药物滥用、肥胖和饮食失衡等）和社会心理问题（辍学、骚扰和暴力等），强调了对同性恋或双性恋青少年进行教育、医疗帮助和心理疏导等干预措施的重要性。

Understanding a child's or adolescent's sexual and emotional development is an essential part of any comprehensive pediatric evaluation. For youth who are or might be gay, lesbian, or bisexual (**GLB**), such understanding is particularly important. GLB youth as a group have the same health and developmental needs as all youth, and their sexual orientation is part of the spectrum of human sexuality. However, they encounter distinct developmental challenges and can have additional physical and mental health needs related to their orientation and others' reaction to it. Their sexual orientation is often different from that expected by family, peers, and society (although expectations have been changing in many contexts), and they must cope with peer rejection, bullying, or family nonacceptance more frequently than most youth. Although the majority of GLB adolescents grow up physically and mentally healthy, they are at increased risk for certain health problems as a result of these stresses and the epidemiology of health threats such as HIV and other sexually transmitted infections (STIs). Pediatric clinicians are key in monitoring for such issues, supporting healthy development, and intervening when necessary to prevent or treat the problems for which GLB youth are at increased risk.

Sexual orientation refers to an individual's attraction to others based on sex or gender. It encompasses emotional and erotic desires, physiologic arousal, sexual behavior, sexual identity, and social role. As sexuality develops, youth can be oriented entirely toward a particular sex or gender, or more than one, to various degrees on a continuum. **Homosexuality** involves orientation toward people of one's same sex or gender, and **bisexuality** involves orientation toward males and females. **Gay** is a common term for homosexual males and females; **lesbian** refers to homosexual females. Some do not fit these categories and use other terms to describe themselves. Those unsure of their orientation are **curious** or **questioning**. The term **young men who have sex with men**

(**YMSM**) is sometimes used in the research literature to denote male youth who engage in sexual activity with other males, regardless of how they identify themselves.

PREVALENCE OF HOMOSEXUALITY AND BISEXUALITY IN YOUTH

Some junior high and high school students self-identify as gay, lesbian, or bisexual. Some who do not identify as GLB report same-sex attraction, fantasies, or behavior. Some are unsure of their sexual orientation. Certainty about sexual orientation tends to increase through adolescence with sexual experience, although one can be aware of one's orientation without having had sexual partners. Those who fear nonacceptance may try to suppress or deny their orientation. Consequently, various aspects of orientation—attraction, behavior, and identity—may not be consistent in an individual and may change during development. Not all youth with homosexual attraction or experience identify as "gay," consistent in part with reluctance about having or revealing a gay identity and underscoring the differences among attraction, behavior, and identity. A report providing national estimates of the number of high school students with GLB identity in 2015 found that across 25 states and 19 large urban school districts, a median of 2.7% said they were gay/lesbian, 6.4% said they were bisexual, and 4.0% reported being unsure of their sexual orientation.

DEVELOPMENT OF SEXUAL ORIENTATION IN CHILDHOOD AND ADOLESCENCE

Sexual orientation development appears to begin prenatally and continue through childhood and adolescence and into adulthood. Both gender role behavior in childhood and sexual orientation in puberty and adolescence are partly influenced by prenatal genetic and neuroendocrine factors. Sociocultural and psychological factors also influence sexual development. A gay or lesbian sexual orientation is sometimes preceded developmentally in childhood by **nonconforming gender expression**, or variation from population averages in expression of **gender-related behavior** such as activities, interests, styles, and other attributes recognized as masculine or feminine, such as toy preferences and preference for playmates of a particular gender. Although childhood gender nonconformity is not experienced by all gay or lesbian people—and not all children with nonconforming gender role behavior grow up to be gay or lesbian—nonconformity is not uncommon (particularly among males) and leads many gay or lesbian people to feel different from peers in childhood, even before sexual desire or identity emerges. Depending on the setting, gender-nonconforming children may experience ostracism, bullying, or family nonacceptance. These reactions to gender nonconformity can lead to later difficulty with gender-related self-esteem and long-term mental health problems.

Less frequently, gay or lesbian sexual orientation in adolescence is preceded by childhood **gender variant identity**, a phenomenon in which the gender identity of an individual at any age differs from phenotypic sex and assigned sex at birth (see Chapter 135).

STIGMA, RISK, AND RESILIENCE

Homosexuality has been documented across cultures and historical periods. However, its meaning and acceptance vary greatly with social context. Although gay people are now generally more visible and accepted than previously, youth are often exposed to antihomosexual attitudes. For many GLB youth, revealing their sexual orientation ("coming out") to family, peers, healthcare providers, and others is a significant step. Specific racial/ethnic, religious, and other demographic groups may experience distinct developmental stressors. For example, black youth report feeling less comfortable than white peers with a gay identity and less comfortable disclosing it.

Some GLB youth experience difficulty coping with **stigma**. A longitudinal study that investigated **bullying** and **victimization** among youth from 5th through 10th grade found that the girls and boys that identified as GLB in 10th grade were more likely than their peers to report that they had been bullied and victimized across grades. GLB youth may be perceived by others as different before they themselves have any GLB attraction or experience, or identify as GLB. Even when not overtly threatened, GLB youth frequently encounter negative attitudes that force them to hide at a time when acceptance holds great developmental significance. Family nonacceptance, feeling unsafe due to school harassment, and peer bullying related to sexual orientation elevate risk in GLB adolescents for depression, anxiety, substance abuse, suicidal thoughts and attempts, and social problems such as truancy, dropping out, running away, and homelessness. Mental health problems, sexual risk taking, or substance use may increase exposure to HIV and other STIs. Stigma may also impede access to healthcare in some communities. Thus, along with factors influencing exposure and susceptibility to health threats, stigma partly mediates elevated risk for health and mental health problems in GLB youth.

Nevertheless, most GLB youth are resilient, with good physical and mental health despite pervasive stress. Family connectedness and school support and safety are important protective factors against depression, suicidal thoughts and attempts, and substance abuse. GLB antiharassment policies and organizations such as **genders and sexualities alliances** (also sometimes called gay-straight alliances) and antibullying programs are associated with increased school safety for GLB youth. It is therefore important to reduce stigma, support acceptance, and promote resilient coping.

HEALTH
Depression and Suicidality

Compared to their heterosexual peers, GLB youth and those who are not sure of their sexual orientation have higher prevalence of suicidality. Family rejection, bullying, and other victimization motivated by homophobia account statistically for increased depression and suicidal thoughts and attempts in GLB adolescents. Suicidal thoughts or attempts are highest during the interval following recognition of same-sex

attraction or a same-sex sexual experience but prior to self-acceptance as gay.

Sexually Transmitted Infections

The epidemiology of STIs, related to specific sexual practices as well as prevalence of certain STIs in GLB communities, informs recommended counseling, screening, and treatment strategies. Anal intercourse has been shown to be the most efficient route of infection by hepatitis B (Chapter 385), cytomegalovirus (Chapter 282), and HIV (Chapter 302). Oral-anal and digital-anal contact can transmit enteric pathogens, such as hepatitis A. Unprotected oral sex also can lead to oropharyngeal disease in the receptive partner and gonococcal and nongonococcal urethritis in the insertive partner. Certain STIs, particularly ulcerative diseases, such as syphilis and herpes simplex virus infection, facilitate spread of HIV.

Among U.S. adolescents and young adults, YMSM, and especially black YMSM, continue to face the greatest prevalence of HIV/AIDS. Although possible, female-to-female sexual transmission of HIV is inefficient, and females who only engage in sex with females are less likely than other youth to acquire an STI. However, boys and girls who identify as gay or lesbian may engage in sexual activity with partners of the other sex, so counseling and screening for all types of STIs are still relevant.

Substance Abuse

Compared with their heterosexual peers, GLB youth appear to use alcohol and other substances at higher rates, including more binge drinking and earlier onset and more rapid trajectory of substance use. More substantial substance use may be greatest in youth who do not identify as GLB but have same-sex attractions or engage in same-sex sexual behavior.

Obesity and Disordered Eating

Compared with heterosexual girls, lesbian and bisexual girls are generally more likely to be obese or overweight. In contrast, young gay and bisexual males are more likely to have body image concerns and to restrict eating or engage in compensatory weight loss strategies compared to heterosexual boys. Binge eating may also be more common in GLB youth.

Psychosocial Problems

Academic underachievement, truancy, and dropping out of school are frequently associated in GLB adolescents with homophobic victimization, harassment, violence, and feeling unsafe at school. Studies suggest that youth who eventually identify as GLB have higher rates than other youth of experiencing child abuse and of running away or being kicked out of their homes. GLB young people are overrepresented among homeless and runaway populations across the United States, which can expose them to drugs, sexual abuse and other health risks.

RECOMMENDATIONS FOR CARE
Evaluation

The goal of GLB pediatric care is physical health, social and emotional well-being, and healthy development. Physicians should provide nonjudgmental care to all adolescents, including those who are GLB or questioning (see Chapter 133, Table 133.1). They should receive the age-appropriate history, examination, and anticipatory guidance recommended for adolescents in general. With some exceptions noted later, the physical examination and laboratory evaluation of GLB and questioning adolescents are the same as for any teenager. However, providers should appropriately screen for special potential medical and psychosocial threats to GLB teenagers' health.

A nonjudgmental healthcare environment is important, with open communication and a positive relationship with youth and families. In the waiting room, written material about sexual orientation, support groups, and community resources will signal openness to discussing sexuality. Registration forms recognizing the possibility of same-gender parents signal a safe setting (e.g., forms can list parent/guardian #1, parent/guardian #2). Sexual history questions should avoid heterosexual assumptions (e.g., "Are you dating someone?" vs "Do you have a boyfriend/girlfriend?"). This is important at all ages. For example, asking a 6 yr old boy if he has a girlfriend may convey an unsupportive message if he discovers later that he would like a boyfriend. Explaining confidentiality and incorporating into each adolescent visit private time with no parent in the room (see Chapter 137) may facilitate discussing sexual orientation, as may use of appropriate health history forms such as the American Medical Association's Guidelines for Adolescent Prevention Services Questionnaire.

Clinicians should remember that any youth might be GLB whether or not they are identified or perceived as such, so clinicians should not presuppose a particular orientation. Competency in conveying sensitivity, acceptance, and respectfulness; effective communication skills; and appropriate attention to privacy and confidentiality (including practices related to billing and record requests) are fundamental to providing high-quality care. While remaining attuned to youth's preferences, explicit or implied, for discussing sexual orientation, providers can tactfully take the lead, if necessary, regarding any pressing areas of clinical concern.

Medical and Sexual Health

STIs are covered in Chapter 146, but issues specific to GLB youth are included here. Use of latex condoms for fellatio, and dental dams and cut-open latex condoms for anilingus and cunnilingus, should be discussed with adolescents. Recommendations also include use of latex condoms for sexual appliances. In addition, it is important to emphasize that people who have been using alcohol or other drugs are at increased likelihood for engaging in riskier sexual activity. It is important not to assume that a gay boy or lesbian girl who does not identify as bisexual has not had sex with someone of a different sex or gender. For example, lesbians can still have an unplanned pregnancy. Therefore, prevention counseling about unintended pregnancy is relevant to all adolescents. Similarly, youth who identify as heterosexual and whose attractions are not to those of the same sex or gender may still have sexual activity with a partner of the same sex or gender.

Although vaccination against hepatitis A and B is recommended for all children, it is particularly recommended that nonvaccinated adolescent males who are having sex or are likely to have sex with males receive catch-up vaccines. The same recommendation applies to the human papillomavirus (HPV) vaccine for males. The Centers for Disease Control and Prevention (CDC) recommends that males who are engaging in sexual activity with males have annual testing for HIV, hepatitis A, hepatitis B, syphilis, urethral gonorrhea and chlamydia (if engaging in insertive oral or anal intercourse), oral gonorrhea (if engaging in receptive oral intercourse), and rectal gonorrhea and chlamydia (if engaging in receptive anal intercourse).

Mental Health

Awareness of mental health and social problems is important when caring for GLB youth, as for all youth. Clinicians should monitor for depression, suicidality, anxiety, and substance abuse and know their community's mental health resources. Minor psychosocial problems might be handled by referral to a support group for patients (e.g., GLSEN, formerly known as the Gay, Lesbian and Straight Education Network) or for parents and others (e.g., Parents, Families and Friends of Lesbians and Gays). In some communities, agencies and organizations serving the GLB community can help with social, educational, vocational, housing, and other needs.

Individuals or families who harbor negative attitudes may inquire about mental health treatment to avert or change a homosexual or bisexual orientation. However, a GLB orientation is not an illness, and leading health organizations, including the American Academy of Pediatrics, American Academy of Family Physicians, Society for Adolescent Health and Medicine, American Academy of Child and Adolescent Psychiatry, and American Medical Association, have concluded that such change is neither possible nor warranted. It is important to distinguish between a GLB orientation, which is not a mental illness, and mental health problems (e.g., depression) for which GLB youth are at elevated risk. While understanding different families' values, clinicians must recognize the morbidity and mortality associated with stigma and attempt to foster physical and emotional health. Individual or family therapy might be indicated.

Clinicians should also monitor for specific stressors, such as bullying and other homophobic victimization, family nonacceptance, and abuse. Failure to confront harassment constitutes tacit assent.

Anticipatory guidance, referral, and substance abuse treatment should be considered for the subset of GLB youth who use alcohol, drugs, or tobacco, some of whom may be using these to manage painful feelings related to conflicts over their sexuality.

Adolescents with serious psychiatric symptoms, such as suicidality, depression, and substance abuse, should be referred to mental health specialists with competency in treating GLB adolescents. It is essential to know how to recognize and manage psychiatric emergencies such as suicidal thoughts and attempts (see Chapter 40).

Bibliography is available at Expert Consult.

Chapter 135
Transgender Care
Walter O. Bockting
第一百三十五章
跨性别的护理

中文导读

本章根据跨性别青少年群体容易产生的性别焦虑和不良心理特点，指出针对该群体进行护理的特殊性以及可能出现的护理障碍，并强调医疗卫生人员在面对此类特殊群体时，应当具备有效的沟通能力，提高临床护理能力及诊断评估能力，并根据儿童和青少年的整体发展采取个性化的治疗措施，如支持性治疗、青春期抑制、女性化或男性化激素治疗和变性手术等。

Transgender individuals have a gender identity that differs significantly from the sex they were assigned at birth (see Chapter 133). They may experience **gender dysphoria**, defined as clinically significant distress or impairment in social, school/occupational, or other important areas of functioning associated with incongruence between one's experienced/expressed gender and assigned gender, for at least 6 mo in duration. **Gender-affirming care** has been shown to alleviate gender dysphoria and may include psychological evaluation and supportive therapy, puberty suppression, feminizing or masculinizing hormone therapy, and surgery. Such care is guided by the Standards of Care for **transsexual**, **transgender**, and **gender-nonconforming** people set forth by the World Professional Association for Transgender Health (WPATH). In addition, the Endocrine Society has issued practice guidelines for endocrine treatment to alleviate gender dysphoria.

Transgender and gender-nonconforming children and adolescents have increased vulnerability to mental health concerns because of social stigma attached to gender nonconformity. Moreover, transgender and gender-nonconforming children and adolescents may present with general health concerns unrelated to their gender identity or gender expression, but may experience barriers to care that include a lack of cultural competence on the part of healthcare providers or the healthcare systems in which they practice. Therefore, to serve the youth and their families adequately, attention to both cultural and clinical competency is critical and should be improved. The American Psychological Association and the American Association of Child and Adolescent Psychiatrists have published practice guidelines to promote improved access to competent care.

CULTURAL AND CLINICAL COMPETENCE
Cultural competence refers to the ability to communicate effectively with patients from various backgrounds. This includes appropriate assessment and clinical documentation of both gender identity (What is your current gender identity?) and sex assigned at birth (What sex were you assigned at birth [on your original birth certificate]?), use of preferred names and pronouns, and availability of all-gender bathrooms. It also includes recognition of and respect for gender diversity: children and adolescents may identify as girl, boy, boygirl, girlboy, transgender, genderqueer, nonbinary, gender fluid, gender questioning, or any other way in which they may describe their gender identity and expression (see Chapter 133). Particularly with children and adolescents, it is imperative not to label prematurely a young person's gender identity, but rather allow ample time for them to explore their gender identity and expression.

Clinical competence in transgender care refers to training and experience in providing gender-affirming care to facilitate gender identity development, alleviate any gender dysphoria, and promote resilience in the face of stigma. Care should ideally be provided by an interdisciplinary team or, alternatively, in consultation with other providers involved in the child or adolescent's care. This may include primary care providers, pediatric endocrinologists, and mental health professionals. The WPATH Standards of Care recommend that providers be competent in working with children and adolescents; be able to screen for coexisting mental health concerns; be knowledgeable about gender-nonconforming identities and expressions; and be knowledgeable and engaged in continuing education about the assessment and treatment of gender dysphoria.

GENDER LITERACY
For both providers and patients (child or adolescent and family), an up-to-date understanding of gender diversity is key. Much is yet to be learned about transgender identity development, but we do know that gender is not necessarily *binary*, and transgender and gender-nonconforming children and adolescents may identify and express their gender identity along a spectrum. The implication for care is that not all these children and adolescents need to change their gender role from male to female or female to male, and are in need of early medical interventions. Certainly, for some transgender and gender-nonconforming children and adolescents, these interventions are medically necessary

and lifesaving, and evidence to date indicates that for those who meet criteria for a DSM-5 diagnosis of gender dysphoria, treatment appears safe and effective in reducing gender dysphoria and optimizing mental health and well-being. Others, however, do not identify with the gender binary (i.e., do not identify as male or female, but rather as an alternative gender) and need a more individualized approach that may or may not include changes in gender role and/or any of the available medical interventions. For all young people, it is imperative to support them in the process of identity exploration and tolerate any ambiguity and uncertainty, as well as evaluate and treat their concerns in light of their overall child and adolescent development.

ASSESSMENT

The *Diagnostic and Statistical Manual of Mental Disorders, Fifth Edition* (DSM-5) outlines criteria for a diagnosis of gender dysphoria in children as well as in adolescents and adults (see Table 133.2). For children, these criteria must include a strong desire or insistence to be of the other gender (or some alternative gender that differs from one's assigned gender). For adolescents, this may include a marked incongruence between one's experienced/expressed gender and (anticipated) primary and/or secondary sex characteristics; a strong desire for the sex characteristics of the other gender (or some alternative gender that differs from one's assigned gender), and/or a strong desire to be treated as another gender.

There is considerable variation in the clinical presentation, severity, and persistence of gender dysphoria among children and adolescents. It is therefore important to obtain a history of gender identification and expression and monitor ongoing identity exploration and development. Coexisting mental health concerns of anxiety, depression, nonsuicidal self-injury, suicidal ideation, and suicide attempts are not uncommon and should be assessed. There also is a higher prevalence of autism spectrum disorder among children and adolescents presenting with gender dysphoria.

TREATMENT

Transgender and gender-nonconforming children and adolescents can benefit greatly from a nonjudgmental and empathetic stance, patient education about gender diversity and the available options to alleviate gender dysphoria and affirm gender identity, access to community resources, and family support. Attention to behavioral problems and therapy for any mental health concerns caused by gender nonconformity and the attached social stigma should be incorporated into the treatment plan.

Treatment of gender dysphoria may include psychotherapy to reduce distress related to gender dysphoria or any other psychosocial difficulties. *Gender nonconformity in and of itself is not pathologic.* In addition, it is not ethical to try to change gender identity and expression to become more congruent with sex assigned at birth, because this has proved unsuccessful, particularly in the long term. Instead, psychotherapy (by a professional trained in transgender health) should support the unfolding process of identity exploration and development and assist the patient and family to manage any uncertainty and anxiety about the eventual outcome. Options to affirm gender identity include changes in gender role and expression, puberty suppression, feminizing or masculinizing hormones, and surgery. Changes in gender role may include changes in name and pronouns.

Puberty suppression with GnRH analogs, a reversible early medical intervention to reduce dysphoria by preventing the development of unwanted sex characteristics, is available as early as Tanner Stage 2. Feminizing or masculinizing **hormone therapy**, only partially reversible, is available and should be tailored to the somatic, emotional, and mental development of the adolescent. **Masculinizing chest surgery**, irreversible, is available preferably after ample experience living in a gender role congruent with the adolescent's gender identity. **Breast augmentation** is available, particularly after feminizing hormones have reached their maximum impact on breast growth. Hormone therapy or chest/breast surgery is indicated in patients with persistent, well-documented gender dysphoria who have the capacity to make a fully informed decision and to consent for treatment. **Genital surgery** (phalloplasty, metoidioplasty, vaginoplasty), irreversible, is available after living for a least 12 mo in a gender role congruent with the adolescent's gender identity, and preferably after the legal age of majority to give consent for medical procedures has been reached. For all these options, informed consent and support from family are critically important.

Early medical interventions have shown great promise in reducing gender dysphoria and optimizing psychosocial adjustment and well-being, but much remains unknown, particularly about the long-term effects of puberty suppression. Moreover, gender identity and expression should be evaluated within the larger context of identity and human development, especially during the formative years of childhood and adolescence.

Many transgender people choose hormone therapy and do not undergo surgery of breast/chest or genitals. The implications for fertility and options for fertility preservation should be discussed and considered before hormone therapy and surgery. Indeed, there are transgender individuals who elect to have children and nurse the child after birth. Rather than using the term *breastfeeding*, the term *chest feeding* may be preferred. When transgender adults seek primary healthcare, attention must be focused on gender- as well as sex organ–specific preventive screening (e.g., Pap smear, mammography, prostate exam).

FAMILIES

Family support is an important resource for transgender and gender-nonconforming youth and has been shown to buffer the negative impact of stigma on mental health. Family support also is a prerequisite for initiation of puberty suppression, feminizing or masculinizing hormone therapy, or any surgery before the age of legal majority has been reached. Providers are encouraged to include family in all aspects of treatment, while understanding that family members may be at different points in the process of coming to terms with having a transgender or gender-nonconforming loved one. Family members may benefit from online and community resources to educate themselves about gender diversity and to connect with similar others. Transgender and gender-nonconforming children and adolescents as well as their families are encouraged to learn as much as possible to be able to make fully informed decisions, in consultation with clinically competent transgender care providers, about the available behavioral and medical treatment options to affirm gender identity.

Bibliography is available at Expert Consult.

Chapter 136
The Epidemiology of Adolescent Health Problems

Gale R. Burstein

第一百三十六章
青少年健康问题的流行病学

中文导读

本章介绍了青少年的主要健康问题及流行趋势，指出了影响青少年发病和死亡的主要因素不是先天性疾病或传染病，而是不良行为导致的各类健康问题，如吸烟、饮酒、少女妊娠、性传播疾病和药物滥用等。通过比较青少年在青春发育早期、中期、晚期的心理和行为发育特点，揭示了青少年健康问题在不同发育阶段的差异，并分析了导致差异的原因，如贫穷、不良环境、获得医疗保健的机会不足、个人行为因素以及教育不公平等。

Adolescence is the first period of life where the major determinants of morbidity and mortality are *behavioral* rather than congenital or infectious. As adolescents make the transition from childhood to adulthood, they establish **behaviors** that affect both their current and future health. Adolescence is a time of immense **biologic, psychological, and social change** (see Chapter 132). Many of the psychological changes have a biologic substrate in the development and eventual maturation of the central nervous system, particularly the frontal lobe areas responsible for executive functioning (Fig. 136.1). In addition to cognitive development, there are both risk and protective factors for adverse adolescent health behaviors that are dependent on the social environment as well as the mental health of an adolescent (Table 136.1).

Many adolescents continually confront the task of making healthy choices while struggling with impulsivity that can lead to unintentional consequences, such as injuries, sexually transmitted infections (STIs), or drug overdoses. Adolescents are also challenged with adopting behaviors that will affect their future adult health, such as eating nutritiously, engaging in physical activity, and choosing not to use tobacco. Environmental factors, such as family, peers, school, community, and religiosity, also contribute to adolescents' health and risk behaviors. The U.S. Centers for Disease Control and Prevention (CDC) **Youth Risk Behavior Surveillance Survey**, a school-based survey of a nationally representative sample of U.S. high school students, demonstrates that youth begin engaging in behaviors that place their health at risk during

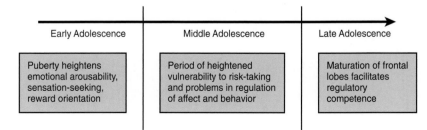

Fig. 136.1 It has been speculated that the impact of puberty on arousal and motivation occurs before the maturation of the frontal lobes is complete. This gap may create a period of heightened vulnerability to problems in the regulation of affect and behavior, which might help to explain the increased potential in adolescence for risk taking, recklessness, and the onset of emotional and behavioral problems. *(From Steinberg L: Cognitive and affective development in adolescence, Trends Cogn Sci 9:69–74, 2005.)*

Table 136.1	Identified Risk and Protective Factors for Adolescent Health Behaviors	
BEHAVIOR	**RISK FACTORS**	**PROTECTIVE FACTORS**
Smoking	Depression and other mental health problems, alcohol use, disconnectedness from school or family, difficulty talking with parents, minority ethnicity, low school achievement, peer smoking	Family connectedness, perceived healthiness, higher parental expectations, low prevalence of smoking in school
Alcohol and drug misuse	Depression and other mental health problems, low self-esteem, easy family access to alcohol, working outside school, difficulty talking with parents, risk factors for transition from occasional to regular substance misuse (smoking, availability of substances, peer use, other risk behaviors)	Connectedness with school and family, religious affiliation
Teenage pregnancy	Deprivation, city residence, low educational expectations, lack of access to sexual health services, drug and alcohol use	Connectedness with school and family, religious affiliation
Sexually transmitted infections	Mental health problems, substance misuse	Connectedness with school and family, religious affiliation

Adapted from McIntiosh N, Helms P, Smyth R, editors. *Fofar and Arneil's textbook of pediatrics*, ed 6, Edinburgh, 2003, Churchill Livingstone, pp 1757–1768; and Viner R, Macfarlane A: Health promotion, *BMJ* 330:527–529, 2005.

Table 136.2	Leading Causes of Death Among 15-19 Yr Olds by Gender, United States, 2014*				
	MALE		**FEMALE**		
LEADING CAUSES OF DEATH	**Cause of Death**	**Mortality Rate per 100,000 Population**	**Cause of Death**	**Mortality Rate per 100,000 Population**	
#1	Accidents (unintentional injuries)	24.9	Accidents (unintentional injuries)	10.1	
#2	Intentional self-harm (suicide)	13.0	Intentional self-harm (suicide)	4.2	
#3	Assault (homicide)	11.2	Malignant neoplasms	2.5	

*Based on data from Heron M: Deaths: leading causes for 2014, *Natl Vital Stat Rep* 65(5), 2016.

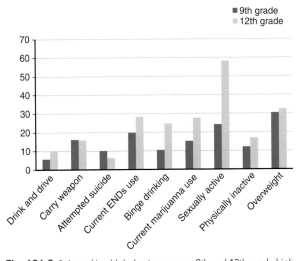

Fig. 136.2 Selected health behaviors among 9th and 12th grade high school students. ENDs, Electronic nicotine delivery system. *(Data from Centers for Disease Control and Prevention: 1991–2015 High school youth risk behavior survey data. http://nccd.cdc.gov/youthonline.)*

adolescence (Fig. 136.2).

Although according to the 2015 CDC National Health Interview Survey (https://www.cdc.gov/nchs/nhis/shs/tables.htm), a probability sample survey conducted annually, an estimated 82% of 12-17 yr olds report excellent or very good health, 11% reported limitation in usual activities due to one or more chronic conditions, 10% missed 6-10 school days in the past year, 6% are uninsured, 6% have no usual place

of healthcare, 10% have asthma, 12% have respiratory allergies, 10% have a learning disability, 14% have attention-deficit/hyperactivity disorder, and 18% take prescription medications routinely. In 2014 the mortality rate among adolescents 15-19 yr of age was 45 deaths per 100,000 population. While varying by gender, the leading **causes of death** overall among adolescents 15-19 yr of age are (1) unintentional injuries; (2) suicide; and (3) homicide (Table 136.2).

Within the adolescent population, **disparities in health** occur. Adolescent health outcomes and behaviors vary among populations that can be defined by race or ethnicity, gender, education or income, disability, geographic location (e.g., rural or urban), or sexual orientation. Health disparities result from multiple factors, including poverty, environmental threats, inadequate access to healthcare, individual and behavioral factors, and educational inequalities (Table 136.3).

ACCESS TO HEALTHCARE

Adolescents in the United States make fewer visits to physicians for ambulatory office visits than any other age group; school-age children and adolescents are more likely than younger children to have unmet health needs and delayed medical care. Adolescents who actually receive preventive care may still not have access to **time alone with their provider** to discuss confidential health issues such as STIs, HIV, or pregnancy prevention. Less than half (40%) of adolescents have time alone with their healthcare provider during a preventive healthcare visit; sexually experienced teens report sexual health discussions more often than nonsexually experienced teens, but the frequency is still low at 64% and 33.5% for sexually experienced females and males, respectively.

Young adults 18-24 yr are more likely to be insured with the 2010 Patient Protection and Affordable Care Act (**ACA**). Currently, the ACA permits children to receive benefits from their parents' health plans through age 26 yr. *Healthy People* provides science-based, 10-yr national objectives for measuring and improving the health of all Americans by establishing benchmarks and monitoring progress over time. The

Table 136.3	Adolescent Health Outcomes by Race/Ethnicity, United States, 2010–2012				
OUTCOME	**WHITE**	**BLACK**	**AI/AN**	**API**	**HISPANIC**
Deaths*	43.5	62.3	49.7	23.1	38.1
Births[†]	17.3	34.9	27.3	7.7	38.0
Obese[‡]	12.4	16.8	15.9	5.5[§]	16.4
Asthma[‡]	22.1	27.8	17.7	17.7[§]	22.5
Depressed[‡]	28.6	25.2	34.9	22.9[§]	35.3
Chlamydia*	775.2	4,200.8	2,229.6	267.9[§]	1,067.0
Gonorrhea*	94.4	1,218.5	393.8	37.6[§]	150.6
HIV*	1.8	36.2	4.9	2.8[§]	7.0

*2015 Rates per 100,000 15-19 yr old population by race/ethnicity.
[†]2014 Rates of births in per 1,000 15-19 yr old females by race/ethnicity.
[‡]Percent high school students reporting health outcome in 2015.
[§]Rates of Asian-only race.
AI/AN, American Indian or Alaska Native; API, Asian or Pacific Islander; HIV, human immunodeficiency virus.

Healthy People 2020 agenda includes 11 adolescent-specific objectives with a goal of improving the healthy development, health, safety, and well-being of adolescents and young adults over the next 10 yr (Table 136.4). This science-based initiative is centered around a framework for public health prevention priorities and actions to improve the health status of U.S. youth.

Bibliography is available at Expert Consult.

Table 136.4	*Healthy People 2020* Adolescent Health (AH) Objectives

- **AH-1**: Increase the proportion of adolescents who have had a wellness checkup in the past 12 months
- **AH-2**: Increase the proportion of adolescents who participate in extracurricular and out-of-school activities
- **AH-3**: Increase the proportion of adolescents who are connected to a parent or other positive adult caregiver
  AH-3.1: Increase the proportion of adolescents who have an adult in their lives with whom they can talk about serious problems
  AH-3.2: Increase the proportion of parents who attend events and activities in which their adolescents participate
- **AH-4**: (Developmental) Increase the proportion of adolescents and young adults who transition to self-sufficiency from foster care
- **AH-5**: Increase educational achievement of adolescents and young adults
  AH-5.1 *(Leading Health Indicator)*: Increase the proportion of students who graduate with a regular diploma 4 years after starting 9th grade
  AH-5.2: Increase the proportion of students who are served under the Individuals with Disabilities Education Act who graduate high school with a diploma
  AH-5.3: Increase the proportion of students whose reading skills are at or above the proficient achievement level for their grade
  AH-5.4: Increase the proportion of students whose mathematics skills are at or above the proficient achievement level for their grade

- **AH-5.5**: Increase the proportion of adolescents who consider their school work to be meaningful and important
- **AH-5.6**: Decrease school absenteeism among adolescents due to illness or injury
- **AH-6**: Increase the proportion of schools with a school breakfast program
- **AH-7**: Reduce the proportion of adolescents who have been offered, sold, or given an illegal drug on school property
- **AH-8**: Increase the proportion of adolescents whose parents consider them to be safe at school
- **AH-9**: (Developmental) Increase the proportion of middle and high schools that prohibit harassment based on a student's sexual orientation or gender identity
- **AH-10**: Decrease the proportion of public schools with a serious violent incident
- **AH-11**: Reduce adolescent and young adult perpetration of, as well as victimization by, crimes
  AH-11.1: Decrease the rate of minor and young adult perpetration of violent crimes
  AH-11.2: Decrease the rate of minor and young adult perpetration of serious property crimes
  AH-11.3: (Developmental) Decrease the percentage of counties and cities reporting youth gang activity
  AH-11.4: (Developmental) Reduce the rate of adolescent and young adult victimization from crimes of violence

From US Department of Health and Human Services: *Healthy People 2020,* available at: https://www.healthypeople.gov/2020/topics-objectives/topic/Adolescent-Health/objectives.

Chapter **137**
Delivery of Healthcare to Adolescents

Gale R. Burstein

第一百三十七章
青春期卫生保健

中文导读

　　基于青少年死亡和残疾的发生可通过行为干预来预防，以及医疗保健在干预过程中发挥着重要作用的原则。本章强调每个社区都应建立全面的卫生保健系统，以确保为青少年提供全面和高质量的护理；医疗保健提供方应满足青少年的发展需要，特别是在生殖健康、心理健康、口腔健康和用药方面给予指导，并向所有青少年提供连续的、保密的、负担得起的医疗卫生服务。

Healthcare providers play an important role in nurturing healthy behaviors among adolescents, because the leading causes of death and disability among adolescents are preventable. Adolescence provides a unique opportunity to prevent or modify health conditions arising from behaviors that develop in the 2nd decade of life and that can lead to substantial morbidity and mortality, such as trauma, cardiovascular and pulmonary disease, type 2 diabetes, reproductive health disease, and cancer (see Chapter 132, Table 132.4).

Health systems in each community should be in place to ensure comprehensive and high-quality care to adolescents. **Health insurance coverage** that is affordable, continuous, confidential, and not subject to exclusion for preexisting conditions should be available for all adolescents and young adults. **Comprehensive, coordinated benefits** should meet the developmental needs of adolescents, particularly for reproductive, mental health, dental, and substance abuse services. **Safety net providers and programs** that provide confidential services, such as school-based health centers, federally qualified health centers, family planning services, and clinics that treat sexually transmitted infections (**STIs**) in adolescents and young adults, need to have assured funding for viability and sustainability. **Quality-of-care** data should be collected and analyzed by age so that the performance measures for age-appropriate healthcare needs of adolescents are monitored. **Affordability** is important for access to preventive services. Family involvement should be encouraged, but **confidentiality** and adolescent consent are critically important. **Healthcare providers**, trained and experienced in adolescent care, should be available in all communities. Healthcare providers should be adequately compensated to support the range and intensity of services required to address the developmental and health service needs of adolescents. The development and dissemination of provider education about **adolescent preventive health guidelines** have been demonstrated to improve the content of recommended care (Table 137.1). The ease of recognition or expectation that an adolescent's needs can be addressed in a setting relates to the **visibility and flexibility** of sites and services. Staff at sites should be approachable, linguistically capable, and culturally competent. Health services should be coordinated to respond to goals for adolescent health at the local, state, and national levels. The coordination should address service financing and delivery in a manner that reduces disparities in care.

Although most adolescents in the United States have seen a healthcare provider in the past year and report a usual source of healthcare, adolescents are less likely to receive **preventive care** services. According to the 2011 National Health Interview Survey, an estimated 90% of 12-17 yr old U.S. adolescents had 1 or more contacts with a healthcare professional in the past year, 98% identify a usual source of care at a physician's office or clinic, and 17% made at least 1 emergency department visit in the past year. Uninsured adolescents are the least likely to receive care. In 2015, 63% of people under age 19 yr were covered at some point during the year by private insurance, and 43% of children had public health insurance at some point during 2015. However, even among adolescents who are fully insured with a usual source of care, most do not receive preventive healthcare. An analysis of claims data from a large Minnesota health plan with approximately 700,000 members found that among patients age 11-18 yr who were enrolled for at least 4 yr between 1998 and 2007, few received preventive care visits. One third of adolescents had no preventive care visits from age 13 through 17 yr, and another 40% had only a single such visit. Nonpreventive care visits were more frequent in all age-groups, averaging about 1 per yr at age 11 yr, climbing to about 1.5 per yr at age 17 yr. Among older adolescents, females had both more preventive care and more nonpreventive care visits than did males.

The **Patient Protection and Affordable Care Act (ACA)**, enacted in March 2010, has expanded access to both commercial health plans

Table 137.1	Bright Futures/American Academy of Pediatrics Recommendations for Preventive Healthcare for 11-21 Yr Olds
	PERIODICITY AND INDICATIONS
HISTORY	Annual
MEASUREMENTS	
Body mass index	Annual
Blood pressure	Annual
SENSORY SCREENING	
Vision	At 12 yr and 15 yr visits or if risk assessment positive
Hearing	Screen with audiometry, including 6,000 and 8,000 Hz high frequencies once at 11-14 yr, once at 15-17 yr, and once at 18-21 yr.
DEVELOPMENTAL/BEHAVIORAL ASSESSMENT	
Developmental surveillance	Annual
Psychosocial/behavioral assessment	Annual
Depression screening	Annual for 12 yr and older
Tobacco, alcohol, and drug use assessment	If risk assessment positive
PHYSICAL EXAMINATION	Annual
PROCEDURES	
Immunization*	Annual
Hematocrit or hemoglobin	If risk assessment positive
Tuberculin test	If risk assessment positive
Dyslipidemia screening	Once at 9-11 yr, and once at 17-21 yr
STI screening	If sexually active
HIV screening[†]	Once between ages 15 and 18 yr Discuss and offer at earlier age and annually if risk assessment positive.
Cervical dysplasia screening[‡]	Beginning at age 21 yr
ORAL HEALTH	Annual; refer to dental home
ANTICIPATORY GUIDANCE	Annual[§]

*Schedules per the Advisory Committee on Immunization Practices, published annually at http://www.cdc.gov/vaccines/schedules/hcp/index.html and http://redbook.solutions.aap.org/SS/Immunization_Schedules.aspx.

[†]CDC recommends universal, voluntary HIV screening of all sexually active people, beginning at age 13 yr. The American Academy of Pediatrics recommends offering routine HIV screening to all adolescents at least once by 16-18 yr of age and to those younger if at risk. US Preventive Services Task Force recommends offering routine HIV screening to all adolescents age 15 yr and older at least once and to those younger if at risk. Patients who test positive for HIV should receive prevention counseling and referral to care before leaving the testing site.

[‡]Screening for cervical cancer, April 2012, US Preventive Services Task Force. http://www.uspreventiveservicestaskforce.org/uspstf/uspscerv.htm.

[§]Refer to specific guidance by age as listed in *Bright Futures* guidelines.
HIV, Human immunodeficiency virus; STI, sexually transmitted infection.
Adapted from Hagan JF, Shaw JS, Duncan PM, editors: *Bright Futures: guidelines for health supervision of infants, children, and adolescents*, ed 4, Elk Grove Village, IL, 2017, American Academy of Pediatrics.

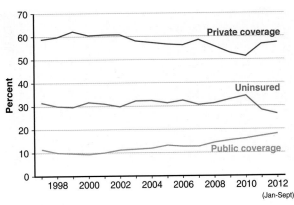

Fig. 137.1 Percentage of adults age 19-25 yr with health insurance by coverage type and percentage uninsured at the time of the interview: United States, 1997–September, 2012. *Note:* Estimates for 2012 are based on data collected in January through September. Data are based on household interviews of a sample of the civilian noninstitutionalized population. *(Data from CDC/NCHS, National Health Interview Survey, 1997–2012, Family Core Component.)*

services free of any cost sharing, deductibles, or copayments. In states that have expanded Medicaid coverage, all adults with incomes <133% of the federal poverty level are eligible to enroll.

The complexity and interaction of physical, cognitive, and psychosocial **developmental processes** during adolescence require sensitivity and skill on the part of the health professional (see Chapter 132). Health education and promotion, as well as disease prevention, should be the focus of every visit. In 2017 the American Academy of Pediatrics (AAP) in collaboration with the U.S. Department of Health and Human Services, Health Resources and Services Administration, Maternal and Child Health Bureau, published the 4th edition of *Bright Futures: Guidelines for Health Supervision of Infants, Children, and Adolescents*, which offers providers a strategy for delivery of adolescent preventive health services with screening and counseling recommendations for early, middle, and late adolescence (Table 137.2). *Bright Futures* is rooted in the philosophy of preventive care and reflects the concept of caring for children in a "medical home." These guidelines emphasize effective partnerships with parents and the community to support the adolescent's health and development.

The Centers for Disease Control and Prevention (CDC) Advisory Committee on Immunization Practices (ACIP) currently recommends routine **adolescent vaccines** for universal administration beginning at the 11-12 yr old visit, or as soon as possible, (a) tetanus–diphtheria–acellular pertussis vaccine (Tdap), (b) the meningococcal conjugate vaccine (MCV4) with a booster at age 16 yr, and (c) the human papillomavirus (HPV) series (see Chapter 197). ACIP recommends annual influenza vaccination and hepatitis A virus (HAV) vaccination to adolescents and young adults who have not previously received the HAV vaccine series if immunity against HAV is desired or for those at increased risk for infection, such as men who have sex with men (MSM), injection drug users (IDU), and those with chronic liver disease or clotting factor disorders, or who live in areas that target older children for HAV vaccine.

The time spent on various elements of the screening will vary with the issues that surface during the assessment. For **gay and lesbian youth** (see Chapter 134), emotional and psychological issues related to their experiences, from fear of disclosure to the trauma of homophobia, may direct the clinician to spend more time assessing emotional and psychological supports in the young person's environment. For youth with **chronic illnesses or special needs**, the assessment of at-risk behaviors should not be omitted or deemphasized by assuming they do not experience the "normal" adolescent vulnerabilities.

Bibliography is available at Expert Consult.

and Medicaid for young adults age 19-26 yr (Fig. 137.1). From June 2010 through June 2012, the proportion of young adults with insurance increased from 65.7% to 73.8%. Currently, ACA provisions require that commercial health plans (1) continue dependent coverage to 26 yr, regardless of the young adult's financial or dependent status, marriage, or educational enrollment; (2) mandate university and college student health plans to enhance consumer protections for students; (3) provide financial assistance for young adults to enroll into health insurance exchanges with incomes ranging from 133–399% of the federal poverty level in **Medicaid expansion states**; and (4) offer preventive healthcare

Table 137.2 | Adolescent Screening Recommendations

Universal Screening	11-14 YR OLD VISIT Action	15-17 YR OLD VISIT Action	18-21 YR OLD VISIT Action
Cervical dysplasia*	N/A	N/A	Pap smear all young women at 21 yr visit
Depression	Adolescent depression screen beginning at 12 yr visit	Adolescent depression screen	Adolescent depression screen
Dyslipidemia	Lipid screen once at 9-11 yr	Lipid screen once at 17-21 yr	Lipid screen once at 17-21 yr
Hearing	Once at 11-14 yr Audiometry, including 6,000 and 8,000 Hz high frequencies	Once at 15-17 yr Audiometry, including 6,000 and 8,000 Hz high frequencies	Once at 18-21 yr Audiometry, including 6,000 and 8,000 Hz high frequencies
HIV[†]	Selective screening (see below)	HIV test once at 15-18 yr	HIV test once at 15-18 yr
Tobacco, alcohol, or drug use	Tobacco, alcohol, or drug use screen	Tobacco, alcohol, or drug use screen	Tobacco, alcohol, or drug use screen
Vision	At 12 yr visit Objective measure with age-appropriate visual-acuity measurement using HOTV or Lea symbols, Sloan letters, or Snellen letters	At 15 yr visit Objective measure with age-appropriate visual-acuity measurement using HOTV or Lea symbols, Sloan letters, or Snellen letters	N/A

Selective Screening	Risk Assessment (RA)	11-14 YR OLD VISIT Action If RA+	15-17 YR OLD VISIT Action If RA+	18-21 YR OLD VISIT Action If RA+
Anemia	+ on risk screening questions	Hemoglobin or hematocrit	Hemoglobin or hematocrit	Hemoglobin or hematocrit
Dyslipidemia (if not universally screened at this visit)	+ on risk screening questions and not previously screened with normal results	Lipid profile	Lipid profile	Lipid profile
HIV[†]	+ on risk screening questions	HIV test	HIV test (if not universally screened at this visit)	HIV test (if not universally screened at this visit)
Oral health (through 16 yr visit)	Primary water source fluoride deficient	Oral fluoridation supplementation	Oral fluoridation supplementation	N/A
STIs • Chlamydia • Gonorrhea • Syphilis	Sexually active females Sexually active males and + on risk screening questions Sexually active and + on risk screening questions	Chlamydia and gonorrhea NAAT (use tests appropriate for population and clinical setting) Syphilis test	Chlamydia and gonorrhea NAAT (use tests appropriate for population and clinical setting) Syphilis test	Chlamydia and gonorrhea NAAT (use tests appropriate for population and clinical setting) Syphilis test
Tuberculosis	+ on risk screening questions	Tuberculin skin test	Tuberculin skin test	Tuberculin skin test
Vision at other ages	+ on risk screening questions at 11, 13, and 14 yr visits	Objective measure with age-appropriate visual-acuity measurement using HOTV or Lea symbols, Sloan letters, or Snellen letters	Objective measure with age-appropriate visual-acuity measurement using HOTV or Lea symbols, Sloan letters, or Snellen letters	Objective measure with age-appropriate visual-acuity measurement using HOTV or Lea symbols, Sloan letters, or Snellen letters

*Screening for Cervical Cancer. April 2012. U.S. Preventive Services Task Force. http://www.uspreventiveservicestaskforce.org/uspstf/uspscerv.htm.

[†]Centers for Disease Control and Prevention recommends universal, voluntary HIV screening of all sexually active people, beginning at age 13 yr. American Academy of Pediatrics recommends routine HIV screening offered to all adolescents at least once by 16-18 yr of age and to those younger if at risk. U.S. Preventive Services Task Force recommends routine HIV screening offered to all adolescents age 15 yr and older at least once and to those younger if at risk. Patients who test positive for HIV should receive prevention counseling and referral to care before leaving the testing site.

NA, Not applicable; NAAT, nucleic acid amplification test; STIs, sexually transmitted infections.

Adapted from Hagan JF, Shaw JS, Duncan PM, editors: *Bright Futures: guidelines for health supervision of infants, children, and adolescents*, ed 4, Elk Grove Village, IL, 2017, American Academy of Pediatrics; and Bright Futures/American Academy of Pediatrics: Recommendations for Preventive Pediatric Health Care (Periodicity Schedule), 2017. https://www.aap.org/en-us/Documents/periodicity_schedule.pdf.

137.1 Legal Issues

Gale R. Burstein

The rights of an individual, including those of adolescents, vary widely between nations. In the United States, the right of a minor to consent to treatment without parental knowledge differs between states and is governed by **state-specific minor consent laws**. Some consent laws are based on a minor's status, such as minors who are emancipated, parents, married, pregnant, in the armed services, or mature. In some states, minors can be considered *emancipated* if they are or have served in the armed services or are living apart from parents and are economically independent through gainful employment. A *mature minor* is a minor who is emotionally and intellectually mature enough to give informed consent and who lives under the supervision of a parent or guardian. Courts have held that if a minor is mature, a physician is not liable for providing beneficial treatment. There is no formal process for recognition of a mature minor. The determination is made by the healthcare provider.

Some minor consent laws are based on services a minor is seeking, such as emergency care, sexual healthcare, substance abuse, or mental healthcare (Table 137.3). All 50 states and the District of Columbia explicitly allow minors to consent for their own health services for **STIs**. Approximately 25% of states require that minors be a certain age (generally 12-14 yr) before they can consent for their own care for STIs. No state requires parental consent for STI care or requires that providers notify parents that an adolescent minor child has received STI services, except in limited or unusual circumstances.

Minors' right to consent for **contraceptive services** varies from state to state. Almost 50% of states and the District of Columbia explicitly authorize all minors to consent for their own contraceptive services; and 50% of states permit minors to consent for their own contraceptive services under specific circumstances, such as being married, a parent, currently or previously pregnant, over a certain age, or a high school graduate, or per physician's discretion.

A minor's right to consent for **mental healthcare** and **substance abuse** treatment services vary by state and age of minor, whether care is medical vs nonmedical (e.g., counseling), and whether care is delivered as an inpatient vs outpatient basis. Minor consent laws often contain provisions regarding confidentiality and disclosure, even when general state consent laws do not have such provisions.

The **confidentiality** of medical information and records of a minor who has consented for his or her own *reproductive healthcare* is governed by numerous federal and state laws. Laws in some states explicitly protect the confidentiality of STI or contraceptive services for which minors have given their own consent and do not allow disclosure of the information without the minor's consent. In other states, laws grant physicians discretion to disclose information to parents.

The confidentiality of medical information and records of a minor who has consented for his or her own healthcare is also governed by numerous federal and state laws. Laws in some states explicitly protect the confidentiality of STI, contraceptive, or mental health services for which minors have given their own consent, and do not allow disclosure of the information without the minor's consent. In other states, laws grant physicians discretion to disclose information to parents. Title X and Medicaid both provide confidentiality protection for family planning services provided to minors with funding from these programs.

Federal regulations issued under the Federal Health Insurance Portability and Accountability Act of 1996, known as the **HIPAA Privacy Rule**, defer to state and "other applicable laws" with respect to the question of whether parents have access to information about care for which a minor has given consent. Thus, both the state laws that either prohibit or permit disclosure of confidential information and the federal Title X and Medicaid laws that protect the confidentiality of care for adolescents are important under the HIPAA Privacy Rule in determining when confidential information about health services for minors can be disclosed to parents.

Billing for confidential services is complex. Commercial health plans send home an **explanation of benefit (EOB)** to the primary insured or the primary beneficiary, listing services rendered by the provider and reimbursed by the health plan. An EOB documenting that confidential health services were rendered to their adolescent dependent that is received by a parent may disclose those services. In addition, copayments automatically generated with certain billing codes for office visits and medications can be a barrier for adolescents receiving care, including treatment.

Providers may elect to establish a policy of discussing with their adolescent patients when medical records and other information will

Table 137.3	Types of Minor Consent Statutes or Rules of Common Law That Allow for Medical Treatment of a Minor Patient Without Parental Consent
LEGAL EXCEPTIONS TO INFORMED CONSENT REQUIREMENT	**MEDICAL CARE SETTING**
The "emergency" exception	• The child is suffering from an emergent condition that places his or her life or health in danger. • The child's legal guardian is unavailable or unable to provide consent for treatment or transport. • Treatment or transport cannot be safely delayed until consent can be obtained. • The professional administers only treatment for emergent conditions that pose an immediate threat to the child.
The "emancipated minor" exception	• Married • Economically self-supporting and not living at home • Active-duty status in the military • In some states, a minor who is a parent or pregnant • Some states might require a court to declare the emancipation of a minor.
The "mature minor" exception	Most states recognize a mature minor, in which a minor, usually ≥14 yr, displays sufficient maturity and intelligence to understand and appreciate the benefits, risks, and alternatives of the proposed treatment and to make a voluntary and reasonable choice on the basis of that information. States vary or whether a judicial determination is required.
Exceptions based on specific medical condition (state laws vary)	Minor seeks: • Mental health services • Pregnancy and contraceptive services • Testing or treatment for HIV infection or AIDS • Sexually transmitted infection testing and treatment • Drug and alcohol addiction treatment

Data from American Academy of Pediatrics: Consent for emergency medical services for children and adolescents, *Pediatrics* 128:427–433, 2011.

be disclosed and developing a mechanism to alert office staff as to what information in the chart is confidential. For legal and other reasons, a chaperone should be present whenever an adolescent female patient is examined by a male physician.

Bibliography is available at Expert Consult.

137.2 Screening Procedures
Gale R. Burstein

INTERVIEWING THE ADOLESCENT
The preparation for a successful interview with an adolescent patient varies based on the history of the relationship with the patient. Patients (and their parents) who are going from preadolescence to adolescence while seeing the same provider should be guided through the transition. Although the rules for confidentiality are the same for new and continuing patients, the change in the **physician–patient relationship**, allowing more privacy during the visit and more autonomy in the health process, may be threatening for the parent as well as the adolescent. For new patients, the initial phases of the interview are more challenging given the need to establish rapport rapidly with the patient in order to meet the goals of the encounter. Issues of **confidentiality and privacy** should be explicitly stated along with the conditions under which that confidentiality may need to be altered, that is, in life- or safety-threatening situations. For new patients, the parents should be interviewed with the adolescent or before the adolescent to ensure that the adolescent does not perceive a breach of confidentiality. The clinician who takes time to listen, avoids judgmental statements and the use of street jargon, and shows respect for the adolescent's emerging maturity will have an easier time communicating with the adolescent. The use of open-ended questions, rather than closed-ended questions, will further facilitate history taking. (The closed-ended question, "Do you get along with your father?" leads to the answer "yes" or "no," in contrast to the question, "What might you like to be different in your relationship with your mother?" which may lead to an answer such as, "I would like her to stop always worrying about me.")

The **goals** of the interview or clinical encounter are to establish an information base, identify problems and issues from the patient's perspective, and identify problems and issues from the perspective of the clinician, based on knowledge of the health and other issues relevant to the adolescent age-group. The adolescent should be given an opportunity to express concerns and the reasons for seeking medical attention. The adolescent as well as the parent should be allowed to express the strengths and successes of the adolescent, in addition to communicating problems.

The effectiveness of an interview can be compromised when the interviewer is distracted by other events or individuals in the office, when extreme time limitations are obvious to either party, or when there is expressible discomfort with either the patient or the interviewer. The need for an **interpreter** when a patient is hearing impaired or if the patient and interviewer are not language compatible provides a challenge but not necessarily a barrier under most circumstances (see Chapter 11). Observations during the interview can be useful to the overall assessment of the patient's maturity, presence or absence of depression, and the parent–adolescent relationship. Given the key role of a successful interview in the screening process, adequate training and experience should be sought by clinicians providing comprehensive care to adolescent patients.

PSYCHOSOCIAL ASSESSMENT
A few questions should be asked to identify the adolescent who is having difficulty with **peer relationships** (Do you have a best friend with whom you can share even the most personal secret?), **self-image** (Is there anything you would like to change about yourself?), **depression** (What do you see yourself doing 5 yr from now?), **school** (How are your grades this year compared with last year?), **personal decisions** (Are you feeling pressured to engage in any behavior for which you

do not feel you are ready?), and an **eating disorder** (Do you ever feel that food controls you, rather than vice versa?). *Bright Futures* materials provide questions and patient encounter forms to structure the assessments. The **HEADS/SF/FIRST** mnemonic, basic or expanded, can be useful in guiding the interview if encounter forms are not available (Table 137.4). Based on the assessments, appropriate counseling or referrals are recommended for more thorough probing or for in-depth interviewing.

PHYSICAL EXAMINATION
Vision Testing
The pubertal growth spurt may involve the optic globe, resulting in its elongation and myopia in genetically predisposed individuals (see Chapter 636). Vision testing should therefore be performed to detect this problem before it affects school performance.

Audiometry
Highly amplified music of the kind enjoyed by many adolescents may result in hearing loss or tinnitus (see Chapter 654). A hearing screening is recommended by the *Bright Futures* guidelines for adolescents who are exposed to loud noises regularly, have had recurring ear infections, or report problems.

Table 137.4	Adolescent Psychosocial Assessment: HEADS/SF/FIRST Mnemonic

Home. Space, privacy, frequent geographic moves, neighborhood

Education/School. Frequent school changes, repetition of a grade/in each subject, teachers' reports, vocational goals, after-school educational clubs (e.g., language, speech, math), learning disabilities

Abuse. Physical, sexual, emotional, verbal abuse; parental discipline

Drugs. Tobacco, electronic cigarettes or vaping devices, alcohol, marijuana, inhalants, "club drugs," "rave" parties, others; drug of choice, age at initiation, frequency, mode of intake, rituals, alone or with peers, quit methods, number of attempts

Safety. Seat belts, helmets, sports safety measures, hazardous activities, driving while intoxicated

Sexuality/Sexual Identity. Reproductive health (use of contraceptives, presence of sexually transmitted infections, feelings, pregnancy)

Family and Friends
Family: Family constellation; genogram; single/married/separated/divorced/blended family; family occupations and shifts; history of addiction in first- and second-degree relatives; parental attitude toward alcohol and drugs; parental rules; chronically ill, physically or mentally challenged parent
Friends: Peer cliques and configuration ("preppies," "jocks," "nerds," "computer geeks," cheerleaders), gang or cult affiliation

Image. Height and weight perceptions, body musculature and physique, appearance (including dress, jewelry, tattoos, body piercing as fashion trends or other statement)

Recreation. Sleep, exercise, organized or unstructured sports, recreational activities (television, video games, computer games, internet and chat rooms, church or community youth group activities [e.g., Boy (BSA)/Girl Scouts; Big Brother/Sister groups, campus groups]). How many hours per day, days per week involved?

Spirituality and Connectedness. Use HOPE* or FICA[†] acronym; adherence, rituals, occult practices, community service or involvement

Threats and Violence. Self-harm or harm to others, running away, cruelty to animals, guns, fights, arrests, stealing, fire setting, fights in school

*HOPE, Hope or security for the future; organized religion; personal spirituality and practices; effects on medical care and end-of-life issues.
[†]FICA, Faith beliefs; importance and influence of faith; community support.
From Dias PJ: Adolescent substance abuse: assessment in the office, *Pediatr Clin North Am* 49:269–300, 2002.

Blood Pressure Determination

Criteria for a diagnosis of hypertension are based on age-specific norms that increase with pubertal maturation (see Chapter 449). An individual whose blood pressure (BP) exceeds the 95th percentile for his or her age is suspect for having hypertension, regardless of the absolute reading. Those adolescents with BP between the 90th and 95th percentiles should receive appropriate counseling relative to weight and have a follow-up examination in 6 mo. Those with BP above the 90th percentile should have their BP measured on 3 separate occasions to determine the stability of the elevation before moving forward with an intervention strategy. The technique is important; false-positive results may be obtained if the cuff covers less than two thirds of the upper arm. The patient should be seated, and an average should be taken of the 2nd and 3rd consecutive readings, using the change rather than the disappearance as the diastolic pressure. Most adolescents with BP elevation have labile hypertension. If BP is below 2 standard deviations (SD) for age, anorexia nervosa and Addison disease should be considered.

Scoliosis

See Chapter 699.

Approximately 5% of male and 10–14% of female adolescents have a mild curvature of the spine. This is 2-4 times the rate in younger children. Scoliosis is typically manifested during the peak of the height velocity curve, at approximately 12 yr in females and 14 yr in males. Curves measuring >10 degrees should be monitored by an orthopedist until growth is complete.

Breast Examination

See Chapters 141 and 556.

Visual inspection of the young and middle adolescent female adolescent's breasts is performed to evaluate progression of sexual maturation and provide reassurance about development.

Scrotum Examination

Visual inspection of the young and middle adolescent male testicles is performed to evaluate progression of sexual maturation and provide reassurance about development. The peak incidence of germ cell tumors of the testes is in late adolescence and early adulthood. Palpation of the testes may have an immediate yield and should serve as a model for instruction of self-examination. Because varicoceles often appear during puberty, the examination also provides an opportunity to explain and reassure the patient about this entity (see Chapter 560).

Pelvic Examination

See Chapter 563.

Laboratory Testing

The increased incidence of iron-deficiency **anemia** after menarche directs the performance of a hematocrit annually in females with moderate to heavy menses. The reference standard for this test changes with progression of puberty, as estrogen suppresses erythropoietin (see Chapter 474). Populations with nutritional risk should also have the hematocrit monitored. Androgens have the opposite effect, causing the hematocrit to rise during male puberty; sexual maturity rating (SMR) 1 males have an average hematocrit of 39%, whereas those who have completed puberty (SMR 5; see Chapter 132) have an average value of 43%. **Tuberculosis (TB)** testing is important in adolescents with risk factors, such as an adolescent with HIV, living in the household with someone with HIV, the incarcerated or homeless adolescent, adolescents from a country where TB is common, or those with other risk factors, because puberty has been shown to activate this disease in those not previously treated. **Hepatitis C virus (HCV)** screening should be offered to adolescents who report risk factors, such as IDU, received blood products or organ donation before 1992, or long-term hemodialysis. Almost 10% of all HCV cases reported to CDC in 2015 were among 15-24 yr olds. CDC HCV surveillance data demonstrates that from 2006 to 2014, the number of reported HCV infections among females of reproductive age (15-44 yrs) doubled. Nearly half of those cases were among females 15-30 yrs of age. Two thirds (67%) of those with a known risk factor reported intravenous drug use.

Sexually active adolescents should undergo screening for **STIs** per CDC guidelines, regardless of symptoms (see Chapter 146). There are clear indications for chlamydia and gonorrhea screening of females ≤24 yr old, but less sufficient evidence to support routine screening in young men. Based on feasibility, efficacy, and cost-effectiveness, evidence is insufficient to recommend routine chlamydia screening in all sexually active young men. However, screening of sexually active young males should be considered in clinical settings associated with high prevalence of chlamydia (e.g., adolescent clinics, correctional facilities, sexually transmitted disease clinics) and should be offered to all young MSM. **HIV** screening should be discussed and offered at least once to all adolescents aged 15-18 yr and to younger and older adolescents who are at increased risk. Routine screening of adolescents who are asymptomatic for certain STIs (e.g., syphilis, trichomoniasis, herpes simplex virus, HPV) is not recommended. However, young MSM and pregnant adolescent females might require more thorough evaluation for all sexually transmitted diseases. Because cervical cancer incidence is low and complications from procedures may outweigh benefits of screening adolescent females, cervical cancer screening should not begin until age 21 yr.

Bibliography is available at Expert Consult.

Chapter **138**
Transitioning to Adult Care

Cynthia M. Holland-Hall, Gale R. Burstein, and Lisa K. Tuchman

第一百三十八章
青少年到成年的过渡保健服务

中文导读

本章介绍了保健服务从青少年过渡到成年的重要性，指出成功过渡能改善健康状况和提高生活质量，而过渡管理不善则会造成健康损害甚至疾病恶化。另外，本章介绍了儿科专业学会的指南和指导方针，帮助卫生服务提供者了解医疗保健转型的关键要素，包括制定过渡政策、定期评估、提供沟通服务和制定长期护理计划等。

The importance of successfully transitioning the care of adolescents with **special healthcare needs (SHCN)** from pediatric to adult services has been recognized for more than 2 decades. Successful transition is associated with improved health outcomes and quality of life; poorly managed transition may lead to loss of a medical home and worsening of chronic disease control and previous care.

The American Academy of Pediatrics, in conjunction with other key professional societies, published detailed, comprehensive guidelines for incorporating transition services into the **medical home** for all adolescents, regardless of the presence or absence of SHCN. These guidelines are based on expert opinion because the evidence on transition outcomes is limited. This clinical report emphasizes that **transition** encompasses much more than simply the transfer of care to another provider. The guidelines go beyond recommendations for the pediatric medical home by providing guidance and practice-based resources for implementing elements of transition support in family medicine and internal medicine practices. This includes providing assistance for the patient in adapting to an adult model of healthcare delivery. Table 138.1 represents the key elements of healthcare transition. Tools to assist providers with these steps are available online from the National Center for Health Care Transition Improvement (www.gottransition.org).

The process begins with the development of a transition policy and its dissemination to all families of young adolescents, ensuring that families understand that transition planning will be an element of health maintenance and chronic care management visits throughout the adolescent years. By middle adolescence, a transition plan should be developed with the youth and family caregivers and updated at subsequent visits until the patient is ready for implementation of the adult care model in early adulthood. Periodic **readiness assessments** are key to plan and anticipate challenges. Critical to the transition process is **skills training** for the adolescent in communication, self-advocacy, and self-care. Some youth with SHCN depend on caregivers for navigating the healthcare system on their behalf, and it is not realistic to expect

Table 138.1	Key Elements of the Transition of Healthcare Process

- **Written transition policy** to be shared with youth, families, providers, and staff, explaining the process and the responsibilities of all team members
- **Transitioning youth registry** to track the progress of each patient through the transition process
- **Longitudinal readiness checklists** assessing the youth's ability for independence, self-management, and communicating with the adult healthcare system, as well as the family's readiness to assist the patient in achieving these goals
- **Written transition plan** documenting the steps to be conducted to meet the needs identified in the readiness assessment, as well as identifying appropriate adult care resources
- For youth with SHCN, expanded transition services, including attention to insurance, entitlements, guardianship, and vocational needs, in addition to adult subspecialty care
- Appropriate communication between the pediatric and adult medical home and subspecialists, including a **portable medical summary** and care plan delivered to the patient and caregivers
- Transfer of care, within the 18-21 yr old range, to adult providers, to whom pediatric providers continue to serve as a resource until transition is complete

increased independence. For these youth, addressing guardianship, long-term care planning, and advanced directives are important. **Care coordination** has been found to facilitate navigation and engagement in an adult-oriented health system, especially for adolescents with SHCN. The goal is to help all youth maximize their potential as they become young adults.

Bibliography is available at Expert Consult.

Chapter 139
Violent Behavior

Michael N. Levas and
Marlene D. Melzer-Lange

第一百三十九章
暴力行为

中文导读

　　本章首先介绍了青少年暴力和危险行为的种类（自残、人际暴力、集体暴力）、流行病学特征和发生原因；其次，通过分析青少年暴力的危险因素，发现贫困、与犯罪同龄人的联系、教育水平低、与成人或榜样的关系破裂、有暴力或受害史以及某些心理健康障碍的青少年更容易发展为有暴力倾向者；最后，提出了针对有暴力行为或有受害史的青少年进行评估、治疗和预防的方法。

Violence is recognized by the World Health Organization (WHO) as a leading worldwide public health problem. WHO defines **violence** as "the intentional use of physical force or power, threatened or actual, against oneself, another person, or against a group or community that either results in or has a high likelihood of resulting in injury, death, psychologic harm, maldevelopment or deprivation" (see Chapter 14). Youths may be perpetrators, victims, or observers of violence (or any combination of the 3 roles), with varying severity of impact on the individual, family, and larger community. Risk factors for youth violence include poverty, relative social disadvantage, war, substance abuse, mental health disorders, and poor family functioning.

EPIDEMIOLOGY

In 2015, **homicide** in the United States was the 3rd leading cause of death for 10-24 yr olds, totaling 4,979 deaths, which were largely males (87%) killed by a handgun (90.1%). The 2015 homicide rate for teens ages 12-17 yr was 3.1/100,000 youth, down 65% from 8.4/100,000 youth in 1993. WHO reports that other than the United States, where the youth and young adult homicide rate was 11 per 100,000, most countries with homicide rates above 10 per 100,000 are developing nations or countries with rapid socioeconomic changes. In the United States the prevalence of behaviors that contribute to violence has not decreased since 1999; fighting, weapon carrying, and gang involvement remain prevalent among youth. Gang-related homicides among youth in 5 major U.S. cities are more likely to involve young (15-19 yr) males (80%), racial/ethnic minorities (73%), and a firearm (90%) in comparison to homicides unrelated to gang activity. In addition, gang homicides are more likely to occur in public places, in the afternoon/evening hours, and rarely are related to drug trade/use. Furthermore, the rate of homicide in youth had been declining but showed an increase in 2015 (Fig. 139.1).

Adolescent reports of **physical fighting** have decreased from 42% in 1991 to 23% in 2015. Violence at U.S. schools remains a significant

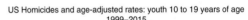

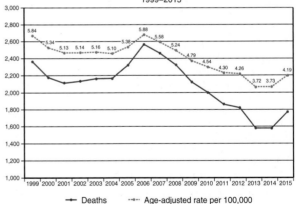

Fig. 139.1 Homicides and age-adjusted rates: youth age 10-19 yr, United States, 1999–2015. *(Data from Centers for Disease Control and Prevention, National Center for Injury Prevention and Control, Web-based Injury Statistics Query and Reporting System [WISQARS], 1999–2015. http://www.cdc.gov/ncipc/wisqars.)*

problem, however, with 7.8% of students reporting being in a physical fight on school property 1 or more times in the preceding 12 mo. The 2015 Youth Risk Behavior Surveillance System reported 16.2% of youths overall carried a weapon such as a gun, knife, or club in the last 30 days; 4.1% carried the weapon to school; and 6.0% reported being threatened or injured with a type of weapon on school property. Males are more likely than females to carry a gun or weapon and therefore may need more support and engagement at home and at school. **Weapon carrying** is highest among white males overall, which may begin as early as 9th grade. These violence-related behaviors at school affect the general students' perception of safety. More than 5.6% of students did not go to school on 1 or more days in the preceding 30 days because they felt it was unsafe. School-based prevention programs initiated at the elementary school level have been found to decrease violent behaviors in students. Increased surveillance of students is warranted both on and around school property to improve student safety.

Dating violence (or intimate partner violence) occurs between 2 people in a close relationship and can be physical (punching, kicking, hitting, shoving), emotional (shaming, bullying, controlling, stalking), or sexual (forcing partner to engage in a sexual act when he/she does not consent to it). Incidents of dating violence often occur during the adolescent years, with 22.4% of women and 15% of men experiencing some type of partner violence between the ages of 11 and 17 yr. The highest prevalence rates are seen in black students and older students. It may start with teasing, name calling, or shaming but often progresses electronically, as frequent calls, texting, or posting sexual pictures of a partner on social media. Risk factors for being a victim of dating violence includes those who use alcohol, believe dating violence is acceptable, have lack of parental supervision, or have a friend who is in a violent relationship. Most teens do not report the behaviors due to fear of retaliation from the partner. Teens who are victims of dating violence are more likely to experience decreased school performance, have thoughts about suicide, use drugs and alcohol, develop an eating disorder, experience depression, and are more likely to be victimized during college. School-based prevention programs that address attitudes and behaviors linked with dating violence, such as **Safe Dates** and **Dating Matters**, offer training experiences to change social norms among teens.

ETIOLOGY

WHO places youth violence in a model within the context of 3 larger types of violence: self-inflicted, interpersonal, and collective. **Interpersonal violence** is subdivided into violence largely between family members or partners and includes child abuse. **Community violence** occurs between individuals who are unrelated. **Collective violence** incorporates violence by people who are members of an identified group against another group of individuals with social, political, or economic motivation. The types of violence in this model have behavioral links, such that child abuse victims are more likely to experience violent and aggressive interpersonal behavior as adolescents and adults. Overlapping risk factors for the types of violence include firearm availability, alcohol use, and socioeconomic inequalities. The benefit to identifying common risk factors for the types of violence lies in the potential for intervening with prevention efforts and gaining positive outcomes for more than 1 type of violent behavior. The model further acknowledges 4 categories

that explore the potential nature of violence as involving physical, sexual, or psychological force, and deprivation.

The social-ecologic model of public health focuses on both population-level and individual-level determinants of health and their respective interventions. On the individual level, there may be 2 types of antisocial youth: life course persistent and limited. **Life course–limited offenders** have no childhood aberrant behaviors and are more likely to commit *status* offenses such as vandalism, running away, and other behaviors symbolic of their struggle for autonomy from parents. **Life course–persistent offenders** exhibit aberrant behavior in childhood, such as problems with temperament, behavioral development, and cognition; as adolescents they participate in more *victim-oriented* crimes. The existence of **adverse childhood events** foretells future health issues and subsequent violence. This hypothesis proposes that precursors such as child abuse and neglect, a child witnessing violence, adolescent sexual and physical abuse, and adolescent exposure to violence and violent assaults predispose youths to outcomes of violent behavior, violent crime, delinquency, violent assaults, suicide, or premature death. This public health model also emphasizes the community environment and other external influences. An additional common paradigm for high-risk violence behavior poses a balance of risk and protective factors at the individual, family, and community levels.

CLINICAL MANIFESTATIONS

The identified risk factors for youth violence include poverty, association with delinquent peers, poor school performance or low education status, disconnection from adult role models or mentors, prior history of violence or victimization, poor family functioning, childhood abuse, substance abuse, and certain mental health disorders. The most common disorders associated with **aggressive behavior** in adolescents are mental retardation, learning disabilities, moderately severe language disorders, and mental disorders such as attention-deficit/hyperactivity disorder (ADHD) and mood disturbances. The link between severe mental illness and violent behaviors is strongest for those with coexisting alcohol or substance abuse or dependence.

Inability to master prosocial skills such as the establishment and maintenance of positive family/peer relations and poor resolution of conflict may put adolescents with these disorders at higher risk of physical violence and other risky behaviors. **Conduct disorder** and **oppositional defiant disorder** are specific psychiatric diagnoses whose definitions are associated with violent behavior (Table 139.1). They occur with other disorders such as ADHD (see Chapter 49) and increase an adolescent's vulnerability for juvenile delinquency, substance use or abuse, sexual promiscuity, adult criminal behavior, incarceration, and antisocial personality disorder. Other co-occurring risk factors for youth violence include use of anabolic steroids, gang tattoos, belief in one's premature death, preteen alcohol use, and placement in a juvenile detention center.

Table 139.1	Oppositional Defiant Disorder, Conduct Disorder, and Juvenile Delinquency	
PSYCHIATRIC DISORDER LABELS		
Oppositional Defiant Disorder	**Conduct Disorder**	**Legal Label Juvenile Delinquency**
Recurrent pattern of negativistic, defiant, disobedient, and hostile behavior toward authority figures that has a significant adverse effect on functioning (e.g., social, academic, occupational)	Repetitive and persistent pattern of behavior that violates the basic rights of others or major age-appropriate societal norms or rules	Offenses that are illegal because of age; illegal acts
Examples: losing temper; arguing with adults; defying or refusing to comply with request or rules of adults; annoying behavior; blaming others; being irritable, spiteful, resentful	Examples: physical fighting, deceitfulness, stealing, destruction of property, threatening or causing physical harm to people or animals, driving without a license, prostitution, rape (even if not adjudicated in the legal system)	Examples: single or multiple instances of being arrested or adjudicated for any of the following: stealing, destruction of property, threatening or causing physical harm to people or animals, driving without a license, prostitution, rape
Diagnosed by a mental health clinician	Diagnosed by a mental health practitioner	Adjudicated in the legal system

From Greydanus DE, Pratt HD, Patel DR, et al: The rebellious adolescent, *Pediatr Clin North Am* 44:1460, 1997.

DIAGNOSIS

The assessment of an adolescent at risk or with a history of violent behavior or victimization should be a part of the health maintenance visit of all adolescents. The answers to questions about recent history of involvement in a physical fight, carrying a weapon, or firearms in the household, as well as concerns that the adolescent may have about personal safety, may suggest a problem requiring a more in-depth evaluation. The **FISTS** mnemonic provides guidance for structuring the assessment (Table 139.2). The additional factors of physical or sexual abuse, serious problems at school, poor school performance and attendance, multiple incidents of trauma, substance use, and symptoms associated with mental disorders are indications for evaluation by a mental health professional. In a situation of acute trauma, assault victims are not always forthcoming about the circumstances of their injuries for fear of retaliation or police involvement. Stabilization of the injury or the gathering of forensic evidence in sexual assault is the treatment priority; however, once this is achieved, addressing a more comprehensive set of issues surrounding the assault is appropriate.

Table 139.2	FISTS Mnemonic to Assess an Adolescent's Risk of Violence

F: Fighting (How many fights were you in last year? What was the last?)
I: Injuries (Have you ever been injured? Have you ever injured someone else?)
S: Sex (Has your partner hit you? Have you hit your partner? Have you ever been forced to have sex?)
T: Threats (Has someone with a weapon threatened you? What happened? Has anything changed to make you feel safer?)
S: Self-defense (What do you do if someone tries to pick a fight? Have you carried a weapon in self-defense?)

The FISTS mnemonic is adapted with permission from the Association of American Medical Colleges. Alpert EJ, Sege RD, Bradshaw YS: Interpersonal violence and the education of physicians, *Acad Med* 72:S41–S50, 1997.

TREATMENT

In the patient with acute injury secondary to violent assault, the treatment plan should follow standards established by the American Academy of Pediatrics model protocol, which includes the stabilization of the injury, evaluation and treatment of the injury, evaluation of the assault circumstance, psychological evaluation and support, social service evaluation of the circumstance surrounding the assault, and a treatment plan on discharge that is designed to protect the adolescent from subsequent injury episodes, prevent retaliation, and minimize the development of psychological disability. Victims as well as witnesses of violence are at risk for posttraumatic stress disorder and future aggressive or violent behavior. Utilizing a **trauma-informed care** approach enables providers to help these victims and witnesses so that they can develop linkages to recovery and resilience. **Hospital-based violence intervention programs** have shown success by supporting youth who have sustained a violent injury in the emergency department, hospital, or community.

Multiple treatment modalities are used simultaneously in managing adolescents with persistent violent and aggressive behavior and range from cognitive-behavioral therapy involving the individual and family to specific family interventions (parent management training, multisystemic treatment) and pharmacotherapy. Treatment of comorbid conditions, such as ADHD, depression, anxiety, and substance abuse, appears to reduce aggressive behavior.

PREVENTION

The WHO recognizes a multifactorial approach to prevention: parenting and early childhood development strategies; school-based academic and social skills development strategies, strategies for young people at higher risk of or already involved in violence, and community-and society-level strategies (Table 139.3). **Parenting and early childhood development approaches** concentrate on working with families to provide nonviolent parenting through home visitation and parent groups as well as teaching coping strategies and nonviolent conflict resolution for all children and families. **School-based social skills development strategies** focus on students' families and peer relationships, especially those with the potential to trigger aggressive or violent responses. Solutions include

Table 139.3	WHO Youth Violence Prevention Strategies: Effectiveness by Context	
STRATEGIES	**CONTEXT/PROGRAMS**	**EFFECTIVENESS**
Parenting and early childhood development strategies	Home visiting programs	?
	Parenting programs	+
	Early childhood development programs	+
School-based academic and social skills development strategies	Life and social skills development	+
	Bullying prevention	+
	Academic enrichment programs	
	Dating violence prevention programs	+
	Financial incentives for adolescents to attend school	?
	Peer mediation	+/−
	After-school and other structured leisure-time activities	?
Strategies for young people at higher risk of, or already involved in, violence	Therapeutic approaches	+
	Vocational training	?
	Mentoring	?
	Gang and street violence prevention programs	?
Community- and society-level strategies	"Hot spots" policing	+
	Community- and problem-oriented policing	+
	Reducing access to and the harmful use of alcohol	+
	Drug control programs	+
	Reducing access to and misuse of firearms	+
	Spatial modification and urban upgrading	+
	Poverty deconcentration	+

+, Promising (strategies that include 1 or more programs supported by at least 1 well-designed study showing prevention of perpetration and/or experiencing of youth violence, or at least 2 studies showing positive changes in key risk or protective factors for youth violence).
?, Unclear because of insufficient evidence (strategies that include 1 or more programs of unclear effectiveness).
+/−, Unclear because of mixed results (strategies for which the evidence is mixed; some programs have a significant positive effect and others a significant negative effect on youth violence).
From World Health Organization (WHO) Library Cataloguing-in Publication Data, Preventing youth violence: an overview of the evidence, 2015.

improving skills in coping or problem solving in bullying, peer mediation, dating violence prevention, and after-school programs. **Strategies for young people at higher risk of, or already involved in, violence** include therapeutic mental health approaches, crime victim services, vocational training, mentoring, and gang intervention. These youth are at highest risk for repeat injury or incarceration. **Community- and societal-level approaches** include broader advocacy and legislative actions, as well as changing the cultural norm toward violent behaviors.

A specific prevention strategy can incorporate several approaches, such as the handgun/firearm prevention recommendations that include gun-lock safety, public education, and legislative advocacy. Other efforts are directed toward establishing a national database to track and define the problem of youth violence. The **National Violent Death Reporting System** collects and analyzes violent death data from 40 states and aims to improve surveillance of current trends, to share information state to state, to build partnerships among state and community organizations, and to develop and implement prevention and intervention programs. The Centers for Disease Control and Prevention characterizes specific successful prevention programs and summarizes program content on its website (www.cdc.gov).

Bibliography is available at Expert Consult.

Chapter **140**
Substance Abuse
Cora Collette Breuner

第一百四十章
药物滥用

中文导读

　　本章主要介绍了药物滥用的种类、流行水平、治疗、预后和预防；介绍了吸食或滥用乙醇、烟草/电子烟、大麻、吸入剂、致幻剂、可卡因、安非他命、兴奋剂、麻醉药和浴用盐的药理机制、临床表现、诊断和治疗方法。面对青少年药物滥用的问题，社会应建立相应的行为规范，通过行为节制来减少药物滥用带来的健康危害，从而保障青少年的身心健康。

Although varying in percentages by nation and culture, a substantial proportion of adolescents will engage in the use of a wide range of substances, including alcohol, tobacco, natural and synthetic marijuana, opiates, and stimulants. Their reactions to and the consequences of these exposures are influenced by a complex interaction among biologic and psychosocial development, environmental messages, legality, and societal attitudes. The potential for adverse outcomes even with occasional use in adolescents, such as motor vehicle crashes and other injuries, is sufficient justification to consider any drug use in adolescents a considerable risk.

Individuals who initiate drug use at an early age are at a greater risk for becoming addicted than those who try drugs in early adulthood. Drug use in younger adolescents can act as a substitute for developing age-appropriate coping strategies and enhance vulnerability to poor decision-making. First use of the most commonly used drug (alcohol) occurs before age 18 yr, with 88% of people reporting age of first alcohol use at <21 yr old, the legal drinking age in the United States. Interestingly, inhalants have been identified as a popular first drug for youth in 8th grade (age 13-14 yr).

When drug use begins to negatively alter functioning in adolescents at school and at home, and risk-taking behavior is seen, intervention is warranted. Serious drug use is a pervasive phenomenon and infiltrates every socioeconomic and cultural segment of the population. It is one of the costliest and most challenging public health problems facing all societies and cultures. The challenge to the clinician is to identify youths at risk for substance abuse and offer early intervention. The challenge to the community and society is to create norms that decrease the likelihood of adverse health outcomes for adolescents and promote and facilitate opportunities for adolescents to choose healthier and safer options. Recognizing those drugs with the greatest *harm*, and at times focusing on *harm reduction* with or without abstinence, is an important modern approach to adolescent substance abuse (Figs. 140.1 and 140.2).

ETIOLOGY
Substance abuse has multifactorial origins (Fig. 140.3). Biologic factors, including genetic predisposition, are established contributors. Behaviors such as rebelliousness, poor school performance, delinquency, and

criminal activity and personality traits such as low self-esteem, anxiety, and lack of self-control are frequently associated with or predate the onset of drug use. Psychiatric disorders often coexist with adolescent substance use. Conduct disorders and antisocial personality disorders are the most common diagnoses coexisting with substance abuse, particularly in males. Teens with depression (see Chapter 39.1), attention deficit disorder (Chapter 49), anxiety (Chapter 38), and eating disorders (Chapter 41) have high rates of substance use. The determinants of adolescent substance use and abuse are explained using numerous theoretical models, with factors at the individual level, the level of significant relationships with others, and the level of the setting or environment. Models include a balance of risk and protective or coping factors contributing to individual differences among adolescents with similar risk factors who escape adverse outcomes.

Risk factors for adolescent *drug use* may differ from those associated with adolescent *drug abuse*. Adolescent *use* is more commonly related to social and peer factors, whereas *abuse* is more often a function of psychological and biologic factors. The likelihood that an otherwise normal adolescent would experiment with drugs may depend on the availability of the drug to the adolescent, the perceived positive or otherwise functional value to the adolescent, the perceived risk associated with use, and the presence or absence of restraints, as determined by the adolescent's cultural or other important value systems. An adolescent who abuses drugs may have genetic or biologic factors coexisting with dependence on a particular drug for coping with day-to-day activities.

Specific historical questions can assist in determining the severity of the drug problem through a rating system (Table 140.1). The type of drug used (marijuana vs heroin), the circumstances of use (alone or in a group setting), the frequency and timing of use (daily before school vs occasionally on a weekend), current mental health status, and general functional status, including sleep habits and screen use, should all be considered in evaluating any child or adolescent found to be using a drug. The stage of drug use/abuse should also be considered (Table 140.2). A teen may spend months or years in the experimentation phase trying a variety of illicit substances, including the most common drugs: cigarettes, alcohol, and marijuana. Often it is not until regular use of drugs resulting in negative consequences (problem use) that the teen

is identified as having a problem, either by parents, friends, teachers, or a healthcare provider. Certain protective factors play a part in buffering the risk factors as well as assisting in anticipating the long-term outcome of experimentation. Having emotionally supportive parents with open communication styles, involvement in organized school activities, having mentors or role models outside the home, and recognition of the importance of academic achievement are examples of the important protective factors.

EPIDEMIOLOGY

Alcohol, cigarettes, and marijuana are the most commonly reported substances used among U.S. teens (Table 140.3). The prevalence of substance use and associated risky behaviors vary by age, gender, race/ethnicity, and other sociodemographic factors. Younger teenagers tend to report less use of drugs than do older teenagers, except for inhalants (in 2016, 4.4% in 8th grade, 2.8% in 10th grade, 1.0% in 12th grade). Males have higher rates of both licit and illicit drug use than females, with greatest differences seen in their higher rates of frequent use of smokeless tobacco, cigars, and anabolic steroids. For a number of years, black 12th graders have reported lifetime, annual, 30-day, and daily

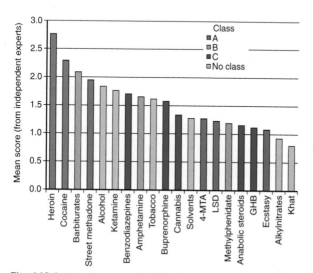

Fig. 140.1 Mean harm scores for 20 substances as determined by an expert panel based on 3 criteria: physical harm to user; potential for dependence; and effect on family, community, and society. Classification under the Misuse of Drugs Act, when appropriate, is shown by the color of each bar. Class A drugs are deemed potentially most dangerous; class C least dangerous. *(From Nutt D, King LA, Saulsbury W, et al: Development of a rational scale to access the harm of drugs of potential misuse, Lancet 369:1047–1053, 2007.)*

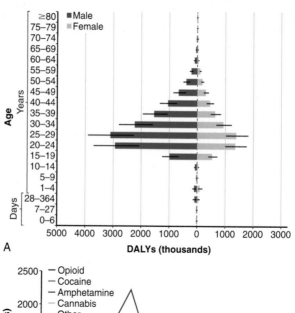

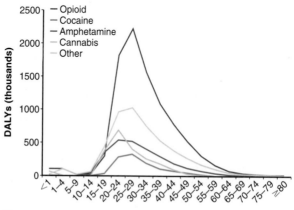

Fig. 140.2 Total burden (DALYs) of drug dependence by age and sex in 2010. **A,** DALYs attributable to drug dependence, by age and sex. **B,** DALYs attributable to each type of drug dependence by age. DALYs, Disability-adjusted life years. *(From: Degenhardt L, Whitford HA, Ferrari AJ, et al: Global burden of disease attributable to illicit drug use and dependence: findings from the Global Burden of Disease study 2010, Lancet 382:1569, 2013.)*

Table 140.1	Assessing the Seriousness of Adolescent Drug Abuse		
VARIABLE	**0**	**+1**	**+2**
Age (yr)	>15	<15	
Sex	Male	Female	
Family history of drug abuse		Yes	
Setting of drug use	In group		Alone
Affect before drug use	Happy	Always poor	Sad
School performance	Good, improving		Recently poor
Use before driving	None		Yes
History of accidents	None		Yes
Time of week	Weekend	Weekdays	
Time of day		After school	Before or during school
Type of drug	Marijuana, beer, wine	Hallucinogens, amphetamines	Whiskey, opiates, cocaine, barbiturates

Total score: 0-3, less worrisome; 3-8, serious; 8-18, very serious.

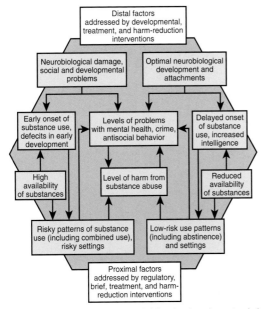

Fig. 140.3 Protection and risk model for distal and proximal determinants of risky substance use and related harms. *(From Toumbourou JW, Stockwell T, Neighbors C, et al: Interventions to reduce harm associated with adolescent substance use, Lancet 369:1391–1401, 2007.)*

Table 140.2	Stages of Adolescent Substance Abuse
STAGE	**DESCRIPTION**
1	Potential for abuse • Decreased impulse control • Need for immediate gratification • Available drugs, alcohol, inhalants • Need for peer acceptance
2	Experimentation: learning the euphoria • Use of inhalants, tobacco, marijuana, and alcohol with friends • Few, if any, consequences • Use may increase to weekends regularly • Little change in behavior
3	Regular use: seeking the euphoria • Use of other drugs, e.g., stimulants, LSD, sedatives • Behavioral changes and some consequences • Increased frequency of use; use alone • Buying or stealing drugs
4	Regular use: preoccupation with the "high" • Daily use of drugs • Loss of control • Multiple consequences and risk taking • Estrangement from family and "straight" friends
5	Burnout: use of drugs to feel normal • Polysubstance use/cross-addiction • Guilt, withdrawal, shame, remorse, depression • Physical and mental deterioration • Increased risk taking, self-destructive, suicidal

prevalence levels for nearly all drugs that were lower than those for white or Hispanic 12th graders. That is less true today, with levels of drug use among blacks more similar to the other groups.

The distribution of annual marijuana use by race/ethnicity varies by grade level. In all 3 grades, prevalence is highest among Hispanic students. Differences in prevalence across the groups are proportionately largest in 8th grade (13% for Hispanics, 7.8% for whites), somewhat smaller in 10th grade (27% for Hispanics, 24% for whites), and negligible in 12th grade (37% for Hispanics, 35% for whites). Blacks fall between whites and Hispanics in 8th and 10th grade but are slightly below them in 12th grade (35%).

The number of 12th graders who report using any of the prescription psychotherapeutic drugs, including amphetamines, sedatives (barbiturates), tranquilizers, and narcotics other than heroin, decreased in 2016 (Table 140.4). Prevalence was 18.0%, 12.0%, and 5.4% for lifetime, annual,

and 30-day use, respectively, indicating that a substantial portion of adolescents still use prescription drugs nonmedically. Rural adolescents were 26% more likely than urban adolescents to have used prescription drugs nonmedically. Use was associated with decreased health status, major depressive episode(s), and other drug use (marijuana, cocaine, hallucinogens, inhalants) and alcohol use. In a large-scale study of 16,209 adolescent exposures to prescription drugs, 52.4% were females, and the mean age was 16.6 yr. The 5 most frequently misused or abused drugs were hydrocodone (32%), amphetamines (18%), oxycodone (15%), methylphenidate (14%), and tramadol (11%). Many of these drugs can be found in the parents' home, some are over-the-counter (OTC) drugs (dextromethorphan, pseudoephedrine), whereas others are purchased from drug dealers at schools and colleges. Teen users of nonmedical opioids use other substances concurrently. Most frequently, teens combine

Text continued on p. 1124

| Table 140.3 | Trends in Annual Prevalence (%) of Use of Various Drugs for Grades 8, 10, and 12 Combined |

	1991	1992	1993	1994	1995	1996	1997	1998	1999	2000	2001	2002	2003	2004	2005
Any illicit drug[c]	20.2	19.7	23.2	27.6	31.0	33.6	34.1	32.2	31.9	31.4	31.8	30.2	28.4	27.6	27.1
Any illicit drug other than marijuana[c]	12.0	12.0	13.6	14.6	16.4	17.0	16.8	15.8	15.6	15.3‡	16.3	14.6	13.7	13.5	13.1
Any illicit drug including inhalants[c]	23.5	23.2	26.7	31.1	34.1	36.6	36.7	35.0	34.6	34.1	34.3	32.3	30.8	30.1	30.1
Marijuana/hashish	15.0	14.3	17.7	22.5	26.1	29.0	**30.1**	28.2	27.9	27.2	27.5	26.1	24.6	23.8	23.4
Synthetic marijuana	—	—	—	—	—	—	—	—	—	—	—	—	—	—	—
Inhalants	7.6	7.8	8.9	9.6	**10.2**	9.9	9.1	8.5	7.9	7.7	6.9	6.1	6.2	6.7	7.0
Hallucinogens	3.8	4.1	4.8	5.2	6.6	7.2	6.9	6.3	6.1	**5.4**‡	**6.0**	4.5	4.1	4.0	3.9
LSD	3.4	3.8	4.3	4.7	5.9	**6.3**	6.0	5.3	5.3	4.5	4.1	2.4	1.6	1.6	1.5
Hallucinogens other than LSD	1.3	1.4	1.7	2.2	2.7	3.2	3.2	3.1	2.9	**2.8**‡	**4.0**	3.7	3.6	3.6	3.4
Ecstasy (MDMA),[d] original	—	—	—	—	—	3.1	3.4	2.9	3.7	5.3	**6.0**	4.9	3.1	2.6	2.4
MDMA, revised	—	—	—	—	—	—	—	—	—	—	—	—	—	—	—
Salvia	—	—	—	—	—	—	—	—	—	—	—	—	—	—	—
Cocaine	2.2	2.1	2.3	2.8	3.3	4.0	4.3	**4.5**	**4.5**	3.9	3.5	3.7	3.3	3.5	3.5
Crack	1.0	1.1	1.2	1.5	1.8	2.0	2.1	**2.4**	2.2	2.1	1.8	2.0	1.8	1.7	1.6
Other cocaine	2.0	1.8	2.0	2.3	2.8	3.4	3.7	3.7	**4.0**	3.3	3.0	3.1	2.8	3.1	3.0
Heroin	0.5	0.6	0.6	0.9	1.2	**1.3**	**1.3**	1.2	1.3	**1.3**	0.9	1.0	0.8	0.9	0.8
With a needle	—	—	—	—	0.7	0.7	0.7	0.7	0.7	0.5	0.5	0.5	0.5	0.5	0.5
Without a needle	—	—	—	—	0.9	0.9	1.0	0.9	1.0	**1.1**	0.7	0.7	0.6	0.7	0.7
OxyContin	—	—	—	—	—	—	—	—	—	—	—	2.7	3.2	3.3	3.4
Vicodin	—	—	—	—	—	—	—	—	—	—	—	6.0	**6.6**	5.8	5.7
Amphetamines[c]	7.5	7.3	8.4	9.1	10.0	10.4	10.1	9.3	9.0	9.2	9.6	8.9	8.0	7.6	7.0
Ritalin	—	—	—	—	—	—	—	—	—	—	**4.2**	3.8	3.5	3.6	3.3
Adderall	—	—	—	—	—	—	—	—	—	—	—	—	—	—	—
Methamphetamine	—	—	—	—	—	—	—	—	**4.1**	3.5	3.4	3.2	3.0	2.6	2.4
Bath salts (synthetic stimulants)	—	—	—	—	—	—	—	—	—	—	—	—	—	—	—
Tranquilizers	2.8	2.8	2.9	3.1	3.7	4.1	4.1	4.4	4.4	**4.5**‡	**5.5**	5.3	4.8	4.8	4.7
OTC cough/cold medicines	—	—	—	—	—	—	—	—	—	—	—	—	—	—	—
Rohypnol	—	—	—	—	—	1.1	1.1	1.1	0.8	0.7	**0.9**‡	0.8	0.8	**0.9**	0.8
GHB[b]	—	—	—	—	—	—	—	—	—	**1.4**	1.2	1.2	1.2	1.1	**0.8**
Ketamine[b]	—	—	—	—	—	—	—	—	—	**2.0**	1.9	**2.0**	1.7	1.3	**1.0**
Alcohol	67.4	66.3‡	59.7	60.5	60.4	60.9	**61.4**	59.7	59.0	59.3	58.2	55.3	54.4	54.0	51.9
Been drunk	35.8	34.3	34.3	35.0	35.9	36.7	**36.9**	35.5	36.0	35.9	35.0	32.1	31.2	32.5	30.8
Flavored alcoholic beverages	—	—	—	—	—	—	—	—	—	—	—	—	—	**44.5**	43.9
Alcoholic beverages containing caffeine	—	—	—	—	—	—	—	—	—	—	—	—	—	—	—
Any vaping	—	—	—	—	—	—	—	—	—	—	—	—	—	—	—
Vaping nicotine	—	—	—	—	—	—	—	—	—	—	—	—	—	—	—
Vaping marijuana	—	—	—	—	—	—	—	—	—	—	—	—	—	—	—
Vaping just flavoring	—	—	—	—	—	—	—	—	—	—	—	—	—	—	—
Dissolvable tobacco products	—	—	—	—	—	—	—	—	—	—	—	—	—	—	—
Snus	—	—	—	—	—	—	—	—	—	—	—	—	—	—	—
Steroids	1.2	1.1	1.0	1.2	1.3	1.1	1.2	1.3	1.7	1.9	2.0	2.0	1.7	1.6	1.3

Continued

	2006	2007	2008	2009	2010	2011	2012	2013	2014	2015	2016	2017	2016–2017 CHANGE	PEAK YEAR–2017 CHANGE Absolute Change	PEAK YEAR–2017 CHANGE Proportional Change[a]	LOW YEAR–2017 CHANGE Absolute Change	LOW YEAR–2017 CHANGE Proportional Change[a]
Any illicit drug[c]	25.8	24.8	24.9	25.9	27.3	27.6	27.1	28.6‡	27.2	26.8	25.3	26.5	+1.2	-0.7	-2.6	+1.2	+4.6
Any illicit drug other than marijuana[c]	12.7	12.4	11.9	11.6	11.8	11.3	10.8	11.4‡	10.9	10.5	9.7	9.4	-0.3	-1.5 ss	-14.2	—	—
Any illicit drug including inhalants[c]	28.7	27.6	27.6	28.5	29.7	29.8	29.0	30.5‡	28.5	28.4	26.3	28.3	+2.0 ss	-0.2	-0.6	+2.0 ss	+7.7
Marijuana/hashish	22.0	21.4	21.5	22.9	24.5	25.0	24.7	25.8	24.2	23.7	22.6	23.9	+1.3 s	-6.2 sss	-20.6	+2.5 sss	+11.8
Synthetic marijuana	—	—	—	—	—	—	8.0	6.4	4.8	4.2	3.1	2.8	-0.4 s	-5.2 sss	-65.4	—	—
Inhalants	6.9	6.4	6.4	6.1	6.0	5.0	4.5	3.8	3.6	3.2	2.6	2.9	+0.2	-7.3 sss	-71.9	+0.2	+8.1
Hallucinogens	3.6	3.8	3.8	3.5	3.8	3.7	3.2	3.1	2.8	2.8	2.8	2.7	0.0	-3.2 sss	-54.1	—	—
LSD	1.4	1.7	1.9	1.6	1.8	1.8	1.6	1.6	1.7	1.9	2.0	2.1	+0.1	-4.3 sss	-67.5	+0.6 ss	+46.1
Ecstasy (MDMA),[d] original	2.7	3.0	2.9	3.0	3.8	3.7	2.5	2.8	—	—	—	—	—	—	—	—	—
MDMA, revised	—	—	—	—	—	—	—	—	3.4	2.4	1.8	1.7	-0.1	-1.6 sss	-48.9	—	—
Salvia	—	—	—	—	3.5	3.6	2.7	2.3	1.4	1.2	1.2	0.9	-0.3 ss	-2.7 sss	-74.2	—	—
Cocaine	3.5	3.4	2.9	2.5	2.2	2.0	1.9	1.8	1.6	1.7	1.4	1.6	+0.2	-2.9 sss	-64.5	+0.2	+12.2
Crack	1.5	1.5	1.3	1.2	1.1	1.0	0.9	0.8	0.7	0.8	0.6	0.7	+0.1	-1.7 sss	-70.7	+0.1	+20.1
Other cocaine	3.1	2.9	2.6	2.1	1.9	1.7	1.7	1.5	1.5	1.5	1.2	1.3	+0.1	-2.7 sss	-66.3	+0.1	+8.8
Heroin	0.8	0.8	0.8	0.8	0.8	0.7	0.6	0.6	0.5	0.4	0.3	0.3	0.0	-1.0 sss	-75.4	0.0	+8.9
With a needle	0.5	0.5	0.5	0.5	0.6	0.5	0.4	0.4	0.4	0.3	0.3	0.2	0.0	-0.5 sss	-69.5	—	—
Without a needle	0.6	0.7	0.6	0.5	0.6	0.5	0.4	0.4	0.3	0.3	0.2	0.2	0.0	-0.9 sss	-81.4	0.0	+6.5
OxyContin	3.5	3.5	3.4	3.9	3.8	3.4	2.9	2.9	2.4	2.3	2.1	1.9	-0.2	-2.0 sss	-51.6	—	—
Vicodin	6.3	6.2	6.1	6.5	5.9	5.1	4.3	3.7	3.0	2.5	1.8	1.3	-0.5	-5.2 sss	-79.6	—	—
Amphetamines[c]	6.8	6.5	5.8	5.9	6.2	5.9	5.6	7.0‡	6.6	6.2	5.4	5.0	-0.4	-1.6 sss	-24.1	—	—
Ritalin	3.5	2.8	2.6	2.5	2.2	2.1	1.7	1.7	1.5	1.4	1.1	0.8	-0.2	-3.4 sss	-80.5	—	—
Adderall	—	—	—	4.3	4.5	4.1	4.4	4.4	4.1	4.5	3.9	3.5	-0.3	-0.5 s	-10.3	—	—
Methamphetamine	2.0	1.4	1.3	1.3	1.3	1.2	1.0	1.0	0.8	0.6	0.5	0.5	0.0	-3.6 sss	-88.2	—	—
Bath salts (synthetic stimulants)	—	—	—	—	—	—	0.9	0.9	0.8	0.7	0.8	0.5	-0.3 s	-0.4 s	-43.6	—	—
Tranquilizers	4.6	4.5	4.3	4.5	4.4	3.9	3.7	3.3	3.4	3.4	3.5	3.6	+0.1	-1.9 sss	-35.1	+0.2	+7.5
OTC cough/cold medicines	5.4	5.0	4.7	5.2	4.8	4.4	4.4	4.0	3.2	3.1	3.2	3.0	-0.2	-2.4 sss	-44.4	—	—
Rohypnol	0.7	0.8	0.7	0.6	0.8	0.9	0.7	0.6	0.5	0.5	0.7	0.5	-0.2 s	-0.5 sss	-50.4	—	—

Continued

Table 140.3 | Trends in Annual Prevalence (%) of Use of Various Drugs for Grades 8, 10, and 12 Combined—cont'd

	2006	2007	2008	2009	2010	2011	2012	2013	2014	2015	2016	2017	2016–2017 CHANGE	PEAK YEAR–2017 CHANGE Absolute Change	PEAK YEAR–2017 CHANGE Proportional Change[a]	LOW YEAR–2017 CHANGE Absolute Change	LOW YEAR–2017 CHANGE Proportional Change[a]
GHB[b]	0.9	0.7	0.9	0.9	0.8	0.8	—	—	—	—	—	—	—	—	—	—	—
Ketamine[b]	1.1	1.0	1.2	1.3	1.2	1.2	—	—	—	—	—	—	—	—	—	—	—
Alcohol	50.7	50.2	48.7	48.4	47.4	45.3	44.3	42.8	40.7	39.9	36.7	36.7	0.0	-24.7 sss	-40.2	0.0	+0.1
Been drunk	30.7	29.7	28.1	28.7	27.1	25.9	26.4	25.4	23.6	22.5	20.7	20.4	-0.3	-16.5 sss	-44.8	—	—
Flavored alcoholic beverages	42.4	40.8	39.0	37.8	35.9	33.7	32.5	31.3	29.4	28.8	25.3	25.9	+0.5	-18.6 sss	-41.9	+0.5	+2.1
Alcoholic beverages containing caffeine	—	—	—	—	—	19.7	18.6	16.6	14.3	13.0	11.2	10.6	-0.6	-9.1 sss	-46.1	—	—
Any vaping	—	—	—	—	—	—	—	—	—	—	—	21.5	—	—	—	—	—
Vaping nicotine	—	—	—	—	—	—	—	—	—	—	—	13.9	—	—	—	—	—
Vaping marijuana	—	—	—	—	—	—	—	—	—	—	—	6.8	—	—	—	—	—
Vaping just flavoring	—	—	—	—	—	—	—	—	—	—	—	17.2	—	—	—	—	—
Dissolvable tobacco products	—	—	—	—	—	—	1.4	1.4	1.2	1.1	0.9	0.9	0.0	-0.5	-35.1	—	—
Snus	1.3	—	—	—	—	—	5.6	4.8	4.1	3.8	3.6	2.6	-1.0 sss	-3.0 sss	-53.9	—	—
Steroids	1.3	1.1	1.1	1.0	0.9	0.9	0.9	0.9	0.9	1.0	0.8	0.8	0.0	-1.2 sss	-61.3	0.0	+2.9

Notes: "—" indicates data not available; "‡" indicates a change in the question text. When a question change occurs, peak levels after that change are used to calculate the peak year to current year difference.
Values in **bold** equal peak levels since 1991. Values in *italics* equal peak level before wording change. Underlined values equal lowest level since recent peak level.
Level of significance of difference between classes: s = .05, ss = .01, sss = .001.
Any apparent inconsistency between the change estimate and the prevalence estimates for the 2 most recent years is caused by rounding.
[a]The proportional change is the percent by which the most recent year deviates from the peak year (or the low year) for the drug in question. Thus, if a drug was at 20% prevalence in the peak year and declined to 10% prevalence in the most recent year, this would reflect a proportional decline of 50%.
[b]Question was discontinued among 8th and 10th graders in 2012.
[c]In 2013, for the questions on the use of amphetamines, the text was changed on 2 of the questionnaire forms for 8th and 10th graders and 4 of the questionnaire forms for 12th graders. This change also impacted the any illicit drug indices. Data presented here include only the changed forms beginning in 2013.
[d]In 2014, the text was changed on 1 of the questionnaire forms for 8th, 10th, and 12th graders to include "Molly" in the description. The remaining forms were changed in 2015. Data for both versions of the question are presented here.
From Johnston LD, Miech RA, O'Malley PM, et al: Monitoring the Future national survey results on drug use: 1975–2017. Overview, key findings on adolescent drug use. Ann Arbor, 2018, Institute for Social Research, University of Michigan. http://www.monitoringthefuture.org/pubs/monographs/mtf-overview2017.pdf.

Table 140.4 | Commonly Abused Prescription Drugs

NIDA
NATIONAL INSTITUTE
ON DRUG ABUSE

Commonly Abused Prescription Drugs
Visit NIDA at www.drugabuse.gov

National Institutes of Health
U.S. Department of Health and Human Services

Substances: Category and Name	Examples of Commercial and Street Names	DEA Schedule*/How Administered	Intoxication Effects/Health Risks
Depressants			
Barbiturates	*Amytal, Nembutal, Seconal, Phenobarbital:* barbs, reds, red birds, phennies, tooies, yellows, yellow jackets	II, III, IV/injected, swallowed	*Sedation/drowsiness, reduced anxiety, feelings of well-being, lowered inhibitions, slurred speech, poor concentration, confusion, dizziness, impaired coordination and memory/slowed pulse, lowered blood pressure, slowed breathing, tolerance, withdrawal, addiction; increased risk of respiratory distress and death when combined with alcohol*
Benzodiazepines	*Ativan, Halcion, Librium, Valium, Xanax, Klonopin:* candy, downers, sleeping pills, tranks	IV/swallowed	
Sleep Medications	*Ambien (zolpidem), Sonata (zaleplon), Lunesta (eszopiclone)*	IV/swallowed	*for barbiturates*—euphoria, unusual excitement, fever, irritability/life-threatening withdrawal in chronic users
Opioids and Morphine Derivatives**			
Codeine	*Empirin with Codeine, Fiorinal with Codeine, Robitussin A-C, Tylenol with Codeine:* Captain Cody, Cody, schoolboy; (with glutethimide: doors & fours, loads, pancakes and syrup)	II, III, IV/injected, swallowed	*Pain relief, euphoria, drowsiness, sedation, weakness, dizziness, nausea, impaired coordination, confusion, dry mouth, itching, sweating, clammy skin, constipation/ slowed or arrested breathing, lowered pulse and blood pressure, tolerance, addiction, unconsciousness, coma, death; risk of death increased when combined with alcohol or other CNS depressants*
Morphine	*Roxanol, Duramorph:* M, Miss Emma, monkey, white stuff	II, III/injected, swallowed, smoked	*for codeine*—less analgesia, sedation, and respiratory depression than morphine
Methadone	*Methadose, Dolophine:* fizzies, amidone, (with MDMA: chocolate chip cookies)	II/swallowed, injected	*for fentanyl*—80–100 times more potent analgesic than morphine
Fentanyl and analogs	*Actiq, Duragesic, Sublimaze:* Apache, China girl, dance fever, friend, goodfella, jackpot, murder 8, TNT, Tango and Cash	II/injected, smoked, snorted	*for oxycodone*—muscle relaxation/twice as potent analgesic as morphine; high abuse potential
Other Opioid Pain Relievers: Oxycodone HCL Hydrocodone Bitartrate Hydromorphone Oxymorphone Meperidine Propoxyphene	*Tylox, Oxycontin, Percodan, Percocet:* Oxy, O.C., oxycotton, oxyset, hillbilly heroin, percs *Vicodin, Lortab, Lorcet:* vike, Watson-387 *Dilaudid:* juice, smack, D, footballs, dillies *Opana, Numorphan, Numorphone:* biscuits, blue heaven, blues, Mrs. O, octagons, stop signs, O Bomb *Demerol, meperidine hydrochloride:* demmies, pain killer *Darvon, Darvocet*	II, III, IV/chewed, swallowed, snorted, injected, suppositories	*for methadone*—used to treat opioid addiction and pain; significant overdose risk when used improperly
Stimulants			
Amphetamines	*Biphetamine, Dexedrine, Adderall:* bennies, black beauties, crosses, hearts, LA turnaround, speed, truck drivers, uppers	II/injected, swallowed, smoked, snorted	*Feelings of exhilaration, increased energy, mental alertness/increased heart rate, blood pressure, and metabolism, reduced appetite, weight loss, nervousness, insomnia, seizures, heart attack, stroke*
Methylphenidate	*Concerta, Ritalin:* JIF, MPH, R-ball, Skippy, the smart drug, vitamin R	II/injected, swallowed, snorted	*for amphetamines*—rapid breathing, tremor, loss of coordination, irritability, anxiousness, restlessness/delirium, panic, paranoia, hallucinations, impulsive behavior, aggressiveness, tolerance, addiction
			for methylphenidate—increase or decrease in blood pressure, digestive problems, loss of appetite, weight loss
Other Compounds			
Dextromethorphan (DXM)	*Found in some cough and cold medications:* Robotripping, Robo, Triple C	not scheduled/swallowed	*Euphoria, slurred speech/increased heart rate and blood pressure, dizziness, nausea, vomiting, confusion, paranoia, distorted visual perceptions, impaired motor function*

* *Schedule I and II drugs have a high potential for abuse. They require greater storage security and have a quota on manufacturing, among other restrictions. Schedule I drugs are available for research only and have no approved medical use. Schedule II drugs are available only by prescription and require a new prescription for each refill. Schedule III and IV drugs are available by prescription, may have five refills in 6 months, and may be ordered orally. Most Schedule V drugs are available over the counter.*
** *Taking drugs by injection can increase the risk of infection through needle contamination with staphylococci, HIV, hepatitis, and other organisms. Injection is a more common practice for opioids, but risks apply to any medication taken by injection.*

opioids with marijuana, alcohol, cocaine, and tranquilizers, putting them at risk for serious complications and overdose.

CLINICAL MANIFESTATIONS

Although manifestations vary by the specific substance of use, adolescents who use drugs often present in an office setting with no obvious physical findings. Drug use is more frequently detected in adolescents who experience trauma such as motor vehicle crashes, bicycle injuries, or violence. Eliciting appropriate historical information regarding substance use, followed by blood alcohol and urine drug screens, is recommended in emergency settings. Although waning in popularity, the illicit substances known as "club drugs" still need to be considered in the differential diagnosis of a teen with an altered sensorium (Table 140.5). An adolescent presenting to an emergency setting with an impaired sensorium should be evaluated for substance use as a part of the differential diagnosis (Table 140.6). Screening for substance use is recommended for patients with psychiatric and behavioral diagnoses. Other clinical manifestations of substance use are associated with the route of use; intravenous drug use is associated with venous "tracks" and needle marks, and nasal mucosal injuries are associated with nasal insufflation of drugs. Seizures can be a direct effect of drugs such as cocaine, synthetic marijuana, and amphetamines or an effect of drug withdrawal in the case of barbiturates or tranquilizers.

SCREENING FOR SUBSTANCE ABUSE DISORDERS

In a primary care setting the annual health maintenance examination provides an opportunity for identifying adolescents with substance use or abuse issues. The direct questions as well as the assessment of school performance, family relationships, and peer activities may necessitate a more in-depth interview if there are suggestions of difficulties in those areas. Several self-report screening questionnaires also are available, with varying degrees of standardization, length, and reliability. The **CRAFFT mnemonic** is specifically designed to screen for adolescents' substance use in the primary setting (Table 140.7). Privacy and confidentiality must be established when asking the teen about specifics of their substance experimentation or use. Interviewing the parents can provide additional perspective on early warning signs that go unnoticed or disregarded by the teen. Examples of early warning signs of teen substance use are change in mood, appetite, or sleep pattern; decreased interest in school or school performance; loss of weight; secretive behavior about social plans; or valuables such as money or jewelry missing from the home. The use of urine drug screening is recommended when select circumstances are present: (1) psychiatric symptoms to rule out comorbidity or dual diagnoses, (2) significant changes in school performance or other daily behaviors, (3) frequently occurring accidents, (4) frequently occurring episodes of respiratory problems, (5) evaluation of serious motor vehicular or other injuries, and (6) as a monitoring procedure for a recovery program. Table 140.8 shows common tests used for detection by substance, along with the approximate retention time between use and identification in the urine. Most initial screening uses an immunoassay method, such as the enzyme-multiplied immunoassay technique, followed by a confirmatory test using highly sensitive, highly specific gas chromatography–mass spectrometry. The substances that can cause false-positive results should be considered, especially when there is a discrepancy between the physical findings and the urine drug screen result. In 2007 the American of Academy of Pediatrics (AAP) released guidelines that strongly discourage routine home-based or school-based testing.

DIAGNOSIS

The *Diagnostic and Statistical Manual of Mental Disorders* (DSM-5) no longer identifies substance use disorders as those of *abuse* or of *dependence*. A substance use disorder is defined by a cluster of cognitive, behavioral, and physiologic symptoms that indicate that an adolescent is using a substance even though there is evidence that the substance is harming the adolescent. Even after detoxification, a substance use disorder may leave persisting changes in brain circuits with resulting behavioral changes. There are 11 criteria that describe a pathologic pattern of behaviors related to use of the substance, falling into 4 categories:

impaired control, social impairment, increased risk, and pharmacologic criteria. The 1st category, **impaired control**, describes an individual taking increasing amounts of the substance who expresses a persistent desire to decrease use, with unsuccessful efforts. The individual may spend a great deal of time obtaining the substance, using the substance, or recovering from its effects and expresses an intense desire for the drug, usually in settings where the drug had been available, such as a specific type of social situation. The 2nd cluster of criteria (5-7) reflects **social impairment,** including the inability to perform as expected in school, at home, or at a job; increasing social problems; and withdrawing from the family. The 3rd cluster of 2 criteria addresses **increased risk** associated with use of the substance, and the 4th cluster includes 2 criteria addressing **pharmacologic responses** (tolerance and/or withdrawal). The total number of criteria present is associated with a determination of a *mild, moderate,* or *severe* disorder.

These criteria may have limitations with adolescents because of differing patterns of use, developmental implications, and other age-related consequences. Adolescents who meet diagnostic criteria should be referred to a program for substance use disorder treatment unless the primary care physician has additional training in addiction medicine.

COMPLICATIONS

Substance use in adolescence is associated with comorbidities and acts of juvenile delinquency. Youth may engage in other high-risk behaviors such as robbery, burglary, drug dealing, or prostitution for the purpose of acquiring the money necessary to buy drugs or alcohol. Regular use of any drug eventually diminishes judgment and is associated with unprotected sexual activity with its consequences of pregnancy and sexually transmitted infections, including HIV, as well as physical violence and trauma. Drug and alcohol use is closely associated with trauma in the adolescent population. Several studies of adolescent trauma victims have identified cannabinoids and cocaine in blood and urine samples in significant proportions (40%), in addition to the more common identification of alcohol. Any use of injected substances involves the risk of hepatitis B and C viruses as well as HIV (see Chapter 302).

TREATMENT

Adolescent drug abuse is a complex condition requiring a multidisciplinary approach that attends to the needs of the individual, not just drug use. Fundamental principles for treatment include accessibility to treatment; utilizing a multidisciplinary approach; employing individual or group counseling; offering mental health services; monitoring of drug use while in treatment; and understanding that recovery from drug abuse/addiction may involve multiple relapses. For most patients, remaining in treatment for a minimum period of 3 mo will result in a significant improvement.

PROGNOSIS

For adolescent substance abusers who have been referred to a drug treatment program, positive outcomes are directly related to regular attendance in posttreatment groups. For males with learning problems or conduct disorder, outcomes are poorer than for those without such disorders. Peer use patterns and parental use have a major influence on outcome for males. For females, factors such as self-esteem and anxiety are more important influences on outcomes. The chronicity of a substance use disorder makes **relapse** an issue that must always be considered when managing patients after treatment, and appropriate assistance from a health professional qualified in substance abuse management should be obtained.

PREVENTION

Preventing drug use among children and teens requires prevention efforts aimed at the individual, family, school, and community levels. The National Institute on Drug Abuse (NIDA) of the U.S. National Institutes of Health has identified essential principles of successful prevention programs. Programs should enhance *protective factors* (parent support) and reduce *risk factors* (poor self-control); should address all forms of drug abuse (legal and illegal); should address the specific type(s)

Table 140.5 Common Names and Salient Features of Club Drugs Used Recreationally

	MDMA	EPHEDRINE	γ-HYDROXYBUTYRATE	γ-BUTYROLACTONE	1,4-BUTANEDIOL	KETAMINE	FLUNITRAZEPAM	NITRITES	BATH SALTS
Common name	Ecstasy, XTC, E, X, Adam, hug drug, Molly	Herbal Ecstasy, herbal fuel, zest	Liquid Ecstasy, goop soap, Georgia homeboy, grievous bodily harm	Blue nitro, longevity, revivarant, GH revitalizer, gamma G, nitro, insom-X, remforce, firewater, invigorate	Thunder nectar, serenity, pine needle extract, zen, enliven, revitalize plus, lemon drops	K, special K, vitamin K, ket, kat	Roofies, circles, rophies, rib, roche, roaches, forget pill, R2, Mexican valium, roopies, ruffies	Poppers, ram, rock hard, thrust, TNT	White lightning, Ivory wave, Cloud 9, zoom, white rush
Duration of action	4-6 hr	4-6 hr	1.5-3.5 hr	1.5-3.5 hr	1.5-3.5 hr	1-3 hr	6-12 hr	Minutes	2-8 hr
Elimination half-life	8-9 hr	5-7 hr	27 min	ND	ND	2 hr	9-25 hr	ND	Prolonged
Peak plasma concentration	1-3 hr	2-3 hr	20-60 min*	15-45 min	15-45 min	20 min	1 hr	Seconds	Varies
Physical dependence	No	No	Yes	Yes	Yes	No	Yes	No	Yes
Antidote	No	No	No	No	No	No	Yes	No	Treat with benzodiazepine
DEA schedule	I	None	III	None	None	III	IV	None	I
Detection with routine drug screen	Yes†	Yes†	No	No	No	No‡	No‡	No	In progress
Best detection method (time frame)	GC/MS (4 hr-2 days)	GC/MS (4 hr-2 days)	GC/MS (1-12 hr)	GC/MS (1-12 hr)	GC/MS (1-12 hr)	GC/MS (1 day)	GC/MS (1-12 hr)	GC/MS (1-12 hr)	GC/MS (1-12 hr)

*Depends on dose.
†Concentrations that are sufficiently high can give positive results for amphetamine because of cross-reactions.
‡Flunitrazepam can give positive results for benzodiazepines; ketamine can give positive results for phencyclidine.
DEA, U.S. Drug Enforcement Agency, currently reviewing possibility of flunitrazepam being placed into schedule of the U.S. Controlled Substance Act; GC/MS, gas chromatography–mass spectroscopy. Duration, half-life, and peak plasma are probably different after high or sequential doses because of nonlinear kinetics; ND, not determined in humans.
Modified from Ricaurte GA, McCann UD: Recognition and management of complications of new recreational drug use. Lancet 365:2137–2145, 2005.

| Table 140.6 | Most Common Toxic Syndromes |

ANTICHOLINERGIC SYNDROMES

Common signs   Delirium with mumbling speech, tachycardia, dry, flushed skin, dilated pupils, myoclonus, slightly elevated temperature, urinary retention, and decreased bowel sounds. Seizures and dysrhythmias may occur in severe cases.

Common causes   Antihistamines, antiparkinsonian medication, atropine, scopolamine, amantadine, antipsychotic agents, antidepressant agents, antispasmodic agents, mydriatic agents, skeletal muscle relaxants, and many plants (notably jimsonweed and *Amanita muscaria*).

SYMPATHOMIMETIC SYNDROMES

Common signs   Delusions, paranoia, tachycardia (or bradycardia if the drug is a pure α-adrenergic agonist), hypertension, hyperpyrexia, diaphoresis, piloerection, mydriasis, and hyperreflexia. Seizures, hypotension, and dysrhythmias may occur in severe cases.

Common causes   Cocaine, amphetamine, methamphetamine (and its derivatives 3,4-methylenedioxyamphetamine, 3,4-methylenedioxymeth-amphetamine, 3,4-methylenedioxyethamphetamine, and 2,5-dimethoxy-4-bromoamphetamine), some synthetic marijuana, and OTC decongestants (phenylpropanolamine, ephedrine, and pseudoephedrine). In caffeine and theophylline overdoses, similar findings, except for the organic psychiatric signs, result from catecholamine release.

OPIATE, SEDATIVE, OR ETHANOL INTOXICATION

Common signs   Coma, respiratory depression, miosis, hypotension, bradycardia, hypothermia, pulmonary edema, decreased bowel sounds, hyporeflexia, and needle marks. Seizures may occur after overdoses of some narcotics, notably propoxyphene.

Common causes   Narcotics, barbiturates, benzodiazepines, ethchlorvynol, glutethimide, methyprylon, methaqualone, meprobamate, ethanol, clonidine, and guanabenz.

CHOLINERGIC SYNDROMES

Common signs   Confusion, central nervous system depression, weakness, salivation, lacrimation, urinary and fecal incontinence, gastrointestinal cramping, emesis, diaphoresis, muscle fasciculations, pulmonary edema, miosis, bradycardia or tachycardia, and seizures.

Common causes   Organophosphate and carbamate insecticides, physostigmine, edrophonium, and some mushrooms.

From Kulig K: Initial management of ingestions of toxic substances, *N Engl J Med* 326:1678, 1992. ©1992 Massachusetts Medical Society. All rights reserved.

| Table 140.7 | CRAFFT Mnemonic Tool |

- Have you ever ridden in a **C**ar driven by someone (including yourself) who was high or had been using alcohol or drugs?
- Do you ever use alcohol or drugs to **R**elax, feel better about yourself or fit in?
- Do you ever use alcohol or drugs while you are by yourself (**A**lone)?

- Do you ever **F**orget things you did while using alcohol or drugs?
- Do your **F**amily or Friends ever tell you that you should cut down on your drinking or drug use?
- Have you ever gotten into **T**rouble while you were using alcohol or drugs?

From the Center for Adolescent Substance Abuse Research (CeASAR): *The CRAFFT screening interview.* (Copyright John R. Knight, MD, Boston Children's Hospital, 2015.)

| Table 140.8 | Urine Screening for Drugs Commonly Abused by Adolescents |

DRUG	MAJOR METABOLITE	INITIAL	FIRST CONFIRMATION	SECOND CONFIRMATION	APPROXIMATE RETENTION TIME
Alcohol (blood)	Acetaldehyde	GC	IA		7-10 hr
Alcohol (urine)	Acetaldehyde	GC	IA		10-13 hr
Amphetamines		TLC	IA	GC, GC/MS	48 hr
Barbiturates		IA	TLC	GC, GC/MS	Short-acting (24 hr); long-acting (2-3 wk)
Benzodiazepines		IA	TLC	GC, GC/MS	3 days
Cannabinoids	Carboxy- and hydroxymetabolites	IA	TLC	GC/MS	3-10 days (occasional user); 1-2 mo (chronic user)
Cocaine	Benzoylecgonine	IA	TLC	GC/MS	2-4 days
Methaqualone	Hydroxylated metabolites	TLC	IA	GC/MS	2 wk
Opiates					
Heroin	Morphine Glucuronide	IA	TLC	GC, GC/MS	2 days
Morphine	Morphine Glucuronide	IA	TLC	GC, GC/MS	2 days
Codeine	Morphine Glucuronide	IA	TLC	GC, GC/MS	2 days
Phencyclidine		TLC	IA	GC, GC/MS	8 days

GC, Gas chromatography; IA, immunoassay; MS, mass spectrometry; TLC, thin-layer chromatography.

Modified from Drugs of abuse—urine screening [physician information sheet], Los Angeles, Pacific Toxicology. From MacKenzie RG, Kipke MD: Substance use and abuse. In Friedman SB, Fisher M, Schonberg SK, editors: *Comprehensive adolescent health care*, St Louis, 1998, Mosby.

of drug abuse within an identified community; and should be culturally competent to improve effectiveness (Table 140.9). The highest-risk periods for substance use in children and adolescents are during life transitions, such as the move from elementary school to middle school, or from middle school to high school. Prevention programs need to target these emotionally and socially intense times for teens to adequately anticipate potential substance use or abuse. Examples of effective research-based drug abuse prevention programs featuring a variety of strategies are listed on the NIDA website (www.drugabuse.gov), and on the Center for Substance Abuse Prevention website (www.prevention .samhsa.gov).

Bibliography is available at Expert Consult.

140.1 Alcohol

Cora Collette Breuner

Alcohol is the most widely used substance of abuse among America's youth, and a higher proportion use alcohol than use tobacco or other drugs, but the numbers are trending down. According to the 2016 **Monitoring the Future (MTF)** study, 19.9% (down from 27.6%) of 10th graders reported using alcohol in the past 30 days. Early initiation of alcohol use increases the risk for a variety of developmental problems during adolescence and is frequently an indicator of future substance use. Drinking by children, adolescents, and young adults has serious negative consequences for the individuals, their families, their communities, and society as a whole. Underage drinking contributes to a wide range of costly health and social problems, including motor vehicle crashes (the greatest single mortality risk for underage drinkers); suicide; interpersonal violence (e.g., homicides, assaults, rapes); unintentional injuries such as burns, falls, and drowning; brain impairment; alcohol dependence; risky sexual activity; academic problems; and alcohol and drug poisoning. On average, alcohol is a factor in the deaths of approximately 4,300 youths in the United States per year, shortening their life by an average of 60 yr.

According to the Centers for Disease Control and Prevention (CDC) 2015 Youth Risk Behavior Survey (YRBS), 63.2% of students had had at least 1 drink of alcohol on at least 1 day during their life (i.e., ever drank alcohol). The prevalence of having ever drunk alcohol was higher among female (65.3%) than male (61.4%) students; higher among black female (57.9%) and Hispanic female (68.6%) than black male (51.0%) and Hispanic male (63.4%) students, respectively; and higher among female (53.0%) than male (48.9%) 9th graders.

The prevalence of having ever drunk alcohol was higher among white (65.3%) and Hispanic (65.9%) than black (54.4%) students, higher among white female (66.7%) and Hispanic female (68.6%) than black female (57.9%) students, and higher among white male (64.0%) and Hispanic male (63.4%) than black male (51.0%) students.

The prevalence of having ever drunk alcohol was higher among 10th graders (60.8%), 11th graders (70.3%), and 12th graders (73.3%) than 9th graders (50.8%); higher among 11th-grade female (72.1%) and 12th-grade female (75.2%) than 9th-grade female (53.0%) and higher among 10th-grade male (58.8%), 11th-grade male (68.7%), and 12th-grade male (71.5%) than 9th-grade male (48.9%) students.

Multiple factors can affect a young teen's risk of developing a drinking problem at an early age (Table 140.10). One third of high school seniors admit to combining drinking behaviors with other risky behaviors, such as driving or taking additional substances. **Binge drinking** remains especially problematic among the older teens and young adults; 31% of high school seniors report having 5 or more drinks in a row in the last 30 days. Higher use is seen in males (23.8%) than females (19.8%), and whites (24.0%) and Hispanics (24.2%) than in blacks (12.4%). Teens with binge-drinking patterns are more likely to be assaulted, engage in high-risk sexual behaviors, have academic problems, and be injured than those teens without binge drinking patterns.

Alcohol contributes to more **deaths** in young individuals in the United States than all the illicit drugs combined. Among studies of adolescent trauma victims, alcohol is reported to be present in 32–45% of hospital admissions. Motor vehicle crashes are the most frequent type of event associated with alcohol use, but the injuries spanned several types, including self-inflicted wounds.

Alcohol is often mixed with energy drinks (caffeine, taurine, sugars), which can result in a spectrum of alcohol-related negative behaviors. **Caffeine** may counter the sedative effects of alcohol, resulting in more alcohol consumption and a perception of not being intoxicated, thus leading to risk-taking behavior such as driving while intoxicated. In addition, aggressive behavior, including sexual assaults and motor vehicle or other injuries, has been reported. Both alcohol and caffeine overdoses have also been reported.

PHARMACOLOGY AND PATHOPHYSIOLOGY

Alcohol (ethyl alcohol or ethanol) is rapidly absorbed in the stomach and is transported to the liver and metabolized by 2 pathways. The primary metabolic pathway contributes to the excess synthesis of triglycerides, a phenomenon that is responsible for producing a **fatty liver**, even in those who are well nourished. Engorgement of hepatocytes with fat causes necrosis, triggering an inflammatory process (**alcoholic hepatitis**), later followed by fibrosis, the hallmark of **cirrhosis**. Early hepatic involvement may result in elevation in γ-glutamyltransferase (GGT) and serum glutamic-pyruvic transaminase (alanine transaminase). The 2nd metabolic pathway, which is utilized at high serum alcohol levels, involves the microsomal enzyme system of the liver, in which the cofactor is reduced nicotinamide-adenine dinucleotide phosphate. The net effect of activation of this pathway is to decrease metabolism of drugs that share this system and to allow for their accumulation, enhanced effect, and possible toxicity.

Table 140.9	Domains of Risk and Protective Factors for Substance Abuse Prevention	
RISK FACTORS	**DOMAIN**	**PROTECTIVE FACTORS**
Early aggressive behavior	Individual	Self-control
Lack of parental supervision	Family	Parental monitoring
Substance abuse	Peer	Academic competence
Drug availability	School	Anti–drug use policies
Poverty	Community	Strong neighborhood attachment

From National Institute on Drug Abuse: *Preventing drug use among children and adolescents: a research-based guide for parents, educators, and community leaders*, NIH Pub No 04-4212(B), ed 2, Bethesda, MD, 2003, NIDA.

Table 140.10	Risk Factors for a Teen Developing a Drinking Problem

FAMILY RISK FACTORS
- Low parental supervision
- Poor parent to teen communication
- Family conflicts
- Severe or inconsistent family discipline
- Having a parent with an alcohol or drug problem

INDIVIDUAL RISK FACTORS
- Poor impulse control
- Emotional instability
- Thrill-seeking behaviors
- Behavioral problems
- Perceived risk of drinking is low
- Begins drinking before age 14 yr

CLINICAL MANIFESTATIONS

Alcohol acts primarily as a central nervous system (CNS) depressant. It produces euphoria, grogginess, talkativeness, impaired short-term memory, and an increased pain threshold. Alcohol's ability to produce vasodilation and hypothermia is also centrally mediated. At very high serum levels, respiratory depression occurs. Its inhibitory effect on pituitary antidiuretic hormone release is responsible for its diuretic effect. The gastrointestinal (GI) complications of alcohol use can occur from a single large ingestion. The most common is acute **erosive gastritis**, manifesting as epigastric pain, anorexia, vomiting, and heme-positive stools. Less frequently, vomiting and mid-abdominal pain may be caused by acute alcoholic **pancreatitis**; diagnosis is confirmed by the finding of elevated serum amylase and lipase levels.

DIAGNOSIS

Primary care settings provide the opportunity to screen teens for alcohol use or problem behaviors. Brief alcohol screening instruments such as CRAFFT (see Table 140.7) or AUDIT (Alcohol Use Disorders Identification Test, Table 140.11) perform well in a clinical setting as techniques to identify alcohol use disorders. A score of ≥8 on the AUDIT questionnaire identifies people who drink excessively and who would benefit from reducing or ceasing drinking. Teenagers in the early phases of alcohol use exhibit few physical findings. Recent use of alcohol may be reflected in elevated GGT and aspartate transaminase levels.

In acute care settings the **alcohol overdose syndrome** should be suspected in any teenager who appears disoriented, lethargic, or comatose. Although the distinctive aroma of alcohol may assist in diagnosis, confirmation by analysis of blood is recommended. At levels >200 mg/dL, the adolescent is at risk of death, and levels >500 mg/dL (median lethal dose) are usually associated with a fatal outcome. When the level of obtundation appears excessive for the reported blood alcohol level, head trauma, hypoglycemia, or ingestion of other drugs should be considered as possible confounding factors.

TREATMENT

The usual mechanism of death from the alcohol overdose syndrome is **respiratory depression**, and artificial ventilatory support must be provided until the liver can eliminate sufficient amounts of alcohol from the body. In a patient without alcoholism, it generally takes 20 hr to reduce the blood level of alcohol from 400 mg/dL to zero. Dialysis should be considered when the blood level is >400 mg/dL. As a follow-up to acute treatment, referral for treatment of the alcohol use disorder is indicated. Group counseling, individualized counseling, and multifamily educational intervention have proved to be effective interventions for teens.

Bibliography is available at Expert Consult.

140.2 Tobacco and Electronic Nicotine Delivery Systems

Brian P. Jenssen

CIGARETTES

Tobacco use and addiction almost always start in childhood or adolescence, a period when the brain has heightened susceptibility to nicotine addiction. Nearly 90% of adult smokers began smoking before age 18. Factors associated with youth tobacco use include exposure to smokers (friends, parents), tobacco availability, low socioeconomic status, poor school performance, low self-esteem, lack of perceived risk of use, and lack of skills to resist influences to use tobacco.

From 2011–2017, among all US high school students, current use of cigarettes decreased from 15.8% to 7.6%. During the same time period, however, current use of e-cigarettes and hookah (water pipes used to smoke tobacco) increased significantly among middle and high school students. In 2017, e-cigarettes (11.7%) were the most commonly used tobacco product among high school students. Cigars (7.7%) and cigarettes (7.6%) were the second and third most commonly used tobacco

Table 140.11	Alcohol Use Disorders Identification Test (AUDIT)	
		SCORE (0-4)*
1. How often do you have a drink containing alcohol?		Never (0) to more than 4 per wk (4)
2. How many drinks containing alcohol do you have on a typical day?		One or 2 (0) to more than 10 (4)
3. How often do you have 6 or more drinks on 1 occasion?		Never (0) to daily or almost daily (4)
4. How often during the last year have you found that you were not able to stop drinking once you had started?		Never (0) to daily or almost daily (4)
5. How often during the last year have you failed to do what was normally expected from you because of drinking?		Never (0) to daily or almost daily (4)
6. How often during the last year have you needed a first drink in the morning to get yourself going after a heavy drinking session?		Never (0) to daily or almost daily (4)
7. How often during the last year have you had a feeling of guilt or remorse after drinking?		Never (0) to daily or almost daily (4)
8. How often during the last year have you been unable to remember what happened the night before because you had been drinking?		Never (0) to daily or almost daily (4)
9. Have you or someone else been injured as a result of your drinking?		No (0) to yes, during the last year (4)
10. Has a relative, friend, doctor or other health worker been concerned about your drinking or suggested that you should cut down?		No (0) to yes, during the last year (4)

*Score ≥8 = problem drinking.
From Schuckit MA: Alcohol-use disorders, *Lancet* 373:492–500, 2009.

products among high school students, followed by smokeless tobacco (5.5%), hookah (3.3%), and pipe tobacco (0.8%).

Tobacco use is associated with other high-risk behaviors. Teens who smoke are more likely than nonsmokers to use alcohol and engage in unprotected sex, are 8 times more likely to use marijuana, and are 22 times more likely to use cocaine.

Tobacco is used by teens in all regions of the world, although the form of tobacco used differs. In the Americas and Europe, cigarette smoking is the predominant form of tobacco use, followed by cigars and smokeless tobacco; in the Eastern Mediterranean, hookah use is prevalent; in Southeast Asia, smokeless tobacco products are used; in the Western Pacific, betel nut is chewed with tobacco; and pipe, snuff, and rolled tobacco leaves are used in Africa. Cigarette use by teens in low- and middle-income nations is increasing.

PHARMACOLOGY

Nicotine, the primary active ingredient in cigarettes, is addictive. Nicotine is absorbed by multiple sites in the body, including the lungs, skin, GI tract, and buccal and nasal mucosa. The action of nicotine is mediated through nicotinic acetylcholine receptors located on noncholinergic presynaptic and postsynaptic sites in the brain and causes increased levels of dopamine. Nicotine also stimulates the adrenal glands to release epinephrine, causing an immediate elevation in blood pressure, respiration, and heart rate. The dose of nicotine delivered to the user in a cigarette depends on a variety of factors, including puffing characteristics. A smoker typically takes 10 puffs within the span of 5 minutes and absorbs 1-2 mg of nicotine (range: 0.5–3 mg). **Cotinine,** the major metabolite of nicotine, has a biologic half-life of 19-24 hr and can be detected in urine, serum, and saliva.

CLINICAL MANIFESTATIONS

Cigarettes are addictive by design and result in life-shortening diseases in half their long-term users. Each year, approximately 480,000 deaths are attributable to smoking, responsible for 1 of every 5 deaths and 1 of every 3 cancer deaths in the United States. Cigarette smoking has severe adverse health consequences for youth and young adults, including increased prevalence of chronic cough, sputum production, wheezing, and worsening asthma. Smoking during pregnancy increases prenatal and perinatal morbidity and mortality, either causing or exacerbating the risks of preterm birth, low birthweight, congenital malformations, stillbirth, and sudden infant death syndrome (SIDS). **Withdrawal** symptoms, including irritability, decreased concentration, increased appetite, and strong cravings for tobacco, can occur when adolescents try to quit.

ELECTRONIC CIGARETTES (E-CIGARETTES)

E-cigarettes, also known as **electronic nicotine delivery systems (ENDS)**, are handheld devices that produce an aerosol created from a solution of nicotine, flavoring chemicals, propylene glycol, and often other constituents unknown and unadvertised to the consumer. There is wide variability in terminology, product design, and engineering of these products, with alternative names including e-cigs, electronic cigars, electronic hookah, e-hookah, personal vaporizers, vape pens, and vaping devices. The industry continues to develop new products, such as JUUL, which contain nicotine but may not be recognized as a tobacco product by teens. The unique flavors offered in e-cigarette solution, the majority of which are confectionary in nature and appealing to children, have been shown to encourage youth experimentation, regular use, and addiction.

Adverse effects to users include dry cough, throat irritation, and lipoid pneumonia. Nonusers could be impacted by the secondhand and thirdhand aerosol (residual nicotine and other chemicals left on surfaces), which have been shown to contain known toxicants, including nicotine, carcinogens, and metal particles. Rates of acute nicotine poisoning have increased from unintentional exposure of children to the concentrated nicotine–containing e-cigarette solution. Studies of adolescents suggest a strong association between e-cigarette use at baseline and progression to traditional cigarette smoking. E-cigarettes may contribute to subsequent cigarette use through nicotine addiction and social normalization of smoking behaviors.

E-cigarettes are not U.S. Food and Drug Administration (FDA) approved and have not been shown to be safe or effective for smoking cessation treatment. Unless the quality of the evidence improves, adolescent smokers interested in quitting should seek and be referred to evidence-based treatments. In August 2016 the FDA finalized a rule that extends its regulatory authority to all tobacco products, including e-cigarettes, affecting how these products are manufactured, marketed, and sold. It requires manufacturers to report product ingredients and undergo the agency's premarket review to receive marketing authorization. In 2017, however, the FDA delayed implementation of this rule until 2022, allowing e-cigarettes (as of April 2019) to remain on the market without premarket review.

HOOKAH

Hookah (water pipe) smoking uses specially treated tobacco that comes in a variety of flavors. Emerging evidence indicates that hookah may involve comparable health risks to cigarettes, including nicotine dependence. Both human and machine simulation studies of hookah use consistently find that smoke content and user toxicant exposure, including carbon monoxide, tar, and nicotine, are at least comparable to that of cigarettes. Secondhand smoke from hookahs can be a health risk for nonsmokers exposed to harmful toxicants.

TREATMENT

Tobacco prevention interventions delivered in pediatric settings, including individual encounters or connection to educational materials, can reduce the risk for smoking initiation in school-age children and adolescents. Messages should be clear, personally relevant, and age appropriate. Adolescents may be more responsive to messages that emphasize the effects of tobacco use on appearance, breath, and sports performance; lack of benefit for weight loss; monetary cost of tobacco addiction; and deceptive marketing by the tobacco industry.

The approach to smoking cessation in adolescents includes the **5 As** (**ask, advise, assess, assist,** and **arrange**) and use of **nicotine replacement therapy (NRT)** in addicted teens who are motivated to quit. Consensus panels recommend the 5 As, although evidence of efficacy in adolescents is limited. Studies of the NRT patch in adolescents suggest a positive effect on reducing withdrawal symptoms; pharmacotherapy should be combined with behavioral therapy to increase cessation and lower relapse rates. In a limited number of studies, cessation rates of 15% were reported at 3 and 6 mo. NRT is also available as a gum, inhaler, nasal spray, lozenge, or microtab (Table 140.12). Medications such as bupropion and varenicline improve smoking cessation rates in adults but are not FDA approved for use in adolescents <18 yr old. Preliminary studies in adolescents report cessation efficacy with 150 mg of bupropion twice daily. In postmarketing surveillance, suicidal ideation and suicide have been reported among patients taking bupropion and varenicline.

Pediatric clinicians can connect patients to effective behavioral interventions, including telephone, text message, smartphone app, internet, and community-based resources. Free telephone-based treatment (1-800-QUIT-NOW) has been shown to improve smoking cessation rates. Smoke-free TXT, offered by the National Cancer Institute, engages teens to quit smoking using free, daily text messaging. Teens can sign up online (teen.smokefree.gov) or text QUIT to iQUIT (47848). A smartphone-based app, QuitSTART, helps teens track cravings, monitor moods, use cessation tips, and follow quitting attempts. The American Lung Association's **Not-On-Tobacco Program (NOT)** is a nationally recognized best-practice model for teen smoking cessation (see www.lung.org).

Bibliography is available at Expert Consult.

140.3 Marijuana

Cora Collette Breuner

Marijuana (cannabis, pot, weed, hash, grass), derived from the *Cannabis sativa* hemp plant, is the most commonly abused illicit drug. The main active chemical, tetrahydrocannabinol (**THC**), is responsible for its hallucinogenic properties. THC is absorbed rapidly by the nasal or oral routes, producing a peak of subjective effect at 10 min and 1 hr, respectively. Marijuana is generally smoked as a cigarette (reefer, joint) or in a pipe. Although there is much variation in content, each cigarette contains 8–10% THC. Another popular form that is smoked, a "blunt," is a hollowed-out small cigar refilled with marijuana. Marijuana products (hash oil or leaf) can also be used in some vaping devices or hookah pens. **Hashish** is the concentrated THC resin in a sticky black liquid or oil. Although marijuana use by U.S. teens has declined in the last decade, 23.1% of high school students have used marijuana at least once during the previous 30 days, and current marijuana use is highest in black males and high school seniors. About 8% of students report having tried marijuana before age 13, with a range of 4.3–18.5% across various states, indicating the need for early prevention efforts. Adolescents living in states where medical marijuana is legal report a higher use of cannabis "edibles." It is important to recognize that as perceived harm drops, marijuana use increases (Fig. 140.4).

CLINICAL MANIFESTATIONS

In addition to the "desired" effects of elation and euphoria, marijuana may cause impairment of short-term memory, poor performance of tasks requiring divided attention (e.g., those involved in driving), loss of critical judgment, decreased coordination, and distortion of time perception (Table 140.13). Visual hallucinations and perceived body distortions occur rarely, but "flashbacks" or recall of frightening hallucinations experienced under marijuana's influence may occur, usually during

| Table 140.12 | Smoking Cessation Pharmacotherapy Available in the United States | | | | | |

THERAPY BRAND	NAME	STRENGTHS	FDA-APPROVED ADULT DOSING	AVAILABILITY*	STUDIED IN ADOLESCENTS	QUIT DATE
NICOTINE REPLACEMENT THERAPY						
Gum‡	Nicorette	2 mg, 4 mg	The 4-mg strength should be used by patients who smoke ≥25 cigarettes a day; otherwise, 2-mg strength should be used. Wk 1-6: 1 piece every 1-2 hr Wk 7-9: 1 piece every 2-4 hr Wk 10-12: 1 piece every 4-8 hr	OTC*	Yes	
Inhaler	Nicotrol Inhaler	4 mg	6-16 cartridges a day for up to 12 wk	Rx	No	
Lozenge	Commit, Nicorette mini	2 mg, 4 mg	The 4-mg strength should be used by patients who smoke 1st cigarette within 30 min of waking; otherwise, 2-mg strength should be used. Wk 1-6: 1 lozenge every 1-2 hr Wk 7-9: 1 lozenge every 2-4 hr Wk 10-12: 1 lozenge every 4-8 hr	OTC	No	Prior to beginning nicotine replacement therapy
Nasal Spray	Nicotrol NS	0.5 mg/spray	1-2 sprays/hr up to a maximum of 80 sprays per day	Rx	Yes	
Transdermal Patch‡	NicoDerm CQ	7, 14, 21 mg/24 hr	For patients who smoke >10 cigarettes daily: Step 1: one 21-mg patch daily for wk 1-6 Step 2: one 14-mg patch daily for wk 7-8 Step 3: one 7-mg patch daily for wk 9-10 For patients who smoke <10 cigarettes daily: Begin with 14-mg patch daily for 6 wk, followed by 7-mg patch for 2 wk.	OTC	Yes	
NONNICOTINE THERAPY						
Bupropion SR‡	Zyban	150-mg sustained-release tablets	150 mg PO in morning for 3 days, then increase to 150 mg PO bid	Rx	Yes	1 wk after starting therapy
Varenicline	Chantix	0.5-, 1-mg tablets	0.5 mg PO in morning for 3 days; increase to 0.5 mg PO bid for 4 days, then increase to 1 mg PO bid	Rx	No	

*OTC, Over the counter; Rx, prescription product; PO, by mouth (orally); bid, twice daily.
†None is FDA approved for use in patients younger than 18 yr.
‡Generics available.
From JP Karpinski et al: Smoking cessation treatment for adolescents, *J Pediatr Pharmacol Ther* 15(4):249–260, 2010.

stress or with fever.

Smoking marijuana for a minimum of 4 days/wk for 6 mo appears to result in dose-related suppression of plasma testosterone levels and spermatogenesis, prompting concern about the potential deleterious effect of smoking marijuana before completion of pubertal growth and development. There is an antiemetic effect of oral THC or smoked marijuana, often followed by appetite stimulation, which is the basis of the drug's use in patients receiving cancer chemotherapy. Although the possibility of teratogenicity has been raised because of findings in animals, there is no evidence of such effects in humans.

An **amotivational syndrome** has been described in long-term marijuana users who lose interest in age-appropriate behavior; proof of the causative relationship remains equivocal. Chronic use is associated with increased anxiety and depression, learning problems, poor job performance, hyperemesis, and respiratory problems such as pharyngitis, sinusitis, bronchitis, and asthma (see Table 140.13).

The **cannabinoid hyperemesis syndrome** is characterized by recurrent episodes of vomiting associated with abdominal pain and nausea; patients often find relief by taking a hot shower or bath. Cannabis use has been chronic (>1-2 yr) and frequent (multiple times per week). Treatment includes stopping marijuana use, antiemetics, and topical capsaicin.

The increased THC content of marijuana of 5-15–fold compared to that of the 1970s is related to the observation of a **withdrawal syndrome**, occurring 24-48 hr after discontinuing the drug. Heavy users experience malaise, irritability, agitation, insomnia, drug craving, shakiness, diaphoresis, night sweats, and GI disturbance. The symptoms peak by

the 4th day and resolve in 10-14 days. Certain drugs may interact with marijuana to potentiate sedation (alcohol, diazepam) and stimulation (cocaine, amphetamines) or may be antagonistic (propranolol, phenytoin).

Behavioral interventions, including **cognitive-behavioral therapy (CBT)** and motivational incentives, have shown to be effective in treating marijuana dependency.

SYNTHETIC MARIJUANA

Spice, K2, crazy clown, aroma, black mamba, blaze, dream, and funky monkey are some of the common street names for synthetic marijuana, which is a mixture of herbs or plant materials that have been sprayed with artificial chemicals similar to THC, the psychoactive ingredient in marijuana. One active group of chemicals is the **carboxamides,** which are not detected by standard assays to detect THC. In the United States the chemicals in "Spice" are designated a Schedule I controlled substance (as is marijuana) by the Drug Enforcement Administration (DEA), thereby making it illegal to sell, buy, or possess them. Nonetheless, synthetic marijuana is the 2nd most common illicit drug used by high school seniors. More than 10% of high school seniors used synthetic marijuana in the last year.

Synthetic marijuana is mainly used by smoking, or mixed with marijuana, or brewed as a tea for drinking. The chemicals in synthetic marijuana affect the same receptors as THC and produce similar effects as seen in cannabis use, such as relaxation, elevated mood, and altered perception. In addition, sympathomimetic symptoms are quite common and are the cause of significant toxicity. Symptoms of **intoxication**

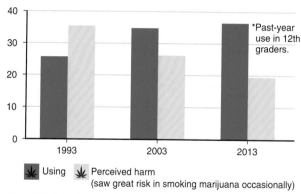

Fig. 140.4 As the perceived harm of marijuana drops, use goes up. The 36.4% using in 2013 equates to about 11 students in the average class. *(From NIH National Institute on Drug Abuse.)*

Table 140.13	Acute and Chronic Adverse Effects of Cannabis Use

ACUTE ADVERSE EFFECTS
- Anxiety and panic, especially in naïve users
- Psychotic symptoms (at high doses)
- Road crashes if a person drives while intoxicated

CHRONIC ADVERSE EFFECTS
- Cannabis dependence syndrome (in about 1 in 10 users)
- Chronic bronchitis and impaired respiratory function in regular smokers
- Psychotic symptoms and disorders in heavy users, especially those with a history of psychotic symptoms or a family history of these disorders
- Impaired educational attainment in adolescents who are regular users
- Subtle cognitive impairment in those who are daily users for 10 yr or more

From Hall W, Degenhardt L: Adverse health effects of non-medical cannabis use, *Lancet* 374:1383–1390, 2009.

include vomiting, tachycardia, hypertension, hyperthermia, confusion, extreme anxiety, profuse sweating, agitation, aggression, dysphoria, hallucinations, seizures, rhabdomyolysis, dystonia, unresponsiveness, confusion, catatonia, "zombie-like" behaviors, and myocardial ischemia. In response to legislation to ban the chemicals in OTC synthetic marijuana products, manufacturers alter and substitute the chemicals in the product, keeping it on the legal market and leaving teens particularly vulnerable to potential health effects.

Synthetic marijuana are not detected by standard toxicology screening but can be identified in specialized laboratories.

Bibliography is available at Expert Consult.

140.4 Inhalants
Cora Collette Breuner

Inhalants, found in many common household products, comprise a diverse group of volatile substances whose vapors can be inhaled to produce psychoactive effects. The practice of inhalation is popular among younger adolescents and decreases with age. Young adolescents are attracted to these substances because of their rapid action, easy availability, and low cost. Products that are abused as inhalants include *volatile*

solvents (paint thinners, glue, e-cigarette solvents known as "dripping," toluene, acetone, refrigerants, gasoline, cleaning fluids, correction fluids), *aerosols* (spray paint, nitrous oxide, hair spray), *gases* (propane tanks, lighter fluid), *nitrites* ("poppers" or "video head cleaner"), and *propellants* used in whipped cream dispensers. The most popular inhalants among young adolescents are glue, shoe polish, and spray paint. The various products contain a wide range of chemicals with serious adverse health effects (Table 140.14). **Huffing**, the practice of inhaling fumes, can be accomplished using a paper bag containing a chemical-soaked cloth, spraying aerosols directly into the nose/mouth, or using a balloon, plastic bag, or soda can filled with fumes. The percentage of adolescents using inhalants has remained stable, with 5.8% of high school students reporting having ever used inhalants. Eighth and 9th graders report highest use, suggesting targeted prevention strategies for this age-group.

CLINICAL MANIFESTATIONS
The major effects of inhalants are psychoactive (Table 140.15). The intoxication lasts only a few minutes, so a typical user will huff repeatedly over an extended period (hours) to maintain the high. The immediate effects of inhalants are similar to alcohol: euphoria, slurred speech, decreased coordination, and dizziness. **Toluene**, the main ingredient in model airplane glue and some rubber cements, causes relaxation and pleasant hallucinations for up to 2 hr. Euphoria is followed by violent excitement; coma may result from prolonged or rapid inhalation. **Volatile nitrites**, such as amyl nitrite, butyl nitrite, and related compounds marketed as room deodorizers, are used as euphoriants, enhancers of musical appreciation, and sexual enhancements among older adolescents and young adults. They may result in headaches, syncope, and light-headedness; profound hypotension and cutaneous flushing followed by vasoconstriction and tachycardia; transiently inverted T waves and depressed ST segments on electrocardiography; methemoglobinemia; increased bronchial irritation; and increased intraocular pressure. There may be dermatologic findings, including perianal/perioral dermatitis ("huffer rash"), frostbite, and contact dermatitis, as well as epistaxis, nasal ulcers, and conjunctivitis.

COMPLICATIONS
Model airplane glue is responsible for a wide range of complications, related to chemical toxicity, to the method of administration (in plastic bags, with resultant suffocation), and to the dangerous setting in which the inhalation occurs (inner-city roof tops). Common neuromuscular changes reported in chronic inhalant abusers include difficulty coordinating movement, gait disorders, muscle tremors, and spasticity, particularly in the legs (Table 140.16). Chronic use may cause pulmonary hypertension, restrictive lung defects or reduced diffusion capacity, peripheral neuropathy, hematuria, tubular acidosis, and possibly cerebral and cerebellar atrophy. Chronic inhalant abuse has long been linked to widespread brain damage and cognitive abnormalities that can range from mild impairment (poor memory, decreased learning ability) to severe dementia. High-frequency inhalant users were significantly more likely than moderate- and low-frequency users to experience adverse consequences of inhalant intoxication, such as behavioral, language, and memory problems. Certain risky behaviors and consequences, such as engaging in unprotected sex or fighting while high on inhalants, were dramatically more common among high-frequency than low-frequency inhalant users. Death in the acute phase may result from cerebral or pulmonary edema or myocardial involvement (Table 140.16).

DIAGNOSIS
Diagnosis of inhalant abuse is difficult because of the ubiquitous nature of the products and decreased parental awareness of the dangers. In the primary care setting, providers need to ask parents if they have witnessed any unusual behaviors in their teen; noticed high-risk products in the teen's bedroom; seen paint on the teen's hands, nose, or mouth; or found paint- or chemical-coated rags. Complete blood count, coagulation studies, and hepatic and renal function studies may identify the complications. In extreme intoxication, a user may manifest symptoms of restlessness, general muscle weakness, dysarthria, nystagmus, disruptive

Table 140.14	Hazards of Chemicals Found in Commonly Abused Inhalants

Amyl nitrite, butyl nitrite ("poppers," "video head cleaner"): sudden sniffing death syndrome, suppressed immunologic function, injury to red blood cells (interfering with oxygen supply to vital tissues)

Benzene (found in gasoline): bone marrow injury, impaired immunologic function, increased risk of leukemia, reproductive system toxicity

Butane, propane (found in lighter fluid, hair and paint sprays): sudden sniffing death syndrome via cardiac effects, serious burn injuries (because of flammability)

Freon (used as a refrigerant and aerosol propellant): sudden sniffing death syndrome, respiratory obstruction and death (from sudden cooling/cold injury to airways), liver damage

Methylene chloride (found in paint thinners and removers, degreasers): reduction of oxygen-carrying of blood, changes to the heart muscle and heartbeat

Nitrous oxide ("laughing gas"), **hexane**: death from lack of oxygen to the brain, altered perception and motor coordination, loss of sensation, limb spasms, blackouts caused by blood pressure changes, depression of heart muscle functioning

Toluene (found in gasoline, paint thinners and removers, correction fluid): brain damage (loss of brain tissue mass, impaired cognition, gait disturbance, loss of coordination, loss of equilibrium, limb spasms, hearing and vision loss), liver and kidney damage

Trichloroethylene (found in spot removers, degreasers): sudden sniffing death syndrome, cirrhosis of the liver, reproductive complications, hearing and vision damage

Table 140.15	Stages in Symptom Development After Use of Inhalants

STAGE	SYMPTOMS
1: Excitatory	Euphoria, excitation, exhilaration, dizziness, hallucinations, sneezing, coughing, excess salivation, intolerance to light, nausea and vomiting, flushed skin and bizarre behavior
2: Early CNS depression	Confusion, disorientation, dullness, loss of self-control, ringing or buzzing in the head, blurred or double vision, cramps, headache, insensitivity to pain, and pallor or paleness
3: Medium CNS depression	Drowsiness, muscular uncoordination, slurred speech, depressed reflexes, and nystagmus or rapid involuntary oscillation of the eyeballs
4: Late CNS depression	Unconsciousness that may be accompanied by bizarre dreams, epileptiform seizures, and EEG changes

CNS, Central nervous system; EEG, electroencephalogram.
From Harris D: Volatile substance abuse, *Arch Dis Child Educ Pract Ed* 91:ep93-ep100, 2006.

Table 140.16	Documented Clinical Presentations of Acute and Chronic Volatile Substance Abuse

Ventricular fibrillation	Muscle weakness
Asystolic cardiac arrest	Abdominal pain
Myocardial infarction	Cough
Ataxia	Aspiration pneumonia
Agitation	Chemical pneumonitis
Limb and trunk uncoordination	Coma
Tremor	Visual and auditory hallucinations
Visual loss	Acute delusions
Tinnitus	Nausea and vomiting
Dysarthria	Pulmonary edema
Vertigo	Photophobia
Hyperreflexia	Rash
Acute confusional state	Jaundice
Conjunctivitis	Anorexia
Acute paranoia	Slurred speech
Depression	Diarrhea
Oral and nasal mucosal ulceration	Weight loss
Halitosis	Epistaxis
Convulsions/fits	Rhinitis
Headache	Cerebral edema
Peripheral neuropathy	Visual loss
Methemoglobinemia	Burns
Acute trauma	Renal tubular acidosis

behavior, and occasionally hallucinations. Toluene is excreted rapidly in the urine as hippuric acid, with the residual detectable in the serum by gas chromatography.

TREATMENT
Treatment is generally supportive and directed toward control of arrhythmia and stabilization of respirations and circulation. Withdrawal symptoms do not usually occur.

Bibliography is available at Expert Consult.

140.5 Hallucinogens
Cora Collette Breuner

Several naturally occurring and synthetic substances are used by adolescents for their hallucinogenic properties. They have chemical structures similar to neurotransmitters such as serotonin, but their exact mechanism of action remains unclear. Lysergic acid diethylamide (**LSD**) and methylenedioxymethamphetamine (**MDMA**) are the most commonly reported hallucinogens used. 251-NBOMe ("N-Bomb") is a new designer drug that interacts with the 5HT-2a receptor and has sympathomimetic and hallucinogenic properties.

LYSERGIC ACID DIETHYLAMIDE
LSD (acid, big "d," blotters) is a very potent hallucinogen that is made from lysergic acid found in ergot, a fungus that grows on rye and other grains. Its high potency allows effective doses to be applied to absorbent paper, or it can be taken as a liquid or a tablet. The onset of action can be 30-60 min, and it peaks at 2-4 hr. By 10-12 hr, individuals return to the predrug state. Among U.S. 12th graders, 4% report trying LSD at least once.

Clinical Manifestations
The effects of LSD can be divided into 3 categories: somatic (physical effects), perceptual (altered changes in vision and hearing), and psychic (changes in sensorium). The common somatic symptoms are dizziness, dilated pupils, nausea, flushing, elevated temperature, and tachycardia.

The sensation of *synesthesia,* or "seeing" smells and "hearing" colors, as well as major distortions of time and self, have been reported with high doses of LSD. Delusional ideation, body distortion, and suspiciousness to the point of toxic psychosis are the more serious of the psychic symptoms. LSD is not considered to be an addictive drug because it does not typically produce drug-seeking behavior.

Treatment

An individual is considered to have a "bad trip" when the sensory experiences causes the user to become terrified or panicked. These episodes should be treated by removing the individual from the aggravating situation and placing him in a quiet room with a calming friend. In situations of extreme agitation or seizures, use of benzodiazepines may be warranted. "Flashbacks" or LSD-induced states after the drug has worn off and tolerance to the effects of the drug are additional complications of its use.

METHYLENEDIOXYMETHAMPHETAMINE

MDMA ("X," Ecstasy, Molly), a phenylisopropylamine hallucinogen, is a synthetic compound similar to hallucinogenic mescaline and the stimulant methamphetamine. Like other hallucinogens, this drug is proposed to interact with serotoninergic neurons in the central nervous system (CNS). It is the preferred drug at "raves," all-night dance parties, and is also known as one of the "club drugs" along with γ-hydroxybutyrate (GHB) and ketamine (see Table 140.5). Between 2009 and 2010, past-year use of MDMA increased among U.S. 8th and 10th graders but then declined in both grades. Nationwide, the prevalence of having ever used MDMA was 8.4% of college students. In 2016, MDMA use by blacks (2.2%) in 12th grade was lower than for Hispanics (2.8%) or whites (3.3%).

Clinical Manifestations

Euphoria, a heightened sensual awareness, and increased psychic and emotional energy are acute effects. Compared to other hallucinogens, MDMA is less likely to produce emotional lability, depersonalization, and disturbances of thought. Nausea, jaw clenching, teeth grinding, and blurred vision are somatic symptoms, whereas anxiety, panic attacks, and psychosis are the adverse psychiatric outcomes. A few deaths have been reported after ingestion of the drug. In high doses, MDMA can interfere with the body's ability to regulate temperature. The resultant hyperthermia in association with vigorous dancing at a "rave" has resulted in severe liver, kidney, and cardiovascular system failure and death. There are no specific treatment regimens recommended for acute toxicity.

Chronic MDMA use can lead to changes in brain function, affecting cognitive tasks and memory. These symptoms may occur because of MDMA's effects on neurons that use serotonin as a neurotransmitter. The serotonin system plays an important role in regulating mood, aggression, sexual activity, sleep, and sensitivity to pain. A high rate of dependence has been found among MDMA users. MDMA exposure may be associated with long-term neurotoxicity and damage to serotonin-containing neurons. In nonhuman primates, exposure to MDMA for only 4 days caused damage to serotonin nerve terminals that was evident 6-7 yr later. There are no specific pharmacologic treatments for MDMA addiction. Drug abuse recovery groups are recommended.

PHENCYCLIDINE

Phencyclidine (**PCP**) (sternyl, angel dust, hog, peace pill, sheets) is an arylcyclohexalamine whose popularity is related in part to its ease of synthesis in home laboratories. One of the by-products of home synthesis causes cramps, diarrhea, and hematemesis. It is a "dissociative drug" that produces feelings of detachment from the surrounding environment and self. The drug is thought to potentiate adrenergic effects by inhibiting neuronal reuptake of catecholamines. PCP is available as a tablet, liquid, or powder, which may be used alone or sprinkled on cigarettes (joints). The powders and tablets generally contain 2-6 mg of PCP, whereas joints average 1 mg for every 150 mg of tobacco leaves, or approximately 30-50 mg per joint. The prevalence of PCP use (hallucinogenic drug) among U.S. 12th graders was 1.3%.

Clinical Manifestations

The clinical manifestations are dose related and produce alterations of perception, behavior, and autonomic functions. Euphoria, nystagmus, ataxia, and emotional lability occur within 2-3 min after smoking 1-5 mg and last for 4-6 hr. At these low doses the user is likely to experience shallow breathing, flushing, generalized numbness of extremities, and loss of motor coordination. Hallucinations may involve bizarre distortions of body image that often precipitate panic reactions. With doses of 5-15 mg, a toxic psychosis may occur, with disorientation, hypersalivation, and abusive language lasting for >1 hr. Hypotension, generalized seizures, and cardiac arrhythmias typically occur with plasma concentrations of 40-200 mg/dL. Death has been reported during psychotic delirium, from hypertension, hypotension, hypothermia, seizures, and trauma. The **coma** of PCP may be distinguished from that of the opiates by the absence of respiratory depression; the presence of muscle rigidity, hyperreflexia, and nystagmus; and lack of response to naloxone. PCP psychosis may be difficult to distinguish from schizophrenia. In the absence of a history of use, the diagnosis depends on urinalysis.

Treatment

Management of the PCP-intoxicated patient includes placement in a darkened, quiet room on a floor pad, safe from injury. Acute alcohol intoxication may also be present. For recent oral ingestion, gastric absorption is poor, and induction of emesis or gastric lavage is useful. Diazepam, in a dose of 5-10 mg orally or 2-5 mg intravenously, may be helpful if the patient is agitated and not comatose. Rapid excretion of the drug is promoted by acidification of the urine. Supportive therapy of the comatose patient is indicated with particular attention to hydration, which may be compromised by PCP-induced diuresis. Inpatient and/or behavioral treatments can be helpful for chronic PCP users.

Bibliography is available at Expert Consult.

140.6 Cocaine

Cora Collette Breuner

Cocaine, an alkaloid extracted from the leaves of the South American *Erythroxylum coca,* is supplied as the hydrochloride salt in crystalline form. With **snorting,** it is rapidly absorbed into the bloodstream from the nasal mucosa, detoxified by the liver, and excreted in the urine as benzoylecgonine. Smoking the cocaine alkaloid (**freebasing**) involves inhaling the cocaine vapors in pipes, or cigarettes mixed with tobacco or marijuana. Accidental burns are potential complications of this practice. With **crack** cocaine, the crystallized rock form, the smoker feels "high" in <10 sec. The risk of addiction with this method is higher and more rapidly progressive than from snorting cocaine. Tolerance develops, and the user must increase the dose or change the route of administration, or both, to achieve the same effect. To sustain the high, cocaine users repeatedly use cocaine in short periods of time known as "binges." Drug dealers often place cocaine in plastic bags or condoms and swallow these containers during transport. Rupture of a container produces a sympathomimetic crisis (see Table 140.6). Cocaine use among U.S. high school students has decreased in the last decade, as noted in the MTF 2016 data, with 3.7% of 12th graders having tried the drug (any route) at least once.

CLINICAL MANIFESTATIONS

Cocaine is a strong CNS stimulant that increases dopamine levels by preventing reuptake. Cocaine produces euphoria, increased motor activity, decreased fatigability, and mental alertness. Its sympathomimetic properties are responsible for pupillary dilation, tachycardia, hypertension, and hyperthermia. Snorting cocaine chronically results in loss of sense of smell, nosebleeds, and chronic rhinorrhea. Injecting cocaine increases risk for HIV infection. Chronic abusers experience anxiety, irritability, and sometimes paranoid psychosis. Lethal effects are possible, especially when cocaine is used in combination with other drugs, such as heroin, in an injectable form known as a "speedball." Cocaine, when taken with alcohol, is metabolized by the liver to produce cocaethylene, a substance that enhances the euphoria and is associated with a greater risk of sudden death than cocaine alone. Pregnant adolescents who use cocaine place their fetus at risk of premature delivery, complications of low birthweight, and possibly developmental disorders.

TREATMENT

There are no FDA-approved medications for treatment of cocaine addiction. CBT has been shown to be effective when provided in combination with additional services and social support. Oral sustained-release dexamfetamine has been shown to be partially effective in adults with cocaine dependence.

Bibliography is available at Expert Consult.

140.7 Amphetamines
Cora Collette Breuner

Methamphetamine, commonly known as "ice," is a nervous system stimulant and schedule II drug with a high potential for abuse. Most of the methamphetamine currently abused is produced in illegal laboratories. It is a white, odorless, bitter-tasting powder that is particularly popular among adolescents and young adults because of its potency and ease of absorption. It can be ingested orally, smoked, needle-injected, or absorbed across mucous membranes. Amphetamines have multiple CNS effects, including release of neurotransmitters and an indirect catecholamine agonist effect. In recent years, there has been a general decline of methamphetamine use among high school students. In the 2012 MTF Study, 1.1% of 12th graders reported using methamphetamine at least once, reflecting a steady decline in use.

CLINICAL MANIFESTATIONS

Methamphetamine rapidly increases the release and blocks the reuptake of dopamine, a powerful "feel good" neurotransmitter (Table 140.17). The effects of amphetamines can be dose related. In small amounts, amphetamine effects resemble other stimulants: increased physical activity, rapid and/or irregular heart rate, increased blood pressure, and

decreased appetite. High doses produce slowing of cardiac conduction in the face of ventricular irritability. Hypertensive and hyperpyrexic episodes can occur as seizures (see Table 140.6). Binge effects result in the development of psychotic ideation with the potential for sudden violence. Cerebrovascular damage, psychosis, severe receding of the gums with tooth decay, and infection with HIV and hepatitides B and C can result from long-term use. A withdrawal syndrome is associated with amphetamine use, with early, intermediate, and late phases (Table 140.17). The early phase is characterized as a "crash" phase with depression, agitation, fatigue, and desire for more of the drug. Loss of physical and mental energy, limited interest in the environment, and anhedonia mark the intermediate phase. In the final phase, drug craving returns, often triggered by particular situations or objects.

TREATMENT

Acute agitation and delusional behaviors can be treated with haloperidol or droperidol. Phenothiazines are contraindicated and may cause a rapid drop in blood pressure or seizure activity. Other supportive treatment consists of a cooling blanket for hyperthermia and treatment of the hypertension and arrhythmias, which may respond to sedation with lorazepam or diazepam. For the chronic user, comprehensive CBT interventions have been demonstrated as effective treatment options.

Bibliography is available at Expert Consult.

140.8 Stimulant Abuse and Diversion
Cora Collette Breuner

In MTF 2016, 6.4% of 12th graders reported using OTC diet pills in their lifetime, and 2.1% in the past 30 days. These include nonprescription stimulants of 2 general types: pseudoamphetamines, usually sold by internet/mail order, and OTC stimulants, primarily diet and "stay-awake" pills. These drugs usually contain caffeine, ephedrine, and/or phenylpropanolamine. Stay-awake pills were used less often in 2016, with 3.6% of 12th graders reporting lifetime use and a 30-day prevalence of 1.7%. Even fewer students indicated use of look-alike products (2.3% lifetime and 0.9% monthly prevalence).

The *misuse* of a stimulant medication, defined as taking a stimulant not prescribed by a health care provider and not in accordance with health

Table 140.17	Signs and Symptoms of Intoxication and Withdrawal		
	OPIATES	**AMPHETAMINES/COCAINE**	**BENZODIAZEPINES**
INTOXICATION			
Behavior	Apathy and sedation; disinhibition; psychomotor retardation; impaired attention and judgment	Euphoria and sensation of increased energy; hypervigilance; grandiosity, aggression, argumentative; labile mood; repetitive stereotyped behaviors; hallucinations, usually with intact orientation; paranoid ideation; interference with personal functioning	Euphoria; apathy and sedation; abusiveness or aggression; labile mood; impaired attention; anterograde amnesia; impaired psychomotor performance; interference with personal functioning
Signs	Drowsiness; slurred speech; pupillary constriction (except anoxia from severe overdose—dilation); decreased level of consciousness	Dilated pupils; tachycardia (occasionally bradycardia, cardiac arrhythmias); hypertension; nausea/vomiting; sweating and chills; evidence of weight loss; dilated pupils; chest pain; convulsions	Unsteady gait; difficulty in standing; slurred speech; nystagmus; decreased level of consciousness; erythematous skin lesions or blisters
Overdose	Respiratory depression; hypothermia	Sympathomimetic symptoms	Hypotension; hyperthermia; depression of gag reflex; coma
Withdrawal	Craving to use; lacrimation; yawning; rhinorrhea/sneezing; muscle aches or cramps; abdominal cramps; nausea/vomiting/diarrhea; sweating; dilated pupils; anorexia; irritability; tremor; piloerection/chills; restlessness; disturbed sleep	Dysphoric mood (sadness/anhedonia); lethargy and fatigue; psychomotor retardation or agitation; craving; increased appetite; insomnia or hypersomnia; bizarre or unpleasant dreams	Tremor of tongue, eyelids, or outstretched hands; nausea or vomiting; tachycardia; postural hypotension; psychomotor agitation; headache; insomnia; malaise or weakness; transient visual, tactile, or auditory hallucinations or illusions; paranoid ideation; grand mal convulsions

From Haber PS, Demirkol A, Lange K, et al: Management of injecting drug users admitted to hospital, *Lancet* 374:1284–1292, 2009.

care provider guidance, has been growing over the past 2 decades, with a surge in prevalence rates of nonprescription stimulant use among both adolescents and young adults in the past 10 years. Nonprescription use of methylphenidate (**MPH**) in 2000 was 1.2%, increasing to 2% for MPH and 7.5% for nonprescription mixed amphetamine salts (**AMPs**) in 2015.

The majority of nonprescription stimulant users reported obtaining the drugs by **diversion**, a process for obtaining the drug from peers. Diversion occurs quite often and can begin in childhood, adolescence, or young adulthood. Lifetime rates of diversion ranged from 16–29% of students with stimulant prescriptions. One survey reported that 23.3% of middle and high school students taking prescribed stimulants had been solicited to divert their medication to others at a rate that increased from middle to high school. It has been shown that 54% of college students prescribed stimulants for attention-deficit/hyperactivity disorder (ADHD) had been approached to divert their medication.

In U.S. college students, nonprescription use of stimulants (Ritalin, Adderall, Dexedrine) is more prevalent among particular subgroups (male, white, members of fraternities/sororities, with lower grade point averages, more likely to use alcohol, cigarettes, marijuana, MDMA, or cocaine) and types of colleges (northeastern region, with more competitive admission standards). Lifetime prevalence of nonprescription stimulant use was 6.9% and past-month prevalence 2.1%. According to a survey of 334 ADHD-diagnosed college students taking prescription stimulants, 25% misused their own prescription medications. Scholastic pressures, including the need to succeed academically, and persistent social and financial demands place many students at an increased risk for misuse of various drugs, especially at the end of school terms. A web-based survey of medical and health profession students found that the most common reason for nonprescription stimulant use was to focus and concentrate during studying.

CLINICAL MANIFESTATIONS

Misuse of stimulants is associated with psychosis, seizures, myocardial infarction, cardiomyopathy, and even sudden death. Intentional misuse of MPH or AMPs in combination with other substances leads to adverse medical consequences. One study revealed an increase in emergency department (ED) visits involving AMP misuse from 862 in 2006 to 1,489 in 2011. Importantly, 14% of the ED visits for stimulant use were associated with cardiovascular (CV) events. Psychosis includes visual hallucinations, delusions, anorexia, flattening of affect, and insomnia mediated by dopaminergic excess. The CV effects include hypertension, arrhythmias, tachycardia, cardiomyopathy, cardiac dysrhythmias, necrotizing vasculitis, and CV accidents. Case reports include serious CV adverse drug reactions (ADRs), sudden death, and psychiatric disorders. Many patients report sleep difficulties (72%), irritability (62%), dizziness and lightheadedness (35%), headaches (33%), stomach aches (33%), and sadness (25%). Other health risks include loss of appetite, weight loss, and nervousness. Many users are involved in heavy episodic alcohol use while using MPH or AMPs. Most users of MPH or AMPs are unaware of these adverse effects and predominantly "feel good" about taking these medications.

Despite reports that MPH misuse is a healthcare issue, >82% of primary care physicians did not suspect misuse of prescribed ADHD medication in one report, and <1% thought that their patients were diverting prescribed ADHD medication. Improved monitoring for malingering and patient misuse may assist stopping diversion of these medications. ADHD diagnosis should be confirmed in those requesting ADHD medication, and they should be screened for use of other drugs.

TREATMENT

Treatment for nonprescription stimulant overdose is similar as that for amphetamine overdose. Haloperidol or droperidol is recommended for acute agitation and delusional behaviors. Phenothiazines are contraindicated and may cause a rapid drop in blood pressure or seizure activity. Hyperthermia may require use of a cooling blanket, and sedation with a benzodiazepine is recommended for treatment of the hypertension and arrhythmias. In those with chronic use, inpatient or outpatient substance abuse interventions utilizing CBT has been shown to be the

most effective treatment option.

Monitoring of the diversion and misuse of pharmaceutical stimulants must be a priority. More data need to be obtained on the prevalence, patterns, and harmful effects in adolescents and young adults.

Bibliography is available at Expert Consult.

140.9 Opiates

Cora Collette Breuner

Heroin is a highly addictive synthetic opiate drug made from a naturally occurring substance (**morphine**) in the opium poppy plant. It is a white or brown powder that can be injected (intravenously or subcutaneously), snorted/sniffed, or smoked. Intravenous (IV) injection produces an immediate effect, whereas effects from the subcutaneous route occur in minutes, and from snorting, in 30 minutes. After injection, heroin crosses the blood-brain barrier, is converted to morphine, and binds to opiate receptors. Tolerance develops to the euphoric effect, and the chronic user must take more heroin to achieve the same intense effect. Heroin use among U.S. teens peaked in the mid-1990s but is resurgent in some suburban communities, as is the use of **prescription opioids** found in the home. Nationwide, 2.9% of high school students report having tried heroin at least once. Highest use is seen in black males, with a growing prevalence in suburban high school students; ranges vary from 0.8% to 5.3% across large urban, suburban, and rural school districts. **Fentanyl** is a more potent opiate and is responsible for many opiate overdoses. *Recreational (illegal) use of prescription opiate medications by oral or injection (dissolving the pill) is a major source of opiate addiction and opiate overdoses.*

CLINICAL MANIFESTATIONS

The clinical manifestations are determined by the purity of the heroin or its adulterants, combined with the route of administration. The immediate effects include euphoria, diminution in pain, flushing of the skin, and pinpoint pupils (see Table 140.17). An effect on the hypothalamus is suggested by the lowering of body temperature. The most common dermatologic lesions are the "tracks," the hypertrophic linear scars that follow the course of large veins. Smaller, discrete peripheral scars, resembling healed insect bites, may be easily overlooked. The adolescent who injects heroin subcutaneously may have fat necrosis, lipodystrophy, and atrophy over portions of the extremities. Attempts to conceal these stigmata may include amateur tattoos in unusual sites. Skin abscesses secondary to unsterile techniques of drug administration are usually found. There is a loss of libido; the mechanism is unknown. The chronic heroin user may resort to prostitution to support the habit, thus increasing the risk of sexually transmitted diseases (including HIV), pregnancy, and other infectious diseases. Constipation results from decreased smooth muscle propulsive contractions and increased anal sphincter tone. The absence of sterile technique in injection may lead to cerebral microabscesses or endocarditis, usually caused by *Staphylococcus aureus* or *Pseudomonas aeruginosa*. Abnormal serologic reactions are also common, including false-positive Venereal Disease Research Laboratories and latex fixation tests. Infectious complications are usually not seen with oral prescription opioid use unless the pills are dissolved and injected.

WITHDRAWAL

After ≥8 hr without heroin, the addicted individual undergoes a series of physiologic disturbances over 24-36 hr, referred to collectively as "withdrawal" or the **abstinence syndrome** (see Table 140.17). The earliest sign is yawning, followed by lacrimation, mydriasis, restlessness, insomnia, "goose flesh," cramping of the voluntary musculature, bone pain, hyperactive bowel sounds and diarrhea, tachycardia, and systolic hypertension. Although the administration of methadone is the most common method of detoxification, the addition of **buprenorphine**, an opiate agonist-antagonist, is available for detoxification and maintenance treatment of heroin and other opiates. Buprenorphine has the advantage of offering less risk of addiction, overdose, and withdrawal effects, and can be dispensed in the privacy of a physician's office. Combined with behavioral interventions, it has a greater success rate of detoxification. A combination drug, buprenorphine plus naloxone, has been formulated to minimize abuse during detoxification. Clonidine and tramadol have also been used to manage opioid withdrawal.

Drugs used to treat **opioid use disorder**, a chronic relapsing problem, traditionally include methadone maintenance and buprenorphine. Abuse-deterrent opioid pill formulations (when pain control requires an opioid) include pills resistant to crushing that form a viscous gel when dissolved or pills with a sequestered opioid antagonist (naltrexone).

OVERDOSE SYNDROME

The overdose syndrome is an acute reaction after administration of an opiate. It is the leading cause of death among drug users. The clinical signs include stupor or coma, seizures, miotic pupils (unless severe anoxia has occurred), respiratory depression, cyanosis, and pulmonary edema. The differential diagnosis includes CNS trauma, diabetic coma, hepatic (and other) encephalopathy, Reye syndrome, and overdose of alcohol, barbiturates, PCP, or methadone. Diagnosis of opiate toxicity is facilitated by IV administration of naloxone, 0.01 mg/kg (2 mg is a common initial dose for an adolescent), which causes dilation of pupils constricted by the opiate. Diagnosis is confirmed by the finding of morphine in the serum.

TREATMENT

Treatment of acute heroin overdose consists of maintaining adequate oxygenation and continued administration of **naloxone**, a pure opioid antagonist. It may be given intravenously, intramuscularly, subcutaneously, as a nasal spray, or by endotracheal tube. Naloxone has an ultrarapid onset of action (1 min) and duration of action of 20-60 min. Naloxone is often available in the field, carried by first responders. Take-home naloxone may also be given to drug users, their family, or friends; such programs have been effective in treating overdoses. If there is no response, other etiologies for the respiratory depression must be explored. Naloxone may have to be continued for 24 hr if methadone, rather than shorter-acting heroin, has been taken. Admission to the intensive care unit is indicated for patients who require continuous naloxone infusions (rebound coma, respiratory depression) and for those with life-threatening arrhythmias, shock, and seizures.

Bibliography is available at Expert Consult.

140.10 Bath Salts
Cora Collette Breuner

Bath salts refers to a group of previously OTC, but now illicit, substances containing 1 or more synthetic chemicals similar to **cathinone**, an amphetamine-like stimulant found in the khat plant. The bath salts, marketed under brand names (e.g., Lunar Wave, Cloud Nine, Vanilla Sky), are sold online or in drug paraphernalia stores as a white or brown crystalline powder and can be ingested, inhaled, or injected. The most current information about teen use of bath salts is from the 2016 MTF survey of 8th, 10th, and 12th graders, who report use of 0.9%, 0.8%, and 0.8%, respectively. The synthetic cathinones found in bath salts include methylone, mephedrone, and 3,4-methylenedioxypyrovalerone (MDPV), all of which are chemically similar to amphetamines and MDMA (Ecstasy).

CLINICAL MANIFESTATIONS

The chemicals in bath salts raise brain dopamine levels, causing the user to feel a surge of euphoria, with increased sociability and sex drive. In addition, the user may experience a surge in norepinephrine, causing reactions such as an elevated heart rate, chest pain, vasoconstriction, diaphoresis, hyperthermia, dilated pupils, seizures, arrhythmias, and high blood pressure. Users also experience psychiatric symptoms such as aggressive behavior, panic attacks, paranoia, psychosis, delirium, self-mutilation, and hallucinations caused by elevated serotonin levels. Intoxication from bath salts may cause **excited delirium syndrome**, which includes dehydration, rhabdomyolysis, and kidney failure.

TREATMENT

Treatment of overdose should be directed at specific complications but often includes benzodiazepines or propofol for agitation and other neuropsychiatric manifestations. The synthetic cathinones in bath salts are highly addictive, triggering intense cravings in those who consume them frequently. This may result in dependence, tolerance, and strong withdrawal symptoms, as seen in other highly addictive substances. The sale of 2 of the synthetic cathinones, mephedrone and MDPV, is illegal in the United States.

Bibliography is available at Expert Consult.

Chapter **141**

The Breast
Cynthia M. Holland-Hall

第一百四十一章
乳房

中文导读

本章介绍了青春期女性乳房正常发育、变异和乳腺疾病，提供了青春期乳房发育成熟度的评定量表。

本章针对青春期男性乳房发育相关的疾病，产生的原因、临床特征、治疗和预后做了简单介绍，强调乳房的定期视诊检查应该成为青少年常规体格检查的组成部分。

Breast development is often the first visible sign of puberty in the adolescent female. Pediatric practitioners must be able to distinguish normal breast development, including normal variants, from pathologic breast disorders. Visual inspection of the breast tissue should routinely be a component of the young adolescent's general physical examination. Breast development during puberty is described using the **Sexual Maturity Rating (SMR)** scale, progressing from SMR 1 to SMR 5 as the breast becomes more mature (see Chapter 132, Fig. 132.2).

FEMALE DISORDERS
See Chapter 566.

MALE DISORDERS
Pubertal gynecomastia occurs in up to 65% of healthy adolescent males (see Chapter 603). Although this finding has long been attributed to a transient imbalance of estrogen and androgen concentrations, this biochemical imbalance has not been clearly demonstrated. Recent studies suggest that elevations of insulin-like growth factor (IGF)-I may have a stronger association. Onset typically is between 10 and 13 yr, peaking at SMR 3-4. Careful physical examination is essential to distinguish between **true gynecomastia**, characterized by a discrete disk of palpable glandular tissue under the nipple-areolar complex, and **pseudogynecomastia**, characterized by more diffuse, bilateral adiposity of the anterior chest wall. Physiologic gynecomastia regresses spontaneously in up to 90% of adolescents within 18-24 mo. Reassurance and continued observation are recommended in most patients; surgery may be indicated in severe or persistent cases. No medical therapies for gynecomastia have been approved for use in adolescents by the U.S. Food and Drug Administration. Small, noncontrolled trials of antiestrogens, such as tamoxifen, appear promising, but more evidence is needed. Conditions associated with nonphysiologic gynecomastia include endocrine disorders, liver disease, neoplasms, chronic disease, and trauma. Although dozens of medications are implicated as possible causes of gynecomastia, convincing evidence exists only for a few, including several antiandrogens and other exogenous hormones, antiretrovirals, and histamine$_2$ receptor blockers. Calcium channel blockers, certain antipsychotics, proton pump inhibitors, lavender, and tea tree oil may be causative. Among drugs of abuse, alcohol, opioids, and anabolic steroids may be associated with gynecomastia, but minimal evidence supports an association with marijuana or amphetamines.

Other breast pathology in males is uncommon. Benign masses such as neurofibromas, lipomas, and dermoid cysts have been reported in the male breast. Males with Klinefelter syndrome have an elevated risk of breast cancer (see Chapter 601), but this malignancy is otherwise exceedingly rare in adolescents.

Bibliography is available at Expert Consult.

Chapter **142**
Menstrual Problems
Krishna K. Upadhya and Gina S. Sucato

第一百四十二章
月经

中文导读

　　本章介绍了正常月经及各种月经紊乱（月经延迟、月经不规则、月经过多和经期疼痛等）的表现与特征；从病史、体格检查、实验室诊断等方面介绍了少女闭经、异常子宫出血、经前综合征及经前烦躁等症状的特点和临床表现，及针对性的治疗和预防措施，强调通过改善饮食和生活行为习惯进行经期调节，必要时及时就医并接受药物干预。

See also Chapter 565.

Menstrual disturbances, including delayed onset, irregularity, heavy flow, and pain, occur in 75% of females during adolescence. Menstrual problems vary in presentation. For adolescents with minor variations from normal (Table 142.1), an explanation of symptoms and reassurance may be all that is needed. Severe dysmenorrhea or prolonged menstrual bleeding can be not only frightening, but a cause of persistent morbidity requiring more aggressive management, potentially including referral to a specialist in adolescent gynecology.

NORMAL MENSTRUATION

Data from many countries, including the United States, suggest that the average age of menarche, or first menses, varies according to ethnic origin and socioeconomic status. There is often a close concordance of the age at menarche between mother and daughter, suggesting that genetic factors are determinants in addition to individual factors such as weight, exercise level, and chronic medical conditions. The age of menarche has declined in countries and populations experiencing improved nutritional standards and other living conditions. In U.S. females, the average age of menarche, 12.5 years, has been relatively stable over the last few decades; it is slightly older for non-Hispanic whites, and slightly younger for non-Hispanic blacks and Hispanic Americans.

Menarche typically occurs within 2-3 yr of the onset of breast budding (**thelarche**), which is the 1st sign of puberty in most females. Menarche usually occurs during breast **sexual maturity rating** (SMR; i.e., Tanner stage) 4. Periods gradually become more regular, initially with longer cycle lengths ranging between 21 and 45 days. The older the age at which menarche occurs, the longer it takes for consistently ovulatory cycles to be established. However, for most adolescents, by 3 yr after menarche, menstrual cycles are similar to that of adults: between 21 and 35 days long.

MENSTRUAL IRREGULARITIES

In young adolescents, many variations in menstruation are explained by **anovulation** that results from immaturity of the hypothalamic-pituitary-ovarian axis governing menstrual cyclicity. Significant deviations from normal should prompt a search for organic pathology in a logical and cost-effective manner. An accurate menstrual history is an important, but often lacking, 1st step toward a diagnosis. At menarche, all patients should be encouraged to track their periods, which several free smartphone and tablet applications can facilitate.

Previously, a range of terms has been used to describe abnormal menstrual bleeding. These include "menorrhagia" to indicate regularly occurring bleeding that was excessive in amount or duration, and "metrorrhagia" to indicate irregular bleeding between periods. Such terms are imprecise, confusing, and not linked to any specific underlying pathology. **Abnormal uterine bleeding (AUB)** is the preferred term for uterine bleeding that is abnormal in regularity, volume, frequency, or duration. AUB is further specified by adding terms that describe the bleeding as heavy *menstrual* bleeding, or *intermenstrual* bleeding. A qualifying letter is added to indicate the etiology of the abnormal bleeding. Of the 9 categories of etiologies, the 3 most relevant to adolescents are **ovulatory dysfunction** (AUB-O), previously referred to as "dysfunctional uterine bleeding" and discussed in Chapter 142.2; **coagulopathy** (AUB-C); and **not yet classified** (AUB-N).

Table 142.1	Characteristics of Normal Menses*
Cycle length	21-35 days from the 1st day of one period to the 1st day of the next (during 1st 3 yr after menarche can be 21-45 days)
Duration of menses	7 or fewer days
Blood flow	6 or fewer (soaked) pads or tampons per day

*Adolescents with 2 or more cycles outside this range or who skip their period for 3 consecutive mo warrant evaluation.

In addition to a standard medical history noting hospitalizations, chronic illness, and medication use, a complete history for evaluating a patient with menstrual irregularity should include the timing of pubertal milestones, such as onset of pubic and axillary hair and breast development; a detailed patient menstrual history; age of menarche and overall menstrual pattern of mother and sisters; and a family history of gynecologic problems. The complete review of systems should elicit any changes in headache pattern or vision; the presence of galactorrhea; and any changes in skin, hair, or bowel patterns. Changes in diet, level of exercise, and sports participation are also important factors when generating a differential diagnosis. As with all adolescent visits, the patient should be interviewed alone, and the confidential history should assess substance use, consensual sexual activity, forced sexual behavior, abuse, and other psychosocial stressors.

In addition to the basic growth parameters of weight, height, blood pressure, heart rate, and body mass index, a careful review of the patient's growth chart is indicated. Physical examination should document SMR; signs of androgen excess, such as hirsutism or severe acne; and signs suggestive of an eating disorder (see Chapter 41), such as lanugo or knuckle calluses. A careful external genital examination should be performed, but in the absence of sexual activity, an internal pelvic examination is rarely necessary. If being considered for the young adolescent, an internal exam should be performed by a physician with expertise in this age-group using proper equipment and technique. Transabdominal pelvic ultrasound can be a useful adjunct for evaluating anatomic abnormalities in the adolescent; when indicated, MRI can provide greater detail of pelvic anatomy.

Bibliography is available at Expert Consult.

142.1 Amenorrhea

Krishna K. Upadhya and Gina S. Sucato

Amenorrhea, the absence of menstruation, generally requires evaluation at age 15 yr, or if there has been no menstruation within 3 yr of the onset of puberty (**primary amenorrhea**), or if there has been no menstruation for the length of 3 previous cycles in a postmenarchal patient (**secondary amenorrhea**). However, the following caveats exist: lack of any pubertal signs by age 13 yr in a girl should prompt evaluation for pubertal delay; in sexually active patients, or those with other symptoms suggesting pathology, evaluation should be initiated without waiting for 3 missed cycles; in patients whose breast development started between age 8 and 9 yr, observation for >3 yr may be warranted in some cases, given data suggesting that the age of thelarche has decreased but the age of menarche has not. Conversely, expectant management with close follow-up can be considered in a patient whose history, physical examination (showing some signs of pubertal development), and family history suggest constitutional delay of puberty.

The differential diagnosis of amenorrhea is broad (Table 142.2) and requires a careful history and physical exam to guide any necessary diagnostic studies. Key to the evaluation is understanding the timing and tempo of the patient's pubertal milestones. The evaluation of a patient presenting with amenorrhea should begin by ascertaining whether she has ever had any prior menstrual bleeding. Some aspects of the evaluation of both primary and secondary amenorrhea are identical; conditions that can interrupt the menstrual cycle can also prevent menarche. In females with primary amenorrhea, however, genetic and anatomic conditions must also be considered (Table 142.3).

HISTORY AND PHYSICAL EXAMINATION

Important elements of the history include dietary intake, exercise level, and a thorough review of any ongoing symptoms, including fever, headache, vision changes, chronic respiratory or gastrointestinal (GI) complaints, changes in bowel history, galactorrhea, changes in hair or nails, excessive body hair, severe acne, unexplained musculoskeletal complaints, and changes in vaginal discharge (which can disappear in females who are hypoestrogenic for reasons such as poor caloric intake).

Any underlying medical conditions and the adequacy of their control should be noted, as well as the presence of any renal or skeletal anomalies, some of which may be associated with reproductive system anomalies. Medications, particularly those for psychiatric conditions, should be documented. Family history of menarcheal age, eating disorders (see Chapter 41), and **polycystic ovary syndrome (PCOS**; see Chapter 567) should be elicited. A thorough social history is necessary, especially concerning the presence or absence of sexual activity or abuse (see Chapter 16.1).

Physical examination should begin with careful attention to growth chart trajectories. In addition to a search for undiagnosed systemic disease, clues to an eating disorder, thyroid disease, or hyperandrogenism should be sought. The exam should assess for body mass index, orthostatic pulses, blood pressure, abnormal dentition, anosmia or hyposmia (suggestive of Kallmann syndrome; see Chapter 601.2), parotid enlargement, thyroid gland palpation, hepatosplenomegaly or other abdominal mass, lymphadenopathy, presence or absence of breast tissue (by palpation, not inspection), and SMR (see Chapter 132). Skin examination should note any lanugo, dry or doughy skin, loss of hair from scalp or eyebrows, striae, acanthosis nigricans, or acne. The genital exam should note SMR and appearance of the vagina, which should be pink and moist; thin, dry, reddened mucosa suggests estrogen deficiency. The clitoral width should be <1 cm. In the patient with primary amenorrhea, vaginal patency can be assessed painlessly using a slender saline-moistened swab and careful avoidance of the hymen. If physical assessment of the cervix and uterus is not tolerated, a pelvic ultrasound is advisable in patients with primary amenorrhea, followed by MRI if more detail is needed.

LABORATORY STUDIES

A urine pregnancy test, serum levels of prolactin, thyroid-stimulating hormone, and follicle-stimulating hormone (FSH) are reasonable to measure in all patients presenting with amenorrhea (Fig. 142.1). Elevation of FSH (>30 mIU/mL) in an amenorrheic female suggests ovarian insufficiency, and if confirmed with repeat testing, should be followed with a pelvic ultrasound, karyotype, and specialist referral. Diagnostic tests in the patient presenting with amenorrhea should be tailored to her history and physical exam (Table 142.4).

In patients with signs of androgen excess (e.g., severe acne or hirsutism) or other physical stigmata associated with PCOS (rapid pubertal weight gain, acanthosis nigricans) consider measuring levels of 17-hydroxyprogesterone (17-OHP) (collected in the morning, approximately 8 AM), free and total testosterone, dehydroepiandrosterone sulfate (DHEAS), and androstenedione. PCOS affects up to 15% of females; diagnostic criteria for adolescents are controversial but include variations of menstrual irregularity (ranging from amenorrhea to AUB) and physical or biochemical evidence of androgen excess. The interpretation of polycystic ovarian morphology identified on ultrasound in adolescents can be challenging, and an ultrasound is not necessary for diagnosis in adolescents.

With the exceptions of pregnancy, constitutional delay, and imperforate hymen, conditions causing primary amenorrhea are associated with reduced fertility; thus their diagnosis may cause profound emotional responses in patients and families. Therefore, before ordering studies to confirm these diagnoses (e.g., karyotype, MRI of reproductive anatomy), the clinician should carefully consider the implications and

Table 142.3	Additional Causes of Primary Amenorrhea

Physiologic/constitutional delay
Anatomic abnormalities
  Müllerian agenesis
  Imperforate hymen
  Transverse vaginal septum
Genetic disorders
  46,XY disorders of sexual development (e.g., androgen insensitivity syndrome, 5α-reductase deficiency, 17α-hydroxylase deficiency)
  Mixed gonadal dysgenesis (associated with a number of different chromosome patterns)
  Turner syndrome (resulting from 45,X or a variety of mosaic or other abnormal karyotypes)
  Genetic hypogonadotropic hypogonadism (e.g., X-linked Kallmann syndrome)

Table 142.2	Causes of Amenorrhea (Primary or Secondary)

Pregnancy (regardless of history can cause primary or secondary amenorrhea)
Functional hypothalamic causes (stress, weight loss, undernutrition, high levels of exercise, energy deficit even at normal weight)
Female athlete triad (inadequate energy intake, amenorrhea, and low bone density)
Eating disorders
Premature ovarian insufficiency (autoimmune, idiopathic, galactosemia, or secondary to radiation or chemotherapy)
Hypothalamic and/or pituitary damage (e.g., irradiation, tumor, traumatic brain injury, surgery, hemochromatosis, midline central nervous system defects such as septooptic dysplasia, autoimmune pituitary hypophysitis)
Thyroid disease (hyper- or hypo-; hypothyroidism more likely to be associated with increased bleeding)
Prolactinoma
Systemic disease (e.g., inflammatory bowel disease, cyanotic congenital heart disease, sickle cell disease, cystic fibrosis, celiac disease)
Hyperandrogenism (polycystic ovary syndrome, nonclassic congenital adrenal hyperplasia, adrenal tumor or dysfunction)
Drugs and medications (e.g., illicit drugs, atypical antipsychotics, hormones)
Turner syndrome (including mosaicism)

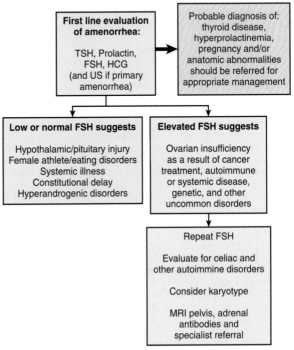

Fig. 142.1 Initial diagnostic testing to evaluate amenorrhea. *FSH,* Follicle-stimulating hormone; *HCG,* human chorionic gonadotropin; *LH,* luteinizing hormone; *MRI,* magnetic resonance imaging; *US,* ultrasound.

Table 142.4	Laboratory Tests to Evaluate Patients With Abnormal Uterine Bleeding

Total and free testosterone*
Liver, kidney, and thyroid function studies
Complete blood count with platelets
Urine pregnancy test (regardless of history)
Nucleic acid amplification test (NAAT) or other equivalent testing
    for *Chlamydia*, gonorrhea, and *Trichomonas*
Prothrombin time and partial thromboplastin time
Ferritin level
Von Willebrand factor antigen, ristocetin cofactor, and factor VIII[†]
    activities
Pelvic ultrasound (if bleeding persists despite treatment)

*In patients with signs or symptoms suggestive of polycystic ovary syndrome, such as acne, hirsutism, obesity, acanthosis nigricans, and a history of infrequent menses.

[†]Any abnormalities should be followed with a ristocetin-induced platelet aggregation and von Willebrand factor multimers. Testing in the 1st 3 days of menses and before any estrogen treatment is started minimizes the chances of false-negative tests. Repeat testing can be warranted in patients for whom there is a high pretest suspicion.

be prepared to refer to specialists with experience managing the long-term treatment of such diagnoses.

In patients presumed to have hypothalamic amenorrhea, based on prepubertal luteinizing hormone (LH) and low FSH levels using an ultrasensitive assay and consistent history and physical exam, MRI of the brain is not necessary in all patients. However, MRI should be considered for patients presenting with a headache history that is a change from baseline, persistent emesis, change in thirst, urination, or vision, elevated prolactin or galactorrhea, or other neurologic symptoms.

TREATMENT

Treatment for amenorrhea varies widely depending on the underlying cause. Many diagnoses require referral to clinicians in specialties such as endocrinology, adolescent medicine, gynecology, and other surgical subspecialists; often, collaboration with other disciplines such as psychology or nutrition is also indicated. For patients with **PCOS**, the mainstay of treatment is suppression of ovarian androgens (typically with combined hormonal contraception, i.e., estrogen and progestin) and lifestyle modifications to decrease obesity and insulin resistance. Patients with abnormal glucose tolerance may benefit from the addition of metformin. Spironolactone, an androgen receptor blocker, can also be used to reduce androgen effects, including hirsutism. Because of the high prevalence of **metabolic syndrome** in PCOS, evaluation of comorbid diabetes and hyperlipidemia with periodic lipid screening and oral glucose tolerance testing should be considered, particularly for obese patients, those with familial risk factors, and those with other signs such as acanthosis nigricans and hypertension. For patients with eating disorders or other conditions of energy imbalance that render them hypoestrogenic, normalizing weight and improving nutritional status are the keys to treatment. Initiation of hormonal therapy is not recommended routinely in these patients. However, for those who remain amenorrheic after a trial of nutritional and activity modification, short-term use of **transdermal estrogen therapy** (E2) may be considered to protect bone health. For females with amenorrhea based on ovarian insufficiency (or absence), exogenous hormones are required for all pubertal development. Experts recommend starting at age 10-12 yr with low-dose transdermal estrogen, progressing to increased doses of estrogen and cyclic progestin. Continued maintenance therapy can be accomplished with higher-dose combination products, as found in typical combined hormonal contraceptive pills, patches, and rings.

For patients with **secondary amenorrhea**, use of hormones to bring on monthly bleeding (e.g., with combined hormonal contraception) in the absence of a clear indication (e.g., PCOS, contraception) is not recommended, because this will mask the patient's subsequent menstrual

pattern. However, in patients with normal postpubertal estrogen levels, progesterone can be useful to periodically (every 4-12 wk) induce shedding of the endometrial lining to avoid buildup and subsequent heavy menses. One commonly used regimen is medroxyprogesterone, 10 mg daily for the 1st 12 days of the month.

Bibliography is available at Expert Consult.

142.2 Abnormal Uterine Bleeding

Krishna K. Upadhya and Gina S. Sucato

Abnormal uterine bleeding (AUB) is a broad term used to describe any menstrual bleeding pattern that is outside what is considered physiologic. Clinicians are encouraged to categorize the abnormal pattern based on the patient's complaint, which will usually be menses that are irregular (AUB/**IMB: intermenstrual bleeding**) or heavy (AUB/**HMB: heavy menstrual bleeding**).

IRREGULAR MENSTRUAL BLEEDING

The American Academy of Pediatrics (AAP) advocates treating menstrual status as a *vital sign* at routine visits. Although menses are frequently irregular in the early postmenarcheal years, further evaluation is necessary when menstrual patterns vary too widely from what is normal for age. Even in the 1st postmenarcheal year, menses should not be less frequent than every 45 days. Menses become increasingly regular with age, and by 3 years after menarche typically occur every 21-35 days, lasting 3-7 days. An adolescent's personal cycle duration is usually established by age 19 or 20 yr.

Adolescents rarely present with complaints of unusually short or light menses. However, short, light, or infrequent menses should be evaluated similarly to secondary amenorrhea. Females whose menses are excessive are much more likely to come to attention for AUB.

In the early postmenarcheal years, the most common cause of AUB in adolescents is anovulation caused by immaturity of the hypothalamic-pituitary-ovarian axis. In the absence of a mid-cycle surge of LH to stimulate ovulation, there is no corpus luteum production of progesterone. Without the stabilizing effects of progesterone on the endometrial lining, there is increased risk of irregular bleeding. Irregular bleeding because of anovulation, in the absence of anatomic, systemic, or endocrinologic disease, is categorized as **AUB caused by ovulatory dysfunction** (AUB-O; previously referred to as dysfunctional uterine bleeding). Although it is the most common cause of abnormal menstrual bleeding in adolescents, AUB-O is a diagnosis of exclusion. In generating a differential diagnosis, it is important to remember that most conditions that lead to amenorrhea can cause anovulation first, and anovulation is a key risk for heavy irregular bleeding. Table 142.5 lists the causes of AUB.

Unscheduled bleeding during the use of hormonal contraception frequently occurs, particularly with progestin-only methods. Common causes include medication nonadherence, interacting medications (prescribed or over-the-counter), and smoking. Patients should be reassured such bleeding is benign and not an indication to stop an otherwise satisfactory contraceptive method.

HEAVY AND PROLONGED MENSTRUAL BLEEDING

Irregular bleeding, particularly that resulting from anovulation, can be long and heavy (Table 142.5). However, in patients who have regular, cyclic menses that are long and/or heavy, particularly if menses are heavy from the onset of menarche, a hematologic cause should be strongly considered. **Von Willebrand disease** and coagulation disorders are found in up to 13% and 20%, respectively, of women with heavy menstrual bleeding; prevalence goes up significantly among women with bleeding severe enough to warrant hospitalization. Other symptoms suggestive of bleeding disorders include *flooding* (changing a pad or tampon more than hourly), passing clots larger than 1 inch in diameter, menses longer than 7 days, a history of hemorrhagic ovarian cysts, excessive bleeding from wounds or postoperatively, and first-degree relatives with heavy menses or epistaxis requiring medical treatment.

LABORATORY FINDINGS

Table 142.4 lists laboratory tests to be considered in patients with long, heavy bleeding. Females with persistent heavy bleeding despite negative testing should be referred to a hematologist for testing for platelet function disorders, factor deficiencies, and other less common disorders. In the initial evaluation, rapidity of blood loss in conjunction with the hemoglobin establishes the **severity of the bleeding: mild** (hemoglobin > 10 g/dL), **moderate** (hemoglobin 8-10 g/dL), or **severe** (hemoglobin < 8 g/dL).

TREATMENT

In **mild** bleeding, iron supplementation is recommended, and the patient should keep a menstrual calendar to follow the subsequent flow patterns. Nonsteroidal antiinflammatory drugs (NSAIDs; e.g., naproxen) are more effective than placebo in treating heavy bleeding and also would help treat any concurrent dysmenorrhea. Active bleeding typically responds well to cycling with any combined hormonal contraceptive (containing estrogen and progestin) method starting with twice-daily dosing if needed until bleeding stops. Patients with estrogen contraindications can be treated with progestins alone, such as medroxyprogesterone or norethindrone acetate, 10 mg orally (PO) per day, either continuously or for 12 days per month. The latter regimen will be followed by monthly bleeding.

With **moderate** anemia, any of the hormonal regimens above can be used. However, it may be necessary to start with 3-4 combined oral contraceptive (COC) pills (or 3-4 doses of medroxyprogesterone 10 mg) per day, with additional medication to control nausea. The dose can

usually be tapered to daily dosing over the next 2 wk. Patients with ongoing rapid bleeding, syncope or lightheadedness, or hemodynamic instability should be treated in the hospital, as should most patients with a hemoglobin of <8 g/dL.

Patients with **severe** anemia should be treated with 1 of the hormone tapers described above, in addition to fluid or blood products as indicated; it is advisable to draw necessary laboratory studies before transfusion. Patients with emesis or other significant symptoms may be treated initially with conjugated estrogens, 25 mg intravenously (IV) every 4-6 hr for 1-2 days. A COC or progestin regimen should be added within the 1st day because progestin is needed to stabilize the endometrial lining and can be used as maintenance therapy after hospital discharge. In the exceptionally rare case of a patient whose bleeding cannot be controlled hormonally, options for gynecologic interventions include intrauterine Foley balloon placement or uterine packing to tamponade the uterus mechanically. Dilation and curettage, performed frequently in adult women, is almost never indicated in adolescents and can increase blood loss in women with bleeding disorders.

Hormonal treatment for AUB should continue for at least 3-6 mo, depending on the patient's age, prior menstrual history, and severity of presentation, before reassessing the need for ongoing therapy. Additional options for maintenance therapy include combined hormonal transdermal patches and vaginal rings; depot medroxyprogesterone acetate, 150 mg intramuscularly (IM) or 104 mg subcutaneously (SC) every 3 mo; and placement of a levonorgestrel intrauterine device (IUD), depending on the patient's concurrent need for long-term contraception. For patients who choose to avoid hormonal therapy, tranexamic acid, 1,300 mg PO

Table 142.5	Causes of Irregular Menstrual Bleeding/Abnormal Uterine Bleeding (AUB)	
CAUSES OF AUB	**EXAMPLES**	**FEATURES**
Immature hypothalamic-pituitary-ovarian axis (AUB-O)	Patient within 2 yr of menarche	Painless; patient responds to hormonal treatment.
Weight changes, disordered eating, or excessive exercise	Anorexia nervosa, bulimia, weight gain or loss of more than 10 pounds from any etiology	Weight loss more frequently results in lighter, less frequent menses.
Endocrinologic causes	Thyroid disease, polycystic ovary syndrome (PCOS)	Bleeding typically increases with hypothyroidism and decreases with PCOS and hyperthyroidism.
Complication of pregnancy	Threatened abortion, postpartum or postabortal endometritis	History of sexual activity and/or pregnancy
Infection	Cervicitis, condyloma, pelvic inflammatory disease	Bleeding is usually not heavy and may occur with sexual intercourse.
Trauma	Sexual assault, straddle injuries	History will be evident in patients of menstruating age unless there is cognitive disability.
Vaginal foreign body	Toilet paper, broken condoms, tampons	Associated with odor and vaginal discharge, but usually not heavy bleeding.
Hematologic causes	Von Willebrand disease, platelet function disorder, thrombocytopenia (idiopathic thrombocytopenic purpura, drug induced), hemophilia carriage, clotting factor deficiency, leukemia	Bleeding is heavy and/or long and frequently regular, may present at menarche, and may be accompanied by a suggestive family history (hysterectomy, uterine ablation, cautery for epistaxis) or physical exam (ecchymoses, petechiae).
Medications	Estrogens, progestins, (in pills, patches, rings, injections, implants, and intrauterine devices), androgens, drugs that cause prolactin release (estrogens, phenothiazines, tricyclic antidepressants, metoclopramide), anticoagulants (heparin, warfarin, aspirin, NSAIDs), SSRIs	Affect the hypothalamic-pituitary-ovarian axis, endometrial lining, platelets, or coagulation pathway.
Anatomic	Partial obstruction of vagina or uterus causing asynchronous bleeding; cervical or endometrial polyps or myomas; hemangioma; uterine vascular malformation; genital/reproductive tract cancer	Most of these entities are extremely rare, especially reproductive tract cancers.
Systemic disease	Celiac disease, rheumatoid arthritis, Ehlers-Danlos syndrome	Accompanied by other signs of the condition.

3 times daily, can be used for up to the 1st 5 days of menses in patients who do not have an increased risk of thrombosis.

For young women with bleeding disorders, formulation of a long-term treatment plan is best done in collaboration with the patient's hematologist. Females with a known bleeding disorder may be up to 5 times more likely to develop heavy menstrual bleeding. Therefore, it can be helpful while the patient is still premenarcheal to put a proactive plan in place in the event of acute heavy menstrual bleeding, which can occur with a patient's first menstrual period.

Bibliography is available at Expert Consult.

142.3 Dysmenorrhea

Krishna K. Upadhya and Gina S. Sucato

Dysmenorrhea, painful uterine cramps that precede and accompany menses, occur in up to 90% of women age 17-24. Although dysmenorrhea is frequently severe enough to interfere with school and other activities, many adolescents undertreat their symptoms, and fewer still seek medical care for relief.

Dysmenorrhea may be primary or secondary. **Primary dysmenorrhea**, characterized by the absence of any specific pelvic pathologic condition,

Table 142.6	Differential Diagnosis of Dysmenorrhea in Adolescents*	
	PRESENTATION	**DIAGNOSIS**
Primary	Crampy pelvic pain may be accompanied by aching/heaviness in lower back and upper thighs, nausea, emesis, diarrhea, headache, mastalgia, fatigue, and dizziness; symptoms begin at or shortly before onset of menstrual flow and last 1-3 days.	Normal physical exam; internal exam only for sexually active adolescents. Ultrasound can be reserved for those patients with atypical presentations (e.g., onset at menarche) or those whose pain does not respond to NSAIDs and hormonal therapy.
Endometriosis and adenomyosis[†]	**Increasingly severe dysmenorrhea despite adequate therapy;** pain exacerbated during menses can occur acyclically as well.	Increased risk in patients with obstructive anomalies and possibly bleeding disorders; however, most teenagers with endometriosis have normal anatomy and bleeding indices; diagnosis is made visually during surgery. *Found in up to 69% of adolescents who underwent laparoscopy for persistent pelvic pain.*
Müllerian anomalies with partial outflow obstruction	**Pain begins at or shortly after menarche** and occurs with bleeding; presence of **known renal tract anomaly** (often coexists with müllerian anomaly).	Pelvic ultrasound will demonstrate uterine anomalies (e.g., rudimentary uterine horn); MRI may be required to identify some lesions (e.g., obstructed hemivagina). *Found in 8% of adolescents who underwent laparoscopy for persistent pelvic pain.*
Pelvic inflammatory disease	Abrupt onset of dysmenorrhea more severe than baseline in a sexually active adolescent; presentation can range from mild discomfort to acute abdomen.	Clinical diagnosis made by findings of uterine or adnexal tenderness on bimanual pelvic examination (see Chapter 146); supporting features include dysuria, dyspareunia, **vaginal discharge,** fever, and increased white blood cell count.
Pregnancy complication	Coincident pain and bleeding may be misdiagnosed as dysmenorrhea.	Urine test positive for human chorionic gonadotropin.

****Bold** entries indicate "red flags" for diagnosis.
[†]Adenomyosis is the presence of endometrial tissue within the uterine myometrium.

Table 142.7	Treatment for Dysmenorrhea		
	MEDICATION	**REGIMEN**	**COMMENTS**
NSAIDs for up to 5 days)	Ibuprofen, 200 mg Naproxen sodium, 275 mg Celecoxib (cyclooxygenase [COX]-2 inhibitor)*	2 tablets PO q 4-6 hr 550 mg loading dose, then 275 mg PO q 6 hr 400 mg, then 200 mg PO q 12 hr prn pain	Over-the-counter Patients may prefer the equivalent 550 mg PO q 12 hr dosing regimen. Can be used for patients with von Willebrand disease.
Hormonal contraception	Combined oral contraceptive pills or vaginal ring Progestin-only methods	Continuous hormone regimens (vs standard 21 hormone days followed by 7 placebo days) may offer better relief but may increase the risk of unscheduled intermenstrual bleeding. DMPA 150 mg IM or 104 mg SC q 3 mo; levonorgestrel intrauterine device for up to 5 yr; etonogestrel implant for up to 3 yr	The data favoring rings and pills over the combined hormone patch for this indication are sparse; treatment can be based on patient preference. DMPA has potential side effects of weight gain and interference with expected bone density increase during adolescence, as well as a higher discontinuation rate than LARC methods.
Gonadotropin-releasing hormone agonist	Depot leuprolide	11.25 mg IM q 3 mo	Consider for patients with presumed endometriosis not responsive to hormonal methods; add-back hormones are recommended to prevent bone loss.

*This medication may cause serious cardiovascular and gastrointestinal events. Use with caution in patients with impaired renal or liver dysfunction, heart failure, or a history of GI bleeding or ulcer. Full prescribing information can be found at: http://www.accessdata.fda.gov/drugsatfda_docs/label/2011/020998s033,021156s 003lbl.pdf.
  DMPA, Depot medroxyprogesterone acetate; LARC, long-acting reversible contraceptive; NSAIDs, nonsteroidal antiinflammatory drugs.

is by far the more commonly occurring form, accounting for approximately 90% of cases. After ovulation, withdrawal of progesterone results in synthesis of prostaglandins by the endometrium, which stimulates local vasoconstriction, uterine ischemia and pain, and smooth muscle contraction, explaining both uterine and GI symptoms. Because of the association with ovulation, primary dysmenorrhea typically presents at least 12 mo after menarche.

Secondary dysmenorrhea results from underlying pathology, such as anatomic abnormality, or infection, such as pelvic inflammatory disease. However, the most common cause of secondary dysmenorrhea in adolescents is **endometriosis**, a condition in which implants of endometrial tissue are found outside the uterus, usually near the fallopian tubes and ovaries. Often, other family members have endometriosis. Although characteristically there is severe pain at menses, adolescents can present with noncyclic pain as well.

Although primary dysmenorrhea is almost always the cause, a careful history and physical examination are required for adolescents who present with pelvic pain. An internal pelvic exam is not required in females who are not sexually experienced and whose presentation is consistent with primary dysmenorrhea. Constipation can vary cyclically in many females, especially those with irritable bowel syndrome, and often significantly contributes to the pain. **Mittelschmerz**, brief severe pain with ovulation, occurs at mid-cycle and can explain what initially appeared to be noncyclic pelvic pain. Table 142.6 lists the differential diagnosis and "red flags" for secondary dysmenorrhea. Ovarian cysts, a frequent concern of families, are usually transient and painless.

Treatment for primary dysmenorrhea is aimed at preventing or decreasing prostaglandin production. The mainstay of treatment is prostaglandin synthetase inhibition with NSAIDs (Table 142.7) beginning at, or preferably the day before, menstruation. High doses of around-the-clock treatment are rarely needed for more than the 1st 2 days. More data are needed to make specific treatment recommendations regarding exercise, but females should be reassured that participation in usual sports and extracurricular activities is not only permissible but a benchmark of adequate treatment.

For those adolescents whose pain does not respond to optimally dosed NSAIDs, or who also require contraception, the currently available forms of hormonal contraception will improve dysmenorrhea. A number of trials have investigated adjuvant treatments including heat, aromatherapy, acupressure, acupuncture, transcutaneous nerve stimulation, herbal remedies, yoga, and dietary supplements; however, the mainstay second-line treatment is hormones. The mechanisms are not fully delineated but are presumed to include elimination of progesterone production from the corpus luteum for those methods that prevent ovulation, and decreased prostaglandin production from the diminished endometrial lining. Up to 3 cycles may be required to appreciate the full benefit. Methods and regimens that eliminate a placebo interval may provide better relief. Females whose pain persists despite more than 3 mo of adequate hormonal therapy require further evaluation and treatment.

Bibliography is available at Expert Consult.

142.4 Premenstrual Syndrome and Premenstrual Dysphoric Disorder

Krishna K. Upadhya and Gina S. Sucato

Premenstrual dysphoric disorder (PMDD) is a depressive disorder that is distinguished from other depressive disorders by its timing. Symptoms of anxiety and depressed mood begin in the luteal phase of the menstrual cycle (i.e., in the 2nd half, after ovulation) and improve within a few days after the onset of menses. PMDD causes significant distress and functional impairment and may be accompanied by physical and behavioral symptoms. PMDD occurs in 2–6% of menstruating females worldwide. Based on a large body of scientific evidence, it has been included in the *Diagnostic and Statistical Manual of Mental Disorders, Fifth Edition* (DSM-5) as a distinct, treatment-responsive,

depressive disorder (Table 142.8). PMDD is distinguished from **premenstrual syndrome (PMS)**, which has similar timing and occurs in up to 30% of adolescents, by the severity and consequences of the affective symptoms. Premenstrual symptoms are precipitated by ovulation; symptoms recur in the luteal phase and should disappear at the end of menstruation. Up to half of women who report PMS do not meet diagnostic criteria for PMDD when symptoms are rated prospectively. Consequently, use of a menstrual calendar to document symptoms prospectively is necessary, because it is important to distinguish PMDD from anxiety, depression, or another mental health disorder, the symptoms of which are exacerbated cyclically but occur throughout the cycle.

Treatment success is gauged by improvement in patient symptoms. In mild cases of PMS, adolescents may have adequate relief following education about the relationship of symptoms to the menstrual cycle and instruction on stress management techniques, including exercise. There is not strong evidence supporting the effectiveness of most combined hormonal contraceptive methods for PMS, particularly in adolescents. However, some experts suggest this treatment option for those patients who also have dysmenorrhea or contraceptive needs.

The treatment option for severe PMS and PMDD with the most supportive evidence is use of selective serotonin reuptake inhibitors

---

Table 142.8	Criteria for Premenstrual Dysphoric Disorder

A. In the majority of menstrual cycles, at least 5 symptoms must be present in the final week before the onset of menses, start to *improve* with a few days after the onset of menses, and become *minimal* or absent in the week post menses.

B. One (or more) of the following symptoms must be present:
  1. Marked affective lability (e.g., mood swings; feeling suddenly sad or tearful, or increased sensitivity to rejection).
  2. Marked irritability or anger or increased interpersonal conflicts.
  3. Marked depressed mood, feelings of hopelessness, or self-deprecating thoughts.
  4. Marked anxiety, tension, and/or feelings of being keyed up or on edge.

C. One (or more) of the following symptoms must additionally be present, to reach a total of 5 symptoms when combined with symptoms from criterion B above.
  1. Decreased interest in usual activities (e.g., work, school, friends, and hobbies).
  2. Subjective difficulty in concentration.
  3. Lethargy, easy fatigability, or marked lack of energy.
  4. Marked change in appetite; overeating; or specific food cravings.
  5. Hypersomnia or insomnia.
  6. A sense of being overwhelmed or out of control.
  7. Physical symptoms such as breast tenderness or swelling, joint or muscle pain, a sensation of "bloating," or weight gain.
Note: The symptoms in criteria A-C must have been met for most menstrual cycles that occurred in the preceding year.

D. The symptoms are associated with clinically significant distress or interference with work, school, usual social activities, or relationships with others (e.g., avoidance of social activities; decreased productivity and efficiency at work, school, or home).

E. The disturbance is not merely an exacerbation of the symptoms of another disorder, such as major depressive disorder, panic disorder, persistent depressive disorder (dysthymia), or a personality disorder (although it may co-occur with any of these disorders).

F. Criterion A should be confirmed by prospective daily ratings during at least 2 symptomatic cycles. (*Note:* The diagnosis may be made provisionally prior to this confirmation).

G. The symptoms are not attributable to the physiological effects of a substance (e.g., a drug of abuse, a medication, other treatment) or another medical condition (e.g., hyperthyroidism).

From *Diagnostic and Statistical Manual of Mental Disorders, Fifth Edition* (Copyright 2013), American Psychiatric Association, pp 171–172.

(SSRIs), which are first-line therapy for adult women. In contrast to the treatment of depression, SSRIs can be rapidly effective for PMDD and thus can be prescribed either continuously or intermittently, beginning at ovulation (or whenever in the luteal phase symptoms begin) and ending when symptoms resolve. Adolescents can be prescribed the standard doses used for adults, such as fluoxetine, 20 mg PO daily.

Bibliography is available at Expert Consult.

Chapter **143**
Contraception
Tara C. Jatlaoui, Yokabed Ermias, and Lauren B. Zapata

第一百四十三章
避孕

中文导读

本章首先介绍了意外怀孕对青少年的心理和健康损害。其次，介绍了适合青少年采用的避孕措施，如避孕套、放置宫内避孕器、注射黄体酮、口服避孕药、结合激素避孕、皮肤药贴、植入阴道环及紧急避孕使用的一些药物。第三，针对常用的避孕药物，逐一列举并介绍了主要的禁忌证和适用范围，最后，强调青少年在采取安全性行为的前提下，进行避孕咨询，并根据自身情况选择适当的避孕措施。

The untoward consequences of sexual activity, including unintended pregnancy (see Chapter 144) and sexually transmitted infections (STIs; Chapter 146), are experienced by adolescents at unacceptably high rates. Adolescents often do not seek reproductive healthcare until 6-12 mo after initiating sex; many will become pregnant and/or acquire an STI during this interval. Early and appropriate counseling and educational interventions with adolescents, including direct discussion of unwanted pregnancy and STI prevention, can decrease risky sexual behavior; adolescents who plan sexual initiation are 75% more likely to use contraception at sexual debut. Therefore, appropriate counseling and provision of contraception as warranted are a critical component in comprehensive healthcare for adolescents.

CONTRACEPTIVE EFFECTIVENESS

To decrease rates of unintended pregnancy, the American Academy of Pediatrics (AAP) and American College of Obstetricians and Gynecologists (ACOG) recommend adolescents use the most effective forms of reversible contraception. Comparing typical effectiveness of contraceptive methods the chart illustrates a tiered system of contraceptive methods ranging from more effective to less effective methods (Fig. 143.1). These tiers are categorized by **typical-use failure rates**, which reflect the effectiveness of a method for the average person who may not consistently use the method or may not always use the method correctly (Table 143.1). For example, for oral contraceptive pills, the typical-use failure rate is 7%, whereas the *perfect-use* failure rate is <1%. **Tier 1** methods, the most effective, include those with failure rates of <1 pregnancy per 100 women in a year of typical use, and reversible Tier 1 methods include intrauterine devices (IUDs) and implants. **Tier 2** methods have failure rates of 4-7 pregnancies per 100 women in a year of typical use and include injectable contraception, oral contraceptive pills, contraceptive patch, and vaginal ring. **Tier 3** methods have failure rates of >13 pregnancies per 100 women per year of typical use and include the male and female condom, the diaphragm, withdrawal, the sponge, fertility awareness–based methods, and spermicides.

143.1 Contraceptive Use
Tara C. Jatlaoui, Yokabed Ermias, and Lauren B. Zapata

SEXUAL ACTIVITY

According to the Youth Risk Behavior Surveillance System 2015, 41.2% of U.S. high school students had ever had sexual intercourse and approximately one-third reported being currently sexually active.

Although U.S. teens and European teens have similar levels of **sexual**

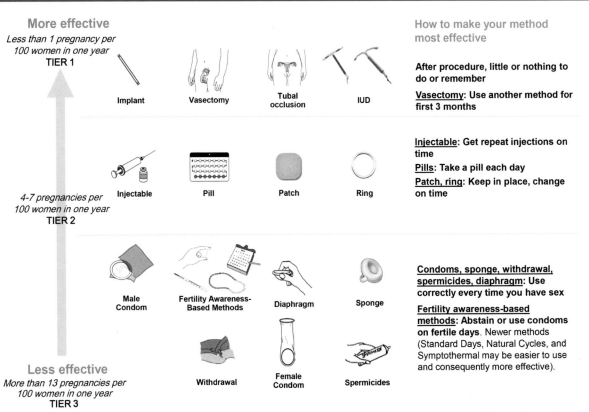

Fig. 143.1 Effectiveness of contraceptive methods. *(From Trussell J, Aiken ARA, Micks E, Guthrie K. Contraceptive efficacy, safety, and personal considerations. In Hatcher RA, Nelson AL, Trussell J, et al, eds. Contraceptive technology, ed 21, New York, 2018, Ayer Company Publishers p. 102.)*

Table 143.1	Efficacy of Contraceptives			
	FAILURE RATE*			**SOME ADVERSE EFFECTS AND DISADVANTAGES**
METHOD	**Typical Use**	**Perfect Use**	**SOME ADVANTAGES**	
Implant Nexplanon	0.1%	0.1%	Convenience; long-term contraception; no patient compliance required; rapid return of fertility after removal	Irregular bleeding; removal complications
Intrauterine devices (IUDs)			Convenience; long-term contraception; no patient compliance required; rapid return of fertility after removal	Rare uterine perforation; risk of infection with insertion; anemia
ParaGard T380A	0.8%	0.6%	Effective for 10 yr; nonhormonal	Irregular/heavy bleeding and dysmenorrhea
Mirena	0.1%	0.1%	Decreased menstrual bleeding and dysmenorrheal	Irregular bleeding in 1st 3-6 mo, followed by amenorrhea; ovarian cysts
Liletta	0.1%	0.1%	Decreased menstrual bleeding and dysmenorrheal	Irregular bleeding in 1st 3-6 mo; ovarian cysts
Kyleena	0.2%	0.2%	Smaller T-frame and narrower insertion tube	Irregular bleeding in 1st 3-6 mo; ovarian cysts; amenorrhea in 13% of users after 1 yr
Skyla	0.4%	0.3%	Smaller T-frame and narrower insertion tube	Irregular bleeding in 1st 3-6 mo; ovarian cysts; amenorrhea in only 6% of users after 1 yr
Sterilization Female	0.5%	0.5%	Long-term contraception; no patient compliance required	Potential for surgical complications; regret among young women; reversal often not possible and expensive
Male	0.15%	0.1%	Long-term contraception; no patient compliance required	Pain at surgical site, regret among young men; reversal often not possible and expensive
Injectable Depo-Provera	4%	0.2%	Convenience; same as progestin-only oral contraceptives	Delayed return to fertility, irregular bleeding and amenorrhea; weight gain; may decrease bone mineral density

Continued

Table 143.1	Efficacy of Contraceptives—cont'd			

METHOD	FAILURE RATE*		SOME ADVANTAGES	SOME ADVERSE EFFECTS AND DISADVANTAGES
	Typical Use	Perfect Use		
Combination oral contraceptives	7%	0.3%	Protection against ovarian and endometrial cancer, PID, and dysmenorrhea	Increased rate of thromboembolism, stroke, and myocardial infarction in older smokers; nausea; headache; contraindicated with breastfeeding
Progestin-only oral contraceptives	7%	0.3%	Protection against PID. iron-deficiency anemia, and dysmenorrhea; safe in breastfeeding women and those with cardiovascular risk	Irregular, unpredictable bleeding; must take at same time every day
Transdermal Evra	7%	0.3%	Convenience of once-weekly application; same benefits as combination oral contraceptives	Dysmenorrhea and breast discomfort may be more frequent than with oral contraceptives; application site reactions; detachment; increased estrogen exposure compared to oral contraceptives
Vaginal NuvaRing	7%	0.3%	Excellent cycle control; rapid return to fertility after removal; convenience of once-monthly insertion	Discomfort; vaginal discharge
Diaphragm with spermicide	17%	16%	Low cost; may reduce risk of cervical cancer	High failure rate; cervical irritation; increased risk of urinary tract infection and toxic shock syndrome; some require fitting by healthcare professional; may be difficult to obtain; available only by prescription
Condom without spermicide				
Female	21%	5%	Protection against STIs; covers external genitalia; OTC	High failure rate; difficult to insert; poor acceptability
Male	13%	2%	Protection against STIs, OTC	High failure rate; allergic reactions; poor acceptability; breakage possible
Withdrawal	20%	4%	No drugs or devices	High failure rate
Sponge	14-27%	9-20%	OTC; low cost; no fitting required; provides 24 hr of protection	High failure rate; contraindicated during menses; increased risk of toxic shock syndrome
Fertility awareness–based methods	15%	-	Low cost; no drugs or devices	High failure rate; may be difficult to learn; requires relatively long periods of abstinence
Standard Days method	12%	5%		
TwoDay method	14%	4%		
Ovulation method	23%	3%		
Symptothermal method	2%	0.4%		
Spermicide alone	21%	16%	OTC	High failure rate; local irritation; must be reapplied with repeat intercourse; increased risk of HIV transmission
No method	85%	85%	-	—

*Risk of unintended pregnancy during first year of use; data from Trussel J, et al: In Hatcher RA et al: *Contraceptive technology.* ed 21, New York, 2018, Ayer Company Publishers.
STIs, Sexually transmitted infections; PID, pelvic inflammatory disease; OTC, over the counter.
Adapted from *The Medical Letter:* Choice of contraceptives. *Med Lett* 57(1477):128, 2015.

activity and ages of **sexual debut**, U.S. teens are less likely to use contraception and less likely to use the most effective methods. Teen pregnancy rates have been declining worldwide as a result of delayed initiation of sexual activity and increased contraceptive use. Despite declines, the United States still had the highest 2013 teen birthrate in the Western industrialized world, with 26.5 live births per 1,000 females aged 15-19 yr (Fig. 143.2). This is almost 1.5 times higher than the 2013 teen birthrate in the United Kingdom, which has the highest rate in Western Europe, and almost 8 times higher than the teen birthrate in Switzerland, which has the lowest rate in Western Europe. In 2011, of the 574,000 teen pregnancies in the United States, 75% were unintended, indicating an unmet need for reliable, effective contraception that teens will correctly and consistently use.

USE OF CONTRACEPTION AMONG TEENS

According to the National Survey of Family Growth, 2011–2013, virtually all sexually experienced teens have used some method of contraception in the past. The most commonly used method by teenage females is the *condom*, followed by withdrawal (both least effective methods) and then the pill (a moderately effective method). IUDs and implants, the most effective reversible methods, are only used by 4.3% of female contraceptive users age 15-19 yr. Use of contraception at **first sex** has greatly increased over the last 50 yr. As of 2010, the condom is the most common method used at first sex, reported by >75% of males and females. Factors associated with contraception use at first sex include increasing age among teens up to age 17 yr; time spent in college; and planning their sexual debut.

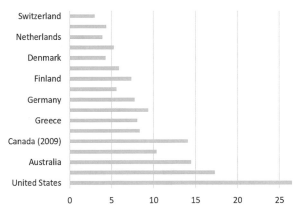

Fig. 143.2 Teen birthrates in high-income countries, 2013. Live births per 1,000 females age 15-19 yr. *(Data from United Nations Statistical Division. Demographic Yearbook 2014, New York, http://unstats.un.org/unsd/demographic/products/dyb/dyb2014.htm, and Martin JA, Hamilton BE, Osterman MJK, et al: Births: final data for 2013, Natl Vital Stat Rep 64(1):1–68, 2015.)*

More than half of sexually experienced female teens are currently using the most effective reversible contraceptives or moderately effective contraceptive methods. U.S. teens' use of hormonal methods at last intercourse is less frequent compared to teens in other developed countries: 52% of U.S. teens, 56% of Swedish 18-19 yr olds, 67% of French 15-19 yr olds, 72% of British 16-19 yr olds, and 73% of Canadian 15-19 yr olds use hormonal methods. A higher likelihood of female current contraceptive use is associated with older age at sexual initiation, aspirations for higher academic achievement, acceptance of one's own sexual activity, and a positive attitude toward contraception. Despite the importance of dual protection to protect against both unwanted pregnancy and STIs, only 21.3% of sexually active female U.S. teens are using condoms in addition to another, more effective contraceptive method.

Bibliography is available at Expert Consult.

143.2 Contraceptive Counseling

Tara C. Jatlaoui, Yokabed Ermias, and Lauren B. Zapata

The health screening interview during the adolescent preventive visit offers opportunities to identify and discuss unsafe sexual practices among all adolescents and to identify and reinforce safe sexual behaviors, including abstinence (see Chapter 137). Adolescents with medical conditions, either chronic or acute, are particularly vulnerable to having sexual and reproductive health omitted from their visits, although they have similar sexual health and contraceptive needs as healthy adolescents (see Chapter 734). Their comorbidities or concurrent medication use may make unintended pregnancy an increased health risk and may also reduce contraceptive options. The **U.S. Medical Eligibility Criteria for Contraceptive Use** outlines medical conditions associated with increased risk for adverse health events as a result of pregnancy and also provides recommendations for who can safely use specific contraceptive methods.

The goals of counseling with adolescents are to (1) understand adolescent experiences, preferences, perceptions, and misperceptions about pregnancy and use of contraceptives; (2) help adolescents put unprotected intercourse risk in a personal perspective; (3) educate adolescents about the various methods available using information that is medically accurate, balanced, and provided in a nonjudgmental manner; and (4) help adolescents choose a safe and effective method

that can either be provided on site or be easily obtained through prescription or by referral. Counseling should include a review of all contraceptive methods available that the adolescent can use safely (see U.S. Medical Eligibility Criteria), starting with the most effective methods. **Long-acting reversible contraception** (IUDs and implants) is a safe and effective option for many adolescents, including those who have not been pregnant or given birth. The adolescent should be counseled about method effectiveness using typical-use failure rates. It is important to ask about use of **withdrawal** because 60% of female teens have used it for contraception and it has a typical-use failure rate of 20%. **Abstinence** should also be discussed as an option even if teens have engaged in sexual intercourse in the past. Situational abstinence may be the best option if they do not have another method available at a particular time.

Necessary concepts to address while discussing individual methods include how effective the method is, how long the method works, what behaviors are required for correct and consistent use, what side effects may be seen, any noncontraceptive benefits of the method (e.g., reduced menstrual bleeding, protection from STIs), and what signs or symptoms of complications should prompt a return visit. Reviewing common side effects allows teens to anticipate and cope with any changes with reassurance and may avoid method discontinuation. Weighing the possibility of certain side effects with the possibility of an unintended pregnancy may also help with the conversation. It is also important to address any specific misperceptions teens may have for certain contraceptives regarding side effects, effectiveness, or any other concept discussed.

Once an adolescent chooses a method, the provider and adolescent should discuss clear plans on correct and consistent use of the chosen method and strategies for appropriate follow-up (Table 143.1). Providers should help the adolescent consider potential barriers to correct and consistent use (e.g., forgetting to take a pill daily) and develop strategies to deal with each barrier (e.g., use of reminder systems such as daily text messages or phone alarms). The provider should assess whether the teen understood the information discussed and may confirm by asking the teen to repeat back key concepts.

The U.S. Selected Practice Recommendations for Contraceptive Use provides guidance for providers regarding when to start contraception, how to be certain the woman is not pregnant at contraception initiation, and what examinations and tests are recommended before initiating contraception. Generally, women may start a contraceptive method other than an IUD at any time, and an IUD may be placed when a provider is reasonably certain that a woman is not pregnant. Most women do not require any exams or tests before initiating contraception. A pelvic examination is only required for placement of an IUD, unless otherwise indicated. STI screening is appropriate at IUD placement once sexual activity has begun, but most women do not require additional screening if they have been recently screened according to CDC sexually transmitted disease (STD) treatment guidelines. Gonorrhea and chlamydia screening using a self- or provider-collected vaginal swab or urine sample is recommended unless symptoms require a pelvic exam. IUD placement should not be delayed to receive screening results. ACOG guidelines recommend that the female teen should first visit a gynecologist between age 13 and 15 yr, unless necessary at an earlier age. This visit aims to establish rapport, educate the patient and parents or guardian on healthy sexual development, and provide routine preventive services. Cervical cancer screening is not recommended until age 21.

Providers should offer confidential services to adolescents and observe all relevant state laws and legal obligations (e.g., notification or reporting of sexual abuse). Chapter 137 discusses confidentiality and consent issues related to contraceptive management. Providers should also encourage adolescents to involve parents or guardians in their healthcare decisions, while giving parents clear information on their teen's right to confidentiality, privacy, and informed consent. All services should be provided in a youth-friendly manner, meaning that they are accessible, equitable, acceptable, appropriate, comprehensive, effective, and efficient. Resources are available that describe ways to ensure a **teen-friendly** reproductive health visit.

Bibliography is available at Expert Consult.

143.3 Long-Acting Reversible Contraception

Tara C. Jatlaoui, Yokabed Ermias, and Lauren B. Zapata

Long-acting reversible contraception (**LARC**) includes 4 **levonorgestrel (LNG)** IUDs, the **copper (Cu)** IUD, and the etonogestrel subdermal implant. LARC methods are the only Tier 1 methods that are reversible (see Fig. 143.1). Considered "forgettable" contraception, LARC does not require frequent office or pharmacy visits and does not depend on user compliance for effectiveness. In the Contraceptive CHOICE Project in St. Louis, MO, >9,000 women were given the contraceptive method of their choice at no cost and were followed for 2-3 yr. The failure rates among women who used oral contraceptive pills, transdermal patch, or vaginal ring were >20 times higher than the failure rates for women using a LARC method. Acceptance, continuation, and satisfaction in this project were also higher among adolescents using LARC compared with adolescents using non-LARC methods. *ACOG and AAP support the use of LARC methods for adolescents.* The U.S. Medical Eligibility Criteria supports safe use of both IUDs and implants for adolescents and nulliparous women. Implants are considered category 1 for all ages, and IUDs are considered category 2 for women <20 yr old and for nulliparous women (Table 143.2).

INTRAUTERINE DEVICES

IUDs are small, flexible, plastic objects introduced into the uterine cavity through the cervix. They differ in size, shape, and the presence or absence of pharmacologically active substances. In the United States, 5 IUDs are currently approved by the Food and Drug Administration (FDA): the CuT380A (Paragard) and 4 LNG IUDs (Liletta, Kyleena, Mirena, and Skyla). The effectiveness of the Cu IUD is enhanced by the copper ions released into the uterine cavity, with possible mechanisms including inhibition of sperm transport and prevention of implantation; this IUD is effective for at least 10 yr.

The LNG IUDs also have various actions, from thickening of cervical mucus and inhibiting sperm survival to suppressing the endometrium. LNG IUDs are effective for at least 3 and 5 years. All IUDs have typical-use failure rates of <1% (see Fig. 143.1).

Common misconceptions of IUDs among healthcare providers are that IUDs cause infections, infertility, and generally are not safe for teens or nulliparous women to use; these misconceptions are a barrier to teens accessing these highly effective and acceptable methods. IUDs do not increase risk of infertility and may be inserted safely in teens as well as nulliparous women (category 2; see Table 143.2).

Although early studies suggested an increased risk for upper genital tract infection, theoretically as a result of passing a foreign body through the cervix, newer work has refuted these earlier concerns. Therefore, clinicians are encouraged to consider use of IUDs in adolescents despite relatively high prevalence rates of STIs in this population. Teens should be screened for gonorrhea and chlamydia at or before IUD placement, although placement should not be delayed if results have not returned and there are no signs of current infection (e.g., purulent discharge, erythematous cervix). If STI testing is positive with an IUD in place, the patient may be treated without removing the IUD if she wants to continue the method. Evidence from 2 systematic reviews did not find

Table 143.2	Categories of Medical Eligibility Criteria for Contraceptive Use

Category 1: A condition for which there is no restriction for the use of the contraceptive method.
Category 2: A condition for which the advantages of using the method generally outweigh the theoretical or proven risks.
Category 3: A condition for which the theoretical or proven risks usually outweigh the advantages of using the method.
Category 4: A condition that represents an unacceptable health risk if the contraceptive method is used.

benefit in routinely administering misoprostol to women undergoing routine IUD placement to decrease pain or improve provider ease of insertion. A paracervical block with lidocaine may reduce patient discomfort during placement and, along with other medications (e.g., NSAIDs, anxiolytics), may be considered on an individual patient basis, but these are not routinely recommended.

IMPLANTS

Currently, one contraceptive implant is available in the United States. Originally FDA approved in 2006, the single rod that releases 60 μg/day of **etonogestrel** has been updated to a radiopaque rod with a new inserter. This **progestin-only method** keeps etonogestrel at steady serum levels for at least 3 yr and primarily works to inhibit ovulation. Similar to the levonorgestrel IUD, the progestin acts on the uterus to cause an atrophic endometrium and thicken cervical mucus to block sperm penetration; its typical-use failure rate is also <1% (see Fig. 143.1). Unlike the IUD, no pelvic exam is required for insertion. A trained provider can quickly place or remove the implant in the upper arm under local anesthesia. Common side effects include amenorrhea, irregular bleeding, or infrequent bleeding, and less often, prolonged or frequent bleeding. One potential unique complication of this method relates to localized infection and other side effects after implantation, such as bleeding, hematoma, or scarring, and if inserted too deeply into the muscle, neural damage or migration; however, these events are rare, occurring in <1% of patients. Minor side effects, such as bruising or skin irritation, are more common but most often resolve without treatment.

Bibliography is available at Expert Consult.

143.4 Other Progestin-Only Methods

Tara C. Jatlaoui, Yokabed Ermias, and Lauren B. Zapata

Several progestin-only contraceptive methods are available and include the LNG IUDs and implant (see Chapter 143.3), as well as an injectable and progestin-only pills. These methods do not contain estrogen and may be useful for teens with contraindications to estrogen (Table 143.3) and are considered generally safe for use in teens (category 1 or 2; see Table 143.2). Progestins thicken cervical mucus to block sperm entry into the uterine cavity as well as induce an atrophic endometrium leading to either amenorrhea or less menstrual blood loss; the implant and injectable additionally suppress ovulation. Teens should be provided anticipatory counseling regarding bleeding irregularities that may normally occur in the 1st 3-6 mo of hormonal contraception use.

DEPO-PROVERA

An *injectable progestin,* depot **medroxyprogesterone acetate (DMPA,** Depo-Provera) is a Tier 2 contraceptive method available as a deep intramuscular (IM) injection (150 mg), or as a subcutaneous (SC) injection (104 mg) with typical-use failure rates of 4% (see Table 143.1). Both preparations must be readministered every 3 mo (13 wk) and act to inhibit ovulation. DMPA is particularly attractive for adolescents who have difficulty with compliance, are intellectually or physically impaired, and are chronically ill or have a condition for which estrogen use is not recommended. Common concerns with DMPA include bleeding changes, bone effects, and weight gain. After 1 yr of use, 50% of DMPA users develop amenorrhea, which may be an added advantage for teens with heavy menstrual bleeding, dysmenorrhea, anemias, or blood dyscrasias, or for those with impairments that make hygiene difficult. Although studies have demonstrated bone mineral density (BMD) loss in adolescents, potentially increasing their risk for osteoporosis later in life, other studies have found that BMD is recovered after discontinuation of this method, and it is thus considered safe for use in this population. Healthcare providers may want to consider a contraceptive containing estrogen in teens who are already at high risk for low BMD, such as those receiving chronic corticosteroid therapy or those with

| Table 143.3 | Conditions Classified as Category 3 and 4 for Combined Hormonal Contraceptive Use |

CATEGORY 4

Complicated valvular heart disease
Current breast cancer
Severe decompensated cirrhosis
Deep venous thrombosis/pulmonary embolism (acute; history, not on anticoagulation or on established therapy for at least 3 mo with higher risk recurrence; major surgery with prolonged immobilization)
Complicated diabetes with nephropathy, retinopathy, neuropathy, or other vascular disease or duration of diabetes >20 yr
Migraine with aura
Hypertension (blood pressure >160/100 mm Hg) or hypertension with vascular disease
Ischemic heart disease (history of or current)
Hepatocellular adenoma
Malignant liver tumor
Peripartum cardiomyopathy (diagnosed <6 mo prior or with moderately or severely impaired cardiac function)
Postpartum <21 days
History of cerebrovascular accident
Systemic lupus erythematosus with positive antiphospholipid antibodies
Thrombogenic mutations
Viral hepatitis (acute or flare)

CATEGORY 3

Past breast cancer with no evidence of disease for 5 yr
Breastfeeding and <1 mo postpartum
Deep venous thrombosis/pulmonary embolism (history of DVT/PE with lower risk recurrence)
Gallbladder disease (current, medically treated)
History of malabsorptive bariatric surgery
History of cholestasis and past combined oral contraceptive–related
Hypertension (adequately controlled or blood pressure <160/100 mm Hg)
Peripartum cardiomyopathy with mild impairment or >6 mo
Postpartum 21-42 days with other risk factors for venous thromboembolism
Drug interactions (Ritonavir-boosted protease inhibitors; certain anticonvulsants; rifampin or rifabutin)

From Curtis KM, Tepper NK, Jatlaoui TC, et al: U.S. medical eligibility criteria for contraceptive use, 2016, *MMWR Recomm Rep* 65(RR-3):1–104, 2016.

eating disorders (see Chapter 726). Although the FDA issued a black box warning in 2004, AAP and ACOG do not recommend limiting DMPA use to 2 yr for all women and do not recommend routine BMD screening for females using DMPA. Early weight gain may be predictive of progressive gain over time; thus those teens gaining weight in the 1st 3-6 mo should consider another method.

PROGESTIN-ONLY PILLS

Progestin-only oral contraceptive pills (**POPs**) are available for the adolescent in whom the use of estrogen is potentially harmful, such those with active liver disease, replaced cardiac valves, or hypercoagulable states (see Table 143.3). POPs (**mini pills**) are quickly effective after 2 days of initiation in thickening cervical mucus, but are less reliable in inhibiting ovulation. Effects are short-lived, and pill-taking must be punctual, which may be difficult for teens. If a pill is >3 hr late from normal time, an unintended pregnancy may occur. POPs have a typical-use failure rate of 7% (see Table 143.1). Acceptance by adolescents is limited by the necessity of taking the pill at the same time daily and bleeding irregularities, including amenorrhea and breakthrough bleeding.

Bibliography is available at Expert Consult.

143.5 Combined Hormonal Contraceptives

Tara C. Jatlaoui, Yokabed Ermias, and Lauren B. Zapata

Combined hormonal contraceptives (**CHCs**) are methods that include an estrogenic substance in combination with a progestin; methods available in the United States include several formulations of combined oral contraceptives (**COCs**), a transdermal patch, and a vaginal ring. The major mechanism of action of the **estrogen-progestin** combination is to prevent the surge of luteinizing hormone and thereby inhibit ovulation. Additional effects to the reproductive tract include thickening of the cervical mucus, which prevents sperm penetration, and thinning of the endometrial lining, which may decrease menstrual blood loss. Typical-use failure rates for all CHCs are the same at 7%.

The COCs, patch, and vaginal ring are classified together as CHCs in the U.S. Medical Eligibility Criteria for Contraceptive Use, and recommendations mostly consider estrogen exposure for a given condition or characteristic (see Table 143.3). Venous thromboembolism, hepatic adenomas, myocardial infarction, and stroke are some of the more serious potential complications of exogenous estrogen use. These serious adverse events are exceedingly rare in adolescents. Even though teenage smokers who use oral contraceptives have more than twice the risk of myocardial infarction, the likelihood of its occurrence is very small, and thus clinically insignificant, compared to the risk of dying from other pregnancy-related complications.

COMBINED ORAL CONTRACEPTIVES

Oral contraceptive pills (OCs) can be either COCs or progestin-only pills and are commonly referred to as "the pill." The pill is one of the most common contraceptive methods used among women of all ages. To decrease risk of pregnancy and increase continuation, providers are encouraged to provide OCs at the time of patient presentation to start immediately rather than waiting for next menses, as long as the provider is reasonably sure that the patient is not pregnant. Providers are also encouraged to provide up to 13 pill packs at a time, based on evidence that more pill packs given is associated with higher continuation rates. Advanced provision of emergency contraceptive pills is also recommended should patients miss pills and have unprotected sex. The effectiveness of COCs depends on compliance, and unfortunately, adolescents may forget to take a pill each day. Figs. 143.3 and 143.4 list the rules for missed pills or following vomiting or diarrhea.

COCs contain 50, 35, 30, 25, or 20 μg of estrogenic substance, typically **ethinyl estradiol**, and as many as 10 progestins have been available in the United States for combined pills. Multiple preparations are available to help select the formulation that satisfies an individual patient, with minimal side effects.

COCs can be packaged as 28-day *monophasic* pills, which contain the same dose of active pills for 21 or 24 days, followed by 7 or 4 days of placebo pills, respectively. Monophasic formulations are also available for extended cycles of 91 days or 1 yr so that withdrawal bleeding does not occur each month, but at the end of each extended cycle. **Extended cycling** of monophasic COCs for adolescents has some anticipated benefits associated with increased ovarian activity suppression and may decrease failure rates. Other advantages include diminished frequency of hormonal withdrawal (premenstrual) effects, including headaches and migraines, mood changes, and heavy monthly bleeding. The most common side effect of extended-cycle OCs is intermenstrual bleeding and/or spotting, with the total days of bleeding over the 1st yr of treatment being similar for extended-cycle users and users following a 28-day cycle regimen. The unscheduled bleeding pattern diminishes over time. *Multiphasic* pill packs contain various levels of estrogen and progestin for 21 active pills and contains 7 placebo pills. Multiphasic formulations are not available for extended-cycle use. Providers can refer to the U.S. Selected Practice Recommendations for Contraceptive Use to counsel patients on how to manage late or missed COCs.

The short-term adverse effects of COCs, such as nausea and weight gain, often interfere with compliance in adolescent patients. These effects are usually transient and may be overshadowed by the beneficial effects

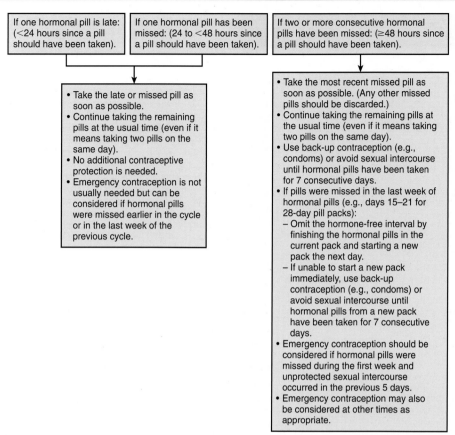

| If one hormonal pill is late: (<24 hours since a pill should have been taken). | If one hormonal pill has been missed: (24 to <48 hours since a pill should have been taken). | If two or more consecutive hormonal pills have been missed: (≥48 hours since a pill should have been taken). |

- Take the late or missed pill as soon as possible.
- Continue taking the remaining pills at the usual time (even if it means taking two pills on the same day).
- No additional contraceptive protection is needed.
- Emergency contraception is not usually needed but can be considered if hormonal pills were missed earlier in the cycle or in the last week of the previous cycle.

- Take the most recent missed pill as soon as possible. (Any other missed pills should be discarded.)
- Continue taking the remaining pills at the usual time (even if it means taking two pills on the same day).
- Use back-up contraception (e.g., condoms) or avoid sexual intercourse until hormonal pills have been taken for 7 consecutive days.
- If pills were missed in the last week of hormonal pills (e.g., days 15–21 for 28-day pill packs):
  – Omit the hormone-free interval by finishing the hormonal pills in the current pack and starting a new pack the next day.
  – If unable to start a new pack immediately, use back-up contraception (e.g., condoms) or avoid sexual intercourse until hormonal pills from a new pack have been taken for 7 consecutive days.
- Emergency contraception should be considered if hormonal pills were missed during the first week and unprotected sexual intercourse occurred in the previous 5 days.
- Emergency contraception may also be considered at other times as appropriate.

Fig. 143.3 Recommended actions after late or missed combined oral contraceptives. *(From Curtis KM, Jatlaoui TC, Tepper NK, et al. U.S. selected practice recommendations for contraceptive use, 2016, MMWR Recomm Rep 65(RR-4):1–66, 2016, Fig 2, p 28.)*

of a shortened menses and the relief of dysmenorrhea. The inhibition of ovulation or the suppressant effect of estrogens on prostaglandin production by the endometrium makes COCs effective in preventing dysmenorrhea (see Chapter 142). Acne may be worsened by some and improved by other oral contraceptive preparations (see Chapter 689). The pills with nonandrogenic progestins are particularly effective in reducing acne and hirsutism. **Drospirenone**, a progestin with antimineralocorticoid activity, has been shown to reduce premenstrual symptomatology, but the potential for hyperkalemia as a side effect eliminates patients with renal, liver, or adrenal diseases and patients taking certain medications.

As of 2011, the FDA has concluded that drospirenone-containing OCs may be associated with a higher risk of venous thromboembolism (VTE) than other progestin-containing pills. Although no studies have provided consistent estimates of the comparative risk of VTE between OCs that contain drospirenone and those that do not, or accounted for patient characteristics that may affect VTE risk, there has been a 3-fold increased risk of VTE reported for drospirenone compared with products containing levonorgestrel or other progestins. As a result, the FDA is requiring that labeling be revised for the OCs marketed under the Beyaz, Safyral, Yasmin, and Yaz brands. Despite the risk of VTE with all OCs, the absolute risk remains lower than the risk of developing VTE during pregnancy or the postpartum period.

TRANSDERMAL PATCH

The transdermal patch (Ortho Evra or Xulane) releases 20 μg ethinyl estradiol and 150 μg norelgestromin daily and is applied to the lower abdomen, buttocks, or upper body, excluding the breasts. It is worn continuously for 1 wk and changed weekly for a total of 3 wk, then no

patch is worn for the 4th week, at which time bleeding occurs (see Table 143.1). Limited studies in adolescents suggest higher rates of partial or full detachment compared to adults, with high patient satisfaction and 50–83% continuation rates from 3-18 mo of use (Fig. 143.5). As with other combined hormonal methods, the patch is a Tier 2 contraceptive. Providers can refer to the U.S. Selected Practice Recommendations to counsel patients on how to manage delayed application or detachment of the patch.

VAGINAL RING

The vaginal contraceptive ring (NuvaRing) is a flexible, transparent, colorless vaginal ring that measures about 2.1 inches in diameter and is inserted into the vagina by the patient. It releases 15 μg ethinyl estradiol and 120 μg etonogestrel per day and remains in place for 3 weeks, during which time these hormones are absorbed. If the ring is accidentally expelled or removed for intercourse, it should be reinserted; however, if it is out of place ≥48 hr, a backup method of contraception should be used (Fig. 143.6). As with other combined hormonal methods, the vaginal ring is a Tier 2 contraceptive. Providers can refer to the U.S. Selected Practice Recommendations to counsel patients on how to manage delayed insertion or reinsertion with the vaginal ring.

CONTRAINDICATIONS

Contraindications to the use of estrogen-containing methods include those conditions for which CHCs pose an unacceptable health risk (category 4) in the U.S. Medical Eligibility Criteria for Contraceptive Use (see Table 143.3): current breast cancer, severe cirrhosis, acute deep venous thrombosis/pulmonary embolism or history of DVT/PE with higher risk for recurrence, major surgery with prolonged immobilization,

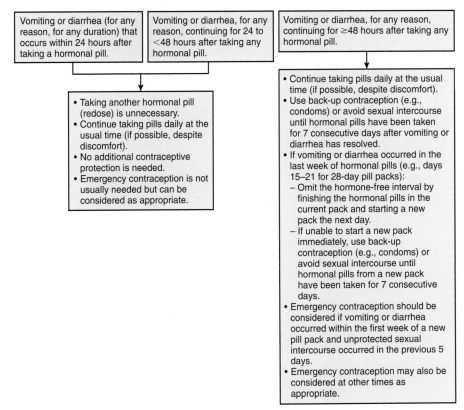

Fig. 143.4 Recommended steps after vomiting or diarrhea while using combined oral contraceptives. *(From Curtis KM, Jatlaoui TC, Tepper NK, et al. U.S. selected practice recommendations for contraceptive use, 2016, MMWR Recomm Rep 65(RR-4):1–66, 2016, Fig 5, p 30.)*

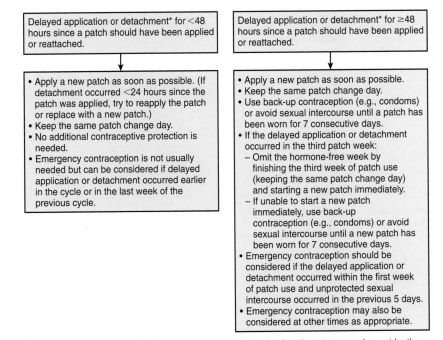

*If detachment takes place but the woman is unsure when the detachment occurred, consider the patch to have been detached for ≥48 hours since a patch should have been applied or reattached.

Fig. 143.5 Recommended actions after delayed application or detachment with combined hormonal patch. *(From Curtis KM, Jatlaoui TC, Tepper NK, et al. U.S. Selected practice recommendations for contraceptive use, 2016, MMWR Recomm Rep 65(RR-4):1–66, 2016, Fig 3, p 28.)*

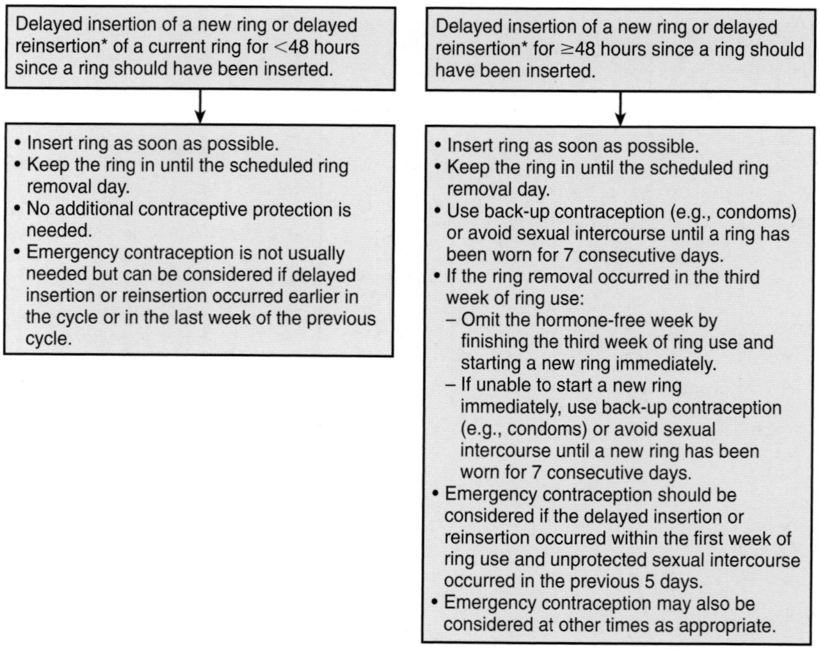

Delayed insertion of a new ring or delayed reinsertion* of a current ring for <48 hours since a ring should have been inserted.	Delayed insertion of a new ring or delayed reinsertion* for ≥48 hours since a ring should have been inserted.

• Insert ring as soon as possible.
• Keep the ring in until the scheduled ring removal day.
• No additional contraceptive protection is needed.
• Emergency contraception is not usually needed but can be considered if delayed insertion or reinsertion occurred earlier in the cycle or in the last week of the previous cycle.
	• Insert ring as soon as possible.
	• Keep the ring in until the scheduled ring removal day.
	• Use back-up contraception (e.g., condoms) or avoid sexual intercourse until a ring has been worn for 7 consecutive days.
	• If the ring removal occurred in the third week of ring use:
	  – Omit the hormone-free week by finishing the third week of ring use and starting a new ring immediately.
	  – If unable to start a new ring immediately, use back-up contraception (e.g., condoms) or avoid sexual intercourse until a new ring has been worn for 7 consecutive days.
	• Emergency contraception should be considered if the delayed insertion or reinsertion occurred within the first week of ring use and unprotected sexual intercourse occurred in the previous 5 days.
	• Emergency contraception may also be considered at other times as appropriate.

*If removal takes place but the woman is unsure of how long the ring has been removed, consider the ring to have been removed for ≥48 hours since a ring should have been inserted or reinserted.

Fig. 143.6 Recommended actions after delayed insertion or reinsertion with combined vaginal ring. *(From Curtis KM, Jatlaoui TC, Tepper NK, et al. U.S. selected practice recommendations for contraceptive use, 2016, MMWR Recomm Rep 65(RR-4):1–66, 2016, Fig 4, p 29.)*

diabetes with nephropathy, retinopathy or neuropathy, migraines with aura, stage II hypertension, vascular disease, ischemic heart disease, hepatocellular adenoma or malignant liver tumors, multiple risk factors for cardiovascular disease, peripartum cardiomyopathy, postpartum <21 days, complicated solid-organ transplantation, history of cerebrovascular accident, systemic lupus erythematosus with positive antiphospholipid antibodies, thrombogenic mutations, and complicated valvular heart disease. The initial history taken before prescribing CHCs should specifically address these risks. The U.S. Medical Eligibility Criteria provides contraceptive safety guidance with >1,800 recommendations for >120 medical conditions or characteristics.

Bibliography is available at Expert Consult.

143.6 Emergency Contraception
Tara C. Jatlaoui, Yokabed Ermias, and Lauren B. Zapata

Unprotected intercourse at mid-cycle carries a pregnancy risk of 20–30%. At other times during the cycle, the risk is 2–4%. The risk may be reduced or eliminated by interventions known collectively as emergency contraception (**EC**) up to 120 hr after unprotected intercourse or contraceptive failure. Table 143.4 lists the indications for use of EC. EC methods include the Cu IUD and emergency contraceptive pills, which include ulipristal acetate, levonorgestrel (LNG), and COCs following the Yuzpe method. Although the mechanism of action of the Cu IUD as EC is unclear, all emergency contraceptive pills work to delay ovulation and are effective only for intercourse that occurs before administration. Initiation of a regular contraceptive method is necessary to prevent pregnancy for any intercourse that occurs for the remainder of the cycle and for future cycles. If pregnancy has already occurred, emergency contraceptive pills will not cause an abortion or have teratogenic effects on the fetus.

Table 143.4	Possible Indications for Emergency Contraception

HIGH RISK SEXUAL ACTIVITY
No contraception during intercourse
Rape
Coitus interruptus
Intoxication (alcohol, drugs)

CONTRACEPTION FAILURES
Condom breaking, spillage, leaks, removal by male (purposeful)
Dislodgement, breaking of diaphragm, female condom, cervical cap
Expulsion of IUD
Spermicide failure to melt before coitus

DELAYED OR MISSED CONTRACEPTION
2 consecutive missed days of combined oral contraceptive
1 missed day of progestin only oral contraceptives
> 2-week late injection of depot medroxyprogesterone
≥ 2 day late start of vaginal ring or patch cycle

OTHER
Exposure to teratogens in absence of contraception

Teens can access EC information through a hotline at 1-888-NOT-2-LATE to obtain EC pills over the counter (OTC). AAP recommends advance provision of EC pills for teens who are or may become sexually active. A follow-up appointment is also recommended to determine the effectiveness of treatment and to diagnose a possible early pregnancy. The visit also provides an opportunity to counsel the adolescent, explore the situation leading up to the unprotected intercourse or contraceptive failure, test for STIs, offer HIV testing, and initiate continuing contraception when appropriate. Pap smear screening is not initiated until age 21.

COPPER IUD

The CuT380A (Paragard) is FDA approved for EC and has been shown to be >99% effective if used within 5 days (120 hr) after unprotected sex. The additional benefit of using the Cu IUD for EC is it also provides long-term reversible contraception.

ULIPRISTAL ACETATE

This formulation is available for EC and was FDA approved in 2010 for use up to 120 hr after unprotected sex. Ulipristal acetate is available only by prescription regardless of age. A few studies have shown it to be more effective than LNG at and beyond 72 hr. If starting regular contraception after taking ulipristal acetate, it is recommended to start or resume hormonal contraception no sooner than 5 days after taking ulipristal, to avoid a potential interaction and its decreased effectiveness. If starting a method requires an extra visit (e.g., IUDs, implant, Depo-Provera), starting the method at the time of ulipristal may be considered, weighing the risk of decreasing the effectiveness of ulipristal with the risk of not starting a contraceptive method.

LEVONORGESTREL

In 2013 the FDA approved the emergency contraceptive drug **Plan B** One-Step as an OTC option for all women of childbearing potential. Experience in adolescent women demonstrates more effective use of EC with advance provision, and it is not associated with more frequent unprotected intercourse or less condom or pill use. Nausea and vomiting are uncommon side effects, and in a recent comparison, LNG proved more effective at preventing pregnancy than the Yuzpe method.

The **Yuzpe method** has been replaced by the more effective LNG pills but may be useful for women who already have COCs at home and are in need of EC. For EC, pills consist of COCs totaling 200 μg ethinyl estradiol and 2.0 mg norgestrel or 1.0 mg levonorgestrel. This method is effective in reducing the risk of pregnancy by 75%. The most common side effects are nausea (50%) and vomiting (20%), prompting some clinicians to prescribe or recommend antiemetics along with the COCs.

Bibliography is available at Expert Consult.

143.7 Dual Protection

Tara C. Jatlaoui, Yokabed Ermias, and Lauren B. Zapata

Dual protection refers to contraceptive use that protects against STIs/HIV as well as pregnancy. Although correct and consistent condom use with every act of sexual intercourse provides dual protection, providers should encourage adolescents to use condoms for STI/HIV protection along with a more effective method for pregnancy protection.

CONDOMS

This method prevents sperm from being deposited in the vagina. No major side effects are associated with the use of a condom. The risk of HIV may have increased the use of condoms among adolescents, with 46.2% of high school students in 1991 reporting using a condom at last sexual intercourse increasing to 56.9% in 2015. The main advantages of condoms are their low price, availability without prescription, little need for advance planning, and, most important for this age-group, their effectiveness in preventing transmission of STIs, including HIV and human papillomavirus (HPV). The typical-use failure rate for male condoms is 13%. For the most effective dual protection, **male latex condoms** are recommended as protection against STIs, and should be used with an effective contraceptive method for adolescents, such as a LARC. According to the National Survey of Family Growth, only 21.3%

of females used another contraceptive method along with a condom at last sex during the past 12 mo.

A **female condom** is available OTC in single-size disposable units. It is a 2nd choice over the male latex condom because of the complexity of properly using the device, its high typical-use failure rate of 21%, and the lack of human studies demonstrating its effectiveness against STIs. Most adolescents would require intensive education and hands-on practice to use it effectively.

Bibliography is available at Expert Consult.

143.8 Other Barrier Methods

Tara C. Jatlaoui, Yokabed Ermias, and Lauren B. Zapata

DIAPHRAGM, CERVICAL CAP, AND SPONGE

These methods have few side effects but are much less likely to be used by teenagers. Typical use failure rates exceed 14%. The **cervical cap** and **sponge** have lower failure rates in nulliparous women, while the **diaphragm** has similar rates among nulliparous and parous women. Adolescents tend to object to the messiness of the jelly or the insertion of a diaphragm interrupting the spontaneity of sex (to be inserted before sex and left in for several hours afterward), or they may express discomfort about touching their genitals.

143.9 Other Contraceptive Methods

Tara C. Jatlaoui, Yokabed Ermias, and Lauren B. Zapata

SPERMICIDES

A variety of agents containing the spermicide **nonoxynol-9** are available as foams, jellies, creams, films, or effervescent vaginal suppositories. They must be placed in the vaginal cavity shortly before intercourse and reinserted before each subsequent ejaculation to be effective. Rare side effects include contact vaginitis. Some concern surrounds the vaginal and cervical mucosal damage observed with nonoxynol-9, and the overall impact on HIV transmission is unknown. The finding that nonoxynol-9 is gonococcicidal and spirocheticidal has not been substantiated in randomized clinical trials. Spermicides should be used in combination with other barrier methods because their typical-use failure rate alone is 21%.

WITHDRAWAL

The pregnancy risk for use of withdrawal as a contraceptive method is probably underestimated in adolescents, and high typical-use failure rate of 20% should be specifically addressed with young adolescents; especially since 60% of teens have used withdrawal for contraception.

FERTILITY AWARENESS–BASED METHODS

These include the Standard Days method, basal body temperature method, and Billings method and may also include combinations as well. Since fertility awareness methods are based on regular ovulatory cycles, which are less common in teens, these should be used with caution.

LACTATIONAL AMENORRHEA METHOD

The lactational amenorrhea method may be a highly effective, temporary contraceptive method if the following criteria are met: (1) no return of menses, (2) the infant is <6 mo old, and (3) exclusively breastfeeding.

Bibliography is available at Expert Consult.

Chapter **144**
Adolescent Pregnancy
Cora Collette Breuner

第一百四十四章
少女怀孕

中文导读

本章基于流行病学趋势强调少女妊娠问题的严重性，从妊娠给少女带来的生理变化、心理影响、临床表现、并发症以及社会风险等角度，探讨了少女妊娠对母亲和胎儿的双重影响；本章还分别介绍了少年母亲和少年父亲的社会人口学特征、心理、社会问题，以及导致少女怀孕相关的强奸和性侵犯等犯罪问题；最后介绍了基于循证依据的预防少女怀孕的策略和方法。

EPIDEMIOLOGY

There has been a trend of decreasing teen births and pregnancies since 1991 (Figs. 144.1 and 144.2). Teen birthrates in the United States are at a historic low secondary to increased use of contraception at first intercourse and use of dual methods of condoms and hormonal contraception among sexually active teenagers. Despite these data, the United States continues to lead other industrialized countries in having high rates of adolescent pregnancy, with >700,000 pregnancies per year. Nonetheless, the National Survey of Family Growth (NSFG) 2006–2010 revealed that less than one third of 15-19 yr old females consistently used contraceptive methods at last intercourse.

The improvement in U.S. female teen birthrates is attributed to 3 factors: more teens are delaying the onset of sexual intercourse, are using some form of contraception when they begin to have sexual intercourse, and are using long-lasting contraceptive agents such as injections, implants, and intrauterine devices (IUDs).

Most pregnancies among U.S. adolescents are **unintended** (unwanted or mistimed); 88% of births to teenagers 15-17 yr old were the result of unintended pregnancies. Birthrate statistics underestimate actual adolescent pregnancy rates because the birthrate numerator includes the number of actual births per 1000 individuals in that age-group, but the pregnancy rate includes actual births, abortions, and best estimates of fetal loss per 1,000 adolescents in that age-group.

The abortion rate among adolescents 15-19 yr old was 14.3 per 1,000 females and accounted for 16.2% of all abortions in 2008. During the decade 1999–2008, the abortion rate decreased by 20.7% among adolescents 15-19 yr old, with a 5.8% decrease noted from 2004–2008.

ETIOLOGY

In industrialized countries with policies supporting access to protection against pregnancy and sexually transmitted infections (**STIs**), older adolescents are more likely to use hormonal contraceptives and condoms, resulting in a lowered risk of unplanned pregnancy. Younger teenagers are likely to be less deliberate and logical about their sexual decisions,

and their sexual activity is likely to be sporadic or even coercive, contributing to inconsistent contraceptive use and a greater risk of unplanned pregnancy. Better personal hopes for employment and higher educational goals are associated with lowered probability of childbearing in most groups. In nonindustrialized countries, laws permitting marriage of young and mid-teens, poverty, and limited female education are associated with increased adolescent pregnancy rates.

CLINICAL MANIFESTATIONS

Adolescents may experience the traditional symptoms of pregnancy: morning sickness (vomiting, nausea that may also occur *any* time of the day), swollen tender breasts, weight gain, and amenorrhea. Often the presentation is less classic; headache, fatigue, abdominal pain, dizziness, and scanty or irregular menses are common presenting complaints.

In the pediatric office, some teens are reluctant to divulge concerns of pregnancy. Denial of sexual activity and menstrual irregularity should not preclude the diagnosis in face of other clinical or historical information. An unanticipated request for a complete checkup or a visit for contraception may uncover a suspected pregnancy. Pregnancy is still the most common diagnosis when adolescents present with secondary amenorrhea.

DIAGNOSIS

Table 144.1 provides classic symptoms, laboratory tests, and physical changes in the diagnosis of pregnancy.

On physical examination, the findings of an enlarged uterus, cervical cyanosis (**Chadwick sign**), a soft uterus (**Hegar sign**), or a soft cervix (**Goodell sign**) are highly suggestive of an intrauterine pregnancy. A confirmatory pregnancy test is always recommended, either *qualitative* or *quantitative*. Modern **qualitative** urinary detection methods are efficient at detecting pregnancy, whether performed at home or in the office. These tests are based on detection of the beta subunit of human chorionic gonadotropin (**hCG**). Although claims for nonprescription home pregnancy tests may indicate 98% detection on the day of the

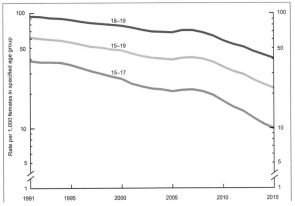

Fig. 144.1 Birthrates for females age 15-19, by age group: United States, 1991–2015. Rates are plotted on a logarithmic scale. For each age group, differences are significant (p < 0.05) from 1991–2015, 2007–2015, and 2014–2015. *(From Martin JA, Hamilton BE, Osterman MJK, et al: Births: final data for 2015,* Natl Vital Stat Rep 66(1), 2017, *Division of Vital Statistics, National Center for Health Statistics, National Vital Statistics System, Natality. Access data table at http://www.cdc .gov/nchs/data/databriefs/db259_table.pdf#1.)*

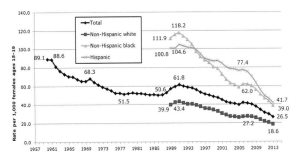

Fig. 144.2 Birthrates (per 1,000) for femals ages 15-19, by race and Hispanic origin: Selected years, 1960–2014. Differences in teen childbearing across the race and Hispanic-origin groups have narrowed from 1991 to 2015. In 1991, there was a difference of 77 births per 1,000 teenagers age 15-19 between the lowest rate (27.3 for Asian Pacific Islander [API] females) and the highest rate (104.6 for Hispanic females), compared with a difference of 28 births between the lowest rate (6.9 for API females) and the highest rate (34.9 for Hispanic females) in 2015. From 2014 to 2015, the birthrate for females age 15-19 declined 10% for API (to 6.9), 9% for non-Hispanic black (31.8), 8% for both non-Hispanic white (16.0) and Hispanic (34.9), and 6% for American Indian or Alaska Native (AIAN) (25.7) females. Since 2007, declines in teen birthrates have ranged from 41% for non-Hispanic white females to 54% for Hispanic females. Since 1991, declines have ranged from 63% for non-Hispanic white females to 75% for API females. Data for 2014 are preliminary. *(Data for 1960 from National Center for Health Statistics: Health, United States, 2001 with urban and rural health chartbook, Hyattsville, MD, 2001, Table 3; data for 1970–2011 from Martin JA et al: Births: final data for 2011, Natl Vital Stat Rep 62(1), 2013, http://www.cdc.gov/nchs/ data/nvsr/nvsr62/nvsr62_01.pdf; data for 2012 from Martin JA et al: Births: final data for 2012, Natl Vital Stat Rep 62(9), 2013, http:// cdc.gov/nchs/data/nvsr/nvsr62/nvsr62_09.pdf; data for 2013 from Martin JA et al: Births: preliminary data for 2013, Natl Vital Stat Rep 63(2), 2014, http://www.cdc.gov/nchs/data/nvsr/nvsr63/nvsr63_02.pdf.)*

1st missed menstrual period, sensitivity and accuracy vary considerably. Office or point-of-care tests have increased standardization and generally have increased sensitivity, with the possibility of detecting a pregnancy within 3-4 days after implantation. However, in any menstrual cycle, ovulation may be delayed, and in any pregnancy, the day of implantation may vary considerably, as may rate of production of hCG. This variability,

Table 144.1	Diagnosis of Pregnancy Dated from First Day of Last Menstrual Cycle

CLASSIC SYMPTOMS

Missed menses, breast tenderness, nipple sensitivity, nausea, vomiting, fatigue, abdominal and back pain, weight gain, urinary frequency.

Teens may present with unrelated symptoms that enable them to visit the doctor and maintain confidentiality.

LABORATORY DIAGNOSIS

Tests for human chorionic gonadotropin in urine or blood may be positive 7-10 days after fertilization, depending on sensitivity.
Irregular menses make ovulation/fertilization difficult to predict.
Home pregnancy tests have a high error rate.

PHYSICAL CHANGES

2-3 wk after implantation: cervical softening and cyanosis.
8 wk: uterus size of orange.
12 wk: uterus size of grapefruit and palpable suprapubically.
20 wk: uterus at umbilicus.
If physical findings are not consistent with dates, ultrasound will confirm.

along with variation of urinary concentration, may affect test sensitivity. *Consequently, each negative test should be repeated in 1-4 wk if there is a heightened suspicion of pregnancy.* The most sensitive pregnancy detection test is a serum **quantitative** βhCG radioimmunoassay, with reliable results within 7 days after fertilization. This more expensive test is used primarily during evaluations for ectopic pregnancy, to detect retained placenta after pregnancy termination, or in the management of a molar pregnancy. It is used when serial measurements are necessary in clinical management.

Although not used for primary diagnosis of pregnancy, pelvic or vaginal **ultrasound** can be helpful in detecting and dating a pregnancy. Pelvic ultrasound will detect a gestational sac at about 5-6 wk (dated from last menstrual period) and vaginal ultrasound at 4.5-5 wk. This tool may also be used to distinguish diagnostically between intrauterine and ectopic pregnancies.

PREGNANCY COUNSELING AND INITIAL MANAGEMENT

Once the diagnosis of pregnancy is made, it is important to begin addressing the psychosocial, as well as the medical, aspects of the pregnancy. The patient's response to the pregnancy should be assessed and her emotional issues addressed. It should not be assumed that the pregnancy was unintended. Discussion of the patient's options should be initiated. These options include (a) releasing the child to an adoptive family, (b) electively terminating the pregnancy, and (c) raising the child herself with the help of family, father of the baby, friends, and/or other social resources. Options should be presented in a supportive, informative, nonjudgmental fashion; for some young women, they may need to be discussed over several visits. Physicians who are uncomfortable in presenting options to their young patients should refer their patients to a provider who can provide this service expeditiously. Pregnancy terminations implemented early in the pregnancy are generally less risky and less expensive than those initiated later.

Other issues that may need discussion are how to inform and involve the patient's parents and the father of the infant; implementing strategies for insuring continuation of the young mother's education; discontinuation of tobacco, alcohol, and illicit drug use; discontinuance and avoidance of any medications that may be considered teratogenic; starting folic acid, calcium, and iron supplements; proper nutrition; and testing for STIs. Especially in younger adolescents, the possibility of **coercive sex** (see Chapter 145) must be considered and appropriate social work/ legal referrals made if abuse has occurred, although most pregnancies are not a result of coercive sex. Patients who elect to continue their pregnancy should be referred as soon as possible to an adolescent-friendly obstetric provider.

Risk factors for teen pregnancy include growing up in poverty, having parents with low levels of education, growing up in a single-parent family, fewer opportunities in their community for positive youth involvement, neighborhood physical disorder, foster care (are more than twice as likely to become pregnant than those not in foster care), and having poor performance in school (see later, Psychosocial Outcomes/ Risks for Mother and Child).

The Importance of Prevention

Teen pregnancy and childbearing bring substantial social and economic costs through immediate and long-term impacts on teen parents and their children. In 2010, teen pregnancy and childbirth accounted for at least $9.4 billion in costs to U.S. taxpayers for increased healthcare and foster care, increased incarceration rates among children of teen parents, and lost tax revenue because of lower educational attainment and income among teen mothers.

ADOLESCENT FATHERS

Those who become fathers as adolescents also have poorer educational achievement than their age-matched peers. They are more likely than other peers to have been involved with illegal activities and with the use of illegal substances. Adult men who father the children of teen mothers are poorer and educationally less advanced than their age-matched peers and tend to be 2-3 yr older than the mother; any combination of age differences may exist. Younger teen mothers are more likely to have a greater age difference between themselves and the father of their child, raising the issue of coercive sex or statutory rape (see Chapter 145).

Male partners have a significant influence on the young woman's decision/desire to become pregnant and to parent her child. Sensitively and appropriately including the male partner in discussions of family planning, contraception, and pregnancy options may be a useful strategy in improving outcomes for all. This can only be successful if the young female patient is willing to have her partner involved in such discussions.

MEDICAL COMPLICATIONS OF MOTHERS AND BABIES

Although pregnant teens are at higher-than-average risk for some complications of pregnancy, most teenagers have pregnancies that are without major medical complications, delivering healthy infants. The miscarriage/stillbirth risk for adolescents is estimated at 15-20%. In the United States, elective pregnancy termination rates peaked from 1985-1988 at 41-46%, decreasing since then to approximately 30% in 2008. Teen mothers have low rates of age-related chronic disease (diabetes or hypertension) that might affect the outcomes of a pregnancy. They also have lower rates of twin pregnancies than older women. They tolerate childbirth well with few operative interventions. However, compared with 20-39 yr old mothers, teens have higher incidences of low birthweight infants, preterm infants, neonatal deaths, passage of moderate to heavy fetal meconium during parturition, and infant deaths within 1 yr after birth. The highest rates of poor outcomes occur in the youngest and most economically disadvantaged mothers. *Gastroschisis,* although rare, has a much higher incidence in infants of teen mothers, for reasons that are unclear. Teen mothers also have higher rates of anemia, pregnancy-associated hypertension, and eclampsia, with the youngest teens having rates of pregnancy-associated hypertension higher than the rates of women in their 20s and 30s. The youngest teens also have a higher incidence of poor weight gain (<16 lb) during their pregnancy. This correlates with a decrease in the birthweights of their infants. Poor maternal weight gain also has correlated strongly with teens' late entrance into prenatal care and with inadequate utilization of prenatal care. Sexually active teens have higher rates of STIs than older sexually active women.

Globally, many young women who become pregnant have been exposed to violence or abuse in some form during their lives. There is some evidence that teenage women have the highest rates of **violence** during pregnancy of any group. Violence has been associated with injuries and death as well as preterm births, low birthweight, bleeding, substance abuse, and late entrance into prenatal care. An analysis of the Pregnancy Mortality Surveillance System indicates that in the United States 1991–1999, homicide was the 2nd leading cause of injury-related deaths in pregnant and postpartum women. Women age 19 yr and younger had the highest pregnancy-related homicide rate (see Chapter 139).

Ectopic pregnancy occurs in 1–2% of conceptions and is more common in women with a previous history of an ectopic pregnancy, pelvic inflammatory disease, prior appendicitis, infertility, in utero exposure to diethylstilbestrol, and possibly an IUD. Most ectopic pregnancies are in the fallopian tube (tubal pregnancy). Manifestations include vaginal spotting after a missed menstrual period that may progress to more intense vaginal bleeding (suggestive of spontaneous abortion); vaginal bleeding is absent in 10–20%. Abdominal pain is associated with distention of the fallopian tube; tubal rupture results in more intense pain, hemorrhagic shock, and peritonitis. Some women have nonspecific abdominal complaints and are misdiagnosed with gastroenteritis. Cervical motion and adnexal tenderness (and adnexal mass) may be present. **Transvaginal sonography** (not transabdominal) is the diagnostic test of choice to detect an ectopic pregnancy and reveals an adnexal mass and no uterine pregnancy. Nonetheless, some women will have pregnancy of unknown location by transvaginal sonography; approximately 20% of these will have an ectopic pregnancy. Measurement of sensitive quantitative serum βhCG levels together with transvaginal sonography has value in diagnosing an ectopic pregnancy. If the initial βhCG is above the *discriminatory zone* (level at which one expects an intrauterine pregnancy) but on transvaginal sonography there is no intrauterine pregnancy, there may be an ectopic pregnancy or an abnormal uterine pregnancy. In addition, if the βhCG is below the discriminatory level (usually <3000 mIU/mL) with no definitive diagnosis by sonography, serial βhCG testing should be performed every 48 hr. In a normal uterine pregnancy, βhCG levels should increase approximately 50% every 48 hr; declining levels may suggest a miscarriage or an ectopic pregnancy. Some would perform a dilation and curettage and check for products of conception or follow serial βhCG levels. If there are no products of conception or if βhCG levels plateau or increase, an ectopic pregnancy is present. Treatment of unstable or advanced patients is usually by laparoscopic surgery or by laparotomy. Because of early detection, many patients remain stable *(unruptured)*. Stable patients with an unruptured ectopic pregnancy may be treated with single-dose, or more often multidose, methotrexate to induce abortion. Contraindications to methotrexate in a stable patient include size of the ectopic mass (>3.5 cm) and embryonic cardiac motion.

Prematurity and low birthweight increase the perinatal morbidity and mortality for infants of teen mothers. These infants also have higher-than-average rates of sudden infant death syndrome (see Chapter 402), possibly because of less use of the supine sleep position or cosleeping, and are at higher risk of both intentional and unintentional injury (see Chapter 16). One study showed that risk of homicide is 9-10 times higher if a child born to a teen mother is not the mother's firstborn compared with the risk to a firstborn of a woman age 25 yr or older. The perpetrator is often the father, stepfather, or boyfriend of the mother.

After childbirth, **depressive symptoms** may occur in as many as 50% of teen mothers. Depression seems to be greater with additional social stressors and with decreased social supports. Support from the infant's father and the teen's mother seems to be especially important in preventing depression. Pediatricians who care for parenting teens should be sensitive to the possibility of depression, as well as to inflicted injury to mother or child; appropriate diagnosis, treatment, and referral to mental health or social agencies should be offered and facilitated.

PSYCHOSOCIAL OUTCOMES/RISKS FOR MOTHER AND CHILD
Educational Issues

Pregnancy and birth are significant contributors to high school dropout rates among girls. Only about 50% of teen mothers receive a high school diploma by age 22, whereas approximately 90% of women who do not give birth during adolescence graduate from high school. Mothers who have given birth as teens generally remain 2 yr behind their age-matched peers in formal educational attainment at least through their 3rd decade. Maternal lack of education limits the income of many of these young

Table 144.2	2012 American Academy of Pediatrics Clinical Guidelines: Care of Adolescent Parents and Their Children
GUIDELINE	**INTERVENTIONS**
Create a medical home for adolescent parents and their children.	Involve both adolescent mothers and coparenting father. Emphasize anticipatory guidance, parenting, and basic childcare skills, especially for teen dads.
Provide comprehensive, multidisciplinary care.	Access community resources such as special Supplemental Nutrition Program for Women, Infants, and Children. Provide medical and developmental services to low-income parents and children. Facilitate coordination of services.
Contraceptive counseling.	Emphasize condom use. Encourage long-acting contraceptive methods.
Encourage breastfeeding.	Support breastfeeding in home, work, and school settings.
Encourage high school completion.	
Assess risk of domestic violence.	
Encourage adolescent parenting.	Work with other involved adults such as grandparents to encourage developmental growth of adolescent as parent as well as optimize infant developmental outcomes.
Adapt counseling to developmental level of adolescent.	Utilize school-, home-, and office-based interventions. Consider use of support groups.
Awareness and monitoring of developmental progression of infant and adolescent parent.	Advocate for high-quality community resources for adolescents, including developmental resources, childcare, and parenting classes. Facilitate access to Head Start and education resources for individuals with disability.

Data from Pinzon JL, Jones VF; Committee on Adolescence and Committee on Early Childhood: Care of adolescent parents and their children, *Pediatrics* 130(6): e1743–e1755, 2012.

families (see Chapter 1).

The children of teenage mothers are more likely to have lower school achievement and to drop out of high school, have more health problems, and face unemployment as a young adult.

Substance Use
See also Chapter 140.

Teenagers who abuse drugs, alcohol, and tobacco have higher pregnancy rates than their peers. Most substance-abusing mothers appear to decrease or stop their substance use while pregnant. Use begins to increase again about 6 mo postpartum, complicating the parenting process and the mother's return to school.

Repeat Pregnancy
In the United States, approximately 20% of all births to adolescent mothers (age 15-19) are second order or higher. Prenatal care is begun even later with a 2nd pregnancy, and the 2nd infant is at higher risk of poor outcome than the 1st birth. Mothers at risk of early repeat pregnancy (<2 yr) include those who do not initiate long-acting contraceptives after the index birth, those who do not return to school within 6 mo of the index birth, those with mood disorders, those receiving major childcare assistance from the adolescent's mother, those who are married or living with the infant's father, those having peers who were adolescent parents, and those who are no longer involved with the baby's father and who meet a new boyfriend who wants to have a child. To reduce repeat pregnancy rates in these teens, programs must be tailored for this population, preferably offering comprehensive healthcare for both the young mother and her child (Table 144.2). Healthcare providers should remember to provide positive reinforcement for teen parenting successes (i.e., compliment teen parents when they are doing a good job).

Children Born to Teen Mothers
Many children born to teen mothers have behavioral problems that may be seen as early as the preschool period. Many drop out of school early (33%), become adolescent parents (25%), or, if male, are incarcerated (16%). Explanations for these poor outcomes include poverty, parental learning difficulties, negative parenting styles of teen parents, maternal depression, parental immaturity, poor parental modeling, social stress,

Table 144.3	Common Components of Most Successful Evidence-Based Programs to Prevent Teen Pregnancy

- Information is provided about the benefits of abstinence.
- Information is provided about contraception for those who are already sexually active.
- Information is provided about the signs and symptoms of STIs and how to prevent STIs.
- Interactive sessions on peer pressure are presented.
- Teenagers are taught communication skills.
- Programs are tailored to meet the needs of specific groups of young people (e.g., young men or young women, cultural groups, younger or older teens).

Adapted from Suellentrop K: *What works 2011–2012: curriculum-based programs that help prevent teen pregnancy*, Washington, DC, National Campaign to Prevent Teen and Unplanned Pregnancy. http://www.c-hubonline.org/sites/default/files/resources/main/What_Works_0.pdf.

exposure to surrounding violence, and conflicts with grandparents, especially grandmothers. Continued positive paternal involvement throughout the child's life may be somewhat protective against negative outcomes. Many of these poor outcomes appear to be attributable to the socioeconomic/demographic situation in which the teen pregnancy has occurred, not solely to maternal age. Even when socioeconomic status and demographics are controlled, infants of teen mothers have lower achievement scores, lower high school graduation rates, increased risk of teen births themselves, and, at least in Illinois (where records include age of birth mother), a higher probability of abuse and neglect.

Comprehensive programs focused on supporting adolescent mothers and infants utilizing life skills training, medical care, and psychosocial support demonstrate higher employment rates, higher income, and less welfare dependency in participating adolescents.

PREVENTION OF TEEN PREGNANCIES
Adolescent pregnancy is a multifaceted problem that requires multifactorial solutions. The provision of contraception and education about fertility

risk from the primary care physician is important, but insufficient to address the problem fully. Family and community involvement are essential elements for teen pregnancy prevention. Strategies for primary prevention (preventing 1st birth) are different from the strategies needed for secondary prevention (preventing 2nd or more births). Over the last 30 yr, many models of teen pregnancy prevention programs have been implemented and evaluated. Table 144.3 lists the common components of many successful evidence-based programs.

Abstinence-only sexual education aims to teach adolescents to wait until marriage to initiate sexual activity but, unfortunately, does not mention contraception. Abstinence education is sometimes coupled with "virginity pledges" in which teenagers pledge to remain abstinent until they marry. Other educational programs emphasize HIV and STI prevention and in the process prevent pregnancy, whereas others include both abstinence and contraception in their curricula. Sex education and teaching about contraception do not lead to an increase in sexual activity. Teenagers who participate in programs with **comprehensive** sex education components generally have lower rates of pregnancy than those exposed solely to abstinence-only programs or no sex education at all.

In many U.S. communities, programs that engage youth in community service and that combine sex education and youth development are also successful in deterring pregnancy. Programs vary in their sites of service from schools to social agencies, health clinics, youth organizations, and churches. Programs must be tailored to the cultural background, ethnicity, age-group, and gender of the group being targeted for the prevention services.

Secondary prevention programs are fewer in number. In the United States, some communities have tried to "pay" young mothers not to become pregnant again, but these efforts have not always been fruitful. **Home visiting** by nurses has been successful in some areas, and many communities have developed "Teen Tot" Clinics that provide a "one-stop shopping model" for healthcare for both the teen mother and the baby in the same site at the same time. Both programs have reported some successes.

In the practice setting, the identification of the sexually active adolescent through a confidential clinical interview is a first step in pregnancy prevention. The primary care physician should provide the teenager with factual information in a nonjudgmental manner and then guide the teenager in the decision-making process of choosing a contraceptive (see Chapter 143). The practice setting is an ideal setting to support the teenager who chooses to remain abstinent. When a teenager does become pregnant and requires prenatal care services, healthcare providers should remember that the pregnant teenager is an adolescent who has become pregnant, not a pregnant woman who happens to be an adolescent.

Bibliography is available at Expert Consult.

Chapter **145**

Adolescent Sexual Assault

Allison M. Jackson and Norrell Atkinson

第一百四十五章
青春期的性侵犯

中文导读

　　本章将性侵犯定义为一种暴力行为而不是性行为，通过介绍性侵犯的流行病学特点和容易受到性侵犯的高危人群，将强奸分为几种类型：熟人强奸、陌生人强奸、约会强奸、同性强奸以及毒品促成的强奸等。本章还针对性侵犯结局和健康损害，介绍了其实验室检测和评估方法，建议青少年在遭遇性侵犯后及时就医，医护人员应在保护青少年的前提下提供医疗护理，并在适当的情况下收集和记录侵犯的证据。

Sexual assault is an act of violence that may or may not involve rape. Rape, also an act of violence, is not an act of sex. Rape is historically defined as coercive sexual intercourse involving physical force or psychological manipulation of a female or a male. Recognizing that sexual intercourse is not a requirement for the definition, the U.S. Department of Justice (DOJ) defines rape as "the penetration, no matter how slight, of the vagina or anus with any body part or object, or oral penetration by a sex organ of another person, without the consent of the victim."

EPIDEMIOLOGY

Exact figures on the incidence of rape are unavailable because many rapes are not reported. It is estimated that 1 in 5 women and 1 in 71

Table 145.1	Adolescents at High Risk of Rape Victimization

MALE AND FEMALE ADOLESCENTS

Drug and alcohol users
Runaways
Those with intellectual disability or developmental delay
Street youths
Transgender youth
Youths with a parental history of sexual abuse
Sex trafficking

PRIMARILY FEMALES

Survivors of prior sexual assault
Newcomers to a town or college

PRIMARILY MALES

Those in institutionalized settings (detention centers, prison)
Young male homosexuals

Table 145.2	Types of Nonstranger Rape

ACQUAINTANCE RAPE

Most common form of rape for adolescents age 16-24 yr.
Assailant may be a neighbor, classmate, or friend of the family.
Victims are more likely to delay seeking medical care, may never report the crime (males > females), and are less likely to proceed with criminal prosecution even after reporting the incident(s).

DATE RAPE

Assailant is in an intimate relationship with the victim.
May be associated with intimate partner violence.
Assailant may engage in more sexual activities than other men his age and often has a history of aggressive behavior toward women.

SEXUAL ABUSE

All sexual contact or exposure between an adult and a minor, or when there is a significant age or developmental difference between the youth.
The assailant may be a relative, close family friend, or someone of authority.

STATUTORY RAPE

Sexual activity between an adult and an adolescent under the age of legal consent, as defined by individual state law.
Based on the premise that below a certain age or beyond a specific age difference with the assailant, an individual is not legally capable of giving consent to engage in sexual intercourse.
The intent of such laws is to protect youth from being victimized, but they may inadvertently lead a teenager to withhold pertinent sexual information from a clinician for fear that her sexual partner will be reported to the law.

MALE RAPE

Same-sex rape of males.
More prevalent in institutional settings.
Males are less likely than females to report rape and less likely to seek professional help.

GANG RAPE

See Table 145.3.

men will be raped in their lifetime. Females exceed males as reported rape victims, but male rape may be more underreported than female rape. In 2010 the DOJ National Crime Victimization Survey reported that the annual rates of **sexual victimization** per 1,000 persons were 4.1 for ages 12-17 yr and 3.7 for 18-34 yr. Between 1995 and 2013 the rate of rape and sexual assault was highest for adolescent females between ages 18 and 24 yr. The National Survey of Children's Exposure to Violence (NatSCEV 2014), revealed that 12.9% of 14-17 yr olds experienced any sexual victimization in the past year, 21.7% had experienced any sexual victimization in their lifetime; and 4.2% experienced **sexual assault** in the past year and 10.2% in their lifetime. This survey also demonstrated how other experiences with violence compound the risk for sexual victimization. Youth with a history of maltreatment by a caregiver were 4 times more likely to experience sexual victimization and >4 times more likely to experience sexual victimization if they had any witness to violence. Among older adolescents age 18-24 yr, the rate of rape and sexual assault was 1.2 times higher for those not enrolled in college than those in college. Further, several studies of youth in the juvenile justice system demonstrate a particularly high prevalence of prior sexual victimization of girls in the juvenile justice system.

Rape occurs worldwide and is especially prevalent in war and armed conflicts. The World Health Organization estimates that rape and domestic violence are responsible for 5–16% of healthy years of life lost by females of reproductive age.

Female adolescents and young adults have the highest rates of rape compared to any other age-group. The normal developmental growth tasks of adolescence may contribute to this vulnerability in the following ways: (1) the emergence of independence from parents and the establishment of relationships outside the family may expose adolescents to environments with which they are unfamiliar and situations that they are unprepared to handle; (2) dating and becoming comfortable with one's sexuality may result in activities that are unwanted, but the adolescent is too inexperienced to avoid the unwanted actions; and (3) young adolescents may be naïve and more trusting than they should be (see Chapter 132). Many teens are technologically competent, which gives sexual perpetrators access to unsuspecting vulnerable populations who were previously beyond their reach. Social media, chat rooms, and online dating sites represent a major risk for adolescents, resulting in correspondence with individuals unknown to them or protective family members, while simultaneously providing a false sense of security because of remote electronic communications. A determined perpetrator can obtain specific information to identify the adolescent and arrange for a meeting that is primed for sexual victimization.

Some adolescents are at higher risk of being victims of rape than others (Table 145.1).

TYPES OF RAPE

Rape and sexual assault can occur in a variety of circumstances (Tables 145.2 and 145.3). A victim can be sexually assaulted or raped by someone they know or a by stranger, though more often the assailant is someone known to the victim. Understanding those circumstances allows for a more trauma-sensitive approach and may impact the medical management and response to the patient. The circumstances and relationship of the assailant to the victim may impact if, when, and how a patient discloses. The gender of the victim may also affect disclosure; transgendered people and males are uniformly less likely to disclose rape/sexual assault than females. The gender of the assailant may be the same or different than the victim's, and there may be one or more than one perpetrator. In any scenario the sexual assault/rape can be facilitated by threats or coercion, physical force, or drugs.

Acquaintance rape, the most common form of rape, is committed by a person known to the victim outside of the family. If the known assailant is a family member, caregiver, or someone in a position of authority, it would be considered **sexual abuse**. The victim–assailant relationship may cause conflicting loyalties in families, and the teen's report may be received with disbelief and/or skepticism by the family. Adolescent acquaintance rape differs from adult acquaintance rape because weapons are less often used, and victims are less likely to sustain physical injuries.

Date rape is sexual violence perpetrated by a person in an intimate relationship with the victim. These victims may be new to a specific environment (college freshman, newcomer to a town or high school) and lack strong social support. Victims may have difficulty establishing boundaries or limits with their partner and in some cases may be intoxicated when the incident takes place. The assailant may interpret passivity as assent and deny the charge of coercion or force, and he may also be intoxicated at the time of the assault.

Table 145.3	Types of Stranger Rape

SEX TRAFFICKING AND COMMERCIAL SEXUAL EXPLOITATION OF CHILDREN (CSEC)
The average age of recruitment into CSEC is between 12 and 13 yr.
The assailant(s) can be the pimp (acquaintance) or the john/"date" (stranger).
Victims often have a history of child maltreatment.
Fear of the pimp results in reluctance to disclose.

DRUG-FACILITATED RAPE
Alcohol is the most common drug associated with sexual victimization.

GANG RAPE
When a group of males rapes a solitary female victim.
May be part of a ritualistic activity or rite of passage for some male groups (e.g., gang, college fraternity), or may be displaced rage on the part of the assailants.
Victims may fear retaliation or confrontation with assailants.
Victims may desire or require relocation.

Drug-facilitated rape may involve illicit and/or legal substances. The opportunity for acquaintance and date rape may be greater with individuals under the influence of alcohol. Even more predatory is the furtive administration of pharmaceuticals to potential victims. In these scenarios, date rape drugs such as γ-hydroxybutyric acid (GHB), flunitrazepam (Rohypnol), and ketamine hydrochloride are the leading agents used for these illegal purposes, but may also include alcohol, benzodiazepines, stimulants, barbiturates, opiates, and other drugs (see Chapter 140). Their pharmacologic properties make these drugs effective for this use because they have simple modes of administration, are easily concealed (colorless, odorless, tasteless), have rapid onset of action with resulting induction of anterograde amnesia, and have rapid elimination because of a short half-life. Detection of these drugs requires a high index of suspicion and medical evaluation within 8-12 hr, prompting specific testing because routine toxicology screening is insufficient.

Acquaintance and date rape victims often experience long-term issues of trust, self-blame, and guilt, resulting in lost confidence in judgment concerning future relationships. Survivors are nearly always ashamed of the incident and are less likely to report the rape. They are also typically reluctant to talk about the rape to family, friends, or a counselor and may never heal from the psychological scars that ensue. For those adolescents who are LGBTQ, the shame and reluctance to disclose the rape may be even greater.

The **commercial sexual exploitation of children (CSEC)**, also known as **sex trafficking**, is a more complex form of sexual victimization and is considered a form of child abuse (see Chapter 15). Sex trafficking is federally defined as the recruiting, harboring, transporting, providing, obtaining, patronizing, or soliciting of an individual through the means of force, fraud, or coercion for commercial sex. While a pimp often personally recruits victims, he may use others to recruit. These youth may experience physical and sexual assault by the pimp as well as the "johns." Many of these youth have a history of child maltreatment, increasing their vulnerability to this form of abuse. Fear of the consequences of disclosure and the survival skills acquired often yield a very guarded presentation in the healthcare setting.

Male rape generally refers to same-sex rape of males. Specific subgroups of young men are at high risk of being victims of rape (see Table 145.1). Male rape that occurs outside of institutional settings typically involves coercion of the male teen by someone considered an authority figure, either male or female. Male rape victims often experience conflicted sexual identity about whether they are homosexual. Issues of loss of control and powerlessness are particularly bothersome for male rape victims, and these young men usually have symptoms of anxiety, depression, sleep disturbance, and suicidal ideation.

Stranger rape occurs less frequently within the adolescent population and is similar to adult rape. There can be a variety of scenarios for stranger rape (see Table 145.3). Nevertheless, such rapes frequently occur with abduction, use of weapons, and increased risk of physical injuries. These rapes are more likely to be reported and prosecuted.

CLINICAL MANIFESTATIONS

The adolescent's acute presentation following a rape may vary considerably, from histrionics to near-mute withdrawal. Even if they do not appear afraid, most victims are extremely fearful and very anxious about the incident, the rape report, examination, and the entire process, including potential repercussions. Because adolescents are between the developmental lines of childhood and adulthood, their responses to rape may have elements of both child and adult behaviors. Many teens, particularly young adolescents, may experience some level of cognitive disorganization.

Adolescents may be reluctant to report rape for a variety of reasons, including self-blame, fear, embarrassment, or in the circumstances of drug-facilitated rape, uncertainty of event details. Adolescent victims, unlike child victims who elicit sympathy and support, often face intense scrutiny regarding their credibility and inappropriately misplaced societal blame for the assault. This view is baseless and should not be used during an evaluation of any teenage victim, including acquaintance rape.

When adolescents do not report a rape, they may present at a future date with concerns for pregnancy, symptoms of or concerns for a sexually transmitted infection (STI), and symptoms of posttraumatic stress disorder (see Chapter 38), such as sleep disturbances, nightmares, mood swings, and flashbacks. Other teens may present with psychosomatic complaints or difficulties with schoolwork; all adolescents should be screened for possible sexual victimization at most health examination visits.

INTERVIEW AND PHYSICAL EXAMINATION

The purpose of the adolescent medical evaluation following a sexual assault is to provide medical care for the teen and to collect and document evidence of the assault when applicable. Although many teens delay seeking medical care, others present to a medical facility within 72 hr (or up to 96 hr depending on the protocol used) of the rape, at which time forensic evidence collection should be offered to the patient. Experienced clinicians with training and knowledge of forensic evidence collection and medical-legal procedures should complete the rape evaluation or supervise the evaluation when possible.

The clinician's responsibilities are to provide support, obtain the history in a nonjudgmental manner, conduct a complete examination without retraumatizing the victim, and collect forensic evidence. The clinician must complete laboratory testing, administer prophylaxis treatment for STIs and emergency contraception, arrange for counseling services, and file a report to appropriate authorities in accordance with the law. It is not the clinician's responsibility to decide whether a rape has occurred; the legal system will make that determination.

Ideally, a clinician trained in forensic interviewing should obtain the history. In all cases, the history should be obtained by asking *only* open-ended questions to obtain information about (1) what happened; (2) where it happened; (3) when it happened; and (4) who did it. After obtaining a concise history, including details of the type of physical contact that occurred between the victim and the assailant, the clinician should conduct a thorough and complete physical examination and document all injuries. Clinicians should provide sensitive, nonjudgmental support during the entire evaluation, as the adolescent victim has experienced a major trauma and is susceptible to retraumatization during this process. Each component of the evaluation should be explained in detail to the victim, allowing the adolescent as much control as possible, including refusal to complete any part or all of the forensic evidence collection process. It is often useful to permit a trusted supportive person, such as a family member, friend or rape crisis advocate, to be present during the evaluation if that is the adolescent's wish.

The examining clinician should be familiar with the **forensic evidence collection** kit prior to initiating the examination. In the United States, each state's forensic evidence kit is different, but most include some or all of the following components: forensic evidence of semen deposits detected by a fluorescent lamp with a wavelength near 490 nm (many

Woods lamps are inadequate); swabs of bite mark impressions to collect genetic markers (DNA, ABO group); swabs of any penetrated orifice or body surface where saliva may be present; and documentation of acute cutaneous injuries using body diagram charts and photographs with visible standard measurements. Areas of restraint should be carefully inspected for injuries; these areas include extremities, neck, and the inner aspect of the oral mucosa, where a dentition impression may be seen.

The genital examination of a female rape victim should be undertaken with the patient in the lithotomy position. The prone knee-chest position may be used as an exam-clarifying technique, specifically to evaluate the posterior rim of the hymen. The genital exam of a male rape victim should be undertaken with the patient in supine position. The clinician's exam should include careful inspection of the entire pelvic, genital, and perianal areas. The clinician should document any acute injuries such as edema, erythema, petechiae, bruising, hemorrhage, or tearing. Aqueous solution of toluidine blue (1%), which adheres to nucleated cells, may be used during the acute examination to improve visualization of microtrauma in the perianal area. Any disruption to the superficial epidermis will allow for dye uptake and thus cannot differentiate between disruption of the skin from trauma, irritation, or infection. Additionally, a colposcope may be used to provide magnification and photo documentation of injuries.

LABORATORY DATA

When adolescents present for medical care within 72-96 hr of a sexual assault, a forensic evidence collection kit should be offered to the patient. Regardless of an adolescent's decision to have evidence collection completed, medical care, including physical examination, laboratory testing (Table 145.4), and prophylactic therapies, should be offered to the patient. Follow-up evaluations should be scheduled to repeat these laboratory studies.

Table 145.4	Laboratory Evaluation of Sexual Assault

WITHIN 8-12 HR (IF INDICATED BY HISTORY)
Urine and blood for date rape drugs (GHB, Rohypnol, ketamine)

WITHIN 24 HR (IF INDICATED BY HISTORY)
Blood for comprehensive toxicology screen (for other classes of drugs)

WITHIN 72 HR (OR UP TO 96 HR DEPENDING ON THE PROTOCOL USED)
Forensic evidence kit
Pregnancy test
Hepatitis B screen (hepatitis B surface antigen, surface antibody, and core antibody)
Syphilis (rapid plasma reagin [RPR], Venereal Disease Research Laboratories [VDRL])
HIV infection
Bacterial vaginosis (BV) and candidiasis: point-of-care testing and/or wet mount with measurement of vaginal pH and KOH application for whiff test
Trichomonas vaginalis: nucleic acid amplification tests (NAATs) by urine or vaginal specimen or point-of-care testing (DNA probes) from vaginal specimen
Chlamydia and *Neisseria gonorrhoeae*: nucleic acid amplification testing (NAATs) at sites of penetration or possible penetration:
  1. *N. gonorrhoeae*: oropharynx, rectum, urine*
  2. *Chlamydia*: urine,* rectum

*Dirty urine sample may be used as alternate for genital swab.
From Centers for Disease Control and Prevention: Sexually transmitted diseases: treatment guidelines 2015, *MMWR Recomm Rep* 64(RR-3):1–140, 2015, and Updated guidelines for antiretroviral postexposure prophylaxis after sexual, injection drug use, or other nonoccupational exposure to HIV—United States, 2016.

TREATMENT

Treatment includes **prophylactic antimicrobials** for STIs (see Chapter 146) and emergency contraception (see Chapter 143). The Centers for Disease Control and Prevention (CDC) reports that trichomoniasis, bacterial vaginosis, gonorrhea, and chlamydial infection are the most frequently diagnosed infections among women who have been sexually assaulted. Antimicrobial prophylaxis is recommended for adolescent rape victims because of the risk of acquiring an STI and the risk of pelvic inflammatory disease (Table 145.5). A two- or three-drug antiretroviral regimen for HIV **postexposure prophylaxis (PEP)** must be considered and an infectious disease specialist consulted if higher transmission risk factors are identified (e.g., knowing that the perpetrator

Table 145.5	Postexposure Prophylaxis (PEP) for Acute Sexual Assault Victims

ROUTINE
Recommended Regimen for STI Prophylaxis
Ceftriaxone 250 mg intramuscularly
plus
Azithromycin 1g orally in a single dose
plus
Metronidazole 2 g orally in a single dose *or*
Tinidazole 2 g orally in a single dose

*Pregnancy Prophylaxis**
Levonorgestrel (Plan B) 1.5 mg orally in a single dose
OR
Ulipristal acetate (Ella) 30 mg is effective for up to 120 hr.

Human Papillomavirus (HPV)
Assess HPV vaccine history; to unimmunized, administer initial vaccine at initial exam, with 2 follow-up doses at 1-2 mo and at 6 mo if >15 yr old *or* a single follow-up dose at 6-12 mo if ≤15 yr old

AS INDICATED
All persons offered PEP should be prescribed a 28-day course of a two- or three-drug antiretroviral regimen.

Human Immunodeficiency Virus (HIV)[†]
Preferred regimen:
  Tenofovir 300 mg and fixed-dose combination emtricitabine, 200 mg (Truvada) once daily
  plus
  Raltegravir 400 mg twice daily *or*
  Dolutegravir 50 mg daily[‡]
Alternative regimens available (The National Clinicians Consultation Center is a resource for providers prescribing PEP, reachable at 1-888-448-4911.)

Hepatitis B virus (HBV)
Specific indications for vaccine, immunoglobulin and/or booster dependent upon assailant's status

*Provided for patients with negative urine pregnancy screen. In addition, antiemetic (Compazine, Zofran) can be prescribed for patients receiving emergency contraception.
[†]HIV PEP is provided for patients with penetration and when the assailant is known to be HIV-positive or at high risk because of a history of incarceration, intravenous drug use, or multiple sexual partners. If provided, laboratory studies must be drawn before administration of medication (HIV, CBC, LFTs, BUN/Cr, amylase, lipase), and follow-up must be arranged.
[‡]Dolutegravir has been associated with neural tube defects if the exposure occurs within the first trimester of pregnancy. Therefore it should be avoided in pregnant patients or those at risk for becoming pregnant. U.S. Department of Health and Human Services, U.S. Food & Drug Administration. Julica, Tivicay, Triumeq (dolutegravir): FDA to evaluate potential risk of neural tube birth defects. May 18, 2018. https://www.fda.gov/safety/medwatch/safetyinformation/safetyalertsforhumanmedicalproducts/ucm608168.htm.
Data from Centers for Disease Control and Prevention: Sexually transmitted diseases: treatment guidelines 2015, *MMWR Recomm Rep* 64(RR-3):1–140, 2015, and Updated guidelines for antiretroviral postexposure prophylaxis after sexual, injection drug use, or other nonoccupational exposure to HIV—United States, 2016.

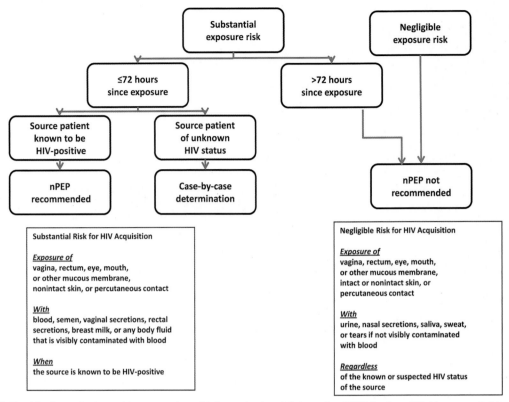

Fig. 145.1 Algorithm for evaluation and treatment of possible human immunodeficiency virus (HIV) infection. nPEP, Nonoccupational postexposure prophylaxis. *(From Seña AC, Hsu KK, Kellogg N, et al: Sexual assault and sexually transmitted infections in adults, adolescents, and children,* Clin Infect Dis *61(Suppl 8):S859, 2015.)*

is HIV-positive, significant mucosal injury of the victim) to prescribe a triple-antiretroviral regimen (Fig. 145.1). Similar considerations should be made for possible exposure to the hepatitis B virus in vaccinated/unvaccinated individuals. Clinicians should review the importance for patient's compliance with medical and psychological treatment and follow-up care.

At the time of presentation, the clinician should address the need for follow-up care, including psychological counseling. Adolescent victims are at increased risk of posttraumatic stress disorder, depression, self-abusive behaviors, suicidal ideation, delinquency, substance abuse, eating disorders, and sexual revictimization. It is important for the adolescent victim and parents to understand the value of timely counseling services to decrease these potential long-term sequelae. Counseling services should be arranged during the initial evaluation, with follow-up arranged with the primary care physician to improve compliance. Counseling services for family members of the victim may improve their ability to provide appropriate support to the adolescent victim. Caution parents not to use the assault as a validation of their parental guidance, as it will only serve to place blame inappropriately on the adolescent victim.

PREVENTION
Primary prevention may be accomplished through education of preadolescents and adolescents on the issues of rape, healthy relationships, internet dangers, and drug- and alcohol-facilitated rape. Prevention messages should be targeted to both males and females at high schools and colleges. Particular emphasis on prevention efforts during college orientation is highly recommended. High-risk situations that may increase the likelihood of a sexual assault (use of drugs or alcohol) should be discouraged. **Secondary prevention** includes informing adolescents of the benefits of timely medical evaluations when rape has occurred. Individual clinicians should ask adolescents about past experiences of forced and unwanted sexual behaviors and offer help in dealing with those experiences. The importance of prevention cannot be overstated because adolescents are disproportionately affected by rape, and they are particularly vulnerable to long-term consequences.

Bibliography is available at Expert Consult.

Chapter **146**
Sexually Transmitted Infections

Gale R. Burstein

第一百四十六章
性传播性疾病

中文导读

　　本章介绍了在有性经历的青少年中罹患性传播性疾病的流行现状和高危人群特征，通过分析性传播疾病的病原生物体特点、主要的并发症和临床表现，指出尽管性传播疾病是由特定病原体引起的，但大多数患者是无症状的，只能通过实验室检测发现。预防和控制性病感染的方法在于对青少年进行教育、筛查、早期诊断及治疗。

Age-specific rates of many sexually transmitted infections (**STIs**) are highest among sexually experienced adolescents and young adults, after controlling for sexual activity. Although some STI pathogens present as STI syndromes with a specific constellation of symptoms, most are asymptomatic and only detected by a laboratory test. The approach to prevention and control of these infections lies in education, screening, and early diagnosis and treatment.

ETIOLOGY

Any adolescent who has had oral, vaginal, or anal sexual intercourse is at risk for acquiring an STI. Not all adolescents are at equal risk; physical, behavioral, and social factors contribute to the adolescent's higher risk (Table 146.1). Adolescents who initiate sex at a younger age, youth residing in detention facilities, youth attending sexually transmitted disease (STD) clinics, young men having sex with men, and youth who are injection drug users are at higher risk for STIs. Risky behaviors, such as sex with multiple concurrent partners or multiple sequential partners of limited duration, failure to use barrier protection consistently and correctly, and increased biologic susceptibility to infection, also contribute to risk. Although all 50 states and the District of Columbia explicitly allow minors to consent for their own sexual health services, many adolescents encounter multiple obstacles to accessing this care. Adolescents who are victims of sexual assault may not consider themselves "sexually active," given the context of the encounter, and need reassurance, protection, and appropriate intervention when these circumstances are uncovered (see Chapter 145).

EPIDEMIOLOGY

STI prevalence varies by age, gender, and race/ethnicity. In the United States, although adolescents and young adults ages 15-24 yr represent

Table 146.1	Circumstances Contributing to Adolescents' Susceptibility to Sexually Transmitted Infections

PHYSICAL
Younger age at puberty
Cervical ectopy
Smaller introitus leading to traumatic sex
Asymptomatic nature of sexually transmitted infection
Uncircumcised penis

BEHAVIOR LIMITED BY COGNITIVE STAGE OF DEVELOPMENT
Early adolescence: have not developed ability to think abstractly
Middle adolescence: develop belief of uniqueness and invulnerability

SOCIAL FACTORS
Poverty
Limited access to "adolescent-friendly" healthcare services
Adolescent health-seeking behaviors (forgoing care because of confidentiality concerns or denial of health problem)
Sexual abuse, trafficking, and violence
Homelessness
Drug use
Young adolescent females with older male partners
Young men having sex with men

From Shafii T, Burstein G: An overview of sexually transmitted infections among adolescents, *Adolesc Med Clin* 15:207, 2004.

25% of the sexually experienced population, this age-group accounts for almost 50% of all incident STIs each year. Adolescents and young adults <25 yr of age have the highest reported prevalence of **gonorrhea** (see Chapter 219) and **chlamydia** (see Chapter 253); among females and males, rates are highest in the 15-24 yr old age-groups (Fig. 146.1). In 2015, females age 20-24 yr had the highest reported chlamydia rate (3,730 per 100,000 population), followed by females 15-19 yr of age (2,994/100,000). The reported 2015 chlamydia rate for 15-19 yr old females was almost 4 times higher than for 15-19 yr old males. Chlamydia is common among all races and ethnic groups; Blacks, Native American/Alaska Native, and Hispanic females are disproportionately affected. In 2015, non-Hispanic black females 20-24 yr of age had the highest chlamydia rate of any group (6,783), followed by black females 15-19 yr of age (6,340). Data from the 2007–2012 National Health and Nutrition Examination Survey (NHANES) estimated the prevalence of chlamydia among the U.S. population was highest among African Americans (Fig. 146.2).

Reported rates of other bacterial STIs are also high among adolescents and young adults. In 2015, 20-24 yr old females had the highest (547/100,000) and 20-24 yr old males had the second highest **gonorrhea rates** (539/100,000) compared to any other age/sex group (see Chapter 219). Gonorrhea rates among 15-24 yr old males and females increased between 2014 and 2015. **Syphilis rates** are increasing at an alarming rate, especially among males, accounting for >90% of all primary and secondary syphilis cases. Of those male cases, **men who have sex with men (MSM)** account for 82% of male cases when the gender of the sex partner is known. Males age 20-24 yr have the 2nd highest rate of primary and secondary syphilis among males of any age-group (36/100,000); whereas rates among males 15-19 yr old (8/100,000) are

much lower. Female primary and secondary syphilis rates are much lower than male rates (5/100,000 among 20-24 yr olds; 3/100,000 among 15-19 yr olds) (see Chapter 245). **Pelvic inflammatory disease (PID)** rates are highest among females age 15-24 compared with older women.

Adolescents also carry a large burden of viral STIs. U.S. youth are at persistent risk for **HIV infection** (see Chapter 302). In 2015, youth age 13-24 yr accounted for 22% (8,807) of all new HIV diagnoses in the United States, with most (81%) occurring among gay and bisexual males. Of those new infections, 55% (4,881) were among blacks, 22% (1,957) among Hispanic/Latinos, and 17% (1,506) among whites. Only 10% of high school students have been tested for HIV. Among male students who had sexual contact with other males, only 21% have ever been tested for HIV.

Human papillomavirus (HPV) is the most frequently acquired STI in the United States. According to NHANES, prevalence of HPV vaccine types 6, 11, 16, and 18 (**4vHPV**) declined between the prevacccine (2003–2006) and vaccine (2009–2012) eras: from 11.5% to 4.3% among females age 14-19 yr and from 18.5% to 12.1% among females age 20-24 (see Chapter 293).

Herpes simplex virus type 2 (HSV-2) is the most prevalent viral STI (see Chapter 279). NHANES data show that among 14-19 yr olds, HSV-2 seroprevalence has remained low (<2%, in 1999–2010 surveys). In addition, according to NHANES, HSV-1 seroprevalence among 14-19 yr olds has significantly decreased, from 39% in 1999–2004 to 30% in 2005–2010, indicating less orolabial infection in this age-group. Studies have also found that genital HSV-1 infections are increasing among young adults. Youth who lack HSV-1 antibodies at sexual debut are more susceptible to acquiring a genital HSV-1 infection and developing symptomatic disease from primary genital HSV-2 infection. Increasing oral sex among adolescents and young adults also has been suggested as a contributing factor in the rise in genital HSV-1 infections.

PATHOGENESIS

During puberty, increasing levels of estrogen cause the vaginal epithelium to thicken and cornify and the cellular glycogen content to rise, the latter causing the vaginal pH to fall. These changes increase the resistance of the vaginal epithelium to penetration by certain organisms (including *Neisseria gonorrhoeae*) and increase the susceptibility to others (*Candida albicans* and *Trichomonas*; see Chapter 310). The transformation of the vaginal cells leaves columnar cells on the ectocervix, forming a border of the 2 cell types on the ectocervix, known as the squamocolumnar junction. The appearance is referred to as **ectopy** (Fig. 146.3). With maturation, this tissue involutes. Prior to involution, it represents a unique vulnerability to infection for adolescent females. The association of early sexual debut and younger gynecologic age with increased risk of STIs supports this explanation of the pathogenesis of infection in young adolescents.

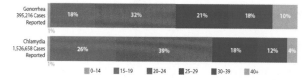

Most Reported Chlamydia and Gonorrhea Infections Occur among 15–24-Year-Olds

| | 0–14 | 15–19 | 20–24 | 25–29 | 30–39 | 40+ |

Fig. 146.1 Proportion of reported gonorrhea and chlamydia cases by age, United States, 2015. (*Adapted from Centers for Disease Control and Prevention: Reported STDs in the United States.* https://www.cdc.gov/nchhstp/newsroom/docs/factsheets/STD-Trends-508.pdf.)

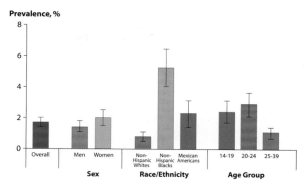

NOTE: Error bars indicate 95% confidence intervals.

Fig. 146.2 Chlamydia prevalence among persons age 14-39 yr by sex, race/ethnicity, and age-group, National Health and Nutrition Examination Survey, 2007–2012. (*From Centers for Disease Control and Prevention: Sexually transmitted disease surveillance, 2015.* https://www.cdc.gov/std/stats15/slides/chlamydia.pptx.)

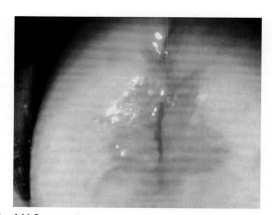

Fig. 146.3 Cervical ectopy. (*From Seattle STD/HIV Prevention Training Center, University of Washington, Claire E. Stevens.*)

Table 146.2	Routine Laboratory Screening Recommendations for Sexually Transmitted Infections in Sexually Active Adolescents and Young Adults

CHLAMYDIA TRACHOMATIS AND NEISSERIA GONORRHOEAE

- Routine screening for *C. trachomatis* and *N. gonorrhoeae* of all sexually active females aged <25 yr is recommended annually.
- Routinely screen sexually active adolescent and young adult MSM at sites of contact for chlamydia (urethra, rectum) and gonorrhea (urethra, rectum, pharynx) at least annually regardless of condom use. More frequent screening (i.e., at 3-6 mo intervals) is indicated for MSM who have multiple or anonymous partners or who have sex with illicit drug use.
- Consider screening for *C. trachomatis* of sexually active adolescent and young adult males annually who have a history of multiple partners in clinical settings with high prevalence rates, such as jails or juvenile corrections facilities, national job training programs, STD clinics, high school clinics, or adolescent clinics.

HUMAN IMMUNODEFICIENCY VIRUS (HIV)

- HIV screening should be discussed and offered to all adolescents at least once by age 16-18 yr and throughout young adulthood in healthcare settings. HIV risk should be assessed annually for >13 yr and offered if HIV risk factors identified.
- Routinely screen sexually active adolescent and young adult MSM at least annually regardless of condom use. More frequent

screening (i.e., at 3-6 mo intervals) is indicated for MSM who have multiple or anonymous partners or who have sex with illicit drug use.

SYPHILIS

- Syphilis screening should be offered to sexually active adolescents reporting risk factors, including MSM.
- Routinely screen sexually active adolescent and young adult MSM at least annually regardless of condom use. More frequent screening (i.e., at 3-6 mo intervals) is indicated for MSM who have multiple or anonymous partners or who have sex with illicit drug use.
- Providers should consult with their local health department regarding local syphilis prevalence and associated risk factors that are associated with syphilis acquisition.

HEPATITIS C VIRUS (HCV)

- Screening adolescents for HCV who report risk factors, i.e., injection drug use, receipt of an unregulated tattoo, received blood products or organ donation before 1992, received clotting factor concentrates before 1987, long-term hemodialysis.
- Given the high HCV prevalence among young injection drug users, screening should be strongly considered.

MSM, Men who have sex with men; STD, sexually transmitted disease.
From Centers for Disease Control and Prevention. https://www.cdc.gov/std/tg2015/screening-recommendations.htm.

SCREENING

Early detection and treatment are primary **STI control** strategies. Some of the most common STIs in adolescents, including HPV, HSV, chlamydia, and gonorrhea, are usually asymptomatic and if undetected can be spread inadvertently by the infected host. **Screening** initiatives for chlamydial infections have demonstrated reductions in PID cases by up to 40%. Although federal and professional medical organizations recommend annual chlamydia screening for sexually active females <25 yr old, according to the National Center for Quality Assurance, in 2015 among sexually active 16-20 yr old females, approximately 42% of commercial health maintenance organization (HMO) members and 52% Medicaid HMO members were tested for chlamydia during the previous year. The lack of a dialog about STIs or the provision of STI services at annual preventive service visits to sexually experienced adolescents are missed opportunities for screening and education. Comprehensive, confidential, reproductive health services, including STI screening, should be offered to all sexually experienced adolescents (Table 146.2).

COMMON INFECTIONS AND CLINICAL MANIFESTATIONS

STI syndromes are generally characterized by the location of the manifestation (vaginitis) or the type of lesion (genital ulcer). Certain constellations of presenting symptoms suggest the inclusion of a possible STI in the differential diagnosis.

Urethritis

Urethritis is an STI syndrome characterized by inflammation of the urethra, usually caused by an infectious etiology. Urethritis may present with urethral discharge, dysuria, urethral irritation, or meatal pruritus. Urgency, frequency of urination, erythema of the urethral meatus, and urethral pain or burning are less common clinical presentations. Approximately 30–50% of males are asymptomatic but may have signs of discharge on diagnosis. On examination, the classic finding is mucoid or purulent discharge from the urethral meatus (Fig. 146.4). If no discharge is evident on exam, providers may attempt to express discharge by applying gentle pressure to the urethra from the base distally to the meatus 3-4 times. *Chlamydia trachomatis* and *N. gonorrhoeae* are the most commonly identified pathogens. *Mycoplasma genitalium* has been

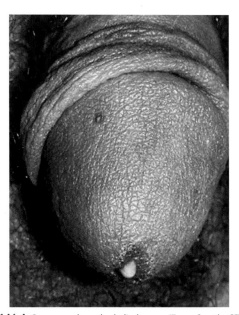

Fig. 146.4 Gonococcal urethral discharge. *(From Seattle STD/HIV Prevention Training Center, University of Washington, Connie Celum and Walter Stamm.)*

associated with urethritis, but data supporting *Ureaplasma urealyticum* have been inconsistent. *Trichomonas vaginalis* can cause nongonococcal urethritis (NGU), but the prevalence varies. HSV-1, HSV-2, and Epstein-Barr virus (EBV) are also potential urethritis pathogens in some cases. Sensitive diagnostic *C. trachomatis* and *N. gonorrhoeae* tests are available for the evaluation of urethritis. However, other pathogens can be considered when NGU is not responsive to treatment, although commercial diagnostic tests are not available for males. Noninfectious causes of urethritis include urethral trauma or foreign body. Unlike in females, urinary tract infections (UTIs) are rare in males who have no genitourinary medical history. In the typical sexually active adolescent male, dysuria and urethral discharge suggest the presence of an STI unless proven otherwise.

Epididymitis

The inflammation of the epididymis in adolescent males is most often associated with an STI, most frequently *C. trachomatis* or *N. gonorrhoeae*. The presentation of unilateral scrotal swelling and tenderness, often accompanied by a hydrocele and palpable swelling of the epididymis, associated with the history of urethral discharge, constitute the presumptive diagnosis of epididymitis. Males who practice insertive anal intercourse are also vulnerable to *Escherichia coli* infection. **Testicular torsion**, a surgical emergency usually presenting with sudden onset of severe testicular pain, should be considered in the differential diagnosis (see Chapter 560). The evaluation for epididymitis should include obtaining evidence of urethral inflammation by physical exam, Gram stain of urethral secretions, urine leukocyte esterase test, or urine microscopy. A *C. trachomatis* and *N. gonorrhoeae* **nucleic acid amplification test (NAAT)** should be performed.

Vaginitis

Vaginitis is a superficial infection of the vaginal mucosa frequently presenting as a vaginal discharge, with or without vulvar involvement (see Chapter 564). **Bacterial vaginosis, vulvovaginal candidiasis,** and **trichomoniasis** are the predominant infections associated with vaginal discharge. Bacterial vaginosis is replacement of the normal hydrogen peroxide (H_2O_2)–producing *Lactobacillus* species vaginal flora by an overgrowth of anaerobic microorganisms, as well as *Gardnerella vaginalis, Ureaplasma,* and *Mycoplasma*. Although bacterial vaginosis is not categorized as an STI, sexual activity is associated with increased frequency of vaginosis. Vulvovaginal candidiasis, usually caused by *C. albicans*, can trigger vulvar pruritus, pain, swelling, and redness and dysuria. Findings on vaginal examination include vulvar edema, fissures, excoriations, or thick curdy vaginal discharge. Trichomoniasis is caused by the protozoan *T. vaginalis*. Infected females may present with symptoms characterized by a diffuse, malodorous, yellow-green vaginal discharge with vulvar irritation or may be diagnosed by screening an asymptomatic patient. Cervicitis can sometimes cause a vaginal discharge. Laboratory confirmation is recommended because clinical presentations may vary and patients may be infected with >1 pathogen.

Cervicitis

The inflammatory process in cervicitis involves the deeper structures in the mucous membrane of the cervix uteri. Vaginal discharge can be a manifestation, but cervicitis frequently is asymptomatic, Patients also present with complaints of irregular or postcoital bleeding. Two major diagnostic signs characterize cervicitis: (1) a purulent or mucopurulent endocervical exudate visible in the endocervical canal or on an endocervical swab specimen (e.g., swab sign; Fig. 146.5), called **mucopurulent cervicitis** or cervicitis, and (2) sustained endocervical bleeding easily induced by gentle passage of a cotton swab through the cervical os, signifying friability. Cervical changes associated with cervicitis must be distinguished from cervical ectopy in the younger adolescent to avoid the overdiagnosis of inflammation (Fig. 146.6; see Fig. 146.3). The pathogens identified most frequently with cervicitis are *C. trachomatis* and *N. gonorrhoeae,* although no pathogen is identified in most cases. HSV is a less common pathogen associated with ulcerative and necrotic lesions on the cervix.

Pelvic Inflammatory Disease

PID encompasses a spectrum of inflammatory disorders of the female upper genital tract, including **endometritis, salpingitis, tuboovarian abscess,** and **pelvic peritonitis,** usually in combination rather than as separate entities. *N. gonorrhoeae* and *C. trachomatis* predominate as the involved pathogenic organisms in younger adolescents (see Chapters 219 and 253), although PID should be approached as multiorganism etiology, including pathogens such as anaerobes, *G. vaginalis, Haemophilus influenzae,* enteric gram-negative rods, and *Streptococcus agalactiae*. In

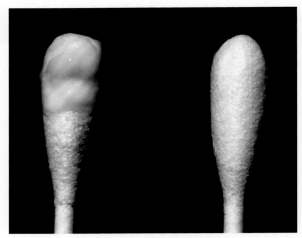

Fig. 146.5 Mucopurulent cervical discharge positive swab test. *(From Seattle STD/HIV Prevention Training Center, University of Washington, Claire E. Stevens and Ronald E. Roddy. http://www2a.cdc.gov/stdtraining/ready-to-use/pid.htm.)*

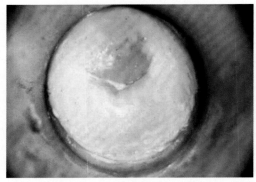

Fig. 146.6 Inflamed cervix caused by gonococcal cervicitis. *(From Centers for Disease Control and Prevention: STD clinical slides. http://www.cdc.gov/std/training/clinicalslides/slides-dl.htm.)*

addition, cytomegalovirus, *Mycoplasma hominis, Ureaplasma urealyticum,* and *M. genitalium* may be associated with PID. PID (tuboovarian abscess) has rarely been reported in virgins and is usually caused by *E. coli* and associated in some patients with obesity and possible pooling of urine in the vagina.

PID is difficult to diagnose because of the wide variation in the symptoms and signs. Many females with PID have subtle or mild symptoms, resulting in many unrecognized cases. Healthcare providers should consider the possibility of PID in young, sexually active females presenting with vaginal discharge or abdominal pain.

The clinical diagnosis of PID is based on the presence of at least 1 of the minimal criteria, either cervical motion tenderness, uterine tenderness, or adnexal tenderness, to increase the diagnostic sensitivity and reduce the likelihood of missed or delayed diagnosis. Providers should also consider that adolescents are the population in whom PID is typically diagnosed and thus should have a low threshold for initiating empirical treatment. In addition, the majority of females with PID have either mucopurulent cervical discharge or evidence of white blood cells (WBCs) on a microscopic evaluation of a vaginal fluid–saline preparation. If the cervical discharge appears normal and no WBCs are observed on the wet prep of vaginal fluid, the diagnosis of PID is unlikely, and alternative causes of pain should be investigated. Specific, but not always practical, criteria for PID include evidence of endometritis on biopsy, transvaginal sonography or MRI evidence of thickened, fluid-filled tubes, or Doppler evidence of tubal hyperemia or laparoscopic evidence of PID.

Genital Ulcer Syndromes

An **ulcerative lesion** in a mucosal area exposed to sexual contact is the unifying characteristic of infections associated with these syndromes. These lesions are most frequently seen on the penis and vulva but also occur on oral and rectal mucosa, depending on the adolescent's sexual practices. HSV and *Treponema pallidum* (syphilis) are the most common organisms associated with genital ulcer syndromes.

Genital herpes, the most common ulcerative STI among adolescents, is a chronic, lifelong viral infection. Two sexually transmitted HSV

types have been identified, HSV-1 and HSV-2. The majority of cases of recurrent genital herpes are caused by HSV-2. However, among young women and MSM, an increasing proportion of anogenital herpes has been HSV-1. Most HSV-2–infected persons are unaware of their diagnosis because they experience mild or unrecognized infections but continue to shed virus intermittently in the genital tract. Therefore, most genital herpes infections are transmitted by asymptomatic persons who are unaware of their infection.

Although the initial herpetic lesion is a vesicle, by the time the patient presents clinically, the vesicle most often has ruptured spontaneously, leaving a shallow, painful ulcer (Fig. 146.7*A*), although recurrences are generally less intense and painful (Fig. 146.7*B*). Up to 50% of first genital

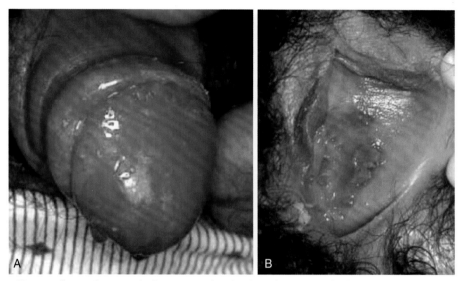

Fig. 146.7 A, Initial herpes infection showing multiple erosions with polycyclic outlines surrounded by an erythematous halo and associated with intense pain. **B,** Erosions surrounded by an erythematous halo. Clinical signs and symptoms of recurrences are usually less intense than those of initial infection. *(From Martín JM, Villalón G, Jordá E: Update on treatment of genital herpes, Actas Dermosifiliogr 100:22–32, 2009, Figs 1 and 2.)*

Table 146.3	Signs, Symptoms, and Presumptive and Definitive Diagnoses of Genital Ulcers		
SIGNS/SYMPTOMS	**HERPES SIMPLEX VIRUS**	**SYPHILIS (PRIMARY)**	**CHANCROID**
Ulcers	Vesicles rupture to form shallow ulcers	Ulcer with well-demarcated indurated borders and a clean base (chancre)	Unindurated and undermined borders and a purulent base
Painful	Painful	Painless*	Painful
Number of lesions	Usually multiple	Usually single	Multiple
Inguinal lymphadenopathy	First-time infections may cause constitutional symptoms and lymphadenopathy.	Usually mild and minimally tender	Unilateral or bilateral painful adenopathy in >50% Inguinal bubo formation and rupture may occur.
Clinical suspicion	Typical lesions; positive HSV-2 type-specific serology test	Early syphilis: typical chancre plus reactive nontreponemal test (RPR, VDRL) and no history of syphilis, or 4-fold increase in quantitative nontreponemal test in person with history of syphilis; positive treponemal EIA with reactive nontreponemal test (RPR, VDRL) and no prior history of syphilis treatment	Exclusion of other causes of ulcers in the presence of (a) typical ulcers and lymphadenopathy, (b) typical Gram stain, and (c) history of contact with high-risk individual (prostitute) or living in an endemic area
Definitive diagnosis	Detection of HSV by culture or PCR from ulcer scraping or aspiration of vesicle fluid	Identification of *Treponema pallidum* from a chancre or lymph node aspirate on dark-field microscopy	Detection of *Haemophilus ducreyi* by culture

*Primary syphilitic ulcers may be painful if they become co-infected with bacteria or 1 of the other organisms responsible for genital ulcers.

DFA, Direct fluorescent antibody; EIA, enzyme immunoassay; HSV, herpes simplex virus; PCR, polymerase chain reaction; RPR, rapid plasma reagin; VDRL, Venereal Disease Research Laboratories.

Data from Centers for Disease Control and Prevention: Sexually transmitted diseases: treatment guidelines, *MMWR* 64(RR-3), 2015. https://www.cdc.gov/std/tg2015/default.htm.

herpes episodes are caused by HSV-1, but recurrences and subclinical shedding are much more frequent for genital HSV-2 infection.

Syphilis is a less common cause of genital ulcers in adolescents than in adults. **Lymphogranuloma venereum** caused by *C. trachomatis* serovars L1-L3 is uncommon, although outbreaks do occur in MSM. In these circumstances, proctitis or proctocolitis is the usual manifestation. HIV is often present in affected men. Unusual infectious causes of genital, anal, or perianal ulcers in the United States and other industrialized countries include chancroid and donovanosis.

Table 146.3 presents the clinical characteristics differentiating the lesions of the most common infections associated with genital ulcers, along with the required laboratory diagnosis to identify the causative agent accurately. The differential diagnosis includes Behçet disease (see Chapter 186), Crohn disease (Chapter 362), aphthous ulceration, and **acute genital ulcers** caused by cytomegalovirus (Chapter 282) or Epstein-Barr virus (Chapter 281). Acute genital ulcers often follow a flu or mononucleosis-like illness in an immunocompetent female and is unrelated to sexual activity. The lesions are 0.5-2.5 cm in size, bilateral, symmetric, multiple, painful, and necrotic, and are associated with inguinal lymphadenopathy. This primary infection is also associated with fever and malaise. The diagnosis may require Epstein-Barr virus titers, or polymerase chain reaction (PCR) testing. Treatment is supportive care including pain management.

Genital Lesions and Ectoparasites

Lesions that present as outgrowths on the surface of the epithelium and other limited epidermal lesions are included under this categorization of syndromes. HPV can cause genital warts and genital-cervical abnormalities that can lead to cancer (see Chapter 293). **Genital HPV** types are classified according to their association with cervical cancer. Infections with low-risk types, such as **HPV types 6 and 11**, can cause benign or low-grade changes in cells of the cervix, genital warts, and recurrent respiratory papillomatosis. High-risk HPV types can cause cervical, anal, vulvar, vaginal, and head and neck cancers. **High-risk HPV types 16 and 18** are detected in approximately 70% of **cervical cancers**. Persistent infection increases the risk of cervical cancer. **Molluscum contagiosum** and **condyloma latum** associated with secondary syphilis complete the classification of genital lesion syndromes.

As a result of the close physical contact during sexual contact, common ectoparasitic infestations of the pubic area occur as **pediculosis pubis** or the papular lesions of **scabies** (see Chapter 688).

HIV Disease and Hepatitis B

HIV and hepatitis B virus (HBV) present as asymptomatic, unexpected occurrences in most infected adolescents. High vaccination coverage rates among infants and adolescents have resulted in substantial declines in acute HBV incidence among U.S.-born adolescents. Risk factors identified in the history or routine screening during prenatal care are much more likely to result in suspicion of infection, leading to the appropriate laboratory screening, than are clinical manifestations in this age-group (see Chapters 302 and 385).

DIAGNOSIS

Most often, adolescents infected with viral and bacterial STI pathogens do not report symptoms suggestive of infection. With the use of very sensitive, noninvasive chlamydia and gonorrhea NAAT, providers are finding that most genital infections in females as well as many males are asymptomatic. A thorough sexual history is key to identifying adolescents who should be screened for STIs and for identifying those who require a laboratory diagnostic evaluation for an STI syndrome.

When eliciting a sexual health history, discussions should be appropriate for the patient's developmental level. In addition to questions regarding vaginal or urethral discharge, genital lesions, and lower abdominal pain among females, one should ask about prior treatment of any STI symptoms, including self-treatment using nonprescription medications. **Dyspareunia** is a consistent symptom in adolescents with **PID**. Providers must ask about oral or anal sexual activity to determine sites for specimen collection.

Urethritis should be objectively documented by evidence of inflammation or infectious etiology. Patient complaint without objective clinical or laboratory evidence does not fulfill diagnostic criteria. Inflammation can be documented by (a) observing urethral mucopurulent discharge, (b) ≥2 WBCs per high-power field on microscopic examination of Gram stain urethral secretions, (c) urine microscopic findings of ≥10 WBCs per high-power field of first-void urine specimen, or (d) a positive urine leukocyte esterase test of a first-void specimen. Laboratory evaluation is essential to identify the involved pathogens to determine treatment, partner notification, and disease control. *C. trachomatis* and *N. gonorrhoeae* NAATs of a urine specimen are recommended. The presence of gram-negative intracellular diplococci on microscopy obtained from a male urethral specimen confirms the diagnosis of gonococcal urethritis.

An essential component of the diagnostic evaluation of vaginal, cervical, or urethral discharge is a chlamydia and gonorrhea NAAT. NAATs are the most sensitive chlamydia and gonorrhea tests available and are licensed for use with urine, urethral, vaginal, and cervical specimens. Many of the chlamydia NAATs are approved by the U.S. Food and Drug Administration (FDA) to test patient-collected vaginal swabs in the clinical setting and liquid cytology specimens. Female vaginal swab specimens and male first-void urine are considered the optimal specimen types. Female urine remains an acceptable chlamydia and gonorrhea NAAT specimen, but may have slightly reduced performance when compared with cervical or vaginal swab specimens. Urine is the recommended specimen for male urethral infection. Gonorrhea and chlamydia NAATs perform well on rectal and oropharyngeal specimens and can be performed by clinical laboratories that have completed the appropriate verification studies to obtain Clinical Laboratory Improvement Amendments (CLIA) approval, which includes most clinical laboratories.

Evaluation of adolescent females with **vaginitis** includes laboratory data. Traditionally, the cause of vaginal symptoms was determined by pH and microscopic examination of the discharge. However, CLIA-waived point-of-care vaginitis tests are available. Using pH paper, an elevated pH (i.e., >4.5) is common with bacterial vaginosis or trichomoniasis. Because pH testing is not highly specific, discharge should be further examined. For microscopic exam, a slide can be made with the discharge diluted in 1-2 drops of 0.9% normal saline solution and another slide with discharge diluted in 10% potassium hydroxide (KOH) solution. Examining the saline specimen slide under a microscope may reveal motile or dead *T. vaginalis* or clue cells (epithelial cells with borders obscured by small bacteria), which are characteristic of **bacterial vaginosis**. WBCs without evidence of trichomonads or yeast are usually suggestive of cervicitis. The yeast or pseudohyphae of *Candida* species are more easily identified in the KOH specimen (Fig. 146.8). The sensitivity of microscopy is approximately 50% and requires immediate evaluation of the slide for optimal results. Therefore, lack of findings does not eliminate the possibility of infection. More sensitive point-of-care vaginitis tests include the OSOM Trichomonas Rapid Test (Sekisui Diagnostics, Lexington, MA), an immunochromatographic capillary flow dipstick technology with reported 83% sensitivity. The OSOM BVBLUE Test (Sekisui) detects elevated vaginal fluid sialidase activity, an enzyme produced by bacterial pathogens associated with bacterial vaginosis, including *Gardnerella*, *Bacteroides*, *Prevotella*, and *Mobiluncus*, and has a reported 90% sensitivity. Both tests are CLIA waived, with results available in 10 min.

Clinical laboratory–based vaginitis tests are also available. The Affirm VPIII (Becton Dickenson, San Jose, CA) is a moderate-complexity nucleic acid probe test that evaluates for *T. vaginalis*, *G. vaginalis*, and *C. albicans* and has a sensitivity of 63% and specificity >99.9%, with results available in 45 min. Some gonorrhea and chlamydia NAATs also offer an assay for *T. vaginalis* testing of female specimens tested for *N. gonorrhoeae* and *C. trachomatis*, considered the gold standard for *Trichomonas* testing.

Objective signs of vulvar inflammation in the absence of vaginal pathogens, along with a minimal amount of discharge, suggest the possibility of mechanical, chemical, allergic, or other noninfectious irritation of the vulva (Table 146.4).

The **definitive diagnosis of PID** is difficult based on clinical findings alone. Clinical diagnosis is imprecise, and no single historical, physical,

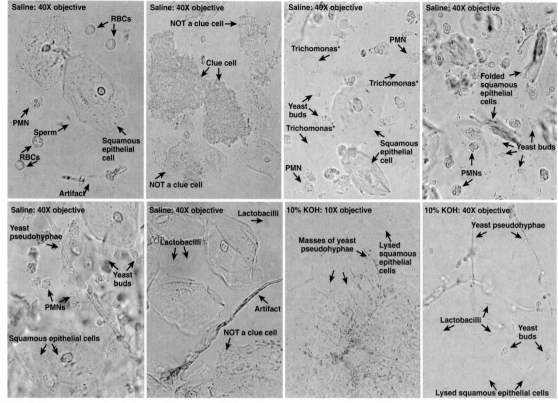

Fig. 146.8 Common normal and abnormal microscopic findings during examination of vaginal fluid. KOH, Potassium hydroxide solution; PMN, polymorphonuclear leukocyte; RBCs, red blood cells. (*From* Adolescent medicine: state of the art reviews, *vol 14, no 2, Philadelphia, 2003, Hanley & Belfus, pp 350–351.)*

or laboratory finding is both sensitive and specific for the diagnosis of acute PID. Clinical criteria have a positive predictive value of only 65–90% compared with laparoscopy. Although healthcare providers should maintain a low threshold for the diagnosis of PID, additional criteria to enhance specificity of diagnosis, such as transvaginal ultrasonography, can be considered (Table 146.5).

Cell culture and polymerase chain reaction (PCR) are the preferred **HSV tests.** Viral culture sensitivity is low, and intermittent viral shedding causes false-negative results. NAATs, including PCR assays for HSV DNA, are more sensitive and increasingly available for diagnosing genital HSV. The Tzanck test is insensitive and nonspecific and should not be considered reliable.

Accurate type-specific **HSV serologic assays** are based on the HSV-specific glycoproteins G2 (HSV-2) and G1 (HSV-1). Both laboratory-based point-of-care tests are available. Because almost all HSV-2 infections are sexually acquired, the presence of type-specific HSV-2 antibody implies anogenital infection. The presence of HSV-1 antibody alone is more difficult to interpret because of the frequency of oral HSV infection acquired during childhood. Type-specific HSV serologic assays might be useful in the following scenarios: (1) recurrent genital symptoms or atypical symptoms with negative HSV cultures; (2) a clinical diagnosis of genital herpes without laboratory confirmation; and (3) a patient with a partner with genital herpes, especially if considering suppressive antiviral therapy to prevent transmission.

For **syphilis testing,** nontreponemal tests, such as the rapid plasma reagin (RPR) or Venereal Disease Research Laboratories (VDRL), and treponemal testing, such as fluorescent treponemal antibody absorbed tests, the *T. pallidum* passive particle agglutination (TP-PA) assay, and various enzyme and chemiluminescence immunoassays (EIA/CIA), are recommended. However, many clinical laboratories have adopted a

Table 146.4	Pathologic Vaginal Discharge
INFECTIVE DISCHARGE	**OTHER REASONS FOR DISCHARGE**
COMMON CAUSES	**COMMON CAUSES**
Organisms	Retained tampon or condom
Candida albicans	Chemical irritation
Trichomonas vaginalis	Allergic responses
Chlamydia trachomatis	Ectropion
Neisseria gonorrhoeae	Endocervical polyp
Mycoplasma genitalium	Intrauterine device
Conditions	Atrophic changes
Bacterial vaginosis	
Acute pelvic inflammatory disease	**LESS COMMON CAUSES**
Postoperative pelvic infection	Physical trauma
Postabortal sepsis	Vault granulation tissue
Puerperal sepsis	Vesicovaginal fistula
	Rectovaginal fistula
LESS COMMON CAUSES	Neoplasia
Ureaplasma urealyticum	Cervicitis
Syphilis	
Escherichia coli	

From Mitchell H: Vaginal discharge—causes, diagnosis, and treatment, *BMJ* 328:1306–1308, 2004.

reverse sequence of screening in which a treponemal EIA/CIA is performed first, followed by testing of reactive sera with a nontreponemal test (e.g., RPR). A positive treponemal EIA or CIA test can identify both *previously treated and untreated or incompletely treated syphilis*. False-positive results can occur, particularly among populations with

Table 146.5	Evaluation for Pelvic Inflammatory Disease (PID)

2015 CDC DIAGNOSTIC CRITERIA

Minimal Criteria
- Cervical motion tenderness
  or
- Uterine tenderness
  or
- Adnexal tenderness

Additional Criteria to Enhance Specificity of the Minimal Criteria
- Oral temperature >38.3°C (101°F)
- Abnormal cervical or vaginal mucopurulent discharge*
- Presence of abundant numbers of WBCs on saline microscopy of vaginal secretions*
- Elevated ESR or C-reactive protein
- Laboratory documentation of cervical *Neisseria gonorrhoeae* or *Chlamydia trachomatis* infection

Most Specific Criteria to Enhance the Specificity of the Minimal Criteria
- Transvaginal sonography or MRI techniques showing thickened, fluid-filled tubes, with or without free pelvic fluid or tuboovarian complex, or Doppler studies suggesting pelvic infection (e.g., tubal hyperemia)
- Endometrial biopsy with histopathologic evidence of endometritis
- Laparoscopic abnormalities consistent with PID

Differential Diagnosis (Partial List)
- Gastrointestinal: appendicitis, constipation, diverticulitis, gastroenteritis, inflammatory bowel disease, irritable bowel syndrome
- Gynecologic: ovarian cyst (intact, ruptured, or torsed), endometriosis, dysmenorrhea, ectopic pregnancy, mittelschmerz, ruptured follicle, septic or threatened abortion, tuboovarian abscess
- Urinary tract: cystitis, pyelonephritis, urethritis, nephrolithiasis

*If the cervical discharge appears normal and no WBCs are observed on the wet prep of vaginal fluid, the diagnosis of PID is unlikely, and alternative causes of pain should be investigated.
ESR, Erythrocyte sedimentation rate; WBCs, white blood cells.
Adapted from Centers for Disease Control and Prevention (CDC). https://www.cdc.gov/std/tg2015/screening-recommendations.htm.

low syphilis prevalence. Persons with a positive treponemal screening test should have a standard nontreponemal test with titer (RPR or VDRL) to guide patient management decisions. If EIA/CIA and RPR/VDRL results are discordant, the laboratory should perform a different treponemal test to confirm the results of the initial test. Patients with discordant serologic results by EIA/CIA and RPR/VDRL testing whose sera are reactive by TP-PA testing are considered to have past or present syphilis; if sera is TP-PA nonreactive, syphilis is unlikely (Fig. 146.9).

Rapid HIV testing with results available in 10-20 min can be useful when the likelihood of adolescents returning for their results is low. Point-of-care CLIA-waived tests for whole blood fingerstick and oral fluid specimen testing are available. Clinical studies have demonstrated that the rapid HIV test performance is comparable to those of EIAs. Because some reactive test results may be false positive, every reactive rapid test must be confirmed.

TREATMENT

See Part XVI for chapters on the treatment of specific microorganisms and Tables 146.6 to 146.8. Treatment regimens using nonprescription products for candidal vaginitis and pediculosis reduce financial and access barriers to rapid treatment for adolescents, but potential risks for inappropriate self-treatment and complications from untreated more serious infections must be considered before using this approach. Minimizing noncompliance with treatment, notifying and treating the sexual partners, addressing prevention and contraceptive issues, offering available vaccines to prevent STIs, and making every effort to preserve fertility are additional physician responsibilities.

Chlamydia- and gonorrhea-infected males and females should be retested approximately 3 mo after treatment, regardless of whether they believe that their sex partners were treated, or whenever persons next present for medical care in the 12 mo following initial treatment. Once an infection is diagnosed, partner evaluation, testing, and treatment are recommended for sexual contacts within 60 days of symptoms or diagnosis, or the most recent partner if sexual contact was >60 days, even if the partner is asymptomatic. Abstinence is recommended for at least 7 days after both patient and partner are treated. A test for pregnancy should be performed for all females with suspected PID because the test outcome will affect management. Repeat testing 3 mo after treatment is also recommended for *Trichomonas* infection.

Diagnosis and therapy are often carried out within the context of a **confidential** relationship between the physician and the patient. Therefore, the need to report certain STIs to health department authorities should be clarified at the outset. Health departments are Health Insurance Portability and Affordability Act (HIPAA) exempt and will not violate confidentiality. The health department's role is to ensure that treatment and case finding have been accomplished and that sexual partners have been notified of their STI exposure. **Expedited partner therapy (EPT)**, the clinical practice of treating sex partners of patients diagnosed with chlamydia or gonorrhea, by providing prescriptions or medications to the patient to take to the partner without the healthcare provider first examining the partner, is a strategy to reduce further transmission of infection. In randomized trials, EPT has reduced the rates of persistent or recurrent gonorrhea and chlamydia infection. Serious adverse reactions are rare with recommended chlamydia and gonorrhea treatment regimens, such as doxycycline, azithromycin, and cefixime. Transient gastrointestinal side effects are more common but rarely result in severe morbidity. Most states expressly permit EPT or may allow its practice. Resources for information regarding EPT and state laws are available at the Centers for Disease Control and Prevention website (http://www.cdc.gov/std/ept/).

PREVENTION

Healthcare providers should integrate **sexuality education** into clinical practice with children from early childhood through adolescence. Providers should counsel adolescents regarding sexual behaviors associated with risk of STI acquisition and should educate using evidence-based prevention strategies, which include a discussion of abstinence and other risk reduction strategies, such as consistent and correct condom use. The U.S. Preventive Services Task Force recommends **high-intensity behavioral counseling** to prevent STIs for all sexually active adolescents. The HPV vaccine (Gardasil 9) is recommended for 11 and 12 yr old males and females as routine immunization. Catch-up vaccination is recommended for females age 13-26 and for males age 13-21 who have not yet received or completed the vaccine series; males age 22 through 26 may be vaccinated.

Bibliography is available at Expert Consult.

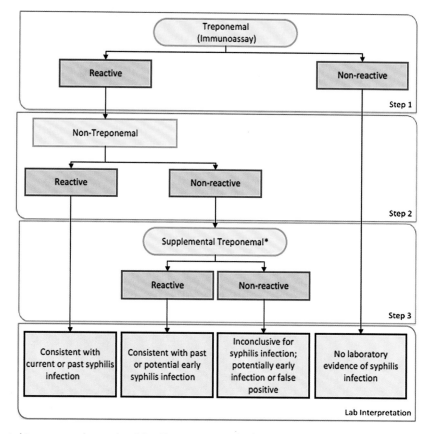

The supplemental treponemal test should utilize a unique platform and or antigen, different than the first treponemal test.

Fig. 146.9 Centers for Disease Control and Prevention (CDC) recommended algorithm for reverse-sequence syphilis screening: treponemal test screening followed by nontreponemal test confirmation. *(From Association of Public Health Laboratories: Suggested reporting language for syphilis serology testing, 2015.)*

Table 146.6	Management Guidelines for Uncomplicated Bacterial STIs in Adolescents and Adults	
PATHOGEN	**RECOMMENDED REGIMENS**	**ALTERNATIVE REGIMENS AND SPECIAL CONSIDERATIONS**
Chlamydia trachomatis	Azithromycin 1 g orally once *or* Doxycycline 100 mg orally twice daily for 7 days	**For pregnancy:** Azithromycin 1 g orally once **Alternative regimens:** Erythromycin base 500 mg orally 4 times daily for 7 days *or* Erythromycin ethylsuccinate 800 mg orally 4 times daily for 7 days *or* Levofloxacin 500 mg orally once daily for 7 days *or* Ofloxacin 300 mg orally twice daily for 7 days

Continued

Table 146.6	Management Guidelines for Uncomplicated Bacterial STIs in Adolescents and Adults—cont'd	

PATHOGEN	RECOMMENDED REGIMENS	ALTERNATIVE REGIMENS AND SPECIAL CONSIDERATIONS
Neisseria gonorrhoeae (cervix, urethra, and rectum)	Ceftriaxone 250 mg IM in a single dose *plus* Azithromycin 1 g orally once	Single-dose injectable cephalosporin regimens (other than ceftriaxone 250 mg IM) that are safe and effective against uncomplicated urogenital and anorectal gonococcal infections include ceftizoxime 500 mg IM, cefoxitin 2 g IM with probenecid 1 g orally, and cefotaxime 500 mg IM *plus* Azithromycin 1 g orally once *Alternative if unable to offer IM:* Cefixime 400 mg orally in a single dose *plus* Azithromycin 1 g orally in a single dose **If patient is allergic to azithromycin:** Doxycycline 100 mg orally twice daily for 7 days may be substituted for azithromycin as the 2nd antimicrobial. **Severe cephalosporin allergy:** Gemifloxacin 320 mg orally *plus* azithromycin 2 g orally in a single dose *or* Gentamicin 240 mg IM *plus* oral azithromycin 2 g orally in a single dose
N. gonorrhoeae (pharynx)	Ceftriaxone 250 mg IM in a single dose *plus* Azithromycin 1 g orally once	**No recommended alternative therapy** Possibly gemifloxacin *plus* azithromycin as above for cervix, urethra, rectum Patients treated with an alternative regimen should return 14 days after treatment for a test of cure using either culture or NAAT.
Treponema pallidum (primary and secondary syphilis or early latent syphilis, i.e., infection <12 mo)	Benzathine penicillin G 2.4 million units IM in a single dose	**Penicillin allergy:** Doxycycline 100 mg orally twice daily for 14 days, *or* tetracycline 500 mg orally 4 times daily for 14 days. Limited data suggest ceftriaxone 1-2 g daily either IM or IV for 10-14 days. *or* Azithromycin 2 g orally in a single dose has been effective. but treatment failures have been documented.
T. pallidum (late latent syphilis or syphilis of unknown duration)	Benzathine penicillin G 7.2 million units total, administered as 3 doses of 2.4 million units IM each at 1 wk intervals	**Penicillin allergy:** Doxycycline 100 mg orally twice daily for 28 days, *or* tetracycline 500 mg orally 4 times daily for 28 days, with close serologic and clinical follow-up
Haemophilus ducreyi (chancroid: genital ulcers, lymphadenopathy)	Azithromycin 1 g orally in a single dose *or* Ceftriaxone 250 mg IM in a single dose *or* Ciprofloxacin 500 mg orally twice daily for 3 days *or* Erythromycin base 500 mg orally 3 times daily for 7 days	
C. trachomatis serovars L1, L2, or L3 (lymphogranuloma venereum)	Doxycycline 100 mg orally twice daily for 21 days	**Alternative:** Erythromycin base 500 mg orally 4 times daily for 21 days *or* Azithromycin 1 g orally once weekly for 3 wk

IM, Intramuscularly; IV, intravenously; NAAT, nucleic acid amplification test.
 Adapted for Centers for Disease Control and Prevention: Sexually transmitted diseases: treatment guidelines, *MMWR* 64(RR-3), 2015. https://www.cdc.gov/std/tg2015/default.htm.

Table 146.7	Management Guidelines for Uncomplicated Miscellaneous Sexually Transmitted Infections in Adolescents and Adults	

PATHOGEN	RECOMMENDED REGIMENS	ALTERNATIVE REGIMENS AND SPECIAL CONSIDERATIONS
Trichomonas vaginalis	Metronidazole 2 g orally in a single dose *or* Tinidazole 2 g orally in a single dose	Metronidazole 500 mg orally twice daily for 7 days
Phthirus pubis (pubic lice)	Permethrin 1% cream rinse applied to affected areas and washed off after 10 min *or* Pyrethrins with piperonyl butoxide applied to affected areas and washed off after 10 min Launder clothing and bedding	Malathion 0.5% lotion applied for 8-12 hr and washed off *or* Ivermectin 250 μg/kg orally, repeat in 2 wk
Sarcoptes scabiei (scabies)	Permethrin 5% cream applied to all areas from the neck down, washed off after 8-14 hr *or* Ivermectin 200 μg/kg orally, repeated in 2 wk Launder clothing and bedding	Lindane (1%) 1 oz of lotion or 30 g of cream in thin layer to all areas of body from neck down; wash off in 8 hr

Adapted from Centers for Disease Control and Prevention: Sexually transmitted diseases: treatment guidelines, *MMWR* 64(RR-3), 2015. https://www.cdc.gov/std/tg2015/default.htm.

Table 146.8	Management Guidelines for Uncomplicated Genital Warts and Genital Herpes in Adolescents and Adults

PATHOGEN	RECOMMENDED REGIMENS	ALTERNATIVE REGIMENS AND SPECIAL CONSIDERATIONS
HUMAN PAPILLOMAVIRUS (HPV)		
External anogenital warts (penis, groin, scrotum, vulva, perineum, external anus, and perianus)	**Patient applied:** Imiquimod 3.75% cream self-applied to warts at bedtime nightly for up to 16 wk; wash off after 6-10 hr *or* Imiquimod 3 5% cream self-applied to warts at bedtime 3 times weekly for up to 16 wk; wash off after 6-10 hr *or* Podofilox 0.5% solution or gel self-applied to warts twice daily for 3 consecutive days each wk followed by 4 days of no therapy. May be repeated for up to 4 cycles. *or* Sinecatechins 15% ointment self-applied 3 times daily for up to 16 wk. Do not wash off after use, and avoid genital, anal, and oral sexual contact while ointment is on skin. **Provider-administered:** Cryotherapy with liquid nitrogen or cryoprobe. Repeat applications every 1-2 wk. *or* Surgical removal either by electrocautery, tangential excision with scissors or scalpel, or by carbon dioxide (CO_2) laser *or* Trichloroacetic acid (TCA) or bichloracetic acid (BCA) 80–90%; small amount applied only to warts and allowed to dry, when white "frosting" develops; can be repeated weekly.	**Provider administered:** Podophyllin resin 10–25% in a compound tincture of benzoin applied to each wart and then allowed to air-dry; thoroughly wash after off 1-4 hr; can be repeated weekly. Systemic toxicity has been reported when podophyllin resin was applied to large areas of friable tissue and was not washed off within 4 hr. Many persons with external anal warts also have intraanal warts and might benefit from inspection of anal canal by digital examination, standard anoscopy, or high-resolution anoscopy.
Cervical warts	Cryotherapy with liquid nitrogen *or* Surgical removal *or* TCA or BCA 80–90% solution Management should include consultation with a specialist.	
Vaginal warts	Cryotherapy with liquid nitrogen; avoid cryoprobe use. *or* Surgical removal *or* TCA or BCA 80–90%; small amount applied only to warts and allowed to dry, when white "frosting" develops; can be repeated weekly.	
Urethral meatal warts	Cryotherapy with liquid nitrogen *or* Surgical removal	
Intraanal Warts	Cryotherapy with liquid nitrogen *or* Surgical removal *or* TCA or BCA 80-90% applied to warts. A small amount should be applied only to warts and allowed to dry, at which time a white "frosting" develops. Can be repeated weekly	Management of intraanal warts should include consultation with a specialist.
HERPES SIMPLEX VIRUS (HSV; GENITAL HERPES)		
First clinical episode	**Treat for 7-10 days with 1 of the following:** Acyclovir 400 mg orally 3 times daily Acyclovir 200 mg orally 5 times daily Valacyclovir 1 g orally twice daily Famciclovir 250 mg orally 3 times daily	Consider extending treatment if healing is incomplete after 10 days of therapy
Episodic therapy for recurrences	**Treat with 1 of the following:** Acyclovir 400 mg orally 3 times daily for 5 days Acyclovir 800 mg orally twice daily for 5 days Acyclovir 800 mg orally 3 times daily for 2 days Valacyclovir 500 mg orally twice daily for 3 days Valacyclovir 1,000 mg orally once daily for 5 days Famciclovir 125 mg orally twice daily for 5 days Famciclovir 1,000 mg orally twice daily for 1 day Famciclovir 500 mg orally once, then 250 mg twice daily for 2 days	Effective episodic treatment of recurrences requires initiation of therapy within 1 day of lesion onset or during the prodrome that precedes some outbreaks. The patient should be provided with a supply or a prescription for the medication with instructions to initiate treatment immediately when symptoms begin.
Suppressive therapy to reduce frequency of recurrences	**Treat with 1 of the following:** Acyclovir 400 mg orally twice daily Valacyclovir 500 mg orally once daily* or 1 g orally once daily Famciclovir 250 mg orally twice daily	All patients should be counseled regarding suppressive therapy availability, regardless of number of outbreaks per year. Since the frequency of recurrent outbreaks diminishes over time in many patients, providers should periodically discuss the need to continue therapy.

*Valacyclovir 500 mg once daily might be less effective than other valacyclovir or acyclovir dosing regimens in patients who have very frequent recurrences (i.e., ≥10 episodes per year).

Adapted from Centers for Disease Control and Prevention: Sexually transmitted diseases: treatment guidelines, *MMWR* 64(RR-3), 2015. https://www.cdc.gov/std/tg2015/default.htm.

Chapter **147**
Chronic Overlapping Pain Conditions

Thomas C. Chelimsky and
Gisela G. Chelimsky

第一百四十七章
多种慢性疼痛

中文导读

　　本章主要介绍了一组医学上无法解释、可影响身体多个部位、没有明确病理生理原因、表现为疼痛症状与精神共患的异常综合征（COPCs），这种疾病常表现为多种症状叠加的状态，如功能性胃肠疾病的青少年出现头晕、恶心、疲劳和睡眠障碍等。此外，本章还介绍了青少年中COPCs的流行趋势、临床特征、精神并发症、发病诱因和疾病自然病程等。

In chronic overlapping pain conditions (**COPCs**), several painful symptoms affecting different body systems coexist without clear underlying pathophysiology. Other terms for COPCs include **medically unexplained symptoms**, **functional somatic syndromes** (FSS), and **central sensitivity syndromes**. These disorders are probably highly prevalent; for example, 2 COPCs, irritable bowel syndrome (IBS) and migraine, *each* affect 10–20% of the population. Pediatric COPC studies usually focus on populations with 1 painful condition (headaches) and their psychiatric comorbidities, rather than somatic comorbidities. The overlap of these disorders with psychiatric conditions has led both the public and the medical specialists to dichotomize these disorders artificially into "physical," by implication, "real" disorders; and "psychological," by implication, "not real" disorders. This classification ignores the unity of brain and body and hinders progress in understanding these disorders. COPC connotes a nonassumptive neutral position, appropriately attributing no assumed pathophysiology to the disorder, in contrast to other terms, such as "medically unexplained syndrome," subtly suggesting a psychological process, more strongly implied in the term "functional."

PREVALENCE
The prevalence of COPCs is unknown, ranging from 20% to >50% depending on which symptom is being assessed and how much overlap exists across disorders. A large study from 28 countries (about 400,000 participants) found a prevalence of headache of 54%, stomachache 50%, and backache 37%, occurring at least once a month for at least 6 mo.

Females had a higher prevalence of having all 3 complaints when compared to males; the prevalence increased with age. These three pain syndromes, headache, stomach-ache and backache, frequently coexist.

IBS and chronic abdominal pain affect 6–20% of children and adolescents. Idiopathic musculoskeletal pain affects about 16% of schoolchildren age 5-16 yr and is often associated with sleep disturbances, headache, abdominal pain, daytime tiredness, and feeling sad (see Chapter 193). Migraines present >6 mo occur in about 8% of the population (children and adolescents <20 yr) (see Chapter 613.1). **Fibromyalgia** is present in 1.2–6% (see Chapter 193.3). The prevalence of chronic disabling fatigue increases during adolescence from about 1.9% at age 13 to 3% at 18 yr (see Chapter 147.1). As with most COPCs, fibromyalgia has many comorbid disorders, such as sleep disturbance, fatigue, headache, sore throat, joint pain, and abdominal pain. The American College of Rheumatology definition of fibromyalgia incorporates some of these comorbid conditions.

SYMPTOM/DISORDER OVERLAP
Diagnostic criteria of many of these disorders overlap with one another, making differentiation between two disorders more of a semantic issue rather than a clinical differentiation. **Chronic fatigue syndrome (CFS)**, clinically the most concerning symptom, shares many of the diagnostic criteria with fibromyalgia. Patients with a single pain condition, such as fibromyalgia, CFS, IBS, multiple chemical sensitivity (MCS), headaches, or temporomandibular joint disorder (TMJD), will typically have another disorder. This overlap of symptoms may reflect a shared pathophysiology, possibly a central nervous system (CNS) dysfunction, as was implied in the prior term "central sensitization syndrome". A CNS pathophysiology would also explain the "invisibility" of these disorders to usual screening tools that most often target an end organ.

This chapter was made possible with the support of an Advancing Healthier Wisconsin 5520298 grant.

COPCs also harbor many symptoms that are not strictly "pain," although they may be equally or more disabling. Adolescents seen in a tertiary referral center with a **functional gastrointestinal disorder (FGID)** also manifest dizziness, chronic nausea, chronic fatigue and sleep disturbance, as well as migraines. Up to 50% of adolescents complain of weekly fatigue, and 15%, daily fatigue.

Migraine headaches are frequently associated with anxiety and depression. **Anxiety** also predicts the persistence of migraine headaches. Sleep disturbance and migraine also interact closely. Poor sleep can trigger a migraine or a migraine cluster; migraine headache itself disturbs sleep. Juvenile fibromyalgia is associated with sleep disturbances such as prolonged sleep latency, frequent awakening, less total sleep time, and periodic limb movements. Adult patients with IBS also have sleep disturbances, correlating with anxiety, depression, and stress.

The comorbidities of **hypermobility Ehlers-Danlos (hEDS)** and **postural orthostatic tachycardia syndrome (POTS)** have been significant. Patients with hEDS may complain of widespread and sometimes debilitating pain with or after activity, severe fatigue, handwriting difficulties, "cracking" of joints, joint swelling, joint dislocation, subluxation, or back pain. The chronic pain reduces exercise tolerance, with poorer quality of life and an ever-worsening cycle because exercise is a key piece of management. Patients with FGID may also have hEDS, fibromyalgia, chronic pains, and higher somatizations scores than those with organic gastrointestinal (GI) disorders.

Diagnosis of **pediatric POTS** requires an increase in heart rate >40 beats/min in the 1st 10 min of upright tilt test associated with orthostatic symptoms. POTS is also associated with multiple comorbidities, including sleep disruption, chronic pain, Raynaud-like symptoms, GI abnormalities, and less frequently headaches, syncope, and urinary complaints. Patients with both POTS and hEDS usually have more migraines and syncope than those with POTS alone. The prevalence of comorbid disorders in children with COPC is identical whether they have POTS or hEDS.

PSYCHIATRIC COMORBIDITIES
Many of these disorders have significant psychiatric comorbidities. Juvenile fibromyalgia is associated with anxiety disorders and major mood disorders. Children with medically unexplained symptoms generally have more anxiety and depression than children with other chronic disorders. Other associations include disruptive behaviors, symptom internalization, fearfulness, greater dependency, hyperactivity, and concern about sickness.

PREDISPOSING FACTORS
Female gender and older age (adolescence) increase the risk of COPCs. Certain conditions (e.g., headache) are more common in males or have similar prevalence across genders during childhood, but the prevalence in females increases after puberty. Trauma or posttraumatic stress disorder increases psychological comorbidities in juvenile fibromyalgia. Some studies suggest that anxiety predisposes to chronic pain. A population-based study following children from 18 mo to 14 yr of age suggested that maternal psychological distress in early childhood and depressive and pain complaints in preadolescence increase the risk of recurrent abdominal pain at age 14. Postinfectious IBS is an identifiable risk factor for new-onset anxiety, depression, and sleep disruption in adults. Children with recurrent abdominal pain often have parents with abdominal pain. It is unclear if this association is caused by a common environmental/genetic factor or a learned behavior of the child imitating the parent.

NATURAL HISTORY
The natural history of COPC is not well known. Chronic disabling fatigue in the general adolescent population persists 2-3 yr in about 25% of patients, but only 8% of youth affected at age 13 still had the complaints at ages 16 and 18. A meta-analysis suggests that the prognosis of CFS in children is usually good, with a small minority having persistent disabling symptoms. The patient's belief in an underlying physical disorder and the presence of psychiatric comorbidities predicts a poorer outcome.

In a study of children with FGID, the outcome depended on specific variables. Those who perceived their abdominal pain as more threatening,

with high levels of pain catastrophization and little capacity to cope with pain because of reduced activity levels, had a poorer outcome. This "high pain dysfunctional profile" subgroup was predominantly female (70%) with a mean age of 12.2 yr. Two thirds of this subgroup still complained of FGID at follow-up, vs about one third of those in the other groups. These groups included a "high pain adaptive profile" group with similar pain levels but better adaptive skills and less catastrophization, predominantly slightly younger (11.8 yr) females, and a "low pain adaptive profile" group, slightly younger (11.1 yr), with equal males and females but less abdominal pain, better coping mechanisms, and less impairment of daily activities. In the high pain dysfunctional profile group, 41% had both FGID and nonabdominal chronic pain at follow-up, vs 11% in the high pain adaptive and 17% in the low pain adaptive group. Another study following children age 4-16.6 yr with IBS demonstrated resolution of symptoms in 58%, usually without medication. The differences between these studies may result from the age of the groups, with better outcome in the younger patients, as well as the number of comorbidities and psychological profile.

PROPOSED PATHOPHYSIOLOGY
There may be dysfunction in the hypothalamic-hypophyseal-adrenal axis, circadian patterns, autonomic responses, some aspects of CNS processing, the inflammatory immune response, and the musculoskeletal system. Vagal tone measured by heart rate variability is decreased in some children with FGID symptoms and in children with COPCs. Alterations in the autonomic nervous system may affect the immune system, as well as circadian patterns. The stress response may increase muscle tone, which in turn leads to body aches and tension headaches. In fibromyalgia the cortisol response is altered, with lower cortisol levels on awakening and throughout the day. **Orthostatic intolerance** from autonomic abnormalities may also contribute to poor concentration from brain hypoperfusion and blood pooling in the lower extremities.

The pathophysiology has been better studied in myalgic encephalomyelitis (ME)/CFS (Chapter 147.1). ME/CFS has been associated with joint hypermobility, orthostatic intolerance, decreased range of motion, and reduced activity. These patients demonstrate excessive glial activation resulting in neuroexcitation, neuroinflammation, and possibly neurodegeneration. These features may contribute to the cognitive issues and fatigue present in this disorder.

Neuroinflammation and other changes in processing may lead to abnormal descending inhibitory pain pathways, resulting in distal pain and "central sensitization." The malfunction of descending antinociceptive pathways allows pain to spread in the body, associated with increased activity of the nociceptive facilitator pathways. These facilitator pathways are further activated by psychological factors, such as catastrophization, depression, lack of acceptance, and hypervigilance. Other signals such as pressure, sound, heat, and cold are also aberrantly processed, with activation of areas of the brain that are typically activated only by acute pain stimuli, such as the insula, prefrontal cortex, and anterior cingulate cortex, as well as some regions usually not involved in pain processing.

TREATMENT
As general rules, *chronic pain should never be treated with opioids*, and *cognitive-behavioral therapy (CBT) and a gradually progressive exercise program constitute the cornerstones of treatment*. The complex comorbid nature of COPCs typically requires a multidisciplinary approach. Since neither CBT nor exercise will have any effect in the absence of full patient engagement and understanding, the team must include the family and the patient, a pain psychologist with experience in CBT, a physical therapist, and the primary care physician. Depending on comorbid conditions, rheumatology, neurology, or gastroenterology may have important roles for symptom management and possible alternative diagnosis. Depending on the initial symptomatology, the differential diagnosis should include inflammatory bowel disease, celiac disease, juvenile idiopathic arthritis, systemic lupus erythematosus, dermatomyositis, autoinflammatory disorders, Fabry disease, porphyrias, hereditary sensory-autonomic neuropathies, and Ehlers-Danlos syndrome.

When a thorough evaluation for a structural cause of symptoms is unrevealing, an important next step is patient and family **education**. This should include the common presentation, the expectation that "markers" for these types of disorders would typically be absent, and the presence of solid management tools with high probability of improvement. Families and patients need to receive encouragement to stop seeking a "magic diagnosis and cure" and to begin the path to full recovery. Without this step, critical patient engagement in the treatment will not occur. In our practice, we sometimes call *functional* disorders a problem of "software," in contrast to *structural* issues that would involve "hardware." We explain that successful management must change the software, not just mask symptoms. Approaches that accomplish such a goal include CBT, and a rehabilitative program that may require physical therapy, vigorous exercise program with interval training, meditation, and/or yoga. Patients are often deconditioned and may need to start with a very low level of physical activity. In addition, their exercise tolerance may be significantly hampered by an orthostatic intolerance syndrome (e.g., POTS). For these reasons, we frequently recommend starting with a *water aerobics* program, which provides several benefits: (1) very low gravitational force, so the patient can be set up for success, working only on conditioning and not simultaneously fighting an orthostatic challenge; (2) builds both limb and core strength; and (3) gentle on joints for those with arthralgias or a hypermobility syndrome. When water is unavailable, we recommend starting with a recumbent exercise program such as a recumbent stationary bike. In both circumstances, we then slowly introduce upright aerobic activities on land over 2-3 mo. Strength exercises are also useful. A Cochrane Review in adults with painful disorders showed exercise to have minimal side effects, to improve functionality, reduce pain, and improve quality of life. Patients with fibromyalgia who undergo a 3 mo multidisciplinary program with twice-weekly physical therapy and CBT benefited in function and physical activity level, and most importantly continued to exercise regularly at 1 yr follow-up. Pharmacologic interventions have less impact than nonmedical treatments.

When children are missing school or are homebound, it is important to work closely with the school to encourage reentry to school. This may require modifying the school schedule initially, starting with fewer hours at school, and providing extra time for homework on days that the children are not feeling well.

Although medications such as tricyclic antidepressants are often added to the treatment, the improvement with these medications for chronic pain is minimal, and the side effects need to be considered. Nonetheless, **amitriptyline** is often used because it helps in treating headaches and abdominal pain and improves sleep quality, a critical element to manage any chronic pain condition.

Bibliography is available at Expert Consult.

147.1 Chronic Fatigue Syndrome

Mark R. Magnusson

Chronic fatigue syndrome (**CFS**), also known as **myalgic encephalomyelitis (ME)**, is a complex, diverse, and debilitating illness characterized by chronic or intermittent fatigue accompanied by select symptoms and occurring in children, adolescents, and adults. The combination of fatigue and other symptoms interferes significantly with daily activities and has no identified medical explanation (Fig. 147.1). The fatigue does not require exertion by the patient, nor does rest relieve it. Some consider **postexertion malaise,** or worsening of the fatigue with additional symptoms after mental or physical exertion and lasting >24 hr, to be characteristic of CFS. A definitive causal agent or process has not been identified, although the differential diagnosis includes infectious, inflammatory, metabolic, genetic, and autoimmune diseases. Our understanding of this condition is largely from studies of adults and adolescents, with limited descriptions of chronic fatiguing illnesses in younger children.

The illness was formally defined in 1988 as *chronic fatigue syndrome* because persistent unexplained fatigue was considered the principal

and invariable physical symptom. A variety of other names have been used to describe the illness, including chronic mononucleosis, chronic Epstein-Barr virus (EBV) infection, postinfection syndrome, and immune dysfunction syndrome. Several case definitions have been developed and are in use in both clinical care and research (Table 147.1).

The Institute of Medicine (IOM) 2015 recommendations apply to all ages and include a special focus on pediatrics. The IOM suggested new diagnostic criteria and a new name, **systemic exertion intolerance disease (SEID)**, to emphasize the postexertion malaise criterion and better understand the illness (Table 147.2). The most recent expert consensus report (June 2017) from the International Writing Group for Pediatric ME/CFS provides a primer for diagnosis and management.

EPIDEMIOLOGY
Based on worldwide studies, 0.2–2.3% of adolescents or children have CFS. Most epidemiology studies use the 1994 definition. CFS is more prevalent in adolescents than in younger children. The variation in CFS prevalence estimates may result from variations in case definition, study methodology and application, study population composition (specialty vs general practice or general population), and data collection (parent, self-reporting vs clinician evaluation). Gender distribution in children differs from that in adults, with a more equal distribution in children <15 yr old, while remaining 2-3–fold higher in females 15-18 yr old. Few studies have reported the incidence of CFS among children <10 yr old, leading to uncertainty in this group. In adolescents in The Netherlands, the pediatrician-diagnosed incidence of CFS/ME was 0.01%, and in the United Kingdom, 0.5%.

PATHOGENESIS
Although etiology and pathophysiology of CFS are unknown, some patients and clinicians correlate the onset with a recent episode of a viral illness such as infectious mononucleosis (10–12%) (EBV; see Chapter 281). A pathophysiologic relationship of CFS to infection is suggested because the symptoms and biologic markers elicited by the nonspecific innate host responses to infections in general are present in CFS. CFS-like illness after infectious mononucleosis is not predicted by viremia or altered host response to EBV infection but is associated with the severity of the primary infection. A wide variety of other candidate viral infections have been associated with postinfectious fatigue syndromes, particularly in adolescents and adults. There are ongoing efforts to determine if infections with these or other agents may produce the illness.

Similarities between CFS symptoms and those experienced by patients with autoimmune and other inflammatory disorders suggests primary perturbation of immune function in the pathogenesis of CFS. Hypo- and hypergammaglobulinemia, immunoglobulin subclass deficiencies, elevated levels of circulating immune complexes, altered helper/suppressor lymphocyte ratios, natural killer cell dysfunction, elevated cytokines, and monocyte dysfunction have been reported in adult patients with CFS. These findings have not been consistent among studies. CFS patients as a group differ from healthy controls, but most laboratory values of the immune parameters are not outside the normal range.

Autonomic nervous system (ANS) changes are suggested by the **orthostatic intolerance** (OI) experienced by some patients with CFS. OI syndromes with circulatory dysfunction include **neutrally mediated hypotension** and **postural orthostatic tachycardia syndrome** (POTS) (see Chapter 147) have been observed in some patients with CFS and could contribute to the syndrome. The pathophysiology of these manifestations among adolescents with CFS is unclear, but in postinfectious states could be associated with unreplenished fluid and electrolyte losses associated with acute infection or immune-mediated injury (autoantibodies directed against ANS).

Because the widespread musculoskeletal pain in CFS is similar to **fibromyalgia** (see Chapter 193.3), and because some consider these to be overlapping syndromes, fibromyalgia and CFS may share similarities in pathogenesis. Other hypotheses under investigation for the biologic basis of CFS involve alterations in energy metabolism (e.g., mitochondrion, particularly as related to exercise intolerance and postexertion malaise), alterations in sleep, the stress response, hypothalamic-pituitary

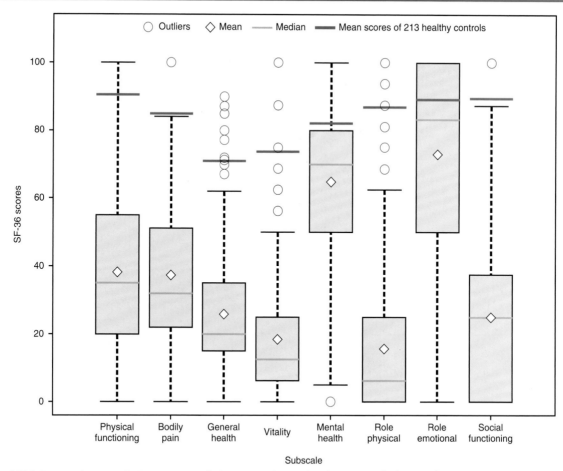

Fig. 147.1 Functional status* of 471 patients enrolled in CDC Multisite Clinical Assessment† of ME/CFS§—United States, September 2015. *Measured by box plots of scores in the 8 subscales of Short-Form Health Survey (SF-36) scores (25th and 75th percentile at *bottom* and *top* of box). SF-36 scores range from 0-100, with higher scores indicating better functioning. †https://www.cdc.gov/cfs/programs/clinical-assessment/index.html. §ME/CFS (myalgic encephalomyelitis/chronic fatigue syndrome) patients show significant impairment, particularly in vitality and physical functioning subscale scores, but with preservation of mental health and emotional role functioning. *(From Unger ER, Lin JMS, Brimmer DJ, et al: CDC Grand Rounds: Chronic fatigue syndrome—advancing research and clinical education, MMWR 65(50-51):1434–1438, 2016.)*

axis. Understanding CFS has proved so challenging because it likely represents more than 1 underlying pathophysiology. Current studies and guidelines are attempting to stratify or subgroup patients to address this possibility.

CLINICAL MANIFESTATIONS

The dominant symptom expressed by adolescents and adults is a substantial reduction or impairment in the ability to engage in preillness levels of activity, accompanied by fatigue (see Fig. 147.1). In younger children, who often do not spontaneously report symptoms, exertion induces behavioral changes, manifested by a lack of their usual energy and reduced participation in activities. In adolescents, fatigue and postexertion malaise may lead to decreased participation in school, family activities, and social exchange.

Cognitive impairment includes reported difficulties in concentrating, which are common and indicated by reduced participation in school, difficulty keeping up with homework, and drop in grades. Sleep may be impaired, and nonrestorative sleep is common. Other sleep complaints include difficulty falling asleep and staying asleep, whereas diagnosed sleep disorders, including restless legs syndrome, parasomnias, and sleep apnea, are less common. Myalgia and arthralgia may accompany fatigue and altered sleep. Sore throat and cervical lymph node tenderness can

occur but may be part of an inciting illness. Adolescents also have increased reports of headache, abdominal pain, nausea, and sensitivity to light and sound with amplified pain.

Patients diagnosed with CFS in primary care practices are more likely to report abrupt onset of their symptoms, often as part of an initial virus-like illness, whereas gradual onset is more common in those identified in population-based studies. School absenteeism is a major social issue. In one study, two thirds of adolescents missed >2 wk over a 6 wk observation period, and one third required home tutoring. Unlike school phobia, inactivity due to CFS persists on the weekends and during holidays the same as it does during the school week.

Although fatigue and accompanying symptoms are subjective, the magnitude of impairment of each component can be measured by questionnaires addressing pain and function or, in the case of suspected orthostatic instability, by recording routine supine and standing heart rate and blood pressure measurement's. Fatigue cannot be dismissed as a minor ailment. It generally manifests as lassitude, profound tiredness, intolerance of exertion with easy fatigability, and general malaise.

Abnormal physical examination findings are conspicuously absent, providing both reassurance and consternation for the patient, family, and physician. The presence of "alarm symptoms" such as weight loss, chest pain with exertion, paresthesia, dry mouth and eyes, fevers, diarrhea,

Table 147.1	Overview of Current Case Definitions for Systemic Exertion Intolerance Disease (SEID) and Past Definitions of Chronic Fatigue Syndrome or Myalgic Encephalomyelitis

SYMPTOM	SEID	CFS	ME
Fatigue and impairment of daily function	≥ 6 mo	≥ 6 mo	≥ 6 mo
Sudden onset	Yes	Yes	
Muscle weakness			Yes
Muscle pain		Yes	
Postexertional symptoms	Yes	Yes	Yes
Sleep disturbance	Yes		Yes
Memory or cognitive disturbances	Yes		Yes
Autonomic symptoms			Yes
Sore throat		Yes	
Lymph node involvement		Yes	
Cardiovascular symptoms	Yes		
Headaches		Yes	
Arthralgias		Yes	Yes

CFS, Chronic fatigue syndrome; ME, myalgic encephalomyelitis.
Data from Institute of Medicine: Beyond Myalgic Encephalomyelitis/Chronic Fatigue Syndrome Redefining an Illness. Washington, DC, National Academies Press 2015; Jason L, Evans M, Porter N, et al: The development of a revised Canadian myalgic encephalomyelitis chronic fatigue syndrome case definition. Am J Biochem Biotechnol 6:120 135, 2010; Reeves WC, Wagner D, Nisenbaum R, et al: Chronic fatigue syndrome—a clinically empirical approach to its definition and study. BMC Med 3:19, 2005.

Table 147.2	Criteria for Diagnosis of Myalgic Encephalomyelitis/Chronic Fatigue Syndrome (ME/CFS)

Patient has each of the following 3 symptoms at least half the time, to at least a moderately severe degree:
- A substantial reduction or impairment in the ability to engage in preillness levels of occupational, educational, social, or personal activities that persists for >6 mo and is accompanied by fatigue, which is often profound, is of new or definite onset (not lifelong), is not the result of ongoing excessive exertion, and is not substantially alleviated by rest.
- Postexertional malaise*
- Unrefreshing sleep*

Plus at least 1 of the 2 following manifestations (chronic, severe):
- Cognitive impairment*
- Orthostatic intolerance

*Frequency and severity of symptoms should be assessed. The diagnosis of ME/CFS should be questioned if patients do not have these symptoms at least half of the time with moderate, substantial, or severe intensity.
From Institute of Medicine: *Beyond myalgic encephalomyelitis/chronic fatigue syndrome: redefining an illness,* Washington, DC, 2015, National Academies Press.

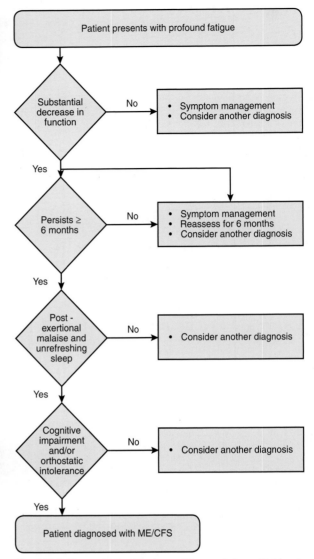

Fig. 147.2 Diagnostic algorithm for myalgic encephalomyelitis/chronic fatigue syndrome (ME/CFS). *(From Institute of Medicine: Beyond myalgic encephalomyelitis/chronic fatigue syndrome: redefining an illness, Washington, DC, 2015, National Academies Press.)*

cough, night sweats, and rash is uncommon and warrants consideration of a diagnosis other than CFS.

DIAGNOSIS

There are no pathognomonic signs or diagnostic tests for CFS. The diagnosis is clinically defined based on inclusion and exclusion criteria (Fig. 147.2). The diagnostic criteria are applicable to adults and adolescents >11 yr old because of the current requirement for a self-generated history. Whereas duration of symptoms is 3- 6 mo, depending on age, symptom management should not wait until this criterion is met.

CFS is difficult to diagnose in children, who may have difficulty describing their symptoms and articulating their concerns. Sole reliance on parental history can be fraught with confusion because parents may also struggle to interpret their children's symptoms and feelings in providing accurate historical information. A combination of child and parent reporting is most effective. It is important to document the child's activity levels and worsening of symptoms after physical or mental endeavors. Changes in participation in hobbies and family or other social activities can help identify the impact of CFS on function.

The diagnosis of CFS can be established only after other medical and psychiatric causes of fatigue and other symptoms, many of which are treatable, have been excluded. These include medical conditions presenting with chronic symptoms, such as hypothyroidism, adrenal insufficiency, respiratory and food allergies, sleep apnea, narcolepsy, substance abuse, posttraumatic stress disorder, adverse drug reactions, and obesity. A previously diagnosed medical condition with incomplete or uncertain resolution that may explain fatigue needs be considered.

Certain illnesses (e.g., fibromyalgia), amplified pain, and depression share similar symptoms with CFS but are not exclusionary diagnoses. These should be considered in the differential diagnosis in select cases. There is concern that CFS might be mistaken for readily identifiable psychiatric disorders such as anxiety and mood disorders, but evidence supports differences in their clinical presentation from CFS. CFS should not be diagnosed in persons with prior diagnosis of major depressive disorder with psychotic or melancholic features, bipolar affective disorders, schizophrenia of any subtype, delusional disorders of any subtype, dementia of any subtype, eating disorder of any type, or alcohol or other substance abuse within 2 yr before the onset of the chronic fatigue or any time thereafter.

Although evaluation of each patient should be individualized, initial laboratory evaluation should be limited to screening laboratory testing sufficient to provide reassurance of the lack of significant medical illness. Further evaluation should be directed primarily toward excluding treatable illnesses that may be suggested by the history, symptoms, signs, or physical exam findings present in specific patients.

MANAGEMENT

Management of CFS is based on relief of the core and most disruptive symptoms in the individual patient. The diagnostic criterion of 6 mo duration of illness should not delay evaluation and symptom management, since these may be initiated as soon as the child or adolescent presents with a CFS-like picture. Problems with sleep can be addressed by encouraging patients to adopt good sleep habits using standard sleep hygiene techniques. It may be beneficial to refer the patient to a sleep medicine specialist for the identification and treatment of sleep disorders and disturbances. Once pain is found not to be related to other specific disease of illness, nonpharmacologic treatment is indicated.

One of the nonpharmacologic approaches to pain management, **cognitive-behavioral therapy** (CBT), may also assist patient in managing and coping with CFS. Through explanation and changes in perception of the illness, CBT may help patients and their families develop coping skills and provide emotional support. Improved methods of coping may allow some improved function while living with the illness.

Comorbid psychiatric conditions such as anxiety require appropriate evaluation and intervention. Guided graded-exercise therapy may be beneficial and added to CBT.

While the overall goal is to help patients with CFS tolerate activity, children and adolescents with CFS should limit physical or mental efforts that result in aggravated symptoms. Return to school should be initiated gradually and systematically with the goal return to full-time attendance. Home tutoring, cyberschool, and partial attendance can be interim steps. Parents and clinicians can work with teachers and school administrators to define appropriate expectations for attendance and performance for children with CFS. Because of the crucial importance of learning socialization skills, even brief attendance in school or participation in school activities should be encouraged, remembering that too rapid remobilization usually exacerbates symptoms and should be avoided.

Continued **empathy and support** by the treating physician are crucial in maintaining a physician–parent–patient relationship that is conducive to managing this illness. Careful attention must be directed to family dynamics to identify and resolve family problems or psychopathology that may be contributing to children's perception of their symptoms.

PROGNOSIS

The natural history of CFS is highly variable, and patients and families understand that the symptoms will wax and wane. Children and adolescents with CFS appear to have a more optimistic outcome than adults, typically with an undulating course of gradual improvement over several years. Overall, a good functional outcome has been reported in up to 80% of patients. Poor prognostic factors include gradual onset, increased school absenteeism, lower socioeconomic status, chronic maternal health problems, and untreated comorbid individual and family psychiatric disorders. Favorable prognostic factors include patient control of the rehabilitation program, with continuing support from health professionals and family members, and improvement in orthostatic intolerance.

Bibliography is available at Expert Consult.

Immunology
免疫学

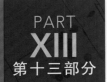

Section 1
Evaluation of the Immune System
第一篇
免疫系统评估

Chapter 148
Evaluation of Suspected Immunodeficiency

Kathleen E. Sullivan and Rebecca H. Buckley

第一百四十八章
可疑免疫缺陷评估

中文导读

本章主要介绍了对可疑免疫缺陷的初步评估和高级检测手段。初步评估包括免疫缺陷临床特征识别、病史、体格检查、家族史，以及血细胞计数和分类、各类免疫球蛋白水平等初筛实验；高级检测包括抗原特异性抗体、IgG亚类、B细胞和B细胞亚类计数、T细胞和T细胞亚类计数、T细胞功能、NK细胞计数和功能、吞噬细胞功能和黏附分子表达、补体CH50和AH50等检测。

Primary care physicians must have a high index of suspicion to diagnose immune system defects early enough to institute appropriate treatment before irreversible damage develops. Diagnosis can be difficult because most affected patients do not have abnormal physical features. The most typical manifestation of immunodeficiency in children is *recurrent sinopulmonary infections*. Although infections are common in children in general, an infection exceeding the expected frequency and usually involving multiple sites can suggest immunodeficiency. A single, severe, opportunistic, or unusual infection can also be the presentation of an immunodeficiency (Table 148.1). Increasingly recognized is the co-occurrence of autoimmune disease or inflammatory conditions and recurrent infections. Newborn screening for T-cell lymphopenia has been instituted in most states; this has led to the identification of some infants with immunodeficiency before any clear manifestations but is limited to T-cell deficiencies. Additional clues to immunodeficiency include failure to thrive with or without chronic diarrhea, persistent infections after receiving live vaccines, and chronic oral or cutaneous candidiasis (Tables 148.2 and 148.3).

With >300 distinct primary immunodeficiencies, in order to focus the diagnostic approach and appropriate testing. it is often useful to consider 5 categories: T-cell disorders, B-cell and antibody disorders, complement disorders, phagocytic disorders, and natural killer cell

Table 148.1	Predisposition to Specific Infections in Humans		
PATHOGEN	**PRESENTATION**	**AFFECTED GENE/ CHROMOSOMAL REGION**	**COMMENTS**
BACTERIA			
Streptococcus pneumoniae	Invasive disease	*IRAK4, MyD88, C1QA, C1QB, C1QC, C4A+C4B, C2, C3*	Also susceptible to other encapsulated bacteria
Neisseria	Invasive disease	C5, C6, C7, C8A, C8B, C8G, C9, properdin	Recurrent disease common
Burkholderia cepacia	Invasive disease not pulmonary colonization	*CYBB, CYBA, NCF1, NCF2*	Also susceptible to staphylococcal and fungal infections
Nocardia	Invasive disease	*CYBB, CYBA, NCF1, NCF2*	Also susceptible to staphylococcal and fungal infections
Mycobacteria	Usually nontuberculous mycobacteria	IL12B, IL12RB1, IKBKG, IFNGR1, IFNGR2, STAT1 (loss of function)	Also susceptible to *Salmonella typhi* infections
VIRUSES			
Herpes simplex virus	Herpes simplex encephalitis	*TRAF3, TRIF, TBK, UNC93B1, TLR3, STAT1*	Age of onset is typically outside the neonatal period.
Epstein-Barr virus	Severe infectious mononucleosis, hemophagocytic syndrome	*SH2DIA, XIAP, ITK, CD27, PRF1, STXBP2, UNC13D, LYST, RAB27A, STX11, AP3B1*	Fulminant infectious mononucleosis, malignant and nonmalignant lymphoproliferative disorders, dysgammaglobulinemia, autoimmunity
Papillomavirus	Warts	*RHOH, EVER1, EVER2, CXCR4, DOCK8, GATA2, STK4, SPINK5*	Warts are often progressive despite therapy.
Global susceptibility to viral infection	Severe, progressive viral infections	All types of severe combined immune deficiency, *IFNAR2*	Presentation depends on virus and infected organ
FUNGI			
Candida	Mucocutaneous candida	*AIRE*, STAT1 (gain of function), *CARD9, STAT3, IL17F, IL17RC, IL17RA, ACT1*	*AIRE* deficiency is associated with endocrinopathies, STAT1 (GOF) is associated with autoimmunity
Dermatophytes	Tissue invasion	*CARD9*	Autosomal recessive
Aspergillus	Deep infections	*CYBB, CYBA, NCF1, NCF2*	
Environmental fungi	Deep infections	*CYBB, CYBA, NCF1, NCF2, GATA2,* STAT1 (gain of function), *CD40L*	

Table 148.2	Characteristic Clinical Patterns in Some Primary Immunodeficiencies	
FEATURES		**DIAGNOSIS**
IN NEWBORNS AND YOUNG INFANTS (0-6 mo)		
Hypocalcemia, unusual facies and ears, heart disease		22q11.2 deletion syndrome, DiGeorge anomaly
Delayed umbilical cord detachment, leukocytosis, recurrent infections		Leukocyte adhesion defect
Persistent thrush, failure to thrive, pneumonia, diarrhea		Severe combined immunodeficiency
Bloody stools, draining ears, atopic eczema		Wiskott-Aldrich syndrome
IN INFANTS AND YOUNG CHILDREN (6 mo to 5 yr)		
Recurrent staphylococcal abscesses, staphylococcal pneumonia with pneumatocele formation, coarse facial features, pruritic dermatitis		Hyper-IgE syndrome, PGM3 deficiency
Persistent thrush, nail dystrophy, endocrinopathies		Autoimmune polyendocrinopathy, candidiasis, ectodermal dysplasia
Short stature, fine hair, severe varicella		Cartilage hair hypoplasia with short-limbed dwarfism
Oculocutaneous albinism, recurrent infection, hemophagocytic syndrome		Chédiak-Higashi syndrome, Griscelli syndrome, Hermansky-Pudlak syndrome

disorders (Table 148.4 and Fig. 148.1).

The initial evaluation of immunologic function includes a thorough history, physical examination, and family history (Table 148.5). Over 10 immunodeficiencies are X-linked, and a growing number are autosomal dominant with variable expressivity and/or incomplete penetrance. Close attention to physical signs of autoimmune disease or end-organ effects from recurrent infections should be noted. The history of infections should include the age of onset, severity, involved locations, and assessment of the underlying microbial cause. Viral, bacterial, fungal, and mycobacterial infections all require distinct arms of the immune system for eradication; therefore identification of microbiologic causes of infection can be extremely helpful in defining the deficiency states in people with primary immunodeficiencies.

Most immunologic defects can be excluded at minimal cost with the proper choice of screening tests, which should be broadly informative,

reliable, and cost-effective (Table 148.6 and Figs. 148.2 and 148.3). A complete blood count (CBC) with differential is the initial study if neutropenia is a consideration but is less recognized as a screening test for T-cell defects. Lymphopenia is seen the majority of T-cell defects. If an infant's neutrophil count is persistently elevated in the absence of any signs of infection, a leukocyte adhesion deficiency should be suspected. Normal lymphocyte counts are higher in infancy and early childhood than later in life (Fig. 148.4). Knowledge of normal values for absolute lymphocyte counts at various ages in infancy and childhood is crucial in the detection of T-cell defects. Additional clues from the CBC include absence of Howell-Jolly bodies, which argues against congenital asplenia. Normal platelet size or count excludes Wiskott-Aldrich syndrome. When immunodeficiency is suspected, obtaining IgG, IgA, IgM, and IgE levels can be a useful strategy, since antibody defects are the most common type of immunodeficiency. Immunoglobulin levels must be interpreted

| Table 148.3 | Clinical Aids to the Diagnosis of Immunodeficiency |

SUGGESTIVE OF B-CELL DEFECT (HUMORAL IMMUNODEFICIENCY)

Recurrent bacterial infections of the upper and lower respiratory tracts

Recurrent skin infections, meningitis, osteomyelitis secondary to encapsulated bacteria (*Streptococcus pneumoniae. Haemophilus influenzae. Staphylococcus aureus. Neisseria meningitidis*)

Paralysis after vaccination with live-attenuated poliovirus

Reduced levels of immunoglobulins

SUGGESTIVE OF T-CELL DEFECT (COMBINED IMMUNODEFICIENCY)

Systemic illness after vaccination with any live virus or bacille Calmette-Guérin (BCG)

Unusual life-threatening complication after infection with benign viruses (giant cell pneumonia with measles; varicella pneumonia)

Chronic oral candidiasis after age 6 mo

Chronic mucocutaneous candidiasis

Graft-versus-host disease after blood transfusion

Reduced lymphocyte counts for age

Low levels of immunoglobulins

Absence of lymph nodes and tonsils

Small thymus

Chronic diarrhea

Failure to thrive

Recurrent infections with opportunistic organisms

SUGGESTIVE OF MACROPHAGE DYSFUNCTION

Disseminated atypical mycobacterial infection, recurrent Salmonella infection

Fatal infection after BCG vaccination

CONGENITAL SYNDROMES WITH IMMUNODEFICIENCY

Ataxia-telangiectasia: ataxia, telangiectasia

Autoimmune polyglandular syndrome: hypofunction of 1 or more endocrine organs, chronic mucocutaneous candidiasis

Cartilage-hair hypoplasia: short-limbed dwarfism, sparse hair, neutropenia

Wiskott-Aldrich syndrome: thrombocytopenia, male gender, eczema

Chédiak–Higashi syndrome: oculocutaneous albinism, nystagmus, recurrent bacterial infections, peripheral neuropathies

DiGeorge syndrome (22q deletion syndrome): unusual facies, heart defect, hypocalcemia

SUGGESTIVE OF ASPLENIA

Heterotaxia. complex congenital heart disease, Howell-Jolly bodies on blood smear, sickle cell anemia

From Kliegman RM, Lye PS, Bordini BJ, ET AL, editors: *Nelson pediatric symptom-based diagnosis*, Philadelphia, 2018, Elsevier, p 750.

| Table 148.4 | Characteristic Features of Primary Immunodeficiency |

CHARACTERISTIC	PREDOMINANT T-CELL DEFECT	PREDOMINANT B-CELL DEFECT	GRANULOCYTE DEFECT	CYTOLYTIC DEFECT	COMPLEMENT DEFECT
Age at onset of infection	Early onset, usually 2-6 mo	Onset after maternal antibodies diminish, usually after 5-7 mo, later childhood to adulthood	Early onset most frequently	Childhood onset generally	Onset at any age
Specific pathogens involved	Bacteria: common gram-positive and gram-negative bacteria and mycobacteria	Bacteria: pneumococci, streptococci, staphylococci, *Haemophilus, Campylobacter, Mycoplasma*	Bacteria: staphylococci, *Serratia, Salmonella,* mycobacteria	None usually	Bacteria: encapsulated organisms (C1, C4, C2, C3), *Neisseria* (FP, FD, FH, FI, C3, C5, C6, C7, C8, C9)
	Viruses: CMV, EBV, adenovirus, parainfluenza 3, varicella, enterovirus	Viruses: enterovirus*	None generally	CMV, EBV	None generally
	Fungi: *Candida* and *Pneumocystis jiroveci*	Fungi and parasites: *Giardia*, Cryptosporidia	Fungi and parasites: *Candida, Nocardia, Aspergillus*	None generally	None generally
Affected organs	Extensive mucocutaneous candidiasis, lungs, failure to thrive, protracted diarrhea	Recurrent sinopulmonary infections, chronic gastrointestinal symptoms, malabsorption, arthritis, enteroviral meningoencephalitis*	Skin: abscesses, impetigo, cellulitis. Lymph nodes: suppurative adenitis. Oral cavity: gingivitis, mouth ulcers. Internal organs: abscesses, osteomyelitis	Hemophagocytic syndrome can affect any organ.	Deep or systemic infections
Special features	Graft-vs-host disease caused by maternal engraftment or nonirradiated blood transfusion. Postvaccination disseminated BCG or varicella. Autoimmunity common in mild-moderate T-cell defects	Autoimmunity. Lymphoreticular malignancy: lymphoma, thymoma	Prolonged attachment of umbilical cord, poor wound healing		SLE (C1, C4, C2), Glomerulonephritis (C3), atypical hemolytic-uremic syndrome (FH, FI, MCP, C3, FB)

*X-linked (Bruton) agammaglobulinemia.

BCG, Bacille Calmette-Guérin; CMV, cytomegalovirus; EBV, Epstein-Barr virus; SLE, systemic lupus erythematosus.

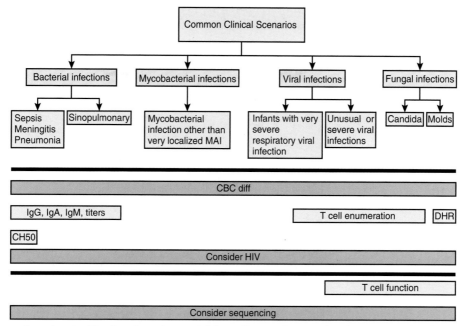

Fig. 148.1 Diagnostic testing algorithm for primary immunodeficiency diseases. Common clinical scenarios are listed at the *top*. The 1st tier of testing is listed below each category between the *dark lines*. The 2nd tier of testing is located below the 2nd *dark line*. CBC, Complete blood count; DHR, dihydrorhodamine; MAI, *Mycobacterium avium-intracellulare* infection.

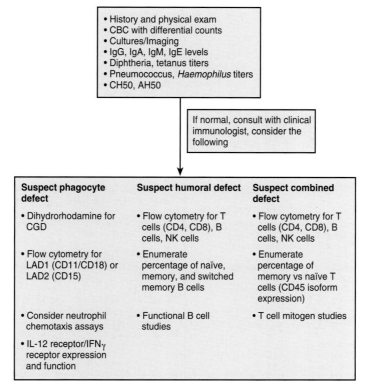

Fig. 148.2 Initial workup and follow-up studies of patients with suspected immunodeficiency. Consultation with a clinical immunologist is recommended to guide advanced testing and interpret results. CBC, Complete blood count; CGD, chronic granulomatous disease; LAD, leukocyte adhesion defect; NK, natural killer cell; IL, interleukin; IFN, interferon. *(From Kliegman RM, Lye PS, Bordini BJ, et al, editors:* Nelson pediatric symptom-based diagnosis, *Philadelphia, 2018, Elsevier, p 753.)*

Table 148.5	Special Physical Features Associated With Immunodeficiency Disorders

CLINICAL FEATURES	DISORDERS
DERMATOLOGIC	
Eczema	Wiskott-Aldrich syndrome, IPEX, hyper-IgE syndromes, hypereosinophilia syndromes, IgA deficiency
Sparse and/or hypopigmented hair	Cartilage-hair hypoplasia, Chédiak-Higashi syndrome, Griscelli syndrome
Ocular telangiectasia	Ataxia-telangiectasia
Oculocutaneous albinism	Chédiak-Higashi syndrome
Severe dermatitis	Omenn syndrome
Erythroderma	Omenn syndrome, SCID, graft-vs-host disease, Comel-Netherton syndrome
Recurrent abscesses with pulmonary pneumatoceles	Hyper-IgE syndromes
Recurrent organ granulomas or abscesses, lung, liver, and rectum especially	CGD
Recurrent abscesses or cellulitis	CGD, hyper-IgE syndrome, leukocyte adhesion defect
Cutaneous granulomas	Ataxia telangiectasia, SCID, CVID, RAG deficiency
Oral ulcers	CGD, SCID, congenital neutropenia
Periodontitis, gingivitis, stomatitis	Neutrophil defects
Oral or nail candidiasis	T-cell immune defects, combined defects (SCIDs); mucocutaneous candidiasis; hyper-IgE syndromes; IL-12, -17, -23 deficiencies; *CARD9* deficiency; STAT1 deficiency
Vitiligo	B-cell defects, mucocutaneous candidiasis
Alopecia	B-cell defects, mucocutaneous candidiasis
Chronic conjunctivitis	B-cell defects
EXTREMITIES	
Clubbing of nails	Chronic lung disease caused by antibody defects
Arthritis	Antibody defects, Wiskott-Aldrich syndrome, hyper-IgM syndrome
ENDOCRINOLOGIC	
Hypoparathyroidism	DiGeorge syndrome, mucocutaneous candidiasis
Endocrinopathies (autoimmune)	Mucocutaneous candidiasis
Diabetes, hypothyroid	IPEX and IPEX-like syndromes
Growth hormone deficiency	X-linked agammaglobulinemia
Gonadal dysgenesis	Mucocutaneous candidiasis
HEMATOLOGIC	
Hemolytic anemia	B- and T-cell immune defects, ALPS
Thrombocytopenia, small platelets	Wiskott-Aldrich syndrome
Neutropenia	Hyper-IgM syndrome, Wiskott-Aldrich variant, CGD
Immune thrombocytopenia	B-cell immune defects, ALPS
SKELETAL	
Short-limb dwarfism	Short-limb dwarfism with T- and/or B-cell immune defects
Bony dysplasia	ADA deficiency, cartilage-hair hypoplasia

ADA, Adenosine deaminase; ALPS, autoimmune lymphoproliferative syndrome; CGD, chronic granulomatous disease; CVID, common variable immunodeficiency; IPEX, X-linked immune dysfunction enteropathy polyendocrinopathy; SCID, severe combined immunodeficiency.
From Goldman L, Ausiello D: *Cecil textbook of medicine,* ed 22, Philadelphia, 2004, Saunders, p 1599.

Table 148.6	Initial Screening Immunologic Testing of the Child With Recurrent Infections

COMPLETE BLOOD COUNT, DIFFERENTIAL, AND ERYTHROCYTE SEDIMENTATION RATE

Absolute lymphocyte count (normal result rules against T-cell defect)

Absolute neutrophil count (normal result rules against congenital or acquired neutropenia and [usually] both forms of leukocyte adhesion deficiency, in which elevated counts are present even between infections)

Platelet count (normal result excludes Wiskott-Aldrich syndrome)

Howell-Jolly bodies (absence rules against asplenia)

Erythrocyte sedimentation rate (normal result indicates chronic bacterial or fungal infection unlikely)

SCREENING TESTS FOR B-CELL DEFECTS

IgG, IgA, IgM (low in most antibody defects)

Isohemagglutinins (low in agammaglobulinemia)

Antibody titers tetanus, diphtheria, *Haemophilus influenzae*, and pneumococcus (low in most antibody defects)

SCREENING TESTS FOR T-CELL DEFECTS

Absolute lymphocyte count (normal result indicates T-cell defect unlikely)

Flow cytometry to examine for the presence of naïve T cells (CD3$^+$CD45RA$^+$ cells)

SCREENING TESTS FOR PHAGOCYTIC CELL DEFECTS

Microscopy (abnormal in some neutropenias)

Respiratory burst assay (abnormal in chronic granulomatous disease)

SCREENING TEST FOR COMPLEMENT DEFICIENCY

CH_{50} (nearly absent in classical pathway and terminal component deficiencies)

AH_{50} (nearly absent in alternative pathway and terminal component deficiencies)

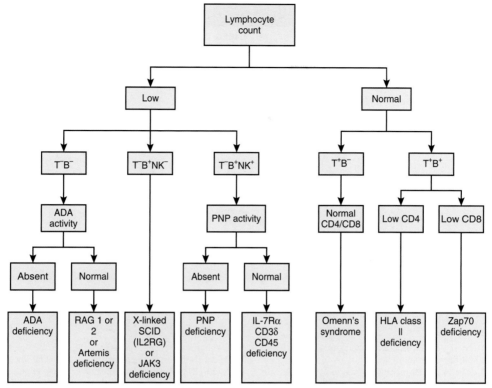

Fig. 148.3 Algorithm for evaluating the most common deficiencies of cell-mediated immunity. ADA, Adenosine deaminase; PNP, purine nucleoside phosphorylase. *(From Leung DYM, Szefler SJ, Bonilla FA, et al, editors: Pediatric allergy: principles and practice, ed 3, St Louis, 2016, Elsevier, p 68.)*

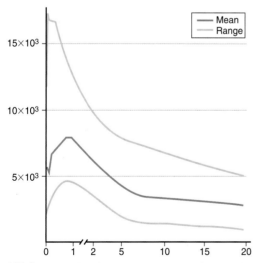

Fig. 148.4 Absolute lymphocyte counts in a normal individual during maturation. *(Data graphed from Altman PL: Blood and other body fluids. Prepared under the auspices of the Committee on Biological Handbooks, Washington, DC, 1961, Federation of American Societies for Experimental Biology.)*

within the context of age-specific normative data.

ADVANCED TESTING

Additional testing should be focused based on the phenotype and suspected category of immune deficiency (Table 148.7; see Figs. 148.2

and 148.3). For patients with recurrent sinopulmonary infections in whom an antibody defect is suspected, further attention to antibody testing may be revealing. In addition to Ig levels, responses to vaccines should also be pursued in this setting. A small but significant subset of patients with antibody deficiencies will have normal Ig levels but abnormal function, as detected by poor responses to vaccines. When hypogammaglobulinemia is identified, it is important to determine whether it is primary or secondary. Patients receiving corticosteroids or who have protein-losing states (nephrosis, protein-losing enteropathy) often have low serum IgG concentrations but produce normal responses to vaccines. Thus, if Ig levels are low, it is crucial before starting immune globulin replacement therapy that antibody titers to vaccines are measured. Antibody titers are not interpretable after the patient has received a blood transfusion, fresh-frozen plasma, or immune globulin therapy.

One useful test for B-cell function is to determine the presence and titer of **isohemagglutinins**, or natural antibodies to type A and B red blood cell polysaccharide antigens. This test measures predominantly IgM antibodies. Isohemagglutinins may be absent normally in the first 2 yr of life and are always absent if the patient is blood type AB.

Because most infants and children are immunized with diphtheria-tetanus-pertussis (dTP), conjugated *Haemophilus influenzae* type b, and pneumococcal conjugate vaccine, it is often informative to test for specific antibodies to diphtheria, tetanus, *H. influenzae* polyribose phosphate, and pneumococcal antigens. If the titers are low, measurement of antibodies to diphtheria or tetanus toxoids before and 2-8 wk after a pediatric dTP or dT booster is helpful in assessing the capacity to form IgG antibodies to protein antigens. To evaluate a patient's ability to respond to polysaccharide antigens, antipneumococcal antibodies can be measured before and 4-8 wk after immunization with 23-valent unconjugated pneumococcal polysaccharide vaccine in patients ≥2 yr old. Antibodies detected in these tests are of the IgG isotype. These antibody studies can be performed in several different laboratories, but

Table 148.7	Laboratory Tests in Immunodeficiency	
SCREENING TESTS	**ADVANCED TESTS**	**RESEARCH/SPECIAL TESTS**
B-CELL DEFICIENCY		
IgG, IgM, IgA, and IgE levels	B-cell enumeration (CD19 or CD20)	Advanced B-cell phenotyping
Isohemagglutinin titers		Biopsies (e.g., lymph nodes)
Ab response to vaccine antigens (e.g., tetanus, diphtheria, pneumococci, *Haemophilus influenzae*)	Ab responses to boosters or to new vaccines	Ab responses to special antigens (e.g., bacteriophage φX174), mutation analysis
T-CELL DEFICIENCY		
Lymphocyte count	T-cell subset enumeration (CD3, CD4, CD8)	Advanced flow cytometry
Chest x-ray examination for thymic size*	Proliferative responses to mitogens, antigens, allogeneic cells	Enzyme assays (e.g., ADA, PNP)
TRECs	22q11.2 deletion analysis	Mutation analysis
		T-cell activation studies
PHAGOCYTIC DEFICIENCY		
WBC count, morphology	Adhesion molecule assays (e.g., CD11b/ CD18, selectin ligand)	Mutation analysis
		Macrophage functional testing
Respiratory burst assay	Mutation analysis	
COMPLEMENT DEFICIENCY		
CH$_{50}$ activity	AH$_{50}$, activity	Specific component assays

*In infants only.

Ab, Antibody; ADA, adenosine deaminase; C, complement; CH, hemolytic complement; G6PD, glucose-6-phosphate dehydrogenase; HLA, human leukocyte antigen; Ig, immunoglobulin; MPO, myeloperoxidase; NADPH, nicotinamide adenine dinucleotide phosphate; PNP, purine nucleoside phosphorylase; TRECs, T-cell receptor rearrangement excision circle; WBC, white blood cell; φX, phage antigen.

it is important to choose a reliable laboratory and to use the same laboratory for pre- and postimmunization titers.

Patients with defective B-cell maturation due to a class-switching defects produce neither IgA nor IgG antibodies normally. IgM is normal or elevated. Vaccine responses are uniformly low. If antibody responses to vaccines are normal and the IgG level is low, studies should be performed to evaluate the possible loss of immunoglobulins through the urinary or gastrointestinal tract (nephrotic syndrome, protein-losing enteropathies, intestinal lymphangiectasia). Another common confounder is the use of rituximab or corticosteroids, leading to hypogammaglobulinemia. Very high serum concentrations of 1 or more Ig classes suggest HIV infection, chronic granulomatous disease, chronic inflammation, or autoimmune lymphoproliferative syndrome.

IgG subclass measurements are seldom helpful in assessing immune function in young children with recurrent infections. They are strongly developmentally regulated with highly variable production in early childhood. It is difficult to know the biologic significance of the various mild to moderate deficiencies of IgG subclasses, particularly when completely asymptomatic individuals have been described as totally lacking IgG1, IgG2, IgG4, and/or IgA1 because of Ign heavy-chain gene deletions. Many healthy children have been described as having low levels of IgG2 but normal responses to polysaccharide antigens when immunized. In older children and adults, a low IgG2 maybe an antecedent finding before evolving into **common variable immunodeficiency (CVID)**. Specific vaccine responses are usually much more useful than IgG subclass determinations.

Patients found to be **agammaglobulinemic** should have their blood B cells enumerated by flow cytometry using dye-conjugated monoclonal antibodies to B-cell–specific CD antigens (usually CD19 or CD20). Normally, approximately 5–10% of circulating lymphocytes are B cells. B cells are absent in X-linked agammaglobulinemia (XLA) and in several very rare autosomal recessive conditions, but they are usually present in CVID, IgA deficiency, and hyper-IgM syndromes. This distinction is important, because children with hypogammaglobulinemia from XLA and CVID can have different clinical problems, and the 2 conditions clearly have different inheritance patterns. Patients with CVID have more problems with autoimmune diseases and lymphoid hyperplasia. Molecular testing for XLA and other B-cell defects (see Chapter 150.1) is indicated in cases without a family history to aid genetic counseling.

T cells and T cell subpopulations can be enumerated by flow cytometry using dye-conjugated monoclonal antibodies recognizing

CD antigens present on T cells (i.e., CD2, CD3, CD4, and CD8). This is a particularly important test to perform on any infant who is lymphopenic, because CD3$^+$ T cells usually constitute 70% of peripheral lymphocytes. Regardless of molecular type, infants with SCID are unable to produce T cells, so are lymphopenic at birth. The flow cytometry for infants suspected of having SCID should also include monoclonal antibodies to naïve (CD45RA) and memory (CD45RO) T cells. In normal infants, >95% of the T cells are CD45RA$^+$ (naïve) T cells. If the infant has SCID, there could be transplacentally transferred maternal T cells detected by flow cytometry, but they would be predominantly CD45RO$^+$ T cells. SCID is a pediatric emergency that can be successfully treated by hematopoietic stem cell transplantation in more than 90% of cases if diagnosed before serious, untreatable infections develop. Normally, there are about twice as many CD4$^+$ (helper) T cells as there are CD8$^+$ (cytotoxic) T cells. Because some severe immunodeficiencies have phenotypically normal T cells, tests of T-cell function can be helpful. T cells can be stimulated directly with **mitogens** such as phytohemagglutinin, concanavalin A, or pokeweed mitogen. After 3-5 days of incubation with the mitogen, the proliferation of T cells is measured. Other stimulants that can be used to assess T-cell function in the same type of assay include antigens (*Candida*, tetanus toxoid) and allogeneic cells.

Natural killer (NK) cells can be enumerated by flow cytometry using monoclonal antibodies to NK-specific CD antigens, CD16 and CD56. NK function is assessed by killing of target cells and flow cytometry for CD107a, a marker of degranulation.

Chronic granulomatous disease should be suspected if a patient has recurrent staphylococcal abscesses or fungal infections. It can be evaluated by screening tests measuring the neutrophil respiratory burst after phorbol ester stimulation. **Leukocyte adhesion defects** (LAD) can be easily diagnosed by flow cytometric assays of blood lymphocytes or neutrophils, using monoclonal antibodies to CD18 or CD11 (LAD1) or to CD15 (LAD2). **Neutrophil defects** are most often associated with neutropenia or morphologic abnormalities visible by microscopy. Therefore, a combination of a CBC with differential, microscopic evaluation, and the flow cytometric approaches previously described often yields a diagnosis. The same is not true for **macrophage defects**, which are usually associated with susceptibility to mycobacteria, and testing requires advanced functional analyses or sequencing.

When invasive infection with encapsulated organisms or *Neisseria* leads to a suspicion of a complement defect, a **CH$_{50}$ test** should be obtained. This bioassay measures the intactness of the entire complement pathway and yields abnormal results if classical pathway or terminal components are missing. Genetic deficiencies in the complement system often have a CH50 that is almost absent, although the most frequent cause of a slightly low CH50 is improper transport of the specimen. Complement proteins are highly labile and must be transported on ice. Specific factor assays are available at reference laboratories. Rare causes of neisserial susceptibility include alternative pathway defects, and the

test for these deficiencies is the **AH₅₀ test.** Identifying the specific component deficiency in the mode of inheritance is important for genetic counseling. Properdin deficiency is X-linked, and other deficiencies are autosomal recessive or autosomal dominant.

Bibliography is available at Expert Consult.

Section 2
The T-, B-, and NK-Cell Systems

第二篇

T，B和NK细胞系统

Chapter 149

Lymphocyte Development and Function

Kathleen E. Sullivan and Rebecca H. Buckley

第一百四十九章

淋巴细胞发育和功能

中文导读

本章主要介绍了胎儿淋巴细胞生成、生后淋巴细胞行为，以及T、B和NK细胞发育遗传异常。淋巴细胞生成中具体描述了T细胞发育和分化、B细胞发育和分化、NK细胞发育以及淋巴细胞编排；生后淋巴细胞行为中描述了CD4 T细胞亚类、生后各类免疫球蛋白水平的变化、抗原特异性抗体产生能力，以及淋巴器官发育；淋巴细胞发育遗传异常包括不同的细胞免疫学机制。

Defense against infectious agents is secured through a combination of anatomic physical barriers, including the skin, mucous membranes, mucous blanket, and ciliated epithelial cells, and the components of the immune system. The **immune system** of vertebrates integrates 2 fundamental response mechanisms. **Innate (natural) immunity** is rapid and utilizes receptors encoded in the germline. The innate defenses comprise cell-intrinsic responses to viral infections, leukocyte responses to pathogens, and soluble mediators such as complement proteins. **Acquired (adaptive) immunity** is specific to T and B cells. These cells

undergo DNA recombination to generate receptors and require an education process to minimize autoreactive cells. In addition, there are lymphocyte subsets that are innate in nature and either do not require DNA recombination or utilize a single recombination event to generate a monospecific receptor.

LYMPHOPOIESIS IN THE FETUS
Pluripotential hematopoietic stem cells first appear in the yolk sac at 2.5-3 wk of gestational age, migrate to the fetal liver at 5 wk gestation,

and later reside in the bone marrow, where they remain throughout life (Fig. 149.1). Lymphoid stem cells develop and differentiate into T, B, or natural killer (NK) cells, depending on the organs or tissues to which the stem cells traffic. Development of the **primary lymphoid organs**—thymus and bone marrow—begins during the middle of the 1st trimester of gestation and proceeds rapidly. Development of the **secondary lymphoid organs**—spleen, lymph nodes, tonsils, Peyer patches, and lamina propria—soon follows. These organs serve as sites of differentiation of T, B, and NK lymphocytes from stem cells throughout life. Both the initial organogenesis and the continued cell differentiation result from the interaction of a vast array of lymphocytic and micro-environmental cell surface molecules and proteins secreted by the involved cells. **Clusters of differentiation (CD)** refer to cellular protein (Table 149.1), whereas **cytokines** and **chemokines** refer to soluble mediators of immune function (Table 149.2).

T-Cell Development and Differentiation

The primitive thymic rudiment is formed from the ectoderm of the 3rd branchial cleft and endoderm of the 3rd branchial pouch at 4 wk gesta-tion. Beginning at 7-8 wk, the right and left rudiments fuse in the midline. Bloodborne T-cell precursors from the fetal liver then begin to colonize the perithymic mesenchyme at 8 wk gestation and move into the thymus at 8.0-8.5 wk. The earliest cells to enter the thymus are found in the subcapsular region and do not express CD3, CD4, CD8, or either type of T-cell receptor (TCR). These lymphoid cell precursors are triggered to proliferate and become thymocytes through interactions with the thymic stroma. The cells are arrested at this stage until they productively rearrange the β-chain locus of the TCR. The β chain then pairs with the surrogate pre-T α chain. This tests the function of the β chain, and if signaling occurs, β-chain rearrangement ceases. CD4 and CD8 are then expressed simultaneously (i.e., they are double-positive thymocytes). Fetal cortical thymocytes are among the most rapidly dividing cells in the body and increase in number by 100,000-fold within 2 wk after stem cells enter the thymus. As these cells proliferate and mature, they migrate deeper into the thymic cortex. The double-positive thymocytes begin efficient rearrangement of the α-chain locus. TCR gene rearrangement occurs by a process in which large, noncontiguous blocks of DNA are spliced together. **V (variable)**, **D (diversity)**, and **J (joining)** blocks exist in families of minimally different segments. Random combinations of the segments account for much of the enormous diversity of TCRs that enables humans to recognize millions of different antigens. TCR gene rearrangement requires the presence of **recombinase-activating genes**, *RAG1* and *RAG2,* as well as other recombinase components.

As immature cortical thymocytes begin to express TCRs, the processes of positive and negative selection take place. **Positive selection** occurs in immature thymocytes, recognizing major histocompatibility complex (MHC) antigens present on cortical thymic epithelial cells. Some cells are selected to mature into CD4 or CD8 single-positive cells. **Negative selection** occurs next in the thymic medulla on medullary thymic epithelial cells. Autoreactive T cells undergo apoptosis and die. T cells begin to emigrate from the thymus to the spleen, lymph nodes, and appendix at 11-12 wk of embryonic life and to the tonsils by 14-15 wk. They leave the thymus via the bloodstream and are distributed throughout the body, with the heaviest concentrations in the paracortical areas of lymph nodes, the periarteriolar areas of the spleen, and the thoracic lymph duct. Recent thymic emigrants co-express the CD45RA isoforms and CD62L (L-selectin).

Rearrangement of the TCR locus during intrathymic T-cell develop-ment results in the excision of DNA and the excised elements form circular episomes as a by-product. These **TCR recombination excision circles** can be detected in T cells that are recent thymic emigrants. TCR recombination excision circles detected in dried-blood spots collected from infants shortly after birth is the test used for newborn screening for severe combined immunodeficiency (SCID). By 12 wk gestation, T cells can proliferate in response to plant lectins, such as phytohemag-glutinin and concanavalin A. Antigen-specific T cells have been found by 20 wk gestation. **Hassall corpuscles (bodies),** which are swirls of terminally differentiated medullary epithelial cells, are first seen in the

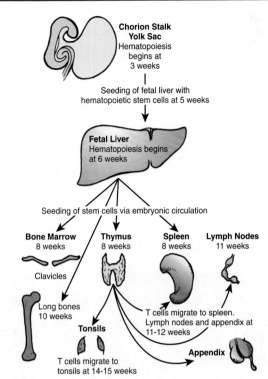

Fig. 149.1 Migration patterns of hematopoietic stem cells and mature lymphocytes during human fetal development. *(From Haynes BF, Denning SM: Lymphopoiesis. In Stamatoyannopoulis G, Nienhuis A, Majerus P, editors: Molecular basis of blood diseases, ed 2, Philadelphia, 1994, Saunders.)*

thymic medulla at 16-18 wk of embryonic life.

B-Cell Development and Differentiation

B-cell development begins in the fetal liver by 7 wk gestation. Fetal liver CD34 stem cells are seeded to the bone marrow of the clavicles by 8 wk of embryonic life and to that of the long bones by 10 wk (see Fig. 149.1). As B cells differentiate from primitive stem cells, they proceed through stages that are marked by the sequential rearrangement of immunoglobulin gene segments to generate a diverse repertoire of antigen receptors. The early **pro-B cell** is the first descendent of the pluripotential stem cell committed to B-lineage development, and in this stage the heavy chain locus rearranges first. In the early pro-B cell, D-J rearrangements are made on both chromosomes. In the late pro-B cell, the V segment rearranges to a D-J gene segment. The next stage is the **pre-B cell**, during which immunoglobulin (Ig) light-chain genes are rearranged. The **pre-B cell** is distinguished by the expression of cytoplasmic μ heavy chains but no **surface IgM (sIgM)**, because Ig light chains are not yet produced. Next is the **immature B-cell** stage, during which the light-chain genes have already been rearranged, and sIgM but not sIgD is expressed. Immature B cells leave the bone marrow for secondary lymphoid organs. The last stage of antigen-independent B-cell development is the **mature naïve B cell,** which co-expresses both sIgM and sIgD. Pre-B cells can be found in fetal liver at 7 wk gestation, sIgM+ and sIgG+ B cells at 7-11 wk, and sIgD+ and sIgA+ B cells by 12-13 wk. By 14 wk of embryonic life, the percentage of circulating lymphocytes bearing sIgM and sIgD is the same as in cord blood and slightly higher than in the blood of adults.

Antigen-dependent stages of B-cell development are those that develop after the mature B cell is stimulated by antigen in secondary lymphoid organs. Once antigen stimulation has occurred, the mature B cells can become memory B cells or plasmablasts. Both outcomes require the presence of T-cell help.

Table 149.1	CD Classification of Some Lymphocyte Surface Molecules	
CD NUMBER	**TISSUE/LINEAGE**	**FUNCTION**
CD1	Cortical thymocytes; Langerhans cells	Lipid antigen presentation to TCRγδ cells
CD2	T and NK cells	Binds LFA-3 (CD58); alternative pathway of T-cell activation
CD3	T cells	TCR associated; transduces signals from TCR
CD4	T-helper cell subset	Receptor for HLA class II antigens; associated with p56 *lck* tyrosine kinase
CD7	T and NK cells and their precursors	Mitogenic for T lymphocytes
CD8	Cytotoxic T-cell subset; also on 30% of NK cells	Receptor for HLA class I antigens; associated with p56 *lck* tyrosine kinase
CD10	B-cell progenitors	Peptide cleavage
CD11a	T, B, and NK cells	With CD18, ligand for ICAMs 1, 2, and 3
CD11b, c	NK cells	With CD18, receptors for C3bi
CD16	NK cells	FcR for IgG
CD19	B cells	Regulates B-cell activation
CD20	B cells	Mediates B-cell activation
CD21	B cells	C3d, also the receptor for EBV; CR2
CD25	T, B, and NK cells	Mediates signaling by IL-2
CD34	Stem cells	Binds to L-selectin
CD38	T, B, and NK cells and monocytes	Associates with hyaluronic acid
CD40	B cells and monocytes	Initiates isotype switching in B cells when ligated
CD44	Bone marrow stromal and many other cells	Matrix adhesion molecule
CD45	All leukocytes	Tyrosine phosphatase that regulates lymphocyte activation; CD45R0 isoform on memory T cells, CD45RA isoform on naïve T cells
CD56	NK cells	Mediates NK homotypic adhesion
CD62L	Marker for recent thymic emigrants Also found on other leukocytes	Cell adhesion molecule
CD69	T cells and NK cells	Early activation marker
CD73	T and B cells	Associates with AMP
CD80	B cells	Co-stimulatory with CD28 on T cells to upregulate high-affinity IL-2 receptor
CD86	B cells	Co-stimulatory with CD28 on T cells to upregulate high-affinity IL-2 receptor
CD117	Pro-B cells, double-negative thymocytes	Receptor for stem cell factor
CD127	T cells	Mediates IL-7 signaling
CD132	T, B, and NK cells	Mediates signaling by IL-2, IL-4, IL-7, IL-9, IL-15, and IL-21
CD154	Activated CD4+ T cells	Ligates CD40 on B cells and initiates isotype switching
CD278	T cells	Interacts with B7-H2

AMP, Adenosine monophosphate; EBV, Epstein-Barr virus; ICAMs, intracellular adhesion molecules; IL, interleukin; LFA, leukocyte function–activating antigen; NK, natural killer; TCR, T-cell receptor.

There are 5 **immunoglobulin isotypes**, which are defined by unique heavy chains: IgM, IgG, IgA, IgD, and IgE. IgG and IgM, the only complement-fixing isotypes, are the most important immunoglobulins in the blood and other internal body fluids for protection against infectious agents. IgM is confined primarily to the intravascular compartment because of its large size, whereas IgG is present in all internal body fluids. IgA is the major protective immunoglobulin of external secretions—in the gastrointestinal, respiratory, and urogenital tracts—but it is also present in the circulation. IgE, present in both internal and external body fluids, has a major role in host defense against parasites. Because of high-affinity IgE receptors on basophils and mast cells, however, IgE is the principal mediator of allergic reactions of the immediate type. The significance of IgD is still not clear. There are also **immunoglobulin subclasses**, including 4 subclasses of IgG (IgG1, IgG2, IgG3, and IgG4) and 2 subclasses of IgA (IgA1 and IgA2). These subclasses each have different biologic roles. Secreted IgM and IgE have been found in as young as 10 wk gestation, and IgG as early as 11-12 wk.

Even though these B-cell developmental stages have been described in the context of B-cell ontogeny in utero, it is important to recognize that the process of B-cell development from pluripotential stem cells goes on throughout postnatal life. Plasma cells are not usually found in lymphoid tissues of a fetus until about 20 wk gestation, and then only rarely, because of the sterile environment of the uterus. Intestinal lymphoid development occurs relatively late. Peyer patches have been found in significant numbers by the 5th intrauterine mo, and plasma cells have been seen in the lamina propria by 25 wk gestation. Before birth there may be primary follicles in lymph nodes, but secondary follicles are usually not present.

A human fetus begins to receive significant quantities of maternal IgG transplacentally at around 12 wk gestation, and the quantity steadily increases until, at birth, cord-blood serum contains a concentration of IgG comparable to or greater than that of maternal serum. IgG is the only class to cross the placenta to any significant degree. All 4 IgG subclasses cross the placenta, but IgG2 does so least well. A small amount of IgM (10% of adult levels) and a few nanograms of IgA, IgD, and IgE are normally found in cord blood serum. Because none of these proteins crosses the placenta, they are presumed to be of fetal origin. These observations suggest that certain antigenic stimuli normally cross the placenta to provoke responses, even in uninfected fetuses. Some atopic infants occasionally have IgE antibodies to antigens, such as egg white, to which they have had no known exposure during postnatal life, suggesting that synthesis of these antibodies could have been induced in the fetus by antigens ingested by the mother.

Natural Killer–Cell Development
NK cell activity is found in human fetal liver cells at 8-11 wk of gestation. NK lymphocytes are also derived from bone marrow precursors. Thymic processing is not necessary for NK-cell development, although NK cells have been found in the thymus. After release from bone marrow, NK cells enter the circulation or migrate to the spleen, with very few NK cells in lymph nodes. In normal individuals, NK cells represent 8–10% of lymphocytes. Certain tissues harbor large numbers of NK cells.

Unlike T and B cells, NK cells do not rearrange antigen receptor genes during their development but are defined by their functional capacity to mediate non–antigen-specific cytotoxicity. NK cells have killer inhibitory receptors that recognize certain MHC antigens and inhibit the killing of self tissues. NK-activating receptors recognize stress protein, and the balance of activating and inhibitory receptor engagement determines the action of the NK cells. If a viral infection drives down MHC class I expression, the loss of inhibitory function drives cytotoxicity. High levels of stress proteins, typically seen in viral infections, can also activate cytotoxicity.

Lymphocyte Choreography
The main functions of T cells are to signal B cells to make antibody, to kill virally infected cells or tumor cells, and to activate macrophages for intracellular killing. The subset of **regulatory T cells** (Tregs), is critical in the prevention of autoimmune responses. T cells are activated by antigen presented by **antigen-presenting cells (APCs)**. These are usually dendritic cells, macrophages, or B cells. For high-affinity binding of T cells to APCs, several molecules on T cells, in addition to TCRs, bind to molecules on APCs or target cells. The CD4 molecule binds directly to MHC class II molecules on APCs. CD8 on cytotoxic T cells binds the MHC class I molecule on the target cell. Lymphocyte function–associated antigen 1 (**LFA-1**) on the T cell binds a protein called **ICAM-1** (intracellular adhesion molecule 1), designated **CD54**, on APCs. CD2 on T cells binds LFA-3 (CD58) on the APCs. With the adhesion of T cells to APCs (the immunologic synapse), **T-helper (Th)** cells are stimulated to make interleukins and upregulate cell surface molecules, such as the CD40 ligand (CD154), that provide help for B cells, and cytotoxic T cells are stimulated to kill their targets. A key safety net to ensure appropriate activation of T cells in the setting of a true threat is the requirement for co-stimulation of the T cells. APCs that have encountered a pathogen express CD80 and CD86. Engagement of these molecules provides the 2nd, co-stimulatory, signal. Without co-stimulation, the T cell will be rendered *anergic*, or nonfunctional.

In the **primary antibody response**, native antigen is carried to a lymph node draining the site, captured by complement, taken up by specialized cells called **follicular dendritic cells (FDCs)**, and expressed on their surfaces. Mature B cells bearing sIgM specific for that antigen then bind to the antigen on the surfaces of the FDCs. If the affinity of the B-cell sIgM antibody for the antigen present on the FDCs is sufficient, and if other signals are provided by activated T cells, the B cell develops into a memory B cells or antibody-producing plasma cell. The signals from activated T cells include several cytokines (IL-4, IL-5, IL-6, IL-10, IL-13, and IL-21) that they secrete (see Table 149.2) and a surface T-cell molecule, the CD40 ligand or CD154, which, on contact of the activated CD4$^+$ T cell with the B cell, binds to CD40 on the B-cell surface. Binding of CD40 on B cells by CD154 on T cells in the presence of certain cytokines causes the B cells to undergo proliferation and to initiate

immunoglobulin synthesis. In the primary immune response, only IgM antibody is usually made, and most of it is of relatively low affinity. Some B cells become memory B cells during the primary immune response. The **secondary antibody response** occurs when these memory B cells again encounter that antigen. Developing memory B cells switch their Ig genes so that IgG, IgA, and/or IgE antibodies of higher affinity are formed on a secondary exposure to the same antigen. Plasma cells form, just as in the primary response; however, many more cells are rapidly generated, and IgG, IgA, and IgE antibodies are made. In addition, genetic changes in Ig genes (somatic hypermutation) lead to increased affinity of those antibodies.

The exact pattern of isotype response to antigen in normal individuals varies, depending on the type of antigen and the cytokines present in the microenvironment. Both class switching and somatic hypermutation are completely dependent on T-cell help. Thus, T cells represent a kind of gatekeeper for specific antibody production.

POSTNATAL LYMPHOCYTE BEHAVIOR
Virtually all T cells in cord blood bear the CD45RA (naïve) isoform, and a dominance of CD45RA over CD45RO T cells persists during childhood. After mid-adulthood, the CD45RO (memory) T cells predominate. CD4 T cells can be further subdivided according to the cytokines they produce when activated. **Th1 cells** produce interleukin (IL)-2 and interferon (IFN)-γ, which promote cytotoxic T-cell or delayed hypersensitivity types of responses, whereas **Th2 cells** produce IL-4, IL-5, IL-6, IL-13, and IL-21 (see Table 149.2), which promote B-cell responses and allergic sensitization, **Th17** cells produce IL-17, and **Tregs** produce IL-10 (Fig. 149.2). Differentiation into these memory subsets is dictated by the cytokine milieu regulating specific transcription factors and epigenetic changes. In vivo, these subsets are largely stable but in some circumstances can change to a different subset. The importance of these subsets is that memory cells respond to antigen more quickly and are primed to produce the cytokines most likely to drive pathogen clearance.

Newborn infants have increased susceptibility to infections with gram-negative organisms because IgM antibodies, powerful **opsonins** that enhance phagocytosis, do not cross the placenta. The other major opsonin, C3b, is also lower in newborn serum than in adults. These factors probably account for impaired phagocytosis of some organisms by newborn polymorphonuclear cells. Maternally transmitted IgG

Table 149.2	Common Cytokines	
CATEGORY	**CYTOKINE**	**FUNCTION**
Interferons	IFN-α	Antiviral defense
	IFN-β	Antiviral defense
	IFN-γ	Antiviral defense
Innate responses	TNF	Regulates endothelial adhesion molecules for recruitment of neutrophils; activates macrophages for killing
	IL-1β	Drives the inflammatory response, fever
	IL-12	Polarizes T cells toward Th1; activates NK cells
Lymphocyte regulation	IL-2	Key growth factor for T cells
	IL-4	Polarizes T cells toward Th2
	IL-6	Growth factor for B cells
	IL-7	T-cell homeostatic factor
	IL-10	Growth factor for B cells, immunosuppressive
	IL-12	Polarizes T cells toward Th1, activates NK cells
	IL-17	Polarizes T cells toward Th17, stimulates antimicrobial peptide expression
	IL-21	Supports B-cell class switching

IL, Interleukin; NK, natural killer; Th, T-helper cell; TNF, tumor necrosis factor.

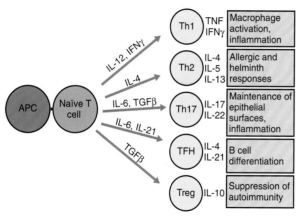

Fig. 149.2 T-cell differentiation into memory subsets is tightly regulated by cytokines. Specific subsets have distinct roles in host defense. APC, Antigen-presenting cell; IFN, interferon; IL, interleukin; Th, T-helper cell; TFH, follicular helper T cell; TGF, transforming growth factor; TNF, tumor necrosis factor.

antibodies serve quite adequately for most gram-positive bacteria, and IgG antibodies to viruses offer protection against those agents. Because there is a relative deficiency of the IgG2 subclass in infancy, antibodies to capsular polysaccharide antigens may be deficient. Because premature infants have received less maternal IgG by the time of birth than full-term infants, their serum opsonic activity is low for all types of organisms.

Neonates begin to synthesize antibodies of the IgM class at an increased rate very soon after birth in response to the immense antigenic stimulation of their new environment. Premature infants appear to be as capable of doing this as are full-term infants. At about 6 days after birth, the serum concentration of IgM rises sharply. This rise continues until adult levels are achieved by approximately 1 yr of age. Cord serum from noninfected normal newborns does not contain detectable IgA. Serum IgA is normally first detected at around the 13th day of postnatal life but remains low throughout infancy. Cord serum contains an IgG concentration comparable to or greater than that of maternal serum. Maternal IgG gradually disappears during the 1st 6-8 mo of life, while the rate of infant IgG synthesis increases (IgG1 and IgG3 faster than IgG2 and IgG4 during the 1st yr) until adult concentrations of total IgG are reached and maintained by 7-8 yr. IgG1 and IgG4 reach adult levels first, followed by IgG3 at 10 yr and IgG2 at

12 yr. The serum IgG level in infants usually reaches a low point at about 3-4 mo of postnatal life. The rate of development of IgE generally follows that of IgA.

After adult concentrations of each of the 3 major immunoglobulins are reached, these levels remain remarkably constant for a normal individual. The capacity to produce specific antibodies to protein antigens is intact at birth, but infants cannot usually produce antibodies to polysaccharide antigens until after 2 yr of age unless the polysaccharide is conjugated to a protein carrier, as is the case for the conjugate *Haemophilus influenzae* type b and *Streptococcus pneumoniae* vaccines.

The percentage of NK cells in cord blood is usually lower than in the blood of children and adults, but the absolute number of NK cells is approximately the same because of the higher lymphocyte count. The capacity of cord blood NK cells to mediate target lysis in either NK-cell assays or antibody-dependent cellular cytotoxicity assays is about two-thirds that of adults.

Lymphoid Organ Development
Lymphoid tissue is proportionally small but rather well developed at birth and matures rapidly in the postnatal period. The thymus is largest relative to body size during fetal life and at birth is ordinarily two-thirds its mature weight, which it attains during the 1st yr of life. It reaches its peak mass, however, just before puberty, then gradually involutes thereafter. By 1 yr of age, all lymphoid structures are mature histologically. Absolute lymphocyte counts in the peripheral blood also reach a peak during the 1st yr of life (see Fig. 149.2). The spleen, however, gradually accrues its mass during maturation and does not reach full weight until adulthood. The mean number of Peyer patches at birth is one-half the adult number, and gradually increases until the adult mean number is exceeded during adolescent years.

INHERITANCE OF ABNORMALITIES IN T-, B-, AND NK-CELL DEVELOPMENT
More than 300 immunodeficiency syndromes have been described. Specific molecular defects have been identified for most diseases. Most are recessive traits with X-linked, autosomal dominant loss of function, and autosomal dominant gain of function also is seen. Defects include those associated with absence of a cell type, either a lineage (e.g., absence of T cells in SCID), absence of a subset of cells (e.g., absence of Tregs in immune dysregulation, polyendocrinopathy, X-linked syndrome), or dysfunction of a cell (e.g., the hemophagocytic lymphohistiocytosis disorders). In some cases, multiple cell types are affected, and in some syndromes, excess of a certain cell type or function disrupts the critical balance needed for immune homeostasis.

Bibliography is available at Expert Consult.

Chapter **150**
Primary Defects of Antibody Production

Kathleen E. Sullivan and
Rebecca H. Buckley

第一百五十章
原发性抗体产生缺陷

中文导读

　　本章主要介绍了X连锁无丙种球蛋白血症、普通变异免疫缺陷、选择性IgA缺陷、IgG亚类缺陷、免疫球蛋白重链和轻链缺失、婴儿暂时性低丙种球蛋白血症、类别转换缺陷，以及X连锁淋巴增殖性疾病。具体描述了X连锁无丙种球蛋白血症的遗传发病机制、临床表现和诊断、普通变异免疫缺陷的遗传发病机制和临床表现，以及选择性IgA缺陷的临床表现；具体描述了X连锁和常染色体隐性遗传高IgM综合征的遗传发病机制、临床表现和治疗；具体描述了X连锁淋巴增殖性疾病的发病机制和临床表现；详细阐述了B细胞缺陷的治疗。

Of the primary immunodeficiency diseases, those affecting antibody production are the most prevalent. Selective absence of IgA is the most common defect, with rates ranging from 1 in 333 to 1 in 18,000 persons among different races and ethnicities. Patients with antibody deficiency are usually recognized because they have recurrent infections with encapsulated bacteria, predominantly in the upper and lower respiratory tracts. Some individuals with selective IgA deficiency or infants with transient hypogammaglobulinemia may have few or no infections. These conditions have a complex and likely polygenic inheritance, as do the common variable immunodeficiency (CVID) syndromes. The gene defects for many primary antibody deficiency disorders have been identified (Table 150.1) and localized (Fig. 150.1). Sometimes the defect is not in the B cell itself but in T cells, which are required for complete B-cell function. Some disorders are caused by unknown factors or are secondary to an underlying disease or its treatment (Table 150.2).

X-LINKED AGAMMAGLOBULINEMIA

Patients with X-linked agammaglobulinemia (**XLA**), or **Bruton agammaglobulinemia**, have a profound defect in B-lymphocyte development resulting in severe hypogammaglobulinemia, an absence of circulating B cells, small to absent tonsils, and no palpable lymph nodes.

Genetics and Pathogenesis

The abnormal gene in XLA maps to q22 on the long arm of the X chromosome and encodes the B-cell protein tyrosine kinase **Btk** (Bruton tyrosine kinase). Btk is a member of the Tec family of cytoplasmic

protein tyrosine kinases and is expressed at high levels in all B-lineage cells, including pre-B cells. Some pre-B cells are found in the bone marrow, but the percentage of peripheral blood B lymphocytes is <1%. The percentage of T cells is increased, ratios of T-cell subsets are normal, and T-cell function is intact. The thymus is normal.

Seven **autosomal recessive defects** have also been shown to result in **agammaglobulinemia with an absence of circulating B cells** (see Table 150.1), including mutations in the genes encoding (1) the μ heavy chain gene; (2) the Igα and (3) Igβ signaling molecules; (4) B-cell linker adaptor protein (BLNK); (5) the surrogate light chain, λ5/14.1; (6) leucine-rich repeat-containing 8 (LRRC8); and (7) the p85α subunit of phosphatidylinositol-3 kinase. These are rare but are clinically indistinguishable from the X-linked form.

Clinical Manifestations

Most boys afflicted with XLA remain well during the first 6-9 mo of life by virtue of maternally transmitted IgG antibodies. Thereafter, they acquire infections with extracellular pyogenic organisms, such as *Streptococcus pneumoniae* and *Haemophilus influenzae*, unless they are given prophylactic antibiotics or immunoglobulin therapy. Infections include sinusitis, otitis media, pneumonia, or, less often, sepsis or meningitis. Infections with *Mycoplasma* are also particularly problematic. Chronic fungal infections are seen; *Pneumocystis jiroveci* pneumonia rarely occurs. Viral infections are usually handled normally, with the exceptions of hepatitis viruses and enteroviruses. There were several examples of **paralysis** when live polio vaccine was administered to these patients, and

Table 150.1	Genetic Basis of the Most Common Primary Antibody Deficiency Disorders	
GENE	**PHENOTYPE**	**DISORDER**
BAFFR	CVID	Hypogammaglobulinemia
CD19	CVID	Hypogammaglobulinemia
CD20	CVID	Hypogammaglobulinemia
CD21	CVID	Hypogammaglobulinemia
CD81	CVID	Hypogammaglobulinemia
CTLA4	CVID	Hypogammaglobulinemia, pronounced lymphoproliferation and autoimmunity
ICOS	CVID	Hypogammaglobulinemia, autoimmunity, neoplasia
LRBA	CVID	Hypogammaglobulinemia, pronounced lymphoproliferation and autoimmunity
NFKB2	CVID	Hypogammaglobulinemia, autoimmunity
NFKB1	CVID	Hypogammaglobulinemia, autoimmunity
PIK3CD	CVID	Hypogammaglobulinemia, adenopathy
PI3KR1 (AD)	CVID	Hypogammaglobulinemia
TNFRSF13B	CVID	Hypogammaglobulinemia, low penetrance of disease
Unknown	CVID	Hypogammaglobulinemia, autoimmunity Majority of patients with CVID have no known gene defect.
Unknown	IgG subclass deficiency	Variable association with infection
Unknown	Specific antibody deficiency	Normal immunoglobulin levels with poor vaccine responses
Unknown	Transient hypogammaglobulinemia of infancy	Vaccine responses are usually preserved, and most children outgrow this by age 3 yr.
Unknown	Selective IgA deficiency	Low or absent IgA; low concentrations of all immunoglobulins and of switched memory B cells in CVID
BLNK	Agammaglobulinemia	Absence of antibody production, lack of B cells
BTK	Agammaglobulinemia	Absence of antibody production, lack of B cells, X-linked agammaglobulinemia
CD79A	Agammaglobulinemia	Loss of the Igα required for signal transduction, absence of antibody production, lack of B cells
CD79B	Agammaglobulinemia	Loss of the Igβ required for signal transduction, absence of antibody production, lack of B cells
IGHM	Agammaglobulinemia	Loss of the Ig heavy chain, absence of antibody production, lack of B cells
IGLL1	Agammaglobulinemia	Loss of the surrogate light chain, absence of antibody production, lack of B cells
PI3KR1 (AR)	Agammaglobulinemia	Loss of signal transduction through the B-cell receptor, absence of antibody production, lack of B cells
TCF3	Agammaglobulinemia	Loss of a key transcription factor for B-cell development, absence of antibody production, lack of B cells
AID	Class switch defect	Failure to produce IgG, IgA, and IgE antibodies
CD40	Class switch defect	Failure to produce IgG, IgA, and IgE antibodies, *Pneumocystis* and *Cryptosporidium* susceptibility
CD154	Class switch defect	Failure to produce IgG, IgA, and IgE antibodies, *Pneumocystis* and *Cryptosporidium* susceptibility
INO80	Class switch defect	Failure to produce IgG, IgA, and IgE antibodies
MSH6	Class switch defect	Failure to produce IgG, IgA, and IgE antibodies, malignancy
UNG	Class switch defect	Failure to produce IgG, IgA, and IgE antibodies
SH2D1A	X-linked lymphoproliferative disease	Various phenotypes including hypogammaglobulinemia
XIAP	X-linked lymphoproliferative disease	Various phenotypes including hypogammaglobulinemia
CD27	EBV lymphoproliferation	Memory B-cell deficiency Hypogammaglobulinemia
NEMO	Anhidrotic ectodermal dysplasia with immunodeficiency	Phenotype highly variable but includes specific antibody deficiency and CVID

CVID, Common variable immunodeficiency; EBV, Epstein-Barr virus.

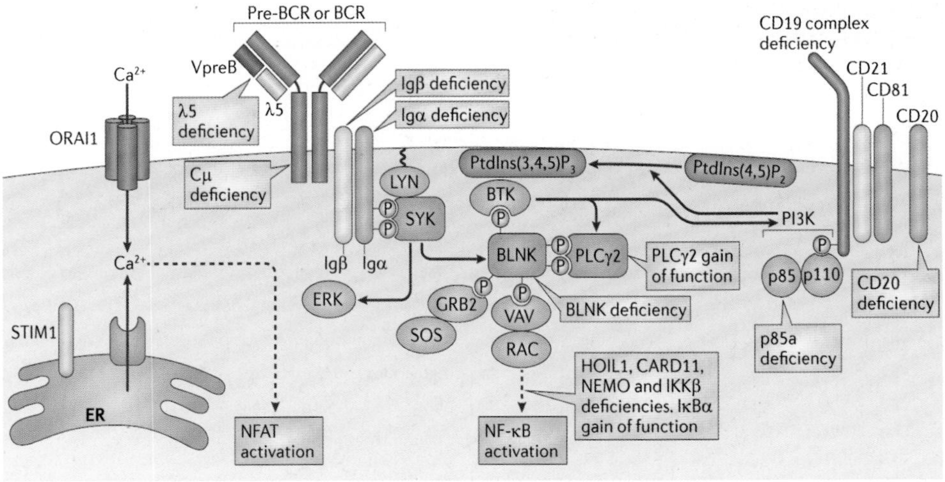

Fig. 150.1 The pre-B cell receives proliferation and differentiation signals through the pre–B-cell receptor (BCR) and the co-receptors Igα and Igβ. Signaling from the pre-BCR involves the immunoreceptor tyrosine-based activation motifs (ITAMs) of the co-receptors Igα and Igβ, which scaffold and activate the tyrosine kinase SYK. SYK either activates the extracellular signal–regulated kinase (ERK) pathway or phosphorylates (P) (together with LYN) the adaptor protein B-cell linker (BLNK) and Bruton tyrosine kinase (BTK), leading to the activation of phospholipase Cγ2 (PLCγ2) and the phosphoinositide-3 kinase (PI3K) pathway. Defects in this pathway affect the pre-BCR (in Cμ or pseudo light-chain λ5), the pre-BCR signal transduction molecules Igα and Igβ, the downstream molecules BTK, BLNK, and PI3K, components of the co-stimulatory CD19 complex (CD19, CD21, and CD81), and the B-cell marker CD20. The BCR triggers the canonical nuclear factor-κB (NF-κB) pathway through the scaffolding protein CARD11 and activation of the IκB kinase (IKK) complex (comprising IKKα, IKKβ, and NEMO [NF-κB essential modulator]). IKK activation leads to the phosphorylation and degradation of NF-κB inhibitor-α (IκBα) and the subsequent release of the p50-p65 NF-κB heterodimer, which then translocates to the nucleus to regulate gene transcription (not shown). Following antigen binding to antigen receptors (e.g., BCR), endoplasmic reticulum Ca²⁺ stores are depleted, STIM1 is activated, and ORAI1 Ca²⁺ release-activated Ca²⁺ channels open, resulting in store-operated Ca²⁺ entry. This influx results in activation of the transcription factor NFAT (nuclear factor of activated T cell). The *dashed arrows* indicate downstream signaling events. ER, Endoplasmic reticulum; PAD, primary antibody deficiency; PtdIns(4,5)P₂, phosphatidylinositol-4,5-bisphosphate; PtdIns(3,4,5)P₃, phosphatidylinositol-3,4,5-trisphosphate. (*From Durandy A, Kracker S, Fischer A. Primary antibody deficiencies. Nat Rev Immunol 13:521, 2013*).

Table 150.2	Other Conditions Associated With Humoral Immunodeficiency
GENETIC DISORDERS	
T-cell defects	Most T-cell defects can have a secondary deficit in immunoglobulin.
Complex syndromes	Transcobalamin II deficiency and hypogammaglobulinemia, Wiskott-Aldrich syndrome, ataxia telangiectasia, etc.
Chromosomal anomalies	Chromosome 18q– syndrome 22q11.2 deletion Trisomy 8, trisomy 21
SYSTEMIC DISORDERS	
Malignancy	Chronic lymphocytic leukemia Immunodeficiency with thymoma T-cell lymphoma
Metabolic or physical loss	Immunodeficiency caused by hypercatabolism of immunoglobulin Immunodeficiency caused by excessive loss of immunoglobulins and lymphocytes
ENVIRONMENTAL EXPOSURES	
Drug induced	Antimalarial agents Captopril Carbamazepine Glucocorticoids Fenclofenac Gold salts Imatinib Penicillamine Phenytoin Sulfasalazine
Infectious diseases	Congenital rubella Congenital infection with cytomegalovirus Congenital infection with *Toxoplasma gondii* Epstein-Barr virus Human immunodeficiency virus

chronic, eventually fatal, central nervous system (CNS) infections with various echoviruses and coxsackieviruses have occurred in a significant number of patients. An enterovirus-associated **myositis** resembling dermatomyositis has also been observed. **Neutropenia**, typically seen at diagnosis when infected, can be associated with *Pseudomonas* or staphylococcal infections.

Diagnosis

The diagnosis of XLA should be suspected if **lymphoid hypoplasia** is found on physical examination (minimal or no tonsillar tissue and no palpable lymph nodes), and serum concentrations of IgG, IgA, IgM, and IgE are far below the 95% confidence limits for appropriate age- and race-matched controls; total immunoglobulins are usually <100 mg/dL. Levels of natural antibodies to type A and B red blood cell polysaccharide antigens (isohemagglutinins) and antibodies to antigens given during routine immunizations are abnormally low in XLA, whereas they are typically normal in transient hypogammaglobulinemia of infancy. Flow cytometry is an important test to demonstrate the **absence of circulating B cells**, which will distinguish XLA from most types of CVID, the hyper-IgM syndrome, and transient hypogammaglobulinemia of infancy.

COMMON VARIABLE IMMUNODEFICIENCY

CVID is a syndrome characterized by hypogammaglobulinemia. Serum IgG must be <2 standard deviations below the age-adjusted norms, with low IgA and or IgM levels. CVID patients may appear similar clinically to those with XLA in the types of infections experienced and bacterial etiologic agents involved, except that enterovirus meningoencephalitis is rare in patients with CVID (Table 150.3). In contrast to XLA, the sex distribution in CVID is almost equal, the age at onset is later, and infections may be less severe. CVID is the most common of the antibody defects.

Table 150.3	Main Phenotypes of Primary Antibody Deficiencies	
PHENOTYPE	**MAIN CLINICAL FEATURES**	**MAIN B-CELL FEATURES**
Agammaglobulinemia	Bacterial infections (in respiratory tract) and enterovirus infections	Absence of CD19 B cells
Combined variable immunodeficiency (CVID)	Bacterial infections (in respiratory tract and gut), autoimmunity, cancer, and increased risk of granuloma	Highly variable; may see decreased memory B cells
Class switch defects	Bacterial and opportunistic infections	Decreased frequency of memory B cells
Selective IgA deficiency	Most often asymptomatic	Normal
IgG subclass deficiency	Frequent bacterial infections; diagnosis after age 2 yr	B-cell subsets normal
Selective polysaccharide antibody deficiency	Bacterial infections (after age 2 yr)	Normal IgG (including IgG2 and IgG4) levels, normal B-cell subsets

Genetics and Pathogenesis

CVID is a phenotypic diagnosis with a polygenic inheritance in most cases. Genes known to produce the CVID phenotype when mutated include *ICOS* (inducible co-stimulator) deficiency, *SH2D1A* (responsible for X-linked lymphoproliferative disease [XLP]), *CD19, CD20, CD21, CD81, BAFF-R* (B-cell–activating factor of the tumor necrosis factor family of receptors), *TACI* (transmembrane activator, calcium modulator, and cyclophilin ligand interactor). These mutations in aggregate account for <10% of all cases of CVID. With rare exceptions, management of CVID does not depend on a genetic diagnosis. In the setting of atypical infections or autoimmunity, pursuing a genetic diagnosis can be useful because some genetic etiologies can have a poor prognosis and transplantation should be considered.

Despite normal numbers of circulating B cells in many patients and the presence of lymphoid cortical follicles, blood B cells from CVID patients do not differentiate normally into immunoglobulin-producing cells. They may have a deficiency of switched memory B cells.

Clinical Manifestations

The serum immunoglobulin and antibody deficiencies in CVID are associated with recurrent sinopulmonary infections. Repeated pulmonary infections may produce bronchiectasis. Sepsis and meningitis with encapsulated bacteria occur more frequently than in the general population. Patients with recurrent infections as their only manifestation typically have a normal life expectancy and do well with immunoglobulin replacement. The presence of autoimmune disease or lymphoproliferation confers a poor prognosis. Patients with CVID often have autoantibody formation and normal-sized or enlarged tonsils and lymph nodes; about 25% of patients have splenomegaly. CVID has also been associated with a spruelike enteropathy with or without nodular lymphoid hyperplasia of the intestine. Other autoimmune diseases include alopecia areata, hemolytic anemia, thrombocytopenia, gastric atrophy, achlorhydria, and pernicious anemia. Lymphoid interstitial pneumonia, intestinal lung disease, pseudolymphoma, B-cell lymphomas, amyloidosis, and noncaseating sarcoid-like granulomas of the lungs, spleen, skin, and liver also occur. There is an increased risk of lymphomas.

SELECTIVE IgA DEFICIENCY

An isolated absence or near absence (<5 mg/dL) of serum and secretory IgA is the most common well-defined immunodeficiency disorder, with a disease frequency as high as 0.33% in some populations. Patients may be asymptomatic or may develop sinopulmonary or gastrointestinal (GI) infections (especially *Giardia*). IgA deficiency is also associated with celiac disease and autoimmune disorders. The diagnosis cannot be made until about 4 yr of age, when IgA levels should be matured to adult levels.

The basic defect resulting in IgA deficiency is unknown. Phenotypically normal blood B cells are present. This defect also often occurs in pedigrees containing individuals with CVID. Indeed, IgA deficiency may evolve into CVID. IgA deficiency is noted in patients treated with the same drugs associated with producing CVID (phenytoin, D-penicillamine,

gold, and sulfasalazine), suggesting that environmental factors may trigger this disease in a genetically susceptible person.

Clinical Manifestations

Infections occur predominantly in the respiratory, GI, and urogenital tracts. Bacterial agents responsible are the same as in other antibody deficiency syndromes. Intestinal giardiasis is common. Serum concentrations of other immunoglobulins are usually normal in patients with selective IgA deficiency, although IgG2 (and other) subclass deficiency has been reported.

Serum antibodies to IgA are reported in as many as 44% of patients with selective IgA deficiency. These antibodies can cause nonhemolytic transfusion reactions. Washed erythrocytes (frozen blood would have this done routinely) or blood products from other IgA-deficient individuals should be administered to patients with IgA deficiency. Many intravenous immune globulin (IVIG) preparations contain sufficient IgA to cause reactions. However, administration of IVIG, which is >99% IgG, is not indicated because most IgA-deficient patients make IgG antibodies normally.

IgG SUBCLASS DEFICIENCIES

Some patients have deficiencies of 1 or more of the 4 subclasses of IgG despite normal or elevated total IgG serum concentration. Some patients with absent or very low concentrations of IgG2 also have IgA deficiency. Other patients with IgG subclass deficiency have gone on to develop CVID, suggesting that the presence of IgG subclass deficiency may be a marker for more generalized immune dysfunction. The biologic significance of the numerous moderate deficiencies of IgG subclasses that have been reported is difficult to assess. IgG subclass measurement is not cost-effective in evaluating immune function in the child with recurrent infection. The more relevant issue is a patient's capacity to make specific antibodies to protein and polysaccharide antigens, because profound deficiencies of antipolysaccharide antibodies have been noted even in the presence of normal concentrations of IgG2. IVIG should not be administered to patients with IgG subclass deficiency unless they are shown to have a deficiency of antibodies to a broad array of antigens.

IMMUNOGLOBULIN HEAVY- AND LIGHT-CHAIN DELETIONS

Some completely asymptomatic individuals have been documented to have a total absence of IgG1, IgG2, IgG4, and/or IgA1 as a result of gene deletions. These patients illustrate the importance of assessing specific antibody formation before deciding to initiate IVIG therapy in IgG subclass–deficient patients.

TRANSIENT HYPOGAMMAGLOBULINEMIA OF INFANCY

A common laboratory finding in infants, transient hypogammaglobulinemia represents developmental delay in the production of immunoglobulin. It is thought to occur in as many as 1:1000 children. Most infants begin to produce IgG in the 1st 3 mo of life, and the quantity produced increases throughout infancy. For reasons incompletely understood, a small number of infants either begin late or do not increases their production as expected. This condition will resolve with no intervention but represents a source of diagnostic confusion. A key distinction is that responses to vaccines are usually preserved in this condition, whereas in the others, responses will be low to absent.

CLASS SWITCH DEFECTS

The **hyper-IgM syndrome** is genetically heterogeneous and characterized by normal or elevated serum IgM levels associated with low or absent IgG, IgA, and IgE serum levels, indicating a defect in the class switch recombination (CSR) process. Causative mutations have been identified in the CD40 ligand gene on the X chromosome and 3 genes on autosomal chromosomes: the activation-induced cytidine deaminase (**AID**) gene, the uracil DNA glycosylase gene (**UNG**), and the **CD40** gene on chromosome 20. Distinctive clinical features permit presumptive recognition of the type of mutation in these patients, thereby aiding proper choice of therapy. All such patients should undergo molecular analysis to ascertain the affected gene for purposes of genetic counseling, carrier detection, and decisions regarding definitive therapy.

X-Linked Hyper-IgM Caused by Mutations in CD40 Ligand Gene

X-linked hyper IgM is caused by mutations in the gene that encodes the CD40 ligand (CD154, CD40L), which is expressed on activated T-helper (Th) cells. Boys with this syndrome have very low serum concentrations of IgG and IgA, with a usually normal or sometimes elevated concentration of polyclonal IgM; may or may not have small tonsils; usually have no palpable lymph nodes; and often have profound neutropenia.

Genetics and Pathogenesis

The B cells are actually normal in this condition; the defect is in the T cells. CD40L is the ligand for CD40, which is present on B cells and monocytes. CD40L is upregulated on activated T cells. Mutations result in an inability to signal B cells to undergo isotype switching, and thus the B cells produce only IgM. The failure of T cells to interact with B cells through this receptor-ligand pair also causes a failure of upregulation of the B-cell and monocyte surface molecules CD80 and CD86 that interact with CD28/CTLA4 on T cells, resulting in failure of "crosstalk" between immune system cells.

Clinical Manifestations

Similar to patients with XLA, boys with the CD40 ligand defect become symptomatic during the 1st or 2nd yr of life with recurrent pyogenic infections, including otitis media, sinusitis, pneumonia, and tonsillitis. They have marked susceptibility to *P. jiroveci* pneumonia and can be neutropenic. Lymph node histology shows only abortive germinal center formation with severe depletion and phenotypic abnormalities of follicular dendritic cells. These patients have normal numbers of circulating B lymphocytes, but a decreased frequency of CD27+ memory B cells. Circulating T cells are also present in normal number and in vitro responses to mitogens are normal, but there is decreased antigen-specific T-cell function. In addition to opportunistic infections such as *P. jiroveci* pneumonia, there is an increased incidence of extensive verruca vulgaris lesions, *Cryptosporidium* enteritis, subsequent liver disease, and an increased risk of malignancy.

Treatment

Because of the poor prognosis, the treatment of choice is an HLA-identical hematopoietic stem cell transplant at an early age. Alternative treatment for this condition is monthly infusion of IVIG. In patients with severe neutropenia, the use of granulocyte colony-stimulating factor has been beneficial.

Autosomal Recessive Hyper-IgM
Genetics and Pathogenesis

In contrast to patients with the CD40L defect, B cells from these patients are not able to switch from IgM-secreting to IgG-, IgA-, or IgE-secreting cells, even when co-cultured with normal T cells. The defects are all B cell intrinsic. The most common autosomal recessive defect in a gene that encodes AID. AID deaminates cytosine into uracil in targeted DNA, which is followed by uracil removal by UNG. Severely impaired CSR was found in 3 hyper-IgM patients reported to have UNG deficiency. Their clinical characteristics were similar to those with AID deficiency, with increased susceptibility to bacterial infections and lymphoid hyperplasia. Histologic examination of the enlarged lymph nodes reveals the presence of giant germinal centers (5-10 times > normal) filled with highly proliferating B cells. Autosomal recessive hyper-IgM can be caused by defects in CD40. Clinical manifestations included recurrent sinopulmonary infections, *P. jiroveci* pneumonia, and *Cryptosporidium parvum* infections, very similar to the manifestations seen in X-linked hyper IgM syndrome.

Clinical Manifestations

Concentrations of serum IgG, IgA, and IgE are very low in AID, UNG, and CD40 deficiencies. In contrast to the CD40 ligand defect, however, the serum IgM concentration in patients with AID deficiency is usually markedly elevated and polyclonal. Patients with AID and UNG mutations have lymphoid hyperplasia, are generally older at age at onset, do not have susceptibility to *P. jiroveci* pneumonia, often do have isohemagglutinins, and are much less likely to have neutropenia unless it occurs on an autoimmune basis. They have a tendency, however, to develop autoimmune and inflammatory disorders, including diabetes mellitus, polyarthritis, autoimmune hepatitis, hemolytic anemia, immune thrombocytopenia, Crohn disease, and chronic uveitis.

Treatment and Prognosis

With early diagnosis and monthly infusions of IVIG, as well as good management of infections with antibiotics, patients with AID and UNG mutations generally have a more benign course than do boys with the CD40L or CD40 defects. CD40 deficiency is rare but appears to mimic the manifestations of CD40L quite closely.

X-LINKED LYMPHOPROLIFERATIVE DISEASE

There are two types of X-linked lymphoproliferative disease (Table 150.4). They have distinct clinical features but share a susceptibility to **Epstein-Barr virus (EBV)** and the development of **hemophagocytic lymphohistiocytosis (HLH)**.

Genetics and Pathogenesis

The defective gene in **XLP type I** was localized to Xq25, cloned, and the gene product was initially named SAP (SLAM-associated protein), but is now known officially as SH2D1A. SLAM (signaling lymphocyte activation molecule) is an adhesion molecule that is upregulated on both T and B cells with infection and other stimulation. The absence of SH2D1A can lead to an uncontrolled cytotoxic T-cell immune response to EBV. The SH2D1A protein associates permissively with 2B4 on natural killer (NK) cells; thus selective impairment of 2B4-mediated NK-cell activation also contributes to the immunopathology of XLP.

XLP type 2 is caused by a mutation in *XIAP* (X-linked inhibitor of apoptosis protein). Disease manifestations are similar to XLP. The precise role of this protein in the susceptibility to EBV has not been elucidated.

Clinical Manifestations

Affected males are usually healthy until they acquire EBV infection. The mean age of presentation is <5 yr. There are 3 major clinical phenotypes: (1) fulminant, often fatal, infectious mononucleosis (50% of cases); (2) lymphomas, predominantly involving B-lineage cells (25%); and (3) acquired hypogammaglobulinemia (25%). A less common manifestation is CNS vasculitis. There is a marked impairment in production of antibodies to the EBV nuclear antigen, whereas titers of antibodies to the viral capsid antigen have ranged from absent to greatly elevated. XLP has an unfavorable prognosis. Unless there is a family history of XLP, diagnosis before the onset of complications is difficult because affected individuals are asymptomatic initially.

Table 150.4	Features of SAP (SH2D1A) and XIAP Deficiency	
FEATURE	**SAP DEFICIENCY (XLP)**	**XIAP DEFICIENCY**
CLINICAL MANIFESTATIONS		
HLH	Yes	Yes
Hypogammaglobulinemia	Yes	Yes
Lymphoma	Yes	No
Aplastic anemia	Yes	No
Vasculitis	Yes	No
GENETICS		
Causative gene	SH2D1A	XIAP
Genetic locus	Xq25	Xq25
Encoded protein	SAP	XIAP
Effect of mutation	Reduced, absent protein expression	Reduced, absent or truncated protein
IMMUNE CELL FUNCTIONS		
Natural killer T (NKT) cell cytotoxicity/degranulation	Reduced	Normal
NKT cell number (blood)	Absent	Variable
Restimulation-induced death	Reduced	Increased
Memory B-cell numbers	Reduced	Not reported
TREATMENT OPTIONS		
HLH	Immunosuppression and/or chemotherapy (etoposide) Consideration of rituximab	Immunosuppression and/or chemotherapy (etoposide)
Humoral deficiency	Intravenous IgG infusions	Consider rituximab for EBV-positive cases Intravenous IgG infusions
Lymphoma	Standard chemotherapy	
Curative therapy	Stem cell transplantation	Stem cell transplantation

EBV, Epstein-Barr virus; HLH, hemophagocytic lymphohistiocytosis; SAP, SLAM-associated protein; XIAP, X-linked inhibitor of apoptosis protein.
From Rezaei N, Mahmoudi E, Aghamohamadi A, et al: X-linked lymphoproliferative syndrome: a genetic condition typified by the triad of infection, immunodeficiency and lymphoma, *Br J Haematol* 152:14, 2010.

In 2 pedigrees reported, boys in one arm of each pedigree were diagnosed with CVID, whereas those in the other arms had fulminant infectious mononucleosis. The family members with CVID never gave a history of infectious mononucleosis. All affected members of each pedigree had the same distinct *SH2D1A* mutation, however, despite the different clinical phenotypes. Because the *SH2D1A* mutation was the same but the phenotype varied in these families, XLP should be considered in all males with a diagnosis of CVID, particularly if there is more than 1 male family member with this phenotype.

Bibliography is available at Expert Consult.

150.1 Treatment of B-Cell Defects
Kathleen E. Sullivan and Rebecca H. Buckley

Except for the CD40 ligand defect and XLP, for which stem cell transplantation is recommended, judicious use of antibiotics to treat documented infections and regular administration of immunoglobulin are the only effective treatments for primary B-cell disorders. The most common forms of replacement therapy are either intravenous or subcutaneous immune globulin (IVIG or SCIG). Broad antibody deficiency should be carefully documented before such therapy is initiated. The rationale for the use of IVIG or SCIG is to provide missing antibodies, not to raise the serum IgG or IgG subclass level. The development of safe and effective immunoglobulin preparations is a major advance in the treatment of patients with severe antibody deficiencies, although it

is expensive and there have been national shortages. Almost all commercial preparations are isolated from normal plasma by the Cohn alcohol fractionation method or a modification of it. Cohn fraction II is then further treated to remove aggregated IgG. Additional stabilizing agents such as sugars, glycine, and albumin are added to prevent reaggregation and protect the IgG molecule during lyophilization. The ethanol used in preparation of immunoglobulin inactivates HIV, and an organic solvent/detergent step inactivates hepatitis B and C viruses. Some preparations are also nanofiltered to remove infectious agents. Most commercial lots are produced from plasma pooled from 10,000 to 60,000 donors and therefore contain a broad spectrum of antibodies. Each pool must contain adequate levels of antibody to antigens in various vaccines, such as tetanus and measles. However, there is no standardization based on titers of antibodies to more clinically relevant organisms, such as *S. pneumoniae* and *H. influenzae* type b.

The IVIG and SCIG preparations available in the United States have similar efficacy and safety. Rare transmission of hepatitis C virus has occurred in the past, but this has been resolved by the additional treatment step. There has been no documented transmission of HIV by any of these preparations. *IVIG or SCIG at a dose of 400 mg/kg per month* achieves trough IgG levels close to the normal range. Higher doses are indicated in patients with chronic or severe respiratory infections. Systemic reactions may occur, but rarely are these true anaphylactic reactions. Neutropenia associated with B-cell defects has responded to granulocyte colony-stimulating factor.

Bibliography is available at Expert Consult.

Chapter **151**

Primary Defects of Cellular Immunity

Kathleen E. Sullivan and Rebecca H. Buckley

第一百五十一章
原发性细胞免疫缺陷

中文导读

本章主要介绍了染色体22q11.2缺失综合征、T细胞激活缺陷、慢性黏膜皮肤念珠菌病，以及自身免疫多内分泌腺病念珠菌病外胚层发育不良。具体描述了染色体22q11.2缺失综合征的遗传发病机制、临床表现和治疗；描述了T细胞受体信号通路和导致T细胞激活缺陷的遗传基础；分别具体描述了慢性黏膜皮肤念珠菌病和自身免疫多内分泌腺病念珠菌病外胚层发育不良的遗传发病机制和临床表现。

Defects in cellular immunity, historically referred to *T-cell defects*, comprise a large number of distinct immune deficiencies. The manifestations usually include prolonged viral infections, opportunistic fungal or mycobacterial infections, and a predisposition to autoimmunity. To facilitate conceptualization of this large and complex category, this chapter describes immunodeficiencies where the defect primarily affects T cells and those where the defect alters function of many cell types. Chapter 152.1 describes severe combined immunodeficiency (SCID). These disorders are further approached clinically by considering whether or not nonhematologic features are present.

CHROMOSOME 22Q11.2 DELETION SYNDROME
Chromosome 22q11.2 deletion syndrome is the most common of the T-cell disorders, occurring in about 1 in 3,000 births in the United States. Chromosome 22q11.2 deletion disrupts development of the 3rd and 4th pharyngeal pouches during early embryogenesis, leading to hypoplasia or aplasia of the thymus and parathyroid glands. Other structures forming at the same age are also frequently affected, resulting in anomalies of the great vessels (right-sided aortic arch), esophageal atresia, bifid uvula, congenital heart disease (conotruncal, atrial, and ventricular septal defects), a short philtrum of the upper lip, hypertelorism, an antimongoloid slant to the eyes, mandibular hypoplasia, and posteriorly rotated ears (see Chapters 98 and 128). The diagnosis is often first suggested by hypocalcemic seizures during the neonatal period.

Genetics and Pathogenesis
Chromosome 22q11.2 deletions occur with high frequency because complex repeat sequences that flank the region represent a challenge for DNA polymerase. This condition is inherited in an autosomal dominant fashion and occurs with comparable frequency in all populations. Within the deleted region, haplosufficiency for the TBX1 transcription factor appears to underlie the majority of the phenotype. The phenotype is highly variable; a subset of patients has a phenotype that has also been called **DiGeorge syndrome**, **velocardiofacial syndrome**, or **conotruncal anomaly face syndrome**.

Variable hypoplasia of the thymus occurs in 75% of the patients with the deletion, which is more frequent than total aplasia; aplasia is present in <1% of patients with 22q11.2 deletion syndrome. Slightly less than half of patients with complete thymic aplasia are hemizygous at chromosome 22q11.2. Approximately 15% are born to diabetic mothers. Another 15% of infants have no identified risk factors. Approximately one third of infants with complete DiGeorge syndrome have **CHARGE association** (*c*oloboma, *h*eart defect, choanal *a*tresia, growth or developmental *r*etardation, *g*enital hypoplasia, and *e*ar anomalies including deafness). Mutations in the chromodomain helicase DNA-binding protein 7 (CHD7) gene on chromosome 8q12.2 are found in approximately 60–65% of individuals with CHARGE syndrome; a minority have mutations in *SEMA3E*.

Absolute lymphocyte counts are usually only moderately low for age. The CD3 T-cell counts are variably decreased in number, corresponding to the degree of thymic hypoplasia. Lymphocyte responses to mitogen stimulation are absent, reduced, or normal, depending on the degree of thymic deficiency. Immunoglobulin levels are often normal, but there is an increased frequency of IgA deficiency, low IgM levels, and some patients develop progressive hypogammaglobulinemia.

Clinical Manifestations
Children with partial thymic *hypoplasia* may have little trouble with infections and grow normally. Patients with thymic *aplasia* resemble

patients with SCID in their susceptibility to infections with low-grade or opportunistic pathogens, including fungi, viruses, and *Pneumocystis jiroveci*, and to graft-versus-host disease from nonirradiated blood transfusions. Patients with complete DiGeorge syndrome can develop an atypical phenotype in which oligoclonal T-cell populations appear in the blood associated with rash and lymphadenopathy. These atypical patients appear phenotypically similar to patients with **Omenn syndrome** or maternal T-lymphocyte engraftment.

It is critical to ascertain in a timely manner whether an infant has thymic aplasia, because this disease is fatal without treatment. A T-cell count should be obtained on all infants born with primary hypoparathyroidism, CHARGE syndrome, and conotruncal cardiac anomalies with syndromic features. Some infants are being identified by newborn screening for SCID and when 22q11.2 deletion is suspected, a calcium level should be obtained at the time of T-cell evaluation. The 3 manifestations with the highest morbidity in early infancy are profound immunodeficiency, severe cardiac anomaly, and seizures from hypocalcemia. Thus an early focus on these concerns is warranted even before the diagnosis is confirmed. Affected patients may develop autoimmune cytopenias, juvenile idiopathic arthritis, atopy, and malignancies (lymphomas).

Treatment

The immunodeficiency in thymic aplasia is correctable by cultured unrelated **thymic tissue transplants**. Some infants with thymic aplasia have been given nonirradiated unfractionated bone marrow or peripheral blood transplants from a human leukocyte antigen–identical sibling, with subsequent improved immune function because of adoptively transferred T cells. Infants and children with low T-cell counts but not low enough to consider transplantation should be monitored for evolution of immunoglobulin defects. Infections in these patients are multifactorial. Their anatomy may not favor drainage of secretions; they have a higher rate of atopy, which may complicate infections; and their host defense may allow persistence of infections. Interventions range from hand hygiene, probiotics, prophylactic antibiotics, and risk management to immunoglobulin replacement for those who have demonstrated defective humoral immunity.

T-CELL ACTIVATION DEFECTS

T-cell activation defects are characterized by the presence of normal or elevated numbers of blood T cells that appear phenotypically normal but fail to proliferate or produce cytokines normally in response to stimulation with mitogens, antigens, or other signals delivered to the TCR, owing to defective signal transduction from the TCR to intracellular metabolic pathways (Fig. 151.1). These patients have problems similar to those of other T-cell–deficient individuals, and some with severe T-cell activation defects may clinically resemble SCID patients (Table 151.1). In some cases, susceptibility to a single pathogen or a limited number of pathogens dominates the clinical phenotype. Susceptibility to Epstein-Barr virus, cytomegalovirus, and papillomavirus is common in this set of T-cell defects. Most individuals with significant T-cell activation defects will require a hematopoietic stem cell transplant. Although each infection may be manageable early in life, the long-term prognosis is not favorable in many of these conditions.

CHRONIC MUCOCUTANEOUS CANDIDIASIS

Chronic mucocutaneous candidiasis (**CMC**) is a syndrome characterized by impaired immune responsiveness to *Candida*. Some of the known gene defects with CMC have **autoimmune polyendocrinopathy syndrome type 1** (**APS1**, or autoimmune polyendocrinopathy-candidiasis–ectodermal dystrophy [**APECED**]). One of the other genetic types of CMC is associated with autoimmunity and predisposition to other infections (*STAT1* gain-of-function mutations). However, most of the

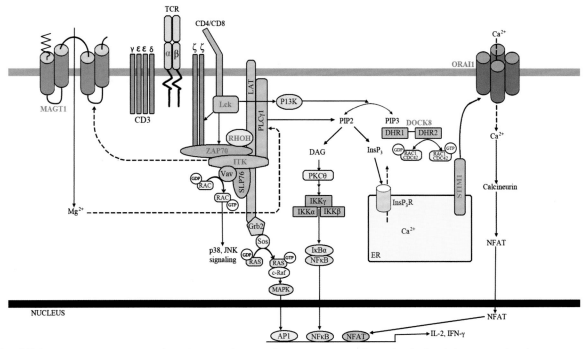

Fig. 151.1 Schematic representation of signaling through the T-cell receptor–CD3 complex. Molecules for which mutations have been associated with partial defect of T-cell development and impaired T-cell function are indicated in *red* and highlighted in **boldface**. AP1, Activator protein 1; DHR, DOCK-homology region; Grb2, growth factor receptor-bound protein 2; IKK, IκB kinase; JNK, c-Jun N-terminal kinase; MAPK, mitogen-activated protein kinase; NFAT, nuclear factor of activated T cells; NFκB, nuclear factor κB; PI3K, phosphoinositide-3 kinase; PIP3, phosphatidylinositol (3,4,5)-triphosphate. *(From Notarangelo L: Partial defects of T-cell development associated with poor T-cell function, J Allergy Clin Immunol 131:1299, 2013.)*

Table 151.1	Genetic Basis of Primary Cellular Immunodeficiency Diseases	
GENE PRODUCT	**EFFECT ON T CELLS**	**INFECTION SUSCEPTIBILITY**
Lck	↓↓ CD4 CD8	Viral infections predominantly
CD8α	↓↓ CD8 deficiency	Viral infections predominantly
ZAP-70	CD8 deficiency	Viral infections predominantly
RhoH	↓ Naïve CD4+ cells	Warts
ITK	↓ Naïve CD4+ cells Absence of NKT cells	Epstein-Barr virus
22q11.2 deletion	Thymic hypoplasia (DiGeorge syndrome, velocardiofacial syndrome)	Highly variable
CD3γ and ε	CD3 deficiency	Viral infections predominantly
TRAC	TCR-αβ T-cell deficiency	Similar to SCID
Coronin-1A	↓↓ CD4 ↓↓ CD8	Similar to SCID
MST1/STK4	↓ Naïve T cells Low number of recent thymic emigrants, restricted T-cell repertoire	Warts
AIRE	APECED, chronic mucocutaneous candidiasis, parathyroid and adrenal autoimmunity	Candida
TBX1	Thymic hypoplasia	Similar phenotype with 22q11.2 deletion

AIRE, Autoimmune regulator; APECED, autoimmune polyendocrinopathy-candidiasis–ectodermal dysplasia; Ig, immunoglobulin; ITK, IL-2–inducible tyrosine kinase deficiency; MST1, macrophage-stimulating factor 1; NKT, natural killer T; RhoH, Ras homology family member H; SCID, severe combined immunodeficiency; STK4, serine threonine kinase 4; TCR, T-cell receptor; TRAC, T-cell receptor α chain constant region; ZAP-70, zeta-associated protein 70.

specific genetic types of CMC have isolated susceptibility to *Candida*. These types of CMC relate to defects in the Th17 cell pathway. Autosomal recessive deficiency in the interleukin-17 receptor A (IL-17RA) chain, and an autosomal dominant deficiency of the cytokine IL-17F are both associated with predisposition to *Candida*. Other immunodeficiencies in which *Candida* occurs in the context of other infections also affect the Th17 cells. Another CMC genetic type, caused by mutations in *CARD9*, has a strong predisposition to *Candida* but also to other fungi.

Although the underlying gene defects are varied, the clinical presentation of CMC is usually similar. Symptoms can begin in the 1st mo of life or as late as the 2nd decade. The disorder is characterized by chronic and severe *Candida* skin and mucous membrane infections. Patients rarely develop systemic *Candida* disease, except as noted below. Topical antifungal therapy can provide limited improvement early in the course of the disease, but systemic courses of azoles are usually necessary; antifungal resistance often develops later in life. The infection usually responds temporarily to treatment, but it is not eradicated and recurs. Patients with *CARD9* gene mutations have a more severe fungal susceptibility than typical CMC patients. Two described patients with *CARD9* mutations had fungal sepsis in addition to CMC; deep tissue dermatophyte infections were also present.

AUTOIMMUNE POLYENDOCRINOPATHY-CANDIDIASIS–ECTODERMAL DYSPLASIA

Patients with this syndrome present with CMC and autoimmune polyendocrinopathy, usually developing hypoparathyroidism and Addison disease before adulthood. Additional features include male and female hypogonadism, chronic active hepatitis, alopecia, vitiligo, pernicious anemia, enamel hypoplasia, type 1 diabetes, asplenia, malabsorption, interstitial nephritis, hypothyroidism, hypopituitarism, and Sjögren syndrome. APECED, or APS1, is caused by a mutation in the autoimmune regulator *(AIRE)* gene (see Table 151.1). The gene product, AIRE, is expressed at high levels in purified human thymic medullary stromal cells and is thought to regulate the cell surface expression of tissue-specific proteins such as insulin and thyroglobulin. Expression of these self proteins allows for the negative selection of autoreactive T cells during their development. Failure of negative selection results in organ-specific autoimmune destruction.

Bibliography is available at Expert Consult.

Chapter **152**

Immunodeficiencies Affecting Multiple Cell Types

Jennifer R. Heimall, Jennifer W. Leiding, Kathleen E. Sullivan, and Rebecca H. Buckley

第一百五十二章
影响多种细胞类型的免疫缺陷

中文导读

本章主要介绍了重症联合免疫缺陷、联合免疫缺陷、固有免疫缺陷、细胞或联合免疫缺陷的治疗，以及伴自身免疫或淋巴增殖性免疫失调。详细阐述了重症联合免疫缺陷；具体描述了软骨毛发发育不全、WAS综合征、共济失调毛细血管扩张症和常染色体显性遗传高IgE综合征；具体描述了INFγ-IL12通路缺陷、IRAK4和MyD88缺陷、NK细胞缺陷、病毒和真菌感染固有免疫应答缺陷；具体描述了自身免疫淋巴增生综合征、X连锁免疫失调多内分泌腺病肠病综合征、CLTA4与LRBA缺陷，以及其他信号通路缺陷等。

The manifestations of immune deficiencies that affect multiple cell types range from profound to mild; these conditions can present with severe infection, recurrent infections, unusual infections, or autoimmunity. The most profound disorder is severe combined immunodeficiency. Other combined immunodeficiencies include defects of innate immunity and defects leading to immune dysregulation; the latter category is typically associated with profound autoimmunity. Combined immunodeficiencies are characterized by a predisposition to viral infections, and the innate immunodeficiencies are susceptible to a range of bacteria.

152.1 Severe Combined Immunodeficiency

Kathleen E. Sullivan and Rebecca H. Buckley

Severe combined immunodeficiency (**SCID**) is caused by diverse genetic mutations that lead to absence of T- and B-cell function. Patients with this group of disorders have the most severe immunodeficiency.

PATHOGENESIS

SCID is caused by mutations in genes crucial for lymphoid cell development (Table 152.1 and Fig. 152.1). All patients with SCID have very small thymuses that contain no thymocytes and lack corticomedullary distinction or Hassall corpuscles. The thymic epithelium appears histologically normal. Both the follicular and the paracortical areas of the spleen are depleted of lymphocytes. Lymph nodes, tonsils, adenoids, and Peyer patches are absent or extremely underdeveloped.

CLINICAL MANIFESTATIONS

SCID is included in the newborn screening program in many states. Thus, infants are identified prior to symptoms, which has dramatically improved the survival of infants with SCID. A few genetic types of SCID are not detected by newborn screening, and there are a few states where newborn screening for SCID is not yet performed.

When infants with SCID are not detected through newborn screening, they most often present with **infection**. Diarrhea, pneumonia, otitis media, sepsis, and cutaneous infections are common presentations. Infections with a variety of opportunistic organisms, either through direct exposure or immunization, can lead to death. Potential threats include *Candida albicans, Pneumocystis jiroveci,* parainfluenza 3 virus, adenovirus, respiratory syncytial virus (RSV), rotavirus vaccine, cytomegalovirus (CMV), Epstein-Barr virus (EBV), varicella-zoster virus, measles virus, MMRV (measles, mumps, rubella, varicella) vaccine, or bacille Calmette-Guérin (BCG) vaccine. Affected infants also lack the ability to reject foreign tissue and are therefore at risk for severe or fatal **graft-versus-host disease (GVHD)** from T lymphocytes in nonirradiated blood products or maternal immunocompetent T cells that crossed the placenta while the infant was in utero. This devastating presentation is characterized by expansion of the allogeneic cells, rash, hepatosplenomegaly and diarrhea. A 3rd presentation

Table 152.1	Genetic Basis of SCID and SCID Variants			
DISEASE	**INHERITANCE**	**PRESUMED PATHOGENESIS**	**ADDITIONAL FEATURES**	**TREATMENT**
Reticular dysgenesis	AR	Impaired mitochondrial energy metabolism and leukocyte differentiation	Severe neutropenia, deafness. Mutations in adenylate kinase 2	GCSF, HSCT
Adenosine deaminase deficiency	AR	Accumulation of toxic purine nucleosides	Neurologic, hepatic, renal, lung, and skeletal and bone marrow abnormalities	HSCT, PEG-ADA, gene therapy
IL-2Rγ deficiency	X-linked	Abnormal signaling through by IL-2 receptor and other receptors containing γc (IL-4, -7, -9, -15, -21)	None	HSCT
Jak3 deficiency	AR	Abnormal signaling downstream of γc	None	HSCT
RAG1 and RAG2 deficiency	AR	Defective V(D)J recombination	None	HSCT
Artemis deficiency	AR	Defective V(D)J recombination, radiation sensitivity	*DCLERE1C* gene defects	HSCT
DNA-PK deficiency	AR	Defective V(D)J recombination	None	HSCT
DNA ligase IV deficiency	AR	Defective V(D)J recombination, radiation sensitivity	Growth delay, microcephaly, bone marrow abnormalities, lymphoid malignancies	HSCT
Cernunnos-XLF	AR	Defective V(D)J recombination, radiation sensitivity	Growth delay, microcephaly, birdlike facies, bone defects	HSCT
CD3δ deficiency	AR	Arrest of thymocytes differentiation at CD4⁻CD8⁻ stage	Thymus size may be normal	HSCT
CD3ε deficiency	AR	Arrest of thymocytes differentiation at CD4⁻CD8⁻ stage	γ/δ T cells absent	HSCT
CD3ζ deficiency	AR	Abnormal signaling	None	HSCT
IL-7Rα deficiency	AR	Abnormal IL-7R signaling	Thymus absent	HSCT
CD45 deficiency	AR		None	HSCT
Coronin-1A deficiency	AR	Abnormal T-cell egress from thymus and lymph nodes	Normal thymus size. Attention deficit disorder.	HSCT

AR, Autosomal recessive; GCSF, granulocyte colony-stimulating factor; HSCT, hematopoietic stem cell transplantation; IL, interleukin; Jak3, Janus kinase 3; PEG-ADA, polyethylene glycol-modified adenosine deaminase; RAG1, RAG2, recombinase-activating genes 1 and 2; V(D)J, variable, diversity, joining domains.

(Adapted from Roifman, CM. Grunebaum E: Primary T-cell immunodeficiencies. In Rich RR, Fleisher TA, Shearer WT, et al, editors: *Clinical immunology,* ed 4. Philadelphia, 2013, Saunders, pp 440–441.)

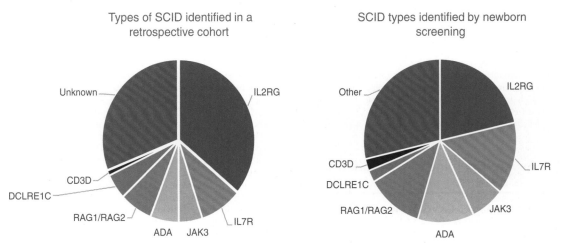

Fig. 152.1 Relative frequencies of the different genetic types of severe combined immunodeficiency (SCID). ADA, Adenosine deaminase; IL-7R, interleukin 7 receptor; JAK, Janus kinase; RAG, recombinase-activating gene.

is often called **Omenn syndrome**, in which a few cells generated in the infant expand and cause a clinical picture similar to GVHD (Fig. 152.2). The difference in this case is that the cells are the infant's own cells.

A key feature of SCID is that almost all patients will have a low lymphocyte count. A combination of opportunistic infections and a persistently low lymphocyte count is an indication to test for SCID. The diagnostic strategy both for symptomatic infants and those detected by newborn screening is to perform flow cytometry to quantitate the T, B, and natural killer (NK) cells in the infant. The CD45RA and CD45RO markers can be helpful to distinguish maternal engraftment and Omenn syndrome. T-cell function is also often assessed by measuring proliferative responses to stimulation.

All genetic types of SCID are associated with profound immunodeficiency. A small number have other associated features or atypical features that are important to recognize. Adenosine deaminase (ADA) deficiency can be associated with pulmonary alveolar proteinosis and chondroosseous dysplasia. Adenylate kinase 2 (AK2) deficiency causes a picture referred to as **reticular dysgenesis** where neutrophils, myeloid cells, and lymphocytes are all low. This condition is also often associated with deafness.

TREATMENT

SCID is a true pediatric immunologic emergency. Unless immunologic reconstitution is achieved through hematopoietic stem cell transplantation (**HSCT**) or gene therapy, death usually occurs during the 1st yr of life and almost invariably before 2 yr of age. *HSCT in an infant prior to infection is associated with a 95% survival rate.* ADA-deficient SCID and X-linked SCID have been treated successfully with gene therapy. Early trials of gene therapy were associated with a risk of malignancy, but this has not been seen in trials with new vectors. ADA-deficient SCID can also be treated with repeated injections of polyethylene glycol–modified bovine ADA (**PEG-ADA**), although the immune reconstitution achieved is not as effective as with stem cell or gene therapy.

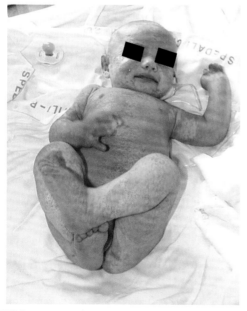

Fig. 152.2 Typical clinical features in an infant with Omenn syndrome. Note generalized erythroderma with scaly skin, alopecia, and edema. *(From Leung DYM, Szefler SJ, Bonilla FA, et al, editors: Pediatric allergy: principles and practice, ed 3, Philadelphia, 2016, Saunders, p 82).*

GENETICS

The 4 most common types of SCID are the X-linked form, caused by mutations in *CD132*; autosomal recessive *RAG1* and *RAG2* deficiencies; and *ADA* deficiency. Additional forms are listed in Table 152.1. For X-linked SCID and ADA deficiency, gene therapy exists, but genetic counseling is the most compelling reason for genetic sequencing to identify the gene defect. Several specific gene defects are associated with increased sensitivity to radiation and chemotherapy, and their early identification can lead to a better transplant experience.

Sequencing is often done by requesting a SCID gene panel. There are certain laboratory features that predict specific gene defects. When both T cells and B cells are low, often a gene encoding a protein involved in V(D)J recombination is the cause. Similarly, certain cytokine receptor defects are associated with specific lymphocyte phenotypes.

Hypomorphic mutations in genes most often associated with SCID can lead to varied phenotypes. This condition is often referred to as *leaky SCID*, referring to the mutation being "leaky" for some lymphocyte development. Leaky phenotypes range from the dramatic Omenn syndrome phenotype to later-onset immunodeficiency, granulomas, and autoimmunity.

Bibliography is available at Expert Consult.

152.2 Combined Immunodeficiency

Kathleen E. Sullivan and Rebecca H. Buckley

Combined immunodeficiency (**CID**) is distinguished from SCID by the presence of low but not absent T-cell function. CID is a syndrome of diverse genetic causes. Patients with CID have recurrent or chronic pulmonary infections, failure to thrive, oral or cutaneous candidiasis, chronic diarrhea, recurrent skin infections, gram-negative bacterial sepsis, urinary tract infections, and severe varicella in infancy. Although they usually survive longer than infants with SCID, they fail to thrive and often die before adulthood. Neutropenia and eosinophilia are common. Serum immunoglobulins may be normal or elevated for all classes, but selective IgA deficiency, marked elevation of IgE, and elevated IgD levels occur in some cases. Although antibody-forming capacity is impaired in most patients, it is not absent.

Studies of cellular immune function show lymphopenia, deficiencies of T cells, and extremely low but not absent lymphocyte proliferative responses to mitogens, antigens, and allogeneic cells in vitro. Peripheral lymphoid tissues demonstrate paracortical lymphocyte depletion. The thymus is usually small, with a paucity of thymocytes and usually no Hassall corpuscles.

CARTILAGE-HAIR HYPOPLASIA

Cartilage-hair hypoplasia (CHH) is an unusual form of **short-limbed dwarfism** with frequent and severe infections. It occurs with a high frequency among the Amish and Finnish people.

Genetics and Pathogenesis

CHH is an autosomal recessive condition. Numerous mutations that cosegregate with the CHH phenotype have been identified in the untranslated RNase MRP (*RMRP*) gene. The RMRP endoribonuclease consists of an RNA molecule bound to several proteins and has at least 2 functions: cleavage of RNA in mitochondrial DNA synthesis and nucleolar cleaving of pre-RNA. Mutations in *RMRP* cause CHH by disrupting a function of *RMRP* RNA that affects multiple organ systems. In vitro studies show decreased numbers of T cells and defective T-cell proliferation because of an intrinsic defect related to the G1 phase, resulting in a longer cell cycle for individual cells. NK cells are increased in number and function.

Clinical Manifestations

Clinical features include short, pudgy hands; redundant skin; hyperextensible joints of hands and feet but an inability to extend the elbows completely; and fine, sparse, light hair and eyebrows. Infections range from mild to severe. Associated conditions include deficient erythrogenesis, Hirschsprung disease, and an increased risk of malignancies. The bones radiographically show scalloping and sclerotic or cystic changes in the metaphyses and flaring of the costochondral junctions of the ribs. Some patients have been treated with HSCT.

WISKOTT-ALDRICH SYNDROME

Wiskott-Aldrich syndrome is an X-linked recessive disorder characterized by atopic dermatitis, thrombocytopenic purpura with normal-appearing megakaryocytes but small defective platelets, and susceptibility to infection.

Genetics and Pathogenesis

The Wiskott-Aldrich syndrome protein (WASP) binds CDC42H2 and Rac, members of the Rho family of guanosine triphosphatases. WASP controls the assembly of actin filaments required for cell migration and cell-cell interactions.

Clinical Manifestations

Patients often have prolonged bleeding from the circumcision site or bloody diarrhea during infancy. The thrombocytopenia is not initially caused by antiplatelet antibodies. **Atopic dermatitis** and **recurrent infections** usually develop during the 1st yr of life. *Streptococcus pneumoniae* and other bacteria having polysaccharide capsules cause otitis media, pneumonia, meningitis, and sepsis. Later, infections with agents such as *P. jiroveci* and the herpesviruses become more frequent. Infections, bleeding, and EBV-associated malignancies are major causes of death.

Patients with this defect uniformly have an impaired humoral immune response to polysaccharide antigens, as evidenced by absent or greatly diminished isohemagglutinins, and poor or absent antibody responses after immunization with polysaccharide vaccines. The predominant immunoglobulin pattern is a low serum level of IgM, elevated IgA and IgE, and a normal or slightly low IgG concentration. Because of their profound antibody deficiencies, these patients should be given immunoglobulin replacement regardless of their serum levels of the different immunoglobulin isotypes. Percentages of T cells are moderately reduced, and lymphocyte responses to mitogens are variably depressed.

Treatment

Good supportive care includes appropriate nutrition, immunoglobulin replacement, use of killed vaccines, and aggressive management of eczema and associated cutaneous infections. HSCT is the treatment of choice when a high-quality matched donor is available and is usually curative. Gene-corrected autologous HSCT has resulted in sustained benefits in 6 patients.

ATAXIA-TELANGIECTASIA

Ataxia-telangiectasia is a complex syndrome with immunologic, neurologic, endocrinologic, hepatic, and cutaneous abnormalities.

Genetics and Pathogenesis

The ataxia-telangiectasia mutation (*ATM*) gene encodes a protein critical for responses to DNA damage. Cells from patients, as well as from heterozygous carriers, have increased sensitivity to ionizing radiation, defective DNA repair, and frequent chromosomal abnormalities.

In vitro tests of lymphocyte function have generally shown moderately depressed proliferative responses to T- and B-cell mitogens. Percentages of CD3 and CD4 T cells are moderately reduced, with normal or increased percentages of CD8 and elevated numbers of γ/δ T cells. The thymus is very hypoplastic, exhibits poor organization, and lacks Hassall corpuscles.

Clinical Manifestations

The most prominent clinical features are progressive **cerebellar ataxia, oculocutaneous telangiectasias, chronic sinopulmonary disease**, a high incidence of malignancy, and variable humoral and cellular immunodeficiency. Ataxia typically becomes evident soon after these children begin to walk and progresses until they are confined to a wheelchair, usually by age 10-12 yr. The telangiectasias begin to develop at 3-6 yr. The most frequent humoral immunologic abnormality is the selective absence of IgA, which occurs in 50–80% of these patients. IgG2 or total IgG levels may be decreased, and specific antibody titers may be decreased or normal. Recurrent sinopulmonary infections occur in approximately 80% of these patients. Although common viral infections have not usually resulted in untoward sequelae, fatal varicella has occurred. The malignancies associated with ataxia-telangiectasia are usually of the lymphoreticular type, but adenocarcinomas also occur. Unaffected carriers of mutations have an increased incidence of malignancy.

Therapy in ataxia-telangiectasia is supportive.

AUTOSOMAL DOMINANT HYPER-IgE SYNDROME

This syndrome is associated with early-onset atopy and recurrent skin and lung infections.

Genetics and Pathogenesis

The autosomal dominant hyper-IgE syndrome is caused by heterozygous mutations in the gene encoding signal transducer and activator of transcription 3 (STAT-3). These mutations result in a dominant negative effect. The many clinical features are caused by compromised signaling downstream of the interleukin (IL)-6, type I interferon, IL-22, IL-10 and epidermal growth factor (EGF) receptors.

Clinical Manifestations

The characteristic clinical features are staphylococcal abscesses, pneumatoceles, osteopenia, and unusual facial features. There is a history from infancy of recurrent staphylococcal abscesses involving the skin, lungs, joints, viscera, and other sites. Persistent pneumatoceles develop as a result of recurrent pneumonia. Patients often have a history of sinusitis and mastoiditis. *Candida albicans* is the 2nd most common pathogen. Allergic respiratory symptoms are usually absent. The pruritic dermatitis that occurs is not typical atopic eczema and does not always persist. There can be a prominent forehead, deep-set wide-spaced eyes, a broad nasal bridge, a wide fleshy nasal tip, mild prognathism, facial asymmetry, and hemihypertrophy, although these are most evident in adulthood. In older children, delay in shedding primary teeth, recurrent fractures, and scoliosis occur.

These patients demonstrate an **exceptionally high serum IgE concentration**; an elevated serum IgD concentration; usually normal concentrations of IgG, IgA, and IgM; pronounced blood and sputum eosinophilia; and poor antibody and cell-mediated responses to neoantigens. Traditionally, IgE levels >2000 IU/mL confirm the diagnosis. However, IgE levels may fluctuate and even decrease in adults. In neonates and infants with the pruritic pustular dermatosis, IgE levels will be elevated for age and are usually in the 100s. In vitro studies show normal percentages of blood T, B, and NK lymphocytes, except for a decreased percentage of T cells with the memory (CD45RO) phenotype and an absence or deficiency of T-helper type 17 (Th17) cells. Most patients have normal T-lymphocyte proliferative responses to mitogens but very low or absent responses to antigens or allogeneic cells from family members. Blood, sputum, and histologic sections of lymph nodes, spleen, and lung cysts show striking eosinophilia. Hassall corpuscles and thymic architecture are normal. Therapy is generally directed at prevention of infection using antimicrobials and immunoglobulin replacement.

DOCK8 DEFICIENCY

Deficiency of DOCK8 (dedicator of cytokinesis 8) is an autosomal recessive condition that most often presents with impressively severe eczema in infancy and toddlerhood. **Cutaneous viral infections** and **susceptibility to CMV, EBV, and cryptosporidia** are common (Fig. 152.3). The infectious susceptibility tends to worsen over time, as do the laboratory features of immune dysfunction, most often low T-cell counts and poor proliferative function. Although these patients can survive to adulthood without transplantation, they suffer many complications and their quality of life is often poor. For this reason, most patients are now transplanted early in life to avoid the later complications.

Bibliography is available at Expert Consult.

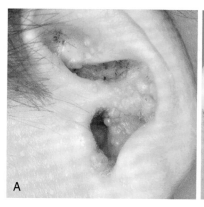
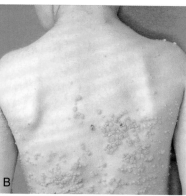

Fig. 152.3 Extensive sheets of molluscum on the ear (**A**) and trunk (**B**). *(From Purcell C, Cant A, Irvine AD: DOCK8 primary immunodeficiency syndrome, Lancet 386:982, 2015.)*

152.3 Defects of Innate Immunity

Jennifer R. Heimall and Kathleen E. Sullivan

The innate immune system is the earliest responding feature of host defense in vertebrates. Components include the physical barrier function of the skin and mucosal surfaces, complement, neutrophils, macrophages, dendritic cells (DCs), NK cells, and their associated cytokines. The activation of innate immunity is critically reliant on a group of **pattern recognition receptors (PRRs)** that respond to host infections or tissue damage within minutes. These receptors are all germline encoded and are therefore able to be expressed in all cells, where they serve as critical monitors for the presence of **pathogen-associated molecular patterns (PAMPs)**.

INTERFERON-γ RECEPTORS 1 AND 2, IL-12 RECEPTOR β₁, AND IL-12P40 DEFECTS

Among the best-described defects of innate immunity are those associated with susceptibility to nontuberculous mycobacteria. These defects are associated with abnormalities in the interferon-gamma (IFN-γ)–IL-12 signaling axis.

Pathogenesis

Interleukin-12 is a cytokine secreted by macrophages, neutrophils, and DCs in response to infection with mycobacterial and other microbes. IL-12 then binds to receptors on NK cells and T cells to stimulate secretion of IFN-γ. IFN-γ is critical in the activation of phagocyte secretion of tumor necrosis factor alpha (TNF-α) and destruction of the phagocytosed microbe. IFN-γ activates phagocytes via binding of IFN-γ receptor 1 (IFN-γR1) which is found in a homodimerized form associated with Janus-associated kinase-1 (Jak1) that recruits and binds IFN-γ receptor 2 (IFN-γR2) which is associated with Janus-associated kinase-2 (Jak2). Jak1 and Jak2 are then transphosphorylated, which leads to phosphorylation of IFN-γR1 and subsequent docking of signal transducer and activator of transcription 1 (STAT1). Phosphorylated STAT1 then homodimerizes and translocates to the cell nucleus to induce gene transcription. Deficiency of any of these components has a significant impact on phagocyte activation.

Clinical Manifestations

IFN-γR1 deficiency leads to impaired IFN-γ binding and signaling and inability to form mature granulomas and indicates a risk of **susceptibility to *Mycobacteria*** species and *Salmonella*. There are both autosomal recessive (AR) and autosomal dominant (AD) forms of this defect. In the AR form are both partial and complete defects. In the complete AR form, patients present with early onset of disseminated *Mycobacteria*, and some have been reported to present with nontyphoid *Salmonella* or *Listeria monocytogenes*. Treatment should be directed at the presenting

infection, with multiple antimicrobial agents used without interruption. HSCT has been used once mycobacterial disease is controlled but requires conditioning to permit the myeloid engraftment necessary to correct the underlying disease. In the partial AR form, IFN-γR1 deficiency remains associated with disseminated *Mycobacteria* and *Salmonella* infections but is managed with symptomatic treatment of infections and consideration of IFN-γ therapy to induce higher serum IFN-γ levels. The AD form is also a partial defect in IFN-γ signaling and most often presents with *Mycobacteria* osteomyelitis, although *Salmonella* and *Histoplasma* infections have also been described. Similar to the partial AR defect, these patients are able to be managed with antimicrobial therapy of infections and supplemental IFN-γ injections. Deficiency of IFN-γR2 is an AR defect that also has partial and complete forms. The complete form is a phenocopy to complete IFN-γR1, presenting with early-onset, severe, and disseminated mycobacterial infections. Treatment involves uninterrupted multidrug therapy for the infections and consideration for HSCT. A partial form of IFN-γR2 also presents with mild but potentially disseminated *Mycobacteria* or *Salmonella* infections, which can be controlled with antibiotic therapy that can be stopped once the infection is resolved.

Deficiencies of the IL-12 receptor (IL-12R) components have also been described as inherited in an AR fashion, with defects in both the IL-12p40 chain as well as the shared IL-12/IL-23Rβ₁, causing impaired IFN-γ secretion and resultant susceptibility to *Mycobacteria* and *Salmonella*. Both forms of IL-12R defects are characterized by relatively mild disease, with some ability to form granulomatous lesions in response to *Mycobacteria* infections. These defects can usually be managed with antimicrobials and supplemental IFN-γ. Partial defects in STAT1, inherited in an AD fashion, are associated with *Mycobacteria* susceptibility, whereas complete AR defects in STAT1 are associated with mycobacterial susceptibility as well as defects in responses to IFN-α and IFN-β, leading to fulminant herpesvirus infections. Other defects associated with poor production of IFN-γ leading to increased *Mycobacteria* susceptibility include AR inherited defects in **ISG-15**, which is associated with *Mycobacteria*-induced brain calcifications, and **RORγC** deficiency, which leads to a lack of IL-17–producing T cells, in addition to lack of IFN-γ production. RORγC defects are associated with an increased risk of candidiasis in addition to *Mycobacteria* infections. Defects in **Tyk2**, inherited in an AR fashion, generally present with susceptibility to intracellular bacteria, fungi and viruses. AD mutations in interferon regulatory factor 8 (*IRF8*) are also associated with impaired IL-12 production by the CD1-DCs, leading to increased risk of recurrent mycobacterial infection, which can be treated with antimicrobial therapy.

IL-1R–ASSOCIATED KINASE 4 DEFICIENCY AND MYELOID DIFFERENTIATION FACTOR 88

Toll-like receptors (**TLRs**) are the best described of the PRRs in humans, and deficiencies almost uniformly cause infection susceptibility.

Pathogenesis

Among those expressed on the cell surface, TLRs 1, 2, and 6 bind lipoproteins and are important in defense to bacteria and fungi, TLR4 binds lipopolysaccharides and has an important role in defense from gram-negative bacteria as well as the fusion protein of RSV. TLR5 binds flagellin, found in many bacterial organisms. The remaining TLRs (3, 7, 8, and 9) are expressed intracellularly, respond to nucleic acids and are initiators of the host response for viral defense. When bound to their PAMP, TLRs activate an intracellular signaling cascade that in most cases utilizes myeloid differentiation primary response gene 88 (MyD88) and IL-1R–associated kinase 4 (IRAK4). TLR4 also signals using the Toll/IL-1R domain-containing adaptor-inducing interferon-B (TRIF). Both MyD88 and TRIF can lead to activation of the nuclear factor (NF)-κB pathway via the IKK complex to induce proinflammatory cytokine production. The IKK complex is composed of IKKα and IKKβ, and IKKγ (NF-κB essential modulator, or NEMO).

Clinical Manifestations

IRAK4 and *MYD88* deficiencies have identical features and are associated with deep infections such as pneumonia, meningitis, or sepsis with encapsulated organisms early in life. The main organisms recovered from patients are *Staphylococcus aureus*, *Streptococcus pneumoniae*, *Haemophilus influenzae*, and *Pseudomonas aeruginosa*. This is one of the few types of immunodeficiency where clostridial infections are also seen with increased frequency. Most patients have an improved infection risk after adolescence. Therapy has generally focused on education of parents and clinicians to the life-threatening nature of the infections with encouragement of timely cultures and empirical antibiotic use. These patients may have a **blunted febrile response**, and clinical features of infection may be subtle.

Among the first-described defects of TLR signaling were X-linked mutations in *NEMO*, which causes a broad range of clinical manifestations, with most demonstrating a poor inflammatory response. NEMO is typically considered in the category of combined immunodeficiency because of its impact on both innate and adaptive immune responses. Severely affected patients may present with disseminated *Mycobacteria* infections, severe infections from encapsulated organisms such as *S. pneumoniae* or other opportunistic infections. In addition to the infectious phenotype, these patients characteristically have conical or peg-shaped teeth, hypohydrosis, and hypotrichosis from anhidrotic ectodermal dysplasia (EDA). Patients should be treated with immunoglobulin replacement, antibiotic prophylaxis with trimethoprim/sulfamethoxazole, azithromycin, and/or penicillin VK. HSCT is a treatment consideration, but myeloid lineage engraftment is needed to fully correct the underlying immunodeficiency.

NATURAL KILLER CELL DEFICIENCY

NK cells are the major lymphocytes of the innate immune system. NK cells recognize virally infected and malignant cells and mediate their elimination. Individuals with absence or functional deficiencies of NK cells are rare, and they typically have susceptibility to the herpesviruses (including varicella-zoster virus, herpes simplex virus (HSV), CMV, and EBV) as well as papillomaviruses. A number of gene defects are associated with these isolated abnormalities in NK cells. Autosomal recessive CD16 gene mutations were described in 3 separate families and altered the first immunoglobulin-like domain of this important NK cell activation receptor. Patients with these mutations have NK cells that are functionally impaired and have clinical susceptibility to **herpesviruses**. AD deficiency of NK cells occurs in individuals with mutations in the **GATA2 transcription factor**. These patients also have cytopenias and very low numbers of monocytes. They have extreme susceptibility to **human papillomavirus** (HPV) as well as mycobacteria, the latter presumably from the monocytic defect. They are at risk for alveolar proteinosis, myelodysplasia, and leukemia. AR mutations in the *MCM4* gene have been identified in a cohort of patients who had growth failure and susceptibility to herpesviruses. Therapeutically, patients should

be maintained on antiviral prophylaxis, and HSCT has been successful in certain cases.

DEFECTS IN INNATE RESPONSES TO VIRAL INFECTION

Defects in both the JAK-STAT signaling pathways and the TLR signaling pathways have been implicated in patients with increased susceptibility to severe viral infections. AR defects in STAT1 cause a complete lack of response to INF-γ and IFN-α/β, affecting the function of T and NK cells as well as monocytes, leading to disseminated mycobacterial infections as well as severe herpesvirus infections, including recurrent **HSV encephalitis** and EBV-driven lymphoproliferative disease. In these patients, lifelong antibiotic therapy to protect from *Mycobacteria* and antiviral therapy for herpesviruses is recommended, and HSCT should be considered. Defects in STAT2, inherited in an AR fashion, lead to poor T- and NK-cell responses to IFN-α and IFN-β, leading to increased viral susceptibility, in particular development of **disseminated vaccine strain measles** with central nervous system (CNS) involvement despite development of normal vaccine titers. The interferon response factor 7 (IRF7) is important in induction of IFN-α/β via the both the MyD88-dependent and independent pathways of TLR signaling. AR defects in IRF7 have been associated with severe respiratory distress with influenza A infection in a patient with otherwise normal vaccine responses and T- and B-cell populations.

HSV-1 encephalitis has been associated with a group of defects in TLR signaling that lead to decreased production of IFN-α/β/λ causing impaired immunity to HSV-1 but not other viral infections. The first described was deficiency of UNC93B1, a protein involved in trafficking of the TLRs 7 and 9 and inherited in an AR fashion. Subsequently, defects in TLR3 and TRIF as well as the other TLR pathway signaling molecules tumor necrosis factor (TNF), receptor–associated factor 3 (TRAF3), and tank-binding kinase 1 (TBK1) were described to lead to decreased production of IFN-α/β/λ and an associated risk of sporadic HSV-1 encephalitis that can be recurrent. The symptoms were controlled with acyclovir prophylaxis.

DEFECTS IN INNATE RESPONSES TO FUNGI

Although **chronic mucocutaneous candidiasis (CMC)** can be seen in association with CID, T-cell disorders, and hyper-IgE syndromes, there are also innate defects known to cause CMC (see Chapter 151). The most common include AD gain-of-function mutations in *STAT1*, where an increased response to IFN-α/β/γ leads to decreased Th17 differentiation. In addition to CMC, these patients also have increased susceptibility to bacterial, fungal, and HSV viral infections; autoimmunity; and enteropathy. Patients with CMC are managed with antifungal, antibacterial, and acyclovir prophylaxis, and HSCT should be considered as a treatment option. Mutations in the IL-17RA and IL-17F have also been described to increase risk of CMC; IL-17RA and IL-17F deficiencies are also associated with *S. aureus* folliculitis, likely from impaired skin β-defensin production. Treatment includes **fluconazole** and sulfamethoxazole/trimethoprim prophylaxis. TRAF3-interacting protein 2 (TRAF3IP2) interacts with IL-17RA on binding of IL-17; AR mutations in TRAF3IP2 have been described in patients with CMC, blepharitis, folliculitis, and macroglossia. CMC is also seen in 25% of patients with IL-12RB1 and IL12p40 defects. Invasive fungal infections, including invasive **dermatophyte infections** and *Candida* brain abscesses, have been seen in addition to CMC in patients with AR inherited defects in CARD9. CARD9 leads to NF-κB–induced cytokine production in response to fungal PAMPS that bind to C-type lectin receptors, including Dectin 1, Dectin 2, and MINCLE. Both granulocyte-macrophage colony-stimulating factor (GM-CSF) and G-CSF have been successfully used to control refractory brain lesions, and once identified, these patients should be maintained on fluconazole prophylaxis.

Bibliography is available at Expert Consult.

152.4 Treatment of Cellular or Combined Immunodeficiency

Kathleen E. Sullivan and Rebecca H. Buckley

Good supportive care, including prevention and treatment of infections, is critical while patients await more definitive therapy (Table 152.2). Having knowledge of the pathogens causing disease with specific immune defects is also useful.

Transplantation of major histocompatibility complex (MHC)–compatible sibling or rigorously T-cell–depleted haploidentical (half-matched) parental hematopoietic stem cells is the treatment of choice for patients with fatal T-cell or combined T- and B-cell defects. The major risk to the recipient from transplants of bone marrow or peripheral blood stem cells is GVHD from donor T cells. Patients with less severe forms of cellular immunodeficiency, including some forms of CID, Wiskott-Aldrich syndrome, cytokine deficiency, and MHC antigen deficiency, reject even HLA-identical marrow grafts unless chemoablative treatment is given before transplantation. Several patients with these conditions have been treated successfully with hematopoietic stem cell transplantation after conditioning.

More than 90% of patients with primary immunodeficiency transplanted with HLA-identical related marrow will survive with immune reconstitution. T-cell–depleted haploidentical-related marrow transplants in patients with primary immunodeficiency have had their greatest success in patients with SCID, who do not require pretransplant conditioning or GVHD prophylaxis. Of patients with SCID, 92% have survived after T-cell–depleted parental marrow is given soon after birth when the infant is healthy, without pretransplant chemotherapy or posttransplant GVHD prophylaxis. Bone marrow transplantation remains the most important and effective therapy for SCID. In ADA-deficient and X-linked SCID, there has been success in correcting the immune defects with ex vivo gene transfer to autologous hematopoietic stem cells. Gene therapy has also been successful in the Wiskott-Aldrich syndrome. Initial protocols of gene therapy for X-linked SCID resulted in **insertional mutagenesis** with the development of leukemic-like clonal T cells or lymphoma in some patients. Modification of the gene therapy protocol has greatly reduced the risk of insertional mutagenesis.

152.5 Immune Dysregulation With Autoimmunity or Lymphoproliferation

Jennifer W. Leiding, Kathleen E. Sullivan, and Rebecca H. Buckley

Primary immunodeficiency diseases characterized by immune dysregulation, autoimmunity, and autoinflammation are monogenic defects of the immune system. These complex multisystem diseases often have a progressive phenotype with organ-specific autoimmunity, specific infectious susceptibility, and lymphoproliferation.

AUTOIMMUNE LYMPHOPROLIFERATIVE SYNDROME

Autoimmune lymphoproliferative syndrome (**ALPS**), also known as Canale-Smith syndrome, is a disorder of abnormal lymphocyte apoptosis leading to polyclonal populations of T cells (double-negative T cells), which express CD3 and α/β antigen receptors but do not have CD4 or CD8 co-receptors (CD3$^+$ T-cell receptor α/β^+, CD4$^-$CD8$^-$). These T cells respond poorly to antigens or mitogens and do not produce growth or survival factors (IL-2). The genetic deficit in most patients is a germline or somatic mutation in the *FAS* gene, which produces a cell surface receptor of the TNF receptor superfamily (TNFRSF6), which, when stimulated by its ligand, will produce programmed cell death (Table 152.3). Persistent survival of these lymphocytes leads to immune dysregulation and autoimmunity. ALPS is also caused by other genes in the Fas pathway (*FASLG* and *CASP10*). In addition, ALPS-like disorders are associated with other mutations: RAS-associated autoimmune

Table 152.2	Infection in the Host Compromised by B- and T-Cell Immunodeficiency Syndromes		
IMMUNODEFICIENCY SYNDROME	**OPPORTUNISTIC ORGANISMS ISOLATED MOST FREQUENTLY**	**APPROACH TO TREATMENT OF INFECTIONS**	**PREVENTION OF INFECTIONS**
B-cell immunodeficiencies	Encapsulated bacteria (*Streptococcus pneumoniae, Staphylococcus aureus, Haemophilus influenzae,* and *Neisseria meningitidis*), *Pseudomonas aeruginosa, Campylobacter* spp., enteroviruses, rotaviruses, *Giardia lamblia, Cryptosporidium* spp., *Pneumocystis jiroveci, Ureaplasma urealyticum,* and *Mycoplasma pneumoniae*	IVIG, 200-800 mg/kg Vigorous attempt to obtain specimens for culture before antimicrobial therapy Incision and drainage if abscess present Antibiotic selection on the basis of sensitivity data	Maintenance IVIG for patients with quantitative and qualitative defects in IgG metabolism (400-800 mg/kg every 3-5 wk) In chronic recurrent respiratory disease, vigorous attention to postural drainage In selected cases (recurrent or chronic pulmonary or middle ear), prophylactic administration of ampicillin, penicillin, or trimethoprim-sulfamethoxazole
T-cell immunodeficiencies	Encapsulated bacteria (*S. pneumoniae, H. influenzae, S. aureus*), facultative intracellular bacteria (*Mycobacterium tuberculosis,* other *Mycobacterium* spp., and *Listeria monocytogenes*); *Escherichia coli; P. aeruginosa; Enterobacter* spp.; *Klebsiella* spp.; *Serratia marcescens; Salmonella* spp.; *Nocardia* spp.; viruses (cytomegalovirus, herpes simplex virus, varicella-zoster virus, Epstein-Barr virus, rotaviruses, adenoviruses, enteroviruses, respiratory syncytial virus, measles virus, vaccinia virus, and parainfluenza viruses); protozoa (*Toxoplasma gondii* and *Cryptosporidium* spp.); and fungi (*Candida* spp., *Cryptococcus neoformans, Histoplasma capsulatum,* and *P. jiroveci*)	Vigorous attempt to obtain specimens for culture before antimicrobial therapy Incision and drainage if abscess present Antibiotic selection on the basis of sensitivity data Early antiviral treatment for herpes simplex, cytomegalovirus, and varicella-zoster viral infections Topical and nonadsorbable antimicrobial agents frequently are useful	Prophylactic administration of trimethoprim-sulfamethoxazole for prevention of *P. jiroveci* pneumonia Oral nonadsorbable antimicrobial agents to lower concentration of gut flora No live virus vaccines or bacille Calmette-Guérin vaccine Careful tuberculosis screening

IVIG, Intravenous immune globulin.
From Stiehm ER, Ochs HD, Winkelstein JA: *Immunologic disorders in infants and children,* ed 5, Philadelphia, 2004, Saunders.

REQUIRED

1. Chronic (>6 months), nonmalignant, noninfectious lymphadenopathy, splenomegaly or both
2. Elevated CD3+TCRαβ+CD4-CD8- DNT cells (≥1.5% of total lymphocytes or 2.5% of CD3+ lymphocytes) in the setting of normal or elevated lymphocyte counts

ACCESSORY

Primary

1. Defective lymphocyte apoptosis (in 2 separate assays)
2. Somatic or Germline pathogenic mutation in *FAS*, *FASLG*, or *CASP10*

Secondary

1. Elevated plasma sFasL levels (>200 pg/mL) OR elevated plasma interleukin-10 levels (>20 pg/mL) OR elevated serum or plasma vitamin B 12 levels (>1500 ng/L) OR elevated plasma interleukin-18 levels >500 pg/mL
2. Typical immunohistological findings as reviewed by an experienced hematopathologist
3. Autoimmune cytopenias (hemolytic anemia, thrombocytopenia, or neutropenia) AND elevated immunoglobulin G levels (polyclonal hypergammaglobulinemia)
4. Family history of a nonmalignant/noninfectious lymphoproliferation with or without autoimmunity

*A *definitive* diagnosis is based on the presence of both required criteria plus one primary accessory criterion. A *probable* diagnosis is based on the presence of both required criteria plus one secondary accessory criterion.

From Petty RE, Laxer RM, Lindsley CB, Wedderburn LR, editors: Textbook of pediatric rheumatology, ed 7, Philadelphia, 2016, Elsevier, Box 46-2.

lymphoproliferative disorder (RALD), caspase-8 deficiency, Fas-associated protein with death domain deficiency (FADD), and protein kinase C delta deficiency (PRKCD). These disorders have varying degrees of immunodeficiency, autoimmunity, and lymphoproliferation.

Clinical Manifestations

ALPS is characterized by **autoimmunity, chronic persistent or recurrent lymphadenopathy**, splenomegaly, hepatomegaly (in 50%), and hypergammaglobulinemia (IgG, IgA). Many patients present in the 1st yr of life, and most are symptomatic by age 5 yr. Lymphadenopathy can be striking (Fig. 152.4). Splenomegaly may produce hypersplenism. Autoimmunity also produces anemia (Coombs-positive hemolytic anemia) or thrombocytopenia or a mild neutropenia. The lymphoproliferative process (lymphadenopathy, splenomegaly) may regress over time, but autoimmunity does not regress and is characterized by frequent exacerbations and recurrences. Other autoimmune features include urticaria, uveitis, glomerulonephritis, hepatitis, vasculitis, panniculitis, arthritis, and CNS involvement (seizures, headaches, encephalopathy).

Malignancies are also more common in patients with ALPS and include Hodgkin and non-Hodgkin lymphomas and solid-tissue tumors of thyroid, skin, heart, or lung. ALPS is one cause of Evan syndrome (immune thrombocytopenia and immune hemolytic anemia).

Diagnosis

Laboratory abnormalities depend on the lymphoproliferative organ response (hypersplenism) or the degree of autoimmunity (anemia, thrombocytopenia). There may be lymphocytosis or lymphopenia. Table 152.3 lists the criteria for the diagnosis. Flow cytometry helps identify the lymphocyte type (see Fig. 152.4). Functional genetic analysis for the *TNFRSF6* gene often reveals a heterozygous mutation.

Treatment

Rapamycin (sirolimus) will often control the adenopathy and autoimmune cytopenias. Malignancies can be treated with the usual protocols used in patients unaffected by ALPS. Stem cell transplantation is another possible option in treating the autoimmune manifestations of ALPS.

IMMUNE DYSREGULATION, POLYENDOCRINOPATHY, ENTEROPATHY, X-LINKED SYNDROME

This immune dysregulation syndrome is characterized by onset within the 1st few wk or mo of life with watery diarrhea (autoimmune enteropathy), an eczematous rash (erythroderma in neonates), insulin-dependent diabetes mellitus, hyperthyroidism or more often hypothyroidism, severe allergies, and other autoimmune disorders (Coombs-positive hemolytic anemia, thrombocytopenia, neutropenia). Psoriasiform or ichthyosiform rashes and alopecia have also been reported.

Immune dysregulation, polyendocrinopathy, enteropathy, X-linked (**IPEX**) syndrome is caused by a mutation in the *FOXP3* gene, which encodes a forkhead-winged helix transcription factor *(scurfin)* involved in the function and development of CD4+CD25+ regulatory T cells (Tregs). The absence of Tregs may predispose to abnormal activation of effector T cells. Dominant gain-of-function mutations in *STAT1* and other gene mutations (Table 152.4) produce an IPEX-like syndrome, also associated with compromised Tregs.

Clinical Manifestations

Watery diarrhea with intestinal **villous atrophy** leads to failure to thrive in most patients. Cutaneous lesions (usually eczema) and insulin-dependent diabetes begin in infancy. Lymphadenopathy and splenomegaly are also present. Serious bacterial infections (meningitis, sepsis, pneumonia, osteomyelitis) may be related to neutropenia, malnutrition, or immune dysregulation. Laboratory features reflect the associated autoimmune diseases, dehydration, and malnutrition. In addition, serum IgE levels are elevated, with normal levels of IgM, IgG, and IgA. The diagnosis is made clinically and by mutational analysis of the *FOXP3* gene.

Treatment

Inhibition of T-cell activation by cyclosporine, tacrolimus, or sirolimus with corticosteroids is the treatment of choice, along with the specific care of the endocrinopathy and other manifestations of autoimmunity. These agents are typically used as a bridge to transplant. HSCT is the only possibility for curing IPEX.

CYTOTOXIC T-LYMPHOCYTE ANTIGEN 4 (CTLA4) DEFICIENCY

Patients with CTLA4 deficiency have lost the ability to maintain immune tolerance, leading to a disease characterized by autoimmunity and multiorgan lymphocytic infiltration of lymphoid and nonlymphoid organs. CTLA4, also known as CD152, is a protein receptor that is expressed on activated T cells. It acts as an immune checkpoint, downregulating immune responses, on T-cell activation. CTLA4 deficiency is inherited in a haploinsufficient manner.

Autoimmune cytopenias, **lymphoid infiltration of lymphoid and nonlymphoid organs**, granulomatous disease, hypogammaglobulinemia, and recurrent respiratory infections are key features. Nonlymphoid organs most often affected with lymphoid infiltration are the brain and gastrointestinal (GI) tract. The immune phenotype of CTLA4-deficient patients includes reduced naïve T cells (CD4+CD45RA+CD62L+), loss of circulating B cells, and reduced Treg expression. Treatment is symptom specific, although use of abatacept, a CTLA4-Ig fusion protein, has alleviated disease-specific symptoms in several patients. When refractory to therapy, *HSCT has led to remission of symptoms and cure of disease.*

LIPOPOLYSACCHARIDE (LPS)-RESPONSIVE BEIGE-LIKE ANCHOR PROTEIN (LRBA) DEFICIENCY

Homozygous mutations in *LRBA* cause a syndrome of early-onset hypogammaglobulinemia, autoimmunity, lymphoproliferation, and inflammatory bowel disease.

LRBA is a member of the pleckstrin homology-beige and Chédiak-Higashi–tryptophan–aspartic acid dipeptide (PH-BEACH-WD40) protein family. Much is unknown about the function of LRBA. However, in normal T cells, LRBA co-localizes with CTLA4 within recycling endosomes, suggesting that LRBA may play a specific role in the

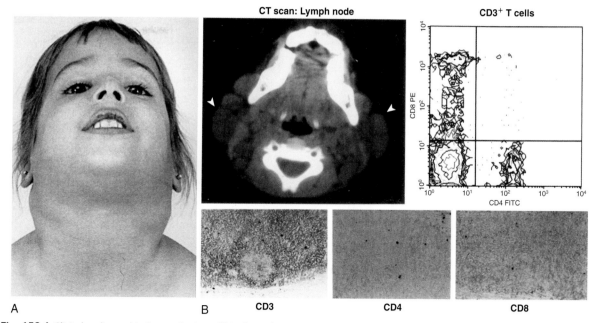

Fig. 152.4 Clinical, radiographic, immunologic, and histologic characteristics of the autoimmune lymphoproliferative syndrome. **A,** Front view of the National Institutes of Health patient. **B,** *Top middle,* a CT scan of the neck is shown demonstrating enlarged preauricular, cervical, and occipital lymph nodes. *Arrowheads* denote the most prominent lymph nodes. The *top right* panels show the flow-cytometric analysis of peripheral blood T cells from a patient with autoimmune lymphoproliferative syndrome (ALPS), with CD8 expression on the vertical axis and CD4 on the horizontal axis. The *lower left quadrant* contains CD4⁻CD8⁻ (double-negative) T cells, which are usually present at <1% of T cells expressing the αβ T-cell receptor. The *bottom panels* show CD3, CD4, and CD8 staining on serial sections of a lymph node biopsy specimen from a patient with ALPS, and also show that large numbers of DNCD3⁺ CD4⁻CD8⁻ (double-negative) T cells are present in the interfollicular areas of the lymph node. (Adapted from Siegel RM, Fleisher TA: The role of Fas and related death receptors in autoimmune and other disease states, J Allergy Clin Immunol 103:729–738, 1999.)

regulation of recycling endosomes. Homozygous mutations in *LRBA* abrogate LRBA protein expression.

Immune dysregulation consisting of enteropathy, autoimmune cytopenias, granulomatous-lymphocytic **interstitial lung disease**, **lymphadenopathy**, and hepatomegaly or splenomegaly are the most common manifestations. Other, less common symptoms of immune dysregulation include cerebral granulomas, type 1 diabetes mellitus, alopecia, uveitis, myasthenia gravis, and eczema. Growth failure occurs in many patients, complicated especially by enteropathy. Bacterial, fungal, and viral infections have been reported in about 50% of patients. The immune phenotype is variable but can consist of reduced T-cell quantities (CD3⁺), elevated double-negative T cells (CD3⁺CD4⁻CD8⁻), normal T-cell proliferation to mitogens and antigens, reduced Treg numbers (CD4⁺CD25⁺FoxP3⁺), reduced NK cells (CD56⁺), and reduced B cells (CD19⁺). Immunoglobulin quantities are also variable, with hypogammaglobulinemia occurring most frequently.

The focus of therapy is treatment of the immunodysregulatory features with immunosuppression. Corticosteroids, immunoglobulin replacement, mycophenolate mofetil, tacrolimus, rapamycin, budesonide, cyclosporine, azathioprine, rituximab, infliximab, and hydroxychloroquine have all been used with mixed success. Abatacept has been successful in treating the immunodysregulatory features. HSCT has been successfully performed in LRBA-deficient patients as well.

ACTIVATED PHOSPHOINOSITIDE 3-KINASE (PI3K) δ SYNDROMES

These syndromes are primary immunodeficiencies that cause a spectrum of immunodeficiency, lymphadenopathy, and senescent T cells. PI3K molecules are composed of a p110 catalytic subunit (p110α, p110β, or p110δ) and a regulatory subunit (p85α, p55α, p50α, p85β, or p55γ). PI3Ks convert phosphatidylinositol 4,5-bisphosphate to phosphatidylinositol 3,4,5-triphosphate (PIP₃), an important second messenger.

Autosomal dominant gain-of-function mutations in *PIK3CD*, the gene that encodes for the catalytic unit, p110δ, leads to hyperactivated PI3Kδ signaling. AD mutations in *PI3KR*, the gene that encodes the regulatory subunit (p85α, p55α, and p50α) of PI3Ks are associated with the same phenotype. Defects in this pathway lead to a syndrome of chronic lymphoproliferation and T-cell senescence.

Early-onset respiratory tract infections, noninfectious lymphadenopathy, and hepatosplenomegaly are the most common features. A large proportion of patients develop early-onset **bronchiectasis** as a result of recurrent pneumonia. Persistent, severe, or recurrent herpesvirus infections are also common. **Lymphadenopathy** often starts in childhood and localizes to sites of infection. However, lymphadenopathy may be diffuse and is usually associated with chronic CMV or EBV viremia. **Mucosal lymphoid hyperplasia** of the respiratory and GI tracts is also frequent. Histologically, lymph nodes show atypical follicular hyperplasia. **Autoimmune cytopenias** are the most frequent autoimmune manifestation, but others include glomerulopathies, autoantibody-mediated thyroid disease, and sclerosing cholangitis. Early-onset lymphoma, as early as the 2nd yr of life, have been reported as well and are a major cause of mortality. Growth impairment affecting weight and height and developmental delay with mild cognitive impairment also may occur.

The immunophenotype consists of reduced naïve T cell (CD3⁺CD4⁺) and B-cell counts (CD19⁺) and normal NK cell counts (CD56⁺). More specifically, reduced numbers of recent thymic emigrants (CD3⁺CD4⁺CD45RA⁺ CD31⁺) with increased effector memory cytotoxic T-cell counts (CD3⁺ CD8⁺CCR7⁻CD45RA⁺/⁻), increased transitional B cells (CD19⁺IgM⁺CD38⁺), and reduced nonswitched memory B cells (CD19⁺IgD⁺CD27⁺) and class-switched memory B cells (CD19⁺IgD⁺CD27⁺) are hallmark. Immunoglobulin levels are variable, but typically there are increased serum quantities of IgM, reduced or normal IgG, and reduced or normal IgA.

Treatment is symptom specific but can include antimicrobial

Table 152.4	Clinical and Laboratory Features of IPEX and IPEX-Like Disorders				
	IPEX	**CD25**	**STAT5B**	**STAT1**	**ITCH**
AUTOIMMUNITY					
Eczema	+++	+++	++	++	++
Enteropathy	+++	+++	++	++	++
Endocrinopathy	+++	++	+	++	++
Allergic disease	+++	+	+	++	++
Cytopenias	++	++	++	−	
Lung disease	+	++	+++		+++
INFECTIONS					
Yeast	−	++	−	+++	−
Herpes virus	−	+++ (EBV/CMV)	++ (VZV)	++	−
Bacterial	+/−	++	++	++	+
Associated features	None	None	Growth failure	Vascular anomalies	Dysmorphic growth failure
Serum immunoglobulins	Elevated	Elevated or normal	Elevated or normal	Low, normal, or high	Elevated
Serum IgE	Elevated	Normal or elevated	Normal or elevated	Normal or mildly elevated	Elevated
CD25 expression	Normal	Absent	Normal or low	Normal	Not tested
CD4⁺CD45RO	Elevated	Elevated	Elevated	Normal or high	Not tested
FOXP3 expression	Absent or normal	Normal or low	Normal or low	Normal	Not tested
IGF-1, IGFBP-3	Normal	Normal	Low	Normal	Not tested
Prolactin	Normal	Normal	Elevated	Normal	Not tested

CMV, Cytomegalovirus; EBV, Epstein-Barr virus; IGF-1, insulin-like growth factor 1; IGFBP-3, insulin-like growth factor–binding protein 3; IPEX, immune dysregulation, polyendocrinopathy, enteropathy, X-linked; VZV, varicella-zoster virus; ITCH, ubiquitin ligase deficiency.
From Verbsky JW, Chatila TA: Immune dysregulation, polyendocrinopathy, enteropathy, X–linked (IPEX) and IPEX–related disorders: an evolving web of heritable autoimmune diseases, *Curr Opin Pediatr* 25:709, 2013.

prophylaxis and immunoglobulin replacement. Various immunosuppressive agents (e.g., rituximab, rapamycin) have been used to treat the lymphoproliferative disease and autoimmune cytopenias that are often present. HSCT has also been successfully performed in those refractory to medical therapy.

SIGNAL TRANSDUCER AND ACTIVATOR OF TRANSCRIPTION (STAT) PATHWAY DEFECTS
The Janus kinase (JAK)-STAT signal transduction pathway is used for signal transduction by type 1 and type 2 cytokine receptors within most hematopoietic cells. Cytokines bind to their cognate receptor, triggering JAK-STAT pathways, ultimately leading to the upregulation of genes involved in the immune response against many pathogens. There are 4 JAK proteins (Jak1, Jak2, Jak3, Tyk2) and 6 STATs (1-6). Mutations in several JAKs and STATs cause immunodeficiency. Table 152.5 includes diseases affecting STAT proteins characterized by immune dysregulation. Chronic immunosuppression is necessary for control of STAT defects. Ruxolitinib, a JAK-STAT inhibitor, has been used with some success. With the advent of JAK-STAT immunomodulating therapies, more treatment options will be available to patients.

NUCLEAR FACTOR-κB PATHWAY DEFECTS
The NF-κB pathways consists of canonical (NF-κB1) and noncanonical (NF-κB2) pathways. On cellular activation, both pathways lead to activation and translocation of NF-κB proteins into the nucleus, where they initiate downstream inflammatory responses. Defects in many proteins in both pathways have been described. Table 152.6 describes immune defects of the NF-κB pathways that cause symptoms of immune dysregulation or autoimmunity. Treatment of NF-κB defects includes prevention of infections and replacement of immunoglobulin and has included HSCT.

TETRATRICOPEPTIDE REPEAT DOMAIN 7A (TTC7A) DEFICIENCY
Combined immunodeficiency with T-cell and B-cell defects had long accompanied hereditary **multiple intestinal atresia**. Mutations in *TTC7A* are causative of the combined intestinal and immunologic defects.

TTC7A is involved in cell cycle control, cytoskeletal organization, cell shape and polarity, and cell adhesion. Deficiency of TTC7A is inherited in an autosomal recessive manner. Multiple intestinal atresia with disruption of intestinal architecture is a universal feature. Often, early-onset severe enterocolitis occurs concurrently. Immunodeficiency with severe T-cell lymphopenia has been described; B- and NK-cell defects are variable. T-cell proliferative responses are also abnormal. Severe hypogammaglobulinemia is common. Treatment includes removal of atretic areas of the intestine and antimicrobial prophylaxis in immunodeficient patients. Bowel transplant has also been performed with some success.

DEFICIENCY OF ADENOSINE DEAMINASE 2 (DADA2)
Deficiency in ADA2 is a cause of early **vasculopathy, stroke**, and immunodeficiency. DADA2 is secondary to autosomal recessive mutations in cat-eye syndrome chromosome region 1 (*CECR1*), mapped to chromosome 22q11.1. ADA2 is important in purine metabolism converting adenosine to inosine and 2′-deoxyadenosine to 2′-deoxyinosine. The pathogenesis is not exactly known, but ADA2 is mostly secreted by myeloid cells, and deficiency leads to upregulation of proinflammatory genes and increased secretion of proinflammatory cytokines. DADA2 is characterized by chronic or recurrent inflammation with elevated acute-phase reactants and fever. Skin manifestations include livedo reticularis, maculopapular rash, nodules, purpura, erythema nodosum, Raynaud phenomenon, ulcerative lesions, and digital necrosis. CNS involvement is variable but can include transient ischemic attacks and ischemic or hemorrhagic stroke. Peripheral neuropathy is also common. GI manifestations include hepatosplenomegaly, gastritis, bowel perforation, and portal hypertension. Nephrogenic hypertension is common and can be associated with glomerulosclerosis or amyloidosis. Immunodeficiency consists of hypogammaglobulinemia and variable decreases in IgM.

Treatment with chronic long-term corticosteroids and anti-TNF-α agents have shown modest control of disease manifestations. HSCT has been successful in 2 patients as well.

Bibliography is available at Expert Consult.

| Table 152.5 | | Defects of STAT Proteins Associated With Immunodysregulation | | |

PROTEIN	LOF/GOF	AUTOIMMUNE OR INFLAMMATORY COMPLICATIONS	OTHER CHARACTERISTICS	IMMUNOPHENOTYPE
STAT1	GOF	IPEX-like enteropathy, enteropathy, endocrinopathy, dermatitis, cytopenias	Infections CMC Viral infections NTM Dimorphic mold Respiratory bacterial	Variable lymphopenia, hypogammaglobulinemia, abnormal T-cell function, reduced Th17 expression
STAT3	GOF	Early onset enteropathy, severe growth failure, lymphoproliferation, autoimmune cytopenias, inflammatory lung disease, type 1 diabetes, dermatitis, arthritis	Respiratory tract infections Herpes viral infections T-cell LGL leukemia NTM	Increased DNT (CD3⁺CD4⁻CD8⁻) Hypogammaglobulinemia T-cell lymphopenia B-cell lymphopenia
STAT5B	LOF	Severe growth hormone resistant growth failure, lymphocytic interstitial pneumonitis, atopic dermatitis	Respiratory tract infections Viral infections	Lymphopenia Reduced Treg cells Reduced γδ T cells Reduced NK cells

STAT, Signal transducer and activator of transcription; GOF, gain of function; LOF, loss of function; IPEX, immunodysregulation, polyendocrinopathy, enteropathy, X-linked; CMC, chronic mucocutaneous candidiasis; NTM, nontuberculous mycobacteria; DNT, double-negative T cell.

| Table 152.6 | | Defects of Nuclear Factor-κB Pathways Associated With Immune Dysregulation | | |

PROTEIN	INHERITANCE	AUTOIMMUNE OR INFLAMMATORY COMPLICATIONS	OTHER MANIFESTATIONS	IMMUNOLOGIC PHENOTYPE
IKBKG (NEMO)	XL	Colitis	Ectodermal dysplasia Osteopetrosis Lymphedema Bacterial infections Opportunistic infections DNA viral infections	Hypogammaglobulinemia Hyper IgM Hyper IgA Hyper IgD Poor antibody responses Decreased NK cell function Decreased TLR responses
NF-κB1	AD	Pyoderma gangrenosum Lymphoproliferation Cytopenia Hypothyroidism Alopecia areata Enteritis LIP NRH	Atrophic gastritis Squamous cell carcinoma Respiratory tract infections Superficial skin infections Lung adenocarcinoma Respiratory insufficiency Aortic stenosis Non-Hodgkin lymphoma	Hypogammaglobulinemia IgA deficiency
NF-κB2	AD	Alopecia totalis Trachyonychia Vitiligo Autoantibodies: thyroid peroxidase, glutamate decarboxylase, thyroglobulin Central adrenal insufficiency	Viral respiratory infections Pneumonias Sinusitis Otitis media Recurrent herpes Asthma Type 1 Chiari malformation Interstitial lung disease	Early-onset hypogammaglobulinemia Low vaccine responses Variable B-cell counts Low switched memory B cells (CD19⁺CD27⁺IgD⁻) Low marginal zone B cells (CD19⁺CD27⁺IgD⁺)

XL, X-linked; AD, autosomal dominant; LIP, lymphocytic interstitial pneumonitis; NRH, nonregenerative hyperplasia.

Section 3
The Phagocytic System

第三篇
吞噬细胞系统

Chapter **153**
Neutrophils
Thomas D. Coates
第一百五十三章
中性粒细胞

中文导读

本章主要介绍了吞噬细胞炎症反应、血细胞生成、中性粒细胞成熟，以及中性粒细胞功能。具体描述了吞噬细胞系统的构成和功能；血细胞生成中具体描述了淋系、髓系造血过程和细胞因子对粒单核细胞生成的影响；中性粒细胞成熟中具体描述了骨髓微环境对中性粒细胞的支持与中性粒细胞的动力学；中性粒细胞功能则具体描述了中性粒细胞迁移、杀菌过程及其机制，以及与此相关的中性粒细胞功能异常疾病。

THE PHAGOCYTIC INFLAMMATORY RESPONSE

The phagocyte system includes both granulocytes (neutrophils, eosinophils, and basophils) and mononuclear phagocytes (monocytes and tissue macrophages). Neutrophils and mononuclear phagocytes share primary functions, including the defining properties of large-particle ingestion and microbial killing. Phagocytes participate primarily in the innate immune response but also help initiate acquired immunity. Mononuclear phagocytes, including tissue macrophages and circulating monocytes, are discussed in Chapter 154.

Neutrophils provide the rapid effector arm of the innate immune system. They circulate in the bloodstream for only about 6 hr (Table 153.1), but on encountering specific chemotactic signals, they adhere to the vascular endothelium and transmigrate into tissues. There they ingest and kill microbes and release chemotactic signals to recruit more neutrophils and to attract dendritic cells and other initiators of the acquired immune response.

HEMATOPOIESIS

The hematopoietic progenitor system can be viewed as a continuum of functional compartments, with the most primitive compartment composed of very rare **pluripotential stem cells**, which have high self-renewal capacity and give rise to more mature stem cells, including cells that are committed to either lymphoid or myeloid development (Fig. 153.1). Common lymphoid progenitor cells give rise to T- and

Table 153.1	Neutrophil and Monocyte Kinetics
NEUTROPHILS	
Average time in mitosis (myeloblast to myelocyte)	7-9 days
Average time in postmitosis and storage (metamyelocyte to neutrophil)	3-7 days
Average half-life in the circulation	6 hr
Average total body pool	6.5×10^8 cells/kg
Average circulating pool	3.2×10^8 cells/kg
Average marginating pool	3.3×10^8 cells/kg
Average daily turnover rate	1.8×10^8 cells/kg
MONONUCLEAR PHAGOCYTES	
Average time in mitosis	30-48 hr
Average half-life in the circulation	36-104 hr
Average circulating pool (monocytes)	1.8×10^7 cells/kg
Average daily turnover rate	1.8×10^9 cells/kg
Average survival in tissues (macrophages)	Months

From Boxer LA: Function of neutrophils and mononuclear phagocytes. In Bennett JC, Plum F, editors: *Cecil textbook of internal medicine*, ed 20, Philadelphia, 1996, Saunders.

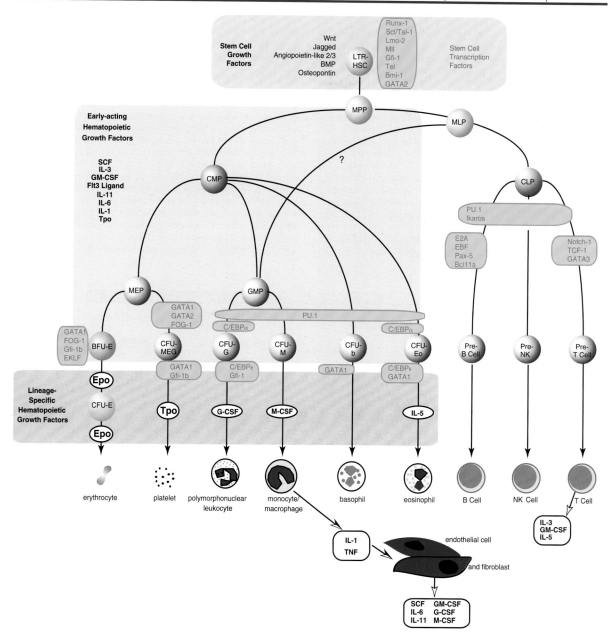

Fig. 153.1 Major cytokine sources and actions and transcription factor requirements for hematopoietic cells. Cells of the bone marrow microenvironment, such as macrophages, endothelial cells, and reticular fibroblastoid cells, produce macrophage, granulocyte-macrophage, and granulocyte colony-stimulating factors (M-CSF, GM-CSF, G-CSF), interleukin-6 (IL-6), and probably stem cell factor (SCF) (cellular sources not precisely determined) after induction with endotoxin (macrophage) or IL-1/tumor necrosis factor (TNF) (endothelial cells and fibroblasts). T cells produce IL-3, GM-CSF, and IL-5 in response to antigenic and IL-1 stimulation. These cytokines have overlapping actions during hematopoietic differentiation, as indicated, and for all lineages, optimal development requires a combination of early-acting and late-acting factors. Transcription factors important for survival or self-renewal of stem cells are shown in *red* at the *top*, whereas stages of hematopoiesis blocked after the depletion of indicated transcription factors are shown in *red* for multipotent and committed progenitors. *(From Nathan & Oski's hematology and oncology of infancy and childhood, ed 8, vol 2, Philadelphia, 2015, Elsevier, p 10.)*

B-cell precursors and their mature progeny (see Chapter 149). Common myeloid progenitor cells eventually give rise to committed single-lineage progenitors of the recognizable precursors through a random process of lineage restriction in a stepwise process (see Chapter 473). The capacity of lineage-specific committed progenitors to proliferate and differentiate in response to demand provides the hematopoietic system with a remarkable range of response to changing requirements for mature blood cell production.

The proliferation, differentiation, and survival of immature hematopoietic progenitor cells are governed by hematopoietic growth factors, a family of glycoproteins (see Chapter 473). Besides regulating proliferation and differentiation of progenitors, these factors influence the survival and function of mature blood cells. During granulopoiesis and monopoiesis, multiple cytokines regulate the cells at each stage of differentiation from pluripotent stem cells to nondividing, terminally differentiated cells (monocytes, neutrophils, eosinophils, and basophils). As cells mature, they lose receptors for most cytokines, especially those that influence early cell development; however, they retain receptors for cytokines that affect their mobilization and function, such as granulocyte and macrophage colony-stimulating factors. Mature phagocytes also express receptors for chemokines, which help direct the cells to sites of inflammation. Chemokine receptors such as CXCR4 and its ligand SDF-1 play a key role in retention of developing myeloid cells within bone marrow.

NEUTROPHIL MATURATION AND KINETICS

The process of intramedullary granulocyte maturation involves changes in nuclear configuration and accumulation of specific intracytoplasmic granules. The bone marrow microenvironment supports the normal steady-state renewal of peripheral blood neutrophils through the generation of growth and differentiation factors by stromal cells. Growth factors such as granulocyte colony-stimulating factor (G-CSF) and granulocyte-macrophage colony-stimulating factor (GM-CSF) not only stimulate cell division, but also induce the expression of transcription factors that regulate the biosynthesis of functional components of the neutrophil, such as granule proteins. The transcription factor PU.1 is essential for myelopoiesis, both as a positive regulatory element and as a suppressor of GATA1, a transcription factor that directs nonmyeloid differentiation. Other transcription factors, such as Runx1 (AML1), c-myb, CDP, C/EBPα, C/EBPγ, and MEF, are expressed in the myeloblast and

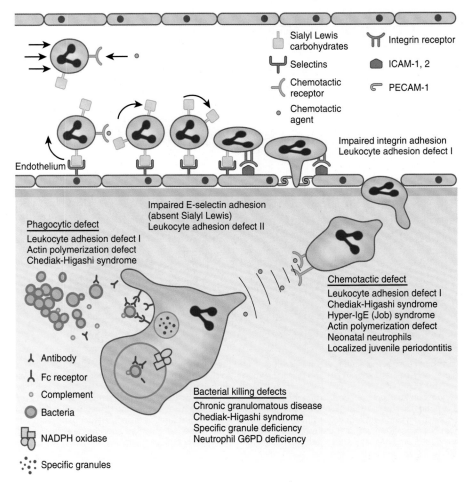

Fig. 153.2 The neutrophil-mediated inflammatory response and associated neutrophil dysfunction syndromes. Circulating neutrophils loosely attach to endothelium via selectins and roll along the vessel wall until they arrive at the site of infection. Inflammatory monokines, interleukin-1 (IL-1), and tumor necrosis factor (TNF) activate endothelial cells to express E- and P-selectins. E- and P-selectins serve as counter-receptors for neutrophils sialyl Lewis X and Lewis X to cause low-avidity neutrophil rolling. Activated endothelial cells express ICAM-1, which serves as a counter-receptor for neutrophil β₂-integrin molecules, leading to high-avidity leukocyte spreading and the start of transendothelial migration at the infection site. Neutrophils invade through the vascular basement membrane with the release of proteases and reactive oxidative intermediates, causing local destruction of surrounding tissue at sites of high concentrations of chemotactic factors, and migrate to the site of infection, where they ingest and kill the bacteria. (*Modified from Kyono W, Coates TD: A practical approach to neutrophil disorders, Pediatr Clin North Am 49:929, 2002.*)

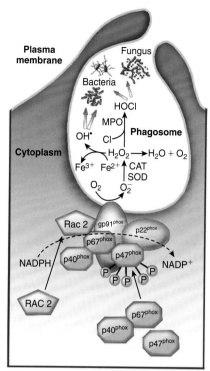

large oval nucleus, a sizable nucleolus, and a deficiency of granules. **Promyelocytes** acquire peroxidase-positive azurophilic (primary) granules, and then **myelocytes** and **metamyelocytes** acquire specific (secondary) granules; tertiary granules and secretory vesicles develop in the final stage of neutrophil maturation.

NEUTROPHIL FUNCTION

Neutrophil responses are initiated as circulating neutrophils flowing through the postcapillary venules detect low levels of chemokines and other chemotactic substances released from a site of infection. The sequence of events as the neutrophil moves from circulating in the blood to the encounter and destruction of bacteria is carefully orchestrated by a series of biochemical events, defects of which are associated with genetic disorders of neutrophil function (Fig. 153.2). In fact, these disorders of neutrophil function lead to our understanding of the cell biology of phagocyte function. A subset of circulating neutrophils loosely adheres to the endothelium through low-affinity receptors called **selectins** and rolls along the endothelium, forming the marginated pool. Soluble effectors of inflammation trigger subtle changes in surface adhesion molecules on endothelial cells at the site of infection. The rolling of neutrophils allows more intense exposure of neutrophils to activating factors such as tumor necrosis factor or interleukin-1 (Fig. 153.2). Exposure of neutrophils to these same activating factors induces qualitative and quantitative changes in the family of β_2-integrin adhesion receptors (the CD11/CD18 group of surface molecules), leading to tight adhesion between neutrophils and endothelial cells at the site of inflammation and ultimately to transmigration of the neutrophil into the tissue.

Once through the endothelium, the neutrophil senses the gradient of chemokines or other chemoattractants and migrates to sites of infection. **Neutrophil migration** is a complex process involving rounds of receptor engagement, signal transduction, and remodeling of the actin microfilaments composing in part the cytoskeleton. Actin polymerization-depolymerization occurs in approximately 8 sec cycles and drives cyclic extension and retraction of the actin-rich lamella at the front of the neutrophil. Receptors at the leading edge of the lamella detect the gradient of attractant and follow microorganisms, then ingest and destroy them. When the neutrophil reaches the site of infection, it recognizes pathogens by means of Fc immunoglobulin and complement receptors, Toll-like receptors, fibronectin receptors, and other adhesion molecules.

The neutrophil ingests microbes that are coated by **opsonins**, serum proteins such as immunoglobulin and complement component **C3**. The pathogens are engulfed into a closed vacuole, the **phagosome** (Fig. 153.3), where 2 cellular responses essential for optimal microbicidal activity occur concomitantly: degranulation and activation of nicotinamide-adenine dinucleotide phosphate (NADPH)–dependent oxidase. Fusion of neutrophil granule membranes with the phagosome membrane delivers potent antimicrobial proteins and small peptides into the phagosome.

Assembly and activation of NADPH oxidase occur at the phagosome membrane as well (see Fig. 153.3), generating large amounts of superoxide (O_2^-) from molecular oxygen, which in turn decomposes to produce hydrogen peroxide (H_2O_2) and singlet oxygen. **Myeloperoxidase**, a major azurophil granule component, catalyzes the reaction of H_2O_2 with ubiquitously present chloride ions to create hypochlorous acid (HOCl) in the phagosome. H_2O_2 and HOCl are potent microbicidal agents that break down and clear pathogens from sites of infection.

In addition, neutrophils secrete a wide variety of cytokines and chemokines that recruit more neutrophils to fight the infection, attract monocytes and macrophages that possess both microbicidal and scavenger functions, and promote antigen presentation to help initiate the adaptive immune response. Also, the reactive oxidants can inactivate chemotactic factors and may serve to terminate the process of neutrophil influx, thereby attenuating the inflammatory process. Finally, the release of reactive oxygen species, granule proteins, and cytokines can also damage local tissues, leading to the classic signs of inflammation or to more permanent impairment of tissue integrity and function.

Bibliography is available at Expert Consult.

Fig. 153.3 Nicotinamide adenine dinucleotide phosphate (NADPH) oxidase components and activation. On activation of phagocytic cells, the 3 cytosolic components *(red)* of the NADPH oxidase (p67^{phox}, p47^{phox}, and p40^{phox}), plus the small guanosine triphosphatase (GTPase) protein Rac2, are translocated to the membrane of the phagocytic vacuole. The p47^{phox} subunit binds to the flavocytochrome$_{b558}$ membrane component *(blue-green)* of the NADPH oxidase (gp91^{phox} plus p22^{phox}). The NADPH oxidase catalyzes the formation of superoxide by transferring an electron from NADPH to molecular oxygen (O_2), thereby forming the superoxide free radical. The unstable superoxide anion is converted to hydrogen peroxide, either spontaneously or by superoxide dismutase (SOD). H_2O_2 can follow different metabolic pathways into more potent reactive oxidants, such as OH* or HOCl) or degradation to $H_2O + O_2$. *(Adapted from Stiehm ER, Ochs HD, Winkelstein JA: Immunologic disorders in infants and children, ed 5, Philadelphia, 2004, Saunders, p 622.)*

promyelocyte, and some of these are required for azurophil granule protein expression. As cells enter the myelocyte stage, Runx1 and myb are downregulated, whereas PU.1 and C/EBPε expression rises to initiate terminal differentiation.

Granulocytes survive for only 6-12 hr in the circulation, and therefore daily production of 2×10^4 granulocytes/μL of blood is required to maintain a level of circulating granulocytes of 5×10^3/μL (see Table 153.1). The relatively small peripheral blood pool includes the rapidly interchanging circulating and marginating pools; the latter provides entrance into the tissue phase, where neutrophils may survive for hours or days. The circulating pool is fed and buffered by a much larger marrow population of mature neutrophils and myeloid precursors, representing the marrow reserve and proliferating pools, respectively. Proliferation of myeloid cells, encompassing approximately 5 mitotic divisions, takes place only during the first 3 stages of neutrophil development, in myeloblasts, promyelocytes, and myelocytes. After the myelocyte stage, the cells terminally differentiate into nondividing, maturing metamyelocytes, bands, and neutrophils.

Neutrophil maturation is associated with nuclear condensation and lobulation and the sequential production of characteristic granule populations. A **myeloblast** is a relatively undifferentiated cell with a

Chapter 154

Chapter 154
Monocytes, Macrophages, and Dendritic Cells

Richard B. Johnston Jr.

第一百五十四章
单核细胞、巨噬细胞和树突状细胞

中文导读

本章主要介绍了单核吞噬细胞发育、激活、功能活性、树突状细胞以及单核吞噬细胞或树突状细胞功能异常。具体描述了单核细胞的发育和分类、组织特异性巨噬细胞的来源与功能分类；具体描述了巨噬细胞的经典激活途径和替代激活途径；具体描述了应对感染时的巨噬细胞功能；具体描述了树突状细胞的分类、成熟过程与功能；细胞功能异常中介绍了慢性肉芽肿病、脂质贮积病、INFγ-IL12通路缺陷、组织细胞增多症和累及IL-1的自身炎症性疾病。

Mononuclear phagocytes (monocytes, macrophages) are distributed across all body tissues and play a central role in maintaining immunologic and metabolic homeostasis. They are essential for innate host defense against infection, tissue repair and remodeling, and the antigen-specific adaptive immune response. No human has been identified as having congenital absence of this cell line, probably because macrophages are required to remove primitive tissues during fetal development as new tissues develop to replace them. Monocytes and tissue macrophages in their several forms have variable morphology, surface markers, and transcriptional profiles but common functions, particularly phagocytosis (Table 154.1). Dendritic cells (DCs) are specialized derivatives of this mononuclear phagocyte system that develop from myeloid cell precursors or monocytes themselves.

DEVELOPMENT

Monocytes develop more rapidly during bone marrow hematopoiesis and remain longer in the circulation than do neutrophils (see Table 153.1). The **monoblast** is the first recognizable monocyte precursor, followed by the **promonocyte**, with cytoplasmic granules and an indented nucleus, and finally the fully developed monocyte with cytoplasmic granules filled with hydrolytic enzymes. The transition from monoblast to mature circulating monocyte requires about 6 days.

Three major subsets of human monocytes can be identified on the basis of surface antigens: CD14^{++} CD16$^-$ *classical* monocytes that constitute the majority of total monocytes in the resting state; the more mature CD14^{++} CD16$^+$ *proinflammatory* (*intermediate*) monocytes, which produce proinflammatory hormone-like factors termed **cytokines**, such as tumor necrosis factor-α (TNF-α), in response to microbial stimuli; and *nonclassical* (*regulatory*) monocytes (CD14$^+$ CD16^{++}) that promote

wound healing. Monocytes from these subsets migrate into tissues in response to localized inflammation or injury and provide proinflammatory host defense or antiinflammatory responses and wound healing.

Tissue (organ)-specific macrophages arise from macrophage progenitors that develop in the yolk sac and fetal liver before hematopoiesis occurs in the bone marrow. These cells maintain their population through self-renewal. Tissue macrophages can also be populated to some extent by circulating monocytes. Monocytes or macrophages at sites of active inflammation mature into proinflammatory (M1) macrophages or proresolving (M2) macrophages. In ongoing tissue injury or inflammation, many (perhaps most) of the macrophages will express a mix of the properties of the classic types.

Table 154.1	Principal Sites of Macrophages in Tissues

Liver (Kupffer cells)
Lung (interstitial and alveolar macrophages)
Connective tissue, adipose tissue, and interstitium of major organs and skin
Serosal cavities (pleural and peritoneal macrophages)
Synovial membrane (type A synoviocytes)
Bone (osteoclasts)
Brain and retina (microglial cells)
Spleen, lymph nodes, bone marrow
Intestinal wall
Breast milk
Placenta
Granulomas (multinucleated giant cells)

Whether embryonic or blood derived, tissue macrophages are directed by organ-specific factors to differentiate into macrophages characteristic of that organ. Embryonic progenitors or monocytes in the liver become **Kupffer cells** that bridge the sinusoids separating adjacent plates of hepatocytes. Those at the lung airway surface become large ellipsoid **alveolar macrophages**, those in the bone become **osteoclasts**, and those in brain or retina become **microglia**. All macrophages, however, have at least 3 major functions in common: phagocytosis, presentation of antigens to lymphocytes, and enhancement or suppression of the immune response through release of a variety of potent cytokines. At sites of inflammation, monocytes and macrophages can fuse to form **multinucleated giant cells**; these cells maintain the antimicrobial functions of macrophages.

ACTIVATION

The most important step in the maturation of tissue macrophages is the conversion from a resting to a more functionally active cell, a process driven primarily by certain cytokines and microbial products. *Macrophage activation* is a generic term, with the functional characteristics of an activated macrophage population varying with the cytokine or other stimulus (microbial, chemical) to which the population has been exposed. **Classical activation** refers to a response to infection that is driven by specifically activated T-helper (Th) type 1 (Th1-type) lymphocytes and natural killer (NK) cells through their release of interferon-γ (IFN-γ). TNF-α secreted by activated macrophages amplifies their activation, as does bacterial cell wall protein or endotoxin through Toll-like receptors (TLRs). **Alternative activation** is driven by Th2-type lymphocytes through release of interleukin-4 (IL-4) and IL-13, cytokines that regulate antibody responses, allergy, and resistance to parasites. Alternatively activated macrophages may have particular functional advantages, such as in wound healing and immunoregulation. In the traditional context of host defense, the term *activated macrophage* indicates that the "classically activated" cell has an enhanced capacity to kill microorganisms or tumor cells. These macrophages are larger, with more pseudopods and pronounced ruffling of the plasma membrane, and they exhibit accelerated activity of many functions (Table 154.2). Considering the variety of macrophage activities essential to the maintenance of homeostasis, it seems likely that so-called classically activated, M1-type, and alternatively activated, M2-type, macrophages are extremes of a continuum of physiologic functions expressed by these long-lived cells in response to the specific task at hand.

Classical macrophage activation is accomplished during infection with intracellular pathogens (e.g., mycobacteria, *Listeria*) through crosstalk between Th1 lymphocytes and antigen-presenting macrophages mediated by the engagement of a series of ligands and receptors on the 2 cell types, including class II major histocompatibility complex (MHC)

Table 154.2	Upregulated Functions in Macrophages Activated in Response to Infection

Microbicidal and tumoricidal activity
Phagocytosis (of most particles) and pinocytosis
Phagocytosis-associated respiratory burst (O_2^-, H_2O_2)
Generation of nitric oxide
Chemotaxis
Glucose transport and metabolism
Membrane expression of MHC, CD40, TNF receptor
Antigen presentation
Secretion:
   Complement components
   Lysozyme, acid hydrolases, and cytolytic proteinases
   Collagenase
   Plasminogen activator
   Interleukins, including IL-1, IL-12, and IL-15
   TNF-α
   Interferons, including IFN-α and IFN-β
   Antimicrobial peptides (cathelicidin, defensins)
   Angiogenic factors

H_2O_2, Hydrogen peroxide; IFN, interferon; IL, interleukin; MHC, major histocompatibility complex; O_2^-, superoxide anion; TNF, tumor necrosis factor.

molecules and CD40 on macrophages and CD40 ligand on Th1 cells, and through secretion of cytokines. Macrophages encountering microorganisms release IL-12, which stimulates T cells to release IFN-γ. These interactions constitute the basis of cell-mediated immunity. IFN-γ is an especially important macrophage-activating cytokine; it is currently used as a therapeutic agent.

FUNCTIONAL ACTIVITIES

Numerous functions are upregulated when the macrophage is activated in response to infection (see Table 154.2). Of importance are the ingestion and killing of *intracellular* pathogens such as mycobacteria, *Listeria*, *Leishmania*, *Toxoplasma*, and some fungi. Killing of the ingested organisms of any kind depends heavily on products of the *respiratory burst* (e.g., hydrogen peroxide) and on nitric oxide, and release of these metabolites is enhanced in activated macrophages. Whether activated or not, splenic and hepatic macrophages are essential for clearing the bloodstream of *extracellular* pathogens such as pneumococci.

The capacity to undergo diapedesis across the endothelial wall of blood vessels and to migrate to sites of microbial invasion is essential to monocyte function. Chemotactic factors for monocytes include complement products and chemotactic peptides (**chemokines**) derived from neutrophils, lymphocytes, and other cell types. Phagocytosis of the invading organisms can then occur, influenced by the presence of opsonins for the invader (antibody, complement, mannose-binding and surfactant proteins), the inherent surface properties of the microorganism, and the state of activation of the macrophage.

Monocytes migrating to intestinal mucosa are modified by stromal factors so that they lose innate receptors for microbial products such as endotoxin, and they do not effectively produce proinflammatory cytokines. They retain, however, the capacity to ingest and kill microbes. They have been modified during evolution to allow the absence of inflammation typical of normal intestinal mucosa despite its constant exposure to huge numbers of microbes and their inflammatory by-products.

Macrophages play an essential role in the disposal of damaged and dying cells, helping resolve the inflammatory response and heal wounds. Brain microglia demonstrate these functions particularly well. In conditions such as stroke, neurodegenerative disease, and tumor invasion, these cells can become activated, surround damaged and dead cells, and clear cellular debris. Macrophages lining the sinusoids of the spleen are especially important in ingesting aged or autoantibody-coated erythrocytes or platelets; splenectomy is used to manage autoimmune cytopenias. In the process of **efferocytosis**, macrophages in inflammatory sites can recognize changes in phosphatidylserine on the membrane of neutrophils undergoing apoptosis, and these can be removed before they spill their toxic contents into the tissue. Macrophages also remove the extracellular traps exuded by inflammatory neutrophils, thus reducing the risk of autoimmunity. Macrophages can be identified early in fetal development, where they function to remove debris as one maturing embryonic tissue replaces another; in the brain, microglia prune synapses opsonized with C1q. Macrophages are also important in removing inorganic particles, such as elements of cigarette smoke, that enter the alveoli.

Macrophages are involved in the induction and expression of adaptive immune responses, including antibody formation and cell-mediated immunity. This depends on their capacity to break down foreign material, then present individual antigens on their surface as peptides or polysaccharides bound to MHC class II molecules. Monocytes, B lymphocytes, and most effectively, DCs, also present antigens to T cells for the specific immune response. Activated macrophages express increased MHC class II molecules, and antigen presentation is more effective.

The heightened capacity of activated macrophages to synthesize and release various hydrolytic enzymes and microbicidal materials contributes to their increased killing capacity (see Table 154.2). The macrophage is an extraordinarily active secretory cell shown to secrete >100 distinct substances, including cytokines, growth factors, and sterol hormones, placing it in a class with the hepatocyte. Because of the profound effect of some of these secretory products on other cells and the large number and widespread distribution of macrophages, this network of cells can be viewed as an important endocrine organ. IL-1 illustrates this point.

Microbes and microbial products, burns, ischemia–reperfusion, and other causes of inflammation or tissue damage stimulate the release of IL-1, mainly by monocytes, macrophages, and epithelial cells. In turn, IL-1 elicits fever, sleep, and release of IL-6, which induces production of acute-phase proteins.

The complex relationship between mononuclear phagocytes and cancer is becoming more clear. Macrophages have been demonstrated to kill tumor cells by ingestion and by means of secreted products, including lysosomal enzymes, nitric oxide, oxygen metabolites, and TNF-α. In contrast, M2-type **tumor-associated macrophages (TAMs)** can stimulate growth of tumors through secretion of growth and angiogenic factors such as vascular endothelial growth factor (VEGF), promote metastasis, and inhibit T-cell antitumor immune responses. TAMs are currently targets of clinical trials studying attempts to reprogram them to antitumor macrophages or otherwise blunt their tumor-supportive capacity.

As traumatic damage and infection subside, the macrophage population shifts toward playing an essential role in tissue repair and healing through removal of apoptotic cells and secretion of IL-10, transforming growth factor-β, lipoxins, and the "specialized proresolving mediators," omega-3 fatty acid–derived resolvins, protectins, and maresins.

DENDRITIC CELLS

Dendritic cells are a type of mononuclear phagocyte found in blood, lymphoid organs, and all tissues. DCs are specialized to capture, process, and present antigens to T cells to generate adaptive immunity or tolerance to self-antigens. Human monocytes can be induced to differentiate into DCs in some circumstances, particularly inflammation. DCs express retractable dendritic (branched) extensions and potent endocytic capacity but are a heterogeneous population from the standpoint of location, surface markers, level of antigen-presenting activity, and function. Single-cell RNA sequencing has defined 6 human DC subtypes; but 2 major functional types of DCs can be identified: *conventional* DCs, which include Langerhans cells in the epithelial surfaces of skin and mucosa, dermal or interstitial DCs in subepithelial skin, and interstitial DCs in solid organs; and *plasmacytoid* DCs, sentinels for viral infection and principal source of antiviral IFN-α and IFN-β.

DCs migrating from the bloodstream enter skin, epithelial surfaces, and lymphoid organs where, as immature cells, they internalize self and foreign antigens. Microbial products, cytokines, or molecules exposed in damaged tissue ("danger signals" or "alarmins") induce DC maturation, with upregulation of cytokine receptors and MHC class II and co-stimulatory molecules that expedite cell-cell binding. Stimulated DCs in the periphery migrate to lymphoid organs, where they continue to mature. They function there as the most potent cells that present antigens to T lymphocytes and induce their proliferation, activities that are central to the antigen-specific adaptive immune response. Macrophage IL-10 acts to suppress DC maturation during resolution of inflammation.

DCs from cancer patients have been used in an attempt to control their cancer. The patient's DCs are amplified and matured from blood monocytes or marrow progenitor cells by cytokines, exposed to antigens from the patient's tumor, then injected into the patient as a "vaccine" against the cancer.

ABNORMALITIES OF MONOCYTE-MACROPHAGE OR DENDRITIC CELL FUNCTION

Mononuclear phagocytes and neutrophils from patients with **chronic granulomatous disease (CGD)** exhibit a profound defect of phagocytic killing (see Chapter 156). The inability of affected macrophages to kill ingested organisms leads to abscess formation and characteristic granulomas at sites of macrophage accumulation beneath the skin and in the liver, lungs, spleen, and lymph nodes. IFN-γ is used to prevent infection in CGD patients and to treat the decreased bone resorption of **congenital osteopetrosis**, which is caused by decreased function of osteoclasts. Genetic deficiency of the CD11/CD18 complex of membrane adherence glycoproteins (**leukocyte adhesion defect 1**), which includes a receptor for opsonic complement component 3, results in impaired phagocytosis by monocytes (see Chapter 156).

The monocyte-macrophage system is prominently involved in **lipid storage diseases** called sphingolipidoses (see Chapter 104). In these conditions, macrophages express a systemic enzymatic defect that permits accumulation of cell debris that they normally clear. Resistance to infection can be impaired, at least partly because of impairment in macrophage function. In **Gaucher disease**, the prototype for these disorders, the enzyme glucocerebrosidase functions abnormally, allowing accumulation of glucocerebroside from cell membranes in Gaucher cells throughout the body. In all locations the Gaucher cell is an altered macrophage. These patients can be treated with infusions of the normal enzyme modified to expose mannose residues, which bind to mannose receptors on macrophages.

The cytokine IL-12 is a powerful inducer of IFN-γ production by T cells and NK cells. Individuals with inherited deficiency in macrophage receptors for IFN-γ or lymphocyte receptors for IL-12, or in IL-12 itself, undergo a severe, selective susceptibility to infection by nontuberculous mycobacteria such as *Mycobacterium avium* complex or bacille Calmette-Guérin (see Chapter 152). About half these patients have had disseminated *Salmonella* infection. These abnormalities are grouped as **defects in the IFN-γ–IL-12 axis**.

Monocyte-macrophage function has been shown to be partially abnormal in various clinical conditions. Cultured mononuclear phagocytes of newborns are more readily infected than adult cells by HIV-1 and measles virus. Macrophages from newborns release less granulocyte colony-stimulating factor (G-CSF) and IL-6 in culture, and this deficiency is accentuated in cells from preterm infants. This finding supports the observations that G-CSF levels are significantly decreased in blood from newborns, and that the marrow granulocyte storage pool is diminished in infants, particularly preterm infants. Mononuclear cells from newborns produce less IFN-γ and IL-12 than do adult cells, and macrophages cultured from cord blood are not activated normally by IFN-γ. This combination of deficiencies would be expected to blunt the newborn's response to infection by viruses, fungi, and intracellular bacteria.

More than 100 different subtypes of the **histiocytoses** have been organized into 5 major groups based on clinical, pathologic, genetic, and other features. These rare disorders are characterized by accumulation of macrophages or DCs in tissues or organs. "Histiocyte" is a histologic term and not cell specific, but it has been retained because of its long usage to identify the classic members of this family. Familial and secondary **hemophagocytic lymphohistiocytosis** is characterized by uncontrolled activation of T cells and macrophages, with resultant fever, hepatosplenomegaly, lymphadenopathy, pancytopenia, marked elevation of serum proinflammatory cytokines, and macrophage hemophagocytosis (see Chapter 534). The familial form usually presents in the 1st yr of life. Up to 5% of children with systemic-onset juvenile rheumatoid arthritis develop an acute severe complication termed **macrophage activation syndrome**, with persistent fever (rather than typical febrile spikes), hepatosplenomegaly, pancytopenia, macrophage hemophagocytosis, and coagulopathy, which can progress to disseminated intravascular coagulation and death if not recognized (see Chapter 180).

Two genetic autoinflammatory diseases result from dysregulation of the mononuclear phagocyte–produced proinflammatory cytokine IL-1. In **neonatal-onset multisystem inflammatory disorder**, monocytes overproduce IL-1. In **deficiency of the IL-1 receptor antagonist**, normal activity levels of IL-1 go unopposed. In both conditions, patients present in the 1st few days or weeks of life with pustular or urticarial rash, bony overgrowth, sterile osteomyelitis, elevated erythrocyte sedimentation rate, and other evidence of systemic inflammation. The recombinant IL-1 receptor antagonist anakinra is effective treatment for both these disorders (Chapter 188).

Bibliography is available at Expert Consult.

Chapter **155**
Eosinophils
Benjamin L. Wright and Brian P. Vickery

第一百五十五章
嗜酸性粒细胞

中文导读

　　本章主要介绍了嗜酸性粒细胞的病理生理和嗜酸性粒细胞增多相关性疾病。具体描述了嗜酸性粒细胞的分化、嗜酸性粒细胞特异性颗粒、过敏和炎症状态下嗜酸性粒细胞的迁移过程，以及IL-15对嗜酸性粒细胞的影响；具体描述了过敏性疾病、感染性疾病、高嗜酸性粒细胞综合征，以及其他嗜酸性粒细胞增多性疾病；描述了酸性粒细胞增多的原因和高嗜酸性粒细胞综合征的分类。

Eosinophils are distinguished from other leukocytes by their morphology, constituent products, and association with specific diseases. Eosinophils are nondividing, fully differentiated cells with a diameter of approximately 8 μm and a bilobed nucleus. They differentiate from stem cell precursors in the bone marrow under the control of T-cell–derived interleukin-3 (IL-3), granulocyte-macrophage colony-stimulating factor (GM-CSF), and especially IL-5. Their characteristic membrane-bound specific granules stain bright pink with eosin and consist of a crystalline core made up of major basic protein (MBP) surrounded by a matrix containing the eosinophil cationic protein (ECP), eosinophil peroxidase (EPX), and eosinophil-derived neurotoxin (EDN). These basic proteins are cytotoxic for the larval stages of helminthic parasites and are also thought to contribute to much of the inflammation associated with chronic allergic diseases such as asthma (see Chapter 169).

Eosinophil MBP, ECP, and EPX are also present in large quantities in the airways of patients who have died of asthma and are thought to inflict epithelial cell damage leading to airway hyperresponsiveness, although recent studies indicate the role of these granule proteins may be more nuanced and not purely destructive. Eosinophil granule contents also contribute to eosinophilic endomyocardial disease associated with the hypereosinophilic syndrome. MBP has the potential to activate other proinflammatory cells, including mast cells, basophils, neutrophils, and platelets. Eosinophils have the capacity to generate large amounts of the lipid mediators platelet-activating factor and leukotriene C₄, both of which can cause vasoconstriction, smooth muscle contraction, and mucus hypersecretion (Fig. 155.1). Eosinophils are a source of a number of proinflammatory cytokines, including IL-1, IL-3, IL-4, IL-5, IL-9, IL-13, and GM-CSF. They have also been shown to influence T-cell recruitment and immune polarization in inflammatory settings. Thus, eosinophils have considerable potential to initiate and sustain the inflammatory response of the innate and acquired immune systems.

Eosinophil migration from the vasculature into the extracellular tissue is mediated by the binding of leukocyte adhesion receptors to their ligands or counterstructures on the postcapillary endothelium. Similar to neutrophils (see Fig. 153.2), transmigration begins as the eosinophil selectin receptor binds to the endothelial carbohydrate ligand in loose association, which promotes eosinophils rolling along the endothelial surface until they encounter a priming stimulus such as a chemotactic mediator. Eosinophils then establish a high-affinity bond between integrin receptors and their corresponding immunoglobulin-like ligand. Unlike neutrophils, which become flattened before transmigrating between the tight junctions of the endothelial cells, eosinophils can use unique integrins, known as very late antigens (VLA-4), to bind to vascular cell adhesion molecule (VCAM)-1, which enhances eosinophil adhesion and transmigration through endothelium. Eosinophils are recruited to tissues in inflammatory states by a group of chemokines known as **eotaxins** (eotaxin 1, 2, and 3). These unique pathways account for selective accumulation of eosinophils in allergic and inflammatory disorders. Eosinophils normally dwell primarily in tissues, especially tissues with an epithelial interface with the environment, including the respiratory, gastrointestinal (GI), and lower genitourinary tracts. The life span of eosinophils may extend for weeks within tissues.

IL-5 selectively enhances eosinophil production, adhesion to endothelial cells, and function. Considerable evidence shows that IL-5 has a pivotal role in promoting eosinophilpoeisis. It is the predominant cytokine in allergen-induced pulmonary late-phase reaction, and antibodies against IL-5 (mepolizumab, reslizumab, benralizumab), decrease sputum eosinophils and reduce exacerbations in a subset of patients with asthma. Eosinophils also bear unique receptors for several chemokines, including RANTES (regulated on activation, normal T-cell expressed and secreted), eotaxin, and monocyte chemotactic proteins 3 and 4. These chemokines appear to be key mediators in the induction of tissue eosinophilia.

DISEASES ASSOCIATED WITH EOSINOPHILIA

The **absolute eosinophil count** (AEC) is used to quantify peripheral blood eosinophilia. Calculated as the white blood cell (WBC) count/μL × percent of eosinophils, it is usually <450 cells/μL and varies diurnally,

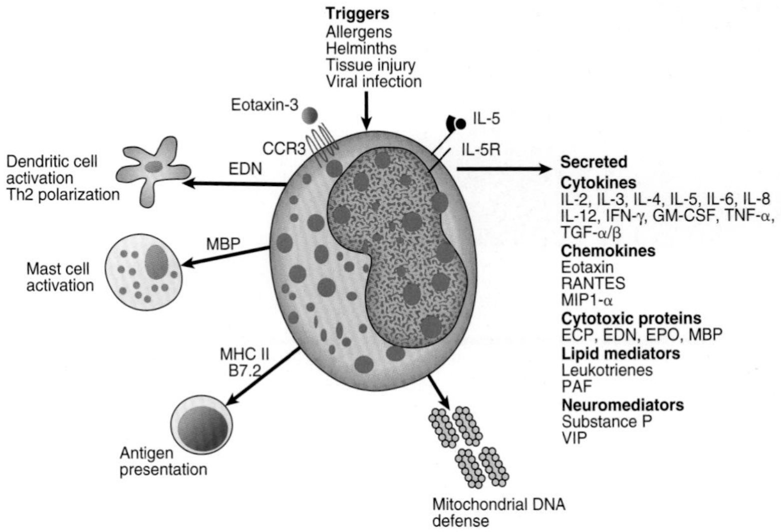

Fig. 155.1 Schematic diagram of an eosinophil and its diverse properties. Eosinophils are bilobed granulocytes that respond to diverse stimuli, including allergens, helminths, viral infections, allografts, and nonspecific tissue injury. Eosinophils express the receptor for IL-5, a critical eosinophil growth and differentiation factor, as well as the receptor for eotaxin and related chemokines (CCR3). The secondary granules contain four primary cationic proteins designated eosinophil peroxidase (EPO), major basic protein (MBP), eosinophil cationic protein (ECP) and eosinophil-derived neurotoxin (EDN). All 4 proteins are cytotoxic molecules; also, ECP and EDN are ribonucleases. In addition to releasing their preformed cationic proteins, eosinophils can release a variety of cytokines, chemokines and neuromediators and generate large amounts of LTC4. Lastly, eosinophils can be induced to express MHC class II and co-stimulatory molecules and may be involved in propagating immune responses by presenting antigen to T cells. *(From Leung YM, Szefler SJ, Bomilla FA, Akdis CA, Sampson HA: Pediatric allergy principles and practice, ed 3, Philadelphia, 2016, Elsevier, p 42.)*

with eosinophil numbers higher in the early morning and diminishing as endogenous glucocorticoid levels rise.

Many diseases with allergic, infectious, hematologic, autoimmune, or idiopathic origins are associated with moderate (AEC 1,500-5,000 cells/μL) or severe (AEC >5,000 cells/μL) eosinophilia in peripheral blood (Table 155.1). These disorders may range from mild and transient to chronic and life threatening. Importantly, blood eosinophil numbers do not always reflect the extent of eosinophil involvement in tissues and degranulation products may more accurately reflect disease activity. Because prolonged eosinophilia is associated with end-organ damage, especially involving the heart, patients with persistently elevated AECs should undergo a thorough evaluation to search for an underlying cause.

Allergic Diseases

Allergy is the most common cause of eosinophilia in children in the United States. Patients with allergic asthma typically have eosinophils in the blood, sputum, and/or lung tissue. **Hypersensitivity drug reactions** can elicit eosinophilia, and when associated with organ dysfunction (e.g., DRESS [drug rash with eosinophilia and systemic symptoms]), these reactions can be serious (see Chapter 177). If a drug is suspected of triggering eosinophilia, biochemical evidence of organ dysfunction should be sought, and if found, the drug should be discontinued. Various skin diseases have also been associated with eosinophilia, including atopic dermatitis/eczema, pemphigus, urticaria, and toxic epidermal necrolysis.

Eosinophilic gastrointestinal diseases are important emerging allergic causes of eosinophilia in tissue and, in some cases, peripheral blood (see Chapter 363). In these conditions, eosinophils are recruited to esophagus, stomach, and/or intestine, where they cause tissue inflammation and clinical symptoms such as dysphagia, food aversion, abdominal pain, vomiting, and diarrhea. Treatment options include allergen elimination diets and swallowed or inhaled corticosteroids.

Infectious Diseases

Eosinophilia is often associated with invasive infection with multicellular helminthic parasites, which are the most common cause in developing countries. Table 155.1 includes examples of specific organisms. The level of eosinophilia tends to parallel the magnitude and extent of tissue invasion, especially by larvae such as **visceral larva migrans** (see Chapter 324). Eosinophilia often *does not* occur in established parasitic infections that are well contained within tissues or are solely intraluminal in the gastrointestinal tract, such as *Giardia lamblia* and *Enterobius vermicularis* infection.

In evaluating patients with unexplained eosinophilia, the dietary history and geographic or travel history may indicate potential exposures to helminthic parasites. It is frequently necessary to examine the stool for ova and larvae at least 3 times. Additionally, the diagnostic parasite stages of many of the helminthic parasites that cause eosinophilia never appear in feces. Thus, normal results of stool examinations do not absolutely preclude a helminthic cause of eosinophilia; diagnostic blood tests or tissue biopsy may be needed. *Toxocara* causes visceral larva migrans usually in toddlers with pica (see Chapter 324). Most young children are asymptomatic, but some develop fever, pneumonitis, hepatomegaly, and hypergammaglobulinemia accompanied by severe eosinophilia. Isohemagglutinins are frequently elevated, and serology can establish the diagnosis.

Two fungal diseases may be associated with eosinophilia: aspergillosis in the form of **allergic bronchopulmonary aspergillosis** (see Chapter 264.1) and **coccidioidomycosis** (see Chapter 267) following primary infection, especially in conjunction with erythema nodosum. HIV infection can also be associated with peripheral eosinophilia.

Hypereosinophilic Syndrome

The idiopathic hypereosinophilic syndrome is a heterogeneous group of disorders characterized by sustained overproduction of eosinophils.

Table 155.1	Causes of Eosinophilia

ALLERGIC DISORDERS
Allergic rhinitis
Asthma
Acute and chronic urticaria
Eczema
Angioedema
Hypersensitivity drug reactions (drug rash with eosinophilia and systemic symptoms [DRESS])
Eosinophilic gastrointestinal disorders
Interstitial nephritis

INFECTIOUS DISEASES
Tissue-Invasive Helminth Infections
Trichinosis
Toxocariasis
Strongyloidosis
Ascariasis
Filariasis
Schistosomiasis
Echinococcosis
Amebiasis
Malaria
Scabies
Toxoplasmosis

Other Infections
Pneumocystis jirovecii
Scarlet fever
Allergic bronchopulmonary aspergillosis (ABPA)
Coccidioidomycosis
Human immunodeficiency virus (HIV)

MALIGNANT DISORDERS
Hodgkin disease and T-cell lymphoma
Acute myelogenous leukemia
Myeloproliferative disorders
Eosinophilic leukemia
Brain tumors

GASTROINTESTINAL DISORDERS
Inflammatory bowel disease
Peritoneal dialysis
Chronic active hepatitis
Eosinophilic gastrointestinal disorders:
    Eosinophilic esophagitis
    Eosinophilic gastroenteritis
    Eosinophilic colitis

RHEUMATOLOGIC DISEASE
Rheumatoid arthritis
Eosinophilic fasciitis
Scleroderma
Dermatomyositis
Systemic lupus erythematosus
IgG4-related disease
Eosinophilic granulomatosis with polyangiitis (Churg-Strauss vasculitis)

IMMUNODEFICIENCY/IMMUNE DYSREGULATION DISEASE
Hyperimmunoglobulin E syndromes
Wiskott-Aldrich syndrome
Graft-versus-host disease
Omenn syndrome
Severe congenital neutropenia
Autoimmune lymphoproliferative syndromes (ALPS)
Immune dysregulation, polyendocrinopathy, X-linked (IPEX)
Transplant rejection (solid organ)

MISCELLANEOUS
Thrombocytopenia with absent radii
Hypersensitivity pneumonitis
Adrenal insufficiency
Postirradiation of abdomen
Histiocytosis with cutaneous involvement
Hypereosinophilic syndromes
Cytokine infusion
Pemphigoid

The 3 diagnostic criteria for this disorder are (1) AEC >1,500 cells/µL persisting for 6 mo or longer or at least on 2 occasions or with evidence of tissue eosinophilia; (2) absence of another diagnosis to explain the eosinophilia; and (3) signs and symptoms of organ involvement. The clinical signs and symptoms of hypereosinophilic syndrome can be heterogeneous because of the diversity of potential organ (pulmonary, cutaneous, neurologic, serosal, GI) involvement. Eosinophilic endomyocardial disease, one of the most serious and life-threatening complications, can cause heart failure from endomyocardial thrombosis and fibrosis. Eosinophilic leukemia, a clonal myeloproliferative variant, may be distinguished from idiopathic hypereosinophilic syndrome by demonstrating a clonal interstitial deletion on chromosome 4q12 that fuses the platelet-derived growth factor receptor-α (*PDGFRA*) and FIP1-like-1 (*FIP1L1*) genes; this disorder is treated with imatinib mesylate, a tyrosine kinase inhibitor, which helps target the fusion oncoprotein (Fig. 155.2).

Therapy is aimed at suppressing eosinophilia and is initiated with corticosteroids. Imatinib mesylate may be effective in FIP1L1-PDGFRA–negative patients. Hydroxyurea or interferon-alfa may be beneficial in patients unresponsive to corticosteroids. Specific anti–IL-5 monoclonal antibodies (mepolizumab) target this cytokine, which has a central role in eosinophil differentiation, mobilization, and activity. With therapy, the eosinophil count declines and corticosteroid doses may be reduced. For patients with prominent organ involvement who fail to respond to therapy, the mortality is about 75% after 3 yr.

Miscellaneous Diseases

Eosinophilia is observed in many patients with primary immunodeficiency syndromes, especially hyper-IgE syndrome, Wiskott-Aldrich syndrome, and Omenn syndrome (see Chapters 148 and 152). Eosinophilia is also frequently present in the syndrome of thrombocytopenia with absent radii and in familial reticuloendotheliosis with eosinophilia. Eosinophilia can be found in patients with Hodgkin disease, as well as in acute lymphoid and myeloid leukemia. Other considerations include GI disorders such as ulcerative colitis, Crohn disease during symptomatic phases, chronic hepatitis, eosinophilic granulomatosis with polyangiitis (Churg-Strauss vasculitis), and adrenal insufficiency.

Bibliography is available at Expert Consult.

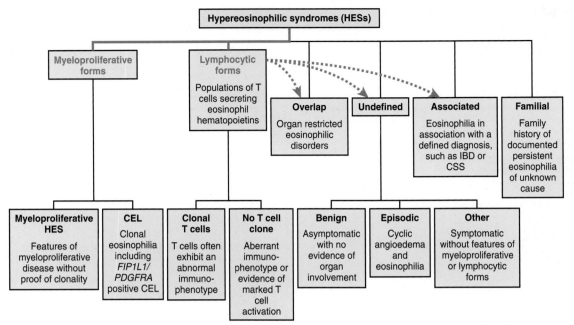

Fig. 155.2 Revised classification of hypereosinophilic syndromes. Changes from the previous classification are indicated in *red*. *Dashed arrows* identify hypereosinophilic syndrome (HES) forms for which at least some patients have T-cell–driven disease. Classification of myeloproliferative forms has been simplified, and patients with HES and eosinophil hematopoietin–producing T cells in the absence of a T-cell clone are included in the lymphocytic forms of HES. CEL, Chronic eosinophilic leukemia; CSS, Churg-Strauss syndrome; IBD, inflammatory bowel disease. *(From Simon HU, Rothenberg ME, Bocher BS, et al: Refining the definition of hypereosinophilic syndrome, J Allergy Clin Immunol 126:47, 2010.)*

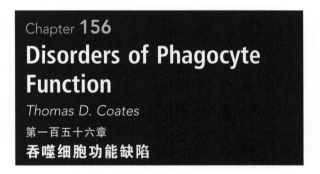

Chapter **156**

Disorders of Phagocyte Function

Thomas D. Coates

第一百五十六章
吞噬细胞功能缺陷

中文导读

　　本章主要介绍了白细胞黏附缺陷、Chediak-Higashi综合征、髓过氧化物酶缺陷以及慢性肉芽肿病。具体描述了白细胞黏附缺陷的分类、遗传发病机制、临床表现、实验室检测、治疗和预后；具体描述了Chediak-Higashi综合征的遗传发病机制、临床表现、实验室检测和治疗；具体描述了髓过氧化物酶缺陷的临床表现、实验室检测和治疗；详细描述了慢性肉芽肿病的遗传发病机制、临床表现、实验室检测、治疗、遗传咨询和预后。

Neutrophils are the first line of defense against microbial invasion. They arrive at the site of inflammation during the critical 2-4 hr after microbial invasion to contain the infection and prevent hematogenous dissemination. This well-orchestrated process is one of the most interesting stories in modern cell biology. In fact, much of our knowledge about neutrophil function derives from studies done in patients with genetic errors in neutrophil function. These critical functions and their associated disorders are depicted in Fig. 153.2. Children with phagocytic dysfunction present at a young age with recurrent infections that often involve unusual organisms and are poorly responsive to treatment.

Primary defects of phagocytic function comprise <20% of immunodeficiencies, and there is significant overlap in the presenting signs and symptoms between phagocytic disorders and lymphocyte and humeral disorders. Children with phagocytic defects present with deep tissue infection, pneumonia, adenitis, or osteomyelitis rather than bloodstream infections (Tables 156.1 and 156.2 and Fig. 156.1). A few clinical features point to phagocyte defects rather than other immunodeficiencies, but correct diagnosis relies on highly specialized laboratory tests.

Chemotaxis, the direct migration of cells into sites of infection, involves a complex series of events (see Chapter 153). Disorders of adhesion or granule abnormalities can have intermediate or profound motility defects, and the propensity to infections is related to a combination of these functional deficits. One family with recessively inherited neutrophil actin dysfunction demonstrated that a pure severe chemotactic defect can result in fatal recurrent infection. Defective in vitro chemotaxis of neutrophils can be detected in children with various clinical conditions. However, unless chemotaxis is essentially absent, it is difficult to establish whether frequent infections arise from a primary chemotactic abnormality or occur as secondary medical complications of the underlying disorder. Dental infection with *Capnocytophaga* is associated with a clear neutrophil motility defect that resolves when the infection is eliminated.

Motility defects present with significant skin and mucosal infections. Tender cutaneous nodular lesions may also be present and characteristically do not contain neutrophils. In fact, presence of a true abscess makes the diagnosis of a significant chemotactic defect less likely.

Laboratory tests of chemotaxis are biologic assays and have high variability except in the most experienced hands. The assays must be done on freshly obtained blood and are affected by many factors related to blood sampling itself. It is best to assay other features of the suspected disorder, such as surface marker expression, to establish a specific diagnosis.

LEUKOCYTE ADHESION DEFICIENCY

Leukocyte adhesion deficiency types 1 (LAD-1), 2 (LAD-2), and 3 (LAD-3) are rare autosomal recessive disorders of leukocyte function. LAD-1 affects about 1 per 10 million individuals and is characterized by recurrent bacterial and fungal infections and depressed inflammatory responses despite striking blood neutrophilia (Table 156.3). The neutrophils have significant defects in adhesion, motility, and ability to phagocytose bacteria.

Genetics and Pathogenesis

LAD-1 results from mutations of the gene on chromosome 21q22.3 encoding CD18, the 95-kDa β_2-leukocyte transmembrane integrin subunit. Normal neutrophils express 4 heterodimeric adhesion molecules: LFA-1 (CD11a/CD18), Mac-1 (CD11b/CD18, also known as CR3 or iC3b receptor), p150,95 (CD11c/CD18), and $\alpha_1\beta_2$ (CD11d/CD18). These 4 transmembrane adhesion molecules are composed of unique extracellular α_1 encoded on chromosome 16, and they share a common β_2 subunit (CD18) that links them to the membrane and connects them to intracellular signal transduction machinery. This group of leukocyte integrins is responsible for the tight adhesion of neutrophils to the endothelial cell surface, egress from the circulation, and adhesion to iC3b-coated microorganisms, which promotes phagocytosis and particulate activation of the phagocyte nicotinamide adenine dinucleotide phosphate (NADPH) oxidase. Some mutations of CD11/CD18 allow a low level of assembly and activity of integrin molecules, resulting in retention of some neutrophil integrin adhesion function and a moderate phenotype.

Because of their inability to adhere firmly to intercellular adhesion molecules 1 (ICAM-1) and 2 (ICAM-2) expressed on inflamed endothelial cells (see Chapter 153), neutrophils cannot transmigrate through the vessel wall and move to the site infection. Furthermore, neutrophils that do arrive at inflammatory sites fail to recognize microorganisms opsonized with complement fragment **iC3b**, an important stable opsonin formed by the cleavage of C3b. Therefore, other neutrophil functions such as degranulation and oxidative metabolism normally triggered by iC3b binding are also greatly compromised in LAD-1 neutrophils, resulting in impaired phagocytic function and high risk for serious and recurrent bacterial infections.

Monocyte function is also impaired, with poor fibrinogen-binding function, an activity that is promoted by the CD11/CD18 complex.

Table 156.1	Infections and White Blood Cell Defects: Features That Can Be Seen in Phagocyte Disorders						

SEVERE INFECTIONS		RECURRENT INFECTIONS		SPECIFIC INFECTIONS		UNUSUALLY LOCATED INFECTIONS	
Type of Infection	Diagnosis to Consider	Site of Infection	Diagnosis to Consider	Microorganism	Diagnosis to Consider	Site of Infection	Diagnosis to Consider
Cellulitis	Neutropenia, LAD, CGD, HIES	Cutaneous	Neutropenia, CGD, LAD, HIES	*Staphylococcus epidermidis*	Neutropenia, LAD	Umbilical cord	LAD
Colitis	Neutropenia, CGD	Gums	LAD, neutrophil motility disorders	*Serratia marcescens, Nocardia, Burkholderia cepacia*	CGD	Liver abscess	CGD
Osteomyelitis	CGD, MSMD pathway defects	Upper and lower respiratory tract	Neutropenia, HIES, functional neutrophil disorders	*Aspergillus*	Neutropenia, CGD, HIES	Gums	LAD, neutrophil motility disorders
		Gastrointestinal tract	CGD, MSMD pathway defects (salmonella)	Nontuberculous mycobacteria, BCG	MSMD pathway defects, SCID, CGD		
		Lymph nodes	CGD, MSMD pathway defects (mycobacteria)	*Candida*	Neutropenia, CGD, MPO		
		Osteomyelitis	CGD, MSMD				

BCG, Bacille Calmette-Guérin; CGD, chronic granulomatous disease; HIES, hyper-IgE syndrome; LAD, leukocyte adhesion deficiency; MSMD, mendelian susceptibility to mycobacterial disease; SCID, severe combined immunodeficiency.
From Leung DYM: *Pediatric allergy principles and practice*, ed 2, Philadelphia, 2010, Saunders, p 134.

Table 156.2	Clinical Disorders of Neutrophil Function		
DISORDER	**ETIOLOGY**	**IMPAIRED FUNCTION**	**CLINICAL CONSEQUENCE**
DEGRANULATION ABNORMALITIES			
Chédiak-Higashi syndrome (CHS)	Autosomal recessive; disordered coalescence of lysosomal granules; responsible gene is *CHSI/LYST*, which encodes a protein hypothesized to regulate granule fusion	Decreased neutrophil chemotaxis, degranulation, and bactericidal activity; platelet storage pool defect; impaired NK function, failure to disperse melanosomes	Neutropenia; recurrent pyogenic infections; propensity to develop marked hepatosplenomegaly as a manifestation of hemophagocytic syndrome
Specific granule deficiency	Autosomal recessive; functional loss of myeloid transcription factor arising from a mutation or arising from reduced expression of *Gfi-1* or *C/EBPε*, which regulates specific granule formation	Impaired chemotaxis and bactericidal activity; bilobed nuclei in neutrophils; defensins, gelatinase, collagenase, vitamin B_{12}–binding protein, and lactoferrin	Recurrent deep-seated abscesses
ADHESION ABNORMALITIES			
Leukocyte adhesion deficiency 1 (LAD-1)	Autosomal recessive; absence of CD11/CD18 surface adhesive glycoproteins ($β_2$-integrins) on leukocyte membranes most commonly arising from failure to express CD18 messenger RNA	Decreased binding of iC3b to neutrophils and impaired adhesion to ICAM-1 and ICAM-2	Neutrophilia; recurrent bacterial infection associated with a lack of pus formation
Leukocyte adhesion deficiency 2 (LAD-2)	Autosomal recessive; loss of fucosylation of ligands for selectins and other glycol conjugates arising from mutations of GDP-fucose transporter	Decreased adhesion to activated endothelium expressing ELAM	Neutrophilia; recurrent bacterial infection without pus
Leukocyte adhesion deficiency 3 (LAD-1 variant syndrome)	Autosomal recessive; impaired integrin function arising from mutations of *FERMT3*, which encodes kindlin-3 in hematopoietic cells; kindlin-3 binds to β-integrin and thereby transmits integrin activation	Impaired neutrophil adhesion and platelet activation	Neutrophilia, recurrent infections, bleeding tendency
DISORDERS OF CELL MOTILITY			
Enhanced motile responses; FMF	Autosomal recessive gene responsible for FMF on chromosome 16, which encodes for a protein called pyrin; pyrin regulates caspase-1 and thereby IL-1β secretion; mutated pyrin may lead to heightened sensitivity to endotoxin, excessive IL-1β production, and impaired monocyte apoptosis	Excessive accumulation of neutrophils at inflamed sites, possibly the result of excessive IL-1β production	Recurrent fever, peritonitis, pleuritis, arthritis, amyloidosis
DEPRESSED MOTILE RESPONSES			
Defects in the generation of chemotactic signals	IgG deficiencies; C3 and properdin deficiency can arise from genetic or acquired abnormalities; mannose-binding protein deficiency predominantly in neonates	Deficiency of serum chemotaxis and opsonic activities	Recurrent pyogenic infections
Intrinsic defects of the neutrophil, e.g., LAD, CHS, specific granule deficiency, neutrophil actin dysfunction, neonatal neutrophils	In the neonatal neutrophil there is diminished ability to express $β_2$-integrins, and there is a qualitative impairment in $β_2$-integrin function	Diminished chemotaxis	Propensity to develop pyogenic infections
Direct inhibition of neutrophil mobility, e.g., drugs	Ethanol, glucocorticoids, cyclic AMP	Impaired locomotion and ingestion; impaired adherence	Possible cause for frequent infections; neutrophilia seen with epinephrine arises from cyclic AMP release from endothelium
Immune complexes	Bind to Fc receptors on neutrophils in patients with rheumatoid arthritis, systemic lupus erythematosus, and other inflammatory states	Impaired chemotaxis	Recurrent pyogenic infections
Hyper-IgE syndrome	Autosomal dominant; responsible gene is *STAT3*	Impaired chemotaxis at times; impaired regulation of cytokine production	Recurrent skin and sinopulmonary infections, eczema, mucocutaneous candidiasis, eosinophilia, retained primary teeth, minimal trauma fractures, scoliosis, and characteristic facies

Continued

Table 156.2	Clinical Disorders of Neutrophil Function—cont'd		
DISORDER	**ETIOLOGY**	**IMPAIRED FUNCTION**	**CLINICAL CONSEQUENCE**
Hyper-IgE syndrome–AR	Autosomal recessive; more than 1 gene likely contributes to its etiology	High IgE levels, impaired lymphocyte activation to staphylococcal antigens	Recurrent pneumonia without pneumatoceles sepsis, enzyme, boils, mucocutaneous candidiasis, neurologic symptoms, eosinophilia
MICROBICIDAL ACTIVITY			
Chronic granulomatous disease (CGD)	X-linked and autosomal recessive; failure to express functional gp91^{phox} in the phagocyte membrane in p22^{phox} (AR) Other AR forms of CGD arise from failure to express protein p47^{phox} or p67^{phox}	Failure to activate neutrophil respiratory burst, leading to failure to kill catalase-positive microbes	Recurrent pyogenic infections with catalase-positive microorganisms
G6PD deficiency	<5% of normal activity of G6PD	Failure to activate NADPH-dependent oxidase; hemolytic anemia	Infections with catalase-positive microorganisms
Myeloperoxidase deficiency	Autosomal recessive; failure to process modified precursor protein arising from missense mutation	H_2O_2-dependent antimicrobial activity not potentiated by myeloperoxidase	None
Rac2 deficiency	Autosomal dominant; dominant negative inhibition by mutant protein of Rac2-mediated functions	Failure of membrane receptor–mediated O_2^- generation and chemotaxis	Neutrophilia, recurrent bacterial infections
Deficiencies of glutathione reductase and glutathione synthetase	AR; failure to detoxify H_2O_2	Excessive formation of H_2O_2	Minimal problems with recurrent pyogenic infections

AMP, Adenosine monophosphate; AR, autosomal recessive; C, complement; CD, cluster of differentiation; ELAM, endothelial-leukocyte adhesion molecule; FMF, familial Mediterranean fever; G6PD, glucose-6-phosphate dehydrogenase; GDP, guanosine diphosphate; ICAM, intracellular adhesion molecule; IL-1, interleukin-1; NADPH, nicotinamide adenine dinucleotide phosphate; NK, natural killer.
Adapted from Curnutte JT, Boxer LA: Clinically significant phagocytic cell defects. In Remington JS, Swartz MN, editors: *Current clinical topics in infectious disease,* ed 6, New York, 1985, McGraw-Hill, p 144.

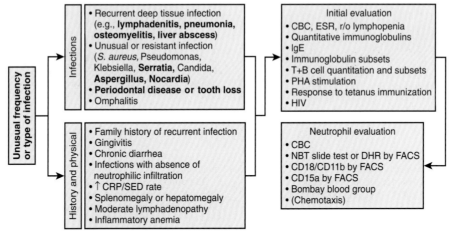

Fig. 156.1 Algorithm for clinical evaluation of patients with recurrent infections. Shown are the evaluations that can be done in a routine clinical laboratory. The complete blood count (CBC) can detect marked leukocytosis in leukocyte adhesion deficiency (LAD) and giant granules of Chédiak-Higashi syndrome may be seen on the smear. Chemotaxis and all other neutrophil functions assays require highly specialized research laboratories. CD, Cluster of differentiation; CRP, C-reactive protein; DHR, dihydrorhodamine; ESR, erythrocyte sedimentation rate; FACS, fluorescence-activated cell sorter; HIV, human immunodeficiency virus; IgE, immunoglobulin E; NBT, nitroblue tetrazolium; PHA, phytohemagglutinin. *(Adapted from Dinauer, MC, Coates TD, Disorders of neutrophil function. In Hoffman R, Benz EJ, Silberstein LE, Helsop H, Weitz J, Anastasi J, editors: Hematology: basic principles and practice, ed 6, Philadelphia, 2012, Saunders.)*

Consequently, such cells are unable to participate effectively in wound healing.

Children with **LAD-2** share the clinical features of LAD-1 but have normal CD11/CD18 integrins. Features unique to LAD-2 include neurologic defects, cranial facial dysmorphism, and absence of the erythrocyte ABO blood group antigen (**Bombay** phenotype). LAD-2 (also known as **congenital disorder of glycosylation IIc (CDG-IIc)**) derives from mutations in the gene encoding a specific guanosine diphosphate (GDP)-L-fucose transporter of the Golgi apparatus. This abnormality prevents the incorporation of fucose into various cell surface glycoproteins, including the carbohydrate structure sialyl Lewis X that is critical for low-affinity rolling adhesion of neutrophils to vascular endothelium. This is an important initial step necessary for subsequent integrin-mediated activation, spreading, and transendothelial migration. Infections in LAD-2 are milder than that in LAD-1.

LAD-3 is characterized by a **Glanzmann thrombasthenia**–like

Table 156.3	Leukocyte Adhesion Deficiency Syndromes				
LEUKOCYTE ADHESION DEFICIENCY (LAD)	**TYPE 1 (LAD-1)**	**TYPE 2 (LAD-2 or CDG-IIc)**	**TYPE 3 (LAD-3)**	**E-SELECTIN DEFICIENCY**	**Rac2 DEFICIENCY**
OMIM	116920	266265	612840	131210	602049
Inheritance pattern	Autosomal recessive	Autosomal recessive	Autosomal recessive	Unknown	Autosomal dominant
Affected protein(s)	β_2-Integrin common chain (CD18)	Fucosylated proteins (e.g., sialyl-Lewis^x, CD15s)	Kindlin 3	Endothelial E-selectin expression	Rac2
Neutrophil function affected	Chemotaxis, tight adherence	Rolling, tethering	Chemotaxis, adhesion, superoxide production	Rolling, tethering	Chemotaxis, superoxide production
Delayed umbilical cord separation	Yes (severe phenotype only)	Yes	Yes	Yes	Yes
Leukocytosis/ neutrophilia	Yes	Yes	Yes	No (mild neutropenia)	Yes

CDG-IIc, Congenital disorder of glycosylation IIc, OMIM, Online Mendelian Inheritance in Man.
From Leung DYM: *Pediatric allergy principles and practice*, ed 2, Philadelphia, 2010, Saunders, p 139.

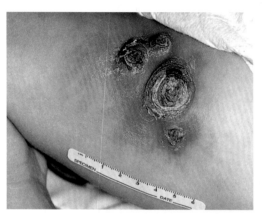

Fig. 156.2 Skin infection of a patient with leukocyte adhesion deficiency type 1. Failure to form pus, inability to demarcate the fibrotic skin debris, and limited inflammation. *Enterococcus gallinarium* was cultured from the wound. *(From Rich RR: Clinical immunology principles and practices, ed 4, Philadelphia, 2013, Saunders, p 273).*

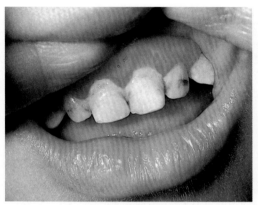

Fig. 156.3 Oral pathology in a patient with leukocyte adhesion deficiency type 1. Gingivitis and severe periodontitis are hallmarks of LAD-1. *(From Rich RR: Clinical immunology principles and practices, ed 4, Philadelphia, 2013, Saunders, p 273.)*

bleeding disorder, delayed separation of the umbilical cord, and serious skin and soft tissue infections similar to those seen in LAD-1, and failure of leukocytes to undergo β_2- and β_1-integrin–mediated adhesion and migration. Mutations in *KINDLIN3* affect integrin activation.

Clinical Manifestations

Patients with the severe clinical form of LAD-1 express <0.3% of the normal amount of the β_2-integrin molecules, whereas patients with the moderate phenotype may express 2–7% of the normal amount. Children with severe forms of LAD present in infancy with recurrent, indolent bacterial infections of the skin, mouth, respiratory tract, lower intestinal tract, and genital mucosa. Significant neutrophilic leukocytosis, often >25,0000/mm^3, is a prominent feature. They may have a history of delayed separation of the umbilical cord, usually with associated infection of the cord stump. The presence of significant omphalitis is an important feature that distinguishes these rare patients from the 10% of healthy infants who can have cord separation at age 3 wk or later. Skin infection may progress to large chronic ulcers with polymicrobial infection, including anaerobic organisms (Fig. 156.2). The ulcers heal slowly, need months of antibiotic treatment, and often require plastic surgery grafting. Severe gingivitis can lead to early loss of primary and secondary teeth (Fig. 156.3). Infected areas characteristically have very little neutrophilic infiltration.

The pathogens infecting patients with LAD-1 are similar to those affecting patients with severe neutropenia (see Chapter 157) and include *Staphylococcus aureus* and enteric gram-negative organisms such as *Escherichia coli*. These patients are also susceptible to opportunistic infection by fungi such as *Candida* and *Aspergillus*. Typical signs of inflammation, such as swelling, erythema, and warmth, may be absent. Pus does not form, and few neutrophils are identified microscopically in biopsy specimens of infected tissues. Despite the paucity of neutrophils within the affected tissue, the circulating neutrophil count during infection typically exceeds 30,000/μL and can surpass 100,000/μL. During intervals between infections, the peripheral blood neutrophil count may chronically exceed 12,000/μL. LAD-1 genotypes with only moderate, rather than absent, amounts of functional integrins at the surface of the neutrophil have significantly reduced severity and frequency of infections compared with children with the severe form, although gingival disease is still a prominent feature.

Laboratory Findings

The diagnosis of LAD-1 is established most readily by flow cytometric measurements of surface CD11b/CD18 in stimulated and unstimulated neutrophils. Neutrophil and monocyte adherence, aggregation, chemotaxis, and iC3b-mediated phagocytosis demonstrate striking abnormalities. However, these assays are not clinically available. Delayed-type hypersensitivity reactions are normal, and most individuals have normal specific antibody synthesis, although some patients have impaired T-lymphocyte–dependent antibody responses. The diagnosis of LAD-2 is established by flow cytometric measurement of sialyl Lewis X (CD15) on neutrophils. It is important to note that the flow cytometric assays are not done the same as the more common lymphocyte subset analysis and require specialized approaches to detect levels of surface expression, especially to detect milder phenotypes.

TREATMENT

Treatment of LAD-1 depends on the phenotype, as determined by the level of expression of functional CD11/CD18 integrins. Early allogeneic hematopoietic stem cell transplantation (HSCT) is the treatment of choice for severe LAD-1 (and LAD-3). One patient was successfully treated with ustekinumab, an inhibitor of interleukins 12 and 23. Other treatment is largely supportive. Patients can be maintained on prophylactic trimethoprim/sulfamethoxazole (TMP/SMX) and should have close surveillance for early identification of infections and initiation of empirical treatment with broad-spectrum antibiotics. Specific determination of the etiologic agent by culture or biopsy is important because of the prolonged antibiotic treatment required in the absence of neutrophil function.

Some LAD-2 patients have responded to fucose supplementation, which induced a rapid reduction in the circulating leukocyte count and appearance of the sialyl Lewis X molecules, accompanied by marked improvement in leukocyte adhesion.

PROGNOSIS

The severity of infectious complications correlates with the degree of β_2-integrin deficiency. Patients with severe deficiency may die in infancy, and those surviving infancy have a susceptibility to severe life-threatening systemic infections. Patients with moderate deficiency have infrequent life-threatening infections and relatively long survival.

CHÉDIAK-HIGASHI SYNDROME

Chédiak-Higashi syndrome (CHS) is a rare autosomal recessive disorder characterized by increased susceptibility to infection caused by defective degranulation of neutrophils, a mild bleeding diathesis, partial oculocutaneous albinism, progressive peripheral neuropathy, and a tendency to develop a life-threatening form of **hemophagocytic lymphohistiocytosis** (see Chapter 534.2). CHS is caused by a fundamental defect in granule morphogenesis that results in abnormally large granules in multiple tissues. Pigmentary dilution involving the hair, skin, and ocular fundi results from pathologic aggregation of melanosomes. Neurologic deficits are associated with a failure of decussation of the optic and auditory nerves. Patients exhibit an increased susceptibility to infection that can be explained only in part by defects in neutrophil function. The patients have progressive neutropenia as well as abnormalities in natural killer (NK) function, again related to granule dysfunction.

Genetics and Pathogenesis

LYST (for lysosomal traffic regulator), the gene mutated in CHS, is located at chromosome 1q2-q44. The LYST/CHS protein is thought to regulate vesicle transport by mediating protein-protein interaction and protein-membrane associations. Loss of function may lead to indiscriminate interactions with lysosomal surface proteins, yielding giant granules through uncontrolled fusion of lysosomes with each other.

Almost all cells of patients with CHS show some oversized and dysmorphic lysosomes, storage granules, or related vesicular structures. Melanosomes are oversized, and delivery to the keratinocytes and hair follicles is compromised, resulting in hair shafts devoid of pigment granules. This abnormality in melanosomes leads to the macroscopic impression of hair and skin that is lighter than expected from parental coloration. The same abnormality in melanocytes leads to the partial ocular albinism associated with light sensitivity.

Beginning early in neutrophil development, spontaneous fusion of giant primary granules with each other or with cytoplasmic membrane components results in huge secondary lysosomes with reduced contents of hydrolytic enzymes, including proteinases, elastase, and cathepsin G. This deficiency of proteolytic enzymes may be responsible for the impaired killing of microorganisms by CHS neutrophils.

Clinical Manifestations

Patients with CHS have light skin and silvery hair and frequently complain of solar sensitivity and photophobia that is associated with rotary nystagmus. Other signs and symptoms vary considerably, but frequent infections and neuropathy are common. The infections involve mucous membranes, skin, and respiratory tract. Affected children are susceptible to gram-positive bacteria, gram-negative bacteria, and fungi, with *Staphylococcus aureus* being the most common offending organism. The **neuropathy** may be sensory or motor in type, and ataxia may be a prominent feature. Neuropathy often begins in the teenage years and becomes the most prominent problem.

Patients with CHS have prolonged bleeding times with normal platelet counts, resulting in impaired platelet aggregation associated with a deficiency of the dense granules containing adenosine diphosphate and serotonin.

The most life-threatening complication of CHS is the development of an accelerated phase characterized by pancytopenia, high fever, and lymphohistiocytic infiltration of liver, spleen, and lymph nodes. The onset of the accelerated phase, which can occur at any age, is now recognized to be a genetic form of hemophagocytic lymphohistiocytosis. This occurs in 85% of patients and usually results in death.

Laboratory Findings

The diagnosis of CHS is established by finding large inclusions in all nucleated blood cells. These can be seen on Wright-stained blood films and are accentuated by a peroxidase stain. Because of impaired egress from the bone marrow, cells containing the large inclusions may be missed on peripheral blood smear but readily identified on bone marrow examination. The patients have progressive neutropenia and abnormal platelet, neutrophil, and NK function.

Treatment

High-dose ascorbic acid (200 mg/day for infants; 2,000 mg/day for adults) may improve the clinical status of some children in the stable phase. Although controversy surrounds the efficacy of ascorbic acid, given the safety of the vitamin, it is reasonable to administer ascorbic acid to all patients.

The only curative therapy to prevent the accelerated phase is HSCT. Normal stem cells reconstitute hematopoietic and immunologic function, correct the NK cell deficiency, and prevent conversion to the accelerated phase, but cannot correct or prevent the neuropathy. If the patient is in the accelerated phase with active hemophagocytic lymphohistiocytosis, HSCT often fails to prevent death.

MYELOPEROXIDASE DEFICIENCY

Myeloperoxidase (MPO) deficiency is an autosomal recessive disorder of oxidative metabolism and is one of the most common inherited disorders of phagocytes, occurring at a frequency approaching 1 per 2,000 individuals. MPO is a green heme protein located in the azurophilic lysosomes of neutrophils and monocytes and is the basis for the greenish tinge to pus accumulated at a site of infection.

Clinical Manifestations

MPO deficiency is usually clinically silent. Rarely, patients may have disseminated candidiasis, usually in conjunction with diabetes mellitus. Acquired partial MPO deficiency can develop in acute myelogenous leukemia and in myelodysplastic syndromes.

Laboratory Findings

Deficiency of neutrophil and monocyte MPO can be identified by histochemical analysis. Severe MPO deficiency can cause the dihydrorhodamine (DHR) flow cytometric assay for chronic granulomatous disease (CGD) to be falsely positive. Unlike CGD, eosinophils in severe MPO deficiency will still reduce DHR and yield a normal reaction.

Table 156.4	Classification of Chronic Granulomatous Disease					

COMPONENT AFFECTED	INHERITANCE	SUBTYPE*	FLAVOCYTOCHROME b SPECTRUM	NBT SCORE (% Positive)	INCIDENCE (% of Cases)
gp91^{phox}	X	X91^0	0	0	60
		X91$^-$	Low	80-100 (weak)	5
		X91$^-$	Low	5-10	<1
		X91$^+$	0	0	1
p22^{phox}	A	A220	0	0	4
		A22$^+$	N	0	<1
p47^{phox}	A	A470	N	0†	25
p67^{phox}	A	A670	N	0	5
		A67$^+$	N	0	<1
p40^{phox}	A	A40$^-$	N	100	<1

NBT, Nitroblue tetrazolium.

*In this nomenclature, the first letter represents the mode of inheritance (X-linked [X] or autosomal recessive [A]), whereas the number indicates the *phox* component that is genetically affected. The superscript symbols indicate whether the level of protein of the affected component is undetectable (^{0}), diminished ($^-$), or normal ($^+$), as measured by immunoblot analysis.

†Can be weakly positive.

From *Nathan & Oski's hematology and oncology of infancy and childhood*, ed 8, Philadelphia, 2015, Elsevier, p 833.

Treatment

There is no specific therapy for MPO deficiency. Aggressive treatment with antifungal agents should be provided for candidal infections. The prognosis is usually excellent.

CHRONIC GRANULOMATOUS DISEASE

Chronic granulomatous disease is characterized by neutrophils and monocytes capable of normal chemotaxis, ingestion, and degranulation, but unable to kill **catalase-positive microorganisms** because of a defect in the generation of microbicidal oxygen metabolites. CGD is a rare disease, affecting 4-5 per 1 million individuals; it is caused by 4 genes: 1 X-linked and 3 autosomal recessive in inheritance (Table 156.4).

Genetics and Pathogenesis

Activation of the phagocyte NADPH oxidase requires stimulation of the neutrophils and involves assembly from cytoplasmic and integral membrane subunits (see Fig. 153.3). Oxidase activation initiates with phosphorylation of a cationic cytoplasmic protein, p47^{phox} (47-kDa phagocyte oxidase protein). Phosphorylated p47^{phox}, together with 2 other cytoplasmic components of the oxidase, p67^{phox} and the low-molecular-weight guanosine triphosphatase Rac2, translocates to the membrane, where they combine with the cytoplasmic domains of the transmembrane flavocytochrome b$_{558}$ to form the active oxidase complex. The flavocytochrome is a heterodimer composed of p22^{phox} and highly glycosylated gp91^{phox}. The gp91^{phox} glycoprotein catalyzes electron transport through its NADPH-binding, flavin-binding, and heme-binding domains. Defects in any of these NADPH oxidase components can lead to CGD.

Approximately 65% of patients with CGD are males who inherit their disorder as a result of mutations in *CYBB*, an X-chromosome gene encoding gp91^{phox}. Approximately 35% of patients inherit CGD in an autosomal recessive fashion resulting from mutations in the *NCF1* gene on chromosome 7, encoding p47^{phox}. Defects in the genes encoding p67^{phox} (*NCF2* on chromosome 1) and p22^{phox} (*CYBA* on chromosome 16) are inherited in an autosomal recessive manner and account for approximately 5% of cases of CGD.

The CGD phagocytic vacuoles lack microbicidal reactive oxygen species and remain acidic, so bacteria are not killed or digested properly (Fig. 156.4). Hematoxylin-eosin–stained sections from patients' tissues show multiple granulomas that give CGD its descriptive name.

Clinical Manifestations

Although the clinical presentation is variable, several features suggest the diagnosis of CGD. Any patient with recurrent pneumonia, lymphadenitis, hepatic, subcutaneous, or other abscesses, osteomyelitis at

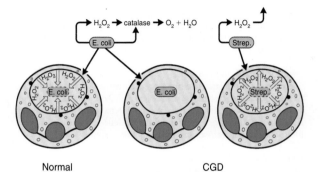

Fig. 156.4 Pathogenesis of chronic granulomatous disease (CGD). The manner in which the metabolic deficiency of the CGD neutrophil predisposes the host to infection is shown schematically. Normal neutrophils stimulate hydrogen peroxide (H$_2$O$_2$) in the phagosome containing ingested *Escherichia coli*. Myeloperoxidase is delivered to the phagosome by degranulation, as indicated by the *closed circles*. In this setting, H$_2$O$_2$ acts as a substrate for myeloperoxidase to oxidize halide to hypochlorous acid and chloramines that kill the microbes. The quantity of H$_2$O$_2$ produced by the normal neutrophil is sufficient to exceed the capacity of catalase, an H$_2$O$_2$-catabolizing enzyme of many aerobic microorganisms, including *Staphylococcus aureus*, most gram-negative enteric bacteria, *Candida albicans*, and *Aspergillus*. When organisms such as *E. coli* gain entry into CGD neutrophils, they are not exposed to H$_2$O$_2$ because the neutrophils do not produce it, and the H$_2$O$_2$ generated by microorganisms themselves is destroyed by their own catalase. When CGD neutrophils ingest streptococci, which lack catalase, the organisms generate enough H$_2$O$_2$ to result in a microbicidal effect. As indicated (*middle*), catalase-positive microbes such as *E. coli* can survive within the phagosome of the CGD neutrophil. (*Adapted from Boxer LA: Quantitative abnormalities of granulocytes. In Beutler E, Lichtman MA, Coller BS, et al, editors: Williams hematology, ed 6, New York, 2001, McGraw-Hill, p 845.*)

multiple sites, a family history of recurrent infections, or any infection with an unusual catalase-positive organism requires evaluation. Other clinical features include chronic colitis or enteritis, gastric outlet or ureteral obstruction from granulomas, or bloodstream infection caused by *Salmonella*, *Burkholderia cepacia*, or *Candida*.

The onset of clinical signs and symptoms usually occurs in early infancy, although a few patients with very rare CGD subtypes have presented later in life. The attack rate and severity of infections are exceedingly variable; however, the infection incidence decreases in the 2nd decade, coincident with maturation of the lymphocyte and humoral immunity. The most common pathogen is *S. aureus*, but any catalase-positive microorganism may be involved. Other organisms frequently causing infections include *Serratia marcescens, B. cepacia, Aspergillus, Candida albicans, Nocardia,* and *Salmonella*. There may also be increased susceptibility to mycobacteria, including the bacille Calmette-Guérin vaccine. Pneumonia, lymphadenitis, osteomyelitis, and skin infections are the most common illnesses encountered. Bacteremia or fungemia occurs but is much less common than focal infections and usually only occurs when local infections have been inappropriately treated for long periods. Patients may have sequelae of chronic infection, including anemia of chronic disease, poor growth, lymphadenopathy, hepato-splenomegaly, chronic purulent dermatitis, restrictive lung disease, gingivitis, hydronephrosis, esophageal dysmotility, and pyloric outlet narrowing. Perirectal abscesses and recurrent skin infections, including folliculitis, cutaneous granulomas, and discoid lupus erythematosus, also suggest CGD.

Granuloma formation and inflammatory processes are a hallmark of CGD and may be the presenting symptoms that prompt testing for CGD if they cause pyloric outlet obstruction, bladder outlet or ureter obstruction, or rectal fistulas and granulomatous colitis simulating Crohn disease. More than 80% of CGD patients have positive serology for Crohn disease. Persistent fever, especially with splenomegaly and cytopenia warrants an evaluation for secondary macrophage activation syndrome. This has been seen in CGD and may require treatment with corticosteroids and discontinuation of interferon-γ treatment.

Laboratory Findings

The diagnosis is most often made by performing flow cytometry using DHR to measure oxidant production through its increased fluorescence when oxidized by hydrogen peroxide (H_2O_2). The nitroblue tetrazolium dye test is frequently cited in the literature but is now only rarely used clinically. The X-linked carrier state is usually easily diagnosed in the mother by DHR fluorescence through a bimodal response to stimulation. It is important to test the mother as some extremely lyonized carriers with <5% positive cells may have chronic clinical problems as well. Ideally, at least the first patient in a kindred should have DNA analysis to facilitate prenatal diagnosis and for genetic counseling purposes.

A few individuals have been described with apparent CGD caused by severe glucose-6-phosphate dehydrogenase deficiency, leading to insufficient NADPH substrate for the phagocyte oxidase. The erythrocytes of these patients also lack the enzyme, leading to chronic hemolysis.

Treatment

HSCT is the only known cure for CGD, although gene therapy has been transiently successful in a few patients and is the topic of active research. HSCT transplant for all patients with CGD is strongly recommended if a suitable sibling or unrelated donor can be identified. The long-term outcome for survival late into adulthood is not good, even in the hands of experienced CGD physicians.

Patients with CGD should be given daily oral TMP/SMX because it reduces the number of bacterial infections. A placebo-controlled study found that interferon-γ 50 μg/m² 3 times/wk significantly reduces the number of hospitalizations and serious infections, although the mechanism of action is unclear. Itraconazole (200 mg/day for patients weighing >50 kg and 100 mg/day for patients <50 kg and ≤5 yr old) administered prophylactically reduces the frequency of fungal infections.

Management of infection is dramatically different than in normal children. CGD patients are always at risk for deep-seated, indolent bacterial infections that can become widespread if not treated properly. They also develop the same kinds of infections that occur in normal children, so determination of the appropriate treatment can be difficult. The erythrocyte sedimentation rate (ESR) can be quite helpful. If the child does not have a deep-seated infection, the ESR will be normal or will normalize within several days with standard management. If it does not, however, a search for deep tissues is warranted, as is

consideration of empirical antibiotics. Cultures should be obtained, but are usually negative. Because all neutrophil functions in CGD except killing are normal, there is often an exuberant inflammatory reaction to a very small number of organisms. Thus, blood cultures and direct cultures of biopsy samples are usually negative unless there are many organisms. Most abscesses require surgical drainage for therapeutic and diagnostic purposes. Prolonged use of antibiotics is required even for common bacterial infections. A simple pneumonia may require 6-8 wk or more of parenteral antibiotics. Infections should be treated for at least 1 wk past normalization of ESR to prevent recurrence. Severe pneumonias can be cleared completely but may require many months of parenteral antibiotics. Especially because cultures are often not helpful, many support an "antibiotic sensitivity by sedimentation rate response" approach to treatment. The ESRs are often 40-80 mm/hr or more with severe infection and will drop monotonically over a week or so after starting antibacterial drugs. It is important to check the ESR daily or every other day because of moderate variability in this test, and changes in treatment need to be based on trends rather than individual values. If there is a clear downward trend over 3-10 days, continue with antibacterials alone. If this is not the case, parenteral voriconazole should be added to cover *Aspergillus*. Failure of the ESR to drop suggests another antimicrobial approach needs to be tried. This sequential addition of antimicrobials offers some insight into the nature of the infection. If both antibacterials and antifungal are started at the same time, one cannot know what caused a response.

Because of the rarity of this disorder, it is critical to seek counsel from someone with significant direct experience with management of several CGD patients. Granulocyte transfusions have been used, but their benefit is unclear. The ESR should be regularly monitored in well patients and whenever they appear ill. A high ESR itself is usually not enough to trigger treatment. However, in the presence of symptoms, one should search for sources at least by contrast CT of the sinus, chest, and abdomen. If the patient is unstable or has very high fevers, *B. cepacia* should be considered and empirically covered. This organism can cause septic shock quickly, unlike the usual smoldering infections seen in CGD. The patient can be treated with antibiotics until the ESR is normal and radiographic evidence of infection has been cleared, if possible. The overall incidence of infection decreases in the 2nd decade of life as nonneutrophil immunity matures, but increased risk of infection is lifelong.

Corticosteroids may be useful for the treatment of children with antral and urethral obstruction or severe granulomatous colitis. Corticosteroids can also be helpful in pneumonia to shrink granulomas in the lung and promote drainage. Short (4-6 days) pulses of 1-2 mg/kg of prednisone are recommended, with rapid taper to avoid long-term side effects and risk of fungus. Pulses can be repeated if clinical effect has not been achieved.

Genetic Counseling

Identifying a patient's specific genetic subgroup by DNA analysis is useful primarily for genetic counseling and prenatal diagnosis. In X-linked CGD, all possibly affected females should be tested by DHR to exclude carrier state. Diagnosis by DNA is strongly recommended in suspected carriers with normal DHR who are related to a known proband, because rarely DHR testing is normal in obligate carriers. Counseling is best done by a physician who has direct knowledge of the clinical manifestations of CGD.

Prognosis

The overall mortality rate for CGD is about 2 patient deaths per year per 100 cases, with the highest mortality among young children. The development of effective infection prophylaxis regimens, close surveillance for signs of infections, and aggressive surgical and medical interventions have improved the prognosis.

Bibliography is available at Expert Consult.

Chapter 157
Leukopenia
Thomas F. Michniacki and
Kelly J. Walkovich

第一百五十七章
白细胞减少症

中文导读

本章主要介绍了中性粒细胞减少症和淋巴细胞减少症。具体描述了中性粒细胞减少症的临床表现、实验室检测、获得性中性粒细胞减少症、遗传性中性粒细胞减少症、未分类中性粒细胞减少性疾病以及治疗；其中获得性中性粒细胞减少症包括感染相关、药物诱导、营养相关、免疫相关、骨髓疾病继发和网状内皮隔离继发的中性粒细胞减少症；遗传性中性粒细胞减少症包括原发性粒细胞生成障碍、分子处理性疾病、囊泡运输性疾病、代谢性疾病和免疫功能异常疾病相关中性粒细胞减少；淋巴细胞减少症具体描述了获得性和遗传性淋巴细胞减少症。

Leukopenia refers to an abnormally low number of white blood cells (WBCs) in the circulating blood secondary to a paucity of lymphocytes, granulocytes, or both. Because there are marked developmental changes in normal values for WBC counts during childhood (see Chapter 748), normal ranges must be considered in the context of age. For newborns, the mean WBC count at birth is high, followed by a rapid fall beginning at 12 hr through the 1st wk of life. Thereafter, values are stable until 1 yr of age, after which a slow, steady decline in the WBC count continues throughout childhood until adult values are reached during adolescence. Evaluation of patients with leukopenia begins with a thorough history, physical examination, and at least 1 confirmatory complete blood count with differential. Further evaluation then depends on whether the leukopenia represents a decreased number of neutrophils, lymphocytes, or both cell populations (Table 157.1). Treatment depends on the etiology and clinical manifestations of the leukopenia.

NEUTROPENIA
Neutropenia is defined as a decrease in the absolute number of circulating segmented neutrophils and bands in the peripheral blood. The **absolute neutrophil count (ANC)** is determined by multiplying the total WBC count by the percentage of segmented neutrophils plus bands. Normal neutrophil counts must be stratified for age and race. Neutrophils predominate at birth but rapidly decrease in the 1st few days of life. During infancy, neutrophils constitute 20–30% of circulating leukocyte populations. Near-equal numbers of neutrophils and lymphocytes are found in the peripheral circulation at 5 yr of age, and the characteristic 70% predominance of neutrophils that occurs in adulthood is usually attained during puberty. For white children >12 mo old, the lower limit of normal for the ANC is 1,500/μL; for black children >12 mo old, the

lower limit of normal is 1,200/μL. The relatively lower limit of normal in blacks likely reflects the prevalence of the Duffy negative (Fy−/−) blood group, which is enriched in populations in the malarial belt of Africa and is associated with ANCs 200-600/μL less than those who are Duffy positive.

Neutropenia may be characterized as **mild** (ANC 1,000-1,500/μL), **moderate** (ANC 500-1,000/μL), or **severe** (ANC <500/μL). ANC <200 is also termed **agranulocytosis**. This stratification aids in predicting the risk of pyogenic infection in patients who have neutropenia resulting from disorders of bone marrow production, because only patients with severe neutropenia have a significantly increased susceptibility to life-threatening infections. Neutropenia associated with monocytopenia, lymphocytopenia, or hypogammaglobulinemia increases the risk for infection compared to isolated neutropenia. *Patients with neutropenia caused by increased destruction (e.g., autoimmune) may tolerate very low ANCs without increased frequency of infection,* because of their often robust ability to generate additional neutrophils from their functioning marrow when needed.

Acute neutropenia evolves over a few days and is often a result of rapid neutrophil use and compromised neutrophil production. **Chronic neutropenia** by definition lasts longer than 3 mo and arises from reduced production, increased destruction, or excessive splenic sequestration of neutrophils. The etiology of neutropenia can be classified as either an acquired disorder or extrinsic insult (Table 157.2) or more rarely an inherited, intrinsic defect (Table 157.3).

Clinical Manifestations of Neutropenia
Individuals with neutrophil counts <500/μL are at substantial risk for developing infections, primarily from their endogenous flora as well as

Table 157.1	Diagnostic Approach for Patients With Leukopenia

EVALUATION	ASSOCIATED CLINICAL DIAGNOSES
INITIAL EVALUATION	
• History of acute or chronic leukopenia	
• General medical history including prior serious, recurrent or unusual infections and malignancy	Congenital syndromes (severe congenital neutropenia, cyclic neutropenia, Shwachman-Diamond, Wiskott-Aldrich, Fanconi anemia, dyskeratosis congenita, glycogen storage disease type Ib, disorders of vesicular transport, GATA2 haploinsufficiency, and primary immunodeficiencies)
• Physical examination: stomatitis, gingivitis, dental defects, warts, lymphedema, congenital anomalies	
• Spleen size	Hypersplenism
• History of drug exposure	Drug-associated neutropenia
• Complete blood count with differential and reticulocyte counts	Neutropenia, aplastic anemia, autoimmune cytopenias
IF ANC <1,000/μL	
Evaluation of Acute-Onset Neutropenia	
• Repeat blood counts in 3-4 wk	Transient myelosuppression (e.g., viral)
• Serology and cultures for infectious agents	Active or chronic infection with viruses (e.g., EBV, CMV), bacteria, mycobacteria, rickettsia
• Discontinue drug(s) associated with neutropenia	Drug-associated neutropenia
• Test for antineutrophil antibodies	Autoimmune neutropenia
• Measure quantitative immunoglobulins (IgG, IgA, IgM, IgE), lymphocyte subsets	Neutropenia associated with disorders of immune function
IF ANC <500/μL ON 3 SEPARATE TESTS	
• Bone marrow aspiration and biopsy, with cytogenetics	Severe congenital neutropenia, cyclic neutropenia, Shwachman-Diamond syndrome, myelokathexis; chronic benign or idiopathic neutropenia; reticular dysgenesis
• Glucocorticoid stimulation test	Chronic benign or idiopathic neutropenia, some autoimmune neutropenias
• Serial CBCs (3/wk for 6 wk)	Cyclic neutropenia
• Exocrine pancreatic function	Shwachman-Diamond syndrome
• Skeletal radiographs	Shwachman-Diamond syndrome, cartilage-hair hypoplasia, Fanconi anemia
IF ALC <1000/μL	
• Repeat blood counts in 3-4 weeks	Transient leukopenia (e.g., viral)
IF ALC <1000/μL ON 3 SEPARATE TESTS	
• HIV-1 antibody or RNA test	HIV-1 infection, AIDS
• Quantitative immunoglobulins (IgG, IgA, IgM, IgE), vaccine titers, lymphocyte subsets	Congenital or acquired disorders of immune function
IF THERE IS PANCYTOPENIA	
• Bone marrow aspiration and biopsy	Bone marrow replacement by malignancy, fibrosis, granulomata, storage cells; aplastic anemia
• Bone marrow cytogenetics and flow cytometry	Myelodysplasia, leukemia
• Vitamin B_{12} and folate levels	Vitamin deficiencies

ALC, Absolute lymphocyte count; ANC, absolute neutrophil count; CBC, complete blood count; CMV, cytomegalovirus; EBV, Epstein-Barr virus.

Table 157.2	Causes of Neutropenia Extrinsic to Marrow Myeloid Cells

CAUSE	ETIOLOGIC FACTORS/AGENTS	ASSOCIATED FINDINGS
Infection	Viruses, bacteria, protozoa, rickettsia, fungi	Clinical features and laboratory findings of the infectious agent
Drug induced	Phenothiazines, sulfonamides, anticonvulsants, penicillins, aminopyrine	Usually none; occasional hypersensitivity reaction (fever, lymphadenopathy, rash, hepatitis, nephritis, pneumonitis, aplastic anemia) or antineutrophil antibody
Immune neutropenia	Alloimmune, autoimmune	Myeloid hyperplasia with left shift in bone marrow (may appear to be "arrest" at metamyelocyte or band stage)
Reticuloendothelial sequestration	Hypersplenism	Anemia, thrombocytopenia
Bone marrow replacement	Myelofibrosis, malignancy (leukemia, lymphoma, metastatic solid tumor, etc.)	Anemia, thrombocytopenia, marrow fibrosis, malignant cells in bone marrow sites of extramedullary hematopoesis
Cancer chemotherapy or radiation therapy	Suppression of myeloid cell production	Anemia, thrombocytopenia, bone marrow hypoplasia

from nosocomial organisms. However, some patients with isolated chronic neutropenia may not experience many serious infections, probably because the remainder of the immune system remains intact or because neutrophil delivery to tissues is preserved, as in autoimmune neutropenias. In contrast, children whose neutropenia is secondary to acquired disorders of production, as occurs with cytotoxic therapy, immunosuppressive drugs, or radiation therapy, are likely to develop serious bacterial infections because many arms of the immune system are markedly compromised and the ability of the marrow to robustly generate new phagocytes is impaired. Neutropenia associated with additional monocytopenia or lymphocytopenia is more highly associated with serious infection than neutropenia alone. The integrity of skin and mucous membranes, the vascular supply to tissues, and nutritional status also influence the risk of infection.

The most common clinical presentation of profound neutropenia includes fever, aphthous stomatitis, and gingivitis. Infections frequently associated with neutropenia include cellulitis, furunculosis, perirectal inflammation, colitis, sinusitis, warts, and otitis media, as well as more serious infections such as pneumonia, deep tissue abscess, and sepsis. The most common pathogens causing infections in neutropenic patients are *Staphylococcus aureus* and gram-negative bacteria. Isolated neutropenia does not heighten a patient's susceptibility to parasitic or viral infections or to bacterial meningitis but does increase the risk of fungal pathogens causing disease. The usual signs and symptoms of local infection and inflammation (e.g., exudate, fluctuance, regional lymphadenopathy) may be diminished in the absence of neutrophils because of the inability to form pus, but patients with agranulocytosis still experience fever and feel pain at sites of inflammation.

Laboratory Findings

Isolated absolute neutropenia has a limited number of causes (see Tables 157.2 to 157.5). The duration and severity of the neutropenia greatly influence the extent of laboratory evaluation. Patients with chronic neutropenia since infancy and a history of recurrent fevers and chronic gingivitis should have WBC counts and differential counts determined 3 times/wk for 6-8 wk to evaluate for periodicity suggestive of **cyclic neutropenia**. Bone marrow aspiration and biopsy should be performed on select patients to assess cellularity and myeloid maturation. Additional marrow studies, such as cytogenetic analysis and special stains for detecting leukemia and other malignant disorders, should be obtained for patients with suspected intrinsic defects in the myeloid progenitors and for patients with suspected malignancy. Selection of further laboratory tests is determined by the duration and severity of the neutropenia and the associated findings on physical examination (see Table 157.1).

Acquired Neutropenia
Infection-Related Neutropenia

Transient neutropenia often accompanies or follows **viral infections** and is the most frequent cause of neutropenia in childhood (Table 157.4). Viruses causing acute neutropenia include influenzas A and B, adenovirus, respiratory syncytial virus, enteroviruses, human herpesvirus 6, measles, rubella, and varicella. Parvovirus B19 and hepatitis A or B may also cause neutropenia, but are more often associated with pure red cell aplasia or multiple cytopenias, respectively. Viral-associated acute neutropenia often occurs during the 1st 24-48 hr of illness and usually persists for 3-8 days, which generally corresponds to the period of viremia. The neutropenia is related to virus-induced redistribution of neutrophils from the circulating to the marginating pool. In addition, neutrophil sequestration may occur after virus-induced tissue damage or splenomegaly.

Significant neutropenia also may be associated with severe bacterial, protozoal, rickettsial, or fungal infections (see Table 157.4). **Bacterial sepsis** is a particularly serious cause of neutropenia, especially among younger infants and children. Premature neonates are especially prone to exhausting their marrow reserve and rapidly succumbing to bacterial sepsis.

Chronic neutropenia often accompanies infection with Epstein-Barr virus, cytomegalovirus, or HIV and certain immunodeficiencies such as X-linked agammaglobulinemia, hyper IgM syndrome and HIV. The neutropenia associated with AIDS probably arises from a combination of viral bone marrow suppression, antibody-mediated destruction of neutrophils, and effects of antiretroviral or other drugs.

Drug-Induced Neutropenia

Drugs constitute a common cause of neutropenia (Table 157.5). The incidence of drug-induced neutropenia increases dramatically with age; only 10% of cases occur among children and young adults. The majority of cases occur among adults >65 yr, likely reflecting the more frequent use of multiple medications in that age-group. Almost any drug can cause neutropenia. The most common offending drug classes are antimicrobial agents, antithyroid drugs, antipsychotics, antipyretics, and antirheumatics. Drug-induced neutropenia has several underlying mechanisms—immune-mediated, toxic, idiosyncratic, hypersensitivity, idiopathic—that are distinct from the severe neutropenia that predictably occurs after administration of antineoplastic drugs or radiotherapy.

Drug-induced neutropenia from immune mechanisms usually

Table 157.3	Acquired Disorders of Myeloid Cells	
CAUSE	**ETIOLOGIC FACTORS/AGENTS**	**ASSOCIATED FINDINGS**
Aplastic anemia	Stem cell destruction and depletion	Pancytopenia
Vitamin B₁₂, copper, or folate deficiency	Malnutrition; congenital deficiency of B₁₂ absorption, transport, and storage; vitamin avoidance	Megaloblastic anemia, hypersegmented neutrophils
Acute leukemia, chronic myelogenous leukemia	Bone marrow replacement with malignant cells	Pancytopenia, leukocytosis
Myelodysplasia	Dysplastic maturation of stem cells	Bone marrow hypoplasia with megaloblastoid red cell precursors, thrombocytopenia
Prematurity with birthweight <2 kg	Impaired regulation of myeloid proliferation and reduced size of postmitotic pool	Maternal preeclampsia
Chronic idiopathic neutropenia	Impaired myeloid proliferation and/or maturation	None
Paroxysmal nocturnal hemoglobinuria	Acquired stem cell defect secondary to mutation of *PIGA* gene	Pancytopenia, thrombosis (hepatic vein thrombosis)

Table 157.4	Infections Associated With Neutropenia
Viral	Cytomegalovirus, dengue, Epstein-Barr virus, hepatitis viruses, HIV, influenza, measles, parvovirus B19, rubella, varicella, HHV-6
Bacterial	*Brucella*, paratyphoid, pertussis, tuberculosis (disseminated), tularemia, Shigella, typhoid; any form of sepsis
Fungal	Histoplasmosis (disseminated)
Protozoan	Malaria, leishmaniasis (kala-azar)
Rickettsial	*Anaplasma* (formerly *Ehrlichia*) *phagocytophilum*, psittacosis, Rocky Mountain spotted fever, typhus, rickettsialpox

develops abruptly, is accompanied by fever, and lasts for about 1 wk after the discontinuation of the drug. The process likely arises from effects of drugs such as propylthiouracil or penicillin that act as haptens to stimulate antibody formation, or drugs such as quinine that induce immune complex formation. Other drugs, including the antipsychotic drugs such as the phenothiazines, can cause neutropenia when given in toxic amounts, but some individuals, such as those with preexisting neutropenia, may be susceptible to levels at the high end of the usual therapeutic range. Late-onset neutropenia can occur after rituximab therapy. Idiosyncratic reactions, for example to chloramphenicol, are unpredictable with regard to dose or duration of use. Hypersensitivity reactions are rare and may involve arene oxide metabolites of aromatic anticonvulsants. Fever, rash, lymphadenopathy, hepatitis, nephritis, pneumonitis, and aplastic anemia are often associated with hypersensitivity-induced neutropenia. Acute hypersensitivity reactions such as those caused by phenytoin or phenobarbital may last for only a few days if the offending drug is discontinued. Chronic hypersensitivity may last for months to years.

Once neutropenia occurs, the most effective therapeutic measure is withdrawal of nonessential drugs, particularly drugs most commonly associated with neutropenia. Usually the neutropenia will resolve soon after withdrawal of the offending drug. If the neutropenia fails to improve with drug withdrawal and the patient is symptomatic with infection or stomatitis, subcutaneous administration of recombinant human granulocyte colony-stimulating factor (filgrastim, 5 μg/kg/day) should be considered. Drug-induced neutropenia may be asymptomatic and noted only as an incidental finding or because of regular monitoring of WBC counts during drug therapy. For patients who are asymptomatic, continuation of the suspected offending drug depends on the relative risks of neutropenia vs discontinuation of a possibly essential drug. If the drug is continued, blood counts should be monitored for possible progression to agranulocytosis.

Neutropenia usually and predictably follows the use of anticancer drugs or radiation therapy, especially radiation directed at the pelvis or vertebrae, secondary to cytotoxic effects on rapidly replicating myeloid precursors. A decline in the WBC count typically occurs 7-10 days after administration of the anticancer drug and may persist for 1-2 wk. The neutropenia accompanying malignancy or following cancer chemotherapy is frequently associated with compromised cellular immunity and barrier compromise secondary to central venous lines and mucositis, thereby predisposing patients to a much greater risk of infection (see Chapter 205) than found in disorders associated with isolated neutropenia. Patients with chemotherapy/radiation-related neutropenia and fever must be treated aggressively with broad-spectrum antibiotics.

Nutrition-Related Neutropenia

Poor nutrition can contribute to neutropenia. Ineffective myelopoiesis may result in neutropenia caused by acquired dietary copper, vitamin B_{12}, or folic acid deficiency. In addition, megaloblastic pancytopenia also can result from extended use of antibiotics such as trimethoprim/sulfamethoxazole that inhibit folic acid metabolism and from the use of phenytoin, which may impair folate absorption in the small intestine,

or from surgical resection of the small intestine. Neutropenia also occurs with starvation and marasmus in infants, with anorexia nervosa, and occasionally among patients receiving prolonged parenteral nutrition without vitamin supplementation.

Immune-Mediated Neutropenia

Immune-mediated neutropenia is usually associated with the presence of circulating antineutrophil antibodies, which may mediate neutrophil destruction by complement-mediated lysis or splenic phagocytosis of opsonized neutrophils, or by accelerated apoptosis of mature neutrophils or myeloid precursors.

Alloimmune neonatal neutropenia occurs after transplacental transfer of maternal alloantibodies directed against antigens on the infant's neutrophils, analogous to Rh-hemolytic disease. Prenatal sensitization induces maternal IgG antibodies to neutrophil antigens on fetal cells. The neutropenia is often severe and infants may present within the 1st 2 wk of life with skin or umbilical infections, fever, and pneumonia caused by the usual microbes that cause neonatal disease. By 7 wk of age, the neutrophil count usually returns to normal, reflecting the decay of maternal antibodies in the infant's circulation. Treatment consists of supportive care and appropriate antibiotics for clinical infections, plus granulocyte colony-stimulating factor (G-CSF) for severe infections without neutrophil recovery.

Mothers with autoimmune disease may give birth to infants who develop transient neutropenia, known as **neonatal passive autoimmune neutropenia**. The duration of the neutropenia depends on the time required for the infant to clear the maternally transferred circulating IgG antibody. It persists in most cases for a few weeks to a few months. Neonates almost always remain asymptomatic.

Autoimmune neutropenia (AIN) of infancy is a benign condition with an annual incidence of approximately 1 per 100,000 among children between infancy and 10 yr of age. Patients usually have severe neutropenia on presentation, with ANC <500/μL, but the total WBC count is generally within normal limits. Monocytosis or eosinophilia may occur but does not impact the low rate of infection. The median age of presentation is 8-11 mo, with a range of 2-54 mo. The diagnosis is often evident when a blood count incidentally reveals neutropenia in a child with a minor infection or when a routine complete blood count is obtained at the 12 mo well-child visit. Occasionally, children may present with more severe infections, including abscesses, pneumonia, or sepsis. The diagnosis may be supported by the presence of antineutrophil antibodies in serum; however, the test has frequent false-negative and false-positive results, so the absence of detectable antineutrophil antibodies does not exclude the diagnosis, and a positive result does not exclude other conditions. Therefore the diagnosis is best made clinically based on a benign course and, if obtained, a normal or hyperplastic myeloid maturation in the bone marrow. There is considerable overlap between AIN of infancy and "chronic benign neutropenia."

Treatment is not generally necessary because the disease is only rarely associated with severe infection and usually remits spontaneously. Low-dose G-CSF may be useful for severe infections, to promote wound healing following surgery, or to avert emergency room visits or hospi-

Table 157.5	Forms of Drug-Induced Neutropenia		
	IMMUNOLOGIC	**TOXIC**	**HYPERSENSITIVITY**
Paradigm drugs	Aminopyrine, propylthiouracil, penicillins	Phenothiazines, clozapine	Phenytoin, phenobarbital
Time to onset	Days to weeks	Weeks to months	Weeks to months
Clinical appearance	Acute, often explosive symptoms	Often asymptomatic or insidious onset	May be associated with fever, rash, nephritis, pneumonitis, or aplastic anemia
Rechallenge	Prompt recurrence with small test dose	Latent period; high doses required	Latent period; high doses required
Laboratory findings	Antineutrophil antibody may be positive; bone marrow myeloid hyperplasia	Bone marrow myeloid hypoplasia	Bone marrow myeloid hypoplasia

talizations for febrile illnesses. Longitudinal studies of infants with AIN demonstrate median duration of disease ranging from 7-30 mo. Affected children generally have no evidence or risk of other autoimmune diseases.

AIN in older children can occur as an isolated process, as a manifestation of other autoimmune diseases, or as a secondary complication of infection, drugs, or malignancy. In primary AIN, low circulating neutrophil counts are the only hematologic finding, and associated diseases or other factors that cause neutropenia are absent. Secondary AIN associated with immune dysregulation or other factors is more often identified in older children and is less likely to remit spontaneously. AIN is distinguished from other forms of neutropenia by the demonstration of antineutrophil antibodies (with caveats previously discussed) and myeloid hyperplasia on bone marrow examination. The most common antineutrophil antibody targets are human neutrophil antigens 1a, 1b, and 2.

Treatment of AIN relies on management of any underlying disorders. In addition, judicious use of appropriate antibiotics for bacterial infections and regular dental hygiene are generally beneficial, as is family and primary care provider education. Infections tend to be less frequent in AIN than with the corresponding degree of neutropenia from other causes, probably because tissue delivery of neutrophils is greater than that in conditions resulting from impaired production. Prophylactic antibiotics may be helpful for the management of recurrent minor infections. For patients with serious or recurrent infections, G-CSF is generally effective at raising the ANC and preventing infection. Very low doses (<1-2 μg/kg/day) are usually effective, and administration of standard doses can lead to severe bone pain from marrow expansion.

Neutropenia Secondary to Bone Marrow Replacement

Various acquired bone marrow disorders lead to neutropenia, usually accompanied by anemia and thrombocytopenia. Hematologic malignancies, including leukemia, lymphoma, and metastatic solid tumors, suppress myelopoiesis by infiltrating the bone marrow with tumor cells. Neutropenia may also accompany aplastic anemia, myelodysplastic disorders, or preleukemic syndromes, which are characterized by multiple cytopenias and often macrocytosis. Treatment requires management of the underlying disease.

Neutropenia Secondary to Reticuloendothelial Sequestration

Splenic enlargement resulting from intrinsic splenic disease (storage disease), portal hypertension, or systemic causes of splenic hyperplasia (inflammation or neoplasia) can lead to neutropenia. Most often the neutropenia is mild to moderate and is accompanied by corresponding degrees of thrombocytopenia and anemia. The reduced neutrophil survival corresponds to the size of the spleen, and the extent of the neutropenia is inversely proportional to bone marrow compensatory mechanisms. Usually the neutropenia can be corrected by successfully treating the underlying disease. In select cases, splenectomy may be necessary to restore the neutrophil count to normal, but results in increased risk of infections by encapsulated bacterial organisms. Patients undergoing splenectomy should receive appropriate preoperative immunizations and may benefit from antibiotic prophylaxis after splenectomy to help mitigate the risk of sepsis. Splenectomy should be avoided in patients with common variable immunodeficiency (CVID), autoimmune lymphoproliferative disease, and other immunodeficiency syndromes because of the higher risk of sepsis.

Inherited Neutropenia

Intrinsic disorders of proliferation or maturation of myeloid precursor cells are rare. Table 157.6 presents a classification based on genetics and molecular mechanisms; select disorders are discussed next.

Primary Disorders of Granulocytopoiesis

Cyclic neutropenia is an autosomal dominant congenital granulopoietic disorder occurring with an estimated incidence of 0.5-1 cases per 1 million population. The disorder is characterized by regular, periodic oscillations, with the ANC ranging from normal to <200/μL, mirrored by reciprocal cycling of monocytes. Cyclic neutropenia is sometimes termed *cyclic hematopoiesis* because of the secondary cycling of other blood cells, such as platelets and reticulocytes. The mean oscillatory period of the cycle is 21 days (±4 days). During the neutropenic nadir, many patients develop malaise, fever, oral and genital ulcers, gingivitis, periodontitis, or pharyngitis, and occasionally lymph node enlargement. More serious infections occasionally occur, including pneumonia, mastoiditis, and intestinal perforation with peritonitis leading to life-threatening clostridial sepsis. Before the availability of G-CSF, approximately 10% of patients developed fatal clostridial or gram-negative infections. Cyclic neutropenia arises from a regulatory abnormality involving early hematopoietic precursor cells and is almost invariably associated with mutations in the neutrophil elastase gene, *ELANE*, that lead to accelerated apoptosis as a result of abnormal protein folding. Many patients experience abatement of symptoms with age. The cycles tend to become less noticeable in older patients, and the hematologic picture often begins to resemble that of chronic idiopathic neutropenia.

Cyclic neutropenia is diagnosed by obtaining blood counts 3 times/wk for 6-8 wk. The requirement for repeated blood counts is necessary because some of the elastase mutations overlap with those in patients who have **severe congenital neutropenia**. Demonstrating oscillation or a lack thereof in the blood counts helps to identify the patients' risk for progression to **myelodysplastic syndrome (MDS)/acute myelogenous leukemia (AML)**, a risk that is only associated with severe congenital neutropenia. The diagnosis can be confirmed with genetic studies demonstrating a mutation in *ELANE*. Affected patients with neutrophil nadirs <200/μL are treated with G-CSF, and their cycle of profound neutropenia changes from a 21-day period with at least 3-5 days of profound neutropenia to 9-11 days with 1 day of less profound neutropenia. The dose needed to maintain nadirs >500/μL is usually 2-4 μg/kg/day administered daily or every other day.

Severe congenital neutropenia (SCN) is a rare, genetically heterogeneous, congenital granulopoietic disorder with an estimated incidence of 1-2 cases per 1 million population. The disorder is characterized by an arrest in myeloid maturation at the promyelocyte stage in the bone marrow, resulting in ANCs consistently <200/μL and may occur sporadically, with autosomal dominant or recessive inheritance. The **dominant** form is caused most often by mutations in *ELANE*, which accounts for 60–80% of SCN cases, whereas **recessive** forms arise from mutations in *HAX1* (the form also known as **Kostmann disease**) or *G6PC3* (encoding a myeloid-specific isoform of glucose-6-phosphatase). *HAX1* mutations may be associated with neurologic deficits, and *G6PC3* with heart defects, urogenital abnormalities, and venous angiectasia. In addition to severe neutropenia, peripheral blood counts generally show monocytosis and many also exhibit eosinophilia; chronic inflammation may lead to secondary anemia and thrombocytosis. Patients who have SCN experience frequent episodes of fever, skin infections (including omphalitis), oral ulcers, gingivitis, pneumonia, and perirectal abscesses, typically appearing in the 1st few mo of life. Infections often disseminate to the blood, meninges, and peritoneum and are usually caused by *S. aureus*, *Escherichia coli*, and *Pseudomonas* species. Without filgrastim therapy, most patients die of infectious complications within the first 1-2 yr of life despite prophylactic antibiotics.

More than 95% of SCN patients respond to filgrastim treatment with an increase in the ANC and a decrease in infections. Doses required to achieve an ANC >1000/uL vary greatly. A starting dose of filgrastim at 5 μg/kg/day is recommended; the dose should be gradually increased, if necessary, as high as 100 μg/kg/day to attain an ANC of 1,000-2,000/μL. The 5% of patients who do not respond to filgrastim or who require high doses (>8 μg/kg/day) should be considered for hematopoietic stem cell transplantation (HSCT). Besides infections, patients with SCN are at risk for developing MDS associated with monosomy 7 and AML. For this reason, regular monitoring with blood counts and yearly bone marrow surveillance, including karyotyping and fluorescence in situ hybridization, should be performed on all SCN patients. Although clonal cytogenetic abnormalities may spontaneously remit, their appearance should be considered a strong indication for HSCT, which is much more likely to be successful before progression to MDS/AML.

Table 157.6	Intrinsic Disorders of Myeloid Precursor Cells

SYNDROME	INHERITANCE (GENE)	CLINICAL FEATURES (INCLUDING STATIC NEUTROPENIA UNLESS OTHERWISE NOTED)
PRIMARY DISORDERS OF MYELOPOIESIS		
Cyclic neutropenia	AD (ELANE)	Periodic oscillation (21-day cycles) in ANC
Severe congenital neutropenia	AD (primarily ELANE, also GFI and others)	Risk of MDS/AML
	AR (G6PC3, HAX1) (HAX1 = Kostmann syndrome)	G6PC3: cardiac and urogenital anomalies, venous angioectasias; HAX1: neurologic abnormalities, risk of MDS/AML
	XL (WAS)	Neutropenic variant of Wiskott-Aldrich syndrome
DISORDERS OF MOLECULAR PROCESSING		
Shwachman-Diamond syndrome	Ribosomal defect: AR (SBDS, DNAJC21, EFL1, SRP54)	Pancreatic insufficiency, metaphyseal dysostosis, bone marrow failure, MDS/AML
Dyskeratosis congenita	Telomerase defects: XL (DKC1), AD (TERC), AR (TERT)	Nail dystrophy, leukoplakia, abnormal and carious teeth, lacey reticulated hyperpigmentation of the skin, bone marrow failure
DISORDERS OF VESICULAR TRAFFICKING		
Chédiak-Higashi syndrome	AR (LYST)	Partial albinism, giant granules in myeloid cells, platelet storage pool defect, impaired NK cell function, HLH
Griscelli syndrome, type II	AR (RAB27a)	Partial albinism, impaired NK cell function, neurologic impairment, HLH
Cohen syndrome	AR (COH1)	Partial albinism, pigmentary retinopathy, developmental delay, facial dysmorphism
Hermansky-Pudlak syndrome, type II	AR (AP3B1)	Cyclic neutropenia, partial albinism, HLH
p14 deficiency	Probable AR (MAPBPIP)	Partial albinism, decreased B and T cells
VPS45 defects	AR (VPS45)	Neutrophil dysfunction, bone marrow fibrosis, nephromegaly
DISORDERS OF METABOLISM		
Glycogen storage disease, type 1b	AR (G6PT1)	Hepatic enlargement, growth retardation, impaired neutrophil motility
Methylmalonic/propionic acidemias	AR Mutase or cobalamin transporters/ propionyl coenzyme A carboxylase	Ketoacidosis, metabolic stroke, depressed consciousness
Barth syndrome	XL (TAZ1)	Episodic neutropenia, dilated cardiomyopathy, methylglutaconic aciduria
Pearson syndrome	Mitochondrial (DNA deletions)	Episodic neutropenia, pancytopenia; defects in exocrine pancreas, liver, and kidneys
NEUTROPENIA IN DISORDERS OF IMMUNE FUNCTION		
Common variable immunodeficiency	Familial, sporadic (TNFRSF13B)	Hypogammaglobulinemia, other immune system defects
IgA deficiency	Unknown (Unknown or TNFRSF13B)	Decreased IgA
Severe combined immunodeficiency	AR, XL (multiple loci)	Absent humoral and cellular immune function
Hyper-IgM syndrome	XL (HIGM1)	Absent IgG, elevated IgM, autoimmune cytopenias
WHIM syndrome	AD (CXCR4)	Warts, hypogammaglobulinemia, infections, myelokathexis
Cartilage-hair hypoplasia	AR (RMRP)	Lymphopenia, short-limbed dwarfism, metaphyseal chondrodysplasia, fine sparse hair
Schimke immunoosseous dysplasia	Probable AR (SMARCAL1)	Lymphopenia, pancytopenia, spondyloepiphyseal dysplasia, growth retardation, renal failure
X-linked agammaglobulinemia	Bruton tyrosine kinase (Btk)	Agammaglobulinemia, neutropenia in ~25%

AD, Autosomal dominant; AML, acute myelogenous leukemia; ANC, absolute neutrophil count; AR, autosomal recessive; HLH, hemophagocytic lymphohistiocytosis; MDS, myelodysplastic syndrome; XL, X-linked.

Disorders of Molecular Processing

Shwachman-Diamond syndrome (SDS) is an autosomal recessive disorder classically characterized by neutropenia, pancreatic insufficiency, and short stature with skeletal abnormalities. SDS is most commonly caused by proapoptotic mutations of the *SBDS* gene, which encodes a protein that plays a role in ribosome biogenesis and RNA processing. The initial symptoms are usually steatorrhea and failure to thrive because of malabsorption, which usually develops by 4 mo of age, although the gastrointestinal symptoms may be subtle in some patients and go unrecognized. Patients have also been reported to have respiratory problems with frequent otitis media, pneumonia, and eczema. Virtually all patients with SDS have neutropenia, with the ANC periodically <1000/μL. Some children have defects in chemotaxis or in the number or function of B, T, and natural killer (NK) cells that may contribute to the increased susceptibility to pyogenic infection. The diagnosis of SDS is based on clinical phenotype; approximately 90% of patients have

mutations identified in *SBDS* with additional mutations now recently discovered in *DNAJC21*, *EFL1*, and *SRP54*. SDS may progress to bone marrow hypoplasia or MDS/AML; cytogenetic abnormalities, particularly isochromosome i(7q) and del(20q), often precede conversion to MDS, so bone marrow monitoring is warranted. Treatment includes pancreatic enzyme replacement, plus G-CSF in patients with severe neutropenia.

Dyskeratosis congenita, a disorder of telomerase activity, most often presents as bone marrow failure rather than isolated neutropenia. The classic phenotype also includes nail dystrophy, leukoplakia, malformed teeth, and reticulated hyperpigmentation of the skin, although many patients, particularly young ones, do not exhibit these clinical features.

Vesicular Trafficking Disorders

This group of rare **primary immunodeficiency syndromes** (see Table 157.6) derives from autosomal recessive defects in the biogenesis or trafficking of lysosomes and related endosomal organelles. As a result, the syndromes share phenotypic characteristics, including defects in melanosomes contributing to partial albinism, abnormal platelet function, and immunologic defects involving not only neutrophil number, but also the function of neutrophils, B lymphocytes, NK cells, and cytotoxic T lymphocytes. The syndromes share a high risk of hemophagocytic lymphohistiocytosis (HLH) as a result of defects in T and NK cells.

Chédiak-Higashi syndrome, best known for the characteristic giant cytoplasmic granules in neutrophils, monocytes, and lymphocytes, is a disorder of subcellular vesicular dysfunction caused by mutations in the *LYST* gene, with resultant giant granules in all granule-bearing cells. Patients have increased susceptibility to infections, mild bleeding diathesis, progressive peripheral neuropathy, and predisposition to life-threatening HLH. The only curative treatment is HSCT, but transplant does not treat all aspects of the disorder.

Griscelli syndrome type II also features neutropenia, partial albinism, and a high risk of HLH, but peripheral blood granulocytes do not show giant granules. Patients often have hypogammaglobulinemia. The disorder is caused by mutations in *RAB27a*, which encodes a small guanosine triphosphatase that regulates granule secretory pathways. The only curative treatment is HSCT.

Disorders of Metabolism

Recurrent infections with neutropenia are a distinctive feature of **glycogen storage disease (GSD) type Ib**. As in classic **von Gierke disease** (GSDIa), glycogen storage in GSDIb causes massive hepatomegaly and severe growth retardation. Mutations in glucose-6-phosphate transporter 1, *G6PT1*, inhibit glucose transport in GSDIb, resulting in both defective neutrophil motility and increased apoptosis associated with neutropenia and recurrent bacterial infections. Treatment with G-CSF can correct the neutropenia but does not correct the underlying functional neutrophil defects.

Neutropenia in Disorders of Immune Dysfunction

Congenital immunologic disorders that have severe neutropenia as a clinical feature include X-linked agammaglobulinemia (XLA), CVID, the severe combined immunodeficiencies, autoimmune lymphoproliferative syndrome, hyperimmunoglobulin M syndrome, WHIM (warts, hypogammaglobulinemia, infections, myelokathexis) syndrome, GATA2 haploinsufficiency, and a number of even rarer immunodeficiency disorders (see Table 157.6).

Unclassified Neutropenic Disorders

Chronic benign neutropenia of childhood represents a common group of disorders characterized by mild to moderate neutropenia that does not lead to an increased risk of pyogenic infections. Spontaneous remissions are often reported, although these may represent misdiagnosis of AIN of infancy, in which remissions often occur during childhood. Chronic benign neutropenia may be sporadic or inherited in either dominant or recessive form. Because of the relatively low risk of serious infection, patients usually do not require any therapy.

Idiopathic chronic neutropenia is characterized by the onset of neutropenia after 2 yr of age, with no identifiable etiology. Patients with an ANC persistently <500/μL may have recurrent pyogenic infections involving the skin, mucous membranes, lungs, and lymph nodes. Bone marrow examination reveals variable patterns of myeloid formation with arrest generally occurring between the myelocyte and band forms. The diagnosis overlaps with chronic benign and AINs.

Treatment

The management of acquired transient neutropenia associated with malignancies, myelosuppressive chemotherapy, or immunosuppressive chemotherapy differs from that of congenital or chronic forms of neutropenia. In the former situation, infections sometimes are heralded only by fever, and sepsis is a major cause of death. Early recognition and treatment of infections may be lifesaving (see Chapter 205). Therapy of severe chronic neutropenia is dictated by the clinical manifestations. Patients with benign neutropenia and no evidence of repeated bacterial infections or chronic gingivitis require no specific therapy. Superficial infections in children with mild to moderate neutropenia may be treated

with appropriate oral antibiotics. In patients who have invasive or life-threatening infections, broad-spectrum intravenous antibiotics should be started promptly.

Subcutaneously administered G-CSF can provide effective treatment of severe chronic neutropenia, including SCN, cyclic neutropenia, and chronic symptomatic idiopathic neutropenias. Treatment leads to dramatic increases in neutrophil counts, resulting in marked attenuation of infection and inflammation. Doses range from 2-5 μg/kg/day for cyclic, idiopathic, and autoimmune neutropenias, to 5-100 μg/kg/day for SCN. The long-term effects of G-CSF therapy include a propensity for the development of moderate splenomegaly, thrombocytopenia, and rarely vasculitis; only patients with SCN are at risk for MDS/AML.

Patients with SCN or SDS who develop MDS or AML respond only to HSCT; chemotherapy is ineffective. HSCT is also the treatment of choice for aplastic anemia or familial HLH.

LYMPHOPENIA

The definition of **lymphopenia**, as with neutropenia, is age dependent and can have acquired or inherited causes. **The absolute lymphocyte count (ALC)** is determined by multiplying the total WBC count by the percentage of total lymphocytes. For children <12 mo old, lymphopenia is defined as an ALC <3,000 cells/μL. For older children and adults, an ALC <1,000 cells/μL is considered lymphopenia. In isolation, mild to moderate lymphopenia is generally a benign condition often detected only in the evaluation of other illnesses. However, severe lymphopenia can result in serious, life-threatening illness. Lymphocyte subpopulations can be measured by flow cytometry, which uses the pattern of lymphocyte antigen expression to quantitate and classify T, B, and NK cells.

Acquired Lymphopenia

Acute lymphopenia is most often a result of infection and/or is iatrogenic from lymphocyte-toxic medications and treatments (Table 157.7). Microbial causes include viruses (e.g., respiratory syncytial virus, cytomegalovirus, influenza, measles, hepatitis), bacterial infections (e.g., tuberculosis, typhoid fever, histoplasmosis, brucellosis), and malaria. The mechanisms behind infection-associated lymphopenia are not fully elucidated but probably include lymphocyte redistribution and accelerated apoptosis. Corticosteroids are a common cause of medication-induced lymphopenia, as are lymphocyte-specific immunosuppressive agents (e.g., antilymphocyte globulin, alemtuzumab, rituximab), chemotherapy drugs, and radiation. In most cases, infectious and iatrogenic causes of acute lymphopenia are reversible, although full lymphocyte recovery from chemotherapy and lymphocyte-specific immunosuppressive agents may take several months to years. Prolonged lymphopenia (Table 157.7) may be caused by recurrent infection; persistent infections, mostly notably HIV; malnutrition; mechanical loss of lymphocytes through protein-losing enteropathy or thoracic duct leaks; or systemic diseases

Table 157.7	Causes of Lymphocytopenia
ACQUIRED	
Infectious diseases	AIDS, hepatitis, influenza, sepsis, tuberculosis, typhoid
Iatrogenic	Corticosteroids, cytotoxic chemotherapy, high-dose PUVA, immunosuppressive therapy, radiation, thoracic duct drainage
Systemic diseases	Hodgkin disease, lupus erythematosus, myasthenia gravis, protein-losing enteropathy, renal failure, sarcoidosis
Other	Aplastic anemia, dietary deficiencies, thermal injury
INHERITED	
Aplasia of lymphopoietic stem cells	Cartilage-hair hypoplasia, ataxia-telangiectasia, SCID, thymoma, Wiskott-Aldrich syndrome

PUVA, Psoralen and ultraviolet A irradiation; SCID, severe combined immunodeficiency.

such as lupus erythematosus, rheumatoid arthritis, sarcoidosis, renal failure, lymphoma, and aplastic anemia.

Inherited Lymphopenia

Primary immunodeficiencies and bone marrow failure syndromes are the main cause of inherited lymphopenia in children (see Table 157.7). Primary immunodeficiency may result in a severe quantitative defect, as in XLA and severe combined immunodeficiency (SCID), or a qualitative or progressive defect, as in Wiskott-Aldrich syndrome and CVID. XLA is characterized by a near-absence of mature B cells because of a mutation in *BTK* that results in a dysfunctional tyrosine kinase. SCIDs

are a genetically heterogeneous group of disorders characterized by abnormalities of thymopoiesis and T-cell maturation. Newborn screening for severe T-cell deficiency, by analysis of T-cell receptor excision circles from dried blood spot Guthrie cards, aids in the rapid identification and treatment of infants with SCID and other T-cell disorders. Quantitative defects in lymphocytes can also be appreciated in select forms of inherited bone marrow failure such as reticular dysgenesis, SCN secondary to *GFI1* mutation, and dyskeratosis congenita.

Bibliography is available at Expert Consult.

Chapter **158**

Leukocytosis

Thomas F. Michniacki and
Kelly J. Walkovich

第一百五十八章

白细胞增多症

中文导读

　　本章主要介绍了中性粒细胞增多症和其他类型的白细胞增多症。中性粒细胞增多症中具体描述了急性获得性中性粒细胞增多症、慢性获得性中性粒细胞增多症和终生中性粒细胞增多症；其他类型的白细胞增多症中具体描述了单核细胞增多症、嗜酸性粒细胞增多症、嗜碱性粒细胞增多症、淋巴细胞增多症以及发生这些白细胞增多症的常见原因。

Leukocytosis is an elevation in the total leukocyte or white blood cell (WBC) count that is 2 SD above the mean for age (see Chapter 748). It is most often caused by elevated numbers of neutrophils (i.e., neutrophilia), although marked increases in monocytes, eosinophils, basophils, and lymphocytes can be seen. Before extensive evaluation, it is important to assess for spurious elevations in the WBC count caused by platelet clumping (secondary to insufficient sample anticoagulation or the presence of EDTA-dependent agglutinins), high numbers of circulating nucleated red blood cells (RBCs), and the presence of cryoglobulins by review of the peripheral smear.

Malignancy, namely leukemia and lymphoma, is a primary concern for patients with leukocytosis. For discussion of WBC elevation caused by immature leukocytes in acute and chronic leukemias, see Chapter 522. Nonmalignant WBC counts exceeding 50,000/μL have historically been termed a **leukemoid reaction**. Unlike leukemia, leukemoid reactions show relatively small proportions of immature myeloid cells, consisting largely of band forms, occasional metamyelocytes, and progressively rarer myelocytes, promyelocytes, and blasts. Leukemoid reactions are

most often neutrophilic and are frequently associated with severe bacterial infections, including shigellosis, salmonellosis, and meningococcemia; physiologic stressors; and certain medications.

The presence of a **left shift**, defined as having >5% immature neutrophils in the peripheral blood, is consistent with marrow stress. Higher degrees of left shift with more immature neutrophil precursors are indicative of serious bacterial infections and may be a dire sign of depletion of the bone marrow reserve pool of neutrophils. Marked left shift may occasionally be encountered with trauma, burns, surgery, acute hemolysis, or hemorrhage.

NEUTROPHILIA

Neutrophilia is an increase in the total number of blood neutrophils that is 2 SD above the mean count for age (see Chapter 748). Elevated absolute neutrophil counts represent disturbances of the normal equilibrium involving bone marrow neutrophil production, migration out of the marrow compartments into the circulation, and neutrophil destruction. Neutrophilia may arise either alone or in combination with enhanced mobilization into the **circulating pool** from either the bone marrow storage compartment or the peripheral blood **marginating pool**, by impaired neutrophil egress into tissues, or by expansion of the circulating neutrophil pool secondary to increased granulocytopoiesis. Myelocytes are not released to the blood except under extreme circumstances.

Acute Acquired Neutrophilia

Neutrophilia is usually an acquired, secondary finding associated with inflammation, infection, injury, or an acute physical or emotional stressor (Table 158.1). Bacterial infections, trauma (especially with hemorrhage), and surgery are among the most common causes encountered in clinical practice. Neutrophilia may also be associated with heat stroke, burns, diabetic ketoacidosis, pregnancy, or cigarette use.

Drugs commonly associated with neutrophilia include epinephrine, corticosteroids, and recombinant growth factors such as recombinant human granulocyte colony-stimulating factor (G-CSF) and recombinant human granulocyte-macrophage colony-stimulating factor (GM-CSF). Epinephrine causes release into the circulation of a sequestered pool of neutrophils that normally marginate along the vascular endothelium. Corticosteroids accelerate the release of neutrophils and bands from a large storage pool within the bone marrow and impair the migration of neutrophils from the circulation into tissues. G-CSF and GM-CSF cause acute and chronic neutrophilia by mobilizing cells from the marrow reserves and stimulating neutrophil production.

Acute neutrophilia in response to inflammation and infections occurs because of release of neutrophils from the marrow storage pool. The postmitotic marrow neutrophil pools are approximately 10 times the size of the blood neutrophil pool, and about half of these cells are bands and segmented neutrophils. Exposure of blood to foreign substances such as hemodialysis membrane activates the complement system and causes transient neutropenia, followed by neutrophilia secondary to release of bone marrow neutrophils. Reactive neutrophils often have toxic granulation and Döhle bodies present.

Chronic Acquired Neutrophilia

Chronic acquired neutrophilia is usually associated with continued stimulation of neutrophil production resulting from persistent inflam-matory reactions or chronic infections (e.g., tuberculosis), vasculitis, postsplenectomy states, Hodgkin disease, chronic myelogenous leukemia, chronic blood loss, sickle cell disease, some chronic hemolytic anemias, and prolonged administration of corticosteroids (see Table 158.1). Chronic neutrophilia can arise after expansion of cell production secondary to stimulation of cell divisions within the mitotic precursor pool, which consists of promyelocytes and myelocytes. Subsequently, the size of the postmitotic pool increases. These changes lead to an increase in the marrow reserve pool, which can be readily mobilized for release of neutrophils into the circulation. The neutrophil production rate can increase greatly in response to exogenously administered hematopoietic growth factors, such as G-CSF, with a maximum response taking at least 1 wk to develop.

Lifelong Neutrophilia

Congenital or acquired asplenia is associated with lifelong neutrophilia. Some patients with trisomy-21 also have neutrophilia. Uncommon genetic disorders that present with neutrophilia include leukocyte function disorders such as leukocyte adhesion deficiency and Rac2 deficiency (see Chapter 156) and systemic disorders such as familial cold urticaria, periodic fever syndromes, and familial myeloproliferative disease (see Table 158.1). Rare patients with an autosomal dominant hereditary neutrophilia have been reported.

Evaluation of persistent neutrophilia requires a careful history, physical examination, and laboratory studies to search for infectious, inflammatory, and neoplastic conditions. The leukocyte alkaline phosphatase score of circulating neutrophils can differentiate chronic myelogenous leukemia, in which the level is uniformly almost zero, from reactive or secondary neutrophilia, which features normal to elevated levels.

ADDITIONAL FORMS OF LEUKOCYTOSIS
Monocytosis

The average absolute blood monocyte count varies with age, which must be considered in the assessment of monocytosis. Given the role of monocytes in antigen presentation and cytokine secretion and as effectors of ingestion of invading organisms, it is not surprising that many clinical disorders give rise to monocytosis (Table 158.2). Typically, monocytosis occurs in patients recovering from myelosuppressive chemotherapy and is a harbinger of the return of the neutrophil count to normal. Monocytosis is occasionally a sign of an acute bacterial, viral, protozoal, or rickettsial infection and may also occur in some forms of chronic neutropenia and postsplenectomy states. Chronic inflammatory conditions can stimulate sustained monocytosis, as can preleukemia, chronic myelogenous leukemia, and lymphomas.

Table 158.1	Causes of Neutrophilia	
TYPE	**CAUSE**	**EXAMPLE**
Acute acquired	Bacterial infections	
	Surgery	
	Acute stress	Burns, diabetic ketoacidosis, heat stroke, postneutropenia rebound, exercise
	Drugs	Corticosteroids, epinephrine, hematopoietic growth factors, lithium
Chronic acquired	Chronic inflammation	Inflammatory bowel disease, rheumatoid arthritis, vasculitis, cigarette exposure
	Persistent infection	Tuberculosis
	Persistent stress	Chronic blood loss, hypoxia, sickle cell and other chronic hemolytic anemias
	Drugs	Corticosteroids, lithium; rarely ranitidine, quinidine
	Other	Postsplenectomy, tumors, Hodgkin disease, pregnancy, Sweet syndrome
Lifelong	Congenital asplenia	
	Hereditary disorders	Familial cold urticaria, hereditary neutrophilia, leukocyte adhesion deficiencies, periodic fever syndromes

Table 158.2	Causes of Monocytosis	
CAUSE	**EXAMPLE**
Infections	
Bacterial infections	Brucellosis, subacute bacterial endocarditis, syphilis, tuberculosis, typhoid
Nonbacterial infections	Fungal infections, kala-azar, malaria, Rocky Mountain spotted fever, typhus
Hematologic disorders	Congenital and acquired neutropenias, hemolytic anemias
Malignant disorders	Acute myelogenous leukemia, chronic myelogenous leukemia, juvenile myelomonocytic leukemia, Hodgkin disease, non-Hodgkin lymphomas, preleukemia
Chronic inflammatory diseases	Inflammatory bowel disease, polyarteritis nodosa, rheumatoid arthritis, sarcoidosis, systemic lupus erythematosus
Miscellaneous	Cirrhosis, drug reaction, postsplenectomy, recovery from bone marrow suppression

Eosinophilia

Eosinophilia is defined as an absolute eosinophil count >1500 cells/μL. The majority of eosinophilic conditions are reactive, including infections (especially parasitic diseases), connective tissue disorders, allergic and hyperinflammatory diseases, pulmonary disorders, and dermatologic conditions. Hypereosinophilic syndrome and systemic mastocytosis are additional important causes of an elevated eosinophil count. However, persistent eosinophilia can also herald a malignancy such as leukemia, lymphoma, or carcinoma.

Basophilia

Basophilia is defined as an absolute basophil count >120 cells/μL. Basophilia is a nonspecific sign of a wide variety of disorders and is usually of limited diagnostic importance. Basophilia is most often present in hypersensitivity reactions and frequently accompanies the leukocytosis of chronic myeloid leukemia.

Lymphocytosis

The most common cause of lymphocytosis is an acute viral illness, as part of the normal T-cell response to the infection. In infectious mononucleosis, the B cells are infected with the Epstein-Barr virus, and the T cells react to the viral antigens present in the B cells, resulting in **atypical lymphocytes** with characteristic large, vacuolated morphology. Other viral infections classically associated with lymphocytosis are cytomegalovirus and viral hepatitis. Chronic bacterial infections such as tuberculosis and brucellosis may lead to a sustained lymphocytosis. Pertussis is accompanied by marked lymphocytosis in approximately 25% of infants infected before 6 mo of age. Thyrotoxicosis and Addison disease are endocrine disorders associated with lymphocytosis. Persistent or pronounced lymphocytosis suggests acute lymphocytic leukemia.

Bibliography is available at Expert Consult.

Section 4
The Complement System

第四篇
补体系统

Chapter 159
Complement Components and Pathways
Richard B. Johnston Jr.

第一百五十九章
补体成分和活化途径

中文导读

　　本章主要介绍了补体成分、补体活化经典和凝集素途径、旁路途径、膜攻击复合物、控制机制以及宿主防御参与。补体成分包括补体血清成分、膜调节蛋白和膜受体。分别具体描述了经典途径、凝集素途径和旁路途径的活化顺序及初始活化过程；具体描述了膜攻击复合物的形成过程；具体描述了C3抑制剂和血清蛋白等补体活化调节机制；具体描述了补体参与机体抗感染防御和炎症机制。

Complement is an exquisitely balanced, highly influential system that is fundamental to the clinical expression of host defense and inflammation. The complement system also has the capacity to perform functions beyond host defense, such as promoting phagocytic removal of dying cells, molecular debris, and weak or superfluous synapses during brain formation. Complement components and receptors function within individual cells and can stabilize intracellular homeostasis. However, complement activation can also cause harm and has been implicated in many illnesses.

The complement system, an essential component of innate and adaptive immunity, is broadly conceptualized as (1) the classical, lectin, and alternative **pathways**, which interact and depend on each other for their full activity; (2) the **membrane attack complex** (C5b6789), formed from activity of any pathway; (3) cell membrane **receptors** that bind complement components or fragments to mediate complement activity; and (4) a large array of serum and membrane **regulatory proteins** (Table 159.1 and Fig. 159.1). The circulating components and regulators together comprise approximately 15% of the globulin fraction and 4% of the total proteins in serum. The normal concentrations of serum complement components vary by age (see Chapter 748); newborn infants have mild to moderate deficiencies of all components.

After C1423, complement nomenclature is logical and consists of only a few rules. Fragments of components resulting from cleavage by other components acting as enzymes are assigned lowercase letters (a, b, c, d, e); with the exception of C2 fragments, the smaller piece that is released into surrounding fluids is assigned the lowercase letter a, and the major part of the molecule, bound to other components or to some part of the immune complex, is assigned letter b, such as C3a and C3b. Components of the alternative pathway, B and D, have been assigned uppercase letters, as have the control proteins I and H, which downregulate both pathways. **C3**, and especially its major fragment **C3b**, is a component of both classical and alternative pathways.

Complement is a system of interacting proteins. The biologic functions of the system depend on the interactions of individual components, which occur in sequential, cascade fashion. Activation of each component, except the 1st, depends on activation of the prior component or components in the sequence. Interaction occurs along the 3 pathways (Fig. 159.2): the **classical pathway**, in the order antigen–antibody–C142356789; the **lectin** (carbohydrate-binding) **pathway**, in the order microbial carbohydrate–lectin (mannose-binding lectin [MBL] or ficolin)–MBL-associated serine protease–C42356789; and the **alternative pathway**, in the order activator–C3bBD–C356789. Antibody accelerates the rate of activation of the alternative pathway, but activation can occur on appropriate surfaces in the absence of antibody. The classical and the alternative pathways interact with each other through the ability of both to activate C3.

Activation of the early-acting components of complement (C1423) results in the generation of a series of active enzymes, C1, C42, and C423, on the surface of the immune complex or underlying cell. These enzymes cleave and activate the next component in the sequence. In contrast, the interaction among C5b, C6, C7, C8, and C9 is nonenzymatic and depends on changes in molecular configuration.

CLASSICAL AND LECTIN PATHWAYS

The classical pathway sequence begins with fixation of C1, by way of C1q, to the Fc, non–antigen-binding part of the antibody molecule after antigen-antibody interaction. The C1 tricomplex changes configuration, and the C1s subcomponent becomes an active enzyme, "C1 esterase." Certain bacteria, RNA viruses, and the lipid A component of bacterial endotoxin can activate C1q directly and trigger the full complement cascade.

As part of the **innate immune response**, broadly reactive "natural" antibodies and C-reactive protein, which reacts with carbohydrate from microorganisms and with dying cells, can substitute for specific antibody in the fixation of C1q and initiate reaction of the entire sequence. Endogenous agents, including uric acid crystals, amyloid deposits, DNA, and components of damaged cells such as apoptotic blebs and mitochondrial membranes, can activate C1q directly. In this case, however, the ligand-C1q complex interacts strongly with the inhibitors C4-binding protein and factor H, allowing some C3-mediated opsonization and phagocytosis but limiting the full inflammatory response typically triggered by microbes. C1q synthesized in the brain and retina fixes to superfluous synapses, which then can be cleared through C1q receptors on microglia, clearing the way for fresh synapses to populate the developing nervous system.

There are 4 recognition molecules in the lectin pathway: **mannose-binding lectin** (MBL) and **ficolins** 1, 2, and 3. MBL is the prototype of the collectin family of carbohydrate-binding proteins (**lectins**) that are believed to play an important part in innate, nonspecific immunity; its structure is homologous to that of C1q. These lectins, in association with **MBL-associated serine proteases** 1, 2, and 3 (**MASPs** 1, 2, 3), can

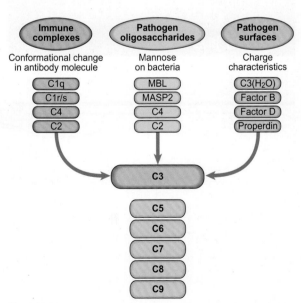

Fig. 159.1 Activation of the complement cascade. The classical pathway is activated primarily by antibody, whereas the mannose-binding lectin and alternative pathways are activated directly by pathogens. In each case, the activation arm leads to cleavage of C3. *(From Leung DYM, editor: Pediatric allergy principles and practice, ed 2, Philadelphia, 2010, Saunders, p 121.)*

Table 159.1	Constituents of the Complement System

SERUM COMPONENTS THAT ARE THE CORE OF THE COMPLEMENT SYSTEM
Classical pathway: C1q, C1r, C1s, C4, C2, C3
Alternative pathway: factor B, factor D
Lectin pathway: Mannose-binding lectin (MBL), ficolins 1/2/3, MBL-associated serine proteases (MASPs) 1/2/3
Membrane attack complex: C5, C6, C7, C8, C9
Regulatory protein, enhancing: properdin
Regulatory proteins, downregulating: C1 inhibitor (C1 INH), C4-binding protein (C4-bp), factor H, factor I, vitronectin, clusterin, carboxypeptidase N (anaphylatoxin inactivator)

MEMBRANE REGULATORY PROTEINS
CR1 (CD35), membrane cofactor protein (MCP; CD46), decay-accelerating factor (DAF, CD55), CD59 (membrane inhibitor of reactive lysis)

MEMBRANE RECEPTORS
CR1 (CD35), CR2 (CD21), CR3 (CD11b/CD18), CR4 (CD11c/CD18), C3a receptor, C5a receptor, C1q receptors, complement receptor of the immunoglobulin superfamily (CRIg)

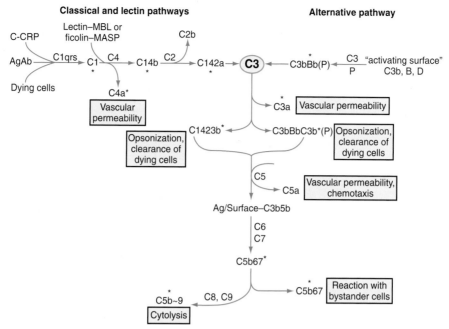

Fig. 159.2 Sequence of activation of the components of the classical and lectin pathways of complement and interaction with the alternative pathway. MBL, Mannose-binding lectin; MASP, MBL-associated serine protease. Activation of C3 is the essential target. Functional activities generated during activation are enclosed in *boxes*. The multiple sites at which inhibitory regulator proteins (*not shown*) act are indicated by *asterisks*, emphasizing the delicate balance between action and control in this system that is essential for host defense yet capable of profound damage to host tissues. Ab, Antibody (immunoglobulin G or M class); Ag, antigen (bacterium, virus, tumor or tissue cell); B, D, I, P, factors B, D, I, and properdin; C-CRP, carbohydrate–carbohydrate-reactive protein; C4-bp, C4-binding protein; MBL, mannose-binding lectin; MASP, MBL-associated serine protease.

bind to mannose, lipoteichoic acid, and other carbohydrates on the surface of bacteria, fungi, parasites, and viruses. There, MASPs then function like C1s to cleave C4 and C2 and activate the complement cascade. The peptide C4a has weak "anaphylatoxin" activity and reacts with mast cells to release the chemical mediators of immediate hypersensitivity, including histamine. C3a and C5a, released later in the sequence, are potent anaphylatoxins, and C5a is also an important chemotactic factor. Fixation of C4b to the complex permits it to adhere to neutrophils, macrophages, B cells, dendritic cells, and erythrocytes. MASP-2 can activate clotting by generating thrombin from prothrombin, which could prevent microbial spread.

Cleavage of C3 and generation of C3b is the next step in the sequence. The serum concentration of C3 is the highest of any component, and its activation is the most crucial step in terms of biologic activity. Cleavage of C3 can be achieved through the **C3 convertase** of the classical pathway, C142, or of the alternative pathway, C3bBb. Once C3b is fixed to a complex or dead or dying host cell, it can bind to cells with receptors for C3b (complement receptor 1 [**CR1**]), including B lymphocytes, erythrocytes, and phagocytic cells (neutrophils, monocytes, and macrophages). Efficient **phagocytosis** of most microorganisms, especially by neutrophils, requires binding of C3 to the microbe. The severe pyogenic infections that frequently occur in C3-deficient patients illustrate this point. The biologic activity of C3b is controlled by cleavage by **factor I** to iC3b, which promotes phagocytosis on binding to the **iC3b receptor (CR3)** on phagocytes. Further degradation of iC3b by factor I and proteases yields C3dg, then C3d; C3d binds to CR2 on B lymphocytes and thereby serves as a co-stimulator of antigen-induced B-cell activation.

ALTERNATIVE PATHWAY

The alternative pathway can be activated by C3b generated through classical pathway activity or proteases from neutrophils or the clotting system. It can also be activated by a form of C3 created by low-grade,

spontaneous reaction of native C3 with a molecule of water, a "tickover" that occurs constantly in plasma. Once formed, C3b or the hydrolyzed C3 can bind to any nearby cell or to factor B. **Factor B** attached to C3b in the plasma or on a surface can be cleaved to Bb by the circulating protease **factor D**. The complex C3bBb becomes an efficient C3 convertase, which generates more C3b through an amplification loop. **Properdin** can bind to C3bBb, increasing stability of the enzyme and protecting it from inactivation by **factors I and H**, which modulate the loop and the pathway.

Certain "activating surfaces" promote alternative pathway activation if C3b is fixed to them, including bacterial teichoic acid and endotoxin, virally infected cells, antigen–immunoglobulin A complexes, and cardiopulmonary bypass and renal dialysis membranes. These surfaces act by protecting the C3bBb enzyme from the control otherwise exercised by factors I and H. Rabbit red blood cell membrane is such a surface, which serves as the basis for an assay of serum alternative pathway activity. Conversely, sialic acid on the surface of microorganisms or cells prevents formation of an effective alternative pathway C3 convertase by promoting activity of factors I and H. In any event, significant activation of C3 can occur through the alternative pathway, and the resultant biologic activities are qualitatively the same as those achieved through activation by C142 (see Fig. 159.2).

MEMBRANE ATTACK COMPLEX

The sequence leading to cytolysis begins with the attachment of C5b to the C5-activating enzyme from the classical pathway, C4b2a3b, or from the alternative pathway, C3bBb3b. C6 is bound to C5b without being cleaved, stabilizing the activated C5b fragment. The C5b6 complex then dissociates from C423 and reacts with C7. C5b67 complexes must attach promptly to the membrane of the parent or a bystander cell, or they lose their activity. Next, C8 binds, and the C5b678 complex then promotes the addition of multiple C9 molecules. The C9 polymer of at least 3-6 molecules forms a transmembrane channel, and lysis ensues.

CONTROL MECHANISMS

Without control mechanisms acting at multiple points, there would be no effective complement system, and unbridled consumption of components would generate severe, potentially lethal damage to the host. At the 1st step, **C1 inhibitor (C1 INH)** inhibits C1r and C1s enzymatic activity, and thus the cleavage of C4 and C2. C1 INH also inhibits MASP-2, factors XIa and XIIa of the clotting system, and kallikrein of the contact system. Activated C2 has a short half-life, and this relative instability limits the effective life of C42 and C423. The alternative pathway enzyme that activates C3, C3bBb, also has a short half-life, although it can be prolonged by the binding of properdin (P) to the enzyme complex. P can also bind directly to microbes and promote assembly of the alternative pathway C3 convertase.

Serum contains the enzyme carboxypeptidase N, which cleaves the N-terminus arginine from C4a, C3a, and C5a, thereby limiting their biologic activity. Factor I inactivates C4b and C3b; factor H accelerates inactivation of C3b by factor I; and an analogous factor, C4-binding protein (**C4-bp**), accelerates C4b cleavage by factor I, thus limiting assembly of the C3 convertase. Three protein constituents of cell membranes—**CR1**, membrane cofactor protein (**MCP**), and decay-accelerating factor (**DAF**)—promote the disruption of C3 and C5 convertases assembled on those membranes. Another cell membrane–associated protein, **CD59**, can bind C8 or both C8 and C9 and thereby interfere with insertion of the membrane attack complex (C5b6789). The serum proteins **vitronectin** and **clusterin** can inhibit attachment of the C5b67 complex to cell membranes, bind C8 or C9 in a full membrane attack complex, or otherwise interfere with the formation or insertion of this complex. Vitronectin also promotes macrophage uptake of dying neutrophils. The genes for the regulatory proteins factor H, C4-bp, MCP, DAF, CR1, and CR2 are clustered on chromosome 1.

PARTICIPATION IN HOST DEFENSE

Neutralization of virus by antibody can be enhanced with C1 and C4 and further enhanced by the additional fixation of C3b through the classical or alternative pathway. Complement may therefore be particularly important in the early phases of a viral infection when antibody is limited. Antibody and the full complement sequence can also eliminate infectivity of at least some viruses by the production of typical complement "holes," as seen by electron microscopy. Fixation of C1q can opsonize (promote phagocytosis) through binding to the phagocyte C1q receptor.

C4a, C3a, and C5a can bind to mast cells and thereby trigger release of histamine and other mediators, leading to vasodilation and the swelling and redness of inflammation. C5a can enhance macrophage phagocytosis of C3b-opsonized particles and induce macrophages to release the cytokines tumor necrosis factor and interleukin-1. C5a is a major chemotactic factor for neutrophils, monocytes, and eosinophils, which can efficiently phagocytize microorganisms opsonized with C3b or cleaved C3b (iC3b). Further inactivation of cell-bound C3b by cleavage to C3d and C3dg removes its opsonizing activity, but it can still bind to B cells. Fixation of C3b to a target cell can enhance its lysis by natural killer cells or macrophages.

Insoluble immune complexes can be solubilized if they bind C3b, apparently because C3b disrupts the orderly antigen-antibody lattice. Binding C3b to a complex also allows it to adhere to C3 receptors (CR1) on red blood cells, which then transport the complexes to hepatic and splenic macrophages for removal. This phenomenon may at least partially explain the immune complex disease found in patients who lack C1, C4, C2, or C3.

The complement system serves to link the innate and adaptive immune systems. C4b or C3b coupled to immune complexes promotes their binding to antigen-presenting macrophages, dendritic cells, and B cells. Coupling of antigen to C3d allows binding to CR2 on B cells, which greatly reduces the amount of antigen needed to trigger an antibody response.

Neutralization of endotoxin in vitro and protection from its lethal effects in experimental animals require C1 INH and later-acting components of complement, at least through C6. Finally, activation of the entire complement sequence can result in lysis of virus-infected cells, tumor cells, and most types of microorganisms. Bactericidal activity of complement has not appeared to be important to host defense, except for the occurrence of *Neisseria* infections in patients lacking later-acting components of complement (see Chapter 160).

Bibliography is available at Expert Consult.

Chapter **160**

Disorders of the Complement System

第一百六十章

补体系统疾病

中文导读

　　本章主要介绍了补体系统评估、补体成分遗传缺陷、补体控制蛋白缺陷、继发性补体疾病以及补体疾病治疗。具体描述了总溶血补体活性CH50和旁路途径活性AH50；具体描述了经典途径中11个补体缺陷和旁路途径中因子D和因子B缺陷；补体控制蛋白缺陷中具体描述了因子I缺陷、因子H缺陷、C4结合蛋白缺陷、备解素缺陷和遗传性血管性水肿；继发性补体疾病描述了慢性膜增殖性肾小球肾炎、镰状细胞病、肾病综合征、创伤和其他疾病；治疗中描述了遗传性血管性水肿、aHUS和PNH的治疗，以及其他对症治疗。

160.1 Evaluation of the Complement System

Richard B. Johnston Jr.

Testing for **total hemolytic complement activity (CH$_{50}$)** effectively screens for most of the common diseases of the complement system. A normal result in this assay depends on the ability of all 11 components of the classical pathway and membrane attack complex to interact and lyse antibody-coated sheep erythrocytes. The dilution of serum that lyses 50% of the cells determines the end-point. In **congenital deficiencies** of C1 through C8, the CH$_{50}$ value is 0 or close to 0; in C9 deficiency the value is approximately half-normal. Values in the acquired deficiencies vary with the type and severity of the underlying disorder. This assay does not detect deficiency of mannose-binding lectin (MBL), factor D or B of the alternative pathway, or properdin (Fig. 160.1). Deficiency of factor I or H permits persistence of the classical and alternative pathway convertase and thus consumption of C3, with reduction in the CH$_{50}$ value. When clotted blood or serum sits at room temperature or warms, CH$_{50}$ activity begins to decline, leading to values that are falsely low but not zero. It is important to separate the serum and freeze it at −70°C (−94°F) by no more than 1 hr after blood draw.

In **hereditary angioedema**, depression of C4 and C2 during an attack significantly reduces the CH$_{50}$. Typically, C4 is low and C3 normal or slightly decreased. Concentrations of C1 inhibitor protein will be normal in 15% of cases; but C1 acts as an esterase, and the diagnosis can be established by showing increased capacity of the patient's sera to hydrolyze synthetic esters.

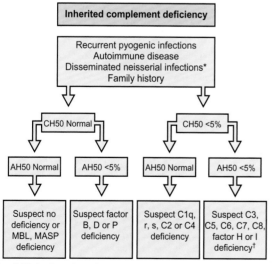

Fig. 160.1 Flow chart for the evaluation of inherited complement deficiencies using hemolytic screening assays for the classical (CH50) and alternative pathways (AH50). For each assay, the entire activation pathway, including the membrane attack complex, is required for lysis. MASP, MBL-associated serine protease; MBL, mannose-binding lectin. *Gonococcal and meningococcal. †C9 deficiency may have up to 30% normal CH50 with low AH50. (*Adapted from Rich RR, Fleisher TA, Shearer WT, et al, editors: Clinical immunology: principles and practice, ed 4, Philadelphia, 2012, Saunders, p 262.*)

A decrease in serum concentration of both C4 and C3 suggests activation of the *classical pathway* by immune complexes. Decreased C3 and normal C4 levels suggest activation of the *alternative pathway*. This difference is particularly useful in distinguishing nephritis secondary to immune complex deposition from that caused by **NeF** (nephritic factor). In the latter condition and in deficiency of factor I or H, factor B is consumed and C3 serum concentration is low. Alternative pathway activity can be measured with a relatively simple and reproducible hemolytic assay that depends on the capacity of rabbit erythrocytes to serve as both an activating (permissive) surface and a target of alternative pathway activity. This assay, **AP$_{50}$**, detects deficiency of properdin, factor D, and factor B. Immunochemical methods can be used to quantify individual components and split products of all 3 pathways, guided by results of the screening hemolytic assays.

A defect of complement function should be considered in any patient with recurrent angioedema, autoimmune disease (especially SLE), chronic nephritis, hemolytic-uremic syndrome, or partial lipodystrophy, or with recurrent pyogenic infections, disseminated meningococcal or gonococcal infection, or a 2nd episode of bacteremia at any age. A previously well adolescent or young adult with meningococcal meningitis caused by an uncommon serotype (not A, B, or C) should undergo screening for a late-component or alternative pathway deficiency with CH$_{50}$ and AP$_{50}$ assays.

Bibliography is available at Expert Consult.

160.2 Genetic Deficiencies of Complement Components

Richard B. Johnston Jr.

Congenital deficiencies of all 11 components of the classical–membrane attack pathway and of factors D and B and properdin of the alternative pathway are described in Table 160.1. All components of the classical and alternative pathways except properdin and factor B are inherited as autosomal recessive co-dominant traits. Each parent transmits a gene that codes for synthesis of half the serum level of the component. Deficiency results from inheritance of 1 null gene from each parent; the hemizygous parents typically have low normal CH$_{50}$ levels and no consequences of the partial deficiency. Properdin deficiency is transmitted as an X-linked trait. Factor B is an autosomal recessive non–co-dominant trait.

Most patients with primary **C1q deficiency** have systemic lupus erythematosus (SLE); some have an SLE-like syndrome without typical SLE serology, a chronic rash with underlying vasculitis, or membrano-proliferative glomerulonephritis (MPGN). Some C1q-deficient children have serious infections, including septicemia and meningitis. Individuals with **C1r, C1s, combined C1r/C1s, C4, C2,** or **C3 deficiency** also have a high incidence of autoimmune syndromes (see Table 160.1), especially SLE or an SLE-like syndrome, without an elevated antinuclear antibody level.

C4 is encoded by 2 genes, *C4A* and *C4B*. **C4 deficiency** represents absence of both gene products. Complete deficiency of only C4A, present in approximately 1% of the population, also predisposes to SLE, although C4 levels are only partially reduced. Patients with only C4B deficiency may be predisposed to infection. A few patients with **C5, C6, C7,** or **C8 deficiency** have SLE, but recurrent meningococcal infections are much more likely to be the major problem.

Table 160.1	Complement Defects			

DISEASE	GENETIC DEFECT/ PRESUMED PATHOGENESIS	INHERITANCE	FUNCTIONAL DEFECT	ASSOCIATED FEATURES
C1q deficiency	Mutation in *C1QA, C1QB, C1QC*: classical complement pathway components	AR	Absent CH_{50} hemolytic activity; defective activation of the classical pathway, diminished clearance of apoptotic cells	SLE, infections with encapsulated organisms
C1r deficiency	Mutation in *C1R*: classical complement pathway component	AR	Absent CH_{50} hemolytic activity; defective activation of the classical pathway	SLE, infections with encapsulated organisms
C1s deficiency	Mutation in *C1S*: classical complement pathway component	AR	Absent CH_{50} hemolytic activity; defective activation of the classical pathway	SLE, infections with encapsulated organisms
C4 deficiency	Mutation in *C4A, C4B*: classical complement pathway components	AR	Absent CH_{50} hemolytic activity; defective activation of the classical pathway, defective humoral immune response to carbohydrate antigens in some patients	SLE, infections with encapsulated organisms
C2 deficiency	Mutation in *C2*: classical complement partway component	AR	Absent CH_{50} hemolytic activity; defective activation of the classical pathway	SLE, infections with encapsulated organisms, atherosclerosis
C3 deficiency	Mutation in *C3*: central complement component	AR, gain-of-function AD	Absent CH_{50} and AH_{50} hemolytic activity; defective opsonization, defective humoral immune response	Infections; glomerulonephritis, aHUS with gain-of-function mutations
C5 deficiency	Mutation in *C5*: terminal complement component	AR	Absent CH_{50} and AH_{50} hemolytic activity; defective bactericidal activity	Neisserial infections
C6 deficiency	Mutation in *C6*: terminal complement component	AR	Absent CH_{50} and AH_{50} hemolytic activity; defective bactericidal activity	Neisserial infections
C7 deficiency	Mutation in *C7*: terminal complement component	AR	Absent CH_{50} and AH_{50} hemolytic activity; defective bactericidal activity	Neisserial infections
C8 α-γ deficiency	Mutation in *C8A, C8G*: terminal complement components	AR	Absent CH_{50} and AH_{50} hemolytic activity; defective bactericidal activity	Neisserial infections
C8b deficiency	Mutation in *C8B*: terminal complement component	AR	Absent CH_{50} and AH_{50} hemolytic activity. defective bactericidal activity	Neisserial infections
C9 deficiency	Mutation in *C9*: terminal complement component	AR	Reduced CH_{50} and AH_{50} hemolytic activity; deficient bactericidal activity	Mild susceptibility to neisserial infections
C1 inhibitor deficiency	Mutation in *C1NH*: regulation of kinins and complement activation	AD	Spontaneous activation of the complement pathway with consumption of C4/C2; spontaneous activation of the contact system with generation of bradykinin from high-molecular-weight kininogen	Hereditary angioedema
Factor B	Mutation in *CFB*: activation of the alternative pathway	AD	Gain-of-function mutation with increased spontaneous AH_{50}	aHUS
Factor D deficiency	Mutation in *CFD*: regulation of the alternative complement pathway	AR	Absent AH_{50} hemolytic activity	Neisserial infections
Properdin deficiency	Mutation in *CFP*: regulation of the alternative complement pathway	XL	Absent AH_{50} hemolytic activity	Neisserial infections
Factor I deficiency	Mutation in *CFI*: regulation of the alternative complement pathway	AR	Spontaneous activation of the alternative complement pathway with consumption of C3	Infections, neisserial infections, aHUS, preeclampsia, membranoproliferative glomerulonephritis
Factor H deficiency	Mutation in *CFH*: regulation of the alternative complement pathway	AR	Spontaneous activation of the alternative complement pathway with consumption of C3	Infections, neisserial infections, aHUS, preeclampsia, membranoproliferative glomerulonephritis
MASP-1 deficiency	Mutation in *MASP1*: cleaves C2 and activates MASP-2	AR	Deficient activation of the lectin activation pathway, cell migration	Infections, 3MC syndrome

AD, Autosomal dominant; aHUS, atypical hemolytic-uremic syndrome; AR, autosomal recessive; SLE, systemic lupus erythematosus; XL, X-linked; 3MC, previously Carnevale, Mingarelli, Malpuech, and Michels syndromes.

From Kliegman RM, Lye PS, Bordini BJ, et al, editors: *Nelson pediatric symptom-based diagnosis*, Philadelphia, 2018, Elsevier, Table 41.11, p 765.

There are at least 2 possible reasons for the concurrence of complement component deficiencies, especially C1, C4, C2, or C3 deficiency, and autoimmune–immune complex diseases. First, deposition of C3 on autoimmune complexes facilitates their removal from the circulation through binding to complement receptor 1 (CR1) on erythrocytes and transport to the spleen and liver. Second, the early components, particularly C1q and C3, expedite the clearance of necrotic and apoptotic cells, which are sources of autoantigens.

Individuals with **C2 deficiency** carry the risk of life-threatening septicemic illnesses, usually caused by pneumococci. However, most have not had problems with other increased susceptibility to infection, presumably because of the protective function of the alternative pathway, particularly if enhanced by pneumococcal and *Haemophilus influenzae* immunization. The genes for C2, factor B, and C4 are situated close to each other on chromosome 6, and a partial depression of factor B levels can occur in conjunction with C2 deficiency. Persons with a deficiency of both proteins may be at particular risk. One percent of European Caucasians carry 1 null gene for C2.

Because C3 can be activated by C142 or by the alternative pathway, a defect in the function of either pathway can be compensated for, at least to some extent. Without C3, however, opsonization of bacteria is inefficient, and the chemotactic fragment from C5 (C5a) is not generated. Some organisms must be well opsonized in order to be cleared, and genetic **C3 deficiency** has been associated with recurrent, severe pyogenic infections caused by pneumococci, *H. influenzae*, and meningococci.

More than half the individuals reported to have congenital **C5, C6, C7, or C8 deficiency** have had meningococcal meningitis or extragenital gonococcal infection. **C9 deficiency** is most often reported in individuals of Japanese or Korean descent. C9-deficient individuals retain about one-third normal CH_{50} titers; some have had *Neisseria* disease. In studies of patients ≥10 yr old with systemic meningococcal disease, 3–15% have had a genetic deficiency of C5, C6, C7, C8, C9, or properdin. Among patients with infections caused by the uncommon *Neisseria meningitidis* serogroups (X, Y, Z, W135, 29E, or nongroupable; but not A, B, or C), 33–45% have an underlying complement deficiency. It is not clear why patients with a deficiency of one of the late-acting components have a particular predisposition to *Neisseria* infections. It may be that serum bacteriolysis is uniquely important in defense against this organism. Many persons with such a deficiency have no significant illness.

A few individuals have been identified with **deficiency of factor D or Factor B** of the alternative pathway, all with recurrent infections, most often neisserial or pneumococcal. Hemolytic complement activity and C3 levels in their serum were normal, but alternative pathway activity was markedly deficient or absent.

Mutations in the structural gene encoding MBL or polymorphisms in the promoter region of the gene result in pronounced interindividual variation in the level of circulating MBL. More than 90% of individuals with **MBL deficiency** do not express a predisposition to infection. Those with a very low level of MBL have a predisposition to recurrent respiratory infections in infancy and to serious pyogenic and fungal infections if there is another underlying defect of host defense. MBL-associated serine protease (**MASP**)-2 deficiency has been reported with SLE-like symptoms and recurrent pneumococcal pneumonia. Homozygous **ficolin-3 deficiency** has been associated with repeated pneumonia since early childhood, cerebral abscesses, and bronchiectasis.

Bibliography is available at Expert Consult.

160.3 Deficiencies of Plasma, Membrane, or Serosal Complement Control Proteins
Richard B. Johnston Jr.

Congenital deficiencies of 5 plasma complement control proteins have been described (see Table 160.1). **Factor I deficiency** was reported originally as a deficiency of C3 resulting from hypercatabolism. The

1st patient described had suffered a series of severe pyogenic infections similar to those associated with agammaglobulinemia or congenital deficiency of C3. Factor I is an essential regulator of both pathways. Its deficiency permits prolonged existence of C3b as a part of the C3 convertase of the alternative pathway, C3bBb. This results in constant activation of the alternative pathway and cleavage of more C3 to C3b, in circular fashion. Intravenous infusion of plasma or purified factor I induced a prompt rise in serum C3 concentration in the patient and a return to normal of C3-dependent functions in vitro, such as opsonization.

The effects of **factor H deficiency** are similar to those of factor I deficiency because factor H assists in dismantling the alternative pathway C3 convertase. A trigger event such as infection initiates uninhibited continuous activation of the alternative pathway, which consumes C3, factor B, total hemolytic activity, and alternative pathway activity. Patients have sustained systemic infections due to pyogenic bacteria, particularly *Neisseria meningitidis*. Many have had glomerulonephritis or **atypical hemolytic-uremic syndrome** (aHUS) (see Chapter 538.5). Mutations in genes encoding membrane cofactor protein (MCP, CD46), factors I or B, C3, or the endothelial antiinflammatory protein thrombomodulin, or autoantibodies to factors H or B, are also associated with aHUS. The majority of patients with factor H deficiency and aHUS, typically <2 yr old, develop end-stage renal disease, and many die.

The few patients thus far reported as having **C4-binding protein deficiency** have approximately 25% of the normal levels of the protein and no typical disease presentation, although one patient had angioedema and Behçet disease.

Persons with **properdin deficiency** have a striking predisposition to *N. meningitidis* meningitis. All reported patients have been male. The predisposition to infection in these patients demonstrates clearly the need for the alternative pathway in defense against bacterial infection. Serum hemolytic complement activity is normal in these patients, and if the patient has specific antibacterial antibody from immunization or prior exposure, the need for the alternative pathway and properdin is greatly reduced. Several patients have had dermal vasculitis or discoid lupus.

Hereditary angioedema occurs in persons unable to synthesize normal levels of functional C1 inhibitor (C1 INH). In 85% of affected families, the patient has markedly reduced concentrations of inhibitor, averaging 30% of normal; the other 15% have normal or elevated concentrations of an immunologically cross-reacting but nonfunctional protein. Both forms of the disease are transmitted as autosomal dominant traits. C1 INH suppresses the complement proteases C1rs and MASP-2 and the activated proteases of the contact and fibrinolysis systems. In the absence of full C1 INH function, activation of any of these proteases tips the balance toward the protease. This activation leads to uncontrolled C1 and kallikrein activity with breakdown of C4 and C2 and release of bradykinin, which interacts with vascular endothelial cells to cause vasodilation, producing localized, nonpitting edema. The biochemical triggers that induce attacks of angioedema in these patients are not well understood.

Swelling of the affected part progresses rapidly, without urticaria, itching, discoloration, or redness and often without severe pain. Swelling of the intestinal wall, however, can lead to intense abdominal cramping, sometimes with vomiting or diarrhea. Concomitant subcutaneous edema is often absent, and patients have undergone abdominal surgery or psychiatric examination before the true diagnosis was established. Laryngeal edema can be fatal. Attacks last 2-3 days and then gradually abate. They may occur at sites of trauma, especially dental, after vigorous exercise, or with menses, fever, or emotional stress. Attacks begin in the 1st 5 yr of life in almost half of patients, but are usually not severe until late childhood or adolescence. **Acquired C1 INH deficiency** can occur in association with B-cell cancer or autoantibody to C1 INH. SLE and glomerulonephritis have been reported in patients with the congenital disease (for treatment see Chapter 160.5).

Three of the membrane complement control proteins—CR1, MCP (CD46), and decay-accelerating factor (DAF)—prevent the formation of the full C3-cleaving enzyme, C3bBb, which is triggered by C3b deposition. CD59 (membrane inhibitor of reactive lysis) prevents the full development of the membrane attack complex that creates the "hole."

Paroxysmal nocturnal hemoglobinuria (PNH) is a hemolytic anemia that occurs when DAF and CD59 are not expressed on the erythrocyte surface. The condition is acquired as a somatic mutation in a hematopoietic stem cell of the *PIGA* gene on the X chromosome. The product of this gene is required for normal synthesis of a glycosylphosphatidylinositol molecule that anchors about 20 proteins to cell membranes, including DAF and CD59. One patient with **genetic isolated CD59 deficiency** had a mild PNH-like disease despite normal expression of membrane DAF. In contrast, **genetic isolated DAF deficiency** has not resulted in hemolytic anemia (for treatment see Chapter 160.5).

Bibliography is available at Expert Consult.

160.4 Secondary Disorders of Complement
Richard B. Johnston Jr.

Partial deficiency of C1q has occurred in patients with severe combined immunodeficiency disease or hypogammaglobulinemia, apparently secondary to the deficiency of IgG, which normally binds reversibly to C1q and prevents its rapid catabolism.

Chronic membranoproliferative glomerulonephritis can be caused by nephritic factor (NeF), an IgG autoantibody to the C3-cleaving enzyme of the classical pathway (C4b2a) or alternative pathway (C3bBb). NeF protects the enzyme from inactivation and promotes consumption of C3 and decreased concentration of serum C3. Pyogenic infections, including meningitis, may occur if the serum C3 level drops to <10% of normal. This disorder has been found in children and adults with dense-deposit disease or partial lipodystrophy. Adipocytes are the main source of factor D and synthesize C3 and factor B; exposure to NeF induces their lysis. The IgG NeF that inhibits the classical pathway C3 convertase has been described in acute postinfectious nephritis and in SLE. The consumption of C3 that characterizes poststreptococcal nephritis and SLE could be caused by this factor, by immune complex activation, or by both.

Newborn infants have mild to moderate reductions in all plasma components of the complement system. Opsonization and generation of chemotactic activity in serum from full-term newborns can be markedly deficient through either the classical or the alternative pathway. Complement activity is even lower in preterm infants. Patients with severe chronic cirrhosis of the liver, hepatic failure, malnutrition, or anorexia nervosa can have significant deficiency of complement components and functional activity. Synthesis of components is depressed in these conditions, and serum from some patients with malnutrition also contains immune complexes that could accelerate depletion.

Patients with **sickle cell disease** have normal activity of the classical pathway, but some have defective function of the alternative pathway in opsonization of pneumococci, in bacteriolysis and opsonization of *Salmonella,* and in lysis of rabbit erythrocytes. Deoxygenation of erythrocytes from patients with sickle cell disease alters their membranes to increase exposure of phospholipids that can activate the alternative pathway and consume its components. This activation is accentuated during painful crisis. Children with **nephrotic syndrome** may have decreased serum levels of factors B and D and subnormal serum opsonizing activity.

Immune complexes initiated by microorganisms or their by-products can induce complement consumption. Activation occurs primarily through fixation of C1 and initiation of the classical pathway. Formation of immune complexes and consumption of complement have been demonstrated in lepromatous leprosy, bacterial endocarditis, infected ventriculojugular shunts, malaria, infectious mononucleosis, dengue hemorrhagic fever, and acute hepatitis B. Nephritis or arthritis can develop as a result of deposition of immune complexes and activation of complement in these infections. In SLE, immune complexes activate C142, and C3 is deposited at sites of tissue damage, including kidneys and skin; depressed synthesis of C3 is also noted. The syndrome of recurrent urticaria, angioedema, eosinophilia, and hypocomplementemia secondary to activation of the classical pathway may be caused by

autoantibody to C1q and circulating immune complexes. Circulating immune complexes and decreased C3 have been reported in some patients with dermatitis herpetiformis, celiac disease, primary biliary cirrhosis, and Reye syndrome.

Circulating bacterial products in **sepsis** or tissue factors released after severe **trauma** can initiate activation of the classical and alternative pathways, leading to increased serum levels of C3a, C5a, and C5b-9 and systemic inflammatory response syndrome (SIRS) and multi-organ failure. C5a and its receptors, particularly on neutrophils, appear to be central to the pathogenesis of SIRS. Intravenous injection of iodinated roentgenographic contrast medium can trigger a rapid and significant activation of the alternative pathway, which may explain the occasional reactions that occur in patients undergoing this procedure.

Burns can induce massive activation of the complement system, especially the alternative pathway, within a few hours after injury. Resulting generation of C3a and C5a stimulates neutrophils and induces their sequestration in the lungs, leading to shock lung. Cardiopulmonary bypass, extracorporeal membrane oxygenation, plasma exchange, or hemodialysis using **cellophane membranes** may be associated with a similar syndrome as a result of activation of plasma complement, with release of C3a and C5a. In patients with **erythropoietic protoporphyria** or **porphyria cutanea tarda**, exposure of the skin to light of certain wavelengths activates complement, generating chemotactic activity. This chemotactic activity leads to lysis of capillary endothelial cells, mast cell degranulation, and the appearance of neutrophils in the dermis.

Some tumor cells can avoid complement-mediated lysis by overexpressing DAF, MCP, CD59, CR1, or factor H, or by secreting proteases that cleave tumor-bound C3b. Microorganisms have evolved similar evasive mechanisms; for example, HIV-1 particles budding from infected cells acquire the membrane proteins DAF and CD59, and staphylococci can produce multiple complement inhibitors.

Bibliography is available at Expert Consult.

160.5 Treatment of Complement Disorders
Richard B. Johnston Jr.

No specific therapy is available at present for genetic deficiencies of the components of the classical, alternative, and lectin complement pathways. Much can be done, however, to protect patients with any of these disorders from serious complications; and specific treatment is available for 3 disorders caused by control-protein deficiencies: hereditary angioedema, aHUS, and PNH.

Management of **hereditary angioedema** starts with avoidance of precipitating factors, usually trauma. Infusion of C1 INH concentrate (nanofiltered **C1-esterase inhibitor**) was approved by the U.S. Food and Drug Administration (FDA) for use in children in 2016. An inhibitor of kallikrein (**ecallantide**) that blocks bradykinin production and an antagonist of the bradykinin receptor (**icatibant**) are approved in the United States for use in adolescents and adults for long-term prophylaxis, preparation for surgery or dental procedures, or treatment of acute attacks. The synthetic androgen **oxandrolone** increases the level of functional C1 INH several-fold and is approved for cautious use in children. Antihistamines, epinephrine, and corticosteroids have no effect.

Lanadelumab, a selective inhibitor of kallikein, has potential as a prophylactic agent. **Eculizumab**, a humanized monoclonal antibody to C5, prevents generation of the membrane-attack complex C5b9 and is an effective treatment for **PNH** and **aHUS**.

Effective supportive management is available for other primary diseases of the complement system, and identification of a specific defect in the complement system can have an important impact on management. Concern for the associated complications, such as autoimmune disease and infection, should encourage vigorous diagnostic efforts and earlier institution of therapy. Individuals with SLE and a complement defect generally respond as well to therapy as do those without complement deficiency. With the onset of unexplained fever, cultures should be obtained and antibiotic therapy instituted more quickly and with less stringent indications than in a normal child.

The parent or patient should be given letters describing any predisposition to systemic bacterial infection or autoimmune disease associated with the patient's deficiency, along with the recommended initial approach to management, for possible use by school, camp, or emergency department physicians. The patient and close household contacts should be immunized against *H. influenzae*, *Streptococcus pneumoniae*, and *N. meningitidis*. High titers of specific antibody might opsonize effectively without the full complement system, and immunization of household members could reduce the risk of exposing patients to these particularly threatening pathogens. *Repeat immunization of patients is advisable since complement deficiency can be associated with a blunted or shorter-lived antibody response than normal.*

Heparin, which inhibits both classical and alternative pathways, has been used to prevent "postpump syndrome."

Bibliography is available at Expert Consult.

Section 5
Hematopoietic Stem Cell Transplantation
第五篇
造血干细胞移植

Chapter 161
Principles and Clinical Indications of Hematopoietic Stem Cell Transplantation

Rachel A. Phelan and David Margolis

第一百六十一章
造血干细胞移植原则和临床适应证

中文导读

本章主要介绍了造血干细胞移植的原则，HLA相同同胞供体造血干细胞移植和临床适应证。具体描述了急性淋巴细胞白血病、急性髓性白血病、慢性髓系白血病、幼年粒单核细胞白血病、非幼年粒单核细胞白血病骨髓增生异常综合征、非霍奇金淋巴瘤和霍奇金病、获得性再生障碍性贫血、遗传性骨髓衰竭综合征、地中海贫血、镰状细胞病、免疫缺陷疾病和遗传代谢性疾病等适应证及其移植效果。

Allogeneic (from a donor) or **autologous** (from the same individual) hematopoietic stem cells have been used to cure both malignant and nonmalignant disorders. **Autologous** transplantation is employed as a rescue strategy after delivering otherwise lethal doses of chemotherapy with or without radiotherapy in children with hematologic malignancies such as relapsed lymphoma or selected solid tumors (e.g., neuroblastoma, brain tumors). **Allogeneic** transplantation is used to treat children with genetic diseases of blood cells, such as hemoglobinopathies, primary immunodeficiency diseases, various inherited metabolic diseases, and bone marrow failure. Allogeneic transplant is also used as treatment for hematologic malignancies, such as leukemia and myelodysplastic syndromes. Bone marrow had represented the only source of hematopoietic progenitors employed. Growth factor (granulocyte colony-stimulating factor)–mobilized peripheral blood hematopoietic stem cells and umbilical cord blood hematopoietic progenitors have now also been regularly used in clinical practice to perform hematopoietic stem cell transplantation (**HSCT**).

An HLA-matched sibling was once the only type of donor employed. Currently, matched unrelated volunteers, full-haplotype mismatched family members, and unrelated cord blood donors have been largely employed to transplant patients lacking an HLA-identical relative.

Protocols for allogeneic HSCT consist of 2 parts: the preparative regimen and transplantation itself. During the **preparative conditioning regimen**, chemotherapy, at times associated with irradiation, is administered to destroy the patient's hematopoietic system and to suppress the immune system, especially T cells, so that graft rejection is prevented. In patients with malignancies, the preparative regimen also serves to significantly reduce the tumor burden. The patient then receives an intravenous infusion of hematopoietic cells from the donor. Less aggressive conditioning regimens, known as **reduced-intensity conditioning regimens**, are also used in pediatric patients. These regimens are mainly immunosuppressive and aim at inducing a state of reduced immune competence of the recipient to avoid the rejection of donor cells.

The immunology of HSCT is distinct from that of other types of transplant because, in addition to stem cells, the graft contains mature blood cells of donor origin, including T cells, B cells, natural killer cells, and dendritic cells. These cells repopulate the recipient's lymphohematopoietic system and give rise to a new immune system, which helps eliminate residual leukemia cells that survive the conditioning regimen. This effect is known as the **graft-versus-leukemia (GVL) effect.**

The donor immune system exerts its T-cell–mediated GVL effect through alloreactions directed against histocompatibility antigens displayed on recipient leukemia cells. Because some of these histocompatibility antigens are also displayed on tissues, however, unwanted T-cell–mediated alloreactions may ensue. Specifically, donor alloreactive cytotoxic CD8⁺ effector T cells may attack recipient tissues, particularly the skin, gastrointestinal (GI) tract, and liver, causing acute **graft-versus-host disease (GVHD)**, a condition of varying severity that in some cases can be life threatening or even fatal (see Chapter 163).

The success of allogeneic HSCT is undermined by diversity between donors and recipients in major and minor histocompatibility antigens. The **human leukocyte antigens (HLA)**, including HLA-A, HLA-B, and HLA-C major histocompatibility complex (MHC) class I molecules, present peptides to CD8⁺ T cells, whereas the HLA-DR, HLA-DQ, and HLA-DP MHC class II molecules present peptides to CD4⁺ T cells. There are 100s of variant forms of each class I and class II molecule, and even small differences can elicit alloreactive T-cell responses that mediate graft rejection and/or GVHD. Disparities for HLA-A, -B, -C, or -DRB1 alleles in the donor-recipient pair are independent risk factors for both acute and chronic GVHD. There is also increasing evidence that HLA-DQ and HLA-DP may play a role, prompting some transplant centers to also explore matching at these alleles.

Minor histocompatibility antigens derive from differences between the HLA-matched recipient and donor in peptides that are presented by the same HLA allotype. These antigens result from polymorphisms of non-HLA proteins, differences in the level of expression of proteins, or genetic differences between males and females. An example of the latter is represented by the H-Y antigens encoded by the Y chromosome, which can stimulate GVHD when a female donor is employed to transplant an HLA-identical male recipient. Thus, from this evidence, it is clear that GVHD may occur even when the donor and recipient are HLA identical.

The preferred donor for any patient undergoing HSCT is an HLA-identical sibling. Because polymorphic HLA genes are closely linked and usually constitute a single genetic locus, **any pair of siblings has a 25% chance of being HLA identical**. Thus, also in view of the limited family size in the developed countries, <25–30% of patients in need of an allograft can receive their transplant from an HLA-identical sibling. This percentage is even lower in patients with inherited disorders since affected siblings will not be considered donor candidates.

HSCT FROM AN HLA-IDENTICAL SIBLING DONOR

Allogeneic HSCT from an HLA-compatible sibling is the treatment of choice for children with hematologic malignancies and various congenital or acquired diseases (Table 161.1). Best results are achieved in patients with congenital or acquired nonmalignant disorders because the risk of disease recurrence is low and the cumulative transplantation-related mortality is lower than in children receiving transplants for hematologic malignancies.

ACUTE LYMPHOBLASTIC LEUKEMIA

Allogeneic HSCT is used for pediatric patients with acute lymphoblastic leukemia (**ALL**), either in the 1st complete remission when a child is considered to be at high risk of leukemia recurrence (e.g., those carrying poor-risk cytogenetic characteristics or with high levels of minimal residual disease), or in 2nd or further complete remission after previous marrow relapse. ALL is the most common indication for HSCT in childhood. Several patient-, donor-, disease-, and transplant-related variables may influence the outcome of patients with ALL given an allogeneic HSCT. The long-term probabilities of **event-free survival (EFS)** for patients with ALL transplanted in the 1st or 2nd complete remission is 60–70% and 40–60%, respectively. Inferior results are obtained in patients receiving transplants in more advanced disease phases. The use of **total body irradiation (TBI)** during the preparative regimen offers an advantage in terms of better EFS compared to a regimen consisting of cytotoxic drugs alone (Fig. 161.1), but it can induce more long-term side effects. This has prompted more investigation into TBI-sparing alternatives. Less intensive GVHD prophylaxis is also associated with a better outcome. Bone marrow is generally still the preferred source of stem cells to be employed for transplantation, although this differs among transplant centers.

Although the main benefit for allogeneic HSCT recipients with leukemia derives from the GVL effect displayed by immunocompetent cells, disease recurrence remains the main cause of treatment failure. The risk of failing to eradicate leukemia is influenced by many variables, including disease phase, molecular lesions of tumor cells, and disparity for major or minor histocompatibility antigens in the donor/recipient pairs. To overcome the hurdle of tumor elusion caused by HLA loss on malignant cells, the use of non–HLA-restricted **chimeric antigen receptors (CARs)** has been proposed. This therapeutic strategy is based on genetic reprogramming of T cells through artificial immune receptors that reproducibly and efficiently redirect the antigen specificity of polyclonal T lymphocytes toward target antigens expressed by leukemic cells. When expressed by T cells, CARs mediate antigen recognition and tumor cytolysis in an MHC-unrestricted fashion and can target any molecule (protein, carbohydrate, or glycolipid) expressed on the surface of tumor cells, thus bypassing one of the major tumor escape mechanisms based on the downregulation of MHC molecules. CARs are composed of an extracellular specific antigen-binding moiety, obtained from the variable regions of a monoclonal antibody, linked together to form a single-chain antibody (scFv), and of an intracellular signaling component derived from the ζ chain of the T-cell–receptor (TCR)–CD3 complex. The addition to the *CAR* gene construct of co-stimulation signals and cytokines promoting T-cell expansion and survival improves the antitumor efficiency of the engineered T cells and their survival in the tumor milieu. Gamma retrovirus and lentiviruses are usually used to transduce CARs into T lymphocytes to be employed in the clinical setting. These vectors have been shown to efficiently infect T lymphocytes,

Table 161.1	Indications for Allogeneic Hematopoietic Stem Cell Transplantation for Pediatric Diseases

MALIGNANCY

Acute lymphoblastic leukemia (ALL)
  First complete remission for patients at very high risk of relapse
  T-cell immunophenotype and poor response to corticosteroid therapy
  Not in remission at the end of the induction phase
  Marked hypodiploidy (<43 chromosomes)
  Minimal residual disease at the end of consolidation therapy
High-risk infant ALL
  Second complete remission
  Third or later complete remission
Acute myeloid leukemia in 1st complete remission or in advanced-disease phase
Philadelphia chromosome–positive chronic myeloid leukemia
Myelodysplastic syndromes
Hodgkin and non-Hodgkin lymphomas
Selected solid tumors
  Metastatic neuroblastoma
  Rhabdomyosarcoma refractory to conventional treatment
  Very-high-risk Ewing sarcoma

ANEMIAS

Severe acquired aplastic anemia
Fanconi anemia
Paroxysmal nocturnal hemoglobinemia
Congenital dyskeratosis
Diamond-Blackfan anemia
Thalassemia major
Sickle cell disease
Shwachman-Diamond syndrome

IMMUNOLOGIC DISORDERS

Variants of severe combined immunodeficiency
Hyper-IgM syndrome
Leukocyte adhesion deficiency
Omenn syndrome
Zap-70 kinase deficiency
Cartilage-hair hypoplasia
PNP deficiency
CD40 ligand deficiency
MHC class II deficiency
Wiskott-Aldrich syndrome
Chédiak-Higashi syndrome
Kostmann syndrome (infantile malignant agranulocytosis)
Chronic granulomatous disease
Autoimmune lymphoproliferative syndrome
X-linked lymphoproliferative disease (Duncan syndrome)
IPEX syndrome
Interleukin-10 receptor deficiency
Hemophagocytic lymphohistiocytosis
Interferon-γ receptor deficiency
Griscelli disease
Granule deficiency

OTHER DISORDERS

Selected severe variants of platelet function disorders (e.g., Glanzmann thromboasthenia, congenital amegakaryocytic thrombocytopenia)
Selected types of mucopolysaccharidosis (e.g., Hurler disease) or other liposomal/peroxisomal disorders (e.g., Krabbe disease, adrenoleukodystrophy)
Infantile malignant osteopetrosis
Life-threatening cytopenia unresponsive to conventional treatments

IPEX, Immune dysregulation, polyendocrinopathy, enteropathy, X-linked; MHC, major histocompatibility complex; PNP, purine nucleoside phosphorylase.

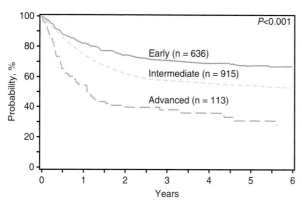

Fig. 161.1 Survival after HLA-matched sibling donor hematopoietic stem cell transplantation for acute lymphoblastic leukemia (ALL), age <18 yr, 2004–2014. *Early,* first complete remission (CR1); *Intermediate,* second or greater complete remission (CR2+); *Advanced,* active disease. (From D'Souza A, Zhu X: Current uses and outcomes of hematopoietic cell transplantation (HCT), CIBMTR Summary Slides, 2016. http://www.cibmtr.org.)

integrate into the host genome, and produce robust expression of the gene in human T cells and their progeny.

ACUTE MYELOID LEUKEMIA

Allogeneic HSCT from an HLA-identical sibling is largely employed as postremission treatment of pediatric patients with acute myeloid leukemia (**AML**). Children with AML in 1st complete remission who are given allogeneic HSCT as consolidation therapy have a better probability of EFS than those treated with either chemotherapy alone or autologous transplantation. Results obtained in patients given HSCT from an HLA-identical sibling after either a TBI-containing or a chemotherapy-based preparative regimen are similar, the probability of EFS being in the order of 70%. Therefore, for AML, conditioning regiments generally omit the use of TBI because of associated long-term side effects. Children with acute promyelocytic leukemia in molecular remission at the end of treatment with chemotherapy and all-*trans*-retinoic acid, or with AML and translocation t(8;21); inversion of chromosome 16 (inv16), translocation t(16;16), or normal cytogenetics and presence of *NPM1* or *CEPBα* mutation are no longer considered eligible for allogeneic HSCT in 1st complete remission in view of their improved prognosis with alternative treatments. Studies suggest restricting the use of HSCT to those patients with poor molecular lesions, such as FLT3-internal tandem duplication or mixed-lineage leukemia abnormalities, or with high levels of minimal residual disease at the end of induction therapy. Approximately 40–60% of pediatric patients with AML in the 2nd complete remission can be rescued by HSCT.

CHRONIC MYELOGENOUS LEUKEMIA

For many years, allogeneic HSCT has been considered the only proven curative treatment for children with Philadelphia-positive (Ph+) chronic myelogenous leukemia. Leukemia-free survival of chronic myelogenous leukemia patients after an allograft is 45–80%. The phase of disease (chronic phase, accelerated phase, blast crisis), recipient age, type of donor employed (related or unrelated), and time between diagnosis and HSCT are the main factors influencing the outcome. The best results are obtained in children transplanted during the chronic phase from an HLA-identical sibling within 1 yr from diagnosis. Unlike other forms of pediatric leukemia, infusion of donor leukocytes can reinduce a state of complete remission in a large proportion of patients experiencing leukemia relapse.

Treatment with the specific BCR-ABL tyrosine protein kinase inhibitors (imatinib mesylate, dasatinib, nilotinib), targeting the enzymatic activity of the BCR-ABL fusion protein, has modified the natural history of the disease and thus the indications for transplantation. The indication for HSCT in this population is thus evolving and is generally reserved for patients with a poor response to tyrosine kinase inhibitors or those who do not tolerate their side effects.

JUVENILE MYELOMONOCYTIC LEUKEMIA

Juvenile myelomonocytic leukemia (**JMML**) is a rare hematopoietic malignancy of early childhood, representing 2–3% of all pediatric leukemias. JMML is characterized by hepatosplenomegaly and organ infiltration, with excessive proliferation of cells of monocytic and granulocytic lineages. Hypersensitivity to granulocyte-macrophage colony-stimulating factor (GM-CSF) and pathologic activation of the RAS-RAF-MAP (mitogen-activated protein) kinase signaling pathway play an important role in the pathophysiology. JMML usually runs an aggressive clinical course, with a median duration of survival for untreated children of <12 mo from diagnosis. Rare patients with *CBL1* or *N-RAS* mutations can survive for years without an allograft.

HSCT is able to cure approximately 50–60% of patients with JMML. Patients who receive a transplant from an unrelated donor have comparable outcome to those given HSCT from an HLA-compatible related donor. Cord blood transplantation represents a suitable alternative option. Leukemia recurrence is the main cause of treatment failure in children with JMML after HSCT, with the relapse rate as high as 40–50%. Because children with JMML frequently have massive spleen enlargement, splenectomy has been performed before transplantation. However, spleen size at the time of HSCT and splenectomy before HSCT do not appear to affect the posttransplantation outcome. Unlike in CML, donor leukocyte infusion is not useful to rescue patients experiencing disease recurrence; a 2nd allograft can induce sustained remission in approximately one third of children with JMML relapsing after a 1st HSCT.

MYELODYSPLASTIC SYNDROMES OTHER THAN JUVENILE MYELOMONOCYTIC LEUKEMIA

Myelodysplastic syndromes are a heterogeneous group of clonal disorders characterized by ineffective hematopoiesis leading to peripheral blood cytopenia and a propensity to evolve toward AML. HSCT is the treatment of choice for children with **refractory anemia with excess of blasts (RAEB)** and for those with RAEB in transformation (RAEB-t). The probability of survival without evidence of disease for these children is 65–70%. It is still unclear whether patients with myelodysplastic syndromes and a blast percentage >20% benefit from pretransplantation chemotherapy. HSCT from an HLA-identical sibling is also the preferred treatment for all children with refractory cytopenia. Transplantation from an alternative donor is also employed in children with refractory cytopenia associated with monosomy 7, complex karyotype, life-threatening infections, profound neutropenia, or transfusion dependency. For children with refractory cytopenia, the probability of EFS after HSCT may be as high as 80%, disease recurrence being rarely observed. This observation has provided the rationale for testing reduced-intensity regimens in these patients.

NON-HODGKIN LYMPHOMA AND HODGKIN DISEASE

Childhood non-Hodgkin lymphoma (NHL) and Hodgkin disease (HD) are very responsive to conventional chemoradiotherapy, but some patients have refractory disease or are at high risk for relapse. HSCT can cure a proportion of patients with relapsed NHL and HD and should be offered early after relapse, while the disease is still sensitive to therapy. If an HLA-matched donor is available, allogeneic transplantation can be offered to patients with NHL to take advantage of the GVL effect. Patients with sensitive disease and limited tumor burden have favorable outcomes, with EFS rates of 50–60%. Studies also suggest that patients with relapsed or refractory HD do well after autologous HSCT, with EFS of 50–60%. HD patients may also benefit from a GVL effect when given an allograft.

ACQUIRED APLASTIC ANEMIA

Because the probability of long-term survival for a matched-*sibling* bone marrow transplant (BMT) is reproducibly >80% for children and young adults, BMT is the treatment of choice for children and young adults with acquired severe aplastic anemia. Historically, the treatment of choice for children and young adults without an HLA-matched sibling has been intensive immunosuppression. Because the outcomes of matched *unrelated donor* transplant for children with acquired aplastic anemia have improved to probability of survival rates >75%, the use of unrelated donor HSCT upfront *without* prior immunosuppressive therapy is being considered more frequently; 2-year overall survival can be as high as 96% in upfront, matched unrelated donor recipients.

For patients who do not have a matched-sibling donor or well-matched unrelated donor, historically the transplant options were very disappointing. Fortunately, there is hope in current studies looking at haploidentical transplant for this disease. Although numbers are small, the use of posttransplant cyclophosphamide has shown significant improvement over prior experiences. There is hope that all children and young adults who need a transplant for severe aplastic anemia will have the opportunity to do well with a BMT.

INHERITED BONE MARROW FAILURE SYNDROMES

Fanconi anemia and dyskeratosis congenita are genetic disorders associated with a high risk of developing pancytopenia. **Fanconi anemia (FA)** is an autosomal recessive disease characterized by spontaneous chromosomal fragility, which is increased after exposure of peripheral blood lymphocytes to DNA cross-linking agents, including clastogenic compounds such as diepoxybutane, mitomycin C, and melphalan. Patients with FA, besides being at risk for pancytopenia, show a high propensity to develop clonal disorders of hematopoiesis, such as myelodysplastic syndromes and AML. HSCT can rescue aplastic anemia and prevent the occurrence of clonal hematopoietic disorders. In view of their defects in DNA repair mechanisms, which are responsible for the chromosomal fragility, FA patients have an exquisite sensitivity to alkylating agents and radiation therapy. Thus, they must be prepared for the allograft with reduced doses of cyclophosphamide and only judicious use of radiation. Many FA patients were once successfully transplanted after receiving low-dose cyclophosphamide and thoracoabdominal irradiation. However, the use of this regimen is associated with an increased incidence of posttransplantation head and neck cancers. Low-dose cyclophosphamide combined with fludarabine has been very well tolerated in patients with FA who have a matched-related donor. The addition of low-dose TBI and antithymocyte globulin (ATG) for those with an unrelated donor has shown similar success. Currently, the 5-yr overall survival is >90% in patients with FA who receive HSCT before the transformation to hematologic malignancy. Because of their underlying disorder, however, patients with FA must be monitored closely in the years after transplant to assess for late effects, including secondary malignancies and endocrinopathies.

Allogeneic HSCT remains the only potentially curative approach for severe bone marrow failure associated with **dyskeratosis congenita**, a rare congenital syndrome characterized also by atrophy and reticular pigmentation of the skin, nail dystrophy, and leukoplakia of mucous membranes. Results of allograft in these patients have been relatively poor, with 10-yr survival of 20–30%, because of both early and late complications, reflecting increased sensitivity of endothelial cells to radiotherapy and alkylating agents.

THALASSEMIA

Conventional treatment (i.e., regular blood transfusion and iron-chelation therapy) has dramatically improved both the survival and the quality of life of patients with thalassemia, changing a previously fatal disease with early death to a chronic, slowly progressive disease compatible with prolonged survival. However, HSCT remains the only curative treatment for patients with thalassemia. In these patients the risk of dying from transplant-related complications depends primarily on patient age, iron overload, and concomitant hepatic viral infections. Adults, especially when affected by chronic active hepatitis, have a poorer outcome than children. Among children, 3 classes of risk have been identified on the basis of 3 parameters: regularity of previous iron chelation, liver enlargement, and presence of portal fibrosis. In pediatric patients without liver disease who have received regular iron chelation (class 1 patients), the probability of survival with transfusion independence is >90%, whereas for patients with low compliance with iron chelation and signs of severe liver damage (class 3 patients), the probability of survival has been 60%.

With improvements in supportive care and conditioning regimens, even patients with more advanced liver disease have had excellent outcomes (Fig. 161.2). The most effective pharmacologic combinations (e.g., including cyclosporine and methotrexate) should be employed to prevent GVHD. The outcome of patients transplanted from an unrelated donor has been reported similar to that of HLA-identical sibling recipients. The increased use of umbilical cord blood and haploidentical donors in this population is being explored to expand the number of patients eligible for HSCT. Also, advancements in gene therapy are being made in thalassemia in early trials, which may eventually change the approach to this disease.

SICKLE CELL DISEASE

Disease severity varies greatly among patients with sickle cell disease, with 5–20% of the overall population suffering significant morbidity from vasoocclusive crises and pulmonary, renal, or neurologic damage. Hydroxyurea, an agent favoring the synthesis of fetal hemoglobin, reduces the frequency and severity of vasoocclusive crises and improves the quality of life for patients with sickle cell disease; however allogeneic HSCT is the only curative treatment for this disease at this time. Although HSCT can cure homozygous hemoglobin S, hemoglobin Sβ0, or hemoglobin SC disease, selecting appropriate candidates for transplantation is difficult. Patients with sickle cell disease may survive for decades, but some patients have a poor quality of life, with repeated hospitalizations for painful vasoocclusive crises and central nervous system (CNS) infarcts. The main indications for performing HSCT in patients with sickle cell disease are history of strokes, MRI of CNS lesions associated with impaired neuropsychologic function, failure to respond to hydroxyurea as shown by recurrent acute chest syndrome, and/or recurrent vasoocclusive crises, severe anemia, or osteonecrosis. The results of HSCT are best when performed in children with an HLA-identical sibling, with a probability of cure of 80–90%. However, the use of alternative donor transplants in this population, including matched unrelated donors and haploidentical donors, is being investigated through a number of clinical trials and may increase the number of patients eligible to undergo potentially curative HSCT. Reduced-intensity and reduced-toxicity regimens are also being explored to further decrease transplant-related morbidity and mortality, although graft failure remains an important issue in this patient population.

IMMUNODEFICIENCY DISORDERS

HSCT is the treatment of choice for children affected by severe combined immunodeficiency (SCID), as well as for other inherited immunodeficiencies, including Wiskott-Aldrich syndrome, leukocyte adhesion deficiency (LAD), and chronic granulomatous disease (see Table 161.1). With an HLA-identical sibling, the probability of survival approaches 100%, with less favorable results for patients transplanted from an HLA–partially matched relative. Some children with SCID, mainly those without residual natural killer activity or maternal T-cell engraftment, may be transplanted without receiving any preparative regimen, the donor lymphoid cells usually being the only elements that engraft. Sustained donor engraftment is more difficult to achieve in children with Omenn syndrome, **hemophagocytic lymphohistiocytosis**, or LAD.

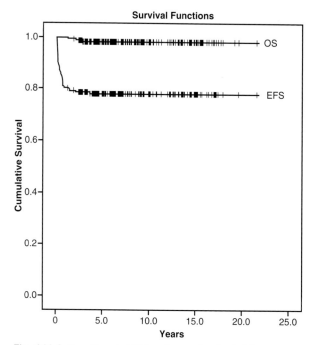

Fig. 161.2 Overall survival (OS) and event-free (graft failure) survival (EFS) after hematopoietic stem cell transplantation in children ≥1 yr from transplant for β-thalassemia major. *(From Chaudhury S, Ayas M, Rosen C, et al: A multicenter retrospective analysis stressing the importance of long-term follow-up after hematopoietic cell transplantation for β-thalassemia, Biol Blood Marrow Transplant 23(10):1695–1700, 2017.)*

Life-threatening opportunistic fungal and viral infections occurring before the allograft adversely affect the patient's outcome after HSCT. Because of this, patients with the most severe immunodeficiencies must be transplanted as early as possible to prevent infectious complications.

INHERITED METABOLIC DISEASES

Inherited metabolic diseases are a broad group of diseases that result from the accumulation of substrate within tissues caused by dysfunction of the lysosome or peroxisome. The use of HSCT has been established for a variety of inherited metabolic diseases, including mucopolysaccharidosis type 1 (Hurler syndrome) and adrenoleukodystrophy (ALD). Although some of these diseases are treatable with exogenous enzyme replacement therapy, the clinical manifestations of disease tend to progress over time, especially disease in the CNS, where enzyme is unable to be reliably delivered. It is thought that undergoing HSCT results in the engraftment of microglial cells that are able to provide new enzyme to the areas where enzyme replacement therapy, if available, cannot have a substantial impact. Multiple studies have shown significantly improved outcomes for patients who are diagnosed with their underlying conditions relatively early and are able to undergo HSCT expeditiously, before significant damage from accumulated substrate that may be irreversible.

Bibliography is available at Expert Consult.

Chapter **162**

Hematopoietic Stem Cell Transplantation From Alternative Sources and Donors

Rachel A. Phelan and David Margolis

第一百六十二章
替代供体来源造血干细胞移植

中文导读

　　本章主要介绍了无关供体移植、脐带血移植、半相合移植、供体抗受体NK细胞同种反应性以及自体造血干细胞移植。无关供体移植具体描述了移植配型；具体描述了脐带血移植的优点、不利因素和结果；具体描述了半相合移植的优势、移植物处理和结果；具体描述了供体抗受体NK细胞同种反应性的发生机制及其益处；具体描述了自体造血干细胞移植的干细胞来源和移植适应证。

Two thirds of patients who need allogeneic hematopoietic stem cell transplantation (HSCT) do not have an available HLA-identical sibling. Alternative sources of hematopoietic stem cells (HSCs) are being increasingly used and include **matched unrelated donors, unrelated umbilical cord blood,** and **HLA-haploidentical relatives**. Each of these 3 options has advantages and limitations, but rather than being considered competing alternatives, they should be regarded as complementary strategies to be chosen after a careful evaluation of the relative risks and benefits in the patient's best interest. The choice of the donor will depend on various factors related to urgency of transplantation, patient-, disease-, transplant-related factors, center experience, and physician preference.

UNRELATED DONOR TRANSPLANTS

One of the most widely used strategies for children who need an allograft and do not have an available HLA-identical sibling is to identify an unrelated HLA-matched donor in a registry (Fig. 162.1). Worldwide international registries include almost 27 million HLA-typed volunteer donors. HLA-A, -B, -C class I loci, and the DRB1 class II locus are the HLA loci most influencing outcome after HSCT from an unrelated volunteer. Other class II loci (namely, DQB1 and DP1 loci), as well as KIR haplotypes, are also being increasingly considered when choosing a donor, although their impact on outcome is less well studied.

Although in the past serologic (low-resolution) typing was used for HLA-A and HLA-B loci, currently the unrelated donors are selected

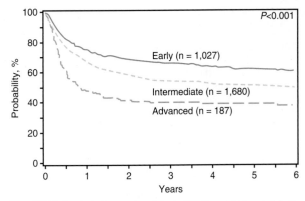

Fig. 162.1 Survival after unrelated donor HCT for acute lymphoblastic leukemia (ALL), age <18 yr, 2004–2014. *Early,* first complete remission (CR1); *Intermediate,* second or greater complete remission (CR2+); *Advanced,* active disease. *(From D'Souza A, Zhu X: Current uses and outcomes of hematopoietic cell transplantation (HCT), CIBMTR Summary Slides, 2016. http://www.cibmtr.org.)*

using high-resolution (allelic) molecular typing of loci HLA-A, -B, -C, and -DRB1. Less stringent HLA typing is required for cord blood units, where only HLA-A, -B, and -DRB1 are used. The chance of finding an HLA-matched unrelated donor depends on the frequency of the HLA phenotype, which is closely linked to the ethnic origin of the registry donors. Data from the National Marrow Donor Program (NMDP) donor registry and banked cord blood units estimated that essentially every patient in need of a transplant would be able to find a donor in a timely fashion, despite the recipient's race/ethnic group, donor availability, and cell dose. However, many of those patients may not have access to an "ideal" graft, defined as HLA matching of 8/8 for bone marrow and 6/6 for cord blood. It is also estimated that an additional 5.5 million donors will be added to the registry by 2017, making it even more likely for a potential, and more ideal, donor to be identified.

Initially, HLA polymorphism and the intrinsic limitations of conventional (i.e., serologic) HLA-typing techniques unfavorably affected the accuracy of matching, thus increasing rejection rates and the incidence of acute and chronic graft-versus-host disease (GVHD). The advent of both high-resolution molecular HLA classes I and II typing coupled with progress in the prophylaxis and treatment of GVHD has resulted in a reduction of transplantation-related mortality and improvement in outcome. Indeed, outcomes from a fully matched unrelated volunteer donor are now similar to those of HSCT from an HLA-identical sibling. The outcomes of haploidentical transplantation are similarly reaching that of matched unrelated donors as well as matched sibling donors.

Although a single locus disparity in patients with leukemia may be seen as beneficial by a reduction in the relapse rate caused by the graft-versus-leukemia (GVL) effect, in patients with nonmalignant disorders in whom GVL is not beneficial, optimal results are obtained only when a donor matched at the allelic level with the recipient is selected. In general, a single HLA disparity in the donor-recipient pair, irrespective of whether antigenic or allelic in nature, predicts a greater risk of nonleukemia mortality; multiple allelic disparities at different HLA loci have an additive detrimental effect and are associated with an even worse outcome. To reduce the risk of acute GVHD, **ex vivo T-cell depletion of the graft** has been employed, with variable efficacy. Studies are looking at selectively depleting donor α/β T cells, which are the T cells that drive GVHD, while preserving the T cells and natural killer (NK) cells, which may be responsible for GVL and protection from infection.

Although the majority of patients who have required a matched unrelated donor transplant have received a bone marrow or peripheral stem cell graft, for patients who urgently need a transplant, the time required to identify a suitable donor from a potential panel, establish eligibility, and harvest the cells may lead to relapse and failure to transplant. For this subset of patients who urgently need a transplant, attention has focused on unrelated cord blood and HLA-haploidentical, mismatched family donors.

UMBILICAL CORD BLOOD TRANSPLANTS

Umbilical cord blood transplantation (UCBT) is a viable option for children who need allogeneic HSCT. UCBT offers the advantages of absence of risks to donors, reduced risk of transmitting infections, and for transplants from unrelated donors, immediate availability of cryopreserved cells, with the median time from start of search to transplantation only 3-4 wk. Compared with bone marrow transplantation (BMT), the advantages of UCBT are also represented by lower incidence of chronic GVHD and the possibility of using donors showing HLA disparities with the recipient. Despite these advantages, the large experience gained over the last 2 decades has demonstrated that UCBT patients may be exposed to an increased risk of early fatal complications, mainly because of a lower engraftment rate of donor hematopoiesis, delayed kinetics of neutrophil recovery, and lack of adoptive transfer of pathogen-specific memory T cells. Transfer of donor-derived, memory T cells significantly contributes to early immunologic reconstitution of children after unmanipulated allogeneic bone marrow or peripheral blood stem cell transplantation.

Concerning the issues of engraftment and hematopoietic recovery, it has been demonstrated that an inverse correlation exists between the number of nucleated cord blood cells infused per kilogram recipient body weight and the risk of dying for transplantation-related causes. In particular, engraftment is a major concern when the nucleated cells are $<2.5 \times 10^7$/kg of recipient body weight. Since a cord blood unit usually contains between 1×10^9 and 1.8×10^9 cells, it is not surprising that UCBT has been less frequently employed for adolescents or adults with body weight >40 kg. Indeed, it can be estimated that only 30% of the UCB units available in the bank inventory could suffice for a 75 kg patient, according to the recommended threshold cell dose. Efforts have focused on approaches capable of increasing the number of UCB cells to be transplanted. Selection of the richest cord blood units, infusion of 2 units in the same recipient (i.e., double UCBT), and transplantation of ex vivo expanded progenitors have been explored to improve the results of UCBT, opening new scenarios for a wider application of the procedure. The results of these studies have been mixed, with one large study demonstrating no survival advantage for children and adolescents that receive double UCBT.

The long-term results of UCB transplants are similar to those after transplantation from other sources of HSCs for pediatric hematologic malignancies. In patients with hematologic malignancies, recipients of UCBT may be transplanted from donors with greater HLA disparities, receive 1-log fewer nucleated cells, have delayed neutrophil and platelet recovery, and show reduced incidence of GVHD compared with children given BMT from unrelated donors. In one study, there were similar rates of acute GVHD, but significantly less chronic GVHD in patients who received UCBT. Nevertheless, both the relapse rate and the overall survival probability did not differ in unrelated UCBT or BMT pediatric recipients. Thus, in the absence of an HLA-identical family donor, unrelated UCBT can be considered a suitable option for children with malignant and nonmalignant disorders. Results of UCBT have been of particular interest in children with certain nonmalignant disorders to proceed to transplant quickly and prevent further progression of disease. An additional benefit is the potential for lower rates of GVHD, which serves no benefit in a patient receiving a transplant for a nonmalignant disorder.

HAPLOIDENTICAL TRANSPLANTS

HSCT from an HLA-haploidentical (**haplo-HSCT**) donor offers an immediate source of HSCs to almost all patients who fail to find a matched donor, whether related or unrelated, or a suitable cord blood unit. Indeed, almost all children have at least 1 haploidentical–3 loci mismatched family member who is promptly available as donor. The few patients who reject the haploidentical transplant also have the advantage of another immediately available donor within the family. Moreover, this may represent an approach that would be attractive in the global health setting, where more sophisticated donor registries and cell-processing techniques are unavailable.

Efficient T-cell depletion of the graft has been demonstrated to prevent acute and chronic GVHD even when using haploidentical parental bone marrow differing at the 3 major HLA loci. This can be done ex vivo or in vivo with the use of chemotherapeutic agents before and after cell infusion. The use of **posttransplant cyclophosphamide** is one such in vivo technique now being widely incorporated into haploidentical transplant regimens. The benefits of T-cell depletion were first demonstrated in transplantation of children with severe combined immunodeficiency (SCID). More than 300 transplants in SCID patients using haploidentical donors have been performed worldwide, with a high rate of long-term partial or complete immune reconstitution.

The elimination of mature T cells from the graft, necessary for preventing GVHD in a context of great immune genetic disparity, results in recipients being unable to benefit from the adoptive transfer of donor memory T lymphocytes that, through their peripheral expansion, are the main factor responsible for protection from infections in the 1st few mo after transplantation. A state of profound immunodeficiency lasts for at least 4-6 mo after transplantation in haplo-HSCT recipients. Sophisticated strategies of adoptive infusions of T-cell lines or clones specific for the most common and life-threatening pathogens (Epstein-Barr virus [EBV], human cytomegalovirus, *Aspergillus*, adenovirus) have been successfully tested in a few pilot trials, to protect the recipients in the early posttransplant period.

Selective approaches of graft manipulation in haploidentical and unrelated donor transplant have also been developed. In particular, promising results have been obtained through a negative depletion of T lymphocytes carrying the α/β chains of the T-cell receptor, which are believed to be the mediators of GVHD. B lymphocytes are also depleted to prevent EBV-related lymphoproliferative disease. Through this approach the patient can benefit from the adoptive transfer of committed hematopoietic progenitors, mature NK cells and γ/δ+ T cells, which can confer a protection against life-threatening infections as well as provide a GVL effect.

The outcomes of haplo-HSCT have been more extensively reported in adults than in children. The reported probability of survival at 3-4 yr after a haplo-HSCT in children with acute leukemia ranged from 18–48%. Survival was influenced by many factors, most importantly the state of remission at transplantation, with poorer outcomes in children with myeloid leukemias than in those with lymphoid leukemia. In haplotype-mismatched parent-to-child HSCT, patients with acute leukemia grafted from the mother had reduced relapse rates compared with recipients of paternal grafts, translating into better event-free survival.

For many years the absence of the T-cell–mediated GVL effect has been considered as rendering the recipients of a T-cell–depleted allograft more susceptible to leukemia relapse. However, it has been demonstrated that a GVL effect displayed by donor NK cells can compensate for this lack of T-specific alloreactivity when an HLA-disparate NK-alloreactive relative is employed as a donor.

DONOR VERSUS RECIPIENT NK-CELL ALLOREACTIVITY

Natural killer cells are the first lymphocytes derived from the donor to recover after allogeneic HCT. Donor vs recipient NK-cell alloreactivity derives from a mismatch between donor NK clones, carrying specific inhibitory receptors for self–major histocompatibility complex (MHC) class I molecules, and MHC class I ligands on recipient cells. NK cells are primed to kill by several activating receptors, which play an important role in the NK cell–mediated GVL effect. Human NK cells discriminate allelic forms of MHC molecules via **killer cell immunoglobulin-like receptors (KIRs),** which are clonally distributed with each cell in the repertoire bearing at least 1 receptor that is specific for self-MHC class I molecules. Because NK cells co-express inhibitory receptors for self-MHC class I molecules, autologous cells are not killed. When faced with mismatched allogeneic targets, NK cells sense the missing expression of self–class I alleles and mediate alloreactions. In mismatched transplants, there are many donor recipient pairs in which the donor NK inhibitory

cells do not recognize the recipient's class I alleles as self. Consequently, the donor NK cells are not blocked and are activated to lyse the recipient's lymphohematopoietic cells.

Haplo-HSCT trials demonstrate that MHC class I mismatches, which generate an alloreactive NK-cell response in the graft-vs-host direction, eradicate leukemia cells, improve engraftment, and protect from T-cell–mediated GVHD. The potential for donor vs recipient NK-cell alloreactivity, which can be predicted by standard HLA typing, is increasingly being examined when selecting the donor of choice. Although the importance of KIR haplotype in transplants other than haploidentical transplantation has still not been fully elucidated in the pediatric population, its role in preventing GVHD as well as relapse has been shown to be increasingly beneficial in the adult population.

AUTOLOGOUS HEMATOPOIETIC STEM CELL TRANSPLANTATION

Autologous transplantation, using the patient's own stored marrow, is associated with a low risk of life-threatening transplant-related complications, although the main cause of failure is disease recurrence. Bone marrow was once the only source of stem cells employed in patients given an autograft. In the past few years, the vast majority of patients treated with autologous HSCT receive hematopoietic progenitors mobilized in peripheral blood by either cytokines alone (mainly granulocyte colony-stimulating factor) or by cytokines plus cytotoxic agents. A CXCR4 antagonist (plerixafor) can be extremely effective in mobilizing hematopoietic progenitors in the periphery. Compared with bone marrow, the use of peripheral blood progenitors is associated with a faster hematopoietic recovery and a comparable outcome. A major concern in patients with malignancies given autologous HSCT is represented by the risk of reinfusing malignant cells with the graft; tumor progenitors contained in the graft can contribute to recurrence of the original malignant disease. This observation has provided the rationale for **tumor purging** using elaborate strategies aimed at reducing or eliminating tumor contamination of the graft.

Autologous HSCT is employed primarily for selected children with relapsed lymphomas and select solid tumors (Table 162.1).

Patients with sensitive lymphomas and minimal tumor burden have favorable outcomes after autologous HSCT, with disease-free survival rates of 50–60%, whereas high-risk patients with bulky tumor or poorly responsive disease have a poor outcome, with survival rates of 10–20%.

Autologous HSCT in patients with high-risk neuroblastoma is associated with a better outcome than conventional chemotherapy. A Children's Oncology Group (COG) study demonstrated further survival advantage by performing 2 sequential, or **tandem,** transplants that use different chemotherapeutic agents. Because of these improved outcomes, tandem autologous transplants are now considered the standard recommended treatment. In these patients, posttransplantation infusion of a monoclonal antibody directed against a molecule (GD2) expressed on the surface of neuroblastoma cells confers a protection against the risk of tumor recurrence.

For children with brain tumors at high risk of relapse, or resistant to conventional chemotherapy and irradiation, the dose-limiting toxicity for intensifying therapy is myelosuppression, thus providing a role for stem cell rescue. Several studies provide encouraging results for patients with different histologic types of brain tumors treated with autologous HSCT.

Bibliography is available at Expert Consult.

Table 162.1	Indications for Autologous Hematopoietic Stem Cell Transplantation for Pediatric Diseases

- Relapsed Hodgkin or non-Hodgkin lymphoma
- Stage IV or relapsed neuroblastoma
- High-risk, relapsed, or resistant brain tumors
- Stage IV Ewing sarcoma
- Life-threatening autoimmune diseases resistant to conventional treatments

Chapter **163**

Graft-Versus-Host Disease, Rejection, and Venoocclusive Disease

Rachel A. Phelan and David Margolis

第一百六十三章

移植物抗宿主病、排斥和静脉阻塞性疾病

中文导读

　　本章主要介绍了急性移植物抗宿主病、慢性移植物抗宿主病、植入失败以及静脉阻塞性疾病。急性移植物抗宿主病具体描述了病因、发病机制、临床表现、分级、预防和治疗手段；慢性移植物抗宿主病具体描述了危险因素、发病机制、临床表现和治疗；具体描述了植入失败的分类、发生原因、诊断以及治疗；描述了静脉阻塞性疾病的表现、危险因素、预防和治疗。

A major cause of mortality and morbidity after allogeneic hematopoietic stem cell transplantation (HSCT) is **graft-versus-host disease (GVHD)**, which is caused by engraftment of immunocompetent donor T lymphocytes in an immunologically compromised host who shows histocompatibility differences with the donor. These differences between the donor and the host may result in donor T-cell activation against either recipient major histocompatibility complex (MHC) antigens or minor histocompatibility antigens. GVHD is usually subdivided in 2 forms: **acute GVHD**, which occurs within 3 mo after transplantation, and **chronic GVHD**, which, although related, is a different disease, occurring later and displaying some clinical and pathologic features that resemble those observed in selected autoimmune disorders (e.g., systemic sclerosis, Sjögren syndrome).

ACUTE GRAFT-VERSUS-HOST DISEASE

Acute GVHD is caused by the alloreactive, donor-derived T cells contained in the graft, which attack nonshared recipient's antigens on target tissues. A 3-step process generates the clinical syndrome. First, conditioning-induced tissue damage activates recipient antigen-presenting cells, which present recipient alloantigens to the donor T cells transferred with the graft and secrete **cytokines**, such as interleukin (IL)-12, favoring the polarization of T-cell response in the type 1 direction. Second, in response to recipient antigens, donor T cells become activated, proliferate, expand, and generate cytokines such as tumor necrosis factor (TNF)-α, IL-2, and interferon (IFN)-γ. In the 3rd step of the process, these cytokines cause tissue damage and promote differentiation of cytotoxic CD8⁺ T cells, which, together with macrophages, kill recipient cells and further disrupt tissues.

Acute GVHD usually develops 2-8 wk after transplantation. The primary manifestations depend on the sites of involvement and may include an erythematous maculopapular rash (Figs. 163.1 and 163.2), persistent anorexia, vomiting and/or diarrhea, and liver disease with increased serum levels of bilirubin, alanine transaminase (ALT), aspartate transaminase (AST), and alkaline phosphatase (ALP). Diagnosis may benefit from skin, liver, or gastrointestinal (GI) biopsy for confirmation. Endothelial damage and lymphocytic infiltrates are seen in all affected organs. The epidermis and hair follicles of the skin are damaged, the hepatic small bile ducts show segmental disruption, and there is destruction of the crypts and mucosal ulceration of the GI tract. Grade I acute GVHD (skin rash alone) has a favorable prognosis and often requires no treatment, or topical treatment alone. Grade II GVHD is a moderately severe multiorgan disease requiring immunosuppressive therapy. Grade III GVHD is a severe multiorgan disease, and grade IV GVHD is a life-threatening, often fatal condition (Table 163.1).

The standard **pharmacologic prophylaxis** of GVHD after an unmanipulated allograft relies mainly on posttransplant administration of immunosuppressive drugs, such as cyclosporine or tacrolimus or combinations of either with methotrexate or prednisone, anti–T-cell antibodies, mycophenolate mofetil (MMF), and other immunosuppressive agents. Infusion of cyclophosphamide on days +3 and +5 after transplantation has been proposed as a strategy to deplete alloreactive donor T lymphocytes that become activated after exposure to recipient antigens. This approach has been successful in patients undergoing haploidentical transplantation. Pretransplantation infusion of either antithymocyte globulin (ATG) or monoclonal antibodies (mAbs) such as alemtuzumab is largely used to modulate alloreactivity of donor T cells, in particular

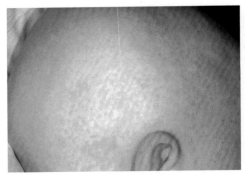

Fig. 163.1 Acute graft-versus-host disease. Involvement of the scalp, ears, palms, and soles is common. *(From Paller AS, Mancini AJ, editors: Hurwitz clinical pediatric dermatology, ed 5, Philadelphia, 2016, Elsevier, p 577.)*

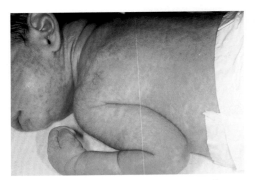

Fig. 163.2 Acute graft-versus-host disease. Almost confluent eruption of erythematous macules and papules in an immunodeficient neonate treated with extracorporeal membrane oxygenation (ECMO) and transfusion of nonirradiated blood. *(From Paller AS, Mancini AJ, editors: Hurwitz clinical pediatric dermatology, ed 5, Philadelphia, 2016, Elsevier, p 577.)*

in patients given the allograft from either an unrelated donor or a partially matched relative. An alternative approach, which has been widely used in clinical practice, is the removal of T lymphocytes from the graft (**T-cell depletion**). Other approaches, through clinical trials, are being used to selectively remove the α/β T cells, which are thought to be responsible for the development of GVHD, while preserving the γ/δ T cells in order to sustain GVL and the ability to fight infection. Any form of GVHD prophylaxis in itself may impair posttransplantation immunologic reconstitution, increasing the risk of infection-related deaths. Traditional T-cell depletion of the graft is also associated with an increased risk of leukemia recurrence in patients transplanted from an HLA-identical sibling or an unrelated volunteer.

Despite prophylaxis, significant acute GVHD develops in approximately 30% of recipients of HSCT from matched siblings and in as many as 60% of HSCT recipients from unrelated donors. These numbers are estimates, and the actual risk of acute GVHD is highly variable depending on several factors. Risk for development of GVHD is increased by diagnosis of malignant disease, older donor and recipient age, and in patients given an unmanipulated allograft, GVHD prophylaxis including only 1 drug. The most important risk factor for acute GVHD is the presence of disparities for HLA molecules in the donor-recipient pair.

Acute GVHD is usually initially treated with glucocorticoids; approximately 40–50% of patients show a complete response to corticosteroids. The risk of transplantation-related mortality is much higher in patients who do not respond to corticosteroids than in those showing a complete response. Promising results in children with steroid-resistant acute GVHD have been obtained using **mesenchymal stromal cells**, which are able to blunt the inflammatory response associated with acute GVHD. MMF, pentostatin, or mAbs targeting molecules expressed on T cells or cytokines released during the inflammatory cascade (including infliximab and etanercept targeting TNF, and tocilizumab targeting IL-6), which underlies the pathophysiology of GVHD, have been used in patients with steroid-resistant acute GVHD. There are no clear data showing the superiority of one of these approaches over the others. **Extracorporeal photopheresis** is another second-line treatment for GVHD and is most efficacious for skin GVHD. A patient's peripheral blood is exposed to a photosensitive compound and then exposed to ultraviolet light. The cells are then reinfused into the patient. It is thought that this process results in an increase in apoptosis of lymphocytes responsible for GVHD as well as the upregulation of antiinflammatory cytokines and regulatory T cells.

Table 163.1	Clinical Staging and Grading* of Graft-Versus-Host Disease (GVHD)			
STAGE	**SKIN (ACTIVE ERYTHEMA ONLY)**	**LIVER (BILIRUBIN)**	**UPPER GI**	**LOWER GI (STOOL OUTPUT/DAY)**
0	No active (erythematous) GVHD rash	<2 mg/dL	No or intermittent nausea, vomiting, or anorexia	Adult: <500 mL/day or <3 episodes/day Child: <10 mL/kg/day or <4 episodes/day
1	Maculopapular rash <25% BSA	2-3 mg/dL	Persistent nausea, vomiting or anorexia	Adult: 500-999 mL/day or 3-4 episodes/day Child: 10-19.9 mL/kg/day or 4-6 episodes/day
2	Maculopapular rash 25-50% BSA	3.1-6 mg/dL		Adult: 1000-1500 mL/day or 5-7 episodes/day Child: 20-30 mL/kg/day or 7-10 episodes/day
3	Maculopapular rash >50% BSA	6.1-15 mg/dL		Adult: >1500 mL/day or >7 episodes/day Child: >30 mL/kg/day or >10 episodes/day
4	Generalized erythroderma (>50% BSA) plus bullous formation and desquamation >5% BSA	>15 mg/dL		Severe abdominal pain with or without ileus or grossly bloody stool (regardless of stool volume)

*Overall clinical grade (based on most severe target organ involvement):
  Grade 0: no stage 1-4 of any organ.
  Grade I: stage 1-2 skin without liver, upper GI, or lower GI involvement.
  Grade II: stage 3 rash and/or stage 1 liver and/or stage 1 upper GI and/or stage 1 lower GI.
  Grade III: stage 2-3 liver and/or stage 2-3 lower GI, with stage 0-3 skin and/or stage 0-1 upper GI.
  Grade IV: stage 4 skin, liver, or lower GI involvement, with stage 0-1 upper GI.
  GI, Gastrointestinal; BSA, body surface area.
  From Harris AC, Young R, Devine S, et al: International, multicenter standardization of acute graft-versus-host disease clinical data collection: a report from the Mount Sinai Acute GVHD International Consortium, Biol Blood Marrow Transplant 22:4–10, 2016.

CHRONIC GRAFT-VERSUS-HOST DISEASE

Chronic GVHD develops or persists >3 mo after transplantation and is the most frequent late complication of allogeneic HSCT with an incidence of approximately 25% in pediatric patients. Chronic GVHD is the major cause of nonrelapse mortality and morbidity in long-term HSCT survivors. Acute GVHD is recognized as the most important factor predicting the development of the chronic form of the disease. The use of matched unrelated volunteers as donors and use of peripheral blood as the stem cell source have increased the incidence and severity of chronic GVHD. Other factors that predict occurrence of chronic GVHD include older donor and recipient ages, female donor for male recipient, diagnosis of malignancy, and use of total body irradiation (TBI) as part of the preparative regimen.

Chronic GVHD is a disorder of immune regulation characterized by autoantibody production, increased collagen deposition and fibrosis, and clinical symptoms similar to those seen in patients with autoimmune diseases (Table 163.2). The predominant cytokines involved in the pathophysiology of chronic GVHD are usually type II cytokines such as IL-4, IL-5, and IL-13. IL-4 and IL-5 contribute to eosinophilia, B-cell hyperactivity with elevated IgM, IgG, and IgE titers. Associated mono-clonal gammopathies indicate clonal dysregulation. Chronic GVHD is dependent on the development and persistence of donor T cells that are not tolerant to the recipient. Maturation of transplanted stem cells within a damaged thymus could lead to errors in negative selection and production of cells that have not been tolerized to recipient antigens and are therefore autoreactive or, more accurately, **recipient reactive**. This ongoing immune reactivity results in clinical features resembling a systemic autoimmune disease with lichenoid and sclerodermatous skin lesions, malar rash, sicca syndrome, arthritis, joint contractures, bronchiolitis obliterans, and bile duct degeneration with cholestasis.

Patients with chronic GVHD involving only the skin and liver have a favorable course (Figs. 163.3 and 163.4). Extensive multiorgan disease may be associated with a very poor quality of life, recurrent infections associated with prolonged immunosuppressive regimens to control GVHD, and a high mortality rate. Morbidity and mortality are highest in patients with a **progressive onset** of chronic GVHD that directly follows acute GVHD, intermediate in those with a **quiescent onset** after resolution of acute GVHD, and lowest in patients with **de novo onset** in the absence of acute GVHD. Chronic GVHD can be classified as mild, moderate, or severe depending on extent of involvement. Single-agent prednisone is standard treatment at present, although other agents, including extracorporeal photopheresis, MMF, anti-CD20 mAb, and pentostatin, have been employed with variable success. Treatment with imatinib mesylate, which inhibits the synthesis of collagen, has been effective in some patients with chronic GVHD and sclerotic features. As a consequence of prolonged immunosuppression, patients with chronic GVHD are particularly susceptible to infections and should

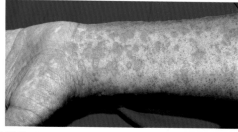

Fig. 163.3 Chronic graft-versus-host disease (GVHD), lichenoid. After bone marrow transplantation, this boy had acute GVHD and subsequently developed cutaneous scaling papules and plaques typical of lichen planus. *(From Paller AS, Mancini AJ, editors: Hurwitz clinical pediatric dermatology, ed 5, Philadelphia, 2016, Elsevier, p 577.)*

Table 163.2	Clinical Findings in Chronic Graft-Versus-Host Disease
ORGAN SYSTEM	**SYMPTOMS AND SIGNS**
Systemic	Immunodeficiency and recurrent infections
Skin	Lichen planus, scleroderma, hyperpigmentation or hypopigmentation, erythema, freckling, ichthyosis, ulcerations Flexion contractures Vaginal scars Onycholysis Nail loss
Hair	Alopecia; scarring or nonscarring
Mouth	Sicca syndrome, lichen planus, depapillation of tongue with variegations, scalloping of lateral margins, xerostomia, mucocele
Joints	Diffuse myositis/tendonitis, arthritis, contractures
Eyes	Decreased tearing, injected sclerae, scarring conjunctivitis, keratopathy
Liver	Increased enzymes, cholestasis, hepatomegaly, cirrhosis
Gastrointestinal	Failure to thrive, malabsorption, chronic diarrhea Esophageal strictures
Lung	Cough, dyspnea, wheezing Bronchiolitis obliterans, chronic rales, pneumothorax, fibrosis
Hematology	Thrombocytopenia, eosinophilia, Howell-Jolly bodies (splenic dysfunction)

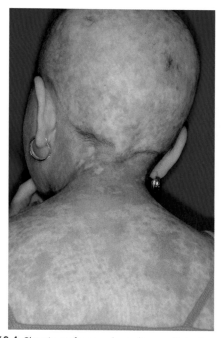

Fig. 163.4 Chronic graft-versus-host disease. Note the extensive alopecia of the scalp with dyschromia and numerous sclerodermatous plaques of the scalp and back. *(From Paller AS, Mancini AJ, editors: Hurwitz clinical pediatric dermatology, ed 5, Philadelphia, 2016, Elsevier, p 579.)*

receive appropriate antibiotic prophylaxis, including trimethoprim/sulfamethoxazole (TMP/SMX). Chronic GVHD resolves in most pediatric patients but may require 1-3 yr of immunosuppressive therapy before the drugs can be withdrawn without the disease recurring. Chronic GVHD promotes the development of secondary neoplasms, in particular in patients with Fanconi anemia, and has a significant impact on quality of life.

GRAFT FAILURE

Graft failure is a serious complication exposing patients to a high risk of fatal infection. **Primary graft failure** is defined as failure to achieve a neutrophil count of $0.5 \times 10^9/L$ after transplantation. **Secondary graft failure** is loss of peripheral blood counts following initial transient engraftment of donor cells. Causes of graft failure after autologous and allogeneic transplantation include transplantation of an inadequate stem cell dose (more frequently observed in children given cord blood transplantation) and viral infections such as with cytomegalovirus or human herpesvirus type 6, which are often associated with activation of recipient macrophages. Graft failure after allogeneic transplantation, however, is mainly caused by immunologically mediated rejection of the graft by residual recipient-type T cells that survive the conditioning regimen.

Diagnosis of graft failure resulting from immunologic mechanisms is based on examination of peripheral blood and marrow aspirate and biopsy, along with molecular analysis of chimerism status. Persistence of lymphocytes of host origin in allogeneic transplant recipients with graft failure indicates immunologic rejection. The risk of immune-mediated graft rejection is higher in patients given HLA-disparate, T-cell–depleted grafts, reduced-intensity conditioning regimens, and transplantation of low numbers of stem cells, and in recipients who are sensitized toward HLA antigens or, less frequently, minor histocompatibility antigens. Allosensitization develops as a consequence of preceding blood product transfusions and is observed particularly in recipients with aplastic anemia, sickle cell disease, and thalassemia. In HSCT for nonmalignant diseases, such as mucopolysaccharidoses, graft failure is also facilitated by the absence of previous treatment with cytotoxic and immunosuppressive drugs. In thalassemia, graft failure is promoted by expansion of recipient hematopoietic cells. GVHD prophylaxis with methotrexate, an antimetabolite, and antiinfective prophylaxis with TMP/SMX or ganciclovir may also delay engraftment.

Treatment of graft failure usually requires removing all potentially myelotoxic agents from the treatment regimen and attempting a short trial of hematopoietic growth factors, such as granulocyte colony-stimulating factor. A 2nd transplant, usually preceded by a highly immunosuppressive regimen, is frequently employed to rescue patients experiencing graft failure. High-intensity regimens are generally tolerated poorly if administered within 100 days from a 1st transplant because of cumulative toxicities, but this risk must be balanced with the risk of infection from prolonged neutropenia and lymphocytopenia.

VENOOCCLUSIVE DISEASE

Hepatic venoocclusive disease (**VOD**), also known as **sinusoidal obstruction syndrome**, presents with hepatomegaly, right upper quadrant tenderness, jaundice, and weight gain from fluid retention and ascites. It results from endothelial damage within the liver, which can then progress to multiorgan dysfunction. Onset is usually within 30 days of transplantation, with an incidence of approximately 15%, depending on the intensity of the conditioning protocol. Risk factors include young age, prior hepatic disease (fibrosis, cirrhosis), abdominal radiation, repeated transplantations, neuroblastoma, osteopetrosis, and familial hemophagocytic lymphohistiocytosis. The severe form of VOD has a high mortality rate (>80%) without treatment.

Prophylaxis has traditionally used ursodeoxycholic acid and occasionally heparin; only **defibrotide** has demonstrated some efficacy in preventing and treating VOD. A phase 3 study demonstrated improvement in survival and response rate to VOD in patients treated with defibrotide. Defibrotide is a combination of porcine oligodeoxyribonucleotides that reduces procoagulant activity and enhances fibrinolytic properties of endothelial cells. Defibrotide is U.S. Food and Drug Administration (FDA) approved for the treatment of VOD in adult and pediatric patients with renal or pulmonary dysfunction after HSCT. Defibrotide is often used as prophylaxis in Europe, with data showing efficacy, but this use is not yet approved in the United States.

Bibliography is available at Expert Consult.

Chapter **164**

Infectious Complications of Hematopoietic Stem Cell Transplantation

Anna R. Huppler

第一百六十四章

造血干细胞移植感染并发症

中文导读

本章主要介绍了造血干细胞移植后不同阶段的感 染并发症以及不同病原感染。具体描述了移植后早期中性粒细胞不足所致感染并发症及其病原、后期T细胞数量与功能缺陷所致感染及病原；具体描述了侵袭性真菌病，主要包括播散性念珠菌病和侵袭性肺曲霉菌病，及其临床、影像学和实验室诊断依据，药物预防与治疗；具体描述了CMV感染、EBV相关移植后淋巴增生性疾病，以及播散性腺病毒感染的危险因素、临床表现、预防和治疗。

Hematopoietic stem cell transplantation (HSCT) recipients experience a transient but profound state of immune deficiency. The risk of infection depends on the stage after transplantation (pre- vs postengraftment), ongoing immunosuppression, disruption in barrier functions (indwelling catheters, graft-versus-host disease [GVHD], mucositis) and preexisting infections (Fig. 164.1). Management approaches may include the use of prophylactic antimicrobials, preemptive antimicrobials for infection prior to symptomatic disease, or antimicrobial treatment of documented or suspected infection.

Immediately after transplantation, the absence or paucity of neutrophils (**neutropenia**) renders patients susceptible to bacterial and fungal infections. Consequently, most centers start antipseudomonal and antifungal prophylaxis during the conditioning regimen. Despite these prophylactic measures, the majority of patients will develop fever and signs of infection in the early posttransplantation period. The common pathogens include enteric gram-negative bacteria and fungi. An indwelling central venous line, routinely employed in all children given HSCT, is a significant risk factor for infection. Staphylococcal species and *Candida* are the most frequent pathogens in catheter-related infections (see Chapter 206). Multidrug-resistant strains of *Pseudomonas aeruginosa* and *Klebsiella pneumoniae* are an emerging problem, with prevalence highly variable among centers. Severe lower respiratory tract disease

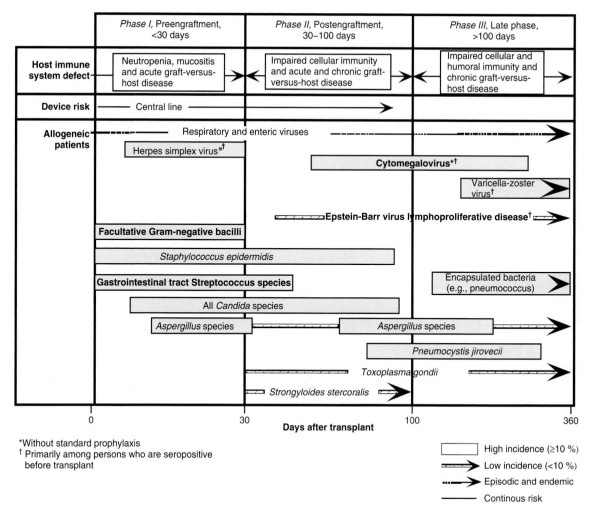

Fig. 164.1 Phases of opportunistic infections among allogenic HSCT recipients. *(From Centers for Disease Control and Prevention: Guidelines for preventing opportunistic infections among hematopoietic sickle cell transplant recipients, MMWR 49(RR-10):1–128, 2000.)*

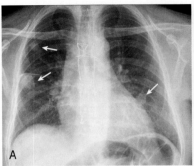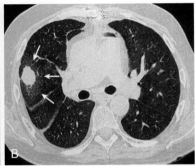

Fig. 164.2 Angioinvasive aspergillosis. **A,** Posteroanterior radiograph shows multiple nodules in the lungs *(arrows)*. **B,** CT section at the level of the intermediary bronchus shows a nodule surrounded by a halo of ground-glass attenuation *(arrows)*. *(From Haaga JR, Boll DT, editors: CT and MRI of the whole body, ed 6, vol 1, Philadelphia, 2017, Elsevier, p 933.)*

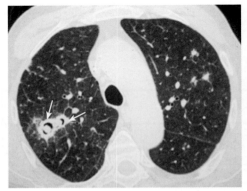

Fig. 164.3 Angioinvasive aspergillosis. CT section at the level of the lower trachea shows a consolidation with an eccentric cavitation and air crescent sign *(arrows)*. This finding in this neutropenic patient is highly diagnostic of angioinvasive aspergillosis. *(From Haaga JR, Boll DT, editors: CT and MRI of the whole body, ed 6, vol 1, Philadelphia, 2017, Elsevier, p 933.)*

caused by seasonal respiratory viruses, such as influenza, respiratory syncytial virus (RSV), parainfluenza virus, and human metapneumovirus, can occur during the pre- or postengraftment phase. Published guidelines from the Infectious Disease Society of America and the U.S. Centers for Disease Control and Prevention (CDC) address the management of fever and neutropenia after HSCT.

HSCT recipients remain at increased risk of developing severe infections even after the neutrophil count has normalized because of prolonged depression in T-cell number and function. The manifestations of GVHD, as well as the associated immunosuppressive therapy, are additional risk factors for fungal and viral opportunistic infections. After umbilical cord blood transplant (UCBT), infections are the consequence of both slow neutrophil engraftment and donor T-cell naïveté. In haploidentical transplantation, T-cell depletion results in an increased risk of infection in the first 4-6 mo. Recipients of this type of transplantation, as well as those receiving UBCT, do not have the benefit of adoptive transfer of donor-derived, antigen-experienced T cells. For HSCT recipients after engraftment, invasive fungal disease, herpesviruses, and adenovirus infections represent life-threatening complications that significantly affect outcomes. Additional pathogens to consider include nontuberculous mycobacteria, BK virus, *Clostridium difficile*, and norovirus.

Invasive fungal disease (IFD) remains a significant cause of infectious morbidity and mortality in allogeneic HSCT recipients. Empirical treatment for IFD is considered for HSCT patients with persistent fever despite 96 hr of broad-spectrum antibiotic treatment. The most common organisms are *Aspergillus* and *Candida* species. Infections also occur with non-*Aspergillus* molds, including *Mucor* and *Rhizopus* species (among other agents of mucormycosis), *Fusarium*, and *Scedosporium* species. *Pneumocystis jiroveci* is a unique, noncultivatable cause of fungal pneumonia in immunocompromised patients. Despite prompt and aggressive administration of potent antifungal agents, proven cases of IFD carry case fatality rates of 20–70%. IFD can present early after transplant, although there is a shift toward presentation of infection in the postengraftment period in the presence of GVHD. The risk of developing IFD is mainly influenced by history of previous fungal infection, duration of neutropenia, use of corticosteroid therapy, mucosal tissue damage (GVHD, posttransplant CMV infection, viral respiratory tract infections), and for candidiasis, presence of central venous catheters.

Disseminated candidiasis presents frequently as a central venous catheter–associated infection. However, up to 50% of patients with disseminated candidiasis do not present with positive blood cultures. Patients with and without candidemia can have infection of normally sterile organs, including liver, spleen, kidney, brain, heart, and eye. Mortality rates in pediatric series range from 10–25%. **Echinocandins** (micafungin, caspofungin) are the initial drugs of choice for candidiasis in immunocompromised patients.

The most common presentation of invasive **aspergillosis** is pulmonary aspergillosis. The upper airway mucosa (nose and sinuses) can also be a site of initial infection. Infection progresses from lung or sinus sites by direct extension across tissue or angioinvasion resulting in hematogenous dissemination to brain and other organs. The earliest imaging finding is classically 1 or more small pulmonary nodules (Figs. 164.2 and 164.3). As a nodule enlarges, the dense central core of infarcted tissue may become surrounded by edema or hemorrhage, forming a hazy rim known as the *halo sign*. When bone marrow function recovers, the infarcted central core may cavitate, creating the *crescent sign*. Unfortunately, radiographic signs, including the halo sign, crescent sign, and cavitation, have low sensitivity in pediatric patients. Clinical criteria are used to diagnose proven or probable IFD, requiring direct or indirect microbiologic data. Direct, culture-based diagnosis requires invasive procedures, such as sinus endoscopy or lung biopsy. Indirect measures, known as *fungal biomarkers*, are used in adult HSCT patients to screen or diagnose for aspergillosis. Fewer data are available for pediatric patients, and currently no major guidelines support routine use of fungal biomarkers to diagnose IFD in immunocompromised children. **Galactomannan** from serum or bronchoalveolar lavage fluid is a promising adjunct to current diagnostic strategies because of a high negative predictive value for aspergillosis; however, lack of detection of mucormycosis limits its utility as a single diagnostic test. Other tests used in adult patients, such as $(1{\rightarrow}3)$-β-D-glucan, are insufficiently studied for routine use in pediatric patients.

Fungal infection prevention includes isolation of the patient in a laminar airflow or positive pressure room. Universal prophylaxis to prevent *Pneumocystis* pneumonia is advocated until the return of T-cell function in HSCT patients; the primary agent for prophylaxis is trimethoprim/sulfamethoxazole. Alternative agents are pentamidine, dapsone, and atovaquone. For prevention and treatment of other IFD, liposomal amphotericin B, azole compounds (itraconazole, voriconazole, posaconazole) and echinocandins (caspofungin, micafungin) are used. **Voriconazole** represents the treatment of choice for adult patients with invasive aspergillosis, but achieving adequate trough levels can be challenging in young children. The agents of mucormycosis are resistant to most azole and echinocandin medications, which makes liposomal **amphotericin B** the initial drug of choice. IFD often does not respond satisfactorily to antifungal agents alone, and infection may persist until immune function recovers.

Herpesviruses, including cytomegalovirus (CMV), Epstein-Barr virus (EBV), herpes simplex virus (HSV1 and HSV2), and varicella-zoster virus (VZV) are pathogens that can cause significant disease after HSCT. Because herpesviruses can establish latency in the human host, symptomatic infection can occur from viral reactivation as well as acquisition from the donor or de novo infection. Baseline susceptibility to disease and viremia before symptom development can be established with laboratory monitoring (pretransplant donor-recipient serology, posttransplant viral load monitoring) and can inform decisions on prophylactic and preemptive antiviral treatment.

CMV infection remains the most common and potentially severe viral complication in patients receiving allogeneic HSCT. Risk factors for CMV viremia include recipient seropositivity, UCBT, and acute GVHD. The period of maximal risk for CMV disease is 1-4 mo after transplantation. Late presentation of CMV disease is associated with GVHD. Until CMV-specific T-cell responses develop months after transplant, CMV infection may result in a variety of syndromes, including fever, leukopenia, thrombocytopenia, hepatitis, pneumonitis, retinitis, esophagitis, gastritis, and colitis. CMV pneumonia has been reported to occur in up to 15–20% of bone marrow transplant recipients, with a case fatality rate of 85% in the absence of early treatment. Tachypnea, hypoxia, and nonproductive cough signal respiratory involvement. Chest radiography often reveals bilateral interstitial or reticulonodular infiltrates, which begin in the periphery of the lower lobes and spread centrally and superiorly. Gastrointestinal CMV involvement may lead to ulcers of the esophagus, stomach, small intestine, and colon with complications of bleeding or perforation. Fatal CMV infections are often associated with persistent viremia and multiorgan involvement.

CMV disease has largely been prevented through prophylaxis or preemptive approaches. Prophylaxis is based on administration of antiviral drugs to at-risk transplanted patients for a median duration of 3 mo after transplantation. The major drawbacks of this approach are drug toxicity, late CMV disease after withdrawal of prophylaxis, potential unnecessary treatment of patients who would not have reactivated CMV infection, and low cost-effectiveness. Preemptive therapy aims at treating only patients who experience CMV reactivation and thus are at risk of developing overt disease; it starts on detection of CMV in blood but before symptom development. The major drawback of this strategy is the need of serial monitoring of CMV by polymerase chain reaction (PCR) in blood. First-line therapy is usually ganciclovir, with foscarnet as an alternative for resistant strains or ganciclovir intolerance.

EBV-related posttransplant lymphoproliferative disease (PTLD) is a major complication in HSCT and solid-organ transplantation. In patients receiving HSCT, selective procedures of T-cell depletion–sparing B lymphocytes and use of HLA–partially matched family and unrelated donors are risk factors for the development of PTLD. PTLD usually presents in the first 4-6 mo after transplantation as high-grade, diffuse, large-cell B-cell lymphomas that are oligoclonal or monoclonal. High EBV viral loads in blood by PCR predict development of PTLD. Standard treatment of PTLD includes the reduction of immunosuppression, monoclonal antibodies directed against CD20 on B cells (rituximab), or cytotoxic chemotherapy. Prophylactic strategies with rituximab for EBV-positive recipients during conditioning for HSCT have also been employed. Histologic diagnosis of PTLD is required to assess for the emergence of neoplasms in which cells are CD19$^+$ but CD20$^-$, thus eliminating susceptibility to rituximab.

Disseminated adenovirus infection is a life-threatening complication of HSCT recipients. Clinical manifestations include fever, hepatitis, enteritis, meningoencephalitis, and pneumonia. Young children or recipients of donor cells naïve to adenovirus (T-cell–depleted grafts or UCBT) are at particular risk of developing this complication. Diagnosis is based on the demonstration of high viral loads by PCR in blood or recovery of virus in tissue biopsies. Pharmacologic treatment of adenovirus infections is with the antiviral cidofovir, which has significant renal toxicity and limited potency at controlling viral replication. Alternative delivery systems for this drug, such as enterally available prodrugs, are currently being investigated in research settings. Recovery of immune system function is associated with improved survival with disseminated adenovirus infection.

In immunocompromised hosts, severe viral infections, including PTLD and adenovirus infection, originate from a deficiency of virus-specific **cytotoxic T lymphocytes** (CTLs). This finding provides the rationale for developing strategies of adoptive cell therapy to restore virus-specific immune competence. Multiple protocols are under development and available at some centers for the rapid generation of specific CTL lines of donor or third-party origin.

Bibliography is available at Expert Consult.

Chapter 165

Late Effects of Hematopoietic Stem Cell Transplantation

Rachel A. Phelan and David Margolis

第一百六十五章

造血干细胞移植的晚期影响

中文导读

　　本章主要介绍了造血干细胞移植对内分泌的影响、心血管影响、继发肿瘤、移植物抗宿主病、其他影响和特殊考虑因素。具体描述了晚期影响的危险因素；对内分泌的晚期影响包括生长受抑、甲状腺功能减退症、不育以及骨骼健康问题等；心血管影响包括代谢综合征、心肌病和动脉粥样硬化等；描述了继发肿瘤的类型和危险因素；其他影响包括肺功能、肾脏、牙齿、胃肠道和精神心理的影响；儿童和遗传病患者等须考虑相应特殊因素。

Pediatric hematopoietic stem cell transplantation (HSCT) is considered standard-of-care treatment for a number of malignant and nonmalignant conditions. Treatment generally involves exposure to chemotherapy and occasionally radiation to encourage engraftment of donor stem cells and prevent donor and recipient rejection. The period of time immediately after transplant is associated with the risk for a number of serious acute complications, including profound immunosuppression and subsequent risk for infection, graft-versus-host disease (GVHD), and organ toxicities. Fortunately, significant progress has been made in supportive care strategies to reduce the risk of acute complications and treat them more effectively if they do arise. This has resulted in a growing number of pediatric patients who are now long-term survivors following HSCT. The estimated total number of HSCT survivors in 2009 was 108,900, and this is expected to increase 5 times by 2030 to 502,000. Of these survivors, approximately 14% (64,000) in 2030 will have received a transplant in childhood (<18 yr of age).

Exposure to chemotherapy, radiation, or both places patients at similar long-term risks as the pediatric cancer population; the high doses and types of chemotherapy and radiation often amplify the risk for issues such as ovarian failure/infertility and neurocognitive difficulties. Total body irradiation (TBI) has been shown to increase dramatically the risk for late complications after transplant. In addition, late effects may be additive if the patient received therapy before HSCT for their underlying malignancy. Moreover, the indication for transplant in pediatric patients is not always related to malignancy, but rather an underlying immunodeficiency, bone marrow failure syndrome, or metabolic disorder. These patients are potentially at risk for late effects related to this underlying disease alone and require different types of monitoring.

Essentially, every organ system can be impacted by the long-term effects of therapy, and each must be considered when undergoing late effects surveillance (Table 165.1). As a result of growing evidence of the importance of lifelong care for HSCT survivors, multiple groups have published recent consensus guidelines to help in caring for this patient population. As the field of survivorship continues to expand, *we recommend the following reference for real-time evidence-based recommendations from the* **Children's Oncology Group**: http://survivorshipguidelines.org.

ENDOCRINE EFFECTS

Children given HSCT before puberty may develop **growth impairment**, precluding achievement of the genetic target for adult height. The decrease in growth velocity is similar for boys and girls and is more frequently observed in patients given TBI as part of the preparative regimen. Chronic GVHD and its treatment with corticosteroids may also contribute to growth impairment.

Growth impairment of patients given TBI is mainly a result of direct damage of cartilage plates and to the effect of TBI on the hypothalamic-pituitary axis, which leads to an inappropriately low production of **growth hormone** (GH). GH deficiency is susceptible to at least partial correction through administration of hormonal replacement therapy. Annual growth evaluation should be performed in all children after HSCT. Children showing a decreased growth velocity should be further investigated through evaluation of bone age and secretion of GH in response to pharmacologic stimulus.

The use of TBI during the preparative regimen involves the thyroid

Table 165.1	Summary of Late Effects After Hematopoietic Stem Cell Transplantation (HSCT) in Childhood

EXPOSURE	LATE EFFECT*	EXPOSURE	LATE EFFECT*
HSCT experience in general	Dental abnormalities Renal toxicity Hepatic toxicity Low BMD Avascular necrosis Increased risk of second cancers Adverse psychosocial/quality-of-life effects Mental health disorders, risk behaviors Psychosocial disability caused by pain or fatigue	**PRETRANSPLANTATION EXPOSURES (Not Listed Above)**	
		Anthracycline/anthraquinone	Cardiac toxicity Therapy-related AML/MDS
		Bleomycin	Pulmonary toxicity
		Cytarabine	Neurocognitive deficits Leukoencephalopathy
		Methotrexate	Neurocognitive deficits Leukoencephalopathy Renal toxicity Low BMD
TRANSPLANTATION CONDITIONING		Corticosteroid	Cataract Low BMD Avascular necrosis
Alkylating agent	Cataract (busulfan) Pulmonary fibrosis (busulfan) Renal toxicity Urinary tract toxicity Gonadal dysfunction Therapy-related AML/MDS Bladder cancer	Cranial radiation‡	Neurocognitive deficits Leukoencephalopathy Cerebrovascular disease Cataract Craniofacial abnormalities Dental abnormalities, xerostomia GH deficiency Hypothyroidism thyroid nodule Increased obesity Precocious puberty Brain tumor
Epipodophyllotoxin** DNA intersecting and cross-linking agents (i.e., platinum, heavy metal) TBI†	Therapy-related AML/MDS Ototoxicity Renal toxicity Gonadal toxicity Neurocognitive deficits Leukoencephalopathy Cataract Dental abnormalities GH deficiency Hypothyroidism, thyroid nodule Pulmonary toxicity Breast tissue hypoplasia Cardiac toxicity Renal toxicity Gonadal dysfunction Uterine vascular insufficiency Diabetes Dyslipidemia Musculoskeletal growth problems Second cancers	Spinal radiation (in addition to cranial dose)	Cardiac toxicity Scoliosis/kyphosis, musculoskeletal problems
		AFTER TRANSPLANTATION (Not Listed Above)	
		Chronic GVHD	Xerophthalmia Xerostomia, dental abnormalities Pulmonary toxicity Gastrointestinal strictures Genitourinary strictures Skin and joint changes Immunodeficiency Second cancers, especially skin, oral, cervical, lymphoma
		Tyrosine kinase inhibitor	Acute cardiac toxicity reported, but not known to cause late cardiotoxicity
		OTHER EXPOSURES	
		Blood transfusions	Hepatitis C, HIV

AML/MDS, Acute myeloid leukemia/myelodysplastic syndrome; BMD, bone mineral density; GH, growth hormone; GVHD, graft-vs-host disease; HIV, human immunodeficiency virus.

*Focused on those late effects that can develop or persist even after cessation of therapy.

†At given total dose, risks greater for single-fraction vs fractionated total body irradiation (TBI); single-fraction myeloablative TBI (>500 cGy) now rarely used.

‡Effects listed are those more likely to be associated with doses used in HSCT survivors (e.g., those given for leukemia treatment, <25 Gy); late effects are more likely if TBI also given.

**Include etoposide, teniposide.

From Chow EJ, Anderson L, Baker KS, et al: Late effects surveillance recommendations among survivors of childhood hematopoietic cell transplantation: a Children's Oncology Group report, *Biol Blood Marrow Transplant* 22:783–784, 2016.

gland in the irradiation field and may result in **hypothyroidism**. Younger children are at greater risk of developing hypothyroidism. Chemotherapy-only preparative regimens have far fewer adverse effects on normal thyroid function. The site of injury by irradiation is at the level of the thyroid gland rather than at the pituitary or hypothalamus. Therapy with thyroxine is very effective for overt hypothyroidism. The cumulative incidence of hypothyroidism increases over time, underscoring the importance of annual thyroid function studies.

Gonadal hormones are essential for normal pubertal growth, as well as for development of secondary sexual characteristics. A significant proportion of patients receiving TBI-containing preparative regimens as well as high doses of alkylating agents show delayed development of secondary sexual characteristics, resulting from primary ovarian or testicular failure. Laboratory evaluation of these patients reveals elevated follicle-stimulating hormone and luteinizing hormone levels with depressed estradiol and testosterone serum levels. These patients benefit

from careful follow-up with evaluation of annual sexual maturity rating (Tanner) scores and endocrine function. Supplementation of gonadal hormones is useful for primary gonadal failure and is administered with GH to promote pubertal growth. **Infertility** during adulthood remains a common problem of these children, especially those undergoing traditional myeloablative conditioning for HSCT. The use of reduced-intensity regimens may result in sparing fertility in a large proportion of patients, although conditioning regimens vary and studies are limited.

Bone health of HSCT survivors can also be impacted by hormonal changes as well as lifestyle practices, such as inadequate exercise and/or dietary intake of vitamin D. Prior exposures, including corticosteroid use, can result in changes to bone density as well as predispose to the development of avascular necrosis. Dual-energy x-ray absorptiometry (DXA) scans are routinely incorporated into the care of those patients at risk for low bone mineral density.

CARDIOVASCULAR EFFECTS

Survivors of childhood HSCT are at risk for the future development of cardiovascular complications. This population can be prone to developing **metabolic syndrome** (dyslipidemia, hypertension, diabetes mellitus, obesity), especially those with a history of TBI exposure and subsequent hormonal derangements. Prior exposures such as anthracycline chemotherapy and chest radiation further increase the risk for **cardiomyopathy** as well as **atherosclerosis**. As a result, routine anthropometric, imaging, and laboratory screening should be performed in survivors of childhood HSCT to assess and monitor their cardiovascular health.

SECONDARY MALIGNANCY

The overall risk of developing a secondary form of cancer is significantly higher after HSCT than in the general population. Although few studies have specifically analyzed pediatric patients, available evidence indicates that the cumulative incidence of 2nd malignancies shows a slight, but continuous, tendency to increase over time. The development of myelodysplastic syndrome as well as secondary leukemias must be considered in survivors of HSCT. Several other types of secondary tumors have been identified in patients given HSCT. The most frequently diagnosed neoplasms are thyroid carcinoma, brain tumors, and epithelial cancers. Young age, male gender, use of TBI during the preparative regimen, chronic GVHD, and an intrinsic genetic predisposition to develop cancer (Fanconi anemia) have been reported to be risk factors for development of secondary malignancies after HSCT. Routine physical exams, including yearly skin in exams in those that received TBI are important in the care of these patients.

GRAFT-VERSUS-HOST DISEASE

In the posttransplant period, multiple studies have shown that quality of life is severely impacted by the presence of GVHD, which is an issue that is also unique to HSCT (see Chapter 163).

OTHER EFFECTS

HSCT patients can also experience complications related to their pulmonary function, renal function, dental health, and gastrointestinal system, often related to prior exposures as well as their conditioning regimen. It is also important to note that long-term survivors must be monitored for psychological issues because of their prior and current underlying health conditions. They may need extra assistance with school and vocational attainment. These patients are also often at higher risk for depression and anxiety; yearly psychosocial assessments can identify survivors who need additional therapy or psychotropic medication. Parents may also have posttraumatic stress from the experience.

SPECIAL CONSIDERATIONS

Certain patient populations who undergo HSCT are at increased risk for late effects. Young children appear to be at a heightened risk for late complications related to TBI, especially those related to growth, thyroid function, and neurocognition. Patients with an **underlying genetic condition** must also be monitored more closely for specific consequences of therapy, such as specific secondary malignancies in the Fanconi anemia population caused by an underlying DNA repair defect and patients with sickle cell anemia and thalassemia who are predisposed to iron overload.

Bibliography is available at Expert Consult.

Elsevier (Singapore) Pte Ltd.
3 Killiney Road, #08-01 Winsland House I, Singapore 239519
Tel: (65) 6349-0200; Fax: (65) 6733-1817

This English Adaptation of Nelson Textbook of Pediatrics, 21E by Robert M. Kliegman, Joseph W. St. Geme Ⅲ, Nathan J. Blum, Samir S. Shah, Robert C. Tasker, Karen M. Wilson was undertaken by Hunan Science & Technology Press and is published by arrangement with Elsevier (Singapore) Pte Ltd.

Nelson Textbook of Pediatrics, 21E by Robert M. Kliegman, Joseph W. St. Geme Ⅲ, Nathan J. Blum, Samir S. Shah, Robert C. Tasker, Karen M. Wilson 由湖南科学技术出版社进行改编影印，并根据湖南科学技术出版社与爱思唯尔（新加坡）私人有限公司的协议约定出版。

尼尔森儿科学Nelson Textbook of Pediatrics, 影印中文导读版,（张金哲，王天有等改编）
ISBN：978-7-5710-0730-0

图书在版编目（CIP）数据

尼尔森儿科学 ：第 21 版 ：影印中文导读版 ：汉、英文 上册 ／（美）罗伯特 M. 克利格曼（Robert M. Kliegman）等主编 ；张金哲, 王天有等编译. — 长沙 ：湖南科学技术出版社, 2020.10

（西医经典名著集成）

ISBN 978-7-5710-0730-0

Ⅰ．①尼… Ⅱ．①罗… ②张… ③王… Ⅲ．①儿科学－汉、英文 Ⅳ．①R72

中国版本图书馆 CIP 数据核字（2020）第 157308 号

著作权合同登记号 18-2020-187

西医经典名著集成
NIERSHEN ERKEXUE

尼尔森儿科学 第 21 版 影印中文导读版 上册

主　　编：[美]罗伯特 M. 克利格曼（Robert M. Kliegman），[美]约瑟夫 W. St. 盖门（Joseph W. St. Geme Ⅲ），
　　　　　[美]内森 J. 布卢姆（Nathan J. Blum），[美]萨米尔 S. 沙阿（Samir S. Shah），
　　　　　[美]罗伯特 C. 塔斯克（Robert C. Tasker），[美]凯伦 M. 威尔逊（Karen M. Wilson）

编 译 者：张金哲，王天有等
责任编辑：李　忠
出版发行：湖南科学技术出版社
社　　址：长沙市湘雅路 276 号
　　　　　http://www.hnstp.com
印　　刷：长沙德三印刷有限公司
　　　　　（印装质量问题请直接与本厂联系）
厂　　址：宁乡市城郊乡东沩社区东沩北路 192 号
邮　　编：410600
版　　次：2020 年 10 月第 1 版
印　　次：2020 年 10 月第 1 次印刷
开　　本：787mm×1092mm　1/16
印　　张：84
字　　数：4960 千字
书　　号：ISBN 978-7-5710-0730-0
定　　价：1100.00 元（上、中、下册）